PEDIATRIC EMERGENCY MEDICINE

PEDIATRIC EMERGENCY MEDICINE

Concepts and Clinical Practice

SECOND EDITION

EDITOR

ROGER M. BARKIN, MD, MPH, FAAP, FACEP
Vice President for Pediatric and Newborn Programs
  Columbia-HealthONE
Professor of Surgery, Division of Emergency Medicine
University of Colorado Health Sciences Center
Denver, Colorado

ASSOCIATE EDITORS

Grace L. Caputo, MD, MPH, FAAP
Pediatric Residency Program Director
Maricopa Medical Center
Phoenix, Arizona

David M. Jaffe, MD, FAAP, FACEP
Associate Professor of Pediatrics
Director, Division of Emergency Medicine
Washington University School of Medicine
Medical Director, Emergency Services
St. Louis Children's Hospital
St. Louis, Missouri

Jane F. Knapp, MD, FAAP, FACEP
Director, Division of Emergency Medical Services
The Children's Mercy Hospital
Professor of Pediatrics
Department of Pediatrics
University of Missouri Kansas City School of Medicine
Kansas City, Missouri

Robert W. Schafermeyer, MD, FAAP, FACEP
Director, Division of Education
Associate Chair, Department of Emergency Medicine
Carolinas Medical Center
Charlotte, North Carolina
Clinical Professor of Emergency Medicine and Pediatrics
University of North Carolina School of Medicine
Chapel Hill, North Carolina

James S. Seidel, MD, PhD, FAAP
Chief, Division of General and Emergency Pediatrics
Harbor-UCLA Medical Center
Professor of Pediatrics
UCLA School of Medicine
Torrance, California

CONSULTING EDITOR

Peter Rosen, MD, FACEP
Director of Education
Department of Emergency Medicine
Director, Emergency Medicine Residency Program
Professor of Clinical Medicine
Assistant Director, Department of Emergency Medicine
University of California at San Diego Medical Center
San Diego, California

with 375 illustrations

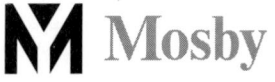

St. Louis Baltimore Boston Carlsbad Chicago Naples New York Philadelphia Portland
London Madrid Mexico City Singapore Sydney Tokyo Toronto Wiesbaden

161046

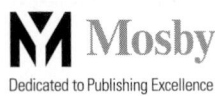

Mosby

Dedicated to Publishing Excellence

A Times Mirror
Company

Publisher: Anne S. Patterson
Editor: Kathryn H. Falk
Developmental Editor: Carolyn M. Kruse
Project Manager: Carol Sullivan Weis
Production Editor: David Stein
Manufacturing Manager: Dave Graybill

NOTE: The indications for, and dosages of, medications recommended conform to practices at the present time. References to specific products are incorporated to serve only as guidelines; they are not meant to exclude a practitioner's choice of other, comparable drugs. Many oral medications may be given with more scheduling flexibility than implied by the specific time intervals noted. Individual drug sensitivity and allergies must be considered in drug selection. Adult doses are provided as a gauge of the maximum dose commonly used.

Every attempt has been made to ensure accuracy and appropriateness. New investigations and broader experience may alter present dosage schedules, and it is recommended that the package insert of each drug be consulted before administration. Often there is limited experience with established drugs for neonates and young children. Furthermore, new drugs may be introduced, and indications for use may change. This rapid evolution is particularly noticeable in the use of antibiotics and cardiopulmonary resuscitation. The clinician is encouraged to maintain expertise concerning appropriate medications for specific conditions.

Printed in the United States of America
Composition by Graphic World, Inc.
Printing/binding by Maple Vail Book Mfg Group

Mosby–Year Book, Inc.
11830 Westline Industrial Drive
St. Louis, Missouri 63146

International Standard Book Number 0-8151-1002-2

96 97 98 99 00 / 9 8 7 6 5 4 3 2 1

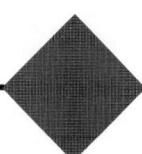

Contributors

THOMAS J. ABRUNZO, MS, MD, MPH, FAAP, FACEP
Director, Pediatric Emergency Services
St. Joseph's Hospital
Clinical Associate Professor of Pediatrics
University of South Florida College of Medicine
Tampa, Florida
49 Ear, Nose, and Throat Disorders

EVALINE A. ALESSANDRINI, MD
Assistant Professor of Pediatrics
University of Pennsylvania School of Medicine
Division of Emergency Medicine
The Children's Hospital of Philadelphia
Philadelphia, Pennsylvania
52 Gastrointestinal Disorders

SUSAN McCLELLAN ASCH, MD, PhD
Pediatrician
Stillwater Medical Group, PA
Stillwater, Minnesota
2 Pediatric Emergency Department Environment
41 Radiation Exposure

DAVID T. BACHMAN, MD
Director, Pediatric Emergency Services
Maine Medical Center
Portland, Maine
Associate Professor of Pediatrics
University of Vermont
Burlington, Vermont
54 Hematologic and Oncologic Disorders

JILL M. BAREN, MD
Assistant Professor of Surgery (Emergency Medicine)
Assistant Professor of Pediatrics
Yale University School of Medicine
Adult and Pediatric Emergency Departments
Yale-New Haven Hospital
New Haven, Connecticut
11 Emergency Management of Respiratory Distress and
Failure

ROGER M. BARKIN, MD, MPH, FAAP, FACEP
Vice President for Pediatric and Newborn Programs
Columbia-HealthONE
Professor of Surgery, Division of Emergency Medicine
University of Colorado Health Sciences Center
Denver, Colorado
13 Shock
15 Fluid and Electrolyte Balance
54 Hematologic and Oncologic Disorders
56 Neurologic Disorders

BARBARA A. BARLOW, MD, FACS, FAAP
Professor of Clinical Surgery
College of Physicians and Surgeons
Columbia University
Chief of Pediatric Surgery
Harlem Hospital Center
New York, New York
4 Emergency Medical Services for Children

THEODORE M. BARNETT, MD, FAAP
Attending Physician
Pediatric Emergency Medicine
Assistant Professor of Pediatrics
Section of Emergency Medical Services
The Children's Mercy Hospital
Kansas City, Missouri
45 Child Abuse and Neglect
58 Psychiatric and Behavioral Disorders

ROBERT A. BELFER, MD
Assistant Professor of Pediatrics
Medical College of Pennsylvania and
Hahnemann University School of Medicine
St. Christopher's Hospital for Children
Philadelphia, Pennsylvania
52 Gastrointestinal Disorders

LYNNE M. BERRY, MD
Fellow
Department of Pediatrics
Division of Neonatology
Harbor-UCLA Medical Center
Torrance, California
17 Newborn Resuscitation

MANANDA S. BHENDE, MD, FAAP, FACEP
Attending Physician, Emergency Department
Children's Hospital of Pittsburgh
Associate Professor of Pediatrics
University of Pittsburgh School of Medicine
Pittsburgh, Pennsylvania
56 Neurologic Disorders

DOUGLAS A. BOENNING, MD
Associate Medical Director
Emergency Medical Trauma Center
Children's Hospital National Medical Center
Washington, District of Columbia
52 Gastrointestinal Disorders

JOHN R. BOWER, MD
Assistant Professor
Departments of Pediatrics and Microbiology/Immunology
Children's Hospital Medical Center of Akron
Northeastern Ohio Universities College of Medicine
Akron, Ohio
55 Infectious Disorders

SHARON A. BRENNAN, MD
Fellow
Pediatric Hematology/Oncology
Department of Pediatrics
Yale University School of Medicine
New Haven, Connecticut
54 Hematologic and Oncologic Disorders

RICHARD J. BRILLI, MD
Associate Professor of Clinical Pediatrics
University of Cincinnati
Clinical Director, Pediatric Intensive Care Unit
Fellowship Director, Pediatric Critical Care Medicine
Children's Hospital Medical Center
Cincinnati, Ohio
15 Fluid and Electrolyte Balance

DENA R. BROWNSTEIN, MD, FAAP
Assistant Professor of Pediatrics
Department of Pediatrics
University of Washington
Emergency Services
Children's Hospital and Medical Center
Seattle, Washington
*26 Foreign Bodies of the Gastrointestinal Tract and
    Airway*

DAVID J. BURCHFIELD, MD
Associate Professor
Departments of Pediatrics and Physiology
Division of Neonatology
University of Florida College of Medicine
Gainesville, Florida
18 Acute Distress in the Neonate and Postnatal Period

RICHARD M. CANTOR, MD, FAAP, FACEP
Associate Professor
Departments of Emergency Medicine and Pediatrics
University Hospital
Syracuse, New York
13A Venous and Arterial Access

JULIO CASTILLO, MD
Assistant Professor of Pediatrics
Emory University
Attending Physician
Egleston Children's Hospital
Atlanta, Georgia
60 Urinary and Renal Disorders

JAMES M. CHAMBERLAIN, MD
Assistant Medical Director
Emergency Medical Trauma Center
Children's National Medical Center
Washington, District of Columbia
52 Gastrointestinal Disorders

LEON CHAMEIDES, MD, FAAP
Director, Pediatric Cardiology
Connecticut Children's Medical Center
Clinical Professor
University of Connecticut School of Medicine
Hartford, Connecticut
14 Dysrhythmias

NORMAN C. CHRISTOPHER, MD
Coordinator, Pediatric Emergency Medicine
Departments of Emergency Medicine and Pediatrics
MetroHealth Medical Center
Cleveland, Ohio
 7A Block of the Upper Extremities
13A Venous and Arterial Access
23A Tube Thoracostomy

FELTON E. COMBEST, MD, FAAP, FACEP
Director, Acute Care
Health First
Memphis, Tennessee
60 Urinary and Renal Disorders

**EDWARD E. CONWAY, JR., MD, MS, FAAP, FCCP,
    FCCM**
Associate Professor of Pediatrics, Critical Care and
    Anesthesiology
Albert Einstein College of Medicine
Director of Pediatric Critical Care Fellowship Program
Associate Director, PCCM
Division of Critical Care
Children's Medical Center at Montefiore
Bronx, New York
*6 Emergency Department and Intensive Care Unit
    Interface*

ARTHUR COOPER, MD, MS, FACS, FAAP, FCCM
Associate Professor and Chief
Pediatric Surgical Critical Care
College of Physicians and Surgeons of Columbia
    University
Harlem Hospital Center
New York, New York
 4 Emergency Medical Services for Children
23 Thoracic Trauma
24 Abdominal Trauma

MITCHELL B. CORDOVER, MD, FACEP
Vice President, Medical Affairs
Spectrum Healthcare Services
St. Louis, Missouri
10 Legal Issues

JAMES D'AGOSTINO, MD
Assistant Professor
Departments of Emergency Medicine and Pediatrics
SUNY Health Science Center at Syracuse
Syracuse, New York
7 Pain Control, Analgesia, and Sedation

L.A. DANDREA, MD, FAAP
Associate Director, Pediatric Emergency Medicine
Children's Medical Center of Northwest Ohio
Toledo, Ohio
9 Continuous Quality Improvement

EARL R. DIXON, MD
Fellow, Pediatric Emergency Medicine
Department of Pediatrics
Division of Critical Care
Le Bonheur Children's Medical Center
University of Tennessee
Memphis, Tennessee
60 Urinary and Renal Disorders

MARGARET DOLAN, MD, FAAP
Associate Professor of Pediatrics
Department of Pediatrics
Children's Medical Center
Medical College of Virginia
Richmond, Virginia
20 Head Trauma

M. DENISE DOWD, MD, MPH
Assistant Professor of Pediatrics
Division of Emergency Medicine
Children's Hospital Medical Center
University of Cincinnati College of Medicine
Cincinnati, Ohio
3 Injury Prevention and Control

JAMES E. DUFORT, MD, FAAP
Pediatrician
St. Paul, Minnesota
57 Orthopedic Disorders

KIMBERLY H. EDWARDS, MD
Fellow, Department of Pediatric Emergency Medicine
The Children's Hospital of Alabama
Birmingham, Alabama
46 Allergic and Immunologic Disorders

LISA S. ETZWILER, MD
Director, Pediatric Emergency Services
St. John's Mercy Medical Center
Assistant Clinical Professor of Pediatrics
St. Louis University School of Medicine
Attending Physician, Division of Emergency Medicine
Cardinal Glennon Children's Hospital
St. Louis, Missouri
28 Hand and Wrist Injuries

ROBERT A. FELTER, MD, FAAP
Chairman, Department of Pediatrics
TOD Children's Hospital
Western Reserve Care System
Youngstown, Ohio
55 Infectious Disorders

PAULA C. FINK, MD
Clinical Assistant Professor of Pediatrics
University of Minnesota
Department of Pediatrics
Children's Health Care, Minneapolis
Minneapolis, MN
57 Orthopedic Disorders

LAURA S. FITZMAURICE, MD, FAAP, FACEP
Chief, Emergency Medicine Section
Department of Pediatrics
The Children's Mercy Hospital
Associate Professor of Pediatrics
University of Missouri – Kansas City
Kansas City, Missouri
19 Approach to Multiple Trauma

GEORGE L. FOLTIN, MD, FAAP, FACEP
Director, Pediatric Emergency Medicine
Bellevue Hospital Center/New York University Medical
    Center
Assistant Professor of Clinical Pediatrics
New York University School of Medicine
New York, New York
4 Emergency Medical Services for Children
23 Thoracic Trauma
24 Abdominal Trauma

SUSAN M. FUCHS, MD, FAAP
Associate Professor of Pediatrics
Department of Pediatrics
University of Pittsburgh School of Medicine
Attending Physician
Emergency Department
Children's Hospital of Pittsburgh
Pittsburgh, Pennsylvania
56 Neurologic Disorders

MARIANNE GAUSCHE, MD, FAAP, FACEP
Associate Professor of Medicine
University of California – Los Angeles School of Medicine
Director, Emergency Medical Services
Harbor-UCLA Medical Center
Department of Emergency Medicine
Torrance, California
25 Genitourinary Trauma
59 Respiratory Disorders

JAVIER A. GONZALEZ DEL REY, MD, FAAP
Assistant Professor of Pediatrics
Department of Pediatrics
Division of Emergency Medicine
University of Cincinnati College of Medicine
Cincinnati, Ohio
56 Neurologic Disorders

MARC H. GORELICK, MD
Assistant Professor of Pediatrics and Epidemiology
Division of Emergency Medicine
University of Pennsylvania School of Medicine
Philadelphia, Pennsylvania
52 Gastrointestinal Disorders

M. LOIS HALL, MD, FAAP
Emergency Physicians, P.A.
Bloomington, Minnesota
Emergency Department
Unity Medical Center
Minneapolis, Minnesota
36 Electrical and Lightning Injuries

JIM R. HARLEY, MD, MPH
Assistant Clinical Professor
Department of Pediatrics
University of California—San Diego
Emergency Department
Children's Hospital and Health Center
San Diego, California
35 Near Drowning

LISA SINCLAIR HART, MD
Assistant Professor of Pediatrics
University of Maryland School of Medicine
Baltimore, Maryland
52 Gastrointestinal Disorders

MARY FRAN HAZINSKI, RN, MSN, FAAN
Clinical Specialist
Division of Trauma
Departments of Surgery and Pediatrics
Vanderbilt University Medical Center
Nashville, Tennessee
13 Shock

DEBORAH PARKMAN HENDERSON, RN, MA
Co-Director, National EMSC Resource Alliance
Harbor-UCLA Medical Center
Torrance, California
*1 Approach to the Pediatric Patient in the Emergency
    Department*
8 Death of a Child

MARTIN I. HERMAN, MD, FAAP, FACEP
Assistant Professor
Department of Pediatrics
Division of Critical Care
University of Tennessee—Memphis
Emergency Department
Le Bonheur Children's Medical Center
Memphis, Tennessee
60 Urinary and Renal Disorders

AMY L. HERTZ, MD, FAAP
Assistant Professor
Department of Pediatrics
Division of Critical Care
University of Tennessee—Memphis
Associate Director of Emergency Services
Le Bonheur Children's Medical Center
Memphis, Tennessee
60 Urinary and Renal Disorders

DEE HODGE III, MD, FAAP, FACEP
Director Emergency Medical Services
Department of Emergency Medicine
Children's Hospital Oakland
Assistant Clinical Professor of Pediatrics
University of California—San Francisco School
    of Medicine
Oakland, California
*27 Management Principles—Musculoskeletal and Soft
    Tissue Injuries*

HAROLD J. HOFSTRAND, MD, PhD, FACEP
Emergency Medical Specialist
Department of Emergency Medicine
St. Mary's Medical Center
Duluth Clinic, Ltd.
Adjunct Associate Professor of Physiology
Associate, Hypothermia Laboratory
University of Minnesota School of Medicine
Duluth, Minnesota
39 Accidental Hypothermia and Frostbite

DOUGLAS HOLTZMAN, MD
Pediatric Emergency Fellow
Department of Pediatric Emergency Medicine
Kosair Children's Hospital
University of Louisville School of Medicine
Louisville, Kentucky
56 Neurologic Disorders

WARREN L. HUTCHESON, MD, MPH
Assistant Professor
Department of Pediatrics
Division of Critical Care
University of Tennessee—Memphis
Emergency Department
Le Bonheur Children's Medical Center
Memphis, Tennessee
60 Urinary and Renal Disorders

ALSON S. INABA, MD, FAAP
Attending Physician and Pediatric Emergency Medicine
Fellowship Director
Kapiolani Medical Center for Women and Children
Assistant Professor of Pediatrics
University of Hawaii
John A. Burns School of Medicine
Medical Director, Hawaii Poison Center
Honolulu, Hawaii
32 Emergency Care of Minor Wounds

DANIEL J. ISAACMAN, MD, FAAP
Associate Professor of Pediatrics
Eastern Virginia School of Medicine
Chief, Division of Pediatric Emergency Medicine
Children's Hospital of the King's Daughters
Norfolk, Virginia
56 Neurologic Disorders

EUGENE IZSAK, MD
Director, Pediatric Emergency Medicine
Children's Medical Center of Northwest Ohio
Toledo, Ohio
9 Continuous Quality Improvement

J. LEIGH JACKSON, MD
Attending Physician
Department of Pediatric Emergency Medicine
Rhode Island Hospital/Hasbro Children's Hospital
Providence, Rhode Island
31 Ankle and Foot Injuries

MARK JOFFE, MD, FAAP
Director, Emergency Medicine
St. Christopher's Hospital for Children
Associate Professor of Pediatrics
Temple University School of Medicine
Philadelphia, Pennsylvania
29 Upper Extremity Injuries

CARDEN JOHNSTON, MD, FAAP
Professor of Pediatrics
Department of Pediatrics
University of Alabama—Birmingham
Birmingham, Alabama
46 Allergic and Immunologic Disorders

RAYMOND B. KARASIC, MD, FAAP, FACEP
Emergency Department
Children's Hospital of Pittsburgh
Associate Professor
Department of Pediatrics
University of Pittsburgh School of Medicine
Pittsburgh, Pennsylvania
56 Neurologic Disorders

TERRY P. KLASSEN, MD, MSc, FRCPC
Associate Professor
Department of Pediatrics
University of Manitoba
Winnipeg, Manitoba
Canada
47 Cardiovascular Disorders

BRUCE L. KLEIN, MD, FAAP
Associate Medical Director
Emergency Medical Trauma Center
Children's National Medical Center
Washington, District of Columbia
52 Gastrointestinal Disorders

JOHN G. KNEPPER, MD, FAAP
Assistant Professor
Department of Pediatrics
Division of Critical Care
University of Tennessee—Memphis
Emergency Department
Le Bonheur Children's Medical Center
Memphis, Tennessee
60 Urinary and Renal Disorders

MARY A. LETOURNEAU, MD, FAAP
Assistant Professor of Pediatrics
University of Southern California
Director, Division of Emergency and Transport Medicine
Children's Hospital Los Angeles
Los Angeles, California
59 Respiratory Disorders

MARILYN M. LI, MD, FRCP(C), FAAP
Associate Professor of Pediatrics
University of Ottawa
Children's Hospital of Eastern Ontario
Division of Emergency Medicine
Ottawa, Ontario
Canada
47 Cardiovascular Disorders

KATHLEEN A. LILLIS, MD
Chief, Division of Emergency Medicine
Children's Hospital of Buffalo
Assistant Professor of Pediatrics and Emergency
    Medicine
State University of New York at Buffalo
Buffalo, New York
52 Gastrointestinal Disorders

JAMES G. LINAKIS, PhD, MD, FAAP
Assistant Professor of Pediatrics
Division of Pediatric Emergency Medicine
Brown University School of Medicine
Emergency Department
Rhode Island Hospital/Hasbro Children's Hospital
Providence, Rhode Island
31 Ankle and Foot Injuries

JACALYN S. MALLER, MD, FAAP
Clinical Assistant Professor of Pediatrics
University of Pennsylvania School of Medicine
Emergency Department/Primary Care
Children's Hospital of Philadelphia
Philadelphia, Pennsylvania
51 Eye Disorders

KARIN A. McCLOSKEY, MD, FAAP
Associate Professor of Pediatrics
Division of Pediatric Emergency Medicine
University of Texas Southwestern Medical Center
    at Dallas
Dallas, Texas
5 Interhospital Transport

FRANCISCO A. MEDINA, MD, FAAP
Medical Director
Department of Pediatric Emergency Medicine
Baptist Hospital of Miami
Miami, Florida
22 Neck and Spinal Cord Trauma

LARRY BRUCE MELLICK, MD, MS, FAAP, FACEP
Chief of Service and Chairman
Department of Emergency Medicine
Associate Professor of Pediatrics and Emergency
    Medicine
Director of Pediatric Emergency Medicine
Loma Linda University Medical Center
Loma Linda, California
2 Pediatric Emergency Department Environment

MARILYN F. A. MELLOR, MD
Consultant in Pediatric Emergency Medicine
Department of Pediatric and Adolescent Medicine
Mayo Medical Center
Rochester, Minnesota
38 Heat-Induced Illnesses

MARLENE D. MELZER-LANGE, MD, FAAP
Associate Professor, Department of Pediatrics
Medical College of Wisconsin
Emergency Medicine Section
Children's Hospital of Wisconsin
Milwaukee, Wisconsin
53 Gynecologic and Obstetric Disorders

THOMAS T. MYDLER, MD, FAAP
Attending Physician
Baptist Medical Center
Kansas City, Missouri
43 Specific Toxins

DANIEL W. OCHSENSCHLAGER
Associate Professor of Pediatrics
Medical Director, Emergency Medical Trauma Center
Children's National Medical Center
Washington, District of Columbia
35 Near Drowning
52 Gastrointestinal Disorders

TIMOTHY J. O'CONNOR, MD, FAAP
Assistant Professor of Pediatrics
Director, Division of Pediatric Emergency Medicine
Department of Pediatrics and Adolescent Medicine
University of South Alabama
Mobile, Alabama
21 Facial Trauma

JAMES A. O'DONNELL II, MD, FAAP
Assistant Professor, Department of Pediatrics
Division of Critical Care
University of Tennessee—Memphis
Associate Director for EMS and Trauma
Emergency Department
Le Bonheur Children's Medical Center
Memphis, Tennessee
60 Urinary and Renal Disorders

JULIAN B. ORENSTEIN, MD, FACEP, FAAP
Assistant Professor
Emergency Medicine and Pediatrics
Fairfax Hospital
Fairfax, Virginia
52 Gastrointestinal Disorders

RICHARD A. ORR, MD
Associate Professor of Anesthesiology/Critical Care
    Medicine and Pediatrics
University of Pittsburgh School of Medicine
Associate Director, Pediatric Intensive Care
Medical Director, Pediatric Transport
Children's Hospital of Pittsburgh
Pittsburgh, Pennsylvania
5 Interhospital Transport

JAMES F. PADBURY, MD
Professor of Pediatrics
UCLA School of Medicine
Chief, Division of Neonatology
Harbor-UCLA Medical Center
Torrance, California
17 Newborn Resuscitation

RUTH ANN PARISH, MD, FAAP
Clinical Associate Professor
Department of Pediatrics
University of Washington School of Medicine
Children's Hospital Medical Center
Seattle, Washington
37 Thermal Injury

MARY D. PATTERSON, MD
Director, Pediatric Emergency Department
The Bowman-Gray School of Medicine
Winston-Salem, North Carolina
52 Gastrointestinal Disorders

RONALD I. PAUL, MD, FAAP
Medical Director, Emergency Department
Kosair Children's Hospital
Associate Professor of Pediatrics
University of Louisville School of Medicine
Louisville, Kentucky
56 Neurologic Disorders

WASSAM M. RAHMAN, MD, FAAP
Medical Director
Pediatric Emergency Medicine
Children's Hospital of the King's Daughters
Assistant Professor of Pediatrics
Eastern Virginia Medical School
Norfolk, Virginia
21 Facial Trauma

MICHAEL RECHT, MD, PhD
Fellow, Pediatric Hematology/Oncology
Department of Pediatrics
Yale University School of Medicine
New Haven, Connecticut
54 Hematologic and Oncologic Disorders

JULIA A. ROSEKRANS, MD, FAAP, FACEP
Consultant in Pediatric and Adolescent Medicine
Section Head, Pediatric Emergency Medicine
Pediatric Residency Program Director
Mayo Graduate School of Medicine
Assistant Professor of Pediatrics
Department of Pediatric and Adolescent Medicine
Mayo Medical School
Mayo Medical Center
Rochester, Minnesota
33 Animal and Human Bites
48 Dermatologic Disorders

ALFRED SACCHETTI, MD, FACEP
Research Director
Our Lady of Lourdes Medical Center
Camden, New Jersey
Assistant Clinical Professor
Emergency Medicine
Thomas Jefferson University
Philadelphia, Pennsylvania
15 Fluid and Electrolyte Balance

RICHARD A. SALADINO, MD
Assistant Professor of Pediatrics
Harvard Medical School
Assistant in Medicine
Department of Medicine
Division of Emergency Department
Children's Hospital
Boston, Massachusetts
50 Endocrine and Metabolic Disorders

JOHN P. SANTAMARIA, MD, FACEP, FAAP
Director, Wound and Hyperbaric Center
Attending Physician, Pediatric Emergency Services
St. Joseph's Hospital
Clinical Associate Professor of Pediatrics
University of South Florida School of Medicine
Tampa, Florida
49 Ear, Nose, and Throat Disorders

ANTHONY J. SCALZO, MD, FAAP, ACMT
Professor of Pediatrics
Department of Pediatrics
Division of Emergency Medicine and Toxicology
Saint Louis University Health Sciences Center
Cardinal Glennon Children's Hospital
St. Louis, Missouri
44 Inhalation Injuries

SUZANNE SCHUH, MD, FRCP(C), FACEP (PEM)
Associate Professor of Pediatrics
University of Toronto
Emergency Department
The Hospital for Sick Children
Toronto, Ontario
Canada
59 Respiratory Disorders

JAMES S. SEIDEL, MD, PhD, FAAP
Chief, Division of General and Emergency Pediatrics
Harbor-UCLA Medical Center
Professor of Pediatrics
UCLA School of Medicine
Torrance, California
  1 Approach to the Pediatric Patient in the Emergency Department
  11 Emergency Management of Respiratory Distress and Failure
  12 Cardiopulmonary Resuscitation

VIDYA SHARMA, MD, FAAP
Associate Professor of Pediatrics
University of Missouri
Section of Emergency Medicine
The Children's Mercy Hospital
Kansas City, Missouri
43 Specific Toxins

LANCE SIEGER, MD
Chief, Division of Hematology/Oncology
Professor of Pediatrics
Harbor-UCLA Medical Center
Torrance, California
16 Blood, Blood Components, and Transfusion Reactions

ROBERT M. SILLS, DO, FAAP
Attending Physician, Pediatric Emergency Medicine
Department of Emergency Medicine
St. John's Hospital and Medical Center
Detroit, Michigan
36 Electrical and Lightning Injuries

ANGELA SIRNICK, MD, FRCP
Assistant Professor
University of Ottawa
Department of Pediatrics
Children's Hospital of Eastern Ontario
Ottawa, Ontario
Canada
53 Gynecologic and Obstetric Disorders

KATHLEEN M. SMITH, MD, FAAP
Clinical Assistant Professor of Pediatrics
University of Washington — Seattle
Pediatric Emergency Medicine Attending
Department of Emergency Medicine
Mary Bridge Children's Hospital
Tacoma, Washington
40 High Altitude Illness and Dysbarism

DEBORAH L. SMITH-WRIGHT, MD
Director of Pediatrics — Twin Cities Unit
Department of Pediatrics
Shriner's Hospital for Crippled Children
Minneapolis, Minnesota
57 Orthopedic Disorders

CARL D. STEVENS, MD, MPH
Department of Emergency Medicine
Harbor-UCLA Medical Center
Assistant Clinical Professor
UCLA School of Medicine
Torrance, California
3 Injury Prevention and Control

MARY P. SWEENEY, MD
Assistant Professor
Department of Pediatrics
Division of Critical Care
University of Tennessee — Memphis
Emergency Department
Le Bonheur Children's Medical Center
Memphis, Tennessee
60 Urinary and Renal Disorders

MILTON TENENBEIN, MD, FRCP(C), FAAP, FAACT
Director of Emergency Services
Children's Hospital, Winnipeg
Director, Manitoba Poison Control Centre
Professor of Pediatrics and Pharmacology
University of Manitoba
Winnipeg, Manitoba
Canada
42 General Management Principles for Poisoning

THOMAS E. TERNDRUP, MD, FACEP
Associate Professor
Director, Pediatric Emergency Department
Departments of Emergency Medicine and Pediatrics
State University of New York Health Science Center
   at Syracuse
Syracuse, New York
7 Pain Control, Analgesia, and Sedation

SUSAN B. TORREY, MD, FAAP
Instructor of Pediatrics
Harvard Medical School
Assistant in Medicine
Children's Hospital
Boston, Massachusetts
30 Lower Extremity and Pelvic Injuries

SUSAN B. TULLY, MD, FAAP
Professor of Pediatrics
UCLA School of Medicine
Director, Ambulatory and Emergency Pediatrics
Department of Pediatrics
Olive View-UCLA Medical Center
Sylmar, California
34 Venomous Animal Bites and Stings

MICHAEL G. TUNIK, MD, FAAP
Associate Director
Pediatric Emergency Medicine
Bellevue Hospital Center/New York University Medical
   Center
Assistant Professor of Clinical Pediatrics
New York University School of Medicine
New York, New York
4 Emergency Medical Services for Children

YEHESKEL WAISMAN, MD
Director, Unit of Emergency Medicine
Schneider Children's Medical Center of Israel
Lecturer, Sackler Faculty of Medicine
Tel Aviv University
Tel Aviv, Israel
52 Gastrointestinal Disorders

DAVID G. WARD, MD
Assistant Professor
Associate Director of Medicine/Pediatric Training
Departments of Pediatrics and Medicine
Division of Critical Care
University of Tennessee — Memphis
Emergency Department Staff Attending
Le Bonheur Children's Medical Center
Memphis, Tennessee
60 Urinary and Renal Disorders

GARY S. WASSERMAN, DO, FAAP, FAACT
Chief, Section of Clinical Toxicology
Director of Poison Control Center
Division of Emergency Medical Services
The Children's Mercy Hospital
Professor of Medicine
Department of Pediatrics
Children's Mercy Hospital
Kansas City, Missouri
43 Specific Toxins

LISE K. WATTERS, MD, FRCP(C)
Emergency Pediatrician
Children's Hospital of Eastern Ontario
Assistant Professor
Department of Pediatrics
University of Ottawa
Ottawa, Ontario
Canada
47 Cardiovascular Disorders

JOSEPH A. WEINBERG, MD
Director of Emergency Services
Le Bonheur Children's Medical Center
Associate Professor, Department of Pediatrics
Division of Critical Care
University of Tennessee—Memphis
Memphis, Tennessee
60 Urinary and Renal Disorders

WILLIS A. WINGERT, MD, FAAP
Professor Emeritus of Pediatrics, Emergency Medicine,
    and Family Medicine
University of Southern California School of Medicine
Los Angeles, California
34 Venomous Animal Bites and Stings

JOSEPH L. WRIGHT, MD, MPH, FAAP
Assistant Medical Director
Emergency Medical Trauma Center
Children's National Medical Center
Assistant Professor of Pediatrics and Emergency
    Medicine
School of Medicine and Health Sciences
George Washington University
Washington, District of Columbia
52 Gastrointestinal Disorders

CHRISTOPHER WUERKER, MD
Attending Physician
Emergency Department
Highland General Hospital
Oakland, California
32 Emergency Care of Minor Wounds

DONALD DEMETRIOS ZUKIN, MD, FACEP, FAAP
Departments of Emergency Medicine
Oakland Children's Hospital
Highland General Hospital
Clinical Assistant Professor
University of California—San Francisco
San Francisco, California
32 Emergency Care of Minor Wounds

Dedication

To the many physicians, nurses, and other health professionals whose knowledge, clinical expertise, and pursuit of excellence have served children well.

To my wife, Suzanne, and sons, Adam and Michael, who have taught me the importance of dedication to excellence in patient care, supported and endured me through this endeavor, and provided perspective to my life.

To children who continue as our partners in pursuing excellence and whom we hope will benefit from the skill and expertise of practitioners of pediatric emergency medicine.

RMB

To my husband, Gary Gwozdzik, whose constant support, encouragement, and gentle wisdom are the core of all my accomplishments; and to my son, Spenser Paul, whose development parallels that of this book.

GLC

To my first teachers, Seymour and Lucille Jaffe; to my mentors, Stephen Ludwig and Gary Fleisher, who made it possible for me to explore my interest in pediatric emergency medicine; to the fellows who have inspired me to continue to ask good questions; and to the children using emergency services who may benefit from this work.

DMJ

To my seven sibs—Mary, James, Lucy, Clara, William, Benedict, and Thomas. They taught me a lot about love, life, and pediatrics.

JFK

To the children and families who have helped us understand the importance of care and compassion; to my faculty and residents for their support and dedication to the children we serve; to my wife, An-ping, and my children, Christina, David, Matthew, and Joseph, for their love and support; and to my mom, Virginia, for her love and guidance as I studied and chose to pursue medicine as a career.

RWS

To my mentors, Marietta Voge, Ph.D., who taught me about science and life and Joseph W. St. Geme Jr., M.D., who shared his knowledge, philosophy and love with all that were fortunate enough to have come under his tutelage.

JSS

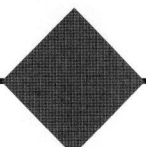

Preface

The biology of children is unique, reflecting the rapid evolution of the infant developmentally and physiologically. Pediatric emergency medicine draws on the expertise of pediatrics and emergency medicine in forming the foundation of a growing body of clinical expertise. Identification and stabilization of emergently ill children presenting for care are the focus of the specialty, but the perspective of the clinician must be comprehensive, often caring for more routine and self-limited conditions.

The uniqueness of pediatric emergency medicine lies in the urgency of intervention to prevent morbidity and mortality, the special requirements of the delivery setting, and the breadth of medical and traumatic problems that require attention. The diversity of physiologic and emotional responses to illness broadens the diagnostic evaluation and differential considerations. Parental concern, observation, and reaction may further complicate the therapeutic plan.

A continuum of care and expertise of the prehospital system, emergency department, inpatient service, and discharge planning must work flawlessly in optimizing outcome.

Pediatric Emergency Medicine: Concepts and Clinical Practice reflects the rapid growth of this new specialty. It brings together a uniquely talented group of clinicians who practice pediatric emergency medicine in pediatric, general, teaching, and community hospitals throughout the country. Many come from initial training in pediatrics, whereas others are from emergency medicine, surgery, and nursing; many have received formal training in both pediatrics and emergency medicine. The contributors are involved in expanding knowledge, technologies, and research that will provide the basis for the evolution of the specialty.

Although individual, institutional, and geographic bias exists in our daily practice, we have tried to present widely accepted diagnostic and management guidelines that consider possible time and resource constraints, incomplete databases, and inadequacy of follow-up in the patient care environment in which we practice.

Bringing together the expertise of these practitioners while presenting the material in an accessible format has drawn upon the experience of many. Throughout, topics are formatted in parallel fashion to allow you, the reader, to quickly retrieve information that is relevant to a presenting sign, symptom, or diagnostic entity. Procedures are described in the relevant chapter and cross-referenced throughout. We have divided the book into medical and traumatic conditions, with the remaining parts of the text being easily accessible through the table of contents, index, and page headings. Outlines at the beginning of each chapter include page numbers to facilitate access to the vast array of information.

New material has been added since the first edition to reflect the expansion of knowledge. We have further emphasized resuscitation, fluid and electrolyte management, and legal issues in the practice of pediatric emergency medicine. New diagnostic entities and updated clinical and physiologic principles have been incorporated throughout the text.

We have enjoyed the challenge of chronicling pediatric emergency medicine based upon the uniqueness of a specific area of information, the importance of the specialty, and the frequency of presentation. We hope that this book will continue to provide a foundation for study and practice by an expanding generation of practitioners in pediatric emergency medicine during a period of growth that will stimulate us to achieve even greater heights of clinical practice and exploration of knowledge.

The body of expertise encompassed within these pages should provide a framework for all clinicians to allow children and parents to expect consistency of access and excellence of care. We shall all face this challenge with enthusiasm, knowledge, and commitment.

ROGER M. BARKIN, M.D.

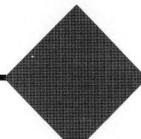

Acknowledgments

The physicians, nurses, paramedics, and other practitioners have created the specialty of pediatric emergency medicine. Their competency, skill, patience, experience, concerns, and sensitivity molded this book.

Peter Rosen, through his leadership, mentoring, and perspective, has served as a model for many of us during the process of learning. His impact is evident.

We are obviously grateful to the editors and authors who have contributed and graciously participated in the evolution of this text. The Department of Surgery at the University of Colorado Health Sciences Center, the Department of Emergency Medical Services of Denver General Hospital, and Columbia-HealthONE in Denver have provided an environment of support and encouragement that has made these efforts both possible and gratifying.

Kathy Falk, Laurel Craven, Carol Weis, David Stein, Carolyn Kruse, and a host of other editors at Mosby have moved this book to completion with frequent reminders, close monitoring, a tight time-frame, superb editing, and a sense of humor. Adam Barkin reviewed many of the galleys and page proofs. Kathi Thompson made it move smoothly through its many steps, monitoring progress and coordinating communication and editing, while balancing many other responsibilities.

We would also like to thank our readers who will synthesize the insights provided by this text and use it with expertise and confidence in the care of our pediatric patients.

RMB

I would like to acknowledge Stephen Ludwig and Gary Fleisher, who first taught me as mentors and now continue to encourage me as friends and colleagues; and to the residents and fellows I have trained—they are the source of my professional inspiration and growth.

GLC

On behalf of the chapter authors, I would like to acknowledge the clerical and administrative contributions of Majda Avsenik, Fatima Almeida, Irene Fischer, Paula Zimmerle, Veronica Hammond, Joanne Taggart, and David Kazimer.

DMJ

I would like to acknowledge the work of my secretary, Carla Taylor, and my valued colleagues in Pediatric Emergency Medicine who helped in the preparation of this book.

JFK

I want to personally thank all of our contributors for their expertise and writings that will help all of us in our daily practices. I also wish to thank Marge Garthwaite, my secretary over the past several years, for providing technical guidance on the manuscripts. I thank my colleagues and residents of the Carolinas Medical Center for their support and encouragement. And last, I wish to thank Dr. John A. Marx, Chairman of our Department, and Dr. Harry Nurkin, CEO of Carolinas Medical Center, for their commitment to the importance of education and patient care.

RWS

Special thanks to my colleague, Deborah Parkman Henderson, RN, MA, for her help with the manuscript and her many years of collaboration.

JSS

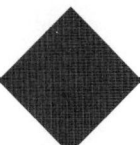

Contents

PEDIATRIC EMERGENCY MEDICINE

CARING FOR CHILDREN

Approach to the Pediatric Patient in the Emergency Department

James S. Seidel • Deborah Parkman Henderson

The initial encounter between emergency department personnel and a child and his or her caretakers often sets the tone for the entire visit. There are many pressures because children and caretakers experience a variety of emotions that may be reflected in their behavior and response to emergency department personnel. To ensure optimal care, emergency care providers should always consider a child within the context of the family and have a good understanding of how to approach both caretakers and pediatric patients in this stressful environment. Approaching families in the emergency department requires focusing on the differences in children at various ages and stages of development and on general principles for use in facilitating the provision of emergency care to the family.

Approximately 25% to 35% of patients seen in many emergency departments are in the pediatric age group. Most of these visits are for problems that the child or caretaker perceives as requiring more urgent care than is available at most physicians' offices, pediatric clinics, and Health Maintenance Organizations. About 3% to 5% of these visits represent true medical and surgical emergen-

cies. In these cases, the child could suffer permanent disability or death without immediate intervention. Many visits to the emergency department, however, are clearly for problems that could be best managed elsewhere and do not represent true emergencies. Emergency care providers must understand that, at present, emergency departments provide health care for a population with a wide spectrum of injuries and illnesses. The emergency department has also become the only resource for patients who are unable to access primary health care because of financial or social barriers.

The emergency department staff is faced with a broad array of pediatric patients who need care; these patients are generally accompanied by parents or caretakers. Triage decisions must be made on the basis of a short history, vital signs, and a brief physical assessment. In addition to being able to make these quick evaluations and provide therapies for medical and surgical problems, the emergency nurse and physician must have the knowledge, attitudes, and skills to rapidly evaluate the patient-caretaker relationship. A certain amount of anxiety and fear should be anticipated. The fears experienced by parent and child often include the following:

1. Fear of the unknown: what will happen next and what procedures may be performed
2. Fear of pain or loss
3. Fear of isolation and separation
4. Fear of strangers caring for the child
5. Fear of the unfamiliar environment with strange machines and equipment

There may also be a difference between the perceived needs of the caretaker or parent and those of the caregivers — the physician and nurse. The goals and objectives of each group need to be met. The caretaker and child need information, nurturing, and understanding. Caregivers need information, cooperation, and understanding. The following basic principles can facilitate the examination and treatment of children:

1. *Remain calm and confident.* Speak with a calm, soft voice. Be confident and maintain control of the situation by taking charge and being gently assertive.
2. *Establish rapport with the parent or caretaker and the child.* A child's anxiety often reflects what he or she feels or sees in the parent. Speak directly to the parent and child; ask them how they are doing several times during the visit. A brief conversation with the parent or caretaker about a nonmedical topic improves rapport and establishes good contact. Avoid the use of technical and medical terms.
3. *Be direct and honest.* If there is something that the parent, caretaker, or child needs to do, tell them what it is directly. Do not lie or mislead, and do not say that something will not be painful when you know that it will be.
4. *Keep the child and caretaker informed.* Many caretakers consider the lack of information to be the most stressful factor in visiting the emergency department. Avoid surprises by telling the child and caretaker what you are going to do: what, where, and how. Describe procedures and sensations: "I am going to wipe your arm with a wet, cool piece of cotton. It probably feels cold to you. Now I am going to . . ." Provide children with methods they can use to relieve their distress: "The medicine may taste icky for a few minutes, but you can wash it down with water."
5. *Assign one caregiver to the child if possible.* The patient and parent or caretaker often feel more comfortable when the same physician and nurse care for them throughout the course of the visit.
6. *Do not separate the parent or caretaker and child.* Parents can often be helpful, even in the most stressful and anxiety-producing situations. However, an adolescent may wish not to have the caretaker in the room.
7. *Make as many observations as possible without touching the patient.* Physical assessment can usually be done by careful observation. Valuable information may also be gained about the parent-child relationship.
8. *Be kind, and provide feedback and reassurance.* The caregiver's attitude toward the parent and child is expressed verbally and nonverbally. Give reassurance frequently during the visit, and always provide hope (of whatever kind possible). Children especially appreciate reassurance, rewards, and praise after a painful procedure.

Each developmental stage has been described in various ways in the literature, although the stages cannot be differentiated with absolute precision. The child's developmental level affects the family and the interaction between each member of the family and emergency care providers. A general description of theories of child development and age-appropriate emergency department interventions is shown in Table 1-1. Emergency care personnel may find it useful to consider these developmental stages when assessing and caring for children.

EARLY INFANCY (0 TO 6 MONTHS)

Developmental Issues

During the birth process, a transition takes place. The newborn baby begins breathing air, but although he or she is separated physically, the child is still wholly dependent on caretakers for sustenance. The neonate requires food, comfort, shelter, love, and attention, and when these needs are not met, the child cries. Because discomfort is generalized rather than differentiated, it is not always a simple task for the caregiver to determine what the child needs. As parents bond with their child, a rhythm and understanding naturally develop. As parents meet their child's basic needs, the child begins to develop a sense of trust.

Neonates' undeveloped musculature prevents them from lifting their heads and turning over, and they generally sleep a lot, although the sleep may not be when and where the parents wish. The egocentrism of neonates keeps them attuned largely to their bodily needs, but they respond to some degree to the environment and can fix their eyes for short periods on bright, shiny toys, moving objects, and on the faces of individuals in their field of vision.

Caretakers may need to meet some of their own basic needs during this period; they often require comfort because they may be very anxious and concerned about their tiny, vulnerable child. Most parents of infants under 6 weeks of age are just adapting to the new member of the family and may not be able to trust their own instincts and abilities, even when they have several other children.

After 6 weeks of age, children are increasingly able to respond to their environment and achieve limited control. They begin to smile and interact with caretakers by making cooing sounds and following them with their eyes. They begin to reach for objects, even though they may not be able to grasp them yet. Around 4 months of age, infants turn over, usually much to the caretakers' surprise. This, and their increasing ability to support themselves while sitting up, give them more control over their positioning. This may be a more rewarding period for parents than the newborn period, but until about 6 months of age, children are still very helpless and require a remarkable amount of work and attention. Parents are often exhausted because most babies wake up several times during the night for feedings.

Physical Examination

From birth to about 6 or 9 months of age, approaching and examining the infant is usually a simple task. Much of the physical examination consists of observation. The examination should be performed with the child on the parent's lap or in an adult's arms. A quiet room in which the caretaker can sit in a chair holding the child is ideal but not always an easy location to find in a busy emergency depart-

TABLE 1-1. Ages and Stages of Children

	Birth-18 mo	19 mo-2 yr	3 yr-5 yr	6 yr-11 yr	12 yr-18 yr
Theories of child development					
Erikson	Trust vs. mistrust	Autonomy vs. shame and doubt	Initiative vs. guilt	Industry vs. inferiority	Identity vs. role confusion
Freud	Oral-sensory	Anal	Phallic	Latency	Genital
Piaget	Sensori-motor egocentrism	Preoperational, beginnings of perceptual constancy	Preoperational, prelogical reasoning	Concrete operations	Formal operations
Task mastery	Differentiate self and non-self	Toilet training	Use of language	Logic	Abstract thinking
Pain perception	Physical but possibly not cognitive pain perceived, in younger patients	Primarily egocentric: "Here and now" May see pain as punishment	Pain as punishment Overextension of causality Fear and fantasy	Beginning of understanding of true causality Fear of destruction and death	Concept of emotional and physical pain Understanding of root causes of pain
Suggested interventions	1. Involve caretaker in care of child. 2. Keep child warm. 3. Keep room quiet. 4. Provide comfort measures (e.g., pacifier). 5. Keep child on caretaker's lap during physical examination. 6. Return child to caretaker as soon as possible after procedures; allow caretaker to comfort child.	1. Prepare caretaker for procedures. 2. Tell caretaker that he or she may assist in normal care. 3. Give child a familiar toy or blanket as a transitional object. 4. Use child's name. 5. Restrain child as little as possible. 6. Avoid covering child's face. 7. Describe sensations and talk with child during the procedures. 8. Praise, smile, and have a cheerful attitude.	1. Explain procedure *immediately before* performing it. 2. Allow child to see and touch samples of equipment. 3. Be honest: "This will sting." 4. Use simple distractions and talk to child. 5. Allow child to see under bandages. 6. Use praise, decorated adhesive bandages, and small rewards.	1. Explain procedures beforehand. 2. Enlist cooperation. 3. Ask about simple preferences. 4. Give alternatives (e.g., child may yell but not move.) 5. Identify sensations and personnel. 6. Use distraction and counting games. 7. Include child in discharge instructions. 8. Use rewards, stickers, badges, and praise.	1. Give *full* explanations. 2. Encourage child's participation. 3. Allow time for questions. 4. Provide *privacy*. Child may want to exclude parents. 5. Avoid teasing and embarrassing child. 6. Allow as much control as possible. 7. Provide discharge instructions to patient. 8. Reassure child that his or her behavior was appropriate.

ment. Assess the bonding of the infant with the caretaker or parent. The examiner observes whether the infant makes eye contact with the caretaker and responds to voices, startles with loud sounds, and is generally aware of the environment. The examiner also observes whether the child can be consoled when crying. It is a good idea to determine whether the infant arouses by himself or herself while asleep or whether he or she needs additional stimulation. The child should be able to suck on a bottle or nipple, and all four extremities should move normally. The examiner also notes whether the skin color is normal, mottled, or cyanotic.

The infant is kept with the caretaker during the active portions of the physical examination. The least invasive assessments are done first; the examiner listens to the heart and chest and then palpates the abdomen and head. Examinations requiring bright lights in the eyes and ears are saved for last. Fever (above 38° C) or inconsolable crying must be explained. The cause of crying may be hidden; sometimes there is a foreign body in the eye or a string around a digit on the hands or feet. The uncovered body of the infant is observed for normal development (Table 1-2).

LATE INFANCY (6 TO 18 MONTHS)

Developmental Issues

During the first 6 to 9 months of life, infants become increasingly aware of their environment and other people. As they become more aware of the separation between themselves and others, they also become aware of the differences between their familiar caretakers and other strangers. From 9 months until 18 months of age, stranger anxiety is common. At this age, no matter how kind and approachable a person is, he or she is likely to be perceived as an enemy. This should never be taken personally. In late infancy, a good general rule is to accept the child's fear and hostility as normal behavior.

Until about 1 year of age, the infant does not begin to develop perceptual constancy, so if the parent is not visible to them at any moment, the parent simply stops existing. For this reason, it is important to keep the caretaker with the child as much as possible and to return him or her to the caretaker as quickly as possible if separation is necessary.

Physical Examination

The emergency physician should have an understanding of normal physical development when evaluating any child. It is generally good practice to obtain measures of weight, length, and head circumference on every infant. Standardized charts are available to plot these parameters (see Appendix A). If the infant is below the 5th percentile for age, the examiner plots the parameter to the 50th percentile line and determines the chronologic age for which that number is normally found. For example, a 6-month-old girl is found to weigh 5.6 kg. This is below the 5th percentile for age and at the 50th percentile for a 3-month-old baby. Some general rules follow:

1. The birth weight of most infants doubles within 5 months and triples within a year.

TABLE 1-2. Screening Developmental Milestones

Age	Milestones
Newborn	Lies flexed.
	Turns head from side to side.
	Fixates to light and close objects.
	Has a visual preference for the human face.
1 mo	Has more-extended legs.
	Lifts chin.
	Smiles responsively.
	Follows a moving object.
4 mo	Lifts head and chest upward.
	Lacks Moro reflex.
	Rolls front to back.
	Reaches for objects.
	Coos, says "ah," and laughs.
6 mo	Sits unsupported.
	Resists the pull of a toy.
	Bears some weight on legs.
	Turns to a voice.
	Responds more to emotion.
	Babbles.
9 mo	Bears weight.
	Crawls.
	Cruises holding on to furniture.
	Plays pat-a-cake.
	Tries to find a hidden object.
	Responds to name.
	Says nonspecific "Mama-Dada."
	Imitates speech.
1 yr	Walks holding a hand.
	Has a pincher response.
	Plays simple games (i.e., ball).
	Has three simple words other than "Mama."
2 yr	Walks up and down stairs.
	Jumps and runs well.
	Climbs on furniture.
	Puts three words together.
	Handles spoon well.
	Listens to stories.
	Observes pictures.
3 yr	Goes up stairs.
	Rides a tricycle.
	Stands momentarily on one foot.
	Knows age.
	Counts three objects.
	Knows first and last names.
6 yr	Balances on one foot.
	Hops.
	Can heel-toe walk.
	Knows colors.
	Counts to 10.
	Speaks sentences of at least 10 syllables.

2. The average length of a neonate is 50 cm. The length of most infants increases by 30 cm (10 to 12 inches) within the first year.

3. The head circumference of an infant increases by 2 cm per month for the first 3 months and by 1 cm a

month for the next 3 months; thereafter, it increases by ½ cm a month (see Appendix A-1).

Another developmental milestone is the development of dentition. Deciduous teeth (baby teeth) begin to erupt at 5 to 9 months. Eruption proceeds with four teeth per 4 months until all 20 teeth are in place. A 1-year-old infant, for instance, will have six to eight teeth.

Physical examination should include a careful examination of the head, noting the size, shape, symmetry, and status of the fontanelles. The posterior fontanelle varies in size; it is usually about 1 inch in width at the widest opening, and it closes at about 4 months. The anterior fontanelle diminishes in size after 6 months, with closure between 9 and 18 months. If it remains open after this, further investigation is necessary. Pulsations may be felt during palpation normally, but the anterior fontanelle should never be tense and full.

It is also important to assess intellectual and emotional development, and any delays should be noted for referral. There are many ways to consider the child's development (Table 1-1). As in early infancy, it is best to examine the older infant on the caretaker's lap. The examiner begins with the noninvasive examination (i.e., chest and abdomen) and completes the examination with parts that may be uncomfortable for the infant. Normal pulse, respiration, and blood pressure vary with age.

TODDLERHOOD (18 MONTHS TO 3 YEARS)

Developmental Issues

Toddlers are curious children who delight in exploring their environment. This characteristic is easily observed in a well child or in one who has only minor ailments. A toddler will run around the room, looking in drawers and under tables and chairs, and is generally interested in everything. It is unusual for this age child to be withdrawn and quiet. Toddlers are developing a much greater sense of their own autonomy and are beginning to be able to meet some of their own needs and care for themselves. They have developed a pincer grasp and can therefore obtain objects within their reach and bring them to their mouths. They are able to eat most of their food by themselves and hold and drink from a cup and may have very pronounced likes and dislikes. They are also beginning toilet training at this age, allowing them even more independence from their caretakers. Most important of all, perhaps, they are learning to walk and explore their world by themselves.

The new-found independence of toddlers may be hard for parents to accept, and a period of negotiation and renegotiation of limits ensues, reaching its height at about the age of 2 years. Because of the toddler's independence and mobility, traumatic injuries become a major cause of emergency department visits. Parents may feel very responsible (and they may be indirectly or directly responsible) for their child's injury; this issue must be carefully addressed by anticipatory guidance and by discussion of their feelings of responsibility after such an event has occurred.

During this stage, perceptual constancy becomes well developed. Toddlers are better able to accept the absence of a parent if necessary and can be aided in this acceptance with the use of a transitional object such as a blanket or familiar toy. They can play games such as peek-a-boo without being afraid that the person no longer exists and delight in this activity. They are also beginning to talk and can answer simple questions about the location of their pain, pointing with their fingers. Encouraging them to make simple decisions relating to their care may help. Because of the developing independence of the toddler, the decision to use any type of restraints must be carefully considered. Parents should not be asked to assist in restraining their child.

Physical Examination

During toddlerhood (Table 1-1), there is a deceleration in the rate of growth. The average toddler gains about 2.5 kg in weight and 12 cm in length; head circumference increases by only 2 cm during the entire second year of life. The toddler's appetite may decrease when compared with that during infancy. Dental hygiene and caries become an issue, so examination of the mouth should include assessment of the teeth, gums, and palate. There is a mild lordosis, and the child may appear to have a protuberant abdomen. Speech becomes important and an ever-present word is "no." During this stage, the child is more ambulatory, and the parental concerns often involve perceived orthopedic problems such as toeing in and out, which are generally due to normal curvatures of the bones of the lower extremities.

PRESCHOOL YEARS (3 TO 6 YEARS)

Developmental Issues

Preschool children have gained control of their environment to a large extent. They can play with blocks, make drawings, generally dress themselves, and brush their own teeth. Just as the major advance for toddlers was their ability to move into and grasp the physical world, the major advance in the preschool-age child is the ability to move into the world of the mind. Communication skills move rapidly forward, and some prelogical reasoning develops.

Along with the nascent ability to reason comes the ability to fantasize, and children at this age may develop inexplicable fears and nightmares. This may have a significant impact on care in the emergency department; preschool children overextend the concept of causality and may believe (without telling anyone) that their illnesses and injuries are related in some way to perceived or real misbehavior. Injury to another family member may be felt by a preschool child to be the direct result of wishing them ill. Emergency department personnel should address these concerns, asking the preschooler directly what he or she thinks caused the injury or illness and giving brief, simple, concrete explanations when possible.

To prevent fantasies from becoming unmanageable, the preschool child should also be given information regarding treatments immediately before the procedure rather than long in advance so that there will not be sufficient time to develop frightening fantasies. The preschool child should also be allowed to handle some of the simple objects used in his or her care, such as medicine cups, tongue blades, and cotton swabs. During short procedures, the preschool child can often be distracted with counting games, small toys, or conversation. Adhesive bandages are essential after a procedure or when an injection has been given because preschool children may believe that they will continue to lose blood through the injection site. All explanations should be carefully adjusted to the developmental level of the child. The tendency is for health care providers to overestimate rather than underestimate the preschool child's ability to understand.

Physical Examination

Gains in weight and stature generally are constant during the preschool years (3, 4, and 5 years) with a 2-kg and 6- to 8-cm gain per year. The child appears to become lean, which may be mistaken for weight loss by the parent or caretaker. The lordosis and protuberant abdomen are less pronounced. The 20 primary teeth should all have erupted by 2½ years of age, and the face has relatively more growth than the cranium. There is a refinement of gross and fine motor skills. Language becomes more prominent, and sentences become longer and more coherent. Lymph nodes may begin to be palpable.

SCHOOL-AGE YEARS (6 TO 11 YEARS)

Developmental Issues

School-age children assume many adult characteristics. They are able to move around independently and have some basic reasoning powers. They can ride bicycles, run, jump, hop, skip, and write. They are also industrious and interested in learning. This may also be a period of relative calm for parents, when children become interested and involved in their school work and activities. The way that the child is performing in school is an important assessment for health care providers. The examiner asks whether the child has problems paying attention in class and is learning at the appropriate level. It is important to determine whether there are any problems in relating to peers. The child, not just the parent, should be asked questions when the medical history is obtained.

School-age children want to participate in their care and should be encouraged to make choices when possible, such as in which hand to insert an intravenous line or whether they would like to sit up or lie down. They also respond well to specific instructions about their behavior such as, "You may make as much noise as you want, if you hold your hand still." Explanations should be given well before the procedure. The older school-age child should also be included in the conversations regarding treatment plans when instructions are given for care at home. Rewards should be given after a procedure and can include stickers, small toys, and praise. Even when a child has struggled and fought, the examiner can give credit for trying.

Physical Examination

As in the earlier age group, growth is steady until the prepubescent growth spurts, which occur at age 10 years in girls and 12 years in boys. The spine straightens, but scoliosis may be a problem in late childhood and early adolescence. Some parents may be concerned about the child's posture because the child may appear flat footed or knock-kneed. Most of the sinuses, including the frontal sinuses, are now aerated. The first permanent teeth erupt at 6 to 7 years, and the shedding of the primary deciduous teeth occurs in the same order as their eruption. The permanent teeth erupt at about four teeth per year. The lymphatic glands are often larger than in early childhood, and the tonsils may appear relatively enlarged until they reach their nadir at 7 to 8 years of age. As the child approaches adolescence, the musculature becomes more prominent, and the body habitus slowly evolves into one that more closely resembles an adult. The bony growth plates are still not fused, and longitudinal growth will continue.

ADOLESCENCE (12 TO 18 YEARS)

Developmental Issues

Adolescence is a period of rapid growth. Early adolescents exist solidly in the world of children; in later adolescence, these children join the adult world. They learn to think and reason abstractly and become aware of their sexuality. Parents may be fascinated and frightened by the new changes in their child. Hearing a son's voice change, helping a daughter cope with menarche, and teaching children how to drive an automobile are only a few of the remarkable experiences of parents at this stage. In this brief and often confusing transition to full adulthood, one child may have many adult characteristics and yet remain childlike; another may not appear to have grown as much, and yet be capable of adult responsibilities and activities.

During the examination of the adolescent child, privacy should be maintained when possible. The adolescent is modest and is easily embarrassed by teasing or by any suggestion that he or she has not acted appropriately. If an adolescent child does not want a caretaker present during the examination or procedures, the caretaker should be encouraged to leave. It may be best to include both parent and child when any information is provided regarding the injury or treatment, but confidentiality may be required in some instances. In certain states it is illegal to give parents of adolescents information concerning certain subjects such as pregnancy, drug abuse, or sexually transmitted diseases, including HIV status, without the permission of the patient.

Physical Examination

During adolescence, major physical and emotional growth occur. It is the period of development in which there is the highest rate of growth. Physical maturation occurs at different times in the sexes, beginning at 10 years of age in girls and 12 in boys. Some individuals in both sexes may have delayed growth, and as long as they are following a sequential pattern of physical and sexual development, there is generally no need to be concerned. Emergency physicians should be familiar with the normal stages of sexual development and the sequence of growth in adolescents (Fig. 1-1).

In early adolescence, girls are larger than boys; this reverses in mid-to-late adolescence when boys experience their growth spurts and become more muscular. Physical

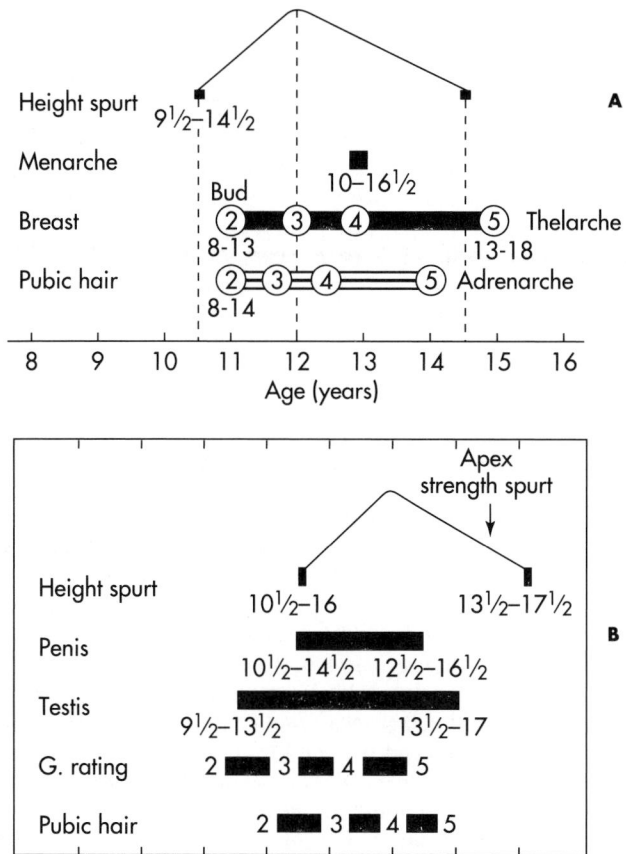

FIG. 1-1. A, The normal sequence of sexual maturation of an average girl. **B,** The normal sequence of sexual maturation of an average boy. Numbers refer to Tanner stage of sexual development. (*From Marshall WA and Tanner JM:* Arch Dis Child *45:13, 1970.*)

and psychosocial milestones are not always achieved at the predicted age. With puberty, there are major changes in vital signs. The pulse and respiratory rates are lower and systolic blood pressure higher.

Although minor and major trauma and behavioral emergencies are the most common reasons for visits to emergency departments by adolescent patients, adolescents are also concerned with physical appearance, including scars, skin care, and any abnormality that might set them apart

from their peers, as well as problems related to sexuality, pregnancy, and sexually transmitted diseases. Attention should be directed to these concerns.

The physical examination should be done in private and should include a complete examination, including the genitalia. It may be necessary to have a chaperone in the room if the chief complaint demands a complete genital examination.

SUMMARY

The emergency department staff must be aware of the developmental and physical stages of growth of pediatric patients, as well as be sensitive to the needs of both the patient and caretaker. When possible, it is important to consider the entire family as the patient and involve family members in the care of the patient in the emergency department. These key family members or caretakers should also be present when instructions for home or follow-up care are provided by the staff. When appropriate, older children or adolescents should be included in discussions of the treatment plan and be allowed to participate in decisions concerning care.

Emergency departments generate fear and anxiety in pediatric patients and their caretakers; good (and frequent) verbal and nonverbal communication is important to establish; rapport should be maintained. With kindness, patience, empathy, and understanding, emergency personnel can decrease the amount of stress experienced, facilitate the care of young patients and their families, and improve compliance.

Bibliography

Aquilera DC: *Crisis intervention: the theory and methodology,* ed 6, St. Louis, 1990, Mosby.

Bates B: *A guide to the physical examination,* Philadelphia, 1986, JB Lippincott.

Behrman RE, editor: *Nelson textbook of pediatrics,* ed 15, Philadelphia, 1996, WB Saunders.

Cormier WH and Cormier LS: *Interviewing strategies for helpers,* Monterey, Calif, 1985, Brooks/Cole Publishing.

Dixon SL: *Working with people in crisis: theory and practice,* St. Louis, 1979, Mosby.

Gellert E: *Psychosocial aspects of pediatric care,* New York, 1978, Grune & Stratton.

Hoekelman RA, editor: *Primary care pediatrics,* St. Louis, 1997, Mosby.

Piaget J and Inhelder B: *The psychology of the child,* New York, 1969, Basic Books.

Ross DM and Ross SA: *Childhood pain: current issues, research, and management,* Baltimore, Md, 1988, Urban & Schwarzenberg.

Tanner JM: *Growth at adolescence,* Oxford, England, 1962, Blackwell Scientific Publications.

Pediatric Emergency Department Environment

Larry Bruce Mellick • Susan McClellan Asch

Emergency pediatrics has only recently emerged figuratively from the hospital dungeons to which it traditionally was consigned, moving from "the pit" to "the front door of the hospital." Many authors have described the unique technical requirements of children's acute medical and trauma services, particularly as they differ from adult services, but few have dealt with the specific ways in which pediatric emergency departments must fit into their communities and meet the needs of their staff.[1-4] All of these factors must be addressed in designing the emergency department, if the department is to deliver acute care that is responsive to the needs of a community's children.

The pediatric patient is seen in a variety of emergency department settings, commonly representing over one third of all patients seen. Often the pediatric patient is integrated into the general emergency department with equipment and supplies to evaluate and care for the youngster but without a specific section and staff for children. Increasingly, general emergency departments have physically segmented an area for pediatric patients, allowing for personnel, equipment, and space conducive to caring for the younger patient population. Simultaneously, for major resuscitation activities these departments allow team integration and take advantage of the expertise and responsiveness of the entire emergency department staff. Children's hospitals with emergency departments typically focus exclusively on the needs of children within their entire triage, evaluation, and treatment areas.

As the emergency physician, nurse, and hospital planner evaluate their needs, whether during palliative construction and reorganization or during the building of an emergency department, the specific requirements of caring for children should be an integral part of the planning process. Although many of the issues parallel those associated with caring for adults, some are unique and require special emphasis. Nevertheless, the process provides an opportunity to provide for the special needs of children within the population served (i.e., to control the environment, to reduce threatening stimuli on patients, and to prevent "psychic numbing" of the staff).[5]

In planning or assessing a pediatric emergency environment the initial patient-focused questions that must be asked are the following: who are the patients, what are their health-care needs, and which of these needs is the department expected to meet? Factors that may be manipulated in response to these defined needs are physical space and its layout; personnel skill mix, number, and scheduling; and policies and procedures (i.e., planned behavior patterns of emergency staff and ancillary services) (see box on p. 9).

EXTERNAL COMPONENTS

The pediatric patient population that relates to a particular emergency department may be defined in terms of its own demographics: size, age, ethnicity, socioeconomic status, general health patterns, and special problems.

Size

The size of the population refers to the number of patients in the "cachement" area of the hospital who may use the emergency department for primary acute or emergency stabilization and treatment, secondary (referred) evaluation and definitive care, and for special procedures (e.g., minor orthopedic evaluation and treatment, suturing of lacerations, gastrostomy appliance replacement, intravenous [IV] starts, rabies vaccine administration, "sepsis work-ups," and lumbar punctures).

Population size is an important determinant of potential emergency department patient volumes. Adequate space is important to support efficient service in the waiting, triage, and treatment areas, as well as to support efficient patient flow. To ensure maximal program efficiency, the lay-out planning for this space requires input from those who are involved in the day-to-day treatment of patients. The space plan should ideally match the current needs and those expected in the future. Beyond specific medical necessities, the planning process should also reflect how many people (multiple health professionals and patients and accompanying relatives and friends) will conceivably use the space at the same time (or in rapid succession).

Patient volume is also a significant determinant of the number and mix of staff needed in the department at any one time. Space and equipment used by the staff such as charting and computer workstations, telephones, scales, bathrooms, break rooms, and lockers should be planned to handle staff numbers at peak periods.

Department efficiency and the quality of patient care will also be enhanced by careful planning. It is useful to break down the work process for each staff category to determine the components of their jobs and plan adequate space and efficient work-space ergonomics. For example, having the ward secretary frequently travel away from the workstation to pick up laboratory results, charts, or other paperwork from a tube station or computer printer, abandons the telephone, adds to nonproductive time, and may result in work-related injuries from repetitive motions.

Age

The age distribution of the emergency department population creates different needs for facilities. Typically, the majority of patients are infants or toddlers and specific environmental adaptations are required to accommodate these younger children. If, however, more than half of the children expected in the department are school age or adolescent, the physical plant, equipment, and staff orientation should be geared to these age groups and their emergency needs, as well as to those of infants and toddlers. Children and teenagers need chairs to sit on, books and magazines to read, and electronic entertainment of various sorts in waiting and minor treatment areas. The population is more likely to present with sports injuries necessitating particular surgical and orthopedic equipment. They require less restraint and more privacy, which may mean larger gowns or pajamas, curtains, and standing scales, in addition to the table scales and papoose boards needed for younger children.

Ethnicity

The ethnicity of the population refers to its specific cultural attributes and needs that may impact care, such as language barriers requiring interpreters between staff and patients; unique cultural health practices (e.g., coining), which must be understood; and norms of child care (the biologic parents may not be the primary caregivers or decision-makers in some cultural groups).

Other factors that may vary widely regionally, ethnically, and socioeconomically are norms for noise levels and physical violence. Construction of barriers between patients and between patients and staff may be needed for potential patterns of behavior. Bulletproof glass around staff space and restricted access doors into treatment areas may be seen as unnecessary and unfriendly in suburban Minnesota but may be expected and required in some urban areas. Conversely, since intimate, personal, and social distances differ regionally, the amount of individual space people require will differ.[6] Waiting room seating, registration and triage desk width, and examination room arrangement should also be considered in these cultural characteristics.

Additionally, subcultural differences between regions of the country; rural, urban, and suburban dwellers; and different socioeconomic groups must be understood by planners. In some regions of the country, physically separating one patient family from another by placing them in individual examination rooms to wait would be regarded as desirable privacy and protection from the diseases of others; in other regions, it would lead to feelings of entrapment and isolation.[7]

Sociocultural factors in emergency department planning are best addressed by involving representatives of the patient and staff groups that will be using the space. It is important that they be involved in designing the basic physical plant from the beginning, with ample opportunity to do conceptual walk-throughs of the entire patient-flow process (including details such as registration desk height and width and line-of-sight, sound from triage nurse to waiting room, play area, security points, and patient-care areas). This is necessary because subcultural differences are intuitively well known to their members, but these norms are seldom expressed formally, despite their importance.[8]

Emergency department personnel and staffing must also be responsive to the ethnic and subcultural characteristics of the patient population. The potential need for interpreters must be considered; in addition, staff who are ethnically, regionally, and socioeconomically similar to the patient population will enhance communications. For example, if the patient populations' caretakers speak in dialects such as Cajun, "Brooklynese," or "Harvard Yard," communication will be facilitated if the staff in high-visibility positions speak the same or a mutually comprehensible vernacular.

Sociocultural compatibility of staff and patients will help avoid the unconscious violation of subgroup norms. Inquiring in detail about the sexual activity of a 12-year-old might be highly appropriate for medical care for some ethnic and socioeconomic groups but irrelevant and a gross violation of norms for another subgroup, bewildering and embarrassing the child, angering the parents, and producing no useful medical information. Instructions such as "three times a day" must be interpreted identically by staff and patients. The instruction "take one with dinner" can only be correctly interpreted if both the giver and receiver of the instructions agree on what, when, and how often "dinner" is. Speaking the same subcultural language as the patients is crucial for health-care providers. If this is not achieved through staff background, it will need to be addressed through staff training in cultural diversity.

Socioeconomic and General Health Status

Socioeconomic status and general health status of the potential emergency department population will lead to different needs for physical facilities, staff, and policies. In a population with tenuous child health status, where seeking medical care late is the norm, more facilities for acute resuscitation may be needed. Further, if few acute patients have personal physicians, personnel and facilities for providing well-child care may be necessary. For populations with severe material deprivation, personnel (e.g., social service) and materials to assist in providing basic subsistence needs—food, clothing, and shelter—may be necessary.

Conversely, for a population where general health status is good, personal physicians are readily available, and poverty is rare, the facilities needed may only need to complement those provided elsewhere, and the staff must communicate with consulting and referring physicians on a frequent and prompt basis. This may mean, for example, increased facilities for sophisticated or invasive diagnostic procedures, as well as the need to provide funds for interior decor embellishments and equipment.

The parents of both poor and affluent children are asking the same question: "Is this a safe environment for my children, and will they receive the help they need in this setting?" The things on which the patients' parents and personal physicians base their judgment, as well as the needs of the children, may be noticeably different for diverse socioeconomic groups and health status levels.

Special Problems

Other external components of the emergency system that must be considered in planning the pediatric emergency department are preexisting relationships with referring and consulting physicians (on-going and episodic), existing community health-care facilities, community health-

care seeking patterns and expectations, managed care expectations and contractual relationships, perspectives of prehospital emergency care providers, and the physical environment of the hospital and the department. The physical facilities, personnel, outreach planning, and policies must reflect these as well.

Other community health-care facilities can be evaluated in terms of their number, proximity, competency, and interrelationships, as well as existing plans for community health care and product lines. For example, if the state health department plans to open a clinic in a nearby impoverished area to provide basic well-child care and social services, the children's emergency department may be able to refer patients to these facilities and serve as a back-up for those clinics when sick children are encountered. If, on the other hand, a local HMO opens a well-appointed urgent-care center in a feeder suburb for your hospital, you may need to develop an easily accessed emergency transport link with them and provide for acceptance, late hours, and urgent-care patient referrals of acutely ill children.

Prehospital Emergency Medical Services (EMS) is another component that should be planned for in the pediatric emergency department. Physically, if the department operates as medical control and receives ambulances, space for radio, operator, and supporting materials (protocol books or computer) must be available. EMS services may have particular preferences (e.g., loading dock style vs. covered garage). Storage for equipment, drug restocking, telephone access, desk space, coffee, and other amenities are valued by EMS personnel. Additionally, unencumbered space for movement of gurneys from the ambulance into the department without excessive maneuvering is also essential.

The local physical environment will also impinge on planning the emergency department itself. Because of the need for highly visible ambulatory patient and EMS access, the department must be located on the outer edge of the hospital. This means that climate, neighborhood type, and external spatial arrangements (i.e., type of street access, building sizes, parking, and proximity to other institutions) will dictate certain decisions in planning. Extensive weather barriers in certain climates and security barriers in particular neighborhoods have their own logic, but all of these needs must be considered early in planning.

INTERNAL COMPONENTS

The emergency department is a focal access point for patients, concurrently serving as a central resource for personnel and equipment in the stabilization of all patients. The first part of this chapter reviews personnel, facilities, and external components of the emergency department caring for children. Similar planning must also occur *within* the emergency department and hospital.

To ensure a patient- and family-centered focus, a number of relevant internal environments must be adapted. Physical, educational, sociologic, psychologic, emotional, professional, academic, design, and clinical factors have an impact on pediatric patients, their families, and their health-care providers. Optimal communication with the patient's primary care physician must be assured.

Physical

Body temperature regulation and control are important issues and one of the most easily overlooked aspects of pediatric care. Rapid heat loss and its metabolic impact on the child must be carefully monitored and prevented. Heat lamps, warmed IV solutions, commercial warming blankets, and heated blankets should be standard in all emergency departments. Thermostatic control of resuscitation rooms must not be overlooked. Severely hypothermic patients should have more aggressive treatment modalities available such as peritoneal lavage, bladder irrigation, and cardiopulmonary bypass.

The auditory environment can have significant impact on the pediatric patient and parents. A certain level of privacy for the staff is necessary because normal laughter and extraneous comments can be misunderstood by parents and caretakers. The noise and sounds of the emergency department can be frightening and stressful to the child; protection must be afforded. In general, private rooms are often useful. Finally, faulty departmental acoustics can interfere with communication, patient care, and physical examinations.

Surroundings that are aesthetic and soothing are ideal for children. Nevertheless, finding the right balance for wall motifs and decorations that do cause a sense of dissonance to the pediatric age and ethnic spectrum is a challenge. A colorful and tasteful pediatric decor is generally ideal but should simultaneously remain acceptable to a larger spectrum of preferences. Another important aspect of the physical environment is a mutual visual access between patients, families, and staff. This must be balanced with the need for limitation of staff interruptions by parents approaching caretakers for conversation, as well as patient privacy.

The management of the tactile aspect of pediatric care is without doubt an important part of the child's physical environment. Rough or brusque handling, cold hands, or a less-than-polished approach to the patient will lessen the effectiveness and success of the evaluation.[9] While management must remain efficient, the interaction is more successful when the child is slowly desensitized to touch and examination equipment. Playful conversation before and during the examination, distracting the child when appropriate, careful timing of the touch, and beginning the examination at the feet away from the face are less threatening. Warm hands, which have been recently washed, are necessary for both infection control and patient comfort.

Adequate pain control is another important, but frequently overlooked aspect of the pediatric patient's physical environment. Appropriate sedation policies and practices are mandatory for both pediatric and general emergency departments. Training in an appropriate spectrum of pain control options should also be an emergency medicine standard.[10]

Attention to and planning for comfort of the patient and family is another recognized area for emphasis. There should be adequate treatment room space for chairs, stools, and comfortable seating. Emergency department temperature control not only protects against unwanted patient heat loss but preserves the family's physical comfort. Easily accessible sources for fluids and nutrition also make the emergency department visit generally more comfortable. Access to diapers and formula when needed should be an expected amenity. Other patient comforts should include interesting and distracting activities as provided by child-life volunteers, as well as children's videos.

Sociologic, Psychologic, and Emotional

High priority must be given to the creation of an atmosphere of friendliness, kindness, caring, and concern for patients and their families. There is no place for a perfunctory, cold, or militant approach by health-care providers caring for children and their families. Nevertheless, enormous amounts of patience and forbearance may often be necessary for young and needy families.

Appropriate support resources for victims of child abuse, rape, or violent crime or those facing bereavement should be available. Patient representatives, child-life workers and volunteers, hospital chaplains, sexual assault response teams, and social workers are critical emergency department resources.

The staff must understand the different emotional needs and developmental levels of their patients. Skillful interfaces with a spectrum of patient ages and age-specific fears and anxieties are necessary for successful pediatric evaluations. An awareness by the health-care staff that children own a range of different temperaments is also useful.

Support for the emergency department staff's emotional needs is also important. Critical incident stress debriefing, defusing after resuscitations, and counseling and mental health support are important elements in the emotionally demanding and exacting environment of emergency medicine; pediatric patients often exacerbate these stresses.

Educational

The emergency department is a potentially superb educational environment for patients, parents, and visitors and a strong educational perspective is also a giving orientation. Many educational moments exist, and therefore the emergency medicine team can have positive impacts on human lives. Adolescents and alcohol-related injuries, accidental ingestions, appropriate care access and utilization, vaccinations, accidents and safety, and appropriate discipline are just a few of the educational areas potentially addressed. An educational topic commonly required at the onset and throughout an emergency department visit is an understanding of the triage process. Patients and their parents frequently need reassurance that their health-care needs will be met in a timely and appropriate fashion.

Many educational tools are currently available and include educational videos in the waiting room or patient rooms, wall posters with the latest safety warnings, holding telephone message systems, informational brochures and pamphlets, hospital-specific or computerized discharge instructions, and follow-up telephone calls. Both the nursing and physician staff have significant educational roles and impacts.

Training and Research

Emergency departments frequently serve as training sites for prehospital personnel, nursing students, medical students, residents, and other health-care professionals in training. The participation of trainees in the delivery of medical care to emergency department patients requires awareness and sensitivity. Research protocols are often initiated to address specific clinical issues. This environment requires specific sensitivity. Awareness and attention must address the fact that there is a patient behind the disease, the importance of adequate trainee supervision, the patient's right to privacy, and parental concerns about their child being included in research or being used for training purposes. Other issues in training programs involve the interface between patients and often overworked residents, disputes over admissions or stonewalling, delays in patient work-ups, and teaching discussions in the family's presence. Although the benefits of academic programs to the patients, trainees, and all health-care professionals in training is incalculable, every effort should be made to ensure that this environment strongly affirms our patients and families.

Professional

The emergency department environment should provide the highest levels of health-care professionalism. The emergency department represents one of the most highly visible components of the Medical Center to the community and attention to delivering a first class, professional environment has broader benefits than simply a local reputation. The spectrum of areas requiring the highest standards of professionalism includes dress and appearance, demeanor, sensitivity to patient expectations, personal hygiene and handwashing, clean and uncluttered waiting rooms and patient care areas, communication and interviewing skills, emotional and verbal discipline, the establishment of therapeutic relationships, and competence in physical and developmental assessments.

Emergency Department Design

An in-depth discussion of emergency department design issues requires a separate chapter. Nevertheless, the design of an emergency department is an environment that has a strong impact on health-care delivery. Geographically separate entrances for ambulatory and ambulance patients prevent potentially dangerous mixing of traffic into the emergency department. Waiting rooms must be planned to provide a safe, but comfortable environment for children and their families, as well as an ability to separate children with highly contagious diseases. The total number of patient rooms available for effective patient flow and timely delivery of care is just one of many important design issues. Design considerations that find the best juxtaposition of privacy and patient monitoring are extremely important. Nursing stations should generally be open work areas that are constructed to provide an adequate compromise between maximal visual and auditory conditions for patient monitoring against staff privacy, which allows necessary conversations and minimization of work distractions and intrusions. While physician work areas should be in close proximity to patient-care areas these workstations are best enclosed to allow for private discussions and medical dictations. Internal relationships between rooms and their roles are very important. Trauma and resuscitation rooms and their critically ill patients should be in close proximity

to nursing stations. Rooms where conscious sedation is frequently administered should also be in close proximity to the nursing work areas. Infectious disease rooms must be strategically located to minimize exposure of other patients to infectious agents. Emergency department observation units need to be in close proximity to allow efficient patient care in both areas by responsible attending physicians. Attention to staff comfort and necessary amenities that affect efficient job performance have long-term benefits. Staff members should have separate areas for eating and drinking away from the view of patients and their families. Finally, design attention to necessary amenities for waiting family members and friends such as isolated smoking locations, grief rooms, children's play areas, telephone booths, and snack machines requires thoughtful consideration.

Clinical Environment

The emergency department must be certain that appropriate age- and size-specific equipment and monitoring capabilities are provided and that manuals and references are available to assure timely intervention. The American Academy of Pediatrics and the American College of Emergency Physicians have developed guidelines that should be reviewed in establishing a responsive emergency department and are outlined in the box on pp. 13-14.[11]

Ancillary services require special attention, including respiratory therapy administration of nebulization treatments, provision for home nebulization therapy, laboratory drawing and processing of specimens, a pharmacy, and radiology equipment. Forms may require adaptations so that growth charts, parental information sheets, immunization consents, and so on are all available. Follow-up procedures and specific policies and procedures such as those reporting child abuse and caring for minors in the absence of consent need to be developed.

Consultation services specifically for children must be arranged and schedules provided to assure availability of pediatric medical and surgical subspecialists on a timely basis. A quality improvement program should be developed (see Chapter 9). Agreements and transport protocols should be developed early to provide for transfer of patients with unique clinical problems.

Personnel must be trained and motivated. Emergency physicians and nurses have become increasingly well trained and experienced through formal residency and continuing education programs. The formal training of pediatric emergency physicians and nurses is now in its adolescence; certification for physicians is now a reality with the establishment by the American Board of Pediatrics and the American Board of Emergency Medicine of the subboards in pediatric emergency medicine in 1991. Training of pediatric subspecialty nurses and EMS professionals is less formalized, but prolonged orientation periods, programs such as Advanced Pediatric Life Support (APLS) and Pediatric Advanced Life Support (PALS), and apprenticeship experiences have enhanced expertise.

The morale and motivation of all staff is a vital component of the internal environment that cannot be ignored. Often the resources to care for children have been short-changed, but the commitment to kids is real throughout the

Pediatric Equipment Guidelines

The following supplies and equipment are recommended by the American College of Emergency Physicians for pediatric patients in a general emergency department (ED).

An emergency cart or other system to house supplies, equipment, and drugs for a designated pediatric resuscitation area should be available.

Monitoring devices

Blood pressure cuffs (neonatal, infant, child, adult—arm, thigh)
ECG monitor-defibrillation/cardioverter with pediatric and adult-sized paddles and hard copy recording capability
End-tidal P_{CO_2} monitor and/or pediatric CO_2 detector
Otoscope/ophthalmoscope/stethoscope
Pediatric monitor patches
Pulse oximeter with pediatric adapter
Sphygmomanometer and Doppler ultrasound blood pressure devices
Thermometer (hypothermia)
Central venous pressure monitoring equipment

Vascular access supplies and equipment

Arm boards (infant, child, and adult sizes)
Blood gas kits
Butterfly needles (19-25 g)
Catheter-over-needle devices (16-24 g)
Central venous catheters (3-8 Fr)
Infusion pumps, drip or volumetric, with microinfusion capability, with appropriate tubing and connectors
Intraosseous needles (16, 18 g)
IV administration sets and extension tubing
IV fluid/blood warmer
IV solutions: In addition to standard solutions, the following should be readily available to the ED for the care of pediatric patients
    D10W
    D5W 0.2% NS
Umbilical vein catheters (feeding tubes size 5 Fr may be used)
Vascular access supplies utilizing the Seldinger technique

Respiratory equipment and supplies

Bag-valve-mask resuscitator, self-inflating (child and adult)
Clear oxygen masks
    Standard and non-rebreathing (neonatal, infant, child, adult)
Endotracheal tubes
    Uncuffed sizes: 2.5, 3.0, 3.5, 4.0, 4.5, 5.0 mm
    Cuffed sizes: 5.5, 6.0, 6.5, 7.0, 7.5, 8.0 mm
Stylets for endotracheal tubes (pediatric and adult)
Laryngoscope handle (pediatric)
Laryngoscope blades
    Curved: 2, 3
    Straight or Miller: 0, 1, 2, 3
Pediatric Magill forceps
Nasopharyngeal airways
    Sizes: 12, 16, 20, 24, 28, 30 Fr
Nasal cannulae (child and adult)
NG tubes
    Sizes: 6, 8, 10, 12, 14, 16 Fr

Oral airways
    Sizes: 0, 1, 2, 3, 4, 5
Suction catheters
    Sizes: 6, 8, 10, 12, 14, 16 Fr
Tracheostomy tubes
    Shiley tube sizes: 00, 0, 1, 2, 3, 4, 6

Medications

Activated charcoal
Adenosine
Antidotes immediately available:
    Cyanide kit
    Flumazenil
    Methylene blue
    Naloxone
Antipyretics
Atropine
Barbiturates
Benzodiazepines
Beta-agonist (commonly albuterol) for inhalation
Beta-blockers
Bretylium
Calcium chloride
Dextrose
Dexamethasone
Diphenhydramine
Dopamine
Epinephrine (1:1,000 and 1:10,000)
Furosemide
Glucagon
Hydrocortisone
Insulin
Isoproterenol
Lidocaine
Magnesium sulfate
Mannitol
Methylprednisolone
Narcotics
Neuromuscular blocking agents
    Succinylcholine
    Pancuronium and/or vecuronium
Potassium chloride
Phenytoin
Procainamide
Racemic epinephrine for inhalation
Sodium Bicarbonate
Verapamil

Related supplies/equipment

Medication chart, tape, or other system to assure ready access to information on proper per-kilogram dose for resuscitation drugs and equipment sizes.

Miscellaneous equipment

Infant scale and older child scale
Infant formulas, dextrose in water with various nipple sizes
Heating source, overhead warmer preferred

Continued.

Pediatric Equipment Guidelines—cont'd

Medical photography capability
Oral rehydrating solution, such as Pedialyte, Ricelyte
Pediatric restraining devices

Specialized pediatric trays
Cricothyrotomy including needle cricothyrotomy
Lumbar puncture
Newborn kit:
  Umbilical vessel cannulation supplies
  Meconium aspirator
Obstetric pack
Peritoneal lavage

Tube thoracostomy and water seal drainage
Thoracotomy tray with chest tubes
  Sizes: 8-40 Fr
Urinary catheterization
  Sizes: 5-12 Fr
Venous cutdown

Fracture management devices
Femur splint (child and adult)
Semi-rigid neck collars (child and adult)
Spinal immobilization board

American College of Emergency Physicians: Pediatric equipment guidelines, *Ann Emerg Med* 25:307, 1995.

---

health-care system. A truly creative and special emphasis on children will enhance patient care and staff enthusiasm and morale. Those special little touches such as decorations, staff clothing, furniture, and entertainment clearly declare that the department is child centered and the environment welcomes children. Furthermore, this attention to decor is reassuring to parents. Their reassurance is based on the assumption that the emergency department paying attention to these touches has most likely made the important clinical preparations for pediatric emergency care.

SUMMARY

An understanding of both the internal and external pediatric emergency department environments allows physician and nursing staffs to provide more effective care of children. The planning and implementation process in making the emergency department environments responsive and conducive to children is essential as hospitals increase their commitment to children. Physicians, nurses, prehospital personnel, and others must all contribute to this process and participate in its growth and formalization.

References

1. Seidel JS and Henderson DP, editors: *Emergency medical services for children: a report to the nation,* Washington DC, 1991, National Center for Education in Maternal and Child Health.
2. Mayer T: Initial evaluation and management of the injured child. In Mayer TA: *Emergency management of pediatric trauma,* Philadelphia, 1985, WB Saunders.
3. *Hospital care of children and youth,* AAP Committee on Hospital Care, 1985, Elk Grove, Ill.
4. Schwartz GR: Psychological and behavioral responses of hospital staff involved in the care of the critically ill, *Crit Care Med* 2(1):48, 1974.
5. Schwartz GR: Psychic numbing in the emergency department, *Emerg Med Serv* 4(1):31, 1975.
6. Hall TE: *The silent language,* New York, 1959, Fawcett.
7. Hall TE: *The hidden dimension,* New York, 1966, Doubleday.
8. Roethlisberger FJ and Dickson WJ: *Management and the worker,* Philadelphia, 1964, JS Wiley.
9. Mellick LM, Lau K: Pearls and pitfalls of pediatric assessment: secrets for approaching children in the emergency department, *Emerg Med Rep* 15(3):19-30, 1994.
10. ACEP policy statement: the use of pediatric sedation and analgesia, *Ann Emerg Med,* 22:626, 1993.
11. ACEP policy statement: pediatric equipment guidelines, *Ann Emerg Med* 25:307, 1995.

3

Injury Prevention and Control

M. Denise Dowd • Carl D. Stevens

Childhood injury is one of the most pressing public health problems in industrialized and developing countries. In the United States, injuries cause more deaths in individuals aged 1 to 19 years than all diseases combined. Nearly 16 million injured children are treated in emergency departments each year, representing 40% of all visits. Approximately 600,000 children are hospitalized each year and the annual cost of childhood injury is estimated at $13.8 billion.[1,2] In countries where the major infectious diseases of childhood have been controlled, injury prevention offers the greatest opportunity to reduce childhood death and disability after the perinatal period. Indeed, trends suggest that improvements in child mortality statistics cannot be achieved without significant advances in injury control.[3]

Physicians and nurses who provide pediatric emergency care play a pivotal role in childhood injury prevention. New trends in causes can be detected by emergency care providers; this is particularly important for nonfatal injuries, for which surveillance systems are nonexistent or incomplete. Emergency care providers also serve as advocates and opinion leaders and are important participants in the political and legislative initiatives crucial to the establishment of effective injury-prevention programs. Finally, in the tertiary or post-event phase, pediatric emergency care providers and the emergency medical services system become the main determinants of outcome for severely injured children.

Although injury has always accounted for a large proportion of childhood morbidity and mortality, it is only fairly recently that injury prevention has been identified as an urgent public health issue.[3] Two main factors have contributed to this awareness. The first is a growing appreciation of the enormous burden that injury places on the nation's health, both in absolute terms and in comparison with other categories of disease. This increasing concern over injury culminated in the publication of "Injury in America," a landmark report issued in 1985 by the National Research Council, which described the magnitude of the problem, pointing out that more potential years of productive life are lost to injury each year than to heart disease, cancer, and stroke.[4] The 1989 report, "Cost of Injury in the United States," further highlighted the huge economic burden that injuries place on our country: $180 billion in 1988.[2] These reports focused the attention of the public and Congress on the problem of trauma, establishing injury prevention as a priority of national public health policy.

A second and equally important factor that spurred the advancement of injury prevention was the evolution of a sound theoretic framework that permitted organized scientific study of the problem. Over the past 4 decades, the work of several investigators has produced a fundamental change in the way that injuries and their causes are perceived.[3,5-7] Traditionally, injuries have been attributed to *accidents,* a term that implies that randomness or fate plays a major role in their cause and infers that prevention efforts are futile. The modern era of injury prevention began more than 4 decades ago when Dr. William Haddon and others rejected this view and focused instead on the observable and predictable elements in the events that produce injuries, stressing that detailed study of these events might reveal common themes that would in turn suggest strategies for preventing them.[6,7]

In 1949, a seminal paper authored by Dr. John Gordon introduced the concept of injury epidemiology. Dr. Gordon patterned the epidemiologic behavior of injury on a paradigm used in the understanding of infectious diseases.[5] Haddon further developed a powerful conceptual framework for studying injury-producing events that identified several levels at which preventive strategies can be implemented. Haddon's model has the following three main aspects:

1. It recognizes that the etiologic agent common to all injuries is a transfer of energy from objects or the environment to the victim and that the basis of injury prevention is blocking or modifying this transfer of energy.[8]
2. The model points out that injuries, like diseases, result from interactions between the host, etiologic agent, vehicles and vectors, and environment. Thus injuries can be prevented by altering any of these factors to disrupt the chain of events leading to the injury (Table 3-1).

TABLE 3-1. Injury Epidemiology

Model	Infectious disease	Injury
Host	Patient with malaria	Child pedestrian struck by car
Etiologic agent	*Plasmodium vivax*	Mechanical energy
Vehicle or vector	Anopheline mosquito	Automobile
Environmental factors	Breeding conditions for mosquitoes; housing design	Roadway design, crosswalks, lighting

Data from Gordon JE: *Am J Public Health* 39:504, 1949; Haddon W: *Public Health Rep* 95:411, 1980.

3. The model focuses the analysis of injuries on the events that surround them. During each phase, opportunities to prevent the injury or reduce its severity are present. Haddon divides these events into the following discrete temporal phases:
   a. The *pre-event phase,* during which the conditions that cause the injury-producing energy transfer are set up.
   b. The *event phase,* in which the energy transfer or release takes place
   c. The *post-event phase,* in which acute medical care and rehabilitation can alter the long-term impact of the injury on the victim.

Combining these three aspects, Haddon described a matrix that can be used to analyze events that result in injury (Fig. 3-1). The strength of the matrix is that it partitions the complex circumstances that surround an injury into manageable *cells* and allows a systematic search for preventive interventions within each cell.

For example, bicycle crashes are an important source of injury morbidity and mortality, resulting in more than 320,000 emergency department visits and nearly 900 deaths in the United States each year.[9,10] Using Haddon's matrix, the search for prevention strategies begins in Cell 1, with host factors in the *pre-event* phase. This includes interventions that alter behavioral characteristics of the bicyclist to reduce the likelihood of a crash. Educational interventions to promote safer riding habits fall into this cell. Interventions of this type, which demand a sustained behavioral change to be effective, often fail to produce major reductions in injury rates, despite their intuitive attractiveness. In Cell 2, the vehicle or *vector* is the bicycle. Laws mandating that bicycles be made more visible to motorists fall into this category, and indeed statutes in most states require new bicycles to have reflectors on the wheels. Cell 3 includes changes to the physical environment that would result in fewer bicycle crashes. Building bike paths that are separate from automobile traffic is such an example. A law prohibiting children from riding bicycles on the street after dark would fall into Cell 4 because it is a change in the social or cultural environment. Interventions that act by preventing the occurrence of the injury-producing event are termed *primary* prevention strategies. Primary prevention seems attractive because it has the potential to block injury completely, but it can be difficult to implement because it often demands major changes in the environment or new legislative action. Also, even the most effective primary prevention programs do not stop all injury-producing events, so additional measures are needed to reduce damage from events that do occur.

	Host (victim)	Vector or vehicle	Environment: Physical	Environment: Sociocultural
Pre-event	1	2	3	4
Event	5	6	7	8
Post-event	9	10	11	12

FIG. 3-1. Haddon's matrix for analysis of injury-producing events and identification of prevention strategies. (*Data from Haddon W:* Public Health Rep *95:411, 1980.*)

Next, in the *event* phase, secondary prevention strategies are invoked. These interventions assume that the potentially injurious event will occur and attempt to reduce the likelihood or severity of injury by modifying the transfer of energy to the victim during the event. For example, the host can be altered or *packaged* to prevent injury or reduce its severity.[7,8] Programs that promote the use of bicycle helmets are an example that fall in Cell 5. Again, the effectiveness of this intervention depends on a sustained behavioral change.[11-14] In Cell 6, bicycles can be built with fewer protruding parts that produce injury in crashes.

In the *post-event* phase, so-called tertiary prevention strategies are invoked to limit the impact of injuries on the victims. Many potential solutions of this type deal with the social or cultural environment. Examples include programs that improve the ability of the emergency medical services system to stabilize and transport injured children and designation of pediatric trauma centers equipped to provide optimal acute care and rehabilitation. Also included in this phase are scientific advances that improve the medical care of the traumatized child—from initial resuscitation through rehabilitation.

Although the matrix was initially used for the analysis of automobile crash injuries, it can be adapted to a wide

Years of potential life lost ages 0-19 yr., USA 1986

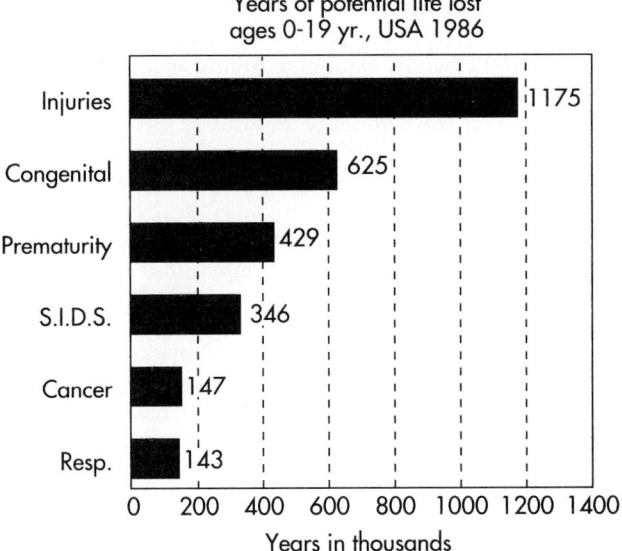

FIG. 3-2. Total years of potential life lost by children resulting from fatal injuries compared with other causes of death. Numbers indicate thousands of years of life lost among U.S. children in 1986, based on life expectancy of 65 years. *S.I.D.S.,* Sudden infant death syndrome; *Resp.,* Respiratory disease. (*Modified from Division of Injury Control, Center for Environmental Health and Injury Control, Centers for Disease Control:* Am J Dis Child *144:627, 1990.*)

TABLE 3-2. Causes of Fatal Injury: US Individuals 0-19 Years of Age, 1990

Causes	Number	Percent (%)
Motor vehicle		
Occupant	5,495	25.6
Pedestrian	1,441	6.7
Motorcycle	303	1.4
Other	1,861	8.7
Firearm		
Homicide	2,852	13.3
Suicide	1,476	6.9
Other	629	2.9
Drowning	1,626	7.8
Homicide, non-firearm	1,412	6.6
Fire and burns	1,201	5.6
Suicide, non-firearm	767	3.6
Poisoning, unintentional	304	1.4
Falls	275	1.2
Other	1,834	8.5
All injuries	21,476	100

Data from Centers for Disease Control: *Injury mortality: national summary of injury mortality data 1984-1990,* Atlanta, 1993, US Department of Health and Human Services.

variety of situations. Use of the matrix facilitates an orderly search for prevention strategies. Above all, the model attributes the cause of injury not to chance or fate but to a definable set of conditions and events that can be modified to decrease the frequency or severity of injuries. Thus with his matrix, Haddon contributed a philosophy and a methodology to the field of injury prevention.

EPIDEMIOLOGY OF CHILDHOOD INJURY

Early work in childhood injury prevention was severely hindered by the lack of adequate information on the scope and nature of the problem. Available data focused on fatal injuries, and even these statistics, which had been collected by law enforcement and other regulatory agencies, were not in a form that could be used for epidemiologic research. By necessity then, the first projects undertaken by injury-prevention researchers were descriptive studies that sought to identify and develop high-quality data sources and prioritize areas for intervention. Although accurate data are far from complete, the literature now contains detailed descriptive data on fatal childhood injuries and greatly improved information on nonfatal injuries.[1,15-17]

Fatal Injuries

Injury is the leading cause of death for children in the United States, accounting for approximately 40% of deaths among children from age 1 to 4 years and nearly 70% of deaths from age 5 to 19.[1,16,17] Injury deaths also account for a far greater loss of potential years of productive life than any other category of childhood disease (Fig. 3-2). Table 3-2 summarizes the major causes of fatal childhood injuries

in the United States, based on published data from the National Center for Health Statistics, compiled from 1990 death certificates.[10] Motor vehicle–related trauma is consistently the most common cause of mortality, followed by deaths from injuries from firearms.

An examination of the 1990 US injury mortality rates reveals that the causes are related to age (Fig. 3-3). In children younger than 5 years, non-firearm homicides (child abuse), fires and burns, and drowning cause the most deaths, closely followed by motor vehicle–occupant injuries. From age 5 to 9, motor vehicle–occupant and –pedestrian deaths predominate as the leading causes of death. Motor vehicle–occupant deaths continue to predominate in the 10- to 14-year age group. Older teenagers, 15 to 19 years of age, have injury rates far greater than the other age groups. Motor vehicle–occupant deaths and firearm-related homicides and suicides take the most lives in this age group.

These statistics reflect exposure to the hazards of childhood such as riding in or driving motor vehicles and access to firearms and identify particular age-related vulnerabilities such as child abuse for infants and fires and drowning for toddlers. The most frequent causes of injury death rank differently than they do in data for nonfatal injury. Still, the study of injury-death rates focuses on injuries with the greatest severity; for this reason, study remains crucial so that prevention efforts can be targeted to population groups at the greatest risk. These incidence rates are but a snapshot from the latest available data. It is important to be aware of trends over time, as they help us predict and plan for future prevention and control measures.

Injury mortality rates for US children and adolescents, by age group, 1990

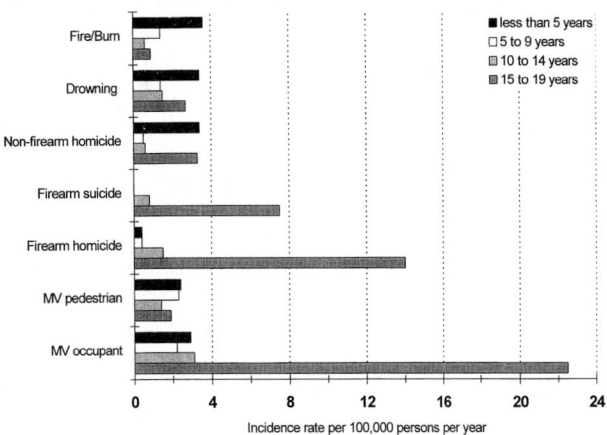

FIG. 3-3. Cause- and age-specific mortality rates for the leading causes of injury death among children and adolescents, United States, 1990. Motor vehicle–occupant includes drivers and passengers; homicides include child abuse. (*Data from Centers for Disease Control:* Injury mortality: National Summary of Injury Mortality Data 1984-1990, *Atlanta, 1993, US Department of Health and Human Services.*)

Nonfatal Injuries

Because data on nonlethal injuries are less complete than those for fatalities, the true incidence of injuries serious enough to bring children to medical attention is unknown. However, studies suggest that the magnitude of the problem is vast and that childhood injuries resulting in fatalities represent only a fraction of all childhood injuries.[1,17-20]

Most of the published statistics relating to nonfatal injuries are derived from data on injured children seen in hospital emergency departments. These data are then linked with census estimates of the population of the areas served by the surveyed hospitals to obtain an approximation of injury incidence rates. A few population-based studies have been conducted either by telephone survey or as part of the National Health Interview Survey.[9,21]

Using the first approach, Gallagher and co-workers set up a surveillance system to detect all childhood injuries that resulted in an emergency department visit, hospital admission, or death in a defined population in Massachusetts.[18] During 1 year, the incidence of such injuries was 2,239 per 10,000 (i.e., approximately one child in five suffered an injury of this severity). For each traumatic death in this study, there were 45 hospital admissions and 1,300 emergency department visits. Other studies from Ohio and Washington have found comparable rates of injury requiring emergency care or hospitalization or causing fatalities.[19,20] These studies point out that death and hospitalizations are the "tip of the iceberg" and highlight the importance of understanding the patterns of childhood injury treated in the emergency department.

The International Classification of Diseases-version 9 (ICD-9) classifies injuries according to their nature (e.g., femur fracture, cerebral concussion, or laceration) and external cause (e.g., motor vehicle crash, pedestrian struck by

motor vehicle, or fall). Although both types of information are important, statistics on the external causes provide insight into the events leading to injuries and are therefore more useful in planning prevention strategies. In general, information on the nature of injuries is easier to collect because a diagnosis is documented on emergency department or inpatient medical records and because most hospitals enter a discharge diagnosis into the Uniform Hospital Discharge Data Set using the ICD-9 "N Code" for injuries.[22] Researchers have had more difficulty in assembling statistics on the external causes of nonfatal injury, largely because hospital and emergency department records often contain little or no description of the injury-producing event. Data collection can be facilitated by increasing the use of the ICD-9 External Cause of Injury Codes (E-Codes) in hospital data sets.[15] Prevention oriented injury surveillance and research depends on classification of the injury by E-code, which is equivalent to assigning a mechanism of injury. Unfortunately, this type of coding is infrequently performed on injury cases discharged from the emergency department and completed on less than half of all injury hospitalizations.[23]

Still, emergency care providers can greatly ease the task of injury epidemiologists by carefully documenting in the medical record the circumstances that lead to significant injuries and advocating the use of ICD-9 E codes. E-coding of all hospital and emergency department discharges has been identified as a high priority data need and has been recommended for widespread implementation by the Institute of Medicine (Report on Emergency Medical Services for Children), Centers for Disease Control, and in the Healthy People 2000.[24-26] E-coding is much more consistent in places where it is mandated by state law; it is usually required for hospitalizations only.

The absence of a national surveillance system has forced researchers to rely on data from regional population-based studies to identify the major causes of nonfatal injuries in children and target them for prevention.[17] Such extrapolation has some risk because differences in causes of childhood injury exist from region to region and from time to time.[16,27]

Some of the most detailed information on nonfatal childhood injuries appeared in the reports of Gallagher, Guyer, and others, which dealt with data collected from 1979 to 1982 by the Massachusetts Statewide Childhood Injury Prevention Project.[17,18,28] As mentioned, the Massachusetts surveillance program was designed to detect all childhood injuries that resulted in an emergency department visit, hospital admission, or death. Their report highlighted the fact that injuries that result in the greatest numbers of deaths are not necessarily the same ones that are most likely to bring children into the emergency department or require hospitalization. The most obvious difference was the predominance of falls as a cause of nonfatal injury. Falls result in relatively few fatalities but produce by far the greatest number of injuries requiring medical attention in children younger than 12 years of age. Sports-related and motor vehicle–occupant injuries ranked next in frequency, and both exhibit a predictable pattern that reflects increasing exposure to these risks with age.

It is important that local injury prevention priorities be based on up-to-date local information. The emergency department offers a unique and underused data opportunity to describe community nonfatal injury rates. Emergency department and EMS databases have been proposed as potential surveillance tools.[29] Much work remains in the development of this potentially very useful means of injury surveillance.

CHOOSING INJURY-PREVENTION PRIORITIES

The Division of Injury Control of the Centers for Disease Control recommends that five factors be considered when deciding which injuries should receive the highest priority for prevention efforts.[1] These are incidence, severity, and economic costs of the injuries and the expense and likelihood of success of the proposed interventions. This type of analysis should balance the burden that a class of injuries imposes on society with the economic and political feasibility of reducing that burden.

Weighing the Burden: Incidence, Severity, and Cost

When setting prevention priorities, it is important to use the best incidence data available from the locale where the intervention is to be carried out. However, most states and counties lack formal systems for collecting data on injuries. In areas where no local data are available, choices of prevention priorities must be based on incidence statistics collected in demographically similar settings.

After the most common causes of injury in a geographic area are known, the next consideration is the severity of the injuries resulting from each cause. This approach makes intuitive sense, and indeed, the most common causes of fatal injuries are often targeted first in injury-control programs. However, such an approach risks ignoring causes such as falls, which account for the greatest number of injuries requiring emergency care in children. Hospitalization rate for a given injury is a simple and available way to measure severity of injury.

More sophisticated measures of severity such as the Injury Severity Score (ISS), an anatomically based scale adapted by Baker from the older Abbreviated Injury Scale (AIS), were developed to standardize severity estimates for automotive injuries.[30-33]

Physiologically based scales that estimate injury severity based on initial vital signs and level of alertness are also in use; Champion's Trauma Score is the best known example.[34,35] In addition, Tepas and others have developed the Pediatric Trauma Score, which incorporates anatomic and physiologic data and is designed for use in the prehospital setting to identify children with injuries severe enough to warrant transport to a designated pediatric trauma center.[36] These scales are useful in evaluating the performance of organized trauma care systems by comparing predicted with observed outcomes, specifically, differences in mortality rates for patients with injuries of similar severity.[37,38] However, since these measures of severity have been validated against the relatively rare outcome of death, their usefulness is limited. A challenge for the future will be to develop measures that help predict more common, nonfatal outcomes or disability status.[25]

The economic cost imposed on society by different classes of injuries is an important consideration when evaluating proposed control measures. Direct and indirect costs should be taken into account. Direct costs include all medical resources consumed while treating the child, from prehospital care through rehabilitation. Indirect costs are the loss to society of the economic output of the injured person, usually calculated by estimating the expected value of wage earnings lost during the period of disability or up to age 65 in the case of fatal injuries. For each cause, the relative magnitude of direct and indirect costs depends on the duration of a disability. For example, because they are so common, falls and sports injuries generate the greatest direct costs, more than four times that of motor vehicle–occupant injuries. However, most injuries of this type do not result in long-term disability, so the indirect costs are fairly modest. In contrast, vehicular injuries are more likely to result in permanent disability or death and therefore have very high indirect costs because of the loss of potential wages. Causes such as submersion injuries, which often result in death or full recovery, produce mainly indirect costs.

Weighing the Interventions: Efficacy, Feasibility, and Cost

In deciding which alternate injury-control strategy is appropriate, the proposed interventions must be evaluated to estimate their likelihood of success and costs. Injury-prevention strategies fall into three broad categories.[1] The first category includes interventions that exert their effect by inducing individuals to voluntarily change their patterns of behavior to reduce the likelihood of injury. In general, interventions in this group consist of education or publicity programs. The second category includes interventions that mandate safer patterns of behaviors through legislation. The third group consists of modifications of the physical environment or equipment to prevent injuries or reduce their severity. Strategies for this last group do not depend on changes in behavior or habits for their effectiveness.

Comprehensive injury-control programs use all three types of interventions. However, the cumulative experience of injury-prevention researchers suggests that sustained changes in the public's behavior are very difficult to accomplish, and for this reason, interventions of the third type usually offer the greatest certainty of success.[7] Legally mandated changes in behavior have the next-best track record among the three strategies. Despite their intuitive appeal, educational and publicity programs that promote safer behavior have not been as successful.

The evolution of automobile restraint systems illustrates this point. Since 1968, all new cars sold in this country have been equipped with seat belts. However, despite many publicity campaigns designed to increase their use, only a minority of drivers and passengers wore seat belts until the mid-1980s when mandatory restraint laws went into effect in many states. These laws produced measurable increases in seat belt use and reductions in injury rates, but even with the laws, restraint use remained far from universal.[39,40] This led in turn to an intervention of the third type, with regulations now requiring that new cars be equipped with passive restraint systems that do not depend on driver behavior for effectiveness; significant reductions in vehicular injury are to be anticipated.

It is probably valid to rank the three categories of injury-control strategies in order of likelihood of success. However, it is critical to bear in mind that each intervention must be objectively evaluated in the field to determine its effectiveness. There has been a tendency to rely on intuition rather than evidence when planning injury-control projects. In particular, communities often respond to proven hazards with educational efforts directed at reducing high-risk behaviors, rather than modifying the physical environment or injury vectors to reduce danger. This approach has resulted in many ineffective and even harmful interventions.

There is no better illustration of this point than Robertson's classic studies of high school–based driver-education programs. The first study showed that the frequency of fatal automobile crashes involving teenage drivers was highest in states that had the most high school students enrolled in driver-education programs.[41] Next, Robertson focused on Connecticut, where reduced funding had forced cancellation of public school driver-education programs in some but not all counties.[42] He found that there were more automobile crashes involving teenage drivers in the counties where driver education continued than in those where it had been stopped. The explanation for this apparent paradox was that more 16- and 17-year-olds obtained driver's licenses where driver education was offered, and therefore exposure to the inherent hazard of teenage drivers was higher in these areas. In other words, any beneficial effect that the courses may have had on driver behavior was more than offset by the increased risk of putting more 16- and 17-year-olds behind the wheel. This illustrates the importance of objectively evaluating the impact of injury prevention programs before committing large amounts of resources to them.

Cost of Prevention

The choice of prevention strategies affects the cost of injury-control programs. In general, interventions that alter the physical environment are more likely to succeed and have the highest short-term costs. For example, child pedestrian injuries might be reduced through educational programs on how to cross streets safely, by increasing the number of crosswalks and pedestrian signals, or by building pedestrian overpasses and separating sidewalks from traffic with barriers. In the short run, the educational intervention would be least expensive, but it would probably also be least effective because of the proven difficulty of inducing behavioral change. The overpass and barrier approach has a much higher short-term cost but also has a far greater likelihood of significantly reducing pedestrian injuries. Whether the costs of the more effective intervention would be justified in the long run depends on local conditions, including the incidence of child pedestrian injuries, the resources available for injury control, and the political feasibility of undertaking large projects intended to reduce injuries. Thus although the science of injury epidemiology provides useful information about the effectiveness of different prevention strategies, deciding which intervention to implement involves a careful analysis of the expected costs and benefits in the context of local political and demographic conditions.

SUCCESSFUL INJURY-PREVENTION PROGRAMS

In the past two decades, researchers have built a sound theoretic and methodologic foundation for childhood injury prevention. However, it is only very recently that health policy makers have become aware of the problem and made funding for large-scale research and demonstration projects available. From 1978 to 1982, the Division of Maternal and Child Health of the Department of Health and Human Services sponsored childhood injury-prevention demonstrations in Massachusetts, Virginia, and California.[43] Since 1987, major funding has been available through the Centers for Disease Control for Injury Prevention Center grants and investigator-initiated projects. As noted from the previous discussions of the Massachusetts data, the information provided by these early projects helped define the problem of childhood injury in quantitative terms and highlighted the areas in which prevention efforts are most urgently needed. Based on this information, many community-based intervention projects that target specific causes of injury have been undertaken, and preliminary results of these efforts are beginning to appear in the literature.[44,45]

By their nature, many interventions are expected to produce measurable decreases in injury rates only after several years. This is especially true for educational interventions that act by gradually modifying the behavior of the population at risk. In such cases, the initial success of the program must be measured by tracking proxy measurements such as increases in the lower-risk *behavior* that the intervention promotes, and following up with measurements of changes in injury rates. An example is the program undertaken in Seattle to decrease the rate of head injuries in bicyclists by increasing the use of helmets.[14] A thorough evaluation consisted of establishing the effectiveness of bicycle helmets in reducing head injury,[12] measuring increased helmet use after the intervention,[14] and ultimately, documenting the change in outcome of interest: a decrease in head injuries related to bicycle crashes.[46]

In a few cases, it has been possible to demonstrate decreases in the incidence of targeted injuries as a result of a legally mandated change in the environment that is implemented quickly and is broadly enforced, thereby rapidly reducing the risk of injury for many people.

In 1969, a study conducted by the New York City Department of Health found that falls from apartment building windows were a major cause of death in children, accounting for 12% of unintentional injury deaths in the city.[47] In response, the Department initiated a prevention program that attacked the problem on several fronts.[48] The project began with a public education program entitled, "Children Can't Fly," which increased awareness of the problem through door-to-door outreach, community groups, and media campaigns. Installation of window guards was offered free-of-charge to apartment residents with children. Using a voluntary reporting system in hospital emergency departments, in addition to death certificates and police reports, the program was able to document a 50% reduction in fall injuries and deaths as a result of an intensive pilot program in the Bronx. The Health Department quickly sought to consolidate this gain and extend it to the rest of the boroughs by sponsoring an amendment to the city's Health Code requiring landlords to install window guards in any apartment in which children under the age of 10 resided. This regulation was opposed by landlords' groups and subsequently was challenged in the state Supreme Court, where it was upheld. This example illustrates a powerful approach to injury control, which is to first demonstrate the efficacy of an intervention with an intensive pilot project in a limited area and then extend the protection to everyone through legislation. Environmental modifications such as window guards obviate the need to effect sustained behavioral changes in those at risk.

Another success story is that of child passenger restraint laws. Between 1977 and 1985, laws mandating the use of approved child-restraint devices for infants and toddlers riding in automobiles were implemented in all 50 states.[49] In several states, the impact of the new laws was studied using a before-and-after design, and these studies demonstrated significant reductions in injury rates when the restraints were properly used. In Tennessee, the first state to require child restraints, implementation of the law was followed by a rapid increase in the rate of restraint use and a 50% reduction in motor vehicle mortality rates for children younger than 4 years of age.[50] In California, more sophisticated statistical techniques failed to demonstrate a reduction in mortality rates but did show reductions in both the rate and severity of injuries to toddlers.[51,52] More recently, data from Michigan have confirmed an important effect of restraint legislation on childhood injury rates.[53,54] The reported rate of restraint use by children involved in crashes rose from 12% before the law to 51% after it was implemented, and reductions in the number of injuries per crash and the total number of injured children requiring hospitalization were convincingly demonstrated. Nationally, there has been a gradual decline in motor vehicle–occupant fatalities among infants and children aged 0 to 4 years, despite the increase in miles being driven. From 1975 to 1993 there has been a 30% drop in the death rate for children and infants aged 0 to 4 years.[55]

FUTURE DIRECTIONS FOR CHILDHOOD INJURY PREVENTION

The childhood injury-prevention movement has made enormous strides in the past two decades; the coming years pose even greater challenges. Chief among these, now that the scientific foundation has been laid, is the need to change the field's focus from description to action. Although the data available on childhood injury are by no means complete or adequate, it is critical that the existing knowledge be applied in the form of large-scale, community-based interventions that reduce the burden of injury on society. Failing to do this risks loss of the momentum and public visibility of injury-prevention and control efforts.

To make this transition, the strategies known to work—infant car seats, automobile air bags, residential smoke detectors, swimming pool fences, delayed licensure for teenage drivers, apartment window guards, child-proof containers, to name but a few—will have to be implemented more broadly and rapidly than they have been. In addition, new strategies must be developed for emerging causes of injury death and disability, for example, firearm- and violence-related injuries. For this to occur injury patterns must be understood in terms of person, place, and time; risk factors must be assessed through analytic epidemiologic methods and prevention strategies must be implemented and rigorously evaluated.

Emergency care physicians, nurses, and prehospital providers are in an excellent (and natural) position to actively participate as practitioners and leaders in injury prevention and control. As clinicians they can take a "prevention" oriented history when caring for an injured child, ascertain risk factors, and practice injury prevention counseling in the emergency department. As researchers, they can form rewarding and productive collaborative relationships with public health practitioners and community groups. They can help develop emergency department databases as injury surveillance tools useful in setting injury prevention priorities, ascertaining trends and evaluating interventions. As administrators they can support and encourage ICD-9 E-coding for all emergency department and hospital discharges. As advocates they can be a strong voice in the community and support legislative initiatives needed to protect children from injury.

An immediate area of concern for emergency care providers is tertiary prevention. This means looking carefully for ways to improve each aspect of the care that seriously injured children receive in the post-event phase, from the arrival of prehospital providers on the scene through rehabilitation. To ensure optimal outcomes, specific standards for pediatric trauma care must be defined and validated, and educational programs must be directed at paramedics, nurses, physicians, and rehabilitation professionals to allow compliance with these standards. This is especially true in rural areas, where long distances preclude the transport of all seriously injured children to pediatric trauma centers. Following the example of other activists, emergency care providers should think globally about injury prevention and act locally to improve areas for which they have responsibility.

References

1. Division of Injury Control, Center for Environmental Health and Injury Control, Centers for Disease Control: Childhood injuries in the United States, *Am J Dis Child* 144:627, 1990.
2. Rice DP, Mackenzie EJ, et al: *Cost of injury in the United States: a report to Congress*, San Francisco: Institute for Health and Aging, University of California and Injury Prevention Center, The Johns Hopkins University, 1989.
3. Baker SP, O'Neill B, Karpf RS: *The injury fact book*, Lexington, Ky, 1984, DC Heath & Co.
4. National Research Council, Committee on Trauma Research: *Injury in America: a continuing public health problem*, Washington, DC, 1985, National Academy Press.
5. Gordon JE: The epidemiology of accidents, *Am J Public Health* 39:504, 1949.

6. Haddon W: A logical framework for categorizing highway safety phenomena and activity, *J Trauma* 12:193, 1972.
7. Haddon W: Advances in the epidemiology of injuries as a basis for public policy, *Public Health Rep* 95:411, 1980.
8. Haddon W: Energy damage and the ten countermeasure strategies, *J Trauma* 13:321, 1973.
9. Burt CW: Injury-related visits to hospital emergency departments: United States, 1992, *Advance Data, National Center for Health Statistics,* 261:8, 1995.
10. Centers for Disease Control. Injury Mortality: *National summary of injury mortality data, 1984-1990,* Atlanta, 1993, National Center for Health Statistics.
11. Nakayama DK, Pasieka KB, Gardner MJ: How bicycle-related injuries change bicycling practices in children, *Am J Dis Child* 144:928, 1990.
12. Thompson RS, Rivara FP, Thomson DC: A case-control study of the effectiveness of bicycle safety helmets, *N Engl J Med* 320:1361, 1989.
13. Cushman R, Down J, MacMillan N, Waclawik H: Bicycle-related injuries: a survey in a pediatric emergency department, *Can Med Assoc J* 143:108, 1990.
14. DiGuiseppi CG, Rivara FP, Koepsell TD, et al: Bicycle helmet use by children: evaluation of a community-wide helmet campaign, *JAMA* 262:2256, 1989.

Epidemiology of Childhood Injury

15. Guyer B, Berenholz G, Gallagher SS: Injury surveillance using hospital discharge abstracts coded by external cause of injury (E code), *J Trauma* 30:470, 1990.
16. Waller AE, Baker SP, Szocka A: Childhood injury deaths: national analysis and geographic variations, *Am J Public Health* 79:310, 1989.
17. Guyer B, Ellers B: Childhood injuries in the United States: mortality, morbidity, and cost, *Am J Dis Child* 144:649, 1990.
18. Gallagher SS, Finison K, Guyer B, Goodenough S: The incidence of injuries among 87,000 Massachusetts children and adolescents: results of the 1980-81 statewide injury prevention program surveillance system, *Am J Public Health* 74:1340, 1984.
19. Fife D, Barancik JI, Chaterjee BF: Northeastern Ohio Trauma Study. II. Injury rates by age, sex, and cause, *Am J Public Health* 74:473, 1984.
20. Rivara FP, Calonge N, Thompson RS: Population-based study of unintentional injury incidence and impact during childhood, *Am J Public Health* 79:990, 1989.
21. Klauber MR, Barrett-Connor E, Hofstetter CR, Micik SH: A population-based study of nonfatal childhood injuries, *Prev Med* 15(2):139, 1986.
22. National Center for Health Statistics: *International classification of diseases: clinical modification,* rev 9, Ann Arbor, Mich, 1980, Commission on Professional and Hospital Activities.
23. Hall MJ, Owings MF: *Hospitalizations for injury and poisoning in the United States, 1991. Advance data from vital and health statistics; 252.* Hyattsville, Maryland, 1984, National Center for Health Statistics.
24. Centers for Disease Control. External Cause of Injury Coding in Hospital Discharge Data-United States, 1992. *MMWR* 41(15): 249, 1992.
25. Durch JS and Lohr KN, editors: *Emergency Medical Services for children,* Division of Health Care Services Institute of Medicine Report, Committee on Pediatric Emergency Medical Services, Washington, DC, 1993, National Academy Press.
26. US Public Health Service: Healthy People 2000: National Health Promotion and Disease Prevention Objectives. Washington, DC, US Department of Health and Human Services, US Public Health Service, 1990, DHHS publication No. (PHS) 91-50213.
27. Baker SP and Waller AE: *Childhood injury state-by-state mortality facts,* Baltimore, 1989, Johns Hopkins Injury Prevention Center.
28. Guyer B and Gallagher SS: An approach to the epidemiology of childhood injuries, *Pediatr Clin North Am* 32:5, 1985.
29. Garrison HG, Runyan CW, Tintinalli JE, et al. Emergency department surveillance: an examination of issues and a proposal for a national strategy, *Ann Emerg Med* 24:849, 1994.

Choosing Injury-Prevention Priorities

30. Baker SP, O'Neill B, Haddon W, et al: The injury severity score: a method for describing patients with multiple injuries and evaluating emergency care, *J Trauma* 14:187, 1974.
31. Baker SP and O'Neill B: The injury severity score: an update, *J Trauma* 16:882, 1976.
32. Greenspan L, McLellan BA, Greig H: Abbreviated injury scale and injury severity score: a scoring chart, *J Trauma* 25:60, 1985.
33. Joint Committee on Injury Scaling: *The abbreviated injury scale: 1980 revision,* Arlington Heights, Ill, 1980, The American Association for Automotive Medicine.
34. Champion HR, Sacco WJ, Carnazzo AJ, et al: Trauma score, *Crit Care Med* 9:672, 1981.
35. Champion HR, Sacco WJ, Copes WS: A revision of the trauma score, *J Trauma* 29:623, 1989.
36. Tepas JJ, Ramenofsky ML, Mollitt DL, et al: The pediatric trauma score as a predictor of injury severity: an objective assessment, *J Trauma* 28:425, 1988.
37. Cales RH: Trauma mortality in Orange County: the effect of implementation of a regional trauma system, *Ann Emerg Med* 13:1, 1984.
38. Boyd CR, Tolson MA, Copes WS: Evaluating trauma care: The TRISS Method, *J Trauma* 27:370, 1987.
39. Chorba TL, Reinfurt D, Hulka BS: Efficacy of mandatory seat belt use legislation, *JAMA* 260:3593, 1988.
40. Orsay EM, Turnbull TL, Dunne M, et al: Prospective study of the effect of safety belts on morbidity and health care costs in motor vehicle accidents, *JAMA* 260:3598, 1988.
41. Robertson LS and Zador PL: Driver education and fatal crash involvement of teenaged drivers, *Am J Public Health* 68:959, 1978.
42. Robertson LS: Crash involvement of teenaged drivers when driver education is eliminated from high school, *Am J Public Health* 70:599, 1980.

Successful Injury-Prevention Programs

43. Alpert JJ and Guyer BG: Foreword, *Pediatr Clin North Am* 32:1, 1985.
44. National Committee for Injury Prevention and Control: Injury prevention: meeting the challenge, *Am J Prev Med* 5(Suppl):63, 1989.
45. Guyer B, Gallagher SS, Chang BH, et al: Prevention of childhood injuries: evaluation of the Statewide Childhood Injury Prevention Program (SCIPP), *Am J Public Health* 79:1521, 1989.
46. Rivara FP, Thompson DC, Thompson RS, et al: The Seattle children's bicycle helmet campaign: effects on helmet use and head injury admissions, *Pediatrics* 93:567-569, 1994.
47. Bergner L, Mayer S, Harris D: Falls from heights: a childhood epidemic in an urban age, *Am J Public Health* 61:92, 1971.
48. Spiegel CN and Lindaman FC: Children can't fly: a program to prevent childhood morbidity and mortality from window falls, *Am J Public Health* 67:1143, 1977.
49. Agran P, Castillo D, Winn D: Childhood motor vehicle occupant injuries, *Am J Dis Child* 144:653, 1990.
50. Decker MD, Dewey MJ, Hutcheson RH, et al: The use and efficacy of child restraint devices: the Tennessee experience, 1982 and 1983, *JAMA* 252:2571, 1984.
51. Guerin D and MacKinnon DP: An assessment of the California child passenger restraint requirement, *Am J Public Health* 75:142, 1985.
52. Agran PF, Dunkle DE, Winn DG: Effects of legislation on motor vehicle injuries to children, *Am J Dis Child* 141:959, 1987.
53. Wagenaar AC and Webster DW: Preventing injuries to children through compulsory automobile safety seat use, *Pediatrics* 78:662, 1986.
54. Margolis LH, Wagenaar AC, Liu W: The effects of a mandatory child restraint law on injuries requiring hospitalization, *Am J Dis Child* 142:1099, 1988.
55. National Highway Traffic Safety Administration: *Traffic safety facts,* 1993, Washington DC, 1994, US Department of Transportation.

CHAPTER

4

Emergency Medical Services for Children

Prehospital Care

GEORGE L. FOLTIN • MICHAEL G. TUNIK

Federal interest in emergency medical services for children (EMSC) has been evident since 1985 in the EMSC Demonstration Grant Program, which has been sponsored and supported through the efforts of Senator Inouye and the advocacy of pediatrician, Dr. Cal Sia, both of Hawaii. Passage of legislation made funding available through the Department of Health and Human Services, Bureau of Maternal and Child Health and Resources Development. Projects were set up in Alabama, California, New York, and Oregon for the purpose of improving emergency medical services for children and to integrate the care into preexisting EMS systems. Since that time, an additional 38 states have received funding for basic implementation grants in EMSC. MCHB has also funded 17 specific "Tar-

geted Issue Grants" and established grants for planning and post-implementation. Major goals for the EMSC projects are to develop strategies, programs, and resources that can be shared nationally and provide expertise and outreach for surrounding states and regions.[1,2] Other organizations have also targeted resources and personnel toward improved EMSC.[3]

EMSC, as envisioned by the federal government, consists of the following six phases of care: prevention, system access, field treatment, emergency department care, inpatient services, and rehabilitation. Each phase contains several of the components addressed in the EMS act of 1973 that functioning together under the umbrella of the Medical Home encompass the entire spectrum of care for a child requiring emergency services and exist within the already established EMS system. These phases of care reside in different, usually independent agencies, which comprise the EMS system that variably interface on a region-to-region basis. Although the scope of care described within EMSC involves the entire health care system, this chapter concentrates on the needs of children within the prehospital phase including prevention, field treatment, and mechanisms of primary referral to subspecialty centers (trauma centers and pediatric critical care centers).

HISTORIC PERSPECTIVE

Pioneering Efforts

A confluence of events and observations within the fields of surgery and medicine took place in the 1960s resulting in the development of Emergency Medical Service Systems in this country in the 1970s. Trauma surgeons had used a systems approach to treat wounded soldiers in Korea and Vietnam that consisted of rapid transport and early definitive care. This approach resulted in a significant improvement in the survival of American soldiers compared with previous wars.[4] These surgeons observed that victims of vehicular trauma in the United States were receiving inadequate care and had an extremely high mortality rate, especially when compared with the wounded soldiers they had cared for in Asia. The publication in 1966 of the milestone paper "Accidental Death and Disability: The Neglected Disease of Modern Society" through the National Academy of Sciences explicitly delineated the inadequacies of emergency care as it existed in this country.[5]

In 1966, Pantridge and Geddes published the results of their insightful work demonstrating that early defibrillation of adults with ventricular dysrhythmias, prior to arrival at a hospital, improved survival.[6] The pioneering work that

---

Components of an EMS System

Consumer participation
Consumer education
Access to care
Public safety agencies
Personnel
Training
Facilities
Communications
Transportation
Transfer of patients
Critical care units
Medical record keeping
Disaster linkage
Mutual aid agreements
Independent review (QI)
Medical control

Institute of Medicine Report on Emergency Medical Services for Children Findings

Problems with the overall EMS system that affect children as well as adults:

- Many communities still lack 911 systems.
- Enhanced 911 is operating in only a few communities.
- Data sets are not uniform and usually lack true outcome measures.
- Physician involvement in EMS is often lacking in many communities.

Problems that reflect deficiencies specific to pediatrics:

- Lack of proper equipment to care for patients of all sizes and ages.
- Lack of protocols and education to care for infants and children.
- Lack of involvement in the EMS system of health professionals with both pediatric and EMS expertise.
- Lack of research into optimal paradigms, approaches, and modalities to care for children in all phases of EMS.
- Lack of regionalization of care for critically ill and injured children. Many communities around the country have already made major inroads into solving these problems; many others have just started the process.

---

subsequently followed resulted in the creation of a nonphysician technician, the paramedic, who could defibrillate and intubate adults in the prehospital setting.[5] These events stimulated the development of a systems approach to emergency medical services that resulted in significant improvement and integration of the prehospital and hospital phases of emergency medical care. Communities around the country during the late 1960s and early 1970s developed various components of an EMS system (see box above).

Federal Involvement

The federal Emergency Medical Services Act of 1973 (PL 93-154) provided funding and guidelines for the development of EMS systems throughout the United States. Populations of patients that would benefit from specialized care at regional hospitals within an integrated EMS system were identified. The seven types of patients identified were trauma, cardiac, burn, spinal cord injury, poisoning, psychiatric, and neonatal.[4] The legislation required local and state agencies to integrate and improve the 16 components of a fully functioning EMS system (see box above). These components were found in a variety of independent agencies such as hospitals, ambulances, and municipal services. Regional and state EMS programs to this day depend on the ability of these organizations to work interdependently.[1,3]

WHAT ABOUT THE CHILDREN?

Surgeons, cardiologists, and anesthesiologists involved in the original EMS system planning were founders of the new field of emergency medicine in the early 1970s and were adult oriented. Although infants and children were being cared for within the EMS system, their special needs were not specifically identified or addressed. Children's special needs within EMS were often overlooked.[1,7,8]

Care of neonates, however, was targeted. Neonatologists focusing on their unique population created the first non-

military setting in which the process of regionalization, specialty transport, and secondary transport were successfully utilized.[4]

A 1993 study of the Institute of Medicine reviewed EMSC, adopting the philosophy that EMSC must not be fragmented, but rather be an integral part of the already existing EMS system and connected to a comprehensive system of child care. Therefore primary care, prevention, and rehabilitation should be linked "seamlessly" to EMSC. It noted that emergency care has improved for both children and adults, but emergency care and the systems for care have not to date improved for children to the extent that they have for adults. Although there is yet much to improve for both adults and children, the gap is wider for children.

Identified deficiencies can be divided into issues for the entire EMS system that adversely affect children and issues specific to children (see box above). The Institute of Medicine (IOM) panel outlines recommendations to correct these problems (see box on p. 25).

CHILDREN ARE DIFFERENT

Epidemiology

The nature of illness and injury encountered by the EMSC system should dictate the training, equipment, protocols for treatment, triage, and transfer, as well as the capabilities of the transport program. Several studies have looked at the epidemiology of prehospital illness and injury

Recommendations of Institute of Medicine Report

Education and training

Educate the public in:

- Injury prevention
- Recognition of childhood emergencies
- First aid and CPR
- Appropriate use of EMS

Educate health professionals in:

- Emergency care of infants and children
- Use of pediatric skills and equipment

State and localities should develop and maintain specific guidelines to ensure education and training for all levels of providers.

Appropriate organizations and accrediting bodies should ensure and require that appropriate programs and curricula exist to ensure education and training in the emergency care of children at all levels from first responder to subspecialty physicians.

Putting essential tools in place

State regulatory agencies should require that emergency departments and transport vehicles have available and maintain equipment and supplies appropriate for emergency care of children.

State regulatory agencies should address the issues of categorization and regionalization as well as the integration of EMSC into EMS.

Planning, evaluation, and research

States and other relevant bodies should require ICD-9-CM E-codes for injury diagnoses.

States should implement a program to collect, analyze, and report the elements of a uniform national data set.

Linkage of patient data from prehospital care to hospital disposition should be implemented.

Research in EMSC should be expanded and encouraged, especially in the areas of:

- Clinical aspects of emergencies and emergency care
- Indices of severity of illness and injury
- Patient outcomes and outcome measures
- System organization, configuration, and operation
- Effective approaches to education and training

Federal and state agencies and funding

Congress should direct the Secretary of the Department of Health and Human Resources to:

1. Establish a federal center or office to conduct, oversee, and coordinate activities related to planning and evaluation, research, and technical assistance in EMSC.
2. Establish a national advisory council for this center. Members should include representatives of federal agencies, state and local governments, the health care community, and the public at large.

Congress should fund $30 million each year for 5 years to support the activities of the federal center and the state agencies related to EMSC.

States should:

1. Establish a lead agency to identify specific needs in EMSC and to address the mechanisms to meet these needs.
2. Establish a statewide advisory council for this agency. Members should include representatives of relevant state and local agencies, the health care community, and the public at large.

---

and demonstrated similar patterns. Children account for 5% to 10% of all ambulance runs but comprise 25% to 30% of all Emergency Department visits.[7-11] The acuity level for pediatric prehospital problems is lower than for adults with approximately 0.3% to 0.5% of transported children requiring tertiary care; 5% involve life- or limb-threatening problems.[7,8,11]

Children usually present in a bimodal age distribution, with most frequent contacts for ages less than 2 and older than 10. Younger children most frequently present with medical problems; above age 2 years, trauma predominates. Approximately 50% of all pediatric contacts are for traumatic events, with motor vehicle–related trauma (occupant, pedestrian, or bicycle struck) being the leading cause. Other common traumatic etiologies include drowning, burns/inhalation injury, intoxications, choking/suffocation, and penetrating trauma due to firearms. Of nontraumatic problems, presenting problems frequently include respiratory conditions (stridor, lower airway disease, apnea); seizures; altered mental status; pregnancy related, prehospital births; and abdominal pain.[7,9] Most children require transport between the hours of noon and midnight.[9]

The Medical Model

Sudden cardiac arrest in adults is a primary event occurring as a result of underlying cardiac disease. Children predominantly suffer cardiac arrest as a late, secondary event resulting from respiratory failure, central nervous system (CNS) insufficiency, or cardiovascular collapse from a variety of etiologies. Adults presenting in cardiac arrest often have a ventricular dysrhythmia. For children presenting in cardiac arrest the predominant dysrhythmia is asystole, which has a poor outcome regardless of patient age or underlying cause. Therefore children who suffer out-of-hospital cardiopulmonary arrests have greater than a 90% mortality.[7-13] Children who suffer in-hospital cardiopulmonary arrest fare slightly better, while children suffering a respiratory arrest have a survival rate of 60% to 70%.[14-18]

Improved outcome in cardiac arrests from prehospital intervention has been one of the outstanding successes for EMS for adults but not for children.[19] It has been suggested that since cardiac arrest is rarely a primary event in children, a more appropriate marker for quality prehospital care of critically ill children is the measure of outcome for prearrest situations related to respiratory failure and shock

TABLE 4-1. Causes of Death in Children

Causes	Age 0-14 yr	Age 14-24 yr	Total
Motor vehicle	3,400	15,000	18,900
Drowning	1,250	1,300	2,550
Fire, burns	1,200	500	1,700
Poisoning, suffocation	520	750	1,270
Firearms	230	600	830
TOTAL	6,600	18,650	25,250

Adapted from Matlack ME: Current problems in the management of pediatric trauma. In Haller JA Jr, editor: *Emergency medical services for children: report on the ninety-seventh Ross conference on pediatric research,* Columbus, Ohio, 1989, Ross Laboratories.

states.[8] Bystander CPR and prehospital intervention have been shown effective in pediatric near-drowning and foreign body aspiration.[20-22]

The Trauma Model

Trauma is the number one killer of children less than 19 years of age, resulting in over 20,000 deaths a year[23] (Table 4-1). The data available that examine the delivery of care for pediatric trauma are discouraging, revealing unnecessary delays in prehospital transport and definitive treatment, as well as lack of focus on injury prevention. Preventable patient mortality in children already injured has been reported by multiple investigators. Ramanofsky argues that as many as 50% of pediatric trauma deaths could probably have been prevented and were due to deficiencies in the EMS response.[24] Seidel reported that the number of trauma deaths for children was greater than for adults especially in areas without a pediatric center available to accept transports.[25] Recent work by Cooper, examining population-based data in New York State, demonstrated that 80% of all trauma deaths in children occurred in the field and were never even treated in a hospital.[26]

Children traumatized in rural areas are least likely to benefit from an EMS response due to large sparsely populated areas that EMS must cover. This often means dealing with prolonged response and transport times because of distance, difficult environmental conditions, and rough terrain. Life-threatening injuries occur infrequently in any given location in a rural setting; however, 70% of all highway fatalities occur on rural roads. Prehospital and hospital staff working in rural areas will be required to manage children with injuries *as severe* as any managed in a regional trauma center but on an infrequent basis. Children are the least likely to be served by adequately trained medical personnel (emergency medical technician, paramedic, physician, nurse).[27]

Pediatric Trauma Centers

Care of the severely injured child requires a coordinated, multispecialty team approach that begins the moment of injury and continues until the child is fully recovered.[28] The development of regionalized care for pediatric trauma victims began in the 1970s.[29] However, until recently there has been limited national attention paid to the care of the injured child. The special needs of children have been outlined.[30] There is clear evidence for improved outcomes for traumatized adults cared for in regionalized trauma centers.[31,32] The outcome for children cared for in regional pediatric critical care/trauma centers has been evaluated by several investigators.[25,33,34] Further study on the impact of regionalized pediatric trauma care still needs to be performed.

The Pediatric Model for Prehospital Advanced Life Support

Two models have shaped the philosophies of prehospital care—the trauma model and the medical model—both based on data collected on adult patients. The driving force for emergency medical care of the adult, both in the field and the hospital, is the rapid delivery of advanced life support (ALS) immediately to prevent or reverse sudden cardiac death. As trauma care systems evolved, it was recognized that the approach of spending time at the scene to assure an adequate airway and to obtain IV access and cardiac monitoring was detrimental to trauma patients, who if they were critically injured required a definitive operation. This led to the concept of the "golden hour" and the current philosophy of rapid transport for these patients to a regional trauma center. Those systems that do deliver ALS to traumatized patients now do so en route; prehospital interventions must not lengthen transport time.

It is optimal to develop a paradigm for treatment of the pediatric patient based on the epidemiology of pediatric illness and injury, with outcome data to support the prehospital intervention chosen. Data do not exist that demonstrate improved outcome to justify the delay in transport while administering ALS to children in the field, whether it is for status epilepticus, poisoning, or vascular instability from dehydration. This is not to suggest children should be denied ALS in the prehospital setting, but rather, as in the adult trauma patient, priorities must be maintained. Two landmark studies deserve mention. Seidel suggested that the availability of a receiving hospital with expertise in pediatric care appeared to affect outcome more than the quality of the prehospital care.[25] Quan demonstrated the value of early prehospital airway management and ventilation in pediatric patients, supporting the consensus of the pediatric emergency medicine community that skill in airway management and intubation by prehospital providers can improve outcome.[22]

However, certain realities affect pediatric prehospital care. The majority of prehospital personnel, whether ALS and basic life support (BLS) providers, have inadequate pediatric training even in BLS skills and knowledge base.[22,35] Prehospital providers do not get constant exposure to critically ill and injured children.[36] Many systems have only recently started acquiring appropriate equipment for pediatric care.

Systems that are in the process of developing their pediatric capabilities cannot expect the field personnel to suddenly feel comfortable with children. Rather it must be understood that the system will evolve in its pediatric capabilities as its field personnel gain experience with children. If the teachers provide a positive mindset and create an attitudinal change in the prehospital provider, this will persist even if the technical skills do not. Constant continuing medical education in pediatric skills is a necessity in any EMS system that plans to deliver appropriate pediatric care. Although the investment is high for manpower and training, the majority of pediatric patients require short-term intervention of which prehospital care is a crucial link. The cost to society and the family for lack of an adequate EMS response is much higher.[37]

In New York City this continuing education has resulted in an approach termed *conservative yet permissive*. This approach is conservative since the BLS principles of keeping the child warm and rapid transport to an appropriate facility are stressed as the primary priority. The approach is permissive in that paramedics have standing orders that permit intubation based on their judgment and that *all other ALS interventions* are permitted en route or if there is an unavoidable transport delay at the scene or en route, from an extrication problem or traffic congestion. It is from those systems that perform prehospital ALS on children and study their efforts that optimal approaches will be developed.

This model might be modified in a setting where a long transport time is anticipated due to long distance from the patient scene to the receiving hospital. Valuable time is more likely to be committed to further stabilize the patient before transport. This is more often the case in a rural setting. The vast majority of prehospital providers in this country are BLS providers, with ALS providers being concentrated in the urban and suburban communities.

PREHOSPITAL CARE FOR CHILDREN

Personnel

Problems in the education, training, equipping, and medical control of prehospital personnel have been identified.* The average EMT or paramedic rarely provides care for truly critical children and sporadically used skills are not well maintained. Although constant retraining has been demonstrated to improve skill and knowledge retention,[38,39] many communities do not yet offer even initial training. The appropriate array of equipment sizes is often not available. Specific protocols may not exist for pediatric prehospital care, reflecting a lack of pediatric expertise in both on-line and off-line medical control Not surprisingly, therefore, prehospital providers generally regard critical pediatric calls as their most stressful encounters.

It is clear that progress is being made in numerous communities. Many are addressing the described problems through improved EMSC programs. Certainly the resources available have increased considerably in the last 10 years.[40]

Education and Training

Before the summer of 1994 the national model for education and training of prehospital personnel did not reflect the pediatric emergencies encountered in the field nor did it emphasize the skills needed. Of the 100 to 120 hours

required for EMT training, only 3 hours were allocated for pediatrics in the Department of Transportation (DOT) curriculum, and of the 1,000+ hours needed for paramedic training, an average of 15 hours was spent in pediatric didactic training. In one published survey, 40% of the programs devoted less than 10 hours.[25]

Pediatric didactic material often focuses on illness or injury that cannot and should not be diagnosed in the field rather than concentrating on recognition of conditions where prehospital interventions may make a difference. The current DOT paramedic curriculum guidelines still require education in meningitis and Reye syndrome, which although important, cannot be diagnosed in the field. Another area that is lacking in most training programs is clinical time spent in an emergency department or on a pediatric unit. Such "hands-on" experience is invaluable as it allows the trainee to assess and treat patients under direct supervision.

In 1990, NHTSA sponsored an EMS consensus workshop to establish national priorities in EMS training for the future. Key priorities included changing the curriculum from a diagnosis-based approach to an assessment-based approach to training. Particular emphasis is placed on pediatric skills and training that prepare prehospital providers for infants and children by integrating information throughout the curricula. Topics that need to be taught in an assessment-based manner are summarized in the box on p. 28.[3,41,42]

A national blueprint for all levels of prehospital care providers was released in 1993[43] and a new national EMT-B curriculum was released in the summer of 1994,[44] both with a much-improved pediatric section. Revision of the Paramedic, EMT-Intermediate, and First Responder National Standard Curriculums are all underway. It is expected that these and future curriculum products should have a profound effect in improving the care of children nationally.

Equipment

Appropriate equipment to care for ill and injured children is necessary for all prehospital vehicles. Minimum equipment standards for BLS, ALS, and critical care transportation of children need to be developed and adopted on a national level. Although equipment lists for prehospital pediatric care exist, many systems still lack the equipment and training to utilize this equipment[19,22,23] (see box on pp. 29-30).

MANAGEMENT

Treatment of children at the scene and during transport depends on the training of prehospital providers (assessment skills and technical skills), predetermined protocols for allowable interventions, appropriate equipment on the ambulance, availability of direct medical control, and the setting (urban vs. rural). Prehospital care protocols (see box on pp. 31-33), equipment (see box on pp. 29-30), and personnel training (see box on p. 34) should be adequate for assessment, stabilization, and triage decisions to be performed. Guidelines for prehospital care of children, including treatment and triage protocols, and equipment lists have been developed.[45-47]

---

* References 7, 8, 9, 12, 13, 20, 22, 24, 25.

Essential Prehospital Pediatric Topics

Assessments of life-threatening conditions
Respiratory distress or failure
Circulatory compromise or failure
Multiple trauma
Altered mental status

Skills
BLS
Oxygen delivery
Suctioning
Assisted ventilation (mouth-to-mask or bag-valve-mask)
C-spine or spinal immobilization
Airway adjuncts, sizing and use

ALS
Endotracheal intubation
Vascular access: IV, IO
Medications: IV, IO, IM, PR
NG tube placement
Defibrillation

Diagnostic etiologies
Upper vs lower airway obstruction
Foreign body aspiration
Shock (nontraumatic)
Sudden infant death syndrome (SIDS)
Near drowning
Poisoning
Status epilepticus
Trauma or shock
Head trauma or increased intracranial pressure (ICP)
Neonatal complications
Child abuse
Anaphylaxis

Transport

Transport of the critically ill or injured child is a vital component of an effective EMS system,[33] including transport to a hospital emergency service (primary transport) and when warranted, interhospital transport (secondary transport) (see Chapter 5). The current status of specialized transport for children has its origins in the transportation of the trauma victim, as well as the high risk neonate.[34] Specialty transport for nontraumatized children developed in 1975 in Ohio.[46] In 1980, the American Academy of Pediatrics (AAP) produced guidelines for the regionalization of neonatal care.[48]

The majority of prehospital transports utilize ground ambulances; the standards were developed in the early 1970s.[49-52] Ambulance designs were developed that reflected differing approaches to the flexibility of the modular ambulance body and the ability to walk through from the driver's cab to the passenger care area. In certain clinical conditions it may be preferable to allow the parent to stay with the child to provide comfort and prevent agitation. However, if the child's condition should deterio-

rate en route, the presence of the parent in the patient care area of the ambulance may obstruct the delivery of optimal care. Therefore a design that allows a connection between the passenger and driver's compartments seems warranted.

Protection of children during transport, in case of a collision involving the ambulance, was not addressed by the DOT ambulance design standards.[49-51] Adult prehospital providers and passengers may be restrained in a sitting position, using lap seat belts; a patient on a stretcher may be immobilized with chest, hip, and leg restraints while the stretcher is fixed in position to the floor of the ambulance passenger compartment. Current guidelines do not include the provision of child safety–seat restraints as part of standard ambulance design.

A third issue for ambulance design is the provision of a warm environment in the passenger compartment of the ambulance. This is ensured during neonatal transport using a double-walled transport isolet. For critically ill or injured older infants and young children it may be difficult to provide a sufficiently warm ambulance environment in cold climates; failure to maintain a neutral thermal environment can significantly compromise resuscitation and stabilization efforts.

Guidelines and voluntary standards[52-54] have also been developed within the industry for air ambulances; however, these have not specifically addressed the special needs of children. Guidelines from the AAP[44,55] and consensus from a national leadership conference on Pediatric Interhospital Critical Care Transport[56] recently focused on the special needs of children. Further work is needed to delineate areas not adequately addressed.

Triage

The purpose of field triage is to allow patients to be transported to a facility that has been categorized and designated as capable of meeting their emergent needs. Triage decisions are often based on the initial assessment with on-line medical control or through established criteria such as a trauma score.

Specific criteria for traumatized children have been developed. The Pediatric Trauma Score is a numeric score, assigned according to severity of injury by field personnel.[24] Children with a score of 8 or less require treatment in a trauma center (see later discussion). Although work on pediatric trauma triage is in its early stages, it is well ahead of triage of children with medical problems. Predetermined criteria for medical triage have been proposed[36]; however, prospective study of medical triage criteria is still necessary. Very few systems currently triage children for trauma or medical problems. Preliminary studies[26,33] suggest that whether medical or traumatic, children have improved outcomes when triaged and transported to tertiary care facilities.

Communication

Essential to the prehospital phase of emergency care is the provision of on-line medical control by direct communication between the prehospital provider and a base station medical expert who may be a physician or in some systems a specially trained nurse. With some notable

Text continued on p. 33.

American College of Emergency Physician (ACEP) Minimum Pediatric Prehospital Equipment Guidelines

Although there is currently no federally mandated list of minimum equipment for BLS or ALS, most states have passed legislation as to what equipment is either required or allowed within their systems. Early on there were equipment lists promulgated by the American Academy of Orthopedic Surgeons along with the original EMT curriculum design. Equipment and medications are currently approved by state regulatory agencies, legislation, and local medical control.

The ACEP published a 1988 policy statement concerning ALS skills, medications, and equipment. This existing Board policy addresses the optimal equipment and medications for the ALS provider. Within it are the equipment and medications necessary to provide care for the pediatric patient within the EMS system. The attached document re-emphasizes the minimum equipment needs for the proper care of the pediatric patient within the EMS system.

The EMS system has many classification levels of prehospital emergency care technicians. BLS refers to the basic EMT level as defined by the DOT. ALS refers to the EMT levels above basic, and these classification levels are highly variable across the nation with respect to skills, training, and capabilities within their own system. ALS is defined by the skills enumerated in the Prehospital Advanced Life Support: Skills, Medication and Equipment document published in the *Annals of Emergency Medicine*, 17:1109; 1988.

The EMS system must meet the diverse needs of the people and regions it serves. Because of differences in length of transport time or distances traveled, the needs for additional equipment, skills, or medication may differ from region to region. For example, long transport times may require humidified oxygen or an IV infusion control device. Extra monitoring devices for glucose measurement or pulse oximetry may be desirable in some cases for selected transports.

Pediatric emergency care is an integral component of the overall EMS system. As such, the EMS system must provide for the proper care of children, especially for those under age 12. Just as hazardous materials management, disaster management, and other special rescue and transport needs dictate equipment to be carried by the rescue and transport vehicles, so too the ACEP suggests that the following minimum equipment guidelines be used by EMS medical control to guide decisions on equipment selections, adding additional equipment or medications deemed appropriate for individual systems or as required by state regulations.

There are state-by-state variations in both legislation and the types of patients transported within those states. ACEP has recommended generic lists for BLS and ALS with these constraints in mind. Ongoing research in EMS may require changes to some of these recommendations in the future.

For the sake of clarity, the document is broken down into BLS minimum equipment lists and a neonatal section. However this document is to be taken as a whole, with the neonatal section being a component of the BLS and ALS minimum lists.

Many systems have continued to improvise and use adult equipment for the transport of children. The response of manufacturing and equipment suppliers to pediatric needs allows a much more appropriate selection of equipment for the care of critically ill and injured children within the emergency medical system.

It is important that appropriate education and training be completed by the EMT and EMT paramedic before using any of these equipment items and medications and that appropriate quality assurance programs exist to evaluate the items and medications used by the EMT and EMT paramedic.

BLS MINIMUM EQUIPMENT LIST

Equipment

Oxygen Tank with Tubing	With humidified source for long transport times
Oral Airways	Sizes 0-5
Nasopharyngeal Airways with Lubricant	12-30F or equivalent sizes in mm
Self Inflating Bags w/oxygen reservoir	250, 500, 2000 ml bags
Oxygen Masks	Infant, Child, Adult
Nasal Cannulas	Infant, Child, Adult Sizes 1-3
Masks for Bag-Valve-Mask	
Stethoscope	
Blood Pressure Cuffs	Infant, Child, Adult
Portable Suction Unit	
Suction Catheters (flexible & rigid)	6F to 14F
Back Board for Spinal Immobilization	Short and long board
Sand Bags or equivalent for Neck Immobilization	
Towel Rolls/Blanket Rolls/or equivalent	
Rigid Extrication Collar (for over 2 year olds)	Infant, Child, Small, Medium, Adult
Femur Splint	Designed for Pediatric Patients
Burn Pack	Standard Pack; Towels or Gel Burn Sheet Acceptable
Thermal Absorbent Blanket	
Equipment Sizing Tape or Equipment/Age/Weight Chart	

Continued.

Supplies

Adhesive Tape	Gauze Rolls
Alcohol Sponges	Gauze Sponges
Arm Boards (various sizes)	Protective Eyewear, and Gloves, Masks
Povidone-Iodine Prep Pads	Scissors
Elastic Bandages	Tincture of Benzoin
Extra Batteries & Bulbs for Equipment Needs	Tongue Blades
Flashlight, Bulb, Batteries	

ALS MINIMUM EQUIPMENT AND MEDICATION LIST

Equipment

BLS Minimum Equipment and Supplies plus:

Monitoring:

Transport Monitor — Battery Operated with 3 or 4 Leads

Defibrillator w/4.25 and 8 cm paddles (or paddle adapter) and pads capable to dial down to appropriate watt-sec for pediatric patients. When replacing current equipment, new equipment should have settings below 25 watt-sec.

Monitoring Electrodes

Equipment and Drug Dosage Tape and age weight chart

Chem Strip for Glucose and Analyzer

Airway:

Laryngoscope Handle with Extra Batteries and Bulbs

Laryngoscope Blades-Straight and/or Curved, #'s 0,1,2,3

Stylets — Pediatric Sizes

Endotracheal Tubes
   Uncuffed Range 3.0-5.5 mm
   Cuffed Range 5.0-8.0 mm

Magill Forceps (Rachevsky)

Lubrication (Water Soluble)

Nasogastric Tube, Sizes 5F to 18F

Vascular Access:

Intravenous Catheter of Choice (16 gm-22 gm)

Intraosseous Needles of Choice

Tourniquet/Rubber Bands

3-Way Stopcocks or adapter that allows administration of additional fluids or medications

Syringes-various sizes

Blood Sample Tubes

Intravenous Tubing, Burritol

Tuberculin Syringes

Intravenous Solutions:

Normal Saline or Lactated Ringer's

D5W (diluent)

Sodium Chloride-Bacteriostatic, for injection

Water-Bacteriostatic, for injection

Medications	*Concentration*
Atropine Sulphate	0.1 mg/ml
Bicarbonate, Sodium	8.4% (1.0 mEq/ml)
Diazepam or Analeptic of Choice	5 mg/ml
Epinephrine	1:1000 (1 mg/ml)
Epinephrine	1:10,000 (0.1 mg/ml)
Lidocaine Hydrochloride (IV)	10 mg/ml
Naloxone Hydrochloride-Adult	1.0 mg/ml
Pain Medication per Medical Control	
D50 (Dextrose 50 + Water and Diluent)	
Inhalant Beta Adrenergic Agent (commonly Albuterol)	
Activated Charcoal	

RESUSCITATION EQUIPMENT AND SUPPLIES FOR THE NEWBORN MINIMUM EQUIPMENT GUIDELINES

BLS for newborn:

Oxygen Cylinder

Stethoscope

Bulb Syringe

Portable Suction

Suction Catheters (5F-10F Range)

Resuscitation Bag (≤ 750 ml [250 ml or 500 ml])

Face Mask (Infant) (Premature and Newborn Sizes)

Gauze

Sterile Scissors

Thermal Absorbent Blanket and Head Cover

Cord Clamps

Appropriate Heat Source for Ambulance Compartment

ALS for newborn:

Basic Life Support Minimum for Newborn plus:

Endotracheal Tube Uncuffed (3.0-4.0 mm)

Endotracheal Tube Stylet (6f)

Laryngoscope (Straight Blades 0 and 1)

Infusion Set, Microdrip Unit

From American College of Emergency Physicians, 1992.

Pediatric Prehospital Protocols

RESPIRATORY ARREST
* Airway positioning, suction, cervical immobilization if indicated.
* Assisted ventilations with BVM device.
+ Perform ET intubation.
* **Transport.**
+ Administer naloxone 2.0 mg via ET, or IM
+ NG or orogastric tube for abdominal distension.

Medical control contact for the following interventions:
+ Obtain vascular access IV to KVO.
# Obtain vascular access IO infusion.
+ Administer naloxone 2.0 mg IV or IO.
* **Transport decision.**

OBSTRUCTED AIRWAY
For pediatric patients who are unconscious or *cannot* breathe, cough, speak, or cry:
* BLS obstructed airway procedures:
< 1 yr back blows/chest thrusts.
> 1 yr abdominal thrusts.
+ Perform direct laryngoscopy.
+ Attempt to remove the foreign body with pediatric Magill forceps. (If an enlarged epiglottis is visualized, use protocol for epiglottitis.)
* USE HIGH PRESSURE BVM VENTILATION.
+ Perform ET intubation (only when other methods of airway control and ventilation are not effective).
Transport.
Needle cricothyrotomy (if child cannot be ventilated or intubated).
+ NG or orogastric tube for abdominal distension.
Transport decision.

STRIDOR (CROUP/EPIGLOTTITIS/FOREIGN BODY)
Respiratory distress
* Help to maintain position of comfort (sitting).
* Avoid procedures (blood pressure, IV line placement)
* Keep caregiver with child.
* Oxygen by face mask or blow by.
* **Transport decision.**

NONTRAUMATIC CARDIAC ARREST
* Assisted ventilations with BVM; 100% oxygen.
* Begin cardiac compressions.
+ Perform ET intubation.
* **Transport.**
* ALS intercept en route (BLS).
+ Cardiac monitoring, record and evaluate ECG strip.
+ Begin an IV, #IO infusion of 0.9% NS.
+ NG or orogastric tube for abdominal distension.

Asystole
+ Epinephrine 0.1 mg/kg 1:1000 via ET.
+ Epinephrine 0.01 mg/kg 1:10,000 IV or IO first dose, 0.1 mg/kg 1:1000 IV or IO subsequent doses.

+ 25% Dextrose 0.5 gm/kg IV (#IO) bolus.
+ Glucagon 1.0 mg IM, IV or #IO.
+ Naloxone 2.0 mg IV (#IO) bolus, or via ET or IM.
+ Sodium bicarbonate 1.0 mEq/kg, IV (#IO) bolus.
+ Atropine sulfate 0.01 mg/kg, IV (#IO) bolus, or via ET (minimum dose 0.1 mg, maximum dose 10 mg).

Ventricular fibrillation
+ Defibrillate at 2 watt-sec/kg.
+ Repeat defibrillation 4 watt-sec/kg × 2.
+ Epinephrine 0.1 mg/kg 1:1000 via the ET tube or Epinephrine 0.01 mg/kg 1:10,000 IV or #IO first dose, 0.1 mg/kg 1:1000 IV (#IO) subsequent doses.
+ Repeat defibrillation 4 watt-sec/kg.
+ Lidocaine 1 mg/kg IV, #IO.
+ Repeat defibrillation 4 watt-sec/kg.
+ Bretylium 5 mg/kg IV (#IO) initial dose, 10 mg/kg next 2 doses.

Pulseless electrical activity
+ Epinephrine 0.1 mg/kg 1:1000 via the ET tube.
+ Epinephrine 0.01 mg/kg 1:10,000 IV or #IO first dose. 0.1 mg/kg 1:1000 IV, #IO subsequent doses.
+ Begin rapid IV (#IO) infusion of 0.9% NS, 20 ml/kg.
# Needle decompression of tension pneumothorax.
* **Transport decision.**

WHEEZING/ASTHMA
* Help maintain position of comfort (sitting).
* Avoid procedures (blood pressure, IV line placement).
* Keep caregiver with child.
* Oxygen by face mask or blow by.
+ Beta-2 agonist of choice: Albuterol via acorn nebulizer 0.15-0.30 ml of 0.5% Albuterol in 2.5 ml saline/children < 2 years, over 5 to 15 min.
0.30-0.50 ml of 0.5% Albuterol in 2.5 ml saline/children ≥ 2 years, over 5 to 15 min.
In patients 1 year of age or older with severe respiratory distress or respiratory failure (cyanosis, altered mental status [lethargic], severe retractions):
+ Epinephrine 0.01 mg/kg (0.01 ml/kg of a 1:1,000 solution), SC (Max. dose is 0.3 ml.)
* **Transport.**

Medical control contact for the following interventions:
If the child develops or remains in severe respiratory distress or respiratory failure:
+ Epinephrine 0.01 mg/kg (0.01 mg/kg of a 1:1,000 solution), SC.
+ 0.3 ml of 0.5% albuterol in 2.5 ml saline, continuous nebulization.
+ Begin an IV infusion of 0.9% NS to KVO
Transport decision.

ANAPHYLACTIC REACTION
For children with hives (red, itchy rash) and history of contact with allergen (Insect sting, food or oral drug)

Continued.

Pediatric Prehospital Protocols—cont'd

Respiratory distress/wheezing
* Help to maintain position of comfort (sitting).
* Avoid procedures (blood pressure, IV line placement).
* Keep caregiver with child.
* Oxygen by face mask or blow by.
+ Beta-2 agonist of choice: Albuterol via acorn nebulizer
   0.15-0.30 ml of 0.5% Albuterol in 2.5 ml saline children
     < 2 years
   0.30-0.50 ml of 0.5% Albuterol in 2.5 ml saline children
     ≥ 2 years

Severe respiratory distress (cyanosis, altered mental status [lethargic], severe retractions) or swelling of tongue or lips, hoarseness or stridor
+ Epinephrine 0.01 mg/kg (0.01 ml/kg of 1:1,000 solution), SC (maximum dose 0.3 ml.)
* **Transport.**

Respiratory failure/arrest, airway obstruction, or decompensated shock
+ Perform ET intubation.
+ Epinephrine 0.01 mg/kg (0.1 mg/kg of a 1:1000 solution) via ET
If ET intubation cannot be accomplished:
+ Epinephrine 0.01 mg/kg (0.01 ml/kg of a 1:1,000 solution) SC (maximum dose 0.3 ml).
* **Transport.**
+ NG or orogastric tube for abdominal distension.

Medical control contact for the following interventions:
+ Begin an IV (#IO) infusion of 0.9% NS.
+ Shock, begin rapid IV (IO) infusion of 0.9% NS 20 ml/kg. Repeat as necessary.
+ Epinephrine 0.01 mg/kg (1.0 ml/kg of a 1:100,000 solution) IV (#IO) slowly.
Transport decision.

ALTERED MENTAL STATUS
* Airway positioning, suction, cervical immobilization if indicated.
* Oxygen 100% by simple face mask.
* Administer oral glucose for known diabetic with intact gag reflex.
Transport.
+ Glucagon 1.0 mg IM.
+ IV infusion of 0.9% NS.
+ 25% Dextrose 0.5 gm/kg IV bolus.
If no change in neurologic function:
+ Naloxone 2.0 mg IV or IM
Transport decision.

Medical control contact for the following interventions:
IO infusion of 0.9% NS.
+ Naloxone 2.0 mg, IO.
+ 25% Dextrose 0.5 gm/kg IO.
+ ET intubation.

STATUS EPILEPTICUS
For pediatric patients in status epilepticus (ongoing seizures on arrival of EMS):
* Airway positioning, suction, cervical immobilization if indicated.
* Oxygen 100% by simple face mask.
* Hold head (extremities) to prevent injury.
Transport.
+ Glucagon 1.0 mg IM.
+ Begin an IV infusion of 0.9% NS.
# Begin an IO infusion of 0.9% NS.

Medical control contact for the following interventions:
25% Dextrose 0.5 gm/kg, IV (#IO) bolus
Diazepam 0.2 mg/kg, IV (#IO) bolus (rate of administration may not exceed 1.0 mg/min)
Do not continue IV administration of Diazepam, if seizures have stopped.
If unable to establish IV, administer Diazepam 0.5 mg/kg per rectum.
Transport decision

TRAUMATIC/HYPOVOLEMIC SHOCK
Decompensated traumatic/hypovolemic shock:
* Airway positioning, suction, cervical immobilization if indicated.
* Oxygen 100% by simple face mask.
* Assisted ventilations with BVM device.
Transport.
+ Begin rapid IV infusion of 0.9% NS, 20 ml/kg

Medical control contact for the following interventions:
Begin rapid IO infusion of 0.9% NS, 20 ml/kg.
Repeat 0.9% NS, 20 ml/kg rapid IV (#IO) infusion.
Begin rapid IV (#IO) infusion of 0.9% NS, 20 ml/kg via a second large bore IV or IO.
Transport decision.

TRAUMATIC CARDIAC ARREST
* Airway positioning, suction, cervical immobilization if indicated.
* Oxygen 100% by simple face mask.
* Assisted ventilations with BVM device.
* Begin CPR
Transport.
+ ET intubation.
+ Begin rapid IV infusion of 0.9% NS, 20 ml/kg.
# Begin rapid IO infusion of 0.9% NS, 20 ml/kg.
+ Orogastric tube for abdominal distention.
# Needle thoracostomy for possible tension pneumothorax.

Medical control contact for the following interventions:
+ Repeat 0.9% NS, 20 ml/kg, rapid IV (IO) infusion.
+ Insert second IV or #IO; rapid infusion of 0.9% NS, 20 ml/kg.
+ Epinephrine 0.01 mg/kg 1:10,000 IV or #IO first dose. 0.1 mg/kg 1:1000 IV (#IO) subsequent doses.
+ Epinephrine 0.1 mg/kg (0.1 ml/kg of a 1:1000 solution), ET.
Transport decision.

NEWBORN

* During delivery, suction the mouth and nose as the newborn's head delivers.
* After delivery, wrap the newborn in absorbent towel or blanket.
* Position the newborn supine.
* Suction the mouth; + if thick meconium is present, perform ET intubation and tracheal suctioning.
* Suction the nose.
* Stimulate the newborn (vigorous drying of the skin).
* Clamp and cut the umbilical cord (leave 2-inches of cord above the abdomen).
* Assess respiratory efforts: * if shallow, slow, or absent, assist ventilations with a BVM and 100% oxygen.
* **ASSESS HEART RATE:**
  If <60/min:
* Begin CPR and continue assisted ventilations with BVM; after 30 seconds to 1 minute of CPR, reassess heart rate.
+ Perform ET intubation if heart rate <60/min. Assist ventilations for 30 sec to 1 min via ET.
* **Transport.**
+ Administer epinephrine 0.01-0.03 mg/kg via ET tube if no improvement in heart rate.
+ Administer epinephrine 0.1 mg/kg via ET tube. if no improvement in heart rate
  If 60-80/min:
* Continue assisted ventilations for 30 sec to 1 min
+ Perform ET intubation if no improvement in heart rate
  Assist ventilations for 30 sec to 1 minute via ET.
* **Transport.**
+ Administer epinephrine 0.01-0.03 mg/kg via ET tube if no improvement in heart rate
+ Administer epinephrine 0.1 mg/kg via ET tube if no improvement in heart rate

If 80-100/min and rising:
* Give blow by oxygen, continue stimulation.
* Reassess heart rate after 30 seconds, * If <100, assisted ventilations with BVM and 100% oxygen.
* **Transport.**
  If >100 min:
* Assess skin color (central), if cyanosis, * Give blow by oxygen.
* **Transport.**
+ Orogastric tube for abdominal distention

Medical control contact for the following interventions:
+ Insert IV or #IO; rapid infusion of 0.9% NS, 20 ml/kg.
+ Administer epinephrine 0.01-0.03 mg/kg via IV or #IO.
+ Glucagon 1.0 mg IM.
+ 10% Dextrose 0.5 gm/kg IV (#IO) bolus.
Transport decision.

POISONING/INGESTION
* Stabilize airway and ventilations as needed.
* Oxygen 100% by simple face mask if needed.
* History of what, when, how much and how poisoning occurred
* Bring in medication bottle or container of substance ingested
Transport.

Medical control contact for the following interventions:
Contact regional poison center or base station for management.
+ Obtain IV access.
+ Activated charcoal 1 gm/kg PO.
+ Glucagon 1.0 mg IM or IV.
# Begin IO infusion of 0.9% NS.
+ 25% Dextrose 0.5 gm/kg IV (#IO) bolus.
+ Naloxone 2.0 mg IV (#IO) or IM
+ Sodium bicarbonate 1.0 meq/kg IV (#IO) bolus
+ Atropine sulfate 0.01 mg/kg IV (#IO)

* BLS procedure; + ALS procedure; # Advanced Intervention may not be applicable to all EMS systems. *BVM,* Bag-valve-mask; *ET,* endotracheal; *ETT,* endotracheal tube; *IM,* intramuscular; *IV,* intravenous; *IO,* intraosseous; *KVO,* keep vein open; *PR,* per rectum; *SC,* subcutaneously; *NS,* normal saline; *NG,* nasogastric.
NOTE: All equipment sizing, weight estimates, and drug dosing should be calculated using a length-based resuscitation tape.

---

exceptions (i.e., Pittsburgh, San Francisco, and the Maryland Institute for Emergency Medical Service Systems [MIEMSS]), very few systems provide adequate on-line medical control to meet the special needs of children.

THE MEDICAL HOME, PREVENTION, AND SYSTEM ACCESS

Prevention

Emergency and intensive care to treat critically ill and injured children is expensive in terms of personal anguish and societal cost.[11,57,58] Prevention is the least expensive intervention possible and has the best outcome. A 1995

EMS leadership conference sponsored by NHTSA has issued a report stating that all EMS systems should be involved in identifying, developing, improving, and supporting successful prevention mechanisms.[58]

The key to prevention is education. Parents, children, the lay public, pediatricians, family physicians, emergency medicine physicians, nurses, and prehospital care providers should be involved in this area by delivering anticipatory information concerning prevention in many areas (see box on p. 34).[37,59] Parents can be taught CPR, how to recognize significant illness and injury, what to do initially for specific medical emergencies, when to call for help ("911"), and what to do until help arrives.

Minimum Standards for Education and Training of Prehospital Health Care Providers

Emergency medical technicians (EMTs)

Knowledge

Anatomic and physiologic differences
Psychologic and developmental issues
Pediatric physical assessment
Pediatric vital signs
Spectrum of illness and injury requiring emergency care
Recognition and management of respiratory distress and failure
Recognition and management of pediatric shock and trauma
Treatment of pediatric medical and surgical emergencies
Recognition and reporting of child abuse
Recognition and management of SIDS
Critical-incident stress debriefing

Skills

Infant and child cardiopulmonary resuscitation
Infant and child BLS maneuvers for obstructed airway
Infant and child airway/ventilation management
Pediatric vital signs determination
Pediatric PSAG use
Pediatric extrication and spinal immobilization

Paramedics

Knowledge

Need for pediatric ETT placement
Need for pediatric NG tube placement
Need for pediatric IV and IO access
Need for defibrillation and cardioversion
Need for needle thoracostomy and cricothyrotomy
Dosage and administration of drugs in pediatric emergencies
Dosage and administration of fluids in pediatric emergencies

Skills

Pediatric ETT placement
Pediatric NG tube placement
Pediatric IV and IO access
Pediatric defibrillation and cardioversion
Pediatric needle thoracostomy and cricothyrotomy
Pediatric PR Valium technique

Modified from Education and Training of Professionals and the Public. In Seidel JS and Henderson DP, editors: *Emergency medical services for children: a report to the nation.* Washington DC, 1991, National Center for Education in Maternal and Child Health.

Prevention of Critical Injury in EMSC

Child restraints in motor vehicles
Infant seats, booster seats, seat belts

Burn prevention
Smoke detectors, limit hot water temperature

Bicycle safety
Bicycle helmets, educational programs

Drowning
Mandatory pool fencing, education

Poisoning
Safety caps, limit container size, education

Falls
Mandatory window guards, education

medical system, as well as allows early planning for rehabilitation and other needs after discharge.[60]

Access to Care

In many regions a "911" telephone system exists and provides direct access to the EMS system. Parents, caretakers, schools, and so on should be familiar with this number and it's correct use.[5] Physicians should provide information for parents regarding when they should contact the physician's office vs. 911, as well as which emergency departments are most appropriate for children. A call to "911" for a minor ailment can cause potentially life-threatening delays in the EMS response to a serious injury requiring emergent care. Some regions are now using an "enhanced 911" (911e) program that automatically provides the EMS system with the address. This valuable addition to 911 technology belongs in every community. Unfortunately, many regions do not yet even have a 911 program in place.

Activating the 911 system elicits an ambulance dispatch that should be medically directed and coordinated. In some regions a two-tiered system exists composed of BLS and ALS units. The type of unit dispatched, as well as the priority of the call, should be based on predetermined guidelines developed by regional medical control physician(s).[61] Standardized dispatch protocols should include standard prearrival instructions, allowing the dispatcher to deliver optimal care. Adult-oriented ambulance dispatching should be optimally supplemented by pediatric guidelines to adequately triage pediatric calls[62] such as has been implemented in San Francisco. Minimal research has been performed to determine the optimal dispatch protocols for children.[10]

REGIONALIZATION OF CARE

In 1978, Los Angeles developed guidelines for prehospital care of pediatric emergencies, a pediatric equipment list for prehospital care providers, a curriculum for the education of paramedics in pediatric emergencies, and

The Medical Home

Under ideal circumstances every child has an identified primary care provider who is involved with the child and family before, during, and after entry into the EMSC system. This has been termed as *the medical home.* Continuity of care improves communication between the family and plans for integration of EMSC into the existing EMS system. Through this work, guidelines for a two-tiered system involving both emergency departments approved for pediatrics (EDAPs) and pediatric critical-care centers (PCCCs) were developed. EDAPs are emergency facilities that provide basic emergency services and voluntarily meet minimum standards for staffing, education, equipment, supplies, and protocols, as appropriate for the initial care and stabilization of critically ill and injured children. PCCCs must meet EDAP criteria and in addition have specialized pediatric services including a pediatric ICU and dedicated pediatric medical and surgical specialists.[11]

Other regions have also been active in improving EMSC in their regions through a systems' approach (Mobile, Alabama; New York City; and Milwaukee).[8,24] The MIEMSS, a model for a successful and fully integrated EMS/trauma system, was one of the first to incorporate pediatric trauma–receiving hospitals.[34]

FUTURE DIRECTIONS

Prehospital care now includes a wide variety of treatment plans and modalities performed in the prehospital phase of medical care; yet the only interventions that have been demonstrated to improve outcome for adults are bystander CPR, early defibrillation, and functional trauma systems of care.[6,20,63] There is preliminary evidence that resuscitation of children in the prehospital phase of care improves outcome. Work by Rivara[64] and Quan[22] demonstrates that control of the airway and provision of adequate ventilation are critical to the survival of children suffering multiple trauma and near drowning.

Studies are needed to determine which system approaches and what interventions will result in the most benefit for children in the prehospital setting. For example, intraosseous (IO) infusion has been suggested as a useful procedure in the prehospital phase of care to gain emergent vascular access in children. Studies do demonstrate that this procedure can be successfully utilized in the prehospital setting[65-67]; however, studies demonstrating that IO infusion improves outcome for children have not yet been performed.

A plan for reporting findings of research on pediatric resuscitation in a standardized manner, including templates and essential data points, has recently been published as the Pediatric Utstein Style.[68] This document offers a matrix that includes prehospital, hospital, and long-term outcome measures. It is hoped this standardized approach will allow comparison of studies and foster interinstitutional cooperation.

As trauma systems develop nationally, the pediatric component will clearly become visible. The 1992 AMA-EMS Commission published guidelines for the categorization of hospitals into various levels of care based on their pediatric capabilities[69] have been modified by the AAP.[70]

To be effective in integrating EMSC into EMS, those expert in the care of critically ill or injured children need to be involved in EMS planning (see box above). The future of EMSC depends on involvement of these individuals, funding for EMSC, and documentation that the integration of EMSC into EMS improves the quality of care and outcome for children.

Chain of Survival for Children Who Require EMS

Parents or school
Public
Primary care physician (medical home)
"911" operators and medical dispatchers
Prehospital personnel: first responder, EMT, or
    paramedic
Medical control physicians: on- or off-line
Emergency department physicians and nurses
Inpatient physician, nurse, etc
Secondary transportation team
Pediatric critical care or trauma center
Rehabilitation team

The Pediatric Trauma System

ARTHUR COOPER • BARBARA A. BARLOW

The early care of the injured child is a complex undertaking that involves the participation of many prehospital, medical, nursing, and allied health professionals, all of whom can lay legitimate claim to the title of "pediatric traumatologist" in their respective disciplines (see box on p. 36). Pediatric trauma care is truly a *team* effort that requires the best efforts of *all* team members if optimal recovery of the child is to be assured; there is no place for "turf battles" or "power struggles" when the care, perhaps even the life, of a child is what is at stake. Overall direction should be the responsibility of the most qualified and experienced physician available, who usually is a trauma surgeon with extensive experience in the management of childhood injuries.[71]

The seriously injured child is best cared for in a hospital with a strong institutional, financial, and moral commitment to comprehensive care of injured children and their families that participates fully in the regional EMS system.[72] Most full-service general, university, or children's hospitals meet these criteria. If transport times are not prohibitive, seriously injured children should be preferentially transported by properly trained and equipped prehospital personnel to these facilities, in accordance with regional policies and protocols and formally-established interinstitutional transfer agreements based on guidelines such as those shown in the box on p. 36. Indeed, there is a growing body of evidence that seriously injured children do fare better in organized trauma systems in which there is emphasis on the special needs of children, including the pediatric ICU.[73-78] The requirements for establishing and maintaining such systems have been widely disseminated.[79-82]

A key responsibility of every emergency physician is to understand the capabilities and limitations of the emergency medical and trauma care system responsible for field stabilization, emergency transport, and initial evaluation

---

Components of the Pediatric Trauma Team

Emergency Medical Services
Emergency Service
Trauma Service
Anesthesiology Service
Critical Care Service
Rehabilitation Service
Trauma Clinic
Injury Prevention Program

Possible Indications for Transfer to a Trauma Center with Pediatric Expertise

History of injury
Patient thrown from a moving vehicle
Falls from >15 feet
Extrication time >20 minutes
Passenger cabin invaded >12 inches
Death of another passenger
Accident in a hostile environment (heat, cold water, etc.)

Anatomic injuries
Combined system injury
Penetrating injury of the groin or neck
Three or more long bone fractures
Fractures of the axial skeleton
Amputation (other than digits)
Persistent hypotension
Severe head trauma
Maxillofacial or upper airway injury
CNS injury with prolonged loss of consciousness, posturing, or paralysis
Spinal cord injury with neurologic deficit
Unstable chest injury
Blunt or penetrating trauma to the chest or abdomen
Burns, flame, or inhalation

System considerations
Necessary service or specialist not available
No beds available
Need for pediatric ICU care
Multiple casualties
Family request
Paramedic judgment
Severity scores: Champion Trauma Score 12 or less; or Revised Trauma Score 11 or less; or Pediatric Trauma Score 8 or less

From Harris BH, Barlow BA, Ballantine TV, et al: American Pediatric Surgical Association principles of pediatric trauma care, *J Pediatr Surg* 27:423-426, 1992.

---

and resuscitation of the pediatric trauma victim. The fact that 80% of pediatric trauma deaths occur before admission to the hospital—and that EMS system personnel are called to assist in resuscitating most of them—suggests that reducing the toll of what has been called "the neglected disease of modern society" will require particular emphasis on improving the quality of pediatric prehospital care.[83-86] Several excellent teaching programs for prehospital providers have now been developed and are available for nationwide distribution, designed to meet the needs of a variety of environments, both urban and rural.[87-90] Fortunately, great strides have been made toward specific incorporation of protocols and equipment for pediatric trauma in prehospital emergency care systems nationwide during the last several years; more than 40 states now have active EMSC programs.

The fundamental philosophy of early pediatric trauma care is threefold:

1. Priority attention to the airway, breathing, and circulation.
2. Prompt recognition and treatment of immediately life-threatening chest injuries.
3. Rapid transport to definitive care, both from the field to the hospital, and from the emergency department to the intensive care unit or operating room.

The basic principles governing emergency management of the pediatric trauma victim therefore are no different than for the child who presents with respiratory, circulatory, or cardiopulmonary failure of any etiology. Typically, the multiply injured child presents with soft tissue obstruction of the upper airway and respiratory compromise due to closed head injury; however, if internal organ injuries have also occurred, the child may present in respiratory failure and shock, which must be treated expeditiously and simultaneously. Thus, together with the *Advanced Trauma Life Support Course* of the American College of Surgeons, a key development in pediatric trauma resuscitation has been the creation and dissemination of the *Pediatric Advanced Life Support Course* of the American Heart Association and American Academy of Pediatrics.[91,92] While this course does not focus exclusively on trauma-related issues, it does address the two major causes of preventable death in childhood trauma—respiratory failure and shock[93,94]; moreover, it presents a conceptual framework that reinforces the cognitive knowledge and psychomotor skills required to resuscitate the critically injured child and relates them specifically to pediatric trauma resuscitation.

The treatment paradigm on which these courses are based neither mandates nor encourages creation of a separate system for pediatric trauma care. On the contrary, the skills required to initiate resuscitation of the injured child are well within the range of any properly trained emergency medical technician, emergency physician, emergency nurse, or trauma surgeon; however, continuing education and training in pediatric trauma resuscitation are highly desirable for all medical professionals to maintain and improve these skills. Reliance on BLS techniques in the earliest phases of trauma resuscitation, particularly in the field, has repeatedly been found superior (in terms of outcome) to untimely provision of ALS modalities (other than definitive airway management in blunt trauma) in adults as well as children.[95-102] This has proved a hard lesson for many EMS systems, emergency physicians, and trauma surgeons in recent years, but underscores the axioms that (1) patients who present in decompensated or hypotensive shock, but without signs of external bleed-

Abbreviated Injury Scale

The Abbreviated Injury Scale (AIS) consists of a lengthy numerical series of precise injury descriptors unique to the various organs, organized by body system, and categorized by injury subtype and severity, the initial purpose of which was to allow vast amounts of motor vehicle–crash data to be analyzed by computer. Designed by the Committee on Injury Scaling of the American Association of Automotive Medicine, now called the Association for the Advancement of Automotive Medicine, the focus of the AIS, through its 1980 revision, was on blunt motor vehicle-related injuries; more recent revisions include specific codes for penetrating injuries as well. In its 1990 revision, each body injury is assigned a unique 7-digit "AIS code," where (1) the first digit represents one of nine general body regions (head, face, neck, thorax, abdomen and pelvic contents, spine, upper extremity, lower extremity and pelvic bones, unspecified); (2) the second digit refers to type of body structure injured; (3) the next two digits refer to the specific body structure injured, and the nature of the injury; (4) the next two digits (those to the left of the decimal point) refer to the type and degree of injury sustained by each region and structure, assigned in numerical succession; and (5) the last digit (to the right of the decimal point) refers to the severity of the injury (1 = minor, 2 = moderate, 3 = serious, 4 = severe, 5 = critical, 6 = virtually unsurvivable, 9 = unknown). The last digit to the right of the decimal point is called the "AIS score" and is used to calculate the Injury Severity Score. Conversion tables are available to translate ICD-9-CM codes into AIS codes and scores.

Example: Major Splenic Laceration: 544226.4

where 5 = body region (abdomen), 4 = subtype of injury (organ), 42 = structure injured (spleen), 26 = type and degree of injury (laceration more damaging than two others listed, less damaging than one other listed), and 4 = severity code (severe but not critical; usually not by itself immediately life-threatening).

Adapted from Association for the Advancement of Automotive Medicine: *The abbreviated injury scale — 1990 revision*, Des Plaines, Ill, 1990, Association for the Advancement of Automotive Medicine.

Injury Severity Score

The Injury Severity Score (ISS) attempts to assess the overall severity of a particular traumatic event by summing the squares of the highest AIS score (last digit severity code) from each of the three body regions with the highest AIS scores. The highest possible ISS is 75, based on the assumption that the patient who sustains critical injury (severity code = 5) to three body regions (sum of squares = 25 + 25 + 25 = 75) will not likely survive; any injury with a severity code of 6 in any body region automatically receives a score of 75.

Example: **Prior Unconsciousness, Spleen Laceration, Femur Fracture**

The AIS scores are 2, 4, and 3; thus the ISS is 4 + 16 + 9 = 29.

Adapted from Baker SP, O'Neill B, Haddon W, et al: *J Trauma* 14:187-196, 1974.

---

ing or tension pneumothorax, nearly always have life-threatening injuries requiring prompt and definitive surgical control of internal bleeding, and (2) volume replacement, however vigorous, cannot keep pace with uncontrolled hemorrhage.

Trauma scores are a vitally important tool in pediatric trauma care and serve three important functions: (1) field triage, (2) quality management, and (3) epidemiologic surveillance; however, to be useful, a score must be valid, reliable, and practical.[103] Anatomic scores (e.g., the Abbreviated Injury Scale [AIS][104] and Injury Severity Score [ISS][105]) are used primarily for quality management and epidemiologic surveillance (see boxes above) and can be translated from the ICD-9-CM[106] nature and etiology of disease codes (N- and E-codes). Physiologic scores (e.g.,

the Champion Trauma Score [TS][107] and Revised Trauma Score [RTS][108]) are more frequently used for field triage (see boxes on p. 38), but may be used with anatomic scores in combination (TRISS)[109] for purposes of quality management, particularly outcome analysis. Although each of these indices has been used in children, none has proved ideal; for this reason, two scores have been developed that attempt to combine the best features of each: the Modified Injury Severity Score (MISS) and the Pediatric Trauma Score (PTS), each of which has been prospectively validated.[110-114] Of the two, the PTS appears somewhat easier to use; thus while its advantages have not consistently proved decisive in relation to other scores,[115,116] it seems to encourage safer triage practices, is acceptable for field use, has proven useful in outcome analysis, and carries the endorsement of both the American Pediatric Surgical Association and the American College of Surgeons Committee on Trauma (see Chapter 19).[72,82]

Assuring high quality care is the most important reason for establishing an organized pediatric trauma system[117]; the key component is a regular case review conference in which all team members participate, focusing on a detailed evaluation of system and human error.[118] Trauma registries also constitute a unique and powerful tool for quality management, particularly if the data are population based and can be pooled into national or regional banks that allow results to be compared with those of comparable centers. The National Pediatric Trauma Registry, which focuses on long-term disability as well as short-term outcome, has been especially successful in this latter regard.[119] Since the aim of quality management is to improve the effectiveness of trauma care, use of objective criteria to identify preventable mortality and morbidity is helpful.[120] No consensus has yet emerged as to the ideal method, but the PTS, the MISS, the AIS, and TRISS analysis have all been used successfully in children for this purpose.[114,121-124] Whatever index is chosen, however, the quality management

Pediatric Trauma Score

	+2	+1	−1
Size (kg)	>20	10-20	<10
Airway	Normal	Maintained	Unmaintained
Systolic blood pressure (mm Hg)	>90	50-90	<50
Central nervous system	Awake	Obtunded	Coma
Open wound	None	Minor	Major
Skeletal trauma	None	Closed	Open-Multiple

From Tepas JJ, Mollitt DL, Talbert JL, et al: *J Pediatr Surg* 22:14-18, 1987.

Champion Trauma Score

Glasgow Coma Scale score	Systolic BP (mm Hg)	Respiratory rate (breaths/min)	Respiratory effort	Cap refill	Coded value
14-15					5
11-13	>89	10-24			4
8-10	70-89	25-34			3
5-7	50-69	>34		Normal	2
3-4	0-49	1-9	Normal	Delayed	1
	Pulse	None	Retractive	None	0

From Champion HR, Sacco WJ, Carnazzo AJ, et al: *Crit Care Med* 9:672-676, 1981.

Revised Trauma Score

Glasgow Coma Scale score	Systolic BP (mm Hg)	Respiratory rate (breaths/min)	Coded value
13-15	>89	10-29	4
9-12	76-89	>29	3
6-8	50-75	6-9	2
4-5	1-49	1-5	1
3	0	0	0

From Champion HR, Sacco WJ, Copes WS, et al: *J Trauma* 29:623-629, 1989.

process must take place within the context of the trauma system as a whole—the *first* priority of which must be to ensure that children who require pediatric prehospital, emergency medical, and trauma center care can get it whenever and wherever it is needed.

Optimal pediatric trauma care requires all the system elements (see box on p. 39) that comprise the trauma center with pediatric expertise; yet the *essential* element and driving force behind all successful pediatric trauma programs is an organized, dedicated but fully integrated Pediatric Trauma Service directed by a knowledgeable, committed surgeon who assumes personal responsibility for overseeing the quality of pediatric trauma care at the host institution and in the regional trauma system.[125] This surgeon need not be a pediatric surgeon but must have training and experience in pediatric trauma that is equal to the task[126-129], and must function in a hospital where appropriate pediatric emergency and critical care resources are in place and all other trauma center criteria have been met for optimal outcome to be achieved.[70-78] Unfortunately, given the relative scarcity both of pediatric surgeons interested in trauma and trauma surgeons interested in pediatrics, quality trauma care is still a luxury far too few of our nation's children currently enjoy.[130] All physicians caring for children therefore must become vigorous advocates for pediatric injury prevention, both primary and secondary, as well as prepare themselves as thoroughly as possible for the day when the life of a critically injured child lies in their hands.

Components of Trauma Center with Pediatric Expertise

Full-service general/children's hospital
Institutional commitment to pediatric trauma
Organized, integrated pediatric trauma service
Responsible surgeon director
Qualified, trained physicians and nurses
Dedicated pediatric ED/ICU areas
Properly equipped OR/ED/ICU facilities
Weekly case review conference
Active quality management program
Community outreach/injury prevention programs

References

Prehospital Care

1. Luten RC: Emergency medical services for children projects. In Luten RC and Foltin G, editors: *Pediatric resources for prehospital care*, ed 2, Elk Grove Village, Ill, 1990, American Academy of Pediatrics.
2. Shaperman J and Backer TE: Introduction. In *Emergency medical services for children innovation bank*, ed 3, Washington, DC, 1991, National Maternal and Child Health Clearinghouse.
3. History of emergency medical services for children. In Seidel JS and Henderson DP, editors: *Emergency medical services for children: a report to the nation*, Washington, DC, 1991. National Center for Education in Maternal and Child Health.

Historic Perspective

4. Boyd DR: The history of emergency medical services (EMS) systems in the United States of America. In Boyd DR, Edlich RF, Micik S, editors: *Systems approach to emergency medical care*, Norwalk, Conn, 1983, Appleton & Lange.
5. Mustalish A: Emergency medical services: twenty years of growth and development, *NY State J Med* 86;414, 1986.
6. Pantridge JF and Geddes JS: Cardiac arrest after myocardial infarction, *Lancet* 1:807, 1966.

What About the Children?

7. Seidel JS: EMS-C in urban and rural areas: the California experience. In Haller JA Jr, editor: *Emergency medical services for children: report of the ninety-seventh Ross conference on pediatric research*, Columbus, Ohio, 1989, Ross Laboratories.
8. Foltin G, Salomon M, Tunik M, et al: Developing prehospital advanced life support for children: the New York City experience, *Pediatr Emerg Care* 6:141, 1990.

Children are Different

9. Tsai A and Kallsen G: Epidemiology of pediatric prehospital care, *Ann Emerg Med* 16:284, 1987.
10. Seidel JS: The six T's of emergency medical services for children: triage, time, treatment, transportation, tertiary care, and training. In Barkin RM, editor: Pediatrics in the emergency medical services system, *Pediatr Emerg Care* 6:72, 1990.
11. Systems approach to care of ill and injured children. In Seidel JS and Henderson DP, editors: *Emergency medical services for children: a report to the nation*, Washington, DC, 1991, National Center for Education in Maternal and Child Health.
12. Applebaum D: Advanced prehospital care for pediatric emergencies, *Ann Emerg Med* 14:7, 1985.
13. Eisenberg M, Bergner L, Hallstrom A: Epidemiology of cardiac arrest and resuscitation in children, *Ann Emerg Med* 12:672, 1983.
14. Torphy DE, Minter MG, Thompson BM, et al: Cardiopulmonary arrest and resuscitation of children, *Am J Dis Child* 138:1099, 1984.
15. Orlowski JP: Cardiopulmonary resuscitation in infants and children, *Emerg Med Clin North Am* 1:3, 1983.

16. Lewis JK, Minter MG, Eshelman SK, et al: Outcome of pediatric resuscitation, *Ann Emerg Med* 5:297, 1983.
17. Ludwig S, Kettrick RG, Parker M: Pediatric cardiopulmonary resuscitation, *Clin Pediatr* (Phila) 23 (2) :71, 1984.
18. Zaritsky A, Nadkarni V, Getson P, et al: CPR in children, *Ann Emerg Med* 16:1107, 1987.
19. Eisenberg MS, Bergner L, Hallstrom A: Cardiac resuscitation for the community: importance of rapid provision and program planning, *JAMA* 241:1905, 1979.
20. Luten RC, Foltin G, Pons P: Access to optimal care. In Luten RC and Foltin G, editors: *Pediatric resources for prehospital care*, ed 2, Elk Grove Village, Ill, 1990, American Academy of Pediatrics.
21. Bushore M: Prehospital care for victims of submersion, *Pediatrics* 86:625, 1990.
22. Quan L, Wentz KR, Gore EJ, et al: Outcome and predictors of outcome in pediatric submersion victims receiving prehospital care in King County, Washington, *Pediatrics* 86:586, 1990.
23. Matlack ME: Current problems in the management of pediatric trauma. In Haller JA Jr, editor: *Emergency medical services for children: report on the ninety-seventh Ross conference on pediatric research*, Columbus, Ohio, 1989, Ross Laboratories.
24. Ramenofsky ML, Luterman A, Quindlen E, et al: Maximum survival in pediatric trauma: the ideal system, *J Trauma* 24:818, 1984.
25. Seidel JS, Hombein M, Yoshiyama K, et al: Emergency medical services and the pediatric patient: are the needs being met? *Pediatrics* 73:769, 1984.
26. Cooper A, Barlow B, Davidson L, et al: Epidemiology of pediatric trauma: importance of population-based statistics, *J Pediatr Surg* 27:149, 1989.
27. National Highway and Transportation Administration: *EMS services, program update*, March, 1989, Washington, DC.
28. Harris B: Creating pediatric trauma systems, *J Pediatr Surg* 24:149, 1989.
29. Harris BH and Schwaitzberg SD: Evolution of care of the injured child. In Nyhus L, editor: *Surgery annual*, Norwalk, Conn, 1988, Appleton & Lange.
30. Committee on Trauma, American College of Surgeons: Planning pediatric trauma care. In *Resources for optimal care of the injured patient*, Chicago, 1990, American College of Surgeons.
31. Shackford SR, Hollingworth-Friedlund P, Cooper GF, et al: The effect of regionalization upon the quality of trauma care as assessed by concurrent audit before and after the institution of a trauma system: a preliminary report, *J Trauma* 26:812, 1986.
32. Cales RH: Trauma mortality in Orange County: the effect of implementation of a regional trauma system, *Ann Emerg Med* 13:1, 1984.
33. Pollack MM, Alexander SR, Clarke N, et al: Improved outcome from tertiary pediatric intensive care: a statewide comparison of tertiary and nontertiary facilities, *Crit Care Med* 19:150, 1991.
34. Haller JA, Shorter N, Miller D, et al: Organization and function of a regional pediatric trauma center: does a system of management improve outcome? *J Trauma* 23:691, 1983.
35. Seidel JS: Emergency medical services and the pediatric patient: are the needs being met? II. Training and equipping emergency medical services providers for pediatric emergencies, *Pediatrics* 78:808, 1986.
36. Simon JE: Current problems in the management of pediatric trauma. In Haller JA Jr, editor: *Emergency medical services for children: report on the ninety-seventh Ross conference on pediatric research*, Columbus, Ohio, 1989, Ross Laboratories.
37. Education and training of professionals and the public. In Seidel JS and Henderson DP, editors: *Emergency medical services for children: a report to the nation*, Washington, DC, 1991, National Center for Education in Maternal and child Health.

Prehospital Care for Children

38. Foltin G, Tunik M, Kulberg, A, et al: EMT ventilation of infant mannequins: a comparison of mouth-to-mouth and bag-valve-mask techniques, *Ped Emerg Care* 4:295, 1988.
39. Foltin G, Tunik M, Cooper A, et al: Educational parameters necessary for successful pediatric intubation by paramedics, Unpublished data.
40. Henderson DP, Seidel JS, editors: EMSC Product Catalogue, 1995, National EMSC.

41. Luten RC: Educational overview. In Luten RC and Foltin G, editors: *Pediatric resources for prehospital care*, ed 2, Elk Grove Village, Ill, 1990, American Academy of Pediatrics.

42. Brownstein D: Educational courses for prehospital care. In Luten RC and Foltin G, editors: *Pediatric resources for prehospital care*, ed 2, Elk Grove Village, Ill, 1990, American Academy of Pediatrics.

43. *National emergency medical services education and practice blueprint*, National Registry of EMTs, Columbus, Ohio, 1993.

44. *EMS injury prevention curriculum* (in print).

Management

45. Luten RC, Foltin G, Pons P: Access to optimal care. In Luten RC and Foltin G, editors: *Pediatric resources for prehospital care*, ed 2, Elk Grove Village, Ill, 1990, American Academy of Pediatrics.

46. *Emergency medical services for children*, Institute of Medicine Report, Washington, DC, 1993, National Academy Press.

47. Dieckmann R: The EMS-EMSC continuum. In Dieckmann R, editor: *Pediatric emergency care systems: planning and management*, Baltimore, 1992, Williams & Wilkins.

48. American Academy of Pediatrics, Committee on Hospital Care: Guidelines for air and ground transportation of pediatric patients, *Pediatrics* 78:943, 1986.

49. US Department of Transportation, National Highway Safety Traffic Administration: *Ambulance design criteria*, Washington, DC, 1973, Committee on Ambulance Design Criteria and National Research Council.

50. US Department of Transportation and General Services Administration (GSA): *Federal specification—ambulance KKK-A-18221974, emergency medical care surface vehicle*, Washington, DC, 1974, GSA, Specifications and Consumer Information Distribution Section.

51. US Department of Transportation and General Services Administration (GSA): *Federal specification—ambulance KKK 1822-C, emergency medical care surface vehicle*, Washington, DC, 1988, GSA, Specifications and Consumer Information Distribution Section.

52. Weigand JV: Prehospital ground transportation: system structure and requirements. In Roush WR, editor: *Principles of EMS systems*, Dallas, 1989, American College of Emergency Physicians.

53. US Department of Transportation, National Highway Traffic Safety Administration and the American Medical Association Commission of EMS: *Air ambulance guidelines*, ed 2, Washington, DC, The Administration and The Association.

54. American Society of Hospital Based Emergency Aeromedical Services (ASHBEAMS): *Interim safety guidelines*, 1987, California.

55. Task force on interhospital transport: *Guidelines for air and ground transport of neonatal and pediatric patients*, Elk Grove Village, Ill, 1993, American Academy of Pediatrics.

56. Pediatric Interhospital Critical Care Transport: *Consensus of a national leadership conference*, Sun Valley, Idaho, March, 1990.

The Medical Home, Prevention, and System Access

57. Division of Injury Control, CDC: Childhood injuries in the United States, *Am J Dis Child* 144:627, 1990.

58. Injury Prevention: strategies for change. In Seidel JS and Henderson DP, editors: *Emergency medical services for children: a report to the nation*, Washington, DC, 1991, National Center for Education in Maternal and Child Health.

59. Losek JD, Hennes H, Glaeser P, et al: Prehospital care of the pulseless, nonbreathing pediatric patient, *Am J Emerg Med* 5:270, 1987.

60. Sia C: The medical home: closing the circle of care. In Seidel JS and Henderson DP, editors: *Emergency medical services for children: a report to the nation*, Washington, DC, 1991, National Center for Education in Maternal and Child Health.

61. *Clawson JJ*: Emergency medical dispatching. In Roush WR, editor: *Principles of EMS systems*, Dallas, 1989, American College of Emergency Physicians.

62. Pon S, Foltin G, Tunik M, et al: Utilization of prehospital care by pediatric patients in New York City, *Pediatr Emerg Care* 5:286, 1989 (abstract).

Future Directions

63. Trauma Care Systems Planning and Development Act of 1990, House of Representatives, 101st Congress, PL-101-59070.

64. Rivara FP, Maier RV, Mueller BA, et al: Evaluation of potentially preventable deaths among pedestrian and bicycle fatalities, *JAMA* 261(4):566, 1989.

65. Seigler RS, Teldenburg FW, Shealy R: Prehospital intraosseous infusion by emergency service personnel: a prospective study, *Pediatrics* 84:173, 1989.

66. Smith Rj, Keseg DP, Manley LK, et al: Intraosseous infusion by prehospital personnel in critically ill pediatric patients, *Ann Emerg Med* 17:491, 1988.

67. Miner WF, Comeli HM, Bolte RC, et al: Prehospital use of intraosseous infusion by paramedics, *Pediatr Emerg Care* 5:5, 1989.

68. Zaritsky A, Nadkari V, Hazinski MF, et al: Recommended guidelines for uniform reporting of pediatric advanced life support: the pediatric utstein style. *Ann Emerg Med* 487-503, 1995.

69. AMA commission on EMS: Pediatric emergencies (excerpt from guidelines for categorization of hospital emergency capabilities), *JAMA* 85:879, 1990.

70. Committee on pediatric emergency medicine: Guidelines for emergency care facilities, *Pediatrics* 96:526, 1995.

The Pediatric Trauma System

71. Haller JA: Emergency medical services for children: what is the pediatric surgeon's role? *Pediatrics* 79:576-581, 1987.

72. Harris BH, Barlow BA, Ballantine TV, et al: American Pediatric Surgical Association: principles of pediatric trauma care, *J Pediatr Surg* 27:423-426, 1992.

73. Haller JA: Toward a comprehensive emergency medical system for children, *Pediatrics* 86:120-122, 1990.

74. Pollack MM, Alexander SR, Clarke N, et al: Improved outcomes from tertiary center pediatric intensive care: a statewide comparison of tertiary and nontertiary facilities, *Crit Care Med* 19:150-159, 1991.

75. Nakayama DK, Copes WS, Sacco W: Differences in trauma care among pediatric and nonpediatric trauma centers, *J Pediatr Surg* 27:427-431, 1992.

76. Hall JR, Reyes HM, Meller JL, et al: Traumatic death in urban children, revisited, *Am J Dis Child* 147:102-107, 1993.

77. Cooper A, Barlow B, DiScala C, et al: Efficacy of pediatric trauma care: results of a population-based study, *J Pediatr Surg* 28:299-305, 1993.

78. Cooper A, Barlow B, DiScala C, et al: *The pediatric trauma patient in the adult trauma system: results of a population-based study*, Tripartite Meeting of the New York Surgical Society, the Philadelphia Academy of Surgery, and the Boston Surgical Society, New York, 1993, The Society.

79. Ramenofsky ML and Morse TS: Standards of care for the critically injured pediatric patient, *J Trauma* 22:921-933, 1982.

80. Harris BH: Creating pediatric trauma systems, *J Pediatr Surg* 24:149-152, 1989.

81. Ramenofsky ML: Emergency medical services for children and pediatric trauma system components, *J Pediatr Surg* 24:153-155, 1989.

82. Anonymous: Pediatric trauma care. In American College of Surgeons Committee on Trauma: *Resources for optimal care of the injured patient: 1993*, Chicago, 1993, American College of Surgeons.

83. Cooper A, Barlow B, Davidson L, et al: Epidemiology of pediatric trauma: importance of population-based statistics, *J Pediatr Surg* 27: 149-154, 1992.

84. Gausche M, Seidel JS, Henderson DP, et al: Pediatric deaths and emergency medical services (EMS) in urban and rural areas, *Pediatr Emerg Care* 5:158-162, 1989.

85. National Academy of Sciences: Accidental death and disability: the neglected disease of modern society, Washington, DC, 1966, *the Academy.*

86. Institute of Medicine, National Academy of Sciences: Emergency medicine services for children, Washington, DC, 1993, The Academy.

87. Eichelberger MR and Stossel-Pratsch G: *Pediatric emergencies*, Englewood Cliffs, NJ, 1992, Brady.

88. Brownstein D, Monaghan S, Bennett R, editors: *Pediatric prehospital care*, Seattle, 1989, Washington State Emergency Medical Services for Children.

89. Elling R and Cooper A, editors: *Pre-hospital pediatric care course student manual*, Albany, 1991, New York State Department of Health.

90. Foltin G, Tunik M, Cooper A, et al, editors: *Teaching resource for instructors of prehospital pediatrics*, Arlington, Va, 1996, National Center for Education in Maternal and Child Health.

91. American College of Surgeons Committee on Trauma: *Advanced trauma life support course for physicians 1993 student manual*, Chicago, 1993, The College.

92. American Heart Association and American Academy of Pediatrics: *Textbook of pediatric advanced life support*, Dallas, 1994, The Association.

93. McKoy C and Bell MJ: Preventable traumatic deaths in children, *J Pediatr Surg* 18:505-508, 1983.

94. Dykes EH, Spence LJ, Young JG, et al: Preventable pediatric trauma deaths in a metropolitan region, *J Pediatr Surg* 24:107-111, 1989.

95. Border JR, Lewis FR, Aprahamian C, et al: Prehospital trauma care—stabilization or scoop and run, *J Trauma* 23:708-711, 1983.

96. Smith JP, Bodai BI, Hill AS, et al: Prehospital stabilization of critically injured patients: a failed concept, *J Trauma* 25:65-70, 1985.

97. Pons P, Honigman B, Moore EE, et al: Prehospital advanced trauma life support for critical penetrating wounds to the thorax and abdomen, *J Trauma* 25:825-832, 1985.

98. Lewis FR: Prehospital intravenous fluid therapy: physiologic computer modeling, *J Trauma* 26:804-811, 1986.

99. Pepe PE, Wyatt CH, Bickell WH, et al: The relationship between total prehospital time and outcome in hypotensive victims of penetrating injuries, *Ann Emerg Med* 16:293-297, 1987.

100. Martin RM, Bickell W, Pepe PE, et al: Prospective evaluation of preoperative fluid resuscitation in hypotensive patients with penetrating truncal injury: a preliminary report, *J Trauma* 33:354-362, 1992.

101. Bickel WH, Wall MJ, Pepe PE, et al: Immediate versus delayed fluid resuscitation for hypotensive patients with penetrating torso injuries, *N Engl J Med* 331:1105-1109, 1994.

102. Ramenofsky ML, Luterman A, Curreri PW, et al: EMS for pediatrics: optimum treatment or unnecessary delay? *J Pediatr Surg* 18:498-504, 1983.

103. Wesson DE, Spence LJ, Williams JI, et al: Injury scoring systems in children, *Can J Surg* 30:398-400, 1987.

104. Association for the Advancement of Automotive Medicine: The abbreviated injury scale—1990 revision, Des Plaines, Ill, 1990, The Association.

105. Baker SP, O'Neill B, Haddon W, et al: The injury severity score: a method for describing patients with multiple injuries and evaluating emergency care, *J Trauma* 14:187-196, 1974.

106. U.S. Department of Health and Human Services: *International classification of diseases*, rev 9, Clinical Modification, ed 5, vol 1-3, Washington, DC, 1995, U.S. Department of Health and Human Services.

107. Champion HR, Sacco WJ, Carnazzo AJ, et al: Trauma score, *Crit Care Med* 9:672-676, 1981.

108. Champion HR, Sacco WJ, Copes WS, et al: A revision of the trauma score, *J Trauma* 29:623-629, 1989.

109. Boyd CR, Tolson MA, Copes WS: Evaluating trauma care: the TRISS method, *J Trauma* 27:370-378, 1987.

110. Mayer T, Matlak ME, Johnson DG, et al: The modified injury severity scale in pediatric multiple trauma patients, *J Pediatr Surg* 15:719-726, 1980.

111. Mayer T, Walker ML, Clarke P: Further experience with the modified injury severity score, *J Trauma* 24:31-34, 1984.

112. Tepas JJ, Mollitt DL, Talbert JL, et al: The pediatric trauma score as a predictor of injury severity in the injured child, *J Pediatr Surg* 22:14-18, 1987.

113. Tepas JJ, Ramenofsky ML, Mollitt DL, et al: The pediatric trauma score as a predictor of injury severity: an objective assessment, *J Trauma* 28:425-429, 1988.

114. Ramenofsky ML, Ramenofsky MB, Jurkovich GJ, et al: The predictive validity of the pediatric trauma score, *J Trauma* 28:1038-1042, 1988.

115. Kaufmann CR, Maier RM, Rivara RP, et al: Evaluation of the pediatric trauma score, *JAMA* 263:69-72, 1990.

116. Nayduch DA, Moylan J, Rutledge R, et al: Comparison of the ability of adult and pediatric trauma scores to predict pediatric outcome following major trauma, *J Trauma* 31:452-458, 1991.

117. Nakayama DK, Saitz EW, Gardner MJ, et al: Quality assessment in the pediatric trauma care system, *J Pediatr Surg* 24:159-162, 1989.

118. Ramenofsky ML, Luterman A, Quindlen E, et al: Maximum survival in pediatric trauma: the ideal system, *J Trauma* 24:818-823, 1984.

119. Tepas JJ, Ramenofsky ML, Barlow B, et al: National pediatric trauma registry, *J Pediatr Surg* 24:156-158, 1989.

120. Wesson DE, Williams JI, Salmi LR, et al: Evaluating a pediatric trauma program: effectiveness versus preventable death rate, *J Trauma* 28:1226-1231, 1988.

121. Zordludemir U, Ergoren Y, Yucesan S, et al: Mortality due to trauma in childhood, *J Trauma* 28:669-671, 1988.

122. Dykes EJ, Spence LJ, Bohn DJ, et al: Evaluation of pediatric trauma care in Ontario, *J Trauma* 29:724-729, 1989.

123. Eichelberger MR, Mangubat EA, Sacco WS, et al: Comparative outcomes of children and adults suffering blunt trauma, *J Trauma* 28:430-434, 1988.

124. Eichelberger MR, Mangubat EA, Sacco WJ, et al: Outcome analysis of blunt injury in children, *J Trauma* 28:1109-1117, 1988.

125. Cooper A, Barlow B: The surgeon and emergency medical services for children, *Pediatrics* 96:184-188, 1996.

126. Knudson MM, Shagoury C, Lewis FR: Can adult trauma surgeons care for injured children? *J Trauma* 32:729-739, 1992.

127. Fortune JB, Sanchez J, Graca L, et al: A pediatric trauma center without a pediatric surgeon: a four-year outcome analysis, *J Trauma* 33:130-139, 1992.

128. Rhodes M, Smith S, Boorse D: Pediatric trauma patients in an "adult" trauma center, *J Trauma* 35:384-393, 1993.

129. Bensard DD, McIntyre RC, Moore EE, et al: A critical analysis of acutely injured children managed in an adult level I trauma center, *J Pediatr Surg* 29:11-18, 1994.

130. Harris BH: Summary of the 1988 American Pediatric Surgical Association Trauma Committee questionnaire, personal communication, May 1989.

5

Interhospital Transport

Karin A. McCloskey • *Richard A. Orr*

IMPORTANCE OF APPROPRIATE INTERHOSPITAL TRANSPORT

Pediatric interhospital transport has become increasingly important because of sophistication and regionalization of pediatric tertiary care centers, especially pediatric intensive care units (PICU). Children with illnesses or injuries that were previously devastating can now often be saved by increasingly sophisticated interventions. However, most children do not become ill or injured close to a pediatric referral center; they are often many miles and hours away. The care received during initial prehospital and hospital stabilization and resuscitation and during interhospital transport has a tremendous impact on the ultimate outcome and the ability of a PICU to fulfill its potential.

The practical aspects of ensuring appropriate interhospital transport of the pediatric patient must be considered when planning a comprehensive EMS system. Because transport for a mild-to-moderate illness or injury is less complicated, issues in transport of the critically ill child are emphasized.

ADVANCE PREPARATION

The efficiency of interhospital transport can be improved by developing a plan of action before a patient actually needs to be transported. A list of receiving hospitals and the phone numbers should be attached to the emergency department telephone or should be posted nearby. Even if all children are transferred to the same hospital, at least one backup number should be provided in case a tertiary care center is at capacity. If transport services are not provided by the hospitals listed, the referral list should include contacts for transport systems with pediatric capabilities.

Pediatric code cards should be easily accessible, either in a crash cart or posted on a wall (not inside a drawer with other documents). A pediatric resuscitation equipment pack or a room containing such equipment should be prepared in advance. If local ambulance services might be used for interhospital transport, appropriately sized equipment must be available for pediatric patients. Pediatric Advanced Life Support (PALS) training for EMTs is an excellent part of advance preparation for pediatric transport.

If a local ambulance with an accompanying nurse or physician from the referring hospital may be utilized, equipment lists and management protocols should be established in advance. While preparing for transport of a critically ill child, for instance, an accompanying physician anticipating possible intubation may need ET tubes and a laryngoscope, as well as tape, Benzoin, extra batteries and bulbs, a stylet, suction equipment and catheters, and a nasogastric (NG) tube. Nurses accompanying a patient on transport should not be expected to perform interventions they would not perform unsupervised in the hospital.

Administrative issues must also be considered. Predetermined protocols or contracts between the two hospitals should address transport payment for unfunded patients. If a patient must be transferred out of state because of proximity of tertiary care or lack of in-state facilities, administrative considerations may arise related to consent, licensure of transport personnel, and insurance. If the receiving hospital does not provide a transport team, logistic and financial arrangements may be needed for use of a third hospital's transport team.

The American Academy of Pediatrics (AAP) manual entitled *Emergency Medical Services for Children: The Role of the Primary Care Provider* provides detailed information on transport issues for the practitioner.[1]

MODE OF TRANSPORT

Options for interhospital transport include transfer via private automobile, local ambulance with or without additional hospital personnel, all-age (usually adult oriented) critical care transport teams, and specialized (i.e., neonatal, pediatric, and cardiac) transport teams. All alternatives may not be available. Very stable patients with negligible potential for deterioration during transport can be easily and inexpensively transferred via car or ambulance. Most ambulance systems are designed for initial stabilization and transfer to the nearest hospital, not for long-distance transport of hospital-stabilized patients. Furthermore, the scientific literature and common anecdotal experience indicate that many ambulance personnel are not trained, experienced, or comfortable in the management of the critically ill child.[2-5]

If an all-age transport team, usually traveling by helicopter, is to be considered, several factors must be taken into account. First, many of these teams are designed for the transport of the adult cardiac or trauma patient; often the team's base hospital may itself refer critically ill children to other centers. Team training and ongoing experience in the care of pediatric patients may be limited. In other cases, team members may be quite proficient and experienced in taking care of children. Advance investigation can clarify this issue and determine the need for provision of alternate options. In addition, it is difficult to perform some procedures in the helicopter (i.e., replacement of ET tubes or IV lines) when an adult is the patient; it is virtually impossible when small children are involved.

A specialized pediatric team is sometimes the best choice to care for critically ill children, even when it takes slightly longer to arrive than an all-age helicopter team. Many pediatric teams have access to helicopter transport, and many do not choose to use it. However, for the critically ill pediatric patient, the level of care during the relatively unstable transport time should be the major concern. A referring hospital uncomfortable with management of a sick child can maintain contact with the receiving hospital for any questions related to care, as well as provide access to the laboratory (blood gas levels), radiology (chest x-ray) studies, and anesthesiology or surgery (for airway maintenance) services. A transport team inexperienced with a sick child has access to none of those resources. It is tempting to think that everyone can breathe easier once the child leaves the emergency department, but that may not be in the best interest of the patient. Except for certain victims of multiple trauma, there is no evidence that speed of transfer, without regard for the level of care in transit, is beneficial to the critically ill pediatric patient.

In addition to experience in the care of children, dedicated pediatric and neonatal teams routinely carry a full range of sizes of equipment and medications for pediatric patients. Monitors are specifically designed to work on small patients. Continuity of care is also improved over the situation in which a patient is transferred from one hospital to another by a team from a third hospital.

No widely accepted standards exist at this time to determine when a critical-care transport team, or a physician on that team, is needed for an individual patient.[6-8] The Pediatric Risk of Mortality (PRISM) score does not predict the need for a team.[8] One study has shown that patients who are intubated at the time of the initial referral or who have unstable vital signs, especially if under 1 year of age, will probably need major procedures or high-level pharmacologic intervention during transport.[9] Orr showed that four simple pretransport variables (blood pressure, respiratory rate, level of consciousness, and oxygen requirement) accurately predicted in-hospital mortality.[10] In addition, major interventions performed by the transport team increased with the probability of in-hospital mortality. Several hospitals use some form of patient status classification system in deciding team use or team composition.

Until more specific data are available, reasonable criteria for use of a critical care transport team include:

1. Any patient with anticipated ICU admission on arrival at the receiving hospital. (If the patient needs that level of care on arrival, it is likely that he or she will also need it during transfer.)
2. Any patient with a potential for significant respiratory or neurologic deterioration (e.g., asthma, croup, or altered mental status) during the anticipated time of transport.
3. Any patient resuscitated from a life-threatening event that may recur (i.e., seizure with apnea or respiratory or cardiac arrest).

PREPARING FOR THE TRANSPORT TEAM

After the transport decision has been made and a team is on the way, the referring hospital should continue active management of the patient's condition. Emergent interventions should be performed and not deferred for arrival of the team.

There are several actions the referring hospital can take to expedite transition of care to the transport team. The patient's parents can be asked to sign a consent to transport, specifying the receiving hospital and the mode of transport. Many pediatric teams ask that the parents stay at the referring hospital to personally sign a consent and provide additional patient information. Copies of all hospital records and x-ray studies can be prepared in advance; phone numbers to call for pending laboratory results should be noted. If blood products might be needed during transfer, they can be ordered before the team's arrival. IV lines and tubes can be additionally secured for transport because the taping job suitable for a patient lying on a stretcher may not be adequate for one being moved. Transport teams should be able to replace lines and tubes if needed; however, they prefer not to have to in a moving vehicle. The spine and any fractures should be stabilized before the team's arrival.

These actions can reduce the time the transport team spends preparing for departure. After the team arrives, additional help is welcomed when referring hospital staff offer to assist the team in navigating the environment of an unfamiliar hospital. However, the team will usually be able to function independently, without tying up critical emergency department personnel.

COMMUNICATIONS

Communication in both directions between the referring and receiving hospitals is essential in facilitating patient transfers. Both hospitals should keep written records of information and recommendations exchanged.

The referring hospital is responsible for providing reasonable information needed to offer stabilization advice and to make a decision about the optimal mode of transport. Personnel should be able to provide updates on the patient's condition. They are responsible for written communication in the form of complete medical records detailing the patient's condition and care before transfer. The referring hospital is responsible for choosing a mode of transport that will at least maintain the level of care available before and during transfer, as well as defining a receiving hospital that can properly care for the patient's condition.[11,12] Appropriate personnel should be available to the transport team to answer questions. If problems occur with a transport team, the team's medical director should be notified so that similar problems can be avoided in the future.

The receiving hospital is responsible for providing timely access via telephone for stabilization advice and notification of availability (or lack thereof) of a bed or a transport team for the patient. A physician should remain easily accessible for advice about ongoing management. An equally important part of the communication process is posttransport follow-up.

When the receiving hospital's transport team is used, it must be mobilized within a reasonable period of time. If that is not possible (e.g., because of weather conditions or multiple simultaneous transport requests), the team is responsible for notifying the referring hospital of the anticipated delay. The team should provide a self-contained mobile intensive care environment, with personnel experienced in handling complications of the patient's condition or treatment. When the team arrives at the referring hospital, it is expected to assume primary responsibility for the patient's care.

Communication between multiple hospital personnel based in different environments during a crisis is difficult and stressful. The referring hospital cannot always follow every recommendation of the receiving hospital; the receiving physician cannot always give optimal advice without seeing the patient, and transport teams cannot arrive immediately and depart within minutes. It is important to try to maintain open communications while keeping the best interests of the patient in mind.

TRANSPORT GUIDELINES

In 1993, the AAP published a manual on *Guidelines for Air and Ground Transport of Neonatal and Pediatric Patients.* This document addressed organization of a pediatric interfacility transport service, communications in the dispatch center, administrative issues, transport system personnel, team composition and training, quality improvement, safety, vehicles, equipment and medications, outreach education, the transport system database, and air medical physiology. The guidelines were specifically written for any team transporting children, not just for dedicated pediatric teams. Personnel criteria focus on training and experience in pediatric transport rather than on educational degrees of team members. Skills defined in detail as necessary for pediatric transport include cognitive skills, procedural skills, communication skills, and "other" (physical stamina, personality characteristics, and so on) skills.[13]

The Commission on Accreditation of Air Medical Services (CAAMS) was established in 1991 as an independent board with representation from a variety of medical organizations whose members are involved in air medical transport. CAAMS developed a rigorous voluntary accreditation process to set a basic quality standard of care for air transport systems. As of January, 1996, 36 programs have been accredited through this process, which could ultimately lead to improved care for patients of all ages.

LEGAL ISSUES

Legal responsibilities during patient transfer operate on a continuum, with increasing involvement in the patient's care meaning greater responsibility. At most intermediate points of the continuum, both the referring and receiving hospitals share some level of responsibility.

Clearly all responsibility lies with the referring hospital until a second center is contacted. Likewise, virtually full responsibility shifts to the receiving hospital after the patient arrives there. However, under the Omnibus Reconciliation Act (OBRA), the referring hospital is considered responsible for the medical integrity of the receiving hospital.[11,12] The intermediate points are less clearly defined. The Joint Commission for the Accreditation of Healthcare Organizations (JCAHO) mandates that "a hospital is capable of instituting essential lifesaving measures and implementing emergency procedures that will minimize further compromise of the condition of any infant, child or adult being transported."[14] Hospitals that choose to examine and treat all patients with critical conditions should follow standard pediatric resuscitation guidelines and be equipped to provide intensive care for several hours, if necessary, until specialized transport services are available.[15,16]

When the receiving hospital offers solicited advice, it bears responsibility for that advice. The referring hospital is obligated to carry out the advice to the best of its ability or to document sound reasons for not doing so. The referring hospital is primarily responsible for the choice of a mode of transport, although in agreeing with that choice the receiving hospital shares some responsibility. For that reason, the receiving physician may attempt to change the mode of transport if he or she considers it dangerous. If unable to influence the mode of transport, the receiving physician should document the details of the attempt.

When a transport team from the receiving hospital assumes care of the patient, primary responsibility shifts to that hospital. Any major conflicts in patient care arising before the team's physical departure from the referring hospital should be resolved at the attending physician level when possible. If a transport team from a third hospital (neither the referring nor the receiving hospital) is used, assignment of responsibility can be difficult. Generally the hospital with primary control over the patient's care at a given time will carry the most responsibility. Any advice given or received in this situation should be especially well documented.

Pediatric transport provides the potential for rapid referral to pediatric tertiary care centers. Preparation and planning must facilitate rapid and appropriate response that reflects the child's clinical needs. A carefully planned, high quality transport continuum has the potential for tremendous impact on long-term morbidity and mortality.

References

Advance Preparation

1. The American Academy of Pediatric Committee on Pediatric Emergency Medicine: *Emergency medical services for children: the role of the primary care provider,* Elk Grove Village, Ill, 1992, The Academy.

Mode of Transport

2. Aijian P, Tsai A, Knopp R, et al: Endotracheal intubation of pediatric patients by paramedics, *Ann Emerg Med* 18(5):489, 1989.
3. Seidel JS: A needs assessment of advanced life support and emergency medical services in pediatric patient: state of the art, *Circulation* 74:IV, 1986.
4. Seidel JS: Emergency medical services and the pediatric patient: are the needs being met? II. Training and equipping emergency medical services providers for pediatric emergencies, *Pediatrics* 78:808, 1986.
5. Seidel JS, Hornbein M, Yoshiyama K: Emergency medical services and the pediatric patient: are the needs being met? *Pediatrics* 73(6):769, 1984.
6. Kissoon N, Frewen TC, Kronick JB, et al: The child requiring transport: lessons and implications for the pediatric emergency physician, *Pediatr Emerg Care* 4:1, 1988.
7. McCloskey K, King WD, Byron L: Pediatric critical care transport: is a physician always needed on the team? *Ann Emerg Med* 18:247, 1989.
8. Orr R, Venkataraman S, Cinoman M, Hogue B, Singleton C, McCloskey K: Pretransport pediatric risk of mortality (PRISM) score underestimates the requirement for intensive care or major interventions during interhospital transport, *Crit Care Med* 22:1:101-107, 1994.
9. McCloskey K, Faries G, King W, et al: Variables predicting the need for major interventions during pediatric critical care transport, *Pediatr Emerg Care* 8:1, 1992.

10. Orr R, Vemlataraman S, McCloskey K, Brandestein M, Janosky J: Four simple pretransport variables accurately predict inhospital mortality, *Crit Care Med* 23:224, 1995.

Communications

11. *Omnibus Budget Reconciliation Act of 1989.* Sec., 6018 42 USC and 1395cc (West Supp. 1990).
12. Omnibus Reconciliation Act of 1980: *Medicare and Medicaid related provisions, summary and analysis,* Camp Hill, Penn, 1981, Hospital Association of Pennsylvania.

Transport Guidelines

13. Guidelines for Air and Grounds Transport of Neonatal and pediatric patients: *American Academy of Pediatrics Task Force on Interhospital transport,* Elkgrove Village, Ill, 1993, The Academy.

Legal Issues

14. Joint Commission for the Accreditation of Healthcare Organizations: *Accreditation manual for hospitals,* Chicago, 1986, The Commission.
15. Orr RA and McCloskey KA: Mobilizing critical care for interhospital and intrahospital transport. In Lumb PD, Shoemaker WC, editors: *Critical care: state of the art,* Fullerton, Calif, 1990, Society of Critical Care Medicine.
16. George JE: General legal principles. In *Law and emergency care,* St Louis, 1980, Mosby–Year Book.

## 6

Emergency Department and Intensive Care Unit Interface

Edward E. Conway Jr.

The overall goal of pediatric emergency medicine training is to produce an individual who is clinically proficient in the practice of pediatric emergency medicine, with emphasis on the acutely ill and injured child; who is competent in teaching pediatric emergency medicine; who is experienced in research; and who is familiar with administrative issues.[1] As the specialty has grown, standards have been established. The Pediatric Emergency Medicine Curriculum Subcommittee of the American Academy of Pediatrics has recently revised its curriculum statement.[1] The current fellowship training period is 3 years for those who have completed pediatric training and 2 years for those trained in adult emergency medicine.[2] In addition, there is a board-sanctioned certification examination in pediatric emergency medicine.

Pediatric critical care is another relatively new subspecialty, also with established standards and a board-sanctioned certification examination. The overall goal of training in pediatric critical care medicine is to produce an individual who demonstrates competence in the practice of pediatric critical care medicine with a particular emphasis on the critically ill infant and child, the ability to teach this knowledge to others, proficiency in performing and interpreting research, and a familiarity with administrative issues.

While each of these subspecialties embodies its own core of knowledge, a thorough understanding of general pediatrics is essential to success in either field; tremendous overlap exists.[1,3] The underlying tenet of both subspecialties is the recognition, stabilization, and management of the critically ill or injured infant, child, or adolescent. Practitioners in both fields must recognize and understand the pathophysiology, management, and outcome of organ system disorders that include cardiovascular, pulmonary, cardiopulmonary and central nervous system resuscitation, trauma, as well as infectious disease, neurologic and neurosurgical, hematology, oncology, metabolic and endocrine, renal, gastrointestinal, and toxicology problems. These practitioners should also understand the pharmacology, actions, indications, utilization, complications, and contraindications of current pharmacologic agents used in the management of critically ill pediatric patients.

Emergency physicians and critical care practitioners share many of the same daily frustrations.[4] The intensivist must balance the need for beds (from the emergency department, hospital units, outside referrals, and surgery) against bed availability. The emergency physician must

triage patients with less severe complaints, to wait at times for a protracted period for an actual physical site in which to be evaluated.[5] There is little published data concerning the amount of time pediatric patients requiring critical care spend in the emergency department. One published adult study found the mean emergency department length of stay for critically ill patients was 145 minutes, with a maximum length of stay of 655 minutes.[5] Another adult study found that 4.1% of all emergency patients were critically ill (defined as those who needed to be admitted directly to the ICU or surgery, along with those who died in the emergency department), and their mean length of stay in the emergency department was 1.1 days.[6] Pediatric data suggest that the mean length of stay is most likely somewhere between these two extremes.

A review of admissions to a 14-bed Pediatric Critical Care Unit, which is University affiliated with a catchment area of over 1 million patients, during 1994 demonstrated that 251 of 650 total admissions (39%) originated in the emergency department (unpublished data, Conway, 1995). One hundred and fifteen of these patients (46%) required intubation and mechanical ventilation, 71 of these patients (66%) were under 5 years of age, and eight had tracheostomies. The major indications for intubation and mechanical ventilation were respiratory failure, status epilepticus, toxic ingestions, trauma, and cardiovascular instability.

Pediatric respiratory disorders account for a majority of pediatric emergency department visits and for approximately 20% to 30% of all pediatric hospitalizations. Respiratory failure is also the leading cause of admission to PICUs, accounting for almost 50% of the total admissions.[7] The infant and child are particularly vulnerable to respiratory failure and frequently require intubation and mechanical ventilation as demonstrated by these data. Therefore the emergency medicine physician should be familiar with the indications, complications, and techniques of both intubation and the initiation of mechanical ventilation. Rotations in pediatric critical care units are required in 38 of 56 pediatric emergency medicine fellowship programs (68%) and 13 of 56 require rotations in anesthesia (23%).[8]

The interface between the emergency department and the intensive care unit must be seamless and provide a mechanism to maintain ongoing support and intervention for the critically ill patient. Training programs must facilitate communication, sharing of expertise, and continuity of care.

References

1. Baker MD: Pediatric emergency medicine fellowship curriculum statement, *Pediatr Emerg Care* 9(1):60, 1993.
2. Seidel JS: Fellowship training in pediatric emergency medicine for graduates of emergency medicine residencies, *Pediatr Emerg Care* 11(2):72, 1995.
3. Task Force on Guidelines, Society of Critical Care Medicine: Guidelines for program content for fellowship training in critical care medicine, *Crit Care Med* 20(6):875, 1992.
4. Conn AT: Critical care in the emergency department: stress within the system, *Crit Care Med* 21(7):952, 1993.
5. Fromm RE et al: Critical care in the emergency department: a time-based study, *Crit Care Med* 21(7):970, 1993.
6. Mullner M, Sterz FR, Laggner AN: Critical care in the emergency department: Saving intensive care unit facilities, *Crit Care Med* 22(5):896, 1994.
7. Gregory GA: Respiratory failure in the child, *Clin Crit Care Med* 3:7, 1981.
8. Abramo TJ: Pediatric emergency medicine fellowship programs, *Pediatr Emerg Care* 11(2):133, 1995.

Pain Control, Analgesia, and Sedation

Thomas E. Terndrup • James D'Agostino

Reception and reaction to noxious or painful stimuli are beneficial in avoiding real or potential danger and essential to human learning and development. Although pain occurs daily, when pain is thought to be severe or prolonged, medical care is often sought. Recent estimates conclude that 40% or more of the world's population experiences *severe* pain each year, varying from several hours to weeks in duration.[1] Further, millions of patients throughout the world suffer repetitive, episodic, or daily from such chronic pain conditions as arthritis, migraine, malignancy, and low back pain. Emergency physicians and pediatricians must be constantly sensitive to painful conditions and consider active pain control measures, particularly in comatose, mentally challenged, and preverbal patients.

Assessment of pain is made especially difficult in children who may deny pain, fearing further medical intervention, particularly when confronted with an unknown practitioner in the emergency department. The presentation of painful conditions varies as a function of the child's development. Infants demonstrate pain reaction as a change in behavior, irritability, crying, inconsolableness, or fussiness.[2,3] Toddlers may describe pain quality in sensory (e.g., aching, hurting), affective (e.g., awful, killing), or evaluative

(e.g., uncontrollable, horrible) terms.[4] Overt pain in pediatric emergency department patients is commonly secondary to minor trauma and infections, parenteral injections, or procedural manipulation. Covert etiologies for pain in children must be vigorously evaluated during emergency department visits to reduce further suffering and mistaken diagnoses.

Patients with the same underlying pathophysiology may have widely divergent pain severity and medication requirements.[5,6] Children may appear in similar distress whether the diagnoses are life threatening or benign (e.g., the abdominal pain in intussusception vs. colic may produce similar behavioral changes). Observer-estimated severity and individually rated perception of pain is highly variable, making assessment and management decisions difficult.[7-9] Unless deeply comatose, patients with acute pain are almost always anxious, which heightens the perception of painful stimuli.[10,11] Anxiety may be a substantial part of every emergency department visit for children, even those without painful conditions.[2,3,12-14] Therefore it is important to control both pain and anxiety in these children.

Pain may be the most common reason for emergency department visits and is a frequent reason to seek medical care in any outpatient setting.[15,16] It may be the presenting sign of malignancy, particularly unexplained bone pain in children, and has been associated with otherwise unexplainable deaths in patients with sickle-cell vasocclusive crisis.[17-19] Pain as part of a generalized stress response produces a series of neurophysiologic changes that result in increased pituitary, adrenal, and pancreatic hormone activity that may disrupt protein and carbohydrate metabolism.[20] In addition, pain heightens the risk of cardiac dysrhythmias and impaired organ perfusion. Intense pain may lead to increased respiratory, thrombotic, cardiovascular, and immunologic complications.[1] Appropriate treatment reduces these complications and may improve outcome.[21-23]

Despite the importance of pain to overall health, there is still no instrument, test, or physiologic change by which we can objectively measure pain.[24] Yet we all know that pain exists, both by personal experience and observation of patient suffering. Despite recognition of the presence and importance of pain, numerous investigators have documented inadequate pain control in various environments in which children are treated. These sites include postoperative wards, neonatal intensive care units, medical wards, and emergency department settings.[6,22,25-30] There has been repeated documentation of a much lower rate of opioid and other potent analgesic use in children, in comparison with adult patients with the same diagnoses. The health-care community, nurses, physicians, and others caring for children must change their behavior in favor of satisfactory pain control, not in just achieving satisfactory complication rates.[31]

The specialties of emergency medicine and pediatrics have unique opportunities for teaching, education, and research in the area of pain evaluation and management.[9,32] Pediatricians and emergency physicians see a wide variety of patients with acute and chronic pain, creating an opportunity to teach ideal pain control methods and evaluate management strategies. Children in emergency departments who suffer from pain or require analgesia have been the subject of few systematic investigations, despite the fact that they represent 30% or more of the overall emergency patient population. Unfortunately, undertreatment of children's pain appears no less common in emergency departments than in other clinical settings.[25,29,30,33]

Beyond providing a perspective on pain control, analgesia, and sedation, several developments require special emphasis. Pain assessment methods in research studies have generally adopted validated tools, with an increased attention to developmentally appropriate scales. Pharmacologic advances have included several studies on the use of midazolam, fentanyl, ketamine, ketorolac, and topical anesthetics. Furthermore, monitoring standards for children undergoing sedation for procedures have been clarified.[34,35]

DEFINITIONS

Pain is defined by the International Association for the Study of Pain as "an unpleasant sensory and emotional experience associated with actual or potential tissue damage, or described in terms of such damage."[36] Pain-control measures include psychologic and medicinal techniques used to produce *analgesia* (i.e., to relieve or reduce nociception [pain perception]) and *sedation* (i.e., to induce a state of reduced awareness). Medications that act at opioid receptors are agonists if they reduce nociception, whereas opioid antagonists oppose the actions of opioids and reduce cardiorespiratory depression while enhancing nociception. Narcotics are analgesic agents that produce stupor, insensibility, or sound sleep, whereas *nonnarcotics* are analgesic agents without these side effects.[37,38]

Acute pain serves as a warning of a potential insult to organ function, facilitates the diagnosis of disease by its location and character, and is often associated with objective physical signs of sympathetic nervous system activation (i.e., tachycardia, increased arterial blood pressure, diaphoresis, and mydriasis). *Chronic pain* is a persistent or recurring pain associated with prolonged disease; it serves no useful purpose for the patient and is often associated with no objective signs of autonomic hyperactivity.[15,36] These patients often have sleep and appetite disturbances and somatic preoccupations.

PATHOPHYSIOLOGY

There are no specific pain sensation "organs," only free nerve endings and a plexiform network of afferent fibers in skin, adipose, fascia, and perivascular tissue.[11] Nerve fiber types carrying pain messages are large, myelinated A alpha fibers and small, unmyelinated C fibers.[11] Sharp, localized, so-called first pain is transmitted predominantly by A alpha fibers. These high-threshold mechanoreceptors cause well-localized discriminative sensation. Dull, diffuse pain messages are transmitted by C fibers when recruitment of nociceptors is sufficiently strong.[39] Thermal, chemical, mechanical, and electrical stimulation causes activation of both fibers through polymodal receptors.[8] Also, tissue injury releases various substances, including histamine, serotonin, and bradykinin, which can activate these fibers.[40] Substance P, a polypeptide, may be the major neurotransmitter in various polymodal nociceptors.[8]

Sensory fibers pass primarily from the dorsal root ganglia and synapse with ascending neurons in the dorsal spinal horn. Fibers that do not terminate in the spinal cord ascend as the ventrolateral funiculus or via the spinothalamic tract. Visceral sensation proceeds along the parasympathetic or sympathetic chains, while afferents converge on the same dorsal horn neurons at certain somatic areas, causing typical patterns of referred pain.[11]

The discovery of opiate receptors in the limbic and periaqueductal structures was instrumental in identifying the body's endogenous opioids, endorphins.[41] Endorphins, such as beta-endorphin, leucine enkephalin, and dynorphin, are 20 to 30 times more potent than morphine. At least four types of opiate receptors have been identified in the CNS.[11,20] The mu and delta receptors, primarily located in the cerebral cortex and limbus, cause respiratory depression, analgesia, euphoria, and physical dependence. Two mu receptors have been identified. The first, mu-1, is predominantly responsible for analgesic activity, whereas the other, mu-2, produces respiratory depression and physical dependence. The kappa receptor, located primarily in the spinal cord, causes spinal analgesia, mild sedation, and myosis. The sigma receptor induces hallucinations and dysphoria. The effects of various opioid drugs and neurotransmitters can be conceptualized by analysis of their agonist and antagonist activity at these receptors.[11,20]

Modulation of pain sensation occurs at three levels. At the spinal level, it occurs by intense activation of A fibers (by vibration, pressure, or electrical stimulation), which increases the threshold for sensibility through C fibers.[42] Endogenous and exogenous opioids act in the *midbrain* and medulla to increase the inhibitory output of neurons synapsing with enkephalin-containing interneurons that cause presynaptic inhibition of nociceptive neurons. Hypnosis, biofeedback, and other psychotherapies modulate *cortical influences* on pain perception.[8,11] In newborn rats, morphine produces much less analgesia but greater respiratory depression compared with 2-week-old rats.[43] This suggests that mu-2 receptors are more prevalent or sensitive than mu-1 receptors in newborn rats. Development of specific opioids that act preferentially at mu-1 receptors may enhance clinical practice by producing adequate analgesia and reducing the risk of respiratory depression, especially in children.

ASSESSMENT OF PAIN

Clinical pain is a complex, multifaceted experience in which subjective, behavioral, and physiologic responses

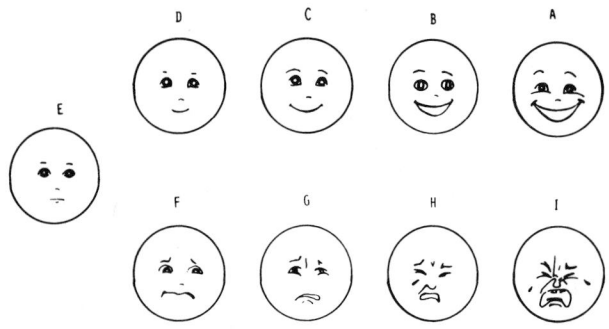

FIG. 7-1. The faces scale is scored by instructing the child to point to the face that best represents how he or she is currently feeling. This scale allows self-reporting by children 5 years and older. Face E is thought to represent a neutral pain affect. To assess treatment effects, a reduction in pain affect is associated with the selection of earlier alphabetical faces, while an increase in pain affect is associated with the selection of later alphabetical faces. *(From McGrath PA: Pain in children: nature, assessment and treatment, 1990, Guilford Publications.)*

of patients contribute to our assessment techniques.[24] The *subjective* component requires verbal and nonverbal input from the child. It is assessed using direct questions, self-rating scales, and derivatives of self-rating, such as pain drawings or projective tests.[44] The *behavioral* component assesses parameters thought to be related to pain severity (e.g., crying, brow furrowing, motor response), whereas *physiologic* measures are objective indexes of pain-related parameters (e.g., increase in heart rate, decrease in oxygen saturation).[24,45]

Several measurement tools have reliably allowed researchers to assess pain in adults and in children older than 7 years. These include the use of cognitive (i.e., self-reported; e.g., visual analogue scale [VAS], poker chip tool, and the faces [Fig. 7-1], Oucher, and thermometer scales) and behavioral scales (Children's Hospital of Eastern Ontario Pain Scale [CHEOPS])[46-50] (Table 7-1). Validation of these instruments has been performed in hospitalized patients or children undergoing repeated invasive procedures, such as bone marrow aspiration or lumbar puncture. Preliminary data from pediatric emergency department patients analyzing observer-rated global distress using VAS and CHEOPS scores appear encouraging, but await further validation studies before widespread use is appropriate.[9,51,52]

REASONS FOR INADEQUATE PAIN CONTROL

Many factors contribute to poor pain control by health professionals, including fear of inducing complications or masking diagnoses by opioids, inability to accurately and reproducibly measure pain, difficulty in interpreting treatment success or failure, failure to appreciate the existence or severity of pain, and a lack of standardized clinical teaching and textbook information about pain and its management. Young nurses and physicians are frequently reminded of the hazards of opioids and sedatives, and yet important therapeutic use may go unaddressed.[2,9,43,53]

In children, additional factors interfering with optimal pain management include improper dosage and administration of analgesics, special techniques required to assess pain in preverbal patients, fear of inducing opioid dependency, an erroneous perception that neonates and infants do not sense or remember pain, difficulty of achieving venous access, and the expectation that children cry during evaluation and treatment.[3,7,12,29,52] Rapidly following stabilization of vital signs and resuscitation, minimizing the suffering while children undergo various diagnostic and therapeutic procedures should be part of routine educational and health management practices.

Childhood pain management and research have only recently received attention, and the first comprehensive textbook on children's pain is only roughly 10 years old. Children's pain research has focused on the age of pain perception, the development of measurement or assessment scales, the psychologic management of pain, and the investigation of the efficacy and safety of medications.* Neonates perceive pain, have reduced distress when measures to reduce pain perception are undertaken, and have the neuroanatomic capacity to remember noxious stimuli.[22] Many pain assessment tools have been developed for use with toddlers and preverbal children, but their applicability in the emergency department is largely untested. Although children benefit from distraction and other psychologic techniques during repeated procedures (e.g., bone marrow aspiration), no investigation of these measures in acute, untrained emergency department children has been performed.[57,58] Many investigators have demonstrated inadequate pain control in hospitalized children.[6,22,25-29] Children with similar diagnoses and undergoing the same procedures are far less likely than adults to receive analgesia or sedation.[25,29,30]

DEVELOPMENTAL RESPONSE TO PAIN

Components of Pain

Clinical pain consists of three components: cognitive, behavioral, and physiologic.[49] Alternatively, pain may be conceptualized as the combined effect of the sensation of and reaction to a painful experience. Children's understanding of and response to pain depends on their developmental concepts of health and illness.[59] Childhood developmental levels of understanding and reaction to pain may be summarized by age (Table 7-2). Pain assessment and control in children must take these developmental stages into account. For example, infants are unable to localize pain and demonstrate a generalized stress response to painful stimuli. Toddlers can localize pain and often see illness as punishment for something they have said or done. Guided use of these facts for reassurance of the patient and family can improve psychologic management of pain in the emergency department.

Assessing the Efficacy of Treatment

Many methods have been suggested for age-dependent pain assessment. Infant assessment methods include behavioral scales (e.g., crying characteristics, body move-

* References 22, 24, 43, 44, 54-56.

TABLE 7-1. Behavioral Definitions and Scoring of CHEOPS*

Item	Behavior	Score	Definition
Cry	No cry	1	Child is not crying.
	Moaning	2	Child is moaning or quietly vocalizing, silent cry.
	Crying	2	Child is crying, but the cry is gentle or whimpering.
	Scream	3	Child is in a full-lunged cry; sobbing; may be score with complaint or without complaint.
Facial	Composed	1	Neutral facial expression.
	Grimace	2	Score only if definite negative facial expression.
	Smiling	0	Score only if definite positive facial expression.
Child verbal	None	1	Child not talking.
	Other complaints	1	Child complains, but not about pain (e.g., "I want to see mommy" or "I am thirsty").
	Pain complaints	2	Child complains about pain.
	Both complaints	2	Child complains about pain and about other things (e.g., "It hurts; I want mommy").
	Positive	0	Child makes any positive statement or talks about other things without complaint.
Torso	Neutral	1	Body (not limbs) is at rest; torso is inactive.
	Shifting	2	Body is in motion in a shifting or serpentine fashion.
	Tense	2	Body is arched or rigid.
	Shivering	2	Body is shuddering or shaking involuntarily.
	Upright	2	Child is in a vertical or upright position.
	Restrained	2	Body is restrained.
Touch	Not touching	1	Child is not touching or grabbing at wound.
	Reach	2	Child is reaching for but not touching wound.
	Touch	2	Child is gently touching wound or wound area.
	Grab	2	Child is grabbing vigorously at wound.
	Restrained	2	Child's arms are restrained.
Legs	Neutral	1	Legs may be in any position but are relaxed; includes gentle swimming or serpentine-like movements.
	Squirming/kicking	2	Definitive uneasy or restless movements in the legs and/or striking out with foot or feet.
	Drawn up/tensed	2	Legs tensed and/or pulled up tightly to body and kept there.
	Standing	2	Standing, crouching, or kneeling.
	Restrained	2	Child's legs are being held down.

From McGrath PJ, Johnson G, Goodman JT, et al: CHEOPS: A behavioral scale for rating postoperative pain in children. In Fields HL, Dubner R, Cervero F, editors: Advances in pain research and therapy, New York, 1985, Raven Press.
*The CHEOPS scale is scored by an observer at critical time points during evaluation and treatment. The score is determined by adding the score for each item listed. Scores range from 4 to 13.

TABLE 7-2. Developmental Sequence of Pain Perception and Reaction in Children

Age	Perception	Reaction
Newborn-6 mo	No understanding	General stress response, withdrawal, crying, physiologic response*
6 mo-1½ yr	Fear of painful situation	Screaming, restlessness, localization, physiologic response
1½-6 yr	Illogical and egocentric perception	Reality distortion, fantasies, poor time appreciation
7-10 yr	Cause-and-effect, understanding verbal description possible	Physiologic response
11-17 yr	Logical perception, abstraction	Deception, bravado to hide pain

*Physiologic response to pain is generally associated with tachycardia, increased arterial blood pressure, mydriasis, and diaphoresis.

ments, facial expression) and physiologic changes.[24,44] Preschooler methods include self-report scales (e.g., facial drawings, Oucher, poker chip tool) and behavioral scales (e.g., CHEOPS and procedural ratings). School-age to adult methods include self-report scales (VAS, pain questionnaires, numeric ratings) and behavioral scales (procedural ratings).[44]

Although these scales represent a significant improvement in pain assessment over traditional empiric observations,[27,45,48] there are several drawbacks that prevent their unrestricted use with acutely injured children in the emergency department. Use of behavioral scales requires training of observers to reduce interobserver variability.[44,45] Self-report scales generally require practice, although some have been validated for use with children after surgery before and after analgesia.[26,48] The content validity (i.e., whether the scale actually measures pain severity), repeatability, precision, and accuracy of any emergency department childhood pain rating scale must be studied before specific recommendations for its use can be made. There are no studies of emergency department patients that have systematically addressed the issues of validity and accuracy of pain scales in children.

Parental and Environmental Influences

The impact of parental or caretaker presence on children's behavioral response during anxiety-provoking procedures has not been adequately investigated. Although opinions regarding the presence or absence of parents during procedures vary, several issues are clear. First, parents and children prefer to remain together.[60,61] Second, there is a risk of physical and psychologic injury to any caregiver observing an invasive procedure (e.g., from vasovagal syncope). Third, anxious parents may adversely influence the child's emotional response to procedures.[62] Often, spending a few moments with parents before initiating a procedure may make them useful allies in reducing the child's anxiety. Until further data are available on emergency department patients, offering a chair to one parent with self-contained anxiety may decrease separation problems. Unilateral exclusion of caretakers from the child's bedside for common procedures by departmental policy or practice is restrictive and not in the best interest of the child.

Children should be isolated from combative, intoxicated, and acutely ill or injured patients.[63] It is unacceptable to unnecessarily expose a child to scenes that increase their anxiety. Physicians and parents have a duty to protect children from potential physical, sexual, or psychologic harm. Whenever possible, separate entry and waiting areas should be designed into modern emergency department facilities.

Preparation of parents is critical when recruiting them to assist in allaying their child's anxiety. However, infants younger than 6 months and many children older than 12 years may be treated successfully without parents in the room. Stranger and separation anxiety begins at about 6 months of age and is generally characterized as sudden crying, inconsolableness, and clinging to parents. A calm, relaxed health professional reassures both child and caregivers. Equipment and needle hiding may reduce anxiety, although some children want to see the needle or suture material before its use. Using familiar, friendly terms, such as *squirt gun* for irrigation or *tight hugging* for a Papoose restraint, may allay fears and increase cooperation. Using experiential-based, particularly unfriendly terms to characterize procedures, such as bee sting for local anesthesia infiltration, may heighten fears. Distraction using storytelling, music, deep breathing, and counting have been effective in reducing self-reported and behaviorally assessed pain.

NONPHARMACOLOGIC APPROACHES

Psychologic Measures

Multiple psychologic techniques, including adequate preparation, careful explanation, distraction, hypnosis, and minimization of separation anxiety (e.g., reassurance), can be successfully used in children to decrease pain perception. These methods facilitate fantasy play, encourage a sense of self-control, decrease separation anxiety, and facilitate cooperation.[3,27,45,64] Children who understand the need for anesthetic infiltration have less distress than those who do not.[65] Injection pain may be modulated by distraction (e.g., headphones with music) in children as early as 4 years.[66] Systematic preparation, rehearsal, and supportive care before surgery results in greater hospitalization satisfaction and reduced anxiety compared with less comprehensive preparation.[67] Other psychologic approaches to modulate pain and anxiety include soothing of infants, preparation of equipment before placing the child in the procedure area, behavioral distraction, hypnosis, and kinesthetic methods (e.g., rocking, patting) in older children.[55,57,58]

A short period of effective restraint on a Papoose board or with sheeting seems less hazardous than an extended period struggling with an uncooperative, ineffectively restrained toddler.[2,12,29] Inadequate immobilization may encourage further struggling because of a "positive-feedback" mechanism, whereas thorough immobilization may decrease further struggling by negative reinforcement. Using psychologic and pharmacologic techniques that decrease anxiety significantly improves the child's hospital experience without substantially increasing physician time.

Hypnosis and Transcutaneous Nerve Stimulation

In 49 children with cancer, a significant reduction in pain associated with bone marrow aspiration was obtained by using hypnotic and nonhypnotic coping techniques.[58] The pain associated with lumbar puncture was reduced only through hypnosis. Patients with acute trauma or illness may be in a heightened, suggestible state, allowing easier hypnotic induction.[68] However, most psychologic evidence and timeliness of care suggest that nonhypnotic coping strategies are preferred by most emergency clinicians.

There are probably limited applications of transcutaneous nerve stimulation for the pediatric patient in the emergency department. Despite its well-documented efficacy for painful conditions,[69-73] only one emergency department trial has been performed.[74]

PHARMACOLOGIC APPROACHES

Traditional routes of drug administration are oral (PO) or per rectum (PR) for mild pain and anxiety problems and intramuscular (IM) or intravenous (IV) routes for moderate-to-severe pain and titratable sedation. Other routes of drug administration include transmucosal (either sublingual or intranasal), inhalational, transdermal, and intraosseous.

Although PO administration is painless and convenient, the reliability of absorption and relative contraindications (e.g., head injury) may limit emergency department applicability to hemodynamically and neurologically stable children with mild pain or anxiety who are not vomiting. Although less convenient, administration of mild analgesics and potent sedatives may be effective PR.[75] Diazepam, midazolam, methohexital, acetaminophen, chloral hydrate, and thiopental can be reliably given PR.[76-84] Although IM remains the most common route of administration of potent analgesics, it is painful and may result in unreliable absorption.[7,12] The preferred method of rapid, titratable drug delivery is intravenously. IV administration facilitates the rapid onset of activity and controlled titration of effects.[7,43] However, insertion of an IV line in a struggling toddler may be much more stressful than a single IM injection. Transmucosal administration of sedatives and analgesics has become fairly popular recently and has been used successfully with butorphanol, ketamine, fentanyl, and midazolam.

Other considerations in the use of sedative and analgesic pharmacotherapy in children include the ability to reverse serious side effects, dosing based on a measured weight, and the question of whether local or regional anesthesia will suffice over systemic analgesics or sedatives. Reversal of CNS and respiratory depression from opioids, using naloxone, is specific and effective therapy.[85] Naloxone has a short half-life, typically 20 to 30 minutes, and requires repeated dosage or infusion when reversing opioids with a longer duration of action.[86] The benzodiazepine antagonist, flumazenil (Mazicon), may enhance the safety profile for deep sedation with benzodiazepines.[87] Although there is limited experience with flumazenil in children, it appears beneficial in adults in suspected benzodiazepine overdose.[88] One report indicates rapid (less than 1 minute) reversal of midazolam sedation with 0.1 to 0.2 mg of flumazenil in over 600 children undergoing bronchoscopy.[89] In another study, children receiving flumazenil awoke approximately four times faster following midazolam anesthesia compared with the placebo group.[90] The use of flumazenil in children has been reviewed.[91]

The dosing of *all* potent analgesics and sedatives should be based on a measured weight, whenever possible. Failure to do so will increase the likelihood of dosing errors and side effects, and may be associated with reduced clinical efficacy. When measured weight is not immediately available, the use of body-length-based estimation of weight appears accurate in children between 3.5 and 25 kg in weight.[92] The use of local anesthesia, rather than systemic sedative and opioid analgesics, requires application of proper local anesthetic techniques, additional psychologic preparation of the child, and gentle physical restraint in the uncooperative child.

Developmentally, infants younger than 1 month of age are more sensitive to morphine-induced respiratory depression and have prolonged elimination and decreased clearance compared with adults.[93,94] However, once infants are older than 3 months, lower plasma fentanyl concentrations result from more-rapid plasma clearance.[95] Children with hypovolemia appear just as susceptible as infants and adults to the vasodilating properties of morphine.[43] Infants may be particularly susceptible to benzodiazepine-induced respiratory depression and apnea.[96] Clinical experience with ketamine, midazolam, and methadone is virtually unreported in ambulatory settings for children younger than 1 year. For infants, the use of more traditional agents such as morphine and chloral hydrate may suffice for most noncritical clinical problems.

Preoperative Sedation Trials

There is a large database obtained from preoperative sedation trials in children. This data may be used to provide information on the relative safety and efficacy of pharmacologic agents in children. Not unlike preoperative studies, the most common purpose of emergency department sedation in children is to enhance patient cooperation, facilitating the performance of relatively painless procedures, such as the repair of an uncomplicated laceration after local anesthesia or for neuroimaging procedures. A substantial minority of children will undergo painful procedures, such as fracture reduction or burn wound debridement, which require analgesia. These children often are best treated with agents that possess both analgesic and sedative/anxiolytic properties to enhance cooperation during the performance of the procedure. However, children enrolled in preoperative sedation trials cannot be compared without consideration of important differences between them and children undergoing emergency department procedures. Children in emergency settings have little time for psychologic preparation, may have a full stomach, often have been acutely injured, and may have taken medications that influence sedation regimens. However, there are some parallels for the stable child who is given brief psychologic preparation and requires mild-to-moderate sedation (e.g., child with a forehead laceration). The child may benefit from administration of a short-acting sedative by demonstrating increased cooperation and reduced anxiety during procedures.[97]

Oral agents, or combinations of agents studied in preoperative children, include chloral hydrate, midazolam, diazepam, pentobarbital, and ketamine. These agents have been reported as efficacious for preoperative sedation in children. In a study of 248 children, midazolam (0.4 to 0.6 mg/kg) and chloral hydrate (25 or 50 mg/kg) administered PO, moderately decreased anxiety in children younger than 5 years.[98] Children given chloral hydrate (75 mg/kg) experienced a large decrease in anxiety. In 21 children undergoing dental treatment, chloral hydrate (75 mg/kg) was compared with 50 mg/kg of chloral hydrate plus 25 mg of promethazine.[99] All children were restrained in a Papoose board and given 50% nitrous oxide. Successful sedation occurred in 89% of the group receiving promethazine and in 72% of the group that did not. Emesis occurred in 14% of the group receiving promethazine and 48% of those who did not. In a preoperative study, 339 children were randomized to chloral hydrate, diazepam, alprazolam, midazolam, or placebo.[100] Chloral hydrate (40 mg/kg) produced more sedation at induction and was more palatable than other agents. Another study examined 149 children who received diazepam (0.5 mg/kg), trimeprazine (4 mg/kg), pentobarbital (3 mg/kg), or placebo.[101] All treatment groups produced better sedation than placebo. The trimeprazine group had prolonged waking times but less emesis and distress in the recovery unit. In an outpatient surgery study, 159 children received meperidine (1.5 mg/kg) plus diazepam (0.2 mg/kg), and atropine (0.02 mg/kg) or placebo.[102] The treatment group had reduced crying and secretions, without an increase in recovery time. Oral meperidine (3 mg/kg) resulted in better sedation and cooperation than IM morphine (0.1 mg/kg) when both were given with pentobarbital (4 mg/kg) to 67 children before surgery.[103] Forty children with congenital heart disease were premedicated with PO ketamine (10 mg/kg) or IM morphine (0.1 mg/kg) after trimeprazine (3 mg/kg).[104] Cooperation and arousal were comparable after 20 minutes. No serious sequelae were reported.

Children who suffer from repeated emesis, have other contraindications to oral medication, or have a full stomach may require rectal administration of sedation. Sixteen children received midazolam (0.3 mg/kg) in 5-ml saline PR.[81] Successful sedation (i.e., calm, drowsy) occurred in 87% of children at 20 minutes. The depth of sedation correlated closely with plasma levels. Diazepam (0.5 mg/kg), morphine (0.15 mg/kg), and scopolamine hydrobromide (Hyoscine, an anticholinergic agent) (0.01 mg/kg) dissolved in propylene glycol produced satisfactory sedation in 20 children before surgery.[77] Peak levels of diazepam were observed at 30 to 40 minutes, and no respiratory depression was observed. Rectal diazepam (0.5 mg/kg) in solution but not as a suppository has also been successfully used for sedation for neuroradiologic imaging and control of seizures.[75,76,78,105] Methohexital cannot be recommended at this time because of an unacceptable frequency of airway obstruction. Chloral hydrate is available in rectal suppositories, and absorption appears adequate.[84]

Data on the use of oral transmucosal fentanyl, PR methohexital, and intranasal midazolam or ketamine for sedating children for outpatient surgery appear favorable. In an unblinded preoperative trial, 59 children were randomized to placebo, meperidine (1.5 mg/kg) plus diazepam (0.2 mg/kg), or PO transmucosal fentanyl citrate (15 to 20 μg/kg).[106] Treatment groups had similarly effective sedation and reduction of anxiety. Facial pruritus (80%) and emesis (37%) occurred frequently in the fentanyl group. Thirty children were randomized to 2% or 10% solution of 25 mg/kg PR methohexital for preoperative induction.[107] Higher serum levels and sedation were seen in the 2% group, and airway obstruction occurred in 7% of children. Thirty-seven children were randomized to an intranasal solution of midazolam (0.2 or 0.3 mg/kg) or placebo for preoperative sedation.[108] Both treatment groups were significantly more sedated than control, without substantial respiratory or hemodynamic changes. Eighty-six children, aged two to five years, were given ketamine (6 mg/kg) nasally in a preoperative study. These children were compared to 62 similarly aged patients who received IM promethazine and meperidine (1 mg/kg of each agent). Sedation was rated as excellent in 48 (56%) and as adequate in 19 (22%) patients in the ketamine group and nine (15%) and 12 (19%), respectively, in the promethazine-meperidine group.[109]

Recovery Criteria and Monitoring

The level of sedation and analgesia required for most children in an emergency department is a function of the patient and the intended procedure. The intensity of monitoring is dictated by the expected depth of sedation. Conscious sedation is a "minimally depressed level of consciousness that retains the patient's ability to maintain a patent airway independently and continuously, and respond appropriately to physical stimulation or verbal command."[34] Deep sedation is a "controlled state of depressed consciousness or unconsciousness from which the patient is not easily aroused, which may be accompanied by a partial or complete loss of protective reflexes. This includes the inability to maintain a patent airway independently and respond purposefully to physical stimulation or verbal command."[34] In general, emergency department patients require conscious or transient deep sedation. During deep sedation, they should be monitored continuously, while conscious sedation patients may be monitored at frequent, regular intervals.[34,110,111] Assessment of respiratory rate, pulse oximetry, Glasgow Coma Scale (GCS) scores, heart rate, and arterial blood pressure at frequent intervals facilitates early identification of excessively sedated children and those meeting discharge criteria.[112,113] The routine use of a pulse oximeter in these children promotes rapid clinical detection of otherwise inapparent hypoxemia.[112,114,115]

There is an increased emphasis on documentation of the child's physiologic and mental status during clinical procedures performed in hospital settings, regardless of where they are performed.[34,114] Proper documentation should include a general health evaluation, time of last meal or oral intake, monitoring of physiologic signs during the procedure, and the condition of the child at the time of discharge from the emergency department. The adoption of a flow sheet for use in all children receiving sedation for procedural issues may facilitate improved monitoring and documentation. Recovery criteria for outpatient surgical centers could easily be adapted for sedated emergency department children. Discharge criteria after sedation should include the ability to maintain an airway, move all limbs, respond to verbal commands, and sit on the stretcher unassisted for 5 seconds or longer.[114,116] Side effects of general anesthesia may be more common in children than adults. In 16,700 children entering the recovery room from 1985 to 1988, a decrease in blood pressure of greater than 20% of baseline values was observed in over 50% of cases.[116] However, only 72 of 8,995 (0.8%) of children undergoing outpatient surgery at the Children's Hospital National Medical Center required hospital admission.[116] Most of these children were admitted for protracted emesis (36%) or "croup" (11%).

Nonnarcotic Analgesics

Ibuprofen and acetaminophen are the most widely prescribed analgesics in children[117] (Table 7-3).

Aspirin has analgesic, antipyretic, and antiinflammatory effects, although the latter effect requires sustained high dosages.[118] Aspirin produces analgesia by blocking the formation of prostaglandins, mediating pain in the peripheral nervous system.[118] Salicylates are extensively metabolized by the liver. About 10% of the parent compound is eliminated by the kidneys, more if the urine is alkaline. Common side effects include gastritis, emesis, hepatotoxicity, tinnitus, anaphylaxis, exacerbation of asthma, and potentiation of the effects of oral anticoagulants combined with irreversible platelet dysfunction, possibly causing bleeding. Aspirin administration has been strongly associated with

TABLE 7-3. Comparison of Nonnarcotic Agents in Common Clinical Use in Children

Agent	Dose (mg/kg)	Maximum initial dose (mg)	Interval (hr)	Route*
Acetaminophen	10-15	1,000	4	PO, PR
Aspirin	10-15	1,000	4	PO, PR
Ibuprofen	5-10	800	6	PO
Ketorolac	0.5-1.0	60†	6	IM, IV, PO

*Preferred route of administration is listed first.
†10 mg for PO.

Reye syndrome when given during varicella or influenza-like illness,[119] and its use has been reduced substantially since this association was made. Enteric-coated aspirin reduces gastrointestinal side effects but may interfere with absorption.[120,121]

Acetaminophen has analgesic and antipyretic properties equipotent to aspirin but possesses no antiinflammatory effects. Analgesia is produced in the CNS by inhibition of prostaglandin synthetase.[118] Acetaminophen is extensively metabolized in the liver by sulfonation and glucuronidation. Side effects are uncommon, but overdoses exceeding 140 mg/kg may result in renal and hepatic injury.[85] Onset of action after oral or rectal administration of aspirin or acetaminophen is generally 30 minutes, whereas duration of action is 3 to 4 hours.[83] The analgesic effects of either may be enhanced with the addition of codeine.[122,123] A study of 127 children with fever suggested that ibuprofen may be a more effective antipyretic than acetaminophen when both were given at a dose of 10 mg/kg.[124]

The class of compounds termed *nonsteroidal antiinflammatory drugs* (NSAIDs) generally have more potent analgesic and antiinflammatory actions than aspirin or acetaminophen. The NSAIDs are inhibitors of prostaglandin biosynthesis.[125-132] Of the many NSAIDs available, the largest experience is with ibuprofen, which has been available in pediatric formulations in the United Kingdom since 1972.[133] Side effects of NSAIDs include renal and hepatic dysfunction, gastrointestinal irritation or bleeding, potentiation of effects of anticoagulants, reversible platelet function inhibition, and allergic reactions. Ibuprofen decreases renal blood flow; reversible renal failure has been reported in a hypovolemic child treated with ibuprofen.[134] In addition, NSAIDs have demonstrated potent analgesic effects in renal colic.[135,136] Ketorolac has potent analgesic effects and is the only parenteral NSAID available for use in the United States.[137] In double-blind trials of adult patients, 60 mg of ketorolac was equivalent to 12 mg of morphine, without comparable sedation.[138] Most adult-based studies have repeatedly demonstrated the efficacy and safety of ketorolac, although one emergency department trial failed to show a narcotic sparing effect in patients with pain from sickle cell crises.[139,140]

Similar efficacy and safety data are rapidly appearing for PO, IM, and IV ketorolac in children. Like many agents used in children, the Food and Drug Administration has not approved ketorolac for use in children less than 16

years of age. A preoperative study of 90 children undergoing bilateral myringotomy, mean age of 2.6 years, compared the postoperative analgesic effects of oral acetaminophen (10 mg/kg) or oral ketorolac (1 mg/kg) when given 30 minutes before anesthesia. Compared with placebo and the acetaminophen groups, the ketorolac group had lower postoperative pain scores and required less postoperative analgesic medication.[141] Both titration and bolus ketorolac groups had comparable postoperative analgesia to morphine in 92 children from 3 to 12 years of age.[142] Children who received IV ketorolac (0.9 mg/kg) had similar pain scores to those receiving IV morphine (0.1 mg/kg) when examined postoperatively.[143] Children who received ketorolac had significantly less nausea and vomiting. Elimination half-lives of ketorolac in children were similar to those reported in adults in 10 children studied after minor surgery.[144] Cautions have been raised over excessive bleeding, particularly in association with repeated use of ketorolac. Initial dosage guidelines have remained unchanged, while subsequent dosing has been reduced, particularly in elderly patients.

Narcotic Analgesics

Narcotics' actions (Table 7-4) are mediated through binding to specific opioid receptors in the spinal cord and brain. Selection of specific narcotic agents should be based on the required duration of action, dose, route of administration, patient's weight and clinical stability, and the use of narcotic potentiators. Intermittent monitoring for hypoventilation, oxygen desaturation, and cardiorespiratory depression is essential.

Morphine sulfate is a potent narcotic acting at opiate receptors in the CNS. The narcotic is metabolized in the liver; morphine undergoes O- and N-demethylation, followed by conjugation and renal excretion of these metabolites. It also has analgesic, sedative, anxiolytic, and euphoric effects.[53] Potent narcotics are indicated for moderate-to-severe pain and are contraindicated in hemodynamically or neurologically unstable children, unless provision for airway and ventilatory assistance has been addressed. In unstable children, these agents may be given IV by slow infusion, with titration to desired effects accompanied by continuous bedside monitoring. Side effects include nausea, emesis, hypotension, sedation, miosis, constipation, potentiation of biliary colic, and respiratory depression.[5,43] Morphine, when contrasted with meperidine, has a longer half-life, much less CNS toxicity, no myocardial depression, and a clearance unaffected by renal or hepatic disease.

Children younger than 2 months of age are particularly susceptible to respiratory depression.[43] In addition, morphine has a prolonged elimination half-life and decreased clearance in infants younger than 1 month of age.[93] When administered to hypovolemic patients, morphine may cause significant hypotension, particularly when given with potent sedatives.[43] However, two recent reports indicate that morphine may be safely used, both during the routine treatment of children in the emergency department[145] and in sick premature neonates.[146]

Fentanyl (Sublimaze) is a rapidly acting, very potent synthetic narcotic with a half-life of about 90 minutes;

TABLE 7-4. Comparison of Narcotic Analgesic Agents in Common Clinical Use in Children*

Agent	Dose (mg/kg)	Maximum initial dose (mg)	Route	Duration (hr)
Morphine	0.1	10	IV, SC, IM	3-4
Meperidine	1	100	IV	2-3
	2	125	IM, PO	3-4
Fentanyl	0.001	0.01†	IV, IM	0.5-0.8
Codeine	1-2	90	PO, IM	3-4
Methadone	0.1	20	PO, IM, IV	4-12

*These agents induce equivalent respiratory depression and sedation when administered in the recommended equipotent dosages. Preferred route of administration is listed first.
†0.005 mg/kg.
SC, Subcutaneous.

potency is approximately 100 times that of morphine.[147,148] It blocks nociceptive stimuli without hemodynamic compromise, histamine release, or exacerbation of bronchospasm, making it the anesthetic of choice in many centers for trauma and cardiac patients.[149] Like morphine, fentanyl in infants has a prolonged half-life of elimination.[95] Infants older than 3 months of age have a greater clearance of fentanyl, reducing risks for prolonged duration of effects.

Although fentanyl is increasingly recommended, few emergency department studies involving children have been reported.[147,150-152] Three (0.2%) of 2,000 children became apneic after receiving 2 to 3 μg/kg IV and required ventilatory assistance. In 84 adult emergency department patients, fentanyl had a serious complication rate of only 1% (hypotension or respiratory depression).[152] In addition to the usual narcotic side effects, fentanyl may also induce chest wall rigidity (potentially interfering with assisted ventilation), vomiting, seizures, and facial pruritus.[153-155]

The transmucosal route of administration using fentanyl citrate in a candy matrix (lollipop) is effective for analgesia.[156] In a nonblinded trial, thirty children were given oral transmucosal fentanyl (10 to 20 μg/kg) before undergoing laceration repair in an emergency department.[150] Sedation/pain control was rated as "good to excellent" in 83% of patients. One child (3.3%) experienced a transient oxygen desaturation, 63% had pruritus, and 33% vomited. A single-blind study compared oral transmucosal fentanyl to IM *m*eperidine, *p*romethazine, and *c*hlorpromazine (MPC) in 39 children undergoing laceration repair.[157] Both medications had equal efficacy in decreasing activity behavior during laceration repair and no serious side effects were reported. The fentanyl group had excessive vomiting (45%), while prolonged tiredness occurred in 37% of patients in the MPC group. These data provide useful preliminary data on the use of oral fentanyl for sedation for laceration repair.

Although the use of fentanyl and midazolam for orthopedic injuries has been reported from one emergency department, caution in their combination is recommended.[158,159] Hypoxemia (92%) and apnea (50%) in

healthy volunteers were reported when fentanyl and midazolam are used in combination.[160] Management of these findings must be implemented. Although rare, 78% of the deaths associated with the use of midazolam were respiratory in nature. Further, in 57% of these adverse case reports, an opioid, most commonly fentanyl or meperidine, was also administered with midazolam.

Meperidine is a synthetic narcotic with few advantages over morphine.[32] There is a relatively small therapeutic range in which analgesia is achieved and above which toxicity occurs.[3,33] High levels of the principal metabolite, normeperidine, may produce tremors, disorientation, and convulsions.[161] Unlike other opioids, meperidine produces a tachycardia when given intravenously.[149] Perhaps its only distinct advantage over morphine is that it is well absorbed PO, with a bioavailability of 50% to 75%. When combined with narcotic potentiating agents, such as hydroxyzine or promethazine, its sedative and possibly analgesic effects are enhanced.[162] It should generally be avoided in the ongoing management of pain because of the increased risk of seizures associated with repeated administration.

Codeine is a commonly administered oral opioid for moderate pain and antitussive effects. Its analgesic potency is increased when administered with acetaminophen or NSAIDs.[122,123,131] Codeine has an oral bioavailability of 60%, with a plasma elimination half-life of 2 to 3 hours.[163] Typical opioid side effects are seen with equipotent dosages of codeine, commonly producing nausea, vomiting, sedation, and constipation.[43] Oral morphine has a potency of one sixth that of parenteral morphine, whereas meperidine given PO has half the potency of the parenteral preparation.

Mixed agonist-antagonist opioids (e.g., pentazocine [Talwin], nalbuphine, butorphanol, and sufentanil) have been developed to reduce the euphoria, respiratory depression, analgesic "ceilings," and dependency seen with standard opioids.[164] Analgesia is produced by agonist action on specific (kappa) receptors, whereas the ceiling on respiratory depression occurs with antagonism of the other (mu) receptors. Although some experience is reported in the anesthesia literature, the use of these newer agents in emergency department patients has not been systematically described.[164-168]

Hydromorphone, hydrocodone, oxycodone, and propoxyphene are semisynthetic agents with limited applicability for pediatric emergency department patients. Oxycodone is a potent oral analgesic with some secondary euphoria. Because of its potent analgesic action, excellent bioavailability, prolonged duration of action, and limited sedation and euphoria, methadone may be useful in patients with chronic pain exacerbation.[2,167]

Sedatives

Sedatives (Table 7-5) decrease activity and blunt responsiveness and are therefore useful in performing procedures requiring patient cooperation. Painful interventions commonly require a combination of sedatives, plus analgesics.

Current sedatives recommended for use in children in the emergency department include chloral hydrate; benzodiazepines, such as diazepam and midazolam; antihista-

TABLE 7-5. Comparison of Sedative Agents in Common Clinical Use in Children

Agent	Dose (mg/kg)	Maximum initial dose (mg)	Route*	Duration (hr)
Diazepam	0.1-0.2	10	IV	1-3
	0.3-0.5	10	PR, PO	2-4
Midazolam	0.05-0.1	5	IV	0.3-0.8
	0.3-0.5	10	PO, IN†, PR	0.5-1.5
Chloral hydrate	50-80	2000	PO, PR	2.5-3.0

*Preferred route of administration is listed first. IV administration, when utilized, should be by slow infusion over 3 to 5 minutes.
†Intranasal drops.

mines (hydroxyzine and promethazine); and the phenothiazine, chlorpromazine. Whereas opioids have sedative properties, these sedatives do not have analgesic properties, and some may actually increase nociception if used without analgesia.[162]

Chloral hydrate has been used as a sedative and hypnotic agent for over 100 years. It remains the most common pediatric sedative for radiologic imaging.[168] Chloral hydrate's activity is secondary to a rapidly formed metabolite, trichloroethanol, produced by alcohol dehydrogenase. Plasma half-life is 4 to 12 hours, and the onset of action is generally 20 to 30 minutes. Although variable, the duration of action is usually 2 to 3 hours until the patient is alert, when given at a dose of 50 to 80 mg/kg. Previous dosage recommendations of 35 to 50 mg/kg may be inadequate for many children, unless it is administered with promethazine or other sedative agents.[99] Usually given orally, it is also effective when given rectally but is contraindicated in hepatic failure.[169]

Concerns have been raised over the use of chloral hydrate in children, especially in critically ill children. Two metabolites, trichloroacetic acid and trichloroethanol, accumulated in tissues or had an excessively prolonged half-life in critically ill newborns.[170] In addition, the onset and duration of action of chloral hydrate, recently reported to be 30 minutes and 92 minutes,[171] may limit its use in emergency department patients.

Doses of 70 to 100 mg/kg of chloral hydrate have been associated with oxygen desaturation in wheezy infants recovering from bronchiolitis.[172] However, doses as high as 120 mg/kg have been described for sedating children for imaging studies.[173] Three percent (11 children) of these children, some who also received IV pentobarbital, had hypoxia detected and all recovered with airway positioning or supplemental oxygen.

All *benzodiazepines* appear to exert their effects by inhibition of gamma-aminobutyric acid (GABA) receptors in the CNS.[174,175] Benzodiazepines have sedative, hypnotic, amnestic, anticonvulsant, and respiratory depressant effects.[176] When given rapidly IV or in large doses, highly lipophilic benzodiazepines rapidly enter the CNS. They may induce cardiorespiratory depression or apnea.[174-177]

Midazolam, a short-acting, water-soluble benzodiazepine, may be given PO, PR, IM, or IV. Midazolam causes less phlebitis compared with diazepam when given IV.[178] Lorazepam, an effective first-line anticonvulsant (see Chapter 56), generally performs poorly as a sedative.[179-182] Trials of pediatric sedation using diazepam or midazolam PO, PR, and IV have reported generally efficacious and safe results.

Nasally, orally, or rectally administered midazolam appears safe and efficacious for reducing distress and anxiety in children undergoing laceration repair. In an emergency department study of 55 children with lacerations, oral midazolam (0.2 mg/kg) reduced the anxiety score significantly in 70% of children.[97] Fifty-nine children in a randomized, double-blind, placebo-controlled study were significantly less anxious and distressed after nasal midazolam (0.4 mg/kg).[183] A retrospective chart review of 42 children receiving nasal midazolam demonstrated some evidence of increased efficacy in doses of 0.3 mg/kg.[184] In a double-blind emergency department trial, 54 anxious children undergoing laceration repair were given either nasal (0.25 mg/kg) or oral (0.5 mg/kg) midazolam. Both groups had significantly less anxiety compared to baseline, but there were no differences between oral or nasal administration.[185] Children given 0.45 mg/kg of rectal midazolam were adequately sedated in 63% of cases, vs. 13% of placebo controls.[186]

In combination with other agents, nasal midazolam is also effective. One emergency department study compared intranasal midazolam (0.2 mg/kg) and sufentanil (75 μg/kg) with IM MPC for sedation in 42 children undergoing laceration repair.[187] No adverse effects were recorded, and sedation as judged by behavioral scores with sufentanil and midazolam was as effective as IM MPC.[185] Time to recovery and discharge was longer with MPC. When combined with ketamine (5 mg/kg), midazolam (0.56 mg/kg) resulted in a success rate of 83% in 30 children undergoing computerized tomography.[188]

The studies of midazolam listed above have found no evidence of serious cardiorespiratory complications or oxygen desaturation. Although appealing for children with vomiting or resistance to take oral medication, the reduced efficacy with rectal administration of midazolam may be related to reduced plasma concentrations.[189] Administration of nasal drops is painful, may increase a child's anxiety, and is not tolerated by some children. Paradoxical agitation following midazolam administration is regularly reported. This disinhibition phenomena is distressing, typically following an otherwise effective sedation experience, and usually resolves within 15 minutes without specific therapy.

Methohexital is an ultra-short-acting barbiturate that may be administered IV, IM, or PR.[190] In eight children undergoing radiographic scanning procedures, methohexital (10 mg/kg IM) produced effective sedation in 87% of children within 5 minutes.[191] Repeat sedation was required in 87% of the children undergoing procedures lasting 22 to 90 minutes. In 20 children before surgery, plasma methohexital levels after 25 mg/kg PR correlated well with plasma levels after parenteral administration.[192] Plasma methohexital levels of more than 2 μg/ml resulted in uni-

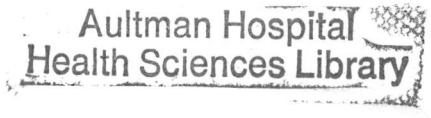

form loss of consciousness within 15 minutes. However, airway obstruction was observed in 7% of 30 children receiving the same dose PR,[107] and thus the agent cannot be recommended at this time for routine emergency department sedation. Methohexital has also been reported as effective for sedation of pediatric oncology, radiologic imaging, and dental procedures in children.[193-195] However, 7 of 132 (5.3%) procedures in oncologic patients required suctioning or bag-mask ventilation.[191] One recent emergency department report of rectal methohexital use reviewed the charts of 26 children who received between 20 and 25 mg/kg for a variety of common emergency department procedures.[196] Three (12%) children suffered from oxygen desaturation, and one required bag-mask ventilation. However, for procedures that require transient deep sedation (e.g., cardioversion or shoulder relocation), methohexital given IV may be an alternative.

Pentobarbital has been reported as effective for sedating children for outpatient imaging studies when administered IM or IV.[197] Pentobarbital had an overall success rate of 97% given either IM or IV, and was associated with an increased risk of oxygen desaturation and airway obstruction when given IV. The reference dosage is 3 mg/kg IV, especially for use in CT scans and imaging procedures. Similarly, rectal thiopental was reported as effective in 96% of 462 children undergoing radiologic imaging.[198] However, it was associated with oxygen desaturation in 11% of cases and a 34% incidence of other complications.

Hydroxyzine is an H_1-receptor antagonist with sedative, antiemetic, antispasmodic, and antihistaminic effects.[162,199] The recommended dose is 1 mg/kg PO or IM, with a maximum dose of 50 mg. The primary indications are for antiemesis and potentiation of analgesia and sedation in combination with opioids. Chlorpromazine is a prototype phenothiazine with sedative, amnestic, antimotion-sensation, and antihistaminic effects.[162] The dose is 1 mg/kg IM or PO; maximum dose is 50 mg. There is conflicting information concerning the ability of phenothiazines to potentiate opioid analgesia.[200] However, phenothiazines do appear to reduce the nausea and vomiting associated with isolated opioid administration. Chlorpromazine has alpha-blocking properties and may induce hypotension or seizures in susceptible patients.[201] Promethazine is also an H_1-receptor antagonist sharing some phenothiazine properties.[162] It has potent antiemetic, antihistaminic, sedative, and antimotion-sensation effects.[200] It appears to potentiate opioid analgesia, without increasing susceptibility to hypotension and seizures. Cautions with any of these agents include enhanced sedative effects when given with other sedative agents, including opioids, barbiturates, and ethanol.

Other Systemic Agents and Techniques

There is no indication for general anesthesia to be used in the emergency department unless an operating theatre is a component of it. Certain agents that are useful in the emergency department but do not easily fit into the above categories are discussed below.

Ketamine. Ketamine is a unique anesthetic that induces a state of electrophysiologic dissociation between the cortical and limbic systems and produces a state of dissocia-

tive anesthesia.[202] It induces analgesia, amnesia, mild sedation, immobilization, and bronchodilation. Ketamine does not appear to impair protective reflexes, but random or purposeful movements are frequently observed in patients after administration.[203] The onset of action is 1 to 2 minutes, with dissociation continuing for 15 to 30 minutes. Recovery gradually occurs within 90 minutes, although disequilibrium may last for several hours.[202,203] Side effects include hypersalivation, vomiting, emergent reactions, nightmares, laryngospasm, hypertension, tachycardia, and increased intracranial pressure.

Unfortunately, there are many relative contraindications to ketamine. They include upper or lower respiratory infection, procedures involving the posterior pharynx, cystic fibrosis, age younger than 3 months, head injury, increased intracranial pressure, acute glaucoma or globe penetration, uncontrolled hypertension, congestive heart failure, arterial aneurysm, allergy or previous adverse reaction to ketamine, acute intermittent porphyria, and thyrotoxicosis.[202,203] Ketamine, in a dosage of 1 to 1.5 mg/kg IV, has been reported as beneficial for sedation for endotracheal intubation in asthmatic children in respiratory failure[204] because it is a bronchodilator.

Clinical experience with ketamine for anesthesia, including brief outpatient procedures, is extensive outside of the emergency department.[202,203] In one emergency department series, 30 children were given up to 2 mg/kg IM ketamine.[205] All children achieved dissociation, although three required repeat doses of half of the original dose. In 52 cases in children and adults (ages 5 to 67 years) given up to 2 mg/kg of ketamine with diazepam, one patient had excessive restlessness during recovery, and one had a "very unpleasant dream."[206] One report of 108 children receiving ketamine (4 mg/kg with atropine IM) for brief emergency department procedures demonstrated adequate analgesia, immobility, and sedation in 97% of patients.[110] Adverse reactions reported were vomiting (6%) and one episode of transient laryngospasm. A double-blind, placebo (flavored syrup)-controlled trial in 30 children with lacerations reported that PO ketamine (10 mg/kg) resulted in significantly greater patient tolerance to lidocaine injection and suturing.[207] No serious complications or significant change in physiologic signs was observed compared to presedation values. Finally, 29 children were randomized to IM ketamine (4 mg/kg with atropine) or MPC for emergency department sedation.[208] The ketamine-treated group had a shorter time to onset of sedation (3 vs. 18 minutes), shorter time to discharge (85 vs. 113 minutes), and lower observed rated behavioral distress.

Ketamine is a very interesting agent; limited reporting of its use in the emergency department hampers widespread use.[209] If serious complications are reported, with more extensive experience, it is important to balance these with the excellence of ketamine in children for a variety of short, outpatient procedures.[210]

Propofol and Etomidate. Propofol is an alkylphenol, IV anesthetic with antiemetic, antipruritic, anticonvulsant, anxiolytic, hypnotic, and analgesic properties.[211] Propofol's onset is immediate and is so rapidly cleared from the plasma that an IV infusion is required to maintain any clinical effects. Side effects of propofol include pain at the site of injection and the occurrence of involuntary or semi-purposeful movements. In doses that produce loss of consciousness, decreases in mean arterial blood pressure and apnea may occur.[212]

Etomidate is another ultra-short-acting sedative hypnotic anesthetic. It has a rapid onset and short duration of action, and its main advantage is the relative lack of hypotension associated with the induction of anesthesia. There is no reported clinical experience with either propofol or etomidate in the emergency department.

It is worth noting that several trials of propofol have been performed in children. In two neuroimaging trials, a total of 119 children received propofol (1 to 2 mg/kg) followed by a propofol infusion or a comparative dose of barbiturates or ketamine.[213,214] Spontaneous respiration was maintained in all patients at these dosages and the incidence of oxygen desaturation to less than 90% was no different between the two groups (propofol 5% and barbiturates 4%) studied. Time to full consciousness and to home discharge was significantly shorter in the propofol group.[213] Compared to ketamine, propofol produced hypotension in 70% of children undergoing cardiac catheterization.[215] Recovery time in the propofol group was significantly less, mean 24 minutes vs. 139 minutes.

Nitrous Oxide. Nitrous oxide (N_2O) is an inhalation anesthetic that induces analgesia when administered in a 30% to 50% concentration.[216] Because N_2O has a low solubility in blood and is carried in solution unbound to hemoglobin, it is excreted unchanged from the lungs. Thus it is rapid and short acting. Several prehospital and emergency department trials of a self-administered mixture of 30% to 70% N_2O and oxygen have reported favorable results in adults and children.[217-220] Good-to-excellent relief from pain of musculoskeletal trauma, laceration repair, incision and drainage of abscesses, venous cannulation, abdominal pain, chest pain, burn injury, and back pain has been demonstrated in emergency department patients, including some children.[217-220] Side effects are generally mild and include lightheadedness, drowsiness, nausea, emesis, and excitement. Contraindications include altered level of consciousness, severe maxillofacial injuries, chronic obstructive pulmonary disease, acute pulmonary edema, decompression sickness, shock, pneumothorax, bowel obstruction, and major chest injury.[217]

In a controlled emergency department trial, 34 children undergoing laceration repair were given 30% N_2O in oxygen.[52] Compared with 100% oxygen, those given N_2O had significant improvements in CHEOPS pain scores without important side effects. All children were continuously monitored by a second physician during N_2O administration. In 165 cases of elective surgery, nonsedated children were given 50% or 70% N_2O before venous cannulation.[219] Little or no pain was felt by 59% and 84% of the treatment groups, respectively, whereas 30% of the control group had evidence of pain. However, 28% of the group receiving 70% N_2O had mild side effects (i.e., excitement, restlessness, and opisthotonos). In a large retrospective report of 3,000 "uncomfortable procedures" in children in an office setting, N_2O produced effective analgesia.[220] Only nine patients vomited while receiving N_2O in this study.

Meperidine, Promethazine, and Chlorpromazine (MPC). MPC is an IM drug combination that has been used for sedation and analgesia in children for nearly 40 years.[221] The onset of action is usually 20 to 30 minutes, with a variable but often prolonged duration of action.[222,223] Serious side effects reported with this combination include dystonia, prolonged sedation, respiratory depression, and after IV use, cardiac arrest.[221,224,225] The frequency of serious cardiorespiratory depression in unselected emergency department patients appears to be less than 1%,[222] whereas it's efficacy for various outpatient procedures is about 70%.[49] This agent may produce significant neurologic depression that should be viewed as deep sedation; it should be administered with continuous monitoring. Contraindications include multiple trauma, hypoxemia, underlying neurologic abnormalities, and head injury.[222] Despite concerns about its continued use, it is the most frequently used agent for pediatric sedation.[129,151,226,227] A review of MPC has concluded that it is an unsound medication, with a high rate of therapeutic failure and serious adverse reactions.[228] The AAP recommended that practitioners carefully weigh alternative sedative choices, and provide careful monitoring and patient selection when using MPC.

Several emergency department trials are particularly important because they have attempted to compare intramuscular MPC with other sedative/analgesic agents. These studies are valuable because they allow practitioners to judge the effects of a well known standard that they have experience with to less known or utilized alternatives. As mentioned above, nasal sufentanil plus midazolam or IM ketamine compares favorably to intramuscular MPC, and both have an improved onset and duration profile.[185,208] Rectal thiopental (25 mg/kg) vs. intramuscular MPC was reported in 29 selected children in an emergency department.[229] Thiopental resulted in significantly deeper sedation at 15 and 30 minute time points, compared to MPC. The mean Glasgow Coma Scores in the thiopental group were 7 and 6 at these time points, respectively. This level of sedation is typically unnecessary for laceration repair and is generally not required. A recent comparison of PO fentanyl lollipops (10 to 15 µg/kg) to intramuscular MPC for conscious sedation enrolled 40 children in a single blind study.[157] The activity score of the MPC group demonstrated less movement during repair, but no differences were found in CHEOPS scores between groups. Sedation was considered excellent or good in 75% and 70% of the fentanyl and MPC groups, respectively.

Patient-Controlled Analgesia (PCA). Using a programmable infusion pump, PCA allows the patient to deliver IV analgesic agents on demand, within safe dosage parameters established by the physician.[230] This is safe and efficacious in adults and children.[230-255] For children with pain from cancer, sickle cell crisis, or surgery, patient satisfaction with pain control is improved.[231-234] Total narcotic doses and side effects are generally reduced utilizing PCA compared with intermittent IM or IV injection.[234] No emergency department trials of PCA have been reported to date, although patients with painful sickle cell crisis or renal colic seem to be potential candidates.

TABLE 7-6. Comparison of Local Anesthetics in Common Clinical Use

Agent	Concentration (%)	Maximum total dose*	Relative potency	Duration of action†
Bupivacaine	0.25-0.75	7	8	Intermediate
Lidocaine	0.5-2.0	4	3	Short
Mepivacaine	1.0	5-7	2.4	Long
Procaine	0.5-2.0	15	1	Short
Tetracaine	1.0-2.0	2	8	Short

*Maximum safe dose is in mg/kg of body weight. Administration with epinephrine approximately doubles the total safe dosage.
†This is the relative duration of action.

Local Anesthesia

Topical anesthesia using *t*etracaine (0.5%), *a*drenaline (epinephrine 1:1000), and *c*ocaine (11.8%), known as *TAC*, has significantly simplified local anesthesia for children with lacerations.[236] Many authors have reported effectiveness comparable with lidocaine infiltration, although efficacy is best on facial areas.[237-243] Wound complications are not increased, and the necessity to restrain and sedate children is reduced because of the relative absence of pain during wound anesthesia.[49,244,245] The application technique is important to maximize efficacy and reduce complications.[245-249] Improved results may be achieved by pooling a small amount of TAC in a dependent portion of the wound before applying the remainder of the dose with a saturated piece of cotton ball (not gauze, which absorbs) into the depth of the wound.[250] Because cocaine absorption has been documented after TAC application, measures to limit systemic exposure may include using a single 3 ml or smaller dose, avoiding mucosal contact, formulating a TAC gel, and limiting the duration of application to less than 20 minutes.[246,251,252] Significant side effects associated with TAC use have included seizures and death, but these have always been associated with inappropriate application to mucous membranes or extensive areas of abrasion/burn.[246,247,249] Contraindications to its use include cholinesterase deficiency, significant hepatic disease, and, on burns, extensive abrasions, highly contaminated wounds, mucous membranes, digits, penis, or pinna of the external ear.[236] Cocaine, cocaine and epinephrine, TAC at half its standard concentration, and TAC with half the standard concentration of cocaine are also effective.[239,243,253]

The duration of TAC application vs. effectiveness was recently studied in 400 children with superficial lacerations.[254] Application times of less than 20 minutes were associated with reduced effectiveness, regardless of laceration location, and efficacy was 97% after 31 minutes. An important alternative to TAC solution for topical anesthesia of lacerations is *l*idocaine (4%), *e*pinephrine (0.1%), and *t*etracaine (0.5%), known as LET.[255] In a double-blind, randomized study in 171 children requiring laceration repair, the efficacy and duration of anesthesia was no different than standard TAC solution.[255] Because there is no cocaine in LET, this alternative offers the advantages of reduced costs, record keeping, storage simplification, and possibly reduced toxicity. Bupivacaine (0.48%) and norepi-

nephrine (1:26,000) may be an equally effective topical anesthetic agent.[256]

A eutectic mixture of local anesthetic (EMLA) containing prilocaine and lidocaine produces good topical anesthesia in intact skin. Unfortunately, at least 60 minutes of application are required before adequate local anesthesia occurs,[257] reducing emergency department utility with the present formulation. In 114 children with application times of 20 minutes or longer, there were no differences in pain reduction unless the mixture was applied for more than 60 minutes.[257] In a single-blind study of 58 children after premedication injection, EMLA applied for 60 minutes or longer produced a significant reduction in pain scores for IV catheter insertion.[256] EMLA is useful in reducing pain associated with lumbar puncture and puncture of SC drug reservoirs.[258,259] Ethyl chloride spray reduces venipuncture pain in adults but not as effectively as intradermal lidocaine.[260]

In a recent, single-blind study of 32 children with extremity lacerations, EMLA (0.15 gm/kg) provided successful anesthesia in 85% of patients compared with 45% for TAC.[261] However, adequate wound anesthesia required an average of 26 minutes longer for the EMLA patients. Further clinical study of topical anesthesia of uncomplicated lacerations in children is warranted because of the reduced effectiveness of these agents in nonfacial lacerations and the contraindications at end-arteriole sites and mucous membranes, which account for a significant number of pediatric soft tissue injuries.

Infiltrative techniques (Table 7-6) using lidocaine remains the standard technique for local anesthesia. Two types of "caine" anesthetics exist. The esters include procaine, tetracaine, and benzocaine. The amides include lidocaine and bupivacaine. Allergies are uncommon, often reflecting a reaction to the pain and stress or the preservative, methylparaben, which is not generally present in single-dose or cardiac lidocaine. There is no cross-hypersensitivity between the amide and ester group agents.

Lidocaine (Xylocaine) may be administered topically or infiltrated SC to produce peripheral nerve blockade. Onset of action after direct infiltration is almost instantaneous, lasting 20 to 60 minutes. Regional nerve block has an onset within 4 to 6 minutes, with a duration of effect of 75 minutes. Generally, 3 to 5 mg/kg of lidocaine is administered, not to exceed 300 mg as a single injection. Epinephrine produces vasoconstriction, prolonging the duration of action and allowing doses up to 5 to 7 mg/kg to be administered. However, epinephrine may delay healing and lower resistance to infection; its use should be avoided when wounds have a high risk of infection or when tissue viability or vascularity is compromised or questionable. It may be useful in prolonging the effect of regional blocks (not in fingers or toes) and in decreasing bleeding while suturing. Lidocaine 1% contains 10 mg/ml.

Using the smallest suitable needle, gentle pressure and slow infiltration of the local anesthetic are very important for reducing pain.[262] When lidocaine is given with bicarbonate, a reduction in infiltration pain may also occur by neutralizing the normally acidic pH to 7.0.[263,264] In 25 healthy adults, lidocaine, with and without epinephrine, and mepivacaine were associated with significantly reduced infiltration pain when buffered anesthetics were used. No reduction in efficacy was observed.[263] When buffered compared with unbuffered lidocaine was used, 91 adults with lacerations had significant reduction in pain scores.[265] There was significant reduction in self-rated infiltration pain in 24 subjects when sodium bicarbonate, 0.1 mEq/ml (1:10 by volume), was added to lidocaine; shelf-life of the solution is approximately one week.[264]

Although epinephrine concentrations decline approximately 25% each week after neutralization of lidocaine, no significant clinical differences in vasoconstriction were reported during the first week of mixing these two agents.[266] Heating the lidocaine up to 42° C and injecting slowly reduces pain.[267]

Bupivacaine (Marcaine) has a rapid onset of action, similar to lidocaine, but the duration of anesthesia is nearly 4 times as long. Although no dosage data is available for children, the normal maximum adult dosage of bupivacaine is 175 mg without epinephrine or 225 mg with epinephrine. Infiltration of the wound edges with bupivacaine (0.25%) reduces postoperative pain in children after a herniorrhaphy and might be beneficial for some emergency department applications.[268,269]

Regional anesthesia may reduce the need for conscious sedation but requires patient cooperation. Commonly, pediatric emergency department patients require digital, distal extremity, and facial nerve blocks (see Appendix, p. 67). An excellent review of the technique of these blocks is available.[270]

Minidose Bier block may be preferable to local hematoma blocks for reducing the pain associated with fracture reduction.[271,272] Minidose Bier block uses half the usual dose of lidocaine used for regional anesthesia and may reduce the toxicity associated with anesthesia of the arm at or below the elbow. Using 1.5 mg/kg or a maximum of 100 mg, at 0.5% concentration, the IV is inserted near the site of injury. After the affected arm is elevated for 30 seconds, a sphygmomanometer is rapidly inflated to 50 mm Hg above the systolic blood pressure. After assuring no leaks in the system, the arm is lowered and lidocaine is injected. After approximately 15 minutes, an additional 0.5 mg/kg of lidocaine may be used if anesthesia is still not effective. Monitoring of heart rate, pulse oximetry, and blood pressure should be performed with resuscitative equipment at the bedside.

RECOMMENDATIONS

Even minor procedures in children often cause considerable anxiety and contribute to the pain experienced.[12] Moderate-to-severe distress from simple venipuncture was experienced by 64% of children younger than 6 years of age.[273] Hospitalized children may perceive blood tests as the most difficult part of their care.[27,274] In adolescent oncology patients, invasive procedures may be considered worse than the disease itself.[55] As advocates for children, pediatric emergency physicians should err on the side of providing pain control and sedation early and often.

Our current recommendations for emergency department pediatric sedation and analgesia are derived from both clinical experience and a view of the literature (Table 7-7). There are a wide array of clinical issues that will dictate choices for individual patients but most important are the patient's severity of pain, the patient's clinical cardiorespiratory and neurologic stability, and the anticipated depth of sedation and analgesia required for the intended intervention or procedure. The duration of the procedure, relative contraindications to certain agents, and the presence or absence of an IV catheter will dictate which agents should be used and by which route of administration.

The majority of children requiring *analgesia* alone are those with minor infections or trauma. For children who are undergoing procedures associated with little additional pain, sedation may be required to reduce anxiety and improve patient cooperation. These patients include those with uncomplicated lacerations and requiring neuroimaging. When the anticipated procedure may produce more than minor pain, as in the case of some complex laceration repairs or a difficult foreign body extraction, some analgesia should also be provided. Common indications for providing sedation plus analgesia routinely are fracture reductions, abscess incision and drainage, and burn wound debridement.

Many children requiring *sedation* are appropriately treated without the need to establish vascular access. However, for children likely to require deep sedation or in severe pain, an IV catheter allows for titration of clinical effects, repeated dosing, and an emergency access line in case of complications. Single IM injections may be used for children who will likely not require further parenteral analgesia or sedation or in whom waiting until vascular access can be obtained will extend the period of suffering excessively. Once an IV catheter is in place, there is no need to administer sedative or analgesic medications by other routes of administration.

When choosing *sedative and analgesic agents*, the pediatric emergency physician must keep in mind the dual objectives of safety and efficacy. Although potent sedative and analgesic agents are widely available, their routine use at doses producing significant cardiorespiratory depression for minor procedures such as uncomplicated laceration repair appears unwarranted. The beneficial effects of these agents must be weighed against their expected complications, and in relation to the objective of sedation and analgesia for each child. Clinical experience and literature clearly indicate that sound environmental and psychologic management contributes substantially to the beneficial aspects of emergency department care for children.

References

1. Benedetti C: Acute pain: a review of its effects and therapy with systemic opioids. In Benedetti C, Chapman CR, Giron G, editors: *Advances in pain research and therapy,* vol 14, Opioid analgesia: recent advances in systemic administration, New York, 1990, Raven Press.
2. Selbst SM: Managing pain in the pediatric emergency department, *Pediatr Emerg Care* 5:56, 1989.
3. Thompson A and Frader J: Pain management in children. In Paris PM and Stewart RD, editors: *Pain management in emergency medicine,* West Hartford, Conn, 1987, Appleton & Lange.

TABLE 7-7. Recommended Sedative and Analgesic Agents for Pediatric Emergency Department Patients

Indication	Agent	Route	Initial dosage (mg/kg)	Maximum initial dosage
Analgesia				
Mild-moderate	Acetaminophen	PO, PR	10-15	1,000 mg
Moderate	Ibuprofen	PO	10	800 mg
Severe	Morphine sulfate	IV, SC	0.1	10 mg
	Ketorolac	IM, IV	0.5-1.0	60 mg
	Meperidine	IM	2	100 mg
	plus promethazine	IM	1	50 mg
Sedation				
Moderate	Midazolam	PO, PR, IN	0.5	10 mg
	Chloral hydrate	PR, PO	50-80	2,000 mg
Deep	Midazolam	IV	0.1	5 mg
	Diazepam	IV	0.2	10 mg
Analgesia and sedation				
No IV	Morphine	IM	0.1	10 mg
	plus midazolam	IM	0.1	5 mg
	Ketamine*	IM	4	8 mg/kg
	Meperidine	IM	2	50 mg
	plus promethazine	IM	1	25 mg
	plus chlorpromazine (MPC)	IM	1	25 mg
With IV	Morphine	IV	0.1	10 mg
	Morphine	IV	0.1	10 mg
	plus midazolam	IV	0.1	5 mg
	Fentanyl	IV	0.001-0.002	0.005 mg/kg

*Atropine is often given in the same syringe to reduce excess secretions associated with ketamine.
IN, Intranasal drops.

4. Wilkie DJ et al: Measuring pain quality: validity and reliability of children's and adolescents' pain language, *Pain* 41:151, 1990.
5. Leonard F: Pain control: anesthesia and analgesia. In Rosen P et al, editors: *Emergency medicine: concepts and clinical practice,* St. Louis, 1985, Mosby–Year Book.
6. Osgood PF and Szyfelbein SK: Management of burn pain in children, *Pediatr Clin North Am* 36:1001, 1989.
7. Paris PM: Pain management in the child, *Emerg Med Clin North Am* 5:699, 1987.
8. Levine J: Pain and analgesia: the outlook for more rational treatment, *Ann Intern Med* 100:269, 1984.
9. Paris PM: No pain, no pain, *Am J Emerg Med* 7:660, 1989.
10. Fields JL: Neurophysiology of pain and pain modulation, *Am J Med* 77(3A):2, 1984.
11. Goodman CE: Pathophysiology of pain, *Arch Intern Med* 143:527, 1983.
12. Selbst SM and Henretig FM: The treatment of pain in the emergency department, *Pediatr Clin North Am* 36:965, 1989.
13. Loveridge CE, West N, Solomon R: Children in pain: the emergency department response, *Top Emerg Med* 11(3):73, 1989.
14. LeBaron S and Zelter L: Assessment of acute pain and anxiety in children and adolescents by self-reports, observer reports, and a behavior checklist, *J Consult Clin Psychol* 52:729, 1984.
15. Frolund F and Frolund C: Pain in general practice: pain as a cause of patient-doctor contact, *Scand J Prim Health Care* 4:97, 1986.
16. Crook J, Rideout E, Browne G: The prevalence of pain complaints in a general population, *Pain* 18:299, 1984.
17. Miser AW et al: Pain as a presenting symptom in children and young adults with newly diagnosed malignancy, *Pain* 29:85, 1987.
18. Jonsson OG et al: Bone pain as an initial symptom of childhood acute lymphoblastic leukemia: association with nearly normal hematologic indexes, *J Pediatr* 117:233, 1990.
19. Parfrey NA, Moore W, Hutchins GM: Is pain crisis a cause of death in sickle cell disease? *Am J Clin Pathol* 84:209, 1985.
20. Anand KJS and Carr DB: The neuroanatomy, neurophysiology, and neurochemistry of pain, stress and analgesia in newborns and children, *Pediatr Clin North Am* 36:795, 1989.
21. Anand KJS, Sippell WG, Aynsley-Green A: Randomized trial of fentanyl anaesthesia in preterm babies undergoing surgery: effects on the stress response, *Lancet* 10:62, 1987.
22. Anand KJS and Hickey PR: Pain and its effects in the human neonate and fetus, *N Engl J Med* 317:1321, 1987.
23. Williamson PS and Williamson ML: Physiologic stress reduction by a local anesthetic during newborn circumcision, *Pediatrics* 71:36, 1983.
24. McGrath PA, deVeber LL, Hearn MT: Multidimensional pain assessment in children. In Fields HL et al, editors: *Advances in pain research and therapy,* vol 9. New York, 1984, Raven Press.
25. Schechter NL, Allen DA, Hanson K: Status of pediatric pain control: a comparison of hospital analgesic usage in children and adults, *Pediatrics* 77:11, 1986.
26. Szyfelbein SK, Osgood PF, Carr DB: The assessment of pain and plasma beta-endorphin immunoactivity in burned children, *Pain* 22:173, 1985.
27. Jay SM et al: Assessment of children's distress during painful medical procedures, *Health Psychol* 2(2):133, 1983.
28. Loeser JD: Pain in children. In Tyler DC and Krane EJ, eds: *Advances in pain research and therapy,* vol 15, Pediatric pain, New York, 1990, Raven Press.
29. Selbst SM and Clark M: Analgesic use in the emergency department, *Ann Emerg Med* 19:1010, 1990.
30. Schecter NL: The undertreatment of pain in children: an overview, *Pediatr Clin North Am* 36:781, 1989.

31. Walco GA, Cassidy RC, Schechter NL: Pain, hurt, and harm: the ethics of pain control in infants and children, *N Engl J Med* 331:541-544, 1994.
32. Paris PM and Stewart RD: *Pain management in emergency medicine,* Norwalk, Conn, 1988, Appleton & Lange.
33. Wilson SE and Pendleton JM: Oligoanalgesia in the emergency department, *Am J Emerg Med* 7:620, 1989.
34. American Academy of Pediatrics, Committee on Drugs: Guidelines for monitoring and management of pediatric patients during and after sedation for diagnostic and therapeutic procedures, *Pediatrics* 89:1110-1115, 1992.
35. U.S. Department of Health and Human Services, Public Health Service, Agency for Health Care Policy and Research: *Acute pain managementin infants, children, and adolescents: operative and medical procedures,* Quick reference guide for clinicians, DHHS Pub. No. (AHCPR) 92-0019. Silver Spring, Md, 1992, AHCPR Clearinghouse.

Definitions

36. American Pain Society: Principles of analgesic use in the treatment of acute pain and chronic cancer pain, ed 2, *Clin Pharm* 9:601, 1990.
37. *Stedman's medical dictionary,* ed 25, Baltimore, 1990, Williams & Wilkins.
38. Lloyd-Thomas AR: Pain management in paediatric patients, *Br J Anaesth* 64:85, 1990.

Pathophysiology

39. Cross SA: Pathophysiology of pain, *Mayo Clin Proc* 69:375-383, 1994.
40. Yaksh TL and Hammond DL: Peripheral and central substates involved in the rostral transmission of nocioceptive information, *Pain* 13:1, 1982.
41. Pat CB and Snyder SH: Opiate receptor: demonstration in nervous tissue, *Science* 179:1011, 1973.
42. Melzack R and Wall PD: Pain mechanisms: a new theory, *Science* 150:971, 1965.
43. Yaster M and Deshpande JK: Management of pediatric pain with opioid analgesics, *J Pediatr* 113:421, 1988.

Assessment of Pain

44. Beyer JE and Wells N: The assessment of pain in children, *Pediatr Clin North Am* 36:837, 1989.
45. Ross DM and Ross SA: *Childhood pain: current issues, research, and management,* Baltimore, 1988, Urban & Schwarzenberg, Inc.
46. Martin LVH: Postoperative analgesia after circumcision in children, *Br J Anaesth* 45:1263, 1982.
47. Pothmann R: Comparison of the visual analog scale (VAS) and a Smiley Analog Scale (SAS) for the evaluation of pain in children. In Tyler DC and Krane EJ, editors: *Advances in pain research and therapy,* vol 15, Pediatric pain, New York, 1990, Raven Press.
48. Aradine CR, Beyer JE, Tompkins JM: Children's pain perception before and after analgesia: a study of instrument construct validity and related issues, *J Pediatr Nurs* 3:11, 1988.
49. McGrath PJ and Unruh AM: Pain in children and adolescents. In *Pain research and clinical management,* vol 1, New York, 1987, Elsevier Science Publishing Co, Inc.
50. Bieri D et al: The Faces Pain Scale for the self-assessment of the severity of pain experienced by children: development, initial validation, and preliminary investigation for ratio scale properties, *Pain* 41:139, 1990.
51. Terndrup TE, et al: A prospective analysis of intramuscular meperidine, promethazine, chlorpromazine in pediatric emergency department patients, *Ann Emerg Med* 20:31, 1991.
52. Gamis AS, Knapp JF, Glenski JA: Nitrous oxide analgesia in a pediatric emergency department, *Ann Emerg Med* 18:177, 1989.

Reasons for Inadequate Pain Control

53. Yaster M, Deshpande JK, Maxwell LG: The pharmacologic management of pain in children, *Pediatrics* 15(10):14, 1989.
54. Johnston CC: Pain assessment and management in infants, *Pediatrician* 16:16, 1989.
55. Kuttner L: Management of young children's acute pain and anxiety during invasive medical procedures, *Pediatrician* 16:39, 1989.
56. Siegel LJ and Smith KE: Children's strategies for coping with pain, *Pediatrician* 16:110, 1989.

57. Wall VJ and Womack W: Hypnotic versus active cognitive strategies for alleviation of procedural distress in pediatric oncology patients, *Am J Clin Hypn* 31:181, 1989.
58. Zeltzer L and LeBaron S: Hypnosis and nonhypnotic techniques for reduction of pain and anxiety during painful procedures in children and adolescents with cancer, *J Pediatr* 101:1032, 1982.

Developmental Response to Pain

59. McGrath PJ and Craig KD: Developmental and psychological factors in children's pain, *Pediatr Clin North Am* 36:823, 1989.
60. Bauchner H, Vinci R, Waring C: Pediatric procedures: do parents want to watch? *Pediatrics* 84:907, 1989.
61. Gonzalez JC et al: Effects of parent presence on children's reactions to injections: behavioral, physiological, and subjective aspects, *J Pediatr Psychol* 14:449, 1989.
62. Bevan JC, et al: Preoperative parental anxiety predicts behavioural and emotional responses to induction of anaesthesia in children, *Can J Anaesth* 37:177, 1990.
63. Goldman A: Child oriented emergency department design. In Fleisher CR and Ludwig S, editors: *Textbook of pediatric emergency medicine,* ed 1, Baltimore, 1983, Williams & Wilkins.

Nonpharmacologic Approaches

64. Bogetz MS: Anesthesia for pediatric outpatient surgery, *Pediatrician* 16:45, 1989.
65. Kissoon N, McGrath PA, Glebe D: Children's understanding of the need for painful procedures in the emergency room modifies their response to pain, *Pediatr Emerg Care* 5:284, 1989.
66. Fowler-Kerry S and Lander JR: Management of injection pain in children, *Pain* 30:169, 1987.
67. Visintainer MA and Wolfer JA: Psychological preparation for surgical pediatric patients: the effect on children's parents' stress responses and adjustment, *Pediatrics* 56:187, 1975.
68. Wain HJ and Amen DG: Emergency room use of hypnosis, *Gen Hosp Psychiatry* 8:19, 1986.
69. Chapman CR and Benedetti C: Analgesia following transcutaneous electrical stimulation and its partial reversal by a narcotic antagonist, *Life Sci* 21:1645, 1977.
70. Pertovaara A and Kemppainen P: The influence of naloxone on dental pain threshold elevation produced by peripheral conditioning stimulation at high frequency, *Brain Res* 215:426, 1981.
71. Sloan JP et al: Multiple rib fractures: transcutaneous nerve stimulation versus conventional analgesia, *J Trauma* 26:1120, 1986.
72. Wynn Parry CB and Girgis F: The assessment and management of the failed back. II. *Int Disabil Stud* 10:25, 1988.
73. Arter OE and Racz GB: Pain management of the oncologic patient, *Semin Surg Oncol* 6(3):162, 1990.
74. Ersek RA: Relief of acute musculoskeletal pain using transcutaneous electrical stimulation, *JACEP* 6:300, 1977.

Pharmacologic Approaches

75. Choonara IA: Giving drugs per rectum for systemic effect, *Arch Dis Child* 62:771, 1987.
76. Dulac O et al: Blood levels of diazepam after single rectal administration in infants and children, *J Pediatr* 93:1039, 1978.
77. Lindahl S, Olsson A-K, Thomson D: Rectal premedication in children: use of diazepam, morphine and hyoscine, *Anaesthesia* 36:376, 1981.
78. Franzoni E, Carbone C, Lambertini A: Rectal diazepam: a clinical and EEG study after a single dose in children, *Epilepsia* 24:35, 1983.
79. De Jong PC and Verburg MP: Comparison of rectal to intramuscular administration of midazolam and atropine for premedication of children, *Acta Anaesthesiol Scand* 32(6):485, 1988.
80. Dochy M: Double blind comparative study with intrarectal administration of midazolam, intramuscular administration of diazepam: preliminary results, *Acta Anaesthesiol Belg* 38(3s):45, 1987.
81. Saint-Maurice C et al: The pharmacokinetics of rectal midazolam for premedication in children, *Anesthesiology* 65:536, 1986.
82. Quaynor H, Corbey M, Bjorkman S: Rectal induction of anaesthesia in children with methohexitone: patient acceptability and clinical pharmacokinetics, *Br J Anaesth* 57(6):573, 1985.
83. Lovejoy FH: Aspirin and acetaminophen: a comparative view of their antipyretic and analgesic activity, *Pediatrics* 62(suppl):904, 1978.

84. Shimoyama M, Mizuguchi T, Yorozu S: Premedication in children: a clinical trial of bromazepam and chloral hydrate suppositories, *Masui* 39:64, 1990.

85. Goldfrank LR et al: *Toxicologic emergencies,* ed 3, Norwalk, Conn, 1986, Appleton-Century-Crofts.

86. Barsan WG et al: Duration of antagonistic effects of nalmefene and naloxone in opiate-induced sedation for emergency department procedures, *Am J Emerg Med* 7:155, 1989.

87. Sage DJ, Close A, Boas RA: Reversal of midazolam sedation with anexate, *Br J Anaesth* 59:459, 1987.

88. Spivey WH, Roberts JR, Derlet RW: A clinical trial of escalating doses of Flumazenil for reversal of suspected benzodiazepine overdose in the emergency department, *Ann Emerg Med* 22:1813, 1993.

89. Baktai G, Szekely E, Marialigeti T, Kovacs L: Use of midazolam and flumazenil in paediatric bronchology, *Cur Med Res Opinion* 12:552-559, 1992.

90. Jones RD, Lawson AD, Andrew LJ, Gunawardene WM, Bacon-Shone J: Antagonism of the hypnotic effect of midazolam in children: a randomized, double-blind study of placebo and flumazenil administered after midazolam-induced anaesthesia, *Br J Anaesth* 66:660-666, 1991.

91. Sugarman JM, Paul RI. Flumazenil: a review, *Pediatr Emerg Care* 10:37-43, 1994.

92. Lubitz DS et al: A rapid method for estimating weight and resuscitation drug dosages from length in the pediatric age group, *Ann Emerg Med* 17:576, 1988.

93. Lynn AM and Slattery JT: Morphine-pharmacokinetics in early infancy, *Anesthesiology* 66:136, 1987.

94. Lynn AM, Opheim KE, Tyler DC: Morphine infusion after pediatric cardiac surgery, *Crit Care Med* 12:863, 1984.

95. Singleton MA, Rosen JI, Fisher DM: Plasma concentrations of fentanyl in infants, children and adults, *Can J Anaesth* 34:152, 1987.

96. Bean JD and Rogers MC: Anesthetic considerations and pain management in the pediatric intensive care unit. In *Textbook of pediatric intensive care,* Baltimore, 1987, Williams & Wilkins.

97. Hennes HM, et al: The effect of oral midazolam on anxiety of preschool children during laceration repair, *Ann Emerg Med* 19:1006, 1990.

98. Saarnivaara L, Lindren L, Klemola UM: Comparison of chloral hydrate and midazolam by mouth as premedicants in children undergoing otolaryngological surgery, *Br J Anaesth* 61:390, 1988.

99. Houpt MI, et al: Comparison of chloral hydrate with and without promethazine in the sedation of young children, *Pediatr Dentistry* 7:41, 1985.

100. Anderson BJ et al: Oral premedication in children: a comparison of chloral hydrate, diazepam, alprazolam, midazolam and placebo for day surgery, *Anaesth Intensive Care* 18:185, 1990.

101. Van der Walt JH et al: The perioperative effects of oral premedication in children, *Anaesth Intensive Care* 18:5, 1990.

102. Brzustowicz RM et al: Efficacy of oral premedication for pediatric outpatient surgery, *Anesthesiology* 60:475, 1984.

103. Nicolson SC et al: Comparison of oral and intramuscular preanesthetic medication for pediatric inpatient surgery, *Anesthesiology* 71:8, 1989.

104. Stewart KG et al: Oral ketamine premedication for paediatric cardiac surgery: a comparison with intramuscular morphine (both after oral trimeprazine), *Anaesth Intensive Care* 18:11, 1990.

105. Knudsen FU: Plasma-diazepam in infants after rectal administration in solution and by suppository, *Acta Paediatr Scand* 66:563, 1977.

106. Nelson PS et al: Comparison of oral transmucosal fentanyl citrate and an oral solution of meperidine, diazepam, and atropine for premedication in children, *Anesthesiology* 70:616, 1989.

107. Laishley RS, O'Callaghan AC, Lerman J: Effects of dose and concentration of rectal methohexitone for induction of anaesthesia in children, *Can Anaesth Soc J* 33(4):427, 1986.

108. Wilton NCT et al: Intranasal midazolam premedication in pre-school children, *Anesth Analg* 67:S260, 1988.

109. Weksler N, Ovadia L, Muati G, Stav A: Nasal Ketamine for paediatric premedication, *Can J Anaesth* 40;119-121, 1993.

110. Green SM, Nakamura R, Johnson NE: Ketamine sedation for pediatric procedures. I. A prospective series, *Ann Emerg Med* 19:1024, 1990.

111. Committee on Drugs, Section on Anesthesiology: Guidelines for the elective use of conscious sedation, deep sedation, and general anesthesia in pediatric patients, *Pediatrics* 76:317, 1985.

112. Cote CJ, Rolf N, Liu LMP, et al: A single-blind study of combined pulse oximetry and capnography in children, *Anesthesiology* 74:980-987, 1991.

113. Casteel HB, Fiedorek SC, Kiel EA: Arterial blood oxygen desaturation in infants and children during upper gastrointestinal endoscopy. *Gastrointest Endosc* 36:489-493, 1990.

114. Sacchetti A, Schafermeyer R, Gerardi M, et al: Pediatric analgesia and sedation, *Ann Emerg Med* 23:237-250, 1994.

115. Patel RI et al: Pediatric outpatient anesthesia: a review of postanesthetic complications in 8995 cases, *Anesthesiology* 65:A435, 1986.

116. McConachie IW, Day A, Morris P: Recovery from anaesthesia in children, *Anaesthesia* 44:986, 1989.

117. Drwal-Klein LA, Phelps SJ: Antipyretic therapy in the febrile child, *Clin Pharm* 11:1005-1021, 1992.

118. Amadio P: Peripherally acting analgesics, *Am J Med* 77(3A):17, 1984.

119. Hurwitz ES: The changing epidemiology of Reye's syndrome in the United States: further evidence for a public health success, *JAMA* 260:3178, 1988.

120. Halpern LM: Analgesia drugs in the management of pain, *Arch Surg* 112:861, 1977.

121. Beaver WT: Combination analgesia, *Am J Med* 17:38, 1984.

122. Bentley KC and Head TW: The additive analgesic efficacy of acetaminophen, 1000 mg, and codeine, 60 mg, in dental pain, *Clin Pharmacol Ther* 42(6):634, 1987.

123. Forbes JA et al: Analgesic effect of naproxen sodium, codeine, a naproxen-codeine combination and aspirin on the postoperative pain of oral surgery, Pharmacotherapy 6(5):211, 1986.

124. Walson PD et al: Ibuprofen, acetaminophen, and placebo treatment of febrile children, *Clin Pharmacol Ther* 49:9, 1989.

125. Moore PA, Acs G, Hargreaves JA: Postextraction pain relief in children: a clinical trial of liquid analgesics, *Int J Clin Pharmacol Ther Toxicol* 23(11):573, 1985.

126. Frame JW et al: A comparison of ibuprofen and dihydrocodeine in relieving pain following wisdom teeth removal, *Br Dent J* 166(4):121, 1989.

127. Aghababian RV: Comparison of diflunisal and acetaminophen with codeine in the management of grade 2 ankle sprain, *Clin Ther* 8(5):520, 1986.

128. Muncie HL Jr, King DE, DeForge B: Treatment of mild to moderate pain of acute soft tissue injury: diflunisal vs. acetaminophen with codeine, *J Fam Pract* 23(2):125, 1986.

129. Indelicato PA: Comparison of diflunisal and acetaminophen with codeine in the treatment of mild to moderate pain due to strains and sprains, *Clin Ther* 8(3):269, 1986.

130. Jain A et al: A double-blind study of diflunisal and codeine compared with codeine or diflunisal alone in postoperative pain, *Clin Pharmacol Ther* 43(5):529, 1988.

131. Turek MD and Baird WM: Double-blind parallel comparison of ketoprofen, acetaminophen plus codeine, and placebo in postoperative pain, *J Clin Pharmacol* 28:S23, 1988.

132. Minotti V et al: Double-blind evaluation of analgesic efficacy of orally administered diclofenac, nefopam, and acetylsalicylic acid plus codeine in chronic cancer pain, *Pain* 36(2):177, 1989.

133. Ibuprofen vs. acetominophen in children, *Med Lett Drugs Ther* 31:109, 1989.

134. Van Biljon G: Reversible renal failure associated with ibuprofen in a child: a case report, *S Afr Med J* 76:34, 1989.

135. Jonsson PE et al: Intravenous indomethacin and oxycone-papaverine in the treatment of acute renal colic: a double-blind study, *Br J Urol* 59(5):396, 1987.

136. Persson NH et al: Comparison of a narcotic (oxicone) and a nonnarcotic anti-inflammatory analgesic (indoprofen) in the treatment of renal colic, *Acta Chir Scand* 151(2):105, 1985.

137. Oostechirck W et al: A double-blind single dose comparison of intramuscular ketorolac and pethidine in the treatment of renal colic, *J Clin Pharmacol* 30:336, 1990.

138. Yee JP et al: Comparison of intramuscular ketorolac and morphine sulfate for analgesia of pain after major surgery, *Pharmacotherapy* 6:253, 1986.

139. Wright SW, Norris RL, Mitchell TR: Ketorolac for sickle cell vaso-occlusive crisis pain in the emergency department: lack of a narcotic-sparing effect, *Ann Emerg Med* 21:925-928, 1992.

140. Sevarino FB, Sinatra RS, Paige D, Ning T, Brueel SJ, Silverman DG: The efficacy of intramuscular ketorolac in combination with intravenous PCA morphine for postoperative pain relief, *J Clin Anesth* 4:285-288, 1992.

141. Watcha MF, Ramirez-Ruiz M, White PF, Jones MB, Laguereula RG, Terkonda RP. Perioperative effects of oral ketorolac and acetaminophen in children undergoing bilateral myringotomy, *Can J Anaesth* 39;649-654, 1992.

142. Maunuksela EL, Kokki H, Bullingham RES: Comparison of intravenous ketorolac with morphine for postoperative pain in children, *Clin Pharmacol Ther* 52:436-443, 1992.

143. Watcha MF, Jones MB, Laguereula RG, Schweiger C, White PF: Comparison of ketorolac and morphine as adjuvants during pediatric surgery, *Anesthesiology* 76:368-372, 1992.

144. Olkkola KT, Maunuksela EL: The pharmacokinetics of postoperative ketorolac tromethamine in children, *Br J Pharmacol* 31:182-184, 1991.

145. Woolard DJ, Terndrup TE: Sedative-analgesic agent administration in children: analysis of use and complications in the emergency department, *J Emerg Med* 12:453-461, 1994.

146. Quinn MW, Wild J, Dean HG, et al: Randomised double-blind controlled trial of effect of morphine on catecholamine concentrations in ventilated pre-term babies, *Lancet* 342:324-327, 1993.

147. Billmire DA, Neale HW, Gregory RO: Use of IV fentanyl in the outpatient treatment of pediatric facial trauma, *J Trauma* 25:1079, 1985.

148. Cartwright P, et al: Ventilatory depression related to plasma fentanyl concentrations during and after anesthesia in humans, *Anesth Analg* 62:966, 1983.

149. Rayburn RL: Ventilatory therapy, anesthesia, and respiratory support. In Mayer TA: *Emergency management of pediatric trauma*, Philadelphia, 1985, WB Saunders Co.

150. Schutzman SA, Burg J, Liebelt E, Strafford M, Schechter N, Wisk M, Fleisher G: Oral transmucosal fentanyl citrate for premedication of children undergoing laceration repair, *Ann Emerg Med* 24:1059-1064, 1994.

151. Hawk W et al: Conscious sedation of the pediatric patient for suturing: a survey, *Pediatr Emerg Care* 6:84, 1990.

152. Chudnofsky CR et al: The safety of fentanyl use in the emergency department, *Ann Emerg Med* 18:635, 1989.

153. Neidhart P et al: Chest wall rigidity during fentanyl- and midazolam-fentanyl induction: ventilatory and haemodynamic effects, *Acta Anaesthesiol Scand* 33:1, 1989.

154. Rawal N and Wennhager M: Influence of perioperative nalbuphine and fentanyl on postoperative respiration and analgesia, *Acta Anaesthesiol Scand* 34:197, 1990.

155. Hertzka RE et al: Fentanyl-induced ventilatory depression: effects of age, *Anesthesiology* 70:213, 1989.

156. Stanley TH, Hague B, Mock DL, et al: Oral transmucosal fentanyl citrate (lollipop) premedication in human volunteers, *Anesth Analg* 69:28, 1989.

157. Schutzman SA, Liebelt E, Wisk M, Burg J: A comparison of oral transmucosal fentanyl citrate and intramuscular meperidine, promethazine, and chlorpromazine for conscious sedation in children, *Acad Emerg Med* 2:428, 1995. (abstract)

158. Bergman I, Steeves M, Burckart G, Thompson A: Reversible neurologic abnormalities associated with prolonged intravenous midazolam and fentanyl administration, *J Pediatr* 119:644-649, 1991.

159. Graff KJ, Kennedy RM, Jaffe DM: Conscious sedation for orthopedic injuries in children, *Am J Dis Child* 147:426, 1993.

160. Bailey PL, Pace NL, Ashburn MA, Moll JB, East KA, Stanley TH: Frequent hypoxemia and apnea after sedation with midazolam and fentanyl, *Anesthesiol* 73:826-830, 1990.

161. Goetting MG and Thirman JM: Neurotoxicity of meperidine, *Ann Emerg Med* 14:1007, 1985.

162. Terndrup TE: Sedative-hypnosis. In Barsan WG, Jastremski MS, Syverud SA, editors: *Emergency drug therapy*, Orlando, Fla, 1990, WB Saunders.

163. Guay DR et al: Pharmacokinetics of codeine after single- and multiple-oral dose administration to normal volunteers, *J Clin Pharmacol* 27(12):983, 1987.

164. Zola EM and McLeod DC: Comparative effects and analgesic efficacy of the agonist-antagonist opioids, *Drug Intell Clin Pharm* 17:411, 1983.

165. Borgeat A et al: Comparison of propofol and thiopental/halothane for short-duration ENT surgical procedures in children, *Anesth Analg* 71:511, 1990.

166. Bailey PL et al: Differences in magnitude and duration of opioid-induced respiratory depression and analgesia with fentanyl and sufentanil, *Anesth Analg* 70:8, 1990.

167. Tobias JD, Schleien CL, Haun SE: Methadone as treatment for iatrogenic narcotic dependency in pediatric intensive care unit patients, *Crit Care Med* 18:1292, 1990.

168. Keeter S et al: Sedation in pediatric CT: national survey of current practice, *Radiology* 175:745, 1990.

169. Lambert GH et al: Direct hyperbilirubinemia associated with chloral hydrate administration in the newborn, *Pediatrics* 86:277, 1990.

170. Mayers DJ, Hindmarsh KW, Sankaran K, Gorecki DKJ, Kasian GF: Chloral hydrate disposition following single-dose administration to critically ill neonates and children, *Dev Pharmacol Ther* 16:71-77, 1991.

171. Ronchera CL, Marti-Bonmati L, Poyatos C, Vilar J, Jimenez NV: Administration of oral chloral hydrate to paediatric patients undergoing magnetic resonance imaging, *Pharm Weekbl* [Sci] 14:349-352, 1992.

172. Mallol J, Sly PD: Effect of chloral hydrate on arterial oxygen saturation in wheezy infants, *Pediatr Pulmonol* 1988;5:96-99.

173. Hubbard AM, Markowitz RI, Kimmel B, Kroger M, Bartko MB: Sedation for pediatric patients undergoing CR and MRI, *J Comput Assist Tomogr* 1992;16:3-6.

174. Greenblatt DJ, Shader RI, Abernethy DR: Current status of benzodiazepines. I, *N Engl J Med* 309:354, 1983.

175. Greenblatt DJ, Shader RI, Abernethy DR: Drug therapy. current status of benzodiazepines. II, *N Engl J Med* 309:410, 1983.

176. Smith DE and Wesson DR: *The benzodiazepines: current standards for medical practice*, Norwell, Mass, 1985, MTP Press Limited.

177. Booker PD, Beechy A, Lloyd-Thomas AR: Sedation of children requiring artificial ventilation using an infusion of midazolam, *Br J Anaesth* 58(10):1104, 1986.

178. Reves JG et al: Midazolam: pharmacology and uses, *Anesthesiology* 62:310, 1985.

179. Cornejo G, Araneda LB, Gallardo F: Use of lorazepam as premedication for apprehensive children, *J Pedodontics* 9:136, 1985.

180. Van de Velde A, Schneider I, Camu F: A double-blind comparison of the efficacy of lorazepam FDDF vs. placebo for anesthesia premedication in children, *Acta Anaesthesiol Belg* 38(3):207, 1987.

181. Ponnudurai R and Hurdley J: Bromazepam as oral premedication: a comparison with lorazepam, *Anaethesia* 41(5):541, 1986.

182. Peters CG and Brunton JT: Comparative study of lorazepam and trimeprazine for oral premedication in paediatric anaesthesia, *Br J Anaesth* 54:623, 1982.

183. Theroux MC, West DW, Corddry DH, et al: Efficacy of intranasal midazolam in facilitating suturing of lacerations in preschool children in the emergency department, *Pediatrics* 91:624-627, 1993.

184. Yealy DM, Ellis JH, Hobbs GD, Moscati RM: Intranasal midazolam as a sedative for children during laceration repair, *Am J Emerg Med* 10:584-587, 1992.

185. Connors KM, Terndrup TE: Nasal versus oral midazolam for sedation of anxious children undergoing laceration repair, *Ann Emerg Med* 24:1074-1079, 1994.

186. Shane SA et al: Efficacy of rectal midazolam for the sedation of preschool children undergoing laceration repair, *Ann Emerg Med* 24 (6):1065, December 1994.

187. Bates BA, Schutzman SA, Fleisher GR. A comparison of intranasal sufentanil and midazolam to intramuscular meperidine, promethazine, and chlorpromazine for conscious sedation in children, *Ann Emerg Med* 24:646-651, 1994.

188. Loudon A and Reddy VG: Nasal midazolam and ketamine for paediatric sedation during computerised tomography, *Acta Anaesthesiol Scand* 38:259-261, 1994.

189. Malinovsky JM, Lejus C, Servin F, et al: Plasma concentrations of midazolam after IV, nasal or rectal administration in children, *Br J Anaesth* 70:617-620, 1993.

190. Bjorkman S et al: Pharmacokinetics of IV and rectal methohexitone in children, *Br J Anaesth* 59(12):1541, 1987.

191. Forbes RB et al: Pharmacokinetics of intramuscular methohexital in children, *Anesth Analg* 70:S109, 1990.

192. Liu LMP et al: Methohexital plasma concentrations in children following rectal administration, Anesthesiology 62:567, 1985.

193. Schwanda AE, Freyer DR, Sanfilippo DJ, et al. Brief unconscious sedation for painful pediatric oncology procedures. Intravenous methohexital with appropriate monitoring is safe and effective, Am J Pediatr Hem Onc 15:370-376, 1993.

194. Ewah B and Carr C: A comparison of propofol and methohexitone for dental chair anaesthesia in children, Anaesthesia 48:260-262, 1993.

195. Manuli MA and Davies L: Rectal methohexital for sedation of children during imaging procedures, Am J Radiol 160:577-580, 1993.

196. Bowers RM, Gossett CW, Hobbs GD: Rectally administered methohexital for pediatric sedation in the emergency department (abstract), Acad Emerg Med 2:428, 1995.

197. Pereira JK, Burrows PE, Richards HM, Chuang SH, Babyn PS: Comparison of sedation regimens for pediatric outpatient CT, Pediatr Radiol 1993;23:341-344.

198. Glasier CM, Stark JE, Brown R, James CA, Allison JW: Rectal thiopental sodium for sedation of pediatric patients undergoing MR and other imaging studies, Am J Neuroradiol 1995;16:111-114.

199. Hupert C, Yacoub M, Turgeon LR: Effect of hydroxyzine on morphine analgesia for the treatment of postoperative pain, Anesth Analg 59:690, 1980.

200. McGee JL and Alexander MR: Phenothiazine analgesia: fact or fantasy? Am J Hosp Pharm 36:633, 1979.

201. Chodoff P and Domino EF: Comparative pharmacology of drugs used in neuroleptanalgesia, Anesth Analg 44:558, 1965.

202. White PF, Way WL, Trevor AJ: Ketamine: its pharmacology and therapeutic uses, Anesthesiology 56:119, 1982.

203. Green SM and Johnson NE: Ketamine sedation for pediatric procedures. II. Review and implications, Ann Emerg Med 19:1033, 1990.

204. L'Hommedieu CS and Arens JJ: The use of ketamine for emergency intubation of patients with status asthmaticus, Ann Emerg Med 1987;16:568-571.

205. Dailey RH et al: Ketamine dissociative anesthesia: emergency department use in children, JACEP 8:57, 1979.

206. Caro DB: Trial of ketamine in an accident and emergency department, Anesthesia 29:227, 1974.

207. Qureshi FA, Mellis PT, McFadden MA: Efficacy of oral ketamine for providing sedation and analgesia to children requiring laceration repair, Pediatr Emerg Care 11 (2):93-97, April 1995.

208. Petrack EM, Marx CM, Wright MS, Lubitz D: Intramuscular ketamine is superior to meperidine, promethazine, and chlorpromazine for pediatric emergency department sedation, Acad Emerg Med 2:358-359, 1995. (abstract)

209. Epstein FB: Ketamine dissociative sedation in pediatric emergency medical practice, Am J Emerg Med 11:180-182, 1993.

210. Smith JA, Santer LJ: Respiratory arrest following intramuscular ketamine injection in a four year old child, Ann Emerg Med 22:613-615, 1993.

211. Biebuyck JF, Phil D: The nonhypnotic therapeutic applications of propofol, Anesthesiology 80;642-656, 1994.

212. Cauldwell CB, Fisher DM: Sedating pediatric patients: is Propofol a panacea? Radiology 186:9-10, 1993.

213. Bloomfield EL, Masaryk TJ, Caplin A, et al: Intravenous sedation for MR imaging of the brain and spine in children: Pentobarbital versus propofol, Radiology 186:93-97, 1993.

214. Kain ZN, Gaal DJ, Kain TS, Jaeger DD, Rimar S: A first-pass cost analysis of propofol versus barbiturates for children undergoing magnetic resonance imaging, Anesth Analg 79:1102-6, 1994.

215. Lebovic S, Reich DL, Steinberg LG, Vela FP, Silvay G: Comparison of propofol versus ketamine for anesthesia in pediatric patients undergoing cardiac catheterization. Anesth Analg 74:490-494, 1992.

216. Thal ER et al: Self-administered analgesia with nitrous oxide, JAMA 242:2418, 1979.

217. Amey BD, Ballinger JA, Harrison EE: Prehospital administration of nitrous oxide for control of pain, Ann Emerg Med 10:247, 1981.

218. Flomenbaum N et al: Self-administered nitrous oxide: an adjunct analgesic, JACEP 8:95, 1979.

219. Henderson JM et al: Administration of nitrous oxide to pediatric patients provides analgesia for venous cannulation, Anesth 72:269, 1990.

220. Griffin GC, Campbell VD, Jones R: Nitrous oxide-oxygen sedation for minor surgery: experience in a pediatric setting, JAMA 245:2411, 1981.

221. Smith C, Rowe RD, Vlad P: Sedation of children for cardiac catheterization with an ataractic mixture, Can Anes Soc J 5:35, 1958.

222. Terndrup TE, Cantor RM, Madden CM: Intramuscular meperidine, promethazine, and chlorpromazine: analysis of use and complications in 487 pediatric emergency department patients, Ann Emerg Med 18:528, 1989.

223. Saravia ME, Currie WR, Campbell RL: Cardiopulmonary parameters during meperidine, promethazine, and chlorpromazine sedation for pediatric dentistry, Anesth Prog 34:92, 1987.

224. Nahata MC, Clotz MA, Krogg EA: Adverse effects of meperidine, promethazine, and chlorpromazine for sedation in pediatric patients, Clin Pediatr (Phila) 24:558, 1985.

225. Cohen GH et al: Decorticate posture following 'cardiac cocktail': a transient complication of sedation for catheterization, Pediatr Cardiol 2:251, 1982.

226. Ros SP: Outpatient pediatric analgesia: a tale of two regimens, Pediatr Emerg Care 3:228, 1987.

227. Stambaugh JE and Wainer IW: Drug interaction: meperidine and chlorpromazine, a toxic combination, J Clin Pharmacol 21:140, 1981.

228. American Academy of Pediatrics, Committee on Drugs: Reappraisal of lytic cocktail/demerol, phenergan, and thorazine (DPT) for sedation of children, Pediatrics 95:598-602, 1995.

229. O'Brien JF, Falk JL, Carey BE, Malone LC: Rectal thiopental compared with intramuscular meperidine, promethazine, and chlorpromazine for pediatric sedation, Ann Emerg Med 20:644-647, 1991.

230. Graves D et al: Patient-controlled analgesia, Ann Intern Med 99:360, 1983.

231. Miser AW, Miser JS, Clark BS: Continuous intravenous infusion of morphine sulfate for control of severe pain in children with terminal malignancy, J Pediatr 96:930, 1980.

232. Cole TB et al: Intravenous narcotic therapy for children with severe sickle cell pain crisis, Am J Dis Child 140:1255, 1986.

233. Miser AW et al: Continuous subcutaneous infusion of morphine in children with cancer, Am J Dis Child 137:383, 1983.

234. Hendrickson M et al: Postoperative analgesia in children: a prospective study of intermittent intramuscular injection versus continuous intravenous infusion of morphine, J Pediatr Surg 25:185, 1990.

235. Bennett R et al: Patient-controlled analgesia, Ann Surg 195:700, 1982.

236. Bonadio WA: TAC: a review, Ped Emerg Care 5:128, 1989.

237. Bonadio WA and Wagner V: Efficacy of TAC topical anesthetic for repair of pediatric lacerations, Am J Dis Child 142:203, 1988.

238. Anderson AB et al: Local anesthesia in pediatric patients: topical TAC versus lidocaine, Ann Emerg Med 19:519, 1990.

239. Bonadio WA and Wagner V: Half-strength TAC for selected dermal lacerations in children, Clin Pediatr (Phila) 27:495, 1988.

240. Schatter DJ: Clinical comparison of TAC anesthetic solutions with and without cocaine, Ann Emerg Med 14:1077, 1985.

241. Hegenbarth MA et al: Comparison of topical tetracaine, adrenaline, and cocaine anesthesia with lidocaine infiltration for repair of lacerations in children, Ann Emerg Med 19:63, 1990.

242. White WB, Iserson KV, Criss E: Topical anesthesia for laceration repair: tetracaine versus TAC, Am J Emerg Med 4:319, 1986.

243. Ernst AE et al: Comparison of tetracaine, adrenaline, and cocaine with cocaine alone for topical anesthesia, Ann Emerg Med 19:51, 1990.

244. Pierluise GJ and Terndrup TE: Influence of topical anesthesia on sedation of pediatric emergency department patients with laceration, Pediatr Emerg Care 5:211, 1989.

245. Pryor GJ, Kilpatrick WR, Opp DR: Local anesthesia in minor lacerations: topical TAC vs. lidocaine infiltration, Ann Emerg Med 9:568, 1980.

246. Dailey RH: Fatality secondary to misuse of TAC solution, Ann Emerg Med 17:159, 1988.

247. Daya MR, Burton BT, Schleiss MR, DiLiberti JH: Recurrent seizure following mucosal application of TAC, Ann Emerg Med 17:646, 1988.

248. Mofenson HC and Caraccio TR: Tack up a warning on TAC, Am J Dis Child 143:519, 1989.

249. Wehner D and Hamilton GC: Seizures following topical application of local anesthetics to burn patients, Ann Emerg Med 13:456, 1984.

250. Lyman JL and McCabe JB: Improving the effectiveness of TAC application, Ann Emerg Med 13:642, 1984.

251. Fitzmaurice LS et al: TAC use and absorption of cocaine in a pediatric emergency department, Ann Emerg Med 19:515, 1990.

252. Altieri M, Bogema S, Schwartz RH: TAC topical anesthesia produces positive urine tests for cocaine, *Ann Emerg Med* 19:577, 1990.

253. Bonadio WA and Wagner V: Efficacy of tetracaine-adrenaline-cocaine topical anesthetic without tetracaine for facial laceration repair in children, *Pediatrics* 86:856, 1990.

254. Ordog GJ, Ordog C: The efficacy of TAC (tetracaine, adrenaline, and cocaine) with various wound-application durations, *Acad Emerg Med* 1:360-363, 1994.

255. Schilling CG, Bank DE, Borchert BA, Klatzko MD, Uden DL: Tetracaine, epinephrine, and cocaine (TAC) versus lidocaine, epinephrine, and tetracaine (LET) for anesthesia of lacerations in children, *Ann Emerg Med* 25:203-208, 1995.

256. Smith GA, Strausbaugh SO, Harbeck-Weber C: Comparison of topical anesthetics without cocaine to tetracaine-cocaine and lidocaine infiltration during repair of laceration, *Pediatrics* 97:301, 1996.

257. Hallen B, Olsson GL, Uppfeldt A: Pain-free venepuncture: effect of timing of application of local anaesthetic cream, *Anesthesia* 39:969, 1984.

258. Kapelushnik J et al: Evaluating the efficacy of EMLA in alleviating pain associated with lumbar puncture: comparison of open and double-blinded protocols in children, *Pain* 42:31, 1990.

259. Halperin DL et al: Topical skin anesthesia for venous, subcutaneous drug reservoir and lumbar punctures in children, *Pediatrics* 84:281, 1989.

260. Armstrong P and McKeown D: Ethyl chloride and venipuncture pain: a comparison with intradermal lidocaine, *Can J Anaesth* 37:656, 1990.

261. Zempsky WT, Karasic RB: Superiority of EMLA compared with TAC for topical anesthesia of extremity wounds in children (abstract), *Acad Emerg Med* 2427, 1995.

262. Edlich RF et al: Performance of disposable needle syringe systems for local anesthesia, *J Emerg Med* 5:83, 1987.

263. Christoph RA et al: Pain reduction in local anesthetic administration through pH buffering, *Ann Emerg Med* 17:117, 1988.

264. McKay W, Morris R, Mushlin P: Sodium bicarbonate attenuates pain on skin infiltration with lidocaine, with or without epinephrine, *Anesth Analg* 66:572, 1987.

265. Bartfield JM et al: Buffered versus plain lidocaine as a local anesthetic for simple laceration repair, *Ann Emerg Med* 19:1387, 1990.

266. Stewart JH et al: Neutralized lidocaine with epinephrine for local anesthesia: IId, *J Dermatol Surg Oncol* 16:842, 1990.

267. Waldbilig DK, Quinn JV, Stiell IG, et al: Randomized double-blind controlled trial comparing room temperature and heated lidocaine to digital nerve block, *Ann Emerg Med* 26:677, 1995.

268. Fell D et al: Paediatric postoperative analgesia: a comparison between caudal block and wound infiltration of local anaesthetic, *Anaesthesia* 43:107, 1988.

269. Langer JC, Shandling B, Rosenberg M: Intraoperative bupivacaine during outpatient hernia repair in children: a randomized double blind trial, *J Pediatr Surg* 22:267, 1987.

270. Copan LM, Patel KP, Turndorf A: Regional anesthesia. In Roberts JR and Hedges JR, editors: *Clinical procedures in emergency medicine*, Philadelphia, 1985, WB Saunders Co.

271. Abbaszadegan H and Jonsson U: Regional anesthesia preferable for Colles' fracture: controlled comparison with local anesthesia, *Acta Orthop Scand* 61:348, 1990.

272. Farrell RG, Swanson SL, Walter JR: Safe and effective IV regional anesthesia for use in the emergency department, *Ann Emerg Med* 14:239, 1985.

Recommendations

273. Fradet C et al: A prospective survey of reactions to blood tests by children and adolescents, *Pain* 40:53, 1990.

274. Goldberger J, Gaynard L, Wolfer J: Helping children cope with health-care procedures, *Contemp Pediatr* 3:141, 1990.

Appendix 7A: Blocks of the Upper Extremities

NORMAN C. CHRISTOPHER

For all except the most complex and extensive injuries, local infiltration into the wound margins provides adequate anesthesia for most procedures. However, this type of anesthesia is often less complete, more painful to administer, requires a larger volume of anesthetic, and may result in distortion of the involved soft tissues. Knowledge of the sensory innervation of the hand, aseptic technique, and the ability to perform a detailed physical examination of the hand are necessary.

DIGITAL BLOCK

Each finger is supplied by two sets of sensory nerves, the dorsal and palmar digital nerves, derived from either the ulnar and median nerves (palmar digital nerves) or the radial and ulnar nerves (dorsal digital nerves). Each of the sensory branches are easily accessed at the level of the web space, the intermetacarpal space, or along the digital shaft. Because the palmar branches innervating the middle three digits innervate the palmar, as well as the dorsal, aspects of the fingers (including the nail bed and the finger tip), infiltration of the dorsal branches is not required to achieve complete anesthesia of these digits.[1] Regarding the thumb and fifth finger, application of this technique is usually quite painful, and the resulting anesthesia is often incomplete (each of the four sensory branches must be blocked to achieve full anesthesia). Because of these factors, a more proximal regional block (at the level of the wrist) is often more desirable when anesthesia of either the thumb or fifth finger is required.[2]

Indications

- Repair/debridement of finger lacerations or amputations.
- Reduction of phalangeal fracture or dislocation.
- Incision and drainage of felon, paronychia.
- Removal of fingernails, repair of injured nail bed.

Technique

A careful neurologic examination of the injured finger(s) should be completed and documented in the chart before any procedure; abnormal findings should be discussed with the patient before instilling anesthetic agents.

The chosen infiltration site is cleaned with povidone-iodine solution. Either lidocaine (1% or 2% solution) or mepivacaine (2% solution) may be used. A 5 ml syringe and a 25- or 27-gauge needle should be used. Because of the risk of excessive distal vasoconstriction, epinephrine should be avoided in all digital blocks. The preferred needle insertion site is on the volar surface of the web space, directing the needle as in Fig. 7A-1, *A*. Injection on the palmar surface or on the ulnar and radial surfaces of each digit is more painful and is best avoided. Between 0.5 and 2 ml of the chosen anesthetic agent is infiltrated, first forming a wheal to block the dorsal digital nerve and then redirecting the needle to anesthetize the palmar branch. The anesthetic bolus should be directed toward the palmar surface of the metacarpal head, and a palpable mass of anesthetic agent should be felt on that surface of the hand. A slow rate of infiltration reduces distension of the adjacent soft tissues and lessens the pain. Vigorous rubbing of the injection sites after infiltration helps disperse the anesthetic agent and hastens the onset of action. A similar approach is used on the opposite side of the digit.

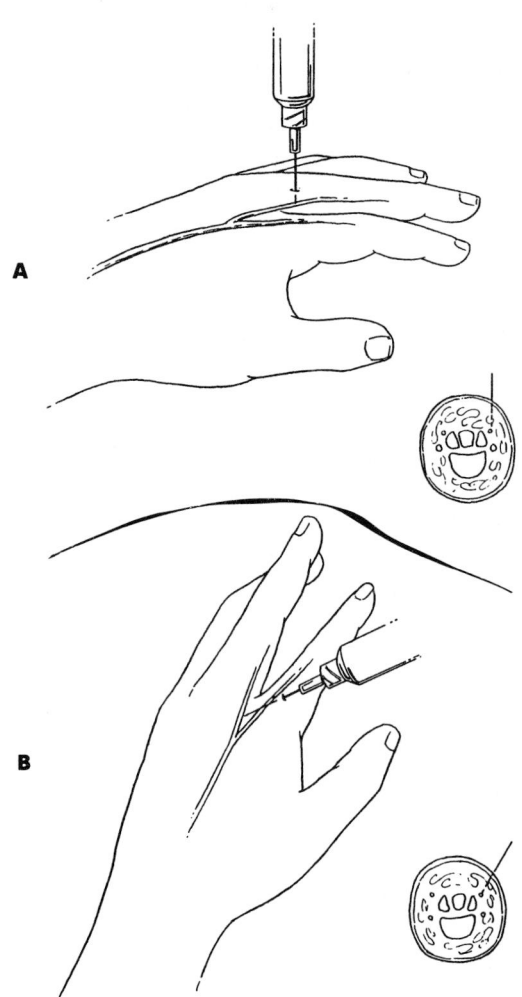

FIG. 7A-1. Digital block. **A,** After preparing the insertion site in a sterile fashion, insert the needle into the volar surface of the web space, directing the needle as shown in the insert. **B,** Alternative method for achieving digital block. (*Courtesy Kathleen M. Digney and The MetroHealth Medical Center, Cleveland, Ohio.*)

An alternative approach involves infiltration of the digital nerves as they enter the shaft of the involved digit. The needle is inserted at a 45-degree angle from the dorsal surface of the hand (Fig. 7A-1, *B*). First the dorsal digital nerve is blocked by infiltration of a wheal of anesthetic below the skin. The needle is then advanced while continuing to inject anesthetic solution until a wheal forms on the volar surface of the proximal digit.

Complications

- Arterial injection with distal vasoconstriction, vasospasm, and ischemia.
- Infection.
- Inadvertent administration of epinephrine, resulting in vasoconstriction and distal ischemia.
- Vasovagal response.
- Allergic reactions.

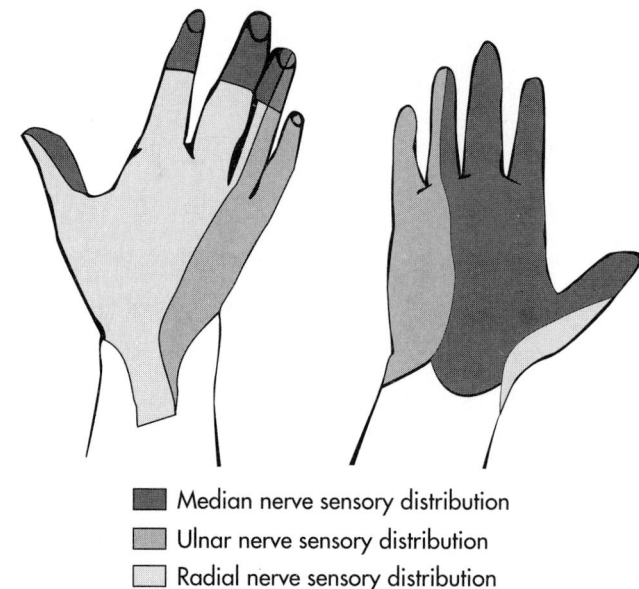

■ Median nerve sensory distribution
■ Ulnar nerve sensory distribution
□ Radial nerve sensory distribution

FIG. 7A-2. Wrist block. Distribution of sensory innervation of the hand. See code. (*Courtesy Kathleen M. Digney and The MetroHealth Medical Center, Cleveland, Ohio.*)

WRIST BLOCK

Knowledge of the topographic anatomy and of the sensory and motor innervation of the hand is required. The expected distributions of the median, radial, and ulnar nerves are shown in Fig. 7A-2. Each of these nerves is readily accessible from the volar side of the wrist and lies adjacent to readily identifiable structures. The major indication for a nerve block at the level of the wrist is the presence of an injury involving or crossing several sensory distributions (large lacerations of the hand, involvement of multiple digits, "road rash" or burns involving a large surface area of the hand). Regional anesthesia administered at this level is slower in onset than that after a digital block.

The chosen injection site should be prepared and cleansed. In most cases, a 3 to 5 ml syringe is adequate, and a 25- or 27-gauge needle should be used. Similar precautions regarding the use of epinephrine apply; it should be avoided. Complications are similar to those described for digital nerve blocks.

MEDIAN NERVE BLOCK

The median nerve lies directly below and lateral (radial) to the palmaris longus tendon (Fig. 7A-3, *A*). When this tendon is absent (as it is in 20% of the general population), the location of the median nerve may be approximated by measuring about 1 cm medially (ulnar) from the flexor carpi radialis. The palmaris longus tendon is best located by having the patient flex the wrist against resistance with the hand held tightly together in a fist (Fig. 7A-3, *B*). Once located, the injection site is cleansed as described previously. A ½-inch 25- or 27-gauge needle is advanced perpendicular to the volar surface of the wrist on the radial side of the palmaris longus tendon until the needle is felt to

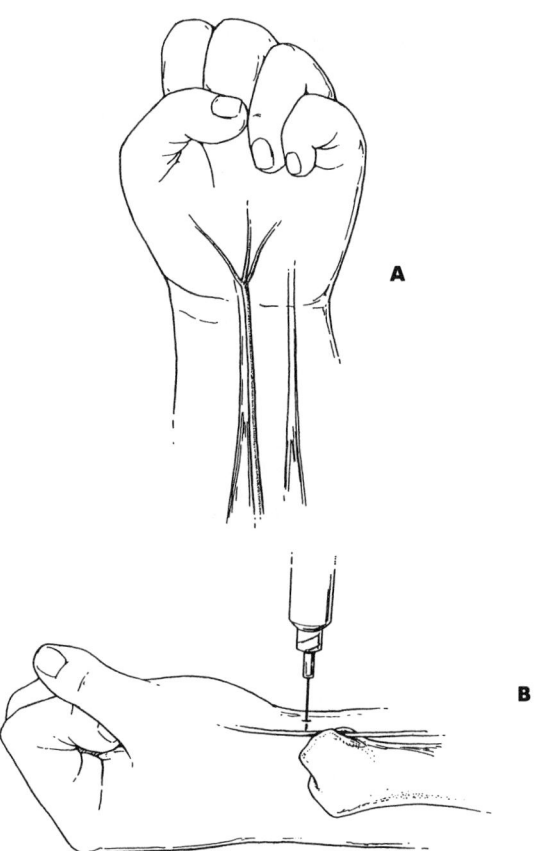

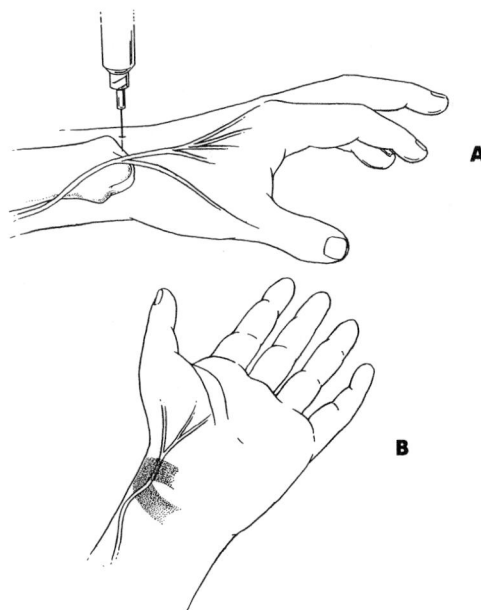

FIG. 7A-4. Radial nerve block. **A,** Preferred injection site for the radial nerve. **B,** Supplemental anesthesia of the smaller peripheral branches of the radial nerve. (*Courtesy Kathleen M. Digney and The MetroHealth Medical Center, Cleveland, Ohio.*)

FIG. 7A-3. Median nerve block. **A,** The position of the median nerve relative to the palmaris longus tendon and to the flexor carpi radialis tendon. **B,** Injection site for achieving median nerve block. (*Courtesy Kathleen M. Digney and The Metro-Health Medical Center, Cleveland, Ohio.*)

enter through the deep retinaculum. The operator should carefully withdraw through the syringe before injecting the anesthetic solution to minimize the risk of intravascular injection. If the anesthetic is injected into the *suprafacial* (subcutaneous) tissue space, only the superficial branch of the median nerve will be innervated, resulting in a poor anesthetic result. Between 2 to 5 ml of anesthetic is usually required to fully anesthetize the median nerve. Intraneural injection is not necessary nor is it desired—infiltration of the surrounding and adjacent soft tissues is adequate. If infiltration is met with high resistance, it may be assumed that a flexor tendon sheath has been inadvertently entered. Merely withdrawing and repositioning the needle remedies the situation.

RADIAL NERVE BLOCK

The major distal trunk of the radial nerve fails to extend into the wrist or hand but rather branches into several smaller peripheral nerves, which together innervate the dorsum of the hand (Fig. 7A-4, A). Block of the superficial branches of the radial nerve requires that anesthetic solution be infiltrated in a field adjacent to and encompassing

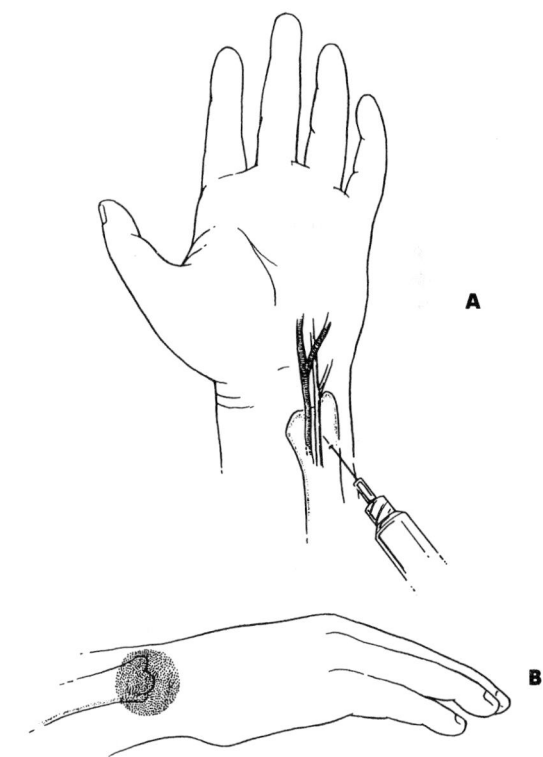

FIG. 7A-5. Ulnar nerve block. **A,** Anesthetic is injected to the radial aspect of the flexor carpi ulnarias tendon. **B,** Supplemental field block at the level of the ulnar styloid will anesthetize the smaller dorsal sensory branch of the ulnar nerve. (*Courtesy Kathleen M. Digney and The MetroHealth Medical Center, Cleveland, Ohio.*)

the expected course of these sensory nerves. Between 2 to 5 ml of anesthetic solution is injected at the level of the proximal palmar crease, just distal to the radial styloid and lateral to and at the same depth as the palpable radial pulse. Further superficial injection is required in a horseshoe distribution along the radial surface of the wrist (Fig. 7A-4, *B*). Caution should be used to avoid intravascular injection of the anesthetic solution.

ULNAR NERVE BLOCK

The ulnar nerve lies just lateral (radial) and deep to the flexor carpi ulnaris (FCU) tendon, its course closely approximating that of the ulnar artery. The FCU tendon inserts on the easily identified pisiform bone just distal to the distal palmar crease on the ulnar surface of the hand. Anesthetic is injected into the subfascial soft tissues at a site just radial to the FCU tendon. Caution should be taken to avoid injury to the adjacent ulnar artery.

An alternative approach is to insert the needle horizontally into the lateral surface of the ulnar aspect of the wrist at the level of the proximal palmar crease (Fig. 7A-5, *A*). Anesthetic solution should be injected below the FCU tendon at a depth that varies with the patient's size, with the needle directed toward the distal surface of the ulnar styloid.

Similar to the radial nerve, the ulnar nerve produces a smaller dorsalsensory branch that courses superficially just distal to the ulnar styloid in the dorsum of the wrist. If anesthesia of the dorsum of the fifth finger or of the dorsal surface of the ulnar side of the hand is required, then a field block at the level of the ulnar styloid is indicated (Fig. 7A-5, *B*).

References

1. Orlinsky M, Dean E: Local and topical anesthesia and nerve blocks of the thorax and extremities. In Roberts JR, Hedges JR, editors: *Clinical procedures in emergency medicine*, edz, Philadelphia, 1991, WB Saunders.
2. Carter PR: Common hand injuries and infections: a practical approach to early treatment, Philadelphia, 1983, W Saunders.

8

Death of a Child

Deborah Parkman Henderson

Mother, mother, I feel sick.
Send for the doctor, quick, quick, quick.
Doctor, doctor, shall I die?
Yes, my dear, and so shall I.
How many carriages shall I have?
One, two, three, four. . .
Skipping rhyme, 1800s

Most families today are wholly unprepared for the death of a child. Sudden death, whether from trauma or illness, comes as a tremendous shock; even a chronically ill child's death may come as a shock because there may have been several close calls before the death. Coping with the death of a child can also be particularly difficult for health-care professionals. The focus of medical education and training is on keeping patients alive; few residency programs allocate significant time to crisis counseling training.[1-3] In the emergency setting, even professionals experienced in coping with crisis situations can feel overwhelmed by the need first to deliver technical expertise and direction during an attempted resuscitation and then to provide support and comfort for the family when death occurs. Professionals may feel that they have failed in some way and may be in need of comforting themselves after such a painful and exhausting event.[4,5] Their own fears about death may also be brought to the surface.[6] An organized approach can

assure that all appropriate documentation is completed and necessary referrals are made (see box on p. 72).[7] Advance preparation through educational programs and effective use of community resources can greatly improve the care of families needing support during the initial stages of grief.

EPIDEMIOLOGY

The majority of deaths of infants (younger than 1 year of age) are from "natural" causes, such as SIDS, prematurity, congenital anomalies, and infections. As children grow and go out into the world, traumatic injury becomes the leading cause of death. Falls, motor-vehicle injuries, drowning, burns, and smoke inhalation are the most common causes of death for children older than 1 year; motor-vehicle deaths strongly predominate in the teenage years.[8] Each type of death presents a unique constellation of problems for families and for caregivers, but there are also many commonalities.

PREHOSPITAL CARE

Many children pronounced dead in urban and rural emergency departments were probably brought there by prehospital providers.[9] When a child is found lifeless in the prehospital setting, the first question for providers is whether to initiate CPR. In most EMS regions, providers are required to initiate CPR unless death is indisputable; the usual guidelines defining death are postmortem rigidity or lividity, decapitation, decomposition, or incineration.[10] Some EMS systems have developed protocols allowing providers some judgment calls.[11] Because the death of a child is a particularly sensitive incident, explicit protocols detailing circumstances in which death may be pronounced in the field should be developed for prehospital personnel. Prehospital personnel should also have training in how to provide support for the family when death is pronounced on-site.[12]

When a child is critically ill, rapid transport to the nearest appropriate facility will be necessary, and immediate action can be taken to try to save the child's life. Even when there is almost no possibility of resuscitation, as in the case of a child who has been apneic for an extended period, prehospital providers may decide to initiate CPR and transport the child to a health-care facility. In some cases, this results from the provider's (or the parents') reluctance to accept the death of the child. The availability of professional support available in the hospital may also be a consideration.[13]

Helpful Interventions After a Death in the Emergency Department

Initial contact with the family

- Introduce yourself; use their names *and* the child's name.
- Give accurate, honest information.
- Offer whatever privacy you can.
- Meet the family's physical needs; show them the location of bathroom, water, and tissues.
- Do not eliminate all hope while resuscitation is still underway.
- Ask about the need for clergy or religious rites.
- Continue to give *brief, frequent* updates.

Informing the family of the child's death

- Inform family as soon as possible.
- Sit down with the family.
- Use the words *death* or *died*.
- Give a *brief* explanation of the cause of death.
- Show the family that you care, and acknowledge their pain.
- Allow the family to express their emotions.
- Address the issues of pain and guilt.
- Allow sufficient time for questions.

Viewing the dead child

- Ask each family member separately if he or she wants to be with the child.
- Warn the family in advance about tubes and wires.
- Stay with the family for a short time initially, then check back with them.
- Allow as much time as is needed for the family to stay with their dead child.
- Check periodically to see whether the family is ready to leave.
- One staff member should remain in room with the child as the family leaves.

Most common questions asked by family members

1. *Most common, often unstated, question:* Was it my or our fault in some way?
2. Was there pain?
3. Why? (There is no appropriate answer.)
4. What will happen to the child now?
5. What should I or we tell children or siblings?
6. Should the children attend the funeral?
7. May we take our baby home? (Remember that parents have had full responsibility until now.)

Conclusion

- Discuss the possibility of organ donation.
- Explain to the family the necessity for or desirability of an autopsy.
- Provide written information about mortuaries and referrals for support.
- Complete all paperwork: release of the body, death certificate, organ donation, etc.
- Give the family the name of a staff member whom they can call if they have questions later.

Once resuscitation is underway, most parents maintain the panic-stricken hope that the child will survive, regardless of the child's condition. A brief explanation about treatment and transport should be given to them at the earliest moment possible. When there is sufficient personnel, this can be done by those not actively involved in the resuscitation. It is well known, however, that the prospect for a good outcome in cardiopulmonary arrest of children is dismal, and parents should not be given false hope.[10,14] Parental guilt is common, and parents should be reassured that it was not their fault, if this is appropriate.[15] In any case, providers should be careful not to add to a caretaker's sense of guilt. A brief history should be elicited, the position of the child noted, and a rapid assessment of the environment made. The possibility that nonaccidental trauma has occurred is a consideration, but the child's caretakers must not under any circumstances be treated with suspicion; judgmental or leading questions should be scrupulously avoided.[10]

Prehospital providers also care for patients under difficult conditions. They rarely have control over the immediate environment, and when a child is ill or injured, they are therefore often in charge of a multiple-casualty incident. Those needing care may include the child, the child's parents, siblings, other relatives, and sometimes concerned bystanders. It may be difficult to cope simultaneously with the psychosocial needs of the family members and the medical needs of the child. A calm family friend or other bystander may sometimes be of help; additional support should be called in if the scene is too chaotic. In most cases, rapid evacuation solves the problem. One or two family members should be allowed to accompany the child if there is room.

HOSPITAL CARE

Some of the most useful information about the way families respond to the death of a child, as well as helpful interventions, may be found in interviews with family members who have experienced such a loss.[16] If the family is not at the hospital when the child is brought in, informing them by telephone of the child's condition is the first step. While resuscitation is still underway, the parents should be told that the child is critically ill and that they must come to the hospital immediately.

Depending on the response of the parents, it may be possible to obtain some basic information such as the name of the child's physician, any history of illness, and the time of the child's last meal. Encourage the parents to find another person to drive, whenever possible, and recommend that they drive slowly. Ask if there is anyone else who they want to notify. At this point, parents rarely ask more questions about the child; if they do, simply tell them that they must come in as soon as possible and that giving information over the telephone may be too time consuming. It helps to be direct and give them the name of a specific staff person to ask for on arrival. Always repeat essential information, such as the name of the hospital, to make sure they understand.

When parents arrive in the acute-care setting, they should be shown to a quiet, private room. This may not be available, so any location away from the public may be used, such as an office, physician sleeping room, or even a corner of the waiting room.[7] Family members list privacy as a high priority; it is embarrassing for many people to display emotion in public.[16,17] Assign one person as liaison and slowly give the family some information about the child's condition. A brief statement is most helpful: "When your daughter was brought in, she was not breathing on her own and her heart was not beating. We are doing CPR and giving medications, but we are not seeing any improvement." This gives a clear picture, without totally eliminating hope. Giving accurate information, however painful, allows the family to prepare for the possibility of the child's death. Meeting the family's physical needs is a priority. Offer water or coffee, tissues, and a telephone; also indicate the location of the bathroom. If there is no staff member who can stay with the family in the waiting area, make sure the family receives updated information every few minutes.[18] Remember that 5 minutes can seem like an interminable period to parents waiting for news.[19] Many families are comforted by their religion; the clergy should be called if spiritual support is desired. If clergy is unavailable and the parents want a religious ceremony performed, a staff member with similar beliefs may be of assistance.

EMOTIONAL CARE OF THE PATIENT

When a child is dying, the medical focus can be so compelling that the child's emotional needs are overlooked. A dying child should be treated first and foremost as a living human being. Part of the focus on medical intervention, even when death appears to be inevitable, may be reluctance to admit such a defeat. Children 3 years old may have some understanding of the meaning of death, and even the most conservative thought is that children gain a clear understanding of the finality of death from 5 to 9 years of age.[20,21] Health-care professionals should be especially aware of this when a child is conscious and dying. Talking to the patient and providing an opportunity to talk about his or her fears may help to lessen the child's terrifying isolation.[22]

FAMILY PRESENCE IN THE TREATMENT ROOM

There are many arguments for and against family presence in the treatment room. Each emergency department should have a general policy addressing this issue, but many times the decision must be made on the basis of clinical judgment. Some parents are terrified and are unable to handle even minor trauma; others seem able to handle major trauma with relative ease. In a study of family members who were allowed to be present during the entire attempted resuscitation, 94% said they would participate again, and 35% felt they had a *right* to be in the treatment room during resuscitation. Most of the resuscitations in this study were unsuccessful, yet 64% of the family members felt they had actually been of help to the patient.[23] Because the family may be unaware that this could be their last chance to see their child alive, health-care professionals should very carefully consider their role in separating parent and child. Emergency department personnel might ask themselves how they would feel if it were their child. If family members are to be allowed in the room, one staff member should be in charge, walking in with the family, explaining procedures, and assisting them in departing.

INFORMING THE FAMILY

When a child dies, the family must be informed immediately. Preferably, they should be given this information by the highest level of professional available, usually the emergency physician.[24] A physician-nurse-social worker (or clergy) team is ideal to provide support. When parents are informed of a child's death, the word dead or *died* must be used; any other term is subject to misinterpretation. When parents are told the child is "gone," their response may be, "Gone where?" Euphemisms such as *passed on* and statements such as "We were not able to resuscitate your child" are often met with similar confusion. After the family has been told of the child's death, offering your presence—simply being available to absorb emotions—may be the most helpful intervention of all.[18,25] Show the family that you care, listen to them, and acknowledge their pain; their needs should be the focus. Most professionals want to do more, however, often because they need to feel useful. In attempting to comfort the family, there are several pitfalls that should be carefully avoided:

1. Do not say, "I know how you feel," because you really do not.
2. Do not tell the family that they can have other children, which assumes that children are interchangeable.
3. Do not inform them that they will feel better in a few weeks or months; they are desperately trying to survive the pain of the next few minutes.

A question frequently asked at this point is "Why did this happen?" This is best left unanswered because it is a philosophic question and the family will have to answer it for themselves. The most appropriate answer may be simply an expression of shared concern, "I wish I had an answer for you."[26]

THE GRIEVING PROCESS

Parents may react in many ways, according to their emotional makeup, culture, previous experiences, and relationship with the child.[27] Allow them to express their emotions without judgment; the grieving process takes many forms.[18] Each family member may respond differently; fathers may express their grief outwardly to a lesser extent and may be less able to ask for support.[24] They may also convert emotion to activity, whereas most mothers show more outward signs of grief and withdraw.[15] Some cultures consider public expression of grief as inappropriate, while others encourage unrestrained display of emotions, even to the point of physical self-abuse.[28,29] Personnel should be aware of the customs and rituals of the cultures they are likely to encounter in their area to understand grief reactions and intervene appropriately when necessary.

Elizabeth Kübler-Ross described grieving as a process that evolves in stages: denial, anger, bargaining, depression and, ultimately, acceptance.[30] These stages should be loosely interpreted; the sequence can progress irregularly, moving toward acceptance at times, with retreats into earlier stages at other times. The patient (if time allows), members of the family, and friends experience a variety of emotions but do not consistently progress systematically through these stages. The sudden death of a child does not allow for preparation, so health-care personnel rarely see the parents get past denial and anger, no matter if the death occurred in the prehospital setting, emergency department, acute-care center, or intensive care unit.

Health-care professionals are very concerned about bringing comfort to the family, as well as easing their own distress. As a result, families are sometimes encouraged to show signs of acceptance of the child's death sooner than they are able.[24] The process of grieving, however, takes its own time. It can be disturbing to listen to a mother who insists that her child is breathing or to a father who wants resuscitation to continue when there is no longer any reasonable hope. Denial is powerful and protective for these parents. It is only when denial persists over a period of time (days or weeks) that there should be concern. In the emergency setting, reality must be presented gently and consistently. Anger may be directed at health care professionals, other family members, God, and sometimes, the child. These emotions are part of the grieving process.

Parents may obsessively review the events before the child's death; this should be accepted as normal behavior and a means of moving toward acceptance.[18] They also will have many spoken and unspoken questions. There is almost always concern about whether the child suffered. If the child was unconscious on arrival, parents can be reassured that there was, as far as is known, no suffering. If it is known that there was pain, parents will often accept an indirect but honest answer: "It is hard to know how much pain a patient feels in these circumstances." If they continue to press for more information, questions should be answered as sensitively and straightforwardly as possible.

Guilt

Family members *invariably* feel responsible in some way for the child's death, even if there is no conceivable connection between their actions and the child's death.[19] Reassure parents that they were not in any way responsible, if this is the case. Parents who have some blame, as when there was inadequate supervision of the child, may obtain some comfort from recognizing that they did not intend harm. These parents will gradually have to accept their responsibility and learn to forgive themselves for making a mistake with such devastating consequences. It is essential to be supportive and nonjudgmental.

Holding the Dead Child

After the family's need for information has been satisfied, ask each parent separately whether they want to hold the child. Although not seeing the child's body may prolong grief, it is unwise to pressure reluctant family members; accept each person's decision.[18] Give them a general description of how the child looks; because many pediatric deaths are coroner's cases, give explicit instructions about not removing tubes and wires, when applicable. The child should be "cleaned-up" before being viewed. Parents should then be allowed to hold their child as long as they want to; this may last as long as a few minutes or several hours. The family may want to unwrap their child or clean his or her face or body; they should be allowed to do so when there are no legal barriers. Offer the parents a lock of the child's hair to keep, if they wish.[31,32] The parents should be reminded occasionally to let a staff member know when they are ready to leave because they may feel awkward about this. As they leave the area, one staff member should stay with the child while another helps the parents to the exit. Parents worry about leaving their child alone.

RELATED ISSUES

Organ Donation

Organ donation must be addressed when appropriate; health-care professionals are mandated to approach the family about this unless there are specific, well-documented reasons not to do so. Some states have legislation requiring health care providers to address this issue with families.[7] Despite the need, there is often hesitation about broaching the subject. Parents who have decided to donate their child's organs, however, have seen it as something positive resulting from their tragedy. When the question of organ donation is raised, it should be approached very gently and with utmost respect for the decision made. In some cases, a regional organ-procurement agency will come to the hospital to discuss this issue with the family.

Autopsy

When the death is a coroner's case, an autopsy is usually required. Autopsies may be advisable in cases that are (1) a result of trauma; (2) unexpected, including suspected SIDS; or (3) "suspicious, obscure, or otherwise unexplained."[7] In cases in which the coroner decides that an autopsy is not necessary and the emergency department physician wishes to have it performed, the family should be carefully approached for permission. Sometimes the statement that this may be of assistance to other families may be helpful; parents may also want to have some answers themselves.[32] The personal physician should be notified of the child's death and should be responsible for informing the family of the autopsy results.[7]

Siblings

Parents' questions of how to inform siblings of the child's death and whether to allow the siblings to see the dead child and attend the funeral are difficult to answer. There is much controversy about when young children should be included, but most experts agree that siblings must be informed honestly; when children are old enough to make choices, perhaps at 4 or 5 years of age, they should be allowed to make a decision themselves about whether they should attend the funeral.[21] The choice of whether siblings should see the dead child in the emergency department is complex; if the family has strong feelings one way or another, their decision must be respected.

Summary

What more can be done? Remember that you *cannot* make the parents feel any better. You *can* help by showing a caring attitude and making sure that the process flows as smoothly as possible. Forms must be filled out for release of the body and for autopsy; mortuary arrangements must be considered. Parents' ability to process information is very limited after the death of a child, and they will be unable to assimilate lengthy explanations or plan for anything other than the next few minutes.[1] It is useless therefore to inform parents how they will feel in a month or a year or to attempt to explain the grief process. Many parents find comfort with others who have experienced such a loss, so referrals to support groups such as the National SIDS Alliance (800-221-SIDS) may be given in written form.[1] Allow the family to take one small step at a time with ongoing support.

Effective intervention by emergency personnel in the death of a child can initiate the process of grieving, but additional questions will arise, so the family should be given the name of someone in the emergency department whom they can call for questions. The primary physician should also be notified of the death if this has not been done and the family referred for follow-up.[33]

ADVANCE PREPARATION IN THE EMERGENCY DEPARTMENT

To improve the care of grieving families in the emergency department, advance preparation can be helpful. Support teams and bereavement protocols can be set up, and written materials can be obtained from local resources such as the National SIDS Foundation and other support groups. The availability of clergy for referrals can be ascertained. Protocols and procedures for organ procurement can be developed, and a list of the local mortuaries and price lists can be made.[34] Emergency department personnel should become familiar with the state and local laws pertaining to sudden death, including the need for reporting to law enforcement departments, Child Protective Services, and the coroner's office or other agencies.[7]

Emergency department personnel are well aware of their need for education about death and dying; lack of training is perceived as a major factor in lack of confidence in death counseling.[2,35] Training and continuing-education programs should incorporate lectures and seminars; experiential learning, such as role playing and preceptoring, may also be used.[36] Regional organ-procurement agencies and child protective services are often willing to provide these educational programs.[2] Additional learning occurs with each experience; the degree of confidence in the ability to handle these situations is directly related to the frequency of such encounters.[1]

EFFECT ON HEALTH-CARE PROFESSIONALS

The death of a child takes a toll on emergency department and prehospital personnel. A sense of sadness for the loss along with frustration and a feeling of failure is experienced.[37] A pause for processing the event should be taken before returning to patient care; completing charts and cleaning the treatment room can serve this purpose. Talking about the death may help defuse emotions.[4]

The tendency to look for scapegoats is often present after the death of a child; this should be recognized as a way of venting anger and frustration; more constructive ways of expressing emotion should be found. Personnel working in emergency settings have found many ways of coping; discussing the death as a group, sharing experiences and emotions in a casual way, and using humor are all ways of allowing the healing process to begin. When the event is particularly overwhelming or involves the child of a staff member, professional intervention may be necessary, such as a critical-incident stress debriefing.[38]

CRITICAL-INCIDENT STRESS MANAGEMENT

The need for professional intervention depends on the degree of trauma experienced. Emergency personnel have rated the death of a child as the most critical of possible events, equal to the death of a co-worker.[38,39] The death of a child may bring to the surface their fears for their own children, concerns about their own mortality, survival guilt, or the anger and frustration that society is unable to protect the most vulnerable of its members. There may also be underlying discomfort that the profession they have chosen was impotent in the face of such a calamitous event.

The long-term psychologic effects of experiencing critical incidents have been recognized and described for many years, but it is only within the last two decades that the value of timely intervention for stress has been recognized. Mental health professionals are now routinely called in to assist with critical-incident stress management during disasters and other high-profile emergencies.

Critical-incident stress management is a useful format for handling the emotions resulting from a critical incident such as the death of a child. Emergency departments should have a program of peer training by mental health professionals, and be prepared to offer services adequate to assist personnel involved in critical incidents. The following two specific types of interventions are useful for coping with the death of a child.

Defusing. Defusing should take place within 12 hours after the critical incident; it is a brief (30 to 45 minute) informal meeting managed by peer support personnel or a mental health professional. A defusing allows brief ventilation of reactions to an incident, and may eliminate the need for a formal debriefing.[38]

Debriefing. A critical-incident stress debriefing (CISD) is a structured, confidential meeting that is offered after 24 hours and before 72 hours after a critical incident when personnel have been adversely affected by the event. The CISD team usually consists of four members including mental health professionals and trained peer counselors. The process begins with an introduction and explanation of ground rules. This is followed by the fact-finding phase in which each group member describes the incident from his/her own perspective, allowing participants to see the event as a whole. Group members are then encouraged to progress through three phases, describing their thoughts, reactions, and symptoms. In the next phase, CISD team members provide participants with information about stress reactions, what to expect, and how to alleviate symptoms. The process concludes with a "re-entry phase" in which any additional comments may be made, and CISD team members make a summary statement. Handouts with the telephone numbers of team members are given out, and team members are available for additional questions after the meeting.[38]

Emergency department managers can prevent some of the most damaging effects of stressful events by assuring adequate staffing, calling in additional help when needed, and encouraging emergency department personnel to take time for meals and breaks. It is important to remember that emergency personnel may also experience extreme stress from long term exposure to a moderate or low level of stress.[38] Above all, emergency department personnel should be made aware of the signs and symptoms of acute stress, and emergency department management should assure the availability of a CISD team prepared to cope with stressful events.

Emergency personnel should be as well prepared for the death of a child as they are for pediatric resuscitation. Advance planning should include development of protocols and procedures, training, preceptoring, and critical-incident stress management strategies.

Coping with the death of a child in the emergency department is a painful and challenging experience, but one that can provide a profound respect for humanity and the value of life.

References

1. Tolle SW, Elliot DL, Hickam DH: Physician attitudes and practices at the time of patient death, *Arch Intern Med* 144:2389, 1984.
2. Schmidt TA and Tolle SW: Emergency physicians' responses to families following patient death, *Ann Emerg Med* 19(2):125, 1990.
3. Greenberg LW, Ochsenschlager D, Cohen GJ, Einhorn AH, O'Donnell R: Counseling parents of a child dead on arrival: a survey of emergency departments, *Am J Emerg Med* 11(3):225, 1993.
4. Mandell F, McClain M, Reece RM: Sudden and unexpected death: the pediatricians response, *Am J Dis Child* 141:748, 1987.
5. Friedman GR, Franciosi RA, Drake RM: The effects of observed sudden infant death syndrome (SIDS) on hospital staff, *Pediatrics* 64(4):538, 1979.
6. Linn BS, Maravec J, Zeppa R: The impact of clinical experience on attitudes of junior medical students about death and dying, *J Med Ed* 57:684, 1982.
7. Committee on Pediatric Emergency Medicine: Death of a child in the emergency department, *Am Acad Ped* 93(5):861, 1993.

Epidemiology

8. Micik S, Yuwiler J, Walker C: *Preventing childhood injuries: a guide for public health agencies,* San Marcos, Calif, 1987, North County Health Services.

Prehospital Care

9. Gausche M, Seidel JS, Henderson DP, et al: Pediatric deaths and emergency medical services (EMS) in urban and rural areas, *Pediatr Emerg Care* 5(3):158, 1989.
10. American Academy of Orthopaedic Surgeons: *Emergency care and transportation of the sick and injured,* Menasha, Wis, 1987, The Academy.
11. Department of Health Services: *Los Angeles County Prehospital Care Manual,* Los Angeles, 1990, The Department.
12. Reigel, M and Barnes, D: A sensitive solution, *Emergency* 26(2):44, 1994.
13. Limerick S: Family and health-professional interactions, *Ann NY Acad Sci* 533:145, 1988.
14. American Heart Association and the American Academy of Pediatrics: *Textbook of pediatric advanced life support,* 1990, The Association.
15. Rando A: *Parental loss of a child,* Champaign, Ill, 1986, Research Press.

Hospital Care

16. Segal S, Fletcher M, Meekison WG: Survey of bereaved parents, *Can Med Assoc J* 134:38, 1986.
17. Lenaghan P: *Nursing interventions after sudden death in the ED,* Emergency Nurses Association Scientific Assembly, Boston, 1987 (abstract).
18. Dubin WR and Sarnoff JR: Sudden unexpected death: interventions with the survivors, *Ann Emerg Med* 15(1):54, 1986.
19. Hamilton G: Sudden death in the ED: telling the living, *Ann Emerg Med* 17(4):382, 1988.

Emotional Care of the Patient

20. Yalom I: *Existential psychotherapy,* New York, 1980, Basic Books.
21. National Institute of Mental Health, US Department of Health and Human Services, Public Health Service, Alcohol, Drug Abuse, and Mental Health Administration: *Talking to children about death,* DHHS Pub No (ADM)80-838, 1980.
22. Seravalli EP: The dying patient, the physician, and the fear of death, *N Engl J Med* 319(26):1728, 1988.

Family Presence in the Treatment Room

23. Doyle CJ, Post H, Burney RE, et al: Family participation during resuscitation: an option, *Ann Emerg Med* 16(6):673, 1987.

Informing the Family

24. Frader JE and Sargent J: Sudden death or catastrophic illness: family considerations. In Fleisher GR and Ludwig S, eds: *Textbook of pediatric emergency medicine,* Baltimore, 1983, Williams & Wilkins.
25. Walker KL: Easing the pain of bereaved parents, *Nursing 86,* April 1986, p 49.
26. Gutheil TG, Bursztajn H, Brodsky A: Malpractice prevention through the sharing of uncertainty, *N Engl J Med* 311:1, 1984.

The Grieving Process

27. daSilva G: Awareness of Hispanic cultural issues in the health care setting, *Childrens Health Care* 131:1, 1984.
28. Kleinman A: Selected issues in treating the Chinese patient, *Hospital physician* (7)58, 1982.
29. Thomas JD: Gypsies and American medical care, *Ann Emer Med* 102:842, 1985.
30. Kübler-Ross E: *On death and dying,* New York, 1969, Macmillan Publishing Co.
31. Hutti MH: Perinatal loss: assisting parents to cope, *J Emerg Nurs* 14(6):338, 1988.
32. Jezierski M: Infant death: guidelines for support of parents in the emergency department, *J Emerg Nurs* 15(6):475, 1989.

Related Issues

33. Breaking the worst news: when a child dies suddenly, *Emerg Med* March 30, 1989, p 74.

Advance Preparation in the Emergency Department

34. Merritt TA, Bauer WI, Hasselmeyer EG: Sudden infant death syndrome: the role of the emergency room physician, *Clin Pediatr* (Phila) 14(12):1095, 1975.
35. Coolican M, Vassar E, Grogan J: Helping survivors survive, *Nursing 89* August 1989, p 53.
36. Tolle SW, Cooney TE, Hickman DH: Program to teach residents humanistic skills for notifying survivors of a patient's death, *Acad Med* 64(9):505, 1989.

Effect on Health-Care Professionals

37. Soreff SM: Sudden death in the emergency department: a comprehensive approach for families, emergency medical technicians, and emergency department staff, *Crit Care Med* 7(7):321, 1979.

Critical-Incident Stress Management

38. Mitchell JT and Bray GP: *Emergency services stress,* Englewood Cliffs, NJ, 1990, Prentice-Hall.
39. Burns C and Harm NJ: Emergency nurses' perceptions of critical incidents and stress debriefing, *J Emerg Nurs* 19(5):431-436, 1993.

Continuous Quality Improvement

Eugene Izsak • L.A. Dandrea

ENSURING QUALITY IN THE EMERGENCY DEPARTMENT

The practice of setting standards for medical quality in the United States began early in the twentieth century. In 1907 the Flexner Report and the American Medical Association were instrumental in shutting down a large number of medical diploma mills. In 1914 Ernest Codman, M.D. delivered an address at the Frank H. Martin Clinical Congress of Surgeons of North America[1]:

"I am called eccentric for saying in public that hospitals if they wish to improve:

- Must find out what their results are
- Must analyze these results to find their strong and weak points
- Must compare the results with those of other hospitals
- Must care for what cases they can care for well and avoid attempting to care for those cases for which they are not qualified to care for
- Must assign the cases to members of the staff for better reasons than seniority, the calendar, or temporary convenience
- Must welcome publicity not only for their successes but their errors, so that the public may give them their help when it is needed
- Must promote members of the staff on a basis which gives due consideration to what they can do and accomplish for their patients

Such opinions will not be eccentric a few years hence."

Avedis Donabedian, in the mid-1960s, outlined three fundamental components in the evaluation of health care: structure—facilities, personnel, equipment, and services; process—the delivery of medical care; and outcome—which are measures of the results of care such as cost, satisfaction and effectiveness.[1]

With the creation of The Joint Commission on Accreditation of Hospitals (JCAH) in the 1950s, major advances in quality assurance have been made. First, there were implicit reviews such as morbidity and mortality reviews that enabled hospitals to demonstrate the delivery of optimal patient care. Next, in 1975, JCAH required institutions to demonstrate that quality was optimal by a process of continual review using explicit and measurable criteria in audits that were care focused and retrospective. This gave way in 1979 to Quality Assurance (QA) standards that focused on the care of individual practitioners. These standards focused on problem areas. In 1985, the standards were again amended to require a systematic, ongoing monitoring and evaluation of patient care. To this aim the "10-step process" (see box on p. 78) was developed, which is more or less a road map in assuring quality in the clinical setting.[2]

Other attempts at assuring quality have met with mixed results. Some of these have yielded useful data about problematic areas and have pointed out areas and individuals of concern; however, the data generated are sometimes late, subjective, or dealt with ineffectively[3] (see box on p. 78).

The QA process remains an important aspect of managing quality in the health-care setting today. The Joint Commission on Accreditation of Healthcare Organizations (JCAHO), formerly the JCAH, now requires that QA systems actually focus on improving the overall quality of health care, rather than just monitoring to assure quality. Thus, the 1992 JCAHO Accreditation Manual changed its focus from QA to Continuous Quality Improvement (CQI).[4]

TOTAL QUALITY MANAGEMENT AND CONTINUOUS QUALITY IMPROVEMENT

CQI is both a philosophic and a methodologic process based on the work of J. Edwards Deming, Joseph Juran, and Walter Shewhart. The philosophy of CQI is contrasted to traditional management styles. Traditional management used authority, inspection, crisis management, and blame to root out problems with producing a good or service. Essentially, if something went wrong it was the manager's responsibility to find out "who" was to blame. This method of management looked at the worker as the cause of deviation from the expected and not at the process itself. Deming contended that 85% of problems are due to faults in the system and not the individual worker.[1] The basic assumption of traditional management is that the system is sound; therefore it is the manager's job to root out the "bad apples" when problems arise.[5]

Traditional QA programs looked to identify bad outcomes and avoid them in the future. This process got rid of the "bad apples" but failed to improve the system as a whole.

The CQI process attempts to continually move the mean in a positive or improved direction by improving the system as a whole (Fig. 9-1).

10-Step Process

1. Assign responsibility.
2. Delineate scope of care.
3. Identify major aspects of care.
4. Identify indicators.
5. Establish thresholds for evaluation.
6. Collect and organize data for each established indicator.
7. Evaluate care.
8. Take actions to solve identified problems and to improve care.
9. Assess actions and document improvement.
10. Communicate information to appropriate parties.

Methods of Medical Quality Assurance

1. Professional credentialing.
2. Mortality and morbidity review.
3. Criteria audits.
4. Autopsy.
5. Tissue audits.
6. Utilization review.
7. Patient satisfaction surveys.
8. Incident reporting.
9. Coroner investigations.
10. Hospital accreditation.
11. Practice guidelines.
12. Random audits.
13. Occurrence screening.
14. Total quality management or continuous quality improvement.

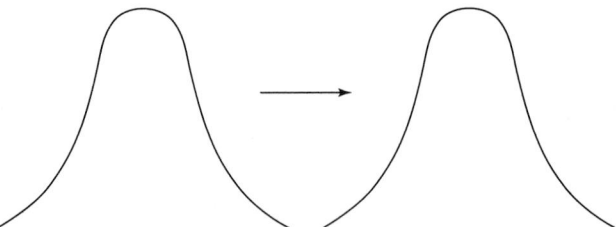

FIG. 9-1. The CQI process shifts the entire curve to the right (improvement) rather than focusing on the outlyers (bad apples).

CQI is best understood by reviewing the philosophies of J. Edwards Deming who believed that managers needed to recognize the customers' needs and work toward constantly improving the products or services they supplied and to use a statistical approach in the process of improvement. Deming felt that improving quality would lower costs because there would be less spent on correcting mistakes and more efficient use of time, materials, and personnel, thereby improving productivity. He also felt that the worker is an important part of the success of the process and not the cause of its problems.[5]

Deming's philosophy can be summarized by his 14 points:

1. Create constancy of purpose for improvement.
2. Adopt a new philosophy of allowing zero defects.
3. Cease dependence on inspection as a means of eliminating poor quality.
4. End the practice of awarding business on price alone.
5. Improve service continuously.
6. Institute training.
7. Institute leadership.
8. Drive out fear.
9. Breakdown barriers between staff.
10. Eliminate posters and slogans.
11. Eliminate numeric quotas—use statistical methods.
12. Remove barriers to pride in workmanship.
13. Provide ongoing training and retraining.
14. Take action to accomplish the transformation by defining management's commitment to quality.

THE CQI APPROACH

A basic precept in CQI is that the process is statistically driven. In other words, hard data lead us through the steps of CQI. The four steps are generally adapted from the Shewhart cycle and are known as the Plan, Do, Check, and Act (PDCA) cycle. Simply stated, during this cycle a process needing to be fixed will be studied and a plan for change is made. Following implementation of these customer-driven changes,[3] data are collected to ascertain the effects of the change. The check process compares original data with the new data to see if progress toward the improvement goal has been made. Finally, the entire process and data are used to continually refine and improve the system to further meet the customers' expectations.

The CQI process can best be broken down to the following seven-step process[7]:

The CQI philosophy begins to answer some very fundamental questions in the production of goods and services. First, what is quality? This can be defined as meeting or exceeding the customers' expectations.[6] Note that this definition is driven by the consumer and not the supplier of the goods or service. The Japanese auto manufacturers outmaneuvered the US manufacturers by building cars that the American public wanted, not what the manufacturer wanted. The Japanese realized that quality is a perception and is based on the interaction between the customer and the product.

Second, who is the customer? This can be defined as whoever is next in the process. In this regard, customers may be internal, such as emergency physicians are customers of the triage nurse, or external, such as our patients and their families.[3] Put another way a customer is "any entity, whether an individual or institution, that has a stake in the operations or product of the process and that customers' concerns and requirements define quality."[1]

1. *Reason for improvement.* This is the decision on what to fix and why. Obviously, there are many problems that need resolution. A team identifies a problem that not only needs improvement but that also has a significant impact on the customer. Potential problems may be identified through ongoing audits, QA indicators, surveys of customers (GAP analysis), or brainstorming. Once this step is finished, the CQI team will have focused on one problem for resolution that has the greatest impact on customer satisfaction. The process must be further broken down to its component steps to better understand how the job under investigation is performed. Finally, an indicator must be selected that measures the "production" of the current process, as well as its efficiency or lack thereof.

An example of a theme or set of problems that might be identified in the emergency medicine setting would be throughput time of patients. Through brainstorming this major problem could be broken down to its various components. During this step, flow charting is used to define how the job is currently done and finally an indicator is developed to track progress. In this example, time from triage to discharge is determined.

2. *Current situation.* The objective of this step is for the CQI team to select a specific problem and establish a target for improvement. The focus is now even further narrowed from what needs improvement to a specific problem that will accomplish this improvement. The team also collects and analyzes data to determine the validity of the problem.

The next step is to determine the causes for the majority of the problem. A Pareto analysis, based on the rule that 80% of the problems are due to 20% of the causes, gives insight to which causes will do the most for solving the problem. The Pareto chart helps to graphically illustrate this concept (Fig. 9-2).

Finally, a problem statement is drafted that clearly states the issues and "what" is wrong. This statement does not imply solution but instead states the team's findings. Solutions are formulated in later steps. The statement focuses on the differences between the current and improved situation. It must be stated in a specific and positive manner, avoiding ambiguities and highlighting how the customer is affected.

In the example chosen, throughput time, the team will focus on the various components that make up this rather broad topic. Using the Pareto chart, 80% of the wait can be attributed to the first three steps in the throughput process.

3. *Analysis.* It is during this step that the causes of the problem are identified. A useful tool for this is the cause and effect or fishbone (Ishikawa) diagram. This provides a meaningful picture of the potential causes of the problem (effect) and how they relate to each other. Most causes can be grouped under the five general areas of management, materials, methods, machines, and manpower (or people) and are known as assignable causes and have the ability to be corrected. Chance causes are those we have no control over but are often identified in old-style QA programs. Once the total picture is finished, it is time to identify the most significant causes of the variances that are verified using data gathered. This ensures that those chosen are truly significant.

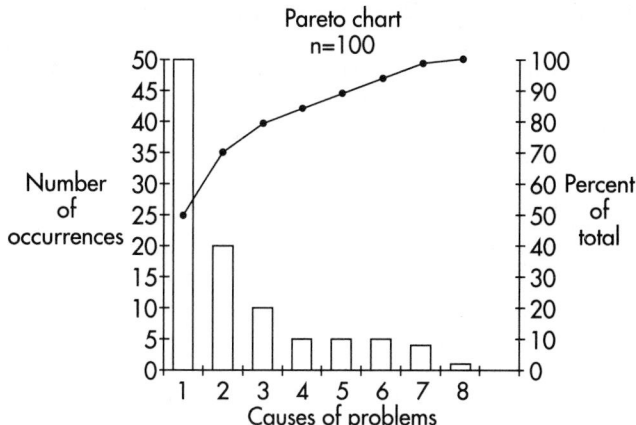

FIG. 9-2. Pareto Chart based upon the rule that 80% of the problems are due to 20% of the causes.

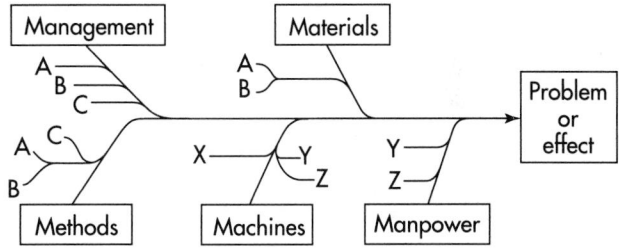

FIG. 9-3. Ishikarta (fishbone) diagram demonstrating contributing factors of a problem or effect.

The fishbone diagram for our example might look something like Fig. 9-3. This diagram is generated by the group to ensure all the root causes are identified.

4. *Countermeasures.* During this phase the team identifies countermeasures or proposed solutions aimed at correcting the root causes of the problem identified. These countermeasures must attack the root causes, meet customer's demands, and be cost-effective. Various tools are available to help during this step. One tool, the countermeasure matrix, helps define the relationship between problem and proposed solutions in a meaningful way. Other useful tools are the barrier and aid analysis, as well as a cost-estimation analysis. The final objective of this step is to develop an action plan noting the tasks that need to be completed to map out the steps in implementing the countermeasure.

This step might be termed the strategic plan, where all the implementation problems are identified and potential cost benefits are analyzed. A "road map" to implementation is produced to better effect the proposed change.

5. *Results.* During this step the team confirms that the implemented solution has indeed accomplished what it was supposed to do. Using the same indicator developed in step 1 the team compares results generated after implementation of the countermeasure to the earlier results. Data are displayed using various types of graphs, including

a control chart that helps make sure that continued problem resolution occurs.

In essence, if throughput time has been decreased this should be easily measured by comparing new data with the previously collected data in step 1.

6. *Standardization.* Once the results step has proven that there was success in correcting the problem, the standardization step now implements the countermeasure into the system. This is done by retraining the work force, revising processes, and changing standards. Periodic checks are established to monitor progress and to ensure there is no slippage from the stated objectives.

Basically stated, if the "fix" works, it should be introduced into the system at large; however, if there was no demonstrable improvement, then the group must look back to earlier steps.

7. *Future plans.* It is during this step that the team not only plans actions on remaining problems but also evaluates its own effectiveness in using the CQI process. Asking such questions as "'What was done well? What could be improved? What could be done differently?'" the team is better able to build on its experience with the CQI process.

The seven steps of the CQI process not only look for problems in the system rather than singling out the individual worker as the problem but also use and value the individuals intimate with the processes that need attention. It is management's job to be sure the team has the training, resources, and freedom to accomplish the task of quality improvement.

References

1. Siegel DM and Crocker PJ: *Continuous quality improvement for emergency departments,* Dallas, 1994, ACEP.
2. Booth FV McL: ABCs of quality assurance, *Crit Care Clin* 9:477, 1993.
3. Wolff AM: A review of methods used for medical quality assurance in hospital: advantages and disadvantages, *J Qual Clin Prac* 14:85, 1994.
4. The Joint Commission on Accreditation of Healthcare Organizations: *Comprehensive accreditation manual for hospitals,* Oakbrook Terrace, Ill, 1994, The Commission.
5. Mayer TA: Industrial models of continuous quality improvement, *Emer Med Clin N Am* 10:523, 1992.
6. McBurney BH and Schultz C: Defining quality services in a general pediatric unit, *J Nurs Care Qual* 7:51, 1993.
7. Klepcyk JC: Total quality management: defining a process for quality improvement, *Top Hosp Pharm Manage* 12:26, 1993.

Legal Issues

Mitchell B. Cordover

WHAT ARE LEGAL ISSUES?

There are three broad areas of legal risk in the practice of medicine. Medical malpractice liability is the most common concern. In the unique and intimate interaction between doctor and patient, however, physicians have general liability as well. This general liability includes such acts as intentionally causing the patient emotional distress, assaulting him or her, or abridging his or her rights. There are also state and federal statutes that specify the physician's responsibility to the patient and to the health of the public at large. Fines and other repercussions of breaking the law represent a statutory liability. Although "legal issues" may show up in the course of a malpractice action, they are sufficiently distinct from "risk management issues" and they warrant separate discussion.

Under the law, a duty is owed to any potential plaintiff to act in a prudent and reasonable manner. If you fail to de-ice your front steps, it can be argued that you failed your duty to the mailman who slips on them. In medicine this includes not only the responsibility to practice within the community standard of medical care but also to know and respect the rights and prerogatives of the patient. In pediatrics, these include the rights of parents. Parental consent, emancipation, competence, and so on are all questions of general liability.

There is a rich body of public health law covering everything from reporting dog bites to testing for AIDS. The Emergency Medical Treatment and Active Labor Act (EMTALA) subsumes all of the relevant sections of the Social Security Act passed as parts of the (Consolidated) Omnibus Budget Reconciliation Acts (COBRA) between 1985 and 1990. Along with its regulations, EMTALA is a detailed legal mandate that establishes the rights of patients to emergency care. It is a federal law, but it has found its way into state actions by providing clear definitions about the responsibility of staff and facilities. It is one of the most significant forces shaping the provision of emergency medicine in modern times.

Legal decisions are seldom simple. The court must make decisions about the interpretation and applicability of the law as it applies to each situation. Each set of facts is more or less unique, and disagreements often arise about whether one or another legal precedent fits the facts of the case at issue. While this chapter cannot offer a firm and reliable set of protective rules, it can provide an introduction to the legal theories that are the substance of the arguments.

In truth, knowing the law is not complete protection. Which arguments a jury will find compelling and where its sympathy will lie are matters that are far less predictable than the law. Two pieces of advice seem germane: Consider what the lay public will think of what you do, and the surest way to win is to avoid the courtroom in the first place.

THE DUTY TO TREAT, THE RIGHT TO REFUSE

One can only be sued by a party to whom one has a duty or responsibility.[1,2] The emergency physician has a duty to see and treat everyone in the emergency department. When does the duty to treat outweigh the right of a parent to give or withhold consent? Does it outweigh the right of a minor patient to request or refuse care? What is the duty to protect children? How vulnerable is the doctor to allegations of medical battery while protecting an unwilling patient?

Generally, the emergency physician has a duty to any individual who presents for examination or treatment of a medical condition.[3] There are cases where the doctor was held liable for a patient in the department without his knowledge.[4] It can be argued that the physician knows or SHOULD KNOW about everyone present. Emergency physicians do not have the same luxury as those practicing in private offices, who can accept or refuse to enter into a doctor-patient relationship.

The duty to examine and treat extends to patients in the department who are waiting for their private physician. While it can be argued that such a patient was under the care of another physician, as though in the waiting room of a private office, duty is always seen as resting with the hospital and thus with the physician responsible for seeing emergency patients.[5] Federal law requires the hospital to provide a screening examination (see EMTALA).

The safest practice might be to know the vital signs and chief complaint of these patients, even when they decline your care to wait for their private physician. Whether or not they are charged for an emergency department visit, it is well worth noting on their chart that they were in no acute distress. It is doubtful that one can escape liability by avoiding the patient altogether.

Patients have the right to refuse your care while awaiting their private doctor.[6-8] However, the decision to refuse will only relieve you of liability if it is an informed one,[9-11] and it will not be considered so without input from a health practitioner. It can be alleged that if the patient had known how serious his or her condition was he or she would have been seen by the emergency department physician rather than wait.

Adult patients have the right to refuse medical care for themselves[12] and within limits for their children. This is true even for lifesaving interventions, although the court is likely to overturn the rights of the parents if the well-being of a child is at risk.[6] As a rule if a person is otherwise competent, refusing medical care does not define that person as incompetent.[7] Because only competent parents have the presumptive right to decide about their children's care, it is key to determine who is competent.

Competence

For the purposes of medical decision making, competence is defined as the ability to fully appreciate the nature of one's condition, the diagnostic and therapeutic options available, and the consequences of these options, including no intervention.[6,9,10,13] It is an entirely clinical standard. There is no alcohol level or drug test that defines one as incompetent, although it may be more difficult to argue that a patient was competent in the face of a recent elevated alcohol level.

A determination of competence can be difficult. For example, does an inebriated parent who can parrot back your words fully appreciate the alternatives when they angrily refuse care for a child who has a potentially disfiguring laceration? Getting a second opinion on competence is worthwhile. This need not be from a psychiatrist. A fellow physician, nursing supervisor, or staff nurse can help

serve to support the determination. Obviously, documentation is critical here.

Certain conditions automatically define one as incompetent. There is a duty to protect patients who attempt suicide,[14] are psychotic, or *clinically* disabled by intoxication, trauma, and so on, regardless of their protestations.[6,15-17] Likewise, medically incompetent parents cannot direct the emergency medical care of their children.[6] The issue of who can act in the parent's place is discussed below.

Leaving Against Medical Advice

With the exception that the state can intervene in the best interests of the child, competent adults can sign themselves and their children out of the emergency department against medical advice. Because the parent's decision only shields the doctor from liability if it is a fully informed choice, documenting the following is essential:

1. The determination that the parent is clinically competent.
2. The options available to the patient and the warnings associated with refusing care.
3. The signature of the person who witnessed your warnings.
4. The nature of the patient's (parent's) response.

The signature on the warnings may prevent the parent from later denying he or she was informed. A signed blanket statement about leaving against advice, however, will not withstand a detailed challenge about what the patient actually understood.[18]

However useful the paper work may be, it is the quality of the patient evaluation and the appropriateness of care that are most important in determining any legal outcome.

Always involve family and friends in an attempt to influence the parents. It can be useful for family members to witness the warnings. On the practical level, they may support your recommendations and prevent the patient from leaving. In court, they represent credible witnesses because they are not defendants. The nurse should make a separate and corroborating note specifying the nature of the warnings.

Competent adults also have rights over medical information about themselves and their children. While no one can require the abridgment or falsification of the medical record, they can limit the distribution of that record.[6,19] Adults can refuse the doctor permission to discuss their personal condition with their spouse, but both parents have the right to know about their children. Whether a biologic parent has the right to clinical information about a child no longer in his or her custody is not clear. In most instances, there is no reason not to inform the estranged parent unless the guardian instructs you otherwise.

The Rights of Minors

Minors are incompetent by law.[6,20] They have no right to consent or withhold consent for treatment. Most state laws allow them to request or refuse intervention only under very specialized circumstances. The age of consent varies widely from state to state. Although it is not clear whether a request from a minor triggers the federal mandate to perform a screening medical examination and subsequent stabilization (EMTALA), if it did the federal requirement would supersede state laws. It is wise to provide every patient with a complaint-appropriate screening examination, whether or not they are of age to legally consent to care.

"In loco parentis" (in the position of the parent) is a very useful legal concept in emergency pediatrics. Naturally, the biologic parents are in loco parentis, when available. In their absence, relatives do not necessarily take their place. States vary in who they allow to act as temporary legal guardian in the case of a medical emergency.[21,22] In all states, however, legal guardianship may be assigned by the court or temporarily assigned to an adult by the parent through a written note.[6,10,15] When the school nurse or baby-sitter presents a handwritten note from mom, it represents the assignment of "in loco parentis." The best practice is, of course, to document a reasonably diligent search for a true parent.[23]

There is always somebody in loco parentis.[24] As a last resort, the state (through the courts) maintains the right to intervene on behalf of the child.[6,25] In most places, that right is conferred to an agency such as Family Services or, in the case of an emergency, to a treating physician. In most hospitals, that right has been delegated to an "administrator on call." Last, the EMTALA statute gives the hospital the duty to examine and stabilize any person if they request or if "a request is made on their behalf" for medical care. There is no mention of guardianship.

Both practically and legally, there is seldom an excuse for withholding care from a minor.[10,24,25] If a parent is not available or the guardianship of a presenting adult is in question, physicians themselves may act on behalf of the child or may have the hospital administrator take responsibility. The parent may refuse financial responsibility for a visit they did not personally approve, although some states have doctrines that hold them financially liable. This financial consideration does not mitigate the duty to provide care or change the standard of the care delivered. It may come to a choice between a complaint about treating a child without permission or a jury trial about a bad outcome. It has been reported that no physician has been successfully sued for providing care without parental permission for over 30 years.[10,24]

Teenagers often refuse care when they are brought in by their parents. It is common for a parent to demand drug testing on their child, which the child subsequently refuses. Two separate questions of duty are embodied in this situation. The emergency physician does not have a duty to provide any test that a layman demands. A physician's license gives him or her a special right to order laboratory tests. Unlicensed patients do not have the right to demand a specific work-up. Drug testing should be done only for medical reasons.[26]

Second, except in certain defined circumstances, an underage person does not have the legal right to refuse the care requested for them by a competent guardian (otherwise, no child would ever receive an injection). However, in obtaining the guardians' permission to treat, it may be important to carefully warn them that drawing blood on an uncooperative and struggling person may cause some minor injury. Likewise, for urinary catheterizing the patient.

An informed consent in this circumstance is advisable, even if the same procedure would not require one otherwise.[26,27]

There are statutes in every state allowing the use of restraining force on incompetent patients and children.[28] There is a trend in some jurisdictions to recognize certain minors as "mature" and thus able to request care without being legally "emancipated." Likewise, there is a growing sentiment in pediatrics to provide older teens with a level of respect and autonomy that goes contrary to drawing blood and urine against the patient's will. This faction would warn against the loss of confidence the teenage patient would experience and the possible loss of the patient from the health-care system. However good this rationale may be, this is the law in very few locations.[27]

Whether you or the parent is acting in loco parentis, one's duty is to act reasonably and in the minor's best behalf. This will be measured by determining that the risk to the patient of performing a certain test or intervention is clearly outweighed by its benefits. For example, a reasonable parent might refuse an intravenous pyelogram (IVP) on a minor with sudden onset of flank pain. If we are acting in the place of the parent, we may be called on to explain why we performed an IVP, if an allergic reaction occurs.[6,27]

Limitations of the Rights of Parents

The reverse situation is also true. Parents do not have an unchallenged right to withhold lifesaving therapy from their children.[6] The Supreme Court has dealt with this issue. State courts have the right to intervene into the special relationship between a parent and child on behalf of the child. Child labor laws are the most common example of this. This rule applies in the face of religious preferences (e.g., the Jehovah's Witness conviction about blood transfusions).

In these cases, the physician must usurp the position of the parent.[29-32] Most hospitals have experience in and are already well-organized for this eventuality. Admitting suspected victims of child abuse, initiating IV therapy, or even giving antibiotics to meningitis cases against the protest of parents are not uncommon occurrences. Federal law specifically requires the protection of handicapped children.[33] While the hospital administrator and attorney may ultimately need to obtain a court order, one need not withhold emergent therapy while awaiting the slow turning of the wheels of the legal system.

Emancipated Minors

There is a class of minors that have the right to consent or withhold consent for treatment of themselves and their children.[17] They are usually referred to as "emancipated." While not perfectly consistent from state to state, the usual elements of emancipation are married and living independently; or pregnant or the primary caretaker of a minor child; or a member of the United States military living out of the parent's home; or living away from home *and* self-sufficient. In some states, this last circumstance makes a minor eligible for emancipation, but a court order is required to make the patient fully emancipated.[6,25,34]

There was a time when every state agreed that minors could be treated for conditions involving pregnancy, venereal disease, and birth control without the involvement of their parent. The last decade has seen a strong conservative trend in regard to matters in women's reproductive rights and public health. It is well worth researching your state's position on these three controversial issues.

Presumed Consent

An important doctrine in the emergency department is "Presumed Consent."[15,35-36] Patients that are unconscious or incompetent or children whose parents are not present (outside of the issue of in loco parentis) may be treated without hesitation[6,21] for a medical emergency. As an outgrowth of the "reasonable man" theory of law, we can presume that a reasonable person would want us to intervene on their best behalf, when they are unable to tell us otherwise.[17]

Most courts have adopted a very broad and generous definition of emergency. Virtually any condition that has the potential of becoming a threat to life, limb, or any bodily function can be treated as an emergency under presumed consent.

Even if the parents are known to have refused care for their child in the past, or if the guardian is not present or is incompetent, one may presume that they would take the "reasonable" course of action. It is, of course, important for the emergency department staff to check with a patient's relatives' or parents' personal effects to be sure that there are no written instructions about the parents' preferences. If, while alert and competent, a legal guardian (or parent) records *in writing* that he or she does not want resuscitation, blood transfusions, intubation, or so on for the child, then that choice must be acknowledged. Whether the physician should accept the word of a family member or not is a matter of circumstance and the credibility of the informant. Where there is such doubt or the written decision is not in the best interest of the child, the pediatrician in the emergency department should take steps to ensure that the decision is a fully informed one. One might remind the adult of the permanent consequences of certain decisions. One can always pull an endotracheal tube later, but once the patient is dead the subsequent choices are nonexistent.

A patient's permission to treat can be quite specific. While the patient does not have the right to design his or her own diagnostic and therapeutic course, the emergency physician does have a duty to treat the patient *to the extent to which the patient will allow them to treat*. If, for example, a patient who requires hospitalization for IV therapy will accept only outpatient antibiotics, and if outpatient therapy is a viable (if not ideal) alternative, then the patient has a right to opt for it. Once again, careful documentation may be protective.

The patient need not sign out against medical advice to choose among reasonable alternatives. To make an informed choice, however, the nature and likelihood of the consequences will have to be made clear to him or her.[9] From the practical point of view, close follow-up of a patient choosing a less prudent alternative is advisable, to limit the possibility of a bad outcome.

STATUTORY LIABILITY: REPORTING

Legislatures and courts of virtually every state have confirmed the importance of patient confidentiality. There are situations, however, where the reporting of certain information is required by state or federal law. In general, this reporting serves a compelling public interest such as public health, the protection of children, the maintenance of vital statistics, or law enforcement. Reporting mechanisms vary among states and localities, but there is a high degree of consistency about what is reported.

Abuse

In pediatrics, surveillance for child abuse is part of the public trust. For those working in general emergency departments, however, elder abuse, the abuse of patients in nursing homes and psychiatric facilities, and the abuse of other defenseless persons are also reportable. Spouse abuse may also require reporting as a crime of violence under different statutes. In most states, failure to report abuse is itself a misdemeanor and punishable by fine.[37]

Child abuse is usually reportable to an agency specifically responsible for child protective services.[38,39] This can be the local sheriff, Family Services, or some other designated agency. As mentioned, it is public policy that suspected abuse be reported liberally and that reporters acting in good faith are protected from liability for any inconvenience or defamation of reputation the report may entail.[40] Malicious or knowingly falsified reports are, of course, a source of liability.[41-43] Such allegations would depend on the plaintiff being able to prove intent.

Bites

Local rules about reporting dog bites are equally inconsistent.[22,44] Many counties maintain a system where official forms or even preaddressed postcards are kept in the emergency department, police department, and other locations. Reporting dog bites is a remnant of a rabies surveillance system that may soon be of greater importance. While human rabies has become a rare disease in most of the United States, there has been a resurgence in wild animal rabies in several regions. In addition, dog bites themselves are a serious injury, especially to children. The control of stray and savage animals is as essential a public service as is monitoring for disease.

Reporting other animal bites is also mandated in most locations.[45] This is a far more important part of the infectious disease surveillance system at this time. Bats, skunks, raccoons, foxes, rodents, and feral cats represent the largest reservoir of mammal zoonoses.

Other Wounds

All gunshot wounds require a report to the local police, including accidental wounds. This separate requirement is not to be confused with the requirement that both penetrating and nonpenetrating injuries resulting from acts of violence or criminal activity must also be reported. Failure to report is usually a misdemeanor punishable by fine.

Some states, but not all, maintain a burn registry. Massachusetts, for example, is considering requiring the registration of burns as small as 5% of body surface area.

Deaths

The reporting of deaths varies somewhat depending on the decedent and the manner of death. Generally, deaths in a hospital or under medical supervision (e.g., hospice) only require reporting through the hospital or hospice administration and the filing of a death certificate for the purpose of vital statistics. Death of a fetus greater than 20 weeks' gestation outside of medical supervision often requires reporting to the medical examiner. In many locales, however, immediate reporting of fetal demise is not necessary and may not even require a standard death certificate until a gestational age of viability. There is always a time limit on filing death certificates. It is well worth learning the rules in your state.

The medical examiner's (or coroner's) office must be notified immediately of any death occurring outside of medical supervision. Needless to say, cases of sudden infant death syndrome (SIDS) are reportable under these and other statutes concerning the SIDS registry. Those who expire shortly after arrival in the emergency department must be reported. Patients that are well known to have a serious illness or who die of an obvious mechanism must also be reported, but it is advisable to contact the attending physician first. He or she may agree to sign a death certificate and thus testify as to the cause of death. The medical examiner may then at his or her discretion release the case.

It is unusual for the emergency physician to complete and sign the death certificate unless the cause of death is perfectly clear. A death certificate is a legal document certifying the cause and manner of death and listing contributing conditions. With the exception of certain kinds of trauma, the pediatric emergency physician is seldom in a position to testify to this. There is nothing specifically prohibiting the emergency physician from completing the death certificate, but more commonly the private physician or medical examiner fulfills this responsibility.

Some states require the reporting of all abortions as well as still births.[46,47] Poisoning and lead poisoning particularly may be reportable in your locale. Nationally, adverse events following childhood vaccinations are reportable. Of special interest are reactions to DPT, measles, mumps, rubella, DT, and both the Salk and Sabin polio vaccines. Anaphylactic and anaphylactoid reactions, encephalopathies (usually within 7 days of vaccination), and seizure (also within 7 days) are specifically mentioned. The acquisition of paralytic poliomyelitis in nonimmunodeficient patients following vaccination is reportable as well.[48]

Communicable Diseases

Certain diseases are reportable to the local department of public health and through them to state and national agencies. Best known are the sexually transmitted diseases. In most facilities, it is the laboratory that is responsible for this. Consequently, it is essential that you submit laboratory specimens to confirm the disease or otherwise undertake to report the occurrence to the laboratory yourself so it can be passed to the Department of Health. Sexually transmitted diseases include genital chlamydia, genital herpes, genital warts, pelvic inflammatory disease, chancroid, lymphogranuloma venereum, syphilis, and gonorrhea. Less commonly remembered are the diseases of children. Ophthalmia neonatorum, neonatal herpes (onset within 30 days of birth), congenital syphilis, and rectal gonorrhea are also reportable as venereal diseases.[49] The latter would also be reportable as suspected child abuse.

While states have the responsibility of gathering public health data, the Centers for Disease Control have published a list of national data requirements and periodically make recommendations for disease surveillance. The box on p. 86 is a representative example. There may be some additional items in your specific locale.

A communicable disease that is both venereal and blood borne but which has proven to be immensely controversial in reporting is human immunodeficiency virus (HIV) infection and its acute clinical form, acquired immunodeficiency syndrome (AIDS). There has been substantial legal activity over reporting requirements, so that they vary widely from state to state. Many states require the reporting of cases such that the identification of the reported individual is impossible.[50,51] Others allow full reporting and case tracking, but use extraordinary means to maintain patient confidentiality.

Almost all states offer confidential and anonymous HIV testing. This service is often accompanied by requirements to provide the tested individual with special counseling and printed material regarding the sensitivity and specificity of the test along with recommendations for further action if the test is positive. Informed consent to perform the test is often required.[50]

STATUTORY LIABILITY, CIVIL RIGHTS

The Federal Civil Rights Act of 1964 specifically prohibits discrimination based on race, color, religion, sex, or national origin in access to health-care services. This is a requirement above and beyond the requirements of the EMTALA.

In addition, the Federal Rehabilitation Act of 1973 and the Americans with Disabilities Act require that hospitals that accept federal funds be accessible to handicapped patients and staff. Reasonable accommodations must be made for wheelchair-bound, hearing impaired, and mentally challenged patients. Some states have their own civil rights statutes that create additional protected classes of patients. Age and sexual orientation, for example, may also be protected.

While not protected by statute, those who do not speak English may also require reasonable accommodation in gaining access to health-care services.[6] It would be unrealistic to expect a facility to maintain translators for every language. Defending the standard of care would be difficult, however, if a good faith effort was not made to effect translation, or somehow facilitate an adequate history and physical examination. In the case of deaf patients, an exchange of written communications can substitute for a sign-language translator.[6]

STATUTORY IMMUNITY

The Good Samaritan statute was designed to encourage physicians (and others) to provide assistance in emergency situations by removing the threat of malpractice suit. While all states have Good Samaritan laws, the degree of protection varies slightly. In general, the law protects physicians from liability for damages that result from acts or omissions, in circumstances where: (1) assistance is rendered free of charge, (2) there is an emergency circumstance, (3) it is outside of the doctor's usual practice, and (4) the physician has no preexisting duty to the patient. Services

Reportable Diseases: Communicable Disease Surveillance System

Amebiasis
Animal bite
Anthrax
Aseptic meningitis
Babesioses
Brucellosis
Bordetella
Campylobacteriosis
Chicken pox
Cholera
Diphtheria
Encephalitis (all types)
Epidemic staphylococcus
Food-borne poisonings
　　Botulism
　　Mushrooms
　　Mineral or inorganic (lead)
　　Staphylococcal
　　Scombroid
　　Other
Giardiasis
HIB meningitis
HIB other
Viral hepatitis (all types)
Kawasaki disease
Legionnaire disease
Hansen disease
Leptospirosis
Listeriosis
Lyme disease
Malaria
Measles
Meningococcal meningitis
Meningococcal other
Mumps
Pertussis
Plague (*Yersinia pestis*)
Poliomyelitis
Psittacosis
Rabies (human or animal)
Reye syndrome
Rickettsia
　　Rickettsialpox
　　Typhus
　　Rocky Mountain spotted fever
　　All other
Rubella (congenital or not)
Salmonella (typhoid, paratyphoid, other)
Shigellosis
Tetanus
Toxic shock syndrome
Toxoplasmosis
Trichinosis
Tuberculosis (any site, any type)
Tularemia
Yersiniosis (enteric)

must be rendered in good faith and without gross negligence.[52,53]

There are two considerable loopholes in this protection. There are court precedents in some states that establish that illness is not considered the kind of emergency for which the law was designed. By the same token, the entire hospital can be considered the physician's usual workplace.[54] A number of courts have limited the protection specifically to rendering aid in traumatic accidents. In response, there are states that have specifically included the response to inhospital resuscitations into their version of the Good Samaritan law.

The other area of weakness in the Good Samaritan laws is in the definition of "gross negligence." Gross negligence involves willful and wanton disregard for another's well being. For emergency physicians or any doctor acting within his or her specialty, the difference between ordinary negligence (failure to act with the skill and caution that other physicians in the community would exercise in the same or similar circumstances) and gross negligence is subtle. A physician that routinely treats trauma knew or *should have known* in the extreme argument, that pulling a patient from a burning car without neck protection might have resulted in a spinal injury. The more subtle the distinction between gross and ordinary negligence in a particular case, the more likely the physician will be subject to a jury trial, with its inconvenience, expense, and uncertainty.

The best use of the Good Samaritan law is to keep a physician out of court in the first place. The courts can award a "summary judgment" to a Good Samaritan: to wit, on the basis of law, the defendant may not be held liable.

Good Samaritan laws might be useful in defending emergency physicians who respond to cardiopulmonary arrests, pediatric emergencies, or other calls outside the department under certain circumstances. Some states (e.g., Michigan) have specifically included this in the statute. However, in requesting that the judge dismiss the case on the basis of Good Samaritan law, if the plaintiff can raise a credible question to whether the physician had a preexisting duty to respond to such events, such "questions of fact" (rather than of law) would routinely be submitted to the jury. Important considerations in determining whether this question has substance is whether the physician's (or group's) contract specifies a duty to respond beyond the emergency department and whether the physician billed for the services rendered.

Parenthetically, the physician responding outside of the emergency department is still liable for the patients in the department and those who may be brought in during his or her absence.

All this is not to suggest that there is no protection afforded by the Good Samaritan act or that health-care professionals should not render help. The law was developed to allow the exercise of the moral obligation to provide aid in a narrow set of circumstances.

Many states provide specific statutory immunity to physicians participating in public health programs. Immunization programs, volunteer primary care projects, neighborhood health clinics, and sexually transmitted disease clinics are often included in these protections.[55]

EMTALA

In 1986, Congress added to its annual Consolidated Omnibus Budget Reconciliation Act (COBRA) amendments that were designed to prevent the practice of "patient dumping." There was some concern that private hospitals were transferring indigent patients to less capable public hospitals for financial reasons. Alternatively, specialized and private hospitals were refusing to accept the transfer of indigent patients from smaller facilities.

In an attempt to ensure that emergency departments would serve equitably as the health-care system safety net, COBRA '86 defined a detailed statutory duty for hospitals and physicians. Since that time there have been a number of additions and refinements. The statute is now referred to as the EMTALA to eliminate confusion with other social legislation passed under the COBRA (or OBRA) name. On July 22, 1994, the final regulations took effect.

The law has had profound and far-reaching effects. It is a civil law associated with fines of up to $50,000 and withdrawal of eligibility from the Medicare program. It is an important vehicle by which the "right to health care" has been established.

EMTALA creates three duties for the hospital and the physician responsible for seeing emergency patients. Each patient must be screened, stabilized, and (if necessary) provided with an "appropriate" transfer.

Medical Screening Requirement

The plain language of the law states that:

> if any individual (whether or not eligible for benefits under this title [Medicare]) comes to the emergency department and a request is made on the individual's behalf for examination or treatment for a medical condition, the hospital must provide for an appropriate medical screening examination within the capability of the hospital's emergency department, including ancillary services routinely available to the emergency room to determine whether or not an emergency medical condition . . . exists. (§1867(a))

While this seems simple enough, it has required substantial clarification through court precedent and regulation.

Patients are considered to have "come to" the emergency department if they enter the hospital campus anywhere. They need not come to the emergency department proper. This includes hospital-owned ambulances in the field. If the patient is in a nonhospital-owned ambulance on the hospital grounds, they have come to the hospital. If they are in a nonhospital-owned ambulance and in the field, they have *not* triggered the EMTALA requirements for the hospital, even if the ambulance crew contacts the hospital by radio.[54]

There was a brief time when a single court precedent suggested that radiotelemetry contact did indeed establish an EMTALA duty to a patient. This has since been clarified by the same courts and finally by regulation. Telemetry does not trigger EMTALA.[56]

An emergency department is any area of the hospital that accepts unscheduled outpatient visits and treats emergencies within its capability to do so. The word "hospital" includes rural primary care hospitals as well.[57] This is a very broad definition and its exact scope has yet to be established. Clearly, one need not call an area "the emergency department" for patients to have rights under the law. Presenting the facility to the public as one which has emergency capabilities (e.g., accepting ambulance traffic) might be enough to define the hospital as having an emergency department.

At the time of this writing, there is no case on point which establishes whether a visit to a hospital's urgent care clinic triggers EMTALA. Hospital policies will be essential in defining whether an ambulatory service treats "emergencies." Policies that mandate the transfer of emergency patients to an emergency department may be of help in excluding hospital outpatient services from the purview of EMTALA.

The language of this part of the law is considered to be inclusive; that is, rather than relieving a hospital of the responsibility to provide medical care that might be beyond its capability, it is interpreted to mean that the emergency department is responsible to provide any and all services routinely available within its full capability.

An emergency medical condition is defined in both statute and regulations. It is:

> a medical condition manifesting itself by acute symptoms of sufficient severity (including severe pain) such that the absence of immediate medical attention could reasonably expect it to result in placing the health of the individual (or with respect to a pregnant woman, the health of the woman or her unborn child) in serious jeopardy, serious impairment to bodily functions, or serious dysfunction of any bodily organ or part; or with respect to a pregnant woman who is having contractions—that there is inadequate time to effect a safe transfer to another hospital before delivery, or that transfer may pose a threat to the health or safety of the woman or the unborn child. (§1867(e)(1)(A)-(B)(ii))

As explained later in the statute, "delivery" includes expulsion of the placenta. (§1867(e)(B)(3))

An appropriate medical screening examination is required on patients who present for "examination" *or* "treatment." This covers patients who are sent to the hospital by their private physician to receive medications in the emergency department. Requesting examination or treatment is not restricted to the patient.

Patients have the right to refuse examination or treatment. The hospital is deemed to have met the requirement of the law if the patient leaves against medical advice or refuses services after being informed of the risks and benefits of refusal. The law suggests that "the hospital shall take all reasonable steps to secure the individual's (or person's) written informed consent to refuse. . ." (§1867(b)(2))

The regulation suggests that the hospital may lose this protection if it allows the patient to leave or transfers him or her against the patient's best interests by using an "improper" suggestion. Specifically mentioned as improper is warning the patients that treatment at the present hospital would involve a large hospital bill or that treatment at a public hospital would be free or less expensive. Clearly, in the course of enforcement, agencies will pay special attention to whether such transfers were coerced and whether they were, in fact, "not in the best interests of the patient."[58]

EMTALA applies to psychiatric patients and facilities as well. Particularly, psychiatric facilities that offer 24-hour services and treat people who are not currently enrolled patients are included. The hospital need not take ambulances to be included in the law.

Who is qualified to perform an appropriate medical screening examination is a question that has only partially been clarified by the new regulations. The hospital governing body must determine and record in a written policy what type of personnel is qualified to perform this initial screening. Ironically, the regulations also state that this decision is not binding on the Department of Health and Human Services (DHHS). The agency may, in some instances, decide that a medical screening examination was *not* appropriate because the condition of an *individual patient* required the expertise of a physician.[59] The regulations suggest that for an examination to be appropriate, it must be sufficient to decide whether or not an individual has an emergency medical condition. Retrospectively, the agency can decide that an appropriate medical screening examination required a physician or even "further examination" by a specialist (see below).

The hospital has the right to decide that a nurse may perform the appropriate medical screening examination, but they live with the risk that DHHS will second-guess them in the event of a bad outcome. The hospital would also have to be sure that this kind of emergency screening examination was within the scope of practice of the state's Nurse Practice Act.

The new regulations provide that the Healthcare Financing Administration (HCFA), acting as the enforcement arm of Congress in implementing this law, will consult with the local Peer Review Organization (PRO) to determine whether an appropriate examination was performed, whether the patient had an emergency medical condition, and whether he or she was appropriately stabilized.[60] In practice this has added physician input to HCFA's decisions. HCFA can, of course, initiate an investigation without first consulting with the PRO.

Whoever performs the appropriate medical screening examination, regulations suggest that all patients will be screened similarly, without regard to their ability to pay or other factors that may arise in the registration process.[61] In a widely used court precedent, an appropriate medical screening examination was defined as that examination that other patients would have received under the same or similar circumstances. Thus a bad outcome does not presume the absence of an appropriate medical screening examination. Missing a diagnosis is not an EMTALA violation.[62,63]

The language of the act suggests that:

a participating hospital may not delay provision of an appropriate medical screening examination . . . or further medical examination and treatment . . . in order to inquire about the individual's method of payment or insurance status. (§1867(h))

As clarified in the regulations, the hospital may continue with the "reasonable registration processes," so long as the information received in registration does not affect the ability of patient to access care.[61] This suggests that an appropriate medical screening examination can be divided into segments. If someone determines that immediate intervention is not required, then registration may proceed. This implies, but does not enforce, the use of a triage nurse system or at the least, a set of well-defined medical conditions that require the patient to be shown to the treatment area without delay for registration.

Further Examination and Stabilizing Treatment Requirement

If a patient does have an emergency medical condition, the hospital is further required to provide:

within the staff and facilities available at the hospital for such further medical examination and such treatment that may be required to stabilize the medical condition OR

for transfer of the individual to another medical facility in accordance with subsection (C). (§1867(b)(1)(A-B))

This provision also seems simple on the surface. In practice, several questions have arisen. The staff and facilities available at the hospital include all departments and services routinely available. The hospital has an independent responsibility under this act to maintain a list of physicians who are available to the emergency department for further examination and stabilization. While not every physician need be on the list, every service at the hospital should be represented.

Even if, by tradition, a certain service was not previously available to the emergency department, if it is available in the *hospital,* it must be made available to the emergency department. If, on the other hand, a service is not routinely available anywhere in the hospital, (including a physician in that specialty visiting his private patients on the floor) then the hospital can claim it is not "within its staff and facilities."

To stabilize is

to provide such medical treatment of the condition as may be necessary to assure, with reasonable medical probability, that no material deterioration of the condition is likely to result from or occur during the transfer. . .

A patient is stabilized if, to a reasonable degree of medical certainty given the information available at the time, no harm would likely result because of or occur during the transfer of the individual from the facility. A woman is in active labor if she is having any contractions. She and the unborn child are not stabilized until delivery (including the placenta).

The term *stabilize* is based on the safety of a patient in transfer. The law defines transfer to include patient discharge. Thus a patient is stable if at the time there is reasonable medical probability that they will not imminently deliver or come to foreseeable harm.

The risk of this definition is that it is retrospective. However, HCFA and the courts have consistently refused to use EMTALA as a substitute for malpractice law. If a patient is discharged and harm comes to them on the basis of medical negligence, nonnegligent error in judgment, or happenstance, it does not necessarily trigger EMTALA.

A physician may be found guilty if he or she certifies that a patient is stable for transfer he knew or "should have known" that they were not. While not widely used, this establishes a more challenging standard. The potential exists for future use of this law as the means of imposing a standard of care.

Transfer Requirement

If a patient has been stabilized, the hospital has fulfilled its responsibilities under EMTALA. This law does not address the transfer of stable patients. It does provide a detailed list of requirements for the transfer of individuals who have not been stabilized; if any requirements are not met, the transfer is illegal. This is referred to as "strict liability."

To be "appropriate," a transfer must be at the patient's signed written request after being informed of the hospital's obligation to treat and the risks of transfer **or** the medical benefits of transfer must reasonably outweigh the risks to the individual (and, as appropriate, the unborn child) **and** a physician has signed a certification that

> based upon the information available at the time of transfer, the medical benefits reasonably expected from the provision of appropriate medical treatment to another medical facility outweigh the increased risks to the individual and . . . the unborn child. (§1867 (c)(1)(A)(ii))

If a physician is not physically present in the emergency department at the time of transfer, another "qualified medical person" may sign the certification after consulting with a physician who, by law, must subsequently countersign it. This does not imply that the patient is stable, only that the transfer is in the patient's best medical interest.

The person certifying the transfer must be specific in recording the reasons for and risks of the transfer. In general, the intent of the law included promoting "uphill" transfers. Access to more sophisticated medical facilities and staff at the receiving hospital is invariably an acceptable reason for transfer. The patient's desire to be treated by his or her own physician at another facility or to be in a facility covered by their insurance plan are weak reasons but could be acceptable if the risk of transfer is quite low.

Before transfer, the transferring hospital is required to provide any and all "medical treatment within its capacity which minimizes the risks to the individual's health and . . . the health of the unborn child" (§1867 (c)(2)(A)). Touch-and-go transfers fail to meet both the appropriate medical screening examination and the appropriate transfer requirements.

The transferring hospital must also

> effect [the transfer] through qualified personnel and transportation equipment, as required including the use of necessary and medically appropriate life support measures during the transfer. (§1867(c)(2)(D))

This could be a private vehicle, under unusual circumstances such as a closed hand injury.

All medical records; observation of signs and symptoms; preliminary diagnosis; record of treatment provided; results of tests, x-ray studies, and other interventions while in the facility; and a copy of the written consent or certification to transfer must accompany the individual to the receiving hospital. The receiving facility must accept the case and confirm that it has available space and qualified personnel to appropriately treat the transferred patient.

Both transferring and receiving hospitals are obliged to keep a complete log of all patients who present to the emergency department, and if they were treated, eloped, left against medical advice, or transferred. They must further maintain records of all transferred patients for no less than 5 years.

Under the heading of "nondiscrimination" there is statutory language requiring hospitals with specialized capabilities and facilities to accept patients in transfer if they have

capacity. The regulations define capacity as adequate space, personnel, and equipment. The facility's ability to expand to accept patients in excess of its usual capacity may be considered.[64] This may include physicians on call, surgery capacity that is available with the use of on-call teams, and special care unit beds and nursing staff that could be expanded. It generally does not imply the need to mobilize staff reserved for disasters. In common parlance, unfairly refusing to accept patients in transfer is referred to as reverse dumping.

The receiving hospital must provide the same level of service as it would if the patient had presented to the emergency department from the community. Arriving through transfer triggers all of the requirements of EMTALA.

In the commentaries to the regulations, HCFA notes it will take into account the need of the patient for the recipient hospital's specialized capability, as well as the capacity of the transferring facility in judging cases of reverse dumping.

A receiving facility need not accept a patient if the transferring hospital has the ability of providing adequate treatment.[65] There need not be a formal department at the transferring hospital in order for it to have that ability. Specifically mentioned in the commentary on the regulations is that a facility need not accept a transfer of an uncomplicated delivery or simple fracture solely on the basis of the transferring facilities not having a formal obstetric or orthopedic department.

The large number of alleged violations that attest to the danger of refusing to accept a transfer notwithstanding, the regulations recognize and provide some protection against "uphill dumping."

In the text of EMTALA, "transfer" is defined as:

> the movement, (including the discharge) of an individual outside a hospital's facilities at the direction of any person employed by (or affiliated or associated directly or indirectly, with) the hospital, but does not include such a movement of an individual who (A) has been declared dead, or (B) leaves the facility without the permission of any such person. (§1867(e)(4))

The mention of patient discharge in the definition of "transfer" has been a point of controversy. There had been concerns that the strict transfer provisions of the law and the risk of civil fines would apply to every emergency patient discharged from the hospital.

However, the transfer requirements of the law are only germane to patients who are not stabilized.[66] The court's scrupulous avoidance of using this federal statute for litigating malpractice actions[67,68] limits the applicability of the transfer definition to patients who are discharged while unstable, where such discharge was not the result of alleged physician negligence. What remains are patients who are discharged from the emergency department by doctors who knew they required further stabilization or transfer and had wanton disregard for their clinical condition.

On the other hand, the utility of this definition is that it eliminates the possibility of circumventing the law by dumping patients "to the street" rather than transferring them. It also allows the law to regulate "transfers disguised as discharges." An unstable patient cannot be discharged with the intent of having him or her proceed directly to another facility to obtain this further care.

Enforcement

EMTALA is a civil statute. There is a $50,000 fine to physicians or hospitals for breaking the law and a $25,000 fine for hospitals with fewer than 100 beds. This fine is applied to *each* violation. There is no limitation on the number of violations that can be found within each case. Typically, there are several.

The physician who is responsible for examining, treating, or transferring emergency patients is the one subject to the law. Physicians on call are also subject to fine.

In addition to failing to perform an appropriate medical screening examination, failing to stabilize, performing an inappropriate transfer, and so on, HCFA can enforce three additional areas of the statute. A physician who signs a certificate stating that the medical benefits of transfer outweigh its risks is in violation if he or she knows or *should have known* that this was not the case. Moreover, a physician who misrepresents an individual's condition or other information (including a hospital's obligation to examine, stabilize, and transfer) is subject to not only fine, but to exclusion from participation in Medicare.

To be fined, HCFA need not prove any malpractice or even harm to the patient, only that the physician was liable for the conduct found to be in violation of the law. Exclusion from Medicare is reserved by regulation for violations that are gross and flagrant in nature or repeated in regard to physicians.[68]

The statute provides relief for physicians working in the emergency department if a patient requires the services of a physician listed by the hospital as being on call to the emergency department and the patient is transferred without being fully stabilized because that physician failed or refused to appear within a reasonable period of time. In that case the liability rests with the on-call physician. To have this protection, the transferring physician must record the name and address of the on-call physician on the transfer record.[3,69]

The enforcing agency for EMTALA is the HFCA. It has identified agencies within each state to perform reviews. Reviews grow out of complaints made by patients or, more often, by hospitals complaining against one another. It is ironic that in such cases, counterclaims usually occur and both hospitals are reviewed. State inspectors may present to the hospital without prior warning. The hospital is obliged to maintain a log of all patients received or transferred out. Medical records for these patients must be kept for 5 years, and inspectors have the right to unearth violations for that period.

Identification of violations usually results in a letter identifying the violations, informing the hospital of the possibility of fine and exclusion from the Medicare program, and requesting evidence that the problem has been or will be remedied. A follow-up survey may take place.

Any violation that will result in the imposition of sanctions must first be evaluated by a PRO.[60] States contract with one or more PROs to do this. The PRO must provide a report specifying whether the patient involved had an emergency medical condition or whether he or she had

been stabilized and may opine about whether the means of transport were appropriate and safe. HCFA may accept or reject the state's recommendations.

If the violations represent a threat to the health and safety of individuals in the community, it can report its findings to the Office of the Inspector General and recommend that termination from Medicare participation take place within 23 days. Otherwise, termination takes place 90 days from the date of notice. The Office of the Inspector General must provide written notice of suspension of the hospital 23 days before the decision becoming effective and the hospital then has eight days to correct the deficiencies or refute the report.

All of these decisions rest with an administrative law judge and are subject to federal court appeal. It is unusual for violations to proceed to court, since the vast majority of them are settled by the hospital providing HCFA with a remediation plan to insure future adherence to the law.

Any individual who suffers personal harm as a direct result of a hospital's violation of EMTALA may sue the hospital for those damages. Although the case may be tried in federal court, recovery is governed by the personal injury laws of the state, with all of its applicable damage caps, rules of evidence, and so on. The statute of limitations on these suits is 2 years (rather than the 5 years for civil fines). This represents an unusual risk, since the plaintiff need not prove liability or malpractice. If the hospital has been found in violation, plaintiffs need only prove damages to collect.[70]

Likewise, medical facilities who suffer financial loss as a result of an illegal transfer may also obtain these damages in a state civil action.

MEDICAL MALPRACTICE ACTIONS

Malpractice is medical negligence and the basic elements of the law of negligence apply. Understanding these elements can help physicians avoid being sued.

To successfully sue for malpractice, the plaintiff must prove that (1) the defendant had a duty to the patient, (2) the duty was breached, (3) the patient suffered damages, and (4) the alleged breach was a substantial contributing factor to the plaintiff's loss (to wit, its "proximate cause"). These actions are civil suits. There are few hard and fast rules. Whether the facts of a case conform with these elements of the law must be argued.[2]

Duty

As mentioned, the physician working in an emergency department has a duty to any and all patients present.[4] A doctor-patient relationship is assumed when the patient enters the emergency department. Many facilities have policies regarding how long a patient should wait for a private physician before the emergency staff must intervene. Some departments require the emergency physician to promptly see every patient, even if they are to be fully evaluated and treated by another staff member.

It is generally accepted that the emergency physician's duty to the patient stops when another physician takes over the case. This may happen within the department (e.g., the trauma surgeon actively takes control) or when the patient leaves the department under the control of an attending physician (e.g., is admitted).[71] Liability becomes much less clear if the emergency physician reinserts himself back into the case by providing telephone orders or treating the patient orders on the inpatient floor.

The emergency physician may be held liable if he or she turns patient care over to a practitioner who is impaired or represents a clear danger to the patient.

Other duties can be alleged that are not precisely malpractice but often appear in the context of a malpractice suit. Since the damages to the patient are identical, the distinction becomes moot. For example, physicians can be sued for failure to properly supervise nurse practitioners or even nurses. Doctors who employ nurse practitioners or other doctors are responsible for the actions of their employees under the doctrine of vicarious liability. These and other allegations are only distantly related to medical decisions.[2]

Breach of Duty

In medical malpractice, the common breach of duty is a breach in the "standard of medical care." This is defined as that degree of skill and caution practiced by physicians of similar training in the same or similar circumstances.[2,67,72] Generally, one cannot judge a pediatrician by the standards of a neurosurgeon. While the rules vary from state to state, there has been a strong tort reform movement toward requiring experts testifying to the standard of care to have a similar specialty as the defendant and emergency department experience. For the most part, the standard is a national one; it is difficult to suggest that regions should account for variance in the standard of care. The specifics of the locale, however, can be argued. Rural vs. urban or academic vs. small community facility may reasonably account for differences in practice.

Because there is no specific legal standard of care for any one patient, the standard against which the defendant is measured is argued in court for each case. This is usually done through expert witnesses. Each side presents experts who give their opinion about what a prudent physician would have done in the circumstances at issue.

The standard of care is not *ideal* care. It is hard to suggest that physicians must all practice perfect textbook medicine. Moreover, the standard cannot be judged retrospectively. A bad outcome does not necessarily imply negligence. Clinical decisions must be judged from the perspective of what was known and knowable at the time.[2]

Loss to the Plaintiff

The plaintiff must demonstrate losses, referred to as "damages," to collect in a malpractice suit. Damages are divided into three types.

"Special" damages include actual expenditures such as medical expenses (past and projected) or economic losses such as lost wages, loss of future income, and so on. These are often sizable. Agencies that pay medical or other expenses may have rules that require the plaintiff to reimburse them if plaintiff collects a judgment for these expenses. This drives the plaintiff's demand higher. It is ironic that in many states, even if there is no such lien on the judgment, a jury may not be allowed to hear that all expenses have been paid, according to certain rules of evidence.

Pain and suffering along with loss of pleasure of life, loss of consortium (sexual availability), and so on represent a second class of damages referred to "noncompensatory." Recent tort reform legislation in various states has capped noncompensatory damages.

A third area of potential loss is punitive damages. Punitive damages are intended to punish the malfeasor. There is often no limitation to these damages, although a figure three times the special damages is often mentioned in product liability cases.

Many insurance companies do not provide coverage for punitive damages. Some states specifically prohibit such coverage. This makes claims for punitive damages somewhat dangerous and intimidating to the defendant. The threat of punitive damages is commonly used by plaintiff attorneys to promote the early settlement of a case.

The need for punitive damages must be proven in court. The defendant must have acted with knowing, willful, and wanton disregard for the patient's safety.[2,6] It is a difficult legal standard to meet. To prove negligence, the plaintiff must show that the physician made an error in judgment or procedure that other physicians would not have made. To be found liable for punitive damages, the physician must have known that his or her actions would injure the patient or have shown utter disregard of the consequences. As a result, such claims are seldom presented to the jury and are rarely found against physicians.

In many states, juries may apportion damages among all of the defendants found to be liable in the case. Thus it is possible for any one defendant to pay only a small percentage of the jury verdict. However, many states have a "joint and several" liability rule that allows the plaintiff to collect all of a judgment from any of the defendants. Thus one doctor can be found 10% liable but be forced to pay all of the judgment. He must then pursue the other defendants to try to collect their portion.[73]

Joint and several liability forces many physicians who are peripheral to a case to settle rather than face the possibility of paying a disproportionate portion of the damages. This is a special problem if some codefendants are underinsured or if a very large verdict threatens to be higher than insurance limits.

Proximate Cause

The proximate cause element of the law is a powerful defense tool. The plaintiff must prove that the defendant's actions were a substantial contributing cause to the adverse outcome. The more severe the disease and inevitable the outcome, the greater the time between the outcome and intervention, and the more peripheral the outcome is to the original complaint, the less likely the plaintiff can prove proximate cause.

In addition, even if a physician's action or omission contributed to a bad outcome, if the missed diagnosis, or consequence is so rare that it could not have been foreseen, then causation is not established.[2]

The proximate cause argument is independent of the standard of care. Negligence that is not associated with the alleged loss is not legal malpractice. It should be noted, however, that this legal point is most useful in getting a judge to dismiss the case at the close of the plaintiff's presentation. Attorneys suggest that the "there was an error but so what" defense is difficult to make before a jury.

A subsequent act of malpractice does not mitigate a prior act. One may not argue therefore that missing a diagnosis is less culpable because it was subsequently missed by others. (Although it can be argued that if subsequent specialists missed the diagnosis, it may not have fallen below the standard of care for the defendant to have done so.) In fact, the first error in a case is often said to have "set the ball rolling" by misleading subsequent care givers. This is a difficult argument to counter if the first visit is by a more highly specialized practitioner.

RISK MANAGEMENT

Risk management programs are designed to reduce the losses associated with being sued for medical malpractice or for any other reason. Malpractice suits are expensive and unpredictable, so it stands to reason that programs tend to focus on prevention. There are so many programs that it can be difficult to discuss them in an organized way. It is possible to use the elements of the law itself to analyze this field.

Suits are usually founded on a real loss to the patient. Thus one essential risk management goal is to prevent a bad outcome. This approach is designed to protect the *patient*. Since it is not possible to predict every outcome, many risk management programs also focus on the plaintiff's need to demonstrate a breach in the standard of care. Documentation, patient-return/follow-up practices, and specialty consultation are the thrust of this aspect of risk control and are focused on the physicians protecting *themselves*. Doctor/patient communication is considered an essential part of protecting oneself. Last, risk management programs may try to sculpt the work environment into a system within which the physician is able to protect the patient and himself or herself through the use of policies, practice guidelines, and protocols.

Protect the Patient

Substantial educational attention is given to the prevention of bad patient outcomes. This approach is attractive to doctors, since they are already committed to it. Knowing medicine does not seem to be enough, however. Most suits arising from an emergency department visit (all ages) are for failure to diagnose. This is divided almost evenly between failure to do a thorough history and physical examination and failure to do tests that are readily available in the department. Recall that the largest group of suits are for missed fractures and missed foreign bodies in wounds, problems that are usually avoidable with x-ray studies. More catastrophic cases are often founded on failure to do a lumbar puncture.[74-76]

This is not to minimize the importance of an attentive history and physical examination. It is one of the great misconceptions of risk management that "defensive testing" will protect one from suit. There is no duty to order tests that are not indicated. The tests that are protective are the ones that prevent a bad outcome, and they are almost invariably guided by the indications revealed by history and physical examination. For example, decision making is not guided by the complete blood count in most instances, but by clinical impression.[77]

Even suits that allege a failure or delay in treatment are often related to a delay in reaching a diagnosis in the emergency department. It is ironic that many allegations of delay in the treatment of meningitis in the emergency department represent a physician waiting for test results to return.

Protecting the patient may include consultations, prolonged emergency department observation, or follow-up returns to the emergency department. While there is some self-protective element in doing this, it should first be motivated by reducing the chance of a bad patient outcome. This is not defensive but prudent for the patient's sake.

In court, an expert witness will testify that the standard of care is up-to-date and researched-based rather than personal, habitual, or anecdotal. Defensible medicine must be well informed. However, it is not usually a failure in knowledge that leads to suits from the emergency department but a failure in diagnostic orientation and therapeutic promptness. The theme of risk management programs of this type is therefore "dig for the diagnosis."

Protect Yourself

Documentation is also a common focus in risk management programs. Plaintiff attorneys may be reticent to prosecute a case where a good standard of care is well documented. Once in court, the chart is an inescapable factor and always to the benefit of one or the other side of the dispute.[78,79]

Juries need not accept the plaintiff's position that "if it wasn't written it wasn't done." However, testimony may be seen as merely self-serving if not supported by a medical record developed concurrent with the case. This is true for both the defense's and plaintiff's testimony. If the chart is created before knowledge of a bad outcome, it has even greater credibility.

The chart serves to prove the standard of care. In the emergency department this includes an adequate complaint-focused history and physical examination, use of consultants and tests, and continuity of care (including patient instructions). More difficult to show is a reasonable differential diagnosis. Even more than the other aspects of the standard, this depends on the generous use of the pertinent negatives in the chart. Pertinent negatives suggest that a condition or finding was considered but not found. It is easier to defend a case arising from a problem if the usual signs and symptoms were noted on the chart as being absent.

It is not realistic or wise to try to list the entire differential diagnosis on the chart. The process of ruling out possibilities is subtle and often unconscious for the experienced practitioner. Many possibilities are moved lower on the differential list in the first moments of observing a child. One wants to avoid being accused of not considering such possibilities because they were dismissed before the charting process. Instead, it is more economical (and more tactically flexible for the defense) to note negative findings for signs and symptoms associated with the most threatening parts of the differential diagnosis. A great many suits have been dropped or won based on the presence of a note about the child being an alert and interactive child with a supple neck.

An area of frequent controversy is the timing and content of telephone consultations. It is worthwhile to record all of the attempts to reach a consultant, if there is a delay. It is indispensable in a dispute to accurately record what was discussed. If all laboratory data and physical findings were communicated or a treatment plan agreed on, it should be so noted. Disagreements over the facts with subsequent treaters among defendants can damage the credibility of all involved.

Entering the time things were done can be useful for the defense. It is constructed for every case. It is always better for it to grow from documented times than from the plaintiff's memory.

It is essential that the chart be treated like the legal document that it is. All charts should be dated and signed and maintained in their original or appropriately amended fashion in a protected environment.

A chart can be changed at any time, but many states have statutes specifically precluding altering the chart *with the intention to deceive.* This risk is eliminated by noting the date and time and then signing the addendum. Likewise, corrections should be made with a single line through the incorrect area and "error" written in. Anything obscured on the chart may be questioned.

If the chart should extend on to additional pages, it is well advised to make a note at the bottom of each page that another page follows. This will support the defendant's claim that a more complete record was kept.

There are specific JCAHO requirements for medical records.[79] In addition, Medicare has established a standard for medical records for reimbursement purposes that experts are relying on as a legal standard. These records include the following elements:

- Chief complaint
- History of present illness
- Review of systems (limited)
- Past medical history
- Socioeconomic considerations
- Family history
- Laboratory results
- Treatments and procedures
- Consultations
- Diagnostic assessment
- Disposition plan

Legibility is a common problem in defending the chart. The document is often enlarged and hung or projected before a jury. The use of familiar abbreviations is easily explained in testimony. A messy and illegible chart may give the jury the impression that the care was rushed and disorganized. Dictated charts tend to be longer, more complete, and of course easier to read. They look more "professional." In general, they are easier to defend in court. Likewise, a legible and organized chart is easier to defend than a scribbled one.[80]

Beyond practicing and documenting good medicine, the factor that is most protective of malpractice suits is patient communication.[71,81] Most medical errors and even error-associated injuries do not result in suits. It is commonly believed that in addition to severity of the outcome, the factor that distinguishes these from the cases that generate a claim is patient communication. Patients are more likely to forgive inconveniences and misunderstandings in an environment that they perceive as friendly and safe and more willing to think well of a practitioner they perceive as caring and concerned.

Most patients cannot tell if their doctor is technically competent and define good quality care by their own criteria. These include the doctor seeming to care, the nurses answering their questions, the staff involving the patient's family or private doctor, prompt pain relief, and the sense of cleanliness and organization of the emergency department. Waiting times and outcome are lower on the list of priorities.[82] Thus our clients are judging us by standards other than those we use on ourselves and which we may not be emphasizing in our practice.

Typically, this part of risk management promotes dress code, correct body language, listening skills, and the use of common social symbols to give the impression of caring and concern. The "therapeutic team" is a technique by which the physician learns the patient's reasons for seeking medical care, clarifies his limitations and the ambiguity of the diagnosis (if appropriate), and recruits the patients into the therapy by requiring participation through changes in diet, activities, follow-up, and so on. It is intended to manage patients' expectations and prevent them from abrogating all responsibility for their care and therefore for their outcome.

Patient compliance, vigilance of symptoms, return for a worsening condition, and adequate follow-up are all made more likely by careful and concerned personal communications.[28] Communication should include written discharge instructions, since patients are less likely to precisely recall what you said in a time of crisis.[18] Legal considerations in pediatric emergency medicine have become progressively important and complex. A thorough understanding of the legal aspects of practice is essential medical information.

References

The Duty to Treat, the Right to Refuse

1. Campion FX: Negligence, *Resident and Staff Physician,* 39(8):49-52, 1993.
2. Prosser: *Torts,* ed 6, 1987, West Publishing.
3. The Emergency Medical Treatment and Active Labor Act (EMTALA)—42 U.S.C.S. §1395dd.
4. Lazzara v Dreyer Medical Clinic, 120 Ill App. dd 721 in re 458 N.E. 2d 958 [Physician responsible for patients in ER not seen.]
5. The Emergency Medical Treatment and Active Labor Act (EMTALA)—42 U.S.C.S. §1867 (a) [Duty rests with hospital and physician responsible.]
6. Oade C: Healthcare decision making, patient autonomy, & professional responsibility, *Health Law Practice* Release No. 1, Ch 8, 1994.
7. Bouvia v Superior Court, 225 Cal. Rptr. 297, 179 Cal. App. 3d 1127 (1986): in re Retter [Competent adults have the right to accept or refuse care.]
8. Massachusetts Patient Bill of Rights, MGL. Ch 111 §70E(h) [Patient right to refuse examination.]
9. Campion FX: Informed consent, *Resident and Staff Physician,* 39(9): 101-106, 1993.
10. Tsai A, Schafermeyer RW, et al: Evaluation and treatment of minors: reference on consent, *Ann Emerg Med* 22(7):1211-1217, 1993.
11. MGL. Ch 111 §70 (1) [Right to informed consent.]
12. In re Farrell, 108 N.J. 335 529 A. 2d 404 (1987) [Adults refusing care are not incompetent per se.]
13. Siegal D: Patient consent. In Henry G: Emergency medicine risk management: a comprehensive review, Dallas, 1991, American College of Emergency Physicians.

14. In re Farrell, 529 A 2d 404, 410 (1987) [A state has the duty to prevent suicide, preserve life, safeguard the medical profession, protect third parties.]
15. McKelway C: *Emergency medicine and the law,* Mansfield, Mass, 1988, Massachusetts American College of Emergency Physicians.
16. MGL. Ch 123 §12 [Obligation to protect psychiatrically incompetent patients.]
17. 35 Pa. Stat. §10101 & 10102 also 13 Del. Code §707(a) [Emancipated minors can give consent for their child.]
18. Buccata WR: Emergency department medical record. In Henry G: *Emergency medicine risk management: a comprehensive review,* Dallas, 1991, American College of Emergency Physicians.
19. 49 Pa Code §16.61(A)(i) [Patient right or privacy over their own information and may forbid disseminating it.]
20. MGL. Ch 112, §12f[Presumed consent in an emergency; minors are not competent.]
21. V.A.M.S. 431.061.1 (A list of who may act as a minor's guardian.)
22. *Physicians guide to Missouri law.* Missouri State Medical Association: Jefferson City, Mo, 1987, The Association.
23. Danner D: The informed consent doctrine, some practical guidelines, *Forum* 1:4, 1991.
24. Cordover M: Whose case is this, anyway? A Short primer on liability, *Emergency Department Law* 19: 7, 1994.
25. Medical Legal Subcommittee, ACEP Board of Directors: *Physician Statement on Treatment of Minors,* Dallas 1991, American College of Emergency Physicians.
26. Howell v Standard Oil Company, 405 U.S. 251, 92S. C.T. 885 1992 [Courts are in parens patriae toward incompetent patients. They should favor treatment.]
27. Henry G: Common sense, *Ann Emerg Med* 20: 319-320, 1991.
28. V.A.M.S. §563.061.5 [You can use restraining force on a minor or incompetent, especially to prevent suicide.]
29. Crouse Irving Memorial Hospital Inc v Paddock, 127 Misc. 2d 101, 485 N.Y.S. 2d 443 (Sup. 1985) [Parent may not refuse a blood transfusion that endangers a fetus on religious grounds.]
30. Custody of a Minor, 378 Mass. 732, 393 N.E. 2d 836 (1979) [Parents do not have authority to refuse care for their children, if there's evidence that it will help.]
31. Md Fam. Law Code Ann. §5-203(B)(1) [Parents cannot refuse life-saving care on religious grounds.]
32. N.J. Stat. Ann. 30: 4C-6 and 9: 6-11 [Parents can martyr themselves but not their children for a religious conviction.]
33. Federal Child Abuse, Prevention and Treatment Act, 1984.
34. Cf. Annot., 32 A.L.R. 1d 1055 [Elements of emancipation.]
35. V.A.M.S. 431.063 (Presumed consent.)
36. Kritzer v Citron, 101 Cal. App. 2d 33 224 p. 2d 808 150 [Implied consent exists in an emergency.

Statutory Liability: Reporting

37. MGL Ch 112, §12a [Report all gun wounds or penetrating wounds secondary to a criminal act. Fine of $50-$100 for failure.]
38. V.A.M.S., §210.115 [A fine to not report child abuse.]
39. Revised Statutes of Missouri 198.070 [A misdemeanor not to report child abuse.]
40. V.A.M.S. §210.125.4 [Immunity from suit for reporting child abuse.]
41. V.A.M.S. §210.125.4§3-8 [Immunity for reporting unless reported in bad faith, which is a misdemeanor.]
42. Staff A: Court backs doctors who report suspected child sexual abuse, Oct. *Emergency Department Law* 7(13): 145, 1995.
43. MGL. Ch 119, §51a [Fine of $1,000 for failure to report child abuse.]
44. MGL. Ch 112, §122 [Report all dog bites.]
45. Requirement and definition of reportable contagious diseases, *MMWR* 37(13): 1988.
46. MGL. Ch 49, §9 [Report 20 week or 350 gram fetal demise.]
47. V.A.M.S. §193.165.1-6 [Report 20 week or 350 gram fetal demise.]
48. 42 U.S.C. §3aa-5 (Supp. 1987) [Requirement to report immunization reactions.]
49. Code of Massachusetts Requirements Ch 105 §300.100 et al (List of reportable diseases.)
50. 1986 Massachusetts HIV Testing Confidentiality and Informed Consent Law, MGL. Ch 111, §70F [No test disclosure of results without informed consent.]
51. Sherer R: The physician's use of the HIV antibody test, the need for consent, counseling, confidentiality, and caution, *JAMA* 259: 264-265, 1988.

Statutory Immunity

52. MGL. Ch 112, §12U [Good samaritan law; also immunity if doing CPR.]
53. V.A.M.S. §537.037 [You can treat children without parental consent as a good samaritan.]
54. MGL. Ch 112, §12b [Good samaritan is not useful in the course of a normal job.]
55. Vernon's Annotated Missouri Statutes (V.A.M.S). §578.353 [Doctors are immune while working in public clinics and giving immunizations.]

EMTALA

56. Johnson v University of Chicago, 1992 U.S. App. 7th Cir 1992 (Levis 25096) [Radio telemetry does not trigger EMTALA.]
57. Interim final rules, EMTALA: *Federal Register* 59(119): June 22, 1994. (32083 & 32098).
58. Interim final rules, EMTALA: *Federal Register* 59(119): June 22, 1994 (32101-2).
59. Interim final rules, EMTALA: *Federal Register* 59(119): June 22, 1994 (32092).
60. EMTALA §111867(d)(3) (PRO involved in investigation.)
61. Interim final rules, EMTALA: Federal Register 59(119): June 22, 1994 (32099). (No difference in care based on registration information.)
62. Mitchell v Candler, No. CV 491-258, 1992 WL-96310 1992 U.S. Dist. [Definition of appropriate medical screening examination, EMTALA not to be used as a federal malpractice statute.]
63. Cordover M: What's new With OBRA, *Emergency Department Law* 7: 1,7, 1995.
64. Interim final rules, EMTALA: *Federal Register* 59(119): June 22, 1994 (32100). (See 42 CFR 482.55.) (Excess capacity is part of a hospital's capacity to stabilize.)
65. Interim final rules, EMTALA: *Federal Register* 59(119): June 22, 1994 (32105). (No responsibility to accept patient if transferring facility has capacity.)
66. Interim final rules, EMTALA: Federal Register 59(119): June 22, 1994 (32104) (EMTALA only applies to unstable patients.)
67. Staff: Hospital not liable for misdiagnosis under EMTALA, Suit dismissed, 17 (20):159, 1995.
68. Interim final rules, EMTALA: Federal Register 59(119): June 22, 1994 (32110) (Exclude doctors from medicare only for gross, repeated or flagrant violations.)
69. Frew S: *Patient transfers:* how to comply with the law, Dallas, 1991, American College of Emergency Physicians.
70. Frew S: COBRA/EMTALA—new risks for emergency medicine and of managed care, Emergency Physician Legal Bulletin, 5(2 & 3): 1995.

Medical Malpractice Actions

71. Relinquishing responsibility: *Emergency Department Law* 5(7):1993. (Also see Rodriques v The Hiriam Hospital, R.I. Sup Ct, No 91-380—appeal 4/20/93.)
72. Bauerman C: Malpractice and civil law. In Henry G: *Emergency medicine risk management Id.*
73. Silverstein C: Joint and several liability. In Henry G: Emergency medicine *risk management Id.*

Risk Management

74. Sites R: Emergency department closed malpractice claims: Ohio, *Perspectives in Healthcare Risk Management* (10) No. 2, Ohio Hospital Association.
75. Holbrook J et al: A computerized audit of 15,009 emergency department records, and *Ann Emerg Med* 19:139-144, 1990.
76. Cordover M and Gatewood J: Claims analysis, Spectrum Emergency Care, unpublished.
77. Young GP: CBC or not CBC: that is the question, *Ann Emerg Med* 15(3):367, 1986.
78. Orlikoff J and Vanegunas A: Malpractice prevention and liability control for hospitals, Chicago, 1988, American Hospital Association.
79. Joint Commission on Accreditation of Healthcare Organizations, 1994: *Accreditation manual for hospitals, 1: 1994.*
80. V.A.M.S. §538.225.1 [Definition of the standard of care.]
81. Little N: Effective communications, your best defense, *Diagnosis* 12:1988. Aug. 1988: 12.
82. Bursch A: Emergency department satisfaction: what really counts? *Ann Emerg Med* 22(3):586-591, 1993.

PART

II

RESUSCITATION

Emergency Management of Respiratory Distress and Failure

Jill M. Baren • James S. Seidel

Respiratory complaints are one of the most common reasons for seeking care in a pediatric emergency department, and respiratory illness is a major cause of poor outcomes in children.[1] Children are prone to develop respiratory distress and failure more often than adults for a variety of reasons; the most important are listed in the box on p. 96 on the left.[2,3] Inadequate respiratory function, regardless of etiology, leads to inadequate gas exchange (hypoxemia and hypercarbia), poor perfusion, acidosis, myocardial dysfunction, shock, and ultimately respiratory failure.[4] Early recognition of poor respiratory function is essential because timely intervention is necessary for a good outcome.[4]

In a respiratory emergency, assessment occurs simultaneously with management. This chapter discusses both assessment and emergent management of respiratory distress and failure from a general perspective; specific respiratory problems are discussed elsewhere.

PHYSIOLOGY

Respiration is the mechanical process of moving gases into and out of the conducting airways (trachea, bronchi, bronchioles), facilitating gas exchange that occurs at the level of the alveoli. It is a two-part process consisting of oxygenation and ventilation. Oxygenation provides the necessary substrate, oxygen (O_2), to the tissues of the body; ventilation eliminates carbon dioxide (CO_2), the metabolic end-product of cellular function.

Three pathophysiologic processes can interfere with normal gas exchange: impaired alveolar ventilation, ventilation-perfusion mismatch, and impaired diffusion.[5]

Impaired Alveolar Ventilation. Both the nervous system and the muscles of respiration must be intact for effective ventilation to occur.[5] Loss of neurologic or muscular control leads to hypoventilation, reduced tidal volume, and failure to eliminate CO_2 (hypercarbia) with subsequent respiratory failure.

Ventilation-Perfusion Mismatch. Under normal circumstances, ventilation and perfusion of the lung are equally matched across all pulmonary segments. If there is a change in the concentration of the alveolar gas mix, (i.e., decreased concentration of inspired O_2 or excess CO_2 production), there is also a change in alveolar ventilation and the subsequent concentration of O_2 and CO_2 in the blood.[5] Similarly, any condition that decreases blood flow to pulmonary segments (pulmonary embolus, vasoconstriction) will also result in a ventilation-perfusion mismatch and subsequent change in arterial O_2 or CO_2 concentration.[5]

Reasons for Increased Susceptibility to Respiratory Emergencies in Infants and Children

1. Obligate nose breathing, higher metabolic requirements, inefficient immune system in young infants. Anatomic components of large tongue, small mandible, and soft epiglottis.
2. Smaller diameter of airways—easily occluded and collapsible, greater resistance to airflow.
3. More compliant, unstable chest wall due to anatomic configuration of ribs, cartilage, and diaphragms.
4. More immature musculature—easy fatigability of diaphragm, which is a major muscle of respiration, and poor control of upper airway patency particularly during sleep.
5. Behavioral immaturity—unable to verbalize distress; prone to foreign body aspiration.

Clinical Correlates of Impaired Alveolar Gas Exchange

Impaired alveolar ventilation

Central neurologic causes: Coma, head trauma, status epilepticus, narcotic or other sedative-hypnotic overdose

Peripheral neurologic causes: Spinal cord injury, botulism, neuromuscular diseases

Ventilation-perfusion mismatch

Changes in ventilation: High altitude (decreased inspired oxygen), atelectasis, pneumothorax, bronchospasm (asthma, bronchiolitis, allergic reaction), excess CO_2 production (burns, glucose administration)

Changes in perfusion: Pulmonary embolus, congenital cardiac lesions (shunting), hypoxic vasoconstriction

Impaired diffusion

ARDS, meconium aspiration, pulmonary edema, pneumonia, interstitial fibrosis

---

Impaired Diffusion. Gases diffuse across the alveolar membrane from an area of high concentration to an area of low concentration. However, diffusion also depends on the properties of the alveolar-capillary membrane itself. If the membrane becomes abnormally thickened or if the entire cross-sectional area of the pulmonary capillary bed is reduced, diffusion will be impaired.[5]

A summary of clinical situations that correspond to these three processes can be found in the box at the right.

DEFINITIONS

Minute ventilation (MV), defined as the total volume of gas inspired per minute, is the product of tidal volume (TV) and respiratory rate (RR). MV must be kept adequate to meet the metabolic demands of the tissues.[4]

$$MV = TV \times RR$$

Since normal TV (volume of gas inspired during one breath) remains relatively constant throughout life at 6 to 8 ml/kg, maintenance of adequate MV is usually accomplished by an increase in RR (tachypnea); changes in TV may ultimately occur.[4,5] Therefore respiratory distress can be defined as a compensated state in which normal gas exchange is maintained at the expense of an increased work of breathing.[5] An early component of respiratory failure is an increase in MV_1 presenting as tachypnea. This is a response to increasing demands for ventilation and oxygenation. The physical work of breathing normally consumes 2% to 3% of total O_2 consumption, potentially increasing to 50% during respiratory distress.

When adequate MV cannot be maintained because of impaired oxygenation, ventilation, or both, respiratory failure ensues. This inability to meet the metabolic demands of the body's tissues is rarely a sudden event (except in the case of acute airway obstruction by a foreign body) and is usually preceded by respiratory distress and an increased work of breathing.[1]

One factor that further complicates the development of respiratory distress in infants and children is that their proportionally small airways produce a markedly increased resistance to air flow, particularly when traumatized or inflamed.[3] Resistance across a narrowed airway is inversely proportional to the radius of the airway to the fourth power.

$$1/r^4$$

One ml of edema in the normal trachea of 4 to 5 cm reduces the cross-sectional area by 75% and increases the resistance to air flow sixteen-fold. Thus the smaller the airway, the greater is the functional resistance when it is obstructed (Fig. 11-1).

ETIOLOGY

The etiologies of respiratory distress and failure are among the most common causes of life-threatening illness in children.[1] Respiratory compromise plays a dominant role in children who ultimately experience a cardiopulmonary arrest.[4] The causes are myriad and many are listed in the box on p. 97. A detailed discussion of these various entities appears elsewhere in the text.

DIAGNOSTIC FINDINGS

The signs and symptoms of respiratory distress in children may be subtle. Older children are able to complain of shortness of breath, chest pain, or other symptoms that younger children and infants cannot verbalize. Complaints related to the respiratory system are common in any emergency department that sees children.[1] All children with respiratory complaints, however mild, should have a rapid and thorough evaluation.[1] The questions one needs to consider are the following:

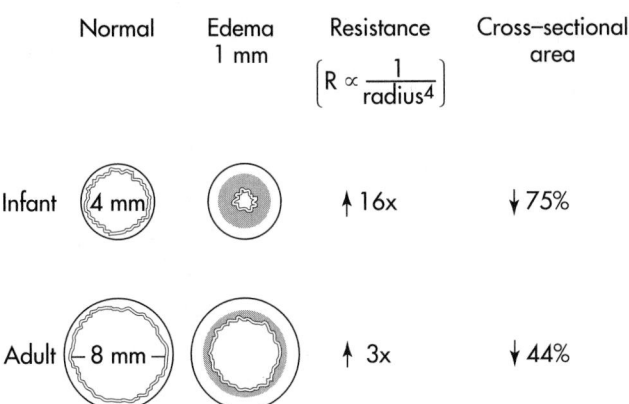

Normal	Edema 1 mm	Resistance $\left[R \propto \dfrac{1}{radius^4}\right]$	Cross−sectional area
Infant (4 mm)		↑ 16x	↓ 75%
Adult (8 mm)		↑ 3x	↓ 44%

FIG. 11-1. Effects of edema on airway resistance in the infant versus the adult. Normal airways are represented on the left, edematous airways (with 1 mm of circumferential edema) on the right. Resistance to flow is inversely proportional to the *fourth* power of the lumen radius for laminar flow and to the *fifth* power for turbulent flow. The net result is a 75% decrease in cross-sectional area and a 16-fold increase in resistance in the infant versus 44% and threefold in the adult during quiet breathing. Turbulent flow in the child (e.g., crying) would increase the work of breathing 32-fold. (*From Coté CJ and Todres ID: The pediatric airway. In Coté CJ et al, editors: A practice of anesthesia for infants and children, ed 2, Philadelphia, 1993, WB Saunders.*)

Common Causes of Respiratory Distress and Failure in Children

Infection: Bronchiolitis, croup, epiglottitis, pneumonia
Foreign body aspiration
Intrinsic: Asthma, reactive airways disease, bronchiolitis, croup
Environmental: Submersion injury, smoke inhalation, toxin exposure
Trauma: Pneumothorax, hemothorax, pulmonary contusion
Cardiac: Congestive heart failure
Neuromuscular diseases
Congenital anomalies
Metabolic disease with acidosis

- Are there signs of increased work of breathing?
- Is the patient in potential respiratory failure, or in danger of progressing to respiratory failure?
- Do the signs and symptoms suggest a problem with the upper airway, lower airway, or is there a nonrespiratory cause, such as severe acidosis, for the observed respiratory problems?

Initially, vital signs should be taken and interpreted according to age (Table 11-1). Next, evaluate the degree of tachypnea; remember that it is the initial compensatory mechanism for preserving MV. Assess the adequacy of TV by observing chest rise or abdominal excursion; listen bi-

TABLE 11-1. Vital Signs by Age

Age	Respirations (breaths per min)	Pulse (beats per min)	Blood pressure (systolic: mm Hg)
Newborn	30-60	100-160	50-70
1-6 wks	30-60	100-160	70-95
6 mon	25-40	90-140	80-100
1 yr	20-40	90-130	80-100
3 yrs	20-30	80-120	80-110
6 yrs	12-25	70-110	80-110
10 yrs	12-20	60-90	90-120

laterally for breath sounds. If TV is decreased, then the compensatory tachypnea may not provide sufficient MV for adequate gas exchange. The patient may be tiring and will progress from respiratory distress to respiratory failure if there is no intervention. Signs of increased work of breathing in the pediatric patient are summarized in the box on p. 98.

Note all noises associated with respiration, as they may help to localize the etiology of the problem. For instance, sounds produced by a partially obstructed upper airway include stridor, stertor (snoring), or gurgling.[6,7] Wheezing, rhonchi, and rales generally signify lower airway pathology. Grunting, an ominous sign of impending respiratory failure, is produced by partial closure of the glottis on expiration in an attempt to provide positive end-expiratory pressure to keep the terminal airways open.[4] Auscultate the lungs in both axillae and then at the apices and bases. Check for the quality of the breath sounds and symmetry of air entry.

When assessing a patient in respiratory distress or failure, it is important to also examine other organ systems. Poor oxygenation may be reflected by pale or cyanotic skin color, lethargy, or agitation. Poor perfusion may result in delayed capillary refill or altered mental status. An abnormal cardiac examination (e.g., murmurs) may also provide clues to the origin of the respiratory distress.[8] Overall general appearance of the child (posture, level of alertness, responsiveness to parents) is exceedingly important to note. Remember that the tissues of the brain have a high O_2 consumption, and hypoxia can result in altered mental status.[4]

MANAGEMENT

Treatment of a respiratory emergency proceeds simultaneously with assessment. The goal is to restore adequate oxygenation and ventilation.[5] If severe respiratory distress or respiratory failure is present and the patient cannot maintain a patent or effective airway, immediate assistance is required with mouth-mouth, mouth-mask, bag-valve-mask (BVM) ventilation or endotracheal tube (ET) intubation.[4] Never delay the decision to secure the airway while awaiting laboratory tests or radiographs; the diagnosis of respiratory failure is based on clinical parameters and intervention must often be decided empirically.[1,9]

If the airway is maintainable, allow the patient to stay in a position of comfort. Do not remove children from the

Signs of Increased Work of Breathing in Pediatric Patients

Tachypnea

Nasal flaring

Retractions (subcostal, intercostal, supraclavicular)

Accessory use of neck muscles

Head bobbing

Change in inspiratory/expiratory ratio (normally equal to one)

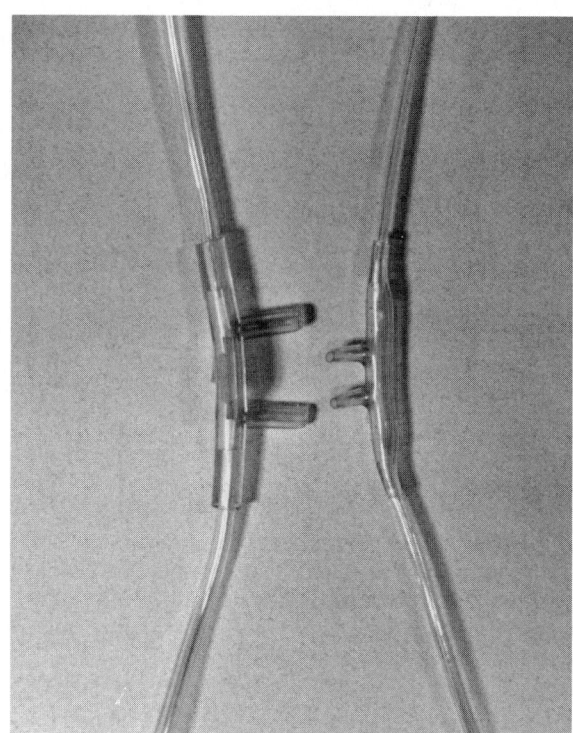

FIG. 11-2. Nasal cannulae: adult and child.

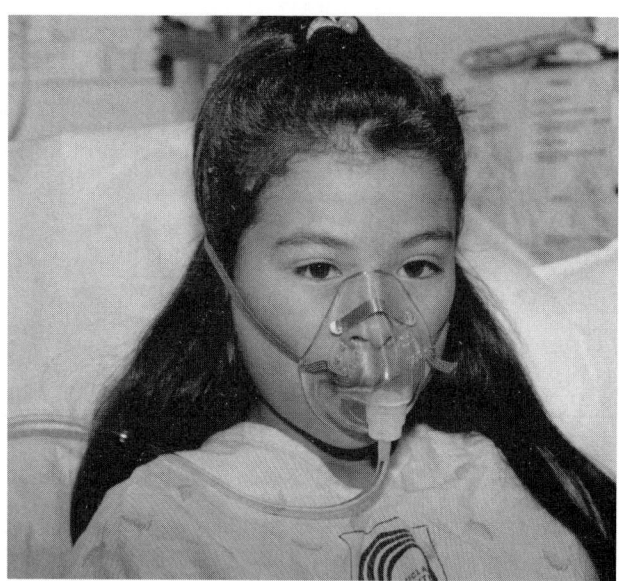

FIG. 11-3. Use of a standard child-size O$_2$ mask.

arms of a parent of caretaker as this may exacerbate anxiety and respiratory distress.[6] Deliver O$_2$ in the highest concentration possible. An increase in the O$_2$ content delivered to the tissues may provide enough of a safety margin to prevent progression to respiratory failure.[5] Available O$_2$ delivery systems for spontaneously breathing patients include nasal cannula (Fig. 11-2), masks (Fig. 11-3), or blow-by using O$_2$ tubing held near the mouth and nose. Remember, although nasal cannula may be better tolerated by some patients, significantly humidified O$_2$ can not effectively be delivered by this system and the nares may become dry after extended use. A non-rebreathing mask, a special adaptation of a regular O$_2$ mask, allows for a maximal concentration of delivered O$_2$ (Fig. 11-4).[4] Face tents (Fig. 11-5) are better tolerated by some children because they do not impede the visual field and are more comfortable. They also allow for the delivery of humidified O$_2$. Use any O$_2$ delivery device that is best tolerated by the patient. Never force an uncooperative pediatric patient to accept an airway adjunct, as it will increase anxiety and distress; try alternating.[4] Table 11-2 lists examples of available O$_2$ delivery systems and the concentration of O$_2$ they deliver based on entrainment of room air and flow rate.

If these measures fail to prevent the worsening of respiratory distress, it may be necessary to provide additional airway support through the use of basic airway positioning maneuvers (see Chapter 12) and then if necessary various artificial airways.[4] Both oropharyngeal and nasopharyngeal airways are available. They both keep the soft tissues of the oropharynx from collapsing against the posterior pharyngeal wall, causing additional airway obstruction in already compromised patients. Both of these adjuncts may be used in concert with BVM ventilation.[1,4]

Oropharyngeal airways (OPAs) are used in unconscious patients (they are contraindicated in conscious or semiconscious patients), since they are poorly tolerated otherwise. They also prevent intubated patients from biting and occluding the ET tube. An OPA will have the proper fit if the flange is held at the corner of the child's mouth and the tip reaches the child's jaw; if it is too small there is a good chance that the tongue will be forced posteriorly onto the pharynx, obstructing the airway.[4] It is inserted by holding the tongue down with a tongue depressor or by inverting the OPA, using the curved portion to hold down the tongue and rotating it 180 degrees into place.[4]

Nasopharyngeal airways (NPAs) are better tolerated in conscious or semiconscious patients and can serve as a conduit for nasotracheal suctioning.[4] The proper size NPA is determined by holding one end next to the tip of the child's nose and noting if the other end falls at the tragus of the child's ear.[4] Use a lubricant and careful technique when inserting the NPA; aim posteriorly and guide the NPA along the floor of the nasopharynx until it is completely in position.[4] The position of both OPA and NPA

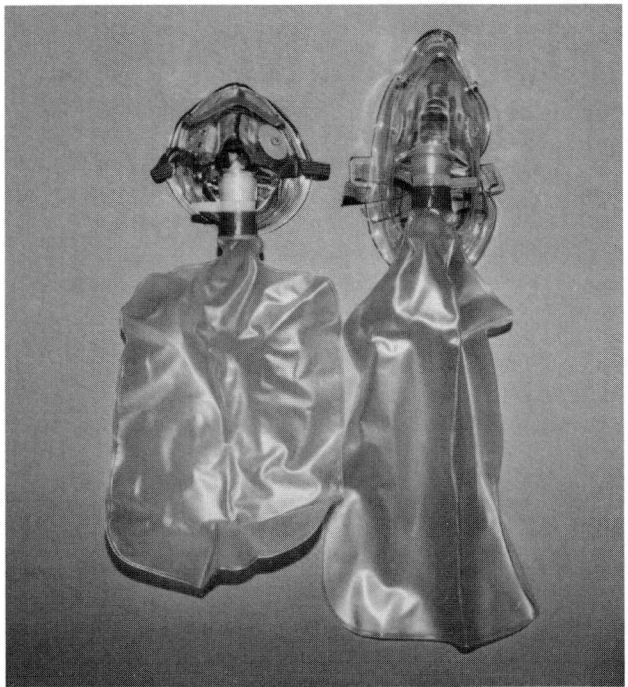

FIG. 11-4. Non-rebreathing O_2 masks that can deliver 90% to 100% O_2. If valves are not present in the mask system, then 60% O_2 will be delivered.

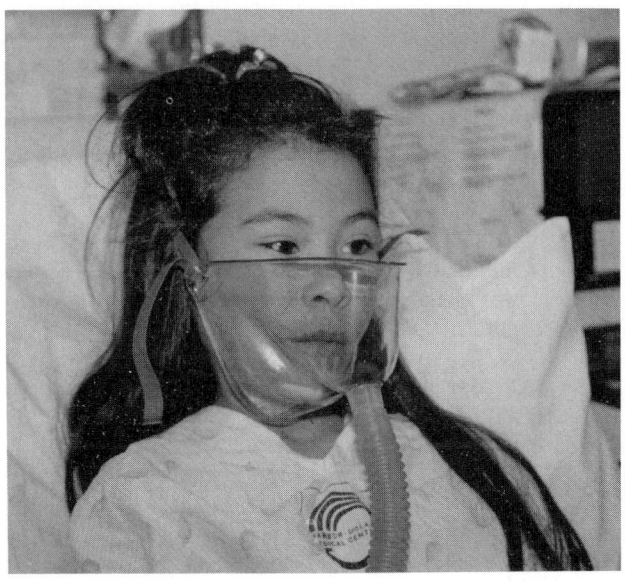

FIG. 11-5. Use of a face tent in an older child.

adjuncts need to be frequently assessed to assure that airway patency is maintained.

The laryngeal mask airway has been useful as an adjunct in controlled environments and may have a role in the prehospital and emergency department. Further studies are necessary.[10,11]

Medication delivery and additional diagnostic tests may also be an important part of the management of children

TABLE 11-2. Available O_2 Delivery Systems

Device	Room air entrainment	Concentration of O_2	Flow needed
Simple mask	Yes	30%-60%	6-10 L/min
Partial rebreather	Yes	50%-60%	10-12 L/min
Non-rebreather	No	Up to 95%	10-12 L/min
Venturi mask	Yes	Variable but predictable	Variable
Face tent/shield	Yes	Up to 40%	10-15 L/min
Oxygen hood	No	80%-90%	10-15 L/min
Oxygen tent	Yes	30%-50%	10-15 L/min
Nasal cannula	Yes	Variable	Up to 4 L/min

with respiratory distress. Any patient with a potentially unstable airway should be accompanied by a physician capable of advanced airway management at all times.[1] Patients with respiratory emergencies should be reassessed frequently, with special attention directed toward level of consciousness, respiratory rate and effort, patency of upper airway, heart rate, color, and peripheral perfusion.[1]

Noninvasive monitoring with pulse oximetry provides continuous evaluation of arterial O_2 saturation. Pulse oximetry can provide early detection of respiratory deterioration, but there are several limitations to its use. Pulse oximetry provides no information on the adequacy of ventilation and does not correctly reflect O_2 saturation when there is elevated CO_2 or methemoglobinemia present.[4] In addition, unless the hemoglobin or hematocrit is known, the oxygen carrying capacity of the blood cannot be determined and the practitioner may be lulled into believing that the situation is not critical because of an adequate oxygen saturation. Low perfusion states such as shock will not allow detection of the pulse signal and therefore limit the use of the oximeter in this setting.[4]

Exhaled CO_2 level may be measured noninvasively with end-tidal CO_2 detectors. These detectors can provide verification of correct ET tube placement. If no CO_2 is detected then esophageal intubation is likely.[4] Interpretation of the end-tidal CO_2 may be confusing in the setting of cardiopulmonary arrest. Lack of detection may indicate improper tube placement but is more likely a result of markedly decreased pulmonary blood flow and resultant low CO_2 tension. Infants with small tidal volumes may require special sized detectors for accurate reflection of the CO_2 level. CO_2 detection can also be performed continuously via nasal cannula systems or in line with the ET tube in mechanically ventilated patients.[4]

In some instances a more accurate analysis of ventilation and oxygenation is required (e.g., impending respiratory failure or patients with chronic pulmonary conditions), and it may be necessary to obtain an arterial blood gas (ABG). The ABG also provides information on the patient's metabolic status.[4] After adjustments in therapy are made, patients can still be continuously monitored by noninvasive techniques.

Indications for Intubation

Acute respiratory failure
- $Po_2 < 60$ mm Hg or $Sao_2 < 93\%$ or $Fio_2 > 0.6$ (sea level)
- $Pco_2 > 50$ mm Hg (acutely)
- Apnea
- Hypoventilation

Airway protection
- Neurologic dysfunction (seizure, ingestion, coma)
- Loss of protective airway reflexes (gagging, coughing)
- Inability to control copious secretions (CHF, ARDS, infection)
- Upper airway obstruction, airway edema, trauma
- Ingestion
- Airway edema, trauma, burns

Decrease the work of breathing
- Hemodynamic instability
- Metabolic acidosis
- Severe bronchospasm

Therapeutic intervention
- Hyperventilation for increased ICP
- Emergency drug administration with no vascular access
- Pulmonary toilet

Mechanical Ventilation

As discussed, infants and children in respiratory distress are particularly vulnerable to respiratory failure and may require airway support with mechanical ventilation. Therefore emergency physicians should be familiar with the indications, contraindications, techniques, and complications for intubation and mechanical ventilation.

Intubation and mechanical ventilation of patients in respiratory failure will protect airway patency, reduce the work of breathing, improve gas exchange, and allow the physician to control ventilation. Patients may also be intubated for additional therapeutic reasons that may not primarily involve the respiratory system. (See the box above for a complete list of indications for intubation.) The decision to proceed with emergency intubation is made on a clinical assessment of the presence of respiratory failure and not based on laboratory tests or radiographs, although this data may certainly support such a decision.[9]

It is important to emphasize that advanced airway management should be executed as smoothly as possible to avoid complications. Therefore one should proceed with basic airway support measures such as positioning, suctioning, and use of airway adjuncts and BVM ventilation before rushing toward intubation. Each of these procedures performed correctly will help to set the stage for a correctly and successfully performed intubation. For a description of the technique of ET intubation, selection of equipment, and pharmacologic adjuncts to facilitate intubation including rapid sequence intubation, see Chapters 12 and 19.

There are no contraindications to performing ET intubation in patients who require ventilatory support except in the case of chronically ill children or their parents who have already expressed a desire to avert or terminate resuscitative measures. The use of a particular technique may be contraindicated in certain patients. For example, patients with severe facial or airway trauma may require cricothyrotomy or tracheostomy as opposed to orotracheal or nasotracheal intubation. Advanced airway procedures are described in Chapter 12.

Complications that can occur during intubation include esophageal intubation, bronchial intubation (right more frequently than left), aspiration of gastric contents, dental trauma, retropharyngeal hematoma, laryngospasm with subsequent failure to intubate, apnea, hypoxemia, hypercarbia, cardiovascular instability with hypotension and dysrhythmias, and even cardiopulmonary arrest.[12,13] Even if intubation has been successfully performed, the application of positive pressure ventilation may result in barotrauma (pneumothorax), hypotension, and cardiovascular instability.[12]

Signs that indicate successful endotracheal intubation are visualization of the ET tube as having passed through the vocal cords, auscultation of symmetric breath sounds over both lung fields, symmetric rise of the chest with assisted ventilation, condensation in the ET tube, and overall clinical improvement of the patient.[4] It may be useful to additionally confirm placement with an end-tidal CO_2 device. Remember that the auscultation of breath sounds over the abdomen may be unreliable for predicting tube placement in all cases. In older children and adolescents one should not hear breath sounds over the abdomen if the tube is in the trachea, but in younger children breath sounds may be present diffusely over the chest and abdomen and do not necessarily indicate correct or incorrect tube placement. If an intubated patient deteriorates, it is essential to assure that the ET tube is correctly positioned and not occluded.

Initial mechanical ventilator settings should be chosen based on the clinical scenario at hand and will also depend on the type of ventilator chosen (pressure vs. volume).[13] Pressure-limited ventilators are used primarily in those under 10 kg, delivering a mechanical breath until a preset pressure is reached. The volume delivered reflects the resistance and compliance of the respiratory system. Volume limited ventilators in older children provide a preset volume, often incorporating a high pressure safety pop-off valve. A good starting point for volume ventilation is a minute ventilator of 10 to 15 ml/kg, an inspiratory time of 0.5 to 1.56 seconds, Fio_2 100%, an age-appropriate respiratory rate, and a positive-end expiratory pressure (PEEP) of 3 to 5 cm H_2O.[14] Inadequate oxygenation at this level should prompt an immediate search for complications of intubation or positive pressure ventilation.[15] (See section in this chapter pertaining to home ventilators.) Postintubation assessment should include signs of adequate ventilation (chest-rise, breath sounds) and oxygenation (color, pulse oximetry), as well as an ABG approximately 10 to 15 minutes after intubation. A chest radiograph should be obtained to document correct and optimal placement.

Subsequent modifications that may improve oxygenation include measuring the Fio_2, tidal volume (volume-limited respirator), peak inspiratory pressure (pressure-limited ventilator), inspiratory time, or PEEP. PEEP levels under 10 cm H_2O do not generally impair cardiac output.

Complications of ventilation may include barotrauma (pneumothorax, pneumomediastinum, pneumopericardium, pneumoperitoneum), decreased cardiac output (secondary to impaired venous return), decreased splanchnic and renal blood flow, gastric stress ulcers, and nosocomial pneumonia.

Obstructed Airway (See Chapter 59)

An obstructed airway resulting from foreign-body aspiration is most often found in children under 5 years of age; 90% of the deaths occur in this age group and 65% in infants. The most commonly aspirated foreign bodies include peanuts, coins, discs, food such as hot dogs, and small toys. Airway obstruction should always be suspected if there is sudden onset of respiratory distress.

Management. When the infant can cry, or when the child can speak and cough, no attempt should be made to remove the object; it should be removed in a controlled manner, preferably in the operating room or endoscopy suite. The child should be allowed to maintain a position of comfort and given supplemental oxygen as tolerated by mask, nasal cannula, or blow-by. If the patient deteriorates, has an ineffective cough, increased stridor, respiratory difficulty, or becomes unconscious, the following procedures should be used:

INFANTS LESS THAN 1 YEAR OF AGE
The rescuer should:

- Straddle the infant over an arm, making sure that the infant's head is lower than the trunk. Hold the infant securely on the forearm and rest this forearm on the thigh.
- Apply 5 hard back blows between the scapulae with the heel of the hand.
- If this fails to dislodge the foreign body, the infant should be turned over, with the head in a dependent position, and give 5 chest thrusts using 2 fingers in the midsternum.
- Open the mouth to see if a foreign body can be seen. If present, remove it with a McGill forceps.

If the Infant Loses Consciousness
- Open the airway using the chin-lift and look for a foreign body.
- Attempt assisted ventilation with a bag-valve-mask device
- If the airway can not be maintained, intubate the trachea.

CHILDREN OLDER THAN 1 YEAR OF AGE
If the child is conscious, the rescuer should:

- Stand behind the victim and place the hands in the midline about the level of the navel. One hand should be made into a fist, with the thumb side of the first resting against the abdomen.
- The fist is grasped with the other hand and pressed into the patient's abdomen with a quick upward motion. Each thrust should be a separate and distinct maneuver.
- Repeat the maneuver until the foreign body is dislodged or the patient becomes unconscious

If the Child Becomes Unconscious
- Position face up on his or her back.
- Open the airway and remove the foreign object if visualized
- Attempt assisted ventilation
- If there is no improvement or rescue breathing can not be accomplished, kneel or straddle the child and place the heel of one hand on the child's abdomen in the midline just about the level of the navel, avoiding the rib cage. The other hand is placed on top of the first hand in a hand position similar to that used for chest compressions in the adult.
- Press the abdomen in a rapid upward thrust in a series of five thrusts.
- If a foreign body can be visualized in the oropharynx it can be removed manually under direct visualization using the fingers or a forceps.

Severe obstruction may require cricothyrotomy or emergency tracheostomy. These techniques should be reserved for practitioners who are trained and capable of successfully obtaining an airway.

Children With Special Health-Care Needs[16]

Children with special health care needs are considered an underserved population that receive emergency care. This population is increasing because of improvements in the care of very small premature infants, improved pediatric intensive care, and the transfer of these children from the inpatient setting to home and the local community. It is important that emergency physicians have an understanding of the needs of these patients and what resources are necessary. Children with tracheostomies or on home ventilation programs are in need of specific focus.

The parents and caretakers of technically dependent children often are well versed in the child's history, medical problems, and care. They are an excellent resource for the emergency department staff in assessment and care of these patients. If time permits, the primary care provider can also be called for information about the child's normal state. Vital signs of these children may often be out of the normal range for age. The caretaker should be able to tell if the respirations or heart rate have changed in frequency or quality. Likewise, the color of the skin may normally be dusky or cyanotic. Many caretakers will carry a card with the problems and baseline vital signs with them.

Tracheostomy Tubes. There are several different types of tubes that are in common use. The reference number on the wings tube and on the package will indicate the size of the tube. The tube may have a cuff on the end that can either be a balloon cuff or a foam cuff. Neonatal tubes do not have cuffs because the narrow diameter of the trachea forms a sufficient seal around the tube.

Although there are different types of tubes, they work basically in the same manner. A *single cannula* is present in all neonatal and most pediatric tubes. *Double cannula* (Fig. 11-6) tubes have two parts: an inner cannula and outer cannula. This type of tube is found in sizes 4 to 8 Fr. The removable inner tube is the passage way for airflow and for removal of secretions. The external tube is inserted into the trachea and maintains the opening in the airway when the inner cannula is removed for cleaning. The inner can-

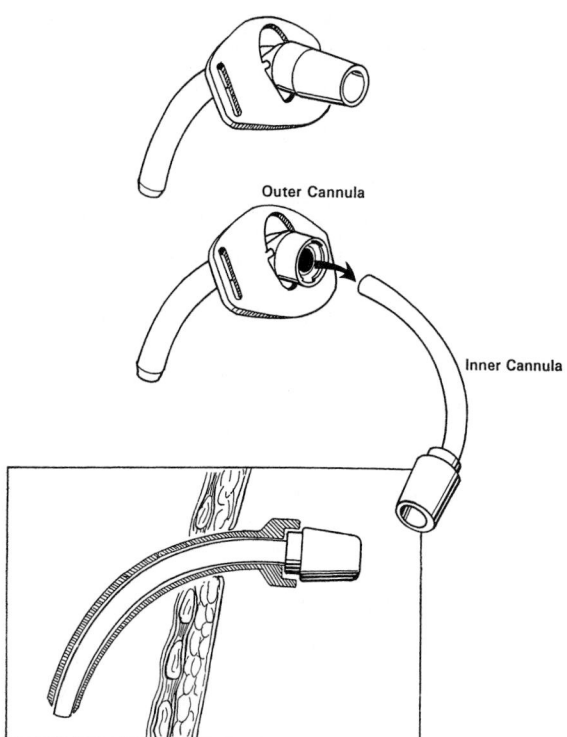

FIG. 11-6. A double cannula tracheostomy tube. (*From Rushton B: Children with special health care needs. In Seidel JS, Henderson DP, editors:* Prehospital care of pediatric emergencies, *Boston, 1996, Barlett and Jones.*)

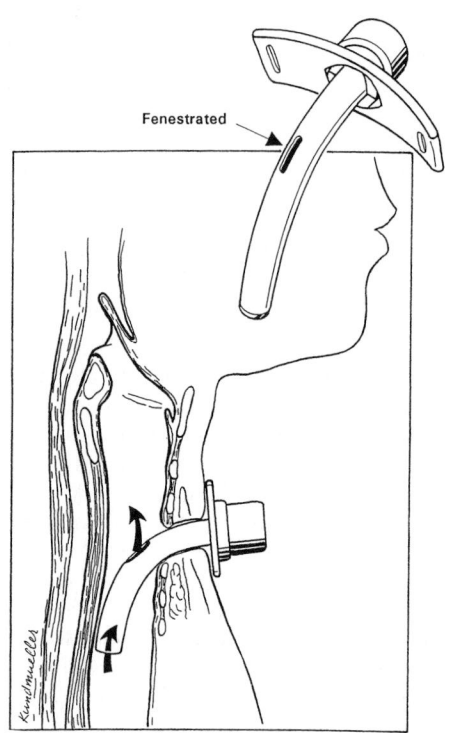

FIG. 11-7. A fenestrated tracheostomy tube. (*From Rushton B: Children with special health care needs. In Seidel JS, Henderson DP, editors:* Prehospital care of pediatric emergencies, *Boston, 1996, Barlett and Jones.*)

nula must be in place for mechanical ventilation of the patient. A *fenestrated cannula* has a small hole in the cannula that allows air to be directed past the vocal cords through the mouth and nose. A decannulation plug attaches to the outer cannula of this tube and blocks airflow through the tracheostomy tube, thus redirecting breathing through the fenestration tube, out the nose and mouth. This type of tube allows for normal respiration and facilitates speech (Fig. 11-7)

Respiratory failure rapidly ensues when the tracheostomy tube is misplaced or obstructed. If there are no spontaneous respirations or severe respiratory distress is present, suction the tube using 2 to 5 ml of normal saline (depending on the size of the patient), and attempt mechanical ventilation with a BVM device. The inner cannula of the tube must be removed to attach a BVM device. If there is resistance, do not attempt to force a suction catheter down the tube. If the tube has an inner cannula, remove it, clean it, and reinsert it or a new one. If the tube does not have an inner cannula, or if replacement fails to clear the airway, the tracheostomy tube must be removed. Be sure to deflate the cuff before removing the tube. Assisted ventilation or blow-by oxygen may be given over the stoma.

If the tube becomes dislodged, it should be replaced. Small tubes have flexible cannulae, and an obturator must be used for insertion. The replacement procedure is as follows:

- If the tube is cuffed, test the balloon by inflating the cuff.

- Place the child supine and place a small towel roll under the shoulders.
- Insert the obturator into the tube.
- Grasp the top of the tube with the thumb and forefinger and insert the tube through the stoma, pointing the tube inferiorly.
- If insertion is difficult, a water soluble lubricant can be applied to the outside of the tube before insertion.
- Remove the obturator.
- Inflate the cuff.
- Give 100% oxygen by blow-by.
- Listen for breath sounds.
- Secure the tube with ties.

The most common complication of tube insertion is anterior dissection of the trachea. This may occur when force is used while inserting the tube against resistance. *Do not push against resistance.*

An ET tube may be inserted through the stoma if a tracheostomy tube is not available. Any bleeding or trauma to the stoma or trachea must be evaluated by a head and neck surgeon.

Children at Home on Ventilators. Children who are cared for at home with mechanical ventilation often will come into the emergency department with the caretakers, including the nurses who attend to them at home. They are valuable sources of information and often know all of the details about the airway and ventilator settings of the child. They may carry a diary that accurately documents the care of the child.

These children may present to the emergency department because of respiratory distress, airway obstruction, pneumothorax, or infection. A systematic approach to assessment is similar to any other child. Remember the reasons for deterioration of a child on a respirator include the pneumonic DOPE:

- **D**islodged tube
- **O**bstructed airway
- **P**neumothorax (pneumomediastinum)
- **E**quipment failure

In this population, pneumonia can also be a major problem, as can a false channel in the trachea, caused by misplacement of a tracheostomy tube.

Clinical assessment of the patient in respiratory distress or impending respiratory failure may be challenging, especially in the very young. Attention to the subtle signs of respiratory illness will allow for early intervention that may prevent a catastrophic event and outcome.

References

1. Thompson AE: Respiratory distress. In Fleisher GR and Ludwig S, editors: *Textbook of pediatric emergency medicine*, Baltimore, 1993, Williams and Wilkins.
2. Berry FA and Yemen TA: Pediatric airway in health and disease, *Ped Clin NA* Feb 41(1):153, 1994.
3. Dickison AE: The normal and abnormal pediatric upper airway, *Clin Chest Med* Oct 8(4):583, 1987.
4. American Heart Association: *Textbook of pediatric advanced life support*, Dallas, 1994, The Association.
5. Anas NG: Respiratory failure. In Levin DL and Morriss FC, editors: *Essentials of pediatric intensive care*, St. Louis, 1990, Quality Medical Publishing.
6. Bank DE and Krug SE: new approaches to upper airway disease, *Emer Med Clin NA* May 13 (2):473-487, 1995.
7. Cressman WR and Myer CM: Diagnosis and management of croup and epiglottitis, *Ped Clin NA* Apr 41(2):265-276, 1994.
8. DiCarlo JV and Steven JM: Respiratory failure in congenital heart disease, *Ped Clin NA* Jun 41 (3):525-542, 1994.
9. Schuster DP: A physiologic approach to initiating, maintaining, and withdrawing mechanical ventilatory support during acute respiratory failure, *Am J Med* 88:268, 1990.
10. Benumof JL: Laryngeal mask airway, *J Anesthesiology* 77:843, 1992.
11. Reinhart DJ and Simmons G: Comparison of placement of laryngeal mask airway with endotracheal tube by paramedics and respiratory therapists, *Ann Emerg Med* 24:260, 1994.
12. Franklin C, Samuel J, Hu TC: Life threatening hypotension associated with emergency intubation and the initiation of mechanical ventilation, *Am J Emerg Med* 12 (4):425, 1994.
13. Grum CM and Morganroth ML: Initiating mechanical ventilation, *J Int Care* 3 (3):6, 1988.
14. Kanter RK, Blatt SD, Zimmerman JJ: Initial mechanical ventilator settings for pediatric patients: clinical judgment in selection of tidal volume, *Am J Emerg Med* 5 (2):113, 1987.
15. Strieter RM and Lynch JP: Complications in ventilated patients, *Clin Chest Med* 1:127, 1988.
16. Rushton B: Children with special health care needs. In Seidel JS and Henderson DP, editors: *Prehospital care of pediatric emergencies*, Boston, 1996, Barlett and Jones.

## 12

Cardiopulmonary Resuscitation

James S. Seidel

Cardiac arrest in the pediatric patient is generally caused by deterioration due to respiratory or circulatory failure (Fig. 12-1). The outcomes from resuscitation of cardiopulmonary arrest are dismal in the pediatric age group because of the relatively long periods of anoxia and poor perfusion.[1-5] This is particularly true if the child is pulseless and not breathing in the field and fails to have return to spontaneous circulation on arrival in the emergency department. Approximately 10% to 28% of the patients who are apneic and pulseless will have return to spontaneous circulation in the emergency department but only 10% of these patients will survive discharge from the hospital. Practically all of these will be severely neurologically handicapped.[5] One study showed a 0.05% normal survival rate after being pulseless and apneic.[6] Although outcomes are improved when the arrest was witnessed, bystander CPR initiated, and rapid transport to an emergency department occurs, some patients who are pulseless and not breathing cannot be successfully resuscitated. We must remember that the word *resuscitation* is derived from the Latin word *resuscitare:* to revive from death. A better word, often used by Peter Safar, is *reanimation,* which derives from the Latin: *anima-breath-life-soul.* If resuscitation is successful, a person has literally been revived from death.[7] Unfortunately, the pediatric resuscitation literature is confusing and cardiopulmonary arrest is often poorly defined. Therefore the public may expect that if advanced cardiac life support is administered properly, the outcome will be good. For the majority of patients this is not the case. Patients with witnessed respiratory arrests or sudden cardiac dysfunction may be more easily resuscitated than patients who have cardiopulmonary failure after deterioration from respiratory distress or shock.

During cardiopulmonary arrest, vital organs are not perfused. The brain and the myocardium are particularly sensitive to the lack of oxygen because of the absence of substrate for aerobic metabolism. Without adequate circulation and ventilation, the oxygen in the blood is rapidly consumed and cannot be replenished. The compensatory mechanisms for poor respiration and circulation—tachypnea, increased work of breathing, increased systemic vascular resistance, and tachycardia—fail after a period of time and lead to hypopnea, bradycardia, and eventually, apnea.

There are many underlying causes of cardiopulmonary collapse in the pediatric patient. The most commonly encountered causes include the following:

- *Upper respiratory:* airway obstruction, croup, epiglottitis, foreign body, suffocation, strangulation, and trauma
- *Lower respiratory:* pneumonia, asthma, bronchiolitis, foreign-body aspiration, near drowning, smoke inhalation, and pulmonary edema
- *Infection:* sepsis and meningitis
- *Cardiac disorders:* congenital heart disease, myocarditis, pericarditis, and rhythm disturbances
- *Shock:* hypovolemia with dehydration, cardiogenic, and distributive
- *Neurologic:* meningitis, encephalitis, stroke, head trauma, and hypoxia
- *Trauma/environment:* hypovolemia, hypothermia, hyperthermia, and submersion injury
- *Metabolic:* hypoglycemia, hypocalcemia, and hyperkalemia
- Near sudden infant death syndrome (SIDS)

The common pathway to cardiopulmonary arrest from the conditions listed previously is respiratory failure or shock. Other chapters deal with the recognition of disease processes that may lead to respiratory and circulatory failure.

The chain of survival for those at risk for cardiopulmonary arrest can be improved by prevention or early intervention for the ill or injured child. The chain requires the following:

- Early recognition of a problem by the caregiver
- Early activation of emergency medical services (EMS)
- Appropriate and timely assessment and triage by the emergency department
- Early definitive care (Fig. 12-2)

For those who suffer a cardiopulmonary arrest, outcomes may be improved by early bystander CPR and early activation of the EMS system.[5,8,9]

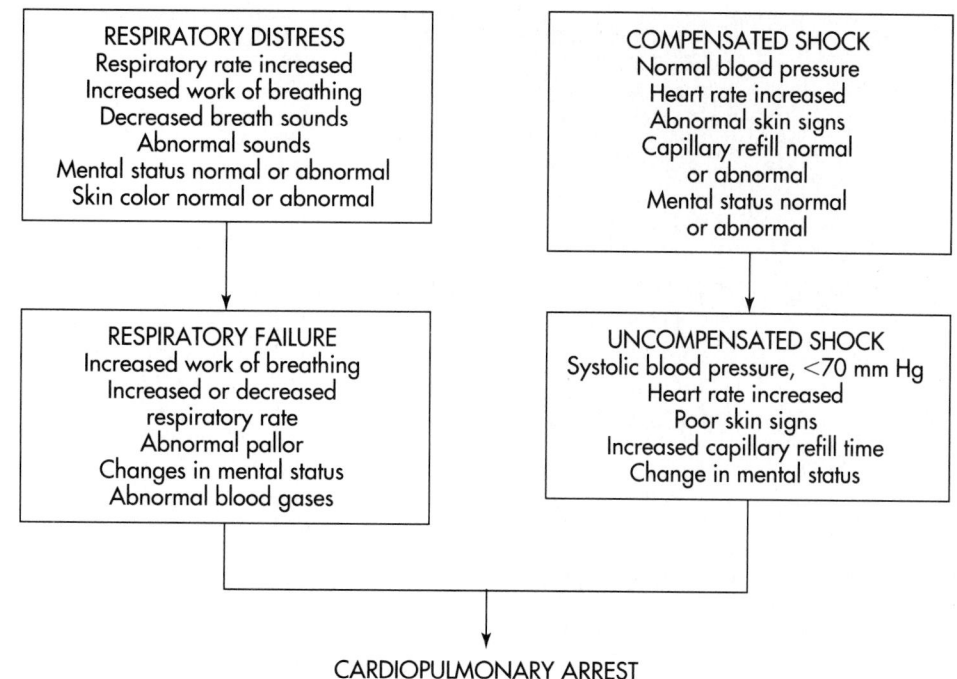

FIG. 12-1. Pathway to cardiopulmonary arrest in the pediatric patient.

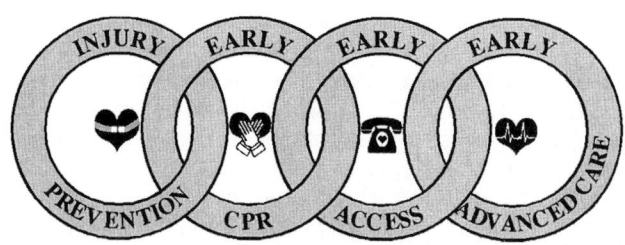

FIG. 12-2. The chain of survival for pediatric patients includes: prevention of illness and injury, early initiation of CPR, early access to appropriate emergency care, and early advanced specialty care. *(From Seidel JS and Henderson DP, editors: Prehospital care of pediatric emergencies, Boston, 1996, Jones and Barlett.)*

RESUSCITATION MANAGEMENT

Management of cardiopulmonary arrest requires the knowledge and psychomotor skills of a team of health professionals.[10] Basic life support (BLS) techniques precede and are often done concurrently with advanced life support (ALS). After every intervention the patient must be reassessed before proceeding with additional interventions or more advanced life support skills. Many health-care providers have difficulty retaining the knowledge and psychomotor skills required to offer BLS or ALS.[11,12] Therefore it is important that CPR be reviewed periodically for all those who care for children in various health-care settings. The present standards and guidelines for CPR include specific attention to the airway, breathing, and circulation.

Airway and Breathing

1. *Establish unresponsiveness.* This may be accomplished by vocal cues—calling the child's name—or by physical cues such as shaking the child. Care should be taken to provide stability for the spine if trauma is suspected.

2. *Open the airway.* Remember that the airway of infants and children is higher, more anterior, and smaller than in adults. The airway is easily obstructed by the relatively large tongue and the block of palatal tissue. Place the airway in a neutral position by using a slight head tilt and chin lift or jaw thrust. If there is a suspicion of trauma, the cervical spine must be protected; therefore only the jaw thrust should be used while the head is held in a neutral position. These maneuvers will align the airway and move the tongue and palatal tissues away from the posterior wall of the pharynx. If the airway remains obstructed, it should be repositioned and then maneuvers for an obstructed airway should be attempted.

3. After any intervention it is important to *reassess the patient.* The movement of air can be assessed by looking for chest rises or abdominal excursions, listening for air movement, and feeling for breathing by placing one's face close to the patient's.

4. If respiration is absent, *rescue breathing must be immediately begun.* With increasing concerns about disease transmission, this may be accomplished at first by mouth-to-mask ventilation using pocket masks. All rooms in the emergency department should be equipped with masks for rescue breathing. The mask ideally should have a port for oxygen and a one-way valve to protect the rescuer from infection (Fig. 12-3). If a bag-valve-mask (BVM) device is available, resuscitation may be initiated with a mask and this device. With both mouth-to-mask and BVM ventilation, it is important that there is adequate inspiratory time. This is best accomplished by allowing 1 to

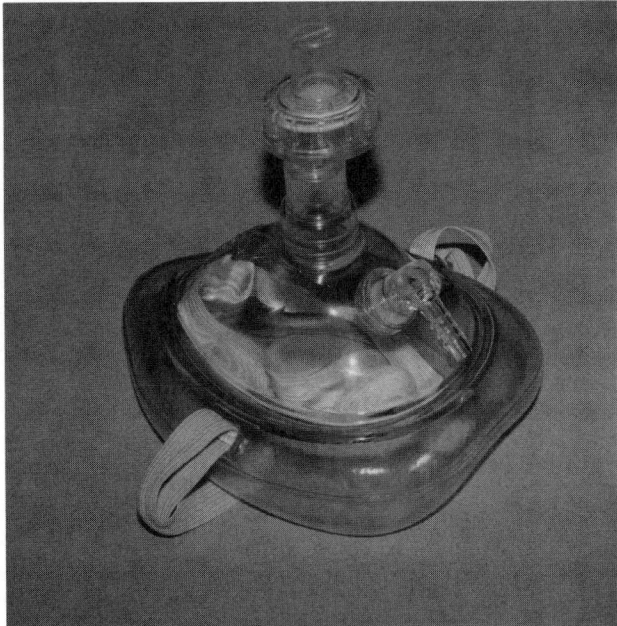

FIG. 12-3. A pocket mask with a one-way valve that can be used to initiate rescue breathing. The port on the side of the mask can be used to attach oxygen tubing.

TABLE 12-1. Endotracheal (ET) Tube and Suction Catheter Sizes by Age

Age	ET tube size (mm)	Suction catheter size
Premature	2.5	5 F
Newborn	3.0-3.5	6-8 F
1-6 mon	3.5-4.0	8 F
7-12 mon	4.0-4.5	8-10 F
18 mon	4.0-4.5	8-10 F
3 yrs	4.5-5.0	10 F
6 yrs	5.0	10 F
8 yrs	5.5-6.0	10 F
10 yrs	5.5-6.0	10 F
12 yrs	6.0-7.0	10 F
15 yrs	6.5-8.0	10-14 F

2 seconds for inspiration.[13] The bag device should be able to deliver 100% O_2 and have an adequate reservoir. There is evidence to suggest that very small bags with 250 ml reservoirs may not deliver adequate tidal volumes, even to small infants.[14] Remember the tidal volume remains relatively constant throughout life at 6 to 8 ml/kg.

5. *Compress the bag slowly* and effectively, giving adequate inspiratory time, watching for the chest rises, and assessing breath sounds during ventilation. A mnemonic to remember this can be used by having the rescuer slowly say "squeeze, relax, relax."[15]

Endotracheal Intubation

Endotracheal (ET) intubation is indicated for the following:

- Control and protection of the airway
- Prolonged mechanical ventilation
- Hyperventilation
- Improved oxygen delivery and ventilation

Before attempting intubation, it is important to have all the necessary equipment and support staff present. A respiratory therapist may provide expertise and experienced hands to help manage the airways. Because the airway is relatively cephalad and the epiglottis floppy and U shaped, pediatric intubation is best achieved by using a straight Miller blade.

All intubation trays should be equipped with Miller blades, numbers 0 to 2. A curved blade may be used in older children and adolescents. Hyperventilate the patient with 100% O_2 before intubation. The correct tube size may be selected by using the Broselow tape[16] (Fig. 12-4), matching the tube size to the diameter of the fifth finger or

nail bed of the fifth finger, or by using the following formula:

$$\text{Size of ET tube} = \frac{\text{Age in years} + 16}{4}$$

Tube sizes that are 0.5 mm smaller and larger than the estimated tube size should also be readily available at bedside along with the appropriate size suction catheters (Table 12-1). The proper length of insertion may be estimated to be that the position of the tube at the lips in centimeters is equal to three times the size of the endotracheal tube in millimeters. The light source on the blade should be checked before intubation and all supplies for securing the tube should be at the bedside. A stylet may be used to help keep the shape of the tube during intubation, but the tip of the stylet must not extend beyond the tip of the tube. Alternatively, tubes kept cold on ice will also retain their stiff shape. The patient's head should be maintained in the neutral position with a slight chin lift and head tilt. If trauma is suspected, spinal stabilization should be maintained and a jaw thrust employed to open the airway and put it in a more neutral position. Cricoid pressure (the Sellick maneuver) may be used as an adjunct maneuver during endotracheal intubation. This is accomplished by applying pressure to the cricoid cartilage with a finger.

The Sellick maneuver will help close the esophagus and prevent aspiration during intubation, as well as move the airway into a more posterior position for easier visualization.

Blind nasotracheal intubation is relatively safe in a hypoventilating older patient who has spontaneous respirations. The nasotracheal tube may also be introduced under direct visualization.

After the ET tube is in place, the chest should be auscultated in the axillae to make sure that breath sounds are equal on both sides of the chest. The chest rise with ventilation should also be symmetric on both sides. The tube should then be secured with tape and a radiograph taken to verify proper tube position. Inspiratory time becomes less of an issue once the airway is managed with an ET tube, but there is a tendency to hyperventilate patients even when this is not necessary for resuscitation. End-tidal CO_2 monitoring can be used to verify tube placement. Dispos-

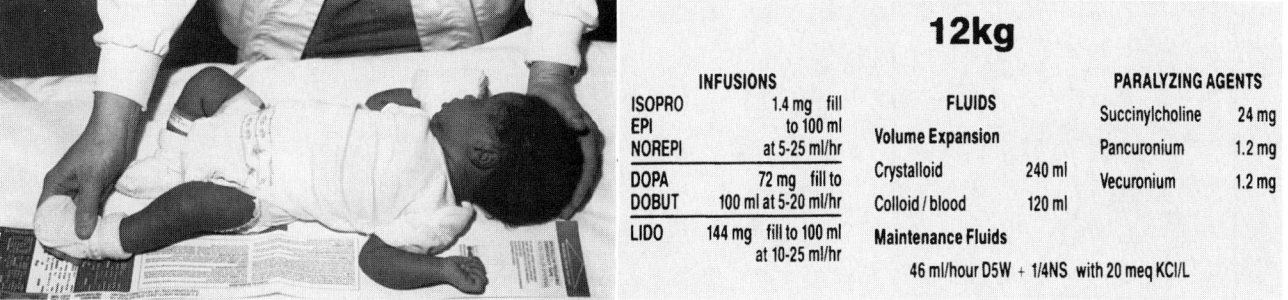

		12kg				
INFUSIONS			**FLUIDS**		**PARALYZING AGENTS**	
ISOPRO	1.4 mg fill to 100 ml at 5-25 ml/hr		**Volume Expansion**		Succinylcholine	24 mg
EPI					Pancuronium	1.2 mg
NOREPI			Crystalloid	240 ml	Vecuronium	1.2 mg
DOPA	72 mg fill to 100 ml at 5-20 ml/hr		Colloid / blood	120 ml		
DOBUT			**Maintenance Fluids**			
LIDO	144 mg fill to 100 ml at 10-25 ml/hr		46 ml/hour D5W + 1/4NS with 20 meq KCl/L			

FIG. 12-4. The Broselow tape can be used as a rapid method for generating drug and fluid doses, as well as ET tube, and suction catheter sizes. The tape uses the principle that length correlates with body surface area and weight. The patient is measured with the tape in the supine position and the line on which the foot of the patient reaches contains the precalculated drug doses and equipment sizes appropriate for the patient.

able end-tidal CO_2 monitors are available and have been used in CPR. These devices use an indicator that changes color in the presence of expired CO_2. If the device is purple, there is perfusion and the tube is probably in the trachea; if it is brown or yellow, one should check the tube position and CPR technique. Remember that an equivocal or negative test may be an indication of poor perfusion as well as a misplaced tube.[17] They are now available for use in infants/children who have small tidal volumes.

Cricothyrotomy may be indicated as a temporizing measure in children over 3 years of age when acute upper airway obstruction cannot otherwise be relieved. It is, however, rarely needed. If unable to ventilate a child on an emergent basis, a 14- to 16-gauge catheter over the needle may be inserted into the cricothyroid membrane. The adapter from a 3-mm nasotracheal or ET tube may be inserted into the Luer adapter of the catheter for application of oxygen and positive pressure for a limited period of time. Commercially available kits are available for this procedure but there is very limited experience with their efficacy and safety.

Patients with pure respiratory arrests unassociated with trauma often respond rapidly to bag-and-mask or mouth-to-mouth (or mouth-to-mouth and nose) ventilation. Pocket masks with a one-way valve are also available and optimally should be used to initiate rescue breathing (see Fig. 12-3). However, if there is no response within 60 seconds, intubation should be considered. Respiratory arrests complicated by such findings as cyanosis and hypotension usually require intubation. Prophylactic intubation of nontraumatized patients in the emergency department is rarely indicated because of concern about depression of respirations secondary to pharmacologic management of such problems as seizures or agitation with sedating agents. Intubate when appropriate. Ultimately, individual judgment must determine the need for intubation, considering the patient's condition, progression of disease, potential therapeutic maneuvers, and personnel and equipment availability. Rapid sequence induction (see Appendix to Chapter 19) may need to be considered.

Foreign Bodies

The presence of a foreign body may impede ventilation. For a complete discussion of foreign body removal, see Chapter 26.

Circulation

If circulation is not established during an asystolic arrest, ventilation will not be effective in exchanging CO_2 for O_2. When a pulse cannot be palpated in a large central artery, central artery, cardiac activity can be assumed to be inadequate or ineffective. A pulse should be assessed by palpation of the carotid artery. In children under 1 year of age, however, the neck may be short and chubby, making palpation of the artery difficult without hyperextending the neck. In these infants, alternate sites include the brachial and femoral arteries. If the pulse is absent, there is severe, symptomatic bradycardia, or there are signs of poor perfusion, chest compressions should be initiated.[18] Remember that heart sounds heard over the apex of the heart represent precordial activity, not a perfusing pulse.

The mechanism by which blood is circulated during chest compressions in the pediatric patient is not completely understood. There is evidence to suggest that in the initial phases, the heart is compressed and blood is pumped into the systemic circulation by this direct compression. After about 10 minutes, however, the distortion of the chest wall may inhibit any further direct compression of the contents of the thorax.[19,20] The thoracic-pump theory of chest compression may also play a role in the circulation of blood during CPR in the pediatric patient. This theory postulates that the increases in the intrathoracic pressure generated by the compressions cause the flow of blood from the lungs, through the heart and into the systemic circulation. Blood within intrathoracic structures is at a higher pressure during compression than in extrathoracic vessels; blood flow occurs. Retrograde blood flow into the venous system is inhibited by the thin-wall veins that collapse with the increased intrathoracic pressures. In contrast, the thicker arteries maintain their patency. The heart is thus a conduit for blood and not an active pump.[21,22]

The heart in the pediatric patient is positioned in the thoracic cage in the same position as in the adult.[23] Chest compression should thus be delivered over the mid to lower third of the sternum at a rate of 100 compressions/min in children and at least 100 times/min in infants. However, there are conflicting data related to the ideal rate of cardiac compressions. High compression pressure and rate may improve cardiac output but consistent studies are not available. Each compression and relaxation phase should be of equal duration, and the fingers or hand should

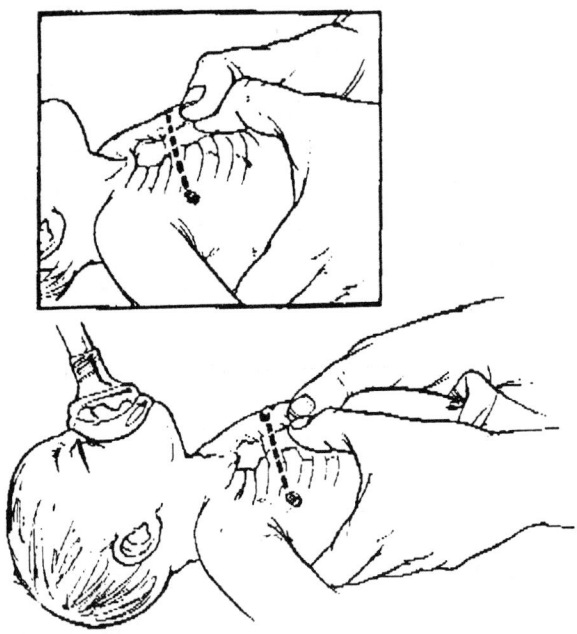

FIG. 12-5. Hand position for chest encirclement technique for external chest compressions in neonates. Thumbs are side-by-side over the mid-sternum. In the small newborn, thumbs may need to be superimposed. (*From American Heart Association:* Textbook of pediatric advanced life support, *Dallas, 1988, 1990, The Association.*)

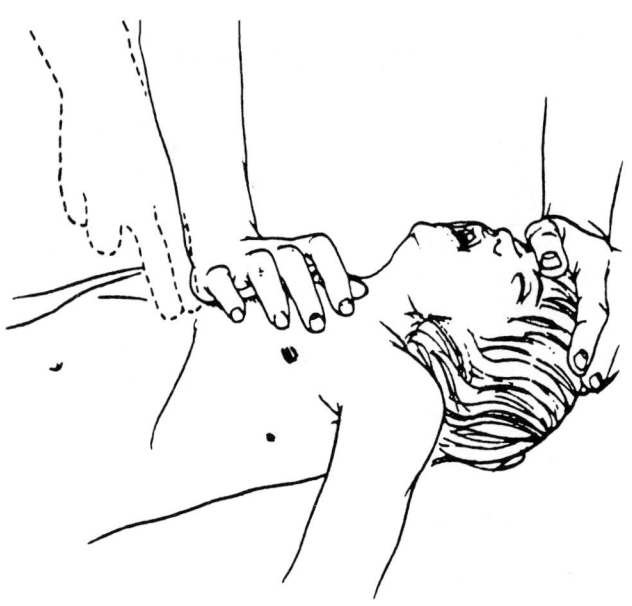

FIG. 12-6. Locating the correct position of the hand in chest compression in the child. (*From American Heart Association:* Textbook of pediatric advanced life support, *Dallas, 1988, 1990, The Association.*)

TABLE 12-2. Summary of BLS Maneuvers in Infants and Children

	Infant	Child
Airway	Head-tilt/chin-lift Jaw-thrust	Head-tilt/chin-lift Jaw-thrust
Breathing		
Initial	Two breaths at 1.0-1.5 sec/breath	Two breaths at 1.0-1.5 sec/breath
Subsequent	20 breaths/min	20 breaths/min
Circulation		
Pulse check	Brachial/femoral	Carotid
Compression area	Lower third of sternum	Lower third of sternum
Compression technique	2-3 fingers	Heel of one hand
Depth	Approximately ⅓ to ½ of depth of chest	Approximately ⅓ to ½ of depth of chest
Rate	At least 100/min	100/min
Compressions:Ventilation ratio	5:1 (pause for ventilation)	5:1 (pause for ventilation)
Foreign-body airway obstruction	Back blows/chest thrusts	Heimlich maneuver

Modified from American Heart Association: *Textbook of pediatric advanced life support,* Dallas, 1994, The Association.

not be removed from the chest during the relaxation phase. Each compression should be smooth; the movement should not be abrupt or jerky. In the newborn and young infant, chest compressions can be done by using two fingers placed on the sternum just below the nipple line. Another approach is the hand encircling technique, using both thumbs for compression (Fig. 12-5). In the older child the heel of the palm is placed on the sternum, two finger breadths above the xiphoid process (Fig. 12-6). Although there is some evidence that simultaneous chest compres-sions and ventilation may increase blood flow, this effect is only transient and may not be important in the pedi-atric patient.[24] The ratio of chest compressions to ven-tilation in both single and multiple rescuers is five to one. In the newborn the ratio is 3 to 1. A summary of BLS in infants and children is shown in Table 12-2. Data indicate that survival during in-hospital CPR may be improved with interposed abdominal counterpulsation. The optimal use of this technique in children requires further study.[25]

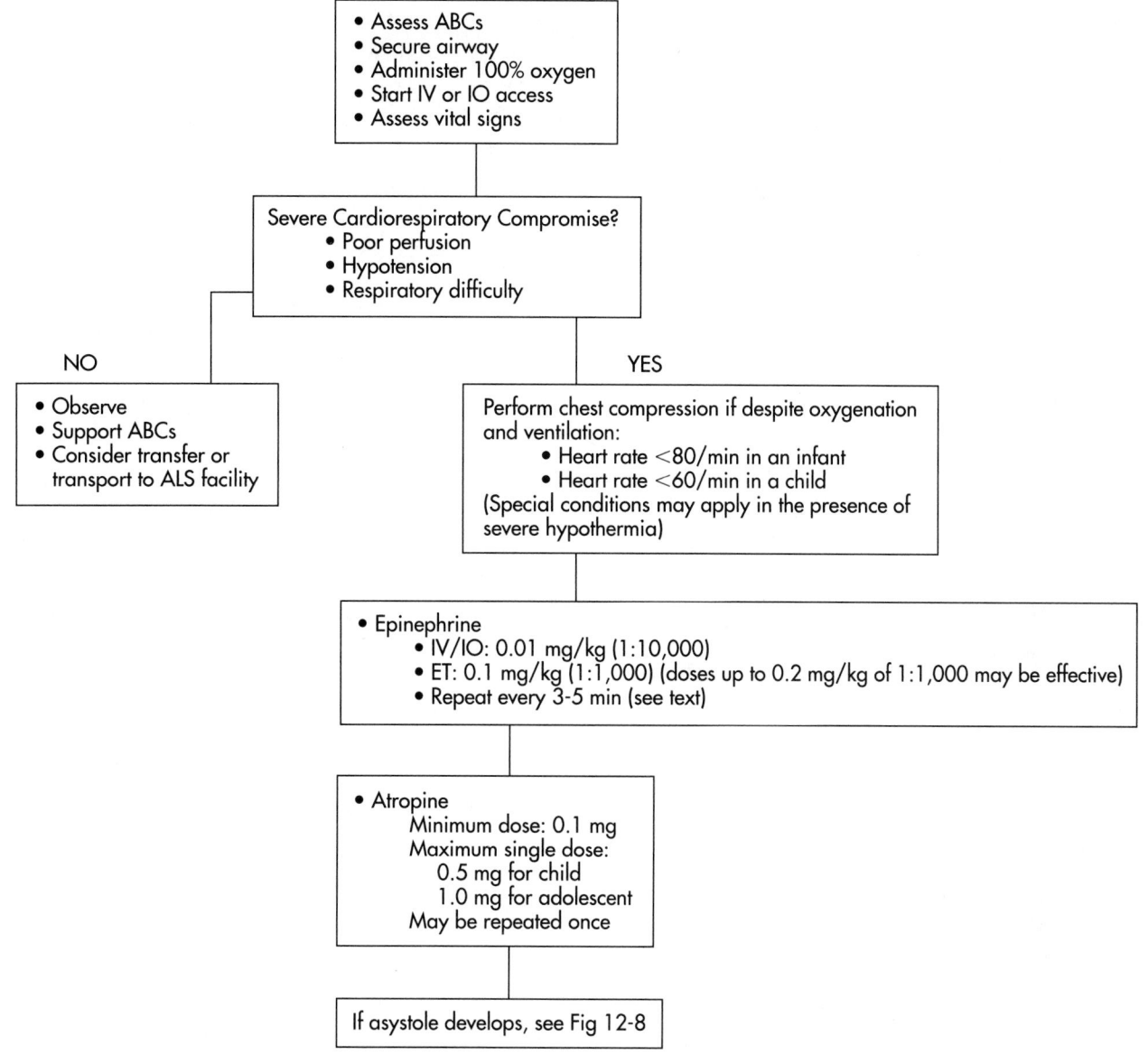

FIG. 12-7. Bradycardia decision tree. *ABCs,* Airway, breathing, and circulation; *ALS,* advanced life support; *ET,* endotracheal; *IO,* intraosseous; *IV,* intravenous. (*From* JAMA 268:2266, 1992.)

Rhythm Disturbances

The assessment and management of specific rhythm disturbances are discussed in Chapter 14. The management of bradycardia and nonperfusing rhythms is shown on the decision trees in Figs. 12-7 and 12-8. Treat all symptomatic patients with bradycardia. Pulseless cardiopulmonary arrest may be due to asystole, ventricular tachycardia, ventricular fibrillation, or pulseless electrical activity (PEA). Assisted ventilation with advanced airway management techniques, as well as chest compressions, should be started immediately. This rhythm is generally seen when the myocardium is "sick" (denied sufficient oxygen or has severe intracellular acidosis), is "constricted" as in tamponade or tension pneumothorax, or does not have sufficient venous return to generate a pulse, as in hypovolemia. If PEA is suspected, identify and treat the causes. These include the following:

- Hypoxia
- Severe acidosis
- Hypovolemia
- Tension pneumothorax
- Cardiac tamponade
- Idioventricular rhythms

Pulseless ventricular tachycardia and fibrillation are two nonperfusing rhythms that are more common in pediatrics than previously suspected.[26] Treat them with immediate defibrillation. If these rhythms go untreated, they will progress to asystole and the outcome will be poor (see Chapter 14). Ventilate the patient with 100% O_2, begin chest compressions, and prepare all necessary equipment. Although all defibrillators deliver transthoracic energy if used properly, each machine is different and thus one should be familiar with the machine in your work area. Know how the machine in your emergency department

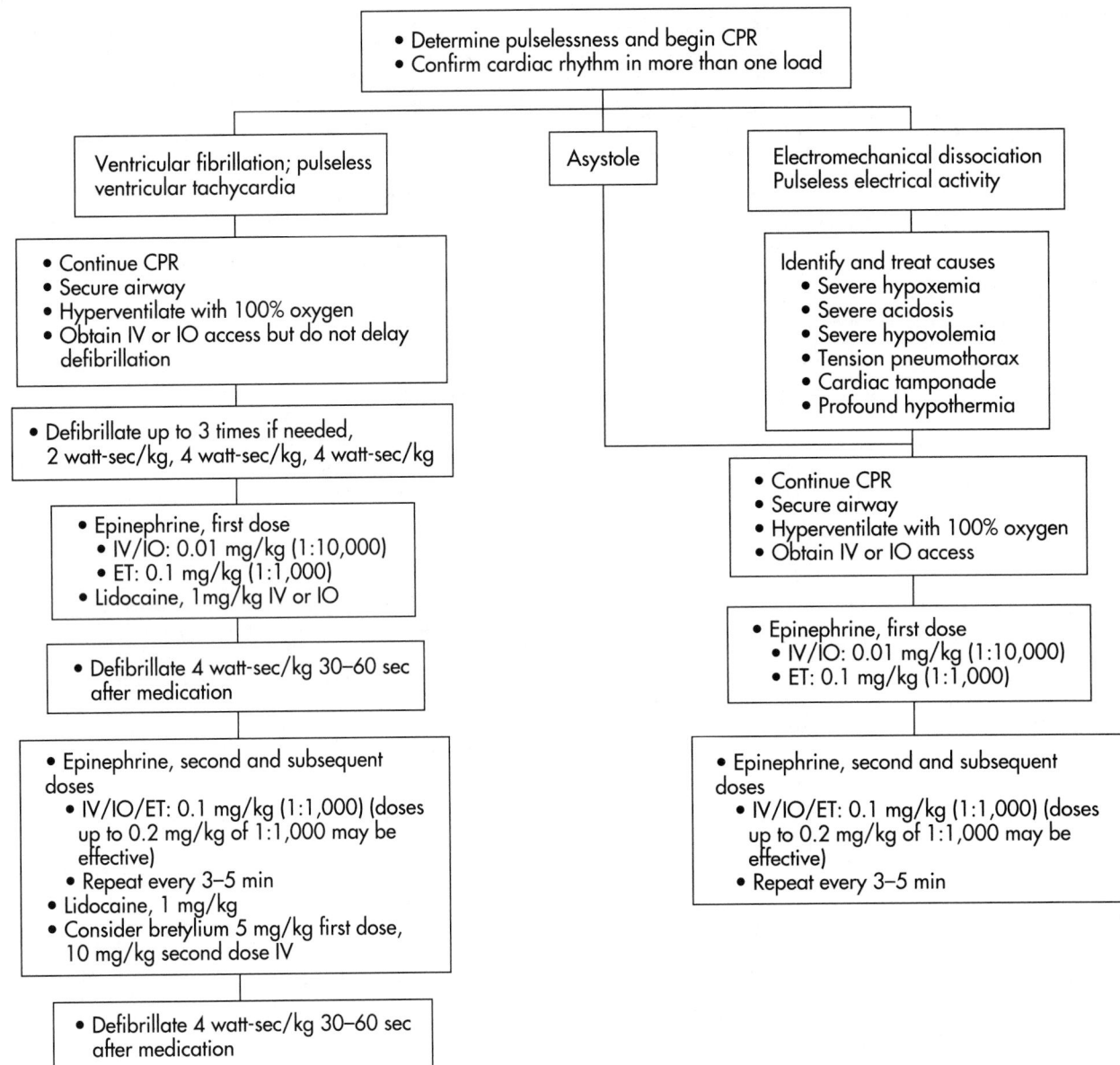

FIG. 12-8. Asystole and pulseless arrest decision tree. *CPR,* Cardiopulmonary resuscitation; *ET,* endotracheal; *IO,* intraosseous; *IV,* intravenous. (*From* JAMA 268:2266, 1992.)

functions: how to turn it on, how it charges the paddles, changes the energy dose, and synchronizes or desynchronizes the discharge. Both ventricular fibrillation and pulseless ventricular tachycardia require defibrillation. Make sure that the synchronize function on the defibrillator is not activated for these rhythms.

For defibrillation to be successful sufficient passage of electrical current must be delivered to the heart. One must depolarize enough of the myocardium to allow for the return of a spontaneous synchronous depolarization of the heart muscle and a perfusing pulse. Flow of current depends on the delivered energy (watt-sec) and the transthoracic impedance. Many factors influence impedance, including paddle size and placement, type of gel used on the paddles, configuration of the chest wall, time interval be-

tween energy dosing, and the skill of the ALS provider in use of a defibrillator.[27]

There is little data available about the optimal dose for defibrillation of infants and children. The American Heart Association recommends 2 watt-sec/kg for the first delivered energy dose (maximum 200 watt-sec) and 4 watt-sec/kg for subsequent doses (maximum delivered energy 360 watt-sec). The paddle size should approximate the size of the palm of the patient. Pediatric paddles are recommended for patients under 10 kilograms, but adult-size paddles may be used on infants using the back-front paddle position and in older children (≥ 10 kg) using standard placement. Various substances may be used for an electrode interface with the skin. These include: electrode cream, gel (not sonographic gel), saline-soaked pads, and self-adhesive

---

Use of the Defibrillator

1. Attach appropriate paddles: pediatric or adult.
2. Apply conductive material to the paddles.
3. Turn on the power.
4. Select the appropriate energy dose for defibrillation or cardioversion.
5. For cardioversion, engage the synchronous mode button and check the monitor to make sure that each QRS complex is marked signifying the machine is in the synchronous mode.
6. For defibrillation, **DO NOT** engage the synchronous mode button.
7. Place paddles on the appropriate areas of the chest.
8. Clear the area to ensure that no personnel is in contact with the patient or gurney.
9. Apply firm pressure to the paddles and discharge the energy dose.
10. Recheck the rhythm on the monitor.
11. Palpate the pulses.
12. Repeat as per protocol.

---

defibrillation pads. Defibrillation is not indicated for treatment of asystole. Make sure that everyone is clear from the gurney when discharging the energy from the paddles (see box above). Inform those in attendance that you are about to discharge the paddles by saying "one—I am clear, two—Are you clear? three—Is everyone clear?"

Supraventricular tachycardia (SVT) generally occurs in infants but may be seen in older children with structural abnormalities of the conducting system of the heart. Assess the hemodynamic stability of the patient. If vital signs are *stable*, attempt vagal maneuvers such as ice to the entire face or placing the infant in a knee-chest position. Start an IV line, and if possible, consult a pediatric cardiologist. Many cardiologists prefer to rapidly digitalize the stable patient with SVT; however, other drugs such as adenosine may be used.

Adenosine is the drug of choice for SVT. It must be given as a very rapid IV push because it is metabolized rapidly by red blood cells. It produces a transient atrioventricular block and terminates the reentry rhythm. It has a half-life of 10 seconds and has almost no side effects. A long pause in rhythm may be seen on the ECG or monitor before conversion to a normal sinus rhythm. The dose is 0.1 mg/kg rapidly (maximum single dose is 12 mg).[18] This may be repeated. Verapamil has been used in children over 1 year of age (see Chapter 14). Treat pediatric patients with SVT who are *unstable* and have an IV line in place with adenosine. If IV access cannot be rapidly achieved, treat with synchronized cardioversion at 0.5 watt-sec/kg. If this fails to produce a sinus rhythm, repeat cardioversion with 1 watt-sec/kg.

Medication and Fluid Therapy

If adequate ventilation, oxygenation, and chest compressions fail to restore cardiac function and ventilation, medi-cations and fluids may be necessary (Table 12-3). Medications and fluids are used during resuscitation to:

- Increase myocardial perfusion
- Increase the reload on the heart muscle
- Correct hypoxemia
- Stimulate myocardial contraction
- Provide more forceful cardiac contraction
- Increase the heart rate
- Decrease the afterload
- Suppress abnormal rhythms
- Correct acidosis

Fluid Administration. Shock and circulatory collapse may be the primary etiology of cardiopulmonary arrest; an initial volume load of 20 ml/kg of isotonic crystalloid should be considered. The type of fluid used—isotonic saline or lactated Ringer's solution—depends on institutional preference. Blood may be required in the trauma patient who has significant blood loss. Fluid should be given by rapid infusion IV or IO push as fast as possible. Several fluid boluses may be required when there is circulatory collapse.

Vascular Access. During resuscitation, vascular access is essential for the infusion of fluids and medications and for obtaining diagnostic blood specimens. Although certain drugs such as *l*idocaine, *e*pinephrine, *a*tropine, and *n*aloxone (easily remembered by the mnemonic *LEAN*) can be given via the tracheobronchial tree using an ET tube, the exact dosage for ET tube administration is not known. The blood levels achieved via the ET route are not as high or sustained as when these drugs are given intravenously or via the intraosseous route.[28,29] However, during an asystolic arrest, it is reasonable to give the first dose of epinephrine down the ET tube while attempts are made in securing an intravenous or intraosseous line. Use at least 10 times the standard dose of epinephrine, or 0.1 mg/kg (0.1 ml/kg of a 1:1,000 solution) for ET installation. Doses as high as 0.2 mg/kg may be useful. Dilute the drug in at least 2 ml of normal saline and either inject via a feeding tube put down the ET tube or instill it directly into the ET tube. This should be followed with positive pressure ventilation to assure distribution into the lower airway.

No more than 1 to 2 minutes should be spent in an initial attempt at IV access.[30] If a line can not be rapidly instituted, the intraosseous route should be used.[31]

Remember that fluids may have to be pushed, since the flow rates are much slower than through intravenous lines.[32] After the intraosseous line is in place, others can continue attempts for venous access through a central or peripheral approach. Practically all drugs and fluids that can be given intravenously can be given via intraosseous access. Dilute hypertonic solutions, such as 50% dextrose or sodium bicarbonate 1:1 with saline or water.

Pharmacologic Agents. The most important functions of medications during CPR are to restore myocardial blood flow to the critical level, to restore the ability of the heart to function as a pump, and to increase cerebral perfusion.[33-36]

Epinephrine. Epinephrine is the most important drug used in CPR of the newborn and pediatric patient. The alpha effects of epinephrine are important in increasing coronary blood flow and perfusion to the brain. Epineph-

TABLE 12-3. Primary and Secondary Measures in Resuscitation

Drug availability	Dose/route	Indications	Adverse reactions	Comments
Adenosine (Adenocard) (3 mg/ml)	0.1 mg/kg rapid IV push (maximum 12 mg/dose)	SVT	Hypotension, chest pain, dyspnea, dysrhythmia, heart block	Monitor carefully; do not use in second or third degree heart block, or sick sinus syndrome
Albuterol (Proventil, Ventolin) soln (inhalation) (0.5%-5 mg/ml)	Inhalation 0.03 ml/kg/dose (maximum: 0.5-1.0 ml/dose) diluted in 2 ml saline	Bronchoconstriction	Tachycardia, nausea	Beta-2 agonist
Atropine (0.1, 0.4, 1.0 mg/ml)	0.01-0.03 mg/kg/dose (minimum: 0.1 mg/dose) (adult: 0.6-1.0 mg/dose; maximum 2 mg) q 5 min prn IV, ET, IO	Bradycardia, asystole, ↑ vagal tone Heart block (temporary)	Tachycardia, dysrhythmias, anticholinergic	Parasympatholytic; use 2-3 times dose ET
Bicarbonate, sodium (NaHCO₃) (8.4%-50 mEq/50 ml) (7.5%-44.5 mEq/50 ml)	1 mEq/kg/dose q 10 min prn IV, IO	Metabolic acidosis Hyperkalemia	Metabolic alkalosis, hyperosmolality, hypernatremia	Dilute 1:1 with D5W or sterile water; incompatible with calcium, catecholamine infusion; monitor ABG
Bretylium (50 mg/ml)	5 mg/kg/dose IV followed prn by 10 mg/kg/dose q 15 min IV up to 30 mg/kg	Ventricular dysrhythmias refractory to lidocaine	Hypotension (orthostatic), bradydysrhythmias	Blocks adrenergic nerve endings; do not give ET
Calcium chloride (10%-100 mg/ml) (1.36 mEq Ca⁺⁺/ml)	20-30 mg (0.2-0.3 ml)/kg/dose (maximum: 500 mg/dose) q 10 min prn IV slowly	Hyperkalemia Calcium channel blocker OD	Rapid infusion causes bradycardia, hypotension Extravasation—necrosis	Inotropic; monitor; use caution with digitalized patient; probably no benefit in asystole or electromechanical dissociation
Crystalloid 0.9% NS, LR, D5W, 0.9% NS, D5WLR	20 ml/kg over 20-30 min IV	Hypovolemia		Monitor volume status
Defibrillation	1-2 watt-sec/kg (adult: 200 watt-sec/kg)	Ventricular fibrillation		Use correct paddle size and paste; cardioversion (0.5-1.0 watt-sec/kg)
Dexamethasone (Decadron) (4, 24 mg/ml)	0.15-0.60 mg/kg/dose IM, IV	Croup, asthma, meningitis		Delayed onset
Dextrose (D50W-0.5 gm/ml)	0.5-1.0 gm (2-4 ml D25W or 1-2 ml D50W)/kg/dose IV	Hypoglycemia, with coma or seizure		Draw glucose; if possible use D25W
Diazepam (Valium) (5 mg/ml)	0.2-0.3 mg/kg/dose (maximum: 10 mg/dose) IV	Status epilepticus	Respiratory depression	Also begin maintenance medication; may give higher dose rectally (0.5 mg/kg PR)
Diazoxide (Hyperstat) (15 mg/ml)	1-3 mg/kg q 4-24 hr IV	Hypertension	Hypotension, hyperglycemia	Monitor (very prompt onset)
Digoxin (0.1, 0.25 mg/ml)	Premie: 0.01-0.02 mg/kg TDD IV 2 wk-2 yr: 0.03-0.05 mg/kg TDD IV Newborn and >2 yr: 0.04 mg/kg TDD IV. ½ TDD initially, then ¼ q 4-8 hr IV × 2	Congestive heart failure Supraventricular tachycardia	Dysrhythmia, heart block, vomiting	Monitor ECG; may also load PO in nonarrest situation; if mild CHF, may give PO without loading

TDD, Total digitalizing dose.

TABLE 12-3. Primary and Secondary Measures in Resuscitation—cont'd

Drug availability	Dose/route	Indications	Adverse reactions	Comments
Dopamine (200 mg/5 ml)	Low: 2-5 μg/kg/min IV Mod: 5-20 μg/kg/min IV High: >20 μg/kg/min IV	Cardiogenic shock (moderate dose) Maintain renal perfusion	Tachycardia, bradycardia, vasoconstriction (increase with higher doses)	Beta adrenergic; avoid in hypovolemic shock; may use in combination with isoproterenol or levarterenol (norepinephrine)
Dobutamine (Dobutrex) (vial: 250 mg)	2-15 μg/kg/min IV	Cardiogenic shock	Tachycardia	Beta adrenergic; positive inotropic; may be synergistic with dopamine or isoproterenol
Epinephrine (1:10,000) (0.1 mg/ml)	Initial: 0.01 mg (0.1 ml) (1:10,000)/kg/dose (max: 10 ml/dose) IV Second or ET: 0.1 mg (0.1 ml) (1:1,000)/kg/dose q 3-5 min prn	Ventricular standstill Ventricular fibrillation (fine)	Tachycardia, dysrhythmia, hypertension, decreased renal and splanchnic blood flow	Alpha and beta—adrenergic; inotropic; not effective if acidotic; higher doses may be effective
Epinephrine (1:1,000) (1 mg/ml)	0.01 ml/kg/dose SC (maximum: 0.35 ml/dose) q 10-20 min SC × 3 prn	Reactive airway disease	Tachycardia, headache, nausea	Rarely used because of side effects; may use for ET or second IV dose (above and text)
Epinephrine racemic (Vaponefrin) (2.25% solution)	0.25-0.75 ml/dose by inhalation	Croup, airway edema	Tachycardia, palpitations, dysrhythmia, nausea, vomiting, rebound stridor	Monitor; observe over time
Fentanyl (Sublimaze, Innovar) (50 μg/ml)	1-5 μg/kg/dose IV, IM	Analgesia	Respiratory depression, apnea, muscle rigidity, bradycardia, nausea, vomiting, cardiac arrest	Monitor; be prepared to manage the airway
Furosemide (Lasix) (10 mg/ml)	1 mg/kg/dose q 6-12 hr IV up to 6 mg/kg dose; may repeat q 2 hr prn	Fluid overload, pulmonary edema, cerebral edema	Hypokalemia, hyponatremia, prerenal azotemia	Reduce dosage in newborn to q 12 hr; if no response in urine output in 30 min, repeat; do not use if hypovolemic
Glucagon (1 mg [1 unit]/ml)	0.03-0.1 mg/kg/dose q 20 min prn IV, SC, IM	Beta-blocker overdose		Not adequate as only glucose support in neonate; inotropic
Hydralazine (Apresoline) (20 mg/ml)	0.1-0.2 mg/kg/dose q 4-6 hr IV/IM	Hypertension	Tachycardia, tachyphylaxis	Prompt onset
Hydrocortisone (Solu-Cortef) (100, 250, 500 mg)	Asthma: 4-5 mg/kg/dose q 6 hr IV	Adrenal failure Asthma		May be detrimental in shock (controversial)
Isoproterenol (1 mg/5 ml)	0.05-1.5 μg/kg/min Begin at 0.1 μg/kg/min and increase q 5-10 min prn	Bradycardia or heart block (S/P atropine)	Tachydysrhythmias	Beta adrenergic; avoid in hypovolemic shock; do not use with digoxin
Lidocaine (1%-10 mg/ml) (2%-20 mg/ml)	1 mg/kg/dose q 5-10 min IV, ET up to 5 mg/kg, then 20-50 μg/kg/min	Ventricular dysrhythmias Cardiac arrest caused by ventricular fibrillation	Hypotension, bradycardia with block, seizures	↓ Automaticity; for ET administration give 1:1 dilution
Lorazepam (Ativan) (2, 4 mg/ml)	0.05-0.10 mg/kg/dose IV (maximum: 4 mg/dose); may repeat	Status epilepticus	Respiratory depression	Longer acting than diazepam
Methylprednisolone (Solu-Medrol) (40, 125, 500, 1,000 mg)	Asthma: 1-2 mg/kg/dose q 6 hr IV	Adrenal failure Asthma		May be detrimental in shock (controversial)

Continued.

TABLE 12-3. Primary and Secondary Measures in Resuscitation—cont'd

Drug availability	Dose/route	Indications	Adverse reactions	Comments
Midazolam (Versed) (1, 5 mg/ml)	0.035 mg/kg/dose titrated up to total dose 0.15 mg/kg (maximum: 5 mg) IV	Sedation	Respiratory depression, hypotension, bradycardia	Monitor; be prepared to manage the airway
Morphine (8, 10, 15 mg/ml)	0.1-0.2 mg/kg/dose (maximum: 15 mg/dose) q 2-4 hr IV	Pulmonary edema Tetralogy spell Reduce preload and afterload Analgesic	Hypotension, respiratory depression	Antidote; naloxone (Narcan)
Naloxone (Narcan) (0.4 mg/ml) (1 mg/ml)	0.1 mg/kg/dose (maximum: 0.8 mg) IV, ET; if no response in 10 min give 2 mg IV	Narcotic overdose, ? septic shock		Give empirically in suspected opiate overdose; may be given ET
Nitroglycerin (Nitrostat, Nitro-Bid) (0.5, 0.8, 5, 10 mg/ml)	IV 0.5-20 µg/kg/min	Pulmonary edema, angina pectoris, perioperative hypertension	Hypotension, headache, nausea, vomiting, palpitations	Contraindicated with hypotension, increased ICP, hypovolemia, cardiac tamponade, pericarditis, inadequate cerebral circulation
Nitroprusside (50 mg/vial)	0.5-10 µg (average: 3 µg)/kg/min IV	Hypertensive emergency Afterload reduction	Hypotension, nausea, vomiting, cyanide poisoning	Monitor closely; light sensitive
Oxygen	100% mask, ET	Hypoxia Major injury	Toxicity not a problem with acute short-term use	Use high flow (3-6 L/min); monitor ABG
Pancuronium (Pavulon) (1, 2 mg/ml)	0.04-0.1 mg/kg/dose IV; may repeat 0.01-0.02 mg/kg/dose q 20-40 min IV prn	Muscle relaxation	Tachycardia	Rapid onset; support respirations; lower dose in newborn
Phenobarbital (65 mg/ml)	15-20 mg/kg load IV/IM (adult: 100 mg/dose q 20 min prn × 3), then 5 mg/kg/24 hr PO, IV, IM	Seizures	Sedation	If not controlled after load, repeat 10 mg/kg/dose IV; administer <1 mg/kg/min IV; IM erratically absorbed
Phenytoin (Dilantin) (50 mg/ml)	15-20 mg/kg load IV slowly, then 5-10 mg/kg/24 hr PO, IV q 12-24 hr	Seizures	Hypotension, bradycardia when given too fast; cerebral disturbance	Do not give faster than 0.5 mg/kg/min; dilute in normal saline
	1.25 mg/kg/dose IV q 5 min up to a total loading dose of 15 mg/kg	Dysrhythmia		
Succinylcholine (20 mg/ml)	1 mg/kg/dose IV	Muscle relaxation	Dysrhythmia Hypotension	Must be able to control ventilation
Vecuronium (Norcuron) (10 mg/ml)	0.08-0.1 mg/kg/dose IV	Non-depolarizing muscle blockade	Profound skeletal muscle weakness, respiratory arrest	Monitor; only to be used by persons with advanced airway management skills
Verapamil (Calan, Isoptin) (2.5 mg/ml)	0.1-0.3 mg/kg/dose (maximum: 5 mg/dose) IV; may repeat in 30 min	SVT	Dizziness, hypotension, bradycardia, A-V block	Monitor; contraindicated in patients <1 yr or with ventricular dysfunction, sick sinus syndrome, 2nd or 3rd degree heart block, atrial fibrillation or flutter

TDD, Total digitalizing dose.

rine increases myocardial contractility, systemic vascular resistance, and the automaticity of the heart. Few patients currently survive when two rounds of medication are given without myocardial response, and studies suggest that the standard doses of epinephrine currently recommended may be too small.[18,37-39] The Pediatric Subcommittee of the American Heart Association Committee on Emergency Cardiac Care currently recommends 0.01 mg/kg for the first dose of a 1:10,000 dilution, with subsequent doses for cardiac standstill of up to 0.1 mg/kg (using a 1:1000 dilution) for asystolic cardiac arrest.[29-31] Successful therapy with return to spontaneous circulation using high dose epinephrine (0.2 mg/kg) was found in a small sample size of children after a witnessed cardiac arrest with CPR initiated in a short period of time.[37] These data, however, do not suggest that high dose epinephrine is effective in the resuscitation of all asystolic arrests in the pediatric population. The optimum dose of epinephrine for ET use has not been determined. The response to standard doses given to animals in shock was erratic and unpredictable.[38] Give the standard dose of 0.01 mg/kg IV or IO for symptomatic bradycardia.

Atropine. Atropine is a parasympatholytic drug that accelerates the atrial pacemakers and atrioventricular (AV) conduction. It should be used for symptomatic bradycardia due to vagal stimulation, such as after ET intubation, or symptomatic bradycardia with AV block. The recommended dose is 0.02 mg/kg ET, IV, IO with a maximum single dose of 0.5 mg for an infant and 1 mg for a child. The minimum dose of atropine is 0.1 mg because of the association of paradoxical bradycardia with low doses.[39] Remember that bradycardia may be the result of poor oxygenation and ventilation, and airway management is always paramount in any resuscitation. Although it has been suggested that atropine may be of benefit in asystolic effect, there are no conclusive studies to suggest its use in resuscitation.[40] Atropine will cause dilatation of the pupils, so this may alter the ability to follow this neurologic sign during the early stages of the patient's clinical course.

Calcium. In healthy myocardial tissue, calcium enhances cardiac contractility but in the hypoxic heart, it can not actively be pumped out of the cell and the influx of calcium ions may lead to rapid cell death. Calcium was originally used during resuscitation because of data from patients undergoing open heart surgery on a pump. These patients required calcium therapy to start their hearts. Both retrospective and prospective studies primarily in adults have failed to demonstrate any benefit of calcium therapy during cardiopulmonary arrest and in fact, it may be detrimental.[41-43] Calcium is only indicated for documented hypocalcemia, hyperkalemia, hypermagnesemia, and calcium channel blocker overdose. Calcium is available as a chloride (10%) or gluconate (10%). The chloride preparation contains three times the amount of available calcium and is the drug of choice as it produces predictable levels of elemental calcium. The recommended dose is 5 to 7 mg/kg of elemental calcium, or 0.2 to 0.25 ml/kg of 10% calcium chloride. Infuse the drug slowly (maximum of 100 mg/min) to avoid significant bradycardia or arrest, especially in those receiving digoxin. Monitor serum calcium levels during therapy.

Sodium Bicarbonate. Severe disturbances of acid-base balance usually accompany cardiopulmonary arrest. It was hypothesized that giving a base during resuscitation would improve the pressor response of epinephrine and improve outcome. There is evidence to suggest that this is not true. In fact, the administration of bicarbonate in cardiopulmonary arrest may actually increase the intracellular carbon dioxide and promote cellular dysfunction. Acidosis does not seem to impair the pressor response of epinephrine and intracellular acidosis may protect the heart from damage because of an influx of calcium ions.[44-46] Sodium bicarbonate may be harmful if given before the establishment of adequate ventilation to remove carbon dioxide. The use of sodium bicarbonate during CPR may actually inhibit cardiac contractility so it should not be used until perfusion is restored. The use of base may also be considered if there is prolonged cardiac arrest with severe acidosis unresponsive to routine therapy, tricyclic antidepressant overdose and hyperkalemia. The recommended dose is 1 mEq/kg IV or IO with subsequent doses of 0.5 mEq/kg every 10 minutes of continued arrest or monitored acid-base status.

Glucose. Hypoglycemia may accompany trauma, respiratory failure, shock, sepsis, and many other illnesses. Small infants are particularly prone to this abnormality because of the lack of adequate glycogen stores. Hypoglycemia may effect myocardial and cerebral function. High blood sugars have been associated with poor recovery after myocardial infarction.[47,48] A bedside glucose test is helpful in the evaluation of hypoglycemia and hyperglycemia. If there is profound hypoglycemia with a glucose of less than or equal to 40 mg/dl, give glucose at a dose of 0.5 gm/kg 25% dextrose in water for intravenous and intraosseous infusions. If 50% dextrose is used, dilute 1:1 with water. A bolus of any solution with 5% dextrose at 10 ml/kg will also provide 0.5 gm/kg of dextrose.

Isoproterenol. The only indication for isoproterenol therapy is hemodynamically significant bradycardia caused by heart block that is unresponsive to atropine. Make sure that the patient is adequately ventilated and is not hypovolemic before administering this drug. Isoproterenol has a very short half-life and must be given by continuous infusion. The starting dose is generally 0.1 µg/kg/min. It is titrated until the desired effect is achieved, and rates up to 1 µg/kg/min may be required.

Infusions. *Epinephrine infusions* are helpful for patients who have suffered ischemic hypoxic insults and are hypotensive and unstable after resuscitation. The infusion rate is 0.05 to 1 µg/kg/min. Higher initial doses (up to 15 µg/kg/min) may be required until a response is seen. The infusion should then be adjusted to deliver the standard dose. Doses below 0.3 µg/kg/min are associated primarily with beta-adrenergic effects; higher doses with an alpha effect. Remember that epinephrine infusions cause a decrease in blood flow to abdominal organs and the kidney and should be used with caution with hypovolemia. The half-life is about 2 minutes and thus the rate can be easily adjusted. Fluid resuscitation should precede the use of an epinephrine infusion in the patient in shock.

Dobutamine is a selected inotrope that is helpful in patients who show signs of poor perfusion with or without a normal blood pressure. The drug increases heart rate and cardiac contractility and may cause mild peripheral vasodilatation. It may be particularly useful in those with cardiogenic shock. The dose is 2 to 15 μg/kg/min.

Dopamine may not be as useful as epinephrine or dobutamine in patients with poor myocardial and peripheral perfusion. It has an advantage over other inotropic agents, however, because of its actions on the renal and splanchnic perfusion. The dose is 5 to 20 μg/kg/min. The renal effects are found with low doses (<3 μg/kg/min) and cardiac effects at higher doses. It may be particularly helpful in septic shock. The half-life is very short; therefore a constant infusion is necessary for the drug to have an effect on perfusion. Like other inotropic agents it may produce tachycardia, hypertension, and rhythm disturbances.

Sodium Nitroprusside. Sodium nitroprusside is a very potent vasodilator that has effects on both the arterial and venous vessels. It is rapidly metabolized by red blood cells and thus a constant infusion is needed to maintain its effects. It is used in the treatment of severe hypertension and heart failure that is unresponsive to diuretic therapy. The drug reduces blood pressure and thus afterload by peripherally dilating the peripheral vessels, thereby decreasing both afterload and preload and the work and oxygen consumption of the myocardium. The drug must be given intravenously and has a rapid onset of action within 1 to 2 minutes after initiation of the infusion. The initial dose is 0.3 to 0.5 μg/kg/min, which may be titrated to the desired endpoint. Monitor the patient carefully for changes in pulse and blood pressure as toxicity may occur suddenly. Take particular caution when using this infusion along with diuretics. Most infusions can easily be made up using the rule of sixes (see Appendix C).

Lidocaine and bretylium may be required to treat rhythm disturbances. These drugs and electrotherapy are discussed in Chapter 14. It should be mentioned, however, that defibrillation is not indicated for the treatment of asystole.

Pacing. Pediatric patients with heart block unresponsive to therapy may require pacing. This may be done transvenously or via the esophagus. These techniques have been successful in stabilizing the patient until a permanent pacemaker can be implanted.[49,50]

Ancillary Data. During the period of resuscitation, a variety of laboratory tests and other procedures should be performed in addition to those necessary to evaluate the patient's underlying condition. Generally, a complete blood count (CBC) is required, optimally with immediate availability of a hematocrit. Chemistries should include electrolytes, BUN, creatinine, glucose, calcium, and phosphorus. ABG levels are routinely done along with oximetry; type and crossmatch is useful. A chest radiograph, ECG, and ongoing cardiac and oximetry monitoring are essential. Remember pulse oximetry is not reliable in severe circulatory compromise and may only be useful in post-resuscitative care. End-tidal CO_2 monitoring can help the assessment of perfusion during CPR. The nature and quantity of output from a nasogastric tube and urinary catheter should be determined.

Psychologic Support. Support for the child and entire family is essential throughout the entire resuscitation. In the child who is successfully resuscitated, time should be taken to calm and reassure the child who has been separated from his or her parents and is in a strange environment. A member of the health-care team should be assigned to provide the family with information, explanations, and emotional support. The decision to allow parents to stay with the child during the resuscitation must be personalized, based on the child's medical condition and state of consciousness and the emotional status of the family.

If the child dies, support and compassion are needed as outlined in Chapter 8. Most parents will want to touch and hold the child after he or she has been made presentable. All health professionals involved in the child's care must be allowed to decompress, expressing their own feelings, often in an environment that allows for review of the team efforts.[51,52] Ultimately, a formal management review should be done once clinical, management, and autopsy information is available and analyzed.

Cardiopulmonary arrest in the pediatric patient is rarely a sudden event. Outcomes may best be improved by preventing cardiopulmonary failure and arrest. This will be best accomplished through public education, improving emergency medical services for children, and provision of optimal definitive care.

POST-RESUSCITATION

After successful resuscitation it is important to continue to offer supportive care and constant monitoring and reassessment of the clinical status of the patient. The goal is to prevent further ongoing damage and organ failure. Although a return to spontaneous circulation may occur, there is no guarantee of a good outcome and many patients will remain in irreversible shock or in a permanent vegetative state. Continually monitor the following parameters:

- Ventilation
- Oxygenation
- Work of breathing, if there is spontaneous respiration
- Ventilator settings, if mechanical ventilation is used
- Pulses
- Blood pressure
- Cardiac rhythm
- Urine output
- Core temperature

Blood gases and other laboratory tests can be ordered as needed. Search for a precipitating cause of the cardiopulmonary arrest and treat it accordingly. Give IV fluids with glucose as appropriate.

Most children who have had a potentially catastrophic event such as a cardiopulmonary arrest will benefit from pediatric intensive care. Minute-to-minute assessment by skilled pediatric intensive care nurses and physicians may improve outcomes. Arrange a critical care transport to a pediatric tertiary care facility. This may be accomplished by air or ground transport, depending on the weather and resources available in the region (see Chapter 5).

It is helpful for all parties who have participated in a resuscitation to meet soon after the incident and openly discuss the resuscitation. Topics for discussion may include the following:

- General impressions on how things went
- How the resuscitation team functioned
- What could have been done differently
- What went well

If the outcome has not been optimal, it is important for those involved to remember that the process is one of reanimation and that the expectation is that very few children will survive intact. Health professionals may feel inadequate and guilty if a resuscitation is not successful and a more formal critical stress debriefing may be required (see Chapter 8).

References

1. O'Rourke PP: Outcome of children who are apneic and pulseless in the emergency room, *Crit Care Med* 14:466-468, 1986.
2. Eisenberg M, Berger L, Hallstrom A: Epidemiology of cardiac arrest and resuscitation in children, *Ann Emerg Med* 12:672-674, 1983.
3. Torphy DE, Minter MG, Thompson BM: Cardiorespiratory arrest and resuscitation of children, *Am J Dis Child* 138:1099, 1984.
4. Ludwig S, Kettrick RC, Parker M: Pediatric cardiopulmonary resuscitation, *Clin Pediatr* 23:71-75, 1984.
5. Teach SJ, Moore PE, Fleisher GR: Death and resuscitation in the pediatric emergency department, *Ann Emerg Med* 25:799-803, 1995.
6. Rainer TH, Gordon MW, Robertson CE, Cusack S: Evaluation of outcome following cardiac arrest in patients presenting to two Scottish emergency departments, *Resuscitation* 29:33-39, 1995.
7. Safar P: Reanimatology—the science of resuscitation, *Crit Care Med* 10:134-136, 1982.
8. Cummins R, Eisenber M, Hallstrom A, Litwin P: Survival of out-of-hospital cardiac arrest with early initiation of CPR, *Am J Emerg Med* 3:114-118, 1985.
9. Kellerman A, Hackman B, Somes G: Dispatcher assisted CPR, *Circulation* 1989;80:1231-1239.
10. Quan L and Seidel JS, editors: *Instructors manual: pediatric advanced life support*, Dallas, 1995, American Heart Association.
11. Kaye W and Mancini M: Retention of CPR skills by physicians, registered nurses and the general public, *Crit Care Med* 14:620-622, 1986.
12. Bossaert L: *CPR: cardiopulmonary resuscitation in Belgium.* An evaluation of CPR education and CPR performance by the lay public, Antwerpen, Belgium, 1991, Universiteit Antwerpen Department Geneeskunde.
13. Melker R and Banner WJ: Ventilation during CPR: two rescuer standards reappraised, *Ann Emerg Med* 14:397, 1985.
14. Terndrop TE, Kanter RK, Cherry RA: A comparison of infant ventilation methods performed by prehospital personnel, *Ann Emerg Med* 18:607, 1989.
15. Gausche M and Henderson DP: *Advanced airway management student manual*, Los Angeles, 1994, Pediatric Airway Project.
16. Lubitz DS, Seidel JS, Chameides L, et al: A rapid method for estimating weight and resuscitation drug doses from length in the pediatric age group, *Ann Emerg Med* 17:576-581, 1988.
17. Bhende MS and Thompson AE: Evaluation of an end-tidal CO_2 detector during pediatric cardiopulmonary resuscitation, *Pediatrics* 95:395-399, 1995.
18. Chameides L and Hazinski MF: *Textbook of pediatric advanced life support*, Dallas, 1994, American Heart Association.
19. Dean JM, Koehler RC, Michael JR, et al: Age-related changes in chest geometry during cardiopulmonary resuscitation, *J Appl Physiol* 62:2212-2219, 1987.
20. Schleien CL, Berkowitz ID, Traystman R, Rogers MC: Controversial issues in cardiopulmonary resuscitation, *Anesthesiology* 71:133-149, 1989.
21. Niemann JT, Rosborough J, Hausknecht M, et al: Cough CPR. Documentation of systemic perfusion in man and in an experimental model: a window to the mechanism of blood flow in external CPR, *Crit Care Med* 8: 141-146, 1980.
22. Chandra NC, Beyar R, Halparin HR, et al: Vital organ perfusion during assisted circulation by manipulation of intrathorasis pressure, *Circulation* 84:279-286, 1991.
23. Orlowski JP: Optimum position for external cardiac compression in infants and young children, *Ann Emerg Med* 15:667-673, 1986.
24. Berkowitz ID, Chantarojanasiri T, Koehler RC, et al: Blood flow during cardiopulmonary resuscitation with simultaneous compression and ventilation in infant pigs, *Pediatr Res* 26:558-564, 1989.

25. Sack JB, Kesselbrenner MB, Bregman D: Survival from in-hospital cardiac arrest with interposed abdominal counterpulsation during cardiopulmonary resuscitation, *JAMA* 267:379-385, 1992.
26. Mogayzel C, Quan L, Graves JR, et al: Out-of-hospital ventricular fibrillation in children and adilescents:causes and outcomes, *Ann Emerg Med* 25:484-491, 1995.
27. Kerber RE, Grayzel J, Hoyt R, et al: Transthoracic resistance in human defibrillation: influence of body weight, chest size, serial shocks, paddle size, and paddle contact pressure, *Circulation* 63:676-682, 1981.
28. Zaritsky A: Selected topics and controversies in pediatric cardiopulmonary resuscitation, *Crit Care Clin* 4:735-750, 1988.
29. McGonigle LF, Coe JY, Timinsky T: Intraosseous epinephrine is efficacious in hypoxic piglets. Sixty-third scientific session, Dallas, 1990, American Heart Association.
30. Kanter RT, Zimmerman JJ, Strauss RN: Pediatric emergency intravenous access: evaluation of a protocol, *Am J Dis Child* 140:132-134, 1982.
31. Fiser DH: Intraosseous infusion, *N Engl J Med* 322:1579-1581, 1990.
32. Hodge D, Delgado-Paredes C, Fleisher G: Intraosseous infusion flow rates in hypovolemic "pediatric" dogs, *Ann Emerg Med* 16:305-307, 1987.
33. Paradis NA, Martin GB, Rivers EP, et al: Coronary perfusion pressure and the return of spontaneous circulation in human cardiopulmonary resuscitation, *JAMA* 263:1106-1113, 1990.
34. Ralston SH, Voorhees WD, Babbs CF: Intrapulmonary epinephrine during prolonged cardiopulmonary resuscitation: improved regional blood flow and resuscitation in dogs, *Ann Emerg Med* 13:79-86, 1984.
35. Berkowitz ID, Gervais H, Schleien CL, et al: Epinephrine dosage effects on cerebral and myocardial blood flow in an infant swine model of cardiopulmonary resuscitation, *Anesthesiology* (In press.)
36. Brown CG and Werman HA: Adrenergic agonists during cardiopulmonary resuscitation, *Resuscitation* 19:1-16, 1990.
37. Goetting MG and Paradis NA: High dose epinephrine improves outcomes from pediatric cardiac arrest, *Ann Emerg Med* 10:22-26, 1991.
38. Barton C and Callaham M: High dose epinephrine improves the return of spontaneous circulation rates in human victims of cardiac arrest, *Ann Emerg Med* 20:722-725, 1991.
39. Paradis NA, Martin GB, Rosenberg J, et al: The effect of standard and high dose epinephrine on coronary perfusion pressure during prolonged cardiopulmonary resuscitation, *JAMA* 265:1139-1144, 1991.
40. Coon GA, Clinton JE, Ruiz E: Use of atropine for brady-asystolic cardiac arrest. *Ann Emerg Med* 10:462-467, 1981.
41. Steuven HA, Thompson BM, Aprahamian C, et al: Lack of effectiveness of calcium chloride in refractory asystole, *Ann Emerg Med* 14:630-632, 1985.
42. Harrison EE and Amey BD: Use of calcium in electromechanical dissociation, *Ann Emerg Med* 13:844, 1984.
43. Dembo DH: Calcium in advanced life support, *Crit Care Med* 19:358, 1981.
44. Kitakaze M, Weisfeldt ML, Marban E: Acidosis during early reperfusion prevents myocardial stunning in perfused ferret hearts, *J Clin Invest* 82:920-926, 1988.
45. Paradis NA, Goetting MG, Rivers EP, et al: The effect of pH on the change in coronary perfusion pressure after epinephrine during CPR in human beings, *Ann Emerg Med* 19:458, 1990.
46. Graf H, Leach W, Arrieff AI: Evidence for a detrimental effect of bicarbonate therapy in hypoxic lactic acidosis, *Science* 227:754-756, 1984.
47. Nakikimura K, Fleisher JE, Drummond JC, et al: Glucose administration before cardiac arrest worsens neurologic outcome in cats, *Anesthesiology* 72:1005-1011, 1990.
48. Zaritsky A: Pediatric resuscitation pharmacology, *Ann Emerg Med* 22:445-455, 1993.
49. Rhodes LA, Walsh EP, Saul JP: Programmed atrial stimulation via the esophagus for managemnent of supraventricular arrhytmias in infants and children, *Am J Cardiol* 74:353-356, 1994.
50. Gillette PC, Zeigler VL, Winslow AT, Kratz JM: Cardiac pacing in neonates, infants and preschool children, *Pace Pacing Clin Electrophysiol* 15:2046-2049, 1992.
51. Soreff SM: Sudden death in the emergency department: a comprehensive approach for families, emergency medical technicians and emergency department staff, *Crit Care Med* 7(7):321, 1979.
52. Mitchell JT and Bray GP: *Emergency services stress.* Englewood Cliffs, NJ, 1990, Prentice-Hall.

13

Shock

Mary Fran Hazinski • Roger M. Barkin

Shock is a condition of sustained and progressive circulatory dysfunction that results in inadequate delivery of oxygen and substrates to meet tissue metabolic demands. Shock may be the end result of hemorrhage, severe dehydration, progressive heart failure, or sepsis. It may also complicate the care of the child with pulmonary failure, drug toxicity, electrolyte or acid-base imbalance, or multiorgan system failure.

Shock may be associated with normal, low, or high cardiac output, but in all forms of shock the cardiac output is inadequate to sustain effective tissue perfusion and organ function. If systemic perfusion and oxygen delivery are not promptly restored and maintained, organ system failure and death will result.

PATHOPHYSIOLOGY

Factors Affecting Cardiac Output

Effective cardiovascular function requires adequate systemic arterial oxygen content, appropriate heart rate, adequate intravascular volume relative to the vascular space, good myocardial function, appropriate systemic and pulmonary vascular resistances, reasonable metabolic rate, effective tissue use of oxygen, and normal capillary permeability. When shock is present, any or all of these elements may be abnormal.

Cardiac output is the volume of blood ejected by the heart each minute; it is the product of heart rate and stroke volume. Inadequate intravascular volume, myocardial dysfunction, or excessive systemic or pulmonary vascular resistances can reduce stroke volume. If either heart rate or stroke volume decreases without a commensurate and compensatory increase in the other component, cardiac output will fall. If the arterial oxygen content is extremely low, the metabolic rate is extremely high, or cardiac output is inappropriately distributed to tissues, even a high cardiac output may be inadequate. Therefore all elements of cardiopulmonary function must be supported to optimize oxygen delivery and use.

During childhood, heart rate is more rapid and the stroke volume is smaller than during adult life.[1] For this reason, the cardiac output depends on an appropriate heart rate, and a fall in heart rate will likely result in a commensurate fall in cardiac output.[2] Several years ago, studies performed in animal models suggested that infants were unable to increase stroke volume[3]; now it is clear that stroke volume may be increased during infancy and childhood but that heart rate continues to exert the most significant impact on cardiac output.[2,4]

Heart Rate. The child's heart rate must be appropriate for the child's clinical condition.[2,5] Tachycardia should be observed in the child with cardiorespiratory distress; a normal heart rate in such a child is inappropriate and will likely be associated with inadequate cardiac output and systemic perfusion. Bradycardia is an ominous sign in the critically ill child with shock or respiratory failure and frequently indicates impending arrest. Hypoxia is a common cause of bradycardia in children.[2,5] As a result, airway patency, oxygenation, and ventilation must be constantly assessed and supported as needed.

An extremely high heart rate may also result in shock. Supraventricular tachycardia (SVT) or ventricular dysrhythmias may result in inadequate ventricular diastolic filling time and a fall in stroke volume. Since the left coronary artery perfuses the left ventricle only during diastole, severe curtailment of diastolic filling time may result in left ventricular subendocardial ischemia and a further compromise in cardiac performance. In general a heart rate exceeding 200 to 220/min in the infant, or a ventricular rate exceeding 160 to 180/min in the child will compromise cardiovascular function, and symptoms of congestive heart failure or shock may develop. Once SVT causes signs of shock, intravenous adenosine or synchronized cardioversion must be provided on an urgent basis.[2]

Stroke Volume. The child's stroke volume may be altered by conditions affecting ventricular preload, compliance, contractility, and afterload. Each of these variables must be evaluated and optimized in the treatment of the shock.

Ventricular Preload and Compliance. *Ventricular preload* refers to the presystolic stretch of ventricular fibers. The Frank-Starling Law of the Heart describes the linear relationship between the presystolic length of isolated normal myocardial fibers and the tension generated by fibers during contraction (Fig. 13-1); as myocardial fiber length is increased, the tension generated by myocardial fibers and the stroke volume generated by the ventricles increase. Since the length of myocardial fibers cannot be conveniently measured in the clinical setting, right or left ventricular end-diastolic pressure (RVEDP or LVEDP) is measured to evaluate trends in the ventricular preload. The VEDP is frequently referred to as the *filling pressure* of the ventricle. Volume administration increases the VEDP or filling pressure, stretching ventricular fibers (see *Point A to B*, Fig. 13-1). This increase in preload should result in an increase in stroke volume and cardiac output.

Central venous or right atrial pressure is equal to the RVEDP in the absence of tricuspid valve stenosis. In the absence of mitral valve disease, the pulmonary artery wedge pressure (PAWP) will reflect the LVEDP if the catheter tip is wedged in a proper location in the lung and the transducer is appropriately zeroed, leveled, and calibrated. In the presence of a high positive end-expiratory pressure or extreme tachycardia the PAWP may be higher than the LVEDP.[6]

Clinical assessment may enable relatively accurate estimation of the central venous pressure (CVP) and RVEDP.[7] If the cardiac silhouette is small on the chest radiograph and hepatomegaly and systemic edema are absent, it is unlikely that the child's CVP or RVEDP is high. Conversely, in the presence of a high CVP and RVEDP, systemic edema and hepatomegaly are likely to be observed, and the cardiac silhouette may be large on the chest radiograph (cardiothoracic ratio >0.5).

Although systemic edema may be associated with a high CVP, it may also be observed in the child with a normal or

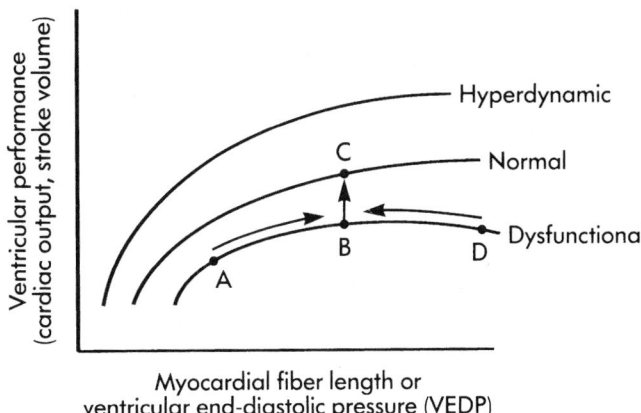

FIG. 13-1. Frank-Starling Curve. In the laboratory description of the Frank-Starling Law (using isolated normal myocardial fibers), an increase in the end-diastolic myocardial fiber length increased the tension generated by the myocardial fiber. In the clinical setting, measurement of end-diastolic fiber length is impossible, so the ventricular end-diastolic pressure (VEDP) is increased to produce improvement in stroke volume or cardiac output. To a point, an increase in VEDP will produce an improvement in cardiac output (A → B); this increase in VEDP is accomplished through judicious titration of intravenous fluid. The clinician must also recognize that a family of myocardial function curves exists; the patient's myocardial function may be characterized as normal, dysfunctional, or hyperdynamic. If the myocardium is dysfunctional, it generally requires a higher VEDP than the normal myocardium to maximize cardiac output. In addition, excessive volume administration can produce a decrease in cardiac output and myocardial performance if the ventricle is dysfunctional (B → D). In this case, administration of a diuretic or vasodilator may improve cardiac output (D → B). Correction of acid-base imbalances, reduction in afterload, or administration of inotropic medications may improve myocardial function so that cardiac output increases without need for further increase in VEDP (B → C). If the patient's myocardial function is hyperdynamic, cardiac output will be high even at low VEDP. (*Courtesy William Banner, Jr, MD; from Hazinski MF: Cardiovascular disorders. In Hazinski MF, editor: Nursing care of the critically ill child, ed 2, St Louis, 1992, Mosby.*)

low CVP and increased capillary permeability or hypoalbuminemia. Therefore systemic edema is not invariably associated with a high CVP and RVEDP.

It is impossible to evaluate the LVEDP from clinical assessment.[7,8] Although pulmonary edema develops once the LVEDP reaches 20 to 25 mm Hg, pulmonary edema may also develop at a normal or low LVEDP if pulmonary capillary permeability is increased. Since the left atrium does not contribute and the left ventricle contributes minimally to the cardiac silhouette on a chest radiograph, moderate left atrial and ventricular dilation may not be detected radiographically.

There is often a significant discrepancy between the RVEDP and the LVEDP, particularly in the presence of septic shock, congenital heart disease, or pulmonary hyper-

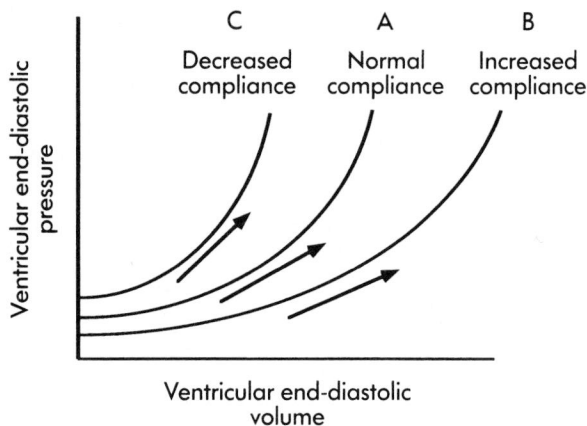

FIG. 13-2. Ventricular compliance is illustrated by a ventricular end-diastolic pressure-volume curve. The slope of a tangent to the curve (*arrows* – dP/dV) represents the stiffness of the ventricle at a given filling pressure. Ventricular compliance changes with age (compliance is lower, or the compliance curve is shifted to the left in the fetus or young infant), cardiovascular disease, and drug therapy. In the normal ventricle (*curve A*), a low ventricular end-diastolic volume is associated with a low VEDP. As the ventricle is filled, smaller changes in volume produce exponentially greater rises in end-diastolic pressure. When the ventricle is dysfunctional or hypertrophied (*curve C*), ventricular compliance is reduced, and even a small increase in ventricular end-diastolic volume will produce a rise in VEDP. Vasodilator therapy can increase ventricular compliance (*curve B*), so that greater ventricular volume can be tolerated without a rise in VEDP; in this manner, the stroke volume can be increased without increasing the VEDP. (*Courtesy William Banner, Jr, MD; from Hazinski MF: Cardiovascular disorders. In Hazinski MF, editor: Nursing care of the critically ill child, ed 2, St Louis, 1992, Mosby.*)

tension. As a result, placement of a pulmonary artery catheter may be necessary to evaluate trends in the LVEDP in response to shock therapy.

It is important to note that the relationship between VEDP and volume administration is not a linear one; it will be influenced by ventricular compliance, or distensibility. *Compliance* is defined as the change in ventricular volume (in ml) for a given change in pressure (in mm Hg) or dV/dP.[9] Fluid administration to the patient with a compliant ventricle may produce minimal change in VEDP, although stroke volume may increase (Fig. 13-2). If the ventricle is noncompliant (stiff), even a small amount of fluid administration may result in a significant increase in VEDP.[10]

The optimal filling pressure for patients with shock is unknown. Certainly, a CVP or PAWP that is normal or low (<5 to 8 mm Hg) is inappropriate and should be treated. Although it is commonly accepted that a dysfunctional ventricle is noncompliant and requires higher filling pressure than the normal ventricle, limited data exist to support this concept in the treatment of adults and children in shock.[11-13] A single study evaluating the relationship between LVEDP and cardiac output in septic adult patients

demonstrated a significant improvement in cardiac output when the LVEDP was increased from <5 to 8 mm Hg to 10 to 12 mm Hg. Little improvement was documented, however, when the LVEDP was increased beyond 12 mm Hg.[13] In children with septic shock, aggressive fluid resuscitation has been linked with improved survival; although the PAWP was not correlated with survival, fluid resuscitation resulted in a mean PAWP of 11.5 mm Hg.[11] These limited data suggest that improvement in cardiac output and systemic perfusion is most likely when the LVEDP is increased to approximately 12 mm Hg.

Fluid administration resulting in an increase in the LVEDP to extremely high levels (i.e., 15 to 18 mm Hg or higher) may not be beneficial and may increase the likelihood of development of cardiogenic pulmonary edema. In any patient in shock, fluid administration should be carefully titrated to determine the right (or left) ventricular filling pressures associated with optimal systemic perfusion and end-organ function in that patient.

Administration of vasodilators increases ventricular compliance. As a result, the stroke volume and cardiac output may improve during volume administration without development of a high VEDP (see *Curve B*, Fig. 13-2).

Ventricular Contractility. Ventricular contractility refers to the speed (efficiency) of ventricular contraction and the force generated by the ventricular fibers during contraction. When ventricular contractility improves, the ventricular fibers contract in a shorter period of time, reducing the time required for ventricular ejection and increasing the time available for ventricular filling. As a result, when ventricular contractility improves, stroke volume increases.

The most reliable method of evaluating ventricular contractility at the bedside is through echocardiographic evaluation of the left ventricular shortening fraction (LVSF), using the following formula[14]:

$$LVSF = \frac{(LV\ end\text{-}diastolic\ dimension - LV\ end\text{-}systolic\ dimension)}{LV\ end\text{-}systolic\ dimension} \times 100$$

The normal shortening fraction in children is approximately 28% to 44%,[14] and a reduced shortening fraction is associated with decreased ventricular contractility.

Other indices of ventricular contractility include the ejection fraction and the rate of ventricular peak pressure development; these may be estimated through echocardiography or nuclear imaging or determined during cardiac catheterization. If invasive monitoring or angiography is performed, a left ventricular end-systolic pressure/volume curve may be generated (using the PAWP and echocardiographic evaluation of left ventricular volume). The slope of the curve is directly related to ventricular contractility. The velocity of circumferential fiber shortening may be evaluated to monitor ventricular contractility, but this index is also affected by heart rate and ventricular preload and afterload.

Ventricular contractility may be depressed by infection, hypoxia, electrolyte or acid-base imbalance, drug toxicity, or congenital heart disease. It may be improved with correction of these factors or administration of inotropic agents (these are presented later in the chapter).

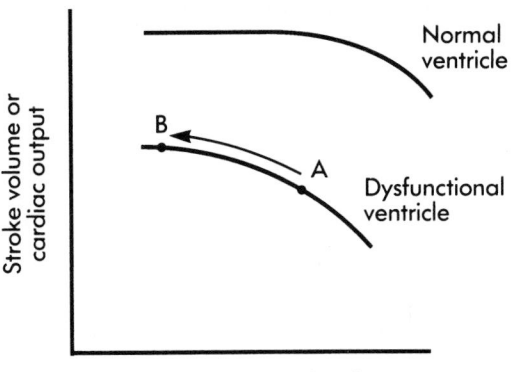

FIG. 13-3. Effects of afterload on ventricular function. The normal ventricle will maintain stroke volume despite a moderate rise in afterload (such as an increase in systemic vascular resistance). Severe increases in afterload, however, can ultimately compromise ventricular function and result in a fall in stroke volume and cardiac output (see *Normal ventricle curve*). The dysfunctional ventricle will be much more sensitive to an increase in afterload, and even a relatively small increase in afterload may substantially reduce myocardial performance. Administration of vasodilators may reduce afterload sufficiently so that stroke volume and cardiac output increase (see A → B). *(Courtesy William Banner, Jr, MD; from Hazinski MF: Cardiovascular disorders. In Hazinski MF, editor: Nursing care of the critically ill child, ed 2, St Louis, 1992, Mosby.)*

Ventricular Afterload. Afterload is the impedance to ventricular ejection. Ventricular afterload is the sum of all forces opposing ventricular emptying and is also described as ventricular wall stress.[15] The greater the afterload, the greater the work and oxygen consumption of the ventricle to maintain cardiac output. Even a normal afterload may provide excessive impediment to ventricular ejection if myocardial function is poor (Fig. 13-3) and may be associated with reduced stroke volume and cardiac output.

The major determinants of afterload or wall stress include: (1) ventricular lumen radius; (2) the thickness of the ventricular wall (hypertrophy decreases afterload); and (3) the ventricular ejection pressure (intracavity pressure). These are related in the following formula[15]:

$$\text{Ventricular wall stress} = \frac{\text{Intracavitary pressure} \times \text{chamber lumen radius}}{2 \times \text{Chamber wall thickness}}$$

In the normal patient, left and right ventricular ejection pressures are equal to the systemic and pulmonary arterial pressures, respectively. In turn, these pressures are determined by blood flow and resistance. Therefore it is often assumed that afterload will be determined primarily by the impedance provided by the pulmonary and systemic arterial circulations (i.e., systemic and pulmonary vascular resistances). This assumes, however, that there is no ventricular outflow tract obstruction and no significant changes in cardiac output, ventricular size, or wall thickness. Pulmonary and systemic vascular resistances cannot be mea-

sured, but they may be calculated using measurements obtained with a thermodilution or fiberoptic pulmonary artery catheter or Doppler echocardiography (Table 13-1). These calculations are subject to error, particularly if inaccurate estimates or calculations of cardiac output are used.

Ventricular afterload may be increased in association with pulmonary or aortic stenosis, or as the result of systemic vasoconstriction or pulmonary hypertension. Pulmonary arterial constriction may develop or may be exacerbated by alveolar hypoxia, acidosis, alveolar distension, or hypothermia[16]; thus these conditions should be avoided in the child with pulmonary hypertension.

Vasodilators may be administered to manipulate vascular resistances in the patient with shock. Such therapy may be particularly useful in the presence of myocardial dysfunction.

OXYGEN DELIVERY

Oxygen delivery is the product of arterial oxygen content (hemoglobin concentration × 1.34 ml oxygen carried by each gram of oxyhemoglobin × hemoglobin saturation) and cardiac output. Normal arterial oxygen content is 18 to 20 ml oxygen/dl blood. The normal *cardiac output* in the child varies with age and averages 200 ml/kg/min in the infant, 150 ml/kg/min in the child, and 100 ml/kg/min in the adolescent.[1] *Oxygen delivery* averages 36 to 40 ml/kg/min in the infant, 27 to 30 ml/kg/min in the child, and 18 to 20 ml/kg/min in the adolescent. *Oxygen consumption* averages 10 to 14 ml/kg/min in infants beyond the neonatal period and 5 to 8 ml/kg/min in children.[17]

If either arterial oxygen content or cardiac output falls without a commensurate and compensatory increase in the other component, oxygen delivery will fall. When cardiovascular function is good, cardiac output increases as a compensatory response to any fall in arterial oxygen content (e.g., with development of anemia or mild hypoxemia). However, if cardiovascular dysfunction is present, such compensation may fail to occur. Furthermore, if oxygen content falls dramatically (as in the case of severe anemia or hemorrhage), even a high cardiac output may fail to maintain oxygen delivery. When cardiac output falls, oxygen content usually does not increase, so oxygen delivery will fall.

Oxygen delivery in the adult is typically four times the oxygen consumption, and the difference between oxygen delivery and supply provides an oxygen reserve. If oxygen delivery falls slightly, oxygen consumption can increase and tissue oxygenation and organ function may be maintained. However, once oxygen delivery falls beyond a critical point, further decreases in oxygen delivery will be associated with reduced tissue oxygen consumption and reduced tissue oxygenation.

Oxygen consumption is very high during childhood because the metabolic rate is high in children. This is particularly true during the newborn period and infancy.[1] For this reason, the young child requires a higher cardiac output and oxygen delivery per kilogram body weight than the adult (Table 13-2) and may develop signs of organ system failure if cardiac output falls or if it is distributed inappropriately.

Under some conditions, including sepsis and malignant hyperthermia, oxygen consumption may become supply

TABLE 13-1. Calculation of Systemic and Pulmonary Vascular Resistance

$$\text{Resistance} = \frac{\text{Pressure drop across system}}{\text{Flow through system}}$$

Systemic vascular resistance

$$\text{Systemic Vascular Resistance (in Wood Units)} = \frac{\text{Mean arterial pressure} - \text{Mean RA pressure (mm Hg)}}{\text{Cardiac output (L/min)}}$$

Note: This equation yields the *SVR in Wood Units* (units). Normal values are listed below. To convert these units to units of absolute physical resistance (dynes-sec-cm^{-5}), multiply the Wood Units by 80.

To normalize SVR for body surface area, *Systemic Vascular Resistance INDEX Units* (SVRI) are calculated. The above equation is utilized, with the substitution of Cardiac Index (L/min/m^2 BSA). In effect, the SVRI is the SVR (in Wood Units) multiplied by the child's body surface area. Normal values are listed below.

Age	Absolute SVR (Wood units)*	SVR index*
Infant	35-50 units	10-15 Index units
Toddler	25-35 units	20 Index units
Child	15-25 units	15-30 Index units

Pulmonary vascular resistance

$$\text{Pulmonary Vascular Resistance (in Wood Units)} = \frac{\text{Mean PA pressure} - \text{LA pressure (mm Hg)}}{\text{Cardiac output (L/min)}}$$

Note: This equation yields the *PVR in Wood Units* (units). Normal values are listed below. To convert these units to units of absolute physical resistance (dynes-sec-cm^{-5}), multiply the Wood Units by 80.

To normalize PVR for body surface area, *Pulmonary Vascular Resistance INDEX Units* (PVRI) are calculated. The above equation is utilized, with the substitution of Cardiac Index (L/min/m^2 BSA). In effect, the PVRI is the PVR (in Wood Units) multiplied by the child's body surface area. Normal values are listed below.

Age	Absolute PVR (Wood units)*	PVR index*
Infant	25-40 units	7-10 Index units
Child	0.5-4 units	1-3 Index units

From Hazinski MF: Cardiovascular disorders. In Hazinski MF, editor: *Nursing care of the critically ill child*, ed 2, St. Louis, 1992, Mosby.
*To convert these units to dynes-sec-cm^{-5}, multiply by 80.
BSA, Body surface area.

TABLE 13-2. Cardiac Output, Oxygen Delivery, and Oxygen Consumption in Infants and Children

Age (wt/BSA)	Cardiac output (CO)* (ml/min)	Oxygen delivery† (Do$_2$)		Oxygen consumption (V̇o$_2$)	
		(ml/min)	(ml/min/m^2)	(ml/min)	(ml/min/m^2)
Newborn (3.2 kg/0.2 m^2)	700-800	133-200	665-1000	36-54	180-270
6 mo (8 kg/0.42 m^2)	1000-1600	200-280	476-667	70-100	167-238
1 yr (10 kg/0.5 m^2)	1300-1500	260-300	520-600	85-110	170-220
2 yr (13 kg/0.59 m^2)	1500-2000	300-400	508-678	91-123	154-208
4 yr (17 kg/0.71 m^2)	2300-2375	460-475	648-669	110-150	155-211
5 yr (19 kg/0.77 m^2)	2500-3000	500-600	649-779	115-170	149-221
8 yr (28 kg/0.96 m^2)	3400-3600	680-720	708-750	150-208	156-200
10 yr (35 kg/1.1 m^2)	3800-4000	760-800	690-727	190-250	122-227
15 yr (50 kg/1.4 m^2)	5000-6000	1200	857	300-400	120-200

Reproduced from Hazinski MF: Hemodynamic monitoring of children. In Daily EK, editor: *Bedside hemodynamic monitoring*, ed 5, St. Louis, 1994, Mosby.
*Cardiac index (CI) for children: 3.0-4.5 L/min/m^2.
†Assuming a hemoglobin concentration of 15 gm/dl and normal arterial oxygen content.

dependent. As a result, any fall in oxygen delivery will result in a reduction in oxygen consumption and tissue oxygenation and may contribute to the development of metabolic acidosis. In patients with supply-dependent oxygen consumption, oxygen delivery should be supported at levels greater than normal, since normal oxygen delivery will still be inadequate to ensure effective tissue oxygenation (Fig. 13-4).

When oxygen delivery is limited or consumption is abnormal, any unnecessary increase in oxygen demand may

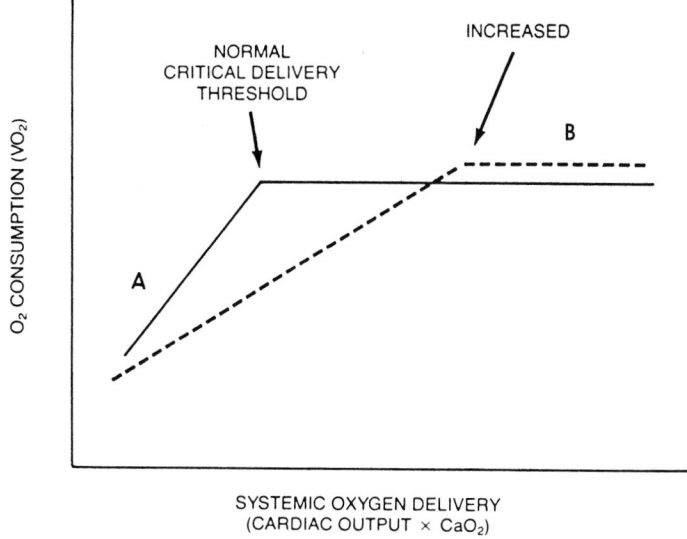

FIG. 13-4. Theoretic relationship between oxygen delivery and oxygen consumption. In normal tissues *(solid line)*, oxygen delivery far exceeds oxygen consumption, so a significant fall in systemic oxygen delivery can be tolerated without any change in oxygen consumption (tissue oxygen extraction merely increases). However, eventually a profound fall in oxygen delivery will reach a critical delivery threshold; further compromise in oxygen delivery will then result in a proportional fall in oxygen consumption. In patients with adult respiratory distress syndrome (ARDS) and patients with sepsis *(broken line)*, oxygen consumption is thought to be far more supply-dependent than in the normal population. In these patients, even a small reduction in oxygen delivery may force a fall in oxygen consumption. For this reason, medical therapy is aimed at increasing oxygen delivery to ranges above "normal" during the treatment of ARDS or sepsis. *(From Schumaker PT and Samuel RW:* Crit Care Clin *5:255, 1989; Hazinski MF: Cardiovascular disorders. In Hazinski MF, editor:* Nursing care of the critically ill child, *ed 2, St Louis, 1992, Mosby.)*

result in further patient deterioration. Therefore conditions that increase oxygen consumption (e.g., cold stress or infection) should be avoided or promptly treated. The treatment of shock must always focus on maximization of oxygen delivery through support of arterial oxygen content and cardiac output. In addition, oxygen demand must be minimized.

ETIOLOGY

Classification

Conventionally, shock is categorized according to the etiologic mechanism (see box on p. 124). Shock caused by inadequate intravascular volume relative to the vascular space is known as *hypovolemic shock*. Shock resulting from impairment of myocardial function is referred to as *cardiogenic shock*. Shock associated with inappropriate distribution of blood flow and increased capillary permeability is called *distributive shock*, and *septic shock* is the best example of this form of shock. Such a classification system may be helpful because it indicates the initial therapy required. However, this classification system is inadequate when the patient demonstrates late or progressive shock, since the patient, at that point, is likely to demonstrate cardiovascular dysfunction, aspects of inappropriate intravascular volume, severe myocardial dysfunction, and maldistribution of blood flow. The classification is also mislead-

ing for patients with septic shock, since sepsis produces elements of hypovolemic and cardiogenic shock, in addition to the complications of maldistribution of blood flow. Finally, any patient in shock is likely to develop some myocardial dysfunction. Thus all aspects of cardiovascular function and oxygen delivery must be skillfully supported during the treatment of any form of shock.

Hypovolemic Shock

Hypovolemic shock is the most common type of shock encountered in the pediatric population. It is defined as shock associated with a reduction in the intravascular volume relative to the vascular space. Dehydration and trauma are the most common causes of hypovolemic shock in children. Hypovolemia may also result from a redistribution of blood volume or increased capillary permeability, such as after burns or with sepsis.

Pathophysiology. If the intravascular volume loss is mild or moderate, compensatory adrenergic responses may enable redistribution of blood flow, diverting flow from the mesenteric, renal, and skin circulation to the heart and brain. Reduced renal perfusion stimulates the renal-angiotensin-aldosterone systems, resulting in renal sodium and water retention; this mechanism may help restore intravascular volume over a period of time. Hypotension will not be observed unless or until fluid loss is rapid and severe. Thus a normal blood pressure may be observed in

Etiologic Classification of Shock

Hypovolemic
1. Hemorrhage
   a. External: laceration
   b. Internal: ruptured spleen or liver, vascular injury, fracture (neonate: intracerebral/intraventricular hemorrhage)
   c. Gastrointestinal: bleeding ulcer, ruptured viscus, mesenteric hemorrhage
2. Plasma loss
   a. Burn
   b. Inflammation or sepsis: leaky capillary syndrome
   c. Nephrotic syndrome
   d. Third spacing: intestinal obstruction, pancreatitis, peritonitis
3. Fluid and electrolyte loss
   a. Acute gastroenteritis
   b. Excessive sweating (cystic fibrosis)
   c. Renal pathology
4. Endocrine
   a. Adrenal insufficiency, adrenal-genital syndrome
   b. Diabetes mellitus
   c. Diabetes insipidus
   d. Hypothyroidism (myxedema coma)

Cardiogenic
1. Myocardial insufficiency
   a. Dysrhythmia: bradycardia, atrioventricular block, ventricular tachycardia, supraventricular tachycardia
   b. Cardiomyopathy: myocarditis, ischemia, hypoxia, hypoglycemia, acidosis
   c. Drug intoxication
   d. Hypothermia
   e. Congenital heart disease, including patent ductus arteriosus (PDA)-dependent lesion such as coarctation of the aorta or critical pulmonary stenosis

Distributive (Vasogenic)
1. High or normal resistance (increased venous capacitance)
   a. Septic shock
   b. Anaphylaxis
   c. Barbiturate intoxication
2. Low resistance, vasodilation: CNS injury (i.e., spinal cord transection)

From Barkin RM and Rosen P: *Emergency pediatrics*, ed 4, St. Louis, 1994, Mosby.

the child with mild or moderate hypovolemic shock. Significant blood volume loss (20% to 25%) or severe dehydration is required before hypotension develops.

Compensatory mechanisms occur at a price, however, and cannot be maintained indefinitely. Systemic vasoconstriction increases left ventricular afterload and myocardial oxygen consumption. Tachycardia may produce impaired subendocardial blood flow and increased myocardial oxygen consumption, which may ultimately contribute to the development of myocardial ischemia. If renal and mesenteric blood flow is significantly compromised, ischemia may develop, and renal or hepatic failure may result.

A relative hypovolemia may develop in patients with sepsis, vasodilation from other causes (e.g., spinal shock or ingestion of beta-adrenergic drugs), or third-spacing of fluids. When this occurs, the increase in vascular space or the redistribution of blood flow results in inadequate ventricular preload, excessive perfusion of some vascular beds, and inadequate perfusion of other tissues. Although no absolute fluid or blood loss has occurred, volume administration is necessary to ensure that the intravascular volume is adequate relative to the vascular space.

Cardiogenic Shock

Cardiogenic shock occurs when impaired myocardial function compromises cardiac output. This form of shock is observed most commonly after cardiovascular surgery or with inflammatory diseases of the heart, including cardiomyopathy and myocarditis. Cardiogenic shock may also develop in children with severe forms of obstructive congenital heart disease (e.g., hypoplastic left heart, severe aortic stenosis, and hypoplastic right ventricle) or it may be caused by drug toxicity or severe electrolyte or acid-base imbalances.

Myocardial dysfunction can complicate any form of shock and is present early in septic shock. For this reason, cardiogenic shock is the final common pathway of virtually all forms of inadequately treated shock.[18]

Pathophysiology. When cardiogenic shock is present, myocardial function limits cardiac output. In the early stages of cardiogenic shock, compensatory mechanisms are activated to redistribute blood flow and retain intravascular volume and perfusion of vital organs. Adrenergic responses produce tachycardia and peripheral vasoconstriction and constriction of the splanchnic arteries. Blood flow is diverted from the skin, kidneys, and gut to maintain flow to the heart and brain.[15]

If these compensatory mechanisms are sufficient, blood pressure may be maintained. However, tachycardia and systemic arterial constriction will increase myocardial oxygen consumption. In addition, reduction in gut and kidney blood flow may produce hepatic, mesenteric, or renal ischemia or failure. For these reasons, the compensatory mechanisms can not be maintained indefinitely.

Decreased renal perfusion stimulates the renal angiotensin-aldosterone systems, resulting in increased sodium and water retention. Unless hypovolemia is present initially, this fluid retention may contribute to a relative hypervolemia.

If the mean arterial pressure or pulse pressure falls, stimulation of the baroreceptors in the carotid sinuses and aortic arch is reduced. This reduced baroreceptor activity removes inhibition from the vasomotor center in the medulla, resulting in increased sympathetic nervous system stimulation.

If myocardial dysfunction progresses, cardiac output and systemic blood pressure will fall. Myocardial ischemia then exacerbates myocardial dysfunction. In addition, the development of multisystem organ ischemia and failure results in the release of proteins, enzymes, and lactic acid that further compromises cardiovascular function. At this point, mortality is very high.

Septic Shock

Sepsis and its complications affect nearly 500,000 patients annually, with a mortality of approximately 25%.[19] Sepsis requires colonization with an organism, clinical evidence of infection, and signs of a host response. Confirmation of infection with positive blood cultures (indicating a bacteremia) is not necessary for the diagnosis of sepsis or septic shock.[20] Approximately half of all cases of sepsis result from gram-negative infections, although sepsis and septic shock may be associated with gram-positive infection, viruses, or fungi.[19]

Patients at greatest risk for the development of sepsis include those at the extremes of age (i.e., young infants, children, and the elderly); those with invasive catheters, surgical incisions, or wounds or burns; immunocompromised patients; and those receiving chronic antibiotic therapy. Many of these risk factors are present in the seriously ill or injured child or any child with a chronic disease.

The infectious agent triggering the development of sepsis and its complications may be nosocomial. The most common nosocomial infections reported in pediatric patients include cutaneous infections, bacteremias, and lower respiratory tract infections, with an equal distribution of both gram-positive and gram-negative infections.[21] As many as half of all children hospitalized in pediatric intensive care units longer than 35 days develop nosocomial infections, and the risk of infection increases with the use of invasive monitoring and support devices.[22] Such infections may be prevented with proper handwashing by hospital personnel before and after every patient contact, appropriate sterile and aseptic technique during catheter insertion and tubing changes, and proper sterilization of respiratory-therapy equipment.

The immunocompromised patient frequently develops sepsis from normal bacterial flora inhabiting the skin, pharynx, or gastrointestinal tract. Cutaneous infections often develop in this manner, and aspiration of pharyngeal secretions may produce a gram-negative pneumonia.

Under normal conditions, the gastrointestinal mucosa is impermeable to gram-negative bacteria. However, mucosal injury caused by shock, trauma, burns, or sepsis may make the mucosa permeable to gram-negative bacteria or its endotoxin. Translocation of gram-negative bacteria or endotoxin also is thought to occur in malnourished patients and those receiving only parenteral nutrition.[23,24] This bacterial or endotoxin translocation may complicate the course of gram-positive, viral, or fungal infections, contributing to the development of signs of gram-negative septic shock in the patient with critical illness or infection.[25]

Pathophysiology. Sepsis is a disease of intermediary metabolism, induced by infectious agents and resulting from the formation or activation of mediators and protein systems. This cascading series of events results in vasodilation, maldistribution of cardiac output, increased capillary permeability, myocardial dysfunction, and organ system ischemia and failure.

The septic cascade may unfold over the course of several days or be telescoped into a period of several hours. Once the septic cascade is activated, simple treatment of the causative infection may not be sufficient to restore adequate systemic perfusion and organ function.

Although the pathophysiology of gram-negative sepsis is more completely understood than the progression of gram-positive, viral, or fungal sepsis, it is likely that most elements of the septic cascade are similar, regardless of the causative organism.

Sepsis begins with an infection that triggers the inflammatory response. This inflammatory response causes vasodilation and increased capillary permeability designed to deliver blood flow and white blood cells (particularly neutrophils) to the site of infection. When sepsis is present, the inflammatory response is not contained, but it becomes generalized, resulting in widespread vasodilation and increased capillary permeability. Activation of and damage to cell walls (particularly white blood cells and endothelial cells) results in release of mediators that further stimulate the immune response. Progressive vasodilation and increased capillary permeability produce maldistribution of blood flow.

Key mediators involved in the gram-negative septic cascade include endotoxin (and lipopolysaccharide), tumor necrosis factor, interleukin-1 (IL-1) and other interleukins, platelet activating factor, nitric oxide, the arachidonic acid metabolites, and myocardial depressant factors.[26-30]

Endotoxin. A major progenitor of the gram-negative septic cascade is endotoxin; endotoxin administration can replicate virtually all of the systemic effects associated with gram-negative sepsis, and serum levels of endotoxin are inversely related to survival.[31] Endotoxin is a component of the cell wall of gram-negative bacteria and is liberated during gram-negative infection. Endotoxin is also liberated when gram-negative bacteria die.[32] This explains the deterioration often observed in septic patients after successful bacterial destruction by antibiotic therapy.

Lipopolysaccharide. The active component of the endotoxin is a lipopolysaccharide (LPS) consisting of a polysaccharide and a lipid-A core. This lipid-A core is common to all gram-negative bacteria, regardless of type.[30,33] A monoclonal antibody to the gram-negative lipid-A core has been developed and may be effective in limiting the effects of endotoxin in some patients with gram-negative sepsis (see Management).[34,35]

Endotoxin and LPS stimulate or release several chemical mediators, including histamine, serotonin, protein cascades, and tumor necrosis factor (TNF). In addition, the complement system and Hageman factor are activated, with initiation of the coagulation, fibrinolytic, and bradykinin systems. Endotoxin also stimulates the endothelium, producing further vasodilation and increased capillary permeability. The endothelium itself becomes a secretory organ, releasing or activating additional mediators, which influence vascular tone and permeability, and platelet activating factor, which influences platelet adhesion. The result of this mediator activation is the maldistribution of blood flow.[26-30,33]

Tumor Necrosis Factor. TNF is a secretory product of the monocyte-macrophage system, which received its name when it was noted to produce hemorrhagic necrosis of tumors. TNF clearly plays an important role in the perpetuation of the septic cascade. In fact, many of the responses triggered by endotoxin are thought to be mediated by TNF, and administration of TNF results in the development of a clinical picture identical to gram-negative septic shock. TNF is probably also involved in the systemic response to other types of infection. TNF levels rise within hours after exposure to endotoxin, before the temperature, white blood cell count, or adrenal hormone levels rise.[36]

TNF reproduces or mediates virtually all of the effects of endotoxin. TNF, in turn, stimulates the release of IL-1 and arachidonic acid, and acts synergistically with the interleukins, the complement system, and other mediators of the septic cascade that will affect vascular tone and permeability and platelet function. TNF is cytotoxic to the endothelium, and it contributes to the development of disseminated intravascular coagulation.

A monoclonal antibody to TNF has been developed, and clinical trials are underway to determine its efficacy in the treatment of septic patients.[37-39] In addition, a recombinant TNF receptor has been developed that may bind TNF and limit its effects.[40]

Interleukin-1. IL-1 is a polypeptide hormone that is similar to TNF. It is made by neutrophils, monocytes, and erythrocytes and it stimulates the inflammatory response. IL-1 promotes release of TNF, other interleukins, platelet activating factor, and the eicosanoids (vasoactive products of arachidonic acid metabolism). IL-1 acts synergistically with TNF in its effects on vascular endothelium and the microcirculation. A recombinant receptor antagonist to IL-1 has recently been developed and may modulate the effects of IL-1 during the septic cascade.[27,37,41]

Platelet Activating Factor. Platelet activating factor (PAF) is a phospholipid produced by a variety of cells, including endothelium and leukocytes during the inflammatory response. The effects of PAF are very similar to those of endotoxin/lipopolysaccharide at very low PAF concentrations.[42,43] PAF probably serves to prime cells and to amplify the systemic inflammatory response.

Several PAF receptor antagonists have been isolated that appear to provide some protective effect when administered to animal models of gram-negative sepsis.[43] PAF can be removed using continuous arteriovenous hemofiltration.[44] The clinical significance of these observations remains to be determined.

Nitric Oxide. Nitric oxide (NO) is thought to be an endothelium-derived relaxant factor, a potent modulator of vascular tone and permeability.[45] NO is normally produced continually by endothelium; it regulates leukocyte adhesion and also affects adhesion of platelets and monocytes. High levels of NO are present in septic patients and contribute to the vasodilation and increased capillary permeability observed.[46] Modulation of nitric oxide levels is now being attempted through administration of nitric oxide synthase inhibitors.[45]

Arachidonic Acid. Arachidonic acid is a normal constituent of cell membranes that is released into the cells during the development of sepsis. It is subsequently metabolized intracellularly through two major pathways, the cyclooxygenase and the lipoxygenase pathways with resultant formation of other lipid mediators.

Arachidonic acid metabolism through the cyclooxygenase pathway results in the formation of prostaglandins, prostacyclins, and thromboxanes. Most prostaglandins are vasodilators, although some are vasoconstrictors, and all reduce platelet aggregation. Thromboxanes are vasoconstrictors that increase platelet aggregation. Arachidonic acid metabolism through the lipoxygenase pathway results in the formation of leukotrienes and other vasoactive substances that constrict airways and vessels.[15] These lipid mediators are all vasoactive substances, called *eicosanoids*, which exacerbate the maldistribution of blood flow and alteration in platelet activity that is present in the microcirculation. As a result, within a single tissue bed, some areas may receive excessive blood flow, whereas other areas are ischemic.

The eicosanoids have been implicated in the development of sepsis-induced pulmonary injury and other microcirculatory disruptions that contribute to multisystem organ failure.[47] Blocking of arachidonic acid metabolism by the administration of ibuprofen and other nonsteroidal antiinflammatory agents has been successful in limiting the development of adult respiratory distress syndrome (ARDS) in adult patients with septic shock.[48] A multicenter clinical trial is currently underway.

Complement System. The complement system serves to opsonize (coat) bacteria, rendering it susceptible to phagocytosis. However, activation of this system includes stimulation of the clotting cascade; thus thrombocytopenia or disseminated intravascular coagulation may result, contributing to microcirculatory obstruction or bleeding.

Myocardial Depressant Factor. Myocardial function is abnormal in patients with sepsis. Early in the septic process ventricular ejection fraction may fall as low as 20%.[49] This decrease in function is thought to be the result of circulating endotoxin, TNF, and specific myocardial depressant factors, and may also be associated with the reduction in serum ionized calcium observed in septic patients.[50]

The compensatory ventricular response during sepsis is an increase in ventricular compliance. As long as intravascular volume remains adequate, the compliant ventricle may be able to maintain a reduced but adequate stroke volume in the face of a reduced ejection fraction through dilation with an increase in ventricular end-diastolic volume. This dilation, coupled with an increase in heart rate and a fall in systemic vascular resistance, typically results in a cardiac output that is much higher than normal. In fact, the likelihood of patient survival has been linked with the development of ventricular dilation.[30,49-51] When the septic condition is treated effectively, cardiac output, heart rate, and ventricular compliance return to normal, generally within 24 hours.

In summary, the septic cascade is triggered by an infection and byproducts of the infectious organism. The inflammatory response becomes widespread, and mediators are activated and released with resultant depression of myocardial function, widespread vasodilation, increased capillary permeability, and maldistribution of blood flow. If skilled treatment is not instituted promptly, refractory shock and multisystem organ failure result.

Spinal (Neurogenic) Shock

Spinal (neurogenic) shock can develop after spinal cord injury, producing a relative hypovolemia caused by vasodilation associated with loss of sympathomimetic vascular tone. This cause of shock should be considered in the pediatric trauma victim with spinal cord injury if hypotension persists despite adequate volume resuscitation and ongoing hemorrhage has been ruled out (see Chapter 19).

DIAGNOSTIC FINDINGS

The child with inadequate cardiac output demonstrates signs of inadequate blood flow to some tissue beds and some evidence of organ system failure. The extremities may feel cool (they cool in a peripheral to proximal fashion), although excessive skin blood flow may be present in patients with septic or spinal shock. Capillary refill time is often prolonged, despite a warm ambient temperature, and the skin may have a mottled appearance. Urine output is decreased if renal perfusion is compromised and will be less than 2 ml/kg/hr in infants, less than 1 ml/kg/hr in children, and less than 0.5 ml/kg/hr in adolescents. Liver enzymes may be elevated if hepatic perfusion is reduced. The development of a metabolic acidosis indicates that blood flow to some tissues is inadequate to support total aerobic metabolism. Hypotension is often not present until shock is severe.

The child's level of consciousness and responsiveness provides valuable information about the child's severity of illness. The normal infant should orient to faces, provide eye contact, and track bright objects across a visual field. The normal child is alert and reluctant to be separated from parents or examined by strangers. The critically ill infant or child is often extremely irritable, and lethargy indicates severe deterioration in the level of consciousness. A decreased response to painful stimulation is abnormal in the infant or child of any age and usually indicates severe cardiorespiratory or neurologic compromise.[17]

*Hypo*glycemia may be observed in seriously ill or injured infants and may be associated with cardiovascular or neurologic deterioration. Infants have high glucose needs and low glycogen stores that may be rapidly depleted during periods of stress. *Hyper*glycemia has been linked with poor survival in older children with trauma or shock[52]; this high glucose level may result from gluconeogenesis or excessive glucose administration. Both hypoglycemia and hyperglycemia can be detrimental; thus the serum glucose concentration should be closely monitored and a normal serum glucose level supported. Excessive glucose administration should be avoided.

Vital signs should be evaluated in light of the child's clinical condition. Normal vital signs are not always appropriate vital signs in the seriously ill or injured child.[17] Such a child is often tachycardic and tachypneic. Hypotension may be only a late (and preterminal) sign of shock in the child.

As a general rule, the typical normal systolic blood pressure for a child older than 1 year of age may be estimated by adding 90 mm Hg to twice the patient's age in years; this corresponds to the 50th percentile blood pressure for the child's age. A systolic pressure equal to or less than 70 mm Hg plus twice the child's age in years is considered hypotensive, since this blood pressure corresponds to the 5th percentile systolic blood pressure for age[2] (see Appendix A-2).

Hypovolemic Shock

The clinical signs observed in the child with hypovolemic shock are those of inadequate systemic perfusion associated with evidence of intravascular fluid loss or redistribution of blood volume. The child demonstrates tachycardia, peripheral vasoconstriction, cool extremities, delayed capillary refill, and oliguria (see Chapter 12).

If the child and the ambient temperature are warm, capillary refill time can be correlated with fluid status. Capillary refill time of less than 1.5 to 2 seconds is normal, although a minimal fluid deficit of less than 5% may be present with a normal capillary refill time. If the refill time is 1.5 to 3 seconds, a 5% to 10% deficit is likely to be present, and a refill time over 3 seconds is associated with a deficit over 10%.[53]

Metabolic acidosis may also be present. The CVP and PAWP will be ≤5 to 8 mm Hg, and the cardiac silhouette is typically small (certainly not enlarged) on chest radiograph. Hypotension is only observed as a very late sign of significant intravascular volume loss.[2]

Clinically significant dehydration is associated with weight loss. Fluid intake and output records (or reports from parents or primary caretakers) will reveal a history of inadequate fluid intake or excessive fluid losses. The child with significant dehydration demonstrates dry mucous membranes, a sunken fontanelle (in infants), and poor skin turgor. The serum blood urea nitrogen (BUN) and urine specific gravity are usually elevated. The serum sodium concentration and osmolality will be affected by the type of dehydration present and the severity of the dehydration.

Moderate *isotonic dehydration* compromises peripheral perfusion once the young child has lost approximately 5% to 10% of body weight or approximately 100 ml/kg. Hypotension is observed in the presence of severe isotonic dehydration, associated with losses greater than 15% of body weight or 150 ml/kg.

Because body water constitutes a smaller percentage of body weight in older children and adults than in young children, a compromise in systemic perfusion is observed in the adolescent with isotonic dehydration once the fluid equivalent of 5% to 7% of body weight is lost acutely, and

TABLE 13-3. Classification of Hemorrhagic Shock in Pediatric Trauma Patients Based on Systemic Signs

System	Very mild hemorrhage (<15% blood volume loss)	Mild hemorrhage (15% to 25% blood volume loss)	Moderate hemorrhage (25% blood volume loss)	Severe hemorrhage (40% blood volume loss)
Cardiovascular	Heart rate normal or mildly increased	Tachycardia	Significant tachycardia	Severe tachycardia
	Normal pulses	Peripheral pulses may be diminished	Thready peripheral pulses	Thready central pulses
	Normal BP	Normal BP	Hypotension	Significant hypotension
	Normal pH	Normal pH	Metabolic acidosis	Significant acidosis
Respiratory	Rate normal	Tachypnea	Moderate tachypnea	Severe tachypnea
CNS	Slightly anxious	Irritable, confused	Irritability or lethargy	Lethargy
		Combative	Diminished pain response	Coma
Skin	Warm, pink	Cool extremities, mottling	Cool extremities, mottling or pallor	Cold extremities, pallor or cyanosis
	Capillary refill brisk	Delayed capillary refill	Prolonged capillary refill	Prolonged capillary refill
Kidneys	Normal urine output	Oliguria, increased specific gravity	Oliguria, increased BUN	Anuria

Modified from American College of Surgeons Committee on Trauma: *Advanced trauma life support student manual,* Chicago, 1993, American College of Surgeons; Fleisher GR and Ludwig S: *Textbook of pediatric emergency medicine,* ed 2, Baltimore, 1988, Williams & Wilkins; Sand T, Pieper P, Hazinski MF: Pediatric trauma. In Hazinski MF: *Nursing care of the critically ill child,* ed 2, St. Louis, 1992, Mosby.

hypotension is observed if fluid totaling 7% to 10% of body weight is lost.

Hypotonic dehydration is associated with a proportionately greater loss of sodium than free water, so the serum sodium falls. The resultant fall in serum osmolality produces an acute extravascular fluid shift and further loss of intravascular volume. As a result, fluid loss is primarily from the intravascular compartment, so a compromise in systemic perfusion is observed after even small quantities of fluid loss. The child with hyponatremic dehydration demonstrates poor peripheral perfusion with a fluid loss equivalent to 5% to 7% of body weight (a deficit of 50 to 75 ml/kg), and hypotension is typically observed if the fluid loss is equal to approximately 10% of body weight (a deficit of 100 ml/kg). The adolescent with hyponatremic dehydration may demonstrate a compromise in peripheral perfusion after a fluid loss equivalent to approximately 3% to 5% of body weight, and hypotension is likely to be observed once the fluid loss equals approximately 5% to 7% of body weight.

Hypernatremic dehydration results when the free water deficit is proportionately greater than the deficit of sodium. As a result, the serum sodium concentration rises. This results in an acute increase in the serum osmolality and a shift of free water into the vascular space. For this reason, the child with hypernatremic dehydration is likely to maintain intravascular volume and systemic perfusion despite relatively large quantities of fluid loss. A compromise in systemic perfusion is not likely to be observed in the child with hypernatremic dehydration until severe dehydration is present, with a fluid loss equivalent to more than 10% of body weight. Hypotension is not likely to be associated with hypernatremic dehydration until the fluid loss approximates 15% or more of body weight (or >7% to 10% of body weight loss in the adolescent). Thus hypotension in the dehydrated child with hypernatremia indicates the presence of a substantial fluid deficit.

To appreciate the significance of any blood loss sustained by the pediatric patient, the child's circulating blood volume should be calculated. Blood lost or drawn for laboratory analysis should be added and considered as a percentage of the child's total blood volume. Normal blood volume is higher per kilogram body weight in infants and children than in adults. The blood volume of the premature neonate averages 90 to 105 ml/kg; the blood volume in term newborns averages 85 ml/kg; the blood volume in children 1 to 11 months of age averages 75 ml/kg; beyond 1 year of age, the circulating blood volume averages 65 to 75 ml/kg in children. In adults, the blood volume averages 55 to 57 ml/kg.

Acute blood loss (hemorrhage) typically does not produce a compromise in the child's peripheral perfusion until 15% to 20% of intravascular volume is lost (an acute intravascular or blood loss of 12 to 16 ml/kg). Tachycardia and peripheral vasoconstriction may be the only evidence of hemorrhage in the pediatric trauma patient. An acute loss of 10% of blood volume may be marked by a pulse increase of 20 beats per minute (bpm), and a 20% deficit is associated with an increase of 30 bpm. Hypotension in the supine position is not observed until blood loss totals approximately 20% to 25% of intravascular volume (Table 13-3). Orthostatic changes may be observed at smaller blood volume losses. Once hypotension develops, cardiovascular collapse is imminent, and rapid intravascular volume expansion must be provided.

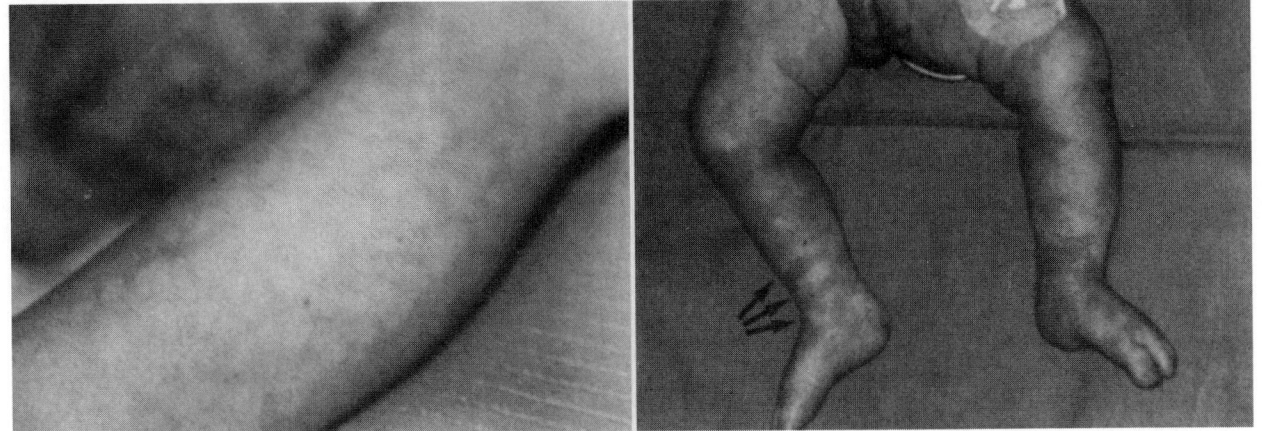

FIG. 13-5. Mottling of skin in children with poor systemic perfusion. **A,** Mottling of skin color often indicates inadequate tissue oxygenation; this may result from hypoxemia or poor systemic perfusion. This child developed myocardial dysfunction and signs of cardiogenic shock. **B,** Mottled skin color is often associated with other signs of compromise of skin perfusion, including delayed capillary refill. The skin over this infant's right ankle was blanched using three fingers *(arrows)*, and the skin failed to reperfuse for more than 5 seconds. This infant suffered from septic shock. *(Courtesy Susan Luck, MD; from Hazinski MF: Cardiovascular disorders. In Hazinski MF, editor:* Nursing care of the critically ill child, *ed 2, St Louis, 1992, Mosby.)*

Comparison of the transcutaneous and arterial oxygen tensions have been helpful in determining the presence of volume deficit in hypovolemic adult trauma patients. If the patient is adequately resuscitated, the transcutaneous oxygen tension should be at least 80% of the arterial oxygen tension. In the presence of hypovolemia, however, the transcutaneous oxygen tension will be less than the arterial oxygen tension, suggesting reduced skin perfusion and the need for volume resuscitation.[54]

Redistribution of blood volume and systemic vasodilation may produce signs of poor systemic perfusion in the absence of evidence of volume loss. For example, children with hepatic failure demonstrate a relative hypovolemia associated with ascites and hepatorenal syndrome. Burn patients demonstrate increased capillary permeability and loss of intravascular volume immediately after a burn. The septic patient may also demonstrate systemic edema associated with capillary leak and further intravascular volume loss. In these patients, some evidence of extravascular fluid movement (i.e., ascites, systemic edema, or fluid loss to dressings over burns) is usually observed.

Cardiogenic Shock

The child with cardiogenic shock demonstrates signs of inadequate systemic perfusion despite the presence of adequate intravascular volume or even hypervolemia. Adrenergic compensatory mechanisms typically divert blood flow from the kidneys, gut, and skin in an attempt to maintain effective blood flow to the heart and brain. This form of shock is generally associated with low cardiac output. The child's extremities will be cool to touch (they will cool in a peripheral to proximal fashion), with delayed capillary refill. The skin may have a mottled appearance (Fig. 13-5).

Evidence of a high CVP, including hepatomegaly and periorbital edema, is typically present in uncomplicated cardiogenic shock. Evidence of pulmonary edema may be noted on clinical assessment (i.e., respiratory distress, reduced lung compliance during hand ventilation, or frothy pink sputum suctioned from an endotracheal tube) or chest radiograph. The cardiac silhouette is usually enlarged on the chest radiograph. If myocardial function is severely compromised, peripheral pulses may be diminished in intensity (dampened) or they may vary in intensity (pulsus alternans).

If cardiac output is calculated through Doppler echocardiography or thermodilution technique, a fall in cardiac output may be detected. If the mixed venous oxygen saturation is continuously monitored (through use of a fiberoptic pulmonary artery catheter), a fall in mixed venous oxygen saturation is observed when the cardiac output falls.

Signs of low cardiac output and cardiogenic shock may be identical to signs of tamponade. Therefore if cardiogenic shock is suspected in the postoperative cardiovascular surgical patient or in any child at risk for the development of pericardial effusion, tamponade should be ruled out through use of an echocardiogram (Fig. 13-6). Specific signs of tamponade, such as pulsus paradoxus, may be impossible to detect in the tachypneic or hypotensive infant or child.

Septic Shock

Although sepsis and its complications produce a progressive cascade of effects, several clinical stages of this process have been described by a consensus panel of physicians,[20] and these stages have been clinically validated in adult patients.[55,56] Application of these consensus terms has also been proposed for pediatric patients (Table 13-4).[57]

Systemic Inflammatory Response Syndrome. Sepsis is thought to begin as the *systemic inflammatory response syndrome* (SIRS). This syndrome is a nonspecific response

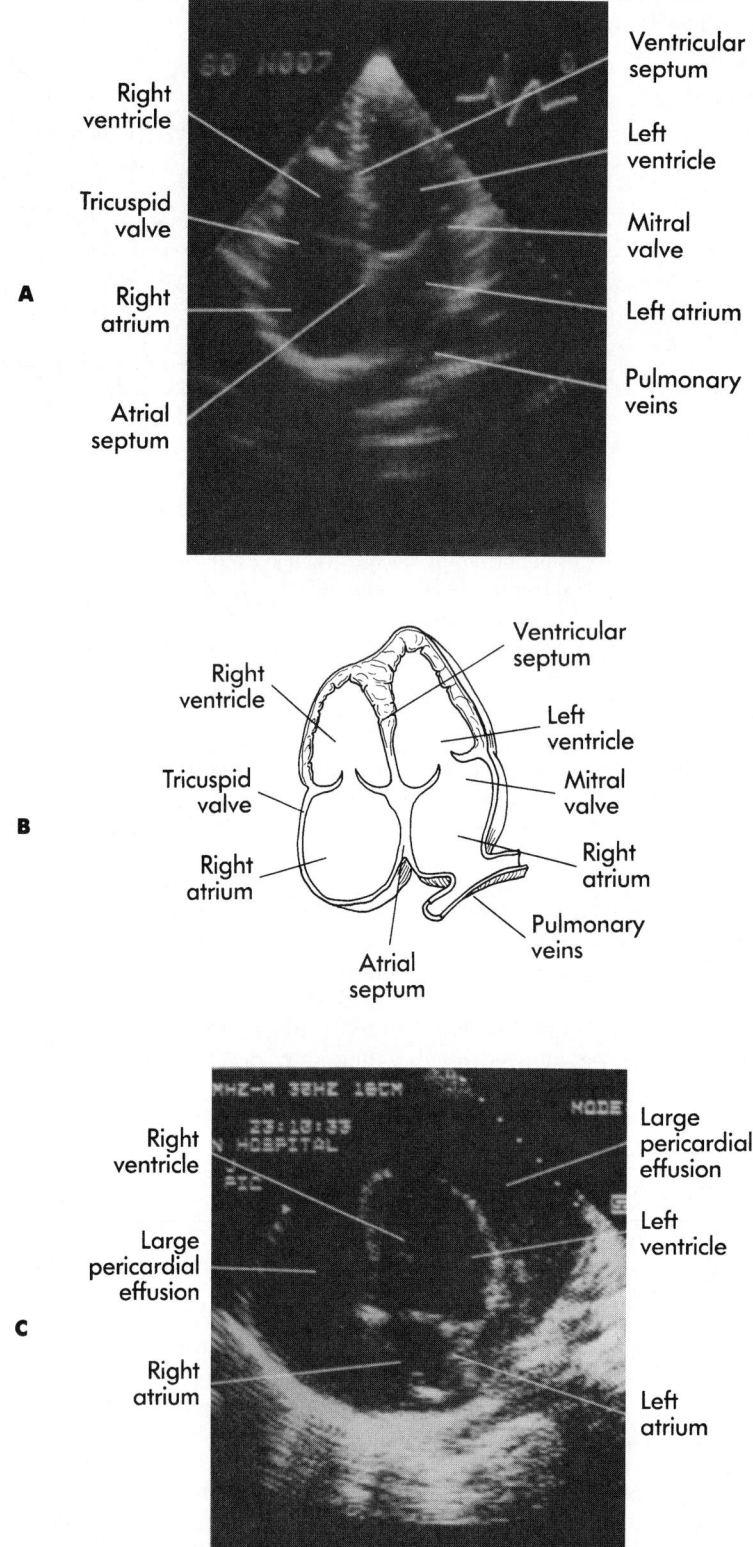

FIG. 13-6. Pediatric two-dimensional echocardiography. **A,** Four-chambered view. The transducer is placed at the apex of the heart, so that all four cardiac chambers, both AV valves, and the atrial and ventricular septa can be viewed. **B,** Schematic representation of the structures viewed. **C,** Identical four-chamber view demonstrates extremely large pericardial effusion that produced cardiac tamponade. *(Illustration by Marilou Kundemueller; echocardiograms courtesy William Berman, Jr, MD; from Hazinski MF: Cardiovascular disorders. In Hazinski MF, editor:* Nursing care of the critically ill child, *ed 2, St Louis, 1992, Mosby.)*

TABLE 13-4. Pediatric Sepsis and Septic Shock Classification and Terminology

Term	Definition	Clinical signs
Sepsis	Suspected infection with signs of the systemic inflammatory response syndrome (SIRS)	Evidence of infection (positive cultures *not* required) Fever or hypothermia Tachycardia Tachypnea, respiratory alkalosis, or increased ventilatory support requirements Possible peripheral vasodilation
Severe sepsis	Sepsis plus signs of altered organ perfusion	Evidence of infection (positive cultures *not* required) Tachycardia Tachypnea, respiratory alkalosis, or increased ventilatory support requirements Fever or hypothermia Possible peripheral vasodilation Altered organ function: 　Altered mental status 　Reduced ventricular ejection fraction 　Pulmonary failure (increased work of breathing, intrapulmonary shunting, or respiratory acidosis) 　GI/hepatic dysfunction (paralytic ileus, GI ulceration or bleeding, coagulopathy, elevation in liver enzymes) 　DIC 　Oliguria or renal failure
Septic shock	Sepsis with hypotension despite fluid therapy or normotension maintained with vasopressors	As above, with hypotension or lactic (metabolic) acidosis Possible multisystem organ failure

to a variety of insults including trauma, burns, or infection. SIRS is present when the patient demonstrates two or more of the following criteria: fever ($>38°$ C) or hypothermia ($<36°$ C), tachycardia, tachypnea or respiratory alkalosis (P_{CO_2} <32 mm Hg), or a white blood cell count $<4,000/mm^3$, $>12,000/mm^3$, or with greater than 10% bands. The demonstration of these "classic" clinical signs may be altered by the patient's age, immune function, and clinical condition. The young infant will often demonstrate hypothermia, rather than fever, and leukopenia, rather than leukocytosis. Since the presence of neutrophils are necessary for the development of fever during infection, the neutropenic patient may demonstrate normothermia or hypothermia. If the patient's respiratory function is supported by mechanical ventilation, tachypnea or respiratory alkalosis may not be detected; in fact, the patient's ventilatory support requirements may increase.

Sepsis. Sepsis is present when there is evidence of SIRS with suspected infection.[20,56,57] Positive blood cultures are not necessary for the diagnosis, but suspicion of infection is required. For example, if the oncology patient presents with an erythematous and draining central venous catheter insertion site or a trauma victim develops a high fever with pulmonary congestion several days after injury, it is highly likely that an infection is present.

The child may demonstrate evidence of peripheral vasodilation. Skin may appear flushed and may feel warm.

Severe Sepsis. Severe sepsis is present when the patient demonstrates evidence of sepsis plus signs of altered organ perfusion.[20,55,56] Altered organ perfusion is detected when signs of organ-system failure are observed. The organ system involved should be separate from the site of suspected infection. This important distinction will enable separation of signs of severe sepsis from those which appear with pneumonia and associated respiratory failure.

The patient with severe sepsis demonstrates evidence of infection (e.g., inflamed wound or pneumonia on chest radiograph), tachycardia, tachypnea, respiratory alkalosis or increased ventilatory support requirements, as well as fever or hypothermia and signs of altered organ function. These signs may include altered mental status, reduced myocardial ejection fraction, pulmonary failure, gastrointestinal dysfunction, or oliguria (urine output less than 1 ml/kg/hr).

Signs of pulmonary failure include increased work of breathing and intrapulmonary shunting. It is important to distinguish simple pneumonia (associated with isolated pulmonary symptoms and fever) from severe sepsis. If severe sepsis is associated with a pneumonia, signs of additional organ system failure should be present. The development of associated ARDS is indicated by the presence of hypoxemia with a P_{O_2} <70 mm Hg (while breathing room air), a PAWP <18 mm Hg (to distinguish from cardiogenic pulmonary edema), and bilateral pulmonary infiltrates on chest radiograph.

Signs of gastrointestinal dysfunction may include an elevation in liver enzymes or the development of a paralytic ileus. Gastrointestinal hemorrhage or ulceration may also be observed. If liver failure is present, coagulopathies may develop or worsen.

Very often, the child with severe sepsis demonstrates evidence of peripheral vasodilation and increased skin blood flow. In addition, peripheral pulses may be bounding, and the diastolic blood pressure may fall.

Septic Shock. The development of septic shock is heralded in the adult patient by the development of hypotension (a systolic blood pressure < 90 mm Hg) despite fluid therapy or normotension, which is maintained only by vasopressor therapy. Since children tend to develop hypotension only late in the course of any shock, septic shock should be recognized when the child develops a metabolic acidosis or a rise in serum lactate, decreased intensity of peripheral pulses, and mottled skin. The skin may be either warm or cool and capillary refill may be delayed. Certainly, if hypotension develops, septic shock is present and progressive. The mortality of septic shock associated with hypotension may be as high as 40% to 60%.[11,20,55-57]

Additional Signs of Sepsis. The child with sepsis generally develops a high cardiac output associated with an increase in heart rate and a fall in systemic vascular resistance. This high cardiac output will be maintained provided the child's intravascular volume remains adequate. Echocardiography may reveal a reduction in ventricular ejection fraction and left ventricular dilation. If the mixed venous oxygen concentration is monitored continuously (through use of a fiberoptic pulmonary artery catheter), a transient fall in SvO_2 may be briefly observed early in septic syndrome or shock as the child's oxygen consumption increases. However, in general the SvO_2 will rise because cardiac output and oxygen delivery rises. An additional reason for an increase in SvO_2 is a reduction in oxygen consumption by some tissue beds as blood is shunted through the tissues. Despite the fact that some tissue beds may be ischemic, overall oxygen extraction does not increase, so the SvO_2 initially remains high.[58]

Warm vs. Cold Septic Shock. Years ago the terms *warm* and *cold* were used to describe patients with septic shock. Warm shock was thought to be associated with peripheral vasodilation and hyperdynamic cardiovascular function with a high cardiac output. Cold shock was thought to be a preterminal condition, associated with a fall in cardiac output and peripheral vasoconstriction. These terms are outdated and should no longer be used.

It is now clear that most patients with septic shock have a high cardiac output and a low systemic vascular resistance.[51] Cardiac output only falls to levels below normal if the patient has severe underlying cardiovascular dysfunction or if fluid administration is inadequate to maintain intravascular volume.[51] Septic patients who developed "cold" cardiogenic shock in the past probably received inadequate volume resuscitation. With successful and liberal fluid resuscitation, cardiac output will be initially high and should return to normal within 24 hours. If the cardiac output and heart rate remain high and systemic vascular resistance remains low despite therapy for longer than 24 hours after the development of hypotension, resuscitation has not been successful, the septic cascade continues to produce maldistribution of blood flow, and the risk of patient mortality is high.[51]

Spinal (Neurogenic) Shock

The child with spinal (neurogenic) shock demonstrates signs of spinal cord injury and hypotension despite adequate volume replacement and absence of ongoing hemorrhage. The skin is typically warm, dry, and flushed. Since the loss of sympathetic nervous system vascular tone produces expansion of the vascular space, signs of a relative hypovolemia, including a low central venous or pulmonary artery wedge pressure, will be observed. Pulmonary edema may also develop if aggressive fluid therapy has been provided.

Ancillary Data

Lactic acidosis may be the most sensitive indicator of inadequate systemic perfusion. The development of a metabolic acidosis or a rise in the serum lactate concentration indicates the presence of inadequate tissue oxygenation.

Evaluation of the child's ventilation and oxygenation should be made whenever shock is present, utilizing arterial blood gas analysis and ongoing monitoring. In addition, evaluation of the child's electrolytes, glucose, BUN, creatinine, liver functions, calcium, phosphorus, and cardiac enzyme concentrations may help determine the cause of the shock or treatment needed.

Hematologic evaluation is necessary if nontraumatic hemorrhage or disseminated intravascular coagulation (DIC) is apparent. This evaluation should include a complete blood count, platelets, coagulation tests (i.e., prothrombin time [PT], partial thromboplastin time [PTT], and bleeding time), and DIC screen (i.e., fibrinogen and fibrin-split products). Hemoglobin and hematocrit may be artificially normal in the face of an acute decrease in intravascular volume; unless volume resuscitation is provided with whole blood, the child's hematocrit will eventually fall. A blood sample should be sent for type and crossmatch when the child is admitted; this procedure may reduce the time required to obtain crossmatched blood if it is needed.

A chest x-ray study should be performed to evaluate cardiac size and exclude pneumonia, pneumothorax, and pulmonary edema. An arterial blood gas (ABG) analysis enables evaluation of the progression of acidosis and identification of diffusion and ventilation problems associated with respiratory distress. Continuous oximetry enables evaluation of hemoglobin saturation, and also indicates the loss of peripheral pulses (although this device should never be used as a pulse check). ECG and echocardiography should be selectively performed to evaluate the cardiac function and eliminate dysrhythmias, effusion, and inflammation as contributing conditions to low cardiac output.

Microbiologic evaluation should be performed as appropriate when infection is suspected. Cultures of blood and urine should be obtained as needed, and a Gram stain should be available immediately on these cultures. Evaluation of spinal fluid, stool, and joints may be needed.

MANAGEMENT

Early recognition and therapy are the keys to the survival of the pediatric patient in shock. Therefore recognition of signs of poor systemic perfusion is essential. Supportive therapy will then be required to optimize each aspect of cardiovascular and pulmonary function. Throughout therapy, it is imperative that the bedside clinician evaluate patient response to therapy and watch for evidence of further deterioration and development of multisystem organ failure.[15]

The goals of the treatment of shock are maximization of oxygen delivery and minimization of oxygen demand. The airway, oxygenation, and ventilation must be supported. Reduction of oxygen demand requires the treatment of pain. Fear also increases oxygen consumption; care must be taken to reassure the child, and keep parents nearby, if possible. In addition, the child should be kept warm, and shivering must be prevented. Blood components (and, perhaps, intravenous fluids) should be warmed before administration to young infants or those with hypothermia.[15]

The child in shock should be resuscitated wherever the shock is detected. Once systemic perfusion is restored, transfer to a pediatric intensive care unit is advised. However, during resuscitation, continuous evaluation and support of cardiopulmonary function must be provided. Hemodynamic monitoring should be instituted, and volume and inotropic support provided as needed. Throughout shock therapy, the warmth of the child's extremities, capillary refill, quality of peripheral pulses, level of consciousness and responsiveness, urine output, oxygenation, ventilation, and acid-base status should be assessed.

All sources of fluid intake and output should be carefully totaled and recorded hourly (and more frequently as needed). Monitoring of the volume of urine output and urine specific gravity is useful in determining the child's response to fluid therapy. A urinary catheter should be inserted if shock is present, unless the patient has sustained pelvic trauma and urethral tear is suspected.

Airway and Ventilation

Initial therapy for any unstable patient requires evaluation of airway patency and ventilation. The child should be positioned to support maximal airway patency, and the effectiveness of ventilation should be constantly evaluated. Supplemental oxygen is administered at 3 to 6 L/min by mask, head hood, or bag-valve-mask ventilation as needed. If the child is not ventilating, initial bag-mask support may temporize until the decision to intubate is made.

Children in shock should be intubated electively before respiratory deterioration or arrest complicates shock management. Too often, advanced therapy is sabotaged by neglect of relatively simple but significant aspects of therapy: establishment and maintenance of an adequate airway and support of effective ventilation.

Intubation should be considered in children with respiratory arrest or apnea, airway obstruction (or significant risk of obstruction, as in the child with facial burns), hypoxemia, hypoventilation, hypercarbia, or increased intracranial pressure. In general, physiologic indications for intubation include an arterial oxygen tension (Po_2) <50 mm Hg (at sea level) with an Fio_2 of 0.5 or greater, a carbon dioxide tension (Pco_2) of greater than 50 mm Hg (unless this is a chronic condition or a compensatory response to metabolic alkalosis), and evidence of an increas-

---

Quantification of Pulmonary Insufficiency

Oxygenation indices:

1. Po_2/Fio_2 normally >180-200 mm Hg
   (e.g., patient Po_2 = 80 mm Hg with Fio_2 of 1.0 yields a Po_2/Fio_2 of 80 mm Hg)

2. $$\frac{\text{Mean airway pressure} \times Fio_2 \times 100}{Po_2}$$
   Normally <25-50 mm Hg

Alveolar-arterial oxygen gradient (A-a O_2 gradient):

= Alveolar (A) oxygen tension − arterial (a) oxygen tension

= $PAo_2 - Po_2$

= $Fio_2 \times$ (barometric pressure − 47 mm Hg) − $Pco_2/0.8$

Normally 15 mm Hg

---

ing intrapulmonary shunt. Calculation of the shunt uses the formulas in the box above.

Once mechanical ventilatory support has been established, it is imperative that the health-care team evaluate the effectiveness of ventilatory support. Sudden deterioration in the intubated child is most often the result of tube *d*isplacement or migration, tube *o*bstruction, *p*neumothorax air leaks, or *e*quipment failure ("DOPE").[2]

ARDS may complicate the management of the patient with shock. ARDS is characterized by increased capillary permeability, pulmonary edema with progressive hypoxemia, increased intrapulmonary shunting, and decreased compliance. If ARDS is present or significant pulmonary lung edema develops during the course of therapy, ventilation with supplementary oxygen and positive end-expiratory pressure (PEEP) is necessary.

In general the PEEP is titrated to minimize the inspired oxygen concentration and risk of oxygen toxicity. However, high peak and end-expiratory pressures may result in barotrauma. As a result, the optimal PEEP is the minimal PEEP required to maintain *maximal oxygen delivery*, typically a Po_2 >60 mm Hg (and a hemoglobin saturation >60%) with an Fio_2 <0.5 if possible. The optimal PEEP will also be associated with reduced intrapulmonary shunting and will probably result in maximal lung compliance.[59] If PEEP is provided, it should be maintained throughout all aspects of pulmonary care (especially during hand ventilation and suctioning).

Circulation

Heart Rate. The child's heart rate must be adequate to support effective cardiac output and systemic perfusion. Bradydysrhythmias and extreme tachydysrhythmias should be promptly treated (see the box on p. 134 and Chapter 14). Pharmacologic therapy, pacing, or synchronized DC cardioversion may be required.

Collapse rhythms result in a loss of all pulses. The most common ECG findings associated with loss of pulses in-

Most Common Pediatric Dysrhythmias

Heart (QRS) rate too slow for clinical condition
QRS duration (width) normal
   Sinus bradycardia
   Junctional rhythm
   Heart block
QRS duration (width) prolonged
   SVT with aberrant ventricular conduction
   Ventricular rhythm
   Heart block

Heart (QRS) rate too fast for clinical condition
QRS duration (width) normal
   Sinus tachycardia
   Supraventricular tachycardia (SVT)
QRS duration (width) prolonged
   SVT with aberrant ventricular conduction
   Ventricular tachycardia

Collapse (pulseless) rhythms
   Electromechanical dissociation
   Ventricular tachycardia
   Ventricular fibrillation
   Asystole

From Hazinski MF: Cardiovascular disorders. In Hazinski MF, editor: *Nursing care of the critically ill child*, ed 2, St Louis, 1992, Mosby.

clude asystole, electromechanical dissociation (EMD), ventricular tachycardia, and ventricular fibrillation. Regardless of the ECG findings present, cardiopulmonary resuscitation, including cardiac compression, must be performed when loss of pulses is identified. In addition, potential causes of reversible EMD, including hypoxemia, severe acidosis, tension pneumothorax, and hypovolemia, must be corrected.[2] See Chapter 12 for review of cardiopulmonary resuscitation.

Volume Resuscitation. Volume resuscitation is designed to restore intravascular volume relative to the vascular space and to optimize ventricular preload. The specific fluid selected and the route of administration will be determined by the child's clinical condition.

Intravenous Access and Hemodynamic Monitoring. To begin shock resuscitation, establishment of intravenous access is required. At least one and preferably two large-bore venous catheters should be inserted. If intravenous access cannot be achieved in infants and young children, an intraosseous needle should be inserted and intraosseous fluid and drug administration provided.[2]

Unless uncomplicated dehydration or mild hypovolemic shock is present, insertion of a central venous (monitoring) catheter is extremely helpful. Several multilumen catheters are available in pediatric sizes that enable simultaneous monitoring of CVP and administration of fluids.

An intraarterial line should also be inserted once initial stabilization has been achieved. This enables reliable, con-

tinuous evaluation of the arterial pressure. Noninvasive oscillometric blood pressure monitoring devices may not accurately measure low or rapidly falling blood pressures and may overestimate the blood pressure in the patient in shock.[60] Sphygmomanometry may also yield inaccurate blood pressure measurement; typically cuff pressure measurements in shock patients underestimate the systolic blood pressure (cuff measurements are lower than the intraarterial pressure).[61]

Insertion of a pulmonary artery catheter should be considered whenever the child demonstrates shock that is unresponsive to initial volume and vasoactive drug support. A pulmonary artery catheter with thermodilution cardiac output thermistor or fiberoptic for continuous monitoring of mixed venous oxygen saturation may be particularly helpful if precise tracking of hemodynamic parameters is desired. This may be necessary in the care of the child with shock or multisystem organ failure. In fact, use of the pulmonary artery catheter and calculation of hemodynamic parameters (including cardiac output, vascular resistances, stroke volume, and stroke work index) provide detailed information about the patient response to therapy and can be very helpful in the titration of volume and vasoactive drug therapy.

Intravenous Fluid Selection and Distribution
Crystalloids and Colloids. Isotonic crystalloids or colloids will be administered during stabilization of the child in shock. As a rule, isotonic crystalloids (0.9% normal saline or lactated Ringer's) are utilized during volume resuscitation, and blood products are provided if blood loss has occurred.

If the heart rate is adequate and signs of hypervolemia are absent, fluid therapy begins with a bolus of 20 ml/kg, administered as quickly as possible. Fluid boluses should be repeated as needed until systemic perfusion improves. If the hematocrit level is satisfactory and several fluid boluses are required, both colloids and crystalloids may be administered in an approximate 3:1 or 4:1 ratio of crystalloids to colloids.[62]

Since isotonic fluids are distributed throughout the extracellular space, only approximately 25% of isotonic fluids can be expected to remain in the vascular space following administration. Interstitial movement of isotonic fluids may result in the development of systemic or pulmonary edema, so the development of edema should be anticipated (and respiratory function supported, as needed). *Hypotonic* fluids should be avoided during shock resuscitation, since the portion of the hypotonic fluid that is water will be distributed throughout the total body water, with only 8% or less of the volume remaining in the vascular space.[62]

The relative merits of crystalloids vs. colloids in the resuscitation of hypovolemic shock continue to be debated.[63-65] Typically both are used in resuscitative efforts. Crystalloids have the advantage of low cost and ready availability. Colloids tend to remain in the vascular space for hours longer than crystalloids. During those hours, they can create an intravascular oncotic force, stimulating fluid movement into the vascular space. As a result, colloids may expand the intravascular volume more efficiently than an equal volume of administered crystalloid.[64] Patients may develop sensitivity reactions to albumin or other colloids, and it is important to note that, although colloids remain in the vascular space longer than crystalloids, they will also ultimately be distributed throughout the extracellular space.

Treatment of Dehydration. Treatment of the child with dehydration requires restoration of adequate systemic perfusion, calculation and replacement of estimated fluid and electrolyte deficits, replacement of ongoing fluid losses, and administration of required maintenance fluids. It is important to note that calculation and replacement of the fluid and electrolyte deficit should be accomplished after intravascular volume and systemic perfusion have been restored. Replacement of the deficit on an hourly basis is inappropriate if shock is present.

If *hypernatremic* dehydration is present, bolus fluid administration should be provided only if needed to restore adequate systemic perfusion. Generous fluid administration beyond that needed for shock resuscitation may result in a rapid fall in the serum sodium and osmolality (since even normal saline will be relatively hypotonic for the hypernatremic child), with resultant neurologic complications. In these patients, the serum sodium concentration should be lowered gradually and should not be allowed to fall more than 1 mEq/hr. If extreme hypernatremia is present (serum sodium concentration exceeding 170 mEq/L), dialysis may be required to enable controlled reduction in the serum sodium concentration.

In any patient with dehydration, the serum sodium and electrolyte concentration should be closely monitored during fluid resuscitation and replacement. Normal serum electrolytes should be restored and maintained. See Chapter 15 for further information about the care of the child with dehydration.

Fluid Therapy for Septic Shock. Patients in septic shock may require a large volume of administered fluid to restore and maintain systemic perfusion. More than 40 ml/kg may be administered during the first hour of volume resuscitation, and 100 to 200 ml/kg or more may be required during the first several hours of therapy. In fact, rapid volume administration, particularly during the first hour of therapy, has been linked with improved survival in hypotensive pediatric patients in septic shock.[11]

Blood and Blood Component Therapy. Administration of blood or blood component therapy will be necessary if significant blood loss has occurred or if severe coagulopathies are present. The presence of a "normal" hematocrit does not rule out the possibility of hemorrhage; the hematocrit typically falls in the patient who has sustained whole blood loss only after intravascular fluid shift or replacement of the blood loss with crystalloids or colloids.

In general, 10 ml/kg boluses of type-specific packed (p)-RBC or 20 ml/kg boluses of type-specific whole blood are administered to patients in shock who have sustained hemorrhage. Whole blood is useful for treatment of massive ongoing hemorrhage but is generally unavailable routinely, having been replaced by p-RBC; p-RBC are particularly appropriate in the treatment of blood loss or anemia associated with hypervolemia. Blood should be administered as quickly as possible to restore systemic perfusion. A blood warmer and micropore filter should be used during blood transfusions.

If crossmatched blood is not available, type-specific blood can generally be obtained within 10 to 15 minutes after delivery of a clot to the blood bank. O-negative blood can be used under emergency conditions. It should be reserved for those patients in profound hemorrhagic shock who are unresponsive to crystalloid administration.

Transfusion for the child with chronic anemia and shock must be accomplished carefully to prevent hypervolemia and further deterioration in myocardial function. Administration of an infusion of p-RBC at a rate averaging 3 to 5 ml/kg/hr over several hours may be well tolerated, particularly if preceded and followed by administration of diuretics. If severe anemia is associated with severe hypervolemia and myocardial dysfunction, an exchange transfusion may be required.

If a coagulopathy is present, blood component therapy should be administered to prevent or treat hemorrhage. Indications for and dosages of blood components are summarized in Table 13-5, as well as Chapters 16 and 54.

Evaluation of Patient Response to Fluid Therapy. The goal of volume resuscitation is the restoration of adequate intravascular volume relative to the vascular space. During volume therapy, the child's systemic perfusion must be closely monitored. A positive response to volume administration includes a decrease in heart rate; correction of hypotension; and improvement in the warmth of extremities, the quality of peripheral pulses, the child's general color, and the briskness of capillary refill. In addition, the child's urine volume should increase. As shock is successfully treated, the child's level of consciousness should improve. *If the child's neurologic function fails to improve or deteriorates during shock therapy, neurologic complications or inadequate resuscitation should be ruled out.*

Throughout volume resuscitation, the health care team should attempt to determine the central venous pressure (and, possibly, the PAWP) associated with optimal systemic perfusion and urine output. This optimal pressure may change in the same patient during the course of therapy (associated with changes in myocardial function), but it may serve as a useful guide during initial resuscitation.

The development of systemic edema should be anticipated during volume resuscitation, particularly when crystalloids are utilized or capillary permeability is increased (e.g., in the patient with septic shock). Pulmonary edema may *not* be observed if pulmonary lymphatic flow increases proportionately with pulmonary extravascular fluid movement.[65] The development of pulmonary edema should be anticipated, however, and ventilatory support with supplementary oxygen and PEEP should be planned.

If the patient fails to respond to initial volume administration, placement of a central venous or pulmonary artery catheter should be considered. Some improvement in systemic perfusion should be apparent once the CVP or PAWP reaches 10 to 12 mm Hg. If systemic perfusion remains inadequate despite these ventricular "filling" pressures, hypovolemia has been corrected and other causes of shock should be considered including myocardial dysfunction, tension pneumothorax, pericardial tamponade, sepsis, or closing of the ductus arteriosus in neonates with a ductal-dependent lesion (e.g., coarctation of aorta in newborns). Shock unresponsive to volume therapy requires

TABLE 13-5. Pediatric Blood Component Therapy

Problem	"Classic" coagulation panel abnormalities	Blood component	Quantity
Acute blood loss	Hematocrit <40 (infants)	Whole blood*	To replace loss give 10-20 ml/kg;
	<30 (children)	P-RBCs	10 ml/kg should raise Hct 10 points
Chronic anemia	Hematocrit <15% to 20% Hemoglobin <5-7 gm/dl Patient symptomatic	P-RBCs If frequent or multiple transfusions are required, or history of febrile reactions, consider leukocyte-poor RBCs (buffy coat removed to prevent reactions with WBCs)	Administer *slowly*: 3 ml/kg/hr (consider diuretics)
Anemia in child with T-cell immune deficiency	Hematocrit <40 (infants) <30 (children) (consider patient baseline)	If time and patient consideration allows, consider irradiated blood cells	As above (see acute blood loss)
Thrombocytopenia	↓ platelets (isolated) ↑ template bleeding time Clot formation but lack of clot retraction	Platelets	1 U/5 kg (maximum: 10 U)
Thrombocytopathia	Normal or only slightly decreased platelet count template bleeding time Clot formation but lack of clot retraction	Platelets	1 U/5 kg (maximum: 10 U)
Disseminated intravascular coagulation (DIC)	↓ fibrinogen and platelets (lower than expected) ↑ PT, PTT ↑ fibrin split products	Treat cause If fibrinogen <50, cryoprecipitate plus FFP should be given. If fibrinogen >50 FFP alone may be effective	Fresh frozen plasma (FFP): 10 ml/kg Cryoprecipitate: 1 bag/5 kg Titrate to achieve improvement in fibrinogen and platelet count
DIC with purpura fulminans	As above with evidence of peripheral embolic phenomena	Administer FFP to restore levels of antithrombin III, then heparin	FFP: 10 ml/kg Heparin: Load: 25-50 U/kg Maintenance: 15-25 U/kg/hr Titrate to achieve rise in fibrinogen and platelet count and fall in PTT
Hemophilia A	Bleeding ↓ factor VIII activity	Purified factor VIII	Severe life-threatening bleeding or major surgery: 50 U/kg or continuous infusion of 2 U/kg/hr to maintain factor VIII activity at 100% Minor bleeding: 25 U/kg

Continued.

correction of acid-base or electrolyte imbalances and vasoactive drug therapy.

Acid-Base and Electrolyte Imbalances

Hypoxemia, metabolic acidosis, and electrolyte imbalances will depress myocardial function, and they must be corrected. As noted, during resuscitation of the child in shock, oxygen is administered and mechanical ventilatory support is usually indicated.

Correction of Acidosis. Metabolic acidosis results from inadequate tissue perfusion and subsequent anaerobic metabolism. Whenever shock is present, metabolic acidosis is treated most effectively by support of adequate oxygenation and ventilation and by restoration of effective systemic perfusion. Hyperventilation and resultant hypocarbia and respiratory alkalosis will correct the serum pH of the patient in shock or cardiopulmonary arrest more efficiently than bicarbonate administration. In fact, bicarbonate administration to adult patients with congestive heart failure and metabolic acidosis actually decreases arterial oxygen tension and myocardial oxygen consumption and oxygen extraction.[66] The use of buffering agents during cardiopulmonary resuscitation is controversial and there is no evidence that it improves survival.

TABLE 13-5. Pediatric Blood Component Therapy–cont'd

Problem	"Classic" coagulation panel abnormalities	Blood component	Quantity
Lack of coagulation factors in general†	↑ PT, PTT, thrombin time ↓ fibrinogen Slow clot formation	FFP	10 ml/kg
Heparin excess‡	↑ ↑ PTT, thrombin time, and template bleeding time PT may be slightly ↑ Platelet count normal (initially) Slow clot formation	Protamine sulfate (titrated to correct thrombin time)	1 mg/kg (slowly); 1 mg IV each 100 U Heparin given concurrently; 0.5 mg IV each 100 U Heparin given in previous 30 min, and so on; maximum: 50 mg/dose (slowly)
Protamine sulfate excess‡	↑ ↑ PTT, thrombin time, and template bleeding time PT may be slightly ↑ Platelet count normal (initially) Slow clot formation	When protamine is titrated and thrombin time does not improve, heparin may be administered	Heparin IV: 50 U/kg Infusion: 10-15 U/kg/hr
Effects of aspirin (ASA)	↑ template bleeding time	Platelets	1 U/5 kg (maximum: 10 U)

From Hazinski MF: Cardiovascular disorders. In Hazinski MF, editor: *Nursing care of the critically ill child*, ed 2, St. Louis, 1992, Mosby.
*Generally unavailable; largely replaced by p-RBC.
†Usually, this condition results from a complex function of dilution and lack of replacement during surgery, inability of the liver to compensate, and occasionally from excessive loss of plasma protein (large proteins) via chest tubes.
‡The only way to distinguish between these two problems is through protamine sulfate titration—see the third column.

The buffering action of sodium bicarbonate will result in the formation of carbon dioxide and may increase central nervous system acidosis. Therefore bicarbonate should not be administered until effective ventilation has been established. The dose may be calculated at 1 mEq/kg or determined by the base deficit as follows[2]:

$$mEq\ NaHCO_3 = base\ deficit \times kilogram\ body\ weight \times 0.3$$

Use of carbon dioxide consuming buffers (e.g., tromethamine, or TRIS buffer) may be considered in the presence of combined metabolic and respiratory acidosis, but these agents may produce hyperkalemia and hypoglycemia, so should be used with caution.[67]

Salts of organic acids (including lactate contained in lactated Ringer's solution) may also act as buffers. However, these buffers must be metabolized to exert their effect, so they will probably not be helpful in the treatment of shock associated with poor systemic perfusion.[68]

Correction of Electrolyte Imbalance

Glucose. Hypoglycemia may develop rapidly in the critically ill or injured infant because the infant has high glucose needs and low glycogen stores. If glucose is needed, however, continuous infusion is preferred to intermittent bolus therapy. In fact, hyperglycemia has been linked to poor outcome in children with head injury, although it is unclear if the poor outcome is caused by idiopathic hyperglycemia or excessive glucose administration.[52]

Sodium. Acute or severe alterations in the serum sodium concentration should be avoided during fluid therapy. Acute changes in serum sodium produce changes in serum osmolality, which result in fluid shifts into and out of the vascular and interstitial spaces. Such fluid shifts are associated with neurologic complications including seizures, cerebral edema, and intracranial hemorrhage.[69]

Potassium. Alterations in serum potassium concentration may affect cardiac conduction and rhythm. However, children are far less sensitive than adults to minor changes in the serum potassium concentration. Hypokalemia may result from inadequate potassium administration during volume therapy or from excessive potassium losses caused by drug therapy (e.g., furosemide). The serum potassium concentration will fall in the presence of alkalosis; this represents an intracellular shift of potassium and will be corrected when the pH is normalized. True hypokalemia should be treated with an infusion of potassium chloride at a dose equivalent to 0.5 to 1 mEq/kg/dose, administered over several hours.

Hyperkalemia may result from excessive potassium administration or reduced potassium excretion (e.g., in renal failure). The serum potassium concentration will also rise when acidosis develops; this rise in serum potassium is caused by a shift of potassium from the intracellular to the vascular space, and the serum potassium will fall when the serum pH is corrected.

Calcium. Both the ionized and total calcium concentration should be monitored during shock therapy, and documented hypocalcemia should be treated. The serum ionized calcium concentration is often low (<4.5 mEq/L) in children with septic shock.[50] Since ionized calcium precipitates with phosphate, the serum ionized calcium concentration will often fall following administration of citrate-phosphate-dextran-preserved bank blood. A reduction in ionized calcium concentration also occurs when the pH rises. Hypocalcemia may also be associated with hypomagnesemia; a low serum magnesium concentration (<1.5

to 2.5 mEq/L) may be the cause of refractory hypocalcemia (and hypokalemia), and often must be treated before the calcium and potassium concentrations can be normalized.

Documented hypocalcemia is treated with administration of calcium chloride, 20 to 25 mg/kg (0.2 to 0.25 ml/kg). Calcium should be administered slowly (no faster than 100 mg/minute); bolus administration of calcium may produce bradycardia and dysrhythmias. Calcium should not be routinely administered during cardiopulmonary resuscitation, since cardiac arrest results in intramyocardial pooling of calcium.[2]

Hypercalcemia may be observed in children with some malignancies, including acute lymphocytic leukemia, lymphomas, and soft tissue sarcomas. These malignant cells often secrete a parathormone-like substance, which stimulates bone reabsorption and release of calcium and rapid cell turnover.[70] Although mild hypercalcemia (total serum calcium below 15 mg/dl) is not life-threatening, extreme hypercalcemia (total serum calcium approaching 19 to 20 mEq/L) may produce renal and cardiovascular complications. In the presence of significant hypercalcemia, the kidneys are unable to concentrate urine, and profound diuresis may produce hypovolemia. Hypercalcemia can usually be treated with hydration (normal saline infusion) and diuretic therapy. Calcitonin administration (3 to 6 MRC U/kg IV or IM every 6 hr) may occasionally be required.[70]

Vasoactive Drug Therapy

General Principles and Preparation. If oxygenation, ventilation, heart rate, and intravascular volume are appropriate, and myocardial function and systemic perfusion remain poor, vasoactive drug therapy with inotropes is indicated. Inotropic agents are not helpful in the treatment of hypovolemic shock unless or until intravascular volume has been restored. These drugs are extremely useful in the treatment of cardiogenic and distributive shock (including septic or spinal shock) or in any progressive shock condition when myocardial function is impaired.

The goals of vasoactive drug therapy in the treatment of shock will be to increase heart rate if it is too slow for clinical condition, to increase cardiac output if it is inadequate, to redistribute cardiac output if it cannot be increased, and to increase cardiac contractility.[15] It is important to note that these drugs may improve systemic perfusion and organ function by increasing or redistributing blood flow without an improvement in blood pressure. However, if significant hypotension is present, it will be necessary to increase blood pressure and blood flow.

Before any vasoactive drug is administered the proposed effects of the drug should be determined, and the clinical or physiologic criteria that will be used to monitor the effectiveness of therapy must be established. For example, dopamine may be administered to increase renal blood flow and urine output, to increase heart rate, or to increase blood pressure. It is important to determine the goals of therapy at the outset, so drug dose can be titrated to desired effects.

Vasoactive drugs have a very short half-life, so are administered by continuous infusion. The drug may be diluted to either standard concentrations (e.g., 400 µg/ml,

TABLE 13-6. Classification of Beta-agonist Agents

Effector organ	Mechanism/effect		
	Alpha	Beta$_1$	Beta$_2$
Heart	—	—	Increase
Rate	—	Increase	—
Contractility	—	Increase	—
Conduction velocity	—	Increase	—
Arterioles	Constrict	—	Dilate
Veins	Constrict	—	Dilate
Lungs—bronchiolar smooth muscles	Constrict	—	Dilate

600 µg/ml, and so on) or variable concentrations based on body weight. Use of standard concentrations reduces the likelihood of dilution errors, since consistent concentrations are always mixed. The disadvantage of standard concentrations is that individual doses must be calculated for every patient and every infusion rate. If variable concentrations of the drug are utilized, each patient receives a unique dilution of the drug calculated on the basis of body weight; then 1 ml/hr infusion of the drug dilution will provide either 1 or 0.1 µg/kg/min of the drug. An advantage of this type of dilution is that the drug dose provided is readily determined. A disadvantage of this form of dilution is that a different concentration and dilution of drug is prepared for each patient, thus increasing the likelihood of error during formulation. In addition, relatively large volumes of fluid will be administered to small infants if high doses of the drug are required. The "Rule of Sixes" for mixing variable concentrations of continuous infusion medications is listed in the box on p. 140.

Vasoactive drugs must be carefully titrated, and the patient response to therapy must be carefully assessed. The correct dose of any vasoactive drug can only be determined at the bedside after careful evaluation of patient response to therapy. The pharmacokinetics (relation between drug dose and plasma concentration) and pharmacodynamics (relation between drug concentration and drug effect) of these drugs will be affected by patient age and clinical condition. Pharmacokinetics are more likely to be determined by the child's underlying clinical condition and hepatic and renal function than by the patient's age.[2,71,72]

Sympathomimetic Drugs and Inotropes. Sympathomimetic drugs are provided to stimulate particular adrenergic receptors. The receptors targeted will be determined by the child's heart rate, peripheral perfusion, blood pressure, and urine output. The effects of receptor activation are summarized in Table 13-6. Typical dosages and clinical and side effects of sympathomimetic drugs have been provided in Table 13-7. It is important to remember that each patient will demonstrate an individual response to each drug. Vasoactive drugs should be titrated to provide maximal therapeutic effects with minimal side or toxic effects. General suggestions for the use of sympathomimetic drugs are listed in the box on p. 140. Often a combination of

TABLE 13-7. Suggested Doses and Actions of Sympathomimetic and Other Inotropic Drugs

Drug	Dose	Effects	Cautions
Dobutamine	2-15 μg/kg/min	Selective beta-adrenergic effects; increases cardiac contractility and also increases heart rate (this latter effect is variable). Beta$_2$ effects produce peripheral vasodilation. No dopaminergic or alpha-adrenergic effects	Extreme tachydysrhythmias have been reported (particularly in infants); hypotension may develop; may produce pulmonary venoconstriction.
Dopamine	2-5 μg/kg/min	Dopaminergic effects predominate (including increase in glomerular filtration rate and urine volume)	Can produce extreme tachydysrhythmias; can result in increase in pulmonary artery pressure; inhibits thyroid stimulating hormone (TSH) and aldosterone secretion.
	5-20 μg/kg/min	Dopaminergic effects persist and beta$_1$ effects are seen (especially an increase in heart rate)	
	>20 μg/kg/min	Alpha-adrenergic effects dominate	
Epinephrine	0.05-0.5 μg/kg/min and titrate	Endogenous catecholamine, which produces alpha, beta$_1$ and beta$_2$ adrenergic effects; at low doses, beta$_1$ effects dominate.	Will increase myocardial work and oxygen consumption at any dose; splanchnic constriction will occur at even low doses.
	0.2-0.3 μg/kg/min	Alpha-adrenergic effects dominate.	
Isoproterenol	0.05-1.5 μg/kg/min	Beta-adrenergic effects; beta$_1$ effects may result in rapid increase in heart rate; beta$_2$ effects may produce peripheral vasodilation and also may effectively treat bronchoconstriction.	Monitor for tachydysrhythmias, hypotension. Will increase myocardial oxygen consumption.
Norepinephrine	0.1 μg/kg/min and titrate	Endogenous catecholamine with alpha- and beta-adrenergic effects; produces potent peripheral and renal vasoconstriction; can increase blood pressure.	May produce tachydysrhythmias, increased myocardial work, and increased oxygen consumption; may result in hepatic and mesenteric ischemia.
Amrinone	0.75 mg/kg (Load—slowly); 5-10 μg/kg/min	Nonadrenergic inotropic agent that produces phosphodiesterase inhibition and increase in intracellular cyclic AMP; intracellular calcium uptake also is delayed. These effects result in improved cardiac contractility and vasodilation.	Monitor for dysrhythmias (especially accelerated junctional rhythm, junctional tachycardia, and ventricular ectopy); may produce hypotension (especially if patient is hypovolemic), liver and gastrointestinal dysfunction, thrombocytopenia, and abdominal pain; experience in children is limited and recent.

Adapted from Hazinski MF: *Crit Care Nurs Clin North Am* 2:309, 1990.

pressor agents is needed. Such combination therapy may produce more significant improvement in cardiac output, systemic perfusion, or distribution of blood flow than will occur when any of the drugs is used separately. However, it is imperative that changes in drug dosage be made carefully. Preferably, the dose of only one drug should be changed at any one time, so the effects of the change on systemic perfusion can be evaluated. When infusions are begun or the infusion rate is changed, the "dead space" in the tubing must be considered, and it may be necessary to temporarily increase the infusion rate to ensure timely delivery of the medication to the patient.

Dopamine is a popular drug for the management of pediatric patients in shock, particularly in the presence of oliguria. Low-dose dopamine therapy may result in improved renal perfusion and urine output and mesenteric perfusion through activation of dopaminergic receptors.

Dobutamine is particularly useful in the treatment of myocardial failure, provided the child's blood pressure is acceptable. Since dobutamine produces peripheral vasodilation in addition to an increase in cardiac contractility, it is not the drug of choice for the patient with hypotension.

Epinephrine may be extremely effective in the treatment of symptomatic bradycardia unresponsive to oxygen

Rule of Sixes for Preparing Variable Concentrations of Vasoactive Drugs

I. For drugs infused in doses of 1 μg/kg/min (or multiples):
   A. Multiply weight (in kg) by 6; place this number of milligrams of drug in solution *totaling* 100 ml
   B. Then 1 ml/hr delivers 1 μg/kg/min

II. For drugs infused in doses of 0.1 μg/kg/min (or multiples):
   A. Multiply weight (in kg) by 0.6; place this number of milligrams of drug in solution *totaling* 100 ml
   B. Then 1 ml/hr delivers 0.1 μg/kg/min

III. For any concentration of a drug:

$$\text{Rate (ml/hr)} = \frac{\text{weight (kg)} \times \text{dose (μg/kg/min)} \times 60 \text{ min/hr}}{\text{concentration (μg/ml)}}$$

From Hazinski MF: Cardiovascular disorders. In Hazinski MF, editor: *Nursing care of the critically ill child*, ed 2, St. Louis, 1992, Mosby.

Suggested Uses of Sympathomimetic and Inotropic Drugs

Goals of sympathomimetic drug therapy
To increase heart rate if it is too slow for clinical condition
To increase cardiac output if it is inadequate
To redistribute cardiac output if it cannot be increased
To increase cardiac contractility

Treatment of bradycardia
Treat cause (correct hypoxia, ensure ventilation)
Epinephrine (drug of choice if bradycardia is hypoxic or ischemic in origin)
Atropine
Isoproterenol (useful if heart block present)
Dopamine
Consider pacing

To improve myocardial function
Epinephrine
Dobutamine (not recommended if hypotension or decreased SVR is present)
Dopamine
Amrinone (not recommended if hypotension or decreased SVR is present)
Consider use of vasodilator if intravascular volume adequate

Treatment of septic shock
Epinephrine
Norepinephrine
Dopamine

To improve renal perfusion
Dopamine (low dose)

From Hazinski MF: Cardiovascular disorders. In Hazinski MF, editor: *Nursing care of the critically ill child*, ed 2, St. Louis, 1992, Mosby.

therapy, or in the treatment of hypotension. Epinephrine may also be extremely effective in increasing mean arterial pressure and improving myocardial function in patients with septic or spinal (neurogenic) shock. Since these drugs invariably reduce splanchnic blood flow, the addition of low-dose dopamine should be considered to maintain renal blood flow and urine output.

Amrinone is a noncatecholamine inotrope that increases ventricular contractility by inhibiting phosphodiesterase (so cyclic AMP accumulates intracellularly). In addition, it increases intracellular calcium concentration and delays calcium uptake. Although pediatric experience with amrinone is limited, it does appear to be effective in the treatment of severe congestive heart failure or cardiogenic shock in the absence of hypotension. Side effects of the drug include hypotension, thrombocytopenia, gastrointestinal dysfunction, and dysrhythmias. Volume expanders should be readily available when infusion is initiated.

Vasodilators. Vasodilators are frequently administered to the patient in shock to reduce impedance to ventricular ejection. However, most vasodilators dilate both arteries and veins, so they may potentially reduce ventricular preload and afterload. Therefore if selective reduction in afterload is desired, it may be necessary to administer intravenous fluid to maintain ventricular preload during the infusion of the vasodilators.

Vasodilators may improve ventricular compliance, so they enable the ventricle to accept more end-diastolic volume without a significant rise in pressure. Increased ventricular compliance increases stroke volume without a further increase in ventricular end-diastolic pressure. These drugs may be particularly useful in the treatment of myocardial failure.

The typical dosages, effects, and side effects of vasodilators and antihypertensives used in the treatment of children are provided in Table 13-8. Before initiation of any vasodilator therapy, the child's intravascular volume must be assessed, and volume expanders should be readily available for administration if hypotension develops.

Evaluation of Response to Vasoactive Drug Therapy. Evaluation of patient response to vasoactive drug therapy must consider the purpose of each drug administered and the underlying patient condition. A positive response to these drugs will result in improved end-organ perfusion and function and correction of metabolic acidosis. Hypotension should also be corrected. If drug therapy targets a specific receptor activity or specific organ perfusion (e.g., low-dose dopamine therapy designed to activate dopaminergic receptors and produce improved renal perfusion), those specific effects should be observed.

TABLE 13-8. Pediatric Vasodilator and Antihypertensive Therapy

Drug	Dose	Effects	Cautions
Amrinone (Inocor)	0.75 mg/kg (loading dose—give *slowly*) 5-10 µg/kg/min	Nonadrenergic inotropic agent that produces phosphodiesterase inhibition and an increase in intracellular cyclic AMP. Intracellular calcium uptake is also delayed. These effects result in increased cardiac contractility and arterial and venous dilation	Can produce profound hypotension, especially if patient is hypovolemic; can also produce hepatic and gastrointestinal dysfunction, abdominal pain, and thrombocytopenia; monitor for dysrhythmias, particularly junctional tachycardia and ventricular ectopy
Captopril (Capoten)	PO: 0.3-0.5 mg/kg/ dose q 6-12 hr	Inhibits angiotensin converting enzyme, resulting in increased sodium excretion and vasodilation	May produce hypotension; may titrate up to 6 mg/kg/24 hr
Diazoxide (Hyperstat)	IV: 1-3 mg/kg/dose (maximum: 10 mg/ kg/dose) May give PO	Nondiuretic cogener of thiazide diuretics. Relaxes arterial smooth muscle causing vasodilation	Increases blood glucose; contraindicated if hypersensitivity to thiazides; may affect phenytoin metabolism and protein-bound substances; may produce nausea, vomiting, flushing; monitor BP
Enalapril (Vasotec)	IV: 5-10 µg/kg/dose q 8-24 hr	Inhibits angiotensin converting enzyme; results in increased sodium excretion and vasodilation	May produce hypotension; pediatric experience is limited
Esmalol (Brevibloc)	IV: 50-300 µg/kg/min (begin at 50 µg/kg/ min and titrate)	Beta₁ adrenergic blocker with selective cardiac effects	May produce hypotension bradycardia; effects will not be apparent for *30 min after infusion begins* so titrate carefully (half-life: 9 min); may compromise myocardial function; do not mix with other drugs; pediatric experience is limited
Hydralazine (Apresoline)	PO: 0.75-3.0 mg/kg/ 24 hr every 6-12 hr IV/IM: 0.1-0.2 mg/kg/ dose	True arterial dilator	Monitor for hypotension, reflex tachycardia, or lupus-like syndrome
Isoproterenol (Isuprel)	IV: 0.05-1.5 µg/kg/ min	Beta₁ and beta₂ adrenergic effects produce vasodilation	Usefulness may be limited by tachydysrhythmias; will increase myocardial O₂ consumption
Labetalol (Normodyne, Transdate)	IV: 0.25 mg/kg may double dose twice to maximum of 1 mg/ kg/dose (total maximum of 3 doses: 4 mg/kg)	Alpha₁ and beta₁ adrenergic blocker; produces fall in blood pressure	Monitor for hypotension and bradycardia, and ventricular dysrhythmias; dilute as per manufacturer's instructions; pediatric experience is limited
Minoxidil (Loniten, Minoxidil)	PO: 0.2-1.0 mg/kg/24 hr (may be given in a single daily dose, and dose may be increased)	Direct peripheral vasodilator	May cause severe edema and is associated with hypertrichosis (may be undesirable for use in girls); pediatric experience is limited
Nifedipine (Adalat, Procardia)	PO/Sublingual: 0.25-0.50 mg/kg/dose	Calcium channel blocker	Monitor for hypotension, signs of decreased myocardial function, flushing, nausea, headache
Nitroglycerin	IV: 1-5 µg/kg/min Ointment: 0.5 cm, changed q 2-6 hr (to increase effective dose, change more frequently)	Systemic and pulmonary vasodilator, venodilator; may be effective in treatment of pulmonary hypertension	Can produce hypotension, headaches; drug is absorbed by polyvinyl chloride tubing

Continued.

TABLE 13-8. Pediatric Vasodilator and Antihypertensive Therapy—cont'd

Drug	Dose	Effects	Cautions
Phentolamine (Regitine)	IV: 0.05-0.1 mg/kg/ dose (repeat q 5 min as necessary)	Alpha-adrenergic blocker with direct effects on vascular smooth muscle so vasodilation results	Monitor for hypotension; tolerance can develop rapidly, so short-term use as advised; gastrointestinal dysfunction may develop
Propranolol (Inderal)	PO: 0.5-3.0 mg/kg/ 24 hr IV: 0.15-0.25 mg/kg	Beta-blocker primarily administered to children with cyanotic heart rate disease and hypercyanotic spells	Monitor for hypotension, bradycardia, and evidence of myocardial dysfunction
Reserpine (Sandril, Serpasil)	PO: 0.02-0.04 mg/kg/ dose q 12 hr	Alpha-adrenergic blocker (results in vasodilation); most frequently used in treatment of hypertension following repair of coarctation of the aorta	Rarely used in children in shock; monitor for hypotension; may have sedative effects and may produce nausea, vomiting
Sodium nitroprusside (Nipride, Nitropress)	IV: 0.5-10 μg/kg/min	Systemic and pulmonary artery and venous dilator	Monitor for hypotension and thrombocytopenia; metabolites include thiocyanate and cyanide (monitor levels if therapy is required for >48 hrs); light sensitive
Tolazoline (Priscoline)	IV: 1-2 mg/kg/hr	Alpha-adrenergic blocker that may act at histamine receptors; primarily used in neonates	Monitor for hypotension, thrombocytopenia, and gastrointestinal bleeding

From Hazinski MF: Cardiovascular disorders. In Hazinski MF, editor: *Nursing care of the critically ill child*, ed 2, St. Louis, 1992, Mosby. Sources: Ingelfinger JR: Systemic hypertension. In Adams FH, Emmanouilides GC, Riemenschneider TA, editors: *Moss' heart disease in infants, children, and adolescents*, ed 4, Baltimore, 1989, Williams & Wilkins; data from Springhouse Corporation: *Handbook of pediatric drug therapy,* Springhouse, Penn, 1990, Springhouse.

Minimization of Oxygen Demand

When shock is present and oxygen delivery is limited, oxygen demand should be minimized. Pain, fever, and anxiety can all increase oxygen demand and should be prevented and treated if they develop. Cold stress will increase the neonate's oxygen consumption, and must be avoided. All children should be kept warm and pain-free. Sedation and possible pharmacologic paralysis (with analgesia) may be necessary to minimize the work of breathing.

Support of Gastrointestinal and Renal Function

Throughout the treatment of shock, end-organ perfusion and function must be supported. Ultimately, the best method of improving end-organ function will be successful treatment, with improvement in cardiac output and its distribution, maximization of oxygen delivery, and limitation of oxygen demand.

Urine output should be closely monitored. Oliguria is often a symptom of prerenal failure and should improve when systemic perfusion is restored to adequate levels. Furosemide (Lasix) may be administered to encourage urine output, but should not be administered repeatedly in the face of prerenal failure. Urine output may also improve with the administration of mannitol (0.15 to 0.25 gm/kg/ dose) or low dose dopamine (0.5 to 5 μg/kg/min IV). If oliguria or anuria persists after restoration of adequate intravascular volume and renal perfusion, acute tubular acidosis or other types of renal failure should be suspected. Dialysis may be required in the face of unresponsive hyperkalemia, acidosis, or symptomatic hypervolemia.

Fluid intake and output must be meticulously monitored. Excessive fluid output should be replaced by a fluid of equivalent electrolyte concentration and volume. Causes of excessive urine output may include the development of diabetes insipidus or hypercalcemia.

Gastrointestinal function must be maintained. A nasogastric tube should be inserted if development of a paralytic ileus results in gastric distension. Nutritional support should be planned as soon as possible. Provision of adequate nutrition may not only reduce the risk of infection and septic shock, but may hasten patient recovery from critical illness. When any critically ill or injured patient is hospitalized, plans should be made to ensure adequate nutritional support from the day of admission. Too often, it is assumed that the patient will be rapidly extubated and able to eat, and several days elapse before parenteral alimentation or tube feedings are provided.

Antibiotics

If signs of sepsis or septic syndrome are present, specimens should be obtained for culture and gram stain from suspected sites of infection. Broad-spectrum antibiotics are usually prescribed until culture results identify a causative organism. Selection of the broad-spectrum antibiotics will be determined by the suspected site of infection, the patient's underlying condition, likelihood of resistant organisms, and typical hospital and unit pathogens. If the patient is immunocompromised, the possibility of fungal or viral infections must be considered. Both gram-positive and gram-negative coverage are typically provided unless or until a gram stain or culture results help to identify an organism. Once antibiotics are prescribed, they must be administered on time, and peak and trough levels of aminoglycoside drugs must be monitored.

Mediator-Specific Therapy for Sepsis

With the exception of endotoxin, all identified mediators of the septic cascade are endogenous lipids or proteins that normally exert some protective effect during infection or inflammation. During sepsis, however, these mediators are found in extremely high concentrations. They no longer exert discrete protective effects; instead, their effects become diffuse and destructive. Thus a logical approach to treatment of sepsis is the elimination of endotoxin/lipopolysaccharide and the modulation of the levels or effects of endogenous proinflammatory mediators. However, in order for sepsis and septic shock to develop, a variety of protective systems must fail. Therefore as a general rule the septic patient has a complex illness that is unlikely to respond to any single therapy.

The major impediment to the clinical study of mediator-specific therapies continues to be an inability to stratify the severity of illness in septic patients. If the severity of illness varies widely in the study population, it is likely that mediator levels will also vary widely. To date, no single mediator-specific therapy has resulted in improvement in outcome in an entire study population, although several studies have documented improvement in subsets of patients after mediator-specific therapy.[27-30,37,39,40-45,73] Future research is likely to focus on strategies to enable early recognition of patients at high risk for the development of septic shock, prompt determination of mediator levels, and combinations of mediator-specific therapies.[55]

Several of the proinflammatory mediators identified during sepsis have also been implicated in the pathogenesis of increased cerebral blood flow and increased intracranial pressure following head trauma. As a result, successful modulation of the effects of these mediators will likely have wide ranging applicability.

Steroids

The efficacy of steroid administration in the treatment of sepsis continues to be debated.[74] Animal models suggest that a combination of steroids and antibiotics is more effective in the treatment of sepsis than antibiotics alone, but no clinical trial has been able to document a reduction in mortality associated with steroid administration.[75,76] Although these clinical trials have been criticized on the basis of patient selection (failure to separate patients with gram-positive from gram-negative sepsis), they provide strong evidence against the routine use of steroids in the treatment of sepsis.

Recently, however, steroid administration to children with meningitis has been shown to reduce auditory sequelae. In addition, administration of steroids 20 to 30 minutes prior to the first dose of antibiotics has been associated with improvement in both neurologic and auditory function in one study of children with meningitis.[77] These data suggest that the timing of steroid administration is crucial, and that steroid administration prior to bacterial lysis may exert some protective effect. This issue requires further study.

It is important to note that steroid administration may be lifesaving if adrenal cortical insufficiency may be virtually identical to many of the signs of septic shock. Although adrenal insufficiency produces hyponatremia and hyperkalemia, these abnormalities may be masked during fluid resuscitation. Adrenal insufficiency may be congenital in origin, or it may result from infection, adrenal hemorrhage associated with shock, or from autoimmune disease. If adrenal insufficiency is suspected, a plasma cortisol level should be drawn. Normal serum free cortisol levels in children range from 2 to 27 μg/dl; a level near or exceeding 20 μg/dl should be present in any child with shock or critical illness with adequate adrenal cortical function. Pending the cortisol results, a single dose of cortisol (1 to 5 mg/kg) may be administered; if adrenal insufficiency is present, even one dose should improve blood pressure and systemic perfusion.

A 23-hour infusion of methylprednisolone has now become standard for the initial therapy of patients with spinal cord injury. This therapy is based on a multicenter study of patients 13 years of age and older, sponsored by the National Acute Spinal Cord Injury Study (NASCS), which showed improvement in motor function and proprioception after use of the drug.[78] To initiate therapy, a bolus of 50 mg/kg is administered intravenously within 8 hours of the injury, followed by an infusion of 5.4 mg/kg/hr for 23 hours (see Chapter 22).

Maintenance of End-Organ Perfusion

Blocking Arachidonic Acid Metabolism. Administration of ibuprofen may block arachidonic metabolism and, hence, block the formation of cytokines, which may contribute to microcirculatory disruption and organ system failure. A pilot study documented the effectiveness of ibuprofen in reducing mortality and reversing ARDS in adult patients with septic shock.[33] Results of a multicenter clinical trial are awaited.

Alteration in Neutrophil Function. Neutrophils play a primary role in the inflammatory response, which may be protective during infection but destructive during sepsis. Drugs that modulate the harmful effects of neutrophils may well be helpful in the prevention of multisystem organ failure following shock. Pentoxifylline reduces polymorphonuclear leukocyte adhesiveness and sludging in animals following fluid resuscitation of hemorrhage. It also increases tissue oxygen availability and whole body oxygen consumption in laboratory animal shock models.[79,80] Additional properties of this drug that may make it a useful adjunct to shock therapy include its ability to increase red blood cell deformability, decrease red blood cell and platelet aggregation, decrease blood viscosity, decrease plasma fibrinogen levels, increase fibrinolysis, and decrease prostaglandin synthesis. It may also inhibit release of tumor necrosis factor.[80] The potential effects of pentoxifylline offer promising applications but require confirmation through pediatric clinical trials.

Patients with severe neutropenia are at high risk for infection and possible sepsis. The synthesis and function of white blood cells is increased by colony-stimulating factors (CSFs), which are normally released from leukocytes or macrophages in response to infection. Two of these CSFs, made with recombinant protein technology, are now commercially available. Administration of granulocytemonocyte CSF (GM-CSF) or granulocyte CSF (G-CSF) can correct neutropenia and neutrophil dysfunction, and may reduce the incidence of sepsis in neutropenic patients.[81] GM-CSF is administered prophylactically after chemotherapy beginning 1 day after the last dose of chemotherapy to prevent the development of or reduce the severity of chemotherapy-induced neutropenia. G-CSF is used after bone marrow transplantation (sensitivity reactions and reactivation of autoimmune diseases have been reported in association with this therapy).[81]

Modulation of Endorphins. Naloxone administration has been advocated for the treatment of septic patients because it is an opiate antagonist and can block some of the actions of endogenous opiates and endorphins. Although naloxone has been shown to increase blood pressure in septic animals and humans, there is no evidence that it improves survival of septic patients.

Mechanical Circulatory Assist Devices

Pneumatic Military Antishock Trousers. Pneumatic military antishock trousers (MAST) theoretically provide an autotransfusion by compressing the venous beds in the legs and abdomen. However, there is no evidence that this device is effective in the treatment of hemorrhagic shock associated with major pediatric trauma,[2] so it is rarely used in children. MAST may be helpful in the management of unstable pelvic fractures, however. Complications include acidosis, ventilatory and renal compromise, and reduced visibility of the patient.

Intraaortic Balloon Pumping. Intraaortic balloon pumping (IABP) has been utilized successfully in the treatment of adults with myocardial failure. The IABP is an elongated balloon that is most commonly threaded in a retrograde fashion into the thoracic aorta (balloons are occasionally inserted into the pulmonary artery for patients with severe right ventricular failure). Balloon inflation is timed with the patient electrocardiogram, and a pediatric balloon, pediatric cassette, and helium inflation of the balloon are required to enable synchrony of balloon inflation with the rapid heart rate of the child. The balloon inflates during ventricular diastole, augmenting diastolic pressure and mean arterial pressure. IABP will also improve coronary artery blood flow. Deflation of the balloon immediately prior to ventricular systole augments the efficiency of ventricular ejection. The IABP has only been utilized in a limited number of children, with a low survival rate (combined survival rate of approximately 34%).[82,83] Further research is needed to perfect pediatric balloon design and to refine criteria for the use of the device in children.

Extracorporeal Membrane Oxygenation. Extracorporeal membrane oxygenation (ECMO) provides support of cardiopulmonary function using an external cardiopulmonary bypass with a membrane oxygenator. This system can provide temporary cardiac or pulmonary support for infants or children with reversible cardiac or respiratory failure. Support of both cardiac and pulmonary function can be provided using venoarterial ECMO. If cardiac function is good, oxygenation and carbon dioxide removal may be provided using veno-venous ECMO. Although heparin-impregnated circuits are available, they have not yet been perfected, so anticoagulation is necessary. Complications during ECMO can be significant and include bleeding, mechanical failures, and central nervous system bleeding. Criteria for use of ECMO in children have not yet been established, and further evaluation of this therapy in children is required.[15]

Ventricular Assist Devices. Although a variety of ventricular assist devices (VADs) are currently available for use in adult patients, most are unsuitable for pediatric use because they require displacement of excessive blood volume to fill the device reservoir. Centrifugal VADs are relatively simple and inexpensive and do not require any filling volume. The centrifugal VAD uses a conical head that rotates and forces blood centrifugally into the outflow tubing. This provides nonpulsatile blood flow, so a constant mean arterial pressure is achieved. Thromboembolic complications and organ system effects of nonpulsatile blood flow limit the use of these devices to short periods. Experience with VADs in children is limited.[15,84]

Abdominal Compression. When shock is associated with severe right ventricular failure or high right atrial pressure postoperatively (as may be observed following a Fontan or similar procedure), intermittent abdominal compression may improve pulmonary blood flow and systemic perfusion. Abdominal compression is provided through use of MAST trousers, or by placement of a 1 to 2 L ventilator reservoir bag (attached to a mechanical ventilator) under an abdominal wrap. The abdominal compression occurs when the MAST trousers or the reservoir bag is inflated to modest pressures. It is not necessary to synchronize inflations with mechanical ventilatory support. Intermittent abdominal compression will elevate right atrial pressure and may improve right ventricular function or pulmonary blood flow and systemic perfusion without the need for large volume infusions and their attendant complications.[15] A positive response to abdominal compressions includes an improvement in systemic perfusion and urine output.[85,86]

Additional Supportive Care

Specific diagnostic or therapeutic procedures may be indicated as adjuncts to the care of the child in shock. For example, computed tomography abdominal scans may aid in the location of sources of abdominal bleeding in the child with abdominal trauma. Refer to the appropriate chapters if procedures such as peritoneal lavage (see Chapter 24) or pericardiocentesis, thoracentesis, or chest tube insertion (see Chapter 23) are required. Patients failing to respond to resuscitation efforts must be rapidly reevaluated to identify associated complicating conditions. Mechanical conditions that may result in cardiovascular collapse include tension pneumothorax or pericardial tamponade. Additional conditions that must be considered include multiple organ failure, myocardial injury or ischemia, anoxic insult, or severe head injury. Uncontrolled sepsis or ongoing blood loss may be difficult to reverse.

Disposition

All patients with shock require immediate admission to a critical care unit and consultation from appropriate specialists. If shock is unresponsive to initial volume and inotropic support, or if multisystem organ failure develops, consideration should be given to transfer of the child to a pediatric intensive care unit or a unit staffed by pediatric intensivists.

References

Pathophysiology

1. Rudolph AM: *Congenital diseases of the heart*, Chicago, 1974, Year Book.
2. Chameides L and Hazinski MF, editors: *Textbook of pediatric advanced life support*, ed 2, Dallas, 1994, American Heart Association.
3. Friedman WF: The intrinsic physiologic properties of the developing heart. In Friedman WF, editor: *Neonatal heart disease*, New York, 1973, Grune and Stratton.
4. Clyman RI, Teitel D, Padbury J: The role of beta-adrenoreceptor stimulation and contractile state in the preterm lamb's response to altered ductus arteriosus patency, *Pediatr Res* 23:316, 1988.
5. Hazinski MF: Nursing care of the critically ill child: the 7-point check, *Pediatr Nurs* 11:453, 1985.
6. Hazinski MF: Hemodynamic monitoring of children. In Daily EK and Schroeder JS: *Principles of bedside hemodynamic monitoring*, ed 4, St. Louis, 1989, Mosby.
7. Shippy CR, Appel PL, Shoemaker WC: Reliability of clinical monitoring to assess blood volume in critically ill patients, *Crit Care Med* 12:107, 1984.
8. Eisenberg PR, Jaffe AS, Schuster DP: Clinical evaluation compared to pulmonary artery catheterization in the hemodynamic assessment of critically ill patients, *Crit Care Med* 12:549, 1984.
9. Perloff WH: Physiology of the heart and circulation. In Swedlow DB and Raphaely RC, editors: *Cardiovascular problems in pediatric critical care. Clinics in critical care medicine*, vol 10, New York, 1986, Churchill Livingstone.
10. Schlant RC, Sonnenblick EH, Gorlin R: Normal physiology of the cardiovascular system. In Hurst JW, editor: *The heart, arteries, and veins*, ed 7, New York, 1990, McGraw-Hill.
11. Carcillo JA, Davis AL, Zaritsky A: Role of early fluid resuscitation in pediatric septic shock, *JAMA* 266:1242, 1991.
12. Rackow EC, et al: Fluid resuscitation in circulatory shock: a comparison of the cardiorespiratory effects of albumin, hetastarch, and saline solutions in patients with hypovolemic and septic shock, *Crit Care Med* 11:839, 1983.
13. Packman MI and Rackow EC: Optimum left heart filling pressure during fluid resuscitation of patients with hypovolemic and septic shock, *Crit Care Med* 33:165, 1983.
14. Meyer RA: Echocardiography. In Adams FH, Emmanouilides GC, Riemenschneider, editors: *Moss' heart disease in infants, children, and adolescents*, Baltimore, 1989, Williams & Wilkins.
15. Hazinski MF: Cardiovascular disorders. In Hazinski MF, editor: *Nursing care of the critically ill child*, ed 2, St. Louis, 1992, Mosby.
16. Schreiber MD, Heyman MA, Soifer SJ: Increased arterial pH, not decreased $Paco_2$ attenuates hypoxia-induced pulmonary vasoconstriction in newborns, *Pediatr Res* 20:113, 1986.

Oxygen Delivery

17. Hazinski MF: Children are different. In Hazinski MF, editor: *Nursing care of the critically ill child*, ed 2, St. Louis, 1992, Mosby.

Etiology

18. Perkin RM and Levin DL: Shock in the pediatric patient, I, *J Pediatr* 101:163, 1982.
19. National Center for Health Statistics: annual summary of births, marriages, divorces, and deaths: United States, 1988, Hyattsville, MD, *US Department of Health and Human Services, Public Health Service, Centers for Disease Control*, 37, Number 13, 1989.
20. American College of Chest Physicians and Society of Critical Care Medicine. Consensus Conference Committee: definitions for sepsis and organ failure and guidelines for the use of innovative therapies in sepsis, *Crit Care Med* 20:864, 1992.
21. Jarvis WR: Epidemiology of nosocomial infections in pediatric patients, *Pediatr Infect Dis J* 6:344, 1987.
22. Millikin J, et al: Nosocomial infections in a pediatric intensive care unit, *Crit Care Med* 16:233, 1988.
23. Fink MP: Gastrointestinal mucosal injury in experimental models of shock, trauma, and sepsis, *Crit Care Med* 19:627, 1991.
24. Crouser ED and Dorinsky PM: Gastrointestinal tract dysfunction in critical illness; pathophysiology and interaction with acute lung injury in adult respiratory distress syndrome/multiple organ dysfunction syndrome, *New Horiz* 2:476, 1994.
25. Danner RI, et al: Endotoxemia in human septic shock, *Chest* 99:169, 1991.
26. Abraham E, editor: Sepsis: cellular and physiologic mechanisms, *New Horiz* 1:1, 1993.
27. Giroir BP: Mediators of septic shock; new approaches for interrupting the endogenous inflammatory cascade, *Crit Care Med* 21:780, 1993.
28. Hazinski MF: Mediator-specific therapies for the systemic inflammatory response syndrome, sepsis, severe sepsis, and septic shock; present and future therapies, *Crit Care Nurs Clin North Am* 6:309, 1994.
29. Bone RC: Sepsis and its complications; the clinical problem, *Crit Care Med* 22:S8, 1994.
30. Parillo JE: Pathogenetic mechanisms of septic shock, *New Engl J Med* 115:1471, 1994.
31. Suffredini AF, et al: The cardiovascular response of normal humans to the administration of endotxin, *N Engl J Med* 321:280, 1989.
32. Schenep JL and Mogan KA: Genetics of endotoxin release during antibiotic therapy in experimental gram-negative bacterial sepsis, *J Infect Dis* 150:380, 1984.
33. Parillo JE (moderator), et al: Septic shock in humans: advances in the understanding of pathogenesis, cardiovascular dysfunction, and therapy, *Ann Intern Med* 113:227, 1990.
34. Ziegler EJ, et al: Treatment of gram-negative bacteremia and septic shock with a HA-JA human monoclonal antibody against endotoxin; a randomized, double-blind, placebo-controlled trial, *New Engl J Med* 324:429, 1991.
35. Greenman RL, et al: A controlled clinical trial of E5 murine monoclonal IgM antibody to endotoxin in the treatment of gram-negative sepsis, *JAMA* 266:1097, 1991.
36. Michie HR, et al: Detection of circulating tumor necrosis factor after endotoxin administration, *New Engl J Med* 318:1481, 1988.
37. Suffredini AF: Current prospects for the treatment of clinical sepsis, *Crit Care Med* 22:S12, 1994.
38. Tracey KJ, et al: Anti-cachectin/TNF monoclonal antibodies prevent septic shock during lethal bacteraemia, *Nature* 330:662, 1987.
39. Fisher CH, Opal SM, Dhainaut JF, et al: Influence of an anti-tumor necrosis factor monoclonal antibody on cytokine levels in patients with sepsis, *Crit Care Med* 21:318, 1993.
40. Ashkenazi A, Marsters SA, Capon DJ, et al: Protection against endotoxic shock by a tumor necrosis factor receptor immunoadhesion, *Proc Natl Acad Sci U S A* 88:10,535, 1991.
41. Fisher CJ, Slotman GJ, Opal SM, et al: Initial evaluation of human recombinant interleukin-1 receptor antagonist in the treatment of sepsis syndrome; a randomized, open-label, placebo-controlled multicenter clinical trail, *Crit Care Med* 22:12, 1994.
42. Shapiro L and Gelfand JA: Cytokines and sepsis: pathophysiology and therapy, *New Horiz* 1:13, 1993.
43. Koltai M, Hosford D, and Braquet PG: Platelet-activating factor in septic shock, *New Horiz* 1:87, 1993.
44. Ronco C, Lupi A, Galloni E, et al: Removal of platelet activating factor in experimental continuous arteriovenous hemofiltration, *Crit Care Med* 23:99, 1995.
45. Fink MP, editor: Nitric oxide, *New Horiz* 3:1, 1995.
46. Sibbald WJ, Fox G, Martin C: Abnormalities of vascular reactivity in the sepsis syndrome, *Chest* 100 (suppl):155S, 1991.
47. Royall J and Levin DL: Adult respiratory distress syndrome in pediatric patients, I: clinical aspects, pathophysiology, pathology, and mechanisms of lung injury, *J Pediatr* 112:169, 1988.
48. Bernard GR, et al: Effects of a short course of ibuprofen in patients with severe sepsis, *Am Rev Resp Dis* 137:138A (abstract).
49. Natanson C, et al: Gram-negative bacteremia produces both severe systolic and diastolic cardiac dysfunction in a canine model that simulates human septic shock, *J Clin Invest* 78:259, 1986.
50. Zaritsky A, et al: CPR in children, *Ann Emerg Med* 16:10, 1987.
51. Parker MM, et al: Serial cardiovascular variables in survivors and nonsurvivors of human septic shock: heart rate as an early predictor of prognosis, *Crit Care Med* 15:923, 1987.

Diagnostic Findings

52. Michaud LJ, et al: Elevated initial blood glucose levels and poor outcome following severe brain injuries in children, *J Trauma* 31:1356, 1991.
53. Seevedra JM, et al: Capillary refill (skin turgor) in the assessment of dehydration, *Am J Dis Child* 145:296, 1991.
54. Buntain WL, Lynch FP, Ramenofsky ML: Management of the acutely injured child, *Adv Trauma* 2:43, 1987.
55. Bone RC: Sepsis and its complications: the clinical problem, *Crit Care Med* 22:S8, 1994.
56. Rangel-Frausto MS, Pittet D, Costigan M, et al: The natural history of the systemic inflammatory response syndrome (SIRS); a prospective study, *JAMA* 273:117, 1995.
57. Hazinski MF, Iberti TJ, MacIntyre NR, et al: Epidemiology, pathophysiology and clinical presentation of gram-negative sepsis, *Am J Crit Care* 2:224, 1993.
58. Dantzker D: Oxygen delivery and utilization in sepsis, *Crit Care Med* 5:81, 1989.

Management

59. Royall J and Levin DL: Adult respiratory distress syndrome in pediatric patients, II: Management, *J Pediatr* 112:335, 1988.
60. Hutton P, et al: An assessment of the Dinamap 845, *Anesthesiology* 39:261, 1984.
61. Cohn JN: Blood pressure measurement in shock; mechanism of inaccuracy in auscultatory and palpatory methods, *JAMA* 199:118, 1967.
62. Rainey TG and Read CA: Pharmacology of colloids and crystalloids. In Chernow B, editor: *The pharmacologic approach to the critically ill patient*, ed 3, Baltimore, 1994, Williams & Wilkins.
63. Rackow EC, et al: Fluid resuscitation in circulatory shock: a comparison of the cardiorespiratory effects of albumin, hetastarch, and saline solutions in patients with hypovolemic and septic shock, *Crit Care Med* 11:839, 1983.
64. Shoemaker WC: Comparison of the relative effectiveness of whole blood transfusions and various types of fluid therapy in resuscitation, *Crit Care Med* 4:71, 1976.
65. Virgilio RW, Rice CL, Smithe DE: Crystalloid vs colloid resuscitation: is one better? A randomized clinical study, *Surgery* 85:129, 1979.
66. Bersin RM, Chatterjee K, Arieff AI: Metabolic and hemodynamic consequences of sodium bicarbonate administration in patients with heart disease, *Am J Med* 87:7, 1989.
67. Gazmuri RJ, et al: Cardiac effects of carbon dioxide-consuming and carbon dioxide-generating buffers during cardiopulmonary resuscitation, *J Am Coll Cardiol* 15:482, 1990.
68. Oh MS and Carroll HJ: Electrolyte and acid-base disorders. In Chernow B, editor: *The pharmacologic approach to the critically ill patient*, ed 3, Baltimore, 1994, Williams & Wilkins.
69. Arieff AI: Hyponatremia, convulsions, respiratory arrest, and permanent brain damage after elective surgery in healthy women, *N Engl J Med* 314:1529, 1986.
70. Whitlock D, Whitlock J, Coates TD: Hematologic and oncologic emergencies requiring critical care. In Hazinski MF, editor: *Nursing care of the critically ill child*, ed 2, St. Louis, Mosby.
71. Zaritsky A and Chernow B: Catecholamines inotropic medications, vasopressor agents. In Chernow B, editor: *The pharmacologic approach to the critically ill patient*, ed 3, Baltimore, 1994, Williams & Wilkins.
72. American Academy of Pediatrics Committee on Drugs: Emergency drug doses for infants and children, *Pediatrics* 81:462, 1988.
73. Moldawer LL: Biology of proinflammatory cytokines and their antagonists, *Crit Care Med* 22:S3, 1994.
74. Sjolin J: High-dose corticosteroid therapy in human septic shock: has the jury reached a correct verdict? *Circ Shock* 35:139, 1991.
75. Bone RC, et al: A controlled clinical trial of high-dose methylprednisolone in the treatment of severe sepsis and septic shock, *N Engl J Med* 317:653, 1987.
76. Hinshaw L and Veterans Administration Systemic Sepsis Cooperative Study Group: Effect of high-dose glucocorticoid therapy on mortality in patients with clinical signs of systemic sepsis, *N Engl J Med* 317:659, 1987.
77. Odio CM, et al: The beneficial effects of early dexamethasone administration in infants and children with bacterial meningitis, *N Engl J Med* 324:1525, 1991.

78. Bracken MB, Shepard MJ, Collins WF et al: A randomized controlled trial of methylprednisolone or naloxone in the treatment of acute spinal-cord injury, *N Engl J Med* 322:1045, 1990.
79. Waxman K, et al: Pentoxifylline in resuscitation of experimental hemorrhagic shock, *Crit Care Med* 19:728, 1991.
80. Haupt MT: Pentoxifylline and the microcirculation in hemorrhagic shock (editorial), *Crit Care Med* 19:100, 1991.
81. Groopman JE, Scadden DT: Hematopoietic growth factors; biology and clinical application, *N Engl J Med* 321:1449, 1989.
82. Veasy LG, Blalock RC, Orth JL: Intra-aortic balloon pumping in infants and children, *Circulation* 68:1095, 1983.
83. Webster HW and Veasy LG: intraaortic balloon pumping in children, *Heart Lung* 14:548, 1985.
84. Pennington DG and Termuhlen DF: Mechanical circulatory support: device selection, *Cardiac Surgery: State of the Art Reviews* 3:1, 1989.
85. Guyton RA, et al: Right heart assist by intermittent abdominal compression after surgery for congenital heart disease, *Circulation* 72 (suppl II):II-97, 1985.
86. Heck HA and Doty DB: Assisted circulation by phasic external lower body compression, *Circulation* 64 (suppl II):II-118, 1981.

Appendix 13A: Venous and Arterial Access

NORMAN C. CHRISTOPHER   •   RICHARD M. CANTOR

Venous access is required when volume resuscitation or administration of parenteral medications is necessary, and in the potentially unstable patient who may require more aggressive therapy in the event of deterioration. Available approaches for gaining peripheral venous access include percutaneous techniques or direct visualization through a cutdown. The latter technique is increasingly being replaced by intraosseous access. Although low volume or poor perfusion states will significantly complicate the procedure, especially in small children or in those with significant subcutaneous fat stores, in most clinical settings peripheral access may be achieved relatively quickly. Central venous access should be considered if the central circulation is compromised, such as during cardiac arrest, when the circulatory time will be prolonged.

PERCUTANEOUS PERIPHERAL VEIN CATHETERIZATION

Indication

In the acute setting, IV catheters are used for the delivery of resuscitative medications, antibiotics, and volume expanders. In the less dynamic scenario, they enable provision of maintenance fluids for patients unable to maintain adequate hydration or those restricted from oral intake in general. In children under 5 years of age, it is essential that a volume-limiting device is used in-line to avoid excessive fluid administration.

Relevant Anatomy

Cannulation should always be directed at the largest available peripheral vessel. If difficulty is anticipated because of the patient's size or a paucity of visible or palpable vessels, it is appropriate for the most experienced available practitioner to be involved early in the process. The veins of the upper extremity are generally the easiest to cannulate and should be considered first. One should choose the most distal site whenever possible, as this allows for increased mobility of the extremity and for repeated attempts at a more proximal site if the initial attempts fail. The dorsal veins of the hands, the basilic veins, the cephalic veins, and the axillary veins should be carefully inspected and palpated. Lower extremity vessels appropriate for peripheral access include those of the dorsum of the feet and the saphenous veins at the ankles. The veins of the scalp may be accessed in younger children but usually require that the surrounding hair be shaved (Fig. 13A-1). Caution should be used to avoid inadvertently cannulating the temporal artery or one of its branches.

Whichever site is chosen, there are a few principles that should be followed when attempting to establish an IV access in the pediatric patient. Always anticipate the need for adequate restraint for all pediatric patients; even the

most calm child will demonstrate a flight response when experiencing pain. In this regard, it is also advisable to restrain (tape down) the extremity chosen for access. It is extremely difficult to secure the hand or foot of a screaming and struggling child with an IV catheter dangling precariously from the skin. In other words, "make your first shot your best shot." Many clinicians also feel that there is no such thing as too much tape when it comes to securing a carefully placed catheter; even the most lethargic infant will magically discover the most facile way to remove an IV. Another feature of infant IVs is the lack of a demonstrable flashback within the IV tubing; do not assume that the absence of blood return indicates improper placement. Rather, flush the catheter and check for infiltrative swelling instead to measure successful cannulation. Representative anatomic diagrams for scalp veins and extremity IV sites with immobilization are contained in Figs. 13A-1 and 13A-2.

Equipment

All necessary equipment should be at the patient's bedside before beginning the procedure. If phlebotomy is also required, the necessary equipment should be collected to facilitate collection of the appropriate samples after venous access is achieved. Preparation of the patient and family should include an explanation of the indications for the procedure, a brief overview of the technique and possible related complications, and the possible need for gentle restraints. Parents who are able to support their child during the procedure should be allowed and encouraged to assist according to their level of comfort.

Plastic catheters have a long half-life and in general, a 22 or 24 gauge should be chosen for use in infancy, whereas older children may be more appropriately catheterized with 20 gauge equipment. Butterfly or scalp vein needles, although uncommonly used, are available in sizes ranging from 19 to 17 gauge. Additional supplies should include

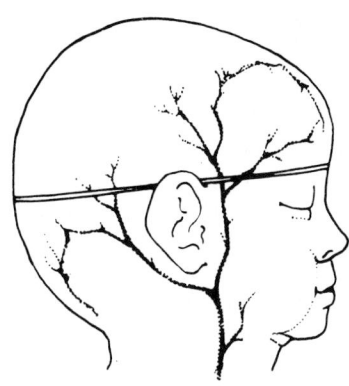

FIG. 13A-1. Location of scalp veins. Rubber band used for tourniquet. (*From Barkin RM and Rosen P: Emergency pediatrics, ed 4, St Louis, 1994, Mosby.*)

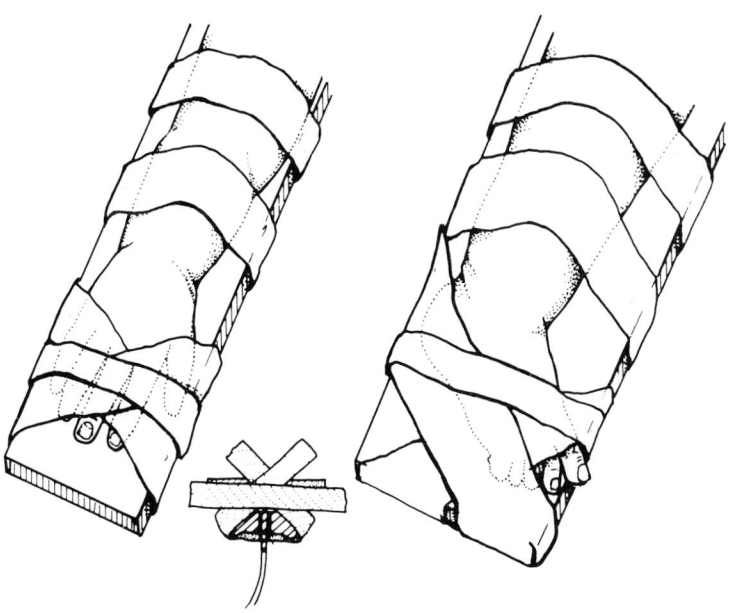

FIG. 13A-2. Immobilization of extremity for percutaneous venous puncture. Scalp vein needle taping. (*From Barkin RM and Rosen P: Emergency pediatrics, ed 4, St. Louis, 1994, Mosby.*)

pretorn tape (¼.½, 1, and 2 inch varieties), alcohol pads, sterile gauze, and material to protect the protruding segment of the catheter (half of plastic medicine cup, catheter container, Kerlix). Armboards of appropriate length are mandatory. Normal saline flush should generally be drawn up before insertion.

Technique

With rare exceptions, the same techniques utilized for IV placement in the adult are applicable, especially in the use of veins within the distal extremities. Some differences need to be pointed out, however. It is not unusual for the ambient temperature within most medical settings to be cool, causing profound distal vasoconstriction in the infant. It may be helpful to warm the chosen extremity with a heated moist towel. Since many of the veins in small infants are more palpable than visible, one can increase the potential for visualization by swabbing the hand or foot with alcohol. This will accentuate any surface irregularity caused by an underlying vein, especially when viewed in a tangential manner. Another method used to facilitate dilation of a vein is gentle surface abrasion or tapping over the chosen vein. Proper positioning and manipulation of the light source may produce shadows and better illuminate a potential site for cannulation.

The child should be positioned so the practitioner has comfortable access to the chosen cannulation site. The extremity (and when necessary, the child) should be carefully and comfortably secured to minimize movement during the procedure. Failure to properly immobilize the chosen site will inevitably result in failure (see Fig. 13A-2). A tourniquet should be placed proximally at a pressure that approximates 10 to 15 mm Hg less than the systolic pressure. Higher tourniquet pressures will occlude arterial flow and significantly lessen venous filling of distal peripheral veins. The catheter should be inserted into the chosen site using a standard over-the-needle catheter device and antiseptic technique. Infant IVs may not routinely have a demonstrable flashback within the catheter; do not assume that the absence of a blood return indicates improper placement. After insertion, remove the tourniquet. Once placement is confirmed by documenting easy flow of saline through the catheter, the device should be carefully secured to the skin with tape and the extremity fully mobilized.

To access a scalp vein in an infant (see Fig. 13A-1), it may be necessary to shave the overlying skin to both expose the vein and provide an adherent surface for the application of tape. Apply a circumferential tourniquet around the head at the level of the forehead, preferably with a rubber band. Insert a catheter into the most proximal portion of the vein and advance caudally. Remove the tourniquet and infuse a flush solution. If the proximal scalp blanches, remove the IV because it is likely that an artery has been inadvertently entered.

PERCUTANEOUS CENTRAL VEIN CATHETERIZATION

Indication

Use of the femoral, external jugular, internal jugular, and subclavian veins for central venous access in the pediatric population may be necessary in a variety of clinical scenarios. In the profoundly dehydrated patient they provide a mechanism for rapid volume expansion, but it is important to recognize that the flow rate is directly proportional to the gauge of the catheter and inversely related to the catheter length. In the traumatized patient, central venous catheters may be used in the replacement of depleted whole blood components. Indwelling pressure monitoring catheters for both CVP and pulmonary arterial wedge pressure measurement are often introduced into the central circulation through these sites. In the emergency department the most common methods of access involve the external jugular and femoral veins.

The flow rate of infusate is directly proportional to the internal diameter of the catheter and inversely proportional to its length. As the radius of the catheter increases, the resistance to flow decreases by the fourth power of the change in the radius.

To avoid complications, sterile technique should be used. Local anesthetics should be provided for the awake patient and when time permits. The child should be properly positioned and restrained. Complications, especially pneumothoracic, should be anticipated.

Relevant Anatomy

The *femoral vein* lies ¼ to ½ cm medial to the femoral artery in most children. In the pulseless patient, the location of the femoral artery may be approximated at the point midway between the anterior iliac crest and the symphysis pubis and is easiest to access at a level just distal to the femoral crease. The vein is just medial to the artery.

The *external jugular vein* is readily visible when the infant is placed in the Trendelenburg position. It usually overlies the belly of the sternocleidomastoid bundle. The external jugular vein is made more obvious when the child cries or initiates a Valsalva maneuver, increasing the intrathoracic pressure and causing distension of the vein. Because of the large number of valves and the tortuosity of this vessel, it is sometimes difficult to advance a guide-wire or a longer catheter through the length of the external jugular vein as it courses toward the subclavian vein.

The location of the *internal jugular vein* is relatively constant, coursing just lateral and slightly anterior to the ipsilateral carotid artery. The internal jugular vein is easiest to locate and access as it emerges below the apex formed at the origin of the two heads of the sternocleidomastoid muscle, and as it courses toward its junction with the subclavian vein. Similar to the external jugular vein, the relative diameter of the internal jugular veins is affected greatly by intrathoracic pressure during the Valsalva procedures and by placing the patient in Trendelenburg position. Prolonged palpation of the adjacent carotid artery may cause reflex constriction of the internal jugular vein, and should be avoided during attempts at cannulation of the latter.

The *subclavian veins* are consistently located posteriorly to the medial third of the clavicle after crossing above the first rib. The veins are valveless and their diameter and volume are not greatly affected by the position of the patient or by changes in intrathoracic pressure. Severely turning the patient's head to the opposite side or placing a pillow between the clavicles will make the surface anatomy more obvious but may also change the anatomic relationship between the first rib and clavicle, resulting in compression of the underlying vein as the shoulders retract. The right subclavian vein is more commonly chosen than the left vein, as the pleural cap is usually lower on the right side and the thoracic duct is on the left. The course of the left subclavian vein relative to the superior vena cava is more direct and may make navigation of the left subclavian vein easier than the right.

Equipment

Regardless of the point of entry, equipment needs are remarkably similar. In the emergency setting, it is unusual to have the luxury of adequate time necessary for the placement of indwelling cardiopulmonary monitoring equipment. In this regard the most commonly used piece of equipment is a basic catheter-over-the-needle apparatus connected to a large-bore syringe. Catheter sizes may range from 22 to 18 gauge, depending on the age of the child. If necessary, these may be replaced with more sophisticated wire-inserted devices at a later time, usually in the pediatric intensive care unit. Basic supplies should include povidone-iodine solution, scalpel with holder, sterile drapes, IV tubing with T-connector, 3-way stop-cock, and occlusive dressing materials. Commercially available central venous catheter kits are available using guide-wire techniques.

Technique: Femoral Vein

The lower extremities and pelvis of an active child must be adequately restrained. The hips should be abducted and externally rotated. As previously described, locate and mark the location of the femoral vein at a point ¼ to ½ centimeter medial to the pulsation of the femoral artery. Sterilize the area with povidone-iodine solution, and establish a sterile field. Attach a 2-inch 20 gauge angiocatheter to a 10- to 20-ml syringe and hold it parallel to the vessel at a 30-degree angle to the horizontal (Fig. 13A-3). Advance the catheter until there is a vigorous blood return into the syringe under gentle suction. At this point, slide the catheter into the vessel over the needle, remove the stylet, and reattach the syringe with flush. Once appropriate placement is confirmed, flush the catheter and secure it in place. Using local anesthesia, a silk suture is used to secure the catheter to the surrounding skin and a sterile occlusive dressing is placed.

If required, the angiocatheter may be replaced with a longer singleported or multiported catheter by directing an appropriately-sized guide-wire through the catheter lumen into the femoral vessel. The angiocatheter is removed and the replacement catheter placed into the vessel over the guide-wire. Placement of a catheter into a supradiaphragmatic position requires that radiography be obtained to confirm the catheter's location.

Complications are minimal if the proper technique is adhered to. Incidental puncture of the femoral artery can be remedied by direct pressure over the vessel. Decompression of the bladder will simplify the procedure and minimize risk of bladder puncture.

Advantages of this technique include accessibility of this site in a critically ill child (monitoring equipment, airway interventions, and CPR have little effect on achieving

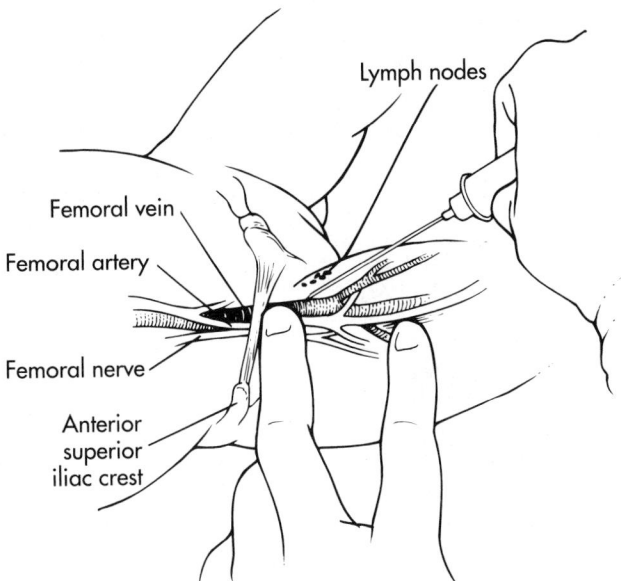

FIG. 13A-3. Percutaneous femoral vein insertion.

femoral venous access, but may prohibit successful insertion of either subclavian or internal/external jugular catheters) and increased mobility of the head and neck without risk to the patency of the catheter.

Technique: External Jugular Vein

The infant should be placed on the examination table in a supine position with the head angled downward approximately 30 degrees from horizontal. The head should be rotated 75 to 90 degrees to the contralateral side and hyperextended approximately 25 to 30 degrees to improve visualization of the external jugular vein (Fig. 13A-4). The latter position also increases tension in the sternocleidomastoid bundle, helping to stabilize the vessel for cannulation. Hyperextension or excessive rotation of the head and neck may result in collapse of the vein and should be avoided. The child should be gently secured to avoid harm to the child or the chosen vessel during the procedure.

The site should be cleansed with povidone-iodine solution and a sterile field should be established. A 22 gauge angiocatheter attached to a 3- or a 5-ml syringe should be inserted into the vein as it crosses over the belly of the sternocleidomastoid muscle. When there is a brisk blood return into the syringe, the catheter should be carefully advanced into the vein, while withdrawing the stylet from the catheter. After flushing the catheter with normal saline, it should be secured.

Complications are unusual if the proper technique is used. There are no adjacent arterial or neural structures, and the pleural dome is distant to the proper insertion site. Bleeding from a failed attempt should be tamponaded with light pressure over the vein.

Technique: Internal Jugular Vein

Position the infant and prepare the insertion site as described in the section on external jugular venous insertion. Visualize a triangle formed by the bellies of the sternal and clavicular branches of the sternocleidomastoid

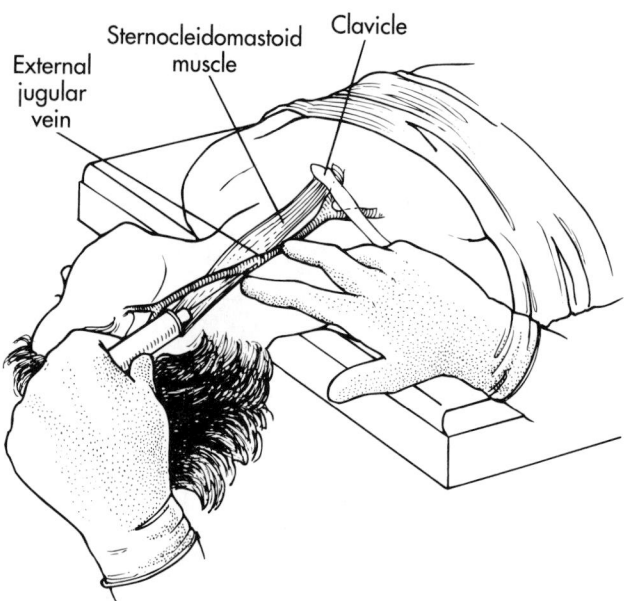

FIG. 13A-4. Percutaneous external jugular vein puncture.

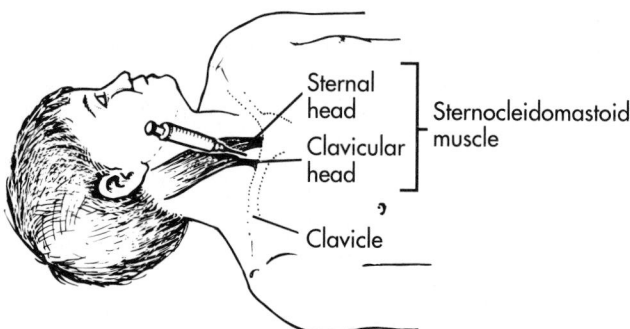

FIG. 13A-5. Percutaneous internal jugular vein insertion. (*From Barkin RM and Rosen P:* Emergency pediatrics, *ed 4, St Louis, 1994, Mosby.*)

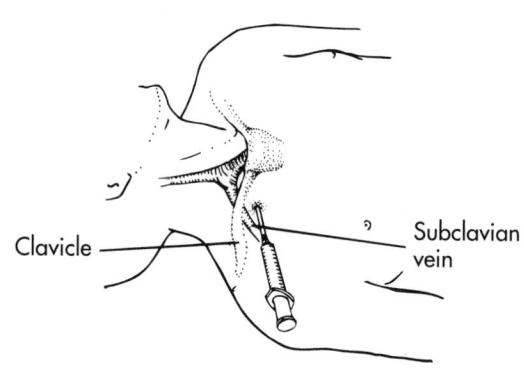

FIG. 13A-6. Percutaneous subclavian vein insertion. (*From Barkin RM and Rosen P:* Emergency pediatrics, *ed 4, St Louis, 1994, Mosby.*)

muscle—the clavicle forms the base of this triangle. For the *medial approach,* insert a catheter-syringe apparatus into the apex of this triangle at a 45-degree angle in the caudad direction. Be careful to direct the needle at the *ipsilateral* nipple (Fig. 13A-5). Some operators will locate the vein first by using a small-gauge locator needle to mark the insertion site and angle. Such a technique minimizes the risk of inadvertent carotid artery puncture with the larger catheter needle. Using constant gentle aspiration, the vein should be entered after only 1 to 2 cm of penetration. If unsuccessful, withdraw the needle to a subcutaneous level and redirect in a more lateral approach (in no way favor the medial aspect). All needle punctures should be made lateral to the carotid artery pulse. Once inserted into the internal jugular vein, the catheter may be secured in place or a longer catheter system may be inserted, using a guide-wire–assisted technique. For the *posterior approach,* the needle is inserted at the lateral edge of the sternocleidomastoid muscle approximately one third of the way from the clavicle to its insertion site at the mastoid process. The needle is directed at an angle of 30 to 45 degrees to the skin and toward the sternal notch. If blood return is not accomplished after inserting the needle 1 to 2 cm, it should be withdrawn and redirected. The *anterior approach* is difficult in children, and the complication rate is higher than with the other approaches. Except in the very experienced operator, this approach should be avoided.

Complications of internal jugular cannulation include inadvertent arterial puncture and pleural puncture with subsequent development of a pneumothorax. The procedure is complicated in children whose surface landmarks are difficult to define, in children undergoing multiple procedures in the head and neck region, and in children who require CPR.

Technique: Subclavian Vein

The child should be placed in the Trendelenburg position with a small towel roll placed underneath the shoul-

ders between the scapulae near the base of the occiput. Caution should be used not to overextend the neck. The insertion site should be cleaned with povidone-iodine solution, and a sterile field established. Local anesthesia should be used in the awake child.

Using a scalpel blade, create an entry point at the juncture of the medial and distal thirds of the clavicle near the depression created by the deltoid and the pectoralis major muscles. Insert a needle through this point and direct it toward the juncture of the first rib and clavicle, and ultimately toward the sternal notch (Fig. 13A-6). Allowing the needle to deviate from the inferior margin of the clavicle will increase the risk of inadvertent puncture of the pleura. Advance the needle underneath the clavicular rim until gentle suction produces an adequate blood return. At this point, the needle may serve as a conduit for the insertion of a guide-wire that will permit the placement of a more lengthy or multiported catheter. Cautiously cover the exposed needle hub when the aspirating syringe is removed to minimize risk of air aspiration and embolism. Development of ventricular ectopy during insertion of the guide-wire implies irritation of the myocardium coincident with its placement into the cardiac chambers. When this occurs, the guide-wire should be withdrawn to an extracardiac position. When proper positioning is confirmed clinically and radiographically, secure the catheter to the skin with a silk suture tie and an occlusive sterile dressing.

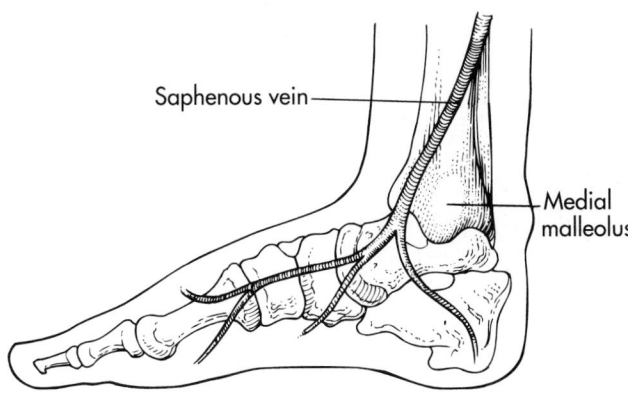

FIG. 13A-7. Saphenous vein cutdown.

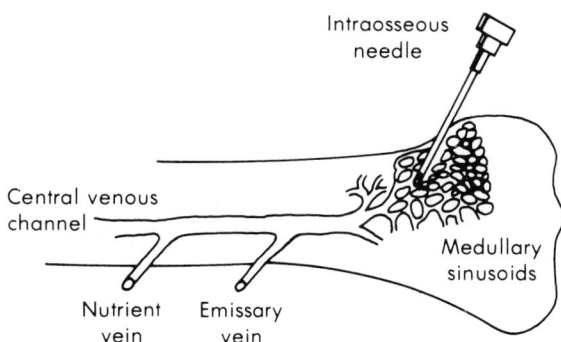

FIG. 13A-8. Venous drainage from marrow of long bone with intramedullary needle in place. (*From Barkin RM and Rosen P:* Emergency pediatrics, *ed 4, St Louis, 1994, Mosby.*)

Complications

Complications common to all (except femoral vein) the central venous access approaches include pneumothorax, hematoma formation, and infection. The jugular and sub-clavian approaches may lead to the development of apical pneumothoraces. A chest x-ray study is usually obtained after catheter insertion. Penetration of the femoral space has been associated with the development of septic arthritis and femoral head osteomyelitis.

SAPHENOUS VEIN CUTDOWN

Indication

The saphenous vein provides a consistently available site for venous access in even the smallest of infants. In the setting of CPR, its location is sufficiently removed from the region of chest compressions to provide an undistracted approach. Most emergency physicians are already familiar with this common and readily available procedure.

Relevant Anatomy

The greater saphenous vein is the body's longest, running subcutaneously throughout its course. It begins at the ankle (where it is most accessible) and crosses 1 cm anterior to the medial malleolus, proceeding along the anteromedial axis of the leg. Its most superficial aspect is at the ankle, where it lies adjacent to the saphenous nerve. At this point, it is exposed with only minimal blunt dissection.

Equipment

Most institutions stock standardized cutdown trays. Their contents contain drapes and gauze (4 × 4 and 2 × 2), hemostats (curved and Kelley), scalpel blades (no. 11 or 15), assorted scissors, needle holders, forceps, syringes, and flush solutions. Catheters of choice include 3-0 or 5-0 French CVP catheters, or standard over-the-needle types (16 to 20 gauge). In addition, material for venous isolation (ties) and line security (3-0 silk) should be provided.

Technique (Fig. 13A-7)

Initially fill the catheter with standard flushing solution. Choose a catheter with a beveled end when dealing with smaller patients. If not available, create a 30- or 45-degree bevel by trimming the end with a scissor. The leg and foot should be externally rotated and secured to a long armboard. Sterilize the medial maleolar circumference and drape to create a surgical field. Palpate the medial malleolus of the tibia and anterior tibial tendon, between which lies the vein itself. In this location, make approximately a 2-cm transverse incision anterior to the malleolar prominence. Bluntly dissect the subcutaneous tissue with a curved hemostat in a cephalad direction, paralleling the course of the vein. The vein lies directly within the tissue overlying the fascia. Once the vein is isolated, pass two silk sutures underneath. Tie the distal suture and secure its ends with a clamp. Loosely knot the proximal tie.

While applying traction to the distal tie, use a scalpel blade to create a wall flap for introduction of the catheter. It may be useful to hook the flap by using a previously bent tip of a 22 gauge needle. It is now possible to insert the beveled catheter into the venostomy site. When advanced to its final cephalad position, the catheter is secured by firmly knotting the proximal tie. The entire catheter is then affixed to the skin by suturing. It may be helpful to flush the catheter during insertion to facilitate easy advancement.

Complications

When performed properly, complications are quite rare. They include local bleeding, infection/phlebitis, sensory nerve damage, and inadvertent loss of the catheter into the vein itself.

INTRAOSSEOUS NEEDLE INSERTION

Indication

When confronted with life-threatening emergencies in the pediatric patient, the administration of resuscitative medication requires rapid access to the central circulation. Even the most skilled practitioner encounters great difficulties when attempting to obtain vascular access in the critically ill pediatric patient. Undue amounts of time are often spent attempting to cannulate distal vasculature that, in the patient near death, may be almost invisible. During the past decade, the intraosseous route of injection has been demonstrated to be a quick and readily established mechanism for the administration of resuscitative drugs

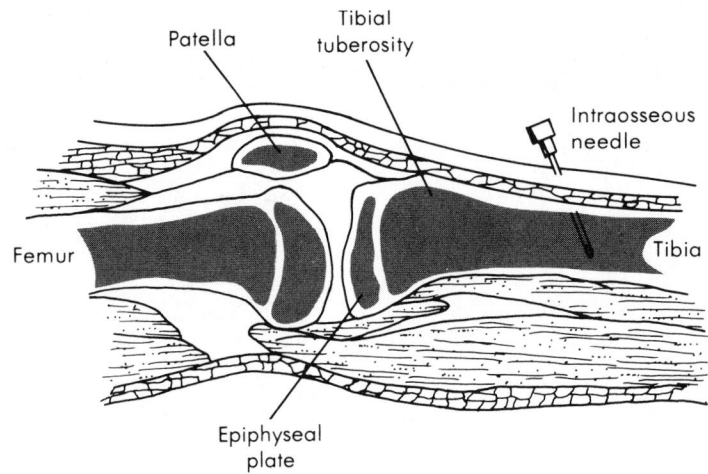

FIG. 13A-9. Intraosseous insertion of needle. (*From Barkin RM and Rosen P:* Emergency pediatrics, *ed 4, St Louis, 1994, Mosby.*)

and fluids. It remains a viable alternative to direct IV cannulation and is recommended in most pediatric references as an alternative route to be used in emergency resuscitative procedures.

Relevant Anatomy

Anatomic and radiographic studies have demonstrated the presence of a rich venous drainage system that parallels the potential space contained within the bone marrow. In the child under the age of five, long-bone marrow contains spacious venous sinusoids that have been demonstrated to drain into larger venous channels that conduct medications and fluids into the IV system (Fig. 13A-8). In many studies there has been the demonstration of a parallel human dynamic response to medications given by the intramedullary route as compared with the IV route. The marrow has also been shown to accept volume flow rates of 600 ml/hr when subjected to gravity infusion alone.

The preferred site of intraosseous infusion in infants and children remains the proximal tibia. Use of the sternum should be avoided in the child because of its small diameter and the increased potential for accidental full-thickness puncture. Additionally, the presence of sternal needle may interfere with effective cardiopulmonary resuscitative efforts. Other possible locations that may be used in the infant child include the distal femur and the medial malleolus.

Equipment

The beauty of the intraosseous route remains the simplicity of equipment that is necessary for success. The first requirement is the provision of a large-bore (approximately 16 gauge) metal needle that contains a stylet. The stylet facilitates easy passage through the periosteum into the bony cortex. Rosenthal, Osgood, and Silverman needles are routinely used by hematologists.

Specialized pediatric, 16 gauge bone marrow-infusion needles are presently marketed. In situations where the aforementioned equipment is not available, some authors have reported success with the use of 19 gauge butterfly

needles, bone marrow needles, and comparatively sized spinal needles. A distinct disadvantage of these remains the potential for inadvertent bending of the needle when confronted with the rigidity of the bony cortex, as well as the absence of a stylet in butterfly needles.

Technique

As previously mentioned, the beauty of this procedure remains its simplicity and expeditious achievement. The skin at the site of puncture should be prepared in a sterile manner. Anesthesia may be omitted in the full-arrest setting. In infants and children a point two finger breadths below the tibial tuberosity should be chosen for insertion. Care should be taken to direct the needle distally to avoid inadvertent damage to the epiphyseal growth plate. A strong downward pressure in a rotary manner should be provided to facilitate entrance into the bony cortex (Fig. 13A-9). The practitioner will notice an easily percepted drop in resistance when the cortex is entered. Once this position is achieved, the stylet may be withdrawn and a syringe with or without a T-connector may be used. Confirmation of adequate placement remains the ability to aspirate marrow content and the absence of infiltrative evidence at the insertion site.

Complications

Significant complications associated with short-term intraosseous access procedures are uncommon, although infiltration may produce complications such as compartment syndrome. Fat embolism has never been reported. Potential structural complications include extravasation of fluids into subcutaneous tissue, full perforation of both the proximal and distal periosteal margins, subcutaneous abscess formation with concomitant osteomyelitis, and epiphyseal injury.

Results and Interpretation

The ability to aspirate bone marrow contents provides strong evidence for proper placement of the intraosseous needle. However, aspiration may result in occlusion of the needle. With administration and installation of resuscitative fluids/drugs, the absence of an infiltrate or compartment syndrome provides adequate evidence for proper placement. It is important to mention that any and all resuscitative medications have been reported in literature to be amenable to intraosseous infusions.

UMBILICAL VEIN CATHETERIZATION

Background

The umbilical vein provides consistent, simple, and rapid access to the central circulation in ill newborns through the middle or the end of the second week of life. The umbilical vein delivers oxygenated blood from the placenta via the ductus venosus to the inferior vena cava and to the right atrium. In the first week after delivery, the cord begins to dry, the umbilical vessels thrombose, and the ductus venosus constricts. When the latter has occurred, it is difficult or impossible to pass an umbilical venous catheter into the central circulation above the liver or diaphragm, limiting the operator's ability to monitor central pressures or to deliver medications or fluids at this level.

Equipment

Cutdown tray (or equivalent)
Povidone-iodine solution
3.5 or 5.0 French umbilical catheters
Three-way stopcock with syringe
Umbilical tape
Adhesive tape

Technique

If the umbilical stump is dried, place a moist, warm gauze around it to soften the tissue. Loosely tie a length of umbilical tape around the base of the cord to allow the operator a mechanism to achieve hemostasis if the umbilical vessels bleed when exposed. Cleanse the umbilicus with povidone-iodine solution and establish a sterile field. The umbilical stump is trimmed with a scalpel in the horizontal plane to expose fresh tissue and to allow identification of the umbilical vein and arteries. The arteries are easily identified by their thick, constricted, muscular walls. The umbilical arteries rarely bleed freely after the stump is cut in this manner. The umbilical vein is identified, and an assistant exposes its lumen by gently grasping opposing sides with hemostats or forceps (without teeth). Because of the large size of the umbilical vein and the lack of muscular tone of its wall, it is often not necessary to have an assistant to complete the procedure. The operator may hold the umbilical stump between the thumb and index finger of his nondominant hand, putting slight tension on the umbilicus to expose the vein's lumen. The umbilical catheter is advanced into the lumen of the vein in a sterile fashion to a premeasured length so the lumen tip is positioned beyond the ductus venosus. The catheter should advance without resistance and with minimal force. Free return of blood with gentle aspiration on a syringe will document proper placement of the catheter. A plain radiograph should be obtained to confirm the placement of the catheter at or above the level of the diaphragm. For emergent placement,

it is necessary to advance the catheter only until free flow into the vessel is possible (usually only 5 to 6 cm). When properly placed, the catheter is secured by tightening the umbilical tape around the stump; a pursestring suture is placed in the umbilical stump to further secure the catheter in the vessel's lumen. A securing bridge is constructed to further secure the catheter in its proper position (Fig. 13A-10).

Complications

Complications of umbilical venous catheter insertion may include hemorrhage, vessel perforation, air embolism, and ischemia of the extremities or of intraabdominal organs if the catheter is malpositioned into a terminal vessel. False tracking of the vessel lumen is unusual when cannulating the umbilical vein, but it occurs frequently when attempting umbilical artery catheterization. The child should be monitored for any infectious and thrombotic complications.

RADIAL ARTERY CATHETERIZATION

Indication

The placement of a peripheral arterial catheter in the radial artery is indicated when the clinical scenario dictates the need for frequent blood gas sampling or continuous monitoring of the arterial pressure. In addition to the radial artery, other peripheral access sites include the radial, ulnar, temporal, and posterior tibial arteries.

Relevant Anatomy

The provider can easily palpate the radial artery proximal to the transverse wrist crease located on the palm or surface of the wrist. The point of maximal impulse is often medial to the styloid process of the radius. A modified Allen test is usually performed to assess the adequacy of collateral flow from the ulnar artery before attempting access to the radial artery. This test is best achieved by simultaneous compression of both the ulnar and radial arteries, after which sequential release of pressure on a unilateral basis will provide a resumption of distal circulation in the adequately vascularized child. Note: Hyperextension of the fingers during the Allen test may result in a false-positive test.

Equipment

The equipment necessary for cannulation of the radial artery essentially mimics the equipment used in the insertion of a peripheral venous catheter. In most infants a 22 gauge catheter-over-needle will suffice for both the provision of fluids and access to the peripheral arterial circulation. In most clinical settings, suture material is not necessary to adequately immobilize and secure the catheter to the wrist.

Technique (Fig. 13A-11)

The emergency physician may locate the radial artery by palpating the point of maximal impulse at the distal wrist. If difficulty is encountered, a fiber-optic light may be placed under the wrist of small infants, which will facilitate location of the radial artery. The wrist is then dorsiflexed to 45 to 60 degrees and the hand and the lower forearm are

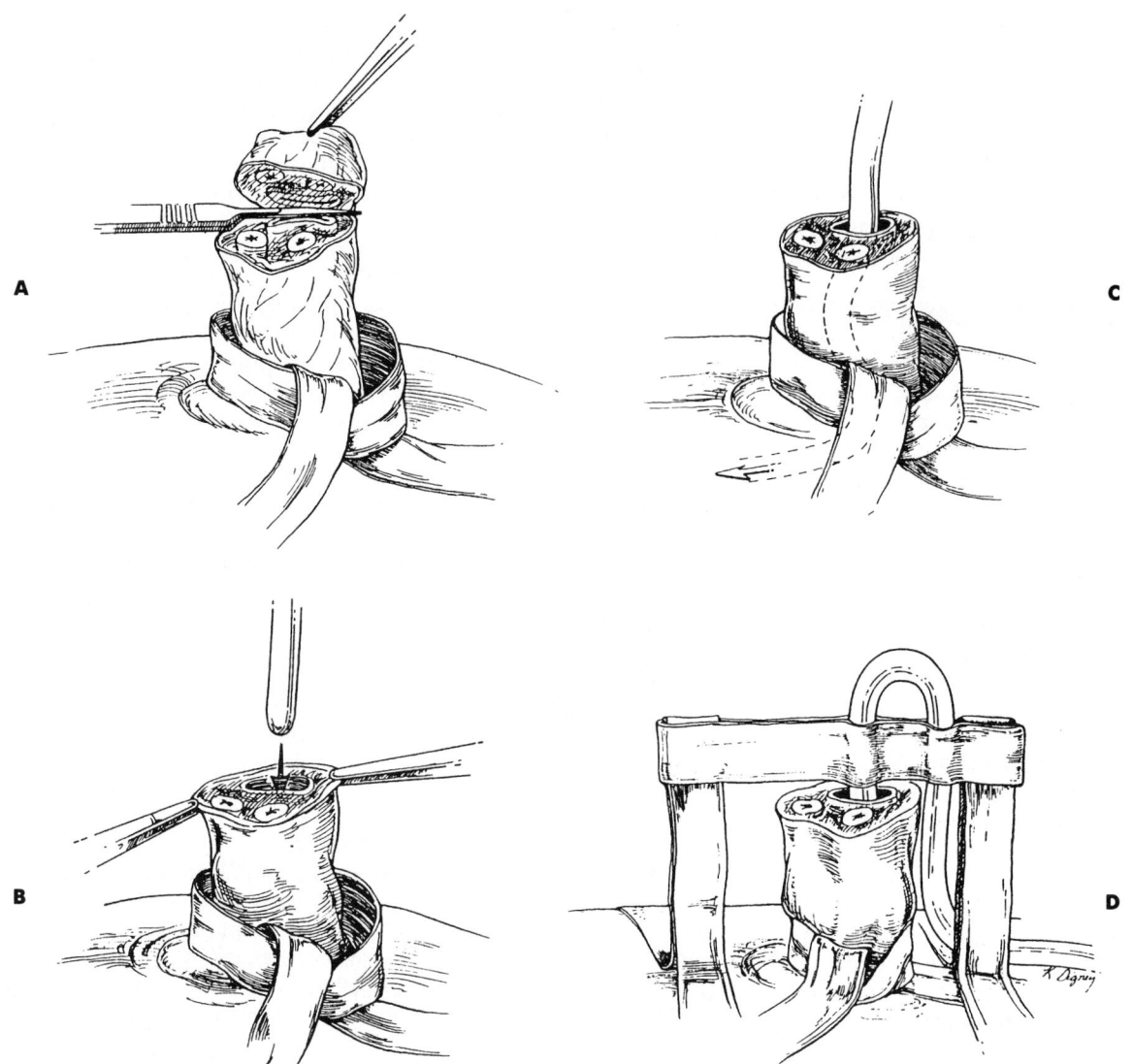

FIG. 13A-10. Umbilical vein catheterization. **A,** Expose the underlying umbilical vein and arteries. The umbilical tape should be securely fastened at the base of the umbilical stump. **B,** Expose the lumina of the umbilical vein. **C,** Advance the umbilical catheter into the lumina of the vein in a sterile fashion. **D,** A technique for securing the umbilical catheter in the umbilical vein.

secured to a board. Dorsiflexion is best maintained at the wrist by the insertion of a roll of gauze underneath. Secure the hand, wrist, and lower forearm to the board taking care to leave all fingers exposed so peripheral circulation may be continually assessed. The overlying skin is then scrubbed with an antiseptic solution and, at the provider's discretion, a local anesthetic may be used without epinephrine.

Puncture the skin at the site of maximal pulsation with the 22 gauge catheter tip. The catheter should be advanced at a 30-degree angle until blood appears in the hub. This indicates adequate puncture of the anterior wall of the artery. At this point, advance the catheter slowly until blood appears in the needle. After lowering the needle carefully to an approximate 10-degree angle, the catheter may be advanced slowly over the needle into the lumen of the artery. Remove the needle, attach the catheter to a T-connector, and close the system with a continuous intravenous infusion. The puncture site may now be covered with antibiotic ointment and a pressure dressing and adhesive tape applied. It is prudent at this point to remove the gauze and reposition the wrist in a more anatomic position.

Complications

Establishment of an indwelling arterial catheter is always accompanied by risks of localized or generalized infection, air or particulate embolization, inadvertent injection of a sclerosing solution, and thrombosis of the artery.

ARTERIAL BLOOD SAMPLING

Indication

Sampling of arterial blood remains the standard of care when applied to the management of the critically ill infant

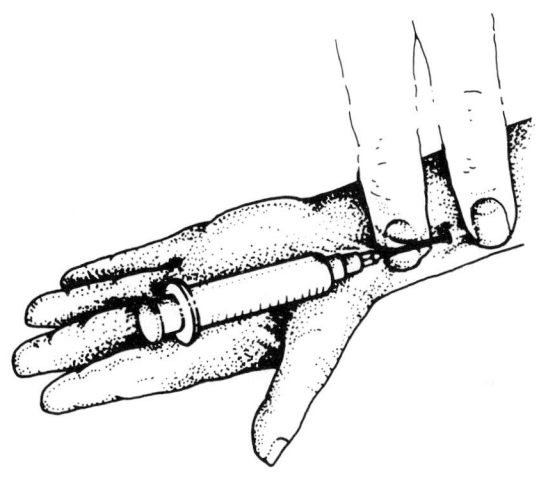

FIG. 13A-11. Radial artery cannulation. (*From Barkin RM and Rosen P: Emergency pediatrics, ed 4, St Louis, 1994, Mosby.*)

or child. Precise measurements of arterial partial oxygen pressures are more reliable than pulse oximetry when performed in the emergency setting. Traditionally acceptable sites available for arterial sampling in the pediatric patient include the radial, brachial, posterior tibial, and dorsalis pedal arteries. Puncture of the femoral artery has been associated with the development of femoral head osteomyelitis; its use is therefore recommended only as a last alternative.

Relevant Anatomy

The radial artery remains the most popular site for arterial sampling in the pediatric patient for a multitude of reasons, including ease of sterilization and compression, absence of contiguous venous structures, and the availabil-

ity of a collateral circulatory supply. The point of maximal pulsation of the radial artery may be palpated just proximal to the transverse wrist crease. This also represents the most superficial component of its overall course. In difficult cases the arterial pathway may be identified by the use of a transilluminator, if available.

Equipment

Necessary supplies include povidone-iodine solution/alcohol for sterilization, a 23 or 25 gauge butterfly needle, and a heparinized syringe for collection.

Technique

Most providers prefer to manually hold the wrist in extension; others are more comfortable with affixing the joint in extension to an arm board with tape. The area is sterilized with alcohol or povidone-iodine and after ascertaining the point of maximal pulsations, the needle is directed at a 30- to 45-degree angle into the subcutaneous tissue. It is advisable to provide negative pressure during the procedure, since in infancy auto-return of blood may not occur. If no blood return occurs before the meeting of bony resistance, it is recommended that the needle be slowly withdrawn in an attempt to reenter the arterial lumen. Once the sample is obtained, the needle is withdrawn, and light pressure is applied for 3 to 5 minutes to prevent residual bleeding.

Complications

Percutaneous radial artery catheterization may produce temporary occlusion of the radial artery and significant compromise of hand perfusion. Therefore hand circulation must be closely monitored after catheter insertion, and the catheter should be removed if evidence of hand ischemia develops. Complications may include arterial or nerve damage, hematoma formation, or infection.

Dysrhythmias

Leon Chameides

Irregularities of cardiac rhythm are very common in the pediatric age group. Most are benign. Significant rhythm disturbances that interfere with cardiac output or are precursors of life-threatening events are infrequent. The challenge facing the physician is in differentiating between the two—to aggressively treat life-threatening rhythm disturbances and to be reassuring and avoid treating those that are not. This chapter reviews the clinical evaluation and *acute* management of some of the more commonly encountered rhythm disturbances; it is not intended as a comprehensive review of all rhythm disturbances or their chronic management. For further evaluation and *chronic* management, the child should be referred to a pediatric cardiologist.

MONITORING METHODS

Evaluation of rhythm disturbances should always begin with an evaluation of peripheral pulses. This not only provides information about rate and regularity, but also provides qualitative and clinically useful information about the adequacy of cardiac output and peripheral vascular resistance.

All children who are critically ill or have an unstable cardiovascular system should have continuous electrocardiographic monitoring. The most commonly used monitoring lead (MCL1) is a modified chest lead. The positive electrode is placed in the usual V_1 position, the negative electrode near the left shoulder, and a third electrode acting as a ground, in a more remote area of the body. The physician should be thoroughly familiar with potential artifacts that may be caused by muscle twitching, alternating current, electrical interference from nearby electronic equipment, and loose electric connections. Diagnostic and treatment decisions should never be based solely on a tracing but must be correlated with the patient's clinical state and physical findings. A complete analysis of complex rhythm disturbances requires a 12- or 13-lead electrocardiogram (ECG). The heart rate may be determined by palpating a central or peripheral pulse, from the cardiac tachometer, or by analyzing an electrocardiographic paper recording. The tachometer may give a false reading if the sensitivity is improperly set. It may double the heart rate if T waves are tall and counted as R waves, or it may underestimate the rate if the R wave is small.

To count the heart rate from a paper recording when the rate is regular, calculate the number of seconds between successive R waves and divide into 60. The ECG grid (Fig. 14-1) is divided into lines separated by 0.04 seconds and bolder lines of 0.2 seconds (5 × 0.04). If the RR interval is 0.2 seconds, the rate is 300 (60/0.2); if it is 1.0 second, the rate is 60 (60/1.0). If the rate is irregular, an average rate may be obtained by counting the number of R waves in a given period of time (i.e., 3.0 seconds, and multiplying by 20).

THE NORMAL RHYTHM

The heart rate is fastest at birth and diminishes as the heart and the autonomic nervous system mature. Normal infants at rest usually have heart rates between 100 and 180 beats/min. The healthy child less than 10 years of age rarely has a sustained rate less than 70 or more than 140 beats/min. These are general guidelines and must be adapted to the individual clinical situation, but if the sustained heart rate is outside these limits an explanation should be sought. The normal heart rate is variable and may increase (sinus tachycardia) with anxiety, fever, pain, acute blood loss, chronic anemia, and any other insult that necessitates an increased cardiac output. The heart rate may decrease (sinus bradycardia) as a result of vagal stimulation that may occur with hypoxia, breath holding, vigorous sucking, or suctioning of the nasopharynx. Sinus dysrhythmia, a phasic variation in heart rate, is common in

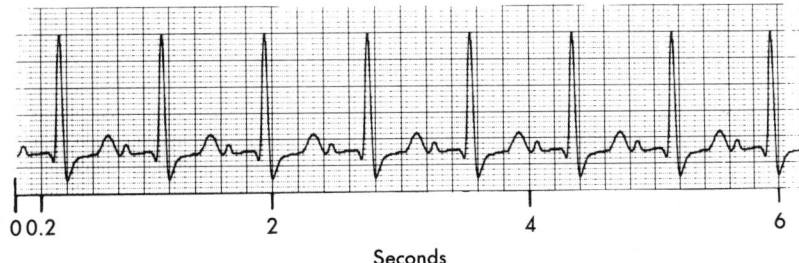

FIG. 14-1. Heart rate can be calculated by counting the number of beats in 2 seconds and multiplying by 30; the number in 4 seconds and multiplying by 15; or the number in 6 seconds and multiplying by 10. Another way is to measure the RR interval and divide into 60.

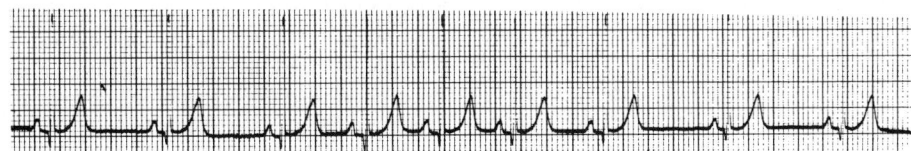

FIG. 14-2. Sinus dysrhythmia. Note that the irregularity is due to RR variation. Each R wave is preceded by a normal P wave and the PR interval is constant.

children. It is eliminated by the increased circulating catecholamines that accompany anxiety, exercise, and fever. If an irregular pulse is palpated, examination of an ECG may be necessary to determine whether it is due to a sinus dysrhythmia. In sinus dysrhythmia (Fig. 14-2) there is RR variation but the sequence of depolarization remains normal and the PR interval is constant.

MECHANISM OF DYSRHYTHMIA GENERATION

Cellular electrophysiologic studies have demonstrated two clinically significant mechanisms for the genesis of dysrhythmias: abnormalities in impulse formation (e.g., abnormal or enhanced automaticity) and abnormalities in impulse propagation (e.g., reentry and block).

Automaticity

The normal heartbeat has an intrinsic hierarchy of pacemaker activity. Impulses generated by the most rapidly depolarizing pacemaker, the sinus node, discharge subsidiary pacemakers before they reach threshold. If the sinus node fails to generate spontaneous activity or if the activity fails to propagate to surrounding cells, a subsidiary pacemaker in the atrium, atrioventricular (AV) node, or His-Purkinje system with an intrinsically slower discharge rate determines the heart rhythm. These subsidiary pacemakers can sometimes produce an accelerated rhythm leading to an ectopic tachycardia.

Reentry

Reentry is clinically the more important mechanism of dysrhythmia genesis. For reentry to occur, two pathways with unequal conducting/refractory properties must be present. The propagating impulse fails to die out after a normal activation; finds the second pathway, which is no longer refractory; and reexcites the area (Fig. 14-3). Such an electrical reentry circuit may be present within any portion of the heart including the sinus node, the AV node, the His-Purkinje system, or an accessory pathway. The reexcitation may last only one beat (e.g., a premature ventricular contraction [PVC] before the sinus node is reset, or it may continue for some time (e.g., an episode of supraventricular tachycardia [SVT]).

The most common accessory pathway bypasses the AV node and its stabilizing influence on ventricular conduction. This pathway makes it possible for the ventricle, or a part of the ventricle, to be preexcited. Electrophysiologic investigations, epicardial mapping, surgical findings, and anatomic studies have shown that there are several possible pathways by which part or all of the ventricle can be activated earlier than expected. By far the most common type is an accessory AV pathway or bundle of Kent. When activation of the ventricles takes place via two pathways, a fusion QRS complex results whose configuration depends on the contribution of each of the two activation fronts. The classic surface ECG representation of a Kent bundle bypass tract is the Wolff-Parkinson-White (WPW) conduction disturbance, which consists of a short PR interval (usually < 0.12 seconds), a delta wave, and a widened QRS complex (often > 0.12 seconds) (Fig. 14-4). In infants the changes are often subtle and may be recognized only retrospectively. As already noted, its exact form and width depends on the amount of ventricular muscle activated over the accessory AV pathway.[1]

HEMODYNAMIC CONSEQUENCES OF DYSRHYTHMIAS

Many interrelated factors affect hemodynamic function when an irregularity of cardiac rhythm is present. The most important ones include the heart rate, the patient's

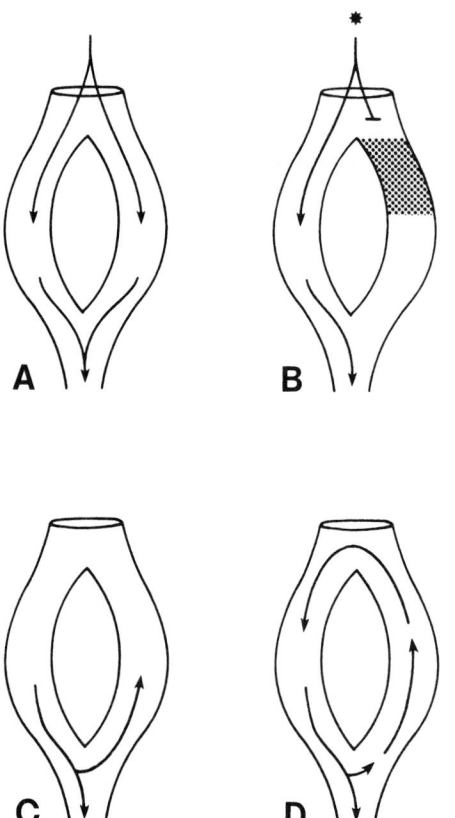

FIG. 14-3. Reentry depends on the availability of two pathways with different conduction times or refractory periods. **A,** Normal propagation of an impulse via both pathways. **B,** A premature beat finds one pathway blocked because it has not yet recovered from the previous depolarization, but the other pathway with a shorter refractory period propagates the impulse. **C,** If, when the impulse reaches the confluence of the two pathways, the other pathway has recovered or there is unidirectional block the impulse can be propagated in a retrograde direction. **D,** A reentrant or reciprocating tachycardia is now possible.

age, the duration of the rhythm disturbance, and the presence of underlying heart disease. When the heart beat originates from a focus other than the sinus node (ectopic beat), the normal AV depolarization sequence may be lost. This results in a diminished stroke volume caused by loss of the atrial contribution. If the heart rate is normal, cardiac output is not impaired by the occasional premature beat because the stroke volume of the next beat is increased. In contrast, very slow or very rapid heart rates usually result in a diminished cardiac output, especially if normal AV depolarization sequence is disturbed. Very young infants are additionally handicapped because they have a limited ability to adapt to a diminished cardiac output by a change in stroke volume; the main compensatory mechanism is increasing the heart rate. If the dysrhythmia is of long duration, with a very rapid or very slow heart rate, secondary ventricular dysfunction (thought by some to be due to diminished coronary blood flow) further

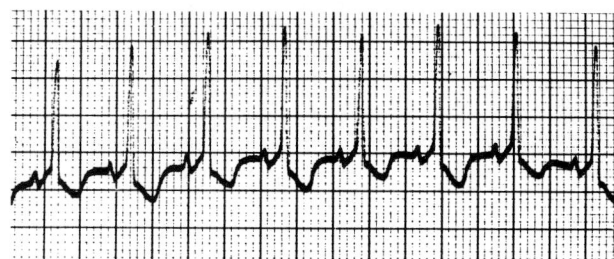

FIG. 14-4. Wolff-Parkinson-White (WPW) conduction disturbance in a 6-week-old infant with SVT. Note the short PR interval (0.04 sec), the delta wave, and the wide QRS (0.12 sec).

depresses the cardiac output, which normalizes only with restoration of a regular sinus rhythm.

Infants and children with underlying heart disease (especially those with an already increased end-diastolic ventricular volume resulting from previous palliative surgical procedures, residual atrioventricular valve regurgitation, or large left-to-right shunts) may be unable to compensate by changes in stroke volume and therefore tolerate the sudden onset of a slow or a rapid heart rate very poorly.

Clinical manifestations of a diminished cardiac output depend on its degree but may include syncope or presyncope, fatigue, diaphoresis, and dizziness; infants may feed poorly and be irritable. Physical evidence of vascular compensation for a low cardiac output is manifested by impaired peripheral perfusion associated with cool extremities, weak pulses, mottled skin, and hypotension. In infants, clinical findings may be primarily respiratory secondary to compromised left ventricular contractility; tachypnea, dyspnea, intercostal retractions, and grunting may be noted.

PREMATURE BEATS

Premature Atrial Contractions

Premature atrial contractions (PACs) result from premature depolarization of an atrial focus. They are common in infants and children and are benign.

Electrocardiographic Features (Fig. 14-5). The P wave is premature as compared to the underlying rhythm and, because it originates in the atrium, has a different configuration than the sinus beats. The QRS-T waves are usually normal; occasionally the P wave occurs so early that it finds the AV node still refractory from the previous beat and is therefore blocked. At other times, ventricular conduction may be aberrant due to one of the bundle branches being refractory and results in a wide QRS wave.

Clinical Features. Children with PACs may complain that the heart "stops" or of a fluttering sensation in the chest. In the absence of heart disease, PACs have no clinical significance unless they initiate an episode of SVT.

Acute Management. Reassurance.

Premature Ventricular Contractions

PVCs result from either premature depolarization of a ventricular focus or reentry. A fixed coupling interval (i.e., the interval between a normal sinus beat and the PVC is repetitive and fixed) may be seen if it is due to reentry.

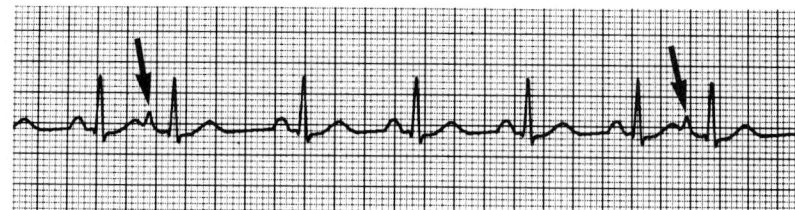

FIG. 14-5. Atrial premature beat. Note that QRS is similar but P wave is different in the premature beat (2 and 7) compared to the regular sinus beats.

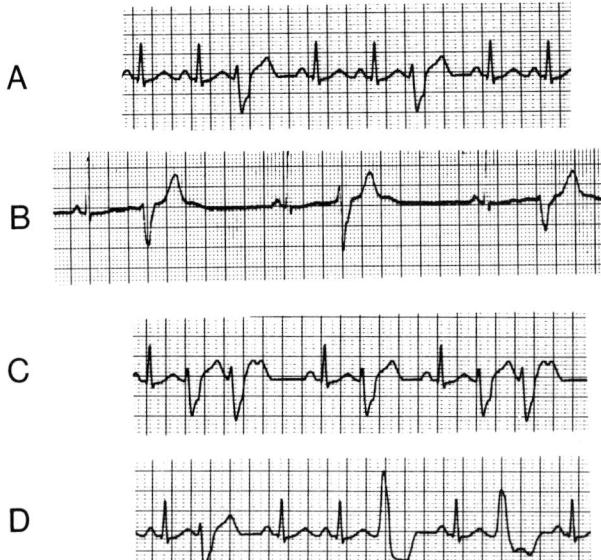

FIG. 14-6. A, Uniform premature ventricular beats. Note prematurity of the beat, wide QRS (0.10 sec), negative T wave, and compensatory pause. **B,** Ventricular bigeminy. **C,** Ventricular couplet. **D,** Multiform ventricular premature beats.

PVCs are not uncommon in infants and children and, in the presence of a structurally and functionally normal heart, are benign.

Electrocardiographic Features (Fig. 14-6). The QRS complex occurs prematurely, has a different configuration from the normally conducted beats, is usually but not always prolonged in duration (>0.08 seconds in infants and >0.09 seconds in children), and the T wave is usually opposite in direction to the QRS. A PVC is usually followed by a compensatory pause that may be full (i.e., the sum of the RR beats surrounding the PVC is equal to twice the normal RR interval) or it may be partial. PVCs that have the same shape in the same lead are called *uniform*, whereas those with varying shapes are called *multiform*. Fusion complexes, with a P wave preceding the QRS that looks like a combination of a normal beat and a PVC, are not considered multiform. *Ventricular bigeminy* is a regularly irregular rhythm in which every other beat is a PVC. *Ventricular trigeminy* is a regularly irregular rhythm in which every third beat is a PVC. A *couplet* is defined as two consecutive PVCs.

Clinical Features. In otherwise healthy children without underlying heart disease, uniform PVCs are benign even if they occur in a bigeminal or trigeminal pattern.[2] Light exercise usually abolishes them or at least does not increase their frequency. If PVCs are multiform, occur in couplets, or increase in frequency with exercise, an underlying cardiac abnormality should be ruled out even though such "complex" ventricular ectopy may also be benign.[3] Cardiac abnormalities that may be associated with PVCs include the prolonged QT interval syndrome (see below), cardiomyopathy (hypertrophic as well as dilated), myocarditis, arrhythmogenic right ventricular dysplasia, postoperative state (especially tetralogy of Fallot), Ebstein's malformation of the tricuspid valve, mitral valve prolapse, pulmonary vascular obstructive disease (Eisenmenger complex), and cardiac tumors. In acutely ill children, PVCs may be caused by hypoxia, acidosis, hypoglycemia, potassium abnormality (hypokalemia or hyperkalemia), and medications including digitalis, the phenothiazines, and the sympathomimetics.

THE TACHYDYSRHYTHMIAS
Supraventricular Tachycardia

SVT is the most common symptomatic dysrhythmia in infants and children and can occur anywhere along the pediatric age span from fetus through adolescence. SVT is most commonly due to a reentry circuit that may be associated with a WPW conduction disturbance, but can be caused by enhancement of an atrial automatic focus. SVT secondary to WPW often appears in the first year of life and may then not recur until late childhood.[4] Obversely, it has been conclusively demonstrated that the WPW of infancy may disappear with growth and maturation. SVT in the WPW syndrome occurs when at least three conditions are satisfied: (1) a premature beat that may be atrial, junctional, or ventricular initiates the episode of tachycardia; (2) the premature beat occurs at a time when conduction over the AV node and the bypass tract is dissociated; and (3) when the premature beat is conducted over one pathway from its chamber of origin, the other pathway must be excitable to permit initiation of a circuit movement.

Electrocardiographic Features (Fig. 14-7). The heart rate can vary widely. Very rapid rates (as high as 300 beats/min) can occur in infants, whereas rates in adolescents are more likely to be in the 120 to 160 beats/min range. QRS complexes are narrow in over 90% of children with SVT. This makes it easier to differentiate SVT from VT in children than in adults: a tachydysrhythmia with a wide QRS should be assumed to be ventricular in origin.[5] Differentiating SVT from sinus tachycardia (ST), especially

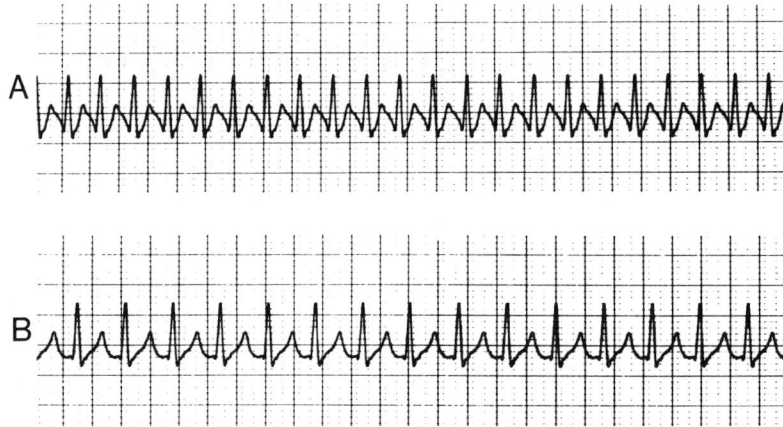

FIG. 14-7. **A,** SVT in an infant. Note the heart rate of 260 BPM, narrow QRS, and indefinite P waves. **B,** SVT in a 13-year-old. Heart rate is 180 BPM.

in infants, can be a more difficult task. Rate can be helpful, since infants with ST are unlikely to have a heart rate that exceeds 220 beats/min, whereas 60% of infants with SVT have a rate above 230 beats/min.[6] Other clues may be derived from a lack of beat-to-beat variability in SVT, and the abnormal P wave axis in the vast majority of infants with SVT. Retrospectively the diagnosis may be deduced from response to therapy. SVT converts abruptly in response to antidysrhythmic therapy, whereas ST does not respond to such therapy and the rate slows gradually when its cause is treated.

P waves are visible in about half the children with SVT but may be superimposed on the end of the T wave or buried within the QRS. Since the atria are activated in a retrograde manner, the P wave axis is most commonly in the superior quadrant (inverted in leads II, III, and aVF and upright in I and aVL).

A high percentage of infants and approximately 25% of children with SVT have a WPW conduction disturbance on the postconversion ECG. During SVT, antegrade conduction usually proceeds via the AV pathway, and the QRS is therefore normal in appearance.

Clinical Features. Although SVT may occur in children with congenital heart disease, especially Ebstein's malformation of the tricuspid valve or as a late sequela of cardiac surgery (especially correction of atrial septal defects and atrial reorientation procedures [Senning and Mustard] for transposition of the great arteries), the vast majority of children with SVT have a structurally normal heart. Symptoms of congestive heart failure and low cardiac output are most likely to be present in newborns, infants, and children with especially rapid heart rates as well as those with underlying congenital cardiac anomalies.

The vast majority of patients with SVT are uncomfortable but clinically stable. Chest pain is common, especially during conversion to sinus rhythm. It should, however, be noted that most chest pain in adolescents is noncardiac in origin.[7]

Acute Therapy. Infants and children with manifestations of shock should be treated immediately with electric cardioversion using an initial energy dose of 0.5 to 2.0 watt-sec/kg. Subsequent doses may be doubled. Hemody-

namically stable children with SVT may be treated with a variety of methods including maneuvers to increase vagal tone, and medications (adenosine, digoxin, or verapamil).

Maneuvers to increase vagal tone should be tried but, with the exception of the diving reflex, are rarely effective in infants. Vagal tone may be increased by the Valsalva maneuver (in infants by gentle upward pressure on the diaphragm) and unilateral carotid massage. Gagging and eyeball pressure should not be used, since the former may produce vomiting and lead to aspiration, and the latter can cause serious retinal damage. The diving reflex is a particularly effective vagal stimulant in infants. In eliciting it, the ECG should be continuously monitored, since occasionally a short period of asystole may be produced. A wash cloth is immersed in cold ice slush, wrung out, and without warning placed on the infant's face covering the mouth and the nose for 15 to 30 seconds.

If vagal maneuvers are not effective, medications are given. Digoxin is the medication with the longest history of use in converting SVT and is both effective and safe. Its major drawback is that conversion takes time; however, this is acceptable in the stable patient. Although digoxin can be given intravenously, the oral route is safer. A total loading dose of 30 μg/kg is used; 15 μg/kg IV is given at once and the remainder is divided into two doses given 4 to 5 hours apart. The patient should be monitored until conversion to a regular sinus rhythm has been documented. Digoxin is best avoided in treating episodes of SVT associated with WPW in children above the age of approximately eight years. Digoxin prolongs conduction over the AV pathway but in some patients may shorten the antegrade refractory period of the bypass tract and thus may encourage antegrade conduction over the latter, if its refractory period is sufficiently short. This can be dangerous in the presence of atrial fibrillation, which is more likely to develop in the teenage years.[8]

Adenosine is the drug of choice for terminating acute episodes of SVT in infants and children because of its effectiveness and safety.[9-12] Adenosine is an endogenous nucleoside that causes a temporary block through the AV pathway and therefore interrupts any reentry circuit that involves the AV node. The major advantage of adenosine is

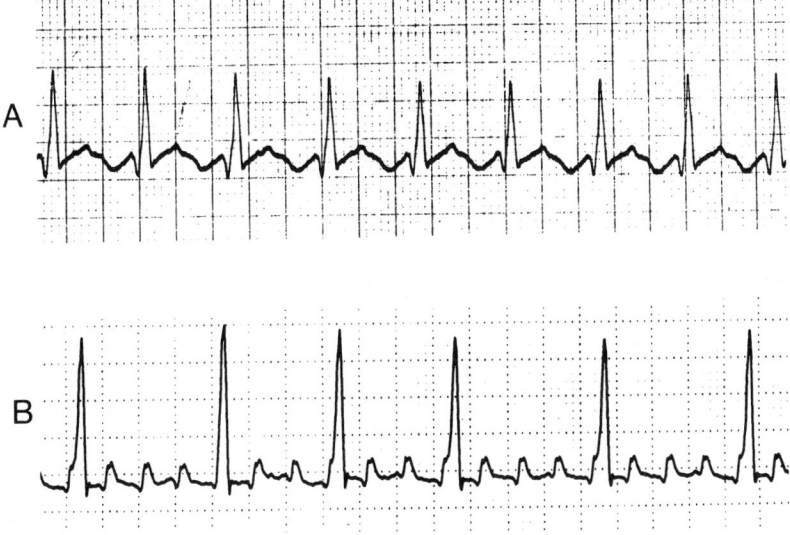

FIG. 14-8. A, Atrial flutter with concealed flutter waves and a heart rate of 105 BPM.
B, Atrial flutter with atrial rate of 300 BPM and a ventricular rate of 78 BPM.

that its half-life is only 10 seconds; side effects are transient and minimal. It should be used with caution in children with sinus node dysfunction or with severe reactive airway disease. Adenosine may be used in patients with WPW and does not interfere with other cardiac drugs. With continuous electrocardiographic monitoring, 0.1 mg/kg should be given as a rapid intravenous bolus followed immediately by a fluid flush. If there is no effect, the dose may be doubled; the maximum dose is 12 mg. Failure to convert must be differentiated from a recurrence of the SVT. If even one sinus beat develops before the SVT resumes, a nonsustained response has been obtained and a higher dose of adenosine is unlikely to be more effective.

Verapamil, a calcium channel blocker, exerts its antidysrhythmic effect by slowing conduction and prolonging the effective refractory period in the AV pathway. Its negative inotropic effect can cause serious myocardial depression, bradycardia, asystole, hypotension, and apnea. Because of the prevalence of these side effects in infants, verapamil should *not* be used in children under a year of age, or who have congestive heart failure or are receiving beta-blocking drugs. Care must also be exercised in patients with a bypass tract. Verapamil should be given slowly with constant and careful electrocardiographic and hemodynamic monitoring. The dose is 0.1 to 0.3 mg/kg (not to exceed a total of 5 mg).

ATRIAL FLUTTER

Atrial flutter is an atrial dysrhythmia without involvement of the AV node that is thought to be caused by local reentry. Very rapid atrial rates (approximately 300 beats/min) can rarely be transmitted to the ventricles; the ventricular rate is slower because of a variable AV block.

Electrocardiographic Features (Fig. 14-8). Atrial flutter is characterized by the presence of "flutter waves" with a sawtooth appearance, usually best seen in leads II, III, aVF, and V_1. The typical waves may not be apparent in

every lead in which case all 13 leads should be carefully examined. Occasionally, flutter waves may not be obvious in any lead and the ECG resembles that of SVT. If atrial flutter is suspected, the ventricular rate can be slowed by producing a transient AV block with vagal stimulation or administration of adenosine; flutter waves then become obvious. The QRS is normal in configuration but may be variable in rate. The ventricular rate may approach 300 beats/min in infants or may be slower with 2:1 or 3:1 AV block.

Clinical Features. In the fetus and young infant, atrial flutter can occur without associated heart defects.[13] In contrast, most older children with atrial flutter have an underlying heart abnormality. In a collaborative study of 380 patients between the ages of 12 months and 25 years with atrial flutter, Garson[14] reported that only 7.6% had a normal heart. Of the patients, 60.4% had repaired congenital heart disease, 13.3% had palliated congenital heart disease, 7.6% had unoperated congenital heart disease, 6.2% had congestive cardiomyopathy, and 4.9% had other cardiac abnormalities. The most common prior surgical procedures were correction of atrial septal defect, Mustard or Senning procedure for transposition of the great arteries, and repair of tetralogy of Fallot.

Symptoms of atrial flutter are similar to those of SVT and are related to the ventricular rate. Infants tolerate atrial flutter poorly because the AV node is capable of very rapid conduction; therefore infants may present with extremely rapid ventricular rates that may cause shock or congestive heart failure. Older children tolerate atrial flutter better and may be asymptomatic or complain of palpitations, dizziness, dyspnea, or syncope.

Acute Therapy. Atrial flutter is very responsive to electric synchronized cardioversion. Clinical improvement may also be obtained by producing a higher degree of AV block with digoxin. Caution must be taken if there is evidence of sinus node dysfunction.

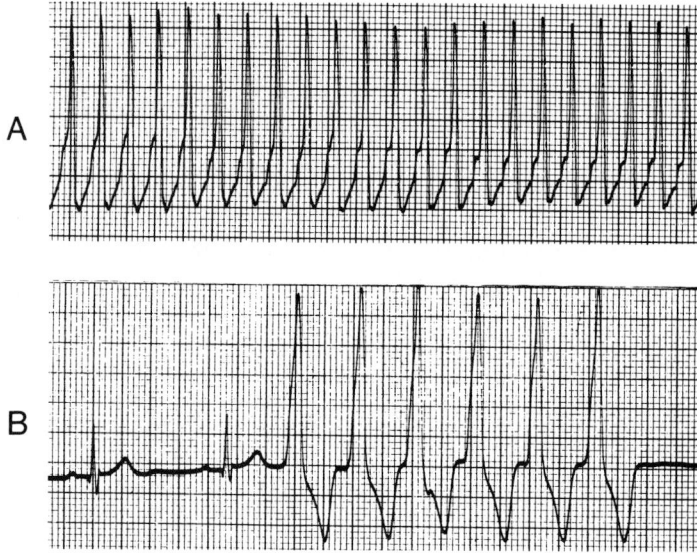

FIG. 14-9. A, Ventricular tachycardia in a symptomatic infant. The heart rate is 300 BPM.
B, VT in an asymptomatic teenager with a heart rate of 150 BPM.

Other useful medications in the control of atrial flutter include quinidine and amiodarone but their use should be under the supervision of a pediatric cardiologist familiar with these medications and their possible side effects.

VENTRICULAR TACHYCARDIA

Ventricular tachycardia (VT) is an uncommon dysrhythmia in the pediatric age group.

Electrocardiographic Features (Fig. 14-9). VT is defined as three successive extrasystoles of ventricular origin. If the VT terminates spontaneously after fewer than 30 beats, it is called "nonsustained" VT. The ventricular rate is variable, but usually exceeds 120 beats/min. As in isolated PVCs, the QRS duration is wide in older children but may be narrow in infants. AV dissociation is usually present, but retrograde conduction can produce 1:1 capture. *Torsades de pointes* is a VT characterized by progressive changes in amplitude and polarity of the QRS complexes so QRS complexes appear to be twisting around the isoelectric line. Although most episodes terminate spontaneously, some may degenerate to ventricular fibrillation (VF).

For proper evaluation of VT, the QT interval, especially of the beat preceding its onset, should be measured. The QT interval is roughly equal to the duration of the cardiac action potential and represents the period between earliest ventricular activation and completion of ventricular recovery (ie., depolarization plus repolarization). The QT interval is best measured in lead II from the onset of the q wave to the end of the T wave or U wave, if one is present. Since the length of the QT interval is inversely related to the heart rate, a corrected QT (QTc) is calculated using Bazett's formula (QTc = QT/the square root of the RR interval). In most normal children the QTc is shorter than 0.44 seconds; a QTc >0.50 seconds is definitely abnormal.

Clinical Features. The box on p. 163 lists some of the known causes of VT in infants and children.

Ventricular hamartoma involving Purkinje cells has been successfully treated by excision in infants with incessant VT.[15] Right ventricular dysplasia is a cardiomyopathy of unknown origin that mainly involves the right ventricle. It is often familial and may cause episodic VT with a left bundle branch block.[16]

In 1957, Jervell and Lange-Nielsen[17] described four siblings with bilateral sensorineural deafness, a long QT interval, and sudden death. Prolonged QT interval with sudden death but without deafness has been described as an autosomal dominant familial disorder and is known as the Romano-Ward syndrome. VT in this disorder is often induced by increased sympathetic stimulation and emotional stress, such as fright or startling noises. The available evidence strongly suggests that the lengthening of the QT interval is neurogenic in origin. VT associated with electrolyte imbalance and many medications is often preceded by a prolonged QT interval. It is currently not clear whether the torsades de pointes VT caused by medications such as quinidine[18] and procainamide is related to an idiosyncratic reaction, a critical drug dose, or a critical prolongation of the QT interval.[19]

The electrophysiologic effects of phenothiazines and tricyclic antidepressants are similar to those of quinidine-like antidysrhythmic drugs. Several phenothiazine derivatives, especially thioridazine and less commonly chlorpromazine and trifluoperazine, produce a dose-dependent prolongation of the QT. Idiosyncratic reactions to these drugs may also play a role in the initiation of the dysrhythmia. Prolongation of the QTc by toxic doses of tricyclic antidepressant drugs is due mainly to prolongation of the QRS.

Acute Therapy

Hemodynamically Stable Patient. Specific therapy should be used if the cause of the VT is identified (see box on p. 163). In addition, the following successive steps should be taken until the VT ceases.

1. Lidocaine, 1.0 mg/kg IV, followed by an infusion of 20 to 40 µg/kg/min.
2. Procainamide, 1 mg/kg IV every 3 to 5 minutes for 15 doses (total of 15 mg/kg over about 1 hr) or until sinus rhythm occurs, is often successful. Careful monitoring of blood pressure is necessary, since too rapid infusions may lead to hemodynamic collapse for which colloid infusion is occasionally necessary. When control is achieved, oral or nasogastric propranolol, 1 mg/kg, should be given every 6 hr and procainamide discontinued.[20]

Causes of Ventricular Tachycardia

Ventricular hamartoma
Right ventricular dysplasia
Acute myocarditis
Congenital prolonged QT interval
Metabolic disturbances
  Electrolyte imbalance
    Hypokalemia
    Hypocalcemia
    Hypomagnesemia
  Liquid protein/starvation diet
Drug toxicity/sensitivity
  Antidysrhythmic agents
    Quinidine
    Disopyramide
    Procainamide
    Flecainide
    Encainide
    Amiodarone
    Sotalol
  Digitalis
  Sympathomimetics
  Phenothiazines
    Thioridazine (Mellaril)
    Chlorpromazine
    Trifluoperazine
  Tricyclic antidepressants
    Imipramine
    Amitriptyline
  Organophosphate insecticide

If the VT is of the torsades de pointes type, procainamide should not be given. Instead, a temporary pacemaker should be inserted and the atrium or ventricle overdriven.

Hemodynamically Unstable Patient. After a bolus of lidocaine, electrical DC cardioversion should be immediately performed using 0.5 to 2.0 watt-sec/kg of energy. If ineffective, the electrical dose may need to be increased. Semiconscious patients should receive an amnestic sedative or, preferably, a short-acting anesthetic.

VENTRICULAR FIBRILLATION

VF is an uncommon dysrhythmia in children. In a study of the terminal rhythm in infants and children, Walsh and Krongrad[21] found that only 6% had VF and not a single episode occurred in a child who did not have congenital heart disease. A more recent study[22] concluded that the incidence of VF in children and adolescents with prehospital cardiac arrest is much higher at 19%.

Electrocardiographic Features (Fig. 14-10). The organized cardiac rhythm is replaced by an undulating line that may be coarse or fine. It should be noted that a similar pattern may be due to a loose electrocardiographic connection.

Clinical Features. VF is a series of disorganized depolarizations not associated with a cardiac output and therefore presents as a cardiopulmonary arrest. The electrocardiographic diagnosis should always be confirmed by absence of a pulse.

Acute Therapy. The initial acute therapy, while awaiting the defibrillator, is directed at cardiopulmonary resuscitation including establishing an airway, ventilation and oxygenation, and chest compressions (see Chapter 12). Electric defibrillation is the definitive therapy, performed up to three times in quick succession using 2, 4, and 4 watt-sec/kg. If this is not successful, give epinephrine, 0.01 mg/kg IV, and perform defibrillation using 4 watt-sec/kg. If still not successful, give lidocaine, 1 mg/kg IV, before another defibrillation attempt. Bretylium, 5 mg/kg IV, may be helpful before defibrillation is again attempted.[23]

THE BRADYDYSRHYTHMIAS

Episodic and asymptomatic bradycardia in infants and children is commonly associated with vagal stimulation. Acute onset symptomatic bradycardia is usually due to hypoxemia, acidosis, and a low cardiac output. Chronic sustained bradycardia is either acquired or due to congenital AV block.

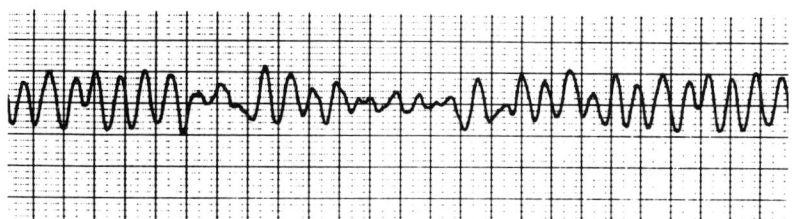

FIG. 14-10. Ventricular fibrillation.

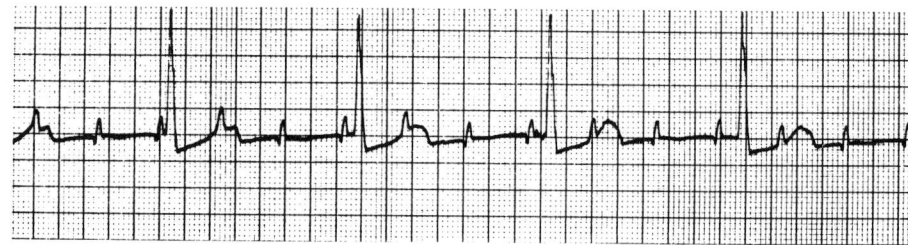

FIG. 14-11. Congenital complete heart block. Note that there is no relationship between P and QRS waves. The atrial rate is 125 BPM and the ventricular rate is 42 BPM.

COMPLETE HEART BLOCK

Complete heart block may be associated with congenital heart disease, may occur as an isolated congenital lesion, or may be acquired as part of a systemic disorder. The most common structural heart abnormality associated with AV block is L-transposition of the great arteries with ventricular inversion. When complete heart block occurs without structural heart disease, there is a high association with maternal connective tissue disease, especially maternal lupus erythematosus.[24] Positive immunofluorescent studies of fetal atrial tissue have identified SS-A/Ro or SS-B/La antibodies as the cause of the inflammatory reaction that leads to the block.[25] When transplacental anti-Ro or anti-La antibodies are present, congenital heart block approaches 100%.[24] Conditions in which AV block may be acquired include Lyme disease, myocarditis, Rocky Mountain spotted fever, certain muscular dystrophies, myotonic dystrophy, and Kearns-Sayre syndrome (progressive external ophthalmoplegia and bifascicular block).

Electrocardiographic Features (Fig. 14-11). P waves are normal in appearance and rate. QRS may be narrow or wide depending on the site of the block. Ventricular rate varies widely and is directly related to the level of the block; the lower the block, the slower the heart rate. Since there is no conduction from atria to ventricles, there is no relationship between P and QRS waves.

Clinical Features. Many children with congenital complete heart block are asymptomatic. Symptoms may, however, include easy fatigability, shortness of breath, syncope, and presyncope. Risk factors associated with symptoms include a persistently low heart rate (mean daytime junctional rate less than 50 beats/min), presence of associated cardiac defects, a prolonged QT interval, and a wide QRS complex.[26,27]

Acute Therapy. The heart rate can sometimes be increased with intravenous atropine (0.03 to 0.06 mg/kg) or an isoproterenol infusion (0.05 to 0.5 µg/kg/min), but the most reliable acute therapy is transvenous ventricular pacing. Transcutaneous pacing may be helpful as a temporary measure while preparations are being made for transvenous pacing.

Acute Onset Bradycardia

Bradycardia in critically ill infants and children is associated with hypoxemia, acidosis, and a low cardiac output. In this setting it is usually the result of AV block and an idioventricular rhythm and is often a preterminal event.

Acute Therapy. Acute therapy includes all the steps of cardiopulmonary resuscitation including adequate ventilation, oxygenation, chest compressions, and resuscitative medications.

DYSRHYTHMIAS ASSOCIATED WITH CARDIAC CONTUSION

Virtually all types of rhythm disturbances can occur in patients with nonpenetrating cardiac injury. The location of the injury may influence the type of dysrhythmia present but electrocardiographic changes lack both specificity and sensitivity. Rhythm disturbances may be due to the often accompanying hypovolemia, hypotension, hypoxia, and acidosis rather than the contusion; sometimes a significant cardiac contusion may be present without any electrocardiographic changes.

DYSRHYTHMIAS AFTER CARDIAC SURGERY

Even when the cardiac rhythm is normal in the immediate postoperative period after corrective cardiac surgical procedures, rhythm disturbances may develop a number of years later. For example, atrial flutter may develop years after correction of an atrial septal defect[28] or after the Fontan procedure[29]; sinus node dysfunction is common following one of the atrial switch procedures (Mustard or Senning procedures) for transposition of the great arteries; and premature ventricular contractions are sometimes seen following correction of a tetralogy of Fallot.[30]

Cardiac dysrhythmias have become a major long-term complication of atrial reorientation procedures (Mustard and Senning procedures) for transposition of the great arteries.[31,32] The cause of the dysrhythmias has been postulated to be due to damage to the sinus node or interruption of atrial conduction pathways. The prevalence of sinus rhythm progressively decreases as the postoperative period increases.[33] Dysfunction of the sinus node causes a subsidiary pacemaker—atrial, or more commonly junctional—to take over at a slower rate (Fig. 14-12). Episodic atrial tachydysrhythmias including SVT and atrial flutter[34] may also be seen. The Joint Commission on Pacing of the American College of Cardiology and the American Heart Association[35] has recommended that in a child with the potential for sinus node dysfunction, even in the absence of symptomatic bradycardia, a temporary pacemaker should be implanted before treatment with any drug that could suppress the sinus node, especially quinidine.[36] Late onset premature ventricular beats, VT, and rarely sudden death

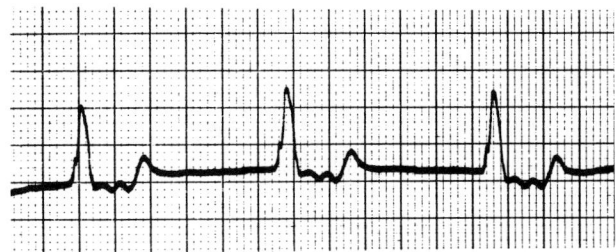

FIG. 14-12. Sinus node dysfunction in a 7-year-old boy who underwent Mustard procedure for transposition of the great arteries in infancy. The QRS is wide; the rate is 52 BPM. P wave after each QRS represents retrograde depolarization of the atrium.

have been documented years after correction of tetralogy of Fallot.[30,35] It has been difficult to establish whether these dysrhythmias are a part of the natural history of the defect, the consequence of the surgical repair, or due to residual hemodynamic abnormalities.

References

1. Durrer D, Schuilenburg RM, Wellemns HJJ: Preexcitation revisited, *Am J Cardiol* 25:690, 1970.
2. Jacobsen JR, Garson A, Gillette PC, et al: Premature ventricular contractions in normal children, *J Pediatr* 92:36, 1978.
3. Yabek SM: Ventricular arrhythmias in children with an apparently normal heart, *J Pediatr* 119:1, 1991.
4. Perry JC, Garson A: Supraventricular tachycardia due to Wolff-Parkinson-White syndrome in children: early disappearance and late recurrence, *J Am Coll Cardiol* 16:1215, 1990.
5. Garson A, Gillette PC, McNamara DG: Supraventricular tachycardia in children: clinical features, response to treatment, and long-term follow up in 217 patients, *J Pediatr* 98:875, 1981.
6. Fisher DJ, Gross DM, Garson A: Rapid sinus tachycardia: differentiation from supraventricular tachycardia, *Am J Dis Child* 137:164, 1983.
7. Selbst SM, Ruddy RM, Clark BJ, et al: Pediatric chest pain: a prospective study, *Pediatrics* 82:319, 1988.
8. Sterba R, Maloney JD: Atrial fibrillation in adolescents with Wolff-Parkinson-White syndrome. *Proceedings of the Second World Congress on Pediatric Cardiology*, New York, 1985, Springer-Verlag.
9. Greco R, Musto B, Arienzo V, et al: Treatment of paroxysmal supraventricular tachycardia in infancy with digitalis, adenosine-5'-triphosphate, and verapamil: a comparative study, *Circulation* 66:504, 1982.
10. Overholt ED, Rheuban KS, Gutgesell HP, et al: Usefulness of adenosine for arrhythmias in infants and children, *Am J Cardiol* 61:336, 1988.
11. Rossi AF, Burton DA: Adenosine in altering short term treatment of supraventricular tachycardia in infants, *Am J Cardial* 64:685, 1989.
12. Till J, Shinebourne EA, Rigby ML, et al: Efficacy and safety of adenosine in the treatment of supraventricular tachycardia in infants and children, *Br Heart J* 62:204, 1989.
13. Rowland TW, Mathew R, Chameides L, et al: Idiopathic atrial flutter in infancy: a review of eight cases, *Pediatrics* 61:52, 1978.
14. Garson A, Bink-Boelkens M, Hesslein PS, et al: Atrial flutter in the young: a collaborative study of 300 cases, *J Am Coll Cardiol* 6:871, 1985.
15. Garson A, Gillette P, Titus J, et al: Surgical treatment of ventricular tachycardia in infants, *N Engl J Med* 310:1443, 1984.
16. Nava A, Thiene G, Canciani B, et al: Familial occurrence of right ventricular dysplasia: a study involving nine families, *J Am Coll Cardiol* 12:1222, 1988.
17. Jervell A, Lange-Nielsen F: Congenital deaf-mutism, functional heart disease with prolongation of the QT interval and sudden death, *Am Heart J* 54:59, 1957.
18. Barton CW, Dick M, Rosenthal A: Quinidine syncope in children, *J Am Coll Cardiol* 5:429, 1985.
19. Surawicz B, Knoebel SB: Long QT: good, bad or indifferent? *JACC* 4:398, 1984.
20. Zeigler VL, Gillette PC, Crawford FA, et al: New approaches to treatment of incessant ventricular tachycardia in the very young, *J Am Coll Cardiol* 16:681, 1990.
21. Walsh CK, Krongrad E: Terminal cardiac electrical activity in pediatric patients, *Am J Cardiol* 51:557, 1983.
22. Mogayzel C, Quan L, Graves JR, et al: Out-of-hospital ventricular fibrillation in children and adolescents: causes and outcome, *Ann Emerg Med* 25:484, 1995.
23. Guidelines for cardiopulmonary resuscitation and emergency cardiac care: Part IV pediatric advanced life support, *JAMA* 268:2266, 1992.
24. Chameides L, Truex RC, Vetter V, et al: Association of maternal systemic lupus erythematosus with congenital complete heart block, *N Engl J Med* 297:1204, 1977.
25. Litsey SE, Noonan JA, O'Connor WN, et al: Maternal connective tissue disease and congenital complete heart block demonstration of immunoglobin in cardiac tissue, *N Engl J Med* 312:98, 1985.
26. Taylor PV, Taylor KF, Norman A, et al: Prevalence of maternal Ro(SS-A) and La(SS-B) autoantibodies in relation to congenital AV block, *Br J Rheumatol* 27:128, 1988.
27. Dewey RC, Capeless MA, Levy AM: Use of ambulatory electrocardiographic monitoring to identify high-risk patients with congenital complete heart block, *N Engl J Med* 316:835, 1987.
28. Pinsky WW, Gillette PC, Garson A, et al: Diagnosis, management, and long-term results of patients with congenital complete atrioventricular block, *Pediatrics* 6:728, 1982.
29. Bink-Boelkens M, Velvis H, Homan van der Heide JJ, et al: Dysrhythmias after atrial surgery in children, *Am Heart J* 106:125, 1983.
30. Chandar JS, Wolff GS, Garson A, et al: Ventricular arrhythmias in postoperative tetralogy of Fallot, *Am J Cardiol* 65:655, 1990.
31. Weber HS, Hellenbrand WE, Kleinman CS, et al: Predictors of rhythm disturbances and subsequent morbidity after the Fontan operation, *Am J Cardiol* 64:762, 1989.
32. Clarkson PM, Barrat-Boyes GB, Meutze JM: Late dysrhythmias and disturbances of conduction following Mustard operation for complete transposition of the great arteries, *Circulation* 53:519, 1976.
33. Deanfield JE, Macarey FJ, Bull C, et al: Arrhythmia and late mortality after Mustard and Senning operations for transposition: a 7-year prospective study, *Circulation* 74(suppl II):II-50, 1986.
34. Hayes CJ, Gersony WM: Arrhythmia after the Mustard operation for transposition of the great arteries: a long term study, *JACC* 7:133, 1986.
35. Vetter VL, Tanner CS, Horowitz LN: Inducible atrial flutter after the Mustard repair of complete transposition of the great arteries, *Am J Cardiol* 61:428, 1988.
36. Frye RL, Collins JJ, DeSanctis RW: Guidelines for permanent cardiac pacemaker implantation, May 1984, *Circulation* 70:331A, 1984.

## 15

Fluid and Electrolyte Balance

Alfred Sacchetti • Richard J. Brilli • Roger M. Barkin

Infants and children have a high metabolic water turnover and a larger body surface area for weight. These differences make them particularly vulnerable to diseases that produce dehydration. Diarrhea and its associated fluid losses are the leading cause of infant mortality in the world and account for 10% of preventable postneonatal deaths in the United States.[1]

PATHOPHYSIOLOGY

Total Body Water and Fluid Compartments

Fluid balance is closely regulated and controlled by multiple homeostatic factors. The total body water (TBW) of children varies with age, as does its distribution within the body's intracellular fluid (ICF) and extracellular fluid (ECF) compartments. The ECF, representing 20% to 25% of the body weight, consists of intravascular or plasma fluid (5%), interstitial fluid (15%), and transcellular fluid (1% to 3%), the latter including gastrointestinal secretions and spinal, intraoccular, peritoneal, and synovial fluid. The intravascular fluid is the circulating blood volume and ranges from 8% (80 ml/kg) in infants to 5% (50 ml/kg) in adults. Body fluid compartments and their variations with age are summarized in Table 15-1. The differential gradients between compartments determine the distribution of fluid between the ECF and ICF and are controlled by physical factors such as ion concentration and osmolality.

TBW is a reflection of intake, absorption, and excretion. The regulation of water in both fluid compartments is continuously modulated by several unique mechanisms. Intake is controlled by the availability of water and a child's thirst. In infants, water availability is controlled for them, whereas older children with free access to fluids determine their own intake. Thirst is regulated by the hypothalamus and possibly the renin-angiotensin system.

Water loss in children also varies with age (Table 15-2). Urinary losses range from 40 to 60 ml/kg/24 hrs, fecal losses 10 to 20 ml/kg/24 hr, and insensible losses 10 to 40 ml/kg/24 hr. Antidiuretic hormone (ADH) regulates renal urinary volume and concentration via effective osmotic pressure in the ECF. ADH increases the permeability of the renal collecting ducts to water, increasing reabsorption of filtered water and decreasing water excretion. Insensible water losses include water converted in metabolic reactions, water lost through the respiratory tract, and water lost through evaporation from skin. Increased basal metabolism rates will increase water utilization and insensible water loss. The most common cause of increased insensible water loss is fever, which may elevate the daily fluid requirements by 7 ml/kg/24 hr for each degree rise in temperature above 37.2° C (99° F). Water loss may also be affected by humidity and ambient temperature. Increased losses by any of these mechanisms requires additional fluid intake to prevent a negative water balance and dehydration. Caloric needs generally parallel water requirements and for most clinical circumstances the number of calories required per day is equal to the number of milliliters of water required for the 24-hour period.

Fluid losses create different deficits in the ECF and ICF compartments, depending on the length of time during which the dehydration evolved. In acute dehydration, approximately 60% of fluid is lost from the ECF, while the remaining 40% comes from the ICF. In longer dehydration processes, a greater percentage of fluid loss is contributed by the ICF compartment. Table 15-3 presents the relationship between dehydration duration and fluid compartment contribution.

In addition to fluid loss, fluid excess can also occur in children. Extracellular fluid increases may result from either water or salt retention. Excessive TBW accumulates in extravascular compartments and produces peripheral edema and ascites. The total body sodium controls the TBW and not the specific plasma sodium concentration. Therefore a child with a serum sodium of 130 mEq/ml may still be total body sodium overloaded. Another source of edema in children is hypoproteinemic states.

TABLE 15-1. Body Fluid Compartments by Age

	Premie	Newborn	1 yr	3 yr	9 yr	Adult
Weight (kg)	1.5	3	10	15	30	70
Body surface area (m²)	0.15	0.2	0.5	0.6	1	1.7
TBW (%)	80	78	65			60
ECF (%)	50	45	25			20
ICF (%)	30	33	40			40

Adapted from Finberg L, Keavath RE, Fleischman AR: *Water and electrolytes in pediatrics*, Philadelphia, 1982, WB Saunders.
TBW, Total body weight; *ECF*, extracellular fluid; *ICF*, intracellular fluid.

TABLE 15-2. Maintenance Water Loss Components (ml/kg/24 hr)

	Age group			
Component	0-6 mo	6 mo-5 yr	5-10 yr	Adolescent
Insensible	40	30	20	10
Urinary	60	60	50	40
Fecal	20	10	—	—
Total	120	100	70	50

Adapted from Winter RW: *Principles of pediatric fluid therapy*, ed 2, Boston, 1982, Little, Brown.

TABLE 15-3. Rapidity of Evolution of Dehydration and Compartment Fluid Source

	Portion of fluid lost (%)	
Period of evolution of dehydration	From ECF	From ICF
Rapid: less than 2 days	75	25
Average: 2 to 7 days	60	40
Long: more than 7 days	50	50

Water and Electrolyte Requirements

Water requirements for children vary by weight and body surface area. Maintenance fluid for children is generally calculated in groups of 10 kg with decreasing requirements for increasing weights. Calculation of maintenance fluids are as follows:

Children <10 kg	100 ml/kg/24 hr
Children 11-20 kg	1,000 ml + 50 ml/kg/24 hr for each kg over 10 kg
Children >20 kg	1,500 ml + 20 ml/kg/24 hr for each kg over 20 kg
Adults	2,000 to 2,400 ml/24 hr

Beyond water and calories, normal metabolism also consumes electrolytes, all of which require replacement. Each body compartment requires a specific number and type of cations and anions for normal cellular integrity and transmembrane potentials.

These solutes also control the distribution of water between the different cellular compartments. Sodium is the primary extracellular cation (interstitial, intravascular, and plasma), and potassium is the main intracellular cation. Like water, daily electrolytes are a function of a child's age and weight. Daily electrolyte requirements are as follows:

Sodium	3 mEq/kg/24 hr (max: 80 mEq/24 hr)
Potassium	2 mEq/kg/24 hr (max: 40 mEq/24 hr)

Osmolality

The intracellular and extracellular compartments are in a state of carefully maintained equilibrium. Water is free to move between compartments, and this movement is determined by the osmotic pressure of each compartment. Osmotic pressure is determined by the number of particles in each compartment and is independent of the weight, type, or valence of the particles. The relative hydration status of the different body compartments is then determined by the concentration of the different osmotically active particles. The unit of measure for osmolality is the osmole, defined as one gram molecular weight of a nondissociable substance. Under the normal physiologic parameters present in the body, the concentration of osmotic particles is small and easiest measured in one-thousandth of an osmole or milliosmoles.

Osmotic forces determine water distribution in the body. Normal plasma or extracellular osmolality is determined by the sodium concentration, glucose, and blood urea nitrogen and ranges between 285 to 295 mOsm. The plasma osmolality can be approximated through the following:

$$\text{Plasma osmolality} = 2 \times (\text{Na}^+) + \left(\frac{\text{Glucose}}{18}\right) + \left(\frac{\text{BUN}}{2.8}\right)$$

Intracellular osmolality is determined by potassium, phosphates, and proteins and is normally equal to extracellular osmolality.

Plasma osmolality is closely regulated by osmoreceptors located in the hypothalamus. When these receptors detect an increase in ECF osmolality, they initiate the synthesis, transport, and release of arginine vasopressin (ADH). ADH increases permeability of the renal tubules to water, allowing free water absorption and urinary concentration. The absorbed free water dilutes the concentration of ECF osmotic particles and decreases the plasma osmolality. As the ECF osmolality drops, free water moves back into the ICF maintaining total body fluid balance. Additional osmoreceptors are located in the thirst center of the hypothalamus. As ECF hyperosmolality produces cellular dehydration in these cells, thirst is perceived and water consumption increased.[7,8]

Regulation of plasma osmolality does not function in isolation but interacts with the mechanisms to control total body and intravascular volume (see Sodium homeostasis). It is the combination of plasma osmolality, intravascular volume, blood pressure, and adrenergic tone that works to determine the kidney's handling of solutes and water.

In the normal state, equal osmolality between the ICF and ECF maintains normal water equilibrium between compartments. In pathologic conditions this balance is offset by an excess or deficit of an osmotic particle causing water to pass from the hyposmolar to the hyperosmolar compartment. An example of this can be seen in severe hyperglycemia in which excess ECF glucose dramatically raises the plasma osmolality. Water is drawn from the ICF compartment to the ECF compartment producing intracellular dehydration.[24]

ELECTROLYTE AND ACID-BASE HOMEOSTASIS

Acid-Base Homeostasis

Acid-base homeostasis is essential to maintain normal cellular function. Acid-base status is defined in terms of the concentration of hydrogen ions (H^+) and expressed as the negative logarithm of this concentration (equivalents per liter or pH). Acids may be defined as substances that raise the H^+ concentration in a solution. As the number of H^+ increase the fluid becomes more acidic and the pH decreases. The converse is true for a substance that is a base. In the human body, H^+ concentration is maintained as a balance between the ionized and nonionized forms of carbonic acid. Carbonic acid is also in equilibrium with its components water and carbon dioxide.

$$H^+ + HCO_3^- \rightarrow H_2CO_3 \rightarrow H_2O + \text{dissolved } CO_2$$

The mathematical relationship between these molecules and pH is described by the Henderson-Hasselbalch equation:

$$pH = pKa + \log\left(\frac{\text{base}}{\text{acid}}\right)$$

$$pH = pKa + \log\frac{(HCO_3^-)}{H_2CO_3}$$

The normal human pH ranges between 7.36 and 7.44.

The renal and respiratory systems provide compensation for acute and chronic alterations in acid-base status. The kidney's compensation is through excretion of H^+ and HCO_3^-, while CO_2 levels are controlled through changes in minute ventilation by the lungs. The kidney responds relatively slowly to pH changes taking 24 to 48 hours to adjust hydrogen and bicarbonate ion excretion in the urine. In contrast the respiratory tract responds quickly to rapid shifts in pH by adjusting respiratory rate or tidal volume. These compensatory mechanisms allow the body to maintain a constant pH. If excess H^+ is produced, the equilibrium of the carbonic acid equation will be shifted to the right resulting in more production of CO_2.

This equilibrium can also be driven by removal of substrate from either side of the equation. Hyperventilation will decrease carbon dioxide tension, pull the equilibrium to the right, and decrease hydrogen ion concentration. These effects are the basis for the Kussmaul respirations seen in diabetic ketoacidosis. Additional acid-base buffering capacity is provided by serum proteins and hemoglobin, which may absorb excess H^+.[6]

The pH of arterial blood defines acid-base balance. Acidemia is present when an abnormally low pH occurs in the blood. Alkalemia is present when an abnormally high pH is present in the blood. The tendency to produce acidemia is called *acidosis* and to produce alkalemia is termed *alkalo-sis*. For example a P_{CO_2} greater than normal is termed *respiratory acidosis* and may be the primary imbalance or a compensation for metabolic alkalosis. An elevated serum pH occurring as a result of bicarbonate excess would be termed an *alkalemia* secondary to a *metabolic alkalosis*. A given primary process will be countered by a secondary or compensatory process in which the body attempts to reverse the change in pH and return the acid-base balance back to normal. Children with dehydration and a primary metabolic acidosis will hyperventilate to lower their P_{CO_2} and produce a respiratory alkalosis. This compensatory process never fully corrects the primary process so the measured pH will generally indicate which process is the primary derangement. In the metabolic acidosis/respiratory alkalosis example, the measured pH would be less than 7.4 and reflect the acidosis as the primary process.

The H^+ along with other cations, predominately sodium and potassium, must be paired with a negative anion to maintain electrical neutrality. These anions are primarily chloride and bicarbonate. In the serum, because of the presence of organic acids, phosphates, and sulfates there is a difference between measured cations and anions. This difference, termed the *anion gap*, represents the amount of unmeasured H^+ in the serum that is present to maintain electrical neutrality. The anion gap is calculated:

$$\text{Anion gap} = (Na^+ + K^+)\,mEq - (Cl^- + HCO_3^-)\,mEq$$

The normal anion gap is 8 to 12 mEq/L. The gap is usually normal in diseases such as diarrhea in which the metabolic acidosis results from a loss of bicarbonate ion through the gastrointestinal tract or the kidneys. It increases with excessive production of organic acids (ketones in diabetic ketoacidosis), lactic acid (shock, sepsis, congestive heart failure [CHF], and starvation), toxins (salicylates, methanol, and ethylene glycol), or renal failure. A useful mnemonic for remembering entities that produce a large anion gap with metabolic acidosis is *MUDPILES: m*ethanol, *u*remia, *d*iabetic ketoacidosis, *p*araldehyde, *i*soniazid, *i*buprofen, or *i*nhalants (H_2S,CN,CO) or *i*ron overdose, *l*actic acidosis, *e*thanol or *e*thylene glycol, and *s*alicylates, *s*tarvation, or *s*olvents (benzene or toluene).

Alterations in acid-base status may represent simple abnormalities or a balance of compensatory mechanisms as noted above. Mixed metabolic and respiratory disorders are common. The characteristic changes in the plasma components for mixed acid-base problems are noted in Table 15-4.

Metabolic Acidosis. Metabolic acidosis results from either an increase in hydrogen ions or a decrease in bicarbonate. As the pH falls from a metabolic acidosis, tachypnea develops in an attempt to create a respiratory alkalosis by exhaling CO_2. Initial P_{CO_2} may decrease 1 to 1.5 times the reduction in HCO_3^- in an attempt to maintain a neutral pH. As the acidosis worsens, cardiac dysrhythmias and cellular dysfunction develop.

Specific correction of the underlying condition is the optimum treatment to halt the generation of the excess hydrogen ion. Intravascular volume must be maintained with intravenous fluid infusions to insure perfusion. If euvolemia is maintained and the HCO_3^- falls acutely below 10 mEq/L, additional bicarbonate should be administered

TABLE 15-4. Acid-Base Responses

Problem	pH	Primary process	Compensatory change
Metabolic acidosis	Decreases	$\downarrow HCO_3^-$	$\downarrow P{CO_2}$ (hyperventilation) ($P{CO_2}$ decreases 1.2 mm Hg for each 1 mEq/L HCO_3^- fall)
Metabolic alkalosis	Increases	$\uparrow HCO_3^-$	$\downarrow P{CO_2}$ (hypoventilation) ($P{CO_2}$ increases 0.7 mm Hg for each 1 mEq/L HCO_3^- rise)
Respiratory acidosis	Decreases	$\uparrow P{CO_2}$	$\uparrow HCO_3^-$ (bicarbonate retention) (HCO_3^- rises 0.1 mEq/L for each 1 mm Hg rise $P{CO_2}$)
Respiratory alkalosis	Increases	$\downarrow P{CO_2}$	$\downarrow HCO_3^-$ (bicarbonate excretion) (HCO_3^- falls 0.2 mEq/L for each 1 mm Hg fall $P{CO_2}$)

to correct the serum HCO_3^- to at least 12 to 15 mEq/L. The initial correction should replace a maximum of *one half* the calculated deficit. The deficit is calculated as follows:

$$\text{Deficit mEq } HCO_3^- = \text{Weight (kg)} \times \text{base deficit} \times 0.5$$

$$\text{Base deficit} = \text{mEq/L desired} - \text{mEq/L observed}$$

Serial monitoring should be used in any patient receiving bicarbonate therapy. Caution should be used in the intravenous administration of any bicarbonate; slow correction is indicated. The neutralization of the excess H^+ depends on the creation of carbonic acid, its dissociation into water and CO_2, and the exhalation of the CO_2. If the bicarbonate is administered quicker than the patient can exhale the newly formed CO_2, an excess of CO_2 will form and actually worsen the situation. The excess CO_2 is then free to diffuse into the central nervous system where it will reform carbonic acid and paradoxically lower the pH. Whenever possible, bicarbonate is best administered as an infusion and not a bolus.

By the same token, patients must be able to sufficiently hyperventilate to rid themselves of the excess CO_2 formed with HCO_3^- administration. Critically ill patients unable to maintain the proper ventilation should be intubated and mechanically hyperventilated before administration of HCO_3^-.

Metabolic Alkalosis. Metabolic acidosis results from an increase in bicarbonate levels or an excessive loss of hydrogen ions. The body is ill-equipped to handle a primary metabolic alkalosis, since few natural conditions produce this problem. Symptoms of metabolic alkalosis include muscle cramps, weakness, paresthesia, seizures, hyperreflexia, tetany, and dysrhythmias. The $P{CO_2}$ will increase 0.5 to 1.0 mm Hg for each mEq/L increase in HCO_3^-.

Primary treatment of the causative condition may require restoration of intravascular volume or stopping of a causative medication such as a diuretic. If alkalosis is severe with a pH of 7.7 (lower if symptomatic), it may be treated with either acetazolamide (Diamox) or ammonium chloride. If the potassium is normal the dose of acetazolamide is 5 mg/kg/24 hr q 6 to 24 hr (adult: 250 to 375 mg/24 hr) PO or IV. The dose of ammonium chloride is (NH_4Cl) 150 to 300 mg/kg/24 hr q 6 hr (adult: 8 to 12 gm/24 hr). PO may also be used.

Respiratory Acidosis. Primary respiratory acidosis results from alveolar hypoventilation and CO_2 retention. As the carbon dioxide level increases, carbonic acid is produced and the pH falls. Treatment of acute primary respiratory acidosis is correction of the underlying cause of the ventilation problem, such as asthma, pneumonia, or drug ingestion. If the process cannot be quickly reversed, then artificial ventilatory support will be needed. A primary respiratory acidosis is never corrected by administration of bicarbonate since this will only worsen the problem.

Respiratory Alkalosis. Primary respiratory alkalosis is caused by acute hypoxia, specific toxins such as aspirin, or acute anxiety. Caution should be used whenever the diagnosis of psychogenic hyperventilation is made and it should be reserved as a diagnosis of exclusion in unfamiliar patients. Treatment of true hyperventilation is through correction of the underlying problem and not administration of organic acids. Psychogenic hyperventilation can be managed through rebreathing of exhaled CO_2 to raise the plasma carbon dioxide. This should only be accomplished with a non-rebreather mask using supplemental O_2 administration. Rebreathing exhaled gases with a device such as a paper bag should be avoided as this has been shown to lead to hypoxia, as well as hypercarbia.

Mixed Acid-Base Disturbances. In assessing acid-base problems the primary process will produce the pH deviation, while the body's compensatory response will try to return the pH back to 7.40. Since the driving force is the abnormal pH, the compensatory mechanism will never overcorrect the pH. Hence the pH will always point to the primary underlying process. In a primary acidosis, the pH will always be less than 7.35, while in a primary alkalosis, the pH will always be above 7.45. This is why determination of the pH is necessary for determination of the cause of an acid-base disturbance. Mixed acid-base disturbances occur when more than one primary process is involved. To assess mixed acid-base disturbances an acidemia or alkalemia must be determined by assessing the patient's pH, arterial $P{CO_2}$, and measured serum bicarbonate. For each primary acid-base disturbance an expected compensation can be calculated (Table 15-4). Using these values the expected compensatory changes can be calculated. If these values do not correlate with those determined for the patient, a second primary acid-base disturbance is acting. As an example, consider an acute aspirin ingestion with an

TABLE 15-5. Concentration of Electrolytes in Gastrointestinal Fluids (mEq/L)

Fluid source	H^+	Na^+	K^+	Cl^-	HCO_3^-
Gastric	90	20-80	5-20	100-150	—
Pancreas	—	120-140	5-40	50-120	90
Small intestine	—	100-140	15-40	90-130	25
Diarrhea	—	10-90	10-80	10-110	45

arterial pH of 7.46, a P_{CO_2} of 24 mm Hg, and an HCO_3^- of 16 mEq/L. The alkalemic pH would indicate an alkalosis and the P_{CO_2} of 24 mm Hg would imply a primary respiratory alkalosis. The low bicarbonate might simply represent the normal compensation to the respiratory alkalosis. However, the expected HCO_3^- for a patient with an acute lowering of the P_{CO_2} to 24 mm Hg can be calculated as:

The drop in P_{CO_2} is 40 mm Hg − 24 mm Hg = 16 mm Hg

Using Table 15-5 the expected compensation in HCO_3^- would be:

$$\text{Expected } HCO_3^- = 0.2 \text{ mEq/L for every 1 mm Hg drop in } P_{CO_2}$$
$$= 0.2 \times 16 = 3.2 \text{ mEq/L}$$

This would imply that the serum bicarbonate in this patient should have fallen from a normal of 24 mEq/L to 20.8 mEq/L (24 mEq/L − 3.2 mEq/L) if only a primary respiratory alkalosis were present. Since the measured value was 16 mEq/L, it indicates that an additional primary acidosis is present along with the respiratory alkalosis.

Electrolyte Abnormalities

Beyond water and calories, normal metabolism also consumes solutes. The two major cations, sodium and potassium, are the primary determinants of the distribution of water between the ECF and ICF spaces. These compartments depend on active transport of potassium into cells and sodium out of cells by an energy-requiring process. Sodium is the major extracellular cation and is essential for maintenance of intravascular volume and cellular transmembrane potentials. Potassium is the major intracellular cation, which along with sodium maintains cellular transmembrane potentials. Concentrations of these anions fluctuate with water and fluid shift. Rapid or extreme changes in either of these ions can produce significant problems in infants and children. Some electrolyte changes may be detected clinically; however, most will require some evaluation of the patient's serum or plasma.

Sodium Homeostasis. Sodium is the primary extracellular cation and is the major determinant of both ECF volume and serum osmolality. Because of its location as an extracellular ion, sodium is very susceptible to changes resulting from acute solute or water losses.

Normal sodium balance is maintained through thirst and control of urinary sodium excretion. Hormonal, oncotic, and hydrostatic pressures all combine to maintain the total body sodium and water content within a relatively narrow range. It is not the serum sodium but the total body sodium that controls the ECF volume.

Sodium is maintained in the extracellular fluid through the actions of a membrane Na-K ATPase pump. This pump uses adenosine triphosphate to actively pump sodium against a concentration gradient from the intracellular space to the ECF. The Na-K exchange transports 3 Na^+ ions for every 2 K^+ ions leading to a relative negative intracellular charge in relation to the extracellular space. Normal intracellular sodium levels are approximately 20 to 40 mEq/L compared with the 135 to 150 mEq/L found in the extracellular compartment. As a consequence, a cell need only open Na^+-specific channels to allow sodium to follow both an electrical, as well as a concentration, gradient into the interior of the cell.[6]

The body monitors sodium content indirectly through the intravascular volume and osmolality. Afferent sensors are located in the atria, right ventricle, pulmonary interstitia, aorta, carotid arteries, kidneys, and the central nervous system. These receptors detect predominately vascular filling pressures and increase or decrease the amount of sodium retention by the kidneys accordingly. A decrease in intravascular pressure is interpreted by the afferent receptors as a loss in extracellular volume and prompts a cascade of urinary sodium retaining actions.[7,8]

Direct neuronal control of the kidney increases active reabsorption of sodium in renal tubules. The juxtaglomerular cells of the kidney produce and secrete the enzyme renin in response to a decrease in glomerular arteriole pressure. Renin converts angiotensinogen to angiotensin I. Angiotensin I is further converted to angiotensin II by a converting enzyme located in the lungs. Angiotensin II has two major actions: stimulation of sodium resorption in the early proximal tubule of the kidney and increased secretion of aldosterone from the adrenal cortex. Aldosterone diffuses into tubular cells in the kidney where it binds with specific receptors on the nuclear chromatin. This binding enhances production of messenger RNA for the synthesis of aldosterone-induced proteins (AIP). A number of different AIPs are produced but at least one is believed to be the Na-K ATPase pump of the renal cell basal membrane. The net effect of aldosterone's action is an increase in renal absorption of sodium and renal secretion of potassium.[7] In addition, angiotensin II is a direct-acting arteriolar vasoconstriction and a stimulant for the release of norepinephrine.

When sodium is lost through pathologic processes such as vomiting or diarrhea, a decrease in ECF volume occurs, triggering these conservation mechanisms.

In contrast, when intravascular pressure is elevated and ECF volume is interpreted as increased, these systems are dampened and factors to increase sodium excretion are produced, the most potent of these hormones being atrial natriuretic factor or peptide. Produced by the atria of the heart and right ventricle this small peptide is a potent vasodilator and inhibitor of sodium reabsorption.

Hyponatremia. Since sodium is the predominant determinant of serum osmolality, any significant hyponatremia must also include significant hyposmolality as well. Low plasma sodium concentrations may exist in all states of hydration. Hyponatremia with a normal or increased ECF volume most commonly occurs as a result of excessive free-water ingestion relative to salt intake. Alternatively,

Abnormalities of Sodium Homeostasis

Hyponatremia
A. Normal or increased total body sodium*
  1. Primary polydipsia
  2. Hypotonic feedings
  3. Reset osmostat
    a. Psychosis
    b. Pregnancy
    c. Quadriplegia
  4. CHF
  5. Cirrhosis
  6. Hypoalbuminemia
    a. Nephrotic syndrome
    b. Malnutrition
  7. Hypokalemia
  8. Renal failure
  9. SIADH
    a. Secondary to pulmonary disease, head trauma, drugs, hypoglycemic and antineoplastic medications
  10. Hypothyroidism
B. Decreased total body sodium*
  1. Volume depletion
    a. Gastrointestinal losses
      1. Vomiting
      2. Diarrhea
      3. Tube draining
      4. Third spacing, i.e., pancreatitis or peritonitis
    b. Renal losses
      1. Diuretics
      2. Hypoaldosteronism/adrenal hyperplasia
      3. Na^+-wasting nephropathy
      4. Renal tubular acidosis
    c. Skin losses
      1. Burns
      2. Cystic fibrosis
    d. Cerebral salt wasting
    e. Decreased salt intake

Hypernatremia
A. Normal or increased total body sodium*
  1. Abnormal salt intake
    a. Salt ingestion
    b. Hypertonic NaCl or $NaHCO_3$ administration
B. Decreased total body sodium*
  1. Abnormality in water regulation
    a. Excessive loss
      1. Increased insensible losses
      2. Respiratory infections
      3. Burns
      4. Lack of access to water
  2. Gastrointestinal losses
    a. Diarrhea (loss may be isotonic but replacement is hypertonic)
    b. Vomiting
    c. Osmotic diarrhea
  3. Renal water loss
    a. Diabetes insipidus (central and nephrogenic)
    b. Osmotic diuretics (mannitol)
    c. Urinary tract obstruction
  4. Hypothalamic abnormalities
    a. Primary hypodipsia
    b. Essential hypernatremia
    c. Intracellular water transfer
      1. Seizures
      2. Exercise
      3. Rhabdomyolysis

Pseudohyponatremia
A. Normal osmolality states
  1. Severe hyperlipidemia
  2. Severe hyperproteinemia
B. Elevated osmolality states
  1. Hyperglycemia
  2. Mannitol, urea, glycerol administration

*Total body sodium controls TBW not sodium concentration. As total body Na^+ increases, TBW also increases.

abnormalities in the normal osmolality homeostasis mechanisms may result from inappropriate antidiuretic hormone secretion, a reset osmostat or inability of the kidneys to excrete free water or reabsorb filtered sodium. As opposed to states of excess total body free water, hyponatremia secondary to excessive sodium losses generally results in a decrease in total body fluid volume.[7,12]

The most common causes of euvolemic hyponatremia is excess free-water ingestion. In older children this may result from primary polydipsia, while in infants it is usually secondary to maternal feeding of hyponatremic solutions. Other causes include the syndrome of inappropriate antidiuretic hormone (SIADH), diuretic use, CHF, hypothyroidism, chronic renal failure, nephrotic syndrome, adrenal insufficiency, tricyclic antidepressants, and hypokalemia. The causes of hyponatremia are listed in the box above.

Hypovolemic hyponatremia results when isotonic fluid is lost but inadequately replaced with a relatively salt poor solution. Hyponatremic dehydration can occur from vomiting, diarrhea, renal losses, and diuretic use.[13]

Pseudohyponatremia occurs when the serum sodium concentration is low, but the serum osmolality is normal or elevated. In these cases another solute has replaced the sodium ion to maintain serum osmolality. Examples of pseudohyponatremia occur with severe hyperlipidemia, severe hyperproteinemia, hyperglycemia, and mannitol or urea administration. In hyperglycemic states the serum sodium level may fall 1.6 mEq/L for each 100 mg/dl rise in the serum glucose level.[14]

The management of hyponatremia is determined by the patient's underlying pathophysiology. Patients with life-threatening manifestations of hyponatremia should receive intravenous (IV) 3% saline solution (0.5 mEq/ml) at the rate of 4 ml/kg over 10 minutes to a maximum of 10 ml/kg over 1 hour. The administration of hypertonic saline requires close monitoring of the serum sodium levels. In stable patients whose hyponatremia is secondary to water intoxication and not a sodium deficit, treatment may be limited to only water ingestion restriction.

In moderately symptomatic patients, furosemide 1 mg/kg/dose IV may be administered. During the subsequent diuresis, urinary sodium, potassium, and chloride concentrations can be measured and replaced milliequivalent for milliequivalent. Replacement can be with either normal saline solution or 3% saline with 20 mEq/L of potassium chloride added to the solution. In patients over 8 years of age whose hyponatremia is the result of chronic severe SIADH, demeclocycline may be useful. See the box on p. 186 for a further discussion on the management of hypotonic dehydration.

Hypernatremia. Hypernatremia is defined as a serum sodium greater than 145 mEq/L. The normal body defense mechanisms against hypernatremia is the release of ADH and the development of increased thirst. Both appear to be modulated by osmoreceptors in the hypothalamus. Thirst is the predominant protector against the development of hypernatremia. Hypernatremia virtually never develops in an alert cognitive individual with access to water and a normal thirst mechanism. However, infants and small children do not have such ad lib access to water and even with intact regulatory systems may develop hypernatremia.[7]

The most common cause of hypernatremia in children is acute hypotonic fluid loss as a result of vomiting or diarrhea. In these instances the TBW is depleted and the child becomes hypovolemic with decreased Na^+ and water excretion in the urine. In contrast, excessive salt intake, either accidental or intentional, can produce hypernatremia with a normal or increased TBW content.[9] Urinary sodium excretion in these patients will be elevated, and they may exhibit signs of total body fluid overload such as CHF. A single tablespoon of salt administered to an infant can raise the plasma sodium concentration up to 70 mEq/L. Intentional salt poisoning should be considered with unexplained hypernatremia. The causes of hypernatremia are summarized in the box on p. 171.

In patients with hypertonic dehydration, the amount of free-water deficit must be estimated based on the serum sodium concentration.[10] As a rule a free-water deficit of 4 ml/kg can be expected for every mEq/L of sodium over 145 mEq/L.[11]

Clinically, hypernatremia presents with predominately neurologic symptoms. Lethargy, weakness, altered mental status, irritability, and seizures may all be seen. Most of the symptoms result from the abnormally high sodium concentrations in the extracellular fluid drawing water from brain cells and producing an intracellular dehydration. To counteract this effect the brain cells will increase synthesis of small organic and amino acids. These osmolytes will increase intracellular osmolality in an attempt to maintain intracellular volume.[11] When again exposed to free water, these osmotically active particles can lead to overhydration of the brain cell and severe neurologic sequelae. Additional findings with hypernatremia include muscle cramps, depressed deep tendon reflexes, and respiratory failure.

Management of severe hypernatremia is through a slow decrease in sodium concentration with replacement of hypotonic electrolyte solutions. Rapid correction of hypernatremia produces devastating cerebral edema as free water flows rapidly into dehydrated hyperosmolar brain cells. Seizures, permanent neurologic damage, and death can occur with too rapid a restoration of serum sodium levels. Patients in shock may require immediate resuscitation with a 10 to 20 ml/kg bolus of isotonic saline. Once the shock state has been addressed the fluid management should be sharply curtailed and a very slow rehydration performed. In patients whose hypernatremia is the result of sodium overload, no dehydration is present and treatment can be accomplished through administration of a diuretic and oral replacement of free water.[6] See the box on p. 187 for a discussion of the management of hypertonic dehydration.

Potassium Homeostasis. Potassium is the primary intracellular cation and essential for the control of intracellular volume and osmolality. Potassium's role in the homeostasis of the intracellular compartment roughly parallels that of sodium in the extracellular compartment. Because of its intracellular location, serum potassium levels are very poor indicators of the body's total potassium stores; only 1.5% to 2.0% of the total body potassium is extracellular. Normal intracellular potassium concentrations are approximately 140 mEq/L compared with extracellular levels of 4 to 5 mEq/L. Electrical neutrality of the intracellular fluid is maintained by phosphates and proteins. Intracellular potassium stores are maintained though the Na-K ATPase pump located on the cell membrane. As noted above, ATP is used to pump Na^+ out of the cell against both a chemical and electrical gradient, while at the same time moving K^+ against a similar concentration gradient into the cell. The cations are exchanged in a 3:2 ratio of Na^+ to K^+. Potassium is essential for maintaining resting membrane potentials and the transmission of neuronal impulses but also plays a role in protein and glycogen synthesis.[6,7]

Potassium balance is maintained through a combination of electrophysiologic and endocrine activities. Plasma potassium concentrations respond directly to increases or decreases in total body potassium levels. As the plasma level increases potassium diffuses passively into cells. Conversely, as K^+ levels fall potassium passively diffuses back out of cells offsetting the drop in plasma levels. When potassium is lost in a process such as gastroenteritis total body potassium stores are depleted and not just extracellular potassium. Pathologic processes may also affect the transcellular movement of potassium directly producing plasma potassium levels opposite those of total body stores.

The activity of the Na-K ATPase pump is the primary determinant of potassium homeostasis. The pump itself responds to a number of different chemical and hormonal stimuli.

Renal excretion of potassium is the major determinant of resting plasma K^+ concentrations. Aldosterone appears to be the primary determinant of this K^+ homeostasis by regulating the activity of the Na-K ATPase pump in the basolateral membrane of the kidney and regulating Na^+ and K^+ channels in the luminal membrane. Aldosterone promotes potassium loss through decreasing its absorption from the lumen of the kidney's tubules in exchange for reabsorption of sodium.

Catecholamines, especially beta 2-adrenergic stimulation, increase the activity of the Na-K pump with enhanced K^+ uptake predominately in skeletal muscle. Alpha stimulation decreases pump activity to a lesser degree. Insulin produces similar effects on the Na-K ATPase pump activity but also stimulates movement of potassium into the liver. This effect on K^+ is independent of glucose movement. Since beta-agonists also stimulate release of insulin, some of the effects of the catecholamines and insulin may overlap. The action of both of these agents responds to a specific potassium load rather than maintenance of baseline plasma concentrations.

Another determinant of plasma potassium concentrations is the extracellular pH. As the plasma hydrogen ion concentration rises it diffuses across the cell membrane into the intracellular compartment and is buffered. Since chloride ions cannot diffuse readily into cells, an equivalent number of positive cations must be displaced back into the extracellular space to maintain electrical neutrality. Both sodium and potassium ions move across the cellular membrane, but since the concentration of potassium is so much greater in the intracellular compartment the loss of potassium ions is much higher. In general a rise or fall of the pH of 0.1 units will change the plasma potassium concentration an average of 0.5 mEq/L with a range of 0.2 to 1.7 mEq/L.[5,7]

Exercise produces a release of potassium from skeletal muscle cells and a local increase in plasma potassium levels. Hyperosmolality also increases plasma potassium (0.4 to 0.8 mEq/L for every 10 mosmol/kg) through passive movement of potassium with water shifts from the intracellular to extracellular compartment. This phenomenon, termed *solvent drag*, then exposes the potassium to renal loss resulting in a total body potassium deficit in the face of a normal or elevated plasma K^+ concentration.[7]

Hypokalemia. Hypokalemia results from either a decreased intake or increased loss of potassium. The causes of hypokalemia are listed in the box on p. 174.

Because potassium is well absorbed from the GI tract and potassium is relatively common in most diets, decreased intake is usually only a problem when an extraneous substance binds the potassium and prevents absorption. The most common cause of this is clay ingestion, which can be common in some areas of the southeastern United States.

Plasma hypokalemia can appear with normal total body potassium if the K^+ is shifted intracellularly. The most common causes of such transcellular movements include metabolic alkalosis, insulin administration, and beta-adrenergic activity. Pseudohypokalemia can occur if blood specimens containing large numbers of metabolically active cells are permitted to remain at room temperature for any period of time. Usually associated with myeloid leukemias, this is generally termed "leukocyte larceny" and may involve plasma glucose and oxygen as well.[15]

Gastrointestinal loss is the most common source of total body potassium loss. Urinary losses may result from diuretic use or mineralocorticoid excess. Excessive aldosterone usually results from an aldosterone-secreting tumor, hypersecretion of renin, Cushing disease, or congenital adrenal hyperplasia. Potassium–wasting adrenal hyperplasia results from defective 17-alpha hydroxylase or 11-beta hydroxylase. Both of these defects produce an excess of a

mineralocorticoid with significant aldosterone-like actions. Other causes of hypokalemia include Bartters syndrome and excessive licorice ingestion. Glycyrrhetinic acid, a steroid in licorice, has slight aldosterone-like actions but also inhibits the enzyme 11-beta hydroxysteroid dehydrogenase, which can then mimic a primary hyperaldosteronism like state.[8]

Hypomagnesemia prevents effective renal conservation of potassium and is a common cause of hypokalemia unresponsive to potassium replacement.[16] Salt-wasting nephropathies, increased sweat loss, vitamin B-12 or folic acid therapy, and dialysis are other causes of hypokalemia.

Hypokalemia is clinically manifest primarily in muscle cell dysfunction. Skeletal muscle weakness or paralysis, ileus, and cardiac dysrhythmias are all common presentations. In severe cases, rhabdomyolysis can even result. Renal abnormalities include impairment of acidification, concentration, bicarbonate absorption, and sodium reabsorption. ECGs demonstrate delayed depolarization of myocardial cells with flat or absent T waves and in extreme cases the formation of U waves.

The immediate treatment of hypokalemia is potassium supplementation. If the serum potassium is only slightly depressed and the patient is not vomiting, then an oral potassium suspension of 0.2 to 0.3 mEq/kg may be attempted. More severe cases of hypokalemia, in the range of less than 3.0 mEq/L, can be treated with infusions of 0.1 to 0.2 mEq/kg/hr of KCl supplementing a primary IV infusion. If the patient is on digitalis or has myocarditis, treatment should be done cautiously. If life-threatening dysrhythmias are noted, potassium may be given IV at 0.2 to 0.3 mEq K^+/kg/hr. Dysrhythmias may also be treated with rapid magnesium sulfate infusions to offset the slow rate of potassium administration. The typical $MgSO_4$ bolus is 25 to 50 mg/kg diluted in 25 to 50 ml of normal saline solution. All potassium infusions must be controlled by an IV pump and rates in excess of 0.1 mEq/kg/hr should be delivered through a central venous catheter in a monitored setting. If burning presents a problem with peripheral infusions a small amount of lidocaine may be injected into the tourniqueted vein before delivery of the potassium.[17]

Hyperkalemia. Because the kidney secretes potassium efficiently, hyperkalemia is a less common but much more serious problem than hypokalemia. The most common causes of hyperkalemia are listed in the box on p. 174.

Potassium supplementation is the most frequent cause of hyperkalemia. Generally seen in adults, this is becoming more common in children as the result of increasing interest in herbal preparation rich in potassium.

Plasma hyperkalemia secondary to movement of potassium from the intracellular to the extracellular compartment is a common cause of hyperkalemia. Insulin deficiency and hyperosmolality may combine to produce large extracellular shifts of potassium as with hyperglycemia and diabetes mellitus. Metabolic acidosis and severe exercise can raise plasma levels as can certain drugs, including digitalis, succinylcholine, spironolactone, and cyclosporine. Pseudohyperkalemia occurs when intracellular potassium leaks into the serum of a blood sample as a result of red cell hemolysis.[8]

Decreased urinary excretion of potassium occurs commonly in patients with renal failure and is a major source of

Abnormalities of Potassium Homeostasis

Hypokalemia

A. Decreased intake
1. Low K$^+$ foods
2. Persistent vomiting
3. Clay ingestion
B. Extracellular to Intracellular shifting
1. Alkalosis
2. Beta-adrenergic stimulation
3. Insulin excess
4. B$_{12}$-Folic acid administration
5. Hypokalemic paralysis
6. Hypothermia
C. Increased gastrointestinal losses
1. Diarrhea
2. Vomiting
3. NG tube suction
D. Urinary losses
1. Diuretics
2. Excess aldosterone
a. Adrenal hyperplasia:
17-alpha hydroxylase deficiency
11-beta hydroxylase deficiency
b. Adenoma/carcinoma
c. Hyperreninism
3. Salt-wasting nephropathies
4. Hypomagnesemia
5. Drug therapy:
Amphotericin B, L-dopa
6. Polyuria
E. Dialysis
F. Periodic paralysis—hypokalemic form

Pseudohypokalemia

A. Leukocyte larceny

Hyperkalemia

A. Increased potassium intake (oral/parenteral)
B. Intracellular to extracellular shifting
1. Acidosis
2. Insulin deficiency
3. Hyperosmolality
a. Hyperglycemia
b. Mannitol administration
4. Beta-receptor blockade
5. Severe exercise
6. Periodic paralysis—hyperkalemic form
7. Drugs
a. Digitalis
b. Succinylcholine
c. Arginine
8. Tissue catabolism
C. Decreased urinary excretion
1. Renal failure
a. Chronic
b. Acute
c. Obstructive uropathy
2. Hypoaldosteronism
a. Renin-angiotensin abnormality
1. ACE inhibitor
2. NSAID
b. Decreased synthesis
1. Adrenal hyperplasia 21-hydroxylase deficiency
2. Primary adrenal insufficiency
c. Others
1. Heparin
2. Isolated hypoaldosteronism
d. Aldosterone resistance
1. Potassium-sparing diuretics
2. Pseudohypoaldosteronism
3. Renal tubular acidosis
4. Selective potassium secretory defect

acute decompensation. Dehydration with reduced renal blood flow can result in significant hyperkalemia but usually only occurs in severely dehydrated children. Hypoaldosterone can occur from a number of sources. Decreased renin-angiotensin activity can result from converting enzyme inhibitors, hypervolemia, and NSAIDs. Congenital adrenal hyperplasia usually associated with a 21-hydroxylase deficiency is the most common pediatric cause of a salt-wasting inborn error of metabolism.

Other causes of hyperkalemia include potassium-sparing diuretics, heparin use, primary adrenal insufficiency, and urinary obstruction.

Clinically, hyperkalemia produces symptoms of muscle weakness, fatigue, depressed deep tendon reflexes, paralysis, and confusion. Prominent peaked T waves may be seen on ECG and in severe cases a widened QRS complex and bradycardia. Complete loss of QRS morphology and the appearance of a sine wave pattern may appear in patients with severe potassium toxicity.

Treatment of hyperkalemia depends on the patient's symptoms and the cause of the elevated potassium. Patients whose hyperkalemia has developed over an extended period are better able to tolerate the high plasma potassium concentration than those who develop hyperkalemia acutely. Unstable patients require immediate aggressive treatment with an IV bolus of a 10% solution of calcium chloride (0.2 to 0.3 ml) (20 to 30 mg)/kg/dose, maximum 5 ml or 500 mg/dose. Such a bolus will restore normal cardiac activity within minutes. A second bolus may be required in patients with potassium levels in excess of 8 mEq/L. Calcium therapy should be immediately followed with a glucose load of 0.5 to 1 gm/kg followed by 1 unit of insulin for every 4 gm of glucose infused. It may be repeated every 10 to 30 minutes. In patients who are not

---

Treatment of Life-Threatening Hyperkalemia

- Cardiac monitor
- Vascular access
- Calcium chloride (10%) 0.2 ml/kg IV bolus.
    May be repeated if insufficient response in 10 minutes
    Avoid in patients in which digoxin toxicity is a possibility
- Dextrose 0.5 to 1.0 gm/kg IV followed by 1 unit of regular insulin IV for every 4 gm of glucose infused.
    May be repeated every 30 minutes.
- Sodium Bicarbonate 0.5-1.0 mEq/kg
    Use with caution in patients in CHF
- Albuterol nebulization (0.5 ml of 20% solution with 5 ml saline)
- Polystyrene sulfonate (Kayexelate)

Disorders of Calcium Homeostasis

Hypocalcemia
A. Hypoparathyroidism
    Decreased PTH
    Ineffective PTH response
B. Vitamin D deficiency
C. Hyperphosphatemia
D. Pancreatitis
E. Malabsorption states
    Malnutrition
F. Drug therapy
    Anticonvulsants
G. Hypomagnesemia

Hypercalcemia
A. Hyperparathyroidism
B. Vitamin D Intoxication
C. Malignancy
D. Prolonged immobilization
E. Diuretics
    Thiazides

---

overtly fluid overloaded or at risk for congestive heart failure a sodium bicarbonate bolus of 0.5 to 1.0 mEq/kg may be administered to raise the extracellular pH and drive the potassium into the intracellular space. Beta-adrenergic agents may lower plasma potassium concentrations; nebulized albuterol solutions can be used to acutely treat hyperkalemic patients in whom vascular access is unachievable but is not adequate as a sole agent. Once cardiovascular stability has been restored excess potassium can be bound through administration of a potassium-binding resin such as polystyrene sulfonate (Kayexelate). Kayexelate is an ion-exchange resin and may be given as 1 gm/kg/dose q 4-6 hours, preferably mixed with 70% sorbitol PO (by NG tube) or PR. For newborns, give 1 gm/kg/dose with Kayexelate dissolved in 10% dextrose to make a 25% solution. The box above summarizes the treatment of life-threatening hyperkalemia (also see Chapter 60).

In patients whose hyperkalemia is the result of an obstructive uropathy, hyperkalemia quickly resolves once the obstruction is relieved and normal urine flow is established. Digitalis associated hyperkalemia accompanied by life-threatening dysrhythmias can be managed through the administration of digoxin-specific antibody fragments (see Chapter 42).[18] Patients with excess total body potassium and nonreversible renal failure will require some form of dialysis.

Calcium Homeostasis. Calcium regulation is under tight hormonal control involving the intestines, bone, and kidneys. The vast majority of total body calcium is bound with phosphorus in bone as hydroxyapatite, but it is plasma-ionized calcium concentration that is regulated by the body.

In the plasma, calcium exists as the divalent cation, Ca^{++}. Forty percent of ionized calcium is bound to protein, mostly albumin; 10% complexed with citrate, bicarbonate, or phosphate; and 50% as free-ionized Ca^{++}. It is this free-ionized calcium that is physiologically most active. Plasma calcium and phosphate metabolism are directly linked and vary inversely with the concentration of each other.

Because it is the ionized calcium that is physiologically active, low serum calcium levels can be well tolerated in the face of concomitant low albumin levels. Normal plasma calcium levels range between 8.8 to 10.8 mg/dl and the normal phosphate levels range between 2.9 to 5.4 mg/dl. Elevation of plasma pH will increase albumin binding of ionized calcium; decreases in pH lower albumin binding.[19]

As free-ionized calcium levels fall, the parathyroid glands secrete parathyroid hormone (PTH). PTH works to increase plasma calcium levels but requires adequate amounts of vitamin D to function effectively. In the presence of sufficient vitamin D, PTH stimulates bone resorption with the release of calcium phosphate. Concurrently, PTH stimulates the kidneys to increase calcium resorption while promoting phosphate excretion; raising plasma calcium with little to no change in plasma phosphate concentrations. If vitamin D is present it is converted to 1,25 dihydroxycholecalciferol or calcitriol by the kidney. Calcitriol increases intestinal absorption of both calcium and phosphate further increasing plasma calcium levels. Although PTH stimulates phosphate excretion, calcitriol decreases urinary loss of phosphate. Plasma hypophosphatemia stimulates calcitriol production but not PTH release. Calcitriol is also an inhibitor of further PTH release providing a negative feedback loop. Thus hypophosphatemia produces an increase in plasma phosphates but little or no change in plasma calcium levels.

Ionized calcium is essential for both proper neuronal and muscle function. Abnormalities of calcium concentration are generally manifest by muscle and CNS symptoms.

Hypocalcemia. Hypocalcemia generally produces symptoms of increased muscle and neuron irritability. Causes of hypocalcemia are listed in the box above.

Hypocalcemia may result from dietary deficiencies of either calcium or vitamin D. In addition, defects in any portion of vitamin D metabolism or activity will also result in a decrease in ionized calcium. Causes to be considered for abnormal calcitriol metabolism include anticonvulsant therapy, malabsorption syndromes, and lack of sunlight exposure. Because of its negative feedback loop on vitamin D, hyperphosphatemia will also lower plasma calcium concentrations directly. In chronic renal failure patients, this may lead to pseudohyperparathyroidism and chronic hypocalcemia. Noncalcitriol-mediated hypocalcemia may result from defects in parathyroid hormone synthesis or release. Hypoparathyroidism may be acquired or congenital. Other causes of hypocalcemia include hypomagnesemia, rhabdomyolysis, and soft tissue precipitation in pancreatitis.

Clinically, hypocalcemia produces neuromuscular irritability with weakness, paresthesia, fatigue, cramping, and altered mental status. Life-threatening signs include seizures, laryngospasm, and cardiac dysrhythmias. Severe hypocalcemia will produce a prolonged QT interval on the ECG. Hypocalcemia may be detected by carpal pedal spasm after arterial occlusion of an extremity for 3 minutes (Trousseau's sign) or percussion of the facial nerve with muscle twitching (Chvostek's sign). If the calcium deficiency is extended, chronic skeletal findings may be present that include joint swelling of the ankles, wrists, and chostochondral junctions. The prominent appearance of the sternum with this condition is the so-called "rosary bead sign" of rickets.

Emergency treatment of hypocalcemia consists of prompt calcium replacement with 0.5 to 1.0 ml/kg of a 10% solution of calcium gluconate or 0.2 ml/kg of a 10% solution of calcium chloride administered over approximately 5 minutes. A second bolus may be indicated in patients experiencing cardiac dysrhythmias or seizures and should be followed with an infusion of calcium gluconate 500 mg/kg/24 hr (5 ml of 10% calcium gluconate solution) usually in 4 to 6 separate doses. Intravenous calcium can produce hypotension and bradycardia so it should be administered with caution and cardiac monitoring. Bolus therapy of calcium can also worsen digitalis-induced cardiac dysrhythmias. A 10% solution of calcium gluconate contains 100 mg/ml of salt with each gram of salt containing 90 mg (4.5 mEq) of calcium. Oral maintenance therapy can be accomplished with 200 to 500 mg/kg/dose of calcium gluconate every 6 hours.

Hypercalcemia. Hypercalcemia may result from either underlying endocrine abnormalities or an occult malignancy. The box on p. 175 lists the causes of hypercalcemia.

Excessive calcium ingestion will not usually lead to hypercalcemia; decreased intestinal absorption and renal excretion limit plasma calcium levels. Hormonal abnormalities, including either excessive parathyroid hormone or vitamin D will both produce hypercalcemia. In PTH excess there will be evidence of extensive bone resorption with lytic lesions and demineralization on x-ray examination. By contrast, vitamin D-induced hypercalcemia results from overabsorption of calcium and produces abnormal soft tissue calcifications and elevated phosphate levels. Since cortical bone requires some degree of stress for maintenance and new bone formation, prolonged immobilization

will result in reabsorption of bone and hypercalcemia. Malignancy-produced hypercalcemia is more common in adults than children but may be seen in cases involving metastasis to bone and PTH or hormone-secreting tumors.

Symptoms of hypercalcemia may be similar to those of hypocalcemia, including weakness, irritability, lethargy, seizures, and coma. Abdominal cramping, anorexia, nausea, vomiting, polyuria, and polydipsia may be noted. Urinary concentration defects in conjunction with decreased intake can produce severe dehydration. Ectopic calcifications, including renal calculi and pancreatitis, can produce painful conditions. Shortening of the QT interval may be seen on ECG examination.

Treatment of hypercalcemia states is aimed at restoration of normal circulating volumes, as well as finding the underlying cause. Fluid resuscitation with a bolus of normal saline, 10 to 20 ml/kg should be administered immediately in any child in shock. Continued overhydration at 1.5 to 2 times maintenance fluid therapy should continue while beginning treatment to promote calcium excretion. Loop diuretics should be administered (furosemide; 1 mg/kg/dose) only after adequate fluid hydration. In malignancy-induced hypercalcemia, treatment with mithramycin is generally employed.[19]

Although theoretically IV phosphates should produce a decrease in ionized calcium levels, administration of these agents should be avoided acutely since ectopic calcifications and sudden death have been reported.

Magnesium Homeostasis. Magnesium is an essential co-factor for many enzymes and protein synthesis systems, including both DNA and ATP synthesis. Although mostly bound in either bone (65%) or protein (34%), only 1% of ionized magnesium remains in the extracellular fluid and up to 30% of this is protein bound. Free-ionized magnesium does have some membrane effects generally operating as an intracellular divalent cation. Normal serum magnesium levels range between 1.5 and 2.5 mEq/L but poorly reflect total body magnesium. Low levels are consistent with hypomagnesemia; however, normal levels may exist in the face of total body magnesium depletion. Magnesium homeostasis is maintained through renal excretion and absorption and seems to parallel potassium maintenance. Conditions that promote potassium loss such as diuretics, aldosterone, and stress will also result in decreased renal magnesium reabsorption. Consequently, many critically ill patients are magnesium depleted and up to 65% of all intensive care unit admissions may require acute magnesium replacement.[20,21]

Hypomagnesemia. Hypomagnesemia results from either increased renal excretion or decreased gastrointestinal absorption. The box on p. 177 lists the causes of abnormal magnesium homeostasis. Diuretics, chronic stress, and hyperadrenergic states are primary causes of renal magnesium loss. Malabsorption and increased gastrointestinal loss are frequent causes of total body magnesium depletion.

Clinically hypomagnesemia may be very subtle and difficult to detect. Anorexia, nausea, weakness, malaise, depression, and nonspecific psychiatric symptoms have all been reported. Because free magnesium does have electrochemical effects on neuronal and muscle cell membranes,

---

Disorders of Magnesium Homeostasis

Hypomagnesemia

A. Increased urinary loss
   1. Diuretic use
   2. Renal tubular acidosis
   3. Hypercalcemia
   4. Chronic adrenergic stimulants
B. Gastrointestinal
   1. Malabsorption syndromes
   2. Diarrhea/vomiting
   3. Severe malnutrition
   4. Short bowel syndromes
      a. Enteric fistula
C. Endocrine
   1. Diabetes mellitus
   2. PTH disorders
   3. Hyperaldosterone states

Hypermagnesemia

A. Renal failure
B. Excessive administration
   1. Eclampsia/preeclampsia states
   2. Cathartics
   3. Enemas

---

signs similar to hypocalcemia may be present. There is evidence that hypomagnesemia secondary to chronic beta-agonist use in asthmatics may contribute to severe bronchospastic episodes. Hypomagnesemic patients may have hyperreflexia, carpopedal spasm, clonus, and frank tetany.[22] Electrocardiographically, both atrial and ventricular ectopy may be present and hypomagnesemia has been shown to be a cause of torsades de pointes.[23]

Initial treatment of symptomatic hypomagnesemia is prompt replacement. Because up to 99% of magnesium is intracellular, replacement therapy must be tailored for prolonged replacement of a total body deficit. Bolus therapy can begin with 25 to 50 mg/kg of $MgSO_4$ diluted in 25 to 100 ml of a normal saline solution. In extreme conditions this may be given as a direct IV bolus but more commonly is infused over 20 to 30 minutes. Maintenance therapy consists of 100 to 200 mg/kg/24 hr as part of the patient's IV therapy.

Hypermagnesemia. The kidneys are extremely efficient in excreting magnesium and under conditions of normal intake, hypermagnesemia only occurs with severe renal failure. Extraneous administration of magnesium is the other major cause of hypermagnesemia. Magnesium sulfate therapy for toxemia of pregnancy has been known to produce hypermagnesemia in newborns; in older children overly aggressive use of magnesium-containing enemas or cathartics may elevate total body magnesium levels. Use of magnesium-containing antacids produces significant hypermagnesemia in renal dialysis patients. Causes of hypermagnesemia are listed in the box above.

Clinically, hypermagnesemia presents with depressed deep tendon reflexes, lethargy, confusion, and in extreme cases, respiratory failure. Treatment of elevated magnesium depends on the patient's renal function. In patients with functioning kidneys, forced diuresis with saline loading and a loop diuretic will rapidly return serum magnesium levels to normal. In unstable patients, administration of a calcium gluconate bolus, 0.5 to 1.0 ml/kg of 10% solution, can antagonize magnesium's effects. Patients with renal failure will require dialysis to remove excess total body magnesium.

DEHYDRATION

Fluid, electrolyte, and acid-base balance is maintained within a very narrow range by multiple compensatory mechanisms. Effective as these mechanisms are they can be overwhelmed in various disease conditions, resulting in severe morbidity and even mortality.

Dehydration is a diminution of the ECF volume, resulting from an imbalance of fluid and solute intake and output. Although dehydration is described in terms of the ECF compartment, it is important to remember that because of water's free movement any ECF dehydration includes a related degree of ICF dehydration.

Classification

Electrolyte disturbances are a major component of the metabolic abnormalities associated with dehydration. Categories of dehydration reflect serum sodium concentration. Isotonic (isonatremic) dehydration occurs with parallel losses of sodium and water from the extracellular fluid space producing a serum sodium level in the normal range. Hypertonic dehydration occurs as a result of a greater water than sodium loss producing a serum sodium above 145 mEq/L. Hypotonic dehydration occurs when salt losses exceed water losses and is defined by serum sodium less than 130 mEq/L.

Pathophysiology

Multiple diseases may lead to dehydration. Some disease states produce dehydration directly through increases in fluid or solute losses while others produce dehydration indirectly by interfering with adequate fluid or solute intake.

A common cause in children of inadequate intake leading to dehydration is respiratory illness. The anorexia associated with an illness itself can lead to enough of a decrease in feeding to produce dehydration. Respiratory distress may produce feeding problems by limiting the child's ability to both drink and breathe simultaneously. Deficits in fluid intake are amplified because of greater insensible losses associated with their tachypnea and any fever that may be present. Normal daily respiratory water losses may range from 40 ml/kg/24 hr in an infant to 10 ml/kg/24 hr in an adolescent. An increase in respiratory rate of 50% can double these losses through evaporative fluid loss and increased metabolism.[2] Dehydration associated with tachypnea and poor feeding may also occur in children with cyanotic congenital heart disease, anatomic malformations, primary pulmonary pathology, and CNS lesions.

In the absence of other underlying problems, children who are unable to tolerate adequate oral intake often develop a water deficit in excess of their solute deficit. Because the insensible water losses associated with respiration contain few solutes, these patients may develop hypernatremic dehydration.

Children with vomiting may have both insufficient fluid intake and excessive upper gastrointestinal fluid loss. The type of dehydration will reflect the etiology of the vomiting and the composition of the lost fluid. The concentration of electrolytes in gastrointestinal fluids is shown in Table 15-5.

A child with gastric outlet obstruction such as pyloric stenosis or duodenal hematoma will have emesis fluid composed of gastric secretions, containing a high concentration of H^+ and a low concentration of sodium. This produces an associated metabolic alkalosis and normal to high serum sodium. If vomiting persists in these children, a secondary lactic acidosis (due to hypoperfusion) may develop, exacerbating the initial metabolic alkalosis.

Without an anatomic upper gastrointestinal obstruction, children will generally vomit gastric and duodenal fluids. Duodenal secretions are rich in HCO_3^-. When vomiting-induced dehydration occurs in these children, a metabolic acidosis usually is present as a result of the HCO_3^--rich duodenal emesis.

Vomiting in children is typically infectious in origin and usually caused by a virus. As a viral agent invades the mucosal cells of the upper gastrointestinal tract, it disrupts the normal sodium and osmotic intracellular balance. ICF is lost, producing cellular fluid depletion. An ileus develops with resultant abdominal distension and further vomiting.

Reduced caloric intake associated with vomiting and inadequate fluid intake will produce a starvation catabolic state. Stored energy sources such as glycogen are mobilized and in small children quickly consumed. Fat becomes the primary source of calories for children in this state with short-chain hydrocarbon groups produced from long-chain fatty acids. As these acids are consumed, betahydroxybuterate and acetoacetate accumulate and an equilibrium with acetone develops. The ketonemia produces further vomiting worsening the dehydration. Starvation ketosis occurs in children even with mild dehydration, and those clinicians who can smell acetone will be able to detect this odor on the breath of these children.

Diarrhea is another source of fluid and electrolyte loss in gastrointestinal illness–related dehydration. The specific etiology of the diarrhea will influence the type of fluid and the duration of the illness. Toxin-producing bacteria, such as *Vibrio cholera* and enterotoxigenic *Escherichia coli*, cause a sodium- and chloride-rich diarrhea as a result of malabsorption and intestinal mucosal secretion. Invasive bacteria may destroy intestinal mucosa causing bloody diarrhea that contains high concentrations of sodium and bicarbonate. Viral enteritis produces a loss of villous epithelium cells in the small intestinal mucosa, which results in decreased absorption of salts and water.[1,25] Table 15-5 outlines the electrolyte concentration of diarrheal fluid.

Abnormalities in renal function may produce excessive electrolyte and water losses. Excessive osmotic loads to the kidneys may exceed the concentration gradients surrounding the renal tubules and prevent reabsorption of filtered water. Such osmotic drag results when an osmotically active particle, such as glucose, remains in the renal tubules and prevents the passive movement of water back from the lumen.[7] Dehydration may also result from loss of normal homeostatic hormonal mechanisms both within and external to the kidney. For example, absence of the hormone aldosterone removes the stimulus for sodium reabsorption creating a urine rich in Na^+ and inappropriately dilute.

Diagnostic Findings

A careful history will help determine the severity of illness and shed light on its etiology. Historic information should include any previous known weights for comparison with the child's present weight. For children with vomiting or diarrhea the relation to meals, amount and content of emesis or stool, presence of blood or bile, timing, and number of episodes should all be determined. The child's intake, including number, size, and content of feedings, should be established. Ultimately, the frequency and volume of urination is an excellent parameter to assess hydration status. Parents of infants routinely monitor diaper changes noting both changes in frequency or weight. Underlying medical problems may contribute to the child's condition.

Physical findings may be very variable in these patients. Evidence of acute fluid overload is generally evidenced by peripheral edema, elevated blood pressure, distended neck veins, and possibly congestive heart failure.

Dehydration is much more difficult to detect solely on physical examination, and few or no physical signs may be present.[26] Tables 15-6 and 15-7 summarize the characteristics associated with dehydration in children. In general these findings are very specific but not very sensitive. If physical findings are present, they may accurately indicate dehydration in a child. However, the absence of physical findings does not necessarily indicate normal hydration. Many dehydrated children continue to have tears, moist mucosal membranes, and even good skin turgor.[27] Tachycardia and tachypnea are early signs of mild-to-moderate dehydration but may be difficult to clearly document in an irritable, crying child. Hypotension is a very specific but a very late sign of dehydration. Children have excellent compensatory mechanisms for intravascular volume depletion and will maintain their blood pressures until frank shock develops. Orthostatic vital signs may be useful in older children, although they must be interpreted in the context of clinical signs and symptoms. Older children have decreased ECF compared to infants and may manifest their signs of dehydration earlier than infants.

The type of dehydration may also effect the physical diagnosis of the problem. Children with hypernatremic dehydration preserve extracellular volume and develop clinical signs of compromise later in the course of their illness. Children with hyponatremia have the opposite presentation and manifest physical signs earlier in their illness.[28]

Ancillary Data. In many children with specific hormonal or electrolyte abnormalities the history and physical exami-

TABLE 15-6. Signs of Dehydration

Clinical findings*	Fluid deficit (%)		
	Mild (≤5%)	Moderate (10%)	Severe (15%)
Mental status	Alert	Irritable	Lethargic
Eyes	Normal	Sunken	Glassy
Fontanelle	Normal	Flat	Sunken
Mucous membranes	Normal	Dry	Very Dry
Tears	Normal	Decreased	Absent
Thirst (drinks)	Normal	Eagerly	Poorly
Skin (pinch retraction)	Immediately	Slowly	Absent
Capillary refill†	<2 sec	2-3 sec	>3 sec
Urination (number wet diapers)	Normal	Fewer	None
Systolic BP	Normal	Normal‡	Abnormal
Heart rate	Normal	Rapid‡	Rapid

*Significant dehydration may be present in the absence of these findings.
†May be affected by external factors such as room temperature.
‡Orthostatic changes often present.

nation may suggest the type of problem, but it may not be truly identified until laboratory data are available. This is particularly true of electrolyte abnormalities in which the overlap of signs and symptoms is so great that clinical differentiation may not be possible. Weakness or fatigue, for example, can be caused by an excess or a deficit of most measurable serum cations. Children with metabolic errors or hormonal imbalances may be identified on physical examination if a classic syndrome is present, such as diabetic ketoacidosis. However, problems with more subtle presentation may go undetected until revealed by unexpected laboratory abnormalities. The box on p. 180 summarizes the role of commonly used laboratory tests in the evaluation of children with dehydration.

The routine use of laboratory studies to search for rare or atypical presentations of diseases should be discouraged in the emergency department. These tests are indicated in seriously ill children, those requiring admission, those in whom extended emergency or observation management is planned, and those not responding to treatment. Laboratory data are also indicated in patients in whom the treating physician suspects a problem based on an historic or physical finding.

An elevated serum blood urea nitrogen (BUN) is frequently regarded as indicative of dehydration but is an extremely poor indicator of hydration status. Children with vomiting or those receiving protein-poor clear liquids may not develop an increase in BUN despite significant extracellular fluid loss. A 50% decrease in glomerular filtration rate results in only a doubling of BUN and total anuria increases BUN just 1 mg %/hr.[29] The upper limit for normal BUN in infants and children is 18 mg/dl; however, in patients with a clinical picture of dehydration the upper limit of 10 mg/dl is more appropriate. Appropriate rehydration will normally result in a 50% decrease in the BUN level during the first day of treatment if there is no underlying renal problem. Serum creatinine levels are primarily

TABLE 15-7. Clinical Findings by Types of Dehydration

	Isotonic	Hypotonic	Hypertonic
Serum Sodium (mEq/L)	130-150	<130	>150
Physical signs			
Skin			
Color	Gray	Gray	Gray
Temperature	Cold	Cold	Cold
Turgor	Poor	Very poor	Fair
Feel	Dry	Clammy	Thick, doughy
Mucous membrane	Dry	Dry	Parched
Sunken eyeballs	+	+	+
Depressed anterior fontanelle	+	+	+
Mental status	Lethargic	Coma/seizure	Irritable/seizure
Increased pulse	+ +	+ +	+
Decreased blood pressure	+ +	+ + +	+

+, + +, + + + Relative prominence of finding.

used to assess renal function. An elevated creatinine level associated with other indications of dehydration may reflect renal dysfunction. Serum bicarbonate levels are used to assess the acid-base status as well as degree of dehydration. The presence of a decreased serum bicarbonate level, in conjunction with an increased anion gap, may indicate the presence of a lactic acidosis, secondary to hypoperfusion. Other causes of an elevated anion gap must also be considered as outlined in Table 15-8. Abnormally elevated serum glucose levels in conjunction with metabolic acidosis may indicate unsuspected diabetes mellitus.

Laboratory Studies

1. *Serum sodium:* Determines osmolar classification of dehydration. Does not predict degree of fluid deficit nor does it determine total body water content.
2. *Serum potassium:* May reflect total body potassium but is very susceptible to modulation by external stimuli.
3. *BUN:* As an isolated test not sensitive for hydration status, but in conjunction with elevated BUN/creatinine ratio, decreased urine output, and high urine osmolality, it may indicate dehydration.
4. Serum bicarbonate: Reflects metabolic acidosis. Sensitive indicator of severity of dehydration and indicator of tissue perfusion or abnormal losses.
5. *ABG:* Additional measure of metabolic acidosis and associated respiratory compensation. In shock states may provide information about adequacy of ventilation.
6. Creatinine: Reflects renal function and not hydration status.
7. Urinalysis: Specific gravity may reveal degree of dehydration. The presence of glucose, protein, ketones, and bile may indicate underlying problem.
8. *Serum/urine osmolality:* Indicates degree of water excess or deficit but does not reflect TBW content. Most useful when used in conjunction to identify source of a problem. For example, low serum osmolality and high urine osmolality found in SIADH secretion.
9. *Urine electrolytes:* Useful to determine inappropriate excretion of sodium in light of serum sodium concentration. Similar to osmolality in identifying source of problem.

TABLE 15-8. Common Sources of Metabolic Acidosis

Condition	Increased anion gap	Normal gap
Diabetic ketoacidosis	Yes	No
Lactic acidosis	Yes	No
Inborn errors of metabolism	Yes	No
Renal failure	+/−	+/−
Ingestions	+/−	+/−
Renal tubular acidosis	No	Yes
Diarrhea without shock	No	Yes

Assessment of the urine can be useful in the evaluation of dehydrated children. The presence of urine with a specific gravity greater than 1.030 may confirm ECF depletion. Monitoring urine specific gravity during management is an excellent technique to assess the efficacy of the rehydration process. A discrepancy between urine specific gravity and state of dehydration is indicative of a significant abnormality in sodium or osmotic homeostasis.[7] Children with diabetes insipidus may be profoundly dehydrated, yet produce urine with low specific gravity, while a child with the SIADH secretion will have the opposite findings. Urinary osmolality and electrolytes are useful in defining where in the homeostatic process the abnormality lies.

Many complex metabolic problems will not be clearly identified with the laboratory studies returned in the emergency department. In these patients it is advisable to obtain 1 to 2 extra serum specimens for use by consultants before initiation of specific therapy.

Management

Clinical assessment and laboratory evaluation enable one to assess the severity and etiology of dehydration and to qualitatively determine the amount of fluid required for repair. The quantitative amount and type of fluid required to treat a child involve calculation of the patient's fluid and solute deficit, any ongoing losses, and maintenance requirements. The emergency management of rehydration process may be divided into two phases, emergent stabilization and repletion.

Many patients can receive rehydration without specific calculation of deficit solute requirements, since they may have a minimal deficit and only require an initial bolus and minimal replacement fluids. However, patients with more severe illness, especially those requiring hospitalization, should receive calculated fluid and electrolyte therapy. The different phases of fluid management are presented in the box on p. 181.

If actual weight loss by the patient is not available, a clinical assessment estimating the percent of dehydration can be used to determine the total body water deficit. Table 15-5 contains the physical findings associated with different levels of dehydration. Again caution must be exercised in that children may be more dehydrated than revealed solely by use of these physical findings. If a previous, recent weight is known, then the degree of dehydration can be calculated directly as follows:

$$\% \text{ Dehydration} = (1 - [\text{present wt/known prior wt}]) \times 100\%$$

The fluid and solute lost during the dehydration process is from the extracellular space initially, followed by equilibration and losses from the intracellular space.[5] The duration of dehydration determines the type of solute and water deficit. Fluids lost from the ECF compartment contain primarily sodium, while fluids lost from the ICF compartment contain a high concentration of potassium. Brief periods of dehydration draw fluid predominantly from the extracellular compartment with a high sodium loss. Prolonged periods of dehydration produce greater intracellular fluid and potassium losses (see Table 15-3).

Initial emergency management of dehydration involves prompt restoration of circulating blood volume in conjunction with therapy for the underlying process. Restoration of normal hydration can be accomplished either enterally or parenterally; however, when hemodynamic instability is present, parenteral management is preferred.

Initial Parenteral Therapy. Vascular access may be difficult in dehydrated children and often is the rate limiting

Phases of Response to Dehydration Management

Phase	Therapeutic plan	Pattern of response
I. Up to ½ hr Restoration of vascular volume	20 ml/kg D5W 0.9% NS or D5WLR over 20-30 min; may repeat	Improved vital signs Increased urine flow Improved state of consciousness
II. ½-9 hr Partial restoration of ECF deficit and acid-base status	⅓ maintenance daily fluids ½ deficit fluids	Gain in body weight Stabilization of vital signs Improved urine flow Partial restoration of normal acid-base status
III. 9-25 hr Restoration of ECF, ICF, and acid-base status	⅔ maintenance daily fluids ½ deficit fluids	Sustained gain in body weight Fall in BUN (50% in 24 hr) Sustained urine flow Improved electrolytes
IV. 25-48 hr Total correction of acid-base, electrolytes, and volume	Ongoing parenteral ± oral hydration Maintenance fluids and replacement of ongoing losses	Sustained gain in body weight Normal electrolytes
V. 2-14 days Restoration of caloric and protein deficits	Ongoing oral support	Steady gain in body weight Plasma constituents normal

step in pediatric resuscitation. Selection of an IV access site is a matter of personal preference with common sites being the dorsum of the hand, antecubital fossa, and foot. In dehydrated children the external jugular is a large vein that often remains patent despite severe fluid losses. In children diagnosed with shock, time should not be wasted on extended searches for peripheral veins or cut downs. If vascular access cannot be readily accomplished in these children, an intraosseus needle should be placed as discussed in Chapter 13.

The amount and rate of parenteral fluid replacement depends on the degree of dehydration and the patient's clinical stability. For patients with hemodynamic instability, emphasis is on restoration of plasma volume. Patients in shock should receive a 20 ml/kg bolus of isotonic fluid (a crystalloid solution such as 0.9% normal saline [NS] or [LR] lactated Ringer's) administered by rapid IV push. If there is no clinical improvement following this first bolus, a second 20 ml/kg bolus should be administered rapidly.[28,30] If a third 20 ml/kg bolus is needed, it should be given more slowly, generally infused over 30 minutes. Hemodynamic status must be reassessed, underlying complicating medical conditions (septic shock, hemorrhage, capillary leakage with third space fluid sequestration, or heart failure) excluded, and if indicated intravascular monitoring initiated. If the etiology of plasma volume depletion is acute hemorrhage, then an infusion of packed red cells may be indicated in addition to crystalloid infusions to stabilize the patient as discussed in Chapter 13.

Although experimental and reserved for investigational purposes, studies have reported the successful use of 7% hypertonic saline solution (HSS) to treat shock secondary to acute blood loss and sepsis.[31] For shock associated with trauma this modality may be applicable, especially for those with intracranial or thoracic injuries. As a hypertonic agent, HSS acts by drawing interstitial fluid from the extravascular compartment into the vascular space preserving circulating blood volume and potentially improving perfusion. However, in dehydration states such fluid shifts may be disastrous, producing ventricular bleeding and other organ injuries; HSS should be regarded as experimental and reserved for specific research protocols.

Continuous monitoring of severely dehydrated children is necessary during the early resuscitation phase. In addition to frequent vital signs such patients should have either indwelling urinary catheters or urine bags to monitor urine production. Children in shock may develop acute tubular necrosis with anuria due to impaired glomerular filtration rate and are at risk of pulmonary edema with aggressive resuscitation. Careful auscultation of the chest and a chest radiograph (looking for cardiomegaly) may allow early recognition of congestive heart failure. This may be most important for the child who receives > 60 ml/kg of fluid in 1 hour but produces little or no urine. Clinical improvement should be evident in children receiving bolus therapy as their intravascular volume expands and tissue perfusion improves. The initial fluid bolus will quickly redistribute to the extravascular compartments and a maintenance infusion will be required for a more gradual rehydration of the child.

Isotonic solutions of 0.9% normal saline or lactated Ringer's are generally the preferred initial resuscitation fluids. LR has the advantage of bicarbonate production as the lactate is metabolized by the liver. In severe shock states perfusion of the liver may be diminished with limited conversion of lactate to bicarbonate. In these instances a

TABLE 15-9. Composition of Common Parenteral Fluids (mEq/L)

Fluid	Na$^+$	K$^+$	Cl$^-$	HCO$_3$$^-$
D5W	0	0	0	0
0.9% NS	154	0	154	0
0.45% NS	77	0	77	0
0.2% NS	34	0	34	0
3% NS	513	0	513	0
Lactated Ringer's (LR)	130	4	109	28*
25% Albumin	140	0	110	0
Plasmanate (5% Albumin)	110	2	50	0

*Contained as lactate but converts to bicarbonate when circulated through the liver. This may assist in the correction of metabolic acidosis and limit the patient's chloride load.

sodium citrate solution may be prepared for long-term infusion. Unlike the lactate ion, the citrate ion is converted to bicarbonate peripherally and is not dependent on hepatic perfusion. Table 15-9 contains the composition of traditional parenteral hydration solutions. Hypotonic solutions should not be given as bolus resuscitation fluid. Less severely dehydrated children may receive their initial 20 ml/kg bolus over 20 to 30 minutes. These children will also demonstrate a redistribution of bolus fluids and require subsequent maintenance infusions for complete therapy.

Repletion and Maintenance Phase of Resuscitation. Administration of maintenance therapy with deficit replacement should be initiated after hemodynamic stabilization. The composition of maintenance fluids and electrolytes is determined by the degree of dehydration and the state of extracellular tonocity. As a general rule, children are rehydrated over a 24-hour period with half of fluid and solute deficits administered during the first 8 hours of therapy. When calculating fluid needs for a dehydrated child, it must be remembered that only half the deficits are replaced in the first 8 hours and that maintenance fluids are infused uniformly over a full 24 hours. Generally, it is easiest to calculate the maintenance therapy and replacement therapy separately and then combine the two to determine the final fluid requirements. In cases of hypertonic dehydration, fluid replacement is performed more slowly and the total replacement occurs over 48 rather than 24 hours. It is essential to monitor the clinical and laboratory response throughout the infusion process. Urine output and urine specific gravity are excellent parameters to monitor a patient's progress along with clinical response and laboratory studies.

Fluid Deficits. Replacement therapy begins with specific calculation of the child's fluid deficits. If a recent prior weight is known, then the fluid deficit can be calculated directly as the difference in the child's normal weight and present weight. The assumption in this calculation is that over a brief time frame, all of the child's weight loss will be the result of fluid losses and not muscle mass or fat.

$$\text{Fluid deficit (liters)} = \text{normal wt (kg)} - \text{present wt (kg)}$$

If no recent weight is known, then the fluid deficit can be determined by clinically assessing the child's degree of dehydration and then calculating the appropriate volume of fluid loss. Table 15-6 summarizes the clinical characteristics associated with the different degrees of dehydration. Children felt to be 10% dehydrated would weigh 10% less than their normal weight or their present weight would be 90% of their normal weight. Calculation of the fluid deficit based on clinical assessment is as follows:

$$\text{Present wt} = \text{normal wt} - (\% \text{ dehydration} \times \text{normal wt})$$

rearranging to solve for the normal baseline weight yields:

$$\text{Normal wt} = \text{present wt} \times (100/[100 - \% \text{ dehydration}])$$

Once the normal weight is calculated the fluid deficit can be determined by simply subtracting the present weight from the normal weight.

For example, calculation of the fluid deficit in a child estimated to be 10% dehydrated and weighing 9 kg in the emergency department would be:

$$\text{Present wt} = \text{normal wt} - (10\% \text{ dehydration} \times \text{normal wt})$$

solving for the normal baseline weight yields:

$$\text{Normal wt} = \text{present wt} \times (100/[100 - 10])$$

$$\text{Normal wt} = 9 \text{ kg} \times 100/90$$

$$\text{Normal wt} = 9 \text{ kg} \times 1.11$$

$$\text{Normal wt} = 10 \text{ kg}$$

The normal baseline weight of this child would be about 10 kg.

The fluid deficit is then determined:

$$\text{Fluid deficit (Liters)} = \text{normal wt (kg)} - \text{present wt (kg)}$$

$$\text{Fluid deficit (Liters)} = 10 \text{ kg} - 9 \text{ kg} = 1 \text{ kg}$$

$$\text{Fluid deficit (Liters)} = 1,000 \text{ ml}$$

Solute Deficit. Once the volume of fluid has been determined the solute composition of the fluid can be calculated.

Sodium loss is composed predominately of the solute lost from the sodium-containing ECF compartment. This amount is determined by multiplying the sodium concentration in the ECF times the ECF's contribution to the total fluid deficit. More simply the sodium loss is the amount of sodium contained in the ECF that was lost in dehydration. The percent of fluid lost from the ECF compartment is determined by the duration of the dehydrating process as noted in Table 15-3. Calculation of the sodium loss then becomes:

$$\text{Sodium loss} = \text{fluid deficit} \times \text{percent from ECF} \times \text{Na}^+ \text{ concentration in ECF}$$

In *isonatremic* dehydration this sodium loss then represents the total sodium that must be replaced with the isotonic fluid deficit.

If the child is *hyponatremic*, an additional calculation must be made to account for the sodium deficit over and above that which occurred with the isonatremic dehydration. To determine this added sodium deficit the observed serum sodium is subtracted from the ideal serum sodium and multiplied times the size of the sodium-containing extracellular space (60% of the healthy body weight).

$$Na^+ \text{ deficit} = (\text{ideal } Na^+ - \text{observed}) \times \text{healthy body wt} \times \text{body space for } Na^+$$

For patients with *hypernatremic* dehydration, there is usually a water loss in excess of sodium loss (free water deficit). In these patients it is the free water and not the sodium deficit which must be calculated. The total fluid deficit is divided into free water loss and solute-containing loss. Free water loss is estimated using 4 ml/kg water deficit for every 1 mEq/L of sodium greater than 145 mEq/L. This is the amount of deficit fluid replacement that is given solute free.

$$\text{Free water deficit (ml)} = (\text{observed sodium} - 145 \text{ mEq/L}) \times 4 \text{ ml/kg} \times \text{wt (kg)}$$

The free water deficit is then subtracted from the total fluid deficit to calculate the amount of the fluid loss that actually contains solute.

$$\text{Solute-containing fluid} = (\text{total fluid deficit} - \text{free water deficit})$$

Electrolyte losses are then calculated as if they are contained in only the solute-containing portion of the fluid deficit.

Potassium losses are calculated in the same manner as sodium losses except the intracellular fluid compartment space is used as the potassium-containing compartment (40% normal body weight). The calculation for potassium loss is:

$$\text{Potassium loss} = \text{fluid loss} \times \text{percent from ICF} \times K^+ \text{ concentration in ICF}$$

Once sodium and potassium requirements have been calculated, corresponding anions must be determined. The selection of the anion depends upon the circumstances of the dehydration. If only chloride salts are used, a hyperchloremic metabolic acidosis will often occur. Salts from weak organic acids such as sodium acetate, sodium lactate, or sodium citrate may be used to provide some buffering capacity and decrease the patient's chloride load in the patient with existing acidosis. All are converted to bicarbonate.

For brief rehydration periods, administration of calcium, magnesium, and other trace elements may be omitted. Caloric replacement is generally provided by using a 5% dextrose solution as part of the rehydration solution. Such preparations provide approximately 200 calories per liter of fluid, which is well below the caloric needs of a dehydrated child. Since the rehydration process should be completed within 24 to 48 hours, such a caloric deficit is usually tolerated. If extended hydration without oral feedings is required for a prolonged period, parenteral hyperalimentation may be required.

Rate of Rehydration. Most children who are not severely dehydrated can be managed in the emergency department and discharged. Treatment of moderately dehydrated children can be accomplished with a 10 to 20 ml/kg bolus of a 0.9% NS or LR crystalloid solution infused over a 30 to 60 minute time frame. This therapy is particularly useful in children with vomiting and ketosis. The rapid intravascular expansion seems to reduce the ketonemia and permit the resumption of oral feedings. Frequently children with intractable vomiting are able to drink and eat without difficulty following a single intravenous fluid bolus. Some clinicians will add dextrose to their initial bolus solutions in mildly dehydrated children to help reduce the gluconeogenesis and treat the ketonemia.

Once a fluid bolus has been administered oral feedings may be attempted. Oral electrolyte/glucose solutions are generally the first fluids attempted and if tolerated may be advanced in the emergency department. Clear liquid fluids must be regarded as only a test and not an extended therapy.[26,32]

Patients requiring repletion therapy are generally not candidates for simple emergency department rehydration and frequently require either an observation unit or overnight hospital admission. Once the total fluid deficits and total solute deficits have been determined the specific resuscitation fluid regimen can be constructed. In its simplest form the rehydration solution can be calculated by adding all of the solute deficits to the total volume deficit and combining this with the maintenance fluid requirements. The standard dextrose and saline solution which is closest to the desired composition is selected and modified to fit the clinical situation. Table 15-9 lists the commonly used intravenous solutions. To provide the desired sodium concentration select an available solution or one that is slightly hypotonic and add sodium as either bicarbonate, lactate, acetate, or citrate to obtain the desired tonicity. Potassium is generally easily added as either a chloride or phosphate salt.

In isotonic and hypotonic dehydration one half of the deficits are replaced in the first 8 hours while the remaining half is replaced during the next 16 hours. Emergency and replacement fluid management is summarized in the box on p. 181.

In determining fluid management for a child the maintenance therapy must also be provided and is added to the replacement therapy as it would be supplied over 24 hours. Calculation of the total fluid requirements would then be summarized as:

Total replacement would be:

$$\text{1st 8 hours} = (\tfrac{1}{3} \text{ of maintenance}) + (\tfrac{1}{2} \text{ deficit})$$

$$\text{Next 16 hours} = (\tfrac{2}{3} \text{ of maintenance}) + (\tfrac{1}{2} \text{ deficit})$$

However, children diagnosed with hypertonic dehydration should receive replacement fluid therapy slowly to avoid cerebral edema. Fluid replacement should generally take place over 48 hours rather than 24 hours and the serum Na^+ should be lowered approximately 15 mEq/L/24 hrs.

Adjustment for Resuscitation Fluids. Some clinicians will subtract bolus resuscitation fluids from deficit replacement calculations prior to determining replacement therapy; others forego this modification. Ongoing losses may require an upward adjustment of infusion rates and even more meticulous monitoring of the clinical response.

Once the maintenance and deficit fluids and solutes have been calculated the specific dehydration therapy can be determined. These calculations are easiest if the solutes and fluids are determined separately and then combined for the different treatment segments. The box on p. 184 summarizes the management of the dehydrated child.

Summary of Parenteral Management of Moderate or Severely Dehydrated Child

Initial care

1. History, physical examination (including weight): confirm dehydration and need for parenteral therapy.
2. Vascular access after initial airway and ventilatory stabilizations.
3. Baseline laboratory studies: electrolytes, BUN, glucose, creatinine, UA (dipstick and specific gravity).
4. Determine type of dehydration: isotonic, hypotonic, hypertonic
5. Bolus 10-20 ml/kg of LR or 0.9% NS. May repeat.

Replacement therapy and maintenance

1. Calculate fluid deficit, p. 182.
2. Calculate solute deficits, p. 182.
3. Calculate maintenance fluids, p. 167.
4. Calculate maintenance solutes, p. 168.
5. Formulate and administer replacement and maintenance therapy
   1st 8 hours = (⅓ of maintenance needs) + (½ deficit needs)
   Next 16 hours = (⅔ of maintenance needs) + (½ deficit needs)

Categories of Dehydration

Isotonic Dehydration. Isotonic dehydration occurs when the sodium concentration of the patient's acute fluid losses is essentially equal to that of their normal serum sodium. The measured serum sodium on these patients will appear normal (130 to 150 mEq/L) although on physical examination they may exhibit overt signs of dehydration. Children with moderate to severe dehydration will be tachycardic with a decreased blood pressure and cool dry skin with poor perfusion. Mental status changes include lethargy; sunken eyes and a depressed anterior fontanelle may be found on physical examination. Table 15-7 summarizes the physical findings of isotonic dehydration.

Initial fluid resuscitation of a shocky child with isotonic dehydration begins with 20 ml/kg of either LR or 0.9% NS. Additional boluses may be required. Once the child is stabilized, repletion therapy can be calculated. Sodium replacement therapy in isotonic dehydration is limited to acute sodium losses plus maintenance therapy. The box on p. 185 presents an example of the management of isotonic dehydration.

Hypotonic Dehydration. In hypotonic dehydration the serum sodium is less than 130 mEq/L as a result of increased sodium losses and limited sodium replacement. Because sodium is the major determinant of the ECF compartment and the intravascular volume, these patients become symptomatic with lesser degrees of dehydration. Signs of shock, including tachycardia, hypotension, coma, poor skin turgor, and a mottled appearance, may appear with only moderate dehydration in patients with hy-

ponatremic dehydration. Table 15-7 summarizes the physical findings of hypotonic dehydration.

The initial treatment of shock in patients with hypotonic dehydration remains unchanged, 20 ml/kg of either LR or 0.9% NS. Calculation of repletion therapy in these children includes maintenance needs, sodium losses, and a sodium deficit. This deficit represents the additional sodium that must be administered to the child to raise the serum sodium back to the normal range. The box on p. 186 presents an example of the management of hypotonic dehydration.

Hypertonic Dehydration. Children with hypertonic dehydration have a serum sodium concentration of greater than 150 mEq/L. These patients have acute fluid losses and despite their hypernatremia are total body sodium depleted. This type of dehydration is a consequence of the deficit in free water beyond the loss of sodium-containing fluids. These patients may undergo a greater degree of dehydration without manifesting overt clinical findings. Hypotension and tachycardia are late findings. The skin is frequently thick and doughy with preservation of the normal skin turgor. Neurologically, these children are irritable and seizures are common. Table 15-7 summarizes the findings of hypertonic dehydration.

Children with hypertonic dehydration and shock should be resuscitated with either 20 ml/kg of LR or 0.9% NS. Calculation of the repletion therapy includes their sodium losses and the amount of water lost, which contained no sodium. This so-called solute-free water must be added to the total fluid volume replacement therapy calculations for the patient. Therapy must be administered over 48 rather than 24 hours to avoid acute cerebral edema with significant neurologic consequences. The box on p. 187 contains an example of the acute management of a child with hypertonic dehydration.

Enteral Therapy

Not all dehydrated children require parenteral fluid therapy or have access to facilities with parenteral capabilities. Experience by the World Health Organization (WHO) has demonstrated that even children in shock may be successfully resuscitated with only enteral hydration. This approach has been shown very effective, although it has not been widely accepted by physicians in the United States.[33,34]

Physiology. The basis for modern enteral rehydration is an improved understanding of how the gut handles fluid and electrolytes in normal and pathologic states. Water is absorbed passively from the intestinal lumen following an actively established concentration gradient. Enterocytes lining the intestinal mucosa create a hypertonic environment in a lateral intercellular space into which they secrete solutes. This space then serves as the osmotic gradient to draw water from the intestinal lumen. The solutes follow a concentration gradient into the intestinal capillaries dragging along any absorbed water.[35,36]

The absorption of solutes for the intercellular space occurs through either passive diffusion or osmotic drag. This carrier-mediated transport is an energy dependent process and the primary mechanism for solute absorption. It is used to establish the electrochemical or concentration gradients needed for passive or solvent drag absorption.

Example: Isotonic Dehydration

A child with vomiting and diarrhea who weighed 10 kg 5 days before, now presents to the emergency department with a weight of 9 kg. Laboratory results include: serum $Na^+ - 140$ mEq/L, $K^+ - 3.8$ mEq/L, $HCO_3^- - 10$ mEq/L, BUN -24 mg/dL. At the time of arrival, the patient received a 150 ml bolus LR. No hemodynamic instability was noted. Calculation of the patient's fluid needs are as follows:

Maintenance therapy

Water requirements = 100 ml/day for each of 9 kg or 900 ml

Na^+ requirements 3 mEq/kg = 27 mEq

K^+ requirements 2 mEq/kg = 18 mEq

Fluid deficit = Premorbid weight − present weight

= 10 kg − 9 kg = 1 kg (1,000 ml)

Na^+ loss (because fluid loss occurring over 5 days is 60% from ECF, which is primary reservoir of sodium):

Na loss = (ECF Na^+ concentration) × (60% of fluid deficit)

= (140 mEq/1 L) × (0.6 × 1 L) = 84 mEq in 1L fluid deficit

K^+ loss (because fluid loss occurring over 5 days is 40% from ICF, which is primary reservoir of potassium):

K^+ loss = (ICF K^+ concentration) × (40% of fluid deficit)

= (150 mEq/L) × 0.4 L = 60 mEq in 1 L fluid deficit

24-hour requirements = maintenance + deficits

Fluids (ml) + 900 ml + 1000 ml = 1900 ml

Sodium (mEq) + 27 + 84 mEq = 111 mEq

Potassium (mEq) + 18 + 60 = 78 mEq

Fluid schedule

The fluid is administered in a step-wise fashion with ½ the deficit given over the first 8 hours and the remainder over the next 16 hours.

First 8 hr = ⅓ maintenance + ½ deficits

= ⅓ (900 ml + 27 mEq Na^+ + 18 mEq K^+) + ½ (1000 ml + 84 mEq Na^+ + 60 mEq K^+)

= (300 ml + 9 mEq Na^+ + 6 mEq K^+) + (500 ml + 42 mEq Na^+ + 30 mEq K^+)

= 800 ml H_2O + 51 mEq Na^+ + 36 mEq K^+

The emergency bolus may be subtracted from the 24-hour requirements but not all clinicians include this additional calculation.

A readily available starting solution for this patient is D5W 0.45% NS with 20 mEq KCl/L to run at 100 ml/hr for 8 hours. This solution would give the child 55 mEq Na^+ over the first 8 hours. One third of the sodium may be administered as $NaHCO_3$ or NaAcetate if there is significant acidosis [$HCO_3^- < 10$ mEq/L or pH < 7.1].

Second 16 hr = ⅔ maintenance + ½ deficits = (600 ml H_2O + 18 mEq Na^+ + 12 mEq K^+) + (500 ml + 42 mEq Na^+ + 30 mEq K^+)

= 1100 ml H_2O + 60 mEq Na^+ + 42 mEq K^+

A readily available solution is D5W 0.45% NS + 20 mEq of KCl/L to run at 68 ml/hr for 16 hours. This solution contains 85 mEq Na^+ and calculated needs are 60 mEq; however, as long as one monitors the therapy, 0.45% NS is probably adequate for this early recovery phase of replacement. Even though the potassium deficit is greater than the 20 mEq/L in the solution, higher concentrations tend to burn the patients and are poorly tolerated.

Sodium is absorbed from the intestinal lumen by both an electrochemical gradient and an active transport system. As with all cells in the body, the enterocytes of the small and large intestines are equipped with a Na-K ATPase pump. This pump actively transports Na^+ from the interior of the cell to the lateral intercellular space in exchange for K^+, in a 3:2 ratio. Such a pump creates a Na^+ poor, negatively charged intracellular space. Sodium in the intestinal lumen then passively enters the cell following both a concentration and electrochemical gradient. The absorbed Na^+ is then pumped out into the intercellular space where it passively follows another gradient into the intestinal capillaries. Such a system accounts for only about 20% of the absorbed sodium in the small bowel.[35]

Sodium is also absorbed through a substrate-dependent carrier system. In this system sodium is absorbed in conjunction with the absorption of another substrate through a membrane-carrier protein. The most commonly used transport substrates are the monosaccharides such as glucose. The absorbed substrate is also pumped out of the cell into a lateral intercellular space that represents another osmotic source for water absorption. Water flowing into this space creates a solvent drag that pulls additional sodium from the intestinal lumen.

Sodium is also absorbed in a sodium-hydrogen exchange system that secretes protons in exchange for sodium ions. This system is independent of the substrate transport protein and is enhanced by the presence of luminal bicarbonate ion.

In pathologic conditions the intestinal absorption of sodium and glucose is disrupted leading to clinical dehydration. Bacterial or secretory diarrhea (cholera type) tend to produce luminal secretion of sodium and little uncoupling of the sodium carrier transport system. Osmotic or viral type diarrhea tends to have little secretion but a greater disruption of sodium absorption mechanisms. This is why the fecal sodium content of viral diarrhea is less than that of bacterial infections. In theory enteral hydration should be more effective in bacterial than viral diarrhea because enteral feedings theoretically reduce secretions. Clinically this difference has not proven significant.

Management. Modern enteral rehydration is based on the linkage of sodium transport and glucose absorption in the gut. If the intestines are presented with a high sodium

Example: Hypotonic Dehydration

A 16-month-old baseline 11 kg child presents to the emergency department with a history of 2 days of gastroenteritis. Physical examination reveals a child, approximately 10% dehydrated, who is a candidate for parenteral hydration.

Laboratory results include: Serum $Na^+ - 110$mEq/L; $K^+ - 4.5$ mEq/L; $HCO_3^- - 13$ mEq/L; BUN-30 mg/dl.

Maintenance therapy

50 ml/day for each kg above 10 kg plus 1000 ml = 1050 ml

Na^+ **requirements** = 3 mEq/kg = 33 mEq/1050 ml

K^+ **requirements** = 2 mEq/kg = 22 mEq/1050 ml

Fluid deficit = 10% of body weight
$$= 0.10 \times 11 \text{ kg} = 1100 \text{ ml}$$

Na^+ loss and deficit

Since the diarrhea occurred over 2 days, 75% of the loss is from the ECF and 25% from the ICF. ECF is primary reservoir for sodium.

Na^+ loss = (ECF Na^+ concentration) × (75% of 1.1 L fluid deficit)

Na^+ loss = (140 mEq/l L) × (0.75 × 1.1 L)

Na^+ loss = 115 mEq

However, since the patient is hyponatremic, there is additional Na^+ deficit that must be corrected. This deficit is calculated:

Na^+ deficit = (ideal Na^+ − observed Na^+) × weight × ECF body space

Na^+ deficit = (135 − 110) × 11 kg × 0.6

Na^+ deficit = 25 mEq/L × 11 kg × 0.6

Na^+ deficit = 165 mEq

Total additional sodium needed = Na^+ loss + Na^+ deficit

115 mEq + 165 mEq = 280 mEq

K^+ loss

K^+ loss is mainly from ICF and 25% of fluid deficit is from the ICF, which is the primary reservoir for potassium.

K^+ **loss** = (ICF K^+ concentration) × (25% of fluid deficit)

$$= (150 \text{ mEq/L}) \times (0.275)$$
$$= 41 \text{ mEq}$$

24-hour requirements = maintenance + deficits

Fluids (ml) = 1050 + 1100 = 2150 ml

Sodium (mEq) = 33 + 115 + 165 = 313 mEq

Potassium (mEq) = 22 + 41 = 63 mEq

Fluid schedule

First 8 hr = ⅓ maintenance + ½ deficits

= ⅓ (1050 ml + 33 mEq Na^+ + 22 mEq K^+) + ½ (1100 ml + 280 mEq Na^+ + 41 mEq K^+)

= (350 ml + 11 mEq Na^+ + 7 mEq K^+) + (550 ml + 140 mEq Na^+ + 20 mEq K^+)

= 900 ml H_2O + 151 mEq Na^+ + 27 mEq K^+ =

A readily available starting solution would be D5W 0.9% NS and adding 20 mEq of KCl/L to run at 110 ml/hr for 8 hours. This therapy will deliver 139 mEq of Na^+ over 8 hours. Close monitoring is essential. A solution with a higher concentration of potassium is usually poorly tolerated because of pain.

Second 16 hr = ⅔ maintenance + ½ deficits (same as for 8 hours)

= (700 ml H_2O + 22 mEq Na^+ + 15 mEq K^+) + (550 ml + 140 mEq Na^+ + 20 mEq K^+)

= 1250 ml + 162 mEq Na^+ + 35 mEq K^+

A readily available solution would be D5W 0.9% NS + 20 mEq of KCl/L to run at 78 ml/hr for 16 hours. This therapy would deliver 192 mEq of Na^+. Clinical response will need to be closely monitored.

Children with significant hypertonic dehydration are not candidates for observation unit management and should be admitted to the hospital for a gradual hydration course.

---

solution containing an available supply of substrate (glucose), then adequate absorption should be possible. In practice, such rehydration solutions contain a minimum of 60 mEq/L along with 2 to 2.5 g/dL of glucose. This is in contrast to the 45 to 50 mEq/L of sodium contained in the typical maintenance oral electrolyte solutions. Table 15-10 contains the composition of common oral solutions used to treat dehydration.

The success of oral hydration depends on excluding patients with severe volume depletion, shock, lethargy, acute abdominal findings, intestinal obstruction, significant sodium derangements, or underlying medical conditions. Close monitoring of intake and output is essential, and the clinical response must be evaluated. Enteral feedings may be continued unless it is clearly a failure based upon deterioration, excessive ongoing losses, or poor compliance with the regimen (see box on p. 187). If this approach is not successful, parenteral IV therapy should be initiated.

TABLE 15-10. Composition of Enteral Hydration Solutions

Solution	Glucose (g/dl)	Na^+	K^+ (mEq/L)	Cl^-	Base (HCO_3^-/citrate)
Rehydration solutions					
WHO solution	2.0	90	20	80	30
Rehydralyte	2.5	75	20	65	30
Common oral fluids					
Pedialyte	2.5	45	20	35	30
Lytren	2.0	50	25	45	30
Ricelyte	3.0	50	25	45	10
Infalyte	1.9	50	25	45	34
Gatorade	2.0	50	20	50	34
Coca Cola*	10.0	3	0.2		13

*Not routinely recommended in infants.

Example: Hypertonic Dehydration

A 2-week-old infant presents to the emergency department with a history of 1 day of poor breastmilk intake. Weight yesterday at a well-baby visit was 4 kg; today the child weighs 3.4 kg. Laboratory studies include: serum $Na^+ - 155$ mEq/L; $K^+ - 4.5$ mEq/L; $HCO_3^- - 13$ mEq/L.

Maintenance therapy
100 ml/day for first 10 kg = 340 ml
Na^+ requirements = 3 mEq/kg × 3.4 kg = 10 mEq
K^+ requirements = 2 mEq/kg × 3.4 kg = 7 mEq

Fluid deficit = 4.0 − 3.4 = 0.6 liters
Free water deficits = [observed Na^+ − ideal Na^+ (145 mEq/L)] × 4 ml/kg × wt (kg) = (155 − 145) × 4 ml/kg × 4 kg = 160 ml

Na^+ deficit (The illness is less than 3 days duration. Therefore the fluid lost is 75% from the ECF and 25% the ICF. Primary sodium reservoir is ECF.)
Na^+ loss = (ECF Na^+ concentration) × (75% of solute fluid deficit*)
    = (140 mEq/L) × (0.75 × 0.440 L)
    = 46 mEq

NOTE: Solute containing deficit = Total fluid deficit − free water deficit
    = 600 ml − 160 ml = 440 ml

K^+ deficit (primary potassium reservoir is ICF):
K^+ loss = (ICF K^+ concentration) × (25% of solute fluid deficit)
    = (150 mEq/L) × (0.25) × .440 Liter
    = 16 mEq

48-hour requirements = maintenance + deficits
Total deficits: Fluid (ml) = 340 ml + 160 ml (free) + 440 (solute) = 940 ml
Sodium (mEq) = 10 + 46 = 56 mEq
Potassium (mEq) = 7 + 16 = 23 mEq

Fluid schedule
The fluid is administered in a step-wise fashion over 48 hours. One half the deficit is given in the first 24 hours then the remainder in the next 24.
First day fluids = Maintenance + ½ deficits
First day fluids = (340 ml + 10 mEq Na^+ + 7 mEq K^+) + ½ (600 ml + 46 mEq Na^+ + 16 mEq K^+)
First day fluids = 640 ml H_2O + 33 mEq Na^+ + 15 mEq K^+

In general practice (and after the calculations are done), the usual fluid that is required to rehydrate the child with hypertonic dehydration is either D5W 0.2% NS or D5W 0.45% NS because it would appear that the *rate* not the type of fluid is important. Studies have demonstrated that D5W, D5W 0.2% NS, or D5W 0.45% NS are all acceptable if infused at a conservative rate, correcting deficits over 48 hours.

*(600 ml fluid deficit − 160 free water deficit)

Failure of Enteral Feedings

1. Circulatory collapse
2. Increasing deficit or deterioration
3. Intractable vomiting
4. Clinical deterioration
5. Failure to achieve clinical rehydration within 8 hours

Realistically the only two solutions applicable for rehydration of dehydrated children are the WHO formulation and Rehydralyte. Since the majority of dehydration-producing diarrhea in third world countries is bacterial in origin and contains a higher sodium concentration, the WHO solution also contains a higher sodium concentration. Some authors believe that in non-third world nations in which viral infections cause most infant diarrhea, the 75 mEq/L solution is the better rehydration solution.[35,36]

Enteral rehydration is performed similar to parenteral hydration but is delivered over a more extended 4- to 12-hour treatment schedule. Enteral hydration is also generally limited to children without marked hemodynamic instability. The WHO recommendation for enteral hydration uses 80 ml/kg of a rehydration solution over a 4-hour period. Following initial hydration, the child is reassessed and if still dehydrated the regimen is repeated over the subsequent 4 hours. Emesis (volume for volume) and stool volume should be estimated and added to the replacement volume on an hourly basis. An alternate approach is to calculate the child's fluid deficit and administer twice this volume during 6 to 12 hours. A third approach is to calculate the child's deficit and estimated maintenance requirements for 12 hours and administer these fluids over 12 hours. Finally, in the simplest approach the child may be permitted to drink ad lib a rehydration solution totaling no greater than 200 ml/kg in 24 hours.

Regardless of the protocol employed, rehydration is provided through frequent repeated feedings of the child and close monitoring. Initial feedings should begin with a minimum of 10 ml/kg and increase as tolerated. If vomiting is persistent, smaller more frequent aliquots should be administered. Vomiting itself is not a contraindication to enteral rehydration.

If a child will not drink and retain the rehydration solution, traditional parenteral therapy may be instituted or fluids administered through a nasogastric tube. Alternately, a 10 ml syringe may be used to administer repeated 2 to 5 ml fluid boluses orally. The bolus must be delivered slowly enough to allow the child to swallow and not aspirate. This approach is very effective in children with a viral stomatitis who will not feed because of pain on feeding even after some topical anesthetic has been attempted.

Once normal fluid volume is restored, maintenance solutions are begun and the child's diet is liberalized. An oral rehydration protocol is contained in the box on p. 188. Because of the time frame involved with oral rehydration this treatment may not be completed in the emergency department and may require an observation or in-patient facility after stabilization.

Oral Hydration Protocol

1. Emergency department management

Initial assessment

Establish dehydration

No contraindications

Shock

Intractable vomiting

Voluminous diarrhea unable to be matched with oral volume

Intestinal obstruction

Short bowel syndromes

Rehydration

a. 100 ml/kg over 4 hr period **or**
b. Deficit volume × 2 over 6-12 hours **or**
c. Deficit + 12 hr maintenance over 12 hours **or**
d. Ad lib feedings to max 200 ml/kg/24 hr

If vomiting occurs decrease feeding aliquots in 5-10 ml increments.

Small amounts of vomiting are not a contraindication to enteral therapy. Add 10 ml/kg for each diarrhea stool seen in emergency department.

If child refuses to feed actively, passive enteral therapy can be instituted

a. NG tube
b. Repeated 2-5 ml syringe boluses to back of mouth

2. Continued care

Rehydration successful: Discharge

Begin maintenance feedings

Breast fed:

Resume breast feeding

Oral electrolyte solution ad lib supplementation

Formula fed: Prior treatment with clear liquids

Resume feedings with soy-based formula

Oral electrolyte solution ad lib supplementation

May consider ½ strength formula

Gradual reintroduction of milk-based formula

Formula fed: No prior clear liquid treatment

Resume formula feedings (may consider brief course of soy-based formula)

Oral electrolyte solution ad lib supplementation

Solid food:

Resume feeding with BRAT diet (Oral electrolyte solution ad lib supplementation.)

Diarrhea and some vomiting may still be present even with successful rehydration.

5-10 ml/kg supplementation with each diarrhea bowel movement.

Rehydration unsuccessful:

Consider parenteral hydration trial/reattempt oral feedings

Admit

Admission Criteria

1. Shock/unstable vital signs
2. Persistent vomiting of significant volume after rehydration
3. Uncontrolled diarrhea
4. Inability to provide home treatment
5. Unreliable home situation
6. Inability to feed in emergency department
7. Hospitalization for nondehydration causes

DISPOSITION

Disposition of children presenting with dehydration must be individualized. The child's present condition, underlying pathology, parenteral capabilities, and social situation must be considered. Obviously any child presenting in shock will require hospital admission, as will severely dehydrated children who have not responded to initial IV bolus therapy. Children who do respond to bolus therapy and demonstrate the ability to tolerate oral fluids may be discharged with close follow-up.

Most rehydration can be accomplished in 2 to 4 hours with rapid rehydration, reintroduction of oral feedings, and discharge. Some children may require slower hydration or a brief period of continued parenteral therapy after the initial boluses. These children may be candidates for observation unit management. The box above lists criteria for admission to the hospital for treatment of dehydration.

Discharge management of dehydrated children should encourage oral fluid intake. Clear liquids as a discharge diet should be limited since they do not decrease vomiting or diarrhea and only lead to protein starvation.[38] Rice-based clear liquid diets may be used and have been shown to decrease diarrhea volume but should not replace the resumption of normal feedings.[37] Resumption of feedings if tolerated results in the resolution of diarrhea and return to normal caloric balance.

In breast-fed infants, prompt resumption of feeding is recommended. Intestinal lactase deficiency may have developed in formula-fed infants who have been placed on clear liquids for more than 1 day, and feedings should be resumed with a consideration of soy-based formula. Milk-based formula can then be reintroduced gradually into the feeding over the next week.

Children who are on a solid food diet may resume eating as soon as rehydration is completed. The traditional BRAT diet (*Bananas, Rice, Applesauce,* and *Toast*) is still recommended by some as the best initial diet.

Many children's symptoms persist after discharge and any child requiring rehydration therapy should have some form of follow-up arranged at the time of discharge.

References

Pathophysiology

1. Laney DW and Cohen MB: Approach to the pediatric patient with diarrhea, *Gastroenterol Clin North Am* 22(3): 499-516, 1993.

2. Boineau FG and Lewy JE: Estimation of parenteral fluid requirements, *Pediatr Clin North Am* 37(2): 257-263, 1990.
3. Stock JA, Packer MG, Kaplan GW: Pediatric urology facts and figures. Data useful in the management of pediatric urologic paitents, *Urol Clin North Am* 22(1): 205-19, 1995.
4. el Dahr SS and Chevalier RL: Special needs of the newborn infant in fluid therapy, *Pediatr Clin North Am* 37(2):323-36, 1990.
5. Meyers A: Fluid and electrolye therapy for children, *Curr Opin Pediatr* 6(3): 303-9, 1994.
6. Hill LL: Body composition, normal electrolyte concentrations and maintenance of normal volume, tonicity and acid base metabolism, *Pediatr Clin North Am* 37(2):241-255, 1990.
7. Rose BD: Clinical physiology of acid-base and electrolyte disorders, ed 4, New York, 1994, McGraw-Hill.
8. Finberg L, Kravath RE, Hellerstein S: Water and electrolytes. In *Pediatrics: physiology, pathology and treatment*, Philadelphia, 1993, WB Saunders.
9. Conley SB: Hypernatremia, *Pediatr Clin North Am* 37(2): 365-72, 1990.
10. Meadow R: Non-accidental salt poisoning, *Arch Dis Child* 68(4):448-52; 1993.
11. Molteri KH: Initial management of hypernatremic dehydration in breast-fed infant, *Clin Ped* 33(12):731-740, 1994.
12. Sterns RH: Severe hyponatremia: the case for conservative management, *Crit Care Med* 20(4):534-9; 1992.
13. Sonnenblick M, Friedlander Y, Rosin AJ: Diuretic-induced severe hyponatremia. Review and analysis of 129 reported patients, *Chest* 103(2):601-6; 1993.
14. Harris GD and Fiordalisi I: Physiologic management of diabetic ketoacidemia. A 5-year prospective pediatric experience in 231 episodes, *Arch Pediatr Adolesc Med* 148(10):1046-52; 1994.
15. Sacchetti AD, Grynn J, Pope A, Vasso S: Leukocyte larceny: Spurious hypoxemia confirmed with pulse oximetry, *J Emerg Med* 8:567-569; 1990.
16. Whang R, Whang DD, Ryan MP: Refractory potassium repletion. A consequence of magnesium deficiency, *Arch Intern Med* 152(1):40-5; 1992.
17. Kruse JA, Clark VL, Carlson RW, Geheb MA: Concentrated potassium chloride infusions in critically ill patients with hypokalemia. *J Clin Pharmacol* 34(11):1077-82; 1994.
18. Woolf AD, Wenger T, Smith TW, Lovejoy FH Jr: The use of digoxin-specific Fab fragments for severe digitalis intoxication in children, *N Engl J Med* 326(26):1739-44; 1992.
19. Bilezikian JP: Management of acute hypercalcemia, *N Engl J Med* 326(18):1196-203; 1992.
20. Rubeiz GJ, Thill-Baharozian M, Hardie D, Carlson RW: Association of hypomagnesemia and mortality in acutely ill medical patients, *Crit Care Med* 21(2):203-9; 1993.
21. Lum G: Hypomagnesemia in acute and chronic care patient populations, *Am J Clin Pathol* 97(6):827-30, 1992.
22. Sydow M, Crozier TA, Zielmann S, Radke J, Burchardi H: High-dose intravenous magnesium sulfate in the management of life-threatening status asthmaticus, *Intensive Care Med* 19(8):467-71, 1993.
23. Warden T, Sacchetti AD, Klodnicki W: Magnesium Sulfate Termination of Torsades de Pointes Following Failure of Cardioversion (letter). *Am J Emerg Med* 7:126-127, 1989.
24. Bonadio WA: Pediatric diabetic ketoacidosis: pathophysiology and potential for outpatient management of selected children, *Pediatr Emerg Care* 8(5):287-90, 1992.
25. Fox R, Leen CL, Dunbar EM: Acute gastroenteritis in infants under 6 months old, *Arch Dis Child* 65(9):936-8, 1990.
26. Kellen RJ: The management of diarrheal dehydration in infants using parenteral fluids, *Pediatr Clin North Am* 37(2):265-86, 1990.
27. Saavedra JM, Harris GD, Li S, et al: Capillary refilling (skin turgor) in the assessment of dehydration, *Am J Dis Child* 145(3):296-8, 1991.
28. DeBruin WJ, Greenwald BM, Notterman DA: Fluid resuscitation in pediatrics, *Crit Care Clin* 8(2):423-38, 1992.
29. Bonadio WA, Hennes HH, Machi J, Madagame E: Efficacy of measuring BUN in assessing children with dehydration due to gastroenteritis, *Ann Emerg Med* 18(7):755-7, 1989.
30. Richards L, Claeson M, Pierce NF: Management of acute diarrhea in children: lessons learned, *Pediatr Infect Dis J* 12(1):5-9, 1993.
31. Younes RN, Aun F, Accioly CQ, et al: Hypertonic solutions in the treatment of hypovolemic shock: a prospective, randomized study in patients admitted to the emergency room, *Surgery* 111(4):380-5; 1992.
32. Brown KH: Dietary management of acute childhood diarrhea: optimal timing of feeding and appropriate use of milks and mixed diets, *J Pediatr* 118(4 (Pt 2)):S92-8; 1991.
33. Avery ME and Snyder JD: Oral therapy for acute diarrhea. The underused simple solution, *N Engl J Med* 323(13):891-4; 1990.
34. Duggan C, Santosham M, Glass RI: The management of acute diarrhea in children: oral rehydration, maintenance, and nutritional therapy, *MMWR* 41(RR-16):1-20, 1992.
35. Casteel HB and Fiedorek SC: Oral rehydration therapy, *Pediatr Clin North Am* 37(2):295-311, 1990.
36. Grisanti KA and Jaffe DM: Dehydration syndromes. Oral rehydration and fluid replacement, *Emerg Clin North Am* 9(3):565-88, 1991.

Disposition

37. Molina S, Vettorazzi C, Peerson M, et al: Clinical trial of glucose oral rehydration solution (ORS), rice dextrin-ORS, and rice flour ORS for the management of children with acute diarrhea and mild or moderate dehydration, *Pediatrics* 95(2):191-7, 1995.
38. Bezerra JA, Stathos TH, Duncan B, et al: *Pediatrics* 90(1):1-4, 1992.

## 16

Blood, Blood Components, and Transfusion Reactions

Lance Sieger

Most patients who are acutely ill or who have suffered minor traumatic injuries do not require the transfusion of whole blood, blood cellular components, or blood products in the emergency department. It is important, however, for the emergency physician and the other personnel in the emergency department to have a full understanding regarding the indications and correct manner of use of these products in the acute care setting as outlined in this chapter.

INDICATIONS FOR TRANSFUSION THERAPY

Red Cells

The primary function of red cells in the human body is to deliver oxygen to body tissues, and therefore one needs a sufficient quantity of red cells to prevent tissue hypoxia. In pediatrics, the volume of red cells required to prevent tissue hypoxia varies with age because of the presence of different types of hemoglobin in the red cells at different ages. Fetal blood present in intrauterine and early extrauterine life has an oxygen dissociation curve distinctive from that of adult hemoglobin (Hgb A).[1] The oxygen dissociation curve of the blood is also affected by the level of red cell 2,3-diphosphoglycerate (2,3-DPG) and by the blood pH. Fetal hemoglobin (Hgb F) does not bind as much 2,3-DPG as Hgb A; this appears to be the major reason a newborn infant's blood possesses an oxygen-hemoglobin dissociation curve that is shifted to the left compared with a normal adult's blood. There is a progressive decline in blood oxygen affinity during the first 6 months of life that does not precisely correlate with either the decline in the percentage of fetal hemoglobin or the 2,3-DPG content of the neonate's blood.[1] Acidosis also decreases the affinity of oxygen to both Hgb F and Hgb A. The fact that these differences between the red cells found in early postnatal life and at older ages are physiologically important is demonstrated by the differences between the mean hemoglobin values of newborns (17gm/dl) and prepubertal children (13 gm/dl).

The absolute level of the hemoglobin or hematocrit values can also be misleading as a measure of tissue oxygenation. Patients with chronic anemias (e.g., chronic hemolytic anemias or longstanding iron deficiency anemia) may tolerate their anemia with few ill effects, since their total blood volume is normal or high, and may appear grossly normal, albeit quite pale, with hemoglobin values as low as 5 gm/dl. These patients often demonstrate near normal vital signs, are usually ambulatory, and may be brought in to see a physician because of a trivial problem unrelated to their underlying anemia. On the other hand, patients with similar levels of hemoglobin after acute blood loss (e.g., acute gastrointestinal [GI] hemorrhage) can be hypotensive and tachycardiac. This can be explained by chronic cardiovascular compensation (i.e., increased cardiac output), normal or increased blood volume, and higher levels of 2,3-DPG in the blood of the chronically anemic patient. Other patients can be profoundly tissue hypoxemic despite normal levels of hemoglobin because the hemoglobin may have a low level of oxygen saturation. This can occur with acute and chronic pulmonary disease, cyanotic congenital cardiac disease, methemoglobinemia, and carbon monoxide poisoning. The patients with chronic conditions are usually polycythemic, and may be particularly hemodynamically unstable with even mild anemias.

The major indication for emergency transfusion of red blood cells (RBCs) is massive blood loss. Although massive blood loss is usually due to hemorrhage, a unique pediatric indication is splenic sequestration of red cells, which can occur in small children with sickle cell disease. Severe hemolysis can also cause profound and acute anemia. Restoration of intravascular volume is the primary treatment goal of the patient who sustains acute blood loss. This is usually accomplished with fluid and crystalloid administration.[2] RBC transfusion is usually indicated only if a patient sustains a whole blood loss exceeding 30% to 35% of his or her estimated blood volume, providing he or she had a normal hemoglobin level prior to that loss.[3] For the patient who is acutely anemic as a result of hemolysis, transfusion of red cells rather than nonblood products can be lifesaving.

Replacement of Red Cells. At pediatric medical centers, the most frequently used blood product is packed RBC (p-RBC). The type of blood products used in the emergency department is dependent on the patient mix utilizing emergency services (i.e., emergency trauma vs chronic medical conditions). When the decision has been made to give a transfusion, p-RBC are almost always the best choice. Because there are so few indications for whole blood, many blood banks do not stock it. Whole blood transfusion may be useful in the neonate or small infant, for whom exchange transfusion may be a more efficient method of normalizing the blood volume and hematocrit, particularly for cases of subacute or chronic blood loss. When whole blood is not available, exchange transfusions can be performed using p-RBC with small additions of normal saline or fresh frozen plasma (FFP). This is not an emergency procedure. The disadvantages of the latter are it requires exposure to more than one donor and it is very time-consuming.

Active bleeding is better managed by component therapy than by whole blood. The dose of p-RBC for infants and children is based on the patient's weight, which is an indirect measurement of blood volume (70 to 80 ml/kg). The maximal volume should be 10 mg/kg or 1 unit of blood (approximately 350 ml), whichever is less. In the presence of profound anemia (hemoglobin < 5 gm/dl), a smaller volume should be given. An easily remembered rule of thumb is when the recipient's hemoglobin is < 5 gm/dl, the transfused volume should be

$$\text{Patient's Hgb (gm)} \times \text{lb of weight} = \text{volume of blood}$$

Because all blood cell transfusion products contain some white cells and can therefore potentially cause graft vs host (GVH) disease, it is necessary to use irradiated products to transfuse immunosuppressed patients (e.g., patients receiving chemotherapy and patients with acquired and hereditary immunodeficiency syndromes).[4]

In urgent situations when one cannot wait for any blood typing, O-negative red cells may be ordered from the blood bank. Under all other circumstances, type-specific blood that has been crossmatched with the patient's blood and tested for reactions to major and minor red cell antigens should be used.

Platelets

Platelets are the cellular component of the blood that interact with plasma and endothelial factors to preserve vascular integrity and terminate hemorrhage when that vascular integrity is interrupted. The normal range of platelet counts in the neonate, child, and adult is 150,000 to 450,000/mm^3, but profoundly low platelet counts are associated with many pathologic states.[5] The platelets are bone marrow–derived. Low platelet numbers are due to increased destruction, decreased production, acute loss (e.g., severe acute hemorrhage), or a combination of the three. Increased destruction of platelets occurs in otherwise healthy children; it is most commonly due to immune destruction (e.g., idiopathic thrombocytopenic purpura [ITP]) or, less commonly in children, can be associated with adverse drug reactions. Childhood ITP is usually a benign self-limited disease following a viral illness, and only rarely results in life-threatening complications.[5] For this reason, platelet transfusions are rarely indicated for ITP. Furthermore, they are usually not effective in raising the platelet count, since the antibody is directed against a common antigen present on the platelet membrane of almost all platelets. In the presence of severe and life-threatening bleeding, platelet transfusions can be used despite their low therapeutic efficacy for ITP. Pharmacologic intervention, particularly with intravenous immunoglobulin, is the treatment of choice for life-threatening ITP.[6,7]

Bleeding caused by decreased numbers and production of platelets can become serious and life-threatening. This is an indication for transfusion of allogeneic platelets. Although there is still some controversy as to whether prophylactic (i.e., in the absence of clinically apparent hemorrhage) platelet transfusions are efficacious and their use justified in thrombocytopenia from decreased production, most hematologists would advocate prophylactic platelet transfusions when the platelet count is less than 10,000/mm^3 or when the platelet count is less than 20,000/mm^3 in the presence of fever.[8,9] After multiple platelet transfusions, some patients become alloimmunized, and intravenous gamma globulin is of questionable efficacy for this cohort of patients.[10]

Patients with hereditary qualitative defects of platelet function are rarely seen, but can present with severe and life-threatening hemorrhage.[11,12] This group of disorders, known collectively as *thrombasthenias*, responds to allogeneic platelets, so that platelet transfusions usually control clinically severe bleeding. Since the cause of these abnormalities is a deficiency of common membrane component or components, they can form antibody to normal platelets.[13] Therefore it is best to reserve platelet transfusions only for serious bleeding, and not for mucous membrane and mild GI bleeding, which are most commonly manifested by patients with thrombasthenia.

An acquired qualitative defect of platelet function is caused by aspirin and aspirin-containing compounds.[14] This does not usually result in serious bleeding; however, when it does, the defect can usually be overcome by administration of non-aspirin–treated allogeneic platelets. These normal platelets release adenosine diphosphate (ADP); this ADP can affect normal aggregation in the aspirin-treated platelets, thus resulting in normal hemostasis. Other patients with acquired qualitative platelet disorders and a severe bleeding diathesis (e.g., uremic patients) ordinarily respond to transfused allogeneic platelets.

Replacement of Platelets. Platelets are ordinarily obtained from random donors of whole blood by differential centrifugation techniques or by apheresis. Random donor platelet concentrates are commonly stocked in blood banks throughout the United States. Although federal guidelines in the United States require at least 5.5×10^{10} platelets/pack of concentrate, optimum techniques should produce an average yield of at least 7.0×10^{10} platelets/pack.[16] Based on body weight, a dosage 1 unit/10 kg of body weight for random platelet units (units separated from one unit of whole blood) can be used or 1 apheresis unit for up to a 90 kg individual. Based on body surface area, a dosage of 4 random units/M^2 of body surface area can be used or a dose of 0.5 apheresis unit/M^2. Either of these doses can be used to increase the platelet count by about 50,000/mm^3 in the absence of increased destruction.[16] Since even normal autologous platelet lifespan is only about 10 days, this rise will be relatively short-lived (i.e., days rather than weeks).

TABLE 16-1. Human Factor VIII Replacement Products

Product	Manufacturer	Concentration*	Storage
Cryoprecipitate†	Local blood banks	<1	Stored at −30° C
Bioclate‡	Baxter for Centeon	3000§	Stable at room temperature for 2 years
Helixate‡	Bayer for Centeon	3000§	Stable at room temperature for 3 months
Kogenate‡	Bayer	3000§	Stable at room temperature for 3 months
Recombinate‡	Baxter-Hyland	3000§	Stable at room temperature for 2 years
Alphanate†	Alpha	3000§	Stable at room temperature for 2 months
Coagulation FVIII, Method M	Baxter for American Red Cross	2000§	Refrigerate
Hemophil-M	Baxter-Hyland	2000§	Refrigerate
Monoclate-P	Centeon	3000§	Stable at room temperature for 6 months
Humate-P†	Centeon	2	Stable at room temperature for 6 months
Koate-HP†	Bayer	50§	Stable at room temperature for 6 months
Profilate-OSD	Alpha	8	Stable at room temperature for 3 months

*Concentration in u Factor VIII: C per mg protein.
†Contains therapeutic amounts of von Willebrand Factor.
‡Factor VIII is human recombinant product, but final preparation contains small amounts of virally inactivated nonrecombinant human albumin.
§Excluding added human albumin.

Hemostasis after platelet transfusion is best assured by giving platelets from multiple non-aspirin–taking donors. Increasingly available even in emergency situations, single donor platelet packs obtained by apheresis may be useful for patients who have developed antiplatelet antibodies after multiple transfusions. Platelet membranes possess HLA and ABO antigens, but not Rh antigens. Because there is some red and white cell contamination in standard platelet packs (although lesser contamination in apheresis units), it is optimal to use Rh-negative platelet donors for Rh-negative individuals, especially for girls and women of childbearing age who can be potentially immunized to Rh antigens from even a small volume exposure of Rh-positive red cells. Thus platelet-rich plasma can actually sensitize the recipient to HLA, ABO, Rh, leukocyte, and white cell antigens, even in small doses and with leukocyte filtering (although the latter diminishes the chances of sensitization significantly).[17] Viable white cells are present in p-RBC units and can cause GVH disease. For this reason, irradiated platelets should be used for the immunosuppressed recipient, since complete removal of white cells from platelet packs is not physically possible at this time, even with leukocyte filtering.[4] Although ABO matching of donor and recipients is not mandatory for platelet transfusions, posttransfusion platelet increments may be suboptimal when ABO-incompatible platelets, particularly A platelets to O recipients, are given.[18]

PLASMA COMPONENTS

Plasma components are given to patients in emergencies either as volume expansion or for replacement of critical plasma elements, primarily the coagulation factors. Thawed FFP can be used, since it has all the major acellular components of whole blood (i.e., whole blood minus the red cells and platelets). Although FFP is excellent as a volume expander, fractionated plasma products are probably a better choice. FFP contains all the blood's major coagulation components, but the volume required to restore coagulation factors to normal is excessive compared to that required by concentrates and is a major drawback if the

patient is already normovolemic. For this reason, various plasma concentrates have been developed, including cryoprecipitate, factor VIII concentrates, and prothrombin concentrates.[19-21] More recently, recombinant products have been developed, and the first of these are now available in the United States and in most of the world.[18] Patients who require immediate volume replacement usually present with evidence of circulatory collapse. Unless the hematocrit is profoundly low or there is continuous hemorrhage, volume expanders are more efficacious than whole blood particularly for mild to moderate shock.[9,22] This allows for complete crossmatching of the patient and donor blood, rather than administration of O-negative or type-specific blood. Plasma and plasma product replacement can be customized for the patient even in emergency situations.[22]

Plasma Component Therapy

The major plasma products used in pediatric emergencies, other than 5% albumin or other similar plasma protein fractions, are thawed gamma globulin, the factor VIII–containing concentrates, and the factor IX–containing concentrates. The latter two are manufactured by several different companies, but are all relatively comparable with respect to efficacy when equivalent doses of factor VIII or factor IX are used. Tables 16-1 and 16-2 list the concentrates that are presently available in the United States. The manufactured factor VIII concentrates generally do not possess von Willebrand factor. An exception is Humate P, which contains both factor VIII and von Willebrand factor. FFP is prepared from whole blood and frozen within 8 hours of phlebotomy.[9] The total volume per unit is typically 200 to 250 ml, and each milliliter contains 1 unit of each coagulation factor contained in normal plasma. FFP is used for hemostasis in patients with multiple coagulation factor deficiencies (e.g., severe hepatic failure) for whom volume is not a limiting factor. It can also be used for the bleeding patient with congenital coagulopathy for whom no concentrates are available or who lack a specific diagnosis of deficiency type.[9,22] Each bag of cryoprecipitate contains approximately 80 to 100 U of factor VIII coagulant

TABLE 16-2. Human Factor IX Replacement Products

Product	Manufacturer	Concentration*	Storage
Alphanine SD†	Alpha	190	Stable at room temperature for 3 months
Mononine†	Centeon	160+	Stable at room temperature for 1 month
Konyne 80	Bayer	1	Stable at room temperature for 1 month
Profilnine-SD	Alpha	4.5	Stable at room temperature for 3 months
Proplex T	Baxter-Hyland	47	Refrigerate
Bebulin	Immuno-U.S.	2	Refrigerate

*U Factor IX: C/mg protein.
†Contains only Factor IX.

(VIII:C), 100 to 200 mg fibrinogen, and some factor XIII activity in a volume of 9 to 16 ml.[9,21] Cryoprecipitate also contains von Willebrand factor. For most significant coagulopathies that are due to pure factor deficiency without sepsis and without ongoing disseminated intravascular coagulation, a dose of coagulation concentrates of 20 to 30 U/kg stops clinical hemorrhaging, although higher doses may be necessary for open wounds or in preparation for surgery.

ADVERSE REACTIONS TO BLOOD AND PLASMA PRODUCTS

Since no human blood product is probably entirely safe, the physician must always weigh the risks associated with transfusion therapy against the benefits to the recipient. A New Zealand study of the outcomes of 440,000 transfusions showed that there were 1,500 acute transfusion reactions (an incidence of 0.34%). The vast majority of these were from red cells, with extremely small incidences of reactions to plasma, stable plasma proteins, and platelet-rich plasma.[23] During a 24 year period at Children's Hospital of Boston, 3.6% of 297,561 transfusions were associated with some form of reaction. Of these, 41.2% were febrile non-hemolytic, 58.3% were urticarial, and the remainder were delayed hemolytic reactions.[24]

Immediate transfusion reactions to p-RBC are almost always due to ABO incompatibility, leukoagglutinins, or contaminants (e.g., endotoxin).[25,26] The vast majority of ABO incompatibility problems are due to human error. Chills, fever, and tachycardia are the most common symptoms associated with immediate hemolytic transfusion reactions resulting from ABO incompatibility. Abdominal and lower back pain are less frequent. Severe and life-threatening symptoms include hypotension, shock, and renal failure. If any of these signs or symptoms are noted, the transfusion should be interrupted immediately, and blood samples obtained from the patient for retyping and recrossmatching, as well as for other laboratory tests. Laboratory confirmation includes evidence of hemoglobinemia, hemoglobinuria, and a positive direct antiglobulin test. Spherocytes may be seen on the peripheral blood film. Supportive care should be instituted to normalize blood pressure and maintain urine output. If the anemia is still profound, O-negative blood can be given while the patient's blood is being retyped, and then type-specific blood can be infused.

Most patients with severe immediate transfusion reactions not resulting from mismatched blood give a history of previous transfusion or other exposure to blood products, or have had one or more pregnancies. Only in exceptional cases should blood be given to the patient who has not been recently typed. Since any p-RBC given to a person who is of unknown or questionable blood type should be O negative, there should be no ABO incompatibility problems. Most ABO incompatibility problems can be traced to clerical errors or errors of patient identification. Therefore it is imperative that no unlabeled blood be sent to the blood bank, and that correct labels be applied to samples as soon as they are obtained. If there is any question as to the correct labeling of the sample, O-negative p-RBC should not be given until another blood sample is drawn from the patient. Once the patient's blood type is correctly determined, type specific p-RBC can be used, while a pretransfusion sample is used for crossmatching. Blood-typing can be performed in minutes, but crossmatching is a more difficult procedure and cannot be completed in less than about 20 minutes. When FFP must be urgently administered to a patient of unknown blood type, FFP from a blood type AB, Rh positive (i.e., AB positive) donor is optimal, since this FFP contains no antibodies against A, B, or Rh antigens.

Delayed transfusion reactions typically occur 3 to 10 days after a previously alloimmunized patient receives a transfusion of entirely compatible p-RBC and may be associated with some or all of the same symptoms as acute transfusion reactions. Less commonly, hemolysis is noted several weeks after a transfusion as a result of primary immunization. These delayed transfusion reactions occur in approximately 1 in 1,600 transfusions and are usually directed against Rh, Kidd, Duffy, Kell, and MNSS system antigens to which the patient was previously sensitized.[26,27] The delayed transfusion reaction is thus an amnestic response, and can vary from mild to severe. Usually the hemolysis is milder than that associated with ABO incompatibility. Delayed transfusion reactions are more commonly associated with heavily transfused patients (e.g., thalassemics) and should be strongly suspected in these patients when they demonstrate a more rapid decline in their hemoglobin level compared to their baseline status.

Nonhemolytic transfusion reactions are usually nonlife-threatening, but are often associated with fever and urticaria. These reactions occur in 2% to 3% of transfusion recipients and are usually due to leukocyte or plasma proteins to which the patient is hypersensitive, although they can result from drugs or food consumed by the donor.[28] Treatment includes antihistamines and corticosteroids after stopping the transfusion. Occasionally, the reactions can be quite severe, and epinephrine and other pressors may be necessary to counteract circulatory collapse and normalize blood pressure. These reactions can be minimized by use of leukocyte filters and washed or frozen RBC.[17] Anaphylaxis is rare but may occur in transfusion recipients with immunoglobulin A (IgA) deficiency; they can present with anaphylaxis after infusion of only 10 ml of blood. Approximately 1 in 700 persons is deficient in IgA as characterized by a serum level of IgA less than 0.05 mg/ml, no deficiency of other immunoglobulins, and otherwise normal cellular and humoral immunity; however, anaphylactic reactions in transfused recipients are reported to occur in only 1:20,000 to 1:300,000 transfusions.[26] Many large U.S. blood banks maintain lists of IgA-deficient donors. If these patients are identified (e.g., by Medic Alert bracelet) they should receive IgA-deficient products (e.g., washed p-RBCs or thawed frozen RBCs) and avoid plasma products.

An additional reaction is the donor leukoagglutinin-associated transfusion reaction. Donor blood, particularly from previously pregnant women or from previously transfused donors, may contain these antibodies. The antibodies appear to be directed against either HLA determinants or granulocyte specific antigens. The reaction of the antibody and the recipient's granulocytes may cause aggregation of granulocytes in vivo or activation of complement. Both are associated with intravascular leukostasis. These reactions can cause fever and neutropenia, and in severe cases are associated with profound respiratory distress with pulmonary edema resulting from severe pulmonary vascular leakage.[28] The onset of respiratory distress can occur in minutes to hours after the transfusion. Treatment is good supportive care. Usually symptoms subside within 2 days with full recovery in most cases. Blood donors who possess significant leukoagglutinins should be excluded from future blood donation.

Massive blood transfusions, including exchange transfusions, can be lifesaving in the appropriate situation. The usual definition of massive transfusion is replacement of greater than one blood volume in a 24-hour period (four units of whole blood in a 30 kg child). The common indications for massive replacement in the pediatric patient are multiple traumatic injuries, severe coagulopathy, or severe GI bleeding. Adverse effects of massive blood replacement include alterations of pH, hyperkalemia, hyperphosphatemia, hypocalcemia, hypothermia, coagulation abnormalities, and altered hemoglobin function.[29] Although the pH of stored blood decreases over time, massive blood replacement is associated with alkalosis because of the metabolism of citrate to bicarbonate. Blood stored even for long periods of time (more than 3 weeks) rarely has a total extracellular potassium level exceeding 7 mEq/unit, so that the amount of potassium is potentially toxic only to small children or to patients with decreased renal function.[30] Hypokalemia is more common during resuscitative efforts due to exogenous bicarbonate given to patients who have a mild metabolic alkalosis from the citrate-to-bicarbonate metabolism.[31] Citrate is added to stored blood to bind calcium and prevent clotting. Any excess citrate is generally rapidly metabolized by the liver, and citrate intoxication associated with massive blood replacement does not appear to be toxic.[32] Although ionized calcium levels do decrease in rapidly transfused patients, clinically significant hypocalcemia is rarely seen, and intravenous calcium replacement can result in hypercalcemia and death.[33] Massive transfusion of cold blood can have numerous adverse effects. These include hypothermia, which can result in significant cardiac dysrhythmias as well as metabolic aberrations.[34,35]

A potentially more severe problem, and one that has aroused public anxiety, is the transmission of acquired immunodeficiency syndrome (AIDS) caused by human immunodeficiency virus (HIV) and other infections. The risk of HIV transmission by transfusion of screened blood components has recently been estimated to be 0.0025/unit (2 in 80,630), with an upper 95% confidence bound of 0.0078%.[36] This is because there is a window period averaging 45 days but rarely as long as 6 months, during which recently HIV infected donors may remain seronegative using ELISA or Western blot examinations.[37] Blood used for transfusion is also screened for hepatitis B and C, and this has significantly reduced the risk of hepatitis transmission, although a window period exists in these diseases during which period blood from a seronegative donor can transmit the disease.[38] Many donors are seropositive for cytomegalovirus (CMV), but most blood banks provide CMV seronegative blood by special request for neonates and other patients at high risk for clinically significant CMV infection. Various blood products produced from pooled human plasma (e.g., factor VIII and factor IX concentrates, AT III) are now heat-treated, so that the risk of HIV transmission has been virtually eliminated. These products have been hazardous with respect to hepatitis transmission. Gamma globulin for intravenous administration has been associated with transmission of hepatitis C.[39] This was a defect in the manufacturing process, and the products now available should be free of this contamination.

References

1. Delivoria-Papadopolous M, Roncevic NP, Oski FA: Postnatal changes in oxygen transport of term, premature, and sick infants: the role of red cell 2,3-diphosphoglycerate and adult hemoglobin, *Pediatr Res* 5:235, 1971.
2. Velanovitch VC: Crystalloid vs. colloid fluid resuscitation: a metaanalysis of mortality, *Surgery* 105:65, 1989.
3. Stehling L and Simon TL: The red blood cell transfusion trigger. Physiology and clinical studies, *Arch Pathol Lab Med* 118:429, 1994.
4. Anderson KC and Weinstein HJ: Transfusion associated graft-versus-host disease, *N Engl J Med* 323:315, 1990.
5. Beardsley DS: Platelet abnormalities in infancy and childhood. In Nathan DG and Oski FA, editors: *Hematology of infancy and childhood*, ed 4, Philadelphia, 1992, WB Saunders.
6. Blancehette VS, Luke B, Andrew M, et al: A prospective randomized trial of high-dose intravenous globulin G therapy, oral prednisone therapy, and no therapy in childhood acute immune thrombocytopenic purpura, *J Pediatr* 123:990, 1993.
7. Albayrak D, Islek I Kalayci A, et al: Acute immune thrombocytopenic purpura: a comparative study of methylprednisolone and intravenously administered immune globulin, *J Pediatr* 125:1004, 1994.

8. Beutler E: Platelet transfusions: The 20,000/mcL trigger, *Blood* 81:1411, 1993.
9. Fresh-frozen plasma, cryoprecipitate, and platelets administration practice guidelines. Development Task Force of the College of American Pathologists: practice parameter for the use of fresh-frozen plasma, cryoprecipitate, and platelets, *JAMA* 271:777, 1994.
10. Lee EJ, Norris D, Schiffer CA: Intravenous immune globulin for patients alloimmunized to random donor platelet transfusion, *Transfusion* 27:245, 1987.
11. Rao AK: Congenital disorders of platelet function, *Hematol Oncol Clin North Am* 4:65, 1990.
12. Coller BS, Seligsohn U, Peretz H, et al: Glanzmann thrombocytopenia: new insights from an historical perspecive, *Semin Hematol* 31:301, 1994.
13. Levey-Toledano S, Tobelem G, Legrand C, et al: Acquired IgG antibody occurring in a thrombasthenic patient: its effect on human platelet function, *Blood* 51:1065, 1978.
14. Roth GJ and Majerus PW: The mechanism of the effect of aspirin on human platelets. I. Acetylation of a particular fraction protein, *J Clin Invest* 56:624, 1975.
15. Rintels PB, Kenney RM, Crowley JP: Therapeutic support of the patient with thrombocytopenia, *Hematol Oncol Clin North Am* 8:1131, 1994.
16. Hanson SR and Slichter SJ: Platelet kinetics in patients with bone marrow hypoplasia: evidence for a fixed platelet requirement, *Blood* 66:1105, 1985.
17. van Marwijk Kooy M, van Prooijen HC, Moes M, et al: Use of leukocyte depleted platelet concentrates for the prevention of refractoriness and primary HLA alloimmunization: a prospective, randomized trial, *Blood* 77:201, 1991.
18. Lee EJ and Schiffer CA: ABO compatibility can influence the results of platelet transfusion: results of a randomized trial, *Transfusion* 29:384, 1989.
19. Lusher JM: Transfusion therapy in congenital coagulopathies, *Hematol Oncol Clin North Am* 8:1167, 1994.
20. Menache D: New concentrates of factors VII, IX, and X. In CK Kasper, editor: *Recent advances in hemophilia care*, New York, 1990, Alan R. Liss.
21. Poon M-C: Cryoprecipitates: Uses and alternatives, *Transfus Med Rev* 7:180, 1993.
22. Labadie LL: Transfusion therapy in the emergency department, *Emerg Med Clin North Am* 11:379, 1993.
23. Henderson RA and Pinder L: Acute transfusion reactions, *N Z Med J* 110:509, 1990.
24. Kevy SV: Red cell transfusion. In Nathan DG and Oski FA, editors: *Hematology of infancy and children*, ed 4, Philadelphia, 1992, WB Saunders.
25. Hogman CF: Immunologic transfusion reactions, *Acta Anaesthesiol Scand Suppl* 89:4, 1988.
26. Jeter EK and Spivey MA: Noninfectious complications of blood transfusions, *Hematol Oncol Clin North Am* 9:187, 1995.
27. Ness PM, Shirey RS, Thoman SK, et al: The differentiation of delayed serologic and delayed hemolytic transfusion reactions: incidence, long term serologic findings, and clinical significance, *Transfusion* 30:688, 1990.
28. Ausley MB Jr: Fatal transfusion reactions caused by donor antibodies to recipient leukocytes, *Am J Forensic Med Pathol* 8:287, 1987.
29. Rudoloph R and Boyd CR: Massive transfusion: complications and their management, *South Med J* 83:1065, 1990.
30. Linko K and Tigerstedt I: Hyperpotassemia during massive blood transfusions, *Acta Anaesthesiol Scand*, 28:220, 1984.
31. Carmichael D, Hosty T, Kastl D, et al: Hypokalemia and massive transfusion, *South Med J* 77:315, 1984.
32. Howland WS, Bellville JW, Zucker MB, et al: Massive blood replacement. V. Failure to observe citrate intoxication, *Surg Gynecol Obstetr* 105:529, 1957.
33. Wolf PL, McCarthy LJ, Hafleigh B: Extreme hypercalcemia following blood transfusions combined with intravenous calcium, *Vox Sang* 19:544, 1970.
34. Reuler JB: Hypothermia: pathophysiology, clinical settings, and management, *Ann Intern Med* 89:519, 1979.
35. Collins JA: Problems associated with the massive transfusion of stored blood, *Surgery* 75:274, 1974.
36. Donahue JG, Nelson KE, McAllister HA, et al: Transmission of HIV by transfusion of screened blood, *N Eng J Med* 323:1709, 1990.
37. Petersen LR, Satten GA, Dodd R, et al: Duration of time from onset of human immunodeficiency virus type 1 infectiousness to development of detectable antibody, *Transfusion* 34:283, 1994.
38. Vrielink H, van der Poel C, Reesink H, et al: Transmission of hepatitis C virus by anti-HCV-negative blood transfusion. Case report. *Vox Sang* 68:55, 1995.
39. CDC: Outbreak of hepatitis C associated with intravenous immunoglobulin administration—United States, October 1993-June 1994, *MMWR* 43:505, 1994.

NEWBORN EMERGENCIES

Newborn Resuscitation

Lynne M. Berry • James F. Padbury

An organized and physiologically appropriate approach to depressed newborns is essential for all who attend to them and their mothers. Only 0.5% to 1% of all term infants require vigorous resuscitation (positive pressure ventilation for more than 1 minute); at earlier stages of gestation nearly all infants require some type of supportive care.[1] The ABCs of optimal newborn resuscitation for these infants are discussed in this chapter.

THE ABCs OF RESUSCITATION

A common approach to evaluating the depressed infant at birth is based on the time-honored Apgar assessment of the degree of newborn depression (Table 17-1).[2] Although scoring various parameters focuses the attention of the health-care provider on the status of the newborn, the Apgar score neither correlates closely with the degree of acid-base disturbance at birth nor intuitively suggests a sequential, physiologically appropriate approach to resuscitative efforts.[3] For these reasons, assessment and interven-

tion based on the ABCs of resuscitation are more useful (see box on p. 198). Supportive efforts begun in one category before appropriate steps in the preceding category (e.g., cardiac massage before breathing) may not be physiologically appropriate and may adversely affect the success of the resuscitative efforts. A systematic approach is essential (Fig. 17-1). One caveat to this rule is that temperature control (discussed under Extras) must be initiated at the outset for all infants. This is particularly important for the very-low-birth-weight (VLBW) infant.

Anticipation

A variety of perinatal risk assessment schemes have been developed to help predict adverse outcome.[4-6] These consider both historic problems and those that develop with advancing gestation. Risk factors that develop intrapartum usually have a more direct impact on newborn outcome than those evident before labor and are categorized into maternal, uteroplacental, and fetal factors (see box on p. 198). It is important to recognize these problems for several reasons. First, early recognition allows time to assemble a full team of providers to care for both mother and infant. Second, early recognition may allow provision of specific, physiologically appropriate resuscitation. For example, if the fetal source of hemorrhage from a vasa praevia is recognized, low titer O-negative whole blood may be required. If intrauterine growth retardation has been noted, a physician/nurse practitioner should be present at the delivery because of the high incidence of intrapartum asphyxia. Finally, anticipation affords the certainty that equipment of correct size (e.g., masks and endotracheal [ET] tubes) is assembled in the area where the delivery is to occur.[7]

TABLE 17-1. Apgar Score

Sign	0	1	2
		Score	
Heart rate	Absent	Slow (< 100/min)	> 100/min
Respirations	Absent	Slow, irregular	Good; crying
Muscle tone	Limp	Some flexion	Active motion
Reflex irritability	No response	Grimace	Vigorous
Color	Blue or pale	Acrocyanosis	Completely pink

ABCs of Neonatal Resuscitation

A Anticipation
  Assessment
  Airway
B Breathing
C Circulation
D Drugs
E Extras
  Evaluation

Assessment

When a depressed infant is born, it is important to make a rapid general assessment while initiating the resuscitation. The newborn with micrognathia caused by the Pierre Robin syndrome may be difficult to ventilate with a bag and mask or to intubate, but the staff may be able to extend the neck to the "sniffing" position and achieve adequate airway patency. The newborn who has a scaphoid abdomen caused by diaphragmatic hernia may suffer massive gastric distention or perforation if overventilated with a bag and mask. Prompt placement of a nasogastric feeding tube for gastric decompression and ET intubation minimizes further compromise of the infant's respiratory status. If the infant has several malformations incompatible with prolonged survival, vigorous resuscitative efforts may be ended and attention directed toward helping the family cope with the tragedy.

Airway

The airway of the newborn infant is at best precarious. Anatomically, all newborns have a short neck, relative macroglossia, and a tendency toward airway obstruction when the neck is overly extended or flexed. The respiratory system of the newborn is fluid-filled in utero and must be cleared to initiate effective respiration. Finally, passage and aspiration of meconium may further compromise the airway.

A good approach starts with *assessment and airway control.* In the depressed infant or the infant who is not responding to initial resuscitation, consider whether there is a congenital malformation of the airway causing obstruction (see box on p. 199). Useful clues to these diagnoses

---

Risk Factors for the Depressed Newborn

I. Maternal factors
  A. Labor
    1. Fetal distress
    2. Cephalopelvic disproportion/abnormal presentation (e.g., face, compound, breech)
    3. Cord accidents, prolapse, or occlusion
    4. Obstetric manipulations
    5. Traumatic or precipitous delivery
    6. Dysfunctional labor
  B. Cardiopulmonary
    1. Hypotension
      a. Supine hypotension syndrome
      b. Anesthesia (e.g., epidural)
      c. Hemorrhage
    2. Hypoxia (e.g., general anesthetic)
    3. Underlying disease
  C. Drugs
    1. General anesthetics
    2. Local anesthetics in excessive amounts (e.g., paracervical scalp infiltration)
    3. Parenteral medications
      a. Opiates
      b. Sedatives
      c. Benzodiazepines
      d. MgSO$_4$
  D. Infection (e.g., chorioamnionitis)
II. Uteroplacental factors
  A. Abruptio placentae
  B. Placenta previa
  C. Vasa praevia
  D. Toxemia
  E. Diabetes
III. Fetal factors
  A. Prematurity
  B. Postmaturity
  C. Congenital anomalies
  D. Deviant fetal growth

---

include the presence of stridor and the quality of the cry. The infant with congenital subglottic stenosis has severe stridor, which is relieved by placement of an ET tube and returns promptly with the tube's removal. Vocal cord paralysis produces an abnormal cry.

Check for excessive secretions (amniotic fluid, cervical mucus, or meconium) obstructing the posterior pharynx. Secretions can be easily cleared by turning the head to one side and suctioning the buccal pouch, while avoiding stimulation of the posterior pharynx.[8] Excessive pharyngeal stimulation may produce vagal-mediated dysrhythmias and apnea[9]; several breaths with a bag and mask can correct this response.

Meconium staining of the amniotic fluid complicates 10% to 18% of all pregnancies and is associated with a pneumonia/aspiration syndrome in 10% to 30% of the infants from these deliveries.[10] Early reports suggested that meconium staining of the amniotic fluid and potential

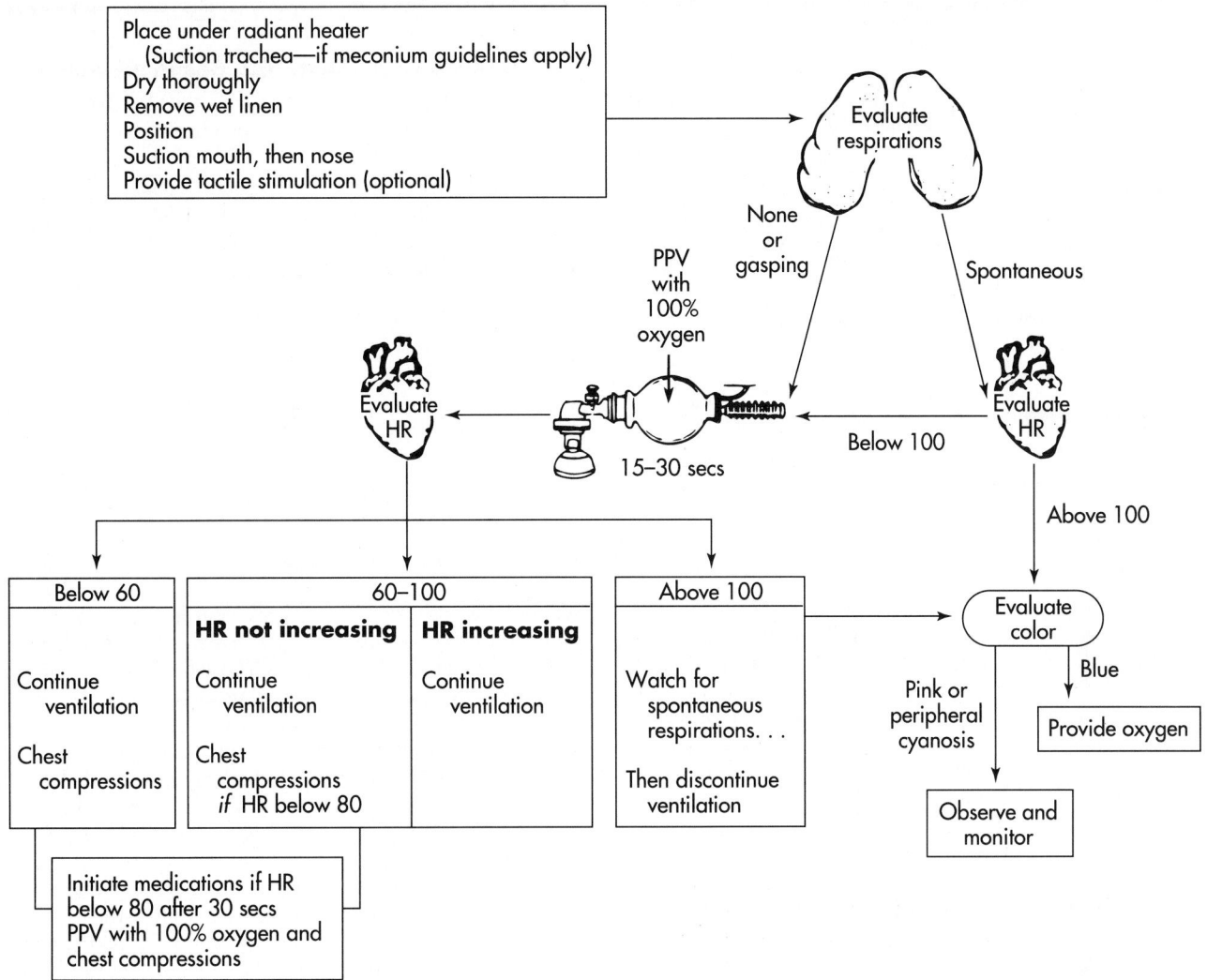

FIG. 17-1. Overview of resuscitation in the delivery room. (*From* Textbook of neonatal resuscitation, *1994, American Heart Association.*)

Congenital Airway Obstruction

Choanal atresia
Posterior pharyngeal web
Micrognathia/macroglossia
Congenital goiter
Cystic hygroma
Thyroglossal duct cysts
Brachial cleft cysts
Vocal cord paralysis
Laryngeal web
Subglottic stenosis
Subglottic tumors (e.g., hemangiomas, tracheal cysts)

---

meconium aspiration are best managed aggressively.[11] This approach includes fetal monitoring whenever meconium passage is detected, suctioning of the oropharynx before delivery of the thorax, and tracheal intubation with suctioning when thick, particulate meconium is observed. This also applies to any severely depressed infant. The absence of meconium in the posterior pharynx does not preclude meconium in the trachea, so intubation is required.[11] This approach may reduce, but not eliminate, the incidence and severity of meconium aspiration and related abnormalities.[7,11] Although this approach has gained widespread acceptance, recent guidelines have been proposed for more selective management of these infants.[12] Iatrogenic respiratory complications after ET intubation may affect as many as 2% of intubated newborns.[13] Therefore oropharyngeal suctioning before delivery is recommended for infants who have meconium-stained amniotic fluid. ET intubation is reserved for depressed infants, those who have thick, particulate meconium, or those who will require positive pressure ventilation.[7,12]

An algorithm developed at Harbor-UCLA Medical Center uses several clinical factors in determining appropriate therapy for resuscitation of the infant with meconium staining: the nature of meconium passed, the presence or absence of fetal distress as evidenced by intrapartum fetal heart rate monitoring, and the condition of the infant at birth (Fig. 17-2). In this approach, infants with lightly

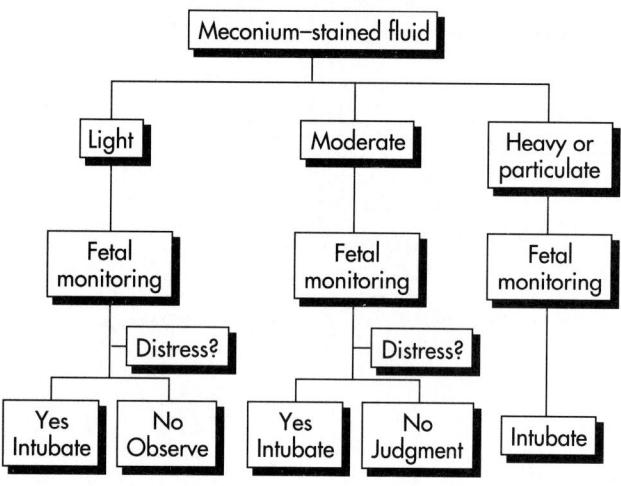

FIG. 17-2. Algorithm for determining appropriate therapy for children born with meconium staining.

Endotracheal Tube Size Based on Weight

Birth weight (gm)	ET tube size (internal diameter mm)
< 1,000	2.5
1,000-2,000	2.5-3.0
2,000-3,000	3.0-3.5
> 3,000	3.0, 3.5, 4.0

Equipment for ET intubation

Laryngoscope and blades: Miller size 0 and 1 straight blades

Suction catheters: 6 and 8 French

Bulb syringes

DeLee suction trap

Meconium aspirator

---

stained amniotic fluid who are vigorous at birth are not intubated unless they are depressed. Infants with moderately stained fluid are intubated if depressed at birth or if significant fetal distress is noted during intrapartum monitoring. Infants with heavy, particulate meconium; fetal distress; or depression are intubated for direct tracheal suctioning before initiation of positive pressure ventilation. For suctioning we use one of the many available adapters that attach directly to the ET tube. Controversy persists as to whether a selective approach to infants in need of ET intubation, taken in an effort to avoid iatrogenic complications, will be associated with an unnecessarily high incidence of preventable aspiration syndromes and other morbidities.[7,10,11]

Positive pressure ventilation (PPV) with 100% oxygen must be initiated in any infant having an initial heart rate below 100 beats/min at birth or bradycardia after suctioning of the airway. Difficulties in providing bag-valve-mask resuscitation may be due to several factors, including the anatomy of the newborn's neck and pharyngeal structures. It is particularly easy to obstruct the airway with undue downward pressure on the mandible or excessive flexion of the neck. The proper position of the head and neck is in the midline and slightly extended. Placing the fingertips under the chin attempting to position the mandible anteriorly, as in an adult, is usually unsuccessful because pressure on the redundant tissues in the submental triangle results in airway occlusion. Proper assessment of the adequacy of ventilation is key to successful bag-mask ventilation. In all infants, the heart rate is the built-in monitor of ventilation adequacy. Breath sounds are also useful. One must be sure to auscultate high in the axilla to avoid the highly transmitted tracheal and pharyngeal sounds heard over the anterior chest, especially with an adult-size stethoscope. Chest excursions may be difficult to assess during resuscitation. If bradycardia does not respond to initial attempts at ventilation, all steps should be reassessed: Is the bag delivering room air or 100% oxygen? Is air reaching the alveoli? If there is no rapid improvement in heart rate after 30 to 45 seconds of *adequate* bag-mask ventilation, intubation is indicated (see the box above). Correct ET tube size can be estimated from birth weight. Orotracheal intubation using direct laryngoscopy is challenging in the neonate because secretions often impair visualization of the upper airway and because of the anatomic constraints of the infant's anatomy. Digital intubation, which entails using the nondominant index finger to guide the ET tube through the larynx is less traumatic and requires no visualization. This technique has been recently rediscovered but has not yet gained widespread acceptance.[14] Once in place, the ET tube must be secured to prevent its entry into the mainstem bronchi or its accidental removal. A convenient method for estimating the insertion distance of the ET tube is to use the formula: total centimeters to the gum line = 6 + the estimated weight of the infant. An alternative technique, which may be superior to bag-mask ventilation, is use of a laryngeal mask airway.[15]

Breathing

During the transition to extrauterine life, the infant absorbs approximately 30 ml/kg of lung fluid, inflates its alveoli, forms a functional residual capacity (FRC), deposits a critical layer of surfactant throughout the alveolar spaces, and initiates spontaneous respiratory efforts.[16,17] In the vigorous infant, absorption of lung fluid probably begins with the onset of labor and is completed with the "vaginal squeeze." Studies have suggested that in these infants spontaneous recoil and large negative intrathoracic pressure with vigorous respiratory efforts almost completely inflate the lung and form an FRC with the first few breaths.[18,19] The depressed infant may have copious residual lung fluid and demonstrate a substantial "opening pressure phenomenon" with poor formation of its FRC. The opening pressure is the minimum transpulmonary pressure below which air is unable to enter the lung. The formation of the FRC is important for gas exchange and indicates the point at which the physical characteristics of the lung have changed sufficiently to allow the lung to remain inflated. To provide optimal initiation of ventilation in depressed infants, inflate the lungs gradually to a peak pressure of 20 to 40 cm H_2O for 3 to 5 seconds once or twice and then inflate at an average rate of 40 breaths/min (30 to 60 breath/min may be required) using a prolonged inflation period (approximately 1 second).[18,19] This technique should be continued until onset of adequate spontaneous respiratory efforts. If bag-mask ventilation is required for more than 2 minutes, an orogastric tube should be placed to prevent gastric or intestinal overdistension. If there is no improvement in heart rate, one should check mask application and mask size, raise peak inspiratory pressure, check tube placement, and intubate or reintubate with the next size ET tube, in that order. Prevent the inherent tendency to ventilate too rapidly (more than 60 breaths/min), which does not promote adequate lung expansion in this early transition period. There is no strict relationship to the peak inspiratory pressure necessary for infants of different birth weights.[18] As a rule, one uses "just enough" by starting at lower (20 cm H_2O) pressures and working up (30 to 40 cm H_2O) in order to avoid pneumothorax. It is also characteristic that peak inspiratory pressure requirements drop after this initial transition period.

Two types of equipment are available to ventilate an infant. The most commonly available bag is self-inflating; many institutions have modified this to allow attachment of an airway pressure manometer near the ET tube connector. The other general type is the anesthesia bag, which must be filled intermittently by entrapment of a continuous gas flow. The anesthesia bag gives the operator more control over peak inspiratory pressure, end tidal pressure, rate of ventilation, and duration of inspiration and expiration; however, its complexity makes it useful only in very experienced hands.

Circulation

At delivery, myocardial performance dramatically increases, systemic vascular resistance increases, and fetal shunts close.[20] In the depressed newborn, the first priority is providing adequate oxygenation and ventilation. This ventilation reverses the reflex bradycardia that accompanies hypoxia/asphyxia. Conversely, therapy directed toward improving circulation, before establishing airway control and ventilation, postpones effective resuscitation. If bradycardia (rate less than 100 beats/min) continues for more than 30 to 60 seconds after adequate ventilation including intubation, cardiac massage should be initiated. The most effective cardiac massage in newborns is performed with the hands placed circumferentially around the chest, with the thumbs overlying the midsternum, rather than the one-hand, two-finger technique.[21] The next priority is assessing the infant's circulation. This assessment may be particularly difficult in the VLBW infant, in whom "normal" means that aortic pressure may be as low as 20 mm Hg.[22] With practice, one can develop a sense of "sufficiency" of pulses and perfusion assessed by capillary filling over the forehead or sternum. One can also *anticipate* most clinical situations in which a severely contracted intravascular compartment is likely to accompany neonatal asphyxia, including fetal hemorrhage from an avulsed cord or velamentous insertion, as well as severe maternal hypotension

---

caused by placenta previa, abruptio placentae, umbilical cord prolapse, fetus-to-fetus transfusion, or severe Rh isoimmunization.[23] In these instances one should consider volume expansion early. The volume expanders available to the clinician are listed in the box above.

Unfortunately, the use of fresh heparinized residual placental (actually fetal) blood is often overlooked. When it is properly anticipated, large collection syringes can be heparinized to provide a final concentration of 3 to 5 U/ml. The blood is collected by direct umbilical vein puncture after sterile preparation of the cord before delivery of the placenta. Blood so obtained, when administered to the infant through small, readily available microaggregate filters, is effective in reversing shock and is associated with limited bacterial contamination.[24] Low-titer O-negative blood should be readily available and may also be enormously beneficial at delivery. For the severely affected Rh-isoimmunized fetus, whole blood or packed cells should be available for early administration in the delivery room, postponing exchange transfusion to a later, elective, and less chaotic moment.

Volume expansion should be administered in 10 ml/kg increments to those infants with clinically evident volume contraction, followed by reassessment. In other infants, one should postpone excessive volume expansion (more than 20 ml/kg) until objective assessments of the circulation, such as intraarterial pressure monitoring, are established (as described in the section on Extras); this is to prevent unnecessary and at times deleterious fluid overload.

Drugs

Drug therapy is an important part of the resuscitative effort but, like circulation, should be preceded by the ABCs. Access to the circulation may be accomplished by several techniques. Umbilical venous catheterization is easily achieved. An umbilical tape should be tied securely around the base of the cord to prevent bleeding or air embolism, and a sterile feeding tube or umbilical vessel catheter, a stopcock, syringes, a sterile scalpel blade, and occasionally a curved iris forceps should be used to facilitate insertion. The umbilical tape is tied firmly at the base of the cord below the reflection of the skin. The cord is prepared briefly and then cut transversely 0.5 to 1.0 cm beyond the skin margin. The patulous umbilical vein can usually be differentiated from the thicker-walled contracted umbilical arteries. The catheter is attached to the stopcock and syringe, flushed, and then inserted to a position just adequate to obtain good blood return (5 to 8 cm in

---

Volume Expanders

Normal saline solution
Plasmanate
Residual placental blood
O-negative blood
Maternal blood

term infants). It is then coiled and taped to the abdomen. Excessive blind insertion may lead to infusion of hyperosmolar solutions into terminal hepatic vessels, leading to hepatic necrosis. Placement of an umbilical arterial catheter is more difficult in uncontrolled conditions and adds the greater risk of exsanguination through accidental separation of the tubing (see Chapter 13 Appendix).

Medication should be administered if the heart rate remains below 100 beats/min after adequate ventilation with 100% oxygen and cardiac massage.[25] Epinephrine (0.01 mg/kg of 1:10,000 epinephrine) may be administered via the umbilical artery, via the umbilical vein, or intratracheally. Its administration should be repeated if there is no response. If continued administration of epinephrine appears necessary, one should obtain a blood gas level and consider administration of bicarbonate. Administration of bicarbonate during resuscitation without documentation of the presence of severe acidosis is controversial.[25,26] However, some degree of acidosis accompanies even the normal process of parturition, which may be significantly exacerbated by the factors presented above.[27] Sodium bicarbonate may be administered at 1 to 2 mEq/kg and no faster than 0.5 to 1.0 mEq/kg/min. A blood gas sample should be drawn through the umbilical vein line first. Blood pH may be used to determine the need for additional sodium bicarbonate. Occasionally severe hypercarbia (indicating inadequate ventilation) is present, thus contradicting the dictum of *A* before *B* before *C*, and so on. Therapy at that point should be to recheck and reestablish the appropriate priorities of ABC. Administration of high-dose epinephrine represents a controversial approach to drug therapy during cardiopulmonary resuscitation when there is no apparent response after several doses of epinephrine.[25,26,28] The benefit of this treatment in neonates is unknown.

Table 17-2 includes atropine for completeness. Many investigators believe that the vagally mediated response to hypoxia is a valuable reflex guiding resuscitative efforts and should therefore not be abolished pharmacologically. Naloxone (Narcan) dosage and route are noted in Table 17-2.[29] There is a very high therapeutic/toxic ratio for neonatal naloxone. Maternal administration of naloxone for the presence of fetal distress may be beneficial, although this remains unclear at present.[30] Recent reports also question the utility of calcium administration in the absence of documented hypocalcemia, hypermagnesemia, or hyperkalemia.

Extras

As mentioned earlier, temperature control is one of the critical "extras" that must be initiated at the outset. Hypothermia develops rapidly in the VLBW infant and profoundly affects survival. All infants therefore should be dried and resuscitated under continuous radiant heat, and appropriate efforts should be made to prevent excessive heat loss.

Glucose administration in asphyxiated animal models improves survival and cerebral hemodynamics and decreases severity of histopathologic lesions in the brain.[31,32] In some species, however, the presence of hyperglycemia during hypoxia increases lactate formation, and generation of free radicals may in fact exacerbate cerebral injury.[33] It

TABLE 17-2. Drug Therapy for Resuscitating the Newborn

Drug (how supplied)	Dosage	Route	Amount
Epinephrine (1:10,000)	0.01 mg/kg	IV, ET	0.1 ml/kg
Sodium bicarbonate 4.2% (0.5 mEq/ml)	1-2 mEq/kg	IV	2-4 ml/kg
Naloxone (1.0 mg/ml)	0.1 mg/kg	IV, IM, ET	0.1 ml/kg
Atropine (0.1 mg/ml)	0.01-0.03 mg/kg	IV, IM, ET	0.1-0.3 ml/kg (minimum 0.1 mg/dose)

IV, Intravenous; *IM*, intramuscular; *ET*, endotracheal.

is unclear at present to what extent developmental differences, species, type of protocol, type of ischemia, and timing of substrate (glucose) administration affect this. It is clear, however, that untreated hypoglycemia in the early neonatal period is deleterious. We therefore recommend evaluation and maintenance of euglycemia in the newborn after vigorous resuscitation. Highly concentrated solutions (25% or 50% dextrose) are not recommended because of the risk of intraventricular hemorrhage after administration of hyperosmolar solutions to the VLBW infant. Instead, one should initiate a continuous infusion of 10% dextrose (5% dextrose for infants weighing less than 1,000 gm) in water at 70 to 80 ml/kg/day after resuscitation and during stabilization along with serial monitoring of blood glucose. Electronic cardiorespiratory monitors provide a valuable adjunct in a well-designed resuscitation area. Arterial pressure monitoring is an adjunct to the assessment of the circulatory system. A defibrillator is used only on rare occasions. When it is used, one should begin at 1 watt-sec/kg and double the wattage until the desired response is observed.

Evaluation

After appropriate resuscitative efforts, there is a wide range of considerations, which are broadly categorized under "Evaluation" in the box on p. 203. Attention should be first directed to determine the basis of newborn depression. The cause may be obvious in some instances (e.g., abruptio placentae), or it may become clear at a later date when more data are available or apparent (e.g., neonatal sepsis, major malformation, or maternal drug abuse). One cannot overstate the value of obtaining umbilical arterial blood gas analysis to aid in the evaluation. Umbilical cord blood gas values are generally accepted as the best indicator of fetal asphyxia, although they correlate poorly with Apgar scores.[3] Blood gas evaluation is frequently helpful in sorting out the puzzle in unexpected newborn depression.[34] The other problems that confront the practitioner after severe neonatal asphyxia are the complications involving each major organ system (see box on p. 203). These require evaluation both as they relate to the cause of unexpected neonatal depression and as an anticipatory approach to the multiple organ system disorders that may follow severe perinatal asphyxia.[35]

Extras and Evaluation

Extras

Temperature control
Glucose administration
Electronic monitors
Defibrillator

Evaluation of cause and postnatal complications

Cause

History and physical examination of mother and infant
Cord gases
Sepsis work-up

Metabolic

Hypoglycemia
Hypocalcemia
Hyponatremia

Cardiorespiratory

Congestive heart failure
Persistent fetal circulation
Pneumonia

Gastrointestinal

Necrotizing enterocolitis
Gastric perforation
Stress ulcer

Renal

Transient oliguria
Cortical or medullary necrosis
Renal vein thrombosis

Neurologic

Seizures
Hypoxic-ischemic encephalopathy

SUMMARY

Teamwork is important to the organized and physiologically appropriate resuscitation of the newborn, as described by the ABCs of resuscitation. Establish a team leader who coordinates the resuscitation, delegates tasks, and does not try to perform all the steps mentioned. Follow the ABCs to maintain the most physiologically functional sequence. All persons who attend to mothers and their newborns during or after labor and delivery should be expert in the ABC approach and update their skills on a regular basis. The Neonatal Advanced Life Support (NALS) program of the American Academy of Pediatrics and American Heart Association or other comparable courses provide an opportunity for review of newborn resuscitation. It is hoped that refinement of care to pregnant women will lessen the need for this approach and better identify those fetuses and newborns who may need it.

References

1. MacDonald HM, Mulligan JC, Allen AC, et al: Neonatal asphyxia. I. Relationship of obstetric and neonatal complications to neonatal mortality in 38,405 consecutive deliveries, *J Pediatr* 96:898, 1980.
2. Apgar V: A proposal for a new method of evaluation of the newborn infant, *Anesth Analg* 32:260, 1953.
3. Sykes GS, Molloy PM, Johnson P, et al: Do Apgar scores indicate asphyxia? *Lancet* 1:494, 1982.
4. Hobel CJ, Hyvarinen MA, Okada DM, et al: Prenatal and intrapartum high risk screening, *Am J Obstet Gynecol* 117:1, 1973.
5. Sokol RJ, Rosen MG, Stojkov J, et al: Clinical application of high-risk scoring on an obstetric service, *Am J Obstet Gynecol* 128:652, 1977.
6. Harper RC, Sokal MM, Sokal S, et al: The high-risk perinatal registry, *Obstet Gynecol* 50:264, 1977.
7. Leuthner SR, Janes RD, Hageman JR: Cardiopulmonary resuscitation of the newborn, *Pediatr Clin North Am* 41:893, 1994.
8. Cohen-Addad N, Chatterjee M, Bautista A: Intrapartum suctioning of meconium: comparative efficacy of bulb syringe and De Lee catheter, *J Perinatol* 7:111, 1987.
9. Cordero L and Hon EH: Neonatal bradycardia following nasopharyngeal stimulation, *J Pediatr* 78:441, 1971.
10. Hernandez C, Little BB, Dax JS, et al: Prediction of the severity of meconium aspiration syndrome, *Am J Obstet Gynecol* 169:61, 1993.
11. Gregory GA, Gooding CA, Phibbs RA, et al: Meconium aspiration in infants—a prospective study, *J Pediatr* 85:848, 1974.
12. Cunningham AS, Lawson EE, Martin RJ, et al: Tracheal suction and meconium: a proposed standard of care, *J Pediatr* 116:153, 1990.
13. Linder N, Aranda JV, Tsur M, et al: Need for endotracheal intubation and suction in meconium-stained neonates, *J Pediatr* 112:613, 1988.
14. Hancock PJ and Peterson G: Finger intubation of the trachea in newborns, *Pediatrics* 89:325, 1992.
15. Peterson SJ, Byrne PJ, Molesky MG, et al: Neonatal Resuscitation using the laryngeal mask airway, *Anesthesiology* 80:1248, 1994.
16. Bland RD: Lung liquid clearance before and after birth, *Semin Perinatol* 12:124, 1988.
17. Jansen AH and Chernick V: Onset of breathing and control of respiration, *Semin Perinatol* 12:104, 1988.
18. Boon AW, Milner AS, Hopkin IE: Lung expansion, tidal exchange, and formation of the functional residual capacity during resuscitation of asphyxiated neonates, *J Pediatr* 95:1031, 1979.
19. Milner AD and Vyas H: Lung expansion at birth, *J Pediatr* 101:879, 1982.
20. Teitel DF: Circulatory adjustments to postnatal life, *Semin Perinatol* 12:96, 1988.
21. Todres ID and Rogers MC: Methods of external cardiac massage in the newborn infant, *J Pediatr* 86:781, 1975.
22. Versmold HT, Kitterman JA, Phibbs RH, et al: Aortic blood pressure during the first 12 hours of life in infants with birth weight 610 to 4,220 grams, *Pediatrics* 67:607, 1981.
23. Linderkamp O: Placental transfusion: determinants and effects, *Clin Perinatol* 9:559, 1982.
24. Paxson CL: Collection and use of autologous fetal blood, *Am J Obstet Gynecol* 134:708, 1979.
25. Guidelines for cardiopulmonary resuscitation and emergency cardiac care. Emergency cardiac care committee and subcommittee. American Heart Association Parts I-IX, *JAMA* 268:2171, 1992.
26. Bleske BE, Rice TL, Warren EW, et al: The effect of sodium bicarbonate on the vasopressor effect of high-dose epinephrine during cardiopulmonary resuscitation in swine, *Am J Emerg Med* 11:439, 1993.
27. Modanlou H, Yeh SY, Hon EH, et al: Fetal and neonatal biochemistry and Apgar scores, *Am J Obstet Gynecol* 117:942, 1973.
28. O'Neil BJ, Wilson RF: The controversies in cardiopulmonary resuscitation on high-dose epinephrine still continue, *Crit Care Med* 22:194, 1994.
29. Kauffman RE, Banner W Jr, Blumer JL, et al: Naloxone dosage and route of administration for infants and children: addendum to emergency drug doses for infants and children, *Pediatrics* 86:484, 1990.
30. Chernick V, Manfreda J, De Booy V, et al: Clinical trial of naloxone in birth asphyxia, *J Pediatr* 113:519, 1988.

31. Dawes GS, Jacobsen HN, Mott JC, et al: The treatment of asphyxiated, mature foetal lambs and rhesus monkeys with intravenous glucose and sodium carbonate, *J Physiol* 169:167, 1963.

32. Rosenberg AA and Murdaugh E: The effect of blood glucose concentration on postasphyxia cerebral hemodynamics in newborn lambs, *Pediatr Res* 27:454, 1990.

33. Vannucci RC: Experimental biology of cerebral hypoxia-ischemia: relation to perinatal brain damage, *Pediatr Res* 27:317, 1990.

34. Strickland DM, Gilstrap LC, Hauth JC, et al: Umbilical cord pH and pCO$_2$: effect of interval from delivery to determination, *Am J Obstet Gynecol* 148:191, 1984.

35. Whitelaw A: Intervention after birth asphyxia, *Arch Dis Child* 64:66, 1989.

Acute Distress in the Neonate and Postnatal Period

David J. Burchfield

The emergency department provides treatment of neonates either in response to emergencies in the nursery or obstetric unit or in the care of children born at home or en route to the hospital. It is essential to be aware of common life-threatening problems that the newborn may experience as well as those problems that may occur during the postnatal period.

Acute Distress in the Neonate

Resuscitation of the newborn infant (see Chapter 17) requires prompt identification of apnea, bradycardia, and cyanosis followed by aggressive management. Measures performed to reverse these conditions include maintenance of a patent airway, artificial ventilation, cardiac compressions, and, occasionally, administration of fluids and medications. Despite timely and effective resuscitation, many infants show signs of continued distress, requiring precise diagnosis and management in the postresuscitation period. In most instances, these symptoms can be attributed to either asphyxia or acute respiratory disorders.

Consultation with a pediatrician or neonatologist should be obtained expeditiously; diagnosis of the underlying condition and specific therapy generally cannot be delayed.

ASPHYXIA NEONATORUM

Asphyxia is the failure of the organ of respiration. In the asphyxiated neonate, the organ that failed may have been the placenta prenatally with decreased transplacental gas exchange or the lungs in the postpartum period. Table 18-1 and the box on p. 198 summarize the causes of asphyxia neonatorum.

Pathophysiology. Early in the course of fetal and neonatal asphyxia, cardiac output is maintained; however, the organ distribution of the blood flow changes drastically. Blood flow to the brain, heart, and adrenal glands increases, whereas flow to the skin, muscle, gastrointestinal tract, and kidneys decreases. These alterations in blood flow partially compensate for the hypoxemia in some vital organs.

In addition to the tissue oxygen deprivation caused by uteroplacental insufficiency, the fetus frequently suffers acute blood loss during the asphyxial episode. If incomplete cord compression is the cause or accompanies the asphyxial incident, blood flow increases to the placenta through the thick-walled umbilical arteries. It is pooled there by obstruction of the thin-walled collapsed umbilical veins. This condition can lead to serious hypovolemia. Rapid cord clamping may complicate hypovolemia in the

TABLE 18-1. Factors Predisposing to Asphyxia

Maternal factors	Fetal factors
Hypoxia	Anemia (twin-twin transfusion, fetal-
Anemia	maternal hemorrhage, placenta previa/
Hypotension	abruptio placentae)
Hypertension	Hypotension
Prolapsed, nuchal	Immature lungs (asphyxia, hypoplasia)
knotted cord	

asphyxiated infant through the loss of the beneficial post-partum placental transfusion.

Diagnostic Findings. The infant's mother may have a history of peripartum bleeding, hypotension, cord prolapse, or meconium-stained amniotic fluid. Additionally, the insult may not have occurred in the immediate peripartum period, but hours before birth. This would lead to the presentation of an infant who might be in the recovery phase of asphyxia. Because of the timing of the insult, as well as its severity, the presentation in the newborn infant is quite variable.

Asphyxia can affect all organ systems. Frequently the most obvious signs of perinatal asphyxia are apnea or periodic breathing, pallor, hypotension, metabolic acidosis, and hypovolemia. The heart rate response is variable and often is lower than expected for the degree of hypotension. A murmur of tricuspid insufficiency is occasionally heard at the lower left sternal border, potentially leading to failure of the right side of the heart. Liver parenchymal injury can occur, as can acute renal failure and tubular necrosis.

As described by Sarnat and Sarnat, the state of consciousness and neurologic examination results are highly variable.[1] In stage I encephalopathy, the infant is hyper-alert and easily aroused and has a normal respiratory pattern. Other than jitteriness, the infant has no other abnormal physical findings and chances for full recovery are excellent. In stage II the infant is somnolent and difficult to arouse; however, she or he withdraws from painful stimuli in a purposeful manner. These infants appear to follow one of two courses: They may slowly improve over the first 24 to 48 hours and recover completely, or they may deteriorate between 12 and 36 hours of life and develop seizures, apnea, and loss of spontaneous movement. In stage III hypoxic-ischemic encephalopathy, the infant cannot be aroused and does not withdraw from painful stimuli. Seizures in the first 12 hours of life are common and are frequently difficult to control. Signs of brain stem dysfunction are usually present.

Plasma glucose and electrolyte disturbances frequently complicate the course of perinatal asphyxia. Hypoglycemia may be due to increased glucose use, hyperinsulinemia, or a complication of management in which strict fluid restriction is instituted. Sodium may be low as a result of inappropriate secretion of antidiuretic hormone, and hypocalcemia can be produced by inhibition of parathyroid hormone.

Management. Prevention of perinatal asphyxia is paramount. Vaginal bleeding, prolapsed umbilical cord, severe abdominal pain, hypertension, hypotension, or passage of meconium-stained amniotic fluid requires rapid patient evaluation. Unfortunately, even with the best of care, in utero asphyxia may have already occurred. In other instances, an infant may have been delivered outside the hospital or in the emergency department, where the signs of prenatal distress or the asphyxiating event would be undetected.[2]

Primary management of the infant with birth asphyxia entails prevention of further hypoxia and ischemia caused by respiratory failure and treatment of hypovolemia, metabolic acidosis, and seizure. Secondary management focuses on prevention and treatment of expected complications of asphyxia, such as hypoglycemia, hypocalcemia, cerebral edema, and acute renal failure.

Patients with stage I hypoxic-ischemic encephalopathy need only close observation, including attention to vital signs and serial determinations of blood glucose levels. Hypovolemia, if present, should be corrected with 10 ml/kg of crystalloid.

Infants with stage II to III encephalopathy require more aggressive management. If apnea, periodic breathing, or seizures are present, tracheal intubation and ventilation should be performed.

Acidosis should be corrected carefully with fluid replacement and judicious use of sodium bicarbonate. Rapid administration of sodium bicarbonate has led to intracranial hemorrhage in premature infants and thus should be avoided.[3] The ideal replacement fluid for hypovolemia is crossmatched whole blood because blood is the fluid most likely lost by the infant; type O-negative blood may be substituted because of the time required to obtain crossmatched blood. If blood is not available in a timely manner, normal saline or lactated Ringer's solution can be administered.

In the term neonate, insensible daily water loss is approximately 35 ml/kg. Even if 10% to 12.5% dextrose is used for the original fluid solution, one may see hypoglycemia that requires either an increased maintenance fluid rate or administration of higher glucose concentrations into the central circulation.

Seizures almost always occur in newborns with stage III hypoxic-ischemic encephalopathy and frequently complicate the course of stage II patients. Although seizures are common after birth asphyxia, prophylactic anticonvulsant therapy is not efficacious.[4] If seizures do occur, phenobarbital is the drug of choice as a first-line anticonvulsant. Administration of phenobarbital (20-30 mg/kg IV) for seizures secondary to hypoxic-ischemic brain insults is well tolerated.[5] Additional doses of 10 mg/kg can be administered if seizures are not controlled. Studies in patients with postperinatal asphyxia show that phenobarbital alone at plasma concentrations of 40 μg/ml or less stops seizures in 77% of cases; using higher concentrations adds little benefit.[6] In unresponsive cases, administration of Dilantin 10 to 20 mg/kg IV slowly is recommended.

ACUTE RESPIRATORY DISTRESS

The newborn infant must make an adaptation from respiration using the placenta to respiration using the lungs. Numerous problems affecting respiration can occur during the transition from uterine to extrauterine life.

Respiratory Distress Syndrome

Respiratory distress syndrome (RDS) is probably the most common diagnosis in babies admitted to a neonatal intensive care nursery. RDS affects approximately 1% of all live births in the United States and occurs primarily in premature infants of less than 36 weeks gestation.[7]

Pathophysiology. The underlying cause of RDS is surfactant deficiency. Human surfactant is released into the lung at a mean gestational age of 34 weeks. However, this can be variable; an infant at 28 weeks may have "mature" lungs, whereas another infant at term has surfactant deficiency.

Surfactant acts to lower the surface tension of the lung and prevent atelectasis at end expiration. The effect of the atelectasis caused by surfactant deficiency is alveolar hypoxia leading to hypoxemia and tissue acidosis, conditions that independently can cause inhibition of surfactant production.[8]

Diagnostic Findings. The neonate with RDS exhibits a variable degree of respiratory distress ranging from mild tachypnea without cyanosis to respiratory failure and shock. In most cases, the respiratory distress worsens over the first several hours. The hallmark of the disease is decreased pulmonary compliance produced by alveolar atelectasis. The baby demonstrates signs and symptoms of decreased compliance problem through intercostal, subcostal, and suprasternal retractions and grunting respirations, a sound generated by forced expiration against a partially closed glottis in an effort to maintain functional residual capacity. Tachypnea, nasal flaring, and cyanosis also are usually present.

Hypoxia generally occurs, often accompanied by a mixed metabolic and respiratory acidosis. The hypoxia should improve with administration of supplemental oxygen, unlike cyanotic congenital heart disease in which oxygen administration does not significantly improve Po_2. As the infant works to generate the pressure required to inflate the atelectatic lungs, fatigue may occur and the carbon dioxide tension in the blood gases begins to rise. All of these findings are nonspecific for RDS.

Ancillary Data. The diagnosis is confirmed by a radiograph of the chest, which demonstrates hypoinflation of the lungs (< 7 posterior rib expansion), and a generalized, homogeneous granular appearance of the lung fields (Fig. 18-1). Air bronchograms may be seen extending out into the lung fields away from the hilum. In severe RDS, the lung fields may be "whited out" on chest film, with only the trachea and main bronchi air columns visible.

Management. Management of RDS involves specialized care and treatment of the surfactant deficiency, often in consultation with a pediatrician or neonatologist. The first objective is to reduce environmental stresses by preventing cold injury and avoiding unnecessary manipulation.[9] An intravenous catheter for administration of fluid and glucose should be established to prevent dehydration and hypoglycemia in these small infants.

The mainstay of therapy is supplemental oxygen administration. However, one must be cautious in the use of oxygen, as high arterial oxygen tension in premature infants has been implicated as a contributor to retinal damage.[10,11] Pulse oximetry is a helpful adjunct for determina-

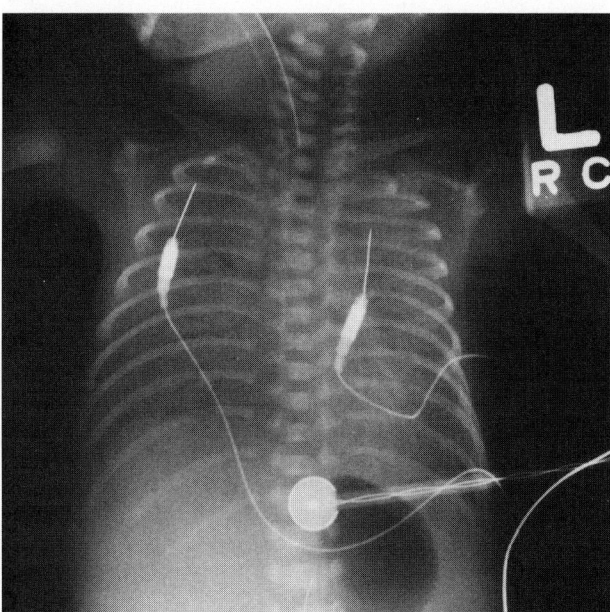

FIG. 18-1. Anteroposterior chest film of a newborn infant with severe hyaline membrane disease.

tion of adequate oxygenation, along with measurement of arterial blood gases. One should attempt to keep the arterial Po_2 between 50 and 70 mm Hg and the oxyhemoglobin saturation between 88% and 95%.

Early tracheal intubation has been advocated by some to prevent further alveolar collapse and decrease the work of breathing.[12] Continuous positive airway pressure (CPAP) administered by special nasal prongs or endotracheal (ET) tube may be a useful adjunct. It is normally begun at 4 to 6 mm H_2O. Severe respiratory distress with respiratory failure may and should be treated with ET intubation. A Pco_2 greater than 55 mm Hg or hypoxemia during high inspired oxygen concentration (> 0.80) is an indication for intubation and mechanical ventilation.

Studies indicate that surfactant replacement, whether human, bovine, or totally artificial surfactant, is safe and efficacious in the treatment of RDS.[13-15] Available data suggest that earlier administration of surfactant in babies less than 30-weeks gestation may have clinical advantages over delayed administration.[16,17]

Meconium Aspiration Syndrome

Pathophysiology. Under normal circumstances the respiratory movements in utero of the near-term fetus cause 600 ml of amniotic fluid to fill the lungs.[18] Under stress, more amniotic liquid may enter the trachea and respiratory tree. Although the amniotic fluid is partially composed of lung liquid, other normal constituents, such as vernix, hair, and sloughed skin, can lead to obstructive lung disease if they are aspirated by the fetus. Blood and meconium, frequently present in the amniotic fluid, can also lead to obstructive lung disease and chemical pneumonitis. Meconium is present in 10% to 20% of all term deliveries, and care should be taken to clear the neonate's airway of thick meconium when it is present.[19,20]

Diagnostic Findings. The infant with meconium aspiration syndrome is often postterm and has either a history of meconium-stained amniotic fluid or signs of meconium staining. The infant has yellow- or green-stained nailbeds and umbilical cord and dried meconium in the ear canals. Respiratory distress may be variable. Grunting and retractions are less prevalent than in RDS and the lungs usually sound coarse. Pulmonary hypertension can accompany this disease process; the heart examination may reveal a right ventricular heave, a loud single-second heart sound, or a murmur of tricuspid insufficiency.

The chest film of an infant with aspiration syndromes is not specific for the material aspirated and usually reveals hyperaerated lung fields caused by air trapping. The lung fields have scattered patchy infiltrates, with occasional lobar atelectasis.

Management. Prevention of aspiration of amniotic contents at birth incorporates a combined approach of clearing the infant's upper airway after delivery of the fetal head and before the delivery of the chest, then repeatedly suctioning the upper airways with a suction bulb immediately after birth. When thick, particulate meconium is present at delivery, immediate tracheal intubation and suctioning of the lower respiratory tract should be attempted. Thin meconium need not be suctioned from the trachea.[21] Individual judgment as to the need for intubation and suctioning of the trachea must be used for the meconium-stained neonate born outside the hospital. If there is severe respiratory distress, intubation is indicated; infants with minimal respiratory distress may not require ventilatory support. Extracorporeal membrane oxygenation (ECMO) provides support to children who do not respond to standard or high-frequency ventilation or adjunctive nitric oxide therapy.

The infant with an aspiration syndrome who has signs of respiratory distress requires consulation with a pediatrician or neonatologist.

Persistent Pulmonary Hypertension

Pathophysiology. Persistent pulmonary hypertension, commonly referred to as persistent fetal circulation (PFC), is a condition in which the pulmonary vascular resistance remains elevated following birth. In utero, the pulmonary vascular resistance of the fetus is greater than systemic vascular resistance. This impedes pulmonary blood flow, causing right ventricular output to be directed via the ductus arteriosus to the aorta and placenta. Under normal circumstances, the lungs expand and pulmonary vascular resistance drops concomitant with the first breath. Pulmonary blood flow increases and the direction of ductus arteriosus blood flow reverses from right-to-left to left-to-right. This increase in pulmonary blood flow also increases left atrial pressure leading to closure of the foramen ovale and prevention of right-to-left shunting at the atrial level. In neonates with persistent pulmonary hypertension, either the initial fall in pulmonary vascular resistance does not occur or constriction of the pulmonary vascular bed occurs sometime shortly after birth. This leads to shunting of deoxygenated blood away from the lungs both through the ductus arteriosus and the foramen ovale.

Diagnostic Findings. Persistent pulmonary hypertension is seen almost exclusively in term or near-term infants. The presenting signs are usually tachypnea and respiratory distress. The infant may have been meconium-stained or may have undergone in utero stress; however, this will be difficult to ascertain. The infant may demonstrate a right ventricular heave, although this may be subtle. Invariably, the second heart sound is not split, resulting from the high pulmonary artery pressure causing early closure of the pulmonary valve. Most commonly, no murmur is auscultated.

Ancillary Data. The chest x-ray may show evidence of pneumonia or meconium aspiration but can be clear with diminished vascular markings. The electrocardiogram is normal.

Because of the presence of right-to-left shunting, venous blood is mixed with arterial blood at the ductus arteriosus. This will lead to differential oxygenation with the upper extremity arteries containing higher oxygen content than the lower extremities. Simultaneously obtained blood gases from the radial artery and a postductal artery (umbilical artery, posterior tibial artery) will typically reveal greater than a 15 mm Hg difference in Po_2. This can be conveniently demonstrated with a peripheral saturation monitor on the right hand and one foot, with the right hand having a 10% to 15% higher reading than the foot.

Management. Immediate management of persistent pulmonary hypertension should include administration of 100% oxygen and establishment of intravenous and intraarterial access. Afterward care should be clustered so as to disturb the patient as little as possible. Intravenous fluids (10% dextrose and water) should be infused at 60 to 80 ml/kg/24 h. Frequently, the patient will remain adequately oxygenated with oxygen administered by hood; however, if the Po_2 should drop into the low 40s, intubation and ventilation are indicated. Sedation and mild hyperventilation may improve oxygenation dramatically; however, no attempts to change seemingly successful therapy should be attempted until the infant has been transferred to a neonatal intensive care unit.

Because some cardiac lesions will also give upper body–lower body differences in saturation (i.e., severe coarctation of the aorta, interrupted aortic arch), these children should be evaluated echocardiographically by a pediatric cardiologist to rule out such lesions.

Upper Airway Obstruction

Upper airway obstruction in the newborn is an uncommon problem; however, when present, it must be diagnosed and managed expeditiously. Upper airway obstruction can be caused by a variety of entities, which are summarized in the box on p. 199.

Diagnostic Findings. Neonates with obstructive upper airway lesions from any cause generally have inspiratory stridor and deep sternal retractions. The infant who breathes with pursed lips and is cyanotic at rest but whose color improves when crying should be suspected of having choanal atresia. The diagnosis is confirmed by an inability to pass a number 5 French size feeding tube down each nostril. Careful inspection of the mandible and palate may reveal micrognathia and the cleft palate seen in the Pierre Robin syndrome, in which the cause of upper airway obstruction is usually the tongue. Airway compromise is occasionally caused by extrinsic compression from a cystic hygroma that presents as a neck mass. Other causes of upper airway obstruction, including vascular rings, tracheal web, and vocal cord paralysis, have no specific physical findings.

Ancillary Data. Many causes of upper airway obstruction can be diagnosed by physical examination; lesions of the glottis and extrathoracic trachea require radiologic and bronchoscopic evaluations that should not be attempted in the emergency department.

Management. In most circumstances, these infants can be positioned, have an oral or nasopharyngeal airway placed, or be intubated. Newborn infants with micrognathia who obstruct their larynx with their tongue generally breathe more easily when placed prone with the chest on several blankets and the head suspended downward. Correct position keeps the tongue falling ventrally away from the larynx and is also helpful in the infant with laryngeal malacia. This temporarily alleviates the obstruction and allows for transfer for an appropriate diagnostic evaluation.

Lower Airway Anomalies

Like upper airway anomalies, lower airway anomalies are rare and seldom cause acute respiratory distress in newborn infants.

Diagnostic Findings. The clinical presentation of the infant with a lower airway anomaly depends on the particular anomaly present and its severity. Generally, newborns with tracheoesophageal fistula have minimal respiratory difficulties and present with spitting all of their feedings. Infants with cystic adenomatoid malformation, congenital lobar emphysema, and bronchogenic cyst frequently are asymptomatic or only mildly symptomatic in the immediate newborn period.

Infants with diaphragmatic hernia or hypoplastic lungs are usually in respiratory distress immediately after birth, when their lungs are required to perform respiratory functions. Many of these infants have such small lung volume that they do not respond to resuscitative efforts. Children with diaphragmatic hernia have a scaphoid abdomen and a displaced cardiac impulse to the right because 90% of diaphragmatic hernias are on the left. Infants with hypoplastic lungs are generally born to mothers who have oligohydramnios. These infants have immediate, severe respiratory distress and subtle features of in utero compression, including compressed nose, narrow head, contractures of the lower extremities, broad and flat hands, and ability to position their legs in the fetal position easily with the legs crossed and knees pulled to the chest.

Ancillary Data. The diagnosis of lower airway anomalies is almost always made by the findings on chest film. Diaphragmatic hernia is characterized by presence of intestinal and abdominal contents in the chest cavity with the heart and mediastinum shifted to the opposite side. Tracheoesophageal fistula is frequently detected by air outlining the esophageal pouch; a feature that accompanies 90%

of cases. A plain chest film after attempted placement of an oral-gastric tube either confirms the esophageal atresia or rules out all but the most rare types of tracheoesophageal fistula. Bronchogenic cyst, congenital lobar emphysema, and cystic adenomatoid malformation of the lung are all diagnosed by chest film and confirmed pathologically at the time of surgery. Hypoplastic lungs may be suggested by the plain film but can only be confirmed at autopsy.

Management. The immediate management of the infant with acute respiratory distress produced by lower airway anomalies is nonspecific and supportive. Infants with frank respiratory failure require tracheal intubation and mechanical ventilation. Bag-mask ventilation should be avoided and an orogastric tube should be placed to prevent gastric distention in children with a diaphragmatic hernia. Infants usually require high-pressure, high-frequency ventilator support to ventilate their small lungs, yet this therapy places them at extremely high risk for pneumothorax.[22] Newer modalities such as nitric oxide and ECMO may have a role.

All infants with lower respiratory anomalies should be transferred to an appropriate neonatal care center after stabilization.

NARCOTIC DEPRESSION

Many women of childbearing age have used drugs regularly. The overall use of illicit drugs has increased and the pattern of drug abuse has changed significantly. The use of cocaine and methamphetamine, drugs that act as strong central nervous system (CNS) stimulants, has risen, whereas the use of narcotics, such as heroin, has declined.[23]

The infant born to a mother who has recently used narcotics, such as heroin, morphine, or meperidine, may suffer acute respiratory distress manifested by apnea. Many of these women do not seek prenatal care and may use drugs during labor to control the pain. Out-of-hospital deliveries are more likely to occur among drug-addicted women.

Diagnostic Findings. Narcotic depression in the infant primarily depends on the time of drug administration before the delivery and the frequency of drug exposure of the fetus. Infants who received intrauterine narcotics within 4 hours of delivery are at highest risk for respiratory depression.[24] However, those infants whose mothers were regular users of narcotics may show minimal or no symptoms of respiratory depression during the immediate neonatal period.

Narcotic depression in the neonate is manifested by apnea or irregular breathing and decreased muscular tone. If no treatment for the apnea is instituted, the infant quickly becomes cyanotic and bradycardic.

Management. The acute management of neonatal narcotic depression focuses on basic resuscitation techniques. Naloxone 0.1 mg/kg should be administered intravenously or endotracheally. Absorption through the intramuscular or subcutaneous route is erratic.[25] Naloxone should only be administered to infants with respiratory depression from suspected narcotic exposure and not to all infants exposed to narcotics. The infant whose mother abused narcotics

---

Causes of Congestive Heart Failure in Neonates

Hypoplastic left ventricle
Coarctation of the aorta
Ventricular septal defect
Truncus arteriosus
Endocardial cushion defect
Aortic stenosis
Patent ductus arteriosus*
Arteriovenous malformations

*Common in premature infants.

---

chronically is less likely to have respiratory depression and naloxone hydrochloride may precipitate drug withdrawal (see Chapter 43).

Postnatal Emergencies

CARDIOVASCULAR DISORDERS
(See Chapter 47)

Cardiovascular diseases in neonates who may appear in the emergency department can be grouped into three categories: (1) structural lesions that lead to congestive heart failure, (2) structural lesions that cause cyanosis, and (3) dysrhythmias.

Congestive Heart Failure

Etiology. The causes of congestive heart failure in order of relative frequency of occurrence are summarized in the box above. Congestive heart failure in the immediate newborn period is primarily due to obstruction to left ventricular outflow (i.e., hypoplastic left heart syndrome, aortic stenosis, coarctation of the aorta). Adequate systemic blood pressure during this time may be maintained through a patent ductus arteriosus (PDA). Poor systemic blood flow may occur in association with closure of the ductus. Dysrhythmias can also lead to congestive heart failure; they are discussed in greater detail below.

Diagnostic Findings. Congestive heart failure in a newborn can be difficult to diagnose. The signs and symptoms are frequently nonspecific and require a thorough physical examination and proper interpretation of ancillary tests to make the diagnosis accurately.

Frequently, the mother consults a physician with complaints about feeding. The infant may be a slow feeder and tire quickly while feeding; paleness and respiratory symptoms may be noted.

A thorough physical examination should reveal evidence of cardiac disease. The infant may have mottled skin and mild to moderate respiratory distress, with retractions, grunting, nasal flaring, and rales revealed on auscultation of the chest.

A careful cardiac examination often demonstrates an active precordium; infants with aortic stenosis usually have a thrill. Evaluation of the pulses is extremely important. Aortic stenosis and hypoplastic left heart syndrome usually are characterized by poor peripheral pulses in all extremities. Coarctation of the aorta is characterized by increased pulses in the upper extremities and absent pulses in the lower extremities, whereas an interrupted aortic arch frequently is characterized by increased pulses in the right upper extremity but poor pulses in the left upper and both lower extremities.

Auscultation of the heart may reveal normal S1 and S2 or an S2 that does not split (hypoplastic left heart). In addition, S3 and S4 may be present. Lesions such as aortic stenosis, ventricular septal defect, and coarctation of the aorta should be accompanied by an easily audible murmur. Auscultation of the cranium through the anterior fontanelle and over the liver to detect arterial-venous malformations should also be performed. Other signs of congestive heart failure include hepatomegaly and peripheral edema. The liver is soft and may have a boggy consistency. The edema is most often seen in the dependent regions, such as the sacral area.

Ancillary Data. The electrocardiogram may provide supporting data for precise anatomic diagnoses of the heart lesion. For instance, infants with ventricular septal defect frequently have a normal electrocardiogram result, whereas those who have hypoplastic left heart usually show poor left ventricular forces in the lateral precordial leads.

The chest film is often helpful. Typically the pulmonary vascular markings radiating from the hilum are increased and interstitial edema is present with fluid in the minor fissure. The heart size is usually enlarged, except in the infant with hypoplastic left heart syndrome, which typically is characterized by a normal-sized heart.

Management. The immediate management of the infant with congestive heart failure is very similar to that of the older child. Oxygen and other ventilatory support should be administered to treat hypoxia. Intravenous access should be obtained. Furosemide 1 mg/kg IV is given to help diuresis and potentially reduce preload. Digoxin therapy is commonly used in chronic cases of congestive heart failure in neonates. For more immediate results from an inotropic agent, one should consider intravenous therapy with dopamine.

Unlike congestive failure in the older child, congestive heart failure in the neonate, particularly in the first week of life, presents some symptoms after the ductus arteriosus closes; reopening this vessel can be lifesaving. Continuous infusion of prostaglandin E_1 at 0.1 µg/kg/min IV may be lifesaving but should be initiated only after appropriate subspecialty consultation.

Cyanotic Heart Disease

Etiology. In most cases cyanotic heart lesions are diagnosed during the newborn nursery stay, usually after several hours have passed since birth. Of these, tetralogy of Fallot and truncus arteriosus may be overlooked in the newborn nursery and these patients may present later to the emergency department. In tetralogy of Fallot cyanosis is caused by impedance of pulmonary blood flow caused by infundibular stenosis and shunting of deoxygenated blood through an overriding aorta. In many cases, the infundibular stenosis is so mild that it does not restrict pulmonary blood flow and cyanosis is not present until the stenosis worsens. In truncus arteriosus, cyanosis is caused by mixing of systemic venous blood with pulmonary venous blood at the ventricular level. Cyanosis is usually mild and the patients commonly present in congestive heart failure when pulmonary artery resistance has dropped to normal postneonatal levels. Other lesions include transposition of the great vessels, tricuspid atresia, total anomalous venous return, and pulmonary atresia.

Diagnostic Findings. The hallmark of cyanotic heart disease is the cyanosis, which is usually unrelated to any signs of respiratory distress. The infants typically appear quite comfortable and may have only minimal tachypnea. Grunting and flaring are uncommon. Typically the pulses are normal and the precordium is quiet. The exception is pulmonary stenosis, which is characterized by a right ventricular lift and a thrill. In many cases, such as transposition of the great vessels and pulmonary atresia, no murmur is heard. However, in other cases, such as those involving tetralogy of Fallot and truncus arteriosus, a murmur is usually heard.

Ancillary Data. The electrocardiogram can provide some useful data for the evaluation of the infant but the results may appear normal or show only minimal changes.

The chest film is very helpful in differentiating between primary pulmonary disease and cyanotic heart disease. In cyanotic heart disease the lung fields are usually clear or have decreased vascular markings. In cyanotic neonates, the absence of pulmonary infiltrates is strong evidence of cyanotic heart disease.

The most important test to confirm a diagnosis of cyanotic heart disease is a comparison of arterial Po_2 while the patient breathes room air and while she or he breathes 100% oxygen. Typically, the Po_2 rises above 100 mm Hg in the child with primary pulmonary disease but remains well below this concentration with cyanotic heart disease.

Management. All patients should receive consultation from a pediatrician and pediatric cardiologist while oxygen is administered and their condition is stabilized. Therapy with prostaglandin E_1 at 0.1 μg/kg/min IV or other modalities may be recommended.

Dysrhythmias

Cardiac dysrhythmias are relatively common, with an incidence of approximately 1% in apparently normal newborns. These rhythm disturbances are rarely serious and are discussed in detail in Chapter 14.

ENDOCRINOLOGIC AND METABOLIC DISORDERS (See Chapter 50)

Endocrinologic emergencies in the neonate primarily encompass the metabolic problems of hypoglycemia and hypocalcemia, ambiguous genitalia, and congenital adrenal hyperplasia. A more prevalent problem, hypothyroidism, is characterized by symptoms that are indolent and is usually diagnosed on routine newborn metabolic screen; therefore, it is not likely to be seen in the emergency department and is not discussed here.

Ambiguous Genitalia/Congenital Adrenal Hyperplasia

Ambiguous genitalia create emotional and physical problems. Assignment of sex of rearing is made at birth, and reversing the parents' mindset later is both traumatic and difficult. Virilization of a genetically determined female may be a clue to congenital adrenal hyperplasia, some forms of which lead to salt wasting and cardiovascular collapse.

Etiology. Congenital adrenal hyperplasia is the most common cause of female virilization and male precocious puberty. It is an autosomal recessive disorder manifested by a deficiency in an enzyme that catalyzes the conversion of cholesterol to aldosterone, cortisol, and estrogen. Cortisol deficiency leads to increased adrenocorticotropic hormone (ACTH) production and hyperplasia of the adrenal gland.

Diagnostic Findings. Ambiguous genitalia in the genetically determined female presents as hypertrophy and enlargement of the clitoris and fusion of the labia, producing a malelike phenotype. In the male, microphallus and septation of the scrotum may produce an appearance similar to that of a clitoris and vagina.

The male with congenital adrenal hyperplasia rarely attracts medical attention in the immediate newborn period because he appears phenotypically normal. This patient may present in a salt-losing crisis with shock, and severe hyponatremia and hyperkalemia, usually late in the first week of life.

The diagnosis of ambiguous genitalia is made by simple observation. The cause of the defect is determined by chromosomal analysis, identification of gonads, and several biochemical markers.

Congenital adrenal hyperplasia should be suspected when any infant exhibits shock, hyponatremia, and hyperkalemia. It may occasionally cause hypoglycemia as well. Diagnosis is confirmed by findings of elevated urinary excretion of 17-ketosteroids and elevated plasma ACTH concentration.

Management. A primary goal is to refrain from speculating on the gender of the baby. It is best to explain to the parents that the child's genitalia are not completely formed and that further tests need to be performed to establish the gender. The pediatric endocrinologist in conjunction with a pediatric urologist will decide the sex of rearing, which may not be the same as the genetic sex.

Salt wasting in congenital adrenal hyperplasia should be treated with aggressive volume replacement and stabilization with isotonic saline solution, followed by intravenous D5W 0.9% normal saline (NS) at 100 to 125 ml/kg/24 hr. If hyponatremia and hyperkalemia are present, the patient should receive desoxycorticosterone acetate (DOCA) 1 mg intramuscularly. In addition, all patients should have steroid replacement with hydrocortisone sodium succinate 50 mg/m² intravenously.

With salt-losing forms of congenital adrenal hyperplasia, patients should be admitted to an intensive care unit for close monitoring and further management.

Hypocalcemia

Etiology. Hypocalcemia is defined as plasma calcium concentration less than 7.0 mg/dl. Hypocalcemia can result from several causes. Early onset hypocalcemia occurs during the first 72 hours of life, primarily in premature infants. Infants who have birth asphyxia and diabetic mothers may also need to be considered.

Late onset neonatal hypocalcemia occurs late in the first week of life and can be due to ingestion of formulas high in phosphates, maternal hyperparathyroidism with resultant suppression of fetal parathyroid activity, congenital hypoparathyroidism, or hypomagnesemia.

Diagnostic Findings. Symptoms in no way predict plasma calcium concentrations. Subtle signs of hypocalcemia include jitteriness and poor feeding. The overt manifestation of neonatal hypocalcemia is tetany, which is manifested by increased muscle activity, twitching, vomiting, carpopedal spasm, and clonus. Laryngospasm, manifested as stridor, can occur. The infant may also have clonic seizures.

Management. Documentation of hypocalcemia should be accomplished before treatment because of the potential for iatrogenic mishaps. In addition to serum calcium concentration, one should obtain magnesium and either serum protein or ionized calcium concentrations.

Administration of calcium gluconate (10%) 100 to 300 mg/kg intravenously (1 to 3 ml/kg at 1 ml/min) is the treatment for hypocalcemic seizures. Slow infusion with careful monitoring is necessary to prevent bradycardia. Continued symptoms can be treated with repeat calcium boluses as described. After control of symptoms, continuous infusion of calcium gluconate should be undertaken with 3 to 5 gm added to each 1 L of fluid.

If hypomagnesemia causes or accompanies hypocalcemia, it should be treated with 0.1 to 0.3 ml/kg of 50% magnesium sulfate intramuscularly. Alternatively, magnesium sulfate, 20 mg/kg IV, can be administered but caution should be exercised due to the side effect of respiratory depression.

Hypoglycemia

Hypoglycemia is defined as a whole blood glucose value less than 30 mg/dl or a plasma glucose level less than 35 mg/dl in the first 3 days of life in a term newborn. After this time, it is defined as less than 40 mg/dl in blood or 45 mg/dl in plasma. In premature infants, hypoglycemia is whole blood glucose level less than 20 mg/dl or plasma level of less than 25 mg/dl.

Etiology. Hypoglycemia is a nonspecific finding in neonates with causes ranging from lack of substrate availability in the low-birth-weight baby to excessive use in the stressed, septic baby. Many disorders associated with hypoglycemia are listed in the box above.

Diagnostic Findings. The maternal history is extremely important in the evaluation of possible neonatal hypoglycemia. Accurate determination of gestational age, glucose intolerance during pregnancy, risk factors for neonatal sepsis, and medication use by the mother are important factors to consider. In addition, information about the labor and delivery may give clues to birth asphyxia or other stresses that could cause hypoglycemia.

Clinical findings vary greatly from one infant to the next. Some infants demonstrate all of the signs that one classically associates with hypoglycemia, including lethargy,

---

Causes of Hypoglycemia in Infancy

Decreased glycogen storage
  Prematurity
  Small for gestational age infant
Metabolic
  Amino acid disorders
  Galactosemia
  Glycogen storage disease
  Mitochondrial enzymopathies
Hyperinsulinism
  Infant diabetic mother
  Insulin-secreting tumor
  Beckwith-Wiedemann syndrome
Other
  Sepsis
  Asphyxia
  Cold stress
  Erythroblastosis
  Polycythemia

---

obtundation, jitteriness, hypotonia, seizures, and apnea. Others may have the same glucose concentration as symptomatic children yet show no symptoms. Whether asymptomatic hypoglycemia causes long-term neurologic sequelae is not known.

The diagnosis is confirmed by plasma glucose level determination; however, the physician should obtain a rapid glucose determination from whole blood (Chemstrip, Dextrostix) while awaiting the confirmatory test.

Management. Treatment of neonatal hypoglycemia is similar to that of hypoglycemia in the older child or adult. If the infant is symptomatic, one should establish an intravenous line immediately and give 0.25 to 0.5 gm/kg of glucose. This can be accomplished by giving 3 to 5 ml/kg of a 10% dextrose solution or 1 to 2 ml/kg of a 25% dextrose solution over 1 to 2 minutes. After this initial "bolus" of glucose, an intravenous infusion of 10% dextrose at 4 ml/kg/hr should be instituted. Glucose concentration must be monitored and further hypoglycemia treated with a repeat bolus of glucose as described previously along with an increase in the continuous infusion rate of 1 ml/hr.

The asymptomatic neonate should also be treated; however, the method of treatment is controversial. If an intravenous line is to be established for another reason, one may follow the steps outlined for the symptomatic neonate. If the infant has a good suck and gag reflex, one may consider frequent oral feedings of formula or glucose water to raise the blood glucose concentration.

Occasionally, the hypoglycemic infant is symptomatic and has no easy intravenous access. In these situations, glucagon 0.1 mg/kg intramuscularly may mobilize hepatic glycogen stores and allow time for peripheral venous or umbilical venous catheterization. However, it is less effective in states of limited substrate availability.

GASTROINTESTINAL DISORDERS

Gastrointestinal emergencies of the neonate include disorders requiring early intervention by a pediatric surgeon, so referrals should be made expeditiously. Esophageal atresia and tracheoesophageal fistula commonly are associated with lower respiratory symptoms in neonates (see Chapter 52).

Abdominal Wall Defects

Abdominal wall defects that should be considered emergencies include omphalocele, gastroschisis, and omphalomesenteric duct. All three defects are uncommon, occurring in 1:2,500 live births. The likelihood that a patient delivered outside the hospital setting will enter the emergency department is minuscule.

Omphalocele and gastroschisis are developmental abnormalities of the intestines in which normal return to the abdominal cavity during foregut rotation does not occur. Associated anomalies are seen in 30% to 50% of children with omphalocele; many of the abnormalities are chromosomal. Gastroschisis has associated intestinal atresia, but no other organ systems appear to be involved.

Management. The rare newborn who enters the emergency department with abdominal wall defects is treated immediately by abdominal decompression with an orogastric tube and covering of the intestines with saline-solution-soaked sterile gauze. The infant can be placed in a sterile plastic bag to the level of the midchest to help minimize the chance of infection and prevent excess insensible water loss. Prophylactic antibiotics should be given. An intravenous infusion of fluid should be administered; rate of administration depends on the degree of dehydration present from evaporative water loss through the defect. Immediate consultation with a pediatric surgeon and administration of fluids are mandatory.

Bowel Obstruction/Perforation

Etiology. Bowel obstruction or perforation can occur at virtually any site along the alimentary tract. Some of the common causes of bowel obstruction and perforation in the neonate are listed in the box above.

Diagnostic Findings. The clinical findings of bowel obstruction vary with the site of the obstruction. High intestinal obstruction presents with emesis both during and between feedings. Emesis is commonly bile-stained, and the discovery of bile-stained emesis in a neonate necessitates an emergency evaluation for bowel obstruction. Abdominal distension is not frequently associated with an upper level bowel obstruction, and a history of passing meconium is commonly obtained.

In lower gastrointestinal obstruction, abdominal distention is the most common finding. The infant may never have passed stool. Vomiting only occurs late in the process. Frequently the infant will have taken feedings without a problem for several days before the symptoms appear.

Ancillary Data. Bilious vomiting in the neonate should be assumed to be a volvulus caused by malrotation until proved otherwise. Projectile vomiting and presence of a mass to the right of midline in the upper abdomen are signs of pyloric stenosis. These require emergency evaluation by a pediatric surgeon and a radiologist experienced

---

Causes of Bowel Obstruction/Perforation in Infancy

Hypertrophic pyloric stenosis
Gastric perforation
Duodenal atresia/web/stenosis
Annular pancreas
Intestinal atresia
Intestinal duplication
Meconium ileus
Malrotation with volvulus
Hypoplastic left colon
Hirschsprung disease
Necrotizing enterocolitis (NEC)
Intussusception
Peritoneal adhesions
Imperforate anus
Ileus

---

with neonatal disorders. A contrast enema, using air or barium, should precede any upper gastrointestinal series. The enema delineates the position of the cecum; a normal position rules out malrotation.

Signs of lower gastrointestinal obstruction also require pediatric surgical evaluation, plain films of the abdomen, and contrast studies.

Management. Acute management of these patients requires immediate decompression, fluid resuscitation, antibiotic prophylaxis, and surgical consultation. The emergency physician should be aware of the infant's ventilatory status because severe abdominal distension can hinder diaphragmatic movement. Fluids should be administered at 100 to 150 ml/kg/24 hr to provide maintenance and ongoing fluid loss replacement. Signs of hypovolemia, such as hypotension or prolonged capillary refill, should be treated vigorously with isotonic crystalloid or colloid fluid boluses of 10 ml/kg. Bolus administration can be repeated as needed.

Antibiotic administration should include coverage for anaerobic infections when evidence of intestinal perforation is present. Surgical consultation and intervention are required.

HEMATOLOGIC DISORDERS (See Chapter 54)

Anemia

Fetal hemoglobin that has a higher oxygen affinity than that of adult hemoglobin is produced in anemia. More red blood cells are present at delivery: hemoglobin in the normal term infant ranges between 13.7 and 20.1 gm/dl. Anemia in the immediate newborn period is therefore defined as a hemoglobin level less than 13.0 mg/dl.

After delivery, the infant is exposed to a high-oxygen environment and red cell production ceases. Hemoglobin values gradually fall over the ensuing 8 to 12 weeks to reach a physiologic nadir of 11.4 ± 0.9 gm/dl. At this point, oxygen delivery to the kidney becomes limited and erythropoiesis resumes.

Etiology. The causes of anemia in the neonate, as in the older child, can be grouped into three major categories: decreased production, increased destruction, and blood loss. Acute blood loss is probably the most common cause of anemia in neonates. The infant can lose blood by several mechanisms. Premature cord clamping can lead to trapping up to 125 ml of blood in the placenta. Abnormal placental channels can lead to fetal-maternal hemorrhage. Abnormal attachment and early detachment of the placenta to the uterus can cause significant maternal and fetal blood loss.

Impaired red cell production is an uncommon cause of anemia in the newborn. It may play a role in anemia associated with congenital viral infections. In addition, vitamin deficiencies can lead to underproduction of red cells. Several congenital red cell anemias exist but are not discussed here in detail.

Increased destruction of red cells may be due to isoimmunization of the mother with antibody production directed against the fetal red blood cell. ABO incompatibility and Rh disease are the most common causes of isoimmunization. In addition, red cells may have rapid turnover caused by inherited defects in the red cell (G6PD deficiency) or abnormal red cell membrane (spherocytosis). Infections, particularly those produced by *Escherichia coli* and TORCHS agents, can cause a hemolytic anemia (see p. 217).

Diagnostic Findings. The acute manifestations of anemia are similar in the neonate to those in the older child; however, they may be less well tolerated. Pallor, tachycardia, and prolonged capillary refill are common. Hypotension is a late manifestation. Jaundice, commonly seen with increased destruction of red cells, is a nonspecific finding in the newborn. Hepatomegaly may be associated with severe hemolytic processes, viral infections, congestive heart failure, or extramedullary hematopoiesis. Signs of congestive heart failure may be present in the infant with chronic anemia, the latter being caused by such conditions as untreated Rh hemolytic anemia.

Ancillary Data. Values for hemoglobin and hematocrit levels vary, depending on the sampling site; capillary values may overestimate the venous hemoglobin level by an average of 3.6 gm/dl. In cases of acute blood loss, the hemoglobin may initially be normal because of contraction of the vascular bed and then fall as interstitial fluid is mobilized into the vascular space to compensate for the acute volume loss.

In general, the diagnosis is confirmed by measuring the hemoglobin or hematocrit level obtained from venous blood and comparing the value to established norms for age. An elevated reticulocyte count suggests increased destruction or blood loss. An abnormal smear may provide evidence of red cell dyscrasia. Jaundice apparent within 24 hours of life or associated with bilirubin values greater than 10 mg/dl may be evidence of increased destruction. A positive direct Coombs' test result is highly sensitive for Rh disease but detects less than 50% of cases of ABO hemolytic anemia.[26]

Management. Treatment with blood transfusions should be reserved for those infants who are hemodynamically unstable or who have respiratory compromise. This instability is more common in infants with acute blood loss as opposed to those with a more chronic cause of anemia. Emergency transfusion can be performed with type O Rh-negative blood, administering 10 to 20 ml/kg over 20 to 30 minutes. If shock is present and blood is not available, colloid or isotonic saline solution may be substituted until blood becomes available.

Infants who have hemolytic anemia may have high-output congestive heart failure and benefit from administration of a diuretic along with slow transfusion of type O Rh-negative red blood cells.

Polycythemia

Polycythemia is defined as a venous hematocrit value greater than 65% in the newborn. Above 65%, blood viscosity increases exponentially.

Etiology. Polycythemia can be due to twin-to-twin transfusion, late clamping of the umbilical cord, and chronic in utero hypoxia. However, most cases have no identifiable cause.

Diagnostic Findings. Although symptoms such as respiratory distress, cyanosis, hypoglycemia, hypocalcemia, seizures, jaundice, and renal vein thrombosis occur in neonates with polycythemia, many infants are asymptomatic.

The diagnosis is confirmed by documenting a venous hematocrit value above 65%. Symptoms probably have more relation to viscosity, which tends to increase as hematocrit increases.

Management. Symptomatic polycythemic patients with hematocrit values greater than 70% usually undergo partial exchange transfusion to achieve a hematocrit value below 60%. Blood should be replaced with isotonic crystalloid.

Long-term follow-up observation of asymptomatic infants has not provided overwhelming evidence that treatment alters the course.[27]

Thrombocytopenia

Thrombocytopenia in infants is defined as a platelet count less than 100,000/mm³. Platelet counts can be low as a result of decreased production, increased destruction, or platelet loss.

Etiology. Decreased platelet production is uncommon in neonates; TORCHS infections are the most common cause (see p. 217). Increased loss is also uncommon and usually occurs after massive blood loss followed by transfusion of packed red blood cells. It is frequently observed after an exchange transfusion.

By far, the most common cause of platelet deficiency is increased destruction by sepsis or congenital infections. Immune thrombocytopenias, disseminated intravascular coagulation, and entrapment within a giant hemangioma (Kasabach-Merritt syndrome) cause thrombocytopenia.

Diagnostic Findings. Petechiae and abnormal bleeding are the hallmarks of thrombocytopenia. Associated findings vary with the cause. Congenital viral infections usually have other clinical manifestations. A giant hemangioma should be readily apparent. Frequently, neonate immune thrombocytopenia can be inferred from a maternal history of thrombocytopenia or of a sibling with PLA-1 antibody–induced thrombocytopenia.

Diagnosis is confirmed by obtaining an arterial or venous platelet count. Diagnostic evaluation should include an assessment for possible sepsis, determination of mother's platelet count, TORCHS infection serologic testing, and examination of the bone marrow for megakaryocytes. Determination of the presence of PLA-1 antigen on maternal platelets can be performed at some centers.

Management. The immediate management of the thrombocytopenic infant is directed toward prevention of bleeding and determination of underlying cause. Immediate determination of sepsis risk, procurement of blood cultures, and initiation of antibiotic administration in patients with disseminated intravascular coagulation are mandatory.

Platelet transfusion should be reserved for the infant who is bleeding or has a platelet count of less than 30,000/mm³. When platelet count is above this value, the patient can be admitted and have serial platelet determinations performed. Transfusion is not helpful for neonatal autoimmune thrombocytopenia because the antibody present rapidly removes these platelets also. In alloimmune thrombocytopenia caused by PLA-1 antibody, PLA-1 negative platelets need to be transfused. Intravenous gamma globulin 500 mg/kg may lead to a significant rise in platelet count in isoimmune and autoimmune thrombocytopenia.[28]

Hyperbilirubinemia

Although jaundice is one of the most common neonatal problems, it only occasionally should be deemed a true emergency. Occasionally jaundice is a symptom of some severe underlying disease process; in other cases it is considered "physiologic."

Pathophysiology. Unconjugated, or indirect, bilirubin is a normal breakdown product of hemoglobin. It binds to albumin and is transported to the liver, where it is conjugated, using the enzyme glucuronyl transferase, and excreted in the bile. During fetal life, glucuronyl transferase activity is low, so the bilirubin stays in the fat-soluble unconjugated form and crosses the placenta for maternal excretion. After birth, several days pass before glucuronyl transferase activity increases to a level where it can conjugate the bilirubin load. This leads to the indirect hyperbilirubinemia so often seen in normal newborn infants and termed *physiologic jaundice.*

Other causes of jaundice in the newborn that should not be considered physiologic are listed in the box above. Of particular importance among these causes of pathologic jaundice is bacterial sepsis, which must always be considered in the differential diagnosis. In addition, direct hyperbilirubinemia is never "physiologic."

Special mention should be made of breast milk and neonatal jaundice. Infants who breast feed have a higher level of physiologic jaundice than matched controls who drink formula.[29] This exaggeration of physiologic jaundice, seen during the first week of life, differs from breast milk jaundice, a syndrome seen in approximately 1% to 2% of breast-fed babies that appears in the second week of life. True breast milk jaundice is probably due to inhibition of hepatic bilirubin uptake, whereas jaundice associated with breast milk is due to calorie deficiency.[29,30]

Diagnostic Findings. Physiologic jaundice peaks on day 4 to 5 of life. The infant appears healthy, is eating well, has

---

Causes of Nonphysiologic Jaundice

Fetal-maternal blood group incompatibility
Sepsis
Polycythemia
Extravasation of blood (bruising, hematoma)
Abnormal red blood cells (spherocytosis, G6PD)
Inborn errors of metabolism (galactosemia, Gilbert disease)
Hypothyroidism
Breast milk jaundice
Direct hyperbilirubinemia

---

no hepatosplenomegaly, but has jaundice of the skin and sclera. Careful examination of liver and spleen size should be performed on all jaundiced infants. Enlargement of these organs may occur in severe hemolytic, processes, sepsis, congestive heart failure, and TORCHS infections.

A careful history to assess the risk factors for sepsis must be undertaken. Usually hyperbilirubinemia is not the only manifestation of bacterial sepsis, and one may find the infant lethargic, poorly perfused, hypotensive, or unable to drink from a bottle.

Ancillary Data. The diagnosis of physiologic jaundice is one of exclusion. The total bilirubin level is usually less than 13 mg/dl, with a direct fraction less than 10% of the total. The physician must evaluate for sepsis on the basis of a careful history and physical examination or cultures especially urine and blood. Hemolytic processes are likely if the reticulocyte count is elevated, an abundance of abnormally shaped cells is present on the peripheral smear, or the direct or indirect Coombs' test result is positive. Bowel obstruction should present additional clinical findings.

Management. Kernicterus, the principle complication of jaundice, appears to be related not only to the absolute bilirubin level, but also to the gestational age, underlying cause of the jaundice, and associated conditions such as asphyxia or presence of medications that displace bilirubin from albumin. For instance, kernicterus in the term, healthy newborn with physiologic jaundice is very rare.[31] However, because kernicterus is irreversible, caution should guide therapy toward prevention. For this reason, another factor should be considered when deciding therapy—the patient's age. Because physiologic jaundice typically peaks on the fourth day of life, one should be more aggressive in treating an infant younger than this to avoid the possibility that a borderline level will rise to a more dangerous level. Table 18-2 contains guidelines for treatment based on the presence or absence of hemolysis or other systemic illness in term infants. Ranges are given to account for a patient's age. Home phototherapy can be considered for select children.[31]

Infants with hemolytic anemia caused by blood group incompatibility need to be treated more aggressively to prevent kernicterus and congestive heart failure. One course of treatment based on the patient's age, weight, and

TABLE 18-2. Guidelines for Treatment of Jaundice

Treatment	Bilirubin level (mg/dl)	
	Well baby, no hemolysis	Sick baby or hemolysis
Phototherapy	17.5-22	13-17.5
Exchange transfusion	25-29	17.5-23.4

Adapted from Newman TB and Maisels MJ: Evaluation and treatment of jaundice in the term newborn: A kinder, gentler approach, *Pediatrics* 89(5):809, 1992.

Signs and Symptoms of Sepsis Neonatorum

Temperature instability
Lethargy
Poor feeding
Tachypnea
Vomiting
Abdominal distension
Jaundice
Petechiae

---

indirect bilirubin level is summarized in Table 18-2. These infants need to be monitored closely; the decision about therapy is based on several factors, including the clinical status of the child, gestational age, bilirubin level, rate of rise, and cause.

Diagnostic evaluation of direct hyperbilirubinemia entails numerous tests, which can be best managed on an inpatient basis.

INFECTIONS (See Chapters 55 and 56)

Bacterial Sepsis and Meningitis

Sepsis in the newborn occurs in 1 to 2/1,000 uncomplicated term births, and the incidence increases with certain peripartum complications, including chorioamnionitis, prolonged or premature (<37 weeks) rupture of membranes, maternal fever, and maternal colonization with group B *Streptococcus*. The bacteria can be acquired before birth and the infant evidences sepsis at birth. Alternatively colonization may occur during passage from the birth canal or later; the result is a delay in the onset of symptoms.

Etiology. During the first 4 to 6 weeks of life, the most common bacteria causing sepsis are organisms that commonly colonize the birth canal, which include group B streptococcus, *E. coli*, and *Listeria monocytogenes*. Group B streptococcus is the most common isolate from the blood of infants with sepsis.

Group B streptococcus and *L. monocytogenes* have similar epidemiologic characteristics. Both can cause early onset sepsis (<72 hours of age) with sepsis predominating or a late onset disease (4 to 14 days), which is usually manifested by meningitis, frequently without sepsis.

Diagnostic Findings. The clinical manifestations of bacterial sepsis are nonspecific (see box above). Respiratory symptoms are especially common in group B streptococcal sepsis.

Ancillary Data. Because the clinical signs of sepsis are nonspecific in the neonate, laboratory support is helpful in establishing a presumptive diagnosis. The complete blood count and differential are valuable but age-dependent. The total leukocyte count averages 18,100 cells/mm³ in healthy neonates with 52% polymorphonuclear neutrophils (PMNs). By 2 weeks of age, the total white blood cell count falls to an average of 11,400 cells/mm³ with a decrease in the number of neutrophils and a subsequent lymphocyte predominance in the differential on blood count. Se-

vere neutropenia (<2,000 PMN/mm³) or neutrophilia (>16,000 PMN/mm³) is worrisome. The ratio of immature granulocytes to total granulocytes can be helpful.[32]

The detection of bacterial antigens in the urine of infants with group B streptococcus and latex agglutination test may also be helpful in diagnosing sepsis. Urine collected by bag may give a false-positive result, requiring repetition with a catheterized specimen. However, a test result can be negative in patients who are septic, and other bacteria not detectable by these rapid methods may be present.

The diagnosis of bacterial sepsis or meningitis is confirmed by blood and cerebral spinal fluid culture. Culture of urine obtained by catheterization or suprapubic aspiration can also be of benefit, especially in neonates outside the immediate newborn period.[33,34] A chest x-ray film is indicated if respiratory symptoms, especially tachypnea, are present. Clinical impression has little reliability in differentiating the septic neonate from one with other disorders.

Management. The management of the neonate who is suspected of having bacterial sepsis or meningitis entails hospitalization and antimicrobial therapy. Generally neonates should be treated prospectively if there are overt signs of infection, laboratory abnormalities, or the child is at high risk (e.g., maternal fever, chorioamnionitis, asphyxia).

Antibiotics acceptable for the empiric treatment of bacterial sepsis in the infant less than 28 days should include coverage for group B streptococcus, *E. coli*, and *L. monocytogenes*. Older infants must be covered for *Haemophilus influenzae* and *Streptococcus pneumoniae*.

Acceptable antibiotic coverage for the infant less than 7 days of age would include a combination of intravenous ampicillin (100 to 200 mg/kg/24 hr) and gentamicin (5 mg/kg/24 hr), or ampicillin and cefotaxime (100 mg/kg/day). Because of the expanded coverage of cefotaxime against *H. influenzae*, its use should be strongly considered for the 4- to 6-week-old patient. Specific therapy should reflect full culture reports. Antibiotics are usually continued for a minimum of 48 hours pending cultures. Treat for 7 to 10 days if the blood culture result is positive or the child remains unstable. Intravenous gamma globulin (0.75 gm/kg) has been advocated by some.

Steroid treatment of the older child with meningitis is recommended to reduce the risks of hearing loss; however, one cannot extrapolate those data to newborn infants.[35]

Clinical Findings in the Congenitally Infected Neonate

Intrauterine growth retardation
Hepatosplenomegaly
Jaundice
Retinopathy
Cataracts
Corneal clouding
Encephalitis
Hearing deficits
Dermal erythropoiesis ("blueberry muffin")
Pneumonia

Congenital Infections

Congenital infections caused by viruses or bacteria are usually acquired transplacentally. Often the infection is subtle and the symptoms are undetectable in the early newborn period. These infections may also cause miscarriages, fetal death, or life-threatening symptoms in the newborn.

Etiology. The organisms that cause congenital infection include the familiar TORCHS agents — *Toxoplasma gondii*, rubella, cytomegalovirus (CMV), herpes simplex virus (HSV-2), and syphilis *(Treponema pallidum)* — as well as human immunodeficiency virus (HIV). Other viruses that cause chronic infection in the fetus and newborn are parvovirus, Epstein-Barr virus, and hepatitis B; they are not discussed in this chapter.

Diagnostic Findings. The infant with a congenital infection may have no signs or symptoms in the early newborn period and come to medical attention several months later with adenopathy, hemorrhagic rhinitis, snuffles, rhagades, and moist, raised plaquelike skin lesions.[36] Only 5% to 10% of CMV infections manifest clinical findings in the neonatal period, although it may be the leading cause of acquired deafness in the United States.[37] The infant born to a mother with acquired immunodeficiency syndrome (AIDS) or AIDS-related complex rarely appears abnormal at birth.

Much overlap exists with the symptoms of the infants with congenital infections, therefore making the diagnosis of the exact cause of the infection difficult (see box above).

Infants with HSV-2 almost always acquire the virus at the time of delivery from their mother with an active genital herpes lesion. The virus has an incubation period of 2 to 40 days with a mean incubation period of 6 days. The emergency physician potentially faces two situations: the asymptomatic newborn infant delivered in the emergency department or outside the hospital to a mother with an active herpes lesion and the 3- to 40-day-old infant who has signs and symptoms of herpes infection, including fever, vesicular rash, irritability, seizures, jaundice, and petechiae. The diagnosis can be readily made if the infant exhibits the classic vesicular skin lesions; these are present in only 50% of cases.[38] Evaluation of the febrile infant less than 2 months of age should always include the maternal history of mode of delivery and possible herpes infection.

Although the infant born to a mother who is seropositive for HIV or hepatitis B is rarely symptomatic at birth, it is imperative to ascertain this history following every delivery because prompt treatment of the newborn may decrease vertical transmission of the virus. A multicenter trial has shown that treatment of the HIV-seropositive mother with zidovudine during pregnancy and labor along with treatment of the newborn with zidovudine for 6 weeks decreased the vertical transmission of HIV from 25.5% in untreated to 8.3% in the treated group.[39] The critical component of the treatment plan (that is, treatment either prenatally or during labor or postnatally) was not ascertained. However, many pediatric immunologists recommend treatment of the baby born to an HIV-seropositive mother for 6 weeks commencing shortly after birth, regardless whether the mother received treatment. Likewise, early treatment of the infant born to a hepatitis B–seropositive mother with hepatitis B immunoglobulin will decrease the vertical transmission of that virus.[40]

Ancillary Data. Presently serologic tests exist for *T. pallidum*, rubella, CMV, *T. gondii*, HSV-2, and HIV. Many laboratories can perform tests for both immunoglobulin G (IgG) and IgM for these organisms. In addition, CMV cultures can be obtained from the urine and HSV-2 from the scraping of a skin lesion, cerebrospinal fluid, and occasionally the nasopharynx. Giemsa stain of scrapings of the base of a skin lesion often show multinucleated cells with viral particles in herpes infections; rapid immunofluorescence techniques can detect herpes virus in skin lesions.

Management. Infants born to a mother with active genital herpes lesion should be hospitalized and have cultures of nasopharyngeal secretions made to test for the virus. Many recommend surface cultures on a baby at 24 hours if there is a history of significant maternal history of herpes. If symptoms of infection are present or a culture grows for the virus, treatment with acyclovir 30 mg/kg/24 hr in three divided doses IV should be initiated. A normal course of 10 days is given if culture findings are positive.

Infants who exhibit signs and symptoms of herpes infection should be admitted to the hospital, preferably to an intensive care unit. Because the clinical signs of systemic herpes infection are so similar to those of bacterial sepsis, one should obtain blood for bacterial culture as well as cerebrospinal fluid for bacterial and viral culture. If skin lesions are present, a scraping deep enough to obtain cells at the base of the lesion should be sent for viral culture and herpes immunofluorescence studies.

Immediate treatment for the remaining congenital infections is primarily supportive. Infants born with syphilis or congenital CMV may have pneumonia. Hydrops fetalis, a condition in which the newborn has edema, ascites, and pleural effusions, is a well-recognized process in congenital syphilis or CMV. These infants have severe respiratory distress requiring respiratory support. Although treatment is available for syphilis, toxoplasmosis, and possibly CMV, treatment can be delayed for specific diagnostic test results. Proven congenital syphilis can be treated with benzathine penicillin G 50,000 units/kg IM as a single dose. A spinal tap should be done before therapy, and if the result is positive, aqueous crystalline penicillin G 50,000 units/kg/24 hr every 12 hours IV or IM for 10 days is appropriate. Some recommend this latter approach for all cases of suspected or proven congenital syphilis.

Organisms that cause congenital viral infections should be considered potentially contagious, and universal precautions should be employed at all times while managing these patients.

Treatment of the infant born to a mother who is seropositive for HIV should begin shortly after birth with zidovudine 2 mg/kg orally every 6 hours. Referral to a pediatrician with expertise in management of these infants is necessary. Infants born to mothers who are hepatitis B seropositive should undergo a thorough bath before receiving hepatitis B immunoglobulin 0.5 ml IM and begin vaccination with hepatitis B vaccine.

NEUROLOGIC DISORDERS

Drug Withdrawal (see Chapter 43)

Overall the incidence of drug abuse in the United States is increasing; abuse of opiates appears to be declining. The increase in drug abuse in the late 1980s and early 1990s appears to be due to cocaine abuse, particularly of crack cocaine. With an increased effort to curtail cocaine importation into the United States, a reemergence of opiate abuse may occur. With this, one can expect to find an increase in the number of infants born to drug-dependent women and thus an increase in the number of infants who suffer drug withdrawal.[41,42]

Diagnostic Findings. Symptoms usually appear 24 to 48 hours after birth, but the onset may be protracted to 2 weeks in newborns exposed to methadone.[43] The hallmarks of infant drug withdrawal are excessive irritability and decreased sleep time, as well as fever, sweating, and diarrhea. Vomiting can be particularly problematic and associated with poor weight gain in the infant. The symptom of most concern is seizures. The risk of seizures increases as the dose of the drug and the duration of drug abuse increase, but seizures remain uncommon and occur in approximately 3% of infants.[44]

Infants exposed to cocaine in utero tend to have small head circumference, jitteriness, irritability, poor eye contact, and vigorous sucking.[42] Seizures are rare.

Ancillary Data. Drug screens are unreliable for the diagnosis of drug withdrawal because the infant usually has metabolized and excreted the drug by the time symptoms occur. Recent work using analysis of hair samples has promise for the detection of cocaine metabolites after the urine concentration has fallen below detectable limits.

Management. Drug withdrawal needs to be aggressively managed because of the risk of seizures and cardiovascular collapse. The infant should be admitted to the hospital and closely monitored. If the history is unreliable, other possible diagnoses, such as sepsis, hypocalcemia, and hypoglycemia, need to be considered.

Some investigators suggest early pharmacologic therapy to treat drug withdrawal in neonates. Paregoric, an opiate itself, as well as benzodiazepam and phenobarbital, is effective in ameliorating some of the symptoms; however, seizures can still occur.[43] Treatment protocol usually entails long-term commitment to therapy, so the emergency physician should not begin therapy for minor symptoms.

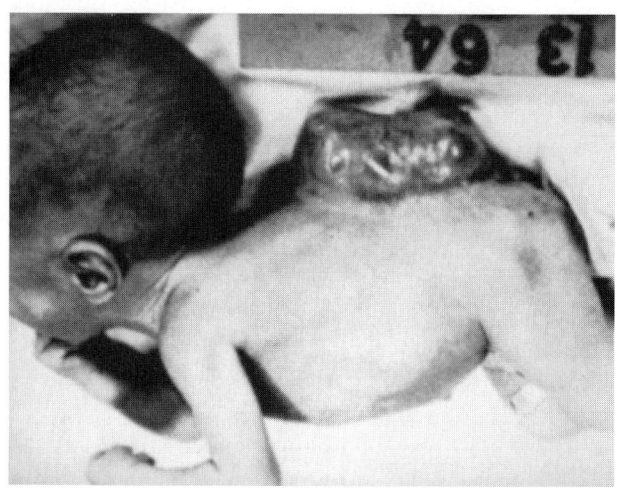

FIG. 18-2. Newborn infant with lumbar meningomyelocele.

Meningitis

The topic of meningitis in the newborn is discussed in detail in Chapter 56.

Meningomyelocele

Etiology. Meningomyelocele is a failure of closure of the neural tube around the fifth week of gestation. It is relatively common, with an incidence of approximately 1 in 500 births.

Diagnostic Findings. The infant with meningomyelocele has an obvious malformation over the spinal column discovered at birth. The defect contains both neural elements and meninges; it is sometimes enclosed in a transparent sac which often ruptures during labor or delivery (Fig. 18-2).

Infants always have associated neurologic deficits that are associated with the level of the defect. Movement of the lower extremities and lack of an anal wink are frequently present.

Meningomyelocele is almost always accompanied by Arnold-Chiari malformation of the brain, which may cause hydrocephalus in the newborn. Occasionally macrocephaly prohibits vaginal delivery.

Many cases of meningomyelocele are diagnosed prenatally through α-fetoprotein screening and subsequent ultrasonography. The diagnosis is readily apparent at birth. Careful examination of the level of neurologic deficits should be performed as well as a careful determination of head circumference for possible hydrocephalus.

Management. Immediate management of the infant with meningomyelocele includes local wound care, prevention of infection, and referral to a pediatrician or neonatologist. The meningomyelocele should be covered with sterile gauze moistened with warmed saline solution. Infants who have meningomyelocele should be treated with broad-spectrum antibiotics, such as ampicillin (100 mg/kg/24 hr q 12 hr IV) and gentamicin (5 mg/kg/24 hr q 12 hr IV).

The family should be counseled that surgery is required to close the defect to prevent infection.

Causes of Neonatal Seizures

Metabolic
    Hypoglycemia
    Hyponatremia
    Hypernatremia
    Hypocalcemia
    Pyridoxine deficiency
Asphyxia/birth trauma
Intracranial hemorrhage
Developmental brain disorder
Meningitis

Seizures (see Chapter 56)

Seizures in the neonate often appear different from those in the older child or adult and frequently are due to causes unique to the neonate.

Etiology. The causes of neonatal seizures are summarized in the box above. In addition to the causes that one sees with first seizures in the older child, several others are unique to the neonate. Among these are birth trauma, narcotic withdrawal, CNS structural abnormalities, inborn errors of metabolism, and pyridoxine deficiency.

Diagnostic Findings. It is vital to obtain information about the mother's prenatal course, labor, and delivery of the infant. Information concerning infection risks, prenatal TORCHS studies, substance abuse, and events suggesting perinatal asphyxia and family history of seizures is important.

The physical examination of the infant with seizures may reveal well-recognized tonic or tonic-clonic activity of the extremities and eyes, but often seizures in neonates are subtle. Findings of subtle seizures include staring spells, prolonged eye deviation, lip smacking, tongue thrusting, bicycling, and apnea.[3]

One should compare growth patterns of the head circumference with length and weight, as relative microcephaly or macrocephaly is a clue to underlying structural brain malformations. The patient's head should be palpated. A bulging fontanelle may be consistent with increased intracranial pressure, as is often seen in meningitis. Examination of the eyes should look for cataracts or corneal clouding, both of which are associated with congenital infections and inborn errors of metabolism.

Serum electrolyte, calcium, magnesium, and glucose concentrations need to be determined as in emergencies involving the older child or adult. Treatment of seizures caused by these imbalances requires correction of the abnormality. Electroencephalography (EEG) may be used to confirm clinical suspicion of a seizure. However, clinical seizures may be unaccompanied by EEG correlation.

Management. Attention must be directed to maintenance of adequate ventilation during the seizure. Oxygen should be given and apnea aggressively managed by tracheal intubation and ventilatory support.

Diagnosis of the underlying cause of the seizure is paramount to management. Correction of hypoglycemia, hypocalcemia, or hypomagnesemia is mandatory. Administration of antibiotics to the septic patient should take place as soon as cultures are obtained.

If the seizure is not due to an immediately correctable cause, treatment with an anticonvulsant is indicated. Phenobarbital 15-20 mg/kg IV loading dose is the most widely used first-line anticonvulsant in neonates. Studies indicate that few patients benefit from plasma concentrations higher than 40 μg/dl.[6] In those instances where phenobarbital is unsuccessful in controlling seizures, phenytoin 10 to 20 mg/kg can be given by slow IV administration. Lorazepam 0.1 mg/kg may also be used for recalcitrant seizures.

Neonates with seizure should be admitted to the hospital, preferably to a pediatric intensive care unit. Close monitoring of cardiorespiratory and neurologic status is important.

RENAL DISORDERS

Acute Renal Failure (see Chapter 60)

Acute renal failure in the neonate is a sudden diminution in renal function with subsequent azotemia. Usually this decrease in renal function is associated with a decrease in urine output, but this is not always the case.

Etiology. As in the older patient, the causes of acute renal failure can be categorized into three major subgroups: prerenal, renal, and postrenal obstruction. Prerenal obstruction is caused by hypoperfusion of the kidney and may be due to hypovolemia, hypotension, hypoxia, or congestive heart failure; it is the most common cause of acute renal failure in newborns.[45] Intrinsic renal causes are numerous and range from renal damage produced by asphyxia to congenital malformations of the kidney and renal damage secondary to drugs or toxins. Postrenal obstructions can be anatomic, as in posterior urethral valves, or physiologic, as in neurogenic bladder.

Diagnostic Findings. The infant may have a history of infrequent urination, edema, blood in the urine, lethargy, or poor appetite. In prerenal azotemia signs of hypovolemia or congestive heart failure may be present. In intrinsic renal disease a history of traumatic labor or delivery (postasphyxia), of maternal diabetes (renal vein thrombosis), or of sibling renal problems (congenital renal anomalies) may be obtained. In postrenal obstruction one may obtain a history of an inadequate stream or dribbling of urine in a newborn male (posterior urethral valves).

Ancillary Data. Acute renal failure in the newborn can be suspected if urine output is less than 0.5 ml/kg/hr or if blood urea nitrogen (BUN) level is greater than 20 mg/dl. Concomitant with this is a rise in serum creatinine; however, in the first few days of life the creatinine level reflects the mother's level and may be falsely elevated in the neonate. By 1 week of age the creatinine level averages 0.4 mg/dl. Hyperkalemia is a late finding in severe acute renal failure.

Other laboratory tests may be helpful in the assessment of renal failure. The fractional excretion of sodium can differentiate prerenal from renal causes of oliguria, with values less than 2 in prerenal and greater than 3 in renal causes.[46]

Causes of Infantile Apnea

Central: apnea of prematurity, particularly <34 weeks, maternal narcotic use, magnesium ingestion before delivery

Metabolic: hypoglycemia, hypocalcemia, hypothermia

Infection: sepsis, pneumonia, meningitis

CNS damage: hemorrhage, hypoxic injury, seizures

Pulmonary: respiratory distress, hyaline membrane disease (HMD), pneumonia, obstruction

---

Response to a fluid challenge is another diagnostic finding that the emergency physician may use to differentiate prerenal from renal causes of oliguria. If no evidence of congestive failure is present, administer 10 ml/kg of isotonic saline solution over 5 to 10 minutes. If there is no urine output within an hour, the fluid bolus can be repeated and followed with furosemide 1.0 mg/kg. If there is still no response, one can assume a renal cause of oliguria, as long as obstruction has been ruled out.

Management. If there is oliguria, the patient should have a urinary catheter placed to rule out urethral obstruction and bladder atony. Any urine collected should be saved for urinalysis and determination of osmolality and fractional excretion of sodium. If prerenal causes are suspected, the underlying cause of the prerenal azotemia should be treated. This would include volume replacement in hypovolemic patients, control of congestive heart failure, and treatment of hypotension. If renal causes are suspected on the basis of either history, laboratory test results, or failure of response to a fluid challenge, then the infant needs to have fluids restricted to insensible water loss, usually 35 ml/kg/day in the term infant. Potassium should be withheld from intravenous fluids.

RESPIRATORY DISORDERS (See Chapter 59)

Respiratory system abnormalities are a common cause of problems in neonates, especially in the first few weeks of life. Often children have been discharged and return to the emergency department in distress.

Apnea

Apnea is defined as the cessation of breathing for 20 seconds, or for less than 20 seconds when associated with symptoms such as bradycardia (<100 beats/min), color change, or altered mental status.

Etiology. Several causes of apnea are known, and the correct diagnosis is critical for the immediate and long-term care of the patient. Some common causes of apnea in infancy are listed in the box above.

Temperature instability, especially overwarming, is an established cause of apnea in premature infants, and the history obtained from the caretaker should include information about this possibility. The incidence of apnea of prematurity is inversely proportional to the gestational age.

It can occur anytime before 44 weeks gestation but is much less likely to present for the first time after 34 weeks gestation.

Diagnostic Findings. The diagnosis of apnea must be made by the history obtained from the caretaker. Specific attention should be directed to observations of color change, limpness, and unresponsiveness, especially if the infant has a history of apnea and was being monitored during the event. Often the monitor alarm sounds for loose leads or for heart rate below the limit selected, although the child is asymptomatic.

The tests to rule out treatable causes of apnea, such as sepsis, hypoglycemia, hypocalcemia, hypoxia, gastroesophageal reflux, and seizures, should include chest x-ray films, pulse oximetry, glucose level, white blood cell count, and, as indicated, levels of electrolytes and calcium, lumbar puncture, and sepsis evaluation.

Management. Infants with the presumptive diagnosis of apnea need to be admitted to the hospital and observed closely. Electronic apnea monitoring is mandatory. A physician with interest in and knowledge of childhood apnea should follow the patient.

Bronchopulmonary Dysplasia

Bronchopulmonary dysplasia (BPD) is an acquired chronic lung disorder found in many newborns who survive modern neonatal intensive care. Most of these infants are premature, suffer from hyaline membrane disease, and have mechanical ventilation. Many of these infants are discharged home with continued oxygen use as well as diuretic and bronchodilator therapy. The emergency physician is not expected to diagnose this disease but may be required to manage an infant with BPD who has acquired an intercurrent illness or decompensation in respiratory status.

Diagnostic Findings. The hallmarks of BPD are hypoxemia and hypercarbia; obtaining an arterial blood gas determination is mandatory. If possible, the chest film should be compared to prior films to determine whether the child has an intercurrent viral or bacterial pulmonary infection.

Because these infants are prone to fluid overload and cor pulmonale, a careful examination of the patient's weight compared to prior weights obtained from the patient's record should be performed.

Management. Hypoxemia should be vigorously treated with supplemental oxygen to obtain a saturation greater than 90% so as to reduce the risk of cor pulmonale. Inappropriate weight gain can be treated with furosemide 1 mg/kg IV or IM. Wheezing can be treated with nebulized albuterol 2.5 to 5.0 mg in 2.5 ml saline solution. Decompensation in the status of an infant with BPD warrants admission and aggressive intervention in the hospital to optimize management and monitor for further decompensation.

Pneumonia

Etiology. Pneumonia in the first month of life is caused by a pathogen acquired either during the birth process or postnatally or by aspiration of oral-gastric contents. The most common bacterial agent to cause pneumonia in the first month of life is group B streptococcus; organisms such as *Chlamydia trachomatis* (especially in the 2- to 4-week-old who has a history of conjunctivitis), *Pneumocystis carinii*, and *Ureaplasma urealyticum* also play a significant role in pneumonia in this age group.[47] Occasionally more than one pathogen is identified. HSV-2, CMV, and respiratory syncytial virus may also cause pneumonia in the neonatal period.

Diagnostic Findings. The symptoms of pneumonia in infancy vary with the causative organism. For instance, the infant with group B streptococcal or herpes simplex pneumonia is usually acutely ill with respiratory distress, shock, and possibly disseminated intravascular coagulation, whereas the infant who has *C. trachomatis* or *U. urealyticum* pneumonia has mild respiratory symptoms of gradual onset. Tachypnea is one of the most reliable signs of pneumonia; however, retractions, rales, adventitious breath sounds, and wheezing may also be present.

Ancillary Data. The chest film confirms the diagnosis of pneumonia as the cause of respiratory distress. It usually demonstrates hyperinflation of the lungs and interstitial or alveolar infiltrates. The chest film of the infant with group B streptococcal pneumonia often cannot be distinguished from that of the infant with hyaline membrane disease; however, after the early peripartum period the likelihood of hyaline membrane disease is small.

A complete blood count and differential can be helpful in distinguishing bacterial from viral or noninfectious causes of pneumonia. In addition, eosinophilia is a common finding in chlamydial pneumonia.

Blood should be obtained for bacterial culture and nasopharyngeal swab or washings for viral, *Chlamydia*, and *Ureaplasma* culture. In addition, nasopharyngeal secretions can be analyzed by fluorescent antibody techniques for rapid diagnosis of *Chlamydia*, herpes simplex, and respiratory syncytial virus infections.

Management. The infant who has pneumonia should be admitted to the hospital and begin antimicrobial therapy while bacterial culture results are pending. The same empiric antibiotic regimen as for presumed sepsis (see Infections/Bacterial Sepsis) can be started until a definitive diagnosis is made.

Supportive therapy, such as use of supplemental oxygen, intravenous fluids, blood pressure support, and mechanical ventilation, must be individualized on the basis of the degree of illness of the patient.

Pneumothorax/Lobar Emphysema

Pneumothorax and lobar emphysema are discussed together because congenital lobar emphysema may lead to pneumothorax and lobar emphysema is often misdiagnosed in the emergency department as pneumothorax.

Etiology. The cause and exact incidence of congenital lobar emphysema are unknown. At surgery or autopsy one lobe of the lung is usually affected.

Spontaneous pneumothorax is common: a reported incidence of 1% to 2% of asymptomatic newborns have small pneumothoraces.[48] Symptomatic spontaneous pneumothorax is much less common but does require symptomatic evaluation, particularly when there is underlying pulmonary disease.

Diagnostic Findings. Lobar emphysema can present in the immediate newborn period but is much more likely to occur between 1 and 4 weeks of life. The primary symptom is progressive dyspnea. On examination the child has some degree of respiratory distress manifested by wheezing, labored breathing, and retractions. An area of hyperresonance may be found over the affected lobe. Pneumothorax can present similar findings, but usually the onset is much more rapid.

Ancillary Data. The diagnosis of either pneumothorax or lobar emphysema is confirmed by chest film; however, one must read the film carefully. The hyperlucent lobe in congenital emphysema may appear so radiolucent that one mistakes it for pneumothorax. If questions about the possibility of pneumothorax in a patient who is not critically ill arise, time should be taken to obtain a lateral decubitus film to verify that the air is extrapleural and layers out along the higher side.

Management. Moderately to severely symptomatic pneumothorax must be treated expeditiously by placement of a thoracostomy tube. In patients who demonstrate hypotension, the air can be aspirated from the chest by needle thoracostomy. This may be done at the second intercostal space in the midclavicular line of anterior axillary line at the level of the nipples. Mildly symptomatic pneumothorax can be admitted to the hospital under close observation.

The treatment of lobar emphysema requires bronchoscopy to remove any potential foreign body, and thoracotomy if symptoms do not abate from removal of foreign bodies. These patients require urgent consultation with a pediatric surgeon experienced in thoracic procedures.

References

Acute Distress in the Neonate

1. Sarnat HB and Sarnat MS: Neonatal encephalopathy following fetal distress, *Arch Neurol* 33:696, 1976.
2. Hagberg B and Hagberg G: Prenatal and perinatal risk factors in a survey of 681 Swedish cases, *Clin Dev Med* 87:116, 1984.
3. Finberg L: The relationship of intravenous infusion and intracranial hemorrhage-a commentary, *J Pediatr* 91:777, 1977.
4. Goldberg RN, Moscosco P, Bauer CR, et al: Use of barbiturate therapy in severe perinatal asphyxia: a randomized controlled trial, *J Pediatr* 109:851, 1986.
5. Donn SM, Grasela TH, Goldstein GW: Safety of a higher dose of phenobarbital in the term newborn, *Pediatrics* 75:1061, 1985.
6. Gilman JT, Gal P, Duchowny MS, et al: Rapid sequential phenobarbital treatment of neonatal seizures, *Pediatrics* 83:674, 1989.
7. Avery ME and Taeusch HW: Hyaline membrane disease. In Avery ME and Taeusch HW, editors: *Schaffer's diseases of the newborn*, ed 5, Philadelphia, 1984, WB Saunders.
8. Klaus M, Fanaroff A, Martin RJ: Respiratory problems. In Klaus M and Fanaroff A, editors: *Care of the high risk neonate*, ed 2, Philadelphia, 1979, WB Saunders.
9. Scopes JW: Metabolic rate and temperature control in the human infant, *Br Med Bull* 22:88, 1966.
10. Patz A, Hoeck LE, De La Cruz E: Studies on the effect of high oxygen administration in retrolental fibroplasia. I. Nursery observation, *Am J Ophthalmol* 35:1248, 1952.
11. Lanmam JT, Guy LP, Dancis J: Retrolental fibroplasia and oxygen therapy, *JAMA* 155:223, 1954.
12. Drew JH: Immediate intubation at birth of the very low-birth-weight infant: effect on survival, *Am J Dis Child* 136:207, 1982.
13. Hallman M, Merritt TA, Jarvenpaa AL, et al: Exogenous human surfactant for treatment of severe respiratory distress syndrome: a randomized prospective clinical trial, *J Pediatr* 106:963, 1985.
14. Horbar JD, Soll RF, Sutherland JM, et al: A multicenter randomized, placebo-controlled trial of surfactant therapy for respiratory distress syndrome. *N Engl J Med* 320:959-965, 1989.

15. Bose C, Corbett A, Bose G, et al: Improved outcome at 28 days of age for very low birthweight infants treated with a single dose of a synthetic surfactant, *J Pediatr* 117:947, 1990.

16. OSIRIS Collaborative Group: Early versus delayed neonatal administration of a synthetic surfactant—the judgement of OSIRIS. *Lancet* 340:1363, 1992.

17. Kattwinkel J, Bloom BT, Delmore P, et al: Prophylactic administration of calf lung surfactant extract is more effective than early treatment of respiratory distress syndrome in neonates of 29 through 32 weeks gestation, *Pediatrics* 92:90, 1993.

18. Duenhoelter JH and Pritchard JA: Fetal respiration: quantitative measurements of amniotic fluid inspired near term by human and rhesus fetuses, *Am J Obstet Gynecol* 125:306, 1976.

19. Gregory GA, Gooding CA, Phibbs RH, et al: Meconium aspiration in infants-a prospective study, *J Pediatr* 85:848, 1974.

20. Falciglia HS: Failure to prevent meconium aspiration syndrome, *Obstet Gynecol* 71:349, 1988.

21. Cardiopulmonary resuscitation (CPR) and emergency cardiac care (ECC). VI: neonatal advanced life support, *JAMA* 255 (CPR issue):2969, 1986.

22. Potter EL: Bilateral renal agenesis, *J Pediatr* 29:68, 1946.

23. Hall JN, Uchman RS, Dominquez R: Trends and patterns of methamphetamine abuse in the United States, Bethesda, Md, 1988, National Institute on Drug Abuse Publication.

24. Bower S and Hull CJ: Comparative pharmacokinetics of fentanyl and afentanil, *Br J Anaesth* 54:211, 1982.

25. Committee on Drugs: Naloxone dosage and route of administration for infants and children: addendum to emergency drug doses for infants and children, *Pediatrics* 86:484, 1990.

Postnatal Emergencies

26. Desjardins L, Blajchman MA, Chintu C, et al: The spectrum of ABO hemolytic disease of the newborn infant, *J Pediatr* 95:447, 1979.

27. Fischer AF and Sunshine P: The thick blood syndrome, *Perinatol Neonat* 8:39, 1984.

28. Brussel JB: Neonatal uses of intravenous immunoglobulin. *Am J Pediatr Hematol Oncol* 12:505, 1990.

29. Maisels MJ, Gifford K, Antle CE, et al: Jaundice in the healthy newborn infant: a new approach to an old problem, *Pediatrics* 81:505, 1988.

30. Follot TA, Ploussard JP, Housset E, et al: Breast milk jaundice: in vitro inhibition of rat liver bilirubinuridine diphosphate glycuronyl transferase activity and Z protein-bromosulfophthalein binding by human breast milk, *Pediatr Res* 10:594, 1976.

31. Meropol SB, Luberti AA, DeJong AR, et al: Home phototherapy: Use and attitudes among community pediatricians, *Pediatrics* 91:97, 1993.

32. Phillips AGS and Hewitt JR: Early diagnosis of neonatal sepsis. *Pediatrics* 65:1036, 1980.

33. Crain EF and Gershel JC: Urinary tract infections in febrile infants younger than 8 weeks of age, *Pediatrics* 86:363, 1990.

34. Voora S, Srinivasan G, Lilien LD, et al: Fever in full term newborns in the first four days of life, *Pediatrics* 69:40, 1982.

35. American Academy of Pediatrics Committee on Infectious Disease: Dexamethasone therapy for bacterial meningitis in infants and children, *Pediatrics* 86:130, 1990.

36. Ikeda MK and Jenson HB: Evaluation and treatment of congenital syphilis, *J Pediatr* 117:843, 1990.

37. Alford CA and Britt WJ: Cytomegalovirus. In Fields BM, Knipe DM, Chanock EM, et al, editors: *Virology,* New York, 1985, Raven Press.

38. Whitley RJ, Nahmias AJ, Soong S, et al: Vidarabine therapy of neonatal herpes simplex virus infection, *Pediatrics* 66:495, 1980.

39. Conner EM, Sperling RS, Gelber R, et al: Reduction of maternal-infant transmission of human immunodeficiency virus type 1 with Zidovudine treatment. Pediatric AIDS Clinical Trials Protocol 076 Study Group, *New Engl J Med* 331:1223, 1994.

40. American Academy of Pediatrics Committee on Infectious Diseases: Section 3: summaries of Infectious Diseases: In Peter G, Halsey NA, Marcuse EK, et al, editors: *1994 Red Book: Report of the Committee on Infectious Diseases,* ed 23, Elk Grove Village, 1994, American Academy of Pediatrics.

41. Rothstein P and Gould JB: Born with a habit, *Pediatr Clin North Am* 21:307, 1974.

42. Bingol N, Fuchs M, Diaz V, et al: Teratology of cocaine in humans, *J Pediatr* 110:93, 1987.

43. Kandall SR, Doberczak TM, Mauer KR, et al: Opiate v. CNS neonatal drug abstinence syndrome, *Am J Dis Child* 137:378, 1983.

44. Zelson C, Rubir E, Wasserman E: Neonatal narcotic addiction, *Pediatrics* 48:178, 1971.

45. Norman ME and Asadi FK: A prospective study of acute renal failure in the newborn infant, *Pediatrics* 63:475, 1979.

46. Jose PA, Stewart CL, Tina LU, et al: Renal disease. In Avery GB, editor: *Neonatology, pathophysiology and management of the newborn,* ed 3, Philadelphia, 1987, JB Lippincott.

47. Stagno S, Bradfield DM, Brown MB, et al: Infantile pneumonitis associated with cytomegalovirus, chlamydia, pneumocystis, and ureaplasma: a prospective study, *Pediatrics* 68:322, 1981.

48. Chernick V and Avery ME: Spontaneous alveolar rupture in newborn infants, *Pediatrics* 32:816, 1963.

PART IV

TRAUMA

Approach to Multiple Trauma

Laura S. Fitzmaurice

Injury is the leading cause of death in children above 9 months of age in the United States,[1] accounting for approximately 22,000 lives lost each year.[2] In addition, 600,000 children are hospitalized and 16 million are seen in emergency departments (ED) across the country.[3] The health care cost is estimated at $158 billion per year nationally, with estimates for initial hospitalization at $5,094 per patient and emergency department visits for injury at $171 per patient.[4] Thus it is important to understand the patterns of pediatric trauma and the specific problems related to the resuscitation of the child. Both the physical and psychologic needs of the child and family must be considered in acute care management. Ideally, a team approach will be used to organize the resuscitation and will provide participants a sense of accomplishment with their particular role in the child's care. From the minor to the most severe injuries, a well-organized approach is essential.

Motor vehicle–occupant injuries are the leading cause of injury death among children up to the age of 19 years in the United States and cause 47% of all injury deaths.[5] The other leading causes of death in descending order are homicide, suicide, drowning, motor vehicle–pedestrian accident, and burns.[6] (Some regional variation exists in the United States.) The death rate for trauma has risen by 1% a year since 1977. For each death from trauma there are at least two cases of permanent disability (50,000 to 100,000 cases), exceeding the years of potential life lost for prematurity and congenital anomalies combined.[7]

Spring and summer are the peak seasons for trauma and the peak occurrences are during daylight hours, particularly when motor vehicle–related.

Male children are injured more frequently, and African-American male children are more often involved in intentional injuries.[8] Bicycle and motor vehicle–pedestrian injuries affect children 6 to 12 and 5 to 9 years of age, respectively, in the majority of circumstances.[9,10] Risk factors for pediatric injury include inadequate supervision, developmental inadequacy to perform the task, inadequate attention to the task, showing off, risk taking, and use of drugs and alcohol[11] (see also Chapter 3).

INJURY SEVERITY MEASURES

Injury severity has been defined by several epidemiologic variables, including trauma scoring systems, numbers of deaths, and length of hospital stay. Mortality has been demonstrated to exhibit a trimodal distribution.[12] *Immediate deaths* are those that occur very shortly after injury, usually at the scene. These represent more than 50% of trauma deaths and are secondary to fatal types of injuries, including decapitation, ventricular rupture, or brain stem

223

TABLE 19-1. Pediatric Trauma Score

Variables	+2	+1	−1
Airway	Normal	Maintainable	Unmaintainable
CNS	Awake	Obtunded/LOC	Coma
Body weight	>20 kg	10-20 kg	<10 kg
Systolic BP	>90 mm Hg	90-50 mm Hg	<50 mm Hg
Open wound	None	Minor	Major
Skeletal injury	None	Closed fracture	Open/multiple fractures

A score of +2, +1, or −1 is given to each variable, then added (range −6 to 12). A score ≤8 indicates potentially important trauma. *LOC,* Loss of consciousness.

TABLE 19-2. Revised Trauma Score

Revised Trauma Score	Glasgow Coma Score	Systolic blood pressure (mm Hg)	Respiratory rate (breaths/min)
4	13-15	>89	10-20
3	9-12	76-89	>29
2	6-8	50-75	6-9
1	4-5	1-49	1-5
0	3	0	0

A score of 0-4 is given for each variable, then added (range, 1-12). A score ≤11 indicates potentially important trauma.

herniation. Trauma centers do not improve the statistics for recovery of these patients. Instead, prevention strategies are invaluable, such as car-seat restraints, bicycle helmets, and smoke detectors. *Early deaths* are those that occur within hours of injury and represent about 30% of the trauma deaths. The usual cause is major internal hemorrhage. Trauma education focusing on early detection and treatment for all acute care providers can help to decrease morbidity and mortality in this category. Trauma center systems, through organization of services and experience of personnel, can decrease this morbidity and mortality. *Late deaths* are those that occur days or weeks after injury and are secondary to infection or multiple organ failure. Ongoing research is needed to help us understand and improve the survival for these patients.

A number of injury severity scoring systems have been developed to assist in triage decisions (see Chapter 4), as well as to monitor progression of the clinical status. The Pediatric Trauma Score is one of these and is based on factors known to increase mortality and morbidity in the pediatric patient (Table 19-1). The points are totaled in each of six categories. The lowest score (−6) represents the most severe injury and the highest score (12) represents the least severe injury. Children with a score ≤8 are considered the most severely injured and should be triaged to a designated trauma center with pediatric critical care capabilities.[13-17] The Revised Trauma Score (Table 19-2) has also been used to define severity of injury from the prehospital environment through the hospital stay. The Revised Trauma Score can be used in both adults and children and has been shown to be a valid predictor of severity.[18-20] The Pediatric Trauma Score has been shown to be a better predictor for emergency department disposition, whereas the Revised Trauma Score has a better predictive value for overall outcome.[21-23] The CRAMS scale is a scoring system developed for field triage based on five components: Circulation, Respiration, Abdomen, Motor, and Speech. It was developed for Emergency Medical Service (EMS) providers as a less complex scale for use in comparison with the Trauma Score to determine major and minor trauma for routing. It has been field tested primarily in adult trauma systems and its applicability to children is unclear.[24]

The Pediatric Glasgow Coma Score (PGCS) (Table 19-3) is a neurologic assessment of the pediatric patient based on

the adult Glasgow Coma Score (GCS) and additionally provides parameters for assessment of younger patients. The PGCS divides categories of assessment to provide for preverbal communication. It is an objective tool in monitoring the child's neurologic function from prehospital care through hospital stay as outlined in Chapter 20. The PGCS was designed for use in trending a patient's neurologic responsiveness over time for a prediction of outcome. A single score does not in itself have predictive value.

The range of scoring is from 3 to 15, where 15 represents a normal neurologic examination result. A PGCS of 13 to 15 represents a mild neurologic defect; 8 to 12 represents a moderate neurologic defect; and <8 represents a severe neurologic defect.

UNIQUE ASPECTS

Although the priorities of history and physical assessment are the same for the child as for the adult, the pediatric trauma patient differs from the adult in many aspects. Whereas adult trauma is predominantly penetrating in nature, blunt trauma represents the major proportion of trauma seen in the pediatric patient. It has traditionally accounted for approximately 80% of all trauma.[25] Penetrating trauma is seen more frequently in urban areas but still represents a minor proportion of the major pediatric trauma patients treated.[26] Children are also noted to have patterns of injury with certain types of trauma that are not seen in the adult. Of major importance are the anatomic and physiologic differences that must be taken into account in the evaluation and management of the injured child.

More than 80% of multiple injuries involve the head and almost 30% of all childhood injury deaths result from a head injury. This is because the head represents a relatively large percentage of the total body mass but is only weakly supported by the muscles of the neck. The combination of these factors plus the thin cranium makes the child especially vulnerable to a primary injury. In addition, the scalp is very vascular with a relatively large surface area creating a potential for significant blood loss leading to shock.

Intracranial pressure is more commonly elevated in children with severe head injuries, but even in those who have an open fontanelle, sudden decompensation can occur because of less cerebrospinal fluid buffering capacity.[27,28] The child with a central nervous system injury has an increased risk of mortality.[29] However, outcome in children

TABLE 19-3. Pediatric Glasgow Coma Score (PGCS)

Glasgow Coma Score (GCS)	Pediatric modification	
Eye opening	**Eye opening**	
≥1 year	*0-1 year*	
4 Spontaneously	Spontaneously	
3 To verbal command	To shout	
2 To pain	To pain	
1 No response	No response	
Best motor response	**Best motor response**	
≥1 year	*0-1 year*	
6 Obeys command		
5 Localizes pain	Localizes pain	
4 Flexion withdrawal	Flexion withdrawal	
3 Flexion abnormal (decorticate)	Flexion abnormal (decorticate)	
2 Extension (decerebrate)	Extension (decerebrate)	
1 No response	No response	
Best verbal response	**Best verbal response**	
>5 years	*2-5 years*	*0-2 years*
5 Oriented and converses	Appropriate words and phrases	Cries appropriately, smiles, coos
4 Disoriented and converses	Inappropriate words	Cries
3 Inappropriate words	Cries/screams	Inappropriate crying/screaming
2 Incomprehensible sounds	Grunts	Grunts
1 No response	No response	No response

A score is given in each category. The individual scores are then added (range 3-15). A score <8 indicates severe neurologic injury.

from head injuries of similar severities is better than that of adults.[30-32] It is difficult to clinically evaluate the combative or unconscious child; reevaluation for changes frequently is vital. Closed head injury is *not* a primary cause of shock in children unless there is an open fontanelle (<15 months); massive intracranial hemorrhage is clinically evident by widely split sutures. Computed tomography (CT) scan is helpful in acute diagnoses for cerebral edema and intracranial hemorrhages. Intracranial pressure monitoring is indicated in those children with severe head injuries as manifested by a GCS of <8.[33,34]

The cervical spine has a high risk potential for injury because of the large head of the child and flexible, weak neck muscles. The ligaments and joint capsules are flexible; contusions and hematomas are more common than fractures. If a fracture occurs, however, it is usually at the level of the occiput, C1, or C2 in children less than 8 years. Children older than 8 years sustain lower cervical spine injuries like those found in adults.[35]

Temperature regulation is a problem in the child. Young children have thin skin, with intrinsically smaller fat stores. They lose heat because of a higher body surface area to mass ratio. Maintenance of body temperature with stress is a problem because of immature hypothalamic control of temperature regulation. Thus there is a need to concentrate on keeping the child warm.

Vital sign ranges of normality change from birth to adolescence along with developmental changes.[36] Determination of body weight or size is important for drug and fluid management (Table 19-4).

The abdominal contents are susceptible to injury because of immature musculature and minimal fat pad offering little protection. The infant/toddler has pelvic organs located in a more abdominal location. The liver and spleen are relatively large and susceptible to injury. Crying and swallowing air may distend the stomach, making the area more susceptible to hematomas and contusions.

The chest wall is flexible, exposing the underlying lung, heart, liver, and spleen to injury without associated external fractures that are common in adults. The child is a diaphragmatic breather and may have more respiratory distress because of impedance to breathing with both abdominal and chest injuries.

The skeleton is an immature structure, and fractures are most likely to occur at the growth plate as described by the Salter-Harris classification. Greenstick and buckle (torus) fractures are also more common in children because of the malleable nature of their growing long bones. The most frequently missed fractures involve the clavicle. surgical neck of the humerus, ulna, radius, ankle, and wrist (see Chapter 27).

Developmental considerations and their psychosocial impact upon the child and family must always be recognized. Parents have a responsibility to the child's well being and have the decision-making role for the child's care. It is important to include the parents in discussions if possible and to keep them informed of the events taking place and procedures done to their child during trauma management. The death of a child from a traumatic injury is a devastating psychologic stress to the family; it is essen-

TABLE 19-4. Vital Signs by Age

Age	Heart rate		Systolic blood pressure		Respiratory rate (breaths/min)	Weight (kg)
	Average (beats/min)	Range	Average (mm Hg)	Range		
Preterm	140	120-180	50	40-60	55-65	2
Term newborn	125	90-170	72	52-92	40-60	3
1 mo	120	110-180	82	60-104	30-50	4
6 mo	130	110-180	94	65-125	25-40	7
1 yr	125	80-160	94	70-118	20-40	10
2 yr	110	80-130	95	73-117	20-30	12
4 yr	105	80-120	91	65-117	20-30	16
6 yr	100	75-115	96	76-116	18-24	20
8 yr	90	70-110	99	79-119	18-22	25
10 yr	80	70-110	102	82-122	16-20	30
12 yr	75	60-110	106	84-128	16-20	40
14 yr	75	60-105	110	84-136	16-20	50

tial to link families with care resources and suggest coping strategies.[37]

PATTERNS OF INJURY

Certain types of injury are commonly seen by those who treat pediatric trauma. Waddell's triad occurs when a child pedestrian is struck by a car. The injuries suffered include a fractured femur secondary to the leg striking the bumper of the car, a chest or upper abdominal injury caused by being thrown on the hood, and a contralateral head injury when the child is thrown clear of the automobile and lands on the pavement. The usual injury triad is to the left side of the body in the United States because of right-side-of-the-road driving.

Bicycle injuries range from minor abrasions and contusions of the extremities occurring when a child falls on the pavement to major blunt abdominal contusions suffered from a child's contact with the bicycle handlebar when he or she is thrown over the bicycle. The duodenal hematoma may present very subtly. Head injuries are very common in those who do not wear helmets and may be severe, depending on the speed of the bicycle. Spoke injuries to the extremities can precipitate a compartment syndrome.

Motor vehicle–occupant injuries are the most common types of major injuries seen in the pediatric patient. Without restraint devices, head and neck injuries are common, as are penetrating injuries from ejection through automobile windows. With lap belt restraints only, contusions and perforations of intraabdominal organs, as well as flexion-extension injuries of the spinal cord, occur.[38,39]

Child safety seats offer the ultimate protection from injury for those less than 4 years of age if the car seat is secured appropriately to the car. The child under 20 pounds should have the car seat facing the rear and not placed in a seat with an airbag. The older child and adolescent are best protected by a combination lap belt and shoulder harness.

The term *child abuse* encompasses patterns of injury related to physical, sexual, and emotional abuse, as well as medical and social neglect. The *battered child syndrome* defines specific injury patterns involving the skin and skeletal system and internal organ damage.[40] The *shaken impact syndrome* is a specific type of physical abuse inflicted on infants less than 1 year of age that may not show external signs of abuse but causes severe neurologic impairment.[41] Sexual abuse affects 1 of every 10 children in the United States.[42] New techniques for examination, including colposcopy, are important for documentation of findings (see Chapter 45). In the event of a traumatic injury, always consider an intentional mechanism, particularly in children with an injury that seems to be more severe than the mechanism presented by the caregiver. Over one fourth of abused and neglected children under 3 months of age have an associated extremity fracture.[43]

Scald burns are the most common type of burn injuries suffered by children.[44] The patterns of the scald represent the area where a splash occurred, and suspicion of abuse should be raised when any child has genital or bilateral extremity scald burns.

If a housefire occurs, signs of smoke inhalation, including carbon monoxide level, are included in the evaluation, in addition to the burn injury. Electrical injuries can be most damaging without much external trauma.

Drownings are more common in locations with areas of warm water or backyard swimming pools. A child can drown in a bathtub or bucket if not supervised.

Firearm injuries have always been a problem, particularly with children who play with a weapon kept at home. There have been increasing injuries both intentional and unintentional with the increase in drug and gang warfare.[45] The air rifle is a more powerful weapon than previously thought because of the improvement in velocity.[46]

THE TEAM APPROACH

The trauma team is made up of highly trained, experienced professionals who manage the patient in the trauma room; a team to support this group in the other areas of the hospital is needed for comprehensive care of the child. Team members in the trauma room should include a physician who is in charge of the overall resuscitation and a physician who manages the airway with the respiratory therapist. Ideally, two other physicians or experienced health professionals are at the bedside to manage procedures, assisted by bedside nurses in making the team function. A documentation nurse is in charge of the nursing personnel in the room. The pharmacist and a fluid nurse manage the fluids and drugs that are needed for resuscitation. Each member of the team should be experienced in the care of the pediatric trauma patient and should update skills as appropriate. Which personnel actually perform these roles depends on the individual institution, but it is wise to use the most experienced critical care personnel without depleting resources from one area so that another team may be mobilized if needed.[47,48]

In addition to the resuscitation team, other members of the trauma team are essential to successful resuscitation. The radiology technician is prepared to perform plain films of the cervical spine, chest, and abdomen/pelvis as necessary and can be the liaison for the CT scan technician. The radiologist also must be aware of and able to expedite procedures as needed (e.g., angiography, CT scan). The laboratory is prepared to run tests immediately and provide blood products expeditiously as needed. The operating room (OR) nurse is invaluable in those instances where surgery is required acutely. The nurse is prepared to set up the operating room suite for the trauma case and alert the needed OR team members. Social services/chaplain should be available for every trauma to offer support services and to act as a patient advocate and liaison between the medical personnel and the family. The nurse manager/nursing supervisor or administrative representative can mobilize extra personnel as needed, obtain inpatient beds, and notify operating room personnel in specific cases. The trauma nurse coordinator oversees all patient care representatives and works with the family throughout the hospital stay to coordinate services.

The prehospital personnel also are a vital part of the team; early communication between the prehospital personnel and the receiving hospital staff provides needed time to prepare for a specific patient. The use of ambulances for children is low as compared to adults. Approximately 10% of prehospital runs are for children, with only about 20% of those transported found to have a severe injury or illness.[49] With such infrequent exposure to the pediatric patient, it is important for the pediatric providers of trauma care to offer courses and lectures pertaining to the care of the pediatric trauma patient.[50] The prehospital provider needs to know not only how to assess, recognize, and treat airway compromise and shock, the most common causes of mortality in the pediatric patient, but also how to access the appropriate care center as quickly as possible. It is important to get to an emergency department while reassessing and treating the airway, breathing, and circulation (ABCs). There has been controversy regarding two views of EMS transport: whether to prolong time in the field to do more patient care ("stay and play") or to quickly move and transport those patients with long transport times ("scoop and run"). Both sides, however, point to the fact that getting to the ED should be a priority.[51,52]

Preparation is in two phases: early and acute. The early preparation includes making sure that each room has

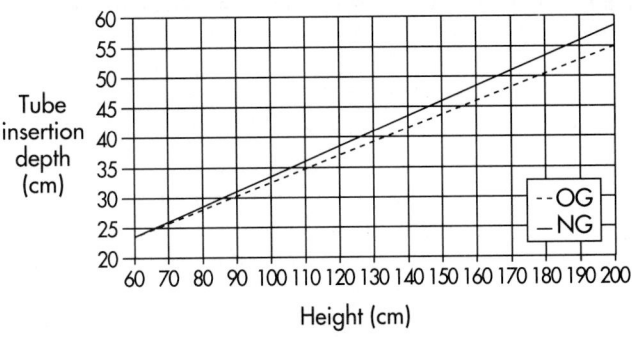

Estimate esophageal length for gastric tube insertion

FIG. 19-1. Graphic representation of recommended tube insertion depths based on patient length. *OG*, Orogastric tube; *NG*, nasogastric tube. (*From Scalzo AJ, Tominack RL, Thompson MN: J Emerg Med 10:581, 1992.*)

equipment appropriate for all ages of pediatric patients, with pediatric size charts readily available (Table 19-5) (Fig. 19-1). The trauma room should be easily accessible to ambulance traffic and large enough for the team to work efficiently. The equipment must be readily accessible, with routine orientation given to new personnel and routine mock trauma simulations performed. A backup plan for more than one trauma patient is essential and should include a call list for extra personnel to access from home as well as from other hospital areas. This plan should be a part of the hospital-wide disaster plan. A paging system for the trauma team members must facilitate rapid mobilization when the prehospital call is received. All members of the trauma team (as well as other hospital staff) should be familiar with the process of caring for the trauma patient as it pertains to them and their roles when a trauma is paged. Key areas such as the laboratory, blood bank, and operating room should be notified with the trauma team members.

The acute preparation follows prehospital notification and includes setting up age-specific equipment and trays for the patient described, universal precautions for team members, and activating the trauma team.

Quality-improvement monitoring of the trauma patient's care is also necessary to ensure adequate peer review and continuing education. Each case is reviewed by the trauma surgeon, the emergency physician, and the trauma nurse coordinator with specific guidelines for areas of concentration. The charts may be reviewed to document completeness, as may videotapes of previous resuscitations. Using videotapes of the resuscitations requires establishing a protocol for use of the tapes as a quality improvement tool with stipulations that they are destroyed after this review or after a set period if not reviewed immediately. A trauma conference is a good educational forum. All members of the health-care team interested in or involved in the care of the trauma patient attend; there is a presentation of cases from the previous month. Teaching points relating to the various types of injuries are made by experts in the field and follow-up evaluation is given on the patient's condition since the initial resuscitation.

TABLE 19-5. Pediatric-specific Equipment

Airway management		Vascular access	Miscellaneous
Premature to 6 mon			
ET tubes	Suction catheters	Overneedle type catheters	Feeding tubes
2.5	5/6 French	24 gauge	5 French
3.0	8 French	22 gauge	8 French
3.5	De Lee suction trap	Scalp veins	Blood pressure cuff
Stylet	Bulb syringe	25 gauge	Neonate
6 French	Neonatal self-inflating bag	23 gauge	Chest tubes
Laryngoscope blades	Premie and newborn masks	Cook single-lumen catheter set	10 French
0 straight	Oropharyngeal airways	3 French	12 French
1 straight	Infant 1	Pediatric side-arm set	16 French
Tracheostomy tubes	Child 2	5.5 French	
00		Umbilical catheters	
0		5 French	
Nasopharyngeal airways		3.5 French	
12 French		Umbilical tape	
14 French		Intraosseous needle	
6 mon to 2 yrs			
ET tubes	Suction catheters	Overneedle type catheters	Foley catheter
3.5	8 French	24 gauge	8 French
4.0	10 French	22 gauge	Feeding tube
4.5	Pediatric bag	Scalp veins	8 French
5.0	Infant mask	25 gauge	Nasogastric tubes
Stylet	Nasopharyngeal airways	23 gauge	8 French
6 French	14 French	21 gauge	10 French
Tracheostomy tubes	16 French	Single-lumen catheter set	Blood pressure cuffs
1	18 French	3 French	Infant
Laryngoscope blades	Oropharyngeal airways	Side-arm set	Child
1 straight	Infant 1	5.5 French	Chest tubes
1.5 straight	Child 2	Double-lumen catheter set	16 French
		5 French	20 French
		Intraosseous needle	24 French
3 to 6 yrs			
ET tubes	Suction catheter	Overneedle type catheter	Foley catheters
5.0	14 French	23 gauge	10 French
5.5	Pediatric nonrebreather mask	20 gauge	12 French
6.0	Child mask	Scalp veins	Nasogastric tubes
Stylets	Pediatric bag	25 gauge	10 French
6 French	Nasopharyngeal airways	23 gauge	12 French
14 French	16 French	21 gauge	Blood pressure cuff
Laryngoscope blades	18 French	Single-lumen catheter set	Child
1.5 straight	22 French	4 French	Chest tubes
2 straight	Oropharyngeal airways	Side-arm sheaths	20 French
2 curved	3	5.5 French	24 French
Tracheostomy tube	4	7.5 French	28 French
2		Triple- or double-lumen catheter set	
		7.0 French	
		Intraosseous needle	

Continued.

AGGRESSIVE PHILOSOPHY

Because the child with multiple injuries has a high potential for rapid deterioration, an aggressive approach must be the foundation for determining treatment priorities. The nature of the acutely ill child may preclude full diagnostic evaluation before initiation of treatment. Delays in treatment may ultimately lead to poor outcome; for example, a tension pneumothorax diagnosed by clinical findings of diminished breath sounds and subcutaneous emphysema in the presence of hemodynamic compromise necessitate decompression and immediate placement of a chest tube without x-ray film confirmation of the diagnosis.

TABLE 19-5. Pediatric-specific Equipment—cont'd

Airway management		Vascular access	Miscellaneous
7 to 10 yrs			
ET tubes	Suction catheter	Overneedle type catheters	Foley catheter
6.0	14 French	20 gauge	12 French
6.5	Adult nonrebreather mask	18 gauge	Nasogastric tubes
7.0 (Cuffed/noncuffed)	Small adult mask	Scalp veins	16 French
Stylet	Adult bag	25 gauge	18 French
14 French	Nasopharyngeal airways	23 gauge	Chest tubes
Laryngoscope blades	24 French	20 gauge	28 French
2 straight	26 French	Single-lumen catheter sets	32 French
2 curved	28 French	3 French	36 French
3 straight	Otopharyngeal airways	5 French	
3 curved	4	Side-arm sheaths	
Tracheostomy tube	5	7.5 French	
3		Triple- or double-lumen catheter set	
		7.0 French	

Note: Additional pediatric surgical instrumentation may be required.

Always assume the most serious diagnosis. Appropriate treatment should be initiated until a particular diagnosis can be excluded. The mechanism and nature of the injury may have an impact on the differential conditions to be considered.

Priorities must be assessed and life-sustaining functions maintained. Frequent and thorough physical examination is essential, requiring removal of clothes. A careful examination does not stop once a single injury has been noted.

Management of the pediatric trauma patient requires treatment based on clinical findings. Assuming the child has a serious injury and assessing the child in a thorough, organized way will result in finding all areas of injury. The physical examination may be unreliable initially if there are several areas of injury. For instance, the child will concentrate on only one bad pain at a time and may respond only to pain from the femur fracture until it is stabilized. Then concentration may focus on the abdominal pain, which may have been persistent but now seems to have become more severe. Information from the prehospital care provider or caretakers at the scene regarding the mechanism of injury is invaluable in giving information for specific injuries.

It is important to follow an organized management protocol such as that advocated by the American College of Surgeons (ACS) in the Advanced Trauma Life Support (ATLS) course. Assessment and management of life-threatening injuries constitute the primary survey; less serious injury assessment and management constitute the secondary survey. During the prioritized assessment, resuscitation takes place. Cardiorespiratory monitoring, oxygen administration, and intravenous fluid therapy are provided during the primary survey. The secondary survey involves a thorough examination of every area of the patient with tube placement in the stomach and bladder as needed; each injured area is documented by external ex-

amination. This is also confirmed by laboratory and radiographic tests.

Frequent reassessments and monitoring after the initial primary and secondary surveys are imperative to identify any changes in the patient's condition. Vital signs are assessed frequently throughout the initial emergency department management and until the child is considered stable.

Pediatric trauma patients also need psychologic support since they may not understand what is happening to them and communication is difficult with toddlers and infants. Because the child is aware of the pain of resuscitation, assigning one person to talk to the child and explain procedures before they are performed is imperative. During the hospital stay the child will need debriefing and follow-up observation to decrease chances of future nightmares and fear of the hospital.

The trauma arrest presents a unique challenge. If the arrest is secondary to penetrating injury, there may be chance of survival if the injury site can be repaired and aggressive resuscitation with rapid OR response occurs. The outcome in a child who has arrested prior to the arrival in the ED as well as one who presents with severe hypotension after blunt trauma is very poor.[53]

Primary Survey

The primary survey is divided into five steps, abbreviated A, B, C, D, and E. The first step is *airway* management and cervical spine control. This encompasses the area from the nose and mouth down to the vocal cords. The child is placed in a "sniffing" position (Fig. 19-2) and either the chin lift or jaw thrust is used to open the airway as in-line stabilization of the cervical spine is maintained. Inspect for foreign bodies in the mouth, as well as broken teeth or facial lacerations. Look for cyanosis and poor perfusion and supply high-flow oxygen by face mask. Palpate the jaw and trachea for deformities and auscultate the upper airway for airflow and turbulence; oral airways are used only for the unconscious child. If a device is needed to open the airway of a conscious child, a nasal airway can be used with minimal discomfort. With the airway open

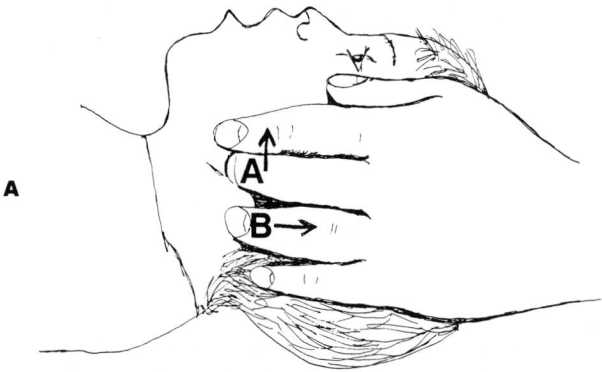

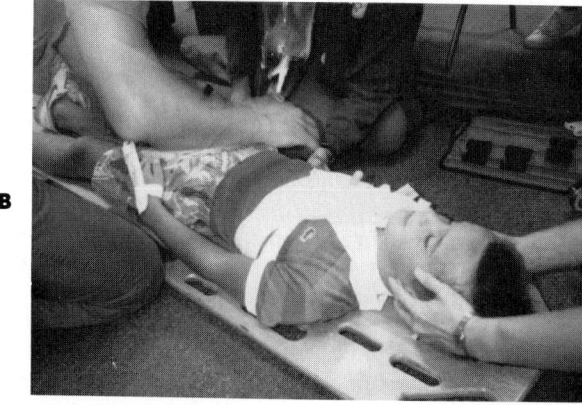

FIG. 19-2. "Sniffing position." **A,** Upward pressure for jaw thrust. **B,** Axial pressure for in-line traction.

and free of any foreign bodies, the child should have secretions suctioned and ventilations supported as necessary with oxygen assistance (Table 19-6).

Intubation may be necessary if the child is neurologically impaired enough to leave the airway unprotected. An objective measurement of this neurologic impairment is the PGCS. A PGCS of <8 constitutes consideration of intubation to maintain an open airway. Rapid sequence induction can be used to aid intubation in a nonflaccid child (see Appendix to this chapter). Needle cricothyrotomy should be considered if the child cannot have oral intubation (Fig. 19-3).

A firm cervical collar with support on each side of the head should be placed on all children with a history of serious injury at the level of the clavicle or above. The cervical collar should be left in place until the physician team leader has evaluated and cleared the cervical spine by radiographs and physical examination.

Assessing *breathing* is the next step. Inspect the chest for abrasions or contusions, as well as the overall color of the patient. Notice any abnormal breathing pattern, such as retractions, splinting, grunting, or flail chest. Palpate the rib cage for any crepitance and note open wounds. Breath sounds are best auscultated under the axillae to minimize the effects of transmitted airway noises. Count the respirations and note unequal, noisy, or decreased breath sounds. Assess the adequacy of ventilations (i.e., chest rise and color) and assist ventilations as necessary (Table 19-7 and Appendix A-2). If the child is not maintaining adequate ventilation, oral intubation may be necessary. The size of the endotracheal tube can be determined by several methods; having chart sizes appropriate for age is the most accurate (see Table 19-5). Nasal intubation is generally not preferred in the acute intubation of a child except for adolescents, with whom a blind nasal approach may be attempted. A preset protocol for intubation is necessary so that all members of the team will anticipate the needs of the intubator.

TABLE 19-6. Summary of Oxygen Assist Devices

Type of breathing device	Oxygen flow rate	Oxygen concentration	Advantages	Disadvantages
Nasal cannula	Up to 4 L/min	25%-40%	No rebreathing of expired air	Can only be used with spontaneous respiration
Simple face mask	6-10 L/min	30%-60%	Higher FIO_2 than cannula	Often not tolerated well by children; spontaneous respiration only
O_2 reservoir mask	10-12 L/min	Up to 95%	Highest FIO_2 of passive methods	Must have tight fit, spontaneous respiration only
Venturi mask	4 L/min 8 L/min	24%-28% 35%-40%	Fixed O_2 concentration	Not carried by EMS; spontaneous respiration only
Pocket mask	10 L/min	50%	Prevents direct oral contact; may be used on apneic patient	Rescuer fatigue; may have poor fit if adult mask used
Bag-valve-mask	12 L/min	40%-90%	Rapid; can get sense of lung compliance; good for apneic or spontaneously breathing patients	Gastric air; must watch tidal volume
O_2-powered breathing device	100 L/min	100%	High O_2 flow with positive pressure	*Not to be used for children!* Insufficient research with pediatric adaptors

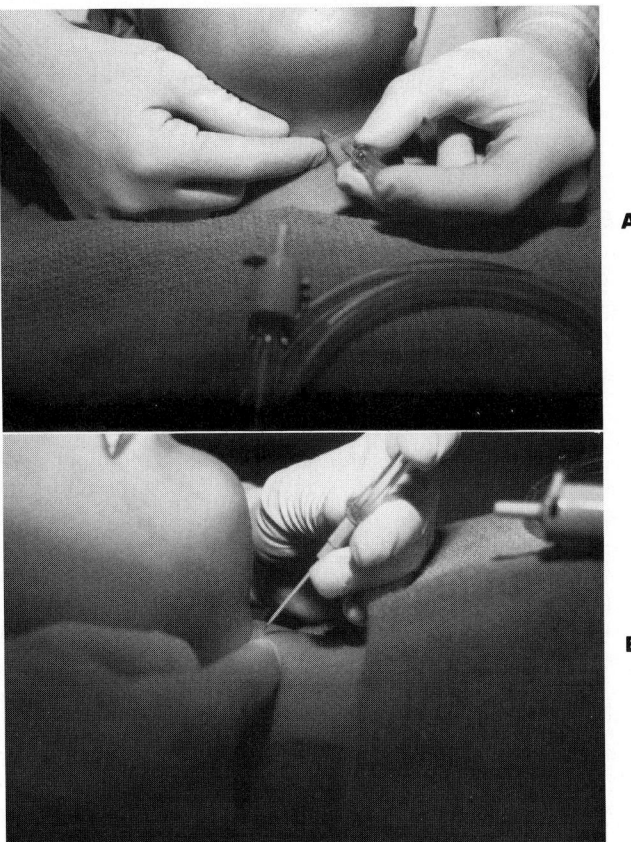

FIG. 19-3. Needle cricothyrotomy. **A,** Needle is inserted through the cricoid membrane. **B,** Needle attached is directed at a 45-degree angle caudally.

TABLE 19-7. Artificial Ventilation Rates

Age	Rate
Infants (birth to 6 mo)	20-25 breaths/min
Toddlers (6 mo to 2 yr)	15-20 breaths/min
Children (2 yr to preadolescence)	15-20 breaths/min
Adolescents	12-16 breaths/min

A life-threatening problem to be evaluated while listening to breath sounds is pneumothorax. Inspection may reveal unequal movements of the chest. With palpation there may be crepitation secondary to subcutaneous emphysema. The trachea is deviated if a tension pneumothorax is present. Auscultation may make the diagnosis with unequal breath sounds. The diagnostic and therapeutic procedure is to insert a 14 gauge needle in the second intercostal space in the midclavicular line and draw air or fluid back into a syringe. The definitive procedure uses a chest tube, which is inserted into the fifth intercostal space in the midaxillary line. Sizes of chest tubes depend on the age and size of the child (see Table 19-5).

Circulation is quickly assessed by using capillary refill of fingers and toes. Visual inspection for any prolongation of normal capillary refill (2 seconds) is noted. Inspect the body for areas of open hemorrhage to be controlled, as well as deformed extremities to be splinted, while the blood pressure and heart rate are determined. Any deformed extremities require pulse and capillary refill checks both proximal and distal to the fracture. The chest and abdomen are palpated for tenderness and guarding, while the examiner attempts to detect liver and spleen injuries. Auscultate the heart and abdomen for abnormalities (i.e., distant heart sounds, tachycardia, decreased or absent bowel sounds). During evaluation for the early signs of shock (tachycardia and prolonged capillary refill), intravenous access is obtained by large-bore peripheral lines. Larger catheters permit greater flow rates. Longer catheters increase resistance. If no peripheral intravenous line can be placed easily, the intraosseous route is used for children less than 6 years of age until the intravascular volume has been repleted enough to place a venous line (see Appendix to Chapter 13). Central venous monitoring may be required in persistently unstable patients.

Fluid management for shock requires rapid isotonic fluid replacement (lactated Ringer's or normal saline solution) in boluses of 20 ml/kg. After three boluses of crystalloid solution are infused for active bleeding, colloid (blood products) is used to improve stability of vascular volume and hemoglobin oxygen–carrying capacity. Blood is infused at a rate of 10 ml/kg as quickly as possible. If completely cross-matched blood is not available, administer type-specific blood. It is usually available 10 to 15 minutes after delivery of a specimen to the blood bank. O-negative blood should be reserved for those patients who are in profound shock. While infusing fluid therapy, use of a fluid warmer decreases the chance of worsening hypothermia and helps prevent loss of body heat.

If a military antishock trousers (MAST) suit is in place, it can be removed one compartment at a time, monitoring the child's blood pressure. (If the blood pressure falls at any time, the compartments are to remain inflated until the blood pressure stabilizes and the procedure is attempted again.) MAST suits do not replace fluid therapy for the management of shock. They are indicated for use only when the child weighs more than 25 to 35 kg or is more than 6 years of age, primarily for pelvic or femur fracture stabilization, although their clinical benefit is controversial. There is little evidence that the MAST suit enhances prehospital outcome more than conventional supportive care does.

Disability or neurologic responsiveness of the child is assessed quickly and frequently. Objective measurement of responsiveness can be obtained through the Alert, Verbal, Pain, Unresponsive (AVPU) system (see p. 238) or the PGCS system (see Table 19-3). The pupillary response and size are also determined. Finally, major spinal cord injury is assessed by gross motor movement or pain to specific areas of the spine to anticipate the need for immobilization and consultation.

Exposure of the child to reveal all possible injuries is important. While removing clothing, it is imperative to remember to take the temperature and cover areas not being directly examined with a warmed sheet or blanket.

The vital signs should be assessed frequently during examination along with the temperature.

Resuscitation Phase

The resuscitation phase, or the technical steps in the care of the child, is performed simultaneously with the primary survey. While controlling the airway, oxygen is administered and the neck immobilized as appropriate.[54] The breathing assessment requires establishment of needed assistance via oxygen through mask or bag-mask ventilation. Invasive procedures to control breathing include endotracheal intubation, needle cricothyrotomy, and chest tube placement. Circulation requires monitoring of vital signs, including capillary refill and temperature, and establishment of intravenous access. If peripheral access is not obtained in three attempts or 90 seconds, an intraosseous line should be considered in the anterior tibia in unstable children less than 3 years of age.

Suggested trauma laboratory determinations include complete blood count (CBC) with differential and platelet counts, electrolytes, blood urea nitrogen (BUN), creatinine, glucose, amylase, liver functions, prothrombin time (PT), partial thromboplastin time (PTT), type and crossmatch for 1 unit of packed red blood cells/10 kg of body weight, arterial blood gas (ABG) levels, and urinalysis. There have been arguments against the use of "trauma panels" for laboratory evaluation in all trauma patients for the reasons of cost efficiency as well as unnecessary tests in certain instances.[55] It is probably better to utilize a critical pathway that can limit laboratory testing based on the patient's presentation and mechanism of injury. Although type and crossmatch have been standard in trauma patients, studies have suggested that a more selective approach may be appropriate. A type and screen may be used when the BP is greater than 100 mm Hg in the prehospital setting, converting to a type and crossmatch if clinical circumstances indicate.[56] Many centers are also performing drug screens on their trauma patients as part of a standard protocol.[57] Fluid resuscitation is given as needed. A urinary catheter should be inserted if the prostate is normal and there is no blood at the urethral meatus; radiographs of the cervical spine, chest, and pelvis should be obtained. Radiographs are concurrently obtained.

While the resuscitation is in progress, a member of the trauma team obtains the patient's history from caregivers and prehospital personnel if appropriate. This history includes the present injury and mechanism if known, as well as the condition of the child when the caregiver first observed him or her after the injury. The past medical history and other important information can be gleaned by the mnemonic AMPLE: *A* represents allergies and immunizations, including the primary immunization status and the tetanus booster status of an older child (see Chapter 55 and Appendix A), and *M* represents medications, including all prescription and over-the-counter (OTC) drugs. Determine when the last dose of medication was given, how large it was, and when the patient is scheduled to have another dose. *P* is past illnesses: chronic illnesses; previous hospitalizations, surgeries, and broken bones/lacerations; bleeding disorders; bone disorders; or immunodeficiency. It is also important at this time to determine the presence of developmental disabilities, including hearing or speech delay. *L* represents last meal; both food and liquid intake should be determined, including quantity and time elapsed since the last meal. *E* represents events preceding the injury. Was the child supervised? Were there witnesses to the event?

Secondary Survey

The secondary survey is a detailed head-to-toe assessment. This is the time to measure lacerations, abrasions, and bruises and document them on the medical record. The back is examined, as well as the front, and tubes are placed wherever needed.

The *head* and *neurologic status* are examined first. Abrasions, contusions, and lacerations of the scalp are noted. Specifically, signs of basilar skull fracture, including raccoon eyes and Battle's sign, are sought. The pupillary size and responsiveness and extraocular movement are checked. Palpation of the skull for pain, crepitance, or deformity is important. The PGCS is repeated and the cranial nerves are assessed.

The *face* and *neck* are examined as a continuation of the head and neurologic examination. The mouth is inspected for broken or misaligned teeth. The ears and nares are inspected for fluid drainage. Hemotympanum, or perforation of the eardrum, is noted. The nares are inspected for alignment of the septum, as well as swelling and drainage. The facial bones are palpated for pain, deformities, or crepitance. Auscultation of the mouth and trachea for airway obstruction is then done. Inspection of the neck for abrasions, contusions, tracheal deviation, and jugular venous distension is important. The cervical collar maintaining in-line stabilization is removed to palpate the cervical spine for deformities and pain after the lateral cervical spine has been reviewed. A gastric tube is then placed either through the nose if there is no evidence of facial trauma or through the mouth if facial trauma is a possibility (see Table 19-6).

The *chest* and *cardiac systems* are examined next. Inspection of the chest assesses equal chest rise, retractions, abdominal breathing, splinting respirations, and paradoxic chest movement. The chest is also inspected for the point of maximal impulse (PMI) and any abnormal coloring, including bruising. The rib cage and sternum are palpated for crepitance and pain. Auscultate the chest for breath sounds, noting unequalness as well as rales, rhonchi, or wheezes. The heart is also auscultated, noting irregular heartbeat as correlated with pulse, heart murmurs, and muffled heart sounds. Radiographs of the chest are made at this time.

The *abdomen* is a difficult area to inspect and requires repeated examinations. Inspect the area for abrasions and contusions; auscultate for bowel sounds in all quadrants before palpation and then palpate for tenderness, as well as size of the liver and spleen. Children swallow air when upset and crying and may have a distended stomach that sounds tympanitic by percussion. With a gastric tube in place, the distension produced by air should be relieved to give a more accurate examination. If the physician is concerned about intraabdominal bleeding, a diagnostic peritoneal lavage may be done. This requires an incision just distal to the umbilicus in the lower quadrant and placement of a catheter by direct visualization or a modified open technique. Normal saline solution is infused with return of fluid from the peritoneal space. If the fluid is grossly bloody or contains >100,000 RBCs/ml, >500 WBCs/ml, or food particles, the child is taken to the operating room. A CT scan of the abdomen may be opted for in the stable pediatric patient and contrast medium is given orally, as well as IV, to enhance visualization of the bowel. The indications and interpretation of the evaluation of the traumatized abdomen are discussed in detail in Chapter 24.

The *pelvis* and *genitalia* are inspected for abnormalities, including contusions and lacerations. The pelvis is palpated for crepitance, instability, and pain. External genitalia are examined for scrotal or labial hematomas. The rectum is examined for bleeding and palpated for muscle tone, and the prostate in the male is also examined. A Foley catheter is inserted if the rectal examination findings are normal and there is no blood at the external meatus of the urethra. If a pelvic fracture is suspected, a Foley catheter is not used until the severity of the fracture is determined.

The *musculoskeletal* system is inspected next for areas of abrasions, contusions, and swelling. All extremities are palpated for pain and crepitance, and neurovascular status is assessed. The patient is rolled to the side as a single unit with the help of several team members to inspect and palpate the back for deformities and pain.

Vital signs and neurologic status are reassessed during the head-to-toe examination, resuscitating as necessary. A Pediatric Trauma Score (see Table 19-1) should be determined during the secondary survey and a PGCS is determined at least four times: at the scene of the injury, on arrival to the emergency department, after resuscitation before release to inpatient care, and with any change in level of consciousness.

Consultants

General surgical colleagues should be intimately involved in the team. The surgical subspecialists required reflect the injuries suffered by the child. An orthopedic surgeon, plastic surgeon, oral surgeon, and neurosurgeon are all necessary consultants to have on call for any multiple trauma.

Staff to provide support in the psychosocial environment of emergency care include social service personnel, a chaplain or someone representing religious services, and a patient advocate for the family as well as the patient.

DISPOSITION

The child who has several traumatic injuries usually is admitted to the hospital; however, if the decision is made to send the child with limited injuries and documented stability home, careful instructions regarding wound care, closed head injury care, and follow-up observation are needed. These should be given to the family more than once with a number to call if any questions arise. If the child is admitted, the severity of injuries dictates whether the child enters the general pediatric floor or the pediatric intensive care unit. Specific guidelines at each hospital should detail decision criteria for floor care vs. intensive care management. If the child requires stabilization of an acute condition in the operating room, he or she is admitted to the operating room/same day surgery and, after recovery and stabilization, usually moves to an intensive care unit for postoperation monitoring.

References

1. Waller A, Baker S, Szocka A: Childhood injury deaths: national analysis and geographic variation, *AJPH* 79(3):310, 1989.
2. Division of Injury Control, Centers for Disease Control: Childhood injuries in the United States, *Am J Dis Child* 144:627, 1990.
3. Guyer B and Ellers B: Childhood injuries in the United States, *Am J Dis Child* 144:649, 1990.
4. Malek M, Chang B, Gallagher SS, et al: The cost of medical care for injuries to children, *Ann Emerg Med* 20(9):997, 1991.
5. Agran P, Castillo D, Winn D: Childhood motor vehicle occupant injuries, *Am J Dis Child* 144:653, 1990.
6. Weesner CL, Hargarten SW, Aprahamian C, et al: Fatal childhood injury patterns in an urban setting, *Ann Emerg Med* 23:231, 1994.
7. Inaba AS and Seward PN: An approach to pediatric trauma—unique anatomic and physiologic aspects of the pediatric patient, *Emerg Med Clin North Am* 9(3):523, 1991.
8. Christoffel KK: Violent death and injury in United States children and adolescents, *Am J Dis Child* 144:697, 1990.
9. Friede AM, Azzara AV, Gallagher SS, et al: The epidemiology of injuries to bicycle riders, *Pediatr Clin North Am* 32(1):141, 1985.
10. Guyer B, Talbot AM, Pless IB: Pedestrian injuries to children and youth *Pediatr Clin North Am* 32(1):163, 1985.
11. Micik S, Yuwiler J, Walker C: *Preventing childhood injuries*, ed 2, San Marcos, Calif, 1987, North County Health Services.

Injury Severity Measures

12. Subcommittee on Advanced Trauma Life Support of the American College of Surgeons Committee on Trauma: *Advanced trauma life support student manual*, Chicago, 1989, American College of Surgeons.
13. Ramenofsky ML, Reynolds EA, Dierking BH: *Pediatric trauma score—a rapid assessment and triage tool for the injured child*, ed 3, Mobile, Ala, 1988, University of South Alabama.
14. Mayer TA: Pediatric care in the general emergency department. In Schwartz GR, Mayer TA, Cayton CG, et al: *Principles and practice of emergency medicine*, ed 3, Philadelphia, 1992, Lea & Febiger.
15. Mayer TA: Pediatric trauma. In Schwartz GR, Mayer TA, Cayton CG, et al: *Principles and practice of emergency medicine*, ed 3, Philadelphia, 1992, Lea and Febiger.
16. Knudson MM, Shagoury C, Lewis F: Can adult trauma surgeons care for injured children? *J Trauma* 32:729, 1992.
17. Harris BH, Barlow BA, Ballantine TV, et al: American Pediatric Surgical Association principles of pediatric trauma care, *J Pediatr Surg* 27(4):423, 1992.
18. Jaffe D and Wesson D: Emergency management of blunt trauma in children, *N Engl J Med* 324(21):1477, 1991.
19. Eichelberger MR, Gotschall CS, Sacco WJ, et al: A comparison of the trauma score, the revised trauma score, and the pediatric trauma score, *Ann Emerg Med* 18(10):1053, 1989.
20. Nayduch DA, Moylan J, Rutledge R, et al: Comparison of the ability of adult and pediatric trauma scores to predict outcome following major trauma, *J Trauma* 31:452, 1991.
21. Kaufmann CR, Maier RV, Rivara FP, et al: Evaluation of the pediatric trauma score, *JAMA* 263(1):69, 1990.
22. Tepas JJ, Ramenofsky ML, Mollitt BL, et al: The pediatric trauma scores are predictor of injury severity: an objective assessment. *J Trauma* 28:425, 1988.
23. Schafermeyer R: Pediatric trauma, *Emerg Med Clin North Am* 11(1):187, 1993.
24. Gormican SP: CRAMS scale: field triage of trauma victims, *Ann Emerg Med* 11(3):132, 1982.

Unique Aspects

25. Ziegler MM: Major trauma. In *Textbook of pediatric emergency medicine*, ed 2, Baltimore, 1983, Williams & Wilkins.
26. Waller AE, Baker SP, Szocka A: Childhood injury deaths: national analysis and geographic variations, *Am J Public Health* 79(3):310, 1989.

27. Kaufman BA and Dacey RG: Acute care management of closed head injury in childhood, *Pediatr Ann* 23(1):18, 1994.
28. Emergency Pediatrics Section, Canadian Pediatric Society: Management of children with head trauma, *Can Med Assoc J* 142(9):949, 1990.
29. Snyder CL, Jain VN, Saltzman DA, et al: Blunt trauma in adults and children: a comparative analysis, *J Trauma* 30(10):1239, 1990.
30. Lang DA, Teasdale GM, Macpherson P, et al: Diffuse brain swelling after head injury: more often malignant in adults than children? *J Neurosurg* 80:675, 1994.
31. Alberico AM, Ward JD, Choi SC, et al: Outcome after severe head injury, *J Neurosurg* 67:648, 1987.
32. Tepas JJ, DiScala C, Ramenofsky ML, et al: Mortality and head injury: the pediatric perspective, *J Pediatr Surg* 25(1):92, 1990.
33. Kasoff SS, Lansen TA, Holder D, et al: Aggressive physiologic monitoring of pediatric head trauma patients with elevated intracranial pressure, *Pediatr Neurosci* 14:241, 1988.
34. Ghajar J and Hariri RJ: Management of pediatric head injury, *Pediatr Clin North Am,* 39(5):1093, 1992.
35. Hill SA, Miller CA, Kosnick EJ, et al: Pediatric neck injuries, *J Neurosurg* 60:700, 1984.
36. American Heart Association Subcommittee on Pediatric Rususcitation: *Textbook of pediatric advanced life support,* Dallas, 1994.
37. Oliver RC and Fallat ME: Traumatic childhood death: how well do parents cope? *J Trauma* 39(2):303, 1995.

Patterns of Injury

38. Orsay EM, Dunne M, Turnbull TL, et al: Prospective study of the effect of safety belts in motor vehicle crashes, *Ann Emerg Med* 19(3):258, 1990.
39. Stylianos S and Harris BH: Seatbelt use and patterns of central nervous system injury in children, *Pediatr Emerg Care* 6(1):4, 1990.
40. Bittner S and Newberger EH: Pediatric understanding of child abuse and neglect, *Pediatr Rev* 2(7):197, 1981.
41. Bruce DA and Zimmerman RA: Shaken impact syndrome, *Pediatr Ann* 18(8):482, 1989.
42. Blumberg ML: Sexual abuse of children—causes, diagnosis and management, *Pediatr Ann* 13(10):753, 1984.

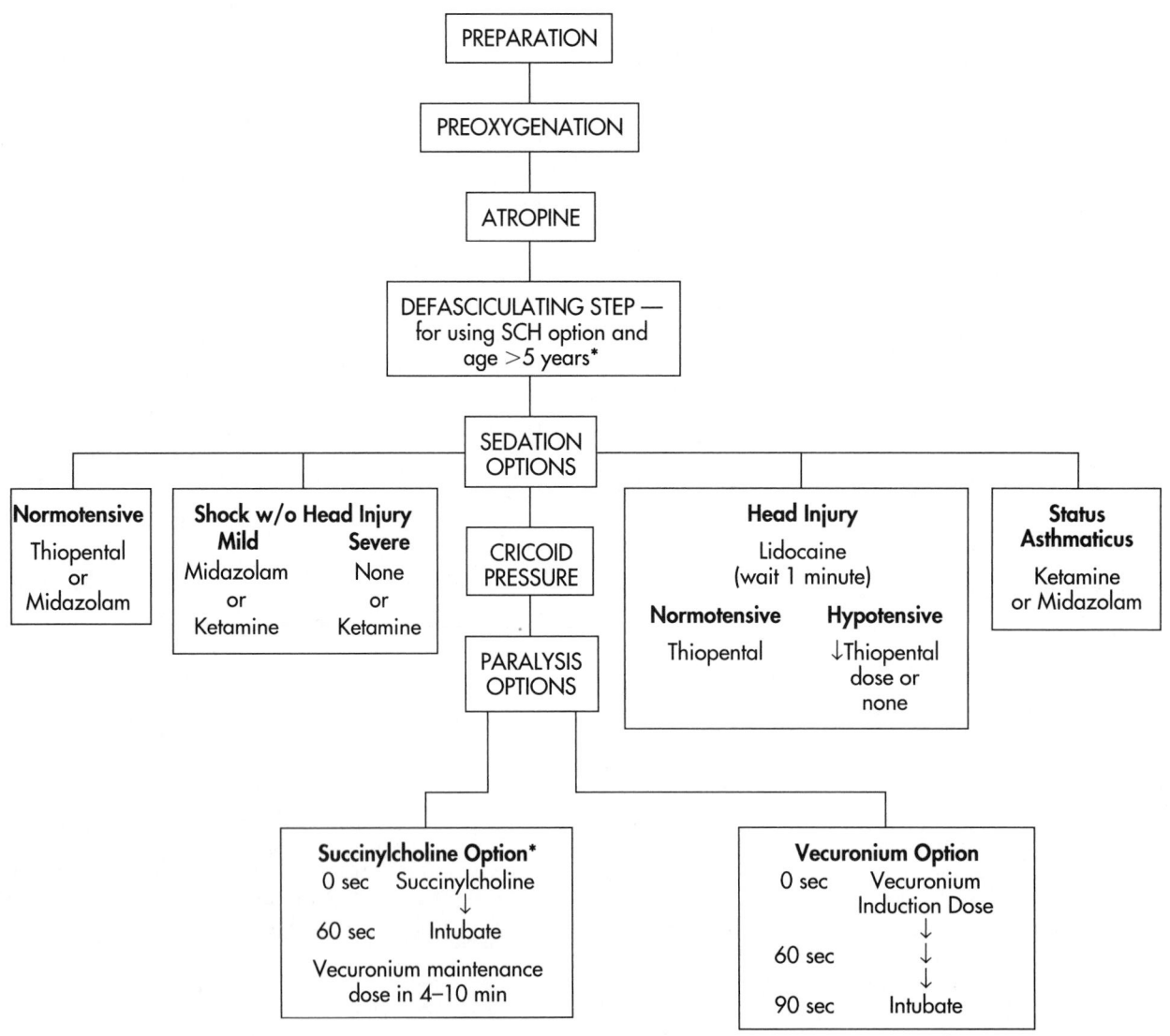

FIG. 19A-1. Suggested sequence for rapid induction in more common clinical situations. (*From Joint Task Force on Advanced Pediatric Life Support: APLS: the pediatric emergency medicine course, ed 2, 1993, American Academy of Pediatrics [Elk Grove, Ill] and American College of Emergency Physicians [Dallas].*)

43. Steward G, Meert K, Rosenberg N: Trauma in infants less than three months of age, *Pediatr Emerg Care* 9:199, 1993.
44. Robinson MD and Seward PN: Thermal injury in children, *Pediatr Emerg Care* 3(4):266, 1987.
45. Barlow B, Niemirska M, Gandhi RP: Ten years' experience with pediatric gunshot wounds, *J Pediatr Surg* 17(6):927, 1982.
46. Myre LE and Black RE: Serious air gun injuries in children: update of injury statistics and presentation of five cases, *Pediatr Emerg Care* 3(3):168, 1987.

The Team Approach

47. Yurt RW: Triage, initial assessment, and early treatment of the pediatric trauma patient, *Pediatr Clin North Am* 39(5):1083, 1992.
48. Singh R, Kissoon N, Singh N, et al: Is a full team required for emergency management of pediatric trauma? *J Trauma* 33(2):213, 1992.
49. Kallsen GW: Epidemiology of pediatric prehospital emergencies. In *Pediatric emergency care systems: planning and management*, Baltimore, 1992, Williams & Wilkins.
50. Committee on Pediatric Emergency Medical Services, Institute of Medicine: Summary. In *Emergency medical services for children*, Washington, DC, 1993, National Academy Press.
51. Ramenofsky ML and Dieckmann RA: Prehospital trauma management. In Dieckmann RA, editor: *Pediatric emergency care systems: planning and management*, Baltimore, 1992, Williams & Wilkins.
52. Ramenofsky ML, Luterman A, Curreri PW, et al: EMS for pediatrics: optimum treatment or unnecessary delay, *J Pediatr Surg* 18(4):498, 1983.

Aggressive Philosophy

53. Hazinski MR, Chahine AA, Holcombe CQ, et al: Outcome of cardiovascular collapse in pediatric blunt trauma, *Ann Emerg Med* 23:1229, 1994.
54. Curran C, Dietrich AM, Bowman MJ, et al: Pediatric cervical-spine immobilization: achieving neutral position? *J Trauma* 39(4):729, 1995.
55. Hooker EA, Miller EB, Hollander JL, et al: Do all trauma patients need early cross matching for blood, *J Emerg Med* 12:447, 1994.
56. Hooker EA, Miller FB, Hollander JL, et al: Do all trauma patients need early cross matching for blood, *J Emerg Med* 12:447, 1994.
57. Gentilello LM, Donovan DM, Dunn CW, et al: Alcohol interventions in trauma centers, *JAMA* 274(13):1043,

Appendix 19A: Rapid Sequence Induction

Rapid sequence induction (RSI) may be indicated for intubation of specific patients to maintain adequate oxygenation, protect the airway, and reduce adverse cardiovascular or intracranial pressure responses to intubation.

A reserve of oxygen is created by preoxygenation should any delays in tube placement occur. The average patient with 30 ml/kg of functional residual capacity uses oxygen at 3 ml/kg/min. The fasciculations associated with succinylcholine are reduced by prior treatment with pancuronium or thiopental, thereby eliminating rises in intracranial, intraocular, and intragastric pressure during the procedure. Pancuronium pretreatment does not reduce the release of potassium in patients with burns or crush injuries.

Relative contraindications to RSI include children who are breathing spontaneously, concern about the intubation being successful, major facial or laryngeal trauma, upper airway obstruction, and distorted facial or airway anatomy.

Technique

The patient's anatomy is initially evaluated, looking for oral or dental abnormalities, evidence of trauma to the neck or face, and systemic abnormalities such as coagulopathy that may create problems. Equipment for the procedure is checked. The patient is then preoxygenated for 4 to 5 minutes by a nonrebreather mask placed without positive pressure. If the patient is hypoventilating, he or she is hyperventilated, while cricoid pressure is maintained. Position the head in a "sniffing" position (see Fig. 19-2).

Atropine 0.02 mg/kg IV (minimum of 0.10 mg/dose) may be given to children <7 years of age to reduce bradycardia.

Then administer pancuronium (Pavulon) or vecuronium (Norcuron) 0.01 mg/kg IV (adolescents 1 mg IV) to reduce fasciculations. Allow 3 to 5 minutes before proceeding with succinylcholine. This step is not necessary in children less than 5 years of age. (An alternative to premedication with pancuronium is to sedate with sodium thiopental 3-5 mg/kg prior to the succinylcholine dose.)

In the presence of significant head injury, administer lidocaine 1.5 mg/kg IV at this time and allow 2 minutes before giving succinylcholine. Sedate the patient with thiopental 3 to 5 mg/kg IV if the patient is not hypotensive or in status asthmaticus. (An alternative for sedation is midazolam 0.1 mg/kg IV up to 5 mg maximum dose or ketamine [1 to 2 mg/kg IV] if no head injury is present.)

Immediately give succinylcholine 1.0 to 2.0 mg/kg IV to adolescents or 2 mg/kg IV to children less than 10 kg and allow 45 to 60 seconds for muscle relaxation. Vecuronium (0.2 to 0.25 mg/kg IV) may be used if succinylcholine is contraindicated or an alternative is preferred.

Cricoid pressure should be continuously maintained.

Orally intubate the patient, verify position, and release cricoid pressure. When the paralysis wears off, administer pancuronium 0.1 mg/kg IV or vecuronium 0.2 mg/kg if needed (Fig. 19A-1).

20

Head Trauma

Margaret Dolan

Head trauma is the leading cause of morbidity in children older than 1 year of age.[1] In the United States each year, 250,000 children between infancy and 14 years are hospitalized and 25,000 children die of or are permanently disabled by head trauma.[2] This death rate is five times that of leukemia, the next leading cause of death in children.

Males sustain head injury twice as often as females and have four times the risk of suffering fatal head injuries.[1,2] Males also have a steadily increasing incidence of head injury from 5 to 25 years of age. The incidence in females generally decreases across the first 15 years of life. Nearly two thirds of deaths caused by head injury occur in the prehospital setting, either at the site of the trauma or in the home after the injury.

PATHOPHYSIOLOGY

Brain injury may be classified clinically as primary or secondary. Primary brain injury occurs at the moment of impact, either by penetration of a foreign body, such as a bullet, knife, or skull fragment (focal injury), or by nonimpact shear forces during acceleration/deceleration events (diffuse injury).[3,4] Acceleration/deceleration injuries are more common than penetrating injuries in childhood, and these phenomena produce shear forces that are greatest at the junction of tissues of different rigidity (gray–white matter interface, skull-brain interface, dura mater–brain interface).[5]

Secondary brain injury occurs after the initial impact or penetrating injury and refers to neuron death due to systemic physiologic responses to the original injury. Because the brain is almost entirely dependent on aerobic metabolism, the final common pathway of secondary injury usually involves interruption of substrate delivery to neurons by hypoxia, ischemia, or both. Hypoxia causes global brain injury because no region of the brain is receiving a preferential supply of oxygen. Ischemia on the other hand may be either focal (e.g., due to occlusion of a single blood vessel), or global (e.g., due to cardiac arrest or reduced cardiac output. Multiple models exist to explain the mechanism(s) of brain injury.[6]

Fig. 20-1 simplifies the complicated and poorly understood relationships involved in secondary brain injury and ultimate neuron death. Experimental studies show that a hypoxic-ischemic event causes damage to some neurons during the primary insult but also triggers a cascade of different pathologic processes that leads to further loss of brain cells later.[7]

Cerebral hypometabolism occurs during ischemia and hypoxia.[8] Hypoventilation associated with brain stem injury or airway instability after head injury contributes to hypercapnia and hypoxia. Systemic hypoperfusion and hypoxia increase anaerobic metabolism in extracerebral tissues, producing systemic acidosis, which may enhance neuron damage during the reperfusion phase.[9]

At the cellular level, substrate absence produces energy failure leading to dysfunction of the ion pumps, depolarization, and influxes of Ca^{++}, Na^+ and Cl^- ions. Accumulation of intracellular Ca^{++} occurs either by influx of extracellular calcium, release of bound or sequestered intracellular calcium, or both. The intracellular accumulation of Ca^{++} is accompanied by loss of "free" intracellular Mg^{++}. Intracellular swelling occurs and if prolonged, results in cell lysis. Glutamate, present in dramatically increased levels during ischemia, opens both calcium and sodium channels promoting cytotoxic (intracellular) swelling and eventual lysis.[10] Some brain regions may be selectively vulnerable to this phenomenon.[11] Preexisting injuries, metabolic status, and cerebral maturation may also influence the sensitivity of the brain to injury.[12]

Membrane phospholipids, oxygen-derived free radical molecules, arachidonate, thromboxanes, and leukotrienes are released early in the course of ischemia. These have been implicated as mediators of neuronal damage or death during the reperfusion phase following ischemia.[13-15]

Cerebral temperature appears to be an important determinant of outcome. Hypothermia may improve or worsen neurologic outcome depending on when it is applied.[16]

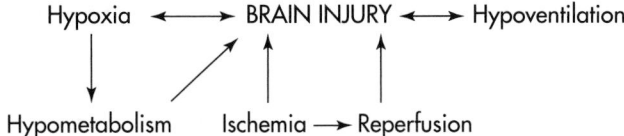

FIG. 20-1. Mechanism of brain injury.

A cascade of neuronal growth factors is induced after brain injury. These growth factors, induced by expression of selective genes, may be important regulators of cell survival.[17]

It is evident therefore that secondary brain injury is mediated by multiple factors that change as the injury evolves. Multiple strategies for brain resuscitation directed at these experimental models have been proposed but remain investigational at this time.[18,19]

The autoregulation of cerebral blood flow is poorly understood but is probably dependent on interacting neurogenic, vasogenic, and myogenic mechanisms.[20] The autoregulatory capacity is also known to be immature in infants and young children. Cerebral blood flow is exquisitely sensitive to arterial P_{CO_2}; decreased P_{CO_2} causes cerebral vasoconstriction, whereas increased P_{CO_2} results in cerebral vasodilatation. When injured, the child's brain may lose its autoregulatory ability and become much more susceptible to fluctuations in systemic blood pressure, resulting in either ischemia or hyperemia.

This unique, "brain-swelling" response of the injured pediatric brain was initially thought to be cerebral edema but is now recognized to be an increase in blood flow, not water content, and has been aptly renamed *cerebral hyperemia*.[3]

The pressure at which the brain is perfused and nourished, *cerebral perfusion pressure* (CPP), is equal to mean arterial, pressure (MAP) minus intracranial pressure (ICP).

$$CPP = MAP - ICP$$

It is important to recall that MAP is preserved in children with poor cardiac output by diverting blood flow from peripheral tissues. Adequate MAP in the presence of signs of increased systemic vascular resistance (pallor, cool extremities, diminished peripheral pulses) may indicate a marginal ability to preserve cerebral perfusion pressure.

The contents of the skull consist predominantly of three components: brain and glial tissue (70%), cerebrospinal fluid (CSF) and interstitial fluid (20%), and blood (10%).[21] An increase in the volume of one component is compensated for by either an enlargement of the cavity or a reduction or displacement of another component according to the Monro-Kellie hypothesis.[22,23] Initial increases in intracranial volume may be compensated for by a downshift of CSF from the skull into the dural sac surrounding the spinal cord. When the volume-buffering capacity of the CSF becomes exhausted, however, the ventricles collapse leaving no room to accommodate further increase in intracranial mass.[24,25] The cranial cavity of a young child (under 2 years of age) is somewhat more elastic than that of an adult. Limited increases in intracranial mass are tolerated

better in these children than in adults because of open fontanelles and the possibility of reopening unfused sutures. Increasing intracranial mass produces ICP increases above the normal of 15 to 20 mm Hg; brain structures swell and interruption of cerebral blood flow begins. If ICP continues to rise, the brain is compressed against the rigid dural folds that support it, blood flow to the brain ceases, and irreversible brain damage occurs. Intracranial pressure elevations are more common in children than adults, occurring in up to 80% of head-injured children.[3] Cerebral hyperemia may play a greater role in children than in adults in the early phases of head injury. When sufficient ICP develops, the skull contents follow the path of the least resistance and herniate into the spinal canal.

Two patterns of herniation occur: (1) central herniation, in which clinically there is an orderly progression of brain stem failure as the brain stem is compressed into the spinal canal, and (2) uncal herniation, in which the perihippocampal gyrus of the temporal lobe, including the uncus from one side of the brain, is compressed by mass effect on that side, resulting in a disorganized progression of brain stem failure. Clinically, uncal herniation is more difficult to recognize and manage since deterioration may be unpredictable and rapid. The earliest signs are deterioration of consciousness (caused by compression of the reticular activating system) followed by unilateral dilated pupil, usually on the side of the herniating brain. The pupillary dilatation results from compression of cranial nerve III by the temporal lobe. In early stages the dilatation is mild and light reflex is preserved; subsequently the pupil becomes unresponsive to light stimulus. As herniation progresses, decerebrate posturing or contralateral extremity hemiparesis occurs, as a result of compression and distortion of the cerebral peduncle. If herniation continues, contralateral pupillary dilatation occurs; it is followed by alteration of respiration, bradycardia, and systemic hypertension (Cushing triad) and, finally, respiratory arrest.[24]

ETIOLOGY

The mechanism of head injury in pediatric populations differs by age.[2] In infants and children less than 2 years of age, head injury usually results from falls from furniture or a caregiver's arms. Falls still account for the greatest frequency of head injury in preschool children: motor vehicle injuries account for nearly one quarter of cases. In school-aged children, the number of injuries caused by motor vehicles, falls, and sports- and recreation-related activities are approximately equal. Motor vehicle-related injuries include those sustained as either passenger, pedestrian, or cyclist. Among adolescents, head injury results from motor vehicle incidents and sports- and recreation-related activity in nearly equal proportions. The severity of sports-related activity is generally much less than that of motor vehicle-associated injury. Motor vehicle-associated head injuries have the greatest morbidity and mortality in all age groups.

Several factors enhance a child's vulnerability to head injury. As pedestrians or cyclists, children are less visible and more likely to be thrown after impact. A child's immature judgment, vulnerability to child abuse, dependency on adult supervision, and exposure to inadequate safety measures in play areas enhance the risk of injury.

Head trauma occurs in 80% or more of severely injured children. Anatomically, the head of the child represents a relatively greater proportion of mass and body surface area. Furthermore, stability largely depends on ligamentous rather than bony integrity. The pediatric brain has a higher water content (88% in a child vs. 77% in an adult) and is thus softer and more susceptible to acceleration-deceleration injury. Brain water content decreases with age, paralleling the myelinization of the brain, which is nearly 90% complete by 3 years of age but not entirely mature until adolescence. The unmyelinated brain is thus more susceptible to shear injuries than surgically treatable lesions.[26] On the other hand this ability of the immature brain to "regrow" itself, referred to as *inherent plasticity,* probably accounts for the fact that children have better outcomes than adults.[26] Infants and young children tolerate increases in ICP better than adults because the cranial sutures are not fused and the thin skull is more compliant than in adults.[3,4]

DIAGNOSTIC FINDINGS

Clinical Findings

A comprehensive approach to the head-injured child begins in the prehospital area and continues through acute hospital management and ultimate rehabilitation. Predetermined protocols facilitate accurate assessment and treatment during the initial moments of care. The history obtained at the scene is critical in determining extent of injury and priorities of care. Often, because of the severity of the injury, the history is obtained from family or bystanders the same time that initial assessments and resuscitative efforts are being made.

If the child fell, it is important to ascertain how far and onto what surface. If the child was involved in a motor vehicle accident, was the child a pedestrian, cyclist, or passenger? If the child was a cyclist, was a helmet worn? If a pedestrian, was the child thrown after impact, how far, and onto what surface of impact? If the injury was due to a direct blow, what was the vector (e.g., baseball bat or fist)? Explanations that are not consistent with the injury severity or the developmental level of the child should be investigated further.

The child's behavior after the injury should be assessed by determining alterations in consciousness, if any, as well as any memory loss or perseverative questioning. Symptoms of possible increased ICP (e.g., vomiting, seizures, weakness, and visual or gait change) should be elicited. Treatment measures initiated since injury should be noted.

The child's past medical history should be briefly reviewed, noting concurrent hyperactivity or epilepsy that might have placed the child at increased risk for head injury, as well as features that might make the injury more serious, such as hydrocephalus, bleeding diathesis, or intracranial malformations. Baseline neurodevelopmental function should be determined. If possible, the time of the child's last meal should be ascertained; and potential airway foreign bodies, such as loose teeth, candy, or food, should be noted.

Child abuse should be suspected in the child with an unexplained injury, a discrepancy among caretakers as to

---

> **Neurologic Examination of the Primary Survey**
>
> Pupil examination: size and reactivity
> Level of consciousness
>   A: Alert
>   V: Responsive to verbal stimulus
>   P: Responsive to painful stimulus
>   U: Unresponsive

---

how the injury occurred, a mechanism of injury inconsistent with the child's developmental level, a delay in seeking medical care, a history of repeated suspicious injuries, or a head injury associated with evidence of other body injury (e.g., old or new bruises on soft tissue areas, welts, and scars or burns).

The familiar ABC mnemonic (airway, breathing, circulation) should be used in the physical assessment of head-injured children. Features of this examination pertinent to head injury are discussed in Chapter 19.

Airway instability can be both a cause and an effect of head injury, especially when associated with unconsciousness. It is essential that an inadequate airway be recognized and relieved. Airway assessment should always be concurrent with cervical spine control if a head injury is present or cervical spine injury cannot be ruled out. Because head injury is commonly associated with hypoventilation, it is important (1) to note the quality of breath sounds and the adequacy of chest rise with spontaneous respirations, and (2) to support respirations as necessary to provide equal bilateral breath sounds and visible chest rise.

Recognition and control of life-threatening hemorrhage and peripheral signs of shock are important to ensure adequate perfusion of the brain. Neurogenic shock is a special circumstance manifested by systemic hypotension in a patient with warm extremities. The clue to the diagnosis is in the presence of associated motor or sensory abnormalities. Hypovolemic shock is rarely found after isolated head injury; other sources must be delineated.

The neurologic examination of the primary survey evaluates the level of consciousness (LOC) and the presence of abnormal pupillary findings. LOC is the best indicator of insufficient perfusion and oxygenation of the brain. Pupil asymmetry is the earliest sign of ICP that has increased above the physiologic 15 to 20 mm Hg.

The LOC examination of pediatric patients follows the mnemonic *AVPU* (see box above). The highest level of consciousness, *A*, is that of the awake verbal child, or in the nonverbal child who watches the examiner's actions, cries spontaneously, or seeks verbal or nonverbal reassurance from the parent or caretaker. *V* denotes a child who is responsive to verbal stimuli; clues to this status in the nonverbal child include behavioral signs of intact hearing and responsiveness such as eye opening, quieting, or calming in response to the parent's or caretaker's voice. Response to painful stimuli only is denoted by *P*. Children of all ages may moan or cry with painful stimulus; children more than 1 year of age withdraw from the stimulus. The letter *U* denotes the child who is unresponsive to any stimulus. The pupillary response is evaluated by the size and equality of the pupils. The frequency of pupil checks and AVPU examination should be dictated by the child's acuity; the unstable head-injured child may need minute-to-minute reassessment to recognize early signs of altered LOC or increasing ICP.

After life-threatening physiologic instability has been recognized and addressed in the primary survey, the secondary survey should identify potentially life-threatening situations and reassess interventions begun in the primary survey. Recognized patterns of injury help the examiner detect occult but potentially lethal injuries. For example, the Waddell triad of injuries to the child pedestrian—chest-abdominal injury, leg injury, and head injury—includes a contrecoup head injury that may be more serious but less obvious than the thorax or leg injury (see Chapter 19).

Crush or impact head injuries associated with parietal skull fractures crossing the groove occupied by the middle meningeal artery should make the examiner suspicious of an epidural hematoma.

Head injuries associated with child abuse may be due to direct blows to the skull or to shaking injuries. The coup injury of shaken baby syndrome (SBS) and other acceleration-deceleration head injuries may be associated with a high cervical spine injury even in the absence of external signs of trauma.[27] Subdural hematoma is the most dangerous injury; it is characterized by coma, convulsions, and increased ICP. It may be associated with fractures if the injury was caused by a direct blow by an adult's hand or impact against a wall or door. Subgaleal hematomas or cephalohematomas after the newborn period may substantiate other findings of suspected child abuse.

Emergency personnel should be aware of the presentation and treatment of birth trauma because of the frequency of home births and the practice of early postpartum discharge from the hospital. Seizures manifested after 48 hours of life are the most common presenting symptom of subarachnoid or subdural hemorrhage produced by birth trauma that may or may not be associated with external signs of trauma, such as cephalohematoma, caput succedaneum, or skull fracture.[28,29]

The neurologic examination of the secondary survey is more detailed than that of the primary survey.[30] The scalp should be carefully examined and lacerations palpated for tenderness or depressed skull fragments. The fontanelle should be evaluated in the infant for signs of increased ICP. Signs of basilar skull fracture such as periorbital hemorrhage ("raccoon eyes"), ecchymosis behind the ear (Battle sign) or eardrum (hemotympanum), or bleeding or clear fluid from the ears or nose should be noted. Extraocular muscle movements and the position of the eyes at rest should be noted, as should spontaneous abnormal eye movements. Motor and sensory function is evaluated by noting first the kind and quality of the child's spontaneous movements and posture. Asymmetry of function may signify midbrain compression associated with uncal herniation. The older child should be asked to move the fingers and toes. Muscle tone should be checked, including that of

the rectum. The awake child should be asked about pain, particularly of the neck. The neck muscles and cervical vertebrae should be palpated for tenderness and step-offs.

Stereotyped posturing should be noted. Decorticate posturing includes flexion of the arms, wrists, and fingers with adducted upper extremities and extension, internal rotation, and plantar flexion of the lower extremities. Decorticate posturing signifies diffuse damage to the cerebral cortex, white matter, or basal ganglia. In decerebrate posturing the rigidity is more pronounced and the arms and legs are extended, signifying more extensive damage down the midbrain. Note distribution (hemiparetic or paraparetic) of any muscular flaccidity or spasticity.

Examination of the response to noxious sensory stimuli, such as pinprick, tests of brain stem function (e.g., "doll's eyes"), corneal reflexes, and cold water calorics, as well as deep tendon and plantar reflex testing should be withheld in cases of head trauma until cervical spine injury has been ruled out. A funduscopic examination should be made to rule out retinal hemorrhages, which may be associated with high-energy acceleration-deceleration events. Retinal hemorrhages are often noted in SBS children from abuse.

Vital signs should be noted initially and followed with each neurologic reassessment. Hypothermia is a frequent complication in multiply injured children and should be prevented if possible. Slow or irregular respirations can be a sign of increasing ICP. The classic Cushing triad is rarely present in its complete form in children and, when present, is frequently a late finding. Very young children may bleed sufficiently into the intracranial cavity to have bradycardia associated with herniation as the first sign of increased ICP.

The secondary survey is completed by evaluating the child using the Glasgow Coma Score (GCS) and its pediatric modification (PGCS) (Table 20-1) to assess younger children, as well as the Pediatric Trauma Score (PTS) (see Table 19-1).[31,32] The GCS does not include a pupil evaluation which must be included on each assessment to completely evaluate the patient. Well-recognized problems exist when attempts are made to apply the GCS to young children with limited verbal skills. As a consequence of these problems, the modified PGCS was developed for children less than 5 years of age (see Table 20-1). A PGCS of 13 to 15 denotes minor injury, 8 to 12 moderate injury, and less than 8 severe injury.

The most important feature of the neurologic examination of head-injured children is serial and frequent reassessment. The initial result serves merely as the baseline against which subsequent results are compared. It is not unusual for head trauma patients to have alternating periods of agitation and depression, but sudden changes may demand immediate therapeutic intervention.

Complications

Shock. In general, shock should never be ascribed to head trauma alone, and other causes should be sought (e.g., bleeding from the abdomen or chest or long-bone fractures). There are, however, some rare exceptions to this rule in childhood. In children less than 1 year of age in whom an epidural hematoma associated with a large fracture develops, the hematoma may expand sufficiently to produce significant blood loss and shock. Young children

TABLE 20-1. Pediatric Glasgow Coma Score (PGCS)

Glasgow Coma Score	Pediatric modification	
Eye opening	**Eye opening**	
≥1 year	**0-1 year**	
4 Spontaneously	Spontaneously	
3 To verbal command	To shout	
2 To pain	To pain	
1 No response	No response	
Best motor response	**Best motor response**	
≥1 year	**0-1 year**	
6 Obeys command		
5 Localizes pain	Localizes pain	
4 Flexion withdrawal	Flexion withdrawal	
3 Flexion abnormal (decorticate)	Flexion abnormal (decorticate)	
2 Extension (decerebrate)	Extension (decerebrate)	
1 No response	No response	
Best verbal response	**Best verbal response**	
>5 years	**2-5 years**	**0-2 years**
5 Oriented and converses	Appropriate words and phrases	Cries appropriately, smiles, coos
4 Disoriented and converses	Inappropriate words	Cries
3 Inappropriate words	Cries/screams	Inappropriate crying/screaming
2 Incomprehensible sounds	Grunts	Grunts
1 No response	No response	No response

PGCS is the sum of individual scores from eye opening, best verbal response, and best motor response. PGCS of 13 to 15 indicates mild head injury; PGCS of 8 to 12 indicates moderate head injury; PGCS of <8 indicates severe head injury.

with large CSF spaces (e.g., hydrocephalus) can lose sufficient blood into the cranial cavity that acute anemia and occasionally shock develop. Occasionally an infant may have such a large subgaleal hematoma that anemia develops, but usually the bleeding is slow and shock does not occur.[32]

Apnea. Posttraumatic apnea is more common in children than in adults. The apnea is probably related to transient impairment of the reticular activating system along the brain stem; it occurs with sudden brain shifts that accompany acceleration/deceleration head trauma. It is usually of short duration and reverses itself spontaneously or with assisted ventilation unless a more serious brain stem or cervical spine injury has occurred. Because of the frequency with which children are known to be eating or sucking on small candies or snack foods at the time of their injury, it is important to rule out foreign body aspiration as a cause of traumatic apnea.

Cortical Blindness and Migraines. Although previously discussed as separate entities, transient blindness after head injury and trauma-induced migraine headache are now discussed as variations of the same manifestation. Cortical blindness is an acute, complete loss of vision that follows head injury in the young and generally resolves within 24 hours without sequelae.[33,34] Various mechanisms have been postulated, including acute focal edema and vasospasm with vascular compromise to the visual cortex. It is now thought to be one of a number of complex temporary alterations of brain function observed to occur

---

Signs and Symptoms of Increased ICP

Headache	Projectile vomiting
Irritability	Dizziness
Lethargy	Visual changes
Seizures	Unsteady gait
Bulging fontanelle	High-pitched cry
Pupillary dilatation	Head tilt
Cushing triad*	

*Cushing triad (bradycardia, increased blood pressure, and irregular respirations or apnea) is rarely present in its complete form in children. Frequently the only observable change in vital signs produced by increased ICP is an isolated bradycardia.
ICP, Intracranial pressure.

---

after minor head injury. Trauma-induced migraine typically begins within minutes to hours of the traumatic event and lasts hours to days. The traumatic incident itself is typically a minor injury. Propranolol (10 to 20 mg TID PO) has been beneficial when tried. Calcium channel blockers might be of theoretic benefit if a vascular cause were substantiated.[35] Impact seizures are considered to be part of the same phenomena.

Increased Intracranial Pressure. The signs of increased ICP are listed in the box above. Since the brain itself has no sensory innervation, most of the sensory symptoms are due to pressure or pain from associated innervated structures such as the dura and meninges. The remaining signs are caused by compression of brain stem or other functional centers. Cheyne-Stokes respirations (cyclic crescendo-decrescendo respirations with a period of apnea between each cycle) are common in increased ICP.

Seizure. Evidence of seizure is common after head trauma in children. A sole impact seizure that occurs immediately after injury has no prognostic significance. Approximately 5% of children hospitalized after head trauma have a seizure within the first week after injury. Nearly 80% of these do not have seizures after the first week. In another 5% of children hospitalized with head trauma seizures develop after the first week. Half of these children eventually stop having seizures; 25% continue to have seizures, but rarely, and another 25% have more than 10 seizures per year. Although seizures occur more commonly in children than adults, the literature is inconclusive as to whether posttraumatic seizures are more common in younger children than in older children.[36,37] The likelihood of seizure development increases with the severity of injury. Children with a PGCS of 3 to 8 upon presentation to the emergency department have an increased risk of posttraumatic seizure.[38] Patients in coma longer than 6 hours have an incidence of seizure approaching 50%.[39]

Posttraumatic seizures are more common after intracranial laceration than after concussion, more common after subdural than epidural injury, more common after depressed skull fractures, and more common in patients with severe brain injury (GCS of 3 to 5).

Posttraumatic Syndrome. The symptoms of the syndrome that may rarely follow mild or moderate head trauma are headache, which can be disabling for some children; irritability; nervousness; inability to concentrate; and behavioral or cognitive impairment.[24,40-43] Motor skills and receptive and expressive language function appear to be more sensitive than intelligence to sustained effects of closed head injury. Evidence suggests that children less than 3 years of age at time of injury may be more vulnerable to persistent expressive language deficits.[44] Sense of smell may also be impaired.[45] Although symptoms can persist for several weeks, most children recover normally. Some observers suggest that posttraumatic functional morbidity, when unaccompanied by physical morbidity, may be an expression of parental overreaction, inadvertently reinforced by the examining physician, and preexisting family dysfunction.[46] Posttraumatic syndrome may be difficult to differentiate from the premorbid state in children with previously undiagnosed attention deficit hyperactivity disorder.

Ancillary Data

Routine laboratory evaluations (e.g., complete blood cell count, type and cross-matching, and electrolytes) are made for significant injuries. Other studies, such as toxicology screens and blood alcohol levels, are done as indicated (see Chapter 42). The use of skull films for pediatric head trauma has been controversial.[47-49] Routine imaging studies of all children with head trauma provide little information. Specific situations do exist in which plain skull films are indicated or are a necessary adjunct to other studies.

In suspected child abuse, skull x-ray films are an essential part of a full skeletal survey. Children who enter the emergency department after head trauma with a nonlocalizing neurologic examination finding but a hematoma that precludes ruling out a depressed skull fracture clinically should have a skull x-ray film. In this instance tangential views are helpful. Skull x-ray films may also detect focal depressions and some fractures, such as stellate fractures and widely separated linear skull fractures not visualized by computed tomography (CT) scan. Children less than 2 years of age with a history of head trauma associated with loss of consciousness, vomiting, or seizures should have skull x-rays in addition to their head CT scan to define potential fractures because of the possibility of subsequent development of a leptomeningeal cyst if a dural tear has occurred with the fracture.

The primary goal of intracranial radiologic imaging in the emergency setting is to determine the need for operative intervention (in the case of intracranial hemorrhage) or to ascertain evidence of increased ICP. In patients with severe head trauma, instability with multiple trauma or head trauma with localizing neurologic examination findings, the most rapid and least invasive imaging modality is the cranial CT scan. Other patients for whom CT scan is indicated include children with posttraumatic seizures, amnesia, progressive headache, alcohol or drug intoxication, unreliable or inadequate history of injury, vomiting more than two or three times or more than 8 hours after injury, loss of consciousness more than 5 minutes after injury, or signs of basilar skull fracture.[39,45,46] However, clinical symptoms are a poor predictor of abnormalities on CT.[50] In the immediate posttraumatic period, intracranial hemorrhage is usually evident on CT scan without use of contrast medium (Fig. 20-2). After 7 to 10 days, extravasated blood may begin breaking down; scanning after this time should be done with and without contrast medium. On CT scan, cerebral hyperemia is manifested as increased density with blurring of the sulci and gray-white margins. Cerebral hyperemia associated with increased ICP appears as obliteration of the cisterns and ventricles (early sign) and shift of the midline structures.

Recently CT imaging of the brain has been compared with magnetic resonance imaging (MRI) scan. Pathologic studies demonstrate that CT scan underestimates the severity of many types of cerebral trauma.[49,51] Occasionally, blood collections located close to the bone may be difficult to visualize on CT scan because of averaging techniques. Small hypothalamic and brain stem infarcts are not resolved by CT scan, and shear injuries of the cerebral white matter, unless hemorrhagic, usually are not identifiable.[52] MRI scan has been found more sensitive than CT scan in detecting nonhemorrhagic intracranial lesions in the acute phase[53,54] and is the definitive procedure to identify diffuse axonal injury (DAI). DAI is the most frequent intraaxial lesion in patients presenting with acute severe trauma associated with immediate loss of consciousness and a negative CT scan.[51] MRI scan has also been reported to detect secondary forms of injury, such as territorial arterial infarction, pressure necrosis from increased ICP, cerebral herniation, and secondary brain stem injury not detected with CT scan.[5] Visualization by MRI scan differentiates

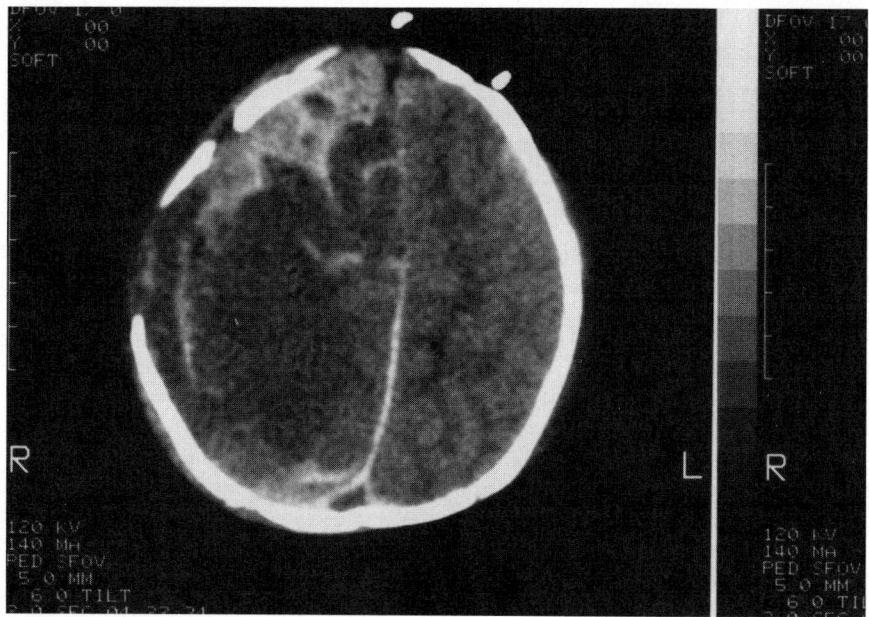

FIG. 20-2. Unenhanced axial CT scan of brain revealing high-density extraaxial collections over the right cerebral hemispheres consistent with both subdural and subarachnoid blood. Diffuse low-density throughout the right brain parenchyma represents edema or infarction. Midline structures have shifted. Right frontoparietal calvarial fracture with missing bone fragments.

subacute and chronic injuries better than does CT scan and does not require the use of contrast to identify chronic subdural hematomas that have become isodense.[53] MRI scan allows a better understanding of the initial mode of brain injury and may be fundamental in preventing secondary lesions, guiding treatment, and predicting outcome.[55] However, because of the lengthy time required for MRI studies compared with CT scans, the need for ferromagnet-compatible equipment on the child being studied, and the monitoring difficulties during the MRI examination, MRI scan appears to be less practical than CT scan at present for evaluating the acutely injured or unstable head-injured child in the emergency setting. Ultimately, an MRI scan should be performed as part of the evaluation of a neurologically stable patient with some severe impairment of consciousness with or without focal deficit.[55]

Ultrasonography has proven helpful in newborns and young infants with open fontanelles and sutures in demonstrating displacement or obstruction of the ventricular system. Ultrasonography requires no radiation exposure. Ultrasonography is performed routinely on newborns who have suffered traumatic births, on premature infants at risk of periventricular or interventricular hemorrhage, and on any infant with open fontanelles and a suspected anatomic abnormality within the skull.

MANAGEMENT

Initial management of all head trauma should be directed toward the recognition and treatment of life-threatening and physiologic instability. Identification and correction of prearrest syndromes (e.g., respiratory failure, shock, and increased ICP) is the goal of the primary survey

and the most effective way to prevent secondary brain injury.

Airway and cervical spine management should be initiated simultaneously in the head-injured child. The airway should be cleared of vomitus and secretions; foreign bodies (e.g., broken teeth or chewing gum) should be removed with a tonsillar suction device. All patients should be placed on a cardiorespiratory monitor. Oxygen (100%) should be supplied by nonrebreather mask and monitored by arterial blood gas or pulse oximetry to maintain the Po_2 greater than or equal to 95 mm Hg. Because adequate minute ventilation is determined by tidal volume and respiratory rate, bag-valve mask assisted ventilation should be initiated if the patient has inadequate spontaneous chest rise or respiratory rate. The patient who requires prolonged assisted ventilation should be intubated.

Cervical spine immobilization should be initiated in all children with significant head injury and in all patients with altered mental status in whom trauma cannot be excluded.

In managing the breathing status of the patient, it is important to note rate, pattern, and mechanics of spontaneous respirations. Life-threatening chest injuries should be suspected in the primary survey if signs of increased work of breathing continue in the presence of 100% oxygen and a stable airway. Chest injuries should be corrected to assure adequate oxygenation and ventilation secondary to brain injury. Slow or irregular respirations can be a sign of increased ICP, and can worsen acidosis. Traumatic apnea is common in children. Central hyperventilation can be seen in children with decerebrate or decorticate posturing.

Unconscious head-injured children who require intubation should be suspected of having rising ICP. Because traumatic intubations increase ICP even further, medications for induction, paralysis and maintenance agents during rapid sequence intubation should be chosen to minimize ICP increases and should afford the examiner opportunity to regain ability to monitor neurologic status within the shortest possible time. Intubations should be carried out quickly by the person most experienced in airway stabilization. Because of the emergency nature of the procedure, an appropriately sized and placed stylet should be used. Orotracheal intubations are preferred for head-injured children because of the possibility of cribriform plate fractures and the difficulties associated with blind nasotracheal intubations in young children. If intubation is initiated before evaluating lateral cervical spine films, spinal immobilization should be maintained throughout the procedure.

Because head-injured children may be combative and may have eaten recently, a rapid-sequence induction technique should be used (see Appendix, Chapter 19). It is important to recognize the clinical signs of poor perfusion in the multiply injured child (delayed capillary refill, pallor, weak distal pulses) and to deliver sufficient resuscitation fluids to the child in hypovolemic shock even if a head injury is serious. Because children desaturate their hemoglobin more rapidly than adults, patients should be preoxygenated for at least 3 minutes with 100% O_2 before intubation is attempted. When intubating head-injured children, with or without paralysis, it is crucial to maintain cricoid pressure (Sellick maneuver) from initiation of sedation until tube placement is secured to prevent aspiration of stomach contents. Lidocaine, 1 to 2.0 mg/kg IV before intubation, may be used to suppress the cough reflex and may exert a direct effect in lowering ICP. An oral airway should be inserted after intubation in the unconscious or semiconscious child to prevent biting on the endotracheal tube.

Management of the circulatory status includes establishing control of life-threatening hemorrhage and identification and aggressive treatment of shock to prevent secondary brain injury caused by hypotension. It is important to deliver sufficient resuscitation fluids to the child in hypovolemic shock even if a head injury is serious. Most head trauma patients with altered consciousness have excessive output of antidiuretic hormone but not usually during the initial resuscitation. There is therefore little reason to restrict fluids during prehospital or emergency department resuscitations.

An abnormal AVPU or pupil-check result in the primary survey signifies the potential for increased ICP and impending cerebral herniation. Hyperventilation via bag-valve-mask or endotracheal tube should be initiated if the patient has inadequate spontaneous respirations or is not breathing. Ventilatory rates should be directed at maintaining the patient's Pco_2 at 20 to 25 mm Hg. Repeated arterial punctures may be avoided by use of an indwelling arterial catheter or an end-tidal CO_2 monitor. The head should be elevated to 15 to 30 degrees above the feet if the patient is not in shock and the cervical spine cleared clinically and radiographically. While the patient is still on a backboard, head elevation can be achieved by placing blanket rolls under the head of the backboard.

Interventions begun during the primary survey should be reassessed during the more detailed secondary survey.

Children with severe head trauma are at risk for sudden intracranial hemorrhage, acute respiratory insufficiency, or brain swelling and herniation from increased ICP. Repeated serial assessments of the patient, including AVPU, pupil check, and evaluation using the PGCS and PTS, should be made for early detection of clinical changes in the patient's status.

Radiologic examination is undertaken when the patient's cardiovascular and respiratory status is stabilized. CT scans may also be performed preoperatively in unconscious patients who require emergency chest or abdominal surgery to rule out intracranial abnormality or elevated ICP.

Pharmacologic agents have limited usefulness in the emergency department management of head trauma or remain controversial. Osmotic agents such as mannitol (0.25 to 0.5 gm/kg) are not used prophylactically but may occasionally be necessary to decrease intracranial pressure not responsive to elevation and hyperventilation. In multiple trauma they should be used only after adequate fluid resuscitation has begun. Fluid and electrolyte management may become very complicated, especially if furosemide is used to enhance the effect of mannitol; therefore this diuretic is usually not used during initial resuscitation. It is crucial to follow serum electrolyte levels and osmolarity carefully in these situations and to monitor volume status and perfusion.

Routine prophylactic use of anticonvulsants in pediatric head injury is unwarranted. In certain instances, where there is potential for gliosis and epileptogenic scar-tissue formation, they may be indicated. Specific injuries include acute subdural hematoma; open, depressed skull fracture with parenchymal damage; or severe head injury (PGCS of ≤ 8).[36,56] Brain contusions have also been considered a site of potential epileptogenic focus. Phenytoin (10 to 20 mg/kg infused at 1 mg/kg/min IV up to a maximum 50 mg/min) is most commonly considered as the prophylactic anticonvulsant.[57] It may reduce posttraumatic seizures in children presenting to the ED with a PGCS of 3 to 8.[38]

Other pharmacologic agents have limited usefulness or remain controversial in ED management of head trauma. Corticosteroids are helpful in reducing the cerebral edema produced by tumors but have little use in head injury and may even compound nitrogen losses associated with head injury.[58] Traditionally, management of head injury with increased ICP in the intraoperative or intensive care setting included barbiturate coma, hypothermia and ICP monitoring via intraventricular catheter or subarachnoid bolts. The efficacy of each of these latter measures is controversial.[45,59-63] Experimental models including the use of mild early cerebral hyperthermia, infusion of free radical scavenger molecules, and gene induction therapy remain investigational at this time.[6]

Management approaches must reflect the severity of the injury, accompanying injuries, preexisting health problems, and clinical judgment. Children with severe head injury are those with a PGCS of 8 or less or a PGCS decrease of 2 points or more not clearly caused by seizures, drugs, or metabolic factors.[64] Other criteria for severe head injury include focal signs on neurologic examination, a penetrating skull injury, palpable depressed skull fracture, or compound skull fracture. Children with severe head injury should have prompt neurosurgical consultation and CT

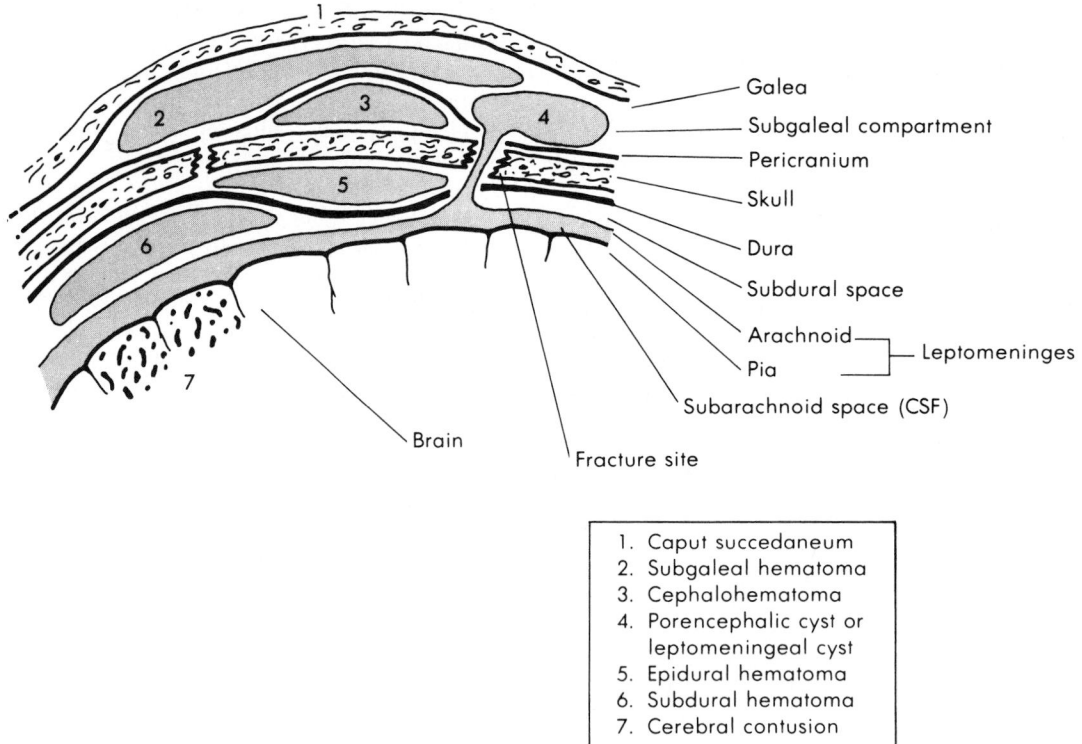

Galea
Subgaleal compartment
Pericranium
Skull
Dura
Subdural space
Arachnoid ⎤
            ⎬ Leptomeninges
Pia ⎦
Subarachnoid space (CSF)
Brain
Fracture site

1. Caput succedaneum
2. Subgaleal hematoma
3. Cephalohematoma
4. Porencephalic cyst or leptomeningeal cyst
5. Epidural hematoma
6. Subdural hematoma
7. Cerebral contusion

FIG. 20-3. Traumatic head injuries. (*From Barkin RM and Rosen P:* Emergency pediatrics, *ed 4, St. Louis, 1994, Mosby.*)

scan (see box on p. 245). The majority of deaths after severe head injury in children are due to a severe impact injury or the development of significant secondary injury. Head injury associated with moderate or severe extracranial injury has poor outcome.[65]

Children with moderate head injury (PGCS of 9 to 12) have generally had a loss of consciousness for 5 minutes or more and manifest progressive lethargy or headaches. They may have posttraumatic amnesia or seizure or have signs of a basal skull fracture.[45] Frequently these children have been involved in multiple trauma or are victims of suspected child abuse. Injuries to other areas such as the chest or abdomen should be identified and treated promptly since they may contribute to morbidity and alter the central nervous system findings. The most important feature of the examination is serial assessment with assignment of a PGCS. CT scan and neurosurgical consultation should be obtained if the child's condition does not improve or deteriorates. Skull x-ray films may identify isolated linear fractures missed by CT scan. Because of the chance of subsequent intracranial hemorrhage or worsening cerebral edema, admission for observation is warranted in most cases of moderate head injury.

Patients with a PGCS of 13 to 15 are classified as having a mild head injury. These children typically have sustained at most a momentary loss of consciousness (>5 minutes), arrive awake, and primarily need a thorough physical examination. They may be asymptomatic or complain of a mild headache or dizziness. Skull x-ray radiographs are generally unnecessary except for the indication previously

described. Careful, thorough neurologic examination is important to rule out focal abnormalities. Children with a PGCS of 15 who have a normal neurological examination rarely have an intracranial hemorrhage.[66] Scalp and facial wounds should be cleaned and sutured as necessary. Tetanus prophylaxis should be updated as indicated. Skull x-ray films are generally unnecessary, except for the indications described. Children who meet these criteria may be discharged from the emergency department to a responsible adult, with medication for headache and a head-injury instruction sheet specifying signs and symptoms to monitor, including those indicative of increasing ICP.

SPECIFIC CLINICAL ENTITIES

Scalp Injuries (Fig. 20-3)

The scalp is richly vascularized; small lacerations can bleed profusely. Although most children can handle this blood loss well, it is important to remember that a blood loss too small to be hemodynamically significant for an adult may produce shock in an infant or child. Scalp bleeding can be controlled by direct pressure, hemostats, or rapid suturing. It is important to ascertain that the skull underneath a laceration is not damaged. If the possibility of a skull fracture exists, direct pressure should be applied over a broad area rather than a small localized area. Scalp wounds should be carefully explored to determine the condition of the skull underneath and to verify that no foreign body is embedded in the wound. The wound should then be scrubbed and irrigated profusely with

Clinical Indications for X-Ray Examinations in Head-Injured Children*

Low-risk group	Moderate-risk group	High-risk group
Possible findings	Possible findings	Possible findings
Asymptomatic	History of change of consciousness at the time of injury or subsequently	Depressed level of consciousness not clearly due to alcohol, drugs, or other cause (e.g., metabolic and seizure disorders)
Headache	History of progressive headache	Focal neurologic signs
Dizziness	Alcohol or drug intoxication	Decreasing level of consciousness
Scalp hematoma	Unreliable or inadequate history of injury	Penetrating skull injury or palpable depressed fracture
Scalp laceration	Age >2 yr (unless injury very trivial)	
Scalp contusion or abrasion	Posttraumatic seizure	
Absence of moderate-risk or high-risk criteria	Vomiting	
	Multiple trauma	
	Serious facial injury	
	Signs of basilar fracture†	
	Possible skull penetration or depressed fracture‡	
	Suspected physical child abuse	
Recommendations	Recommendations	Recommendations
Observation alone; discharge patients with head-injury information sheet (listing subdural precautions) and a second person to observe them	Extended close observation (watch for signs of high-risk group) Consider CT examination and neurologic consultation. Skull series may (rarely) be helpful, if positive, but do not exclude intracranial injury if normal.	Patient is a candidate for neurosurgical consultation or emergency CT examination or both.

From Masters SJ, et al: *New Engl J Med* 316 (2):85, 1987.
*Physician assessment of the severity of the injury may warrant reassignment to a higher-risk group. Any single criterion from a higher-risk group warrants assignment of the patient to the highest-risk group applicable.
†Signs of basilar fracture include drainage from ear, drainage of cerebrospinal fluid from nose, hematotympanum, Battle sign, and "raccoon eyes."
‡Factors associated with open and depressed fracture include gunshot, missile, or shrapnel wounds; scalp injury from firm, pointed object (including animal teeth); penetrating injury of eyelid or globe; object stuck in the head; assault (definite or suspected) with any object; leakage of cerebrospinal fluid; and sign of basilar fracture.
CT, Computed tomography.

saline solution, after which it can be closed with sutures or staples (if less than 2 inches). Patients with scalp injuries should have their tetanus status ascertained and updated as needed.

Caput succedaneum and cephalohematoma, the two extracranial manifestations of birth trauma, are differentiated by location, onset, and duration (Fig. 20-4). Caput succedaneum involves molding of the very pliable neonate skull to fit through the maternal pelvis, with some degree of soft tissue swelling also involved. Cephalohematoma involves subperiosteal bleeding. Caput succedaneum usually crosses suture lines, whereas cephalohematomas are limited by the cranial sutures. Caput succedaneum is present at delivery and resolves in the first days of life; the appearance of cephalohematoma may be delayed by the slow rate of subperiosteal bleeding and resolve spontaneously over a period of 2 weeks to 3 months. X-ray studies of cephalohematomas that have indicated underlying skull fractures are uncommon: such fractures occur in 5% to 25% of patients studied.[28,29] Aspiration attempts are contraindicated in both cephalohematoma and caput succedaneum because of the risk of introducing infection.

Concussion

Concussion is defined as a transient loss of awareness and responsiveness with impaired consciousness.[24] Concussion is a common finding in injuries associated with rapid acceleration-deceleration forces or a sudden blow that deforms the skull sharply. The hallmark of concussion is amnesia, which may be temporary or permanent, retrograde or antegrade. If unconsciousness occurs, it is usually brief. The clinical symptoms associated with concussion are dizziness, headache, and vomiting. Patients are almost always arousable with semiappropriate responses to vigorous stimuli. They may have conjugate or dysconjugate roving eye movements. Pupils are responsive but may spontaneously fluctuate considerably in size. Children with concussion may occasionally have unilateral or bilateral extensor plantar reflexes.[67] No consistent morphologic changes are noted with concussion and no findings are

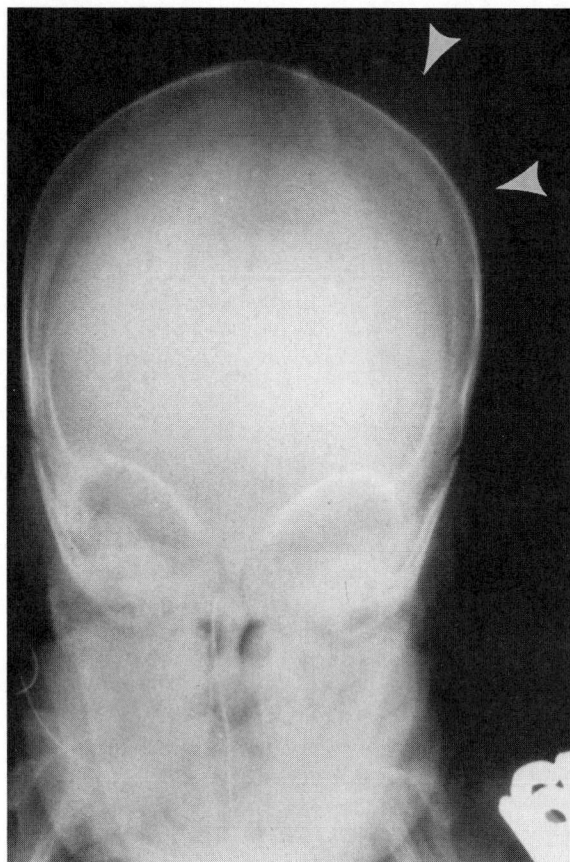

FIG. 20-4. Towne view of the skull revealing focal soft tissue swelling over left parietal convexity confirming clinically suspected cephalohematoma *(white arrowheads)*.

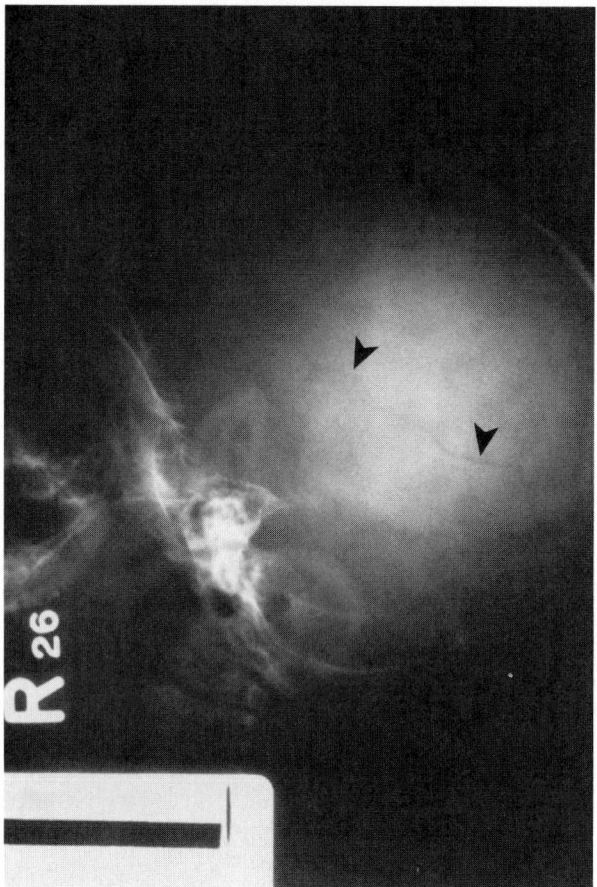

FIG. 20-5. Lateral radiograph of skull revealing extensive curvilinear lucency in the parietooccipital bone crossing the squamosal suture, consistent with acute skull fracture *(black arrowheads)*. Compare this with the normal appearing squamosal suture immediately inferior to the fracture.

seen on CT scan. Plum and Posner point out that concussion is a retrospective diagnosis since it describes a transient state.[24]

Most children with concussion require only acetaminophen analgesia and close observation at home by a responsible adult with good instructions to observe for symptoms of increasing ICP. Children with loss of consciousness longer than 5 minutes, persistent symptoms, or inadequate home observation should have a CT scan and be hospitalized.[48]

Contusion

Contusion is a bruising or tearing of brain tissue and is the most common brain injury found on CT scan. It can be caused by a penetrating foreign body (e.g., a bullet, knife, or other missile). More commonly it is due to bruising from the irregular bony projections within the skull itself or skull fragments after a skull fracture. The contusion may occur at the site of impact (coup injury) or at a site remote from the impact (contrecoup injury). The poles and undersurfaces of the frontal and temporal lobes are the most vulnerable. Signs and symptoms of contusion are unconsciousness, disturbance in strength or sensation, change in visual awareness, or focal neurologic signs (e.g., seizures) that were absent before the injury. CT scans on patients with contusions reveal small focal areas of mixed high and low density.

Direct occipital trauma resulting from falls or blows to the head bear special mention because of the unique anatomy of the posterior fossa. The contents of the posterior fossa have a limited area in which to expand. With trauma and subsequent brain swelling, posterior fossa contents herniate into the spinal canal. This fact must be kept in mind when assessing and managing the child with mild or moderate direct occipital head trauma.[21]

Patients with contusion should have neurosurgical consultation and hospitalization with close observation for signs of worsening brain injury.

Skull Fractures

Linear fractures are disruptions in the integrity of the skull occurring at the point of impact; they are the most common pediatric skull fractures, comprising almost 75% (Fig. 20-5). The parietal bone is the most common fracture site and has associated intracranial lesions in up to 48% of fractures identified.[21] Linear skull fractures often spread at

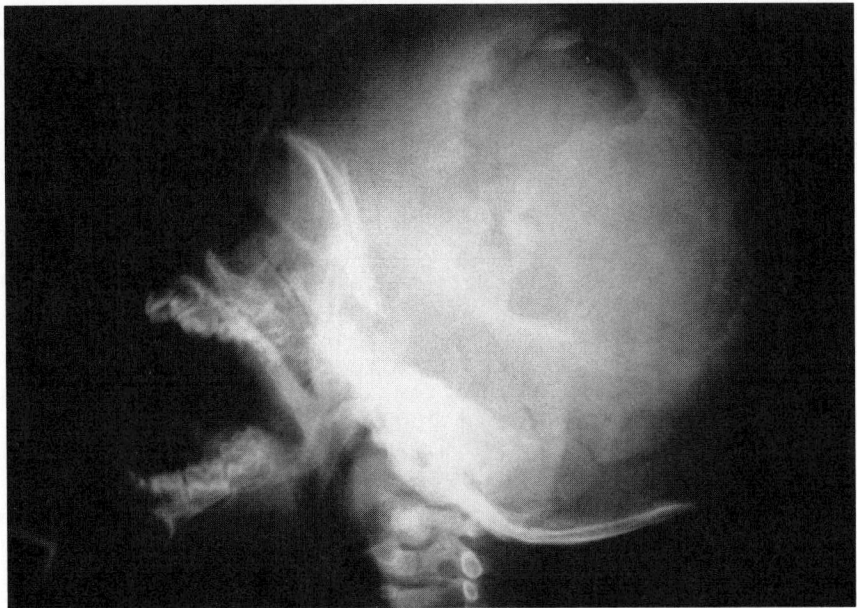

FIG. 20-6. Lateral radiograph of skull revealing lucent defects of varying sizes in the parietal bone corresponding in location to leptomeningeal cyst, after skull fracture with presumed dural tear.

the point of impact, assuming a V-shaped configuration.[68] Usually they do not cross sutures. All patients with skull fractures should have a neurosurgical consultation. Linear fractures that suggest the possibility of an accompanying more serious injury are those that cross the path of the middle meningeal artery and extend into paranasal sinuses or mastoid air cells.

The most common complication of linear skull fracture is subgaleal hematoma, which may develop within days to weeks of an injury. The large fluctuant fluid collection is often mistakenly thought to be CSF when x-ray films demonstrate a linear skull fracture beneath it. The collection should never be aspirated unless there is clear evidence of infection because of the risk of introducing bacteria into the liquefied blood, an excellent medium for bacterial growth. The fluid collection resorbs slowly if left alone.

Several normal variations of the pediatric skull are occasionally misread as skull fractures.[69,70] Vascular grooves differ from fractures in that they generally occur in the anterior third of the bone, run vertically with a gentle posterior curve, and tend to have sclerotic edges. The metopic suture, which often is open, may appear to be a midline fracture. A differentiating point is that the metopic suture crosses the foramen magnum, whereas the midline occipital fracture does not, and the metopic suture frequently has sclerosis on each side of the suture line. Posterior fossa sutures and accessory sutures of the parietal bone are usually horizontal and frequently paired. Soft tissue edema over the site of a suspected fracture may be helpful.

A unique fracture of infants and small children is the "growing fracture" (Fig. 20-6). Such fractures occur in patients less than 2 years of age who are experiencing rapid brain growth.[71] They result from significant head trauma that produces a skull fracture with a dural tear. In the postinjury period, rapid growth of the child's brain is associated with extrusion of brain or a CSF cyst (leptomeningeal cyst) through the dural defect preventing fusion of the fracture margins. This complication is treated neurosurgically. The potential for this uncommon complication mandates neurosurgical follow-up observation for patients less than 2 years of age who have skull fractures associated with significant head trauma.

Depressed skull fractures are the result of a direct, forceful impact. They should be suspected when there is a history of high-energy mechanism of injury. When the blow is over a small area of impact, such as from a hammer or high-heeled shoe, the fracture generally assumes a stellate configuration that is seen on plain films but may be missed by CT scan. Depressed fractures are frequently difficult to delineate on a single view and may require oblique views for diagnosis. The area may appear sclerotic because of overlapping of the fracture fragments; there may be an area of widening between fragments (Fig. 20-7).

Management of depressed skull fractures is neurosurgical and may include intraoperative elevation of the depressed fragment if the depth of depression is deeper than the thickness of the calvarium. Tetanus status should be ascertained and updated as necessary. Depressed skull fractures are frequently associated with brain laceration and occasionally the subsequent development of a seizure focus.

Early and complete surgical management is the mainstay of therapy for open skull fractures and penetrating head injuries. Cultures of the wound should be obtained to guide the selection of antibiotic therapy if an infection

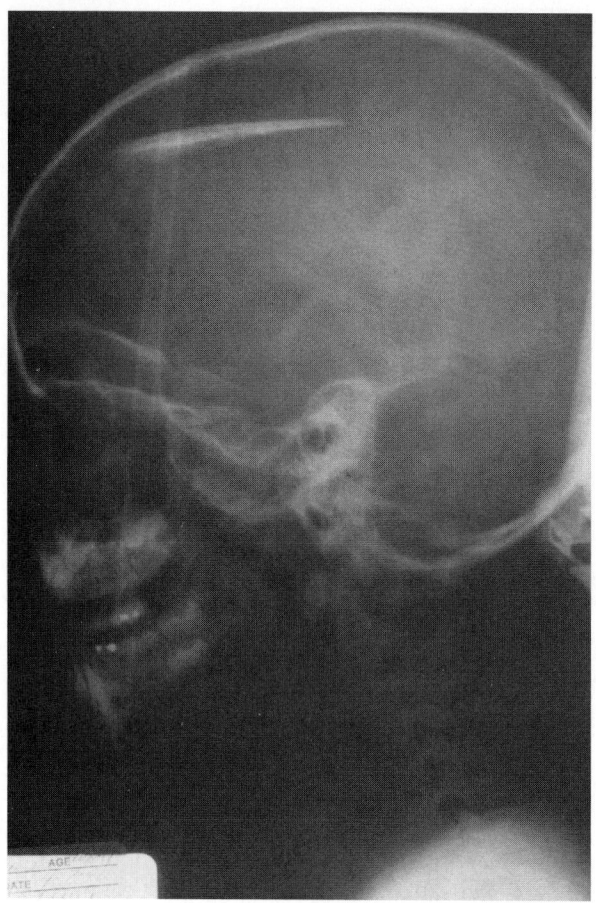

FIG. 20-7. Lateral radiograph of skull revealing linear depressed frontoparietal fracture. Increased density at the fracture site results from overlapping bone fragments.

develops, but routine prophylactic antibiotics remain controversial because of the risk of selecting out a resistant organism.[26]

Basal skull fractures are usually not seen on routine skull films and are best diagnosed by CT scan. Clinically the diagnosis is made by coexisting signs. Hemotympanum (blood visible behind the tympanic membrane) and Battle sign, a purplish discoloration behind the ear, are suggestive of a posterior basal fracture. "Raccoon eyes" (i.e., periorbital bruising) suggests an anterior basal fracture; lack of conjunctival injection helps to exclude other causes of periorbital hyperemia from the diagnosis. Blood or CSF may drain from the nose or ears with basal skull fractures. Up to 21% of patients with a normal mental status and neurologic examination were noted to have an intracranial injury on emergency CT scan.[72]

Management of basal skull fractures is neurosurgical consultation and symptomatic care; frequently no treatment is required in the presence of a normal examination and CT study. Prophylactic administration of antibiotics for basal skull fractures, even with CSF leak, is controversial. There is no clear evidence that prophylactic antibiotics decrease the risk of meningitis in these fractures, and they may predispose to infection by more resistant organisms. Regardless of the initial decision made about using antibiotics, obtaining nose and throat cultures is probably worthwhile if there is evidence of a CSF leak.[46]

Intracranial Hemorrhage

Epidural Hemorrhage. Epidural hemorrhages most commonly occur in the lateral temporal fossa as a result of laceration of the middle meningeal artery or vein secondary to skull fracture. Other possible sites are frontal and occipital hematomas.

Epidural hemorrhages tend to enlarge rapidly, pushing the brain laterally away from the skull, thereby stretching pain-sensitive meninges and blood vessels at the base of the middle fossa. Epidural hemorrhages occasionally tamponade themselves after 30 to 50 ml of blood has accumulated and subsequently act as a unilateral focal mass lesion. More frequently they produce a rapidly progressing uncal syndrome within a few hours or days after injury.

The diagnosis of epidural hemorrhage can be difficult since it often follows seemingly trivial trauma. The classic picture of a brief loss of consciousness with a lucid interval followed by clinical deterioration occurs more often in children than adults but is not consistent.[73] The first symptom in conscious patients is usually headache, followed by alteration of consciousness or agitation and then by uncal syndrome, the earliest signs of which are pupillary changes and hemiparesis. Motor signs occur only late in the course and may include focal or generalized convulsions.

CT scan is the most appropriate diagnostic tool in suspected epidural hemorrhages. Epidural hemorrhages are lens shaped on CT scan and may be limited in children by the attachment of the dura at the suture lines (Fig. 20-8). Fresh blood is demonstrated on the CT scan as an area of increased density, appearing whiter than surrounding tissue.

In the newborn, intracranial hemorrhages associated with birth trauma are most commonly subarachnoid. Because these bleeds in the newborn are of venous rather than arterial origin, they are frequently asymptomatic. The most common symptom associated with either subarachnoid or subdural hemorrhage in the newborn is a seizure that develops after 48 hours of life. Treatment for subarachnoid hemorrhage is supportive (transfusions and anticonvulsants).

Treatment is generally surgical drainage and support.

Subdural Hemorrhages. Subdural hemorrhages are due to venous bleeding, most commonly from disruption of the bridging veins across the dura. Subdural hemorrhages caused by birth trauma may also occur over the lateral aspects of the temporal lobes from tears of the bridging superficial cerebral veins as well as from rupture of the straight or lateral sinus, Galen vein, or inferior sagittal vein. Because the bleeding is not constrained by the tight dura, the clot has more room to expand; consequently subdural hemorrhages are usually associated with a slower time course than epidural hemorrhages. Subdural hemorrhages are rarely associated with fractures but rather with underlying lacerations or brain contusions.

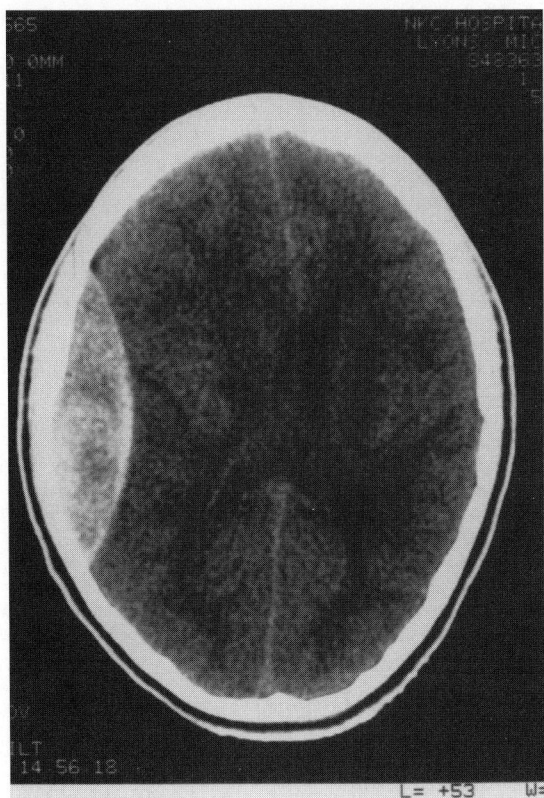

FIG. 20-8. Nonenhanced axial computed tomography scan of brain revealing high-density lentiform extraaxial collection over the right parietal convexity consistent with epidural hematoma. Note resultant shift of midline structures.

Subdural hemorrhages are a classic feature of the shaken baby syndrome (SBS).[55] Some examiners feel that shaking alone does not produce brain injury and that some impact injury is required as well.[74,75] Other examiners have found severe whiplash-shake injury without direct-impact cranial trauma in a group of very young infants. Hemorrhages and contusions of the high cervical spinal cord may contribute to morbidity and mortality in these infants.[22] Emergency personnel should suspect abuse when infants or small children have subdural hemorrhages.

The physical findings of subdural hemorrhage are generally those of increased ICP: full fontanelle, vomiting, lethargy, and irritability. Occasionally in SBS, retinal hemorrhages or even bruising of the pinna may be seen.[76,77]

On CT scan acute subdural hematomas are commonly crescent shaped, spreading diffusely along the inner table of the skull (Fig. 20-9). There may be associated displacement of the underlying brain and midline structures, depending on the size of the collection or the presence of cerebral hyperemia. Contrast enhancement is usually required only in cases of subacute or chronic injury (> 10 days); intracranial collections may have become isodense. In shaken babies, subdural hemorrhages may occasionally be bilateral and located posteriorly in the interhemispheric fissure.

Subdural hemorrhages are managed neurosurgically; symptomatic subdural hemorrhages are treated with serial subdural taps in infants and burr holes in older patients.

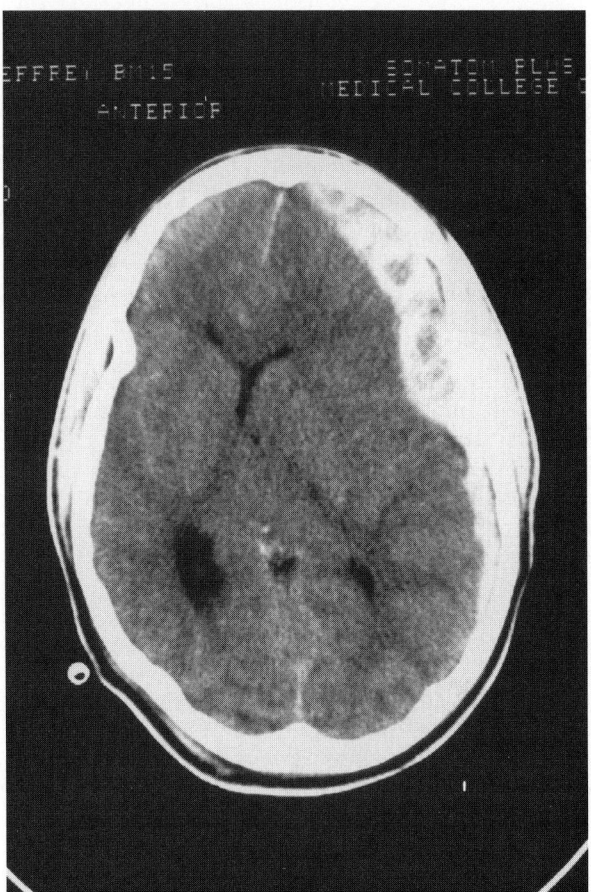

FIG. 20-9. Nonenhanced axial computed tomography scan of brain at level of frontal horns revealing a crescentic hyperdense collection distributed diffusely beneath the left calvarium consistent with subdural hematoma. Shift of midline structures results in mass effect.

DISPOSITION AND PROGNOSIS

The outcome spectrum for head injury is broad, from immediately lethal injury to headache and temporary decline in school performance and extracurricular activities. Return to contact sports after head injury should be decided on an individual basis. Many individuals have significantly reduced scores on neuropsychological testing after head injury, arguing for a return to usual school function before resuming contact sports.[27]

Children with a PGCS of 14 or 15, minor head trauma, and a normal CT scan can usually be observed closely at home by a responsible adult. This generally applies to those who had less than 5 minutes of unconsciousness, a normal examination, no severe or progressive symptoms of headache or vomiting, no evidence of a basilar skull fracture, and a normal skull x-ray. Criteria for hospitalization must be individualized but indications may include:

- Documented, prolonged loss of consciousness
- Coma, altered mental status, or seizure
- Focal neurologic deficit
- Persistent vomiting or severe and persistent headache

- Alcohol or drug intoxication interfering with a reliable examination
- Suspicion of child abuse or unreliable caregiver
- High-risk individuals, including infants and toddlers with difficult examinations and patients with underlying hydrocephalus or coagulopathy.

The outcome for children who have had a severe head injury is generally better than that for adults with the same severity score.[58-61,65,78,79] Children also continue to improve over months and even years after trauma, whereas adults attain their maximum improvement approximately 6 months following injury.[20]

Outcome prediction for children based on GCS has the obvious limitation of which GCS is used—prehospital, emergency department, or intensive care unit. Further, a depressed initial GCS may be due to hypoventilation, hypoxemia, or hypoperfusion if aggressive treatment to prevent secondary brain injury has not been initiated.[79] In general head-injured children who have a PGCS of 8 have no primary intracranial mortality and no long-term sequelae in most studies. Children with PGCS of 6 to 8 can expect to have no primary intracranial mortality. Most regain consciousness within 3 weeks. Behavioral problems and shortened attention span may persist after hospital discharge. Approximately 10% to 20% are left with focal neurologic deficits such as short-term memory problems and delayed response times, especially if the coma persists beyond 3 weeks. Full neuropsychiatric testing is recommended if school difficulty persists.

Children who have a PGCS of 3 to 5 have generally sustained significant impact injury. Death rates in these patients vary from 6% to 35%. Association of the head injury with extracranial trauma is a poor prognostic sign because of the increased possibility of secondary injury caused by hypercarbia, hypoxia, and hypotension.[4,78] Diffuse brain swelling on CT scan correlates with good outcomes in 75% to 85% of these patients but ICP > 40 mm Hg correlates with poor outcome.[59-61,78,79] Presence of a mass lesion on CT scan correlates with poor outcome in some studies.[4,78] Although many of the survivors can return to a school setting, 90% require rehabilitation after discharge and more than half have permanent focal neurologic deficits. Children more than 2 years of age have worse outcomes, perhaps because the effect of the shear forces is worse in the unmyelinated brain or because of immature autoregulation of cerebral blood flow.

Head-injured children who have a PGCS of 3 can expect 50% to 60% mortality from their head injury alone, and survivors have a high likelihood of significant neurologic deficits.

Any family whose child sustains major head injury suffers major stresses; normal family relationships are slowly reestablished if ever. The need for early intervention by social and rehabilitation services is clear, and it is appropriate and important to initiate those contacts in the ED.

References

1. Frankowski RF, Annegers JF, Whitman S: The descriptive epidemiology of head trauma in the United States, *Cent Nerv Syst Trauma* 1:33, 1985.

2. Kraus JF, Rock M, Hemyari P: Brain injuries among infants, children, adolescents and young adults, *Am J Dis Child* 144:684, 1990.

Pathophysiology

3. Bruce DA et al: Pathophysiology, treatment and outcome following severe head injury in children, *Childs Brain* 5:174, 1979.
4. Mayer T and Walker ML: Emergency intracranial pressure monitoring: management of the acute coma of brain insult, *Clin Pediatr (Phila)* 21:391, 1982.
5. Gentry LR, Godersky JC, Thompson B: MR imaging of head trauma: review of the distribution and radiopathologic features of traumatic lesions, *Am J Roentgenol* 150:663, 1988.
6. Dean JM et al: Theories of brain resuscitation. In Rogers M, editor: *Textbook of pediatric intensive care*, Baltimore, 1987, Williams and Wilkins.
7. Gluckman PD and Williams CE: When and why do brain cells die? *Dev Med Child Neurol* 34:1010-1014, 1992.
8. Kochabck PM, Uhl MW, Schoettle RJ: Hypoxic-ischemic encephalopathy: Pathobiology and therapy of the post-resuscitation syndrome in children. In Furhman BP, Zimmerman JJ, editors: *Pediatric critical care*, St. Louis, 1992, Mosby.
9. Siesjkö BK: Acidosis and ischemic brain damage, *Neurochem Pathol* 9:31, 1988.
10. Rothman SM and Olney JW: Glutamate and the pathophysiology of hypoxic-ischemic brain damage, *Ann Neurol* 19:105, 1986.
11. Choi DW and Rothman SM: The role of glutamate neurotoxicity in hypoxic-ischemic neuronal death, *Annu Rev Neurosci* 13:171, 1990.
12. Thordstein M and Kjellmer I: Cerebral tolerance of hypoxia in growth retarded and appropriately-grown newborn guinea pigs, *Pediatr Res* 24:633, 1988.
13. Siesjkö BK: Basic mechanisms of traumatic brain damage, *Ann of Emerg Med* 22(6):959-967, 1993.
14. Povlishock JT: Pathobiology of traumatically induced axonal injury in animals and man, *Ann Emerg Med* 22:980-985, June 1993.
15. White BC and Krause GS: Brain injury and repairing mechanisms: the potential for pharmacologic therapy in closed-head trauma, *Ann Emerg Med* 22:970-979, June 1993.
16. Ginsberg MD, Sternau LL, Globus MT et al: Therapeutic modulation of brain temperature: relevance to ischemic brain injury cerebrovasculature, *Brain Metab Rev* 4:189, 1992.
17. Neuman-Haefalin T, Wiebner C, Vogel P et al: Differential expression of the immediate early genes C-jun, jun-B, and NGFI-B in the rat brain following transient forebrain ischemia, *J Cereb Blood Flow Metab* 14:206, 1994.
18. Goldman H, Morehead M, Murphy: Use of adrenocorticotrophic hormone analog to minimize brain injury, *Ann Emerg Med* 22:1035-1040, June 1993.
19. Doberstein CE, Hovda DA, Becker DP: Clinical considerations in the reduction of secondary brain injury, *Ann Emerg Med* 22:993-1000, June 1993.
20. Kasdon DL: Physiology of the nervous system, Proceedings of the First National Conference on Pediatric Trauma, *Pediatr Emerg Care* 2(2):113, 1986.
21. Bruce DA, Schut L, Sutton L: Neurosurgical emergencies. In Fleischer G and Ludwig S, editors: *Textbook of pediatric emergency medicine*, ed 2, Baltimore, 1988, Williams & Wilkins.
22. Kellie G: An account of the appearances of two of three individuals presumed to have perished in the storm of the third, and whose bodies were discovered in the vicinity of Leith on the morning of the 4th November, 1821, with some reflections on the pathology of the brain, *Trans Med Chir Sci Edinburg* 1:84, 1824.
23. Monro A: *Observations on the structure and function of the nervous system*, Edinburgh, 1783, Creech and Johnson.
24. Plum F and Posner JB: *The diagnosis of stupor and coma*, ed 3, Philadelphia, 1980, FA Davis.
25. Raphaely RC, et al: Management of severe pediatric head trauma, *Pediatr Clin North Am* 27(3):715, 1980.
26. Bell WO: Pediatric head trauma, In Aresman EM, editor *Pediatric trauma: initial care of the injured child*, New York, 1995, Raven Press.

Diagnostic Findings

27. Hadley MN et al: The infant whiplash shake syndrome: a clinical and pathological study, *Neurosurg* 24:4, 1989.

28. Kendall N and Woloshin H: Cephalhematoma associated with fracturing of the skull, *J Pediatr* 41:125, 1952.
29. Zelson C, Lee SJ, Pearl M: The incidence of skull fracture underlying cephalhematomas in newborn infants, *J Pediatr* 85:371, 1974.
30. Teasdale G and Jennett B: Assessment of coma and impaired consciousness: a practical scale, *Lancet* 2:81, 1984.
31. Tepas JJ et al: Pediatric trauma score as a predictor of injury severity in the injured child, *J Pediatr Surg* 22:14, 1987.
32. Shapiro K: Special considerations for the pediatric age group. In *Head injury*, ed 2, Baltimore, 1987, Williams and Wilkins.
33. Haas DC and Laurie H: Trauma-induced migraine: an explanation for the common attacks after mild head injury, review of the literature, *J Neurosurg* 68:181, 1988.
34. Woodward GA: Post-traumatic cortical blindness: are we missing the diagnosis in children, *Pediatr Emerg Care* 6:289, 1990.
35. Duncan CC and Merit LR: Central nervous system: head injury, In Touloukian RJ, editor: *Pediatric trauma*, ed 2, St. Louis, 1990, Mosby.
36. Hahn YS et al: Factors influencing post traumatic seizures in children, *Neurosurg* 22(5):864, 1988.
37. Hahn YS et al: Head injuries in children under 36 months of age, demography and outcome, *Child Nerv Syst* 3:266, 1987.
38. Lewis RJ, Yee L, Inkelis SH et al: Clinical predictors of post-traumatic seizures in children with head injury, *Ann Emerg Med* 22:1114, 1993.
39. Duncan CC and Ment LR: Head injury: management in children, *Conn Med* 53:6, 1988.
40. Hugenholtz H et al: Vomiting in children following head injury, *Child Nerv Syst* 3:266, 1987.
41. Lanser JBK, Jennekins-Schenkel A, Peters ACB: Headache after closed head injury in children, *Headache* 28:176, 1988.
42. Rosenthal BW and Bergman I: Intracranial injury after moderate head trauma in children, *J Pediatr* 115:346, 1989.
43. Rosenthal M: Mild traumatic brain injury syndrome, *Ann Emerg Med* 22(6) 1048-1051, 1993.
44. Ewing-Cobbs L et al: Intellectual, motor and language sequelae following closed head injury in infants and preschoolers, *J Pediatr Psychol* 14:4, 1989.
45. Pons PT: Head trauma. In Barkin RM and Rosen P, editors: *Emergency pediatrics*, ed 4, St. Louis, 1994, Mosby.
46. Casey R, Ludwig S, McCormick MC: Morbidity following minor head trauma in children, *Pediatrics* 78(3):497, 1986.
47. Leonidas JC et al: Mild head trauma in children: when is a roentgenogram necessary? *Pediatrics* 69(2):139, 1982.
48. Masters SJ et al: Skull x-rays after head trauma. Recommendations by a multidisciplinary panel and validation study, *N Engl J Med* 316(2):84, 1987.
49. Zimmerman RA et al: Head injury: early results of comparing CT and high field MR, *Am J Roentgenol* 147:1215, 1986.
50. Dietrich AM, Bowman MJ, Ginn-Pease ME et al: Pediatric head injuries: can clinical factors reliably predict an abnormality on computed tomograph. *Ann Emerg Med* 22:1535, 1993.
51. Bernardi B, Zimmerman RA, Bilanuk LT: Neuroradiologic evaluation of pediatric trauma, *Top Magn Reson Imaging*, 5(3):161, 1993.
52. Han JS, et al: Head trauma evaluated by magnetic resonance and computed tomography: a comparison, *Neuroradiology* 150:71, 1984.
53. Gentry LR et al: Prospective comparative study of intermediate field MR and CT in the evaluation of closed head trauma, *Am J Roentgenol* 150:673, 1988.
54. Cohen RA et al: Cranial computed tomography in the abused child with head injury, *Am J Roentgenol* 146:97, 1986.
55. Sklar EML, Quencer RM, Bowen BC et al: Magnetic resonance applications in cerebral injury, *Radiol Clin NA* 30(2):353, 1992.

Management

56. Lewis RJ, Linton Y, Stanley HI, Glimore D: Clinical predictors of post-traumatic seizures in children with head trauma, *Ann Emerg Med* 22(7):1114-1118, 1993.
57. Tempkin NR and Dikman SS: A randomized double blind study of phenytoin for the prevention of post-traumatic seizures. *N Engl J Med* 323:497, 1990.
58. Ford EG, Jennings LM, Andrassy RJ: Steroid administration potentiates nitrogen losses in head-injured children, *J Trauma* 27:9, 1987.
59. Bruce DA et al: Outcome following severe head injuries in children, *J Neurosurg* 48:677, 1978.
60. Mahoney WF et al: Long term outcome of children with severe head trauma and prolonged coma, *Pediatrics* 71(5):756, 1983.
61. Berger MS et al: Outcome from severe head injury in children and adolescents, *J Neurosurg* 62:194, 1985.
62. Muizelaar JP et al: Cerebral blood flow and metabolism in severely head injured children. 1. Relationship with GCS score, outcome, ICP and PVI, *J Neurosurg* 71:63, 1989.
63. Muizelaar JP et al: Cerebral blood flow and metabolism in severely head injured children. 2. Autoregulation, *J Neurosurg* 71:72, 1989.
64. Jennett B, Teasdale G: Severe head injuries in three countries, *J Neurol Neurosurg Psychiatry* 40:291, 1977.
65. Tepas III JJ et al: Mortality and head injury: the pediatric perspective, *J Pediatr Surg* 25:1, 1990.
66. Davis RL, Mullen N, Makela M et al: Cranial computed tomography scans in the children after minimal head injury with loss of consciousness, *Ann Emerg Med* 24:648, 1994.

Specific Clinical Entities

67. Parish RA et al: The significance of Babinski signs in children with head trauma, *Ann Emerg Med* 14(4):329, 1985.
68. Hubbard A: Pediatric trauma radiology. In Dolan MA and Fitz Maurice L, editors: *Trauma manual for pediatric residents*, Kansas City, 1988, Children's Mercy Hospital.
69. Swischuk L: *Emergency radiology of the acutely ill or injured child*, ed 2, Baltimore, 1986, Williams & Wilkins.
70. Swischuk L: The normal pediatric skull variations and artifacts, *Radiol Clin North Am* 2:277, 1972.
71. Locatelli D et al: Growing fractures: an unusual complication of head injuries in pediatric patients, *Neurochirurgia* 32:101, 1989.
72. Kadisa HA and Schunic JE: Pediatric basilar skull fracture: do children with normal neurologic findings and no intracranial injury require hospitalization, *Ann Emerg Med* 26:37-41, 1995.
73. Schutzman SA, Barnes PD, Mantello M et al: Epidural hematomas in children, *Ann Emerg Med* March 1993, 22:3, 31-37.
74. Duhaime A et al: The shaken baby syndrome, a clinical, pathological and biomechanical study, *J Neurosurg* 66:409, 1987.
75. Bruce DA and Zimmerman RA: Shaken impact syndrome, *Pediatr Ann* 18:8, 1989.
76. Bilmire ME and Myers PA: Serious head injury in infants: accident or abuse? *Pediatrics* 75:340, 1985.
77. Dykes LJ: The whiplash shaken infant syndrome: what has been learned? *Child Abuse Negl* 10:211, 1986.

Prognosis

78. Alberico AA et al: Outcome after severe head injury: relationship to mass lesions, diffuse injury and ICP course in pediatric and adult patients, *J Neurosurg* 67:648, 1987.
79. Kalff R et al: Clinical outcome after head injury in children, *Child Nerv Syst* 5:156, 1989.

Facial Trauma

Wassam M. Rahman • Timothy J. O'Connor

The face is a very sensitive and visible part of the human anatomy. Any disfiguring injury can potentially have long-term physical, cosmetic, and psychologic effects. It is incumbent on the physician treating children with facial trauma to understand the anatomy, physiology, and development of facial structures. Injuries in children differ from those in adults because of differences in anatomy, evolving developmental capabilities, mechanisms of injuries, and potential long-term deformities. Injuries of the head and neck are discussed in Chapters 20 and 22.[1-9]

Dental and soft tissue injuries are very common in children, in contrast to maxillofacial fractures, which are less frequent. Children are more likely to sustain injuries resulting from falls, automobile crashes (as occupants or nonoccupants), burns, abuse, participation in sports, and assault. By adolescence the injury patterns parallel those found in adults.[1-13]

ANATOMY

The growth and development of the face are important considerations in facial trauma. At birth, the skull accounts for most of the head; the face occupies a smaller proportion as compared with that of the adult. The craniofacial proportion in the newborn is 8:1; it is 4:1 at 5 years and 2:1 by adulthood. At 3 months of age the face is approximately 40% of the adult size; it is 70% at 2 years and about 80% at 5.5 years.[14,15] The cranium increases in size four times from birth to adulthood as compared with the face, which increases 12 times its size in the same period.[4] The peak rate of growth of the head and face is between 3 and 5 years of age, with a wide range of variability for the individual facial structures.[6,14,15] As the face becomes more prominent, it is more prone to be injured.

The skeletal anatomy of the face provides the framework to which the overlying soft tissues conform. The anatomy of the face, including the soft tissues, skeletal structure, muscles, and innervation, is shown in Fig. 21-1. When assessing a patient with any injury, the physician must be cognizant of the underlying structural relationships. Any significant injury to the underlying bony structures may result in disfigurement at the time of injury or may become more apparent later in life.[6,16,17]

DIAGNOSTIC FINDINGS

Clinical Findings

Clinical examination of the child may be made difficult by the child's lack of cooperation or inability to communicate.

A history of the mechanism of injury, significant past medical history, immunizations, allergies, interval since last meal, and current medications should be obtained whenever possible. Facial injuries are frequently associated with other cranial, cervical, spinal, thoracic, and abdominal injuries.[18,19]

In the primary survey, adequacy of the airway, cervical spine stabilization, breathing, circulation, and disability or

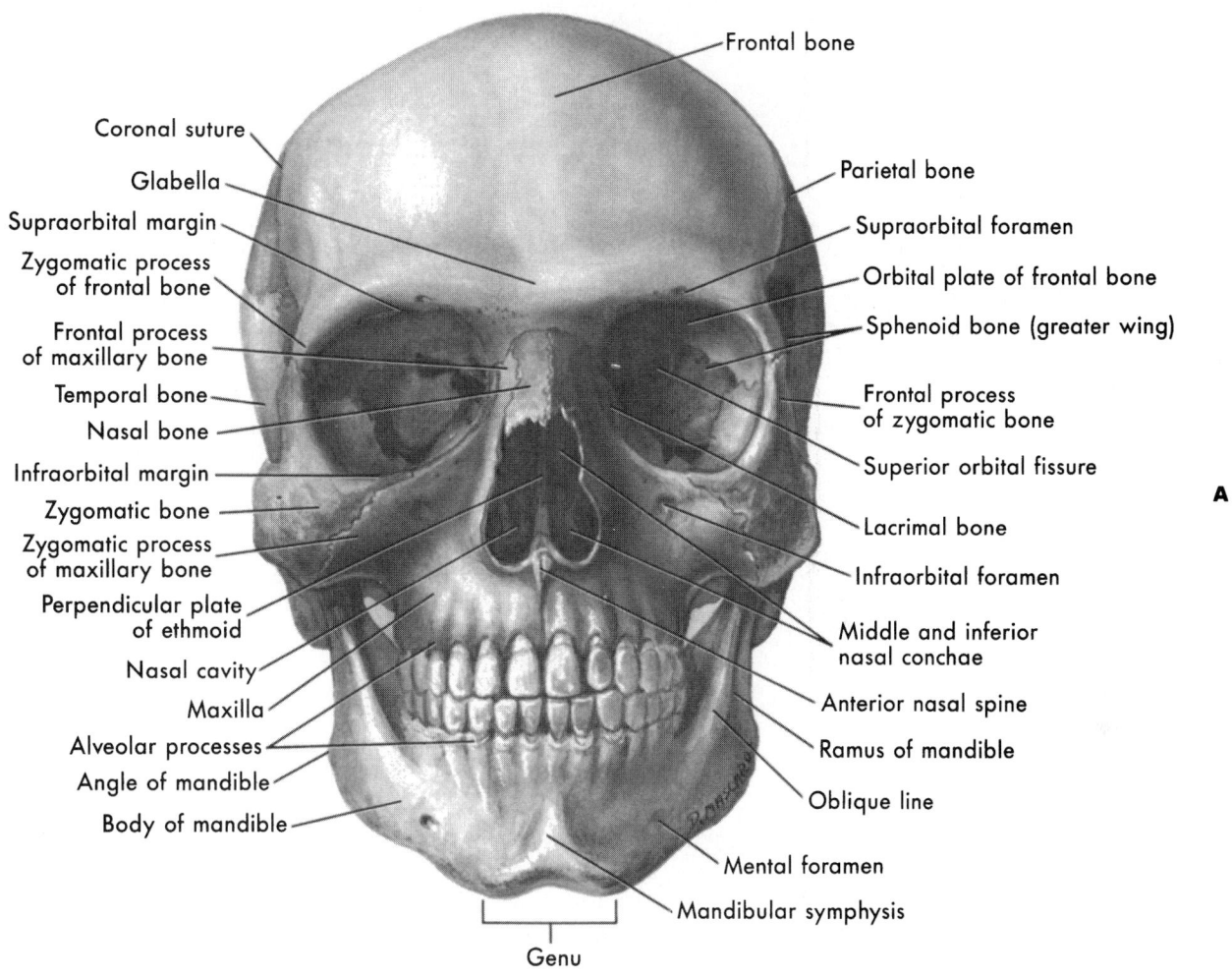

Frontal bone

Coronal suture

Glabella

Supraorbital margin

Zygomatic process
of frontal bone

Frontal process
of maxillary bone

Temporal bone

Nasal bone

Infraorbital margin

Zygomatic bone

Zygomatic process
of maxillary bone

Perpendicular plate
of ethmoid

Nasal cavity

Maxilla

Alveolar processes

Angle of mandible

Body of mandible

Parietal bone

Supraorbital foramen

Orbital plate of frontal bone

Sphenoid bone (greater wing)

Frontal process
of zygomatic bone

Superior orbital fissure

Lacrimal bone

Infraorbital foramen

Middle and inferior
nasal conchae

Anterior nasal spine

Ramus of mandible

Oblique line

Mental foramen

Mandibular symphysis

Genu

A

FIG. 21-1. A, Skull as seen from frontal view. (**A** *reproduced from Seeley RR, Stephens TD, Tate P:* Anatomy and physiology, *St. Louis, 1989, Times Mirror/Mosby College Publishing.*)   *Continued.*

neurologic status of the patient must be assessed and managed before beginning the secondary survey (see Chapter 19). Management of the airway includes suctioning head positioning, chin lift or jaw thrust, and intubation if necessary. Administer oxygen and hyperventilate if necessary with a bag valve mask device. Because of bleeding, secretions, vomitus, and potential foreign bodies in the mouth and hypopharynx, suctioning with a tonsil suction tip or large catheter clears the airway for better air exchange or for visualization of the vocal cords during intubation. When necessary, oral intubation is the preferred method, as nasal intubation may be difficult. A complication of nasal intubation in maxillofacial injury is passage of the endotracheal tube into the cranial vault.[20] In the event of severe facial injury where oral intubation is not possible, an emergency cricothyrotomy should be performed. A tracheostomy may be performed later when the patient is stabilized. The cervical spine should be stabilized with a collar and in-line stabilization[7,21-25] (see box on p. 255).

After the patient has been stabilized, a detailed examination of the face is made as part of the secondary survey (see Figure 21-1).[22] Soft tissue injuries of the face such as lacerations, contusions, presence of foreign bodies, pen-

etrating injuries, and burns must be inspected and evaluated for involvement of underlying muscles, nerves, and glandular and bony tissue injury. Other occult injuries to the cranium and cervical spine must not be overlooked. Facial bones are palpated, looking for step-off, irregularities, crepitus, and abnormalities in contour along all the facial planes, orbits, zygomatic arches, nasal bones, mandible, palate, and alveolar ridges. An ocular examination should include an evaluation of visual acuity, extraocular motion, and corneal and retinal injury. The nasal examination must rule out a septal hematoma. In the dental examination the integrity of the teeth must be evaluated by palpation of individual teeth for instability, displacement, fracture, avulsion, malocclusion, and tenderness. Hemotympanum, CSF rhinorrhea or otorrhea, and periorbital (raccoon eyes) or mastoid ecchymosis (Battle's sign) are diagnostic of occult basilar skull fractures.*

Ancillary Data. The value of standard-view radiographs varies with the cooperation of the child, extent of facial bone development, type of injury, and expertise of the

---

* References 2-6, 22, 24, 26-28.

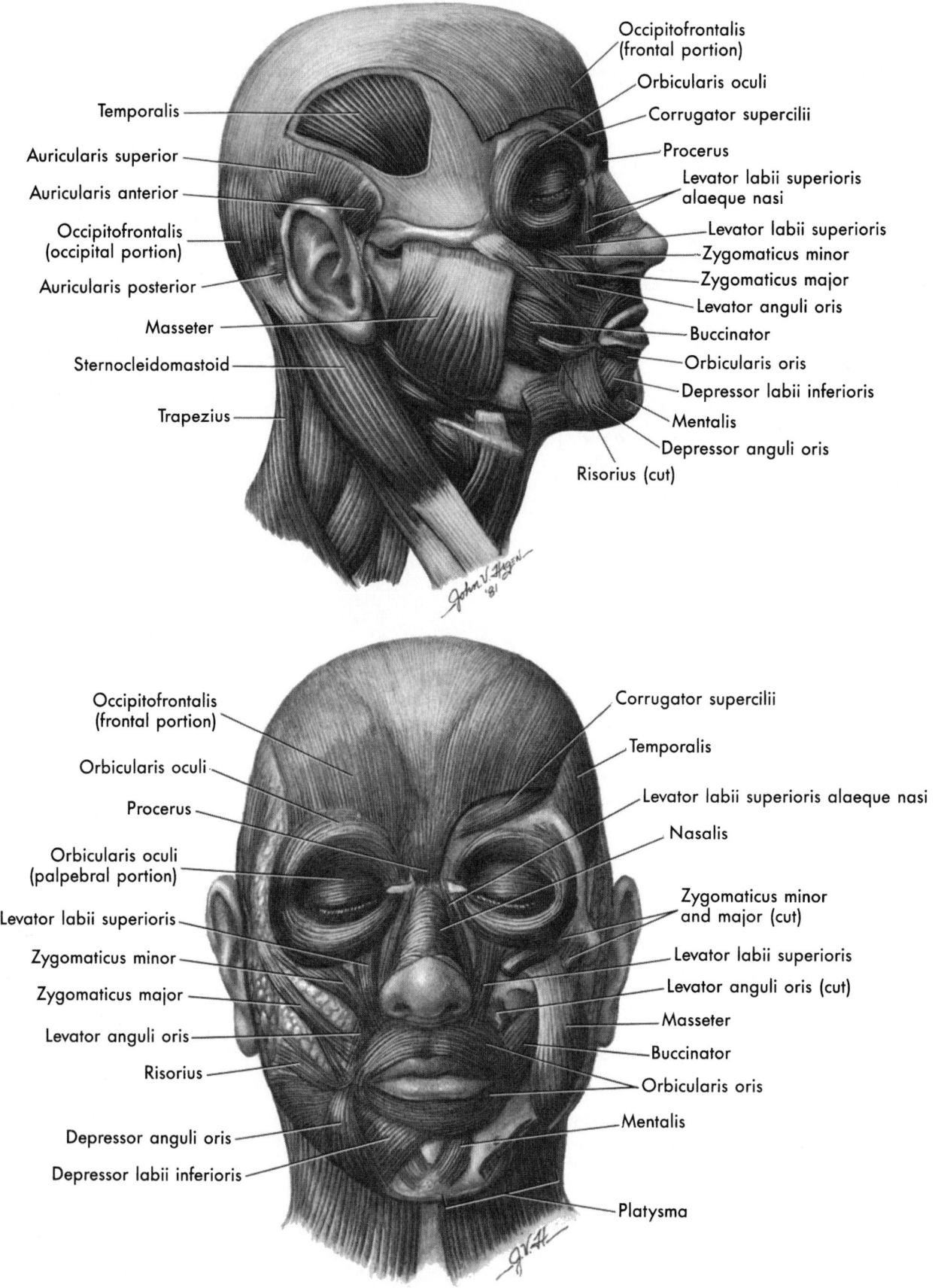

Temporalis

Auricularis superior

Auricularis anterior

Occipitofrontalis
(occipital portion)

Auricularis posterior

Masseter

Sternocleidomastoid

Trapezius

Occipitofrontalis
(frontal portion)

Orbicularis oculi

Corrugator supercilii

Procerus

Levator labii superioris
alaeque nasi

Levator labii superioris

Zygomaticus minor

Zygomaticus major

Levator anguli oris

Buccinator

Orbicularis oris

Depressor labii inferioris

Mentalis

Depressor anguli oris

Risorius (cut)

Occipitofrontalis
(frontal portion)

Orbicularis oculi

Procerus

Orbicularis oculi
(palpebral portion)

Levator labii superioris

Zygomaticus minor

Zygomaticus major

Levator anguli oris

Risorius

Depressor anguli oris

Depressor labii inferioris

Corrugator supercilii

Temporalis

Levator labii superioris alaeque nasi

Nasalis

Zygomaticus minor
and major (cut)

Levator labii superioris

Levator anguli oris (cut)

Masseter

Buccinator

Orbicularis oris

Mentalis

Platysma

FIG. 21-1, cont'd. B, Muscles of facial expression. (**B** *reproduced from Seeley RR, Stephens TD, Tate P:*
Anatomy and physiology, St. Louis, 1989, Times Mirror/Mosby College Publishing.)   *Continued.*

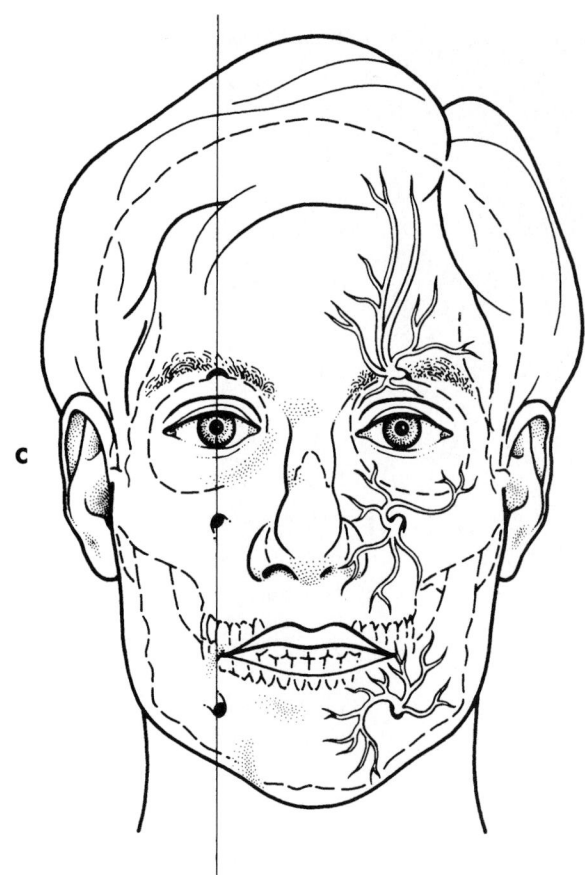

C

Physical Examination of the Face

Airway
Cervical spine
Skull
Soft tissue
Facial bones
   Orbits
     Zygomatic arches
     Nasal bones
     Nasal septum
     Mandible
     Maxilla
     Palate
     Alveolar ridges
     Frontal bones
  Eyes (see section on ocular injuries)
Teeth
Ear canal
Tympanic membrane
Battle's sign
Raccoon eyes
CSF otorrhea
CSF rhinorrhea
Malocclusion
Neurologic examination

FIG. 21-1, cont'd. C, Sensory innervation of anterior aspect of face (trigeminal nerve). Supraorbital, intraorbital, and mental branches are shown. The foramina of bony exit of these nerves lie roughly in a straight line passing through pupil and lateral commissure of lips. (*C reproduced from Rosen P, et al: Emergency Medicine, ed 3, St. Louis, 1992, Mosby.*)

reviewer. Facial radiographs are also of value in detecting radiopaque foreign bodies. The standard plain radiographic views that can be obtained are the Water's, Caldwell, frontal, lateral, Towne, and submentovertex. Of all the views, the Water's view is the most informative (Fig. 21-2).[29-31] Coned-down views of specific bones (i.e., orbits, zygomatic arch, mandible) can be helpful. Computed tomography (CT) scanning is an excellent tool for diagnosing facial fractures along with other cranial abnormalities. A chest, face, and abdominal radiograph should be considered in locating missing avulsed teeth. Table 21-1 summarizes the various views and their diagnostic contributions. Three-dimensional CT scan has not been proven to be helpful.[32]

Plain radiographs of facial trauma can be difficult to interpret. Abnormalities such as air-fluid levels in the sinuses, asymmetry and discontinuance of bone lines, and air in soft tissues may indicate underlying fractures. Table 21-2 correlates the fracture with the most optimal views.

SOFT TISSUE INJURIES (See Chapter 32)

In children, facial tissue heals quickly and is less prone to infection. The aesthetics of outcome in facial injuries is a priority in management. Revisions after primary closure can improve the initial outcome. Potential deformities, follow-up observation, and future management should be discussed at the time of the initial evaluation and must be documented. The management of soft tissue injuries is similar in both adults and children.[4,6,33]

Contusions and Abrasions

Contusions and ecchymoses are managed conservatively by symptomatic local care after ruling out underlying fractures. Ice applied for 20 minutes four times a day for the first 48 hours is usually sufficient. Hematomas rarely require drainage; most resorb without problem. Only hematomas of the external ear and nasal septum must be drained to prevent cartilage deformity.[34-37] Abrasions to the face can be treated conservatively with debridement, local wound care, topical antibiotics, and dressings. All embedded foreign bodies (gravel, glass, splinters, asphalt, etc.) should be removed by picking or scrubbing with a surgical scrub brush to prevent tattooing of the skin after healing. Sedation or local anesthesia may be required during the debridement process.[30,38,39]

Burns (see Chapter 37)

Fifty-four percent of children with burn injuries receive injuries to the face, hands, and neck; 27% of burns involve the face. Usually the potential disfigurement has enormous long-term physical and psychosocial effects on the child. The most frequently burned children are those less than 5

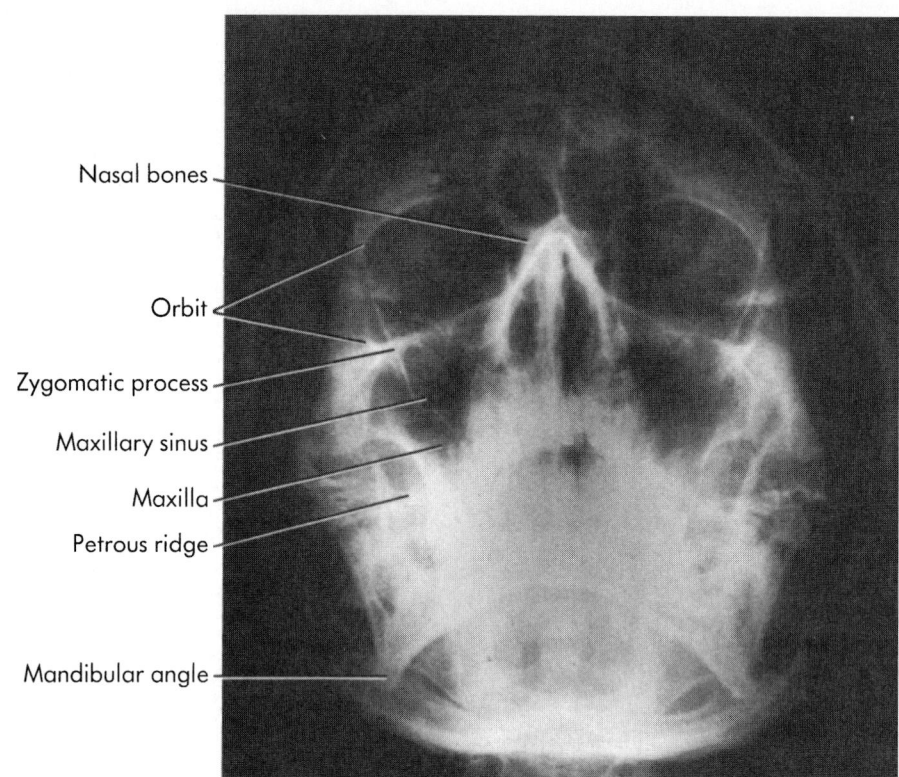

Nasal bones

Orbit

Zygomatic process

Maxillary sinus

Maxilla

Petrous ridge

Mandibular angle

FIG. 21-2. Water's view showing normal facial anatomic landmarks and structures. (*Courtesy Jane Kober, RT. In Ballinger PW: Merrill's atlas of radiographic positions and radiologic procedures, ed 7, St. Louis, 1991, Mosby.*)

TABLE 21-1. Radiologic Techniques for Facial Injuries

Projection	Anatomy defined
Caldwell (posteroanterior)	Frontal bone, anterior ethmoid cells, zygomaticofrontal sutures, frontal sinuses, orbital margin, lateral walls of maxillary sinus, petrous ridges, mandibular rami
Water's	Oblique anterior view of facial bones, orbits, malar bones, zygomatic arches; helpful in the diagnosis of fractures of maxillary sinuses, maxilla, orbital floor, infraorbital rim, zygomatic bones, and arches
Submentovertex	Processes of the mandibular rami, zygomatic arches, base of skull and foramina, petrous pyramid, bony septum, maxillary sphenoidal, and posterior ethmoidal sinuses
Frontal	Orbits, lesser and greater wings of the sphenoids, frontal and ethmoid sinuses, nasal septum, floor of nose, hard palate, mandible, dental arches (upper and lower)
Lateral	Frontal sinuses, lateral walls of orbit, maxilla, mandible, nasal bones
Nasal bones	Maxillary spine, nasal bones
Panoramic	Mandible, teeth, alveolus
Computed tomography	All facial bones except teeth

TABLE 21-2. Optimal Views for Specific Injuries

Injury	View
Nasal	Water's, lateral
Orbital	Caldwell, Water's, lateral, oblique, CT scan
Orbital "blow out"	Water's, Caldwell, CT scan
Zygomaticomaxillary	
Tripod	Water's, CT scan
Zygomatic arch	Towne, Waters, PA, CT scan
Le Fort	CT scan
Mandible	Towne, Caldwell, panoramic CT scan
Alveolar arch	Panoramic
Temporomandibular joint	Oblique, lateral with open and closed mouth views, Towne
Teeth	Panoramic, bite wings

years of age. Scalds are the most common cause, followed by flame (flash), contact, chemical, and electrical injuries. Flame burns are more common in the older child and adult.[1,13,40-44]

The face occupies approximately 7% to 9% of the body surface area at birth; 8.5% at 1 year; 6.5% at 5 years; 5.5% at 10 years; 4.5% at 15 years; and 3.5% in adulthood.[42,45]

After the initial stabilization of the patient, the extent and depth of the burn must be determined. The extent of injury to the airway, eyes, ears, and mouth must be noted.

Injury to the eyes must be evaluated by a fluorescein examination and visual acuity testing. The first-degree (superficial-thickness) burn has pain and redness. Second-degree burns are classified as superficial partial-thickness and deep partial-thickness and are characterized by blister formation. Third-degree (full-thickness) burns involve the whole dermis. Fourth-degree burns involve adjacent soft tissue and bone.

Initial management focuses on securing the airway, breathing, and circulation. After a significant facial burn, rapidly ensuing edema can make maintaining an airway or intubating very challenging. Children who have suffered inhalational injuries are at risk of respiratory compromise. At the scene of the burn, all attempts must be made to remove the offending agent to prevent further skin injury. Cool water or normal saline solution also helps decrease the pain and wound injury. Children with extensive facial burns should be admitted for optimal wound management. Some minor scald burns may be treated on an outpatient basis with close follow-up observation every 2 to 4 days. All major facial wounds must be evaluated by a surgeon. To manage the pain and anxiety, the patient may be given morphine sulfate 0.1 to 0.2 mg/kg/dose and midazolam 0.1 mg/kg/dose IV, as well as other agents discussed in Chapter 7. Broken blisters and debris must be gently debrided. No dressings are applied to facial burns unless the burn is deep.[45] The antibiotic used on wounds is a combination of polymyxin B, bacitracin, neomycin ointment, or silver sulfadiazine.[46,47] Long-term management may include skin grafting, if necessary, and use of elastic pressure masks to minimize hypertrophic scarring.[48]

Oral Electrical Burns. The most common electrical burns in children are those to the mouth caused most frequently by the child's biting into a live electrical wire as noted in Chapter 36.[40,44,49-53] The peak incidence of these injuries is around 2 years of age, paralleling the developmental aptitude of the child and the presence of teeth at this age. The moist oral mucosa contributes to the conduction of electricity and severity of the burn. The heat generated at the site of the burn, by arcing, conduction, and the flash, reaches 3000° Fahrenheit. The resulting damage is to the oral mucosa, vermilion border, commissure, and underlying orbicularis muscle. Injury to the alveolus, tongue, buccal sulcus, and palate has been reported.[51,54] It is unlikely that the child will have any other bodily injury as the electrical energy is dissipated at the area of contact.

The patient exhibits a coagulated, grayish white ulcer with an erythematous base. In a few hours the area becomes edematous. In 3 to 4 weeks the eschar falls off, leaving a slow-healing ulcer. Most commonly the burn occurs at the corners of the mouth. Because of injury to underlying nerves, little pain is associated with this burn. Bleeding may be a late complication, occurring in the first 2 weeks.

Initial management is directed toward controlling any bleeding by pressure or suturing. A topical combination antibiotic may be applied to the wound. There is controversy as to early surgical excision vs. conservative nonsurgical management.[50,51,54-58] More recently, conservative management of oral electrical burns has been advocated, with delayed revision after 6 to 12 months, depending on the extent of the injury. Various fixed and removable splinting devices have been developed to minimize scarring and microstomia.[51,54,59-62]

Good surgical follow-up observation is essential as long-term care is necessary. Hospitalization is required when the child has been electrocuted or severely burned or is unable to take fluids. A soft bland diet, topical antibiotic application, and good oral hygiene ensure a more favorable outcome. The parents must be warned about the possibility of bleeding from the wound during the first 2 weeks after the injury. If this occurs, digital pressure must be applied while the child is being taken to the emergency department. Oral antibiotics against the oral flora may be given for 48 hours. Complications of such injuries include scarring, microstomia, and disruption of the vermilion border.

Lacerations (see Chapter 32)

Lacerations of the face can be disfiguring and must be meticulously repaired to ensure good healing and a favorable cosmetic result. Every attempt must be made to close all facial lacerations. Relatively clean wounds can be sutured within 24 hours of injury with a reasonable margin of protection from infection and dehiscence. Mammalian bites must be handled with extreme care using copious irrigation to prevent infection.

The child must be approached in a manner appropriate to his or her age and development. Explaining the procedure alleviates much anxiety. The presence of the parents must be individualized. Restraining the child may be necessary to prevent excessive movement during the procedure.

Amnesia, sedation, and effective pain management are discussed in detail in Chapter 7 and may be attained by the cautious and monitored use of local anesthesia, benzodiazepines, and narcotics. Local anesthesia for facial lacerations can be achieved by infiltration of 1% or 2% lidocaine with epinephrine (1:100,000 or 1:200,000) if the nose or ear is not involved. The pain of infiltration may be minimized by buffering the solution and using a small-gauge needle (25 to 27 gauge), injecting slowly, and rubbing the site before injection.[63-67] Epinephrine must not be used on the pinna of the ear, tip of the nose, or eyelid. To prevent a toxic effect, the maximum dose of lidocaine is 4 mg/kg without epinephrine, 7 mg/kg with epinephrine.

An alternate, less painful method of local anesthesia for lacerations less than 3 cm is application of a topical solution of tetracaine 1% to 2%, adrenaline 0.05%, cocaine 4% to 11.8% (TAC).[64,66-71] A cotton-tipped applicator or cotton ball soaked with TAC is placed on the wound for 15 minutes. Ten to twenty-five percent of children may require further infiltration of lidocaine. The parents may hold (with gloves) the gauze on the laceration. Complications of TAC include disorientation, seizure, and even death. These complications result from absorption of cocaine through mucous membranes of the mouth and nose. TAC must not be used on areas of the body where epinephrine is contraindicated. It must not be used very close to the eye, as cocaine may cause corneal abrasions.[72]

An alternative to TAC is a topical gel comprised of 4% lidocaine, adrenaline 1:2000, and 0.5% tetracine (LAT). It has been shown to be more cost-effective as compared to TAC.[73,74]

The area adjacent to the wound is prepared with iodophor or chlorhexidine, ensuring that none enters the wound. The wound must be irrigated liberally, employing at least 150 ml/cm of the wound with sterile saline solution through an 18- or 19-gauge needle or 18-gauge angiocath. The field must be draped with sterile towels and be adequately lighted. The wound should be carefully explored for foreign bodies, fractured bone, lacerated muscles, nerves, organs (i.e., parotid gland), and Stensen's and lacrimal duct injuries.

The soft tissue "wrinkle lines" are the lines of minimal tension taking into account the underlying muscles (see Fig. 21-1, *B*). Scars along these lines result in a better cosmetic outcome. Care must be taken to preserve the landmarks for good alignment of the eyebrows, nares, pinnae, and vermilion border of the lips. The edges of the wound are debrided only if devitalized tissue is present; sculpting may assure better skin approximation. Optimal wound healing occurs if aseptic technique is used, the wound is irrigated well, the skin handled gently, and the edges aligned and well opposed. Injuries that should be referred to a plastic surgeon include extensive lacerations; injuries to vessels, nerves, muscle, parotid duct, or gland; associated facial bone fractures; penetrating wounds; and large bite wounds.

Subcutaneous closure with 5-0 absorbable suture (Vicryl) may be necessary in deep lacerations to obliterate the dead space and relieve skin tension. 5-0 or 6-0 gauge nylon (polypropylene) suture is used for repair of the skin. A fast-absorbing gut suture may be used to alleviate the need for suture removal at a later date. (See Chapter 32 for description of skin closure technique.)

A topical antibiotic is applied, the wound dressed, and the parents given wound infection precautions with follow-up observation. Sutures are removed in 3 to 4 days to prevent track marks. At the time of suture removal, the healing wound is reinforced with porous tape strips. The parents must be warned about the weakness of the wound, especially to repeated trauma.[75,76]

The patient's immunization status must be updated. Antibiotics are indicated for mammalian bites. Amoxicillin clavulanate 20 to 40 mg/kg/day TID or cephalexin 50 to 100 mg/kg/day QID for 5 to 7 days is adequate, with close follow-up and observation.[77]

Nasal Lacerations. Lacerations to the nose can result in significant deformity. The edges of the wound and cartilage must be realigned as closely as possible to the original shape for a good cosmetic outcome. An underlying septal hematoma must be evaluated and treated.

Lip Lacerations. All lacerations of the lip must be carefully inspected for involvement of the vermilion (mucocutaneous) border. Further injury to the underlying structures such as teeth, alveolus, oral mucosa, and mandible must be taken into consideration. When repairing a vermilion border laceration, proper alignment is essential for good cosmetic results. Local infiltration of lidocaine with epinephrine can distort the anatomy and blanch the line of distinction necessary for repair. The edges of the mucocutaneous demarcation may be marked with methylene blue applied with a wooden applicator or with a plastic surgery pen marker. A buccal or submental block can be very effective in providing adequate anesthesia without distortion of the anatomy. Avoid debridement of any tissue if possible. Applying the first suture aligning the vermilion border helps keep the tissues aligned while repair is in progress (see Fig. 32-12). Referral to a plastic surgeon is necessary when the border is not clear, when there is extensive tissue avulsion, or when the physician is not comfortable with the procedure. Adequate anesthesia, sedation, and restraint may be necessary to facilitate the procedure. Suture removal should take place in 3 to 4 days.[78,79]

Tongue Lacerations. Lacerations to the tongue are most commonly caused by children biting themselves during a fall. On initial evaluation the tongue and surrounding structures must be carefully examined, looking for dental, mucosal, and other facial injuries. If the teeth are avulsed or fractured, the examiner must make sure that the teeth or any other foreign bodies are not embedded in the tongue. Most minor lacerations that do not cause any significant lateration of the tongue's anatomy or significant discomfort to the patient do not require any repair. Deeper, more extensive lacerations that go through both outer layers, are one half the width of the tongue, involve the tip, or bleed excessively require suturing. Sedation or general anesthesia may be necessary, as local anesthesia is sometimes difficult to administer because of the mobility of the tongue. Airway patency must be maintained with good positioning and adequate suctioning of blood from the mouth.[78,79]

Lidocaine with epinephrine is used for local anesthesia if possible. After local anesthesia, proper visualization of the field is secured by a tacking suture placed through the anterior tip of the tongue for traction, visualization, and repair. Absorbable Vicryl or gut suture should be used to alleviate the need for suture removal. The needle bites must be deep to provide good hemostasis and prevent formation of submucosal hematomas, which impair healing. A buried knot technique is preferred to minimize discomfort from exposed suture. Lacerations of the tongue heal very well after proper closure. Discharge instructions should include maintenance of good fluid intake, a soft bland diet, and half-strength saline (salt water) gargles three to four times a day. Follow-up observation must be encouraged.[78,79]

Oral Mucosal Injuries. Lacerations to the oral mucosa are usually minor. Large lacerations require closure, which may be accomplished by using 4-0 or 5-0 absorbable suture. Half-strength saline (salt water) gargles and topical anesthetics may help relieve discomfort. Underlying orofacial injuries and tooth fragments must be sought. Significant lacerations to the gum may be treated by suturing with appropriate dental follow-up.

Foreign Bodies (see Chapter 26)

Oral Foreign Bodies. Foreign bodies such as pencils, sharp toys, wood splinters, or other objects generally do not cause any significant problems. The object must be removed and large lacerations may be sutured. Lacerations and penetrating wounds of the palate may be associated with retropharyngeal infection or potential underlying vascular injury. One-half-strength saline (salt water) gargles, oral antibiotics, observation, and good follow-up care are all that is necessary for management.[79]

Nasal Foreign Bodies. Children can be injured by a variety of animate and inanimate foreign objects that can fit in their nares. The foreign bodies can be placed by the child or another child or may be iatrogenic (i.e., postsurgical procedure). Most commonly, beads, nuts, seeds, peas, erasers, sponge, paper, or jewelry is found. Once in place, the foreign body causes mucosal edema and inflammation and may result in epistaxis or ulceration. Animate objects such as insects, worms, and larvae have been reported. The length of time the object is in the nose may not be apparent. Consultation is usually prompted by the parent's complaint of the child's having a foul odor despite all attempts to keep the child clean. Purulent malodorous nasal discharge, epistaxis, nasal obstruction, or sneezing may be present. Patients may have concurrent sinusitis or otitis media.

The diagnosis is made by inspection of the nares with an otoscope or nasal speculum. If the clinical findings suggest the presence of a foreign body, but it cannot be identified, posterior rhinoscopy may be performed to look for more posteriorly located objects. Both nares and ear canals must be inspected for other foreign bodies.

Most foreign bodies can be removed without anesthesia or sedation. The child must be restrained in the parent's lap or on an immobilization board. The recommended instruments for the procedure are a headlight to free both hands, nasal speculum, Hartman's or alligator forceps, wire loop, and tonsil suction. A topical vasoconstrictor such as 1% phenylephrine hydrochloride may be used to facilitate the removal. Care must be taken not to cause any mucosal injury or push the foreign body posteriorly as aspiration of the object is a potential complication of the procedure.

Foreign bodies at the nasal opening may be milked out. Care must be taken to avoid pushing the object further back. Another method involves the parent delivering a small puff of air through the child's mouth with occlusion of the contralateral nare. In older children, the foreign body may be removed by having the child blow their nose with one nostril occluded. Removal of animate objects is more difficult and may require referral to a specialist. Antibiotics are not necessary unless there is a concomitant sinusitis or otitis media.[79,80]

Oropharyngeal Foreign Bodies. Foreign bodies such as fish or chicken bones are embedded in the lymphoid tissue of the throat and hypopharynx more commonly in adults. Children are more likely to aspirate peanuts, toys, coins, and other objects. The patient may experience mild pharyngeal discomfort. Direct inspection usually reveals the foreign body. A topical anesthetic is used and the object removed with Magill or alligator forceps. Care must be taken not to allow the foreign body to dislodge into the trachea.[81]

FACIAL FRACTURES

The diagnosis of facial fractures has proved to be quite difficult because of lack of specific physical findings, noncooperation of the child, and the limited value of plain radiographs. Many psychosocial and developmental issues come into play when a child has deforming injuries and must be taken into consideration. By puberty, maxillofacial injuries are diagnosed and managed just as in adults.[7-9,82-93]

Maxillofacial trauma in childhood varies with age and accounts for 5% of all facial trauma in the general population. The most common bone fractured is a nasal bone, followed by mandible, maxilla, orbit, and zygoma.[82-93] Facial fractures before 5 years of age are very uncommon, comprising only one fifth of all pediatric facial fractures. During adolescence, the frequency of facial fractures approaches that during adulthood.*

The causes of children's fractures vary with age and activity. Infants and young children sustain injuries from birth trauma, falls, toys, animal bites, motor vehicle crashes, and abuse. Children above 5 years of age are more likely to sustain facial injuries from motor vehicles (as occupants or pedestrians), bicycles, sporting activities, assault, and airborne objects. In general, fractures produced by falls and play are more common in children and automobile accidents and assaults in adults. Peaks in facial fractures occur in the 5- to 8-year age group and the 10- to 12-year group. The reasons for this pattern are thought to be due to changing bone and overlying architecture, cranial facial proportions, school attendance, exposure to different types of mechanisms of injury, less parental supervision, contact sports, increased independence, and risk taking.[4,82-93]

Injuries to the cranium, brain, neck, thorax, abdomen, and extremities are commonly associated with facial trauma and must be sought.† It must be kept in mind that the pediatric skeleton is growing and bone heals quickly; therefore injuries can affect the normal development of facial bones if untreated.[88,89] The potential effects on abnormal dental development must be taken into consideration.[82,98-100]

The management of complicated facial trauma must preferably use a team approach. Since many different subspecialties may be involved in the management of the various injuries, a coordinated effort and good communication between the emergency department physician, surgeon, neurosurgeon, maxillofacial surgeon, dentist, plastic surgeon, orthopedic surgeon, and other ancillary services assures a good standard of care for the patient.[101]

Children differ from adults because their facial bone architecture is more elastic, less brittle, and less pneumatized (sinuses). Developing bone is more porous and pliable, lending itself to greenstick-type fractures of the zygomatic arch, rather than the shattering-type fractures seen in adults. In children the relationship between body weight and facial size does not allow sufficient inertia on impact to propagate fractures. Infants and children have a larger forehead and cranium, which protect the face, as compared with the mere protruded facies of the adult. The presence of primary teeth and underlying tooth buds gives a greater tooth-to-bone ratio, offering greater elasticity and stability. Fat pads over the upper and lower jaws in children absorb and cushion the underlying structures from external force.‡

Diagnostic Findings

Clinical Findings. Initial evaluation must always address the airway, breathing, and circulation before the secondary survey begins. Often skull and cervical spine inju-

---

* References 2, 4, 7-9, 82-95.
†References 4, 7, 18, 19, 86, 96, 97.
‡References 2, 4, 6, 7, 82, 93.

ries coexist. Care must be taken to stabilize the neck and look for other fractures. A history of the mechanism and circumstances of the injury may help guide the physician's management.

When examining the face, lacerations, bruises, foreign bodies, and abrasions must be noted along with the possibility of underlying fractures and injury to underlying organs (parotid, eye) and tissues (parotid duct, nerves, muscle, teeth, vessels). The examination must proceed in an orderly fashion by palpating the skull, forehead, and orbital rims looking for tenderness, irregularities (step-off) in contour, and crepitus. Eyes are examined, noting limitation of extraocular movement (orbital floor fractures) and palpebral changes (zygomatic and nasoethmoid fractures). Examination of the nose should include external stability, crepitus, and exclusion of a septal hematoma. Palpation of the zygomatic arches and mandible is followed by an intraoral examination for a step-off on the palate indicating a Le Fort's type of fracture, which can also occur without disruption of the mucosa. The stability of the teeth and alveolar ridge should be assessed for tenderness, malalignment, luxations, and avulsions. The severity of the tooth injury (avulsion, luxation) may indicate the possibility of underlying fracture. If the child needs to be orally intubated, the presence of broken or loose teeth or any other oral trauma should be documented on initial laryngoscopy.

The mandibular and maxillary arches are checked for stability and dislocation by lateral pressure and excursion. Fractures of the mandible are suspected when the patient complains of abnormal occlusion. Sublingual hematomas may also indicate that a mandibular fracture is present. The finding of clear fluid rhinorrhea or otorrhea indicates the possibility of CSF leak and underlying skull fracture. Periorbital hematomas (raccoon eyes), Battle's sign, and a hemotympanum raise the possibility of a basilar skull fracture. Neurologic findings such as local anesthesia, hypesthesia, and facial nerve palsies indicate compression or severance of the respective nerve(s) and possibly fractures of the surrounding bony structures. In all cases the physician must be suspicious for the facial manifestations of child abuse. Specific clinical findings are discussed in the sections treating specific fractures.

Leakage of CSF usually results from blunt head and facial trauma that causes a tear in the meninges. The CSF drainage may present as rhinorrhea or otorrhea. The fluid may be clear or serosanguinous. The diagnosis is made by testing the fluid by the glucose oxidase reaction or obtaining a measured glucose level of greater than 50 mg/dl. Most CSF leaks heal spontaneously within 1 week.[27,101-103]

Ancillary Data. In children the diagnosis of fractures may be challenging because of their behavioral and developmental differences from adults.[2,29] Plain radiographs consisting of the Water's, Caldwell, Towne, lateral, frontal, and submentovertex views are helpful when the child is cooperative. Depending on clinical findings and significance of injury, a CT scan can be very useful in delineating facial fractures. Three-dimensional CT scan has not yet been shown to be of value in detecting fractures when compared to conventional two-dimensional CT scanning.[32] A panoramic radiograph of the maxilla, teeth, and mandible is useful in dentoalveolar and mandibular fractures (see Tables 21-1 and 21-2).

Frontal Bone Fractures

The forehead is injured quite commonly because of its prominence in the facial plane. The finding of periorbital ecchymosis (raccoon eyes), Battle's sign, hemotympanum, or CSF rhinorrhea or otorrhea indicates a basilar skull fracture. Evidence of a bony step-off may indicate a depressed skull fracture, which may be diagnosed by Caldwell, Water's, or lateral view radiographs or CT scan. Fractures may extend through the sinuses and orbits. Pseudogrowth of the skull with protrusion of the meninges can be a late complication.

Linear nondepressed fractures are managed conservatively with observation, if necessary. Open reduction is indicated when there is a significant displacement of the bone table, a dural tear with hematoma, frontal lobe contusion with a mass effect, significant cerebrospinal fluid leak, or pneumocephalus.[4,104,105]

Frontal Sinus Fractures

Fractures of the frontal sinuses are uncommon before the teenage years because of the lack of development of the sinuses during childhood. Formation of an abscess adjacent to the fracture site is a possible late complication. These fractures are diagnosed by air-fluid levels on the plain radiographs or by CT scan.

Displaced fractures require removal of the mucous membrane, obliteration of the cavity, or even open reduction. Nondisplaced linear fractures without significant fluid levels may only necessitate observation.[6]

Orbital-zygomatic Fractures

Orbital Floor. Clinically, orbital fractures should be suspected when subconjunctival (especially lateral) or periorbital hemorrhage, midfacial hypesthesia caused by injury of the infraorbital nerve, abnormalities of the orbital rim, buccal hematoma, or unilateral epistaxis produced by bleeding into the maxillary sinus is observed. The eye must be examined for corneal abrasions or intraocular injury.

If diplopia or loss of extraocular motion, especially upward gaze, is noted, an infraorbital floor (blowout) fracture may be present. Blowout fractures of the orbit result from the compressive force of a blunt missile such as a baseball or fist, which causes the already weak orbital floor to drop out, allowing the inferior rectus muscle to herniate down and entrap itself; upward gaze in that eye is lost (Fig. 21-3, A and B). Any restriction in ocular motion or displacement indicates entrapment, edema, and fractures requiring surgical attention.

The diagnosis can be made by noting a disruption of the orbital floor or opacification of the ipsilateral sinus on the Water's view radiograph. The CT scan is the best radiologic technique for diagnosing such fractures. To prevent diplopia, or bony deformity, the floor of the orbit must be repaired by wiring or placement of a mesh by an experienced maxillofacial surgeon.[2,4,6,7,82]

Zygoma. The zygomatic bone is a prominent part of the midface; fractures of this region involve the orbit, maxillary sinus, and orbital floor. As a result of the malleability of the zygomatic bone and the lack of complete development, arch fractures account for only 4.7% of all facial fractures.[85] Usually the fracture of the arch is of the greenstick type. The zygomatic fracture may be isolated, involving the zy-

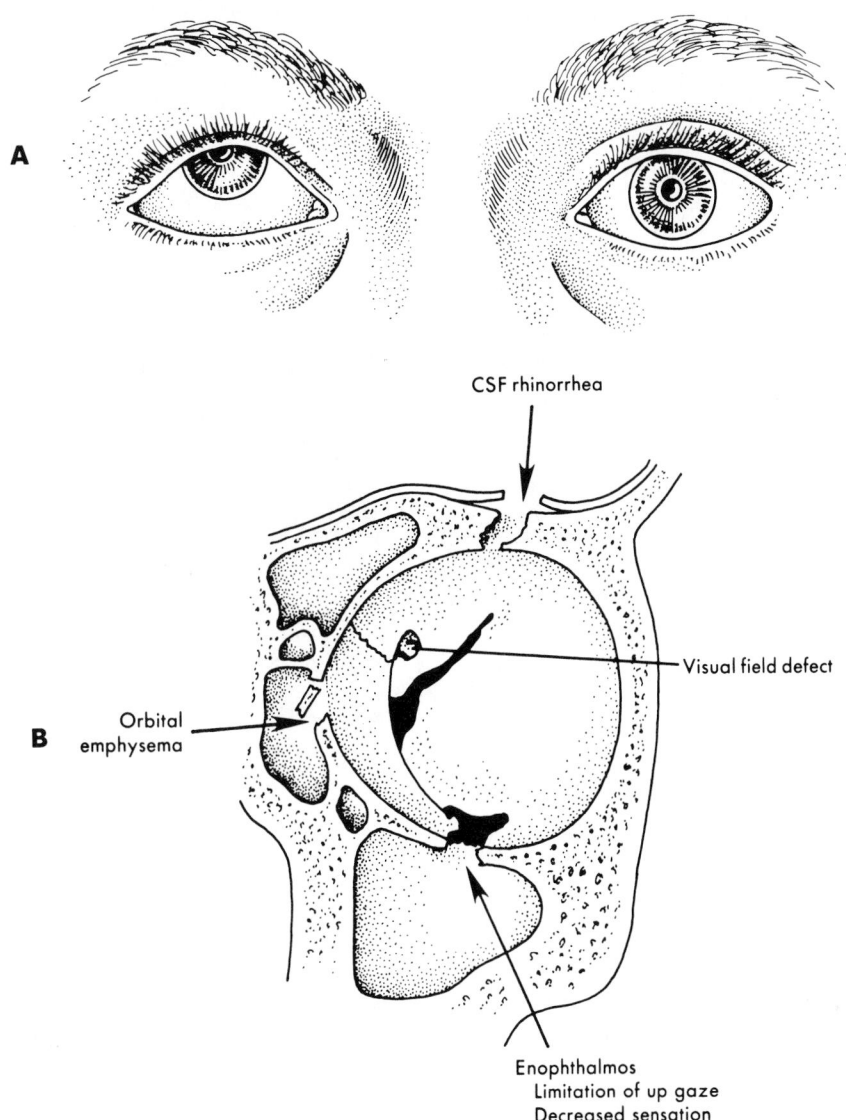

FIG. 21-3. A, Blowout fracture of the left orbit with enophthalmus and limited upward gaze of the left eye. **B,** Problems associated with orbital fractures according to site of fracture. (*From Rosen P, Barkin RM, Sternbach GL:* Essentials of emergency medicine, *St. Louis, 1991, Mosby.*)

gomatic arch, orbital floor, or lateral or medial (rare) orbital walls.

Physical examination reveals swelling, bruising, tenderness, and possibly crepitus over the malar area. A malar fattening may be noted, especially after the swelling has subsided. The finding of trismus usually indicates fracture fragments impinging on the coronoid process of the mandible. This finding can be appreciated by inspection of the cheeks from above. Injury to the zygomaticotemporal branch of the infraorbital branch of the fifth cranial nerve may cause anesthesia or hypesthesia over its distribution. Any neurologic findings related to the cutaneous nerves and ocular findings must prompt evaluation of underlying fractures.

Radiographs showing the Water's, submentovertex, and Caldwell views may be diagnostic. Computed tomography scanning is very helpful in making the diagnosis and guiding management.

Treatment of zygomatic fractures is necessary when the malar eminence is depressed. When the orbital complex is involved, prompt surgical intervention is necessary. Fractures in childhood heal quickly; therefore a delay in the initial recognition and managment can result in facial deformity. The long-term prognosis is good if the fractures are recognized early and managed promptly.[2,4,6,7,82]

Supraorbital Fractures. Discrepancies in the supraorbital ridge, hypesthesia of the distribution of the supraorbital nerve, ptosis, or exophthalmos indicates a supraorbital fracture with orbital roof involvement. Orbital fractures may result in optic nerve injuries or changes in extraocular movement. Orbital and malar fractures may be seen on Caldwell, Water's, and lateral plain radiograph views and definitely are revealed by CT scan.

Significant displacement of the fracture or change in extraocular movement requires exploration and possible bony realignment. Complications of such fractures may

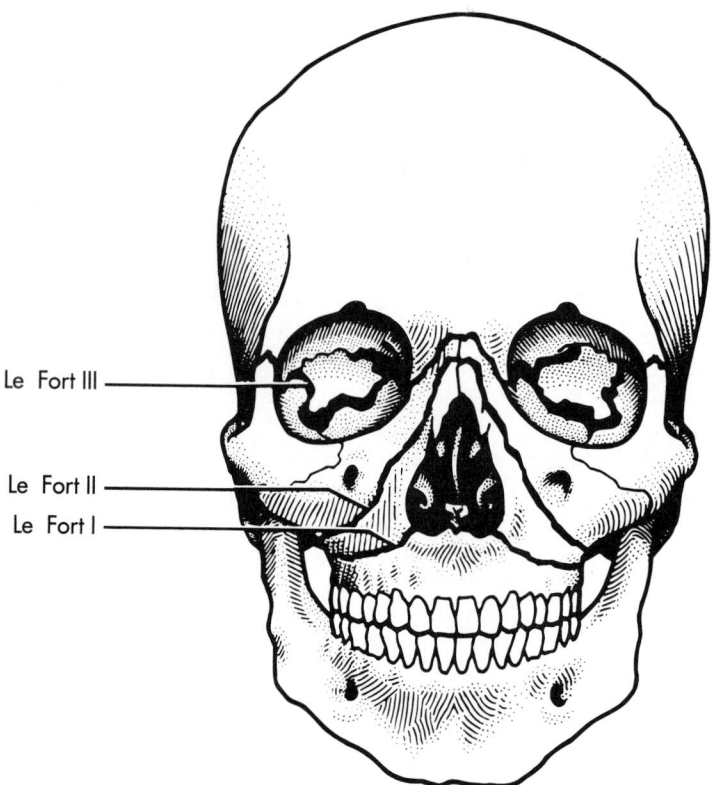

FIG. 21-4. Le Fort classification of maxillary fractures. Le Fort I: palate facial dysjunction. Le Fort II: pyramidal dysjunction. Le Fort III: craniofacial dysjunction.

result in facial deformities and limited extraocular movement.[2,4,6,7]

Maxillary Fractures (Le Fort Type)

Fractures of the maxillary region of the face are rare in children because of the resilience of the facial bones, lack of sinus development, and lack of structural prominence of this area.[85,86,90-92] These fractures are classified according to the horizontal level of the fracture by the system of Le Fort (Fig. 21-4). The Le Fort I fracture is uncommon in children less than 10 years of age and is characterized by a fracture through the lower third of the maxilla, palate, and pterygoid plates. A Le Fort II fracture line is through the nasal bones, floor of the orbit, and pterygoid plates into the pterygomaxillary fossa. When the same fracture extends through the zygomatic arches, resulting in complete separation of the facial bones from the cranium, a Le Fort III is present.

Findings of Le Fort fractures on clinical examination include disruption of the palate, as well as flattening, retrusion, lengthening, swelling, or ecchymosis over the midface. Malocclusion characterized by crossbite, split palate, and open bite may indicate such fractures. Associated basilar skull fractures are also common. Diagnosis of these fractures is by plain radiographs and CT scans.

Referral to a plastic surgeon is necessary. The goal of treatment is to restore the original architecture, occlusion, and facial symmetry.[2,4,7]

Mandibular Fractures

Fractures of the mandible are second to those of nasal bones as the most common facial fractures among children. Greenstick fractures are common because of the presence of subcutaneous tissue fat pads that absorb the impact and the resilience of immature bone. Because the mandible is occupied by unerupted tooth follicles that may be disrupted with trauma, injury to permanent dentition may result. This is an important consideration in diagnosis and management of fractures that may involve dentition.[100]

The history may suggest the location of the fracture incurred. Falls on the chin usually cause symphyseal or parasymphyseal fractures associated with unilateral or bilateral condylar fractures.[28,105,106] Lateral forces cause an ipsilateral angle or body fractures with contralateral condylar or angle fractures. On physical examination the presence of intraoral or extraoral swelling, sublingual hematoma, crepitus, or ecchymosis suggests an underlying fracture. Facial asymmetry, malocclusion, trismus, mandibular shift, open bite, and dental trauma may all be associated with mandibular fractures.[4,6,107]

Diagnosis of these fractures is made on anteroposterior, right and left lateral oblique, and Towne's views. If a fracture is suspected but not apparent on plain films, a panoramic radiograph may be obtained. CT scanning is usually not necessary, as these radiographic techniques are sufficient to make the diagnosis.

Management of mandibular fractures requires referral to a maxillofacial surgeon after initial patient stabilization. Controversy exists over whether closed management is superior.[7,82,108] Factors such as age, dentition (primary, secondary, mixed), site(s), complexity, deforming muscle tension, and association with other fractures determine the management. Most fractures in children managed by closed technique heal well. Open reduction is reserved for fractures resulting in poor jaw movement or malocclusion. A soft diet and observation are all that are needed for unilateral subcondylar fractures, whereas intermaxillary fixation for 2 to 3 weeks is needed for bilateral subcondylar fractures. Ramus, angle, parasymphyseal, and symphyseal fractures are managed by intermaxillary fixation or by various splints. More unstable fractures may require plating.[33,91,97,100,109]

Nasal Contusions and Fractures

Fractures of the nose are the most common facial fracture in children. The nose in the child is less prominent and more cartilaginous than that of the adult; thus it is spared from significant fractures, as the kinetic energy from trauma is distributed across the face. Abnormalities of the nose in adulthood are thought to result from undiagnosed fractures in childhood.[33-35,82,97]

Because of swelling around the nose, clinical diagnosis of a fracture is difficult. On inspection of the nares, the physician must look for a septal hematoma caused by the compression of the septum, the presence of nasal obstruction, or sites of epistaxis. Concomitant injury to other facial structures must be sought.[34,35]

Obtaining nasal radiographs is controversial because of their lack of specificity and sensitivity. In addition, the finding of fractures on nasal radiographs usually does not change the patient's immediate management. Nasal radiographs are indicated only for medicolegal reasons and parental reassurance.[7,34]

Septal Hematoma. As a result of the extensive vascularity of the nose, injury may cause bleeding into the septum. The hematoma must be evacuated immediately to prevent further damage to the cartilage and subsequent deformity. General anesthesia may be needed for younger children; local anesthesia with 4% cocaine or 1% lidocaine may be sufficient in older children.

A vertical incision is made through the mucoperichondrium overlying the septal hematoma, parallel to and usually about 0.5 to 1 cm posterior to the caudal septal margin. Blood is evacuated through the incision; a drain may be inserted into the hematoma cavity. If the hematoma is bilateral, the second incision may be made but should be staggered to the first to avoid a through-and-through defect. An anterior pack is then inserted to reapproximate the mucoperichondrium against the underlying cartilage. Amoxicillin or trimethoprim-sulfamethoxazole are given to prevent potential infection. Close follow-up in 24 to 48 hours is essential.

Complications of an untreated septal hematoma include development of a "saddle nose" deformity through the loss of support from the septum, which gives the bridge of the nose its shape. Other complications include septal necrosis with infection (chondritis), septal perforation, and nasal obstruction.[37,73,80] The management of epistaxis is discussed in Chapter 49.

Specialized follow-up observation of nasal fractures 5 days after injury is recommended. The indications for operative intervention include significant cosmetic deformity and nasal obstruction. Closed reduction is preferable for children less than 15 years of age. There is controversy as to whether open septorhinoplasty causes abnormal facial growth.[4,7,33-35,82]

Nasoethmoid Fractures

Nasoethmoid fractures involve the nasal and lacrimal bones along with the ethmoid labyrinth. Clinical findings include a flattened broad nose and traumatic telecanthus produced by disruption of the medial canthal ligament(s) and resulting in an increase of the intercanthal distance, vertical orbital dystopia secondary to orbital fractures, and findings associated with the other ocular, neurologic, and facial injuries discussed. Fractures of the other facial bones, maxillary sinus(es), superior orbital roof, and skull are often associated with nasoethmoid complex fractures. Along with plain film radiography, axial and coronal CT scanning must be performed to elucidate the extent of the fractures.

Management should be by trained specialists to reduce the fracture(s) to original architecture. This includes redeveloping the contour of the nose, restoring the intercanthal distance, and repairing other facial fractures as needed. Failure to achieve a satisfactory repair can result in significant deformity.[4,6,7,33]

OCULAR INJURIES

Trauma is the leading cause of enucleation of the eye in children; retinoblastoma, infection, inflammation, and congenital disorders are less common underlying conditions. The highest incidence of severe eye injuries occurs in the first and second decades of life.[110,111] Boys are especially at risk, sustaining eye injuries three to four times as often as girls.[3-6,112-115] Children with poor vision in one eye are at increased risk of injuring the well-seeing eye.[116] Motor vehicle collisions, sports injuries, firearms, falls, projectiles, and injuries in the home are important causes of eye injuries in children.[117,118] Eye injuries take a human and financial toll. It is estimated the eye injuries result in up to $200 million in hospital charges and 227,000 hospital days per year in the United States.[119]

Most eye injuries should receive follow-up examination by an ophthalmologist. The emergency physician should be able to provide the initial evaluation and treatment and recognize when immediate consultation is needed. This section first discusses systematic evaluation of eye injuries (Fig. 21-5); a description of specific injuries follows. Orbital fractures and eyelid injuries are discussed in other sections, as well as in Chapter 22.

Anatomy

The external structures of the eye are illustrated in Fig. 21-6. The space between the upper and lower eyelids is the palpebral fissure. When the eye is open, the upper eyelid invaginates between the globe and the roof of the orbit. The tarsus consists of glands and thick connective tissue. It is responsible for maintaining the stiff curved

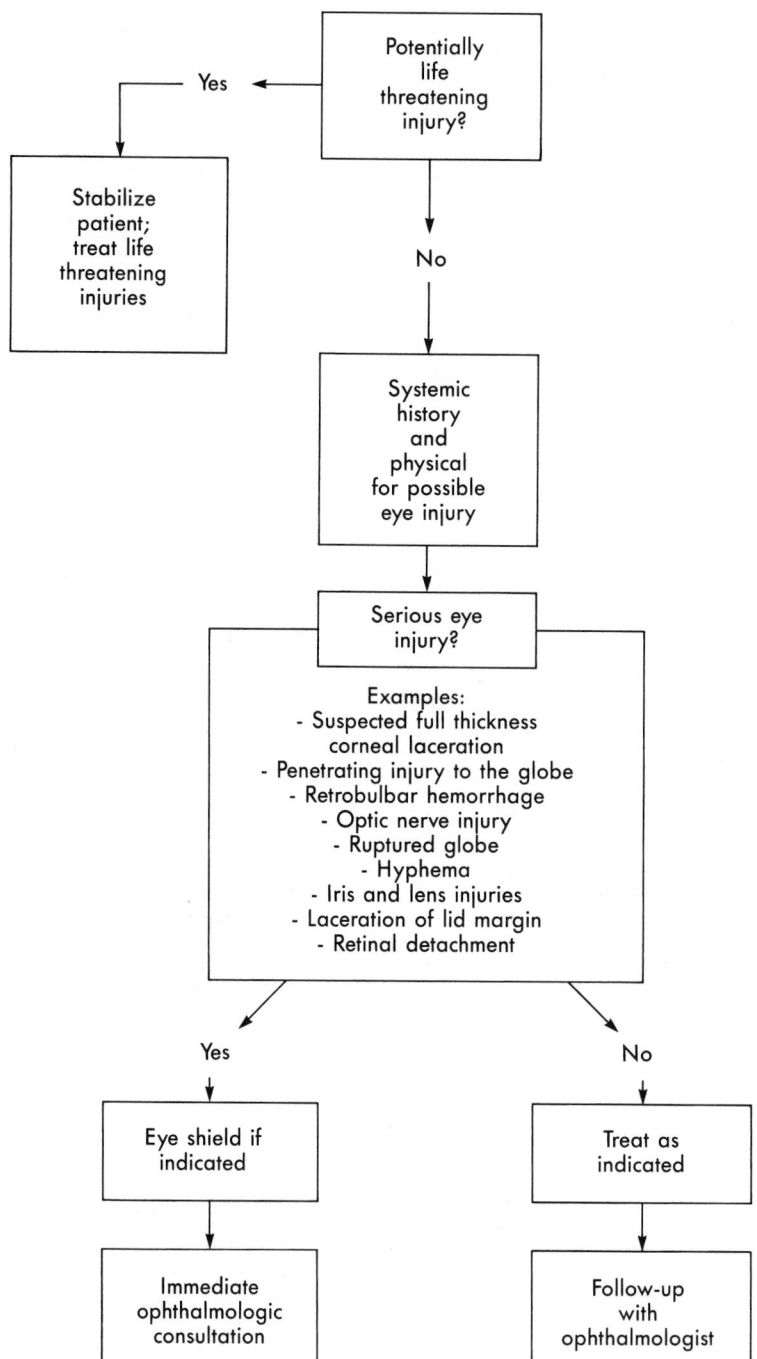

FIG. 21-5. Approach to ocular trauma.

shape of each lid. The tarsal glands open at the lid margins. Thin, loose skin covers the eyelids anteriorly and is continuous with the palpebral conjunctiva on the undersurface of the lid, which in turn is continuous with the bulbar conjunctiva covering the anterior globe up to the periphery of the cornea.

The orbicularis oculi is a circular muscle innervated by cranial nerve VII that serves to close the eye. The levator palpebrae superioris functions to raise the upper eyelid and is innervated by cranial nerve III. The upper eyelid also contains a smooth muscle that helps to raise the eyelid; the superior tarsal muscle is innervated by sympathetic fibers of the superior cervical ganglion.[120]

Six extraocular muscles surround each globe. The superior oblique muscle is innervated by cranial nerve IV and the lateral rectus by cranial nerve VI. The inferior oblique and the remaining rectus muscles (medial, superior, inferior) are innervated by cranial nerve III.[120]

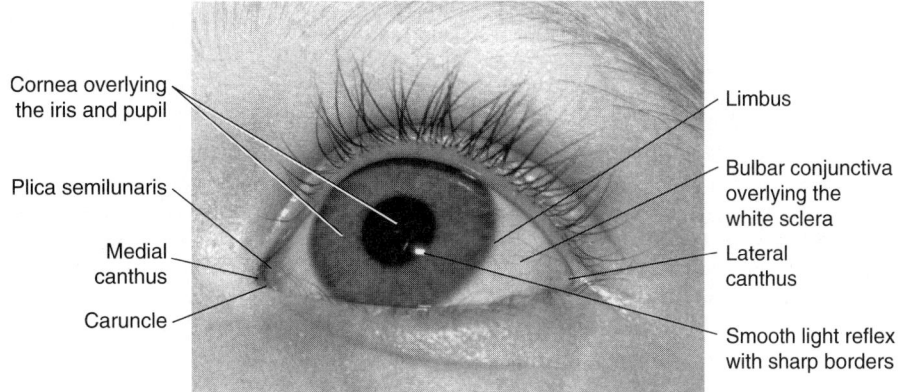

Cornea overlying the iris and pupil

Plica semilunaris

Medial canthus

Caruncle

Limbus

Bulbar conjunctiva overlying the white sclera

Lateral canthus

Smooth light reflex with sharp borders

FIG. 21-6. Anatomy of the eye.

The globe has three layers: an outer fibrous layer, a middle vascular layer, and an inner sensory layer. The outer fibrous layer consists of the sclera and the cornea. The white sclera covers five sixths of the globe and is continuous anteriorly with the cornea. The transparent cornea has a greater curvature than the sclera and this makes the anteroposterior diameter of the globe the longest. The cornea-sclera junction is called the *limbus*.[120]

The middle vascular layer is primarily made up of the choroid, which nourishes the retina. The choroid is continuous anteriorly with the ciliary body, is composed of all three layers, as well as the ciliary muscle, and functions in the control of the shape of the lens. The iris is composed of the vascular and sensory layers, as well as two muscles, the sphincter pupillae and the dilator pupillae. These muscles are innervated by cranial nerve III and sympathetic fibers of the upper thoracic nerves, respectively. The central aperture of the iris, the pupil, is controlled by these two muscles.[120]

The sensory layer of the iris and ciliary body is not sensitive to light. However, the light-sensitive retina makes up the majority of the innermost sensory layer. The rods and cones of the retina are connected to nerve cells that converge to form the optic nerve, which is visible as the optic disk in the posteromedial aspect of the retina. The central artery of the retina branches after it enters through the disk. The central vein exits through the disk.[120]

Diagnostic Findings

Clinical Findings. The history provides a basis for anticipating potential injuries by defining the mechanism of the injury. Pertinent historical questions include the following: When, where, and how did the incident occur? Was eye protection used? Does the patient wear contact lenses or glasses? Was any first aid given? How well can the patient see now compared to his or her preinjury vision? Is there pain, photophobia, or foreign body sensation? Has there been any discharge or excessive tearing? Did the patient have a history of previous eye abnormalities or surgery? What about current medication, allergy, and immunization status?[121]

The components of a systematic physical examination are outlined in the box above. Portions of the examination (e.g.,

---

Physical Examination of the Eye

Visual acuity
Lids and adnexa
Extraocular movements
Conjunctiva
Cornea
Sclera
Anterior chamber
Iris and pupil
Lens
Intraocular pressure
Vitreous
Fundus
Visual fields
Slit-lamp examination

---

intraocular pressure measurement) may be omitted if not indicated. Any omission should be a conscious decision based on an understanding of the patient's problem.[121]

The visual acuity examination is the first and most important component of the eye examination. The patient who has corrective lenses should wear them, if possible, during the acuity examination. Acuity should be tested in each eye separately and then in both eyes. Most children 3 years of age or older can understand and be tested on the "E" chart; those unable to use the chart can be tested on their ability to count fingers, detect hand motions, or fix on and follow a bright object. Useful age-specific acuity levels for screening are as follows: 3-year (20/50), 4-year (20/40), 5-year (20/30). A difference of more than two lines on the chart between the eyes is probably more significant than the absolute acuity and suggests unequal refractive error, amblyopia, or trauma. A topical anesthetic (proparacaine 0.5% [Ophthetic, Ophthaine]) may be needed to ensure an adequate examination.[121]

The lids should be assessed for motion, including raising and lowering, swelling, laceration, and ecchymosis. Foreign bodies, particularly on the inner surface, should be excluded by everting the lids.

Abnormalities of extraocular movements may be due to preexisting conditions, muscle injury or entrapment (in orbital fracture), or cranial nerve injury. The pupils should be equal, round, and equally reactive to light. Irregular pupil shape related to trauma suggests prolapse of the iris. Anisocoria may result from intracranial lesions (bleeding), mydriatic or miotic drugs, third nerve paralysis, and increased intraocular pressure; if it is limited, it may be a normal variant. Miosis, ptosis, and anhydrosis (Horner syndrome) suggest a lesion of the sympathetic pathway.[121] Trauma is the leading cause of acquired oculomotor nerve palsy in children, followed by infection-related, vascular, and neoplastic causes.[122]

The sclera and conjunctiva should be examined for laceration, foreign body, or hemorrhage. The cornea should be smooth, glistening, and clear. Intraocular pressure is normally 10 to 20 mm Hg and should be the same in both eyes (within 1 to 2 mm Hg). It should not be measured if perforation or rupture of the cornea or sclera is suspected.[121,123] The anterior chamber should be examined for blood (hyphema) or pus (hypopyon).

The fundus should be examined next. Unexplained retinal hemorrhages in an infant should suggest shaken baby syndrome (shaken impact syndrome). Papilledema is suggested by blurring of the nasal disk margin, loss of physiologic cupping, disk elevation, and distended, pulseless veins.[121]

Other specific physical findings are related to certain injuries and are discussed in relation to those injuries.

Ancillary Data. Fractures and radiopaque foreign bodies may be identified by plain radiographs. CT scanning, when possible, is preferable for defining small fractures and intraocular foreign bodies. Ultrasonography may analyze ocular structures for rupture of the lens, vitreous hemorrhage, retinal detachment, or intraocular foreign body, particularly intraoperatively.

Eyelid Injuries

An injury of the eyelid must be managed cautiously. First, any underlying injury to the globe should be diagnosed and treated. Lacerations of the lid margin should be referred to an ophthalmologist. Contusion or horizontal laceration may disrupt the levator palpebra, causing ptosis.[124] Careful apposition is essential. Improper repair of lid margin lacerations may lead to deformity (e.g., entropion), leaving the cornea exposed. These complications can be damaging, painful, and cosmetically undesirable.[125] Penetration of the globe should be excluded.

Likewise, lacerations of the medial lid may involve the canalicular system and should therefore be referred, as should any laceration causing ptosis.[125,126]

Interruption of the lacrimal system requires intubation of the lacrimal system and repair of the canaliculus. The medial portion of the lid includes the lacrimal drainage canaliculus, whereas the lacrimal duct runs along the outer third of the upper lid.

Eyelid ecchymoses ("black eyes") are a common consequence of blunt ocular trauma. They require no specific treatment; cool moist compresses may decrease the swelling.[125] Presence of periorbital ecchymoses may also result from basilar skull fracture. A negative history for trauma in the presence of periorbital hematoma may be due to child abuse or metastatic neuroblastoma.[127,128]

Corneal Injuries

Corneal injuries are the most common eye injuries in the emergency department. They commonly result from wind-blown foreign bodies, contact lens injuries, chemical splash injuries, or direct trauma from tree branches or fingertips. Not uncommonly, the patient has accidentally caused the injury with his or her finger. This is especially true of the infant. Indeed, a corneal injury should be part of the differential diagnosis of a "fussy" baby, especially when no other cause is readily apparent.[129]

The eye has several defense mechanisms to prevent injury. The blink reflex is highly effective in preventing most foreign bodies from entering the eye. Bell's reflex rotates the globe upward and outward as the eye closes. As a result, corneal injuries are most common in the inferomedial quadrant. Additionally, increased tearing helps wash foreign bodies from the eye.[129]

Diagnostic Findings. A corneal abrasion implies minimal or no stromal damage. A corneal defect implies stromal tissue loss, and a corneal laceration should be characterized as partial- or full-thickness. Corneal injuries are very painful, and the pain is usually exacerbated by blinking. The patient may complain of excessive tearing. A foreign body or a foreign body sensation may be present.[129]

Central corneal injuries affect visual acuity much more than peripheral corneal injuries. For corneal injuries, a thorough eye examination, including a slit lamp examination, is ideal; however, initial treatment decisions can usually be made without a slit lamp examination and the patient may then be referred to an ophthalmologist the following day. If the patient has symptoms of corneal injury but not history of ocular trauma, herpetic infection should be considered. If it is suspected, check the corneal sensation of both eyes with a wisp of cotton inferiorly or temporally. A relative decreased sensation of the involved cornea associated with a dendritic fluorescein examination suggests herpetic infection.[129]

If there is a clear history of trauma, proparacaine or tetracaine anesthetic may be used to ensure an adequate examination. However, topical anesthetics have no place in the ongoing treatment of corneal injury because they are toxic to corneal epithelium and may predispose the patient to further traumatic injury.[129]

First, examine the cornea without fluorescein. A "ciliary flush" may be seen with injury of the cornea or iris. It appears as a nonblanching pink or red band around the limbus and indicates congested iridial vessels. Epithelial damage may not be evident. Stromal damage may appear as white areas.[129,130]

Ancillary Data. Fluorescence is produced when dilute fluorescein, which is hydrophilic, contacts the hydrophilic stroma in the presence of cobalt blue light. Quenching is produced when concentrated fluorescein does not fluoresce in the presence of cobalt blue light. Both properties of fluorescein are useful in evaluating corneal injuries.[129]

Dilute fluorescein instillation is performed with sterile, single-dose liquid fluorescein or sterile paper strips impregnated with fluorescein. The former may be instilled by asking the supine patient to look up toward his or her eyebrows. The physician then applies gentle downward traction to the lower lid and lets a drop fall into the lower cul-de-sac. For a cooperative patient, the tip of the fluorescein strip is moistened with a drop of sterile ophthalmic irrigation solution. Then with the same positioning, the strip is touched to the pool of tears in the lower cul-de-sac. If the patient is uncooperative, it is helpful to have a syringe filled with premixed fluorescein solution. This can be prepared by dripping irrigation solution over the strip into a sterile container, then aspirating a small amount into a syringe. It is also helpful to orient the child with the blue light before the procedure. Then the lids are retracted and a drop is instilled. The fluorescein may sting briefly. A tissue should be available for wiping excess fluorescein and tears on the face. The cobalt blue light is turned on and the room lights are turned off. The cornea is then visualized in its entirety. Some patients like the blue light and may begin to cooperate. If the patient does not, allowing the parent to hold the child in his or her arms may help to calm the child.[129]

Corneal lesions fluoresce brightly. The staining pattern often confirms the suspected cause. The presence of many linear abrasions suggests a retained foreign body.[129]

The *concentrated fluorescein instillation* (Seidel test) takes advantage of the quenching property of concentrated fluorescein. It is used when full-thickness corneal injury is suspected. The fluorescein strip is touched directly to the site of the injury. If aqueous humor is leading from the anterior chamber, it dilutes the fluorescein and causes a stream of fluorescence at the site of injury in the presence of cobalt blue light.[129]

If available, the slit lamp examination may yield additional information. The presence of "flare and cell" in the anterior chamber indicates traumatic iritis. "Flare" resembles a sunbeam entering a dark room and results from plasma proteins released into the anterior chamber. The individual specks of dust in the sunbeam are called "cell" and represent white blood cells and pigment. Because traumatic iritis may be associated with corneal injuries, a slit lamp examination is indicated for these patients. Traumatic iritis is treated with an intermediate-acting cycloplegic.[129]

Corneal Abrasions. Corneal abrasions result from several causes. The diagnosis is suggested by the history of trauma (usually minor) resulting in a painful, tearing eye. It is confirmed by the fluorescein examination. It is important to search diligently for a retained foreign body and to complete the examination to rule out associated injuries.[129]

Management of corneal abrasions is a five-part process that includes cycloplegia, use of antibiotics, patching, analgesia, and referral to an ophthalmologist for follow-up observation. Homatropine 5% paralyzes the iris and ciliary body for 12 to 24 hours and in doing so relieves inflammation and pain. Ophthalmic antibiotic preparations of gentamicin, tobramycin, bacitracin, or sulfisoxazole are effective for prophylaxis of eye infections in this setting.[129]

After instillation of the cycloplegic and antibiotic, the involved eye should generally be patched. However, if there is concern of retained foreign body or the abrasion is due to a contact lens or vegetable matter (such as from a nylon line lawn trimmer), patching is not recommended due to a greater risk of infection.[131-133]

Semipressure eye patching (Fig. 21-7) is performed with two eye pads and several premeasured strips of tape. The first eye pad is folded in half and placed with the straight edge just under the brow of the closed eye. In smaller children the standard pad may be too large and a customized pad may be cut from it. The first pad is taped or held in place until a second pad (not folded) is placed over the eye. The pads are then taped with several strips from the midforehead to the cheek. The nose and nasolabial fold should not be taped. The patient should feel slight pressure on the eye and should be unable to open the patched eye. If the patient can open the eye, the patch has been applied improperly.[129]

Once the patch is correctly applied, the patient usually feels better but may require oral analgesics for pain. The patient should have follow-up observation by an ophthalmologist within 24 hours.[129]

Corneal Lacerations and Defects. Corneal lacerations usually result from a sharp object hitting the eye. However, because the history may be misleading and corneal lacerations can be self-sealing, the depth of the laceration may be misjudged. Corneal defects, on the other hand, are usually easily seen. The question is whether either of these injuries has extended to the full thickness of the cornea. If a full-thickness injury is confirmed or suspected, emergency ophthalmologic consultation is necessary.[129]

When considering the diagnosis, carefully assess the pupil for irregularities that may be due to prolapse of the iris. Examine the integrity of the anterior chamber. If it appears collapsed (as a result of leakage of aqueous humor), a full-thickness injury has occurred. Unfortunately, a normal-appearing pupil and anterior chamber may be misleading. The self-sealing ability of small lacerations may produce a normal-appearing eye. The Seidel test should be performed but may yield negative findings in cases of sealed full-thickness injuries. The slit lamp examination can often reveal the extent of the laceration.

If there is any suspicion of a full-thickness injury, an eye shield should be placed and an ophthalmologist consulted. If, for some reason, the care of an ophthalmologist will be delayed for several hours, the patient should be hospitalized at strict bedrest. Atropine sulfate (1%) in the eye every 6 hours and an antiemetic should be started as well. Broad-spectrum antibiotic coverage is provided by cefazolin (50 to 100 mg/kg/24 hr q 8 hr [maximum adult dose 4-6 gm/day]) IV and should be started only after consultation with the ophthalmologist.

Superficial Ocular Foreign Bodies

Most foreign bodies in the eye are relatively small in mass and reach the eye with relatively low velocity. Eyelashes and wind-blown pieces of dust fall into this category and cause only superficial damage.

The physician must search for foreign bodies whenever a patient has a history of foreign body presence or corneal abrasion. The symptoms may be identical and the two conditions may coexist. It is often necessary to evert the upper eyelid or even to use double eversion.[121]

Lid eversion and foreign body removal require a topical anesthetic (proparacaine), two cotton-tipped applicators, lid retractor (e.g., Desmarres), and sterile ophthalmic irrigation solution. The procedure is explained to the patient.[129]

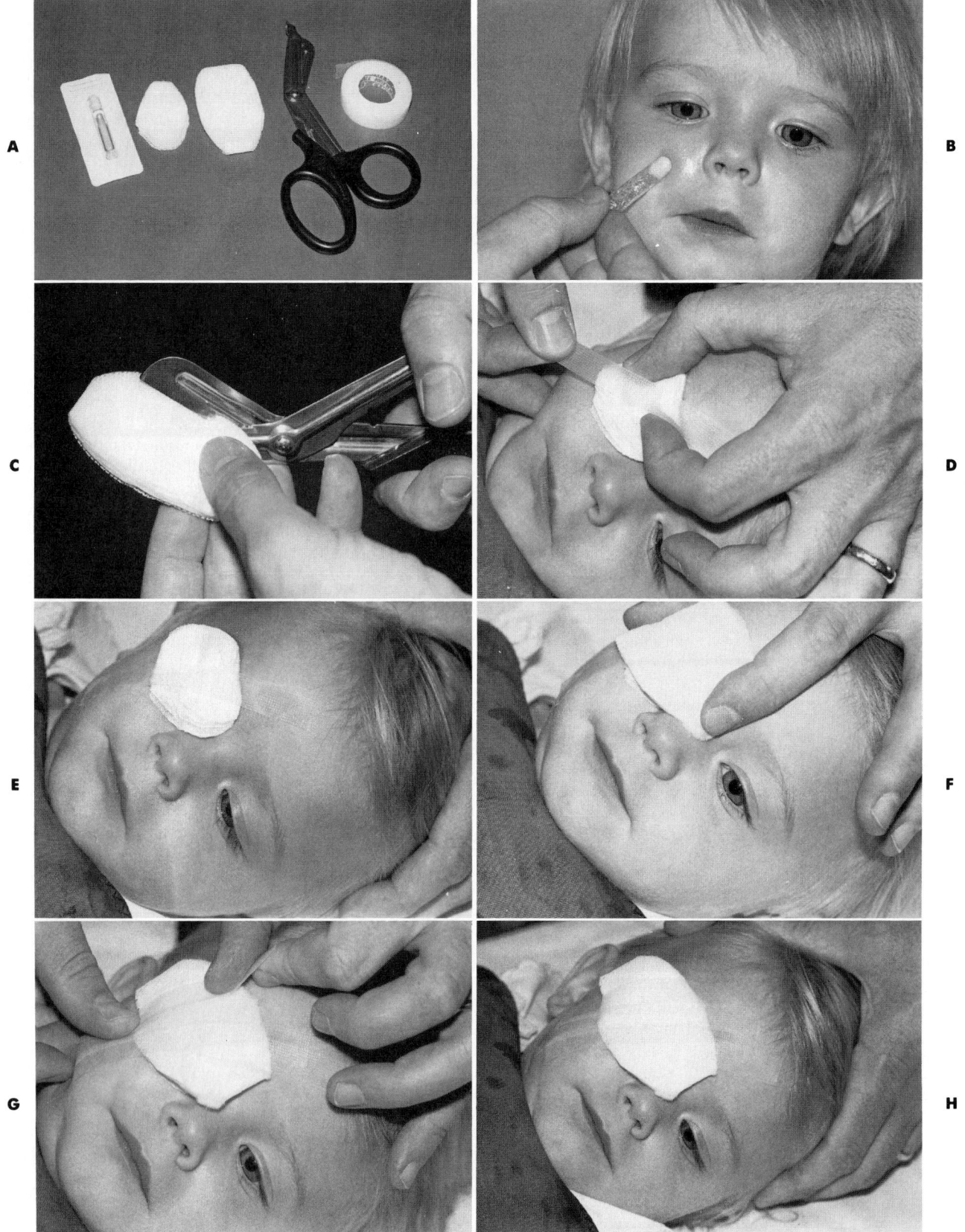

FIG. 21-7. Application of a semipressure patch. **A,** The required equipment is assembled. **B,** Tincture of benzoin is applied. **C,** A customized eye patch is cut from the standard size patch. **D, E,** The restrained child has the first patch taped in place. **F-H,** A second, standard size patch is applied. Care is taken to avoid the nasolabial crease.

A drop of topical anesthetic may be necessary. However, if the patient can cooperate and a corneal abrasion has not yet occurred, the examiner may choose not to use the anesthetic. The dramatic pain relief on removal of the foreign body can reassure both the physician and the patient that treatment has been successful.

Generally, to accomplish single eversion of the right eyelid, the examiner places the right thumb just below the eye. The patient is instructed to look down. As this occurs, the upper eyelashes are easily grasped between the thumb and forefinger. With the left hand, the wooden handle of a cotton-tipped applicator is placed horizontally on top of the upper lid, just above the tarsal plate to act as a fulcrum. Then, in a swift fashion, the right hand flips the lid upward. The lid is everted and the conjunctiva of the upper lid and superior globe is easily inspected. Foreign bodies may be washed away with irrigating solution or gently swabbed away with a second cotton-tipped applicator.[129]

If necessary, double eversion of the upper lid may be accomplished by vertically placing a lid retractor (instead of the cotton-tipped applicator handle) above the tarsal plate before single eversion. After single eversion, the eyelid can be everted further by gentle retraction of the lid retractor.[129]

If the patient's left eye is involved, the examiner's left hand should grasp the eyelashes and the right hand should apply the fulcrum. After removal of the foreign body, the patient should be inspected for a corneal abrasion.[129]

Contact Lens Injuries

Several different injuries may result from or be related to the wearing of contact lenses. Traumatic insertion or removal of contact lenses may result in abrasions of the inferior cornea. Foreign bodies may become trapped under or embedded in a contact lens. Also, patients may wear contact lenses an excessive length of time and get lens overwear syndrome. When this occurs, the hypoxic corneal epithelium die. It sloughs 2 to 4 hours later, causing severe eye pain and all the other symptoms of corneal abrasion. Lens overwear syndrome may occur with soft or hard lens use. This neglect of proper lens use may be unintentional when, for example, a patient has head trauma.

The emergency physician must know how to remove contact lenses from the eyes of these patients safely; this is the first step in treatment. It may be necessary to apply a topical anesthetic (proparacaine HCI ophthalmic solution 0.5%) before removing the lenses. Because soft lenses may be permanently stained by fluorescein, they should be removed before its use.[129,134]

Rigid contact lens removal is most easily accomplished by a special suction cup available for this purpose. The cup is moistened, pressed gently on the center of the lens, and pulled straight off the eye. Care should be taken not to rotate or slide the lens excessively. If such a cup is not available, the soft contact lens removal technique may be used.[129]

To remove soft contact lenses the examiner gently touches the lens with the index finger while the patient is looking up and slides it onto the inferior conjunctiva. Here the lens is pinched and removed.[129]

After the lenses are removed, the evaluation (for foreign bodies and corneal abrasions) and treatment are as previously described. The patient should refrain from wearing the lenses until he or she and the lenses have been examined by an ophthalmologist.[129]

Blunt Ocular Injury

Blunt injury to the eye may occur not only at the site of direct impact but at distant sites because of forces transmitted to the entire globe. Indeed, a direct blow to the eye is not necessary to inflict damage. A rapid deceleration or acceleration (e.g., shock waves of an explosion) may cause injury to the eye.[135]

Blunt injury to the eye may be associated with other closed head trauma. A history of loss of consciousness or other neurologic signs and symptoms should prompt evaluation for serious intracranial injury. After the patient's condition has been stabilized, the evaluation of the eye should continue.[135]

Diagnostic Findings. A thorough history should be taken. Certain symptoms associated with blunt ocular trauma suggest particular problems. If there is history of immediate loss of vision, severe damage to the retina or optic nerve is suggested. Gradual loss of vision, which later returns, suggests a contusion of the optic nerve or vascular occlusion. Photophobia may result from traumatic iritis, whereas diplopia suggests a blowout fracture of the orbit. A retinal tear or vitreous hemorrhage may cause flashes of light or floaters.[135] A history of a blast injury to the eye usually warrants consultation with an ophthalmologist.[136]

The usual ocular examination should be performed. However, if there is concern about rupture of the globe, manipulation should be minimized to prevent extrusion of intraocular contents. Indeed, it may be necessary to defer measurement of intraocular pressure if rupture is suspected. A topical anesthetic may be helpful in performing the examination, and eyelid retraction may be necessary. Once again, testing visual acuity is very important. A penlight should be quickly passed from one pupil to the next to check for an afferent pupillary defect. If the pupil of the injured eye constricts consensually, then dilates with direct light, an afferent pupillary defect exists. If present at all, the defect is usually mild and associated with hyphema, cataracts, or vitreous hemorrhage. An obvious afferent pupillary defect suggests retinal detachment or optic nerve injury.[135] An afferent pupillary defect or a nonreactive pupil or associated facial fractures are predictors of serious eye injury in patients with blunt ocular trauma.[137]

Specific Blunt Ocular Injuries. *Subconjunctival hemorrhages* are of no consequence, but they may be associated with more severe injuries. They appear as bright red hemorrhages that obliterate any underlying blood vessels. They are often localized to one area and occur next to normal-appearing sclera. They resolve in 2 to 3 weeks.[135]

Conjunctival chemosis (swelling) may be a sign of scleral rupture or perforation. Conjunctival crepitus is usually a sign of a blowout fracture of the medial wall of the orbit. It is worsened by nose blowing. It may also result from a compressed air injury to the eye that causes a tear in the conjunctiva.[135]

Hyphema (blood in the anterior chamber) often appears as a layering out of blood in the anterior chamber. In its most severe form, it fills the entire chamber and obscures the iris. This is called a total hyphema or "eight ball" hyphema, because it often is black. In an acute condition hyphema may appear as clouding of the anterior chamber (before settling has occurred).[135]

Before the blood settles in a hyphema, vision is impaired and the anterior chamber shows a diffuse decrease in its detail, sometimes obscuring the pupil. As the blood begins to layer out, a meniscus may form and a blood-aqueous level may form in the inferior chamber angle. Management approaches to a hyphema are somewhat controversial and are focused on preventing rebleeding within 3 to 5 days after the initial injury.[138-145] Intraocular pressure must be carefully assessed and managed. Late complications include secondary glaucoma, corneal blood staining, and optic atrophy. Patients who have sickle hemoglobinopathies are at increased risk of optic atrophy. Hyphema management consists of administration of long-acting cycloplegic (atropine 0.25% to 2%) and bedrest. Hospitalization or close (daily) outpatient follow-up observation is essential. Aminocaproic acid (initial doses of 200 mg/kg/dose [maximum 6 gm] PO followed by 50 to 100 mg/kg/dose q 6 hr PO) is often used to help prevent rebleeding. Patching, shielding, sedation, and administration of topical steroids have also been used.[135,146] Pain should be treated with nonaspirin products; all black patients should be questioned (or tested) concerning sickle cell disease.[147] The anterior chamber drainage angle should be examined by gonioscopy 4 to 6 weeks after injury. Nontraumatic causes of hyphema include leukemia, hemophilia, juvenile kanthogranuloma, and retinoblastonia.[124,131]

Traumatic iritis is the most common iris injury. The patient may have photophobia, blurred vision, or headache. Aqueous "flare and cell" is revealed by slit lamp examination. Traumatic iritis is managed by a short-acting cycloplegic such as homatropine.[135]

Traumatic mydriasis results from damage to the pupillary sphincter and may be transient or permanent. Iris sphincter tears appear as small radial defects of the iris on the pupillary border. Iridodialysis is a disinsertion of the iris root from the ciliary body. No emergency treatment is required, although it may be associated with other injuries, such as hyphema.[135]

Traumatic cataracts result when lens, blunt penetrating, electrical or radiation injury causes hydration and opacification of the gelatinous center.[145] When the contents of the lens leak into the globe, further inflammation of the eye results. Cataracts may develop rapidly or over weeks or months. If they occur rapidly, the ophthalmologist removes them as soon as possible to attenuate secondary glaucoma and inflammation.[135,148] There is preliminary evidence that suggests that intraocular lens implants may be an effective treatment for children with traumatic cataracts.[149,150] CT scanning may be helpful in the prompt diagnosis of traumatic cataracts, especially when examination of the lens is impaired by other injuries of the globe.[151]

Vossius' lenticular ring is a circular ring of pigment seen on the anterior lens capsule after dilatation. It is a sign of blunt ocular trauma and has little consequence.[135]

Subluxation and dislocation of the lens may also be noted. Subluxation occurs when some of the zonules are broken. Dislocation occurs when so many of the zonules are broken that the lens has fallen forward into the anterior chamber or posteriorly into the vitreous cavity. Iridodonesis (trembling iris) may be seen after rapid eye movement if the lens is dislocated. Surgical management of a dislocated lens is urgent if the lens is touching the cornea or is stuck in the pupil, resulting in pupillary block glaucoma.[135] Nontraumatic causes of lens dislocation include congenital causes, Marfan syndrome, homocystinuria, and inflammation.[124]

Scleral rupture is a severe injury often associated with other ocular injury. The eye may feel soft. The anterior chamber may be deeper than normal and bloody chemosis is often present. Areas frequently ruptured include (1) circumferential arcs concentric with limbus, (2) insertion sites of the extraocular muscles, (3) the equator of the globe, and (4) the impact site. The superonasal quadrant is the quadrant most frequently involved.[135] In one study, visual acuity worse than 20/400, decreased intraocular pressure, intraocular pressure less than in the nontraumatized eye, and an afferent pupillary defect were found to be important indicators of an open globe.[152]

Treatment of scleral rupture (see box below) begins with a shield over the eye to prevent pressure to the globe and extrusion of intraocular contents. Antiemetic should be given if the patient is nauseated, because vomiting can cause extrusion of intraocular contests. The patient should be kept on nothing by mouth (NPO) status and the time of last intake recorded. Tetanus should be given if indicated. Finally, after consultation with the ophthalmologist, IV antibiotics (cefazolin 50 to 100 mg/kg/24 hr q 8 hr [maximum 1.5 gm/dose] and gentamicin 3 to 7.5 mg/kg/24 hr q 8 hr [maximum adult dose 5 mg/kg/day]) should be started and the dosage adjusted in relation to serum drug levels.[135] Orbital CT scanning may confirm an open globe in unproven cases but is secondary in importance to consultation with ophthalmology.[124] An alternative would be vancomycin and gentamicin.[153]

Vitreous hemorrhage may be manifested through "floaters," showers of dark specks, or significant visual loss. It causes the fundus to be poorly visible. The red reflex may be absent. There may be a slight afferent pupillary defect; a pronounced defect suggests retinal detachment or optic nerve damage. Isolated vitreous hemorrhage does not require surgical treatment. The patient should keep the head elevated (even during sleep) to allow the blood to settle. Medications that may exacerbate bleeding, such as aspirin, should be avoided. The patient should also be instructed to avoid heavy lifting, straining, and Valsalva maneuvers. The patient should be seen by an ophthalmologist within 24

"SANTA" Therapy for Scleral Rupture

S—Shield the eye
A—Antiemetic (if indicated)
N—NPO
T—Tetanus immunization (if indicated)
A—Antibiotics (after consultation)

hours for isolated vitreous hemorrhage and sooner if optic nerve injury or retinal detachment is suspected.[135]

Retinal tears may lead to detachment, either immediately or months to years later. The patient with a tear may have symptoms of vitreous hemorrhage (which is often associated) or may see flashes of light as a result of traction on the retina. In addition to these symptoms, patients with retinal detachment may complain of a curtain of darkness across the visual field. Since the detachment is not limited to any particular part of the retina, the "curtain" may appear from any direction. A profound loss of vision, an afferent pupillary defect, and a diminished red reflex may all be present.[135]

Retinal detachments are usually separations of the sensory retina from the underlying retinal pigment epithelium, which result from accumulation of fluid in that potential space. The detachment may remain flat, or it may billow toward the vitreous cavity. Detachments that occur superiorly are generally more serious because they may rapidly progress to involve the macula. This may cause permanent loss of central vision. It may be difficult to visualize retinal detachments in the anterior (peripheral) retina with a direct ophthalmoscope. Retinal detachment may appear as a grayish flap of retina out of focus with the optic disk.[154] Traumatic retinal detachments may not be apparent immediately, but almost half are apparent within one month, and most are by two years.[124]

Treatment of retinal tears or detachments in the emergency department includes emergency ophthalmologic consultation, patching of both eyes, patient NPO status, and bed rest pending surgery.[135]

Retinal hemorrhages are common in cases of child abuse.[148,155,156] If abuse is suspected, an ophthalmologic consultation is indicated. The ophthalmologist can document whether the hemorrhages are new, old, or a combination thereof. This may be medicolegally important in a legal case if the defense claims that the hemorrhages were iatrogenic (e.g., caused by chest compressions).

Retinal hemorrhages may be preretinal, intraretinal, or subretinal. Preretinal hemorrhages are bright red and boat-shaped and obscure retinal vessels. Intraretinal hemorrhages also obscure the vessels and appear as bright red blots. Subretinal hemorrhages are dark red or purple, and the overlying retinal vessels are not obscured.[135]

Berlin's edema (commotio retinae, retinal edema) appears as a patchy whitening of the retina and is a sign of chorioretinal trauma. It typically occurs in the retina opposite from the site of impact (contrecoup).[124] It usually resolves without sequelae within 2 weeks. However, if it occurs in the macula, it may leave a macular cyst or hole with permanent loss of central vision.[135]

Choroidal rupture may initially be obscured by vitreous hemorrhage but, as this resolves, appears as a yellow-white curvilinear scar concentric with the disk. If the macula is involved or if subretinal neovascularization occurs, the prognosis worsens.[135]

Fat emboli appear as yellow exudates associated with flame-shaped hemorrhages. They result from long bone fractures and have little ocular significance unless the macula is involved.[135]

Optic nerve injuries may result in permanent total vision loss of the involved eye. One millimeter of the optic nerve is intraocular, 30 mm is intraorbital, 6 mm is fixed in a bony canal, and 10 mm is intracranial. The intracanalicular portion is the most vulnerable to stretching forces (which interrupt the nutrient artery supply) or to transection by bony fragments. Often the patient has visual field abnormalities or severe visual loss with an afferent pupillary defect. High-resolution CT scanning of the orbits with 1.5-mm cuts can help define the injury.[135] Ultrasound, fluorescein angiography and electrodiagnostic tests may also be helpful in making the diagnosis.[157,158]

Treatment of the optic nerve contusion is controversial and may be medical (administration of glucocorticoids) or surgical. Prompt ophthalmologic and neurosurgical consultation is indicated.[135]

Avulsion of the optic nerve from the globe is a rare injury resulting from very forceful injury. It generally results in total permanent vision loss of the involved eye. Currently it cannot be treated.[135]

Retrobulbar hemorrhage is a true ocular emergency. The increased orbital pressure is transmitted to the globe and can produce central retinal artery occlusion. The patient complains of pain and variable amounts of vision loss. The eyelids are tense, proptosis is present, and hemorrhagic swelling of the conjunctiva often occurs. Increased intraocular pressure, decreased ocular motility, and afferent pupillary defect may occur. Emergency ophthalmologic consultation is mandatory.[135]

Maneuvers to minimize damage to the eye include intravenous administration of mannitol, anterior chamber paracentesis, lateral canthotomy, intermittent digital massage (to decrease intraocular pressure) and inhalation of carbon dioxide-enriched air (to induce retinal vasodilatation).[135,159]

Penetrating Injuries

Penetrating injuries are the most frequent eye injuries requiring hospitalization and consideration in all potential cases of eye trauma.[146,160] High-velocity missiles, if small enough, may cause relatively few symptoms until late sequelae develop. Therefore, any penetrating injury or history that suggests penetrating injury should prompt consultation of an ophthalmologist.

Penetrating injuries to the eye usually result from a sharp object or a projectile that comes into contact with the eye. Perhaps the most serious threat to a child's eye is a perforating injury from a BB or pellet gun (Fig. 21-8). These injuries have a poor prognosis and often result in enucleation.[112,161] The gun is often unintentionally fired by the patient or a playmate. The BB often ricochets off another object before hitting the eye.[162] Although other guns can cause even more severe damage, the ready availability of BB guns and the misguided belief of many that they are harmless toys lead to their unique potential for damage. Other common causes of penetrating ocular trauma are striking of steel on steel; knives, razors, glass, and foreign bodies propelled by explosions; lawn mowers; and nylon-line grass trimmers.[163-165] The risk of endophthalmitis increases if the foreign body is not removed within 24 hours.[166]

Diagnostic Findings. The patient's initial symptoms may be mild when the penetrating foreign body is small.

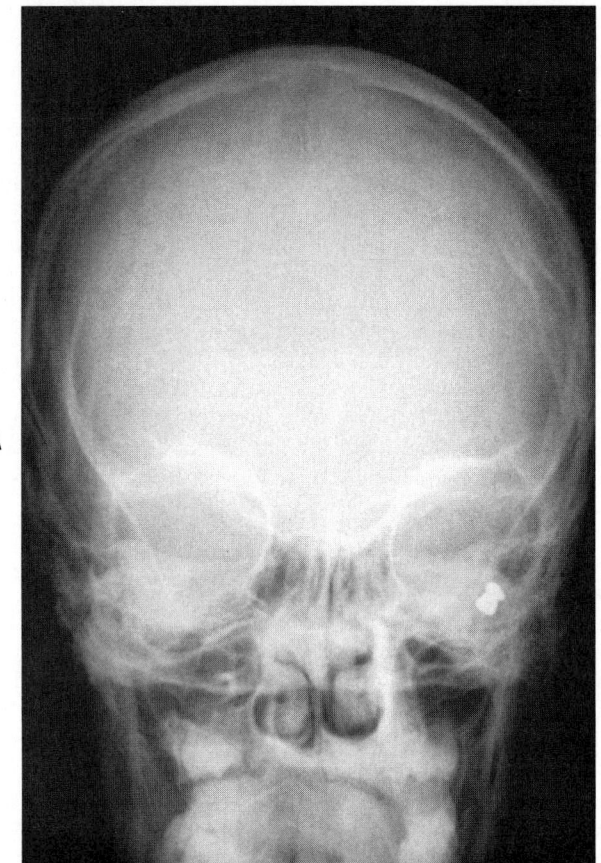

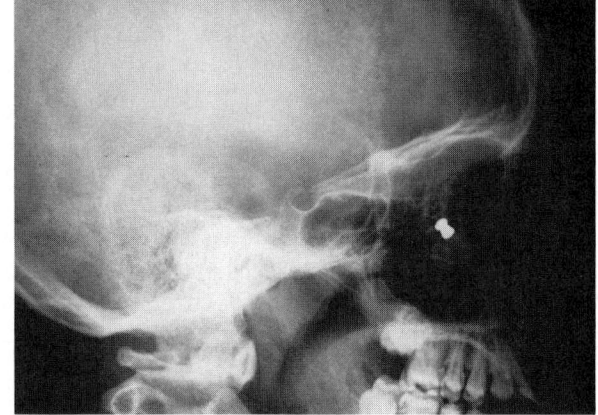

FIG. 21-8. Penetrating injury. **A,** Anteroposterior and **B,** lateral radiographs of the skull showing a metallic pellet from a pellet gun in the orbit.

For instance, a metal sliver caused by filing metal on a grinding wheel may penetrate the globe and yet cause only mild pain and irritation. Although the initial injury to the globe from such an injury may be minimal, the sequelae may be devastating. Other penetrating injuries may have more obvious signs and symptoms. The patient may complain of partial or complete loss of vision, bleeding, and severe pain. Obvious laceration, bleeding, or extruded intraocular contents may be visible. Some of the more common and serious sequelae of penetrating ocular trauma are discussed later.[167]

Management. Emergency department management of penetrating eye injuries generally requires placement of an eye shield (not a semipressure patch) and emergency consultation of an ophthalmologist. Generally, the penetrating foreign body should be removed in the operating room, not the emergency department. Pressure to the eye should be prevented so that leakage of intraocular contents may be minimized. The patient should be prepared, anticipating surgery. Tetanus immunization, antibiotics, and antiemetic should be given as indicated. It must be remembered that some penetrating foreign bodies may have traveled beyond the orbit and into the cranium. Management of these life-threatening injuries takes precedence. CT scanning may be useful in identifying intraocular and intracranial foreign bodies.[167]

Specific Penetrating Ocular Injuries. Traumatic cataracts (discussed in relation to blunt ocular trauma) may also result from penetrating injury.

Intraocular hemorrhage into the vitreous or anterior chamber (hyphema) may occur. Orbital scanning by CT may be necessary to determine the presence of retinal detachment, intraocular foreign body, or other injury hidden by the hemorrhage.[167]

Chorioretinal hemorrhage is a rare consequence of some missile injuries. The bleeding and scarring are generally worse than those associated with choroidal rupture. The prognosis is poor.[167]

Infection of the eye secondary to trauma, traumatic endophthalmitis, occurs in 2% to 7% of patients who sustain significant eye trauma. It may result in irreversible visual loss. Infections by *Bacillus* spp. have a particularly poor prognosis.[166,168]

Prophylaxis is recommended despite lack of good human studies. The antibiotics are often given by topical subconjunctival and systemic routes. Ophthalmologists often obtain cultures for bacteria and fungi from the wound edges and from any foreign body.[169]

Chalcosis is a purulent sterile endophthalmitis that results from release of ions from copper-containing foreign bodies. Siderosis is the insidious toxicity of iron to the retina, lens, and iris that occurs over months to years. Other metals such as aluminum, lead mercury, nickel, and zinc also have their own unique toxic effects.[170] It is therefore important to determine what type of metal has penetrated a patient's eye.[167,171]

Occasionally, the immune system mounts a response against the uveal tract of the traumatized eye; however, it also attacks the nontraumatized eye. This sympathetic ophthalmia may be prevented by enucleation of the severely traumatized eye within 7 to 14 days of the initial injury.[167]

Chemical Injuries

Children may splash everything from gasoline to "super" glue into their eyes. Some of the chemical eye injuries can have devastating consequences, and all efforts should be made to prevent their occurrence. Acid and alkali burns may cause blindness and require emergency treatment before acuity evaluation and full examination. They are ocular emergencies and should be treated as such. If the nature of the substance contacting the eye cannot be ascertained and the patient is symptomatic, emergency irrigation should be started.[129]

Diagnostic Findings. Alkali burns to the eye rapidly penetrate the cornea and cause coagulative necrosis. Lime (plaster and mortar), lye, and ammonia derivatives (fertilizers, refrigerants, and cleansing agents) are the most common agents. Corneal opacification and conjunctival blanching result. Emergency irrigation, as discussed later, is imperative.[129]

Acid burns may be equally devastating and should also receive emergency irrigation. They cause protein precipitation in the corneal epithelium and stroma that is destructive but tends to limit acid penetration of the cornea. For this reason, the prognosis for acid burns is generally a little better than for alkali burns. However, delay in irrigation is a poor prognostic indicator for either type.[129]

Solvents and detergents may cause superficial corneal epithelial injury, conjunctival irritation, and iritis. Patients should receive first-aid eye irrigation as described later. However, if the patients are asymptomatic at arrival in the emergency department and have normal eye examination findings, further irrigation is unnecessary.[129]

Mace and tear gas also cause superficial injury but have the added hazard of propelling foreign bodies toward the eye; hence a search for foreign bodies is indicated. Initial management is described later.[129]

"Super" glues dry very quickly and may cause the eyelids to be glued shut. If gentle traction does not separate the lids, moist saline solution compresses (or alternatively, neosporin ophthalmic ointment) applied for 24 hours usually allows easy separation. Some ophthalmologists recommend early surgical intervention, especially if direct contact with the globe is suspected (e.g., the patient is unable to move the globe freely under the eyelid)[172-174]; However, this is controversial. Consultation with an ophthalmologist is recommended. If "super" glue dries on the cornea and is removed, a corneal abrasion often results and the patient should be treated accordingly.[129]

Management. The sooner the eye is irrigated after exposure to a damaging chemical, the better the prognosis. The local poison control center should have information about the ocular toxicity of a particular substance. However, if there will be any delay in acquiring this information, it is better to begin irrigation immediately. First-aid irrigation at the closest source of water is generally preferable to the delay of a ride to the hospital. Irrigation at home may be accomplished by slowly running tap water into the affected eye for 15 minutes. The patient should then be transported to the emergency department for further evaluation.[129]

When the patient arrives in the emergency department, it is best to assume that home irrigation, though very helpful, may not have been optimal. If the patient has any symptoms at all, the affected eye(s) should be irrigated in the emergency department for an additional 15 minutes as discussed later. If the patient is asymptomatic and has normal eye examination (including fluorescein) findings, further irrigation may not be necessary.[129]

Irrigation of the eye requires at least 1 L of normal saline solution with IV tubing attached, topical anesthetic such as proparacaine, lid retractor, nitrazine paper, and an empty basin. The patient is positioned supine and the basin located where the used irrigation solution will fall. Topical anesthetic is applied. The patient is asked to count fingers as a quick estimate of visual acuity. Conjunctival pH is measured with the nitrazine paper. The upper lid is retracted. The normal saline solution is allowed to flow across the affected eye until the entire liter has been used, usually taking over 10 minutes. For serious alkali and acid burns, irrigation should continue until conjunctival pH equals 7.4 (about 20 minutes). To irrigate the superior cul-de-sac, retract the upper lid and instruct the patient to look down; to irrigate the inferior cul-de-sac, retract the lower lid and ask the patient to look up. Any particulate matter should be swept from the fornices with moist cotton swabs.[129]

After irrigation is completed, a thorough eye examination may be made. If there is any evidence of ocular damage (corneal opacification, conjunctival blanching, increased intraocular pressure), an ophthalmologist should be consulted immediately. Occasionally, emergency anterior chamber paracentesis is necessary to relieve pressure or to remove the toxic substance from the eye. This procedure is best performed by an ophthalmologist.[129]

The patient with severe chemical burns is admitted to the hospital for treatment and observation. Complications of this injury include corneal opacification, ulceration and perforation, glaucoma, cataract, retinal detachment, and adhesions of the eyelid to the globe.[129]

If examination reveals only corneal epithelial damage, the patient may be treated with topical antibiotics, cycloplegic (homatropine 2% to 5%), and patching. He or she should then be seen by an ophthalmologist within 24 hours.[129]

Radiation Injury

Prolonged exposure to sunlight, tanning lamps, or electric arcs without proper eye protection may result in ultraviolet keratitis. Ultraviolet light has deleterious effects on the cornea: the corneal epithelium swells and then cell death gradually occurs. Several hours after exposure, the patient notices a foreign body sensation that progressively worsens. Photophobia, redness, pain, tearing, and blepharospasm also occur. Diffuse punctate staining is seen on fluorescein examination. These injuries are treated similarly to corneal abrasions with cycloplegia, topical antibiotics, and patching (often bilateral). Oral narcotic medication may be needed for analgesia.[129]

Thermal Injury

Thermal injuries to the eye are rare; they are caused by contact with a hot object or liquid. Most produce superficial injury; however, deep injury may occur, especially from some liquids. If the injury is superficial, a corneal abrasion or superficial eschar results. The eschar may be removed with a moist cotton swab, then the eye is treated as for corneal abrasion. If necrosis of the cornea or sclera has occurred, emergency ophthalmologic consultation is indicated.[129]

Thermal burns to the eyelids should generally be treated by an ophthalmologist or a burn specialist. Scarring and contraction of the burned eyelid may expose the cornea. A lubricating eye ointment (e.g., Lacrilube) should be frequently applied. It may be necessary to place a moisture-retaining dressing over the eye.[129]

Prevention

Most ocular injuries are preventable.* For instance, many sports-related injuries can be prevented by improvements in equipment or supervision. Protective face shields on batting helmets could prevent more than one third of baseball-related eye injuries. Most tennis-related eye injuries result from the ball being thrown during unsupervised play, not during a tennis match. Hockey-related injuries also generally occur during unsupervised play.[161] Fireworks continue to cause serious eye injuries resulting in blindness. Bottle rockets are particularly dangerous. Attending public fireworks displays is generally safer than using fireworks at home.[180]

Although sports-related eye injuries are a leading cause of childhood eye injuries, they account for less than one third.[113] In the United States, the sports with the highest risk of eye injury are combative sports: baseball, basketball, hockey, football, soccer, and racquet sports.[181,182] The emergency physician must encourage safe behavior as well as proper use of headgear, seat belts, and other safety features. Lensless eye guards do not provide adequate eye protection.[181] Polycarbonate lenses and frames should be recommended as protective eyewear.[173] Children with poor vision in one eye should use polycarbonate lenses for constant wear.[116] Clearly, prevention is the most effective, least costly, and most efficient means of caring for the eye.

EAR INJURIES

When a patient who has isolated ear trauma enters the emergency department, management is often straightforward. On the other hand, if the patient has multisystem trauma, the injury to the ear may be overlooked. Of course, life-threatening injuries take precedence. However, once stabilization of the patient's condition and initial assessment have been achieved, a careful and thorough examination is mandatory to detect occult injuries of the ear.

Anatomy

The external ear consists of the auricle and the external ear canal. The ear lobe contains skin and underlying connective tissue. Excepting the lobe and the rim of the helix, the skin of the auricle closely adheres to the perichondrium of the auricular cartilage. The external ear canal extends medially to the tympanic membrane.[186]

The tympanic membrane faces interiorly and only slightly laterally in the newborn infant. By adulthood, it faces more laterally. The tympanic membrane separates the external from the middle ear. This cavity contains the malleus, incus, and stapes. The malleus articulates with the tympanic membrane and incus, the incus with the stapes, and the stapes with the oval window. The eustachian tube connects the pharynx with the middle ear cavity, permitting equalization of pressure on both sides of the tympanic membrane.[186]

*References 111-115, 118, 160, 161, 163, 175-185.

Within the petrous portion of the temporal bone lies the inner ear, a bony labyrinth encasing a membranous labyrinth containing endolymph. The fluid between the membranous and bony labyrinths is perilymph. The anterior part of this system is the cochlea, which changes sound vibrations into the nerve impulses that are perceived as hearing. The posterior part of this system contains the bony vestibule and three semicircular canals. The vestibule contains the membranous utriculus and sacculus, and the semicircular canals contain a membranous semicircular duct. This posterior portion of the inner ear is an organ of balance.[186]

Obviously the eighth cranial nerve is closely associated with the inner ear. However, cranial nerves III, IV, V, VI, and VII also have a close anatomic relationship with this area of the temporal bone. The facial nerve (VII) runs in a bony canal between the middle and inner ears. This relationship is important for detection of middle ear damage.[186,187]

Foreign Bodies in the External Ear Canal

Presence of foreign bodies in the external ear is a common occurrence in childhood. Children put foreign bodies into their own ears or those of playmates. Some foreign bodies (e.g., insects) find their own way into the external auditory canal (see Chapter 49).

Diagnostic Findings. It is useful to know how long the foreign body has been present, what it is, and how it entered. This may be a clue to the likelihood of associated infection and tympanic membrane or middle ear damage.

The first step is to examine the foreign body and, if possible, the tympanic membrane. If the tympanic membrane is known to be perforated, irrigation should be avoided. Similarly, if the foreign body is a vegetable substance that might swell when hydrated, avoid irrigation. A clawing insect may cause extreme discomfort and agitation, which may be alleviated by instilling 2% lidocaine hydrochloride into the ear canal. This kills the insect and provides almost instant relief.[188,189] A button battery in the external ear canal is especially dangerous because it may cause burns of the canal or tympanic membrane.[190]

Management. Several methods of management may be attempted.[191,192] The child may need to be restrained or sedated. If the foreign body is small, it may be helpful to use gravity to remove it or move it more laterally in the ear canal. This can be accomplished by putting the head in a horizontal posture with the involved ear downward. Gentle downward traction on the auricle allows the foreign body to "wiggle" out. If the foreign body becomes visible in the most lateral portion of the canal, leave the patient in that position. Then an alligator forceps may be used to grasp the foreign body. Alternatively, a curette or right angle forceps may be slipped behind it to complete the extrication.[193]

A forceps removal may be attempted by direct visualization. This method is most effective with irregularly shaped foreign bodies. Spherical foreign bodies are often difficult to remove with this method. The parents should be warned about possible bleeding. Using the largest speculum that is comfortable allows direct visualization of the foreign body; advance an alligator forceps through the speculum to grab it. The otoscopic speculum, forceps, and foreign body may then be gently removed as a single unit. This may require several attempts but is often successful.

An interesting modification of this technique uses "super" glue on the wooden end of a cotton swab stick. After contacting the foreign body, the stick is held in place for 1 minute so that it may bind to the foreign body. Then it is removed. If the foreign body is very close to the tympanic membrane, it may be possible to attempt irrigation first, provided irrigation is not relatively contraindicated.[193]

Irrigation may be accomplished by using a large syringe with soft, flexible tubing attached (often the tubing of a butterfly with the needle cut off) or a motorized irrigation system (Water Pik). Water temperature should be close to body temperature. A gentle stream should be used. It is sometimes helpful to combine this method with the positioning used in the gravity technique. A kidney-shaped basin catches the runoff. The technique may completely remove the foreign body or make it more accessible to the alligator forceps.[193]

Still another method is the suction approach. Constant wall suction with a suction catheter that fits loosely in the ear canal is recommended. A soft, pliable suction catheter is preferable to a rigid suction device. If the suction catheter cannot "grasp" the foreign body, it may be necessary to modify the tip of the catheter. One method is to create a flange-tipped catheter by inserting a tympanotomy tube into the tip of the catheter. This may be particularly helpful in the removal of spherical objects.[193]

After removal of the foreign body, the ear should be reexamined to ensure that no foreign material remains. Any damage to the tympanic membrane or the external ear canal should be noted, as well as the presence of any infection. Be sure to examine the contralateral ear for the presence of a foreign body. If the foreign body cannot be removed after a reasonable effort, it is best to refer the patient to an ear, nose, and throat (ENT) specialist. The urgency of referral depends on the patient's level of discomfort, the type of foreign body, and the presence of coexisting infection or tympanic membrane perforation.[193,194]

External Ear Trauma

Blunt Trauma. Blunt trauma to the external ear may cause ecchymoses that heal without any therapy. However, if any auricular hematoma forms, it must be evacuated. The hematoma occurs in a plane between the cartilage and the overlying perichondrium, interrupting the cartilaginous blood supply. Necrosis of the normal cartilage leads to formation of new cartilage close to the perichondrium. The new growth is abnormal and excessive in quantity and results in the deformity known as cauliflower (or wrestler's) ear.[187,194,195]

Auricular hematoma presents as a posttraumatic fluctuant or doughy blue mass on the external ear that disrupts the ear's normal architecture. Bilateral auricular hematomas suggest child abuse.[196]

Management consists initially of drainage and then application of a pressure dressing that will prevent reaccumulation.[187,195] An auricular hematoma can be drained with the patient supine. Sedation or restraints may be used as indicated. The area should be prepared and drained. Lidocaine for local anesthesia is effective.[187,195]

Needle aspiration may be attempted first with an 18 gauge or larger needle. However, if the blood has clotted, this technique will probably not be sufficient for evacuation and a 4- to 5-mm incision with a number 15 blade through the skin overlying the hematoma is made. A curved hemostat can break up the clot; direct digital pressure can facilitate squeezing the blood and clot out through the incision. Apply an antibacterial ointment, followed by a pressure dressing. Cotton balls wetted with saline solution can be molded to conform to the shape of the auricle. Then, dry 4 × 4s can be placed behind the ear and lateral to it to make a bulky dressing, which is held in place by a head cap made of surgical tube gauze. A hole should be cut in the cap for the contralateral ear. Other methods, such as stitching the dressing to the ear, have been used with success and may be more practical for a wrestler who wants to continue training.[195-197]

Lacerations, Avulsions, and Abrasions. Lacerations, avulsions, and abrasions of the external ear should be managed with the same principles as other comparable injuries. However, if a full-thickness laceration involves the helix, imprecise repair may result in notching or other deformity. Therefore some lacerations of the ear may require the expertise of a plastic surgeon. However, successful repair of uncomplicated lacerations may be accomplished by the emergency physician if good general wound care is observed.[187,195]

Anesthesia may be provided by a ring block around the base of the ear with 1% lidocaine. Debridement should be conservative. Some surgeons recommend skin-to-skin repair when possible and avoid suturing the cartilage. If sutures must be placed in the cartilage, it is important to remember that cartilage tears easily; sutures should not be close to the edge. Cartilage that is not covered by perichondrium may be resorbed. Sutures should be used sparingly and crossed between fragments (figure-of-eight) to prevent one piece of cartilage from overriding another. An absorbable, white 5-0 suture (Vicryl) is recommended.[187,195]

An alternative to suturing the cartilage as a separate layer is to use through-and-through sutures of monofilament nylon. Although good approximation of the cartilage is usually accomplished, it may be difficult to achieve good skin approximation by this method. Except for lacerations involving only the lobe, a pressure dressing should be applied to prevent formation of auricular hematoma.[187,195]

Significant *avulsion* of skin or perichondrium requires skin grafting and is best handled by a plastic surgeon. Small abrasions may be treated with topical antibiotic ointments.[195,198]

Any patient whose ear cartilage is even temporarily exposed to bacterial contamination may develop chondritis. The ear becomes red, tender, warm, and swollen. *Pseudomonas aeruginosa* is causative in 95% of cases, mixed with *Staphylococcus aureus* in up to 50%. The end stage of this rapidly progressive infection is loss of ear cartilage and a small, deformed pinna.[195] Hospitalization for intravenous antibiotics effective against *Pseudomonas* (ceftazidime 100 to 150 mg/kg/day q 8 hr IV [maximum 6 gm/day]) and *Staphylococcus* (nafcillin 100 to 150 mg/kg/24 hr q 6 hr [maximum 1 gm/dose]) provides the best possibility of preventing major deformity.

Amputations. Amputations of the ear, if complete, should be treated by wrapping the ear in moist, sterile gauze and cooled (but not frozen) until ready for replantation. Incomplete amputation of the ear should not be converted to a complete amputation. The blood supply to the ear is abundant. Even a small pedicle of skin may retain enough blood flow to sustain the partially amputated part.[195]

Burns. Burns of the ear should be treated in consultation with a burn specialist, but the same basic principles of burn management apply. Burns of the external ear canal may result in stenosis. Frostbite injury should be treated by rapid rewarming. Reexposure of the rewarmed ear to cold temperatures should be prevented.[195,199]

Tympanic Membrane Trauma

Trauma to the tympanic membrane may result from rapid changes in ambient pressure, which may be caused by flying, diving, explosives, or the slap of an open hand against the ear (see Chapter 45).[187,200,201] The tympanic membrane may also be perforated by a foreign body introduced through the external ear canal.

The most important aspect of treating injuries of the tympanic membrane is to be sure that they are isolated. The patient should receive thorough cranial nerve examination. The Weber test should be performed. Sound that lateralizes to the uninjured ear when the tuning fork is placed in the center of the forehead suggests sensorineural hearing loss in the traumatized ear. A fistula test should also be performed. To do this, positive pressure is applied to the external ear canal by pushing the tragus against the ear canal and holding it there for 15 seconds. Alternatively, a pneumatic otoscope can be used to apply the pressure. If the patient has nystagmus or vertigo, the test result is positive and suggests a labyrinthine fistula.[2] Mild hearing loss or mild tinnitus after concussive injury is usually transient but should prompt ENT evaluation within 24 hours.[202]

Evidence of cranial nerve (II, IV, V, VI, VII, or VIII) deficit, especially vertigo, nystagmus, positive fistula test result, facial paralysis, moderate to severe hearing loss, or moderate to severe tinnitus, suggests middle or inner ear trauma; urgent ENT consultation is indicated.[202]

Hemotympanum and CSF otorrhea suggest basilar skull fracture, discussed in Chapter 20. If the patient is free of these more severe symptoms, then an isolated injury to the tympanic membrane is the likely diagnosis.

In isolated tympanic membrane injuries pain occurs before perforation but may not be present afterward because of equalization of pressure. The patient may enter the emergency department because of fear of ear damage or because of a slight amount of bleeding from the ear. Often the perforation is an incidental finding of routine examination. The patient may or may not be able to recall the causative incident.[187]

Because the clot that forms after perforation tends to seal the perforation, irrigation or instillation of ear drops is relatively contraindicated in this setting. The examiner should try to ascertain whether a flap of tympanic membrane has been folded medially or laterally onto the tympanic membrane. If so, the patient should be referred to an ENT specialist. Because such flaps prevent healing, it is necessary for the specialist to unfold them. If the tympanic membrane has a simple perforation without folded flaps, it usually heals spontaneously.[203] Smaller and more centrally located perforations heal more readily than large or peripheral ones. The patient should keep the ear dry. Failure to heal within 2 to 3 weeks is cause for referral.[187]

If a perforation does not heal spontaneously, epithelium may grow through it. With time, it may develop into a cholesteatoma. This cystlike mass may expand in the middle ear and destroy adjacent structures. Therefore all tympanic membrane perforations should be reexamined in a few weeks to verify that healing has occurred without complication.[187,204,205] Blast injuries to the ear deserve prolonged follow-up.[206]

Middle and Inner Ear Trauma

Trauma to the middle or inner ear may result in discontinuity of the ossicular chain, labyrinthine damage, facial nerve or chorda tympani damage, or rupture of the oval or round window. Signs and symptoms of these injuries are discussed in the section on tympanic membrane trauma.

Tympanometry may help in diagnosis of ossicular discontinuity if the tympanic membrane is intact by showing an "open-topped" curve. A CT scan or polytomogram may yield additional information.[187,202] Emergency consultation of an ENT specialist is indicated when these injuries are suspected.

DENTAL INJURIES

Injuries to the primary or permanent teeth in the pediatric age group have been reported in up to 50% of all children.[207-213] The types of injuries to teeth vary with the developmental capability of the child. Children are more likely to injure their anterior teeth. Dental trauma in children between infancy and 3 years of age results from falling from or onto furniture, tripping when walking or running, or using strollers or walkers. All these mechanisms of injury reflect the lack of motor coordination or appropriate supervision at this age range. During the early school years, dental injuries are related to playground, bicycle, and pedestrian injuries and other falls. Dental injuries in adolescents are related to sports activities and assaults. Children at risk of dental injury are those who have significant incisal overbite; who have any condition that impairs motor or perceptual skills (e.g., cerebral palsy, visual impairment); or who participate in contact sports. Although boys have a slight predilection toward primary tooth injuries, they clearly are more likely to injure their permanent teeth than girls. It must be kept in mind that child abuse can also cause dental injury at any age. Consideration of the involvement of primary as well as underlying permanent teeth is important in the diagnosis and management of dental injuries in children.[212-217]

Dental Development

The development of the crown and root of teeth is of ectodermal origin beginning at the sixth week of embryonic life. The pulp of the tooth develops from a mesodermal invagination with alveolar bone surrounding the root.[218] The permanent teeth develop under the primary

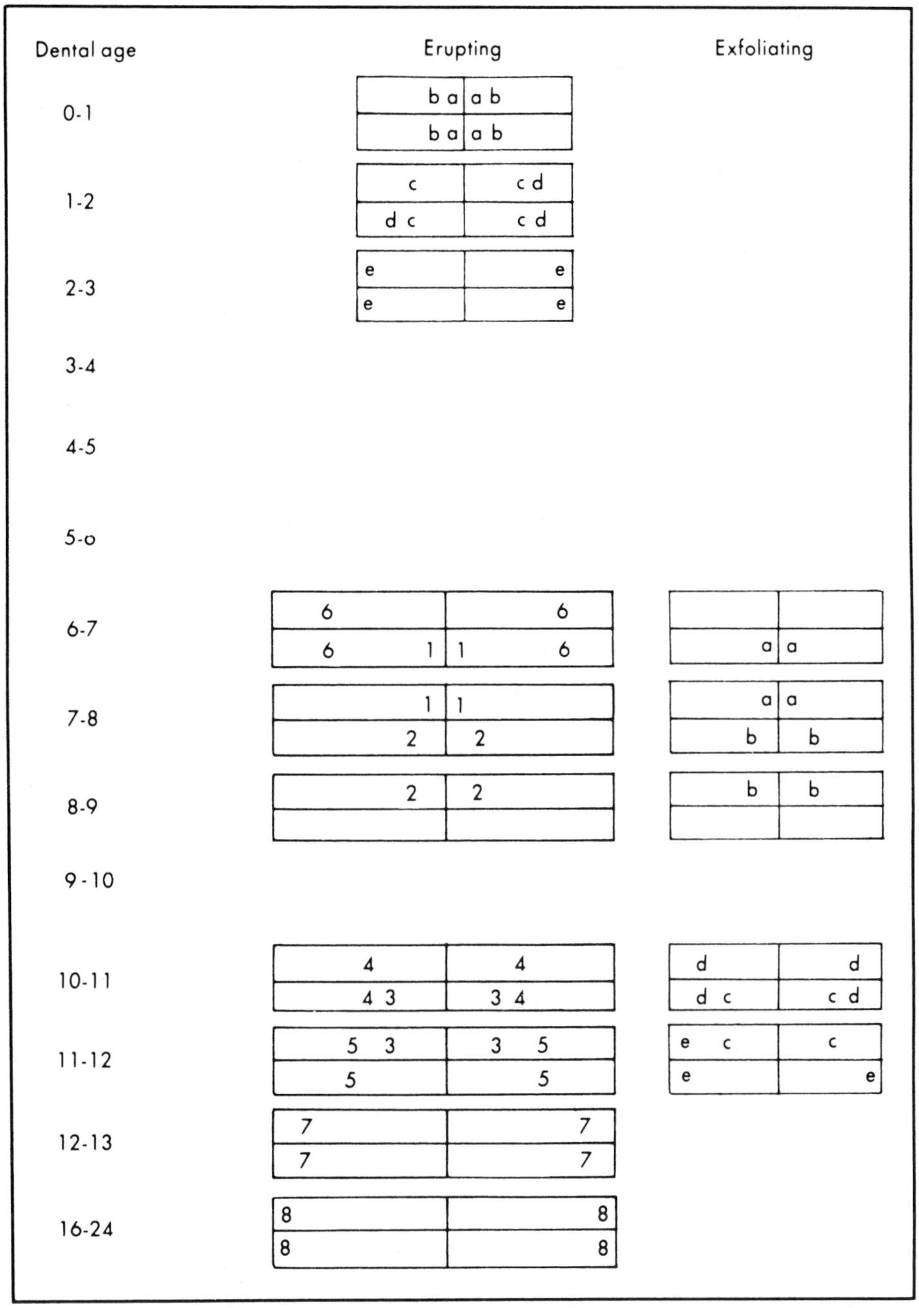

Dental age	Erupting		Exfoliating	
0-1	b a | a b			
	b a | a b			
1-2	c | c d			
	d c | c d			
2-3	e | e			
	e | e			
3-4				
4-5				
5-6				
6-7	6 | 6			
	6 1 | 1 6		a | a	
7-8	1 | 1		a | a	
	2 | 2		b | b	
8-9	2 | 2		b | b	
9-10				
10-11	4 | 4		d | d	
	4 3 | 3 4		d c | c d	
11-12	5 3 | 3 5		e c | c	
	5 | 5		e | e	
12-13	7 | 7			
	7 | 7			
16-24	8 | 8			
	8 | 8			

FIG. 21-9. Most common pattern of dental development. *a-e,* Primary teeth; *1-8,* secondary (permanent) teeth.

dentition and must be considered in patient management.[100,215]

Onset of the eruption of the primary and permanent teeth is important in determining the management of injuries. The first teeth to erupt are the lower incisors at about 6 months of age. Most frequently, teeth erupt in the following sequence: central incisors, 6 to 8 months; lateral incisors, 7 to 9 months; first molar, 12 to 14 months; cuspids, 16 to 18 months; second molar, 20 to 24 months. All 20 of the primary teeth have erupted by 3 years of age (Fig. 21-9). When the child is about 5 to 6 years of age the permanent teeth begin to erupt. The adult complement of 32 teeth should have erupted by ado-

lescence, with the possible exception of the third molars (wisdom teeth).[100,207-211,219-221]

Anatomy

Teeth are embedded in the bone (alveolar bone) of the maxilla and mandible. The tooth is divided into the visible portion called the *crown* and its base, which is below the gingival line, called the *root* (Fig. 21-10). The pulp is in the central part of the tooth, providing the blood circulation and innervation. The dentin overlays the pulp, which in turn is covered by the hard enamel. The gingiva, periodontal ligament, cementum, and alveolar bone hold the tooth

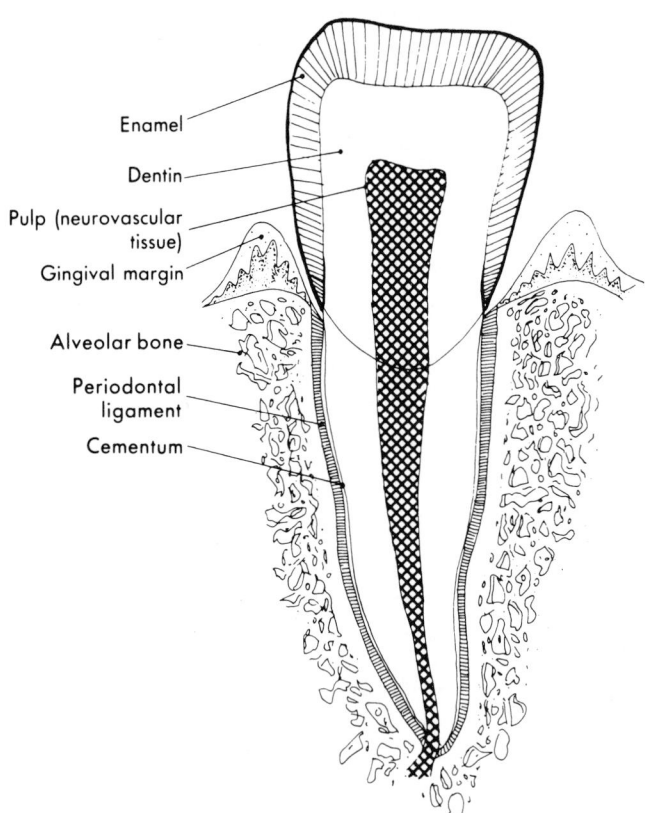

Enamel
Dentin
Pulp (neurovascular tissue)
Gingival margin
Alveolar bone
Periodontal ligament
Cementum

FIG. 21-10. Basic dental anatomy.

in place. Innervation of the teeth is via the superior alveolar nerve for the upper teeth and inferior alveolar nerve for the lower teeth. Blood supply is provided by the maxillary artery inferiorly and anterior superior alveolar artery.

Despite the various numbering systems for teeth, the anatomic name of the tooth should be used to describe the injury (e.g., right upper central incisor). Other anatomic terms used are *labial* or *buccal* to describe the outer surfaces; *palatal* to describe the interior side of the upper teeth; *lingual* to describe the interior surface of the lower teeth; and *occlusal* to describe the bite surfaces of the upper and lower teeth. *Apical* refers to position close to the root and *coronal* to the crown of the tooth.

Diagnostic Findings

A complete history should be obtained to determine the mechanism of injury, concomitant injuries, loss of tissue, immunization status, past medical history (immunodeficiency, cardiac disease, diabetes, musculoskeletal disorders, allergies, social problems), and developmental and neurologic status. An inconsistent history should alert the physician to the possibility of child abuse. Other important parts of the history are the presence or absence of tooth pain, response to thermal stimuli, and normal bite. It is important to determine if the tooth is primary or permanent, since management can vary.

Examination for orofacial trauma should proceed in the fashion described earlier. Evaluation of the airway, breathing, and circulation of the patient must be addressed and

managed before a more cursory secondary survey of the teeth. If oral intubation is indicated, preexisting dental trauma must be documented on initial laryngoscopy. On inspection, the external facial structures should be evaluated for contusions, lacerations, fractures, and dislocations. Evaluation of the gums and alveolar bone must be done to ensure stability of supporting structures. The anatomic relation of the tooth should be noted along with any gross fractures. Each tooth must be examined for mobility and tenderness to touch and thermal stimuli.

Plain radiographs are useful in diagnosing facial bone fractures associated with dental injuries. (See Tables 21-1 and 21-2) Panoramic radiographic views are very helpful when viewing the alveolus, mandible, and specific teeth. Specific bite radiographs taken aid evaluation of specific teeth and are usually made by a dentist.

Specific Dental Injuries

Luxations. Injuries that involve the periodontal ligament and alveolar bone causing a disruption of the supporting structures of the tooth are referred to as *luxations*. Damage to the periodontal ligament causes instability of the tooth, thus targeting the diagnosis and management to the viability of the anchoring structures.

The following terms describe the various luxations. *Concussion* occurs when the tooth maintains its stability with no displacement but may be painful or tender to pressure, percussion, and occlusion. *Subluxation* occurs when the tooth is mobile with less than 2 mm of displacement in its socket but stable with minimal damage to the periodontal ligament. Percussion sensitivity or a change in sensation may be noted by the child. *Intrusion* or traumatic impaction is a condition in which the tooth is impacted into its socket with laceration of the periodontal ligament and possible impingement of the permanent tooth bud. In *extrusion* the tooth is vertically dislodged in the socket with tearing of the periodontal ligament; this must be differentiated from intrusion. Lateral *luxation* occurs when mobility and tearing of the periodontal ligament with buccal, lingual, labial, or lateral displacement are present. In *avulsion* the tooth is completely detached from the alveolar socket with severance of the periodontal ligament and possibly alveolar fracture.

When examining the individual teeth, the physician must look for gross abnormalities and recognize the extent of luxations and fractures. In both primary and permanent teeth bleeding from the tooth or a pinkish color in the center indicates a pulp exposure requiring immediate dental consultation and management.

Management. The main objective in management of dental injuries is to preserve the integrity of erupted or unerupted permanent teeth. Teeth that have been injured are at risk of being devitalized by the disruption of blood flow to the pulp and lack of collateral circulation to the tooth. When the pulp is damaged, reversible hyperemia may occur, precluding necrosis of the root. Rupture of vessels stains the dentin, resulting in darkening of the tooth, which may become evident later. Injury to the periodontal ligament by luxation can lead to resorption of the root, dentoclastic activity, and ultimate destruction of the permanent tooth. Parents must be advised of the potential

TABLE 21-3. Management of Injuries to Primary and Permanent Teeth

Injury	Management
All tooth injuries	General guidelines: 1. Assess extent of injury 2. Seek concomitant injuries 3. Provide good pain management 4. Ensure immunizations are up to date 5. Obtain appropriate radiographs and dental consultation 6. All injuries need follow-up
Concussion (no displacement or fracture of tooth)	Management the same for primary and permanent teeth: 1. Pain management with analgesics 2. Parental reassurance 3. Follow-up with dentist in a few days
Subluxation (mobility without displacement)	Management the same for primary and permanent teeth: 1. Pain management with analgesics 2. No intervention to splinting by a dentist depending on the extent of mobility 3. Dental referral within 24 hours recommended
Intrusion (tooth pushed into socket)	Primary teeth: 1. Immediate dentist referral recommended 2. If intrusion is greater than one-half crown length, reeruption without intervention is likely 3. If tooth is in contact with underlying tooth by radiograph, extraction by dentist is recommended 4. Integrity of underlying tooth bud is primary consideration Permanent teeth: 1. Immediate dental referral 2. Allow tooth to reerupt on its own with close follow-up with dentist
Extrusion (tooth partially out of socket)	Primary teeth: 1. Immediate dental referral 2. With slight extrusion gently reposition tooth 3. If tooth very loose and almost out, extraction is recommended Permanent teeth: 1. Immediate dental referral 2. Aggressive repositioning with splinting by a dentist
Lateral luxation (buccal, lingual, labial, or lateral displacement of tooth)	Primary teeth: 1. Immediate dental referral 2. With minimal displacement or mobility no therapy other than repositioning is recommended 3. Avoid injury to permanent tooth buds Permanent teeth: 1. Immediate dental referral 2. Repositioning and splinting by dentist

Continued.

discoloration. If pulpal injury is undiagnosed, an abscess may form at the root. Pulpal exposure and evulsion of the tooth both require immediate attention. All dental injuries, especially those of primary teeth, can lead to damage of permanent teeth. Good follow-up observation after any dental injury may prevent unnecessary tooth damage (Table 21-3).[212,215,222]

Concussion. In a concussion, there is injury to the supporting structures but the tooth maintains stability without displacement. There is generally no bleeding or mobility of the tooth but there is significant pain to percussion. The parents must be reassured and periodic evaluation by a dentist is recommended. Management is the same for both primary and permanent teeth.[215,216,222]

Subluxation. Subluxation is when there is mobility of the tooth without displacement (lateral luxation, extrusion, intrusion) as a result of damage to the supporting structures. The tooth is in place with obvious mobility. Bleeding may be present at the margin of the gums, a result of damage to the supporting structures. There is discomfort to percussion. Management ranges from no intervention to splinting, depending on the degree of mobility and the age of the patient. Both primary and permanent subluxations are managed the same way. Because of the potential for pulp necrosis, patients must have referral to a dentist the next day with close follow-up.[215,216,222]

Intrusion. Intrusion is when the tooth is pushed into the socket by an axial force. There is obvious "shortening" of

TABLE 21-3. Management of Injuries to Primary and Permanent Teeth—cont'd

Injury	Management

Avulsion (tooth completely displaced from socket)	General guidelines:
	1. Locate tooth as it may be intruded, aspirated, fractured, lost. Obtain radiographs (face, chest, abdomen) as indicated
	2. Differentiate primary from permanent tooth
	3. Immediate dental referral for avulsion of permanent teeth
	4. Permanent teeth must be placed in following transport medium in decreasing order of preference
	    a. Hank's Balanced Salt Solution (Save-A-Tooth)
	    b. Fresh cold milk
	    c. Saline
	    d. Saliva (buccal vestibule)
	    e. Water
	Primary teeth:
	1. Do not replant
	2. Control bleeding
	3. Dental referral as needed
	Permanent teeth:
	1. Extra-oral time less than one hour: replant immediately after removing debris
	2. Extra-oral time greater than one hour: replant tooth after soaking it in Hank's Balanced Salt Solution or a dental fluoride solution for 20-30 minutes
	3. Splinting by dentist
	4. Systemic antibiotics
	5. Chlorhexidine oral rinses
	6. Close follow-up by dentist

Fractures (break in integrity of enamel, dentin, pulp) Crown fractures	General guidelines (see above): 1. Object is to avoid injury to underlying primary tooth and to preserve viability of tooth
Enamel infractions (incomplete break through enamel only)	Management the same for primary and permanent teeth: 1. No treatment necessary 2. Dental referral as needed
Ellis Class I (fracture through enamel only)	Management the same for primary and permanent teeth: 1. No treatment 2. Dental referral to smooth out edges of tooth
Ellis Class II (fracture through enamel or dentin)	Management the same for primary and permanent teeth: 1. Immediate dental referral 2. Preserve integrity of underlying permanent teeth 3. Calcium hydroxide application and repair by dentist
Ellis Class III (fracture through enamel, dentin, and pulp)	Management the same for primary and permanent teeth: 1. Immediate dental referral 2. Calcium hydroxide with subsequent composite repair by dentist
Crown root (fracture involving the crown or root)	Management the same for primary and permanent teeth: 1. Immediate dental referral 2. Primary teeth generally extracted 3. Permanent tooth needs evaluation by dentist for method of treatment based on radiograph
Root (fracture through root)	Management the same for primary and permanent teeth: 1. Immediate dental referral 2. Management dependent on radiographic findings

the intruded tooth with bleeding. Root and alveolar fractures may occur. Usually primary teeth will reerupt depending on the extent of injury and digital and labial pressure placed by the child. In primary teeth, when the intrusion is less than half the crown length, reeruption is likely and no further intervention is indicated. If contact between the primary tooth and underlying permanent tooth bud is confirmed or suspected by radiography, the tooth must be extracted. The intruded tooth is extracted if it does not reerupt in 3 to 4 weeks. Once reerupted, most primary teeth follow normal resorption or replacement. This type of injury requires immediate referral and guidance by a dentist. The integrity of the underlying permanent tooth bud is of prime consideration.[215,222]

Controversy surrounds the exact management of intruded permanent teeth. Allowing the tooth to reerupt on its own or orthodontically extruding the tooth over 3 to 4 weeks seems to be the most popular way to manage these injuries. Immediate referral to a dentist is critical.[215,216,222]

Extrusion. In extrusion, the tooth is shown, by clinical examination or radiograph, to be partially or almost completely out of its socket. As in luxation, the integrity of the supporting structures of the tooth must be evaluated. In primary teeth that are slightly extruded, gentle pressure is applied to reposition the tooth. If the tooth is almost avulsed or very mobile, extraction is preferable. Permanent teeth that are extruded require aggressive supporting repositioning and splinting for best results. In either case, immediate dental referral is recommended with subsequent close follow-up.[215,222]

Lateral Luxation. In primary teeth, the tooth is most commonly displaced lingually, thus decreasing the chance of underlying permanent tooth bud injury. Unless there is extreme mobility in the tooth or the tooth is laterally displaced, no therapy is needed other than repositioning. Immediate dental referral is recommended.

In permanent teeth, lateral luxation requires repositioning and splinting. As with primary teeth, permanent teeth need immediate dental referral.[215,222]

Avulsion. Avulsion is when the tooth is completely knocked out of the alveolar socket. The physician must determine whether the tooth is primary or permanent, as this guides management (see Fig. 21-9). When the patient does not present with the tooth, all efforts must be made to find it. Radiographs must be obtained to rule out the possibility of the tooth being lodged in the airway, lungs, esophagus, stomach, or intruded into the respective alveolar socket or adjacent structure (i.e., sinus, bone, nasal cavity).[215]

Avulsed primary teeth are never replaced. This is due to the potential for pulp necrosis with subsequent inflammation and damage to the underlying permanent tooth bud.[215,223]

The philosophy on the management of avulsed permanent teeth has recently changed.[224] The object of management is to restore the tooth's viability, which is dependent on the vitality of the root periodontal ligament (PDL) cells. The amount of extra oral time, the status of the PDL cells, and the stage of root development are important factors in the success rate of reimplantation. Principles taken into consideration of permanent tooth avulsions include the use of biologic or appropriate storage media; avoidance of further damage to PDL cells; timing to reimplantation; careful handling and cleaning of the tooth prior to reimplantation; splinting; and immediate referral to a dentist with follow-up.[223-227]

Immediately after a tooth has been avulsed it must be replanted. If the tooth is contaminated with debris, rinse off the root with water, saline, or appropriate storage media. Do not scrape the root. If the tooth can not be replanted immediately, it should be kept moist by placing it in the following transport media in decreasing order of preference: (1) Hank's Balanced Salt Solution (H.B.S.S.), also known as Save-A-Tooth; (2) fresh cold milk; (3) saline; (4) saliva (buccal vestibule); or (5) water (if nothing else is available). The tooth must be kept moist at all times.[224-227]

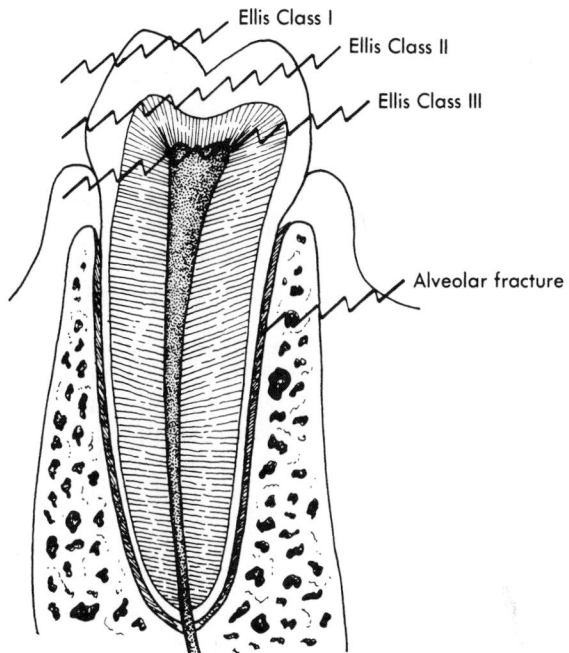

FIG. 21-11. Ellis classification for fractures of anterior teeth.

When the patient presents to the emergency department with a tooth with an extra-oral time of less than one hour, replant the tooth immediately after gently removing debris. If the extra-oral dry time is greater than one hour, soak the tooth in H.B.S.S. or a dental fluoride solution (2% stannous fluoride, sodium fluoride) for 20 to 30 minutes and then replant it.[224-226]

To prevent damage to the PDL cells keep the tooth moist at all times; hold the tooth by the crown, not the root; clean contaminated roots with H.B.S.S., saline, or water; lightly scrub excess debris with a sponge or cotton tip applicator; and never brush, scrape or modify the root.[224]

Before replacing the tooth, the socket can be prepared by lightly aspirating or irrigating out the blood clot (do not enter socket); by separating alveolar bone flaps gently with blunt probe; by manually compressing separated alveolar bone around the reimplanted tooth; and by not curetting or venting the socket.[224]

All avulsions need immediate dental consultation, referral, and follow-up. Splinting to stabilize the tooth and endodontics are done by the dentist. After reimplantation, systemic antibiotics (penicillin or equivalent), chlorhexidine oral rinses, good oral hygiene counseling, analgesics, and reassurance are recommended. Prognosis of the replanted tooth depends on the above mentioned factors. These patients need follow-up with a dentist for a minimum of five years.[224,225]

Dental Fractures. Fractures of the teeth involve a break in the integrity of the tooth and may include surrounding structures; these fractures may involve various layers of the tooth at different levels (i.e., crown, root). The Ellis classification shown in Fig. 21-11 shows how crown fractures are classified. Crown injuries vary in their direction (horizontal, oblique, vertical) and are considered class I, when the fracture line involves only the enamel; class II, when the line is through the enamel and dentin; and class III, when fractures involve the enamel, dentin, and pulp.

Crown-root fractures have an angulated line through the crown and root. Root fractures are apical, midapical, and coronal (closer to the crown). The mobility of the crown reflects the depth of the fracture. Alveolar fractures are often associated with dental trauma, which must be sought. Root fractures are diagnosed by x-ray studies and vary in their severity and prognosis depending on the extent of underlying disruption.[107,215]

Management. Radiograph evaluation by a dentist is very important in the evaluation and management of such injuries. Infractions, nondisplaced fractures (cracks) in the tooth, require no treatment other than dental follow-up. Fractures of the enamel (class I) in primary and permanent teeth require no further treatment other than dental follow-up observation. The sharp edges of the tooth may need to be smoothed down by a dentist to relieve any discomfort.

Crown fractures of the enamel and dentin (class II) in primary and permanent teeth require dental consultation. The exposed tubules in the dentin can be a conduit for bacteria and other irritants to cause inflammation of the pulp. The tooth may have greater thermal sensitivity. A calcium hydroxide coating may be applied along with repair of the tooth with a composite resin.[215,216]

Crown fractures with pulpal exposure (class III) need immediate attention by a dentist. The exposed surface may be covered with calcium hydroxide or a root canal performed, depending on the extent of pulpal exposure and interval since the injury. If the pulp is exposed for more than 6 hours, the possibility of a pulp infection with abscess formation is more likely. An infection in the primary tooth may affect the developing tooth bud and is an important factor in managing such injuries.[215,218,219,225]

Crown-root fractures of primary teeth are generally treated by extraction. In permanent teeth, treatment is predicated on the integrity of the remaining root fragment. Outcome after root canal therapy is better when more of the root is intact. Replacement of the tooth fragment has a poor prognosis. All injuries require immediate dental referral.

Root fractures are diagnosed radiographically and are clinically suspected when there is luxation of the crown. In both primary and permanent teeth the prognosis is better when the fracture line is closer to the apex of the root (apical). The greater the mobility of the tooth, the more likely the fracture is closer to the crown (coronal). The more coronal the fracture, the poorer the prognosis. Both primary and permanent teeth may be extracted if the fracture is more coronal or possibly splinted if the fracture is apical.[215,216]

References

1. Division of injury control, Center for environmental health and injury control, centers for disease control. Childhood injuries in the United States, *Am J Dis Child* 144:627, 1990.
2. Kaban LB: Facial trauma. I. Midface fractures. In Kaban LB, editor: *Pediatric oral and maxillofacial surgery,* Philadelphia, 1990, WB Saunders.
3. Kaban LB: Facial trauma. II. Dentoalveolar injuries and mandibular fractures. In Kaban LB, editor: *Pediatric oral and maxillofacial surgery,* 1990, Philadelphia, WB Saunders Co.
4. Manson PN: Skull and midface injuries. In Mustarde JC and Jackson IT, editors: *Plastic surgery in infancy and childhood,* ed 3, Edinburgh, 1988, Churchill Livingstone.
5. Moos KF and El-Attar: Mandible and dental injuries. In Mustarde JC and Jackson IT, editors: *Plastic surgery in infancy and childhood,* ed 3, Edinburgh, 1988, Churchill Livingstone.
6. Dufresne CR and Manson PN: Pediatric facial trauma. In McCarthy JG, editor: *Plastic surgery: the face,* vol. 2, Philadelphia, 1990 WB Saunders Co.
7. Crockett DM, Mungo RP, Thompson RE: Maxillofacial trauma, *Pediatr Clin North Am* 20:1471, 1989.
8. Hunter JG: Pediatric maxillofacial trauma, *Pediatr Clin North Am* 39:1127, 1992.
9. Hussain K et al: A comprehensive analysis of craniofacial trauma, *J Trauma* 36:34, 1994.
10. Fingerhut L and Kleinman J: Trends and current statistics of childhood mortality, United States, 1900-1985, *Vital Health Stat* 26:1, 1989.
11. Committee on Trauma Research, Commission of Life Sciences, National Research Council. Institute of Medicine. *Injury in America: a continuing public health problem,* Washington DC, 1985, National Academy Press.
12. National Safety Council: *Accident facts: 1988,* Chicago, 1988, National Safety Council.
13. Baker SP, O'Neil B, Ginsburg MJ, et al: *The injury fact book,* ed 2, New York, 1992, Oxford University Press.

Anatomy

14. Scott JH: Further studies on the growth of the human face, *Proc R Soc Med* 52:263, 1959.
15. Enlow DH: *Handbook of facial growth,* ed 2, Philadelphia, 1982, WB Saunders.
16. Precious DS, Delaire J, Hoffman CD: The effects of nasomaxillary injury on the future facial growth, *Oral Surg* 66:525, 1988.
17. Ouster DK and Vargervik K: Maxillary hypoplasia secondary to maxillofacial trauma in childhood, *Plast Reconstruct Surg* 80:491, 1987.

Diagnostic Findings

18. Sinclair D, Schwartz M, Gruss J, et al: A retrospective review of the relationships between facial fractures, head injuries and cervical spine injuries, J Emerg Med 6:109, 1988.
19. Lim LH, Lam LK, Moore MH, et al: Associated injuries in facial fractures: review of 839 patients, Br J Plast Surg 46:635, 1993.
20. Capan LM: Airway management. In Capan LM, Miller SM, Turndorf H, editors: *Trauma anesthesia and intensive care,* Philadelphia, 1991, JB Lippincott Co.
21. American Heart Association: *Textbook of pediatric advanced life support,* Dallas, 1994, American Heart Association.
22. American College of Surgeons: *Advanced trauma life support student manual,* Chicago, 1993, College of Surgeons.
23. Holihan JA, Lubart S, Ellis A, et al: Pediatric trauma resuscitation: nursing aspects. In Eichelberger MR and Pratsch GL, editors: *Pediatric trauma care,* Rockville, Md, 1988, Aspen Publishers.
24. Mayer TA: Evaluation and general management of the injured child. In Mayer TA, editor: *Emergency management of pediatric trauma,* Philadelphia, 1985, WB Saunders.
25. Mazurek A: Anesthesia for the trauma patient. In Touloukian RJ, editor: Pediatric trauma, ed 2, St. Louis, 1990, Mosby.
26. Spicer TE: Facial and soft tissue trauma in childhood. In Mayer TA, editor: Emergency management of pediatric trauma, Philadelphia, 1985, WB Saunders Co.
27. Mealy J: Skull fractures. In Mclaurin RL, Venes JL, Schut L, et al, editors: *Pediatric neurosurgery,* ed 2, Philadelphia, 1989, WB Saunders.
28. Lee CY, McCullum C, Blaustein DI: Pediatric chin injury: occult condylar fractures of the mandible, *Pediatr Emerg Care* 7:160, 1991.
29. Swischuk LE: *Emergency radiology of the acutely ill or injured child,* ed 3, Baltimore, 1994, Williams & Wilkins.
30. Manson PN. Facial injuries. In McCarthy JG, editor: *Plastic surgery,* vol 2, Philadelphia, 1990, WB Saunders.

31. Miller JH and Schatz CJ: Facial and temporal bone trauma. In Swin JL and Stanley P, editors: *Diagnostic imaging in pediatric trauma*, Berlin, 1980, Springer-Verlag.

32. Broumand SR: The role of three-dimensional computed tomography in the evaluation of acute craniofacial trauma, *Ann Plast Surg* 31:488, 1992.

Soft Tissue Injuries

33. Converse JM and Dingman RO: Facial injuries in children. In Converse JM, editor: *Reconstructive plastic surgery*, Philadelphia, 1977, WB Saunders Co.

34. Stucker FJ, Bryarly RC, Shockley WW: Management of nasal trauma in children, *Arch Otolaryngol* 110:190, 1984.

35. East CA and O'Donaghue GO: Acute nasal trauma in children, *J Pediatr Surg* 22:308, 1987.

36. Donaldson JD: Otologic trauma. In Healy GB, editor: *Common problems in pediatric otolaryngology*, Chicago, 1990, Year Book.

37. Rabuzzi DD and Hengeren AS: Complications of nasal and sinus infections. In Bluestone CD, Stool SE, Scheetz M, editors: *Pediatric otolaryngology*, ed 2, Philadelphia, 1990, WB Saunders Co.

38. Stahl RS and Seashore JH: Soft tissue injuries. In Touloukian RJ, editor: *Pediatric trauma*, St. Louis, 1990, Mosby.

39. LaRossa D and Whitaker LA: Soft tissue injuries. In Welch KJ, Randokf JG, Ravitch, et al, editors: *Pediatric surgery*, Chicago, 1986, Year Book.

40. Raine PA and Azmy A: A review of thermal injuries in young children, *J Pediatr Surg* 18(1):21, 1983.

41. East MK, Jones CA, Feller I, et al: Epidemiology of burns in children. In Carvajal HF and Parks DH, editors: *Burns in children: pediatric burn management*, Chicago, 1988, Year Book Medical Publishers, Inc.

42. Mani MM and Rubin WD: Treatment of burns. In Mustarde JC and Jackson IT, *Plastic surgery in infancy and childhood*, ed 3, Edinburgh, 1988, Churchill Livingstone.

43. Libber SM and Stayton DJ: Childhood burns reconsidered: The child, the family, and the burn injury, *J Trauma* 19:670, 1984.

44. Hamond JS and Ward CG: Burns of the head and neck, *Otolaryngol Clin North Am* 16:679, 1983.

45. Lund CC, Browder NC: The estimation of areas of burns, *Surg Gynecol Obstet* 79:352, 1944.

46. Zucker RM: Initial management of the burn wound. In Carvajal HF, Parks DH, editors: *Burns in children: pediatric burn management*, Chicago, 1988, Year Book Medical Publishers, Inc.

47. Wachtel TL: Topical antimicrobials. In Carvajal HF and Parks DH, editors: *Burns in children: pediatric burn management*, Chicago, 1988, Year Book.

48. Housinger TA, Hills J, Warden GD: Management of pediatric facial burns, *J Burn Care Rehabil* 15:408, 1994.

49. Blandford SE: Electrical burns of the mouth in children, *Rocky Mt Med J* 65(6):25, 1968.

50. Fogh-Anderson P and Sorenson B: Electric mouth burns in children: treatment and prevention, *Acta Chir Scand* 131:214, 1966.

51. Palin WE, Sadove AM, Jones JE, et al: Oral electrical burns in a pediatric population, *J Oral Med* 42(1):17, 1987.

52. Pitts W, Pickrell L, Quinn G, et al: Electrical burns of the lips and mouth in infants and children, *Plast Reconst Surg* 44:471, 1969.

53. Thomsen HG, Juckes AW, Farmer AW: Electrical burns to the mouth of children, *Plast Reconst Surg* 35:466, 1965.

54. Salman RA, Glickman RS, Super S: Splint therapy for electrical burns of the oral commissure in children, *J Dent Child* 54:161, 1987.

55. Sadove AM, Jones JE, Lynch TR, et al: Appliance therapy for perioral electrical burns: a conservative approach, *J Burn Care Rehabil* 9:391, 1988.

56. Orgell MG, Brown HC, Woolhouse FM: Electrical burns of the mouth in children: a method for assessing results, *J Trauma* 15:285, 1975.

57. Chasman LR: Electrical burns, *Can Med Assoc J* 97:453, 1967.

58. Mladnick RA: Electrical burns of the mouth in children, *Arch Dermatol* 105:296, 1972.

59. Cooney BM: Conservative management of oral electrical burns: report of a case successfully treated, *Int J Orthop* 24(3-4):12, 1986.

60. Marunick M: Prosthetic management of electrical burns to the oral commissures, *J Mich Dent Assoc* 68:529, 1986.

61. Hartford CE, Kealy GP, Lavelle WE, et al: An appliance to prevent and treat microstomia from burns, *J Trauma* 15:356, 1975.

62. Barone CM, Hulnick SJ, Grigsby de Linde L, et al: Evaluation of treatment modalities in perioral electrical burns, *J Burn Care Rehabil* 15:335, 1994.

63. Selbst SM: Managing pain in the pediatric emergency department, *Pediatr Emerg Care* 5:56, 1989.

64. Selbst SM and Henretig FM: The treatment of pain in the emergency department, *Pediatr Clin North Am* 36:949, 1989.

65. Willcock M: Drugs, dosages and dangers, *Emerg Med* 14:100, 1982.

66. Altman RS, Smith-Coggins R, Ampel LL: Local anesthetics, *Ann Emerg Med* 14:1209, 1985.

67. Zeltzer LK, Jay SM, Fisher DM: The management of pain associated with pediatric procedures, *Pediatr Clin North Am* 36:965, 1989.

68. Pryor GJ, Kilpatrick WR, Opp DR: Local anesthesia in minor lacerations: topical TAC versus lidocaine infiltration, *Ann Emerg Med* 9:568, 1980.

69. Bonadio WA and Wagner V: Efficacy of TAC topical anesthesia for repair of pediatric lacerations, *Am J Dis Child* 142:203, 1988.

70. Nicols FC, Macha P, Farnell MB: TAC topical anesthetic and minor lacerations, *Resid Staff Physician* 33:59, 1987.

71. Hegenbarth MA, Alteri MF, Hawk WH, et al: Comparison of topical tetracaine, adrenaline, and cocaine anesthesia with lidocaine infiltration for repair of lacerations in children, *Ann Emerg Med* 19:63, 1990.

72. Droner SC: Complications of TAC (letter), *Ann Emerg Med* 12:333, 1983.

73. Ernst AA, Marvez E, Nick TG, et al: Lidocaine adrenaline tetracaine gel versus tetracaine adrenaline cocaine gel for topical anesthesia in scalp and facial lacerations in children aged 5 to 17 years, *Pediatrics* 95:255, 1995.

74. Shilling CG, et al: Tetracuine, epinephrine (adrenalin), and cocaine (TAC) versus lidocaine, epinephrine and tetracaine (LET) for anesthesia of lacerations in children, *Ann Emerg Med* 25:203, 1995.

75. Eldich RF, Rodeheaver GT, Morgan RF, et al: Principles of wound management, *Ann Emerg Med* 17:1284, 1988.

76. Stevenson TR and Jurkiewicz MJ: Plastic and reconstructive surgery. In Schwartz SI, Shines GT, Spencer FC, et al, editors: *Principles of surgery*, ed 5, New York, 1989, McGraw-Hill.

77. Callaham M: Controversies in antibiotic choices for bite wounds, *Ann Emerg Med* 17:1321, 1988.

78. Lindsay WK: Lips, tongue and floor of mouth. In Mustarde JC and Jackson IT, editors: *Plastic surgery in infancy and childhood*, ed 3, Edinburgh, 1988, Churchill Livingstone.

79. Maisel RH and Mathog RH: Injuries to the mouth, pharynx and esophagus. In Bluestone CD, Stool SE, Scheetz M, editors: *Pediatric otolaryngology*, ed 2, Philadelphia, 1990, WB Saunders.

80. Maceri DR: Trauma: Nasal trauma. In Krause CJ, editor: *Otolaryngology—head and neck surgery*, St. Louis, 1986, Mosby.

81. McGill TJ: Foreign bodies in the aerodigestive tract. In Fredreckson JM, editor: *Otolaryngology—head and neck surgery*, St. Louis, Mosby.

Facial Fractures

82. Bartlett SP and Delozier III JB: Controversies in the management of pediatric facial fractures, *Clin Plast Surg* 19:245, 1992.

83. Anderson PJ: Fractures of the facial skeleton in children, *Injury* 26:47, 1995.

84. Panagopoilos AP: Management of fractures of the jaws in children, *J Int Coll Surg* 28:806, 1957.

85. Graham GG and Peltier RJ: Management of mandibular fractures in children, *J Oral Surg* 18:416, 1960.

86. McCoy FJ, Chandler RA, Crow ML: Facial fractures in children, *Plast Reconstr Surg* 37:209, 1966.

87. Rowe NL: Fractures of the facial skeleton in children, *J Oral Surg* 26:505, 1968.

88. Bales CR, Randal P, Lehr HB: Fractures of the facial bones in children, *J Trauma* 12:56, 1972.

89. Waite DE: Pediatric fractures of the jaw and facial bones in children, *J Trauma* 12:56, 1972.

90. Reil B and Krantz S: Traumatology of the maxillofacial region in childhood, *J Maxillofac Surg* 4:197, 1976.

91. Kaban LB, Mulliken JB, Murray JE: Facial fractures in children, *Plast Reconstr Surg* 59:15, 1977.

92. Ramba J: Fractures of the facial bones in children, *Int J Oral Surg* 14:472, 1985.
93. McGraw BL and Cole RR: Pediatric maxillofacial trauma: age-related variations in injury, *Arch Otolaryngol Head Neck Surg* 116:41, 1990.
94. Agran PA and Duncle DE: Motor vehicle occupant injuries of children in crash and non-crash events, *Pediatrics* 70:993, 1982.
95. Agran PF, Dunke DE, Winn DG: Motor vehicle childhood injuries caused by non-crash falls and ejections, *JAMA* 253:2530, 1985.
96. Robert R and Shopfnex CE: Plain skull roentgengeons in children with head trauma, *Am J Roentgenol* 114:230, 1972.
97. Thaller SR, Huang V: Midfacial fractures in the pediatric population, *Ann Plast Surg* 29:348, 1992.
98. Ousterhout DK and Vargevik: Maxillary hypoplasia secondary to midfacial trauma in childhood, *Plast Reconstr Surg* 80:491, 1987.
99. Precious DS, Delaire J, Hoffman CD: The effects of nasomaxillary injury on future facial growth, *Oral Surg Oral Med Oral Pathol* 66:525, 1988.
100. Koeng WR, Olsson AB, Pensler JM: The fate of developing teeth in facial trauma: tooth buds in the line of mandibular fractures in children, *Ann Plast Surg* 32:503, 1994.
101. Chuong R, Mulliken JB, Kaban LB, et al: Fragmented care of facial fractures, *J Trauma* 27:477, 1987.
102. Chandler RJ: Traumatic cerebrospinal fluid leakage, *Otolaryngol Clin North Am* 16:623, 1983.
103. Jones DT, McGill TJ, Healy GB: Cerebrospinal fistulas in children, *Laryngoscope* 102:443, 1992.
104. Goldstein FP, Rosenthal SA, Garancis JC, et al: Varieties of growing skull fractures in childhood, *J Neurosurg* (war surgery supplement) 1:81, 1970.
105. Sekhar LN and Scarff TB: Pseudogrowth of skull fractures in childhood, *Neurosurgery* 6:285, 1980.
106. Bertolami CN and Kaban LB: Chin trauma: a clue to associated mandibular and cervical spine injury, *Oral Surg* 53:122, 1982.
107. O'Karinen KS: Clinical mangement of injuries to the maxilla, mandible, and alveolus, *Dent Clin North Am* 39:113, 1995.
108. Klotch D: Use of rigid internal fixation in the repair of complex comminuted mandible fractures, *Otolaryngol Clin North Am* 20:495, 1988.
109. Danforth HB: Mandibular fractures: use of acrylic splints for immobilization, *Laryngoscope* 79:280, 1969.

Ocular Injuries

110. Apt L and Sarin LK: Causes for enucleation of the eye in infants and children, *JAMA* 181:948, 1962.
111. Macewen CJ: Eye injuries: a prospective survey of 5671 cases, *Br J Ophthalmol* 73:888, 1989.
112. LaRoche GE, McIntyre L, Schertzer RM: Epidemiology of severe eye injuries in childhood, *Ophthalmology* 95:1603, 1988.
113. Strahlman E, Elman M, Daub E, et al: Causes of pediatric eye injuries: a population-based study, *Arch Ophthalmol* 108:603, 1990.
114. Niiranen M and Raivoi I: Eye injuries in children, *Br J Ophthalmol* 65:436, 1981.
115. Patel BC: Penetrating eye injuries, *Arch Dis Child* 64:317, 1989.
116. Klein BR and Sears ML: Eye injury, *Pediatr Rev* 13(4):127, 1992.
117. Sastry SM, Paul BK, Bain L, et al: Ocular trauma among major trauma victims in a regional trauma center, *J Trauma* 34(2):223, 1993.
118. Cascairo MA, Mazow ML, Prager TC: Pediatric ocular trauma: a retrospective survey, *J Pediatr Ophthalmol Strabisimus* 31:312, 1994.
119. Tielsch JM and Parver LM: Determinants of hospital charges and length of stay for ocular trauma, *Ophthalmology* 97(2):231, 1990.
120. Hollingshead WH: The ear, orbit, and nose. In *Textbook of anatomy*, ed 3, New York, 1984, Harper and Row.
121. Boyar C: Ocular examination, *Emerg Med Clin North Am* 6:111, 1988.
122. Ing EB, Sullivan TJ, Clarke MP et al: Oculomotor nerve palsies in children, *J Pediatr Ophthalmol Strabismus* 29(6):331, 1992.
123. Arts HA, Eisele DW, Duckert LG: Intraocular pressure as an index of ocular injury in orbital fractures, *Arch Otolaryngol Head Neck Surg* 115:213, 1989.
124. Catalano RA: Eye injuries and prevention, *Pediatr Clin North Am* 40(4):827, 1993.
125. Hague S and Cooling RJ: Ocular trauma, *Practitioner* 22:181, 1988.

126. Wulc AE and Arterberry JF: The pathogenesis of canalicular laceration, *Ophthalmology* 98(8):1243, 1991.
127. Klein BR and Sears ML: Pediatric ocular injuries, *Pediatr Rev* 13(11):422, 1992.
128. Waterhouse W, Enzenauer RW, Parmley VC: Inflammatory orbital tumor as an ocular sign of a battered child, *Am J Ophthalmol* 114(4):510, 1992.
129. Lubeck D and Greene JS: Corneal injuries, *Emerg Med Clin North Am* 6:73, 1988.
130. Elkington AR and Khaw PT: Injuries to the eye, *Br Med J* 297:122, 1988.
131. Deutsch TA: Ocular emergencies in childhood, *Pediatrician* 17:173, 1990.
132. Wedge CI and Rootman DS: Collagen shields: efficacy, safety and comfort in the treatment of human traumatic corneal abrasions and effect on vision in healthy eyes, *Can J Ophthalmology* 27(6):295, 1992.
133. Clinch TE, Robinson MJ, Barron BA, et al: Fungal keretitis from nylon line lawn trimmers, *Am J Opthalmol* 114(4):437, 1992.
134. Turturro MA, Paris PM, Arffa R, et al: Contact lens complications, *Am J Emerg Med* 8:228, 1990.
135. Joondeph BC: Blunt ocular trauma, *Emerg Med Clin North Am* 6:147, 1988.
136. Zerihum N: Blast injuries of the eye, *Topical Doctor* 23:76, 1993.
137. Joseph E, Zak R, Smith S, et al: Predictors of blinding or serious eye injury in blunt trauma, *J Truama* 33(1):19, 1992.
138. Fong LP: Secondary hemorrhage in traumatic hyphema. Predictive factors for selective prophylaxis, *Ophthalmology* 101:1583, 1994.
139. Ng CS, Strong NP, Sparrow JM, et al: Factors related to the incidence of secondary hemorrhage in 462 patients with traumatic hyphema, *Eye* 6 pt 3:308, 1992.
140. Farber MD, Fiscella R, Goldberg MF: Aminocaproic acid versus prednisone for the treatment of traumatic hyphema, *Ophthalmology* 98(3):279, 1991.
141. Volpe NJ, Larrison WI, Hersh PS, et al: Secondary hemorrhage in traumatic hyphema, *Am J Ophthalmol* 112(5):507, 1991.
142. Kearns P: Traumatic hyphema: a retrospective study of 314 cases, *Br J Opthalmol* 75:137, 1991.
143. Little BC and Aylward GW: The medical management of traumatic hyphaema: a survey of opinion among ophthalmologists in the UK, *J Roy Soc Med* 86(8):458, 1993.
144. Deans R, Noel LP, Clarke WN: Oral administration of tranexamic acid in the management of traumatic hyphema in children, *Can J Ophthalmology* 27(4):181, 1992.
145. Hiatt RL: Eye trauma in children, *So Med J* 84(6):747, 1991.
146. Spoor TC: Traumatic hyphema in an urban population, *Am J Opthalmol* 109(6):23, 1990.
147. Bloom JN: Traumatic hyphema in children, *Pediatr Ann* 19:368, 1990.
148. Levy I, Wysenbeek YS, Nitzan M, et al: Occult ocular damage as a leading sign in the battered child syndrome, *Metab Pediatr Syst Ophthal* 13:20, 1990.
149. Koenig SB, Ruttum MS, Lewandowski MF, et al: Pseudophakia for traumatic cataracts in children, *Ophthalmology* 100(8):1218, 1993.
150. Sinskey RM, Stoppel JO, Amin P: Long-term results of intraocular lens implantation in pediatric patients, *J Cataract Refrac Surg* 19:405, 1993.
151. Boorstein JM, Titelbaum DS, Patel Y, et al: CT diagnosis of unsuspected traumatic cataracts in patients with complicated eye injuries: significance of attenuation value of the lens, *Am J Roent* 164(1):181, 1995.
152. Werner MS, Dana MR, Viana MA, et al: Predictors of occult scleral rupture, *Ophthalmology* 101(12):1941, 1994.
153. Shrader SK, Bond JD, Lauter CB, et al: The clinical spectrum of endophthalmitis: incidence, predisposing factors, and features influencing outcome, *J Infect Dis* 162(1):115, 1990.
154. Paton D, Hyman BN, Justice J Jr: Introduction to ophthalmoscopy, Kalamazoo, Mich, 1982, Uphohn.
155. Buys YM, Levin AV, Enzenauer RW, et al: Retinal findings after head trauma in infants and young children, *Ophthalmology* 99(11):1718, 1992.
156. Elner SG, Elner VM, Arnall M, et al: Ocular and associated systemic findings in suspected child abuse, *Arch Ophthalmology* 108:1094, 1990.

157. Talwar D, Kumar A, Verma L, et al: Ultrasonography in optic nerve head avulsion, *ACTA Ophthalmol* 69(1):121, 1991.
158. Cohen HL, Eidelman EM, Kaufman I: Traumatic central retinal artery occlusion: diagnosis by color doppler imaging, *J Ultra Med* 12(7):411, 1993.
159. Culbertson WW: Diagnosis and management of ocular injuries, *Otolaryngol Clin North Am* 16:563, 1983.
160. Sternberg P and Aaberg TM: The persistent challenge of ocular trauma, *Am J Ophthalmol* 107:421, 1989.
161. Nelson LB, Wilson TW, Jeffers JB: Eye injuries in childhood: demography, etiology, and prevention, *Pediatrics* 84:438, 1989.
162. Rudd JC, Jaeger EA, Frietag SK, et al: Traumatically ruptured globes in children, *J Pediatr Ophthalmol Strabismus* 31(5):307, 1994.
163. Lubniewski A, Olk RJ, Grand G: Ocular dangers in the garden: a new menace-nylon lawn trimmers, *Ophthalmol* 95:906, 1988.
164. Williams DF, Mieler WF, Abrams GW, et al: Results and prognostic factors in penetrating ocular injuries with retained intraocular foreign bodies, *Ophthalmology* 95:911, 1988.
165. Baxter RJ, Hodgkins PR, Calder I, et al: Visual outcome of childhood anterior perforating eye injuries: prognostic indicators, *Roy Coll Ophthal* 8:349, 1994.
166. Thompson JT, Parver LM, Enger CL, et al: Infectious endophthalmitis after penetrating injuries with retained intraocular foreign bodies, *Ophthalmology* 100(10):1468, 1993.
167. Lubeck D: Penetrating ocular injuries, *Emerg Med Clin North Am* 6:127, 1988.
168. O'Day DM, Smith RS, Gregg ER, et al: The problem of bacillus species infection with special emphasis on the virulence of bacillus cereus, *Ophthalmology* 88:833, 1981.
169. O'Day DM, Parrish CM: Traumatic endophthalmitis, *Int Ophthalmol Clin* 27:112, 1987.
170. Schwartz JG, Somerset JS, Harrison JM, et al: Eye injuries with metal missiles presenting to an emergency center: a three year study, *Am J Emer Med* 9(4):313, 1991.
171. Lin DT, Webster RG, Abbot RL: Repair of corneal lacerations and perforations, *Int Ophthalmol Clin* 28:69, 1988.
172. Raynor LA: Treatment for inadvertent cyanoacrylate ankyloblepharon: a case report, *Ophthalmol Surg* 17(3):176, 1986.
173. Kimbrough RL: Conservative management of cyanoacrylate ankyloblepharon: a case report, *Ophthalmol Surg* 17(3):176, 1986.
174. Allar RM: Most cyanoacrylate super-glues should be removed promptly (letter), *Ophthalmol Surg* 18(2):156, 1987.
175. Shingleton BJ: Eye injuries, *N Engl J Med* 325:408, 1991.
176. Parver LM, Dannenberg AL, Blacklow B, et al: Characteristics and causes of penetrating eye injuries reported to the national eye trauma system registry, 1985-91, *Public Health Reports* 108(5):625, 1993.
177. Fong LP: Eye injuries in Victoria, Australia, *Med J Austr* 162(2):64, 1995.
178. Dannenberg AL, Parver LM, Fowler CJ: Penetrating eye injuries related to assault, *Arch Ophthalmol* 110(6):849-52, 1992.
179. Cantani A, Bamonte G: Epidemiology of ocular complications of childhood head trauma, *Ped Emer Care* 6(4):271, 1990.
180. American Academy of Pediatrics Committee on injury and poison prevention: Children and fireworks, *Pediatrics* 88(3):652, 1991.
181. Farber AS: Preventing eye injuries. What to tell patients, *Postgrad Med* 89(5):121-2,127-8, 1991.
182. Larrison WI, Hersh PS, Kunzweiler T, et al: Sports-related ocular trauma, *Ophthalmology* 97(10):1265, 1990.
183. Liggett PE, Pince KJ, Barlow W, et al: Ocular trauma in an urban population, *Ophthalmology* 97(5):581, 1990.
184. Nichols CJ, Boldt HC, Mieler WF, et al: Ocular injuries caused by elastic cords, *Arch Ophthalmology* 109(3):371, 1991.
185. Patel BCK and Morgan LH: Work-related penetrating eye injuries, *ACTA Ophthalmologica* 69:377, 1991.

Ear Injuries

186. Hollinshead WH: The ear, orbit, and nose. In *Textbook of anatomy*, ed 3, New York, 1984, Harper & Row.
187. Turbiak WR: Ear trauma, *Emerg Med Clin North Am* 5:243, 1987.
188. O'Toole K, Paris PM, Stewart RD, et al: Removing cockroaches from the auditory canal: controlled trial, *N Engl J Med* 312:1197, 1985.
189. Schittek A: Insect in the external auditory canal—a new way out, *JAMA* 243:331, 1980.

190. Rachlin S: Assault with battery, *N Engl J Med* 311:921, 1984.
191. Brownstein DR and Hodge D, III: Foreign bodies of the eye, ear, and nose, *Pediatr Emerg Care* 4:215, 1988.
192. Cuomo MD, Sobel RM: Concrete impaction of the external auditory canal, *Emerg Med Clin North Am* 5:183, 1987.
193. Fritz S, Kelen GD, Sivertson KT: Foreign bodies of the external auditory canal, *Emerg Med Clin North Am* 5:183, 1987.
194. Pride H and Schwab R: A new technique for removing foreign bodies of the external auditory canal, *Pediatr Emerg Care* 5:135, 1989.
195. Templer J and Renner GJ: Injuries of the external ear, *Otolaryngol Clin North Am* 23:1003, 1990.
196. Manning SC, Casselbrant M, Lammers D: Otolaryngologic manifestations of child abuse, *Int J Pediatr Otorhinolaryngol* 20:7, 1990.
197. Schuller DR, Dankle SD, Strauss RH: A technique to treat wrestler's auricular hematoma without interrupting training or competition, *Arch Otolaryngol Head Neck Surg* 115:202, 1989.
198. Kirsch JP and Amadee RG: Management of external ear trauma, *J Louisiana State Med Soc* 143(10):13, 1991.
199. Ngim RCK: The burned ear (I): an experimental study with the rabbit model to evaluate scalding temperature, surface and histopathologic appearance, and healing responses with depth of injury, *Ann Acad Med Singapore* 21(5):597, 1992.
200. Knapp JF, Sharp RJ, Beatty R, et al: Blast trauma in a child, *Pediatr Emerg Care* 6:122, 1990.
201. Berger G, Finkelstein Y, Harell M: Non-explosive blast injury of the ear, *J Laryngol Oto* 108:395, 1994.
202. Bellucci RJ: Traumatic injuries of the middle ear, *Otolaryngol Clin North Am* 16:633, 1983.
203. Armstrong W: Traumatic perforations of the tympanic membrane: observe or repair, *Laryngoscope* 82:1822, 1972.
204. Hanigan WC, Peterson RA, Njus G: Tin ear syndrome: rotational acceleration in pediatric head injuries, *Pediatrics* 80:618, 1987.
205. Garth, RJN: Blast injury of the auditory system: a review of the mechanisms and pathology, *J Laryngol Otol (Eng)* 108:925, 1994.
206. Wolf, M, Ben-Shoshan, J, Roth Y, et al: Blast injury of the ear, *Mil Med* 156(12)651, 1991.

Dental Injuries

207. Andreasen JO: Challenges in clinical dental traumatology, *Endodont Dent Traumatol* 1:45, 1985.
208. Ravn JJ: Dental injuries in Copenhagen school children, school years 1967-1972, *Community Dent Oral Epidemiol* 2:231, 1974.
209. Andreasen JO: Etiology and pathogenesis of traumatic dental injuries: a clinical study of 1298 cases, *Scand J Dent Res* 78:339, 1970.
210. Gutz DP: Fractured permanent incisors in clinic population, *J Dent Child* 38:94, 1971.
211. O'Neal DW, Clark MV, Lowe JW, et al: Oral trauma in children: a hospital survey, *Oral Surg Oral Med Oral Pathol* 68:691, 1989.
212. Gutmann JL, Gutmann MS: Cause, incidence, and prevention of trauma to teeth, *Dent Clin North Am* 39:1, 1995.
213. Harrington MS, Eberhart AF, Knapp JF: Dentofacial trauma in children, *J Dent Child* 55:334, 1988.
214. Needleman HL: Orofacial trauma in child abuse: types prevalence, management and the dental profession's involvement, *Pediatr Dent* 8:71, 1986.
215. Wilson CF: Management of trauma to primary and developing teeth, *Dental Clin North Am* 39:133, 1995.
216. Josell SD: Evaluation, diagnosis, and treatment of the traumatized patient, *Dent Clin North Am* 39:15, 1995.
217. Andreason JO: Examples and diagnosis of dental injuries. In Andreasen JO, editor: *Traumatic injuries to the teeth*, Philadelphia 1981, WB Saunders.
218. Moore KL: The integumentary system: the skin and related structures. In Moore KL, editor: *The developing human*, Philadelphia, 1988, WB Saunders.
219. Woelfel JB: Terminology. In Woelfel JB, editor: *Dental anatomy: its relevance to dentistry*, ed 4, Philadelphia, 1990, Lea & Febiger.
220. Wolford GD and Mathog RH: Development of teeth and fracture of the jaw in children. In Mathog RH, editor: *Maxillofacial trauma*, Baltimore, 1984, Williams & Wilkins.
221. Dierks EJ: Management of associated dental injuries in maxillofacial trauma, *Otolaryngol Clin North Am* 24:165, 1991.

222. Dumsha TC: Luxation injuries, *Dent Clin North Am* 39:79, 1995.

223. Coccia CT: A clinical investigation of root resorption rates and reimplanted permanent incisors: a five year study. *J Endod* 6:413, 1980.

224. American Association of Endodontists: *Treatment of the avulsed permanent tooth:* recommended guidelines of the American Association of Endodontists, 1995.

225. Trope M: Clinical management of the avulsed tooth, *Dent Clin North Am* 39:93, 1995.

226. Krasner P and Rankow H: New philosophy for the treatment of avulsed teeth, *Oral Surg Oral Med Oral Path* 79:616, 1995.

227. Hiltz J and Trope M: Vitality of human lip fibroblasts in milk, Hanks Balance Salt Solution and viaspan storage media, *Endod Dent Traumatol* 7:69, 1991.

CHAPTER

22

Neck and Spinal Cord Trauma

Francisco A. Medina

More than 10,000 people sustain spinal cord injuries (SCI) annually in the United States, usually from vehicular trauma, significant falls, diving accidents, sporting accidents, or personal assault.[1] Unlike head injuries, cervical spine injuries are rarely diagnosed in children.

During the first decade of life, the most frequent cause of SCI are motor vehicle accidents, followed by firearm injuries.[2] Young children may be injured as pedestrians, as well as passengers.[3] Spinal injuries in pedestrians hit by automobiles occur mainly in children younger than 10 years.[2] The type and degree of injury sustained as a passenger in a motor vehicle depends on several factors, including the age of the victim and passenger restraint among others. Violent shaking by adult caretakers may cause injury with minimal outward signs of abuse, although retinal hemorrhage and intracranial pathology may be evident.[4,5] SCI at the time of birth is associated with breech delivery or intrauterine hyperextension of the neck (the "stargazing neonate").[6]

During the second decade, sports and recreational activities account for 44% of injuries and motor vehicle accidents for 37% of cases.[7-9] Diving injuries are significant as well. Lifeguard personnel must be aware of the potential for spinal injury in the drowning victim. Males have a higher incidence of SCI than females, with a ratio greater than 2:1.[2]

Penetrating SCI from missiles, knife blades, and other sharp objects are reported to be the second most common cause of spinal cord damage in children younger than 14 years.[10] Additionally, there have been isolated reports of electrical injuries and industrial accidents that have resulted in significant spinal injuries.

Up to 40% of patients who sustain SCI die before hospitalization as a result of respiratory failure or concurrent massive head, chest, or abdominal trauma. Eighty percent of patients with severe multiple traumas have neurologic injury, which ultimately determines the prognosis. One tenth of victims are younger than 15 years, one half require hospitalization. Postmortem radiographic studies of victims of traffic accidents have identified 21.1% of the fatal injuries as cervical spine injuries.[11] The social, economic, and psychologic sequelae are catastrophic.

Eighty percent of patients hospitalized for SCI survive with varying degrees of neurologic deficit, including permanent paralysis. When managed appropriately in the prehospital and emergency department settings, the risk of permanent disability may be reduced. Mortality from SCI has decreased by 24% over the last 30 years as a result of improvements in the trauma care system.[12] Underdiagnosis or failure to recognize neurologic abnormalities in children represents the most serious error. This chapter offers the emergency physician dealing with children a review of the important aspects of the anatomy of the pediatric neck and spine; pathophysiology and classification of neck, vertebral, and spinal cord injuries; clinical and radiologic findings of children at different ages; stabilization; treatment; and complications.

ANATOMY AND BIOMECHANICS

The neck contains three major systems: neurologic, respiratory, and cardiovascular. The larynx and trachea are the most anterior of the vital cervical structures and therefore

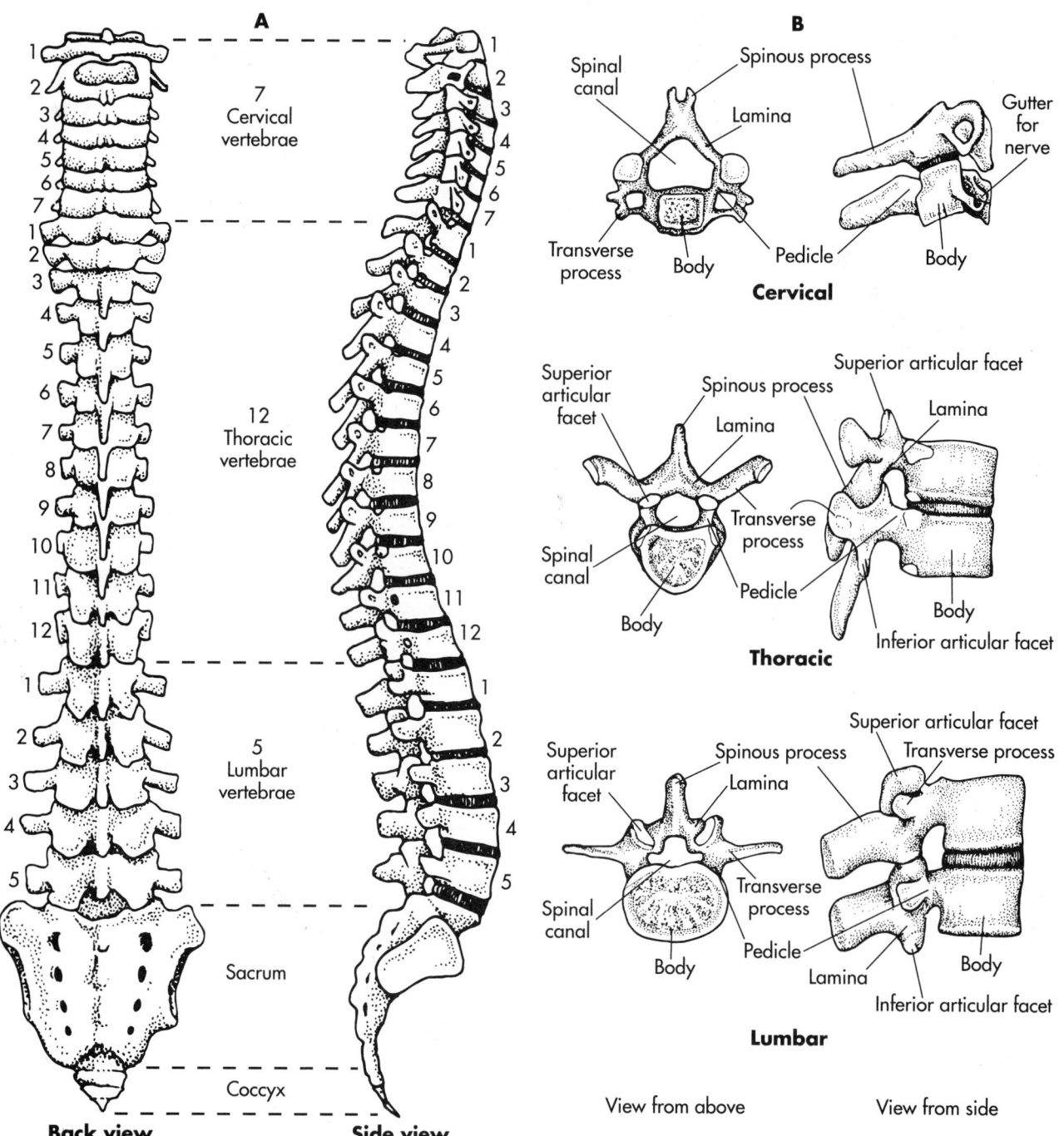

FIG. 22-1. **A,** Vertebral column. **B,** Typical vertebrae. (*From Rosen P et al:* Emergency medicine, *ed 4, St. Louis, 1997, Mosby.*)

are prone to be damaged by blunt or sharp objects. The spinal cord—with the support elements of the neck, including the vertebral bodies, muscles, and ligaments—is the most posterior structure. The esophagus and the major blood vessels lie among these structures. The intimate anatomic relationships found in the neck increase the risk of structural damage, and the initial evaluation and management of neck injuries must be planned and executed well.

The pediatric spine can best be understood by review of the development with increasing age and the several nor-

mal anatomic variants and physiologic adaptations seen in children compared with the adult spine. The pediatric spine exhibits hypermobility, characteristic vertebral configurations, epiphyseal growth plates, synchondrosis, incomplete ossification, and several normal variations and congenital anomalies.

The human spine comprises 33 bony vertebrae: 7 cervical, 12 thoracic, 5 lumbar, 5 sacral (fused), and 4 coccygeal (fused) (Fig. 22-1). Flexible intervertebral disks separate the bony structures, gaining stability through ligamentous attachments.[13] The intervertebral disks are hyaline fibrocartilage and gelatinous material. The central area of the disk, the nucleus pulposus, contains an amorphous gelatinous material. The peripheral annulus fibrosus has an outer layer of collagenous fibers and an inner layer of collagenous fibers mixed with cartilage or fibrocartilage.

In addition to providing basic structural support for the upright torso of the human being, the vertebral column serves as a protective encasement for the spinal cord. It is helpful to think of the spine as two parallel, connected columns: the anterior vertebral bodies and the posterior elements enveloping the neural canal. The anterior column of alternating vertebral bodies and disks is held in alignment by the anterior and posterior longitudinal ligaments. The posterior column protecting the spinal canal consists of pedicles, transverse processes, articulating facets, laminae, and spinous processes. It is held in alignment by the ligamentous structures: supraspinous, interspinous, and infraspinous; the capsular ligaments; and the flava ligaments (Fig. 22-2).

Biomechanical concepts of stability of the spine can be complex and confusing.[14,15] The disruption of one of the columns may cause a mechanically unstable spine, depending on the integrity of the ligamentous structures supporting the involved column. However, if both columns are disrupted at one level, the lesion is considered unstable, and a slight motion may result in a SCI. Spinal cord damage may occur independent of lack of stability of the spine. Unstable injuries have been reported after falls from distances of just a few feet.[16,17] The overall incidence of SCI that occur with vertebral injuries has been reported to be 14%.[18]

Approximately half the spinal canal is occupied by the subarachnoid space with equal volumes in front and behind the spinal cord. The cerebellar tonsils may extend 1 to 2 mm into the cranial end of the posterior subarachnoid space. The epidural space in the cervical spinal canal is narrow and mainly vascular; small amounts of fat and connective tissue are present.

The neural foramina are short canals that allow the cervical nerves to exit anteriolateral from the spinal canal. The dorsal and ventral nerve roots arise along the dorsolateral and ventrolateral aspects of the cord. The dorsal root, posterior and superior to the ventral root, has an enlargement called the dorsal root ganglion that lies posterior to the vertebral artery.

Cervical Spine

At birth, the entire spine forms a single shallow curve, concave to the anterior surface. The cervical spine curve does not become apparent until the head control develops.[19] Voluntary or reflex (from pain) muscular contraction may obliterate the normal cervical lordosis.

There is considerable mobility of the upper segments of the cervical spine, especially the forward movement of the second on the third cervical vertebrae. Movement at this level is common in healthy infants and younger children; Bailey observed that this shift may be as large as 3 mm. Sullivan noted that the third cervical vertebra may shift on the fourth by 3 to 4 mm.[20-23] The most mobile joint space with greatest angular displacement is at C3 to C4 for 3- to 8-year-olds, C4 to C5 for 9- to 11-year-olds, and C5 to C6 for 12- to 15-year-olds.

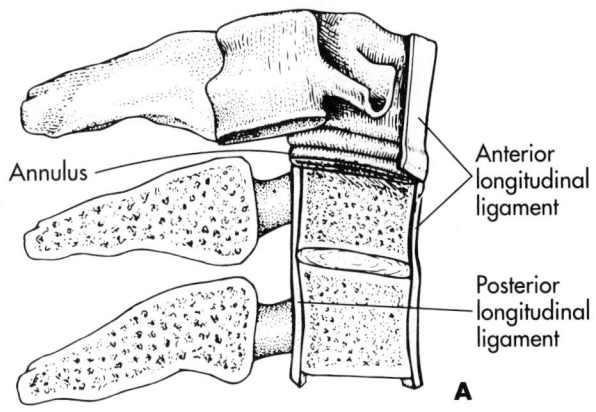

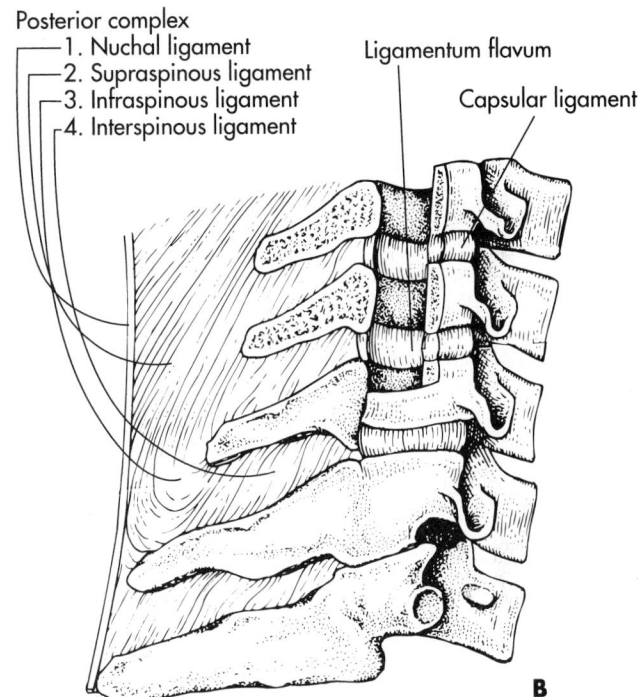

FIG. 22-2. **A,** Ligaments of anterior column. **B,** Ligaments of posterior column. (*From Rosen P et al: Emergency medicine, ed 4, St. Louis, 1997, Mosby.*)

The occipitoatlantoaxial complex presents unique anatomic considerations. The ligamentous structure, the assimilation of the body of C1 to C2 as the dens, and the fact that the articular facets lie in a relatively horizontal plane permit extreme freedom of motion in sagittal flexion and extension at the occipitoatlanto joint and in axial rotation at the atlantoaxial joint.

The *atlas* (C1) moves in union with the occiput. Ossification centers of the atlas vary with age[19] (Fig. 22-3); usually two are present at birth. Each center forms a lateral mass; the neural arch unites posteriorly by 3 to 4 years of age. A third ossification center appears at 1 year and forms the anterior arch, which fuses with the lateral masses by 7 to 10 years.

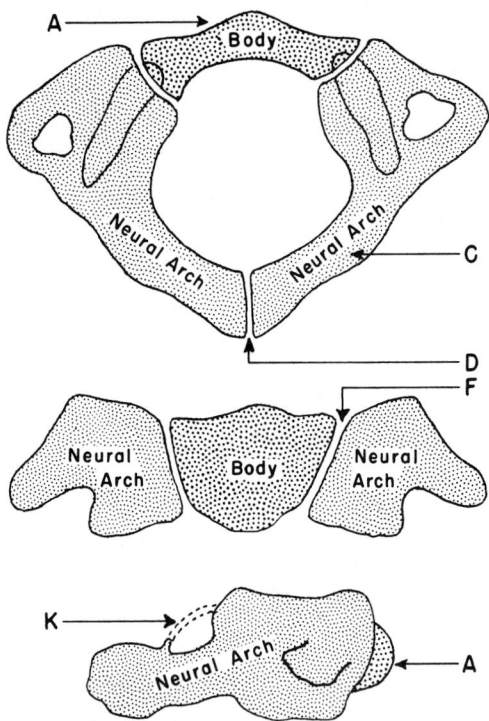

FIG. 22-3. Developmental components of the first cervical vertebra (atlas). *A,* Ossification center for the anterior arch, which may normally appear during the last fetal or the early postnatal months. *C,* Components of the dorsal segment of the neural arch that may appear as ossification centers as early as the third fetal month. *D,* Synchondrosis that binds the neural arch together at its dorsal extremity in the midsaggital plane of the spinous process. Rarely, an independent ossification center may appear in this synchondrosis. *F,* Neurocentral synchondroses that bind the vertebral body (anterior arch in C1) to the neural arches on both sides, which gradually diminish and disappear during last half of childhood. *K,* Ligament that crosses behind superior vertebral notch may ossify to form a superior vertebral foramen in adults. *(Redrawn from Bailey DK: Radiology 59:712, 1952 for Silverman FN: Caffey's pediatric x-ray diagnosis, ed 9, Chicago, 1993, Year Book.)*

The *axis* (C2) has five primary ossification centers (Fig. 22-4).[19] The two centers of the odontoid process fuse at birth and form the base of the dens. The other primary centers are present at birth and form the body and neural arches of the axis. An epiphyseal growth plate separates the odontoid from the axis; it appears as a lucent horizontal line for the first 3 to 6 years. The odontoid (*dens*) process of C2 rests posterior to the anterior arch of C1 and anterior to the transverse atlantal ligament, permitting rotation of the neck.

The cruciate ligament of the occipito-atlanto-axial complex comprises an atlantal transverse portion attached to the lateral masses of the atlas medially by way of insertions on osseous tubercles, and triangular ascending and descending bands that attach to the foramen magnum and body of C2, respectively. The atlantal transverse is the largest, strongest, and thickest ligament of the upper cer-

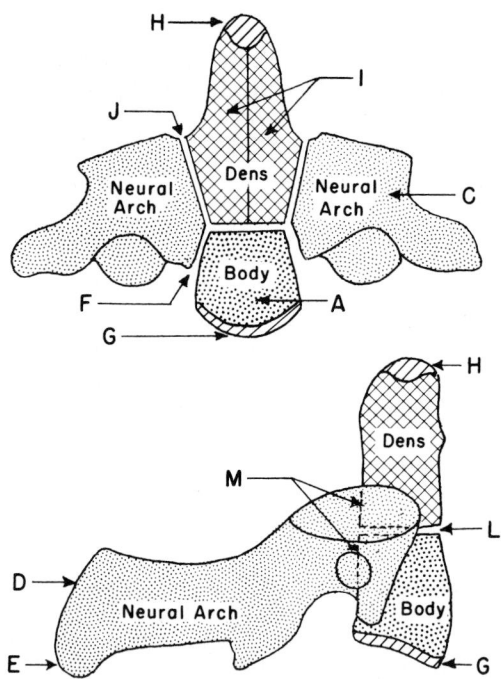

FIG. 22-4. Developmental elements in the second cervical vertebra *(axis). A,* Body, a single ossification center usually appears during the fourth fetal month. *C,* Neural arches appear in paired ossification centers by sixth fetal month. *D,* Neural arches that fuse posteriorly during third and fourth years. *E,* Bifid spinous process. *F,* Neurocentral synchondroses that disappear when the body and pedicles fuse during the fourth to seventh years. *G,* Inferior vertebral ring that ossifies during the late years of childhood and fuses with the body during early life. This ring is not part of an epiphysis and contributes nothing to growth of the vertebral body. *H,* "Summit" ossification center of the odontoid that appears between second and sixth years, then fuses with the main mass of the odontoid at 11 to 12 years. *I,* Odontoid process or dens. Two independent ossification centers appear during the fifth fetal month, then usually fuse during the seventh fetal month. *J,* Synchondroses that bind base of the dens on each side to the neural arches and disappear between 3 and 7 years. *L,* Synchondrosis between the dens and body, which disappears between 3 and 7 years. *M,* Posterior surfaces of dens and body. *(Redrawn from Bailey DK: Radiology 59:712, 1952 for Silverman FN: Caffey's pediatric x-ray diagnosis, ed 9, Chicago, 1993, Year Book.)*

vical spine.[24-26] It is the most important ligamentous structure of the occiput-C1-C2 region and is the main stabilizing component of the ligaments of the atlantoaxial complex. The neck of the odontoid process—constricted where the transverse ligament passes posteriorly, forming a tight band behind the dens and confining this process within the articular notch on the anterior arch of C1—fixes the atlas on the axis, allowing normal atlantoaxial rotation to occur within a 47-degree range of motion and preventing anterior subluxation of C1 on C2.[25,27] The tranverse ligament is nonelastic and rigid[25] and can rupture in the central portion or at the insertions at the lateral masses of C1.[28-30] The

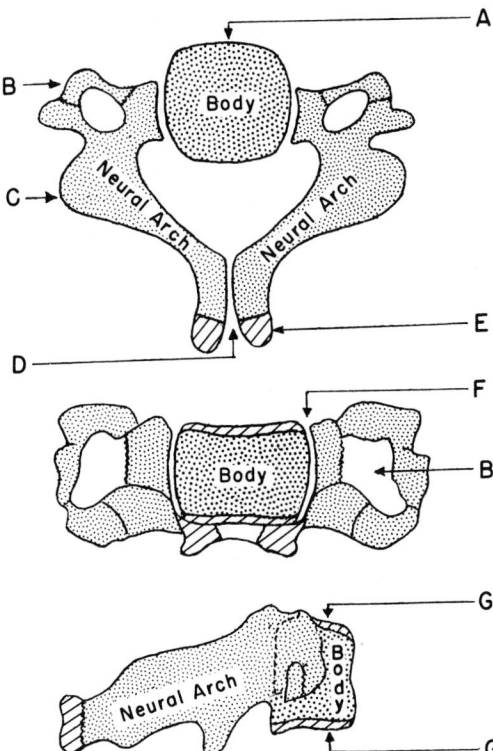

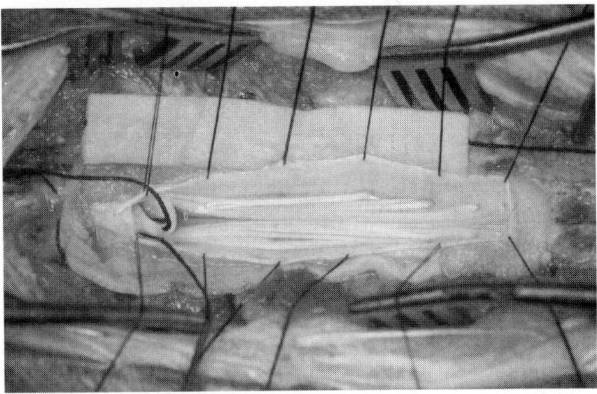

FIG. 22-6. Cauda equina. (*Courtesy Antonio Prats, MD, Miami Children's Hospital, Miami.*)

FIG. 22-5. Developmental parts of typical cervical vertebrae (C3-C7). *A*, Body. *B*, Anterior segment of costal portion of the transverse process, which may develop from a separate center that appears in the cartilage about the sixth fetal month and fuses with the main ossification center of the transverse process by the sixth year. *C*, Neural arches whose ossification centers usually appear by the third fetal month. *D*, Synchondrosis that binds the two sides of the spinous process and usually disappears by the fourth year but may persist 2 or 3 years longer. *E*, Secondary, separate ossification centers in the tips of the two sides of the spinous process. *F*, Neurocentral synchondroses that bind the neural arches to each body on both sides and usually disappear between 3 and 7 years. *G*, Superior and inferior vertebral rings that may begin to ossify as early as 7 years in girls and then fuse with their vertebral body at about 25 years. These rings are not parts of an epiphysis, contribute nothing to vertebral body growth, and have no causal relationship to juvenile kyphosis. (*Redrawn from Bailey DK: Radiology 59:712, 1952 for Silverman FN: Caffey's pediatric x-ray diagnosis, ed 9, Chicago, 1993, Year Book.*)

alar ligaments, which are attached to the dens and occipital condyles, limit the atlantoaxial rotation.[24,27]

Each vertebra of the C2-C7 segment has up to three ossification centers in the newborn (Fig. 22-5), a single large center in the body, and paired centers in the neural arch.[19] Osseous fusion of the posterior ends of the neural arch in the midline of the cervical segments is complete by 6 years of age. Retardation of the closing of the neural arches of the cervical spine (spina bifida occulta) is common but is rarely of clinical significance. Elongation of the anterior tubercle of the transverse process of the C6 may be visible radiographically in direct lateral projections, stimulating a fracture fragment.

Thoracic Spine (T1-T10)

The thoracic spine has considerable stability because of the strong costotransverse and intertransverse ligaments, the splinting effect of the rib cage, and the relative sagittal orientation of the facet joints, which strongly resist rotational forces. The spinal canal has a relatively narrow diameter.

Thoracolumbar (T11-L1) and Lumbar (L2-L5) Spine

The thoracolumbar-lumbar region is more vulnerable to osseoligamentous injuries because of the lack of splinting of the rib cage. The spinal cord terminates as the conus medullaris opposite the L1-L2 vertebral body (Fig. 22-6). The neural elements of the cauda equina are a bundle of peripheral nerves. The spinal canal is wider than the cord.

Sacral and Coccygeal Spine

The sacral-coccygeal area is relatively stable because of the support provided by the pelvic bones and ligaments. The sacral level innervates areas of the perineum, bowel, bladder, and legs. The coccyx is not associated with acute neurologic deficits.

Spinal Cord

The spinal cord extends caudad from the midbrain at the base of the skull to the level of the L1-L2 vertebra. The cervical spinal cord is a nearly cylindrical structure, approximately centered in the subarachnoid space. The diameter of the cord enlarges slightly at the C5-C6 level where the roots of the brachial plexus arise. By virtue of its elastic recoil and plasticity, the spinal cord adapts to changes in the length of the spinal canal within the limitations imposed by the pia mater.[2] Breig demonstrated elongation of the spinal cord in flexion and shortening in extension; individual cord segments change in length by as much as 25%.[31] Beyond this maximal length, further axial tensile forces may disrupt neuronal tissue, leaving the arachnoid and dura in continuity. Further stretching may injure the meninges and transect the spinal cord.

The dentate ligament is a serrated membrane consisting of delicate fibers attached to the cord between the nerve roots. It connects the lateral margin of the cervical cord to the dural sac. The anterior spinal artery runs in a shallow groove on the ventral surface of the spinal cord; a pair of veins is located on the dorsal surface.

The spinal cord comprises gray and white matter. The white matter tracts include the descending tracts: anterior and lateral corticospinal, lateral vestibulospinal, ventrolateral reticulospinal, ventral and dorsal spinocerebellar, and spinothalamic tracts. On the dorsal surface of the cord are the ascending white matter tracts, the dorsal columns of the fasciculus cuneatus and fasciculus gracilis, each separated by the dorsal intermediate sulcus. The spinothalamic tracts along the dorsal surface of the cord and pyramidal tracts along the ventral surface are the most important white matter structures.

The gray matter lies deep to the white matter tracts and consists of ventral and dorsal horns and intermediate gray. The central canal, a small ependymal lined space within the spinal canal, is located in the gray matter.

The relative hypermobility of the cervical area and dorsolumbar junction increases the frequency of SCI in these areas. The horizontal direction of nerve roots in the cervical region, the attachment of the dura mater at the foramen magnum and intervertebral foramina, and the brachial plexus tend to anchor the cervical spine. These features reduce mobility and latitude in elongating the spinal canal. Below, the spinal cord is anchored by the lumbar roots; little anchoring support is present in the thoracic region.

The spinal canal at the atlas is equally occupied by the spinal cord, odontoid process, and free space. Anterior displacement of the atlas on the axis past a distance equal to the anteroposterior diameter of the odontoid places the cord at risk. Because odontoid fracture is the most common osseous injury in young children, it is understandable that many of these patients survive without neurologic disability.[32]

PATHOPHYSIOLOGY

The developmental anatomy influences the pathophysiology of injury. The pediatric spine exhibits incomplete ossification, epiphyseal growth plates, synchondroses, hypermobility, and several normal and congenital variations. Because the immature spine ossifies progressively throughout childhood, younger children tend to sustain avulsions or epiphyseal separations rather than true fractures.

The cervical spine in children is remarkably flexible, facilitating activity patterns. However, this hypermobility does not always protect the skeleton or spinal cord. The child's relatively large and heavy head, weak neck musculature, and hypermobile upper cervical spine increase the risk of injuries from acceleration and torsion forces.[33]

The molecular and electrophysiologic events of neurotransmission failure after SCI are incompletely understood. Generally the spinal cord is not physically disrupted but functionally deranged. Alterations of white and gray matter of the spinal cord are of an ischemic nature.[34] Tissue oxygen tension declines, and vasomotor autoregulation is disrupted. The role of endorphins, free catecholamines, lipid peroxides and free radicals, lysosomal enzymes, and adenosine triphosphatase (ATP-ase) are yet to be defined. It is thought that several events following traumatic injury to the spinal cord lead to cord ischemia and loss of neurologic function. A sudden flux of calcium from the extracellular space to the intracellular space occurs.

The calcium shift causes lipid peroxidation, initiates free radical reactions and alters spinal cord blood flow by way of arachidonic acid metabolism, and increases the activity of calcium-dependent proteases. Also, the increased intracellular calcium compromises the respiratory function of the neuronal mitochondria.[35]

SCI are usually partial or incomplete, associated with an abnormal neurophysiologic state caused by anatomic alteration of the cord or the adjacent skeletal structures. The injury may result from direct primary injury or from a series of secondary insults, the latter often being partially remediable.

The most common cervical spine lesions in children under 8 years of age remain centered in the atlantoaxial region; they include odontoid fracture, atlantoaxial dislocation or subluxation, and hyperextension fracture of the axis because of the enhanced flexibility in this region. These lesions tend to have a smaller percentage of neurologic deficits and pancervical involvement than those of adolescents and adults. The large diameter of the spinal canal at C1 probably accounts for this discrepancy.

Although most pediatric cervical spine fractures are unstable, only a few present with a neurologic deficit.[16,17,36] A study of 97 children with SCI noted that direct compression and disruption by the luxated vertebra or fracture fragments are the most common mechanisms of spinal cord trauma in patients with evidence of osteoarticular injury.[2]

Disruption of the spinal cord may be complicated by extruded disk material, luxated vertebral bodies, and fracture fragments of vertebrae compromising the width of the spinal canal.

Flexion

Hyperflexion is the most common mechanism of injury in spinal trauma. The maximal compressive forces focus on the anterior portion of the vertebral body, causing a simple wedge fracture, while distraction occurs at the posterior elements. Tensile forces applied to the posterior elements cause distraction of the interspinous ligament, ligamentum flavum, and facet capsules. The facet serves as a fulcrum through which compressive forces are exerted on the vertebral body and disk. With flexion, the stretching of the posterior ligamentous complex produces tears or spinous process avulsion. The "clay-shoveler's fracture" is an avulsion fracture of the base of the spinous process of C6, C7, or T1 by posterior distractive forces.

A flexion tear drop fracture is a fracture of the vertebral body with disruption of a large, triangular bony fragment displaced anteriorly from the anteroinferior portion of the vertebral body. This injury commonly involves the posterior structural elements and may be associated with neurologic damage.[14] Ligamentous disruptions may result from variable degrees of subluxation and dislocation of bony cervical spine elements.

The middle and lower cervical spine is commonly injured through a flexion mechanism, sometimes involving rotational forces.

Extension

Hyperextension of the spine creates distractive forces in the anterior longitudinal ligament and compression of the posterior elements. Extension can cause compression and subsequent fracture of the posterior neural arch of C1 or the pedicles of C2 as a result of the weight of the heavy occiput. The latter is known as a "hangman's fracture", described by Wood-Jones in 1913.[37]

Stretching of the anterior longitudinal ligament can produce ligamentous tears at the disk space or at the vertebral body end plate, producing avulsion fractures of the anterior vertebral bodies. These distractive forces are maximal at the C4-C5 level.

Buckling of the ligamentum flavum into the posterior spinal canal can produce central or posterior cord syndromes.

Axial Loading/Vertical Compression

Injuries may be due to forces delivered along the longitudinal axis of the spinal column and transmitted inferiorly from the superior end of the spine or superiorly from the pelvis.

The cervical and lumbar spines straighten at the time of impact from above or below, potentially compressing the nucleus pulposus into the vertebral body with compromise of the anterior spinal canal, causing the anterior cord syndrome. Burst or comminuted fractures of the vertebral body with protrusion of bony fragments into the spinal canal are common in the lower cervical spine and the thoracolumbar junction and are often accompanied by a posterior element fracture.

A Jefferson burst fracture[38] of the anterior or posterior arches of C1 is characterized by bilateral lateral displacement of the articular mass of C1 relative to the lateral margins of C2. It is produced by a vertical compression force transmitted through the occipital condyles to the superior articular surfaces of the lateral masses of the atlas.

Simple wedge fractures of the vertebral bodies may result from compression; they occur with impaction of the superior end plate and impaction and angulation of the anterior margin of the vertebral body.

Rotation

Pure rotational dislocations are not uncommon and are usually caused by muscle pulls not associated with external trauma. Rotational forces concentrate at the facet, where they may cause fracture or dislocation because the coronal orientation of the articular surface offers only moderate resistance to these stresses. Rotational forces may produce unstable articular process fractures in the lumbar region.

Other Mechanisms

A combination of mechanisms may cause spinal injury. The first cervical vertebra is susceptible to fracture by forceful extension, flexion, or axial loading. Simultaneous flexion and rotation of one of the facet joints may cause unilateral posterior facet-joint dislocation. A pillar fracture results from a combination of hyperextension and rotation, causing a fracture of the lateral mass. Fractures of the uncinate process (bony projection from the superior end plate) usually result from extreme lateral bending.

The C2 pedicle fracture is often a bilateral extension injury caused by downward compression of the occiput and atlas against the posterior arch of the axis. This injury may be accompanied by anterior subluxation of C2 on C3, and about 15% of individuals so affected exhibit a neurologic deficit.[39]

Initial Cervical Spine Immobilization

Posttraumatic neck or back pain.

Posttraumatic impaired level of consciousness or inability to give an accurate history. As many as 5% of patients with serious head injury have associated CSI.[41]

Posttraumatic neurologic complaints or deficits, whether stable or progressive.

Multiple-system trauma, with severe associated injuries or shock.

Vulnerability to forces in a traumatic event with a recognized life-threatening potential such as being hit by a car or falling from a significant height or an accident associated with diving (mechanism of injury).

Trauma in a patient with congenital or acquired cervical spine vulnerability such as Down and Klippel-Fiel syndromes or after cervical spine surgery.

Traumatic birth-related SCI. Difficult to diagnose in the newborn and requires careful evaluation.[42,43]

Axial loading in mild flexion is the most common mechanism of injury in football. With the neck slightly flexed, the normal cervical lordosis is lost and the cervical spine becomes a straight column. Impact on the top of the head, such as that which occurs during head-down blocking in football, can then produce axial loading of the cervical spine with excessive energy absorption, fracture or dislocation, and cord injury.[2,40]

DIAGNOSTIC FINDINGS

Cervical Spine Injuries

Any patient with history of a significant injury, evidence of neurologic impairment, or radiologic evidence of abnormality should be evaluated and treated in the emergency department with the presumption that a mechanically and neurologically unstable injury is present (see box above).

The stability of a cervical spine injury is influenced by the nature of the bony injury (Table 22-1). Unstable fractures are associated with disruption of the posterior elements with intact anterior structures, disrupted anterior elements with intact posterior elements, and disruption of both the anterior and posterior structures. Mechanically stable fractures may coexist with neurologic deficits (Table 22-2).[14,15]

Clinical Findings. The classic clinical triad of an upper cervical spine injury comprises pain, cervical muscle spasm, and limitation of neck movement.[38,44,45]

The symptoms of SCI in small children are most of the time not obtainable or easy to evaluate. The complexity of the clinical signs of SCI in children depends on several variables: age, location of the SCI, presence and stability of a spinal fracture, and other system injuries.

The history is essential to the assessment of neck trauma and the evolution of management plans. The history must detail the mechanism and time of injury, the resuscitation at the scene, and any prehospital observations, especially

TABLE 22-1. Classification of Spinal Injuries

Mechanisms of spinal injury	Stability
Flexion	
Wedge fracture	Stable
Clay shoveler's fracture	Stable
Subluxation	Potentially unstable
Bilateral facet dislocation	Always unstable
Flexion tear drop fracture	Extremely unstable
Atlantooccipital dislocation	Unstable
Anterior atlantoaxial dislocation with or without fracture	Unstable
Odontoid fracture with lateral displacement fracture	Unstable
Fracture of transverse process	Stable
Rotation	
Unilateral facet dislocation	Stable
Rotary atlantoaxial dislocation	Unstable
Extension	
Posterior neural arch fracture (C1)	Unstable
Hangman's fracture (C2)	Unstable
Extension tear drop fracture	Usually stable in flexion; unstable in extension
Posterior atlantoaxial dislocation with or without fracture	Unstable
Vertical compression	
Bursting fracture of vertebral body	Stable
Jefferson fracture (C1)	Extremely unstable
Isolated fracture of articular pillar and vertebral body	Stable

From Rosen P et al: *Emergency medicine*, ed 4, St Louis, 1997, Mosby.

TABLE 22-2. Incidence of SCI Associated with Vertebral Injuries

Type of injury	Percentage with neurologic deficit
Fracture of vertebral body only	3
Fracture of posterior element only	19
Fracture of posterior elements and vertebral body	11
Dislocation only	17
Dislocation with fracture of posterior elements	27
Dislocation with fracture of vertebral body	56
Dislocation with fracture of posterior elements and vertebral body	61

Adapted from Riggins RS and Kraus JF: *J Trauma* 17:126, 1977.

changes in neurologic or cardiorespiratory status. After initial stabilization efforts, a full description of the events should be obtained, including the distance of the fall, velocity of moving vehicles, and extent of vehicle damage, as well as other relevant data.

Subjective complaints of head or neck pain, paresthesia, amnesia, or weakness should be recorded. The ability to walk after an accident does not exclude spine or spinal cord trauma; 15% to 20% of patients may be able to walk initially.

Patients with neck pain produced by a rotatory atlantoaxial subluxation often have a history of recent upper respiratory infection and a minor injury.

Physical examination must include vital signs in the initial evaluation. SCI may produce apnea followed by cardiac arrest or profound hypotension and subsequent hypoxic/ischemic encephalopathy with or without a serious traumatic brain injury.[46] The breathing pattern may indicate a loss of diaphragmatic breathing and hypoventilation of apnea with injuries to C3, C4, and C5, which supply the phrenic nerve. Although lower cervical lesions preserve diaphragmatic function, there may be a loss of abdominal and intercostal breathing.

Hypotension may develop with spinal shock as a result of a physiologic sympathectomy (i.e., bradycardia with severe hypotension, warm dry skin with hypotension, and increased capacitance vessel pooling of blood).[47] Hypothermia or hyperthermia may develop with instability of temperature regulation.

Neurologic Evaluation. Neurologic findings may be manifested in a number of clinical patterns. The neurologic examination begins with the observation of the pattern of chest-wall excursion during spontaneous breathing. Visual inspection may demonstrate a "see-saw" respiratory pattern with paralyzed intercostal muscles as a result of cervical or upper thoracic spinal cord injury. Alterations in mental status and level of consciousness are often noted.

A *gross motor* examination of the extremities must determine spontaneous and purposeful movements (Table 22-3). Muscle tone is usually flaccid as a result of lower motor neuron lesions or spinal shock (areflexia). Spasticity, with hyperreflexia may evolve as a sign of upper motor neuron injury. The evaluation of power must compare the strength of upper to lower extremities and right to left. Muscles essential for the maintenance of normal posture usually have bilateral innervation and are not useful in lateralizing weakness. The best rapid examinations are dorsiflexion of the wrist and extension of the forearm or dorsiflexion of the great toe and flexion of the lower leg at the knee, depending on the extremity requiring evaluation. Mass flexion withdrawal movements in response to stimulation may occur in infants with paralyzed limbs and may be indistinguishable from normal movement.

The *upper level of sensory impairment determined by sensory examination* is used for localization of the injury (Fig. 22-7). Light touch tests the ipsilateral posterior spinal column and contralateral anterior column. The anterolateral spinal column is evaluated by means of pain sense (pinprick); position sense tests the ipsilateral posterior spinal column (see Table 22-3).

Deep-tendon and superficial *reflexes* may indicate the level of injury (see Table 22-3). Primitive reflexes such as Babinski's and Hoffmann's reflexes may indicate an upper motor neuron lesion if noted beyond 4 months of age. Rectal tone is important prognostically; if it is present, sacral sparing is implied with subsequent partial or com-

TABLE 22-3. SCI: Motor, Sensory, and Reflex Deficits

Level of lesion	Motor function lost	Sensation lost at and below	Reflex
C2	Breathing	Occiput	
C3	Spontaneous breathing and trapezius	Thyroid cartilage	
C4	function	Suprasternal notch	
C5	Shoulder flexion and abduction	Infraclavicular with or without lateral arm sparing	Biceps brachialis*
C6		Infraclavicular with or without lateral arm, forearm sparing	Brachioradialis*
C7	Elbow and wrist extension	Infraclavicular with sparing as above to middle finger	Triceps*
C8	Small muscles of hand (lumbricales and interossei)	Infraclavicular with sparing as above to little finger	
T1		Infraclavicular with upper extremity sparing to axilla	
T4		Nipple line	
T7	Intercostal and abdominal musculature	Inferior costal margin	Upper abdominal†
T10		Umbilicus	
T12			Lower abdominal†
L1	Hip flexion	Groin	
L2		Anteromedial thigh	
L3	Hip adduction and knee extension	Medial knee	Knee/patellar*
L4	Hip abduction and knee extension	Anterior knee and medial calf	
L5	Foot and great toe dorsiflexion	Lateral dorsum foot and lateral sole foot	
S1	Foot and great toe plantar flexion	Lateral dorsum foot and lateral sole foot	Ankle/Achilles tendon*
S2			
S3	Perianal and rectal sphincter tone	Perianal and rectal sensation	
S4			

From Barkin R and Rosen P: *Emergency pediatrics*, ed 4, St. Louis, 1994, Mosby.
*Deep tendon.
†Superficial.

plete neurologic recovery in up to 30% to 50% of patients. The absence of rectal tone implies only a 2% to 3% chance of partial or complete recovery. The bulbocavernosus reflex elicited when the glans penis is pressed or a urinary catheter is pulled is intact if distinct rectal sphincter contraction occurs. The absence of an intact reflex indicates the presence of spinal shock. Autonomic reflex paralysis produces vasomotor paralysis with flushed, warm, dry skin; loss of temperature regulation (if the lesion is above T8); hypotension; and bradycardia.

Hyperextension of the cervical spine with central cord contusion (central spinothalamic tract) is thought to be the pathophysiology of the "burning hands" syndrome[48] in football players who sustain neck trauma. It is characterized by burning dysesthesias in the hands and fingertips and, occasionally, in the feet after injury.

Paralysis requires assessment, even though its presence may be difficult to define in infants and smaller children. SCIs demonstrate segmental and recognizable patterns of movement of some arm muscles and paralysis of others (see Table 22-3).

The ratio of paraplegic to tetraplegic patients among children younger than 10 years is 1:2.5, whereas in older patients it is 2:1. Mass flexion withdrawal movements may occur in children with paralyzed limbs in response to stimulation and may be indistinguishable from normal movements. Crying in response to these movements may occur.

Complications. Many complications of cervical spinal injury may have acute manifestations in the emergency department and require emergency intervention. Early death after trauma may be associated with airway instability. Aspiration must be avoided, the airway secured, and ventilation and oxygenation supported. However, preexisting spinal injury may be exacerbated by airway-stabilizing maneuvers. Paralysis of intercostal muscles and decreased diaphragmatic function and paralysis often impair ventilation. Neurogenic pulmonary edema may worsen oxygenation.

Spinal shock may accompany injury. Flaccid paralysis, areflexia, priapism, and sensory loss distal to the lesion are noted with impaired temperature control. Hypotension with bradycardia may accompany the loss of sympathetic tone and decreased peripheral vascular resistance. Urine retention or incontinence, paralytic ileus, and gastric stress ulcer are reported.

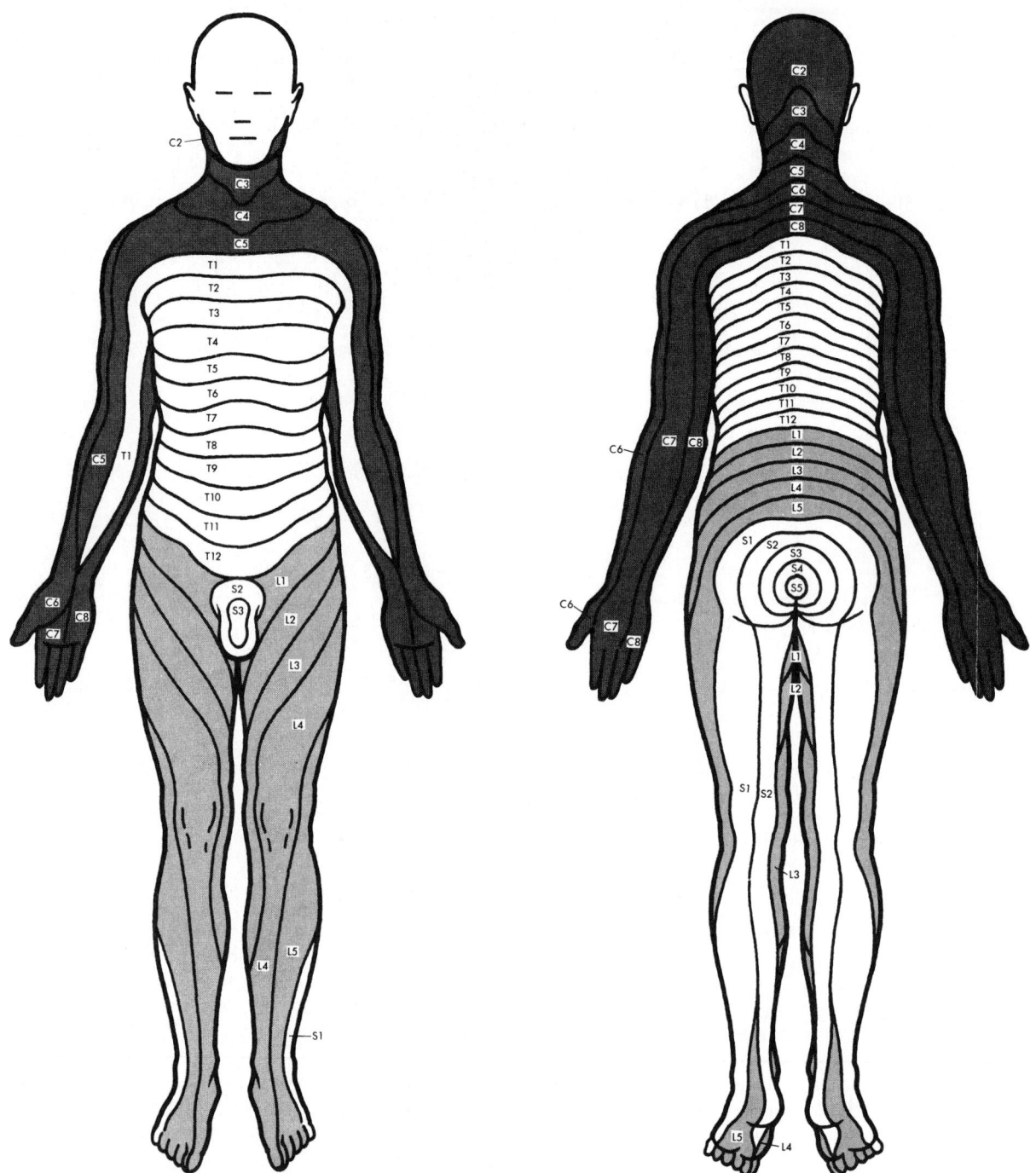

FIG. 22-7. Sensory dermatome. (*From Rosen P et al: Emergency medicine, ed 4, St. Louis, 1997, Mosby.*)

Incomplete spinal cord syndromes may be noted (Fig. 22-8). The *anterior cord* injury is marked by contusion of the anterior cord or laceration/thrombosis of the anterior spinal artery. Such patients have complete paralysis and *hyperalgesia* with preservation of touch and proprioception. This commonly occurs with flexion or vertical compression injuries, whereby the anterior spinal cord is compressed by bony fragments, disk material, or hematoma. *Central cord syndrome* occurs with damage to the central gray matter and the most central regions of the pyramidal and spinothalamic tracts, with preservation of the long white matter tracts. Motor weakness in the arms is greater than that in the legs; variable bladder and sensory involvement is noted. Acute central cervical cord syndrome may result from minor trauma, particularly hyperextension of the neck.[9,49]

The *posterior cord syndrome* is similar to the central cord presentation with loss of proprioception and variable paresis. Injuries are associated with extension and buckling of the ligamentum flavum into the posterior spinal cord.

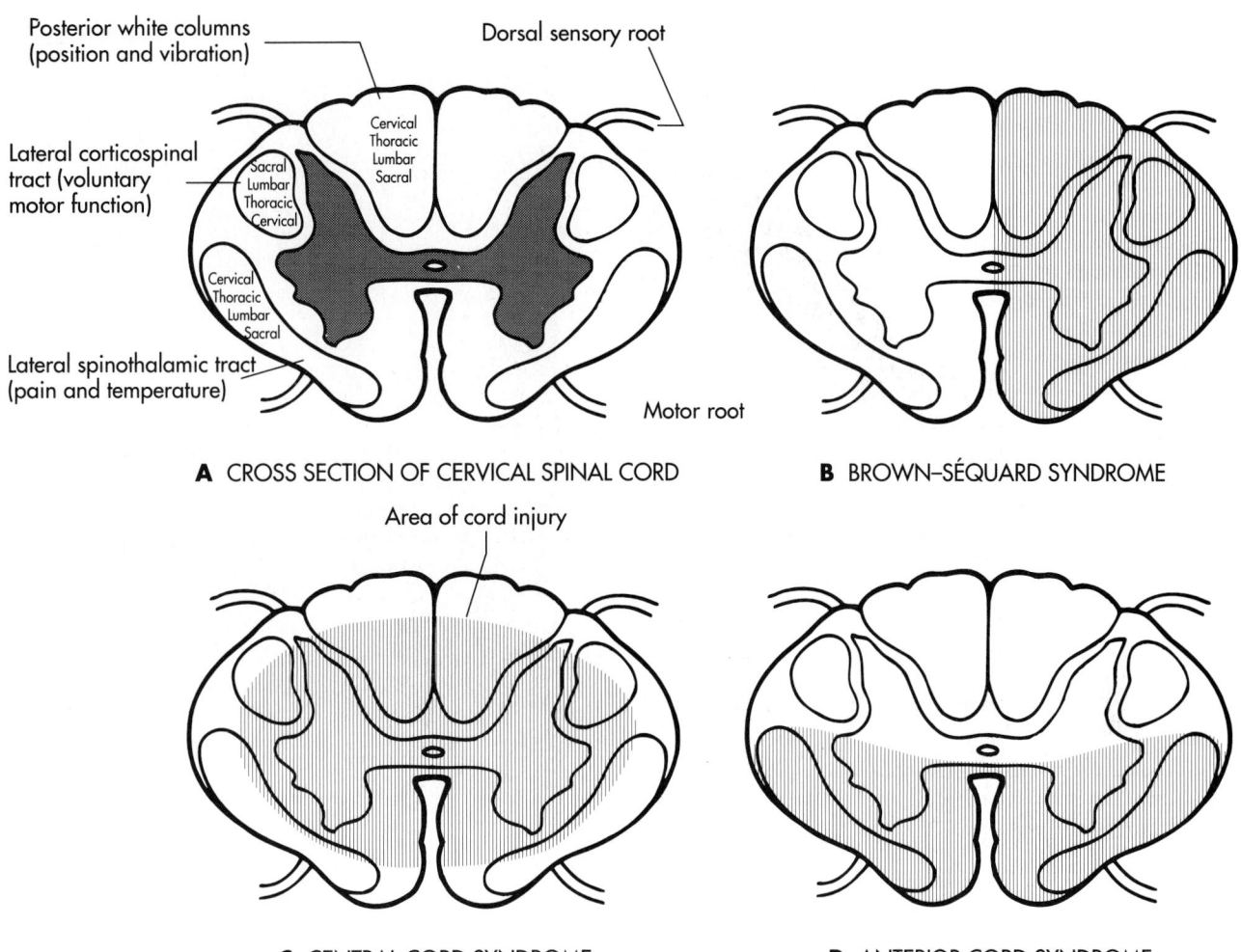

FIG. 22-8. Incomplete spinal cord syndromes. (*From Rosen P et al:* Emergency medicine, *ed 4, St. Louis, 1997, Mosby.*)

Penetrating injuries may produce a cord hemisection that presents as *Brown-Sequard syndrome,* with ipsilateral motor, proprioception, and light-touch deficits; contralateral pain; and temperature impairment. *Horner syndrome* is associated with ptosis, miosis, anhidrosis, facial flushing, and enophthalmos produced by disruption of the cervical sympathetic chain that arises at C7-T1.

Vertical trauma in addition to spinal injury may have associated pelvic fractures and urinary and thoracic injuries.

Acute pulmonary edema has occurred after cervical spine injuries that are not associated with significant head injury. The mechanism is unclear, but it may be the spinal cord injury itself.[50,51]

Unrecognized injuries of the pharynx and esophagus may lead to mediastinitis. Initially no symptoms may be attributed to the esophagus or pharynx. Esophagoscopy is a useful method of diagnosis.

Thoracic duct injury should be considered in instances of penetrating injury to the left supraclavicular region. Thoracic duct fistulization may cause significant fluid and protein loss.

Long-term sequelae may follow cervical spinal injury. Repeated pulmonary or genitourinary infections, psychologic problems, muscle contractions, decubitus ulcers, and progressive spinal deformity (scoliosis, lordosis, or kyphosis) may be noted.

Radiologic Studies. Several radiologic modalities are available with which to study the child with suspected cervical spine injury. Plain radiography is routinely performed in early management. Magnetic resonance imaging (MRI) may demonstrate soft-tissue injuries of the spinal cord, an area in which computed tomography (CT) often falls short. The CT scan has been shown to be superior to MRI in delineating fractures and dislocations (see box on p. 298).

Cervical Spine X-ray Films. Cervical spine radiographs are routinely performed in children with risk factors of cervical spine injury. Studies should generally be obtained in patients with neck pain, tenderness, limitation of movement, significant neck or head injury, involvement in a vehicular accident with head trauma, or symptoms of neurologic impairment including altered level of consciousness or abnormality of reflexes, strength, or sensation. The con-

Indications for Radiography in Spinal Trauma

1. Acute neurologic deficit.
2. Altered mental status secondary to head injury or shock.
3. Intoxication from alcohol or other drugs.
4. Head or back pain.
5. Neck or back tenderness.
6. Unconsciousness.
7. High-risk mechanism of injury
   a. High-speed motor vehicle accident
   b. Fall from >10 feet
   c. Drowning
8. Severe associated injuries
   a. Head or face
   b. Multiple skeletal
9. Competitive pain from a nonspinal injury.

From Keene JG and Daffner RH: Spinal trauma. In Rosen P, Doris PE, Barkin RM, et al: *Diagnostic radiology in emergency medicine*, St. Louis, 1992, Mosby.

TABLE 22-4. Correlation Between Clinical Observations and Positive X-ray Film Results

Number of children	Positive x-ray films	Clinical identification of children with positive study	Clinical variable(s) studied
2133[52]	25	25 (100%)	Neck pain
			Vehicular accident with head trauma
206[51]	59	58 (98%)	Neck pain
			Neck tenderness
			Limitation of neck mobility
			History of neck trauma
			Abnormal reflexes
			Abnormal strength
			Abnormal sensation
			Abnormal mental status

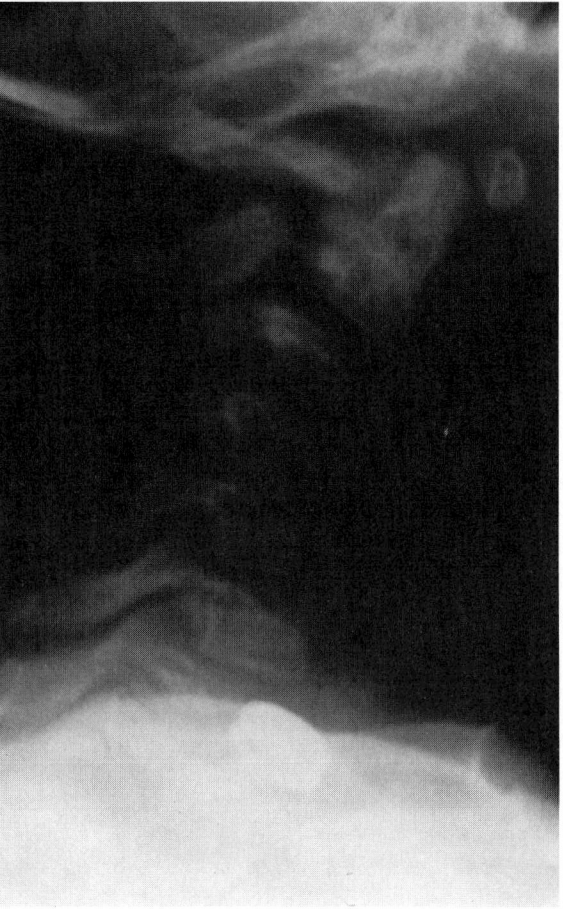

FIG. 22-9. C2 fracture.

Fig. 22-9 shows a radiologic appearance of a C2 cervical spine fracture detected in a 4-month-old who exhibited only neck weakness and had no risk factors on history and physical examination. This injury was later determined to be a result of child abuse.

History and physical examination abnormalities are not always available and may be difficult to obtain in the emergency setting. Studies have shown that the ability of the physician to predict the presence of a cervical spine injury on the basis of history and physical examination alone is only 50%.[55] If the patient is alert and without complaints, immobilization and radiologic examination should be completed if any doubt exists. If the patient is not alert, priorities for resuscitation should be followed with a high degree of suspicion for SCI, appropriate immobilization, and protection of the cervical spine until radiography can be performed.

Interpretation of studies must assure that the films are of adequate quality and the views appropriate for evaluation of the potential injury. Normal embryologic and developmental peculiarities of the cervical spine must be understood. The radiographic studies document, directly, the osseous integrity and, indirectly, the ligamentous and disk stability.

Films must be carefully inspected for evidence of fracture, misalignment, and soft-tissue abnormalities. A source

sequences of overlooking a CSI require this inclusive approach. The findings of retrospective studies in adults and children suggest that a selective approach for a radiologic workup is appropriate in patients without altered mental status or other high-risk factors after the completion of a careful history and physical examination (Table 22-4).[52-54] Nevertheless, some authors have suggested broader guidelines; painless or occult cervical spine injuries exist.

of diagnostic error is the unfamiliarity of many physicians with the appearance of the immature skeleton.[54,56,57]

Many variations of the final development—synchondrosis, hypoplasia of segments, and fusion of the cervical vertebrae—are commonly seen. Block vertebrae (abnormal fusion) should raise suspicion of Klippel-Feil syndrome. Assimilation with complete or partial fusion of the atlas to the occiput may be associated with an Arnold-Chiari anomaly.

The number of cervical spine x-ray views that constitute a complete pediatric cervical spine trauma series is controversial. Assessment using the "minimal" cervical spine trauma series includes the *portable cross-table lateral cervical spine* (PCTLCS), open-mouth odontoid view, and anteroposterior studies. The films should be assessed systematically, with evaluation of the alignment, the bony integrity of each vertebrae, and cartilaginous and soft-tissue spaces.[58,59]

General agreement exists that the initial radiograph should be a PCTLCS with the patient immobilized.[58] However, reported series in adults confirm that evaluations of the cervical spine based on a single PCTLCS are unreliable and have an unacceptable false positive rate of 23% to 26%.[55,60]

Jaffe,[53] in a retrospective study, noted that the PCTLCS detected 95% of cervical abnormalities, 100% in combination with anteroposterior and open-mouth odontoid views. All seven cervical vertebrae must be included. Emphasis should be placed on the need to scrutinize the cervicothoracic junction.[15,61] To visualize C7-T1, it is often necessary, particularly in heavy patients, to have one person hold the patient's head and apply in-line stabilization while another pulls gently down on the arms from the foot of the bed. The "swimmer's" (transaxillary) view may be helpful in visualizing the lower cervical spine if C7-T1 is not visualized on the PCTLCS film.

Alignment should assure the continuity of four continuous curvilinear lines without step-offs (Fig. 22-10). As noted in Fig. 22-10, the lateral cervical spine can be assessed by delineation of the lines of the anterior and posterior vertebral bodies, spinolaminal line and posterior spinal canal, and spinous process tips from C2-C7. The normal lordotic curve is disturbed in 20% of normal patients with spasm; it may also be the only evidence of severe spinal injury.

Vertebrae should be inspected for uniformity, shape, mineralization, and density. Fractures, lines, displacement, subluxation, and dislocation must be excluded. The vertebral bodies have a normal biconcave appearance. The anterior portions of the vertebral bodies of C2, C3, and C4 taper anteriorly and may be confused with compression fractures. Epiphyseal growth plates may resemble fractures. Increased C1-to-C2 interspinous distance may be observed in a normal spine and should not be mistaken for posterior ligamentous disruption.

Pseudosubluxation of C2 occurs anterior to C3—and in rare cases at C3-C4—up to 3 mm in up to 40% of children younger than 8 years. When a C2 anterior displacement on C3 is noted, a posterior cervical line[62,63] (line drawn from the anterior aspect of the spinous process of C1 to the anterior aspect of the spinous process of C3) should miss the anterior aspect of C2 spinal process by less than 2 mm

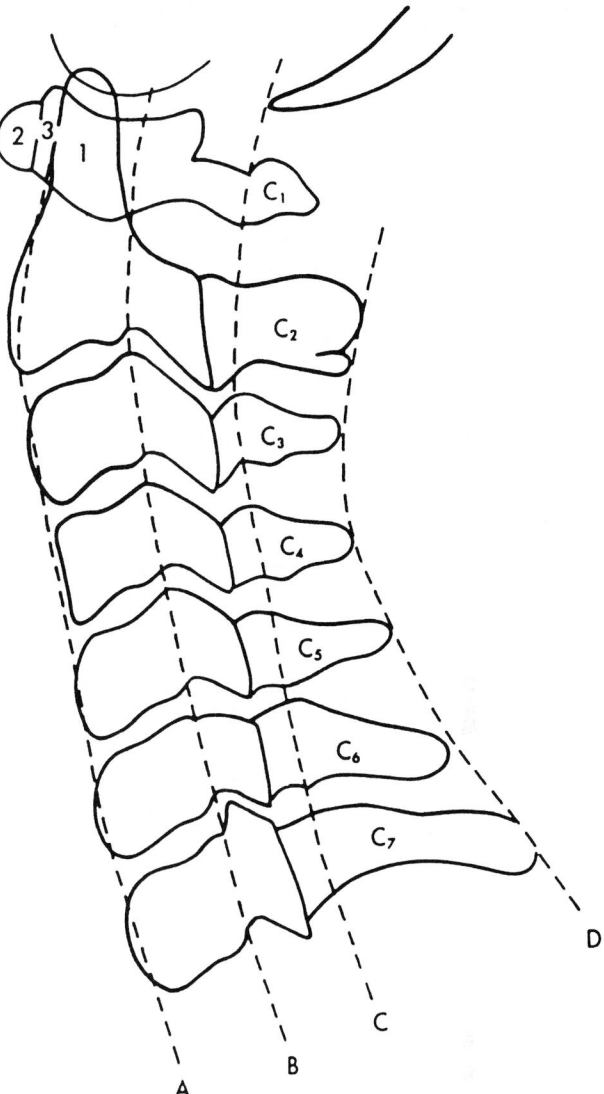

FIG. 22-10. Cervical vertebrae. Lateral cervical spine. *A,* Anterior vertebral bodies. *B,* Posterior vertebral bodies and anterior spinal canal. *C,* Spinolaminal line and posterior spinal canal. *D,* Spinous process tips C2-C7. *1,* Odontoid process of dens of C2; *2,* anterior arch of C1; *3,* predental space between posterior surface of anterior arch of C1 and anterior surface of odontoid process. (*From Barkin RM, Rosen P:* Emergency pediatrics, *ed 4, St. Louis, 1994, Mosby.*)

(1.5 mm is borderline) (Fig. 22-11). If it misses the anterior aspect of the C2 spinous process by 2 mm or more, a hangman's fracture or true subluxation should be suspected.[62] However, even in normal individuals who do not show C2-on-C3 displacement, the posterior cervical line will commonly miss the anterior aspect of C2 spinous process by 2 mm or more.[64]

Soft-tissue spaces must be specifically evaluated. The width of the *prevertebral soft tissue* may change dramatically with respiration (widened during expiration), crying, and flexion or extension of the neck.[39] Large adenoidal tissue can also cause thickening of the prevertebral space.

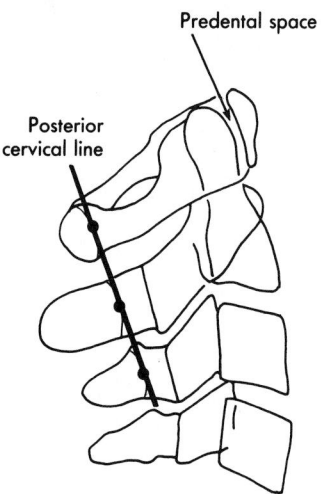

FIG. 22-11. Normal structural relationships of lateral cervical spine. (*From Rosen P, et al:* Emergency medicine, *ed 4, St. Louis, 1997, Mosby.*)

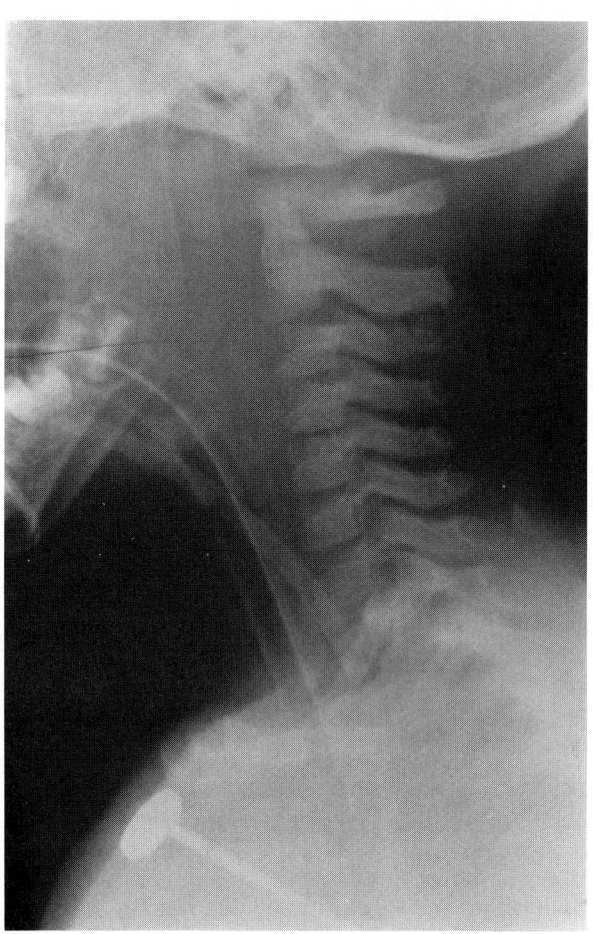

FIG. 22-12. Portable cross-table lateral cervical spine. Soft-tissue changes caused by nasogastric and endotracheal tubes, cervical-collar, and foreign body (C7 spinous process).

Nasogastric and endotracheal tubes may invalidate specific measurements (Fig. 22-12). Soft-tissue swelling may be a result of hemorrhage, abscess, infection, foreign body, tumor, air, or bony injury. Anterior bulging of the prevertebral fat stripe is a good indirect sign of an underlying bony or soft-tissue injury. Normal prevertebral space distances have been defined as 7 mm or less in children and adults anterior to C2,[65] 5 mm or less in children and adults, or less than 40% of the anteroposterior diameter of the C3 and C4 vertebral bodies anterior to C3 and C4. Below the level of C4 the prevertebral space should be less than 14 mm in children younger than 15 years and 22 mm or less in adults, measured between C6 and the trachea because of the presence of the esophagus and the cricopharyngeal muscle.[57,63,65] The presence of air in the prevertebral space is a sign of a rupture of the esophagus or some portion of the airway.

The *predens space* or atlantodental distance (synovial joint between the anterior odontoid surface of C2 on lateral view and the posterior cortex of the anterior arch of C1) may be up to 5 mm in normal children younger than 8 years and less than 3 mm in adults.[66-68] Variations up to 3 mm may be observed with flexion and extension as a result of normal atlantoaxial movement.[68,69] In extension, the anterior arch may appear to ride up over the odontoid so that the posterior two thirds of the anterior arch lies above the tip of the odontoid process. The two margins of the space are normally parallel but may also exhibit a V shape.[70] The space is usually measured at the lower edge of the anterior arch of C1, when it has a V shape. A truly increased predental space suggests atlantoaxial instability, Jefferson fracture, or atlantoaxial rotational subluxation.

The transverse atlantal ligament attaches to the lateral masses of C1 at two tubercles. Isolated avulsion or traumatic disruption of the transverse ligament is extremely rare. Inflammatory disorders can affect the dens and the transverse ligament behind it. Individuals with Down syndrome, Morquio disease, or rheumatoid arthritis commonly demonstrate laxity of the transverse ligament and instability at the atlantoaxial level.[71] This fact is the rationale for the American Academy of Pediatrics recommendation that all children with Down syndrome who participate in Special Olympics activities be screened by means of dynamic cervical radiography.[72] Even in normal children, minimal trauma or the local inflammation of a pharyngitis causing increased atlantoaxial ligamentous laxity may lead to rotatory subluxation of C1-C2.[73-75] The physiologic integrity of the atlantal transverse ligament is reflected by the predens space. A wide or mobile space noted on the PCTLCS raises the suspicion of rupture or incompetence of the transverse ligament.[68,73,76,77] Atlas fractures associated with displacement of lateral masses greater than 7 mm have been considered unstable on the basis of probable ligament rupture.[67,68]

After the transverse ligament ruptures, the support provided by the elastic occiput-C1-C2 ligaments is inadequate to prevent significant displacement of C1 on C2, and minor trauma can cause late neurologic sequelae or sudden death resulting from C1-C2 subluxation.[25,67]

Extension injuries of the cervical spine frequently yield no dramatic radiologic findings. The lateral radiograph may disclose a slight posterior subluxation of one vertebra on

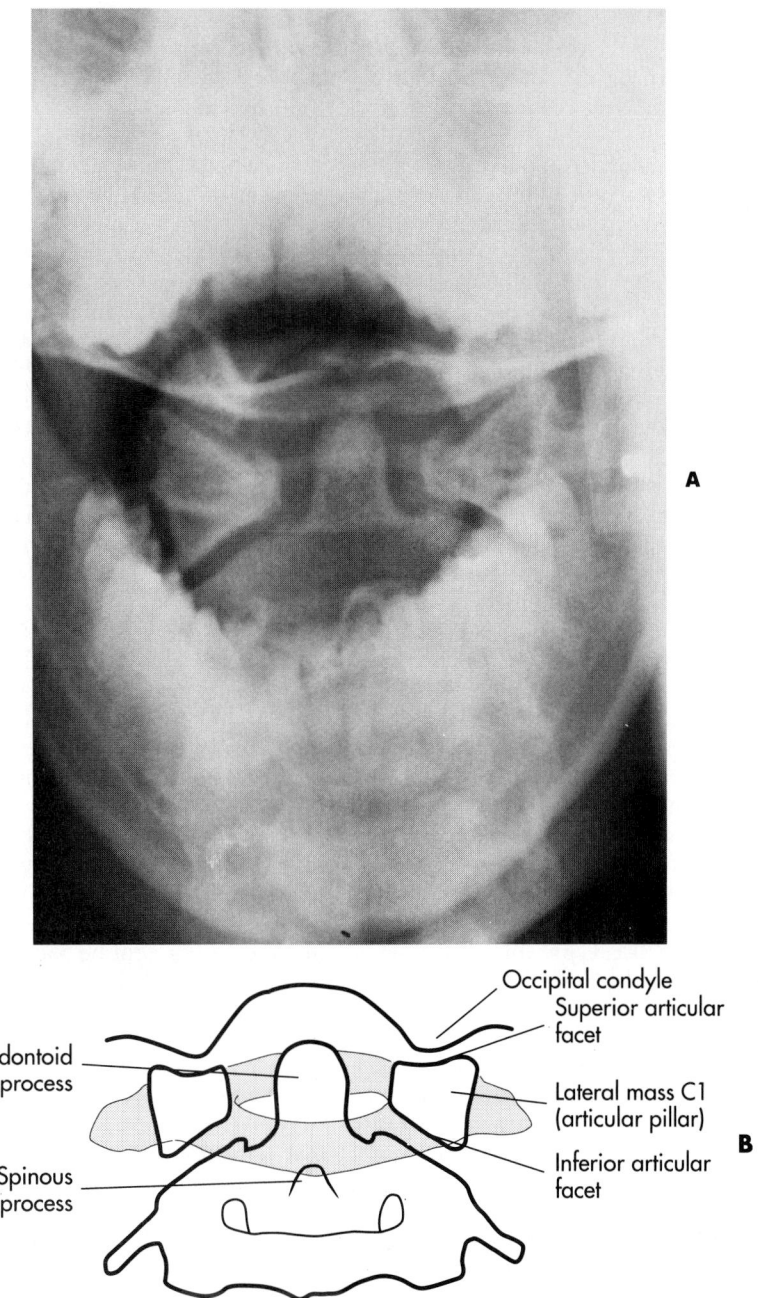

FIG. 22-13. Open-mouth view of C1 and C2. (*From Rosen P, et al:* Emergency medicine, *ed 4, St. Louis, 1997, Mosby.*)

another, a small avulsion of the anterior body, or a prevertebral hematoma.

The *odontoid view* (open-mouth view) allows visualization of the entire odontoid process and the body of C2 (Fig. 22-13). The dens should be centered between the lateral masses of the atlas.

The odontoid can normally vary in radiologic appearance. It is normally inclined posteriorly at an average angle of 17 degrees but can also have a posterior, lordotic curve; an anterior, kyphotic curve; or a slight lateral curve, usually less than 5 degrees. Fractures of the odontoid may be isolated findings or may occur in combination with frac-

tures through the body of the axis. Three basic types exist: Type 1 fractures involve the apex of the dens and are exceedingly rare. Type 2 fractures are the most common, crossing the waist of the dens near its junction with the body of C2. Type 3 odontoid fractures extend into the body of C2.

Slight asymmetry of the space between the dens and the lateral masses of C1 is usually due to minor turning of the head. Patients with findings of bilateral or significant peripheral offset of the lateral masses of C1 on those of C2 should be evaluated for more serious injury—including, for example, a Jefferson fracture.[38] Failure of midline fusion and incomplete development of the arch of the atlas posteriorly are common findings associated with peripheral displacement of the lateral masses of C1 relative to C2 simulating a Jefferson fracture. CT may be necessary to rule out a true fracture.

In terms of experimentally simulated C1 burst fractures with rupture of the transverse ligament, the open-mouth view has also been helpful in determining ligament rupture and instability.[67]

Rotation is the predominant normal motion between the atlas and axis, with the alar ligaments preventing excessive rotation. It has been demonstrated that with a 5-mm anterior displacement of the atlas on the axis, unilateral C1-to-C2 dislocation can occur at 45-degree rotation.[73]

Diversity of accessory bony ossicles may be seen at the apex of the dens and above or below the anterior arch of C1.[78] Calcification may also be noted in those areas, and careful observation should be given to superimposed images such as the styloid process, cervical collar, and foreign bodies. Asymmetry of the lateral masses and facet joints may result from developmental anomalies of the lateral masses of C1 or body and facets of C2. These are called segmentation anomalies and may vary from very minor to severe.

The dens of C2 may show as an odontoid peg (os odontoideum) when it forms a corticated ossicle separated from the body of C2. Frequently it is associated with a secondary hypertrophy of the anterior arch of C1. The origin is not clear[79,80] but may be congenital, a failure of the odontoid to fuse with the body of C2, or a product of nonunion of a fracture and may indicate C1-C2 instability requiring surgical fusion. *Os terminale* or Bergmann's ossicle has been applied to a separate ossification center of the apex of the dens; in infants and children it may appear as a fracture.[79] However, fractures of the odontoid occur more at the base, not frequently at the apex.

Most authors recommend that an anteroposterior film should be obtained and reviewed with special attention to lateral mass fractures. The only injuries that may not be evident on the lateral view but may appear on the anteroposterior views are the isolated oblique pillar fracture and the isolated transverse process fracture.[61,81] However, the findings of a recent retrospective study suggested that the initial anteroposterior film is not helpful in adding to the sensitivity of the lateral and odontoid films in diagnosing CSI.[82]

Views in addition to the "minimal" three-view series considered essential by some physicians include oblique studies, which may show fractures of the pedicle, subluxations, improved images of posterior laminar fractures, and articular mass fractures, and intervertebral foramina and lamina and may allow better assessment of the facet alignment.[83-86] In a prospective study by Freemyer,[87] 33 of 58 high-risk patients undergoing plain roentgenography had one or more fractures, subluxation, or dislocations on tomography. No fractures or dislocations were detected on the five-view series (including obliques) that were not identified or suspected on the "minimal" three-view series, including those injuries reported to be better visualized by the supine obliques. However, the supine oblique did add more specific diagnostic information in two patients. The false-positive rate of the "minimal" cervical spine series has been reported in the range of 18% to 63%.[58,88,89]

The pediatric literature has limited information on the indication for oblique views and current practice varies.[58,59]

Supine oblique rather than erect oblique views are often used in the initial evaluation because no movement of the neck is required. Recommendations regarding the indications for obtaining supine obliques range from routine use in all stable trauma patients with potential cervical spine injuries to selective addition of supine obliques if the findings of the three-view series are negative or questionable.[84,85]

Isolated fractures of vertebral body, spinous or transverse process, lamina, pedicle, or facet can be accurately delineated with flexion-extension views and CT scanning. Pillar views (anteroposterior view with the x-ray beam at a 25-degree angle and the head turned away from the beam) evaluate the lower cervical posterior elements. Atlantoaxial joint stability and ligamentous injuries may be further assessed with flexion-extension views, but only after initial films and consultations are obtained.[90] A physician must be present when these studies are performed.

Disk-space uniformity should be assured. Isolated disk-space narrowing in a child with consistent injury is suggestive of acute disk herniation. Lengthening of the disk space implies disruption of the annulus fibrosis and, possibly, the longitudinal ligaments. Interspinous widening suggests ligamentous damage.

The inferior articular facets above and the superior facets below articulate and must line up in parallel. Unilateral facet injuries usually do not damage the cord but may involve a nerve root. These injuries may be difficult to appreciate on routine radiography, although they may be suspected when failure of the spinous process to align on the anteroposterior radiograph or a slight degree of coupled subluxation of one body on another in the lateral view is observed.

Fractures caused by compression, in contrast to the wedge fractures, may appear radiologically as a symmetrical reduction of the vertebral body height anteriorly and posteriorly.

On roentgenography, by 8 years of age most of the adult patterns have been attained.[22,91] A temporal correlation appears to exist between radiographic evidence of maturation and clinical manifestations of SCI; however, causation is not implied.[8,9]

SCI Without Radiologic Abnormality. SCI without radiologic abnormality (SCIWORA) is more common in children than in adults, particularly injuries that involve the high cervical spine.[92,93] Studies have indicated that the incidence varies between 4% and 66%, accompanied by an incidence of complete cord injury of 40% to 55%.[7,8] The reason for this wide range of reported incidence of SCIWORA is unclear, although it may reflect differences in the age or population of patients studied (hospital vs. rehabilitation). Kewalramani, in an epidemiologic analysis of 16 California counties, found an incidence of 20% of all pediatric spinal injuries, probably most accurately reflecting the true incidence of this syndrome.[94]

Factors contributing to development of SCIWORA in children are unknown at present. However, attention has been given to the anatomic and biomechanical differences and the effects of aging of the spine. Indirect evidence suggests that maturation of the vascular supply to the spinal cord might play a role in a SCI and may account for some of the reported cases of SCIWORA.[9,95] The most common cause is motor vehicle accidents.

The mechanisms proposed for SCIWORA include hyperextension with inward bulging of interlaminar ligaments, reversible disk prolapse, flexion compression of the cord, longitudinal distraction of the cord, and vertebral artery spasm or thrombosis.[9,57,96,97] Depending on the mechanism of neck injury, a combination of these proposed mechanisms may work to produce SCIWORA. It is suspected that flexion compression forces were responsible for the more severe lesions in the younger age group, accounting for the traumatic myelopathy that occurred at C1 to C4 in most complete lesions in the younger patients. However, the younger patients had less severe injuries at C5 to C8, the area in which most older children sustained their lesions.[9]

SCIWORA is a diagnosis of exclusion that should only be made after occult fractures and ligament/disk damage have been ruled out with CT, flexion-extension views under fluoroscopy, and myelography. MRI of the cervical spine is usually necessary to rule out spinal-cord compression. In all of the cases of SCIWORA these tests show no abnormality soon after the injury. Patients with suspected SCIWORA should be considered for high-resolution, thin-section CT and high field strength MRI (Fig. 22-14). However, if there is neurologic sequelae, MRI performed 1 to 3 months after the injury may reveal atrophy of the spinal cord.

History of paresthesia may be the only clinical finding in SCIWORA; children with significant neck trauma and normal neurologic findings should be questioned specifically regarding paresthesia at the time of the accident.[9]

Prognosis in SCIWORA depends on the extent of spinal cord abnormality. Pang and Wilberger[9] recently reported an association of SCIWORA with poor prognosis; 55% of the children with SCIWORA had complete neurologic injuries and 54% had delayed onset of symptoms (range, 30 minutes to 4 days; mean, 1.2 days after injury). Of the lesions, 83% involved the cervical cord, 58% involved children younger than 8 years, and 42% involved children 8 years or older.

The nature of cord injuries is variable. In the subset of 13 patients with delayed onset of neurologic deficit reported by Pang and Wilberger[9], two were complete, 7 central, and 4 partial. Seven of these patients later recalled transient paresthesia at the time of the injury. No associations were identified in age distribution or mechanism of injury to distinguish this group from those patients with immediate cord deficit. In the delayed-paralysis group, paralysis usually develops rapidly once it begins and most frequently culminates in a complete cord lesion.

Missed Spinal Fracture. Despite the extensive radiologic evaluation, some cervical spine fractures are still overlooked, potentially delaying diagnosis. Several explanations for overlooked spinal injuries in children are likely: inappropriate or incomplete views, lack of experience in evaluating infants, failure to distinguish normal anatomy

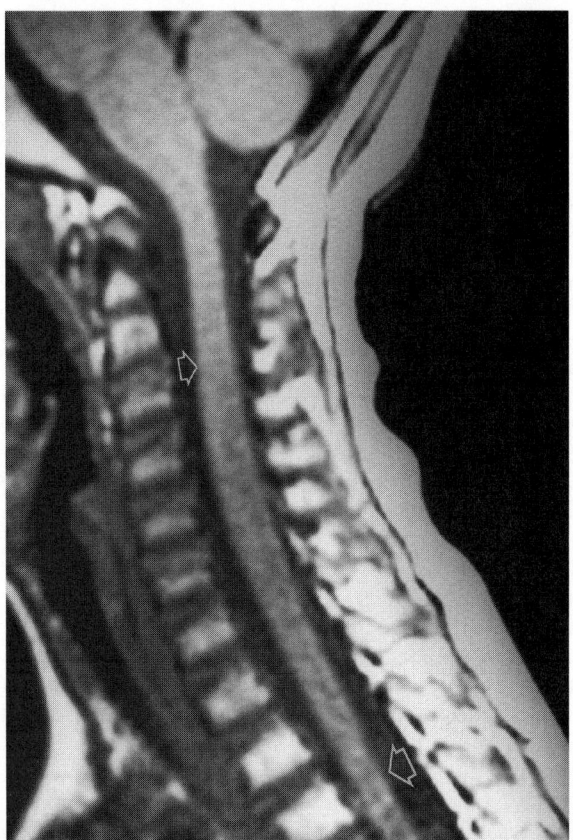

FIG. 22-14. Sagital view magnetic resonance image of the cervical region. T1-weighted image. Spinal cord has an increased signal (bright) *(arrows)*. Normal study in a 2-month-old girl.

from subluxation, significant soft-tissue swelling, and other signs. Under ideal conditions and x-ray exposures, a sensitivity of 95% in detecting cervical spine injuries can be attained with plain x-ray films.[59] The false-negative rate of the cervical spine x-ray has been reported to range from 1.5% to 20%[88,98,99] as detected on CT.

Delay in clearance of the cervical spine of an acutely injured patient leads to unnecessary discomfort from prolonged use of a stiff collar or other uncomfortable technique. Evidence that delayed diagnosis can increase neurologic deficit during resuscitation and the reported occurrence of subtle neurologic signs resulting from minor trauma[49] has led to early completion of cervical spine films in the resuscitative algorithm of trauma patients.[15,49,100-102] However, the use of other available modalities in evaluating the cervical spine should be considered and emphasis on completion of cervical spine films should not be made at the expense of resuscitation.

CT scanning is useful in patients with equivocal or inconsistent radiologic evidence of SCI. The early clearance of the cervical spine in acutely injured blunt-trauma patients by means of plain roentgenography alone is not always possible because of a lack of patient cooperation, the nature of associated injuries, unavailability of equipment, or technical inability to view all the cervical vertebrae in a timely fashion on conventional x-rays. It is therefore important to be able to supplement the plain-film cervical spine series with another diagnostic technique that is accurate, safe, and efficient.

It has been suggested[88] that CT is useful in the evaluation of all patients with equivocal areas on their plain cervical spine x-ray films and for better understanding of complex fractures/dislocations that may result in compromise of the spinal cord.[98] This capacity of CT to rule out suspected areas of pathologic involvement quickly decreases patient evaluation time, expense, and in some cases, length of hospital stay.[58,88]

Some authors suggest that because of the high cost of portable x-ray films and because the quality of these x-ray films is not always optimal, CT scanning may be more economical in the final evaluation of patients.[88] However, despite the technical superiority of CT, the low incidence of cervical spine injury and the lack of availability in some areas make the routine use of CT an impractical screening tool.[52,60] CT is excellent in visualizing paraspinal soft tissues, as well as bone. With contrast augmentation, this imaging technique provides excellent definition of the subarachnoid space, disk abnormalities, and sites of epidural compression. CT scanning has been shown to be more sensitive in delineating bony integrity and position of bone fragments in relation to the spinal canal.[103,104] It has also been shown to reveal more than twice as many cervical spine fractures as plain x-ray films alone.[104] CT should be performed in injuries resulting in neurologic deficit, fractures of the posterior arch of the cervical canal, and fractures in which penetration of fragments into the spinal canal is a clinical consideration.[57,105]

The CT scan of the cervical spine also has limitations. CT resolution does not allow adequate visualization of the cord or nerve roots anywhere but in the upper cervical region.[106] In a study of patients with vertebral burst fractures,[107] 65.2% had acute neurologic deficits; however, no definite correlation existed between radiographic appearance on plain radiography or CT and neurologic status. Neither of these techniques provides a direct image of the nature or extent of cord damage because the internal anatomy of the spinal cord cannot be visualized. Thus the evaluation must be primarily clinical rather than radiographic.

Visualization of the atlantal transverse ligament is inconsistent using CT scanning.[108,109] The transverse plane of CT images makes subtle malalignment difficult to interpret, but sagittal reconstruction can compensate for the deficiency.[110] Small vertebral fractures, axially oriented fractures that fall within the CT slice, and compression fractures may be overlooked.[60,65,110] Acheson has suggested the use of 1.5-mm slices through a vertebra suspected to be damaged to improve the detection of fractures in these cases.[58]

CT images in the axial plane can be reformatted in sagittal, coronal, or oblique planes without additional movement of the patient or additional exposure to radiation, giving more information with less chance of harm to the patient (Fig. 22-15).[111]

Myelography. Myelography, often performed in conjunction with computed tomography, is rarely necessary. It is recommended when clinical signs of cord compression,

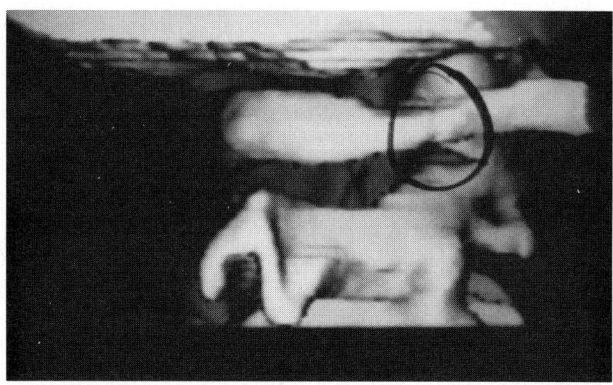

FIG. 22-15. Computer-generated image of the upper cervical spine by CT. Nondisplaced fracture of the right lamina of C1 is noted.

neurologic deficit, or neurologic deterioration are not explained by findings on X-ray films or plain CT.[2] This procedure is associated with adverse reactions including seizures, allergic phenomena, vomiting, headache, pain, and dizziness, even with the newer nonionic contrast agents.[112] Compared with MRI, myelography has several disadvantages: (1) it has a higher frequency of false-negative results, (2) the site of myelographic block may not correspond with the level of the lesion, (3) myelography may fail to demonstrate more than one area of damage, and (4) it cannot define the underlying spinal cord abnormality.[43,113,114]

Other Tests. Somatosensory evoked potentials have been used to diagnose cervical cord lesions.[43] However, cervical responses are typically small and can be difficult to identify even in clinically normal infants.[115] Electromyography and nerve-conduction studies can show anterior horn cell and spinal root lesions, but these abnormalities are not specific to SCI.

Tomography. Tomography has largely been supplanted by CT scanning. It is useful in evaluating fractures in which the fracture line is oriented in the axial plane such as dens fractures and horizontal avulsion of the anterior arch of the atlas.

Magnetic Resonance Imaging. MRI has become the noninvasive imaging modality of choice for almost all diseases of the brain and spinal cord. MRI relies on physical interactions between protons and external magnetic fields. Protons behave as dipoles, aligning themselves in the direction of a strong magnetic field applied to the body. A radio frequency wave burst applied at right angles to the axis of the magnetic field deflects the protons. When the radio frequency current is turned off, the protons "dephase" in the plane of the applied radio frequency and then realign themselves with the field; the times required for these two processes (known as T2 and T1 "relaxations") can be measured.[116-118] Serial images in two or three (axial, sagittal, coronal, or all three) planes are routinely obtained for optimal evaluation of normal anatomic structures and pathologic lesions. Normal and abnormal biologic tissues have different rates of T2 and T1 relaxation and may contain different concentrations of protons. The "spin echo"

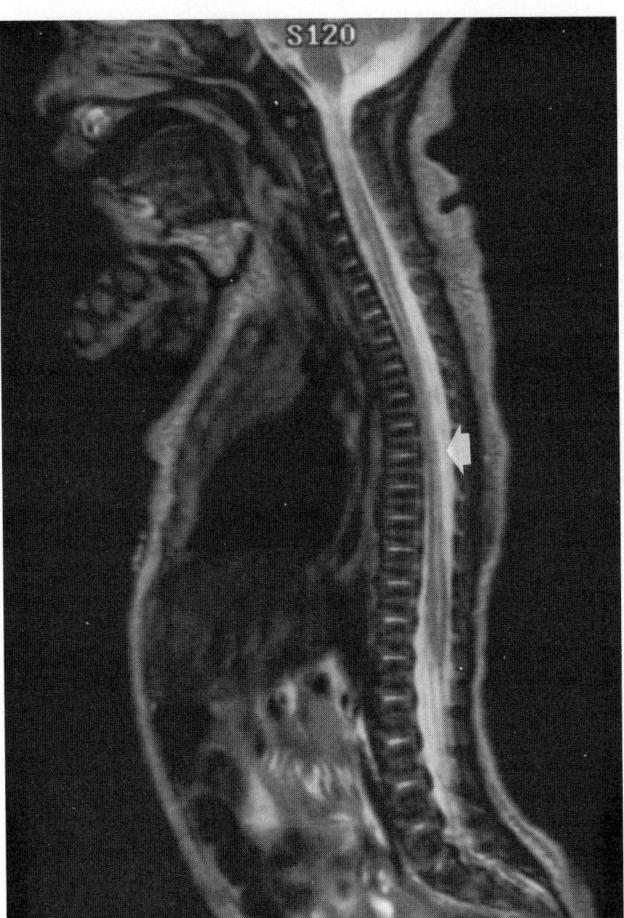

FIG. 22-16. Sagital T2-weighted MRI of the entire spine in a 2 months old female. Cerebral-spinal fluid has an increased signal (bright) (see arrow).

technique of imaging yields important data concerning these tissue differences. An initial radio frequency pulse is applied at 90 degrees to the axis of the magnetic field, followed at a predetermined interval (known as echo time) by a second pulse in a direction 180 degrees from that of the first. These radio frequency pulse cycles are repeated 128 or 256 times at a preset interval (known as the "repetition time"). By varying the echo and repetition times, the operator can obtain radio signals containing additional data relevant to T1 or T2 relaxations or to proton concentration. The resulted scans are referred to as "T1-weighted," "T2-weighted," and "proton-density images," respectively.

The MRI appearance of the vertebral column depends mainly on the signal from the bone marrow (Figs. 22-16 and 22-17, A and B). Fat within the marrow of the vertebral bodies, neural arches, and articular pillars has a moderately intense signal in T1-weighted images. Dense cortical bones surrounding these osseous structures produce a negligible signal. The intervertebral disk structure can also be identified with MRI. The nucleus pulposus and medial portions of the annulus in T2-weighted images produce a relatively bright signal. The collagenous fibers in the pe-

riphery produce little signal in T1- and T2-weighted images. An MRI-sensitive, biologically inert intravenous contrast medium, gadolinium, can be administered to aid detection of lesions invisible or poorly seen on plain MRI scans. Unlike iodinated CT contrast media, which are hazardous in allergic patients, gadolinium is not known to pose any such danger.

The use of MRI in head trauma has been helpful in identifying parenchymal contusion and intracranial hemorrhage.[119-121] Epidural and intramedullary hematomas may yield an intense signal for MRI from methemoglobin after the acute stage and are easily detected in both T1- and T2-weighted images.

Experience with MRI in pediatric trauma and spinal disease is very limited.[28,122-125] MRI is superior to CT in demonstrating spinal cord injury (edema, hemorrhage, compression, and transection) and intervertebral disk herniation and in differentiating extramedullary from intramedullary lesions.[106,116,117] However, CT was superior to MRI in demonstrating osseous injury. T1-weighted spin-echo and gradient recalled acquisition at steady state (GRASS) sequences have proved best for osseous injury, and T2-weighted spin-echo sequence imaging demonstrate spinal cord edema and acute hemorrhage best.

The use of MRI has been described for the assessment of the transverse ligament of the atlas because MRI clearly demonstrates ligaments. Tears of the transverse ligament appear as a loss of anatomic continuity of the ligament. Acute hemorrhage may also be defined. Furthermore, MRI may help select patients prone to nonunion fractures of the odontoid and identify candidates for early surgical stabilization.

Certain patterns of MRI signals are associated with a normal spinal cord signal. The contrast between high-intensity cerebrospinal fluid (CSF) and lower-intensity spinal cord creates a magnificent myelographic effect. T1-weighted images show the cord to have a higher-intensity signal than the CSF in proton density. With T2-weighted images, the CSF has a brighter signal intensity than the spinal cord. Rarely, the dentate ligament or vessels in the subarachnoid space are identified.

MRI may help identify patients prone to nonunion fractures of the odontoid and candidates for early surgical stabilization.[28]

The major drawbacks of the technique are lack of availability, the potential hazard of metal material inside the patient, and the image degradation by metallic collars and resuscitative equipment. These problems will likely be overcome in the near future. Improved "MRI-compatible," pneumatically driven fluidic ventilators are now commercially available. Devices using telemetric or fiberoptic transmission can monitor hemodynamic status at a distance without interfering with MRI signals.[117,126]

Thoracic Spine (T1-T10) Injuries

Clinical Findings. Most thoracic spine injuries are a direct result of flexion or axial stress. Severe multiple trauma may impart energy sufficient to cause a fracture or dislocation. When this occurs, a neurologic deficit may develop because of the relatively narrow diameter of the spinal canal.

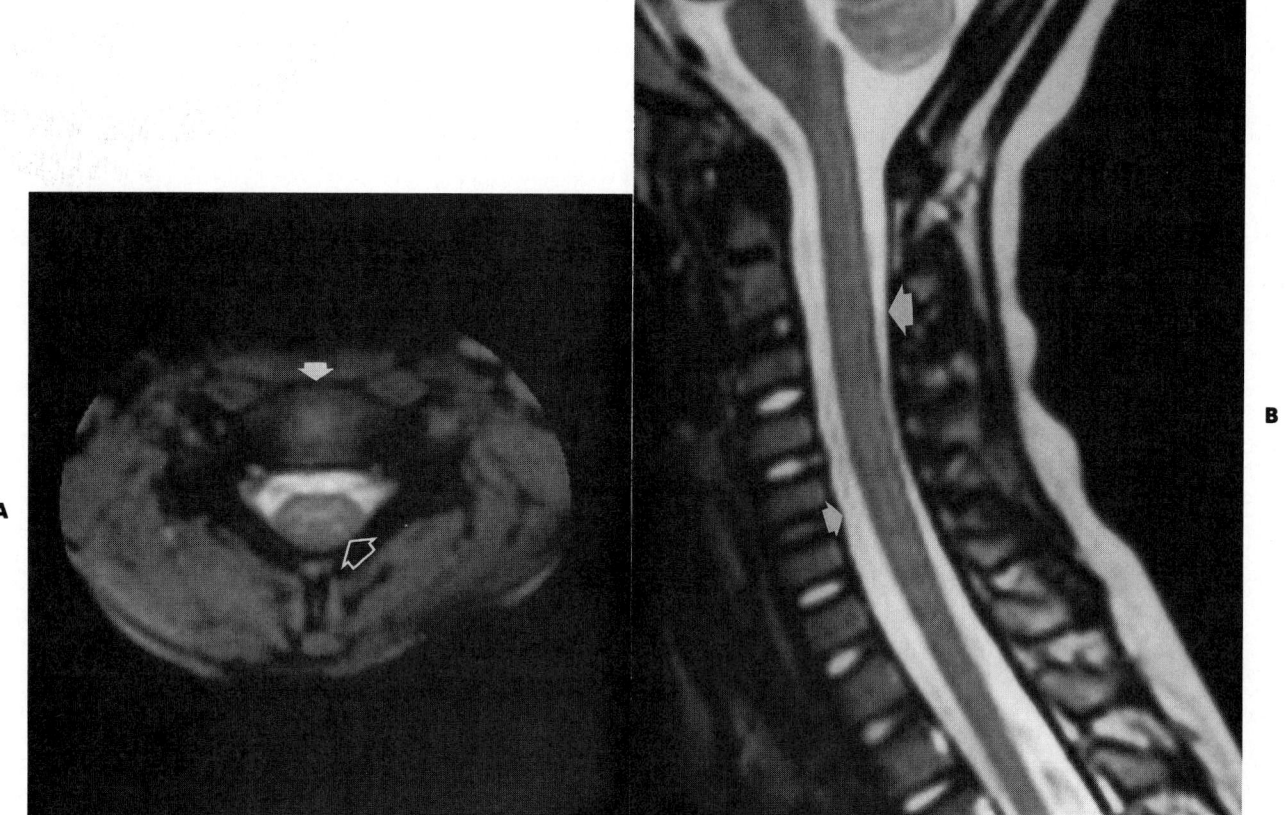

FIG. 22-17. A, Axial T2-weighted MRI through the intervertebral space of C4-C5 in a 2-month-old girl. Spinal fluid has a bright image. *Open arrow,* spinal cord. *White arrow,* intervertebral disc. **B,** Sagittal T2-weighted MRI of the cervical area. Normal study in a 2-month-old girl. Spinal fluid has a bright image *(white arrow).*

Flexion injury usually results in a wedge fracture with collapse of the vertebral body anteriorly and may be accompanied by forward subluxation.

Upper thoracic spinal lesions have been reported in the total absence of osteoarticular injury on plain radiography. A lower cervical supine oblique view may be beneficial in visualizing the cervicothoracic junction. Harris states that the supine oblique views, although slightly distorted because of short target-film distance magnification, are more likely to be of diagnostic quality and to provide more useful information and no patient movement compared with the swimmer's view.[85]

"Longitudinal axial traction" may be the mechanism of such injuries in a number of children who have upper-thoracic spinal cord lesions and total absence of osteoarticular injury on plain radiography.[96,127,128] Widening of the mediastinum may be associated with fractures of T1-T5.

Radiologic Studies. Routine plain film examinations are indicated in conditions paralleling those suggested for cervical spine injury. Initially, cross-table lateral and anteroposterior views should be obtained with the patient immobilized on a firm backboard. The spaces between the vertebral bodies and symmetry of the vertebral structures should be evaluated.

CT has not been found to be reliable in the study of thoracolumbar spinal injury.[129] However, MRI may be a promising technique for the evaluation of these injuries because of the qualities mentioned (Fig. 22-18, *A* and *B*).[112,113,121]

Thoracolumbar (T11-L1) and Lumbar Spine Injuries

Clinical Findings. Excessive stress in flexion or axial loading can cause wedge and burst fractures. Of particular importance are the flexion-distraction or chance fractures of the spine, associated with hyperflexion of the spine about a fixed axis anterior to the vertebral column (Fig. 22-19, *A* and *B*).[130] This lesion is described in children wearing automobile lap belts at the time of injury; concurrent intraabdominal injuries must also be sought.[129,131,132] Children are more susceptible than adults to rotational stresses resulting in unstable fracture-dislocations.

Lumbar disk herniation may be noted after falls on the buttocks. Neurologic signs may mimic those of chronic lumbar disk herniation or may be present as an acute cauda equina syndrome with sphincter dysfunction.

Injuries below the L2 vertebral level affect only the cauda equina and produce monoradicular and polyradicular deficits. Conus medullaris injuries are characterized by

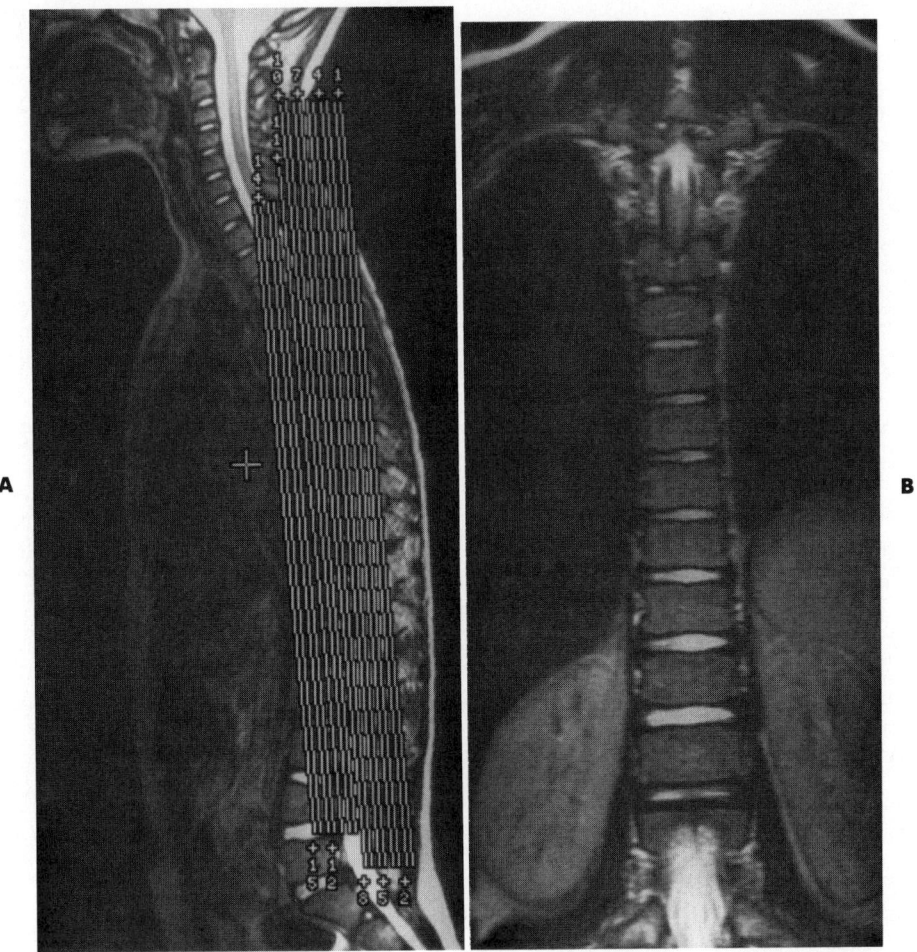

FIG. 22-18. A, Coronal scanning planes of the thoracic region. Serial images in two or three planes are routinely obtained for optimal evaluation of normal or pathologic structures. **B,** Normal thoracic spine anatomy seen in a coronal view T2-weighted magnetic resonance image of a 7-year-old boy.

fecal and urinary incontinence caused by sphincter dysfunction and perineal sensory loss.

Unstable fractures may occur at the junction of the mobile lumbar spine with the relatively immobile thoracic spine. Bone and disk material frequently penetrate into the canal.

Radiologic Studies. Routine radiography may be unnecessary in asymptomatic blunt-trauma patients without clinical neurologic deficits or distracting injuries. Lateral x-ray studies should be obtained initially and followed by anteroposterior views (Figs. 22-20 and 22-21). Most fractures are observed in the T10-L4 region. Fractures at several levels may be seen. Radiologic findings in traumatic disk herniation may include only a narrowing of the intervertebral disk space. MRI is a promising technique in the evaluation of these injuries because of the qualities mentioned (Figure 22-22).[112,113,121]

Sacral and Coccygeal Spine Injuries

Clinical Findings. Generally the severity of sacral fractures reflects the force acting on the lumbar spine or pelvis at the time of the injury. Direct impact to the buttocks may

result in a low transverse fracture of the sacrum or in a coccygeal fracture. Hyperflexion of the lumbar spine and a locked pelvis in a posture of hip flexion can cause transverse fractures of the sacrum with spondylolisthesis. Pelvic fractures are usually associated with vertically oriented sacral fractures.

Neurologic deficit usually manifests as weakness of dorsi and plantar flexion, bowel and bladder dysfunction, and perineal numbness.

Coccygeal fractures are not associated with recognized acute neurologic deficit but are very uncomfortable. Coccydynia, a chronic disabling pain syndrome of the coccygeal area, develops in some patients.

Radiologic Studies. A routine pelvic x-ray study in a multiple-system trauma victim may show a concurrent injury of the spine. MRI may be helpful in the evaluation of these injuries because of the qualities mentioned (Fig. 22-23).[112,113,121]

Neck Injuries

Penetrating injuries produced by gunshot to the neck have a high mortality, and few patients reach the emer-

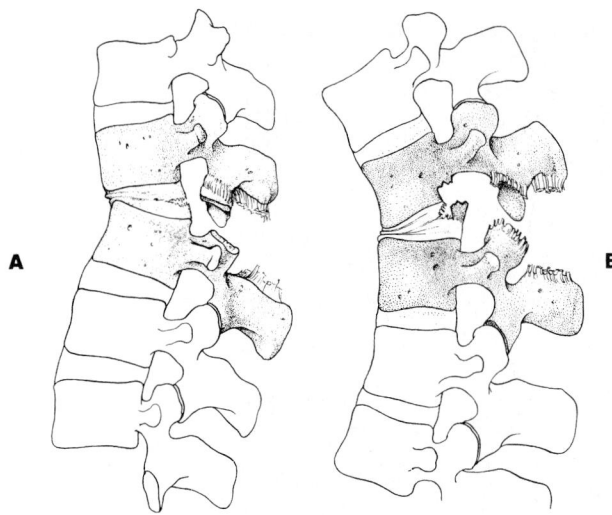

FIG. 22-19. Characteristic spinal injuries associated with seat belts. **A,** Drawing of lateral radiograph that shows fracture of the articular process, laceration of the dorsal segment of intervertebral disk, posterior widening of the contiguous wider vertebral spaces, and ligamentous damage. **B,** Drawing of lateral radiograph with additional avulsion fracture of the dorsal edge of the vertebral body from stress induced by the posterior longitudinal ligament. (From Smith WS and Kaufer H: J Bone Joint Surg 51A:239, 1969.)

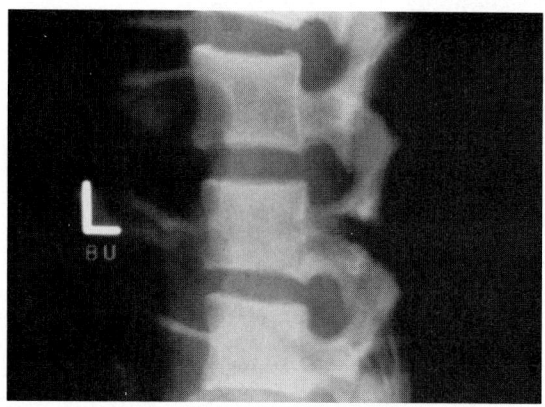

FIG. 22-20. Chance fracture of L3.

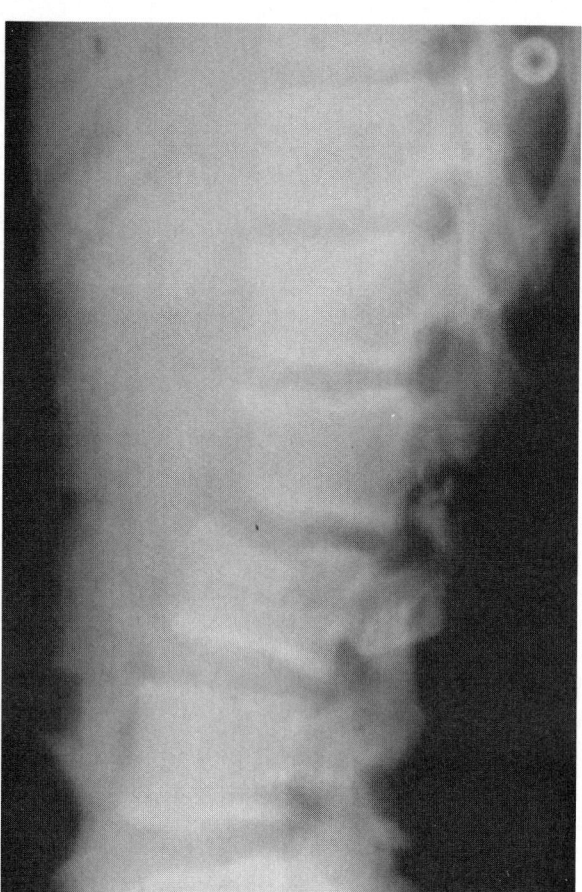

FIG. 22-21. Fracture of L2-L3 with dislocation.

gency department alive. The neck has been divided into three zones: zone I, below the sternal notch; zone II, from the sternal notch to the angle of the mandible; and zone III, above the angle of the mandible. Low-velocity bullets such as the .22-caliber rimfire and some BB guns inflict injuries only within the wound track. Expanding and high-velocity bullets are very destructive to tissue in the neck, even with tangential wounds or without striking a vital structure.

Blunt Neck Injuries. Blunt trauma can cause severe, life-threatening injuries and may be less obvious. Extensive vascular and visceral injury may result. Vascular injury is usually caused by intimal disruption with subsequent thrombosis, with or without embolization. Visceral injuries may include disruption of the trachea or esophagus by the sudden compression of air trapped in their lumina.

SCI may occur in conjunction with penetrating or blunt neck injury. Any evidence of neurologic deficit in these patients should alert the physician to the possibility of an SCI. Nevertheless, brachial plexus injury may be caused by an external pressure hematoma or by a fracture of the clavicle. Injury of the stellate ganglion may result in Horner syndrome. Stridor or alteration in phonation may be seen with injury to the vagus nerve or, specifically, to the recurrent laryngeal branch. Weakness of the trapezius muscle indicates damage to the spinal accessory nerve as it courses through the posterior cervical triangle. Deviation of the tongue toward the injured hypoglossal nerve results when this cranial nerve is damaged in the upper portion of the anterior cervical triangle.

Neck Sprain and Strains

The literature detailing neck sprains and strains in children is limited. Both terms tend to be used indiscriminately and incorporated into the category of spinal column injuries. A sprain is an injury to the ligamentous structure, and a strain is an injury to a muscle-tendon unit. Neither is associated with neurologic abnormalities or potential for spinal cord damage as a result of spinal instability.

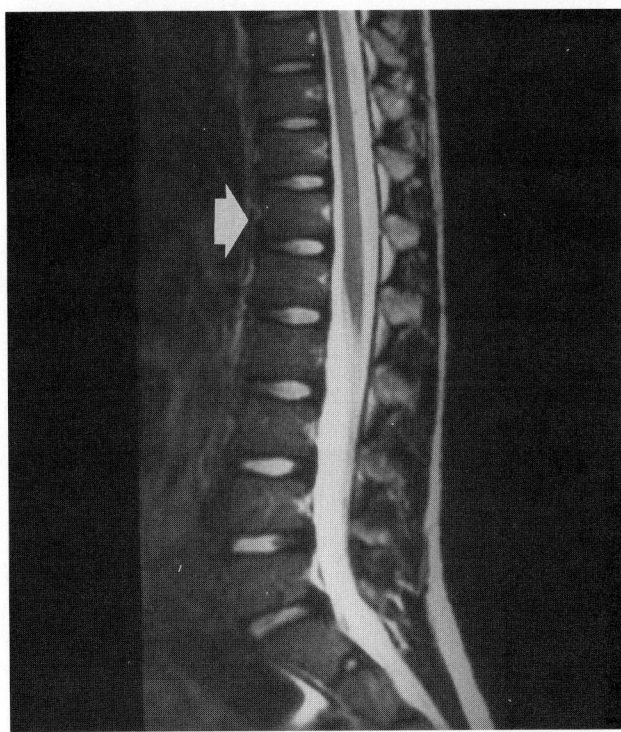

FIG. 22-22. Sagital T-2–weighted magnetic resonance image of the lower thoracic and lumbar area with normal anatomy. *White arrow,* T12.

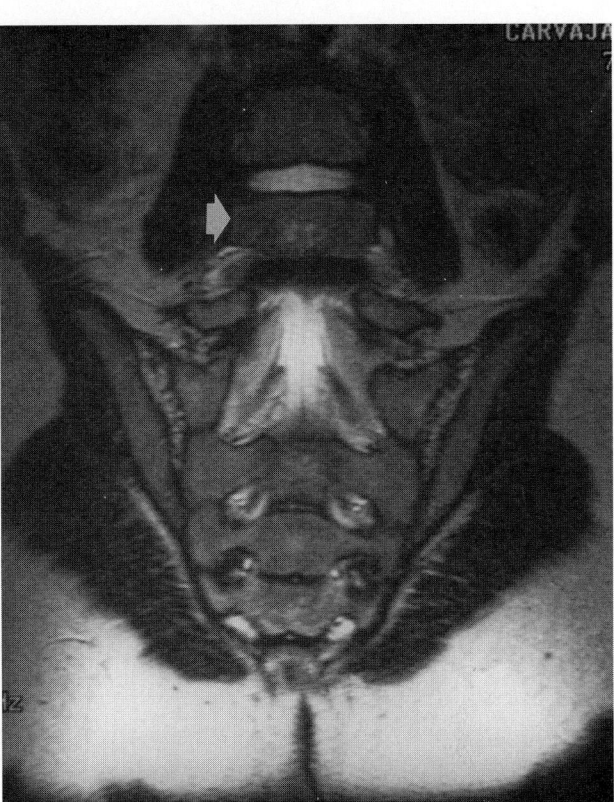

FIG. 22-23. Normal coronal MRI of the lower lumbar and sacrum in a 5-year-old boy. T-2–weighted image. *White arrow,* L5.

There is a tendency to use a more clinical definition in which "cervical strain" is defined as acute trauma-related neck pain and tenderness, with limitation of movement, muscle spasm, rapid recovery with conservative treatment, and absence of evidence of neurologic or radiologic abnormalities (not including transient reversal of the normal cervical lordosis). "Cervical sprain" may have all of these features and radiologic evidence of subluxation on dynamic films.

A large series of spinal injuries in children[8] showed that cervical strain was the dysfunction that caused almost 40% of the admissions for neck injury. Acute sprains of the cervical spine may occur because sudden motion bends the spine; its severity depends on the forces involved and the relative movements of the head and the neck on the torso. Associated injuries such as concussion should always be considered.

Seat belts prevent deadly injuries but may increase the risk of neck sprain. "Whiplash injury" refers to the group of acute sprain symptoms that follow sudden head movement, such as that which occurs in rear-end motor collisions. Bony damage and other serious injuries are excluded in this definition. The injury causes stretching and bruising of the muscles and supporting ligaments, which progress to cervical pain and stiffness, often extending into the shoulders and interscapular region and associated with occipital pain or generalized headache. The onset of symptoms is delayed up to 24 hours in a large proportion of patients.

Treatment relates to rest and muscle relaxation. Nonsteroidal antiinflammatory agents and warm packs are useful initially.

Torticollis is the presence of pain in the muscles of the neck. *Congenital torticollis,* or "wryneck," in infancy has been associated with breech presentation and a traumatic delivery with contusion of the sternocleidomastoid muscle. A hematoma yields fibrosis and a palpable mass of the sternocleidomastoid muscle and a compensatory twisting of the head and neck. Neurologic examination and radiographic findings are normal. Treatment consists of supervised passive neck motion exercises (see Chapter 18).

Traumatic or *spastic torticollis* is an acute neck sprain that can occur after mild trauma sustained in sports, falls, or vehicular accidents. The child may complain of pain in the neck and hold the head to one side in a fixed position similar to that seen in a rotary subluxation of the atlantoaxial joint.

Back Strain

Analysis of disease classification shows that low back pain is the most common musculoskeletal presenting complaint.[133] It is the major cause of disability in young patients. Although most cases are acute in onset and resolution, there is a progression to a refractory condition, the low back pain syndrome.[134]

The lumbosacral and upper-thoracic areas are the most commonly involved. Bilateral back pain is most often seen in adolescents. Physical examination usually reveals spasm and tenderness of the paraspinous muscles and augmentation of the back pain during straight-leg raising, with normal neurologic findings. Radiologic examination reveals normal results for bony abnormalities.

Spinal fractures other than cervical ones may be overlooked. Cervical spine films are usually obtained in the initial management, but the need for thoracic or lumbar spine films may not be apparent until days to weeks later, when the patient continues to complain of back pain. Neurologic deficit may have been overlooked in the initial assessment or may develop secondarily.

DIFFERENTIAL CONSIDERATIONS

Although the history and temporal sequence of events usually define the cause, inconsistent presentations may prompt consideration of other conditions. Trauma-related possibilities include bilateral brachial plexus injury such as that which might occur at birth, nerve root injury, and cauda equina syndrome. Vascular abnormalities may lead to ischemia as a result of thoracic aorta dissection, epidural hematoma, or thromboembolic disease. Spinal tumor may also be causative. Hysterical paralysis or conversion reactions have been reported to mimic acute spinal cord injury (see Chapter 58).

MANAGEMENT

Cervical Spine Injuries

A team approach to cervical spine injuries is essential. Immobilization of the cervical spine with immediate assessment and correction of compromised cardiopulmonary status is always the initial concern in management. Immediate consultation with a neurosurgeon is necessary when cervical spine injuries are suspected. Unfortunately, in approximately 10% of patients who are neurologically intact at initial observation, neurologic deficits develop as a result of manipulation during resuscitation.[18,101]

The goal must be to maintain adequate cardiopulmonary function and spinal immobilization. Implementation of these principles begins in the prehospital setting, at the injury site, with recognition of an actual or potential SCI. In the case of SCI, immobilization is the first step in the treatment and prevention of exacerbation of any injury of the central nervous system resulting from mechanical or vascular disruption. In the evaluation of the airway and the vascular structures, precautions must be taken to avoid doing more damage to existing cervical spine or cord lesions. If the head is held in a deviated position, it must not be corrected by manipulation; the cord may be damaged by vertebral misalignment. Pain and rigidity of the cervical muscles should alert the clinician to the possibility of underlying spine injury.

The health care provider should address the airway and cervical spine immobilization simultaneously. Between 3% and 25% of SCI occurs after the initial insult, during transport or early in management.[100] Movement from a prone to a supine position is performed with a log-rolling maneuver, while one person maintains the patient's head and neck neutrality. The need for prompt airway management may preclude a complete neurologic assessment or appropriate and good-quality cervical spine films.

Immobilization

Proper management at the scene of an accident during the extrication, transport, and evaluation of the trauma victim requires the use of cervical immobilization devices. Some authors believe that immobilization is generally not needed in a crying and fighting child who resists attempts to immobilize the cervical spine and who will move the spine more in the fight over the restraints.[69] It is unlikely that the child would resist strongly if a cervical spine lesion is present. Neck movement may cause or aggravate damage to the spinal cord in an unstable cervical spine.

Gentle efforts should be made to immobilize the crying child with an obviously stiff neck after trauma. Cervical spine neutrality should be maintained with gentle in-line stabilization until immobilization is achieved. If the head is tilted to one direction and the child resists gentle motion toward neutrality, the spine should be immobilized in the original position. The patient should be placed on a spinal board or scoop device and then immobilized with tape on the forehead and sandbags alongside the head and neck; secure binding or strapping of the trunk to the board should be achieved. The patient should be immobilized on the backboard so that the entire board may be log-rolled in the event of emesis. When extrication from a sitting position is required, a short backboard is useful. If a helmet is in place, leave it alone if breathing is adequate, or use recommended helmet-removal techniques if necessary.[135]

Many devices are available with which to achieve immobilization and stabilization of the spine, although studies have shown them to be less than ideal and to do little more than serve as a warning to the physician that a neck injury may be present.[100,136-138] From the adult experience, it is recommended that the head be held in neutral position with sandbags and tape (1 to 3 inches) across the forehead and chin with the patient on a rigid backboard. This technique, in combination with a stiff collar, is considered the most effective immobilization.[100,139] However, this method may not be applicable to pediatric patients because of significant differences in anatomy, size, and equipment design. Useful cervical collars should be semirigid, appropriate in size, and easy to apply and remove, and they should not obstruct the airway. Appropriate cervical immobilization can be achieved with a semihard Stiff-Neck Immobilizing Collar, the Philadelphia collar, or a four-poster collar.

The mechanism of splinting the head and torso to a rigid object appears to be superior in cervical-stabilizing efficacy to the use of a cervical collar. The authors of a recent study compared different methods of cervical immobilization and concluded that the methods involving a short board were far superior to collars in all planes of movement.[139] This finding was later confirmed with radiographic methods.[140]

Airway and Ventilation

Urgent management of the unstable airway is essential. Oxygenation and positive end-expiratory pressure are useful in the management of neurogenic pulmonary edema.[69]

Simultaneous stability of the airways and the cervical spine should be provided. Because many patients require intubation in the field or immediately after arrival in the emergency department, determination of the presence and severity of SCI may not be possible before intubation.

Airway injury may announce itself by obstruction, noisy respiration, suprasternal retraction, subcutaneous emphysema, hemoptysis, voice change, or hypoxia. Complete evaluation of the airway includes examination of the thorax for evidence of pneumothorax, tension pneumothorax, and hemopneumothorax.

Cervical injuries may be associated with an airway obstruction resulting from retropharyngeal hemorrhage or edema, as well as with associated maxillofacial trauma.[141] Bleeding from facial injuries, vomitus, and oral-pharyngeal secretions often contribute to airway obstruction.

Compression of the larynx against the cervical vertebral bodies by a direct blow to the neck may produce a laryngeal fracture with associated airway obstruction. In addition to the symptoms of airway obstruction, the three most common symptoms of laryngeal fracture are subcutaneous emphysema, aphonia, and severe facial pain.[20] The best diagnostic sign of a fractured larynx is the loss of normal anatomic landmarks produced by the laryngeal cartilages.

Early endotracheal intubation should be performed in patients with intercostal or diaphragmatic hypofunction or paralysis. Bag-valve mask ventilation can usually be applied, particularly with gentle cricoid pressure (Sellick maneuver).[142]

Movement of the neck during resuscitation and airway management is of concern in trauma victims with potential spinal injury. Some maneuvers may cause or aggravate a spinal injury by allowing movement regardless of stabilization measures.[143] Studies of a fresh cadaver model with a ligamentous injury to C5-C6 show that the extension of the neck that occurs with an aggressive chin lift, jaw thrust, insertion of an esophageal obturator airway, and oral endotracheal intubation produces potential aggravation of the injury, as demonstrated by anterior subluxation or widening of the disk space.[136,144] Use of a soft cervical collar or a two-piece semirigid collar failed to immobilize the neck effectively and consistently during endotracheal intubation, chin lift, or jaw thrust.[143]

Determination of the safest technique for endotracheal intubation in patients with suspected cervical trauma is controversial.[145-147] Although nasotracheal intubation is classically used, its benefits have not been clearly documented; nor is it easily achieved in younger children, in whom it may be contraindicated.[148,149]

Nasotracheal intubation and orotracheal intubation with in-line manual cervical immobilization are the most frequently recommended techniques in patients with suspected cervical-spine injury. The *Advanced Trauma Life Support* course specifies "in-line manual cervical immobilization," implying that an assistant should effect stabilization during intubation to prevent movement of the cervical spine.[148] Cervical movement during intubation would seem more likely to be detected by manual immobilization than use of a cervical immobilization device alone. If the nasal route is not an option, the choice must be made among cricothyrotomy, creation of a surgical airway, and oral intubation with in-line manual stabilization.[148,149]

Nasotracheal intubation requires a patient who is breathing spontaneously, whether unconscious or conscious; adequate topical anesthesia and verbal reassurance; and the presence of a physician skilled in the technique. Nasotracheal intubation should not be attempted if the possibility of a cribriform plate fracture exists.

Orotracheal intubation with manual cervical immobilization is an alternative in the potentially neck-injured trauma patient.[143] However, it is controversial, and the studies supporting and disproving the safety of this approach are limited by the mobilization of the neck in the presence of cervical instability.[143,146,147,150] Cervical spine movement is reported to be present with the use of curved and straight laryngoscope blades, and the application of cervical traction alone may produce distraction of the cervical spine.[144,151] This technique offers several advantages: Most physicians are comfortable and skilled in its performance, and it requires no specialized equipment.

Techniques involving a flexible fiberoptic bronchoscope or lighted stylet for orotracheal intubation have been reported to reduce neck movement.[152-155] Percutaneous transtracheal ventilation and retrograde intubation are other alternatives that could be performed, but most physicians have no experience with these techniques.[156-158]

Cricothyrotomy is an invasive technique at which many physicians are uncomfortable and unskilled.[159] According to some authors, it is the preferred method of airway management for patients with respiratory arrest and evidence of a spinal injury.[61] Cricothyrotomy requires special equipment and does not provide a definitive airway, although it might provide additional time to establish one. Setting up an appropriate transtracheal ventilation apparatus ahead of time is important for successful cricothyrotomy.[148]

The use of rapid-sequence induction (RSI) technique after a brief neurologic examination in a combative multiple trauma patient may provide the advantages of a smooth oral-intubation[160-163] (see Chapter 19 Appendix). Advantages include precise direct glottic visualization without mobilization of the neck, decreased risk of increased intracranial pressure and hemodynamic and respiratory instability, and decreased trauma to the airways resulting from forceful intubation.[160,161,164] RSI has a high success rate of intubation with fewer attempts and a low risk of hypoxemia. It requires the presence of a physician with experience in the technique and its complications. Its use for pediatric trauma victims is mainly for immediate diagnostic workup and therapy: airway control, respiratory support, and hyperventilation to decrease intracranial pressure and maintain good oxygenation.[160,161] Most of the cases require clinical decisions based on the history, physical examination, and repeat clinical assessment findings.

When it is apparent that the patient requires the use of an RSI technique, the one chosen must provide an effective response with the least possibility of an adverse outcome. Consideration should be given to the benefits and adverse effects of the medications to be used.[160,161,165] In patients with SCI, a hyperkalemic response to succinylcholine may also develop[166]; thus it should be avoided in the acute management of SCI.[166-168] Limited literature is available in which these resuscitation techniques in trauma patients with SCI are evaluated.

Circulation (See Chapter 13)

Hypotension and shock should be treated initially as resulting from hypovolemia; sources of internal hemorrhage with associated injuries must be sought. Excessive administration of crystalloid in the presence of spinal shock may precipitate pulmonary edema.

Once hypovolemia has been corrected, neurogenic shock due to an SCI should be suspected if hypotension persists with bradycardia and warm, flushed, dry skin. Place the patient in the Trendelenburg position. Bleeding from the lower extremities can be controlled and stabilization of a lower spine or pelvic fracture achieved by application and inflation of a pneumatic antishock garment. Decreased sympathetic tone is treated with low-dose norepinephrine (Levophed) drip infusion at 0.1 to 1.0 µg/kg/min IV. Increased parasympathetic tone is managed by administration of atropine at 0.01 to 0.02 mg/kg/dose IV, repeated every 5 to 10 minutes as necessary, used alternately or concurrently with norepinephrine. A nasogastric tube and Foley catheter should be inserted and antacid therapy initiated.

Steroids

A medication has been sought that might decrease the morbidity associated with SCI. Animal studies suggested a role for glucocorticoids, but nonrandomized studies of low-dose steroids have shown unequal benefits, mostly in those with incomplete cord injuries.[169]

The role of glucocorticoids in the management of SCIs has been clarified by the National Acute Spinal Cord Injury Study 2 (NASCIS2).[170] A multicenter study demonstrated that very-high-dose methylprednisolone 50 mg/kg beginning within 8 hours of injury, followed by an infusion of 5.4 mg/kg/hr for 23 hours, improved neurologic function at all levels of injury. However, children younger than 13 years were excluded from the study, as were patients with gunshot wounds, nerve root impairment, or cauda equina syndrome; pregnant women; and patients in whom drug interactions might be problematic. The advantages of methylprednisolone that favor its use over that of other steroids include rapid passage through cell membranes, effective inhibition of neutropenic response to activated complement, and compatibility with anticonvulsants.[171] The mechanism postulated by the investigators to explain the improved recovery is probably related to the ability of high-dose steroids to spare the cord's neurofilament membrane by interfering with lipid peroxidation, which is considered to be a cause of the release of toxins and enzymes that cause further destruction after a SCI.[170]

Significant improvement in motor function and pin prick and touch sensations were seen in patients treated with high-dose methylprednisolone compared with those who were given placebo at 6 weeks and 6 months after injury and it is therefore widely used for children despite the absence of a definitive study in this age group.[170] Neither mortality nor the complications studied showed statistically significant differences when steroids were used. Improvement in function was observed in the patients who had both complete and incomplete motor and sensory loss, although the more severely injured patients improved less.

Naloxone and Gangliosides

Naloxone, an opiate antagonist, may have promise in minimizing the neurologic deficit in a traumatic myelopathy by improving spinal cord blood flow.[172] However, indications for treating patients with naloxone at any time, or methylprednisolone after 8 hours of injury, are not supported by the findings of the NASCIS2 study.[170] Although the effect of the steroids on SCI in children is not known, they may have a similar response; thus this information has been extrapolated for use in children with SCI until new trials are available.

Gangliosides are a complex acidic glycolipid present in the central nervous system. They are a component of the cell membrane. Administration of GM-1 ganglioside may enhance recovery of motor function.[173]

Skeletal Traction and Decompression

When possible, closed reduction and external bracing is the treatment of choice. Traction can be applied with a halo brace or Gardner-Wells, Crutchfield, or Vinke tongs. A neurosurgeon should be involved in the application.

In all cervical injuries with significant subluxation, an attempt should be made to accomplish reduction by skeletal traction. Stable injuries are treated with rigid orthosis. A major neurologic deficit usually implies an unstable spine requiring stabilization. Surgical decompression may be indicated with acute neurologic deterioration, penetrating injuries of the spinal cord, inability to achieve a closed reduction, or presence of a foreign body in the spinal canal.[8,174-176] It may also be necessary for potentially unstable injuries. Unstable cervical spine injuries that are not associated with neurologic deficit may be managed with the halo vest, operative fixation, or, in the presence of other injuries, prolonged skeletal traction.[174-177]

Occipitoatlantal dislocation is a highly unstable injury with profound ligamentous damage that usually occurs in combination with a fracture of the odontoid and is usually fatal. Emergency treatment consists of application of halo traction to maintain anatomic relationships. Fusion of C1-C2 and occipital bone is subsequently effected.

Single fractures of the anterior or posterior arch, or in the lateral masses of C1, are stable fractures. However, confirmatory CT and dynamic radiographic studies should be performed to ensure that the fracture is isolated. Although widely displaced C1 fractures have been assumed to have transverse ligament disruption, this association has not been proved pathologically.[26,38,67,174-176] A Jefferson fracture, although rarely associated with a concomitant neurologic deficit, should be regarded as an unstable injury that usually requires halo-vest immobilization.

Translational dislocations or rotational injuries of the atlas should be evaluated with MRI to determine the most appropriate treatment.[73,178,179] Atlantoaxial dislocations are frequently associated with an odontoid fracture and usually occur in an anterior direction. Initial treatment is with skeletal traction to achieve anatomic reduction. Unilateral rotatory dislocations are usually managed with a rigid orthosis. Translational dislocations usually require a posterior fusion.

C2 pedicle fracture is an unstable injury, and alignment is maintained with halo-vest immobilization until bony union is radiographically demonstrable. In compression fractures with neurologic deficit (not quadriplegic), removal of the destroyed body and disk material and reconstruction with bone grafts and halo-vest support are recommended by some authors.[180] Isolated fractures of a vertebral body without neurologic abnormalities are usually treated with firm orthosis.

Disruption of the atlantal transverse ligament is thought to be an unstable situation that requires surgical fusion.[67,68,73,181] Since atlantoaxial dislocations present the risk of sudden death or late neurologic sequelae,[25,26,73,181] the recommended procedure has been to fuse the C1 and C2 vertebrae.[25,26,73,178]

Ligamentous integrity is also an important consideration in the evaluation of odontoid fractures.[176] The relationship between nonunion of odontoid fractures and transverse ligament injury must be evaluated directly. Although most C2 fractures heal with rigid external immobilization, type 2 fractures of the odontoid with extensive dens displacement usually do not heal spontaneously because of the poor blood supply in this area.[67,174-176] Definitive treatment employs halo-vest immobilization or C1-C2 posterior fusion. Type 3 odontoid fractures can be successfully treated with firm external orthosis.

In cases of cervical sprain, no clear consensus exists on the treatment, which ranges from expectant conservative bedrest variably including immobilization (soft collar) with or without analgesics or muscle relaxants to a carefully supervised program of intensive mobilization. Patients are observed until asymptomatic. Radiographic studies may be repeated to assure the diagnosis and usually are repeated before discharge.

Thoracic Spine (T1-T10) Injuries

Conservative management is usually adequate.[180] Rest in extension is followed by immobilization in a molded orthosis when the anterior vertebral body is collapsed by less than 40% of its normal height. When collapse exceeds 40%, operative intervention is often required for the removal of the bone and disk material from the spinal canal. Progressive kyphosis may develop, particularly after decompressive laminectomy.

Thoracolumbar (T11-L1) and Lumbar (L2-L5) Spine Injuries

Most flexion distraction fractures are treated with bedrest and postural reduction. Neural compression is less likely; if it occurs, it affects the peripheral nerve, which appears to be more tolerant of physical deformation than the spinal cord itself. A highly unstable rotatory fracture/dislocation—a fracture of the body, pedicle, facet, and lamina—is associated with disruption of the anterior and posterior ligamentous, and bone and disk material is frequently retropulsed into the canal. They imply severe trauma, and neurologic deficit is common. Surgery is recommended, even if no dislocation exists, to repair the dura, control epidural hemorrhage and remove compressive elements; it is combined with spinal stabilization.[180,182] Traumatic lumbar disk herniation usually requires laminectomy and discectomy.

Sacral and Coccygeal Spine Injuries

Optimal pelvic reduction and nonsurgical stabilization of the pelvis may be recommended for sacral fractures. Experience with direct operation for neural decompression is limited.[180] Coccygeal injuries are usually managed with observation and symptomatic treatment. Coccydynia is a frustrating complaint for the patient and the physician because treatment is usually unsatisfactory.

Penetrating and Blunt Neck Injuries

Penetrating injuries of the neck involving the platysma or deeper structures or extensive blunt soft-tissue damage require surgical consultation and commonly necessitate inpatient observation.

Vascular neck injuries are a cause of severe bleeding and may result in death. The carotid and vertebral arteries, as well as the jugular veins, may be the source of major bleeding. The large external jugular veins are very superficial and prone to injury by lacerations and stab wounds. Hemorrhage from a penetrating neck wound should be controlled by external direct pressure. Circumferential bandaging, wrapping, or taping is absolutely contraindicated. When the wounding instrument (knife or other object) is found protruding from a neck wound, it should not be removed or otherwise manipulated until appropriate conditions for cervical or thoracic exploration are available. Definitive treatment of vascular injuries is carried out in the operating room.

Hemorrhage may occur externally, or it may be contained in the fascial compartments of the neck. These contained hematomas may cause compression of the trachea, with subsequent airway obstruction. Pulsating hematomas may suggest major underlying vascular injury. A continuous bruit or thrill in the area of the injury is diagnostic of an arteriovenous fistula.

Thrombosis of the vertebral artery may be manifest as brain stem ischemia and cerebellar signs. Thrombosis usually occurs in association with fractures of the transverse process or partial subluxation of the upper cervical spine.[183] Subarachnoid hemorrhage may occur with disruption of the vertebral artery at the base of the skull.

The presence of bubbling, frothing blood in the wound or airway suggests combined tracheal and vascular injury. Major vessel injury in association with disruption of the trachea may produce airway obstruction from aspiration of blood and immediate intubation or cricothyrotomy is necessary.

When a large vein such as the internal jugular is injured, air embolism must be considered. Further embolism is best prevented by transporting the patient supine and applying pressure to the wound. If there is suspicion that embolism is already present, the patient should be placed on his or her left side in a slight Trendelenburg position.

In addition to the rapid blood loss that follows major arterial injuries in the neck, attempts to stop this loss may cause cerebral hypoxia. Digital pressure may result in retention of blood within the fascial compartments of the neck, exerting a strangling pressure on the airways.

Currently half of all deaths in penetrating neck trauma are attributed to SCI or thrombosis of the common or internal carotid arteries leading to central nervous system infarction.[184] Controversy regarding mandatory vs. selective management of penetrating neck wounds remains unresolved. Little data are available related to this injury in children.[185]

Angiography has assumed increasing importance in the evaluation of penetrating neck injuries. The categorization of such injuries by zone has provided a basis for diagnostic and therapeutic decisions making for wounds that penetrate the platysma. Saletta suggested that zone I injuries be studied with an aortogram to visualize the innominate, common carotid, subclavian, and vertebral arteries.[186] Zone II injuries should be explored; zone III should be evaluated with selective carotid arteriography.

Blunt neck injuries may also require arteriography to rule out vascular injuries. Furthermore, laryngotracheal and pharyngoesophageal injuries must be excluded by diagnostic studies, often requiring surgical exploration and intervention with the assistance of an otolaryngologist.

DISPOSITION

Hospitalization in a setting where multidisciplinary care can be provided is mandatory. Policies for neurosurgical consultation and referral and transport of individuals with SCIs should be discussed. It is important to stress that among the few indications for operative neurosurgical intervention in cervical spine injuries are deteriorating neurologic examination results. Repeat neurologic examinations should include evaluation of the mental status, cranial nerves, deep-tendon reflexes, muscle tone and strength, sensation, and cerebellar function.

In very young children, some authors report that mild degrees of cord injury have a better prognosis for return of function, even to normalcy, than in adults.[8,23] Hadley reported a 28% incidence of disability after fractures of the spine, but the report included all levels of the vertebral column (cervical, thoracic, lumbar).[187] Prognosis is partially determined by associated injuries or when progression of a partial neurologic deficit is observed. The long term prognosis of SCIWORA is poor. Patients with severe incomplete and complete lesions do not recover. The initial neurologic status is the major predictor of the extent of recovery.

Some authors have attempted to identify differences between a subpopulation of children 3 years and younger and 4 to 12 years.[7] A larger proportion of the very young were girls who had C1-C2 bone involvement and required surgical stabilization. No differences in neurologic injuries, subluxation alone, and SCIWORA were found.

Many SCI injuries could be prevented by appropriate use of automobile restraints. All 50 states have enacted child passenger-restraint laws requiring young children to be restrained in safety seats or seat belts while riding in automobiles. However, recent studies have shown that as many as 74% of car safety seats are used improperly, resulting in deficient protection and possible consequences of the misuse such as cervical spine injuries.[188-190]

References

1. Trafton PD: Spinal cord injuries, *Surg Clin North Am* 6(1):61, 1982.
2. Kewalramani LS and Tori JA: Spinal cord trauma in children, *Spine* 5:11, 1980.
3. Rivara FP: Traumatic deaths of children in the United States: Currently available prevention strategies, *Pediatrics* 75:456, 1985.
4. Coffey J: Whiplash-induced intracranial and intraocular bleedings, linked with residual permanent brain damage and mental retardation, *Pediatrics* 54:396, 1974.
5. Swischuk LE: Spine and spinal cord trauma in the battered child syndrome. *Radiology* 92:733, 1969.
6. Bresnan MJ and Abrams IF: Neonatal spinal cord transection secondary to intrauterine hyperextension of the neck in breech presentation, *J Pediatr* 84:734, 1974.
7. Ruge JR, Sinson GP, McLone DG, et al: Pediatric spinal injury: the very young, *J Neurosurg* 68:25, 1988.
8. Hill SA, Miller CA, Kosnik EJ, et al: Pediatric neck injuries, *J Neurosurg* 60:700, 1984.
9. Pang D and Wilberger JE: Spinal cord injury without radiological abnormalities in children, *J Neurosurg* 57:114, 1982.
10. Young JS, Burns PE, Bowen AM, et al: *Spinal cord injury statistics: Experience of regional model spinal cord injury systems*, Phoenix, 1988, Good Samaritan Medical Center.
11. Alker GJ Jr, Oh YS, Leslie EV, et al: Post mortem radiology of head and neck injuries in fatal traffic accidents, *Radiology* 114:611, 1985.
12. Ducker TB, Treatment of spinal cord injury, *N Engl J Med* 322:1459, 1990.

Anatomy and Biomechanics

13. Aqup AMR: *Grant's atlas of anatomy*, ed 9, Baltimore, 1991, Williams & Wilkins.
14. Holdworth F: Fractures, dislocations, and fracture-dislocations of the spine, *J Bone Joint Surg* 52:1534, 1970.
15. Babcock JL: Cervical spine injuries: Diagnosis and classification, *Arch Surg* 111:646, 1976.
16. Hubbard DD: Injuries of the spine in children and adolescents, *Clin Orthop* 100:56, 1974.
17. Gaufin LM and Goodman SJ: Cervical spine injuries in infants: Problems in management, *J Neurosurg* 42:179, 1975.
18. Riggins RS and Kraus JF: The risk of neurologic damage with fractures of the vertebrae, *J Trauma* 17:126, 1977.
19. Caffey J: In: Silverman FN and Kuhn JP, editors: *Caffey's pediatric x-ray diagnosis: an integrated imaging approach*, ed 9, St. Louis, 1993, Mosby.
20. Townsend EH and Rowe ML: Mobility of the upper cervical spine in health and disease, *Pediatrics* 10:567, 1952.
21. Cattell HS and Filtzer DL: Pseudosubluxation and other normal variations in the cervical spine in children, *J Bone Joint Surg* 47A:1295, 1965.
22. Bailey DK: The normal cervical spine in infants and children, *Radiology* 59:712, 1952.
23. Sullivan CR et al: Hypermobility of the cervical spine in children: A pitfall in the diagnosis of cervical disorders, *Am J Surg* 95:636, 1958.
24. Driscoll DR: Anatomical and biomechanical characteristics of the upper cervical ligamentous structures: a review, *J Manipulative Physiol Ther* 10:107, 1987.
25. Fielding JW, Cochran GVB, Lawsing JF III, et al: Tears of the transverse ligament of the atlas: A clinical and biomechanical study, *J Bone Joint Surg (Am)* 56:1683-1691, 1974.
26. White AA III and Panjabi MM: The clinical biomechanics of the occipitoatlantoaxial complex, *Orthop Clin North Am* 9:867, 1978.
27. de Oliveria E, Rhoton AL Jr, Peace D: Microsurgical anatomy of the region of the foramen magnum, *Surg Neurol* 24:293, 1985.
28. Dickman CA, Mamourian A, Sonntag VK, et al: Magnetic resonance imaging of the transverse atlantal ligament for the evaluation of atlantoaxial instability, *J Neurosurg* 75:221-227, 1991.
29. Saldinger P, Dvorak J, Rahn BA, et al: Histology of the alar and transverse ligaments, *Spine* 15:257, 1990.
30. Dvorak J, Shneider E, Saldinger P, et al: Biomechanics of the craniocervical region: The alar and transverse ligaments, *J Orthop Res* 6:452, 1988.
31. Breig A: *Biomechanics of central nervous system*, Stockholm, 1960, Almqvist & Wiksell.
32. Steel HH: Anatomical and mechanical considerations of the atlantoaxial articulation, *J Bone Joint Surg* 50A: 1481, 1968.

Pathophysiology

33. Aufdermaur M: Spinal injuries in juveniles: Necropsy findings in twelve cases, *J Bone Joint Surg (Br)* 56:513, 1974.
34. Ducker TB, Salcman M, Perot PL, et al: Experimental spinal cord trauma. I. Correlation of blood flow, tissue oxygen, and neurologic status in the dog, *Surg Neurol* 10:60, 1978.
35. Braughler JM and Hall ED: Effects of multidose methylprednisolone sodium succinate administration on injured cat spinal cord

neurofilament degradation and energy metabolism, *J Neurosurg* 61:290-295, 1984.

36. Weiss MH and Kaufman B: Hangmans fracture in an infant, *Am J Dis Child* 126:268, 1973.

37. Wood-Jones F: The ideal lesion produced by judicial hanging, *Lancet* 53, 1913.

38. Jefferson G: Fracture of the atlas vertebra: Report of four cases, and a review of those previously recorded, *Br J Surg* 7:407-422, 1920.

39. Holdsworth F: Fractures, dislocations, and fractures dislocations of the spine, *J Bone Joint Surg* 52A:1534, 1970.

40. Mueller FO, Blyth CS: Catastrophic head and neck injuries, *Phys Sportsmed* 7:71-74, 1979.

Diagnostic Findings

41. Ducker TG: Head trauma and cervical spine injuries, *Am J Emerg Med* 7(2):248, 1989.

42. Leventhal HR: Birth injuries of the spinal cord, *J Pediatr* 56:447, 1960.

43. Bell HJ and Dykstra DD: Somatosensory evoked potentials as an adjunct to diagnosis of neonatal spinal cord injury, *J Pediatr* 106:298, 1985.

44. Richards PG: Stable fractures of the atlas and axis in children, *J Neurol Neurosurg Psychiatry* 47:781-783, 1984.

45. Roy L and Gibson DA: Cervical spine fusions in children. *Clin Orthop* 73:146-151, 1970.

46. Bohn D, Armstrong D, Becker L, et al: Cervical spine injuries in children, *J Trauma* 30(4):463, 1990.

47. Hachen HJ: Spinal cord injury in children and adolescents: Diagnostic pitfalls and therapeutic considerations in the acute stage, *Paraplegia* 15:55, 1977.

48. Maroon JC: "Burning hands" in football spinal cord injuries, *JAMA* 238:2049-1051, 1977.

49. Chen LS and Blaw ME: Acute central cervical cord syndrome caused by minor trauma, *J Pediatr* 108:96, 1986.

50. Brisman R, et al: Pulmonary edema in acute transection of the cervical spinal cord, *Surg Gynecol Obstet* 139:363, 1974.

51. Kervaliamani LS: Neurogenic gastroduodenal ulceration and bleeding associated with spinal cord injuries, *J Trauma* 19:259, 1989.

52. Rachesky I, Boyce T, Duncan B, et al: Clinical prediction of cervical spine injuries in children, *Am J Dis Child* 141:199, 1987.

53. Jaffe DM, Binns H, Radkowski MA, et al: Developing a clinical algorithm for early management of cervical spine injury in child trauma victims, *Ann Emerg Med* 16:270, 1987.

54. Dietrich AM, Ginn-Pease ME, Bartkowski, et al: Pediatric cervical spine fractures: predominately subtle presentation, *J Pediatr Surg* 26:995-999, 1991.

55. Jacobs LM and Schwartz R: Prospective analysis of acute cervical spine injury: A methodology to predict injury, *Ann Emerg Med* 15:44, 1986.

56. Ehara EK: Cervical spine injury in children: Radiologic manifestations, *Am J Roentgenol* 152:1175-1178, 1988.

57. Apple JS, Kirks DR, Merten DF, et al: Cervical spine fractures and dislocations in children, *Pediatr Radiol* 17:45, 1987.

58. Acheson MB, Livingston RR, Richardson ML, et al: High resolution CT scanning in the evaluation of cervical spine fracture: Comparison with plain film examinations. *Am J Roentgenol* 148:1179, 1987.

59. Vandemark RM: Radiology of the cervical spine in trauma patients: Practice pitfalls and recommendations for improving efficiency and communication, *Am J Roentgenol* 155:465, 1990.

60. Bachulis BL, Long WB, Hynes CD, et al: Clinical indications for cervical spine radiographs in the traumatized patients, *Am J Surg* 153:473, 1987.

61. Hockberger RS and Doris PE: Spinal injury. In Rosen P, Baker FJ, Barkin RM, et al (eds): *Emergency medicine concepts and clinical practice*, ed 4, St. Louis, 1997, Mosby.

62. Swischuk LE: Anterior displacement of C2 in children: physiologic or pathologic? *Radiology* 122:759, 1977.

63. Swischuk LE: Emergency radiology of the acutely ill or injured child, ed 3, Baltimore, 1994, Williams & Wilkins.

64. Fesmire FM and Luten RC: The pediatric cervical spine: Developmental anatomy and clinical aspects, *J Emerg Med* 7:133, 1989.

65. Shaffer MA and Doris PE: Limitations of the cross table lateral view in detecting cervical spine injuries, *Ann Emerg Med* 10:508, 1981.

66. Gerlock AJ, Kirchner SG, Heller RM, Kaye JJ, et al: *The cervical spine in trauma*, Philadelphia, 1978, Saunders.

67. Spence KF Jr, Decker S, Sell KW: Bursting atlantal fracture associated with rupture of the transverse ligament, *J Bone Joint Surg (Am)* 52:543, 1970.

68. Panjabi MM, Thibodeau LL, Crisco JJ III, et al: What constitutes spinal instability?, *Clin Neurosurg* 34:313-339, 1988.

69. Tecklenburg F: Problems in managing cervical spine injuries. In Luten RC, editor: *Problems in pediatric emergency medicine*, New York, 1988, Churchill Livingstone.

70. Bohrer SP et al: "V" shaped predens space, *Skel Radiol* 14:111, 1985.

71. Bland JH: *Disorders of the cervical spine: Diagnosis and medical management*, Philadelphia, 1987, Saunders.

72. American Academy of Pediatrics Committee on Sports Medicine: Atlantoaxial instability in Down syndrome, *Pediatrics* 96:171, 1995.

73. Fielding JW, Hawkins RJ: Atlanto-axial rotatory fixation, *J Bone Joint Surg* 59A:37, 1977.

74. Marar BC and Balachandran N: Non-traumatic atlanto-axial dislocation in children, *Clin Orthop* 92:220, 1973.

75. Clark RN: Diagnosis and management of torticollis, *Pediatric Ann* 5:231, 1976.

76. Hohl M and Baker HR: The atlanto-axial joint: Roentgenographic and anatomical study of normal and abnormal motion, *J Bone Joint Surg (Am)* 46:1739, 1964.

77. Jackson H: The diagnosis of minimal atlanto-axial subluxation, *Br J Radiol* 23:672-674, 1950.

78. Keats TE (editor): *Atlas of normal roentgen variants that may simulate disease*, ed 4, Chicago, 1988, Year Book.

79. Truex RC and Johnson CH: Congenital anomalies of the upper cervical spine, *Orthop Clin North Am* 9:891, 1978.

80. Garber JN: Abnormaleties of the atlas and axis vertebrae: Congenital and traumatic, *J Bone Joint Surg* 46-A:1782-91, 1964.

81. Scher AT: Articular pillar fractures of the cervical spine: Diagnosis on the anteroposterior radiograph, *S Afr Med J* 60:968-969, 1981.

82. Holliman CJ, Mayer JS, Cook RT, et al: Is the Anteroposterior cervical spine radiograph necessary in the initial trauma screening?, *Am J Emerg Med* 9:421-425, 1991.

83. Miller MD, Schweiler JA, Marinez S, et al: Significant new observations on cervical spine trauma, *Am J Roentgenol* 130:659-663, 1978.

84. Doris PE, Wilson RA: The next logical step in the emergency radiographic evaluation of the cervical spine: The five view trauma series, *J Emerg Med* 3:371-385, 1985.

85. Harris JH: *The radiology of acute cervical spine trauma*, Baltimore, 1987, Williams & Wilkins.

86. Abel MS: The exaggerated supine oblique view of the cervical spine, *Skel Radiol* 8:213-219, 1982.

87. Freemyer B, Knopp R, Piche J, et al: Comparison of five-view and three-view cervical spine series in the evaluation of patients with cervical trauma, *Ann Emerg Med* 18:818-821, 1989.

88. Borock EC, Sheryl GA, Gabram MD, et al: A prospective analysis of a two-year experience using computed tomography as an adjunct for cervical spine clearance, *J Trauma* 31:1001, 1991.

89. Streitwieser DR, Knopp R, Wales LR, et al: Accuracy of standard radiographic views in detecting cervical spine fractures, *Ann Emerg Med* 12:538, 1983.

90. Pennecot GF, et al: Traumatic ligamentous instability of the cervical spine in children, *J Pediatr Orthop* 4:339, 1984.

91. Wilberger JE Jr: *Spinal cord injuries in children*, Mount Kisco, NY Futura Publishing, 1986.

92. Dachling P and Pollack IF: Spinal cord injury without radiographic abnormality in children: the SCIWORA syndrome, *J Trauma* 29:654-663, 1989.

93. Dickman CA et al: Spinal cord injuries in children without radiographic abnormalities. *West J Med* 158 (1):67-68, 1993.

94. Kewalramani LW, Orth MS, Kraus JF, et al: Acute spinal cord lesions in pediatric population: Epidemiological and clinical features, *Paraplegia* 18;206, 1980.

95. Choi JU, Hoffman HJ, Hendrick EB, et al: Traumatic infarction of the spinal cord in children, *J Neurosurg* 65:608-610, 1986.

96. Burke DC: Traumatic spinal paralysis in children, *Paraplegia* 11:268, 1974.

97. Cheshire DJ: The pediatric syndrome of traumatic myelopathy without demonstrable vertebral injury, *Paraplegia* 15:74, 1977.

98. Mace SE: Emergency evaluation of the cervical spine injuries: CT versus plain radiographs, *Ann Emerg Med* 14:973, 1985.

99. Shleelauf K, Ross SE, Civil ID, et al: Computed tomography in the initial evaluation of the cervical spine, *Ann Emerg Med* 18:815, 1989.

100. Podolsky S, Baraff LJ, Simon RR, et al: Efficacy of cervical spine immobilization methods, *J Trauma* 23:461, 1983.

101. Rogers WA: Fractures and dislocations of the cervical spine: An end result study, *J Bone Joint Surg* 39A:341, 1957.

102. Seiman LP: Fracture of the odontoid process in young children, *J Bone Joint Surg* 59A:943, 1977.

103. Cacayorin ED, & Kieffer SA: Application of limitations of computed tomography of the spine, *Radiol Clin North Am* 20:185, 1982.

104. Djang WT: Radiology of acute spinal trauma, *Crit Care Clin* 3:495, 1987.

105. Wales LR, Knapp RK, Morishima MS: Recommendations for evaluation of the acutely injury cervical spine: A clinical radiologic algorithm, *Ann Emerg Med* 9:422, 1980.

106. Levitt MA, Flanders AE: Diagnostic capabilities of magnetic resonance imaging and computed tomography in acute cervical spinal column injury, *Am J Emerg Med* 9131-135, 1991.

107. Atlas SW, Regewbogen V, Rogers LF, et al: The radiographic characterization of burst fractures of the spine, *Am J Roentgenol* 147:572, 1986.

108. Burguet JL, Sick H, Dirheimer Y, et al: CT of the main ligaments of the cervico-occipital hinge, *Neuroradiology* 27:112, 1985.

109. Daniels DL, Williams AL, Haughton VM: Computed tomography of the articulations and ligaments at the occipito-atlantoaxial region, *Radiology* 146:709, 1983.

110. Handel SF and Lee Y: Computed tomography of spinal fractures, *Radiol Clin North Am* 19:69, 1981.

111. Harris JH: Radiographic evaluation of spinal trauma, *Orthop Clin North Am* 17:75, 1986.

112. Kieffer SA, Binet EF, Davis DO, et al. Lumbar myelography with iohexol and metrizamide: A comparative multicenter prospective study, *Radiology* 151:665, 1984.

113. Enriquez G, Aso C, Lucaya J et al: Traumatic cord lesions in the newborn infant, *Ann Radiol* 19:179, 1976.

114. Harwood-Nash DC and Fitz CR: Myelography. In *Neuroradiology in infants and children*, vol 3, St. Louis, 1976, Mosby.

115. Cracco JB, Cracco RQ, Graziani LJ: The spinal evoked response in infants and children, *Neurology* 25:31, 1975.

116. Hyman RA and Gorey MT: Imaging strategies for MR of the spine, *Radiol Clin North Am* 26:505, 1988.

117. Masaryk TJ: Spine trauma. In Modic MT, Masaryk TJ, Ross JS, editors: *Magnetic resonance imaging of the spine*, St. Louis, 1993, Mosby.

118. Schaefer DM, Flanders A, Northrup BE, et al: Magnetic resonance imaging of acute cervical spine trauma: Correlation with severity of neurologic injury, *Spine* 14:1090, 1989.

119. Hesselink JR: MR imaging of brain contusions: A comparative study with CT, *Am J Roentgenol* 150:1133, 1988.

120. Kelly AB, Zimmerman RD, Snow RB, et al: Head trauma: Comparison of MR and CT: Experience in 100 patients, *Am J Neuroradiol* 9:639-708, 1988.

121. Gentry LR, Godersky JC, Thompson B, et al: Prospective comparative study of intermediate-field MR and CT in the evaluation of closed head trauma, *Am J Neuroradiol* 9:91-100, 1988.

122. Modic MT, Weinstein MA, Pavlicek W,et al: Magnetic resonance imaging of the cervical spine: Technical and clinical observations, *AJNR* 5:15-22,1984.

123. Norman D, et al: Magnetic resonance imaging of the spinal cord and canal: Potentials and limitations, *AJNR* 5:9, 1984.

124. Lanska MJ, Roessmann U, Wiznitzer M: Magnetic Resonance imaging in cervical cord birth injury, *Pediatrics* 85:760, 1990.

125. Felsberg GJ, et al: Utility of MR imaging in pediatric spinal cord injury, *Pediatr Radiol* 25:131-135, 1995.

126. Smith DS, Askey P, Young ML, et al: Anesthetic management of acutely ill patients during magnetic resonance imaging, *Anesthesiology* 65:710, 1986.

127. Glasauer FE and Cares HL: Traumatic paraplegia in infancy, *JAMA* 219:38, 1972.

128. LeBlanc HJ and Nadel J: Spinal cord injuries in children, *Surg Neurol* 2:411, 1974.

129. Newman KD, Bowman LM, Eichelberger MR, et al: The lap belt complex: Intestinal and lumbar spine injury in children, *J Trauma* 30:1133, 1990.

130. Chance CQ: Note on a type of flexion fracture of the spine, *Br J Radiol* 21:452, 1948.

131. Vandersluis R: The seatbelt syndrome, *Can Med Assoc J* 137:1023, 1987.

132. Reid AB, Letts RM, Black GB: Pediatric chance fractures: Association with intra-abdominal injuries and seatbelt use, *J Trauma* 30:384, 1990.

133. Barton J, Haight RO, Marslan DW, et al: Low back pain in the primary care setting, *J Fam Pract* 3:363, 1976.

134. Vukmir RB: Low back pain: Review of diagnosis and therapy, *Am J Emerg Med* 9:328, 1991.

Management

135. Aprahamian C, Thompson BM, Darin JC: Recommended helmet removal techniques in a cervical spine injured patient, *J Trauma* 24:841, 1984.

136. Huerta C, Griffith R, Joyce SM: Cervical spine stabilization in pediatric patients: Evaluation of current techniques, *Ann Emerg Med* 16:1121, 1987.

137. Sarant G, Chipman L: Early management of cervical spine injuries, *Postgrad Med* 71:164-171, 1982.

138. McCabe JB, Nolan DJ: Comparison of the effectiveness of different cervical immobilization collars, *Ann Emerg Med* 15:50, 1986.

139. Cline JR, Schneidel E, Bigsby E: A comparison of methods of cervical immobilization used in patients extrication and transport, *J Trauma* 7:649, 1985.

140. Graziano AF, Scheidel EA, Clino JR, et al: A radiographic comparison of prehospital cervical immobilization methods, *Ann Emerg Med* 16:1127-1131, 1987.

141. Lewis VL, Manson PN, Morgan RF, et al: Facial injuries associated with cervical fractures: Recognition, patterns, and management, *J Trauma* 25:90, 1985.

142. Sellick BA: Cricoid pressure to control regurgitation of stomach contents during induction of anesthesia, *Lancet* 2:404, 1961.

143. Aprahamian C, Thompson BM, Finger WA, et al: Experimental cervical spine injury model: Evaluation of airway management and splinting techniques, *Ann Emerg Med* 13:584-587, 1984.

144. Majernick TG, Bienick R, Houston JB, et al: Cervical spine movement during orotracheal intubation, *Ann Emerg Med* 13:584, 1984.

145. Rosen P and Wolfe RE: Therapeutic legends of emergency medicine, *J Emerg Med* 7:387, 1989.

146. Joyce SM: Cervical immobilization during orotracheal intubation in trauma victims [editorial], *Ann Emerg Med* 17:88, 1988.

147. Knopp RK: The safety of orotracheal intubation in patients with suspected cervical-spine injury [editorial], *Ann Emerg Med* 19:603, 1990.

148. American College of Surgeons Committee on Trauma: *Advanced Trauma Life Support instructor manual*, Chicago, 1988, American College of Surgeons.

149. Jorden RC and Rosen P: Airway management in the acutely injured. In Moore EE, Eisenman B, Vanway CW III. (editors): *Critical decisions in trauma*, St Louis, 1984, Mosby.

150. Holley J Jorden R: Airway management in patients with unstable cervical spine fractures, *Ann Emerg Med* 18:1237-1239, 1989.

151. Bivins HG, et al: The effect of axial traction during orotracheal intubation of the trauma victim with an unstable cervical spine, *Ann Emerg Med* 17:25-29,1988.

152. Hemmer D, Lee T, Wright BD: Intubation of a child with a cervical spine injury with the aid of a fiberoptic bronchoscope, *Anaesth Intens Care* 10:163, 1982.

153. Ovassapian A, Krejcie TC, Yelich SJ, et al: Awake fiberoptic intubation in the patient at high risk of aspiration, *Br J Anaesth* 62:13, 1989.

154. Vollmer TP, Stewart RD, Paris PM, et al: Use of a lighted stylet for caddied orotracheal intubation in the prehospital setting, *Ann Emerg Med* 14:324, 1985.

155. Ellis DG, Stewart RD, Kaplan RM, et al: Success rates of blind orotracheal intubation using a transillumination technique with a lighted stylet, *Ann Emerg Med* 15:138, 1986.

156. Barriot P, Riou B: Retrograde technique for tracheal intubation in trauma patients, *Crit Care Med* 16:712-713, 1988.

157. Neff CC, Pfister RC, Van Sonnenberg E: Percutaneous transtracheal ventilation: Experimental and practical aspects, *J Trauma* 23:84-90, 1983.

158. Hogan K, Harpur MH, Pollard BJ: Use of a pharyngeal guide to aid intubation with the fiberoptic larygoscope, *Anaesth Intens Care* 12:18, 1984.

159. Megill J, Clinton JE, Ruiz E: Cricothyroidotomy in the emergency department, *Ann Emerg Med* 11:361-364, 1982.

160. Medina F: Rapid sequence induction/intubation in the pediatric emergency department, *Int Pediatr* 4:24, 1989.

161. Yamamoto LG, Yim GK, Britten AG: Rapid sequence anesthesia induction for emergency intubation, *Pediatr Emerg Care* 6:200, 1990.

162. Kuchinski J, Tinkoff G, Rhodes M, et al: Emergency intubation for paralysis of the uncooperative trauma patient, *J Emerg Med* 9:9, 1991.

163. Talucci RC, Shaikh KA, Schwab CW: Rapid sequence induction with oral endotracheal intubation in the multiply injured patient, *Am Surg* 54:185, 1988.

164. Stene JK: Anesthetic management of the shock trauma patient. In Crowley RA (editor): *Trauma care*, vol 1, Philadelphia, 1987, Lippincott.

165. Medina FA: Evaluation of the use of vecuronium for emergency department endotracheal intubation in pediatric trauma victims [abstract], *Ann Emerg Med* 20:484, 1991.

166. Gronert GA, Theye RA: Pathophysiology of hyperkalemia induced by succinylcholine, *Anesthesiology* 43:89, 1975.

167. Albin MS: Resuscitation of the spinal cord, *Crit Care Med* 6:270, 1978.

168. Fraser A, Edmonds-Seal J: Spinal cord injuries: A review of the problem facing the anaesthetist, *Anaesthesia* 37:1084, 1982.

169. Means E, Anderson DK, Waters TR, et al: Effect of methylprednisolone in compression trauma to the feline spinal cord, *J Neurosurg* 55:200, 1981.

170. Bracken MB, Shepard MJ, Collins WF, et al: A randomized controlled trial of methylprednisolone or naloxone in the treatment of acute spinal-cord injury, *N Engl J Med* 322:1405, 1990.

171. Bracken MB, Collins WF, Freeman DF, et al: Efficacy of methylprednisolone in acute spinal cord injury, *JAMA* 251:45-52, 1984.

172. Faden AI, Jacobs TP, Mougey E, et al: Endorphin in experimental spinal injury: Therapeutic effect of naloxone, *Ann Neurol* 10:326, 1981.

173. Geisler FH, Dorsey FC, Coleman WP: Recovery of motor function after spinal cord injury: A randomized, placebo-controlled trial with GM-1 ganglioside, *N Engl J Med* 324:1829, 1991.

174. Dickman CA, Hadley MN, Browner C, et al: Neurosurgical management of acute atlas-axis combination fractures: A review of 25 cases, *J Neurosurg* 70:45-49, 1989.

175. Hadley MN, Dickman CA, Browner CM, et al: Acute traumatic atlas fractures: management and long term outcome, *Neurosurgery* 23:31-35, 1988.

176. Lipson SJ: Fractures of the atlas associated with fractures of the odontoid process and transverse ligament ruptures, *J Bone Joint Surg (Am)* 59:940-943, 1977.

177. Mandabach M, et al: Pediatric axis fractures: Early halo immobilization, management and outcome. *Pediatr Neurosurg* 19 (5):225, 1993.

178. Fielding JW, Hawkins RJ, Ratzan SA, et al: Spine fusion for atlanto-axial instability, *J Bone Joint Surg (Am)* 58:400-407, 1976.

179. Ono K, Yonenobu K, Fuji T, et al: Atlantoaxial rotatory fixation: radiographic study of its mechanism, *Spine* 10:602-608, 1985.

180. Schmidek HH and Sweet WH (editors): *Operative neurosurgical techniques.* New York, 1982, Grune & Stratton.

181. Dickman CA, Hadley MN, Pappas CTE, et al: Cruciate paralysis: A clinical and radiographic analysis of injuries to the cervicomedullary junction, *J Neurosurg* 73:850-858, 1990.

182. Schmidek HH, Gomes FB, Seligson D, et al: Management of acute unstable thoracolumbar (T11-L1) fractures with and without neurologic deficit, *Neurosurgery* 7:30, 1980.

183. Simeone FA, Goldberg HI: Thromboses of the vertebral artery from hyperextension injury to the neck, *J Neurosurg* 229:540, 1968.

184. Sankaran S, Walt AJ: Penetrating wounds of the neck-principles and controversy, *Surg Clin North Am* 57:139-149, 1977.

185. Cooper A, Barlow B, Niemirska M, et al: Fifteen years' experience with penetrating trauma to the head and neck in children, *J Pediatr Surg* 22:24-27, 1987.

186. Saletta JD, Lowe RJ, Lim LT, et al: Penetrating trauma of the neck, *J Trauma* 16:579, 1976.

187. Hadley MN, Zabramski JM, Browner CM, et al: Pediatric spinal trauma: review of 122 cases of spinal cord and vertebral column injuries, *J Neurosurg* 68:18-24, 1988.

188. Bull MJ, Stroup KB, Gerhart S: Misuse of car safety seats, *Pediatrics* 81:98, 1986.

189. Cynechi MJ and Goryl ME: *The incidence and factors associated with child safety seat misuse*, Washington, DC, 1984, National Highway Traffic Safety Administration, US Department of Transportation report DTO HS 806-676.

190. Fuchs S, Barthel J, Flannery AM, et al: Cervical spine fractures sustained by young children in forward facing car seats, *Pediatrics* 84:348, 1989.

Thoracic Trauma

Arthur Cooper • George L. Foltin

Serious thoracic injuries are relatively rare among children. In the United States, only 6% of children admitted to pediatric trauma centers have documented thoracic injuries[1] (Table 23-1); moreover, fewer than 15% of survivors require operative intervention beyond simple tube thoracostomy. Although the mechanism of injury in most cases of serious pediatric chest trauma suggests that many deaths occur before the child reaches the hospital, a significant number occur after arrival. Thus early management and subsequent outcome of serious thoracic injuries in childhood depend on the emergency physician and surgical colleagues experienced in these situations.

EPIDEMIOLOGY

Pediatric chest trauma has received scant attention. Only ten comprehensive reports on the subject have been published in the English-language literature since 1962, one of which reviewed operative cases only; none distinguished between blunt and penetrating injuries, although two additional reports described penetrating chest wounds in pediatric civilian and military casualties.[2-13] The National Pediatric Trauma Registry, founded in 1984, has vastly improved our knowledge of major thoracic injury in childhood, particularly its relation to other types of injury.[1] As with other types of pediatric trauma, blunt injuries predominate (see Table 23-1).

Despite its low overall incidence, serious chest trauma is among the most lethal of all childhood injuries, blunt or penetrating (Table 23-2).[1] Although thoracic injuries themselves are the proximate cause of death in less than 1% of all blunt childhood trauma, multisystem trauma is about 10 times more deadly when associated with chest injury; thus the presence of major thoracic injury serves as a marker of injury severity.[9] Both rib fractures and pulmonary contusions are much more common than is often realized; each occurs in about half of all major blunt trauma cases. By contrast, pneumothorax occurs in no more than 25% of major blunt thoracic injuries, and significant hemothorax only in about 10%. Cardiac, vascular, tracheobronchial, and diaphragmatic injuries occur much less frequently.

The mortality rate attributed to penetrating chest trauma in childhood is similar to that observed for blunt chest trauma; however, death is usually due to concomitant head or abdominal injuries in the latter, whereas it is rarely produced by associated injuries in the former. The vast majority of penetrating thoracic injury deaths, especially from gunshot wounds, are due to hemorrhagic shock resulting from massive hemothorax; however, a significant number, particularly with stab wounds, result from tension pneumothorax. Cardiac tamponade and aortic interruption are responsible for the rest. The causes of morbidity in penetrating chest trauma generally parallel those of mortality; direct violation of the heart and great vessels is encountered far less often in nonfatal cases.

ANATOMY

Certain anatomic characteristics of the pediatric chest contribute to the mortality and morbidity observed in childhood thoracic trauma. The compliance of the cartilagi-

TABLE 23-1. Thoracic Injuries in Selected North American Pediatric Trauma Centers*

	Number (%)
Blunt	1,288 (83)
Penetrating	230 (15)
Other	35 (2)
TOTAL	1,553

From National Pediatric Trauma Registry, 1985-1991.
*Total number of patients in registry: 25,301.

TABLE 23-2. Mortality Caused by Thoracic Injuries in Selected North American Pediatric Trauma Centers

Thoracic injuries	Number (%)
Total blunt	1,288
Deaths	195 (15)
From intrathoracic injuries	27 (14)
From associated injuries	168 (86)
Total penetrating	230
Deaths	33 (14)
From intrathoracic injuries	32 (97)
From associated injuries	1 (3)

From National Pediatric Trauma Registry, 1985-1991.

TABLE 23-3. Mechanisms of Thoracic Injuries in Selected North American Pediatric Trauma Centers

Thoracic injuries	Number (%)
Blunt	
Motor vehicle/occupant	528 (41)
Motor vehicle/pedestrian	423 (33)
Fall	101 (8)
Bicycle	87 (7)
Motorcycle	34 (3)
Other	115 (9)
TOTAL	1,288
Penetrating	
Gunshot wound	138 (60)
Stab wound	75 (33)
Other	17 (7)
TOTAL	230

From National Pediatric Trauma Registry, 1985-1991.

caused by the air swallowing usually associated with pediatric multisystem trauma.

MECHANISM OF INJURY

Blunt Trauma

Blunt trauma accounts for 83% of chest injuries severe enough to warrant treatment in a pediatric trauma center (see Table 23-1).[1] Of these, nearly three fourths are motor vehicle–related; the remainder are caused mostly by falls, bicycles, or motorcycles (Table 23-3).[1] Each of these mechanisms gives rise to recognizable patterns of injury unique to childhood. Femur, torso, and head trauma (Waddell's triad) typically occur when small children are struck by automobiles; head, multiple long bone, and chest wall trauma are characteristic of falls from a height. More recently recognized is a "lap belt" complex of injuries sometimes associated with "blowout" injuries of the diaphragm.[14-17] The mechanisms of blunt injury in childhood are generally less damaging than those in adulthood, explaining the relative infrequency of major *intrathoracic* injury in pediatric blunt trauma.

Penetrating Trauma

Penetrating trauma is responsible for only 15% of serious chest injuries in childhood. Although on the rise among adolescents because of the increasing incidence of gunshot wounds (see Table 23-3), it is still relatively uncommon among younger children.[1] These injuries are less often fatal than in adults, perhaps because fewer children are victims of intentional gunshot wounds at close range. This may also explain the lower incidence of *nonpulmonary* injuries after thoracic penetration in children.

PATTERNS OF INJURY

Whether blunt or penetrating, all intrathoracic structures are liable to injury after severe trauma (Tables 23-4 and 23-5).[1-3,5-13]

nous ribs enclosing the thoracic cavity often allows the kinetic energy associated with forceful impacts to be transmitted to underlying structures without bony injury. Moreover, blows significant enough to cause serious damage to vital intrathoracic organs (i.e., lungs, heart, airways, and blood vessels) can also be absorbed without apparent chest wall injury or even obvious external trauma, bruising, or petechiae. Thus the pediatric patient sustains rib fractures somewhat less often than the adult, and the associated complications of pneumothorax or hemothorax even less commonly. Yet the exceptional mobility of the mediastinum in the younger age groups means that when such injuries occur, the child is at great risk of sudden marked ventilatory and circulatory compromise if tension subsequently develops.

PATHOPHYSIOLOGY

Special physiologic characteristics limit the ability of the child to compensate for respiratory derangements caused by major thoracic injury. The proportionately larger oxygen consumption and smaller functional residual capacity make for greater susceptibility to hypoxia. Reduced pulmonary compliance and greater chest wall compliance dictate a chiefly tachypneic response to this hypoxia. Finally the horizontally aligned ribs and rudimentary intercostal musculature that make the child a diaphragmatic breather also lead to earlier fatigue. This is particularly true if diaphragmatic excursion is limited by concomitant gastric dilation

TABLE 23-4. Frequency of Injury to Intrathoracic Organs in Selected North American Pediatric Trauma Centers

	Blunt (%)	Penetrating (%)	Total (%)
Pneumothorax and hemothorax	486 (38)	148 (64)	634 (41)
Pneumothorax	306 (24)	52 (23)	358 (23)
Pneumohemothorax	110 (9)	55 (24)	165 (11)
Hemothorax	69 (5)	41 (18)	110 (7)
Unspecified	1 (<1)	0 (0)	1 (<1)
Lung	679 (53)	66 (29)	745 (48)
Contusion	630 (49)	33 (14)	663 (43)
Laceration	16 (1)	24 (10)	40 (3)
Unspecified	33 (3)	9 (4)	42 (3)
Heart	60 (5)	29 (13)	89 (6)
Contusion	51 (4)	1 (<1)	52 (3)
Laceration	5 (<1)	19 (8)	24 (2)
Unspecified	4 (<1)	9 (4)	13 (1)
Diaphragm	29 (2)	35 (15)	64 (4)
Fractures	484 (38)	19 (8)	503 (33)
Ribs	453 (35)	17 (7)	470 (31)
Flail chest	15 (1)	1 (<1)	16 (1)
Larynx and trachea	9 (<1)	1 (<1)	10 (<1)
Sternum	7 (<1)	0 (0)	7 (<1)
Open wounds	5 (<1)	48 (21)	53 (3)
Blood vessels	17 (1)	22 (10)	39 (3)
Aorta	11 (1)	3 (1)	14 (1)
Innominate/subclavian artery	1 (<1)	5 (2)	6 (<1)
Superior vena cava	2 (<1)	1 (<1)	3 (<1)
Innominate/subclavian vein	2 (<1)	4 (2)	6 (<1)
Pulmonary	0 (0)	2 (1)	2 (<1)
Intercostal/internal mammary	0 (0)	6 (3)	6 (<1)
Unspecified	1 (<1)	1 (<1)	2 (<1)
Bronchi	5 (<1)	0 (0)	5 (<1)
Esophagus	4 (<1)	3 (1)	7 (<1)
Intrathoracic injuries NOS	24 (2)	6 (2)	30 (2)
TOTAL PATIENTS	1,288	230	1,518

From National Pediatric Trauma Registry, 1985-1991.
NOS, Not otherwise specified.
NOTE: Many children had more than one injury recorded.

Pulmonary

Pulmonary injuries, which consist of contusions and lacerations, are most frequent.[1-3,5-13] The former is more common in blunt trauma, the latter in penetrating trauma; either can result in a hematoma. Large pulmonary lacerations can be identified by a cavitary appearance on chest x-ray film but do not require surgical repair unless associated with ongoing hemorrhage or air leak[18]; they should not be confused with traumatic pneumatocele, a rare sequela of blunt trauma that resolves spontaneously over several weeks.[19,20] Pulmonary hematomas are relatively uncommon because of the high tissue thromboplastin content of lung tissue and the low pressure within the pulmonary circulation; most are rapidly reabsorbed. On rare occasions they progress to lung abscess.

Pulmonary contusions are perhaps the major source of morbidity caused by blunt chest trauma in childhood, especially when they result from crush injury or sudden compressive injury severe enough to cause traumatic asphyxia.[21-26] They are most commonly associated with the more forceful mechanisms of blunt injury, such as motor vehicle accidents and falls from extreme heights, but may also be caused by extremely powerful, direct blows.[27] The principal danger is that the condition may progress to posttraumatic pulmonary insufficiency (PTPI) (adult respiratory distress syndrome [ARDS]). Although most deaths from chest trauma occur during the early phases of hospitalization, ARDS remains the chief cause of late deaths attributed to thoracic injury.

Cardiac

Cardiac injuries are infrequently encountered in the pediatric age groups.[1-3,5-13] The most common problem is myocardial contusion from blunt trauma,[28-31] which is usually self-limited unless ventricular fibrillation occurs after an extremely forceful precordial blow.[32] Myocardial rup-

TABLE 23-5. Frequency and Type of Injury Following Pediatric Thoracic Trauma

Author	N	Pen	Mort	TP	OP	HP	CT	PC	MC	DP	TB	AO	SP	SH	RF	(IS)
Bickford[2]	26	10	3	1	1	6	1		1		3		5	6	9	(3)
Kilman[3]	73	9	5			5	2	29			2	1	27	5	21	(?)
Smyth[5]	94	10	13			15		61		3	5		13	6	45	(10)
Meller[6]	68	40	2			14		3	3	2	1	1	8		6	(?)
Rege[7]	24	3	1			10		3				1			19	(2)
Nakayama[8]	105	3	7	9				56					30	14	52	(16)
Peclet[9]	104	12	27			15		57					13	14	33	(16)
Roux[10]	128	19	8			25		73	1	1			13	31	62	(?)
Rielly[11]	27	8	7			7		6					9	5		
TOTALS	629	111	73	10	1	97	3	288	5	6	11	3	118	81	247	(47)
PERCENTAGE	100	18	12	2	<1	15	<1	46	<1	<1	2	<1	19	13	39	(7)

N, Total cases; *Pen*, penetrating cases; *Mort*, mortality; *TP*, tension pneumothorax; *OP*, open pneumothorax; *HP*, hemopneumothorax; *CT*, cardiac tamponade; *PC*, pulmonary contusion; *MC*, myocardial contusion; *DP*, diaphragmatic injury; *TB*, tracheobronchial injury; *AO*, aortic injury; *SP*, simple pneumothorax; *SH*, simple hemothorax; *RF*, rib fracture; *(IS)*, (isolated rib fracture). There were no instances of flail chest or esophageal injury cited in these reports.

ture, myocardial necrosis with subsequent aneurysm formation, traumatic aortic and mitral insufficiency, and pericardial laceration and fatal cardiac herniation are rare complications of blunt trauma.[33-38] The coronary circulation and conduction system can be irreversibly damaged after blunt precordial trauma.[39,40] Finally, cardiac tamponade occurs occasionally in blunt trauma but is far more common in penetrating trauma.[41]

Great Vessels

Life-threatening injuries to the great vessels of the thorax are rare.[1-3,5-13] Traumatic aortic rupture occurs most frequently, although traumatic avulsion of arch vessels has also been reported[42-45]; they are probably more common than suggested in the literature, as most victims die at the scene or during transport to the hospital.[46,47] Early detection of such injuries is vital for treatment and survival. Injuries to the superior vena cava and pulmonary vessels produced by blunt trauma are known to occur but have not been separately reported in children.

Other Intrathoracic

Injuries to vital organs other than the lungs and heart are relatively uncommon.[1-3,5-13] Of these, traumatic diaphragmatic hernia and tracheobronchial disruption occur most often, with nearly equal frequency.[48-61] Both may have dramatic presentations, marked by severe respiratory distress; either may be overlooked on initial evaluation, particularly small diaphragmatic lacerations caused by penetrating trauma and posterior tracheal lacerations produced by blunt trauma that do not rupture into either pleural cavity. Traumatic intercostal hernias have also been reported to occur after both blunt and penetrating trauma[62-64]; however, they rarely cause serious physiologic derangement unless associated with open pneumothorax. Esophageal perforations are extremely rare.[65]

Rib Fractures

Rib fractures are caused by severe direct blows to the chest.[66-69] Although the incidence of rib fractures associated with severe blunt trauma is probably somewhat higher than often stated, the pliable nature of these structures allows impacting forces to be transmitted directly to underlying tissues in as many as 50% of the cases.[1-3,5-13]

Although rare, sternal fractures and dislocations have also been reported, usually in association with rib and clavicular fractures and cardiac injuries.[70] They are notable chiefly as markers of injury severity.

DIAGNOSTIC FINDINGS

Clinical Findings

The respiratory derangements produced by major intrathoracic trauma (i.e., arterial hypoxemia, tissue hypoxia, and ultimately acidosis and death) necessitate that the child who has potential thoracic injury be evaluated immediately. Unfortunately, the physical signs of thoracic injury, even if severe, are often quite subtle. Respirations may appear shallow rather than labored, especially with coma. Central cyanosis is only apparent in the presence of hemorrhagic shock if the unsaturated blood hemoglobin concentration exceeds 5 gm/dl.

History

The mechanism and time of the injury should be defined, often through information from the patient, observers, and prehospital personnel. This provides invaluable data related to the type and severity of the injury to be anticipated. Routine information about pertinent medical history, tetanus status, allergies, and medication should be sought, but must not delay lifesaving treatment.

Physical Examination

In *primary assessment* of the chest, the emergency physician must exclude injuries that compromise ventilation or oxygenation. The adequacy of gas exchange is assured by confirming the patency of the airway, excluding tracheal deviation, visualizing chest movement, and auscultating breath sounds bilaterally. A history of penetrating trauma additionally mandates a rapid search for sucking chest wounds and paradoxical jugular venous distension. Unilaterally decreased breath sounds with hyperresonance or dullness to percussion, with or without tracheal shift, suggest the development of tension pneumothorax or hemothorax, respectively, both of which must be treated as emergencies. Jugular venous distension may corroborate a clinical diagnosis of tension pneumothorax or cardiac tamponade.

However, the absence of such signs does not necessarily exclude these diagnoses; tension pneumothorax is notorious for the false transmission of breath sounds in children, and neither this condition nor cardiac tamponade exhibits jugular venous distension if the patient is sufficiently hypovolemic.

As soon as practical after the primary assessment and treatment of immediately life-threatening injuries, a *secondary assessment* should search for less urgent conditions. This must include complete exposure of the patient and log rolling, especially in penetrating trauma. Care must be taken to prevent hypothermia, which worsens acidosis, through the use of blankets, an overhead radiant warmer, and warmed intravenous fluids. A careful head-to-toe examination that includes reexamination of the chest is the cornerstone of this phase of the trauma response; attention *must be specifically redirected* to the thorax if there is any history of chest pain or tenderness, abnormal noises, difficulty in breathing, rapid or shallow respiration, central cyanosis, subcutaneous or bony crepitus, hemoptysis, or hemodynamic instability.

Careful inspection and palpation of the chest wall often yield valuable insights regarding the nature of the child's injuries. Point tenderness, palpable bony deformity, crepitus, or subcutaneous emphysema suggests the presence of rib fracture(s). Multiple posterolateral rib fractures indicate flail chest; as many as 30% of these cases may be overlooked in the initial examination. Rib fractures always suggest the possibility of underlying injury; fractures of the upper ribs are commonly associated with injuries to the lungs or great vessels, whereas those of the lower ribs occur with damage to the solid viscera of the upper abdomen (i.e., liver, spleen, and to a lesser extent kidney). Finally, pain referred to the proximal aspect of a rib may indicate a distal fracture that initially was overlooked, whereas upper abdominal tenderness severe enough to mimic peritonitis may result from intercostal nerve injury associated with lower rib fracture.

Ancillary Data

Laboratory Studies. Laboratory evaluation is an integral part of the secondary assessment. Arterial blood gas analysis is of paramount importance in determining the adequacy of ventilation and oxygenation; an increased alveolar-arterial oxygen difference is the most sensitive and specific biochemical means of detecting respiratory abnormalities. However, it must be remembered that the most important determinant of blood oxygen content, assuming that the arterial oxygen tension (Po_2) exceeds 60 mm Hg (hence that the arterial oxygen saturation [SaO_2] exceeds 90%), is the concentration of circulating hemoglobin. Serial hematocrit values offer a better clue to the extent of blood loss than the initial value, since initial values may not immediately be reflected by acute blood loss; however, if physical and vital signs indicate the presence of shock, an initial hematocrit value of 30% or less suggests significant hemorrhage, and 25% or less, massive hemorrhage.[71] Blood type and crossmatch should be obtained early to assure availability of blood products during management.

Radiologic Studies. Radiologic evaluation of the pediatric chest trauma victim constitutes a vitally important part of the overall examination. A supine chest film is integral to the specific trauma series of x-ray studies obtained in every multiply injured child, assuming the patient does not require immediate transport to the operating room. However, the chest x-ray film should never take precedence over resuscitation and treatment of life-threatening thoracic injuries. The hypoxia and hypercarbia that are the inevitable consequences of most such injuries may not leave adequate time for confirmatory radiographs, and the emergency physician must therefore be prepared to act on the basis of clinical judgment alone. However, a chest x-ray film should be obtained once respiratory and circulatory stability has been achieved.

Any collection of air or fluid in the hemithorax after thoracic injury must be considered abnormal and immediately addressed. Abnormal fluid collections must be assumed to be blood. Because of the exceptional mobility of the mediastinum in childhood, every sign of tension must be considered with the utmost urgency. The typical radiographic appearance of some of the more commonly encountered diagnostic entities is illustrated in Fig. 23-1.

Geometry and gravity dictate that small amounts of air and blood "layer out" anteriorly and posteriorly, respectively, on an initial anteroposterior chest film when the child lies flat, making detection of these collections extremely difficult. When the history or physical examination result suggests blunt chest injury, a posteroanterior chest film therefore should be obtained after stabilization with the patient in the upright position. This technique facilitates the diagnosis of small apical pneumothoraces as well as hemothoraces in the costophrenic sulcus.

The supine chest x-ray film often shows a widened mediastinum suggesting aortic rupture, which is extremely rare in children.[72] If there is no other radiographic indication of aortic disruption, the child is hemodynamically stable, the lateral cervical spine x-ray film result is normal, and there are no signs of cervical spine injury, a repeat chest x-ray film, preferably posteroanterior, should be obtained with the child in a semiupright or sitting position, *carefully maintaining the cervical spine in a neutral position.* This may obviate the need for aortography if the result is interpreted as normal; computed tomograms of the aortic arch, even if obtained immediately after intravenous contrast medium administration, are rarely definitive enough to be helpful.

Although the diagnosis of isolated rib fracture may be overlooked on as many as 50% of initial radiographs, roentgen diagnosis by means of rib x-ray studies is expensive, inexact, and difficult in children, whose cartilaginous bones often make such diagnosis impossible. Moreover, such x-ray studies are time-consuming, require repeated painful positioning that is especially poorly tolerated by children, and may be frankly dangerous, since they often preclude

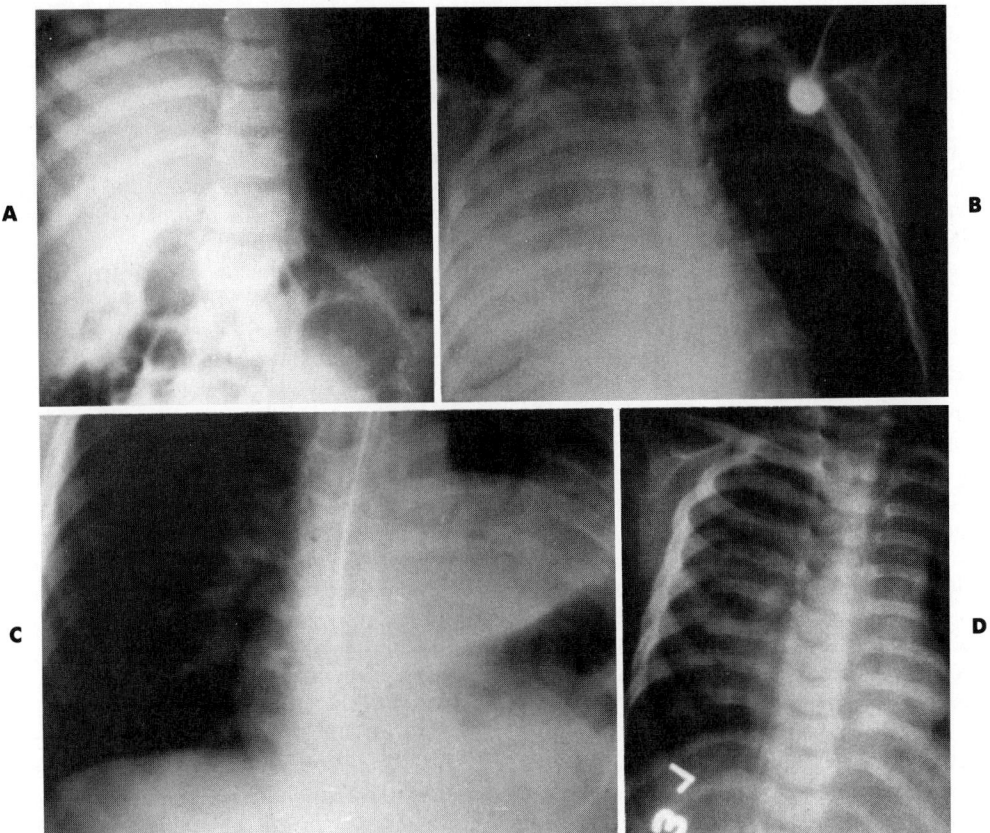

FIG. 23-1. A, Classic radiographic findings of tension pneumothorax from blunt pedestrian motor vehicle trauma that was initially missed in the emergency department. Note the presence of contralateral mediastinal shift. Although the child did not present with respiratory distress, symptoms developed shortly after admission. The child should have undergone immediate needle decompression without waiting for the confirmatory x-ray study. **B,** Classic radiographic findings of massive hemothorax from penetrating wound that lacerated internal mammary artery. Note the presence of the concomitant pneumothorax. **C,** Classic radiographic findings in a child with traumatic left diaphragmatic hernia from blunt pedestrian motor vehicle trauma. Note elevation of the hemidiaphragm, unusual gas shadows in the left inferior hemithorax, and the presence of the nasogastric tube within the chest. **D,** Classic radiographic findings in a child with fractured ribs suggestive of inflicted injury from physical abuse. Note callus formation about the fracture site in the right ninth rib not present about the other fracture sites, indicative of repetitive injuries in different stages of healing.

proper observation and monitoring while adding little information vital to therapy.

Computed tomography (CT) has revolutionized the management of pediatric head, abdominal, and cervical spine trauma. The technique is also useful in airway trauma and is more sensitive than routine supine anteroposterior chest radiography in evaluating multiply injured children.[58,73,74] Although in 40% of multiply injured children detectable thoracic injuries are discovered incidentally on CT scans of the abdomen, lesions requiring immediate treatment are effectively diagnosed with plain x-ray studies. Children who require abdominal scans as victims of motor vehicle–related injuries, falls from heights, or child abuse should have the uppermost abdominal "cuts" visualize, at least those portions of the lower chest directly adjacent to the liver and spleen, to exclude unsuspected intrathoracic injury. If unsuspected abnormality is identified, the CT scan can then be extended cephalad, assuming the integrity of

ventilation, oxygenation, and perfusion can be adequately maintained.

MANAGEMENT

The early management of the child with thoracic injuries requires a physiologic approach. Yet, the basic principles are no different from those for the child who has sustained multisystem trauma of any type. A combined primary assessment and resuscitation phase that gives priority attention to the airway, breathing, and circulation, including bleeding and shock, precedes the detailed evaluation of the patient for signs of major injuries to the head, chest, abdomen, and skeleton performed during a secondary assessment, at which time definitive management of such injuries is first undertaken. However, if there is an injury to the chest that poses such a dire threat to the integrity of ventilation, oxygenation, and perfusion that resuscitative measures will be of no avail until it is addressed, it must be treated immediately upon discovery. Unfortunately, the full extent and consequences of serious thoracic injury often are not recognized upon initial evaluation. This fact underscores the necessity of taking an aggressive approach to resuscitation, the initial minutes of which (as outlined in Chapters 12 and 19) should be guided by consensus protocols of the American Heart Association, American Academy of Pediatrics, American College of Surgeons, and American College of Emergency Physicians.[75-77] Rapid clinical assessment (and reassessment) of ventilation, oxygenation, and perfusion is fundamental to this process to identify and treat any condition that may lead imminently to cardiopulmonary failure.

Initial Resuscitation

Because hypoxia is the fundamental physiologic derangement resulting from chest trauma regardless of cause, most children with major thoracic injuries experience some degree of respiratory insufficiency. The treatment is rapid administration of humidified oxygen at the highest available concentration to areas of the lung with normal ventilation and perfusion. For those with simple respiratory distress (increased rate or work of breathing), it should be given via a nonrebreathing mask if the airway is patent and breathing is spontaneous. Patients in whom upper airway obstruction or frank respiratory failure (cyanosis or overwhelming fatigue in addition to the specified symptoms and signs) develops should have oxygen administered by assisted ventilation, using a bag-valve device attached to either a face mask or, if necessary, an endotracheal tube of the proper size for the child's age. Emergency treatment of immediately life-threatening chest injuries detected by the primary assessment is essential. Nasogastric intubation for gastric decompression is important to minimize dilation and reduce limitation of diaphragmatic motion and risk of pulmonary aspiration.

Tube Thoracostomy and Emergency Thoracotomy

All acute collections of air or blood, regardless of size, require *immediate* drainage by means of *lateral tube thoracostomy*. This alone will prove sufficient treatment for the vast majority of pneumothoraces and hemothoraces, as most such drainage stops shortly after the lung or lungs fully reexpand. In general, it is best to avoid using the site of injury for tube insertion in cases of penetrating trauma, as placement through a contaminated tract may introduce infection into the chest (see Appendix 23A: Tube Thoracostomy). Emergency thoracotomy is usually indicated if there is initial drainage of more than 10 to 15 ml of intrapleural blood/kg of body weight; rapid, continuing blood loss exceeding 2 to 4 ml/kg/hr; or uncontrolled air leak. It is also indicated if food or saliva drains from the chest tube and for all cases of cardiac tamponade, whether the injury is blunt or penetrating.

The chief indications for *emergency department thoracotomy* are cardiac arrest and tamponade caused by penetrating trauma. Although there is no contraindication to open chest cardiac massage in blunt trauma and anecdotal reports have been published suggesting that it may be useful in the child who has measurable vital signs but loses them during the course of resuscitation,[78] the outcome of emergency department thoracotomy in pediatric blunt trauma victims has been dismal.[79-84] External chest compressions, together with control of external hemorrhage and rapid volume restoration, may therefore be the better choice for this group of patients. Pediatric patients with penetrating chest injuries who do not exhibit arrest, tamponade, or decompensated shock but do not respond to initial treatment, including tube thoracostomy, are candidates for urgent thoracotomy in the operating room, not the emergency department.

Emergency department thoracotomy for cross-clamping of the distal thoracic aorta in blunt abdominal trauma associated with profound hemorrhagic shock, as advocated by some emergency physicians and trauma surgeons for use in adults, also has been largely abandoned in children[85] because of a high failure rate caused in part by the abundance of collateral vessels.[86] It is also technically more difficult in children, in whom it may result in avulsion of intercostal vessels and exsanguinating hemorrhage. Finally, no convincing advantage has been demonstrated over direct finger compression of the proximal abdominal aorta via laparotomy, which the vast majority of pediatric victims of blunt abdominal trauma require if they present in decompensated hypotensive shock.

Disposition

Any child who has thoracic injuries and presents in respiratory insufficiency or requires resuscitation in an emergency department should be admitted to a pediatric critical care unit for further treatment. Children who are less ill but have sustained thoracic injuries serious enough to warrant evaluation by an emergency physician should be hospitalized if physical assessment indicates that their injuries have resulted in significant anatomic or physiologic derangement. As a general rule, it is probably safe to proceed with "routine" admission and evaluation if the Pediatric Trauma Score, Champion Trauma Score, Revised Trauma Score, or other trauma score falls within the low-risk category.[87-89] However, children with chest trauma must be considered for triage or transfer to a regional trauma center with pediatric expertise if the mechanism of injury suggests that this level of care may be required or if trauma scores indicate the possibility of life-threatening injury.[90]

SPECIFIC INJURIES

Postresuscitation care of the child with thoracic injuries obviously depends on the type, extent, and severity of the injuries. Most thoracic injuries are limited to the chest wall and therefore can be managed either expectantly or by means of tube thoracostomy. In the unstable patient, additional treatment is required immediately; in the stable patient, definitive therapy will be directed by the appropriate surgical specialist. All patients who are in critical condition must be carefully monitored by means of serial physical and roentgen examinations, oximetry, capnography, and blood gas determinations; serial cardiac enzyme determinations, electrocardiography, and echocardiography are obtained as indicated.

Immediately Life-Threatening Injuries

The patient who has major thoracic injuries is a rapidly evolving pathophysiologic "experiment of nature," challenging the emergency physician (1) to develop a hypoth-

TABLE 23-6. Differential Diagnosis of Immediately Life-Threatening Cardiopulmonary Injuries

	Tension pneumothorax	Massive hemothorax	Cardiac tamponade
Breath sounds	Ipsilaterally decreased	Ipsilaterally decreased	Normal
Percussion note	Hyperresonant	Dull	Normal
Tracheal location	Contralaterally shifted	Midline	Midline
Neck veins	Distended	Flat	Distended
Heart tones	Normal	Normal	Muffled

esis as to whether the respiratory tract, circulatory tract, or both are deranged, and why; (2) to institute a plan of action that will confirm this theory without causing the patient further harm, especially if there is a potential delay in diagnosis; (3) to observe the effects of these efforts and evaluate the results of these interventions; and (4) to be fully prepared to reject previous thinking if proved wrong and rapidly redesign the approach with the detached, dispassionate, yet directed determination required of any true scientist. All this must be done with the greatest sense of urgency, for the injuries may lead to the uncoupling of the mitochondrial energy process of oxidative phosphorylation on which all human life ultimately depends.

Six conditions are so *immediately* life-threatening that particular expertise is required. The differential diagnosis of the three most frequently misdiagnosed cardiopulmonary injuries is summarized in Table 23-6.

Upper Airway Obstruction. In the child trauma victim, posterior displacement of the tongue and epiglottis across the laryngeal inlet may produce obstruction and usually is associated with loss of pharyngeal muscle tone during unconsciousness.[91,92] The pediatric airway is at particular risk because of its narrow intrinsic diameter, propensity to trap foreign matter (blood, mucus, and dental fragments), and greater frequency of severe closed head injury in childhood.

Diagnostic Findings. Partial upper airway closure produced by soft tissue obstruction is recognized by inspiratory gurgling or snoring; complete blockage is manifested by severe rocking chest motions, marked by intercostal and substernal retractions and no gas exchange. These may be absent when an unconscious child has apnea or labored breathing. Failure to establish an adequate airway causes particularly rapid demise of the pediatric trauma patient. The diagnosis of upper airway obstruction is made on solely clinical grounds.

Management. The head should be placed in a neutral position, simultaneously stabilizing the cervical spine and lifting the mandibular block forward by means of a modified jaw thrust. If this fails to relieve the obstruction, the oropharynx should be vigorously suctioned with a rigid Yankauer-type device, with care to prevent lodging particulate matter above the cricoid ring. If effective gas exchange has not yet been achieved, assisted ventilation should be instituted with an oropharyngeal airway and bag and mask, as needed. If the child still cannot be ventilated, foreign body obstruction should be suspected; however, since obstructed airway maneuvers are contraindicated in unconscious children unless concomitant injury to the upper abdomen can be excluded, direct retrieval is the treatment of choice.

If direct laryngoscopy identifies particulate matter, it should be removed by Rovenstein (pediatric Magill) forceps. Although endotracheal intubation of a child whose airway is completely obstructed by particulate matter is controversial, most experts believe that an attempt should be made to intubate "around" a foreign body that cannot be dislodged; intubation should also be attempted if the airway remains obstructed despite absence of a visible foreign body. Only when intubation fails should establishment of a surgical airway be attempted. As in the adult, needle cricothyrotomy with jet ventilation is the preferred approach; emergency tracheostomy or surgical cricothyrotomy is an extremely difficult procedure in small children.

Some authorities advocate routine cricothyrotomy in patients with potential cervical spine injury, but this is rarely necessary. The incidence of cervical spine injury is low. Approximately 350 children per 100,000 annually sustain head injuries, with only 8 of these 350 having cervical spine injuries.[93,94] Those who argue in favor of establishment of surgical airways also cite the "inherent" difficulty of intubation in a child, whose larynx is more anterior and cephalad than that of an adult, when the neck is manually stabilized as the head rests on a flat surface. However, it must be remembered that the prominent occiput of the young child forces the neck into slight flexion when the child is in the supine position[95]; intubation is more easily accomplished when the spine is kept truly neutral by placing a thin layer of padding beneath the child's body or slightly lowering the head of the bed.

Complete anatomic obstruction of the upper airway of the child is a distinctly unusual event. When encountered, it usually is due to blunt injury to the larynx or upper trachea of the type caused by either a direct blow or the rapid deceleration against an outstretched wire or clothesline and is often associated with a hangman's fracture. The larynx and trachea may be either partially or completely shattered or transected, resulting in marked subcutaneous emphysema and crepitus, hematoma about the cartilaginous fracture site, loud gurgling on inspiration, and bloody secretions in the mouth. Emergency endotracheal intubation should be attempted before creation of an artificial airway; use of the fiberoptic laryngoscope may prove invaluable, particularly if an endotracheal tube is first placed over the body of the instrument, permitting it to act as a "guide wire" for intubation once the tracheal lumen has been identified.

A normal lateral cervical spine x-ray film result does not exclude the possibility of injury, either to the bony elements of the cervical spine or to the spinal cord itself; indeed, spinal cord injury without radiographic abnormality (SCIWORA) is known to occur.[96,97] Since the only sure way to exclude the possibility of injury to the bony and neural elements of the spine is complete physical and radiologic examination of a degree rarely possible in the unstable patient, there is no absolute need to obtain a lateral cervical spine x-ray film before intubation in the patient with airway instability. A reasonable clinical approach to such patients during management of the airway is to assume that such an injury is present and to maintain full cervical spine precautions by means of bimanual in-line cervical spine stabilization (or a cervical extrication collar, head immobilizer, and tape) until a definitive evaluation can be performed (see Chapter 22).

Tension Pneumothorax. Tension pneumothorax is caused by accumulation of air behind a one-way "flap-valve" type of defect in the lung or airway and usually is due to the barotrauma sustained when the chest is exposed to a severe compressive blunt force as the glottis is held tightly closed. However, it also may be caused by the sharp end of a fractured rib or penetrating trauma, particularly stab wounds, in which the chest wall defect is not large enough to cause an open pneumothorax.

Diagnostic Findings. Profound respiratory distress, distended neck veins, contralateral tracheal deviation, ipsilateral hyperresonance to percussion, and decreased breath sounds are cardinal signs; sudden circulatory collapse may also develop as the mediastinum shifts away from the side of increased pressure and kinks the superior and inferior vena cava at the thoracic inlets. In most cases, the diagnosis should be made on clinical grounds alone because there rarely is sufficient time to obtain a confirmatory chest x-ray film.

Management. The condition is treated definitively by means of lateral tube thoracostomy, using a large-caliber posteriorly directed chest tube, since it is nearly always accompanied by hemothorax in trauma patients. However, should signs of respiratory or circulatory insufficiency also be present, immediate decompression (by means of an over-the-needle catheter placed percutaneously through the second intercostal space on the midclavicular line, just above the third rib to avoid the intercostal vessels) must first be performed. Only in patients who are fully compensated from *both* the respiratory and circulatory standpoints may the physician delay treatment until a chest x-ray study is obtained. However, should signs of respiratory insufficiency or shock supervene while the physician is waiting for the results of this study, the lesion must be treated without further delay, since the extraordinary mobility of the mediastinum in children promotes rapid development of tension and frank cardiopulmonary failure.

Open Pneumothorax. Sucking chest wounds occur when there is free bidirectional flow of air between the atmosphere and the pleural space; thus, by definition, they cannot occur without concomitant penetration sufficient to result in a loss of a portion of the chest wall that approaches the size of the bronchial lumen. It may be caused by a gunshot or shotgun wound, large knife wound, or blast injury.

Diagnostic Findings. Open pneumothorax produces ineffective gas exchange (resulting from the equilibration of intrathoracic and extrathoracic pressure) as atmospheric air follows the path of least resistance into the thorax. Although it is extremely rare in children, it is especially lethal. It results in paradoxical breathing and near-complete cessation of ventilation and oxygenation as the mediastinum swings to and fro, and both the ipsilateral and contralateral lungs collapse rather than expand on inspiration.

Management. In addition to management of respiratory insufficiency, emergency treatment of open pneumothorax consists of temporary closure of the chest wall and immediate evacuation of entrapped air. In the spontaneously breathing patient, simple occlusion of the defect with Vaseline-impregnated gauze and insertion of a chest tube via a separate tract usually suffice; construction of a "flutter-valve" type of dressing taped on three sides is useful as a temporizing measure only. If the defect is too large to close airtight, positive pressure (i.e., assisted ventilation) is required to assure the adequacy of ventilation and oxygenation. In most such instances, emergency treatment must be followed by urgent thoracotomy for repair of the chest wall; small defects usually will close spontaneously.

Massive Hemothorax. In blunt injury and penetrating trauma caused by gunshot wounds, massive hemothorax is more often due to bleeding from lung parenchyma than from intercostal vessels; in penetrating trauma produced by stab wounds, the reverse is true. However, since most pulmonary disruptions are rapidly self-sealing regardless of cause, massive hemothorax is rare in children and does not occur without the severe type of destruction associated with the extremely sudden, forceful impacts seen in high-speed motor vehicle accidents, falls from extreme heights, and gunshot wounds inflicted at close range.

Diagnostic Findings. As in tension pneumothorax, initial examination reveals respiratory distress and absence of breath sounds on the affected side. Contralateral tracheal deviation is rare, the neck veins usually are flat, the chest is dull to percussion, and the development of shock precedes the development of respiratory failure rather than the reverse. If the hemothorax is caused by a major vascular disruption, signs of tension pneumothorax may coexist with those of decompensated shock.

Management. Massive hemothorax requires urgent treatment by means of tube thoracostomy; evacuation of the pleural space must proceed simultaneously with rapid administration of type-specific or O-negative blood. A large-caliber posteriorly directed chest tube, inserted laterally at nipple level, should be used. It must be of sufficient size to allow free drainage of blood (i.e., about as wide as the intercostal space); a chest x-ray film should be obtained soon after placement to document tube position and lung reexpansion. Thoracotomy for control of bleeding usually is reserved for cases in which the volume of the blood initially evacuated from the hemithorax exceeds 25% of total blood volume or ongoing blood loss exceeds 2% of total blood volume/hour. Control of intrathoracic bleeding may prove difficult and should be undertaken only by a surgeon experienced in the management of thoracic trauma.

Cardiac Tamponade. Cardiac tamponade treated in the emergency department is most commonly caused by stab wounds, since most gunshot-wound victims usually die at the scene or in transport to the hospital; it is an extraordinarily rare sequela of blunt trauma. Sudden hypotensive decompensation ensues once enough blood is contained within the pericardial sac to compromise venous return.

Diagnostic Findings. The presence of a precordial wound suggests the diagnosis, which usually is associated with pronounced tachycardia, muffled heart tones, narrowed pulse pressure, and pulsus paradoxus; distended neck veins are present only when hypovolemia is absent. Echocardiography may provide a noninvasive means of establishing the diagnosis in questionable cases.

Management. Once the diagnosis is confirmed, definitive emergency treatment by means of thoracotomy, pericardiotomy, and direct myocardial repair is required. If a qualified surgeon is not immediately available to the emergency department, the associated myocardial constriction can sometimes be relieved by repeated aspiration of blood from the pericardial sac by means of an indwelling catheter placed at the time of left subxyphoid *pericardiocentesis.* This technique is performed under electrocardiographic control by grasping the large-bore introducing needle near its hub with an alligator clip electrode and watching for atypical ventricular depolarization(s), as the tip of the needle is advanced slowly, under constant aspiration, from the left subxyphoid area toward the tip of left scapula (see Chapter 47).

The patient who has decompensated shock or traumatic arrest with cardiac tamponade caused by penetrating trauma can be saved only by immediate thoracotomy begun in the emergency department; pericardial blood may be clotted in acute tamponade in contrast to chronic pericarditis, and often cannot be decompressed even with a large needle.

Flail Chest. Flail chest occurs when massive blunt trauma to the chest wall causes parallel double fractures of two or more adjacent ribs, with subsequent loss of the bony continuity of the thoracic cage, resulting in "paradoxical" chest wall motion, with inspiratory collapse and expiratory bulge during breathing. Because of the concomitant pulmonary contusion, the small size of the chest cavity, and the proximity of typically posterolateral flail segments to the diaphragm, large injuries are often poorly tolerated by children.

Diagnostic Findings. Although tenderness and crepitus at the fracture sites are usually obvious at the time of initial evaluation and paradoxical chest wall motion is pathognomonic, the diagnosis is often overlooked in the primary survey, since the associated muscle spasm tends both to stabilize and obscure the flail segment.

Management. Immediate treatment aimed at prevention of arterial hypoxemia is supportive. Assisted ventilation, followed by intubation; positive pressure ventilation, including positive end expiratory pressure (PEEP) of 5 to 10 cm H_2O; and, sometimes, neuromuscular blockade are required if the child is incapable of sustained respiratory effort. Narcotic analgesics are rarely necessary because children are remarkably tolerant of the discomfort associated with rib fractures; moreover, respiratory depression may adversely affect the recovery of the patient who is spontaneously breathing or being weaned from ventilatory support. External or internal splinting is unnecessary during any phase of treatment; patients with small flail segments usually do not benefit, and those with more extensive injuries require positive pressure ventilation, which

generally is sufficient to maintain proper alignment of the chest wall.

Potentially Life-Threatening Injuries

Treatment of immediately life-threatening injuries is obviously of greatest concern to the emergency physician. However, there are six potentially life-threatening thoracic injuries; failure to recognize these lesions may lead to a course of therapy that accelerates their progression. The presenting signs are often subtle and are likely to be overlooked on initial physical examination. Repeated examination and ongoing monitoring are therefore essential.

Pulmonary Contusion. Indirect forceful disruption of pulmonary parenchyma may result from direct transmission to underlying lung tissue of the kinetic energy associated with severe blunt impact to the overlying chest wall. Although truly life-threatening pulmonary contusions are encountered infrequently in children, the pliable nature of the chest wall increases the potential for this type of injury; moreover, damage frequently occurs even in the absence of external signs of severe internal thoracic trauma, such as broken ribs.

Diagnostic Findings. The leaky capillary membranes of injured lung tissue promote sequestration of fluid in the interstitial space, but the contracted state of the circulation in the multiply injured child may retard accumulation of this fluid. Thus early detection of the pathognomonic infiltrate by either physical examination (through signs of pulmonary consolidation) or chest x-ray film (by the presence of a patchy radiopacity) usually is difficult. An increased alveolar-arterial oxygen difference is, similarly, a poor early indicator of pulmonary contusion. In the emergency department it is probably best to make the diagnosis presumptively whenever the mechanism of injury suggests that it may be present.

Management. The treatment of pulmonary contusion is expectant. The goal is to prevent clinically significant arterial hypoxemia, using the least possible amount of artificial respiratory support. Intubation must be performed in children who are in respiratory failure, are unconscious and require hyperventilation for control of intracranial pressure, or need general anesthesia for repair of abdominal or skeletal injuries. However, if intubation is required, PEEP of 5 to 10 cm H_2O should be used to maintain functional residual capacity and prevent oxygen toxicity whenever a fraction of inspired oxygen (F_{IO_2}) of 40% or more is needed to maintain an arterial oxygen tension (P_{O_2}) of 70 to 80 mm Hg.

Much has been made of the many similarities between pulmonary contusion ("traumatic wet lung") and PTPI ("shock lung") or ARDS. The natural history of pulmonary contusion is characterized by spontaneous resolution unless PTPI supervenes. Therapies known to be associated with the development of this ARDS, particularly excessive administration of crystalloid fluids, should be avoided.

PTPI in childhood is significantly worsened when there is concomitant aspiration of gastric contents. All intubated multiply injured patients should have vigorous suction once the airway has been established, for diagnosis as well as for treatment. If significant pulmonary aspiration is proved to have occurred, tracheobronchial lavage must be considered, sometimes necessitating rigid bronchoscopy under general anesthesia. Antibiotic coverage must be designed to include treatment for oral and gastric anaerobes. The role of corticosteroids in PTPI or ARDS remains unproved; however, if they are to be given, they must be started as early as possible after injury.

Myocardial Contusion. Myocardial contusion may result from a concussive force applied to the chest, the impact typically being directed centrally and anteroposteriorly, as opposed to laterally or obliquely. Although it is being diagnosed with increasing frequency in the younger age groups, neither its significance nor the most appropriate diagnostic criteria are yet certain; the fact that children are uncommon victims of steering wheel injuries may account for its apparently lower morbidity in pediatric patients. Nevertheless, myocardial dysfunction attributable to the concussive impact has been anecdotally reported; myocardial rupture after contusion in the pediatric age groups has not. Myocardial contusion can and does occur, but its status as a potentially life-threatening thoracic injury in childhood is unclear.

Diagnostic Findings. Symptoms and signs are nonspecific, consisting chiefly of poorly localized chest pain. The diagnosis rests on a battery of specific diagnostic tests, including serial electrocardiography, echocardiography, and determination of myocardial enzymes; radionuclide angiography may also be useful in selected cases. In contrast to adults, children do not commonly have specific electrocardiographic abnormalities or sudden life-threatening ventricular tachydysrhythmias such as multifocal premature depolarizations or ventricular tachycardia; echocardiographic and scintigraphic abnormalities are rare.

Management. Treatment of myocardial contusion consists of continuous observation in a fully monitored environment. Should evidence of myocardial irritability develop, standard antidysrhythmic therapy should be employed; intravenous lidocaine is the agent of choice and is usually successful.

Traumatic Bronchial Disruption. Traumatic bronchial disruption is fortunately rare in childhood. It may be caused by direct shearing when associated with crushing injuries but more often results from severe compression of the chest during expiration against a closed glottis (i.e., a Valsalva maneuver). It nearly always occurs adjacent to the carina and is highly lethal, particularly if undetected. As many as half of these patients die within the first hour after injury.

Diagnostic Findings. The injury usually is associated with ipsilateral tension pneumothorax. In the absence of hemoptysis, the characteristic presenting signs are failure to reexpand the lung or persistence of a large air leak despite adequate treatment of a tension pneumothorax by means of tube thoracostomy. Ultimately, bronchoscopic confirmation may be needed.

Management. Mild bronchial disruptions may require nothing more than tube thoracostomy and supportive care until effective healing occurs. There is no contraindication to intubation in patients with bronchial damage, although it may be precluded if the trachea is also disrupted or is distorted by paratracheal hematoma formation; in such cases, a surgical airway must be established *below* the level of the injury by means of cricothyrotomy or tracheostomy.

Intrathoracic control of the airway is obviously the only hope for survival when there is complete tracheal obstruction or discontinuity below the level of the thoracic inlet. Uncontrollable bleeding and inability to ventilate once an adequate airway has been established constitute the indications for emergency thoracotomy in bronchial injury.

Traumatic Diaphragmatic Hernia. Disruption caused by blunt injury, once considered rare in childhood, is being identified with increasing frequency as part of the "lap belt" complex of injuries described earlier. It is more common on the left than on the right. In left-sided blunt injury, the impacting force typically produces large radial tears in the diaphragm, followed by immediate herniation. Presentation in right-sided blunt injury or penetrating trauma is often delayed; symptoms and signs do not develop until abdominal viscera are drawn into the thorax by the positive-to-negative pressure gradient between these body cavities. Diaphragmatic hernia remains uncommon in penetrating injury but must be considered whenever the torso is violated at a level between the nipples and umbilicus.

Diagnostic Findings. The immediate pathophysiologic effects of traumatic diaphragmatic hernia are not due to the diaphragmatic injury per se, but to the subsequent herniation of abdominal contents into the chest. Thus the time to onset of symptoms and signs usually varies inversely with the size of the rent in the diaphragm. If presentation is acute, the diagnosis is obvious on chest x-ray film. Confusing radiologic findings, including unexplained elevation of the hemidiaphragm, unrelieved acute gastric dilatation, and loculated subpulmonic hemopneumothorax, herald the diagnosis when presentation is delayed.

Management. Direct surgical repair is indicated as soon as the lesion is identified. If the patient's condition is acute, the respiratory status must first be stabilized, usually by means of intubation and positive pressure ventilation. This should be preceded by placement of a nasogastric tube to prevent development of tension pneumoenterothorax.

When a delayed presentation occurs, the diagnosis is usually confirmed fluoroscopically by means of a water-soluble contrast agent, unless further studies are rendered unnecessary by the presence of a nasogastric tube in the thoracic cavity on chest x-ray study. On rare occasions, abdominal exploration may be required to exclude the diagnosis.

Traumatic Rupture of Great Vessels. Rupture of the great vessels after blunt injury is extremely rare in childhood. The most common cause is aortic disruption at the level of the ligamentum arteriosum, which may be associated with aortic dissection. Children with Marfan syndrome are at especially high risk because of the intrinsic weakness of their uncross-linked collagen, whereas the higher elastin content of the connective tissues probably accounts for the relative invulnerability of normal children to this type of injury. As in adults, these injuries are associated with severe deceleration events (e.g., high-speed automobile crashes, falls from extreme heights) that are likely to be fatal at the scene. The injury is often associated with first or second rib injuries.

Diagnostic Findings. Traumatic aortic rupture is suspected clinically when there is a murmur that radiates to the back after an injury involving severe deceleration. However, this murmur is not frequently heard and ultimately the diagnosis rests on the same radiologic criteria used for the adult: (1) widened mediastinum with obliteration of the aortic knob, (2) deviation of the trachea (endotracheal tube) to the right or the esophagus (nasogastric tube) to the left, and (3) presence of an apical pleural cap, particularly if associated with fractures of the first or second ribs. The most common sign encountered is a widened mediastinum; however, as previously noted, this is rarely due to aortic disruption in a child and does not mandate further work-up unless other signs of mediastinal hemorrhage are present, in an appropriate clinical setting. Transesophageal echocardiography is increasingly used in confirming the diagnosis; arteriography is still needed in equivocal cases and is preferred in stable patients as far more detailed information is obtained.

Management. Emergency surgical repair is the treatment of choice and may require cardiopulmonary bypass.[40] Survival is rare unless the condition is immediately recognized and aggressively treated.

Traumatic Esophageal Rupture. Esophageal rupture caused by blunt injury is virtually unknown in childhood, although it can occur. It is believed to result from a blow to the upper abdomen forceful enough to inject gastric contents into the lower esophagus under extremely high pressure, as the cricopharyngeal muscle is held tightly closed in anticipation of the impact.

Diagnostic Findings. Clinically the injury is similar to that observed in the Boerhaave syndrome (postemetic esophageal rupture), which progresses rapidly to mediastinitis, sepsis, and death if unrecognized. It should be suspected if pain or shock disproportionate to the apparent severity of the injury occurs. Communication with the pleural cavity, which results in pneumothorax, may also occur; however, this hastens the diagnosis if a chest tube inserted for treatment drains food or saliva or bubbles equally and continuously throughout the respiratory cycle. "Mediastinal crunch," or Hamman's sign, is rarely heard in the child; thus the only clue to the diagnosis may be the presence of mediastinal emphysema on chest roentgenogram, since the small volume of gas entrapped is unlikely to dissect superiorly as far as the neck, where it could be palpated subcutaneously. The diagnosis is confirmed fluoroscopically by using a water-soluble contrast agent.

Management. Direct transthoracic repair and wide mediastinal drainage are urgently undertaken. If irreparable damage is present, total esophageal exclusion by means of temporary cervical esophagostomy and gastrostomy may be necessary and definitive repair deferred until a later date.

Serious Injuries

The emergency physician must be aware of a number of serious conditions associated with severe injury to the chest that are not immediately or potentially life-threatening. Some of these injuries are self-limited and heal without treatment. However, they cannot be ignored, for they may have serious consequences, not just in terms of unnecessary discomfort, but in terms of possible unrecognized deterioration. These conditions are also important in that they are markers of truly life-threatening intrathoracic or multisystemic trauma.

Simple Pneumothorax. Blunt or penetrating trauma may produce a simple pneumothorax. The former usually causes tearing of the parietal and visceral pleural membranes by the sharp end of a fractured rib; the latter results from violation by a pointed instrument. The injury results from a transpleural laceration of peripheral lung tissue. Unless the parenchymal wound is large, it is usually self-sealing because of the high concentration of tissue thromboplastin in lung tissue and the low pressure within the pulmonary circulation. Assuming that this wound proceeds to spontaneous healing, the entrapped air usually is reabsorbed over the course of several days.

Because of the self-limited nature of the lesion, simple pneumothorax rarely causes life-threatening ventilatory compromise. However, as pneumothorax and hemothorax often coexist in victims of serious chest trauma, appropriate therapy includes upright positioning and placement of a large-caliber posteriorly directed chest tube, even for a simple pneumothorax. Observation or aspiration of small intrapleural air collections, even stable ones, is dangerous to the multiply injured patient and is contraindicated for the child who requires positive pressure ventilation, general anesthesia, or emergency transport. This is particularly true for those patients who must be evacuated by air ambulance.

Simple Hemothorax. A simple hemothorax may result from the same mechanisms of injury that cause simple pneumothorax. However, in these cases the intercostal or internal mammary vessels may be injured as well as the pulmonary parenchyma. Unfortunately, although such bleeding by definition also is self-limited, this injury can rarely be quantified prospectively, since it is difficult to know how fast the patient is bleeding without the benefit of tube thoracostomy. Occasionally, however, such patients present long enough after their injuries (i.e., several hours or days) that one can safely assume that bleeding has stopped.

Collections of blood that are truly small can be reabsorbed by the body and at worst result in mild basilar pleural scarring. However, collections of blood that appear small on upright chest x-ray study may be significant: to be identified radiographically, their volume must approach about 10 ml/kg of body weight. For this reason, most authorities recommend that even "small" collections be drained by means of large-caliber posteriorly directed chest tube(s) placed through the midaxillary line at nipple level. Such treatment also minimizes the chance of subsequent pulmonary restriction produced by "trapped lung" (i.e., tethering and compression by large, organizing intrapleural clots that progress to fibrothorax), unless removed by decortication.

Rib Fractures. Rib fractures are uncommon sequelae of all but serious cases of major blunt trauma in young children. The posterolateral aspects of the middle and lower ribs sustain most of the injuries, as these are the areas most commonly struck by a moving vehicle or injured in a fall. However, they are also the areas most accessible to assailants during child battering, a diagnosis that should be considered whenever a clear-cut history of severe trauma is lacking in a young child with rib fractures, particularly if there are several and in various stages of healing. Greenstick fractures and costochondral separations are not seen on chest x-ray film but may be suspected if there are obvious deformities or areas of exquisite point tenderness or crepitus directly over a rib or costochondral junction; fractures with bony discontinuity on chest x-ray film may yield similar clinical findings.

No specific treatment is indicated for rib fractures beyond that provided for associated injuries. In contrast to the adult, the child rarely experiences enough discomfort to cause splinting or atelectasis. Splints or narcotic analgesics are not recommended. However, intercostal nerve blocks have been used in selected cases for long-term pain control.

Traumatic Asphyxia. Traumatic asphyxia is a rare but striking phenomenon that may be associated with severe blunt injury to the chest. It is due to the transmission of the sudden increase in intrathoracic pressure associated with massive compressive force applied to the chest and the venules of the head, neck, and upper body via the valveless great veins of the thoracic inlet. The resultant acute increase in extrathoracic venous pressure causes the fragile capillaries feeding these venules to rupture, producing petechial hemorrhage in the areas adjacent to the damage. Indeed, the diagnosis is made when petechiae are identified in the conjunctiva, sclerae, scalp, and integument of the upper body.

The same type of petechial hemorrhage visible on external body surfaces also occurs internally, particularly within the brain. As a result, traumatic asphyxia may be associated with transient neurologic findings. The effects of the suffusion injury usually resolve over the course of several days as hemorrhages are resorbed and capillaries are repaired. Thus although the condition itself requires no specific treatment other than supportive care, its presence serves to indicate the extreme severity of blunt forces applied to the chest and mandates an especially diligent search for intrathoracic injury.

Penetrating Injuries

As previously noted, penetrating injuries in children are being encountered in greater numbers than ever before. Since management by experienced surgeons is required, the children should be managed in a trauma center with pediatric capabilities. All penetrating chest wounds are contaminated and must be treated as infected (i.e., by means of intravenous antibiotics); aggressive debridement of penetrating chest wounds, however, is contraindicated because it may result in open pneumothorax. Finally, early involvement of responsible law enforcement agencies is mandatory in all but clearly accidental cases of penetrating trauma in childhood; the initial history is rarely accurate when injuries are intentional.

The problem usually associated with penetrating injuries to the chest is pneumohemothorax. Expeditious treatment by means of tube thoracostomy is required; few such injuries ultimately require thoracotomy for control of bleeding. Should this prove necessary, however, the usual cause is injury to the intercostal vessels, since most parenchymal injuries are self-sealing. Violation of other thoracic viscera, vessels, and airways is uncommon after gunshot and stab wounds in children; when present, however, such violations require immediate surgical repair and must be excluded by means of appropriate radiographic or endoscopic studies if the location and direction of penetration or mis-

sile tract suggest that such injuries could have occurred. Use of the pneumatic antishock garment (PASG) (i.e., military or [or medical] antishock trousers [MAST]), as well as excessive fluid resuscitation, is strictly contraindicated in penetrating thoracic injury, since the rate of bleeding may be seriously accelerated by the associated increase in afterload.[98,99]

Thoracoabdominal injury should be suspected whenever the chest is penetrated at or below the level of the sixth rib or food, chyme, or saliva is recovered from the chest tube. The diagnosis must also be considered if the upper abdomen is penetrated, especially by a missile. In the absence of other indications, laparotomy must be performed if abdominal findings, including tenderness or peritonitis, develop after thoracic penetration or in association with hemopneumothorax, even in the absence of a coexisting abdominal wound. It should be strongly considered if injury trajectory or noninvasive studies (CT, ultrasonography, or fluoroscopy) indicate the possibility of penetrating diaphragmatic injury.

Thoracoabdominal injuries require a special approach to their management. In addition to the tube thoracostomy that is mandatory for all such injuries, laparotomy must be performed for diaphragmatic closure as well as evaluation and possible repair of intraabdominal organs, although less invasive techniques such as laparoscopy or thoracoscopy are increasingly used to exclude diaphragmatic injury in questionable cases.[100] Thoracotomy is required as indicated but precedes laparotomy only for the life-threatening chest injuries of massive hemorrhage, cardiac tamponade, and tracheobronchial disruption. Otherwise, laparotomy for closure of lacerated viscera precedes the "cleansing" thoracotomy that becomes necessary when intestinal contents are found in the chest.

References

1. Cooper A, Barlow B, DiScala C, et al: Mortality and truncal injury: the pediatric perspective, *J Pediatr Surg* 29:33, 1994.

Epidemiology

2. Bickford BJ: Chest injuries in childhood and adolescence, *Thorax* 17:240, 1962.
3. Kilman JW and Charnock E: Thoracic trauma in infancy and childhood, *J Trauma* 9:863, 1969.
4. Sinclair MC and Moore TC: Major surgery for abdominal and thoracic trauma in childhood and adolescence, *J Pediatr Surg* 9:155, 1974.
5. Smyth BT: Chest trauma in children, *J Pediatr Surg* 14:41, 1979.
6. Meller JL, Little AG, Shermeta DW: Thoracic trauma in children, *Pediatrics* 74:813, 1984.
7. Rege VM and Deshmukh SS: Major thoracic trauma in children, *J Postgrad Med* 34:93, 1988.
8. Nakayama DK, Ramenofsky ML, Rowe MI: Chest injuries in children, *Ann Surg* 210:770, 1989.
9. Peclet MH, Newman KD, Eichelberger MR, et al: Thoracic trauma in children: an indicator of increased mortality, *J Pediatr Surg* 25:961, 1990.
10. Roux P and Fisher RM: Chest injuries in children: an analysis of 100 cases of blunt chest trauma from motor vehicle accidents, *J Pediatr Surg* 27:551, 1992.
11. Rielly JP, Brandt ML, Mattox KL, et al: Thoracic trauma in children, *J Trauma* 34:329, 1993.
12. Bellinger SB: Penetrating chest injuries in children, *Ann Thorac Surg* 14:635, 1972.
13. Peterson RJ, Tiwary AD, Kisoon N, et al: Pediatric penetrating thoracic trauma: a five-year experience, *Pediatr Emerg Care* 10:129, 1994.

Mechanism of Injury

14. Agran PF, Dunkle DE, Winn DG: Injuries to a sample of seatbelted children evaluated and treated in a hospital emergency department, *J Trauma* 27:58, 1987.
15. Hoffman MA, Spence LJ, Wesson DE, et al: The pediatric passenger: trends in seatbelt use and injury patterns, *J Trauma* 27:974, 1987.
16. Stylianos S, Termeulen DC, Latchaw LA, et al: Seatbelt injuries in children, *Ann Emerg Med* 20:169, 1988.
17. Newman KD, Bowman LM, Eichelberger MR: The lap belt complex: intestinal and lumbar spine injury in children, *J Trauma* 30:1133, 1990.

Patterns of Injury

18. Sorsdahl OA and Powell JW: Cavitary pulmonary lesions following nonpenetrating chest trauma in children, *Am J Roentgenol* 95:118, 1965.
19. Blane CE, White SJ, Wesley JR, et al: Immediate traumatic pulmonary pseudocyst formation in children, *Surgery* 90:872, 1981.
20. Galea MH, Williams N, Mayell MJ, et al: Traumatic pneumatocele, *J Pediatr Surg* 27:1523, 1992.
21. Schwartz A and Borman JB: Contusion of the lung in childhood, *Arch Dis Child* 36:557, 1969.
22. Levy JL: Management of crushing chest injuries in children, *South Med J* 65:1040, 1972.
23. Bonadio WA and Hellmich T: Post-traumatic pulmonary contusion in children, *Ann Emerg Med* 18:1050, 1989.
24. McEniery J, Hanson R, Grigor W, et al: Lung injury resulting from a nonaccidental crush injury to the chest, *Pediatr Emerg Care*, 7:166, 1991.
25. Haller JA and Donahoo JS: Traumatic asphyxia in children: pathophysiology and management, *J Trauma* 11:453, 1971.
26. Gorenstein L, Blair GK, Shandling B: The prognosis of traumatic asphyxia in childhood, *J Pediatr Surg* 21:753, 1986.
27. Shaw J: Pulmonary contusion in children due to rubber bullet injuries, *Br Med J* 4:764, 1972.
28. Golladay ES, Donahoo JS, Haller JA: Special problems of cardiac injuries in infants and children, *J Trauma* 19:526, 1979.
29. Tellez DW, Hardin WD, Takahashi M, et al: Blunt cardiac injury in children, *J Pediatr Surg* 22:1123, 1987.
30. Langer JC, Winthrop AL, Wesson DE, et al: Diagnosis and incidence of cardiac injury in children with blunt thoracic trauma, *J Pediatr Surg* 24:1091, 1989.
31. Ildstad ST, Tollerud DJ, Weiss RG, et al: Cardiac contusion in pediatric patients with blunt thoracic trauma, *J Pediatr Surg* 25:287, 1990.
32. Dickman GL, Hassan A, Luckstead EF: Ventricular fibrillation following baseball injury, *Phys Sportsmed* 6:85, 1978.
33. Mozzetti MD, Devin JB, Susselman MS, et al: A pediatric survivor of left ventricular rupture after blunt chest trauma, *Ann Emerg Med* 19:386, 1990.
34. Rheuban KS, Tompkins DG, Nolan SP, et al: Myocardial necrosis and ventricular aneurysm following closed chest injury in a child, *J Trauma* 21:170, 1981.
35. Rowland TW: Traumatic aortic insufficiency in children: case report and review of the literature, *Pediatrics* 60:893, 1977.
36. McCrory D, Craig B, O'Kane H: Traumatic mitral valve rupture in a child, *Ann Thorac Surg* 51:821, 1991.
37. Coleman DM, Cox PH, Dyck J et al: Pediatric transesophageal echocardiography in the evaluation of acute disruption of the mitral valve following blunt thoracic trauma: case report, *J Trauma* 36:135, 1994.
38. Senagore A, Senagore PK, Cohle SD, et al: Pericardial laceration and fatal cardiac herniation in an improperly restrained six-month-old infant, *J Pediatr Surg* 21:931, 1986.
39. Cizmarova E, Simkovic I, Masura J: Traumatic coronary occlusion and its consequences in a young child, *Pediatr Cardiol* 9:117, 1988.
40. Marino TA and Langston C: Cardiac trauma and the conduction system: a case study of an 18-month-old-child, *Arch Pathol Lab Med* 106:173, 1982.
41. Bowers P, Harris P, Truesdell S, et al: Delayed hemopericardium and cardiac tamponade after unrecognized chest trauma, *Pediatr Emerg Care* 10:222, 1994.
42. Meyer JA, Neville JF, Hansen WG: Traumatic rupture of the aorta in a child, *JAMA* 208:527, 1969.
43. Meagher DP, Defore WW, Mattox KL, et al: Vascular trauma in infants and children, *J Trauma* 19:532, 1979.
44. Eddy AC, Misbach GA, Luna GK: Traumatic rupture of the thoracic aorta in the pediatric patient, *Pediatr Emerg Care* 5:228, 1989.
45. Schmidt CA and Smith DC: Traumatic avulsion of arch vessels in a child: primary repair using hypothermic circulatory arrest (case report), *J Trauma* 29:248, 1989.
46. Bergman K, Spence L, Wesson DE, et al: Thoracic vascular injuries: a post mortem study, *J Trauma* 30:604, 1990.
47. Eddy AC, Rusch VW, Fligner CL, et al: The epidemiology of traumatic rupture of the thoracic aorta in children: a 13-year review, *J Trauma* 30:989, 1990.
48. Myers NA: Traumatic rupture of the diaphragm in children, *Aust N Z J Surg* 34:123, 1964.
49. Radhakrishna C, Dickinson SJ, Shaw A: Acute diaphragmatic hernia from blunt trauma in children, *J Pediatr Surg* 4:553, 1969.
50. Holgersen LO and Schnaufer L: Hernia and eventration of the diaphragm secondary to blunt trauma, *J Pediatr Surg* 8:433, 1973.
51. Melzig EP, Swank M, Salzberg AM: Acute blunt traumatic rupture of the diaphragm in children, *Arch Surg* 111:1009, 1976.
52. West K, Weber TR, Grosfeld JL: Traumatic diaphragmatic hernia in childhood, *J Pediatr Surg* 16:392, 1981.
53. Brandt ML, Luks FI, Spigland NA, et al: Diaphragmatic injury in children, *J Trauma* 32:298, 1992.
54. Sola JE, Mattei P, Pegoli W, et al: Rupture of the right diaphragm following blunt trauma in an infant: case report, *J Trauma* 36:417, 1994.
55. Myers WO, Leape LL, Holder TM: Bronchial rupture in a child with subsequent stenosis, resection, and anastamosis, *Ann Thorac Surg* 12:442, 1971.
56. Rose E, Schmitt M, Lotte E, et al: Fissures due to tracheobronchial trauma in children based on three observations, *Chir Pediatr* 26:294, 1985.
57. Hancock BJ and Wiseman NE: Tracheobronchial injuries in children, *J Pediatr Surg* 26:1316, 1991.
58. Padler SB, Shandling B, Manson D: Rupture of the thoracic trachea following blunt trauma: diagnosis by CAT scan, *J Pediatr Surg* 26:1320, 1991.
59. Wiener Y, Simansky D, Yellin A: Main bronchial rupture from blunt trauma in a 2-year-old child, *J Pediatr Surg* 28:1530, 1993.
60. Perchinsky M, Long W, Rosoff J, et al: Traumatic rupture of the tracheobronchial tree in a 2 year old, *J Pediatr Surg* 29:1548, 1994.
61. Ford HR, Garnder MJ, Lynch JM: Laryngotracheal disruption from blunt neck injuries: impact of early recognition and intervention on outcome, *J Pediatr Surg* 30:331, 1995.
62. Salter DG and Hopton DS: Traumatic intercostal hernia without penetrating injury in a child, *Br J Surg* 56:550, 1969.
63. Sandrasagra FA, DiEusanio G, Hamilton DI: Traumatic intercostal hernia due to a nonpenetrating injury in a child, *J Pediatr Surg* 14:471, 1979.
64. Forty J and Wells FC: Traumatic intercostal pulmonary hernia, *Ann Thorac Surg* 49:670, 1990.
65. Reino AJ, Jahn AF, Parson J, et al: Traumatic pneumomediastinum in a child secondary to corn chip perforation of the esophagus, *Pediatr Emerg Care* 9:211, 1993.
66. Thomas PS: Rib fractures in infancy, *Ann Radiol* 20:115, 1977.
67. Schweich P and Fleisher G: Rib fractures in children, *Pediatr Emerg Care* 1:187, 1985.
68. Harris GJ and Soper RT: Pediatric first rib fractures, *J Trauma* 30:343, 1990.
69. Garcia VF, Gotschall CS, Eichelberger MR, et al: Rib fractures in children: a marker of severe trauma, *J Trauma* 30:695, 1990.
70. Scudamore CH and Ashmore PG: Spontaneous sternal segment dislocation: a case report, *J Pediatr Surg* 17:61, 1982.

Diagnostic Findings

71. Cooper A, Floyd T, Barlow B, et al: Major blunt abdominal trauma due to child abuse, *J Trauma* 28:1483, 1988.
72. Fleisher AG, David I, Hilfer C, et al: Mediastinal hematoma mimicking aortic rupture, *J Trauma* 21:445, 1986.
73. Ben-Ami T, Rozenman J, Yahav J, et al: Computed tomography in children with esophageal and airway trauma, *J Pediatr Surg* 23:919, 1988.
74. Sivit CJ, Taylor GA, Eichelberger MR: Chest injury in children with

blunt abdominal trauma: evaluation with CT, *Radiology* 171:815, 1989.

Management

75. American Heart Association and American Academy of Pediatrics Working Group on Pediatric Resuscitation: *Textbook of pediatric advanced life support*, Dallas, 1988, American Heart Association.

76. American College of Surgeons Committee on Trauma: *Advanced trauma life support student manual*, Chicago, 1990, American College of Surgeons.

77. American Academy of Pediatrics and American College of Emergency Physicians Joint Task Force on Advanced Pediatric Life Support: *Advanced pediatric life support*, Elk Grove Village and Dallas, 1989, American Academy of Pediatrics and American College of Emergency Physicians.

78. Langer JC, Hoffman MA, Pearl RH, et al: Survival after emergency department thoracotomy in a child with blunt multisystem trauma, *Pediatr Emerg Care* 5:255, 1989.

79. Beaver BL, Colombani PM, Buck JR, et al: Efficacy of emergency room thoracotomy in pediatric trauma, *J Pediatr Surg* 22:19, 1987.

80. Powell RW, Gill EA, Jurkovich GJ, et al: Resuscitative thoracotomy in children and adolescents, *Am Surg* 54:188, 1988.

81. Rothenberg SS, Moore EE, Moore FA, et al: Emergency department thoracotomy in children—a critical analysis, *J Trauma* 29:1322, 1989.

82. Skeikh AA and Culbertson CB: Emergency department thoracotomy in children: rationale for selective application, *J Trauma* 34:323, 1993.

83. Sheikh A and Borgan T: Outcome and cost of open- and closed-chest cardiopulmonary resuscitation in pediatric cardiac arrests, *Pediatrics* 93:392, 1994.

84. Hazinski MF, Chahine AA, Holcomb GW, et al: Outcome of cardiovascular collapse in pediatric blunt trauma, *Ann Emerg Med* 23:1229, 1994.

85. Sankaran S, Lucas C, Walt AJ: Thoracic aortic cross clamping for prophylaxis against sudden cardiac arrest during laparotomy for acute massive hemoperitoneum, *J Trauma* 15:290, 1975.

86. Brotman S, Osta-Granite M, Cox EF, et al: Failure of cross clamping the thoracic aorta to control intra-abdominal bleeding, *Ann Emerg Med* 11:147, 1982.

87. Tepas JJ, Mollitt DL, Talbert JL, et al: The pediatric trauma score as a predictor of injury severity in the injured child, *J Pediatr Surg* 22:14, 1987.

88. Champion HR, Sacco WJ, Carnazzo AJ, et al: Trauma score, *Crit Care Med* 9:672, 1981.

89. Champion HR, Sacco WJ, Copes WS, et al: A revision of the trauma score, *J Trauma* 29:623, 1989.

90. Harris BH, Barlow BA, Ballantine TV, et al: American Pediatric Surgical Association: principles of trauma care, *J Pediatr Surg* 27, 1992.

Specific Injuries

91. Boidon MP: Airway patency in the unconscious patient, *Br J Anaesth* 57:306, 1958.

92. Safar P, Escarraga L, Chang F: Upper airway obstruction in the unconscious patient, *J Appl Physiol* 14:760, 1959.

93. Hubbard DD: Injuries of the spine in children and adolescents, *Clin Orthop* 100:56, 1974.

94. Kewalramani LS, Kraus JF, Sterling HM: Acute spinal-cord lesions in a pediatric population: epidemiological and clinical features, *Paraplegia* 18:206, 1980.

95. Herzenberg JE, Hensinger RN, Dedrick DK, et al: Emergency transport and positioning of young children who have an injury of the cervical spine, *J Bone Joint Surg Am* 71-A:15, 1989.

96. Pang D and Pollack IF: Spinal cord injury without radiographic abnormality in children—the SCIWORA syndrome, *J Trauma* 29:654, 1989.

97. Bohn D, Armstrong D, Becker L, et al: Cervical spine injuries in children, *J Trauma* 30:463, 1990.

98. Mattox KL, Bickell W, Pepe PE, et al: Prospective MAST study in 911 patients, *J Trauma* 29:1104, 1989.

99. Bickell WH, Wall MJ, Pepe PE, et al: Immediate versus delayed fluid resuscitation for hypotensive patients with penetrating torso injuries, *N Engl J Med* 331:1105, 1994.

100. Cooper A: Pediatric trauma (thoracic trauma), *Textbook of penetrating trauma*, Malvern, 1995, Lea & Febiger.

Appendix 23A: Tube Thoracostomy

NORMAN C. CHRISTOPHER

INDICATIONS

The presence of pneumothorax, hemothorax, or hemopneumothorax is indication for the performance of a tube thoracostomy. Recurrent or persistent pleural effusions, chylothorax, or empyema may also require chest tube placement. The degree of clinical symptoms present dictates the urgency with which the emergency physician must respond.

EQUIPMENT

Most centers have prepared "trays" containing instruments required to perform a tube thoracostomy. At the least, the procedure will require local anesthetic and appropriate syringes and needles, sterile dressings and towels, cloth tape, 1-2 large curved (Mayo) and straight (suture) scissors, a scalpel handle with blades (number 10), 2-4 large and medium Kelly clamps, and a needle holder and several packages of 0-0 or 1-0 silk sutures. Appropriate chest tube sizes depend on the intended purpose of the procedure (evacuation of air, serosanguineous fluid, or blood) and the size of the patient (Table 23A-1).

TECHNIQUE

The axillary (lateral) approach will be described. Oxygen should be provided as necessary. The patient should be placed in a supine position with the head of the bed elevated to approximately 30 to 45 degrees and the ipsilateral arm placed over the head and gently secured in that position by a soft restraint or cloth tape (Fig. 23A-1). The insertion site and widely surrounding area of the chest wall should be cleansed with povidone-iodine soap; sterile towels should be draped over the adjacent operative field. The operator and assistant(s) should wear proper barrier garments.

In the awake patient, generous local anesthesia (1% lidocaine with epinephrine) should be infiltrated into the skin, the subcutaneous tissues, the muscle, and the periosteum until maximal local anesthesia is achieved. A linear incision should be made through the skin and subcutaneous tissue *directly over the rib one space below* the target intercostal space (the fourth or fifth intercostal space just

TABLE 23A-1. Appropriate Chest Tube Sizes

Age	Weight (kg)	Chest tube (Fr)
Premature	1	6
Newborn	2-3	6-8
1 mo	4	8
1 yr	10	8-10
2-3 yr	12-14	10
10-12 yr	32-42	12

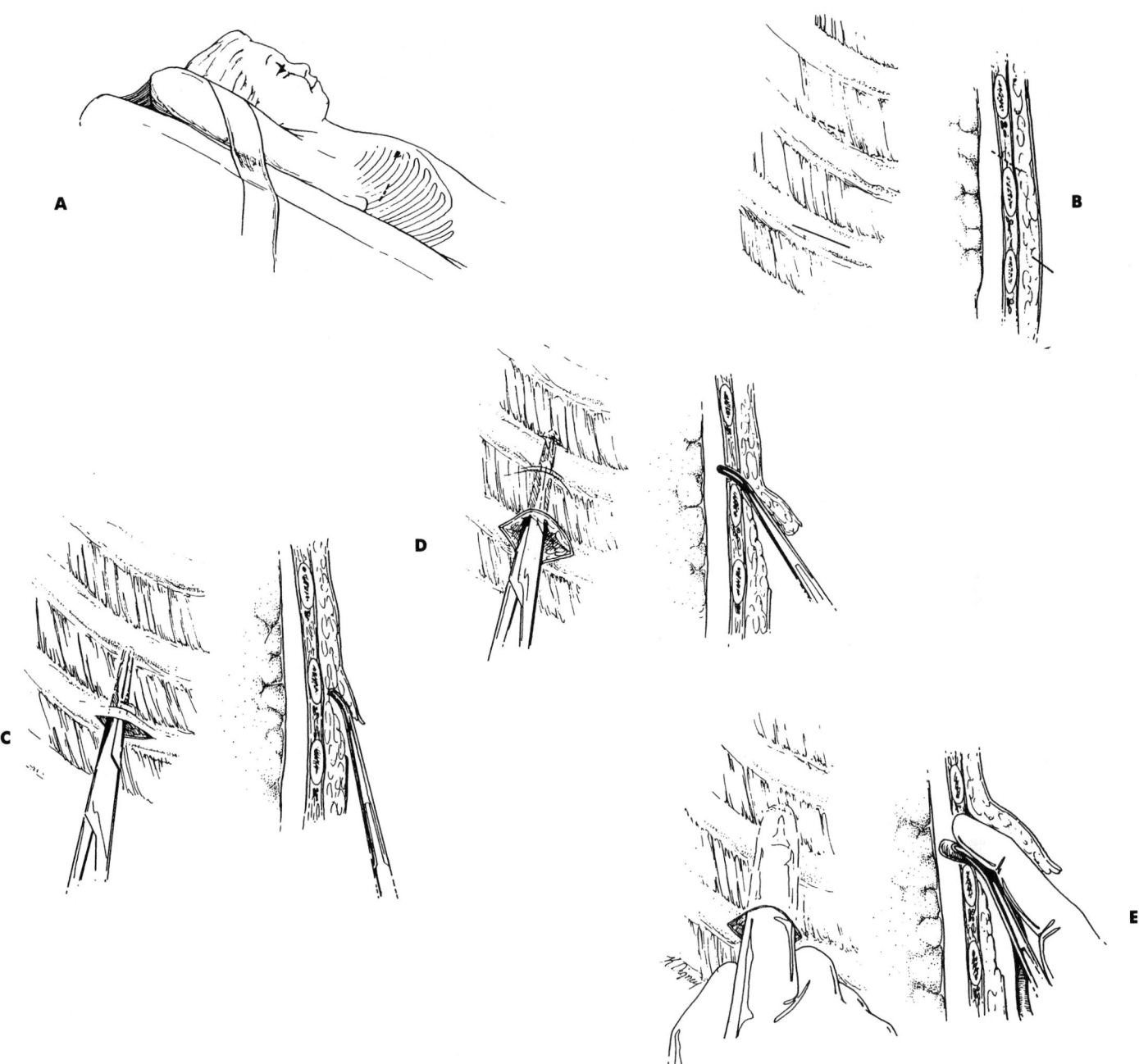

FIG. 23A-1. Tube thoracostomy. **A,** The patient is comfortably positioned and the entrance site identified and sterilely prepared; **B,** The skin incision site is identified over the rib one space below the target intercostal space; **C,** Using a blunt instrument, dissect through the subcutaneous tissues, tunneling over the rib below the target intercostal space; **D,** Penetrate the pleural space with a curved clamp or hemostat; **E,** Using a sterile digit, track through the soft tissues through the underlying pleural space, identify the underlying lung tissue, and guide the thoracostomy tube into the pleural space. A curved hemostat placed into the distal sideport of the thoracostomy tube may serve as a blunt stylet to facilitate the advancement of the chest tube. (*Courtesy Kathleen M. Digney and the MetroHealth Medical Center, Cleveland, Ohio.*)

anterior to the midaxillary line is the preferred site for tube insertion). Bluntly dissect through the underlying subcutaneous tissues to the fascial layer covering the intercostal muscles. A curved clamp or a hemostat is then used to penetrate through the intercostal muscle and into the pleural space. The instrument is directed *over* the upper margin of the rib to avoid the intercostal nerves and vascular bundles lying inferiorly to the rib (see Fig. 23A-1). As the instrument enters the pleural space, a rush of escaping air or fluid is usually heard, indicating a normalizing of intrapleural with atmospheric pressure. A finger should be carefully advanced along the track extending through to the pleural space where the pleura should be easily palpated. The chest tube should be directed toward the apex of the lung and secured tightly with a purse-string suture. The distal end of the thoracostomy tube should be attached to an appropriate suction device, and the insertion site should be dressed in a sterile fashion. Chest radiography should confirm proper placement of the thoracostomy tube.

COMPLICATIONS

A variety of problems may result from insertion, prolonged placement, or physiologic response to the resulting decompression (see box at left).

Abdominal Trauma

George L. Foltin • Arthur Cooper

Serious abdominal injuries are relatively common in childhood; some 8% of children admitted to the pediatric trauma centers of this nation have documented abdominal injuries (Table 24-1).[1] Yet fewer than 15% of children with major abdominal trauma require operative intervention; most are victims of penetrating wounds. Thus early management of serious abdominal injuries in childhood has the most direct impact on survival; *inadequate* resuscitation still remains the leading cause of preventable death.[2,3] Excepting immediately life-threatening pulmonary conditions, there is no other class of injury in which the chances for a successful outcome depend so clearly on the expertise of the first responding emergency physician and team.

EPIDEMIOLOGY

Abdominal trauma follows both head injury and thoracic injury as a cause of traumatic death in childhood, accounting for 6% of the mortality (Table 24-2).[1] However, if a child with severe abdominal injury has suffered concomitant head injury, it becomes more difficult to decide which was causative and which contributory; abdominal injury occurs in approximately 22% of all children with fatal injuries.[1,4] Children suffer serious abdominal injury in a variety of situations; the automobile is clearly the most lethal

agent (Table 24-3).[1] Most of these events result from blunt trauma, the predominant mechanism of injury in children (85% vs. 50% in adults). However, penetrating trauma is becoming more frequent, especially in the urban setting. Males suffer abdominal trauma twice as often as females.

Data accumulated by the National Pediatric Trauma Registry since 1984 have vastly improved understanding of the scope and consequences of major abdominal trauma in childhood in terms of its incidence, mortality, causes, and nature of the injuries (Table 24-4).[1] These data both confirm and amplify the trends demonstrated by numerous studies of pediatric abdominal trauma epidemiology that have been performed in recent years.[5-10] Moreover, review of these statistics indicates that the types of injuries to which children are susceptible are different from those sustained by adults. The special anatomic and physiologic characteristics of the infant and small child and the mechanism of injury dictate the unique patterns of injuries sustained.

ANATOMY

Anatomic features of children predispose to the specific patterns and types of injuries. Children have proportionately larger solid viscera and more protuberant abdomens in relation to the rest of the torso than adults. Flexible, thin, poorly muscled ribs cover less of the abdomen than in adults. Children lack much of the abdominal musculature and body fat typically found in the adult. The relatively large organs, especially the liver, combined with the overall small size of the child, predispose children to multiple rather than single injuries. The overall likelihood of organ disruption with subsequent significant hemorrhage caused by transmission of kinetic energy to the child's smaller body mass when struck by a blunt force is also greater. In addition, flexible ribs readily permit transmission of impact energy to internal organs; significant internal injury may not be accompanied by external marks. In fact, the discovery of fractured ribs in the injured child is an indication of a very significant force and should heighten the clinician's suspicion that serious injury has occurred.

In small children, the bladder is an intraabdominal structure; hence, the bladder is more vulnerable than when protected by a mature pelvis. The dome of a distended bladder in the child is more likely to rupture after a blow to the abdomen than in the adult, although this condition is rare. Thus, the child with a full bladder who sustains blunt abdominal trauma occasionally presents with a large, firm, tender suprapubic mass that disappears when the urinary tract is decompressed by means of a Foley catheter. Fi-

TABLE 24-1. Incidence of Abdominal Injuries in Selected North American Pediatric Trauma Centers*

	Number (%)
Blunt	1,754 (86)
Penetrating	264 (13)
Other	29 (1)
TOTAL	2,047†

From National Pediatric Trauma Registry, 1985-1991.
*Total number of patients in registry: 25,301.
†Percent of total number of patients in registry with abdominal injuries: 8%.

TABLE 24-2. Mortality Caused by Abdominal Injuries in Selected North American Pediatric Trauma Centers

Abdominal injuries	Number (%)
Total blunt	1,754
Deaths	161 (9)
From intraabdominal injuries	35 (22)
From associated injuries	126 (78)
Total penetrating	264
Deaths	15 (6)
From intraabdominal injuries	10 (67)
From associated injuries	5 (33)

From National Pediatric Trauma Registry, 1985-1991.

TABLE 24-3. Mechanisms of Abdominal Injuries in Selected North American Pediatric Trauma Centers

Abdominal injuries	Number (%)
Blunt	
Motor vehicle: occupant	559 (32)
Motor vehicle: pedestrian	472 (27)
Fall	232 (13)
Bicycle	211 (12)
Other	280 (16)
TOTAL	1,754
Penetrating	
Gunshot wound	149 (56)
Stab wound	63 (24)
Other	52 (20)
TOTAL	264

From National Pediatric Trauma Registry, 1985-1991.

nally, as in the adult, fractures of the pelvic ring may be associated with significant retroperitoneal hemorrhage, as well as extraperitoneal rupture of the bladder. However, because of the softer nature of the child's axial skeletal components, these conditions may sometimes occur in the absence of identifiable bony abnormality. This is especially true for retroperitoneal bleeding, which in hemophiliac patients can follow a seemingly trivial episode of blunt trauma to the belly or flank.

PATHOPHYSIOLOGY

The most common physiologic derangement encountered in the child with serious intraabdominal injury is hemorrhagic shock. As discussed in depth in Chapter 13, children have compensatory mechanisms to hemorrhage that allow reflex sympathetic peripheral vasoconstriction and a rapid heart rate. Although hypotension may not occur until up to 30% of circulating volume is lost, it can develop after loss of a relatively small amount of blood, because of the smaller absolute volume of blood.[11] Indeed, children with hemorrhage secondary to trauma may demonstrate diffuse signs common to shock and acidosis rather than findings specific to the abdomen.

Significant gastric dilatation is also a common problem in children with abdominal trauma, and is chiefly the result of crying and air swallowing.[12,13] The severely distended stomach can produce numerous problems. First, respiratory effort may be compromised by interference with motion of the hemidiaphragms. Since children have small diaphragms and are primarily diaphragmatic breathers, this can be significant. Second, risk of pulmonary aspiration of gastric contents is increased, particularly if the stomach is full at the time of impact. Third, circulatory compromise may be caused by distension-induced vagally mediated dampening of the normal tachycardic response that should occur with hypovolemia. This is especially dangerous because the decreased compliance of the myocardium in small children limits its capacity to respond to a decrease in cardiac output by any means other than an increase in heart rate. Fourth, gastric distension confounds examination of the abdomen, even by an experienced physician. The associated abdominal tenderness may also simulate peritonitis; relieved or unrelieved abdominal distension may mimic or mask serious intraabdominal bleeding.

MECHANISM OF INJURY

Blunt Trauma

Injury from blunt trauma is caused by one of three mechanisms (Fig. 24-1).[14] The first is sudden compression of solid abdominal organs against the unyielding spine, resulting in contusion, laceration, or bursting of the organ with subsequent hemorrhage. The second is sudden compression of hollow viscus against the vertebral column, resulting in rupture associated with the sudden increase in luminal pressure. Shearing forces that result in tearing of the posterior attachments or blood supplies of the abdominal viscera, chiefly in victims of rapid deceleration events (e.g., high-speed motor vehicle crashes or falls from extreme heights) constitute the third mechanism.

Penetrating Trauma

Penetrating trauma is due nearly exclusively to gunshot and stab wounds; occasionally injury may result from impalement. Examination of statistics from urban centers reveals a higher percentage of penetrating trauma than the national average.[15-18] Young adolescents primarily comprise this segment, whether as innocent bystanders or as victims of intentional violence or suicide attempts; younger children too are victims. In patients less than 13 years of age, penetrating injuries are likely to be caused by acciden-

TABLE 24-4. Frequency of Injury to Intraabdominal Organs in Selected North American Pediatric Trauma Centers

	Blunt (%)		Penetrating (%)		Total (%)	
Liver	484	(28)	71	(27)	555	(27)
Hematoma/contusion	171	(10)	5	(2)	176	(9)
Laceration, minor	175	(10)	29	(11)	204	(10)
Laceration, moderate	41	(2)	19	(7)	60	(3)
Laceration, major	40	(2)	7	(3)	47	(2)
Other/unspecified	53	(3)	21	(8)	74	(6)
Spleen	522	(30)	25	(9)	547	(27)
Hematoma	134	(8)	1	(<1)	135	(7)
Capsular tear	150	(9)	9	(3)	159	(8)
Deep laceration	63	(4)	8	(3)	71	(3)
Shattered	93	(5)	4	(2)	97	(5)
Other/unspecified	82	(5)	3	(1)	85	(4)
Kidneys	483	(28)	27	(10)	510	(25)
Hematoma/contusion	299	(17)	5	(2)	304	(15)
Laceration	70	(4)	14	(5)	84	(4)
Disruption	21	(1)	3	(1)	24	(1)
Other/unspecified	93	(5)	8	(3)	101	(5)
Gastrointestinal tract	252	(14)	186	(70)	438	(21)
Stomach	16	(<1)	34	(13)	50	(2)
Duodenum	55	(3)	10	(4)	65	(3)
Jejunum/ileum	99	(6)	64	(24)	163	(8)
Colon/rectum	53	(3)	72	(27)	125	(6)
Intestine NOS	29	(2)	6	(2)	35	(2)
Genitourinary tract	76	(4)	21	(8)	97	(5)
Bladder/urethra	67	(4)	9	(3)	76	(4)
Ureters/other	9	(<1)	12	(5)	21	(1)
Pancreas	59	(3)	17	(6)	76	(4)
Blood vessels	48	(3)	49	(19)	97	(5)
Aorta	1	(<1)	8	(3)	9	(<1)
Celiac/mesenteric arteries	11	(<1)	5	(2)	16	(<1)
Inferior vena cava	13	(<1)	11	(4)	24	(1)
Portal/splenic veins	3	(<1)	4	(2)	7	(<1)
Renal arteries	9	(<1)	1	(<1)	10	(<1)
Renal veins	2	(<1)	1	(<1)	3	(<1)
Iliac	6	(<1)	13	(5)	19	(<1)
Other	3	(<1)	6	(2)	9	(<1)
Pelvis	14	(<1)	0	(0)	14	(<1)
Open wounds	44	(3)	112	(42)	156	(8)
Intraabdominal injuries NOS	4	(<1)	3	(1)	7	(<1)
TOTAL PATIENTS	1,754		264		2,018	

From National Pediatric Trauma Registry, 1985-1991.
NOS, Not otherwise specified.
NOTE: Many children had more than one injury recorded.

tal impalement on objects such as scissors or picket fences. In patients more than 13 years of age, 75% of penetrating injuries are knife or handgun wounds inflicted by an assailant. Penetrating trauma carries the highest mortality rate; firearms are the most lethal agents of injury.[1] Children who suffer gunshot injuries are often victims of firearms that are kept in the home by their parents and that the children or their siblings find and use.

PATTERNS OF INJURY

The pattern of injuries reflects the child's unique anatomy and physiology, as well as mechanism of injury. Common patterns of intraabdominal injury are described below.

Motor Vehicle Injury: Pedestrian

Young children who dart out into traffic are commonly hit by a motor vehicle and often struck in the abdomen. Such motor vehicle accidents may cause a specific injury pattern, consisting of closed head injury, intraabdominal injury, and midshaft femur fracture known as Waddell triad.[19] In North America where people drive on the right side of the road, children who dart out onto the road from between parked cars are hit on the left side. Not surprisingly, splenic injury commonly results.

Head and extremity injuries are often obvious and may divert attention from the more subtle findings of intraabdominal injury, which if present is usually the site of sig-

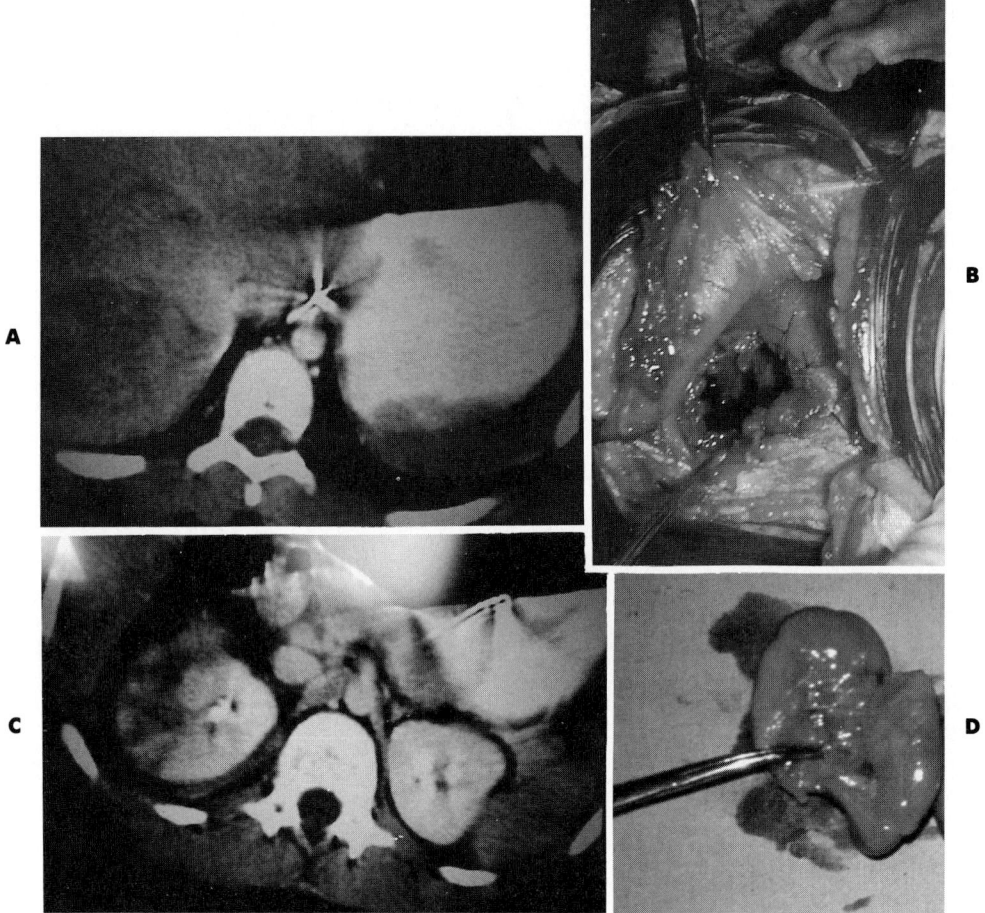

FIG. 24-1. Typical radiographic and clinical appearance of commonly encountered diagnostic entities. **A** and **B,** Subcapsular hematoma of liver following blunt trauma due to motor vehicle–pedestrian injury: tomographic and intraoperative findings. Treatment is mostly nonoperative. **C** and **D,** Stellate fracture of kidney following blunt trauma due to motor vehicle–pedestrian injury: tomographic and intraoperative findings. Treatment is mostly nonoperative.

Continued.

nificant hemorrhage. The common belief that a unilateral femur fracture can result in hypovolemic shock is questionable. The average drop in hematocrit with isolated femur fractures is three to six percentage points, not sufficient to cause hypovolemic shock.[20] Thus, signs of shock associated with a unilateral femur fracture should prompt a search for another source of bleeding, usually found within the abdomen.

Motor Vehicle Injury: Occupant

Unrestrained pediatric passengers in motor vehicle crashes typically are victims of multisystem trauma; head injury is the most common and by far the most lethal injury.[21] However the most frequent site of significant blood loss in these patients is the abdomen, although external bleeding and pelvic fractures can also result in devastating blood loss. Injuries may be associated with accidents involving both crashes and noncrashes (e.g., sudden swerves), particularly if the car door opens inadvertently; crash events outnumber the latter by about five to one.[22] A

higher fraction of serious injuries occurs inside the passenger compartment in crashes.

Among restrained children, there is recent recognition of a "lap belt" complex of injuries, consisting of bursting injuries of solid or hollow viscus, flexion-distraction (Chance type), fractures of the lumbar spine, and, rarely, disruption of the diaphragm.[23-32] All cases reported were characterized by hemorrhagic markings across the abdomen or flanks. This entity was reported to occur in up to 10% of children who were restrained but is thought to occur only when children are made to wear lap belts without an appropriately sized booster seat or improperly fitted three-point restraints that allow the lap belt to ride up and compress the abdomen as the victim submarines into the seat at the time of impact. This injury has not been described in small children properly restrained in appropriate car seats, although cervical spine injuries have recently been reported. Overall, however, restrained children suffer such a lower incidence of head injury than unrestrained children that a child is far bet-

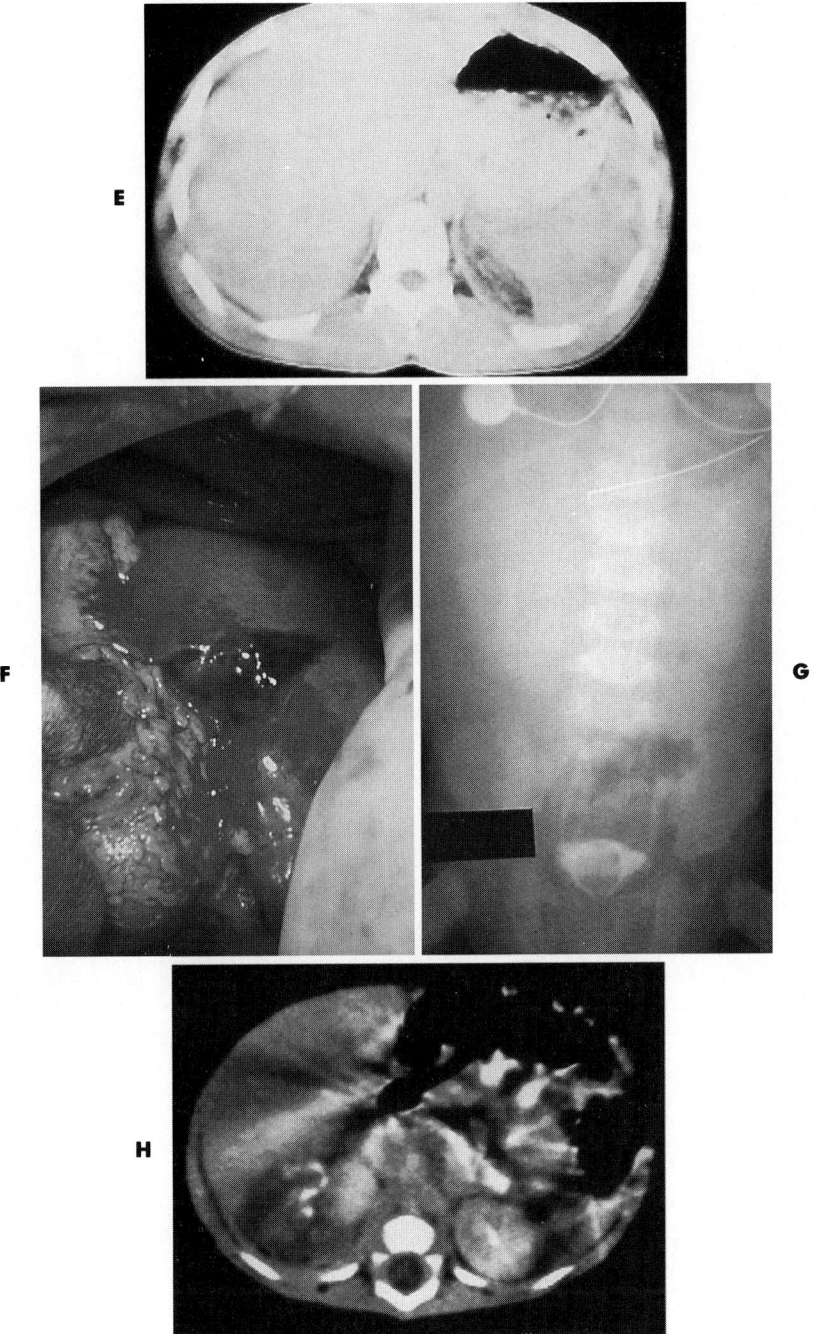

FIG. 24-1, cont'd. E and **F,** Transverse laceration of spleen following blunt trauma due to motor vehicle–pedestrian injury: tomographic and intraoperative findings. Treatment is mostly nonoperative. **G** and **H,** Intraperitoneal extravasation of urine due to rupture of dome of bladder following blunt trauma: urographic and tomographic findings. Treatment requires operative repair.   *Continued.*

ter off restrained, despite the small risk of associated injury.

Bicycle Injury

Head trauma caused by a bicycle injury is the most lethal; abdominal injury also occurs.[33,34] A child may be impaled on a handlebar or land on the abdomen when thrown off a bicycle. The handlebar can lacerate the kidney, spleen, or liver; contuse or inflame the pancreas; rupture the intestine or common bile duct; or cause a duodenal hematoma.[35,36] Perineal straddle and scrotal tearing injuries may also result from forceful impact against the

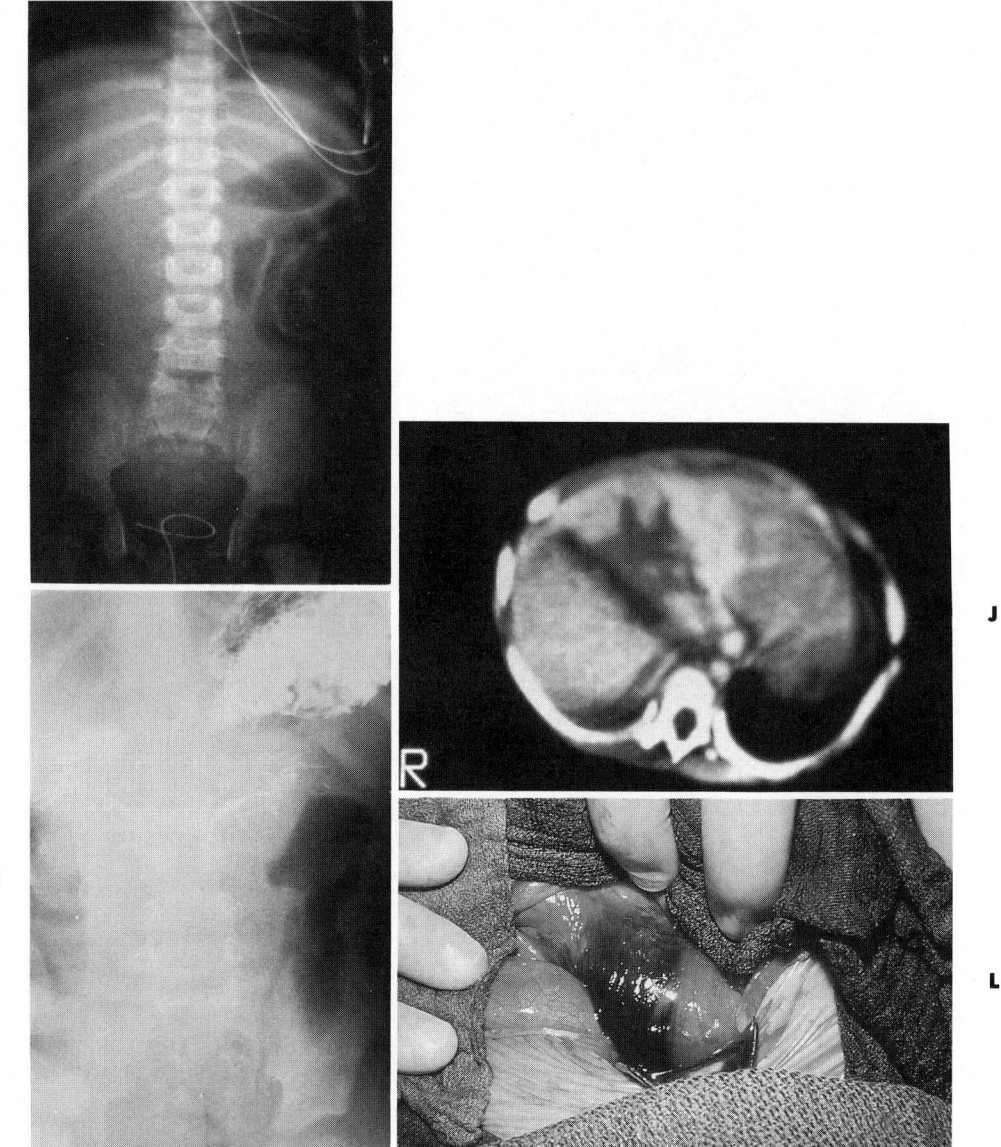

FIG. 24-1, cont'd. I and **J,** Intraparenchymal hematoma of liver following blunt trauma due to child abuse: roentgenographic and tomographic findings. Treatment is mostly nonoperative. **K** and **L,** Intramural hematoma of duodenum following blunt trauma due to child abuse: fluoroscopic and intraoperative findings. Treatment is mostly nonoperative.

Continued.

crossbar; extremity fractures, facial lacerations, and severe abrasions are more often the result of rapid deceleration, shearing, and scraping as body parts leading the fall make contact with the road surface.

Handlebar injuries are particularly dangerous because they are most often viewed as trivial. Most children show no signs of serious injury for several hours and sometimes days, after the impact; the mean elapsed time to onset of symptoms approaches 24 hours. As many as one third are discharged home after an initial evaluation fails to disclose the true nature of the problem. Once identified, however, the magnitude of the insult is soon recognized; the mean length of stay among children who require hospitalization for bicycle handlebar injuries exceeds 3 weeks.[35]

Inflicted Injury

The child who has an intraabdominal injury from child abuse often presents a diagnostic dilemma (see Chapter 52). There is often a delay in appropriate medical attention for the child; the reason given for the visit may obscure the true nature of the injury.[37] In addition, external signs of associated overlying soft tissue damage may be lacking in up to one half of the cases involving the abdomen. Of children with inflicted injuries, less than 5% suffer significant intraabdominal injury. Among these, however, abdominal injury is second only to head injury as a cause of mortality; the vast majority are due to blunt trauma.[38]

The three mechanisms of blunt abdominal injury described above may be observed in a battered child. Crush-

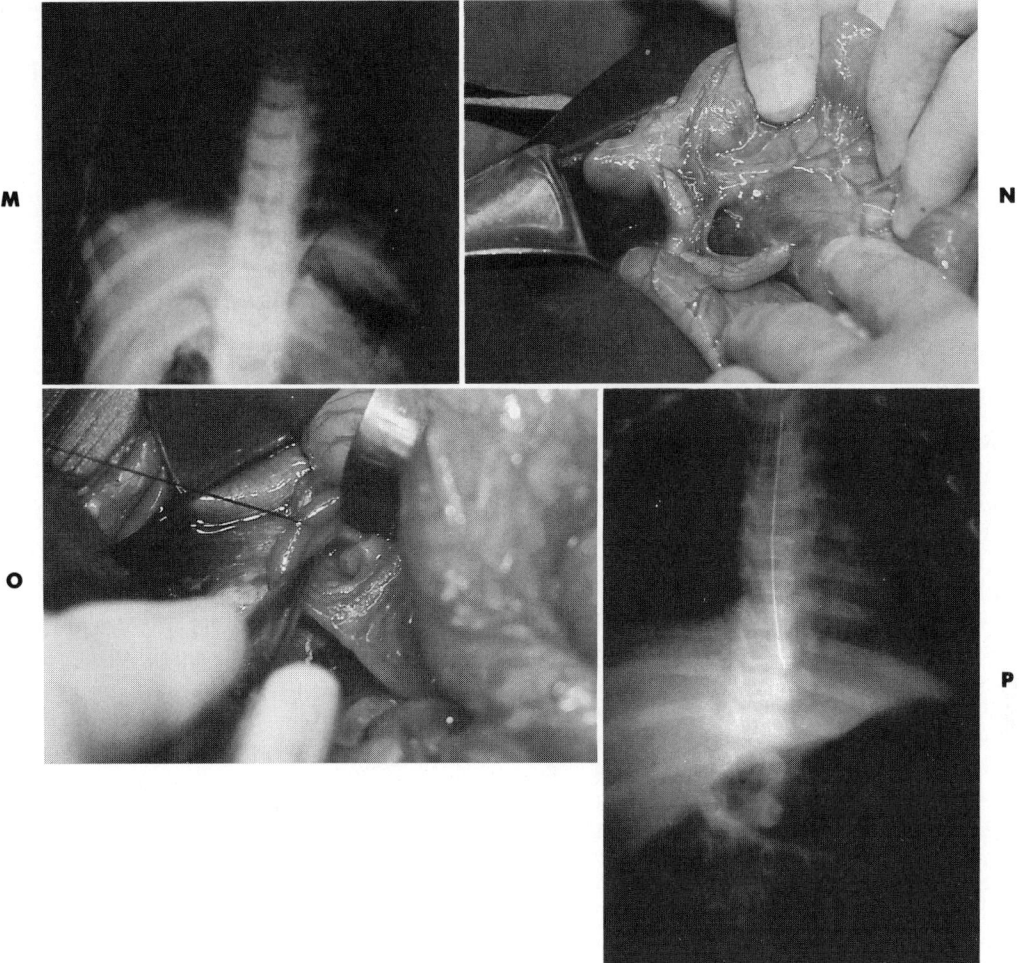

FIG. 24-1, cont'd. M, N, and **O,** Retroperitoneal hematoma and duodenal transection following blunt trauma due to child abuse: roentgenographic and intraoperative findings. Note the presence of both subdiaphragmatic and retroperitoneal gas on plain film. **P,** Gastric dilation following blunt trauma due to motor vehicle–pedestrian injury. Note that gastric dilation remains unrelieved despite passage of nasogastric tube as tube was not advanced fully into stomach.

ing of solid upper abdominal organs against the vertebral column results in massive laceration and uncontrolled hemorrhage after a severe blow to the lower rib cage or midgastric area. Sudden compression of hollow upper abdominal viscera against the vertebral column after a kick or punch to the hypogastric area can cause gastrointestinal (GI) perforation and subsequent peritonitis. Duodenal hematoma can also occur but is rarely lethal. Finally, shearing of the posterior attachments or vascular supply of abdominal viscera may follow being hurled against an object or struck by a blow that supplies a forceful tangential impact. Of these mechanisms, massive injury to the liver accounts for the majority of the deaths.

The delayed presentation of these children makes the injuries particularly lethal. A ruptured viscus, in and of itself, is rarely fatal, unless it is the result of sepsis caused by an especially prolonged delay in the ability to treat peritonitis. Renal and pancreatic injuries seldom require surgery and do not threaten life unless associated with other abdominal injuries, even if there is a significant delay in presentation.

Sports Injuries and Falls

Sports injuries typically are associated with isolated damage to an intraabdominal organ and depend on the magnitude and direction of the force vector. Falling onto the abdomen while sliding into a base, a blow to the abdomen by a football helmet or falling off a sled and striking a tree may produce isolated splenic injury. In like manner, a direct blow to the flank can readily result in renal trauma. However, GI perforations more commonly result from forceful, direct blows from blunt objects such as baseball bats.

Falls, perhaps the most common mechanism of injury in childhood, are an uncommon cause of serious intraabdominal damage. The greater mass of the head in relation to the rest of the body, by the laws of physics, usually leads to a head-first fall, sparing the torso major injury. Thus, falls from heights of 5 to 10 feet commonly result in head injury[39,40] but rarely in intraabdominal injury unless the child happens to fall onto an object that strikes the abdomen or lower thorax. Falls from heights of two stories or above are more hazardous and may be associated with serious intraabdominal injury but seldom are fatal.[41,42] By contrast, falls from heights of five stories or above carry an increasing rate of mortality because of the vertical organ and vascular displacement; falls from the eighth story or above are more likely to cause death and are frequently associated with injuries to several body regions, including the abdomen.[41,42]

DIAGNOSTIC FINDINGS

Clinical Findings

Injury to the abdominal cavity by both blunt and penetrating mechanisms requires specific examination. The diagnosis of children with penetrating abdominal injury actually differs little from that in adults; however, the evaluation of children with blunt abdominal injury presents a special challenge to the emergency physician. First, although children occasionally experience isolated intraabdominal injury, the majority also have significant injuries to the head and extremities that can overshadow the often subtle early findings of intraabdominal injury, especially when combined with the difficulties inherent in obtaining a history in pediatric patients. Second, because most pediatric abdominal trauma victims can be managed nonoperatively, there is a greater reliance on radiologic imaging, physical examination, and ongoing physiologic monitoring, to the virtual exclusion of peritoneal lavage. Finally, hemorrhagic shock caused by major solid organ injury remains a significant source of morbidity and mortality in these patients, especially when diagnosis is delayed. Collectively, these axioms lead to the logical conclusions that evidence of hemodynamic instability not immediately responsive to fluid resuscitation or of peritoneal irritation is a sign that life-threatening intraabdominal injury is likely to be present, that nonoperative management is inappropriate under such circumstances, and that a surgeon experienced in the management of pediatric abdominal injuries should be involved as soon as possible in all cases of serious abdominal trauma.

History. Historical information can aid in evaluation and management of abdominal injuries. Routine data to be obtained include pertinent medical history, tetanus immunization status, allergies, and medications. A history of abdominal pain, bruising or tenderness, distension, or vomiting, particularly when stained with blood or bile, mandates a very thorough abdominal examination. The mechanism and time of injury should be elicited. Information should also be obtained from prehospital personnel (see box above).

The mechanism and nature of the injury must be carefully delineated. For vehicular trauma it is helpful to know the amount of damage to the automobile and what, if any, restraint systems were used. For penetrating injuries the type of weapon, number of shots or stabs inflicted, and blood loss at the scene should be ascertained. Child abuse should be suspected if the history is inconsistent with the injury.

History by Mechanism of Injury

Blunt

Motor vehicle: occupant
Time of injury
Speed of vehicles involved
Condition of vehicle
Location of victim
Type of restraint
Condition of other patients in motor vehicle
Vital signs in field

Motor vehicle: pedestrian
Time of injury
Speed of vehicles
Condition of vehicle
Location of victim
Vital signs in field

Fall
Time of injury
Estimated distance of fall
Position of victim
Surface type
Vital signs in field

Penetrating
Type of weapon
Number of shots or stabs reported
Blood at scene
Vital signs in field

Physical Examination. A careful physical examination, repeated frequently, and serial assessments of vital signs are the key to appreciating the progression of findings associated with intraabdominal injury. Clothes should be removed and inspection completed after stabilization. Peritoneal signs can be masked by an altered mental status caused by drugs or, more often, by head trauma; simple tenderness may also be obscured by pain elsewhere. Signs of peritoneal irritation produced by blood or bowel contents in the abdominal cavity may be among the first appreciated physical findings; abdominal distension may accompany hemorrhage or third spacing. If significant hemorrhage has occurred, abnormal vital signs and perfusion status may be seen early and is indicative of hypovolemia.

Gastric dilatation may confound the abdominal examination by obscuring signs of life-threatening intraabdominal hemorrhage and occasionally causing sufficient abdominal tenderness to simulate peritonitis.

A nasogastric tube should generally be inserted to empty the stomach and, simultaneously, look for blood or bile. Similarly, after determining that the prostate is normal and no blood is present at the tip of the urethra, a Foley catheter should be placed if there is any hint of tenderness or mass in the lower abdomen, as well as for monitoring purposes in cases when there is possible hemodynamic instability. It may not be necessary to place the catheter if the child is clinically stable; one may wait until the child voids spontaneously to obtain a urine specimen.

An abdomen that remains distended and doughy after gastric decompression is clearly an ominous sign suggesting the presence of an intraabdominal catastrophe, particularly if there is hemodynamic instability indicative of intraabdominal bleeding. Fever, marked tenderness, involuntary guarding, and spasm are more common if enteric disruption is present.

If the child is conscious, he or she will be quite agitated and fearful, because of inability to comprehend the events of the accident, the frightening environment, and the presence of strangers surrounding and often restraining him or her. When the examiner is gentle and speaks quietly, more information is obtained.

Inspection. The entire torso, front and back, must be carefully examined for abrasions, tire marks, contusions, lacerations, and signs of deep penetration, as well as abnormal breathing patterns. Tachypnea without retractions can be an early sign of hypovolemia; a rapid, shallow breathing pattern can result from abdominal wall injury or peritoneal irritation.

Auscultation. Auscultation for bowel sounds should be performed over all four quadrants. Although presence of bowel sounds is generally inconsistent with significant injury to hollow viscera, their absence is nonspecific, as ileus typically results from generalized injury to the abdominal compartment.

Percussion. A tympanitic percussion note over the upper abdomen may indicate gastric dilatation caused by swallowed air, whereas a flat percussive note over the lower abdomen may reveal a suprapubic mass produced by a distended urinary bladder. If the examiner elicits tenderness when percussing the abdomen, this is equivalent to rebound tenderness, indicating parietal peritoneal irritation, hence peritonitis.

Palpation. Gentle palpation to appreciate subtle findings of rebound tenderness should be performed, starting away from the areas of pain. Attempting deep palpation early will probably negate the possibility of subsequently obtaining meaningful examination findings.

Complete examination of the abdomen is not limited to the anterior abdominal wall. The flanks and back should be inspected for evidence of contusion, laceration, penetration, and tenderness. The perineum should also be inspected for contusions, lacerations, hematomas, and gross bleeding from the vagina. These are especially important findings in cases of suspected sexual abuse.

Rectal examination should also be part of the examination of every injured child. The presence of gross or occult blood is commonly due to rectal or colonic injury and rarely due to more proximal injury. Tenderness or anterior palpation can result from peritoneal irritation. Sphincter tone should be noted and may be absent in cases of spinal injury or sexual abuse. A boggy or high-riding prostate gland may be a clue to genitourinary or pelvic injury. Blood at the urethra should be noted and evaluated.

The pelvis should be palpated for evidence of instability as well as discontinuity, especially bony prominences such

---

Routine Laboratory Tests

Type and cross-match
Complete blood count
Platelet count
Arterial blood gases
Electrolytes
Blood urea nitrogen
Creatinine
Liver enzymes
Serum/urine amylase
Urinalysis

---

as the anterior superior iliac spines, which commonly are injured in major blunt trauma. The integrity of the pelvic ring may be tested in two ways: (1) by auscultating over one anterior superior iliac spine while gently tapping the other, to determine whether bone conduction is preserved, as it is only when the ring is intact; and (2) by pressing simultaneously on the anterior superior iliac spines to determine whether the pelvic wings "spring" apart as a result of separation of the pubic symphysis. In the absence of such obvious deformities, fractures should be suspected if there is point tenderness, even if it is not associated with a laceration or hematoma, particularly when it is clinically suggested by perineal swelling or discoloration. A careful search for concomitant trauma to the bladder, bladder neck, prostate gland, and urethra is mandatory.

Ancillary Data

Laboratory Studies. Laboratory tests that may be useful in evaluation of the pediatric victim of abdominal trauma are listed in the box above. The most important of these are blood type and cross-match. The hematocrit, although important early in the course of resuscitation as a baseline value, initially may be of limited utility as there generally will not have been adequate time for equilibration to have occurred.[43] *Serial* hematocrits offer a better clue to the extent of blood loss than the initial value. However, if the physical and vital signs indicate the presence of shock, an initial hematocrit of 30% or less suggests significant hemorrhage; 25% or less, massive hemorrhage.[37]

Elevations of the serum concentrations of the hepatic transaminases suggest injury to the liver.[44] An elevated serum amylase concentration indicates an injury to the pancreas and possibly the spleen, which is contiguous with the tail of the pancreas.[45] Urine that is grossly bloody or has 20 or more red blood cells per high-power field (RBCs/ HPF) suggests renal damage and, indirectly, damage to adjacent organs, caused by the high incidence of associated injuries in blunt renal trauma.[46,47] Asymptomatic hematuria is a low-yield indication for radiologic evaluation of children with blunt abdominal trauma, particularly if the injury is seemingly trivial, but may serve to indicate an undiagnosed renal anomaly. It should be noted that myoglobin also may yield positive results on dipstick evaluation of the urine, suggesting a significant crush injury; creatinine phosphokinase should be measured to find out whether the skeletal muscle fraction is elevated.[48]

Radiologic Studies. The specific radiologic trauma series obtained in the emergency department for screening purposes in the seriously injured child includes a supine chest film and combined (when possible) supine abdominal and pelvic roentgenograms, unless the patient's condition is deteriorating and requires immediate transport to the operating room. These studies frequently offer important clues not only to the diagnosis but also to the pattern and severity of intraabdominal injury. For example, fractures of ribs, pelvis, or vertebrae suggest that the force of injury was significant and indicate a need for more definitive imaging studies in the absence of other markers of serious intraabdominal injury. However at no time should x-ray studies take precedence over resuscitation; immediate therapy may be required for treatment of life-threatening injuries. Also, only hemodynamically stable patients should be taken to the radiology department, and then only if the physician accompanies and continuously monitors the child.

The initial screening film often gives evidence of gastric dilatation, which is common in injured children but frequently is normal. Roentgenographic signs of solid visceral injury in the child on supine radiography, as shown in the box above, are (1) ground glass appearance of the abdominal cavity as a whole, suggesting the presence of intraperitoneal blood or urine; (2) medial displacement of the lateral border of the stomach by the spleen marked by the nasogastric tube suggesting splenic laceration or hematoma; and (3) scoliosis, obliteration of the nephric outline(s) and psoas shadow(s), and fractures of the lower ribs, suggesting renal injury. Bleeding from short gastric vessels gives the fundic mucosa a "saw-tooth" appearance.[49]

Signs of hollow visceral injury, unfortunately, are much more subtle; indeed, short of contrast studies, the only clue to duodenal or proximal jejunal hematoma, when a nasogastric tube is in place, may be the relative lack of gas in the distal small intestine, although this is rarely an early sign. Similarly, disruptions of the duodenum or proximal jejunum may be heralded only by tiny retroperitoneal or perinephric gas shadows on the right side of the abdomen, adjacent to and slightly below the liver, which may not be seen, or the ileus, which is a nonspecific finding. The presence of a pneumoperitoneum confirms its presence but is rarely identified on plain x-ray film; it may be detected by air injected via the nasogastric tube used as a radiolucent contrast agent when an upright or left lateral decubitus view is obtained. Radiopaque contrast studies and computed tomography (CT) scanning do not reliably reveal bowel rupture.

Further diagnostic imaging to define the extent of or to rule out major intraabdominal injury is undertaken only if the patient is hemodynamically stable.[50-54] Ultrasonography is useful for evaluation of pancreatic injuries and detection of intraperitoneal hemorrhage, particularly in the splenic and pelvic fossae; CT scan is best for evaluation of liver, kidney, and spleen injuries and, to a lesser extent, GI injuries, particularly in comatose patients, although radiologic diagnosis of GI injuries is less accurate than for other injuries.[55-60] The use of oral and intravenous contrast

---

Chest and Abdominal X-ray Study Findings Suggesting Abdominal Injury

Gastric dilatation
Medially displaced lateral stomach border
Inferiorly displaced transverse colon
Ground glass appearance of abdominal cavity
Blurring of psoas shadow(s)
Associated lower rib fracture(s)
Signs of ileus
Pneumoperitoneum

---

agents increases the sensitivity of the examination. Intramural duodenal hematomas are more easily diagnosed if barium is used as a contrast agent. Water-soluble oral contrast medium should be used for suspected gastric, duodenal, and rectal perforations.

A relative contraindication to radiographic contrast studies is in patients with histories of anaphylactoid reactions to iodinated contrast agents, unless such patients are known to have been successfully pretreated with corticosteroids and antihistamines; nonionic agents are now available. The patient must also lie still and on occasion may need sedation; adequate supervision of ventilation, oxygenation, and perfusion must be maintained throughout the course of the study.

CT scans of the abdomen should be obtained whenever there are signs of internal bleeding such as abdominal tenderness, distension, bruising, or gross hematuria, as well as a history of shock in the field that has responded to volume resuscitation. The study should be obtained if there is a mechanism or pattern of injuries suggesting that significant intraabdominal injury may have occurred.[61] However, they cannot be used solely to predict the need for laparotomy, as this is a clinical decision that is based not on test results but on physiologic status.[62-64] Ultrasonography generally is reserved for those cases in which intraabdominal injury is suspected and CT scan cannot be obtained because of lack of equipment or a history of allergy to iodinated contrast agents; it has been successfully used in screening for intraabdominal injuries.[65,66] Nuclear scans, which remain the "gold standard" for detection of minor splenic and hepatic injuries, are now used chiefly for follow-up evaluation of solid visceral injuries initially detected by CT scan and for cases in which these injuries are strongly suspected but CT scan cannot be obtained and ultrasonography findings are negative.[67,68]

The radiographic diagnosis of blunt renal injuries has undergone especially rapid evolution in recent years. Ultrasonography has become the elective diagnostic study of choice when information is sought about the structural integrity of the kidneys; nuclear renal perfusion scan has become the first-line nonemergency test of renal function. Nonetheless, CT scan of the abdomen, if obtained, serves to rule in or out major abnormalities and generally suffice unless minor injuries beyond the resolution of the scanner are present.[69,70] Finally, although intravenous urography has been largely supplanted by these techniques, it is still used in situations where isolated blunt renal injury is suspected and there are neither clinical findings nor mechanism of injury that suggest that adjacent structures may be damaged. The intravenous urogram may also be useful if the urinalysis reveals significant microscopic hematuria (i.e., 20 or more RBCs/HPF), especially if no other reliable test of renal function is immediately available.[47,71-73] Although the adult literature suggests that the finding of 50 or fewer RBCs/HPF is rarely associated with significant renal abnormality, pediatric studies have suggested this lower number of RBCs to assure identification of congenital urinary tract anomalies as well. Clinical findings and mechanism of injury should be considered.[46] Arteriography is required only for the diagnosis of renal pedicle injury in which specific information regarding vascular anatomy is desired in preparation for urgent operation; such injuries are rare, but this lesion must always be suspected, as hematuria, whether gross or microscopic, may not be present unless the renal parenchyma itself is also damaged.[74,75]

Diagnostic Peritoneal Lavage. Diagnostic peritoneal lavage (DPL) was for many years the procedure of choice for early detection of intraabdominal bleeding in children as well as adults. However, the fact that the decision to operate on patients with hepatic or splenic lacerations is based not on the presence or absence of intraperitoneal blood but on the ongoing transfusion requirement renders use of this technique debatable for most children.[76,77] It is therefore used chiefly for patients in whom the usual diagnostic modalities of serial physical, laboratory, and radiologic evaluation are unavailable or unreliable including those who are unconscious, are grossly intoxicated, or must undergo immediate general anesthesia for repair of life-threatening intracranial or axial skeletal injuries. It has no place in the management of the hemodynamically unstable patient who requires emergency laparotomy for control of intraabdominal bleeding, as the test adds nothing to what is already known and only delays definitive surgical therapy.

Nevertheless, although it (1) is neither organ nor injury specific and (2) cannot reliably assess retroperitoneal injury, DPL is a safe and effective method of detecting intraperitoneal hemorrhage, and is somewhat more sensitive than CT scan.[78] Thus, DPL may be used instead of CT scan or ultrasonography if physicians skilled in nonoperative trauma management are not available or if those responsible for the definitive management of pediatric abdominal trauma prefer this approach. DPL also has a role in children who have sustained injuries in which the integrity of the bowel possibly has been violated, particularly victims of stab wounds in whom findings of wound exploration are positive or equivocal. However, frequent, careful serial examination of the child for signs of peritoneal irritation is probably an equally sensitive test; moreover, it prevents the complications associated with DPL and negates the possibility that later physical or roentgenographic examinations will be confounded by tenderness resulting from the presence of intraperitoneal blood caused by oozing from the puncture site in the abdominal wall or air introduced at the time of peritoneal incision.[79]

Red Blood Cell (RBC) Criteria for Positive Diagnostic Peritoneal Lavage

Type of trauma	RBCs/mm³ in effluent
Blunt	>100,000*
Penetrating stab wound	
Anterior abdomen	>100,000*
Flank or back	>100,000*
Lower chest (? diaphragm)	>5,000

*20,000-100,000 equivocal.

The procedure is best performed after decompression of the stomach and bladder. The open technique is most reliable and safe. The test result is considered positive for intraperitoneal hemorrhage if (1) free blood is aspirated or (2) the effluent obtained from instillation of 10 ml/kg of body weight of 0.9% normal saline or lactated Ringer's (LR) solution into the peritoneal cavity, via a catheter inserted through the lower peritoneal midline under direct visualization, is sufficiently murky to prevent the reading of standard newsprint, or meets the criteria shown in the box above. The integrity of the bowel is considered to have been violated if the effluent contains (1) stool, (2) more than 500 white blood cells per mm³, (3) amylase concentration of more than 175 IU/L, or (4) alkaline phosphatase concentration of more than 6 IU/L.

MANAGEMENT

Emergency management of the injured child for symptoms and signs of abdominal trauma is not undertaken until the integrity of the airway, breathing, and circulation have first been assured and immediately life-threatening chest injuries have been excluded (see Chapter 23). Serial monitoring is essential. Once resuscitation has commenced, and initial stabilization achieved while the primary survey has been performed, a careful head-to-toe examination is undertaken, addressing all organ systems, including the central and peripheral nervous and musculoskeletal systems. To be sure no findings are overlooked, the secondary survey must include both complete exposure of the patient and log-rolling, especially in penetrating trauma (see Chapter 19). However, care must be taken to prevent subsequent development of hypothermia, which worsens acidosis; blankets, an overhead radiant warmer, and intravenous fluids warmed to body temperature may be helpful.

Initial Resuscitation

The initial resuscitation of the child who has abdominal trauma begins in the field and continues in the emergency department. Rapid clinical assessment of ventilation, oxygenation, and perfusion is performed with the purpose of identifying and treating any condition that may lead imminently to cardiopulmonary failure.[80] The initial minutes of resuscitation should be guided by the consensus protocols of the American Heart Association, the American Academy of Pediatrics, the American College of Surgeons, and the American College of Emergency Physicians (see Chapter 19).[81-83]

Priority attention is directed to maintenance of the airway, breathing, and circulation. However, since the limited circulatory reserves of the child require immediate relief from uncontrolled hemorrhage, rapid restoration of hemodynamic stability by means of volume resuscitation is emphasized.[11] Since the chief cause of preventable death in pediatric abdominal trauma has been the failure to recognize and stop internal bleeding in a timely manner, a surgeon with experience in pediatric trauma should be involved as early as possible in the course of resuscitation.[2,3] Most patients in decompensated shock are victims of major intraabdominal hemorrhage; hypotension resulting from isolated intracranial, intrathoracic, pelvic, or axial skeletal injuries is distinctly uncommon.[20]

Principles

The initial resuscitation and stabilization are achieved and the definitive evaluation completed to ascertain the need for operative intervention as a team effort; the focus is not on making an organ-specific diagnosis.[84,85] The child with a suspected intraabdominal injury should initially receive no oral intake, not only because temporary paralytic ileus usually accompanies the type of major blunt abdominal trauma often seen in children but because general anesthesia may be required later. Fluid resuscitation is completed. A nasogastric tube and urinary catheter are inserted as indicated and blood evaluations, including a type and cross-match, are sent for analysis.

Attention then is turned to acute management of whatever abdominal injuries may be present. As noted, fewer than 15% of pediatric blunt trauma victims now require operative management, a change driven largely by the extraordinary power of modern imaging technologies. It must always be remembered that the decision not to operate is always the more difficult one, for it commits both patient and physician to an extended and stressful period of uncertainty before a definite conclusion is reached that operative intervention will not be required.

The decision regarding the need for emergency operation is based on the hemodynamic response to resuscitation and the presence or absence of peritoneal signs as shown in the box above. Immediate operation is generally required if the child is in decompensated shock, circulation cannot be stabilized despite rapid administration of 40 to 60 ml/kg of LR solution with or without whole blood or packed RBCs, or unequivocal peritoneal signs are detected. Urgent operation may be indicated if the transfusion requirement exceeds half the child's normal circulating blood volume after crystalloid resuscitation, hemodynamic stability cannot be achieved or maintained despite seemingly adequate volume resuscitation, or peritoneal signs gradually evolve over a period of 6 to 12 hours. However, a small percentage of children still require late operation because of ongoing hemorrhage associated with an unsuccessful attempt at nonoperative management.

A practical initial approach to management is described in the box at right. An unstable patient who does not respond promptly to volume resuscitation is taken directly

---

Indications for Emergency Operation

Blunt

Hemodynamic instability despite adequate volume resuscitation
Decompensated shock on admission
Transfusion requirement >50% of estimated blood volume
Physical signs of peritonitis
>100,000 RBCs/mm^3 on peritoneal lavage
Bile, bacteria, stool, or >500 WBC/mm^3 on peritoneal lavage
Radiologic evidence of pneumoperitoneum
Radiologic evidence of intraperitoneal bladder rupture
Radiologic evidence of renovascular pedicle injury

Penetrating

All gunshot wounds
All stab wounds associated with evisceration; blood in stomach, urine, or rectum; physical signs of shock or peritonitis; radiologic evidence of intraperitoneal or retroperitoneal gas
Bile, bacteria, stool, or >500 WBC/mm^3 on peritoneal lavage
All suspected thoracoabdominal injuries

RBCs, Red blood cells; *WBCs,* white blood cells.

Triage Guidelines for Emergency Management of Abdominal Trauma

Stable, (−) indications for CT → acute care area
Stable, (+) indications for CT → CT (−) → acute care area
Stable, (+) indications for CT → CT (+) → PICU vs. OR
Unstable, responds well to volume → CT (−) → PICU
Unstable, responds well to volume → CT (+) → PICU vs. OR
Unstable, responds poorly to volume → OR

CT, Computed tomography; *PICU,* pediatric intensive care unit; *OR,* operating room.

---

to the operating room. If the patient has significant head trauma and can be transiently stabilized, rapid-head CT scan is performed on the way to the operating suite. For an unstable patient who responds promptly and unequivocally to volume resuscitation, appropriate x-ray studies are obtained as indicated; then the patient is taken to the pediatric intensive care unit (PICU) for further care. Patients who are stable on presentation, require diagnostic imaging for the reasons outlined, and have a positive CT scan are taken to the PICU for continuing observation and management. After a negative CT scan result patients may be admitted to an acute care unit. Most patients who are managed according to this plan are discharged from the emergency department within 30 minutes and in a hospital bed within 1 hour. Early involvement of surgeons and critical care physicians experienced in the management of pediatric trauma assures high quality of care and a smooth transition for the injured child after emergency department discharge.

Disposition

Any child with abdominal injuries who is in shock or requires resuscitation in an emergency department should be admitted to a PICU for further treatment, whether or not an operation is ultimately performed.[86] Children who are less ill but have sustained injuries serious enough to warrant resuscitation require definitive assessment of the physiologic risk of injury, to ensure that potentially life-threatening injuries are not overlooked. Children should be considered for triage or transfer to a trauma center with pediatric expertise if the mechanism of injury suggests that this level of care may be required or the Pediatric, Revised, or Champion Trauma Score suggests that the injuries sustained are of sufficient magnitude to have caused serious physiologic derangement (see Chapter 19).[87-90] As a general rule, it is probably safe to proceed with routine admission and evaluation if the chosen index falls within the low-risk category.[91]

SPECIFIC INJURIES

Definitive management of the child with abdominal injuries depends on the type, extent, and severity of these injuries. In the unstable patient immediate operative treatment is generally required. In the stable patient definitive therapy is frequently nonoperative, especially with respect to lacerations, hematomas, and extravasations of the spleen, kidneys, and liver. However the term *nonoperative* does not mean "nonsurgical" since many victims of major blunt abdominal trauma do require surgical intervention at some point.[84] Mature surgical judgment is needed to determine whether, or when, surgical intervention will be required, and, if so, what type of operation should be performed.[85]

Blunt Injuries

Liver. Since the advent of the CT scan, the liver has been recognized as the most commonly injured solid organ in cases of blunt pediatric trauma; it is second only to the spleen as a source of major hemorrhage but is the most common source of lethal hemorrhage. Mortality from serious injury is reported to be as high as 10% to 20%, even after admission to a hospital.[92-95]

Diagnostic Findings. Clinical presentation depends on the extent of damage to the organ and ranges from nonspecific abdominal pain to posttraumatic cardiac arrest; however the majority of liver injuries encountered in children are minor and remain undetected unless a liver enzyme or imaging study is obtained.[68,96]

Management. Although the nonoperative management of small capsular lacerations that have ceased active bleeding and self-contained subcapsular hematomas in children is now widely accepted as safe, large stellate lacerations

and subcapsular hematomas that have eroded through Glisson capsule rarely stop bleeding without surgical intervention.[97-102] Nevertheless, children with liver injuries who are not in hypotensive shock and respond promptly to volume resuscitation rarely require laparotomy for control of bleeding, which usually ceases spontaneously.[103] Those who require late laparotomy have transfusion requirements that exceed 50% of estimated circulating blood volume (i.e., 40 ml/kg), during the 24 hours immediately after injury.[104,105] Hemobilia is a recognized late complication of nonoperative management.[106,107]

Most hepatic lacerations that require laparotomy for active bleeding can be managed by means of direct suture repair and drainage, regardless of size. Hepatic resection is rarely indicated, unless it simply completes removal of a nearly transected lobe or segment; prophylactic drainage of the biliary tree is neither necessary nor desirable. Management of retrohepatic venous injuries usually presents the greatest challenge; bleeding from tears in these extremely short veins, which may extend into the retrohepatic vena cava, is often massive and difficult to control. Circulating blood volume should ideally be restored before laparotomy, and certainly before disturbing the clot that invariably forms in the areas adjacent to these injuries. On rare occasions direct suture of these vessels may prove so difficult that it becomes necessary to use a thoracic catheter as a temporary intracaval shunt until vascular repair is accomplished; the use of gauze packs for primary hemostasis occasionally may slow bleeding if all else fails, but must be regarded as a temporizing measure.

Kidneys. After the liver, the kidneys are the solid organs most commonly injured in cases of blunt childhood trauma (see Chapter 25). The fact that the kidneys are well protected by the paraspinous muscles and embedded in fat pads enclosed by tough fascial envelopes means that substantial force is required to injure them, unless there is preexisting renal abnormality. Injuries to less well-protected organs occur in as many as 80% of the cases in which renal injury is present.

Diagnostic Findings. Since the classic findings of renal injury, including flank pain, tenderness, and a mass are difficult if not impossible to elicit in examining a child, the absence of these symptoms and signs in no way excludes the diagnosis of renal trauma. The diagnosis of significant renal injury therefore is heralded by the presence of significant hematuria, which may also result from seemingly inconsequential renal trauma in children with embryologically malformed and misplaced kidneys.[46,71-73] Unfortunately there appears to be no direct correlation between the degree of hematuria and the severity of injury; thus any child who has significant hematuria must be assumed to have sustained serious injury until it is proved otherwise.

Management. Although the long-term results of surgical intervention in the acute stage are good, blunt renal injury does not require operative management unless (1) injury is so severe that direct communication exists between the renal arterioles and the renal calyx, resulting in the presence of bright red hematuria and shock; or (2) the renal pedicle is injured, occasionally causing hypertension or hematuria.[73-75,108-113] With the single exception of the former, in which case exsanguination via the urinary tract can be swift, the tight fascial compartment within which the kidney is situated causes prompt tamponade of renal parenchymal hemorrhage, effectively limiting the amount of blood loss to no more than about 25% of circulating blood volume.[49] Most renal injuries (contusions and small capsular lacerations predominate) are much less severe; rarely, retroperitoneal extravasation may develop when communication exists between the renal calyx, usually at the pelvocaliceal junction, and the perinephric space, and leaks through a rent in Gerota fascia. Although this injury may ultimately require surgical repair, this is rarely necessary in the acute stage, unless there is major disruption or frank transection of a portion of the main collecting system. Most small urinary leaks are self-sealing, particularly if they are parenchymal in origin; direct surgical attack is necessary if the urinoma persists or becomes infected.

Spleen. The spleen is the solid organ most liable to severe damage in childhood, second only to the liver in terms of potential for lethal injury. Fortunately it is also predisposed to spontaneous healing in most cases; recognition of this fact has led to the hypothesis that nonoperative management is possible and the subsequent development of protocols that prove the efficacy of this approach in children.[114]

Diagnostic Findings. Splenic injury often is associated with left upper quadrant pain that radiates to the left shoulder and left upper quadrant tenderness. The diagnosis should also be suspected if there is persistent unexplained leucocytosis or hyperamylasemia. Most often, however, as with liver injury, signs are nonspecific and the injury is diagnosed until an imaging study is obtained.[115]

Management. Nonoperative management is somewhat more successful than it is for hepatic injuries, since the transverse orientation of most splenic parenchymal lacerations, parallel to the blood vessels, and the thicker, more elastic nature of the splenic capsule in childhood promote the spontaneous cessation of bleeding.[114] Although the same caveats that apply to patients in decompensated shock after blunt hepatic injury are applicable to blunt splenic injury,[116,117] transfusion requirements are actually lower for nonoperative management than they are for operative management.[118,119] The vast majority of splenic injuries heal spontaneously on a regimen of limited activity, beginning with 7 to 10 days of strict bed rest. It is essential not to be lulled into a false sense of security: splenic lacerations that have ceased active bleeding and previously contained subcapsular hematomas may subsequently leak or rupture, classically on the third to fifth day after injury. However, whereas the physician who selects a nonoperative course of management must be prepared for an extended period of careful observation, including frequent reexamination, nonoperative management is otherwise safe, as the risk of missed associated injuries is essentially zero.[120,121]

In the rare instance that operation is required, active splenic bleeding is found, and control of hemorrhage proves impossible, a splenic salvage procedure is performed if at all feasible. The incidence of overwhelming postsplenectomy infections in childhood, particularly of encapsulated bacterial organisms (e.g., *Streptococcus pneumoniae, Haemophilus influenzae, Neisseria meningitidis,* *Staphylococcus aureus,* and *Escherichia coli*), remains considerable. The 65-fold increase in the incidence of overwhelming lethal sepsis in children who have undergone splenectomy and decreased actuarial survival vs. a control population stands in stark contrast to the low mortality and minimal morbidity associated with other types of management.[122] Fortunately the results of splenorrhaphy or partial splenectomy (if either the superior or inferior pole of the spleen has been shattered beyond repair) have been as good as those of nonoperative management.[123-125] Care must be taken to ensure that approximately 50% of splenic mass is salvaged to perform the functions of this organ.[126-129] Most important of course is the recognition that splenic salvage procedures should be undertaken only if there is no untoward risk to the life of the child. If splenectomy must be performed, it should be accompanied by omental implantation (autotransplantation) of splenic remnants, fashioned into thin "wafers."[130,131] Finally, any patient in whom splenectomy (partial or complete) is anticipated (or has been performed) should receive vaccine to provide prophylaxis against *S. pneumoniae* as soon as possible before (or after if necessary) operation, even though antibody response may be both inconsistent and impermanent.[132,133]

Pancreas. The pancreas is rarely seriously injured in cases of blunt trauma. Its location deep in the upper abdomen accounts for this relative invulnerability, although its fixed position directly anterior to the vertebral column suggests that when the impact is of sufficient force, it will not be displaced out of harm's way but absorb the full amount of kinetic energy applied to it. As a result, serious injuries to the pancreas tend to be central and consist mainly of moderate to severe pancreatic hematomas and, in severe cases, transection.[134] Disruption of the pancreatic duct is obviously a constant feature of the latter but may also occur in the former. Unless the injury is self-sealing or there is free communication with the lesser peritoneal sac, a pancreatic pseudocyst begins to develop within 3 to 5 days. These capsulized collections of pancreatic secretions and debris form in the lesser sac, causing chronic intermittent attacks of abdominal pain, nausea, vomiting, and weight loss. Chemical peritonitis results immediately after leakage of pancreatic fluid into the peritoneal sac, causing pancreatic ascites. Fortunately, severe injuries such as these are rare; traumatic pancreatitis is more frequently encountered in cases of blunt trauma.[45,135]

Diagnostic Findings. Pancreatic injury is suspected if there is deep epigastric pain radiating to the back or deep tenderness on palpation of the upper abdomen; it is confirmed by the presence of elevated serum or urinary levels of amylase, which, together with other activated pancreatic enzymes, are responsible for both the inflammation and the erosive, necrotizing pancreatic autolysis and chemical peritonitis associated respectively with the more localized and generalized forms of the disease. Unfortunately, even though significant hyperamylasemia is typically observed after instances of serious pancreatic trauma, the serum level does not correlate directly with the severity of the injury.

Management. Treatment of simple traumatic pancreatitis is expectant; it consists of bed and bowel rest, nasogastric decompression as tolerated, intravenous administration of fluids as necessary, and, if pain persists for more than a few days, total parenteral nutrition. Refeeding with clear liquids, followed by a low-fat diet, is allowed when pain and tenderness subside and the serum amylase level falls into the normal range. By contrast, patients who have severe pancreatic injury (i.e., a large, tender epigastric mass complicated by acute peritonitis or pancreatic ascites) are candidates for external surgical drainage of the lesser peritoneal sac or partial resection or repair of lacerated pancreatic ducts.[134] Patients in whom a pancreatic pseudocyst develops require 6 to 8 weeks of complete bowel rest and total parenteral nutrition in preparation for an external or internal drainage procedure (e.g., cyst gastrostomy or cyst jejunostomy Roux-en-Y operation).[136,137]

Alimentary Tract. As a group, solid visceral injuries are far more common than hollow visceral injuries in blunt trauma, the latter occurring in 1% to 5% of children, but ranging as high as 16% in children who have had routine laparotomy after abdominal trauma.[7,79] "Blowout" injuries to the duodenum and proximal jejunum are most frequently encountered.[79,138,139]

Diagnostic Findings. The recognition of bowel injury is often delayed. In most circumstances this reflects the time required for evolution of the signs of peritonitis or obstruction rather than a deficiency of the examiners. Signs of the parietal peritoneal irritation invariably develop within 6 to 12 hours of injury once the integrity of the bowel has been violated; serial examination remains the most reliable indicator of enteric disruption.[37,39] X-ray studies play an adjunctive role. Of course, this method of diagnosis does entail an inherent delay; however, the associated risk is small and entirely acceptable, when balanced against the need to prevent unnecessary laparotomy.

Management. Treatment of GI perforations is relatively straightforward: primary suture repair and nasogastric decompression. Colonic perforations require proximal diversion, if the degree of contamination and inflammation is so great that suture repair cannot safely be performed. By contrast, hematomas of the duodenum or jejunum rarely require operative management. They may cause both intestinal obstruction and, if Vater ampulla is involved, traumatic pancreatitis. Treatment consists of nasogastric decompression and administration of intravenous fluid and electrolytes appropriate for the level of obstruction.[140,142]

Genitourinary Tract. Genitourinary tract injury other than renal trauma is extremely rare in children and is associated only with especially severe blunt injury to the abdomen or pelvis (see Chapter 25). Intraperitoneal rupture of the dome of the bladder, which is an intraabdominal organ in the child when distended, and ureteropelvic junction avulsion are associated with major blunt abdominal trauma.[143-146] Extraperitoneal vesical and urethral injuries are associated with major blunt pelvic trauma (e.g., unstable fractures or crush injuries).

Diagnostic Findings. As intraperitoneal extravasation of urine causes little, if any, peritoneal reaction, the diagnosis of intraperitoneal rupture of the bladder may be missed, especially when secondary to child abuse, until self-dialysis across the peritoneal membrane causes hypochloremic, hyperkalemic metabolic acidosis and azotemia.[147,148] Extra-

peritoneal vesical disruption caused by bone spicules or ligamentous shear should be suspected when any pelvic fracture involves the pubic bones or rami. Urethral injuries, which typically are associated with bloody urethral discharge, inability to void, and a boggy, high-riding prostate revealed on rectal examination, should be similarly considered. Ureteral and bladder injuries require excretory urography for diagnosis. Urethral injuries typically require retrograde urethrography for diagnosis.

Management. Direct operative repair is the treatment of choice, except in extraperitoneal vesical rupture, which should be managed by suprapubic or Foley catheter drainage, plus intravenous antibiotics, until the associated hematoma is resorbed and complete healing occurs in 2 to 3 weeks. Urethral injuries, which in severe pelvic fractures typically occur at or below the urogenital diaphragm and therefore are diagnosed by retrograde cystography, are often managed by means of suprapubic catheter drainage.[149] Treatment of urethral disruption by Foley catheter drainage is usually impossible, as the severed urethral ends are typically separated by several centimeters; it is also undesirable, as such treatment is associated with higher rates of intractable stricture and impotence. Moreover, most pelvic-fracture-related posterior urethral strictures in children whose urethral injuries are managed conservatively are amenable to straightforward transpubic or transperineal repair, as are straddle-injury–related anterior urethral strictures.[150-152]

Retroperitoneum. Significant injuries to upper retroperitoneal structures other than the kidneys, duodenum, and pancreas are confined nearly exclusively to the blood vessels and are quite rare, except in cases of severe deceleration injury and massive physical abuse.[37,49,153,154] They are caused by the shearing effect associated with such injuries and therefore affect the lumbocaval anastomoses, although the cavomesenteric and cavohepatic venous junctions may be involved if the impact is especially forceful. Significant injury to lower retroperitoneal structures other than the bladder and urethral tract also mainly affects the blood vessels and is frequently associated with pelvic fractures. Branches of the iliac vessels are typically involved; venous injuries are more common than arterial injuries.

Diagnostic Findings. Patients with retroperitoneal bleeding due to great vessel injury or severe pelvic fracture are likely to present in hemorrhagic shock. CT scan may be helpful in identifying the extent of injury in the stable patient with an upper retroperitoneal hematoma. The diagnosis of pelvic fracture is confirmed by pelvic roentgenography.

Management. In injuries involving smaller veins, hemorrhage usually is confined to the upper retroperitoneal space and, when seen at laparotomy, presents as small areas of retroperitoneal bruising that are best left undisturbed, as the increased pressure within the retroperitoneal space effectively tamponades further venous bleeding. However, with injuries involving the aorta or great veins, a large upper retroperitoneal hematoma is present and the overlying peritoneal membrane has usually been disrupted, resulting in massive intraperitoneal hemorrhage; prompt control of bleeding and repair of damaged vessels are necessary, although ligation of great veins that are damaged beyond repair is not necessarily lethal, given the abundant collateral vessels. For pelvic injuries, early immobilization of the fracture fragments is critical to hemorrhage control and constitutes the one proven indication for use of the pneumatic antishock garment (PASG), or military (medical) antishock trousers (MAST).[155] However, selective pelvic angiography may be required for individuals who do not respond to external pressure control of retroperitoneal venous or arterial hemorrhage.[156]

Pelvis. Despite the fact that pedestrian motor vehicle trauma involving substantial force accounts for the great majority of pelvic fractures, more than half of these bony injuries may be classified as stable (see Chapter 19). Among the remaining bony injuries, unstable injuries predominate, most of which are undisplaced; crush injuries are rare.[157-162] Nonetheless, crush injuries and unstable fractures, particularly when fragments are displaced, are responsible for most complications. Retroperitoneal hematoma is present in nearly all such injuries, although associated genitourinary and arterial injuries are uncommon. Serious associated injuries such as severe, closed head trauma are present in 80% of pelvic fractures and are typically associated with multiple pelvic and other skeletal injuries;[163,164] they also cause most of the deaths, which occur in 2% to 5% of patients with pelvic fractures.

Diagnostic Findings. As previously stated, the diagnosis of pelvic fracture is made with plain x-rays.

Management. Treatment is chiefly nonoperative, even in high-risk cases, as the associated hematoma produced by venous oozing usually is contained by the peritoneal membrane. However, although transfusion is universally required for children who sustain severe pelvic fractures, emergency operation is required only when hemorrhage is ongoing and cannot be controlled by the PASG or MAST devices and selective pelvic angiography with embolization. In these instances, open reduction with external fixation is the treatment of choice.[165,166]

Diaphragm. Blunt trauma that produces a sudden increase in intraabdominal pressure can result in rupture of the diaphragm. The impacting force typically causes large radial tears that allow abdominal contents to creep into the thoracic cavity, resulting in respiratory embarrassment caused by compression of lung parenchyma. Traumatic diaphragmatic hernia is far more common on the left than on the right side and is being identified with increasing frequency as part of the "lap belt" complex of injuries.[167-172]

Diagnostic Findings. Diagnosis can be difficult, in part because the condition is so rare: as many as 90% of these injuries are overlooked in the initial evaluation. Contusions and abrasions of the upper abdomen and lower chest should raise suspicion of this injury, although rupture can occur in the absence of external markings. Because herniation is immediate in left-sided injury, the onset of symptoms and signs is rapid; however, in right-sided injury the liver prevents sudden extrusion of the bowel into the chest and the presentation typically is late. Breath sounds typically are decreased on the affected side, where bowel sounds may also be heard, and frequently are associated with unusual x-ray study findings, such as (1) unexplained elevation of the hemidiaphragm, (2) unrelieved acute gastric dilatation, (3) localized subpulmonic hemopneumothorax, and (4) presence of a nasogastric tube in the thoracic cavity. If necessary, the diagnosis can be confirmed fluoroscopically by means of a water-soluble contrast agent.

Management. Direct surgical repair is indicated as soon as the lesion is demonstrated.

Abdominal Wall. An injury that lacerates or contuses internal organs can injure the intervening abdominal walls and tissues as well. It is important to differentiate isolated muscle contusions and hemorrhages from those associated with underlying intraabdominal injuries. Trauma to the anterior abdomen involves the rectus abdominus muscles, whereas injury to the lateral abdomen can affect the internal and external oblique as well as the transversalis muscle groups. Posteriorly, muscle groups surrounding the spine are affected; the spine itself may be damaged, and this may often be accompanied by a psoas hematoma, particularly in children with hemophilia, even after minor trauma.[173]

Diagnostic Findings. The diagnosis is made by exclusion, once intraabdominal injury has been ruled out. Ultrasonography may be useful in confirming the diagnosis or in defining the extent of the associated hematoma.

Management. Treatment is supportive. Application of dry heat may provide symptomatic relief and promote more rapid resolution of the hematoma.

Penetrating Injuries

Penetrating injuries in children are being encountered in greater numbers than ever before.[174-176] Management by experienced surgeons obviously is required, and all such children should be referred to a trauma center with pediatric capabilities. All penetrating wounds from below the nipple line to the groin potentially involve the peritoneal cavity; all penetrating wounds are contaminated and considered infected. They must be treated by means of aggressive debridement and intravenous administration of antibiotics. Finally most localities require police department notification in all cases of penetrating injury, particularly gunshot wounds; child protective services must also be involved if there is suggestion of abuse.

The focus of initial treatment is on resuscitation. The physical examination should carefully note the location and size of all entrance and exit wounds, to aid in determining the trajectory of the penetrating instrument and hence the site and extent of damage.[177] Where possible, an emergency intravenous urogram should be obtained at the bedside together with the supine, upright, and cross-table lateral radiographs of the abdomen that must be made in all cases of penetrating trauma. The posteroanterior and lateral chest x-ray films are required to evaluate combined thoracoabdominal injury.

Immediate exploration is warranted for all gunshot wounds, since 85% of them violate the peritoneal cavity. Ninety-five percent injure an organ either directly or as a result of the energy that is dissipated from the projectile as it passes through the abdominal cavity, as described by the formula:

$$KE = \frac{M(V_{en}^2 - V_{ex}^2)}{2g}$$

where KE = kinetic energy, V_{en} = entrance velocity, V_{ex} = exit velocity, M = mass, and g = gravity.[157] Two thirds of stab wounds do not enter the peritoneal cavity;

one third are characterized by visceral injury needing repair. Selective management is acceptable if (1) there are no signs of shock or peritonitis and none develops during the ensuing 12 to 24 hours; (2) there is no blood in the stomach, rectum, or urine; (3) there is no evidence of free or retroperitoneal air on plain x-ray films of the abdomen; and (4) an experienced surgeon who is familiar with selective management and will commit to the frequent serial examinations it requires is available. Exploration, however, is mandated if there is evidence or a history of evisceration; in the former case exposed bowel should be kept moist with saline-solution–soaked gauze sponges and must not be allowed to assume a dependent position. The possibility of thoracoabdominal injury must be kept in mind whenever the upper abdomen is penetrated, particularly if penetration is caused by a missile; if such injury is strongly suspected, laparotomy should be undertaken even in the absence of other indications.

Penetrating thoracoabdominal injuries, when present, require a special approach to their management (see Chapter 23).[178] In addition to the tube thoracostomy mandatory for all such injuries, laparotomy must be performed for diaphragmatic closure as well as evaluation and possible repair of intraabdominal organs. Thoracotomy is required as indicated but precedes laparotomy only for life-threatening chest injury. Otherwise, laparotomy for closure of lacerated viscera precedes the "cleansing" thoracotomy that is necessary only when intestinal contents are found in the chest.

References

1. Cooper A, Barlow B, DiScala C et al: Mortality and truncal injury: the pediatric perspective, *J Pediatr Surg* 29:33, 1994.
2. McKoy C and Bell MJ: Preventable traumatic deaths in children, *J Pediatr Surg* 18:505, 1983.
3. Dykes EH, Spence LJ, Young JG et al: Preventable pediatric trauma deaths in a metropolitan region, *J Pediatr Surg* 24:107, 1989.

Epidemiology

4. Tepas JJ, Ramenofsky ML, DiScala C et al: Mortality of head injury: the pediatric perspective, *J Pediatr Surg* 25:92, 1990.
5. Tank ES, Eraklis AJ, Gross RE: Blunt abdominal trauma in infancy and childhood, *J Trauma* 8:439, 1968.
6. Touloukian RJ: Abdominal trauma in childhood, *Surg Gynecol Obstet* 127:561, 1968.
7. Levy JL and Linder LH: Major abdominal trauma in children, *Am J Surg* 120:55, 1970.
8. Richardson JD, Belin RP, Griffen WO: Blunt abdominal trauma in children, *Ann Surg* 176:213, 1972.
9. Sinclair MC and Moore TC: Major surgery for abdominal and thoracic trauma in childhood and adolescence, *J Pediatr Surg* 9:155, 1974.
10. Wilt EM and Adkins RB: A ten-year experience with blunt trauma to the abdomen in children, *Am Surg* 48:114, 1982.

Anatomy

11. Schwaitzberg SD, Bergman KS, Harris BH: A pediatric model of continuous hemorrhage, *J Pediatr Surg* 23:605, 1988.
12. Cogbill TH, Bintz M, Johnson JA et al: Acute gastric dilatation after trauma, *J Trauma* 27:1113-1117, 1987.
13. Vyas H, Milner AD, Hopkin IE: Face mask resuscitation: does it lead to gastric distention? *Arch Dis Child* 58:373-375, 1983.

Mechanism of Injury

14. Haller JA: Injuries of the gastrointestinal tract in children: notes on recognition and management, *Clin Pediatr* 5:476, 1966.
15. Velcek FT, Weiss A, DiMaio D et al: Traumatic death in urban children, *J Pediatr Surg* 12:375, 1977.
16. Holmes MJ and Reyes HM: A critical review of urban pediatric trauma, *J Trauma* 24:253, 1984.
17. Vane D, Shedd FG, Grosfeld JL et al: An analysis of pediatric trauma deaths in Indiana, *J Pediatr Surg* 25:955, 1990.
18. Cooper A, Barlow B, Davidson L et al: Epidemiology of pediatric trauma: importance of population-based statistics, *J Pediatr Surg* 27:149, 1992.

Patterns of Injury

19. Rang M: *Children's fractures*, ed 2, Philadelphia, 1983, JB Lippincott.
20. Barlow B, Niemirska M, Gandhi R et al: Response to injury in children with closed femur fractures, *J Trauma* 27:429, 1987.
21. Cristoffel KK and Ranz R: Motor vehicle injury in childhood, *Pediatr Rev* 4:247, 1983.
22. Agran PA and Dunkle DE: Motor vehicle occupant injuries to children in crash and noncrash events, *Pediatrics* 70:993, 1982.
23. Agran PF, Dunkle DE, Winn DG: Injuries to a sample of seatbelted children evaluated and treated in a hospital emergency department, *J Trauma* 27:58, 1987.
24. Hoffman MA, Spence LJ, Wesson DE et al: The pediatric passenger: trends in seatbelt use and injury patterns, *J Trauma* 27:974, 1987.
25. Braun PG and Dion Y: Intestinal stenosis following seat belt injury, *J Pediatr Surg* 8:549, 1973.
26. Stylianos S, terMeulen DC, Latchaw LA et al: Seatbelt injuries in children, *Ann Emerg Med* 20:169, 1988.
27. Bull MJ, Stroup KB, Gerhart S: Misuse of car safety seats, *Pediatrics* 81:98, 1988.
28. Stylianos S and Harris BH: Seatbelt use and patterns of central nervous system injury in children, *Pediatr Emerg Care* 6:4, 1990.
29. Newman KD, Bowman LM, Eichelberger MR: The lap belt complex: intestinal and lumbar spine injury in children, *J Trauma* 30:1133, 1990.
30. Hardacre JM, West KW, Rescorla FR et al: Delayed onset of intestinal obstruction in children after unrecognized seatbelt injury, *J Pediatr Surg* 25:967, 1990.
31. Glassman SD, Johnson JR, Holt RT: Seatbelt injuries in children, *J Trauma* 33:882-886, 1992.
32. Tso EL, Beaver BL, Haller JA: Abdominal injuries in restrained pediatric passengers, *J Pediatr Surg* 28:915-919, 1993.
33. Fife D, Davis T, Tate L et al: Fatal injuries to bicyclists: the experience of Dade County, Florida, *J Trauma* 23:745, 1983.
34. Selbst SM, Alexander D, Ruddy R: Bicycle-related injuries, *Am J Dis Child* 141:140, 1987.
35. Sparnon AL and Ford WDA: Bicycle handlebar injuries in children, *J Pediatr Surg* 21:118, 1986.
36. Rohatgi M and Gupta DK: Isolated complete transection of common bile duct following blunt bicycle handlebar injury, *J Pediatr Surg* 22:1029, 1987.
37. Cooper A, Floyd T, Barlow B et al: Major blunt abdominal trauma due to child abuse, *J Trauma* 28:1483, 1988.
38. Klein DM: Central nervous system injuries. In Ellerstein NS, editor: *Child abuse and neglect: a medical reference*, ed 1, New York, 1981, John Wiley & Sons.
39. Selbst SM, Baker MD, Shames M: Bunk bed injuries, *Am J Dis Child* 144:721, 1990.
40. Joffe M and Ludwig S: Stairway injuries in children, *Pediatrics* 82:457, 1988.
41. Barlow B, Niemirska M, Gandhi R: Ten years of experience with falls from a height in children, *J Pediatr Surg* 18:509, 1983.
42. Roshkow JE, Haller JO, Hotson GC et al: Imaging evaluation of children after falls from a height: review of 45 cases, *Radiology* 175:359, 1990.

Diagnostic Findings

43. Ebert RV, Stead EA, Gibson JG: Response of normal subjects to acute blood loss, *Arch Intern Med* 68:578, 1941.
44. Oldham KT, Guice KS, Kaufman RA et al: Blunt hepatic injury and elevated hepatic enzymes: a clinical correlation in children, *J Pediatr Surg* 19:457, 1984.
45. Synn AY, Mulvihill SJ, Fonkalsrud EW: Surgical management of pancreatitis in childhood, *J Pediatr Surg* 22:628, 1987.
46. Lieu TA, Fleisher GR, Mahboubi S et al: Hematuria and clinical findings as indications for intravenous pyelography in pediatric blunt renal trauma, *Pediatrics* 82:216, 1988.

47. Taylor GA, Eichelberger MR, Potter BM: Hematuria: a marker of abdominal injury in children after blunt trauma, *Ann Surg* 208:688, 1988.

48. Mukherji SK and Siegel MJ: Rhabdomyolysis and renal failure in child abuse, *Am J Roentgenol* 148:1203, 1987.

49. Jewett TC: Chest and abdominal injuries. In Ellerstein NS, editor: *Child abuse and neglect: a medical reference,* ed 1, New York, 1981, John Wiley & Sons.

50. Berger PE and Kuhn JP: CT of blunt abdominal trauma in childhood, *Am J Roentgenol* 136:105, 1981.

51. Karp MP, Cooney DR, Berger PE et al: The role of computed tomography in the evaluation of blunt abdominal trauma in children, *J Pediatr Surg* 16:316, 1981.

52. Kaufman RA, Towbin R, Babcock DS et al: Upper abdominal trauma in children: imaging evaluation, *Am J Roentgenol* 142:449, 1984.

53. Mohamed G, Reyes HM, Fantus R et al: Computed tomography in the assessment of pediatric abdominal trauma, *Arch Surg* 121:703, 1986.

54. Kane NM, Cronan JJ, Dorfman GS et al: Pediatric abdominal trauma: evaluation by computed tomography, *Pediatrics* 82:11, 1988.

55. Gorenstein A, O'Jalpin D, Wesson DE et al: Blunt injury to the pancreas in children: selective management based on ultrasound, *J Pediatr Surg* 22:1110, 1987.

56. Haftel AJ, Lev R, Mahour GH et al: Abdominal CT scanning in pediatric blunt trauma, *Ann Emerg Med* 17:684, 1988.

57. Beaver BL, Colombani PM, Fal A et al: The efficacy of computed tomography in evaluating abdominal injuries in children with major head trauma, *J Pediatr Surg* 22:1117, 1987.

58. Taylor GA and Eichelberger MR: Abdominal CT in children with neurologic impairment following blunt trauma: abdominal CT in comatose, children, *Ann Surg* 210:229, 1989.

59. Luks FI, Lemire A, St.-Vil D et al: Blunt abdominal trauma in children: the practical value of ultrasonography, *J Trauma* 34:607-611, 1993.

60. Ford EG and Senac MO: Clinical presentation and radiographic identification of small bowel rupture following blunt trauma in children, *Ped Emerg Care* 9:139-142, 1993.

61. Taylor GA, Eichelberger MR, O'Donnel R et al: Indications for computed tomography in children with blunt abdominal trauma, *Ann Surg* 213:212, 1991.

62. Brick SH, Taylor GA, Potter BM et al: Hepatic and splenic injury in children: role of CT in the decision for laparotomy. *Radiology* 165:643, 1987.

63. Taylor GA, Fallat ME, Potter EM et al: The role of computed tomography in blunt abdominal trauma in children, *J Trauma* 28:1660, 1988.

64. Kohn JS, Clark DE, Isler RJ et al: Is computed tomographic grading of splenic injury useful in the nonsurgical management of blunt trauma? *J Trauma* 36:385-390, 1994.

65. Hoelzer DJ, Brian MB, Balsara VJ et al: Selection and nonoperative management of pediatric blunt trauma patients: the role of quantitative crystalloid resuscitation and abdominal ultrasonography, *J Trauma* 26:57, 1986.

66. Filiatrault D, Longpre D, Patriquin H et al: Investigation of childhood blunt abdominal trauma: a practical approach using ultrasound as the initial diagnostic modality, *Pediatr Radiol* 17:373, 1987.

67. Harris BH, Morse TS, Weidenmier CH et al: Radioisotope diagnosis of splenic trauma, *J Pediatr Surg* 12:385, 1977.

68. Howman-Giles R, Gilday DL, Venugopal S et al: Splenic trauma—nonoperative management and long-term follow-up by scintiscan, *J Pediatr Surg* 13:121, 1978.

69. Karp MP, Jewett TC, Kuhn JP et al: The impact of computed tomography scanning on the child with renal trauma, *J Pediatr Surg* 21:617, 1986.

70. Yale-Loehr AJ, Kramer SS, Quinlan DM et al: CT of severe renal trauma in children: evaluation and course of healing with conservative therapy, *Am J Roentgenol* 152:109, 1989.

71. Cass AS, Luxenberg M, Gleich P et al: Clinical indications for radiographic evaluation of blunt renal trauma, *J Urol* 136:370, 1986.

72. Stalker HP, Kaufman RA, Stedje K: The significance of hematuria in children after blunt abdominal trauma, *Am J Roentgenol* 154:569, 1990.

73. Bass DH, Semple PL, Cywes S: Investigation and management of blunt renal injuries in children: a review of 11 years' experience, *J Pediatr Surg* 26:196, 1991.

74. Kolihova E, Obenbergerova D, Apetaurova B: Total severence of the renal pedicle caused by blunt trauma in children, *Pediatr Radiol* 1:59, 1973.

75. Barlow B and Gandhi R: Renal artery thrombosis following blunt trauma, *J Trauma* 20:614, 1980.

76. Powell RW, Green JB, Ochsner MG et al: Peritoneal lavage in pediatric patients sustaining blunt abdominal trauma: a reappraisal, *J Trauma* 27:6, 1987.

77. Rothenberg S, Moore EE, Marx JA et al: Selective management of blunt abdominal trauma in children—the triage role of peritoneal lavage, *J Trauma* 27:1101, 1987.

78. Mayer DM, Thal EM, Coln D et al: Computed tomography in the evaluation of children with blunt abdominal trauma, *Ann Surg* 217:272-276, 1993.

79. Cobb LM, Vinocur CD, Wagner CW et al: Intestinal perforation due to blunt trauma in children in an era of increased nonoperative treatment, *J Trauma* 26:461, 1986.

Management

80. Trunkey D: Initial treatment of patients with extensive trauma, *N Engl J Med* 324:1259, 1991.

81. American Heart Association and American Academy of Pediatrics Working Group on Pediatric Resuscitation: *Textbook of pediatric advanced life support,* Dallas, 1988, American Heart Association.

82. American College of Surgeons Committee on Trauma: *Advanced trauma life support student manual,* Chicago, 1990, American College of Surgeons.

83. American Academy of Pediatrics and American College of Emergency Physicians Joint Task Force on Advanced Pediatric Life Support: *Advanced pediatric life support,* Elk Grove Village, Ill and Dallas, 1989, American Academy of Pediatrics and American College of Emergency Physicians.

84. Kaufmann CR, Rivara FP, Maier RV: Pediatric trauma: need for surgical management, *J Trauma* 29:1120, 1989.

85. Haller JA: Emergency medical services for children: what is the pediatric surgeon's role? *Pediatrics* 79:576, 1987.

86. Pollack MM, Alexander SR, Clarke N et al: Improved outcomes for tertiary center pediatric intensive care: a statewide comparison of tertiary and nontertiary facilities, *Crit Care Med* 19:150, 1991.

87. Harris BH, Barlow BA, Ballantine TV et al: American Pediatric Surgical Association: principles of trauma care, *J Pediatr Surg* 27:423, 1992.

88. Tepas JJ, Mollitt DL, Talbert JL et al: The pediatric trauma score as a predictor of injury severity in the injured child, *J Pediatr Surg* 22:14, 1987.

89. Champion HR, Sacco WJ, Carnazzo AJ et al: Trauma score, *Crit Care Med* 9:672, 1981.

90. Field categorization of trauma patients (field triage). In American College of Surgeons Committee on Trauma: *Hospital and prehospital resources for optimal care of the injured patient and Appendices A through J,* Chicago, 1986, American College of Surgeons.

91. Jubelirer RA, Agarwal NN, Beyer FC: Pediatric trauma triage: review of 1,307 cases, *J Trauma* 30:1544, 1990.

Specific Injuries

92. Eleiding SC, Aragon GE, Moore EE: Fatal hepatic hemorrhage after trauma, *Am J Surg* 138:883, 1979.

93. Jaufman JM and Burington JD: Liver trauma in children, *J Pediatr Surg* 6:585, 1971.

94. Suson EM, Klotz D, Kottmeier PK: Liver trauma in children, *J Pediatr Surg* 10:411, 1975.

95. Stone HH and Ansley JD: Management of liver trauma in children, *J Pediatr Surg* 12:3, 1977.

96. Vock P, Kehrer B, Tschaeppeler H: Blunt liver trauma in children: the role of computed tomography in diagnosis and treatment, *J Pediatr Surg* 21:413, 1986.

97. Cheatham JE, Smith EI, Tunell WP et al: Nonoperative management of subcapsular hematomas of the liver, *Am J Surg* 140:852-857, 1980.

98. Karp MP, Cooney DR, Pros GA et al: The nonoperative management of pediatric hepatic trauma, *J Pediatr Surg* 18:512, 1983.

99. Grisoni ER, Gauderer MWL, Ferron J et al: Nonoperative management of liver injuries following blunt abdominal trauma in children, *J Pediatr Surg* 19:515, 1984.

100. Giacomantonio M, Filler RM, Rich RH: Blunt hepatic trauma in children: experience with operative and nonoperative management, *J Pediatr Surg* 19:519, 1984.
101. Cywes S, Rode H, Millar AJW: Blunt liver trauma in children: nonoperative management, *J Pediatr Surg* 20:14, 1985.
102. Bass BL, Eichelberger MR, Schisgall R et al: Hazards of nonoperative therapy of hepatic injury in children, *J Trauma* 24:978, 1984.
103. Moulton SL, Lynch FP, Hoyt DB et al: Operative intervention for pediatric liver injuries: avoiding delay in treatment, *J Pediatr Surg* 27:958-963, 1992.
104. Oldham KT, Guice KS, Ryckman F et al: Blunt liver injury in childhood: evolution of therapy and current perspective, *Surgery* 100:542, 1986.
105. Galat JA, Grisoni ER, Gauderer MWL: Pediatric blunt liver injury: establishment of criteria for appropriate management, *J Pediatr Surg* 25:1162, 1990.
106. Lackgren G, Lorelius LE, Olsen L et al: Hemobilia in childhood, *J Pediatr Surg* 23:105, 1988.
107. MacGillivray DC and Valentine RJ: Nonoperative management of blunt pediatric liver injury—late complications: case report, *J Trauma* 29:251, 1989.
108. Jakse G, Putz A, Gassner I et al: Early surgery in the management of pediatric blunt renal trauma, *J Urol* 131:920, 1984.
109. Mandour WA, Lai MK, Linke CA et al: Blunt renal trauma in the pediatric patient, *J Pediatr Surg* 16:669, 1981.
110. Kuzmarov IW, Morehouse DD, Gibson S: Blunt renal trauma in the pediatric population: a retrospective study, *J Urol* 126:648, 1981.
111. Ahmed S and Morris LL: Renal parenchymal injuries secondary to blunt abdominal trauma in childhood: a 10-year review, *Br J Urol* 54:470, 1982.
112. Cass AS: Blunt renal trauma in children, *J Trauma* 23:123, 1983.
113. Cass AS: Renal trauma in multiple-injured child, *Urology* 21:487, 1983.
114. Ein SH, Shandling B, Simpson JS et al: Nonoperative management of the traumatized spleen in children: how and why? *J Pediatr Surg* 13:117, 1978.
115. Saladino R, Lund D, Fleisher G: The spectrum of liver and spleen injuries in children: failure of the pediatric trauma score and clinical signs to predict isolated injuries, *Ann Emerg Med* 20:636-640, 1991.
116. Wesson DE, Filler RM, Ein SH et al: Ruptured spleen: when to operate? *J Pediatr Surg* 16:324, 1981.
117. Pearl RH, Wesson DE, Spence LJ et al: Splenic injury: a 5-year update with improved results and changing criteria for conservative management, *J Pediatr Surg* 24:121, 1989.
118. Consentino CM, Luck SR, Barthel MJ et al: Transfusion requirements in conservative nonoperative management of blunt splenic and hepatic injuries during childhood, *J Pediatr Surg* 25:950-954, 1990.
119. Schwartz MZ and Kangah R: Splenic injury in children after blunt trauma: blood transfusion requirements and length of hospitalization for laparatomy versus observation, *J Pediatr Surg* 29:596-598, 1994.
120. Haller JA, Papa P, Drugas G et al: Nonoperative management of solid organ injuries in children: is it safe? *Ann Surg* 219:625-631, 1994.
121. Morse MA and Garcia VF: Selective nonoperative management of pediatric blunt splenic trauma: risk for associated injuries, *J Pediatr Surg* 29:23-27, 1994.
122. Velanovich V and Tapper D: Decision analysis in children with blunt splenic trauma: the effects of observation, splenorrhaphy, or splenectomy on quality-adjusted life expectancy, *J Pediatr Surg* 28:179-185, 1993.
123. Ratner MH, Garrow E, Valda V et al: Surgical repair of the injured spleen, *J Pediatr Surg* 12:1019, 1977.
124. Mishalany HG, Mahour GH, Andrassy RJ et al: Modalities of preservation of the traumatized spleen, *Am J Surg* 136:697, 1978.
125. Buntain WL and Lynn HB: Splenorrhaphy: changing concepts for the traumatized spleen, *Surgery* 86:748, 1979.
126. Cooney DR, Bearth JC, Swanson SE et al: Relative merits of partial splenectomy, splenic reimplantation, and immunization in preventing postsplenectomy infection, *Surgery* 86:561, 1979.
127. vanWyck DB, Witte MH, Witte CH et al: Critical splenic mass for survival from experimental pneumococcemia, *J Surg Res* 28:14, 1980.
128. Okinaga K, Giebink GS, Rich RH et al: The effect of partial splenectomy on experimental pneumococcal bacteremia in an animal model, *J Pediatr Surg* 16:717, 1981.
129. Karp MP, Guralnick-Scheff S, Schiffman G et al: Immune consequences of nonoperative treatment of splenic trauma in the rat model, *J Pediatr Surg* 24:112, 1989.
130. Velcek FT, Jongco B, Shaftan GW et al: Function of the replanted spleen in dogs, *J Trauma* 22:501, 1982.
131. Velcek FT, Jongco B, Shaftan GW et al: Posttraumatic splenic replantation in children, *J Pediatr Surg* 17:879, 1982.
132. Giebink JS, Folker JE, Kim Y et al: Serum antibody and opsonic responses to vaccination with pneumococcal capsular polysaccharide in normal and splenectomized children, *J Inf Dis* 141:404, 1980.
133. Douglas RM, Paton JC, Duncan SJM et al: Antibody response to pneumococcal vaccine in children younger than five years of age, *J Inf Dis* 148:131, 1983.
134. Smith SD, Nakayama DK, Gantt N et al: Pancreatic injuries in childhood due to blunt trauma, *J Pediatr Surg* 23:610, 1988.
135. Vane DW, Grosfeld JL, West KW et al: Pancreatic disorders in infancy and childhood: experience with 92 cases, *J Pediatr Surg* 24:771, 1989.
136. Dahman B and Stephens CA: Pseudocysts of the pancreas after blunt abdominal trauma in children, *J Pediatr Surg* 16:17, 1981.
137. Warner RL, Othersen HB, Smith CD: Traumatic pancreatitis and pseudocyst in children: current management, *J Trauma* 29:597, 1989.
138. Pokorny WJ, Brandt ML, Harberg FJ: Major duodenal injuries in children: diagnosis, operative management, and outcome, *J Pediatr Surg* 21:613, 1986.
139. Grosfeld JL, Rescorla FJ, West KW et al: Gastrointestinal injuries in childhood: analysis of 53 patients, *J Pediatr Surg* 24:580, 1989.
140. Holgersen LO and Bishop HC: Nonoperative treatment of duodenal hematomata in childhood, *J Pediatr Surg* 12:11, 1977.
141. Winthrop AL, Wesson DE, Filler RM: Traumatic duodenal hematoma in the pediatric patient, *J Pediatr Surg* 21:757, 1986.
142. Jewett TC, Caldarola V, Karp MP et al: Intramural hematoma of the duodenum, *Arch Surg* 123:54, 1988.
143. Brereton RJ, Philp N, Buyukpamukcu N: Rupture of the urinary bladder in children: the importance of the double lesion, *Br J Urol* 52:15, 1980.
144. Merchant WC, Gibbons MD, Gonzales ET: Trauma to the bladder neck, trigone, and vagina in children, *J Urol* 131:747, 1984.
145. Reda EF and Lebowitz RL: Traumatic ureteropelvic disruption in the child, *Pediatr Radiol* 16:164, 1986.
146. Bard JL and Klein FA: Ureteropelvic junction avulsion following blunt abdominal trauma, *J Tenn Med Assoc* 83:242, 1990.
147. Halsted CC and Shapiro SR: Child abuse: acute renal failure from ruptured bladder, *Am J Dis Child* 133:861, 1979.
148. Sawyer RW, Hartenberg MA, Benator RM: Intraperitoneal bladder rupture in a battered child, *Int J Pediatr Nephrol* 8:227, 1987.
149. Glassberg KI, Tolete-Velcek F, Ashley R et al: Partial tears of prostatomembranous urethra in children, *Urology* 13:500, 1979.
150. alRifaei MA, Gaafar S, Abdel-Rahman M: Management of posterior urethral strictures secondary to pelvic fractures in children, *J Urol* 145:535, 1991.
151. Glassberg KI, Kassner EG, Haller JO et al: The radiographic approach to injuries of the prostatomembranous urethra in children, *J Urol* 122:678, 1979.
152. Harshman MW, Cromie WJ, Wein AJ et al: Urethral stricture disease in children, *J Urol* 126:650, 1981.
153. Amin A, Alexander JB, O'Malley KF et al: Blunt abdominal aortic trauma in children: case report, *J Trauma* 34:293-296, 1993.
154. Parks CS and Wesselhoeft CW: Blunt traumatic laceration of the suprahepatic inferior vena cava presenting as abdominal pain and shock in a child: case report, *J Trauma* 38:68-69, 1995.
155. Garcia V, Eichelberger M, Ziegler M et al: Use of military antishock trouser in a child, *J Pediatr Surg* 16:544, 1981.
156. Barlow B, Rottenberg RW, Santulli TV: Angiographic diagnosis and treatment of bleeding by selective embolization following pelvic fracture in children, *J Pediatr Surg* 10:939, 1975.
157. Bryan WJ and Tullos HS: Pediatric pelvic fractures: review of 52 patients, *J Trauma* 19:799, 1979.
158. Reichard SA, Helikson MA, Shorter N et al: Pelvic fractures in children: review of 120 patients with a new look at general management, *J Pediatr Surg* 15:727, 1980.

159. So SKS and Perry F: Injuries and mortality associated with pelvic fractures in children, *J Trauma* 22:641, 1982.

160. Torode I and Zeig D: Pelvic fractures in children, *J Pediatr Orthop* 5:76, 1985.

161. Musemeche CA, Fischer RP, Cotler HB et al: Selective management of pediatric pelvic fractures: a conservative approach, *J Pediatr Surg* 22:538, 1987.

162. Garvin KL, McCarthy RE, Barnes CL et al: Pediatric pelvic ring fractures, *J Pediatr Orthop* 10:577, 1990.

163. Bond SJ, Gotschall CS, Eichelberger MR: Predictors of abdominal injury in children with a pelvic fracture, *J Trauma* 31:1169-1173, 1991.

164. Vasquez WD and Garcia VF: Pediatric pelvic fractures combined with an additional skeletal injury is an indicator of significant injury, *Surg Gynecol Obstetr* 177:468-472, 1993.

165. Tile M: Pelvic fractures, *Orthop Clin North Am* 11:423, 1980.

166. Mears DC and Fu F: External fixation in pelvic fractures, *Orthop Clin North Am* 11:465, 1980.

167. Myers NA: Traumatic rupture of the diaphragm in children, *Aust NZ J Surg* 34:123, 1964.

168. Radhakrishna C, Dickinson SJ, Shaw A: Acute diaphragmatic hernia from blunt trauma in children, *J Pediatr Surg* 4:553, 1969.

169. Holgersen LO and Schnaufer L: Hernia and eventration of the diaphragm secondary to blunt trauma, *J Pediatr Surg* 8:433, 1973.

170. Melzig EP, Swank M, Salzberg AM: Acute blunt traumatic rupture of the diaphragm in children, *Arch Surg* 111:1009, 1976.

171. West K, Weber TR, Grosfeld JL: Traumatic diaphragmatic hernia in childhood, *J Pediatr Surg* 16:392, 1981.

172. Marchildon MB: Unpublished data, 1991.

173. Shirkoda A, Mauro MA, Staab EV et al: Soft tissue hemorrhage in hemophiliac patients: computed tomography and ultrasound, *Radiology* 147:811, 1983.

174. Barlow B, Niemirska M, Gandhi R: Ten years' experience with pediatric gunshot wounds, *J Pediatr Surg* 17:927, 1982.

175. Barlow B, Niemirska M, Gandhi R: Stab wounds in children, *J Pediatr Surg* 18:926, 1983.

176. Ordog GJ, Prakash AP, Wassenberger J et al: Pediatric gunshot wounds, *J Trauma* 27:1272, 1987.

177. Swan KG and Swan RC: *Gunshot wounds: pathophysiology and management*, Littleton, Mass, 1980, PSG Publishing.

178. Barlow B: Penetrating gunshot and knife wounds. In Burg FD, Ingelfinger J, Wald E, editors: *Gellis' and Kagan's current pediatric therapy*, ed 14, Philadelphia, 1993, WB Saunders.

## 25

Genitourinary Trauma

Marianne Gausche

HISTORIC PERSPECTIVE AND EPIDEMIOLOGY

Children suffer from trauma on a daily basis and, while blunt injury is most common, penetrating injury is all too frequent. Nonaccidental trauma rates also have risen. Trauma kills more children each year than any other disease.[1] Multisystem injury is common in children because of their small size and lack of protective musculature and subcutaneous tissue, which allows for a wider distribution of traumatic forces.[2] Of children with multiple injuries, genitourinary (GU) tract injury is second in incidence only to brain injury.[3] Approximately 10% of trauma patients seen in the emergency department have genitourinary injuries; most of these patients are male and two thirds are older than 10 years of age.[4-7]

Pediatric GU trauma victims are a challenge to the emergency physician because injury to the GU tract is rarely visible and the physical findings may be nonspecific.[8] GU tract trauma should be considered in patients with multiple trauma, especially those involving a blow to the flank, deceleration injury (e.g., a fall or motor vehicle accident (MVA), hematuria, a pelvic fracture, or penetrating trauma to the trunk or pelvis).[4,7,9,10] Factors that must be included are the age of the patient, associated injuries, and hemodynamic status.[7,8] Early recognition and appropriate management of patients with GU injury may prevent loss of renal function, reoperation and its complications, increased hospital stays, or death.[7,9,11]

In managing patients with GU injury the clinical status of the patient and the availability of resources must be evaluated.[12] Fig. 25-1 can serve as a guide for this evaluation. This chapter describes, by area of injury, the evalua-

tion and management of the pediatric patient with GU trauma.

RETROPERITONEAL STRUCTURES

Renal Injury

The kidney is injured more often than any other genitourinary structure in children.[9,13] Many patients are multiply injured, requiring aggressive resuscitation.[7,9] Early recognition and appropriate management of severe renal injuries can reduce morbidity and save lives.[7,13]

Pathophysiology. Children are more susceptible to renal injury than adults.[7,9,14] This is due to the larger kidney in relation to body size, lesser protection because of decreased perirenal fat and fascia, weaker anterior abdominal musculature and more flexible thoracic cage, and presence of more lobulations.[14] Preexisting renal abnormality may be found in up to 15% of patients evaluated for renal trauma.[3,7,9,15,16]

The kidney is protected from injury anteriorly by the abdominal viscera and posteriorly by the musculature of the back. The anterior surface of the kidney is crossed by ribs 6 through 10 and the posterior surface by ribs 11 and 12. Because of the kidney's mobility on its vascular pedicle, it can be pushed against the ribs or the vertebrae, causing contusion or laceration.[9]

Mechanism of Injury. More than 80% of renal injuries are secondary to blunt trauma or deceleration injury.[7,9,17-19] The large majority of pediatric renal injuries are due to MVAs, followed by falls, sports injuries, direct blows to the flank, and, in a small percentage of cases, penetrating trauma (Fig. 25-2).[18] Most renal injuries (85%) are minor.[7,9] Lacerations or more moderate injuries comprise 10%; severe injuries, including renal ruptures, fractures, or pedicle injuries, comprise 3% of renal injuries.[7,20]

Pediatric patients who have either a gunshot wound (GSW) or a stab wound (SW) to the abdomen must be evaluated for GU tract injury.[21,22] Scott reports that 6% to 8% of all patients with penetrating trauma to the abdomen have injury to the kidney. Penetrating renal trauma has also been reported as a complication of amniocentesis and must be considered in the newborn with hematuria.[23]

Classification Systems. Although a number of classification systems for renal injuries have been proposed in the past, an organ injury scale has recently been developed to unify such systems for research purposes.[17,24,25] The new scaling system for renal injury is illustrated in Fig. 25-3. Grade I injuries are contusions or hematomas that are

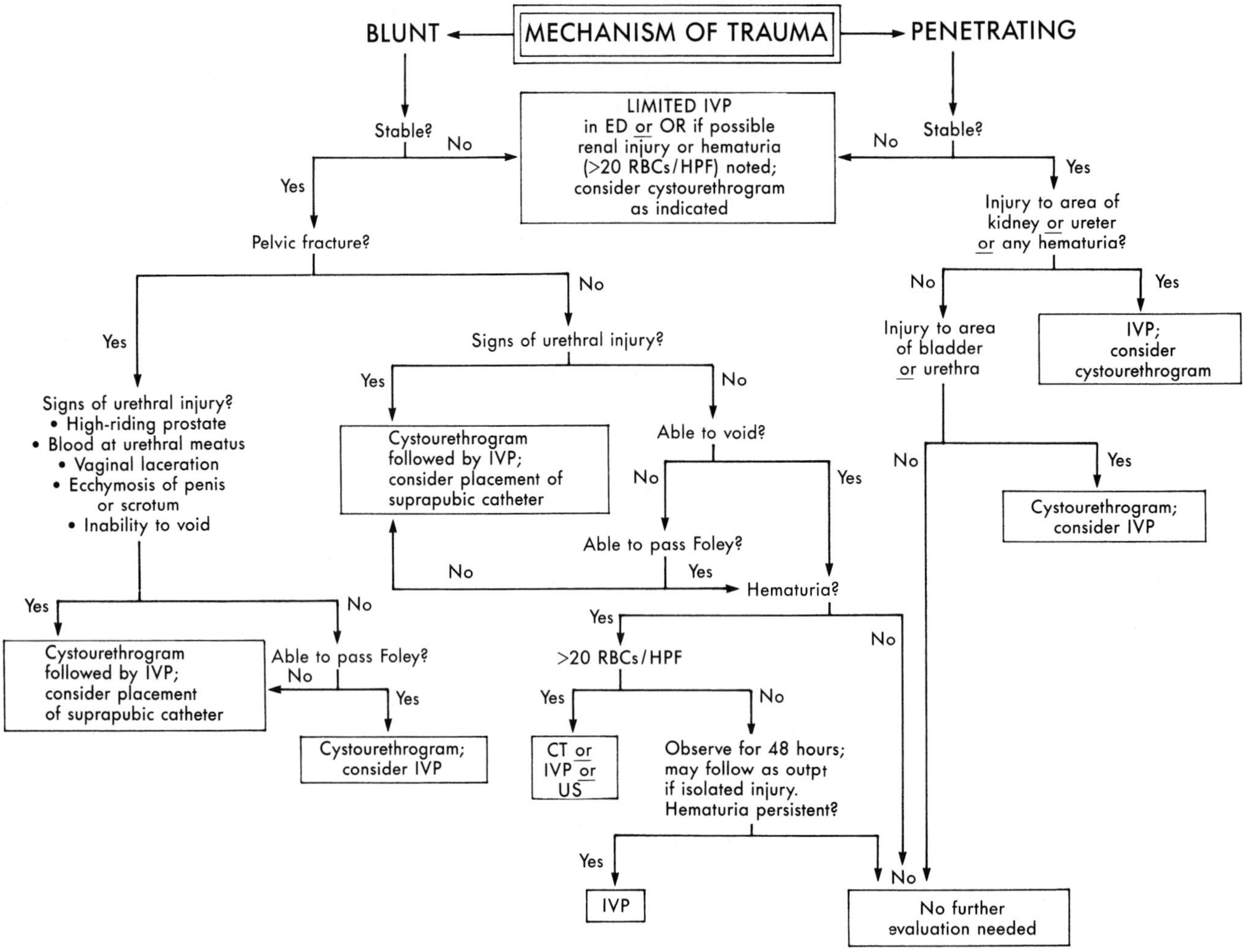

```
                        ┌─────────────────────────┐
              BLUNT ◄───│  MECHANISM OF TRAUMA    │───► PENETRATING
                        └─────────────────────────┘
```

MECHANISM OF TRAUMA

BLUNT ◄─────── → PENETRATING

Stable? ──No──► ┌──────────────────────────┐ ◄──No── Stable?
                 │ LIMITED IVP   │
   Yes   │ in ED or OR if possible │   Yes
    │   │ renal injury or hematuria│   │
Pelvic fracture? │ (>20 RBCs/HPF) noted;   │   Injury to area of
                 │ consider cystourethrogram│   kidney or ureter
                 │ as indicated   │   or any hematuria?
                 └──────────────────────────┘
   Yes   No   No   Yes
    │   │   │   │
Signs of urethral injury?   Signs of urethral   Injury to area   ┌──────────────┐
• High-riding prostate   injury?   of bladder   │ IVP;   │
• Blood at urethral meatus   Yes   No   or urethra   │ consider   │
• Vaginal laceration   │   │   │ cystourethrogram│
• Ecchymosis of penis   ┌─────────────┐ Able to void?   └──────────────┘
  or scrotum   │Cystourethrogram   No   Yes   No   Yes
• Inability to void   │followed by IVP;   │   │   │
                         │consider placement of │   Able to pass Foley? ┌──────────────┐
  Yes   No   │suprapubic catheter│   No   Yes   │Cystourethrogram;│
   │   │   └─────────────┘   │   │   │consider IVP   │
┌──────────────┐ Able to pass Foley?   └──► Hematuria?   └──────────────┘
│Cystourethrogram │ No   Yes   No
│followed by IVP; │   Yes   │   │
│consider placement│ ┌──────────────┐   >20 RBCs/HPF
│of suprapubic   │ │Cystourethrogram;│   Yes   No
│catheter   │ │consider IVP   │   │   │
└──────────────┘   └──────────────┘   ┌──────┐ Observe for 48 hours;
                                            │CT or │ may follow as outpt
                                            │IVP or│ if isolated injury.
                                            │US   │ Hematuria persistent?
                                            └──────┘   Yes   No
                                                        │
                                              ┌─────┐   ┌──────────────────┐
                                              │ IVP │   │ No further   │
                                              └─────┘   │ evaluation needed│
                                                        └──────────────────┘
```

**FIG. 25-1.** Algorithm for evaluating the trauma patient for genitourinary injury.

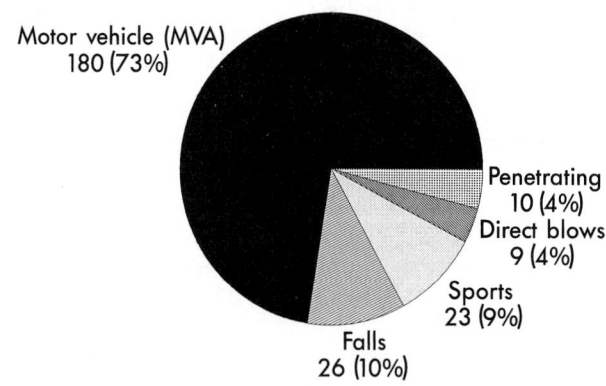

Motor vehicle (MVA)
180 (73%)

Penetrating
10 (4%)

Direct blows
9 (4%)

Sports
23 (9%)

Falls
26 (10%)

*from Cass AS. Urol 1983;21:487.*

**FIG. 25-2.** Renal injury in children: mechanism of trauma.

small, subcapsular, and nonexpanding and may have associated hematuria; urologic study findings are essentially normal. Grade II injuries include hematomas confined to the retroperitoneum and lacerations less than 1 cm in depth that do not result in urinary extravasation. Grade III injuries include lacerations into the perirenal fat greater than 1 cm in depth but not penetrating into the collecting system and having no urinary extravasation. Grade IV injuries include deep lacerations into the collecting system and renal vascular injury with contained hemorrhage.
```

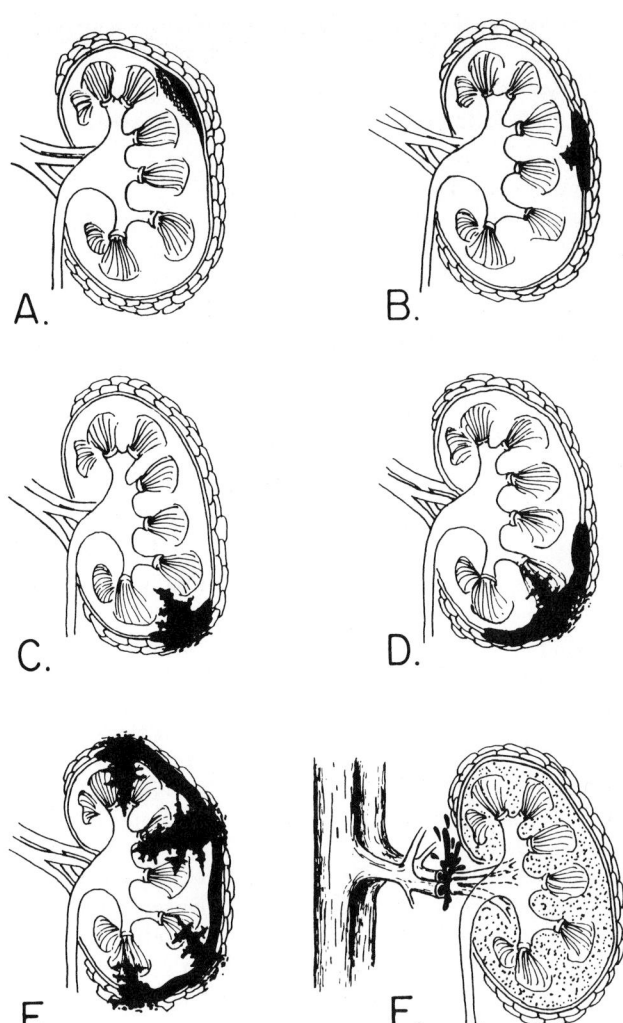

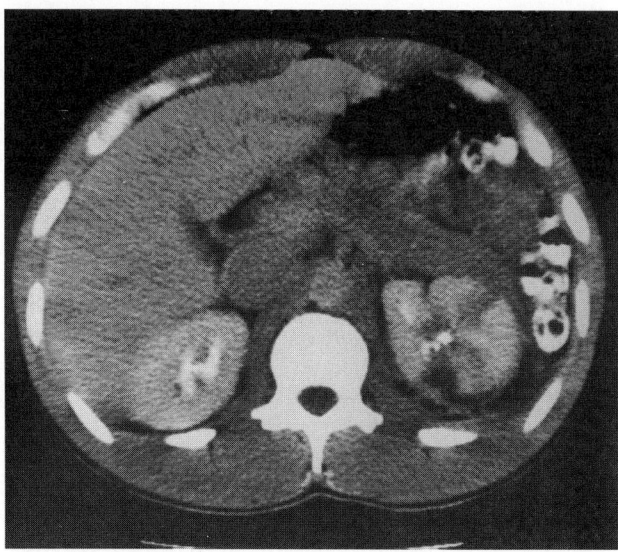

FIG. 25-4. Abdominal computed tomography scan revealing grade V (fracture) injury of the left kidney. (Courtesy Peter N. Bretan, Jr, MD)

FIG. 25-3. Grading of renal injury. **A,** Grade I: contusions, small lacerations. **B,** Grade II: contained lacerations. **C,** Grade III: lacerations into the perirenal fat, but not into the collecting system. **D,** Grade IV: lacerations into the collecting system. **E** and **F,** Grade V: fractured kidney or renal pedicle injury.

Grade V injuries include the shattered or fractured kidney (Fig. 25-4) and renal pedicle injuries that devascularize the kidney.

Diagnostic Findings

Clinical Findings. Injuries that include the head, liver, spleen, intestines, and pancreas are common, occurring in 40% to 70% of patients with blunt renal trauma and 80% of patients with penetrating renal trauma.[3,5,7,16,18,21] The more severe the renal injury, the more likely the patient is to have injured other organs.[18] Signs and symptoms of these associated injuries tend to dwarf those of renal injury. The emergency physician must therefore consider the possibility of concomitant renal injury in all multiple trauma patients.[17,18]

Hematuria occurs in up to 96% of cases.[24] Some authors have noted that the degree of hematuria in blunt trauma patients parallels the severity of injury; others have

not.[22,24,26-28] In particular, it is important to note that up to 50% of patients with renal pedicle injury may not experience hematuria.[20]

The entire clinical picture, including mechanism of injury, severity of associated injuries, and hemodynamic status of the patient, must be considered by the emergency physician in deciding how to investigate hematuria and possible renal injury in the pediatric trauma patient[29-31] (See Fig. 25-1). Sudden deceleration injuries from MVAs, falls, or direct blows to the flank are the most common mechanisms for blunt renal trauma and should alert the clinician to the possibility of underlying renal injury.[7] Although mechanism is an important clue to the actual underlying injury, it is not the sole factor in predicting the severity of injury.[27,29-31]

Signs and symptoms of renal trauma may be specific or subtle. Flank pain, tenderness, or hematoma (Grey Turner sign) or periumbilical ecchymosis (Cullen sign) may indicate urologic trauma or retroperitoneal hemorrhage.[4]

Complications. Within the first few weeks to months after renal trauma, complications such as renal failure secondary to acute tubular necrosis, delayed bleeding, urinary extravasation with sepsis, and abscess formation and hypertension (renin-mediated) may occur.[4,8,9] Delayed complications include hypertension, which can occur years after the traumatic event; arteriovenous fistula; chronic pyelonephritis; hydronephrosis; chronic pain and stone formation; chronic renal insufficiency; and pseudocyst formation.[4,8,9,17] An intravenous pyelogram (IVP) or computed tomography (CT) scan of the abdomen should be performed 3 to 6 months after the renal injury to evaluate renal anatomy.[4]

Ancillary Data. *Urinalysis* should be performed on every multiple-trauma patient as well as those in whom isolated renal injury is suspected. When there is traumatic injury, a urinary catheter should be inserted to obtain urine, once the stability of the pelvis is assured and the genitourinary and rectal examinations are completed. Urinary catheter insertion may cause only a small amount of hematuria (<4 red blood cells/high-powered field [RBCs/HPF]) in most patients.[32]

Assessment for hematuria is probably one of the most well-studied yet controversial aspects of the evaluation of the patient for GU tract injury. Hematuria of >20 RBCs/HPF has been reviewed retrospectively and prospectively and is an indicator of underlying renal injury but is present in many cases of nonsignificant injury as well.[20,28,33-39] Hematuria of >20 RBCs/HPF has been reviewed retrospectively and prospectively and is an indicator of underlying significant renal injury.[20,28,33-36] Nicolaisen prospectively studied 359 patients with blunt (306 [85%]) and penetrating (53 [15%]) injury. This study and others suggest that patients with microscopic hematuria without the presence of shock (systolic blood pressure <90 mm Hg) could be managed without radiographic evaluation, namely by IVP.[37,38] Radiographic evaluation was necessary for patients with gross hematuria, microscopic hematuria and shock, or penetrating trauma.[37] Cass later showed that major vascular injury might be overlooked if Nicolaisen's criteria were strictly applied and concluded that blunt trauma patients with <20 RBCs/HPF could be managed acutely without radiographic evaluation, but those with >20 RBCs/HPF in the urine, with or without shock, should be radiologically evaluated for renal injury.

Penetrating trauma to the trunk is another indication for radiologic evaluation of the genitourinary tract.[21,22,30,37,39-41] Hematuria may be absent in up to 29% of these patients. In addition, Scott found that the absence of physical findings (e.g., as flank mass or abdominal rigidity) did not exclude renal injury in cases of penetrating trauma to the abdomen.[21]

Anuria post trauma should also alert the clinician to a rare but significant injury, namely bilateral renal artery occlusion.[42]

In conclusion, radiographic evaluation of the kidney should be undertaken when the following factors are present: hematuria of >20 RBCs/HPF, microscopic hematuria with shock, gross hematuria, penetrating trauma to the abdomen, physical findings consistent with renal trauma, and a significant mechanism that warrants GU tract evaluation. A patient in whom hematuria develops after a minor mechanism should be considered for radiographic evaluation to rule out underlying congenital abnormality or tumor[15] (See Fig. 25-1).

CT scan of the abdomen has been well studied as a diagnostic modality in the detection of intraabdominal injury in the trauma patient.[16,24,43-55] Its accuracy is high (98%), and it is considered the diagnostic test of choice for the detection of renal injury in the stable pediatric trauma patient.[16,45-47,56]

The main advantage of CT scan over other diagnostic modalities in evaluating renal injury lies in the fact that it can delineate intraabdominal, retroperitoneal, and pelvic injuries simultaneously.* Since CT scan may overestimate the amount of extravasation, extravasation alone should not be used as an absolute indication for surgery.[16,24] CT scan

---

* References 16, 24, 31, 44, 48, 52, 57.

Indications for Abdominal CT Scan in the Evaluation of Genitourinary Injury

Stable patient
Gross hematuria
Microscopic hematuria >20 RBCs/HPF in the multiple trauma patient
Mechanism suggesting intraabdominal or renal injury
IVP result equivocal for injury or indicative of severe injury

CT, Computed tomography; *RBC/HPF,* red blood cells/high-powered field; *IVP,* intravenous pyelogram.

---

may be more practical in the evaluation of renovascular injuries than is arteriography, because of the former's ready availability and delineation of other abdominal anatomy.[24]

Nonionic agents when used as the contrast media decrease minor side effects and adverse reactions. Generally, nonionic contrast media is considered in children younger than 1 year of age, those with previous reactions or allergies to contrast media, as well as children who are unstable or have underlying medical problems including renal disease, diabetes, sickle cell anemia, heart or lung conditions, or dehydration.

The disadvantages of CT scanning are its high cost, lack of availability in all areas, and limited use to the stable pediatric patient.[12,16,54,55] CT scan is cost effective in the multiply injured patient but may not be warranted in cases where an IVP alone would be adequate, that is, in those patients in whom renal injury alone is suspected or only a minor mechanism of injury with subsequent hematuria.[15,16] Pediatric trauma patients who require immediate operative intervention should be evaluated in the operating room (OR) for renal injury by one-shot IVP or angiography, depending on the clinical situation.[30]

There is new interest in evaluating the stable patient with penetrating injury to the flank by CT scan.[24,48] Phillips showed that 52 of 56 patients (92%) suffering penetrating trauma to the flank could be managed nonoperatively after staging by contrast-enhanced CT enema. Presently, most clinicians still use IVP to evaluate renal and ureteral injury in the stable penetrating trauma patient.[9]

Indications for the use of CT scan of the abdomen in the evaluation of renal trauma in the pediatric patient are summarized in the box above.

The *intravenous pyelogram* (IVP) can be performed quickly in the emergency department or on the OR table and can give evidence of contralateral renal presence and function in cases of penetrating injury (see box on p. 359).[17]

However, the one-shot IVP may not show enough detail for interpretation in a significant number of cases; patients may have an allergic reaction to the contrast material; the IVP result may be falsely negative in renal pedicle injuries; and the study correlates to the injuries found at exploration in only 50% to 75% of cases.[8,17,27,43,57-60]

Indications for Emergency Intravenous Pyelogram (or Limited View IVP) in the Evaluation of GU Injury

GU injury alone suspected
Flank pain, hematoma, or ecchymosis
Penetrating trauma to the abdomen
Suspected ureteral injury
Patient too unstable to undergo CT scan for evaluation
Microscopic hematuria >20 RBCs/HPF
Gross hematuria

GU, Genitourinary; *CT*, computed tomography; *RBCs/HPF*, red blood cells/high-powered field.

Overall, the one-shot IVP may provide additional information on renal function that may be helpful in the patient's intraoperative management.[60]

The formal IVP can be reserved for stable patients with minor mechanisms and hematuria or in which isolated GU tract trauma is suspected.

IVP with tomography correlates well with the lesions seen at exploration or with selective angiography.[17] However a patient may be too unstable to undergo the procedure. For situations in which the patient must be rushed to the operating suite for other injuries, a limited view IVP may be helpful in demonstrating the presence of two functioning kidneys.[30,57]

The limited IVP is performed by giving contrast material (2.0 ml/kg [in adult, 100 ml]) of diatrizoate meglumine–diatrizoate sodium (Renograffin-60) or iopamidol/iohexol (1 to 2 ml/kg) and then taking an abdominal flat plate at 5 and 10 minutes.[61] This procedure may be performed in the emergency department or OR, depending on the stability of the patient.

Angiography is technically more difficult and may lead to more complications in the pediatric patient than the adult patient, so it must be reserved for those instances in which a potentially significant injury has not been clearly defined by either IVP or CT scan.[9,13,24] Digital subtraction angiography (DSA) is less invasive and can be performed by intravenous injection of contrast material. DSA and CT scan have virtually replaced angiography in the evaluation of renovascular injury in the pediatric patient.[9,24] As with other modalities, on arteriography, an injury may appear greater than the clinical condition warrants; therefore, operative management must depend on the clinical status of the patient as well.[17,24]

Retrograde pyelography is rarely used in the evaluation of traumatic genitourinary injury.[9] It may be indicated for evaluation of lesions at the level of the renal pelvis, such as ureteropelvic disruptions, if IVP findings are indeterminate.[17]

Ultrasound (US) is used extensively in other countries for the staging of renal trauma.[12,62,63] Although US is less accurate than CT, especially in the detection of renovascular injury, its use in the evaluation of pediatric renal trauma may be justified.[54] Filiatrault found that US in some settings may be preferred to CT scan for the initial evaluation of renal injury because US is readily available in most hospitals, it can be quickly performed, the machine can be transported easily to the emergency department or the intensive care unit, and does not require sedation of the child.

US is excellent for detecting perinephric and intraabdominal fluid collections and may be useful for locating shotgun pellets in the renal parenchyma or collecting system.[9,64]

The disadvantages of US include not providing information on renal function and the quality and interpretation of the test is operator dependent.[65] Because US does not require the use of contrast material or irradiation, for the pregnant trauma patient it may be an alternative method for evaluating renal injury.[64]

Radionuclide studies, in evaluation of renal injury, are used in conjunction with other diagnostic modalities, such as US or IVP.[24] They may be indicated when IVP reveals poor or no visualization of one or both kidneys.[24,66] Chopp staged 24 patients comparing high-dose IVP and renal scanning and found renal scanning more sensitive, 94% vs. 64%, in the detection of significant renal injury. Radionuclide scan results correlated well with results of arteriography.[66] Radionuclide scanning has an advantage over other modalities because it can be used for patients who are allergic to contrast material. Limitations of the radionuclide scan include lack of availability of the procedure 24 hours a day and the need to perform the procedure in an area of the hospital remote from the emergency department. It may be an alternate modality for the evaluation of renovascular injury in the pediatric trauma patient.[9,66]

Magnetic resonance imaging is not used in the evaluation of the GU tract as it has been shown to be inferior to US in the detection of perirenal fluid collections and to be less sensitive than CT in the detection of renal injury.[67]

A standard *trauma panel* is recommended, depending on the severity of trauma: complete blood cell count (CBC); levels of electrolytes, blood urea nitrogen (BUN), creatinine, glucose, and amylase; prothrombin time (PT); partial thromboplastin time (PTT); type; and screen. A hemoglobin (Hgb) may be useful; serial Hgb values are required for patient monitoring. Clinical signs of shock imply that the patient has ongoing blood loss regardless of the level of the Hgb.

A chest radiograph should determine the presence of hemothorax, pneumothorax, contusions, and rib fractures. In addition, lower rib fractures can be associated with genitourinary injury.[28] An anterior-posterior pelvis radiograph may detect pelvic fractures associated with injury to the upper and lower GU tract.[68] Abdominal flat plate or scout radiographs should be made before contrast studies of the GU tract. Findings such as loss of psoas shadows (retroperitoneal blood), abnormal spinal curvature (concave to the side of the injury), and lower rib or transverse process fractures may be clues to underlying renal injury.[6,17,56]

Differential Considerations. Abdominal pain or hematuria associated with multiple trauma may be secondary to a number of intraabdominal or GU tract injuries. A complete trauma examination should help the practitioner in pinpointing the cause of the pain or the hematuria. Hematuria may be secondary to injury in the ureter (rare in blunt trauma), urethra (blood at the meatus or abnormal prostate location), or bladder (pelvic fracture).

Management. The management of renal injury must begin with the assessment and treatment of life-threatening injury first. The basic tenets of trauma care must be followed, including appropriate airway and cervical spine stabilization, ventilatory support as needed, and aggressive volume replacement with crystalloid (20 ml/kg) and blood products (10 ml/kg pRBCs) when shock is present. The source of the blood loss must be investigated quickly, and the kidney and renal pedicle must be considered.

The need for immediate surgery for renal injury depends on the correct staging of the injury, the hemodynamic status of the patient, and other associated injuries.[4,7,9] Cass found that of 36 children with severe renal injury, 89% required laparotomy for associated intraabdominal injury. Immediate surgery is indicated for hemodynamic instability, renal pedicle injury, and expanding retroperitoneal or pulsatile hematoma; surgery, may be indicated for laceration of the kidney with extensive extravasation.[3,24,69,70]

In cases of blunt renal trauma, mild injuries, such as contusions and small lacerations without urinary extravasation, are common (85% of renal injuries are grades I, II, and III). Management of these injuries is conservative. Generally all of these patients do well and do not develop long-term complications.[5,71,72]

The area of controversy lies in the management of moderate to severe renal injuries (grades IV and V).* Some authors advocate early surgical intervention; others do not.[6,7,9,17,72-79] Moderate injuries to the kidney can be managed without early operative intervention, depending on the degree of extravasation, stability of the patient, underlying renal anatomy, and degree of renal impairment.[4,7,9,78,80] The most severe renal injuries, grade V, are rare (3%), and their treatment is less controversial. Exploration and either nephrectomy of the fractured kidney or repair of a renal pedicle injury are recommended in most cases, even though results of revascularization are generally poor.[5,75,76] Conservative management of moderate to severe renal injuries has been challenged because of the high risk of subsequent complications, including hypertension in more than 50% of patients and delayed nephrectomy in more than 40%.[4,7,8,77] Overall, the management of moderate and some severe renal injuries must be individualized. Early consultation with the trauma surgeon, pediatric surgeon, and urologist is paramount to determine the most appropriate course of action for the management of the severely injured patient.[5]

Whitney's study of 81 penetrating renal injuries noted that minor injuries to the kidney could be treated conservatively without operative intervention. All major injuries involving urinary extravasation or hemodynamic instability required surgery.[22,76]

Disposition. All patients with significant renal injury or a significant mechanism of injury should be admitted. Most who have moderate to severe renal injury have other associated injuries that require admission, observation, and, often, surgery.[7] Patients who have a minor amount of hematuria and minor mechanism without associated injuries may be sent home after a period of observation (4 hours).[25] All patients should be reevaluated within 24 hours if they have any degree of hematuria or did not undergo a diagnostic evaluation for their hematuria during their ED visit. If the hematuria persists, an IVP should be performed to rule out structural or functional abnormalities (See Fig. 25-1).

Ureteral Injury

Injury to the ureter is uncommon in children; it occurs in less than 5% of patients who have GU tract injury.[4]

Mechanism of Injury. Injury to the ureter may result from blunt or penetrating trauma.[4,8,9,81,82] The greatest majority of ureteral injuries however are iatrogenic.[4] This type of ureteral injury is less common in children than in adults because lack of pelvic and retroperitoneal fat makes the ureter easier to identify.[9] The distal ureter may be injured during urologic or gynecologic procedures. Colonic and vascular surgery is responsible for injuries to the proximal ureter.

Penetrating trauma is by far the most common external mechanism resulting in ureteral injury.[83] Gunshot wounds are the primary agent of injury in over 90% of cases; stab wounds rarely cause ureteral injury.[4,8,82,83]

Blunt trauma must be massive to cause injury to the ureter.[9,84,85] This is generally demonstrated by avulsion of the ureteropelvic junction.[84] Although this injury is uncommon, ureteral avulsion primarily occurs in children.[84-86] Most often the right ureter is avulsed.[9,84] Children have a greater capacity to flex laterally in the upper and lower spine, causing the ureter to be stretched across the transverse processes or compressed against the lower ribs, resulting in ureteropelvic disruption.[9,85]

Diagnostic Findings

Clinical Findings. Signs and symptoms of ureteral injury are generally absent immediately postinjury. As time passes, nonspecific complaints (e.g., fever, ileus, hematuria, and flank or abdominal pain) may appear as evidence of the ureteral injury.[8] In the case of ureteropelvic disruption, patients may only demonstrate initial hemodynamic instability and may not have a hematoma within Gerota fascia at the time of exploratory laparotomy.[87]

Hematuria is an unreliable sign; it occurs in at most two thirds of patients but may be absent in more than 40% of patients with ureteral injury.[4,9,81] Ureteral injury is often discovered during evaluation for other associated traumatic injuries.[82]

Complications. Complications of ureteral injury are directly related to the delay in making the diagnosis.[4,9,82] Nephrectomy rates increase from 4% to as high as 32% in patients in whom ureteral injury was not recognized for days after the injury.[4,83] Other complications include fistula, stricture, and abscess formation.[8,9]

Ancillary Data. Some authors have reported greater than 90% accuracy of the IVP in detecting injuries to the ureter making IVP the diagnostic test of choice in evaluating injury.[4,8] Brandes et al recently reported on 12 patients with ureteral injury from penetrating trauma. IVP was

---

* References 4, 5, 7, 9, 17, 24, 72-74.

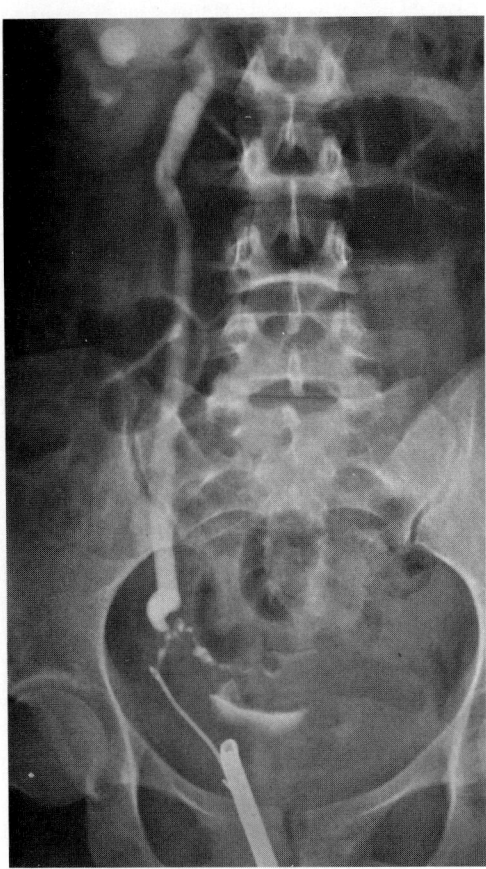

FIG. 25-5. Retrograde pyelogram demonstrates transection of the right ureter (iatrogenic injury) with extravasation of dye into the pelvis. (Courtesy Ines Boechat, MD)

nondiagnostic in 75% of the cases and misleading in one case.[81] The IVP if positive (extravasation) for injury is helpful, but if negative, the clinician must consider exploration of the ureter if there is a high level of suspicion for possible injury.

Retrograde pyelogram, although not useful in the initial evaluation of the trauma patient for GU tract injury, helps to determine the level of injury to the ureter once the injury has been detected by IVP[9] (Fig. 25-5).

CT scan is used in most multiple trauma cases for evaluation of intraabdominal injury. Although it is difficult to evaluate the integrity of the ureter on CT scan, occasionally CT findings may indicate ureteral injury. CT findings of ureteropelvic injury have been described by Kenney; they include medial perirenal space contrast extravasation with no evidence of injury to the renal parenchyma and no further opacification of the ureter distal to the level of injury. Otherwise injury to the ureter may be indicated by the presence of fluid on CT scan in the interfascial, anterior pararenal, and periureteral spaces.[88,89] Exploration of the ureter may be the only reliable way to detect injury.[81]

Obtaining a *urinalysis* for all trauma patients is important in alerting the physician to injury in the genitourinary tract. Since the absence of hematuria is not infrequent in

patients with ureteral injury, the emergency physician must consider the possibility of ureteral injury in evaluating patients who have significant blunt trauma or penetrating injuries to the trunk and pelvis.[4]

Diagnostic Considerations. Injury to the ureter is not infrequently noted late in the patient's course of treatment when being evaluated for fever, sepsis, or abdominal pain.

Management. Emergency department management of the patient with ureteral injury generally focuses on therapy for associated life-threatening injury. When the diagnosis of ureteral injury is made, management is by surgical repair.[4,9,82-86]

Repair of the injured ureter is very successful when the injury is immediately recognized.[9,82] The type of repair of the injured ureter depends on the level of injury.[84,85] Direct anastomosis of the ends can be considered in injuries above the pelvic rim. Other alternatives should be considered when direct anastomosis is not possible, including those outlined by Godec: nephrostomy, cross-abdominal ureteroureterostomy, replacement of ureter with ileum, and autotransplantation on the ipsilateral or contralateral side. Below the pelvic rim, injury to the ureter may be reapproximated to the bladder.[4]

Disposition. All patients with ureteral injury require admission for surgical management.[9]

Bladder Injury

Bladder injuries represent 22% of all urologic injuries.[4] Approximately one fourth of these patients are less than 18 years of age.[90] Associated injuries occur in more than 90% patients with bladder injury and are often the cause of mortality in these patients.[90,91] Pelvic fracture is the most common associated injury, occurring in 73% to 84% of patients.[90,92]

Pathophysiology. The apex and lateral portions of the bladder are well protected within the pelvis; however, bony fragments from a compressed pelvis can cause injury to the bladder. The dome of the bladder is relatively unprotected and can explode when subjected to blunt force, especially when the bladder is full. This latter mechanism is more common in the pediatric age group as a result of the more abdominal position of the bladder.[9]

Mechanism of Injury. Blunt external trauma is the cause of most bladder injury, especially in children.[9,90-92] Cass found 83.5% secondary to traffic collision, 5% to falls, 5% to assault or direct blows, and 1% to sports injury. Penetrating trauma as a cause of bladder injury is less common, occurring in 4% to 14% of all patients.[90,92] Although over 80% of cases of bladder injury with rupture are associated with pelvic fractures, only 19% of pelvic fractures have an associated bladder injury.[91] Bladder rupture may occur with any type of pelvic fracture, no matter how minor the fracture appears.[90] There is a reported increase in the incidence of bladder rupture with anterior arch fractures and this incidence increased proportionately to the number of fractures to the pubic ramus.[93]

Iatrogenic injury and spontaneous rupture of the bladder may occur.[4,9]

High-risk procedures for resultant bladder injury include herniorrhaphy, cystoscopy, and umbilical vessel catheterization.[9]

Diagnostic Findings

Clinical Findings. More than 90% of patients with bladder rupture have hematuria.[4,91] Microscopic hematuria is associated with bladder contusion and gross hematuria with bladder rupture.[90] Gross hematuria in the initial or subsequent bladder effluent indicates urologic injury and must be investigated by cystography even if the urine clears.[40,93,94] Cass found no hematuria in 9% of patients with bladder rupture. Patients may not be able to void, and little or no urine may be obtained when a urinary catheter (Foley) is placed. In acute cases of extravasation, urine causes no peritoneal irritation, so abdominal pain may be absent initially. Generally patients have abdominal or pelvic pain, which may be related to associated intraabdominal injury or pelvic fractures. As time passes, the urine may become infected, resulting in peritoneal irritation, or it may be absorbed, leading to an elevated BUN level in the serum.[95]

Bladder injuries can be divided into contusion, intraperitoneal rupture, extraperitoneal rupture, or a combination of intraperitoneal and extraperitoneal rupture.[4] Cass found in his series of 417 patients with bladder trauma that contusion was common, occurring in 67% of the patients; it was followed by extraperitoneal rupture (18%), intraperitoneal rupture (13%), and both types (2%).

Complications. Mortality rate resulting from bladder rupture has been reported at from 11% to 44%.[90] Cass notes a mortality rate of 20%; a delay in diagnosis increased the rate. Early recognition of bladder injury is vitally important to prevent morbidity and mortality. Other complications include persistent hematuria, sepsis, and renal failure.[90]

Ancillary Data. The radiographic method of choice to diagnose bladder injury is the cystogram.[96,97] The accuracy of a cystogram in determining bladder injury is high: it detects 96% to 100% of injuries.[91,96,97] False-negative cystogram results may occur if the bladder is underfilled or the injury is secondary to penetrating trauma.[8,9] An IVP alone may demonstrate a bladder rupture about 15% of the time; a normal IVP result is insufficient to evaluate bladder injury.[92]

A *CT scan* of the abdomen may be performed on the patient who has multiple traumatic injury when intraabdominal or pelvic injury is suspected; however, CT scan may not be sensitive or specific enough to detect bladder injury.[96] Just as with a cystogram, the bladder must be distended to obtain accurate results on the CT scan.[96] A retrograde CT cystogram is an option to standard cystography and may offer several advantages to conventional cystography in the patient who requires a CT scan of the abdomen and pelvis.[40,98] Advantages include minimizing patient movement and decreasing the number of examinations necessary in the GU tract evaluation.[98] As with standard cystography, the bladder should be adequately distended during the examination. Disadvantages of the procedure are (1) emergency physicians and radiologists lack experience in its use, and (2) interpretation of the results is dependent on the skill of the radiologist.

Contusions may be demonstrated on cystogram by a teardrop shape or elevation of the bladder from perivesical hematoma and by the absence of extravasation of contrast material.[4,92] Extraperitoneal rupture occurs when the bladder is lacerated, often by fragments from pelvic fractures below the level of the pelvic peritoneum. Cystogram and postvoid films reveal a typical "sunburst" appearance of extravasation outside the peritoneal cavity.[4,92] Intraperitoneal rupture occurs with blunt force to the lower abdomen or pelvis when the bladder is full. Cystogram shows extravasation in the peritoneal cavity around the bowel, outlining the intraabdominal organs, or in the pericolic gutters[4,9,95] (Fig. 25-6).

Indications for a *retrograde cystogram* are outlined in the box on p. 363. A cystogram is often preceded by a urethrogram. Urethral injury should always be ruled out before a urinary catheter or feeding tube is placed in the bladder.

The procedure for performing a *cystourethrogram* in children is outlined in the box on p. 363. There are some important points to be made about the procedure that will prevent complications. First, the procedure should be performed fluoroscopically so that the bladder is not overfilled; second, the penis should never be compressed to obtain better filling during the urethrogram portion of the test. In the cases where urethral injury is not suspected and a urinary catheter is placed into the bladder, a voiding cystourethrogram can be made. Once bladder or urethral injury is ruled out, an IVP or CT scan should be performed to evaluate the patient for ureteral and renal injury as indicated.

Urinalysis should be performed for all patients with suspected bladder injury. Hematuria is found in at least 90% of cases and is gross in more than 50% of patients who experience bladder rupture.[90]

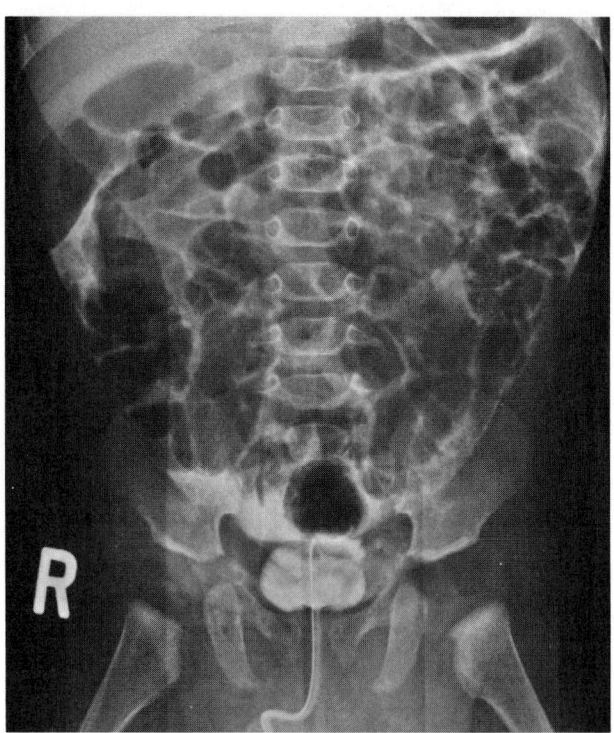

FIG. 25-6. Retrograde cystogram demonstrating intraperitoneal bladder rupture with extravasation in peritoneal cavity and under the liver in a 5-month-old child. (Courtesy Ines Boechat, MD)

Indications for a Cystogram in the Pediatric Trauma Patient

Penetrating trauma when lower GU tract injury is suspected

Pelvic fracture with hematuria, lower abdominal pain, or inability to void

Lower abdominal or perineal trauma with hematuria

Inability to void

Gross hematuria

GU, Genitourinary.

Procedure for Retrograde Cystourethrogram in the Pediatric Trauma Patient

1. Obtain plain film of the pelvis.
2. Place a urinary catheter or feeding tube (no. 5 Fr, newborn, or no. 8 Fr, infant and child) into the urethral meatus, assuming no gross blood is noted.
3. If the catheter can be advanced gently, do so; otherwise stop advancing, pull back slightly, and continue under fluoroscopic guidance. Begin injection of no more than 10 ml of Renograffin-60, watching for extravasation. If there is extravasation in the urethra, stop the procedure and obtain immediate urologic consultation. If there is no extravasation, the catheter may be placed into the bladder.
4. With fluoroscopic guidance, begin further injection of Cystograffin, to fill the bladder until the patient spontaneously voids, has the urge to void, or extravasation is noted. Note: In an adult, the bladder should be filled with at least 300 ml Cystograffin (400 ml is preferable) in order to rule out extravasation.
5. Obtain AP pelvis film with the bladder full.
6. Allow the bladder to drain; then obtain a postdrainage film. A cross-table lateral film may also be helpful to delineate extravasation.

AP, Anteroposterior.

Diagnostic Considerations. In cases of gross hematuria the entire urinary tract should be evaluated, including cystourethrogram followed by CT scan.[96]

Management. Management of bladder injury is the least controversial type of GU tract management, beginning with the principles outlined in Chapter 19.[4] This chapter also assesses injury of the GU tract, including the bladder. Once the type of bladder injury is defined, management is straightforward. Patients with contusions to the bladder, without serious associated injury, may be allowed to void spontaneously and receive close follow-up observation by a urologist.[90] Other patients with contusions and associated injury and those with small extraperitoneal ruptures can

generally be managed by urethral or suprapubic drainage for 7 to 14 days.[3,4,8,9,90-92,95,99]

Suprapubic drainage is preferred by Livne in extraperitoneal ruptures in male infants to preclude the need for long-term catheter drainage. Larger extraperitoneal rupture with extravasation may require surgical debridement of a bone spicule from a pelvic fracture and repair of the bladder laceration.[9,92,100] Patients with intraperitoneal bladder rupture are managed surgically: the ruptured bladder is repaired and adequate vesical drainage assured.[3,8,9,90,91]

DPL may be helpful in determining the presence of intraperitoneal extravasated urine; Rubin measured serum and lavage fluid urea nitrogen and creatinine levels in dogs after urine was instilled into the intraperitoneal cavity. When lavage fluid urea nitrogen and creatinine levels exceeds serum levels, intraperitoneal urine extravasation should be suspected.[95]

Disposition. Patients with contusions and without associated injury may be discharged and followed closely. Caution must be exercised in all such cases to evaluate the patient thoroughly for other injuries as associated injury is high. Admission, operative repair, and supportive care constitute the appropriate management of the multiply injured patient with bladder injury.

EXTERNAL GENITOURINARY STRUCTURES

Urethral Injury

Urethral injury in the pediatric age group is less common than in the adult population because of the flexibility to the pelvis.[101,102]

Pathophysiology. The anterior urethra (bulbar and penile portions) extends from the inferior border of the urogenital diaphragm to the urethral meatus. The anterior urethra in males is injured by direct blows to the perineum or straddle-type injury.[9,103]

The posterior urethra extends from the superior border of the urogenital diaphragm to the neck of the bladder. The posterior male urethra (prostatic and membranous) is injured more frequently than the anterior urethra.[9,104] The membranous urethra may be injured in its path through the urogenital diaphragm, and the prostatic urethra may be injured at its attachment to the posterior surface of the symphysis pubis by the puboprostatic ligaments or at its attachment to the neck of the bladder. Injury to the posterior urethra may occur when the bladder is pulled upward, causing tension and shearing force on the urethra.[103] Blood and urine may be extravasated into the pelvis.

The female urethra is rarely injured.[9,105,106] If the blunt force is severe enough, the female urethra may be injured at its attachment to the bladder neck and vaginal septum (vesicourethrovaginal septum).[9]

Mechanism of Injury. MVAs with direct blows to the perineum are the mechanism of injury in 79% of cases; straddle injuries cause the remainder of injuries.[61,100] Pelvic fractures are found in patients with posterior urethral injury in more than 90% of cases, and urethral injury occurs in 4% to 25% of cases of pelvic fractures.[68,100,101,107,108] Penetrating trauma is far less common but may cause anterior or posterior urethral injury.[104,109]

Diagnostic Findings

Clinical Findings. Patients with urethral injury have difficulty or inability to void.[61] Blood is present at the urethral meatus in more than 90% of patients with urethral injury.[61,103] Physical examination may also reveal abdominal pain or instability of the pelvis with compression. Rectal examination may reveal a high-riding, floating, or boggy prostate.

Anterior urethral injuries result in the extravasation of blood and urine into the scrotum, perineum, or anterior abdominal wall, which can be recognized by edema and discoloration extending into the scrotum.[103] If the extravasation is confined to Buck fascia, edema and discoloration are confined to the penis.[103]

Associated injuries to the skull, spleen, ribs, diaphragm, and extremities have been reported in addition to the most common associated injury, fracture of the pelvis.[100,102]

The female urethra is short and mobile and generally escapes urethral injury.[105] If it is injured, it is usually at its attachment to the bladder neck.[105,106,109] Vaginal lacerations are associated with urethral injury in girls because of the close association of the urethra and the vagina. Therefore, in the female trauma patient inability to void or vaginal bleeding may indicate urethral injury.[105,106]

Complications. Mortality secondary to urethral injury alone is rare.[100] Anterior urethral injuries are less likely to be associated with injuries other than posterior urethral injuries.[102] Traumatic urethrovaginal fistula has been reported in females after blunt injury to the urethra.[110] Mortality rates greater than 30% have been reported in patients with posterior urethral injury and are almost invariably secondary to injuries of other organ systems.[102] Complications after urethral repair may include stricture, diverticula, fistulas, incontinence (2%), and impotence (10%).[9,103]

Ancillary Data. The patient generally is unable to void, the clinician is unable to pass a urethral catheter, and the patient may have blood at the urethral meatus or have gross hematuria.[4] Catheterization of the urethra, when urethral injury is suspected, is contraindicated as the passage of the catheter may change a partial tear to a complete one.[4,9,61] The incidence of partial vs. complete tears is difficult to determine as some of the reported complete tears may have been partial initially.[111] Webster reports that about 66% of the injuries to the prostatomembranous urethra are complete.

Retrograde urethrogram is the radiologic method of choice for diagnosis of urethral injury in the pediatric trauma patient.[40,61,112] Indications for urethrography are outlined in the box above. Extravasation indicates a partial tear (if contrast medium is seen in the bladder) or complete tear (no contrast medium in the bladder).[103] If there is no extravasation, the urinary catheter (Foley) can be gently advanced into the bladder and a cystogram should follow to rule out injury to the urinary bladder.[61]

CT scan is neither sensitive nor specific in detecting urethral injury.[113]

Management. Anterior urethral injury is generally not associated with other severe injuries, so primary repair or in some cases suprapubic drainage with delayed repair is recommended.[102-104] In the case of posterior urethral injury, the management is controversial. Instead of primary

---

Indications for Urethrogram in the Pediatric Trauma Patient
Penetrating trauma when lower GU tract injury is suspected
Lower abdominal or perineal trauma with hematuria
Blood at the urethral meatus
Inability to void
High-riding or boggy prostate indicated by rectal examination
Swelling, ecchymosis, or hematoma of the perineum or penis
Vaginal laceration or bleeding in a multiple trauma patient
Inability to advance a urinary catheter
GU, Genitourinary.

---

repair or splinting, many investigators recommend suprapubic drainage of the bladder followed by repair of the urethral injury several months later when the patient is stable and other pelvic abnormality resolved.* Primary repair of the injured urethra over a silicone (Silastic) catheter or over a Foley catheter[116] has also been done.[102,108,117]

Malek reported on seven boys with posterior urethral injury repaired primarily who were followed for more than 8 years and experienced no stricture or impotence. In contrast, the adult literature reports stricture rates of 69%, impotence rates of 44%, and incontinence rates of 20% after primary realignment of the posterior urethra.[111] Webster in his review of the literature of prostatomembranous urethral injuries recommends immediate surgical intervention with pelvic hematoma evacuation and urethral repair in cases of "severe prostatourethral dislocation" with a "pie-in-the-sky" bladder, concomitant rectal tear, and bladder neck injury, as the bladder neck is important in preserving continence. Otherwise, suprapubic cystostomy and delayed repair are recommended.[111]

Disposition. Patients who have anterior and posterior urethral injury generally require immediate assessment and treatment of associated injuries and prompt urologic consultation. Because of the high rate of injury associated with posterior urethral injury, many of these patients require surgical intervention and intensive care.

Scrotal and Testicular Injury

Trauma to the scrotum and testicles is not uncommon; injury to the testicles requiring surgical intervention is relatively rare in children because of the small size and mobility of the testicles.[9] Testicular torsion, torsion of the testicular appendages, testicular dislocation, epididymitis, hematocele, and testicular rupture have all been reported after trauma to the scrotum.[9,117-125]

Mechanism of Injury. Testicular injury may result from a direct blow to the testicle or a straddle injury in which

---

* References, 3, 100, 102, 103, 107, 111, 114, 115.

the testicle is forced against the hard surface of the symphysis pubis.[9,120,121] Trauma to the testicles and scrotum may result from birth trauma as well.[126] Tiwary's prospective study of 166 male breech deliveries noted that of the 134 infants delivered vaginally, 6.5% had testicular injury; physical examination of up to 30% of these injured infants revealed normal testes up to 4 years later. Other mechanisms of injury have been described, including testicular torsion caused by riding a racing bicycle with a long, narrow saddle and injuries to the scrotum and testis from BMX bicycle handlebars.[123,127] Donovan and Kaplan have reported on two cases of dog bite to the external genitalia in males.[128]

Diagnostic Findings

Clinical Findings. The challenge to the emergency physician in cases of trauma to the scrotum is to determine whether the patient may have suffered testicular dislocation, testicular torsion, or testicular rupture. All of these conditions are rare but must be diagnosed promptly to maintain fertility.[119,123,124]

Approximately 49 cases of traumatic testicular *dislocation* have been reported in the literature.[119] Dislocation of the testis occurs when the testicle is forcibly displaced from its anatomic position, usually as a result of a high-speed motorcycle accident or, in the case of children, of a forcible upward blow to the scrotum, such as occurs in a straddle-type injury.[118] Children are unlikely to dislocate their testes because of a brisk cremasteric reflex, which acts as a protective mechanism against dislocation, and the relative small size of the testes. The patient with testicular dislocation may experience nausea, vomiting, and scrotal pain.[118,119] An empty hemiscrotum or a testis palpated in another location is found by physical examination.[118] The dislocated testis may be found in any of a number of ectopic locations: superior inguinal, pubic, preputial, penile, abdominal, deep inguinal, acetabular, crural, perineal, or compound (testis extruded outside the scrotum).[118] Often the diagnosis is delayed several days or longer because of other associated injuries.[118,119] If closed reduction of the testis is unsuccessful, then surgical intervention to evaluate the integrity of the testis and to place it into normal anatomic position in the scrotum is required.[118] Results of relocation of the testis have been rewarding since spermatic function and fertility have a good chance of being normal.[118]

The exact mechanism that causes the testicle to *torse* after trauma is controversial but may relate to the abnormal relationship between the tunica vaginalis and the testis and epididymis ("bell-clapper" deformity) or a cremasteric reflex that causes rotation of the mobile testis. Although some authors question the role of trauma in causing torsion of the testis, reports of torsion after scrotal trauma provide compelling evidence.[122,123]

Testicular *rupture* is caused by the testis being forced against the pubic bone, tearing the tunica albuginea and allowing extrusion of seminiferous tissue.[120,121] The patient is able to continue with regular activities for several hours, later noting the onset of pain and scrotal swelling.[120,121]

The patient with trauma to the scrotum experiences edema, ecchymosis, and tenderness of the testis on palpation. It is difficult to assess whether pain on palpation of the testis is secondary to soft tissue injury with a hematocele or testicular torsion or rupture. Testicles with a transverse lie that are high-riding may be torsed.[122]

Ancillary Data. Ultrasonography is a valuable tool in the evaluation of the patient with scrotal trauma.[129-133] A number of case reports have shown its accuracy in distinguishing hematoceles and abscesses from testicular ruptures.[132] Radionuclide scan with ^{99m}technetium pertechnetate is the procedure of choice for the evaluation of testicular torsion after trauma.[130]

Differential Considerations. The differential examination for an enlarged and tender scrotum after scrotal trauma is extensive and includes hematoma, hematocele, pyocele, hydrocele, epididymitis, torsion of the testis or testicular appendage, and rupture of the testis (see Chapter 60).[131]

Management. Patients with significant blunt trauma to the testis first require evaluation by ultrasound to evaluate the integrity of the testis, then radionuclide imaging to rule out torsion. All cases of testicular rupture and torsion require urologic consultation and management. If the testicle is found to be viable, the torsion is reduced and bilateral orchiopexy is performed.[122] If the testicle is necrotic at exploration, orchiectomy and contralateral orchiopexy are performed.[126] Testicular rupture is repaired by excision of the necrotic seminiferous tubules as necessary and suturing of the torn tunica albuginea.[121] Orchiectomy may be necessary in 6% to 30% of patients with testicular rupture.[121]

Disposition. When individuals have suffered scrotal trauma and the emergency physician believes that rupture and torsion are unlikely, management entails bedrest and close urologic follow-up observation. Patients with large, tender, or expanding scrotal hematomas have a testicular rupture until proven otherwise; ultrasound is performed to evaluate the nature of the hematoma and integrity of the testis. Testicular torsion requires radionuclide scan and urologic consultation.

Penile Injury

The most common cause of injury to the penis are complications arising from circumcision.[9] Other noniatrogenic causes are falls, sports injuries, direct blows to the perineum, zipper entrapment of the foreskin, and tourniquet injuries.[9,134,135] The large majority of penile injuries are minor abrasions and can be managed expectantly. Rarely, soft tissue injuries of the perineum may include the penis and be extensive, requiring aggressive volume replacement, surgical debridement, and skin grafting.[136] Associated urethral and bladder injury must be considered and evaluated by cystourethrogram, as appropriate. Urinalysis should routinely be performed.

Lacerations involving the penis can be sutured after proper anesthesia.[9] A penile block is performed by injecting 1% lidocaine without epinephrine in a circumferential fashion around the base of the penis.[137] Patients with penile lacerations may have injured the urethra. If marked penile swelling, ecchymosis, or meatal blood is present or the patient is unable to void, a urethrogram is indicated, as is urologic consultation.

Fracture of the penis is uncommon and generally occurs during sexual intercourse when the erect penis is forced

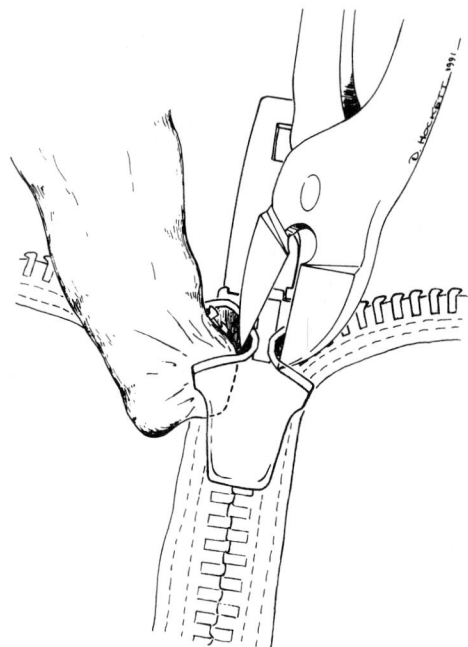

FIG. 25-7. Bone cutter shown cutting the median bar of the zipper, releasing the foreskin entrapment.

against a hard object such as the thigh or pubis of the partner.[138,139] The patient hears a cracking sound, which is followed by pain, swelling, and deformity of the shaft of the penis.[138,139] The fracture occurs in the corpora cavernosa and, rarely, can involve the urethra.[138-140] Management may be conservative but often involves primary surgical repair of the torn corpora.[139,141]

Zipper injuries to the foreskin occur when an uncircumcised male zips up his pants quickly, entrapping the foreskin.[9,134,135,142] The male is often young, between 3 and 6 years of age, and quite uncomfortable on presentation to the ED. The zipper can be easily removed from the foreskin by splitting the median bar of the zipper mechanism with bone cutters (Fig. 25-7).[134,135] The zipper with the fastener intact then falls apart, allowing its removal from the foreskin. This procedure causes very little pain, so local anesthesia is not required; the child may be very anxious and sedation or restraint may be necessary. Another described method requires soaking the part of the zipper on the penis in mineral oil before removal.[143]

Tourniquet injuries may occur in young infants when a band of hair becomes entrapped in the coronal groove.[9] The infant has balanitis, paraphimosis, or cellulitis of the area; injuries to the corpora and urethra may occur.[9]

As with other injuries occurring in children, the emergency physician must always consider the possibility of sexual or physical abuse (see Chapter 45). Children of toilet-training age may be at particular risk for genital injury from frustrated parents or caretakers.[9] Toilet seats may fall or be pushed against the shaft of the penis, or the penis may be bruised when pinched by the parent as a punishment for toilet-training "accidents." Burns to the perineum, unusual mechanisms of injury, physical examination suggesting previous injury, or history elicited from the child or another source of possible abuse constitutes evidence of child abuse and needs to be reported to child protective services and law enforcement agencies.[144]

Perineal Trauma in Girls

Perineal trauma in girls is not uncommon and may present with vulvar hematomas, vaginal tears or lacerations, or urethral, rectal, or bladder injuries.[144-146] It is important that the clinician evaluate the mechanism of trauma and subsequent injuries to estimate the likelihood of whether the injuries were secondary to child abuse.

Straddle injuries from the bar of a bicycle or other object that strikes the perineal area generally are minor.[9,145] At times the force is severe enough to cause a vulvar hematoma.[145] Small vulvar hematomas can be managed with icepack alone. If a hematoma is large enough or continues to increase in size, the area should be incised, the clot removed, and the area packed loosely. Prophylactic broad-spectrum antibiotics are recommended, and the patient should be followed closely. Sitz baths may allow the further drainage of serosanguinous material and increase patient comfort. An x-ray examination of the pelvis should be obtained, looking for fractures. If the patient is unable to void, then a urethrogram followed by a cystogram may be warranted. A suprapubic catheter may be necessary to allow urinary drainage.

Occasionally the vulvar or vaginal area may be injured by a child while masturbating.[145] These injuries are manifested as minor scratches or abrasions that may become secondarily infected. If severe lacerations or bruising is noted, the practitioner must consider sexual abuse as a possibility and the child should be treated and the incident reported to child protective services and law enforcement agencies.[144]

Vaginal trauma may result from penetrating trauma to the perineum or rarely from severe blunt injury to the pelvis.[146,147] Penetrating injuries to the vagina more commonly are caused by objects that penetrate the hymenal opening, generally causing small vaginal tears.[145] If the laceration is large enough or high in the vaginal vault, the child may enter the emergency department in shock.[145] Aggressive fluid resuscitation and repair of the laceration with ligation of the bleeding vessel are needed. If the penetration extends into the peritoneal cavity, the child may have peritoneal signs. The bleeding may also occur in the retroperitoneal space, causing a large retroperitoneal hematoma.[145] For major injuries such as these, the emergency physician must consider concomitant injury to the urethra, bladder, or ureter. Provided the patient can be stabilized with volume replacement, a cystourethrogram followed by IVP can rule out injury to the GU tract. In all cases of severe vaginal penetrating injury, caused by GSW, SW, or foreign bodies, a surgeon should be consulted early in the resuscitation.

Sexual abuse (see Chapter 45) is an ever-increasing problem in our society.[144] It has been estimated that one in five girls is sexually abused during childhood.[145] Fortunately most of the injuries to the female genital tract from sexual abuse are minor. These injuries are caused by rubbing or fondling; physical examination may show swelling, erythema, ecchymoses, or excoriations.[146] Injuries to the perineum that are not adequately explained by the history, a history of possible abuse from the child or other source, or other physical evidence of abuse obligate the care provider to report the incident to child protective and law enforcement services.

Complications of urinary retention, secondary infection, and urinary tract infection may result from minor injuries to the vulva or vagina. More severe injuries may be associated with injury to peritoneal contents and the lower GU tract.

Sexually transmitted disease must be considered in all patients when sexual abuse is suspected. Although prophylactic antibiotics are not recommended for children who disclose that they have been sexually assaulted, documented infection must be treated with the appropriate antibiotic regimen (see Chapter 53).[146]

PELVIC FRACTURES AND INJURY TO THE GENITOURINARY TRACT

GU injury is often associated with pelvic fractures; because of the flexibility of the pelvis in children, they experience less associated GU injury than adults.[101,115] Fractures to the pelvis in children are generally caused by blunt trauma from motor vehicle–pedestrian accidents (see Chapters 27 and 30).[118]

There is about a 4% incidence of bladder rupture and a 6% incidence of renal laceration or contusion. In a report in 1980 of 120 children with pelvic fractures, no cases of urethral injury were noted; one case of posterior urethral disruption was subsequently reported. Perineal, vaginal, and rectal injuries were significant, occurring in 3% to 7% of patients with pelvic fractures.[101] The adult literature reports a higher incidence of pelvic fracture and associated GU tract injury.[112,115,148] Weems' review of 282 pelvic fractures in males found GU injury in 48 patients (17%); bladder injury in 19 patients (6.7%), urethral injury in 20 patients (7.1%), and renal injury in 9 patients (3.2%). Other investigators have found the incidence of lower tract injuries in the male with pelvic fractures to range from 4% to 25%.[100,103,108,148]

Several classifications for pelvic fractures have been used. The classification by Trunkey is most often cited in discussions of pelvic injury, and GU tract injury.[68,149] Type I are crush-type injuries involving three or more major components (rami, ilium, acetabulum, sacrum); type II are unstable, requiring immobilization and including "sprung pelvis" and acetabular fractures; type III are stable, isolated fractures of the pubic rami.[149] Type I fractures had the highest mortality and morbidity rates in Trunkey's study at 21.7% and 69.5%, respectively.

A classification of pelvic fractures in children has not been extensively used. Bryan's review of 52 children with pelvic fractures divided these into four types: type I, iliac wing fractures (8%); type II, acetabular fractures (6%); type III, stable pelvic ring fractures (62%); and type IV, unstable fractures with breaks in the anterior and posterior rings (24%). Type III and type IV pelvic fractures as described by Bryan had significant urologic injury rates of 12% and 42%, respectively. The best predictor of abdominal injury in children with pelvic fractures was multiple fractures to the pelvic ring.[147]

Although any pelvic fracture may be associated with GU tract injury, the most significant of these injuries are associated with anterior arch fractures of the pelvis. Reichard found that all of the patients with bladder injury had anterior ring fractures.

In male patients with a pelvic fracture, the clinician must consider the possibility of lower GU tract injury. If the patient exhibits no signs of anterior or posterior urethral injury, then a urinary catheter may be gently advanced. When there is resistance, a urethrogram should be performed; a cystogram and IVP (or CT scan) is needed if there is no extravasation. A urinary catheter should never be placed when a patient has signs of anterior or posterior urethral injury. Female patients who have pelvic fractures are unlikely to have urethral injury; in the absence of signs of urethral injury, a cystogram alone may be performed, followed by CT scan or IVP (see Fig. 25-1).

Treatment of pelvic fractures include immobilization of the patient in the supine position, restriction of movement as much as possible (oblique views should be avoided during radiographic evaluation), early stabilization of the fracture (external fixator), blood products and angiography as indicated for ongoing blood loss.[150,151]

SUMMARY

GU injury is an important subset of pediatric trauma that must be considered in every case of blunt and penetrating trauma to the trunk and pelvis. The management of GU injury is determined first by the nature of associated injuries and second by the recognition that a GU injury has occurred. Aggressive airway and fluid management is paramount, followed by evaluation of the patient with appropriate diagnostic studies to determine the nature of the injuries. The order of the diagnostic tests depends on the clinical condition of the patient, but, as a general rule, should begin with a cystourethrogram followed by IVP, ultrasound, or CT scan.[40]

References

1. National Center for Health Statistics: *Advance report of final mortality statistics*, 1985, Washington, DC, 1987, U.S. Government Printing Office.
2. Inaba AS: An approach to pediatric trauma: unique anatomic and pathophysiologic aspects of the pediatric patient, *Emerg Clin North Am* 9:523, 1991.
3. Feins NR: Multiple trauma, *Pediatr Clin North Am* 26:759, 1979.
4. Godec CJ: Genitourinary trauma, *Urol Radiol* 7:185, 1985.
5. Monstrey SJM, vanderWerken C, Debruyne MJ, et al: Urological trauma and severe associated injuries, *Br J Urol* 60:393, 1987.
6. Young LW, Wood BP, Linke CA: Renal injury from blunt trauma in childhood: radiological evaluation and review, *Eur Soc Paediatr Radiol* 18:359, 1974.
7. Cass AS: Blunt renal trauma in children, *J Trauma* 23:123, 1983.
8. Guerriero WG: Trauma to the kidneys, ureters, bladder, and urethra, *Surg Clin North Am* 62:6, 1047, 1982.
9. Livne PM and Gonzales ET: Genitourinary trauma in children, *Urol Clin North Am* 12(1):53, 1985.
10. Quinlan DM, Gearhart JP: Blunt renal trauma in childhood. Features indicating severe injury, *Br J Urol* 66:526-531, 1990.
11. Ahmed S and Morris LL: Renal parenchymal injuries secondary to blunt abdominal trauma in childhood: a 10-year review, *Br J Urol* 54:470, 1982.
12. Filiatrault D, Longpre D, Patriquin H et al: Investigation of childhood blunt abdominal trauma: a practical approach using ultrasound as the initial diagnostic modality, *Pediatr Radiol* 17:373, 1987.

Retroperitoneal Structures

13. Mandour WA, Lai MK, Linke CA et al: Blunt renal trauma in the pediatric patient, *J Pediatr Surg* 16:669, 1981.

14. Kuzmarov IW, Morehouse DD, Gibson S: Blunt renal trauma in the pediatric population: a retrospective study, *J Urol* 125:648, 1981.

15. Brower P, Paul J, Brosman SA: Urinary tract abnormalities presenting as a result of blunt trauma, *J Trauma* 18:719, 1978.

16. Karp MP, Jewett TC, Kuhn JP et al: The impact of computed tomography scanning on the child with renal trauma, *J Pediatr Surg* 21:617, 1986.

17. Mendez R: Renal trauma, *J Urol* 118:698, 1977.

18. Cass AS: Renal trauma in multiply-injured child, *Urology* 21:487, 1983.

19. McAleer IM, Kaplan GW, Scherz HC et al: Genitourinary trauma in the pediatric patient, *Urology* 42(5):563-568, 1993.

20. Cass AS, Luxenberg M, Gleich P et al: Clinical indications for radiologic evaluation of blunt trauma, *J Urol* 136:370, 1986.

21. Scott R, Carlton CE, Goldman M: Penetrating injuries of the kidney: an analysis of 181 patients, *J Urol* 101:247, 1969.

22. Whitney RF and Peterson NE: Penetrating renal injuries, *Urology* 7:7, 1976.

23. Cromie WJ, Bates RD, Duckett JW: Penetrating renal trauma in the neonate, *J Urol* 119:259, 1978.

24. Bretan PN and McAninch W: Evaluation of renal trauma: indications for computed tomography and other diagnostic techniques, *Adv Urol* 1:65, 1988.

25. Moore EE, Shackford SR, Pachter HL et al: Organ injury scaling: spleen, liver, and kidney, *J Trauma* 29:1664, 1989.

26. Guice K, Oldham K, Eidie B et al: Hematuria after blunt trauma: when is pyelography useful? *J Trauma* 23:305, 1983.

27. Lieu TA, Fleisher GR, Mahboubi S et al: Hematuria and clinical findings as indications for intravenous pyelography in pediatric blunt renal trauma, *Pediatrics* 82:216, 1988.

28. Klein S, Johs S, Fujitani R et al: Hematuria following blunt abdominal trauma: the utility of intravenous pyelography, *Arch Surg* 123:1173, 1988.

29. Haller JO, Bass IS, Sclafani SJA: Imaging evaluation of traumatic hematuria in children, *Urol Radiol* 7:211, 1985.

30. Sclafani SJA, Becker A, Shaftan GW et al: Strategies for the radiologic management of genitourinary trauma, *Urol Radiol* 7:231, 1985.

31. Kuhn JP: Diagnostic imaging for the evaluation of abdominal trauma in children, *Pediatr Clin North Am* 32:1427, 1985.

32. Sklar DP, Diven B, Jones J: Incidence and magnitude of catheter-induced hematuria, *Am J Emerg Med* 4:14, 1986.

33. Fleisher G: Prospective evaluation of selective criteria for imaging among children with suspected blunt renal trauma, *Pediatr Emerg Care* 5:8, 1989.

34. Kisa E and Schenk WG: Indications for emergency intravenous pyelography (IVP) in blunt abdominal trauma: a reappraisal, *J Trauma* 26:1086, 1986.

35. Fortune JB, Brahme J, Mulligan M et al: Emergency intravenous pyelography in the trauma patient: a reexamination of the indications, *Arch Surg* 120:1056, 1985.

36. Hardeman SW, Husmann DA, Chinn HKW et al: Blunt urinary tract trauma: identifying those patients who require radiological diagnostic studies, *J Urol* 138:99, 1987.

37. Nicolaisen GS, McAninch JW, Marshall GA et al: Renal trauma: re-evaluation of the indications for radiographic assessment, *J Urol* 133:183, 1985.

38. Eastham JA, Wilson TG, Ahlering TE: Radiographic evaluation of adult patients with blunt renal trauma, *J Urol* 148:266-267, 1992.

39. Uehara DT: Indications for intravenous pyelography in trauma, *Ann Emerg Med* 15:266, 1986.

40. Scheneider RE: Genitourinary trauma, *Emerg Clinics North Am* 11(1):137-145, 1993.

41. McAndrew JD, Corriere JN: Radiographic evaluation of renal trauma: evaluation of 1103 consecutive patients, *Br J Urol* 73:352-354, 1994.

42. Stables DP, Fouche RF, De Villiers JP et al: Traumatic renal artery occlusion: 21 cases, *J Urol* 115:229, 1976.

43. Bretan PN, McAninch JW, Federle MP et al: Computerized tomographic staging of renal trauma: 85 consecutive cases, *J Urol* 136:561, 1986.

44. McAninch W and Federle MP: Evaluation of renal injuries with computerized tomography, *J Urol* 128:456, 1982.

45. Kane NM, Cronan JJ, Dorfman GS et al: Pediatric abdominal trauma: evaluation by computed tomography, *Pediatrics* 82:11, 1988.

46. Mohamed G, Reyes HM, Fantus R et al: Computed tomography in the assessment of pediatric abdominal trauma, *Arch Surg* 121:703, 1986.

47. Taylor GA, Fallat ME, Potter BM et al: The role of computed tomography in blunt abdominal trauma in children, *J Trauma* 28:1660, 1988.

48. Lang EK: Intra-abdominal and retroperitoneal organ injuries diagnosed on dynamic computed tomograms obtained for assessment of renal trauma, *J Trauma* 30:1161, 1990.

49. Sandler CM and Toombs BD: Computed tomographic evaluation of blunt renal injuries, *Radiology* 141:461, 1981.

50. Federle MP, Kaiser JA, McAninch JW et al: The role of computed tomography in renal trauma, *Radiology* 141:455, 1981.

51. Sclafani SJA and Becker JA: Radiologic diagnosis of renal trauma, *Urol Radiol* 7:191, 1985.

52. Erturk E, Sheinfeld J, DiMarco PL et al: Renal trauma: evaluation by computerized tomography, *J Urol* 133:946, 1985.

53. Bresler MJ: Computed tomography of the abdomen, *Ann Emerg Med* 15:280, 1986.

54. Karp MP, Cooney DR, Berger PE et al: The role of computed tomography in the evaluation of blunt abdominal trauma in children, *J Pediatr Surg* 16:316, 1981.

55. Yale-Loehr AJ, Kramer SS, Quinlan DM et al: CT of severe renal trauma in children: evaluation and course of healing with conservative therapy, *Am J Roentgenol* 152:109, 1989.

56. Stubbs DM: Emergency radiology of urinary tract injuries, *Am J Emerg Med* 10(3):242-250, 1992.

57. Pollack HM, Wein AJ: Imaging of renal trauma, *Radiology* 172:297, 1989.

58. Guerriero WG, Carlton CE, Scott R et al: Renal pedicle injuries, *J Trauma* 11:53, 1971.

59. Bergen CT, Chan FN, Bodzin JH: Intravenous pyelogram results in association with renal pathology and therapy in trauma patients, *J Trauma* 27:515, 1987.

60. Stevenson J and Battistella FD: The 'one shot' intravenous pyelogram: is it indicated in unstable patients before celiotomy? *J Trauma* 36:6:828-833, 1994.

61. Halsell RD, Vines FS, Shatney CH et al: The reliability of excretory urolography as a screening examination for blunt renal trauma, *Ann Emerg Med* 16:1236, 1987.

62. Wong L, Waxman K, Smolin M et al: The role of IVP in blunt trauma, *J Trauma* 28:502, 1988.

63. Herter GE and Schiff M: Radiologic procedures for the evaluation of urinary tract trauma. In Roberts JR, Hedges JR, editors: *Clinical procedures in emergency medicine*, Philadelphia, 1985, WB Saunders.

64. Frank RG, Gerard PS, Feldhamer L: Serial sonographic evaluation of "buckshot colic" following penetrating gunshot wound, *Urol Radiol* 14:172-176, 1991.

65. Loberant N: Emergency imaging of the urinary tract, *Emerg Clinics North Am* 10(1):59-91, 1992.

66. Chopp RT, Hekmat-Ravan H, Mendez R: Technetium-99m Glucoheptonate renal scan in diagnosis of acute renal injury, *Urology* 15:201, 1980.

67. Leppaniemi AK, Kivisaari AO, Haapiainen RK et al: Role of magnetic resonance imaging in blunt renal parenchymal trauma, *Brit J Urol* 68:355-360, 1991.

68. Bryan WJ and Tullos HS: Pediatric pelvic fractures: review of 52 patients, *J Trauma* 19:799, 1979.

69. Whitaker RH: Urological trauma, *Annals Acad Med* 21(2):258-262, 1992.

70. Baumann L, Greenfield SP, Aker J et al: Nonoperative management of major blunt renal trauma in children: Inhospital morbidity and long-term followup, *J Urol* 148:691-693, 1992.

71. Cheng DLW, Lazan D, Stone N: Conservative treatment of type III renal trauma, *J Trauma* 36:4:491-494, 1994.

72. Scott R, Carlton CE, Ashmore AJ et al: Initial management of non-penetrating renal injuries: clinical review of 111 cases, *J Urol* 90:535, 1963.

73. Cockett ATK, Frank IN, Davis RS et al: Recent advances in the diagnosis and management of blunt renal trauma, *J Urol* 113:750, 1975.

74. Hodges CV, Gilbert DR, Scott WW: Renal trauma: a study of 71 cases, *J Urol* 66:627, 1951.

75. Cass AS and Ireland GW: Management of renal injuries in the severely injured patient, *J Trauma* 12:516, 1972.

76. Sagalowsky AI, McConnell JD, Peters PC: Renal trauma requiring surgery: an analysis of 185 cases, *J Trauma* 23:128, 1983.

77. Cass AS, Luxenberg M, Gleich P et al: Long-term results of conservative and surgical management of blunt renal lacerations, *Br J Urol* 59:17, 1987.

78. Leppaniemi AK, Haapiainen RK, Lehtonen TA: Diagnosis and treatment of patients with renal trauma, *Br J Urol* 64:13, 1989.

79. Waterhouse K and Gross M: Trauma to the genitourinary tract a 5-year experience with 251 cases, *J Urol* 101:241, 1969.

80. Husman DA, Gilling PJ, Perry MO et al: Major renal lacerations with a devitalized fragment following blunt abdominal trauma: A comparison between nonoperative (expectant) versus surgical management, *J Urol* 150:174-177, 1993.

81. Brandes SB, Chelsky MJ, Buckman RF et al: Ureteral injuries from penetrating trauma, *J Trauma* 36(6):766-769, 1994.

82. McGinty D and Mendez R: Traumatic ureteral injuries with delayed recognition, *Urology* 10:115, 1977.

83. Pitts JC and Peterson NE: Penetrating injuries of the ureter, *J Trauma* 21:978, 1981.

84. Laberge I, Homsy YL, Dadour G et al: Avulsion of ureter by blunt trauma, *Urology* 13:172, 1979.

85. Wallijn E, De Sy W, Fonteyne E: Blunt ureteral trauma with perineal urine fistulization: review of the literature, *J Urol* 114:942, 1975.

86. Palmer M, Drago JR: Ureteral avulsion from non-penetrating trauma, *J Urol* 125:108, 1981.

87. Boone TB, Gilling PJ, Husmann DA: Ureteropelvic junction disruption following blunt abdominal trauma, *J Urol* 150:33-36, 1993.

88. Kenney PJ, Panicek DM, Witanowski LS: Computed tomography of ureteral disruption, *J Comput Assist Tomogr* 11:480, 1987.

89. Siegal MJ and Balfe DM: Blunt renal and ureteral trauma in childhood: CT patterns of fluid collections, *Am J Roentgenol* 152:1043, 1989.

90. Cass AS: The multiple injured patient with bladder trauma, *J Trauma* 24:731, 1984.

91. Cass AS: Bladder trauma in the multiple injured patient, *J Urol* 115:667, 1976.

92. Brosman SA and Fay R: Diagnosis and management of bladder trauma, *J Trauma* 13:687, 1973.

93. Hochberg E and Stone NN: Bladder rupture associated with pelvic fracture due to blunt trauma, *Urology* 41(6):531-533, 1993.

94. Fuhrman GM, Simmons GT, Davidson BS et al: The single indication for cystography in blunt trauma, *Am Surg* 59(6):333-336, 1993.

95. Rubin MJ, Blahd WH, Stanisic TH et al: Diagnosis of intraperitoneal extravasation of urine by peritoneal lavage, *Ann Emerg Med* 14:433, 1985.

96. Rehm CG, Mure AJ, O'Malley F et al: Blunt traumatic bladder rupture: the role of retrograde cystogram, *Ann Emerg Med* 20:845, 1991.

97. Carroll PR and McAninch JW: Major bladder trauma: the accuracy of cystography, *J Urol* 130:887, 1983.

98. Lis LE and Cohen AJ: CT cystography in the evaluation of bladder trauma, *J Comput Assist Tomogr* 14(3):386-389, 1990.

99. Richardson JR, Leadbetter GW: Non-operative treatment of the ruptured bladder, *J Urol* 114:213, 1975.

100. Del Villar RG, Ireland GW, Cass AS: Management of bladder and urethral injury in conjunction with immediate surgical treatment of the acute severe trauma patient, *J Urol* 108:581, 1972.

External Genitourinary Structures

101. Reichard SA, Helikson MA, Shorter N et al: Pelvic fractures in children: review of 120 patients with a new look at general management, *J Pediatr Surg* 15:727, 1980.

102. Cass AS and Godec CJ: Urethral injury due to external trauma, *Urology* 11:607, 1978.

103. Morehouse DD: Emergency management of urethral trauma, *Urol Clin North Am* 9:251, 1982.

104. Pontes JE and Pierce JM: Anterior urethral injuries: four years of experience at the Detroit General Hospital, *J Urol* 120:563, 1978.

105. Pode D and Shapiro A: Traumatic avulsion of the female urethra: case report, *J Trauma* 30:235, 1990.

106. Parkhurst JD, Coker E, Halverstadt DB: Traumatic avulsion of the lower urinary tract in the female child, *J Urol* 126:265, 1981.

107. Coffield KS and Weems WL: Experience with management of posterior urethral injury associated with pelvic fracture, *J Urol* 117:722, 1977.

108. Fowler JW, Watson G, Smith MF et al: Diagnosis and treatment of posterior urethral injury, *Br J Urol* 58:167, 1986.

109. Persky L: Childhood urethral trauma, *Urology* 11:603, 1978.

110. Onuora VC, Patil MG, Al-Jasser AN: Missed urological injuries in children with polytrauma, *Injury* 24(9):619-621, 1993.

111. Webster GD, Mathes GL, Selli C: Prostatomembranous urethral injuries: a review of the literature and a rational approach to their management, *J Urol* 130:898, 1983.

112. Uehara DT and Eisner RF: Indications for retrograde cystourethrography in trauma, *Ann Emerg Med* 15:270, 1986.

113. Kane NM, Francis IR, Ellis JH: The value of CT in the detection of bladder and posterior urethral injuries, *Am J Roentgenol* 153:1243, 1989.

114. Glassberg KI, Tolete-Velcek F, Ashley R et al: Partial tears of prostatomembranous urethra in children, *Urology* 13:500, 1979.

115. Weems WL: Management of genitourinary injuries in patients with pelvic fractures, *Ann Surg* 189:717, 1979.

116. Herschorn S, Thijssen A, Radomski SB: The value of immediate or early catheterization of the traumatized posterior urethra, *J Urol* 148:1428-1431, 1992.

117. Malek RS, O'Dea MJ, Kelalis PP: Management of ruptured posterior urethra in childhood, *J Urol* 117:105, 1977.

118. Pollen JJ and Funckes C: Traumatic dislocation of the testis, *J Trauma* 22:247, 1982.

119. Nagarajan VP, Pranikoff K, Imahori SC et al: Traumatic dislocation of testis, *Urology* 22:521, 1983.

120. Zivkovic SM and Janjic G: Traumatic rupture of the testis and epididymis, *J Pediatr Surg* 15:287, 1980.

121. MacDermott JP, Gray BK, Stewart PAH: *Br J Urol* 62:179-181, 1988.

122. Elsaharty S, Pranikoff K, Magoss IV et al: Traumatic torsion of the testis, *J Urol* 132:1155, 1984.

123. Cos LR and Rabinowitz R: Trauma-induced testicular torsion in children, *J Trauma* 22:244, 1982.

124. Cass AS, Ferrara L, Wolpert J et al: Bilateral testicular injury from external trauma, *J Urol* 140:1435, 1988.

125. Jackson JH and Craft AW: Bicycle saddles and torsion of the testis, *Lancet* 983, May 1978.

126. Tiwary CM: Testicular injury in breech delivery: possible implications, *Urology* 34:210, 1989.

127. Sparnon T, Moretti K, Sach RP: BMX handlebar: a threat to manhood? *Med J Aust* 11:587, 1982.

128. Donovan JF and Kaplan WE: The therapy of genital trauma by dog bite, *J Urol* 141:1163, 1989.

129. Miskin M, Buckspan M, Bain J: Ultrasonographic examination of scrotal masses, *J Urol* 117:185, 1977.

130. Friedman G, Rose JG, Winston MA: Ultrasound and nuclear medicine evaluation in acute testicular trauma, *J Urol* 125:748, 1981.

131. Schaffer RM: Ultrasonography of scrotal trauma, *Urol Radiol* 7:245, 1985.

132. Albert NE: Testicular ultrasound for trauma, *J Urol* 124:558, 1980.

133. Anderson KA, McAninch JW, Jeffrey RB et al: Ultrasonography for the diagnosis and staging of blunt scrotal trauma, *J Urol* 130:933, 1983.

134. Flowerdew R, Fishman IJ, Churchill BM: Management of penile zipper injury, *J Urol* 177:671, 1977.

135. Saraf P and Rabinowitz R: Zipper injury of the foreskin, *Am J Dis Child* 136:557, 1982.

136. Kudsk KA, McQueen MA, Voeller GR et al: Management of complex perineal soft-tissue injuries, *J Trauma* 30:1155, 1990.

137. Anesthesia and regional blocks. In Simon RR and Brenner BE, editors: *Procedures and techniques in emergency medicine*, Baltimore, 1982, Williams & Wilkins.

138. Gross M, Arnold TL, Peters P: Fracture of the penis with associated laceration of the urethra, *J Urol* 117:725, 1977.

139. Nymark J, Kristensen JK: Fracture of the penis with urethral rupture, *J Urol* 129:147, 1983.

140. Cendron M, Whitmore KE, Carpiniello V et al: Traumatic rupture of the corpus cavernosum: evaluation and management, *J Urol* 144:987-991, 1990.

141. Jallu A, Wani NA, Rashid PA: Fracture of the penis, *J Urol* 123:285, 1980.

142. Wyatt JJP and Scobie WG: The management of penile zip entrapment in children, *Injury* 25:1:59-60, 1994.

143. Kanegaye JT and Schonfeld N: Penile zipper entrapment: a simple and less threatening approach using mineral oil, *Pediatr Emerg Care* 9(2):90-91, 1993.

144. Johnson CF: Inflicted injury versus accidental injury, *Pediatr Clin North Am* 37:791, 1990.

145. Muram D: Genital tract injuries in the prepubertal child, *Pediatr Ann* 15:616, 1986.

146. Paradise JE: The medical evaluation of the sexually abused child, *Pediatr Clin North Am* 37:839, 1990.

147. Bond SJ, Gotschall CS, Eichelberger MR: Predictors of abdominal injury in children with pelvic fracture, *J Trauma* 31:1169, 1991.

Pelvic Fractures and Injury to the Genitourinary Tract

148. Palmer JK, Benson GS, Corriere JN: Diagnosis and initial management of urological injuries associated with 200 consecutive pelvic fractures, *J Urol* 130:712, 1983.

149. Trunkey DD, Chapman MW, Lim RC et al: Management of pelvic fractures in blunt trauma injury, *J Trauma* 14:912, 1974.

150. Chan L, Nade S, Brooks A et al: Experience with lower urinary tract disruptions associated with pelvic fractures: Implications for emergency room management, *Aust NZ J Surg* 64:395-399, 1994.

151. Davidson BS, Simmons GT, Williamson PR et al: Pelvic fractures associated with open perineal wounds: A survivable injury, *J Trauma* 35(1):36-39, 1993.

MUSCULOSKELETAL AND SOFT TISSUE INJURIES

CHAPTER

26

Foreign Bodies of the Gastrointestinal Tract and Airway

Dena R. Brownstein

The incidence of foreign body ingestion and aspiration is greatest among infants, toddlers, and preschool-aged children, reflecting their natural curiosity, tendency toward oral exploration of their environment, and lack of fully developed dentition. The presentation of children with a foreign body of the gastrointestinal (GI) tract or airway varies greatly. The child may have acute symptoms of airway compromise or esophageal obstruction; vague, chronic complaints of persistent cough or failure to thrive; or no symptoms at all. Given the s
sis must be made in a timely fashion. Pitfalls in emergency department management may include incomplete radiologic evaluation, ascribing symptoms to a medical illness, improper patient transfer within and between facilities, and inappropriate attempts at foreign body removal.[1]

GASTROINTESTINAL FOREIGN BODIES

Foreign body ingestion is common in the pediatric age group. The majority of ingestions occur in children 6 months to 6 years of age; the high-risk period begins when the toddler becomes orally inquisitive and ends with the appearance of the back molars.[2-6] The incidences of foreign body ingestion are approximately equal in males and females.[4,7,8] Less than 50% of these patients have a history of a witnessed or strongly suspected event,[9] and patients may consult a physician hours to months after ingestion.[4,9] Once the diagnosis is made, a good history may reveal that the patient has a past history of similar episodes, or may uncover a variety of psychologic or social risk factors. However, foreign body ingestions often involve children with no risk factors, who ingest easily accessible household items, often in full view of supervising adults.[10]

The natural curiosity of the preschool-aged child results in the ingestion of a wide range of objects; coins are the most popular nonfood ingestant.[2,6,10,12] Small toy parts, buttons, pins, and batteries are but a few of the numerous foreign bodies described in the literature. Unlike adults, children without preexisting esophageal disease rarely have esophageal food bolus impaction.[6] Conversely, the child who has undergone esophageal surgery, as for a tracheoesophageal fistula repair, or who has an esophagus damaged by a prior ingestion of alkali, is at high risk of repeated presentations with food impacted at the site of anatomic narrowing.[13]

Although it is estimated that 80% to 90% of all ingested foreign bodies that reach the stomach pass through the GI tract without significant sequelae, foreign bodies impacted in the esophagus require expeditious removal to prevent serious complications.[4,14,15]

Pathophysiology

Foreign body impaction in the GI tract is a function of the shape and size of the ingested object, the presence of normal or abnormal areas of anatomic narrowing, and impaired motility. Large objects and angulated sharp objects tend to lodge in the esophagus at one of three anatomic sites of narrowing: the inferior edge of the cricopharyngeus muscle, the level of the aortic arch crossing, and the gastroesophageal junction. The majority of impacted foreign bodies are found at the level of the cricopharyngeus in the proximal third of the esophagus.[4,13] Children who have preexisting esophageal disease or surgery are particularly prone to lodging of foreign material in the upper esophagus because of poor motility or stricture.[3] Symptoms and signs such as drooling, refusal to eat or drink, or vomiting reflect partial or complete obstruction of the esophagus. In the thin-walled esophagus, the presence of an impacted foreign body may lead to intramural ulceration, perforation, and hemorrhage.

Most foreign bodies that pass through the esophagus make their way uneventfully through the GI tract. Long, straight, or pointed objects have a greater risk of becoming impacted and have a tendency to lodge at any area of acute angulation. The majority reach the distal small bowel and may cause symptoms and signs of obstruction. Although perforation of the intestine is a rare complication of foreign body impaction, cases of peritonitis have been reported.[4,13-15]

Esophageal Foreign Bodies

Diagnostic Findings. Less than 50% of children who have a retained esophageal foreign body have a history of witnessed or suspected ingestion.[6,9] Although the majority of children present within hours of such ingestion, delays in presentation as long as 6 months have been reported.[16]

Many children with a retained esophageal foreign body are asymptomatic. When present, symptoms and signs depend on the nature of the object ingested, the site at which it has lodged, and the duration of impaction. Complaints may be referred either to the GI tract or to the airway. As the posterior wall of the trachea is compressible, acute symptoms and signs of either ingestion or aspiration of a foreign body may be those of airway compromise: gagging, choking, coughing, and stridor.[2,4-6,17] Such historical symptoms may have resolved on arrival at the emergency department.[17] Other common symptoms and signs of acute ingestion include refusal to feed, increased salivation or drooling, dysphagia, neck or throat pain, vomiting, and foreign body sensation.[3,4] A retained esophageal foreign body should be suspected when any child without prior history of esophageal disease experiences swallowing difficulty.[6]

Although less than 1% of foreign body ingestions result in perforation, major complications usually occur more than 24 hours after impaction.[4] The nature of such complications depends on the site of esophageal perforation but may include mucosal ulceration, pressure necrosis, esophageal perforation, retropharyngeal abscess, mediastinitis, pleural effusions, pneumothorax, lung abscess, and great vessel injury.[4,16,18] Such children may present in extremis, requiring aggressive supportive care for sepsis and cardiopulmonary compromise.

A history of a specific event is not likely to be elicited from children with delayed presentation. Failure to thrive, chronic cough, wheezing, stridor, or recurrent pneumonia caused by airway compression or atelectasis may be the presenting complaint.[16]

Radiologic Studies. Since fewer than 20% of children who have ingested a foreign body have abnormalities revealed by physical examination and a history of ingestion is often not available, radiologic evaluation is a cornerstone of diagnosis.[4] Anteroposterior (AP) and lateral soft tissue neck or chest films that include the cervical esophagus are diagnostic in the case of radiopaque esophageal foreign bodies (Fig. 26-1). Impaction tends to occur at one of three anatomic sites of narrowing in the normal esophagus—the cricopharyngeus, the aortic arch crossing, or the cardioesophageal sphincter—and the majority of retained foreign bodies lodge in the cervical esophagus at the level of the cricopharyngeus.[5,13,18] Coins in the esophagus lodge in the coronal plane on AP or postero anterior (PA) radiographs, whereas those in the trachea are oriented in the sagittal plane.[4]

Unfortunately, plastic and aluminum are not generally radiopaque. When retention of a foreign body in the esophagus is suggested by history or examination and plain films do not contribute useful information, radiologic consultation should be sought. Xeroradiography or computed tomography (CT) scan may allow visualization of low-density objects, and contrast studies under fluoroscopy may also be diagnostic. Contrast media should be chosen to minimize complications in the event of aspiration or leakage into the mediastinum (e.g., inert barium sulfate if pulmonary aspiration is a concern or a water-soluble contrast medium if esophageal perforation is suspected).[4] In institutions with a skilled pediatric endoscopist, direct visualization of the esophagus is preferable to contrast studies when plain films are nondiagnostic but a foreign body is believed present. Endoscopy permits examination for the presence of several foreign bodies, evaluation of esophageal damage, and definitive therapy.

There has been some controversy in recent years regarding the necessity of obtaining radiographic studies in asymptomatic children who have a history of coin ingestion. In several series, which offer conflicting conclusions, radiographs yielded positive findings in 20% to 57% of children who entered the emergency department with a history of coin ingestion.[9,17,19] Although symptomatic children were significantly more likely to have a positive radiograph result, coins were identified in the esophagus in up to 30% of *asymptomatic* children.[8,17,19] Spontaneous passage of the coin into the stomach occurred in 16% to 76% of patients during observation in the emergency department.[8,19] No complications were noted in patients followed expectantly over 12 to 120 hours without intervention.[8,17] Despite the high likelihood that a smooth round foreign body such as a coin will pass spontaneously into the stomach, a fatal complication of esophageal coin retention in a child has been reported.[20]

The small numbers of patients evaluated in the preceding series are insufficient to set policy regarding the need for plain films in all children with a history of coin ingestion. However, given the low incidence of complications associated with impaction of a coin in the first 12 hours

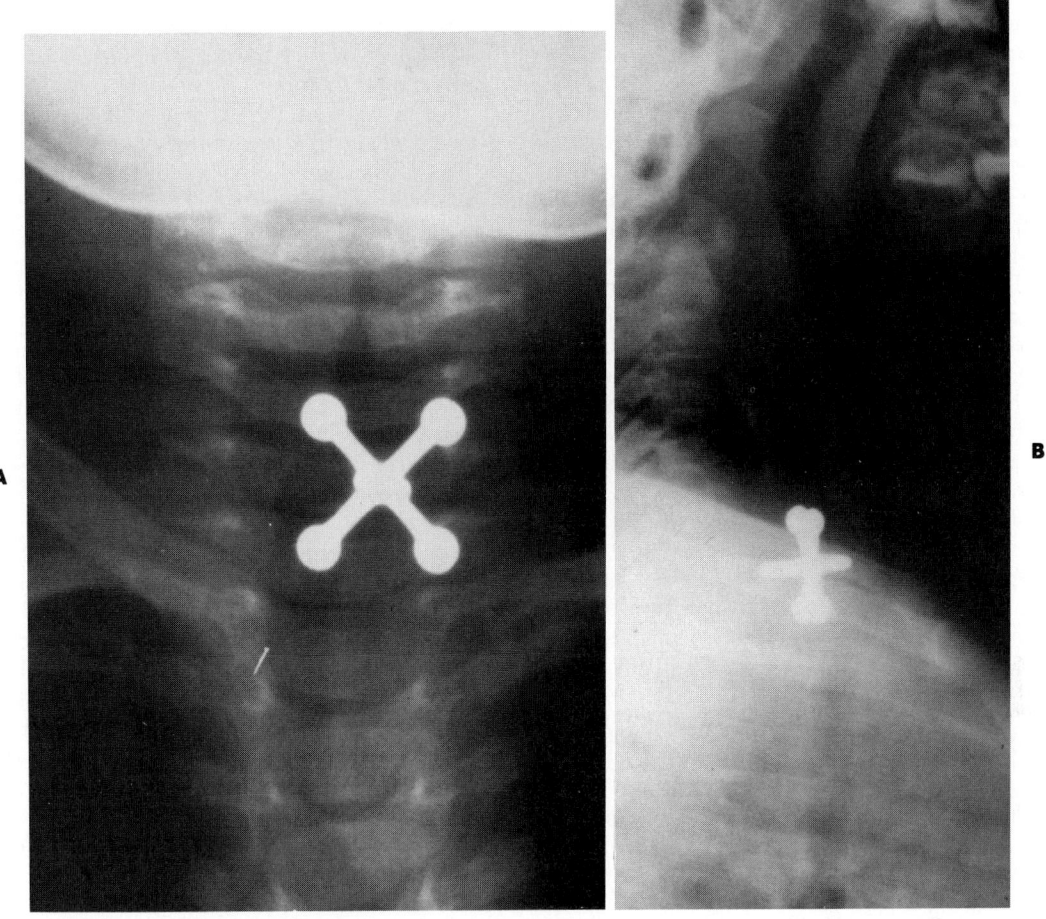

FIG. 26-1. A and **B,** Jack in the esophagus. This 2-year-old girl entered the emergency department with the chief complaint of refusal to look up. Further questioning revealed poor solid food intake. The jack, lodged at the level of the aortic arch crossing, was removed under general anesthesia via rigid endoscopy.

postingestion, it seems both safe and cost-effective to observe asymptomatic children with a coin lodged in the esophagus for up to 12 hours before attempting its removal.[13,14,21] This will provide an opportunity for spontaneous passage of the coin into the stomach, as well as more advantageous conditions for airway management should the child have general anesthesia for endoscopic removal.

The use of a metal detector may provide a useful alternative to radiographs for "screening" asymptomatic children who are believed to have ingested a metallic foreign body,[22,23] either to establish that a foreign body has indeed been ingested or to follow its passage through the gut. Examination with a metal detector does not provide information on the nature of the object ingested, may not identify the presence of multiple foreign bodies, and may not enable the examiner to localize the object to the gastroesophageal junction vs. the stomach.[1,22,23] If a procedure to remove the foreign body is planned, radiographs in two planes should be obtained.

Management. All esophageal foreign bodies must be removed. Techniques used for removal vary with the nature and location of the impacted object, ability to enlist the child's cooperation, presence of complications mandating operative intervention, experience and skills of individual physicians, and institutional custom. Endoscopy, permitting direct visualization and removal of the foreign body and simultaneous examination of the esophagus, is considered by many surgeons and gastroenterologists to be the procedure of choice and is the only safe, nonoperative method of removing sharp or irregular foreign bodies.[2,4,11,24] However, a variety of other techniques have been employed in the emergency department to retrieve esophageal foreign bodies or facilitate their passage into the stomach.

Glucagon. The use of intravenous glucagon (0.03 to 0.1 mg/kg/dose; adult, 1 mg) to promote passage of smooth foreign bodies lodged in the distal third of the esophagus into the stomach has been described. Success rates of 30% to 50% have been reported and attributed to the pharmacologic action of glucagon, which causes relaxation of smooth muscle and reduction of gastroesophageal sphincter tone.[4] Such reports are limited to adult patients and confined largely to impacted boluses of meat.[11] Esophageal food impaction in children is generally seen only in the presence of preexisting esophageal disease and stricture and usually necessitates endoscopic removal. The use of glucagon therefore is rarely applicable to the pediatric patient.

Esophageal Bougienage. Blind attempts to advance esophageal coins into the stomach through the use of bougie dilators have been described.[7,25] The technique, performed by a surgeon skilled in esophageal dilatation, involves passage of a lubricated bougie dilator from the mouth, through the esophagus, and into the stomach in an upright, unsedated patient. This technique carries the risk of airway compression and esophageal perforation and does not permit examination of the esophagus for additional foreign bodies or mucosal damage.[4,26] Given the availability of other safe techniques, use of esophageal bougienage in the emergency department should be viewed skeptically and will rarely be the first choice for foreign body management in children.

Balloon Catheter. The safety and efficacy of the removal of smooth esophageal foreign bodies, particularly those lodged for less than 24 hours, by means of a balloon catheter have been supported by a number of authors.[2-5,17,19,26,27] The technique is well documented by O'Neill[3]:

Esophageal foreign bodies without sharp edges are first identified and localized either on plain roentgenograms or are coated with a small amount of barium swallowed by the patient. Depending on the size of the patient, a 12 to 16 Fr Foley catheter with an intact balloon containing a small amount of contrast material is placed through the nose to a location below the level of the foreign body under fluoroscopic control. This is performed with the patient on his or her side while restrained and unsedated. Once the balloon has been passed beneath the foreign body, it is then inflated sufficiently to move the foreign body upward using approximately 3 to 5 ml of contrast. Then with gentle pressure exerted on the catheter the foreign body is dislodged and the patient quickly turned prone in order to avoid reingestion or aspiration of the foreign body.

Campbell strongly recommends that the catheter be passed orally, to prevent impaction of the foreign body in the nasopharynx on extraction, and that the fluoroscopic table be positioned in a steep head-down position just before withdrawing the catheter to reduce the risk of the foreign body contacting the airway.[27] The technique has been successfully employed for infants as young as 7 months of age, and serious reported complications are rare.[3,27] Safe application of the technique requires adherence to the following guidelines: (1) balloon catheter removal should be attempted only by a skilled physician and staff, with the expertise and equipment to deal with any complications of the technique, including airway obstruction; (2) a single coin is radiologically demonstrated to be present in the esophagus, has been lodged for less than 72 hours, and has caused incomplete obstruction; (3) the child is cooperative and has no respiratory compromise; and (4) no history of prior esophageal disease, foreign body ingestion, or surgery has been elicited.[4]

Reported success rates for balloon catheter removal of esophageal foreign bodies in children vary between 55% and 91%; success rates approach 100% when dislodgment into the stomach is included among positive outcomes.[2,3,17,27] When the procedure is uncomplicated, the child may be discharged from the emergency department with instructions to return for any symptoms or signs of infection, bleeding, perforation, airway compromise, or retained foreign body.

Advantages of the balloon catheter technique include the avoidance of general anesthesia or sedative medications, the outpatient nature of the procedure, and the accessibility of the technique to emergency physicians and radiologists. Objections to the routine use of balloon catheter include the theoretical risks of aspiration, prolonged radiation exposure, overlooking of additional foreign bodies, failure to detect esophageal abnormality, and esophageal perforation.[4,28] In addition, in an era of increased consciousness of the need for proper sedation and analgesia during pediatric procedures, this technique has traditionally relied on physical restraint for cooperation; the use of appropriate sedation should be considered if the child cannot cooperate.

If balloon catheter extraction is to be employed, equipment for emergency airway management, including suction, supplemental oxygen, McGill forceps, laryngoscope, and endotracheal tubes, must be immediately available. The operator must be competent in emergency airway management of children and the patient placed in Trendelenburg position. Endoscopic and surgical backup should be readily available in the event of a complication.

Endoscopy. Endoscopy remains the "gold standard" for the removal of esophageal foreign bodies. It is the safest nonsurgical method of removing sharp or pointed objects lodged in the esophagus. Both rigid and flexible fiberoptic endoscopy have been advocated.[6,13,24,29,30] Endoscopy under general anesthesia permits direct visualization and removal of the foreign body, control of the airway, examination of the esophagus for acute or chronic abnormality, and a search for additional radiolucent swallowed objects. Success rates are high, and complications in the hands of a skilled endoscopist are uncommon.[14,30] Reported complications include cardiopulmonary compromise, esophageal perforation, and bleeding.[14,30] Exposure to a general anesthetic represents an additional inherent risk. In experienced hands, the benefits of endoscopy clearly outweigh the risks of the procedure, which remains the method of choice for the removal of most esophageal foreign bodies.

Although esophageal endoscopy is generally performed by an otorhinolaryngologist or gastroenterologist in the operating suite under general anesthesia, removal of blunt esophageal foreign bodies in children by flexible endoscopy with sedation has been described.[24] Flexible endoscopy under sedation eliminates the risks of general anesthesia and uncontrolled removal via balloon catheter extraction. It has been very effective, especially when coins dislodged into the stomach are considered to be a successful procedure. Use of the technique is limited to skilled endoscopists with ready access to the personnel and equipment necessary for emergency airway management and resuscitation. Acutely symptomatic patients, situations in which the duration of impaction is unknown or prolonged, and foreign bodies that are not smooth or blunt are more likely to lead to complications on removal and are best handled by rigid endoscopy.[24]

Gastric and Intestinal Foreign Bodies

Diagnostic Findings. Symptoms are uncommon when a swallowed foreign body has passed through the gastroesophageal sphincter. Many children present acutely with a history of ingestion or of coughing, choking, or dysphagia that has resolved by arrival in the emergency department. Physical examination findings are likely to be unremarkable. Plain films of the chest and abdomen, taken to rule out the presence of an esophageal foreign body, may reveal a radiopaque object in the stomach. Of such foreign bodies 80% to 90% will pass uneventfully through the GI tract, resulting in no long-term sequelae.[4,14] Perforation occurs in less than 1% of cases, most commonly at a site of anatomic narrowing or acute angulation: the pylorus, duodenum, duodenojejunal flexure, ileocecal valve, or appendix.[13,14] Other rare complications include bowel obstruction and GI hemorrhage, but these are noted less frequently in children than in adults because of the types and quantities of objects ingested.[31]

Radiologic Studies. When an asymptomatic child has a history of foreign body ingestion and imaging of the esophagus has ruled out impaction at that level, plain films of the abdomen may confirm the presence of a radiopaque foreign body in the stomach or intestines. Given the high rate of uneventful passage of subdiaphragmatic foreign bodies through the GI tract and the relatively rare indications for their retrieval, more sophisticated imaging techniques are not indicated in the absence of signs of perforation or obstruction.

Management. A conservative approach of outpatient observation is appropriate for most asymptomatic children.[5,13,15,29,31,32] Indications for removal of foreign bodies in the stomach or proximal duodenum include risk of perforation and failure to progress through the GI tract.[29] Long, slender, pointed objects such as sewing needles or fish, chicken, or meat bones represent the greatest risk for perforation, and some authors advocate endoscopic removal of such objects from the stomach or duodenum on identification.[13,14,29,33,34] Large, blunt foreign bodies and circular objects greater than 5 cm in diameter can become impacted and cause mucosal ulceration.[29]

Cathartics, stool softeners, and special diets have no proven benefit in the management of most foreign bodies.[14,34] If the foreign body is not identified in the stool, repeat radiographs at 2 weeks to exclude lack of progression may be obtained. Most importantly, however, parents should be advised to return for symptoms or signs of obstruction, perforation, or failure of the object to progress: abdominal pain, vomiting, fever, or bloody stool.

If a bone, toothpick, or sewing needle has been ingested, surgical consultation to evaluate the patient for endoscopic removal from the stomach or proximal duodenum should be obtained, because of the higher risk of perforation of such long, pointed objects. Large, blunt objects that do not pass the pylorus within 2 weeks may also warrant surgical input.[14,15,27] Because of the likelihood that foreign bodies of all types will pass without complication, prophylactic laparotomy for removal of asymptomatic intestinal foreign bodies is infrequently indicated.[14,31-33] Serial radiographs to document progression are therefore of questionable value. Surgical consultation should certainly be sought when any symptomatic child returns with abdominal pain, fever, vomiting, or blood per rectum. Water-soluble contrast studies may demonstrate "silent" perforation of a hollow viscus, even in the absence of frank peritonitis.[33]

Button Batteries. The management of button battery ingestions has been the subject of some debate during the last decade. These batteries are widely available in a variety of small electronic products, including watches, cameras, calculators, and hearing aids. The ingestion of 2,320 button batteries was reported to the National Battery Ingestion Hotline between 1983 and 1990. Hearing aid batteries were the type most commonly ingested, and children younger than 5 years of age accounted for 61.8% of cases.[35] Case reports of catastrophic complications of button battery ingestion, including two pediatric deaths associated with esophageal impaction, initially led to recommendations for an aggressive policy of early endoscopic or surgical removal of these batteries, regardless of their location in the gastrointestinal tract. Concerns pertained to the corrosive and toxic qualities of the contents of these batteries, the risk of hollow viscus perforation, and the potential for heavy metal poisoning.

With the accumulation of additional data, it has become apparent that ingested button batteries, other than those that lodge in the esophagus, infrequently cause problems.[34-36] In a large series, over 95% of button batteries passed through the GI tract spontaneously, with transit time of less than 96 hours in 86% of cases.[35] Most patients remain asymptomatic throughout the battery's passage.[29,34,35,37]

This accumulated experience has led to a conservative approach to most battery ingestions. In all cases of suspected battery ingestion, initial radiographs should be obtained to locate the battery and exclude esophageal retention. Disc batteries can be distinguished from coins on plain radiographs by the double-density shadow demonstrated in an AP projection and the rounded edges and presence of a step-off at the junction of the anode and cathode on lateral views.[38]

If the battery is retained in the esophagus, immediate endoscopic removal is mandated. Patients with impacted esophageal batteries develop burns within hours of ingestion; perforations leading to tracheoesophageal fistula formation, erosion into the aorta, and death have been reported.[34-36,39]

The use of a magnet tube or balloon catheter technique has been suggested as an alternative to endoscopy for removal of a battery from the esophagus, especially when a skilled endoscopist is not readily available.[36,40-42] In the presence of caustic or electrical burns, which have been documented as early as 4 hours postingestion, blind removal with a tube or catheter may have greater potential for iatrogenic perforation than endoscopy and precludes assessment of the degree of mucosal damage.[34,35] Further study is needed to document the safety of these techniques and identify appropriate patient selection criteria.

The high failure rate of endoscopic attempts at retrieval of a battery from the stomach or duodenum, anesthetic risk, and lack of significant injury from battery ingestion mitigate against endoscopy when the battery has passed beyond the esophagus.[34-36] Ipecac syrup should not be administered, as it has been shown to be ineffective in expelling batteries from the stomach, and could potentially lead to a gastric foreign body becoming lodged in the esophagus.[35] If the battery has passed the lower esophageal sphincter, asymptomatic patients may be observed at home and the stools strained to document elimination. Symptoms and signs such as vomiting, fever, anorexia, abdominal pain, or bloody stools should prompt repeat radiographs to locate the battery.[34-36] Surgical consultation should be obtained if peritoneal signs are present. If passage of the battery in the stool has not been documented, but the patient remains asymptomatic, follow-up radiographs are necessary only if needed to allay parental concerns.[35] Once a battery has passed the pylorus, failure of progression does not correlate with serious adverse outcome, so endoscopy or laparotomy should be reserved for patients with significant symptoms.[34,35]

Because the transit of larger button batteries is frequently impeded, Litovitz recommends follow-up radiographs at 48 hours for patients who have ingested batteries bigger than 15 mm, and endoscopic removal of those persisting in the stomach.[35] If a child is known to have ingested a 15.6 mm mercuric oxide cell, weekly radiographs may be obtained to determine if the battery is intact. Serum and urine mercury levels should be measured if the cell has split or radioopaque droplets are evident in the gut.[35] Although daily use of cathartics and metaclopramide has been empirically recommended to hasten passage, there are insufficient data to support their use and such treatment therefore cannot be routinely recommended.[34]

AIRWAY FOREIGN BODIES (see Chapter 59)

Foreign body aspiration into the tracheobronchial tree is a major cause of childhood morbidity and mortality. Approximately 75% of all cases of foreign body aspiration occur in children younger than 3 years of age, and hundreds of pediatric choking deaths occur each year in the United States.[13,43-50] The male/female ratio is approximately 2:1.[43-49] The natural curiosity of the toddler, the ubiquitous presence of small food and nonfood objects in the home, and the lack of an efficient grinding surface before the eruption of the back molars explain the high propensity for choking in this age group.

Organic debris is most frequently retrieved on bronchoscopy; peanuts are the most common offending agent.[44-52] In contrast to esophageal foreign bodies, airway foreign bodies are rarely radiopaque.[3,43,51] Respiratory symptoms may be produced by an object lodged anywhere in the airway from the hypopharynx to a segmental bronchus. Although most airway foreign bodies lodge in a mainstem bronchus, tracheal or laryngeal foreign bodies account for 3% to 11% of all those aspirated and are inherently associated with greater morbidity and mortality.[43,44-49,51-53] Slightly less than half of all bronchial foreign bodies are found on the left side of the tracheobronchial tree.[3,43-49,51-53]

Although prevention is clearly the key to management of this problem, the emergency physician is not infrequently called on to provide rapid assessment and intervention for the child with respiratory compromise caused by a foreign body in the airway. Children who have ingested foreign bodies may seek treatment in acute distress or days to months after the aspiration episode, partially reflecting the

location and relative degree of the obstruction. Complete laryngotracheal obstruction is clearly a critical event and can be considered a "prehospital disease"; only those with witnessed aspiration who receive immediate bystander or emergency medical service intervention to relieve the obstruction are likely to benefit from subsequent emergency department care. Children with incomplete obstruction of the upper or lower airway may provide more of a diagnostic dilemma for the emergency care provider and can be inadvertently compromised by delays in diagnosis as well as overzealous intervention in the emergency department.

Diagnostic Findings. The presentation of a child with a foreign body in the airway reflects the location and relative size of the object (i.e., its presence in the trachea vs. the bronchial tree and the percentage of obstruction of the airway). In addition, the nature of the object affects clinical findings. Organic material leads to an acute inflammatory reaction that may not be present when an inert foreign body is inhaled. The diagnosis of an airway foreign body may be obvious when a child presents immediately after a witnessed aspiration event or has the classic triad of acute onset of wheezing, coughing, and absent or diminished breath sounds.[51] However, delayed presentation and inconclusive physical examination findings may make the diagnosis more obscure.

Between 50% and 90% of children with foreign body aspiration have a suggestive history, most commonly of an acute episode of paroxysmal cough.[43,45,46,51] Other common symptoms and signs at the time of aspiration are cyanosis, choking, and dyspnea.[43,46,54] However, delays in presentation for care are common, and the family's and physician's concern about aspiration as a cause of the child's symptoms may diminish as the primary event becomes more distant. Only half of all children are diagnosed correctly in the first 24 hours after an aspiration event; an additional 30% receive the correct diagnosis in the following week.[44,49,51] The remainder may have delays in diagnosis of weeks to years.[44,46,48,49,51,55]

One fourth of children may be asymptomatic at the time of presentation to the emergency department; up to 39% may have no helpful physical examination findings.[43,46] The complete triad of coughing, wheezing, and decreased or absent breath sounds is present in about 40% of cases.[51] Other suggestive physical examination findings are stridor, tachypnea, retractions, rales, and fever.[45-47,51]

The presence of such symptoms and signs, in the absence of a clear-cut history of aspiration or in the case of a delay in presentation, may lead to the misdiagnosis of croup, asthma, pneumonia, or bronchitis[45,47,50,56] (Fig. 26-2, A and B). A combination of history, physical examination results, and radiologic findings leads to the correct diagnosis on the initial emergency department visit in the majority of patients.

Radiologic Studies. The diagnosis of foreign body aspiration must be entertained in any previously well, afebrile child who has a history of acute onset of choking, coughing, or wheezing, as well as the child who has a poorly defined chronic respiratory complaint. Although only 6% to 17% of aspirated foreign bodies are radiopaque, appropriate radiologic studies localize the site of the foreign body in the majority of cases.[44-47,51-53,55-57] A significant number of

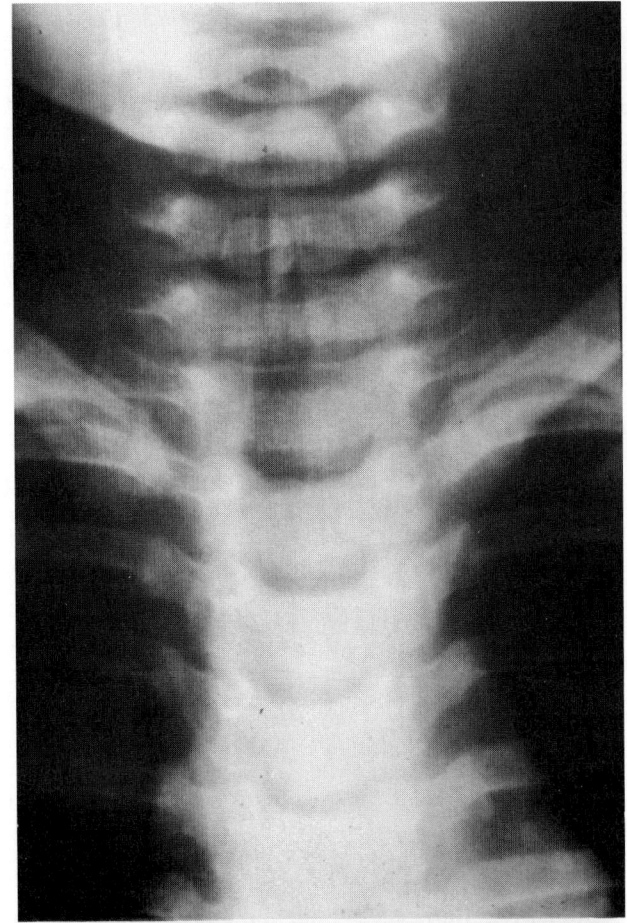

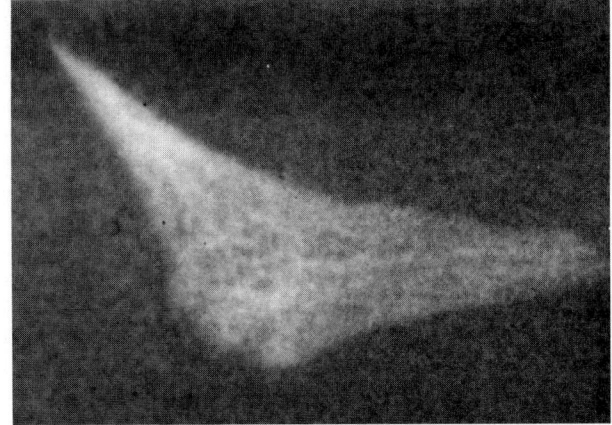

FIG. 26-2. A and **B,** Chicken bone in glottis misdiagnosed as croup. This child was referred by a private physician with the diagnosis of croup made on the basis of stridor, cough, and radiographs of the neck. The bone, lodged in the glottis, was initially overlooked.

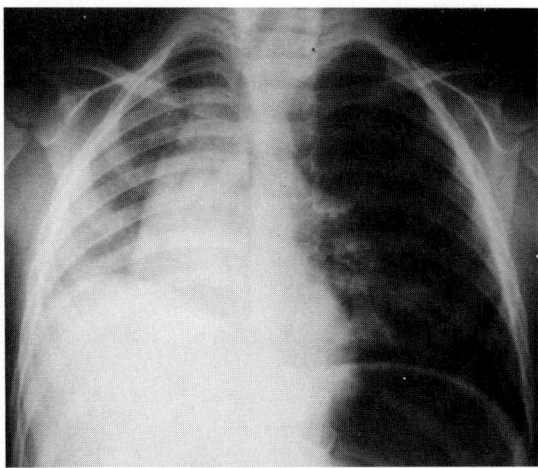

FIG. 26-3. Radiolucent left mainstem bronchus foreign body demonstrated with assisted expiratory film. Unilateral hyperinflation and mediastinal shift are provoked by the forced expiratory maneuver, a function of the "ball-valve" effect of a partially obstructive bronchial foreign body.

children with retained airway foreign bodies, however, have nondiagnostic films.

Radiologic evaluation in the emergency department should start with AP and lateral views of the chest and neck. Although plain films may be interpreted as normal, differential inflation of the affected lung, the most common abnormality identified, may be documented by fluoroscopy, lateral decubitus views, or an assisted expiratory film.[3,43,45,46,51-53] In the latter technique for a supine patient the radiology technician pushes on the epigastrium with a gloved fist, forcing the child to exhale to nearresidual volume. This maneuver accentuates the "ballvalve" effect of a partially obstructive bronchial foreign body, leading to residual hyperinflation of the involved lung and sometimes to mediastinal shift toward the unaffected side (Fig. 26-3). The assisted expiratory technique precludes the increased radiation exposure of fluoroscopy and does not require patient cooperation to obtain full exhalation.

Other indirect signs of an airway foreign body include resorption atelectasis beyond the site of complete bronchial obstruction and the presence of pulmonary infiltrates reflecting an inflammatory reaction.[43-46,51] Esclamodo reported positive findings on chest radiographs in only 42% of children with laryngotracheal foreign bodies, but a 92% rate of positive findings on lateral neck films in the same series, emphasizing the need to direct the examination to the neck when signs of upper airway obstruction are present.[47]

Although CT scan, xeroradiography, and ultrasonography have been advocated for foreign body imaging, their utility has not been demonstrated.[43,58] MRI scanning has recently been suggested for localizing peanuts in the airways.[59] Given the high morbidity associated with delay in diagnosis of an airway foreign body and the limited sensitivity of radiographic studies in identifying this condition, clinical judgment must dictate whether the child should be scheduled for diagnostic bronchoscopy in the absence of radiologic findings.

Management. Initial management of the patient who has aspirated a foreign body must focus on the establishment of adequate oxygenation and ventilation. In the prehospital setting, the conscious child who is able to talk and

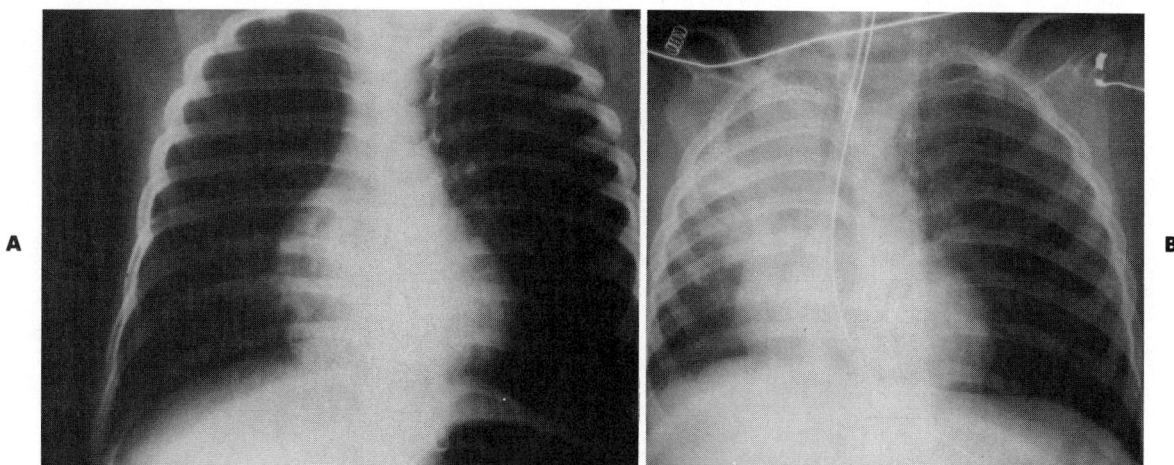

FIG. 26-4. A, AP chest radiograph of an infant with presumed reactive airway disease. **B,** The same patient, after endotracheal intubation, now demonstrating right upper lobe collapse. This 10-month-old infant entered the emergency department in respiratory failure, with poor air entry, faint expiratory wheezing, and a P_{CO_2} of 78 mm Hg. Aggressive bronchodilator treatment was ineffective. Endotracheal intubation resulted in immediate relief of symptoms, by dislodging a foreign body from the trachea into the right upper lobe bronchus. A peanut was recovered through rigid bronchoscopy.

cough should be administered 100% oxygen by whatever device is best tolerated—nasal prongs, face mask, or blow-by—and rapidly transported to a facility capable of performing pediatric bronchoscopy and establishing a surgical airway. In the patient with partial airway obstruction, blind attempts to remove foreign bodies by finger sweeps or to dislodge the foreign body by back blows or abdominal thrusts may cause impaction of the object in the trachea, converting a manageable situation to one that is immediately life threatening.[60]

The 1992 guidelines issued by the American Heart Association suggest age-specific maneuvers for foreign body removal in the case of airway obstruction where an aspiration has been witnessed or is strongly suspected, the patient is apneic and unconscious, or the patient is in rapidly progressive respiratory failure.[61] A series of 5 back blows and chest thrusts is recommended for children younger than 1 year of age, because of potential risk of injury to the abdominal viscera with the Heimlich maneuver. These are repeated as necessary. In children older than 1 year of age, a series of subdiaphragmatic abdominal thrusts is recommended, with the child either in the upright or in the supine position until the foreign body is dislodged.[61]

If these maneuvers fail to produce foreign body expulsion, direct laryngoscopy may permit visualization of a hypopharyngeal, proximal tracheal, or laryngeal foreign body and its removal with McGill forceps. If the foreign body is in the subglottic trachea, orotracheal intubation may be lifesaving, dislodging the object into a mainstem bronchus and converting complete to partial obstruction (Fig. 26-4, A and B). If the foreign body cannot be removed and endotracheal intubation cannot be achieved, needle cricothyrotomy may provide a mechanism to bypass the obstruction and deliver oxygen to the patient.[50,62] Although

emergency tracheotomy or cricothyrotomy may be lifesaving for the child who develops complete obstruction in the hospital setting, the techniques have high associated morbidity in unskilled hands.[6,63]

Fortunately, the majority of children arriving in the emergency department with airway foreign bodies are not in extremis. Administration of supplemental oxygen, establishment of vascular access, and close observation for deteriorating respiratory status are the only emergency department interventions required for most patients. Cardiopulmonary monitoring should be undertaken. If the child is in respiratory distress, determination of arterial blood gases or pulse oximetry in conjunction with capillary blood gases permits evaluation of the adequacy of oxygenation and ventilation during the emergency department course. If a child must be transferred to another facility for definitive management, transport should be performed by emergency medical personnel capable of managing the child's airway in the event of deterioration.

If a pharyngeal foreign body is easily visualized and the child's cooperation can be enlisted, it can safely be removed in the emergency department. In the vast majority of cases, however, airway foreign body removal is best achieved under controlled conditions in an operating suite. Rigid bronchoscopy under general anesthesia is the procedure of choice for removal of most foreign bodies of the trachea or bronchi.[43-46,52,53,55,63] The availability of a ventilating bronchoscope with a fiberoptic telescope system allows visualization, ventilation, and instrumentation to be achieved simultaneously.[60,63] After the foreign body has been removed, careful reexamination of the airway for additional foreign bodies or fragments is facilitated by this system.[43,63] The use of a Fogarty balloon catheter in conjunction with a rigid bronchoscope to facilitate airway foreign body removal has been advocated.[3,53] Foreign bodies at the level of the larynx may be retrieved with the aid of McGill forceps, with subsequent bronchoscopic examination to assess for additional objects in the distal airway.[46,53]

The incidence of postbronchoscopy complications ranges from 2% to 8%, most commonly in relation to foreign body reactions or subglottic edema from the endoscopic procedure.[3,47,52] Though flexible fiberoptic bronchoscopy may be undertaken to confirm the presence of an airway foreign body when the diagnosis is in question, most authors caution against the use of this technique for foreign body removal, because of the inherent potential for further airway compromise, inability to administer anesthetic agents, and greater difficulty in controlling instruments.[3,45,47,54,55,63]

Rarely, a child's airway is so unstable that induction of general anesthesia is not possible, necessitating the use of topical anesthetics and restraints to remove a tracheal or laryngeal foreign body.[60,63] Open thoracotomy may be required for foreign body removal when an object is tightly impacted and bronchoscopic attempts fail.[44,46,55]

References

Gastrointestinal Foreign Bodies

1. Papsin BC and Friedberg J: Aerodigestive-tract foreign bodies in children: pitfalls in management, *J Otolaryngol* 23:102-8, 1994.
2. Binder L and Anderson WA: Pediatric gastrointestinal foreign body ingestions, *Ann Emerg Med* 13:112, 1984.
3. O'Neill JA, Holcomb GW, Neblett WW: Management of tracheobronchial and esophageal foreign bodies in childhood, *J Pediatr Surg* 18:475, 1983.
4. Taylor RB: Esophageal foreign bodies, *Emerg Med Clin North Am* 5:301, 1987.
5. Suita S, Ohgami H, Nagasaki A et al: Management of pediatric patients who have swallowed foreign objects, *Am Surg* 55:585, 1989.
6. Stool SE and Manning SC: Foreign bodies of the pharynx and esophagus. In Bluestone CD and Stool SE, editors: *Pediatric otolaryngology,* vol 2, Philadelphia, 1990 WB Saunders.
7. Bonadio WA, Jona JZ, Glicklich M et al: Esophageal bougienage technique for coin ingestion in children, *J Pediatr Surg* 23:917, 1988.
8. Caravati EM, Bennett DL, McElwee NE: Pediatric coin ingestion: a prospective study on the utility of routine roentgenograms, *Am J Dis Child* 143:549, 1989.
9. Friedman EM: Caustic ingestions and foreign bodies in the aerodigestive tract of children, *Pediatr Clin North Am* 36:1403, 1989.
10. Paul RI, Christoffel KK, Binns HJ et al: Foreign body ingestions in children: Risk of complications varies with site of initial health care contact, *Pediatrics* 91:121-127, 1993.
11. Giordano A, Adams G, Boies L et al: Current management of esophageal foreign bodies, *Arch Otolaryngol* 107:249, 1981.
12. Savitt DL and Wason S: Delayed diagnosis of coin ingestion in children, *Am J Emerg Med* 6:378, 1988.
13. Spitz L: Management of ingested foreign bodies in children, *Br Med J* 4:468, 1971.
14. Henderson C, Engel J, Schlesinger P: Foreign body ingestion: review and suggested guidelines for management, *Endoscopy* 19:68, 1987.
15. Selivanov V, Sheldon GF, Cello JP et al: Management of foreign body ingestion, *Ann Surg* 199:187, 1984.
16. Nussbaum E, Fleming DG, Wood RE et al: Radiological case of the month, *Am J Dis Child* 138:1081, 1984.
17. Hodge D, Tecklenburg F, Fleisher G: Coin ingestion: does every child need a radiograph? *Ann Emerg Med* 14:443, 1985.
18. Nandi P and Ong GB: Foreign body in the oesophagus: review of 2394 cases, *Br J Surg* 65:5, 1978.
19. Schunk JE, Corneli H, Bolte R: Pediatric coin ingestions: a prospective study of coin location and symptoms, *Am J Dis Child* 143:546, 1989.
20. Vella EE and Booth PJ: Foreign body in the oesophagus, *Br Med J* 2:1042, 1965.
21. Marcuse EK and Quan L: Radiograph for coin ingestion (letter), *Ann Emerg Med* 15:511, 1986.
22. Arena L and Baker SR: Use of a metal detector to identify ingested metallic foreign bodies, *AJR Am J Roentgenol* 155:803-4, 1990.
23. Ros SP, Cetta F: Successful use of a metal detector in locating coins ingested by children, *J Pediatr* 120:752-753, 1992.
24. Bendig DW: Removal of blunt esophageal foreign bodies by flexible endoscopy without general anesthesia, *Am J Dis Child* 140:789, 1986.
25. Jona JZ, Glicklich M, Cohen RD: The contraindications for blind esophageal bougienage for coin ingestion in children, *J Pediatr Surg* 23:328, 1988.
26. Behrman RE, Vaughan FC, Nelson WE: *Textbook of pediatrics,* ed 13, Philadelphia, 1987, WB Saunders.
27. Campbell JB, Quattromani FL, Foley LC: Foley catheter removal of blunt esophageal foreign bodies: experience with 100 consecutive children, *Pediatr Radiol* 13:116, 1983.
28. Korcok M: No-confidence vote on catheter removal of foreign bodies (editorial), *JAMA* 247:3304, 1982.
29. Christie DL and Ament ME: Removal of foreign bodies from esophagus and stomach with flexible fiberoptic panendoscopes, *Pediatrics* 57:931, 1976.
30. Webb WA: Management of foreign bodies of the upper gastrointestinal tract: an update, *Gastrointest Endosc* 41:39-51, 1995.
31. Gracia C et al: Diagnosis and management of ingested foreign bodies: a ten-year experience, *Ann Emerg Med* 13:30, 1984.
32. Pellerin D, Fortier-Beaulieu M, Gueguen J: The fate of swallowed foreign bodies: experience of 1250 instances of sub-diaphragmatic foreign bodies in children, *Prog Pediatr Radiol* 2:286, 1969.
33. Paul RI and Jaffe DM: Sharp object ingestions in children: illustrative cases and literature review, *Pediatr Emerg Care* 4:245, 1988.
34. Litovitz TL: Battery ingestions: product accessibility and clinical course, *Pediatrics* 75:469, 1985.
35. Litovitz T and Schmitz BF: Ingestion of cylindrical and button batteries: an analysis of 2382 cases, *Pediatrics* 89:747-757, 1992.
36. Kuhns DW and Dire D: Button battery ingestions, *Ann Emerg Med* 18:293, 1989.
37. Mofenson HC, Greensher J, Caraccio TR et al: Ingestion of small flat disc batteries, *Ann Emerg Med* 12:88, 1983.
38. Maves MD, Lloyd TV, Carithers JS: Radiographic identification of ingested disc batteries, *Pediatr Radiol* 16:154, 1986.
39. Maves MD, Carithers JS, Birck HG: Esophageal burns secondary to disc battery ingestion, *Ann Otol Rhinol Laryngol* 93:364, 1984.
40. Volle E, Hanel D, Beyer P et al: Ingested foreign bodies: removal by magnet, *Radiology* 160:407, 1986.
41. Volle E, Beyer P, Kaufmann HJ: Therapeutic approach to ingested button-type batteries: magnetic removal of ingested button-type batteries, *Pediatr Radiol* 19:114, 1989.
42. Jaffe RB, Corneli HM: Fluroscopic removal of ingested alkaline batteries, *Radiology* 150:585, 1984.

Airway Foreign Bodies

43. McGuirt WF, Holmes KD, Feehs R et al: Tracheobronchial foreign bodies, *Laryngoscope* 98:615, 1988.
44. Hamilton AH, Carswell F, Wisheart JD: The Bristol Children's Hospital experience of tracheobronchial foreign bodies 1977-87, *Bristol Med Chir J* 104:72, 1989.
45. Steen KH, Zimmerman T: Tracheobronchial aspiration of foreign bodies in children: a study of 94 cases, *Laryngoscope* 100:525, 1990.
46. Laks Y and Barzilay Z: Foreign body aspiration in childhood, *Pediatr Emerg Care,* 4:102, 1988.
47. Esclamado RM and Richardson MA: Laryngotracheal foreign bodies in children, *Am J Dis Child* 141:259, 1987.
48. Mantel K and Butenandt I: Tracheobronchial foreign body aspiration in childhood, *Eur J Pediatr* 145:211, 1986.
49. Brown TCK and Clark CM: Inhaled foreign bodies in children, *Med J Aust* 2:322, 1983.
50. Lima JA: Laryngeal foreign bodies in children: a persistent, life-threatening problem, *Laryngoscope* 99:415, 1989.
51. Wiseman NE: The diagnosis of foreign body aspiration in childhood, *J Pediatr Surg* 19:531, 1984.
52. Black RE, Johnson DG, Matlak ME: Bronchoscopic removal of aspirated foreign bodies in children, *J Pediatr Surg* 29:682-684, 1994.

53. Vane DW, Pritchard MD, Colville CW et al: Bronchoscopy for aspirated foreign bodies in children, *Arch Surg* 123:885, 1988.

54. Banerjee A, Subba Rao K, Khanna SK et al: Laryngo-tracheobronchial foreign bodies in children, *J Laryngol Otol* 102:1029, 1988.

55. Weissberg D and Schwartz I: Foreign bodies in the tracheobronchial tree, *Chest* 91:730, 1987.

56. Gyi B, Austin JHM, Eisenberg LD: Radiolucent intratracheal foreign body mistaken for croup in a 9-year-old boy, *Am J Dis Child* 138:749, 1984.

57. Svedstrom E, Puhakka H, Kero P: How accurate is chest radiography in the diagnosis of tracheobronchial foreign bodies in children? *Pediatr Radiol* 19:520, 1989.

58. Cotton E and Yasuda K: Foreign body aspiration, *Pediatr Clin North Am* 31:937, 1984.

59. Imaizumi H, Kaneko M, Nara S et al: Definitive diagnosis and location of peanuts in the airways using magnetic resonance imaging techniques, *Ann Emerg Med* 23:1379-1382, 1994.

60. Holinger LD: Foreign bodies of the larynx, trachea, and bronchi. In Bluestone CD, Stool SE, Scheetz MD, editors: *Pediatric otolaryngology*, Philadelphia, 1990, WB Saunders.

61. American Heart Association: Guidelines for cardiopulmonary resuscitation and emergency cardiac care, *JAMA* 268:2171, 1992.

62. Chameides L and Hazinski MF (editors): *Textbook of pediatric advanced life support*, Dallas, 1994, American Heart Association.

63. Witt WJ: The role of rigid endoscopy in foreign body management, *Ear Nose Throat J* 64:70, 1985.

Management Principles

Dee Hodge III

Musculoskeletal injuries account for 10% to 15% of childhood injuries.[1] In younger children 70% of injuries are related to falls.[2,3] In older children and adolescents sports injuries and motor vehicle accidents predominate.[4] Of multiply traumatized patients, more than half have at least one musculoskeletal injury. The recognition of these injuries by the health-care provider is the key to preventing loss of function and possible deformity while assuring normal growth.

This chapter provides a basic explanation of the mechanisms and types of musculoskeletal injuries seen in children as compared to adults and discusses general management and diagnostic strategies. Specific injuries and their management are discussed in Chapters 28 through 31.

PATHOPHYSIOLOGY

Children have different injuries than adults because of the dynamic nature of the musculoskeletal system of the growing child. The patterns of structural failure vary with the degree of chondroosseous maturation. A brief overview of the development and growth of the skeletal system from conception to maturity is important to understanding the patterns of injuries seen.

Bones form from mesenchymal tissues that first chondrify and then ossify. Two types of ossification are seen in long bones. Endochondral ossification is the integrated replacement of a preexisting cartilage model with osteoid elements. This occurs with cellular proliferation of the physis and results in the lengthening of long bone. Membranous ossification of long bones is due to the formation and modification of bony elements by the periosteum and results in the enlargement of a bone's circumference.[5]

The long bone can be divided into four parts: the shaft of the bone, known as the *diaphysis;* the *metaphysis,* adjacent to the growth plate; the *growth* or *epiphyseal plate,* a radiolucent horizontal line near the end of the bone where longitudinal growth occurs; and the *epiphysis,* which is the end of the bone near a joint and is separated from the metaphysis by the epiphyseal plate (Fig. 27-1).

Besides the cellular components, the microscopic anatomy of cortical bone reveals a collagen matrix embedded with hydroxyapatite crystals. Strength is due to the complex interaction between these mineral crystals and collagen units. In general, the density of bone in children is less than in adults and immature bone is more porous because there are fewer lamellar components. The relatively porous compliant bone often responds to stress by buckling rather than fracturing.

The periosteum of both diaphyseal and metaphyseal bone is thicker in children, serving as a major attachment between the epiphysis and metaphysis. This thickness is beneficial because it is less readily disrupted and has greater osteogenic potential.

The ligaments around major joints are stronger and more resistant to tensile forces than the adjacent epiphyseal plate and perichondral ring. The strength of the ligaments and their attachments makes these the most stable elements of joints in children and accounts for the relative rarity of dislocations in children.[3,5,6] Forces that cause musculotendinous or ligamentous failure in adults often result in apophyseal avulsion or epiphyseal displacement in pediatric patients because of the ligamentous strength when contrasted with that of the periosteum and epiphyseal plate.

TYPES OF INJURY

It is best to approach common injuries by dividing them into two broad categories: macrotrauma (fractures, sprains, strains, and dislocations) and repeated microtrauma (overuse syndromes). One must always consider the possibility of bony injuries in children after mechanisms of force that in an adult would cause only soft tissue injuries.

Fractures

Fractures are any breaks in the continuity of bone or cartilage. They are described in terms of the anatomic location on the bone, the fracture pattern, and the relationship of the fracture fragments to each other (see Fig. 27-1).

Several fracture patterns occur in adults and children (Fig. 27-2). *Transverse fractures* occur when the fracture

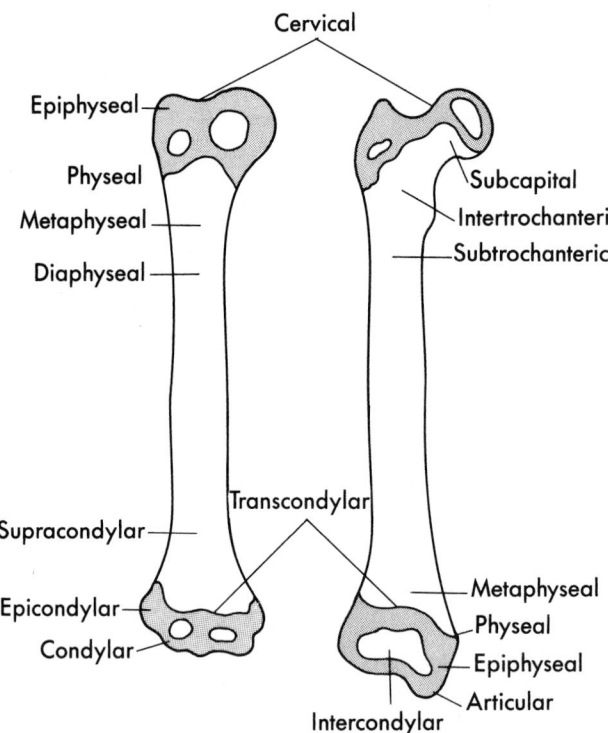

FIG. 27-1. Schematic of humerus (left) and femur (right) from a 10-year-old child showing anatomic locations to localize fractures. (*Redrawn from Ogden JA: Skeletal injury in the child, ed 2, Philadelphia, 1990, WB Saunders.*)

line is at a right angle to the bone. These injuries are due to angulating forces. *Longitudinal fractures* are those of the fracture line along the longitudinal axis of the bone. *Oblique fractures* are angled relative to the longitudinal axis. *Spiral fractures* occur on an oblique fracture line that, in addition, encircles a portion of the shaft. *Impacted fractures* are due to compression injury with crushing of cortical and trabecular bone on both sides of the fracture. *Comminuted fractures* are characterized by several fragments of variable sizes.[7]

Stress fractures in adults occur when normal forces are applied to weakened bone. In children, however, these fractures result when repetitive loading is placed on normal bone until the bone fatigues. These fractures may be difficult to diagnose and may resemble infective or malignant conditions.[8]

Fracture fragments may relate to each other with (1) sideways shift, (2) angulation, (3) overriding, (4) distraction, (5) shortening, and (6) rotation. These relationships may occur singly or in combination.

An *open fracture* is in contact with the external surface of the body. There are three types of open fractures. In type 1 fracture the wound is 1 cm or less and somewhat clean. In type 2 open fractures the wounds are greater than 1 cm and are not characterized by extensive soft tissue damage, flap, or avulsion. Type 3 open fractures are associated with extensive soft tissue trauma or the following

special considerations: open segmental fracture irrespective of wound size, farm injuries, high-velocity and close-range gunshot wounds, open fractures with neurovascular compromise, traumatic amputations, open fractures more than 8 hours old, and mass casualties.[9]

Fractures Unique to Childhood. The elasticity of children's bones allows the bone to deform before breaking.

Cortical or torus fractures are due to impaction forces. Because of the porous nature of metaphyseal bone the response to a compression load is buckling of the bone rather than complete fracture. The site of fracture resembles the torus of a Roman column. These fractures are common, representing 15% of childhood fractures.[6]

A *greenstick fracture* results when force is applied but released before the fracture is completed. The periosteum tears on the fractured side but remains intact on the compression side. The cortical bone deforms but remains intact on the compression (concave) side.

Bending or bowing fractures are due to the propensity of pediatric bone to deform instead of fail. The increase in mineralization characterizing mature bone decreases the amount of deformity it will tolerate before failure. These fractures are most commonly seen in the long bones of the forearm or leg when an angular midshaft fracture of the other bone occurs.[10,11]

Epiphyseal-metaphyseal growth plate fractures account for 10% to 15% of the fractures in children.[6,12] These fractures are most often described by the Salter-Harris classification, which is based on the five fracture types shown in Fig. 27-3.[13] More recent classification systems describe nine fracture types.[14,15] These more detailed classifications are more difficult for the nonorthopedist to remember and are less widely used.

Salter-Harris type I fractures (6% of physeal injuries) extend through the physis; clinical diagnosis is based on tenderness over the physis.[16] They may not be displaced, making them difficult to diagnose radiographically. These are common injuries and should be considered similar to dislocations with tearing of the periosteum when the patient's bony development has not fused at the epiphysis. Type II fractures follow the physeal-metaphyseal interface, extending into the metaphysis. The metaphyseal fragments vary in size. This is the most common physeal-metaphyseal injury pattern: 75% of physeal injuries. Reduction and immobilization of type I and type II injuries for 3 to 4 weeks produce a good result. Type III fractures (8% of physeal injuries) are transverse along the physeal-metaphyseal interface; they then cross the physis, epiphyseal ossification center, and articular cartilage. The epiphyseal fragment is unstable and requires good alignment. Type IV fractures account for 8% of physeal injuries. The fracture line extends from the articular surface to the metaphyseal cortex, traversing the epiphysis, physis, and metaphyseal bone. Surgical intervention to stabilize the fragments is indicated. Type V fractures (1% of physeal injuries) show a linear disruption of the physeal plate with microvascular compromise and a high risk of growth problems.[16] Like type I fractures these may be difficult to diagnose; diagnosis is often made retrospectively. Specific applications of this classification of fractures to the ankle are discussed in Chapter 30.

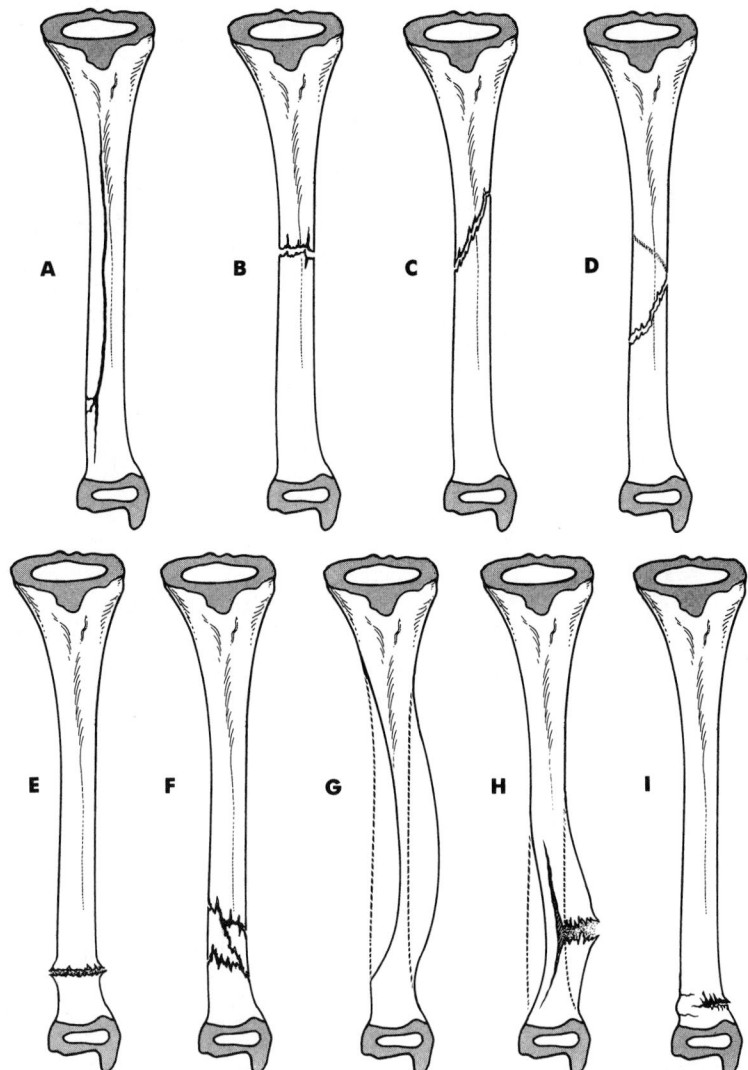

FIG. 27-2. Schematic of tibia (3-year-old child) showing basic types of fractures. **A,** Longitudinal; **B,** transverse; **C,** oblique; **D,** spiral; **E,** impacted; **F,** comminuted; **G,** bending/bowing; **H,** greenstick; **I,** cortical/torus. (*Redrawn from Ogden JA: Skeletal injury in the child, ed 2, Philadelphia, 1990, WB Saunders.*)

Sprains

Sprains describe injury to a *ligamentous structure* and are usually a diagnosis of exclusion in children. Sprains are classified by the following grading system. Grade I sprains are characterized by stretching or microscopic tearing of the ligament. Joint stability is normal and the patient can bear weight. Grade II sprains reveal a partial overt tearing of the ligament, but at least some ligamentous continuity remains. Joint instability, pain, and disability occur. Weight bearing is painful, and there is localized soft tissue hemorrhage and hemarthrosis. Grade III sprains have a total loss of ligamentous continuity; ecchymosis is present. The joint is unstable, extremely painful, and unusable. There is abnormal motion with absolute joint instability, deformity with swelling, and inability to bear weight. Persistent instability may occur without surgical repair.

The signs and symptoms commonly seen with sprains include limitation of motion, swelling, and localized tenderness over the anatomic course of the injured structure. Ligament laxity is best appreciated immediately after injury and before appreciable swelling has occurred.[17-21]

Strains

Strains describe injury to a *muscle-tendon* unit. Grade I or first-degree strains reveal the least disruption, and there is no deficit in the muscle tendon unit. In grade II or second-degree strains partial tearing, bleeding, and spasm occur. Again there is no deficit in the muscle-tendon unit. In grade III or third-degree strains disruption of the muscle-tendon unit is complete. Signs and symptoms of strain include mild to marked local tenderness, bleeding with spasm, and pain in the affected limb; evidence of a

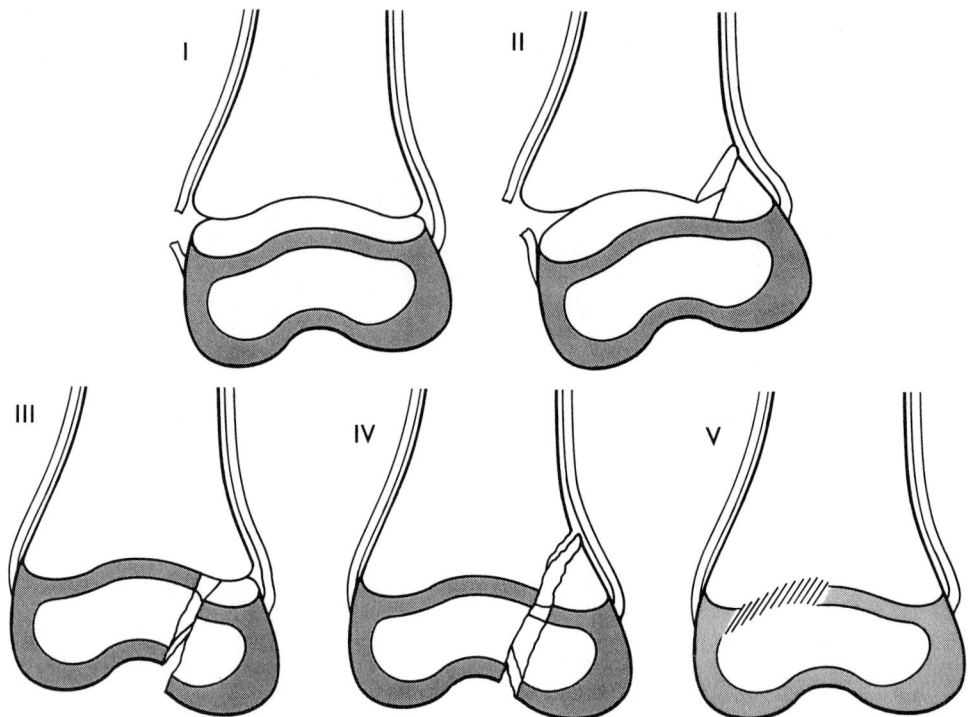

FIG. 27-3. Salter-Harris classification of epiphyseal fractures (see text).

palpable defect; and hematomas that when large are associated with more severe strains. Grade III strains are rare in young children, but tendon avulsion with an attached piece of bone is not uncommon.[19,22]

Dislocations

Dislocations represent displacement of one or more bones of a joint from the original position. These injuries are rare in children because of the relative strength of the ligaments and musculotendinous units around their joints. Fractures are, therefore, more common than dislocations.

DIAGNOSTIC FINDINGS

In the emergency department a comprehensive history and description of the events of the accident provide helpful clues to the severity and type of injury to be suspected. The mechanism and time of injury, neurologic findings (paresthesia or weakness), and subsequent course should be ascertained. The mechanism of injury is particularly important in defining the potential complications and nature of injury. By using the mnemonic *AMPLE* (*A*, allergy; *M*, medication; *P*, past medical history including tetanus immunization status; *L*, time since last meal; *E*, events leading to the accident or injury) one can be assured of obtaining an adequate history.[23] Frequently the injury was not witnessed and the child may be too young or too frightened to give an adequate account. Children rarely complain persistently unless there is abnormality; pseudo-paralysis secondary to pain is common. Pain may also be referred; the classic example is hip problems characterized as knee pain.

Histories inconsistent with the injury should raise the suspicion of child abuse. Up to 10% of musculoskeletal injuries in children younger than 5 years of age may not be accidental (see Chapter 45).

Physical Examination

The evaluation of musculoskeletal injury involves a three-step process that occurs while building a thoughtful and interactive relationship with the child. Obviously, multiple trauma injuries take precedence. The first part of the specific musculoskeletal examination is careful observation. Close attention should be paid to evidence of angulation, deformity, shortening or rotation, and swelling of the injured extremity. Next gentle palpation should be done to find point tenderness. Finally the injured extremity should be moved to examine for crepitus and abnormal movements, using varus, valgus, and anteroposterior stress in several positions of flexion and extension. Evaluation should include the joint above and below the site of injury. Document distal motor function and sensory perception, vascular function, ecchymoses, and swelling; repeat the examination after any manipulation. The absence of pulses distal to an angulated injured extremity requires immediate reduction, if possible.

After initial stabilization treatment must focus on establishment of normal alignment of bones and joints; assurance of tissue perfusion; immobilization; and elevation of the injured extremity, identifying open fractures and neurovascular compromise. Consultation must be obtained as indicated.

Should there be any suggestion of vascular compromise, consultation is mandatory. The absence of a pulse does not always indicate that the vascular status is at risk, nor does the presence of a pulse assure adequate circulation. Severe pain in the forearm or calf, pain with passive stretching of a finger or toe, or a sensory deficit in the distal extremity is a more sensitive indicator of ischemia caused by arterial injury or a compartment syndrome.

Radiographic Evaluation

Plain films are the study of choice in musculoskeletal injury after appropriate splinting, particularly in view of the difficulty of physical examination in children. A minimum of two views at 90 degrees to each other, including the joints on either side of the injury, should be obtained. Other radiographs such as oblique views may be useful to visualize certain joint spaces (e.g., hip, knee, and shoulder) but are not ordered routinely. Comparison views, although often helpful in visualizing areas with multiple ossification centers such as the elbow, are not mandatory and should be obtained selectively. They may be obtained whenever a finding is doubtful.[24,25] Always use an organized approach when evaluating radiographs, looking for subtle changes, such as deformities of the cortex, abrupt angle step-offs, loss of symmetry, soft tissue swelling over the site of injury, obliteration of normal fascial plains, fat pads, and other soft tissue changes.[25,26] Radiographs should be of good technical quality; poor films should never be accepted. Repeating radiographic studies 7 to 10 days after injury is often beneficial in identifying subtle fractures since at this time new callus formation and periosteal reaction are visible.

Physical findings may be at least partially predictive of a fracture. A study of adult patients suggested that specific clinical findings are more commonly associated with positive radiographs: gross signs (deformity, instability, crepitation), point tenderness, ecchymoses or severe swelling of the upper extremity, moderate to severe pain with weight bearing in a hip or thigh, or any positive finding in a knee. Other factors that must be considered in the evaluation include abnormal examination of distal neurovascular or tendon function, open wound associated with musculoskeletal injury, palpable mass, medical history suggestive of an increased risk of fracture (cancer, chronic renal disease), impaired peripheral sensation, altered less of consciousness, or intoxication.[27,28]

The criteria's applicability to pediatric patients has been evaluated, and it appears that although not all of these adult criteria are directly applicable, many are as outlined in the box.[29,30] In applying such guidelines, obviously the impact of potentially missing fractures must be considered since criteria miss some significant injuries.

The age of fractures may be estimated by the following radiographic guidelines:

Resolution of soft tissue findings	4 to 10 days
Periosteal elevation	7 to 14 days
Soft callus	14 to 21 days
Hard callus	21 to 42 days
Remodeling	1 year

Computed tomography (CT) scanning is an adjunctive procedure. It is especially useful in spinal trauma, pelvic

---

Clinical Findings Suggestive of a Positive Extremity Radiograph

Upper extremity	Lower extremity
McConnochie, et al[29]	
Activity not routine	Activity not routine
Bone point tenderness	Bone point tenderness
Gross finding	Knee injury
Pain with motion	Foot injury
Swelling moderate or severe	
Time since injury >6 hr	
Rivera et al[30]	
Gross deformity	Gross deformity
Point tenderness	Pain on motion

---

and acetabular injuries, triplane fractures of the ankle, and sternoclavicular joint injuries.[30]

Magnetic resonance imaging (MRI) studies are increasingly useful in evaluation of musculoskeletal injuries. Because of the enhanced soft tissue contrast resolution this technique is helpful in the evaluation of fibrocartilaginous injuries and in the detection of radiographically occult fractures. The technique is also useful in assessing ligamentous and muscular injuries and currently is most commonly used for examination of the knee to assess meniscus tears.[31-33]

MANAGEMENT

Initially management of musculoskeletal injuries requires assessment and management of life-threatening injuries. Maintaining an adequate airway, assuring cervical spine stabilization, evaluating and maintaining adequate ventilation, and maintaining adequate circulation/perfusion are essential before concentrating on specific musculoskeletal injuries. Prehospital evaluation of musculoskeletal injuries includes distal motor, sensory, and vascular function. Distal function should be evaluated and recorded during the secondary assessment and repeated every 15 minutes during transport.[34]

Prehospital management of musculoskeletal injuries hinges on minimization of the initial swelling and immobilization. To accomplish these, "RICE" (*rest, ice, compression, elevation*) should be applied immediately. A wet elastic wrap should be used both to hold the ice pack in place and to protect the skin. Ice should not be applied directly to the skin. Next compress and elevate the injured site. The affected limb is then immobilized in position to assure that further injury does not occur and to provide some pain relief.[17,19] Distal function should be evaluated and recorded after immobilization.

Analgesia

Relief of pain is a fundamental principle of the management of musculoskeletal injuries. Children's pain is often times treated less vigorously than adults' for many reasons.[35,36] Proper use of conscious sedation and analgesia in the emergency department is an essential part of compassionate medicine and makes the physician's job easier.[37-39] Analgesia with or without sedation is indicated whenever painful manipulations or procedures are anticipated. The outpatient facility must be able to provide emergency life support and equipment for all ages. Monitoring should include continuous observation of color and airway patency. Heart rate and respiratory rate should be monitored, and pulse oximetry is desirable. Oxygen and suctioning equipment should be readily available, as should emergency medications.[40,41] Contraindications to conscious sedation include head trauma, hypotension, need for general anesthesia, and patient condition worse than ASA class II[42-54] (see Chapter 7).

Local analgesia may be achieved for closed reduction by "hematoma blocks," whereby lidocaine 1% to 2% is injected directly into the hematoma overlying a fracture, which requires minimal reduction.

More complete control can be achieved by the "mini" Bier's block, which provides excellent regional analgesia for fracture reduction. In this technique, two intravenous lines should be placed: one in the affected limb and a second in the unaffected limb. A cardiac monitor is placed on the patient. Above the elbow a double-cuff pneumatic tourniquet or two blood pressure cuffs should be placed. The limb should be exsanguinated using a pneumatic splint or Esmarch bandage placed on the affected limb. The upper cuff should be inflated to 200 to 250 mm Hg. A 1.5 to 3 mg/kg volume of a 0.5% solution of lidocaine should be administered intravenously in the affected limb over 30 to 60 seconds. The lower cuff should be inflated to 100 mm Hg above systolic pressure and the upper cuff should then be deflated. Anesthesia is usually satisfactory in 5 to 10 minutes. The tourniquet can be left in place for 60 to 90 minutes after the procedure (or at least 15 minutes after the effusion of lidocaine). To terminate the block, the blood pressure cuff should be slowly deflated. The patient should be observed for at least 1 hour in the emergency department.

Immobilization

Immobilization is the treatment of choice for most musculoskeletal injuries on arrival in the prehospital or emergency department setting. Immobilization accomplishes the following objectives: it decreases pain, risk of converting a minor injury to a major one, risk of blood flow restriction, and chance of neurologic injury; prevents further injury; and controls bleeding. Immobilization should begin immediately, continue until the injury has healed, and be accomplished by splinting or casting. In the emergency department, casting is usually delayed 24 to 48 hours after swelling has subsided.

Splinting can be performed in the position of function with firm materials, slings, and tape and is used primarily as initial treatment to allow rest for an injured area. Acute injuries should be splinted over adequate padding and affixed with cotton or elastic bandages. Swelling during this period can cause neurovascular compromise and needs to be monitored. In some situations, splinting is the definitive therapy.

One joint above and one below should usually be incorporated. Dislocations should be splinted, using the bone above and the one below the affected joint. Fractured extremities should also be splinted to immobilize the joint above and below the fracture. All fractures should be splinted in the position of function. In general the following principles should be adhered to: (1) splints of appropriate size and shape should be used; (2) all bony prominences should be padded to decrease the chance of development of pressure areas; (3) application of fully circular rigid splints or casts should be avoided, because they increase the chance of compartment syndrome or impaired distal function to an acutely injured extremity; (4) splint should not be wrapped in place too tightly; (5) adequate aftercare instructions should be given; and (6) when in doubt, the fracture should be splinted.[55]

Those fractures with obvious deformities should be stabilized in the prehospital setting or emergency department on arrival and before complete evaluation unless sensation or circulation distal to the injury is compromised, as indicated by pain, pallor, pulselessness, paralysis, paresthesias, and pain with passive movement. If neurovascular deficits exist, gentle longitudinal traction in line with the extremity should be effected before immobilization.

Many types of splints are available for different injuries. Inflatable splints are particularly useful in the prehospital setting. Soft splints, such as figure-of-eight or clavicular straps, pillow splints, and Jones' dressings, are appropriate for specific injuries. Rigid splints may be prefabricated, made of Webril and plaster, or fashioned from premade plaster rolls. Some commonly used splints are shown in Fig. 27-4.

Pneumatic antishock trousers may be used as an inflatable splint to stabilize femur fractures. Traction splints such as the Hare's or Thomas' splint may be useful for more prolonged stabilization.

The *long leg splint* extends just below the buttock to 3 inches above the malleoli. When the knee is in full extension this splint is an effective knee immobilizer; it stabilizes distal femur, proximal, and midshaft tibia/fibula fractures when fashioned with the knee in slight flexion, the splint extended to the foot, and the ankle in neutral position of function.

Short leg posterior splints provide initial treatment of simple and displaced fractures of the foot and ankle.[56-58] A sugar tong splint may be preferred in the treatment of acute ankle injuries.[46]

A *sling and swathe* are used in the treatment of injuries of the upper extremity between the sternoclavicular joint and the elbow. The arm is placed at 90 degrees of flexion with a sling and immobilized against the chest by means of a swathe wrapped around the body.

Long arm splints may be employed for fractures of the forearm and distal radius.

Posterior arm splints are used for elbow and forearm injuries, as well as wrist injuries in which forearm rotation and elbow flexion must be eliminated. The splint is applied from the dorsal aspect of the midupper arm, across the olecranon, and down the ulnar aspect of the forearm to the distal palmar flexion crease. Seven to eight layers of plaster are used from the upper part of the humerus across the radial side of the elbow as a cross-support. The elbow should be at 90 degrees of flexion and the forearm in neutral position.

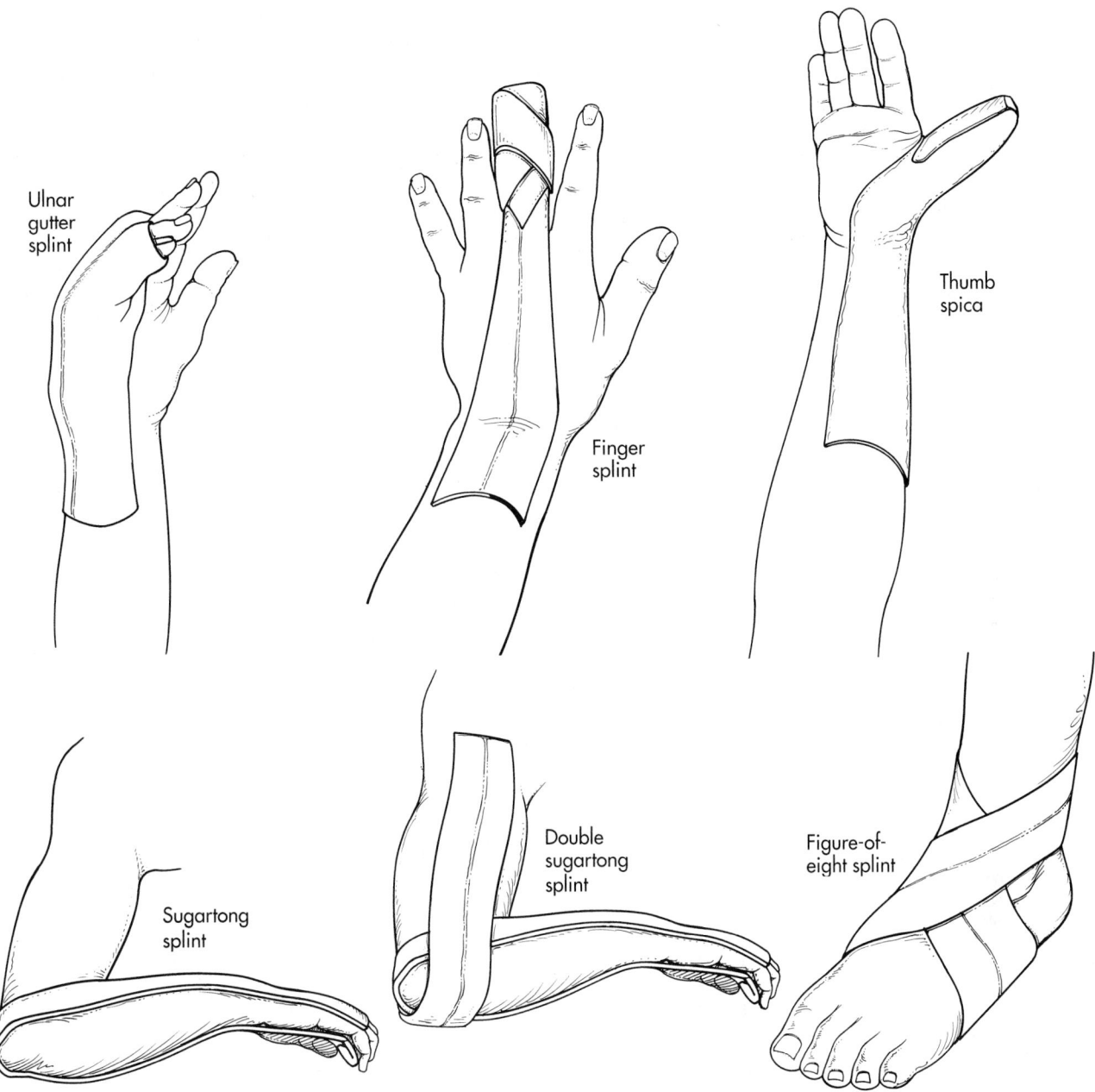

FIG. 27-4. Splint types (see text). (*Redrawn from Orthopedic Casting Laboratory, Inc, 1985.*)

Continued

Sugar tong splint is important for injuries of the forearm and elbow. The *brachial humerus splint* is applied from above the acromioclavicular joint, over the humerus, around the elbow, and up to the axillary splint crease. A collar and cuff provide support. The *forearm splint* extends from the distal palmar flexion crease to the elbow. The plaster is drawn around the elbow to the dorsum of the hand just proximal to the metacarpophalangeal (MCP) joint.

Splints are also used for injuries of the hand and wrist.

In general, the position of function or "hooded cobra" places the wrist in neutral (the long axis of the forearm roughly lines up with the long axis of the thumb), the MCP joints are flexed to about 60 to 70 degrees, the interphalangeal (IP) joints are flexed 10 to 20 degrees, and the thumb is widely abducted. The tips of the fingers must be visible for neurovascular examination.

Special types of hand and wrist splints are also available. The *ulnar gutter splint* is useful for nondisplaced fractures of the fourth and fifth digits. The fingers should be kept at 35 to 40 degrees of flexion at the MCP joint and 20 to 30 degrees at the IP joint. *Dorsal extension splints* are used for nonrotated finger injuries involving the phalanges, metacarpals, MCP, and proximal interphalangeal (PIP) joints. A foam-padded aluminum splint is taped to the dorsum of the hand and wrist and bent to keep the MCP joint at 90

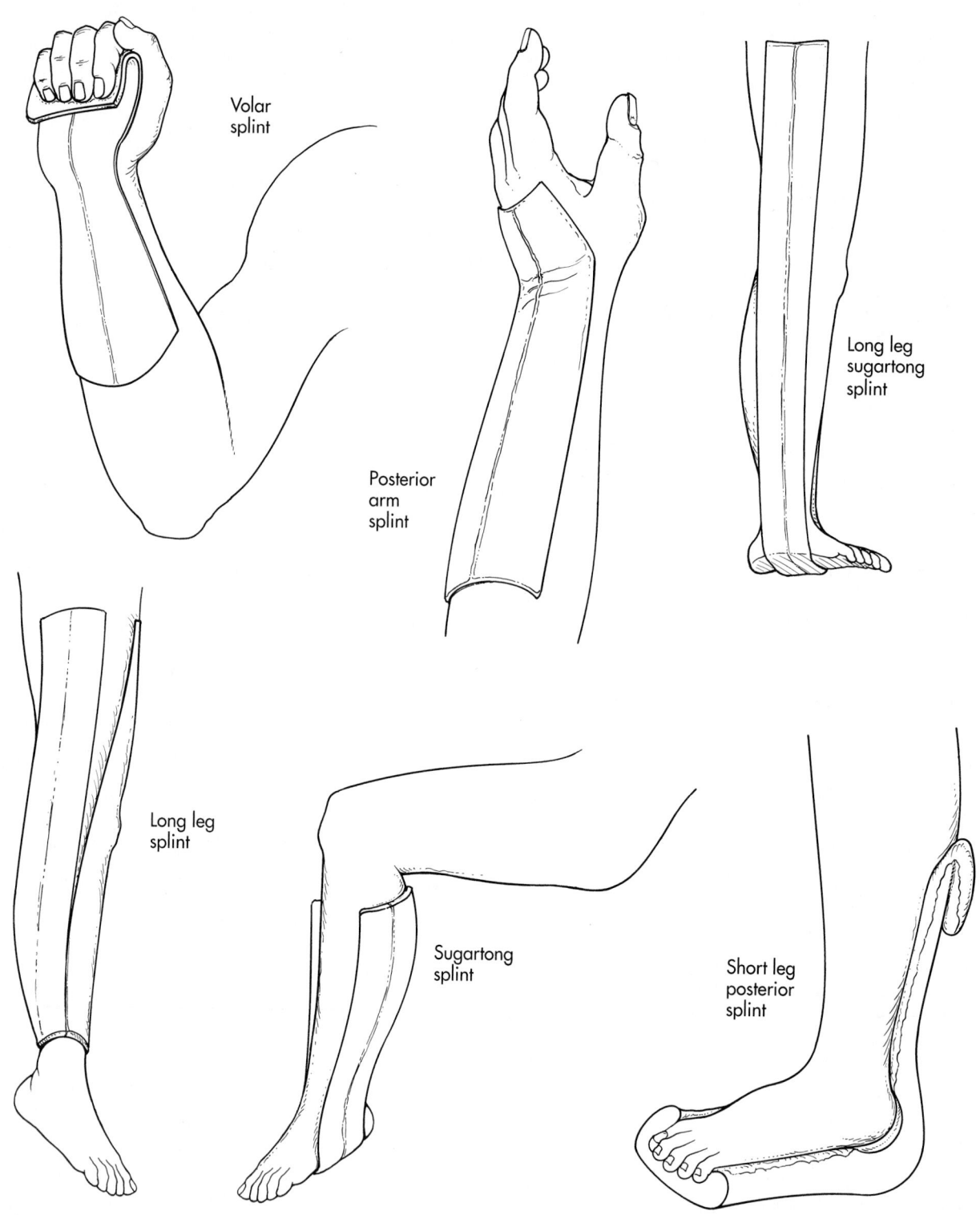

Volar
splint

Posterior
arm
splint

Long leg
sugartong
splint

Long leg
splint

Sugartong
splint

Short leg
posterior
splint

FIG. 27-4, cont'd.

degrees of flexion. The PIP joint is bent to 45 degrees. The *thumb spica* is mandatory for scaphoid fractures and injuries to the thumb. Plaster is cut in half longitudinally into two tails. The splint is applied to the radial aspect of the forearm, and one tail is wrapped around the thenar eminence and onto the palm and hand across the distal palmar crease. The second flap is wrapped around the thumb and up to the base of the nail.

In general, sprains and strains should be elevated, with ice packs applied for 12 to 24 hours. Elevation can reduce swelling and pain. Ice packs are best prepared by crushing ice and placing it with some water in a plastic bag and applied for 15 to 20 minutes every 3 to 4 hours with continuing use of an elastic bandage in between. The elastic ACE bandage, if used, should be rewrapped as necessary if too loose or too tight.

Parents should immediately report any pressure or pain within a cast or splint, increasing blueness, coldness, tingling, swelling, or decreased motion of the toes or fingers. Oral analgesics and antiinflammatory agents may be useful for ongoing care.

Orthopedic Referral

Immediate orthopedic referral should be obtained for any structurally significant fractures, obvious deformity, evidence of neurovascular compromise, open dislocations, and dislocations with neurovascular compromise. Anteroposterior angulation and bayonet apparatus often correct, particularly those in children younger than 2 years. Fractures that are shortened, angulated, rotated, intraarticular, or that cross the growth plate usually need anatomic reduction and referral. Open fractures require antibiotics, debridement, fracture stabilization, and wound coverage.[9] Other injuries that require immediate orthopedic referral include wounds penetrating into a joint space and possible grade III strains.[59,60]

Hospitalization is indicated for patients who have any fracture or dislocation involving potential vascular compromise (supracondylar for humerus and posterior knee dislocation).

Long-Term Sequelae

The long-term sequelae of fractures in children focus on the problems of growth slowdown or arrest. Other problems include disorders of union, which are unusual in children and when seen are associated with Salter type III fractures and open fractures. In delayed union, fracture healing is abnormally slow. Nonunion and malunion occur when fracture alignment is unsatisfactory. Avascular necrosis may be a complication of injury that disrupts blood supply. Improperly managed greenstick fractures, bowing fractures, and Salter type II, III, and IV injuries produce angulation deformities. Shortening may occur with Salter V fractures, and longitudinal growth deformities are especially common sequelae of Salter type II and III fractures. Overgrowth of bone, infection with open fracture, joint stiffness, articular deformity, and posttraumatic arthritis are also seen.

References

1. Ogden JA: *Skeletal injury in the child*, ed 2, Philadelphia, 1990, WB Saunders.
2. Sacks JJ, Smith JD, Kaplan KM et al: The epidemiology of injuries in Atlanta day-care centers, *JAMA* 262:1641, 1989.
3. Williamson DM and Loudon IMR: Why do children break their arms? *Injury* 19:9, 1988.
4. McLain LG and Reynolds S: Sports injuries in high school, *Pediatrics* 84:446, 1989.

Pathophysiology

5. Ogden JA: "Uniqueness of growing bones." In Rockwood CA Jr, Wilkins KE, King RE, editors: *Fractures in children*, vol 3, Philadelphia, 1984, JB Lippincott.
6. Reed MH: Fractures and dislocations of extremities in children, *J Trauma* 17:351, 1977.

Types of Injury

7. Chipman C and Strangeland RG: Basic principles of emergency orthopedics. In Chipman C, editor: *Emergency department orthopedics*, Rockville, Md, 1982, Aspen Publishers.
8. Devas MB: Stress fractures in children, *J Bone Joint Surg* 45B:528, 1963.
9. Scott WP and Grantham SA: The open fracture, *Orthop Review* 14:19, 1985.
10. Blankstein A, Liberty E, Itay S et al: Biomechanical aspect of traumatic bowing of the forearm in children: clinical and radiographic findings also clarified, *Orthop Rev* 14:217, 1985.
11. Mabrey JD and Fitch RD: Plastic deformation in pediatric fractures: mechanism and treatment, *J Pediatr Orthop* 9:310, 1989.
12. Pollen AG: Fractures involving the epiphyseal plate, *Reconstr Surg Traumatol* 17:25, 1979.
13. Salter RB and Harris WR: Injuries involving epiphyseal plates, *J Bone Joint Surg* 45A:587, 1963.
14. Ogden JA: Injury to the growth mechanisms of the immature skeleton, *Skeletal Radiol* 6:237, 1981.
15. Shapiro F: Epiphyseal growth plate fractures-separations: a pathophysiologic approach, *Orthopedics* 5:720, 1982.
16. Rogers LF: The radiography of epiphyseal injuries, *Radiology* 96:289, 1970.
17. Dyment PG: Initial management of minor acute soft tissue injuries, *Pediatr Ann* 17:99, 1988.
18. Garrick JG: Sports medicine, *Pediatr Clin North Am* 33:1541, 1986.
19. Smith RW, Reischl SF: Treatment of ankle sprains in young athletes, *Am J Sports Med* 14:465, 1986.
20. Tursz A and Crost M: Sports-related injuries in children, *Am J Sports Med* 14:294, 1986.
21. Webber A: Acute soft-tissue injuries in the young athlete, *Clin Sports Med* 7:611, 1988.
22. Kellett J: Acute soft tissue injuries-a review of the literature, *Med Sci Sports Exerc* 18:489, 1986.

Diagnostic Findings

23. Worsing RA: Principles of prehospital care of musculoskeletal injuries, *Emerg Med Clinics North Am* 2:205, 1984.
24. Chacon D, Kissoon N, Brown T et al: Use of comparison radiographs in the diagnosis of traumatic injuries of the elbow *Ann Emerg Med* 21:895, 1992.
25. Rang M and Wright J: Pitfalls in fractures, *Pediatr Ann* 18:53, 1989.
26. Resnik CS: Diagnostic imaging of pediatric skeletal trauma, *Radiol Clin North Am* 27:1013, 1989.
27. Rogers LF: *Radiology of skeletal trauma*, vol 1, New York, 1982, Churchill Livingstone.
28. Brand DA, Frazier WH, Kohlhepp WC et al: A protocol for selecting patients with injured extremities who need x-rays, *N Engl J Med* 306:333, 1982.
29. McConnochie KM, Roghmann KJ, Pasternack J et al: Prediction rules for selective radiographic assessment of extremities in children and adolescents, *Pediatrics* 86:45, 1990.
30. Rivera FP, Parish RA, Mueller BA: Extremity injury in children: predictive value of clinical findings, *Pediatrics* 78:803, 1986.
31. Dalenka MK, Boorstein JM, Zlatkin MB: Computed tomography of musculoskeletal trauma, *Radiol Clin North Am* 27:933, 1989.
32. Cohen MD: Clinical utility of magnetic resonance imaging in pediatrics, *Am J Dis Child* 140:947, 1986.
33. Council on Scientific Affairs: Musculoskeletal applications of magnetic resonance imaging, *JAMA* 262:2420, 1989.

Management

34. Deutsch AL and Mink JH: Magnetic resonance imaging of musculoskeletal injuries, *Radiol Clin North Am* 27:983, 1989.
35. Schecter NL: The undertreatment of pain in children: an overview, *Pediatr Clin North Am* 36:781, 1989.
36. Selbst SM and Clark M: Analgesia use in the emergency department (abstract), *Am J Dis Child* 143:434, 1989.
37. Schecter NL: Pain and pain control in children, *Curr Prob Pediatr* 15:1, 1985.
38. Cohen DE and Broennle AM: Emergency department anesthetic management. In Fleisher G and Ludwig S, editors: *Textbook of pediatric emergency medicine*, 3, Baltimore, 1993, Williams & Wilkins.

39. Zeltzer LK, Jay SM, Fisher DM: The management of pain associated with pediatric procedures, *Pediatr Clin North Am* 36:941, 1989.

40. Selbst SM and Henretig FM: The treatment of pain in the emergency department, *Pediatr Clin North Am* 36:965, 1989.

41. American Academy of Pediatrics: Guidelines for elective use of conscious sedation, deep sedation, and general anesthesia in pediatric patients, *Pediatrics* 76:317, 1985.

42. Barclay JK, Hunter KM, McMillan W: Midazolam and diazepam compared as sedatives for outpatient surgery under local analgesia, *Oral Surg* 59:349, 1984.

43. Clark MS, Silverstone LM, Coke JM: Midazolam, diazepam and placebo as intravenous sedatives for dental surgery, *Oral Surg* 63:127, 1987.

44. Taylor MB, Vine PR, Hatch DJ: Intramuscular midazolam premedication in small children, *Anesthesia* 41:21, 1986.

45. Billmire DA, Neale HW, Gregory RO: Use of IV fentanyl in the outpatient treatment of pediatric facial trauma, *J Trauma* 25:1079, 1985.

46. Miller DL and Wall RT: Fentanyl and Diazepam for analgesia and sedation during radiologic special procedures, *Radiology* 162:195, 1987.

47. Hubert C, Yacoub M, Turgeon LR: Effect of hydroxyzine on morphine analgesia for the treatment of postoperative pain, *Anesth Analg* 59:690, 1980.

48. Griffin GC, Campbell VD, Jones: Nitrous oxide-oxygen sedation for minor surgery, experience in a pediatric setting, *JAMA* 245:2411, 1981.

49. Nahata MC, Clotz MA, Krogg EA: Adverse effects of meperidine, promethazine, and chlorpromazine for sedation in pediatric patients, *Clin Pediatr* 24:558, 1985.

50. Ros SP: Outpatient analgesia-a tale of two regimens, *Pediatr Emerg Care* 3:228, 1987.

51. Stambaugh JE and Wainer IW: Drug interaction: meperidine and chlorpromazine a toxic combination, *J Clin Pharmacol* 21:140, 1981.

52. Terndrup TE, Cantor RM, Madden CM: Intramuscular meperidine, promethazine, and chlorpromazine: analysis of use and complication in 487 pediatric emergency department patients, *Ann Emerg Med* 18:528, 1989.

53. Olney BW, Lugg PC, Turner PL et al: Outpatient treatment of upper extremity injuries in childhood using intravenous regional anesthesia, *J Pediatr Orthop* 8:576, 1988.

54. Farrel RG, Swanson SL, Walter JR: Safe and effective IV regional anesthesia for use in the emergency department, *Ann Emerg Med* 14:239, 1985.

55. Shaw DC and Heckman JD: Principles and techniques of splinting musculocutaneous injuries, *Emerg Med Clin North Am* 2:391, 1984.

56. Stover CN: Air stirrup management of ankle injuries in the athlete, *Am J Sports Med* 8:360, 1980.

57. Howes DS and Kaufman J: Plaster splints: techniques and indications, *Am Fam Physician* 30:215, 1984.

58. Halvorson G and Iserson KV: Comparison of four ankle splint designs, *Ann Emerg Med* 16:1249, 1987.

59. Pappas AM: Epiphyseal injuries in sports, *Physician Sports Med* 11:140, 1983.

60. Rang M: *Children's fractures*, Philadelphia, 1983, JB Lippincott.

Hand and Wrist Injuries

Lisa S. Etzwiler

Because the hand is the most frequently injured part of the body in children, medical personnel who care for children must be familiar with hand and wrist injuries.[1-5] The hand is exquisitely designed to provide not only gross movement and powerful strength but delicate motor control and fine touch. The structures controlling these movements are compacted into a small space; even minor trauma may result in a cosmetic or functional defect. Knowledge of the anatomy of the hand and the mechanisms of its injury is essential to provide appropriate treatment for children with hand injuries.

DIAGNOSTIC FINDINGS

To assist in diagnosis and prognosis, the *history* should focus on the mechanism and time of the injury with particular reference to whether it is potentially a clean or dirty wound and the child's immunization status.

The patient's dominant hand should be defined, and any subjective motor or sensory dysfunction since the occurrence of injury should be noted.

Previous injuries, if any, should be determined, as well as past medical history, known allergies, and current medications.

PHYSICAL EXAMINATION[6-8]

Observation

Even in adults, the examination of a painful injury can be difficult. In children, not only is physical examination further hindered by the smaller size of anatomic structures but fear and lack of understanding often contribute to poor cooperation. Observation therefore plays an important role in determining the extent of a child's injuries.

Inspection begins when the patient walks into the room. The way the child positions and uses the hand provides clues to residual function. One good way to gain a child's confidence and simultaneously obtain clinical information is to inspect the other extremity. Although swelling and digital cyanosis may be easy to determine, comparison of the two hands is a quick way to discover subtle deformities that may herald tendon or dislocation injuries.

At rest, a hand with the palm held upward should be slightly flexed at all the interphalangeal (IP) and metacarpophalangeal (MCP) joints. The fingers should be almost parallel; the wrist in this resting position is slightly extended.

Palpation

Swelling and asymmetry are not always obvious to observation alone. Palpation can often localize tenderness, which is a good indicator of injury.

Palpation of the *wrist* should be systematic, beginning on one side and moving across, feeling both rows of carpal bones. Injuries to the wrist bones are rare in children, but at the very least, one should be able to isolate the scaphoid (also known as the *navicular*). It is the largest bone in the proximal row of carpals and sits on the floor of the anatomic snuffbox. When the wrist is held in ulnar deviation, the scaphoid slips out from beneath the styloid process of the radius and can be felt more easily.

The *metacarpals* should each be palpated separately, taking the time to examine the full length of each bone. Fractures occur most often at the neck of the bone where

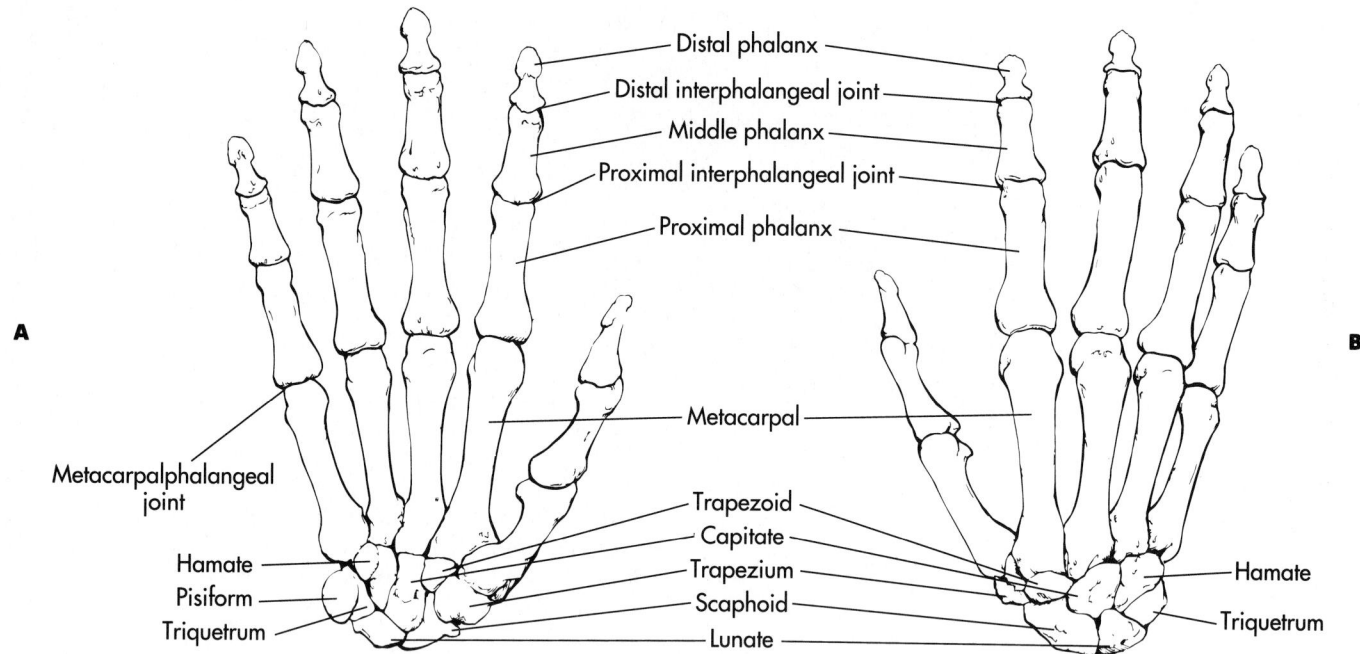

FIG. 28-1. Bones of the right hand. **A,** Palmar surface. **B,** Dorsal surface. (*From Fess EE and Philips CA: Hand splinting, principles and methods, ed 2, St. Louis, 1987, Mosby.*)

the head and shaft meet. Each end should be examined as well for joint tenderness.

The best way to expose the articulations of the metacarpophalangeal joints for palpation is to flex the knuckles.

As with examination of the other bones, all 14 *phalanges* and nine IP joints should be examined for tenderness, swelling, and asymmetry (Fig. 28-1).

Sensation

Three peripheral nerves are responsible for supplying sensation in the hand (Fig. 28-2). The *radial nerve* supplies the dorsal surfaces of the thumb, index, and middle fingers at least as far as their distal IP joints. It also innervates the whole dorsum of the hand lying on the radial side of the third metacarpal. Because the dorsal surface of the web space between the thumb and index finger is supplied almost exclusively by the radial nerve, assessing sensation here is a good way to test for its integrity.

Sensation supplied by the *median nerve* mirrors that of the radial nerve but on the palmar surface of the hand. It may also supply the dorsal surfaces of the distal phalanges of the thumb and first two digits. The best place to test for pure median nerve sensation is on the palmar surface of the tip of the index finger.

The *ulnar nerve* is responsible for innervation of the ulnar surfaces of the hand. This includes both the dorsal and palmar skin surfaces of the terminal two digits and metacarpals. The tip of the little finger provides the best site for sensation testing.

In addition to general testing for sensation, always document the presence or absence of feeling distal to an injury. In children who are old enough to cooperate, testing for *two-point discrimination* can also be performed. This can

be done with the aid of a toothed forceps or a bent paper clip. Distinction of two points at 8 mm or less confirms neuronal integrity. Performing this examination first on the uninjured hand is often helpful in reducing anxiety.

Motor Function

Motor function relies on not only the ability of a muscle or group of muscles to perform but that of nerves and tendons as well. Thus testing for motor function means establishing that all components are functioning.

Muscles of the hand may be intrinsic or extrinsic. *Extrinsic muscles* have their muscle origins and bellies in the forearm. Only their tendons lie within the hand where they insert. Each joint can be tested individually by exerting pressure against the part that the patient is asked to flex or extend. *Intrinsic muscles* lie completely within the hand and may also be tested individually. The lumbricals and interossei that adduct and abduct the fingers are included in this category.

The radial, median, and ulnar *nerves* can be tested for their contribution to motor function just as they can be examined for sensation. Many tests of neuromuscular integrity simultaneously establish tendon functioning.

To test for *radial nerve* function at the level of the wrist, the patient should be instructed to cock the wrist upward in full extension. Next downward pressure should be applied on the dorsum of the patient's hand. If the child is cooperating and strength is intact, it is not possible to push the wrist down. For comparison, the other wrist should be tested as well. (This test also establishes the strength and integrity of wrist extensors.) At the level of the digits, radial nerve intactness is established by examining the fingers for extension at the metacarpophalangeal joints. To do this,

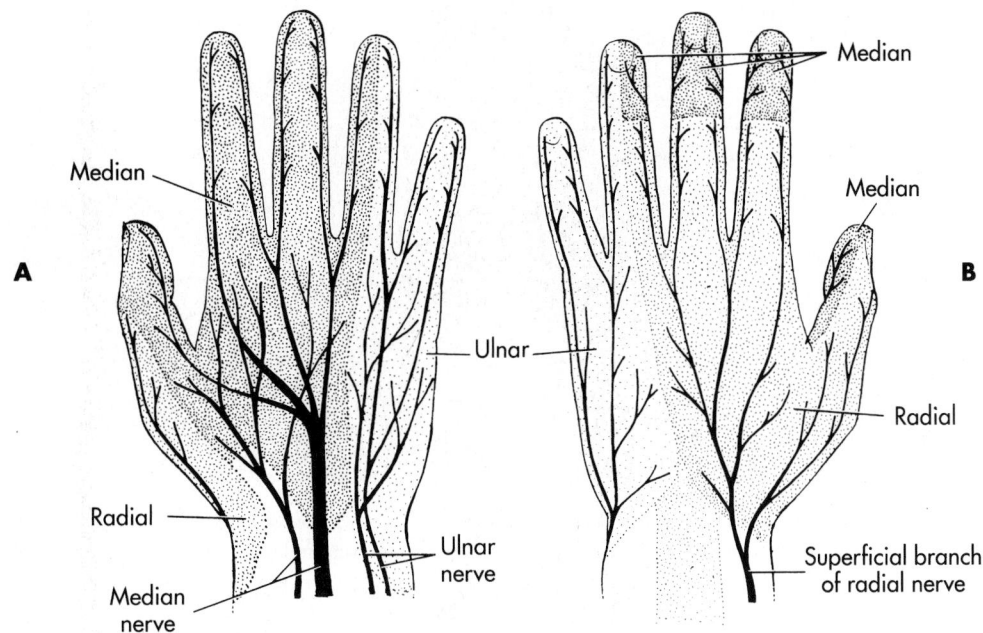

FIG. 28-2. Cutaneous distribution of the nerves of the hand. **A,** Palmar surface. **B,** Dorsal surface. (*From Fess EE and Philips CA:* Hand splinting, principles and methods, *ed 2, St. Louis, 1987, Mosby.*)

first the patient should flex the proximal interphalangeal (PIP) joints to prevent compensatory assistance from the intrinsic muscles of the hand. Then, as the patient resists, downward pressure should be applied on the dorsum of the hand in an attempt to force flexion at the MCP joint.

The *median nerve* supplies the flexor digitorum superficialis, which divides into four tendons and is the primary flexor for each finger's PIP joint. To confirm intactness of the nerve (and each tendon) at the level of the fingers, tell the patient to hold all fingers in extension. The patient should then attempt to flex the finger being tested at the PIP joint. Success establishes that function is intact.

The *ulnar nerve* is responsible for innervating the interossei muscles. The palmar interossei are responsible for finger adduction. To test this, the patient holds his or her extended fingers together. Next, taking two adjacent fingers at a time, attempt to pull the fingers apart while the patient resists. Test each group of neighboring fingers and compare their strength to that of the other side.

Tendons

Extensor tendons should be checked by examining each joint, including the IP joints, separately. Extension testing of the wrist and MCP joints is discussed in the section on radial nerve testing. To isolate extensor function at the IP joints, instruct the patient to flex his or her fingers. Next take hold of the patient's finger just proximal to the joint being examined. If the tendon is intact, the patient will be able to extend the finger from this flexed position. Thumb extension is best tested with the patient's thumb already in extension. He or she should be able to resist pressure to push it into flexion.

Each joint should be checked for *flexor tendon function.* Testing for flexion at the PIP joints is discussed in the sec-

tion on median nerve/flexor digitorum superficialis testing.

To test for flexion of the distal interphalangeal (DIP) joints, which are controlled by the flexor digitorum profundus tendons, first stabilize the MCP and IP joints in extension. Then ask the patient to flex the finger being tested at the DIP joint.

Vascular Integrity

Vascular integrity of the hand is relatively easy to assess and is usually obvious on inspection: warmth and pinkness are reassuring signs. Functional tests of circulation can be performed as well. To assess peripheral circulation, one can test for nailbed capillary refill. With pressure, the nailbed should blanch and then rapidly refill when the pressure is released.

At the level of the wrist one can feel the pulses of the two major arteries that supply the hand, the radial and ulnar arteries. Their presence assures integrity to the level of the wrist. To formally test the influence of these arteries on the circulation of the hand, the *Allen test* can be performed. To begin this examination, the examiner simultaneously compresses both arteries in the patient's hand. Then to facilitate venous drainage, the patient elevates the hand and repeatedly clenches and opens it. When the hand is blanched, the examiner releases the radial artery. If the artery is intact, all five digits should flush as they refill with blood. This test can be repeated to test the ulnar circulation by first releasing the ulnar artery after the hand is blanched.

A variation of the Allen test can be performed to assess integrity of the digital arteries in a specific finger. Both arteries are occluded, venous return is observed, and one artery is then released while observing capillary refill to the digit.

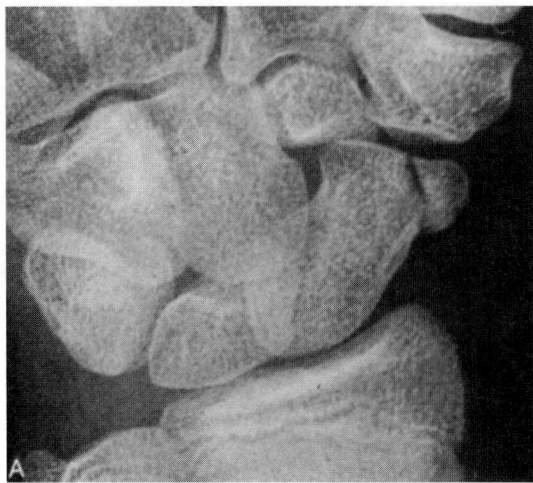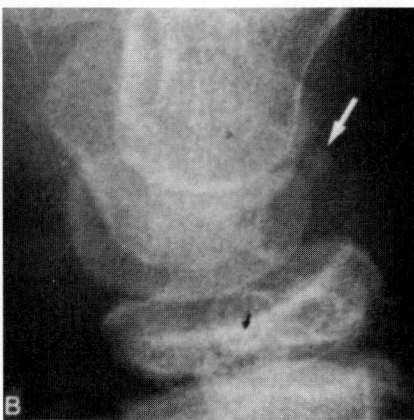

FIG. 28-3. A, Distal scaphoid fracture in a 14-year-old. **B,** Avulsion fracture *(arrow)* of the dorsal scaphoid surface in a 12-year old. These patterns are common before skeletal maturation. *(From Ogden JA: Skeletal injury in the child, ed 2, Philadelphia, 1990, WB Saunders.)*

FRACTURES[1,3,6,8-14]

Fractures may result in a deformity that limits future functioning. Thus, the threshold for referral to an orthopedic surgeon or other hand specialist should be low.

Specifically, all open fractures should be referred, as their treatment requires debridement and antibiotic therapy. When wounds are dirty, preferred treatment includes delayed primary closure. Consultation should also be sought for fractures that involve a joint. If these injuries are not properly reduced, even the smallest intraarticular fractures may cause a significant defect.

Carpal Bone Fractures

Because the carpal bones are largely cartilaginous in the growing years, carpal fractures are rare in childhood. Even so, they can occur in older children. As with adults, the majority of carpal injuries result from injury to the wrist while it is in extension.

Scaphoid (Navicular) Fractures. Just as in adults, the scaphoid is the most commonly fractured carpal bone (Fig. 28-3). This is because of its position as a bridge between the two rows of wrist bones. Prognosis for these fractures is good, for essentially all pediatric scaphoid fractures diagnosed at the time of injury heal with cast immobilization.[3,10]

Mechanism of Injury. These fractures are almost always the result of a fall on an outstretched hand.

Diagnostic Findings. Patients have a subjective complaint of pain in the periscaphoid area with consistent tenderness to palpation over the anatomic snuffbox. Range of motion and strength of the wrist are decreased.

To maximize the profile of the scaphoid, radiologic evaluation should include a scaphoid series: posteroanterior and oblique views of the patient's hand held in a fist with the wrist extended and in mild ulnar deviation. It is not uncommon for the initial film to produce a negative result.

Management. If, despite a negative radiographic study, snuffbox tenderness is found on examination, it should be

assumed that the scaphoid is fractured, and the wrist should be immobilized. In 10 to 14 days, radiographs should be repeated. If the repeat film result is still negative, the cast may then be removed. Other clinicians prefer to immobilize these patients and reexamine them in 2 to 4 days; if there is no tenderness, they assume that there was no significant fracture and merely follow the patient clinically without immobilization.

When radiographic studies reveal nondisplaced fractures, then immobilization is required for 6 to 10 weeks. The cast should include the thumb and extend upward, covering the elbow. If the fracture is displaced, consultation with an orthopedic surgeon is required, as open reduction and internal fixation may be necessary.

Metacarpal Bone Fractures

Although metacarpal bone fractures are uncommon in children, their management is improved if one recalls that finger metacarpals have their epiphyses at the distal end. The thumb's epiphysis is at the proximal end. Occasionally metacarpals have epiphyses at both ends.

Mechanism of Injury. Metacarpal fractures result from a direct blow to the hand. For pediatric patients this typically occurs in an adolescent who has been in a fist fight or has taken out frustration by punching a fixed object such as a wall.

Diagnostic Findings. Pain at the site of injury is common in association with swelling and point tenderness over the fractured bone on palpation. There may also be loss of knuckle prominence. Deformity and angulation with rotation of the fracture's fragments may occur and can be detected by observing the fingers in flexion. Normally in this position all the fingers should point in the same direction. If they do not, or if they overlap or appear deformed in flexion, then rotation is almost certainly present. This should be confirmed by radiographic studies.

In children as in adults, the most commonly fractured metacarpal is that of the little finger. This *boxer's fracture*

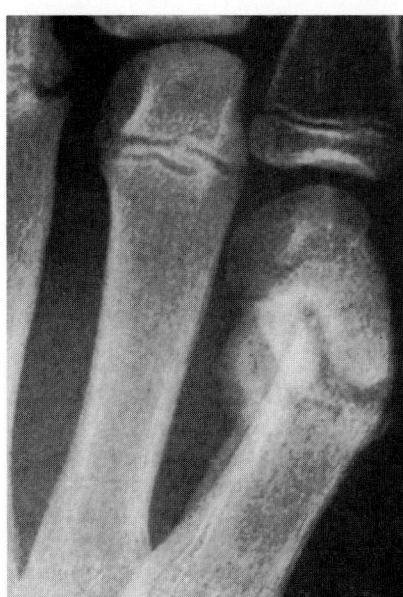

FIG. 28-4. Boxer's fracture: metaphyseal fracture of the fifth metacarpal. *(From Ogden JA: Skeletal injury in the child, ed 2, Philadelphia, 1990, WB Saunders.)*

does not involve the epiphysis but is a fracture of the neck of the metacarpal (Fig. 28-4). *Bennett's fracture* is unusual in children, involving a fracture of the thumb metacarpal base into the joint.

Anteroposterior (AP) and lateral radiologic views of the hand are indicated. Direction and degree of displacement should be determined.

Management. Because they are rarely displaced, most metacarpal shaft fractures heal with closed reduction and immobilization. Generally 3 to 4 weeks of casting is sufficient. The cast should extend from the midforearm to the distal phalanges. To preserve hand function best, the MCP joint should be splinted in 45 to 90 degrees of flexion. The wrist should be placed in mild extension.

If there is displacement or unsatisfactory realignment, open reduction and internal fixation are indicated. Intraarticular fractures involving the physis should be similarly treated. These are rare in children.

For boxer's fracture or its equivalent of the fourth metacarpal, immobilization with an ulnar gutter splint with orthopedic followup is sufficient if there is less than 30 degrees angulation. For angulation greater than 30 degrees, or for neck fractures of the second or third metacarpal with greater than 20 degrees of angulation, reduction is required and orthopedic consultation should be sought.

Fractures through the base of the metacarpal that are displaced radially can be treated by closed reduction and immobilization for 4 weeks. The best known of these is Bennett's fracture, which involves the thumb. Ulnar displaced fractures are unstable, however, and need to be followed with weekly radiographs to ensure continued reduction. If closed methods fail, open reduction and fixation are required.

Phalangeal Fractures

Mechanism of Injury. Phalangeal fractures are the most common fractures in children and usually result from a direct blow to the finger. Typically the blow is caused by the hand or fingers being caught in a door.

Diagnostic Findings. Localized pain accompanies tenderness and swelling on palpation over the site of injury. Rotational deformities may be noted. Normally when the fingers are flexed over the palm, the fingernails all point in the same direction toward the scaphoid tubercle. If they do not, or if they overlap, there may be rotational injury.

When *proximal and middle phalangeal fractures* occur, the border digits are most commonly involved. Radiographs must include at least AP and lateral views. These are usually sufficient for shaft fractures, which are usually nondisplaced. True lateral views are important to guide reduction of fractures such as those involving the neck of the phalanx. These fractures are common in children between the ages of 5 and 10 years of age, particularly in the proximal phalanx, and often include distal fragment displacement. It is important to determine the degree of rotation of these fragments, as they can dorsally rotate up to 90 degrees. The fingernail can be used as a landmark for obtaining appropriate radiographic views. When intraarticular fractures of the head of the proximal or middle phalanx are suspected, oblique views should be taken as well. These fractures may be unicondylar or bicondylar.

Distal phalangeal fractures are generally the result of crush injuries and are nondisplaced. AP and lateral views usually suffice.

Management. Most childhood fractures of the hand heal well and can be treated conservatively. Only 10% require open reduction and internal fixation. As with other fractures, any open or intraarticular wound or rotational deformity requires consultation with a hand specialist or orthopedic surgeon.

Fractures of the *proximal phalanx* heal well with closed reduction and splinting. The most common childhood fracture is a Salter II at the base of the little finger. This fracture, whose distal fragment is usually displaced in the ulnar direction, can be reduced with the aid of a pen or pencil. The pen should be pushed into the web space between the ring and little finger. Then, using it as a fulcrum, pressure should be applied on the distal fragment, pushing it toward the thumb. Reduction should be assessed after immobilization. Rotational deformities are not acceptable. Casting is required for 3 to 4 weeks. Ulnar displaced fractures at the base of the other phalanges can be similarly managed. As discussed, phalangeal neck fractures may have a great degree of distal fragment rotation. In some circumstances, however, closed reduction is possible. If it is, these fractures need to be followed with weekly radiographs as recurrent displacement is not uncommon. Unsuccessful closed reduction requires surgical intervention.

When splinting or casting proximal phalangeal fractures, care should be taken to flex collateral ligaments in an attempt to best preserve hand function. Thus the wrist should be placed in mild extension (about 30 degrees), the MCP joint at 45 to 90 degrees, and the IP joint at about 15 degrees. This is notably different from the "grasp" or "functional" position, which promotes MCP joint extension and IP joint flexion contractures and is no longer advocated.

Special mention is made later of *gamekeeper's thumb*. In the pediatric age group, a Salter III injury of the proximal phalanx typically accompanies this avulsion of the collateral ligament of the thumb.

Most uncomplicated fractures of the *middle phalanx* can be treated by immobilizing them with a neighboring digit in a finger splint or by buddy taping with follow-up in 3 to 5 days. These include Salter I and II fractures without angulation. Care should be taken to identify displaced or angulated fractures, and when found, they should be referred.

Distal phalangeal fractures are usually the result of crush injuries and are rarely displaced.

Splinting in extension with buddy taping and a bulky dressing may be used for tuft fractures and nondisplaced Salter I and Salter II fractures. Salter III fractures, which are more common in adolescents, require referral, as treatment often involves open reduction and fixation. Open fractures and nailbed injuries should be managed as discussed in Chapter 27.

DISLOCATIONS AND LIGAMENTOUS INJURIES

Wrist

Mechanism of Injury. Ligamentous injuries to the wrist are very rare in children but can result from a fall on an outstretched hand.[3,4,6,8-11] These are more common in older children.

Diagnostic Findings. With perilunate dislocations, patients have pain and tenderness in the wrist, often accompanied by minimal swelling or deformity with perilunate dislocation.

These injuries may be diagnosed only after ongoing problems have occurred, and repeated reassessment may be required. Intermittent subluxation of one or more carpal bones should be suspected when a patient complains of persistent pain or a "clicking" sound that is associated with certain wrist movements.

On a true lateral roentgenogram the long finger metacarpal, capitate, lunate, and radius normally line up in a straight line, and the lunate and navicular form an angle no greater than 50 degrees. This normal alignment is disrupted by a dislocation.

Rotary subluxation of the scaphoid should be suspected if routine radiographic film results are negative but tenderness persists in the snuffbox area.

For scaphoid subluxation additional AP views with the wrist in full supination should be taken. Widening of the scaphoid-lunate articulation is diagnostic.

Management. Dislocation and subluxation injuries require referral. For a scaphoid injury, radial deviation of the hand with plaster immobilization for 8 weeks may close the scaphoid-lunate gap. Close monitoring is required. Usually, however, surgery is indicated.

Hand and Fingers

Ligamentous injuries and dislocations of the hand and fingers are also uncommon in children. Because the ends of their bones are still growing, children's ligaments are stronger than their epiphyseal plates. Thus the same force that might cause only a ligamentous injury in an adult produces a fracture in a child.

Mechanism of Injury. Dislocations of the carpometacarpal joint are rare because the compression force responsible for injury usually results in a fracture. Impact occurs at the tip of the digit with the force directed along its axis. MCP joint injuries often result from forced ulnar deviation such as when the fingers are grasped and yanked in athletic play. Finger injuries usually result from a direct blow to the finger.

Diagnostic Findings. The joint deformity is obvious, accompanied by swelling and tenderness. Flexion of the finger is difficult. MCP joint dislocations usually have less angulation than IP joint dislocations. Dimpling of the skin on the palmar side is another indication of injury.

It is important to obtain radiographic studies before attempting any manipulation, since fractures with associated dislocations require surgical referral. As a minimum, AP and lateral films should be obtained. Oblique views may be required, especially for carpometacarpal dislocations, which are particularly difficult to diagnose.

Management. Carpometacarpal joint dislocations usually involve the thumb. These dorsal subluxations are usually reduced quite easily by closed manipulation. While distal traction is applied to the patient's thumb with one hand, the other hand pushes the metacarpal back into place. A thumb spica cast should then be applied and worn for 6 weeks.

The problem associated with these injuries is that they are unstable and often require referral for internal fixation to prevent long-term complications.

MCP joint sprains usually involve the radial collateral ligaments of the ring and little fingers. Immobilization is usually sufficient to treat first- and second-degree sprains of the MCP joint. If the joint is unstable, suggesting a more severe sprain or avulsed ligament, referral and surgery are required.

Dislocations of the MCP joint are rare, but when they occur, the joint is dislocated dorsally. The capsular structure about the joint is very strong; once it is dislocated, a closed reduction, unless performed with general anesthesia, is difficult. Forceful manipulation should be avoided to prevent epiphyseal displacement and damage. Internal repair is usually necessary.

Proximal IP joint dislocations can be posterior or anterior. Posterior (dorsal) dislocations are most common and can often be reduced without anesthesia; however, a digital block may be placed first. Reduction may usually be accomplished by hyperextending the joint while pushing the distal bone into its position from above without pulling.

After reduction the joint should be tested for lateral instability. If instability is present, the joint should be splinted in the straight position for 3 weeks; otherwise immobilization for 7 to 10 days is sufficient. If the dislocation is anterior, then there has been tendon damage and referral for operative repair is required.

DIP dislocations are rare but can be easily reduced and splinted for a short period.

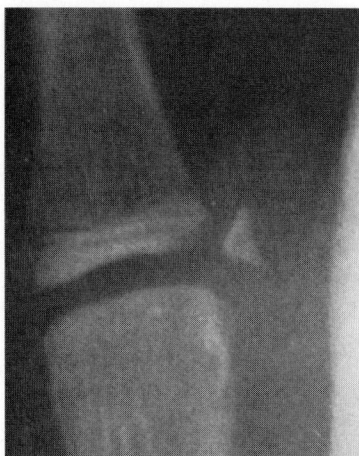

FIG. 28-5. Gamekeeper's thumb in a 12-year-old child. Type 3 avulsion fracture with rotation of the fragment. *(From Ogden JA: Skeletal injury in the child, ed 2, Philadelphia, 1990, WB Saunders.)*

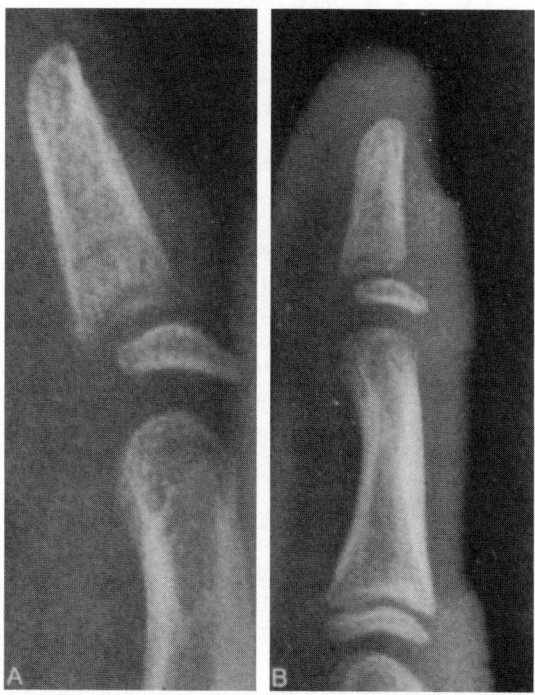

FIG. 28-6. Mallet finger. **A,** Displaced. **B,** Acceptable reduction with hyperextension splint. *(From Ogden JA: Skeletal injury in the child, ed 2, Philadelphia, 1990, WB Saunders.)*

Gamekeeper's or Skier's Thumb

Mechanism of Injury. Gamekeeper's or skier's thumb is an instability of the ulnar collateral ligament of the thumb. It gets its name from the frequency with which it occurred in British gamekeepers, who developed chronic sprains from wringing the necks of game. This injury also occurs when a skier falls on an outstretched hand while still grasping the ski pole. The pole exerts a lever effect on the already hyperextended MCP thumb joint and further exacerbates the injury.

Diagnostic Findings. Tenderness and swelling over the ulnar aspect of the MCP joint of the thumb are noted. Radial deviation of the thumb at the MCP joint exacerbates the pain. Laxity of the joint with stress is found. If the joint is significantly unstable compared to the other side (< 30% to 45%), the ligament may be avulsed and operative repair is necessary.

AP and lateral films are indicated (Fig. 28-5). Avulsion fractures of the proximal phalanx are often present in children and should be ruled out.

Management. With the thumb in extension a thumb spica cast or splint should be worn for 6 weeks. The patient should be followed by an orthopedist or a hand specialist. When an avulsion fragment is present, open reduction and pinning are usually required.

TENDON INJURIES[3,5,6,13,15,16]

In general, children with tendon injuries need to be admitted to the hospital, as the small size of their structures necessitates fine surgical technique for repair. Some injuries are more common in older children and may be initially managed in the emergency room. These are discussed later. "Jersey finger" is also discussed, as this is a frequently overlooked injury.

Mallet Finger

Mallet finger (also known as baseball finger or drooped finger) results from injury to the extensor tendon at its attachment at the DIP joint. It is often associated with a fracture of the dorsal lip of the base of the distal phalanx. Additionally, the tendon may be damaged by a laceration or crush injury.

Mechanism of Injury. Typically the finger is forcibly flexed as a result of a direct blow, when catching a football or striking an object and "jamming" the finger.

Diagnostic Findings. The finger cannot be extended at the distal phalanx because of rupture or laceration of the terminal slip or an avulsion fracture. The distal phalanx of the injured finger is held in flexion, and marked tenderness and swelling are noted at the distal interphalangeal (DIP) joint.

AP and lateral views are required to exclude a chip fracture of the DIP joint. Fractures in adolescents may be Salter III epiphyseal injuries, whereas younger children typically experience Salter I or II fractures.

Management. If a fracture is present but involves no more than 25% of the joint surface and there is no subluxation, it may be splinted in mild hyperextension (Fig. 28-6). Either a dorsal or a volar splint is adequate. Daily tape changes are suggested so that adequate skin care may be provided. These changes should be made with the finger in extension. Consultation and follow-up observation by a specialist should be arranged. If the fracture involves more than 25% of the joint surface or if the joint is subluxed, then referral for operative repair is required.

In older adolescents the injury may occur without a fracture. In these cases the finger should be splinted with the DIP joint in hyperextension for at least 6 weeks. Strict immobilization is necessary to preclude need for operative repair.

Boutonnière Deformity

Disruption of the central slip of the extensor tendon at the PIP joint with concomitant volar subluxation of the lateral bands of the tendon creates a boutonnière deformity.

Mechanism of Injury. The injury may result from either a direct blow or an associated open injury at the PIP joint.

Diagnostic Findings. The DIP joint is held in extension while the PIP is held in flexion. The dorsal PIP joint has overlying tenderness and swelling. Finger films should be obtained to exclude associated fracture.

Management. If there is no associated fracture, the finger should be splinted in extension. Follow-up observation by a specialist should be arranged. Some patients require surgical reattachment of the tendon, especially if initial management was delayed.

Jersey Finger

This avulsion of the flexor digitorum profundus is the most common closed flexion tendon injury in the adolescent athlete. The ring finger is most often affected. Although its management requires referral, it needs to be recognized by emergency physicians.

Mechanism of Injury. This injury occurs when a hyperextension force is applied to the DIP joint while simultaneous attempted flexion of the tendon is occurring. It is most frequently seen in football or rugby players when a finger catches on another player's shirt or jersey, hence the name "jersey finger."

Diagnostic Findings. The patient is unable to flex the DIP joint. The physician should not assume that this inability is secondary to swelling. Pain, swelling, and extensive soft-tissue injury with hemorrhage are present at the DIP joint.

Localized tenderness may occur at the level to which the tendon has retracted, including the PIP joint or within the palm.

AP and lateral radiographs of the finger are required to exclude an associated chip fracture.

Management. Management requires referral for surgical repair.

NERVE INJURIES

Mechanism of Injury. Nerve injuries are usually caused by laceration or crush injury.

Diagnostic Findings. In young children, evaluating sensation is particularly difficult because their apprehension, and lack of understanding inhibit cooperation. Sharp/dull testing can be particularly frightening. Some cooperate with two-point discrimination testing when it is treated as a game. For the very young child lack of sweating or absence of the skin wrinkling in water may be the only clue to nerve damage. Older children usually cooperate with sharp/dull testing and discrimination tests.

Management. A qualified surgeon should always be consulted when these injuries occur. A specific injury of which one should be aware is laceration that involves the flexor surface of the finger. If the digital artery has been injured (identified by pulsating blood flow), it should be assumed that the nerve is also injured because the nerve lies superficial to the artery. The bleeding should be stopped by elevation and pressure. Never clamp the artery, as the nerve may become damaged. In children the digital nerve should be repaired as far as the distal joint and the results are usually excellent.

SOFT TISSUE INJURIES AND INFECTION

Lacerations

Diagnostic Findings. Because many structures are compacted within a small space in the hand, lacerations may involve more than skin and subcutaneous tissue. Thus, the wound must be explored to determine whether the damage includes vessels, nerves, tendons, ligaments, muscle, bones, or joints.

In addition to determining the extent of injury by observation and exploration, sensation, motor function, and vascular sufficiency must be tested. Nerve injury should be assessed as described previously, with attention to examination of the radial, median, and ulnar nerves. The presence or absence of sensation distal to the injury should also be noted. An abnormal attitude of the hand may signal tendon or joint injury. Vascular compromise can be assessed by checking pulses and capillary refill.

Radiographic studies are not usually necessary; however, in some instances the presence of a foreign body needs to be excluded. A common laceration is that which results when the patient falls while holding a drinking glass. Identification and removal of any residual glass fragments are required before suturing.

Management. If the wound is still actively bleeding, direct pressure and elevation should be applied.[6] Using a clamp or deep suture for hemostasis may permanently damage surrounding structures.

Cleaning and repair of the wound can be facilitated by infiltration with lidocaine. This should be done only after sensory testing has been documented. The wound should then be copiously irrigated with a sterile isotonic solution such as normal saline solution under high pressure to provide good debridement. Attaching an 18- or 20-gauge intravenous catheter to a 60-ml syringe provides good pressure and direction while limiting the number of refills. After anesthesia and cleaning, more thorough exploration of the wound is possible and should be repeated before closure.

If the wound is less than 8 hours old, it may be closed. Repair with 4-0 or 5-0 suture on a P3 needle with nylon (Prolene, Ethicon) is usually adequate. Deep sutures should *not* be placed (see Chapter 32).

Children have an uncanny ability to "escape" their dressings, necessitating that one be creative. Small, simple lacerations may require only antiseptic ointment and an adhesive bandage. More extensive injuries may require bulky dressings or a splint to prevent further damage.

The "hooded cobra" is the best position for immobilization when a tendon is involved. The hand should be positioned with the wrist in a neutral position, the MCP joint flexed at approximately 60 degrees, the IP joints in 10 to 20 degrees of flexion, and the thumb in abduction. The dressing directly over the wound should be of nonadherent material such as xeroform gauze. The next layer should be absorbent as well as supportive. Gauze or sponges, which also provide padding, are useful. Using a material such as Kling for the next layer holds other layers in place and contributes to positioning. As the hand is wrapped from the distal end proximally, less tension should be applied. A volar (palmar) splint may also be incorporated.

Tetanus status should be addressed as necessary.

Fingertip Injuries[6,16,17]

Subungual Splinter. Subungual splinters, embedded by fingertip injuries, are usually wooden splinters, but other materials may be present.

Diagnostic Findings. Foreign material is found under the nail but may not be completely embedded. Progressively worsening inflammation and tenderness may be present. If treatment has been delayed, signs of infection may also be found.

Management. Trim the nails as short as possible and clean the hand thoroughly. If a splinter is only partially embedded, it may be possible to grasp an end of the splinter with a tweezers or catch it against the nail and stroke it out from under the nail. Special tweezers are available. Shaving away the nail overlying the foreign material must be done carefully to prevent injury and pain. The best instrument for this purpose is the scalpel blade. To prevent infection, the hand should be soaked three times a day until well healed. Additionally, it may be dressed with antibacterial ointment.

Crush Injury of the Fingertip

Mechanism of Injury. Crush injuries of the fingertip occur when the distal phalanx sustains a blow between two objects. In children it is not uncommon for the fingertip to be slammed in a door.

Diagnostic Findings. The fingertip may be swollen, discolored, and tender, often with a subungual hematoma present as indicated by blood beneath the fingernail. Fracture and laceration, including nailbed injury, may also be present. The nail itself may be completely or partially avulsed.

Finger films need to be taken to exclude an underlying fracture.

Management. For simple injury without associated laceration or hematoma, treatment is straightforward. The finger should be well cleaned and a bulky dressing applied to prevent further trauma. *Tuft fractures* are quite common; a hairpin splint and bulky dressing are all that is necessary to protect the fingertip from further trauma.

If a *subungual hematoma* is present, it is important to evaluate associated injuries, including distal fracture or lacerations of the nailbed. The hematoma should be drained to relieve painful and potentially harmful pressure on the nailbed. To do so, simply place an electric cautery or red-hot paper clip on the nail directly over the hematoma. It usually takes a fraction of a second to burn through the nail and drain the fluid. Gentle pressure on the surrounding nail may facilitate drainage of the fluid.

Some controversy exists over the criteria used to determine whether or not the nail needs to be removed in order to repair a potential nailbed laceration. Many experts have advocated for nail removal if the hematoma exceeds greater than 25% of the nailbed surface. One study shows that long-term nail growth is not compromised as long as there are no underlying fractures and the hematoma covers less than 50% of the nailbed surface.[18] Another paper concludes that the size of the hematoma does not impact long-term growth as long as the complete nail and its borders are intact.[19] A combination of these less invasive approaches (intact nail and borders, no underlying fracture, no limitation of hematoma size) is also advocated[20] and is appealing as it reduces the time, pain, and expense of nail removal. For children, sedation is often required just to place the digital block necessary to perform the procedure.

When there are associated lacerations of the fingertip and nailbed, they need to be repaired; the latter healing poorly by second intention. A good digital block should be placed. Without adequate anesthesia appropriate care is impossible. With the finger anesthetized, the nail should be systematically detached from the nailbed. Taking forceps, slide it under the nail and begin to lift and loosen the adhesions between the nail and its bed. Continue to move the forceps from side to side, working down toward the base. When it has been completely disconnected from its bed, it may be removed by grasping the tip and firmly pulling it out along the axis of the finger. The laceration should be repaired with 6-0 absorbable suture.

If the nail is clean and intact, it may be used as an anatomic tent by placing it back over the repaired nailbed, held in place by sutures. When it is not possible to use the nail, nonadherent material such as Xeroform gauze may be used to cover the nailbed. It may also be held in place with sutures for 7 to 10 days. The finger may then be covered with a bulky dressing, and, if desired, with a splint as well.

Amputations

Hands or Parts. In cases of amputation examine the hand carefully and preserve all viable tissue. The amputated part should be appropriately preserved and cooled. Uncooled tissue survives up to 6 hours and cooled tissue up to 12 hours. When a single digit is involved, successful reimplantation of cooled tissue can occur up to 24 hours after amputation since the fingers essentially contain no muscle tissue.

To preserve the tissue best, it can be wrapped in sterile gauze or towels that have been soaked with Ringer's lactate or saline solution. It is then placed in a plastic bag, which is put in icewater. Care should be taken so that the amputated part does not come into direct contact with ice or become frozen.

Radiographic studies of the hand and parts should be made to determine their integrity. The patient should be immediately referred to a center capable of reimplantation.

Fingertip. Although fingertip amputations are common in children and usually heal well, a hand surgeon should be consulted before management.

Management. Radiographic studies of the finger should be made to determine whether there is bony involvement. If only soft tissue from the tip is involved or missing, the wound will heal well by secondary intention. Good cleaning and debridement should be performed, and a bulky dressing should be applied.

For partial amputations loose approximation with sutures should be attempted and often is successful. It is worth the attempt even if the tissue subsequently becomes necrotic and requires removal. Amputations distal to the insertion of the extensor and flexor tendons of the distal phalanx can usually be adequately managed nonoperatively. The finger should be carefully cleaned, debrided, dressed with ointment and gauze, and immobilized. If the wound is contaminated, antibiotic administration may be started.

For amputations involving injury proximal to the insertion of the extensor and flexor tendons, management requires preservation of the amputated part as previously described with immediate referral to a hand specialist.

Wringer or Degloving Injury[6,8,21]

Mechanism of Injury. With the advent of the electric drier, injuries from a clothes wringer are no longer common; however, other machines or automobile tires can produce the same kind of damage to a limb. Injury is sustained not only from crushing forces but from shearing or burning from the friction of the moving part, as when an extremity is run over by a car.

Diagnostic Findings. Soft tissue swells as a result of edema surrounding damaged tissue. Bleeding into the soft tissues and their compartments may also occur. Overlying skin may be severely abraded or degloved. Fractures, dislocations, or extensive lacerations may coexist.

Although fractures are rare, radiographic studies should be made to determine whether bony damage has occurred.

Management. Because of the risk of compartment syndrome caused by internal bleeding and swelling after initial therapy, management should focus on prevention of neurovascular compromise. The extremity should be examined to determine the extent of injury. After thorough cleaning, a sterile, occlusive dressing should be placed to help control swelling. The extremity should be elevated and the patient should be hospitalized for 24 hours of observation and continuous reassessment of the limb's neurovascular integrity.

If neurovascular compromise develops, a fasciotomy or carpal tunnel decompression may become necessary. Skin slough is common if loss of vascular supply or compartment syndrome has occurred. Skin grafting may be necessary.

Ring on a Swollen Finger

A ring may get stuck on a swollen finger.[6] There is more than one alternative to management.

One approach is first to reduce the swelling. This can be done by cooling the finger in cold water. If this can be managed with the finger elevated as well, it should be attempted. Otherwise the patient can alternate between soaking the finger and elevating it at 5-minute intervals. After 30 minutes mineral oil, petroleum jelly, or other lubricant should be applied to the finger. The ring is then removed by applying steady pressure and pushing it distally.

Another method employs the use of a piece of string that is slipped under the ring. The distal end of the string should then be wrapped in loops around the finger, spiraling the string from the distal finger toward the ring. Once the finger has been wrapped, the proximal end of the string should be grasped firmly and a slow pull exerted. The other hand gently pulls the ring distally as the string unwinds. Alternatively, a Penrose drain may also be used to wrap around the finger. Digital block to lessen pain should be considered.

For emergency cases, uncooperative patients, failure of other methods, or as an alternative, a ring cutter can be used.

Frostbite

Mechanism of Injury. Frostbite occurs when tissues are exposed to excessive cold (see Chapter 39). In children this results from inadequate protection or prolonged duration of exposure. Fingertips are commonly involved.

Diagnostic Findings. Superficial frostbite is present if a wound that initially appears white and doughy becomes red and mildly edematous with rewarming. With deep frostbite the extremity is cyanotic and hard, lacking sensation. Warming produces a mottled rather than a hyperemic appearance. In the hours after rewarming, pain and swelling develop.

Management. The involved areas need to be rapidly rewarmed. When possible, this should be done with warm water (40° to 42° C) for 20 to 30 minutes. The last 10 minutes or so of rewarming may be extremely painful. Hot water should never be used. Likewise, the extremity should never be rubbed with snow, as it may cause more extensive tissue damage.

After rewarming, care should be taken to prevent further injury or infection. If blisters are present, they should remain intact. Most frostbite injuries can be treated on an outpatient basis; however, deep tissue injury involving muscle or bone requires inpatient care.

Infections[6,8,22,23]

Felon

Mechanism of Injury. A *felon* is an infection of the pulp of the distal phalanx. It usually develops after a small puncture wound of the skin; however, often the patient has no recall of a specific injury.[22]

Diagnostic Findings. Spread of infection within the pulp of the finger is limited by the lack of potential space. Therefore, pressure can build up rapidly, leading to further tissue damage from ischemia. The volar aspect of the distal phalanx is red, swollen, indurated, and painful.

Management. Frequently treatment includes hospital admission for initial management, including incision and drainage under general anesthesia, which is followed by intravenous administration of antibiotics.

On occasion, outpatient management is possible with use of a digital block. The wound should then be incised and drained even if there is little evidence of fluctuance.

A longitudinal incision is advocated to avoid iatrogenic complications (e.g., neurovascular compromise and scarring). Drainage prevents further tissue necrosis and infection spread. It is the most important step toward elimination of the infection and may be additionally aided by the placement of a Penrose drain for 48 hours.

Antibiotics such as dicloxicillin (50 mg/kg/24 hr QID PO) or cephalexin (50 mg/kg/24 hr QID PO) should be started. The patient should elevate the hand whenever possible.

After removal of the drain frequent daily warm soaks should be started. There should be close follow-up observation, including checks at 24 and 48 hours.

Eponychia

Mechanism of Injury. The eponychium or cuticle is the flap of epidermis that overlies the base of the nail. In children it is particularly thin and is susceptible to trauma and infection caused by athletic play or finger biting or sucking.

Diagnostic Findings. Swelling, erythema, and swelling are localized to the cuticle.

Management. Healing is rapid, usually in 2 to 3 days of management. The finger should be soaked for 20 minutes three to four times daily. Place the finger in a finger cot (or a finger that has been cut from a rubber glove) filled with antibiotic ointment (Betadine or Neosporin).

Paronychia (see Fig. 32-14)

Mechanism of Injury. Paronychia infection is caused by bacterial inoculum along the side of the nail, often as the result of finger biting, sucking, or a hangnail.

Diagnostic Findings. Swelling, erythema, and tenderness along the nail may extend along its base. There is usually a visible collection of pus under the skin and often under the base of the nail.

Management. A digital block of lidocaine without epinephrine should be placed. An incision should be made in the infected skin at the medial or lateral edge of the nail. If the pus has extended deep to the base of the nail, the involved portion of proximal nail should also be excised. The distal nail may be left in place.

The wound should have antibiotic ointment placed on it and be covered. Frequent warm soaks should occur each day. Oral antistaphylococcal antibiotics such as dicloxicillin or cephalexin may be started.

Tenosynovitis

Mechanism of Injury. Tenosynovitis occurs when a local infection extends into the tendon. Typically there has been a puncture wound into the volar surface of the finger in an area where the tendon sheath lies relatively superficial, such as in the flexor crease.

Diagnostic Findings. Erythema and tenderness are present along the tendon sheath. Pain is often extremely intense over the head of the involved metacarpal.

The finger is held rigidly in a semiflexed position. Passive extension of the DIP joint produces extreme pain.

Management. Hospitalization is usually necessary; consultation with a hand surgeon should be sought.

The hand should be immobilized along the entire length of the tendon and elevated. Incision and drainage may be necessary. High doses of antibiotics such as cephalothin (75 to 150 mg/kg/24 hr q 4-6 hr IV) are administered.

Palmar Space Infections

Mechanism of Injury. Palmar space infections are serious infections of the fascial spaces. They occur when there is extension of infection from a local injury, such as an animal bite, into the midpalmar, thenar, or hypothenar space.

Diagnostic Findings. Swelling, tenderness, and erythema outline the dimensions of the compartment. Finger extension is extremely painful.

Management. The patient needs to be hospitalized. Excision and drainage should be performed by a hand specialist and the hand immobilized and elevated. The patient should have high-dose antistaphylococcal intravenous antibiotics such as cephalothin (75-150 mg/kg/24 hr q 4-6 hr IV) or cefazolin (25 to 100 mg/kg/24 hr q 4-6 hr IV).

Herpetic Whitlow

Mechanism of Injury. Herpetic whitlow is herpes simplex I infection along the borders of the fingernail or beneath it. It is usually acquired from the patient's own oral lesions. Because its treatment differs from that of paronychia, these two entities must be distinguished.

Diagnostic Findings. Herpetic whitlow can usually be distinguished from bacterial paronychia by appearance. The fingertip is red and indurated. Characteristically the lesions along the nail may consist of ulcers or blisters, and serous exudate or crusting may be present. Lesions beneath the nail may be difficult to see. Pain and inflammation may persist for weeks, recovery may be prolonged, and there may be recurrences. The subjective pain is often described as burning. Gram stain of exudate may show giant cells without bacteria. Superinfection by bacteria is possible.

Management. Surgery should be avoided if possible because instruments may actually spread infection. One exception is when multiple subungual lesions are present. Incision and drainage should be used for decompression, the patient should be made comfortable, and the finger should be splinted.

Topical antibacterial ointment may be used to help prevent secondary infection. Topical acyclovir 5% ointment may shorten the course and possibly limit recurrence.

References

1. Wood VE: Fractures of the hand in children, *Orthop Clin North Am* 7:527, 1976.
2. Hastings H and Simmons BP: Hand fractures in children, *Clin Orthop* 188:120, 1984.
3. Simmons BP and Lovallo JL: Hand and wrist injuries in children, *Clin Sports Med* 7:495, 1988.
4. Zaticzny B, Shattuck LJ, Mast TA et al: Sports-related injuries in school-aged children, *Am J Sports* Med 8:318, 1980.
5. Bhende MS, Dandrea LA, Davis HW: Hand injuries in children presenting to a pediatric emergency department *Ann Emerg Med* 22:1519, 1993

Physical Examination

6. Barkin RM and Rosen P: *Emergency pediatrics: a guide to ambulatory care,* ed 4, St Louis, 1994, Mosby.
7. Hoppenfeld S: *Physical examination of the spine and extremities,* East Norwalk, Conn, 1976, Appleton-Century-Crofts.

Fractures, Dislocations, and Ligamentous Injuries

8. Lammers RL and Freemyer BC: Hand. In Rosen P: *Emergency medicine,* ed 3, St Louis, 1992, Mosby.
9. Almquist EE: Hand injuries in children, *Pediatr Clin North Am* 33:1511, 1986.
10. McCue FC, Baugher WH, Kulund DN et al: Hand and wrist injuries in the athlete, *Am J Sports Med* 7:275, 1979.
11. Posner MA: Injuries to the hand and wrist in athletes, *Orthop Clin North Am* 8:593, 1977.
12. Ashkenaze DM and Ruby LK: Metacarpal fractures and dislocations, *Ortho Clin North Am* 23:19, 1992.

Tendon Injuries

13. Ruby LK: Common hand injuries in the athlete, *Orthop Clin North Am* 11:819, 1980.
14. O'Brien ET: Acute fractures and dislocations of the carpus, *Orthop Clin North Am* 15:237, 1977.

15. Stein A, Lemos M, Stein S: Clinical evaluation of flexor tendon funeron in the small finger, *Ann Emerg Med* 19:991, 1990.

Soft Tissue Injury and Infection

16. Reef TC: Avulsion of the flexordigitorum profundus: an athletic injury, *Am J Sports Med* 5:281, 1977.
17. Simon RR and Brenner BE: *Emergency procedures and techniques,* ed 3, Baltimore, 1994, Williams & Wilkins.
18. Simon RR and Wolgin M: Subungal hematoma: Association with occult laceration requiring repair, *Am J Emerg Med* 5:302, 1987.
19. Seaberg DC, Angelos WJ, Paris PM: Treatment of subungal hematomas with nail trephination: a prospective study, *Am J Emerg Med* 9:209, 1991.
20. Chudnofsky CR and Sebastian S: Special wounds: Nail bed, plantar puncture, and cartilage, *Emerg Med Clin North Am* 10:801, 1992.
21. Chamberlain SW and Soltes M: Wringer injuries, *Pediatrics* 28:96, 1961.
22. Kilgore ES, Brown LG, Newmeyer WL et al: Treatment of felons, *Am J Surg* 130:194, 1975.
23. Koch SL: Felons, acute lymphangitis, and tendon sheath infections, *JAMA* 92:1171, 1929.

Upper Extremity Injuries

Mark Joffe

Injuries to the upper extremity are extremely common in childhood and adolescence. Fortunately, a small number of injuries account for the vast majority of patients with significant upper-extremity trauma. The pediatric emergency physician can develop considerable expertise in the diagnosis and treatment of these injuries. Orthopedic consultation and follow-up can then be used appropriately.

CLAVICLE

Clavicular Fractures

The clavicle is the bone most frequently fractured in childhood. It is the only osseous connection between the shoulder and the trunk, extending from the manubrium to the acromion. The clavicle comprises a double curve, convex over the medial two thirds and concave over the lateral third. The point of inflection between the curves, between the middle and lateral thirds, is most often the site of fracture. Incomplete fractures such as greenstick or buckle injuries are more common in the young child; complete

fractures, with or without displacement and angulation, are found in the older child. The medial end is bound to the sternum by strong ligaments. In children younger than 18 years, displacement of the medial clavicle from the sternum almost always results from epiphyseal separation and not true dislocation. Similarly, fracture through the physis rather than rupture of the strong coracoclavicular and acromioclavicular ligaments is the cause of displacement of the lateral end of the clavicle in children.

Mechanism of Injury. Fracture of the clavicle may result from direct or indirect force. It is a common birth injury, found in approximately 0.5% of vertex and 16% of vaginal breech deliveries.[1] Low-energy trauma, including falls of less than 3 feet, account for most clavicular fractures. Medially directed impact to the shoulder or a fall on an extended arm transmits force to the clavicle that can cause fracture. Direct trauma to the clavicle from frontal impact may fracture the clavicle, often in association with rib and thoracic injuries.

Diagnostic Findings. The subcutaneous location of the clavicle makes it relatively easy to examine. Newborns with fractured clavicles are often asymptomatic. Parents may notice the callous that develops at 2 or 3 weeks of life causing a bony prominence over the clavicle. Pseudoparalysis of the arm may be noted in the nursery in babies with clavicular fractures and should not be confused with brachial plexus injuries.

Children with fractures of the clavicle have pain with movement of the upper arm and neck. Fractured clavicles often bow anteriorly, giving an asymmetric appearance on inspection. Local tenderness, swelling, and crepitation at the fracture site enable the examiner to accurately predict the presence of clavicular fracture. An older child with complete fractures and overriding fragments will have downward and inward displacement of the shoulder, will keep the injured arm close to the body, and will support it with the other hand.

The thick periosteum prevents significant displacement of the fracture fragments and reduces the risk of injury to adjacent vessels and nerves. Rarely a subclavian vessel may be damaged; such damage is manifested as swelling, ecchymosis, pulse changes, and, occasionally, a bruit over the involved vessel radiating to the heart.

Radiographic Studies. Radiographs are useful in confirming the diagnosis of clavicular fracture, in determining the degree of angulation or displacement, and ruling out associated bony injuries including fractures of the proximal humerus, rib, coracoid, and acromion. Anteroposterior

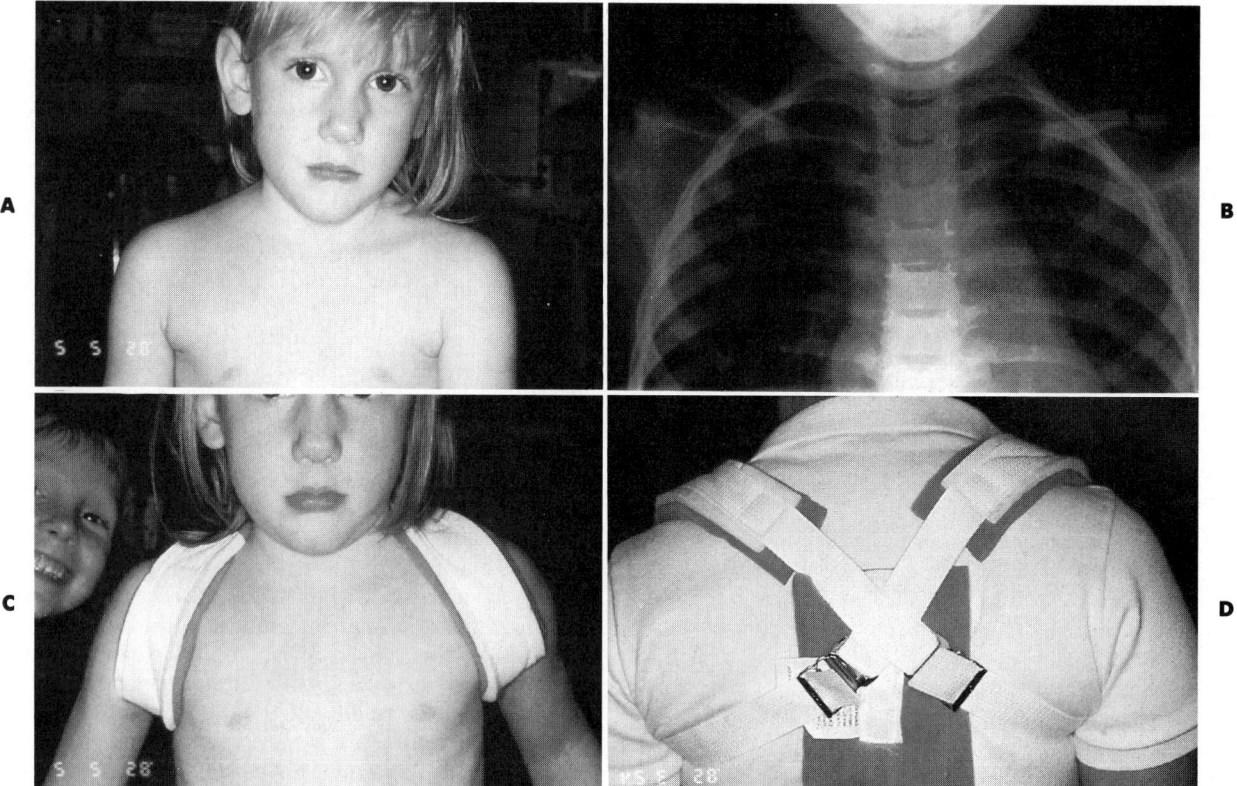

FIG. 29-1. A, Fracture of the clavicle. Note asymmetric appearance of clavicle and the head tilt. **B,** Radiograph shows complete fracture at the intersection of the middle and lateral thirds of the clavicle. **C** and **D,** Proper placement of the figure-of-eight splint.

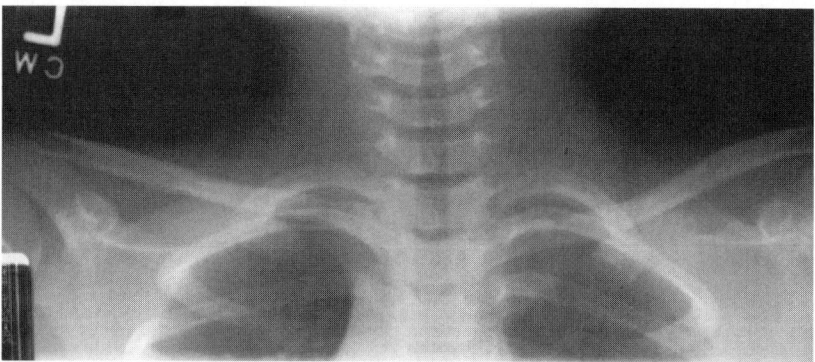

FIG. 29-2. Sternoclavicular fracture/dislocation with superior displacement of medial left clavicle.

views are usually sufficient, but occasionally lordotic views are helpful in visualizing subtle fractures.

Fracture with epiphyseal displacement of the proximal clavicle is rare in childhood and can easily be missed radiographically as a result of overlap of ribs. A Salter I fracture of the distal clavicle is often associated with superior displacement of the metaphysis and can be mistaken for acromioclavicular separation. Coracoid fractures are sometimes noted with this uncommon injury.

Management. The treatment of most clavicular fractures is in the purview of the pediatric emergency physician.

Fractures resulting from birth trauma usually require no treatment, although splinting the arm occasionally reduces pain in the uncomfortable newborn. Parents should be counseled that the bony prominence will be noticeable for 6 to 18 months (Figs. 29-1 and 29-2).

A figure-eight splint helps keep the shoulder in abduction and is usually sufficient for treatment of clavicular fractures. Placement of a sling or sling and swathe are alternatives for shoulder immobilization. Children should wear the splint for a total of 3 to 4 weeks, day and night for the first 2 weeks and during the day only for the remainder. Several manufacturers produce clavicular straps in various sizes, or a figure-eight splint can easily be fashioned from stockinette. The splint must not be applied too tightly, and the neurovascular status of the affected arm should be assessed after the splint is fitted.

Displaced fractures of the clavicle in children older than 6 years may need reduction and must be referred for orthopedic evaluation. Fractures of the proximal clavicle with epiphyseal displacement and fractures of the distal clavicle can be immobilized with a sling and swathe.

Acromioclavicular Sprain/Separation

Young children rarely sustain injury to the acromioclavicular (AC) joint because force applied to the distal clavicle usually results in metaphyseal fracture rather than AC separation. Older children and adolescents, particularly those involved in sports, may fall directly on the shoulder and injure the AC ligaments. Sprain (first-degree) or rupture of the acromioclavicular ligaments (second-degree) can occur alone or in association with disruption of the entire ligamentous complex (third-degree).

Diagnostic Findings. Movement of the upper arm in the presence of AC sprains and separations causes pain. Localization of tenderness at the AC joint requires knowledge of the surface anatomy of the shoulder. In cases of ligamentous rupture, the lateral portion of the clavicle on the affected side is displaced upward compared with the normal side.

Pediatricians unfamiliar with AC injuries may miss the diagnosis radiographically. Careful attention to the distal clavicle may reveal small fracture fragments without the widening of the space between the clavicle and acromion that indicates rupture of the ligaments. When the physical examination suggests AC separation and radiographic findings are normal, the patient should be given a weight to hold (30 gm, or 1 ounce per kilogram of body weight up to 2 kg), which often widens the joint space, enabling the physician to make the diagnosis radiographically. No displacement suggests first-degree AC ligament sprain, less than 1 cm second-degree, and greater than 1 cm of displacement third-degree injury (Fig. 29-3).

Management. First- and second-degree AC separations can be treated with a sling and swathe with orthopedic follow-up. Third-degree AC dislocation may require surgical repair, so consultation with an orthopedist from the emergency department is advisable.

SCAPULAR FRACTURES

The scapula floats freely on the posterior chest wall. Its coracoid and acromial processes and glenoid fossa form the socket in which the proximal humerus articulates. The scapula is especially resilient in childhood, making fracture rare. Direct high-energy trauma and crushing injury are the usual mechanisms of fracture. Children with scapular fractures often have other injuries that take priority. Physical examination of a child with a fracture of the scapula usually reveals local tenderness and swelling, along with inability to move the upper arm. In severely injured children the diagnosis is often made from radiographs obtained for other reasons. Tangential or oblique views are sometimes necessary and should be obtained in selected patients. Most fractures are not displaced and occur along the lateral border involving the acromion, coracoid, or glenoid.

A child with a fracture of the scapula and no other serious injuries may use a sling and swathe for 3 to 4 weeks. Other injuries often require initial stabilization.

SHOULDER

Shoulder Dislocation

Dislocation of the humeral head from the glenoid is rare in young children, but this injury becomes more frequent in the adolescent years with physeal closure. Dislocation is anterior in 95% of cases; posterior and inferior dislocations are uncommon. Newborns with shoulder dystocia can have displaced Salter I fractures of the proximal humerus resembling shoulder dislocation because the unossified epiphysis that remains in the glenoid is not visible radiographically.

Indirect trauma—usually from a fall on an outstretched arm, forcing the shoulder into abduction and extension—results in disruption of the joint capsule. The head of the humerus moves anteriorly and interiorly. Before closure of the physis, this mechanism usually results in humeral fracture rather then dislocation.

Diagnostic Findings. Physical examination of a patient with an anterior dislocation reveals a flattened deltoid muscle on the affected side, with a prominent acromion. The head of the humerus is palpable anterior, inferior, and medial to the glenoid. The patient cannot abduct or externally rotate the arm. Posterior dislocations present with the affected shoulder flattened anteriorly, with the head of the humerus fully posterior.

Fracture of the greater tuberosity may occur. Associated abnormalities of the glenoid include detachment of the labrum, tearing of the anterior capsule and subscapularis muscle, and Hill Sachs compression fracture of the posterior humeral head. The axillary nerve may be injured; its status may be assessed on the basis of sensation over the lateral portion of the shoulder and upper arm with deltoid muscle palsy. Distal vasculature may also be compromised.

Radiographs are useful in confirming the anterior dislocation and ruling out associated fractures. They should be obtained initially and after reduction. Anteroposterior and lateral views demonstrate the dislocation of the humeral head from the glenoid. The humeral head lies inferior to the coracoid process (Fig. 29-4).

Management. Several methods are used to reduce shoulder dislocations. Longitudinal traction on the arm with countertraction and slow external rotation can be used to reduce most of these dislocations if muscle relaxation is achieved. Careful use of narcotic analgesics with benzodiazepines for muscle relaxation can help in this regard. A brute-force approach is painful and increases the tone of the musculature, preventing reduction. Forceful reduction increases the risk of epiphyseal and neurovascular injury. The axillary nerve, which innervates the deltoid, is particularly vulnerable and should be assessed before and after shoulder reduction. A less traumatic method of reduction, often successful with a minimum of discomfort for the patient, involves having the child lie prone on a stretcher. The child is instructed to let the affected arm hang down

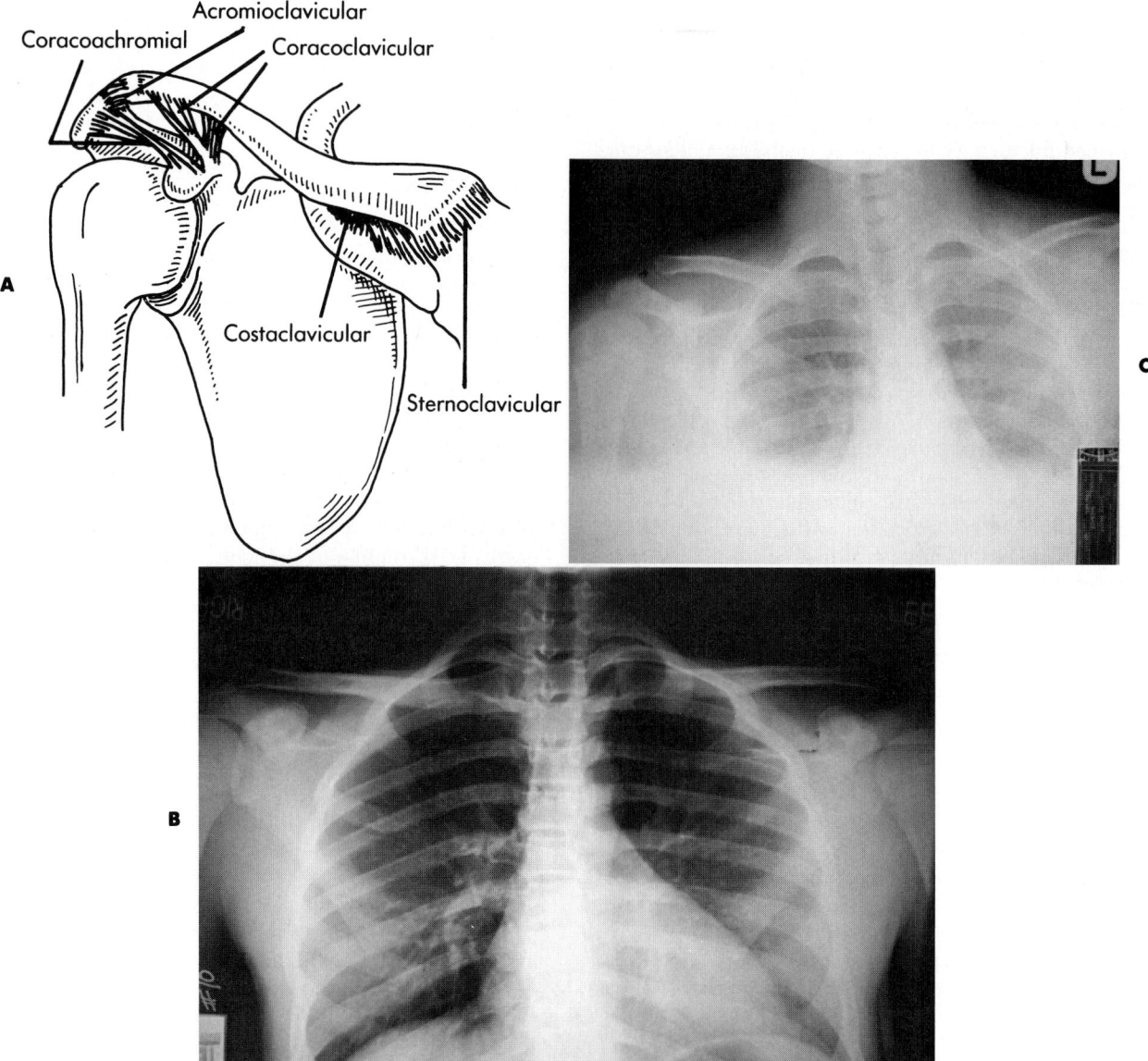

FIG. 29-3. A, Ligaments of the AC joint. **B,** AC separation. Superior displacement of the distal left clavicle indicates disruption of the ligaments of the AC joint. **C,** Fracture of the distal clavicle with superior displacement resembles AC separation. (**A** *from Jackimczyk KC and Goy W: Musculoskeletal trauma. In Rosen P, Doris PE, Barkin RM, et al: Diagnostic radiology in emergency medicine, St Louis, 1992, Mosby.*)

over the side while holding a 10-pound weight. The weight may be taped to the child's hand. The patient is told to relax and is left alone. Five to 10 minutes later the shoulder is usually relocated. After reduction, a sling and swathe or shoulder immobilizer (in internal rotation) is used for 4 weeks to allow healing, which is followed by a rehabilitation program.

Injury to the axillary artery, brachial plexus, or axillary nerve may occur with shoulder dislocation or on reduction. Some patients have recurrent shoulder dislocation; this is more common in children and adolescents. Voluntary dislocation in adolescents is usually associated with psychological and behavioral problems. Surgery is often indicated for recurrences; referral to an orthopedist is necessary after the second episode.

Brachial Plexus Injury

Trauma to the brachial plexus occurs in difficult deliveries and as a complication of injuries of the upper extremity. Advances in obstetrical care have decreased the incidence of traumatic paralysis of the upper extremity.[2] The emergency physician must recognize this problem, which may be encountered in young infants in whom injury is not diagnosed in the nursery or, rarely, in older children with upper-extremity injuries. Traction on the brachial plexus and direct trauma are the causes of the neurologic dysfunc-

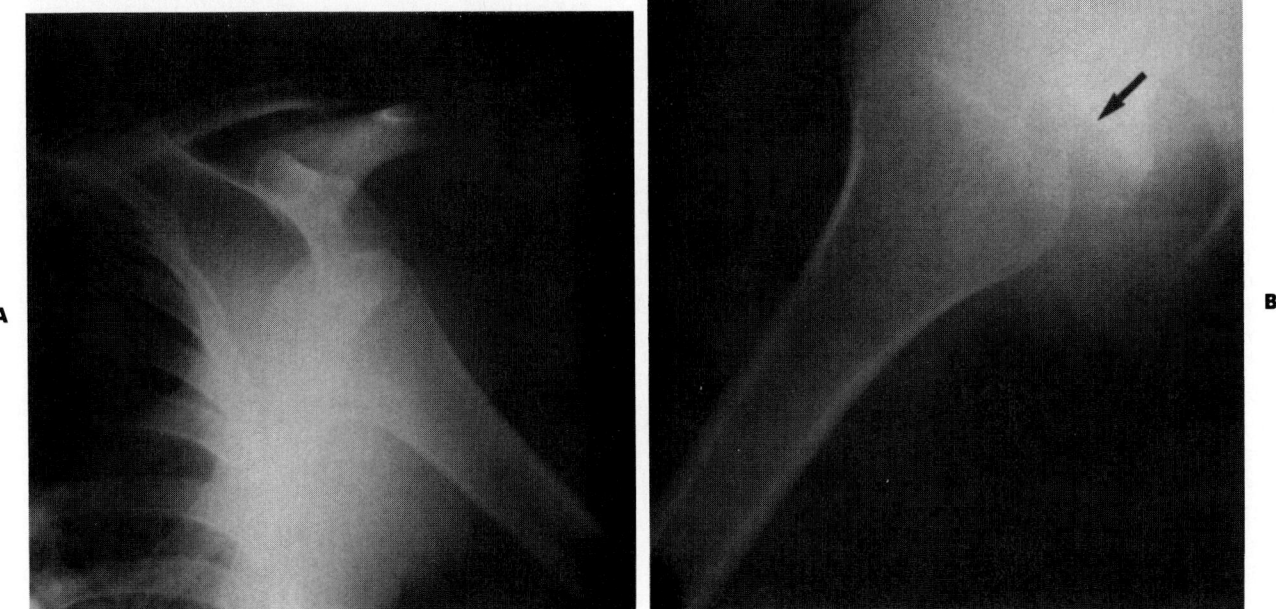

FIG. 29-4. Anterior dislocation of the shoulder becomes more common in adolescence. **A,** Anteroposterior view. **B,** Axillary view demonstrates displacement of the humeral head from the glenoid. Note the humeral head is anterior to the anterior rim of the glenoid fossa. (*From Jackimczyk KC and Goy W: Musculoskeletal trauma. In Rosen P, Doris PE, Barkin RM, et al: Diagnostic radiology in emergency medicine, St Louis, 1992, Mosby.*)

tion. The child has decreased active range of motion, with normal passive range of motion of the affected arm. Assessment of the Moro reflex in infants is useful in detecting the asymmetric function of the arms. The considerable overlap in innervation makes it difficult to localize the lesion to the upper roots (C5, C6), which innervate the shoulder and elbow; lower roots (C7, C8), which innervate the wrist and hand; or a complete injury. This distinction ultimately has little impact on the management or prognosis for these children.

All patients with suspected brachial plexus injury should undergo radiography of the clavicle and shoulder as a means of ruling out bony injury.

Evaluation by a pediatric neurologist and early physical therapy to teach parents range of motion exercises are important to maximize the chances of complete recovery. Approximately 80% of patients have full return of function by 1 year.[3]

Pulled Shoulder

Forceful traction on a child's arm occasionally causes a partial tear in the joint capsule of the shoulder without dislocation. Patients with such injuries have pain with movement of the shoulder and normal radiographic findings.

Treatment with a sling should result in resolution of the pain. Repeat radiography in a patient with persistent pain may reveal a healing Salter I fracture of the proximal humerus.

Rotator Cuff Injury

The term "rotator cuff" refers to the supraspinatus, infraspinatus, and teres minor muscles, which stabilize the shoulder. Strenuous movement, usually related to throwing, can cause partial or complete tearing in this muscle group. The presence of pain with abduction or external rotation of the shoulder and point tenderness over the insertion of the rotator cuff helps establish the diagnosis. Passive range of motion of the shoulder may be normal. Tenderness over the insertion of the rotator cuff into the tuberosities may be noted. Partial tears are associated with abduction weakness, pain, and reduced endurance.

Radiography, including anteroposterior and lateral views of the shoulder, sometimes shows avulsion of bone from the tuberosities where the muscles insert. If significant weakness persists, arthrography may demonstrate leakage of contrast medium from the shoulder joint capsule into the subacromial bursa.

Minor injuries can be treated with immobilization in a sling, passive range of motion exercises, and analgesia. Severe or persistent injury necessitates orthopedic evaluation. Early repair is required for patients with avulsion fractures of the tuberosity.

HUMERUS

Proximal Humeral Epiphyseal Fractures

Epiphyseal fractures are the main type of injury to the proximal humerus in pediatric patients. Salter I fractures are occasionally seen in patients younger than 6 years, sometimes as a consequence of birth trauma in the newborn period. Older children—especially those aged 11 to 15 years who are involved in sports—sustain Salter II fractures. Salter III, IV, and V fractures almost never occur. Proper treatment is especially important because 80% of the longitudinal growth of the humerus occurs at the proximal epiphysis.

Fracture of the proximal humeral epiphysis can result from direct or indirect force. Extension of the arm in an adducted position in an attempt to break a fall is a common mechanism of injury. Some authors believe such injuries are particularly likely when an individual falls backwards with the force transmitted up the humerus, causing anterior and lateral displacement of the metaphysis. Direct trauma to the lateral aspect of the shoulder can also cause this injury.

Diagnostic Findings. The child with a proximal humeral fracture has great disability and tenderness with even slight movement of the arm. Examination shows swelling and local tenderness that may be difficult to differentiate from clavicular tenderness in the hysterical young child. Proximal humeral fractures are seldom markedly displaced, so shortening is usually absent. Attempts to force the arm through range of motion are to be avoided because they cause severe pain and may damage the axillary nerve. Assessment should include a test of deltoid function for evidence of axillary nerve injury.

Anteroposterior and lateral radiographs are necessary to make the diagnosis. The metaphyseal fragment that is often displaced with the epiphysis makes the Salter II fracture in the older child relatively easy to diagnose. Salter I injuries in young children, however, may be more difficult to recognize because so little of the cartilage is ossified. Radiographs must include the entire shoulder girdle for fractures of the distal clavicle and acromion to be identified.

Proximal humeral fractures usually heal quite well, even if some displacement remains. Longitudinal growth impairment is the main complication, especially in children older than 11 years. Varus deformity may occur over time as a consequence of injury to the medial portion of the physis. Injury to the axillary nerve or circumflex can cause deltoid weakness that usually resolves in weeks to months.

Management. Most fractures of the proximal humerus can be treated with a sling and swathe. Displacement is usually minimal, so manipulation is not often necessary. All patients with fractures of the proximal humerus should be seen within 24 hours by an orthopedic surgeon (Fig. 29-5).

Proximal Humeral Metaphyseal Fractures

Fracture of the proximal humeral metaphysis is more frequent than epiphyseal fracture in children 5 to 11 years old. Unicameral bone cysts and other lesions of the proximal humerus are common, and pathologic fractures often occur. The mechanism of injury and clinical presentation are similar to those of proximal humeral epiphyseal fractures. Metaphyseal fractures can usually be distinguished radiographically from epiphyseal injuries. Fractures may be torus, greenstick, or transverse. The strong periosteal sleeve in most cases maintains the fracture fragments in alignment. Significant displacement or angulation must be reduced for optimal healing. The treatment of proximal humeral metaphyseal fractures, including pathologic fractures, is similar to epiphyseal fractures. Steroids should never be injected into bony lesions at the time of pathologic fracture.

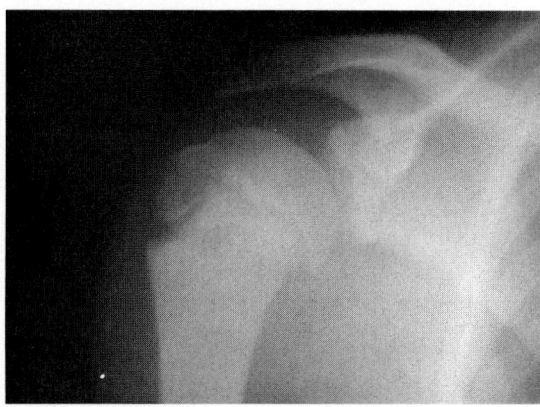

FIG. 29-5. Displaced Salter I fracture of the proximal humerus.

Humeral Shaft Fractures

Fractures of the shaft of the humerus are uncommon because the proximal and distal cartilaginous structures are more likely to fail. The middle third is the most common location of diaphyseal fractures. The location of the fracture relative to the many muscle insertions on the humerus determines the direction and severity of displacement.

Mechanism of Injury. Indirect trauma sustained when a child falls on the elbow or hand causes oblique or comminuted fractures. A spiral fracture suggests a twisting force that, especially in young children, may be the result of child abuse. A fall on an arm, with subsequent twisting of the remainder of the body, may also cause a spiral fracture. Direct impact is likely to cause a transverse, comminuted, or open fracture. Pathologic fracture through a defect in the humeral shaft can occur with a low-energy mechanism such as throwing a ball.

Diagnostic Findings. A child with a fracture of the humeral shaft has swelling, localized tenderness, and sometimes deformity. It is especially important to document rotational deformity. Sensory and motor nerve function should be assessed. The radial nerve, which courses obliquely in the musculospiral groove, is particularly vulnerable to injury. Anesthesia of the dorsum of the hand between the first and second metacarpals and weakness of the wrist and finger extensors suggest injury to the radial nerve.

Shaft fractures are usually obvious on radiography of the humerus, which serve to establish the pattern of fracture and the degree of displacement (Figs. 29-6 and 29-7). The shoulder and elbow should be visualized to rule out other bony injuries.

Treatment of humeral shaft injuries must begin as soon as fracture is suspected. Immobilization in a sling prevents further neurovascular injury from movement of the fracture fragments and should be accomplished before radiography is performed. After diagnosis, a sling and swathe are sufficient in younger children. A long-arm splint from axilla to wrist (sugar tong), with the elbow at 90 degrees, may be more comfortable for the older child. All children with fractures of the humeral shaft should be evaluated within 24 hours by an orthopedic surgeon. Reduction of the override, angulation, and muscular interposition may be necessary.

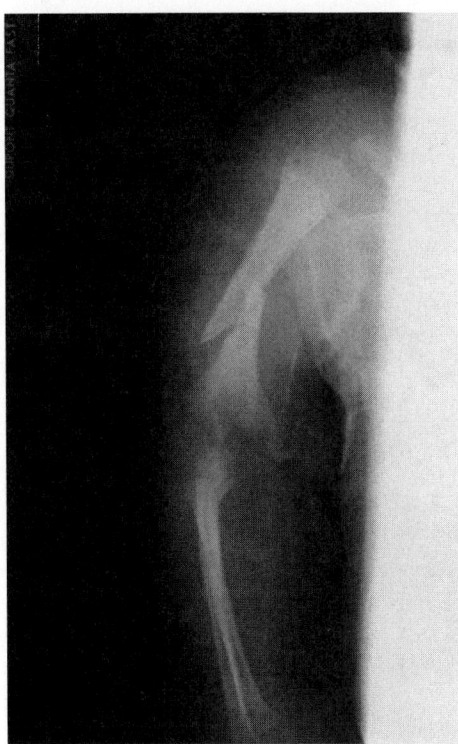

FIG. 29-6. Spiral fracture of humerus in an infant who reportedly caught the arm between slats of a crib. Further evaluation revealed child abuse.

Radial nerve injury occasionally necessitates traction or surgical release of entrapment. The hand and wrist should be splinted in a position of function; close follow-up is necessary to monitor improvement. Paralysis is rarely permanent. Malunion can occur, especially with angulated fractures of the distal shaft.

ELBOW

Supracondylar (Distal Humeral Metaphyseal) Fractures

Supracondylar (distal humeral metaphyseal) fractures are the most frequent elbow fractures in pediatric patients. Children between 3 and 10 years are at greatest risk, and boys outnumber girls. These injuries are probably the most challenging fractures in childhood in terms of diagnosis and treatment. The potential for serious neurovascular complications makes accurate diagnosis and prompt, appropriate treatment crucial.

The elbow joint involves three articulations—between the capitellum and the radial head, the trochlea and the ulna, and the proximal radius and ulna. Six centers of ossification begin ossifying at different times, making radiographic interpretation more difficult (Table 29-1).

Mechanism of Injury. The vast majority of supracondylar fractures result from hyperextension. Extension of the arm to prevent body impact in a fall transmits the force up the forearm to the distal humerus. In extension the force may fracture the supracondylar area, pushing the distal fragment posteriorly and superiorly. The amount of force and conse-

TABLE 29-1. Ossification Centers of the Elbow: Age of Appearance

Capitellum	< 1 year
Radial head	4 to 5 years
Medial epicondyle	4 to 6 years
Trochlea	8 to 10 years
Olecranon	8 to 9 years
Lateral epicondyle	9 to 11 years

quent periosteal stripping from the proximal and distal humeral fragments determine the degree of displacement.

Supracondylar fractures are acute emergencies because of the vulnerability of the arterial blood supply. The brachial artery can be entrapped or kinked at the fracture site. Contusion of the vessel can cause spasm; tight bandaging in an effort to control swelling can further disrupt the vascular supply. Ischemia of the muscles of the forearm causes edema, increased pressure inside the fascial compartment, and further reduction in perfusion. Necrosis of volar muscle and subsequent fibrosis can cause permanent disability, known as "Volkmann contracture."

Diagnostic Findings. Tenderness over the distal humerus and pain with flexion of the elbow suggest supracondylar fracture. The arm is usually held in pronation. Swelling varies considerably with the degree of displacement, associated vascular disruption, and time elapsed since the injury.

Evaluation of distal neurovascular function is more important than examination of the fracture site. Pain, poor perfusion (coolness, capillary refill time longer than 2 seconds), absence of radial pulse, paresthesias, and paralysis (the "five Ps") of the forearm suggest ischemia. A child with elbow injuries who complains of increasing pain in the forearm should be immediately reevaluated. Exacerbation of the pain by passive extension of the fingers is a useful early finding in patients with vascular compromise. The radial pulse can be reconstituted from arterial flow that does not traverse the ischemic compartment and therefore may remain palpable despite significant vascular insufficiency in the forearm. Any child suspected of having vascular compromise should have emergency orthopedic consultation for reduction of a displaced fracture. Sensory and motor function of the radial, ulnar, and medial nerves should be carefully tested.

The incidence of complications of supracondylar fracture has decreased with greater awareness of compartment syndromes and proper emergency care. Infarction of the forearm musculature is complete after 12 to 24 hours of vascular insufficiency. Necrosis, usually in the distribution of the anterior interosseous artery, progresses over 5 to 10 days and is followed by fibrosis and contracture. Volkmann contracture is characterized by fixed flexion of the elbow, pronation of the forearm, flexion of the wrist, extension of the metacarpophalangeal joints, and flexion of the interphalangeal joints.

Neurologic complications in the form of radial, medial, or ulnar nerve injuries occur in 5% to 10% of supracondylar

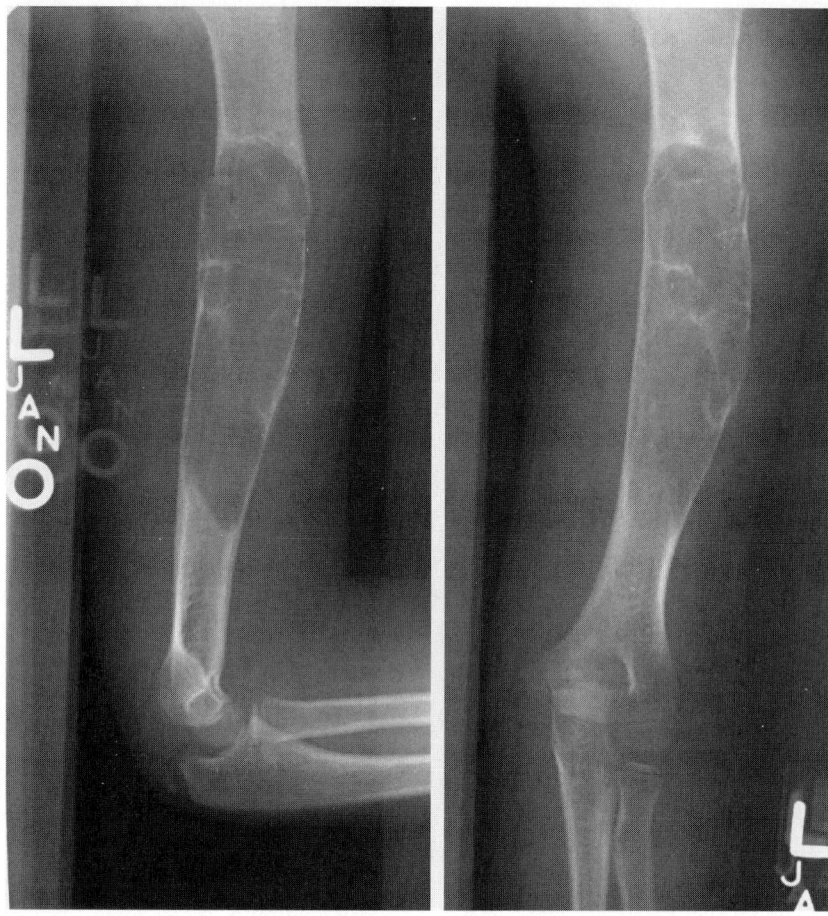

FIG. 29-7. Pathologic fracture through bone cyst of humerus.

fractures. The nerve may be damaged at the time of injury, during fracture reduction, as a result of ischemia (especially median), or by entrapment in fracture callus. Return of full function usually occurs in 6 to 10 weeks.

Changes in the carrying angle, which is the angle of the forearm relative to the humerus, can result from incomplete reduction of even slight degrees of medial or lateral tilt of the distal fragment. Cubitus varus, or "gunstock deformity," is more of a cosmetic than a functional problem. It can be corrected surgically.

Radiologic Studies. The child with an elbow injury and no neurovascular problems should be splinted before radiography is performed. An anteroposterior view in extension and a true lateral radiograph with 90 degrees of flexion should be ordered. Supracondylar fractures with significant displacement are easily diagnosed. A true lateral is extremely important for identifying subtle fractures.

The "fat-pad sign" is a nonspecific sign of injury. The anterior fat pad is normally visible on a lateral radiograph with the elbow flexed to 90 degrees. The posterior fat pad is recessed in the olecranon fossa and should not be visible under normal circumstances (Fig. 29-8, A). Fluid in the elbow joint, such as hemarthrosis with elbow fracture, displaces the anterior and posterior fat pads upward and outward. Radiolucency visible posteriorly and outward dis-

placement of the normal anterior lucency are important radiographic signs of significant elbow injury. The fat-pad sign without an identifiable fracture line is frequently seen in greenstick or nondisplaced supracondylar fracture (Fig. 29-8, B). Radiographs should be carefully inspected for subtle fractures of the radial head, capitellum, trochlea, or olecranon. Immobilization and orthopedic follow-up are important in children with fat-pad sign on elbow radiography but no identifiable fracture. Subsequent radiography usually documents a bony injury.

The anterior humeral line is another radiologic tool in the diagnosis of subtle supracondylar fracture. It is drawn down the anterior margin of the humerus on the lateral view and should intersect the capitellum in its middle or posterior third. Subtle supracondylar fractures can be diagnosed on the basis of the loss of the normal anterior angulation of the capitellum, which results in the anterior humeral line intersecting in its anterior portion. Concomitant fractures of the proximal humerus and distal radius should not be overlooked.

Management. Treatment of supracondylar fracture must start as soon as a child with an elbow injury comes to medical attention (Fig. 29-9). Secondary injury to the soft tissues, nerves, and vessels around the fracture site must be prevented with prompt immobilization of the injured

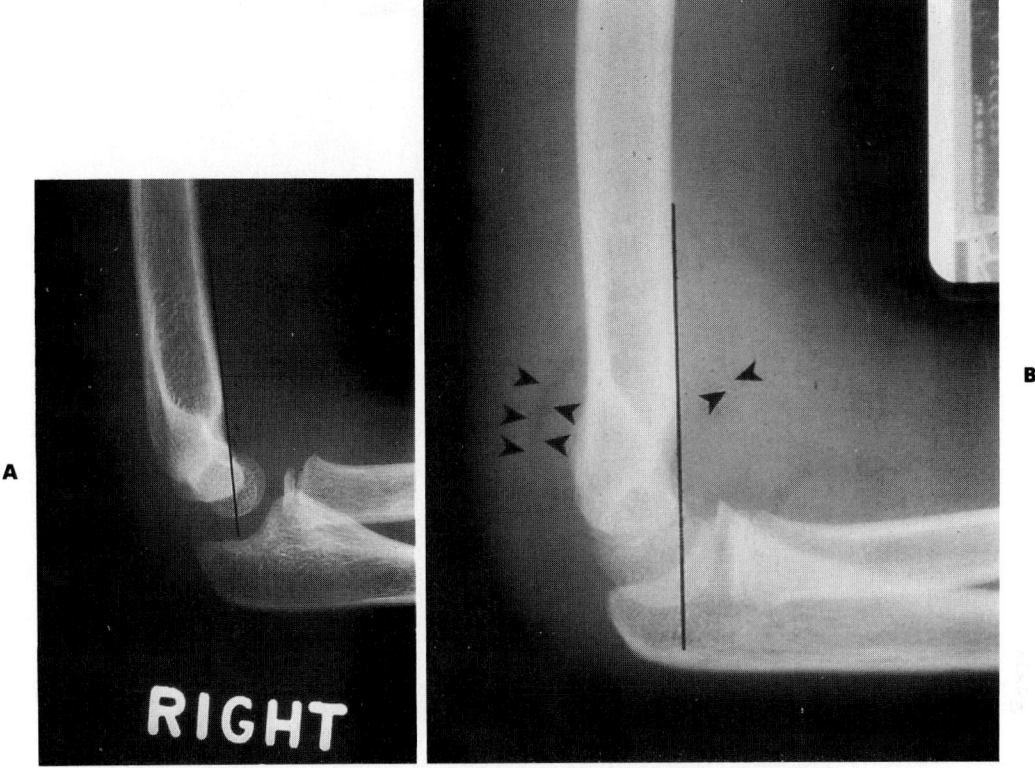

FIG. 29-8. A, Normal lateral radiograph of the elbow. The anterior fat pad is visible adjacent to the humerus, and the posterior fat pad is not seen. **B,** Greenstick supracondylar fracture. The posterior fat pad is visible and the anterior fat pad is displaced anteriorly. Posterior angulation of the distal humerus causes the anterior humeral line to intersect the capitellum in its anterior portion.

arm. Excessive flexion of the elbow can compromise perfusion. The arm should be secured with no more than 20 to 30 degrees of flexion. The position in which the arm is held is usually adequate. Splinting must not be too tight, and the neurovascular status of the injured arm should be reevaluated after immobilization.

Many orthopedic surgeons admit all children with supracondylar fractures, even nondisplaced ones, to observe the progression of swelling and check for vascular compromise over the first 24 to 48 hours. After communication with an orthopedic surgeon, a child with a greenstick or nondisplaced supracondylar fracture and a minimum of swelling can be treated as an outpatient if close follow-up is assured. The arm is immobilized in a posterior splint from axilla to wrist with the elbow slightly flexed and the forearm in a neutral or pronated position. Perfusion is reassessed after splinting. The child must be seen by the orthopedic surgeon within 24 hours of injury.

Children with supracondylar fractures that are at all displaced or involve significant soft-tissue swelling and those for whom follow-up cannot be ensured should be treated as inpatients. Prompt reduction of a displaced fracture minimizes the risk of complications. Many supracondylar fractures, especially oblique ones, are treated with open reduction.

Immediate reduction is necessary if signs of vascular compromise are evident. If symptoms and signs of is-

chemia are severe and an orthopedic surgeon is not immediately available, the fracture can be reduced with traction, supination of the forearm, and direct downward and anterior pressure on the displaced fragment. If after 6 to 8 hours extension of the elbow, reduction of the fracture, and removal of constricting bandages have failed to restore perfusion, fasciotomy and arterial exploration may be necessary.

Lateral and Medial Condylar Fractures

Fractures of the lateral condyle of the distal humerus are common, accounting for about 15% of all elbow fractures. Most such injuries are sustained by children aged 3 to 14 years; 6- to 10-year-old children are at especially high risk.

The mechanism of most lateral and medial condylar injuries involves indirect force. A fall on an outstretched hand with the forearm abducted transmits the energy through the radius to the lateral condyle, which may fail. Traction on an extended, supinated arm with varus stress puts tension on the forearm extensors; this can avulse the lateral condyle. Displacement and rotation of the distal fragment results from the action of the forearm extensors.

Diagnostic Findings. The child with a lateral condylar fracture is usually in severe pain, with impressive swelling and ecchymosis. Careful examination can localize the tenderness to the lateral aspect of the elbow, but this is often difficult in the crying child. The elbow can be rotated, but

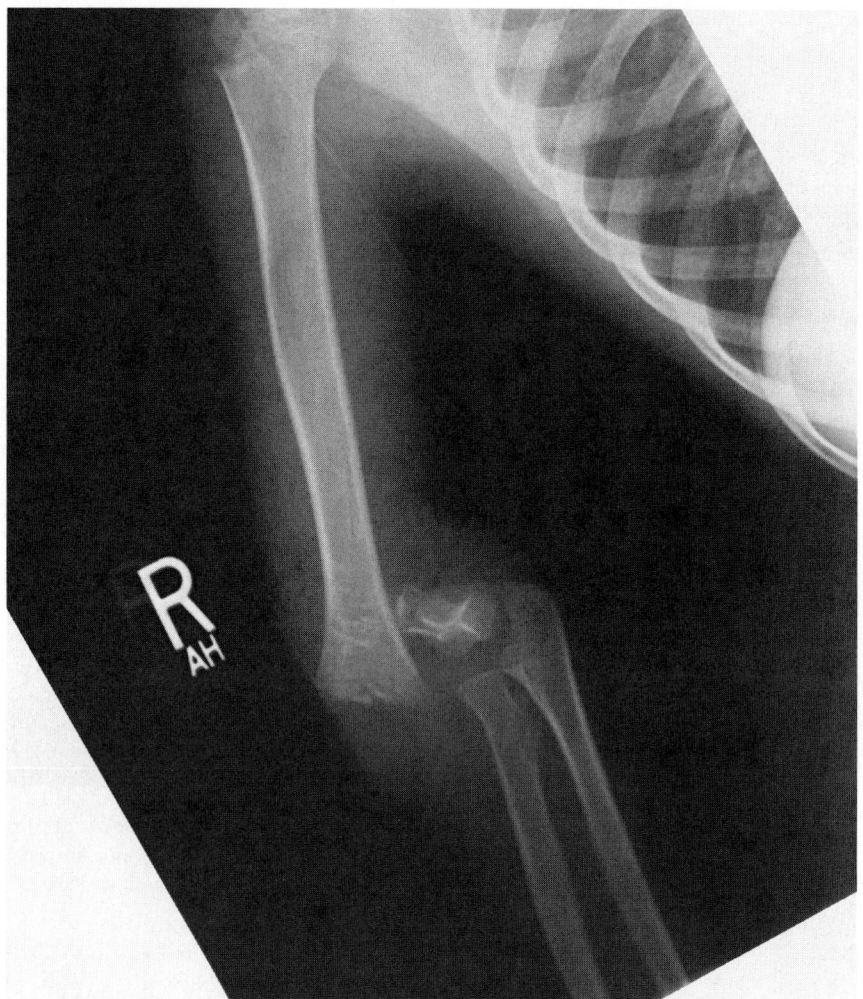

FIG. 29-9. Displaced supracondylar fracture with vascular compromise requires emergency reduction.

rotation causes pain. A minimum of manipulation is best; it is usually obvious that radiography is necessary. The neurovascular status of the forearm and hand must be checked.

Anteroposterior and lateral radiographs are usually sufficient to visualize the fracture and assess the degree of displacement, although an oblique view is sometimes necessary. Condylar fractures are usually of Salter type III or IV. In young children with unossified cartilage, radiographic diagnosis can be difficult. The fracture usually extends into the trochlea but can traverse the capitellum (Fig. 29-10).

Cubitus valgus resulting from growth arrest of the lateral condylar physis is not uncommon, especially in minimally displaced fractures that are not treated aggressively. Progressive cubitus valgus stretches the ulnar nerve around the medial condyle, leading to ulnar neuritis and delayed ulnar nerve palsy.

Management. Displaced lateral condylar fractures are unstable and require prompt attention of an orthopedic surgeon. The degree of displacement is often underestimated, and many fractures become displaced while immobilized as a result of the action of the wrist and finger extensors. A long-arm cast with the elbow at 90 degrees of flexion and the forearm fully supinated is the treatment for nondisplaced fracture. Displaced fractures require open reduction.

Medial Epicondylar Fractures

The flexors of the forearm originate from the medial epicondyle. A valgus strain exerts traction on these muscles, which can avulse and sometimes displace the medial epicondyle. Medial epicondylar injury is relatively common in 7- to 15-year-old children, accounting for 10% of all elbow fractures in childhood. In about half of all cases the elbow is also dislocated.

Children with fractures of the medial epicondyle keep the elbow partially flexed for comfort. Pain occurs with range of motion, especially valgus stress and pronation. Maximum swelling and tenderness can be localized to the medial portion of the elbow. The ulnar nerve, which courses around the medial epicondyle, is often injured, and its function must be tested.

Anteroposterior and lateral radiographs of both elbows are important in making the diagnosis. Displacement of the epicondyle, which ossifies at 4 to 6 years of age, causes

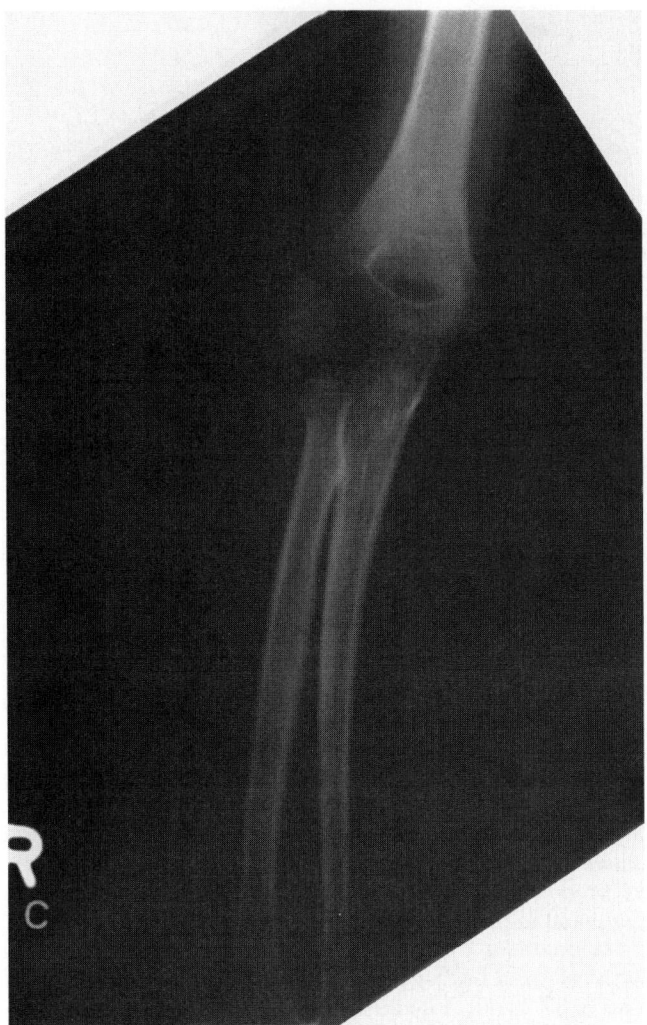

FIG. 29-10. Lateral condylar fracture with displacement and rotation caused by the action of the wrist and finger extensors. These injuries are unstable and require open reduction.

apparent medial widening of the physis on the injured side. The proximal radius may also be fractured (Fig. 29-11).

Treatment with a long-arm cast or open reduction depends on the degree of displacement, which must be determined by an orthopedic surgeon. Ulnar nerve injuries usually resolve, and growth disturbance is rare.

Intercondylar and Transcondylar Fractures

Intercondylar fractures extending downward between the distal humeral condyles occasionally occur in older children. Such "T" fractures are often unstable and require immediate orthopedic consultation. Avascular necrosis of the trochlea can complicate these injuries.

Transcondylar fractures across the entire distal humeral physis can occur, especially in very young children. These injuries are often the result of child abuse. Displaced transcondylar fractures can be difficult to distinguish from elbow dislocations before ossification of the capitellum during the first year of life. The relationship of the radial head to the capitellum is preserved in transcondylar fractures.

The radius and ulna are usually shifted medially compared with the lateral displacement seen in most dislocations of the elbow. An older child is more likely to have Salter II injury with a metaphyseal fragment. Admission to the hospital for monitoring of the distal circulation is advisable. Growth disturbance and neurovascular injuries are rare.

Elbow Dislocation

The elbow has little osseous stability, making it the most commonly dislocated joint in childhood. Elbow dislocations account for 5% of all serious elbow injuries in children, particularly those aged 8 years through adolescence.

The mechanism of most dislocations is a fall on an outstretched hand with partial flexion or extension of the elbow. The force disrupts the joint capsule and, often, one or both of the collateral ligaments, enabling the proximal radius and ulna to be displaced posteriorly. In most children the medial collateral ligament is ruptured and the dislocation is posterior and lateral. Rupture of the lateral collateral or fracture of the lateral condyle can be associated with posteromedial displacement. Pure dislocations without associated fractures are rare in children.

Diagnostic Findings. The child with a dislocated elbow experiences extreme pain, impressive swelling, and restricted motion of the elbow produced by muscle spasm. The arm is partially flexed and often supported by the other hand. Shortening of the forearm is apparent. The tip of the olecranon protrudes posteriorly compared with the uninjured side and becomes more prominent with elbow flexion. The two epicondyles and the tip of the olecranon normally form an isosceles triangle. In a dislocation the sides of the triangle are unequal, whereas in a nondisplaced supracondylar fracture they remain equal.

The most important part of the assessment of any serious elbow injury is an evaluation of the circulatory and neurologic integrity of the distal arm. Ischemia of the forearm musculature is manifested by pain, poor perfusion (coolness, capillary refill time longer than 2 seconds), decreased pulses, paresthesias, and paralysis of the forearm. Increased pain with passive extension of the fingers is a useful indicator of early vascular compromise. Sensory and motor function of the ulnar, median, and radial nerves should also be tested.

Injury to the brachial artery or compression from a large hematoma causes vascular complications in 7% of elbow dislocations, especially when fractures coexist.[4] The incidence of Volkmann contracture, which occurs as often with elbow dislocations as with supracondylar fractures, has decreased because of the increased awareness of compartment syndromes. Damage to the ulnar nerve from stretching or median nerve from entrapment occurs in 22% of elbow dislocations[4] and usually resolves without residua.

Radiography is performed after splinting, except when severe vascular compromise requires immediate reduction. The radial head and olecranon are displaced posteriorly and laterally, without the normal relationship to the capitellum and trochlea. Fracture of the proximal radius, proximal ulna (coronoid or olecranon), medial epicondyle, lateral epicondyle, or distal radius and ulna is usually found. Spontaneous reduction of elbow dislocation is common. Some children are seen after dislocation and reduction, in

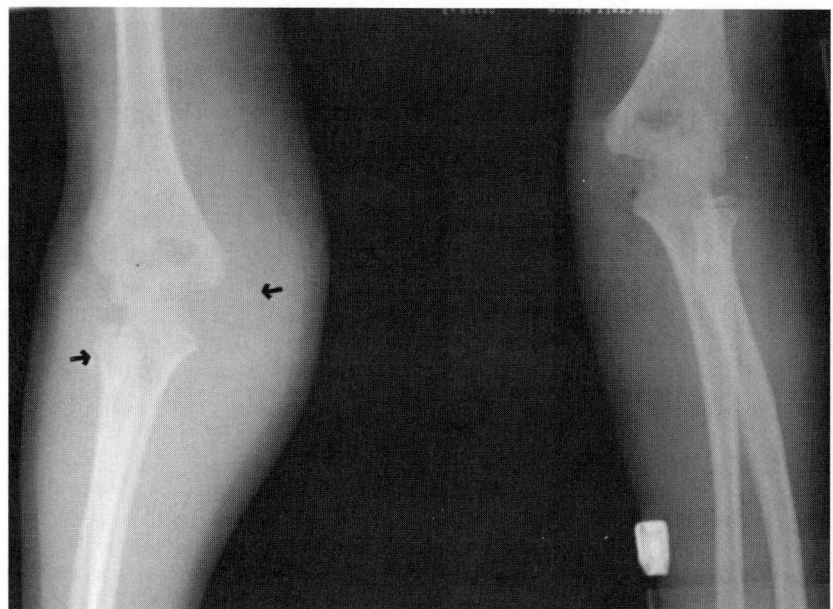

FIG. 29-11. Avulsion of the medial epicondyle. Note the subtle fracture of the radial head.

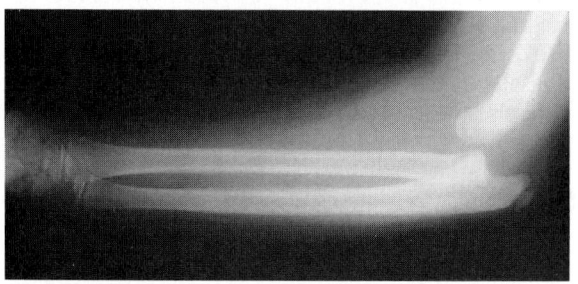

FIG. 29-12. Posterior dislocation of the elbow.

which case the associated fracture is the only radiographic evidence of elbow injury (Fig. 29-12).

Management. Reduction of elbow dislocation is an urgent or emergency measure, depending on the status of the vasculature, and requires orthopedic consultation. Sedation and analgesia are recommended to reduce pain, decrease muscle spasm, and prevent fracture of the radial head with reduction. The patient can be placed prone on a stretcher with the injured arm hanging down. Countertraction and direct pressure, with the thumbs on the olecranon pushing downward and anteriorly, often reduces the dislocation. After reduction the elbow should be flexed with careful attention to the adequacy of the distal circulation. Postreduction radiography is necessary to prove that the reduction is complete and to detect fractures not noted on the initial films or fractures caused by reduction. Hospital admission for observation for vascular compromise is recommended.

Radial Head Subluxation ("Nursemaid's Elbow")

Radial head subluxation, "nursemaid's elbow," "pulled elbow," and "temper tantrum elbow" are all names for a very common injury known since the time of Hippocrates. It accounts for 22% of all upper extremity injuries in children.[5] Most patients are between 6 months and 5 years, with a peak incidence between 1 and 3 years, but injury to younger and older children occurs.[6] The left elbow is more frequently injured because many caretakers prefer to hold the child's left hand in the right hand.

Mechanism of Injury. Abrupt traction on a pronated wrist or hand has long been known to cause subluxation of the radial head. (Fig. 29-13) Anatomic studies have shown that underdevelopment of the radial head is not the reason this injury occurs so frequently in young children. In pronation, longitudinal traction enables the annular ligament to slip over the margin of the radial head and become interposed between the articular surfaces of the radial head and capitellum. Tearing of the annular ligament does not always occur. Supination causes the higher and more flared side of the radial head to push the ligament back to its anatomic position, thereby reducing the subluxation.

Diagnostic Findings. A history of a pull on the arm is not found in as many as half of cases.[6] Falls are occasionally reported as the cause of injury, although the mechanism of such an injury is difficult to understand. Many parents believe they have fractured the child's arm and feel very guilty. They should be reassured and asked about the circumstances of the injury; this often yields information about a pulling mechanism not previously obtained.

The diagnosis can often be made from across the room. A child with radial head subluxation holds the arm partially flexed, pronated, and close to the body. The child will refuse to reach with the injured arm but is usually not distressed[6] when the arm is left undisturbed. Physicians often suspect injury to the shoulder or wrist, especially when a history of a pull is lacking. A slow and nonthreatening approach enables the physician to palpate the clavicle, humerus, radius, and ulna to exclude point tender-

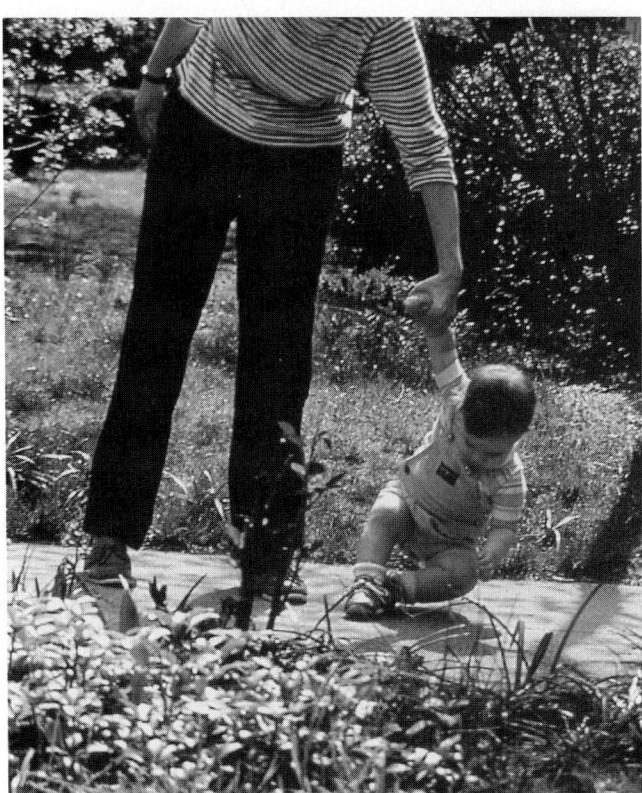

FIG. 29-13. An abrupt pull on the pronated arm causes subluxation of the radial head. Radiographs are normal with nursemaid's elbow and need not be obtained.

ness that would suggest fracture. In one series, tenderness of the radial head was noted in only 16.7% of patients[6], and appreciable swelling is usually absent. The physical examination finding of disuse is often more common and diagnostic than localized tenderness, which is confirmed with reduction of the subluxation. Recurrent subluxation of the radial head occurs in 26% to 39% of cases.[5-7]

Radiography before or after reduction is neither necessary nor desirable in the child when the history and examination are consistent and, upon reduction, function returns. No radiographic abnormality exists. Many radiology technicians have experience in reducing nursemaid's elbow from the supination they require to properly position the injured arm for an anteroposterior view. Radiography is indicated if the child has bony tenderness or no return of function after attempts at reduction.

Management. Reduction of radial head subluxation with prompt return of full function is one of the most satisfying procedures for the pediatric emergency physician. Several effective maneuvers exist; supination is the common component of all. The amount of elbow flexion or extension is probably not important.[8]

The elbow is held with the thumb positioned over the radial head to detect a click. The child's hand is grasped, gently pulled to elbow extension, and then rapidly supinated fully and flexed. Reduction is accomplished with the first maneuver in 69% to 80% of cases.[5,6] If a click is noted, reduction has been successful in more than 90% of cases.

The absence of a click may still be associated with successful reduction in up to 31% of cases.[5] The child should be encouraged to use the injured arm after the maneuver to prove that the reduction is complete. A sling for comfort is seldom needed. Parents should be counseled to lift their children from the axilla or upper arm, not the hand or wrist, to avoid recurrent injury.

Many authors have suggested that return of function is usually immediate and that slow return of function is attributable to delay in seeking care. When studied, however, only 14.3% of patients had immediate return of function, 60% in less than 5 minutes, and 87% in less than 15 minutes.[6] Delayed attempt at reduction was not significantly associated with slow return of function.[5,6] Younger children took longer to resume use of the injured arm than older children.[6]

If no click is appreciated and function does not return in 5 to 10 minutes, another attempt at reduction should be made. Children in whom a click is felt should be given 15 minutes for return of movement before attempts at reduction are repeated. Alternative diagnoses and radiographic evaluation should be considered after two or three unsuccessful attempts.

Olecranon Fractures

Fractures of the olecranon are infrequent in children; they occurred in 6% of all elbow fractures in one series.[9] Direct blows are the cause of olecranon fractures more often than falls on an extended hand and elbow.

Children with olecranon fractures have localized tenderness and restricted motion of the elbow. Except with small fractures of the tip, joint effusion and fat-pad sign are present. Complications are rare because little longitudinal growth occurs at the olecranon. Abnormalities of the radioulnar joint could affect the carrying angle and range of supination-pronation.

A few olecranon fractures at the physeal-metaphyseal interface are not easily visualized radiographically and require clinical diagnosis. The many variations in ossification of the olecranon lead to false-positive interpretations of radiographs. Comparison with the uninjured side can be very useful in these cases (Fig. 29-14).

Treatment of nondisplaced fractures usually involves a long-arm cast with the elbow at 90 degrees for 4 weeks, although incomplete fractures may need only a sling for 3 weeks. Displacement requires early involvement of an orthopedic surgeon.

RADIUS AND ULNA

Radial Head and Neck Fractures

Fractures of the radial head or neck are common after 5 years of age, particularly in 10- to 13-year-old children. Such injuries account for 5% to 10% of elbow fractures in childhood.

The mechanism of injury is usually a fall on an outstretched hand with valgus angulation. If the elbow is at full extension on impact, fracture of the olecranon or ulna also may occur. Partial flexion of the elbow causes the capitellum to drive against the outer portion of the radial head, leading to fractures with lateral or posterior angulation or displacement. The valgus stress may cause associ-

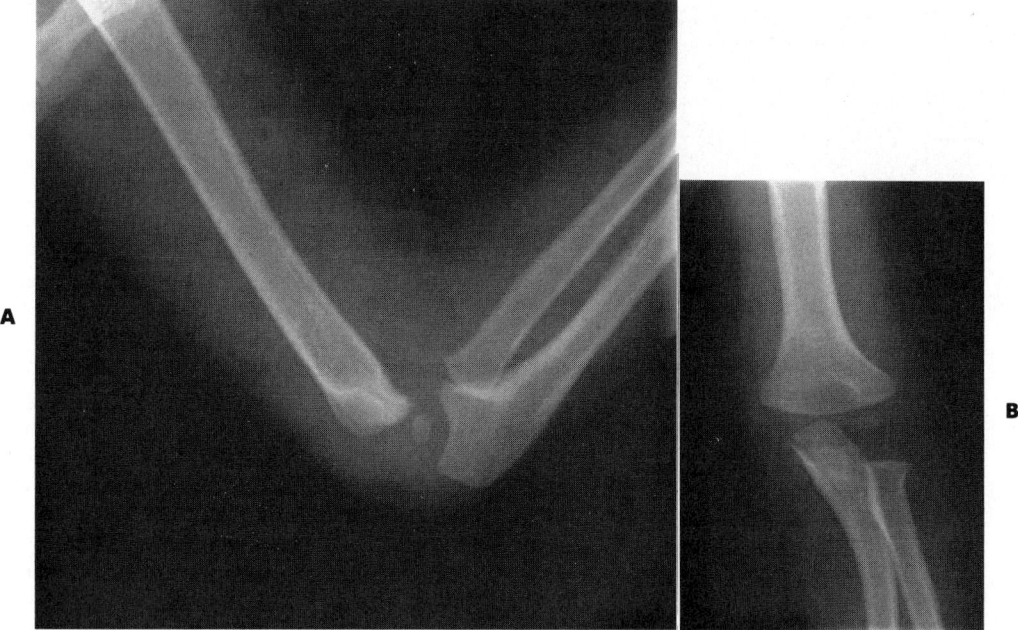

FIG. 29-14. A, Subtle posterior fat-pad sign. **B,** Fracture of the olecranon is visible on the anteroposterior radiograph.

ated injury to the medial epicondyle or medial collateral ligament.

Diagnostic Findings. The injured child holds the elbow in moderate flexion. Both flexion-extension and supination-pronation are restricted. Tenderness over the lateral aspect of the elbow, with ecchymosis, is present. Pain is sometimes noted in the wrist or hand, which also require careful assessment for concomitant injury. Radial nerve function in particular should be tested.

A slight increase in carrying angle is common after fracture of the proximal radius. Range-of-motion exercises aid in more rapid return of full flexion-extension and supination-pronation. The vascular supply of the radial head is limited, and partial avascular necrosis is common after fractures. Premature fusion of the physis may occur, especially as a consequence of displaced fracture.

Most fractures are impaction or greenstick injuries through the metaphysis close to the physeal interface. Radiographically these may resemble epiphyseal injuries (Fig. 29-15). Salter I and II fractures can also occur. Anteroposterior and lateral views are usually sufficient, although different amounts of rotation may be useful in showing the maximum degree of angulation. Dislocation of the elbow or radial head and fractures of the olecranon, ulna, capitellum, medial epicondyle, wrist, and navicular bone have all been associated with fracture of the proximal radius.

Management. Incomplete and minimally displaced fractures can be treated in a long-arm cast with 90 degrees of elbow flexion. Displaced fractures require early orthopedic involvement to ensure adequate reduction.

Monteggia Fracture and Radial Head Dislocation

Isolated dislocation of the radial head is rare. Congenital dislocation is sometimes diagnosed at the time of elbow

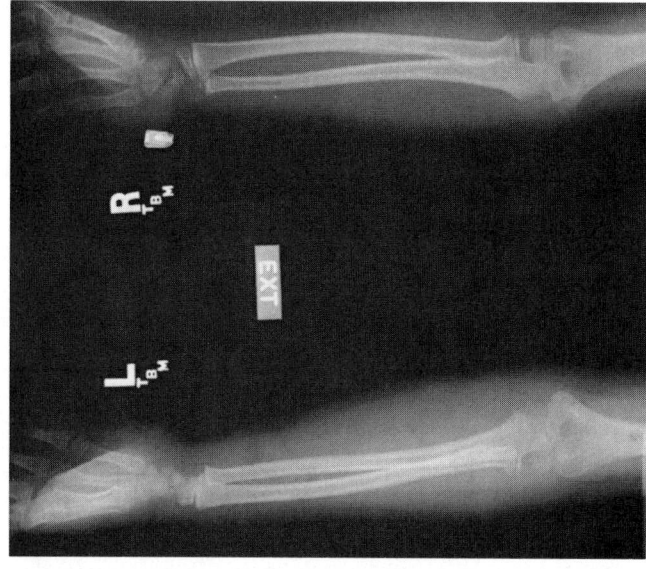

FIG. 29-15. Subtle fractures of the radial head are often found in older children with a fat-pad sign but not obvious fracture.

trauma. Abnormality of the capitellum suggests the dislocation is chronic and probably congenital.

Monteggia first described fracture of the proximal ulna with anterior dislocation of the radial head in 1814. The name "Monteggia fracture" is now given to several types of ulnar fracture and radial head dislocation. Monteggia fractures comprise only 2% of all elbow fractures in children. The dislocation in this injury can easily be overlooked, resulting in serious complications. A physician treating a child with an apparently isolated fracture of the ulna

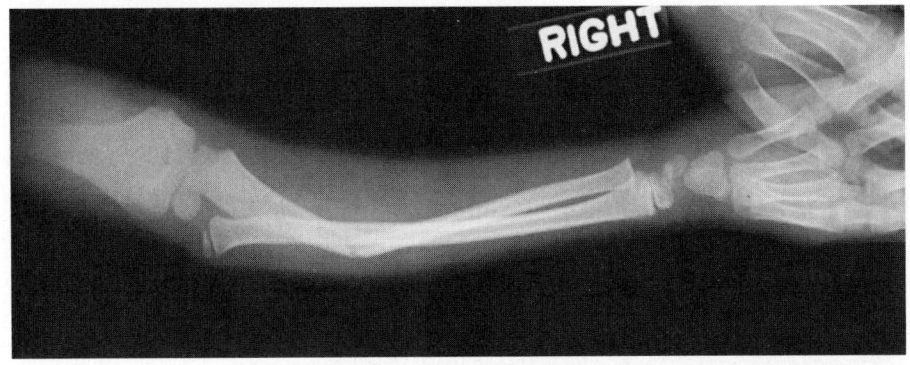

FIG. 29-16. Monteggia fracture/dislocation. Isolated fracture of the ulna is uncommon. Dislocation of the radial head must be suspected. (*From Jackimczyk KC and Goy W: Musculoskeletal trauma. In Rosen P, Doris PE, Barkin RM, et al: Diagnostic radiology in emergency medicine, St Louis, 1992, Mosby.*)

should expect to find an injury to the radius, be it fracture or dislocation, proximally or distally.

Mechanism of Injury. The theories about the mechanism of ulna fracture with dislocation of the proximal radius are numerous, complex, and supported by experimental data. Most authors believe these injuries usually result from a fall on an outstretched hand. Hyperpronation that occurs when the trunk and humerus rotate externally after the hand is fixed on the ground can result in fracture of the ulna, which may then act as a fulcrum to dislocate the radial head. The annular ligament is either torn or displaced over the head of the radius. Other mechanisms, including hyperextension and direct trauma, are probably responsible for the many variations of Monteggia fractures.

Diagnostic Findings. A child with a Monteggia fracture holds the elbow partially flexed and pronated, as does a toddler with subluxation of the radial head. Pain and restricted movement are present with flexion-extension and supination-pronation. Before development of significant soft-tissue swelling the dislocated radial head may be palpable anteriorly.

Tenderness, swelling, and deformity at the site of ulnar fracture may draw attention away from the elbow. Any child with a forearm fracture should be carefully examined for injury to the elbow or wrist.

An unrecognized Monteggia fracture may result in chronic dislocation and impairment of elbow function. A child treated adequately for such an injury usually recovers with no sequelae. Recurrent dislocation is rare. Injury to the posterior interosseous branch of the radial nerve resolves in most cases.

Radiography of the forearm must include the elbow to assess the relationship of the radial head to the capitellum. A line along the axis of the radius should pass through the capitellum on all views. A fracture at the junction of the proximal and middle third of the ulna with overriding fragments is often noted. Transverse, greenstick, and plastic deformation–type fractures have also been associated with dislocation of the radial head. Fracture of the wrist may accompany Monteggia fracture. Inclusion of both the wrist and elbow in all radiographs for forearm injuries will

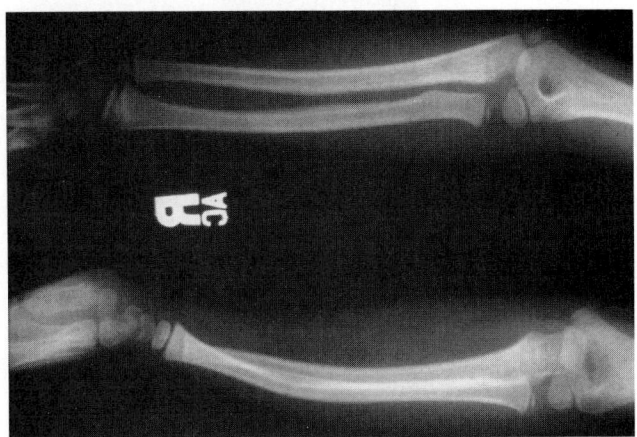

FIG. 29-17. Greenstick fracture of the radius with plastic bowing of the ulna.

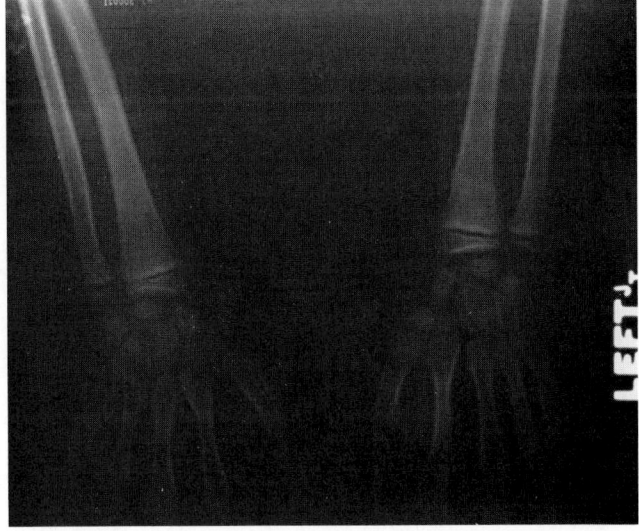

FIG. 29-18. Torus or buckle fracture of the distal radius.

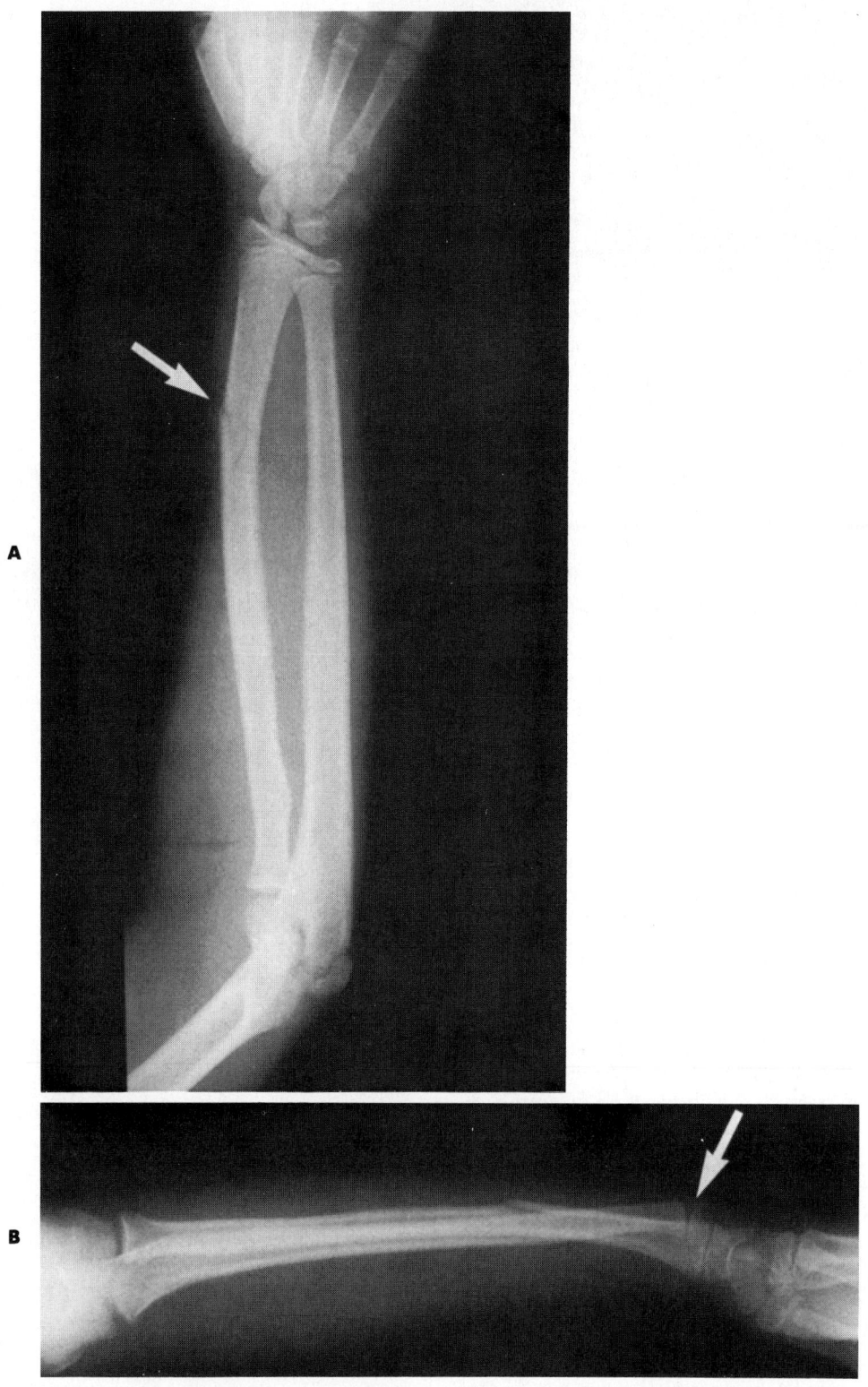

FIG. 29-19. A, Galeazzi fracture, anteroposterior view. A fracture at the junction of the middle and distal thirds of the radius is associated with disruption of the distal radioulnar ligaments. **B,** Lateral view. Note subluxation of the distal radioulnar joint. (*From Jackimczyk KC and Goy W: Musculoskeletal trauma. In Rosen P, Doris PE, Barkin RM, et al: Diagnostic radiology in emergency medicine, St Louis, 1992, Mosby.*)

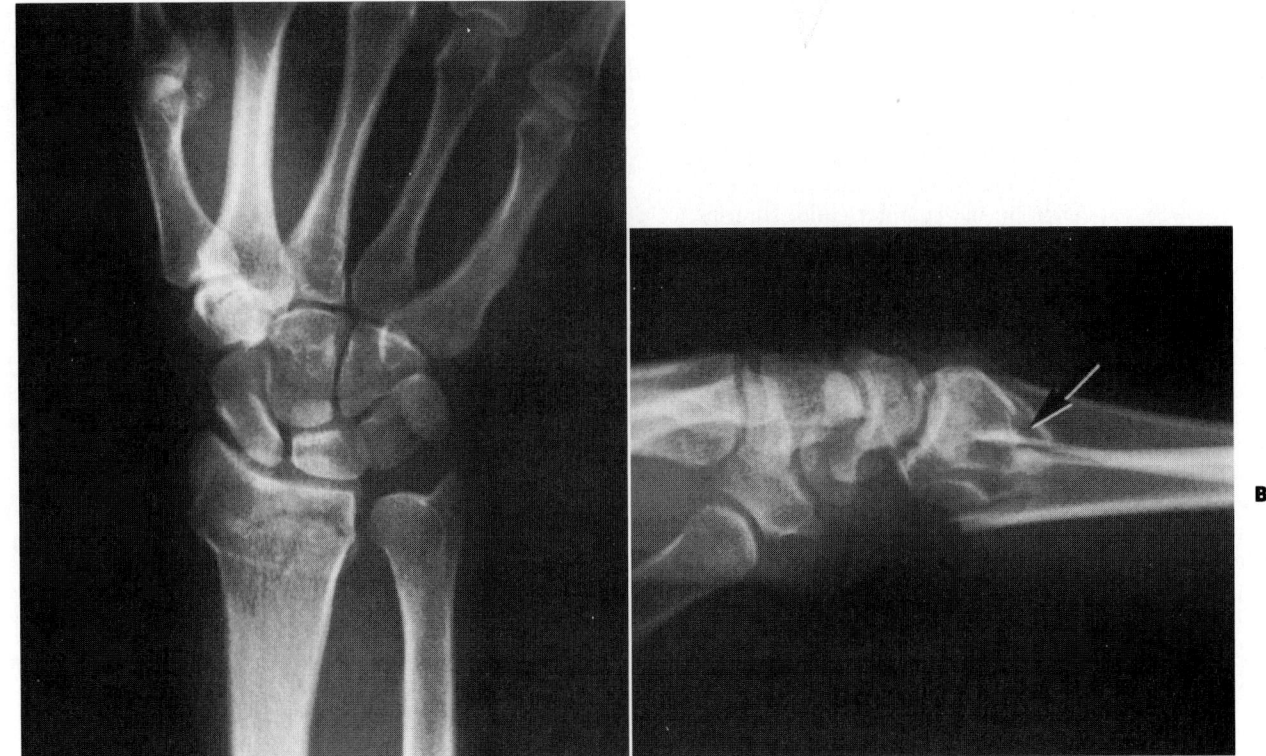

FIG. 29-20. Colles fracture. **A,** Anteroposterior view. **B,** Lateral view shows a fracture with comminuted fragments. The typical dorsal radioulnar angulation is seen. (*From Jackimczyk KC and Goy W: Musculoskeletal trauma. In Rosen P, Doris PE, Barkin RM, et al:* Diagnostic radiology in emergency medicine, *St Louis, 1992, Mosby.*)

help ensure that significant injuries do not go unrecognized (Fig. 29-16).

Management. Reduction of the radial head dislocation and ulnar fracture should be accomplished as soon as an orthopedic surgeon is available. Supination, traction, and direct pressure on the radial head with the elbow at 90 degrees of flexion will reduce the dislocation. Often these maneuvers help reduce the fracture of the ulna. The elbow is then splinted in flexion; repeat radiographs to document the reduction are mandatory. Open reduction may be necessary if the dislocation persists or recurs.

Radial and Ulnar Diaphyseal and Metaphyseal Fractures

Fractures of the forearm from both direct and indirect mechanisms are very common in childhood, second only to fractures of the clavicle. Most of these injuries involve the radius and ulna, which tend to fracture at the same level in children more often than adults.

Sprains of the wrist are distinctly uncommon in children with open epiphyses. A patient with localized tenderness of the wrist and normal radiographs often has a nondisplaced Salter-type fracture or buckle fracture, both difficult to visualize on radiography. A child with an apparent sprain of the wrist should be splinted and referred for follow-up; subsequent radiographs will usually indicate that a fracture is present.

Many different types of fractures of the radius and ulna occur in children. Subtle greenstick or plastic-deformation fractures of the diaphyses of long bones involve a fracture of only one side of the cortex (Fig. 29-17). Torus fractures are noted with a buckling or angulation of the cortex with no visible fracture line, most often involving the metaphysis (Fig. 29-18). If only one of the forearm bones appears fractured, it is very likely that a subtle greenstick or plastic deformation fracture of the other bone is present or that a dislocation of the radial head (Monteggia fracture) or distal radioulnar joint (Galeazzi fracture) exists (Fig. 29-19).

Colles fracture is a transverse fracture of the distal radius with dorsal angulation and loss or reversal of the volar tilt to the distal radial articulating surface (Fig. 29-20). The patient may have an accompanying fracture of the ulnar styloid and usually a Salter II epiphyseal injury. Smith fracture is the reverse of Colles fracture, caused by a blow to the dorsum of the wrist or distal radius with the forearm in pronation.

Barton fracture is a marginal fracture of the dorsum or volar surface of the radius with corresponding dorsal or volar dislocation of the carpal bones. Hutchinson fracture, or "chauffeur fracture," involves the radial styloid process secondary to direct trauma or impact of the styloid process against the navicular bone.

Diagnostic Findings. Localization of point tenderness correlates well with fracture on radiographs. Anteroposterior and lateral radiographs should include the elbow and wrist.

Complications from forearm fractures other than some loss of rotation are infrequent. Unrecognized plastic deformation fractures can result in limited supination-pronation. Compartment syndromes and ischemia seldom occur. The strong and highly osteogenic periosteal sleeve make nonunion unlikely, especially in the younger child. Injuries to the median, ulnar or radial nerves are uncommon. A self-limited neuropraxia almost always resolves in 3 weeks or less.

The potential for longitudinal bone growth disturbances increases with age and distance from the growth plate, especially the distal one, where 80% of forearm growth occurs. The strong and highly osteogenic periosteal sleeve makes nonunion unlikely, especially in young children.

Management. Treatment depends mainly on the type of fracture and alignment. Rotational deformity must be corrected to preserve the range of supination-pronation. Angulated fractures greater than 15 degrees (especially if proximal or in an older child) must be reduced to prevent functional limitation. If both the radius and ulna are broken or dislocated, alignment is more difficult to achieve and maintain; open reduction and internal fixation may be re-

quired. Greenstick fractures require overcorrection or completion of the fracture to prevent subsequent angulation. Colles fractures may be reduced in consultation with an orthopedist. Most forearm fractures can be splinted and referred for evaluation, reduction and immobilization for 4 to 6 weeks.

References

1. Corrigan GE: The neonatal clavicle, *Biol Neonate* 79:2, 1959.
2. Chung SMK and Nessenbaum MM: Obstetrical paralysis, *Orthop Clin North Am* 6:393, 1975.
3. Hardy AE: Birth injuries of the brachial plexus: Incidence and prognosis, *J Bone Joint Surg* 63B:98, 1981.
4. Wheeler DK and Lindscheid RL: Fracture-dislocations of the elbow, *Clin Orthop* 50:95, 1967.
5. Quan L and Marcuse EK: The epidemiology and treatment of radial head subluxation, *Am J Dis Child* 139;1194, 1985.
6. Schunk JE: Radial head subluxation: Epidemiology and treatment of episodes, *Ann Emerg Med* 19;1019, 1990.
7. Illingsworth CM: Pulled elbow: A study of 100 patients, *BMJ* 2:672-674, 1975.
8. Salter RB and Zaltz C: Anatomic investigations of the mechanism of injury and pathologic anatomy of "pulled elbow" in young children, *Clin Orthop* 77:134, 1971.
9. Mahlahn DJ and Fahey JJ: Fractures of the elbow in children, *JAMA* 166:220, 1958.

Lower Extremity and Pelvic Injuries

Susan B. Torrey

Injuries to the lower extremity reflect children's anatomy and exposure to injury. They may present as pain, reduction of joint function, alteration in gait, and a host of nontraumatic conditions (see Chapter 57).

Developmental factors impact on the mechanism of injury. In children the pelvis is more elastic and the presence of cartilaginous structures allows absorption of more energy. In contrast to that of the adult the pediatric pelvic ring has more flexibility and may permit a single fracture to occur in the younger patient. Fractures through the cartilage may result in growth arrest and subsequent inequality in leg length.

The femoral head, neck, and trochanter are largely cartilaginous during most of childhood. Injury can significantly affect the growth potential of the femur. Several arteries supply the femoral head at birth; by 8 years of age this is more limited. The infant hip is more susceptible to infection; vascular injury with avascular necrosis may occur with minimal injury in the older child.

Until 18 months of age the femur is predominantly woven bone, providing the flexibility required during the birth process. The child's femur is quite vascular; the vessels are flexible and resistant to injury. Consequently, fractured femurs in children heal well without the exsanguinating hemorrhage that may be noted in the adult. The distal femur contributes 70% to the growth of the femur and 37% to the growth of the lower extremity. Injury to the distal femoral epiphysis can have a great impact on growth.

The primary blood supply to the proximal tibia and rapidly growing epiphysis is the popliteal artery.[1]

PELVIC FRACTURES

The child has generally suffered blunt trauma from a motor vehicle accident, usually as a pedestrian. The injury occurs most frequently between 1 and 8 years of age. There are often major associated injuries; the mortality rate is as high as 5% because of the nature of the multiple trauma.

Diagnostic Findings

The history commonly involves a major mechanism of injury. Unstable vital signs and associated multiple trauma are common, necessitating resuscitation and stabilization. In the secondary survey the pelvis should be evaluated by grasping each anterior superior iliac spine and rocking the pelvis anteriorly and posteriorly, noting stability of the pelvis and presence of pain. Downward pressure placed on the pubis may similarly produce movement, pain, and crepitus. Fractures of pelvic ring may be isolated in younger children because of its flexibility; older patients usually have an associated fracture, particularly if the fracture is displaced. Classification of pelvic fractures are outlined in Chapter 25.

Fractures without a break in the continuity of the pelvic rim may vary in site. Avulsion fractures are usually associated with athletic activity. They occur through secondary ossification centers before the center is fused with the pelvis. These sites include the anterior superior iliac spine, anterior inferior iliac spine, and iliac tuberosity.

Fractures of the pubis usually result from high-velocity trauma. The sacrum and coccyx can be fractured by direct blunt trauma and are usually diagnosed clinically on the basis of palpation through the rectum. Bowel and bladder incontinence may result from sacral plexus damage.

Since the pelvis is a bony ring, fractures of one part are usually associated with fracture elsewhere in the ring. However, a single break in the pelvic ring can occur in children because of the mobility of the sacroiliac joint and symphysis pubis. Significant displacement is unusual and, if present, indicates that a second fracture is present. Fractures of two ipsilateral pubic rami are most common, but fractures of the symphysis pubis and sacroiliac joint can occur.

Double breaks in the pelvic ring have a high incidence of associated remote and local injuries. Large linear fractures through the acetabulum are stable and associated with pelvic injury. Small fragment fractures and unstable linear fractures are the result of forces transmitted proximally through the femur.

Iliac crest contusion (hip pointer) usually occurs in contact sports as a result of a direct blow to the iliac crest. This produces a tender periosteal hematoma, commonly on the anterior superior iliac crest. Pain is elicited with contraction or stretching of the external oblique muscle.

Among children 40% to 60% have an associated head or neck injury, and 10% have thoracic involvement. Concomitant rectal, abdominal, or vaginal injuries occur in 10% of patients. Bladder and urethral injuries may occur in 10% of children; therefore, a catheter should not be placed if there is blood at the meatus or an abnormal prostate (see Chapter 25).[2,3] Obturator, femoral, and sciatic nerve injuries are infrequent. Blood loss may be significant in older children, although massive hemorrhage is less common in pediatric pelvic fractures. Up to 2,500 ml of hemorrhage is common in adults, proportionately less in children, ultimately determining mortality. Massive retroperitoneal hematoma can occur with shock and vascular collapse.

Radiographic studies of the pelvis should await stabilization of vital signs and management of other life-threatening injuries. Anteroposterior (AP) and frogleg projections are appropriate. There are three secondary ossification centers in the acetabular cavity at puberty, which may be confused as avulsion fractures or loose bodies within the hip joint. They may be distinguished by comparison views of the unaffected side. Selected views of the sacroiliac joint may be appropriate. Angiography may be required to localize the site of massive hemorrhage, if present.

Serial hematocrits may be useful in monitoring.

Management

Prehospital transport and stabilization should be maintained on arrival in the emergency department, requiring presumptive management of the child as a multiple trauma victim. Life-threatening injuries should be managed first (see Chapter 19). Intravenous administration of fluids should be initiated early. The use of pneumatic antishock trousers (MAST) is controversial but may be helpful in the initial stabilization of the patient with a pelvic fracture who is unstable.[4]

Orthopedic referral, bedrest, and early mobilization are generally indicated. Iliac crest contusions require only ice, compression, and rest.

Pelvic fractures with a gravid uterus present a major risk of fetal injury and death. Obstetric consultation is necessary. Fetal distress must be assessed by monitoring scalp pH and heart tones. If there is evidence of distress, an emergency cesarean section may be needed.

All pelvic injuries require consultation with an orthopedic surgeon and a general surgeon if multisystem trauma is suspected. Although avulsion fractures can be managed on an outpatient basis, other injuries commonly require hospitalization.

HIP

Hip Fractures

Hip fractures are rare in children; when present, 75% to 80% are associated with severe trauma. The femoral neck of a child is strong; therefore, in contrast to that of the elderly, high-velocity force, usually from a fall or motor vehicle accident, is required to fracture it. Range noted that the location of a fractured hip correlates with the side of the road on which the cars travel in a given country (i.e., in countries where cars travel in the right lane, most hip fractures are on the left side of the body).[5]

A number of diagnostic entities must be considered in evaluating the child with hip pain or decreased mobility.

Diagnostic Findings. The history should be consistent with the mechanisms described. Attention to fever and constitutional symptoms should help to distinguish other causes when the history is confused or inconsistent.

The examination of the hip must follow patient stabilization. Careful attention should be given to position and length at rest and movement on passive and active testing. The greatest volume in the hip joint can be accommodated when the hip is held in 20 degrees of flexion, abduction, and external rotation; the knee should be positioned this way at rest with a large hematoma or fluid collection present. The range of motion of the hip should be examined by initially placing the hip in flexion. The joint should be rotated internally and externally; then abducted with the hip still in flexion. Subtle limitations in the range of motion in comparison to that of the unaffected joint are important clues to abnormality.

After a high-velocity injury or other injury causing a hip fracture the child will tend to hold the affected hip in flexion and external rotation with some shortening and severe pain. Range of motion is limited. Localized swelling and tenderness are noted, with pain on movement of the leg. Vascular and neurologic status requires careful assessment.

Transepiphyseal injuries are rare, representing less than 8% of hip fractures. The fracture is through the capital femoral epiphyses and requires considerable force. In the adolescent it may actually represent a slipped capital femoral epiphysis.

Transcervical fractures comprise 45% to 50% of hip fractures. Avascular necrosis of the femoral head is most frequently associated with displaced fractures; in 42% to 43% of fractures without displacement avascular necrosis may develop. Cervicotrochanteric fractures occur in 30% to 35% of patients with hip fractures. Avascular necrosis occurs in 20% to 30% of such injuries.[6]

Routine AP and lateral films should be adequate to identify the injury. Standard views may be inadequate if the patient's discomfort limits proper positioning. Comparison views or tomograms may be helpful.

Ancillary data may be necessary if there is a question of infection. Determination of the erythrocyte sedimentation rate or aspiration of the joint may be indicated.[7,8]

Management. Prehospital and emergency department focus must be on stabilization of the patient and evaluation of life-threatening injuries. Subsequently orthopedic injuries may become prominent.

Injuries require immobilization and initial orthopedic evaluation and management. Transepiphyseal injuries may require open reduction and pinning to prevent growth problems or deformity.

Any child who has a hip fracture should be admitted for management by an orthopedic surgeon. Long-term follow-up observation is essential to monitor for avascular necrosis.

Hip Dislocation

Posterior dislocation of the hip, although rare in children, is more common than anterior and obturator dislocation. Fractures are less common.

The acetabulum is very flexible and the ligaments lax in children less than 5 years of age; dislocation can result from simple falls. After the age of 6 years more force is required, frequently that characteristic of motor vehicle or athletic incidents. Posterior dislocations are produced by longitudinal forces applied to the knee with the hip and knee in 90-degree flexion and slight abduction, as when the knee hits the dashboard in a car.

Diagnostic Findings. The severity of the injury can often be determined by the history. Attention should focus on the position of the child at the time of impact and the forces involved in the blow. If the hip is posteriorly dislocated, the leg is internally rotated, adducted, held in flexion, and shortened. Less commonly, in anterior dislocation the leg is externally rotated, abducted, and extended.

Associated fractures, especially of the posterior wall of the acetabulum, are noted.

The sciatic nerve is injured in as many as 10% of patients. Avascular necrosis of the femoral head may follow, particularly if reduction is delayed.

AP and lateral views of the hip identify associated fractures. Computed tomography (CT) scan of the articular surface provides excellent spatial resolution.

Management. Prehospital stabilization should emphasize associated injuries. Rapid transport in a position of relative comfort is essential.

The key to successful management is early diagnosis. Attempts at closed reduction are most successful in the first 8 to 12 hours after injury. Early reduction minimizes the risk of avascular necrosis. The lowest incidence of avascular necrosis is in children younger than 5 years of age.

Reduction without delay can be performed in consultation with an orthopedist. Muscle relaxation, using analgesia and sedation, may be useful. If a long period of time to transfer the patient is necessary, the dislocation is ideally performed early to minimize avascular necrosis. Traction in the line of deformity should be followed by gentle flexion of the hip to 90 degrees and then internal-to-external rotation.

Children should be hospitalized on bedrest. Long-term follow-up observation is essential. Careful neurologic evaluation of the extremity should be performed.

Congenital Hip Dislocation

Congenital hip dislocation is commonly called *congenital dysplasia of the hip* (CDH) or *developmental dysplasia of the hip,* which more accurately reflects the variability of findings.

A hip dislocation is usually noted at birth or immediately thereafter. It occurs more commonly in girls, in firstborn children, and in those with a family history of the condition. It is important to diagnose and treat hip dislocation before the child bears weight.

Parents may note that the child moves one leg differently than the other during diapering or that the legs are asymmetric. On examination the creases of the anterior thigh and buttocks posteriorly are not symmetric. The affected hip has less abduction than normal, and a hip click

may be elicited by passive abduction or adduction. Although radiographs remain the standard for diagnosis, ultrasound serves as a useful confirmatory tool.

The child should be referred to an orthopedic surgeon for ongoing casting and management.

Toxic Synovitis

The inflammatory process of toxic synovitis occurs in toddlers and young children 1½ to 7 years of age, with a peak incidence at 2 years of age. It often follows a respiratory infection by several days to 2 weeks.

The child develops pain in the hip or knee and a limp (see Chapter 57). Minimal or no pain on abduction and external rotation are noted; limitation on range of motion is variable. There is often a low-grade fever.

Radiographic studies should include hip films, which may demonstrate a bulging joint capsule. Aspiration of the joint may be necessary to confirm the diagnosis and exclude others, often under ultrasound visualization. The complete blood cell count (CBC) and erythrocyte sedimentation rate are usually normal or slightly elevated. Rarely, a blood culture and joint aspirate may be useful in excluding other entities.

Management includes symptomatic treatment with nonsteroidal antiinflammatory agents and follow-up observation once joint-threatening injury, neoplasm, and infection have been excluded. Children can usually be managed at home; activities should be limited.

Legg-Calvé-Perthes Disease

Legg-Calvé-Perthes disease is avascular necrosis of the femoral head and usually occurs in children 5 to 9 years of age and is more common in boys. The disease may follow injury to the hip.

A limp and pain in the hip or knee may develop; knee pain represents a common site of referred hip abnormality. There is pain with passive range of motion and limited hip movement, particularly internal rotation and abduction.

Findings on radiographs of the hip may initially be normal. In advanced disease x-ray films often demonstrate a widened joint space between the ossified head and acetabulum and lucencies, ultimately progressing to collapse of the head, increased neck width, and head demineralization (Fig. 30-1). Radionuclide bone scintigraphy can help the physician evaluate the patient for avascular necrosis of the bone.

Management by orthopedic consultants allows minimal weight bearing with the femur abducted to keep the femoral head within the acetabulum.

Slipped Capital Femoral Epiphysis

Obese or rapidly growing adolescent males between 12 and 15 years of age are commonly affected by slipped capital femoral epiphysis (SCFE), or epiphyseal separation of the head of the femur. It often follows an upward blow transmitted through the shaft of the femur. There may be no associated injury.

The onset of symptoms may be acute or gradual. Recent classification schemes also catagorize the epiphysis as stable or unstable. Pain in the hip or referred to the knee or groin is reported. Although the referral of hip pain to the thigh or knee has been well described, the diagnosis of

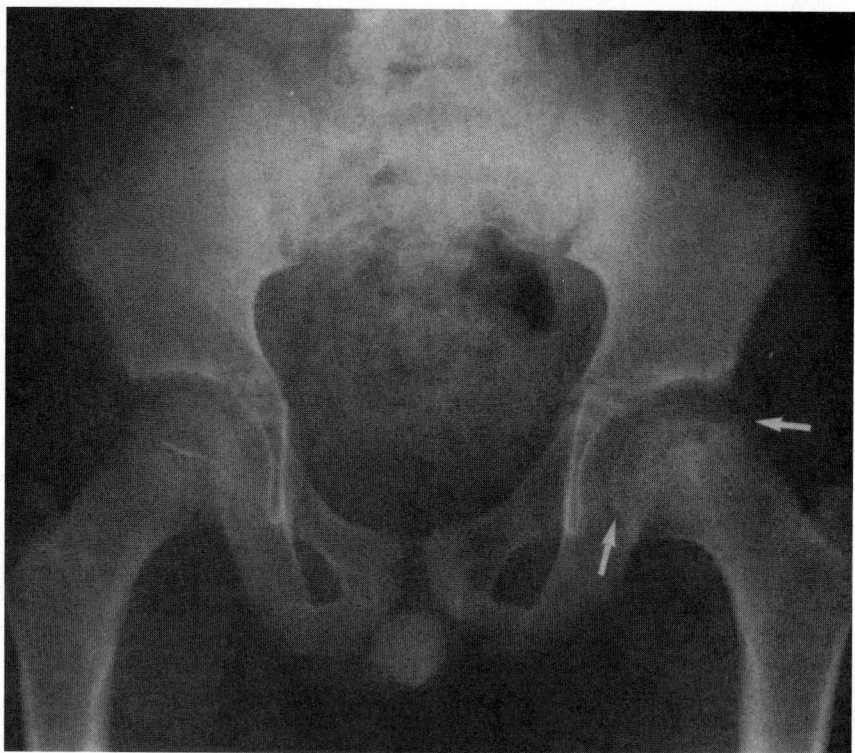

FIG. 30-1. Legg-Calvé-Perthes disease, AP view. Involved femoral head is flattened and mottled (*arrows*). (*From Jackimczyk KC and Goy W: Musculoskeletal trauma. In Rosen P, Doris PE, Barkin RM, et al: Diagnostic radiology in emergency medicine, St. Louis, 1992, Mosby.*)

SCFE is frequently missed when the presenting symptom is thigh pain.[9] Legs may be shortened, externally rotated and adducted. Pain is noted with movement; internal rotation and abduction are limited. The condition may occur bilaterally with impaired weight bearing and limp.

AP and frogleg films of the hip demonstrate an irregular widening of the epiphyseal line (Fig. 30-2). The epiphysis may be displaced, usually downward and posterior. If both hips are affected, this displacement may be difficult to appreciate. However, a line drawn along the lateral edge of the femoral neck on the frogleg view should transect the lateral one quarter of a normal epiphysis; this does not occur with a slipped epiphysis.

A child with a SCFE should be referred to an orthopedic surgeon. Surgical reduction by pinning and immobilization may be required. Since bilateral disease is common, children should be followed closely but prophylactic pinning of the unaffected side is not routinely recommended.[10]

FEMORAL FRACTURES

Fractures of the femur may occur in several locations, reflecting the mechanism of injury. Midshaft fractures of the femur result from direct blows. A motor vehicle-pedestrian accident (bumper injury) often produces the fracture, particularly in children in the first 3 years of life.

Indirect force, usually rotational, may produce a spiral femoral fracture. The child catches his or her foot and falls. Motor vehicle injuries or child abuse may also be caus-

ative, the latter from a twisting force to the thigh. Epiphyseal-metaphyseal fractures may be the result of child abuse (see Chapter 45).

High-mileage long-distance runners may experience femoral stress fractures.

Diagnostic Findings. The history is usually suggestive of the injury; associated trauma, including bruises, other fractures, and organ damage, should be sought. A history inconsistent with the injury suggests child abuse.[11]

The fractured femur is usually obvious. The hip is abducted and flexed, and the thigh is noticeably swollen and deformed. The child is quite uncomfortable; distal neurovascular integrity should be assessed.

Spiral fractures may have less associated swelling and deformity; often they are not suspected until the child refuses to bear weight.

Rarely, fat embolus may develop, usually with concordant injuries to the hip, knee, or pelvis. Significant blood loss may occur but is unusual. The presence of hypovolemia suggests an associated life-threatening injury.

Stress fractures result in insidious onset of symptoms. Aching pain with exercise may be present for weeks. The physical examination may suggest a muscular origin, but the persistence of symptoms should suggest a stress fracture.

A direct blow to the thigh without bony injury may cause a quadriceps contusion, typically in football or soccer. The severity of the injury may increase for 24 to 48 hours, with

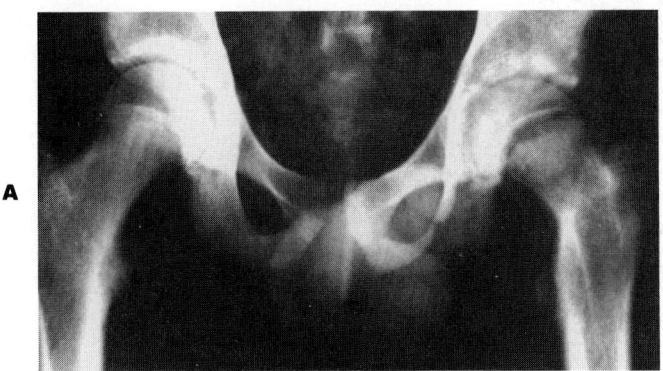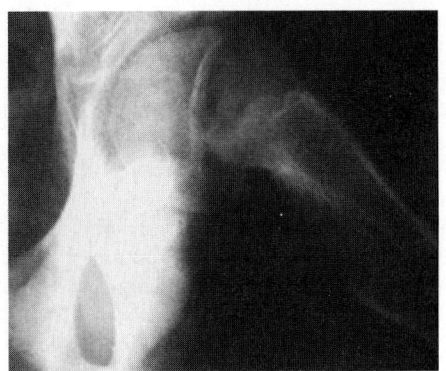

FIG. 30-2. A and **B,** Acute slipped capital femoral epiphysis with moderate displacement. (*From Canale ST and Beaty JB:* Operative pediatric orthopedics, *St. Louis, 1990, Mosby.*)

more swelling and tenderness over the thigh and pain on flexion of the knee. Significant hemorrhage or myositis ossificans may occur.

AP and lateral views of the femur and hip are used in the diagnosis of a fracture. Stress fractures may require a technetium bone scan to confirm the diagnosis.

Management. The location and nature of the injury determines the management of the femoral fracture. Immediate reduction of the fracture with Hare or Thomas traction splinting or another device is appropriate after assessment for associated injuries and stabilization. Management may include traction, internal rod placement, or external fixation.[12] Orthopedic consultation is appropriate and hospitalization is common.

Stress fractures require rest for about 8 weeks and a gradual return to normal activity. Contusions of the quadriceps may be managed by rest, ice, compression, and elevation. Rehabilitation by means of quadriceps stretching and strengthening exercise may facilitate return to normal activity once there is no longer pain on palpation, full range of motion is achieved, and muscle strength is 85% of the uninjured leg.

KNEE

Knee Epiphyseal Fractures

Displacement of the distal femoral or proximal tibial epiphysis may result from injury. Separation of the distal femoral epiphysis is most frequently associated with an indirect blow to the knee. Compression or avulsion can result in separation and fracture of the growth plate. Avulsion may occur with bending of the distal femur against a fixed lower leg or wrenching of the lower leg against a fixed thigh, as when a football player is hit in the side with his foot fixed. A direct blow from a vehicle-pedestrian bumper injury can produce the damage.

The proximal tibial epiphysis may be injured by either direct or indirect force. The direct blow is usually associated with a motor vehicle-pedestrian accident in which the lower leg is forced into abduction or hyperextension against a fixed knee and subsequently separated.

Diagnostic Findings. The history suggests the type of injury. Systematic examination of the knee is necessary.

Begin with the child in a sitting position with the knee flexed to 90 degrees. The bony landmarks of the distal femur and proximal fibula and tibia can be palpated in this position. With the patient supine and the knee fully extended, the patella is examined for pain and movement. The joint can be evaluated for areas of tenderness and presence of an effusion.

Stability of the knee to medial and lateral stress can be assessed as described in the evaluation of ligamentous and meniscus injuries. With the knee flexed, the joint can also be tested for anterior and posterior stability. Strength, sensation, and vascular integrity in the leg and foot should be noted.

Separation of the distal femoral epiphysis produces inability to bear weight. The knee is held in flexion and an effusion evolves rapidly. Point tenderness over the physis may be elicited. Displaced fractures often have associated deformity.

Proximal tibial epiphyseal separation is associated with pain and effusion. Extension and passive flexion are limited by muscle spasm and protective splinting. If the fracture is displaced, a deformity may be palpated. The knee may feel unstable and the fracture separation must be distinguished from ligamentous injury.

A careful neurovascular assessment of the distal extremity must be performed, focusing on vascular impairment, peroneal nerve injury, and, ultimately, growth disturbances, recurrent displacement, and stiffness of the knee.

AP and lateral views of the knee are indicated. Ultimately stress films may be required for the diagnosis, particularly if the primary injury is of the Salter I type.

Management. Prehospital stabilization takes precedence over other priorities in intervention. Once other injuries are stabilized and problems identified, the leg should be immobilized and orthopedic consultation sought to determine ongoing management.

Knee Fractures

Several fractures that do not involve the epiphysis may occur.

Avulsion of the tibial tubercle results from forceful contraction of the quadriceps muscle, often from jumping. There is an increased incidence of avulsion of the tubercle in children with Osgood-Schlatter disease, which must be distinguished.

Osteochondral fractures occur in adolescents and are significant because the fracture fragment may become loose within the joint and cause disability. A direct blow or fall on a flexed knee can cause fracture of the medial or lateral condyles. Endogenous forces, such as rotation and compression, as well as the shearing force involved in a patellar dislocation can also cause fracture.

Fractures of the intercondylar eminence of the tibia are common in 8- to 15-year-olds. They occur with the knee extended, often as a result of falling off a bicycle.

Dislocation is rare and when it occurs is usually associated with a fracture and severe trauma causing ligamentous disruption.

Diagnostic Findings. Children with avulsion of the tibial tubercle usually have swelling and tenderness over the proximal tibia. An effusion may be present, particularly when the joint is involved. A loose fragment of bone may be palpated.

A snap felt or heard after a direct blow or twisting of a flexed knee is common in children with osteochondral fractures. Tenderness and effusion are noted over the knee, but the joint cannot be fully extended.

Fractures of the intercondylar eminence of the tibia demonstrate a painful and swollen knee that cannot bear weight. An anterior draw sign may be present if the medial collateral ligament has been torn.

AP and lateral views of the knee are essential. Intercondylar eminence fractures are best indicated on lateral films; the tibial tubercle is best seen in the lateral projection with the tibia rotated slightly medially. Tunnel views may be helpful. Arthroscopy may be necessary to identify fragments of osteochondral fractures.

Management. Initial stabilization of associated injuries is essential with concurrent immobilization of the affected limb. It is essential to distinguish between an avulsion of the tibial tubercle and Osgood-Schlatter disease, since the former may require an open reduction and pinning. In Osgood-Schlatter disease, there is an avulsion of the anterior surface of the apophysis but no separation between the ossific nucleus of the apophysis and the tibial metaphysis. Dislocations require immediate referral and reduction, usually by internal fixation.

Disposition is a reflection of the injury but generally includes immobilization.

Knee Ligamentous and Meniscus Injuries

In contrast to previous teaching, significant ligamentous injury can occur in the child with open physes.

The medial collateral ligament (MCL) is most commonly affected, frequently in contact sports because of a twisting motion or a blow to the lateral aspect of the knee causing a valgus stress.

The anterior cruciate ligament (ACL) produces severe swelling within hours of the injury, often with complete (third-degree) disruption. This is usually a noncontact injury in children above 8 years of age. The knee experiences forcible hyperextension or sudden deceleration with the foot flexed, causing abduction and external rotation of the leg.

The posterior cruciate ligament (PCL) is less often involved and less severely disrupted. The injury results from a direct blow to the tibia when the knee is flexed, forcing it posterior.

Meniscus injury is uncommon in children but does occur in adolescents. The medial meniscus is more frequently involved. Injury follows a squatting or twisting motion. While the knee is weight bearing and slightly flexed, a twisting motion is applied. Internal rotation injures the medial meniscus, whereas external rotation damages the lateral meniscus.

Diagnostic Findings. A complete examination of the knee is essential in assessing ligamentous injuries. After assessment for deformity, effusion should be sought. A large effusion suggests an intraarticular injury or patellar dislocation. The degree of pain on flexion, extension, and palpation should be noted.

Injuries of the medial collateral ligament (MCL) are associated with tenderness with palpation. The response to stress may be tested by placing the knee in 20 to 30 degrees of flexion with the child supine; then as one hand stabilizes the femur, the other hand grasps the ankle and gently applies valgus (pressure on lateral side) stress. The degrees of the sprain may be determined by the amount of laxity.

ACL damage may have been noted by a loud pop at the time of injury, followed by severe pain, swelling, and effusion. Of tense acute hemarthroses 85% are caused by ACL tears. Laxity of the ACL is best evaluated by the Lachman test. With the patient supine the knee is flexed to 20 to 30 degrees. One hand stabilizes the distal femur while the other grasps the proximal tibia and pulls it anteriorly. Hamstring spasm may interfere with ability to identify excessive anterior movement.

Examination of the patient with a PCL injury reveals posterior knee pain in a stable joint, often with a small effusion. An 8- to 10-mm step-off is identified by palpating the medial and lateral femoral condyles and the anterior tibial plateau with the knee in 90 degrees of flexion.

If the tibia is posteriorly displaced, a complete PCL injury has occurred and this step-off is not appreciated. Since the popliteal artery is located posteriorly, careful evaluation of the vascular status of the distal extremity is essential.

The AP drawer sign may be of further assistance. With the patient supine, hip at 45 degrees, and knee flexed at 90 degrees, the foot is allowed to rest on the table in external rotation. Pushing or pulling may produce a sliding motion, suggestive of a ligamentous injury. If there is increased anterior mobility, ACL instability is present; if there is increased posterior mobility, PCL damage has occurred.

Meniscus injury results in pain on flexion of the joint with an accompanying effusion. The knee may lock in flexion or prevent full extension. There is tenderness over the involved meniscus. The McMurray maneuver is performed when the patient is supine. The foot is held under the arch with one hand and the cup of the knee is held with the other. The knee is flexed and then extended with the leg in internal or external rotation. A clicking or rattling on extension in internal rotation indicates a tear of the lateral meniscus and, on external rotation, involvement of the medial meniscus.[13]

AP, lateral, and sunrise (tangential view of the patella) should be routinely obtained. Small avulsion fragments of the tibial spine should be excluded since these are associated with ACL injuries and require urgent orthopedic consultation. Magnetic resonance imaging is becoming a useful tool in evaluating knee injuries but is rarely required emergently.[14,15]

Management. Initial management should include ice, compression and elevation. Weight bearing should be avoided and both a knee immobilizer and crutches should be used; antiinflammatory agents are prescribed. If there is a hemarthrosis or laxity in the joint, orthopedic consultation is appropriate. Ligamentous or meniscal injury is frequently identified when these signs are vigorously pursued with imaging techniques or arthroscopy.[16]

Patellar Fracture and Dislocation

Because the osseous portion of the patella is surrounded by thick cartilage in children, this fracture is infrequent.

A direct blunt force over the anterior aspect of the knee can fracture the patella. Sudden extension may also cause fracture.

Patellar dislocation is common in adolescent females, in association with internal rotation of the leg, a direct blow to the outer aspect of the knee, or knee flexion occurring with a valgus stress. It may occur with forcible contraction of the quadriceps muscle.

Patellar tendinitis (jumper's knee) occurs frequently in running and jumping sports such as volleyball and basketball. It is associated with microtears where the patellar tendon inserts into the inferior aspect of the patella.

Prepatellar bursitis (wrestler's knee) results from a direct blow to the patella that causes injury to the bursa. Patellofemoral stress syndrome (runner's knee, chondromalacia, peripatellar pain syndrome) affects runners as a result of subchondral stress and synovial inflammation. There may be a deterioration of the articular cartilage of the patella.

Diagnostic Findings. Effusion and tenderness accompany the fracture, which may be palpable. Extension of the knee is limited if the fracture is transverse with complete transection of the extensor tendon. The patient may also lose extensor function through rupture of the patellar or quadriceps tendons or fracture of the tibial tubercle. If the fracture was caused by pressure applied through the femur, such as the knee's hitting a dashboard, examination should also exclude posterior dislocation of the hip.

The patella may be palpated laterally or in normal position. Dislocation is the second most common cause of acute hemarthrosis. Effusion and tenderness over the medial collateral ligament and along the articular surface of the patellar are common. Often subluxation of the patella is reduced spontaneously. The knee "gives out" or buckles. Pain may be reproduced by pushing the patella laterally with the knee flexed at 30 degrees and the foot supported (patellar apprehension). Fracture of the medial border of the patella or osteochondral fracture of the lateral condyle may be associated.

Patellar tendinitis may be associated with subtle onset of pain. Point tenderness at the inferior pole of the patella is elicited on examination. There may be poor flexibility of the quadriceps muscle. Bursitis causes swelling and tenderness over the patella.

Patellofemoral stress syndrome or chondromalacia patella is associated with chronic pain, particularly when the knee is extended against resistance, during uphill running or climbing. The patella may be tender with palpation. The patellar inhibition test result provides a positive diagnosis; it is performed with the child lying supine and the knee fully extended. With the thumb and forefinger on the superior aspect of the patella, it is pushed distally in the trochlear groove. The child then contracts the quadriceps. Pain with movement and crepitation constitute a positive test result.

Routine AP, lateral, and sunrise views should be obtained. Generally, a dislocation is reduced before diagnostic studies are made. The films yield normal findings in patients who have chondromalacia patella.

Management. Dislocations of the patellar are reduced, often by extension of the knee and flexion of the hip (relaxing quadriceps). Slight medial pressure should be applied to the patella. Reduction often is spontaneous.

Generally ice, elevation, and immobilization in extension constitute initial management. Fractures are generally referred for orthopedic consultation after immobilization in extension; dislocations require 6 weeks of immobilization in extension and avoidance of weight bearing.

Rehabilitation is essential and must be individualized. Generally quadriceps strengthening measures are a component of any program.

Osgood-Schlatter Disease

Osgood-Schlatter disease is generally seen in early adolescence in active children 11 to 15 years of age. Boys are more commonly affected. It results from repetitive microscopic injury that produces inflammation of the apophysis of the tibial tubercle and partial avulsion and separation of the tibial tubercle.

Children experience localized swelling, pain, and tenderness over the tibial tuberosity, exacerbated by running and jumping. There may be partial avulsion of the tubercle. Radiographs demonstrate irregularity of the tibial tuberosity and some edema along the posterior surface of the intrapatellar ligament.

Rest, administration of antiinflammatory agents, and stretching exercises should be initiated. (The knee is generally immobilized in extension for 2 to 4 weeks if injury is severe.) Athletic participation is limited only by the child's discomfort. With an avulsion there is a possibility of nonunion or avascular necrosis, requiring surgery at a later date. Orthopedic follow-up and observation are appropriate.

Osteochondritis Dissecans

Boys in the second decade of life are most commonly affected by osteochondritis dissecans. It is characterized by bone necrosis and softening of the overlying cartilage of the proximal tibia. It may be the result of a stress fracture in a susceptible child.

The pain is mild to moderate, chronic, and activity related. Point tenderness over the lesion, thigh atrophy, and perhaps mild joint effusion occur. Radiographic studies should include routine and tunnel views (Fig. 30-3). Scintigraphy may be helpful.

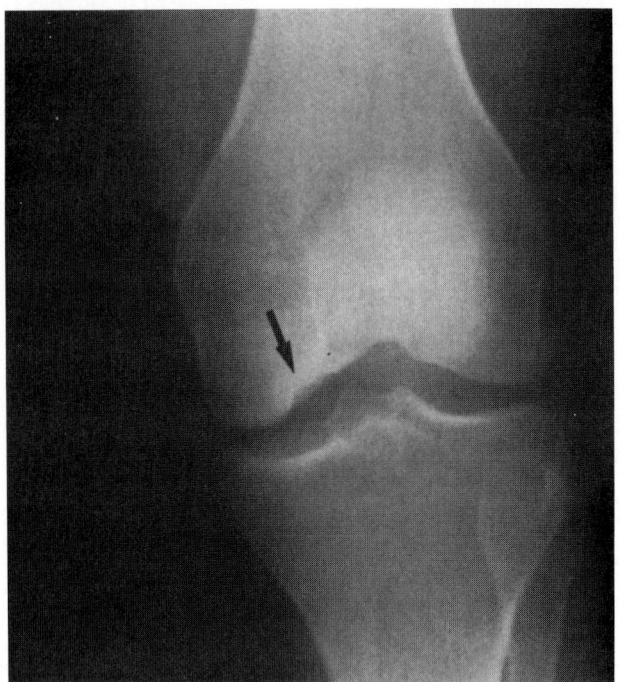

FIG. 30-3. Osteochondritis dissecans, AP view. A shallow concave defect is seen at the joint surface of the medial condyle of the distal femur (arrow). (*From Jackimczyk KC and Goy W: Musculoskeletal trauma. In Rosen P, Doris PE, Barkin RM et al: Diagnostic radiology in emergency medicine, St. Louis, 1992, Mosby.*)

Activity should be limited and orthopedic referral considered.

TIBIA AND FIBULA FRACTURES

Tibia and fibula fractures are the most common injuries to the lower extremity in children. Midshaft fractures heal readily and rarely result in complications. Fractures are classified as incomplete (greenstick) or complete.

Rotational force results in an oblique or spiral fracture, whereas a direct blow or indirect valgus or varus stress causes a distal femur or tibial plateau fracture. An isolated fracture of the tibia most often results from a fall but may be caused by torsion of the foot of a toddler younger than 6 years of age (toddler's fracture). When both the tibia and fibula are broken, the mechanism is most often a motor vehicle accident.

Diagnostic Findings. Findings depend on the nature of the injury. In an incomplete fracture the child may actually bear weight but will certainly limp. If the child can tolerate the examination, point tenderness may localize the injury. Spiral and oblique fractures are usually located at the junction of the middle and distal thirds, the weakest region of the tibia. Tibial shaft fracture associated with a fibular reciprocal fracture is considered eccentric if the fibular site

is subcapital or malleolar. In children eccentric fibular fracture is unusual, possibly because of the greater flexibility of the ligamentous structures anchoring the proximal and distal fibula.

Distal neurovascular injuries (compartment syndrome) are common. If the proximal third of the tibia is fractured, there may be injury at the bifurcation of the anterior and posterior tibial arteries. Associated trauma must also be considered.

AP and lateral radiographs are indicated. In some circumstances initial films may not reveal a fracture in the child with a probable fracture. Repeat films in 7 to 10 days should be obtained to look for a response to these hairline toddlers' fractures.

Management. Life-threatening injuries should be managed. Isolated fibular fractures are managed with a short-leg walking case. Undisplaced tibial fractures can be immobilized in a long leg posterior splint, with the patient bearing no weight and followed as an outpatient for 4 to 6 weeks. Early orthopedic consultation is indicated.

Displaced closed tibial fractures require hospitalization for observation of circulatory status after orthopedic reduction and consultation. Open fractures require immediate consultation.

References

1. Rockwood CA, Wilkins KE, King RE: *Fractures in children*, Philadelphia, 1984, JB Lippincott.
2. Palmer JK, Benson GS, Corriere JN: Diagnosis and initial management of urologic injuries associated with 200 consecutive pelvic fractures, *J Urol* 130:712, 1983.
3. Reichard SA, Helikson MA, Shorter N et al: Pelvic fractures in children review of 120 patients with a new look at general management, *J Pediatr Surg* 15:727, 1980.
4. McSwain NE: Pneumatic anti-shock garment: state of the art, 1988, *Ann Emerg Med* 17:506, 1988.
5. Rang M: *Children's fractures*, ed 2, Philadelphia, 1983, JB Lippincott Co.
6. Jacob R and Niemann K: Fractures of the hip in childhood, *South Med J* 69:629, 1976.
7. Blatt SD, Rosenthal BM, Barnhart DC: Diagnostic utility of lower extremity radiographs of young children with gait disturbances, *Pediatrics* 87:138, 1991.
8. Illingsworth CM: 128 limping children with no fracture, sprain or obvious cause, *Clin Pediatr (Phila)* 17:139, 1978.
9. Ledwith CA and Fleisher GR: Slipped capital femoral epiphysis without hip pain leads to missed diagnosis, *Pediatrics* 89:660, 1992.
10. Loder RT: Slipped capital femoral epiphysis in children, *Curr Opin Pediatr* 7:95, 1995.
11. Taylor MT, Banerjee B, Alper EK: Injuries associated with fractured shaft of femur, *Injury* 25:185, 1994.
12. Tolo VT: External skeletal fixation in children's fractures, *J Pediatr Orthop* 3:435, 1982.
13. Paulos L, Noyes FR, Malek M: A practical guide to the initial evaluation and treatment of knee ligament injuries, *J Trauma* 20:498, 1980.
14. Zobel MS, Borrello JA, Siegel MJ et al: Pediatric knee imaging: patterns of injury in the immature skeleton, *Radiology* 190:397, 1994.
15. Cook PC and Leit ME: Issues in the pediatric athlete, *Orthop Clin North Am* 26:453, 1995.
16. Vahasarja V, Kinnuen P, Serlo W: Arthroscopy of the acute traumatic knee in children. Prospective study of 138 cases, *Acta Orthop Scand* 64:580, 1993.

## 31

Ankle and Foot Injuries

J. Leigh Jackson • James G. Linakis

ANKLE INJURIES

Sprains

Ankle sprains are among the most common sports injuries evaluated in the emergency department. Although many ankle sprains are minor, more severe injuries may lead to chronic instability or degenerative joint disease. Accurate diagnosis and appropriate management are therefore imperative to prevent chronic sequelae and to ensure prompt return of function.

Anatomy. The ankle is a hinge joint formed by three bones, the tibia, fibula and talus, connected by a number of ligaments (Fig. 31-1). The ankle mortise is formed by the distal ends of the tibia and fibula. The talus, which is broader anteriorly than posteriorly, articulates within the mortise. During dorsiflexion the broad anterior aspect is wedged into the mortise, limiting movement to 20 degrees. When the ankle is plantar flexed, the narrower aspect of the talus lies in the mortise, allowing 50 degrees of flexion in this direction as well as some lateral movement.[1]

Three ligaments provide lateral support to the ankle–the anterior talofibular ligament (ATFL), the calcaneofibular ligament (CFL), and the posterior talofibular ligament (PTFL). The ATFL and the CFL together prevent anterior and lateral subluxation of the talus during ankle movement; the PTFL prevents posterior subluxation. Medial support is provided by the deltoid ligament, which has both superficial and deep components. It originates on the medial malleolus and fans out to insert on the medial surface of the navicular, calcaneus, and talus. This ligament is both larger and stronger than the lateral ligaments and protects against eversion stress and medial subluxation.[1]

Mortise stability is maintained by the ligaments of the tibiofibular syndesmosis, which firmly bind the distal tibia and fibula and prevent diastasis during dorsiflexion and eversion.[2] The anterior portion of these ligaments is palpable just proximal to the talus.[1]

Mechanism of Injury. The ankle is more susceptible to inversion injury than eversion injury. The lateral ligaments are weaker than the medial deltoid ligament and thus provide less protection against inversion stress. It is not surprising, therefore, that more than 80% of ankle sprains are inversion injuries with damage to the lateral collateral ligaments.[3]

The ligament most easily injured by inversion stress is the ATFL. Of lateral ligament sprains, 65% are restricted to the ATFL and 20% have concomitant CFL tears. The PTFL is the strongest of the lateral ligaments and is injured only in severe sprains.[2]

Eversion injuries involving the deltoid ligament, although less common, are generally more serious. Eversion stress is more likely to cause a fracture or syndesmotic injury, leading to instability.[4] The syndesmotic ligaments may also be injured with hyperdorsiflexion as the talus is pushed superiorly, separating the tibia and fibula.

Classification of Sprains. Ligamentous ankle sprains are graded according to severity as partially outlined in Chapter 27.

Grade I (mild) sprains have minor ligamentous injury with little swelling and tenderness and minimal loss of function. The patient may be able to walk without a limp.

Grade II (moderate) sprains have a partial tearing of the ligament with diffuse swelling and tenderness and moderate functional loss. The patient has difficulty walking.

Grade III (severe) sprains are marked by complete disruption of the ligament with marked disability, swelling, and tenderness. The patient is unable to bear weight.

Diagnostic Findings. A careful history should be obtained before clinical and radiologic examination (except in cases of obviously deformed and unstable joints, when prompt neurovascular examination is warranted). A good history alone will determine which structures are most likely to be injured and how severe the injury may be.

The history should focus on the mechanism of injury (i.e., what was the position of the foot and how was it stressed?), as well as the time of injury. Patients may report that they heard or felt a snap or pop. It is important to determine whether the child was able to walk or bear weight after the injury and when swelling, pain, or discoloration occurred. Subsequent treatment should be noted. Obviously, prior injury to either ankle and important medi-

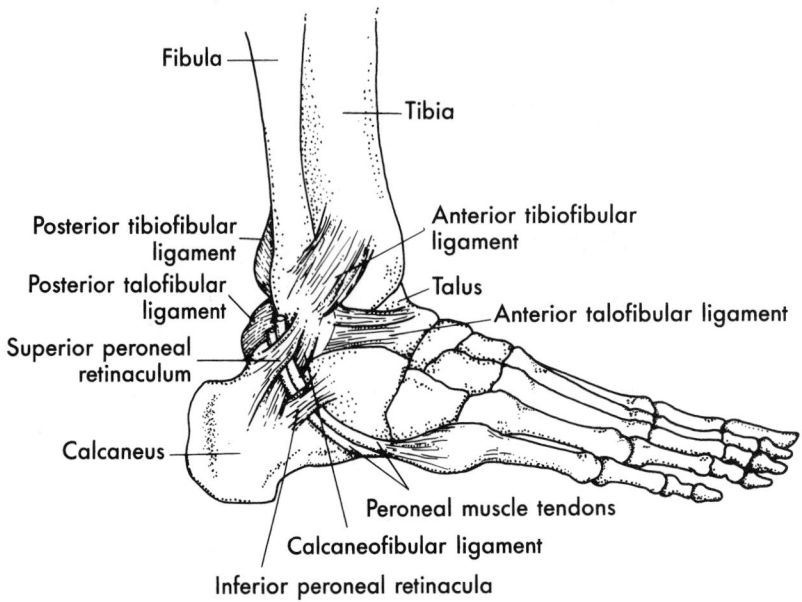

FIG. 31-1. Lateral view of the ankle showing the lateral ligaments (anterior talofibular, calcaneofibular, posterior talofibular), as well as the anterior and posterior tibiofibular ligaments, which contribute to the tibiofibular syndesmosis. (*From Hergenroeder AC: Am J Dis Child 144:809, 1990.*)

cal problems should be discussed. It is important to determine whether abnormalities revealed by examination or x-ray studies may be due to past injury.

The physical examination is most reliable immediately after the injury, before pain, swelling, and muscle spasm make assessment of joint stability more difficult. Comparison of the injured ankle with the normal ankle should be made throughout the examination unless previous problems with the uninjured joint make comparison difficult. The likelihood of a fracture or unstable joint is lower when patients are able to walk without pain or limp.[4]

The ankle should be inspected for deformity, swelling, and discoloration during assessment of neurovascular status by evaluating pulses, capillary refill, and temperature of the distal extremity. Two-point sensory discrimination testing will provide information about sensory status.

The bones, including the entire length of the tibia and fibula and the base of the fifth metatarsal, should be carefully palpated, searching for point tenderness. The anterior portion of the dome of the talus is palpable when the foot is plantar flexed.[1] Particular attention should be paid to evaluation of the tibial and fibular growth plates in children. Palpation should then proceed to evaluation of the ligaments to localize the area of maximal tenderness. Tenderness between the malleoli just proximal to the joint may indicate a syndesmotic injury. Pressing the tibia and fibula together above the joint worsens the pain of a syndesmotic ligament injury.[4] Active and passive range of motion should be assessed.

Ankle stability must be specifically determined. The *anterior drawer sign* tests the stability of the ATFL and should be performed on all patients with a suspected injury to the lateral ligaments (Fig. 31-2, *A*). The test is performed with the ankle at a 90-degree angle. The examiner stabi-

lizes the tibia with one hand while the foot is gently but firmly drawn forward. The test result is considered positive if the talus moves anteriorly more than 3 to 5 mm or if there is asymmetry between the ankles.[2] This test is unlikely to yield positive findings in the acute state because of muscle spasm and swelling.[4] The *talar tilt test* evaluates the integrity of the ATFL and CFL (Fig. 31-2, *B*). The examiner stabilizes the patient's leg and firmly inverts the foot to determine the degree of talar tilt. The degree of tilt is best compared to that of the contralateral side; a 10-degree difference is considered significant.[2] During the acute period there may be false-negative findings caused by muscle spasm and swelling.

Complications. A number of fractures are commonly associated with ankle sprains.

Epiphyseal Injuries. Ankle sprains are uncommon in children with open epiphyseal growth plates. The ligaments are stronger than the bones of the ankle, and undue stress may cause distal tibial or fibular epiphyseal injury.[5] These injuries are discussed in greater detail later in this chapter.

Avulsion Fractures. Avulsion fractures occur in approximately 15% of injuries involving complete ligamentous disruption. They may occur anywhere along the length of the fibula or may involve the malleoli, the talus, or the base of the fifth metatarsal.[4]

Point tenderness over the fracture is present in avulsion fractures, and radiologic examination generally confirms the diagnosis. It should be stressed that ankle films should include the base of the fifth metatarsal since this is a common site of avulsion fractures. Occasionally, the x-ray diagnosis may be complicated by the presence of accessory bones,[4] although generally, accessory bones are round and smooth, whereas avulsed fragments tend to have sharp edges.[4]

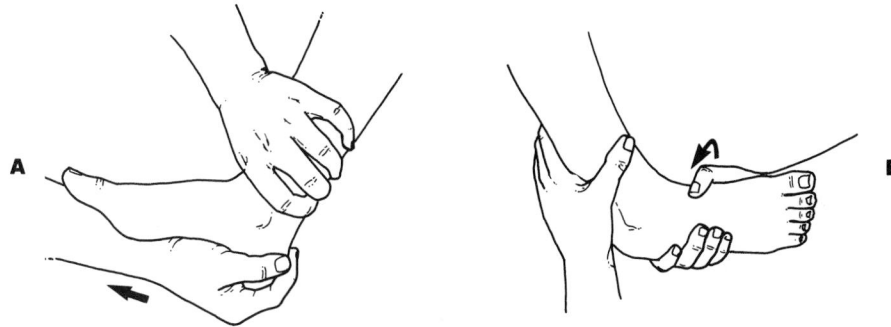

FIG. 31-2. Tests for joint stability (see text for description). **A,** The anterior drawer test. **B,** The talar tilt test. (*From Hergenroeder AC: Am J Dis Child 144:809, 1990.*)

Conservative management of avulsion fractures with immobilization is appropriate unless the avulsed fragment is large or invades the joint space, in which case surgery is required.[4]

Radiographic Studies. Clinical decision rules have been developed to assist emergency physicians in the appropriate use of radiographic studies in adult patients with acute ankle injuries (Ottawa Ankle Rules).[6,7] Although initial testing suggests that these decision rules may be applicable to children, additional testing on a large number of children will be required to validate the rules for pediatric application.[8] Until then radiographs should be obtained in all but the mildest ankle sprains. Diffuse swelling and tenderness may make physical examination unreliable in pinpointing bony point tenderness suggestive of a fracture. In addition, all children with ankle injuries should be evaluated radiographically to rule out epiphyseal injury.

Standard x-ray views of the ankle include anteroposterior (AP), lateral, and mortise views. The mortise view is taken with the ankle internally rotated 15 degrees. This exposes the entire mortise and tibiofibular joint, structures that are obscured by the distal fibula on the AP view. The lateral film should extend to include the base of the fifth metatarsal.[9] Although not routine, comparison views of the normal ankle may be valuable in evaluating possible epiphyseal growth plate injuries in children.

Stress films may be helpful if ligament rupture is suspected but not confirmed clinically. Radiographs of both ankles are made with anterior drawer stress and inversion stress applied. The degree of talar shift is then measured. The accuracy of these tests for the acutely injured ankle has been questioned, however, since muscle spasm may lead to a high incidence of false-negative results unless the tests are performed under anesthesia.[10]

Arthrography may be more effective for diagnosing ligament rupture in acute cases. Contrast material is injected and extraarticular extravasation of the dye is generally indicative of ligament rupture.[11]

Management. Initial management of all grade I and II ankle sprains should follow the RICE protocol: rest, ice, compression, elevation. The goal of treatment is to limit edema and prevent any further soft tissue injury, thereby limiting disability. This regimen should be followed for a minimum of 24 to 48 hours postinjury. The use of aspirin or nonsteroidal antiinflammatory drugs during this period will also help to decrease pain and inflammation.

Rest should include the use of crutches if there is any swelling or pain on weight bearing. Ice should be applied 20 minutes at a time every 2 hours while the patient is awake during the first 24 to 48 hours. The goal of compression is to keep fluid out of the joint space. This can be achieved by the use of an elastic bandage. For more effective compression, Tanner, Harvey, and Poole suggest the use of ¼-inch-thick orthopedic felt cut into a horseshoe shape and applied around the malleolus.[12] An elastic wrap can then be used to hold the horseshoe in place and provide compression. Alternatively, a layer of cotton pads or gauze can be placed around the swollen area and held in place with gauze wrap. An elastic bandage is then used for compression.[13] The ankle should be elevated as much as possible during the first 1 to 2 days after the injury. The patient should be instructed to elevate the ankle to a level above the heart.

There is little role for casting of mild to moderate inversion sprains. Wrapping with early mobilization (as outlined later) is as effective as casting and may lead to shorter recovery time.[4,14] Patients with more severe sprains may require immobilization for comfort. A posterior splint can be used for this purpose for a short period and followed by early mobilization and rehabilitation.[2,13] Air splint and "ski boot" devices may also be useful to facilitate early mobilization.

The treatment of grade III sprains is controversial and best left to the discretion of an orthopedic surgeon. Options include conservative management vs. a surgical approach. Interestingly, among the various types of conservative therapy, most studies have found wrapping and early mobilization superior to casting since they result in a less prolonged period of disability.[14]

Deltoid ligament sprains and syndesmotic injuries are generally more serious in terms of associated injuries and chronic sequelae. Surgical repair is indicated for most of these injuries.[12]

Proper rehabilitation is imperative in all but the mildest ankle sprains to permit more rapid functional recovery and prevent reinjury and chronic ankle instability. The initial step in rehabilitation is early mobilization. Once the swelling has stabilized (usually by 24 to 48 hours), the patient may begin range of motion exercises and Achilles tendon stretches.[4] As soon as the patient is able to bear weight, a semirigid ankle orthosis or air stirrup should be applied. The orthosis provides compression and allows flexion of the ankle while protecting against inversion or eversion. Rehabilitation should continue with activities for strengthening, increasing endurance, and regaining proprioception with ultimate return to functional activities.[12]

Disposition. Most ankle sprains can be appropriately managed by the emergency department physician. Certain injuries require referral to an orthopedic surgeon, including injuries with an unclear diagnosis, eversion injuries, grade III inversion sprains, syndesmotic injuries, and structurally significant fractures. In addition, most ankle injuries require follow-up observation for an appropriate rehabilitation regimen.

Fractures

Ankle fractures are relatively common in the pediatric population, particularly among children who are in the active phases of growth. In fact, the distal tibial physis is one of the weakest components of the ankle joint and is more likely to be disrupted than the adjoining ligaments in a growing child. The Salter and Harris classification system (Fig. 31-3) describes the types and mechanisms of injuries that may occur in the epiphyses[15] (see Chapter 27). In Salter type I and II injuries, subsequent growth disturbance is relatively uncommon, occurring in less than 5% of those sustaining the injury. In Types III and IV, however, growth is more commonly affected; as many as 20% of individuals demonstrate growth deformities. Finally, Salter V fractures, in which the growth plate is crushed, have the poorest prognosis for normal growth of the affected bones.

Diagnosis of Salter fracture types II to V is relatively straightforward radiographically. Clinically, Salter-Harris fractures should be suspected when there is point tenderness of the distal tibia or fibula at, or just proximal to, the medial or lateral malleolus. Salter I fractures may or may not be evident on radiographs, depending on whether physeal separation occurs. If it does not, the injury should be treated as a Salter-Harris fracture whenever malleolar point tenderness exists, regardless of radiographic appearance.

Mechanism of Injury. Injuries to the ankle often result from indirect trauma, generally through a twisting mechanism. Commonly the fixed foot is forcefully everted, inverted, rotated, or flexed, causing severe stress to the ligaments and the physis. According to one survey, adduction injuries resulted more frequently in complicated fractures, and abduction or external rotation injuries more often resulted in Salter type III and type IV injuries.[16] Fractures of the distal tibial physis are most common, comprising nearly 10% of all physeal injuries, although associated fractures through the distal fibular metaphysis or physis may also occur.[17] Isolated fractures through the physis of the distal fibula are uncommon.[17]

Diagnostic Findings. Findings of the physical examination are determined by the extent of the injury. The patient should be examined for obvious deformities and the area(s) of maximal tenderness should be determined. Point tenderness over epiphysis, physis, or metaphysis suggests fracture. Neurovascular status must be assessed and docu-

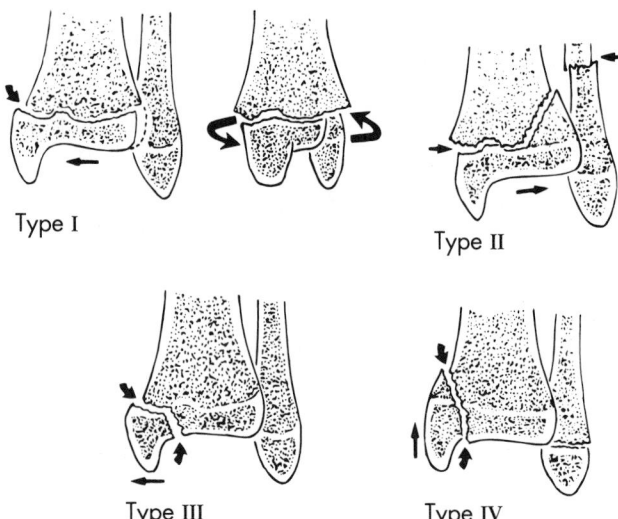

FIG. 31-3. The Salter classification. Type I, Salter I fracture of the distal tibia. The fracture is through the physis. An associated fibular fracture is also shown. Type II, Salter II fracture. The fracture involves a separation of the physis with inclusion of a triangular fragment of the metaphysis. Type III, Salter III fracture. The fracture involves a separation of the physis with inclusion of a vertical fragment of the epiphysis. Type IV, Salter IV fracture. The fracture line passes through the physis and also splits off portions of the metaphysis and the full thickness of the epiphysis. Salter V fracture is not illustrated. (*From Ogden JA, Skeletal injury in the child, ed 2, Philadelphia, 1990, WB Saunders Co.*)

mented; this usually includes evaluation of the peripheral pulses, qualitative assessment of the temperature of the distal extremity, determination of peripheral capillary refill, two-point discrimination, and inspection for evidence of an open wound. Determination of range of motion generally should not be attempted when an individual has an obvious deformity or open injury. In addition to careful examination of the ankle and foot, it is important to inspect the entire lower extremity since twisting injuries to the ankle may be associated with more proximal fibular fractures.[18]

Complications. Fractures involving the distal tibial and fibular growth plates have the potential for significant complications, including growth disturbances resulting in leg length discrepancies, osteoarthritis, and avascular necrosis of the distal tibial physis.[19]

Radiographic Studies. Radiographs should generally include AP, lateral, and oblique views. It must be remembered that nondisplaced Salter I type fractures of the distal fibula or tibia may appear normal radiographically. Consequently, when physical examination discloses point tenderness in the region of the medial or lateral malleolus, this type of fracture should be strongly suspected. Because certain types of ankle fractures are fully apparent only when a combination of radiographic views is available (e.g., the so-called Tillaux's and triplane fractures), all of these views should be obtained when significant injury is suspected. In addition, it is often preferable to include views

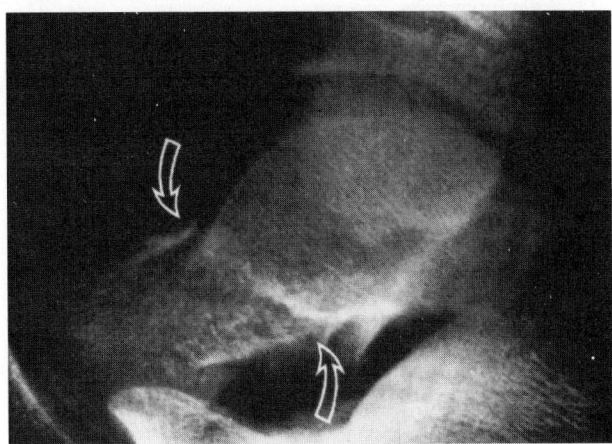

FIG. 31-4. Displaced fracture of the talar neck. (*From Ogden JA:* Skeletal injury in the child, *ed 2, Philadelphia, 1990, WB Saunders.*)

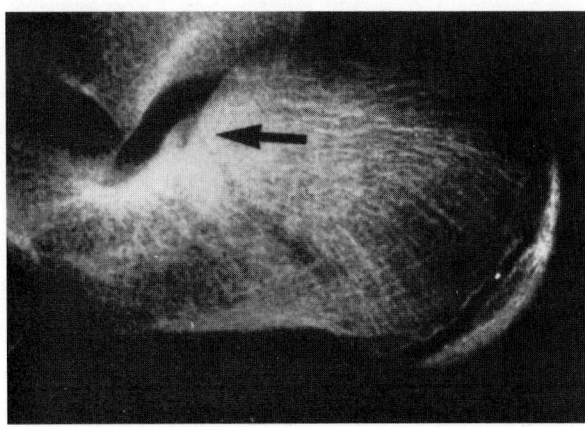

FIG. 31-5. Intraarticular fracture of the calcaneus. (*From Ogden JA:* Skeletal injury in the child, *ed 2, Philadelphia, 1990, WB Saunders.*)

of the entire fibula and tibia, since the mechanism of ankle injury often results in more proximal fibular fractures.

Management. All ankle fractures that potentially involve the epiphyseal growth plate should be referred to an orthopedic surgeon for follow-up observation. This includes children with point tenderness in the area of the lateral or medial malleolus even in the absence of x-ray findings.

Definitive treatment is determined by the specific fracture type. Nondisplaced fractures require immobilization for up to 4 weeks, pain control, and careful follow-up observation. Displaced Salter type I and II fractures are generally treated with closed reduction and no weight bearing in a short leg cast for at least 6 weeks. Rarely, open reduction and fixation are required. Salter type III and IV injuries require open reduction somewhat more frequently, although closed reduction is often effective.

Type I and II fractures have a good prognosis for normal or near-normal growth, whereas more extensive type III and IV displaced fractures are associated with a relatively high frequency of growth deformity.

FOOT INJURIES

Fractures

Mechanism of Injury. Fractures of the bones of the foot are relatively uncommon in children, presumably because of the resiliency and pliability of the child's foot. The majority of pediatric foot fractures are the result of direct trauma, since the forces of indirect (twisting) trauma are primarily transmitted to the distal tibia or fibula. Fractures of the foot, therefore, are generally caused by crush injuries from heavy objects (e.g., dropping a heavy object on the foot or being run over by the wheels of a motor vehicle) or by a fall from a height. Even less commonly, lawn mower blades may cause severe injury to the foot.

Diagnostic Findings. The majority of foot fractures in children are closed fractures; the major exception occurs when the injury results from a lawn mower blade accident. Often foot injuries are associated with marked soft tissue swelling with the potential for neurovascular compromise.

Therefore, the child's circulatory, neurologic, muscular, and skin status should be carefully assessed.

Radiographic evaluation should be directed to the area of concern; certain fractures (e.g., some fractures of the talus or calcaneus) may be especially difficult to image and thus should have radiography performed in consultation with a radiologist.

Specific Injuries

Talar Fractures. Fractures of the talus are uncommon in children, although they may occasionally be diagnosed in the adolescent. The most common injury is a vertical fracture through the neck of the talus (Fig. 31-4). When the fracture is displaced, diagnosis is not difficult, although a nondisplaced fracture can be more subtle. These fractures are characterized by a history of forced dorsiflexion of the foot and swelling and pain over the dorsum of the talus. When they are suspected, AP, lateral, and oblique radiographs should be obtained with the beam centered on the hindfoot.[20]

Talar neck fractures should be referred to an orthopedist for treatment and follow-up care. In nondisplaced or minimally displaced fractures, the injury is treated with immobilization and no weight bearing for 4 to 6 weeks. When the fracture is displaced, it is generally reduced by closed manipulation, although rarely open reduction and internal fixation are required.

Calcaneal Fractures. Although relatively uncommon, fractures of the calcaneus are the most frequent tarsal injuries in children.[21] Children less than 3 years may fracture the calcaneus with relatively minor trauma.[22] The majority of calcaneal fractures reported are the result of a fall from a height, although lawn mower injuries are a comparatively common cause of *open* calcaneal injuries. Spinal injury may be associated with fractures produced by falls. Generally calcaneal fractures do not involve the subtalar joint; however, intraarticular fractures do occasionally occur (Fig. 31-5). On physical examination these injuries are manifested by heel pain with localized swelling and tenderness. Children often refuse to walk or bear weight after trauma to the lower extremity. Radiographically, AP,

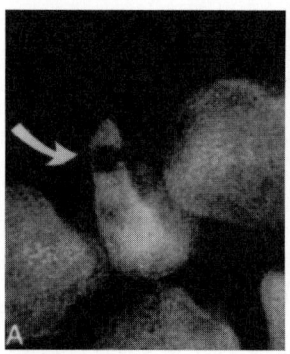
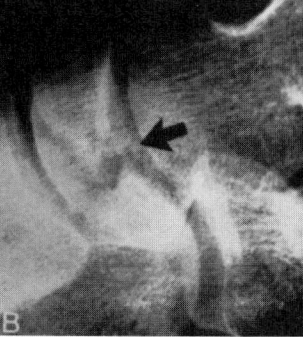

FIG. 31-6. Navicular fractures *(arrows)*. *(From Ogden JA: Skeletal injury in the child, ed 2, Philadelphia, 1990, WB Saunders.)*

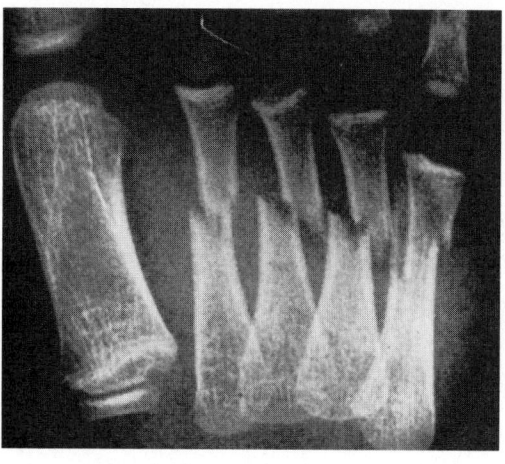

FIG. 31-7. Multiple fractures of the second to fifth metatarsals. *(From Ogden JA: Skeletal injury in the child, ed 2, Philadelphia, 1990, WB Saunders.)*

lateral, and axial views are required for assessment of calcaneal fractures. Bohler's angle, described by the anterior and posterior halves of the superior cortex of the bone, is flattened. Spinal films may be indicated.

Fractures should generally be referred to an orthopedic surgeon for evaluation and treatment. Most fractures require only non–weight-bearing immobilization for 4 to 6 weeks after the initial swelling has subsided.

Calcaneal stress fractures, although rare, have been reported in children and should be considered in the differential diagnosis of a child who refuses to bear weight.

Fractures of the Other Tarsal Bones. Fractures of the navicular (Fig. 31-6), cuboid, and cuneiforms are also quite rare and generally caused by a direct blow or crushing injury. Commonly they are associated with other fractures, thus suggesting a major injury to the foot.

Initial treatment employs use of a compression dressing and elevation to control swelling and subsequent application of a walking cast for approximately 4 weeks.

Metatarsal Fractures. Metatarsal fractures are relatively common in children. Shaft fractures most often result from direct trauma caused by a falling object. Fractures to the proximal metatarsals may also be caused by twisting injuries to the foot. Fractures near the metatarsal base may be associated with an injury to the tarsometatarsal joint. Stress fractures may present as hairline fractures of the base of the metatarsal, often after hiking or jogging.

The first and fifth metatarsals are most frequently involved, and injury to more than one metatarsal is not unusual (Fig. 31-7). Clinically metatarsal fractures exhibit pain, swelling, and ecchymosis over the dorsum of the foot. As with previously described fractures, point tenderness strongly suggests a fracture. Radiographic evaluation should be carried out in three planes (AP, lateral, and oblique) to allow determination of the extent of displacement. Follow-up films may be required to exclude stress fractures.

One area of potential confusion is the proximal, lateral fifth metatarsal. Although avulsion fractures in this region may result from forceful inversion or sudden twisting, it is also frequently the site of a secondary ossification center in children between the ages of 8 and 15 years.[23] Clinical correlation is important in making the distinction, and radiologic consultation may be required.

Treatment of metatarsal fractures generally requires no more than immobilization in a walking cast for 3 to 6 weeks. Displacement is rarely severe enough to require open reduction. Stress fractures may usually be treated with the use of hard-soled shoes.

Phalangeal Fractures. These fractures are usually secondary to direct trauma caused by a crushing blow or by kicking a surface less yielding than the toe itself. Physical examination generally reveals swelling, ecchymosis, and localized tenderness. In most cases reduction is not necessary, although Salter type III fractures are not uncommon and require reduction (often open) if they are significantly displaced.

Most pediatric orthopedic surgeons agree that relatively nondisplaced metaphyseal fractures involving any one of the lateral four toes require little more than symptomatic treatment. This can involve using the adjacent uninjured toes as splints and taping them to the injured toe with gauze placed between the toes to prevent maceration ("buddy taping"). Immobilization in this fashion for 3 weeks is generally adequate, although 5 weeks is appropriate for children engaged in sports.

Fractures of the first toe, on the other hand, require more careful treatment by an orthopedist, since malalignment is more likely to alter the weight-bearing areas of the foot.[17] An injury to the great toe that is of particular concern is the so-called stubbed-toe fracture (Fig. 31-8). Because stubbing often causes minute breaks in the skin that allow bacterial invasion, these fractures, which usually involve the distal physis, are associated with an increased incidence of osteomyelitis. Consequently, according to Ogden, fractures of this particular physis, in *any* of the toes, should generally be treated as open injuries, even in the absence of definite clinical evidence.[17] Thus, prophylactic antibiotics should be started and close follow-up observation and consultation arranged.

Puncture Wounds

Plantar puncture wounds of the foot are generally uncomplicated but may lead to serious sequelae, including

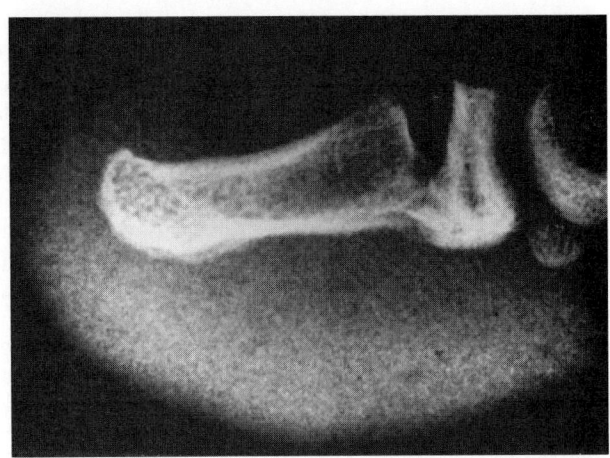

FIG. 31-8. "Stubbed" toe fracture of the distal phalangeal physis. (*From Ogden JA: Skeletal injury in the child, ed 2, Philadelphia, 1990, WB Saunders.*)

cellulitis, osteomyelitis, and septic arthritis, if improperly evaluated and treated. Cellulitis is the most common complication, occurring after 8% to 15% of puncture injuries[24]; osteomyelitis and septic arthritis are less frequent. Thorough evaluation and appropriate management may decrease the incidence of these complications.

Mechanism of Injury. Most puncture wounds of the foot are caused by nails, although a variety of other objects may be responsible (e.g., glass, wood splinters, metal objects). There is seasonal variation, as the majority of these injuries occur during the warmer months of the year.[24] Tennis shoes may be colonized with *Pseudomonas,* which can be inoculated into a puncture wound, increasing the risk of infection.[25]

Diagnostic Findings. Historical information may be helpful in guiding management and identifying risks of complications. It is essential to define when the injury occured since wounds more than 24 hours old have a higher incidence of infection. The nature of the penetrating object and its condition (i.e., dirty or rusty), the mechanism of injury, the immunization status of the patient, and any relevant underlying health problems should be noted.

The physical examination should define the location and depth of the wound and exclude retained foreign bodies. Signs of infection should be sought.

A deep puncture wound penetrating the plantar fascia, contacting bone, or invading a joint space is at higher risk of complications.[26] An injury in the metatarsophalangeal joint area may penetrate more deeply because of the weight-bearing nature of this area. The wound can be gently probed with a blunt-tipped instrument to assess the depth of penetration and the presence of a foreign body. Some foreign bodies, such as pieces of foam insole from a shoe, may not be detected through probing.

Complications. Cellulitis is the most common complication, developing in up to 15% of puncture wounds. *Staphylococcus aureus* is the causative organism in the majority of cases. *Pseudomonas* rarely causes cellulitis after a puncture wound.[24]

The infected wound should be cultured, cleansed, debrided, and irrigated. A radiograph is advisable to rule out a retained foreign body. These infections usually respond well to treatment with an appropriate oral antistaphylococcal antibiotic, but close follow-up observation is recommended. Patients who do not respond to appropriate antibiotic therapy have a high likelihood of a retained foreign body.[24]

Osteomyelitis and septic arthritis are much less common complications (occurring in less than 2% of cases) but are clearly more serious.[24] These deep space infections are usually caused by *Pseudomonas.*[26] The patient typically experiences increasing pain and swelling several days after the injury.[27] Examination reveals tenderness and redness in the area of the puncture wound and around the involved bone or joint. Dorsal foot pain may also be present over the involved bone or joint. Typically there are few systemic signs of infection. The patient may have a normal temperature and white blood cell count.[27] Plain radiographs may not show evidence of periosteal reaction until a minimum of 10 to 14 days after the injury. A bone scan may be necessary to confirm the diagnosis.

Ancillary Data. Culture and gram stain of areas of cellulitis or abscess should be obtained to direct antibiotic management.

Radiography should be employed if there is any question of a retained foreign body, although certain substances (e.g., wood) are not consistently radiopaque. Ultrasound examination or computed tomographic scan may be helpful if the penetrating object is radiolucent.

Management. Appropriate management is guided by the appearance of the wound and depth of penetration. Small, superficial puncture wounds require only surface cleaning. Deeper, larger wounds and those with retained foreign bodies may require more vigorous management, including high-pressure irrigation and debridement.

Debridement is helpful in large wounds when jagged skin edges overlie the puncture tract. This allows better visualization and drainage of the puncture wound and can be performed easily by means of iris scissors or a scalpel blade. More aggressive debridement (coring) into the dermal and subdermal tissue has not been studied adequately to assess its efficacy in decreasing wound complications. Further clinical studies will delineate the indications for this approach (see Chapter 32).

Superficial foreign bodies should be removed with adequate anesthesia. Deeper foreign bodies or more superficial ones that are particularly difficult to locate or remove should be referred to a surgeon. Retained foreign bodies that are overlooked or not completely removed may cause persistent infection.

The use of prophylactic antibiotics in the management of puncture wounds of the foot is controversial. No clear evidence indicates that prophylactic antibiotics decrease the incidence of infectious complications, and it is possible that they may increase the risk of development of gram-negative osteomyelitis.[28] At this time antibiotics are probably best reserved for treating established wound infections or wounds with severe contamination at the time of presentation. Routinely gram-positive coverage provided by cephalosporins or semisynthetic antistaphylococcal pen-

---

Common Causes of Foot Pain in Children

Extrinsic
Ill-fitting shoes (ingrown toenail)
Foreign body

Trauma
Stress fracture
Fracture
Sprain
Achilles tendonitis

Infection/inflammation
Osteomyelitis
Septic arthritis
Juvenile rheumatoid arthritis
Rheumatic fever

Structural
Hypermobile flat foot with tight heel cord
Pes cavus
Congenital problems

Tumors
Osteoid sarcoma
Ewing's sarcoma

Adapted from Gross RH: *Pediatr Clin No Amer* 33:1395, 1986.

---

icillins is indicated. *Pseudomonas* treatment often requires the use of intravenous ceftazidime in children because the use of quinolones in children is not currently recommended. Tetanus immunizations should be updated as necessary.

After the wound has been debrided and irrigated and any foreign body removed, a dry sterile dressing should be applied. If the wound is deep and wide, it can be packed with a gauze wick for 48 hours.[29] The patient should be instructed to keep the wound clean and dry, keep the foot elevated, limit weight bearing, and seek follow-up care from a physician in 48 hours.

Certain puncture wounds require surgical consultation: those with a deep foreign body or one that is difficult to locate or remove and wounds with possible or probable cartilage, bone, or joint space invasion. This is particularly likely when the puncture occurs in the area of the metatarsophalangeal joints.

FOOT PAIN

Foot pain is a relatively common complaint in pediatric patients in the emergency department, particularly those involved in athletics. The more frequent causes of foot pain in children are listed in the box above. Although the majority of patients who enter the pediatric emergency department with foot pain are suffering from sprains or fractures, other acute causes of foot pain must be considered once those are ruled out. The more common causes are discussed here.

Differential Considerations

Ingrown Toenails. Ingrown toenails are more common during adolescence than at any other time, although they do occur in infancy as well.[30,31] Ingrown toenails are the result of irritation by the growing nail of the soft tissues surrounding the nail with a consequent swelling of the tissues and encroachment on the nail. The problem is exquisitely painful and may be exacerbated by wearing tight-fitting shoes and by trimming the nail in an arch pattern, as is commonly done for fingernails.[32] Toenails are preferably left square at the edges (Fig. 31-9).

Treatment depends on the severity of the inflammation and the presence of infection. If ingrowth is minimal, placement of petrolatum gauze under the nail edge, frequent soaks, and use of properly fitting shoes should resolve the inflammation. A digital anesthetic block may be required before manipulation of the nail edge. Treatment should be continued until the distal end of the nail has grown beyond the edge of the nail groove.[31] When infection is present, oral antibiotics are generally sufficient.

In more severe cases where soft tissue hypertrophy is significant, removal of the nail or nail margin and matrix may be indicated. Unfortunately, recurrence of the problem is not unusual.

Achilles Tendonitis and Apophysitis. Although less common than in adults, pain along the Achilles tendon may be seen in children and adolescents involved in sports requiring long-distance running (e.g., cross-country, soccer). Training errors involving inadequate footwear, rapid rate of increase in distance, and hard running surfaces are often at fault.

Examination indicates tenderness along the Achilles tendon with or without swelling or crepitus. In addition, tenderness in the region of the calcaneus represents apophysitis. Apophysitis is an inflammatory injury to the apophysis caused by overuse and repetitive microtrauma.[33] Radiograph results for patients with Achilles tendonitis or calcaneal apophysitis are generally normal.

Treatment of both mild tendonitis and mild apophysitis consists of restricted activity, generally for 1 to 3 months. In individuals with apophysitis, soft heel cups may provide some symptomatic relief. Nonsteroidal antiinflammatory medications may provide some pain reduction but appear not to reduce inflammation significantly in apophysitis. In more severe cases of both maladies, immobilization for 4 to 8 weeks and referral to an orthopedist may be warranted.

Infectious Causes. Osteomyelitis may involve the talus or the calcaneus. Often the child has a history of a puncture wound to the foot. On examination, the child may be febrile and refuses to bear weight on the affected foot. Localized swelling and marked tenderness to palpation are common. The diagnosis may not be evident on plain radiographs, particularly early in the course of the disease, whereas a bone scan is often helpful. Blood cultures may reveal the offending organism, although bone aspiration is generally more reliable.[20] Although less common in other contexts, *Pseudomonas* osteomyelitis is of specific concern in puncture wounds of the foot (classically, through an old tennis shoe).[34] Although pain from the puncture may persist for 3 to 4 days, pain that worsens beyond that point should be considered suggestive of osteomyelitis, and re-

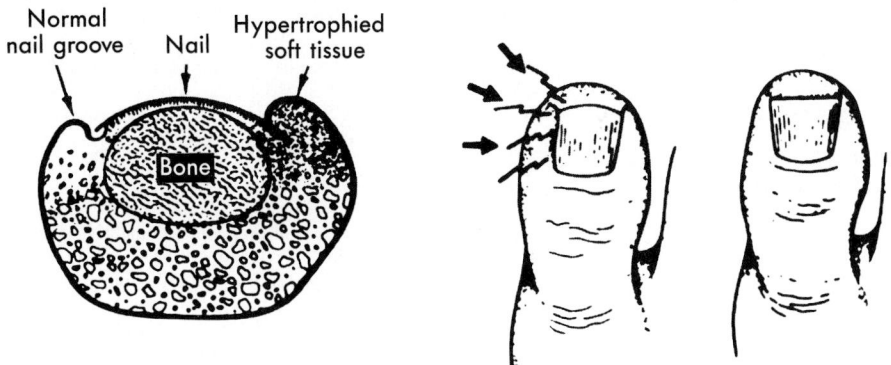

FIG. 31-9. Ingrown toenail. **A,** Crosssection of the distal phalynx of the great toe, demonstrating inflammation of the soft tissue fold, which overlaps the nail. **B,** Nail trimmed by rounding off the edges, allowing the hypertrophied, inflamed soft tissue fold to overlap the nail, causing ingrowth at the distal margin. **C,** Correct way to trim the nail, leaving the edges squared (*A from Crenshaw AH, editor:* Campbell's operative orthopaedics, *ed 8, St. Louis, 1992, Mosby. B and C redrawn from Heifetz CJ:* J Mo Med Assoc 42:213, 1945 for *Crenshaw AH, editor:* Campbell's operative orthopaedics, *ed 8, St. Louis, 1992, Mosby.*)

ferral to an orthopedic surgeon made. Although surgical drainage followed by parenteral administration of antibiotics is often required, some selected cases respond to intravenous antibiotics alone as discussed previously.

Septic arthritis rarely affects the foot except in the context of direct inoculation via a foreign body. When present, an orthopedic surgeon should be consulted since surgical drainage is frequently necessary.

Köhler's Disease. Köhler's disease is a syndrome of pain and swelling localized to the tarsal navicular. It is reported to be a common cause of painful foot in children.[35,36] Clinically patients are typically between 4 and 6 years of age and experience tenderness and swelling over the navicular. The child may walk with a limp. Radiographic findings are relatively nonspecific, showing irregular ossification in some cases but normal ossification in others. Although it is thought to be the result of a chronic trauma-related process. Köhler's disease is not routinely associated with any specific traumatic event or series of events.

Treatment is primarily symptomatic and consists of non–weight-bearing immobilization in a short leg cast for 8 to 10 weeks. The outcome is uniformly excellent.

Diagnostic Evaluation. In the initial evaluation of the child with foot pain it is important to obtain an accurate history describing the initiating event (if any) as well as the duration of symptoms. The child should be asked to locate the pain accurately and characterize it to the best of his or her ability (sharp, dull, throbbing, etc.). Both the patient and parents should be questioned to determine the extent to which the pain restricts normal activities and whether there are any signs or symptoms of an associated systemic illness (e.g., fever or rash).

Examination of the painful foot should first be carried out with the child in a non–weight-bearing position. Active and passive range of motion should be assessed and followed by palpation for localized areas of tenderness. Observation of gait and inspection of the child's shoes are also helpful, since ill-fitting shoes frequently cause foot pain in the pediatric and adolescent age groups.[37] If no obvious cause of the pain is elicited by the examination, radiographs of the foot, generally consisting of weight-bearing AP and lateral views and an oblique non–weight-bearing view, are obtained.[38] These may disclose subtle fractures, effusions, radiopaque foreign bodies, or structural deformities.

References

Ankle Injuries

1. Hoppenfeld S: *Physical examination of the spine and extremities,* Norwalk, Conn, 1976, Appleton-Century-Crofts.
2. Birrer RB: Evaluation and treatment of the injured ankle. In Mellion MB, editor: *Sports injuries and athletic problems,* Philadelphia, 1988, Hanley and Belfus.
3. Brostrom L: Sprained ankles. I. Anatomic lesions in recent sprains, *Acta Chir Scand* 128:483, 1964.
4. Hergenroeder AC: Diagnosis and treatment of ankle sprains—a review, *Am J Dis Child* 144:809, 1990.
5. Conrad EU and Rang MC: Fractures and sprains, *Pediatr Clin North Am* 33:1523, 1986.
6. Stiell IG, Greenberg GH, McKnight RD et al: A study to develop clinical decision rules for the use of radiography in acute ankle injuries. *Ann Emerg Med* 21:384-390, 1992.
7. Stiell IG, Greenberg G, McKnight R et al: Decision rules for the use of radiography in acute ankle injuries, *JAMA* 269:1127-1132, 1993.
8. Chande V: Decision rules for roentgenography of children with acute ankle injuries. *Arch Pediatr Adolesc Med* 149:255-258, 1995.
9. Tanner SM, Harvey JS, Poole B: How to evaluate ankle sprains, *Your Patient Fitness Pediatricians* 2(2):4, 1990.
10. Sauser DD, Nelson RC, Lavine MH: Acute injuries of the lateral ligaments of the ankle: Comparison of stress radiography and arthrography, *Radiology* 148:653, 1983.
11. Brostrom L, Liljedahl SO, Lindvall N: Sprained ankles. II. Arthrographic diagnosis of recent ligament ruptures, *Acta Chir Scand* 129:485, 1965.
12. Tanner SM, Harvey JS, Poole B: Treatment and rehabilitation for ankle sprains, *Your Patient Fitness Pediatricians* 2(3):4, 1990.
13. Awbrey BJ: Foot and ankle injuries. In May HL, Aghababian RV, Fleisher GR, editors: *Emergency medicine,* ed 2, vol 1, Boston, 1992, Little, Brown.
14. Lassiter TE, Malone TR, Garrett WE: Injury to the lateral ligaments of the ankle, *Orthop Clin North Am* 20:629, 1989.

Foot Injuries

15. Salter RB and Harris WR: Injuries involving the epiphyseal plate, *J Bone Joint Surg* 45:587, 1963.
16. Carothers CO and Crenshaw AH: Clinical significance of a classification of epiphyseal injuries at the ankle, *Am J Surg* 89:879, 1955.
17. Ogden JA: *Skeletal injury in the child*, ed 2, Philadelphia, 1990, WB Saunders.
18. Dias LS: Fractures of the tibia and fibula. In Rockwood CA, Wilkins KE, King RE, editors: *Fractures in children*, ed 3, vol 3, Philadelphia, 1991, JB Lippincott.
19. Spiegel PG, Cooperman DR, Laros GS: Epiphyseal fractures of the distal ends of the tibia and fibula. A retrospective study of 237 cases in children, *J Bone Joint Surg* 60A:1046, 1978.
20. Gross RH: Fractures and dislocations of the foot. In Rockwood CA, Wilkins KE, King RE, editors: *Fractures in children*, ed 3, vol 3, Philadelphia, 1991, JB Lippincott.
21. Chapman HG and Galway HR: Os calcis fractures in childhood, *J Bone Joint Surg* 59B:510, 1977.
22. Matteri RE and Frymoyer JW: Fractures of the calcaneus in young children: report of three cases, *J Bone Joint Surg* 55A:1091, 1973.
23. Dameron TB: Fractures and anatomical variation of the proximal portion of the fifth metatarsal, *J Bone Joint Surg* 57A:788, 1975.
24. Fitzgerald RH and Cowan JE: Puncture wounds of the foot, *Orthop Clin North Am* 6:965, 1975.
25. Fisher MC, Goldsmith JF, Gilligan PH: Sneakers as a source of *Pseudomonas aeruginosa* in children with osteomyelitis following puncture wounds, *J Pediatr* 106:607, 1985.
26. Chisholm CD: Plantar puncture wounds: controversies and treatment recommendations, *Ann Emerg Med* 18:1352, 1989.
27. Green NE and Edwards K: Bone and joint infections in children, *Orthop Clin North Am* 18:569, 1987.
28. Graham BS and Gregory DW: *Pseudomonas aeruginosa* causing osteomyelitis after puncture wound of the foot, *South Med J* 77:1228, 1984.
29. Verdile VP, Freed HA, Gerard J: Puncture wounds to the foot, *J Emerg Med* 7:193, 1989.

Foot Pain

30. Lloyd-Davies RW and Brill GC: The etiology and out-patient management of ingrowing toenails, *Br J Surg* 50:592, 1963.
31. Dixon GL: Treatment of ingrown toenail, *Foot Ankle* 3:254, 1983.
32. Pearson HJ, Bury RN, Wapples J et al: Ingrowing toenails: is there a nail abnormality? A prospective study, *J Bone Joint Surg* 69:840, 1987.
33. Micheli LJ and Ireland ML: Prevention and management of calcaneal apophysitis in children: an overuse syndrome, *J Pediatr Orthop* 7:34, 1987.
34. Green NE and Bruno J: *Pseudomonas* infection of the foot after puncture wounds, *South Med J* 73:146, 1980.
35. Waugh W: The ossification and vascularization of the tarsal navicular and their relation to Köhler's disease, *J Bone Joint Surg* 40B:765, 1958.
36. Williams GA and Cowell HR: Köhler's disease of the tarsal navicular, *Clin Orthop* 158:53, 1981.
37. Bleck EE: The shoeing of children-sham or science? *Dev Med Child Neurol* 13:188, 1971.
38. Gross RH: Foot pain in children, *Pediatr Clin North Am* 33:1395, 1986.

32

Emergency Care of Minor Wounds

Donald Demetrios Zukin • Alson S. Inaba • Christopher Wuerker

Soft tissue injuries are common in children and produce minor wounds. Meticulous wound care and repair are necessary to maximize cosmetic and functional outcomes. Table 32-1 summarizes the basic steps in wound care.

ANATOMY

The skin is composed of two layers, the epidermis and the dermis (Fig. 32-1).

The epidermis protects the underlying dermis from infection and desiccation. The dermis, high in collagen, imparts to the skin most of its tensile strength.

The nutrient vessels of the skin arborize into dermal capillaries.

The epidermis is normally without blood vessels, and so is fed solely by the diffusion of nutrients from the dermis.

Below the dermis is the subcutaneous fat, a layer of loose connective tissue and adipose. The large vessels and nerves lie within this layer.

PATHOPHYSIOLOGY

Wound healing is a sequential process that provides temporary protection and eventual restoration of function of the disrupted tissue. The stages of wound healing are coagulation, inflammation, proliferation, and maturation. Coagulation begins immediately after disruption of the tissue. Platelet aggregation mediates the initial hemostasis. Then activation of both the intrinsic and extrinsic clotting systems results in a fibrin meshwork.

Inflammation begins within hours as polymorphic neutrophils invade the disrupted tissue, providing immediate defense against infection. Once the wound is free from invading bacteria, the polymorphonuclear (PMN) leukocytes decrease in numbers.

Responding to chemotactic factors from platelets, monocytes marginate through local vessels made more permeable by mast cell degranulation. The monocytes transform into macrophages and begin debridement of foreign material and necrotic tissue.

The proliferation phase begins when macrophages, stimulated by phagocytosis, release factors that guide the migration and stimulate the proliferation of surrounding fibroblasts. Fibroblasts then produce a web of collagen. Myofibroblasts, linked with the collagen matrix, contract the wound margins. Clinically, this proliferation phase is marked by the presence of healthy pink friable granulation tissue made up of macrophages, fibroblasts, and endothelial cells of advancing capillaries from the wound margins.

In wounds left open to the air, a scab forms, produced by the desiccation of clot and cellular elements. The scab provides limited mechanical protection for the wound and a moist environment for proliferating cells. Epithelial cells from hair follicles, oil and sweat glands, and the adjacent skin migrate beneath the scab to produce a new layer of epidermis.

During maturation, proliferating fibroblasts continue to produce collagen, which is remodeled into increasingly strong, uniform bundles. As the metabolic demands decline, capillary density decreases and the scar loses its bright pink hue.

Optimal wound healing requires good nutritional status including adequate vitamins C and A, which are required for collagen formation. Many drugs interfere with wound healing. Anticoagulants and aspirin inhibit clot formation,

TABLE 32-1. Steps in Wound Care

Step	Hints and cautions
Examine the patient	Include sensory, motor, and perfusion examination.
	Consider child abuse if physical findings are not consistent with the history.
Sedation	Usually not necessary; local anesthesia and papoose immobilization usually suffice.
	All parenteral sedatives have the potential for causing apnea.
Local anesthesia	It is less painful to inject through the wound edge rather than through intact skin.
	The maximum dose is 0.4 ml/kg of 1% lidocaine.
	Raise a wheal at the wound edges.
Irrigation	Normal saline is the irrigation solution of choice.
	Use a 20-ml syringe and an 18-g angiocath.
	Always wear protective mask and goggles.
Topical antisepsis	Apply dilute Betadine solution (*not* the cytotoxic detergent scrub) directly into the open wound, and then paint surrounding intact skin.
Trim the wound edges	Use either a sharp iris scissors or a no. 15 scalpel.
	Never shave the eyebrows.
Close the wound	Use nylon (Ethicon, Dermalon) or prolene for the skin.
	Use Dexon or Vicryl for the deep layer.
	Perform a layered closure on the face whenever possible.
	Never put deep sutures into the hand.
Bandage the wound	Keep the wound clean and covered.
	Splint areas of motion, such as knees, elbows, and hands.
Wound check	For infection-prone wounds have the patient return for a wound check in 2 days (1 day for bites).
Suture removal	Remove sutures relatively early (4 days for facial lacerations) and then reinforce the wound for an additional 1-2 weeks with skin tape.

whereas corticosteroids inhibit cellular immunity and re-epithelialization. The most promising facilitator of wound healing is epidermal growth factor, which accelerates reepithelialization and promotes fibroblast proliferation.

CLASSIFICATION OF SKIN INJURIES

Lacerations

A laceration is simply a cut through the skin. Lacerations that are deep enough to involve dermal capillaries will bleed. If the laceration reaches the layer of subcutaneous fat, the edges of the wound will gape open.

The three main classes of lacerations are shear, tension, and compression.

A *shear* injury is one caused by a sharp object, such as a knife blade or a glass shard. There is little damage to the adjacent tissues. Shear lacerations generally heal the fastest and with the lowest incidence of infection.

A *tension* laceration occurs when stresses cause the skin to rip. An example of a tension injury is the slightly ragged linear laceration on the palm that occurs when a patient falls down on a hard surface and breaks the fall with his hands. In most cases there is not bone directly beneath the surface of the skin. Because of damage to the surrounding soft tissues, tension lacerations heal less quickly than shear lacerations.

A *compression* laceration occurs when the tissue is crushed between a hard surface and an underlying bone. The wound edges are irregular, often with a stellate pattern. Compression lacerations frequently occur when the forehead hits the pavement. Because there is a marked degree of injury to the skin adjacent to the laceration itself, compression injuries heal the most poorly of the three.

Abrasions

An abrasion is an injury in which the upper layers of the skin are scraped away. With superficial abrasions, only the cornified epidermis is lost, and consequently there is transudation of fluid, but little or no bleeding. Abrasions deep enough to involve the dermis itself result in bleeding.

DIAGNOSTIC FINDINGS

The care of the patient as a whole takes precedence over the evaluation treatment of the local wounds. Chapter 19 discusses the general care of the trauma patient.

The patient should be questioned about the past illnesses, present medications, and allergies (particularly to local anesthetics and to antibiotics). Investigate whether a serious medical or psychological disorder may have led to the wound.

The mechanism (cut, fall, crush, bite, or electrical injury) and time of injury should be elicited. When possible, determine the cleanliness of the wound, the amount of blood loss, the history of foreign body sensation, and the degree of paresthesias or impaired motor function distal to the wound. Child abuse must be considered when the history and injury are inconsistent. Tetanus status should be determined.

Wounds should be inspected to determine the depth of the injury and potential involvement of underlying tissues,

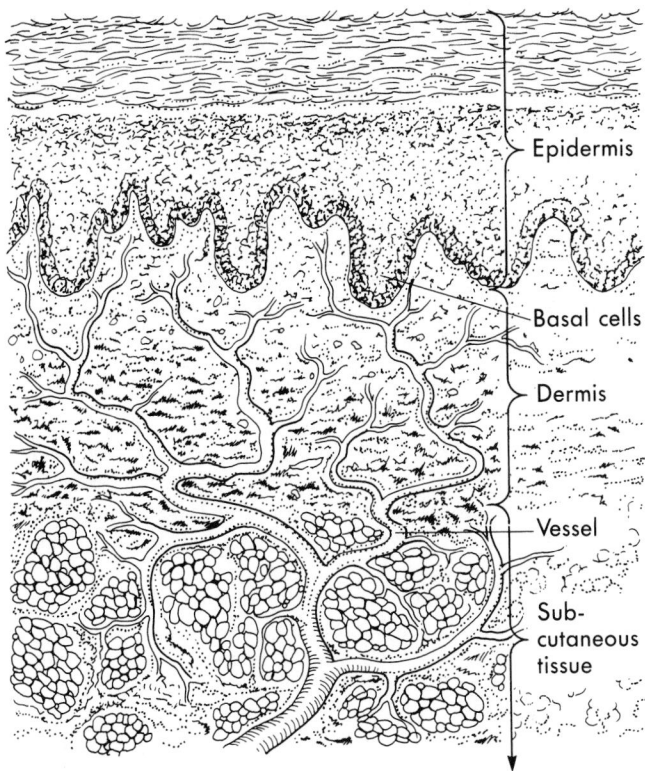

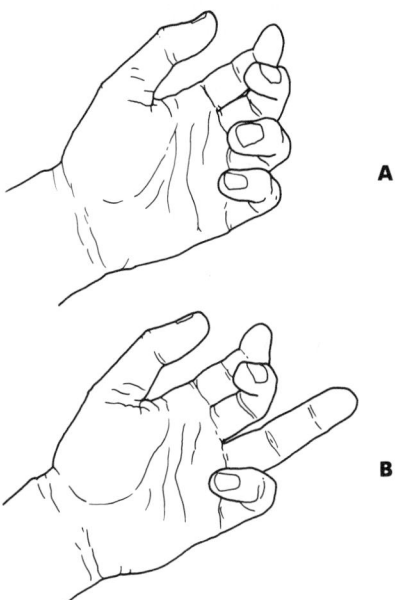

FIG. 32-2. Severed flexor tendon leading to increased extension in the affected digit. **A,** Fingers of a normal, relaxed hand. **B,** The effects of a severed flexor tendon of the fourth digit. (*From Zukin DD, Simon RR: Emergency wound care, Gaithersburg, Md, 1987, Aspen Publishers.*)

FIG. 32-1. The anatomy of the skin (not to scale). The top layer, the epidermis, consists of epithelial cells, and serves to protect the deep tissue from desiccation and infection. The bottom layer, the dermis, contains fibroblasts that produce the collagen that gives the skin its tensile strength. The blood vessels of the skin are contained within the dermis. (*From Zukin DD, Simon RR: Emergency wound care, Gaithersburg, Md, 1987, Aspen Publishers.*)

including vessels, nerves, muscles, tendons, ligaments, bones, joints and ducts. Specific aspects of the wound must be documented, including location, length, depth, nature of the edges, cleanliness, presence of a foreign body, and involvement of underlying structures. The examination often reflects the cooperation and age of the child.

Arterial *circulation* integrity is determined by palpation of peripheral pulses, skin color, temperature, and capillary filling.

Sensory *examination* determines deficits distally and often requires tremendous patience. Deficits may be tested by determinations of distal sensation, often by measurement of two-point discrimination distal to the lesion. A paper clip with the ends separated by 4 to 8 mm is useful in this process. Laceration of the digital artery indicates a high probability of damage to the digital nerve because of the close proximity of these two structures.

The classic examination must be altered for children younger than 5 years of age. The innervation in fingers and hence the normal autonomic tone produces a degree of normal sweating that causes the fingers to be slightly moist. Denervated fingers do not sweat. Running the body of a plastic pen (cleaned first with alcohol to remove all oil) along the volar surface of a normal finger yields a slight degree of drag secondary to the sweat. The pen moves more swiftly across the surface of a denervated finger.

After 15 to 20 minutes in water, skin will normally wrinkle. Denervated skin, however, usually will remain smooth.

Tendons, ligaments, and *muscles* should be tested distal to the injury individually and by muscle group. Hand injuries need special attention. Fig. 32-2, *A,* demonstrates the normal balance between flexion and extension of the fingers in a relaxed hand, termed the "finger cascade." In a significant flexor or extensor tendon injury, this balance is lost. In a flexor tendon injury the finger appears more extended (Fig. 32-2, *B*); in an extensor tendon injury the finger lies abnormally flexed. In cooperative older children the strength of the individual finger flexors (deep and superficial) and of the finger extensors should be documented (see Chapter 28).

In facial lacerations asymmetry of facial expressions, such as ptosis of the lids or loss of the normal forehead skin furrows during upgaze, indicates nerve damage.

X-rays and Scans[1-5]

Wounds that may have retained foreign material (e.g., gravel, broken glass) should be evaluated by x-ray. Glass fragments may not be seen by simple inspection of the wound, but will show up on x-ray more than 90% of the time. Computed tomography and ultrasound can identify wood and other nonradiopaque foreign bodies.

Foreign bodies should be identified and removed.

MANAGEMENT

Although unusual, significant blood loss may require emergency intervention and crystalloid infusion. If hy-

TABLE 32-2. Tetanus Prophylaxis

Tetanus toxoid immunizations	Give tetanus toxoid	Give tetanus immunoglobulin
Clean wounds (clean, superficial abrasions and lacerations)		
Three or more, last within 10 yr	No	No
Three or more, last >10 yr	Yes	No
Fewer than three or unknown	Yes	No
Tetanus-prone wounds (contaminated, deep punctures, tenuous blood supply, extensive lacerations)		
Three or more, last within 5 yr	No	No
Three or more, last >5 yr	Yes	No
Fewer than three or unknown	No	Yes

potension is present, other injuries in addition to soft tissue damage should be sought. Tetanus status should be determined and updated (Table 32-2) (see Chapter 55). Remember that a patient who has not received an adequate primary immunization series may require treatment with both tetanus toxoid and tetanus immunoglobulin.

Masks, gloves, and goggles as the basis of universal precautions are simple means of decreasing the risk of becoming infected with human immunodeficiency virus, as well as viral hepatitis.

Instruments

Only a few basic instruments are required for most wound repairs. The essentials include a needle holder, forceps, a no. 15 scalpel, and scissors.

Needles come straight (for use with the hands), and curved (for use with needle holders). The most commonly used curved needle is the ⅜-inch circle. There are two basic cross-sectional configurations: the taper, which has a circular cross-section, and the cutting needle, which has a triangular-shaped cross-section. A cutting needle facilitates suturing through the skin.

Suture Materials[6-13]

Nonabsorbable Sutures.

Silk.[14] Silk is one of the original nonabsorbable sutures. Silk has several desirable qualities. It lays flat when tied (unlike many synthetic materials). Thus silk is easy to handle. Silk, a braided material, forms a very secure knot.

Silk is not the ideal suture for routine emergency department use. Being a foreign protein, silk engenders a host tissue reaction. Silk sutures have a significantly higher infection rate than synthetic monofilament sutures such as nylon or polypropylene. In one study, although 10^6 bacteria were required to produce a wound in a standard-sized wound, only 10^2 bacteria were needed to cause an infection when silk sutures were present in the wound.[15] The infection-potentiating properties of silk limit its use to clean, uncontaminated wounds in well-perfused parts of the body, such as the face.

Cotton. Cotton possesses many of the qualities of silk. Cotton sutures lie flat, and hold knots well but also have the undesirable attributes of high infection potential and moderate tissue reactivity.[6]

Nylon and Polypropylene.[9] Nylon (Ethilon and Dermalon) and polypropylene (Prolene) are synthetic materials that have significantly lower infection potentials and tissue reactivities than cotton or silk. The low infection potential makes them the sutures of choice for skin closure of most lacerations treated in the emergency department. However, unlike silk and cotton, these materials do not tend to lie flat during suturing, hence the materials are more difficult to handle. Also, the lack of braiding decreases the knot security. Therefore both nylon and polypropylene sutures require four to five "throws" per knot.

Dacron. In experimental wounds, Dacron sutures have an infection potential that is greater than nylon or polypropylene, but less than silk or cotton.[6] Dacron sutures are easier to work with, and they hold knots better than nylon and polypropylene.

Metal. Metal sutures offer many of the advantages of nylon and polypropylene, including low tissue reactivity and low infection potential. Metal, however, is somewhat unwieldy to use and uncomfortable for the patient during healing.

Polybutester (Novafil).[16,17] Polybutester (Novafil) is a flexible, monofilament nonabsorbable suture that is equivalent to nylon or polypropylene in tensile strength and ability to withstand infection. A unique property of polybutester is that it stretches under relatively low tension. This material, therefore, may have an advantage in wounds that tend to swell, such as compression lacerations.

Absorbable Suture Materials

Plain Gut.[6] Plain gut is the original absorbable suture material. The mechanism of absorption is primarily phagocytosis by macrophages. Plain gut sutures maintain their tensile strength for approximately 7 days. Gut will take longer to absorb in poorly perfused areas of the body. Gut has the disadvantage of high tissue reactivity, and increased pyogenicity, compared to synthetic absorbable materials such as polyglycolic acid.

Chromic Gut.[6,18] Treating plain gut with chromium ion yields a suture that retains its tensile strength for approximately 2 to 3 weeks. Like plain gut, chromic gut also has the disadvantages of high pyogenicity and tissue reactivity.

Fast-Absorbing Gut. Baking plain gut sutures produces a material that breaks down within 5 to 7 days. Therefore these sutures can be plucked from the wound at the time of suture removal, rather than cut with scissors. This is an advantage in young children, in whom removal of skin sutures can be as difficult as their original placement.

Because of the theoretical risk of increased pyogenicity, fast-absorbing gut should be used only in clean wounds to well-perfused parts of the body. However in human studies an increased incidence of infection does not appear to be a problem.[19]

Polyglycolic Acid (Dexon) and Polyglactin-10 (Vicryl).[14,20-23] The synthetic absorbable sutures polyglycolic acid (PGA, Dexon), and polyglactin 910 (PG-910, Vicryl) cause less tissue reactivity, and have a lower infection rate than plain or chromic gut.[6] PGA and PG-910 are absorbed

TABLE 32-3. Suture Materials

Material	Properties
Absorbable Sutures	
Vicryl and Dexon (polyglycolic acid)	Lowest infection rates of absorbables because breakdown products inhibit bacterial growth. Lowest tissue reactivity of absorbables. Good tensile strength. Braided, so hold knots well, but make gradual cinching down of ties more difficult. Can take 40 or more days to absorb, but usually lose tensile strength within 14 days. Come both dyed and undyed. For emergency department use, *choose undyed.*
Plain gut	Most tissue reactivity of the absorbables. Higher infection potential than Vicryl or Dexon. Absorbs in 4-8 days, so useful where rapid absorption required, such as inside the mouth.
Chromic gut	Greater tensile strength and lower infection potential than plain gut. Slower absorption than plain gut.
Fast-absorbing gut (Ethicon)	Specifically made for skin sutures in children where suture removal may be difficult. Fast-absorbing gut loses most of its strength by day 5 and can be plucked from the wound without the use of scissors or scalpel.
Nonabsorbable Sutures	
Silk	The standard for all sutures in terms of ease, use, and conformity to tissue contours. Unfortunately silk, being a foreign protein, induces more tissue reaction and has a higher infection potential than nylon or Prolene.
Nylon (Ethylon and Dermalon)	Monofilament. Low tissue reactivity, low infection rate. Suitable for most emergency department wounds. Knots tend to unravel, hence use 4-5 "throws" per knot.
Polypropylene (Prolene)	Monofilament. Similar tissue reactivity and infection potential to nylon, but slightly easier to handle.

by enzymatic hydrolysis, rather than by monophage phagocytosis. Both are braided, and have a fair amount of drag when pulled through the tissues. The drag is lessened by special coatings. Maintenance of tensile strength in vivo for these sutures ranges from as little as only 20% of original strength at 2 weeks to as much as 50% strength at 30 days.[20,21]

Polydioxanone (PDS).[24,25] Polydioxanone, like PGA and PG-910, is degraded primarily by hydrolytic action, and possesses a similar low tissue reactivity. Unlike the other synthetic absorbable suture materials, PDS is a monofilament. Monofilament materials pass more smoothly through tissue, and, in some studies, have a lower infection rate. PDS maintains 58% of its original strength present at 4 weeks and 14% at 8 weeks.

Glycolide Trimethylene Carbonate (GTMC, MAXON).[26] Glycolide trimethylene carbonate (GTMC) is another synthetic, monofilament absorbable suture that is a copolymer of glycolic acid and trimethylene carbonate in a 2:1 ratio. It is degraded in tissues by hydrolysis and phagocytosis. Like PDS, this material maintains about 60% at 28 days and 30% at 42 days.

Table 32-3 summarizes the characteristics of various suture materials.

Hemostasis

The first step to stop bleeding is to apply direct pressure to the wound with a sterile gauze for 10 to 20 minutes. All clots must be removed from the wound before applying the pressure. If this maneuver fails, first the gauze should be moistened with dilute epinephrine solution (0.5 ml 1:1,000 epinephrine mixed with 5 ml sterile saline) and then direct pressure reapplied. Alternatively, the wound should be infiltrated with an appropriate amount of lidocaine with epi-

nephrine. **Epinephrine should not be used in regions such as the fingers and toes, the tip of the nose, and the penis, where ischemic necrosis can occur secondary to constriction of essential arteries.**

When epinephrine is contraindicated, packing the wound with gelfoam, and then applying constant pressure helps control bleeding.

Persistent arterial bleeding in an extremity laceration can be controlled temporarily by placing a blood pressure cuff proximal to the injury and pumping it up to 250 to 300 mm Hg.

In highly vascular regions such as the face and scalp, which continue to ooze blood, perhaps the easiest and most effective way to control bleeding is to suture the wound closed. The intrinsic pressure inside the suture loop is enough to tamponade tiny bleeding vessels.

Persistently bleeding small arteries will need to be clamped and ligated. However, **do not clamp and ligate bleeding arteries in the wrist and hands, or major arteries anywhere in the body.** Rather, maintain local pressure with a gauze and consult with a specialist concerning the possible need for microsurgical reanastomosis.

Hair Removal

In most wounds, even those to the scalp, hair removal is not necessary. Usually, moistening the hair with KY jelly will keep it out of the way.

When hair removal is necessary, hairs should be clipped with a clippers or scissors. Hair should not be removed using a razor, because shaving significantly increases the incidence of wound infections.[27] In one study, shaving the skin before surgery lead to a 5.6% infection rate, compared to 0.6% when the skin was prepared with a depilatory.[28]

The eyebrows should never be shaved or clipped. Eyebrows serve as valuable landmarks for aligning the wound edges during the repair. In addition, eyebrows can take 6 to 12 months to grow back once removed.

Local Anesthesia (see Chapter 7)

Anesthesia, analgesia, and sedation are discussed in detail in Chapter 7. Anesthesia can be achieved through a variety of topical, local, and regional approaches.

Lidocaine (Xylocaine) 1% or 2% is commonly used for most infiltrative and regional anesthesia. Infiltration is achieved by means of a small (25- to 27-gauge) needle injected slowly into the wound margins. Onset of anesthesia is 5 to 15 minutes; duration is 1 to 2 hours. Discomfort may be further reduced by warming the solution to body temperature, and by adding sodium bicarbonate in a 1:10 ratio to the lidocaine to buffer the pH.[29,30] The shelf life of buffered lidocaine is one week. Toxic levels of lidocaine may be achieved with >4 mg/kg of plain lidocaine or >7 mg/kg of lidocaine with epinephrine. Before injection a small amount of 4% lidocaine may be applied topically to decrease pain.

Lidocaine containing epinephrine at a ratio of 1:100,000 may assist with hemostasis but should only be used in areas of good perfusion and *never* on the digits, feet, ear, tarsal plate of the eye, bridge of the nose, nipple or penis.

Regional anesthesia may be achieved by using proper anatomic landmarks but often requires additional local infiltration. It minimizes distortion. The ear may be adequately anesthetized by raising a wheal with lidocaine 1% without epinephrine about the entire base of the ear. This will anesthetize all but the external canal.

Bupivacaine hydrochloride (Marcaine) is an alternative agent with onset of 10 to 30 minutes and a duration of anesthesia of 4 to 6 hours.

Topical mixtures are useful for superficial injuries, particularly in young children. They should not be used on mucosal regions such as the mouth, or when epinephrine is contraindicated. TAC, consisting of topical tetracaine 1%, topical adrenaline (epinephrine) (1:4,000), and cocaine HCl solution 4%, is most effective around the face and inconsistently useful on extremities. For anesthesia, instill 2 to 3 ml of TAC within the inner margins of the laceration until the cavity is filled. An equal amount of TAC is applied using a cotton ball or swab (not gauze) over the wound for 10 to 15 minutes. The individual holding the cotton ball or swab should wear gloves. Lidocaine, epinephrine, and tetracaine (LET) is an effective alternative without the dangers of cocaine absorption.[31] EMLA has also been used effectively for topical anesthesia but requires a 1-hour period before peak effectiveness.

Wound Irrigation

Irrigation is the method of choice for removing bacteria and dirt from wounds. *Normal saline with no additives is the irrigation solution of choice.*

The efficacy of an irrigation system in removing foreign material is directly related to the force of the irrigant stream and the size of the particles being removed. Larger particles are more easily removed than smaller particles. High-pressure irrigation is more efficient than low pressure irrigation.

Irrigation using an asepto or a bulb syringe generates relatively low pressures, on the order of only 0.05 psi (pounds per square inch). Irrigation using a 35-ml syringe fitted with a 19-gauge needle generates intermediate pressures, on the order of 8 psi.[28] Irrigation using a mechanical jet device generates high pressures, on the order of 80 psi. Pressures on the order of 8 psi are needed to remove debris and bacteria from contaminated wounds.[32-36]

For wounds contaminated with bacteria or foreign material the authors recommend using a 35-ml syringe fitted with either an 18-gauge angiocath or a 19-gauge needle, and pressing down firmly on the plunger.

Devices such as the Zerowet Splashshield are available to avoid splashes. The plastic shields are attached to the syringe instead of a needle and the wound is irrigated, holding the shield just above the skin surface.

High-pressure irrigation of contaminated wounds can also be accomplished by placing a 500 to 1000 ml bag of normal saline fitted with blood administration tubing, into a pressure sleeve (the type used to increase the speed of blood administration in hemorrhagic shock). Place an 18-gauge angiocath or Splashshield at the end of the tubing, pump the pressure in the sleeve to 300 mm Hg, and then proceed with the irrigation.

Always wear protective goggles during irrigation. After these procedures, the wound should be reexplored for foreign materials.

Wounds with a glass foreign body need special attention during irrigation and exploration. Retained glass is more likely to be present if the patient has a sensation of a foreign body. Wounds of the head and foot caused by glass are especially likely to have a glass foreign body.[37]

Foreign material in an abrasion must be removed within 24 hours to prevent the creation of permanent traumatic tattoos, particularly in such cosmetically important areas as the face. Anesthesia of the abrasion may be achieved by direct application of a cotton ball/swab to the wound that has been saturated in 4% lidocaine or TAC. The abrasion should then be scrubbed with a scrub brush or toothbrush. A no. 11-blade or 18-gauge needle may be used for material not removed by the scrubbing process.

Wound Antiseptics[38-40]

Wound preparation does not end with irrigation. Proper antiseptics can decrease the incidence of wound infection.

The topical antiseptic agent must effectively destroy bacteria, but without causing tissue damage. Table 32-4 lists the bactericidal efficacy as well as the tissue toxicity of several topical antiseptics.

Isopropyl alcohol, although an effective antiseptic, is highly toxic, essentially fixing the tissues.[41]

The next most damaging agents are detergents. Detergents dissolve the lipid walls of fibroblasts and other cells. In one study, hexachlorophene and povidone iodine aqueous solutions caused little or no cell damage.[37] However, the same agents with detergent (Phisohex and Betadine surgical scrub) caused extensive necrosis. **Therefore no topical agent containing detergent should be used in or near an open wound.**[42]

Many have watched with joy as hydrogen peroxide bubbles away blood stains from scrub suits and white jack-

TABLE 32-4. Antiseptic Agents

Agent	Antibacterial efficacy	Tissue toxicity
Alcohol (70%)	10	10
Betadine surgical scrub*	9	8
Phisohex*	8	8
Hydrogen peroxide	3	5
Quaternary ammonia	6	3
Hexachlorophene solution†	8	2
Betadine prep solution†	9	1
Shur-Clens (Plurionic F-68)	1	0.5
Sterile water	0	0.5
Sterile saline	0	0

*A detergent preparation.
†An aqueous solution.

ets. Unfortunately, this same effervescence takes place in capillaries, leading to a complete standstill in the capillary blood flow when applied to an open wound. Furthermore, peroxide possesses relatively weak antibacterial efficacy.[43] Hence, hydrogen peroxide should not be applied to open lacerations.

Shur-Clens, a nontoxic surface active agent, can be helpful in removing grease from a wound.[44] However, this agent does not possess antibacterial activity.

Povidone-iodine aqueous is a superb antiseptic, with relatively few toxic effects. Numerous studies attest to both the safety and the efficacy of povidone-iodine *solution* (not the cytotoxic detergent scrub) as a topical antiseptic. The antibacterial range of povidone-iodine includes *Staphylococcus aureus, Streptococcus pyogenes, Streptococcus viridans, Klebsiella, Pseudomonas, Proteus,* and *Escherichia coli.*[45] The 1% povidone-iodine solution is as effective as the stock 10% solution in killing bacteria.[46] Emergence of bacterial strains resistant to povidone-iodine is unusual.[45]

Several human studies demonstrate the efficacy of povidone-iodine (applied directly to the open wound just before closure) in decreasing the incidence of surgical wound infections.[47-51]

Of interest to the emergency specialist is a study of 500 consecutive emergency department patients in which Gravett found that the number of wounds with frank pus was 1% in the group treated with povidone-iodine (1% solution = a 1:10 dilution of stock Betadine aqueous solution) vs. 6.2% in those treated with saline (P <0.01).[52]

Local reactions to povidone-iodine are rare. In a study of 500 patients who had povidone-iodine applied directly to open wounds, there were no allergic or other local reactions, and no systemic effects on serum iodine or thyroxine levels.[50] Animal studies demonstrate no differences in wound histology or final tensile strength in wounds treated with povidone-iodine solution compared to placebo.[53] A literature review by Goldenheim concluded that povidone-iodine has "virtually no deleterious effect on wound healing."[54]

The main side effect of chronic iodine use appears to be an alteration of thyroid function tests. Investigators have demonstrated a rise in thyroid stimulating hormone (TSH), but with preservation of total T4 in women using povidone-iodine as a daily douche.[55] Infants born to mothers using the daily douches have had transient elevations of the serum TSH.[56]

Prophylactic Antibiotics[27,47,57-81]

Clinical studies fail to consistently demonstrate a lower wound infection rate in patients treated with prophylactic antibiotics compared to controls.

However, several factors need to be considered in evaluating these studies.

First, the antibiotics must be given promptly. Laboratory experimentation has documented that prophylactic antibiotics need to be administered within 3 hours of the time of the injury in order to be effective.[67] Gently abrading the wound edges with a saline-soaked gauze will extend the period of effectiveness of prophylactic antibiotics.[67]

Second, the study should stratify the patients according to the susceptibility of their wounds to infection before randomization. For example, hand lacerations carry nearly three times the infection potential of facial lacerations.

Third, excessive numbers of patients must not be lost to follow-up. In one study on the efficacy of dicloxacillin for accidental wounds, of 1334 patients more than 1000 were lost to follow-up.[78]

Systemic antibiotics are indicated in selective injuries. Edlich recommends prophylactic antibiotics for highly contaminated wounds, selected foot lacerations, selected animal bites, and wounds sutured closed more than 6 to 8 hours from the time of the injury.[47]

The first dose of antibiotic should be given as soon as possible and should be relatively high. Appropriate agents include first generation cephalosporins such as cephalexin (Keflex), penicillinase-resistant penicillins such as oxacillin and augmentin, and erythromycin.

Penicillin in aqueous solution applied directly to wounds will lower the incidence of wound infection.[59] However, a topical antibiotic is more likely than povidone-iodine to engender allergic sensitization, and to select out resistant bacteria.

Wound Closure

Basic Suturing Techniques. Use a skin hook (made by bending the tip of a 22-gauge needle and inserting a sterile cotton-tipped applicator into the hub) or forceps to manipulate the skin edges. Manipulating the wound edges with the fingers can increase the risk of needlesticks.

The needle should enter the skin at approximately a 90-degree angle. Entering the skin with the needle at a narrow tangent to the plane of the skin will result in a suture loop that has too little tissue at its base, and consequently the edges will invert rather than evert.

Wounds with inverted edges heal more slowly and with a greater potential for scarring than when the edges lay flat or evert flat (Fig. 32-3).

Uplifting the skin edge as the needle enters further increases the amount of tissue at the base of the suture loop. Uplifting the opposite wound edge as the needle exits will cause there to be adequate tissue at the base of the suture loop on that side as well (Fig. 32-4). An alternative is to exit the skin by coursing the needle an extra 2 to 3 mm

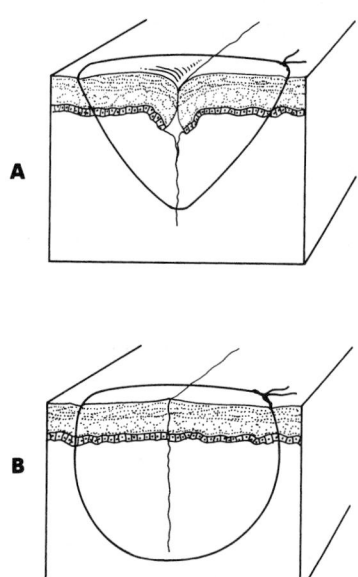

FIG. 32-3. Wound edge inversion and eversion. **A,** The base of the suture loop is not broad enough, and consequently there is inversion of the wound edges. Note that the regenerative basal cells do not come into direct contact with one another. **B,** There is a broad base to the suture loop and the wound edges evert. Notice that the basal epidermal cells do come into contact, thus facilitating healing. (*From Zukin DD, Simon RR: Emergency wound care, Gaithersburg, Md, 1987, Aspen Publishers.*)

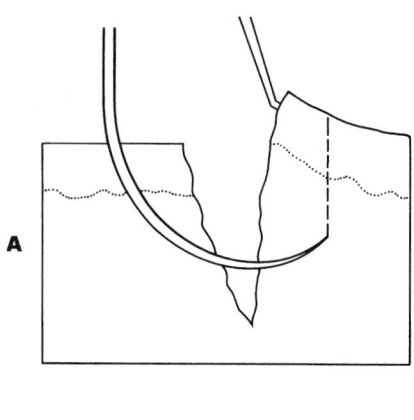

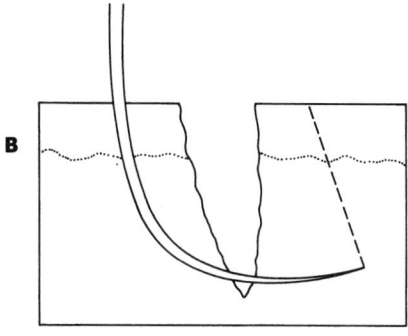

FIG. 32-4. Techniques for exiting the wound. **A,** The edge is uplifted as the needle exits. **B,** The needle courses an extra 2 mm in the deep tissue before being rotated out of the skin; the hatched line indicates the final path the needle will take. (*From Zukin DD, Simon RR: Emergency wound care, Gaithersburg, Md, 1987, Aspen Publishers.*)

in the deep tissue plane before rotating the needle out of the skin (see Fig. 32-4).

Knot Tying (Fig. 32-5). The suture loop should approximate the edges without cutting off the skin's blood supply.

The suture strands must intertwine in opposite directions for the knot to square. Nylon or prolene sutures, in particular, require meticulous knot tying because these materials tend to unravel. With nylon and polypropylene use a total of 4 to 5 "throws" for each knot, double-looping the first throw. With braided material such as Dexon and Vicryl use 3 to 4 throws per knot.

Single vs. Multiple-Layered Closures. The single layer closure is the technique of choice for repairing most of the lacerations to the extremities, trunk, and scalp. **The face, however, often requires both a deep and a superficial layer to insure the best cosmetic outcome.** The deep layer helps to approximate the muscles of facial expression, and also decreases the chances of unsightly pitting in the repaired region.

Suture Placement

Skin Sutures (Top Layer). The more sutures placed per centimeter, the finer the control over the wound edge. **Therefore for facial lacerations, place the skin sutures about 2 mm from the wound edge and about 2 to 3 mm apart** (Fig. 32-6.) **For other areas of the body place the skin sutures about 2 to 4 mm from the edge and 3 to 6 mm apart.** The better the blood supply of the area repaired, the closer together the sutures can be placed.

There are basically two methods for closing a laceration: either start at one end of the wound and work down to the other end, or bisect the wound repeatedly until the wound is closed. Both techniques are acceptable.

When there are definite landmarks, such as the palmar skin creases, the eyebrow, or the vermillion border of the lip, then place the first sutures to align the landmarks.

Close the deep layer with either a buried-knot suture, or a buried horizontal mattress suture (Figs. 32-7 and 32-8). Use absorbable suture material. Because buried sutures tend to increase the possibility of a wound infection, use the minimum number of deep sutures necessary to repair the deep structures.

The Running Suture. In a running suture the suture material is not cut and tied with each stitch. Rather, one ties the first loop in the usual fashion, and then continues across the length of wound without knotting until the very end (Fig. 32-9). The running suture is faster to perform than the interrupted technique. The main risk of the running suture is that if the suture breaks or if the knot unties, the entire repair can be jeopardized.

Vertical Mattress Suture. In areas of the body with little subcutaneous tissue, such as the hands, it often difficult to avoid having the wound edges invert during suturing. The vertical mattress suture holds the edges in apposition,

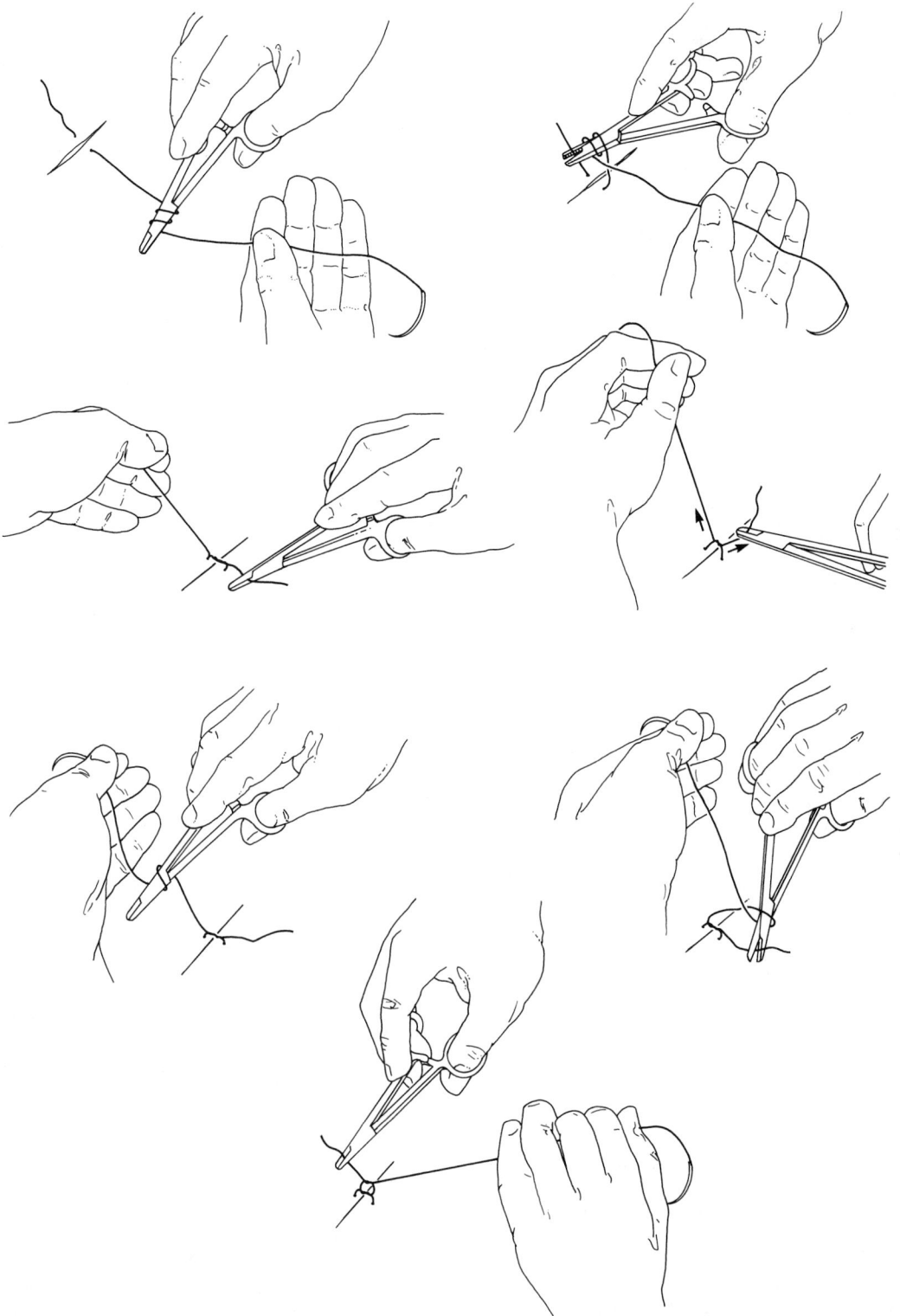

FIG. 32-5. The instrument tie. This pattern is repeated for a total of four to five "throws" per knot when using monofilament suture. (*From Zukin DD, Simon RR:* Emergency wound care, *Gaithersburg, Md, 1987, Aspen Publishers.*)

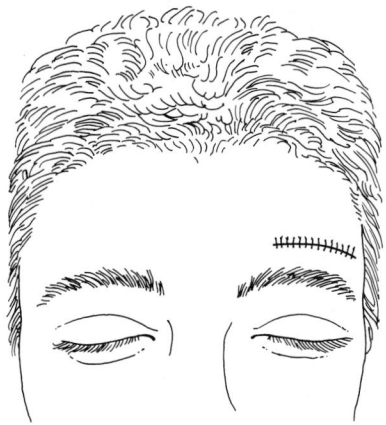

FIG. 32-6. Spacing of sutures. On the face, place the sutures approximately 2 mm from the wound edge and 2 to 3 mm apart. (*From Zukin DD, Simon RR: Emergency wound care, Gaithersburg, Md, 1987, Aspen Publishers.*)

without inversion. The technique is begun the same as a simple skin suture, but after the suture loop is made the skin is reentered about 1 to 2 mm from the wound edge and then tied. (Fig. 32-10).

Corner Stitch (Half-Buried Horizontal Mattress Suture). The corner stitch (also referred to as the half-buried horizontal mattress stitch) is essential for the closure of angulated flaps. The skin is entered and exited directly across from the angulated flap or flaps (Fig. 32-11). The suture loop is made to course within the subcuticular region, which decreases the risk of cutting off the blood supply to the tip of the flap. Use 5-0 or 6-0 nylon or polypropylene and a small needle.

The corner stitch can be used in a purse-string fashion to bring together multiple flaps in a stellate or T-shaped laceration.

Buried Sutures (Bottom Layer). *Muscle tissue and adipose tissue will not hold sutures.* Rather, place sutures in the overlying fascia.

The Buried Knot Suture. This suture loop is constructed such that the knot lies at the bottom, leaving the upper surface that the skin rests upon smooth and flat (see Fig. 32-7).

The Buried Horizontal Mattress Suture. In the buried horizontal mattress, take symmetric bites of tissue from the connective tissue on opposite sides of the wound (see Fig. 32-8).

The Subcuticular Suture. The subcuticular stitch is a running buried suture placed at the dermal-epidermal junction. First enter the skin about 5 mm above the wound, burrowing in the subcuticular plane. Then work down the length of the wound, going side to side. When the wound is closed, again burrow about 5 mm in the subcuticular plane, and then exit the skin. Tape in place the free sutures at either end, and cover the wound itself with Steri-Strips. Dexon-S (uncoated) is an ideal suture for the subcuticular closure.

The subcuticular suture avoids the possibility of skin suture marks, but is more difficult to perform and takes more time than simple interrupted sutures.

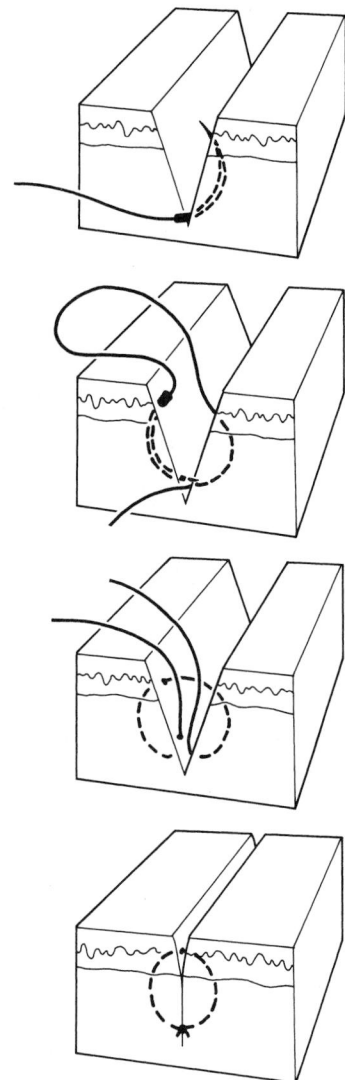

FIG. 32-7. The buried knot suture. (*From Simon RR, Brenner BE: Procedures and techniques in emergency medicine, Baltimore, 1982, Williams & Wilkins.*)

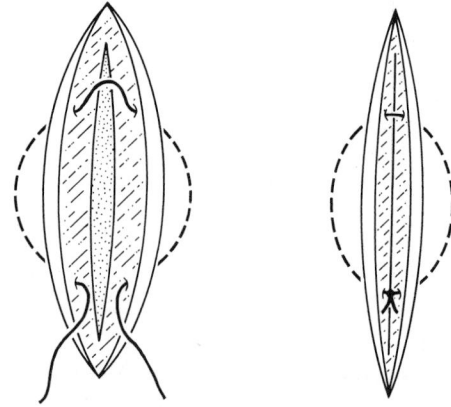

FIG. 32-8. The buried horizontal mattress stitch. See text for details (*From Zukin DD, Simon RR: Emergency wound care, Gaithersburg, Md, 1987, Aspen Publishers.*)

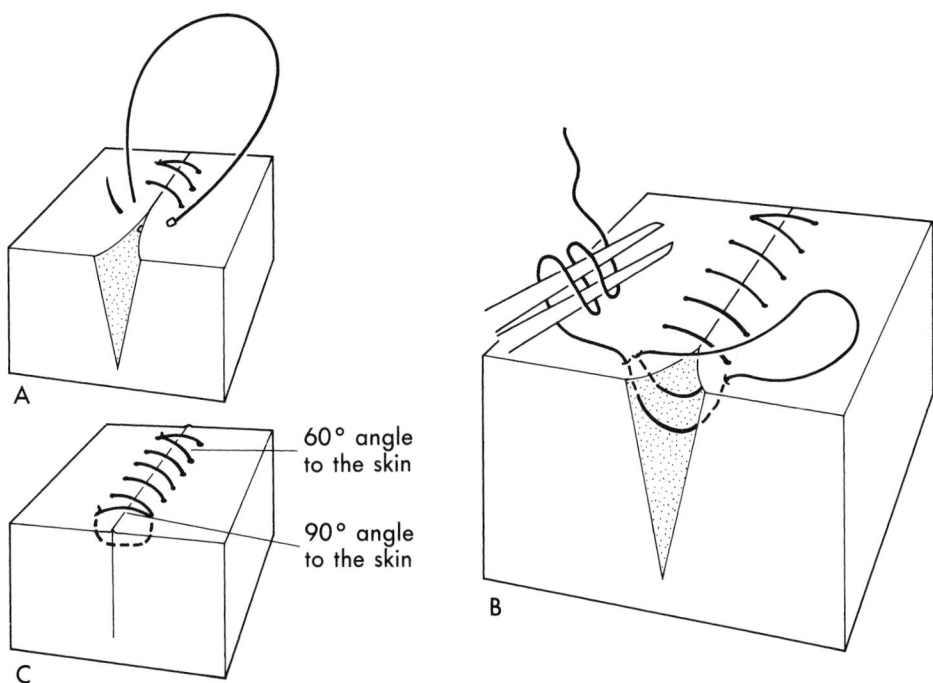

60° angle
to the skin

90° angle
to the skin

FIG. 32-9. The running suture. To complete the repair, knot the suture to itself. (**A** *and* **C** *from Simon RR and Brenner BE: Procedures and techniques in emergency medicine, Baltimore, 1982, Williams & Wilkins;* **B** *from Zukin DD, Simon RR: Emergency wound care, Gaithersburg, Md, 1987, Aspen Publishers.*)

Skin Tape.[82,83] Skin tapes (Steri-Strips, Clearon, and Shur-strips) can be used in place of sutures to repair simple lacerations. In animal studies, contaminated wounds closed with skin tape have a significantly lower incidence of infection than those closed with conventional sutures.[8] Skin tapes also offer the advantage of not causing suture marks, and of not requiring a return visit for removal. Place the skin tape after there is adequate hemostasis; tape will not adhere to a wet skin. **Pretreatment of the adjacent skin with tincture of benzoin significantly increases the sticking power of the tapes.** Parents should be instructed to leave the tapes in place as long as possible.

Do not use skin tape on infants and young children because they tend to peal the tape off. Tape is also impractical for areas of motion such as the elbows or knees, and for areas that may become wet.

Skin Staples. Disposable skin staplers are available for emergency department use. Staples can be placed more rapidly than sutures.

Staples are especially useful for closing small scalp lacerations. When only one or two staples are needed, it is less painful to place the staples rapidly with topical anesthesia alone, rather than first injecting with lidocaine.

Staples, however, afford less control of the skin edges during repair, and therefore should not be used for facial lacerations.

Tissue Adhesives. Although available in Europe and Canada, tissue adhesives are not yet available for routine use in the United States. The two most commonly used adhesives are fibrin glue and cyanoacrylate. In a study of 1500 children, Mizrahi noted excellent cosmetic results using Histoacryl Blau, a butyl cyanoacrylate.[84] Other studies found skin glue to be faster, less painful, and more economical than conventional sutures. The adhesive is particularly useful in clean wounds under 4 cm long of 0.5 cm width. It is applied with a 27-gauge needle and the wound is approximated for about 30 seconds.[85,86]

In using skin glue, first hold the wound edges together. Then apply a thin layer of glue. The glue sets in 1 to 2 minutes. There may be heat production during polymerization. Use extreme caution near the eyes because the glue will adhere to the cornea and lids if it runs into the eye.

Aftercare and Bandaging

After a wound has been repaired, the surrounding skin should be cleansed of any remaining blood or iodine. With some lacerations, those to the hand for example, one may wish to document that the motor examination is still intact. Then the wound should be covered with a nonadherent dressing to protect against invading bacteria.

In a classic experiment Du Mortier demonstrated that 100% of guinea pig lacerations became infected when the wounds were swabbed with *S. aureus* within 6 hours of the injury, 66% at 24 hours, 56% at 48 hours, and 36% at 72 hours. There were no infections in wounds contaminated after 5 days.[87]

In addition to physical protection, proper early wound coverage also serves to speed wound healing. Winter first published the results of experiments showing that semiocclusive bandages increased the rate of reepithelialization in surface abrasions. Material similar to standard Saran Wrap accelerated wound healing by approximately 25% com-

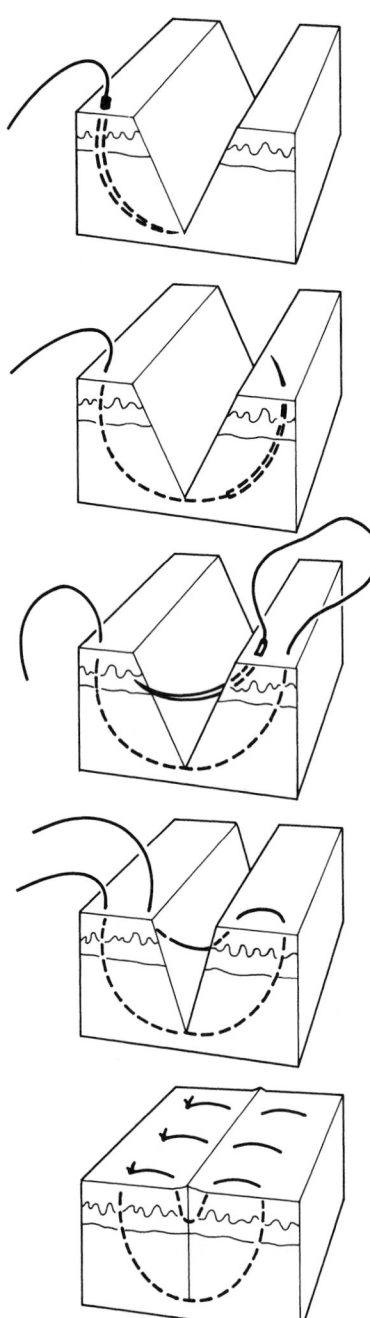

FIG. 32-10. The vertical mattress suture. (*From Simon RR and Brenner BE: Procedures and techniques in emergency medicine, Baltimore, 1982, Williams & Wilkins.*)

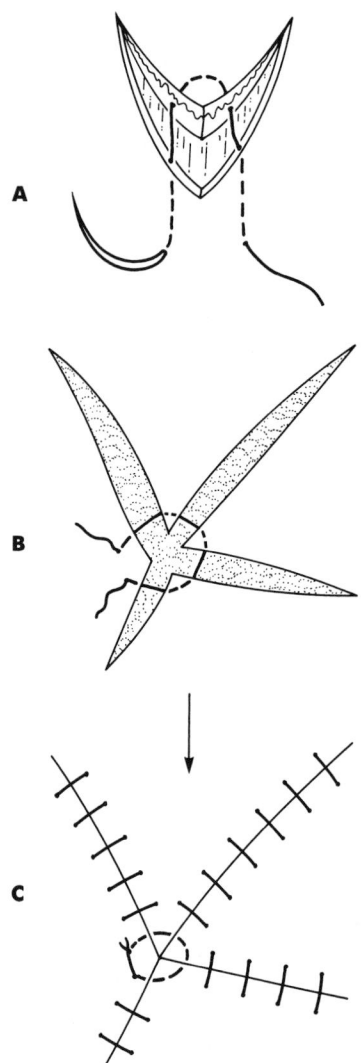

FIG. 32-11. The corner stitch (half-buried horizontal mattress stitch). The buried portion of the stitch, indicated by hatched lines, lies in the subcuticular layer of the skin, just beneath the epidermis. **B** and **C** illustrate the use of the corner stitch to close a stellate laceration. (**A** *from Simon RR and Brenner BE: Procedures and techniques in emergency medicine, Baltimore, 1982, Williams & Wilkins;* **B** *and* **C** *from Zukin DD, Simon RR: Emergency wound care, Gaithersburg, Md, 1987, Aspen Publishers.*)

pared to wounds left open to the air.[88] The protective covering speeds healing by preventing desiccation of fibroblasts and other cells.[89]

Numerous products speed healing, including bandaids, Biobrane, polyurethane film (Op-Site, Tegaderm, and Vigilon), and Duoderm. Antibiotic salves, with or without the "active" antibiotic, also speed healing by protecting against desiccation. Effective salves include Neosporin ointment and Silvadene cream.[90] Bacitracin ointment, less sensitizing than Neosporin, also is probably protective, but has been less extensively studied.

For small lacerations, first dab on Neosporin or Bacitracin ointment and apply an appropriately sized bandaid.

For large wounds use a two-layer bandage, with the bottom layer consisting of a nonadherent dressing such as xeroform gauze or polyurethane film (Op-Site, Tegaderm); and the top layer consisting of sterile 2″ × 2″ or 4″ × 4″ cotton gauze. Cotton gauze alone should not be placed directly against the healing wound, as it will become enmeshed in the eschar.

Suture Removal

Suture removal should be timely enough to avoid suture marks, yet not so soon as to risk dehiscence of the wound.

TABLE 32-5. Suture Chart by Body Area

Region	Suture*	Suture removal†
The face	Skin: 6-0 nylon or prolene	4 days
	Deep: 5-0 Vicryl or Dexon	
The scalp	3-0, 4-0, or 5-0 nylon or prolene	5-7 days
	Galea: 3-0 or 4-0 Vicryl or Dexon	
The hand	5-0 or 6-0 nylon or prolene	Joint 10-14 days, other 7-10 days, no deep sutures
Extremities	Skin: 4-0 or 5-0 nylon or prolene	Joint 10-14 days, other 7-10 days
	Deep: 4-0 Vicryl or Dexon	
The trunk	Skin: 4-0 or 5-0 nylon or prolene	7 days
	Deep: 4-0 Vicryl or Dexon	
Oral mucosa and tongue	6-0 Vicryl or Dexon or 4-0 or 5-0 plain gut	Absorbable

*Skin sutures are those selected to close the upper layer of a two-layer closure. Deep sutures are those selected to close the lower layer of a two-layer closure.
†Because of the low tensile strength of the wound during the first 10-20 days, lacerations, especially on the face and over joints, should be reinforced with skin tape for 1-2 weeks following suture removal. These over joints may benefit from immobilization initially.

Table 32-5 lists times for suture removal by region.

Note that early removal is recommended for the face, because this well vascularized region heals rapidly, and hence also will form suture marks more rapidly. Children both heal faster and form suture marks faster than adults, and therefore need suture removal sooner for a given region. Following early suture removal from any area, skin tape should be applied.

Scar Revision

Certain lacerations, especially those running against the normal skin tension lines, heal with unsightly scars. The scar then contracts and remodels over a period of 6 to 8 months. At the time of initial repair, inform patients about the possibility of scar revision after the scar has finished remodeling. Such revisions can involve excision of the scar or realignment of the scar by Z-plasty. These procedures are usually performed by plastic surgeons.

TREATMENT OF SELECTED INJURIES

Abrasions

An abrasion is an injury in which the outer skin layer is scraped away. With superficial abrasions only the upper, cornified epidermis is removed. There will be little or no bleeding, and regeneration is prompt. With deeper abrasions there is loss of the epidermis, exposing the underlying tissue to infection and desiccation.

Interestingly, abrasions heal more promptly and with fewer infections than burns of equal depth. Whereas pseudomonal infections are common with burns, the same is not true for abrasions. This difference probably stems from the fact that in abrasions, the underlying tissues are relatively uninjured, but in burns there is thermal damage to the tissues beneath the level of frank necrosis.[91]

Evaluation. As with any injury, the sensory and motor status and the perfusion of the affected area should be assessed.

Cleansing of the abrasion is important for two reasons. First, irrigation will flush away bacteria. Second, irrigation will help remove particulate matter imbedded in the wound, which, if not removed, can lead to accidental "tattooing" of the skin.

When irrigation does not remove the foreign material, then abrade the region with a sterile surgical brush or a gauze sponge that has been soaked in saline. Avoid cleansing the abrasion with detergent containing solutions, or with prepackaged scrub brushes with an attached sponges that contains povidone-iodine *detergent.* The detergent (and not the povidone-iodine) can cause severe damage to exposed fibroblasts.

After the wound has been properly cleansed and debrided, cover the abrasion with either an antibiotic ointment such as Bacitracin, or with a nonadherent dressing such as polyurethane film or xeroform gauze (see previous section).

Patients with large or exceptionally deep abrasions should return in 2 days for a wound check, and then every 3 to 4 days to monitor healing.

Scalp Lacerations

The scalp is made up of five layers: skin, subcutaneous, galea, deep loose areolar tissue, and periosteum. Because of the tight adherence of the layers together, scalp lacerations can usually be closed in a single layer.

An extensive system of arterial and venous plexi lies within a thick dermis which accounts for the marked blood loss associated with scalp wounds. Therefore, initial hemostasis is of prime importance. If direct pressure fails, inject the wound with anesthetic containing epinephrine. Ligate large bleeding arteries with 4-0 Vicryl or Dexon. For uncontrolled bleeding from scalping injuries, Rainey clips (wide, flat, plastic compression clamps) provide excellent emergency hemostasis.[92]

Control loose hairs with sterile lubricant or water. When hair removal is necessary, the hair should be clipped and not shaved since shaving increases the incidence of infection.[93] Next, explore for foreign bodies and palpate for bony step-offs indicating a depressed skull fracture. Irrigate with saline. Hematomas are common and should be evacuated. Large lacerations involving the galea should have the galea closed separately using 3-0 or 4-0 absorbable suture to reduce tension on the skin sutures and obliterate potential dead space. Most scalp lacerations can be closed in a single layer. Choose 3-0 or 4-0 nylon or polypropylene suture with a large needle. Cinch down on the sutures with slightly more tension than in other areas of the body, to help control bleeding.

Staples are an effective and expedient alternative to sutures.

Superficial scalp lacerations can be closed using the hair-tie. First lay a long, silk suture in the wound. Next overlay hairs from each side of the wound (twisted into neat bunches). Pull the hair bunches in opposite directions to close the wound, and then tie the silk suture around the hairs.[94]

Antibiotic ointment is sufficient wound covering for most scalp lacerations. Large wounds benefit from pressure dressings to suppress reformation of hematomas.

Patients are allowed to wash their hair gently with mild soap after 2 days. Suture or staples are removed in 1 week.

Forehead Lacerations

As with all head injuries, attention should first be given to evaluation for associated central nervous system (CNS) and neck injury. Wounds above the eyebrows can be anesthetized by supraorbital and supratrochlear nerve blocks at the superior orbital rim. Regional nerve blocks will not distort the tissue to be repaired. Anesthetic with epinephrine is safe in this region and aids in hemostasis. Wounds that may have retained foreign material (e.g., gravel, broken glass) should be evaluated by x-ray.

After adequate anesthesia, explore the wound to determine its extent and the possible presence of foreign bodies. Underlying bone should be palpated for step-offs. Sharp tissue debridement should be limited to obviously devitalized tissue and severely macerated or tattooed epidermis and dermis. The high vascularity in the face and scalp makes infection rare in these areas and allows for successful primary closure of wounds presenting late, even longer than 24 hours.[95]

Perform a layered closure, beginning with approximation of the frontalis fascia using absorbable suture. Areas of moderate tissue loss should be mobilized by undermining the subcutaneous tissue. Use the buried knot or buried horizontal mattress stitch to repair the deep layer. Next close the subcutaneous layer just beneath the skin using 5-0 Vicryl or Dexon. Always align landmarks, such as the forehead furrow marks. Ideally, the subcutaneous sutures should almost completely reapproximate the epidermis, minimizing the tension on the skin sutures. Finally, close the skin with 6-0 nylon, 6-0 polypropylene (Prolene) or 5-0 or 6-0 fast absorbing gut. Place the sutures 1 to 2 mm from the wound edge and 2 to 3 mm apart to insure control of the wound edge. Be meticulous with alignment, tension, and eversion. Bandage the wound in the usual manner. Remove the sutures in 4 days and following suture removal reinforce the wound with skin tapes for an additional 7 to 14 days.

Extensive lacerations, as well as wounds requiring grafting or flaps, are best referred to a surgeon.

Eyebrow Lacerations

Never shave the eyebrows.

The hairs are slow to grow back and the brows are used as landmarks for proper repair. Keep deep sutures to a minimum in the vicinity of the hair follicles. Close the top, taking care to precisely realign the eyebrow. If the patient has dark hair, use blue nylon or Prolene to aid in locating the sutures during removal.

Eyelid Lacerations

Superficial wounds of the eyelid may be closed using a single layer of 6-0 nonabsorbable suture or 6-0 fast-absorbing gut (see previous section). Care should be taken not to suture down to deeper structures such as the tarsal plate. Enter and exit the skin close to the wound edges to avoid inversion of the skin, a common problem with eyelid lacerations.

For both eyebrows and eyelid wounds, perform a careful ocular examination. Any wound that penetrates the tarsal plate or involves the medial canthus should be referred to a specialist. An eccentric pupil is a sign of a perforation of the globe. Always document visual acuity and extraocular movement (EOM) in children old enough to cooperate.

Lip and Cheek Lacerations

In evaluating lip-cheek lacerations there are several points to keep in mind. Remember to inspect the mucosal surfaces, including the sulci, for lacerations. Look for the presence of blood at the Stenson duct, which is a sign of an injury to the parotid gland. Document that there are no loose, fractured, or missing teeth. For lacerations to the cheeks, be sure there is no involvement of ipsilateral facial nerve. Do not use TAC topical anesthetics because toxic amounts of cocaine can be absorbed leading to seizures.

The Vermilion Border. A laceration that involves the vermilion border (the junction of the normal facial skin with the mucosa of the lips) requires exact realignment of the border to achieve the best cosmetic result (Fig. 32-12). Magnification lenses (loops) will aid in the repair of a laceration through the vermillion border. As little as 1 to 2 mm misalignment of the vermillion border will be noticeable after the wound has healed.

Local infiltration of anesthetic, especially with epinephrine, will blanch the skin, obscuring the exact location of the vermilion border. Therefore, before administering anesthetic, use a 23-guage needle to paint a thin line of methylene blue along the vermilion border on each side of the laceration. Allow the methylene blue to dry, and then instill anesthetic. After the skin is numb, use the 23-gauge needle dipped in methylene blue to puncture the skin at the vermilion border on each side of the wound. Irrigate in the usual manner. Using an infraorbital block for the upper lip, or a mental nerve block for the lower lip will avoid the problem of obscuring the landmarks.

Use the first suture (6-0 nylon or prolene) to precisely align the vermillion border, using the methylene blue marks as a guide. Once this crucial suture is in place, leave it untied initially. Then place buried sutures as appropriate to the wound, and close the skin in the usual manner, including the suture at the vermilion border. Do not use

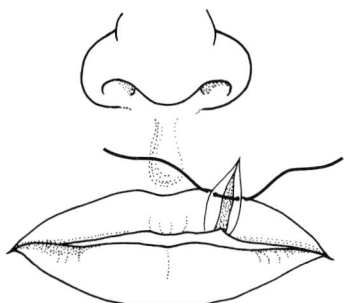

FIG. 32-12. Placement of the initial stitch at the vermilion border during repair of a lip laceration (*From Zukin DD, Simon RR: Emergency wound care, Gaithersburg, Md, 1987, Aspen Publishers.*)

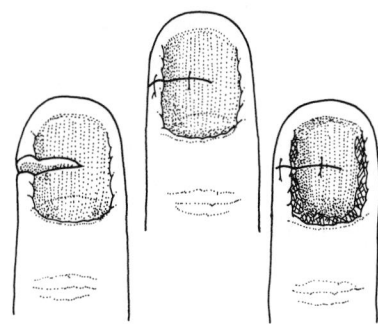

FIG. 32-13. Repair of laceration involving the nailbed and paronychial skin. Notice that the skinfolds are packed with Xeroform gauze to prevent adhesions. (*From Zukin DD, Simon RR: Emergency wound care, Gaithersburg, Md, 1987, Aspen Publishers.*)

fast-absorbing gut sutures for the lip because children tend to chew them out with their teeth.

Through-and-Through Lip or Cheek Lacerations. Small punctures caused by a tooth going through the upper or lower lips to the outside surface usually require only 1 to 2 skin sutures with 6-0 nylon after appropriate skin preparations.

Through-and-through lacerations larger than approximately 0.5 cm require a multilayer closure of the skin, orbicularis oris muscle, and buccal mucosa. After local anesthesia, irrigate the mucosa surface, and prep in the usual manner. Do not allow the child to swallow povidone iodine solution, as this can transiently alter normal thyroid function. Then close the mucosal laceration from inside the mouth using 5-0 absorbable Dexon, Vicryl, or plain gut. The number of mucosal sutures should be adequate to achieve a watertight seal of the mucosa to prevent saliva from leaking to the outside surface of the wound.

After the mucosal surface has been repaired, irrigate the wound a second time from the outside surface, and paint the wound and skin with povidone-iodine aqueous solution to decontaminate the wound. The next layer to be closed is orbicularis oris muscle. Use interrupted stitches of 5-0 Dexon or Vicryl to bring the deep tissue into alignment. Then close the third layer (subcutaneous layer) with 5-0 Vicryl or Dexon, using the buried knot technique. Repair of this subcutaneous layer will bring together the margins of the epidermis, facilitating the final skin closure. Repair the fourth and final layer, the skin itself, using interrupted stitches of 6-0 nylon or Prolene, placed 2 to 3 mm from the wound edges, and 2 to 3 mm apart.

Through-and-through lacerations carry a higher infection rate than lacerations involving the external skin or the oral mucosa solely. Initial studies have shown a benefit from 4 days of oral penicillin (or erythromycin in penicillin-allergic patients) following through-and-through lip lacerations.[73]

Fingertip Injuries

Young children tend to injure their fingertips in doors and windows. Older children are more prone to injury with knives or tools. The fingertip amputation may be complete or partial.

Complete Fingertip Amputation (Guillotine Injuries). For many years complex procedures were advocated to repair fingertip amputations. These procedures included full-thickness skin grafts as well as V-Y advancement flaps. Experimentation, however, has shown superior results when the fingertip is allowed to regenerate naturally.[96-103] Fingertips allowed to heal naturally had greater final length than those treated with grafts.[97] Since the granulation tissue contains neural buds, natural regeneration produces superior sensation compared with amputations treated with grafting or advancement flaps. In one study the group treated with occlusive dressing had a final 2-point discrimination of 4 mm or less, compared with 8 mm in the group treated with grafts.[98] Small protrusions of bone can be left in place.

Therapy of fingertip amputations consists of first irrigating the exposed tissue after local anesthesia. Next apply povidone-iodine solution and finally cover the exposed surface bacitracin ointment plus xeroform gauze and a protective outer bandage. A splint will provide additional protection. The child then returns at 2-day intervals for wound checks. The xeroform gauze need not be pealed off each wound check, only the outer dressing to check for infection.

The prognosis depends upon how much of the tip is lost. When the injury involves just the tip of the finger, but not the fingernail or nailbed, the prognosis is excellent. Injuries involving the nail and nailbed, but sparing the bone, generally heal well, but there may be foreshortening of the digit. Injuries going through the nail, the nailbed, and the distal phalanx, especially those at the base of the nail, heal the most poorly.

Fingertip and Nailbed Lacerations (Fig. 32-13). Lacerations frequently cut through the nail and the nailbed and leave the volar finger pad intact. X-rays will determine if a fracture is present. Frequently there is a blood clot adhering to the open surface of the distal flap. This clot should be removed before closing the wound.

Certain basic principles should be followed concerning nailbed injuries. There should be minimal debridement. The nail should be removed and then the nailbed repaired with 6-0 absorbable suture such as Vicryl or Dexon. Magnification lenses (loops) can aid in the repair of the nailbed.

After repair of the nailbed, lacerations to the skin of the finger can be repaired in the usual manner using 5-0 or 6-0 nylon. The skin folds around the nail margin (the paronychium and eponychium) must not be allowed to form adhesions with the nailbed. The space between the paronychium and eponychium and the underlying nailbed can be preserved by packing this space with xeroform gauze, or by simply replacing the nail itself (after cleansing).

If there is a fracture of the distal phalanx, the patient requires prophylactic antibiotics (cephalosporin or dicloxacillin) as well as splinting. Because of the excellent blood supply to the bone of the distal phalanx, osteomyelitis following fingertip injuries is unusual.

Because the healing of fingertip injuries—amputations in particular—frequently takes weeks or months, it is advisable to arrange for follow-up with an orthopedist or plastic surgeon. Parents should be counseled that the injured finger will never be exactly the same as before the injury.

Paronychia Care

A *paronychia* is a cutaneous abscess located at the lateral aspect of the fingers or toes. The process is usually the result of trauma, often due to an ingrown nail, maceration from sucking or biting the nail or pressure from a tight-fitting shoe. In most cases the pus is located between the nail and the paronychial skin. The affected skin is erythematous, swollen, and tender.

In the case of fingers, extensive incision and drainage are rarely needed. Rather, in the majority of cases if the junction between the nail and the skin (i.e., cuticle) is incised, the pus will freely drain. Drainage can usually be accomplished by placing a no. 11 blade flat on the nail surface, with the tip of the blade pointing toward the abscess cavity. The tip of the blade is then advanced into the abscess, entering below the eponychium and the proximal nail fold; pus then drains out. An extensive incision is not usually required. Finally, the abscess is irrigated with a mixture of saline and povidone-iodine solution (not the cytotoxic detergent scrub). Antibiotics are given only when cellulitis or lymphangitis complicates the paronychia, using such agents as dicloxicillin (50 mg/kg/24 hr QID PO) or cephalexin (25 to 50 mg/kg/24 hr QID PO).

A paronychia of the toes is usually the result of an ingrown toenail and therefore often does not respond to simply opening up the abscess cavity where the nail and paronychial skin join. Rather, a wedge-shaped portion of the adjacent nail should be removed after appropriate anesthesia. The involved portion of the nail is gently elevated using surgical scissors, often after scoring it with a scalpel (Fig. 32-14). Since ingrown nails often recur, the patient may benefit from referral to a podiatrist or an orthopedist for follow-up care (see Fig. 31-9).

Puncture Wounds to the Foot[104]

Puncture wounds to the foot occur when a child steps on a nail or other sharp object. Puncture wounds carry a higher infection rate than lacerations. The increased infection rate most likely results from the introduction of pathogens and particulate matter deep into tissues. An eschar then forms at the top of the puncture site, trapping the

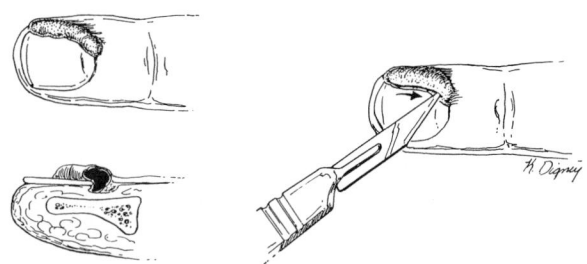

FIG. 32-14. Incision and drainage of paronychial abscess. See text for details. (*Courtesy of Norman Christopher, MD.*)

foreign material below. In addition, the small size of the surface wound impedes irrigation of the deep recesses of the wound.[105]

Initial Evaluation and Management. The patient and parents should be questioned about the injury:

1. When did the puncture occur?
2. What was the depth of the penetration?
3. What type of object caused the wound, and did it break during removal?
4. What type of shoes, if any, was the patient wearing?

Remove debris on the sole before exploring the wound. Soaking the foot in povidone iodine solution may help to loosen surface material.

Simple Puncture Wounds. Since the majority of children who step on nails never seek medical attention, and heal without problems, the incidence of complications is presumably quite low. Therefore patients who present immediately after the injury, whose wounds appear clean, and who do not give a history that part of the object broke off within the foot, can be treated with local irrigation with normal saline followed by a clean covering. Patients are discharged with instructions to return in 48 to 72 hours for a repeat check. Patients reporting continuing symptoms 48 hours postinjury are at a higher risk of complications.[105] Prophylactic antibiotic therapy may predispose to pseudomonas infection. Pseudomonal osteomyelitis of the foot was not described before the discovery of penicillin and its widespread use in puncture wounds.

Complicated Puncture Wounds. Patients with a history of retained foreign material, patients with grossly contaminated wounds, and patients who present with local tenderness 2 to 3 days or more following the injury need more aggressive evaluation and treatment. Most patients with complicated puncture wounds, especially those with prolonged pain, or the history of retained foreign object, should have radiographs of the foot.

Before the wound can be aggressively irrigated, debrided, and explored, anesthesia of the wounded region must first be established, either by local infiltration or by the posterior tibial nerve block. The posterior tibial nerve block provides anesthesia to most of the sole. The block usually is less painful for the patient than direct infiltration at the wound site.

To perform the block, have the patient lie prone and prep the area of the medial malleolus with betadine first,

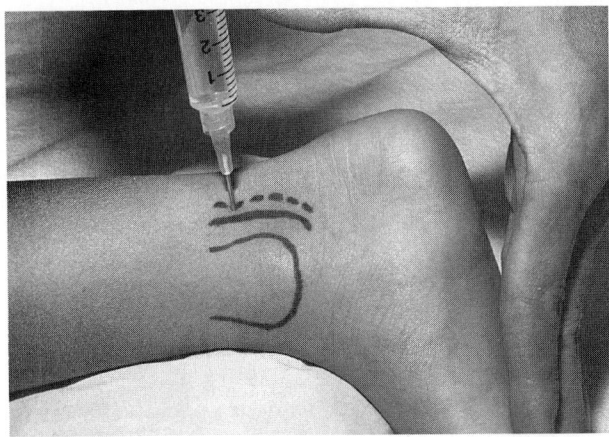

FIG. 32-15. Posterior tibial nerve block. The nerve *(dotted line)* runs posterior and lateral to the posterior tibial artery *(solid line)*, between the achilles tendon and the medial malleolus.

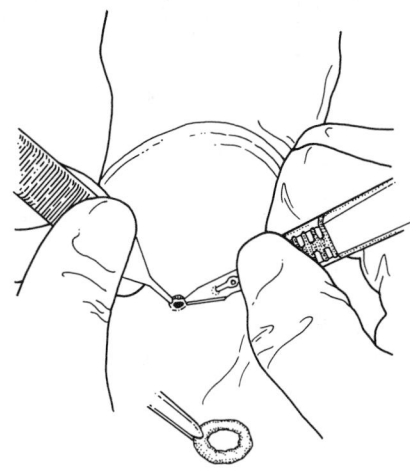

FIG. 32-16. Treatment of a contaminated puncture site. At the top is an excision of a 2 mm rim of tissue using a no. 11 blade. At the bottom is a close-up of the excised tissue. *(From Zukin DD, Simon RR: Emergency wound care, Gaithersburg, Md, 1987, Aspen Publishers.)*

and then alcohol. Then enter the skin just lateral to the posterior tibial artery pulse, at the level of the proximal half of the medial malleolus. The needle will be medial to the Achilles tendon. Advance the needle until it touches the tibia. If paresthesia occurs, pull back 1 to 2 mm and instill 5 ml of anesthetic solution. (Fig. 32-15.) If no paresthesias can be elicited, then instill 5 to 7 ml of anesthesia in a fan-like distribution around the estimated location of the nerve.

Do not use anesthetic with epinephrine. Do not exceed 4 mg/kg of lidocaine (0.4 ml/kg of the 1% solution).

Puncture Wound Debridement and Irrigation. For infected puncture wounds there are several advantages to enlarging the size of the puncture wound. Enlarging the wound will help remove embedded foreign material, such as pieces of foam rubber from the shoes, or strands of material from the patient's socks. Enlarging the wound facilitates irrigation with normal saline. Enlarging the wound also allows for drainage of pus in the cases of infected wounds.

The wound can be enlarged by excising the skin around the puncture using either a no. 11 scalpel blade (Fig. 32-16), or a 4 mm skin biopsy corer. Avoid making the enlargement of the wound greater than 4 to 5 mm, because larger wounds can lead to thick, painful scars on the sole of the foot. A *calgi* swab can be used to culture from within the wound. Surface cultures are not helpful. Gross pus should be examined by Gram stain. Alert the laboratory that *Pseudomonas* is a possible pathogen.

After cultures are taken, irrigate the wound with normal saline, using a 20-ml syringe fitted with an 18-gauge intravenous catheter. Hold the tip of the catheter 4 to 5 mm above the wound rather than inserting the catheter into the wound, to avoid ballooning of the tissue.

Fine forceps can be used to remove small bits of particulate matter from within the wound.

Finally, dab the wound with dilute povidone-iodine solution (not the cytotoxic detergent scrub), and apply a clean dressing. Subsequent therapy depends upon the clinical scenario.

Cellulitis. Cellulitis is the most common complication of puncture wounds to the foot. Patients with cellulitis usually present within 72 hours of the injury complaining of pain at the puncture site.

Physical examination reveals local tenderness and erythema. Fever is uncommon.

After enlargement of the puncture site and copious irrigation, discharge the patient on dicloxacillin or a first-generation cephalosporin, such as cephalexin. Follow-up checks are made at 2 days and 7 days. By the seventh day the patient should be walking without pain. Continued pain raises the question of a bony infection.

Osteomyelitis of the Foot[106-131]

Patients with bony infections usually present 5 days or more after the puncture complaining of local pain and a decreased ability to bear weight on the affected foot. Interestingly, the most common pathogen causing osteomyelitis of the foot following a puncture wound is *P. aeruginosa*. This pathogen is frequently present in the inside of children's tennis shoes.[114] The infections most commonly involve cartilaginous parts of the bone, such as the growth plate.

On examination there may be slight erythema around the puncture site, but drainage of pus or ascending lymphangitis is rare. There is, however, frequently swelling of the dorsal aspect of the foot, even though the injury was to the sole. The dense connective tissue of the sole itself resists swelling.

The complete blood cell count is usually normal, but the erythrocyte sedimentation rate is frequently elevated. X-ray examination may show periosteal new bone if the injury is more than 7 to 10 days old (Fig. 32-17). Children with suspected osteomyelitis of the foot need orthopedic referral for possible operative debridement. The children are then admitted for antibiotic treatment that covers *P. aeruginosa* as well as gram-positive cocci.

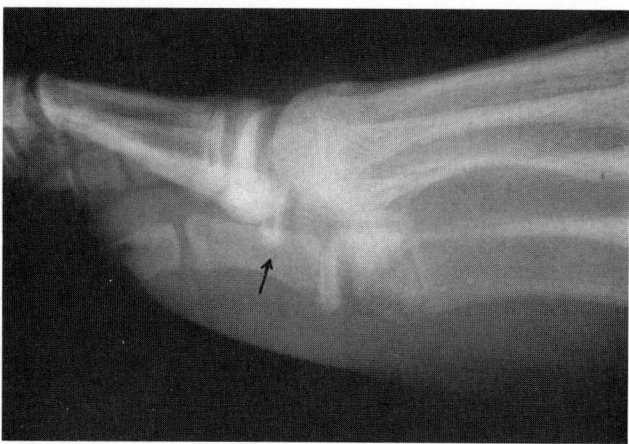

FIG. 32-17. Radiograph showing periosteal new bone in a case of osteomyelitis of the foot following a puncture wound. Cultures in this case were positive for *Pseudomonas aeruginosa.*

References

1. Anderson MA, Newmeyer WL, Kilgore ES Jr: Diagnosis and treatment of retained foreign bodies in the hand, *Am J Surg* 144:63, 1982.
2. Ariyan S: A simple stereotactic method to isolate and remove foreign bodies, *Arch Surg* 112:857, 1977.
3. Bauer AR and Yutani D: Computed tomographic localization of wooden foreign bodies in children's extremities. *Arch Surg* 118:1084, 1983.
4. Cracciolo A: Wooden foreign bodies in the foot, *Am J Surg* 140:586, 1980.
5. Gahhos F and Arons M: Soft-tissue foreign body removal: management and presentation of a new technique, *J Trauma* 24:340, 1984.
6. Edlich RF, Panek PH, Rodeheaver GT et al: Physical and chemical configuration of sutures in the development of surgical infection, *Ann Surg* 177:699, 1972.
7. Swanson NA and Tromovitch TA: Suture materials, 1980: properties, uses and abuse, *Int J Derm* 21:373, 1982.
8. Edlich RF, Tsung M, Rogers W et al: Studies in management of the contaminated wound 1-technique of closure, *J Surg Res* 8:585, 1968.
9. Postlethwait RW: Long-term comparative study of nonabsorbable sutures, *Ann Surg* 171:892-97, 1970.
10. Van Winkle L and Hastings JC: Considerations in the choice of suture material for various tissues, *Surg Gynecol Obstet* 135:113-126, 1972.
11. Von Fraunhofer JA, Storey RS, Masterson BJ: Tensile strength of suture materials, *J Biomed Res* 19:595-600, 1985.
12. Bennett RG: Selection of wound closure materials, *J Am Acad Derm* 18:619-637, 1988.
13. Chu CC and Kizil Z: Quantitative evaluation of stiffness of commercial suture materials, *Surg Gynec Obstet* 168:233, 1989.
14. Mouzas GL and Yeadon A: Does the choice of suture material affect the incidence of wound infection, *Br J Surg* 62:952-955, 1975.
15. Elek SD and Conen PE: The virulence of staphylococcus pyogenes for man-study of the problems of wound Infection, *Br J Exp Pathol* 38:573, 1957.
16. Rodeheaver G, Borzelleca D, Thacker J et al: Unique performance characteristics of novafil, *Surg Gynecol Obstet* 164:230-236, 1987.
17. Rodeheaver GT, Nesbit WS, Edlich RF: Novafil—a dynamic suture for wound closure. *Ann Surg* 204:193-199, 1986.
18. Alexander JW, Kaplan JZ, Altemeier WA: Role of suture materials in the development of wound infection. *Ann Surg* 165:192, 1967.
19. Webster RC, McCollough EG, Giandello PR et al: Skin Wound Approximation With New Absorbable Suture Material, *Arch Otolaryngol* 111:517-519, 1985.
20. Postlethwait R: Polyglycolic Acid Surgical Suture, *Arch Surg* 101:489-494, 1970.
21. Stone I, Fraunhofer JV, Masterson BJ: Mechanical properties of coated absorbable multifilament suture materials, *Obstet Gynecol* 67:737-740, 1986.
22. Rodeheaver G, Thacker J, Owen J: Knotting and handling characteristics of coated synthetic absorbable sutures, *J Surg Res* 35:525-530, 1983.
23. Rodeheaver G, Thacker J, Edlich R: Mechanical performance of polyglycolic acid and polyglactin 910 synthetic absorbable sutures, *Surg Gynecol Obstet* 153:835-841, 1981.
24. Ray J, Doddi N, Regula D et al: Polydioxanone (PDS), a novel monofilament synthetic absorbable suture, *Surg Gynecol Obstet* 153:497-507, 1981.
25. Lerwick E: Studies on the efficacy and safety of polydioxanone monofilament absorbable suture, *Surg Gynecol* 156:51, 1983.
26. Katz A, Mukherjee D, Kaganov A et al: A new synthetic monofilament absorbable suture made from polytrimethylene carbonate, *Surg Gynec Obstet* 161:213-222, 1985.
27. Edlich RF, Rodeheaver GT, Thacker JG et al: *Fundamentals of wound management in surgery-technical factors in wound management,* South Plainfield, NJ; 1977, Chirugecom.
28. Seropian R and Reynolds B: Wound infection after preoperative depilatory versus razor preparation, *Am J Surg* 121:251, 1971.
29. Orlinsky M, Hudson C, Chan L et al: Pain comparison of unbuffered versus buffered lidocaine in local wound infiltration. *J Emerg Med* 10:44, 1992.
30. Brogan GX, Giarrusso E, Hollander JE et al: Comparison of plain, warmed and buffered lidocaine for anesthesia of traumatic wounds, *Ann Emerg Med* 26:121, 1995.
31. Schilling CG, Bank DE, Borchert BA et al: Tetracaine, epinephrine (adrenaline), and cocaine (TAC) versus lidocaine, epinephrine, and tetracaine (LET) for anesthesia of lacerations in children, *Ann Emerg Med* 25:203-208, 1995.
32. Brown LL, Shelton HT, Bornside GH et al: Evaluation of wound irrigation by pulsatile jet and conventional methods, *Ann Surg* 187:170, 1978.
33. Gross A, Cutright DE, Surindar BG et al: Effectiveness of pulsating water jet lavage in treatment of contaminated crushed wounds, *Am J Surg* 124:373, 1972.
34. Rodeheaver GT, Pettry D, Thacker JG et al: Wound cleansing by high pressure irrigation, *Surg Gyn Obstet* 141:375, 1975.
35. Hamer ML, Robson, Krizek TJ et al: Quatitative bacterial analysis of comparative wound irrigation, *Ann Surg* 181:819, 1975.
36. Stevenson TR, Thacker JG, Rodeheaver GT et al: Cleansing the traumatic wound by high pressure syringe irrigation, *JACEP* 5:17, 1976.
37. Montano JB, Steele MT, Watson WA: Foreign body retention in glass caused wounds, *Ann Emerg Med* 21:1360, 1990.
38. Branemark PI, Ekholm R, Albrektsson B et al: Tissue injury caused by wound disinfectants, *J Bone Joint Surg* 49-A:48, 1967.
39. Faddis D, Daniel D, Boyer J: Tissue toxicity of antiseptic solutions: a study of rabbit articular and periarticular tissues, *J Trauma* 17:895, 1977.
40. Lineaweaver W, Howard R, Soucy D et al: Topical antimicrobial toxicity, *Arch Surg* 120:267, 1985.
41. Dzubow LM, Halpern AC, Leyden JJ et al: Comparison of preoperative skin preparations for the face, *J Acad Derm* 19:737-741, 1988.
42. Custer J, Edlich RF, Prusak M et al: Studies in the management of the contaminated wound V. An assessment of the effectiveness of phisohex and betadine surgical scrub solutions. *Amer J Surg* 121:572, 1971.
43. Reed BR and Clark RAF: Cutaneous tissue repair: practical implications of current knowledge, *J Amer Acad Derm* 13:919, 1985.
44. Rodeheaver GT, Kurtz L, Kircher BJ: Pluronic F-68: a promising new skin wound cleanser, *Ann Emerg Med* 9:572, 1980.
45. Huang ET, Reid OJ, Reid C et al: Absence of bacterial resistance to providone-iodine, *J Clin Pathol* 29:752, 1976.
46. Berkelman RL, Holland BW, Anderson RL: Increased bactericidal activity of dilute preparations of povidone-iodine solutions, *Clin Micro* 15:635, 1982.
47. Edlich RF, Kenney JG, Morgan FR et al: Antimicrobial treatment of minor soft tissue lacerations: a critical review, *Emerg Med Clin NA* 4:561-580, 1986.
48. Viljanto J: Disinfection of surgical wounds without inhibition of normal wound healing, *Arch Surg* 115:253, 1980.
49. Gilmore GJ and Sanderson PJ: Prophylactic intra-parietal povidone-iodine in abdominal surgery, *Br J Surg* 62:792, 1975.

50. Sindelar WR, Mason GR: Irrigation of subcutaneous tissue with povidone-iodine solution for prevention of surgical wound infections, *Surg Gynec Obstet* 148:227, 1979.

51. Rogers DM, Blouin GS, O'Leary JP: Povidone-iodine wound irrigation and wound sepsis, *Surg Gynecol Obstet* 157:426, 1983.

52. Gravett A, Sterner S, Clinton JE et al: A trial of povidone-iodine in the prevention of infection in sutured lacerations, *Ann Emerg Med* 16:167-171, 1987.

53. Gilmore OJ, Reid C, Strokon A: A study of the effect of povidone-iodine on wound healing, *Postgrad Med Jour* 53:122, 1977.

54. Goldenheim PD: An appraisal of povidone-iodine and wound healing, *Postgrad Med J* 69 suppl 3:S97-105, 1993.

55. Safram M and Braverman LE: Effect of chronic douching with polyvinylpyrrolidone-iodine on iodine absorption and thyroid function. *Obstet Gynecol* 60:35, 1982.

56. L'Allemand D, Gruters A, Heidemann P et al: Iodine-induced alterations of thyroid function in newborn infants after prenatal and perinatal exposure to povidone-iodine, *J Pediatr* 102:935, 1983.

57. Halasz NA: Wound infection and topical antibiotics, *Arch Surg* 112:1240, 1977.

58. Edlich RF, Madden JE, Prusak M et al: Studies in the management of the contaminated wound: VI. The theraputic value of gentle scrubbing in prolonging the limited period of effectiveness of antibiotics in contaminated wounds, *Am J Surg* 121:688, 1971.

59. Lindsey D, Nava C, Mari M: Effectiveness of penicillin irrigation in control of infection in sutured lacerations, *J Trauma* 22:186, 1982.

60. Glotzer DJ, Goodman WS, Lippman HG et al: Topical antibiotic prophylaxis in contaminated wounds, *Arch Surg* 100:589, 1970.

61. Robson MC, Schmidt D, Heggers JP: Cefamandole therapy in hand infections, *J Hand Surg* 8:560, 1983.

62. Rosen RA: The use of antibiotics in the initial management of recent dog-bite wounds, *Am J Emerg Med* 3:19, 1985.

63. Elenbaas RM, McNabney WK, Robinson WA: Prophylactic oxacillin in dog bite wounds, *Ann Emerg Med* 11:248, 1982.

64. Callaham M: Prophylactic antibiotics in common dog bite wounds: a controlled study, *Ann Emerg Med* 9:410, 1980.

65. Goldstein EJC, Citron DM, Finegold SM: Dog bite wounds and infection: a prospective clinical study, *Ann Emerg Med* 9:508, 1980.

66. Elenbaas RM, McNabney WK, Wa WAR: Evaluation of prophylactic oxacillin in cat bite wounds, *Ann Emerg Med* 13:155, 1984.

67. Edlich RF, Smith QT, Edgerton MT: Resistance of the surgical wound to antimicrobial prophylaxis and its mechanisms of development, *Am J Surg* 126:583, 1973.

68. Grossman JAI, Adams JP, Kunec J: Prophylactic antibiotics in simple hand lacerations, *JAMA* 245:1055, 1981.

69. Haughey RE, Lammers RL, Wagner DK: Use of antibiotics in the initial management of soft tissue hand wounds, *Ann Emerg Med* 10:187, 1981.

70. Roberts AHN and Teddy PJ: A prospective trial of prophylactic antibiotics in hand lacerations, *Br J Surg* 64:394, 1977.

71. Worlock P, Boland P, Darrell J et al: The role of prophylactic antibiotics following hand injuries, *Br J Clin Pract* 34:290, 1980.

72. Boss WK, Brand DA, Acampora D et al: Effectiveness of prophylactic antibiotics in the outpatient treatment of burns, *J Trauma* 25:224, 1985.

73. Steel MT, Riedel C, Robinson WA et al: Prophylactic penicillin for intraoral wounds, *Ann Emerg Med* 18:847, 1989.

74. Altieri M, Brasch L, Getson P: Antibiotic prophylaxis in intraoral wounds, *Am J Emerg Med* 4:507-510, 1986.

75. Goldstein EJ, Reinhardt JF, Murray PM et al: Outpatient therapy of bite wounds. Demographic data, bacteriology, and a prospective, randomized trial of amoxicillin/clavulanic acid versus penicillin +/− dicloxacillin, *Int J Dermatol* 26:123-7, 1987.

76. Skurka J, Willert C, Yogev R: wound infection following dog bite despite prophylactic penicillin, *Infection* 14:134-5, 1986.

77. Day TK: Controlled trial of prophylactic antibiotics in minor wounds requiring suture, *Lancet* 2:1175-1176, 1975.

78. Samson RH and Altman SF: Antibiotic prophylaxis for minor lacerations. Controlled clinical trial, *NY State J Med* 77:1728-1730, 1977.

79. Hutton PAN, Jones BM, Law DJW: Depo penicillin as prophylaxis in care of accidental wounds, *Br J Surg* 65:549-550, 1978.

80. Thirbly RD, Blair J, Thal ER: The value of prophylactic antibiotics for simple lacerations, *Surg Gynecol Obstet* 156:212-216, 1983.

81. Morgan WJ, Hutchinson D, Johnson HM: The delayed treatment of wound of the hand and forearm under antibiotic cover, *Br J Surg* 67:140-141, 1980.

82. Rodeheaver GT, Halverson JM, Edlich RF: Mechanical performance of wound closure tapes, *Ann Emerg Med* 12:203, 1983.

83. Pedersen VM, Jensen BS, Hansen B: Skin closure in abdominal incisions, continuous nylon suture versus steristrip tape suture, *Acta Chir Scand* 147:619-622, 1981.

84. Mizrahi S, Bickel A, Ben-Layish E: Use of tissue adhesives in the repair of lacerations in children, *J Ped Surg* 23:312-313, 1988.

85. Quinn JV, Drzewiecki A, Li MM et al: A randomized, controlled trial comparing a tissue adhesive with suturing in the repair of pediatric facial lacerations, *Ann Emerg Med* 22:1130-1135, 1993.

86. Osmond MH, Klasses TP, Quinn JV: Economic comparision of a tissue adhesive and suturing in the repair of pediatric facial lacerations, *J Pediatr* 126:892-895, 1995.

87. Du Mortier JJ: Resistance of healing wounds to infection, *Surg Gynecol Obstet* 56:762, 1933.

88. Winter GD: Formation of scab and rate of epithelialization of superficial wounds in the skin of the young domestic pig, *Nature* 193:293-294, 1962.

89. Winter GD and Scales JT: Effect of air drying and dressings on the surface of a wound, *Nature* 197:91, 1963.

90. Harkiss KJ: surgical dressings and wound healing, London; 1971, Bradford University Press.

91. Hunt TK and Dunphy FE: *Fundamentals of wound management*, New York, 1979, Appleton-Century-Crofts.

92. Coleman RJ and Rocko RJ: Rapid control of hemorrhage of the scalp in the patient with trauma, *Surg Gynecol Obstet* 166:165, 1988.

93. Alexander JW: The influence of hair-removal methods on wound infection, *Arch Surg* 118:347, 1983.

94. Hoffer ED: Tricks of the trade, *Emerg Med* 16(20):495, 1984.

95. Berk WA, Osbourne DD, Taylor DD: Evaluation of the 'golden period' for wound repair: 204 cases from a third world emergency department. *Ann Emerg Med* 17:496-500, 1988.

96. Ashbell TS, Kleinert HE, Putcha SM et al: The deformed finger nail, a frequent result of failure to repair nail bed injuries, *J Trauma* 7:177, 1967.

97. Douglas BS: Conservative management of guillotine amputation of the finger in children, *Aust Pediatr J* 8:86, 1972.

98. Fox JW, Golden GT, Rodeheaver G et al: Nonoperative management of fingertip pulp amputation by occlusive dressings, *Am J Surg* 133:255, 1977.

99. Allen MJ: Conservative management of finger tip injuries in adults, *Hand* 12:257, 1980. Lamon RP, Cicedro JJ, Frascone RJ et al: Open treatment of fingertip Amputations, *Ann Emer Med* 12:358, 1983.

100. Lamon RP, Cicedro JJ, Frascone RJ et al: Open treatment of fingertip Amputations, *Ann Emer Med* 12:358, 1983.

101. Farrell RG, Disher WA, Nesland RS et al: Conservative management of fingertip amputations, *JACEP* 6:273, 1977.

102. Holm A and Zachariae L: Fingertip lesions. An evaluation of conservative treatment versus free skin grafting, *Acta Orthop Scand* 45:382, 1974.

103. Louis DS, Palmer AK, Burney RE: Open treatment of digital tip injuries, *JAMA* 244:697, 1980.

104. Inaba AS: The rusty nail—and other puncture wounds to the foot, *Contemp Pediatr* 10:138-156, 1993.

105. Schwab RA and Powers RD: Conservative therapy of plantar puncture wounds, *J Emerg Med* 13:291, 1995.

106. Brand RA and Black H: Pseudomonas osteomyelitis following puncture wounds in children, *J Bone and Joint Surg* 56-A:1637, 1974.

107. Chusid MJ, Jacobs MW, Sty JR: Pseudomonas arthritis following puncture wounds of the foot, *J Pediatr* 94:429, 1979.

108. Crissman RK: Punctures through sneakers (letter), *Hosp Pract* 18:21, 1983.

109. Crosby SA and Powell DA: The potential value of the sedimentation rate in monitoring treatment outcomes in puncture wound-related pseudomonas osteomyelitis, *Clin Ortho Rel Res* 88:168, 1984.

110. Das De S and McAllister TA: Pseudomonas osteomyelitis following puncture wounds of the foot in children, *Injury* 12:334, 1981.

111. Edlich RF, Rodeheaver GT, Horowitz JH, et al: Emergency department management of puncture wounds and needlestick exposures, *Emerg Med Clin NA* 4:581, 1986.

112. Elliot SF and Aronoff SC: Clinical presentation and management of pseudomonas osteomyelitis, *Clin Pediatr* 24:566, 1985.

113. Faust RA, Roy WA, Ewin DM et al: Management and tetanus prophylaxis in the treatment of puncture wounds, *Am Surgeon* 38:198, 1972.

114. Fisher MC, Goldsmith JF, Gilligan PH: Sneakers as a source of *Pseudomonas aeruginosa* in children with osteomyelitis following puncture wounds, *J Pediatr* 106:607, 1985.

115. Fitzgerald RH and Cowan JDE: Puncture wounds of the foot, *Ortho Clin NA* 6:965, 1975.

116. Graham BS and Gregory DW: *Pseudomonas aeruginosa* causing osteomyelitis after puncture wounds of the foot, *South Med J* 177:1228, 1984.

117. Green NE and Bruno J: Pseudomonas infections of the foot after puncture wounds, *South Med J* 73:146, 1980.

118. Green NE: Pseudomonas infections of the foot following puncture wounds, *Inst Course Lect* 32:43, 1983.

119. Hagler DJ: *Pseudomonas osteomyelitis:* puncture wounds of the feet (letter), *Pediatrics* 48:678, 1971.

120. Higham M: Infection in a puncture wound after it 'healed,' *Hosp Pract* 18:47, 1983.

121. Houston AN, Roy WA, Faust RA et al: Tetanus prophylaxis in the treatment of puncture wounds of patients in the deep south, *J Trauma* 2:439, 1962.

122. Jacobs RF, Adelman L, Sack CM et al: Management of *Pseudomonas osteochondritis* complicating puncture wounds of the Foot, *Pediatrics* 69:432, 1982.

123. Johanson PH: Pseudomonas infections of the foot following Puncture Wounds, *JAMA* 204:170, 1968.

124. Lang AG and Petterson HA: Osteomyelitis following puncture wounds of the foot in children, *J Trauma* 16:933, 1976.

125. Lynch MC and Dorgan JC: A case of *Pseudomonas aeruginosa* osteomyelitis of the tarsal cuboid following a penetrating wound of the foot in childhood, *Injury* 14:354, 1983.

126. MacKinnon AE: *Pseudomonas osteomyelitis* following puncture wounds, *Postgrad Med* 51:33, 1975.

127. Peterson HS, Tressler HA, Lang AG et al: Fracture conference, puncture wounds of the foot, *Minn Med* 56:787, 1973.

128. Riegler HF and Routson GW: Complications of deep puncture wounds of the foot, *J Trauma* 19:18, 1979.

129. Sanford DD: Puncture wounds of the foot, *Am Fam Phys* 24:119, 1981.

130. Siebert WT, Dewan S, Williams TW: Case report: *Pseudomonas* puncture wound—Osteomyelitis in adults, *Am J Med Sci* 283:83, 1982.

131. Weston WJ: Thorn and Twig-induced pseudotumors of bone and soft tissues, *Br J Radiology* 36:323, 1963.

ENVIRONMENTAL PROBLEMS

CHAPTER

33

Animal and Human Bites

Julia A. Rosekrans

Although the true incidence of animal bites is not known because many bites are minor and treated at home, the Public Health Service has estimated that more than 1 million animal bites requiring medical attention occur annually in the United States.[1,2] Bites that require medical care account for almost 1% of emergency hospital visits, and the majority of patients treated for bite wounds are under 20 years of age. Dogs are responsible for about 85% of all animal bites.

ETIOLOGY

More than 50 million American families own a dog. A survey of families in a suburban pediatric group practice showed that 20% of children had been bitten by a dog at least once. Although stray dogs are feared as a source of biting attacks, family pets or neighbor dogs cause the majority of bites. The highest incidence of bites occurs among school-aged children, with boys being bitten twice as often as girls.[3,4] In colder climates where children spend less time outdoors in the winter, bites are a summertime hazard; but in temperate climates, children are bitten year round. The breed of dog most commonly involved is the

German shepherd, reflecting the popularity of this breed, its tendency to react viciously in some situations, and the bias of observers to identify any large dog as a "shepherd."

Between 1979 and 1988, approximately 200 deaths were related to dog bites. The majority of fatalities occur in children under 10 years of age. The pit bull, which accounts for about 1% of the U.S. dog population, is implicated in over 70% of fatalities; an increasing proportion of fatal attacks by this breed is an alarming trend.

Fatalities generally occur when no adult is present to stop an attack or assist the victim.[5-9] In most cases, the attacking dog has had a previous history of aggressive behavior toward people; the dog frequently outweighs the victim. Although there is little information about the initial events in these attacks, it has been suggested that behavior that appears threatening to the dog, such as poking it with a stick or wandering into its territory, often incites an attack. However, this behavior does not account for the attacks on small infants who are too immature to be threatening and who are most often attacked while sleeping. Although attacks on older children sometimes involve a group of dogs, fatal attacks on infants are usually caused by a single dog who is a family indoor pet.[10-12]

More families own cats than dogs; however, wounds caused by cats need emergency department treatment about one-fourth as often as dog bites. Cat bites and scratches cause less tissue damage but become infected more often than dog bites. Wounds caused by cats occur most often in the home and are found more often in girls than boys.[13]

Human bites are often treated in the emergency department after they have become infected. Although many of our ideas about human bites come from management problems in this group of patients, the group seen for medical care is highly selective and does not present the full spectrum of human bites. The majority of human bites in children are caused by other children; the face, hands, upper extremities, and trunk are the most common sites.[14,15] About 1 in every 600 pediatric visits to pediatric emergency centers is due to a human bite. Although the most common pattern of injury in human bites is a superficial abrasion, the majority of the literature on human bites concerns closed-fist injuries associated with fighting. Human bites may occur during play or as self-inflicted injuries. Bites may also be associated with physical and sexual abuse. Biting activity is higher among disturbed children, including those who are abused or are residents in state mental institutions.

The suspicion of child abuse should be considered in any child with a human bite. A single bite by an adult or multiple bites by other children, which occur if children are poorly supervised, may be indicators for investigation of suspected abuse by appropriate social service agencies. Bruise marks left from a bite can be measured to determine whether the bite was caused by an adult or child. The distance between the center of the canine teeth (third tooth on either side separated by four central incisors) should be measured in centimeters. If the distance is greater than 3 cm, the biter had permanent teeth; if the distance is less than 3 cm, the biter had primary teeth. Bite mark evidence has been admitted in court cases throughout the United States, and attention must be given to collecting forensic documentation in cases of bites in which a crime is suspected.[16]

Rat bites account for approximately 2% of animal bite wounds presenting to the emergency department. Victims are frequently children or adults with mental or physical disabilities. Social service evaluation of victims' homes revealed poor hygiene and frequently other family members who had also been bitten. Reports of wound infections from rat bites are too few to determine the flora likely to be responsible for infections; however, cultures of wounds before treatment showed a group of isolates typical of other mammalian flora. One large series found an infection rate of 2% when wounds were well cleaned. Wounds occurred mainly on the upper extremities and were most often single or multiple punctures.[17-19]

Ferrets are increasingly popular as pets, although they are classified as wild animals. Similar to weasles, they have been used to hunt small game and rodents. Although considered to be docile, playful animals, they are unpredictable and attacks by household ferrets have been reported resulting in very serious mutilation injuries to infants. These animals should not be allowed around young children.[20]

Other animals including pigs, alligators, camels, cougars, wolves, nonhuman primates, squirrels, and hamsters may cause bite wounds.[21-29] Although these bites have not been investigated extensively and statements about infecting organisms cannot be made, wound care is similar to other more familiar bites, with large animals causing crush injuries and small-toothed animals causing deep punctures.

DIAGNOSTIC FINDINGS

Clinical Findings

An animal bite is more complicated than a simple laceration because it involves mechanisms of both a puncture by a contaminated object and a crush injury.[30] A dog's teeth can exert pressures of 200 to 450 pounds per square inch and can penetrate steel plates. Although the majority of bites do not involve any injury other than the skin wound, fractures of underlying bones can occur. Tearing of soft tissue occurs when the animal shakes its head or the victim tries to escape. Large soft tissue defects may be accompanied by vascular or nerve injury. Puncture wounds are frequently deeper than estimated on initial examination; bites can quickly puncture down to a tendon sheath with resulting tenosynovitis.

Because small children are face to face with dogs, 58% of dog bites involve the head and neck. Most injuries occur in the lips, nose, and cheeks; 10% of facial bites in children involve periorbital trauma. Genital injuries have been described in both boys and girls, with serious tissue destruction.[31]

Animal bites to the head may be complicated by intracranial penetration.[32] Young children have a high incidence of bites to the head and their thin skull can be penetrated by the canine teeth of a large dog. Although such injuries may be severe and even fatal, unsuspected cranial punctures can be seen in children with completely normal neurologic examinations.

Cats bite with thin, sharp, needlelike teeth. They produce deep puncture wounds, which are difficult to clean. In addition to the nature of the wound, the frequency with which cat bites are located on victims' hands explains the high rate of serious soft tissue infections from these bites. Not infrequently, cat bites involve a puncture of a finger joint or a tendon sheath and seriously debilitating infections can develop.

Complications

Wound infections are found more frequently in bites on the extremities than in well-vascularized areas such as the scalp. Large extensive wounds seem to have lower infection rates than small wounds; puncture wounds account for as much as 40% of infected wounds, probably because of the difficulty in cleaning a puncture compared with a larger wound, which can be more thoroughly irrigated. Infections occur most often in patients with predisposing conditions such as immunosuppression.[33,34]

Dog bites have a low infection rate of 2% to 5% despite the crushing component of the injury. A wide variety of organisms that come from the animal's saliva rather than the victim's skin flora have been isolated from bite wound cultures. There is a high incidence of infections with *Pasteurella multocida* after bites. *Staphylococcus aureus* is a common secondary infection; coagulase negative staphylococci, streptococci, and some enteric bacteria are also frequently identified. When they are specifically looked for, anaerobic bacteria are also regularly recovered.[35]

Signs of infection usually develop within 72 hours after a bite. Redness, swelling, and tenderness develop around the site of injury with serosanguinous or purulent drainage. Recognition of infection is often difficult, as the crush injury of the wound may also cause swelling and tenderness. Cellulitis with abscess formation may follow a gradually increasing course typical of *S. aureus,* or in the case of streptococcal infection may be rapidly progressive with lymphangitis and systemic signs of fever, chills, and tachycardia. *P. multocida* infections typically show a virulent clinical course, with redness and swelling developing rapidly within the first 12 to 24 hours after the bite. Although temperature is usually normal and lymph node involvement is not common, intense local pain often accompanies this infection.[36,37]

Cats bite and scratch simultaneously with their claws. Because cats frequently lick their paws, their scratches may be inoculated with saliva. Even their scratches have a greater tendency to become infected than scratches from a dog. *P. multocida* is a common bacteria in the saliva of cats and is a frequent cause of infections in these wounds. Approximately 40% of cat bites and scratches become infected despite initial cleaning. Cats can also transmit diseases such as cat scratch fever and tularemia (see Chapter 55). Cat scratch fever is caused by a small, pleomorphic gram-negative bacterium. Regional lymphadenopathy of an extremity occurs an average of 14 days (3 to 50 days) after the scratch (see Chapters 49 and 55).

The human mouth contains many different bacterial species. The most common isolated etiologies of wound infections are *S. aureus*, streptococci, and anaerobes such as *Eikenella corrodens*. A variety of gram-negative organisms have also been cultured from dental scrapings and wounds. Because of experience with the severe consequences of closed-fist injuries, all human bites have a reputation for being easily infected. However, simple bites that are seen and treated soon after the injury and superficial abrasions do not appear to be associated with any higher rate of infection than nonbite lacerations. The most serious infections develop in closed-fist-fighting injuries in which bacteria may be introduced by the puncture of an incisor into the joint space or extensor tendons overlying the metacarpal heads. Because these injuries often occur in people who do not seek medical care quickly and who do not readily volunteer the nature of the injury, the wounds are frequently infected at the time of the presentation to the emergency department.

Concern has been raised about the possibility of transmission of HIV infection through bites, as this virus has been isolated from human saliva. One report has suggested this type of transmission between siblings, but the majority of reports have shown a failure of transmission of HIV virus by biting, and this route of transmission is considered low risk by the Centers for Disease Control.[38,39] Human bites have been implicated in transmission of herpes simplex, which is commonly excreted in respiratory secretions of toddlers. Herpetic whitlow is a well-known hazard among dental workers and is also a common infection from self-inoculation by nail biters.[40] Hepatitis B can also theoretically be transmitted from a human bite.

Because the depth of inoculation of bacteria is difficult to estimate on initial examination, it is important to be suspicious of abscess formation, infections of joints and tendons, and even development of osteomyelitis when inflammation, tenderness, or diminished use of an extremity persists.

Serious infectious complications may follow animal or human bites. Sepsis, meningitis, and endocarditis have been reported, especially in the presence of factors such as malnutrition, splenectomy, or immunosuppression, which increase susceptibility to infection.[41-44] Severe systemic complications of wound infections such as toxic shock syndrome and sepsis, as well as osteomyelitis, septic arthritis, and tenosynovitis due to anaerobic bacteria, have been described.

Ancillary Data

Radiographs should be taken in deep bite wounds in which there is any possibility of fracture. Skull x-ray films are helpful in children with scalp wounds, as bone penetration may not otherwise be suspected. All closed-fist injuries should be evaluated with radiography to document fractures, foreign bodies such as teeth, and air in the joints.

Because of the crushing nature of many dog bites, angiography may be needed to determine the extent of major vessel injury. Angiography should be considered in any bitten extremity in which there is absent or decreased arterial pulse, sensory or motor deficit, a large or expanding hematoma, or active arterial bleeding.[45] Severe dog attacks involving damage to the head and neck may cause suffocation from tracheal trauma or pressure from massive hematoma. Patients with wounds to the neck may suffer damage to carotid arteries leading to cerebral ischemia.

Bite marks thought to involve abuse or the need for law enforcement investigation should be photographed with a small ruler indicating centimeters to provide a scale for reference.

DIFFERENTIAL CONSIDERATIONS

Preschool children may not be able to provide the history of a bite injury, and superficial bites have been mistaken for other conditions such as dermatophyte infections. Differential considerations for bites include any oval-shaped, superficial dermatologic lesion, including fixed drug eruptions, subacute cutaneous lupus erythematosus, pityriasis rosea, and granuloma annulae.[46]

MANAGEMENT

All bites require thorough wound cleaning with judicious debridement of damaged tissue. Povidone-iodine solution provides antibacterial and antiviral activity, which is useful in the presence of a mixed flora inoculum. The solution is preferable to the scrub; solution does not contain detergent compounds, which are painful and can damage uninjured subcutaneous tissue.[47-51]

After cleansing with povidone-iodine solution, all bite wounds should be irrigated with several hundred milliliters of normal saline. The simplest available system in any emergency department for providing high pressure irrigation is an 18- or 19-gauge needle with a 35 ml or larger syringe, which can generate 7 pounds/square inch of pressure. This technique is much more effective for deep cleansing and reducing actual bacterial counts of contaminated wounds than trying to soak the wound or using a low-pressure bulb syringe.

Debridement of all visible devitalized subcutaneous tissue and dermis should be performed carefully on all bite wounds including punctures. Although this procedure helps to reduce the amount of microbial contamination of the wound, it is not always possible in wounds of the face, neck, or hands. Strong consideration must be given to exploration and cleaning in the operating room for all full-thickness wounds of hands, upper extremities, and head and neck. This technique is essential if a joint or tendon may have been bitten, and such wounds should be explored carefully for tendon injury. It is essential to assure that no injury to underlying structures has occurred.

In general most bite wounds are left open; however, primary closure has been successful in areas in which unsightly scarring could otherwise result.[52] Wounds on the face can be sutured using material such as monofilament nylon, which causes little tissue reaction, with minimal placement of subcutaneous absorbable sutures. This technique should be tried only in bites that occurred within a few hours of medical care and only after extremely thorough cleansing and irrigation. Because of the rich blood supply to the face, infection rates there seem to be lower than to other parts of the body.[53-55] Deep puncture wounds, particularly cat bites, which are difficult to clean, should never be closed.

Bites occurring in the periorbital area that potentially involve ocular structures should be referred to an ophthalmologist for specialized care.[56,57] In this area, the lacrimal drainage system must be evaluated and repair instituted quickly. As many as 40% of cat wounds near the eye include corneal abrasions. Because of the dire consequences of periocular infections, these wounds need specialty care.

All patients with bite wounds should be questioned about tetanus immunization status. Because many of the children who are bitten are preschoolers, it is not uncommon to find that their immunization status is deficient or that it is time for the preschool booster (see Chapter 55).

Rabies should be considered in any animal bite. The immunization status of a domestic cat or dog that has bitten someone should be documented in that person's medical record. Behavior at the time of the incident and potential for the animal's exposure to rabies should be recorded. Cats transmit rabies more frequently than dogs in the United States and even a scratch contaminated with saliva could have the potential to transmit rabies. Rabid pet ferrets have been reported in the United States, but no rabies vaccine is available for ferrets. Because the natural history of rabies in the ferret is not known, no quarantine recommendations are available. Killing the ferret and examining the brain for rabies virus antigen is recommended after any ferret bite. Rabbits and rodents (rats, mice, gerbils, hamsters, squirrels) are not known to transmit rabies in the United States. Public health departments require that animal bites be reported; every emergency department should enact procedures to ensure that reporting takes place. Many public health offices are very helpful resources in determining the risk of rabies in a particular community and may also supply or administer rabies vaccine when it is indicated (see Chapter 55).

Despite many carefully designed studies, prophylactic antibiotics have not been shown conclusively to reduce dog bite wound infections. This is hardly surprising, as there is a long lag between the time the wound is inflicted and the time for oral antibiotics to develop adequate tissue levels. A metaanalysis[58] of eight randomized trials indicates that prophylactic antibiotics should be limited to wounds that are at high risk for infection. These include infections on the hands, deep puncture wounds, and wounds in immunocompromised hosts. Studies regarding the efficacy of irrigation of wounds with antibiotics or intravenous administration of antibiotics are inconclusive. Currently, good cleaning and debridement are the most important factors in reducing infection for common small wounds in low-risk patients.[59] Wounds with extensive damage require particular attention to irrigation and debridement. Prophylactic antibiotics are not recommended for superficial dog bites or human bites that have been cleaned properly.[60] On the other hand, antibiotics should be given to all but the most superficial cat scratches because of the difficulty in cleaning puncture wounds and the high rate of associated infection.[61-65]

A wound may be considered high risk for infection based on its location, type, or underlying risk factors in the patient and may benefit from prophylactic antibiotics. All wounds of the hands, wrist, and feet, as well as puncture wounds that cannot be irrigated, are high risk.[66-69] Extensive wounds where devitalized tissue cannot be entirely debrided; wounds involving tendons, joints, or bones; sutured wounds; puncture wounds; crush injuries; and bites in patients with peripheral vascular insufficiency should also be considered high risk. Patients who are asplenic or immunocompromised are at higher risk for developing infections in wounds that appear simple. It may be prudent to administer a first dose of antibiotic intravenously to achieve rapid tissue levels and then continue with oral antibiotic if a patient with a high risk factor will be treated as an outpatient.

Patients who present for care after a wound infection has developed, and patients with cat bites must be treated with antibiotics that cover possible *P. multocida*, streptococcal, and staphylococcal infections. Although *P. multocida* is very sensitive to penicillin, it is relatively resistant to the penicillinase-resistant penicillins and first-generation cephalosporins. This resistance has led to a treatment with a combination of penicillin VK (25 to 50 mg/kg/24 hr QID PO) and dicloxacillin (50 mg/kg/24 hr QID PO). Amoxicillin/clavulanate (30 to 50 mg amoxicillin/kg/24 hr TID PO) eliminates the need for taking two medications but is expensive and causes gastrointestinal upset in some patients. Cefuroxime is effective against the spectrum of possible organisms but is also quite expensive. Although erythromycin is sometimes suggested as an alternative in penicillin-allergic patients, it is not appropriate for bite infections because infections have been reported to occur in some patients. Trimethoprim/sulfa can be used to manage *P. multocida* in patients with a history of penicillin allergy; this does not manage staphylococcal or streptococcal infections. Tetracycline or ciprofloxacin is effective against *P. multocida* but should not be used in growing children younger than 12 years of age.

Elevation and immobilization to reduce tissue swelling are important aspects of bite wound care, especially for wounds of the hands. Any patient treated as an outpatient for a wound that is more than a simple scratch should be reevaluated within 48 hours to observe function of the wounded area and to check for infection. Patients should be advised to return immediately if they develop increasing tenderness or swelling in the wound; red streaking; tender, swollen, regional lymph nodes; or fever and chills. If an infection does not respond to outpatient antibiotic therapy or if there is any suggestion of bacteremia or possible sepsis, intravenous antibiotics (Penicillin G 100,000 units/kg/24 hr q 4 hr IV *and* nafcillin [or equivalent] 100 mg/kg/24 hr q 4 hr IV should be given. Wound discharge and blood should be cultured for both aerobic and anaerobic organisms as outlined and laboratory personnel notified to search for uncommon pathogens such as DF-2 or 11J.[70]

Inpatient care or specialty consultation must be considered in several situations: all bites of the hand unless they are very fresh and superficial; extensive wounds; any wound involving a joint, tendon, cartilage or bone; severely disfiguring wounds; and potentially poor patient compliance.[68,69,71]

PREVENTION

Because the majority of animal bites are caused by pets, families who choose to have pets should follow guidelines to reduce the hazards of interactions between children and animals. Infants should never be left alone with a pet, and preschoolers should be supervised even around their own pets. Families should choose gentle breeds, but must also recognize that bites are often caused by a pet that has never before shown signs of aggressive behavior.[72] Children must be taught to treat animals with respect and to leave them alone when they are eating and sleeping and when they are immature puppies or kittens. Pet owners must keep animals under control and seek professional help when they have pets with behavior problems. The costly damage caused by animals could be ameliorated if children were taught proper behavior toward animals and animal owners maintained responsible attitudes.

References

1. Kizer KW: Epidemiologic and clinical aspects of animal bite injuries, *JACEP* 8:134, 1979.
2. Aghababian RV and Conte JE: Mammalian bite wounds, *Ann Emerg Med* 9:79, 1980.

Etiology

3. Galloway RE: Mammalian bites, *J Emerg Med* 6:325, 1988.
4. Wishon PM and Huang A: Pet-associated injuries: the trouble with children's best friends, *Children Today* May-June, 1989.
5. Winkler WG: Human deaths induced by dog bites, United States, 1974-75, *Public Health Rep* 92:425, 1977.
6. Pinckney LE and Kennedy LA: Traumatic deaths from dog attacks in the United States, *Pediatrics* 69:193, 1982.
7. Borchelt PL, Lockwood R, Beck AM et al: Attacks by packs of dogs involving predation on human beings, *Public Health Rep* 98:57, 1983.
8. Wright JC: Severe attacks by dogs: characteristics of the dogs, the victims, and the attack settings, *Public Health Rep* 100:55, 1985.
9. Sacks JJ, Sattin RW, Bonzo SE: Dog bite-related fatalities from 1979 through 1988, *JAMA* 262:1489, 1989.
10. Viegas SF, Calhoun JH, Mader J: Pit bull attack: case report and literature review, *Tex Med* 84:40, 1988.
11. Baack BR, Kucan JO, Demarest G et al: Mauling by pit bull terriers: case report, *J Trauma* 29:517, 1989.
12. Kneafsey B and Condon KC: Severe dog-bite injuries, introducing the concept of pack attack: a literature review and seven case reports, *Injury* 26:37, 1995.
13. Wright JC: Reported cat bites in Dallas: characteristics of the cats, the victim, and the attack events, *Public Health Rep* 105:420, 1990.
14. Baker MD and Moore SE: Human bites in children: a six-year experience, *Am J Dis Child* 141:1285, 1987.
15. Faciszewski T and Coleman DA: Human bite wounds, *Hand Clin* 5:561, 1989.

16. Gold MH, Roenigk HH, Smith ES et al: Evaluation and treatment of patients with human bite marks, *Am J Forensic Med Pathol* 10:140, 1989.
17. Ordog GJ, Balasubramanium S, Wasserberger J et al: Rat bites: fifty cases, *Ann Emerg Med* 14:126, 1985.
18. Wykes WN: Rat bite injury to the eyelids in a 3-month-old child, *Br J Ophthalmol* 73:202, 1989.
19. McHugh TP, Bartlett RL, Raymond JI: Rat bite fever: report of a fatal case, *Ann Emerg Med* 14:1116, 1985.
20. Paisley JW and Lauer BA: Severe facial injuries to infants due to unprovoked attacks by pet ferrets, *JAMA* 259:2005, 1988.
21. Barnham M: Pig bite injuries and infection: report of seven human cases, *Epidemiol Infect* 101:641, 1988.
22. Flandry F, Lisecki EJ, Domingue GJ et al: Initial antibiotic therapy for alligator bites: characterization of the oral flora of Alligator mississippiensis, *South Med J* 82:262, 1989.
23. Amer Al-Boukai A, El-Din Hawass N, Patel PJ et al: Camel bites: report of severe osteolysis as late bone complications, *Postgrad Med J* 65:900, 1989.
24. Kizer KW: *Pasteurella multocida* infection from a cougar bite: a review of cougar attacks, *West J Med* 150:87, 1989.
25. Cherkasky BL: Roles of the wolf and the raccoon dog in the ecology and epidemiology of rabies in the USSR, *Rev Infect Dis* 10:S634, 1988.
26. Campbell AC: Primate bites in Gibraltar—minor casualty quirk? *Scot Med J* 34:519, 1989.
27. Janda DH, Ringler DH, Hilliard JK et al: Nonhuman primate bites, *J Orthop Res* 8:146, 1990.
28. Magee JS, Steele RW, Kelly NR et al: Tularemia transmitted by a squirrel bite, *Pediatr Infect Dis J* 8:123, 1989.
29. Martin RW, Martin DL, Levy CS et al: Acinetobacter osteomyelitis from a hamster bite, *Pediatr Infect Dis J* 7:364, 1988.

Diagnostic Findings

30. Tuggle DW, Taylor DV, Stevens RJ: Dog bites in children, *J Ped Surg* 28:912, 1993.
31. Redman JF: Genital dog bite injuries in infants and children, *Clinical Pediatrics* 34(6):331, 1995.
32. Wilberger JE and Pang D: Craniocerebral injuries from dog bites, *JAMA* 249:2685, 1983.
33. Marcy SM: Special series: management of pediatric infectious diseases in office practice, *Pediatr Infect Dis* 1:351, 1982.
34. Dire DJ, Hogan DE, Riggs MW: A prospective evaluation of risk factors for infections from dog-bite wounds, *Acad Emerg Med* 1:258-266, 1994.
35. Brook I: Microbiology of human and animal bite wounds in children, *Pediatr Infect Dis* J 6:29, 1987.
36. Brook I: Human and animal bite infections, *J Fam Pract* 28:713, 1989.
37. Weber DJ, Wolfson JS, Swartz MN et al: *Pasteurella multocida* infections: report of 34 cases and review of the literature, *Medicine* 63:133, 1984.
38. Shirley LR and Ross SA: Risk of transmission of human immunodeficiency virus by bite of an infected toddler, *J Pediatr* 114:425, 1989.
39. Tsoukas CM, Hadjis T, Shuster J et al: Lack of transmission of HIV through human bites and scratches, *J Acquir Immune Defic Syndr* 1:505, 1988.
40. Fuortes L and Melson E: Brief report: primary and recurrent herpes simplex infection in a pediatric nurse resulting from a human bite, *Infect Control Hosp Epidemiol* 10:120, 1989.
41. Sackier JM and Daly K: Massive perineal sepsis due to *Bacteroides fragilis*, *J R Coll Surg Edinb* 34:110, 1989.
42. Long WT, Filler BC, Cox E et al: Toxic shock syndrome after a human bite to the hand, *J Hand Surg* 13A:957, 1988.
43. Karody R, Nash N, Bhasin V et al: Toxic shock syndrome due to an infected human bite, *Ann Emerg Med* 17:83, 1988.
44. Minton EJ: *Pasteurella pneumotripica:* meningitis following a dog bite, *Postgrad Med J* 66:125, 1990.
45. Snyder KB and Pentecost MJ: Clinical and angiographic findings in extremity arterial injuries secondary to dog bites, *Ann Emerg Med* 19:983, 1990.

Differential Considerations

46. Gold MH, Roenigk HH, Smith ES et al: Human bite marks—differential diagnosis, *Clin Pediatr* 28:329, 1989.

Management

47. Edlich RF, Spengler MD, Rodeheaver GT et al: Emergency department management of mammalian bites, *Emerg Med Clin* North Am 4:595, 1986.
48. Rest JG and Goldstein EJC: Management of human and animal bite wounds, *Emerg Med Clin North Am* 3:117, 1985.
49. Snyder CC: Animal bite wounds, *Hand Clin* 5:571, 1989.
50. Goldstein EJC: Management of human and animal bite wounds, *J Am Acad Dermatol* 21:1275, 1989.
51. McDonough JJ, Stern PJ, Alexander JW: Management of animal and human bites and resulting human infections, *Curr Clin Top Infect Dis* 8:11, 1987.
52. Maimaris C and Quinton DN: Dog-bite lacerations: a controlled trial of primary wound closure, *Arch Emerg Med* 5:156, 1988.
53. Venter THJ: Human bites of the face—early surgical management, *SA Med J* 74:277, 1988.
54. Datubo-Brown DD: Human bites of the face with tissue losses, *Ann Plast Surg* 21:322, 1988.
55. Morgan JP, Haug RH, Murphy MT: Management of facial dog bite injuries, *J Oral Maxillofac Surg* 53:435, 1995.
56. Herman DC, Bartley GB, Walker RC: The treatment of animal bite injuries of the eye and ocular adnexa, *Ophthalmic Plast Reconstr Surg* 3:237, 1987.
57. Cummings P: Antibiotics to prevent infection in patients with dog bite wounds: a meta-analysis of randomized trails, *Emerg Med* 23:535, 1994.
58. Dire DJ, Hogan DE, Walker JS: Prophylactic oral antibiotics for low-risk dog bite wounds, *Pediatr Emerg Care* 8:194, 1992.
59. Vila-Coro AA, Bonafonte S, del Cotero JNF: Ocular human bite, *Ann Ophthalmol* 21:100, 1989.
60. Rosen RA: The use of antibiotics in the initial management of recent dog-bite wounds, *Am J Emerg Med* 3:19, 1985.
61. Brakenbury PH and Muwanga C: A comparative double blind study of amoxycillin/clavulanate vs placebo in the prevention of infection after animal bites, *Arch Emerg Med* 6:251, 1989.
62. Callaham M: Controversies in antibiotic choices for bite wounds, *Ann Emerg Med* 17:1321, 1988.
63. Levin JM: Erythromycin failure with subsequent *Pasteurella multocida* meningitis and septic arthritis in a cat-bite victim, *Ann Emerg Med* 19:1458, 1990.
64. Feder HM, Shanley JD, Barbera JA: Review of 59 patients hospitalized with animal bites, *Pediatr Infect Dis J* 6:24, 1987.
65. Dellinger EP, Wertz MJ, Miller SD: Hand infections—bacteriology and treatment: a prospective study, *Arch Surg* 123:745, 1988.
66. Dunbar JD: Serious infection following wounds and bites of the hand, *N Z Med J* 8:368, 1988.
67. Lindsey D, Christopher M, Hollenbach J et al: Natural course of the human bite wound: incidence of infection and complications in 434 bites and 803 lacerations in the same group of patients, *J Trauma* 27:45, 1987.
68. Donovan JF and Kaplan WE: The therapy of genital trauma by dog bite, *J Urol* 141:1163, 1989.
69. Turpin IM, Altman DI, Cruz HG et al: Salvage of the severely injured ear, *Ann Plast Surg* 21:170, 1988

Prevention

70. Lauer EA, White WC, Lauer BA: Dog bites—a neglected problem in accident prevention, *Am J Dis Child* 136:202, 1982.
71. Mathews JR and Lattal KA: A behavioral analysis of dog bites to children, *JDBP* 15:44, 1994.
72. Baker MD: Bites and scratches: when pets fight back, *Contemp Pediatr* 6(6):76, 1989.

## 34

Venomous Animal Bites and Stings

Susan B. Tully • Willis A. Wingert

Natural venoms may be characterized according to function and composition into offensive and defensive venoms. *Offensive* venoms are designed to obtain food by immobilizing or killing prey and initiating digestion of the prey's tissue. These venoms usually are secreted at the oral pole, often by modified salivary glands, and are very stable to changes in temperature, moisture, and pH.[1]

Venoms are composed of peptides and proteins of low molecular weight (<100,000), which are rapidly lethal to the prey, as well as a variety of digestive enzymes. Enzymes are required because of a usual lack of masticatory apparatus and the resistant integument of the prey: hair, scales, and feathers. The clinical effect of an offensive venom is paralysis or death due to any combination of neurologic, circulatory, or excretory dysfunction; tissue or organ necrosis occurs secondary to enzyme action. Snake and spider venoms are offensive venoms.

Defensive venoms are designed to drive away predators, invariably causing severe local pain and sometimes a generalized neurologic reaction such as paralysis or dysrhythmias due to the action on the sodium channels of nerves. These venoms generally are secreted by dermal tissues and delivered from the aboral pole or via dorsal spines. The venom lacks digestive enzymes, so tissue necrosis is not prominent. The compounds are characterized by instability to heat and pH changes; a temperature change of 1° C may inactivate them. Almost all marine venoms are considered defensive. A few animal venoms, such as scorpions, include both offensive and defensive venoms.

A venomous animal produces a toxic substance within its own body cells, often in a specific secretory organ. A poisonous animal is one in which stable toxic substances originate outside the body of the animal, but accumulate in the tissue, usually as a result of ingestion of toxic algae or plankton and passage of the toxin through the food chain (e.g., ciguatera or scombroid poisoning). As this chapter deals exclusively with injury by venomous animals, poisonous animals will not be discussed further.

VENOMOUS REPTILES

Of an estimated 45,000 snakebites annually, about 12,000 to 15,000 are by venomous snakes.[2] There have been only 1 to 2 deaths annually since 1990.[3] The venomous snakes in the United States belong to two families: the Crotalidae, or pit vipers, and the Elapidae, or coral snakes. Identifying characteristics of the Crotalidae are vertical, elliptical ("cat's eye") pupils; triangular head; indentation or pit located between the eye and the nostril; and two movable recurved fangs in the upper jaw. The genus *Crotalus*, rattlesnakes, has a series of horny rings (rattles) on the tail, which are lacking in the genus *Agkistrodon*, the copperheads and moccasins. The Elapidae, coral snakes, have round pupils; short, fixed maxillary fangs; a black snout; and a distinctive sequence of ring colors: yellow rings are always adjacent to red rings (many mimics occur).

Snake species are limited geographically. The Elapidae occur only in Arizona and the southern Gulf states. The distribution of the major venomous species by region is indicated in the box on p. 466.[1] About 90% of envenomations occur between April and October, as poikilodermic snakes hibernate in winter months. About 50% of all bites occur in young adult males (18 to 28 years) and most are associated with a high incidence of acute alcohol intoxication. Bites are usually on the extremities: hand and/or finger (80%) and foot and/or ankle (15%). At least 40% are "nonaccidental," caused by careless handling of a known venomous reptile.[4]

Pathophysiology

Crotalid venom consists of two basic components: peptides and enzymes. The low-molecular-weight peptides and polypeptides are responsible for the immediate lethal effects. These proteins damage vascular endothelial cells and lyse cellular plasma membranes. A transient microangiopathic vascular permeability results, with extravasation of plasma, plasma proteins, and erythrocytes into the tissues.[5] Clinically this is manifested by progressive edema and subcutaneous hemorrhage at the site.

Distribution of Venomous Species

Northeast	Copperhead
	Timber rattlesnake
	Massasauga
Midwest	Timber rattlesnake
	Prairie rattlesnake
	Copperhead
South	Eastern diamondback
	Water moccasin (cottonmouth)
	Copperhead
	Eastern coral snake
Rocky Mountains	Prairie rattlesnake
Southwest	Moccasin
	Copperhead (Texas)
	Coral snake (Texas, Arizona)
	Western diamondback
	Sidewinder
	Mojave rattlesnake
West Coast	Pacific rattlesnake

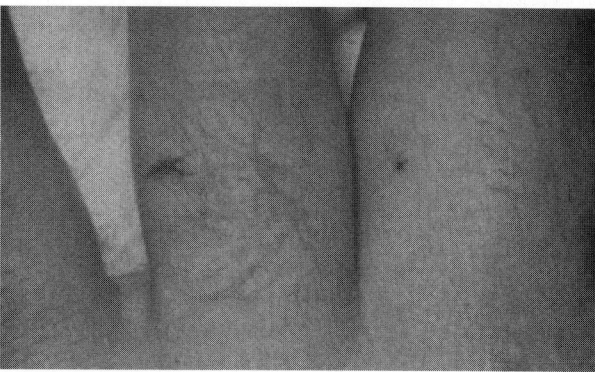

FIG. 34-1. Typical rattlesnake fang marks, with minimal local reaction. (*From Wingert WA, Wainschel J: South Med J 68: 1021, 1975.*)

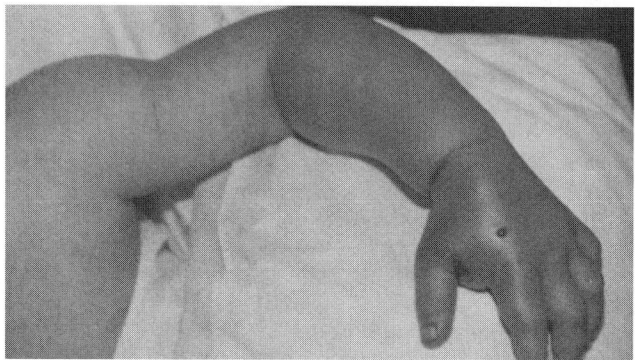

FIG. 34-2. Arm of a 2-year-old child, showing moderate rattlesnake envenomation.

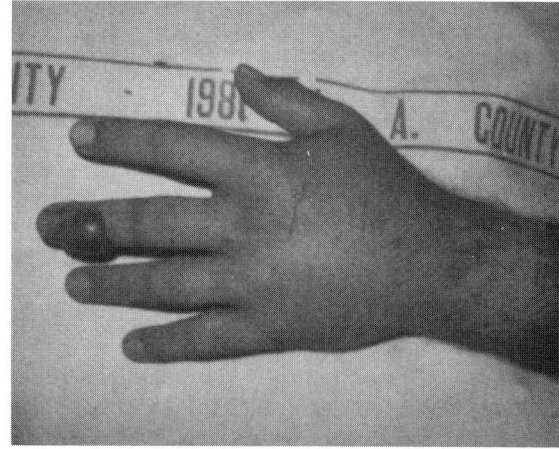

FIG. 34-3. Hemorrhagic bleb at site of severe rattlesnake bite; marks indicate progress of edema.

Tissue destruction, both local and systemic, is caused by various digestive enzymes. Phospholipase A_2, common to all species' venoms, is an esterolytic enzyme, damaging lipid cell membranes of erythrocytes (hemolysis) and the plasma membranes of muscle cells (necrosis). Thrombin-like enzymes split fibrinopeptide A or B from the fibrin molecule, but do not activate factor XIII. Unstable fibrin clots are formed, readily lysed by plasmin. Afibrinogenemia, thrombocytopenia, and increased fibrin split products result, and extensive, uncontrollable hemorrhage may follow.[6]

The severity of the envenomation depends on the quantity of venom injected and the relative toxicity of the venom, as well as host factors, such as the size and age of the victim. The quantity is determined by the size and species of the snake, the number of bites, the irritability of the snake, the length of time the fangs remain imbedded, and the interval since the snake last discharged its venom. Because snakes do not inject all of their venom in a single strike, approximately 20% of bites result in minimal or no envenomation.[4] The most dangerous snakes are the large, aggressive diamondbacks, the highly toxic Southern Pacific and Mojave rattlesnakes, and the neurotoxic coral snake. Copperhead venom is the least toxic; envenomation rarely requires treatment.[7]

Diagnostic Findings

Crotalidae envenomation causes both systemic and local signs and symptoms. The bite causes a brief stinging or burning pain; occasionally no pain is felt (Fig. 34-1). Early and progressive swelling begins at the bite site; rapid progression indicates severe envenomation. The extremity appears tense and shiny, but this edema rarely compromises vascular or nerve supply. Ecchymosis develops around the bite and may extend proximally (Fig. 34-2). As the edema progresses, pain in the extremity may become severe.

Hemorrhagic blebs and bullae develop secondary to extensive edema (Fig. 34-3).

Paresthesias of the scalp, face, and extremities are reported, especially in bites by diamondbacks and Pacific rattlesnakes. A metallic taste occurs early in envenomation

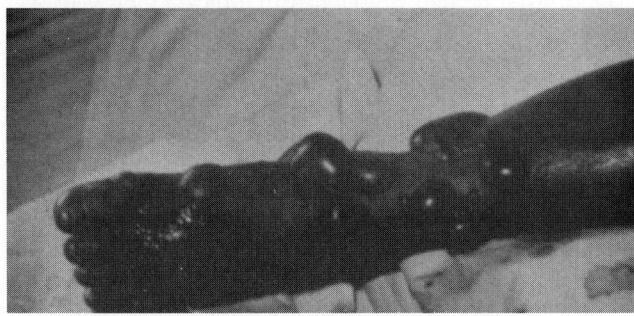

FIG. 34-4. Severe rattlesnake bite, third day, untreated for 24 hours after envenomation. Edema and bullae, lower leg; tissue necrosis, dorsum of foot. (*From Wingert WA, Wainschel J:* South Med J *68:1021, 1975.*)

by diamondbacks and timber and Pacific rattlesnakes. Muscle fasciculations may occur. After envenomation by some species of Mojave rattlesnakes, progressive paralysis occurs, beginning in the cranial nerves.

Signs and symptoms of Elapidae envenomation are primarily neurologic. There may be one or more fang marks in the fingers or toes; blood may ooze. Local swelling is usually not marked. Paresthesias are common. Early symptoms of diplopia, hoarseness, and dysphagia represent cranial nerve palsies. The symptoms may progress to respiratory paralysis.

Complications. Local tissue necrosis may occur at the bite site if the envenomation is inadequately treated (Fig. 34-4). In severe envenomation, hypotension, hypovolemic shock, and pulmonary edema develop secondary to plasma transudation. Renal failure is a late complication, secondary to hemolysis and hypotension. Serum sickness occurs in a large proportion of treated patients, regardless of skin test results.

Ancillary Data. Initial laboratory studies should include a complete blood count with examination of the blood smear for morphologic changes (spherocytosis and pyknocytosis of erythrocytes). Urinalysis may reveal hematuria and proteinuria. The possibility of coagulopathy should be investigated with prothrombin time, partial thromboplastin time, platelet count, fibrin split products, and fibrinogen. Additional baseline studies include electrolytes and serum protein. Creatine phosphokinase elevation is a marker for severe envenomation.

Management

In the prehospital setting, do not incise or suction the fang marks. Remove constrictive clothing and jewelry. Attempt to estimate the length and size of the snake, and identify the type of snake. If species identification is important (in geographic areas where major toxic species overlap), kill the snake with a sharp blow on the neck and transport it in a sealed container to the closest trained person. Immobilize the extremity by splinting or applying an elastic bandage at less than venous pressure. Do not apply a tourniquet. Mark the proximal level of the edema with ink; record the time and transport the victim to a medical facility expeditiously.

TABLE 34-1. Determination of Severity of Envenomation and Therapy Snakebites

Severity	Findings	Initial therapy
None	Fang marks only; no local or systemic signs or symptoms	No skin test/ antivenom
Minimal	Fang marks with slowly progressive local swelling; no systemic symptoms	5 vials (50 ml)
Moderate	History of multiple or provoked bites or bite of large venomous snake or highly toxic species (Mojave, diamondback); fang marks with edema rapidly progressing beyond the bite site; systemic symptoms including metallic taste, parasthesias; laboratory abnormalities	10 vials (100 ml)
Severe	History of bite of highly toxic snake, prolonged imbedding of fangs, and multiple bites; fang marks with very rapidly progressive edema, subcutaneous hemorrhage; severe systemic reaction with muscle fasciculation, hypotension, oliguria; laboratory abnormalities	15 vials (150 ml)

After the patient arrives at the medical facility, obtain a history, particularly including the circumstances of the bite, size of the snake, first aid measures used, time elapsed since the bite, and known allergies to drugs or serum. Verify that the patient was bitten by a poisonous snake by finding one or more fang marks, distinctive puncture wounds with ragged edges, and the presence of characteristic symptoms. Symptoms may be slow to develop, especially in Crotalidae bites; therefore, the patient should be observed for at least 6 hours.[8]

Establish a physiologic baseline by obtaining vital signs and measuring and recording the circumference of the bitten extremity at the leading point of edema and 10 cm proximal to this point.

Grade the severity of envenomation using the schema indicated in Table 34-1. If envenomated, test for horse serum sensitivity as indicated in the antivenom package insert. Note that this skin test is neither highly sensitive nor reliable.

Start two intravenous lines, one line to administer antivenom, the other for life support and additional therapy. If the skin test is negative, administer an adequate amount of neutralizing gamma globulin antibody, depending on the severity of the bite. Crotalid antivenom (Antivenin [Crotalidae] Polyvalent-Wyeth-Ayerst) should be thoroughly dissolved as indicated in the package insert and then diluted 1:4 with 0.45% normal saline. The infusion should be started slowly (15 drops/min); if no reaction occurs, increase the rate and administer the dose over 2 hours. For small children, administer at a rate of 20 ml/kg/hr. The initial dose should be given based on the degree of envenomation (see Table 34-1). The smaller the body of the patient, the larger the initial dose required. Children seem to be more sensitive. Children weighing < 25 kg usually require a 50% larger dose.

Coral snake antivenom (Antivenin [Micrurus fulvius]-Wyeth-Ayerst) is diluted 1:5 with 0.45% normal saline, and administered over 2 hours. The dose is 10 vials for bites of large snakes or those with fangs imbedded, or if there has been a treatment delay of longer than 2 hours. Six vials are an appropriate dose for all others.[9]

If the skin test is positive, or if allergic reaction occurs during infusion of the antivenom, it is prudent to consider the absolute necessity of the treatment, if possible in consultation with a poison control center. If treatment is deemed necessary, pretreatment with H_1 (diphenhydramine) and H_2 (cimetidine) blockers intravenously is appropriate. Start the antivenom infusion at a dilution of 1:10 slowly (10 drops/minute), and observe for signs of anaphylaxis. If no reaction occurs in 20 minutes, the infusion rate may be increased slowly, while continuing close observation of the patient. If no further reaction occurs, the rate, and, if needed to avoid volume overload, the concentration of the solution may be adjusted to deliver the dose over 2 more hours. If anaphylactic reaction still occurs after pretreatment, as indicated earlier, and the patient is severely envenomated, it is possible to titrate with an epinephrine infusion and continue the antivenom; this technique should be performed in consultation with a poison control center.

Even without a positive skin test, one should be prepared to treat anaphylaxis, but severe allergic reactions in children are rare. Most milder ones can be managed with brief discontinuation of the infusion, treatment with diphenhydramine, and resumption of a more dilute infusion when the reaction has subsided.

Monitor the patient's progress and be prepared to treat complications. Follow vital signs, especially blood pressure, as well as fluid intake and output. Hypovolemia is best treated with colloid rather than crystalloid solutions.[10] The choice of colloid (5% albumin, whole blood, or fresh frozen plasma) will depend on the presence of other symptoms, such as coagulopathy. Correct falling hematocrit with packed red blood cells, but do not replace coagulation factors unless active bleeding occurs. Measure the progress of the edema. Mechanical ventilation may be required for coral snake or Mojave rattlesnake bites. Patients with coral snake bites should be observed for 72 hours.

Repeat Crotalidae antivenom at the initial dose every 2 hours until all symptoms have resolved and the swelling no longer progresses. Although antivenom is most efficacious within the first 6 hours after a bite, it may have some effect up to 72 hours, if the patient remains symptomatic.[8] It is important not to undertreat the poisoning. Additional doses of five vials of coral snake antivenom should be given every 2 to 3 hours if neurologic symptoms progress.

Fasciotomy is virtually never indicated. The muscle necrosis seen following a snakebite is the product of the proteolytic enzymes in the venom rather than increased compartmental pressure.[11] Large series of patients have been treated successfully without this mutilating technique.[4]

Administer tetanus prophylaxis if indicated. Prevent secondary infection in severe bites and those who have had nonsterile first aid by administering an antibiotic effective against anaerobic and gram-negative bacteria (ampicillin, amoxicillin, or second-generation cephalosporin).

Serum sickness develops in 7 to 14 days in all patients treated with more than seven vials of antivenom.[12] It may be treated effectively with a short course of prednisone (see Chapter 46).

Possessing a venomous snake without a permit is illegal in most states. Medical personnel should report all illegally possessed reptiles to local police or state fish and game agency.

Exotic Snakes. It is important to determine the species of the snake if possible. Knowledge of the regional habitat is helpful; consultation with experts at a poison control center or zoo may be necessary. Antivenom may be available from the herpetology department of local zoos. The dose varies according to the species of snake. Many antivenoms are polyvalent. Further information may be obtained from Denver Antivenom Index, (800) 332-3037, or Tucson Poison Control Center, (602) 626-6016.

ARTHROPODS

Spiders

Of approximately 18,000 species of spiders, all of which are venomous, only about 50 species have fangs sufficiently long or strong enough to penetrate human epidermis.[13] The toxicity of the venom varies among species: Brown recluse (*Loxosceles reclusa*) and black widow (*Latrodectus*) spiders have highly toxic venom, whereas household spiders (*Lycosa* spp. and others) are much less toxic. The severity of the bite may also depend on the amount of venom discharged. The lesion resulting from a bite, therefore, varies greatly in appearance from a small, red papule to a large, ringlike macule, which may ulcerate. Most spider bites are on the hands. Because spiders bite only once, the presence of more than one bite rules out arachnidism.

The spiders are divided into two groups depending on the typical human reaction to their venom: the neurotoxic spiders, *Latrodectus* genus, and the dermonecrotic spiders, which include all other species.

Neurotoxic Spiders: *Latrodectus*. *Latrodectus*, black widow spider, females are reclusive spiders, building apparently irregular, but actually well-organized, webs in dark recesses, woodpiles, cracks in walls, cellars, and attics. The female rarely leaves the web, but will aggressively defend it when disturbed. Most bites occur when the victim reaches blindly into a web. The female black widow spider is shiny black, measures about 1 to 1.5 cm in diameter, and is distinguished by a red hourglass shape on the ventral abdomen.

Pathophysiology. Proteins in the venom release acetylcholine at myoneural junctions, first causing severe muscle contraction (cramps), and finally exhausting endplate activity with a block of synaptic transmission, resulting in paralysis. Norepinephrine is released from sympathetic nerves, leading to systemic hypertension.[14] Severe envenomation is more common in small children, as they receive a higher dose of venom relative to their size.

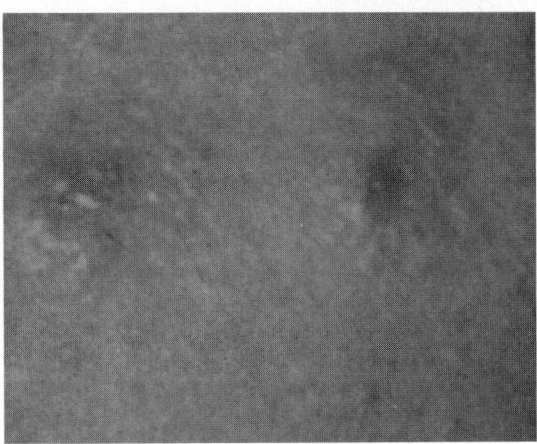

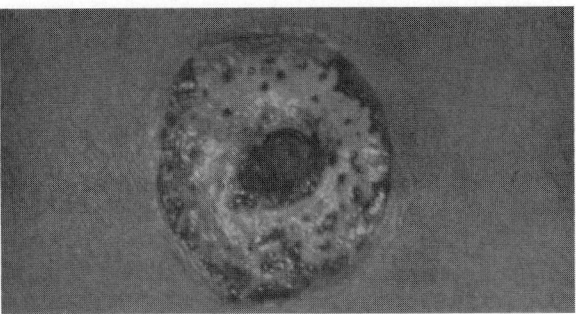

FIG. 34-6. Brown recluse spider bite, thigh; sixth day; large ulcer formation typical of bites on fatty areas.

FIG. 34-5. Black widow spider bite, fang marks 1 mm apart, with early vesiculation.

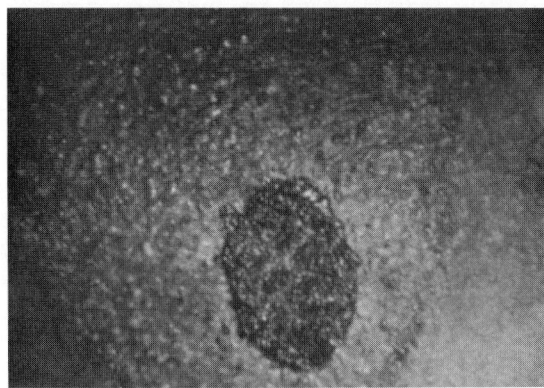

FIG. 34-7. Brown recluse spider bite, tenth day, central eschar surrounded by erythema (target lesion).

Diagnostic Findings. The bite feels like a sharp pinprick, followed by pain radiating up the extremity. Edema is not marked. Occasionally, two small fang marks about ≤ 1 mm apart may be observed (Fig. 34-5). Many nonspecific symptoms have been described after envenomation: headache, dizziness, eyelid edema, faint macular rash, nausea, vomiting, increased perspiration and salivation, and generalized weakness. The pathognomonic symptoms are hypertension with increases in both systolic and diastolic pressures and severe cramping and rigidity of the muscles. Respiratory distress may follow the painful muscle contractions of the thorax if the bite is on the upper extremity. Abdominal pain and rigidity without tenderness to palpation may occur after lower extremity bites. Laboratory studies are not helpful.

Management. Minor envenomations without hypertension or severe cramps may be treated with diazepam intravenously and analgesics. Bites that result in painful muscle contraction or hypertension and those in children under 6 years of age should be treated with Antivenin *Latrodectus* (Lyovac, Merck, Sharp, Dohme), one ampule (2.5 ml) diluted in 50 ml normal saline, intravenously over 20 minutes. A skin test for horse serum sensitivity, included in the package, must be performed before administration of the antivenin. Relief of symptoms occurs rapidly, within 1 to 2 hours, and a second injection is rarely needed.

Dermonecrotic Spiders: *Loxosceles Reclusa* and Others. *Loxosceles reclusa,* the brown recluse spider, and a number of other species of spiders have been implicated in necrotic bites. With the exception of the brown recluse spider, they produce primarily local, with very little systemic, reaction. Brown recluse bites tend to be the most severe, both in local reaction and because systemic reaction is possible. Brown recluse spiders live indoors in closets, trunks, and attics and outdoors in woodpiles and under rocks. The spider, which is often not produced for identification because the bite is painless at first, is 9 to 12 mm in diameter and fawn to brown in color. There is a distinctive violin-shaped marking on the dorsum of the cephalothorax, and there are only six eyes (all others have eight).

Pathophysiology. Brown recluse venom includes protein-activated sphingomyelinase D, which damages the endothelium of local arterioles and venules, lyses erythrocytes, and activates platelets.[15] Subsequent thrombosis results in local infarction. Ongoing necrosis is believed to be due to activation of complement, migration to and lysis of leukocytes in the area, liberating kinins, oxidizing enzymes, and possibly histamine.[16] This persistent autoimmune reaction causes a long-lasting ulcer.

Diagnostic Findings. The bite causes little or no pain and may not be noticed by the victim. One to 2 hours later, a slightly painful erythematous macule or papule forms. The immediate area becomes edematous or slightly cyanotic if the bite is on a finger or toe. The lesion may progress no further and resolve in 5 to 7 days. In more severe envenomations, especially those of the recluse spiders, a vesicle develops, which is surrounded by an ischemic ring, further encircled by an erythematous ring of extravasated blood, the "target lesion." Pain may be severe, and swelling of the entire injured part may be present by 4 to 8 hours. Over the next 3 to 4 days, the central bleb enlarges and becomes necrotic (Figs. 34-6 and 34-7). The resulting ulcer is indolent and may require weeks to heal.[17] Tissue destruction may occur in a funnel-shaped area down to the muscle layer.[18]

The patient may have systemic symptoms of nausea, vomiting, malaise, fever, and chills. Systemic symptoms are proportional to the amount of venom injected and not necessarily to the size of the bite. Rare complications include intravascular hemolysis and disseminated intravascular coagulation.

Management. Minor lesions, usually bites of spiders other than recluse spiders, can be treated with the local application of a potent corticosteroid ointment, three or four times daily. Bites are categorized as severe if the offending species is *L. reclusa* or if a typical vesicular lesion develops. For such severe bites, the leukocyte inhibitor, dapsone (2 mg/kg/24 hr BID PO; adult: 100 mg/24 hr) may be effective in the first 5 days.[19] Antibiotics are indicated for secondary infection. Debridement of the ulcer and plastic repair may be necessary after the necrosis has localized (7 to 10 days).[20] An experimental antivenom developed in rabbits may be effective if given within 48 hours (University of Michigan, Rees and Campbell). A good outcome using hyperbaric oxygen has been reported in uncontrolled human trials, but has not been confirmed by controlled or animal studies.[21,22]

Scorpions

Scorpions occur only in arid regions. The only species dangerous to humans is the sculptured scorpion (*Centruroides* sp.) in the southwestern United States and Mexico. Nearly all reported stings in the United States occur in Arizona, New Mexico, Texas, and Nevada.

Pathophysiology. The venom acts by opening sodium channels at presynaptic nerve terminals, releasing acetylcholine and catecholamines (norepinephrine).[23]

Diagnostic Findings. In all but *Centruroides* stings, the usual symptom is only pain. Marked local hyperesthesia is the pathognomonic finding of sculptured scorpion stings. Symptoms in severe envenomations may include tachycardia, sweating, and marked central nervous system (CNS) stimulation with agitation, numbness, twitching and muscle fibrillation, apparent convulsions, and hypertension. Muscle incoordination and twitching may result in respiratory embarrassment.[24] The venom may be directly cardiotoxic, resulting in dysrhythmias.

Management. For minor stings, cold compresses and local injection of an anesthetic agent may be sufficient. In addition, for *Centruroides* stings, it is appropriate to monitor for several hours for systemic symptoms and to treat them as they occur. Analgesics may be given, but narcotics should be avoided, as they worsen the dysrhythmias. Barbiturates in carefully monitored doses may be used for CNS stimulation and convulsions, and propranolol for tachydysrhythmias. Hypertension can be treated with hydralazine or nifedipine (see Chapter 60).[23,25]

An experimental antivenom manufactured from goat serum is reportedly highly effective, resulting in complete resolution of the symptoms in hours. As the drug is not yet approved by the Food and Drug Administration, its use is limited to Arizona, and common delayed allergic reactions warrant limiting its use to severely envenomated children.[24] It may be obtained from Arizona State University, Tempe, (602) 985-6443.

Other Arthropods

Triatoma. Reduvid bug (assassin bug, kissing bug, "Texas bedbug," or cone-nose bug), specifically *Triatoma protracta*, is a member of the Reduviidae family of arthropods and is most commonly found in the western states. Both nymphal and adult bugs feed on vertebrate blood. The adult is black, about 2.5 cm long and characterized by a long proboscis, which contains sucking mouth parts. Reduvid bugs normally live in the dens of wood rats or opossums, feeding on the blood of these rodents.[26] The bugs are attracted at night by warmth, host odor, carbon dioxide, and artificial light and, therefore, invade residences, especially those located near brush-covered hills or canyons. They emerge from their hiding places in furniture or closets at night, searching for a blood meal.

Diagnostic Findings. The bite is usually in an area of thin integument, such as the lips or eyelid. Bites are initially painless, but are followed by local erythema and itching which last 2 to 4 hours. Foreign proteins in the saliva elicit antibody reactions if the individual is bitten repeatedly. About 5% of persons bitten more than once experience systemic symptoms ranging from itching of the scalp, palms, and soles to severe anaphylaxis. Symptoms tend to increase in severity with each *Triatoma* bite, as sensitization increases.[27]

Management. Treatment of the bite consists of local application of cool compresses, followed by a corticosteroid. Oral antihistamines are given for moderate systemic reactions; oral corticosteroids may be helpful for prolonged urticaria and pruritus. Severe reactions should be managed as any other anaphylactic reaction.

Neither an antivenom nor a vaccine is available for this toxin. Patients with known sensitivity should have an emergency kit with epinephrine immediately available. Potent insect repellents may have some prophylactic value.

Centipedes. Centipedes are elongated, flat, segmented arthropods, varying in size from 2.5 to 35 cm. Each segment has a pair of legs. The head segment bears two fangs, or gnathopods, actually modified legs with poison glands. The last segment is a pseudohead, probably designed to misdirect attacks of predators.

The venom is cytolytic, containing several enzymes, phosphatase, histamine, and serotonin.[28] The venom of most species is not sufficiently toxic to be lethal to humans, although one death due to rhabdomyolysis and renal failure has been reported after envenomation by the giant centipede (*Scolopendra heros*) of the southern and southwestern states.[29]

Symptoms of a bite are burning pain, local swelling, and erythema, along with lymphangitis and regional lymphadenopathy. Systemic symptoms include nausea, dizziness, and fever. The local inflammation usually disappears in 4 to 6 hours, although edema and tenderness may persist or recur for up to 3 weeks. Superficial necrosis may occur at the bite site.

Treatment is symptomatic, consisting of relief of pain by injection of a local anesthetic, or by systemic analgesics, wound cleansing, and tetanus prophylaxis. No antivenom exists or is needed. Antihistamines or corticosteroids may be effective for severe local or systemic reactions.

Millipedes. Millipedes are elongated, cylindrical, segmented animals, 2 to 31 cm long. They differ from centipedes in having two pairs of legs per segment and no venom apparatus, as they are not carnivores. Most species have repugnatorial glands opening on the sides of the body, which secrete defensive toxins, including hydrocyanic acid, phenol, cresol, and quinones.[30]

In humans, this toxin causes contact dermatitis, which may blister and exfoliate. "Mahogany" skin discoloration in the shape of the curled millipede has been confused with abuse.[31] The discoloration is reportedly due to oxidation of quinones.[32] If the poison contacts the eye, severe pain, lacrimation, and blepharospasm occur, followed by conjunctivitis, periorbital edema, and possibly corneal ulceration.[33]

Treatment is removal of the toxin by copious irrigation with water or saline, followed by treatment of the wound as a second-degree chemical burn. Eye injuries should be referred for ophthalmologic consultation.

VENOMOUS MARINE ANIMALS

Toxic marine animals may be either venomous or poisonous. Venomous animals inject their toxin into other animals to cause toxicity, whereas poisonous ones contain a toxin in their tissues that must be ingested by the victim. This chapter deals only with venomous marine animals that can be found near the shore in North America, as these are the most likely to affect children.

Cnidaria (Coelenterata)

The Cnidaria most commonly involved in human poisoning include jellyfish, anemones, and corals.[34] These animals have in common a specialized venom apparatus composed of nematocysts, each containing a small venom-producing cell, inside of which is a "thread," which serves to transfer the venom. The thread is a hollow tube up to 4 mm long, and thousands may be discharged in a single sting. Jellyfish tentacles may be as long as 40 meters; they pose a significant hazard. Even a dead man-of-war or broken tentacles on the beach may still have active nematocysts. In addition, imbedded nematocysts may not discharge all of their venom at once; thus the injury may continue if they are not carefully removed.[35]

Frequent offenders in this group include the Portuguese man-of-war, found throughout tropical and semitropical Atlantic waters along the eastern coast of the United States; and the Pacific Coast bluebottle jellyfish. Corals and anemones are responsible for infrequent envenomations.[34]

Pathophysiology. The venom contains many polypeptides, quaternary ammonium compounds, 5-hydroxytryptamine, histamine, and catecholamines. It is heat stabile from $-90°$ C to $60°$ C over a pH range of 6.0 to 9.5.[36] The severity of the sting is determined by several factors: the specific animal, the amount and relative toxicity of the venom, the general health of the victim and the size of the sting relative to the total surface area of the patient.[37]

Diagnostic Findings. Mild stings are characterized by local reaction, with burning sensations and paresthesias at the site of the sting, sometimes radiating up the involved extremity. Contact with tentacles results in linear wheals and papules surrounded by erythema at the site; these

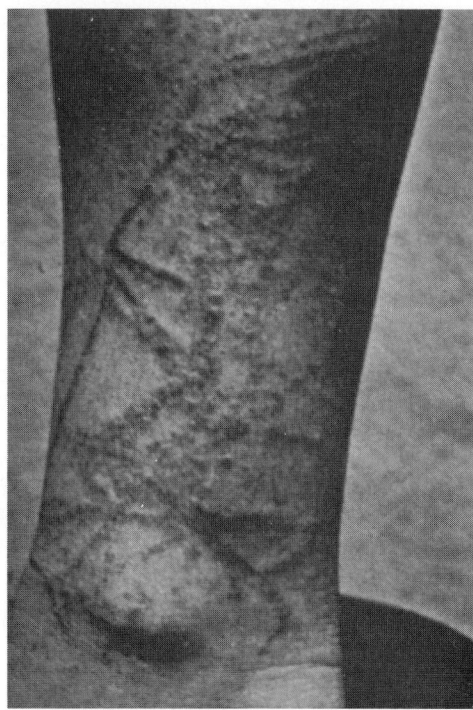

FIG. 34-8. Typical wounds from nematocysts on jellyfish tentacles. (*Courtesy J. Barnes, MD and F.E. Russell, MD.*)

erupt within the first few hours and may last for days (Fig. 34-8). Some stings, especially sea anemone and some jellyfish, may progress to skin necrosis and ulceration. Jellyfish envenomation may result in the production of specific immunoglobulin G and E, persisting for several years and resulting in recurrences of dermatitis.[38]

Severe envenomations may result in systemic symptoms including neurologic symptoms ranging from headache, vertigo, and weakness to seizures, confusion, coma, or paralysis. Severe muscle cramping, especially abdominal and back, nausea, and vomiting may occur. Cardiac dysrhythmias, bronchospasm, laryngeal edema, and respiratory failure occur rarely.[35]

Management. Field management includes bathing the site in seawater, if a detoxicant is not immediately available. Freshwater will induce further toxin discharge. Definitive care involves using detoxicants to inactivate the venom, usually by altering the pH, then removing remaining tentacles. Vinegar (3% to 5% acetic acid) will effectively inactivate nematocysts of most species. Baking soda, in a 50% weight in volume slurry, is preferred for sea nettle stings, and may be effective for the other Cnidaria. These solutions should be applied for 30 minutes, after which the area should be washed clean. Remaining tentacle material and nematocysts are removed by applying a paste of baking soda and scraping with a knife edge or a razor.

General supportive measures are used to treat any resultant local lesions. Topical corticosteroids may relieve local discomfort, and Burow solution soaks may be helpful for ulcerated lesions. Tetanus prophylaxis should be given if indicated, and pain medication may be required. Supportive care is directed at specific systemic symptoms; when there is severe reaction, hospitalization is indicated for observation and care. No specific antivenoms are available for the North American jellyfish, man-of-war, or sea anemones.[35,36]

Echinodermata

The phylum Echinodermata includes about 6,000 species, of which 80 are venomous to humans.[34] Starfish, sea cucumbers, and sea urchins are echinoderms; sea urchins are the major problem for American children.[39] Urchins are small, nonaggressive animals, which are found on beaches, in coral reefs, and on the ocean bottom. They are globular and covered with spines, some of which are venomous and sharp, and others blunt and nonvenomous. Some species have specialized pincerlike venom organs located between the spines, called pedicelleriae, which may attach to the victim and cause continued envenomation. The venom contains serotonin, glycosides, and acetylcholine-like agents. Injuries caused by pedicellariae seem to be more often associated with systemic symptoms than injuries caused by venom-containing spines.[35,36]

In addition, traumatic injury by penetration of the brittle spines may occur without envenomation. Stepping on a sea urchin may result in a puncture wound; and if the spine becomes imbedded, a foreign body reaction and secondary infection may ensue. Granulomas may form, and tattooing can occur from the dye in the colored urchins.[33,35,39]

Diagnostic Findings. The initial reaction, especially with envenomation, is usually severe burning pain, followed rapidly by swelling, redness, and pain in the entire extremity. Systemic symptoms in serious poisoning may include weakness, syncope, paresthesias of the face, and muscle paralysis, especially of the facial muscles and possibly leading to respiratory distress. These symptoms last from 1 to 14 hours. Imbedded spines may be demonstrated by radiography.[35,36]

Management. Immersion in hot water (to 45° C) will provide immediate pain relief. Pincers should be searched for and removed to avoid continued envenomation, and the wound should be thoroughly cleaned. Controversy exists about the advisability of removing imbedded spines. Although it seems sensible to remove easily accessible large spines and those localized by x-ray examination, extensive attempts to remove smaller spines may result in fragmentation and additional tissue damage. Most spines will become resorbed in time, but those lodged near joints or nerves may need to be surgically removed with an operating microscope.[34,40] Antibiotics are indicated if infection develops. Granulomas require excision.

Venomous Fish

Of the more than 200 species of venomous fish, stingrays, catfish, and scorpaenids are most important in North American waters. They envenomate via spines located on their gill covers and dorsal, pectoral, or anal fins.[34] They are nonmigratory, slow swimming bottom dwellers and are found buried in the sand on the ocean floor, on reefs, and in kelp beds. They tend to be well camouflaged and pose risk to those engaging in water sports or fishing. All fish venoms are characterized by marked temperature instability; toxicity is also lost by drying.[36]

Elasmobranch (Stingrays)

Stingrays are the most common offending fish in marine envenomations, accounting for more than 1,500 injuries each year. These flat animals often lie submerged in the sand in shallow coastal waters. The venom organ is arranged on the dorsal surface of the tail. This organ has one to four stingers consisting of a spine containing retroserrate teeth and grooves holding the venom glands and surrounded by an integumentary sheath. The injuries, commonly on the feet and legs and occasionally on the trunk, occur when the victim steps or falls on the ray, provoking it to lash out its tail, burying the barb in the victim resulting in a jagged puncture wound.[40]

Pathophysiology. Both direct trauma and envenomation are responsible for injury. The laceration is often ragged, and pieces of the barb and the integumentary sheath may remain imbedded in the wound, causing secondary infection. The venom contains serotonin, phosphodiesterase, and 5′-nucleotidase.[34,35]

Diagnostic Findings. The predominant symptom is severe pain at the site, accompanied over the next few hours by edema and hemorrhage. The pain peaks in a few hours, but takes days to completely resolve.[34] Systemic symptoms may include severe muscle cramps, nausea, vomiting, diarrhea, weakness, diaphoresis, tachycardia, cardiac dysrhythmias with hypotension, and rarely death. Secondary infections are reportedly common.[41]

Management. Immediate treatment should be directed toward relieving pain and removing and inactivating the venom as quickly as possible. The wound should be copiously irrigated with any available solution, including seawater. Hot water immersion (to tolerance, approximately 45° C, for 1 to 1.5 hours) will provide local pain relief and inactivate the venom.[35] Scrupulous wound care, with copious irrigation, removal of foreign material, and debridement and either suturing loosely or packing open, is important for preventing infection. Anecdotal reports suggest that prophylactic antibiotics (penicillin and a cephalosporin) may prevent secondary infection, although no prospective studies confirm this.[40] Systemic symptoms should be treated supportively.

Scorpaenidae

This group includes the sculpin, lionfish, stonefish, and scorpion fish, all of which are well camouflaged and injure their victims with venomous dorsal, pectoral, and anal spines. In the United States, scorpaenids are primarily found in coastal waters of Florida, California, and Hawaii and along the Gulf of Mexico.[40] Lionfish are popular aquarium fish and account for the majority of reported stings.[41] The severity of the sting varies with the species; stonefish venom is the most potent. The venom is a complex substance; its principal toxin is a heat-labile protein. The venom is probably similar for all of the fish in this group, although potency varies. The venom may remain active as long as 48 hours after the death of the fish.[34]

Diagnostic Findings. The wound immediately becomes ischemic and cyanotic, and pain is intense. The pain may involve the entire extremity, and reaches maximum intensity over 1 to 2 hours. Edema, paresthesias, and tissue necrosis may develop.[40] Systemic symptoms include gastrointestinal discomfort, neurologic complications (seizures, tremors, muscle weakness, and delirium), cardiovascular effects (dysrhythmias, hypotension and hypertension, myocardial ischemia with congestive heart failure), and rarely death.[34,35] Some of these symptoms may represent compensation for the severe pain or the direct cardiotoxic, vasodilatory effects of the venom.[34] Secondary infection, cutaneous granulomas, or indolent ulcers often occur.

Management. Treatment is similar to that described for stingray injuries: hot water immersion to relieve pain and inactivate the venom and careful wound care. An antivenom is available for stone fish envenomation; it may be effective for other scorpion fish envenomations although heat inactivation of the venom is usually effective. It is manufactured in Australia and can be obtained by a physician from Commonwealth Serum Laboratories, 45 Poplar Road, Parkville, 3052, Victoria, Australia.[41]

Catfish

Catfish can be found in both freshwater and saltwater throughout North America. The venom apparatus is similar to Scorpaenidae, and is located on the sharp dorsal and pectoral spines. Most stings occur during fishing and when handling the fish. Symptoms are similar to stingray envenomations, although milder; treatment is similar to that for stingray injuries: immersion in hot water and exploration of the wound for foreign bodies.[34]

References

1. Russell FE: *Snake venom poisoning*, Great Neck, NY, 1983, Scolium International.

Venomous Reptiles

2. Parrish, HM: Incidence of treated snakebites in the United States, *Public Health Rep* 81:269, 1966.
3. Litovitz TL et al: 1992 Annual report of the American Association of Poison Control Centers Toxic Exposure Surveillance System, *Am J Emerg Med* 11:494, 1993.
4. Wingert WA and Chan L: Rattlesnake bites in Southern California and rationale for recommended treatment, *West J Med* 148:37, 1988.
5. Ownby CL: Pathology of rattlesnake envenomation. In Tu AT, editor: *Rattlesnake venoms*, New York, 1982, Marcel Dekker.
6. Cable DM et al: Prolonged defibrination after a bite from a "nonpoisonous" snake, *JAMA* 251:925, 1984.
7. Gold BS and Wingert WA: Snake venom poisoning in the United States: a review of therapeutic practice, *So Med J* 87:579, 1994.
8. Sullivan JB and Wingert WA: North American venomous reptile bites. In Auerbach PS, editor: *Wilderness medicine*, ed 3, St. Louis, 1995, Mosby.
9. Kitchens CS and Van Mierop LHS: Envenomation by the eastern coral snake (*Micrurus fulvius fulvius*), *JAMA* 258:1615, 1987.
10. Schaeffer R et al: Hypotensive and hemostatic properties of rattlesnake venom and venom fractions in dogs, *J Pharmacol Exp Ther* 230:393, 1984.
11. Garfin S et al: The effect of antivenom on intramuscular pressure elevations induced by rattlesnake venom, *Toxicon* 23:677, 1985.
12. Wingert WA and Wainschel J: Diagnosis and management of envenomation by poisonous snakes, *South Med J* 68:1015, 1975.

Arthropods

13. Russell FE: Venomous animal injuries, *Curr Probl Pediatr* 3:1, 1973.
14. Howard BD and Gundersen CB: Effects and mechanisms of polypeptide neurotoxins that act presynaptically, *Annu Rev Pharmacol Toxicol* 20:307, 1980.
15. Gates CA and Rees RS: Serum amyloid P component: its role in platelet activation stimulated by sphingomyelinase D purified from the venom of the brown recluse spider (*Loxosceles reclusa*), *Toxicon* 28:1303, 1990.
16. Berger RS, Adelstein EH, Anderson PC: Intravascular coagulation: the cause of necrotic arachnidism, *J Invest Derm* 61:142, 1973.
17. Berger RS: The unremarkable brown recluse spider bite, *JAMA* 225:109, 1973.
18. Jong V-S, Norment BR, Heitz JR: Separation and characterization of venom components in *Loxosceles reclusa* hydrolytic enzyme activity, *Toxicon* 17:539, 1979.
19. Rees RS et al: Management of brown recluse spider bites, *Plast Reconstr Surg* 68:768, 1987.
20. Erickson T et al: Brown recluse spider bites in an urban wilderness, *J Wilderness Med* 1:258, 1990.
21. Svendsen, FJ: Treatment of clinically diagnosed brown recluse spider bites with hyperbaric oxygen, *J Ark Med Soc* 83:199, 1986.
22. Phillips S, Kohn M, Baker D et al: Therapy of brown spider envenomation: a controlled trial of hyperbaric oxygen, dapsone and cyproheptadine. *Ann Emerg Med* 25:363, 1995.
23. Connor DA and Selden BS: Scorpion envenomation. In Auerbach PS, editor: *Wilderness medicine*, ed 3, St. Louis, 1995, Mosby.
24. Bond GR: Antivenom administration for centroides scorpion stings—risks, benefits, *Vet Human Toxicol* 32:367, 1990.
25. Rimsza ME, Zimmerman DR, Bergeson PS: Scorpion envenomation, *Pediatrics* 66:298, 1980.
26. Hogue CL: Common terrestrial arthropods. In *Natural History Museum of Los Angeles County: the insects of the Los Angeles basin*, Science Series 27:1, 1974.
27. Smith RJ: Venomous animals of Arizona, Bulletin 8245, University of Arizona, 1982, Tucson.
28. Mohammed AA et al: Proteins, lipids, lipoproteins and some enzyme characteristics of the venom extract from the centipede *Scolopendra morsitans*, *Toxicon* 221:371, 1983.
29. Logan DL and Ogden DA: Rhabdomyolysis and acute renal failure following the bite of the giant desert centipede *Scolopendra heros*, *West J Med* 142:549, 1985.
30. Eisner T et al: Defensive secretions of millipedes, *Handbook Exp Pharmacol* 48:41, 1978.
31. Mason G et al: Mysterious lesions: the burning millipede. *Med J Aust* 160:718, 1994.
32. Shpall S and Frieden I: Mahogany discoloration of the skin due to the defensive secretion of the millipede, *Pediatr Dermatol* 8:25, 1991.
33. Minton SA and Bechtel HB: Arthropod envenomation and parasitism. In Auerbach PS, editor: *Wilderness medicine*, ed 3, St. Louis, 1995, Mosby.

Venomous Marine Animals

34. Kizer KW: Marine envenomations, *J Toxicol Clin Toxicol* 21:527, 1983-1984.
35. Rosson CL and Tolle SW: Management of marine stings and scrapes, *West J Med* 150:97, 1989.
36. Wingert WA: Envenomation by poisonous arthropods and marine animals. In Kelley VC, editor, *Brennemann's practice of pediatrics*, ed P-60, Philadelphia, 1987, Harper and Row.
37. Guess HA, Savateer PL, Morris CR: Hemolysis and acute renal failure following a Portuguese man-of-war sting, *Pediatrics* 70:979, 1982.
38. Burnett JW et al: Studies on the serological response to jellyfish envenomation. *J Amer Acad Dermatol* 9:229, 1983.
39. Hodge DW and Tecklenburg FW: Bites and stings. In Fleisher G, Ludwig S, editors: *Textbook of pediatric emergency medicine*, ed 3, Baltimore, 1993, Williams and Wilkins.
40. Auerbach PS: Hazardous marine animals, *Emerg Med Clin North Am* 2:531, 1984.
41. Kizer KW, McKinney HE, Auerbach PS: Scorpaenidae envenomation—a five year poison center experience, *JAMA* 253:807, 1985.

35

Near Drowning

Jim R. Harley • Daniel W. Ochsenschlager

EPIDEMIOLOGY

Drowning is the second most common cause of unintentional injury death in children 5 to 24 years of age and the third most common cause in children 0 to 4 years of age in the United States.[1] In 10 states (Alaska, Arizona, California, Florida, Hawaii, Montana, Nevada, Oregon, Utah, and Washington), drowning surpassed all other causes of injury death in children less than 15 years of age when motor vehicle-related deaths were separated into motor vehicle occupant and motor vehicle-pedestrian injuries.[2] In 1993, there were 4,800 drowning deaths, 2,100 of these were less than age 24 years of age.[1] It is estimated that for every child that drowns there are four hospital admissions. For every hospital admission for near drowning, there are four children seen in emergency departments,[3] although it is estimated that there are 10 "near-miss" events for every emergency department visit.[4] The peak incidence of drowning in children occurs between 1 and 4 years of age. The ages 0 to 4 years accounts for up to 50% of significant submersion injuries.[5] The rates for children older than 10 years of age have declined from 1971 to 1988; infant and toddler rates have changed little.[6] The incidence in males at every age is greater than females. The second incidence peak is at 15 to 24 years of age. Teenage girls have one fifth the drowning rate of teenage boys. Frequently, alcohol or drugs are involved.[5]

Near drowning may result in significant neurologic morbidity. Of children who received cardiopulmonary resuscitation (CPR) in the emergency department, 60% to 100% of the survivors are severely brain damaged. The annual cost of care in a chronic care facility for a severely brain-damaged, near-drowning survivor is approximately $100,000.[3] The annual cost attributed to drowning and near-drowning victims is $384 million.[7]

DEFINITIONS

Drowning generally refers to death from asphyxia within the first 24 hours of submersion in a liquid.

Near drowning is a submersion in which survival is greater than 24 hours regardless of morbidity or mortality.

Secondary drowning is death that occurs 24 hours after submersion due to complications. (It has been suggested that this confusing term be abandoned.) These patients seem well initially, then suddenly deteriorate.

Immersion syndrome describes sudden death after contact with very cold water. The mechanism for this syndrome has been postulated to be intense vagal discharge resulting in cardiac standstill or ventricular fibrillation.

Submersion injury is any submersion that results in hospital admission or death.

Drowning has sometimes been classified theoretically as "classic white cases" and "classic blue cases." Classic white cases refer to those drowning victims who lost consciousness (from seizures, head trauma, stroke) before submersion. The much more common classic blue case occurs when the patient panics and struggles, resulting in a pronounced catecholamine release.[8]

PATHOPHYSIOLOGY

When a person is unexpectedly submersed, there may or may not be a struggle. Small children may sink below the water surface without a struggle. They hold their breath until reflex inspiratory efforts occur. As the victim begins to panic and becomes hypoxic, water may be swallowed into the stomach. Then the patient either aspirates water or has a "dry drowning" in which water does not enter the lung. Drowning without aspiration of fluid occurs in 7% to 10% of victims.[9] The amount of water aspirated is usually small. In 85% of drowning victims, it has been estimated to be much less than 22 ml/kg.[10] The victim becomes unconscious secondary to hypoxia. Hypoxia then leads to cardiac arrest unless there is intervention.

The initial insult is to the lung; most of the secondary effects, particularly involving the brain, result from hypoxemia. Contrary to early suspicions, significant electrolyte imbalance and fluid shifts in submersion injuries do not occur.[11] In animal experiments with dogs, Modell demonstrated that amounts of aspirated water less than 22 ml/kg did not cause significant persistent electrolyte imbalance.[12]

However, in sheep intratracheal instillation of only 1 to 3 ml/kg of freshwater or seawater resulted in an immediate decrease in oxygen saturation.[13]

Although hypoxemia is the final common pathway in all forms of drowning, the mechanisms producing the hypoxemia in saltwater and freshwater are slightly different. In freshwater drowning, the surfactant is inactivated and the alveolar basement membrane is damaged. The resulting alveolitis and transudation of proteinaceous material produces pulmonary edema. The functional loss of surfactant also results in alveolar collapse. In contrast, aspiration of hypertonic seawater results in movement of water from the intravascular space into the alveolar space. Surfactant is diluted and effluted from the alveolar space. In addition, the alveolar basement membrane is damaged.

Alveolar hyaline membranes are formed. The lungs are grossly edematous with local hemorrhages. In rabbits, there are mitochondrial abnormalities of the pulmonary vascular endothelium and alveolar septal bleb formation.[14] Clinically, both freshwater and saltwater aspiration cause pronounced intrapulmonary shunting, decreased lung compliance, ventilation-perfusion mismatch, and often significant bronchospasm. The result of all these effects is hypoxia.

Swimmers who hyperventilate before entering the water significantly lower their Pco_2 level and, in turn, the stimulus to breathe. Thus, after hyperventilation, the victim can become severely hypoxic with an attenuated urge to breathe and may lose consciousness ("shallow water blackout"). A somewhat similar mechanism is a potential danger for long-distance team swimmers who are trained to hold their breath for long periods while doing laps. Prolonged "hypoxic" training can build the patient's tolerance to oxygen deprivation, which can also result in a loss of respiratory drive and sequential loss of consciousness and possible near drowning.[15]

Although chlorine does not seem to affect the prognosis, aspiration of vomitus, sand, mud, and the more than 20 human pathogens found in saltwater can produce a complicating pneumonitis (see Chapter 44).[5]

Hypothermia has several harmful effects on the submersion victim. The rate of heat loss in water is 32 times greater than in air. Children are more likely to become hypothermic than adults because of the greater surface area/body mass ratio and relative decreased amount of insulating fat.[16] Decreased coordination, increased muscle rigidity, clouded sensorium, and decreased duration of breath holding may be noted.[17] Adverse effects of hypothermia include dysrhythmias and exhaustion. Hypothermia plays a role in many drowning deaths. At the sinking of the Titanic in 1912, there were adequate life vests, but few lifeboats. Of the 2,201 passengers, 1,489 died within 2 hours in 0° C water. Only passengers or crew in boats survived (see Chapter 39).[18]

Hypothermia may have beneficial effects on a select few submersion victims. Hypothermia decreases oxygen consumption, basal metabolic rate, and cerebral metabolism. These effects may protect the brain from hypoxic injury. The role of the diving reflex in protecting children during submersion is unknown, but probably is not very active in children and has little influence on the ultimate outcome.[19]

The diving reflex was originally demonstrated in animals (e.g., seals). When the faces of these animals are exposed to cold, a reflex shunting of blood preferentially to the heart and brain with bradycardia occurs.

ETIOLOGY

Over 90% of drownings occur in freshwater even in areas with saltwater beaches. Fifty percent of these freshwater drownings occur in swimming pools; over 90% involve residential pools, frequently a relative's, friend's, or family's own pool. Unattended toddlers simply fall into the swimming pool. Pool drownings are most likely to occur on weekends in the summer months between 4 to 6 p.m. Solar swimming pool blankets (covers that will not support the weight of a person) also have been implicated in neardrowning incidents.[20] Teenage males are more likely to drown in lakes, rivers, and beaches. Use of alcohol and illicit drugs is often associated with these drownings.[8]

Several less common risks for potential drowning exist in the home. Approximately 10% to 24% of all residential drownings occur in the bathtub.[21,22] Usually the victim is an infant who is left in the bathtub with inadequate supervision or an older child with a seizure disorder. Many victims of bathtub drownings have historic or physical findings suggestive of abuse or neglect. In a study of 21 patients treated for near drowning in a bathtub, 67% had evidence of abuse or neglect. Factors associated with nonaccidental submersion include atypical submersion description with inconsistent details, late referral to the hospital, associated history of child abuse, and the child left with an inadequate caregiver.[23] Medical evaluation of bathtub drownings should include a social work consultation and a careful search for other injuries such as suspicious bruises.[24] Each year, an average of 27 children drown in 3 to 5 gallon buckets or pails filled or partially filled with liquid. These children, usually 7 to 15 months of age, fall head first into the bucket and cannot get out. These buckets are large in diameter and do not tip easily even when empty.[25] Children may also drown in hot tubs, spas, and whirlpools. Entrapment of hair or body parts in the suction device of the drains is a major cause of accidents in pools, hot tubs, spas, and whirlpools.[26]

Hyperventilation before underwater swimming can lead to submersion injury. Lowering the Pco_2 by hyperventilation before attempting to swim underwater can lead to cerebral hypoxia and loss of consciousness before the Pco_2 level is high enough to stimulate the urge to breathe.[27] Hypothermia and exhaustion may lead to submersion injuries in even experienced swimmers.

Boating accidents account for approximately 1,200 drownings a year, often related to capsizing, exhaustion, poor preparation and supplies, and inability to swim. The boats are commonly open, less than 16 feet long, and equipped with too few or no personal flotation devices. Two thirds of the drownings are associated with capsizing or flooding the boat. Sixty percent of the deaths associated with scuba (self-contained underwater breathing apparatus) diving are the result of drowning. Inexperience and carelessness are major causes of these deaths. Both cerebral air embolism and decompression sickness can be contributing factors (see Chapter 40).[5]

Factors Associated with Submersion Injuries

Absent or inadequate water barriers
Alcohol
Child abuse or neglect
Entrapment
Exhaustion
Failure to use flotation devices
Head or cervical spine trauma
Hyperventilation
Hypothermia
Illicit drug use
Inability to swim
Inadequate supervision
Scuba diving injuries
Seizures

Important Historic Data

Time of submersion
Time until CPR begun
Preceding trauma
Loss of consciousness
Seizure history
Medications
Drugs/alcohol
Prehospital treatment given

CPR, Cardiopulmonary resuscitation.

Children with seizure disorders have a four to five times greater risk of drowning than the general population. Adequate anticonvulsant drug levels are not completely protective.[28] Circumstances related to swimming such as hyperventilation, photo stimulation, water immersion epilepsy, and exhaustion may precipitate seizures. Risk factors for seizures while swimming are children with mental retardation, recent changes in anticonvulsant medication, or poorly controlled seizures.[29] Although children with seizure disorders should not be prohibited from swimming, they must be closely supervised.[30]

Adolescent boys are most commonly involved in the 700 to 800 diving accidents per year. In 70% of the cases, the water is 4 feet or less in depth. Usually, the victim is unfamiliar with the depth of the water and often the injury occurs after the first dive. Consumption of alcohol is a primary factor in 40% to 50% of these events. Cervical spine and head injuries may result (see box above).[5]

DIAGNOSTIC FINDINGS

The nature of the episode and mechanism of injury must be determined. Evidence of preceding trauma, seizures, intoxication, and exhaustion should be sought. The estimated time of submersion should be obtained as well as the location and condition of the victim when first found and the response to resuscitation. Important facts include being found at the bottom of the pool or body of water, loss of consciousness or confusion, initial apnea or cyanosis, or CPR administered at the scene (see box above, right).

Initially, physical findings vary from none to cardiopulmonary arrest. Vital signs and core temperature must be determined. Abnormal findings may include evidence of respiratory distress such as tachypnea, retractions, cyanosis, rales, rhonci, and wheezing. A neurologic examination should assess for level of consciousness, pupil reaction to light, decerebrate or decorticate posturing, pain response, and verbal and motor response. Traumatic injuries to the neck or other organs should be excluded.

Complications

The hypoxia, acidosis, and hypoperfusion that result from submersion injuries can affect all organ systems. Respiratory insufficiency, aspiration pneumonia, and adult respiratory distress syndrome are seen after near drowning. Coagulation disorders leading to disseminated intravascular coagulation may develop. Hemolysis may occur. Renal failure may result from one or more of the combination of myoglobinuria, hemoglobinuria, hypoxia, acidosis, and hypoperfusion. Brain injury is usually the result of hypoxia, but may be secondary to trauma. Cardiac dysrhythmias and cardiogenic shock are the result of hypoxia and hypoperfusion. Significant electrolyte disturbances are not seen unless the victim drowns in an unusual medium, such as the Dead Sea, or large amounts of water are swallowed by the infant.[31]

Ancillary Data

The most important initial laboratory test is arterial blood gas (ABG), which provides an ongoing guide to respiratory resuscitation and acid-base status. If repeated ABGs are anticipated, then an arterial line should be inserted. Oxygen saturation monitoring by pulse oximetry should be used initially.

Blood should be obtained for complete blood count, electrolytes, serum glucose, blood urea nitrogen, creatinine, liver function tests, and screen for disseminated intravascular coagulation including prothrombin time, partial thromboplastin time, platelets, fibrinogen, and fibrin split products. A baseline urinalysis is also indicated. Several cases of hyponatremia have been reported in patients, particularly infants, who swallowed large volumes of water; electrolytes are usually normal.[10] The blood sugar may be either elevated or depressed in hypothermic patients. Renal failure can occur but is unusual and is suspected to be secondary to hypoxia, acidosis, hypoperfusion, or renal tubular hemoglobin deposits from hemolysis.[31] In selected cases drug screens, type and cross match, and other ancillary tests may be indicated.

A preliminary chest radiograph should be obtained to look for possible associated injuries, barotrauma, and endotracheal tube, nasogastric tube, and central line placement. The initial x-ray film may or may not show the classic fluffy infiltrates associated with aspiration. The appearance of these infiltrates is not correlated with either the severity of

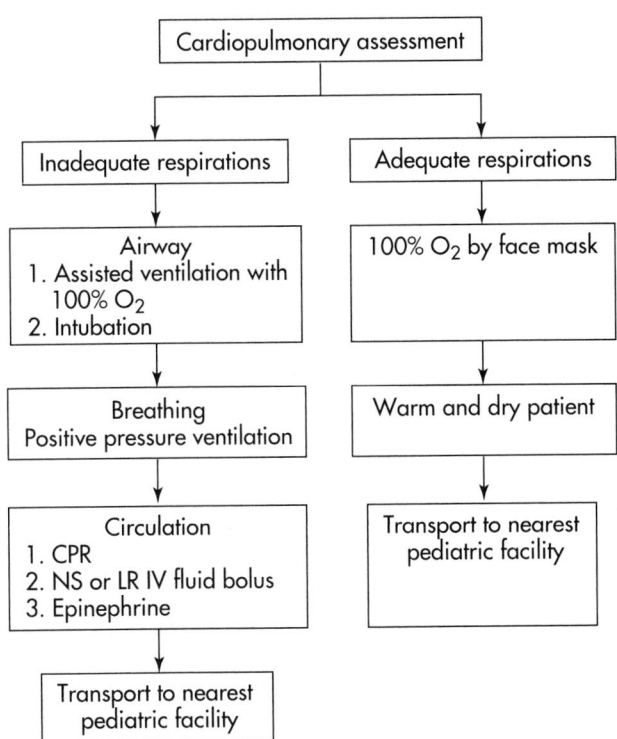

FIG. 35-1. Prehospital management of near drowning.

Prehospital Interventions

100% oxygen administration
Cervical spine immobilization
Intubation
    Airway unmaintainable
    Inadequate respirations
    Cardiopulmonary arrest
    Inadequate assisted ventilation
Venous or intraosseous access
Warming and drying
Nasogastric tube if patient intubated
Cardiac monitoring
Pulse oximetry if available
Epinephrine if patient is in full arrest

---

the hypoxemia or the ultimate prognosis. Serial radiographs may be useful in monitoring progression of infiltrates. A skeletal survey for occult fractures should be considered in a bathtub drowning in which child abuse is suspected.

MANAGEMENT

Prehospital Setting

Treatment at the scene begins with the search, location, and removal of the patient from the water. Medical assistance (911 or equivalent) should be contacted immediately. It is of utmost importance to begin CPR quickly for patients in respiratory or cardiac arrest (Fig. 35-1). The prognosis is directly related to the timeliness and effectiveness of CPR. All patients should receive CPR unless there are obvious signs that death occurred hours before. Properly trained swimmers can perform mouth-to-mouth ventilation in the water. External cardiac massage cannot be performed in the water. Assisted breathing should be initiated as soon as possible. Even untrained people have successfully revived apneic victims with prehospital dispatched phone instructions. If circumstances are suspicious for a potential cervical spine injury, then the neck should be immobilized in a neutral position. There has been some controversy regarding the efficacy of routine administration of the Heimlich maneuver (abdominal thrusts) in drowning resuscitation.[32] The current recommendation is to treat the unresponsive submersion victim the same as any other unresponsive patient. First the airway is examined with cervical spine immobilization if a neck injury is a possibility. If the airway

is open, then breathing and circulation are assessed. If the airway is obstructed, then a chin lift or jaw thrusts (with cervical spine immobilization if injury is suspected) is used to open the airway. If these maneuvers are unsuccessful, then foreign body removal procedures should be used. The Heimlich maneuver should be used only if there is a suspected foreign body or if the rescuer is unable to ventilate with mouth-to-mouth breathing after opening the airway and using a chin lift or jaw thrust.[33,34] Cricoid pressure (Sellick maneuver) may prevent aspiration during CPR and intubation. Chest compressions should be given if the victim is pulseless. Lay CPR recommendations have deemphasized pulse assessment as the determinant on whether to begin chest compressions. If the patient is apneic, chest compressions should be given along with the respirations unless a strong pulse is felt. It is important to continue CPR at the scene, even if the patient seems dead. Oxygen, if available, should be administered.

As mentioned previously, patients with extreme hypothermia, although unconscious, apneic, and with seemingly absent pulse, have been successfully resuscitated with normal neurologic outcomes. To prevent potentially fatal dysrhythmias hypothermic patients should not be aggressively overmanipulated.

Intubation in the field is indicated when (1) the patient is unconscious, to provide an airway and prevent aspiration, (2) the airway cannot be maintained using basic techniques, and (3) prolonged transport time requires maintenance of the airway. Hypothermic patients can be intubated if necessary.

Wet clothing should be removed and the patient kept warm and dry. Peripheral intravenous access should be obtained. Hypotension can be treated with boluses of 20 ml/kg of normal saline or lactated Ringer's solution. All patients with a significant history of near drowning, even if asymptomatic, should be transported to the hospital for evaluation (see box above).

Emergency Department (see box on p. 478)

Respiratory. All symptomatic near-drowning patients should receive oxygen. If the patient is still hypoxic with a

Emergency Department Management

Immobilize neck if cervical spine injury suspected
Vital signs including core temperature
Venous access
Arterial and central lines if indicated
Intubation if indicated
Nasogastric tube if patient intubated
Foley catheter if patient unconscious
Cardiac monitor
Pulse oximetry
Warming and drying if necessary

nonrebreathing face mask, a modern high-flow system that delivers 100% oxygen may be used if available. Persistent hypoxemia suggests the need for positive airway pressure either by continuous positive airway pressure (CPAP), or positive end-expiratory pressure (PEEP).[35] CPAP can be used only on self-ventilating patients and can be provided by either nasal cannula (infants) or mask (adolescents). Intubation is required to administer PEEP. Initially, the positive pressure should be instituted at 5 mm Hg and increased at 2 to 5 mm Hg increments until desired effects are obtained. The success of positive pressure treatment should be monitored with ABG levels and the patient's clinical status. The patient may require endotracheal intubation. Indications for intubation include (1) apnea, (2) unstable airway, (3) prevention of aspiration, (4) excessive work of breathing, (4) neurologic deterioration, and (5) hypoxia or hypercarbia as demonstrated by ABG levels. Although there is no definitive level of hypoxemia or hypercarbia that demands intubation, Po_2 of less than 60 mm Hg or Pco_2 greater than 50 mm Hg on 100% oxygen is a reasonable indication. The decision for intubation, however, must be based on individual considerations.

Bronchospasm may be a prominent feature of near drowning and should be treated with bronchodilators such as selective beta-agonists. Albuterol, 0.15 mg/kg by aerosol, is a useful drug (see Chapter 59). Artificial surfactant has been reported to be of benefit in one case report.[36] Neither corticosteroid nor prophylactic antibiotics have been shown to have a useful effect on immediate respiratory resuscitation.[37,38]

Hypotension. If not previously inserted, an intravenous line should be established for drug administration and the treatment of shock. Hypotension can be the result of several circumstances including ischemic cardiomyopathy, acidosis, central nervous system insult, vascular shunting, associated traumatic injuries with blood loss or cervical spine injury, and hypothermia. Near-drowning victims in cardiopulmonary arrest have been found to have low cardiac indexes, high systemic vascular resistance indexes, increased capillary wedge pressures, and increased pulmonary vascular resistance.[31,39,40] Poor perfusion or hypotension should be treated initially with repeat boluses of either normal saline or Ringer's lactate, 20 ml/kg, with

frequent monitoring. If shock persists, then central lines or even pulmonary artery catheterization is indicated. Infusion of pressor agents may also be necessary if fluid boluses are ineffective and normovolemia is achieved; dobutamine (5 to 20 mg/kg/min) may be used (see Chapter 13).[41]

Hypothermia. Low temperatures can be treated by various methods. However, profoundly hypothermic patients should be treated aggressively with active rewarming techniques (see Chapter 39). Although there are no generally accepted guidelines, patients who are not responding to resuscitation should probably be warmed to 32° C before they are pronounced dead. It may not be possible to rewarm all victims with brain death because brain-dead patients are poikilothermic.[5]

Cerebral Edema

The brain is very sensitive to hypoxemia and acidosis and is the principal secondary organ involved in near drowning. Neurologic sequelae are the most frequent and serious complication of near drowning. Up to 40% of resuscitated patients may have serious neurologic compromise. Currently, the greatest controversy in resuscitation in near drowning involves cerebral resuscitation, particularly the importance of maintaining normal intracranial pressure.[42]

In the 1970s, Conn at Toronto Children's Hospital proposed treatment which included restricting fluids; cooling to a core temperature of 30° C; and using barbiturates, steroids, hyperventilation, diuretics, mannitol, and muscle relaxants.[43] Since that time there has been serious questioning of the usefulness of these various therapies and even the value of intracranial pressure (ICP) monitoring itself. A study of 21 nearly drowned, flaccid, and comatose children showed that increased ICP was related to mortality. However, treatment did not seem to affect mortality. All patients who had an ICP greater than 20 mm Hg and a cerebral perfusion pressure >50 mm Hg died despite vigorous treatment of increased ICP. As could be predicted, 92% of the patients that had an ICP of ≤20 mm Hg and cerebral perfusion pressure (CPP) of ≤50 mm Hg survived. Ten patients died despite this very aggressive treatment regimen, and one patient who died had normal ICP and CPP. Furthermore, increased ICP was not predictive of neurologic residual. In fact, all but one of five brain-damaged survivors had both normal ICPs and CPPs.[44]

In another study of 15 comatose, near-drowning children, ICP was monitored and elevations above 20 mm Hg were treated with hyperventilation, maintaining Pco_2 between 24 and 26 mm Hg, and paralysis. Mannitol and thiopental were also administered if the ICP was elevated. Some patients were cooled to 31.5° C to 34° C. Two of these children survived and seemed normal 6 months later. Five survived but were neurologically impaired. Eight patients died and the ICP in all of them was <20 mm Hg.[45] Corticosteroids, osmotic agents, diuretics, barbiturates, and controlled hypothermia have not been demonstrated to improve either neurologic prognosis or survival. All of these treatment modalities have been associated with complications, particularly increased infection rate.[42,46-48]

It is also generally accepted that ICP does not increase for several hours after the anoxic event and therefore should not be of great concern while the patient is in the emergency department. It is prudent, however, to minimize situations that can increase ICP. The patient's P_{CO_2} should be maintained at about 25 to 30 mm Hg. The patient's head should be elevated to about 30 degrees. Procedures that can increase ICP (e.g., nasogastric tube or Foley catheter placement) should be minimized. Once vascular stability has been achieved, fluids should be restricted to between 50% to 60% of maintenance while keeping the central venous pressure in the range of 8 to 10 mm Hg and urine output between 0.5 and 1.0 ml/kg/hr. Furosemide (Lasix) in a dose of 1 mg/kg IV may be useful. Mannitol 0.5 gm/kg over 30 minutes administered every 3 to 4 hr IV may be given to reduce ICP and used in symptomatic patients. A rebound effect is often noted.

Barbiturates are controversial and there is no evidence that they affect the outcome independent of associated hypothermia. If used, pentobarbital (Nembutal) may be given initially in a dose of 3 to 20 mg/kg IV slowly while monitoring blood and ICP. An intravenous infusion of 1 to 2 mg/kg/hr is used to maintain a level of 25 to 40 μg/ml. Levels above 30 μg/ml are associated with hypotension in about 60% of patients. Intubation and paralysis with a drug such as pancuronium bromide, 0.1 mg/kg IV, may be necessary in some cases to prevent muscle straining (see Chapter 19).

General Measures. Seizures should be controlled with an anticonvulsant such as diazepam 0.3 mg/kg IV or phenytoin 10 to 20 mg/kg IV slowly. Antibiotics and steroids have no beneficial effect and should be reserved for specific indications. Electrolytes and acid-base abnormalities should be corrected.[5]

Supportive and monitoring steps should be initiated concurrently. A nasogastric tube should be placed to aspirate the stomach contents and prevent abdominal distension from ileus and aspiration. Likewise, a Foley catheter should be inserted in seriously ill patients to monitor urinary output and evaluate perfusion. The normal urinary output is approximately 1 ml/kg/hr. Placement of a Foley catheter will also reduce bladder distension if hyperosmotic agents such as mannitol are administered. All seriously ill patients should have continuous cardiac monitoring for potential dysrhythmias.

DISPOSITION

Any patient who is mildly hypoxic or has symptoms such as tachypnea, retractions, wheezing, rales, congestion, tachycardia, cyanosis, or confusion, should be admitted for observation and monitoring. Candidates for intensive care unit (ICU) admission include those with hypothermia <32° C, with depressed mental status, who have persistently abnormal ABG levels, require intubation, require CPAP or PEEP, have unstable cardiovascular status, or have rapidly progressing signs or symptoms. If the hospital does not have an adequate ICU facility, consideration should be given to transporting the patient to a more appropriate institution. A common recommendation is that all near-drowning patients be admitted for observation because of the concern of secondary drowning. This delayed phenomenon has been reported to occur in about 5% of all near-drowning patients.[49] The latent period in one study was less than 4 hours in freshwater drownings and 36 or

---

Hospital Admission Criteria

Tachypnea
Hypoxia
Retractions
Abnormal ABG
Abnormal chest x-ray film
Any neurologic impairment

ABG, Arterial blood gas.

---

more hours in saltwater drownings. This advice has been questioned for patients who have no symptoms after 4 to 6 hours of observation. Pratt found that patients who developed respiratory distress after saltwater submersion did so within 4 hours[50] (see box above).

PROGNOSIS

Accurate prognostic indicators would be useful in the management of near-drowning patients to determine whether aggressive therapy is indicated and to counsel parents on likely outcome. The overall survival rate has been reported to be 75% to 93%, with intact neurologic survival between 58 to 93%.[51] Factors that have been examined include length of submersion time, water temperature, presence of respirations, presence of pulse, pupillary response, level of consciousness, blood pH, provision of immediate CPR, length of time CPR is given, and response to CPR. Although factors such as consciousness or spontaneous respirations before or after resuscitation accurately predict good outcome, there are no completely reliable indicators in the field or in the emergency department to predict poor outcome.[52]

Patients who received immediate resuscitation with CPR and mouth-to-mouth breathing had an improved outcome compared to those who received thoracic or abdominal compression or did not receive any resuscitative efforts.[53] Quan and colleagues demonstrated that prehospital intervention could improve outcome. Aggressive prehospital management resulted in a 32% survival from cardiac arrest. A bad outcome was associated with submersion over 9 minutes or cardiopulmonary resuscitation over 25 minutes.[54]

If cardiotoxic drugs were necessary to establish a perfusing cardiac rhythm, the outcome resulted in death or severe neurologic deficit in all patients.[55] As mentioned earlier, both increased ICP and decreased CPP are associated with poor outcome.[44] Elevated blood sugar is also associated with death or a vegetative state in 68% of the patients.[56] All patients with spontaneous respirations after resuscitation survived and had either little or no neurologic residual.[52]

Brain stem auditory evoked responses (BAER) have been studied in near-drowning patients. Patients who have normal recovery have BAER similar to control subjects. Children who survived in a persistent vegetative state have abnormal BAER within 6 hours of cardiac arrest; however, they became normal at 24 hours. Patients who died had abnormal responses from admission to death.[57]

Serial neurologic examinations will help separate those who will survive intact from those who will not. Bratton and colleagues found that 24 hours after a near-drowning episode, all children with normal recovery had spontaneous, purposeful movements. All children without spontaneous, purposeful movements and normal brain stem function 24 hours after near drowning, died or had severe neurologic impairment.[58]

There have been reports of survival after prolonged submersion in very cold water. A child who had been submerged for 66 minutes in 5° C water survived intact after 2 hours of CPR followed by extracorporeal warming. No precise prognostic indicators are available for hypothermic patients. Of 14 pediatric patients who had core temperatures <33° C and absent vital signs, eight died, two persisted in a vegetative state, and four survived.[59]

When speaking to the parent about the child's prognosis, it is important to realize that the parent is usually suffering from a great deal of guilt. Most pediatric drownings, in fact, occur under preventable circumstances.

PREVENTION

The majority of drowning and near-drowning injuries are preventable.[60] A four-sided fence 1.4 meters high with a self-locking gate will prevent the children from 1 to 4 years of age from entering the water.[61] Proper use of protective fencing is estimated to decrease pediatric submersion incidents by 60% to 80%. Protective fencing should have self-closing and -latching gates and should not include the house as one side of the fence. Unfortunately, many pool owners oppose barrier requirements. The use of a rigid pool cover that prevents entry into the water has not been well studied. Improved supervision will lead to a decreased number of drownings. Small children should never be left alone near any body of water (including bathtubs). All buckets containing water should be emptied immediately after use. Parents should realize that swimming lessons cannot "drownproof" children younger than 4 years of age. Older children should be taught how to swim, but never to swim without supervision. Children should always wear an approved life preserver whenever riding on a boat. Children should be taught the danger of diving in shallow or unknown waters. Adolescents need to understand the danger of drinking and illicit drug use during recreational aquatic activities. Finally, parents and adolescents should be taught CPR. Frequently, the child is rescued from the water by someone who does not know CPR. Wintemute found that in 42% of all pediatric drownings that occurred in the child's own pool, the rescuer did not initiate CPR.[62]

References

Epidemiology

1. National Safety Council: *Accident facts*, Itasca, Ill, 1994, National Safety Council.
2. Waller AE, Baker SP, Szocka A: Childhood injury deaths: National analysis and geographic variations, *Am J Public Health* 79:310, 1989.
3. Wintemute GJ: Childhood drowning and near-drowning in the United States, *Am J Dis Child* 144:663, 1990.

4. Geddis DC: The exposure of pre-school children to water hazards and the incidence of potential drowning accidents, *N Z Med J* 97:223, 1984.
5. Orlowski JP: Drowning, near drowning and ice water submersions, *Pediatr Clin North Am* 34:75, 1987.
6. Brenner RA, Smith GS, Overpeck MD: Divergent trends in childhood drowning rates, 1971 through 1988, *JAMA* 271:1606, 1994.
7. Guyer B and Ellers B: Childhood injuries in the United States: mortality, morbidity, and cost, *Am J Dis Child* 144:649, 1990.
8. Orlowski JP: Adolescent drownings: swimming, boating, diving and scuba accidents, *Pediatr Ann* 17:125, 1987.

Pathophysiology

9. Modell JH: Drowning, *New Eng J Med* 328:253, 1993.
10. Modell JH and Davis JH: Electrolyte changes in human drowning victims, *Anesthesiology* 30:414, 1969.
11. Modell JH: Biology of drowning, *Ann Rev Med* 29:1, 1978.
12. Modell JH and Moya F: Effects of volume of aspirated fluid during chlorinated fresh water drowning, *Anesthesiology* 27:662, 1966.
13. Halmagyi DFJ and Colebatch HJH: Ventilation and circulation after fluid aspiration, *J Appl Physiol* 16:35, 1961.
14. Karch SB: Pathology of the lung in near drowning, *Am J Emerg Med* 4:4, 1986.
15. Higgins P, Seminski J, Pearson RD: Hypoxic lap swimming—a cause of near drowning (letter to the editor), *N Engl J Med* 315:1552, 1986.
16. Bolte RG, Black PG, Bowers RS: The use of extracorporeal rewarming in a child submerged for 66 minutes, *JAMA* 260:377, 1988.
17. Bangs CC: Hypothermia and frostbite, *Emerg Clin North Am* 2:475, 1984.
18. Olshaker JS: Near drowning, *Emerg Clin North Am* 10:339, 1992.
19. Ramey CA, Ramey DN, Hayward JS: Dive Response of children in response to cold water near drowning, *J Appl Physiol Soc* 63:665, 1987.

Etiology

20. Sulkes SB and van der Jagt EW: Solar pool blankets: another water hazard, *Pediatrics* 85:1114, 1990.
21. Quan L, Gore EJ, Wentz K et al: Ten-year study of pediatric drowning and near-drownings in King County, Washington: lessons in injury prevention, *Pediatrics* 83:1035, 1989.
22. O'Carrol PW, Alkon E, Weiss B: Drowning mortality in Los Angeles County, 1976-1984, *JAMA* 260:380, 1988.
23. Kemp AM, Mott AM, Sibert JR: Accidents and child abuse in bathtub submersions, *Arch Dis Child* 70:435, 1994.
24. Lavelle JM, Shaw KN, Seidl T et al: Ten-year review of pediatric bathtub near-drownings: evaluation for child abuse and neglect, *Ann Emerg Med* 25:344, 1995.
25. Mann NC, Weller SC, Rauchschwalbe R: Bucket-related drownings in the United States, 1984 through 1990 [see comments], *Pediatrics* 89:1068, 1992.
26. Shinaberger CS, Anderson CL, Kraus JF: Young children who drown in hot tubs, spas, and whirlpools in California: a 26-year survey, *Am J Public Health* 80:613, 1990.
27. Craig AB: Causes of loss of consciousness during underwater swimming, *J Appl Physiol* 10:583, 1961.
28. Orlowski JP, Rothman DA, Lueders H: Submersion accidents in children with epilepsy, *Am J Dis Child* 136:777, 1982.
29. Pearn J: Epilepsy and drowning in childhood, *Br Med J*:1510, 1977.
30. Pearn JH, Bart R, Yamaoka: Drowning risks to epileptic patients: a study from Hawaii, *Br Med J* 4:1284, 1978.

Complications

31. Hoff B: Multisystem failure: a review with special reference to drowning, *Crit Care Med* 7:310, 1979.

Management

32. Heimlich HJ: Subdiaphragmatic pressure to expel water from the lungs of drowning persons, *Ann Emerg Med* 10:476, 1981.
33. Emergency Cardiac Care Committee and subcommittes AHA: Guidelines for cardiopulmonary resuscitation and emergency cardiac care, IV: Special resuscitation situations, *JAMA* 268:2246, 1992.
34. Rosen P, Stoto M, Harley J: The use of the Heimlich Maneuver in near drowning: Institute of Medicine Report, *J Emerg Med* 13:In press, 1995.

35. Pace HL: Positive end-expiratory pressure (PEEP) in treating salt water near-drowning, *West J Med* 2:165, 1975.
36. McBrien M, Katumba JJ, Mukhtar AI: Artificial surfactant in the treatment of near drowning [letter], *Lancet* 342:1485, 1993.
37. Modell JH, Graves SA, Ketover A: A clinical course of 91 consecutive near-drowning victims, *Chest* 70:127, 1976.
38. Calderwood HW, Modell JH, Ruiz BC: The ineffectiveness of steroid therapy for treatment of fresh-water drowning, *Anesthesiology* 43:642, 1975.
39. Hildehard CA, Hartman AG, Arcenie EL, et al: Cardiac performance in pediatric near drowning, *Crit Care Med* 16:331, 1988.
40. Orlowski JP, Albulleil MM, Phillips JM: The hemodymanic and cardiovascular effects of near drowing in hypotonic, isotonic, and hypertonic solution, *Ann Emer Med* 18: 1989.
41. Chameides L: *Textbook of pediatric advanced life support*, Dallas, American Heart Association, 1990.
42. Bohn DJ, Biggin DW, Smith CR: Influence of hypothermia barbituate therapy and ICP monitoring on morbidity and mortality after near drowning, *Crit Care Med* 14:259, 1986.
43. Conn AW, Edmonds JF, Barker GA: Cerebral resuscitation in near drowning, *Pediatr Clin North Am* 26:691, 1979.
44. Nussbaum E and Galant SP: Intracranial pressure monitoring as a guide to prognosis, *J Pediatr* 102:215, 1983.
45. Frewen TC, Sumalat WO, Han VK: Cerebral resuscitation in pediatric near drowning, *J Pediatr* 106:615, 1985.
46. Conn AW and Barker GA: Fresh water drowning and near water drowning: an update, *Can Anesth Soc* 31:3, 1984.
47. Modell JH: Treatment of near drowning: is there a role for H.Y.P.E.R. therapy, *Crit Car Med* 14:593, 1986.
48. Nussbaum E and Maggi JC: Pentobarbital therapy does not improve neurological outcome in nearly drowned, flaccid-comatose children, *Pediatrics* 81:630, 1988.

Disposition

49. Pearn JH: Secondary drowning in children, *Br Med J* 281:1193, 1980.
50. Pratt FD and Haynes BE: Incidence of "secondary drowning" after submersion, *Ann Emerg Med* 137:1084, 1986.

51. Shaw KN and Briede CA: Submersion injuries, drowning, and near drowning, *Emerg Med Clin North Am* 7:355, 1989.

Prognosis

52. Jacobsen WK, Mason LJ, Briggs BA et al: Correlation of spontaneous respirations and and neurological damage in near-drowning, *Crit Care Med* 11:487, 1983.
53. Kyriacou DN, Arcinue EL, Peek C et al: Effect of immediate resuscitation on children with submersion injury, *Pediatrics* 94:137, 1994.
54. Quan L, Wentz ICR, Gore EJ: Outcome and predictors of outcome in pediatric submersion receiving prehospital care in Kings County, Washington, *Pediatrics* 86:586, 1991.
55. Nussbaum E: Prognostic variables in nearly drowned comatose children, *Am J Dis Child* 139:1058, 1985.
56. Ashwal S, Schneider S, Tomosi L et al: Prognostic implications of hyperglycemia and reduced cerebral blood flow in childhood near drowning, *Neurology* 40:820, 1990.
57. Fisher B, Peterson B, Hicks G: Use of brainstem auditory evoked response testing to assess neurologic outcome following near drowning in children, *Crit Care Med* 20:578, 1992.
58. Bratton SL, Jardine DS, Morray JP: Serial neurologic examinations after near drowning and outcome, *Arch Pediatr Adolesc Med* 148:167, 1994.
59. Biggart MJ and Bohn DJ: Effect of hypothermia and cardiac arrest on outcome of near-drowning accidents in children, *J Pediatr* 117:179, 1990.
60. American Academy of Pediatrics, Committee on Injury and Poison Prevention: Drowning in infants, children and adolescents, *Pediatrics* 92:292, 1993.
61. Nixon JW, Pearn JH, Petrie GM: Childproof safety barriers: an ergonomic study to reduce child trauma due to environmental hazards, *Aust Paediatr J* 15:260, 1979.
62. Wintemute GJ, Kraus JF, Teret SP et al: Drowning in childhood and adolescence: a population-based study, *Am J Pub Health* 77:830, 1987.

## 36

Electrical and Lightning Injuries

M. Lois Hall • Robert M. Sills

Children who are the victims of electrical injury may present clinically with a wide variety of symptoms that vary greatly in degree and type. Each year, an estimated 300 lightning injuries and 100 fatalities occur in the United States.[1] Most lightning injuries go unreported; 70% to 80% of those struck by lightning survive.[2] However, about two thirds of survivors experience permanent sequelae. Fatal outcomes are more often associated with patients who have experienced leg burns, burns to the head, and immediate cardiopulmonary arrest. Most victims of lightning strikes are outdoors for recreational purposes such as hiking, camping, and sports.[3-5]

Accidents resulting from electrical current account for as many as 760 deaths (97% male) annually, 16% of the victims under the age of 20 years and 5% under 10 years of age. Especially at risk are very young children exploring their home environment (see Prevention). The incidence also peaks from 15 to 24 years of age. High-tension wires and industrial accidents play a larger role in injuries to these older groups.[6,7]

PATHOPHYSIOLOGY

The type and severity of injury a patient experiences in an electrical accident depend on the thermal energy generated by the electrical current and the physiologic changes directly caused by the passage of an electric current through the body.[8,9] An electric current is the flow of electrons from an area of higher concentration, called *potential*, to an area of lower potential. This electron flow is governed by the laws of electricity. A review of Ohm's law reminds us that:

$$V = I \times R$$

OR

$$\text{Voltage} = \text{Amperage} \times \text{Resistance}$$

where

V = Voltage is force of electron flow (difference in potential required for a current of 1 amp to flow through a resistance of 1 ohm)

I = Amperage is volume of electrons flowing (unit of intensity produced by 1 V acting through a resistance of 1 ohm)

R = Resistance is degree of hindrance to electron flow (measured in units of electrical resistance, the ohm)

The heat generated by a sustained electrical current is determined by Joule's law:

$$\text{Heat} = I^2 \times R \textbf{ OR } \text{Heat} = \text{Amperage}^2 \times \text{Resistance}$$

Therefore the extent of a patient's injury is determined by the following factors:

1. Tissue resistance of skin and internal body structure
2. Intensity of current (amperage)
3. Pathway of current flow
4. Type of current polarity (AC or DC)
5. Frequency of current
6. Duration of current[10]

Tissue Resistance and Current Intensity (Amperage)

Joule's law states that increased resistance to the passage of a current generates greater heat. Heat is produced as an electric current encounters resistance in the various body structures it traverses between the point of entrance and its exit to ground. This heat may then cause thermal injury to tissues.[8] In addition, according to Ohm's law, resistance is inversely related to the intensity of the current (amperage or I) because it impedes current flow.

Body tissues vary in their electrical resistance capacity in the following order from lesser to greater: nerves, blood vessels, muscle, skin, tendon, fat, and bone.[7] Because the skin is generally the area of initial contact with current, its resistance properties play an important role in the amount of current flow and degree of injury. Skin resistance varies with age, thickness, water content, cleanliness, and type of electric current. Skin with high resistance may result in more thermal damage at the site of the contact with a current, but will impede the intensity of the current. Skin with low resistance may show a lesser degree of thermal damage at the contact site, but still allow for greater passage of current (greater intensity), resulting in more internal damage from heat and flow of electric current.

A newborn's skin is thin and has a high water content, providing very low resistance. Calloused, adult skin may have resistances as high as 1,000,000 ohm. Normal palms have resistance of 40,000 ohm, but resistance drops to a range of 300 to 1,000 ohm when moisture (water or perspiration) is added. Mouth burns in toddlers are exacerbated by the low resistance (<100 ohm) of saliva and moist mucous membranes, allowing the heat of increased current flow to cause severe burns to the lips and oral cavity. Decreased skin resistance of children in bathtubs or pools makes them especially susceptible to injury from electrical exposure, most commonly from appliance cords.[11]

The presence and appearance of entrance and exit wounds on the skin is related to skin resistance and the area of contact. A child electrocuted in a bathtub may have no evidence of skin wounds because of the low resistance of wet skin and the large contact area; yet extensive internal damage may have resulted from internal current flow. Dry skin exposed to a "live-wire" is an example of a smaller area of contact with higher resistance causing thermal skin injury that typically appears as a small, well-defined region of whitish-yellow ischemia and coagulation. Less frequently, electrical contact burns may result in large entrance wounds leading to aseptic necrosis, usually in extremity areas.[12]

Pregnancy

The pathophysiology of electrical injury to the pregnant patient deserves special mention, as certainly pregnancy occurs in the "pediatric age" group. A review of pregnant patients who were victims of household alternating current demonstrated minimal injury to the mothers (only one mother was injured by an electrical burn); fetal death occurred in 11 of the 14 cases, with only one normal pregnancy resulting in the group.[13] The fetus is at higher risk of injury because fetal skin is 200 times less resistant to the passage of current than postnatal skin, and the hyperemic pregnant uterus and amniotic fluid are excellent conductors of electricity. Lighting injury to 11 other pregnant patients resulted in no maternal deaths but 5 fetal or neonatal deaths occurred. The current path in these victims was hand to foot, traversing the uterus. It should be noted that electroconvulsive therapy (ECT) and direct current (DC) cardioversion do not include the uterus in the current path, and the literature supports the safety of these procedures for both mother and fetus. Minor electrical and lightning injuries to the pregnant patient warrant immediate fetal monitoring, ultrasound to assess viability and urgent obstetric consultation and follow-up.[14]

Pathway of Current Flow

Once an electric current penetrates the skin, it tends to flow directly from the point of contact to the ground, which may actually be the ground or another area of the body that completes the circuit. Because internal body tissues have relatively uniform resistances, the current flow tends to travel directly between these points without deflection from anatomic structures, potentially injuring organs on its route.[14] The three principal pathways are (1) hand to hand (mortality rate >60% because of transection of the spinal cord from C-4 to C-8); (2) hand to foot (mortality rate >20% because of current induced dysrhythmias); and (3) foot to foot (mortality rate <5%).[4]

Type of Current Polarity (AC or DC) and Frequency, Intensity, and Duration

Alternating current (AC) means the electron flow changes direction with a certain frequency/second. A perfect example is low-voltage household current alternating at 60 cycles/sec. Human muscle responds to this electrical stimulus with tetanic contraction at a frequency allowing neuromuscular function to remain refractory indefinitely. The victim locks on to the current source via flexor muscle contraction so the duration of contact is longer. High voltage is generally more dangerous and may also throw the victim from the source, decreasing duration of contact but increasing the likelihood of head, spine, and fracture injuries.

Lightning is an example of a direct current (DC), which is massive in energy level (amperage and voltage) and brief in contact, causing a single, strong muscle contraction. Another example is the direct current used medically for defibrillation, countershock, and pacemaking.

Types of Injury Sustained by Electrical Current and Lightning Current

Lightning current may contact a victim in four ways: direct strike, side flash, stride potential, and flash-over phenomenon.[15-17]

Direct strike is the most serious type, as the major pathway of current flow is through the victim. Carrying metal objects such as golf clubs or umbrellas during a thunderstorm greatly increases the chance of a direct strike. When the lightning current discharges from the primary strike area (tree or person) through the air to a nearby victim, it is called a *side flash.*

Stride potential refers to a current that hits the ground, enters through one leg of its victim, and exits through the other leg as it travels because a person has less resistance to flow than the ground. A mortality rate of 30% has been noted in patients with leg burns from stride potential lightning injuries.

Flash-over phenomenon occurs when lightning energy flows outside the body of the victim, usually facilitated by wet clothes, which may actually be blown off the victim. Pathognomonic featherlike skin burns may be found in these circumstances. Partial- and full-thickness thermal burns may also occur as a result of body contact with ignited clothes or other objects. Blunt injury to the head, spine, and major organs should be suspected as lightning strike victims are frequently jolted to the ground or against objects with considerable force due to either the lightning shock wave or a single severe muscle contraction.[5,18]

Commercial high-voltage electrical current has several important characteristics. A victim may experience prolonged exposure to an alternating current because of the muscle "lock-on" phenomenon described earlier. Unlike lightning current, high-voltage electrical current is not as-

TABLE 36-1. Electrical Injury: Clinical Considerations

	Clinical manifestations	Management
General		Extrication; ABCs of resuscitation; immobilize spine
		History: voltage, type of current
		CBC with platelets, electrolytes, BUN, creatinine, glucose
Cardiac	Dysrhythmias: asystole, ventricular fibrillation, sinus tachycardia, sinus bradycardia, PVC, PAC, conduction defects, atrial fibrillation, ST-T wave changes	Treat dysrhythmias
		Cardiac monitor, ECG, and chest x-ray film with suspected thoracic injury
		CPK with isoenzymes if indicated
Pulmonary	Respiratory arrest, acute respiratory distress, aspiration syndrome	Protect and maintain airway
		Mechanical ventilation if indicated, chest x-ray film, ABG level
Renal	Acute renal failure, myoglobinuria	Aggressive fluid management unless CNS injury
		Maintain adequate urine output > 1 ml/kg/hr
		Consider CVP or pulmonary artery pressure monitoring
		Urine myoglobin, urinalysis, BUN, creatinine
Neurologic	Immediate: loss of consciousness, motor paralysis, visual disturbances, amnesia, agitation; intracranial hematoma	Treat seizures
		Fluid restriction if indicated
	Secondary: pain, paraplegia, brachial plexus injury, SIADH, autonomic disturbances, cerebral edema	Consider spine x-ray films, especially cervical
	Delayed: paralysis, seizures, headache, peripheral neuropathy	CT scan of brain if indicated
Cutaneous/oral	Oral commissure burns, tongue and dental injuries; skin burns resulting from ignition of clothes, entrance and exit burns, and arc burns	Search for entrance/exit wound
		Treat cutaneous burns; tetanus status
		Plastic surgery or ENT consult if needed
Abdominal	Viscus perforation and solid organ damage; ileus; abdominal injury rare without visible abdominal burns	NG tube if airway compromise or ileus
		SGOT, SGPT, amylase, BUN, creatinine, CT radiographs as indicated
Musculoskeletal	Compartment syndrome from subcutaneous necrosis limb edema and deep burns	Follow for compartment syndrome
	Long bone fractures, spine injuries	X-ray films and orthopedic/general surgery consultations as indicated
Ocular	Visual changes, optic neuritis, cataracts, extraocular muscle paresis	Ophthalmology consultation as indicated

ABC, Airway, breathing, circulation; *CBC*, complete blood cell count; *BUN*, blood urea nitrogen; *PVC*, premature ventricular contractions; *PAC*, premature atrial contractions; *ECG*, electrocardiogram; *CPK*, creatinine phosphokinase; *ABG*, arterial blood gas; *CNS*, central nervous system; *CVP*, central venous pressure; *CT*, computed tomography; *SIADH*, syndrome of inappropriate secretion of antidiuretic hormone; *ENT*, ear, nose, and throat; *NG*, nasogastric; *SGOT*, serum glutamate oxaloacetate transaminase (aspartate aminotransferase); *SGPT*, serum glutamate pyruvate transaminase (alanine aminotransferase).

sociated with flashover or shock wave. The victim is more likely to experience ventricular fibrillation than asystole.[19]

Direct electrical injury results when current passes through the skin causing entry and exit wounds and frequently extensive underlying tissue damage. *Arc burns* vary in appearance and depth of injury, depending on the proximity of the current to the skin as it externally courses the body. *Flame burns* are direct thermal injuries, which are usually partial thickness if secondary to flashburns and full thickness if they result from ignition of clothing.[18,19]

DIAGNOSTIC FINDINGS

Clinical Findings

After sustaining an electrical injury, patients may present to the emergency department in a variety of clinical states ranging from an asymptomatic appearance to complete cardiopulmonary arrest. The severity of a patient's condition depends on many factors including voltage received, pathway, and type of current. Many injuries incurred from electrical current are initially deceiving. Small cutaneous entry wounds may belie the extensive soft tissue and organ damage that has occurred beneath the surface. Remember, electrical injuries result from the direct effect of current, as well as from the conversion of electrical energy into thermal energy as current passes through the body's tissues. A multitude of types of injuries can therefore be expected and sought (Table 36-1).

Cardiac arrest is the primary cause of immediate death in the electrically injured patient. The major cause of arrest in these patients appears to be the result of malignant dysrhythmias, severe myocardial damage, or respiratory arrest with resultant asphyxia.[14] Cardiac asystole and ventricular fibrillation are important causes of death in the immediate postinjury period. Ventricular fibrillation is more commonly seen in alternating current injures (i.e., household current), whereas the massive direct current of a lightning strike causes a total depolarization of the heart, resulting in asystole.[8] Asystole as the result of a lightning strike is usually brief, but the respiratory depression that also occurs may be prolonged and require aggressive management, as continued hypoxia may accompany resistant ventricular fibrillation.

Cardiac complications occur in between 5% and 54% of electrical exposures and include less malignant dysrhythmias as well.[20-22] Ventricular tachycardia, atrial dysrhythmias, various degrees of heart block, ventricular wall perforation, and myocardial infarction have all been reported.[22-24] Most of the nonfatal rhythm disturbances occur immediately and resolve spontaneously, but their appearance may be delayed up to 12 hours in electrical injuries and 2 weeks in lightning injuries.[24,25] High-voltage and lightning injuries may also result in tachycardia and hypertension, which are thought to be secondary to excess catecholamines.

The most important pulmonary complication of electrical shock is a respiratory arrest. This may occur as a result of respiratory center paralysis or forced tetanic contractions of the muscles of respiration, as well as accompanying ventricular fibrillation and asystole. Respiratory center paralysis that occurs in lightning injury is often prolonged and can outlast cardiac arrest. In fact, the duration of apnea appears to be the critical factor in survival and must, therefore, be managed aggressively even in the clinically dead–appearing patient.[26] Other pulmonary concerns include gastric aspiration, adult respiratory distress syndrome (ARDS), and pulmonary edema.[27,28]

The most frequently involved system in electrical injuries is the nervous system. Many types of neurologic damage occur, and the effects are usually seen in a temporal relationship to the accident. Effects noted as an immediate result of the shock include loss of consciousness, motor paralysis, visual disturbances, amnesia, and intracranial hematomas. Injuries such as these may result from the direct effect of the current or as a result of head trauma when violently thrown from the current source.[29] Neurologic injuries that may present later in the course include paraplegia, brachial plexus injuries, syndrome of inappropriate secretion of antidiuretic hormone (SIADH), diabetes insipidus, hearing loss, neuropathy and seizures.[30,31] Autonomic disturbances such as peripheral edema, cyanosis, peripheral artery spasm, Horner syndrome, and pupillary dysfunction may occur immediately after injury; this possibility is important to remember when considering brain death in electrical shock patients. An entire neurologic evaluation is needed, including caloric and vestibuloocular reflexes to rule out brain death in the face of fixed and dilated pupils.

High-voltage electrical injuries are accompanied by a higher proportion of renal failure than other types of burns. Renal failure may be caused by the direct effect of current on tissue, hypoxic damage to the kidney, or more commonly as a result of excess myoglobin deposition. Myoglobinuria results from the extensive muscle damage caused by the electrical current.[4] This is especially seen in the child who is "locked on" to the current and suffers tetanic muscular contractions with resultant muscular breakdown. It should be considered in patients with urinalysis positive for blood but without red cells visible on microscopic examination. Renal failure is rare with lightning injury, as these patients are usually not "locked on" to the current.

Younger children, particularly those who explore their environment through oral/tactile stimulation, are prone to injury of the oral cavity and lips. This type of injury commonly occurs when a child bites on an electrical cord or sucks on the female end of a live extension cord. Typically, an arc burn occurs between the cord terminals, with the mouth saliva completing the circuit. Intense heat causes coagulation necrosis and liquefaction.[11,32] These lesions are generally painless, as associated neural tissues are destroyed.

Most frequently, oral burns involve the commissure of the lips.[32] A common complication of commissure burns may occur 5 to 14 days after injury in the form of delayed bleeding from the labial artery as healing progresses and nonvital burned tissues (scab or eschar) are sloughed off the lips. The child's parents should be made aware of this possible problem at discharge and be taught how to manage it pending evaluation. The late manifestations of an electrical burn to the mouth include deterioration of the dentition, microstomia, abnormal development of the dental arches, ankyloglossia, speech problems, and labial adhesions.[32]

Massive thermal burns can occur, particularly if clothing has been ignited. However, as stated previously, small entrance and exit wounds are often the case and may mask extensive damage to underlying muscles, nerves, and blood vessels. Tissue that initially appears viable may become edematous, ischemic, and ultimately necrotic. Because the amount of heat produced by traveling current is related to the resistance of the tissue, current passing through bones in the extremities may generate a tremendous amount of heat and cause severe thermal damage to the surrounding soft tissues. As a result of underlying soft tissue damage, swelling of the extremity and compression of neighboring neurovasculature may result in the compartment syndrome.[29] Low-voltage alternating current can induce tetanic muscle contractions so severe that it may cause long-bone fractures, as well as vertebral compression fractures and dislocations. Fractures may also result if a victim is thrown from high-voltage energy sources.[33,34]

Ocular manifestations include cataracts, optic neuritis, optic atrophy, visual defects, and extraocular muscle paresis.[34]

Ancillary Data

Initial evaluation of patients injured by high-voltage electrical current should include complete blood cell count (CBC) with platelets, electrolytes, blood urea nitrogen (BUN), creatinine, urinalysis, and urine myoglobin. Patients with signs suggesting transfer of current through the thorax should have a 12-lead electrocardiogram (ECG) and chest x-ray study. Creatinine phosphokinase (CPK), with isoenzymes, should also be performed if indicated. Cardiac monitoring should be initiated in patients with dysrhythmias, as well as an abnormal ECG or elevated CPK MB levels. Additional radiographic examinations should be obtained as indicated. All patients with a history of loss of consciousness or clinical signs of neck injury should have cervical spine films. Plain skeletal films may be indicated if a fracture is suspected. A computed tomography (CT) scan of the head and abdomen should be performed if significant injury to these areas is suspected. Clinical considerations in electrical injuries are included in Table 36-1.

MANAGEMENT

Initial management of electrically injured patients pertains to prehospital care. Determining the voltage and type of current involved is helpful, and the power company may be of assistance. Extrication of the victim from the source of electrical energy must be approached cautiously so as not to endanger the rescue party. If possible, all electrical current should be shut off, and the rescuer should be well insulated. If wires need to be cut, wooden-handled or insulated cutters should be used. Contrary to popular belief, lightning may in fact strike twice in the same place, and rescuers should consider moving the victim during an ongoing storm.[35] The patient should be immobilized with attention to the spine. Since electrically injured patients can have both medical and traumatic injuries, they should be treated using concepts from both pediatric advanced life support and advanced trauma life support.

As in all emergencies, immediate attention should be given to cardiopulmonary resuscitation (CPR). The airway should be assessed and maintained. Signs of possible airway compromise may be present, such as singed nasal hairs and eyebrows, an unstable cervical spine, loss of consciousness, coma, or an inability to clear secretions. Respiratory effort frequently may be delayed even after resolution of cardiac arrest. Aggressive respiratory management with a bag and mask or intubation should be considered to prevent further hypoxia even in the patient who appears "dead." Patients with cardiac arrest from lightning injury have higher survival rates then those who arrest from other causes and should therefore be treated aggressively. In the case of mass casualties with limited supplies, the most seriously injured patients should be attended to first to prevent further ischemic insult, even if they appear "dead." Unstable dysrhythmias should be treated immediately using current advanced life support protocols.

Once stabilized, the patient should be transported to an appropriate facility. After arrival at the emergency department, repeat assessment of CPR is necessary. A set of vital signs should be obtained and continuous cardiac monitoring should be performed. At least one large-bore IV catheter should be in place. If there is evidence of shock, an initial bolus of 20 ml/kg of an isotonic solution such as lactated Ringer's or normal saline should be given and repeated as indicated.

As stated earlier, electrical burns may be deceptive because underlying soft tissue damage may be extensive without the presence of large surface skin burns, and excessive third spacing of fluids frequently occurs. To prevent ongoing fluid loss and maintain renal diuresis, these patients require much larger fluid volumes than that used to treat plain thermal burns. In one review of electrical burns, 20% of cases exhibited shock secondary to massive third spacing. It is advisable therefore not to base fluid management on a typical surface burn formula but to titrate fluids to urine output.[35] Urinary output should be maintained at greater than 1 ml/kg/hr. Lightning injuries usually do not require this type of fluid management, as extensive, unnoticed soft tissue injury does not often occur. Major central nervous system (CNS) injury is more common in lightning injury; therefore fluid restriction may be ultimately required after initial resuscitation.[36]

Once initial stabilization has taken place, a secondary physical examination should be performed. Cervical spine immobilization should be maintained until radiographic studies and physical examination have confirmed the absence of a fracture. The patient should undergo a complete neurologic examination with attention to the cranial nerves. If indicated, caloric testing and oculocephalic reflexes should be performed if cervical spine injury is not suspected.

An NG tube should be placed to reduce the risk of aspiration pneumonia if abdominal distension occurs or if the patient is unable to protect the airway. A thorough skin examination should identify all entrance and exit wounds. If surface wounds are far apart, more severe internal injuries are likely. Usually, a child with an isolated oral injury does not have an exit wound, since the current is likely to exit via the ground in the cord. Because of the autonomic instability that can occur, the skin of a victim may appear mottled and cyanotic, although this finding is generally transient.

The musculoskeletal system should be examined for occult fractures. All burned extremities should be evaluated for pulse, capillary refill, and motor sensory function. If vascular compromise or compartment syndrome is suspected, fasciotomy may be required and a surgeon should be consulted immediately.

Urinary output should be monitored closely, and if a patient exhibits signs of renal failure, appropriate treatment should be initiated. If myoglobinuria is felt to be the cause of renal failure, urinary alkalinization to keep urine pH ≥ 7.45, and diuretics such as furosemide (1 mg/kg/dose IV) or mannitol (0.5 gm/kg/dose IV) may supplement crystalloid administration to maintain good urine output.

A CT scan of the head is indicated if a patient remains comatose or if intracranial injury is suspected. When signs of impending herniation are present, appropriate treatment should be instituted to minimize increased intracranial pressure. The patient should be intubated immediately and hyperventilated to maintain a P_{CO_2} in the 25 to 30 mm Hg range. The head of the bed may be elevated to 30 degrees, and an osmotic diuretic such as mannitol may be given (0.5 to 1 gm/kg). Cerebral edema can develop over hours to days and should be suspected if deterioration of neurologic status occurs. Intracranial pressure monitoring may be needed in some cases.

Central venous pressure (CVP) monitoring may greatly assist fluid management in the child where central nervous system (CNS) shock or renal disturbances are suspected simultaneously.

Mild thermal burns caused by ignited clothing or the heat generated from the current may be treated like other thermal burns, with application of sterile dressings and antibacterial cream (see Chapter 37). Tetanus prophylaxis, if not current, is indicated. Children who sustain oral injuries should be examined by an oral or plastic surgeon for initial and ongoing evaluation (see Chapter 21). Initial assessment of all significantly burned extremities should involve surgical consultation as complications from edema, necrosis, and vascular compromise may increase over time. In particular, high-voltage injuries require more aggressive evaluation and treatment because of the frequent need for fasciotomy and amputation in these patients.[19,32]

In all but the most minor electrical injuries, children should be admitted and monitored in a hospital experienced in the care of electrical burns. All patients with lightning injuries should be admitted.

The majority of the patients we see are not victims of serious high-voltage injury but of low-voltage household current. These injuries are usually minor and result when a child puts objects into an electrical socket or plays with a frayed extension cord. The literature on the management of these patients is less abundant than that on high-voltage injuries; however, several studies have recommended a less aggressive approach.[21,22,37] Admission for continuous cardiac monitoring in low-voltage–injured asymptomatic patients with a normal ECG is not necessary. One recent study goes even further in stating that an ECG is not required in the absence of loss of consciousness, observed tetany, wet skin, or current flow that crossed the heart region.[37] This article also suggests that CPK and myoglobinuria screening are not necessary after household electrical injuries.

It has become an acceptable practice to observe for a brief period of time those children who sustain a minor household injury; if they remain asymptomatic, they can be discharged home after appropriate local tissue care. This approach assumes that they have none of the above risk factors and will have follow-up care arranged. In only select patients are laboratory studies obtained. Patients with oral commissure burns, extensive thermal burns, and those with entrance and exit wounds not on the same extremity are admitted for observation, laboratory evaluation, and surgical consultation.

Prevention

Prevention is essential. Children should be instructed about the dangers of electrical injuries and ready access to electrical plugs and wires reduced.[38] Flying kites and climbing trees near electrical wires should be avoided. If contact with an electrical source occurs, the patient should be withdrawn from it without exposing the rescuer to potential injury.

Outdoor activities such as mountain hikes and field sports should be planned for early mornings during summer thunderstorm season, since most storms take place between noon and early evening. During lightning storms, children should stay indoors or seek shelter in a building constructed with steel girders, avoiding ungrounded structures like tents, sheds, and cabanas. They should also avoid proximity to metal objects such as bicycles, golf clubs, grandstands, wire fences, and clotheslines.[5] If there is no shelter, youngsters should avoid the highest object in the area, hilltops, open spaces, and bodies of water. They should seek the lowest spot and assume a curled position.[39] If lightning does strike, bystanders should initiate CPR immediately and contact the emergency medical system (EMS).

New technologies such as magnetic directional finders offer the possibility of reducing lightning injuries in the future. These devices, costing several thousand dollars, are able to detect the instantaneous field signal associated with a lightning flash and can locate the site of lightning strikes within a several-mile radius. Another small hand-held device costing several hundred dollars and currently being used at PGA and LPGA tournaments, can identify lightning up to 10 miles away by detecting a change in light intensity in clouds during the daytime. If used during events such as field and golf games, these devices can track the intensity and movement of lightning storms. With approaching storms, players can then be warned and directed to safe shelters.[40]

References

General

1. Duclos PJ, Sanderson LM, Klontz KC: Lightning-related mortality and morbidity in Florida, *Public Health Rep* 105:276, 1990.
2. Cooper MA: Lightning injuries: prognostic signs for death, *Ann Emerg Med* 9:134-138, May, 1980.
3. Miller FE and Peterson D: Abdominal visceral perforation secondary to electrical injury: case report and review of the literature, *Burns* 12(7):505, 1986.
4. Thompson JC and Ashwal S: Electrical injuries in children, *Am J Child* 137:231, 1983.
5. Cwinn AA and Cantrill SV: Lightning injuries, *J Emerg Med* 2:379, 1985.
6. National Safety Council: Accident facts, 1990, final condensed edition, August, 1990.
7. Lee RC, Capelli-Schellpfeffer M, Kelly KM: Electrical injury: a multidisiplinary approach to therapy, prevention, and rehabilitation, *Ann NY Acad Sci* 720, May 1994.

Pathophysiology

8. Esses SI and Peters WJ: Electrical burns, pathophysiology and complications, *Can J Surg* 24(1):11, 1981.
9. Fish R: Electric shock. Part I: physics and pathophysiology, *J Emerg Med* 11 (3):309-12, 1993.
10. Branday JM and DuQuesnay DR: Visceral complications of electrical burn injury, *West Indian Med J* 38:110, 1989.
11. Donly KJ and Nowak A: Oral electrical burns: etiology, manifestations and treatment, *Gen Dent* March-April, 103, 1988.
12. Fish R: Electric shock, Part II: nature and mechanisms of injury, *J Emerg Med* 11 (4):457-62, 1993.
13. Fatovich D: Electric shock in pregnancy, *J Emerg Med* 11 (2):175-177, 1993.
14. Ceddes LA, Bourland JD, Ford G: The mechanism underlying sudden death from electric shock, *Med Instrument* 20(6):1986.
15. Browne BJ and Gaasch WR: Electrical injuries and lightning, *Emerg Med Clin North Am* 10 (2):211-29, 1992.
16. Volinsky JB, Hanson JB, Lustig JV: Picture of the month: denouement and discussion lightning burns, *Arch Ped Adol Med* 148:529-30, 1994.
17. Fontanarosa PB: Electrical shock and lightning strike, *Ann Emerg Med* 22 (2 Pt 2): 378-87, 1993.
18. Epperly TD and Stewart JR: The physical effects of lightning injury, *J Fam Pract* 29(3):267-272, 1989.
19. Burke JE et al: Patterns of high tension electrical injury in children and adolescents and management, *Am J Surg* 133:492, 1977.

Diagnostic Findings

20. Chandra NC and Siu CO: Clinical predictors of myocardial damage after high voltage electrical injury, *Crit Care Med* 18:293, 1990.
21. Fatovitch DM and Lee KY: Household electrical shocks: Who should be monitored? *Med J Aust*, 155, 1991.

22. Cunningham PA: The need for cardiac monitoring after electrical injury, *Med J Aust* 154: 765-766, 1991.

23. Kirchmer J and Larson D: Cardiac rupture following electrical injury, *J Trauma* May 389, 1977.

24. Jensen PT and Thompsen PE: Electrical injury causing ventricular arrhythmias, *Br Heart J:* 57, 279-283, 1987.

25. Lichtenberg R and Drieos D: Cardiovascular effects of lightning strikes, *J Am Coll Cardiol* 21:279-283, 1987.

26. Strasser EJ and Davis RM: Lightning injuries, *J Trauma* 17:315-319, 1977.

27. Diamond TN and Twomey A: High voltage electrical injury, *SA Med J* February 27, 1982.

28. Roland MH and Schein RM: Pulmonary edema associated with electrical injury, *Chest* 97:1248-1250, 1990.

29. Chen C and Yang J: Electrical burns associated with head injuries, *J Trauma* 37(3):195-199, 1994.

30. Jones DT and Ogren FP: Lightning and its effects on the auditory system, *Laryngoscope* 101(8):830-834, 1991.

31. Suematsu N and Matsuura J: Brachial plexus injury caused by electric current through the ulnar nerve, *Arch Orthop Trauma Surg* 108:400, 1989.

32. Wilkinson C and Wood M: High voltage electrical injury, *Am J Surg* 136:69, 1976.

33. Stueland DT and Stramas P: Bilateral humeral fractures from electrically induced muscular spasm, *J Emerg Med* 7:457, 1989.

34. Johnson EV and Kline LB: Electrical cataracts: a case report and review of the literature, *Ophthal Surg* 118(4):283, 1987.

Management

35. Butler ED: Electrical injuries with special reference to the upper extremities, *Am J Surg* 134:95, 1977.

36. Cooper MA: Emergency medicine study guide, *JACEP* 802, 1985.

37. Bailey B and Gaudreault P: Cardiac monitoring of children with household electrical injuries, *Ann Emerg Med* 25(5), 612-617, 1995.

38. Dershewitz RA: Will mothers use free household safety devices? *Am J Dis Child* 133:61-64, 1979.

39. Cherington M, Martorano FJ, Siebuhr L et al: Childhood lightning injuries on the playing field, *J Emerg Med* 12(1):39-41, 1994.

40. Cherington M, Yarnell P, Lammereste D: Lightning strikes: nature of neurological damage in patients evaluated in hospital emergency departments, *Ann Emerg Med* 21(5):575-578, 1992.

Thermal Injury

Ruth Ann Parish

Thermal injuries are relatively common in the United States and around the world. The mechanism of heat transfer to the skin influences the type (and often the severity) of burn. *Scald* burns result from contact with a hot liquid or gas. Most commonly seen in children younger than 3 years of age, these burns may be sharply demarcated as partial- or full-thickness injuries. Direct-flame exposure causes *flame burns*, resulting from ignition of clothing or skin; these are most commonly seen in children older than 2 years of age who play with matches, open fires, or flammable materials. *Contact burns* occur in children who come in contact with a hot object. These burns usually have a well-demarcated border, with either partial- or full-thickness injury. Explosions may cause *flash burns*, resulting in a uniform, partial-thickness burn. *Electrical burns* occur as a result of electric current passing through the skin and tissue structures of the body, usually an extremity. The severity of electrical burn injuries depends on three primary factors: (1) the resistance of skin and internal body structures; (2) the presence of alternating vs. direct current (polarity); and (3) the frequency, intensity, and duration of the stimulus.

EPIDEMIOLOGY

Burns are second only to motor vehicle accidents as a cause of death in children in the United States, with the highest incidence in children younger than 3 years of age. Because of their thinner epidermal layer, infants remain more susceptible than older children to serious burn injuries, and children have a higher mortality rate than adults for the same total body surface area (TBSA) and severity of burn injury.[2,3] Approximately 100,000 children in the United States are hospitalized annually for the treatment of burns, and similar rates, or higher, occur in developing nations.[4-17] In the United States approximately 3.6 million people seek medical treatment for burn injuries annually; half of these visits are for children 15 years of age and younger.[18] A subpopulation of burn victims have been identified in one study as "burn-repeaters," with a growing percentage of children showing more than one burn injury in the past 5 to 10 years.[19] Approximately 3,000 deaths in children occur each year due to burns, and three to four times this number suffer severe and prolonged disability. Most children with burns are seen initially in an emergency department. Before departing for the hospital, family or paramedics may telephone the pediatrician's office or the emergency department for advice on management and transport of the injured child.[2]

Several epidemiologic studies have identified the kitchen as a primary site of burns in the home.[11,12,15,20] Hot foods, water, cookware, and stoves are responsible for the largest number of burns and cases requiring hospital admission for extended treatment.[20]

House fires cause 75% of all fire-related deaths, with the elderly and child-aged victims at highest risk. The male/female ratio varies in different studies from 1.6:1 to 2:1, which is less than the male predominance for most injury-related deaths.[11,18,21-26] A notable exception to this male predominance appears to be the incidence of microwave oven-related burns, in which females predominate 1.3:1.[27] About 2% of residential fire deaths can be attributed to children playing with matches, cigarette lighters, and other ignition sources. (Cigarettes used by adults account for 30% to 45% of these deaths; heating equipment and electrical malfunction are the second and third leading causes.) Death rates are more than twice as high in areas of low per capita income.[26] House fire deaths are most common in the eastern United States, particularly the Southeast, with lower rates in the West. Rates are higher where severe cold is only occasional and heating arrangements are more makeshift.[7,8] The majority of house fire deaths occur at night from December through March.[28,29] Libber and Slayton found that only 18% of children admitted to a regional burn unit were alone during the incident.[22] From the same U.S. data, 76% of the burns occurred indoors; 33% took place outside the child's own home, in less familiar surroundings. Hot water, coffee, and food scalds occur while the child is with an adult; match play commonly occurs with the child alone in the bedroom. Older boys are usually with friends and out of sight of adults when playing with matches and gasoline.

Approximately 5% of fire deaths in the United States are caused by clothing ignition, 75% of these in people age 65 or older.[8] These types of injuries have become rare in children because of legislation regulating flammable fabrics, particularly children's sleepwear.[9,20]

Tap water scalds represented 25% of the hot liquid burns in one study, which also showed that 50% of them occurred in children younger than 5 years of age. The average length of hospital stay for all tap water scalds was 17 days, and the average full-thickness–sized burn was 12% TBSA.[30] Automobile radiator injuries have also been reported recently as a fairly frequent cause of scald injuries in children,[31] and saunas remain the major cause of scald injuries in Finland, according to a recent 30-year review.[32] Prevention of scald injuries by legislation aimed at lowering hot water heater temperatures appears to be effective, both in the United States and Great Britain.[33,34] Child abuse is a well-documented etiology of scald burns in children.[11]

Electrical burns (including household current) severe enough to require emergency department treatment occur in approximately 4,000 cases/year; the majority of these involve children younger than 5 years of age, with injuries to the face and hands.[25] Extension cords are often at fault (111 of 124 electrical mouth burns were found to be due to faulty extension cords).[12] High-voltage electrical injuries are responsible for a relatively small number of burn injuries to children each year, but these are usually quite severe. In one study, 27 patients were admitted to one pediatric burn unit between 1968 and 1974.[35] All were boys, ages 7 to 16 years. Thirteen suffered amputation and two died. Adolescent risk-taking behavior is almost always involved in these injuries (see Chapter 3).

Contact burns occur largely in homes, where young children spend most of their time. The kitchen and bathroom have the largest number of hot surfaces, but electrical appliances and conduits for central heating are found throughout the house. The upsurge in the use of wood stoves for home heating has coincided with an increased incidence of contact burns in young children in the United States.[36]

The decreased mortality rate seen over the past 20 years in burned children is due to quicker use of proper fluid resuscitation, early excision and grafting techniques, and better monitoring for sepsis or serious infection, as well as better treatment for serious respiratory complications of thermal injuries.[37-40] The emergency physician plays a major role in initial, potentially lifesaving management of the child with burn injuries.

PATHOPHYSIOLOGY

Anatomy of the Skin

The epidermis varies greatly in thickness over the human body, with the external horny layer (stratum corneum) occupying approximately one third of this thickness (see Fig. 37-1). The dermis measures 0.5 to 0.7 mm thick and at the dermal-epidermal junctures has shallow ridges, called *rete pegs*, which actually hook the two layers together.

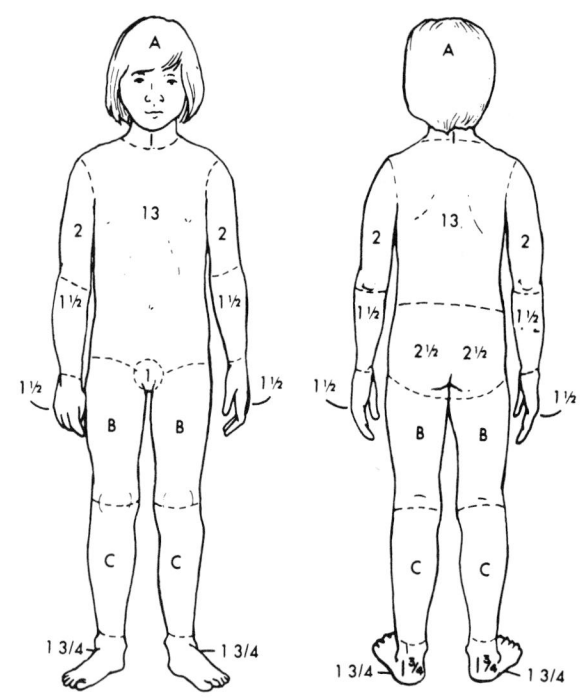

	<1 yr	1 yr	5 yr	10 yr	15 yr	Adult
A: half of head	9½	8½	6½	5½	4½	3½
B: half of thigh	2¾	3¼	4	4¼	4½	4¾
C: half of leg	2½	2½	2¾	3	3¼	3½

FIG. 37-1. Calculation of burn surface area. (*After Lund and Browder. From Barkin RM and Rosen P:* Emergency pediatrics, *ed 4, St. Louis, 1994, Mosby.*)

Domes of subcutaneous fat project into the dermal layer and are visible as yellow spots in a white collagen network when very thick split-thickness skin grafts are removed. Cells capable of regenerating epithelium line the appendages of skin (e.g., hair follicles, sweat and sebaceous glands). Most often, the bulbous ends of hair follicles lie in or just above the summits of the fat domes, and the deepest portions of sweat glands lie beneath and more peripherally in those subcutaneous domes, close to their vertical walls. Pinprick sensation is not destroyed by burns until tissue destruction is great enough to destroy nerve endings lying just superficial to the deepest sweat glands. Epithelium may originate from melanocyte-free sweat glands when melanocyte-rich hair follicles have been destroyed; some burns insensitive to pinprick may still epithelialize from surviving sweat glands.[41]

Surface Area of Burn Injuries

Over the years, numerous scales and indices have been devised to describe the extent of a thermal injury. The seriousness of a thermal injury can be defined by the following factors: extent of the burn, depth of the burn, location, age of the patient, and etiologic factors. The extent of injury is defined by the percent of total body surface area (TBSA) involved. Estimation of TBSA involved is also crucial in calculating the immediate fluid replacement needs of the patient. Even in minor burns, an accurate estimate of TBSA is mandatory.

The "rule of nines" is a reasonably accurate way to estimate TBSA in patients older than 9 years of age. This rule states that each lower extremity is counted as 18% of TBSA (9% anterior surface and 9% posterior surface), each upper extremity as 9%, and the head-neck as 9%. The remaining 1% is allocated to the perineum.[42] For younger children, however, the Lund and Browder chart should be used to correct for the smaller surface area of the lower extremities (Fig. 37-1).[43] A quick assessment may be obtained by using the area of the palm of the hand (minus fingers and thumb) as 1% of the TBSA in a child younger than 5 years. Although data are sparse regarding morbidity associated with thermal injuries in children, most fatal injuries occur in children sustaining a >60% TBSA burn.[44] A minor burn is considered <10% TBSA; moderate-sized burns are 15% to 25% TBSA in adults, or 10% to 20% TBSA in children; and major burns are >25% TBSA in adults or >20% TBSA in children. Significant increases in overall mortality and morbidity occur with >30% TBSA burns.[45]

Depth of Injury

Burns generally have been classified into first-, second- and third-degree burns. In first-degree burns, tissue destruction is superficial, involving only the epidermis. There is local pain, some capillary dilation surrounding the zone of actual thermal injury, and no blister formation. Systemic response is absent or mild. First-degree burns may result from scalding fluids, exposure to ultraviolet light, or flash burns secondary to explosions.

Second-degree burns are divided into superficial and deep partial-thickness injuries. Superficial partial-thickness injuries involve only the epidermis and dermis; wounds appear red and moist, blister formation is present, and touch and pain senses are intact. These injuries will scar minimally and are generally caused by flash, scald, or brief contact with hot object. Deep partial-thickness burns involve the entire epidermis and dermis, leaving only the skin appendages intact. These injuries have a mottled appearance with areas of waxy-white injury. The surface of the burn is dry and anesthetic. A deep partial-thickness injury heals spontaneously in 4 to 6 weeks, but with unstable epithelium, late hypertrophic scarring, and marked contracture formation where the burn crosses a joint. Excision and grafting is the best treatment for such injuries.

Third-degree burns (full-thickness burns) involve destruction of the epidermis, dermis, and subcutaneous tissues. The wounds appear white, red, or black, with or without blisters. Thrombosed blood vessels may be visible. The dry, leathery appearance of the wound is due to destruction of the elasticity of the burned dermal layer. Full-thickness burns require skin grafting if larger than 2 to 3 cm in diameter or if in an area of potential cosmetic deformity. A full-thickness burn is usually caused by flame, high-intensity flash, chemicals, electricity, or prolonged contact with any source of heat.

Location of the burn is an extremely important determinant of severity. Critical areas include eyes, ears, face, hands and feet, and perineum because of the difficulty of care. Other factors influencing severity include age (the very old and very young patients run a higher mortality rate for a given percent TBSA and depth of burn), associated major trauma, inhalation injury, or general health status. The cause of the burn may also be important, for a small burn may be associated with severe inhalation injury; if the wound is secondary to electrical injury, there may be massive soft tissue damage associated with a small cutaneous injury.[35,46]

Severity of Burns

The severity of burns is determined by the depth of the burn, TBSA, location of the injury, age and health of the patient, and associated injuries; these will be the first pieces of information required of the emergency physician in the transfer of a patient to the Burn Center.

Major burns have partial-thickness involvement of >25% TBSA in adults or 15% to 20% in children. Full-thickness burns >10% TBSA are considered in this category. Burns of the hands, face, eyes, ears, feet or perineum are included. Patients with complications of inhalation injury, electrical burns, and burns complicated by fractures or other major trauma must also be considered to have major burns. Preexisting medical conditions or suspicion of child abuse similarly requires aggressive initial management.

Moderate uncomplicated burns may comprise 15% to 25% TBSA in adults and 10% to 15% TBSA in children. A full-thickness burn of 2% to 10% TBSA would also be in this category. *Minor* burns would be those <15% TBSA in adults and <10% in children. A full-thickness burn <2% TBSA would also be minor.

DIAGNOSTIC FINDINGS

A patient history should be obtained if possible. Important features to note are the mechanism of injury, estimated heat of the burning object, length of contact, concurrent trauma, and whether the victim was in closed-space confinement (e.g., a house fire), enhancing the risk of smoke inhalation. The emergency physician would also like to know what first aid measures, if any, were initially applied to the burn.

Generally, there is little doubt regarding the clinical presence of a burn; the clincial assessment of burn victims involves establishing the severity and TBSA of the injury and formalizing a plan for initial fluid resuscitation. One can make some estimate, as mentioned previously, of the depth of burn by the appearance of the wound: Does it appear red and moist, white and waxy, or dry and leathery? These findings help determine long-term management. Distribution of the burn should be noted, particularly if child abuse is suspected. For example, it should be noted if scald burns are at an angle across the legs, indicating that the child was forcibly held down in a tub of hot water.

Complications

In major burns from flame or chemical injury, the victim may sustain significant pulmonary injury from smoke inhalation. Direct inhalation of toxic particles or exposure to hot smoke and air may produce upper or lower airway respiratory distress due to ventilation-perfusion mismatch, consolidation, loss of surfactant, and infection.[47] Carbon monoxide poisoning may be noted and require assessment (see Chapter 44).

Fluid deficit is one of the most common and devastating sequellae of large burns, causing renal failure, myoglobin concentration in the kidneys, hypotensive shock, and cardiovascular collapse. In older children with major burns >70% TBSA, adequate fluid replacement would approach 1 L/hr intravenously. Sepsis and death may result. Forty-seven percent of deaths associated with house fires are children four years of age or younger.

Ancillary Data

Laboratory data obtained in the emergency department is primarily for baseline use. A complete blood count with differential, electrolytes, renal function studies (blood urea nitrogen and creatinine), and possibly liver function tests will aid in managing the patient's shifting metabolic status during the first 2 to 3 days of hospitalization. Oximetry and arterial blood gases may facilitate respiratory management. Urinalysis should also be obtained, with special attention to myoglobin content. Muscle breakdown, which occurs secondary to >30% TBSA burns, will cause accumulation of myoglobin in the kidneys, necessitating even more careful fluid resuscitation of the patient. A chest x-ray examination and carboxyhemoglobin levels should be obtained for baseline purposes and to assess carbon monoxide damage and smoke inhalation injury (see Chapter 44). A type and hold to facilitate later blood availability may be appropriate in patients with major burns. A culture for group A streptococcus should be done if there is evidence of associated disease.

MANAGEMENT

The goal of management is to keep the patient warm, well-hydrated, noninfected, and moderately comfortable.

Prehospital Care

In chemical burns, concentration of the agent and duration of exposure are the main factors that determine the depth and extent of tissue damage. Copious irrigation with any water source will be helpful. Large-volume irrigation with water is preferable to delaying treatment in search of a specific neutralizing solution.

In the case of flame burns, rapidly placing the blazing victim in a supine position will minimize the risk of facial burns, hair ignition, and inhalation injury. Extinguishing the fire is the initial step; having the victim in the supine position will facilitate smothering the flames with rugs, coats, towels, or blankets.

Various factors may influence the extent of tissue damage from electrical burns, including the type and voltage of the circuit, resistance, pathway of transit through the body, and duration of contact. Separating the victim carefully from the electrical source is the essential step, either by cutting the wire with properly insulated instruments, or by switching off power. Rapid institution of cardiopulmonary resuscitation may be necessary in the child who has experienced cardiopulmonary arrest secondary to high-voltage thermal injury.

The use of cool or iced solutions to reduce the pain of a partial-thickness burn may be helpful, but only in burns <20% TBSA and in environmental temperatures >50° F. (Recall that the palm of the hand [minus digits] is approximately 1% TBSA in any human; this may be useful in helping someone else estimate TBSA of a burn over the telephone, if the rule of nines is not helpful.)

Covering a burn can minimize external contamination and also offer pain relief. A clean or sterile sheet provides an excellent covering. Avoid the use of terry cloth if possible to deep partial-thickness or full-thickness burns. Intact blisters should be left unbroken unless they are in flexion creases. Applications of topical medications should be avoided until the victim is in the emergency department. Oral fluids should not be given; children (and adults) with significant thermal injuries may develop ileus, leading to the possibility of vomiting and subsequent aspiration.

Minor and moderate burns (<15% TBSA) may be triaged to the nearest hospital, but burns of >15% TBSA in children, as well as all burns involving the face, hands, and feet, should be triaged when possible to a regional center that can provide rapid stabilization, if no delay in transport would result.

Transport

Two identified phases of transport for the burned child are (1) the initial transfer from the scene of the accident to the nearest medical facility, and (2) referral of the severely burned child from the primary care center to a designated regional burn center.

During *initial transfer*, a clean bedsheet may be used to wrap the victim, after removal of charred clothing or clothing soaked in chemicals. Baseline vital signs such as pulse, blood pressure, and respiratory rate should be noted. An adequate airway must be ensured and oxygen administered universally. If a transit time of longer than 30 minutes is expected, an intravenous line may be necessary in children with >15% TBSA burns.

Oxygen should be administered to all patients involved in thermal injuries where carbon monoxide could be a problem (e.g., flame burns and closed-space injuries). In the unconscious child with either carbon monoxide poisoning or a multisystem injury, an oral airway and adequate ventilation should be obtained. Endotracheal intubation may be advisable, again depending on severity of injury, respiratory status, and length of transport.

All patients with electrical injury should have cardiac monitoring during the initial transport phase; adequate covering (multiple layers of blankets) is also needed to prevent rapid cooling of the patient.

Patients with chemical burns should undergo extensive irrigation of the wound site before initial transport.[48]

Secondary transport of the severely burned child requires adequate preparation. Because major burns require large volumes of intravenous fluid (particularly during the first 8 hours), assuring an adequate amount of fluid is important. The height of the intravenous column may be restricted in an ambulance or airplane; two intravenous sites will most likely be necessary to assure adequate volume replacement if a pump is not available for the transport. A centrally placed (subclavian or internal jugular) line may be needed if the severity of the burn and patient's fluid status warrant. Pain control should be achieved, using morphine sulfate 0.1 to 0.2 mg/kg/dose IV before transport, with appropriate monitoring.

Maintenance of core body temperature is mandatory. Many layers of blankets may be necessary. Airway maintenance needs should be anticipated; if an endotracheal tube may be necessary within a few hours, it is easier to place the tube while on the ground than during flight. Whenever feasible, severely burned children should be accompanied by an experienced nurse, a paramedic, or a physician during secondary transport.

Major (Inpatient) Burns

Any child with >15% TBSA burns; burns of the hands, face, feet, or perineum; and a high suspicion for either smoke inhalation injury or child abuse should be admitted. The child with >15% TBSA burns, whether second or third degree, will need intravenous fluid resuscitation while monitoring urine output and hydration over several days (see preceding section). A team of surgical and medical consultants is required. Fluid resuscitation should be initiated immediately during transport or on arrival at the treating facility as outlined. A nasogastric (NG) tube and Foley catheter are usually indicated for meticulous monitoring. Body temperature should be normalized.

The following guidelines for severely burned children may be useful:

1. Children with second- or third-degree burns >10% TBSA need intravenous fluid resuscitation.
2. Children with >40% TBSA burns need a central line for fluid resuscitation.
3. Children with burns >65% TBSA may need two central access lines for fluid resuscitation.

A number of approaches to fluid resuscitation are possible. Intravenous fluids must be initiated immediately with one or two large-bore catheters. Initial stabilization should include infusion of 20 ml/kg of 0.9% normal saline (NS) or lactated Ringer's solution (LR) over 10 to 30 minutes. After cardiovascular resuscitation, LR solution is used at a rate of 4 ml × kg × % TBSA (70% TBSA = 70) given over the first 24 hours in addition to maintenance rate fluids given as D10W 0.45% NS. Whereas the traditional formula has been to give the first half of these fluid requirements in the first 8 hours of the patient's course, recent data have suggested that children may fare better with that amount given over the first 4 hours, and the remaining half given over the ensuing 20 hours.[49] Whether other studies will confirm the value of this change in the "Baxter Formula" in children remains to be seen. Other parallel approaches to fluid management are acceptable.

As an example, using the traditional Baxter Formula (i.e., the first half of resuscitation requirements given over an 8-hour period), a 15-kg child who sustained a 20% TBSA burn would need:

Maintenance rate fluids (D10W 0.45% NS)

100 ml/kg for first 10 kg + 50 ml/kg for next 10 kg = 1,250 ml over 24 hours, or 52 ml/hr

Resuscitation fluids (LR solution)

4 ml × kg × % TBSA = 4 ml × 15 kg × 20 = 1,200 ml over 24 hours

TOTAL FLUIDS (maintenance *and* resuscitation)

Maintenance   52 ml/hr of D10W 0.45% NS

Resuscitation   75 ml/hr (LR) for first 8 hours (or 150 ml/hr for first 4 hours)
37.5 ml/hr (LR) over next 16 hours (or 30 ml/hr over next 20 hours)

Avoid the addition of potassium chloride to intravenous fluids in the emergency department. Because of massive red blood cell breakdown, these children tend to have high potassium levels initially; in addition renal impairment may develop in children with massive burns. Frequent monitoring of the child's heart rate, respiratory rate, temperature, and blood pressure is mandatory before and during the transport process. Aggressive resuscitation continues throughout this process.[49,50]

Successful fluid resuscitation will result in a normotensive, warm patient with a urine output of >1 ml/kg/hr. All children with >20% TBSA burns should receive nothing by mouth for the first 24 to 48 hours of care to avoid complications of intestinal ileus, which is common in children. An NG tube should also be placed in these children with more severe burns. A central venous catheter may be necessary for patients with major burns with major fluid deficits. Urinary output requires close monitoring.

Twice-daily debridement, eschar removal, and sterile wound dressing with either 1% silver sulfadiazine (Silvadene) or another antibiotic ointment are essential. An absorbent dressing of fine (36 × 44) mesh gauze or 4 × 4 fluffs is applied, using several layers and a roll of gauze to hold the dressing. The face and perineum are usually left open after application of antibiotic cream. At each change, the wound should be cleansed with warm water and debrided, often facilitated by a whirlpool.

The goal is to have viable epithelial tissue formation without areas of avascular tissue; the latter serve as culture media for either *Staphylococcus aureus* (in the first 7 days) or *Pseudomonas aeruginosa* (usually >7 days after the burn occurs) infection. Biologic dressings, such as pigskin (allograft), Biobrane, "artificial skin," and cadaver skin (homograft) should be used only after consulting with a surgeon trained in burn care. Biobrane, a bilayer semisynthetic dressing, may actually decrease pain and healing time in partial-thickness fresh thermal burns.[51] Escharotomy may be indicated with full-thickness circumferential burns of the extremities accompanied by neurovascular compromise. Eschars of the chest may impair ventilation.

Pain medication may be used once vital signs are normalized. Optimally drugs such as morphine or meperidine should be given intravenously. Patient-controlled analgesia may be useful in older children who can be taught this technique. Body temperature should be maintained, and nutrition (intravenous, tube, or oral) considered after stabilization. Tetanus immunization should be updated.

Antibiotics should not be administered prophylactically but rather for specific signs and symptoms of infection after appropriate cultures. Penicillin should be given if there is evidence of group A streptococcal infection to prevent colonization of the burn. Antibiotic therapy should be saved for the child with proven wound infection; it is usually needed only in burn wounds of >20% TBSA and is usually administered on an inpatient basis.[52] For a superficial small (<10% TBSA) burn wound, mupirocin (Bactroban) ointment may be used twice daily to treat a superficial staphylococcal infection, characterized by increased redness around the wound, and a green, soupy-looking appearance.

Peptic ulcer (Curling ulcer) prophylaxis may be initiated early with antacid therapy, cimetadine (20 to 30 mg/kg/24 hr q 6 hr IV or PO), or famotidine (adult dose: 20 to 40 mg q 24 hr PO *or* 20 mg q 12 hr IV).

A burn should be totally epithelialized in 2 to 3 weeks. If wound healing is not occurring by 14 days, a primary excision and grafting are necessary. A superficial partial-thickness injury should be reexamined at 6 weeks for evidence of hypertrophic scarring, which may require the use of a pressure bandage (Jobst stocking). A healed burn may lead to the formation of very thin water blisters, produced as the result of a minor trauma. These blisters, usually <1 cm in diameter, occur 2 to 6 weeks after healing of the wound and leave small open areas that heal without problem in 3 to 5 days if they are kept clean with bland soap and water, and covered with a bland ointment (such as Bacitracin). Healed partial-thickness burn wounds become very dry. A mild lanolin cream (Nivea) or lotion (Vaseline Intensive Care) should be used until the natural skin lubrication mechanisms return, usually in 6 to 8 weeks. The patient should also be warned that sun exposure during wound maturation (up to 6 months after the burn) may cause hyperpigmentation of the wound, which can be permanent. The use of a sunblock (sun protection factor >24) is recommended for healed areas that must be exposed to sunlight. Pruritus may be controlled with diphenhydramine HCl (Benadryl) (5 mg/kg/24 hr QID PO) or hydroxyzine (Atarax) (2 mg/kg/24 hr QID PO). Moisturizing creams are also helpful to alleviate pruritus. Regardless of inpatient vs. outpatient status, the child's tetanus prophylaxis should be updated if the last dose was more than 7 years before the injury.

Psychological support of the patient and family should be provided. Rehabilitation must be considered early.

Minor (Outpatient) Burns

The previous discussion has emphasized the care of the severely burned child (>15 to 20% TBSA). The child with a minor burn (<10 to 15% TBSA) may be treated as an outpatient, assuming that there is a less than a 2 × 2 cm area of deep (deep partial-thickness or full-thickness) burn, no chance for contracture formation, and follow-up with the child's family can be assured (see box). The burn wound can usually heal by intention approximately 1 cm from each side.

Follow-up care should include washing the wound with bland soap and water in a bathtub or shower; patting the wound dry with a clean towel; applying an ointment such as bacitracin, Polymixin B sulfate, or 1% silver sulfadiazene in the case of >5% TBSA injuries; applying a nonstick porous gauze; and wrapping with a gauze roll. This proce-

---

Outpatient Management of Small Burns

At scene of injury
Place under cool water
Wrap wound in clean cloth; get victim to emergency department

Medical management
Administer tetanus prophylaxis
Clean wound using bland soap and water
Shave area of burn, if necessary
Debride dead tissue
Wound care: apply a bland ointment, or nonstick porous gauze and wrap with Kerlix; secure with tape

Follow-up care
Twice daily wash with bland soap and water; repeat steps of wound care (above)
Encourage range of motion to the affected extremity
Return to emergency department, clinic, or supervising physician as needed (daily to once weekly)

From Warden GD: Outpatient management of thermal injuries. In Boswick JA Jr, editor: *The art and science of burn care*, Rockville, Md, 1987, Aspen Publishers.

---

dure should be completed twice a day. Follow-up with the physician may be daily for the first few days to assure that infection does not occur, but may be extended to once a week after the first few days. Tetanus prophylaxis should be administered if the child's last dose was longer than 7 years ago. Blisters should be left intact until they burst spontaneously; the dead skin should then be debrided to keep a viable, vascularized edge to the skin's regrowth area (see box above).

Antibiotics should be reserved for defined infections. For superficial, small burn wounds, mupirocin (Bactroban) ointment may be used twice daily to treat a superficial *S. aureus* infection. Parents of the child with a minor burn should be instructed in vigorous range of motion exercises. Prolonged edema, which may be minimized with vigorous use, is a deterrent to wound healing. Rehabilitation time may be shortened by active exercise.[46]

References

Epidemiology

1. Thompson J and Ashwal K: Electrical burns in children, *Am J Dis Child* 137:231-235, 1983.
2. Otherson HB: Burns and scalds, *Pediatr Ann* 12: 753-760, 1983.
3. Erickson EJ, Merrell SW, Saffle JR et al: Differences in mortality from thermal injury between pediatric and adult patients, *J Ped Surg* 26(7):821-825, 1991.
4. Lari AR, Bang RL, Ebrahim MK et al: An analysis of childhood burns in Kuwait, *Burns* 18(3): 224-227, 1992.
5. Ryan CA, Shankowsky HA, Tredget EE: Profile of the paediatric burn patient in a Canadian burn centre, *Burns* 18(4): 267-272, 1992.
6. Batchelor JS, Vanjari S, Budny P et al: Domestic iron burns in children: a cause for concern? *Burns* 20(1): 74-75, 1994.
7. Feldman KW, Schaller RT, Feldman J et al: Tap water scald burns in children, *Pediatrics* 62: 1-7, 1978.

8. Cickelair GF and Dhaliwal AS: The cause and prevention of electrical burns of the mouth in children, *Plast Reconstr Surg* 58: 206-209, 1976.
9. Kalayi GD: Burn injuries in Zaria: a one year prospective study, *East Africa Med J* 71(5): 317-322, 1994.
10. Hollyoak MA, Muller MJ, Pegg SP: Electric iron contact burns in an Australian paediatric population, *Paediatr Perinat Epidemiol* 8(3): 314-324, 1994.
11. Shugarman R, Rivara FP, Parish RA et al: Contact burns of the hand in children, *Pediatrics* 80: 18-21, 1987.
12. Gupta M, Gupta OK, Goil P: Paediatric burns in Jaipur, India, *Burns* 18(1): 63-67, 1992.
13. Grisolia GA, Pelli P, Pinzauti E et al: [A multicenter epidemiological study of burns of the head in childhood in the period of 1986-1990.] *Pediatria Medica e Chirurgica* 13(6): 585-588, 1991.
14. el Danaf A, Alshlash S, Filobbos P et al: Analysis of 105 patient admitted over a 2-year period to a modern burns unit in Saudi Arabia, *Burns* 17(1): 62-64, 1991.
15. Attalla MF, al-Baker AA, al-Ekiabi SA: Friction burns of the hand caused by jogging machines: a potential hazard to children, *Burns* 17(2): 170-171, 1991.
16. Laing RM and Bryant V: Prevention of burn injuries to children involving nightwear, *N Z Med J* 104(918): 363-365, 1991.
17. Smith T: Accidents, poisoning and violence as a cause of hospital admissions in children, *Health Bull* 49(4): 237-244, 1991.
18. Herndon DN, Rutan RL, Rutan TC: Management of the pediatric patient with burns, *J Burn Care Rehabil* 14(1): 3-8, 1993.
19. Cobb N, Maxwell G, Silverstein P: "Burn repeaters" and injury control, *J Burn Care Rehabil* 13(3): 382-387, 1992.
20. Antoon A and Remensnyder JP: Burns in children, In Boswick JA, editor: *The art and science of burn care*, Rockville, Md, 1987, Aspen Publishers.
21. Moyer CA: The sociologic aspect of trauma, *Am J Surg* 87: 421-430, 1954.
22. Libber SM and Slayton DJ: Childhood burns reconsidered: the child, the family, and the burn injury, *J Trauma* 24: 245-252, 1984.
23. Baker S, O'Neil B, Karpt R: Burns and fire deaths. In *The injury fact book*, Lexington, Mass, 1984, Lexington Books.
24. Bergman AB: Flame-resistant sleepwear: have the birdwatchers gone ape? *Pediatrics* 60: 652-654, 1977.
25. McLoughlin E and Crawford JD: Epidemiology of burns in children, *Pediatr Clin North Am* 22: 62, 1985.
26. Parker DJ, Sklar DP, Tandberg D et al: Fire fatalities among New Mexico children, *Ann Emerg Med* 22(3): 517-522, 1993.
27. Powell EC and Tanz RR: Comparison of childhood burns associated with use of microwave ovens and conventional stoves, *Pediatrics* 91(2): 344-349, 1993.
28. Ballard JE, Koepsell TD, Rivara FP: Association of smoking and alcohol drinking with residential fire injuries, *Am J Epidemiol* 135(1): 26-34, 1992.
29. Hingson R and Howland J: Alcohol and non-traffic unintended injuries, *Addiction* 88(7):877-883, 1993.
30. Baptiste MS and Feck G: Preventing tap water burns, *Am J Public Health* 70:727-729, 1980.
31. O'Neal N, Purdue G, Hunt J: Burns caused by automobile radiators: a continuing problem, *J Burn Care Rehabil* 13(4):422-425, 1992.
32. Zeitlin R, Somppi E, Jarnberg J: Paediatric burns in central Finland between the 1960s and the 1980s, *Burns* 19(5):418-422, 1993.
33. Chapman JC, Sarhadi NS, Watson AC: Declining incidence of paediatric burns in Scotland, *Burns* 20(2):106-110, 1994.
34. Rivara FP: Tap water burn prevention: the effect of legislation, *Pediatrics* 88(3):572-577, 1991.
35. McLoughlin E, Joseph MA, Crawford JD: Epidemiology of high-tension electrical injuries in children, *J Pediatr* 81:62-65, 1976.
36. Yanofsky NN and Morain WD: Upper extremity burns from wood-stoves, *Pediatrics* 73:722-726, 1984.
37. Banco L, Lapidus G, Zavoski R et al: Burn injuries among children in an urban emergency department, *Pediatr Emerg Care* 10(2):98-101, 1994.
38. Smith DL, Cairns BA, Ramadan F et al: Effect of inhalation injury, burn size, and age on mortality, *J Trauma* 37(4):655-659, 1994.
39. Gottschlich MM, Baumer T, Jenkins M et al: The prognostic value of nutritional and inflammatory indices in patients with burns, *J Burn Care Rehabil* 13(1):105-113, 1992.
40. Waller AE, Clarke JA, Langley JD: An evaluation of a program to reduce home hot tap water temperatures, *Aust J Public Health* 17(2):116-123, 1993.

Pathophysiology

41. Zawacki BE: The local effects of burn injury, In Boswick JA, editor: *The art and science of burn care*, Rockville, Md, 1987, Aspen Publishers.
42. Moncrief J: Burns: I. Assessment, *JAMA* 242:72-74, 1979.
43. Lund CC and Browder NC: The estimate of areas of burns, *Surg Gynecol Obstet* 79:352, 1944.
44. Childhood injuries in the United States: report to Congress, *Am J Dis Child* 144:627-646, 1990.
45. O'Neill JA: Evaluation and treatment of the burned child, *Pediatr Clin North Am* 22:407-414, 1975.
46. Warden GD: Outpatient management of thermal injuries. In Boswick JA, editor: *The art and science of burn care*, Rockville, Md, 1987, Aspen Publishers.
47. Hudson DA, Jones L, Rode H: Respiratory distress secondary to scalds in children, *Burns* 20(5):434-437, 1994.

Management

48. Moylan JA: First aid and transportation of burn patients. In Boswick JA, editor: *The art and science of burn care*, Rockville, Md, 1987, Aspen Publishers.
49. Carvajal HF: Fluid resuscitation of pediatric burn victims: a critical appraisal, *Pediatr Nephrol* 8(3):357-366, 1994.
50. Puffinbarger NK, Tuggle DW, Smith EI: Rapid isotonic fluid resuscitation in pediatric thermal injury, *J Pediatr Surg* 29(2): 339-342, 1994.
51. Teepe RG, Burger A, Ponec M: Immunohistochemical studies on regeneration in cultured epidermal autografts used to treat full-thickness burn wounds, *Clin Exp Dermatol* 19(1):16-22, 1994.
52. Dodd D and Stutman HR: Current issues in burn wound infections. *Adv Pediatr Infect Dis* 6:137-162, 1991.

38

Heat-Induced Illnesses

Marilyn F.A. Mellor

Heat illness is a continuum of heat-induced disorders ranging from annoying prickly heat to life-threatening heatstrokes. The majority of patients presenting with heat illness are adults, especially the elderly, but children are also at risk of succumbing to heat stress.

Neonates and infants younger than 2 years of age lack optimal thermoregulatory control.[1,2] In addition, their greater body surface area/mass ratio leads to greater transfer of heat between the environment and their bodies. An infant's metabolic rate peaks at about 5 months of age; high fevers and poor thermoregulation are common in this age group. The ability to dissipate heat through sweating is immature and only completely evolves later. They are vulnerable and depend on others to protect them from extreme heat.

Older children also do not adapt as well as adults to very high temperatures because of physiologic differences. Children do not sweat as much as adults and, as with neonates, they have a greater body surface area/mass ratio than adults. Their ability to dissipate heat peripherally while exercising and to acclimatize to a warm climate is slower than in adults.[3] Children do not instinctively replace their fluid losses or limit exercise in extreme heat. Children, especially toddlers, are at risk of being unable to extricate themselves from high heat environments (e.g., closed cars in the sun).

Teenage and preadolescent athletes are particularly vulnerable to heat illness. They may use poor judgment when exercising in high heat and humidity and frequently do not drink enough to replace their fluid losses. Decreased hydration almost invariably is found with exertional heatstroke. Young athletes are notorious for pushing themselves to their physical limits, with more than a thousand cases of heat exhaustion reported annually among athletes in the United States.[4] Athletes become progressively more susceptible on the third to fourth day of strenuous activity because of cumulative fluid losses from the previous day. Athletes, laborers, and soldiers may exert themselves despite the appearance of physical symptoms.[1,5]

Some childhood chronic diseases, such as cystic fibrosis, quadriplegia, and congenital anhidrosis, may leave patients with a decreased ability to sweat.

Street drugs, including amphetamines and cocaine, can increase heat production, whereas phencyclidine (PCP) and D-lysergic acid diethylamide (LSD) may decrease sweating. Antihistamines, phenothiazines, anticholinergics, diuretics, beta-blockers, alcohol, and others can impair normal sweating.[1,6]

PATHOPHYSIOLOGY

The body is heated either endogenously or exogenously. Physical activity is the main source of increased endogenous heat and can increase heat production several fold. The increased metabolic rate secondary to thyroxine, norepinephrine, and sympathetic stimulation on cells also increases heat production. During fever, endogenous pyrogens stimulate prostaglandins, which reset the hypothalamic thermostat. Normally, fever alone is not a problem, but with an increased temperature set point, the additional heat load may become hazardous. Environmentally produced heat also causes a rise in body temperature, which occurs when external temperatures exceed body temperatures.

Heat illness results when the body can no longer adequately dissipate heat. Heat is lost by (1) conduction, (2) convection, (3) radiation, and (4) evaporation. Of these, the greatest amount of heat loss from the body occurs through radiation, accounting for about 60% of the total loss.[1,7] The effective heat loss from evaporation is approximately 25% and is due mainly to sweating.[1,7] However, this amount is limited by relative humidity; it decreases when the humidity is greater than 75% and is ineffective when it is more than 90%. A core temperature of 37° C (98.6° F) + or − 0.6° C (1° F) can be maintained in a low humidity when the ambient temperatures range from 10° C to 60° C (55° F to 140° F).[1,7]

The hypothalamus contains the thermoregulatory center. The preoptic areas and, to some extent, adjacent areas of the anterior hypothalamus sense increased heat and react accordingly. With increased heat, the hypothalamus lowers the core temperature by three mechanisms:

1. Dilation of cutaneous blood vessels by inhibiting sympathetic centers in the posterior hypothalamus that cause vasoconstriction[7,8]
2. Stimulation of sweating by transmission down the autonomic pathways and through the sympathetic outflow tract to the sweat glands[7,8]
3. Inhibition of heat production from shivering and chemical thermogenesis including decreased release of thyrotropin-releasing hormone[7]

When the core temperature equals or exceeds 40° C (104° F), there is maximal peripheral vasodilation. Sequestration of large volumes of blood with a reduction in effective circulating volume often takes place. Heart rate and force of contraction then increase to maintain cardiac output in the face of this low total peripheral resistance.[1,9]

Splanchnic vasoconstriction correspondingly occurs with decreased blood flow to the gastrointestinal tract, liver, and kidneys, leading to nausea, vomiting, diarrhea, and decreased urinary output. Chemical alterations include increased liver enzymes, blood urea nitrogen, (BUN), and creatinine; hyperkalemia or hypokalemia; hypocalcemia; and changes in blood sugar.[1,5,10-12]

Acute renal failure commonly presents in severe heatstroke, affecting 25% to 30% of patients.[10,12,13] Rhabdomyolysis is a major contributor to renal tubular injury in these cases. Although rhabdomyolysis is seen more often in exertional heatstroke, it can occur in classic heatstroke as well.[6]

With persistence of hyperthermia, central nervous system disturbances take place, including disorientation, seizures, and coma.* Cellular injury can happen at core temperatures of 42° C (114.8° F) and greater.[4,13] Death results from circulatory or respiratory collapse, disseminated intravascular coagulation, major electrolyte imbalances, or cerebral edema. Mortality in hyperthermia is associated with both the degree of temperature and the extent of its duration.[6]

Heat exhaustion and heatstroke can appear very similar. Symptoms unique to heatstroke are a high core temperature (>40° C) and mental status changes (Table 38-1).

TYPES OF HEAT ILLNESS

Prickly Heat

Prickly heat, or miliaria, is an acute inflammatory skin eruption. It is caused by blockage of the eccrine sweat glands secondary to keratinous plugs, maceration, and infection of these pores. Rupture of the duct may occur from back pressure, allowing sweat to seep into the dermis resulting in an inflammatory response. Hot, humid weather most commonly causes the rash to erupt. However, infants who are dressed too warmly can also exhibit prickly heat even during winter.

A maculopapular, erythematous rash with vesicles and intense pruritus is seen in prickly heat. It is generally found on the clothed areas of the body. The affected area is frequently devoid of sweat. A concomitant chronic dermatitis can also occur.

Management. A child with prickly heat should wear light, loose clothing. Maintaining a cool environment is the

* References, 1, 4, 7, 10, 12, 14.

TABLE 38-1. A Comparison: Heat Exhaustion and Heatstroke

Diagnostic findings	Heat exhaustion	Heatstroke
Onset	Gradual	Rapid
Temperature	<40° C	>40° C
CNS	Irritable, headache	Severe headache, disorientation, seizures, coma
Skin	Sweating	Hot, dry or sweating
GI	Nausea, vomiting	Vomiting, diarrhea
Ancillary data		
CBC	Hematocrit ↑	Hematocrit ↑ Platelets ↓
Chemistry	Na+ variable BUN ↑ Glucose ↓	K+ variable, Na+ variable, BUN ↑, glucose ↑, AST ↑, LDH ↑, CPK ↑, Ca++ normal or ↓

CNS, Central nervous system; *GI*, gastrointestinal; *CBC*, complete blood count; *BUN*, blood urea nitrogen; *AST*, aspartate aminotransferase; *LDH*, lactate dehydrogenase; *CPK*, creatinine phosphokinase.

ideal way to avoid this rash and is helpful in relieving it. Cool baths also help alleviate the pruritus. Topical agents, such as talc, other powders, and antibiotics, should be avoided. If the rash becomes diffuse and pustular, systemic antibiotics should be used.

Heat Edema

Heat edema is a dependent swelling of the hands and feet usually occurring at the onset of hot weather. It is self-limiting and spontaneously resolves after being in a cool environment for a period of time. Aldosterone, salt, and water retention are thought to contribute to this condition.

Management. Because heat edema is self-limiting and disappears on its own, diuretics should not be used. Being in a cool environment is the most helpful course of action.

Heat Syncope

Heat syncope is seen during the early phase of heat acclimatization. It is associated with orthostatic hypotension and dehydration. Vasodilation of cutaneous blood vessels with shunting of the blood to peripheral tissues causes heat syncope. Prolonged standing or vigorous activity can worsen it. Heat syncope is also a self-limiting condition.

Syncope, dizziness, visual blurring, and slight tachycardia can be present. Mild dehydration is also seen.

Management. It is essential to remove a child with heat syncope from the heat. Placing the patient in a supine position is helpful. These children are usually mildly dehydrated and can be rehydrated orally. Rest after the syncopal episode should be encouraged.

Heat Cramps

Heat cramps are seen both in unconditioned persons just beginning strenuous work in hot temperatures and in acclimatized individuals who sweat profusely while working vigorously, particularly when thirst is relieved by unsalted fluids. Cramps are normally found in the muscle groups actually used while working but any muscle may be affected. Spasms can occur either during the activity itself or several hours later.

Replacement of fluid losses with hypotonic solutions contribute to the cramping. The exact etiology is unknown, although salt depletion plays a major role in this condition.

Diagnostic Findings. Painful contractions occur in the muscles used while working, most frequently the legs. The cramping often does not appear until after the exercise is over. Normal mental status with a slightly elevated temperature is found.

Differential Considerations. Normal muscle fatigue or hyperventilation may mimic the findings. Hypokalemia and black widow spider bite are more serious problems and need to be included in the differential diagnosis.

Management. Remove the child from the hot environment when cramping occurs. Mild dehydration can be managed with oral replacement of fluids. One teaspoon (4 gm) of NaCl mixed with 500 ml of water should be given over 1 to 2 hours. Severe dehydration should be treated with a 0.9% NS IV bolus of 20 ml/kg run over 1 to 2 hours. Rest is also useful.

Heat Exhaustion

Heat exhaustion is a vague clinical syndrome characterized by headache, nausea, vomiting, lethargy, irritability, thirst, and anorexia. It is the most common heat-related illness seen in athletes.[11] It may be a precursor to heatstroke.

Exposure to high temperatures, excessive sweating, and inadequate replenishment of water and salt are the chief causes. Heat exhaustion is differentiated from heatstroke only by lower core temperatures, usually < 40° C (104° F), and normal mental functioning.

Two types of heat exhaustion can be seen. Most patients experience some combination of both types. *Water-depletion* heat exhaustion results from exposure to high temperatures and insufficient fluid intake. It begins quickly over a few hours. *Salt-depletion* heat exhaustion, in contrast, usually develops over several days, usually in people who adequately replace fluid losses but not salt losses. It is seen more frequently in unacclimatized individuals because of the relatively higher salt content of their sweat.[10,11]

Diagnostic Findings. Thirst, headache, nausea, vomiting, and irritability are common. The temperature may be normal or elevated. Tachycardia and tachypnea are present. Complications of heat exhaustion are impending heatstroke and possible shock, both of which must be closely monitored.

Ancillary Data. Laboratory values that should be obtained include a complete blood count (CBC), electrolytes, blood urea nitrogen (BUN), glucose, and urinalysis. An increased hematocrit can be seen with the CBC. Either hypernatremia or hyponatremia may be present. The BUN is elevated, whereas the glucose is usually decreased. A core temperature will be ≤ 40° C (104° F).

Management. Removal from heat is essential. Fluid replacement is the basic therapy, as patients are always dehydrated.

Mild dehydration can be treated with oral fluids, using either water or an electrolyte solution. If the patient is salt depleted, relatively salty drinks such as tomato juice can be given. Severe isotonic or hypotonic dehydration should be treated with an IV bolus of 0.9% normal saline or lactated Ringer's at 20 ml/kg run over 30 to 60 minutes, followed by a rehydration protocol.

Rest is an important part of therapy in heat exhaustion. The patient may be discharged after a few hours of observation if vital signs are normal, symptoms have subsided, and no metabolic abnormalities are present.

Heatstroke

Heatstroke is a medical emergency characterized by a temperature > 40.6° C (105° F), neurologic dysfunctioning, and often anhidrosis. Heatstroke occurs when the body is unable to dissipate heat, causing loss of temperature control. As a result, there is a rapid rise in core temperature, which is injurious to cells and organs throughout the body. Cellular edema, vacuolization, and widespread hemorrhage may develop.[4] Renal failure, rhabdomyolysis, hepatocellular necrosis, myocardial damage, cerebral edema, and various metabolic abnormalities can also occur. A profound respiratory alkalosis along with metabolic acidosis is common. Hyperventilation and tachycardia are universal.

Heatstroke can be divided into two forms, classic and exertional. *Classic heatstroke* (nonexertional) is seen more commonly in infants and ill children and the elderly. It develops over a period of days, usually coinciding with a heat wave, and presents with nausea, vomiting, headache, and a deteriorating mental status. Most of these patients are severely dehydrated and many have ceased sweating. Hypotension is common.

Exertional heatstroke develops rapidly, usually in young and vigorously exercising individuals who have not acclimatized to a hot environment. A dramatic presentation is seen with central nervous system changes from severe headache to seizures and collapse. Rhabdomyolysis and disseminated intravascular coagulation are often prominent in exertional heatstroke. Marked lactic acidosis may develop early but is not the grave prognostic indicator as that seen in classic heatstroke.

Diagnostic Findings. Rectal or core temperatures > 40° C (104° F); hypotension; mental changes, including severe headache, bizarre behavior, ataxia, seizures, and coma; tachycardia; tachypnea; and profuse or absent sweating can all be seen.

Multiple complications can occur with heatstroke, ranging from simple shivering to death. The patient may become hypotensive and dysrhythmias can occur. Seizures are not uncommon and multiple electrolyte imbalances are found. Acute tubular necrosis, rhabdomyolysis, and hepatic damage occur. In severe heatstroke disseminated intravascular coagulation (DIC) may develop. Coma with persistent neurologic sequelae can also occur.

Ancillary Data. Numerous laboratory studies are appropriate. Arterial blood gas measurement is essential and commonly indicates respiratory alkalosis and a metabolic acidosis. Although controversial, for each degree over 37° C (98.6° F) the values may be adjusted (see Table 39-2) as follows:

pH   ↓ 0.015
P_{CO_2} ↑ 4.4%
P_{O_2} ↑ 7.2%

Electrolyte values can reveal either hyperkalemia or hypokalemia, hypernatremia or hyponatremia. BUN and glucose levels will be elevated. Increased hematocrit; decreased platelets; and elevated aspartate aminotransferase (AST), lactate dehydrogenase (LDH), and creatinine phosphokinase (CPK) can be seen. Calcium can be either normal or decreased. Bleeding times may be prolonged and a DIC screen should be run. An electrocardiogram (ECG) should be obtained and the patient continuously monitored.

Differential Consideration. Meningitis, encephalitis, malaria, typhus, and Rocky Mountain spotted fever are infectious considerations that cause altered mental status and fever. Severe head trauma or drug intoxication may mimic heatstroke.

Diabetic ketoacidosis with infection should be considered. Hypothalmic dysfunction or thyroid storm can cause similar physical manifestations.

Management. Heatstroke is potentially life threatening and requires rapid intervention and ultimately, admission to an intensive care unit. Mortality increases significantly if core temperatures are allowed to remain over 39° C (102° F). Stabilization of the airway is essential. The patient must be removed from the heat and his or her clothes removed to allow for greater cooling of body surfaces.

At the scene, ice packs should be applied to groin, axilla, and neck areas, and the patient should be fanned. In the emergency department, the patient should remain stripped of all clothing and sprayed with lukewarm water while air is blown over him or her from fans until the patient's temperature is below 39° C (102° F).

These patients may or may not be severely dehydrated. In some cases, they may be relatively normovolemic but peripherally vasodilated.[15]

An IV bolus of 0.9% NS at 20 ml/kg should be run over 30 to 60 minutes. Further replacement of fluids and monitoring should reflect the patient's condition. A central venous pressure (CVP) line may be useful in monitoring vascular volume. A Foley catheter and a nasogastric tube should be inserted. Diazepam, 0.2 to 0.3 mg/kg/dose IV, can be given to control shivering.

PREVENTION

Infant deaths resulting from exposure to excessively high temperatures in locked vehicles are both tragic and needless. Closed vehicles in the sun with outside temperatures between 30° C and 40° C (86° F to 104° F) can reach an interior temperature of up to 60° C (140° F) within 15 minutes.[1,3,6] Direct sunlight and inadequate ventilation both contribute to the increased temperature. Infants respond initially by sweating, thus creating a fluid loss. Crying and restlessness increase this fluid loss even more. Eventually, they become unable to dissipate heat by normal methods. Sweating fails, along with other heat-regulating mechanisms, when ambient temperatures far exceed body temperatures for any extended time. Babies younger than 12 months old are the most vulnerable to heated, locked vehicles; but deaths have been reported in children up to 2 years of age in similar situations.[16]

Physicians, coaches, teachers, and parents need to be aware of the dangers involved in strenuous exercising in hot weather. Supervising adults need to be aware that exercising youth need to remain fully hydrated.[11] Adequate fluid preloading, 300 to 500 ml of fluid, and periodic drinking, 150 ml for a 40 kg child every 15 minutes while exercising, should be mandatory during hot weather. Quenching thirst alone does not ensure sufficient fluid replenishment.[4,11,14]

Debate about which liquids are best continues. High-osmolar solutions cause gastric distension and delay emptying and should be avoided. Water and electrolyte preparations are both acceptable. No differences in serum electrolyte concentrations or in rectal temperatures were found in runners drinking an electrolyte solution compared to runners drinking water.[16] Both liquids should be available, plentiful, and palatable so that the young athletes will drink enough to avoid dehydration.

Salt replacement with salt tablets is unnecessary. The average American salted diet has enough sodium to offset deficits in most situations.[4]

Athletic practice sessions should be scheduled for early morning or early evening. Heat exposure should be limited to less than 1 hour per day with periodic breaks.[11] A graduated exercise program should be maintained. Because clothing also affects the ability to dissipate heat, light clothing should be worn.

References

1. Robinson MD and Seward PN: Heat injury in children, *Pediatr Emerg Care* 3:114, 1987.
2. Barkin R and Rosen P, editors: *Emergency pediatrics*, ed 3, St. Louis, 1990, Mosby.
3. Committee on Sports Medicine, American Academy of Pediatrics: Climatic heat stress and the exercising child, *Pediatrics* 69:808, 1982.
4. Callaham M: Heat illness. In Rosen P, editor, *Emergency medicine: concepts and clinical practice*, St. Louis, 1983, Mosby.
5. Knochel JP: Dog days and siriasis: how to kill a football player, *JAMA* 233:513-15, 1975.
6. Nugent SK: Pediatric heatstroke: a case report, *Indiana Med* 80:235-37, 1987.

Pathophysiology

7. Guyton AC: *Textbook of medical physiology*, ed 6, Philadelphia, 1981, WB Saunders.
8. Batt ML and Kiernan JA, editors: *The human nervous system*, ed 4, Philadelphia, 1983, Harper and Row.
9. Hubbard RW: An introduction: the role of exercise in the etiology of exertional heatstroke, *Med Sci Sports Exercise* 22:2-5, 1990.
10. Anderson RJ, Reed G, Knochel J: Heatstroke, *Adv Intern Med* 28:115-40, 1983.
11. O'Donnell TF Jr: Management of heat stress injuries in the athlete, *Orthop Clin North Am* 11:841-55, 1980.
12. Shapiro Y and Seidman DS: Field and clinical observations of exertional heatstroke patients, *Med Sci Sports Exercise* 22:6-14, 1990.
13. Scott J: Heat related illnesses, *Postgrad Med* 85:154-64, 1989.
14. Luckstead EF: Sudden death in sports, *Pediatr Clin North Am* 29:1355-62, 1982.
15. Tek D and Olshaker JS: Heat illness, *Emerg Med Clin North Am* 10:299-310, 1992.

Prevention

16. King K, Negus K, Vance J: Heat stress in motor vehicles: a problem in infancy, *Pediatrics* 68:579-82, 1981.

## 39

Accidental Hypothermia and Frostbite

Harold J. Hofstrand

ACCIDENTAL HYPOTHERMIA

Accidental hypothermia occurs either by cold water immersion or by continuous nonimmersion exposure to a cold environ, the former occurring in the majority of pediatric accidental hypothermia victims.[1] The Centers for Disease Control reports far fewer pediatric hypothermia deaths than adults; drowning victims are categorized differently even though they may have suffered concurrently from hypothermia.[2]

Accidental hypothermia is differentiated from hypothermia related to malfunctioning of the body's heat regulating system. Hypothermia is defined as a core body temperature of 35° C (95° F) or less, and profound hypothermia is generally less than 28° C (82° F). Moderate hypothermia is associated with a temperature of 30° C (86° F) to 32° C (89° F).

The literature on pediatric accidental hypothermia is sparse because of its relative infrequency.[2-4] Much of the information is extrapolated from data about adults. Hypothermia is a special problem for young children and infants, especially the cold water immersion type. Factors that could influence thermoregulatory balance in this group include the following:

1. Large surface area/body weight ratio
2. Minimal subcutaneous fat
3. Thin skin with increased permeability
4. Delayed shivering and inefficient ability to generate heat compared to adult
5. Immature or inappropriate behavioral response to environment

One thermogenic mechanism, however, may be advantageous to infants and young children: a nonshivering cellular heat production mechanism from specialized body cells called "brown fat cells."[5] This mechanism allows for a tripling of heat production by the infant. Brown fat cells are found abundantly in certain infant body fat areas such as the neck and shoulder regions.

The dramatic and fatal complications of cold exposure have been known since the dawn of human experience.[6-8] Heat for our warm-blooded enzyme systems parallels the importance to basic survival of oxygen, food, and water. Our species would not have survived without the ability to maintain a microclimate of approximately 22° C (71° F) next to our relatively hairless body surface.[9] For millennia our ancestors survived by residing in moderate climates. Animal skins and fire "technology" allowed them to live in colder climates. Cold injury has probably claimed more victims over the years of human existence than weapons and war. Ironically, war experiences have contributed to some of our clinical insights and more pervasive treatment questions. Besides recognizing the devastation of the freeze-thaw-freeze cycle on extremities, Baron Larrey, Napoleon's chief surgeon, made the first known observation that severely cold soldiers placed closest to the fire died faster than those placed at a greater distance.[10] The Titanic sinking in April of 1912 in the icy waters (0° C or 32° F) of the North Atlantic revealed the devastatingly fatal power of nondrowning cold water immersion.[11,12] Although rescue boats reached the site within 2 hours, the only survivors of the 2,201 people on board were the 712 who managed to escape the near 0° C (32° F) water temperature without immersion by exiting directly into lifeboats. Almost all of the victims were wearing life jackets and although their deaths were classified officially as drowning, in actuality they died of hypothermia, not drowning.[11]

Pathophysiology

Because most pediatric cold exposure victims have few contributing conditions, such as alcohol or underlying disease, their responses are more likely related to pure hypothermic physiology. The deep rectal and perhaps the tympanic membrane measurements reflect the core temperature.[13] Fig. 39-1 shows a child's temperature profile in its normal homeothermic state. Table 39-1 reflects the common signs and symptoms associated with progressive lowering of core body temperature.

Understanding thermoregulation is critical to understanding hypothermia and its clinical consequences.[5,14,15] Conceptually this is a balance between heat loss and heat production.

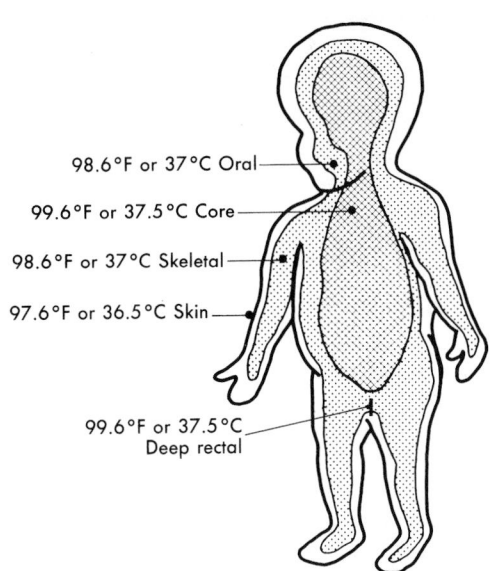

98.6°F or 37°C Oral

99.6°F or 37.5°C Core

98.6°F or 37°C Skeletal

97.6°F or 36.5°C Skin

99.6°F or 37.5°C
Deep rectal

FIG. 39-1. Temperature profile of child in normal homeothermic state. (*Adapted from Pozos RS, Born DO, editors:* Hypothermia: causes, effects, prevention, *Piscataway, NJ, 1982, New Century Publishing.*)

Heat Loss (Fig. 39-2). Although one often hears about cold penetration, heat only flows from hot to cold, and the speed of this heat movement depends on the gradient of the temperature difference. Barriers, such as clothing, can be constructed to slow this process; however, any existing gradient will continue to force the loss of heat. Heat flows in two basic ways: (1) by *radiation* in the form of electromagnetic waves, which can cross a vacuum, accounting for up to 65% of usual heat losses and (2) by *conduction*, which is the movement or transfer of heat from matter to matter. Two additional special types of conduction are important clinically: (1) convection, which is heat flow from matter to moving matter, and (2) evaporation, which is heat flow or transfer as matter changes form.

Even the nonexercising human body in a moderate ambient temperature environment produces more heat than is needed to maintain the body temperature of 37.1° C (98.6° F).[16] Approximately 60% to 80% of the heat produced in this situation is extra and dissipated from the body.[17] This heat can be trapped by appropriate clothing systems, allowing the body to exist comfortably at very low environmental temperatures. Even a mild to moderately cool hypothermic body is capable of producing enough heat to slowly warm back up if this heat can be retained. Heat loss can be either voluntary or involuntary. A human body can voluntarily remove clothing systems to hasten heat loss, or the body involuntarily and automatically controls heat loss by four mechanisms: (1) regulation of blood flow (the heat distribution system of the body), (2) sweating, (3) elimination of warm urine and feces, and (4) exhaled air.

Increased heat loss can be associated with certain problems, such as malnutrition and certain drug ingestions; water and wind are the incredible "thieves of heat." Air is an excellent insulation barrier to heat flow; the more air space that can be trapped within fibers or fabrics, or be-

tween layers of clothing, the better the conductive resistance to heat loss. Heat flow will proceed from a warm body into cold water 20 times faster than into cold air at the same temperature.[5,15,18-20] Conductive heat loss directly into the cold snow or ice environment also occurs faster than heat loss into cold air of the same temperature. A child standing on icy cold ground with bare feet will have a more rapid heat loss directly into the cold ground than into the cold air of the same temperature. The conduction loss to wind or moving water can also play a significant factor in the rate of heat loss.[5,21] The newly warmed air or water adjacent to the warm body is immediately taken away by convection, reestablishing the maximum gradient for conduction.

Windchill temperature is the temperature that would affect the same rate of heat loss without the wind.[22] The temperature rating given in windchill situations does not reflect the temperature of the skin. A child sledding in a winter windchill of −29° C (−20° F) will not freeze tissue if the environmental temperature is actually 2° C (35° F).[23]

Sweat is produced when the core temperature rises significantly. It is the body's natural way of getting rid of heat and is especially effective in the summer. In the warmly dressed child playing outdoors in the winter, however, sweating presents extra problems. If the child generates sufficient heat by exercise, sweating results. Sweating causes an increase in heat loss by reducing the insulating capabilities of the clothing by wetting and by evaporation. Sweat can cause severe winter problems for children in three ways. It can conduct heat away from the body rapidly once it cools because of its fluid nature, it draws additional heat from the warm body if the sweat evaporates from the skin surface, and it reduces the insulating capacity of garments. Keeping the core temperature constant for children is a real challenge in winter. However, because most children can return immediately to warm homes, these physiologic mechanisms have less consequence than in arctic explorers.

Heat Production. The amount of heat an adult needs to generate to maintain the body temperature at 37.1° C (98.6° F) in a room temperature environment is approximately 100 kcal/hr (40 to 60 kcal/m² surface).[9] The ingestion of food, fevers, and cold stress will increase this rate slightly. The two general categories of heat production are (1) voluntary, such as voluntary muscle exercise to increase heat from muscular activity or simply eating food to stoke the metabolic furnace, and (2) involuntary, exemplified by shivering, which is a very efficient and effective means of generating heat.[5] In a 70 kg man, as much as 350 kcal heat/hr can be generated at maximal shivering.[24,25] Also included in this involuntary category is the thermogenesis resulting from the great variety of metabolic reactions that contribute to the body's usual method of heat production.[5]

Certain clinical conditions can lead to decreased heat production such as endocrine insufficiencies, malnutrition, or severe immobilization. Young marathon runners in cooler climates also seem more predisposed to hypothermia than to hyperthermia.[26]

Although the pathophysiology of immersion hypothermia could differ somewhat from that of the nonimmersion, more slowly developing form, little experimental evidence

TABLE 39-1. Signs and Symptoms at Progressive Degrees of Hypothermia*

State of hypothermia	F° core	C° core	Clinical signs and symptoms
Mild	98.6°	37° (oral)	Normal homeothermic state
	99.6°	37.6° (rectal)	
	95°	35°	Maximal shivering and slurred speech
Moderate	89°	32°	Change in level of consciousness
			Change in blood pressure
			Pupils dilated but react to light
			Shivering ceases
			Muscle rigidity and incoordination
	86°	30°	Stuporous state begins
			Many resuscitation drugs inactive
			Respiratory rate decreases
Severe	82°	28°	Bradycardia, up to 50%, refractory to atropine
			Osborne wave possible on ECG
			Decreased minute ventilation
			Voluntary motion ceases
			Cardiac fibrillation threshold on rewarming with stimulation
			Pupils nonreactive to light
	79°	26°	Loss of consciousness
			Areflexic
	77°	25°	No respirations common
			Appears dead with fixed dilated pupils
			Pulmonary edema may occur
			Blood viscosity increases by 173%
			Maximum risk of ventricular fibrillation
	68°	20°	Cardiac asystole common
	64°	18°	Lowest core temperature adult accidental hypothermia victim to survive
	59°	15°	Lowest core temperature infant to survive
	48°	9°	Lowest artificially cooled hypothermia adult patient to recover

Adapted from Pozos RS, Born DO, editors: *Hypothermia: causes, effects, prevention*, Piscataway, NJ, 1982, New Central Publishing.
*Largely extrapolated from adult data unless otherwise indicated.
ECG, Electrocardiogram.

substantiates this theory.[26-30] Animal models for hypothermia are not good, as their more hairy bodies seem to cool and freeze differently than human bodies.[31] The double-blinded studies necessary for understanding physiologic corrections to this altered pathophysiology also are sparse. The pediatric immersion hypothermic victim also has often experienced total submersion, bringing into play additional reflexes ("diving response") that make it difficult to determine which phenomenon has contributed to a particular sign or symptom[29,32] (see Chapter 35).

A human body that drops its core temperature more slowly, as in slow nonimmersion hypothermia, may develop more severe cardiovascular changes, particularly intravascular volume loss.[33-35] If the patient survives the initial few minutes of immersion and does not enter a near-drowning algorithm (see Chapter 35), the respiratory system responses predominate the early phases of immersion hypothermia. Respiratory tidal volume and rate significantly increase (hyperventilation), producing a decrease in arterial Pco_2 and a rapid increase in arterial pH (respiratory alkalosis).[36] The resulting restriction of cerebral blood flow can

further complicate survival by impairing judgment and causing tetanic voluntary muscle contractions, making coordinated movements difficult.[12]

Many changes occur in the cardiovascular system in response to the cold. Cold affects the myocardial conduction cells,[37] contraction cells, and the blood within the intravascular space.[38,39] The volume within the intravascular space is influenced by several factors. Immediate peripheral vasoconstriction shunts blood to the central circulation, somewhat like the application of an imaginary Military Anti-Shock Trousers (MAST) suit.[5] This speculated central volume increase probably triggers pituitary production of antidiuretic hormone causing a cold diuresis phenomenon and volume depletion.[40-42] Eventual depression in renal tubular cell oxidative metabolism with subsequent decreased water and sodium reabsorption causes a continuing decrease in the intravascular volume.[42] Further fluid shifts can occur from intravascular compartment to extravascular compartment by plasma sequestration.[31] Finally, changes occur in blood viscosity (due to mechanisms such as splenic contraction) that increase the hematocrit in

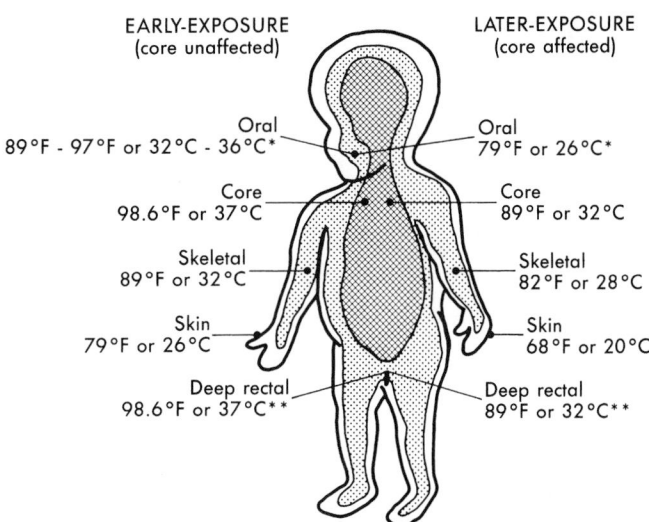

EARLY-EXPOSURE
(core unaffected)

LATER-EXPOSURE
(core affected)

Oral
89°F - 97°F or 32°C - 36°C*

Oral
79°F or 26°C*

Core
98.6°F or 37°C

Core
89°F or 32°C

Skeletal
89°F or 32°C

Skeletal
82°F or 28°C

Skin
79°F or 26°C

Skin
68°F or 20°C

Deep rectal
98.6°F or 37°C**

Deep rectal
89°F or 32°C**

* No correlation with core temperatures
** May not correlate perfectly with thoracic core temperature

FIG. 39-2. Temperature pattern after exposure to increasing degrees of environmental cold. (*Adapted from Pozos RS, Born DO, editors:* Hypothermia: causes, effects, prevention, *Piscataway, 1982, New Century Publishing.*)

an already low flow–low shear state produced by the cold. This viscosity change can be up to 173% of normal at a core temperature of 25° C (77° F).[34]

In addition to rewarming technology,[43] volume reexpansion is clearly one of the most important aspects of therapy in the hypothermic victim. In a prospective controlled study in neonates, administration of intravenous saline before rewarming reduced the mortality rate from 75% to 17%.[44] It appears that the longer it takes for the core temperature to drop significantly, the more profound the eventual intravascular volume loss. Acute immersion hypothermia may not produce the same degree of volume loss as the more slowly generated nonimmersion hypothermia.[45] Other cardiovascular and metabolic problems would still exist at the same low core temperature regardless of exposure mechanism.[28]

Although the physiologic concepts of afterdrop and aftershock are easily defined, they are less easily understood in relationship to the morbidity and mortality of the hypothermic pediatric patient.[5] Afterdrop is the continued decrease in core temperature, even though the patient has been removed from the cold stress and may be under rewarming therapy.[5,46,47] Given additional time, the core temperature will rise again. This sudden change was originally thought to trigger cardiac dysrhythmias, especially ventricular fibrillation. It was also thought to be strictly a human hypothermic response, but it is now believed to be any system's normal response to rewarming and probably is not as dangerous as once thought.[5,47]

Aftershock is the state of depletion of intravascular volume that occurs with rewarming. This occurs through actual volume loss from the intravascular space as described previously or additionally through abnormal vessel tone with the rewarming causing a shocklike state similar to spinal shock. This later mechanism is only speculated. Like

most other hypovolemic and distributive shock states, it requires close monitoring and volume replacement with the progressive rewarming. In contrast to afterdrop, aftershock can contribute significantly to mortality if not appropriately addressed.[5,15,31,48]

Diagnostic Findings

Clinical Findings. The progressive clinical signs and symptoms at various core temperatures are summarized in Table 39-1. Mild hypothermia is arbitrarily defined to that range requiring no hospitalization or special care other than prevention of further heat loss. Even if no external heat is added to the mildly hypothermic body, the victim can recover by his or her own heat generation and physiologic mechanisms when removed from the cold stress. Patients progressing to moderate or severe stages of hypothermia may become physically, mentally, or metabolically incapable of reversing the situation without outside intervention.[31,49]

The severely hypothermic patient appears dead, accounting for the basic rule that resuscitation should continue in the seemingly pulseless, apneic victim until the core temperature is at least 30° C (86° F) or preferably 32° C (89° F).[50,51] Cold patients can still be dead but their status cannot be confirmed until they are rewarmed. Totally frozen extremities can complicate resuscitation if they are thawed at the same time as the core temperature.[52] Commonly described direct complications of severe hypothermia include gastrointestinal (GI) bleeding, acute renal failure, pancreatitis, deep vein thrombosis, disseminated intravascular coagulopathy, pulmonary edema, and probably any organ system failure, given certain conditions.[53-55]

Ancillary Data. Ancillary findings may contribute to the diagnosis and treatment. The most controversial yet impor-

TABLE 39-2. Arterial Blood Gas Correction with Temperature Variations

	ABOVE 37° C Change/° C >37°	BELOW 37° C Change/° C <37°
pH unit	− 0.015 unit	+ 0.015 unit
P_{CO_2} (mm Hg)	+ 4.4%	− 4.4%
P_{O_2} (mm Hg)	+ 7.2%	− 7.2%

tant laboratory parameter is the arterial blood gas (ABG). A controversy has centered around whether the ABG in the hypothermic victim should be corrected or remain uncorrected for the patient's temperature.[56] Recent arguments favor an approach in which the gases are interpreted uncorrected after the blood sample is warmed to 37.1° C (98.6° F) and then analyzed as if it were in a normothermic patient.[31,57-59] Studies show that allowing corrected pH to rise and P_{CO_2} to fall as the temperature decreases or maintaining the uncorrected pH at 7.40 leads to improved ventricular function as measured by cardiac output and decreases the incidence of lactic acidosis and ventricular fibrillation. Corrections, if desired, are 0.0147 pH units per degree Celsius below 37° C, P_{CO_2} correction of 4.4% per degree Celsius temperature reduction and the P_{O_2} drops 7.2% per degree Celsius[61] (Table 39-2).

Acid-base disturbances are common in hypothermia, and the physiologic consequence could be significant. Metabolic acidosis is common from lactic acid buildup and decreased liver metabolism, but mixed acidosis and sometimes even alkalosis can be present. It is not possible to predict which abnormality will be present in a particular situation.[62]

Little evidence demonstrates electrolyte abnormalities directly from hypothermia itself; underlying illness or disease may alter values.[31] Hyperkalemia may become secondary to metabolic acidosis, renal failure, or rhabdomyolysis. Glucose metabolism is generally decreased in hypothermic patients, resulting in hyperglycemia. Prolonged shivering alters blood glucose.[5] If glucose values remain abnormal, diabetes or pancreatitis should be suspected; insulin is ineffective until well above 30° C (86° F). Calcium and magnesium should also be measured.

A full clotting screen (prothrombin time [PT], partial thromboplastin time [PTT], bleeding time), with platelet count and fibrinogen level is necessary. Thrombocytopenia is common; hypercoagulability may exist with a disseminated intravascular coagulation (DIC) syndrome.

Although blood urea nitrogen (BUN) and creatinine are often elevated, they are not particularly useful indicators for acute hypothermia. With severe hypothermia, rhabdomyolysis is often present. There is some correlation between amylasemia and the severity of hypothermia and morbidity in adults, but this correlation has not been substantiated in children.[31] Repeat ABGs, glucose, hematocrit, and potassium should be obtained with every few degrees to 6° F temperature rise in the patient.[50]

Radiography is not particularly diagnostic for acute hypothermia. One needs to remain suspicious of injury poten-

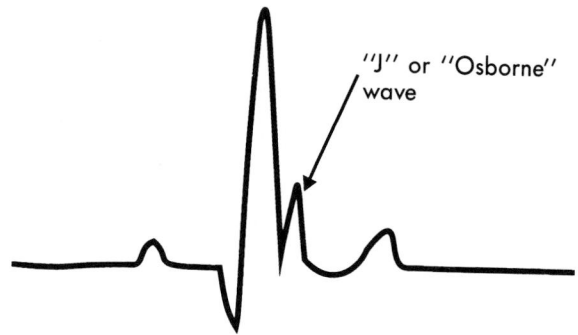

FIG. 39-3. Electrocardiogram demonstrating appearance of "J" or "Osborne" wave.

tial as well as cold insult and order x-ray studies accordingly. The brain usually adapts structurally to hypothermia and to rewarming without swelling so that computed tomography (CT) is not particularly helpful unless there is suspicion of other pathology. Severely frozen extremities may suffer growth plate injuries that have future radiologic considerations.[52]

The only known electrocardiographic (ECG) finding that is pathognomonic of hypothermia occurring near 30° C (86° F) core is the J-wave or Osborne wave.[63] This wave, shown in Fig. 39-3, is a positive deflection on the R-T segment and has been described in pediatric and adult patients.[4]

Bradycardia occurs in all patients in the moderate stages of hypothermia, and other rhythm problems can occur easily.[37,63] Atrial fibrillation is commonly observed; the least problematic usually requires no chemical or electrical therapy for control.[63] The more serious collapse rhythms of ventricular fibrillation or asystole are incompatible with life, and the patient exhibiting these rhythms needs support. These severe rhythm problems are often unmanageable chemically or electrically until the core temperature reaches at least 30° C (86° F); cardiopulmonary resuscitation (CPR) is essential unless bypass or other means are used to support the circulation.

Differential Considerations

The precipitating event is usually overt and hypothermia is easily recognized and measured. For whatever reason, however, if hypothermia is not suspected in an ill or injured patient, the clinical assessment and stabilization could be complicated. Many severe trauma patients are hypothermic.[64] Core temperature should be measured deep rectally with a low reading thermometer that is not embedded in cold stool. Core temperature correlation may be obtained with infrared readings off the tympanic membrane (TM). In dogs, core temperature correlation with thermistor TM measurements has been demonstrated in low ranges.[13] Caution must be used at present with infrared TM measurements in hypothermic patients.

Management

The therapeutic approach to hypothermia is ideally divided into the prehospital and hospital phases.

Prehospital Phase. A basic premise in the prehospital phase management of hypothermia is that no one is dead (although they may look that way) until they are warm and without cardiovascular parameters compatible with life.[40,51,65] Rewarming severely hypothermic victims may actually complicate the resuscitation; there is some protection to staying in the "metabolic icebox," especially during transport to a facility where thawing can be controlled and monitored.[50,66] On arrival at an institution capable of delivering definitive care, thawing can occur rapidly.

Initial assessment should focus on defining associated problems such as a cervical spine or other traumatic injury, hypoglycemia, near drowning, or an inconsistent history suspicious of child abuse/neglect. Immobilization should be completed before transport.

Accurate vital sign measurements are critical.[31,64] Electronic monitoring of rhythm is essential to distinguish bradycardia from collapse, asystole, or ventricular fibrillation. If monitor leads do not adhere to the cold skin, duct tape can be placed over the lead and skin or benzoin can be applied before application of electrodes. It is also possible to puncture a gel foam conventional monitoring pad with small-gauge sterile needles in the unconscious patient. Measuring blood pressure in the field is generally not possible and does not generally change stabilization procedures.

Prehospital personnel should obtain an accurate core temperature reading, if possible; knowledge of core temperature along with electrical rhythm might determine the urgency and type of stabilization and destination for definitive treatment. Drug therapy should be withheld if the core temperature is too low.[15,51] Tympanic temperatures may be close to true core temperatures; however, low ambient temperatures may alter this reading.[13,68] Lacking tympanic thermometers, a low-reading thermometer, placed deep in the rectum (and not embedded in cold stool), is also helpful, although obviously more inconvenient.[5]

An accurate, totally counted 1-minute respiratory rate is helpful because an apneic patient should be intubated and assisted with ventilation and oxygen. A slow, shallow respiratory rate under three breaths/minute may simply reflect the oxygen needs of the "metabolic icebox" or ventilation of little more than the dead space resulting in minimal oxygen delivery. However, patients with these very low rates will likely benefit from increased oxygenation and ventilation, so appropriate measures should be attempted.[31] Oxygenation may be the single most important prehospital issue even if the patient is in the metabolic icebox. Orotracheal intubation with in-line traction, if appropriate, may be the preferred route in apneic pediatric patients. The latter approach depends on the skill of the prehospital team and rigidity of cold tissue. Since most pediatric tracheal intubations are with uncuffed tubes, the problem of cold ambient air in the cuff later expanding and kinking the tube when warmed is much less of a potential problem than in the older patient.

Recent evidence indicates that intubation does not trigger ventricular fibrillation in adult patients.[31] If bag-valve or mouth-to-mask ventilation is used, a nasogastric tube is recommended to prevent distention of the stomach and further compromise respiratory function.

Further heat loss should be prevented. A very cold patient is still likely to be warmer than the cold environment and will still lose heat to that environment unless insulated. All wet clothing should be removed carefully. Significant rewarming of frozen or near frozen limbs should be avoided until cardiovascular and metabolic problems are under control.

Do not consider active means of external rewarming unless that patient is conscious, alert, and shivering. Even then proceed with caution because of the variability of human response. An appropriate rewarming measure is to give humidified oxygen heated to 40° C to 42° C (103° F to 105° F), if available.[69] This procedure basically prevents further respiratory heat loss.[70-73]

Trained personnel should start intravenous lines en route, if this is possible without slowing transport. Frozen or cool extremities, however, make this procedure difficult. The external jugular vein is an excellent choice unless a cervical collar is in place. Room temperature normal saline is a desirable medium. Although there are no reports of intraosseous infusions, this could be an alternative route and more easily established in the unconscious pediatric hypothermic patient 6 years of age or younger in whom intravenous access is not easily achieved.

If a collapse rhythm (ventricular fibrillation or asystole) is electronically verified, CPR should begin, irrespective of core temperature unless there are lethal injuries.[74,75] The cold chest wall may tend to inhibit compressions. Nearly all survivors of severe hypothermia with apnea and collapse rhythms have had CPR.[69,76-81] Bradycardia is probably a physiologic rhythm in the "metabolic icebox."

First-line resuscitation drugs are generally not initiated until the core temperature is greater than 30° C (85° F).[15,51] These medicines are not active at these low ranges, but will accumulate.[82] Defibrillation should also be delayed; however, no definable danger has been demonstrated by giving a series of 1 watt-sec/kg shocks if ventricular fibrillation is present. The cold myocardium is generally resistant to defibrillation but there is individual variation. Bretylium may be a better choice than lidocaine in the hypothermic patient for prophylaxis or treatment of ventricular fibrillation.[83,84] However, there appears to be no need for prophylactic use of bretylium to prevent ventricular fibrillation during intubation attempts.[62,77,85] Magnesium might also be considered.

If there is significantly impaired central nervous system (CNS) function with an accurate core temperature of at least 34° C (93° F), dextrose and naloxone should be given. Although there is some variability, the hypothermic patient with a core temperature greater than 34° C (93° F) who is stuporous often has a concomitant problem.[31]

The prehospital team should notify the correct receiving hospital to allow as much time for preparation for bypass or other means of extracorporeal circulation and rewarming. This time is especially important for hypothermic victims with cardiac arrest.

Hospital Phase. During this phase, the return to normothermia is the primary consideration. Although moderate hypothermia victims have recovered well with all types of core rewarming techniques, the patient with *severe* hypothermia, and especially in cardiac arrest, is probably best resuscitated in facilities with bypass or extracorporeal capabilities.[31]

Initial management should include oxygen, definitive airway stabilization (sometimes, with cold trismus and cold stiff tissue, a fiber-optic intubation may be necessary) intravenous support, and injury and cervical spine precautions. Accurate vital signs and monitoring are essential. Doppler ultrasound may be needed to locate pulses. Remaining clothing should be cut off and wet body parts dried. Truncal heat loss should be prevented by insulation until the definitive method of rewarming has begun. CPR should be continued if there is no electrical activity. Placing a Swan-Ganz catheter may produce more problems than solutions; however, placing a central venous pressure (CVP) line may help evaluate dynamic volume status if the CVP line tip is just above the heart. Aggressive and controlled fluid resuscitation is often required.[15,86] The resuscitation fluid can be warmed by a blood warmer if the rate of infusion is not rapid. Countercurrent in-line warmers and rapid infusion of prewarmed saline and mixtures could possibly be used for rapid transfusions. Normal saline (NS) or D5W 0.9% NS is preferable. Lactated Ringer's solution should not be used because the liver in the "metabolic icebox" does not metabolize lactate well.[87] Arterial lines also may be helpful, especially for repeated blood gases; nasogastric tube and Foley catheter are also inserted.

Frozen extremities, if present, should not be thawed until later in the resuscitation when core temperature is greater than 32° C to 34° C (89° F to 93° F) and when all control measures are in place.[52] The extremity can then be rapidly thawed in 40° C (105° F) water. Initial sterile bath solution may not be advantageous.

Rewarming Techniques. Rewarming techniques can be divided arbitrarily into external rewarming and internal core rewarming.[88-90] For the most severely hypothermic victim in collapse rhythm, extracorporeal techniques (bypass or rewarming hemodialysis) have the greatest efficacy.[91,92] Other core techniques—peritoneal, gastric, rectal, and thoracic cavity lavage and heated intravenous fluids—have been successful in various situations.[93-100]

The advantages of extracorporeal techniques include a rapid return to a normal temperature, reduction of blood viscosity, and the perfusion of the body despite any cardiac instability.[92] Cardiac output is increased directly with increasing vasodilation. This method also likely matches the escalating tissue metabolic needs with the increasing tissue perfusion. Partial bypass can be instituted rapidly by a groin incision and local anesthesia, with little increased morbidity and mortality. Disadvantages include bleeding secondary to heparinization and the need for specific technology. Although some hypothermic infants have been rewarmed successfully using microwaves, this technique is experimental and not recommended.[101] Generally, rewarming is discontinued once the core temperature is approximately 36° C (96° F) to avoid overheating or "after-rise."

Common resuscitation drugs have diminished effectiveness in the severely hypothermic patient except for oxygen. Drugs will likely accumulate and produce potential toxicity after rewarming. Certain drugs such as dopamine may actually have a deleterious effect on extremity survival.

Dysrhythmias. Dysrhythmias are common in adult hypothermic patients, especially with rewarming.[63] They may occur with the same frequency in pediatric victims, although this rate has not been documented. Fortunately, the majority of them are benign and self-correcting with return of normothermia. The atrial dysrhythmias are perhaps the most common, usually converting spontaneously and not requiring drug therapy.[37]

The more serious issue of collapse rhythms and their management is still not totally resolved. Both asystole and ventricular fibrillation are commonly documented.[102-104] In controlled circumstances with adults when good oxygenation and careful continuous monitoring has been achieved, the most common collapse rhythm has been asystole. Recent animal studies have shown that bretylium is a better choice than lidocaine in both prophylaxis and therapy of ventricular fibrillation in hypothermia.[31] Chemical therapies are not advised if the core temperature is less than 30° C (85° F). Although electrical conversion may be unsuccessful below 30° C (85° F), it appears to be rational to attempt three standard defibrillations before resuming CPR. There is no current recommendation on the use of bretylium in humans to prevent prophylactically ventricular fibrillation. Once ventricular fibrillation is documented, bretylium may be the best chemical agent to use,[30,83] although magnesium is a less dangerous alternative and has been successfully used in induced hypothermia fibrillation.[105]

There appears to be no advantage and many potential disadvantages to cardiac pacing. Several cases of ventricular fibrillation have been precipitated by attempts at pacing a cold heart.

Sepsis. Sepsis is an especially important consideration in pediatric patients, who appear to be at greater risk than adults,[106] perhaps due to patient criteria selection more than predisposing factors. It may be due to an impaired immune response.[107] Prophylactic broad-spectrum antibiotics are still recommended after appropriate culturing in patients with moderate or severe hypothermia.

Disposition

The overall outcome of resuscitation is difficult to predict in pediatric or adult patients because of the variability of human physiologic response to the hypothermic state.[48] Mild accidental hypothermia can generally be rewarmed in the field or in the emergency department.[108-110] Moderate and severe hypothermia requires rapid intervention and close monitoring in the hospital environment.[111]

Prognosis. Survival is unlikely if the core temperature is less than 15° C (59° F), serum potassium is more than 10 mEq/L, fibrinogen is less than 50 mg/dl, total environmental exposure is greater than 24 hours, and there is no cardiac rhythm. A recent study indicated that serum potassium might be a very important marker of survival.[112] If the serum level of potassium is greater than 10 mEq/L, survival is unlikely.

Prevention. As with any complex disorder with severe mortality outcomes, prevention is essential. The basis of prevention lies in an understanding of the principles of water safety, winter safety, and heat loss and, above all, supervision by adults. It is equally unfair to the child to impart a fear of the cold, water, or adventure, as cold climates, water sports, and wilderness activities could become important in his or her adult life. A balance is required.[113]

The most significant principles involved in winter clothing systems include the following:

1. It is wise to avoid circumstances that render a clothing system inadequate.
2. Layering allows air trapping (air being an effective insulator), which reduces heat loss by conduction and convection. Layering also allows easier removal or redressing to adjust body core temperature.[16]
3. Wicking primarily involves the movement of sweat (or any water) by special fabrics from the surface of the skin to outer layers of clothing or to the atmosphere.
4. Nonconstriction of garments allows for more air trapping and maximum circulation, which promotes blood (heat) flow and body movement.[114]
5. The body should be protected from the "thieves of heat"—wind and water.[114] Keeping water or snow out, while allowing egress of sweat from the inside is an important property of many fabrics.
6. Access and egress involve the use of zipper systems to vent heat and moisture to the outside and allow urination and defecation to be facilitated.
7. Special attention should be paid to hands, feet, and face because they have special needs and are least protected from the cold.[17]
8. Blocking and trapping of radiation heat should be maximized. Some materials, such as reflecting foil, are useful; foil does not allow moisture to flow out. Remember, radiation often accounts for the greatest percentage of body heat loss.

The victim of cold water immersion has a relatively short time before core temperatures drop.[115] Cold water is a much faster "heat sapping" environment by a factor of at least 20 than either cold air or ice at the same temperature.[19,20]

FROSTBITE

Frostbite occurs almost exclusively in humans,[52] perhaps because the human is still basically a semitropical animal and has not evolved in the same fashion as other warm-blooded mammals residing in cold environments. Frostbite, associated with tissue freezing and vascular disruption, is produced by a significant environmental cold stress associated with a decrease in blood flow to the involved skin and body area.[52] The impaired blood flow does not deliver sufficient heat to the tissue, resulting in freezing injury.[116] Although the skin is an important organ in thermoregulation, under adverse cold conditions it cannot function.[52]

Pathophysiology

Two major mechanisms are involved in the development of frostbite.[116] The first is actual ice crystal formation in the tissues, predominantly in the extracellular space. Although crystal formation appears to disrupt cellular and subcellular anatomy, the major problem is that it draws water from the cells, resulting in intracellular hyperosmolarity reaching toxic levels. The second issue is vascular stasis and abnormal blood flow in the distal parts of the involved skin and surface organ systems. Vasoconstriction, increased blood viscosity, actual freezing, damaged capillary endothelial cells, subsequent increase in capillary permeability and leakage, and arteriovenous shunting will develop after this initial insult.[52] Some of the tissue that survives the direct cold injury may later die from the vascular insufficiency associated with insufficient circulation.

Diagnostic Findings

Frostbite occurs on the most distal or exposed skin areas. The early stage of a freezing injury, frostnip, is a reversible stage of this progressive disorder. Generally, the feeling of intense cold to the part involved with some pain characterizes this early stage. As progressively deeper layers freeze and become involved with vascular stasis, decreased flexibility and movement and total absence of pain and sensation follow. Progression to frostbite (beyond frostnip) occurs in two stages: (1) *superficial frostbite,* which involves the skin and immediate underlying layers of subcutaneous tissue; and (2) *deeper frostbite,* which involves the skin, subcutaneous tissue, and deeper structures, such as muscles, tendons, nerves, and bone.

Findings depend on the depth of the injury and the area involved.[52] Individuals with frostnip experience a sensation of intense cold progressing to pain and numbness; complete loss of sensation does not occur. The skin remains erythematous after warming and capillary refill is generally normal. Superficial frostbite is characterized by no pain or sensation while the area is frozen. Pain starts during the thawing process and becomes progressively more severe. The skin has a white and often paraffin-like appearance, with little or no capillary refill. The affected area becomes edematous and erythematous, purplish, or mottled. Blisters developing in superficial frostbite are generally clear, usually resolving within a week. An eschar could be left, and if it turns black, can be mistaken for gangrene. Deeper frostbite involves no pain while frozen and may remain painless after rewarming if the sensory nerves to the region were damaged. Even after thawing, the color of the affected skin is often grayish and mottled and remains cold without evidence of circulation. Blister formation often does not occur, but when blisters form, they are often hemorrhagic.[52]

Management

A bold therapeutic adventure in the 1950s has become the time-honored and apparently best procedure for treatment of frostbite.[117,118] This treatment is the rapid rewarming or rapid thawing of the frozen body part by immersion in water warmed to between 38° C and 43° C (100° F and 110° F).[119-121] Gradual rewarming by exposure to room temperature or heaters is not only less effective but dangerous and can result in further tissue damage. The worst possible scenario is that the exposed body part is allowed to thaw and then refreeze.[10] In the prehospital wilderness environment, thawing should not be attempted if there is any remote possibility that refreezing could occur. In the hospital environment, other issues such as hypothermia or trauma management are given priority over frostbite therapy. When appropriate following stabilization, rapid thawing in a whirlpool bath is ideal.[52] One can begin the process with nonsterile water; later treatment should be conducted under more aseptic conditions. During rewarming, extremities should not touch the sides or bottom of the rewarming vessel. The process generally takes from 20 to 30 minutes; if deeper structures are involved, up to 1 hour may be required. During this time, the patient may require intravenous analgesia for intense pain.

After the rapid thaw, the basic goals are to salvage as much tissue and achieve as much function as possible.[52,122] These goals are achieved by protecting the area from further injury, preventing infection, aiding circulation, and continuing rehabilitation. Although these therapeutic goals are pursued outside the emergency department, some of them need to be addressed in the department. The first is tetanus prophylaxis and the possible institution of antibiotics at an early stage. Anticoagulation, although seemingly reasonable as a therapeutic approach, has *not* been shown to add any benefit.[52] Vasodilators may be used. Major amputation surgery should be delayed until the demarcating line for tissue nonviability has been determined with certainty.[52,123] Experimental techniques such as thrombolysis and dextran may be of theoretical help at certain stages in selected patients. Hyperbaric oxygen treatment is advocated by some clinicians.

Disposition

The frostbite patient is best managed in a burn unit or a hospital environment where strict use of aseptic technique and knowledge of burn therapy is well understood. Follow-up can be best accomplished in the same manner as with burn victims. In pediatric patients, growth plate injuries have been reported with both digits and long bones after deep frostbite injury.[52] There is no present method to prevent this type of injury, and parents need to be warned of its possibility.

Prevention. Certain body skin areas endure frostbite with less sequelae. Explorers may sacrifice facial frostbite to protect other areas. Special attention must be given to avoiding frostbite on the hands or feet. Although specific clothing systems are designed to prevent frostbite, clear mental functioning is an important factor in avoiding conditions leading to extremity frostbite.[52,122,124]

References

Accidental Hypothermia

1. Corneli HM: Accidental hypothermia: issues for the future, ACEP newsletter: *Peds Emerg Med Section* 2(2):2, 1991.
2. Leads from the MMWR: hypothermia-associated deaths—United States, 1968-1980, *JAMA* 255:307, 1986.
3. Mann TP and Elliot RIK: Neonatal cold injury due to accidental exposure to cold, *Lancet* 2:229-234, 1957.
4. Robinson M and Seward P: Environmental hypothermia in children, *Ped Emerg Care* 4:254, 1986.
5. Pozos RS and Born DO, editors: Hypothermia: causes, effects, prevention, Piscataway, NJ, 1982, *New Century Publishing*.
6. Burton AC and Edholm OG: Man in a cold environment, New York, 1969, *Hafner Publishing*.
7. LeBlanc J: Adaptation of man to cold. In Wang LCH, Hudson JW, editors: *Natural torpidity and thermogenesis*, New York, 1978, Academic Press.
8. LeBlanc J: Man in the cold, Springfield, Ill, 1975, *Charles C Thomas Publishing*.
9. Auerbach PS and Geehr EC, editors: *Management of wilderness and environmental emergencies*, ed 1, New York, 1983, MacMillan.
10. Larrey DJ: *Memoirs of a military surgeon*, vol 2, Baltimore, 1814, Joe Cushing.
11. Mersey Lord (Wreck Commissioner): *Report of a formal investigation into the circumstances attending the foundering on 15 April 1912 of the British steamship "Titanic" of Liverpool after striking ice in or near latitude 41° 46' N, longitude 50° 14' North Atlantic Ocean, whereby loss of life ensued*, London, 1912, HM Stationery Office.
12. Steinman AM and Hayward JS: Cold water immersion. In Auerbach PS, Geehr ED, editors: *Management of wilderness and environmental emergencies*, ed 2, St. Louis, 1989, Mosby.

Pathophysiology

13. Nicholson RW and Iserson KV: Core temperature measurements in hypovolemic resuscitation, *Am Emerg Med* 20:62-66, 1991.
14. Satinoff E, editor: *Thermoregulation*, Stroudsburg, Pa, 1980, Dowden, Hutchinson and Ross Publishing.
15. Pozos RS and Wittmers LE, editors: *The nature and treatment of hypothermia*, Minneapolis, 1983, Univ of Minnesota Press.
16. Horvath SM: Exercise in a cold environment. In Miller DI, editor: *Exercise and sports services reviews*, vol 9, Philadelphia, 1982, Franklin Institute Press.
17. Van de Linde FJG: Heat loss from the head in the cold, *Ann Physiol Anthropol* 5(3):130, 1986, (abstract).
18. Sloan REG and Keatinge WR: Cooling rates of young people swimming in cold water, *J Appl Physiol* 35:371, 1973.
19. Cannon P and Keatinge WR: The metabolic rate and heat loss of fat and thin men in heat balance in cold and warm water, *J Physiol* 154:329, 1960.
20. Witherspoon JM, Goldman RF, Breckenridge JR: Heat transfer coefficients of humans in cold water, *Journal de Physiologie*, extroit due Tome 63(3):459-462, 1971.
21. Siple PA and Passel CF: Measurements of dry atmospheric cooling in sub-freezing temperatures, *Proc Am Phil Soc* 89:177, 1945.
22. Kaufman WC and Bothe DJ: Windchill reconsidered, Siple revisited, *Aviat Space Environ Med* 57:23, 1986.
23. Wilson O and Goldman RF: Role of air temperature and wind in the time necessary for a finger to freeze, *J Appl Physiol* 29(5):658-664, 1970.
24. Iampietro PF, Vaughan JA, Goldman RF et al: Heat production from shivering, *J Appl Physiol* 15(4):632-634, 1960.
25. Myers A, Britten JS, Cowley RA: Hypothermia: quantitative aspects of therapy, *J Am Coll Emerg Phys* 8(12):523-527, 1979.
26. Maughan RH, Leiper JB, Thompson J et al: Rectal temperatures after marathon running, *Br J Sports Med* 19:192, 1985.
27. Hayward JS: The physiology of immersion hypothermia. In Pozos RS, Wittmers LE, editors: *The nature and treatment of hypothermia*, Minneapolis, 1983, Univ of Minnesota Press.
28. Hayward JS: Immersion hypothermia. In Wilkerson JA, editor: *Hypothermia, frostbite and other cold injuries*, Seattle, 1986, The Mountaineers.
29. Keatinge WR: Accidental immersion hypothermia and drowning, *Symp Environmental Problems* 219:183-187, 1977.
30. Mekjavic IB and Bligh J: The pathophysiology of hypothermia, *Int Rev Ergonomics* 1:210, 1987.
31. Danzl DF, Pozos RS, Hamlet MP: Accidental hypothermia. In Auerbach PS, Geehr EC, editors: *Wilderness and environmental emergencies*, ed 2, St. Louis, 1989, Mosby.
32. Sekar TS, MacDonnell KF, Manisirikal P et al: Survival after prolonged submersion in cold water without neurologic sequelae, *Arch Intern Med* 140:775-779, 1980.
33. Epstein M: Water immersion and the kidney: implications for volume regulation, *Undersea Biomed Res* 11(2):113, 1984.
34. Nose H: Transvascular fluid shift and redistribution of blood in hypothermia, *Jpn J Physiol* 32:831, 1982.
35. Swan H: Cessation of circulation in general hypothermia. I. Physiologic changes and their control, *Ann Surg* 138:360, 1953.
36. Cooper KE, Shellagh M, Riben P: Respiratory and other responses in subjects immersed in cold water, *J Appl Physiol* 40:903-910, 1976.
37. Jacob AI, Lichstein E, Ulano SD et al: A-V block in accidental hypothermia, *J Electrocardiol* 11(4):399-402, 1978.
38. Barbour HG, McKay EA, Griffith WP: Water shifts in deep hypothermia, *Am J Physiol* 140:9, 1944.
39. D'Amato HE and Hegnauer AH: Blood volume in the hypothermic dog, *Am J Physiol* 173:100, 1953.

40. Cupples WA, Fox GR, Hayward JS: Effect of cold water immersion and its combination with alcohol intoxication on urine flow rate of man, *Can J Physiol Pharmacol* 58:319, 1980.
41. Kanter GS: Renal clearance of sodium and potassium in hypothermia, *Can J Biochem Physiol* 40:113, 1962.
42. Moyer JH, Morris GC, deBakey ME: Renal functional response to hypothermia and ischemia in man and dog. In Dripps RD, editor: *Physiology of induced hypothermia*, Washington, DC, 1956, National Academy of Science.
43. Kanter GS: Hypothermic hemoconcentration, *Am J Physiol* 214(4): 856-859, 1969.
44. Tafari N and Gentz J: Aspects on rewarming newborn infants with severe accidental hypothermia, *Acta Paediatr Scand* 63:595-600, 1974.
45. Hamlet MP: Fluid shifts in hypothermia. In Pozos RS and Wittmers LE, editors: *The nature and treatment of hypothermia*, Minneapolis, 1983, Univ of Minnesota Press.
46. Golden F and Hervey GR: The mechanism of "afterdrop" following immersion hypothermia in pigs, *J Physiol* 272:26, 1977.
47. Webb P: Afterdrop of body temperature during rewarming: an alternative explanation, *J Appl Physiol* 60:385, 1986.
48. Harnett RM, O'Brien EM, Sias FR et al: Initial treatment of profound accidental hypothermia, *Aviat Space Environ Med* 51:680-687, 1980.

Diagnostic Findings

49. Lilja GP: Emergency treatment of hypothermia. In Pozos RS, Wittmers LE, editors: *The nature and treatment of hypothermia*, Minneapolis, 1983, Univ of Minnesota Press.
50. Zell SC and Kurtz K: Severe exposure hypothermia: a resuscitation protocol, *Ann Emerg Med* 14:339, 1985.
51. Reuler JB: Hypothermia: pathophysiology, clinical settings and management, *Ann Intern Med* 89:519-527, 1978.
52. Smith DJ Jr, Robson MC, Heggers JP: Frostbite and other cold-induced injuries. In Auerbach PS and Geehr EC, editors: *Management of wilderness and environmental emergencies*, ed 2, St. Louis, 1989, Mosby.
53. Maclean D, Murison J, Griffiths PD: Acute pancreatitis and diabetic ketoacidosis in hypothermia, *Br Med J* 2:59, 1974.
54. Mahajan SL, Meyers TJ, Baldini MG: Disseminated intravascular coagulation during rewarming following hypothermia, *JAMA* 245(24):2517-2518, 1981.
55. O'Keefe KM: Non-cardiogenic pulmonary edema from accidental hypothermia: a case report, *Colorado Med* 77(3):106-107, 1980.
56. Thews G: Monograms for the consideration of body temperature in blood gas and pH-measurements, *Anaesthetist* 21:466-472, 1972.
57. Wickstrom P, Ruiz E, Lilja GP et al: Accidental hypothermia, *Am J Surg* 131(5):622-25, 1976.
58. Vassallo S: The blood gases in hypothermia: correct or not? *Wilderness Med Lett* 7(3):5, 1990.
59. Delaney KA, Howland MA, Vassallo S et al: Assessment of acid base disturbances in hypothermia and their physiologic consequences, *Ann Emerg Med* 18:72-82, 1989.
60. Hering JP et al: Influence of pH management on hemodynamics and metabolism in moderate hypothermia, *J Thorac Cardiovasc Surg* 104:1388, 1992.
61. Kelman GR and Nunn JF: Nomograms for correcting of blood P_{O_2}, P_{CO_2} and pH for time and temperature, *J Appl Physiol* 21:1484-1490, 1966.
62. Miller JW, Danzel DF, Thomas DM: Urban accidental hypothermia 135 cases, *Ann Emerg Med* 9(9):456-461, 1980.
63. Trevino A, Razi B, Beller BM: The characteristic ECG of accidental hypothermia, *Arch Intern Med* 127:470-473, 1971.

Differential considerations

64. Luna GK et al: Incidence and effect of hypothermia in seriously injured patients, *J Trauma* 27(9):1014-1018, 1987.

Management

65. Steinman AM: Prehospital management of hypothermia, *Response* 6:18, 1987.
66. Mills WJ Jr: Accidental hypothermia: management approach, *Alaska Med* 22:9, 1980.
67. Weinberg AD: Hypothermia, *Ann Emerg Med* 22:370, 1993.

68. Yaron M et al: Inaccuracy of the infrared tympanic thermometer in emergency dept. *Ann Emerg Med* 21:654, 1992, (abstract).
69. Steinman AM: The hypothermic code: CPR controversy visited, *JEMS* 10:32, 1983.
70. Lloyd EL: Airway rewarming in the treatment of accidental hypothermia: a review, *J Wilderness Med* 1(2):65-79, 1990.
71. Hayward JS and Steinman AM: Accidental hypothermia: an experimental study of inhalation rewarming, *Aviat Space Environ Med* 46:1236, 1975.
72. Hornbein TF, Pavlin E, Chaney RD: Rewarming of hypothermic dogs with use of heated nebulizer ventilation (abstract), *Proc Sci Assem Am Soc Anesth*. San Francisco, CA, 1976.
73. Morrison JB, Conn ML, Hayward JS: Thermal increment provided by inhalation rewarming from hypothermia. *J Appl Physiol* 46(6): 1061, 1979.
74. Danzl DF, Hedges JR, Pozos RS: Hypothermia study group hypothermia outcome score—development and implications, *Crit Care Med* 17:227, 1989.
75. Steinman AM: Cardiopulmonary resuscitation and hypothermia, *Circulation* 74(suppl IV):29-32, 1986.
76. Chipman C: Criteria for cessation of CPR in the emergency department, *Ann Emerg Med* 10:11, 1981.
77. Danzl DF, Pozos RS, Auerbach PS et al: Multicenter hypothermia survey, *Ann Emerg Med* 16:1042, 1987.
78. Maningas PA, DeGuzman LR, Hollenbach SJ et al: Regional blood flow during hypothermic arrest, *Ann Emerg Med* 15:390-396, 1986.
79. Schissler P, Parker MA, Scott SJ: Profound hypothermia: value of prolonged cardiopulmonary resuscitation, *South Med J* 74:474, 1981.
80. Southwick FS and Dalglish PH: Recovery after prolonged asystolic cardiac arrest in profound hypothermia, *JAMA* 243(12):1250-1253, 1980.
81. Steinman AM: The hypothermic code: CPR controversy revisited, *J Emerg Med Serv* 10:32, 1983.
82. Paton BC: Accidental hypothermia, *Pharmacol Ther* 22:331, 1983.
83. Buckley J, Bosch OD, Bacaner MD: Prevention of ventricular fibrillation during hypothermia with bretyllium tosylate, *Anesth Analg* 50:587-593, 1971.
84. Danzl DF, Sowers BM, Vicario SJ: Chemical ventricular defibrillation in severe accidental hypothermia, *Ann Emerg Med* 11:689-699, 1982.
85. Ledingham IM and Mone JG: Treatment of accidental hypothermia: a prospective clinical study, *Br Med J* 280:1102-1105, 1980.
86. Roberts DE: Fluid replacement during hypothermia, *Aviat Space Environ Med* 56:333, 1985.
87. Murray BJ: Severe lactic acidosis and hypothermia, *West J Med* 134(2):162-165, 1981.
88. Collis KJ, Steinman AM, Chaney RD: Accidental hypothermia: an experimental study of practical rewarming methods, *Aviat Space Environ Med* 48:625, 1977.
89. Golden F: Rewarming. In Pozos RS and Wittmers LE, editors: *Nature and treatment of hypothermia*, Minneapolis, 1983, Univ of Minnesota Press.
90. Guild WJ: Centrasel body rewarming for hypothermia—possibilities, problems and progress, *J Royal Naval Med Serv* 26:173, 1976.
91. Bolte RG, Bloch PG, Bowers RS et al: The use of extracorporeal rewarming in a child submerged for 66 minutes, *JAMA* 260(3):377-379, 1988.
92. White FN: Reassessing acid-base balance in hypothermia, a comparative point of view, *West J Med* 138:255, 1983.
93. Brunette DD, Sterner S, Robinson E et al: Comparison of gastric lavage and thoracic cavity lavage in the treatment of severe hypothermia in dogs, *Ann Emerg Med* 16:1222, 1987.
94. Lloyd EL, Mitchell B, Williams JT: Rewarming from immersion hypothermia: a comparison of three methods, *Resuscitation* 5:5, 1976.
95. Iverson RJ, Atkin SH, Jaken MA et al: Successful CPR in a severely hypothermic patient using continuous thoracostomy lavage, *Ann Emerg Med* 19:1335, 1990.
96. Marcus P: Laboratory comparison of techniques for rewarming hypothermic casualties, *Aviat Space Environ Med* 49:692, 1978.
97. Otto RJ and Metzler MH: Rewarming from experimental hypothermia: comparison of heated aerosol inhalation, peritoneal lavage and pleural lavage, *Crit Care Med* 16:869, 1988.

98. Reuler JB and Parker RA: Peritoneal dialysis in the management of hypothermia, *JAMA* 240(21):2289-2290, 1978.

99. Shanks CA: Heat gain in the treatment of accidental hypothermia, *Med J Aust* 2:346-349, 1975.

100. Towne WD, Geiss WP, Yanes HO et al: Intractable ventricular fibrillation associated with profound accidental hypothermia—successful treatment with partial cardiopulmonary bypass, *Med Intelligence* 287(22):1135-1136, 1972.

101. Zhong H, Qinyi S, Mingjiang S: Rewarming with microwave irradiation in severe cold injury syndrome, *Chin Med J* 93(2):119-120, 1980.

102. DaVee TS and Reineberg EJ: Extreme hypothermia and ventricular fibrillation, *Ann Emerg Med* 9(2):100-102, 1980.

103. Lloyd EL and Mitchele B: Factors affecting the onset of ventricular fibrillation in hypothermia, *Lancet* 2:1294, 1974.

104. Nordrehaug JE: Sustained ventricular fibrillation in deep accidental hypothermia, *Br Med J* 284:867, 1982.

105. Buky B: Effect of magnesium on ventricular fibrillation due to hypothermia, *Br J Anaesth* 42:886, 1970.

106. Morris DL and Jande MA: Diagnosis of sepsis in hypothermic patient, *J Clin Research* 30(2):519A, 1982, (abstract).

107. Akriotis V and Biggar WD: The effects of hypothermia on neutrophil function in vitro, *J Leukocyte Biol* 37:51, 1985.

108. Giesbrecht GG, Bristow GK, Uin A et al: Effectiveness of three field treatments for induced mild (33°C) hypothermia, *J Appl Physiol* 63:2375, 1987.

109. Hayward JS, Eckerson JD, Kemma D: Thermal and cardiovascular changes during three methods of resuscitation from mild hypothermia, *Resuscitation* 11:21, 1984.

110. Savard GK, Cooper KE, Veale WL et al: Peripheral blood flow during rewarming from mild hypothermia in humans, *J Appl Physiol* 58(1):4, 1985.

111. Frank DH and Robson MC: Accidental hypothermia treated without mortality, *Surg Gynecol Obstet* 151:379-381, 1980.

112. Schaller MD, Fisher AP, Perrit CH: Hyperkalemia, a prognostic factor during acute severe hypothermia, *JAMA* 264:1842-1845, 1990.

113. Bowman W: Factors influencing human performance in a cold environment, *Wilderness Med Lett* 7(3):10, 1990.

114. Breckenridge JR: Effects of body motion on convection and evaporative heat exchanges through various designs in clothing. In Hollies NRS and Goldman RF, editors: *Clothing comfort,* Ann Arbor, 1977, Ann Arbor Science Publishers.

115. Nunneley SA, Wissler EH, Allan JR: Immersion cooling: effect of clothing and skin fold thickness, *Aviat Space Environ Med* 56:1177, 1985.

Frostbite

116. Jarrett F: Frostbite: current concepts of pathogenesis and treatment, *Rev Surgery* 31:71-74, 1974.

117. Fuhrman RA and Fuhrman GJ: The treatment of experimental frostbite by rapid thawing, *Medicine* (Baltimore) 36:465-487, 1957.

118. Mills WJ, Whaley R, Fish W: Experience with rapid rewarming and ultrasonic therapy, *Alaska Med* 3:28, 1961.

119. Mills WJ Jr and Whaley R: *Frostbite a method of management. Proceedings of the Symposia on Arctic Biology and Medicine. IV. Frostbite,* Fort Wainwright, Alaska, 1964, Arctic Aeromedical Lab.

120. Mills WJ Jr: Out in the cold, *Emerg Med* 134, 1976.

121. Mills WJ Jr: Clinical aspects of frostbite injury. *Proceedings of the Symposia on Arctic Biology and Medicine. IV. Frostbite,* Fort Wainwright, Alaska, 1964, Arctic Aeromedical Lab.

122. Heggers JP, Phillips LG, McCauley RL et al: Frostbite: experimental and clinical evolutions of treatment, *J Wilderness Med* 1(1):27-33, 1990.

123. Gracey L and Ingram D: The diagnosis and management of gangrene from exposure to the cold, *Br J Surg* 55(4):302-306, 1968.

124. Richard A and Butson C: Notes on frostbite, *J Wilderness Med* 1:33-36, 1990.

Additional Readings

Danzl DF, Pozos RS, Hamlet MP: Accidental hypothermia. In Auerbach P, editor: *Wilderness medicine: management of wilderness and environmental emergencies* ed 3, St. Louis, 1995, Mosby.

Dickinson AL: Dressing for the cold, In Auerbach, P, editor: *Wilderness medicine: management of wilderness and environmental emergencies,* ed 3, St. Louis, 1995, Mosby.

McCauley RL, Smith DJ, Robson MC et al: Frostbite and other cold induced injuries, In Auerbach, P, editor: *Wilderness medicine: management of wilderness and environmental emergencies,* ed 3, St. Louis, 1995, Mosby.

Steinman AM and Hayward JS: Cold water immersion. In Auerbach P, editor: *Wilderness medicine: management of wilderness and environmental emergencies,* ed 3, St. Louis, 1995, Mosby.

## 40

High Altitude Illness and Dysbarism

Kathleen M. Smith

Illnesses due to high altitude and dysbarism involve the physiologic adjustments to markedly decreased and excessive ambient pressure. Both emergencies generally occur in areas not easily accessible to emergency medical care.

HIGH ALTITUDE ILLNESS

High altitude illness has been recognized for centuries but was relatively rare until modern times. Mobility and air travel allow the unacclimatized individual who lives at sea level to ascend to high altitude within hours of leaving home.[1,2] Disorders of high altitude occur when the degree of rate of onset of altitude stress exceeds the body's ability to adapt. Altitude-related illnesses are noted above 8,000 feet, the elevation at which most individual's arterial oxygen saturation falls below 90%.[3] The majority of people experience no more than fatigue and mild headaches. Others suffer from a variety of medical problems ranging from relatively benign acute mountain sickness (AMS) to life-threatening pulmonary edema. High altitude illnesses are relatively rapid in onset, affect the young and healthy, and are potentially fatal if not promptly recognized and treated.[4-6]

Hypoxia results from decreased partial pressure of oxygen (PIo_2) at reduced barometric pressures and is the major physiologic consequence of high altitude exposure.[7] The increase in minute ventilation caused by stimulation of the aortic and carotid body receptors compensates only partially for the decreased PIo_2 and a drop in arterial Po_2 occurs.[2,8] Further drops in arterial Po_2 will occur during exercise and sleep. Within 24 hours of ascent, a rise in 2,3-diphosphoglycerate (DPG) facilitates oxygen delivery to the tissues.[9]

A rapid decrease in plasma volume by 10% to 20% occurs within a few hours of ascent to high altitude. Hyperventilation causes a marked increase in insensible fluid losses. Hypoxia impairs the function of the ATP-dependent sodium pump causing fluid shifts from the intravascular space into hypoxic cells and the interstitial space.[9-11] Cardiovascular effects include sinus tachycardia, venoconstriction, pulmonary artery vasoconstriction, and decreased cardiac output. Central nervous system (CNS) hypoxia results in cerebral vasodilation, increased cerebral blood flow, and a slight increase in cerebrospinal fluid (CSF) pressure.[12]

Altitude-related illnesses include AMS, high altitude pulmonary edema (HAPE), high altitude cerebral edema (HACE), and high altitude retinal hemorrhage (HARH) (Table 40-1). Although they are presented as separate entities, these diseases probably represent a continuum of severity of a common underlying pathophysiologic process.[3]

Acute Mountain Sickness

AMS is the most common clinical presentation of high altitude illness. The symptoms include headache, nausea, vomiting, insomnia, fatigue, irritability, and dyspnea on exertion. Males and females are affected equally. The incidence of AMS is highest in the 1- to 20-year age group. AMS rarely occurs below 8,000 feet, but most people are affected above 10,000 feet.[13-16] The onset of AMS generally occurs within 6 to 24 hours after ascent and may last up to 4 days. AMS usually follows vigorous exercise or a night of sleep at high altitude.[13-19]

Pathophysiology. Factors that predispose individuals to high altitude illness include rapid ascent, return of a high altitude resident after a period of low altitude, exercise, preexisting infection or pulmonary disease, and a previous episode of high altitude illness.[20-23] The exact pathophysiologic mechanism is unclear. A number of associated physiologic events have been well documented, including relative hypoventilation, fluid retention, weight gain, cerebral vasodilation, increased CSF pressure, proteinuria, and decreased vital capacity.[2,9,24,25] Individuals who increase their minute ventilation appropriately and have a diuresis at high altitude generally do not suffer from AMS.[9,13,26]

Diagnostic Findings. The clinical manifestations of AMS include tachycardia, ataxia, oliguria despite adequate hydration, and localized rales in 25% to 35% of cases. Headache, nausea, vomiting, lethargy, sleep disturbances, and tinnitus may be noted. A small percentage of patients with severe AMS who continue ascent in spite of illness will develop life-threatening pulmonary edema or cerebral edema.[27]

Severe AMS can lead to HAPE or HACE. Patients with HACE may not have concurrent or preceding HAPE.

TABLE 40-1. High Altitude Illness

	AMS	HAPE	HACE	HARH
Altitude	> 8,000 ft	8,000-14,000 ft	Rarely occurs below 12,000 ft	Occurs in 50% of people at 16,500 ft
Onset (after reaching high altitude)	4-6 hr after reaching high altitude	24-96 hr	48-72 hr	48-72 hr
Diagnostic findings	Headache, nausea, vomiting, lethargy, sleep disturbances, tinnitus, ataxia, tachycardia	Cough, tachypnea, dyspnea on exertion, orthopnea, fever, frothy pink sputum, rales, variable cyanosis, tachycardia	Severe headache, confusion, ataxia, hallucinations, diplopia, papilledema, coma	Decreased visual acuity with macular involvement, dilated retinal vessels, retinal hemorrhages, papilledema
Ancillary data	UA, ABG, electrolytes, chest radiograph	ABG, chest radiograph, ECG, coagulation profile	ABG, electrolytes, coagulation profile, serum osmolality, CT scan of head, if available	None
Differential considerations	Acute renal failure, CHF, dehydration, hypothermia, gastroenteritis, ethanol hangover, concussion, exhaustion, respiratory or CNS infection	Pneumonia, pulmonary contusion, CHF, neurogenic pulmonary edema, uremia, ARDS, narcotic overdose	Head trauma, encephalitis, meningitis, DKA, uremia, encephalopathy, narcotic intoxication	Retinal hemorrhages due to trauma, COPD, congenital cyanotic heart disease, carbon monoxide poisoning
Management:				
Admit	Variable	Yes	Yes	Variable
Oxygen	Yes	Yes	Yes	Variable
Acetazolamide	Prophylactic	Prophylactic	Prophylactic	Probably not effective
Steroids	Controversial	No	Yes	No (unless HACE is present)
Ventilation with PEEP	No	Yes — if severe	Hyperventilation	No

UA, Urinalysis; *ABG,* arterial blood gases; *ECG,* electrocardiogram; *CT,* computed tomography; *CHF,* congestive heart failure; *CNS,* central nervous system; *ARDS,* adult respiratory distress syndrome; *DKA,* diabetic ketoacidosis; *COPD,* chronic obstructive pulmonary disease; *HACE,* high altitude cerebral edema; *PEEP,* positive end-expiratory pressure.

Ancillary Data. Laboratory tests are not indicated for mild AMS. Dehydration and hemoconcentration are more likely to occur with severe AMS. A complete blood count (CBC) will reveal an elevated hematocrit and the specific gravity will be elevated on urinalysis. A chest radiograph evaluation should be performed if rales are present. Chest radiograph findings in severe AMS consist of patchy infiltrates in the peripheral lung fields.[24]

Differential Considerations. The differential diagnosis of AMS includes dehydration, hypothermia, gastroenteritis, ethanol hangover, concussion, acute renal failure, exhaustion, congestive heart failure, and respiratory or CNS infections.[20,24]

Management. AMS is usually a self-limited disease with symptoms that subside within 3 to 5 days. Prevention is key to the management of AMS. Acclimatization is essential with attention to the rate of ascent and initiation of a graded exercise program. Climbers should allow 1 day to ascend 1,000 feet from elevations of 10,000 to 14,000 feet and 2 days to ascend 1,000 feet at elevations greater than 14,000 feet.[2,9,13]

The treatment of AMS is largely symptomatic. Most cases of mild AMS can be managed by rest, analgesics, adequate fluids to avoid dehydration, a high carbohydrate diet, and abstinence from alcohol and tobacco. The recognition of symptoms of AMS should preclude ascent to higher altitude.[14-16,28] The treatment of severe AMS includes oxygen and descent. Prophylaxis is recommended for climbers who have experienced prior episodes of AMS or rescue workers who must make rapid ascents. Acetazolamide has been approved by the FDA for this purpose. It prevents AMS by acting as a diuretic and respiratory stimulant.[28-31] The dose of acetazolamide in children is 5 to 10 mg/kg/24 hr BID PO and the adult dose is 250 mg BID PO. The medication should be started 24 hours before ascent and continued for 2 to 3 days after attaining high altitude.[24,28-31]

Several studies indicate that dexamethasone may be useful in preventing AMS. In one study, climbers taking dexamethasone 4 mg q 6 hr PO starting 48 hours before ascent reported fewer side effects and felt more refreshed than those who took acetazolamide.[32] Another trial concluded that acetazolamide and dexamethasone administered together was more effective in preventing AMS than either drug alone.[33] Until more data is available, dexamethasone is still primarily considered an emergency drug for the treatment of HACE in conjunction with descent and oxygen. There is little experience with its use in children with AMS.[34]

High Altitude Pulmonary Edema

HAPE is an uncommon but potentially fatal form of high altitude illness. It is a unique pulmonary edema of noncardiac origin.[35,36] Initial symptoms include fatigue, nonproductive cough, insomnia, and dyspnea on exertion. Later, symptoms include productive cough, frothy pink sputum, orthopnea, fever, and confusion.[35-37] HAPE rarely occurs below 8,000 ft but affects greater than 10% of individuals above 14,500 ft. The onset of HAPE occurs within 24 to 96 hours after arrival at high altitude.[2,9,37]

Pathophysiology. This high pressure, high permeability edema is caused by alveolar hypoxia secondary to decreased barometric pressure at high altitudes.[37-41] A decline in Po_2 causes hypoxic pulmonary vasoconstriction, peripheral venoconstriction, and fluid retention. The increased pulmonary blood volume in the face of pulmonary hypertension causes pulmonary edema. Individuals who are more prone to altitude illnesses have a blunted ventilatory response to hypoxia and elevated pulmonary artery pressures.[23,42] HAPE occurs more frequently in young adults, adolescents, and children and may be precipitated by exercise at altitude or rapid ascent.[13,21,22,24] One study showed a 4% incidence of HAPE in adults and a 38% incidence in children.[2] It has been reported in children native to high altitude in Leadville, Colorado, and the Andes, who return to high altitude after a visit to a lower altitude.[21,22] Children susceptible to HAPE may have an underlying exaggerated pulmonary vasoreactivity to hypoxia.[43]

Thrombotic complications associated with HAPE are secondary to hemoconcentration and hypercoagulability. Contributing factors include dehydration, polycythemia, cold exposure, constrictive clothing, and venous stasis from prolonged periods of weather-imposed inactivity.

Diagnostic Findings. The clinical findings of HAPE include rales, fever to 102° F, tachypnea with respiratory distress, cyanosis, tachycardia, lethargy, confusion, and ataxia. The complications encountered with HAPE include respiratory failure, venous thrombosis, pulmonary embolism, stroke, and death.[9,21,22]

Ancillary Data. Arterial blood gases reveal a respiratory alkalosis with varying degrees of hypoxia. An electrocardiogram (ECG) demonstrates sinus tachycardia and a right ventricular strain pattern.[10] The CBC shows an elevated hematocrit. Urinalysis reveals an elevated specific gravity and proteinuria.[13] Chest x-ray film usually reveals diffuse patchy infiltrates in both lung fields and a normal cardiac silhouette.[24,44] A coagulation profile may demonstrate hypercoagulability with a decreased partial thromboplastin time and increased fibrinogen.[45-47]

Differential Considerations. Differential considerations include pneumonia, pulmonary contusion, congestive heart failure, neurogenic pulmonary edema, uremia, adult respiratory distress syndrome (ARDS), narcotic overdose, reactive airway disease, carbon monoxide poisoning, pulmonary embolism, and high altitude bronchitis.[20,24]

Management. Early recognition and appropriate treatment of HAPE may be lifesaving. The cornerstones of therapy are descent, rest, and oxygen.

At high altitude, arterial oxygen saturation is on the steep portion of the oxyhemoglobin dissociation curve, so that small changes in altitude can result in large changes in hemoglobin saturation.[2,10] A descent of as little as 1,000 to 2,000 ft can result in great improvements in the patient's condition.

Oxygen administered at 6 to 8 L/min will decrease pulmonary artery pressures, heart rate, and respiratory rate, and improve hemoglobin oxygen saturation.[9,10] End expiratory airway pressure (EPAP) can be delivered via a portable Down mask.[35,48] The clear plastic mask can be strapped to the face to deliver 12.5 cm water and expiratory pressure. EPAP has been recommended by the American Alpine Institute for its use as a temporizing measure during descent. Via alveolar recruitment, EPAP can increase hemoglobin oxygen saturation by approximately 10% and decrease respiratory rate without supplemental oxygen.[35,49] Rarely, intubation and ventilation for HAPE may be required. This support can generally be discontinued once the patient reaches a lower altitude. Portable hyperbaric chambers are used on an experimental basis.[35]

The management of mild to moderate HAPE includes descent to a lower altitude, bed rest, and oxygen. The treatment of severe HAPE includes evacuation to a lower altitude, intubation and ventilation with the use of positive end expiratory pressure, and maintenance intravenous hydration. The patient should be kept warm, since cold stress raises pulmonary artery pressure. Morphine may lessen venous congestion and anxiety but may cause respiratory depression.[20] Diuretics are contraindicated due to the hypovolemia experienced at high altitude.[2,20,24] Nifedipine has been used on an experimental basis as a pulmonary vasodilator. In a study performed by Oelz and colleagues in 1989, six patients with HAPE received 10 mg of nifedipine sublingually followed by 20 mg of slow-release nifedipine every 6 hours during the entire time at high altitude.[49] Patients' symptoms improved, but there was only a minimal improvement in oxygenation. In a randomized, double-blind, placebo-controlled study, Bartsch demonstrated that the prophylactic administration of nifedipine is effective in lowering pulmonary artery pressures and preventing HAPE in susceptible climbers.[50] Digoxin, isoproterenol, steroids, and theophylline are of no proven benefit. Other preventive measures with regard to rates of ascent and the prophylactic use of acetazolamide are the same as in AMS. Avoidance of overexertion when fatigued may prevent HAPE. The overall mortality rate is 11%. The mortality rate without descent is 44%. Descent is the definitive treatment, and all other therapies should be regarded as temporizing measures until descent occurs.[35-37]

High Altitude Cerebral Edema

HACE is the most severe high altitude illness. Symptoms include severe incapacitating headache, ataxia, loss of coordination, confusion, diplopia, emotional lability, and hallucinations. They can progress to lethargy, stupor, coma, and death. HACE rarely occurs below 12,000 feet. Onset is within 2 to 3 days of arrival at altitude.[13,51,52]

Pathophysiology. The pathophysiology of HACE is not completely understood. There is no agreement as to whether HACE is predominantly a vasogenic or cytotoxic form of cerebral edema, or a combination of the two types. The etiology of vasogenic edema is CNS hypoxia, which causes cerebral vasodilation, increased cerebral blood flow, and a slight increase in CSF pressure. CNS hypoxia also plays a role in cytotoxic edema. Hypoxia-mediated compromise of the ATP-dependent sodium pump leads to brain cell dysfunction.[9,49-53]

Diagnostic Findings. Clinical manifestations of HACE include ataxia, headache, nausea, vomiting, altered mental status, papilledema, engorged retinal vessels and hemorrhages, cranial nerve palsies, seizures, abnormal reflexes, paresis, paresthesias, coma, and death.[13] Complications include disseminated intravascular coagulation, venous and sinus thromboses, herniation, permanent neurologic deficits, and death.[9,24]

Ancillary Data. A chest radiograph study should be performed to look for findings of pulmonary edema if rales are present on physical examination. Cranial CT scans in patients with HACE reveal slitlike ventricles and areas of low attenuation. There are no consistent data on CBC, platelet, ABG, and electrolyte findings in HACE. HACE is a rare disease that occurs in isolated areas and patients either recover quickly or die.[2,9,20,54]

Differential Considerations. The differential diagnosis of HACE includes head trauma, subarachnoid hemorrhage, meningitis, encephalitis, diabetic ketoacidosis, uremia, encephalopathy, stroke, carbon monoxide poisoning, and narcotic intoxication.[24]

Management. HACE is potentially fatal if not promptly recognized. Rapid descent and oxygen administration are the major treatment modalities. Severely affected patients require 30 degrees elevation of the head, intubation, and hyperventilation. Intubation is generally performed using rapid sequence induction with intravenous administration of thiopental 2 to 4 mg/kg (if blood pressure is stable), vecuronium 0.2 mg/kg, and lidocaine 1.5 mg/kg (see Chapter 19 Appendix). The patient is hyperventilated to maintain a Pco_2 of 30 to 35 mm Hg. Dexamethasone 4 mg q 6 hr IV may produce dramatic improvement and be useful for prophylaxis. Acetazolamide and osmotic diuretics are not effective in the treatment of HACE.[51,52]

Acclimatization is the key to the prevention of HACE.

High Altitude Retinal Hemorrhage

HARH is characterized by increased dilatation of the retinal veins and arteries, retinal hemorrhages, and papilledema. HARH is a painless condition and patients are usually asymptomatic unless the macula is involved.[33,56] HARH occurs in 50% of climbers who ascend to 16,500 feet, and in 100% of those who ascend to 21,000 feet. The onset of HARH is within 2 to 3 days of arrival at altitude.[55-57]

Pathophysiology. The pathophysiologic mechanisms are the same as those for HACE. The retinal changes may be due to increased retinal venous pressure with exercise, hypoxia-mediated changes in retinal capillary permeability,

and hyperemia of the optic disk. Predisposing factors include previous HARH, rapid ascent, strenuous exercise, and the presence of other high altitude illnesses.[56]

Diagnostic Findings. The clinical findings of HARH include vascular engorgement and tortuosity, retinal hemorrhages and papilledema, and decreased visual acuity. Residual visual deficits are rare. The presence of HARH may be a warning sign of impending cerebral edema.[55-57] Ophthalmoscopy reveals multiple and often bilateral flame-shaped hemorrhages, hyperemia of the optic disc, cotton-wool spots, and dilation and tortuosity of retinal vessels.

Ancillary Data. Laboratory and radiologic studies are not indicated unless HAPE or HACE are present. All patients should have a visual acuity performed.

Differential Considerations. The differential diagnosis of HARH includes retinal hemorrhages associated with other hypoxic conditions such as chronic obstructive pulmonary disease, carbon monoxide poisoning, congenital cyanotic heart disease, closed head trauma, and physical child abuse.[2,13,20]

Management. If visual changes occur, the hemorrhages are most likely to be macular in origin and descent is advised. The patient with HARH should also be monitored for HACE.

Disposition. Prevention is the key to the management of high altitude illnesses. Partial acclimatization for a trip to high altitude (8,000 to 14,000 feet) can be achieved by a 2- to 4-day stay at an altitude of 5,000 to 7,000 feet. For climbs to very high altitude (14,000 to 22,000 feet), an additional 2- to 4-day stay at 10,000 to 12,000 feet is advised. At altitudes above 14,000 feet, climbing at a rate of 1,000 ft/day and resting every other day are useful guidelines.[8]

Air Travel

There are a number of altitude-aggravated illnesses and conditions in children that should be addressed by their physician before traveling to high altitude, particularly when planning a trip on a commercial airline. It is necessary for emergency physicians to be familiar with medical conditions that are aggravated by exposure to elevated altitudes. They should also offer advice on preventive measures to reduce the possibility of an emergency in the air (Table 40-2).

The average commercial aircraft flies at a cabin altitude of 4,500 to 8,000 feet, but cabin altitude may be as high as 8,915 feet due to weather conditions and the presence of other aircraft in the vicinity. In a DC-10 aircraft flying at a cruising altitude of 35,000 feet, the average healthy individual's Po_2 drops from 98 mm Hg at sea level to 65 mm Hg at a cabin altitude of 5,500 feet.[58] In addition to a drop in Po_2, flying causes an expansion of gases within the body producing pain in the middle ear, sinuses, colostomies, and carious teeth.[3] Contraindications to air travel include children with unstable CHF, cyanotic heart disease, pulmonary hypertension, acute pneumonia with borderline oxygen saturations at sea level, pneumothorax or thoracic surgery within the previous 3 weeks, abdominal or eye surgery within the previous 2 weeks, neonates less than 24 hours old, and children who have been scuba diving 12 to 24 hours before the flight.[3,38] Relative contraindications in-

TABLE 40-2. Guidelines for Altitude Travel in Patients With Underlying Disease

Underlying disease	Altitude limit (feet)
Severe congestive heart failure, recent myocardial infarction (less than 4 wk)	2,000
Pulmonary hypertension, congenital or acquired heart disease with cyanosis	4,000
Sickle cell anemia, cor pulmonale, symptomatic coronary artery disease	6,000
Pregnancy and any mild to moderately symptomatic cardiopulmonary disease	8,000

From Foulke GE: Emergencies of high-altitude travel. In Callahan ML, editor: *Current practice of emergency medicine*, ed 2, Philadelphia, 1991, BC Decker.

clude children with sickle cell disease, anemia (Hgb < 7 gm/dl), acute otitis media or sinusitis, and poorly controlled seizures.[59,60] Patients with cardiopulmonary disease are generally considered safe for air travel if their room air Po_2 at sea level is > 67 mm Hg.[38] Twenty percent of patients who have sickle cell disease or sickle-thalassemia will experience vasoocclusive crises in airline cabins pressurized to 5,000 feet. Although some medical experts believe that these patients can fly safely with supplemental oxygen and a medical escort, others believe that commercial air travel is contraindicated for these patients.[3] Most airlines require 24 to 48 hours notice in order to provide supplemental oxygen.

Parents who travel commercially with chronically ill children need to be aware that they are not traveling on an "air ambulance." Medical assistance varies and emergency equipment is limited. All U.S. flight attendants receive basic first aid, but not all of them receive basic cardiopulmonary resuscitation certification. U.S. airline medical supplies generally include epinephrine 1:1,000, diphenhydramine, 50% dextrose, nitroglycerin, syringes, needles, oral airways, a stethoscope, and sphygmomanometer. It may be comforting to the general public to know that a physician may be on board on 40% to 90% of all commercial flights.[61] The incidence of requests for emergency assistance by a physician is approximately 1 in 1,500 flights. The incidence of diversion of an aircraft for a medical emergency is approximately 1 in 10,000 flights.[38]

Prevention is the key to avoiding emergencies in flight. Children with chronic illnesses should have their medications on board with them. Children with respiratory problems should maintain adequate hydration and sit as far as possible from smoking passengers. In general, the overall assessment as to whether a patient is safe to fly needs to be individualized with respect to the patient's need for supplemental oxygen, the safety of being away from medical assistance, and his or her ability to withstand the overall stress of the trip.

DYSBARIC DIVING INJURIES

The popularity of recreational diving has increased dramatically over the past three decades. In 1943, Cousteau

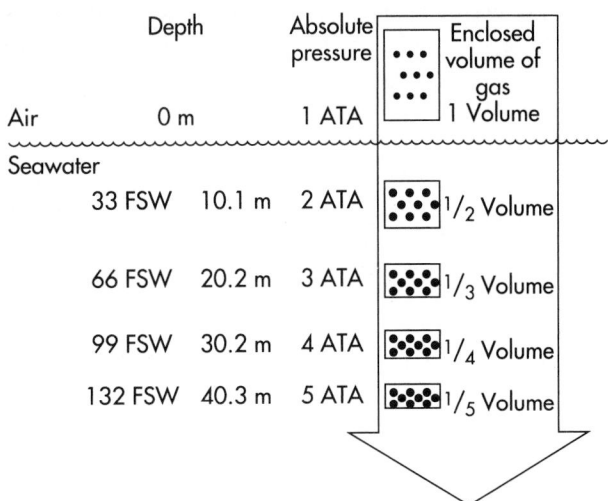

FIG. 40-1. Pressure-volume relationships of enclosed volume of gas as function of depth. Absolute pressure values expressed in atmosphere absolutes. (*From Dembert ML and Keith JF:* Am J Dis Child *140:1145, 1986.*)

and Gagnon devised an apparatus that combined a demand valve breathing regulator with a compressed air cylinder. Self-Contained Underwater Breathing Apparatus (SCUBA) technology paved the way for the development of the recreational diving industry.[62]

Despite its beauty, the underwater world subjects the diver to sudden changes in ambient pressure, the physical demands of swimming in currents, adapting to temperature extremes, and situations that require composure and sound judgment.[63] Drowning is the leading cause of death in sport scuba divers, accounting for 60% of all deaths.[64,65] The remaining diving accidents requiring emergency care are related directly or indirectly to the effects of pressure.

Pressure-related diving syndromes, collectively known as dysbarism, can be divided into the problems caused by the mechanical effects of pressure (i.e., barotrauma) and the problems caused by breathing gases at elevated partial pressures (e.g., gas toxicities and decompression sickness)[62] (Table 40-3).

Diving Physics

Pressure is defined as the force/unit area. At sea level, the depth is 0 feet of sea water (FSW) and the pressure is 1 atmosphere absolute (ATA). When a diver submerges, relatively large changes in pressure are associated with small changes in depth. Therefore ambient pressure is 2.0 ATA at 33 FSW and 6.0 ATA at 165 FSW. Most scuba diving is done at less than 7.0 ATA.[66] The gas-filled organs of the body are affected by pressure, and these effects are based on three fundamental gas laws: Boyle's, Dalton's, and Henry's laws.

Barotrauma is defined as trauma due to barometric pressure changes within body structures. Boyle's law states that with temperature held constant, the volume of a given gas is inversely proportional to the pressure applied on it.

TABLE 40-3. Dysbarism Syndrome: Diagnostic Findings

	Barotrauma				
	Otolaryngolic Dental GI	Pulmonary overpressurization syndrome (POPS)	Arterial gas embolism (AGE)	Nitrogen narcosis	Decompression sickness
Ascent or descent	Both	Ascent	Ascent	Descent	Ascent
Onset	Variable	Before surfacing or at the surface	Within 10 min of surfacing	Variable depths	>10 min after surfacing
Diagnostic findings	Pain in the sinuses, ears, teeth, and abdomen, vertigo, flatulence, hearing impairment	Hoarseness, SC emphysema, dyspnea, cyanosis, neurologic deterioration, hemoptysis	Seizures, visual impairment, aphasia, altered mental status, multiplegia, hemoptysis, chest pain, cardiac arrest	Incoordination, altered mental status, obtundation	Pruritus, lymph node pain, joint pain, vertigo, deafness, paralysis, seizures, headache, respiratory failure, shock
Ancillary data	Electronystagmogram, audiogram	ABG, chest x-ray film	ABG, electrolytes, coagulation profile, chest x-ray film	None	ABG, electrolytes, coagulation profile, UA, ECG, chest x-ray film
Differential considerations	Otitis media, labyrinthitis, sinusitis, head trauma, gastroenteritis	Pulmonary contusion, head trauma, coagulopathy, pneumonitis, spontaneous pneumothorax	Cerebrovascular disease, coronary vascular disease, cerebral AVM or aneurysm, stroke due to cyanotic heart disease, carbon monoxide contamination of air supply	Metabolic derangement, drugs or ethanol intoxication, CNS hemorrhage or infection	Barotrauma, POPS, AGE, exhaustion, dermatitis, muscle strain
Management:					
Admit	Variable	Yes	Yes	Immediate ascent	Yes
Oxygen	No	Yes	Yes	No	Yes
IV hydration	No	Yes	Yes	No	Yes
Recompression	No	Yes	Yes	No	Yes

GI, Gastrointestinal; *SC,* subcutaneously; *ABG,* arterial blood gases; *UA,* urinalysis; *ECG,* electrocardiogram; *AVM,* atrioventricular malformation; *CNS,* central nervous system; *IV,* intravenous.

$$K = PV$$

where K = constant, P = absolute pressure, and V = volume (Fig. 40-1). The greatest volume alterations per change in pressure occur closer to the surface. During an ascent from 33 FSW (2 ATA) to the surface (1 ATA), the lung volume doubles. The lungs will rupture if the diver holds his breath while ascending.[66,67]

The concept of partial pressure is explained by Dalton's law, which states that the total pressure exerted by a mixture of gases is equal to the sum of the partial pressures of the component gases.

$$PT = P \text{ oxygen}_2 + PN_2 + PX$$

where PT = pressure of the total gases; P oxygen$_2$ = partial pressure of oxygen. PN$_2$ = partial pressure of nitrogen; and PX = partial pressure of the other gases.[62,66]

The third basic law of diving physiology is Henry's law, which explains why a more inert gas (nitrogen) dissolves in a diver's body as the ambient pressure increases with un-

derwater descent and is released from the tissue with ascent. Henry's law states that the amount of gas that will dissolve in a liquid at a given temperature is directly proportional to the partial pressure of that gas. Depending on the depth and duration of the dive, the various tissues of the body absorb amounts of nitrogen in excess of that normally present at sea level. Dalton's and Henry's laws explain gas solubility and diffusion as they relate to diving and is important in the study of nitrogen narcosis and decompression sickness.[62,66]

Barotrauma

Barotrauma is the tissue damage that results from inadequate tissue pressure equalization between air-containing cavities and the ambient atmosphere. Barotrauma can be categorized according to whether it occurs during descent or ascent. The body cavities most affected include the ear (inner, middle, and external ear), teeth, paranasal sinuses, GI tract, and thorax.[68,69]

Otolaryngologic and Gastrointestinal

Pathophysiology. Barotrauma *of descent* or "squeeze" occurs when a pressure disequilibrium develops in an enclosed air space as a diver descends underwater and is subjected to increased environmental pressure.[62,66] During descent, if air is unable to enter air-filled structures such as the bowel, which can accommodate volume changes without difficulty, a negative pressure relative to ambient pressure develops. Fluid may be drawn from the intravascular space, causing edema or hemorrhage with pain. Barotrauma to the *external auditory canal* and *middle ear* results in hemorrhage in the canal and middle ear space and tympanic membrane rupture. Inner ear barotrauma results in oval or round window rupture and perilymph fistula. The maxillary and frontal paranasal sinuses may fail to equalize pressure during descent, which results in pain in the sinuses and hemorrhage.

Barotrauma of *ascent* or "reverse squeeze" occurs when the gases in the body, which have equilibrated at depth, expand as ambient pressure decreases with ascent. Reverse squeeze in the middle ear produces pain, hemorrhage, and vertigo. *Dental* barotrauma is caused by air trapped in the teeth from tooth decay and periodontal disease. Expansion of intraluminal *bowel* gas produces abdominal fullness, pain, and flatulence.[62,69]

Diagnostic Findings. The physical findings of barotrauma include blood in the auditory canal, ruptured tympanic membrane, hemotympanum, vertigo, hearing loss, paranasal sinus tenderness, epistaxis, and abdominal distension. Hemotympanum and tympanic membrane rupture are uncommon complications of middle ear squeeze. These findings can lead to a conductive hearing loss that persists for 5 to 7 days. Round or oval window rupture and perilymph fistula are rare complications of barotrauma. Presenting symptoms are vertigo and sensorineural hearing loss (100% of patients). Some degree of permanent sensorineural hearing loss occurs in 88% of these patients.[70,71]

Ancillary Data. Audiograms should be performed on all patients with barotrauma of the middle and inner ear. A significant hearing loss is 50 dB or greater. An electronystagmogram may be used to locate the lesion in the inner ear. (Skin electrodes are placed on the outer canthi of each eye to register horizontal nystagmus and above and below each eye to demonstrate vertical nystagmus; recordings are made in a similar manner to an ECG.) Paranasal sinus x-ray films may show air fluid levels associated with barotrauma of the sinuses.

Differential Considerations. The differential diagnosis includes otitis media, labyrinthitis, sinusitis, head trauma, gastroenteritis, acoustic neuroma, vertebrobasilar insufficiency, and Meniere disease.[62]

Management. Most of the lesions heal spontaneously. The initial treatment of middle ear squeeze consists of abstinence from diving, analgesics, and decongestants.[72] A 10-day course of oral antibiotics should be used to treat tympanic membrane rupture, especially if the rupture occurred while diving in polluted water. Sinusitis that results from sinus barotrauma should also be treated with oral antibiotics for 14 to 21 days. Inner ear barotrauma requires rest and immediate otolaryngologic consultation for possible surgical intervention.[70,71]

Pulmonary Overpressurization Syndrome (POPS).

Pulmonary overpressurization syndrome is the lung rupture that occurs secondary to barotrauma of ascent. The onset is within minutes of surfacing.[62,73,74]

Pathophysiology. POPS occurs when the compressed gas breathed at depth expands on ascent faster than it can be vented from the lung, resulting in overinflation and lung rupture. The release of gas into extraalveolar locations results in pneumomediastinum, subcutaneous emphysema, pneumopericardium, and air embolism.[62,75] Patients with reactive airway disease are particularly susceptible to developing POPS. An asthma attack brought on by extreme exercise, seawater inhalation, or breathing cold, dry air can lead to increased airway resistance upon ascent with subsequent pulmonary barotrauma.[76]

Diagnostic Findings. The clinical manifestations of POPS include hoarseness, subcutaneous emphysema, substernal chest pain, neck fullness, dyspnea, dysphagia, cyanosis, syncope, neurologic deterioration, and hemoptysis. Complications include seizures, neurologic deterioration, cerebral air embolism, pneumomediastinum, pneumopericardium, pneumothorax, pulmonary interstitial emphysema, pneumoperitoneum, shock, and cardiopulmonary arrest from coronary artery air embolism. The development of a pneumothorax while diving is serious, since intrapleural gas that cannot be released to the environment on ascent results in a tension pneumothorax, syncope, shock, and loss of consciousness.

Ancillary Data. A CBC should be performed in patients with significant hemoptysis to look for evidence of anemia. Oximetry demonstrates hypoxemia in the presence of a pneumothorax. An arterial blood gas would show an elevated P_{CO_2} and a decreased P_{O_2} in the presence of a pneumothorax. Radiologic evaluation includes a chest radiograph study to exclude a pneumothorax in any patient with respiratory distress.[62,66,77]

Differential Considerations. Differential considerations include pulmonary contusion, head trauma, dysrhythmia, myocardial infarction, stroke, coagulopathy, pneumonitis, and spontaneous pneumothorax.

Management. Management includes oxygen, bed rest, and restraint from further diving. A needle thoracostomy followed by chest tube placement should be performed in patients with pneumothoraces. Early recompression in a hyperbaric chamber should be performed in any patient whose presenting symptoms include either a rapid neurologic or cardiorespiratory deterioration, which would indicate an arterial gas embolism. A pneumothorax must be recognized and treated with a tube thoracostomy before recompression.[75]

Recompression occurs in a hyperbaric chamber where oxygen is titrated in its administration according to atmospheres of pressure and minutes according to U.S. Navy Decompression tables. Air transport should occur with a helicopter or fixed wing plane flying less than or equal to 1,000 feet or in a plane pressurized to 1 ATA (e.g., Lear jet or Hercules C-130).[66,75]

The three objectives in recompression therapy are to reduce the size of the bubble, promote bubble reabsorption, and to prevent the formation of new bubbles. Reduction in bubble size is accomplished by the increase in ambient pressure, which results in relief of vascular obstruction and the enhancement of tissue reperfusion and oxygenation. Intravascular gas is compressed into a smaller, spherical shape, which allows distal migration and a reduction in the size of the ischemic area. Bubble reabsorption is also enhanced by the increase in ambient pressure as the partial pressure of nitrogen within the bubble exceeds the partial pressure of nitrogen in the surrounding tissues. Breathing 100% oxygen washes out tissue nitrogen and hastens bubble reabsorption by further widening the nitrogen partial pressure difference between the tissue and the bubble. Recompression is performed slowly to avoid the reformation of bubbles. Based on the patient's response to recompression treatment, the treatment tables are modified to provide additional treatment time if necessary. Hyperbaric chamber treatment is performed by diving medicine experts according to U.S. Navy Decompression tables.[66,77]

Arterial Gas Embolism (AGE). Arterial gas embolism is defined as the arterial occlusion caused by the entry of gas bubbles into the systemic circulation via ruptured pulmonary veins. AGE occurs immediately or within 10 minutes of surfacing.

Pathophysiology. AGE usually occurs during a breath-holding ascent in which the expanding intrapulmonic gas is trapped and ruptures the lung. Air passes into the pulmonary veins, heart, and systemic circulation, and the gas bubbles cause arterial occlusion.

Diagnostic Findings. The clinical features of AGE include seizures, visual impairment, aphasia, altered mental status, loss of consciousness, chest pain, abdominal pain, multiplegia or monoplegia, hemoptysis, and cardiac arrest. Complications include anoxic encephalopathy, cardiac arrest, and death.

Ancillary Data. A CBC should be performed to look for anemia with significant hemoptysis. A baseline platelet count, prothrombin time (PT), and partial thromboplastin time (PTT) should be performed, since disseminated intravascular coagulation (DIC) may occur later in the hospital course of patients with AGE. Electrolytes are usually normal at the initial evaluation. An electrocardiogram should be performed to look for myocardial injury and ventricular dysrhythmias. Smith noted an elevated creatinine kinase level in all patients that he studied with AGE. The correlation between serum creatinine kinase activity and neurologic outcome suggests that serum creatinine kinase may be a marker of the size and severity of AGE.[78] A chest x-ray study should be obtained to rule out a pneumothorax before recompression.[73,75] Laboratory tests should not delay a prompt evacuation to a hyperbaric chamber.

Differential Considerations. The differential considerations include cerebrovascular disease, coronary artery vascular disease, cerebral arteriovenous malformation or aneurysm, and a stroke secondary to congenital cyanotic heart disease.[66,68]

Management. The management includes advanced life support stabilization in the emergency department and immediate transfer to a hyperbaric facility. In contrast to prior recommendations, patients should be maintained in a supine, head neutral position in the field and hospital setting. There is no definite benefit associated with placing patients in the Trendelenburg or left lateral decubitus po-

sition. Ventilation is compromised in these positions, and intracranial pressure may increase if the patient is maintained in the Trendelenburg position for 30 to 60 minutes.[38,79,80] The emergency physician should ensure an adequate airway, ventilation, and circulation. All patients should be placed on 100% oxygen. Intubated patients should be hyperventilated to maintain a P_{CO_2} in the 30 to 35 mm Hg range to decrease intracranial pressure. Endotracheal tubes and Foley catheter cuffs must be filled with water to avoid volume changes during recompression. Dysrhythmias caused by bubble embolization into the coronary arteries will be refractory to standard treatment until the bubble resolves with recompression treatment. Intravenous crystalloid with glucose (i.e., D_5W 0.45% NS) should be administered at two-thirds maintenance rates. Hypotension should be treated with vasopressors such as dopamine in doses of 1 to 10 μg/kg/min to increase cardiac output and coronary artery and renal blood flow. Mannitol is not used routinely because of the risk of a rebound increase in intracranial pressure. Mannitol should be reserved only for cases of impending herniation.

Recompression is the definitive treatment for AGE. The patient is usually recompressed at a treatment depth of 60 FSW (2.8 ATA) with the patient breathing 100% oxygen for 20-minute periods. After 75 minutes at 60 FSW, a gradual transition is made to 30 FSW where oxygen and room air breathing are again alternated in order to avoid oxygen toxicity. Subsequently, the patient is slowly brought to sea level pressure. If the patient fails to improve within the first 20 minutes at a treatment depth of 60 FSW, the treatment depth is increased to 165 FSW (6 ATA) in order to reduce the size of the bubbles more effectively.[81] Hyperbaric oxygen improves tissue oxygenation, decreases intracranial pressure, and provides a large diffusion gradient to reabsorb bubbles, which produce the symptoms of AGE.[82]

After treatment, the patient should have a careful neurologic, cardiovascular, and pulmonary examination. Divers who suffer air embolism should not return to diving. Prognosis depends on the duration of CNS ischemia before recompression.[66,75]

Nitrogen Narcosis

Nitrogen narcosis is the narcotic effect similar to that of ethanol intoxication, which is produced when nitrogen and other lipid-soluble gases are breathed at elevated partial pressure. The symptoms include giddiness, uncontrollable laughter, muscular incoordination, and impaired judgment and memory.[68]

Pathophysiology. The progressive intoxicating or anesthetic effect of nitrogen increases with depth. The effects become evident at 80 to 100 FSW and may produce loss of consciousness at 300 to 400 FSW.[62]

Diagnostic Findings. The clinical signs of nitrogen narcosis include muscular incoordination, altered mental status, and obtundation. Complications include diving accidents and their sequelae (i.e., drowning and anoxic encephalopathy).

Ancillary Data. No laboratory or radiologic studies are indicated unless the symptoms do not resolve with ascent. If the patient fails to improve after ascent, an ABG, electrolytes, serum glucose, and alcohol or drug screen may be indicated.[66]

Differential Considerations. Differential considerations include metabolic derangement, drug or ethanol intoxication, and CNS hemorrhage or infection.[66]

Management. Prevention is the key to the management of nitrogen narcosis. Symptoms usually resolve completely with ascent. If deep dives are required, helium should be substituted for nitrogen in the breathing mixture.[77]

Decompression Sickness ("The Bends")

Decompression sickness is a multisystem disorder resulting from the liberation of inert gas bubbles (nitrogen) from saturated tissues when environmental pressure is decreased. During the course of a dive, inert gas accumulates in the body to an extent determined by the depth-time profile of the dive and by the capacities for uptake in the various body compartments.[75] Deeper and longer dives increase the amount of nitrogen absorbed. Once that accumulation exceeds a certain amount, it limits the rate at which the diver can return safely to sea level pressure. If the diver ascends sufficiently slowly, the gas will diffuse out of tissues into blood and escape through the lungs. If the diver returns too fast, the gas will come out of solution as gas emboli in the circulation and as bubbles within tissues. This risk is present at all depths below 10 meters (33 FSW). It is also seen with dives to less than 10 meters in persons who travel by plane within hours of surfacing.[62,63]

Type I (mild) decompression sickness involves the cutaneous, lymphatic, and musculoskeletal systems. Type II (severe) decompression sickness is a more serious illness involving the pulmonary, cardiovascular, and central nervous systems.[69,77]

Pathophysiology. Bubbles released from the tissues by an abnormally rapid reduction in ambient pressure either obstruct blood flow or cause blood chemistry changes, coagulopathy, and tissue damage. The onset usually occurs in 1 to 6 hours after surfacing.[63,66,82]

Diagnostic Findings. The clinical signs of type I decompression sickness include pruritus, skin discoloration, lymph node pain and swelling, periarticular pain, vertigo, tinnitus, and deafness. The clinical signs of type II decompression sickness include nystagmus, paralysis, sensory deficit, seizures, headache, visual impairment, substernal chest pain, cough, dyspnea, respiratory failure, and shock. Although rare in children, decompression sickness usually manifests as type II disease when it does occur. The symptoms seen in children mainly include confusion, behavioral changes, and amnesia. Complications include paralysis secondary to spinal cord venous plexus infarction, DIC, pulmonary edema, and cardiovascular collapse.[62,68,75,82,83]

Ancillary Data. Various laboratory abnormalities are associated with decompression sickness; however, most of them have little relevance with regard to acute management. Two exceptions are a hematocrit and urine specific gravity, since intravascular volume depletion and hemoconcentration are common in severe decompression sickness.[62] A chest x-ray study should be performed in patients with any respiratory symptoms to evaluate for a pneumothorax or pulmonary edema. A magnetic resonance imaging study of the spinal cord may be helpful in the poststabilization period to look for venous plexus infarction.[84]

Differential Consideration. The differential considerations are based on the time of symptom onset. Barotrauma

TABLE 40-4. Differential Diagnosis of Diving Accidents According to Time of Symptom Onset

Time of symptom onset	Differential diagnosis
Predive surface phase (all activities before going and while in the water before descent underwater)	Motion sickness, hyperventilation, physical trauma, near drowning, marine animal encounter
Descent phase	Barotrauma of descent (rarely, alternobaric vertigo), gas mixture problems occasionally
At-depth phase	Physical trauma, marine animal encounter, gas mixture problems occasionally (remember possible effects of nitrogen narcosis at depth)
Ascent phase	Barotrauma of ascent, gas mixture problems most common at this time, decompression sickness rare
Postdive surface phase *Immediate* (within 10 min of surfacing)	AGE until proved otherwise, barotrauma, nondysbaric problems (especially motion sickness)
Delayed (later than 10 min after surfacing)	Decompression sickness, barotrauma or its sequelae, nondysbaric problems (e.g., motion sickness, exhaustion, muscle strains, dermatitis)

From Kizer KW: Dysbaric diving accidents. In: Edlich RF and Spyker DA, editors: *Current emergency therapy—1985*, Gaithersburg, Md, 1985, Aspen Publishers.

of ascent (otolaryngologic, GI, and pulmonary overpressurization syndrome) occur during ascent. Any symptoms occurring within 10 minutes of surfacing indicate AGE until proved otherwise. Symptoms that are delayed longer than 10 minutes after surfacing are due to decompression sickness, barotrauma, motion sickness, dermatitis, muscle strains, or exhaustion[62] (Table 40-4).

Management. Management includes advanced life support measures with 100% oxygen at high flows to facilitate the off-gassing of nitrogen bubbles and to improve oxygenation of damaged tissues. Pneumothoraces should be identified promptly and treated with a thoracostomy tube. Intravenous fluids like normal saline or lactated Ringer's solution should be used to treat the intravascular depletion that accompanies serious decompression sickness. Children should receive a 20 ml/kg fluid bolus of normal saline or lactated Ringer's solution followed by an isotonic glucose and crystalloid solution at a rate that will provide a urine output of 1 to 2 ml/kg/hr.[62] If a cerebral air embolism is suspected, the patient should be placed supine with the head in a neutral position to decrease the chance of gas bubbles traveling to the brain.

Arrangements should be made for immediate transport to a hyperbaric chamber for all patients with decompression sickness. Decompression should be carried out even if therapy is delayed for several hours. In the hyperbaric chamber the patient with type I decompression sickness is brought to an initial treatment depth of 60 FSW (2.8 ATA) where the patient breathes 100% oxygen for 20-minute periods. After 45 minutes, a gradual transition is made to 30 FSW where oxygen and room air breathing are again alternated. Subsequently, the patient is slowly brought to sea level pressure.[80]

The initial treatment guidelines for type II decompression sickness should follow the guidelines previously described for AGE. Recovery is 80% to 90%, depending on the severity of the disease and access to appropriate care.[69,73-75,77,85] The patient should not dive for 4 to 6 weeks after an episode of type I decompression sickness, and at least 4 to 6 months after type II illness. A second type II episode should warrant a critical evaluation of the patient's fitness for further diving.[77]

Disposition. Prevention is the key to the management of diving injuries. Sport diving has no legal age limits, but a candidate must be 15 years old for full certification. Medical considerations for young divers include emotional maturity, ability to learn the physiologic and environmental data needed for safe diving, and the physical strength necessary to handle diving equipment.[63] There is no evidence that increased ambient pressure damages developing bones, but young divers should take shorter, shallower dives to minimize the risk for bone injury.[63,66] Absolute disqualifications for scuba diving include asthma, chronic sinusitis or otitis media, chronic perforations of tympanic membranes, history of spontaneous pneumothoraces, seizures, dysrhythmias, and congenital cyanotic heart disease.[63,86]

Help with the treatment of diving-related incidents may be obtained by contacting the U.S. Diving Accident Network (DAN) at (919)684-8111. Diving medicine experts are available 24 hours a day to provide help with diagnosis, immediate care, and the location of the nearest hyperbaric chamber.[75]

References

High Altitude Illness

1. Hackett PH and Roach RC: Medical therapy of altitude illness, *Ann Emerg Med* 16(9):980-986, 1987.
2. Foulke GE: Altitude related illness, *Am J Emerg Med* 3(3):217-226, 1985.
3. Tso E: High-altitude illness, *Emerg Med Clin North Am* 10(2):231-247, 1992.
4. Mountain RD: High altitude medical problems, *Clin Orthop* 216:50-54, 1987.
5. Dickinson J et al: Altitude-related deaths in seven trekkers in the Himalayas, *Thorax* 38:646-656, 1983.
6. West JB and Lahiri S: *High altitude and man*, Bethesda, Md, 1984, American Physiological Society.
7. King AB and Robinson SM: Ventilation response to hypoxia and acute mountain sickness, *Aerosp Med* 43(4):419-421, 1972.
8. Mathew L et al: Chemoreceptor sensitivity and maladaption to high altitude in man, *Eur J Appl Physiol* 51:137-144, 1983.
9. Auerbach PS and Geehr EC: *Management of wilderness and environmental emergencies*, New York, 1983, Macmillan Publishing.
10. Tintinalli JE, Krome RL, Ruiz E: *Emergency medicine: a comprehensive study guide*, New York, 1988, McGraw-Hill.
11. Nayak NC, Roy S, Narayanan TK: Pathologic features of altitude sickness, *Am J Pathol* 45(3):381-393, 1964.
12. West JB: Human physiology at extreme altitudes on Mount Everest, *Science* 223:784-788, 1984.
13. Jacobson ND: Acute high altitude illness, *Am Fam Pract* 38(3):135-144, 1988.
14. Singh I et al: Acute mountain sickness, *N Engl J Med* 280(4):175-184, 1969.
15. Hackett PH and Rennie D: Rales, peripheral edema, retinal hemorrhage and acute mountain sickness, *Am J Med* 67:214-218, 1979.
16. Hackett PH and Rennie D: Acute mountain sickness, *Semin Respir Med* 5(2):132-140, 1983.
17. Theis MK, Honigman B, Yip R, et al: Acute mountain sickness in children at 2835 meters, *AJDC* 147:143-145, 1993.
18. Honigman B, Theis MK, Koziol-Mclain J et al: Acute mountain sickness in a general tourist population at moderate altitudes, *Ann Intern Med* 118:587-92. 1993.
19. Montgomery AB, Mills J, Luce JM: Incidence of acute mountain sickness at intermediate altitude, *JAMA* 261:732-34, 1989.
20. Murray JF and Nadel JA: *Textbook of respiratory medicine*, Philadelphia, 1988, WB Saunders.
21. Scoggin CH et al: High altitude pulmonary edema in the children and young adults of Leadville, Colorado, *N Engl J Med* 297(23):1269-1272, 1977.
22. Hultgren NH and Marticorena EA: High altitude pulmonary edema: epidemiologic observations in Peru, *Chest* 74:372-376, 1978.
23. Kawashima A et al: Hemodynamic responses to acute hypoxia, hypobaria, and exercise in subjects susceptible to high altitude pulmonary edema, *J Appl Physiol* 67(5):1982-1989, 1989.
24. Barkin R and Rosen P: *Emergency pediatrics: a guide to ambulatory care*, St. Louis, 1990, Mosby.
25. Hackett PH and Rennie D: Fluid retention and relative hypoventilation in acute mountain sickness, *Respiration* 43:321-329, 1982.
26. Gray GW et al: Control of acute mountain sickness, *Aerosp Med* 42(1):81-84, 1971.
27. Hansen JE and Evans WO: A hypothesis regarding the pathophysiology of acute mountain sickness, *Arch Environ Health* 21:666-669, 1970.
28. Hackett PH and Rennie D: The incidence, importance, and prophylaxis of acute mountain sickness, *Lancet* 2:1149-1155, 1976.
29. Sutton JR et al: Effect of acetazolamide on hypoxemia during sleep at high altitude, *N Engl J Med* 301(24):1329-1331, 1979.
30. Greene MK et al: Acetazolamide in prevention of acute mountain sickness: a double blind controlled cross-over study, *Br Med J* 283:811-813, 1981.
31. Larson EB et al: Acute mountain sickness and acetazolamide, *JAMA* 248(3):328-332, 1982.
32. Ellsworth AJ, Larson EB, Strickland D: A randomized trial of dexamethsone and acetazolamide for acute mountain sickness prophylaxis, *Am J Med* 83:1024-30, 1987.
33. Zell SC and Goodman PH: Acetazolamide and dexamethasone in the prevention of acute mountain sickness, *West J Med* 148:541-545, 1988.
34. Gentile DA and Kennedy BC: Wilderness medicine for children, *Pediatrics* 88(5):967-981, 1991.
35. Rabold M: High altitude pulmonary edema: a collective review, *Am J Emerg Med* 7(4):426-433, 1989.
36. Gray GW: High altitude pulmonary edema, *Semin Respir Med* 5(2):141-150, 1983.
37. Schoene RB: High altitude pulmonary edema: pathophysiology and clinical review, *Ann Emerg Med* 16(9):987-992, 1987.
38. Callaham ML: *Current practice of emergency medicine*, Philadelphia, 1991, BC Decker.
39. Schoene RB et al: The lung at high altitude: bronchoalveolar lavage in acute mountain sickness and pulmonary edema, *J Appl Physiol* 64(6):2605-2613, 1988.
40. Hultgren HN et al: Physiologic studies of pulmonary edema at high altitude, *Circulation* 24:393-408, 1964.
41. Koyama S et al: The increased sympathoadrenal activity in patients with high altitude pulmonary edema is centrally mediated, *Jpn J Med* 27(1):10-16, 1988.
42. Naeije R, Melot C, LeJeune P: Hypoxic pulmonary vasoconstriction and high altitude pulmonary edema, *Am Rev Respir Dis* 134:332-333, 1986.
43. Fasules JW, Wiggins JW, Wolfe RR: Increased lung vasoreactivity in children from Leadville, Colorado after recovery from high altitude pulmonary edema, *Circulation* 72(5):957-962, 1985.

44. Vock P et al: High altitude pulmonary edema: findings at high altitude: chest radiography and physical examination, *Radiology* 170:661-665, 1989.

45. Cucinell SA and Pitts CM: Thrombosis at mountain altitudes, *Aviat Space Environ Med* 58:1109-1111, 1987.

46. Nakagawa S, Kubo K, Koizumi T et al: High altitude pulmonary edema with pulmonary thromboembolism *Chest* 103: 948-50, 1993.

47. Bartsch P, Waber U, Haeberli A et al: Enhanced fibrin formation in high altitude pulmonary edema, *J Appl Physiol* 63:752-757, 1987.

48. Schoene RB et al: High altitude pulmonary edema and exercise at 4,400 meters on Mt. McKinley: effect of expiratory positive airway pressure, *Chest* 87(3):330-333, 1985.

49. Oelz O et al: Nifedipine for high altitude pulmonary oedema, *Lancet* 8674(2):1241-1244, 1989.

50. Bartsch P, Maggiorini M, Ritter M et al: Prevention of high-altitude pulmonary edema by nifedipine, *N Engl J Med* 325(18):1284-1289, 1991.

51. Kickinson JG: High altitude cerebral edema: cerebral acute mountain sickness, *Semin Respir Med* 5(3):151-158, 1983.

52. Hamilton AJ et al: High altitude cerebral edema, *Neurosurgery* 19:841-849, 1986.

53. Severinghaus JW et al: Cerebral blood flow in man at high altitude, *Circ Res* 54:274-282, 1966.

54. Clarke C: High altitude cerebral oedema, *Int J Sports Med* 9:170-174, 1988.

55. McFadden MD et al: High-altitude retinopathy, *JAMA* 245(6):581-586, 1981.

56. Sutton R: High altitude retinal hemorrhage, *Semin Respir Med* 5(2):159-163, 1983.

57. Frayser R et al: Retinal hemorrhage at high altitude, *N Engl J Med* 282(21):1183-1184, 1970.

Air Travel

58. Cummins RO: High altitude flights and risk of cardiac stress, *JAMA* 260:3668-3669, 1988.

59. Dan BB: The accidental tourist: medical emergencies in the air, *JAMA* 261(9):1328, 1989.

60. Cummins RO and Schubach JA: Frequency and types of medical emergencies among commercial air travelers, *JAMA* 261:1295-99, 1989.

61. Rodenberg H: Medical emergencies aboard commercial aircraft *Ann Emerg Med* 16:1373-77, 1987.

Dysbaric Diving Injuries

62. Noble J, editor: *Textbook of general medicine and primary care,* Boston, 1987, Little, Brown.

63. Dembert ML and Keith JF: Evaluating the potential pediatric scuba diver, *Am J Dis Child* 140:1135-1141, 1986.

64. Zwingelberg KM, Green JW, Powers K: Primary causes of drowning and near drowning in scuba diving, *The Physician and Sports Med* 14(9):145-151, 1986.

65. Orlowski JP: Adolescent drownings: swimming, boating, diving, and scuba accidents, *Pediatr Ann* 17(2):125-132, 1987.

66. Bove AA and Davis JC: *Diving medicine,* Philadelphia, 1990, WB Saunders.

67. Jarrett AS: Effect of immersion on intrapulmonary pressure, *J Appl Physiol* 20:1261-1266, 1965.

68. Murray JF and Nadel JA: *Textbook of respiratory medicine,* Philadelphia, 1988, WB Saunders.

69. Calder IM: Dysbarism: a review, *Forensic Sci Int* 30:237-266, 1986.

70. Shupak A, Doweck I, Greenberg E et al: Diving-related inner ear injuries, *Laryngoscope* 101:173-179, 1991.

71. Pullen FW: Perilymphatic fistula induced by barotrauma, *Am J Otology* 13(3):270-272, 1992.

72. Brown M, Jones J, Krohmer J: Pseudoephredrine for the prevention of barotitis media: a controlled clinical trial in underwater divers, *Ann Emerg Med* 21:849-852, 1992.

73. Neuman PS: Diving medicine, *Clin Sports Med* 6(3):647-661, 1987.

74. Bruch FR: Pulmonary barotrauma, *Ann Emerg Med* 15(11):1373-1375, 1986.

75. Auerbach PS and Geehr EC: *Management of wilderness and environmental emergencies,* New York, 1983, MacMillan Publishing.

76. Edmonds C, Lowry C, Pennefather J: *Diving and subaquatic medicine,* Oxford, 1992, Butterworth-Heinemann.

77. Arthur DC and Margulies RA: A short course in diving medicine, *Ann Emerg Med* 16:689-701, 1987.

78. Smith RM and Neuman TS: Elevation of serum creatinine kinase in divers with arterial gas embolization, *N Engl J Med* 330(1):19-24, 1994.

79. Krzyzak J: A case of delayed onset pulmonary barotrauma in a scuba diver, *Undersea Biomed Res* 14(6):553-561, 1987.

80. Leitch DR and Green RD: Pulmonary barotrauma in divers and the treatment of cerebral arterial gas embolism, *Aviat Space Environ Med* 57:931-938, 1986.

81. *US Navy Diving Manual,* vol. 1, NAVSEA 0994-LP-001-9010, revision 3, 1993.

82. Garman L: A bubble is born, *Sci News* 118:186-188, 1980.

83. Hallenbeck JM et al: Accelerated coagulation of whole blood and cell-free plasma by bubbling in vitro, *Aerosp Med* 44(7):712-714, 1973.

84. Warren LP, Djang W, Moon R et al: Neuroimaging of scuba diving injuries to the CNS, *AJR* 151:1003-1008, 1988.

85. Pelosi G et al: Decompression sickness: a medical emergency, *Resuscitation* 9:201-209, 1981.

86. Brouhard BH et al: Scuba diving and diabetes, *AJDC* 141:605-606, 1987.

Radiation Exposure

Susan McClellan Asch

Radiation exposure is a problem unfamiliar to most, if not all, practitioners of pediatric emergency care. The experience of Nagasaki and Hiroshima has faded into the past, but the Three-Mile Island and Chernobyl disasters have returned it to public and professional awareness. The issue, however, has never been truly dormant. The potential for radiation exposure from industrial, medical, military, and household sources is a constant problem of modern life. Cosmic rays and in-ground radioactivity have resulted in an annual exposure of 100 mrad/person. Tobacco smoke irradiates the bronchial epithelium of a pack-a-day smoker at 8 to 9 rems/year. Table 41-1 demonstrates some common sources of natural and technologic radiation and the exposure expected from these under routine living conditions.[1]

PATHOPHYSIOLOGY

Young children are particularly vulnerable to radiation effects because of their whole-body preponderance of rapidly dividing cells, similar to those localized largely in the gastrointestinal (GI) and hemopoietic systems of adults.

Radiation can be classified functionally as ionizing or nonionizing radiation. Solar rays, microwaves, and radio waves are sources of nonionizing radiation. Although *nonionizing radiation* can be harmful, it does not produce acute radiation sickness or radioactive contamination and will not be discussed. *Ionizing radiation* can be further subdivided into penetrating or nonpenetrating. It is produced by nuclear weapons and reactors and x-ray machines; material labeled "radioactive" refers to a substance that produces ionizing radiation.

Ionizing radiation comprises alpha and beta particles, gamma rays, and neutrons. Alpha particles are positively charged fragments from heavy radioactive elements (e.g., plutonium, uranium, or radium). Alpha-particle travel is confined to a few centimeters, and biologically, their penetration is limited to approximately the thickness of the epidermis. They are generally not harmful; shielding may be accomplished by a substance no thicker than a sheet of paper or a cornified layer of skin.

Beta particles are electrons. They can travel a few meters, penetrate up to 8 mm, and thus can cause burns. Beta particles are emitted by tritium (^{3}H), the isotope most commonly used in research, as well as ^{14}carbon and phosphorus. Clothing or other material of similar thickness can provide shielding from beta particles.

Gamma rays (e.g., x-rays) have no mass; they are purely electromagnetic radiation, which can penetrate deeply, interacting with each level of tissue through which the ray passes. The chief cause of acute radiation syndrome, they require 1 to 2 inches of lead for adequate shielding. Beta decay from radioisotopes and radiation produced by linear accelerators are also examples of gamma rays.

Neutrons from nuclear reactors, accelerators, and weapons are a type of particulate radiation and can penetrate deeply into tissue because of their lack of electrical charge. Their ability to cause a previously stable atom to become radioactive is the source of fallout when combined with the dispersal effect of a thermonuclear blast.

The key danger from ionizing rays or particles is the conversion of water to free radicals in exposed tissue, resulting in breaks in RNA and DNA strands in that tissue. Because of this effect on genetic material, tissue with rapidly dividing cells is more strongly affected by radiation. The short- and long-term clinical effects are a direct result of interaction of the type of tissue exposed (central nervous system [CNS], GI, genetic, hemopoietic) and the physical properties of the radiation including the following:

1. Type and amount of radiation (the latter expressed as *rads*)*
2. Length of exposure
3. Distance of victim from radiation source
4. Amount and type of shielding
5. Continuous vs. intermittent nature of the radiation exposure

DIAGNOSTIC FINDINGS

Quantifying a particular radiation exposure depends on the contribution of each of the multiple factors described

---

* A rad is a unit of absorbed dose equal to 100 ergs/g of absorbed energy of any type of radiation in any tissue. A *rem* (which is actually equivalent to a rad for gamma and x-rays and B particles) is a *roentgen equivalent man*, a *calculated* radiation unit in which an allowance is made for the actual biologic effect of different radiation types.

TABLE 41-1. Common Sources of Human Radiation

Source	Whole body mrem/yr	Dose rate
Natural		
Background	35	
Air	5	
Building materials	34	
Food	25	
Ground	11	
TOTAL	110	
Technologic		
Coast-to-coast jet flight		5 mrem/roundtrip
Color television		1 mrem/yr
Chest radiograph		10 mrem/film

Linnemann RE: *Background information on radiation*, San Jose, Calif, April 4, 1979.

previously. Clinically, the type of radiation to which the patient has been exposed will be determined by the history of the incident; the dose of exposure can be somewhat predicted by the complex of presenting symptoms. In general, the earlier the onset of symptoms, the greater the amount and length of exposure. Nausea and vomiting, malaise, and possible depression of white cells and platelets are the first clinical signs and symptoms after whole-body irradiation, unless the dose was massive enough to cause CNS damage and cardiovascular collapse. The severity of the symptoms is otherwise not a reliable indicator of the exposure dose or the ultimate prognosis. An approximation of the relationship between the dose received and the clinical laboratory picture presented is shown in Table 41-2.

Experience with therapeutic whole-body irradiation suggests that the absolute lymphocyte count obtained within 48 hours after exposure is a reasonable estimate of ultimate prognosis (in the absence of other significant injuries). If after 48 hours the lymphocyte count is $> 1,200/mm^3$, the prognosis is good; between 300 and $1,200/mm^3$, the prognosis is fair, and $< 300/mm^3$, the prognosis is poor.

Complications

If the radiation exposure victim does not succumb to acute radiation symptoms, many potential sequelae may develop, even with very small doses of radiation. In general, the more quickly the dose is delivered and the greater the body area exposed, the greater the biologic effect. The long-term effects observed in human populations exposed to excessive environmental radiation are of two types: somatic and genetic. Somatic effects include an increased incidence of cancer of many types, cataracts, and decreased life span. The genetic effects present as mutations, which may have a multigenerational effect.[2]

The cancers resulting from acute or chronic radiation exposure have been of many types. Atomic bomb survivors with exposures about 100 rems and children under 10 years of age at exposure show an increased incidence of leukemia, as well as later-onset thyroid and breast cancers. Patients irradiated in childhood for thymic enlargement and tinea capitis have increased incidence of thyroid cancers and

TABLE 41-2. Dose-effect Relationships After Acute Whole-body Irradiation (Gamma Rays)

Whole-body dose (rads)	Clinical and laboratory findings
5-25	Asymptomatic; conventional blood studies are normal; chromosome aberrations detectable
50-75	Asymptomatic; minor depressions of white cells and platelets detectable in a few persons, especially if baseline values established
75-125	Minimal acute doses that produce prodromal symptoms (anorexia, nausea, vomiting, fatigue) in about 10%-20% of persons within 2 days; mild depressions of white cells and platelets in some persons
125-200	Symptomatic course with transient disability and clear hematologic changes in a majority of exposed persons; lymphocyte depression of about 50% within 48 hr
240-340	Serious, disabling illness in most persons with about 50% mortality if untreated; lymphocyte depression of $\geq 75\%$ within 48 hr
500+	Accelerated version of acute radiation syndrome with GI complications within 2 weeks, bleeding, and death in most exposed persons
5,000+	Fulminating course with cardiovascular, GI, and CNS complications resulting in death within 24 to 72 hr

From Mettler FD: *JACEP* 7:302, 1978.
GI, Gastrointestinal; *CNS,* central nervous system.

malignancies of the head and neck, as well as leukemia and functional CNS changes. Women with chest irradiation for postpartum mastitis and during the course of pneumothorax therapy for tuberculosis have a higher incidence of breast cancer. Children of mothers with pelvic irradiation in pregnancy have a higher incidence of leukemia.

In utero exposure (starting at 10 to 19 rads) to the Hiroshima atomic bomb led to small head circumference; mental retardation was seen with in utero exposure to 50 rads or more, with a clear dose-response effect.[3,4]

Genetically, complex chromosomal abnormalities are still found in peripheral lymphocytes of atomic bomb survivors, including those in utero. Because of the low visibility of most mutations, other effects are as yet unknown.

MANAGEMENT

Radiation emergency has four medical objectives:

- To establish airway, breathing, and circulation
- To minimize internal contamination that may increase the patient's later risk of leukemia or other cancer
- To minimize spread of unsealed radioisotope contamination
- To evaluate and treat the acute radiation syndrome

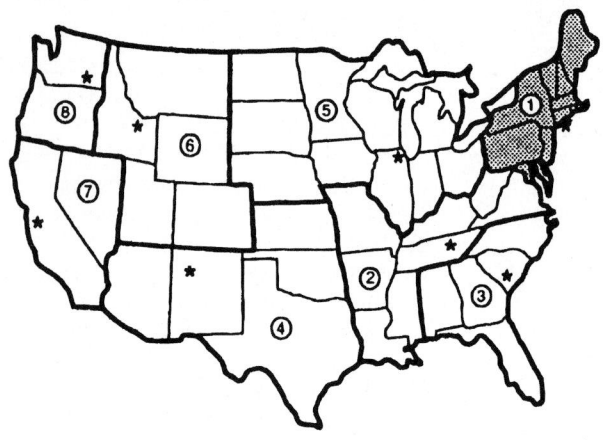

Region	Office	Phone
1	Brookhaven	516-344-2200
2	Oak Ridge	423-576-1005
3	Savannah River	803-725-3333
4	Albuquerque	505-845-4667
5	Chicago	708-252-4800 (or 5731 off hours)
6	Idaho	208-526-1515
7	Oakland	510-637-1794
8	Richland	509-373-3800

FIG. 41-1. United States Department of Energy Radiological Assistance Program Regional Coordinating Offices.

There are two basic types of radiation exposure: irradiation and contamination. Irradiation is simply exposure to a source of radiation, such as gamma or x-ray film, which does not cause the patient to become radioactive. Even a patient who has received a lethal dose does not represent a danger to emergency department or hospital patients, and should receive emergency fluid replacement, much as for a burn, as well as management of specific symptoms.

Contamination is the other type of radiation accident and represents deposition of radioactive material in or on the body (internal or external contamination). Alpha particles, beta particles, and neutrons are the forms of radiation most likely to be encountered in contamination exposures. It is the radiation contamination victim for which the emergency department must make particular preparation.[6] Assistance may be obtained from the Regional Coordinating Offices for Radiological Assistance (Fig. 41-1).

If a patient is radioactive (contaminated), either by dosimeter or by history, the patient should be admitted by a separate entrance to the emergency department. Both internal and external decontamination should be considered. The patient should be covered with a sheet. A room with closed ventilation is ideal to prevent contamination to the rest of the hospital. The morgue or autopsy room is appropriate if emergency equipment can be moved into the rooms. The floor should be covered by plastic or paper sheets.

Personnel in contact with the patient must wear protective clothing to prevent skin and airway contamination.

Surgical caps, gowns, masks, scrub suits, and gloves can be used. Double gowning and gloving are necessary. Plastic shoe covers and rubber laboratory aprons should be available. Prehospital transport personnel should be similarly outfitted. Because most significant contaminants emit medium energy gamma rays, lead aprons are *not* effective protective measures. All staff should be monitored with a radiation detector, with the maximum dose of exposure allowable for personnel at 5 rems. All nonessential personnel should be strictly prohibited, and the area should be clearly marked and security posted if necessary.

The Joint Commission of Accreditation of Hospital Organization requires all hospitals to have a protocol for radiation injuries. A list of specialists familiar with radiation and monitoring should be available. Knowledge of the hospital's means for monitoring exposure (Geiger counter, nuclear medicine machines, and dosimeters) and the personnel needed to interpret the data are necessary. Periodic drills are recommended.[5]

In the event of a nuclear disaster that does not incapacitate the hospital itself, the facility must be prepared to handle many patients with radiation exposure. It should be remembered that a nuclear explosion generates an electromagnetic pulse. The pulse travels a great distance along telephone and electric wires and pipelines. Hospital electronic equipment (automatic clinical laboratories) and computers will be useless. Telephone and computer communication may be down, making contact with other hospitals and authorities impossible. The hospital must be prepared to handle the event with internal resources.[6,7]

External Contamination

Initial attention to respiratory and cardiovascular stability is paramount. The patient should be undressed after obtaining an initial reading. Removing clothing usually results in a 70% to 90% decrease in radiation. The chart used for burn injuries can be used to document radiation readings. The clothing is placed in containers for later radiation analysis and proper disposal. Analysis of metal objects such as watches and belt buckles is particularly valuable for quantifying radioactivity. Swabs are taken from orifices for sampling. The patient is then washed with warm water and soap, being careful not to abrade other skin. Undiluted household bleach can also be used.[8]

If a closed drainage system is not available to prevent environmental contamination, all waste water must be collected and placed in the proper containers. Likewise, all urine, feces, and vomitus should be collected for analysis and disposal. Hair must be shampooed and may need to be carefully trimmed. The patient should not be shaved because of the risk of internal contamination by small lacerations from the razor. Nails should be trimmed and cleaned.

Eyes are irrigated carefully to prevent absorption. After several minutes of cleaning, the radiation control officer should take another reading. The radioactivity level should be less than two times the background. If it is not, internal contamination should be considered. If high results are obtained with more vigorous washing, the area should be placed in a plastic bag until it can undergo more definitive treatment with chelating compounds or other agents under the supervision of radiation experts.

Open wounds should be treated first to prevent washing radioactive material into the site. The wounds should be copiously irrigated with sterile saline after carefully washing all contamination from surrounding skin away from the wound and applying adhesive surgical drapes. Debridement of nonviable tissue and debris is essential. Delayed primary closure is preferred. Burns should be treated in the same manner as a thermal burn. Like electrical burns, these burns are usually minimal at the initial evaluation, but the potential for evolution of greater injury should be kept in mind.

If surgery is necessary, it should be performed immediately, since severely exposed patients will experience increasing difficulty with fluid and electrolyte balance, coagulation disorders, and infection. Foreign objects (metal) should be removed immediately, since they can be highly radioactive.

Internal Contamination

The patient may be known or suspected to have ingested radioactive material. Immediate efforts to prevent absorption and increase elimination are necessary to be effective.

Gastric lavage or emesis is followed by antacids to precipitate heavy metals. Aluminum phosphate gel-star, $BaSO_4$, or $MgSO_4$ is used for $S^{++}Ra$, whereas Prussian blue is used for cesium, thallium, and rubidium. Dilution treatment (3,000 to 4,000 ml in an adult) is useful for ^3H and ^{99}Technetium exposure to produce diuresis. Blocking agents include potassium iodide (300 mg) for radioactive iodide and is useful if given within a few hours of ingestion. Chelation is used for binding metals into complexes. Calcium disodium edetate (EDTA) and penicillamine are indicated for radioactive lead. The zinc or calcium salt of diethylenetriamine pentaacetic acid (DTPA) is recommended for trasuranic metals (1 gm in 500 D5W IV in 30 minutes). Cathartics should also be used to shorten potential absorption.

Inhalation of radioactive particles is more probable in cases of fire or explosion. Inhaled contaminants are removed with multiple bronchopulmonary lavages. Chelation, with 1 gm of DTPA by nebulizer over 15 to 30 minutes, may be performed. Inhaled particles can be coughed up and then swallowed, necessitating further GI contamination. Laboratory studies obtained should include complete blood count (CBC) with platelet count, electrolytes, and coagulation studies.

DISPOSITION

Ultimate disposition of radiation-exposure patients depends on their classification in one of three groups: survival probable, survival possible, and survival improbable. The survival-probable group has no symptoms or mild symptoms that subside within a few hours (such as nausea and vomiting). The initial laboratory studies demonstrate normal leukocyte counts. Exposure is usually less than 200 rads. Unless new symptoms arise or subsequent laboratory studies change, these patients may be discharged if they are adequately decontaminated.

Usually the survival-possible group has been exposed to 200 to 800 rads (LD_{50} for humans is between 300 and 500 rads). Nausea and vomiting are brief, lasting 24 to 48 hours, and are followed by an asymptomatic period. Somewhat later, they will develop thrombocytopenia, granulocytopenia, and lymphopenia. They should be admitted for fluid and electrolyte monitoring if vomiting is severe (antiemetics are often ineffective) and protective isolation precautions if the absolute lymphocyte count at 48 hours is less than 1,200 or 50% of baseline. The exact hematologic abnormalities determine other therapy. Platelet transfusions, antibiotics and antifungals, and bone marrow transplants may have roles in later therapy.

The survival-improbable group (greater than 800 rads of whole-body exposure) experience rapid onset of fulminant nausea, vomiting, and diarrhea. If CNS symptoms appear early, it can be assumed that the patient has been exposed to a very large dose of radiation. Intense fluid and electrolyte therapy may result in initial survival, although the later sequelae of bone marrow aplasia and pancytopenia are uniformly fatal unless bone marrow transplant can be performed. Even so, the prognosis is dismal, and death within 2 to 10 days is usual. Death comes from hemopoietic complications for those who survive the GI and CNS insults. Patients who survive the first 6 weeks are less likely to die from radiation exposure sequelae.

The prognosis, management, and disposition of the ionizing radiation-exposure victim ultimately depends on the type of exposure (irradiation vs. contamination). The bases for estimating the exposure dose and probable prognosis include the following:

1. The type of exposing radiation (alpha, beta, gamma, or neutron)
2. The duration of exposure
3. The distance between the exposing agent and the victim and the amount of exposing agent present (the latter three factors resulting in the exposure dose)
4. The history of exposure
5. The rapidity of onset of symptoms
6. The type of symptoms
7. The initial leukocyte count

Although the initial medical management of the patient is straightforward, the principles and equipment necessary should be planned and assembled well in advance. Guidelines should be readily available within the emergency department. Prompt treatment of the radiation victim and protection of the emergency department staff can both be accomplished in a well-planned system.

References

1. Mettler F: Emergency management of radiation accidents, *JACEP* 7:302, 1978.
2. Barnett MH: The biological effects of ionizing radiation, *Conn Medicine* 43, 1979.
3. Otake M and Schull WJ: In utero exposure to A-bomb radiation and mental retardation, a reassessment, *Br J Radiol* 57:409, 1984.
4. Miller RW and Mulvhill JJ: Small head size after atomic irradiation, *Teratology* 14:355, 1976.
5. Leonard RB and Ricks RC: Emergency department radiation accident protocol, *Ann Emerg Med* 9:462, 1980.
6. Mettler F: Emergency management of radiation accidents, *JACEP* 7:302, 1978.
7. Saenger EL: Radiation accidents, *Ann Emerg Med* 15:1061, 1986.
8. National Council on Radiation Protection and Measurements: *Management of persons accidentally contaminated with radionuclides*, Report No 65, Washington, DC, 1980, NCRP.

PART

VII

POISONING

CHAPTER

42

General Management Principles for Poisoning

Milton Tenenbein

Pediatric emergency toxicology is unique because of its natural division into two distinct components. Young children, aged 1 to 5 years, who innocently ingest a small amount of a single substance, constitute the first group. Members of the second group are adolescents who purposefully ingest larger amounts of one or more substances because of emotional or psychiatric distress. Children between these two age groups are rarely acutely poisoned. Preambulatory infants almost always have the toxicant administered, either by therapeutic misadventure or with malicious intent.

Morbidity and mortality differ between the two groups. The American Association of Poison Control Centers reported an incidence of 27 and 61 deaths per year in children younger than 6 years of age and between 13 to 19 years of age or 27.5 and 523.7 deaths per million exposures respectively.[1] Preschoolers have a lower mortality rate because they are more likely to ingest nontoxic substances (see box on p. 528) or nontoxic amounts of toxic substances. However, management of this age group can be quite taxing because of the vast number of different substances that are ingested.

This chapter reviews the general management of the child taken to the emergency department because of an exposure to a presumed toxic agent. Because approaches to care are evolving rapidly, various methods of gastrointestinal (GI) decontamination are evaluated to reflect contemporary thinking so that the practitioner can make informed therapeutic decisions about these modalities (also see Chapter 43).

PHARMACOKINETICS AND TOXICOKINETICS

"Pharmacokinetics is the study, as a function of time, of all processes which determine a fate of a drug in the organism to which it is administered; in order to establish a model of predictive value."[2] These processes include rates of absorption, distribution, metabolism, and excretion. The term *toxicokinetics* is sometimes used because drugs can behave differently after the ingestion of massive doses. A basic understanding of a few principles will assist with the management of the acutely poisoned patient. Kinetics aid in predicting the need for an intervention to augment the excretion of a toxin, the timing and interpretation of drug concentration determinations, and the explanation for the persistence of clinical toxicity in some overdose patients.

Nontoxic Substances

Pharmaceuticals
Antacids
Antibiotics
Contraceptives
Corticosteroids
Laxatives
Mineral oil
Petrolatum
Vitamins (without iron)
Zinc oxide

Soaps and detergents
Bar soap
Bath foam
Bubble bath
Fabric softener
Hand dishwashing soap
Laundry detergent
Shampoo

Household products
Artificial sweeteners
Ballpoint pen ink
Bath oil
Candles
Crayons
Dehumidifying packets
    (silica gel)
Deodorizers
Fertilizers
Fish bowl additives
Household bleach
Shaving cream
Shoe polish
Thermometers
    (mercury)
Water colors

Cosmetics
Baby product
    cosmetics
Cologne
Deodorants
Eye makeup
Hand lotion
Hair products
Hydrogen peroxide
    (household, 3%)
Lipstick
Perfume
Suntan lotion
Toilet water

Miscellaneous
Chalk
Cigarettes
Clay
Felt tip pens
Glues and paste
Greases
Lubricating oil
Magic markers
Matches
Motor oil
Paint
Pencil lead
Silly putty

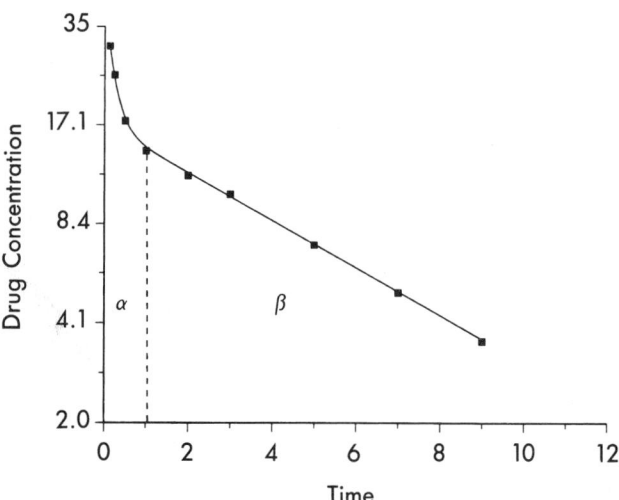

FIG. 42-1. Semilogarithmic plot of plasma concentration vs. time after intravenous dosing of a drug. Concentration falls rapidly during distribution (α phase) and less quickly during metabolism and excretion (β phase). Plasma and tissue drug concentrations are proportionally related during the β phase, during which the former are useful for the prediction of toxicity.

Because drug concentrations in organs and blood are not equal, the lower the amount found in the blood, the greater the apparent volume of distribution. Thus patients poisoned with drugs with lower volumes of distribution are more likely to benefit from procedures that augment excretion. A useful rule is that if the volume of distribution is greater than 1.0 L/kg, it is unlikely that such techniques will be worthwhile. The actual values of specific drugs can be found in pharmacologic texts. Of course a low volume of distribution does not guarantee that any of these procedures will be effective, since other factors such as endogenous clearance and protein binding are also important.

Timing of Blood Concentration Determinations

After administration, a drug is usually absorbed, distributed throughout the body, metabolized, and then excreted. A drug's plasma concentration soon after ingestion is not helpful in predicting toxicity because absorption and distribution are not complete. Distribution is "the act of apportioning or spreading out of a drug in an orderly manner once it reaches the general circulation. It is a state by which a drug is distributed or apportioned to one or more so-called volumes or spaces, tissues, organs, etc."[2] Usually distribution is seen only after intravenous injection of a drug during which the plasma concentration falls rapidly for a short time (Fig. 42-1). Usually it is not seen after oral dosing because, in most cases, it occurs simultaneously with absorption. However, some drugs such as digoxin have a distributive phase even after ingestion (Fig. 42-2). Very high serum digoxin concentrations can be seen (five to ten times the upper limit of the therapeutic range) in asymptomatic patients during the first few hours after oral overdose. After distribution is complete, the fall of plasma

Augmentation of Excretion

Interventions intended to augment the excretion of absorbed poisons include diuresis, dialysis, hemoperfusion, and multiple dose activated charcoal. For any of these to be effective, a significant proportion of the toxin must be in the blood. If, for example, 95% of a drug distributes to lipid-rich organs, cleansing the blood of the remaining 5% would do little to alter the clinical course of a poisoning with such an agent.

A pharmacokinetic value called the *apparent volume of distribution* (often simply called the volume of distribution) helps to predict whether any of these interventions might be helpful. It is the hypothetical volume of body fluid required to dissolve the total amount of a drug at the same concentration found in the blood. It is derived from the following formula:

$$\text{volume} = \text{amount/concentration}$$

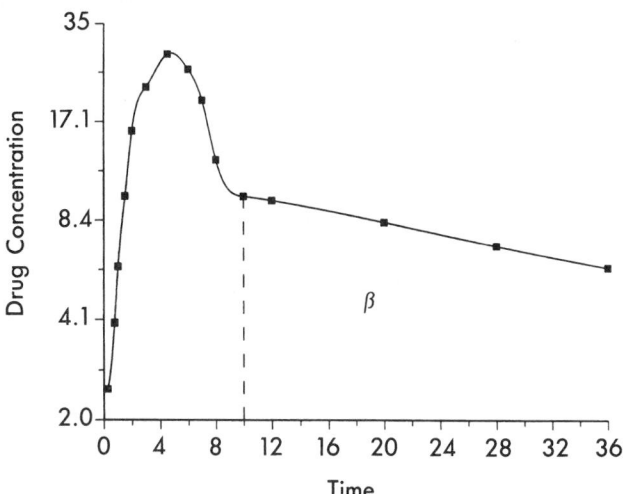

FIG. 42-2. Semilogarithmic plot of plasma concentration vs. time after oral dosing of a drug with a distribution phase. The fall of plasma concentration during the β phase is due to metabolism and excretion of the drug. Only samples obtained during this phase are predictive of toxicity.

concentration is usually slower; this decline represents metabolism and excretion. During this phase there is usually a fixed relationship between plasma and tissue drug concentrations. Thus drug concentrations measured before absorption or distribution is completed are not in equilibrium with body tissues. This is why the acetaminophen and salicylate nomograms begin at 4 and 6 hours, respectively, after ingestion of these drugs.

The timing of drug concentration determinations is complicated by the ingestion of large amounts, since we now deal with toxicokinetics rather than pharmacokinetics. Absorption is typically prolonged, and other processes may be delayed because of early effects of the overdose. For example, circulatory compromise or intestinal ileus could delay various kinetic processes.

Because these and other factors, such as the time of overdose, are unknown, there is often a need to obtain serial blood specimens for drug concentration analysis. During the early stages they may need to be obtained as often as every 1 to 2 hours until a clear trend is established.

Prolonged Symptoms

For some overdose patients, the duration of toxicity is longer than expected. One reason for this prolonged duration involves a principle of toxicokinetics. Large amounts of a drug may saturate processes for its catabolism and excretion. Therefore its half-life during overdose may be longer than after a therapeutic dose. Thus it is not appropriate to subtract half-lives from a drug's plasma concentration until arriving at a nontoxic concentration to predict duration of toxicity because published half-lives only pertain to therapeutic dosing. Phenytoin is an example of prolonged persistence after overdose. In theory it is possible to predict the duration of toxicity using kinetic models. However, the data required to do so are not available because they are

patient specific and not known in the clinical situation. Therefore toxicity may persist for longer than expected, and we cannot predict in whom and for how long.

Overdose with Modified-Release Pharmaceuticals

Modified release pharmaceuticals delay, prolong, sustain, or control the release of drugs within the GI tract.[3] Advantages of modified release pharmaceuticals include decreased variation of plasma drug concentration, resulting in improved efficacy and decreased toxicity, the convenience of fewer doses per day, and improved compliance.[4] Thus the number of these preparations has been increasing, with hundreds of them available.[5] Common modified release drugs include antihypertensives, anticonvulsants, antidysrhythmics, theophylline, iron, and salicylates. The pharmaceutical engineering that confers the modified release property is varied and complex, making the kinetics of each one unique.[3]

Overdose of modified release pharmaceuticals is especially problematic. Most important, toxicity can be delayed and prolonged. Several cases of overdose from modified-release salicylate-preparations with nontoxic serum concentrations at 3 to 10 hours followed by moderate to severe toxicity 10 to 27 hours later have been reported.[6-8] Delayed and prolonged toxicity have also been reported with theophylline.[9-11] Because each modified-release pharmaceutical is unique, its kinetics is unknown. Thus it is important to establish whether the drug is a conventional or a modified-release drug (obtain the trade name whenever possible). When dealing with overdoses of these drugs, patients need to be observed longer with serial serum drug concentration sampling. It is difficult to recommend a specific duration for observation because of the heterogeneity of this group, but 12 to 24 hours is prudent.

THE ACUTELY ILL OVERDOSE PATIENT

As with any other acutely ill patient, first stabilize the airway, breathing, and circulation by providing intubation, ventilation, venous access, and intravascular fluid and pharmacologic support as needed. Management of respiratory and circulatory failure and arrest are described elsewhere in this book (see Chapters 11 and 12). All suspected poisoning patients with a decreased level of consciousness should be treated with oxygen, naloxone, and glucose. Mortality of poisoned patients with vital functions should be less than 1%, and the cornerstone of management is meticulous, supportive care, not prevention of absorption, enhancement of excretion, or antidotal therapy (see box on p. 530).

Acute Toxicologic Syndromes

Expect a set of signs and symptoms, often referred to as a toxidrome, in patients poisoned with a member of various drug groups.[12] These drugs include opioids, cyclic antidepressants, anticholinergics, sympathomimetics, and hallucinogens. It is important to recognize toxidromes when patients acutely ill from poisoning do not have a history of poisoning. Those with specific lifesaving therapies that must be recognized are the opioids, cyclic antidepressants, and cholinergics and are discussed because rapid intervention is critical. The other toxidromes are clinically unimportant because their treatments are nonspecific, they are less frequently life threatening, and presentation as a "pure" toxidrome is uncommon. Because they are frequently associated with drug abuse, they are rarely diagnostic challenges. Each is discussed in Chapter 43.

Opioid Toxidrome. The classic opioid triad consists of decreased level of consciousness, respiratory depression, and miosis.[13] The latter finding is not present in all opiate poisonings (e.g., meperidine and pentazocine). The specific treatment is naloxone (see Chapter 43).

Cyclic Antidepressant Toxidrome. Cyclic antidepressant ingestion is a major contributor to the mortality of acute drug overdose (see Chapter 43). Clinical features of toxicity include decreased level of consciousness, seizures, widened QRS complex, and dysrythmias.[14] Initial treatment with sodium bicarbonate may prevent or reverse life-threatening dysrhythmias.

Cholinergic Toxidrome. The organophosphate and carbamate insecticides are the most important substances that produce this toxidrome.[15] Recognition is important because atropine therapy may be lifesaving (see Chapter 43). Important features are salivation, lacrimation, diaphoresis, respiratory distress attributable to bronchospasm and increased secretions, and a garliclike odor.

THE STABLE OVERDOSE PATIENT

The approach to the stable or stabilized overdose patient includes the traditional components of all patient encounters: history, physical examination, clinical investigations, and management. The latter includes routine supportive care and specific antipoisoning therapy—preventing absorption, enhancing excretion, and administering an antidote (see box at right).

Diagnostic Findings

The obvious questions to ask are: When did it happen and what and how much was taken? The answers to these questions are often difficult to determine. The best way to establish what was taken is to read the label. If the container was not brought in with the patient, send a family member back to retrieve it or phone the home and have it read to you. Although the exact time of ingestion is often unknown, especially in suicide attempts, even approximations can be helpful. For most drug ingestions, except acetaminophen and modified-release pharmaceuticals, if the patient is asymptomatic after 4 to 6 hours, then toxicity is unlikely. Quantification of the ingestion is the most difficult aspect of the history. The ingestors are unreliable sources, whether young children with unintentional ingestions or adolescents who have purposefully overdosed. Always assume that all that cannot be reliably accounted for has been ingested. Assuming the maximum also means that if the container was shared, each child ingested the entire unaccounted for amount. Specific aspects of the physical examination vary with the circumstances of the clinical situation.

Ancillary Data

Specific investigations may be required for various poisonings (see Chapter 43). Examples include blood gases for salicylates, chest radiograph study for hydrocarbons, and

---

> ### Approach to the Overdose Patient
>
> 1. Ensure that airway, breathing, and circulation are satisfactory; stabilize as necessary.
> 2. Administer oxygen, naloxone, and glucose to those patients with an unexplained decreased level of consciousness.
> 3. Obtain history from patient, caretaker, emergency medical service provider, or other accompanying person. What and how much was taken, and when did it occur?
> 4. Examine the patient.
> 5. Obtain studies as required for the specific ingestant(s) of concern. Also obtain specific serum drug concentrations as indicated by the history and physical findings. A drug screen may be necessary, but its results are rarely required on an emergent basis.
> 6. Administer activated charcoal in water to all patients with potentially toxic ingestions presenting within 4 hours of overdose unless a substance not absorbed by activated charcoal has been ingested (see box on p. 531). A nasogastric tube is required for all young children and for those adolescents who will not voluntarily drink it. Concomitant cathartic therapy is not recommended.
> 7. Administer an antidote if indicated.
> 8. Consider admission to hospital.
> 9. Ensure that a psychiatric assessment is obtained for all purposeful overdose patients who are not admitted to the hospital.
> 10. Provide education and poison prevention information for nontoxic ingestions.

---

esophagoscopy for caustics. The issues of when to do a drug screen, a specific serum drug concentration, or an x-ray film of the abdomen pertain to drug ingestions in general.

Drug Screens and Specific Drug Concentrations. Emergency drug screens rarely aid clinical decisions.[16,17] Usually drug screens are ordered when poisoning is suspected as the cause of a decreased level of consciousness, unexplained seizures, or sudden onset of unusual behavior. Specimens of both urine and blood are screened for a large panel of potential toxins. However, results uncommonly aid emergency department clinical decisions.[16,17] One reason for this is their relatively long turnaround time. In addition, the clinical sensitivity of toxic screens is less than acceptable because it is impossible to screen for all potential toxins. Specificity is even less acceptable from both the laboratory and clinical perspectives. Because it is a screening test, laboratory "gold standards" are not used, resulting in the potential for inaccurate identifications. Because toxic screens, by definition, only qualitatively identify the presence of a substance, a cause-and-effect relationship between the presence of a toxin and the clinical findings is not proved. Thus drug screens contribute little to acute

Specific Quantitative Laboratory Analyses Needed on an Emergent Basis
Acetaminophen Salicylate Methanol Ethylene glycol Iron Theophylline Lithium Carbon monoxide

Substances Not Absorbed by Activated Charcoal
Simple ions (e.g., iron, lithium, and cyanide) Strong acids or bases (e.g., hydrochloric acid and sodium hydroxide) Simple alcohols (e.g., ethanol and methanol)

management decisions and are rarely required on an emergent basis.

On the other hand, specific quantitative drug analyses can be helpful. Those needed on an emergent basis (less than 1 hour turnaround time) have specific management interventions based on their results and are listed in the box above.

Radiology. The mnemonic *CHIPS* is often used to help remember radiopaque medications. The letters stand for *c*horal hydrate, *h*eavy metals, *i*ron, *p*henothiazines, and *s*low release (enteric-coated pharmaceuticals).[18] This categorization is based on in vitro investigations; however, additional investigation and clinical experience have demonstrated that an x-ray film of the abdomen is useful only in iron poisoning.[18-20] It can validate that ingestion has occurred and can assess the effectiveness of GI decontamination[21] (Fig. 42-3). Recently, ultrasound has been investigated as a means of identifying the presence of pharmaceutical material within the GI tract. However, additional research and experience are required.[22,23]

SPECIFIC ANTIPOISONING MANAGEMENT
(See Chapter 43)

Preventing Absorption

Ipecac and Gastric Lavage. Prevention of absorption is one of the fundamental principles of acute overdose management. The classic approach has been the use of either syrup of ipecac to induce vomiting or orogastric lavage, one of the so-called gastric-emptying procedures, followed by activated charcoal administration as an adjunctive intervention.[24,25] Since the mid 1980s, research has resulted in a reappraisal and modification of this approach toward using activated charcoal as the sole intervention.[26-35] Although it is fundamentally difficult to prove or disprove the effectiveness of interventions in acute overdose patients, the recent literature dealing with gastric emptying procedures has approached this issue from several perspectives.

One method has been to demonstrate unimpressive prevention of absorption in controlled studies using urinary and drug excretion data and radiologic markers.[28-30] Another approach has been direct evidence of the ineffectiveness using radiologic (see Fig. 42-3) and endoscopic data derived from human volunteer models.[31-33] Most important, however, is the demonstrated lack of impact on patient outcome when these interventions are not used.[34-36]

Gastric lavage is especially worrisome because in addition to its questionable effectiveness, it is associated with the most significant and frequent complications, which occurred at a rate of 3% in one series.[37] The resultant problems include pulmonary aspiration (despite airway protection), cardiorespiratory dysfunction, and esophageal trauma.[36,38]

Charcoal's efficacy has not been demonstrated; it may have only limited benefits. Considering all of the data currently available, I neither use nor recommend syrup of ipecac to induce vomiting or orogastric lavage in the treatment of overdose patients.

Activated Charcoal.[39] Activated charcoal binds toxins to its surface, and being nonabsorbable, the charcoal-toxin complex passes harmlessly through the GI tract. The bond between charcoal and the toxin is reversible, but desorption is minimized by giving large doses of charcoal. Charcoal can be regarded as a universal absorbant, and it is easier to remember what it does not efficiently bind rather than what it does bind (see box above).

The dose of activated charcoal should be as large as can be practically administered. A reasonable guideline is 25 to 50 gm for children younger than 6 years old and 50 to 100 gm for adolescents. Other dose recommendations include 10 times the dose of the ingested toxin or 1.0 gm/kg of patient. The first is impractical, since the dose of the ingestant is rarely known; the second is irrational. Since charcoal is devoid of agonist activity, there is no need to base its dose on the patient's weight. Since the presence of food and digestive juices compete for available charcoal binding sites, this dose is less likely to be effective in young children who would only receive 10 to 15 gm of charcoal by this criterion. Competition for charcoal binding sites by GI contents is supported by the data of Levy and Tsuchiya,[40] which show that the more charcoal, the better the outcome, even at a constant charcoal/drug ratio.

Activated charcoal in water is often recommended to be given to all patients with potentially toxic ingestions within 4 hours of overdose unless a substance found in the box above has been ingested. Generally a nasogastric tube is required for all young children and for those adolescents who will not voluntarily drink it. The only complication is aspiration. Although the mixture is inert, if enough is aspirated, its physical presence can compromise gas exchange. Therefore, caution is required for patients with a decreased level of consciousness, absent gag reflex, or seizures.

Cathartics. Concomitant cathartic administration with charcoal is best avoided. Two reasons often cited for recommending this practice are to prevent charcoal-induced constipation and to hasten the GI transit time so that it will

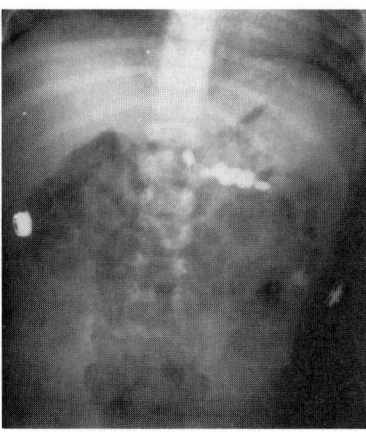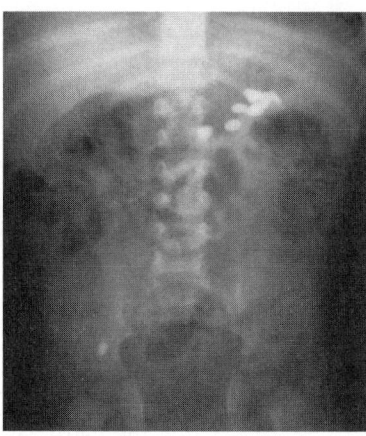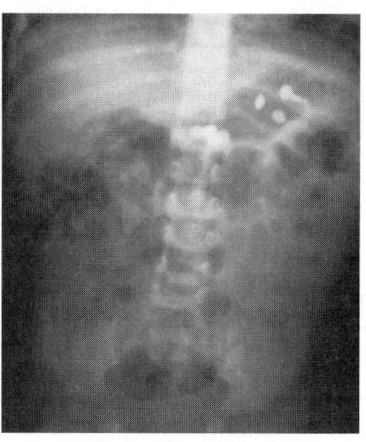

FIG. 42-3. Abdominal radiograph studies of a 17-month-old boy who has ingested ferrous sulfate tablets. *Left,* admission x-ray film shows nine tablets in the stomach. *Center,* the nine tablets remain after administration of syrup of ipecac and three episodes of emesis. *Right,* eight tablets remain after orogastric lavage (one tablet was vomited during the passage of the tube). (*From Tenenbein M:* J Emerg Med *3:133-136, 1985.*)

minimize drug absorption should it desorb from charcoal. Charcoal-induced constipation in the ambulatory patient has not been documented; even if it does occur, diarrhea induction hardly seems a reasonable alternative. Desorption of toxin from charcoal is overcome by administering large charcoal doses. If desorption occurs at all, the amount involved would be relatively small and unlikely to alter the patient's clinical course.

Moreover, at least five human studies do not demonstrate benefit from the addition of cathartics to charcoal.[41-45] A modest treatment effect was demonstrated in a charcoal sorbitol model, the extent of which is of questionable clinical significance.[46] The cathartic sorbitol rapidly produces intense diarrhea and thirst. Aside from discomfort, the fluid lost from the gut stresses the intravascular volume and may decrease renal blood flow, which can reduce renal drug clearance. Large fluid shifts can occur[47] and this cathartic should be avoided in young children.

Whole-Bowel Irrigation. Whole-bowel irrigation can decrease toxin absorption from the GI tract.[32,48-53] It involves the rapid administration of a specialized fluid, polyethylene glycol electrolyte lavage solution (Colyte, GoLYTELY) by nagogastric tube. It should be reserved for situations in which charcoal would be expected to have no or limited benefit, such as ingestion of a large amount of a toxic substance (e.g., many times the lethal dose), late presentation after the overdose, ingestion of a modified release pharmaceutical, and ingestion of a substance not absorbed by activated charcoal. Contraindications include bowel perforation, obstruction, ileus, or GI hemorrhage.

It is best to avoid prior treatment with syrup of ipecac because such patients often do not tolerate the subsequent whole-bowel irrigation. Caution is required in patients with a decreased level of consciousness or otherwise compromised airway. A nasogastric tube is essential because overdose patients will not drink the required volume of irrigation solution. Activated charcoal can be administered immediately before starting whole-bowel irrigation; multiple doses should not be given during the procedure because the polyethylene glycol of the irrigation solution binds to the charcoal, rendering the latter ineffective.[54] A

commode is convenient for both the patient and the nursing staff. The intravenous administration of metoclopramide may be required to control ingestant-or procedural-induced vomiting. The rate of irrigation is 1.5 to 2.0 L/hr for adolescents and adults and 500 ml/hr for toddlers and preschoolers. The end point, which may take several hours to reach, occurs when the rectal effluent is similar in appearance to the infusate.

Other Routes of Exposure. Beside ingestion, other routes of exposure to toxins and noxious agents include dermatologic, ocular, and respiratory. It is important to discontinue exposure as soon as possible. The skin and eye should be flushed with tap water for several minutes. Depending on anatomic considerations, flushing can be achieved by placement of the exposed body part under a running tap, a whole body shower, or by pouring pitchers of water over the exposed area. Eye irrigation is best achieved by using a standard intravenous infusion set, holding the tubing an inch from the eye. Duration of irrigation should be several minutes. In some situations, such as cutaneous exposure to pesticides, it may be necessary for the caregiver to take personal protective precautions such as wearing resistant gloves and aprons.

Hastening Elimination

Diuresis. There is virtually no role for diuresis in the management of the acutely poisoned patient.[55] Theoretically, for diuresis to be effective, the drug must have a small volume of distribution and low protein binding, and a large fraction of the pharmacologically active agent must be excreted in the urine. Salicylate is one of the few poisons that fulfills these criteria. However, diuresis is not without risk in salicylate poisoning, with fluid retention and pulmonary and cerebral edema being specific complications. Moreover, urinary alkalinization is more important than diuresis in the management of salicylate poisoning.[56]

Alkalinization or Acidification of the Urine. Urinary pH manipulation can increase the excretion of weak acids or bases by maintaining the drug in its ionic state within the renal tubule, thereby preventing its reabsorption into the circulation. However, this approach is useful in only a few situations. Urinary alkalinization should be considered for salicylate and phenobarbital poisonings. Urinary acidification has been recommended for phencyclidine, amphetamine, quinidine, and strychnine poisonings. However, acidification of the plasma is not without danger; patients are concurrently at risk for both seizures and rhabdomyolysis. Because of these concerns and because this intervention is unproved, urinary acidification should not be used.

Multiple Dose Activated Charcoal Therapy. The administration of several doses of activated charcoal every few hours enhances the clearance of some drugs from the blood such as phenobarbital and theophylline.[57,58] The chief mechanism is believed to be that of promoting back diffusion of drug from the blood into the gut and has been referred to as GI dialysis.[59] Although interruption of enterohepatic circulation has also been suggested as one of the mechanisms, not all drugs circulate in this way; of those that do, the amounts involved are too small to be clinically significant.

Protocols are empirical, ranging from 10 to 50 gm of charcoal every 1 to 4 hours. Cathartics should not be given with these repeated charcoal doses because of the risk of iatrogenic fluid and electrolyte disturbances. Complications of multiple dose charcoal therapy include intestinal obstruction and pulmonary aspiration.[60] It should be avoided in patients with bowel obstruction or ileus and used cautiously in any patient with an unprotected airway. It should be particularly avoided in patients poisoned by cyclic antidepressants.[61,62] This intervention has not been shown to be clinically beneficial and because complications have been reported, routine use cannot be recommended. The clinician must weigh the theoretical benefits against the risks of complications in individual patients.

Dialysis and Hemoperfusion. Peritoneal and hemodialysis, charcoal, and resin hemoperfusion are methods of enhancing excretion of previously absorbed toxins.[63] They play a limited role in the management of poisoned patients. Peritoneal dialysis is rarely used. Its main strength is that, unlike hemodialysis, it does not require a referral center for its implementation. However, the latter is more effective. Hemodialysis should be considered only for poisonings from agents with a small volume of distribution and low protein binding. In actual practice it should be considered only for salicylate, methanol, ethylene glycol, and phenobarbital. Hemoperfusion is similar to hemodialysis, except that a charcoal or resin cartridge is substituted for the dialysis machine. This removes toxin from the blood by adsorption but unlike dialysis does not correct imbalances of homeostasis. Usually it is used in severe theophylline poisoning; controlled evidence for its efficacy in any poisoning is lacking. The main risk of hemodialysis and hemoperfusion is hemorrhage because of the need for anticoagulation.

Antidotes

Antidote is probably the first word that comes to mind when the word poison is mentioned. The cornerstone of the care of the poisoned patient, however, is meticulous, supportive care. The few antidotes available for the treatment of specific poisonings are listed in Table 42-1 and are discussed in detail in Chapter 43.

TABLE 42-1. Antidotes

Agent	Antidote
Carbon monoxide	Oxygen
Opiates	Naloxone
Acetaminophen	N-acetylcysteine
Methanol	Ethanol and folic acid*
Ethylene glycol	Ethanol
Iron	Deferoxamine
Cyanide	Cyanide antidote kit (Lilly)
Cholinesterase-inhibiting pesticides organophosphates carbamates	Atropine and pralidoxime* atropine
Isoniazid	Pyridoxine
Beta blockers	Glucagon
Sulfonylurea oral hypoglycemics	Diazoxide
Digoxin	Digoxin-specific Fab antibody fragments
Methemoglobinemia inducers	Methylene blue
Dystonia inducers	Benzotropine or diphenhydramine

*Adjunctive agents.

CHILD ABUSE BY POISONING

Child abuse by poisoning has been reviewed elsewhere.[64] Its diagnosis requires a high index of suspicion, since the poisoning is almost always concealed. The usual perpetrator is the mother, and the motivation is usually no different from physical child abuse or Munchausen syndrome by proxy.[64] In the latter situation, abuse often continues after hospitalization. Routine toxic screens should not be the sole evidence for making the diagnosis. The presence and the amount of the toxin should be confirmed by a second assay of "gold standard" stature. After stabilization, management requires the multidisciplinary approach used for other child abuse situations (see also Chapter 45).

References

1. Litovitz TL, Clark LR, Soloway RA. 1993 Annual report of the American Association of Poison Control Centers Toxic Exposure Surveillance System. *Am J Emerg Med* 1994;12:546-584.

Pharmacokinetics and Toxicokinetics

2. Zathurecky L: Progress in developing a standard terminology in biopharmaceutics and pharmacokinetics, *Drug Intell Clin Pharm* 11:281-296, 1977.
3. Ranade VV: Drug delivery systems 5A. Oral drug delivery, *J Clin Pharmacol* 31:2-16, 1991.
4. Kendall MJ and John VA: The role of clinical pharmacology in the development and evaluation of oral controlled-release dosage forms, *Br J Clin Pharmacol* 19:655-675, 1985.
5. Mitchell JF and Pawlicki KS: Oral dosage forms that should not be crushed: 1990 revision, *Hosp Pharm* 25:329-335, 1990.
6. Kwong TC, Laczin J, Baum J: Self-poisoning with enteric-coated aspirin, *Am J Clin Pathol* 80:888-890, 1983.
7. Kaufman FL and Dubansky AS: Darvon poisoning with delayed salicylism: a case report, *Pediatrics* 49:610-611, 1972.
8. Henry AF: Overdoses of entrophen, *Can Med Assoc J* 128:1142, 1983.
9. Robertson NJ: Fatal overdose from a sustained-release theophylline preparation, *Ann Emerg Med* 14:154-158, 1985.
10. Clayton D and Bochner F: Delayed toxicity with slow release theophylline, *Med J Aust* 144:386-387, 1986.

11. Corser BC, Young C, Boughman RP: Prolonged toxicity following massive ingestion of sustained-release theophylline preparation, *Chest* 88:749-750, 1985.

The Acutely Ill Overdose Patient

12. Mofenson HC and Caraccio TR: Toxidromes, *Compr Ther* 11:46-52, 1985.
13. Hoffman JR, Schriger DL, Luo JS: The empiric use of naloxone in patients with altered mental status. A reappraisal, *Ann Emerg Med* 20:246-252, 1991.
14. Braden NJ, Jackson JE, Walson PD: Tricyclic antidepressant overdose, *Ped Clin North Am* 33:287-297, 1986.
15. Zweiner RJ and Ginsburg CM: Organophosphate and carbamate poisoning in infants and children, *Pediatrics* 81:121-126, 1988.

The Stable Overdose Patient

16. Osterloh JD: Utility and reliability of emergency toxicologic testing, *Emerg Med Clin North Am* 8:693-723, 1990.
17. Kellermann AL, Fihn SD, Lo Gerfo JP et al: Impact of drug screening in suspected overdose, *Ann Emerg Med* 16:1206-1216, 1987.
18. Savitt DL, Hawkins HH, Roberts JR: The radiopacity of ingested medications, *Ann Emerg Med* 16:331-339, 1987.
19. Handy CA: Radiopacity of oral nonliquid medications, *Radiology* 98:525-533, 1971.
20. O'Brien RP, McGeehan PA, Helmeczi AW et al: Detectability of drug tablets and capsules by plain radiography, *Am J Emerg Med* 4:302-312, 1986.
21. Staple TW and McAlister WH: Roentgenographic visualization of iron preparations in the gastrointestinal tract, *Radiology* 83:1051-1056, 1964.
22. Amitai Y, Silver B, Leiken JB et al: Detection of tablets in the gastrointestinal tract by ultrasound (abstract), *Vet Hum Toxicol* 32:354, 1990.
23. Anderson AC, Share JC, Woolf AD: The use of ultrasound in the diagnosis of toxic ingestions (abstract), *Vet Hum Toxicol* 32:355, 1990.

Specific Antipoisoning Management

24. Cupit GC and Temple AR: Gastrointestinal decontamination in the management of the poisoned patient, *Emerg Med Clin North Am* 2:15-28, 1984.
25. Rogers GC and Matyunas NJ: Gastrointestinal decontamination for acute poisoning, *Pediatr Clin North Am* 33:261-285, 1986.
26. Greensher J, Mofenson HC, Caraccio TR: Ascendency of the black bottle (activated charcoal), *Pediatrics* 80:949-951, 1987.
27. Vale JA, Meredith TJ, Proudfoot AT: Syrup of ipecacuanha: is it really useful? *Br Med J* 293:1321-1322, 1986.
28. Curtis RA, Barone J, Giacona N: Efficacy of ipecac and activated charcoal/cathartic, prevention of salicylate absorption in a simulated overdose, *Arch Intern Med* 144:48-52, 1984.
29. Tenenbein M, Cohen S, Sitar DS: Efficacy of ipecac-induced emesis, orogastric lavage and activated charcoal for acute drug overdose, *Ann Emerg Med* 16:838-841, 1987.
30. Saetta JP, March S, Gaunt ME et al: Gastric emptying procedures in the self-poisoned patient: are we forcing gastric content beyond the pylorus? *J Royal Soc Med* 84:274-276, 1991.
31. Tenenbein M: Inefficacy of gastric emptying procedures, *J Emerg Med* 3:133-136, 1985.
32. Tenenbein M: Whole bowel irrigation in iron poisoning, *J Pediatr* 111:142-145, 1987.
33. Saetta JP and Quinton DN: Residual gastric content after gastric lavage and ipecacuana-induced emesis in self-poisoned patients: an endoscopic study, *J Royal Soc Med* 84:35-38, 1991.
34. Kulig K, Bar-Or D, Cantrill SV et al: Management of acutely poisoned patients without gastric emptying, *Ann Emerg Med* 14:562-567, 1985.
35. Albertson TE, Derlet RW, Foulke GE et al: Superiority of activated charcoal alone compared with ipecac and activated charcoal in the treatment of acute toxic ingestions, *Ann Emerg Med* 18:56-59, 1989.
36. Merigian KS, Woodard M, Hedges JR et al: Prospective evaluation of gastric emptying in the self-poisoned patient, *Am J Emerg Med* 8:479-483, 1990.

37. Matthew H, Mackintosh TF, Tompsett SL et al: Gastric aspiration and lavage in acute poisoning, *Br Med J* 1:1333-1337, 1966.
38. Thompson AM, Robins JB, Prescott LF: Changes in cardiorespiratory function during gastric lavage for drug overdose, *Hum Toxicol* 6:215-218, 1987.
39. Neuvonen PJ: Clinical pharmacokinetics of oral activated charcoal in acute intoxications, *Clin Pharmacokinet* 7:465-489, 1982.
40. Levy G and Tsuchiya T: Effect of activated charcoal on aspirin absorption in man, *Clin Pharmacol Ther* 13:317-322, 1972.
41. Mayersohm M, Perrier D, Picchioni AL: Evaluation of charcoal-sorbitol mixture as an antidote for oral aspirin overdose, *Clin Toxicol* 11:561-567, 1977.
42. Easom JM, Caraccio TR, Lovejoy FH Jr: Evaluation of activated charcoal and magnesium citrate in the prevention of aspirin absorption in humans, *Clin Pharm* 1:154-156, 1982.
43. Sketris IS, Mowry JB, Czajka PA et al: Saline catharsis: effect on aspirin bioavailability in combination with activated charcoal, *J Clin Pharmacol* 22:59-64, 1982.
44. Neuvonen PJ and Olkkola KT: Effect of purgatives on antidotal efficacy of oral activated charcoal, *Hum Toxicol* 5:255-263, 1986.
45. McNamara R, Aaron CK, Gemborys M et al: Sorbitol catharsis does not enhance efficacy of charcoal in a simulated acetaminophen overdose, *Ann Emerg Med* 17:243-246, 1988.
46. Keller RE, Schwab RA, Krenzelok EP: Contribution of sorbitol combined with activated charcoal in prevention of salicylate absorption, *Ann Emerg Med* 19:654-656, 1990.
47. Farley TA: Severe hypernatremic dehydration after use of an activated charcoal-sorbitol suspension, *J Pediatr* 109:719-722, 1986.
48. Tenenbein M: Whole bowel irrigation as a gastrointestinal decontamination procedure after acute poisoning, *Med Toxicol* 3:77-84, 1988.
49. Tenenbein M, Cohen S, Sitar DS: Whole bowel irrigation as a decontamination procedure after acute drug overdose, *Arch Intern Med* 147:905-907, 1987.
50. Kirshenbaum A, Mathews SC, Sitar DS et al: Whole bowel irrigation vs activated charcoal in sorbitol for the ingestion of modified release pharmaceuticals, *Clin Pharmacol Ther* 46:264-271, 1989.
51. Burkhart KK, Kulig KK, Rumack B: Whole bowel irrigation as treatment for zinc sulfate overdose, *Ann Emerg Med* 19:1167-1170, 1990.
52. Hoffman RS, Smilkstein MJ, Goldfrank LR: Whole bowel irrigation and the cocaine body packer, *Am J Emerg Med* 8:523-527, 1990.
53. Smith SS, Ling LJ, Halstenson CE: Whole-bowel irrigation as a treatment for acute lithium overdose, *Ann Emerg Med* 20:536-539, 1991.
54. Kirshenbaum LA, Sitar DS, Tenenbein M: Interaction between whole bowel irrigation solution and activated charcoal. Implications for the treatment of toxic ingestions, *Ann Emerg Med* 19:1129-1132, 1990.
55. Todd JW: Do measures to enhance drug removal save life? *Lancet* 1:331, 1984.
56. Prescott LF, Balali-Mood M, Critchley JAJH et al: Diuresis or urinary alkalinization for salicylate poisoning? *Br Med J* 285:1383-1386, 1982.
57. Berg MJ, Berlinger WJ, Goldberg MJ et al: Acceleration of the body clearance of phenobarbital by oral activated charcoal, *N Engl J Med* 307:642-644, 1982.
58. Berlinger WJ, Spector R, Goldberg MJ et al: Enhancement of theophylline clearance by oral activated charcoal, *Clin Pharmacol Ther* 33:351-354, 1983.
59. Levy G: Gastrointestinal clearance of drugs with activated charcoal, *N Engl J Med* 307:676-678, 1982.
60. Tenenbein M: Multiple doses of activated charcoal: time for reappraisal? *Ann Emerg Med* 20:529-531, 1991.
61. Goldberg MJ, Park GD, Spector R et al: Lack of effect of oral activated charcoal on imipramine clearance, *Clin Pharmacol Ther* 37:367-371, 1985.
62. Harsch HH: Aspiration of activated charcoal, *N Engl J Med* 314:318, 1986.
63. Peterson RG and Peterson LN: Cleansing the blood. Hemodialysis, peritoneal dialysis, exchange transfusion, charcoal hemoperfusion, forced diuresis, *Pediatr Clin North Am* 33:675-689, 1986.

Child Abuse by Poisoning

64. Tenenbein M: Child abuse by poisoning, *Curr Probl Pediatr* 16:198-206, 1986.

Specific Toxins

Gary S. Wasserman • *Thomas T. Mydler* • *Vidya Sharma*

It is estimated that 95% to 99% of poisoned patients can survive if management is initiated before the onset of significant signs and symptoms regardless of whether the poison is known on presentation. Only a small percentage of poison cases require a specific antidote to reverse the life-threatening effects of the toxin. Permanent toxic sequelae and survival are much improved if symptomatic and supportive treatment is instituted before the patient suffers respiratory or cardiovascular compromise, hypoxemia, metabolic acidosis, or prolonged seizure activity.

When treating any poisoned patient, the principles of stabilization and support are paramount: (1) immediately correct life-threatening problems by use of airway, breathing, and circulation (ABC); (2) prevent further absorption of toxins from the gastrointestinal (GI) tract with the use of emesis or lavage, activated charcoal, and cathartics or whole-bowel irrigation; (3) enhance excretion of toxins already absorbed by the use of diuresis (forced or alkaline) or dialysis and other modalities; (4) administer an antidote if available; and (5) provide symptomatic and supportive care, as they are the cornerstones of management (see Chapter 42).

Initial stabilization must focus on the ABCs. An IV line is established with potentially serious ingestions. Any patient with altered mental status, seizures, or coma generally should receive oxygen at 2 to 10 L/min, dextrose (0.5 to 1 gm [2 to 4 ml D2.5W]/kg/IV]), and naloxone (0.1 mg/kg up to 2 mg, initially IV). A careful history and physical examination are essential. Management of specific clinical presentations such as seizures and altered mental states is discussed in Chapter 56.

GI decontamination remains controversial. Emesis or lavage is unlikely to be beneficial unless performed within 1 to 2 hours of ingestion or if the ingested drug delays gastric emptying. Beyond this time, administration of charcoal is probably the most beneficial approach but also has its skeptics.

Emesis induced by *syrup of ipecac* is reserved for specific recent ingestions that are potentially toxic. It is generally not given to children under 12 months of age; those 1 to 12 years receive 15 ml and older children should receive 30 ml or 1 oz. It should not be given to children who are comatose, have central nervous system (CNS) depression, are experiencing or at risk for convulsions, have no gag reflex, are under 6 months of age, or have a bleeding diathesis. It should also be avoided if ingestion involves a caustic. Ipecac is more likely to be used in the home than in the emergency department. It will delay the use of activated charcoal and other orally administered antidotes.

Lavage is indicated for patients who require stomach decontamination but are not candidates for ipecac. The procedure facilitates gastric emptying and administration of charcoal and cathartics. It is contraindicated for alkaline ingestion. A no. 24 to 42 Fr tube is inserted orally, and the patient is generally tilted slightly to the left side in the Trendelenburg position. Room temperature saline or half normal saline at 100 to 200 ml/pass in adults (10 ml/kg in children) is administered and repeated until the return is clear. Intubation may be helpful in protecting the airway but is rarely necessary in the child with an intact gag reflex.

Activated charcoal may be given orally after lavage, or 60 to 90 minutes after induced emesis. Generally, about 1 gm/kg is given, with adults receiving 50 to 100 gm charcoal and children 15 to 30 gm.

Cathartics are the least effective modality of the common GI decontamination methods. Magnesium citrate, 4 ml/kg to a maximum of 300 ml, or magnesium or sodium sulfate, 250 mg/kg orally (adults up to 30 gm), may speed GI transit and therefore decrease absorption. It is contraindicated in patients with renal failure, severe diarrhea, adynamic ileus, or abdominal trauma. Sorbitol is often mixed with charcoal for smoothness, sweetness, and osmotic catharsis. It is contraindicated in children less than 12 months of age because of fluid and electrolyte disturbances and should not be used in multiple dose regimens. The pediatric dose is not well established, but 1 gm/kg is generally used in a 35% concentration for children (maximum, 50 gm) and 70% for adults (maximum, 150 gm).

Laboratory evaluation should reflect the circumstances of each particular intoxication. A comprehensive toxicology screen or panel (qualitative identification) is best obtained from a urine or gastric specimen, whereas drug levels (quantitative amount) are performed on blood samples. The ordering physician must have a basic understanding of methodology, capabilities, limitations, and therapeutic and toxic ranges, as well as turnaround time to obtain results and approximate expense. Tests should be individualized but may include serum electrolytes, glucose, blood urea nitrogen (BUN), creatinine, liver function studies, and urinalysis. Complete blood count (CBC), blood gases, serum calcium, magnesium, ketone levels, prothrombin time (PT), partial thromboplastin time (PTT), electrocardiogram (ECG), and chest radiograph are also often needed. Fertile females, especially teenagers, should have a pregnancy test.

Differential considerations include many drugs (especially similar drugs in each class); medical, neurologic, surgical, and psychiatric conditions; infections; metabolic abnormalities; and trauma. Also to be considered are the malingerer, factitious illness patient, and "Münchausen by proxy" child.

Consultation with a variety of specialists is ordered according to the skills and experience of each practitioner. The local/regional poison control center should be consulted as appropriate. POISINDEX Information System, Micromedex, Inc, Denver, provides up-to-date information available on microfiche or computer tape/disk.[1]

The specific intoxications discussed were chosen because of their serious morbidity and mortality, as well as pediatric frequency of appearance in the emergency department. Management is clearly changing, and the guidelines of supportive and specific therapy must reflect the rapidly evolving toxicologic literature. Admissions for a toxicologic exposure at Children's Mercy Hospital in Kansas City, Missouri, for a 7-year period (1988 to 1994) revealed 862 patients or 2% of the total medical and surgical admissions. The top 15 categories were as follows:

1. Multiple drugs or chemicals (83)
2. Anticonvulsants (71)
3. Caustics (66)
4. Analgesics (62)
5. Cardiovascular drugs (61)
6. Lead (57)
7. Hydrocarbons (56)
8. Antidepressants (51)
9. Antipsychotics, sedatives, hypnotics (45)
10. Iron (43)
11. Alcohols (38)
12. Cough and cold preparations (34)
13. Bite and sting envenomations (34)
14. Stimulants and street drugs (27)
15. Bronchodilators (24)

Acetaminophen

THOMAS T. MYDLER • GARY S. WASSERMAN

Acetaminophen (paracetamol) is a synthetic opioid analgesic and antipyretic. Acetaminophen has become a common component of medicines and widely used in the health-care industry. Although recommended for childhood fevers in place of aspirin by the Centers for Disease Control (because of a suspected link between the development of Reye syndrome and the use of salicylates in influenza or varicella), large ingestions can lead to severe hepatic damage and death.[2] In 1994, overdoses related to acetaminophen numbered 103,616, of which 73,934 occurred in patients 19 years of age and under.[3]

Acetaminophen (N-acetyl-p-aminophenol, [APAP]) is manufactured in various forms including drops, elixir, chewable and junior tablets, adult tablets, extended relief, suppositories, and in combination in many over-the-counter cold remedies.

Pathophysiology

Absorption from the GI tract of acetaminophen is rapid, ranging from 70 minutes (mean peak plasma concentration) in a fasting individual, to 4 hours when gastric emptying has been slowed.[4,5] Therefore blood levels should not be drawn before 4 hours after administration.

Uniformly distributed throughout most body fluid, acetaminophen has a volume of distribution of approximately 0.75 L/kg. According to Michaelis-Menten (nonlinear saturable) kinetics, 90% of the acetaminophen dose is conjugated by the liver to sulfate or glucuronide, with children younger than 12 years of age primarily using the sulfate pathway.[6,7] Less than 5% is excreted unchanged by the kidney under first-order kinetics.[8] However, it is the metabolism of approximately 5% of the ingested dose by the hepatic cytochrome P-450 mixed function oxidase system to a reactive intermediary, N-acetyl-p-benzoquinoneimine (NAPQI), that probably accounts for the liver toxicity.[9] Normally, glutathione conjugates NAPQI to cysteine and mercapturate compounds.[10] In an overdose, the reactive metabolite NAPQI is formed in such a sufficiently large concentration that the glutathione stores with which it conjugates are unable to detoxify all of the compound, thus leaving enough of the metabolite available to covalently bind with the hepatocyte and produce immediate centrilobular hepatic necrosis. Another explanation for hepatotoxicity is that an overdose of acetaminophen may saturate the sulfate pathway, causing an increase in the amount of toxic intermediate compound.[11] Pathologically, acetaminophen intoxication causes a necrosis of the liver affecting the areas around the central vein.

A number of studies have shown a variation in the susceptibility of individuals to acetaminophen's toxicity.[8,12] Diet, nutritional status, age, chronic liver disease, and the ingestion of other drugs before or along with acetaminophen affect the activity of the cytochrome P-450 pathway and therefore the amount of toxic metabolite formed. For example, phenobarbital stimulates metabolism by the P-450 microsomal system and more severe hepatotoxicity has been described in phenobarbital enhanced hepatic enzyme systems.[13-15] In another study, severe liver damage occurred in only 8% of acetaminophen overdose patients not given antidotal therapy, even though 15% of these patients had acetaminophen levels in a toxic range.[12] Other drugs decrease the toxicity of acetaminophen by maintaining adequate glutathione stores in the hepatocyte to conjugate the probable toxic metabolite NAPQI to cysteine and mercapturate compounds.[10] In children younger than 5 years of age, Rumack reported that only 3 of 55 patients with toxic acetaminophen levels showed signs of elevation in hepatic aminotransferase.[16]

The plasma half-life for therapeutic doses of acetaminophen is approximately 2 to 3 hours and is similar for different ages. In patients with hepatic cirrhosis or intoxications, however, the elimination half-life increases.[16-18] A half-life greater than 4 hours suggests liver toxicity, whereas a half-life greater than 12 hours increases the possibility of hepatic coma.[8] When timing of the ingestion is uncertain, calculation of the half-life can provide an alternative indication of potential toxicity.

Diagnostic Findings

Clinical Findings. The clinical presentation of an acetaminophen overdose occurs in three stages depending on the quantity ingested, time elapsed to initiation of decontamination, and previous health and medical status as mentioned earlier. Initially, the patient exposed to an overdose of acetaminophen will present with little symptomatology. During the first 24 hours after ingestion, children will develop anorexia, nausea, and vomiting; lethargy and diaphoresis may also be noted. Coma or CNS depression early after exposure should make the physician suspicious of other drugs.[13] Because signs and symptoms are not marked in this initial stage, medical management is often delayed or not pursued. This false sense of security is reinforced by the middle stage, 24 to 48 hours postingestion, during which a subclinical increase in hepatic enzymes occurs. For a given toxic plasma level, adults have a higher incidence of hepatic aminotransferase elevation than do children.[17] Subjectively, the patient will be thought to be improving. In the final "hepatic" stage, 3 to 7 days after ingestion, the patient develops a progressive hepatic encephalopathy characterized by vomiting, jaundice, abdominal pain, bleeding, confusion, lethargy, and eventually coma. Hepatic necrosis and failure destroy 60% or more of the hepatocytes in the liver.[19] Other clinical problems occurring in this terminal stage are a severe coagulation disorder, including the possibility of disseminated intravascular coagulation; pancreatitis; and dysrhythmias. It is unclear whether the myocardial damage found during histologic examination is a direct result of acetaminophen

toxicity or hepatic failure. Renal damage may also appear in overdoses, a result of acute tubular necrosis from the toxic metabolite.[20,21]

Ancillary Data. Acetaminophen levels characterize the severity and management of potential intoxications. Based on the peak acetaminophen level 4 or more hours from the time of ingestion, the semilogarithmic nomogram developed by Rumack and Matthew[13,22] (Fig. 43-1) can be used to determine the relative risk of hepatic damage and need for administration of the antidote N-acetylcysteine (NAC). The nomogram is not applicable to chronic or acute-or-chronic exposures. The acetaminophen level is drawn between 4 and 12 hours from the time of ingestion. Therapeutic acetaminophen levels range from 5 to 20 μg/ml. On the nomogram, a line drawn from the 200 μg/ml point at 4 hours postingestion to the 25 μg/ml point at 16 hours postingestion represents those levels above which approximately 60% of adult patients develop elevated (>1,000 units) serum hepatic transaminases.[22] It is imperative, however, that treatment with NAC be instituted within 8 to 12 hours of ingestion for maximum efficacy. The new Tylenol ER (extended relief) preparation is monitored in the same way except that a second level is obtained at least 4 to 6 hours after the first level, and antidotal therapy is instituted if either level is above the "possible hepatic toxicity" line.

Some children who have been given cumulative doses of 150 mg/kg/24 hr of APAP for 2 to 4 days, 8 to 10 larger multiple doses of 400 mg/kg/24 hr over 32 hours, and 174 mg/kg/24 hr over 72 hours, respectively, developed hepatotoxicity that resolved spontaneously.[23-25] Other chronic moderate overdoses were fatal.[26-28] Children with an APAP level in the toxic range on the nomogram related to the last known dosage time should also be treated with NAC.

Extensive serum baseline values (chemistry panel) are required in all patients administered antidotal treatment. Patients who develop signs and symptoms of hepatotoxicity require close monitoring of coagulation ability, renal dysfunction, and cerebral edema from hepatic encephalopathy. Serum glucose levels should be checked regularly for hypoglycemia. Elevated unconjugated bilirubin levels and PT will indicate liver damage before hepatic enzymes may peak. Although serum transaminases usually peak in 3 to 5 days, significant elevations may occur in the first 24 hours.[29]

Differential Considerations

Although numerous poisonings may present with liver toxicity, some of the more common pediatric agents concern amanita mushrooms, certain hydrocarbons, some heavy metals, isoniazid, nonsteroidal antiinflammatory drugs, erythromycin estolate, some anticonvulsants, vitamin A, and steroids.

Management

If the patient presents within 4 to 6 hours after ingestion, gut decontamination should be instituted. However, unless the patient has coingested substances that would slow gastric emptying, late induction of emesis may delay the administration of the antidote NAC within 8 to 12 hours from exposure. It is essential to delineate the time of ingestion, draw acetaminophen levels no earlier than 4

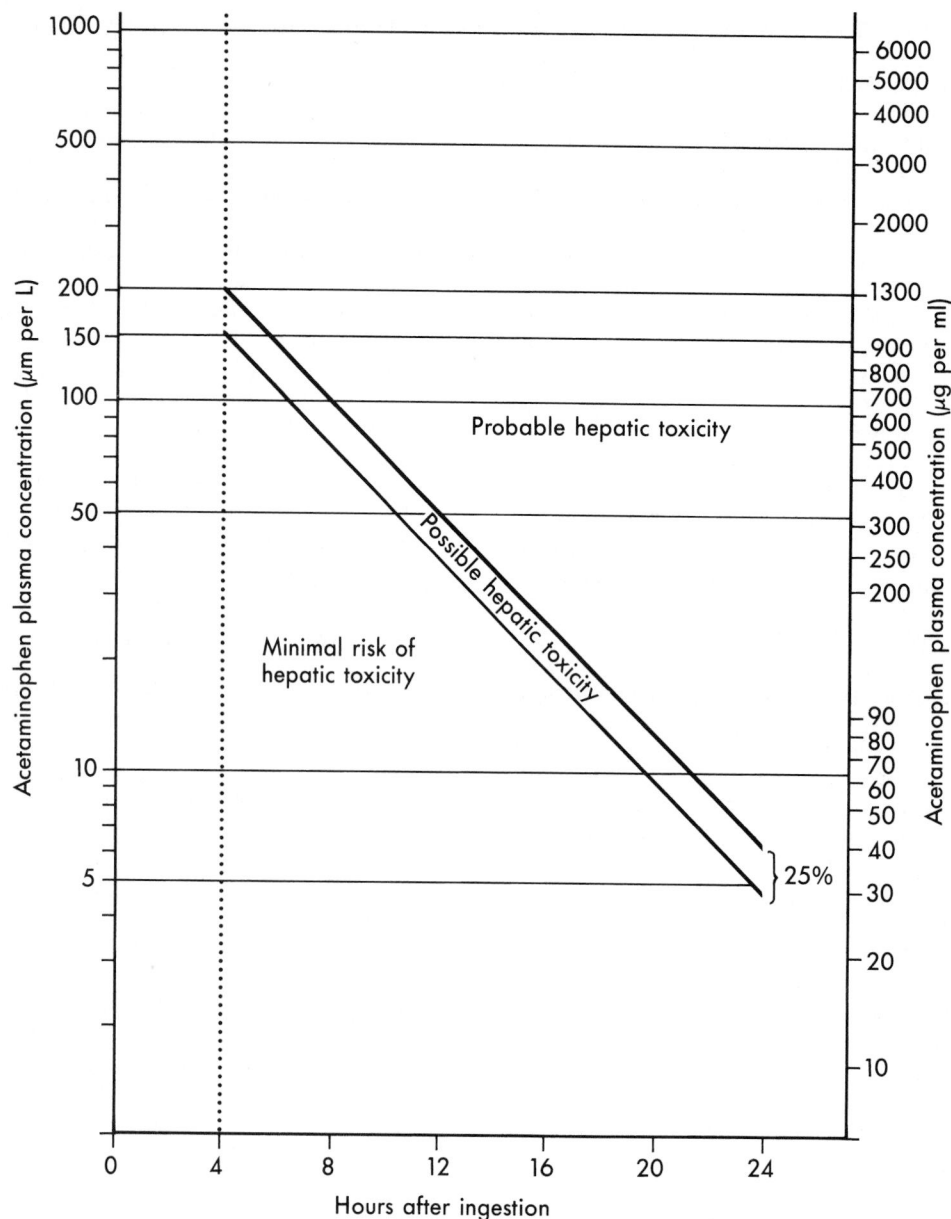

FIG. 43-1. Semilogarithmic plot of plasma acetaminophen levels vs. time. (*Adapted from Rumack RH and Matthews M: Pediatrics 55:871, 1975.*)

hours from exposure, and avoid delay in administration of NAC if indicated.

Controversy surrounds the use of activated charcoal and cathartics in acetaminophen ingestions, as both modalities interfere with the absorption of NAC.[27,28,30-32] Early in the course of an APAP ingestion, the use of charcoal may have been initiated before the administration of antidote; a 2-hour separation between antidote and charcoal is probably sufficient. The gastric lavage may reduce this time period. There is little value in the use of forced diuresis, hemodialysis, or charcoal hemoperfusion in preventing acetaminophen toxicity.[33-35] Vitamin K_1 is administered to patients with elevated PT (1.5 times the normal level); fresh frozen plasma may be needed in severe cases.

NAC, a precursor of glutathione, readily enters hepatocytes to block acetaminophen toxicity. It enhances glutathione stores and acts as a glutathione substitute.[36-38] NAC is the antidote of choice and should be initiated within 8 hours of an acetaminophen overdose for almost 100% effectiveness.[39] Delayed use of NAC resulted in toxicity ranging from 8% to 33% if initiated between 8 and 16 hours after ingestion and 4% to 50% between 16 to 24 hours after ingestion.[39] Only oral NAC (72-hour protocol) is approved for use in the United States, although the pyrogen-free intravenous form (48-hour regimen) is under investigation.[40] In Canada and Europe a 20-hour course of intravenous NAC has been used since the late 1970s.[41] Administration of NAC to children with APAP ingestions of

>200 mg/kg should not be delayed beyond 8 hours postingestion while waiting for a blood level. Treatment with NAC should be instituted based on the plasma level correlated to time after exposure, indicating the potential for hepatotoxicity from the Rumack and Matthew nomogram (see Fig. 43-1). Repeat monitoring of acetaminophen levels for one or two 4-hour intervals allows for the calculation of an APAP half-life. Once a previous result drawn at least 4 hours after ingestion is in or above the possible hepatic toxicity zone, NAC therapy should not be discontinued if a subsequent APAP level falls below this line on the nomogram. Treatment for pregnant adolescents with acetaminophen intoxication should follow the same protocol, as fetal hepatotoxicity is possible and NAC appears to protect both mother and fetus with no known teratogen effects.[42]

The oral loading dose of NAC is 140 mg/kg diluted to a 5% solution mixed in juice or sweet soda drink to mask the rotten egg smell and taste. Maintenance doses are 70 mg/kg every 4 hours for 17 more doses, for a total of 18 doses. If vomiting occurs within 1 hour of ingestion, the dose should be repeated. NAC is available as a 10% (100 mg/ml) or 20% (200 mg/ml) Mucomyst solution. A 5% oral preparation is concocted by mixing the calculated dose volume of Mucomyst with either an equal (if 10%) or three times (if 20%) that volume of drink (i.e., a 10 kg infant requiring a maintenance dose of 70 mg/kg NAC should be given 3.5 ml of 20% Mucomyst mixed with 10.5 ml of dilutant). Side effects from NAC are mainly related to GI distress. Sometimes it is helpful to cover the NAC preparation and have the patient drink it through a straw. Persistent vomiting may require the use of an antiemetic such as metoclopramide (Reglan), 1 mg/kg IV or IM 30 minutes before NAC. Some pediatricians concomitantly administer diphenhydramine (Benadryl) to block potential dystonic reactions from the metoclopramide. If the patient continues vomiting or develops CNS depression, an alternative method of administration is a 30 to 60 minute drip through a nasogastric tube or a radiographically placed duodenal tube.

Disposition

Children whose serum acetaminophen levels are in the "minimal risk of hepatic toxicity" range on the nomogram or in whom ingestion is definitely < 140 mg/kg may be sent home with a recommendation for routine follow-up by their physician. Suicidal gesture-attempt should be excluded. Patients who are potentially hepatotoxic by the nomogram are admitted for antidote therapy, which may be initiated immediately in the emergency department depending on the time after ingestion.

Untreated overdose patients who are asymptomatic and present to the emergency department more than 24 hours after ingestion can be monitored daily as an outpatient or admitted for renal and coagulation observation and hepatic protection. It may be appropriate to begin NAC therapy after more than 24 hours postingestion, but consultation should be sought.

The Rocky Mountain Poison and Drug Center in Denver (1-800-525-6115) has the most experience dealing with unusual and difficult acetaminophen treatment decisions.

If no local toxicology assistance is available, physicians may call for consultation.

Alcohols (Ethanol, Isopropanol, and Methanol) and Ethylene Glycol

THOMAS T. MYDLER • GARY S. WASSERMAN

Because of their ubiquitous presence in the home, the alcohols (ethanol, isopropanol, methanol) and ethylene glycol are responsible for some of the most common intoxications in children, totaling 62,585 exposures in 1994.[43] These substances, along with acetone, are discussed individually, although the signs and symptoms of their toxicity and the treatment for acute intoxications may be similar. Close attention to the patient's history, physical examination, and laboratory analyses will aid in accurate and early diagnosis, thus avoiding some of the long-term complications including respiratory embarrassment and renal failure.

Differential Considerations

Ethanol, methanol, isopropanol, and ethylene glycol all produce similar symptoms in acute intoxication, although the effects of methanol and ethylene glycol are usually delayed until the parent compound is metabolized. Certain findings help differentiate the various alcohols (Table 43-1). Renal failure and ophthalmologic changes, as well as hypocalcemia and oxaluria, are often present with ethylene glycol poisoning. Acetonemia and a sweet ketotic breath suggest isopropanol or acetone intoxication.

Severe metabolic acidosis with a large anion gap distinguishes methanol and ethylene glycol from isopropanol and ethanol poisonings; the latter two alcohols produce more CNS depression but less metabolic acidosis. Acetone also causes a metabolic acidosis and depressed sensorium. The anion gap is equal to the difference between the measured cations of sodium (Na^+) and potassium (K^+) and the measured anions of chloride (Cl^- and bicarbonate (HCO_3^-).

$$[(Na^+) + (K^+)] - [(Cl^-) + (HCO_3^-]$$

Normally, the anion gap in pediatrics is 8 to 14 mEq/L. In the presence of other organic acids, however, this gap is increased (i.e., > 12 to 14 mEq/L). An elevated anion gap with severe metabolic acidosis is characteristic of methanol and ethylene glycol intoxication and in chronic abuse of ethanol. Other etiologies of an increased anion gap with metabolic acidosis can best be recalled with the mnemonic, *MUDPILES* (see Chapter 15):

M Methanol
U Uremia
D Diabetic ketoacidosis
P Paraldehyde, phenformin (no longer available in United States)
I Iron, isoniazid, ibuprofen, inhalants (H_2S, CN, CO)
L Lactic acidosis—secondary to shock, hemorrhage, sepsis, leukemia, pancreatitis
E Ethylene glycol, ethanol—chronic abuse
S Salicylates, solvents (benzenes, toluene)

TABLE 43-1. Alcohol Ingestion and Overdose: Diagnostic Findings

	Ethanol	Isopropyl alcohol	Methanol	Ethylene glycol	Acetone
Toxic dose	0.72 ml/kg 600 mg/kg	0.3 ml/kg 300 mg/kg	0.14 ml/kg 120 mg/kg	0.11 mg/kg 120 mg/kg	0.48 mg/kg 300 mg/kg
Common sources	Beverages, mouth-washes, colognes	Solvents, rubbing alcohol, deicers, antiseptics	Solvents, wind-shield deicer, gas line anti-freeze, Sterno	Solvents, radiator antifreeze	Solvents, nail polish removers
Increased anion gap acidosis	Alcoholic ketoacidosis (chronic abuse)	Absent	Marked	Moderate to marked	Absent
Ketosis	Alcoholic ketoacidosis (chronic abuse)	Marked	Absent	Absent	Marked
Onset of clinical or laboratory abnormalities	Early, within 1 hr	Early, within 1 hr	Delayed, especially if ingested with ethanol	May be delayed, especially if ingested with ethanol	Early, within 1 hr
CNS excitation	Early, mild Seizures from withdrawal	Absent	Seizures	Seizures	Absent
CNS depression	Moderate lethargy, ataxia, coma possible	Severe coma, respiratory depression common	Moderate vertigo, confusion, weakness, coma possible	Moderate lethargy, ataxia, coma possible	Severe coma, respiratory depression common
GI symptoms	Moderate	Common, severe potential GI bleeding	Common, occasionally severe	Common, mild	Moderate
Breath odor	Fruity	Sweet, fruity	None	Sweet	Fruity
Diagnostic clues	Rapid resolution, nystagmus	Prolonged intoxication, nystagmus	Visual symptoms, more sick than intoxicated	Calcium oxalate crystalluria, renal failure, more sick than intoxicated	Prolonged intoxication, hyperglycemia, paresthesias

CNS, Central nervous system; *GI*, gastrointestinal.
Adapted from *Top Emerg Med* 6:33, 1984.

Management

Monitoring vital signs and mental status is essential to the supportive care required in alcohol and ethylene glycol intoxications. Airway management, ventilatory assistance, and cardiovascular support with IV fluids may be needed.

In general, severe intoxications will require GI decontamination (see Chapter 42). The rapid onset of CNS depression in patients exposed to these compounds makes gastric lavage the method of choice. Emesis or lavage contents may be sent to a toxicology laboratory for drug screen analysis.

Those patients who are alert and have ingested ethanol, methanol, or ethylene glycol in the previous 10 minutes may be given syrup of ipecac to induce emesis. Ipecac is not indicated in children exposed to isopropanol or acetone because of rapid absorption and quick progression to CNS depression. Activated charcoal should be administered for ethylene glycol and methanol ingestions; use of charcoal in ethanol and isopropanol ingestions is without confirmed benefit. Supportive care, particularly metabolic concerns, is the mainstay of management.

ETHANOL

Owing to its prevalence in the home, ethanol is a frequent source of intoxication. Of 33,550 ethanol exposures reported in 1994, 11,940 (36%) occurred in children and adolescents younger than 20 years of age. In those children younger than 6 years of age, the greatest number of intoxications resulted from ethanol containing mouthwash.[43]

Common Sources

Besides alcoholic beverages and candies, other common sources of ethanol include mouthwashes, liquid medications (e.g., cold remedies, tonics), and perfumes and colognes.[44] The American Academy of Pediatrics has established a blood level of 25 mg/dl as the maximum concentration of ethanol one dose of an ethanol-containing medication should be able to produce in a child.[45]

Pathophysiology

Ethyl alcohol is well-absorbed from the stomach, small intestine, and respiratory tract. Although the intestine extracts approximately 80% of the oral ethanol dose with the stomach absorbing the remainder, ingestion with foods and factors delaying gastric emptying slow absorption. Most alcohol is absorbed within 30 to 60 minutes. The volume of distribution in children is 0.7 L/kg. Three main enzymatic pathways account for ethanol's metabolism with alcohol dehydrogenase being the major method of breakdown and the rate-limiting step.[46] Ethanol is oxidized to acetaldehyde. The other two pathways include a microsomal ethanol-oxidizing system located in the endoplasmic reticulum and peroxidase-catalase system in the peroxisomes. Only very small amounts are excreted unchanged in the urine and the breath. Following zero order elimination for the most part, children reduce their serum levels up to 28 mg/dl/hr.[47]

Acute intoxication occurs from ethanol's selective effect on the reticular activating system causing CNS depression. The frontal lobes of the brain are sensitive to low concentrations, resulting in alterations of mood and thought processes, whereas higher concentrations in the blood affect the occipital lobe (vision) and cerebellum (coordination). There is also a preferential inhibition of inhibitory neurons at low ethanol concentrations.[48]

Diagnostic Findings

Clinical manifestations of acute ethanol toxicity include motor incoordination, slurred speech, visual disturbance, and ataxia at low doses. At higher doses, neurologic activity becomes generally depressed with a progression from irritability to stupor to coma. A decreased respiratory drive can lead to respiratory arrest, a frequent cause of death in fatal intoxications. Other findings include a flushed face, excessive sweating, and GI distress. Ethanol is a venodilator that decreases preload, afterload, and systemic vascular resistance, as well as a myocardial depressant.[49] In children, hypoglycemia is a major concern after alcohol consumption; nicotinamide adenine dinucleotide (NAD) depletion from ethanol metabolism results in less NAD available for gluconeogenesis. Convulsions are a frequent manifestation of hypoglycemia. Lactic acidosis can also occur from the excessive production of dihydronicotinamide adenine dinucleotide (NADH). The lethal dose of ethanol in children is only 3 gm/kg, about one half the adult lethal dose, and serum levels as low as 50 mg/dl may produce clinically significant effects in the pediatric population.[50]

Ancillary Data. In the intoxicated child, helpful laboratory tests include serum ethanol levels, arterial blood gases, serum electrolytes and glucose, liver function tests, BUN and creatinine, and urinalysis. Other alcohols (isopropanol, methanol, ethylene glycol) should be considered in the analytic evaluation.

Differential Considerations

Acetone, a component of fingernail polish remover, also causes a metabolic acidosis and CNS depression.[51] Other toxicologic causes of CNS depression include a long list of drugs (opioids, barbiturates, sedative/hypnotics, salicylates, clonidine); medical complications include infections, metabolic disease, and trauma.

Management

If less than 30 to 60 minutes has elapsed from the time of ethanol exposure and the patient is awake, syrup of ipecac may aid in gastric decontamination. However, if signs of CNS depression are present or more than 1 hour has elapsed, gastric lavage is prudent. After 90 minutes from the time of exposure, generalized supportive care, including correction of electrolyte abnormalities, dehydration, and metabolic acidosis, is required. Treat acute hypoglycemia with 2 to 4 ml/kg of D25W IV; a 24-hour infusion of 10% dextrose may be needed for continued low glucose levels. Although activated charcoal can absorb ethanol, the amount necessary is so large that its use is impractical in acute ingestions.[52] Hemodialysis increases ethanol clearance by threefold to fourfold, but will not usually be necessary if the patient has normal hepatic and renal function. Unstable teenagers with levels greater than 500 mg/dl and young children with levels over 300 mg/dl may benefit from rapid removal by dialysis.[52] General supportive care is essential.

Disposition

Children need to be protected from complications due to falls, suffocation, aspiration, hypoglycemia, and other metabolic abnormalities. Young children who are relatively asymptomatic with serum levels <50 mg/dl may be discharged to be observed at home; they should maintain their blood sugar by eating and drinking (juice) at frequent intervals for a few hours.[53] Children with significant symptoms or levels >50 mg/dl should be observed until stable for discharge.

ISOPROPANOL

Isopropanol is a widely used solvent in industry and the home; it is a clear, volatile liquid with a burning, bitter taste and aromatic odor. Toxicity can result from inhalation, skin absorption, and ingestion. In 1994, poison control centers reported 22,761 intoxications from isopropanol or rubbing alcohol-related compounds, making it second only to ethanol in this category.[54] The majority of exposures (17,298) are children less than 6 years of age including neonatal intoxications.[55] The most common source of isopropanol is rubbing alcohol, usually in a 70% solution. It is also a frequent component of windshield deicers, glass cleaners, and acne remedies.

Pathophysiology

Intestinal absorption of up to 80% of an oral dose occurs in the first 30 minutes, with complete absorption in 2 hours; this rapid absorption minimizes the effectiveness of gastric decontamination. Significant toxicity has been reported from dermal absorption in rabbits and from inhalation exposure as a result of rubbing alcohol sponge baths.[56-59] The apparent volume of distribution in body water is 0.6 to 0.7 L/kg. Isopropanol is oxidized to acetone by alcohol dehydrogenase, most closely following concentration-dependent (first-order) kinetics with a half-life of 2.5 to 3.2 hours.[60] About 20% of an absorbed dose is excreted unchanged by the kidneys as well as the metabolite, acetone. Further metabolism of acetone to acetate, formate, and finally carbon dioxide is prolonged and may contribute to a mild acidosis, as can lactic acid accumulation from isopropanol-induced hypotension. Hyperglycemia, instead of the hypoglycemia seen in acute ethanol poisoning, has been described.[59,61] The toxic dose of a 70% isopropanol solution is about 1 ml/kg, with as little as 0.5 ml/kg causing symptoms; blood concentrations greater than 125 mg/dl have produced coma.[59,62,63]

Diagnostic Findings

The clinical picture of isopropanol intoxication presents most commonly with GI side effects and CNS depression. Compared to ethanol, isopropanol is more irritating to the GI mucosa, more toxic at comparable levels, and causes more prolonged CNS depression and a less pleasant euphoria/elation. Gastritis, abdominal cramping, vomiting, and hematemesis occur soon after exposure along with headache, ataxia, lethargy, and confusion. Reflexes may become depressed, nystagmus may be present, and pupils are often miotic. Mild intoxication occurs at serum levels of 50 mg/dl, and death has been reported from levels as low as 150 mg/dl in adults.[64] The possible progression to stupor, coma, and respiratory arrest secondary to CNS depression requires careful observation in cases of severe toxicity. Other physical findings include tachycardia, mild hypothermia, and the odor of acetone or isopropanol on the breath.[65,66] Large doses of isopropanol can cause hypotension, a possible result of direct cardiac depression or peripheral vasodilation.[67,68] Cases with both coma and hypotension often have fatal prognoses.[65] Renal tubular necrosis has been reported.[69] Isopropanol produces an osmolal gap; a 50 mg/dl toxic blood level results in an increase of approximately 8 mOsm/kg H_2O. Acetone serum levels continue to rise as isopropanol levels fall; serum acetone contributes to the osmolal gap. In fact, high serum ketones with little or no acidosis is characteristic of isopropyl alcohol exposure. Elevated cerebrospinal fluid (CSF) protein has also been described in acute intoxication.[63]

Management

Supportive therapy is the primary mode of treatment. Hyperglycemia or hypoglycemia may be present, requiring sequential serum glucose levels. Because of the quick onset of CNS depression, inducing emesis with syrup of ipecac is not recommended. However, with the known gastric resecretion of isopropanol, gastric lavage is recommended, especially in cases of large ingestions. The effectiveness of activated charcoal in adsorption of isopropanol has not been established. Forced diuresis is not effective; hemodialysis should be used only in toxic patients with levels over 150 mg/dl in a deteriorating patient, especially in conjunction with liver or kidney failure.[70]

METHANOL

Methanol (wood alcohol) is formed from the destructive distillation of wood. Whether inhaled or ingested, poisoning results from the formation of the toxic metabolites formaldehyde and formic acid. In 1994, 2,171 exposures from a variety of compounds containing methanol occurred; 1,140 patients were younger than 20 years of age. There were 10 associated deaths.[71]

Common Sources

In the household, window washer fluids, antifreezes, and shellacs often contain large amounts of methanol. It is also a component of gasohol and Sterno canned heat. One repeated source of poisoning is the contamination of bootlegged ethanol.[72]

Pathophysiology

Methanol is rapidly absorbed from the GI tract; peak levels occur within 30 to 60 minutes. Toxicity from skin and lung absorption has been described in an 8-month-old child who had a methanol-soaked pad placed on the chest.[73] As with other alcohols, the volume of distribution in total body water is 0.6 L/kg, the highest concentrations being found in the kidney, liver, GI tract, vitreous humor, and optic nerve. The majority (90% to 95%) of elimination occurs through oxidation via alcohol dehydrogenase-forming formaldehyde, the rate-limiting enzyme (with a half-life of 1 to 2 minutes) that is rapidly converted by aldehyde dehydrogenase to formic acid. Oxidation of formic acid to carbon dioxide depends on the availability of folic acid. Highly reactive formaldehyde is approximately 30 times more toxic than methanol, whereas formic acid is six times more toxic. Accumulation of formaldehyde is not detectable, but formic acid becomes the major contributing toxin to the ongoing metabolic acidosis and increased anion gap. A decrease of intracellular NAD/NADH ratio in the oxidation of methanol may stimulate anaerobic glycolysis and lactate production; lactate also appears late in the course as a result of tissue hypoxia and formate-induced inhibition of mitochondrial respiration.[74] Approximately 2% to 5% of methanol is excreted by the kidneys unchanged, and in human oral ingestion, pulmonary excretion can account for small amounts. The lowest recorded toxic lethal dose is 4 ml, with the generally accepted potentially lethal dose equal to 30 ml. Methanol has a serum half-life of 14 to 20 hours in mild toxicity and 24 to 30 hours in severe toxicity.[75] In children, however, methanol seems to have a greatly reduced half-life. With the concurrent administration of ethanol, the serum half-life increases to 30 to 35 hours.[76]

Diagnostic Findings

Symptoms of methanol poisoning may be delayed, with a 12- to 24-hour latent period, because of the slow rate of metabolite formation and accumulation. Unfortunately, this delay frequently leads to a delay in therapy. The most common presentation of intoxication consists of a triad of findings related to the GI tract, eyes, and metabolic acidosis.[77] Nausea and vomiting, epigastric abdominal pain, pancreatitis, and GI bleeding may all be present. One of the most helpful diagnostic symptoms is visual changes consisting of a blurred, cloudy vision similar to "stepping out into a snowfield."[78] Central scotomata and yellow spots may be present, and permanent complete blindness has been frequently described. Fixed and dilated pupils, retinal edema, and constricted visual fields are other signs of ocular toxicity. If visual function is to return to normal, it will occur in the first 6 days postexposure.[79] Patients presenting with normally reactive pupils have not suffered permanent visual loss.

Ancillary Data. The hallmark of significant methanol poisoning is a severe anion gap metabolic acidosis caused by the metabolite, formic acid. Clinically, the degree of acidosis correlates with the mortality rates and severity of visual symptoms; most patients with a serum bicarbonate under 18 mEq/L had methanol blood levels over 50 mg/dl.[80] CNS signs and symptoms of a methanol exposure include headache, vertigo, confusion, slurred speech, and lethargy with progression to coma and seizures. In severe cases, computed tomography (CT) scans of the head and postmortem examinations have shown evidence of infarction in the putamen region, cerebral edema, and optic nerve demyelination. Hyperpnea, bradycardia, myocardial depression, and shock are present in severe intoxications. Other laboratory findings include an elevated mean cell volume (MCV) and osmolal gap (normal 286 ± 4 mOsm/kg H_2O), myoglobinuria and possible acute renal failure, and increased serum amylase. Peak methanol levels below 20 mg/dl are usually associated with relatively asymptomatic individuals; above this level CNS manifestations begin to present. Serious poisonings are indicated by levels greater than 50 mg/dl, ocular toxicity appears with levels over 100 mg/dl, and fatalities occur in untreated patients with levels greater than 150 to 200 mg/dl.

Management

Although methanol is absorbed rapidly, it must be converted to the toxic metabolite to cause CNS depression; therefore, ipecac-induced emesis may be helpful if administered within the first 10 minutes. Activated charcoal should also be administered.

Maintaining a serum ethanol concentration of 100 mg/dl will fully inhibit alcohol dehydrogenase function and formic acid production because of ethanol's approximately ninefold to twentyfold[76,81,82] greater affinity for alcohol dehydrogenase as compared with methanol. Therefore, any patient with peak methanol levels >20 mg/dl, symptomatic with a history of methanol ingestion, acidosis, or considered for hemodialysis should receive ethanol. Ingestion of 1.5 ml of 100% methanol in a child weighing 10 kg would produce a potential maximum peak plasma level of 20 mg/dl; thus an average swallow (2 to 8 ml) would produce a potential maximum peak level of 26 to 105 mg/dl.[82] Ethanol blood concentrations should be maintained just over 100 mg/dl, which is difficult to achieve in the pediatric patient. A loading dose of 7.6 to 10 ml/kg of 10% ethanol in D5W or D5W 0.9% NS should be administered over 30 minutes with a maintenance dose of 1.4 ml/kg/hr.[82] Serum ethanol and glucose levels should be monitored after the loading dose and frequently thereafter (see section on Ethylene Glycol Management). The half-life of methanol is markedly prolonged to 30 to 45 hours with ethanol, necessitating extended intensive care observation.[81]

Hemodialysis is indicated for peak levels >50 mg/dl, renal failure, visual impairment, or metabolic acidosis not correcting with bicarbonate therapy. Maintenance doses of ethanol must be increased to 2.7 to 3.3 ml/kg/hr during dialysis. Because the oxidation of formic acid to carbon dioxide is a folate-dependent pathway, administration of folate in doses of 1 mg/kg (up to 50 mg/dose) IV q 4 hr for a total of six doses has been advocated.[77,82,83] Early suspicion of methanol intoxication and the initiation of therapy are the keys to survival and avoidance of long-term disability.

ETHYLENE GLYCOL

Ethylene glycol is a water-soluble, odorless, sweet-tasting solvent; although colorless, a blue-green indicator dye is often added to it. Ethylene glycol has a bittersweet flavor and produces a warm exothermic reaction when ingested. In 1994, 4,103 exposures, including 34 deaths, were reported to poison control centers, of which 1,529 (37%) occurred in patients under 20 years of age.[84]

Common Sources

Ethylene glycol is a compound frequently used in commercial automotive products such as antifreeze-coolant solutions, windshield deicers, and brake fluid, thus making it commonly found in the home.

Pathophysiology

Rapidly absorbed in the GI tract, ethylene glycol reaches peak levels in 1 to 4 hours postingestion. Like ethanol, it distributes evenly throughout body tissue because of its high water solubility.[85] Ethylene glycol also depresses the CNS; however, the hepatic metabolites, glycoaldehyde, glyoxylate, and oxylate, are responsible for the compound's greatest toxicity. The first step in the breakdown pathway is conversion to glycoaldehyde by alcohol dehydrogenase. Ethanol has a 100-fold greater affinity for alcohol dehydrogenase than ethylene glycol, which explains why ethyl alcohol is used in treatment of acute glycol poisoning.[86,87] Formation of glycolic acid and some lactic acid is the primary cause of the delayed metabolic acidosis, which can occur from 4 to 12 hours after ingestion.[88] Oxalate itself is highly toxic, causing myocardial depression and acute renal tubular necrosis. Fortunately, only 1% of the metabolites are converted to oxalate.

Ethylene glycol has a plasma half-life of 3 to 5 hours and is primarily oxidized to glycoaldehyde, glycolate, and glyoxylate.[89] The minimum lethal dose is approximately 1 to 1.5 ml/kg or 100 ml in the adult.[90]

Diagnostic Findings

Classically, toxicity from ethylene glycol has been described in three chronologic stages. Clinically, however, the patient often presents with less well-defined and distinct symptoms, usually within 4 to 8 hours after exposure, as the amount and severity of the ingestion varies.

Stage 1. CNS depression is the most significant symptom of the first stage. Other abnormal neurologic findings include lethargy, nystagmus, ophthalmoplegia, hypothermia, and ataxia. Mental status deterioration from stupor and convulsions to coma with myoclonic jerks, tetanic contractions, and depressed deep tendon reflexes develops secondary to cerebral edema and meningoencephalitis. Pathologic changes include a deposition of calcium oxalate crystals in the brain, meninges, and vessel walls as well as cytotoxic damage from diffuse petechiae and edema. Papilledema occasionally may be present, although not as often as with methanol poisoning. A low-grade fever, nausea, and vomiting complete the initial presentation, which is similar to that of ethanol. Coma is most common within the first 12 hours of an ingestion.[91-94]

Stage 2. Stage 2 occurs in severe cases; cardiopulmonary findings are the most prominent 12 to 24 hours postingestion. Tachypnea, tachycardia, and mild hypertension develop, progressing to cyanosis, congestive heart failure, and cardiovascular collapse. Death is most common during this stage. Pathologically, in the pleura, lungs, heart, and pericardium petechial hemorrhages can manifest as pulmonary edema, bronchopneumonia, and cardiac dilatation.[91-94]

Stage 3. Two to three days after initial presentation, if the child survives the first two stages, renal insufficiency and possibly renal failure develop. Signs and symptoms include oliguria or anuria, flank pain, and costovertebral angle tenderness. Acute tubular necrosis with proteinuria and hematuria may precede renal failure; however, it is often reversible. Dilatation of the proximal renal tubules and degeneration of tubular epithelium may be seen in the pathologic specimen, possibly resulting from either precipitation of calcium oxalate crystals in the renal tubules or toxicity of the ethylene glycol metabolites.[92,95,96]

Ancillary Data. Laboratory findings are associated with clinical symptomatology. One of the hallmarks of ethylene glycol poisoning is a profound anion gap metabolic acidosis, without evidence of ketoacidosis or lactic acidosis, from the formation of large amounts of organic acid metabolites.[97-99] A rise in the osmolal gap exceeding the normal 10 mOsm/kg water results from a severe ethylene glycol intoxication (50 mg/dl) and should alert the emergency physician to the presence of other osmotically active particles in the plasma, such as ethylene glycol, methanol, ethanol, and isopropanol. This rise may persist, as the metabolite glycolate accumulates in the blood, in spite of decreasing serum ethylene glycol levels.[97,98]

Hypocalcemia, a result of chelation of calcium by oxalate, may cause dysfunction of the myocardium or tetany.[85] Hypomagnesemia and leukocytosis can occur and hyperkalemia and elevated creatine phosphokinase (CPK) secondary to muscle necrosis is often present. Renal toxicity manifests with elevated serum BUN and creatinine levels, and calcium oxalate crystals are a diagnostic clue for ethylene glycol intoxication when found in the urine, usually within 4 to 8 hours after ingestion.[96]

Differential Considerations

As with other alcohols and acetone, CNS depression is a common finding among these various intoxications and other substances, such as barbiturates, opioids, sedative/hypnotics, and clonidine. Other medical problems (infection-meningitis, metabolic disorders, trauma) causing lethargy, sedation, and neurologic deterioration must be considered. Children presenting with anion gaps greater than 20 mEq/L must also be considered for possible methanol poisoning.[99]

Management

Decontamination of the GI tract is indicated. If exposure has occurred within 10 minutes, syrup of ipecac may be administered, assuming the patient does not show any signs of CNS depression. Otherwise, gastric lavage may be indicated as well as activated charcoal therapy. Gastric lavage can be performed if done within 4 hours of ingestion or if multiple substances have been ingested. Because of its high affinity for alcohol dehydrogenase, ethanol should be administered as an antidote in acute ethylene glycol and methanol intoxications. This procedure will block ethylene glycol metabolism and allow excretion of unchanged ethylene glycol in the urine. Ethanol therapy should be administered for signs or symptoms of severe ethylene glycol poisoning or levels of ≥ 20 mg/dl.[100] In the presence of ethanol concentrations of 100 to 200 mg/dl, the half-life of ethylene glycol is prolonged to 17 hours.[89] A loading dose of 7.6 to 10 ml/kg IV of 10% ethanol in D5W or D5W 0.9% NS should be administered over 30 minutes to achieve blood ethanol levels of 100 to 130 mg/dl.[101] A maintenance dose of 1.4 ml/kg/hr of 10% ethanol is required to keep the blood ethanol level at 100 mg/dl.[100] It is difficult to maintain children in the necessary ethanol range; and ethanol-induced hypoglycemia is common, making it essential to frequently monitor blood glucose levels, ideally every 1 to 2 hours by a rapid method. Blood ethylene glycol concentrations greater than 50 mg/dl require initiation of hemodialysis, as do signs of renal insufficiency irrespective of glycol levels. Hemodialysis also requires increased maintenance doses of ethanol 2.7 to 3.3 ml/kg/hr of 10% ethanol to achieve 100 mg/dl.[100,102] Thiamine (100 mg IM or IV) and pyridoxine (100 mg IM or IV) may help decrease oxalate production[94]; therefore, they are administered empirically every 6 hours for 2 days. Forced diuresis may prevent oxalate crystal formation and deposition in the kidney and enhance urinary elimination. The endpoint of ethanol therapy is when the ethylene glycol level approaches 10 mg/dl; the glycolic acid is not detectable; and the ethylene glycol-induced acidosis, osmolal gap, and CNS depression are resolved.[98]

Disposition

An asymptomatic child may be discharged when levels of ethylene glycol are <20 mg/dl. However, CNS, cardiovascular, pulmonary, and renal abnormalities must be investigated.

Anticholinergics

THOMAS T. MYDLER • **GARY S. WASSERMAN**

Anticholinergic toxicity appears in many forms, including atropine and other belladonna alkaloids, phenothiazines, antihistamines, cyclic antidepressants, plants, and mushrooms. Inherent in these substances are their effects on both the peripheral autonomic and central nervous systems through the antagonism of acetylcholine. The American Association of Poison Control Centers national data pertaining to anticholinergics is scattered among many categories and overlaps with other toxic substances listed; exposures to various types of anticholinergics including plants and atropine-containing antidiarrhea and antispasmodic drugs, numbered approximately 6,365 in 1994, of which 3,464 occurred in the group younger than 20 years of age.[103] Three deaths were associated with substances having anticholinergic properties, excluding the cyclic antidepressants, phenothiazines, and antihistamines (see section on Cyclic Antidepressants).

Common Sources

Poisonings from anticholinergics occur from a variety of sources. Mushrooms (*Amanita muscaria* and *Amanita pantherina* are the most infamous), plants (jimsonweed and deadly black nightshade among many others), cyclic antidepressants, antispasmodics, antimotility agents, and over-the-counter sleep aid preparations and cold remedies containing antihistamines are just a few of the substances causing inhibition of normal cholinergic transmissions.

Pathophysiology

Atropine, the prototype of anticholinergics, and other substances with anticholinergic properties competitively inhibit the muscarinic effect of acetylcholine by blocking its action in the autonomic ganglia and at the neuromuscular junctions of the voluntary muscle system.

Production of acetylcholine is unaffected. Atropine is well absorbed from the eye, GI tract, and skin; parenterally; and during inhalation and is distributed throughout the body.[104-106] Atropine also crosses the blood-brain barrier. Elimination occurs through hepatic metabolism and urinary excretion.[107] The half-lives of anticholinergics vary, atropine's being 4 hours.[108] In children, the half-life for atropine is 6.9 ± 3.3 hours.[109]

Toxic doses of anticholinergics vary. For atropine-like medications fatalities occurred with doses as low as 1 mg.[110,111] Diphenhydramine (Benadryl) is toxic in acute doses of more than 5 mg/kg and potentially lethal over 10 mg/kg. Of 184 diphenhydramine pediatric ingestions, 50 were symptomatic. Of these 56% had CNS depression, 18% had CNS stimulation, 42% had tachycardia, 26% had mydriasis, and 18% had hypertension.[112] In children, seizures have been observed from doses of 150 mg of diphenhydramine and fatalities from doses less than 500 mg.[113,114] Antimotility drugs have been linked to deaths, especially in third world countries where they are used extensively in children with diarrhea.[115,116]

Diagnostic Findings

An old axiom often used to describe the classic case of anticholinergic poisoning is "hot as a hare, blind as a bat, dry as a bone, red as a beet, and mad as a hatter." More specifically, toxicity can be divided into peripheral and CNS signs and symptoms.

Peripherally, photophobia, blurred vision, dilated and unreactive pupils, and loss of accommodation are noted. Hot, erythematous skin (especially flushed face and ears), as well as an absence of perspiration are present along with dry mucous membranes.[117] Urinary and GI tract motility are slowed, resulting in urinary retention, constipation, swallowing difficulty, and diminished or absent bowel sounds. Vital signs may all be elevated, causing hypertension, tachycardia or dysrhythmias, tachypnea, and increased body temperature. The last of symptoms relates to the inhibition of perspiration and heat dissipation.[118]

In the CNS, a toxic response to anticholinergic poisoning may have a wide range of findings depending on the other adverse effects of the substance. For example, diphenhydramine may cause sedation in some children but hyperac-

tivity in others.[112,119-122] Among the more common anticholinergic CNS signs and symptoms are psychoses including disorientation, delirium, agitation, and hallucinations, which are often visual. Restlessness and ataxia may be present, as well as hyperreflexia or an extensor plantar response. Dystonic reactions and movement disorders are sometimes seen. Convulsions have been reported in children, and the patient may progress to coma, respiratory collapse, and death.[110,111,113]

Ancillary Data. There is little correlation among the anticholinergic dose, blood concentration, and effect on the child.[123,124] ECG monitoring is necessary for associated dysrhythmias or changes in the wave form (i.e., prolongation of the QT interval and S-T elevation). Radiographs may reveal opaque phenothiazines. An infrequently used screening test for a patient manifesting signs and symptoms of anticholinergic poisoning is the administration of 1% pilocarpine drops into an eye with a dilated pupil; if anticholinergics are present in the body, the pupil will not constrict.[125] Pupils of children who have suffered a neuropathologic event will usually constrict with 1% pilocarpine.

Urine drug screening in general does not isolate most anticholinergic agents. Diphenhydramine and some other antihistamines, as well as the cyclic antidepressants, are the main ones to be identified. Atropine and other belladonna alkaloids, antimotility drugs, and mushrooms are not typically spotted.

Differential Considerations

Besides the numerous causes of anticholinergic poisoning, other etiologies of organic brain syndrome must also be considered including encephalopathies, cerebral vascular accidents, or brain tumors, which also present with unusual behavior and agitation. In children, especially the infant, cardiac output is based on heart rate; therefore, any patient with sepsis, dehydration, or shock may present with tachycardia, tachypnea, elevated body temperature, and altered mental status. In addition, children subjected to trauma, whether accidental or intentional, may demonstrate abnormal neurologic findings from a subdural or subarachnoid bleed.

Management

Management of anticholinergic poisoning is based on clinical evaluation. Continuous cardiac monitoring is essential as is temperature control. Decontamination of the GI tract is important, as gastric emptying can be delayed 12 hours or more (see Chapter 42). Because the emergency physician cannot correlate the expected toxicity with the exposure, gastric lavage is preferred. Activated charcoal should be administered; the use of cathartics in atropine toxicity is controversial. Dialysis does not help eliminate anticholinergics.[126]

Initial management should include specific therapy for toxicity. Seizures often respond to diazepam, 0.2 to 0.3 mg/kg IV, followed by phenobarbital. Dysrhythmias, most commonly from cyclic antidepressant overdose, are managed with sodium bicarbonate 1 to 2 mEq/kg to achieve alkalinization of the blood (pH > 7.5), as well as phenytoin or lidocaine (see section on Cyclic Antidepressants). The antidote physostigmine salicylate (Antilirium) is indicated in patients presenting with life-threatening signs and symptoms (e.g., dysrhythmias, delirium, seizures, severe hypertension, and rarely hyperpyrexia) unresponsive to standard first-line therapies. Physostigmine inhibits acetylcholinesterase, thus promoting the action of acetylcholine.[127] This tertiary amine crosses the blood-brain barrier and thus reverses both central and peripheral effects of anticholinergics.[128] Reversal of dysrhythmias, hypertension, delirium, and coma should be expedient when physostigmine is administered, assuming no irreversible damage already exists.[125,129] The recommended dose for children and adolescents is divided into a therapeutic trial followed by a repeat of the lowest trial dose necessary to ameliorate life-threatening signs.[130] In children, a dose of 0.02 mg/kg IV should be administered slowly (1 to 2 minutes) and readministered in 5-minute intervals until a total dose of 2 mg is attained to establish the optimal effective amount. Because physostigmine may have a delayed effect, 20 minutes should then elapse before more antidote is given. As a therapeutic trial, adolescents should receive 2 mg slow IV push; if no reversal is achieved, a second dose of 1 to 2 mg may be given, followed by a 20-minute interval for the delayed effect of physostigmine. A total dose of 1 to 4 mg slow IV push may be repeated whenever compromising symptoms recur.[127,130]

Signs of physostigmine overdose include excessive tearing, salivation, sweating, pupillary constriction, abdominal cramping, muscular twitching, bradycardia, and hypotension. More frequent side effects of the antidote include nausea and vomiting, probably secondary to restored peristalsis to a slowed gut. Relative contraindications to using physostigmine include asthma, atherosclerotic coronary vascular disease, heart block, hypothyroidism and hyperthyroidism, glaucoma, gangrene, pregnancy, or obstruction of the GI and urinary tract. Reversal of physostigmine can be accomplished with atropine equal to half the total dose of physostigmine that relieved symptoms.

Disposition

Patients who present to the emergency room with signs and symptoms of anticholinergic poisoning should undergo GI decontamination and be admitted for continuous cardiac monitoring and symptomatic and supportive care. Those patients with a history of exposure but without symptoms or signs of toxicity should undergo GI decontamination and be monitored for approximately 4 to 10 hours after exposure before discharge.

Carbamazepine

VIDYA SHARMA • GARY S. WASSERMAN

Carbamazepine (CBZ) (Tegretol) has been used as an antiepileptic agent since 1974. It is structurally related to tricyclic antidepressants and phenytoin, causing signs and symptoms of both these drugs in overdose.[131,132]

In 1994, 6,179 CBZ exposures were reported to the American Association of Poison Control Centers.[133] Thirty-two percent of these cases were children younger than 6 years of age; 4,175 patients were treated at a health-care facility and 15 died.

CBZ is available in liquid (100 mg/5 ml) and tablets of 100 mg (chewable) and 200 mg for oral use; a parenteral form has not been marketed.

Pathophysiology

The oral absorption of CBZ is erratic and slow, with peak concentrations in 4 to 36 hours.[132,134-136] Overdose may delay and prolong absorption by reducing GI motility, thus making clinical presentation unpredictable.[136-138] Therapeutic serum levels range between 4 and 12 μg/ml. CBZ is rapidly distributed into all tissues and is predominantly metabolized to CBZ 10,11-epoxide (CBZE) as well as at least six other metabolites.[139] CBZE, also active as an anticonvulsant,[132] is further broken down to a trans-CBZ-diol metabolite and excreted in the urine.[131,140] The half-life of CBZ is longer after a single dose than with chronic therapy. The elimination half-life after a single dose is 20 to 65 hours in an adult, and approximately 8 to 9 hours in neonates and children.[134,141] Chronic use in adults yields a half-life of 8 to 19 hours.[142]

At this time no minimal toxic or lethal amount of CBZ has been established. An interaction between many drugs and CBZ affects their metabolism and requires verification with an appropriate reference.[132] CBZ crosses the placenta and is also excreted in breast milk.[143,144]

Diagnostic Findings

The most marked physical findings of CBZ poisoning involve the CNS.[145] Plasma concentrations of 14 μg/ml usually correlate with behavioral symptoms such as confusion, excitation, and aggression. Dizziness and ataxia with nystagmus and deviating pupils are also seen at levels exceeding 10 μg/ml. Nausea and vomiting occur early. After some hours, CNS depression is evident, with drowsiness and respiratory depression. In cases of severe toxicity, cardiac rhythm disturbances are noted, including loss of P waves, QRS prolongation, premature ventricular contractions (PVCs), and complete heart block.[135,146-148] Dysrhythmias usually occur with plasma concentrations higher than 40 μg/ml.[131] In severe poisoning the patient may present in coma with fixed and dilated pupils. Reflexes may vary from initial hyperreflexia to progressive hyporeflexia. Anticholinergic symptoms of decreased bowel motility and sinus tachycardia are commonly seen.[145] Patients may also present with seizures, encephalopathy, or other brain stem dysfunction.[149-151] Mild transient hypotension was observed in 4 of 72 patients in the largest known series to date. No correlation was found between CBZ levels and heart rate or ECG findings.[152] Rarely seen are dystonia, hypothermia, or hyperthermia.

Chronic poisoning with CBZ occurs in some patients. Hyponatremia, water intoxication, and inappropriate secretion of antidiuretic hormone are recognized side effects.

Ancillary Data. Blood glucose levels should be measured. In symptomatic patients, a 12-lead ECG should be obtained. To confirm the diagnosis, serum CBZ and sometimes CBZE concentrations can be rapidly determined. In acute overdose, serial serum levels may be helpful. Increased serum levels appear to correlate with prolonged hospitalization, but peak measured CBZ levels revealed a poor correlation with the presence of coma, seizures, or severe respiratory depression.[145] Levels below 40 μg/ml do not seem to reliably predict the severity of toxicity.[145] Levels approaching 30 μg/ml or above have been associated with seizures.[153] Similar to other anticonvulsants, the free drug level is more meaningful than the routine serum concentration which included both the bound (inactive drug) and the free (active) drug.

Differential Considerations

Symptoms of phenytoin, phencyclidine, hypoglycemia, or alcohol abuse may be similar to mild cases of CBZ overdose. Severe cases may mimic a cyclic antidepressant intoxication. Coexistent head trauma should be ruled out.

Management

Management of gastric emptying and decontamination has been outlined in previous sections. Activated charcoal, especially multidose therapy, may increase the total body clearance of CBZ[154]; the risks of charcoal aspiration and intestinal obstruction vs. benefit of serial charcoal doses must be weighed.[155]

Cardiovascular and CNS improvement has been reported with the use of charcoal hemoperfusion, although only a small portion of ingested CBZ (up to 2.4 gm) can be effectively removed.[146,156] Charcoal hemoperfusion is indicated in a patient with dysrhythmias or prolonged coma who fails to respond to supportive care; hemodialysis is not beneficial.

Intravenous fluids are used for hypotension with care to avoid water intoxication from the antidiuretic effect of CBZ. Aggressive supportive care usually results in recovery within 48 hours for most patients; serious complications are associated with coma, aspiration, or hypoxia from prolonged seizures.

Disposition

All patients with a CBZ level over 20 μg/ml and others with significant neurologic symptoms should be admitted for cardiac monitoring and specialty care as needed.

Cardiovascular Drugs

GARY S. WASSERMAN

Cardiovascular drugs comprise a large category of accidental pediatric ingestions (29,325 exposures in 1994; 1.5% of total). These exposures, in order of frequency, are antihypertensives (e.g., clonidine), calcium antagonists (e.g., nifedipine), beta blockers (e.g., propranolol), cardiac glycosides (e.g., digoxin) and nitroglycerin.[156] There were 11,187 exposures in children younger than 6 years of age.[157] There were 90 fatalities in the total category, with 45 from calcium antagonists, 20 from cardiac glycosides, and 12 from beta-blockers.[157]

CLONIDINE

Clonidine hydrochloride is a central and peripheral alpha$_2$-adrenergic agonist used primarily in the treatment of essential hypertension but also for opioid, ethanol, and nicotine withdrawal as well as other disorders.[158-161] It is commonly being prescribed by pediatric psychiatrists and behavioral specialists for attention deficit disorders, rage reactions, and other behavior problems. Clonidine has become the leading cause of poison admissions at many pediatric centers.[162] The prescription belongs to a grandparent in the majority of pediatric cases.[163,164] Naloxone may be an important adjunct to therapy.[162,163] There are no known fatalities to date.

The most common drug is clonidine (Catapres), which is manufactured not only as tablets but also as a 3-day transdermal therapeutic system. The discarded patch has caused toxicity by accidental ingestion.[164,165] Generic clonidine is inexpensive and commonly prescribed.

Pathophysiology

Clonidine is rapidly absorbed, with as little as 0.1 mg causing symptoms as early as 30 minutes postingestion.[163] The half-life is approximately 9 hours and it is renally excreted. Heart rate and vascular tone are decreased by alpha receptor (sympathetic) stimulation in the CNS; other actions are similar to those of opioids.[166] Peripheral alpha$_2$ stimulation and the blocking of norepinephrine reuptake results in paradoxical hypertension.[167] Central effects predominate, whereas peripheral stimulation is transient.

Diagnostic Findings

Children are unusually sensitive to the depressant effects of clonidine. A total of 86 intoxicated children were observed by three separate centers in the United States.[163,168,169] The most common signs and symptoms were decreased level of consciousness (95%), bradycardia (59%), respiratory depression (41%), miosis (38%), hypotension (33%), hypertension (31%), and hypothermia (21%). Less common effects are hypotonia, dysrhythmias, seizures, pallor, and irritability. The majority of patients developed symptoms within 1 hour of ingestion, the longest onset of symptoms being 4 hours, and no patient suffered clinical deterioration more than 4 hours after presentation.[168] Hypotension is frequently a delayed finding, whereas the paradoxic hypertension is usually benign. The most impressive finding is respiratory depression, which may present with a characteristic "periodic gasping or sighing agonal-like" respiratory effort.[163] Most patients recover in 12 to 24 hours.[163]

Ancillary Data. Ancillary testing offers no assistance in diagnosis or management except as indicated for respiratory failure or cardiac dysrhythmia. Clonidine is not usually identified in drug screening and blood levels are not clinically helpful.

Differential Considerations

Clonidine poisoning should be suspected in any child who becomes rapidly somnolent, especially in a child who is with grandparents or other elderly caretaker. Also rather classic is the appearance of the "gasping or sighing agonal-like" respiratory effort, which is usually easily corrected by simple stimulation. Other drugs to suspect are opioids, sedatives-hypnotics, naphazoline, oxymetazoline, tetrahydrozoline, and xylometazoline. Many medical conditions, exhaustion, and closed head trauma could mimic this overdose.

Management

Induction of emesis with syrup of ipecac is contraindicated because of the rapid onset of somnolence or lethargy.[163,168] Lavage, charcoal, and cathartic therapy may be helpful. Maintenance of an adequate airway is critical. Hypotension easily responds to positioning, an intravenous fluid bolus, or low-dose dopamine. Hypertension, if significant, should be treated with a short-acting vasodilator such as nitroprusside, 0.5 to 10 μg/kg/min, and adjusted per response. Hypothermia is usually mild and managed with external rewarming. Bradycardia is responsive to atropine. Respiratory, cardiovascular, and CNS depression often respond for a brief time to simple external stimulation.

Naloxone response is controversial.[162,163,168-172] It is believed that the early use of large doses of naloxone, 0.1 mg/kg IV, or 2 mg boluses to a total dose of 10 mg, and the use of a naloxone drip as needed are necessary to reverse clonidine's opioid effects.[162,163] This regimen has successfully prevented intubation of apneic children. Naloxone especially reverses somnolence but appears to be less effective against bradycardia and hypotension. Two unusual responses to naloxone used in clonidine poisoning have been an increase in blood pressure from a normotensive or already hypertensive baseline and a decrease in hypertension.[163]

Disposition

All young children who ingest clonidine need to be evaluated in a health-care facility and observed for at least 2 to 4 hours postingestion. All symptomatic patients require admission for monitoring and supportive care. Symptoms rarely persist more than 24 hours; admission for longer than 48 hours is usually secondary to intubation complications.

OTHER CARDIOVASCULAR AGENTS

For management of other cardiovascular agents, a cardiologist, medical toxicologist, or poison control center should be consulted for the most recent recommendations. The diagnostic findings, complications, and management of adverse effects of digoxin overdose are discussed in Chapter 47. An important specific antidote is Digibind, the digoxin-specific Fab (fragments of antibodies) derived from sheep immunoglobulin G (IgG). Digibind is the treatment of choice for life-threatening digitalis and digoxin associated dysrhythmias (including cardiac-glycoside-like-plants (e.g., oleander, lily of the valley).[173,174] Digibind also aids in the correction of hyperkalemia when standard therapy fails. Pediatric cardiologists are now using this antidote prophylactically when inpatients are overdosed iatrogenically.

Caustics

GARY S. WASSERMAN

Dorland's Medical Dictionary defines caustic as "burning or corrosive; destructive to living tissues."[175] Many substances burn not by hyperthermia but by corrosion (e.g., lye, phosphorus), reduction (e.g., hydrochloric and nitric acids), salt formation (e.g., acetic and formic acids), desiccation (e.g., sulfuric acid), oxidation (e.g., chromic acid, potassium permanganate), metabolic competition (e.g., oxalic and hydrofluoric acids), vesication (e.g., mustard gas), and nonspecific protoplasmic poisons and lacrimators (e.g., mace).[176] These mechanisms cause direct tissue injury and possibly cellular death.[177-180] Most serious caustic ingestions involve strong acids and alkalis. The initial presentation and treatment are similar whether caustics burn by pH or other properties. Use of the term corrosive burn is confusing because corrosion is a nonspecific process; some authors use this term to mean poisons that cause tissue destruction by contact with mucous membranes.[180]

Caustic substances account for a substantial number of exposures each year. There are potentially a quarter of a million of these exposures annually in the United States; acute fatalities are rare but morbidity is significant.[181] Commonly encountered alkalis are bleach, drain cleaners, lye, dishwasher detergents, oven cleaners, toilet bowl cleaners and disc battery (see Chapter 42). Commonly ingested acids are metal cleaners, rust removers, battery acid, soldering fluxes, swimming pool cleaners, and toilet bowl cleaners.

Pathophysiology

Acids cause a superficial corrosion and coagulation necrosis that limit penetration of the injury due to eschar formation. Alkalies, on the other hand, cause a liquefaction necrosis of fat and protein penetrating deeply into tissues.[182] This difference in the nature of injury allows acids to more likely damage the stomach whereas alkalies damage the esophagus and oropharynx, but this is not always true.[183] Caustic agents start to burn immediately on contact. Caustic burns are categorized as first, second, or third degree at esophagoscopy by a grading system similar to that used to evaluate surface skin burns. The degree of burn depends on many factors, including the type of chemical; concentration; molarity; quantity; time of contact; form of agent such as solid, liquid, or paste; organ system involved; presence or absence of food in the stomach; and relative tone of the pyloric sphincter.[182] These factors determine morbidity and mortality according to depth of tissue destruction and resulting scar formation.

Diagnostic Findings

Caustic ingestion causes immediate and often intense pain, diarrhea, vomiting, hematemesis-melena, respiratory distress, cough, bronchospasm or asphyxia from glottic edema, and cardiovascular collapse from loss of vasomotor tone. For alkali ingestions, there is a statistically significant relationship between endoscopy findings and the symptoms of vomiting, cough, dysphagia, abdominal cramps, and stridor.[183] Drooling is another significant finding, but no single or group of signs and symptoms can identify all patients with potentially serious esophageal burns.[184] Typically after an oral ingestion, the mouth or esophagus is red and ulceration follows within 24 hours. Edema occurs by 48 to 72 hours and destruction may extend through the mucosa, muscle, and even the serosa, causing perforation of the esophagus, stomach, or upper intestine. Fibrotic scar tissue is deposited as healing occurs.

It is impossible to predict whether esophageal or stomach burns are present by either the absence or presence of lesions in the oropharynx or lips. In general, one third of patients with oral burns develop associated esophageal lesions, whereas 10% to 15% of patients with esophageal lesions have no oropharyngeal burns.[185-187] Some asymptomatic patients with no oral burns develop esophageal injuries.[188,189] Substernal, back, or abdominal pains; shock; hemorrhage; coma; and severe drooling may indicate severe burns or visceral perforation.[190]

Complications. Respiratory complications from direct caustic effects can be lethal. Other acute complications are hemorrhage, perforation, dehydration, metabolic acidosis, coagulopathy, hemolysis, hyponatremia, and shock. Late-onset complications are infection, achlorhydria, and stricture formation. Eighty percent of all strictures are noted within 2 months of ingestion and 99% within 1 year. No strictures are formed from first-degree burns; 15% to 30% of second-degree burns develop strictures; and virtually 100% of third-degree burns develop strictures.[191] Approximately 75% of children who develop strictures present with severe respiratory distress secondary to upper airway burns.[191] Circumferential burns are most likely to cause stenosis. Patients who ingest caustic appear to have an increased risk of developing esophageal carcinoma.[192] Families of these patients should be instructed to consult a physician if dysphagia later occurs at any time in that patient's life. The psychologic, physical, developmental, and financial distress of the patients and their families is considerable.

Ancillary Data. Radiographs of the chest and abdomen may yield early clues of mediastinitis, peritonitis, or severe necrosis.[193] Contrast swallow radiographs are not helpful in the acute situation and often underestimate the extent of injury.[194] When button batteries (disk, miniature) are ingested, an x-ray film should be obtained immediately to locate the position and assure that it is beyond the esophagus. The study should be repeated in 4 to 7 days if the battery does not pass, or sooner as indicated by any symptoms of abdominal distress. A battery in the esophagus demands immediate consultation for removal. Blood and urine analysis for heavy metal concentrations may be indicated if the battery is not quickly excreted. Routine hematology and chemistry baseline studies should be obtained in symptomatic patients and blood should be available for transfusion.[179]

Differential Considerations

A variety of etiologies can mimic a caustic ingestion: iron; calcium oxalate plants (e.g., dieffenbachia, philodendron); candies such as peppermint and cinnamon; tablets stuck in the esophagus and other foreign bodies; infections such as herpetic stomatitis, croup, epiglottitis, peritonsillar cellulitis or abscess, and retropharyngeal abscess; gastritis; esophagitis; ulcers; oral trauma; and, rarely, malignancy.

Management

Management of caustic ingestions is aimed at preventing burns or worsening of burns, preventing strictures and other complications. Immediate first aid consists of rinsing the skin with water for 10 to 15 minutes or drinking milk or water (especially for solid caustics) unless respiratory distress is noted or visceral perforation is suspected. Attempts to neutralize with an opposite weak acid or weak base are contraindicated because the chemical reaction of neutralization may release more heat and gas formation.[195] In vitro large volumes of diluent cause little change in temperature or pH of either strong base or acid; antacid buffer is ineffective and may be harmful.[196] Emesis is contraindicated and lavage is rarely indicated except perhaps immediately after the ingestion of a large volume of acid.[197] Contaminated clothing should not be worn until thoroughly washed. The main focus of early treatment is to avoid vomiting.[198] Once at the hospital, patients take nothing by mouth. Respiratory support is important. The major emphasis of management depends on the surgical consultant, the controversies of which are beyond the scope of this section. The surgeon will decide the timing of endoscopy and the need for antibiotics, steroids, esophagoscopy, surgical procedures, and follow-up (see Chapters 42 and 52).

Disposition

The emergency physician needs to decide which patients require surgical consultation. Asymptomatic children exposed to less caustic agents (e.g., household chlorine bleach, mild detergent soaps) with no physical findings may be discharged with home observation for dysphagia, respiratory distress, skin burns, or GI effects, which occur especially within the first 24 hours.

Cyclic Antidepressants

GARY S. WASSERMAN

Antidepressants are prescribed for depression, headaches, chronic pain syndrome, nocturnal enuresis, school phobia, hyperkinesis, and sleep disorders. The antidepressants have been responsible for the largest number of acute drug fatalities, either pediatric or adult, since surpassing aspirin in the 1970s. Antidepressants were involved in 49,533 exposures (2.6% of total) reported by the American Association of Poison Control Centers in 1994.[199] There were 5,419 cases in the group younger than 6 years of age and 9,020 in the group 6 to 19 years of age. There were 175 deaths reported following overdoses: amitriptyline (50 cases), imipramine (25), doxepin (22), desipramine (12), nortriptyline (10), and 13 lithium deaths. The antidepressant category was second to analgesics for the largest number of fatalities in 1994.[199] Accidental or intentional ingestions of the cyclic antidepressants (CAD) must be aggressively treated because CNS depression, seizures, and cardiac dysrhythmias are common causes of death. Treatment of CAD overdose is still evolving and controversial. There are many drugs in this category and new ones are being marketed on a regular basis (Table 43-2).

Pathophysiology

Cyclic antidepressants block the reuptake of norepinephrine into the postganglionic neurons.[200] The three

TABLE 43-2. Common Antidepressants

Generic name	Trade name	Structure	CNS toxicity	Cardiovascular toxicity
Amitriptyline	Elavil	Tricyclic	Strong	Strong
Amoxapine	Asendin	Tricyclic	Strong	Weak
Desipramine	Norpramin	Tricyclic	Strong	Strong
Doxepin	Sinequan	Tricyclic	Strong	Strong
Fluoxetine	Prozac	Miscellaneous	Weak	Weak
Imipramine	Tofranil	Tricyclic	Strong	Strong
Lithium	Eskalith	Miscellaneous	Moderate	Weak
MAO inhibitors	Nardil	Miscellaneous	Weak	Moderate
Maprotiline	Ludiomil	Tetracyclic	Strong	Strong
Nortriptyline	Pamelor	Tetracyclic	Strong	Strong
Sertraline	Zolott	Miscellaneous	Weak	Weak
Trazodone	Desyrel	Heterocyclic	Weak	Weak
Venlafaxine	Effexor	Heterocyclic	Strong	Moderate

major side effects of CADs are responsible for most toxic reactions: (1) anticholinergic, (2) excessive blockade of norepinephrine reuptake at the postganglionic synapse, and (3) direct quinidine-like effects on the myocardium. All CADs are rapidly absorbed from the GI tract, predominately in the alkaline environment of the small intestine. However, absorption may be delayed or prolonged in the overdose situation because of anticholinergic slowing of the GI tract. Tricyclic antidepressants (TCAs) are very lipophilic, having a large volume of distribution of 10 to 50 L/kg and are highly protein bound (70% to 95%).[201] Average half-lives range from 20 to 80 hours and are known to be shorter in children.[200] All CADs are metabolized by the liver, many forming active metabolites (e.g., amitriptyline to nortriptyline, imipramine to desipramine).

Children seem to be more sensitive to toxic effects of the CADs and demonstrate symptoms at relatively low doses. Ingestion of 10 to 20 mg/kg of most CADs risks a moderate to severe poisoning; coma, seizures, and cardiovascular problems can be expected.[201] Ingestion of 35 to 50 mg/kg without treatment will probably result in death. Observation of clinical effects should determine the course of management regardless of dose. A small fraction of some compounds may be excreted in the bile (enterohepatic recirculation). Less than 5% of these compounds are excreted unchanged in the urine.

Diagnostic Findings

Most toxic manifestations of CADs develop within 4 to 6 hours but may be delayed up to 24 hours. Anticholinergic effects are centrally or peripherally mediated. The CNS is stimulated initially causing agitation, irritability, confusion, delirium, hallucinations, and hyperpyrexia. Other CNS effects are hypertension, myoclonus, choreiform movements, muscular twitching, hyperreflexia, hypertonus, nystagmus, parkinson-like symptoms, and seizures. Peripheral effects include urinary retention, dry mucous membranes, mydriasis, constipation, or ileus.

Blocked norepinephrine reuptake causes increased sympathetic tone resulting in tachycardia, hypertension, in-

creased cardiac output, and ventricular dysrhythmia. As norepinephrine is depleted, hypotension occurs as a late and serious sign; extreme drowsiness also develops. Also seen are areflexia, hypothermia, respiratory depression, cyanosis, and coma.

The quinidine-like effects are the most life threatening. These effects include a prolonged QRS duration as well as QT or PR interval, reentry ventricular dysrhythmias, sinus tachycardia, repolarization disturbances, bundle branch blocks, arterioventricula (AV) conduction defects, and bradycardia.[202] Almost any dysrhythmia may occur, including multifocal PVCs, ventricular tachycardia, flutter and fibrillation, T wave flattening or inversion, ST segment depression, complete heart block, or cardiac arrest. Especially deadly because of its resistance to therapy and recurrence is the torsades de pointes (polymorphous or atypical ventricular tachycardia) dysrhythmia.

Miscellaneous toxic effects of the CADs are almost endless, including ataxia, dysarthria, renal failure, bullous cutaneous lesions, vomiting, and pulmonary complications.

Children especially present with seizures, often status epilepticus, coma, and dysrhythmia. Progression from mild lethargy to deep coma, hypotension, seizures, and ventricular dysrhythmias within 30 minutes is not unusual in the emergency department.[203-205] Therefore, suspected CAD ingestions must be given the highest triage priority regardless of emergency department presentation. Life-threatening CNS or cardiac complications usually occur within 6 hours postoverdose.[195,204,206-208] One retrospective study revealed that 28 of 30 intoxicated patients developed seizures within 3 hours of ingestion.[209]

Tricyclic antidepressants (TCAs) cross the placental barrier, but reports of teratogenicity are not conclusive. Neonatal withdrawal effects of rapid breathing, irritability, restlessness, and insomnia for 1 month were reported after one mother's use of imipramine.[210] TCAs were measured in low concentrations in breast milk from women using therapeutic doses but were undetectable in the plasma of the infants.[211]

Ancillary Data. No laboratory test is readily available to make the definitive diagnosis of an antidepressant intoxication. Likewise, there is no single prognostic indicator to predict toxicity. A comprehensive drug screen will identify CADs as well as some of the metabolites. The long half-life may allow identification even days later. An enzyme immunoassay TCA semiquantitation rapid serum level may be helpful if available. Results are reported in nortriptyline equivalents and the antibody cross-reacts with amitriptyline, nortriptyline, imipramine, desipramine, doxepin, and n-desmethyl-doxepin. Other CADs and their metabolites as well as other unrelated drugs may also cross-react.[212,213] Results are best interpreted in terms of compliance or in an effort to differentiate between a therapeutic and toxic exposure. The threshold limit of this test is 150 μg/ml with a therapeutic range of approximately 50 to 250 μg/ml and toxic amount above 500 μg/ml. Fatalities are usually associated with levels over 1,000 μg/ml but blood levels do not reliably predict severity.[214]

Limb-lead QRS duration may be helpful in deciding patients at risk for ventricular dysrhythmias or seizures. Patients are at negligible risk for seizures or ventricular dysrhythmias if the QRS duration is less than 0.10 seconds.[203,215] Seizures may manifest when the QRS is equal or greater than 0.10 seconds whereas ventricular dysrhythmias are seen only when the QRS is equal to or greater than 0.16 seconds.[203] Another study claims there is no statistical difference in risk of experiencing the toxic effects of ventricular dysrhythmias or seizures based upon widening of the QRS complex beyond 0.10 seconds.[216]

Other studies have shown that the patient's level of consciousness is a better predictor of complications after CAD overdose.[217,218] Patients with a Glasgow Coma Scale of 8 or less were at greater risk for complications as compared to a prolonged QRS greater than 0.10 seconds.[217] These complications of seizures, hypotension, dysrhythmias, and respiratory depression occurred shortly after arrival in the emergency department. If the patient was awake when initially seen in the emergency department, the risk of serious complications was low.

Cardiographic criteria identified over 60% of CAD-overdosed patients by use of heart rate, QRS duration, a mean frontal plane terminal 40-msec QRS axis shift, or corrected QT interval.[219] A rightward axis shift between 120 to 270 degrees in the t-40 msec of the QRS complex may show as an "S" wave in lead I and/or aVL or an "R" wave in aVR but requires special measuring equipment and may even be a common normal variant in the pediatric population. ECG parameters cannot exclude the diagnosis of TCA overdose; TCA levels do not correlate with ECG findings.

Treated patients require serial monitoring of electrolytes, magnesium, calcium, blood gases, and renal and liver function studies. Appropriate laboratory studies are ordered as needed. Patients with hypotension, coma, or seizures often have a metabolic acidosis or combined metabolic and respiratory acidosis.[201,205,220] Chest radiographs are helpful to observe for cardiac enlargement or pulmonary edema.[201] Temperature must be closely monitored because of the anticholinergic action.

Differential Considerations

It is not possible to distinguish clinically between intoxication from CADs and any of many other etiologies. Beta blockers, propoxyphene, quinidine, and phenothiazines all slow cardiac conduction, widen QRS complex, and can cause seizures. Procainamide poisoning also mimics the cardiac dysrhythmias of CADs. Poisoning by amphetamines, cocaine, caffeine, chloral hydrate, and lithium as well as abrupt withdrawal from sedative-hypnotic drugs can cause seizures and ventricular dysrhythmias but not prolongation of the QRS complex.[221]

Management

It is not rare for a CAD-intoxicated patient to present to the emergency department in critical condition without a history of an ingestion. Life-support measures are immediately instituted as indicated. The majority of poison centers do not recommend emesis because the onset of symptoms and deterioration can occur rapidly. When the patient is stable, lavage is performed and activated charcoal and a cathartic are administered. Because the anticholinergic effects of CADs cause slow GI motility and delay gastric emptying, GI decontamination is effective many hours postingestion. A small amount of CADs undergo enterohepatic recirculation, which can be absorbed with the use of multiple serial doses of charcoal in the presence of bowel sounds.[201] Do not extubate a patient without removing residual charcoal from the stomach because of reduced gastric emptying.[222]

All suspected CAD intoxications should be placed on a cardiac monitor for at least 4 to 6 hours and have a baseline 12-lead ECG that is repeated as needed. Ventricular dysrhythmias usually respond to alkalinization and phenytoin therapy. Ventricular fibrillation and pulseless ventricular tachycardia are treated immediately with electric cardioversion. Unresponsive dysrhythmias may respond to lidocaine, propranolol, or physostigmine. Contraindicated because of their similar toxic myocardial effects as the CADs are quinidine, disopyramide, and procainamide.[206] Alkalinization definitely has the ability to reverse dysrhythmias.[206,221,223-225] Alkalinization can be achieved either by use of the mechanical ventilator if the patient is intubated or via intravenous sodium bicarbonate.[223,226,227] The blood pH should be maintained between 7.45 and 7.50 and sometimes 7.55 and higher to prevent recurrence of dysrhythmias.[201,223,227,228]

A sodium bicarbonate loading dose of 1 to 2 mEq/kg (maximum of 50 mEq) slow IV push may be necessary followed by an infusion of 1 to 2 ampules (44 mEq each) of sodium bicarbonate/L IV fluids at a rate appropriate for the child's weight.[229] Try not to exceed the sodium content of normal saline. Some researchers believe that sodium itself influences the cardioprotective effects differently from alkalinization.[230,231] Be aware that this sodium load may precipitate hypokalemia by cellular exchange. Sometimes it is difficult to achieve this degree of alkalinization without extra potassium, but be cautious as hyperkalemia worsens dysrhythmia. CADs are not well excreted in the urine, but fluids should be administered at a rate to ensure a good urine output. Blood gases need to be monitored on a regular basis to guide alkalinization therapy.

Phenytoin (Dilantin) is an excellent antidysrhythmic agent for CAD poisoning,[220,232-234] but a poor choice as an anticonvulsant. The usual loading dose of 15 to 20 mg/kg (maximum, 1,200 mg) is administered IV at the very slow rate of 0.5 mg/kg/min and then maintained with 2 mg/kg every 8 to 12 hours to achieve a therapeutic level of 10 to 30 μg/ml, which needs to be measured before each dose. Because phenytoin loading at this slow rate requires 20 to 30 minutes, many physicians prefer to initially load with lidocaine as far as an antidysrhythmic is concerned.

Lidocaine is used by many medical toxicologists as the drug of choice for ventricular dysrhythmias, including ventricular tachycardia or frequent premature ventricular contractions. Lidocaine should also be used after defibrillation to prevent the recurrence of fibrillation. Load with 1 mg/kg/dose and immediately maintain an infusion of 10 to 40 μg/kg/min. Propranolol or bretylium tosylate should be used with caution; consult a toxicologist or cardiologist for assistance, especially in pacing blocks such as torsades. Supraventricular dysrhythmias are usually self-limited and the patient stable; alkalinization and phenytoin, physostigmine, propranolol, or synchronized countershock may be initiated as needed.

Physostigmine (Antilirium), a cholinergic drug that crosses the blood-brain barrier, is capable of reversing CAD toxic effects of coma, delirium, dysrhythmias, seizures, and hypertension, and is less effective against hypotension and hyperpyrexia.[232,235] A physostigmine trial is best indicated for resistant anticholinergic seizures, movement disorders, and delirium.[236] Physostigmine as an antidote may be dangerous and, therefore, used as a third line or last resort agent in patients who fail to respond to more traditional modalities.[205,232] The pediatric dose is 0.5 mg slow IV push over 1 minute and repeated every 5 minutes to a maximum dose of 2 mg (4 to 5 mg for adults). Physostigmine's effective half-life is only 30 to 60 minutes; do not use a constant infusion since physostigmine itself may cause toxicity. Some adverse effects of physostigmine include bradycardia, asystole, heart block, seizures, and vomiting.[237]

Hypotension requires intravenous fluids and Trendelenburg positioning.[238] If hypotension is unresponsive to these maneuvers, administer norepinephrine[201,239]; add one 4 ml vial of 0.1% solution to 1,000 ml of D5W to yield 4 μg/ml dilution and infuse at 0.1 to 0.2 μg/kg/min and increase the rate as needed.

Seizures should be treated with the usual anticonvulsant regimen of benzodiazepines, barbiturates, and others as needed. Resistant convulsions may require physostigmine or skeletal muscle paralysis.

Forced diuresis or hemodialysis is not effective. Hemoperfusion is not usually recommended but may be helpful in the presence of massive overdose with rapid deterioration that is resistant to standard therapy.[240]

Disposition

All children and adolescents with a history of ingestion or suspected overdose must be observed and monitored in the emergency department or holding area for at least 6 hours postingestion, which includes a minimum of 4 hours under medical supervision. Asymptomatic patients showing no anticholinergic signs and having an ECG tracing with a QRS interval less than 0.1 seconds may be discharged after this time period. A TCA level less than 500 μg/ml is another reassuring finding when determining discharge. Adolescents who have attempted suicide are admitted for psychiatric evaluation whenever appropriate. Any patient showing signs or symptoms, including significant sinus tachycardia, is observed for at least 24 hours postingestion or until asymptomatic for 24 hours before discharge. Late fatal dysrhythmias have been known to occur in adults up to 6 days postingestion,[241-244] but larger studies were unable to verify this occurrence.[245,246]

Insecticide Cholinesterase Inhibitors (Organophosphates and Carbamates)

THOMAS T. MYDLER • GARY S. WASSERMAN

As insecticides have grown in use at home and in the agricultural industry, the frequency of toxic exposures has increased. Two classes of pesticides, organophosphates and carbamates, account for the majority of poisonings. In 1994, The American Association for Poison Control Centers reported 21,654 insecticide/pesticide (excluding rodenticide) exposures; most resulted from organophosphates (14,278) and carbamates (6,465) or combinations of these two toxins (911).[247] In children younger than 6 years of age, 9,454 exposures were reported.

Common Sources

Anticholinesterases are often found in compounds used as insecticides. These compounds may be applied as sprays, fogs, or liquid along with fertilizers and herbicides. In order of decreasing toxicity, some common organophosphates are tetraethyl pyrophosphate (TEPP), ethyl parathion (Parathion), diazinon (Spectracide) and malathion (Cythion). Examples of carbamates include aldicarb (Temik), cembofuran (Furaden), propoxur (Baygon), and carbaryl (Sevin). Residues of these compounds often remain on fruits and vegetables. Some lawn treatments and spraying or fogging from unlicensed exterminators are other sources of toxicity via skin absorption.[248]

Several studies have identified ingestion of improperly stored pesticide as the most common route of intoxication in children.[248-250] Although not as common in children, intentional ingestion of insecticides has been described in adults.[251] Exposure can occur via conjunctival and respiratory routes, and several reports describe children suffering intoxication via dermal absorption from clothes and fabrics contaminated with organophosphates, laundered, and then worn.[252-254]

Pathophysiology

Organophosphates and carbamates both act as cholinesterase inhibitors, preventing a breakdown of acetylcholine to choline and acetic acid. The carbamate-cholinesterase bond is reversible (i.e., spontaneous hydrolysis of the complex occurs in vivo), and the clinical effects of carbamate poisoning last little more than 24 hours. In contrast, organophosphates irreversibly bind to the acetylcholinesterase molecules, resulting in phosphorylation and deactiva-

---

Mnemonics for Cholinergic Excess

D	Diarrhea	S	Salivation
U	Urination	L	Lacrimation
M	Miosis	U	Urination
B	Bronchospasm	D	Diarrhea
B	Bradycardia	G	GI complaints
E	Emesis	E	Everything else
L	Lacrimation		(or emesis)
S	Salivation		

GI, Gastrointestinal.

---

tion. The inactivation of cholinesterase by insecticides leads to a rapid accumulation of acetylcholine at the terminal endings of all postganglionic parasympathetic nerves, at both parasympathetic and sympathetic ganglia, and myoneural junctions.[255,256] Because the amount of available acetylcholine at the synapses cannot be measured practically, laboratory analyses measure the concentration of cholinesterase present in the erythrocyte or plasma.

Clinical effects are a product of overstimulation by acetylcholine of the peripheral muscarinic junctions, primarily the postganglionic parasympathetic nerves of smooth muscle, nicotinic receptors of the autonomic ganglia, and the motor end plates of myoneural junctions in skeletal muscle.[257] In organophosphate poisoning, a delayed neurotoxicity described as a Wallerian degeneration can occur primarily in large myelinated fibers resulting in axonal death distally.[258-260] Symptomatically, a peripheral neuropathy develops.

Toxic amounts vary; fatal oral doses of diazinon and malathion are 25 gm and 60 gm, respectively.[251,261] Detoxification occurs via hydroxylation, hydrolysis, and liver conjugation by cytochrome P-450-mediated monooxygenases. Some metabolites are in fact more toxic than parent compounds (e.g., parathion, diazinon, and malathion form oxons).[255]

Diagnostic Findings

The clinical effects of cholinesterase inhibitors result from an excess of acetylcholine.[257] The major differences between the two types of insecticides are carbamates' shorter duration of toxicity (usually 8 to 24 hours) and their poor penetration of the blood-brain barrier, thereby reducing CNS symptoms. Mnemonics can be helpful in describing cholinergic excess (see box above). Symptoms of cholinergic toxicity vary and depend on whether muscarinic or nicotinic effects predominate.

Stimulated parasympathetic (*muscarinic*) receptors lead to miosis; bronchoconstriction with wheezing and tightness of chest; nausea, vomiting, diarrhea, tenesmus, fecal incontinence, increased frequency of urination and urinary incontinence, and excessive lacrimation, salivation, bronchorrhea, and sweating may be noted. The cardiovascular system may develop bradycardia, hypotension, or ventricular tachycardia. Nicotinic (*motor*) findings include excess sympathetic and skeletal muscle stimulation causing muscle twitching, fasciculations, and weakness. Other nicotinic effects include pallor, tachycardia, hypertension, and hyperglycemia. Two retrospective studies in children have found the predominate symptoms used for diagnosis in adults can be confused with normal behavior.[248,262] Because the majority of children in the studies were younger than 3 years of age, incontinence of urine and feces was not a reliable diagnostic sign. Nor was excessive lacrimation diagnostically useful in children who cried frequently as a result of anxiety or pain. Both studies reported a low percentage of patients with muscle fasciculations.

Organophosphates penetrating the blood-brain barrier cause emotional lability, restlessness, tremors, headaches, withdrawal and depression, drowsiness, lethargy, and depressed mental status. In highly toxic exposures, patients can quickly (minutes to hours) progress to ataxia, generalized weakness, coma, convulsions, and depression of respiratory and cardiovascular drive.

In children, lethargy, coma, and stupor are described as the predominate CNS signs associated with organophosphate toxicity.[248,262] Other signs include an odor of garlic from the skin or breath and contact dermatitis. A case report describes intussusception as a possible complication of organophosphate toxicity or subsequent charcoal-laxative therapy[263]; another patient developed an immune complex nephropathy.[264] Symptoms usually develop within several hours after exposure; duration depends on the severity of the intoxication. Children exposed to highly lipophilic organophosphates may demonstrate a marked delay (up to 2 days) in onset of symptoms and persistence for up to 1 month.[265] The classic picture of death is a patient unable to aerate while drowning in his or her own secretions. The route of exposure usually determines the system affected first (e.g., inhalation-pulmonary, ingestion-gastrointestinal). The CNS effects are usually late, indicating a more severe intoxication.

Chronic effects of organophosphate toxicity are well described in adult literature. Polyneuropathy including paresthesias, weakness, and muscle cramps occasionally affecting gait, usually present within 2 weeks of the acute exposure and persist for several months.[260,266,267] Behavioral effects such as drowsiness, emotional lability, depression, irritability, and deficits on various mental performance tests have been described in adults with occupational exposure; long-term neurologic effects in children are not described.[268,269]

Ancillary Data. Two enzymes are deactivated in organophosphate and carbamate poisonings: red blood cell (RBC) (true) cholinesterase and plasma-serum (pseudo) cholinesterase. Although both enzymes are found in nervous tissue and a number of other organs, RBC cholinesterase is less labile and a better index of toxicity. In reality, however, it is not known which poison affects which enzyme(s), so serial levels of both enzymes are often needed. Some laboratories report the levels in international units (IU) of active enzyme, which has a wide range of normal; others report percentage of active enzyme present or inhibited. It is important, therefore, to understand the laboratory methodology when interpreting results.

Classification of acute exposures is most practically based on the percentage of baseline RBC cholinesterase still available: mild (20% to 50%), moderate (10% to 20%), and severe (<10%) intoxications reflect the extent of inhibition of RBC cholinesterase and degree of symptomatology. It is essential to determine the rate of decline, as symptoms tend to develop when baseline RBC cholinesterase levels fall below 50% of so-called normal. Blood samples should be refrigerated and analyzed within 24 to 48 hours. Levels in mild to moderate exposures will return to near baseline within several weeks.

Other laboratory abnormalities include hyperglycemia, glycosuria, albuminuria, and ketoacidosis.[270] Fifty-six percent of children in one report had a blood glucose >150 mg/dl.[262] Leukocytosis with a left shift is common. Prolongation of the prothrombin time was reported in one infant.[271] Electrocardiogram (EEG) changes are similar to those seen with temporal lobe seizures.[272] Reports of atrial and ventricular dysrhythmias have been associated with organophosphate poisoning.[273]

Differential Considerations

A number of diagnoses may be entertained for anticholinesterase exposure, especially in children.[248] Diabetic ketoacidosis, encephalopathy, pneumonia/pneumonitis, airway foreign body, asthma, GI problems, and head trauma can all present with symptoms similar to those found with cholinesterase inhibitors. However, quick onset of effects, number of body systems involved, and the patient's history will rule out most other possibilities.

Management

The main treatment of organophosphate/carbamate intoxication is anticholinergic therapy. Establishing an airway and adequate cardiopulmonary resuscitation are essential. Gastric decontamination with lavage, activated charcoal, and cathartics should be considered. Clothes should be removed and the skin thoroughly cleansed to prevent further absorption; medical personnel should be doubled gloved and gowned. Two separate water and detergent washes remove a total of 91% to 94% of organophosphates, even when performed up to 6 hours after exposure.

Use of the antidote atropine should begin immediately in suspected organophosphate/carbamate exposures, as it will alleviate the parasympathetic (muscarinic and CNS) effects caused by the relative increase in acetylcholine. Atropine competitively blocks acetylcholine at the muscarinic receptors; however, it cannot reverse nicotinic receptor overstimulation. Therefore, muscular weakness will not be reversed and *even the fully atropinized patient will have respiratory muscle impairment.* Correcting cyanosis to the extent possible before atropine use will help prevent cardiac dysrhythmias secondary to hypoxia. The dose of atropine in children 12 years of age and younger is 0.05 mg/kg slow IV push followed by a maintenance dose of 0.02 to 0.05 mg/kg repeated every 5 to 20 minutes until the child is atropinized.[274,275] Atropinization is associated with warm dry flushed skin, dilated pupils, dry mouth (or decreased bronchial secretions in the intubated patient), decreased bowel sounds, and a rapid heart rate. Children older than 12 years of age may be given the adult dose of 1 to 2 mg repeated as necessary.

Although the dose of atropine may be five times the usual dose of other medical emergencies, it is important to realize that a severely intoxicated patient will experience marked atropine refractoriness and that a common cause of treatment failure is inadequate atropinization.[276-278] Atropine maintenance doses should be repeated when the signs of atropine excess appear to be reversing. The average atropine dose for adults during the first 24 hours is 40 mg/24 hr; some patients require much higher doses. Nicotinic receptors (skeletal myoneural junctions and sympathetic ganglia) will not be affected by atropine.

In general, atropinization should be maintained for at least 24 hours, with some tapering of the dose after the first 12 hours, if the clinical condition permits. Lipophilic organophosphates are slowly metabolized and, therefore, require extended treatment with atropine. Carbamates, on the other hand, are reversible cholinesterase inhibitors, and because signs of intoxication are of shorter duration, length of atropinization may be shortened. Adverse effects of atropine include fever, muscle fasciculations, delirium, dry eyes, adynamic bowel, and unresponsive pupils.

Pralidoxime (2-PAM or Protopam) is an effective antidote for some nicotine effects and is used only for *organophosphate* intoxication. A cholinesterase reactivator at the neuromuscular junction, pralidoxime will restore normal skeletal muscle response, thus making it especially effective in reestablishing respiratory muscle and diaphragmatic movement. CNS dysfunction is unaffected, as pralidoxime does not cross the blood-brain barrier. The dose of pralidoxime given after adequate atropinization in children 12 years of age or younger is 25 to 50 mg/kg infused intravenously over 15 to 30 minutes. Adults require 0.5 to 1 gm.[274,275] The dose should be repeated in 1 to 2 hours and then at 6- to 12-hour intervals if cholinergic signs persist. Severe poisoning and highly lipophilic organophosphates may require more frequent dosing.[279]

Adverse effects of this antidote include dizziness, headache, nausea, blurred vision, and muscle weakness. Administration should begin within 36 hours of the acute exposure or the cholinesterase-organophosphate complex may become resistant to reactivation, a process called aging.[280]

Some animal studies have found cholinesterase reactivators (oximes related to pralidoxime) increase the toxicity of carbamates;[281] therefore, in known carbamate poisoning, atropine alone should be used for treatment and pralidoxime should be avoided.[279] However, patients who may become intoxicated from organophosphates but in whom the substance is unknown should receive pralidoxime.[282] Medications contraindicated in organophosphate poisoning include morphine (respiratory depression), methylxanthines (lower seizure threshold), and loop diuretics such as furosemide (increase urine output).[282-284]

Observation of the child should continue in the hospital for 24 to 48 hours after signs and symptoms resolve to ensure cholinergic signs do not recur.[275] Most patients with adequate decontamination and antidotal treatment do well after the first 24 hours.

Disposition

Patients who remain asymptomatic in the emergency department after several hours may be discharged home for observation. All symptomatic patients are admitted usually for 36 to 72 hours.

Iron

GARY S. WASSERMAN

Iron ingestions are common cases in pediatric medicine because iron preparations are abundant, brightly colored, candy coated, or chewable and come in cartoon shapes and fruit flavors. Of 26,462 iron exposures in 1994, 82% occurred in children younger than 6 years of age.[285] The large majority of these ingestions were evaluated in a health-care facility; fortunately only three deaths occurred.[285]

Iron is an essential mineral that causes damage to the CNS, liver, and gastric mucosa. There are four stages of intoxication (see Diagnostic Findings). It is often difficult to remove the iron mass from the stomach. The chelating agent deferoxamine mesylate is the antidote to bind free iron.

Iron is supplied in a huge variety of mineral and vitamin formulations in tablets, capsules, chewables, and liquid tonics. When determining the toxic amount of iron ingested, the "elemental" iron fraction must be calculated (20% of ferrous sulfate, 33% of ferrous fumarate, and 12% of ferrous gluconate). Ferrous sulfate is the most common form.

Children's multiple vitamins with iron usually contain 8 to 18 mg of elemental iron per chewable tablet. Prenatal preparations prescribed during pregnancy are especially potent, commonly having 325 mg ferrous sulfate (65 mg elemental iron) per tablet.

Pathophysiology

Iron is rapidly absorbed by the small intestine, with peak serum iron levels obtained 2 to 6 hours after ingestion. Chewable formulations may increase iron absorption more than nonchewable forms; a 3-hour level was within 90% of the 4- to 5-hour peak.[286] Free unbound iron is very toxic to living tissues; therefore, the body binds it to proteins or other macromolecules. After absorption, iron is converted to the ferric (Fe^{3+}) state and stored in the intestinal mucosa complexed to ferritin. While transported in the blood, iron is complexed to transferrin. The total amount of iron bound by transferrin is the total iron-binding capacity (TIBC). Normal serum iron levels vary from 50 to 150 μg/dl, and the TIBC ranges from 300 to 500 μg/dl. Therefore, no free iron normally circulates in the blood. Iron itself undergoes no biotransformation and has no biologic mechanism for excretion. It may be difficult to remove concretions from the stomach.

Excess iron is directly caustic to the GI mucosa, causing hemorrhage with resulting hypovolemia and shock. Absorbed free iron (exceeding the TIBC) moves into almost any organ (kidneys, brain, lungs, heart), but accumulates mainly in the liver where it concentrates in the mitochondria, disrupting oxidative phosphorylation and other processes not well defined. Free iron causes third-spacing of

fluids by increasing capillary membrane permeability. Lactic acidosis is the result of various factors including hypovolemia and tissue hypoperfusion. Coagulopathy can occur even before hepatic dysfunction because iron can inhibit thrombin. Multiple-organ system failure and death can occur rapidly or be delayed.

Diagnostic Findings

Clinical Findings. Iron poisoning occurs in four clinical stages; fatality can occur during any stage. The *first stage* develops within a few hours of ingestion due to the direct corrosive action on the GI mucosa. This effect is characterized by abdominal pain, vomiting, and diarrhea, which may be bloody. Lethargy, shock, and metabolic acidosis are secondary to blood and fluid losses and tissue hypoperfusion. The *second stage*, known as "the honeymoon" phase of apparent improvement, may be absent or may persist as long as 36 hours. As GI symptoms resolve, toxic amounts of iron are absorbed through the damaged mucosa barrier. The *third stage* occurs early in severe cases or hours after the second stage. Free iron in the tissues disrupts cellular functions causing fluid third-spacing and venous pooling. This stage is known as the shock phase. Also noted are metabolic acidosis, heart failure, renal failure, and hepatic dysfunction (coagulation defects, hypoglycemia).[287,288] Liver necrosis is seen only in fatal or near-fatal intoxications.[289] The *fourth stage* is delayed for days to weeks and results in GI tract scarring from the initial caustic injury. Common sites of obstruction are the gastric outlet or small bowel. Rare complications of iron poisoning are *Yersinia enterocolitica* infection and pneumatosis intestinalis.[290,291]

The minimum toxic and lethal doses of iron are not well established. Previous studies report a lethal dose of elemental iron at 180 mg/kg or greater.[292-295] Children have died from ingestions of 300 to 600 mg of elemental iron (21-month-old) and 750 mg (19-month-old).[296,297] Toxicity generally begins to occur at doses of 20 to 60 mg/kg, but serious outcomes are unlikely at these doses.[298]

Laboratory

Ancillary Data. Laboratory data include baseline values for CBC, glucose, renal and hepatic functions, and blood type and cross if indicated. Blood gases are indicated for severely symptomatic patients. All stools and emesis should be tested for blood although both the hemocult and gastrocult tests may be either falsely positive or falsely negative in conjunction with whole bowel irrigation.[299] A serum iron should be obtained. If a serum iron cannot be determined, an inconsistent guide partially correlating with an iron level > 300 μg/dl is a white blood cell count $> 15,000/mm^3$ and a serum glucose > 150 μg/dl.[300] Serum iron levels should be obtained 2 to 4 hours after ingestion of nonsustained release products. Levels drawn later, as well as levels drawn after deferoxamine therapy, may be falsely low secondary to tissue distribution.

Symptomatology rather than laboratory data should take precedence. TIBC should not be used as the sole basis for initiation of deferoxamine since it is artificially increased in laboratory determinations following iron poisoning. Treatment decisions are best based on absolute serum iron concentration or a positive challenge test.

Concentrated iron tablets may be seen on abdominal radiographs, but visualization of chewable multivitamins with iron is unlikely.[301] A negative x-ray film, especially 2 hours after ingestion, does not exclude iron overdose.[302] Decubitus views or fluoroscopy may be necessary to determine if an iron bezoar is corroding into the gastric lining.

Intravenous deferoxamine binds with free iron to form ferrioxamine, which causes an orange or red *vin rose* color to the urine. A positive deferoxamine challenge may not always be visually detectable.[303]

Differential Considerations

Differential toxic considerations include caustics, other heavy metals, alcohols, salicylates and nonsteroidal antiinflammatory drugs, theophylline, hepatotoxins, and shock conditions.

Management

Ingestions of more than 20 mg/kg elemental iron require gastric emptying; syrup of ipecac, lavage, or both are performed; which approach is more effective is controversial (see Chapter 42). Lavaging with a 1% to 5% sodium bicarbonate solution may aid results by precipitating an insoluble and nonabsorbable iron complex.[304,305] Charcoal is not effective for heavy metals. Cathartics may be used unless the patient is already experiencing diarrhea. Whole bowel irrigation offers perhaps the best means of bowel evacuation.[306] Determining serum iron levels is helpful in patients with a history of ingestion of over 40 to 60 mg/kg. A repeat level during the period of observation ensures that iron levels are not rising.

Concretions forming iron bezoars identified by serial radiographs are especially difficult to remove. A surgical gastrostomy is the method of choice for removing bezoars that burn into the stomach wall.[307,308] A negative kidney, ureter, upper bladder (KUB) radiograph does not preclude a continued rise in serum iron, as dissolved tablets or capsules will not be visualized.

Intravenous fluid boluses should be administered for hypovolemia and shock. Vasopressors are often not successful against the vasodilatory effects of iron. Blood transfusions may be needed.

Deferoxamine mesylate (Desferal) is the only chelating agent recommended for iron and removes free iron from plasma and perhaps iron from tissues; resulting water soluble ferrioxamine is excreted by the kidneys. The preferred route of administration is an intravenous infusion at a rate of 15 mg/kg/hr with a maximum of 6 gm/day; rapid rates may cause hypotension or an anaphylactoid reaction, although the maximum dose and infusion rate have been questioned as being arbitrary and unsupported by clinical data.[309] In less severe cases or in the early aggressive management of stable patients while awaiting iron levels, deferoxamine may be given deep IM in a dose of 90 mg/kg, up to 1 gm every 4 to 8 hours.[310] Oral deferoxamine is of questionable value and may even promote iron absorption; its use is controversial.

Because 11 mg of deferoxamine are required to bind 1 mg of iron, severe intoxications may require larger doses (up to 35 mg/kg/hr IV) than the standard recommendations given earlier.[311] The rate of administration can be in-creased by 5 mg/kg every 20 to 30 minutes or more rapidly as necessary with close observation. There may be a relationship between the dose and duration of therapy with deferoxamine and the rare occurrence of ARDS. Other rarely seen adverse drug effects are ocular toxicity, ototoxicity and associated infections (Yersinia, mucormycosis and sepsis). A serum iron level below the TIBC does not mean that deferoxamine is not indicated; a single iron concentration may not represent peak absorption. Adequate hydration should precede the use of deferoxamine. Furthermore, iron ingestion may alter the TIBC, making the relationship between iron and TIBC less reliable as a predictor of toxicity.[312,313]

The following patients should receive the antidote deferoxamine: (1) a patient who is symptomatic after a potentially toxic ingestion of iron with hematemesis, hypotension, or lethargy regardless of the serum iron and TIBC, (2) any patient whose serum iron concentration exceeds the TIBC, and (3) any patient with a serum iron greater than 300 to 350 µg/dl. Once a patient receives deferoxamine, subsequent serum iron concentrations are falsely depressed.[312] It should also be noted that significantly elevated serum iron levels falsely elevate the TIBC.[312-314] The duration of antidotal therapy varies according to response. Hemodialysis is indicated only for renal failure, as it effectively removes chelated iron but not free iron. Exchange transfusion offers the most potential for iron removal but is limited to severe intoxications that are deferoxamine failures.

Iron-intoxicated pregnant patients are at greater risk to themselves than iron overload is to the fetus because of some placental protection. Deferoxamine is generally indicated in spite of any suspected potential fetal adverse effects; acute short-term use, especially in the third trimester, offers benefits that greatly outweigh potential risks.[315,316]

Supportive therapy involves careful observation for hypovolemia and blood loss, aggressive replacement of fluid losses, and measuring renal and hepatic functions.

Disposition

Patients may be discharged from the emergency department if they remain asymptomatic 4 to 6 hours after ingestion, and laboratory data are within normal limits. Patients with questionable status and serum iron levels >300 to 400 µg/dl, deserve admission and at least one intramuscular dose of deferoxamine. All symptomatic patients (vomiting, diarrhea, epigastric pain, lethargy) are admitted for chelation therapy. Some toxicologists routinely admit (short-term stay) all iron ingestors for 4 to 6 hours of whole bowel irrigation and then discharge those patients with nontoxic serum iron levels.

Opioids (Narcotics)

GARY S. WASSERMAN

Opioids are a group of drugs with opium or morphine-like properties used mostly as analgesics, antitussives, and antidiarrheal agents. Exposure statistics are difficult to analyze since the 1994 American Association of Poison Control Centers National Data Collection System lists opioids in various categories such as narcotics (6,173 exposures), acetaminophen in combination with narcotics (21,029) and aspirin in combination with narcotics (1,147).[317] Children younger than 6 years of age were involved in 22%, 15%, and 16% of these cases respectively. The narcotic analgesic group was responsible for 89 (11.6%) of the 766 total fatalities recorded in 1994.[317] The category of analgesics (acetaminophen, aspirin, narcotics, nonsteroidal antiinflammatory drugs [NSAIDs], and others) is responsible for the largest number of deaths (205) followed by antidepressants (175).[317]

The patient who has overdosed on narcotics classically presents with coma, miosis, and bradycardia. Young children are especially sensitive to the depressive and dysphoric effects of opioids on the CNS. Naloxone (Narcan), a pure narcotic antagonist, is one of the safest antidotes available to the emergency physician.

Common Drugs or Source

Opioids are classified as natural (e.g., opium, paregoric, morphine, codeine), semisynthetic (e.g., heroin, hydromorphone [Dilaudid], oxycodone, hydrocodone), synthetic (e.g., propoxyphene [Darvon], diphenoxylate [Lomotil], meperidine [Demerol], fentanyl [Sublimaze], dextromethorphan, loperamide [Imodium]) and agonist-antagonists (e.g., butorphanol [Stadol], nalbuphine [Nubain], pentazocine [Talwin]).

Pathophysiology

The pharmacokinetics of each opioid are generally similar to morphine, but variations for each type are beyond the scope of this text. In general, opioids have their major effects on the CNS and GI tract, producing analgesia, drowsiness, mood changes, respiratory depression, nausea, vomiting, reduced GI motility, and alterations of endocrine and autonomic nerve systems.[318] At least four opiate-specific stereoreceptors are in the CNS (Table 43-3), as well as cellular actions and other still unknown activities that produce the effects of opioids.[318-321] Pure opiate antagonists, such as naloxone and naltrexone, interact at all four receptor sites and inhibit these effects.[322] The result of these antidotes is thought to be the decrease in the release of neurotransmitters that mediate the transmission of pain impulses.[318] Endorphins are endogenous peptides located in the CNS and are active neurotransmitters to block pain.[319,323] These natural opioids probably affect drug tolerance and withdrawal.[318-321]

In general, opioids are well absorbed via all routes except the skin; they are metabolized by the liver with half-lives of a few hours and excreted by the kidneys.[318] Many have a large first-pass breakdown in the liver, which accounts for the variable response between oral and parenteral administration (e.g., meperidine, morphine).[318] Opioids have low protein bindings, large volumes of distribution, and variable penetration across the blood-brain barrier, depending on their lipid solubility.[318,324] Tolerance and withdrawal patterns also vary among the opioids.

TABLE 43-3. CNS Opiate Receptors

Receptor	Effects	Agonists	Antagonists
Mu	Analgesia Euphoria Respiratory depression Miosis	Morphine-like drugs	Naloxone Naltrexone Pentazocine Nalbuphine Butorphanol
Kappa	Analgesia Miosis Respiratory depression Sedation	Pentazocine Nalbuphine Butorphanol	Naloxone Naltrexone
Sigma	Dysphoria Psychosis	Same as kappa	Same as kappa
Delta	Euphoria Seizures	Morphine-like drugs	Unknown

From Chisholm CD: Opioid (narcotic) poisoning. In Harwood-Nuss A, editor: *The clinical practice of emergency medicine*, Philadelphia, 1991, JB Lippincott.

Diagnostic Findings

Clinical Findings. Signs and symptoms of opioid intoxication are summarized in Table 43-4. Pinpoint pupils are the norm but may not always be present, especially after ingesting meperidine or diphenoxylate with atropine (Lomotil). Hypoxemia, hypoglycemia, and postictal conditions may also prevent miosis. Children younger than 2 years of age are especially sensitive to the depressive effects of opioids: drowsiness, coma, respiratory insufficiency, bradycardia, and seizures. Convulsions, which may be generalized or focal, are also more common with overdoses of meperidine (due to its active metabolite, normeperidine) and propoxyphene.[325,326] Children also can react with a paradoxical excitation and an itchy face. Direct cardiovascular effects are uncommon with a few exceptions. Cardiac conduction disturbances are attributed to the active metabolite, norpropoxyphene.[327,328]

Severe hypotension suggests propoxyphene or another class of drugs. Atypical presentations are summarized in Table 43-5. Narcotics may cause nausea, vomiting, constipation, and urinary retention.

Neonatal narcotic withdrawal is worse after methadone intoxication than after heroin intoxication; symptoms from methadone withdrawal appear between 36 and 72 hours, peak at 72 to 96 hours, and terminate at 2 to 3 weeks of age.[329,330] This time period is about twice as long as any of the other narcotics abused during pregnancy.

Accidental ingestions and abuse of cough preparations are abundant. Acute ingestion of greater than 1 mg/kg of codeine caused mild-to-moderate symptomatology within 30 to 60 minutes in 51% of children, and acute ingestion of >5 mg/kg caused respiratory arrest in 8 of 234 children.[331] The most common findings in decreasing order of occurrence were somnolence, rash, miosis, vomiting, itching, ataxia, and swelling of the skin.[331] The estimated lethal dose for adults is 7 to 14 mg/kg.[332]

TABLE 43-4. Opiate Overdose: Symptom Summary

Clinical presentation	Effect	Treatment
Pinpoint pupils	Stimulation of nerve III nucleus	None
Coma	Agonist at opioid receptors	Naloxone
Respiratory depression	Depression of medullary respiratory center of CNS	Naloxone; assisted ventilation
Bradycardia	Decrease in sympathetic tone; increase in parasympathetic tone	Naloxone
Hypotension	Dilation of peripheral arteriolar and venous blood vessels	Fluids Naloxone
Hypothermia	External cooling; peripheral vasodilation; CNS depression	Rewarming if temperature is less than 90° F
Pulmonary edema	Increase in pulmonary vascular permeability	Positive end expiratory pressure; assisted ventilation as required
Seizures Morphine Meperidine Propoxyphene	Epileptogenic effects of parent compound and metabolites	Naloxone; oxygen; anticonvulsants

CNS, Central nervous system.
From Ellenhorn MJ, Barceloux DG: *Medical toxicology, diagnosis and treatment of human poisoning*, New York, 1988, Elsevier Science.

TABLE 43-5. Atypical Presentations of Narcotic Poisoning

Agent	Prominent/atypical features
Propoxyphene (Darvon)	Rapid, sudden onset of decreased mental status Seizures Marked negative inotropic and chronotropic action Prolongation of PR and QRS Hypotension Psychosis Late recurrence of symptoms Low dose is life threatening (11 mg/kg)
Diphenoxylate (Lomotil)	Initial anticholinergic features (hyperthermia, tachycardia, mydriasis) Delayed onset of toxicity Children at high risk for toxicity
Meperidine (Demerol)	Mydriasis Prolonged half-life of metabolite Seizures Increased muscle tone Tachycardia possible
Pentazocine (Talwin)	Higher doses of naloxone needed to antagonize the kappa/sigma agonist effects Avoid in myocardial infarction

Modified from Chisholm CD: Opioid (narcotic) poisoning. In Harwood-Nuss A, editor: *The clinical practice of emergency medicine*, Philadelphia, 1991, JB Lippincott.

Dextromethorphan (DM), a codeine-related antitussive, is used in many pediatric cold and cough formulations. Adverse effects from overdose of DM are variable but usually mild; usually massive amounts of DM are required to cause serious symptoms. Overdoses from long-acting DM medications are much worse in children and deserve a physician evaluation.[333] DM has no analgesic or addictive properties,[318] but has become a favorite abusive agent of teenagers; fortunately the acute health risks appear to be minimal.[334]

Ancillary Data. Most opioids are easily identified by drug screen; common exceptions are diphenoxylate, loperamide, butorphanol, nalbuphine, and naloxone. Quantitative levels are only of forensic or medicolegal interests. Routine blood studies are drawn to rule out other problems. Cardiac monitoring is necessary for the symptomatic patient. The asymptomatic accidental ingestor may not need ancillary testing.

Differential Considerations

Narcotic intoxication cannot be distinguished from other depressive agents simply by clinical presentation. It is obvious that many medical problems and toxic substances mimic part or most of the signs and symptoms of opioids. A positive naloxone trial offers excellent evidence for a presumptive diagnosis of opioid poisoning. Naloxone is effective against all opioids, whether natural or synthetic, as well as other drugs that occupy opioid receptor sites, such as clonidine. Some drugs, such as propoxyphene, fentanyl, pentazocine, and clonidine, require large doses of naloxone to override their pharmacologic actions. A positive naloxone trial in conjunction with a negative drug screen should make one especially suspicious of clonidine or fentanyl (sublimaze, "China white") and its designer derivatives (e.g., methylfentanyls).

Miosis is typical of only a few poisons: opioids, cholinergics (e.g., physostigmine and cholinesterase inhibitors, organophosphates, and carbamates), some *Amanita muscaria* mushrooms, lobelia plants, clonidine, and chloral hydrate. Children who were seen for acute drug ingestion, especially those in the deeper stages of coma from phenothiazines (72% miotic), ethanol (35%), and barbiturates (31%), manifested miosis rather than the usual mydriasis.[335] This same study reported that only 1% of children with head trauma and 6% of children with CNS infection exhibited miosis.

Management

Ingestions should be treated aggressively with GI decontamination; syrup of ipecac is not recommended because of the potential for early onset of CNS depression from the opioids. All unresponsive patients are administered oxygen and intravenous glucose (and thiamine as indicated) as soon as possible after blood is drawn for analysis. If there is little change in the patient's condition, naloxone is administered, preferably intravenously; but it can also be given intralingually, intramuscularly, subcutaneously, rectally, intraosseously, and through an endotracheal tube.[336] Remember not to confuse the true positive response from the nonspecific stimulatory response often seen in somnolent individuals. The nonspecific response is not nearly so dramatic and only persists for a few minutes. The pediatric dose of naloxone is 0.1 mg/kg up to 20 kg, whereas older children and adolescents are initially given 2.0 mg. These boluses are followed within 2- to 5-minute intervals with subsequent similar doses to a total of 10 mg as needed.[337-339] Naloxone's effective half-life is only 30 to 60 minutes; therefore, patients need to be closely observed for recurrence of depression. If recurrent doses are necessary to stabilize a patient, a naloxone drip can be administered for many hours.[340] For each hour of continuous drip two thirds of the effective total dose originally required to reverse toxicity should be used. The total amount of naloxone should be mixed in the appropriate volume of intravenous fluid to last as many hours as needed. Fifteen minutes after the drip is started, one naloxone bolus is administered equal to one-half the original effective dose to maintain a steady effective amount of antidote.[341] Usually after a 10- to 14-hour continuous drip during the night, the naloxone can be abruptly discontinued and the patient observed for recurrence of toxicity, which should be noted within 1 to 2 hours. The safety and effectiveness of the new long-acting antagonist, nalmefene (Revex), has not been established in children.

Other opioid effects, such as noncardiac pulmonary edema, are managed symptomatically and supportively. With the exception of the few opioids previously mentioned, it is unusual for narcotics to present with hypotension, cardiac dysrhythmia, repetitive seizures, or cardiogenic shock.[342] GI decontamination is recommended for cough preparations with acute ingestions of greater than 5 mg/kg of codeine or 10 mg/kg of DM.

Disposition

All children who ingest solid form narcotic preparations, whether or not symptomatic, should be admitted for at least 24 hours. Ingestions of smaller volumes of liquid cough formulations (codeine, DM) can be observed in the emergency department for 4 to 6 hours. Only those patients who remain totally asymptomatic throughout the observation period should be discharged. All patients who have ingested diphenoxylate and paregoric require admission for 24 to 36 hours.[343] Any patient receiving naloxone should be admitted. Any admitted patient should be symptom-free for at least 12 hours before discharge.

Salicylates

VIDYA SHARMA • GARY S. WASSERMAN

There has been a dramatic decline in the frequency of aspirin ingestion and mortality among children in the United States. The total number of aspirin and aspirin combination ingestions reported by the American Association of Poison Control Centers for 1994 were 19,796; only 36 deaths were reported among all age groups.[344] Many factors have contributed to this decline. In 1966 and 1967, two major pharmaceutical companies voluntarily limited children's chewable aspirin to 36 per bottle and introduced child-resistant caps. The Poison Prevention Packaging Act of 1970 instituted in 1972 resulted in a further decline in aspirin ingestions in young children. In 1980 concern arose regarding the association of aspirin use and Reye syndrome resulting in recommendations to avoid aspirin usage in children with varicella and influenza illness.[345-347] This further reduced the number of children with aspirin ingestions. Despite these reductions, aspirin still accounts for 3.9% of all health-care visits and 5.5% of the deaths from exposures in 1994.[344] Methyl salicylate and other salicylate topical preparations accounted for an additional 9,387 exposures in 1994; 6,741 of these were children younger than 6 years of age; 933 were seen at health-care facilities and one death was reported.[344]

Common Drugs and Source

Over 200 products contain aspirin (acetylsalicylic acid [ASA]).[348] Children's aspirin contains 81 to 162 mg of ASA per tablet, whereas the adult aspirin is either 325 mg (regular strength) or 500 mg (extra strength). Enteric-coated tablets present a particular problem because the 6-hour salicylate level may not represent the peak level, which is usually delayed many hours.[349] Salicylate is also available as chewable tablets, suppositories, chewing gum, and effervescent tablets.

Many topical preparations contain methyl salicylate (Ben Gay, oil of wintergreen). One teaspoon of topically applied salicylic acid may cause systemic toxicity[350]; this amount is the equivalent of 21 adult aspirin tablets or 7,000 mg.[351] As little as 4 ml of ingested oil of wintergreen has caused death, as this agent is particularly toxic, containing 1,365 mg of salicylate/ml.[352]

Pathophysiology

Salicylate intoxication produces respiratory and metabolic derangements. Fluid, electrolyte, and acid-base disturbances result.

Salicylates stimulate the respiratory center of the CNS. This effect is greater than attributable to increased carbon dioxide production alone and may be a direct effect on the medullary center.[353,354] Other effects include the uncoupling of oxidative phosphorylation, resulting in an increase in metabolic rate, compensated by hyperventilation, temperature elevation, and increased glucose utilization. Inhibition of Kreb's cycle enzymes causes elevations in lactic and pyruvic acids.[355] Both lipid and amino acid metabolisms are inhibited, causing elevations in ketones and amino acids. These effects result in metabolic acidosis,

TABLE 43-6. Usual Clinical Manifestations with Various Levels of Severity of Salicylate Intoxication

Symptom category	Types of symptoms expected
Asymptomatic	None
Mild	Mild to moderate hyperpnea, sometimes with lethargy
Moderate	Severe hyperpnea, prominent neurologic disturbances (marked lethargy or excitability,) but not coma or convulsions
Severe	Severe hyperpnea, coma or semicoma, sometimes with convulsions

From Temple AR: Acute and chronic effects of ASA toxicity and their treatment, *Arch Intern Med* 141:366, 1981.

TABLE 43-7. Assessment of the Severity of Salicylate Intoxication Based on the Estimated Dose Ingested

Ingested dose* (mg/kg)	Estimated severity
<150	No toxic reaction expected
150-300	Mild to moderate toxic reaction
300-500	Serious toxic reaction
>500	Potentially lethal toxic reaction

From Temple AR: *Arch Intern Med* 141:366, 1981.
*Number of tablets ingested × mg aspirin/tablet ÷ by patient weight in kg equals the acute ingested dose. If a patient has been receiving aspirin therapeutically during the previous 24 hours, the potential toxicity of the acutely ingested dose will be increased.

which is more prominent in young children. Adults compensate with a respiratory alkalosis.[356] Salicylism may be more toxic to the fetus than the pregnant patient.

Hyperglycemia often occurs; hypoglycemia is seen late in the course of acute salicylate overdose. In animals, CNS hypoglycemia occurred despite normal blood glucose levels.[357] Hypoglycemia occurs by a combination of depletion of glycogen stores, impaired neoglucogenesis, increased tissue glycolysis, and increased use of peripheral glucose.[358,359]

Salicylate intoxication affects fluid and electrolyte balance in many ways. Increased insensible losses through the lung and skin are accompanied by sodium losses via the sweat and sodium and potassium losses via the urine.[360]

Noncardiogenic pulmonary edema has been reported in some cases, but the mechanisms remain unclear.[361] Noninflammatory cerebral edema has been described on autopsy in children.[362] Therapeutic doses and overdose may cause direct hepatotoxicity with resulting inhibition of vitamin K–dependent synthesis of factor VII.[363] Aspirin also decreases the adhesiveness of platelets for their life span, causing increased capillary fragility but rarely bleeding.[364]

Diagnostic Findings

Salicylate toxicity can be divided into mild, moderate, and severe categories, depending on the amount ingested and type of symptoms expected (Tables 43-6 and 43-7).[365]

Metabolic acidosis characterized by deep, driven, normal rate hyperpnea is seen in salicylate toxicity.[366] Dehydration is manifested by tachycardia, prolonged capillary refill, and changes in orthostatic pressure. Electrolyte imbalance consisting of hyponatremia, hypernatremia, hypocalcemia, or hypokalemia may be seen. Elevated temperatures and alterations in blood glucose may occur. Tetany and paresthesias may result from decreased ionized calcium levels. Hyperventilation, dehydration, and neurologic dysfunction are greater with chronic compared to acute toxicity in children.[367]

Nausea, vomiting, and abdominal pain usually occur early. CNS effects range from mild lethargy, confusion, irritability, and disorientation to seizures and coma in severe cases. Tinnitus usually occurs as serum ASA levels approach 30 mg/dl. Bleeding associated with hypothrombinemia and platelet dysfunction and chemical hepatitis have been observed. Allergic patients may note wheezing.

Ancillary Data. A couple of quick bedside tests offer the opportunity for a presumptive diagnosis. The ferric chloride test is a qualitative method that is usually positive 30 minutes after ingestion. Two to three drops of 10% ferric chloride solution are added to 1 ml of urine; a purple color indicates a positive test. One dose of aspirin or salicylate level as low as 20 mg/dl correlates with a positive urine Phenistix test.[368] A positive result is an immediate brownish-purple color on the Phenistix. Phenothiazines may also give a similar result.

For acute ingestions the Done nomogram categorizes the severity of clinical presentations, with a routine level obtained at 6 hours after ingestion (Fig. 43-2). For chronic ingestions, the Done nomogram underestimates toxicity because it does not reflect the enhanced CNS penetration of chronic ASA exposure across the blood-brain barrier.

Depending on the circumstances of the overdose, baseline values for electrolytes, arterial blood gases, BUN, creatinine, glucose, CBC, and urinalysis are useful. Hypoglycemia, sometimes preceded by an initial hyperglycemia, may develop. Potassium deficit may be secondary to acidosis and hyponatremia is noted with inappropriate antidiuretic hormone (ADH). More severe cases may require calcium, liver function tests, and a prothrombin time. Electrolytes, glucose, and blood pH must be repeated at least every 4 hours until the patient is stable or 2 hours after any intervention such as a change in the intravenous fluid composition or rate.

Symptomatic patients require a repeat ASA level at 10 hours after ingestion so as not to miss a peak level from delayed GI absorption. An acetaminophen level is often indicated because histories are notoriously poor. If CSF is available for analysis, it should be compared with the serum level. Normally, the CSF level is virtually nil, but the closer this level approaches the serum value the more salicylate has crossed the blood-brain barrier, indicating a more severe poisoning independent of the serum level itself.[369]

A chest x-ray film should be obtained if lung findings suggest pulmonary edema. A CT scan may show evidence of cerebral edema in those suggestive cases.

Differential Considerations

Salicylate intoxication is the great imitator. Reye syndrome, diabetic ketoacidosis, acute renal tubular acidosis,

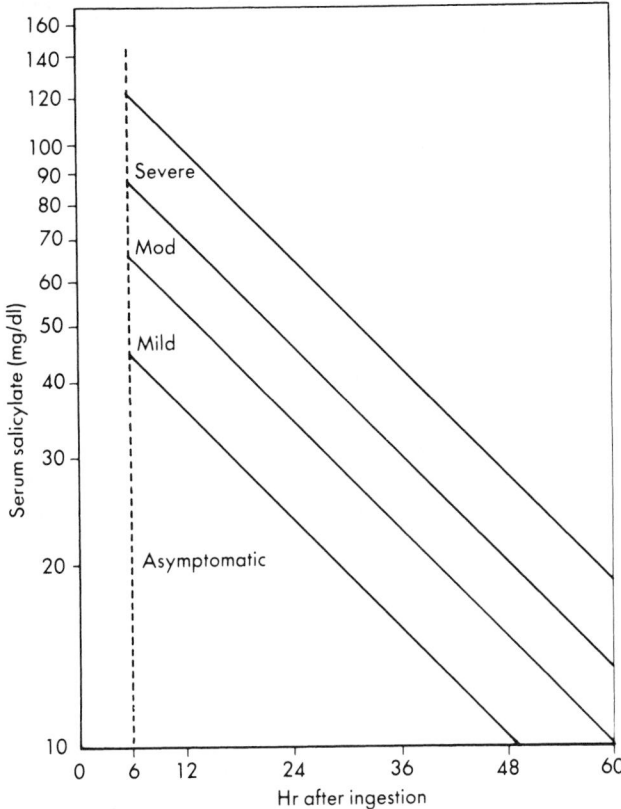

FIG. 43-2. Done nomogram for salicylate poisoning. (*Adapted from Done AK: Pediatrics 62(suppl):895, 1978.*)

pneumonia, encephalitis, meningitis, gastritis, and many others should be considered. Other causes of metabolic acidosis should be excluded.

Management

Consideration for gastric emptying and decontamination are outlined in Chapter 42. Activated charcoal effectively adsorbs ASA.[370] The multiple dose method may enhance elimination of drug already absorbed.[371,372]

Fluid management is crucial in treating salicylate-intoxicated patients. Large volumes of fluid may be needed for initial volume expansion, especially in the first 2 hours. The goal for urinary output is 3 to 6 ml/100 ml maintenance fluid/hr. In children, normal maintenance urinary output is 1 to 2 ml/kg/hr.

Electrolytes should be followed closely, especially potassium, as significant amounts are lost in the urine. After return of adequate urine output, potassium losses must be replaced. This approach also helps achieve urinary alkalinization more rapidly.

Metabolic acidosis must be treated aggressively and early. Decreased serum pH allows ASA to pass more readily into the CSF. Blood pH should be followed closely while correcting metabolic acidosis. If the arterial pH is below 7.2, then a bolus of 1 mEq/kg of sodium bicarbonate may be administered cautiously.[356] In severe cases of salicylate intoxication, 1 to 2 mEq/kg of sodium bicarbonate may be required every 1 to 2 hours to titrate plasma pH to

7.5 in the first 4 to 8 hours.[366] Alkalinization of the urine causes ion trapping and therefore increases salicylate excretion better than forced diuresis.[373] Increased salicylate excretion is seen when urinary pH is over 7.5 and optimally between 8.0 and 8.5.[356] Cerebral or pulmonary edema are contraindications to alkaline diuresis.

Severity of poisoning dictates the aggressiveness of alkaline diuresis.[374] Mild intoxications resolve with standard supportive care, whereas moderate intoxications benefit from an alkaline urine. It is difficult to achieve an alkaline urine in severe poisoning. Initial resuscitation may be undertaken with a solution of D5W 0.45% normal saline (NS) and an addition of 60 mEq/L of $NaHCO_3$. After stabilization and establishment of good urine flow (>2 ml/kg/hr), infuse D5W with 88 to 132 mEq/L of $NaHCO_3$ and 30 mEq/L of KCl at a rate of 3 to 6 ml/kg/hr (2.5 to 4 L/m²/day). A combination of D5W 0.45% NS and 40 to 60 mEq/L of $NaHCO_3$ with 20 to 40 mEq/L of KCl may be used. Alkalinization requires close monitoring of CNS status and serum sodium and potassium levels. Serum calcium should be monitored and if signs of tetany develop, serum glucose administration is mandatory, even if glucose levels are normal, because of the possibility of brain hypoglycemia.[357] Seizures indicate a serious prognosis and are treated with anticonvulsants. Look for metabolic abnormalities that might cause seizures (e.g., hypoglycemia, hypocalcemia, and hypernatremia). If seizures do not resolve immediately with anticonvulsants, consider using glucose and calcium.

Although effective in removing salicylate, dialysis is rarely indicated. Indications for use are a serum salicylate level over 100 to 120 mg/dl for acute ingestions that do not respond to 4 to 8 hours of symptomatic and supportive care, unresponsive metabolic acidosis (pH <7.1), uncontrollable seizures, and severe unresponsive coma.[356] Hyperpyrexia may require external cooling methods. Vitamin K_1 can be given daily intramuscularly or intravenously in a dose of 5 to 10 mg for bleeding diathesis; not all authors advocate this agent prophylactically.

Disposition

A single oral dose of less than 150 mg/kg is not expected to cause serious symptoms and may be managed at home.[360] With ingestions between 150 and 300 mg/kg, young children need gastric decontamination and a serum level at 6 hours after ingestion. Admission for observation or treatment depends on the clinical evaluation in conjunction with the serum level.

Sedatives, Hypnotics, and Antipsychotics: Barbiturates, Benzodiazepines, and Phenothiazines

GARY S. WASSERMAN

The category of sedatives, hypnotics, and antipsychotics totaled 59,532 (3.1% of the total) exposures in the United States in 1994; 7,632 occurred in children younger than 6 years of age, and 6,157 in the 6- to 19-year-old range.[375] Approximately two thirds of all these cases were treated at a health-care facility and 99 deaths occurred. Although these drugs differ pharmacokinetically, the toxic effects are similar and due to progressive CNS depression. These drugs are widely available as anticonvulsants or to treat anxiety, sleep disorders, pain, and other maladies. Symptomatic and supportive care is generally the mainstay of management.

BARBITURATES

Although the benzodiazepines have replaced barbiturates for many therapeutic uses, barbiturate intoxication and abuse remain an important social and medical concern. Of the 4,684 barbiturate exposures in 1994, 1,454 were in the pediatric group; 16 deaths occurred.[375] These poisonings in children are the result of accidental ingestion or the accumulative toxicity of their own anticonvulsant. Poisoning varies with the particular agent. Death may occur within 1 hour, but usually is delayed several hours or days.

Pathophysiology

Barbiturates are classified as long acting (e.g., phenobarbital, mephobarbital), intermediate acting (e.g., amobarbital, butabarbital), short acting (e.g., pentobarbital, secobarbital), and sometimes ultrashort acting (e.g., thiopental, thiamylal) (Table 43-8). The short-acting barbiturates are more lipid soluble (readily diffuse throughout body), bind more readily to protein, have a rapid onset of action, are more rapidly metabolized by the liver, have almost complete reabsorption by the renal tubules, and have a higher pKa. The long-acting drugs exhibit the opposite properties and are primarily renally excreted. Intermediate-acting barbiturates have intermediate properties and are eliminated by both hepatic and renal mechanisms.[376] These drugs inhibit chemical neurotransmission across neuronal and neuroeffector junctions, thus depressing the CNS.

Diagnostic Findings

CNS depression is the classic presentation of barbiturate overdose. Alcohol and other depressants enhance toxicity. Drowsiness is usually the first sign, but may be preceded by a transient period of delirium or excitement. Slurred speech, dizziness, ataxia, and "happy drunk" appearance are common. Stupor may progress through the stages of coma to respiratory or cardiovascular collapse. Pupils are dilated in the milder stages, but constrict as the patient progresses deeper into coma.[377] Hypothermia is the most common abnormal vital sign, but fever can occur. Blisters ("barb burns") occur in 4% to 7% of patients and are mainly located over pressure points.[378]

Complications. Complications of overdose include acute renal tubular necrosis, shock, pulmonary edema, cerebral edema, aspiration pneumonitis, adult respiratory distress syndrome, GI hemorrhage, deep vein thrombosis, cardiac dysrhythmia, rhabdomyolysis, and hypersensitivity reactions such as urticaria, angioedema, asthma, and hepatic necrosis.[379] Permanent sequelae is related to hypoxic damage.

Ancillary Data. Serum barbiturate levels do not necessarily indicate brain tissue concentrations; therefore, clini-

TABLE 43-8. Barbiturate Half-Life

Class	Hours	Examples
Ultra-short acting	1-6+	Thiamylal Thiopental
Short-acting	20-30	Pentobarbital Secobarbital
Intermediate-acting	15-40	Amobarbital Butabarbital
Long-acting	>48	Mephobarbital Phenobarbital

cal status determines treatment decisions. Semiquantitative and quantitative levels for most barbiturates are easy to obtain by immunoassay and mass spectrometry, but barbiturates are frequently not identified qualitatively in routine urine drug screening because of low renal excretion. The short-acting agents begin to cause drowsiness at 6 μg/ml (equal to acute dose of 3 to 5 mg/kg in children) and coma at levels over 20 μg/ml, whereas the patient regains consciousness at 10 to 20 μg/ml on the decline. Long-acting agents are therapeutic at 10 to 40 μg/ml (equal to acute dose of 5 to 20 mg/kg in children), induce coma at 70 μg/ml, are often fatal over 120 μg/ml, and patients regain consciousness at 50 to 90 μg/ml on the decline.[380] Tolerance forces these numbers upward.[381]

An EEG accurately indicates the depth of coma, but is not diagnostic for barbiturates. An isoelectric tracing does not indicate irreversible brain death in this situation. Improved electrical activity precedes improved clinical activity. Arterial blood gas values are necessary to monitor hypercapnia, respiratory acidosis, or failure. Radiographs may reveal intact phenobarbital tablets.[382]

Differential Considerations

Barbiturate poisoning cannot be distinguished by clinical presentation from intoxication by other sedative-hypnotics, alcohols, phenothiazines, opioids, clonidine, carbon monoxide, hydrocarbons, anesthetics, and many other agents that cause coma. The list of medical conditions that cause CNS depression is enormous and head trauma should also be considered.

Management

Considering phenobarbital, the multiple dose charcoal regimen is effective in shortening the half-life and increasing the clearance of drug already absorbed.[383-388] The elimination half-life was reduced from 110 to 20 hours in one study and 110 ± 8 hours to 45 ± 6 hours, and nonrenal clearance increased from 52% to 80% in another study using multiple dose charcoal and cathartic.[384,387] Overdosed patients treated with multiple dose charcoal have shown a reduction in the duration of coma and supportive care required.[383] Another study demonstrated no change in the clinical course (use of ventilator and length of hospital stay) in spite of a shortened half-life using activated charcoal.[386]

Although all barbiturates are partially excreted via the kidneys by forced fluid diuresis, only the long-acting barbiturates are eliminated in sufficient quantity to warrant risking the hazards of cerebral edema, pulmonary edema, or cardiac overload. The half-life of phenobarbital was reduced 61% from 96 hours to 37 hours with forced diuresis.[389] Other than intravenous fluids the most popular agent to augment a forced diuresis is the drug furosemide (Lasix) in a dose of 1 mg/kg body weight every 6 hours. The goal is to achieve a urinary output of 3 to 6 ml/kg/hr. Alkalinization of the urine is likewise only practical to increase the excretion of long-acting barbiturates. This ion-trapping (prevents tubular reabsorption) of phenobarbital results in a five- to ten-fold increase in excretion, depending on the degree of alkalinization.[390] Alkalinization of the urine is most commonly achieved by the administration of sodium bicarbonate to yield a urine pH of 7 to 8 (see section on Salicylates). Intubated patients may be alkalinized mechanically with the respirator.

Hemoperfusion, hemodialysis, and peritoneal dialysis remove barbiturates from the body.[391,392] Long-acting and intermediate-acting barbiturates exhibit less plasma protein binding and less lipid solubility than short-acting agents and, therefore, are extracted in greater quantities. The percentage of short-acting barbiturates extracted by these techniques when compared to total body burden is rather small and usually not worth the risks of these procedures.[393] Hemoperfusion is preferred to hemodialysis in adults, but no data are available regarding these treatments in children. Only the most seriously intoxicated patients who fail to respond to supportive care or who have lethal levels require one of these procedures. Which procedure is best depends on the physician's experience, facility availability, patient's age, and drug dialyzability.

Body heat loss should be prevented; rewarming may be necessary. Coma may be prolonged, and bed pressure sores must be prevented and lubricating drops used to protect the eyes from drying and abrasions.

Disposition

Depending on the degree of sedation, children are admitted for observation and monitoring. Barbiturate serum levels are not as important as the clinical presentation but may be helpful when distinguishing between a potentially serious ingestion that requires hospitalization and a minor poisoning that can be observed at home by reliable caregivers. Asymptomatic patients should be monitored for at least 6 to 10 hours for long-acting preparations and 2 to 4 hours for short-acting barbiturates.

NONBARBITURATE SEDATIVE HYPNOTICS

The management of benzodiazepines, chloral hydrate, phenothiazines, and other nonbarbiturate sedative hypnotics poisonings is similar to the general symptomatic and supportive care of barbiturates.

Benzodiazepines

Benzodiazepines are used as muscle relaxants, anticonvulsants, antianxiety agents, and sedatives. They act on the CNS by potentiating γ-aminobutyric acid (GABA) and, therefore, rendering the postsynaptic receptor sites to be less excitable.[394] Exposures to benzodiazepines are common with 34,940 cases reported in 1994; 4,414 of these occurred in patients younger than 6 years of age.[375] Fortunately when ingested alone, even in large quantities, they do not produce significant toxicity and no fatality has been clearly documented. However, co-ingestion, especially use with other CNS depressants greatly potentiates toxicity as noted by 47 deaths in 1994 in the United States.[375]

Diagnostic Findings. Ataxia, lethargy, and slurred speech are common manifestations of ingestion in children. Hypotension or hypothermia are rarely seen.[395] Bullae may occur similar to those caused by barbiturates.[396] Visual and auditory hallucinations have occurred in children.[397] Semiquantitative serum levels are available to confirm exposure, but are not clinically helpful.[398] Benzodiazepines are presumptively identified by rapid immunoassay methods.

Management. Respiratory depression and coma have been reversed by the antidote flumazenil (Romazicon); onset of effect is 1 to 2 minutes after administering intravenous flumazenil with an effective duration of 1 to 4 hours.[399,400] Initially 0.2 mg (adult) is given and 0.2 to 0.5 mg q 60 seconds is repeated until a response is noted, up to a total cumulative dose of 3 mg or as much as 10 mg. Flumazenil is used in children in doses of 0.02 mg/kg (0.2 mg max).[401] The major contraindications to flumazenil usage are a history of seizures or tricyclic antidepressant co-ingestion. No methods to enhance excretion of benzodiazepines are usually necessary.

Phenothiazines

Phenothiazines are neuroleptic drugs that modify behavior. They are the second most common agent ingested by children in the category of sedatives, hypnotics, and antipsychotics; 1,503 exposures occurred in children younger than 6 years of age and 1,683 in those 6 to 19 years of age. Twenty-four deaths resulted.[375] The phenothiazines have anticholinergic and adrenergic blocking (peripheral vasodilation) and quinidine-like (membrane depressant) effects similar to the cyclic antidepressants, but are less serious in overdose, as they infrequently cause dysrhythmias or severe hypotension. Dopamine receptors are blocked in the CNS.

Phenothiazines are highly protein bound, have a large volume of distribution (average 20 L/kg), and accumulate in lipid tissue resulting in brain levels that may be 10 times the concentration in plasma.[394] They are slowly metabolized in the liver and many of the metabolites are active compounds.

Diagnostic Findings. Dystonic reactions may occur after a single therapeutic dose, chronic therapy, or acute overdose and are noted in about 10% of phenothiazine intoxications.[402] Less common are respiratory depression, coma, seizures, and delirium. Rarely, the neuroleptic malignant syndrome occurs, which consists of hyperthermia, skeletal muscle activity, autonomic disturbances, fluctuating consciousness, and extrapyramidal dysfunction.[403] Rhabdomyolysis, acute renal failure, and death may follow. The toxic dose is not well established, but children appear to be more susceptible. In children, miosis is more common as the level of coma worsens.[377] Extrapyramidal reactions of the acute dystonic types (especially fixed eye gaze;

torticollis; opisthotonus; and face, lip, tongue spasms) are especially common after pediatric exposure.[404] It is not uncommon for these dystonic reactions to be delayed 24 hours after exposure and to recur for 48 to 72 hours or as long as 1 week.

Ancillary Data. Phenothiazines are easily detected in routine urine drug screening. The ferric chloride urine test provides a quick qualitative screen for urine phenothiazines. Phenistix test of the urine also suggests their presence. The Forrest colorimetric test provides quick semiquantitative urine analysis.[405] Blood levels are impractical because they do not correlate with clinical presentation. Many phenothiazines are radiopaque.[406] ECG monitoring is important to observe for mild prolongation of the QT interval, decreased T waves, slurred ST segments, prominent U waves, and other dysrhythmias (see section on Cyclic Antidepressants).

Management

Relief of acute dystonic reactions in children is achieved within 5 minutes with intravenous diphenhydramine (Benadryl) in a dose of 2 mg/kg with a 50 mg maximum.[407] The use of benztropine mesylate (Cogentin) is avoided in pediatric patients because the atropine component often causes worse anticholinergic effects. A reliable second-line drug in young children is a benzodiazepine such as diazepam (Valium) used in a low anticonvulsant dose (0.1 to 0.3 mg/kg IV). Because extrapyramidal reactions tend to recur, children are usually dosed prophylactically with oral diphenhydramine (5 mg/kg/day) every 6 hours for 3 days. Hypothermia is usually mild and responds to passive rewarming. Malignant hyperthermia is a rare complication of pediatric overdose, but requires aggressive therapy with cooling blankets and dantrolene, 1 mg/kg/dose up to 2.5 mg/kg/dose q 6 hr. Techniques such as forced diuresis, dialysis, or hemoperfusion do not effectively enhance the excretion of these drugs. Multiple-dose charcoal regimen may interfere with some GI recirculation but this effect has not been proven.

Substances of Abuse: Cocaine, Phencyclidine, and Sympathomimetics

GARY S. WASSERMAN

Substances of abuse compose a large collection of agents. Statistics are difficult to gather; in 1994 stimulants and street drugs accounted for 29,124 exposures, with 58% of these in the group younger than 20 years of age.[408] There were 18,140 patients treated in health-care facilities; 91 deaths were reported, 56 related to cocaine, 16 to amphetamines, 11 to heroin, 3 to PCP, and 1 each to marijuana and PPA diet aid. Often the street drugs blamed for intoxication are substitute drugs that cause some similar effects ("look-alikes") but contain contaminants and filler.[409] The only constant about drug abuse is that it changes all the time!

Common Drugs or Source

Substances of abuse are divided into five main categories: (1) CNS stimulants (e.g., sympathomimetics, co-caine, amphetamines), (2) hallucinogens (e.g., lysergic acid diethylamide [LSD], psilocybin, mescaline, marijuana, PCP), (3) opioids (e.g., morphine, heroin, codeine, propoxyphene, meperidine, pentazocine, methadone), (4) sedative-hypnotics (e.g., barbiturates, benzodiazepines, alcohol, methaqualone), and (5) inhalants (e.g., solvents, vasodilator-hypoxic agents, tobacco, nitrous oxide, trichlorethylene, butane).

An additional category is the designer drugs, the synthetic chemical modifications of existing abusive agents; these are usually manufactured in makeshift laboratories.[410] Designer drugs are often more potent, cheaper, and technically legal if not identified, evaluated, and scheduled by the Drug Enforcement Agency.[411] Examples are the opioid derivative alpha-methylfentanyl and the methamphetamine modifications called "Ecstasy" and "Eve."[412]

COCAINE

Pathophysiology

Cocaine is readily absorbed via mucous membranes. Be cautious when using TAC (tetracaine, adrenaline, cocaine) solution for facial lacerations. The half-life is 60 to 90 minutes, being rapidly converted by plasma esterases to the metabolites of benzoylecgonine and ecgonine methyl ester. Crack, the smokable free-base form, has a half-life of only minutes. The principal pharmacologic actions are as a local anesthetic, peripheral sympathomimetic, and a potent CNS stimulant.[413] Toxic reactions are mainly related to the respiratory, cardiovascular, and CNS, and may occur at 1 mg/kg.[414]

Diagnostic Findings

Signs and symptoms include tachypnea, cyanosis, dyspnea, respiratory failure, dysrhythmias, hypertension, circulatory failure, excitement, headache, nausea, vomiting, convulsions, hyperthermia, and muscle paralysis. Irritability, anxiety, and paranoia are often seen with the excitation. Chest pain and the fear of dying most likely bring the teenager to the emergency department, whereas young accidental ingestors are hyperactive, fussy, fatigued, or have status epilepticus. Dystonic reactions have also been observed in children and adults.[415] Chronic abuse of cocaine may cause depression and other psychiatric disorders, eating and sleeping problems, and psychologic addiction. Other adverse sequelae associated with cocaine use are myocardial infarction, subarachnoid hemorrhage, aortic dissection, pulmonary edema, renal infarction, cerebral ischemia, rhabdomyolysis, and hepatotoxicity.

Use of cocaine during pregnancy has increased the incidence of abruptio placenta, spontaneous abortion, premature delivery, and intrauterine growth retardation.[416] Exposed newborns may show persistent signs of CNS dysfunction. Breast feeding has caused infant intoxications from both maternal intranasal use of cocaine as well as cocaine applied topically to the nipples.[417] In one study, 15% of cocaine-exposed infants later died of sudden infant death syndrome compared to only 4% of narcotic-exposed infants.[418]

Ancillary Data. Cocaine and its metabolites can be detected in urine and blood for up to 72 hours after use[419] (see box on p. 565). Levels are not clinically useful. Signifi-

Approximate Duration of Detectability of Selected Drugs in Urine

Drug	Approximate duration of detectability*
Amphetamine	48 hr
Methamphetamine	48 hr
Barbiturates	
Short-acting	24 hr
Hexobarbital	
Pentobarbital	
Secobarbital	
Thiamylal	
Intermediate-acting	48-72 hr
Amobarbital	
Aprobarbital	
Butabarbital	
Butalbital	
Long-acting	≥7 days
Barbital	
Phenobarbital	
Benzodiazepines	3 days†
Cocaine metabolites	2-3 days
Benzoylecgonine	
Ecgonine methylester	
Methadone 1,5-dimethyl-3,3-diphenyl-2-ethylidene pyrrolidine (metabolite of methadone)	~3 days
Codeine	48 hr
Morphine	48 hr
Propoxyphene/Norpropoxyphene	6-48 hr
Cannabioids (11-nor-Δ⁹-tetrahydrocannabinol-9-carboxylic acid)	3 days‡ 5 days§ 10 days ‖ 21-27 days¶
Methaqualone	≥7 days
Phencyclidine	~8 days

From Schonberg SK, editor: *Substance abuse: a guide for health professionals*, Elk Grove, Ill, 1988, American Academy of Pediatrics.
*Interpretation of the duration of detectability must take into account many variables, such as drug metabolism and half-life, subject's physical condition, fluid balance and state of hydration, and route and frequency of ingestion. These are general guidelines only.
†Using therapeutic doses.
‡Single use.
§Moderate smoker (4 times/wk).
‖ Heavy smoker (smoking daily).
¶Chronic heavy smoker.

cantly symptomatic cases require an ECG. No specific laboratory work is needed unless indicated such as baseline values, muscle enzymes, and urine for myoglobin. Radiographs may identify body packers.[420]

Management

Management is solely supportive for mild intoxications. More severe findings require corrective measures for respiratory distress, seizures, hypertension, hypotension, dysrhythmias, hyperthermia, and anxiety/psychosis. Ingestors should undergo GI decontamination; syrup of ipecac is probably contraindicated except for asymptomatic "body stuffers" seen soon after ingestion.[421,422] Oxygen and sedation with a benzodiazepine are the initial main strategies for complications. No specific antidote for cocaine overdose exists.

There is no consensus for management guidelines of specific life-threatening manifestations. Tachydysrhythmias may be atrial or ventricular. Atrial tachydysrhythmias unresponsive to observation after oxygen and sedation require cooling if febrile, and a calcium channel blocker should be considered. Ventricular dysrhythmias are more complex. Some toxicologists recommend phenytoin, while others use sodium bicarbonate or lidocaine.[423] Lidocaine is often avoided since it can lower the seizure threshold, may enhance cardiac conduction abnormalities, and is often an adulterant of cocaine. Cardioversion and advanced cardiac life support (ACLS) protocols should be used for unstable dysrhythmias.

Hypertension is usually short lived and causes little mortality.[424,425] After oxygen, and sedation, severe hypertension should be treated with sodium nitroprusside (0.5 to 10 μg/kg/min) or phentolamine (5 to 10 mg IV) or nitroglycerin (start at 10 μg/min), which may improve coronary perfusion.[426] The use of calcium channel blockers, labetalol (beta-blocker with weak alpha-adrenergic activity) and Esmolol (cardioselective beta$_1$-blocker) are controversial, but may be effective in selected cases.[427,428,429,430] The use of propanolol may cause paradoxic hypertension and may worsen induced coronary artery vasospasm.[431] Hypotension is best treated with a direct agonist such as norepinephrine (levarterenol).

Hyperthermia is often associated with fatality and requires aggressive treatment if severe.[432] Less severe cases can be treated conservatively. Agitated patients should be calmed in a dark and quiet area and may require a benzodiazepine such as diazepam (Valium) or midazolam (Versed). Treat seizures aggressively with benzodiazepines, barbiturates or neuromuscular blockers as needed. Cocaine is rapidly metabolized and therefore does not require any procedures to enhance elimination. Monitor the fetus of pregnant patients.

Disposition

Asymptomatic patients may be discharged after observation for a couple of hours. Mildly symptomatic cases can be discharged after reversal of clinical findings and stabilization without drug therapy. All other intoxications are admitted, usually for short-term observation, but many need intensive care monitoring. It is probably prudent to admit for observation all young ingestors whether or not they are symptomatic because of possible delayed absorption from the rock (crack) form and the need to evaluate the child's home environment.

PHENCYCLIDINE

The popularity of phencyclidine (PCP), the *PeaCe Pill*, seems to wax and wane in most communities. It is inexpensive; easy to produce in solid, liquid, and powder forms; and versatile in its use by inhalation, ingestion, or injection. It is often sold under the disguise of another hallucinogen such as an adulterant in other illicit products.

"Shermans" or "Sherms" are popular street names for marijuana boostered by PCP or PCP alone in a joint.[409] Popular street names for PCP are "angel dust," "angel mist," "crystal," "hog," "elephant tranquilizer," "killer weed," and "peace weed." PCP is presently only illegally manufactured.

Pathophysiology

Phencyclidine was originally developed as an anesthetic agent and is related to ketamine, often used in pediatric and oral surgery anesthesia. It is thought to stimulate alpha-adrenergic receptors and potentiate catecholamines.[433] The onset of action is rapid by any route, with maximum effects in 15 to 30 minutes after smoking or 2 to 5 hours after ingestion. The duration of action is approximately 12 to 24 hours or longer,[434] and drug-induced psychosis can persist for weeks; flashbacks can occur. It is highly concentrated in fat and brain tissue and is metabolized in the liver.[435,436]

Diagnostic Findings

Effects from PCP vary according to the dose, ranging from euphoria and emotional lability to stimulation and panic reactions to coma, seizures, rhabdomyolysis, and rarely apnea. Most fatalities are a result of behavioral toxicity, usually violent, rather than a direct overdose effect.[437] The classic emergency department presentation is a combative, wild, super-strong patient with nystagmus. However, in one large study 46% of the patients were alert and oriented when first examined in the emergency department.[438] The major effects from PCP are psychologic (schizophrenia, paranoia, auditory hallucinations, violent behavior), sympathomimetic (tachycardia, hypertension, hyperreflexia), cholinergic (miosis, flushing, diaphoresis), and cerebellar (vertical or horizontal nystagmus, dysarthria, ataxia).[419,439]

Children are intoxicated by accidental ingestion or by passive inhalation when an adult is smoking in close proximity.[438] Poisoned young children are typically fussy, excited, or delirious or may be calm with a blank stare or unresponsive.[440] It is uncommon for hypertension and hyperreflexia to occur in children younger than 5 years of age.[419] The most frequent findings in children are lethargy, nystagmus, and opisthotonos.[441] PCP can cross the placental barrier and has been detected in neonatal urine.[442]

Ancillary Data. PCP is easily identified by drug screening. Blood concentrations correlate better than urine levels to clinical presentation but neither is clinically useful. Other laboratory values (CBC, CPK, electrolytes, BUN, creatinine, and urinalysis) relate to rhabdomyolysis.

Management

Treatment is symptomatic and supportive because there is no antidote for PCP. GI decontamination should be initiated as soon as possible after ingestion because PCP is ion trapped in the stomach fluid. Although PCP has an enterohepatic recirculation that may be adsorbed by serial charcoal usage, the risk of charcoal aspiration probably outweighs any benefits.[443,444] Do not acidify the urine in an attempt to enhance excretion, as an acid urine will precipitate myoglobin and potentiate renal failure if rhabdomyolysis is present. Agitated patients should be kept well hydrated with IV fluids to minimize the hazard of rhabdomyolysis.[445]

The anticonvulsant of choice for seizure control is a benzodiazepine. The acute toxic psychosis is best managed by protecting the patient from harm and minimizing environmental stimulation. "Talk-down" is not effective and should be avoided. Benzodiazepines are the drugs of choice as a knock-down agent. Midazolam (Versed), 0.1 to 0.3 mg/kg with a maximum of 5 to 10 mg, may be advantageous, as it is well absorbed from IM injection.

Be aware that phenothiazines may cause hypotension.[446] Treat hyperthermia with standard cooling methods. Hypertensive crisis is treated with IV nitroprusside, starting with 1 µg/kg/min by infusion and titrating up to 10 µg/kg/min as needed. An alternate antihypertensive is phentolamine in a pediatric dose of 0.05 to 0.1 mg/kg q 5 min until hypertension is controlled and repeated every 1 to 4 hours as needed.[433] Other experts prefer low-dose IV diazoxide or sublingual nifedipine.[447] Localized dystonic reactions are responsive to diphenhydramine, 1 to 2 mg/kg IV to a maximum of 50 mg.[447]

Disposition

Patients who remain asymptomatic for 2 to 4 hours may be discharged. Others are admitted for medical or psychiatric management.

SYMPATHOMIMETICS

Stimulants such as caffeine, amphetamines, and phenylpropanolamine diet aids are responsible for the majority of these cases. In 1994 there were 21,054 of these exposures of which 14,343 were in patients younger than 20 years of age; there were 11,569 health-care visits and 20 deaths.[408] These CNS stimulants share similar pharmacologic properties and will be discussed as a group. Other compounds included are the amphetamine analog diet aids (diethylpropion [Tenuate], phenmetrazine [Preludin], phentermine [Ionamin], ephedrine, pseudoephedrine, methylphenidate [Ritalin]) and beta agonists such as albuterol. Amphetamines are known on the street by a variety of names such as "bennies, black beauties, white crosses, uppers, speed, Christmas trees, pink hearts, robin's eggs, and whites."[409]

Pathophysiology

All of these drugs are readily absorbed from the GI tract. Some are available in sustained-release preparations, which may prolong an intoxication if the gut is not decontaminated. These drugs attain a high concentration in the CNS. They are metabolized in the liver and urinary excretion depends somewhat on pH, as these compounds are basic amines (better excreted in acid media).[448]

Amphetamines cause direct presynaptic catecholamine release, may block catecholamine reuptake, or influence enzymes slowing catecholamine breakdown. Blood pressure elevation is often accompanied by a reflex bradycardia caused by the baroreceptors and results in postural hypotension. Clinical manifestations are a result of a direct effect on adrenergic receptors in muscles and glands, and stimulation of the respiratory center and the cerebrospinal axis.

Diagnostic Findings

Mild intoxications cause restlessness, irritability, insomnia, tremors, hyperreflexia, diaphoresis, dilated pupils, and flushing of the skin. Increased dosage causes confusion, hypertension, tachypnea, mild temperature elevation, and profuse sweating. More severe poisoning causes delirium, hypertensive crisis, dysrhythmias, rhabdomyolysis, and hyperpyrexia leading to seizures, coma, cardiovascular collapse, and death.[447,449-451] Amphetamine psychosis usually occurs in chronic abusers but may occur after a large single dose.[452] Limb deformities, biliary atresia, and other birth defects have been reported from first trimester usage.[453,454] Neonatal withdrawal consisting of sweating, irritability, hypoglycemia, tremors, and seizures have been reported.[455]

Phenylpropanolamine (PPA) is commonly the sympathomimetic in pediatric accidental ingestions; toxicity starts at 6 to 10 mg/kg. Children usually tolerate 2 to 3 times the total daily therapeutic dose (e.g., for PPA, 2 to 6 years: maximum 37.5 mg; 6 to 12 years: maximum 75 mg/24 hr) of any of the cold preparation decongestants.[456] Symptoms are generally seen in acute ingestions of more than 17 mg/kg of PPA.[457] Hypertension is the most common and most serious toxic effect of PPA. Mild hypertension was observed in four adolescent or adult patients who ingested 1.7 to 6.3 mg/kg.[458] Moderate to severe hypertension was seen in children ingesting 10.3 to 50 mg/kg.[458] In the same study, the most severe problems resulted from the sustained-release, long-acting formulations. Rarely, intracerebral hemorrhage has occurred.[459-461] Children in particular suffer psychiatric disturbances including restlessness, aggressiveness, sleep disturbances, hallucinations, acute mania, and other psychotic episodes.[462,463]

Ancillary Data. Most sympathomimetics are readily identified in a comprehensive drug screen. Serum levels are of no practical value. Hypokalemia, elevated creatinine phosphokinase (CPK), and myoglobin should be checked in the agitated patient. Otherwise the laboratory evaluation is dictated by the patient presentation, such as ECG and baseline values. A CT scan is helpful in patients with neurologic deficits, severe headache, or abnormal mental status.

Management

Management is similar to that for the other sympathomimetics covered in this chapter (see box above). Hyperthermia may be the single most lethal complication of stimulant intoxication (amphetamines, cocaine, and derivatives).[464] Mild intoxications require only conservative supportive care. Monitoring blood pressure is essential, as the dominant feature of sympathomimetic overdose is hypertension; treatment should be with nitroprusside or a calcium antagonist. An ECG should be obtained as needed. GI decontaminant is the mainstay of early treatment after hypertension is controlled. Bothersome cardiac palpitations, tremors, and anxiety may respond to propranolol. Ventricular tachycardia and frequent premature ventricular contractions are controlled by IV lidocaine; if this treatment is unsuccessful, propranolol should be administered.[465] Seizures should be treated with a benzodiazepine and then phenobarbital as needed. Hemodialysis or hemoperfusion offers little benefit.

Stimulant Intoxication Management Guidelines (For Amphetamines, Cocaine, and Derivatives)

1. Oxygen
2. Sedation: benzodiazepine
3. Control seizures: benzodiazepine, barbiturate
4. Initiate external evaporative cooling: remove clothes, spray with tepid water, fanning
5. Control muscle rigidity or hyperactivity: neuromuscular paralysis
6. Malignant hyperthermia is muscle cell defect: dantrolene should be used.

Disposition

Patients with mild signs and symptoms may be monitored in the emergency department because toxicity is normally brief. Symptomatic patients need to be observed until toxicity resolves and then may be discharged. Ingestions of sustained-release formulations may require observation for as long as 24 hours or more. Patients with persistent or significant hypertension, dysrhythmias, or CNS stimulation require admission, usually to an intensive care unit for constant monitoring.[466] Psychiatric and neurologic complications require consultation as indicated. Persistent headache or neurologic findings after resolution of hypertension probably indicate an urgent need for a CT scan.[466]

Theophylline

GARY S. WASSERMAN

Theophylline, a methylxanthine related to caffeine, has been an intrinsic component of the management of asthma for over 50 years, although its role has decreased in recent years and no longer indicated for acute bronchodilatation. It is also used to treat apnea of the newborn and bronchopulmonary dysplasia (chronic obstructive pulmonary disease). Because of a narrow margin of safety (therapeutic index) between therapeutic levels and toxicity, many young infants in the 1980s were chronically overmedicated, resulting in severe morbidity and mortality. Toxicity may present as acute (accidental ingestion), subacute (acute overdose while on chronic therapy), or chronic (overmedication accumulation); each varies in presentation and management.[467] Theophylline-induced seizures are difficult to control.[468] In 1994, 35 deaths occurred secondary to theophylline-aminophylline overdoses; there were 4,033 reports of exposure.[469]

There are many theophylline formulations in a variety of concentrations prescribed as tablets, liquids, beaded spansules, capsules, and erratically absorbed suppositories. The sustained-release compounds are especially dangerous because of delayed or prolonged toxicity as a result of an increased absorption half-life.[470] Aminophylline is 79%

to 85% of equivalent anhydrous theophylline (see Chapter 59).

Pathophysiology

Theophylline compounds are well absorbed orally, with peak levels obtained in 1 to 2 hours from liquids and uncoated tablets. Sustained-release formulations differ in their bioavailability and may not peak for more than 12 hours after ingestion.[471] The pharmacokinetics vary widely among patients and cannot be predicted. The volume of distribution averages 0.5 L/kg (higher in premature infants) and protein binding is 60% (lower in newborns).[472] Theophylline is metabolized in the liver (40% to 50%) and excreted by the kidneys (5% to 10% of therapeutic dose unchanged beyond 3 months of age; approximately 50% in neonates). Blood levels follow first-order kinetics at therapeutic doses but mixed first- and zero-order (Michaelis-Menten equation) kinetics in overdose. Clearance rates are age related, with average half-lives of 20 hours in the newborn period, 6 to 7 hours from 1 to 6 months of age, 3.5 to 4 hours from 6 months to 13 years of age, and 4.5 to 5 hours in adults.[473] Fever and infections appear to prolong the half-life. A wide variety of drugs interact: erythromycin, cimetidine, contraceptives, and caffeine decrease metabolism, whereas phenobarbital and phenytoin enhance clearance, just to name a few. Theophylline freely crosses the placenta to the fetus as well as passes into breast milk.

Xanthines relax various smooth muscles (especially bronchi) and cause inotropic and chronotropic effects on the heart while decreasing peripheral vascular resistance.[474] Proposed mechanisms of action in overdose include catecholamine release, prostaglandins inhibition, adenosine receptor antagonism, redistribution of intracellular electrolytes, and inhibition of phosphodiesterase and cyclic guanosine monophosphate metabolism.[474-477] Acute overdose causes electrolyte and acid-base disturbances including hypokalemia, hyperglycemia, hypophosphatemia, and metabolic acidosis.[478]

Death or permanent neurological sequelae from theophylline poisoning are most often secondary to cardiorespiratory arrest or hypoxic encephalopathy as a result of prolonged seizures or dysrhythmias causing hemodynamic compromise.

Diagnostic Findings

Clinical findings of toxicity are mainly confined to the GI, cardiovascular, and central nervous systems. The most common symptoms of toxicity are nausea and vomiting (60% to 100%) and tremulousness and agitation (50%).[479] Cardiac dysrhythmias or seizures usually manifest at different serum levels depending on acute exposure (80 to 100 μg/ml) or chronic buildup (40 to 60 μg/ml).[467] Infants younger than 6 months of age are susceptible to toxic manifestations as the serum concentration approaches 30 μg/ml regardless of the type of intoxication. Seizures may be the initial sign, especially in a chronic overdose where GI symptoms are less common. Seizures are often of the status epilepticus type. They may be focal or generalized, followed by coma, and often result in permanent neurologic sequelae.[467]

Sinus tachycardia is the most frequently seen cardiac effect, occurring in almost 100% of serious poisonings.

Atrial and ventricular premature contractions may occur, but life-threatening dysrhythmias are rare in children. Hypotension and hypokalemia are seen in acute intoxications; hyperkalemia is noted in chronic intoxications where hypotension is less common. Ataxia and visual hallucinations have been observed in pediatric cases.[480] Other effects are headache, insomnia, GI bleeding, diuresis, and hyperthermia. A rare complication is rhabdomyolysis with or without renal failure.[481]

Ancillary Data. Serum levels can be rapidly and accurately obtained by immunoassay. Serial determinations should be performed every 4 hours so as not to miss further absorption, observe peak level, and ensure elimination. Therapeutic levels are 5 to 20 μg/ml, with toxic effects appearing in excess of 20 μg/ml. As a rule, ingestion of 1 mg/kg theophylline raises the serum theophylline level approximately 2 μg/ml.[482] Therefore the acute ingestion of 10 mg/kg or more of theophylline may potentially cause intoxication. The active metabolite, caffeine, may accumulate in the neonate. Bezoar formation can yield additional theophylline peaks.[483] Patients should also be monitored for glucose (acute), calcium (chronic), phosphorus (acute), magnesium (acute), electrolytes, and acid-base imbalance (more common in acute). Leukocytosis is often a result of sympathetic stimulation in acute overdose. Cardiac and respiratory monitoring should be available.

Differential Considerations

Differential considerations mainly concern the many other causes of sympathetic stimulation (e.g., amphetamines, cocaine, phencyclidine, thyroid preparations, other beta-agonists, pheochromocytoma, thyroid storm), as well as anticholinergics, drug withdrawal, hallucinogens, monoamine oxidase (MAO) inhibitors, and other medical conditions (e.g., potassium abnormalities, hypoglycemia, hypocalcemia, Reye syndrome).

Management

GI decontamination (see Chapter 42) is performed after life-threatening problems (e.g., dysrhythmias, seizures, hypotension) are stabilized. Gut decontamination is extremely important, especially if a sustained-release preparation is ingested or a bezoar forms. Activated charcoal binds well to theophylline and the multiple-dose regimen reduces the half-life in overdose by approximately 50%.[484] This serial charcoal GI dialysis is also effective after aminophylline IV administration.[485] Multiple-dose charcoal should be used for mild to moderate chronic poisonings with symptoms, moderate acute ingestions, and severe intoxications managed without hemoperfusion/hemodialysis, although risk vs. benefit must be considered in a patient who is spontaneously vomiting.[473] Use of a cathartic deserves careful observation of serum potassium, as hypokalemia is a common finding after acute intoxication. Whole bowel irrigation is an excellent method to ensure bowel decontamination, especially when a long-acting medication is involved and the level of theophylline is not readily responding to multiple-dose charcoal therapy. If recurrent emesis from gastric hypersecretion is a complication of theophylline, metoclopramide (Reglan), ondansetron, or ranitidine (IV) may be effective[486]; avoid the use of cimetidine, which inhibits theophylline metabolism.

Hypotension is often resistant to fluids and Trendelenburg positioning, as well as primarily beta-adrenergic vasopressors such as dopamine; therefore, a strong alpha-adrenergic vasopressor such as lavarterenol (norepinephrine) is indicated. Propranolol can block the vasodilator effects of theophylline and particularly improves diastolic hypotension.[487] Use of this drug in an asthmatic patient requires cautious observation for bronchospasm but has been administered with safety.[488] Likewise, propranolol or verapamil may be helpful in patients with supraventricular tachycardia and multifocal atrial tachycardia or ventricular tachycardia[489]; lidocaine may also be helpful as well as low-dose B-adrenergic antagonists (i.e., labetalol or esmolol).[490] Seizures are an indication of serious toxicity and are difficult to control. Diazepam or phenobarbital appear to be more effective than phenytoin.[491-493] Barbiturate-induced coma or anesthesia may be necessary. Hypertension rarely requires therapy; a short-acting agent such as nitroprusside can be used.

Hemoperfusion, the procedure of choice to enhance theophylline clearance, may be indicated for status epilepticus or repetitive seizures, hypotension unresponsive to fluids and vasopressors, uncontrollable dysrhythmias, chronic poisonings with theophylline levels >60 μg/ml, or acute intoxications with levels >100 μg/ml.[473,494,495] Charcoal hemoperfusion is probably better than resin types.[496] Hemoperfusion is associated with serious complications such as hypotension, hypocalcemia, platelet consumption and bleeding abnormalities not to mention the technical difficulties of blood-loading the chamber for a child. Modern hemodialysis with the larger catheters being used in children allows for more rapid flows and therefore is extremely effective in as little time as 3 to 4 hours. Peritoneal dialysis is probably not as effective as multiple-dose oral charcoal therapy. Neonates may benefit from exchange transfusion.[497] Regardless of the technique, the end point of extracorporeal removal is a serum level less than 60 μg/ml in an acute exposure or 30 μg/ml in a chronic intoxication, plus the reversal of serious symptoms. Expect a serum theophylline concentration to rebound 5 to 10 μg/ml after discontinuing dialysis.

Supportive care includes cardiac monitoring; observation for rhabdomyolysis; serial monitoring of serum potassium, calcium, magnesium, phosphate, and acid-base; and fluid balance, since a mild diuresis may also occur.

Disposition

Symptoms in conjunction with serum theophylline levels determine aggressiveness of management, including decisions regarding admission and discharge. Levels may be obtained at 2 to 4 hours after exposure, but a second level 4 hours after the first is necessary to ensure that the peak has not been overlooked, especially after ingesting a sustained-release preparation. Patients are observed until the serum theophylline level falls below 20 μg/ml.

References

1. Rumack BH, Hess AJ, Gilman CR, editors: *POISINDEX Systems*, Denver, 1996, Micromedex.

Acetaminophen

2. Ellenhorn MJ and Barceloux DG, editors: *Medical toxicology, diagnosis and treatment of human poisoning*, ed 1, New York, 1988, Elsevier Science.
3. Litovitz TL et al: 1994 Annual report of the American Association of Poison Control Centers national data collection system, *Am J Emerg Med* 13:551-597, 1995.
4. Nimmo J et al: Pharmacological modification of gastric emptying: effects of propantheline and metoclopramide on paracetamol absorption, *BMJ* 1:587, 1973.
5. Prescott LF: Kinetics and metabolism of paracetamol and phenacetin, *Br J Clin Pharmacol* 10:2915-2985, 1980.
6. Miller RP, Roberts RJ, Fischer LJ: Acetaminophen elimination kinetics in neonates, children, and adults, *Clin Pharmacol Ther* 19:284-294, 1976.
7. Slattery JT, Koup JR, Levy G: Acetaminophen pharmacokinetics after overdose, *Clin Toxicol* 18:111-117, 1981.
8. Prescott LF, Roscoe P, Wright N: Plasma paracetamol half-life and hepatic necrosis in patients with paracetamol overdosage, *Lancet* 1:519-522, 1971.
9. Black M: Acetaminophen hepatotoxicity, *Gastroenterology* 78:382-392, 1980.
10. Corcoran GB, Mitchell JR, Vaishnaw YN: Evidence that acetaminophen and n-hydroxyacetaminophen form a common arylating intermediate n-acetyl-p-benzoquinonemine, *Mol Pharmacol* 18:536-542, 1980.
11. Prescott LF: Drug conjugation in clinical toxicology, *Biochem Soc Trans* 12:96-99, 1984.
12. Prescott LF: Paracetamol overdosage. Pharmacological considerations and clinical management, *Drugs* 25:290-314, 1983.
13. Rumack BH and Matthew M: Acetaminophen poisoning and toxicity, *Pediatrics* 55:871-876, 1975.
14. Wright N and Prescott LF: Potentiation by previous drug therapy of hepatotoxicity following panacetamol overdosage, *Scott Med J* 18:56-58, 1973.
15. Mitchell JR et al: Acetaminophen induced hepatic necrosis: I. Role of drug metabolism, *J Pharmacol Exp Ther* 187:185, 1973.
16. Rumack BH: Acetaminophen overdose in young children, *Am J Dis Child* 138:428-433, 1984.
17. Peterson RG and Rumack BH: Age as a variable in acetaminophen overdose, *Arch Intern Med* 141:390-393, 1981.
18. Slattery JT and Levy G: Acetaminophen kinetics in acutely poisoned patients, *Clin Pharmacol Ther* 25:184-195, 1979.
19. Portmann B, Talbut ID, Day DW: Histopathological changes in the liver following a panacetamol overdose: correlation with clinical and biochemical parameters, *J Pathol* 117:169-181, 1975.
20. Curry RW, Robinson JD, Sughrue MJ: Acute renal failure after acetaminophen ingestion, *JAMA* 247:1012-1014, 1982.
21. Gabriel R: Paracetamol induced acute renal failure in the absence of fulminant liver damage, *BMJ* 284:505-506, 1982.
22. Rumack BH et al: Acetaminophen overdose: 662 cases with evaluation of oral acetylcysteine treatment, *Arch Intern Med* 141:382, 1981.
23. Agran PF, Zenk KE, Romansky SG: Acute liver failure and encephalopathy in a 15-month-old infant, *Am J Dis Child* 137:1107, 1983.
24. Swetnam SM and Florman AL: Probable acetaminophen toxicity in an 18-month-old-infant due to repeated overdosing, *Clin Pediatr* 23:104, 1984.
25. Henretig FM et al: Repeated acetaminophen overdosing-causing hepatotoxicity in children, *Clin Pediatr* 28:525, 1989.
26. Nogen AG and Bremmer JE: Fatal acetaminophen overdosage in a young child, *J Pediatr* 92:832, 1978.
27. Hickson GB et al: Apparent intentional poisoning of an infant with acetaminophen, *Am J Dis Child* 137:917, 1983.
28. Blak KV et al: Death of a child associated with multiple overdoses of acetaminophen, *Clin Pharm* 7:391, 1988.
29. Singer AJ, Carracio TR, Mofenson HC: The temporal profile of increased transaminase levels in patients with acetaminophen-induced liver dysfunction, *Ann Emerg Med* 26:49, 1995.
30. Klein-Schwartz W and Oderda GM: Absorption of oral antidotes for acetaminophen poisoning (methionine and n-acetylcysteine) by activated charcoal, *Clin Toxicol* 18:283-290, 1981.
31. North DS, Peterson RG, Krenzelak EP: Effect of activated charcoal on acetylcysteine serum levels in humans, *Am J Hosp Pharm* 38:1022-1024, 1981.

32. Galinsk RE and Levy G: Evaluation of activated charcoal sodium sulfate combination for inhibition of acetaminophen absorption and repletion of inorganic sulfate, *Clin Toxicol* 22:21-30, 1984.

33. Gimson AES, Brand S, Mellor PJ: Early charcoal hemoperfusion in hepatic failure, *Lancet* 2:681-683, 1982.

34. Winchester JF, Geltland MC, Helliwell M: Extracorporeal treatment of salicylate on acetaminophen poisoning, *Arch Intern Med* 141:370, 1985.

35. Rumack BH: Acetaminophen. In Rumack BH, Hess AJ, Gilman CR, editors: *POISINDEX Systems*, Denver, 1996, Micromedex.

36. Slattery JT et al: Dose dependent pharmacokinetics of acetaminophen evidence of glutathione depletion in humans, *Clin Pharmacol Ther* 41:413-418, 1987.

37. Corcoran GB et al: Effects of n-acetylcysteine on the disposition and metabolism of acetaminophen in mice, *J Pharmacol Exp Ther* 232:857-863, 1985.

38. Buckpitt AR, Rollins DE, Mitchell JR: Varying effects of sulfhydryl nucleophiles on acetaminophen oxidation and sulfhydryl adduct formation, *Biochem Pharmacol* 28:2941-2946, 1979.

39. Smilkstein MJ et al: Efficacy of oral n-acetylcysteine in the treatment of acetaminophen overdose: analysis of the national multicenter study (1976-1985), *N Engl J Med* 319:1557-1562, 1988.

40. Smilkstein MJ et al: Acetaminophen overdose: a 48-hour intravenous n-acetylcysteine treatment protocol, *Ann Emerg Med* 20:1058-1063, 1991.

41. Prescott LF et al: Intravenous n-acetylsteine: the treatment of choice for paracetamol poisoning, *BMJ* 2:1097-1100, 1979.

42. Levy G, Garrettson LK, Soda DM: Evidence of placenta transfer of acetaminophen (letter), *Pediatrics* 55:895, 1975.

Ethanol

43. Litovitz TL et al: 1994 Annual report of the American Association of Poison Control Centers national data collection system, *Am J Emerg Med* 13:551-597, 1995.

44. Weller-Fahy ER, Berger LR, Troutman WG: Mouthwash: a source of acute ethanol intoxication, *Pediatrics* 66:302-304, 1980.

45. Committee on Drugs 1983-1984. American Academy of Pediatrics: Ethanol in liquid preparations intended for children, *Pediatrics* 73:405-407, 1984.

46. Lieber CS: Metabolism and metabolic effects of alcohol, *Pediatr Clin North Am* 68:3-31, 1984.

47. Ragan FA Jr, Samuels MS, Hite SA: Ethanol ingestion in children: a five year review, *JAMA* 242:2787-2788, 1979.

48. Minocha A et al: Impairment of cognitive and neuromuscular function by ethanol in social drinkers, *Vet Hum Toxicol* 28:319, 1985.

49. Lang RM et al: Adverse cardiac effects of acute alcohol ingestion in young adults, *Ann Intern Med* 102:742-743, 1985.

50. Litovitz T: The alcohols: ethanol, methanol, isopropanol, ethylene glycol, *Pediatr Clin North Am* 33(2):311-323, 1986.

51. Gamis AS and Wasserman GS: Acute acetone intoxication in a pediatric patient, *Pediatr Emerg Care* 4(1):24-26, 1988.

52. Redetzki HM: Ethanol. In Rumack BH, Hess AJ, Gilman CR, editors: *POISINDEX Systems*, Denver, 1996, Micromedex.

53. Scherger DL et al: Ethyl alcohol (ethanol)-containing cologne, perfume and after-shave ingestions in children, *Am J Dis Child* 142:630-632, 1988.

Isopropanol

54. Litovitz TL et al: 1994 Annual report of the American Association of Poison Control Centers national data collection system, *Am J Emerg Med* 13:551-597, 1995.

55. Mydler TT et al: Two week old infant with isopropanol intoxication, *Pediatr Emerg Care* 9:146, 1993.

56. Martinez TT, Jaeger RW, Decastro FJ: A comparison of the absorption and metabolism of isopropyl alcohol by oral, dermal, and inhalation routes, *Vet Hum Toxicol* 28(3):233-236, 1986.

57. Lewin GA, Oppenheimer PR, Winger WA: Coma from alcohol sponging, *JACEP* 6:165-167, 1977.

58. McFadden SW and Haddow JE: Coma produced by topical application of isopropanol, *Pediatrics* 43:622-623, 1969.

59. Arditi M and Killner MS: Coma following use of rubbing alcohol for fever control, *Am J Dis Child* 141:237-238, 1987.

60. Daniel DR, McAnalley BH, Garriott JC: Isopropyl alcohol metabolism after acute intoxication in humans, *J Anal Toxicol* 5:110-112, 1981.

61. Webster HC et al: Diagnostic clinical osmometry in the unconscious infant, *Crit Care Med* 13:1076-1077, 1985.

62. Mecikalski MB and Depner TA: Peritoneal dialysis for isopropanol poisoning, *West J Med* 137:322-324, 1982.

63. Visudhiphan P and Kaufman H: Increased cerebrospinal fluid protein following isopropyl alcohol intoxication, *N Y State J Med* 71:887-888, 1971.

64. Adelson L: Fatal intoxication with isopropyl alcohol, *Am J Clin Pathol* 38:144-151, 1962.

65. Kelner M and Bailey DN: Isopropanol ingestion: interpretation of blood concentrations and clinical findings, *J Tox Clin Toxicol* 20:497-507, 1983.

66. Lacouture PG et al: Acute isopropyl alcohol intoxication: diagnosis and management, *Am J Med* 75:680-686, 1983.

67. Litovitz T: The alcohols: ethanol, methanol, isopropanol, ethylene glycol, *Pediatr Clin North Am* 33:311-323, 1986.

68. Alcohols and glycols. In Ellenhorn MJ and Barceloux DG, editors: *Medical toxicology, diagnosis and treatment of human poisoning*, New York, 1988, Elsevier Science.

69. Juncos L, Taguchi T: Isopropyl alcohol intoxication: report of a case associated with myopathy, renal failure, and hemolytic anemia, *JAMA* 204:186-188, 1968.

70. Troutman WG: Isopropanol. In Rumack BH, Hess AJ, Gilman CR, editors: *POISINDEX Systems*, Denver, 1996, Micromedex.

Methanol

71. Litovitz TL et al: 1994 Annual report of the American Association of Poison Control Centers national data collection system, *Am J Emerg Med* 13:551-597, 1995.

72. Bennet IV et al: Acute methyl alcohol poisoning: a review based on experiences in an outbreak of 323 cases, *Medicare* 32:431-457, 1953.

73. Kahn A, Blum D: Methyl alcohol poisoning in an 8-month-old boy: an unusual route of intoxication, *J Pediatr* 94:841-843, 1979.

74. Jacobsen D, McMartin KE: Methanol and ethylene glycol poisonings: mechanism of toxicity, clinical course, diagnosis, and treatment, *Med Toxicol* 1:309-334, 1986.

75. Lacoutre PG and Lovejoy FH: Methanol, *Clin Toxicol Rev* 3:1-3, 1981.

76. Alcohols and glycols. In Ellenhorn MJ and Barceloux DG, editors: *Medical toxicology, diagnosis and treatment of human poisoning*, New York, 1988, Elsevier Science.

77. Kulig K et al: Toxic effects of methanol, ethylene glycol, and isopropyl alcohol, *Top Emerg Med* 6(2):15-18, 1984.

78. Becker CE: Acute methanol poisoning: "The blind drunk," Medical Staff Conference, University of California San Francisco, *West J Med* 135:122-128, 1981.

79. Benton CD and Calhoun FP: The ocular effects of methyl alcohol poisoning: report of a catastrophe involving 320 persons, *Am J Ophthalmol* 26:1677-1685, 1952.

80. Swartz RD et al: Epidemic methanol poisoning: clinical and biochemical analysis of a recent episode, *Medicine* 60:373-382, 1981.

81. Palatnick W et al: Methanol half-life during ethanol administration: Implications for management of methanol poisoning, *Ann Emerg Med* 26:202, 1995.

82. Methanol. In Rumack BH, Hess AJ, Gilman CR, editors: *POISINDEX Systems*, Denver, 1996, Micromedex.

83. Noker PE, Eells JT, Tephly TR: Methanol toxicity: treatment with folic acid and 5-formyl tetrahydrofolic acid, *Alcohol Clin Exp Res* 4:378-383, 1980.

Ethylene Glycol

84. Litovitz TL et al: 1994 Annual report of the American Association of Poison Control Centers national data collection system, *Am J Emerg Med* 13:551-557.

85. Litovitz T: The alcohols: ethanol, methanol, isopropanol, ethylene glycol, *Pediatr Clin North Am* 33:311-323, 1986.

86. Freed CR, Bobbitt WM, et al: Ethanol for ethylene glycol poisoning, *N Engl J Med* 304:976-977, 1981.

87. Von Wartburg JP, Bethune JL, Vallee BL: Human liver alcohol dehydrogenase: kinetic and physiochemical properties, *Biochemistry* 3:1775-1782, 1964.

88. Cornish HH: Ethylene glycol. In Doull JM, Kiaassen CD, Amdur MO, editors: *Casarett and Doull's Toxicology. The basic science of poisons*, New York, 1980, MacMillan.

89. Peterson CD et al: Ethylene glycol poisoning: pharmacokinetics during therapy with ethanol and hemodialysis, *N Engl J Med* 304:21-23, 1981.

90. Hurt R: Toxicity of ethylene and propylene glycol, *Ind Eng Chem* 24:361, 1932.

91. Bobbitt WH, Williams RM, Freed CR: Severe ethylene glycol intoxication with multisystemic failure, *West J Med* 144:225-228, 1986.

92. Friedman EA et al: Consequences of ethylene glycol poisoning: report of four cases and review of the literature, *Am J Med* 32:891-902, 1962.

93. Kulig K et al: *Toxic effects of methanol, ethylene glycol, and isopropyl alcohol. Topics in emergency medicine*, 1984, Aspen Systems.

94. Parry MF and Wallch R: Ethylene glycol poisoning, *Am J Med* 57:143-150, 1974.

95. Berman LB, Schreiner GE, Feys J: The nephrotoxic lesions of ethylene glycol, *Ann Intern Med* 46:611-619, 1957.

96. Turk J, Murrell L, Avioli LV: Ethylene glycol intoxication (grand rounds), *Arch Intern Med* 146:1601-1603, 1986.

97. Jacobsen D et al: Anion and osmolal gaps in the diagnosis of ethanol and ethylene glycol intoxication, *Acta Med Scand* 212:17-20, 1982.

98. Cadnaparphornchai P et al: Ethylene glycol poisoning: diagnosis based on high osmolar and anion gaps and crystalluria, *Am J Emerg Med* 10:94-97, 1981.

99. Clay KL, Murphy RC: On the metabolic acidosis of ethylene glycol intoxication, *Toxicol Appl Pharmacol* 39:39-49, 1977.

100. Glycols. In Rumack BH, Hess AJ, Gilman CR, editors: *POISINDEX Systems*, Denver, 1996, Micromedex.

101. McCoy MG et al: Severe methanol poisoning. Application of a pharmacokinetic model for ethanol therapy and hemodialysis, *Am J Med* 67:804-807, 1979.

102. Pappas SL and Silverman M: Treatment of methanol poisoning with ethanol and hemodialysis, *Can Med Assoc J* 126:1391-1394, 1982.

Anticholinergics

103. Litovitz TL et al: 1994 Annual report of the American Association of Poison Control Centers national data collection system, *Am J Emerg Med* 13:551-597, 1995.

104. Cullumbine M, McKee WME, Creasey NM: The effects of atropine sulfate upon healthy male subjects, *Q J Exp Physiol* 40:309-319, 1955.

105. Kradjan WA et al: Serum atropine concentrations after inhalation of atropine sulfate, *Am Rev Respir Dis* 123:471-472, 1981.

106. Huston RL et al: Toxicity from topical administration of diphenhydramine in children, *Clin Pediatr* 29:542-545, 1990.

107. Kalser SC: The fate of atropine in man, *Ann N Y Acad Sci* 179:667-683, 1971.

108. Brown JH: Atropine, scopolamine, and related antimuscarinic drugs. In Gilman AG et al, editors: *The pharmacological basis of therapeutics*, ed 8, New York, 1990, Pergamon Press.

109. Pihlajamaki K et al: Pharmacokinetics of atropine in children, *Int J Clin Pharmacol Ther Toxicol* 24:236-239, 1986.

110. Morton HG: Atropine intoxication: its manifestations in infants and children, *J Pediatr* 14:755-760, 1939.

111. Heath WE: Death from atropine poisoning, *Br Med J* 2:608, 1950.

112. Zavitz M, Lindsay C, McGuigan MA: Acute diphenhydramine ingestion in children (abstract 80), *Vet Hum Toxicol* 31:349, 1989.

113. Wyngaarder JB and Severs MH: The toxic effects of antihistaminic drugs, *JAMA* 145:277-282, 1951.

114. Treibergs J and Lovejoy FH Jr: Diphenhydramine, *Clin Toxicol Rev* 5(7):1-2, 1983.

115. Wasserman GS, Green VA, Wise GW: Lomotil ingestions in pediatrics, *Am Fam Phys* 7:401-406, 1974.

116. Bhutta TI and Tahir KI: Loperamide poisoning in children (letter), *Lancet* 335:363, 1990.

117. Ketchum JS et al: Atropine, scopolamine and ditran: comparative pharmacology and antagonists in man, *Psychopharmacologia* 28:121-145, 1973.

118. Garlington LN and Bailey PJ: Is atropine a poison? *Anesth Analg* 38:254-258, 1959.

119. Jones J, Dougherty J, Cannon L: Diphenhydramine induced toxic psychosis, *Am J Emerg Med* 4:369-371, 1986.

120. Uder DL et al: Antihistamines: a study of pediatric usage and incidence of toxicity, *Vet Hum Toxicol* 26:469-472, 1984.

121. Krenzelok EP, Anderson GM, Mirick M: Massive diphenhydramine overdose resulting in death, *Am J Emerg Med* 11:212-213, 1982.

122. Hestard HE and Tesky DW: Diphenhydramine hydrochloride intoxication, *J Pediatr* 90:1017-1018, 1977.

123. Berghem L et al: Plasma atropine concentrations determined by radioimmunoassay after single dose IV and IM administration, *Br J Anaesth* 52:597-601, 1980.

124. Kradjan WA et al: Atropine serum concentrations after multiple inhaled doses of atropine sulfate, *Clin Pharmacol Ther* 38:12-15, 1985.

125. Lapan D and Smith JW: Atropine coma: physostigmine reversal, *Ariz Med* 34:159-160, 1977.

126. Worth DP et al: Ineffectiveness of haemodialysis in atropine poisoning, *Br Med J* 206:2023-2024, 1983.

127. Rumack BH: Anticholinergic poisoning: treatment with physostigmine, *Pediatrics* 52:449-451, 1973.

128. Slovis TL et al: Physostigmine therapy in acute tricyclic antidepressant poisoning, *Clin Toxicol* 4:451-459, 1971.

129. Greenblatt DJ, Shader RI: Atropine overdose in three children, *Br J Anaesth* 44:750, 1972.

130. Anticholinergic. In Rumack BH, Hess AJ, Gilman CR, editors: *POISINDEX Systems*, Denver, 1996, Micromedex.

Carbamazepine

131. Carbamazepine. In Ellenhorn MJ and Barceloux DG: *Medical toxicology, diagnosis and treatment of human poisoning*, New York, 1988, Elsevier Science.

132. Gilman AG et al: editors: *Goodman and Gilman's the pharmacological basis of therapeutics*, ed 8, New York, 1990, Pergamon Press.

133. Litovitz TL et al: 1994 Annual report of the American Association of Poison Control Centers National Data Collection System, *Am J Emerg Med* 13:551-557, 1995.

134. Morsell PL and Frigerio A: Metabolism and pharmacokinetics of carbamazepine, *Drug Metab Rev* 4:97-113, 1975.

135. Hundt HKL, Aucamp AK, Muller FO: Pharmacokinetic aspects of carbamazepine and its two major metabolites in plasma during overdosage, *Hum Toxicol* 2:607, 1983.

136. Sethna M et al: Successful treatment of massive carbamazepine overdose, *Epilepsia* 30:71-73, 1989.

137. DeZeeun RA et al: An unusual case of carbamazepine poisoning with a near-fatal relapse after two days, *Clin Toxicol* 14:263-264, 1979.

138. Sullivan JB Jr, Rumack BH, Peterson RG: Acute carbamazepine toxicity resulting from overdose, *Neurology* 31:621-624, 1981.

139. Pynnonen S et al: Carbamazepine and 10,11-epoxy carbamazepine levels in children, *Proc Eur Soc Toxicol* 18:192-194, 1977.

140. Eichelbaum M, Tomson T, Tykring G: Carbamazepine metabolism in man: induction and pharmacogenetic aspects, *Clin Pharmacokinet* 10:80, 1985.

141. Rey E et al: Pharmacokinetics of carbamazepine in the neonate and in the child, *Int J Clin Pharmacol Biopharm* 17:90-96, 1979.

142. Levy RH et al: Pharmacokinetics of carbamazepine in normal man, *Clin Pharm Ther* 17:657-668, 1975.

143. Rane A, Bertilsson L, Palmer L: Disposition of placentally transferred carbamazepine (Tegretol) in the newborn, *Eur J Clin Pharmacol* 8:283-284, 1974.

144. Niebyl JR et al: Carbamazepine levels in pregnancy and lactation, *Obstet Gynecol* 53:139-140, 1979.

145. Spiller HA, Krenzelok EP, Cookson E: Carbamazepine overdose: a prospective study of serum levels and toxicity, *Clin Toxicol* 28(4):445-458, 1990.

146. Leshe PJ, Heyworth R, Prescott LF: Cardiac complications of carbamazepine intoxication: treatment by hemoperfusion, *BMJ* 286:1018, 1983.

147. Beerman B, Edhag O, Vallin H: Advanced heart block aggravated by carbamazepine, *Br Heart J* 37:668, 1975.

148. Gaspereth CM: Conduction abnormalities complicating carbamazepine therapy, *Am J Med* 82:381, 1987.

149. Salesman M and Pippenger CE: Acute carbamazepine encephalopathy, *JAMA* 231:915, 1975.

150. Umeda Y and Sakata E: Equilibrium disorders in carbamazepine toxicity, *Ann Otol* 86:318-322, 1977.

151. Kalaawi MH et al: Encephalopathy and brain stem dysfunction in an infant with non-accidental carbamazepine intoxication, *Clin Pediatr* 30:385-386, 1991.

152. Apfelbaum JD et al: Cardiovascular effects of carbamazepine toxicity, *Ann Emerg Med* 25:631, 1995.

153. Nacnab AJ, Birch P, MacReady J: Carbamazepine poisoning in children, *Pediatr Emerg Care* 9:195, 1993.
154. Boldy DAR et al: Activated charcoal for carbamazepine poisoning, *Lancet* 1:1027, 1987.
155. Tenenbein M: Multiple doses of activated charcoal: time for reappraisal? *Ann Emerg Med* 20:529-531, 1991.
156. Gary NE, Byra WM, Eisinger RP: Carbamazepine poisoning: treatment by hemoperfusion, *Nephron* 27:202-203, 1981.

Clonidine

157. Litovitz TL et al: 1994 Annual report of the American Association of Poison Control Centers national data collection system, *Am J Emerg Med* 13:551-557, 1995.
158. Pettinger WA: Clonidine, a new antihypertensive drug, *N Engl J Med* 293:1179, 1975.
159. Gold M et al: Opiate withdrawal using clonidine, *JAMA* 243:343, 1980.
160. Walinder J et al: Clonidine suppression of the alcohol withdrawal syndrome, *Drug Alcohol Depend* 8:345, 1981.
161. Pearce K: Clonidine and smoking (letter), *Lancet* 2:810, 1986.
162. Wasserman GS: Clonidine intoxications (letter), *Vet Hum Toxicol* 31:391, 1989.
163. Bamshad MJ and Wasserman GS: Pediatric clonidine intoxications, *Vet Hum Toxicol* 32:220, 1990.
164. Caravati E and Bennett D: Clonidine transdermal patch poisoning, *Ann Emerg Med* 7:175, 1988.
165. Knapp JF et al: Case 01-1995: A two-year-old female with alteration of consciousness, *Pediatr Emerg Care* 11:62, 1995.
166. Farsang C et al: Possible involvement of an endogenous opioid in the antihypertensive effect of clonidine in patients with essential hypertension, *Circulation* 66:68, 1982.
167. Dollery CT et al: Clinical pharmacology and pharmacokinetics of clonidine, *Clin Pharmacol Ther* 19:11, 1976.
168. Wiley JF et al: Clonidine poisoning in young children, *J Pediatr* 116:654, 1990.
169. Heidemann SM and Sarnaik AP: Clonidine poisoning in children, *Crit Care Med* 18:618, 1990.
170. Kulig K et al: Naloxone for treatment of clonidine overdose, *JAMA* 247:1697, 1982.
171. North DS et al: Naloxone administration in clonidine overdosage, *Ann Emerg Med* 10:397, 1981.
172. Banner W, Lund M, Clawson L: Failure of naloxone to reverse clonidine toxic effect, *Am J Dis Child* 137:1170, 1983.
173. Woolf AD et al: Efficacy of anti-digoxin antibodies in serious pediatric digitalis poisoning (abstract 1), *Vet Hum Toxicol* 32:341, 1990.
174. Woolf AD et al: The post-marketing surveillance study of antidigoxin antibodies in serious digitalis inntoxications *Vet Hum Toxicol* 32:341, 1990 (abstract 3).

Caustics

175. *Dorland's illustrated medical dictionary*, ed 25, Philadelphia, 1974, WB Saunders.
176. Bryson PD, editor: Comprehensive review in toxicology, ed 2, Rockville, Md, 1989, Aspen.
177. Stewart C: Chemical skin burns, *Am Fam Physician* 31:149, 1985.
178. Jelenko C: Chemicals that "burn," *J Trauma* 14:65, 1974.
179. Nelson R, Walson P, Kelly M: Caustic ingestion, *Ann Emerg Med* 12:559, 1983.
180. Klein M: Addressing the controversies of caustic ingestions, *Emerg Med Rep* 4:155, 1983.
181. Litovitz TL et al: 1994 Annual report of the American Association of Poison Control Centers national data collection system, *Am J Emerg Med* 13:551-557, 1995.
182. Wasserman GS and Jazbi B: Poisoning in children. In Jazbi B, editor: *Pediatric otorhinolaryngology: a review of ear, nose, and throat problems in children*, New York, 1980, Appleton-Century-Crofts.
183. Kirsh MM and Ritter FN: Caustic ingestion and subsequent damage to the oropharyngeal and digestive passage, *Ann Thorac Surg* 21:74, 1976.
184. Gorman RL et al: Initial symptoms as predictors of esophageal injury of alkaline ingestions *Vet Hum Toxicol* 31:338, 1989 (abstract 36).
185. Adam J and Birck H: Pediatric caustic ingestion, *Ann Otol Rhinol Laryngol* 91:656, 1982.

186. Buntain W and Cain W: Caustic injuries to the esophagus: a pediatric review, *South Med J* 74:590, 1981.
187. Crain E, Gershel J, Mezey A: Caustic ingestions, *Am J Dis Child* 138:863, 1984.
188. Wason S: The emergency management of caustic ingestions, *J Emerg Med* 2:175, 1985.
189. Cello J, Fogel R, Boland R: Liquid caustic ingestion, *Arch Intern Med* 140:501, 1980.
190. Ritter FN: Lye burns of the esophagus and their treatment, *Adv Otorhinolaryngol* 23:104, 1978.
191. Hoffman R: Caustics and batteries. In Goldfrank LR et al, editor: *Toxicologic emergencies*, ed 5, Norwalk, Conn, 1994, Appleton-Lange.
192. Appelqvist P: Lye corrosion carcinoma of the esophagus: a review of 63 cases, *Cancer* 45:2655, 1980.
193. Martel W: Radiologic features of esophago-gastritis secondary to extremely caustic agents, *Radiology* 103:31, 1972.
194. Howell J: Alkaline ingestions, *Ann Emerg Med* 15:820, 1986.
195. Rumack BH: Caustic ingestions: a rational look at diluents, *Clin Toxicol* 11:27, 1977.
196. Maull KI: Liquid caustic ingestions: an in vitro study of the effects of buffer neutralization, and dilution, *Ann Emerg Med* 14:1160, 1985.
197. Penner GE: Acid ingestion, toxicology and treatment, *Ann Emerg Med* 9:374, 1980.
198. Wasserman R and Ginsburg C: Caustic substance injuries, *J Pediatr* 107:169, 1985.

Cyclic Antidepressants

199. Litovitz TL et al: 1994 Annual report of the American Association of Poison Control Centers national data collection system, *Am J Emerg Med* 13:551-557, 1995.
200. Baldessarini RJ: Drugs and the treatment of psychiatric disorders. In Gilman AG, Rall TW, Nies AS et al, editors: *The pharmacological basis of therapeutics*, ed 8, New York, 1990, Pergamon Press.
201. Frommer DA et al: Tricyclic-antidepressant overdose: a review, *JAMA* 257:521, 1987.
202. Marshall JB and Forker AD: Cardiovascular effects of tricyclic antidepressant drugs: therapeutic usage, overdose, and management of complications, *Am Heart J* 103:401, 1982.
203. Boehnert MT and Lovejoy FH Jr: Value of the QRS duration versus the serum drug level in predicting seizures and ventricular arrhythmias after an acute overdose of tricyclic antidepressants, *N Engl J Med* 313:474, 1985.
204. Bramble MG et al: An analysis of plasma levels and 24 hour ECG recordings in tricyclic antidepressant poisoning: implications for management, *Q J Med* 56:357, 1985.
205. Crome P: Poisoning due to tricyclic antidepressant overdosage: clinical presentation and treatment, *Med Toxicol* 1:261, 1986.
206. Callaham M: Epidemiology of fatal tricyclic antidepressant ingestion: implications for management, *Ann Emerg Med* 14:1, 1985.
207. Pellinen TJ et al: Electrocardiographic and clinical features of tricyclic antidepressant intoxication, *Ann Clin Res* 19:12, 1987.
208. Manoguerra AS: Tricyclic antidepressants, *Crit Care Q* 5:43, 1982.
209. Ellison DW and Pentel PR: Clinical features and consequences of seizures due to cyclic antidepressant overdose, *Am J Emerg Med* 7:5, 1989.
210. Shrand H: Agoraphobia and imipramine withdrawal? *Pediatrics* 70:825, 1982 (letter).
211. Stancer HC and Reed KL: Desipramine and 2-hydroxydesipramine in human breast milk and the nursing infant's serum, *Am J Psychiatr* 143:1597, 1986.
212. Sorisky A and Watson DC: Positive diphenhydramine interference in the EMIT-st assay for tricyclic antidepressants in serum, *Clin Chem* 32:715, 1986 (letter).
213. Labrosse KR and McCoy HG: Reliability of antidepressant assays: a reference laboratory perspective on antidepressant monitoring, *Clin Chem* 34:859, 1988.
214. Hanzlick R: Postmortem tricyclic antidepressant concentrations: lethal vs nonlethal levels, *Am J Forensic Med Pathol* 10:326, 1989.
215. Tokarski GF and Young MJ: Criteria for admitting patients with tricyclic antidepressant overdose, *J Emerg Med* 6:121, 1988.
216. Foulke GE and Albertson TE: QRS interval in tricyclic antidepressant overdosage: inaccuracy as a toxicity indicator in emergency settings, *Ann Emerg Med* 16:160, 1987.

217. Emerson CL, Connors AF, Burma GM: Level of consciousness as a predictor of complications following tricyclic overdose, *Ann Emerg Med* 16:326, 1987.
218. Emerman CL: Tricyclic overdose: consciousness as a predictor of complications, *Ann Emerg Med* 17:381, 1988.
219. Lavoie FW, Gansert GG, Weiss RE: Value of initial ECG findings and plasma drug levels in cyclic antidepressant overdose, *Ann Emerg Med* 19:696, 1990.
220. Pentel PR and Benowitz NL: Tricyclic antidepressant poisoning: management of arrhythmias, *Med Toxicol* 1:101, 1986.
221. Boehnert M: Tricyclic antidepressant poisoning, In Harwood-Nuss A, editor: *The clinical practice of emergency medicine*, Philadelphia, 1990, JB Lippincott.
222. Givens T, Holloway M, Wason S: Pulmonary aspiration of activated charcoal after tricyclic antidepressant overdose, *Vet Hum Toxicol* 32:375, 1990 (abstract 137).
223. Bessen HA et al: Effect of respiratory alkalosis in tricyclic antidepressant overdose, *West J Med* 139:373, 1983.
224. Brown TCK et al: The use of sodium bicarbonate in the treatment of cyclic antidepressant induced arrhythmias, *Anaesth Intensive Care* 1:203, 1973.
225. Hoffman SR and McElroy CR: Bicarbonate therapy for dysrhythmia and hypotension in tricyclic antidepressant overdose, *West J Med* 134:60, 1981.
226. Kingston ME: Hyperventilation in tricyclic antidepressant poisoning, *Crit Care Med* 7:550, 1979.
227. Sasyniuk BI et al: Experimental amitriptyline intoxication: treatment of cardiac toxicity with sodium bicarbonate, *Ann Emerg Med* 15:1052, 1986.
228. Nattel S, Keable H, Sasyniuk BI: Experimental amitriptyline intoxication: electrophysiologic manifestations and management, *J Cardiovasc Pharmacol* 6:83, 1984.
229. Schlesinger JJ and Janz TG: The efficacy of continuous bicarbonate infusion in maintaining an alkaline pH *Ann Emerg Med* 18:916, 1989 (abstract).
230. Pentel P and Benowitz N: Efficacy and mechanism of action of sodium bicarbonate in the treatment of desipramine toxicity in rats, *J Pharmacol Exp Ther* 230:12, 1984.
231. Hedges JR et al: Bicarbonate therapy for the cardiovascular toxicity of amitriptyline in an animal model, *J Emerg Med* 3:253, 1985.
232. Walsh DM: Cyclic antidepressant overdose in children: a proposed treatment protocol, *Pediatr Emerg Care* 2:28, 1986.
233. Hagerman GA and Hanashiro PK: Reversal of tricyclic-antidepressant-induced cardiac conduction abnormalities by phenytoin, *Ann Emerg Med* 10:82, 1981.
234. Mayron R and Ruiz E: Phenytoin: Does it reverse tricyclic-antidepressant-induced cardiac conduct abnormalities? *Ann Emerg Med* 15:876, 1986.
235. Walker WE, Levy RC, Hanenson IB: Physostigmine—its use and abuse, *JACEP* 5:436, 1976.
236. Driggers DA et al: Tricyclic antidepressant overdose, *J Fam Pract* 25:231, 1987.
237. Pentel P and Peterson CO: Asystole complicating physostigmine treatment of tricyclic antidepressant overdose, *Ann Emerg Med* 9:588, 1980.
238. Braden NJ, Jackson JE, Walson PD: Tricyclic antidepressant overdose, *Pediatr Clin North Am* 33:287, 1986.
239. Teba L et al: Beneficial effect of norepinephrine in the treatment of circulatory shock caused by tricyclic antidepressant overdose, *Am J Emerg Med* 6:566, 1988.
240. Comstock TJ, Watson WA, Jennison TA: Severe amitriptyline intoxication and the use of charcoal hemoperfusion, *Clin Pharm* 2:85, 1983.
241. Freeman JW et al: Cardiac abnormalities in poisoning with tricyclic antidepressants, *BMJ* 2:610, 1969.
242. Sedal L et al: Overdosage of tricyclic antidepressants—a report of two deaths and a prospective study of 24 patients, *Med J Aust* 2:74, 1972.
243. Callahan M: Admission criteria for tricyclic antidepressant ingestion, *West J Med* 137:425, 1982.
244. McAlpine SB et al: Late death in tricyclic antidepressant overdose revisited, *Ann Emerg Med* 15:1349, 1986.
245. Pentel P and Sioris L: Incidence of late arrhythmias following tricyclic antidepressant overdose, *Clin Toxicol* 18:543, 1981.
246. Goldberg RJ, Capone RJ, Hunt JD: Cardiac complications following tricyclic antidepressant overdose, *JAMA* 254:1772, 1985.

Insecticide Cholinesterase Inhibitors

247. Litovitz TL et al: 1994 Annual report of the American Association of Poison Control Centers national data collection system, *Am J Emerg Med* 13:551-557, 1995.
248. Zweiner RJ, Ginsburg GM: Organophosphate and carbamate poisoning in infants and children, *Pediatrics* 81:121-126, 1988.
249. DePalma AE, Kwalick DS, Zukerberg N: Pesticide poisoning in children, *JAMA* 211:1979-1981, 1970.
250. Wyckoff DW et al: Diagnostic and therapeutic problems of parathion poisoning, *Ann Intern Med* 68:875-882, 1968.
251. Klemmer HW, Reichert ER, Younger WL Jr: Five cases of intentional ingestion of 25 percent diazinon with treatment and recovery, *Clin Toxicol* 12:435-444, 1978.
252. Clifford NJ, Nies AS: Organophosphate poisoning from wearing a laundered uniform previously contaminated with parathion, *JAMA* 262(12):3035-3036, 1989.
253. Eitzman DV and Wolfson SL: Acute parathion poisoning in children, *Am J Dis Child* 114:397-400, 1967.
254. Warren MC et al: Clothing-borne epidemic: organic phosphate poisoning in children, *JAMA* 184:266-268, 1963.
255. Pesticides. In Ellenhorn MJ and Barceloux DG, editors: *Diagnosis and treatment of human poisoning*, New York, 1988, Elsevier Science.
256. Tafuri J, Roberts J: Organophosphate poisoning, *Ann Emerg Med* 16:193-202, 1987.
257. Namba T et al: Poisoning due to organophosphate insecticides, *Am J Med* 50:475-492, 1971.
258. Barret DS and Oehme FW: A review of organophosphorus ester induced delayed neurotoxicity, *Vet Hum Toxicol* 27:22-37, 1985.
259. Bouldin TW and Cavanagh JB: Organophosphorus neuropathy: I. a teased-fiber study of the spatio-temporal spread of axonal degeneration, *Am J Pathol* 94:241-248, 1979.
260. Senanayake N and Johnson MK: Acute polyneuropathy after poisoning by a new organophosphate insecticide, *N Engl J Med* 306:155-157, 1982.
261. Hassan RM et al: Correlation of serum pseudocholinesterase and clinical course in two patients poisoned with organophosphate insecticides, *Clin Toxicol* 18:401-406, 1981.
262. Sofer S, Asher T, Shahak E: Carbamate and organophosphate poisoning in early childhood, *Pediatr Emerg Care* 5:222-225, 1985.
263. Crispen C et al: Intussusception as a possible complication of organophosphate overdose and/or treatment, *Clin Pediatr* 24:140, 1985.
264. Albright RK, Kram BW, White RP: Malathion exposure associated with acute renal failure, *JAMA* 250:2469, 1983.
265. Borowitz SM: Prolonged organophosphate toxicity in a twenty-six-month-old child, *J Pediatr* 112:302-304, 1988.
266. Vasilescu C, Alexianu M, Dan A: Delayed neuropathy after organophosphorus insecticide (Dipterex) poisoning: a clinical electrophysiological and nerve biopsy study, *J Neurol Neurosurg Psychiatry* 47:543-548, 1984.
267. Senanayake N and Karalliedde L: Neurotoxic effects of organophosphorus insecticides—an intermediated syndrome, *N Engl J Med* 316:761-763, 1987.
268. Savage EP et al: *Chronic neurological sequelae of acute organophosphate pesticide poisoning: a case control study*, US Environmental Protection Agency, 1980, Washington, DC.
269. Korsak RJ and Sato MM: Effects of chronic organophosphate pesticide exposure on the central nervous system, *Clin Toxicol* 11:83-95, 1977.
270. Zadik Z et al: Organophosphate poisoning presenting as diabetic ketoacidosis, *J Toxicol Clin Toxicol* 20:381-395, 1983.
271. Murray JC et al: Prolongation of the prothrombin time after organophosphate poisoning, *Pediatr Emerg Care* 10:289, 1984.
272. Brown HW: Electroencephalographic changes and disturbance of brain function following human organophosphate exposure, *Northwest Med* 70:845-846, 1971.
273. Kiss Z and Fazekas T: Arrhythmias in organophosphate poisonings, *Acta Cardiol* 34:323-330, 1979.
274. Morgan DP: Organophosphates (management/treatment protocol). In Rumack BH, Hess AJ, Gilman CR, editors: *POISINDEX Systems*, Denver, 1996, Micromedex.

275. Mortensen ML: Management of acute childhood poisonings caused by selected insecticides and herbicides, *Pediatr Clin North Am* 33:421-445, 1986.

276. Jordan R and Marx J, editors: Toxic ingestion, *Case Stud Emerg Med* 1:10-11, 1984.

277. Mack R: Toxic encounters of the dangerous kind, *N C Med J* 44:103-105, 1983.

278. Zavon MR: Treatment of organophosphorus and chlorinated hydrocarbon insecticide intoxications, *Mod Treat* 8:503-510, 1971.

279. Morgan DP: Recognition and management of pesticide poisonings, edition Z, Washington, DC, 1982, US Environmental Protection Agency.

280. Taylor P: Anticholinesterase agents. In Gilman AG et al, editors: *The pharmacologic basis of therapeutics*, ed 8, New York, 1990, Pergamon Press.

281. Natoff IL and Reiff B: Effect of oximes on the acute toxicity of anticholinesterase carbamates, *Toxicol Appl Pharmacol* 25:569-575, 1973.

282. Haddad LM: The carbamate, organochlorine, and botanical insecticides; insect repellents. In Haddad LM, Winchester JF, editors: *Clinical management of poisoning and drug overdose*, Philadelphia, 1983, WB Saunders.

283. Johns RJ, Bales PD, Himwich HE: The effects of DFP on the convulsant dose of theophylline, theophylline-ethylenediamine and 8-chlorotheophylline, *J Pharmacol Exp Ther* 101:237-242, 1951.

284. Milby TH: Prevention and management of organophosphate poisoning, *JAMA* 216:2131-2133, 1971.

Iron

285. Litovitz TL et al: 1995 Annual report of the American Association of Poison Control Centers national data collection system, *Am J Emerg Med* 13:551-557, 1995.

286. Hornfeldt CS et al: Rate of absorption of iron from chewable vitamins *Vet Hum Toxicol* 30:375, 1988, (abstract 141).

287. Henriksson P et al: Fatal iron intoxication with multiple coagulation defects and degradation of factor VIII and factor XIII, *Scand J Haematol* 22:235, 1979.

288. Tenenbein M, Kopelow ML, De Sa DJ: Myocardial failure and shock in iron poisoning, *Hum Toxicol* 7:281, 1988.

289. Gleason et al: Acute hepatic failure in severe iron poisoning, *J Pediatr* 95:138, 1979.

290. Milteer RM, Sarpong S, Poydras U: Yersinia entercolitica septicemia after accidental oral iron overdose, *Pediatr Infect Dis J* 8:537, 1989.

291. West KW et al: Pneumatosis intestinalis in children beyond the neonatal period, *J Pediatr Surg* 24:818, 1989.

292. Hoppe JO, Marcelli GMA, Tainter ML: A review of the toxicity of iron compounds, *Am J Med Sci* 230:558, 1955.

293. Thomson J: Two cases of ferrous sulphate poisoning, *Br Med J* 1:640, 1947.

294. McEnery JT: Hospital management of acute iron ingestion, *Clin Toxicol* 4:603, 1971.

295. Engle JP, Polin KS, Stile IL: Acute iron intoxication: treatment controversies, *Drug Intell Clin Pharm* 21:153, 1987.

296. Greenblatt DJ, Allen MD, Koch-Weser J: Accidental iron poisoning in childhood: six cases including one fatality, *Clin Pediatr* 15:835, 1976.

297. Spencer IOB: Ferrous sulphate poisoning in children, *BMJ* 2:1112, 1951.

298. Klein-Schwartz W et al: Assessment of management guidelines: acute iron ingestion, *Clin Pediatr* 29:316, 1990.

299. Tunget CL et al: Iron overdose and detection of gastrointestinal bleeding with the hemocult and gastrocult assays, *Ann Emerg Med* 26:54, 1995.

300. Lacouture PG et al: Emergency assessment of severity of iron overdose by clinical and laboratory methods, *J Pediatr* 99:89, 1981.

301. Everson GW et al: Effectiveness of abdominal radiographs in visualizing chewable iron supplements following overdose, *Am J Emerg Med* 7:459, 1989.

302. Ng CW, Perry K, Martin DJ: Iron poisoning, assessment of radiography in diagnosis and management, *Clin Pediatr* 18:614, 1979.

303. Eisen TF, Lacouture PG, Woolf A: Visual detection of ferrioxamine color changes in urine (abstract 125), *Vet Hum Toxicol* 30:369, 1988.

304. Czajka PA, Konrad JD, Duffy JP: Iron poisoning: an in vitro comparison of bicarbonate and phosphate lavage solutions, *J Pediatr* 98:491, 1981.

305. Czajka PA: Effect of bicarbonate, phosphate, and saline lavage solutions on the dissolution of ferrous sulfate tablets, *Clin Toxicol* 22:447, 1984.

306. Tenenbein M: Whole bowel irrigation in iron poisoning, *J Pediatr* 111:142, 1987.

307. Peterson CD and Fifield GC: Emergency gastrotomy for acute iron poisoning, *Ann Emerg Med* 9:262, 1980.

308. Landsman I et al: Emergency gastrotomy: treatment of choice for iron bezoar, *J Pediatr Surg* 22:184, 1987.

309. Mills KC and Curry SC: Acute iron poisoning, *Emerg Med Clin North Am* 12:397, 1994.

310. Wasserman GS, Martens W, Green VA: Early aggressive treatment of iron poisoning, *Am Fam Physician* 15:125, 1977.

311. Boehnert M et al: Massive iron overdose treated with high-dose deferoxamine infusion *Vet Hum Toxicol* 28:291, 1985 (abstract 5).

312. Tennenbein M and Yatschoff RW: The total iron binding capacity in iron poisoning, *Am J Dis Child* 145:437, 1991.

313. Chyka PA and Brady AY: Elevated ratio of serum iron concentration to total iron binding capacity in assessment of systemic iron poisoning *Vet Hum Toxicol* 31:343, 1989 (abstract 53).

314. Burkhart K et al: The rise in the TIBC after iron overdose *Vet Hum Toxicol* 31:365, 1989 (abstract 143).

315. Strom RL et al: Fatal iron poisoning in a pregnant female, *Minn Med* 59:483, 1976.

316. Blanc P, Hryhorczuk D, Daniel I: Deferoxamine treatment of acute iron intoxication in pregnancy, *Obstet Gynecol* 64:12S, 1984.

Opioids

317. Litovitz TL et al: 1995 Annual report of the American Association of Poison Control Centers national data collection system, *Am J Emerg Med* 13:551-557, 1995.

318. Jaffee JH and Martin WR: Opioid analgesics and antagonists. In Gilman AG et al, editors: *The pharmacological basis of therapeutics*, ed 8, New York, 1990, Pergamon Press.

319. Snyder SH: Opiate receptors in the brain, *N Engl J Med* 296:266, 1977.

320. Thorpe DH: Opiate structure and activity—a guide to understanding the receptor, *Anesth Analg* 63:143, 1984.

321. Goldfrank L, Bresnitz E, Weisman R: Opioids and opiates, *Heart Lung* 12:114, 1983.

322. Bradberry JC and Raebel MA: Continuous infusion of naloxone in the treatment of narcotic overdose, *Drug Intell Clin Pharmacol* 15:945, 1981.

323. Hughes J, Smith TW, Kosterlitz HW: Identification of two related pentapeptides from the brain with potent opioid agonist activity, *Nature* 258:577, 1975.

324. Oldendorf WH et al: Blood-brain barrier penetration of morphine, codeine, heroin, and methadone after carotid injection, *Science* 178:984, 1972.

325. Hershey LA: Meperidine and central neurotoxicity, *Ann Intern Med* 98:548, 1983.

326. Dougherty RJ: Propoxyphene—overdose deaths, *JAMA* 235:2716, 1976.

327. Gary N et al: Acute propoxyphene hydrochloride intoxication, *Arch Intern Med* 121:453, 1968.

328. Bogartz LJ and Miller WG: Pulmonary edema associated with propoxyphene intoxication, *JAMA* 245:259, 1971.

329. Ellenhorn MJ and Barceloux DG: *Medical toxicology, diagnosis and treatment of human poisoning*, New York, 1988, Elsevier Science.

330. Sweet AY: Narcotic withdrawal syndrome in the newborn, *Pediatr Rev* 3(9):285, 1982.

331. von Muhlendahl KE et al: Codeine intoxication in childhood, *Lancet* 2:303, 1976.

332. Baselt RD, editor: *Disposition of toxic drugs and chemicals in man*, ed 2, Davis, Calif, 1982, Biomedical Publications.

333. Delvon KM et al: Toxicity from long-acting dextromethorphan preparations, *Vet Hum Toxicol* 27:296, 1985 (abstract 27).

334. McElwee NE and Veltri JC: Intentional abuse of dextromethorphan (DM) products: 1985-1988 statewide data *Vet Hum Toxicol* 32:355, 1990 (abstract 59).

335. Mitchell AA, Lovejoy FH, Goldman P: Drug ingestions associated with miosis in comatose children, *J Pediatr* 89:303, 1976.

336. Maio RF, Gaukel B, Freeman B: Intralingual naloxone injection for narcotic-induced respiratory depression, *Ann Emerg Med* 16:572, 1987.

337. American Academy of Pediatrics Committee on Drugs: Emergency drug doses for infants and children and naloxone use in newborns: clarification, *Pediatrics* 83:803, 1989.

338. Jefferys DB, Volans GN: An investigation of the role of the specific opioid antagonist naloxone in clinical toxicology, *Hum Toxicol* 2:227, 1983.

339. Moore RA et al: Naloxone—underdosage after narcotic poisoning, *Am J Dis Child* 134:156, 1980.

340. Lewis JM et al: Continuous naloxone infusion in pediatric narcotic overdose, *Am J Dis Child* 138:944, 1984.

341. Goldfrank L et al: A dosing normogram for continuous infusion of intravenous naloxone, *Ann Emerg Med* 15:566, 1986.

342. Chisholm CD: Opioid (narcotic) poisoning. In Harwood-Nuss A, editor: *The clinical practice of emergency medicine*, Philadelphia, 1991, JB Lippincott.

343. Wasserman GS, Green VA, Wise GW: Lomotil ingestions in children, *Am Fam Physician* 11:93, 1975.

Salicylates

344. Litovitz TL et al: 1994 Annual report of the American Association of Poison Control Centers national data collection system, *Am J Emerg Med* 13:551-597, 1995.

345. Centers for Disease Control: Reye's syndrome, Ohio, Michigan, *MMWR* 29:532-539, 1980.

346. Starks KM et al: Reye's syndrome and salicylate use, *Pediatrics* 66:859-864, 1980.

347. Fulginiti VA et al: Aspirin and Reye's syndrome, *Pediatrics* 69:810-812, 1982.

348. Leist ER and Banwell JG: Products containing aspirin, *N Engl J Med* 291:710-711, 1974.

349. Todd PJ et al: Problems with overdoses of sustained-release aspirin, *Lancet* 1:777, 1981.

350. Davies MG, Briff DV, Greaves MW: Systemic toxicity from topically applied salicylic acid, *Br Med J* 1:661, 1979.

351. Johnson PN and Welch DW: Methyl salicylate/aspirin/salicylate/ equivalence: Who do you trust? *Vet Hum Toxicol* 26(4):317-318, 1984.

352. Howie DL, Moriarty R, Breit R: Candy flavoring as a source of salicylate poisoning, *Pediatrics* 75:869-870, 1985.

353. Millhorn DE, Eldridge FL, Waldorp TG: Effect of salicylate and 2,4-dinitrophenol on respiration and metabolism, *J Appl Physiol* 53:925-929, 1982.

354. Brem J et al: Salicylism, hyperventilation, and the central nervous system, *J Pediatr* 83:264-266, 1973.

355. Schwartz R and Landy G: Organic acid excretion in salicylate intoxication, *J Pediatr* 66:658-666, 1965.

356. Salicylates. In Ellenhorn MJ, and Barceloux DG, editors: *Medical toxicology, diagnosis and treatment of human poisoning*, New York, 1988, Elsevier Science.

357. Thurston JH, Pollock PG, Warren SK, et al: Reduced brain glucose with normal plasma glucose in salicylate poisoning, *J Clin Invest* 49:2139-2145, 1970.

358. Cotton EK and Fahlberg V: Hypoglycemia with salicylate poisoning, *Am J Dis Child* 108:171-173, 1964.

359. Arena FP, Dugowson C, Sandex CD: Salicylate induced hypoglycemia and ketoacidosis in a non-diabetic adult, *Arch Intern Med* 138:1153-1154, 1978.

360. Temple AR: Acute and chronic effects of aspirin toxicity and their treatment, *Arch Intern Med* 141:364-369, 1981.

361. Heffner JG and Sahn SA: Salicylate induced pulmonary edema. Clinical features and prognosis, *Ann Intern Med* 95:405-409, 1981.

362. Quint PA and Allman FD: Differentiation of chronic salicylism from Reye's syndrome, *Pediatrics* 74:1117-1119, 1984.

363. Wolfe JD, Metzger AL, Goldstein RC: Aspirin hepatitis, *Ann Intern Med* 80:74-76, 1974.

364. Brantmark B et al: Salicylate inhibition of antiplatelet effect of aspirin, *Lancet* 2:1349, 1981.

365. McGrigan MH: A two year review of salicylate deaths in Ontario, *Intern Med* 147:510, 1987.

366. Snodgrass WR: Salicylate toxicity, *Pediatr Clin North Am* 33(2):381-391, 1986.

367. Gaudrealt P, Temple AR, Lovejoy FH: The relative severity of acute vs chronic salicylate poisoning in children: a clinical comparison, *Pediatrics* 70:566-569, 1982.

368. Johnson PK, Free HM, Free AH: A simplified urine and serum screening test for salicylate intoxication, *J Pediatr* 63:949-953, 1962.

369. Buchanan N, Kundig H, Eyberg C: Experimental salicylate intoxication in young baboons, *J Pediatr* 86:225-232, 1975.

370. Curtis RA, Barone J, Giacona N: Efficacy of ipecac and activated charcoal/cathartic. Prevention of salicylate absorption in simulated overdose, *Arch Intern Med* 144:48-52, 1984.

371. Hillman RJ and Prescott LF: Treatment of salicylate poisoning with repeated oral charcoal, *Br Med J* 291:1492, 1985.

372. Kirshenbaum LA et al: Does multiple-dose charcoal therapy enhance salicylate excretion? *Arch Intern Med* 150:1281-1283, 1990.

373. Prescott LF, Critchley JAJH, Proudfoot AT: Diuresis or urinary alkalinisation for salicylate poisoning? *Br Med J* 286:147, 1983.

374. Linden CH and Rumack BH: The legitimate analgesic: aspirin and acetaminophen. In Hanson W Jr, editor: *Toxic emergencies*, New York, 1984, Churchill Livingstone.

Sedatives, Hypnotics, and Antipsychotics

375. Litovitz TL et al: 1994 Annual report of the American Association of Poison Control Centers national data collection system, *Am J Emerg Med* 13:551-557, 1995.

376. Wasserman GS and Gwin JF: Barbiturates. In Edlich RF and Spyker DA, editors: *Current emergency therapy*, ed 3, Rockville, Md, 1986, Aspen.

377. Mitchell AA, Lovejoy FH, Goldman P: Drug ingestions associated with miosis in comatose children, *J Pediatr* 89:303, 1976.

378. Beveridge GW, and Lawson AAH: Occurrence of bullous lesions in acute barbiturate poisoning, *Br Med J* 1:835, 1965.

379. Mockli G et al: Massive hepatic necrosis in a child after administration of phenobarbital, *Am J Gastroenterol* 84:820, 1989.

380. McCarron MM et al: Short acting barbiturate overdosage. Correlation of intoxication score with serum barbiturate concentration, *JAMA* 248:55, 1982.

381. Baxter PJ, Samuel AM, Cocker J: Exposure to quinalbarbitone sodium in pharmaceutical workers, *Br Med J* 292:660, 1986.

382. Winek CL et al: Sustained-release-barbiturate risk, *Lancet* 2:155, 1967.

383. Neuvonen PJ, Elonen E: Effects of activated charcoal on absorption and elimination of phenobarbitone, carbamazepine and phenylbutazone in man, *Eur J Clin Pharmacol* 17:51, 1980.

384. Berg MJ et al: Acceleration of the body clearance of phenobarbital by oral activated charcoal, *N Engl J Med* 307:642, 1982.

385. Boldy DAR, Vale JA, Prescott PI: Treatment of phenobarbitone poisoning with repeated oral administration of activated charcoal, *Q J Med* 235:997, 1986.

386. Pond SM et al: Randomized study of the treatment of phenobarbital overdose with repeated doses of activated charcoal, *JAMA* 251:3104, 1984.

387. Goldberg MJ and Berlinger WG: Treatment of phenobarbital overdose with activated charcoal, *JAMA* 247:2400, 1982.

388. Gillespie WR et al: Linear systems approach to the analysis of an induced drug process; phenobarbital removal by oral activated charcoal, *J Pharmacokinet Biopharm* 14:19, 1986.

389. Wieth JD: Hemodialysis in barbiturate poisoning, *Int Anesth Clin* 4:359, 1966.

390. Skoutakis VA and Acchiardo SR: Management of acute barbiturate overdose, *Clin Toxicol Consultant* 1:51, 1979.

391. Jacobsen D et al: Pharmacokinetic evaluation of haemoperfusion in phenobarbital poisoning, *Eur J Clin Pharmacol* 26:109, 1984.

392. Zawada ET et al: Advances in the hemodialysis management of phenobarbital overdose, *South Med J* 76:6, 1983.

393. de Broc ME et al: Haemoperfusion—a useful therapy for the severely poisoned patient? *Hum Toxicol* 5:11, 1986.

394. Ellenhorn M and Barceloux D, editors: *Medical toxicology, diagnosis and treatment of human poisoning*, ed 1, New York, 1988, Elsevier Science.

395. Hojer J, Baehrendtz S, Gustafsson L: Benzodiazepine poisoning: experience of 702 admissions to an intensive care unit during a 14 year period, *J Intern Med* 226:117, 1989.

396. Ridley CM: Bullous lesions in nitrazepam overdosage, *BMJ* 3:28, 1971.
397. Vlachos P et al: Lorazepam poisoning, *Toxicol Lett* 2:109, 1978.
398. Cardoni AA: Benzodiazepine overdose. In Edlich RF, Spyker DA, editors: *Current emergency therapy,* ed 2, Rockville, Md, 1985, Aspen.
399. Ashton CH: Benzodiazepine overdose: are specific antagonists useful? *BMJ* 290:805, 1985.
400. Hofer P and Scollo-lavizzari G: Benzodiazepine antagonist R015-1788 in self-poisoning. Diagnostic and therapeutic use, *Arch Intern Med* 145:663, 1985.
401. Wood C et al: Flumazenil—a useful pediatric antidote, *Arch Fr Pediatr* 45:149, 1988.
402. Barry D, Meyskens FL, Becke CE: Phenothiazine poisoning. A review of 48 cases, *Calif Med J* 118:1, 1973.
403. Guze BH and Baxter LR Jr: Neuroleptic malignant syndrome, *N Engl J Med* 313:163, 1985.
404. Lee AS: Drug induced dystonic reactions, *JACEP* 6:351, 1977.
405. Forrest FM, Forrest IS, Mason AS: Review of rapid urine tests for phenothiazine and related drugs, *Am J Psychiatry* 118:300, 1961.
406. O'Brien RP et al: Detectability of drug tablets and capsules by plain radiography, *Am J Emerg Med* 4:302, 1986.
407. Ott DA and Goeden SR: Treatment of acute phenothiazine reaction, *JACEP* 8:471, 1979.

Substances of Abuse

408. Litovitz TL et al: 1994 Annual report of the American Association of Poison Control Centers national data collection system, *Am J Emerg Med* 13:551-557, 1995.
409. Wasserman GS: The drugs on the street where you live, *Emerg Med* 18:139-166, 1986.
410. Ziporyn T: A growing industry and menace: makeshift laboratory's designer drugs, *JAMA* 256:3061, 1986.
411. Hagerty C: Designer Drug Enforcement Act seeks to attack problem at source, *Am Pharm NS* 25:10, 1985.
412. Dowling GP, McDonough III ET, Bost RO: Eve and ecstasy a report of five deaths associated with the use of MDEA and MDMA, *JAMA* 257:1615, 1987.
413. Mofenson HC and Caraccio TR: Cocaine, *Pediatr Ann* 16:864, 1987.
414. Rodgers GC and Matyunas NJ: *Handbook of common poisonings in children,* ed 3, American Academy of Pediatrics; Elk Grove Village, Ill, 1994, p. 143.
415. Choy-Kwong M and Lipton RB: Dystonia related to cocaine withdrawal: a case report and pathogenic hypothesis, *Neurology* 39:996, 1989.
416. Perinatal toxicity of cocaine, *Med Lett* 30:59, 1988.
417. Chaney NE, Franke J, Wadlington WB: Cocaine convulsions in a breast-feeding baby, *J Pediatr* 112:134, 1988.
418. Chasnoff IJ, Burns KA, Burns WJ: Cocaine use in pregnancy: perinatal morbidity and mortality, *Neurotoxicol Teratol* 9:291, 1987.
419. Schonberg SK, editor: *Substance abuse: a guide for health professionals,* Elk Grove Village, Ill, 1988, American Academy of Pediatrics.
420. Beerman R, Nunez D Jr, Wetli CV: Radiographic evaluation of the cocaine smuggler, *Gastrointest Radiol* 11:351, 1986.
421. Linden CH and Rumack BH: Ipecac for ingested drug packets (abstract A-29), *Vet Hum Toxicol* 26:404, 1984.
422. Roberts JR et al: The bodystuffer syndrome, *Am J Emerg Med* 4:24, 1986.
423. Lewin NA, Goldfrank LR, Hoffman RS: Cocaine. In Goldfrank LR et al, editors: *Toxicologic emergencies,* ed 5, Norwalk, Conn, 1994, Appleton & Lange.
424. Bettinger J: Cocaine intoxication: massive oral overdose, *Ann Emerg Med* 9:429, 1980.
425. Schwartz WK and Oderda GM: Management of cocaine intoxications, *Clin Toxicol Consultant* 2:45, 1980.
426. Buegan WC, Lange RA, Kim AS et al: Alleviation of cocaine-induced coronary vasoconstriction by nitroglycerin, *J Am Coll Cardiol* 18:581-586, 1991.
427. Dusenberry SJ, Hicks MJ, Mariani PJ: Labetalol treatment of cocaine toxicity *Ann Emerg Med* 16:235, 1987, (letter).
428. Bessen HA: Treatment of cocaine toxicity, *Ann Emerg Med* 16:922, 1987.
429. Gay GR and Loper KA: The use of labetalol in the management of cocaine crisis, *Ann Emerg Med* 17:282, 1988.

430. Sand IC et al: Experience with esmolol for the treatment of cocaine-associated cardiovascular complications, *Am J Emerg Med* 9:161, 1991.
431. Ramoska E and Sacchetti AD: Propranolol-induced hypertension in treatment of cocaine intoxication, *Ann Emerg Med* 14:1112, 1985.
432. Catravas JD and Waters IW: Acute cocaine intoxication in the conscious dog: studies on mechanisms of lethality, *Pharmacol Exp Ther* 217:350, 1981.
433. Becker CE: Phencyclidine management. In Rumack BH, Hess AJ, Gilman CR, editors: *POISINDEX Systems,* Denver, 1996, Micromedex.
434. Burns RS and Lerner SE: Perspectives: acute phencyclidine intoxication, *Clin Toxicol* 9:477, 1976.
435. Misra AL, Pontani RB, Bartolomea J: Persistence of phencyclidine (PCP) and metabolites in brain and adipose tissue: research communications, *Chem Pathol Pharmacol* 24:431, 1979.
436. Wong LK and Bieman K: Metabolites of phencyclidine, *Clin Toxicol* 9:583, 1976.
437. Burns RS and Lerner SE: Phencyclidine deaths, *JACEP* 7:135, 1978.
438. McCarron MM et al: Acute phencyclidine intoxication: incidence of clinical findings in 1,000 cases, *Ann Emerg Med* 10:237, 1981.
439. Goldfrank L and Osburn H: Phencyclidine (angel dust), *Hosp Physician* 5:18, 1978.
440. Linden CB, Lovejoy FH, Costello CE: Phencyclidine, *JAMA* 234:513, 1975.
441. Welsh MJ and Correa GA: PCP intoxication in young children and infants, *Clin Pediatr* 19:510, 1980.
442. Strauss AA, Modanlou MD, Bosu SK: Neonatal manifestations of maternal phencyclidine (PCP) abuse, *Pediatrics* 68:550, 1981.
443. Aronow R, Miceli JN, Done AK: A therapeutic approach to the acutely overdosed PCP patient, *J Psychedelic Drugs* 12:259, 1980.
444. Picchioni AL and Consroe PF: Activated charcoal—a phencyclidine antidote, or hog in dogs, *N Engl J Med* 300:202, 1979.
445. Lahmeyer HW and Stock PG: Phencyclidine intoxication, physical restraints, and acute renal failure: case report, *J Clin Psychiatry* 44:184, 1983.
446. Morgan JP and Solomon JL: Phencyclidine, clinical pharmacology and toxicity, *Postgrad Med J* 581:783, 1982.
447. Ellenhorn MJ and Barceloux DG, editor: *Medical toxicology, diagnosis and treatment of human poisoning,* New York, 1988, Elsevier Science.
448. Anggard E et al: Pharmacokinetic and clinical studies on amphetamine dependent subjects, *Eur J Clin Pharmacol* 3:3, 1970.
449. Litovitz T: Amphetamines. In Haddad LM and Winchester JF, editors: *Clinical management of poisoning and drug overdose,* Philadelphia, 1983, WB Saunders.
450. Swenson RD, Golper TA, Bennett WM: Acute renal failure and rhabdomyolysis after ingestion of phenylpropanolamine—containing diet pills, *JAMA* 248:1216, 1982.
451. Rampf KW et al: Rhabdomyolisis after ingestion of an appetite suppressant, *JAMA* 250:2112, 1983.
452. Gawin FH and Ellinwood JR EH: Cocaine and other stimulants: actions, abuse, and treatment, *N Engl J Med* 318:1173, 1988.
453. Nelson MM and Forfar JO: Associations between drugs administered during pregnancy and congenital abnormalities of the fetus, *BMJ* 1:523, 1971.
454. Levin JN: Amphetamine ingestion with biliary atresia, *J Pediatr* 79:130, 1971.
455. Larsson G: The amphetamine addicted mother and her child, *Acta Paediatr Scand* 278 (suppl):1, 1980.
456. Olin BR, editor: *Facts and comparisons,* St. Louis, 1988, JB Lippincott.
457. Elkin BR and Spoerke DG: An estimation of the toxicity of nonprescription diet aids from seventy exposure cases, *Vet Hum Toxicol* 25:81, 1983.
458. Larson WL and Rogers A: Overdosage from phenylpropanolamine: experience of the Hennepin Regional Poison Center, *Vet Hum Toxicol* 28:546, 1986.
459. Kase CS et al: Intracerebral hemorrhage and phenylpropanolamine use, *Neurology* 37:399, 1987.
460. Maher LM: Postpartum intracranial hemorrhage and phenylpropanolamine use, *Neurology* 37:1686, 1987.
461. Fallis RJ and Fisher M: Cerebral vasculitis and hemorrhage associated with phenylpropanolamine, *Neurology* 35:405, 1985.

462. Norvenius G, Widerlov E, Lonnerholm G: Phenylpropanolamine and mental disturbances *Lancet* 2:1367, 1979 (letter).

463. Orson J and Bassow L: Over-the-counter cough formulas, *Clin Pediatr* 26:287, 1987.

464. Callaway CW, Clark RF: Hyperthermia in psychostimulant overdose. *Ann Emerg Med* 24:68-76, 1994.

465. King WD, Kohaut EC, Palmisano PA: Phenylpropanolamine toxicity, *The Children's Hospital of Alabama Poison Information Bulletin* 17:1, 1988.

466. Pentel PR, Olson KR: Sympathomimetic poisoning. In Harwood-Nuss A, editor: *The clinical practice of emergency medicine,* Philadelphia, 1991, JB Lippincott.

Theophylline

467. Olson KR et al: Theophylline overdose: acute single ingestion versus chronic repeated overmedication, *Am J Emerg Med* 3:386, 1985.

468. Nakada T et al: Theophylline induced seizures: clinical and pathophysiologic aspects, *West J Med* 138:371, 1983.

469. Litovitz TL et al: 1994 Annual report of the American Association of Poison Control Centers national data collection system, *Am J Emerg Med* 13:551-557, 1995.

470. Minocha A and Spyker DA: Acute overdose with sustained release drug formulations: perspectives in treatment, *Med Toxicol* 1:300, 1986.

471. Robertson NJ: Fatal overdose from a sustained release theophylline preparation, *Ann Emerg Med* 14:154, 1985.

472. Hendeles L and Weinberger M: Improved efficacy and safety of theophylline in the control of airway hyperreactivity, *Pharmacol Ther* 18:91, 1982.

473. Ellenhorn MJ and Barceloux DG: *Medical toxicology, diagnosis and treatment of human poisoning,* ed 1, New York, 1988, Elsevier Science.

474. Vestal RE et al: Effect of intravenous aminophylline on plasma levels of catecholamines and related cardiovascular and metabolic responses in man, *Circulation* 67:162, 1983.

475. Van Dellen RGL: Theophylline, practical application of knowledge, *Mayo Clin Proc* 54:733, 1979.

476. Fredholm BB: Theophylline actions on adenosine receptors, *Eur J Respir Dis* 61:29, 1980 (suppl 109).

477. Fenger M et al: Plasma concentrations of the cyclic nucleotides, adenosine 3′, 5′-monophosphate and guanosine 3′, 5′-monophosphate in healthy adults treated with theophylline, *Pharmacology* 24:215, 1982.

478. Kearney TE et al: Theophylline toxicity and the beta adrenergic system, *Ann Intern Med* 102:766, 1985.

479. Gandreault P, Wason S, Lovejoy FH: Acute pediatric theophylline overdose: a summary of 28 cases, *J Pediatr* 102:474, 1983.

480. Baker MD: Theophylline toxicity in children, *J Pediatr* 109:538, 1986.

481. MacDonald JB, Jones HM, Cowan RA: Rhabdomyolysis and acute renal failure after theophylline overdose, *Lancet* 1:932, 1985.

482. Hendeles L, Weinberger M, Johnson G: Monitoring serum theophylline levels, *Clin Pharmacokinet* 3:294, 1978.

483. Coupe M: Self-poisoning with sustained-release aminophylline: a mechanism for observed secondary rise in serum theophylline, *Hum Toxicol* 5:341, 1986.

484. Gal P, Miller A, McCue JD: Oral activated charcoal to enhance theophylline elimination in an acute overdose, *JAMA* 251:3130, 1984.

485. Berlinger WC et al: Enhancement of theophylline clearance by oral activated charcoal, *Clin Pharmacol Ther* 33:351, 1983.

486. Amitai Y et al: Repetitive oral activated charcoal and control of emesis in severe theophylline toxicity, *Ann Intern Med* 105:386, 1986.

487. Biberstein MP, Ziegler MG, Ward DM: Use of beta-blockade and hemoperfusion for acute theophylline poisoning, *West J Med* 141:485, 1984.

488. Jaffe M et al: Severe albuterol poisoning treated with propranolol *Vet Hum Toxicol* 32:351, 1990 (abstract 44).

489. Taniguichi A, Ohe T, Shimorura K: Theophylline induces ventricular tachycardia in patients with chronic lung disease: Sensitivity to verapamil *Chest* 96:958, 1989, (letter).

490. Weisman RS, Goldfrank LR, Howland MA: Theophylline. In Goldfrank LR et al: *Toxicologic emergencies,* ed 5, Norwalk, Conn, 1994, Appleton & Lange.

491. Kelly HW: Theophylline toxicity. In Jehne JW, Murphy S, editors: *Drug therapy for asthma,* New York, 1987, Marcel Dekker.

492. Hendeles L, Jenkins J, Temple R: Revised FDA labeling guidelines for theophylline oral dosage forms, *Pharmacotherapy* 15:409-427, 1995.

493. Blake KV et al: Relative efficacy of phenytoin and phenobarbital for prevention of theophylline induced seizures in mice, *Ann Emerg Med* 17:1024, 1988.

494. Park GD et al: Use of hemoperfusion in acute theophylline intoxication, *Am J Med* 74:961, 1983.

495. Woo OF et al: Benefit of hemoperfusion in acute theophylline intoxication, *Clin Toxicol* 22:411, 1984.

496. Jeffreys DB et al: Haemoperfusion for theophylline overdose, *BMJ* 280:1167, 1980.

497. Shannon M, Weinberger G, Morris C: Exchange transfusion in the treatment of severe theophylline poisoning, *Pediatr* 89:145, 1992.

Inhalation Injuries

Anthony J. Scalzo

Inhalation injury generally involves the exposure of the respiratory tract to one or more toxic substances (toxicants) with resultant anatomic or physiologic damage. Although these toxicants are primarily gases, volatilized products of combustion and inhaled particulate matter also cause injury. Clearance of particles, either by mucociliary transport, macrophages or translocation to other organs following initial deposition in the respiratory tract, is important in determining toxicity of inhaled agents.[1] However, most fire victims who die immediately do so because of asphyxia.[2,3] In addition, there may be associated thermal injury. Heated air or even inhaled steam has caused injury to the face, nasal or oral cavity, larynx, and rarely to the lower airway.[4-7] Pulmonary edema, adult respiratory distress syndrome (ARDS), and lung dysfunction may complicate thermal injury to the skin in the absence of significant inhalation exposure.[6-14]

Inhalant toxicology has become increasingly complex because of the large number of hazardous gases and environmental pollutants generated by highly industrialized societies. The release of methyl isocyanate gas and over 28 chemical entities/reaction products in the 1984 Bhopal industrial disaster is a dramatic example of our general unpreparedness for large-scale toxic inhalations.[15,16] There were over 3,000 deaths (some estimates of 6,000 to 20,000) and over 100,000 exposures.[15,17] Over 30,000 chemical transportation accidents occurred in 1982 alone, involving both truck and railroad tankers.[18] This has led to an increase in legislation including the Superfund Amendment and Reauthorization Act of 1986, which authorized the EPA to develop emergency response plans both locally and regionally.[19] Yet in 1991, there were 25,800 reports of hazardous materials incidents in the United States.[19] Fortunately, children are rarely involved in occupational chemical exposures; the common pediatric inhalation problems include smoke from house fires, carbon monoxide, hydrocarbon aspiration, and occasionally chlorine.

The increased efficiency of insulation and air tightness of homes and buildings may contribute to an increased concentration of indoor pollutants including passive exposure to cigarette smoke.[20-22]

Regional poison centers can provide protocols for the emergency management of hazardous chemical exposures. Rapid identification of toxins for which antidotal therapy may be initiated is crucial in situations involving, for example, chemical asphyxiants (carbon monoxide, cyanide), methemoglobin (nitrates, nitrites), or inhaled organophosphate insecticides.[18] Comprehensive management of hazardous chemical releases involves prehospital emergency personnel, hazard containment ("HAZMAT") teams, emergency department personnel, a toxicologist, and a specialist in poison information and poison centers. Chemical disasters may be associated with a wide variety of psychologic and psychosocial distress in addition to physiologic injury.[23]

The best management of toxic inhalations is prevention.[15,24,25] Children should be taught to crawl under smoke and place wet cloths over their nose and mouth, and they should be involved in family emergency exit plans. Parents should be encouraged to purchase, install, and maintain smoke detectors in the home.

TYPES OF INHALANTS

Inhaled toxicants may exist in several forms including gases, aerosols, vapors, and liquids with volatile properties such as hydrocarbons, smokes, and dusts. Fumes are a form of aerosol composed of solid particles usually less than 0.1 μm in size arising from chemical reactions or the volatilization of molten metals such as zinc, copper, and nickel.[26] Metal fume fever is an adult occupational disease not seen in children. The inhalant's chemical form, aqueous solubility, pH, particle size, ambient concentration, irritant effects, asphyxiant properties, and ability to combine with biologic substances are all important to its toxicity.[18,24,26,27] Some gases are simple asphyxiants because they displace oxygen but are not biologically active. Carbon dioxide and methane (natural gas) are examples of this type of toxicant. Other gases are chemical or biologic asphyxiants such as carbon monoxide, hydrogen cyanide, or hydrogen sulfide. Table 44-1 displays common types of inhalants and products of combustion that are likely to be encountered in children.

TABLE 44-1. Common Types of Inhalants and Sources

Gases	Smokes	Volatiles and vapors
Formless state of matter composed of molecules moving freely and completely occupying the space of enclosure	Volatilized product of combustion that contains gases and particulate matter (usually carbon) generally less than 0.5 μm to 1 μm in size	Substances that under given ambient pressures or temperatures will volatilize into a gaseous form but normally exist as liquids or solids
Simple asphyxiants Carbon dioxide Methane (natural gas)	**House fires** 1. Wood, cotton, paper, aldehydes (smoke and toxic gases such as carbon monoxide, methane, formic acid) 2. Plastics (cyanide, hydrogen chloride, carbon monoxide, acrolein) 3. Nylon carpeting (ammonia, cyanide) 4. PVC plumbing (phosgene, chlorine, carbon monoxide)	**Aliphatics** Acetone Propane Butane Isobutane (fingernail polish, lighters, aerosol cans)
Chemical or biologic asphyxiants Carbon monoxide Cyanide (heaters, automobile exhaust, house fires) Hydrogen sulfide (sewers)		**Halogenated** Freon (fluorocarbons) Trichloroethylene Trichloroethane (abuse of or exposure to propellants, adhesives, correction fluids)
Respiratory irritants Ammonia Chlorine Formaldehyde (household products, pool products, insulation) Chloramine (mixing ammonia and sodium hypochlorite bleach)	**Cigarettes** Particulate matter Carbon monoxide **Industrial emissions** Numerous gases and particulates **Wood burning stoves and fireplaces**	**Aromatics** Toluene Benzene Xylene (abuse of glues)
Inert and other gases Helium (abuse of party balloons) Nitrous oxide (canned whipped cream)	Carbon monoxide, particulates and if colored fireplace logs—heavy metals **Kerosene heaters** Carbon monoxide and smoke	**Petroleum distillates and mixtures** Gasoline Kerosene Mineral seal oil (aspiration from lamps, furniture polishes)

PATHOPHYSIOLOGY

Inhaled gases, particulate aerosols or a combination of these such as smoke may exert their effects via one or more pathologic mechanisms (Table 44-2). The uptake of toxic gases occurs throughout the entire respiratory system beginning with the nose and nasopharyngeal cavity. Oxygen and carbon dioxide exchange at the pulmonary alveolar level. Whereas gases are breathed directly into the lungs and diffusion is the driving force, particulate matter enters the respiratory tract to varying degrees depending on particle size.[18,26-29] Pulmonary injury can result from the thermal, chemical, or irritant properties of inhalants. Dry air has a low heat capacity and usually only causes thermal damage to the upper airway (e.g., laryngeal burns and edema).[7,30,31] Patients with diffuse and distal airway changes are likely to have suffered a toxic chemical effect from inhalation injury caused by products of combustion.

Injury to the airways may also depend on protective and functional layers of mucous and fluids that line the airway. The mucous layer is generally believed to be thicker in the upper airway than in the more distal airways.[27] Depending on the concentration of the inhaled gas and exposure time, the injury may be variable. Stone[31] identified several temporal stages of pulmonary injury after smoke inhalation: (1) respiratory insufficiency with bronchospasm at 1 to 12 hours after the event, (2) pulmonary edema at 6 to 72 hours after the burn, and (3) bronchopneumonia at greater than 60 hours after the burn.[31]

Anatomic and Physiologic Concerns

The degree of injury is not only dependent on the type of the inhaled gas or particulate aerosol, but also it is related to the anatomic and physiologic state of the pediatric patient. Structure and size of conducting airways, lung volume, and alveolar surface area are just a few of the anatomic features of the respiratory tract that affect deposition and retention of inhaled toxic gases.[27,28,32] Children are unique in that they are undergoing varying degrees of postnatal lung growth and development. Alveoli increase in size from early infancy (40 to 120 μm at 2 months) to adulthood (250 to 300 μm) and in number (20 million at birth to 300 million by 8 years of age).[32] In addition, lung volume increases approximately tenfold from birth (200 ml) to 8 years of age (2.2 L), reaching over 5 L by the second decade of life.[32] Because gases tend to be diluted by radial diffusion due to an increase in lung cross-sectional area, the effect of a given toxic inhalant may vary from the infant to the adult.[27] The increased respiratory rate of the child compared to the adult may also lead to increased uptake of an inhaled toxin at the alveolar level. Children at play or sport have increased minute ventilation and, therefore, increased intake of inhaled pollutants both indoors and outdoors. This factor may be significant in situations such as carbon monoxide poisoning where the lungs are the vehicle for gas entry. In fact, some have reported an increased risk of intoxication and increased symptoms in infants and small children exposed to carbon monoxide.[33-35]

TABLE 44-2. Pathophysiologic Mechanisms of Inhalation Injuries

Inhalation injury	Pathophysiologic mechanism
Upper airway effect	Irritation, tearing, rhinitis, mucosal edema, hyperemia, laryngeal edema and obstruction, tracheitis
Bronchoreactivity-hypersensitivity of airways	Bronchoconstriction, mucosal edema
Chemical pneumonitis	Alveolar transudate or exudate due to mucosal damage, loss of surfactant, or direct chemical effect
Simple asphyxiation	Displacement of oxygen and resultant hypoxemia and anoxia
Pulmonary edema	Usually noncardiogenic
Systemic intoxication	Absorption of toxin such as solvent with resultant effects or interference with physiologic functions (i.e., oxygen transport by carbon monoxide combining with hemoglobin)

TABLE 44-3. Major Toxic Products of Combustion

Systemic toxins	Asphyxiants	Local/pulmonary irritants	
Carbon monoxide	Carbon dioxide	Acetic acid	Hydrogen chloride
Hydrogen cyanide	Methane	Acrolein	Isocyanates
Hydrogen sulfide		Aldehydes (formaldehyde)	Nitrogen oxides
Isocyanates		Ammonia	Phosgene
		Chlorine	

Children may show injury at all levels of the respiratory tract (e.g., nasopharyngeal, tracheobronchial, and pulmonary/alveolar). The mucociliary defense system may remove some particulate matter[27]; the inhalation of toxic gases may result in the destruction of alveolar type I cells and connective tissue proliferation, leading to a thicker barrier impairing physiologic gas exchange.[32] Eventual repair may occur when the thicker alveolar epithelial type II cells form new type I cells, thus restoring the normal alveolar lining.[36]

On a biochemical level, cell injury from inhaled toxins may be enhanced by activated phagocytic cells, which produce reactive oxygen and superoxide species.[37,38] Although hyperoxygen therapy can contribute to this toxicity during the first 4 to 6 hours after exposure to 100% oxygen, most animal species do not demonstrate significant morphologic changes in the structure of alveolar septa.[39]

Physiochemical Properties of Inhaled Toxicants

When considering the inhalation of a toxic gas, diffusion dominates uptake and determines admixture with nontoxic gases such as simultaneously inhaled nitrogen, oxygen, carbon dioxide, and water vapor.[27] The victim usually must take several breaths before sufficient toxin is transported to the alveolus and absorbed; but immediate injury may occur to the conjunctivae, nasal mucosa, and pharynx from certain noxious irritant gases.

Particle size is an important determinant when the inhaled toxin is an aerosol.[28] Deposition in the airway may occur via sedimentation caused by gravity, collision due to drag, diffusion, and electrostatic attraction between particles and the respiratory tract.[27,28] Particle sizes between

0.02 to 10 μm are important for health effects, with particles >10 μm depositing in the large and medium airways and small particles at the alveolar level.[28] From a practical standpoint, this is important in the example of baby powder (talcum) inhalation in which obliteration of small bronchi and obstruction of alveoli may occur because of small particle size (<5 μm).[40]

When a gas is nonirritating, such as methane or carbon dioxide, inhalation of sufficient quantities will exert a toxic effect by displacement of oxygen. These simple asphyxiants may lead to a hypoxic state in closed environments but may respond quickly to pure oxygen inhalation.[18]

Aqueous solubility is an important factor in the injury caused by certain toxic gases. Ammonia (NH_3), with a strong warning odor, may produce acute upper airway symptoms due to high water solubility, whereas hydrogen sulfide (H_2S) can produce injury to both upper and lower airways because of intermediate solubility.[14] Both ammonia and chlorine gas (Cl_2) are classic examples of respiratory irritants that may cause membrane damage and inflammation in the upper respiratory tract because of high water solubility.[41-43]

Systemic absorption of inhaled gases may be required to exert their toxic effect. Hydrogen cyanide (HCN), hydrogen sulfide (H_2S), and carbon monoxide (CO) result in the rapid evolution of cellular anoxia and metabolic acidosis by interfering with the transport or use of oxygen by cells. Systemic effects may occur with inhaled solvents such as toluene, which results in euphoria, disorientation, and narcosis through pulmonary absorption[44,45]; others, such as benzene, exert their specific toxicities via absorption and biotransformation.[29,44]

SPECIFIC INHALATION INJURIES

The emergency department physician should be prepared to manage the common inhalation injuries such as smoke from house fires, CO exposure, and hydrocarbon aspiration.

Smoke Inhalation (see Chapter 37)

Smoke from a house fire is the volatilized product of combustion of any number of substances, most commonly wood, paper, and plastics. Table 44-3 shows some of the major combustion products in smoke.

Thermal injury occurs to both the integument and airway, as well as exposure to particulate matter (soot) and toxic gases. Such gases include pulmonary irritants and systemic toxins such as CO and cyanide. Most victims of structural fires die from smoke inhalation and toxic gases, not thermal burns to the skin.[9,30,46-49] Recognition of cyanide as an important factor in morbidity and mortality from smoke inhalation has stirred some recent controversies regarding the use of cyanide antidotes (e.g., thiosulfate or sodium nitrite).[50,51] One study, however, revealed fatal cyanide levels (> 3 mg/L) in only 31/364 cases and concluded that cyanide poisoning was infrequent.[52] Inhalation injuries in burn patients carry a high mortality and although structural fires account for less than 5% of hospital admissions for burns, they cause more than 45% of burn-related deaths.[9,11] Patients who are responsive to initial therapy are likely to survive at least the first 24 hours. Although a 15-year study of 1,832 burned children revealed that an associated pulmonary injury was present in only 6%, the majority (71%) of the 52 deaths were in these children.[31] The overall incidence of childhood deaths (0 to 14 years of age) from burns was 2.5/100,000 in 1988 in the United States.[53]

Most house fire deaths occur during the night and during the months of December through March[54] when heating systems are most often used[55] and ventilation is limited because of closed windows. Immediate death from smoke inhalation is common in closed space fires; overall the mortality rate is somewhere between 45% and 78%.[6,9] In a study of childhood injury patterns in an urban setting, housefires were the leading cause of death by injury (34%) in 1989-1990.[56] Those patients arriving at the emergency department in full cardiorespiratory arrest are likely to have poor outcomes. Nonetheless, an attempt to secure an endotracheal airway and administer resuscitation medications and fluid boluses may be warranted, especially if the emergency physician is unsure of the duration of exposure and extent of the prehospital care.

Factors Affecting Toxicity

Heat of Gases. The heat of the gases in a fire is a factor causing injury to the upper airway but rarely to the lower respiratory tract. Inhalation of heated air at only 150° C or more may result in injuries to the face, nasal mucosa, oropharynx, and upper airway; but even dry air heated to 500° C and introduced to just below the vocal cords in dogs is cooled to 50° C after reaching the carina.[6,7] However, heat-injury induced edema of the upper airway and supraglottic area may lead to obstruction. Adding moisture to the air increases injury and probable mortality.[7,46] Although, the temperature at the ceiling of a burning room can reach 900° F to 1,100° F, the upper airway including the nasal turbinates is very efficient in heat-decreasing capacity.[3,9] Unfortunately, this does not always prevent serious burn injury to the larynx. Few cases of steam inhalation exist outside of the classic animal experiments by Moritz, Henriques, and McLean in 1945.[7] Because steam has 4,000 times the heat capacity of air, coagulation necrosis of the tracheal and bronchial walls, edema of the lung parenchyma, and pneumonitis may occur.[6,7]

Burn injuries may be seen in children with hot steam vaporizers.[2] Microwaves pose a further danger. For example, we encountered a 22-month-old who sustained an anterior chest wall burn when she "drank" from a cup of hot water super-heated in a microwave oven. The child initially presented with only obvious burns to the skin of the chest and partially to the neck and chin (Fig. 44-1, *A*). There was no drooling, dysphonia, or stridor. Within 1 hour of arrival, however, some mild hoarseness was noted and a radiograph of the airway demonstrated a swollen epiglottis (Fig. 44-1, *B*). Temperatures in microwave ovens can become exceedingly high, and respiratory distress can occur after inhalation of gas from overheated microwave units.[57]

Particulate Matter. In smoke there is particulate matter comprised mostly of carbon particles that may be less than 1 μm in size and inhaled deeply in the lungs.[46] Soot particles by themselves are thought to be nontoxic based on animal experiments, but they may alter pulmonary macrophages by affecting phagocytic function.[30,46] Toxic acids formed in combustion such as acetic and formic acid may adsorb to soot and contribute to mucosal damage.[30] Toxic compounds in the particle phase may be more toxic and filtered smoke is less injurious.[58] Particulate matter deposition with adsorbed toxins may lead to chemical injury and associated tracheobronchitis and pulmonary edema.[6,30]

Toxic Gases. The most common fatal gas from smoke inhalation is CO.[2,5,6] Other toxic gases are hydrogen cyanide; aldehydes, which include acrolein, acetaldehyde, and formaldehyde; ammonia; chlorine; and hydrochloric acid. Cyanide, when present in fire fatalities, is generally associated with significant carboxyhemoglobinemia.[52] Acrolein vapor, a product of the combustion of cotton and wood, can cause severe ocular irritation and pulmonary edema and is a major contributor to pulmonary injury in smoke inhalation.[26] Late development (at 18-month follow-up) of obstructive bronchiolar disease and diffuse bronchiectasis has been reported in a 2-year-old child after prolonged acrolein inhalation due to burning vegetable oil in a kitchen.[59]

Pathophysiology

Upper Airway Obstruction. Thermal injury from smoke inhalation causes upper airway edema. Within hours of exposure to toxic fumes, the mucosa of the upper airway may become denuded and ulcerated with edema and sloughing of epithelial debris.[49] The mucosal covering of the hypopharynx, epiglottis, and other supraglottic structures is loosely attached to underlying tissue, thus leading to swelling and edema.[60] Furthermore, massive edema may develop in upper airway burns before or during fluid administration.[2]

Lower Airway

Irritant Effects of Lower Airways. Certainly, the irritant effects of noxious gases such as methyl isocyanate or chlorine on the conjunctivae, nares, and oropharynx are significant. Respiratory irritants may affect the deposition of particulate matter by causing decreasing airway diameter due to mucosal swelling. Obviously, children have smaller airways than adults, leading to greater resistance to airflow and perhaps earlier and more pronounced signs of respiratory distress. Chemical and particulate matter in smoke may cause bronchoconstriction by stimulating irritant receptors in large airways.[5] Corrosive acids and aldehydes formed by sulphur dioxide and nitrogen oxide result in injury to respiratory cilia and mucosal edema, which may lead to severe airway obstruction.[3,6] Tachypnea induced by

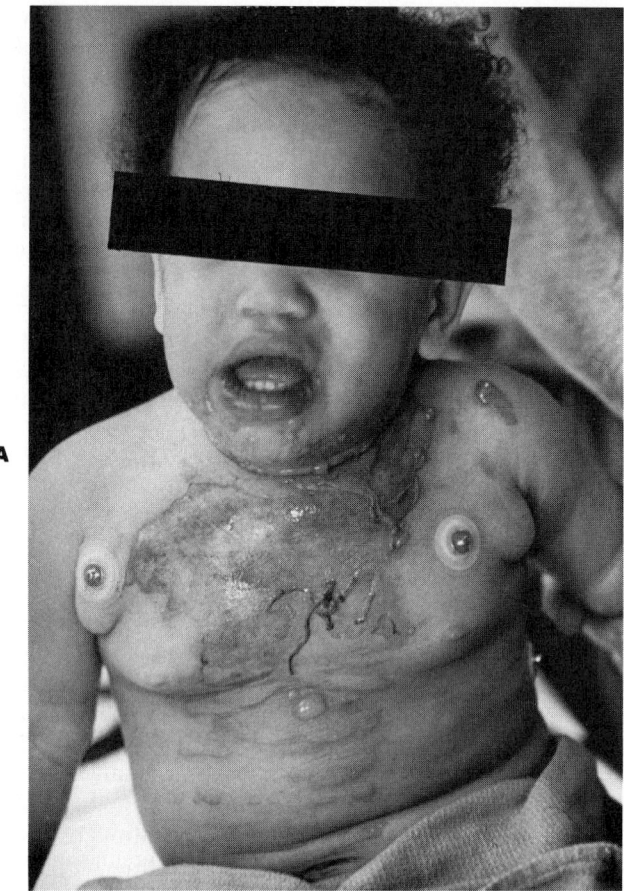

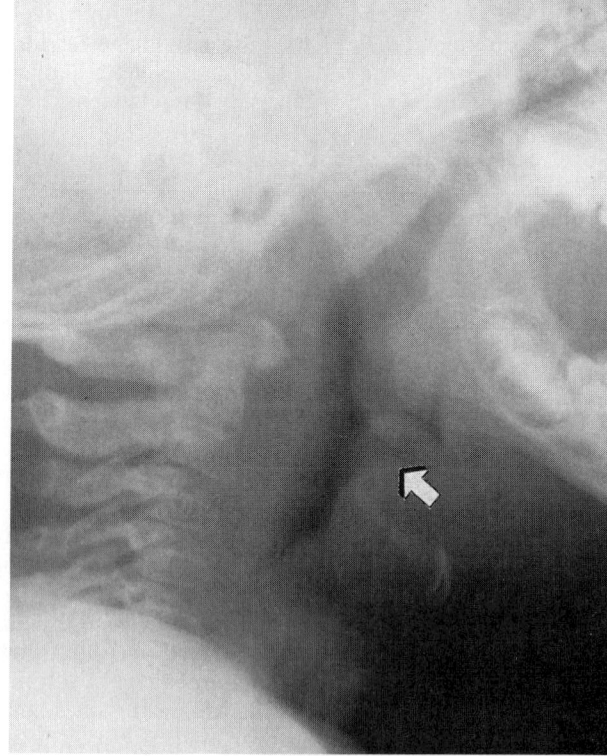

FIG. 44-1. A, Photograph of 22-month-old child showing burn primarily to the anterior chest wall. **B,** Lateral airway radiograph of the same child demonstrating effects of thermal or chemical epiglottitis.

mucosal irritation from toxic fumes and hypoxia may cause further inhalation of smoke and resultant injury.[49] Minute ventilation, the product of respiratory rate (RR) × tidal volume (TV), may be diminished. In children whose breathing is rapid but shallow, hypoventilation may occur. Disturbances in peak flow, forced expiratory volume (FEV), and forced vital capacity (FVC) may occur even before abnormalities and pulmonary edema are apparent on chest radiographs.[6] Lung compliance may decrease because of an increase in lung water.[6,47] Therefore, changes in lung dynamics coupled with development of upper airway obstruction may lead to progressive hypoxemia and respiratory failure in the child.

Alveolar-Capillary Membrane Damage. Smoke is known to destroy alveolar macrophages and the surfactant that type II alveolar epithelial cells produce.[9] Intraalveolar edema and hemorrhage combined with cellular debris and fibrin create a hyaline-like membrane, which may severely impair gas exchange.[6] Pulmonary capillary hyperpermeability appears to be specific to inhalation injury apart from other endothelial damage.[47] Damage to the vascular component of a ventilation-perfusion system may also occur in association with the thermal burns to the skin. Microemboli, burn toxins, effects of resuscitation, and sometimes disseminated intravascular clotting contribute to this vessel injury.[3] A greater than tenfold increase in bronchial blood flow occurs after injury to tracheobronchial tissues, which may contribute to the formation of exudate and interstitial edema.[6]

Pulmonary Infiltrates and Edema. Impaired mucociliary transport, diminished surfactant production, and pulmonary macrophage dysfunction may all contribute to the development of respiratory tract infection, perhaps associated with global suppression of their immune response.[2,9,11,13]

Several hours after inhalation injury there is sloughing of tracheobronchial mucosa, followed by hemorrhage and ultimately alveolar pulmonary edema.[3] In addition, the onset of pulmonary edema may be almost immediate or may occur up to 1 week after inhalation due to the filtration of fluid across damaged alveolar-capillary membranes even in the absence of elevated hydrostatic pressure.[5,49]

Respiratory Failure. Ineffective removal of carbon dioxide or acquisition and delivery of oxygen (O_2) or both may lead to respiratory failure. Evidence from animal research has demonstrated that a pathologic delivery-dependent O_2 consumption develops with combined burn and inhalation injury.[61] This increases the potential for tissue hypoxemia and respiratory failure at the cellular level. When confronting smoke inhalation, the respiratory failure can be both external in the conducting airways to the alveolus or internal, involving diminished delivery of oxygen (i.e., due to CO) or impaired use of oxygen due to cellular toxins (e.g., cyanide).

Asphyxiation. Ambient oxygen concentration may fall to 5% in some fires where oxygen is consumed rapidly in closed spaces.[2] Death occurs in 6 to 8 minutes at oxygen concentrations of 6% or less.[3] The production of methane and carbon dioxide, which displace oxygen, contributes to the asphyxia. Carbon monoxide also adds to asphyxiation by impairing hemoglobin delivery of the remaining oxygen.

Systemic Poisoning. Systemic poisons such as CO and cyanide may be absorbed through the alveoli and exert a major component of fire-related injury.[9,26,30] Cyanide gen-

TABLE 44-4. Initial Findings in 29 Children with Smoke Inhalation and Severe Acute Respiratory Distress

	Bronchospasm	Laryngeal obstruction	Lung consolidation
Patients	18	1	10
Respiratory rate	↑	↑	↑
Respiratory effort	↑	↑	↑
Inspiratory phase	Brief	Prolonged	Prolonged
Expiratory phase	Prolonged	Brief	Brief
Wheezes	+	±	−
Distant breath sounds	±	+	+
Chest radiograph	Normal	Normal	Normal

Adapted from Stone HH: *J Pediatr Surg* 14:48, 1979.
↑, Increased; +, common; −, rare; ±, variable.

eration in fires is of interest because it is generated from numerous modern synthetic materials used in buildings and furnishings. There is a growing concern that cyanide, which is synergistic with CO in causing toxic effects, may contribute to an accelerated death in victims of smoke from fires in modern structures.[30]

Diagnostic Findings. A quick situation-oriented history must acquire relevant details regarding the location of the patient such as in an enclosed area, his or her level of consciousness when found in the fire, and duration of exposure to smoke. Details of the resuscitation at the scene or at a referring hospital, such as the need for artificial ventilation, perfusion status, and amounts of intravenous fluids administered, should be ascertained.

Clinical Findings. Early symptoms due to edema and bronchorrhea may be absent for 24 to 48 hours even in severe mucosal injury.[11] In Stone's study of 101 children with smoke inhalation, serious respiratory distress was noted in 29 children within 12 hours due to bronchospasm, laryngeal edema, or lung consolidation.[31] Table 44-4 depicts the presence or absence of physical findings in the 29 children with life-threatening respiratory distress.

Vital Signs. Inhalation injury and associated thermal burns to the skin can result in significantly altered vital signs that must be monitored. Increased respiratory rate may be due to hypoxia and chemical irritation of the airway, which may be accompanied by an increase in signs of respiratory distress such as retractions, nasal flaring, and grunting, especially in the infant. Bradypnea or apnea may also occur in infants and small children from prolonged hypoxia. Tracheobronchitis, bronchospasm, and areas of lung atelectasis may contribute further to existent hypoxia.[6,9]

Alterations in blood volume with hypertension (as discussed in Chapter 37) due to tissue fluid losses and increased need for fluid resuscitation may exist.[8,12,62,63] In fact, in one study the mean fluid requirement of 3.98 ml/kg/% of total body surface area (% TBSA) burned in patients without inhalation injury increased to 5.76 ml/kg/% TBSA burned in those patients who did have smoke inhalation.[2,64]

Hypertension may be seen in children who suffer thermal injury.[65] A widely variant incidence (10% to 89%) of

blood pressure elevation has been reported in burned children with an ill-defined pathophysiology not necessarily related to increases in circulating catecholamines.[65]

Children, with their large surface area/weight ratio, may lose extensive heat from their body through burn wounds. This loss may be accentuated by the cool ambient temperature of an emergency department trauma room. Maintaining the room temperature at or about 30° C is reported to decrease total energy expenditure of the patient.[11] Some patients may develop elevations in core temperature of 1° C to 2° C due to increased metabolic rate.[11,62]

Upper Airway. The child should be inspected for evidence of thermal burns of the skin or upper airway. Facial burns, burns to the mucous membranes of the nose or mouth, blistering on the hard palate, and singed nasal hairs may be predictive of airway involvement, which may manifest as hoarseness, stridor, or airway obstruction in the first few to 24 hours.* Other signs and symptoms of upper airway involvement may include sore throat, dysphagia, or dysphonia. The clinician must use experience and serial examinations of the airway and lungs for auscultatory findings. These findings include looking for adequate chest rise and inspiratory breath sounds. One review of smoke inhalation injuries states that up to 85% of patients with upper respiratory tract burns have no associated facial burns.[49] Upper airway thermal injury may result in increasing stridor with hypoxemia, excessive secretions in the tracheobronchial tree, posterior pharyngeal swelling, absent or diminished gag reflex, and laryngeal edema leading to obstruction.[9,46,49] Obstructive laryngeal edema may prolong the inspiratory phase of breathing and yield weak or distant breath sounds.

Lower Airway. Lower airway involvement may manifest with cough, bronchorrhea, nasal flaring, grunting, and retractions. Carbonaceous sputum, hoarseness, wheezing, and rales are signs of serious pulmonary involvement but may not always be present.[9] In one study, only 50% of patients with inhalation injury had carbonaceous sputum or signs of bronchospasm.[60] Cyanosis and the presence of rales are poor prognostic signs.[49] Auscultation of the lungs may also reveal areas of absent breath sounds. Nevertheless, it is important to reemphasize that the absence of these abnormal physical findings early on does not exclude the possibility of developing respiratory failure. This point is illustrated by the studies of Blinn et al at a major burn/trauma center who reported in 1988 on a series of 86 patients ranging in age from 2 to 94 years.[67] On admission, 91% had clear lungs to auscultation. In the same study, bronchoscopic findings rated as moderate to severe were present in 99% of the nonsurvivors and only 54.5% of the survivors.

Systemic Poisoning. Signs of systemic poisoning may be related to acidosis and hypoxia. They include headache, nausea, vomiting, dizziness, confusion, and lethargy. The patient may also present with bradycardia, apnea, and coma.

Complications. Those patients who arrive with vital signs to be evaluated and resuscitated may present with a wide variety of complications. Severe complications in-

*References 5, 14, 31, 51, 66-68.

clude cardiac or neurologic dysfunction secondary to CO poisoning.

Bronchospasm, respiratory insufficiency, airway obstruction, loss of surfactant, and atelectasis may be early complications of smoke inhalation.[6,31,47] Destruction of alveoli, edema formation, sloughing of damaged epithelium forming pseudomembranous casts that occlude the airway, and damage to pulmonary capillary endothelium may also occur.[5,6,30]

Bronchiolitis, with an obstructive profile on pulmonary function testing, has been described following inhalational lung injury.[69]

Pneumonia may develop days after the initial insult and carries a high mortality rate.[6,9,14] Bronchopneumonia and infectious pneumonitis are not usually seen immediately postburn, but are sometimes seen days after the initial insult. Stone, in reporting on the management of 101 children with inhalation injury, noted that bronchopneumonia developed in almost all children who lived beyond the third day, with staphylococci cultured from a majority of patients on the fourth day.[31] The infecting organisms are initially penicillin-resistant staphylococci, but later they are predominantly gram negative (*Pseudomonas*) after the first week.[31] Furthermore, the use of prophylactic antibiotics has not been shown to improve outcome, especially with an intact immune system, and are generally not recommended except for topical therapy on associated skin burns.* Early administration of systemic antibiotics has been associated with more pulmonary infections.[6,46] A study in sheep exposed to smoke inhalation showed an increase in nonciliated and ciliated cell counts of injured trachea in cefazolin-treated vs. the placebo-treated group.[71] This study had a small sample size (9 in each group) and at this time further research is needed to determine if this finding applies to humans. Other complications of thermal burns or inhalation include paralytic ileus, transient hyperglycemia and glycosuria, transient neutropenia, and septicemia.[62]

Ancillary Data. The presence of hypoxemia, hypercarbia (rising P_{CO_2}), and elevated carboxyhemoglobin are hallmarks of smoke inhalation.[3] Carboxyhemoglobin saturation should be determined, as unexpectedly high levels may be seen even in children with minimal symptomatology. Arterial blood gases are useful in documenting hypoxemia and hypercarbia. When analyzing arterial blood gases (ABGs), the Sao_2 is calculated based on that level of Po_2 and may overestimate the true physiologically available oxygen. Oxygen content of the blood is primarily from that bound to hemoglobin; the amount of dissolved oxygen as reflected by the Po_2 contributes a negligible amount to the total of about 16 to 20 ml/100 ml blood oxygen content (for example 0.0031 ml/100 ml blood of $O_2 \times 100$ mm Hg $Po_2 = 0.31$ ml of O_2/100 ml blood). Pulse oximetry also overestimates the true oxyhemoglobin saturation in the presence of elevated carboxyhemoglobin (COHb) levels.[72,73] If cooximetry is performed, one can determine percent saturation for oxyhemoglobin (normal), COHb, or even methemoglobin (a form of hemoglobin unable to bind further oxygen).

Metabolic acidosis seen in smoke inhalation may be due to a number of causes including hypoxemia, interference with the cellular energy process by CO and cyanide, and respiratory insufficiency with rising P_{CO_2} levels.[6,26,30,46]

Hematologic and chemistry studies are usually normal unless affected by volume instability. Some have reported neutropenia with the use of silver sulfadiazine topical therapy for thermal burns to the skin.[62] Some have reported hyperglycemia, which may result from the hypermetabolic state seen in burn injuries.[62] Metabolic acidosis may be seen in burn and inhalation patients but require serial monitoring for detection.[9]

The chest radiograph is an insensitive indicator of smoke inhalation injury when obtained immediately or shortly after exposure.* Subsequent radiographs may demonstrate interval development of pulmonary edema (Fig. 44-2) of a nodular, consolidative, or interstitial pattern.[76]

In a study of 62 patients (age range 1½ to 89 years of age) 56 had significant smoke inhalation.[12] Thirty-five had abnormal findings consisting of perivascular haziness, peribronchial cuffing, or mixed alveolar and interstitial edema, the majority being present at 0 to 24 hours after the fire exposure. Infiltrates that appeared more than 48 hours after the injury were associated with positive bacterial cultures of sputum.

An ECG is more likely to reveal abnormalities in adults; some recommend an ECG in any child over 12 years of age.[30,46]

When injury is present, there are early changes in FVC and FEV.[6] Bronchoscopy seems to be more effective in diagnosis and prognosis than ^{133}Xe lung scan alone.[14]

Blood cyanide levels are rarely useful, as therapeutic interventions must usually be made before the assay is available. Those inhalation victims exposed to hydrogen cyanide gas in significant quantities from pyrolysis of certain plastics are likely to die within seconds to minutes.[66] In patients whose acute blood gases reveal marked metabolic acidosis and decreased to absent arteriovenous oxygen tension gradient, cyanide should be considered. Elevated cyanide levels have been reported in survivors of smoke inhalation, although CO usually accounts for most deaths.[66] Several case studies have reported measurable cyanide or carboxyhemoglobin levels in fire victims and some authors have investigated the use of sodium nitrite or sodium thiosulfate as treatment.[50,77] Further studies of the use of sodium nitrite in controlled clinical trials is necessary before its routine use can be recommended in fire victims.

Differential Considerations. The history may be useful in revealing the nature of the combustibles in a fire. A child victim of a fire in a building with a large amount of modern plastics and polyurethane may have inhaled more than the usual concentration of cyanide. Therefore, inquiries about the type of structure, as well as the location of the child in the fire, may be useful.

Management. As in any resuscitation, breathing and circulation are as important to consider as stabilization and evaluation of life-threatening conditions. If the patient is spontaneously breathing, humidified 100% oxygen should be given while further assessments are performed.[3,6,9] The

---

*References 5, 13, 16, 31, 46, 70.

*References 3, 5, 6, 30, 51, 67, 74-76.

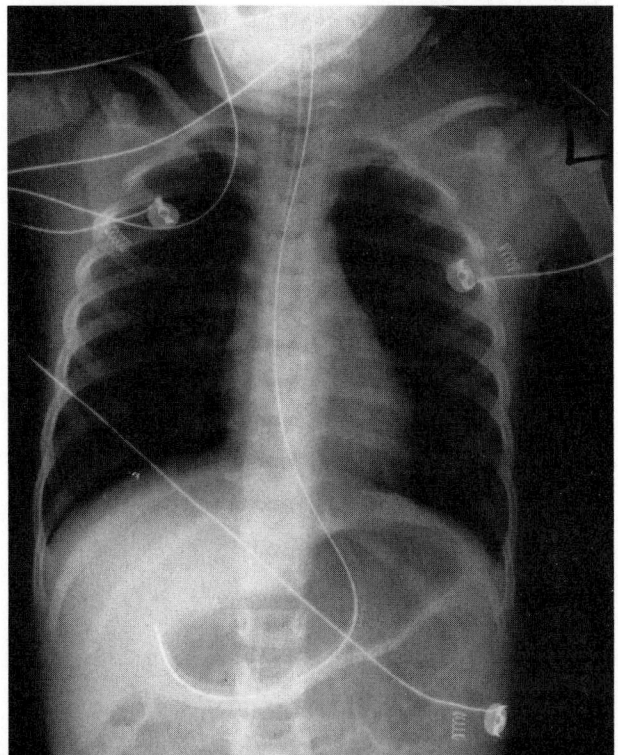

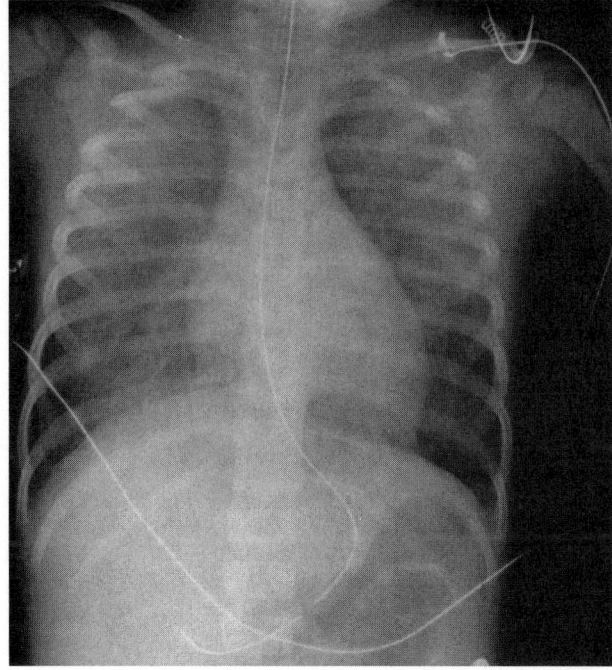

FIG. 44-2. A, Chest radiograph of 3-year-old child obtained 4 hours after resuscitation from cardiopulmonary arrest after smoke inhalation in a house fire. Note the normal appearance of the lung fields at this time. **B,** Chest radiograph of same child obtained 12 hours after exposure demonstrating interval development of pulmonary edema.

half-life of COHb is reduced from 4 or more hours (250 minutes) at room air to 30 to 60 minutes on 100% oxygen as discussed later in this chapter.[49,66]

Humidification of inspired air, which aids in clearing thick casts and preventing secretions from drying, has been used since the famous Coconut Grove fire disaster in 1942.[6] Suctioning of debris, soot, and secretions from the mouth and pharynx is important in maintaining a patent upper airway in children. If the history suggests the likelihood of significant exposure, the child should undergo serial examinations and observation. If the patient is not breathing, artificial ventilation should be administered by standard means with 100% humidified oxygen. Those patients with early signs of respiratory distress are candidates for elective intubation.[2,9,49] These children should be resuscitated with 100% oxygen, intubated, and hyperventilated as needed; their circulation should be supported. Careful inspection with a bright light for soot in the nares or pharynx should be performed along with laryngoscopy, if necessary, to rule out injury to the supraglottic and glottic structures. One should be prepared to place an endotracheal tube at this time if edema of the glottic or supraglottic structures is confirmed. Fiberoptic bronchoscopy is revealing of the severity of injury and somewhat predictive of clinical prognosis.[14,48]

Positive end-expiratory pressure (PEEP) is useful in the management of hypoxemia and respiratory insufficiency and has been recommended by several authors.[2,3,5,6,8,9,30] In a study of smoke inhalation in a sheep model, systemic airway (nutritive) blood flow was preserved and no airway necrosis was seen despite PEEP levels up to 20 cm H_2O.[78] Patients with inhalation injury requiring high pressures may experience barotrauma and oxygen abnormalities after 2 to 4 weeks of mechanical ventilation. Early identification of such patients with ventilatory indices obtained during the initial postburn period may allow for rapid conversion to alternative ventilatory support.[79]

In patients with evidence of wheezing or bronchospasm, aerosolized bronchodilators may be beneficial.[2,30,31]

Resuscitation from shock may be necessary in patients with smoke inhalation. In fact, the presence of inhalation injury may increase fluid requirements above that needed for the thermal injury alone.[64,80] Concurrent injuries must be treated. Furthermore, the inhalation lung is not always protected by fluid restriction, and such limitation of fluid could lead to worsening of intrapulmonary shunt.[8] The elucidation and manipulation of vasoactive mediators, such as thromboxanes, leukotrienes, and various kinins, may afford the clinician more direct therapy.[8,10]

Once circulation has been restored, the clinician should gauge further fluid administration carefully so as to avoid undesirable tissue edema. This tissue edema may manifest as airway obstruction, pulmonary edema, or swelling in injured soft tissues leading to ischemia or tissue hypoxia. Lactated Ringer's solution is usually the fluid of choice in the initial emergency department management.[1,12,63,68] However, some promising research has been performed with hypertonic saline and artificial plasma expanders such as pentastarch and hetastarch in the resuscitation of burn patients (see Chapter 37).[12,81]

Corticosteroids have been evaluated in both animal and human models.[3,31,82] The assumption for their use is that corticosteroids would decrease tracheobronchial inflammation induced by smoke inhalation.[49] However, various authors point to deleterious effects such as increased mortality from sepsis, worsening of airway obstruction, delayed wound healing, and salt and water retention.[3,5,6,31,49] One animal study that investigated attenuation of mortality and lung histopathology by the administration of corticosteroids reported that in animals exposed specifically to pure acrolein vapor, steroids improved survival but did not reduce lung damage.[82] In general, the current consensus is that corticosteroids should not be recommended in smoke inhalation injury.[83] The use of prophylactic antibiotics in patients with smoke inhalation is similarly controversial, and most authors discourage their use.[5,6,9,30,31]

Other adjunctive therapy such as artificial surfactant, antioxidants, and free radical scavengers have been studied.[38] Recently some investigators have explored the use of artificial surfactant in treating wood smoke inhalation. In this study using a rabbit model, Exosurf by instillation was not an effective treatment.[84] No inhibitory effects of vitamin E on leukocyte activation and adhesion to microvascular and macrovascular endothelium could be demonstrated in one study of cigarette smoke effects in animals.[85] However, vitamin C at plasma levels easily achieved in humans by supplementation did demonstrate a protective effect.[85] Whether this can be applied to general smoke inhalation remains to be seen but it is an intriguing concept to consider use of such a simple treatment that may have some benefit.

Recent interest in the use of inhaled nitric oxide (NO) in the management of respiratory failure from a variety of causes has lead to research in animals and some human trials. Inhaled NO has been shown in an animal model of wood smoke inhalation to moderately improve ventilation-perfusion (V/Q) inequalities by selectively causing pulmonary vasodilation of ventilated areas in the absence of bronchodilation.[86]

Management of associated thermal burns to the integument is discussed extensively in Chapter 37. The interaction of thermal injury to the skin and inhalation injury to the lungs may account for an increased mortality rate when both are present.[6,48]

Disposition. To afford the patient the best chance for survival, all children with signs and symptoms of smoke inhalation and concomitant hypoxemia should be admitted to an intensive care unit or a transitional care unit for close observation, monitoring, and therapy. Those children with severe thermal burns or serious inhalation injury should be considered for transfer to a tertiary level pediatric intensive care unit or major burn unit.

The psychologic aspects of the burned child should not be forgotten. The emergency department physician must anticipate the emotional crisis for the family as well as the child.[87] A multidisciplinary team approach involving the physician, nurses, and support personnel such as pastoral counselors and social workers may provide the child with the best chance for recovery.

Carbon Monoxide

Carbon monoxide is the by-product of incomplete combustion of carbon-containing material. An odorless, tasteless, colorless, nonirritating gas (hence no warning properties), it is barely lighter than air (relative specific gravity of 0.97).[66,88] The atmospheric concentration of less than 0.001% causes no known health effects on humans,[2,89] but passive inhalation by children of CO at higher concentra-

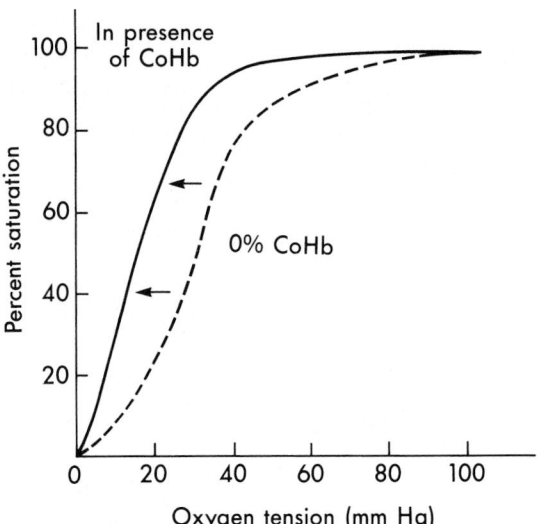

FIG. 44-3. Shift of the hemoglobin/oxygen dissociation curve in the presence of carboxyhemoglobin. (*From Zimmerman SS and Truxal B: Pediatrics 68:215, 1981.*)

tions may occur indoors when adults smoke cigarettes in closed spaces.[21] Adults may have blood COHb levels of 5% to 9%, depending on whether they smoke one pack or more per day.[66] Typical concentrations of CO in home environments where a gas oven is used to provide heat may reach 50 parts per million (ppm) or more, which may be expected to yield an average COHb of 8% or more.[22,66] The buildup of toxic levels of CO may be in part attributed to the airtight insulation of some homes.[89]

The human body also forms CO endogenously during the breakdown of hemoglobin and protoporphyrin heme.[2,88] This process results in a baseline blood level of 0.4% to 0.7% COHb, which may increase tenfold in patients with hemolytic anemia.[66]

Smoke inhalation is commonly associated with CO poisoning, as levels of CO may reach 10% in fires.[66,90] When the child presents with elevated COHb levels after smoke inhalation, it is likely that the true level at the time of exposure was higher. The brief exposure in the prehospital setting to fresh air or oxygen therapy may greatly reduce the apparent blood level of COHb. This reduction may produce a false sense of security about the seriousness of exposure and possible sequelae. Moreover, children presenting with lethargy and syncope (usually not seen in adults until levels of COHb exceed 40%) may have levels as low as 18% to 24%.[3,34,66,91] Children are more susceptible to this form of inhalation toxin because they have a higher metabolic and respiratory rate, leading to greater uptake of CO and a relatively lower hemoglobin compared to adults.[2,34,89] Young infants may be more susceptible to tissue hypoxia because their fetal hemoglobin is already shifted to the left (tighter binding of oxygen) before COHb causes an even greater leftward shift in the dissociation curve[89] (Fig. 44-3). Fetal toxicity is associated with maternal CO exposure.[92]

Carbon monoxide has been reported to be the single leading cause of death by poisoning in the United

States.[18,34,90,93] CO poisoning from smoke inhalation may cause 4,800 deaths per year, and an additional 3,800 may die from accidental or intentional exposure to improperly vented heating systems or automobile exhaust.[90] Many more patients seek medical attention due to CO, but data are less accurate due to the lack of recognition that nonspecific flulike symptoms, headaches, or even personality and memory changes may be due to occult CO poisoning.[34,93-95]

Sources of Exposure. Children are exposed to CO in much the same way as adults, from automobile exhaust, faulty home heating equipment with improper venting, and exposure to closed space fires. Cases of CO poisoning from children riding in the back of vans or pickup trucks have been reported.[96-98] In one study, 89% (25 out of 28) of pediatric cases were due to problems with gas furnaces.[35] Kerosene-powered space heaters or wood burning stoves may be sources of CO poisoning and can be fire hazards.[33,88,93] Other sources include confined spaces such as indoor use of charcoal briquet barbecues or from indoor arenas, department stores, offices, and supermarkets where gas powered equipment may be used with improper venting.[99-101]

Pathophysiology. Carbon monoxide impairs oxygen delivery and utilization. It binds avidly to hemoglobin with an affinity of 230 to 270 times that of oxygen.[66,89] Increasing concentrations of CO gas result in a dramatic rise in hemoglobin saturated by CO, with as little as 0.1% concentration ($\frac{1}{100}$ the concentration in many fires) exposure yielding a COHb level of 60%.[34] Partial saturation of the available hemoglobin with CO also results in tighter binding of the remaining oxygen and hence impaired release at the tissues.[2,5] The uptake of the CO may be related to the alveolar concentration of CO and oxygen, the minute ventilation, and the duration of exposure.[34,102] Carbon monoxide diffuses readily across the alveolar/capillary membrane and, in fact, subtoxic concentrations are used to measure diffusion capacity of the lungs in pulmonary function labs (i.e., diffusing capacity of the lung for carbon monoxide [DLCO]). Once absorbed, about 85% of CO is bound to circulating hemoglobin and of the remainder, myoglobin is a predominant target protein.[66] Carbon monoxide also binds to cytochrome oxidases, thus interfering with cellular oxidative energy metabolism.[5,90] The net result of impaired oxygen delivery, release, and use is tissue and cellular hypoxia. CO poisoning is an important cofactor in the development of inhalation injury by augmenting the ventilation-perfusion mismatch.[103]

Asphyxiation. Direct effects on tissues and organs with high oxygen use such as the brain and heart may contribute to hypoxia. Diminished level of consciousness may result in central respiratory failure or apnea. Although a significant effect on oxygen delivery is due to CO impairing hemoglobin oxygen-carrying capacity to all tissues, there is approximately 10% to 15% of the total body burden of CO bound to extravascular proteins. Binding of CO to myoglobin, reduced cytochromes, guanylate cyclase, and nitric oxide synthase may occur.[104] Cardiotoxicity from the effect of CO on myoglobin may produce diminished cardiac output, hypotension, and resultant decreased oxygen delivery. Myocardial ischemia with S-T segment changes, intraventricular block, extrasystoles, and elevated creatinine phosphokinase (CPK) may occur, especially in those with underlying heart disease.[2] These effects are more common in adults. Crocker and Walker[35] reported two patients out of a series of 28 who had normal electrocardiograms (ECGs) obtained at COHb levels of 18.6% and 36.1%.

Central Nervous System. The central nervous system may also be affected by the hypoxia induced by CO. Specific areas of the brain known to be exceptionally sensitive to hypoxic insult are the globus pallidus, hippocampus, and substantia nigra. Indeed, bilateral necrosis of the globus pallidus with hypodense lesions on computed tomography (CT) imaging is considered by many the characteristic lesion of CO poisoning.[66,105,106] However, basal ganglia infarcts are not always seen in children as they are in adults corresponding to the less common extrapyramidal sequelae of CO in pediatric patients.[95] Cerebral edema, petechia, and hemorrhage may occur secondary to hypoxic-ischemic injury to the cortical white matter.[2,34,95] Demyelinization of white matter, sometimes delayed, and focal damage to the gray matter of the cerebral cortex, thalamus, and cerebellar cortex may be found in CO poisoning.[66,107] Electroencephalograms (EEGs) have shown both diffuse and focal epileptiform discharges, which may represent underlying brain lesions.[95] Neuropsychiatric and behavioral changes ranging from subtle memory loss to severe speech, thought process, or task apraxia have been reported in both adults and children.[34,89,91,95] Cyanide and large amounts of carbon dioxide may exacerbate these effects of CO poisoning by accentuating tissue hypoxia.[90]

Diagnostic Findings. The diagnosis of CO intoxication generally depends on confirming an elevated COHb level in the presence of symptoms and signs consistent with such poisoning. These symptoms and signs, however, may mimic other diseases. Patients who have significant symptomatology can have low COHb levels[29]; an occasional patient with minimal or no symptomatology can have a remarkably elevated blood level of COHb.[91]

Clinical Findings. The emergency physician may see a child who presents with subacute toxicity from exposure to CO slowly over a period of hours to days or may be called on to resuscitate a serious smoke inhalation victim. Subacute poisoning may resemble a flulike syndrome or gastroenteritis, both of which are prevalent in winter months when CO exposure is also common. These symptoms may include headache, nausea, vomiting, malaise, weakness, dizziness, and altered sensorium or syncope.[35,66,93] Infants may present with irritability and lethargy, which may be mistaken for meningitis.

Tachypnea and tachycardia are common, but as the carotid body responds primarily to changes in Po_2 or dissolved oxygen content, the patient may not respond with an increase in minute ventilation early during CO exposure.[5,9,34] Nevertheless, smoke inhalation, a common source of significant CO, may induce hyperventilation and dyspnea initially due to elevated carbon dioxide levels,[9] thereby increasing uptake of more CO gas. When lactic acidosis ensues from the effect of CO on cellular physiology and oxygen use, ventilatory rate[5] and tachycardia[30] may also increase. Hypotension may be caused by and complicate decreased oxygen delivery, in part due to myoglobin dysfunction.[9,66] Cyanosis or paleness may be present, but the classic cherry-red color of the skin and mucous membranes is rare.[2,5,34] When examining the mucous membranes, the clinician may note a coal gas odor to the breath, which is not CO but the associated odor of gases inhaled in smoke.[66] Other reported cutaneous changes include edema, erythema, blistering, burns, bullous formation, and vesiculation, especially in severe cases.[5,108,109]

The neurologic manifestations of CO, such as lethargy and syncope, may be seen in children at lower COHb levels than those associated with such symptoms in adults.[35] As the blood and tissue effects of elevated COHb diminish, the child may start to arouse and become more lucid. Such minor alterations in level of consciousness do not necessarily predict long-term outcome or neuropsychiatric sequelae.[35] However, those children who present with unconsciousness and develop seizures may have significant residual neurologic or behavioral deficits.[89,95] The incidence of delayed neurotoxicity is reported to range from 2% to 30%.[110] Other acute neurologic symptoms include slurred speech, involuntary movements such as posturing and grimacing, agitation and irritability, hyperreflexia, ataxia, muscle weakness, visual changes, seizures, and coma.[34,88,89,95] The clinician should examine the eyes for retinal hemorrhages, which, although not common, may aid in the diagnosis.[34,111] The clinician should also look for red-appearing retinal veins in patients with suspected or documented CO poisoning.[112] This finding, which reverts to normal coloration with treatment, may represent a diminished extraction of oxygen on the venous side.[112]

Complications. The primary cause of complications in CO poisoning is hypoxic injury to organs such as the brain, lungs, heart, and muscle. Pulmonary complications include pulmonary edema, hemorrhage, aspiration pneumonitis, and ARDS.[2,66,89] Pulmonary failure may be complicated not only by cardiovascular compromise but also occasionally by renal dysfunction, although this is rarer in children.[2,89] Myonecrosis, rhabdomyolysis, and resultant myoglobinemia and myoglobinuria may lead to acute renal failure.[89,113]

Cerebral dysfunction may also be accompanied by acute or delayed sensory impairment. Of these, visual field deficits, cortical blindness, auditory damage with hearing loss, and vestibular dysfunction with ataxia may be the most frightening for the child or parent.[2] The young child may look for the comforting sight of a familiar adult, the voice of a parent, and a position of comfort in the parent's lap; however, if these senses are impaired, it may only add to the child's disorientation.

Delayed neurobehavioral effects such as memory loss, personality change, or even psychiatric illness have been described in association with CO poisoning.[34,66,89,90,95] These sequelae may become manifest from 3 days to 4 weeks after initial recovery. In a recent critical review of human outcome studies comparing normobaric oxygen (NBO) with hyperbaric oxygen (HBO), the authors report an alarming incidence of neuropsychologic sequelae of up to 67% after NBO therapy.[114] Delayed neurologic deterioration after anoxia accompanied by a demyelination process may occur rarely after apparent initial recovery.[66] This development may progress to confusion, coma, and death.

Psychometric testing, physical examination, and interview may reveal a number of neuropsychiatric residua of CO. These residua include but are not limited to speech impairment, task apraxia, dysgraphia, object agnosia, amnesia, personality changes with impulsiveness, uncontrollable crying, apathy, depression, easy distractibility, mutism, extrapyramidal or Parkinsonian-like symptoms, seizures, hemiplegia, and urinary or fecal incontinence.[34,66,89,95]

Death due to CO may be immediate at levels of 70% to 80% COHb or more.[34,66] Other toxins in smoke inhalation such as cyanide may contribute to the likelihood of death.[9,90,115]

Ancillary Data. The standard test for CO exposure is the measurement of percent saturation of COHb. Co-oximeters measure the light absorbance of blood to six or more different wavelengths and internally compare this to standard absorbance patterns of known hemoglobin species.[74] With CO poisoning it is important to measure this true hemoglobin saturation with oxygen. Other methods such as standard Corning blood gas analyzers and the like only measure the partial pressure of oxygen and from this calculate the percent hemoglobin oxygen saturation. The clinician should realize that many hospitals use this method. This calculation is not a true measured oxygen saturation. Carboxyhemoglobin levels can be used to document exposure and guide therapy, but there is no consistent correlation between COHb levels and severity of symptoms.[30] Tables comparing percent COHb in blood to clinical signs and symptoms (Table 44-5) lack good correlation in children. At levels normally considered asymptomatic (<10%) for adults, children have displayed symptoms ranging from headache to lethargy at levels of 2% to 5%.[33,93] In one

TABLE 44-5. Correlation of Symptoms with COHb Concentration

Blood COHb concentrations (%)	Symptoms
1-10	Usually no symptoms; slight increase in cardiac output
10-20	Tightness across forehead; slight headache; dilation of cutaneous vessels
20-30	Headache; throbbing in temples
30-40	Severe headache; weakness and dizziness; dim vision; nausea and vomiting; collapse; leukocytosis
40-50	As above, plus increased tendency to collapse, syncope, tachycardia, and tachypnea
50-60	Tachycardia and tachypnea, syncope, Cheyne-Stokes respiration; coma with intermittent convulsions
60-70	Coma with intermittent convulsions; depressed heart action and respirations; death possible
70-80	Weak pulse, depressed respirations; respiratory failure and death

study of 28 pediatric patients exposed to CO, every patient had syncope with levels over 24.3% (mean level of 31.6%).[35] Adult toxicology references note this finding at higher levels, approximately 40% to 50%.[34,66] There is wide individual variance.

Arterial blood gases are not necessary for the measurement of COHb (COHb can be assayed on venous samples), but arterial blood provides accurate measurement of Po_2. The Po_2 may be normal in CO poisoning, and the presence of such a finding in a cyanotic patient should alert the emergency physician to suspect CO.[18,66,89,90] In a canine study by Barker and Tremper,[14] the true oxyhemoglobin and COHb levels were measured by a co-oximeter instrument.

Under varying levels of CO the patient's pulse oximeter saturation (Sao_2) was monitored.[74] At approximately 50% COHb or half of the blood deprived of oxygen-carrying capacity, the pulse oximeter read nearly 95% saturation (Sao_2). In a more recent prospective case study in 16 patients, the researchers found that pulse oximetry was never less than 96% (mean 97.8%) despite arterial COHb levels as high as 44%.[75] Clearly, standard pulse oximetry readings could be misleading to the clinician unaware of this pitfall. Various screening tests for the presence of COHb have been reported but found to be of low sensitivity and specificity when compared to standard laboratory analysis.[116] Therefore, at this time there is no practical substitute for measuring COHb. The presence of hydrogen sulfide, but not methemoglobin, causes interference in the measurement of COHb.[66]

Hematology findings are not specific for CO poisoning but the presence of anemia is a major factor in complicating toxin effect. The normal ratio of oxygen delivery–oxygen consumption is 4:1, as the normal cellular function requires about 5 volume percent (vol %) of oxygen (5 ml oxygen/100 ml blood).[34] When comparing 50% COHb to normal hemoglobin, it appears that the venous point for delivery of this 5 vol % is dangerously low or about 14 mm Hg compared to 40 mm Hg for the normal state.[34] Anemia will also lower this venous point for oxygen release to tissues because of reduced total oxygen content. Carbon monoxide can also affect leukocytes, platelets and the endothelium, inducing a cascade of events involving oxidative injury.[104]

Chemistry may be altered directly by CO toxicity such as acidosis on electrolytes or indirectly as in elevation of creatinine due to myoglobinuric or ischemic-induced acute renal failure.[18,66,89] Carbon monoxide poisoning has presented as apparent ketoacidosis. In one report three members of a family presented with hyperglycemia, acidosis, glycosuria, and ketonuria, but were determined to be suffering from carbon monoxide toxicity after repeat arterial blood gas sampling.[117] Hepatic and muscle injury has been reported[2]; thus one may encounter elevations in transaminases such as aspartate aminotransferase (AST), CPK, and lactate dehydrogenase (LDH). Other blood levels such as glucose should be checked when a child presents with altered mental status.

ECG abnormalities are common in adults with myocardial ischemia induced by CO but are unlikely to be seen in children.[35,89] The most common finding may be simply sinus tachycardia, although one report describes T-wave inversion in a 3-year-old child with a COHb of 29% before treatment with HBO therapy.[115]

Although commonly normal in the emergency department, chest radiographs may reveal abnormalities such as alveolar edema, perihilar haziness with peribronchial cuffing, or a general ground glass appearance.[66,89] CT scan of the brain is usually normal in the emergency setting, but acute changes have been noted in patients within 1 to 6 hours of admission.[90] Low-density lesions of the globus pallidus and deep white matter have been described by CT scanning.[105,106] Magnetic resonance imaging (MRI) may provide more detailed information of cerebral cortex lesions.[107] The main pathologic feature of delayed encephalopathy associated with CO poisoning is a reversible demyelinating process of the cerebral white matter.[107]

Differential Considerations. Many of the clinical and laboratory signs (metabolic acidosis) of CO may be seen in other causes of cellular anoxia such as cyanide or significant methemoglobinemia.[18,24] With methemoglobinemia the diagnosis may be suspected based on history of the characteristic chocolate brown appearance of mucous membranes and blood placed on filter paper.[66]

Management. A nonrebreathing face mask should deliver as close to 100% oxygen as possible. If respiratory failure is present, the patient should be intubated. Oxygen (100%) delivered at 1 atmosphere reduces COHb half-life from 4 to 6 hours to approximately 45 to 60 minutes.[34,66] However, HBO at 3 atmospheres may reduce half-life to 20 or 30 minutes.[9,66] With HBO more oxygen is dissolved in the plasma at higher pressures and may be available for cellular function.[2,34] Controlled prospective clinical trials of HBO are lacking and indications for its use remain controversial.[9,30,89] Nevertheless, numerous clinical reports of HBO exist for CO poisoning and its use is rapidly being liberalized. Some of these reports involve pediatric patients.[35,115,118] Proponents of HBO argue that there are beneficial tissue and organ effects beyond the simple reduction in COHb half-life and that early intervention (less than 6 hours from exposure) would provide the best outcome.[90] It has become apparent that HBO may modify polymorphonuclear cell (PMN)-endothelial interactions and prevent oxidative tissue injury in a number of toxicological conditions including CO poisoning.[119]

Currently, the guidelines for use of HBO are based on the educated opinions of toxicologists and emergency and critical care physicians, since COHb levels in the emergency department may not reflect actual exposure at the scene. If a chamber is available, one should consider using HBO for symptomatic patients (including coma, other neurologic symptoms, and cardiovascular involvement); patients with high COHb levels (over 25% to 40%), recurrent symptoms up to 3 weeks after original treatment with surface oxygen, or symptoms that do not resolve after 6 hours of continuous 100% NBO therapy; and pregnant patients with COHb levels of >15% to 20% or when fetal monitoring shows distress regardless of the COHb level.[34,66,92,107] When compared to the mother, the fetus is more vulnerable to the hypoxic effects of CO.[120] This vulnerability is due to the relative leftward shift in the fetal oxyhemoglobin dissociation curve, which causes fetal arterial oxygen concentration to drop dangerously low after even a small drop in oxygen tension. Toxic effects on the fetus of CO include neurologic dysfunction, decreased birth weight, teratogenicity, and increased fetal death.[120-122] In instances of ill-defined congenital syndromes, including CHARGE association, chronic maternal exposure to CO during fetal life should be investigated.[121] Concern over use of HBO in pregnancy center around possible adverse effects of the fetus such as retinopathy of prematurity, alteration in placental blood flow, and premature closure of the ductus arteriosus. These concerns have generally not been realized in actual practice. Current recommendations indicate that the fetus can tolerate the short duration of hyperoxic exposure during HBO.[120,123] Complications of HBO are rare but include decompression sickness, convulsions, cerebral gas embolism, pneumothorax, tympanic membrane rupture, and complications of transport of critically ill patients.[34,66,124] The limited availability of hyperbaric chambers and the cost of therapy may also be prohibitive in some patients.

Mechanical ventilation for respiratory failure is essential to proper emergency management. Cardiovascular and respiratory monitoring should be instituted and hypotension corrected with available crystalloids. Theoretically, oxygen-carrying blood substitutes such as perfluorochemical emulsions (Fluosol) offer promise for future therapy.[34]

Central nervous system support necessitates a careful and early recognition of hypoxia, respiratory failure, and shock. Consultation with a neurologist and monitoring of the electroencephalogram (EEG) may be helpful. Cerebral edema may be treated with mannitol, diuretics, fluid restriction, and corticosteroids, although the efficacy of the latter is not a proven therapy in CO poisoning.[2,66,125]

Disposition. Criteria for admission after treatment in the emergency department are somewhat based on clinical judgment. However, certain guidelines may be used based on the following: (1) historical criteria—if the patient was initially found stuporous or unconscious, if the elevated COHb was secondary to smoke inhalation in a house fire, if initial vital signs at the scene were abnormal even if they are normal in the emergency department; (2) physical finding criteria—changes in mental status such as persistent or mild confusion, irritability, lethargy; vital sign changes such as tachypnea, tachycardia or hypotension; and (3) laboratory criteria—a carboxyhemoglobin level of >15% to 20% regardless of symptomatology or presence of metabolic acidosis on blood gas analysis or elevated lactate.[66]

Hydrocarbon Aspiration and Solvent Abuse

Hydrocarbons are ubiquitous in our society because of their widely varied use as fuels, solvents, lighter fluids, lubricants, polishes, and household cleaning agents. Incidence figures vary by source from a low of 3.1% of all exposures in children under 6 years of age[126] to an estimated 20% to 25% of childhood poisoning under age 5 years of age.[127] Hydrocarbon ingestion and aspiration may account for 12% to 25% of all poison deaths in children age 5 years and younger.[126,128] Another major factor contributing to the frequency of exposure besides widespread availability is improper storage. In one case review, approximately 33% of 186 cases of hydrocarbon pneumonia were

TABLE 44-6. Saybolt Universal Seconds (SUS) Rating and Aspiration Potential

SUS*	Aspiration potential	Example
>75	Low	Mineral oil, light fuel oil
<60	Moderate	Mineral seal oil,† kerosene
≤35	Very high	Gasoline, naphtha

*Where viscosity is indicated by the rate of flow of the liquid through an orifice of standard diameter.
†Mineral seal oil because of its presence in products like furniture polish has been considered to have high aspiration potential based on availability combined with moderate viscosity.

due to solvents ingested from a beverage container.[127,129]

Hydrocarbons make up a large array of inorganic and organic compounds composed mainly of varying amounts of carbon and hydrogen. Most are derivatives of petroleum distillates, but some are obtained directly from plant sources such as turpentine and pine oils (volatile or essential oils).[130,131] Hydrocarbons can be divided into broad categories based on structural similarities such as straight carbon chain (aliphatics) or cyclic structures (aromatics) incorporating one or more benzene rings.[130] Toluene (glue sniffing) and its parent compound benzene pose risks by ingestion as well as inhalation, as they are absorbed more easily from the gastrointestinal (GI) tract than other hydrocarbons.[130] Therefore, GI ingestion of these agents should be considered an emergency. Deaths have been reported after ingestion of as little as 15 ml of benzene.[131] Aliphatics with substitutions by one or more elements from the halogen series (most commonly chlorine but also fluorine) are termed the halogenated hydrocarbons.[131] These compounds consist of cleaning agents such as carbon tetrachloride (hepatotoxicity), trichloroethylene and trichloroethane (typewriter correction fluids associated with central nervous system [CNS] depression), and fluorinated-chlorinated hydrocarbons (freons) used as refrigerants or propellants (abused by inhalation to induce a high and associated with sudden death).[66,131,132]

The emergency physician must be concerned with the hydrocarbon's aspiration potential, which is directly related to volatility, surface tension, and viscosity. The more volatile a hydrocarbon such as gasoline the more likely it will vaporize to a gas. Surface tension implies adherence of a liquid to a surface, which for the most part is also related to viscosity or resistance to flow. Viscosity is the most important physical characteristic in determining the aspiration potential of a hydrocarbon and is measured standardly through a calibrated orifice with units reported as Saybolt Universal Seconds (SUS).[127] Those agents with low viscosity (<60 SUS) pose a very high risk of aspiration, whereas those agents with viscosity >100 SUS are generally too viscous to be inhaled.[131] Kerosene, naphtha (lighter fluid), and mineral seal oil are of low viscosity and are potential aspiration hazards. Table 44-6 shows the relative order of aspiration potential of some hydrocarbons based on their viscosity coefficients.

Sources of Exposure. Most hydrocarbons are derived from petroleum and a few are derived from the distillation of plant wood, such as pine oil. Sources of childhood unintentional exposures are heating oils such as kerosene, gasoline products, and flammable lighter fluids, which are left in nonsecure containers or in bottles that originally contained beverages.[133-135] In 1988, approximately 30% of the hydrocarbon exposures reported nationally involved gasoline.[131] More recently, a natural disaster resulted in increased use of hydrocarbon or bleach products and a higher percentage of ingestions presenting to a pediatric emergency department.[136] Many lamp and heating oils are scented and attract young children unaware of their dangers. The emergency department physician may take the opportunity to prevent future exposures by inquiring into the presence or lack of safe storage of chemicals such as gasoline in the home.

Hydrocarbons existing as gases, such as methane or butane, have toxic potential as simple asphyxiants. Besides the flammability and risk of fire, these gases may be inhaled unintentionally, leading to hypoxic insults. This potential may extend beyond the immediate patient, as such episodes of hypoxia can affect the fetus of a pregnant adolescent. One case of a newborn with hydranencephaly after maternal butane gas intoxication during the 27th week of pregnancy has been reported.[137]

Passive inhalation of benzene from industrial sources such as gasoline refineries could pose a health hazard if in sufficient concentrations, but the Occupational Safety and Health Administration (OSHA) has strived to control such emissions.[66] The delayed hematopoietic toxicity of benzene, however, is complex and related to biotransformation and bioactivation of the solvent within the human body.[29] These interactions depend on the variables of species, genetics, and age and may therefore strongly influence the toxicity and outcome of such solvent exposure.[29]

Furniture polishes and waxes are sources of mineral seal oil (no longer derived from seals), which has a low volatility but poses a high risk for aspiration because of its low viscosity (< 60 SUS).[126,131] Many pediatricians in emergency medicine are aware of such products as Old English Furniture Polish because of their high content of mineral seal oil.

Mineral spirits used as a solvent and degreaser and household turpentine used as a solvent and paint thinner are both risks for aspiration because of their low viscosity.[66,131] Other agents used as disinfectants and cleaners such as pine oil are toxic by ingestion and aspiration. In one report of 22 cases of pine oil cleaner ingestion, 100% of the children (N = 5) developed CNS depression and three of the five developed acute hydrocarbon pneumonitis.[138]

Heavier oils such as mineral oil found in baby products, skin lubricants, oral laxatives, and rectal enemas have been reported in cases of aspiration and lipoid pneumonia.[126,139,140] These cases have been unexpected because of the low volatility and high viscosity of mineral oil.[85] In addition, mineral oil may be absorbed by the GI tract in small and usually insignificant amounts.[140] However, a case has been reported of a 4-month old with Hirschsprung disease who developed lipoid pneumonia after multiple mineral oil enemas and irrigations of her distal loop of colon via her colostomy stoma.[140] The authors found mineral oil in the peritoneum, lymphatics, and lungs and believed that entry to the abdominal cavity occurred by leak-

age around the stoma. Heavy automotive oils and fluids such as automatic transmission fluid have caused fatal hydrocarbon lipoid pneumonia.[141]

A rare but additional source of exposure to hydrocarbons is intentional poisoning of children by abusive parents. Kempe and others first mentioned this form of child abuse. Since then others have described cases including the report of a 9-month-old infant who developed respiratory arrest after the mother admitted injecting a substance (naphtha) into her son's intravenous line.[142]

Pathophysiology. The toxicity of hydrocarbons varies depending on the type of substance and its aspiration potential. Some agents are toxic if ingested, whereas others pose a high aspiration risk. The ingestion or inhalation of certain hydrocarbons such as turpentine and toluene leads to systemic absorption and CNS effects.[46,66] Pine oil primarily causes toxicity via ingestion, as it is more viscous.[131] Some hydrocarbons such as kerosene, naphtha, and mineral seal oil have a high potential for aspiration because of low viscosity but are poorly absorbed from the GI tract.[131] Aspiration pneumonitis is the most common complication of hydrocarbon ingestion (25% to 40% of cases).[128] Other toxicities include CNS effects such as confusion, weakness, ataxia, cognitive impairment, coma, or decreased ventilatory drive.[128,131] Cardiac dysrhythmias, myocardial dysfunction, and late cardiomyopathy may occur.[130,131,143] Chronic exposure may be associated with toxic effect on the kidneys, liver, and bone marrow, and chlorinated hydrocarbons may cause acute hepatic and renal toxicity.[127]

Initial events on aspiration are irritation of the oral mucosa and tracheobronchial tree and often cyanosis, which is noted within minutes of the event.[131] This brief cyanosis may be due to displacement of alveolar gas by the volatilized hydrocarbon. Bronchospasm may occur, leading to further ventilation-perfusion mismatch.[131] Alveolar edema and hemorrhage may occur as early as 1 hour after kerosene aspiration.[144] Areas of atelectasis may develop, possibly due to reduction in functional surfactant and destruction of airway epithelium and alveolar septa.[131] Chemical pneumonitis with edema, hyperemia, infiltration of leukocytes, and vascular thrombosis are observed.[129] Subsequently, areas of patchy bronchopneumonia may develop. Pulmonary lesions are similar for almost all types of hydrocarbons and may consist of diffuse hemorrhagic exudative alveolitis, bronchiolar necrosis, microabscesses, and later alveolar thickening.[127,129] Hyaline membranes resembling those in neonatal respiratory distress syndrome (RDS) have been seen.[129] Hydrocarbons may cause partial obstruction in airways leading to air trapping phenomena such as emphysematous changes, pneumatoceles, pneumomediastinum, and ultimately pneumothoraces.[126,128] The net result is hypoxia. Lipoid pneumonia is due to aspiration of oil into the tracheobronchial tree. Pathophysiologic changes result from foreign body reactions in the airways, alveolar inflammation or infiltration with lipid-laden macrophages, and the later development of septal fibrosis.[139] Clearance of the aspirate such as mineral oil is poor because of an impaired ciliary escalator mechanism.[139]

Diagnostic Findings

Clinical Findings. The earliest signs in hydrocarbon aspiration may be choking, coughing, and gasping. Children may have initial cyanosis and tachypnea, and within minutes nasal flaring, grunting, and retractions may ensue.[127,129] Symptoms of respiratory distress usually appear within 30 minutes of aspiration but may take up to 2 to 6 hours.[66,129] Crackles, wheezes, and diminished breath sounds may be heard on auscultation. Vomiting has been observed and may result in secondary aspiration. Tachycardia is common and may coincide with significant lung involvement.[128] Dysrhythmias may occur, especially with certain hydrocarbons, but are less common in children.[129]

CNS effects are common and initially may be the most prominent symptom facing the emergency physician. They may precede respiratory symptoms. Children can present to the emergency department with lethargy, sleepiness, headache, difficulty speaking, ataxia, dizziness, seizures, coma, or respiratory paralysis.[127,129,130]

GI effects include nausea, vomiting, abdominal pain, and diarrhea. These effects are likely due to mucosal irritation, although hemorrhage and corrosive effects are rare.[127]

Fever up to 38° C to 39° C may be seen early but does not necessarily coincide with respiratory symptoms.[66,129] Most patients with fever on admission from the emergency department will be afebrile by 24 hours, and the presence of persistent temperature elevation may be associated with bacterial infection.[66]

Renal injury is uncommon but may manifest as acute tubular necrosis, hematuria, proteinuria, glomerulonephritis, and renal tubular acidosis.[66,131] Chronic exposure to toluene has been linked to Goodpasture syndrome.[66] Fatty infiltration of the liver has been described in children, but even in postmortem examination of the liver in fatal aspiration pneumonitis there are often only minor hepatic abnormalities.[129,131] Centrilobular hepatic necrosis, however, may occur with certain chlorinated hydrocarbons such as carbon tetrachloride.[131]

Complications. The most common and serious complication of hydrocarbon ingestion is aspiration and parenchymal lung injury. Respiratory involvement usually progresses over the first 24 hours and subsides between the second and fifth day.[128] Pneumatocele, pneumothoraces, and oxygen toxicity are some of the immediate complications seen in significant hydrocarbon aspiration.[128] Small airway dysfunction with obstruction has been reported in children 10 years after kerosene aspiration pneumonitis.[133] It appears to be related to the severity of the acute insult.

Respiratory failure with intractable hypoxia may occur and can lead to death within 24 hours of aspiration.[128] Cyanosis with increased oxygen requirements may necessitate the use of high PEEP to reduce the intrapulmonary shunt and enhance oxygenation.[127,144] Indeed, the use of PEEP is a standard of care in the ventilatory treatment of hydrocarbon aspiration.

However, barotrauma is a concern, especially with lungs already predisposed to air leak phenomena due to the pathophysiology of hydrocarbon aspiration.[126,144] Although some have achieved success or temporizing effect with high PEEP, children with severe hydrocarbon aspiration may die even 48 hours after admission.[144] Alternatives, such as high frequency jet ventilation (HFJV), have been used in other forms of respiratory failure such as neonatal RDS and meconium aspiration syndrome. Although some

patients have failed a trial of HFJV, a recent report of a child with ARDS secondary to hydrocarbon aspiration highlights the successful use of high-frequency jet ventilation.[126,145] Such techniques are worth consideration, as they may reduce barotrauma. A report of two children with severe respiratory failure due to hydrocarbon aspiration successfully treated with extracorporeal membrane oxygenation (ECMO) suggests that this may be an alternative therapy in some cases.[126]

Other complications of hydrocarbon aspiration related in part to the hypoxic insult are encephalopathy, seizures, and impaired memory.[127,131]

Ancillary Data. Laboratory testing in hydrocarbon aspiration should consist primarily of ABGs, which may reveal significant hypoxemia and usually normal Pco_2 initially.[128] If CNS depression is prominent, there may be a diminished ventilatory drive; hypercarbia can develop rapidly. Unlike CO or methemoglobinemia, hydrocarbon aspiration will not affect the accuracy of pulse oximetry readings. Because hypoxia is the primary result of hydrocarbon aspiration, it is helpful to monitor bedside pulse oximetry in the emergency department.

Hematology may reveal leukocytosis with a left shift even within 1 hour of ingestion, which may last up to 1 week after admission.[127] Intravascular hemolysis has been reported after the ingestion of gasoline.[134]

Chemistry is usually normal but may show ketonuria and glucosuria.[129] An elevated anion gap metabolic acidosis is not common, but can occur with exposure to toluene.[45]

The chest radiograph may show abnormalities within 30 minutes of aspiration or findings may be delayed for hours (Fig. 44-4).[128]

Initially, diagnostic imaging reveals fine mottled densities in the perihilar and midlung, which may coalesce into areas of consolidation.[129] Emphysematous changes may occur on serial radiography along with pneumomediastinum and pneumothoraces. Findings are usually bilateral.[128]

Differential Considerations. The pulmonary infiltrates of hydrocarbon aspiration may be present on the radiograph shortly after presentation. If the history is not supportive of ingestion (i.e., the child was not observed to take hydrocarbon), then infectious pneumonia may be incorrectly diagnosed especially because of early fever. Careful examination noting odor of the breath may help in confirming the diagnosis of hydrocarbon aspiration. Contamination of hydrocarbons with heavy metals or pesticides may complicate the ingestion and require GI decontamination.

Management. Oxygen should be administered to patients with hydrocarbon aspiration. Children who have ingested a hydrocarbon may be agitated or somnolent secondary to hypoxemia from aspiration. Every attempt should be made to maintain oxygenation, which may be monitored by pulse oximetry and ABGs.

Cutaneous decontamination should be performed as some hydrocarbons may be absorbed through the skin or cause a contact irritation.[66] GI decontamination is controversial and may vary among products. Physicochemical and toxicologic properties of the hydrocarbon should be considered. A useful guide to recognizing those hydrocarbons that should *probably* be lavaged is offered by the mnemonic *CHAMP,* where *C* = camphor-containing hydro-

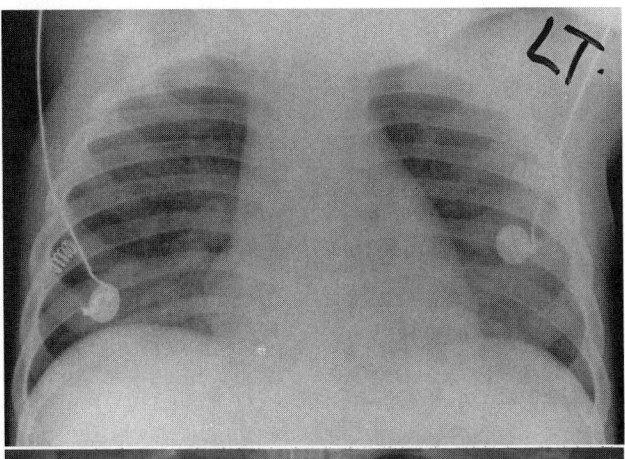

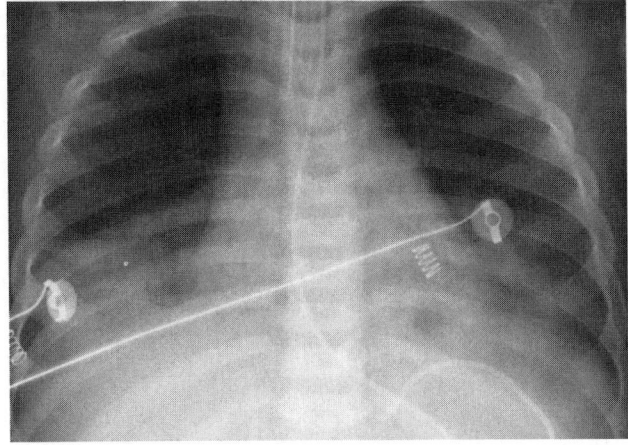

FIG. 44-4. A, Chest radiograph of a 16-month-old child who aspirated mineral seal oil. Note the relatively normal appearance with the exception of a small right basilar infiltrate (2 hrs after ingestion). **B,** Chest radiograph of the same child obtained 17 hours after exposure showing increased bilateral basilar infiltrates.

carbons; *H* = halogenated hydrocarbons (carbon tetrachloride); *A* = aromatic hydrocarbons (benzene); M = heavy metals such as lead, selenium, and cadmium; and *P* = pesticide-containing hydrocarbons. Because of the toxic nature of some of these compounds the patient may benefit from careful gastric emptying.[127,131] However, agents with very low viscosity and insignificant GI absorption or systemic toxicity (gasoline, kerosene, furniture polish, charcoal lighter fluid and mineral spirits) should not be removed by ipecac-induced emesis or gastric lavage because of the possibility of aspiration.[146]

The amount ingested may also aid in determining the need for GI decontamination. One swallow in a child is about 4 ml. If the volume ingested and the content of the hydrocarbon is certain, useful advice may be obtained from poison information specialists. In general, the use of activated charcoal is not recommended unless there is concomitant ingestion of other toxins, or the hydrocarbon contains toxic contaminants such as mentioned earlier. Airway protection as afforded by an endotracheal tube should be considered or dictated by the patient's mental status and

airway reflexes. When liquid hydrocarbons are involved, gastric aspiration and lavage usually can be accomplished with a standard nasogastric tube rather than large bore orogastric hoses.

Airway management may be required for respiratory distress, diminished level of consciousness with associated aspiration hazard, or hypercarbia and hypoxemia. In the child with diminished level of consciousness, regurgitation may readily lead to secondary aspiration of the ingested hydrocarbon. It may be necessary, therefore, to use rapid-sequence induction anesthesia and neuromuscular paralysis to accomplish emergency intubation.[147] When development of ARDS necessitates ventilation with high pressure, a significant air leak may occur around the endotracheal tube. The presence of a cuff, even one that is not inflated, may help diminish this air leak and reduce the demand on the ventilator to provide the given volume.

Ventilator therapy may require the use of PEEP to preserve functional residual capacity (FRC), decrease atelectasis, redistribute alveolar fluid to recruit air spaces, and reduce the required FIo_2 to maintain oxygenation.[127,144] Bronchodilators such as aerosolized albuterol sulfate may be helpful in treating bronchospasm induced by hydrocarbon aspiration, although some investigators believe that no conclusive evidence confirms any benefit.[126,129] Air trapping induced by hydrocarbon aspiration, not relieved by bronchodilators, and exacerbated by positive pressure ventilation and PEEP may lead to complications such as pneumothorax, which can be disastrous.[126,144] Other measures, such as corticosteroids to reduce the inflammatory response and systemic antibiotics, have been considered by some but are not generally felt to be beneficial in hydrocarbon aspiration.[127-129,131]

Disposition. All children who demonstrate respiratory symptoms and signs consistent with aspiration should be admitted for treatment and further monitoring. However, children who may have only coughed briefly (because of the irritant effects) while swallowing the hydrocarbon and who present asymptomatic may be observed in the emergency department for 6 to 8 hours. If monitored pulse oximetry is normal and the child remains asymptomatic over this period, discharge may be appropriate. It may be helpful to wait until the end of the 8-hour period to obtain a radiograph, if indicated at all, in children with minimal or no symptoms, as delaying the study may increase the likelihood of detecting a positive finding. At 8 hours, 92% of patients who eventually develop pulmonary abnormalities exhibit such findings on chest radiographs.[128] Children with positive radiographs should probably be admitted.[131] Even if the patient is minimally symptomatic or asymptomatic, the ingestion of a large amount of hydrocarbon may warrant admission.

If the child survives the immediate hospitalization for acute hydrocarbon aspiration, the prognosis is good. The majority of patients recover without residual effect, although some have reported pulmonary function abnormalities years later.[128,129,133]

Miscellaneous Inhalation Injuries

Chlorine Gas. Chlorine is a yellow-green gas, which is slightly water soluble and about two times as heavy as air.

It has a pungent, irritating odor and is a strong oxidizing agent.[24,66] Sources of exposure for children include accidental releases of chlorine vapor at swimming pools, improper mixing of hypochlorite bleach with acidic cleaning agents, mixing of ammonia and hypochlorite bleach (forming chloramine gas), school chemistry experiments, and industrial or chemical transportation accidents.[43,44,66,148]

The pathophysiology of chlorine involves the formation of hydrochloric and hypochlorous acid on contact with mucous membranes and the destruction of cellular proteins.[66] Pulmonary changes include bronchial and alveolar injury and edema, laryngotracheobronchitis, pulmonary edema, hypoxemia, and thrombi in pulmonary vessels.[44,66,149]

Diagnostic findings on examination include lacrimation, rhinorrhea, conjunctival irritation, cough, sore throat, laryngeal edema, dyspnea, and sometimes hoarseness and stridor.[44] Corneal abrasions and cutaneous burns can occur with direct contact.[66] Symptoms occur within minutes of exposure; hence children displaying no symptoms after possible exposure usually do not need admission.

Complications are generally immediate with severe exposure and include pulmonary edema, ARDS, respiratory failure, and death.[44,66,149] Late sequelae are uncommon and pulmonary function was found to be generally normal at follow-up of 60 patients exposed to chlorine gas from a train derailment.[149] Chronic airflow obstruction, however, has been reported following chlorine and ammonia inhalation.[150]

Laboratory testing should include arterial blood gases, bedside oximetry, and chest radiographs as part of the initial management of symptomatic patients. Humidified oxygen should be administered to relieve hypoxia. In some cases supplemental oxygen may be insufficient to provide adequate oxygenation. Early institution of PEEP in the emergency department may be useful.[151] Pulmonary edema may be treated with standard therapies such as oxygen, PEEP, furosemide, and morphine.[152] Bronchospasm may be treated with inhaled bronchodilators and aminophylline.[66] Skin and eyes should be copiously irrigated with saline. The use of bicarbonate inhalation remains to be clarified. Some animal research and more recent evidence from a study of 86 patients suggest a beneficial effect of inhalation of bicarbonate after exposure to chlorine gas[153,154]; however, others do not recommend its use.[44]

Ammonia. Ammonia is colorless, lighter than air, irritating, extremely water soluble, and alkaline.[26] Sources of ammonia exposure are primarily leakage of pressurized liquid ammonia from tankers involved in transportation incidents. The combustion of wool, silk, and nylon also produces ammonia.[66] Household ammonia products are typically 5% to 10% aqueous solutions, and toxicity is limited to irritation and superficial burns of the mucous membranes.

The pathologic effect of ammonia on respiratory epithelium is liquefaction necrosis at high concentrations and generally irritation of the airway.[41] This irritant property gives the gas an excellent warning effect. Chemical burns of the eyes and skin may occur.[26] Clinical presentation includes partial- and full-thickness burns of the skin, burns

of the upper airway with laryngeal edema requiring immediate intubation, bronchospasm, nausea, vomiting, headache, conjunctivitis, and corneal burns.[41,66] Complications of exposure to ammonia include immediate death at the scene of accidental releases of ammonia fumes and, in less severe but high-dose exposures, persistent airway obstruction, bronchiolitis obliterans, and hyperreactivity of the airways.[41,66,150]

Management of ammonia exposures should begin with administration of oxygen, preferably humidified; assessment of respiratory function with ABGs; oximetry; and radiographs of the chest and airway if indicated. The skin and eyes should be irrigated extensively and fluorescein may be used to uncover corneal epithelial defects. Ophthalmologic consultation should be sought in alkali burns of the cornea, and otolaryngologic or pediatric surgery consultation should be sought for airway burns. Children may be at greater risk for developing upper airway obstruction because of their softer, more narrow airway. All children should be observed for development of stridor, hoarseness, or other signs of obstruction. Treatment, in general, is supportive, although some otolaryngologists recommend the use of corticosteroids to diminish inflammation.[41]

Children should be admitted if they show signs of airway involvement or persistent hypoxemia on laboratory studies and monitoring. Bronchoscopy and pulmonary function tests may be needed to uncover the extent of injury.

Solvent Abuse. Solvent and propellant inhalation abuse is more common than most expect and is an epidemic in England, Canada, and the United States.[66,155] The typical adolescent abuser is a 13- to 15-year-old boy who inhales the material in a group activity and may, for some solvents such as gasoline, be from lower income, rural populations.[66,155] Agents used to acquire an emotional high may exert a direct physiologic effect, such as toluene on the CNS, or indirect effects induced by hypoxia. Hypoxia may yield the desired effects of light-headedness, apparent euphoria, and heightened sexual arousal. Some inhalants such as butane, isobutane, propane, or nitrous oxide displace alveolar oxygen and may cause hypoxia.[66,156] Often these agents are inexpensive and easily obtained due to widespread availability in aerosol sprays used for cooking, cosmetic, or household purposes. Some older children have even experienced light-headedness due to hypoxia after inhaling helium from party balloons.

The inhalation agents most commonly encountered are (1) glues, adhesives, rubber cements, nail polish removers, and correction fluids (e.g., toluene, acetone, benzene, trichloroethylene, and trichloroethane); (2) paints and aerosol propellants (e.g., toluene, trichloroethylene, and fluorocarbons); (3) gasoline; (4) locker room deodorants (e.g., butyl nitrite or isobutyl nitrite, which are used to enhance sexual pleasure by inducing transient hypoxemia via nitrite-induced methemoglobinemia), which include products referred to as "Locker Room" or "Rush" and; (5) other propellants or whipping agents such as nitrous oxide (also abused by adults in anesthetic gas).[44,66,132,152,156] Death due to methemoglobinemia has occurred after inhalation of isobutyl nitrite.[157]

Pathophysiology varies among the agents used for inhalant abuse. Some substances, such as toluene and benzene, exert their toxicity acutely and chronically, including effects on the CNS, liver, and kidneys.[29,44] Gasoline has been associated not only with acute aspiration hazard but also with disorientation, leading to falls and unintentional death or long-term sequelae such as organolead poisoning.[134,155,158] Approximately 15 to 20 breaths of gasoline vapor can produce intoxication for up to 6 hours.[155] Other agents, such as the aliphatic hydrocarbons butane, isobutane, and propane in pure form, can behave as simple asphyxiants and in high concentrations have caused CNS depression, anesthesia, and myocardial susceptibility to catecholamine-induced dysrhythmias in animal models.[156] One report described a 2-year-old child who, after playing with a deodorant aerosol can, developed seizures, apnea, and ventricular tachycardia.[156] Some authors, however, have questioned the causal relationship between the aliphatic hydrocarbon propellant in the aerosol can by pointing out that such cans contain subtoxic levels of butanes when measured directly.[159] Others found no effects when volunteers were monitored continuously by ECG and EEG after being exposed to varied concentrations (ppm) for different lengths of time.[160]

Clinical presentation of adolescents who have abused a solvent may consist of a drunken appearance, with slurred speech, ataxia, euphoria, headache, nausea, vomiting, hallucinations, agitation, violence, syncope, CNS depression, or coma.[44,66,132] Older children and adolescents may also present with delayed organolead poisoning consisting of headache, fatigue, anorexia, insomnia, increased deep tendon reflexes, or severe toxicity with lead encephalopathy, psychosis, cerebellar ataxia, or seizures.[155]

Management of such patients includes provision of high concentration oxygen, assessment for adequacy of ventilation, and decontamination of the skin. Initial assessment may include screening of blood gases, especially methemoglobin if nitrate or nitrite abuse is suspected. Toxicology laboratory screening may be helpful to rule out other drugs of abuse including ethanol. Screening for hepatic effects, renal involvement, or blood dyscrasias from chronic abuse may be indicated. Serum lead levels should be obtained in suspected gasoline sniffers. Acid-base, calcium, potassium, and phosphate imbalance has been reported in solvent abuse and warrants checking in selected cases.[66] Psychiatric and substance abuse counseling should be sought. The emergency physician is in a unique position to direct the patient to appropriate neuropsychiatric care.

Talcum Powder. Talcum powder is generally safe and, if inhaled in small quantities, is effectively removed via the mucociliary escalator mechanism.[161] However, hazards associated with diaper changing, such as an infant or toddler grabbing the open powder container and inhaling large quantities, has been reported in the literature.[40,161-163] Talcum consists of layers of hydrated magnesium silicate and magnesium hydroxide, as well as other components such as zinc stearate, zinc oxide, kaolin, and fragrances.[40] In other commercial preparations cornstarch is the primary ingredient. In 1993, there were 2,939 cases of powder with talc inhalation reported to the American Association of Poison Control Centers (AAPCC) of which 2,621 were by children younger than 6 years of age.[164] No deaths were reported

but there were 37 moderate effect outcomes. In another report, however, a child suffered cardiopulmonary arrest after his tracheostomy tube was occluded accidentally by talcum powder during a diaper change, thus emphasizing the potential hazard of baby powder inhalation.[165]

The pathophysiology of powder inhalation involves airway and interstitial inflammation of small bronchi, bronchioles and alveolar walls, hyalinization with infiltration of mononuclear cells, atelectasis, and emphysematous changes.[40,162] ARDS was reported in a 16-month-old girl who was found playing with a baby powder container.[40]

Clinical presentation is the same as that expected for aspiration of a powder: dyspnea, coughing, choking, tachypnea, cyanosis, tachycardia, wheezing, and vomiting.[161,162] In a study of 138 cases of exposure to poisons during diaper changing, 47% were due to powders and 62% of these children had respiratory symptoms.[161]

Complications of powder inhalation are usually immediate. A child with ARDS recovered without respiratory sequelae.[34] Long-term follow-up using pulmonary function tests are lacking in the literature, except for rare reports of isolated cases of combined restrictive-obstructive defects.[34]

Laboratory testing involves assessing respiratory failure with ABGs and determining changes on chest radiographs. One may see diffuse or coalescing areas of alveolar infiltrates and atelectasis scattered with emphysema.[34]

Treatment of powder inhalation is mainly supportive. Oxygen and respiratory support should be provided as necessary. Steroids have not been shown to be consistently effective.[34,98] Bronchopulmonary lavage may not be successful because of the insolubility of talcum particles in water.[98] Prevention is the most important issue in management. Emergency physicians, pediatricians, and clinicians should educate the parents of young children about the dangers of inhalation from baby powder and other substances for which they are not well informed.

References

1. Newman LS: Pulmonary toxicology. In Sullivan JB, Krieger GR, editors: *Hazardous materials toxicology,* Baltimore, 1992, Williams & Wilkins.
2. Spear RM and Munster AM: Burns, inhalational injury, and electrical injury. In Rogers MC, editor: *Textbook of pediatric intensive care,* Baltimore, 1987, Williams & Wilkins.
3. Trunkey DD: Inhalation injury, *Surg Clin North Am* 58:1133, 1978.
4. Colombo JL, Hopkins RL, Waring WW: Steam vaporizer injuries, *Pediatrics* 67:661, 1981.
5. Fein A, Leff A, Hopewell PC: Pathophysiology and management of the complications resulting from fire and the inhaled products of combustion: review of the literature, *Crit Care Med* 8:94, 1980.
6. Herndon DN et al: Pulmonary injury in burned patients, *Surg Clin North Am* 67:31, 1987.
7. Moritz AR, Henriques FC, McLean R: The effects of inhaled heat on the air passages and lungs, *Am J Pathol* 21:311, 1945.
8. Deitch EA: The management of burns, *N Engl J Med* 323:1249, 1990.
9. Heimbach DM and Waeckerle JF: Inhalation injuries, *Ann Emerg Med* 17:1316, 1988.
10. Demling RH et al: Early lung dysfunction after major burns: role of edema and vasoactive mediators, *J Trauma* 25:959, 1985.
11. Demling RH: Burns, *N Engl J Med* 313:1389, 1985.
12. Demling RH: Fluid replacement in burned patients, *Surg Clin North Am* 67:15, 1987.
13. Moran K, Munster AM: Alterations of the host defense mechanism in burned patients, *Surg Clin North Am* 67:47, 1987.

14. Shirani KZ, Pruitt BA, Mason AD: The influence of inhalation injury and pneumonia on burn mortality, *Ann Surg* 205:82, 1987.

15. Bhopal Working Group: The public health implications of the Bhopal disaster, *Am J Public Health* 77:230, 1987.

16. Chandra H et al: Isolation of an unknown compound, from both blood of Bhopal aerosol disaster victims and residue of tank E-610 of Union Carbide India Limited–chemical characterization of the structure, *Med Sci Law* 34:106, 1994.

17. Varma DR, Guest I: The Bhopal accident and methyl isocyanate toxicity, *J Toxicol Environ Health* 40:513, 1993.

18. Robinson MD and Seward PN: Hazardous chemical exposure in children, *Pediatr Emerg Care* 3:179, 1987.

19. Nadig R: Hazardous materials releases and decontamination. In Goldfrank LR et al, editors: *Toxicologic emergencies*, Norwalk, Conn, 1994, Appleton & Lange.

20. Lebowitz MD: Airway responses of children to environmental irritants, *Pediatr Pulmonol* 1:235, 1985.

21. Lebowitz MD: Influence of passive smoking on pulmonary function: a survey, *Prev Med* 13:645, 1984.

22. Samet JM, Marbury MC, Spengler JD: Respiratory effects of indoor air pollution, *J Allergy Clin Immunol* 79:685, 1987.

23. Bowler RM et al: Psychological, psychosocial, and psychophysiological sequelae in a community affected by a railroad chemical disaster, *J Trauma Stress* 7:601, 1994.

24. Goldfrank LR and Bresnitz EA: Toxic inhalants including cyanide. In Goldfrank LR et al, editors: *Toxicologic emergencies*, Norwalk, Conn, 1990, Appleton & Lange.

25. McLoughlin E, McGuire A: The causes, cost, and prevention of childhood burn injuries, *Am J Dis Child* 144:677, 1990.

Types of Inhalants

26. Kizer KW: Toxic inhalations, *Emerg Med Clin North Am* 2:649, 1984.

27. Menzel DB and Amdur MO: Toxic responses of the respiratory system. In Klaasen CD, Amdur MO, Doull JD, editors: *Casarett and Doull's Toxicology: the basic science of poisons*, New York, 1986, Macmillan.

Pathophysiology

28. Koenig JQ: Pulmonary reaction to environmental pollutants, *J Allergy Clin Immunol* 79:833, 1987.

29. Andrews LS and Snyder R: Toxic effects of solvents and vapors. In Klaasen CD, Amdur MO, Doull JD, editors: *Casarett and Doull's Toxicology: the basic science of poisoning*, New York, 1986, MacMillan.

30. Thom SR: Smoke inhalation, *Emerg Med Clin North Am* 7:371, 1989.

31. Stone HH: Pulmonary burns in children, *J Pediatr Surg* 14:48, 1979.

32. Inselman LS, Mellins RB: Growth and development of the lung, *J Pediatr* 98:1, 1981.

33. O'Sullivan BP: Carbon monoxide poisoning in an infant exposed to a kerosene heater, *J Pediatr* 103:249, 1983.

34. Olson KR: Carbon monoxide poisoning: mechanisms, presentation, and controversies in management, *J Emerg Med* 1:233, 1984.

35. Crocker PJ, and Walker JS: Pediatric carbon monoxide toxicity, *J Emerg Med* 3:443, 1985.

36. Bachofen M and Weibel ER: Basic pattern of tissue repair in human lungs following unspecific injury, *Chest* 65 (suppl):14S, 1974.

37. Fridovich I and Freeman B: Antioxidant defenses in the lung, *Annu Rev Physiol* 48:693, 1986.

38. Youn YK, Lalonde C, Demling R: Oxidants and the pathophysiology of burn and smoke inhalation injury, *Free Radic Biol Med* 12:409, 1992.

39. Crapo JD: Morphologic changes in pulmonary oxygen toxicity, *Annu Rev Physiol* 48:721, 1986.

40. De La Rocha SR and Brown M: Normal pulmonary function after baby powder inhalation causing adult respiratory distress syndrome, *Pediatr Emerg Care* 5:43, 1989.

41. Close LG, Catlin FI, Cohn AM: Acute and chronic effects of ammonia burns of the respiratory tract, *Arch Otolaryngol* 106:151, 1980.

42. Philipp R et al: Domestic chlorine poisoning, *Lancet* 2:495, 1985.

43. Wood BR, Colombo JL, Benson BE: Chlorine inhalation toxicity from vapors generated by swimming pool chlorinator tablets, *Pediatrics* 79:427, 1987.

44. Baselt RC and Cravey RH: *Disposition of toxic drugs and chemicals in man*, Chicago, 1989, Year Book Medical.

45. Fischman CM and Oster JR: Toxic effects of toluene—a new cause of high anion gap metabolic acidosis, *JAMA* 241:1713, 1979.

Specific Inhalation Injuries

46. Parish RA: Smoke inhalation and carbon monoxide poisoning in children, *Pediatr Emerg Care* 2:36, 1986.

47. Head JM: Inhalation injury in burns, *Am J Surg* 139:508, 1980.

48. Thompson PB et al: Effect on mortality of inhalation injury, *J Trauma* 26:163, 1986.

49. Robinson L and Miller RH: Smoke inhalation injuries, *Am J Otolaryngol* 7:375, 1986.

50. Kirk MA, Gerace R, Kulig KW: Cyanide and methemoglobin kinetics in smoke inhalation victims treated with the cyanide antidote kit, *Ann Emerg Med* 22:9, 1993.

51. Perrone J, Hoffman RS: Use of sodium nitrite needs further investigation, *Ann Emerg Med* 24:3, 1994.

52. Barillo DJ, Goode R, Esch V: Cyanide poisoning in victims of fire: analysis of 364 cases and review of the literature, *J Burn Care Rehab* 15:46, 1994.

53. Ruddy RM: Smoke inhalation injury, *Pediatr Clin North Am* 41:317, 1994.

54. Anonymous: Deaths resulting from residential fires-United States, 1991, *MMWR* 43:901, 1994.

55. McLoughlin E and Crawford JD: Types of burns injuries, *Pediatr Clin North Am* 32:61, 1985.

56. Weesner CL et al: Fatal childhood injury patterns in an urban setting, *Ann Emerg Med* 23:231, 1994.

57. Zanen AL, Rietveld AP: Inhalation trauma due to overheating in a microwave oven, *Thorax* 48:300, 1993.

58. Lalonde C et al: Smoke inhalation injury in sheep is caused by the particle phase, not the gas phase, *J Appl Physiol* 77:15, 1994.

59. Mahut B et al: Bronchiectasis in a child after acrolein inhalation, *Chest* 104:1286, 1993.

60. Hunt JR et al: Fiberoptic bronchoscopy in acute inhalation injury, *J Trauma* 15:641, 1975.

61. Demling RH, et al: Oxygen consumption early postburn becomes oxygen delivery dependent with the addition of smoke inhalation injury, *J Trauma* 22:593, 1992.

62. Raine PA and Azmy A: A review of thermal injuries in young children, *J Pediatr Surg* 18:21, 1983.

63. Baxter CR and Waeckerle JF: Emergency treatment of burn injury, *Ann Emerg Med* 17:1305, 1988.

64. Navar PD, Saffle JR, Warden GD: Effect of inhalation injury on fluid resuscitation requirements after thermal injury, *Am J Surg* 150:716, 1985.

65. Popp MB et al: A pathophysiologic study of the hypertension associated with burn injury in children, *Ann Surg* 193:817, 1981.

66. Ellenhorn MJ and Barceloux DG: *Medical toxicology, diagnosis and treatment of human poisoning*, New York, 1988, Elsevier Science.

67. Blinn DL, Slater H, Goldfarb IW: Inhalation injury with burns: a lethal combination, *J Emerg Med* 6:471, 1988.

68. Georgiade GS and Moylan J: Burns. In Mayer TA, editor: *Emergency management of pediatric trauma*, Philadelphia, 1985, WB Saunders.

69. Wright JL: Inhalational lung injury causing bronchiolitis, *Clin Chest Med* 14:635, 1993.

70. Dacso CC, Luterman A, Curreri PW: Systemic antibiotic treatment in burned patients, *Surg Clin North Am* 67:57, 1987.

71. Barrow RE et al: Efficacy of cefazolin in promoting ovine tracheal epithelial repair, *Respiration* 61:231, 1994.

72. Barker SJ and Tremper KK: The effect of carbon monoxide inhalation on pulse oximetry and transcutaneous pO_2, *Anesthesiology* 66:677, 1987.

73. Buckley RG et al: The pulse oximetry gap in carbon monoxide intoxication, *Ann Emerg Med* 24:252, 1994.

74. Teixidor HS et al: Smoke inhalation: radiologic manifestations, *Radiology* 149:383, 1983.

75. Lee MJ and O'Connell DJ: The plain chest radiograph after acute smoke inhalation, *Clin Radiol* 39:33, 1988.

76. Wittram C, Kenny JB: The admission chest radiograph after acute inhalation injury and burns, *Br J Radiol* 67:751, 1994.

77. Baud FJ et al: Elevated blood cyanide concentrations in victims of smoke inhalation, *N Engl J Med* 325:1761, 1991.

78. Stothert JC, Traber L, Traber D: Does positive end-expiratory pressure significantly reduce airway blood flow? *J Trauma* 35:437, 1993.

79. Fitzpatrick JC et al: Predicting ventilation failure in children with inhalation injury, *J Pediatr Surg* 29:1122, 1994.

80. Demling R et al: Effect of graded increases in smoke inhalation injury on the early systemic response to a body burn, *Crit Care Med* 23:171, 1995.

81. Waxman K et al: Hemodynamic and oxygen transport effects of pentastarch in burn resuscitation, *Ann Surg* 209:341, 1989.

82. Beeley MJ et al: Mortality and lung histopathology after inhalation lung injury—the effect of corticosteroids, *Am Rev Respir Dis* 133:191, 1986.

83. Nieman GF, Clark WR, Hakim T: Methylprednisolone does not protect the lung from inhalation injury, *Burns* 17:384, 1991.

84. Feldbaum DM et al: Exosurf treatment following wood smoke inhalation, *Burns* 19:396, 1993.

85. Lehr HA, Frei B, Arfors KE: Vitamin C prevents cigarette smoke-induced leukocyte aggregation and adhesion to endothelium in vivo, *Proc Natl Acad Sci U S A* 91:7688, 1994.

86. Ogura H et al: The effect of inhaled nitric oxide on pulmonary ventilation-perfusion matching following smoke inhalation injury, *J Trauma* 37:893, 1994.

87. Clarke M: Thermal injuries: the care of the whole child, *J Trauma* 20:823, 1980.

88. Kunkel DB: Carbon monoxide part II: updating a silent killer, *Emerg Med* 20:150, 1988.

89. Zimmerman SS and Truxal B: Carbon monoxide poisoning, *Pediatrics* 68:215, 1981.

90. Thom SR and Keim LW: Carbon monoxide poisoning: a review—epidemiology, pathophysiology, clinical findings, and treatment options including hyperbaric oxygen therapy, *Clin Toxicol* 27:141, 1989.

91. Davis SM and Levy RC: High carboxyhemoglobin level without acute or chronic findings, *J Emerg Med* 1:539, 1984.

92. Caravati EM et al: Fetal toxicity associated with maternal carbon monoxide poisoning, *Ann Emerg Med* 17:714, 1988.

93. Baker MD, Henretig FM, Ludwig S: Carboxyhemoglobin levels in children with nonspecific flu-like symptoms, *J Pediatr* 13:501, 1988.

94. Soslow AR, Woolf AD: Reliability of data sources for poisoning deaths in Massachusetts, *Am J Emerg Med* 10:124, 1992.

95. Lacey DJ: Neurologic sequelae of acute carbon monoxide intoxication, *Am J Dis Child* 135:145, 1981.

96. Hampson NB, Norkool DM: Carbon monoxide poisoning in children riding in the back of pickup trucks, *JAMA* 267:538, 1992.

97. Mofenson HC, Caraccio TR: Poisoning by pickup truck, *Pediatrics* 89:1268, 1992.

98. Smith RA, Ball RJ: Carbon monoxide poisoning in two children riding in the back of a van, *Arch Dis Child* 71:482, 1994.

99. Anonymous: Carbon monoxide poisoning associated with a propane-powered floor burnisher—Vermont, 1992, *MMWR* 42:726, 1993.

100. Paulozzi LJ, Satink F, Spengler RF: A carbon monoxide mass poisoning in an ice arena in Vermont, *Am J Public Health* 81:222, 1991.

101. Hampson NB et al: Carbon monoxide poisoning from indoor burning of charcoal briquets, *JAMA* 271:52, 1994.

102. Seger DL, Welch L: Carbon monoxide. In Sullivan JB, Krieger GR, editors: *Hazardous materials toxicology*, Baltimore, 1992, Williams & Wilkins.

103. Barie PS et al: Alterations of pulmonary gas exchange after superimposed carbon monoxide poisoning in acute lung injury, *Surgery* 115:678, 1994.

104. Hardy KR, Thom SR: Pathophysiology and treatment of carbon monoxide poisoning, *Clin Toxicol* 32:613, 1994.

105. Horowitz AL, Kaplan R, Sarpel G: Carbon monoxide toxicity: MR Imaging in the brain, *Radiology* 162:787, 1987.

106. Jones JS, LaGasse J, Zimmerman G: Computed tomographic findings after acute carbon monoxide poisoning, *Am J Emerg Med* 12:448, 1994.

107. Chang KH et al: Delayed encephalopathy after acute carbon monoxide intoxication: MR imaging features and distribution of cerebral white matter lesions, *Radiology* 184:117, 1992.

108. Myers RA, Snyder SK, Majerus TC: Cutaneous blisters and carbon monoxide poisoning, *Ann Emerg Med* 14:603, 1985.

109. Torne R et al: Skin lesions in carbon monoxide intoxication, *Dermatologica* 183:212, 1991.

110. Seger D, Welch L: Carbon monoxide controversies: neuropsychologic testing, mechanism of toxicity, and hyperbaric oxygen, *Ann Emerg Med* 24:242, 1994.

111. Rosenberg NM et al: Retinal hemorrhage, *Pediatr Emerg Care* 10:303, 1994.

112. Jett GK: Red retinal vein (Jett) sign (letter to the editor), *Ann Emerg Med* 13:644, 1984.

113. Wolff E: Carbon monoxide poisoning with severe myonecrosis and acute renal failure, *Am J Emerg Med* 12:347, 1994.

114. Tibbles PM and Perrotta PL: Treatment of carbon monoxide poisoning: a critical review of human outcome studies comparing normobaric oxygen with hyperbaric oxygen, *Ann Emerg Med* 24:269, 1994.

115. Hart GB, et al: Treatment of smoke inhalation by hyperbaric oxygen, *J Emerg Med* 3:211, 1985.

116. Otten EJ, Rosenberg JM, Tasset JT: An evaluation of carboxyhemoglobin spot tests, *Ann Emerg Med* 14:850, 1985.

117. Roshan M, Price DE: Carbon monoxide poisoning presenting as apparent ketoacidosis, *Diabetes Care* 16:956, 1993.

118. Rudge FW: Carbon monoxide poisoning in infants: treatment with hyperbaric oxygen, *South Med J* 86:334, 1993.

119. Tomaszewski CA, Thom SR: Use of hyperbaric oxygen in toxicology, *Emerg Med Clin North Am* 12:437, 1994.

120. Van Hoesen KB et al: Should hyperbaric oxygen be used to treat the pregnant patient for acute carbon monoxide poisoning? *JAMA* 261:7:1039-1043, 1989.

121. Hennequin Y et al: In-utero carbon monoxide poisoning and multiple fetal abnormalities, *Lancet* 341:240, 1993.

122. Koren G et al: A multicenter, prospective study of fetal outcome following accidental carbon monoxide poisoning in pregnancy, *Reprod Toxicol* 5:397, 1991.

123. Brown DB, Mueller GL, Golich FC: Hyperbaric oxygen treatment for carbon monoxide poisoning in pregnancy: a case report, *Aviat Space Environ Med* 63:1011, 1992.

124. Murphy DG et al: Tension pneumothorax associated with hyperbaric oxygen therapy, *Am J Emerg Med* 9:176, 1991.

125. Iberer F et al: Cardiac allograft harvesting after carbon monoxide poisoning. Report of a successful orthotopic heart transplantation, *J Heart Lung Transplant* 12:499, 1993.

126. Scalzo AJ et al: Extracorporeal membrane oxygenation for hydrocarbon aspiration, *Am J Dis Child* 144:867, 1990.

127. Truemper E, De La Rocha SR, Atkinson SD: Clinical characteristics, pathophysiology, and management of hydrocarbon ingestion, *Pediatr Emerg Care* 3:187, 1987.

128. Victoria MS and Nangia BS: Hydrocarbon poisoning: a review, *Pediatr Emerg Care* 3:184, 1987.

129. Klein BL and Simon JE: Hydrocarbon poisonings, *Pediatr Clin North Am* 33:411, 1986.

130. Jaeger RW: *Poisoning emergencies: a primer*, St Louis, 1987, Catholic Hospital Association.

131. Goldfrank LR, Kulberg AG, Bresnitz EA: Hydrocarbons. In Goldfrank LR et al, editors: *Toxicologic emergencies*, Norwalk, Conn, 1990, Appleton & Lange.

132. Watson JM: Solvent abuse by children and young adults: a review, *Br J Addict* 75:27, 1980.

133. Tal A et al: Residual small airways lesions after kerosene pneumonitis in early childhood, *Eur J Pediatr* 142:117, 1984.

134. Banner W and Walson PD: Systemic toxicity following gasoline aspiration, *Am J Emerg Med* 3:292, 1983.

135. Bratton L and Haddow JE: Ingestion of charcoal lighter fluid, *J Pediatr* 87:633, 1975.

136. Quinn B, Baker R, Pratt J: Hurricane Andrew and a pediatric emergency department, *Ann Emerg Med* 23:737-41, 1994.

137. Fernandez F et al: Hydranencephaly after maternal butane-gas intoxication during pregnancy, *Dev Med Child Neurol* 28:355, 1986.

138. Brook MP, McCarron MM, Mueller JA: Pine oil cleaner ingestion, *Ann Emerg Med* 18:391, 1989.

139. De La Rocha SR, Cunningham JC, Fox E: Lipoid pneumonia secondary to baby oil aspiration: a case report and review of the literature, *Pediatr Emerg Care* 1:74, 1985.

140. Rabah R, Evans RW, Yunis EJ: Mineral oil embolization and lipid pneumonia in an infant treated for Hirschsprung's disease, *Pediatr Pathol* 7:447, 1987.

141. Perrot LJ, Palmer H: Fatal hydrocarbon lipoid pneumonia and pneumonitis secondary to automatic transmission fluid ingestion, *J Forensic Sci* 37:1422, 1992.

142. Saulsbury FT, Chobanian MC, Wilson WG: Child abuse: parenteral hydrocarbon administration, *Pediatrics* 73:719, 1984.

143. Anene O, Castello FV: Myocardial dysfunction after hydrocarbon ingestion, *Crit Care Med* 22:528, 1994.

144. Zucker AR, Berger S, Wood LD: Management of kerosene-induced pulmonary injury, *Crit Care Med* 14:303, 1986.

145. Bysani GK, Rucoba RJ, Noah ZL: Treatment of hydrocarbon pneumonitis. High frequency jet ventilation as an alternative to extracorporeal membrane oxygenation, *Chest* 106:300, 1994.

146. Henretig FM: Special considerations in the poisoned pediatric patient, *Emerg Med Clin North Am* 12:549, 1994.

147. Gnauck K et al: Emergency intubation of the pediatric medical patient: use of anesthetic agents in the emergency department, *Ann Emerg Med* 23:1242, 1994.

148. Mrvos R, Dean BS, Krenzelok EP: Home exposures to chlorine/chloramine gas: review of 216 cases, *South Med J* 86:654, 1993.

149. Jones RN et al: Lung function after acute chlorine exposure, *Am Rev Respir Dis* 134:1190, 1986.

150. Weiss SM, Lakshminarayan S: Acute inhalation injury, *Clin Chest Med* 15:103, 1994.

151. Heidemann SM and Goetting MC: Treatment of acute hypoxemia respiratory failure caused by chlorine exposure, *Ped Emerg Care* 7:87-88, 1991.

152. Pino F et al: Effectiveness of morphine in non-cardiogenic pulmonary edema due to chlorine gas inhalation, *Vet Hum Toxicol* 35:36, 1993.

153. Chisholm CD et al: Inhaled sodium bicarbonate therapy for chlorine inhalation injuries, *Ann Emerg Med* 18:466, 1989.

154. Bosse GM: Nebulized sodium bicarbonate in the treatment of chlorine gas inhalation, *Clin Toxicol* 32:233, 1994.

155. Edminster SC and Bayer MJ: Recreational gasoline sniffing: acute gasoline intoxication and latent organolead poisoning, *J Emerg Med* 3:365, 1985.

156. Wason S, Gibler WB, Hassan M: Ventricular tachycardia associated with non-freon aerosol propellants, *JAMA* 256:78, 1986.

157. Bradberry SM et al: Fatal methemoglobinemia due to inhalation of isobutyl nitrite, *Clin Toxicol* 32:179, 1994.

158. Bass M: Sniffing gasoline, JAMA 255:2604, 1986 letter to the editor.

159. McCain HB and Ebrahim AR: Ventricular tachycardia associated with non-freon aerosol propellants, *JAMA* 257:26, 1987 (letter to the editor).

160. Stewart RD et al: Ventricular tachycardia associated with non-freon aerosol propellants, *JAMA* 257:27, 1987 (letter to the editor).

161. McCormick MA et al: Hazards associated with diaper changing, *JAMA* 248:2159, 1982.

162. Wagner TJ and Hindi-Alexander M: Hazards of baby powder? *Pediatr Nurs* 10:124, 1984.

163. Pairaudeau PW et al: Inhalation of baby powder: an unappreciated hazard, *BMJ* 303:58, 1991.

164. Litovitz TL, Clark LR, Soloway RA: 1993 Annual report of the American Association of Poison Control Centers toxic exposure surveillance system, *Am J Emerg Med* 12:546, 1994.

165. Cotton WH and Davidson PJ: Aspiration of baby powder (letter to the editor), *N Engl J Med* 313:1662, 1985.

PART

VIII

DIAGNOSTIC CATEGORIES

CHAPTER

45

Child Abuse and Neglect

Theodore M. Barnett

Child abuse is maltreatment of a child by parents, guardians, or other caregivers. The maltreatment may be direct physical, sexual, or emotional battery; the denial of nutrition or medical care; or failure to provide a safe, nurturing environment. Child abuse presents in many forms. If not detected, it may continue and intensify, ultimately leading to death, permanent physical damage, emotional scarring, or inappropriate development.

Caffey published the first modern medical paper on the abused child in 1946, but the extent of the problem went unrecognized until Kempe et al, in 1962, proposed the term *battered child syndrome* to "characterize a clinical condition in young children who have received serious physical abuse."[1,2] Child abuse is now recognized as a common entity, the most frequent cause of death in infants outside the neonatal period, and a leading cause of morbidity and mortality throughout childhood. As many as 2.5% of American children are abused or neglected each year.[3] The number of reports of child maltreatment continues to increase with time; however, it is unclear whether this increase is a result of better reporting, or if it reflects a true increase in the prevalence of abuse. Because of the frequency of child maltreatment and the increasing patient load in emergency departments, the emergency physician will inevitably see abused or neglected children.

Victims of child abuse may be brought to the emergency department for treatment of physical injuries, inappropriate behavior, failure to thrive, poor home environment, or abandonment. They may be accompanied by parents, police, social workers, or others, with or without a suspicion of abuse. The emergency physician must be aware of the conditions that predispose to abuse and common presenting findings. Appropriate evaluation and treatment must follow recognition. The ultimate goals of recognition and care are to prevent further injury to the child and begin the process of repairing the damage already done.

PHYSICAL ABUSE

Physical abuse refers to the infliction of physical injury upon a child and does not require intent on the part of the abuser. Injury may occur through deliberate attempts to injure the child by a mentally ill caregiver, but more commonly results from excessively harsh punishment or loss of control with anger directed toward the child. Schmitt and Clemmens divide physical abuse into three categories: mild (e.g., infrequent contusions, abrasions), moderate (numerous bruises, burns, an isolated fracture), and severe

Characteristics of the Abused Child

Premature birth
Neonatal separation
Multiple birth
Congenital defects
Mental retardation
Difficult temperament
Conditions interfering with parent-child bonding

Characteristics of the Abusive Caregiver

Aberrant childhood nurture or abuse
Previous loss of child to foster care or avoidable death
Fear of injuring child
Violent behavior toward others
Substance abuser
Mental illness or poor impulse control
Young maternal age
Unrealistic expectations of child

Characteristics of the Abusive Family

Socially isolated with poor support system
Financial stress or unemployment
Marital problems (including spouse abuse)
Inadequate child spacing or unwanted pregnancy
Inadequate housing
Stressful life events

(large burns, internal injuries, multiple fractures, life-threatening injury). The level of abuse noted represents the *minimum* for potential future abuse.[4] Abuse tends to recur if unrecognized and without intervention may well prove fatal.[2]

Predisposing Factors

Certain characteristics of the child increase the likelihood of abuse (see box above).[5-7] Factors that impair parent-child bonding result in emotional devaluation of the child. However, any attribute that marks children as "special" or different may predispose to abuse, presumably because they have less economic, cultural, religious, or emotional value to the abuser.[8,9] The term *vulnerable child syndrome* has been applied to these children.

Similarly, certain characteristics occur more frequently in abusive caregivers (see box above right).[5,6,10-15] Altemeier et al have stressed the importance of the perception of aberrant nurture as opposed to abuse in the life of abusive mothers. A past history of foster care, separation from or failure to "get along with" their own mothers, and a perception that their parents were displeased with or unfairly punished them were significantly more common in the abusive than in the nonabusive mothers.[10] A variety of mental illnesses (particularly depression) and personality disorders (apathetic-futile, childish-dependent, and impulsive), as well as mental retardation have been implicated in abusive parents. Unrealistic expectations of the child are highly correlated with abuse. A lack of knowledge or acceptance of normal childhood development is usually operative, but transference, in which the parent expects the child to act like another person, may also occur. A common example of unrealistic expectations is in toilet training, a stressful period under any circumstances. The parent, particularly if a sibling was toilet trained easily, may expect more than the child is capable of providing. Frustration may occur in both parties, setting the scene for abuse. Unrealistic expectations may also lead to neglect, wherein the parent feels the child can "take care of himself or herself," despite the child's developmental unreadiness to do so.

Finally, abusive families may harbor characteristics that correlate with abuse (see box at right).[5,6,10-17] Social isolation has increased over the past century as society has become more mobile. Families no longer stay in one geographic area and parents can no longer count on other relatives for advice and help in raising children. The increase in single-parent families has led to a further increase in parental isolation and lack of support systems, and may leave a parent with a sense of having nowhere to turn and no one to go to for help. The frustration and anxiety may turn to anger and blame for the child, with the end result of violence.

Many families suffer from the factors listed in the box, but not all of them are abusive. The factors may be chronic, and the family may have adequate coping mechanisms for dealing with them. However, a chronically stressed but nonabusive family may suffer an acute event that does trigger abuse.[16-18] The event may be an exacerbation of an ongoing problem such as a family argument or intoxication, or it may be an entirely new stress such as illness or loss of employment. The family is unable to cope with this additional stress and abuse is the result (Fig. 45-1).

Diagnostic Findings

Clinical Findings. The vast majority of physically abused children are less than 4 years of age.[19] Younger children are at increased risk due to inability to verbally or physically resist, increased time spent in direct contact with caregivers, and greater need for assistance in activities of daily living. As noted above, children with physical or mental handicaps and infants born prematurely are also at greater risk. Boys are more likely to be abused than girls.

The abuser is a related caregiver in 90% of cases, a sibling in 1%, and an unrelated caregiver in the remainder.[4] Abuse occurs across all socioeconomic, ethnic, and cultural groups. Mothers have been reported for abuse more frequently than fathers, but this may be related to the amount of time spent caring for the children and not to an increased proclivity toward abuse.[20,21]

Historic Findings. History in cases of child abuse can come from the child, the abuser, or a witness to the event

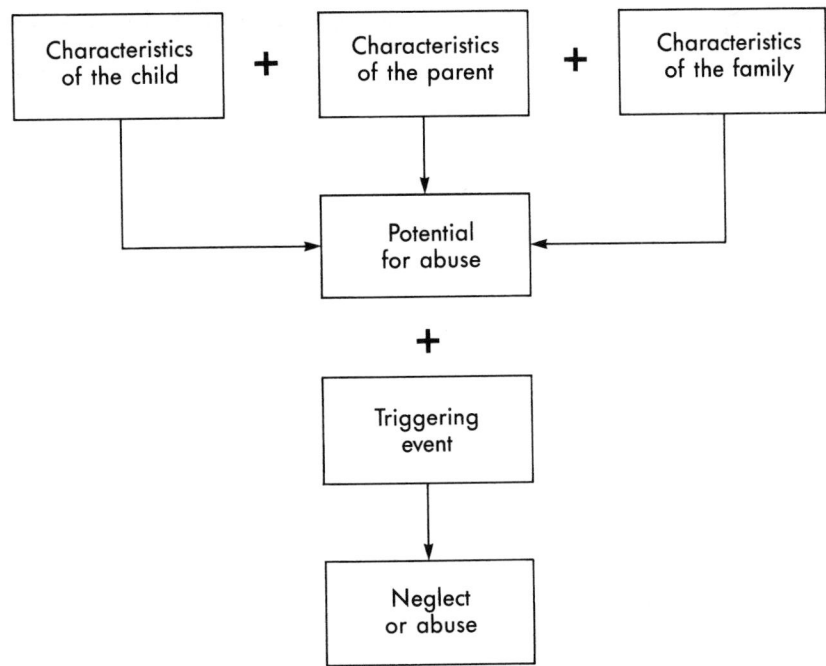

FIG. 45-1. Etiology of child abuse.

or its sequelae. A child who claims to have been injured by a specific adult is usually telling the truth. The examiner should pay attention to the child's specific words and inflection. Coaching of the child to relate a particular history does occur, but is infrequent. In these cases, the child may give the history in a relatively emotionless voice and manner or use words and descriptions well beyond his or her developmental age. Additionally, if the "coach" is in the room, the child will often look to that person for clues on how to react, or for reassurance. Children may report actions by adults that they consider injurious or bad that are not child abuse.[22] This is a result of misinterpretation (e.g., being made to take a bath and normal punishment); rarely, the accusation is made out of spite. Careful questioning will usually lead to the truth.

The abuser will only rarely provide an accurate history of the abuse. In some cases of intentional injury, no history is given at all, but in most some explanation will be offered. If more than one caregiver is questioned, different histories of injury may be given. When no history is offered, further questioning will usually result in a variety of possible explanations. When history is provided, it is often inconsistent with the injuries suffered, as described in the following paragraphs. In either case, these reports are often vague and may bear little similarity to the injuries.[23] In contrast, with unintentional injury, most parents will readily provide a detailed explanation of how the injury occurred.

If more than one caregiver accompanies the child, discrepancies may be noted in their accounts. If there are questions regarding the nature of the event, the caregiver should be interviewed separately. In all cases where the child is old enough to speak, he or she should be interviewed separately as well. A delay in seeking medical care should arouse some concern because many cases of abuse

present late for medical care, a result of lack of concern for the child, inability to recognize the seriousness of injury, or fear of legal action. In unintentional injury, most parents take their child promptly for care. With abuse, the child may be near death or a wound grossly infected before care is sought. If a deliberate attempt is made to cover up the delay, the caregiver may provide a fairly elaborate history of recent illness, particularly in children whose injuries are not visible externally.

Caregivers may claim that injuries were self-inflicted (i.e., due to a fall or deliberate attempt to injure himself or herself). When used to explain multiple injuries of varying ages, the history is often accompanied by comments such as "she falls a lot" or "he's always been clumsy." These stories may be blatantly obvious or quite subtle. Such a history may be inconsistent with a child's development. An example of this is a six-month-old infant suffering trauma from climbing onto a cabinet and falling. A history of recurrent attempts at self-injury can be discounted except in the case of rare illnesses such as Lesch-Nyhan syndrome. The history may also be inconsistent with the severity of injury, as in the child who suffers a severe brain injury while banging his head against a pillow, or with the nature of the injury, as in a child covered with bruises suffered while he was "learning to walk." Parents may also claim their child "bruises easily." Appropriate laboratory studies lay this argument to rest quickly in most cases, but even if the studies are abnormal, the child may still be a victim of abuse.[24,25]

Blame may be deflected onto siblings or other persons. Such stories should be viewed with suspicion. The history may be false, but even if true may suggest some degree of neglect. When possible, interview the alleged abuser or potential witnesses to confirm the story. Alternatively, a history of a dramatic event, such as falling down a flight of stairs, may be offered in explanation of a host of injuries that actually occurred over a period of time. Other common explanations are that injuries were inflicted by other children or during resuscitation attempts.

The history given should be compared to the injuries suffered. The toddler who falls while walking and suffers a fractured femur presents an implausible story. The history may be inconsistent with the severity of injury as in the preceding case, or the distribution of injuries may be discordant. Obtain as much detail as possible in the history in order to bring out inconsistencies. Recurrent or frequent "accidents" should provoke concern. Each incident should be carefully evaluated and previous ones reviewed.

Observe the interaction of the child and caregiver closely. Does the parent act reassuringly and affectionately toward the child, or with hostility? Does the child seem comfortable and happy, or is there fear or suspicion? Negative aspects of the parent-child interaction should increase the level of suspicion that abuse has occurred. An apparently normal interaction does not guarantee that abuse has not occurred. The abuser may not be present, or the child may respond positively in an attempt to gain love, affection, or forgiveness for perceived wrongdoing.

Caregivers accompanying the child to the emergency department may show apathy or diminished concern and anxiety if the injury has been inflicted. This may be readily detectable or carefully concealed. Some will react angrily toward health-care workers, and may try to place blame on them if the child has an adverse outcome. There is substantial overlap among the reactions of parents in inflicted and unintentional injuries, however.

Children may be brought in by law enforcement or social service personnel because of suspected abuse or neglect, criminal activity in the home, delinquency or truancy, and other reasons. These personnel may be able to provide detailed information on the home and child, but more often have limited information. The physician must depend on history from the child, siblings, and examination in most such cases.

Physical Findings. Physical examination findings must be viewed in light of information obtained in the history. Some findings are virtually pathognomonic of child abuse, whereas others may appear innocent until compared to the history provided. A lack of physical findings does not exclude physical abuse. Lesions may be occult (e.g., fractures) or have healed, or abuse may have left no physical signs.

Physical examination of the potentially abused child must be considerate and thorough. Because these children have already been traumatized, time should be taken to listen to them and explain what is to be done and why. If possible, allow time for the child to relax and carry out the examination in a quiet area with minimal interruptions. Record the child's height, weight, and head circumference (if less than 36 months of age). Also note the child's behavior and affect, be it fearful, anxious, depressed, or otherwise altered during the examination. The developmental status of the child should be assessed, as it may provide evidence of the veracity of the history given.

Cutaneous Injuries. Cutaneous lesions are probably the most common and easily recognized signs of physical

TABLE 45-1. Determination of Age of Contusions

Days following injury	Color
0	Red or red-blue
1	↓
2	↓
3	Blue or purple
4	↓
5	Green
6	↓
7	↓
8	Yellow or brown
9	↓
10	↓
14	Normal skin color
21	↓
28	↓

Adapted from Wilson EF: *Pediatrics* 60:751, 1977.

abuse.[26] Included in this category are inflicted contusions, abrasions, lacerations, burns, and hair loss.

Contusions. Contusions are a common result in both accidental and nonaccidental trauma. Identifying lesions resulting from abuse require consideration of morphology, location, distribution, and consistency with history. All lesions should be carefully documented, including location, pattern, shape, and color.[27] Measurements should be recorded when possible. Contusions change in color as they heal (Table 45-1). The depth, location, and amount of bleeding that initially occurs can cause variation in the time course, but the sequence of color change is consistent. Photographs should be taken close to the time of examination to reduce variance with examination findings.[28]

Straight lines are uncommon in nature and in natural injuries; thus, injury from a man-made object should be considered with linear contusions, or with unusual configurations with sharp angles. Certain objects leave a characteristic lesion when a child is struck (Fig. 45-2). When seen early, or if much force is used, these contusions are readily identifiable.[26,29] As time passes, or with less force, the imprint may be less distinct, and more careful inspection will be required to discover its true character. The outline may also be distorted when the point of maximum impact of an object leaves a pale area, whereas adjoining skin shows ecchymosis from capillaries ruptured by blood suddenly forced into them.[30] Human bite marks tend to leave a characteristic ovoid pattern. Abrasions may occur, but the bite is distinguished from that of carnivores by the lack of punctures or lacerations. Size of the marks can be used to separate those caused by other children from adult bites. Dental experts may be able to identify potential perpetrators from the lesions.[31,32] Pinch marks leave a distinctive pair of opposed, crescent bruises.[4]

Skin overlying bony prominences commonly suffers bruising, but other parts of the body are less commonly injured accidentally. Multiple bruises involving the penis, scrotum, vulva, buttocks, or face are probably the result of

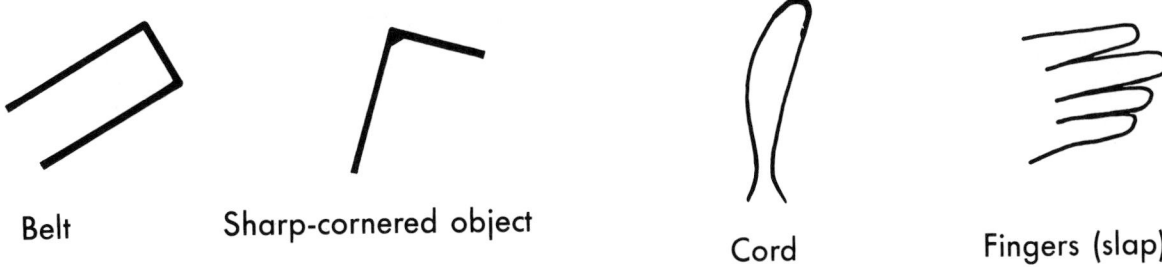

Belt   Sharp-cornered object   Cord   Fingers (slap)

FIG. 45-2. Distinctive contusions.

child abuse.[26,33] Bruises of the inner thighs, inner upper arms, back (other than over spinous processes), or thorax are also unlikely to be from normal injuries.[34] Johnson and Showers found the buttocks and hips, face, arms, back, and thighs to be the most common locations of nonaccidental injury.[35] Bruising of the thorax often occurs when a child is shaken and identifiable finger marks and associated rib fractures may be found. Finger marks are also common on the upper arms from shaking. Bruising of the neck, jaw, and cheek are frequent results of choking, and again may be identifiable as finger marks.

Contusions in multiple stages of healing suggest abuse, and those involving more than one body plane, or occurring bilaterally, are suspicious.[26,35-37] Contusions as a result of falls are typically confined to a single body plane. In the case of tumbling injuries (e.g., falling down stairs), the injuries may occur in several planes, but are usually restricted to bony prominences. In either case, the bruises will all be of the same age.

Abrasions and Lacerations. Electric cords, and other thin instruments used as lashes, have a great potential for breaking the skin. These objects frequently leave combinations of contusions, abrasions, and lacerations after impact, and scarring is common. The lesions typically have the shape shown in (Fig. 45-2), and are easily recognizable.[26,38] Friction from an object or surface causes abrasions. Ropes produce nearly circumferential abrasions, friction burns, or contusions around wrists and ankles in bound children, and abrasions of the neck are the product of hanging or strangulation. Sharp or pointed objects, or blunt objects with sufficient force, cause lacerations or punctures. The injuries may be systematic, such as tattooing with a needle, but more often, no pattern is found.[29] Punctures and open wounds from blunt trauma carry a significant risk of underlying injury.

Burns. As many as 25% of cases of child abuse involve burns, and as many as 39% of childhood burns are a result of abuse, though reported incidences vary widely.[39] Burns are the third leading cause of death in child abuse.[40] More than two burn sites increases the likelihood the burns were inflicted, as does a past history of thermal injury.[41] Abusive burns may take the form of scald, contact, open-flame, chemical, or microwave radiation burns. Reports vary as to whether scalds or contact burns are most common, but scalds tend to produce the more severe injuries.[39,42-46] In 1975, Keen et al reported a series of abusive burns, all of which were minor.[47] Since then, there have been multiple

reports of severe burns, with a significant mortality rate.[39,40,44,45,48] Burns may represent a more premeditated form of aggression in child abuse, with a resulting higher mortality, particularly if unrecognized.[49] Abusers may explain that the child fell, stood, or otherwise initiated contact with the hot object. A detailed history regarding the people involved, environment, objects or substances causing injury is essential. This should include items such as the amount or depth of water in scalds. Comparison of the depth and distribution of the burn to the story provided and the child's development should indicate the true nature of the injury.

As with contusions, some contact burns may be easily identified from the distinctive pattern left behind (Fig. 45-3). This is particularly true of injuries from grills, irons, curling irons, and car cigarette lighters.[29] Cigarettes also leave a distinct pattern when touched to the skin, consisting of a circular crater of burn with the diameter of the cigarette. The depth of the inflicted burn is greater than would be seen from incidental contact with a hot object, the burn is uniform in all directions, and multiple injuries with the same pattern are frequently seen.[41,44,50] Abusive contact burns are most common on the face and dorsum of the hands and feet, distinctly uncommon sites for unintentional injuries.[50] In addition to burns when hot objects are touched to their bodies, children may be pushed or held against a hot surface. The story in such cases is that the child sat or stepped or fell against the surface. Children have the same aversion to being burned that adults do, and will attempt to alleviate contact immediately. A child will not, for example, sit down on a hot stove heating element. Similarly, children will avoid open flames. Full-thickness burns reported from either of these sources are suspicious.

Scald burns can be a result of immersion or splashing with hot liquids, most commonly water. Factors that influence the severity of scalds include temperature of the liquid, duration of exposure, and thickness of the exposed skin. Immersion burns produce a uniform injury to the skin surface exposed to the liquid, and there is a sharp line of demarcation of the burn. Children who are held and immersed rarely have splash or other noncontiguous burns because they are unable to move. If an extremity is immersed, the burn will have a *stocking glove* distribution. The uniformity of the burn makes it most unlikely to result from unintentional immersion. If the exposure is relatively short, the palms and soles may be spared or suffer less injury due to their thickness. The buttocks and perineum

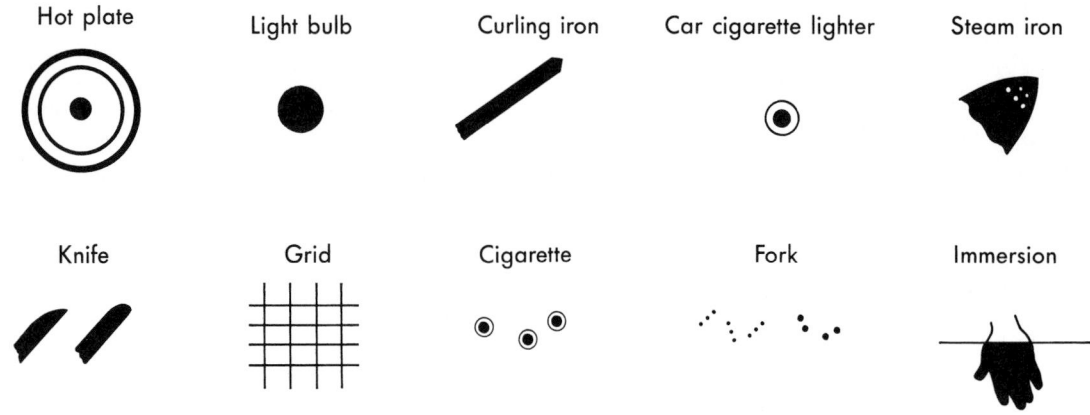

FIG. 45-3. Distinctive burns. *(From Johnson CF: Pediatr Clin North Am 37:807, 1990.)*

are the sites most often affected by abusive immersions, often in response to toilet training "problems."[47,51] If the child is held or placed in hot water, the buttocks alone can be affected, and as the child is placed farther under, the area of involvement spreads to the thighs and waist or trunk. However, unlike the child who is sitting in water when more hot water is added, the legs and feet are relatively spared as the child withdraws from the burning water. Withdrawal can also result in sparing of flexion creases, particularly where the thighs and abdomen meet, as the water cannot contact these areas. When a child is forcefully placed into a container of hot liquid, such as a bathtub, the skin that is in contact with the bottom of the container (which is relatively cooler than the water itself) may be unaffected, creating a doughnut-like burn with sparing of the buttocks. In a similar fashion, the soles or palms may be spared.*

Deliberate splash burns are often difficult to distinguish from their accidental counterparts. In both cases, the burn is usually not uniform and may be noncontiguous. The most useful distinguishing features are a comparison of the description of the incident with the areas affected and the child's development. As liquid splashes onto the skin and runs off, it cools. The area of initial contact can provide a clue to actual events. An "arrowhead"-shaped burn, with its base in the direction from which the liquid came, may be seen where the liquid first struck the skin.[44,46] Isolated splash burns of the buttocks or perineum are quite suspicious.

Alexander et al have reported two cases of abuse involving microwave oven burns.[53] The injuries reported in the first case were a bizarre distribution of full-thickness burns, with relative sparing of subcutaneous tissue between burned dermis, epidermis, and muscle on biopsy. In the second case, the burn was restricted to the back, and the nature of the abuse was discovered from repeated questioning. The burns were sharply demarcated and no charring was noted in either case. Cataract formation and neurologic deficits are potential complications. Biopsy is warranted to establish the diagnosis when doubt exists.

*References 26, 42-45, 47, 48, 50, 52.

Chemical burns occur when a child is immersed, splashed, or forced to ingest a caustic substance, and tend to produce full-thickness injuries. Thermal injury in the form of frostbite can occur as the result of forcing a child to remain outdoors without adequate protection, or from prolonged exposure to ice or snow. These forms of abuse are uncommon.[52]

Hair Loss. Hair pulling or twisting leads to traumatic alopecia, with irregular areas of hair loss, characterized by broken hair, damage to the roots, and possibly open wounds.[26] Hair pulling can also cause subgaleal hematoma, particularly if braids are present.[4]

CNS Injuries. The leading cause of death from child abuse is head injury.[40] These injuries may be inflicted by throwing the child, striking the child with a fist or object, dropping the child, shaking, or a combination of these. Severe accidental head trauma is uncommon in young children, and child abuse must be excluded in any severe intracranial injury in the absence of major trauma.[54-57] Falls while walking or running, or out of bed or from a couch are unlikely to result in skull fracture and will not produce severe intracranial injury.[58,59] As with many abused children, delay in seeking treatment is common, and adds to the morbidity and mortality associated with these injuries. It is not uncommon for nonaccidental head injury victims to die before reaching care.[40,60] Those who do survive have a high incidence of permanent neurologic impairment, ranging from persistent vegetative state, to mental retardation, to focal neurologic defects.[61-64]

Infants with intracranial injury typically present with altered mental status of varying degrees of severity. The child may present completely unresponsive, convulsing, or with focal neurologic deficits. Common complaints include respiratory problems, irritability, poor feeding, and vomiting.[63] Fever and meningismus may be present, further confusing the picture.[64] Injury to other parts of the body may be present, but this is by no means universal, and the injuries are often occult. Child abuse should be included in the differential diagnosis of any child with alteration of consciousness or abnormal neurologic findings.

If the intracranial injury is caused by a direct blow to the head, contusions, open wounds, and fractures are usually found. With inflicted trauma, these injuries are often numerous, and may be present on other parts of the body as well.[4] Multiple or complex skull fractures are associated with abuse, as are fractures with a width of greater than 5 mm.[65]

Some infants and toddlers will present with findings of intracranial injury with no external evidence of head trauma. A substantial number of abusive head injuries are the result not of direct blows, but rather from acceleration-deceleration injuries. The injury results from vigorous shaking, which can be used to admonish the child, in an inappropriate attempt to awaken a comatose child, or from parental frustration aimed at the child (often because of crying).[63] The term *whiplash shaken infant syndrome* has been applied to this kind of injury.[62] Many of these "shaken babies" will have no external signs of head injury. Several authors have disputed that severe intracranial injury can be produced by shaking alone, and postulate that either a combination of shaking and impact or impact alone is responsible for the injury. The lack of external findings is explained by impact with a relatively soft surface, and the deceleration force applied to the brain causes the damage. These authors have dubbed this pattern of injury the *shaken impact syndrome*.[66,67] Other authors have concluded that shaking alone is sufficient to produce the injuries found.[68,69] It is likely that both types of trauma are operative in causing injury. The infant suffering either of these syndromes classically has retinal hemorrhages and subdural hematoma. The subdural hematomas in shake injuries are predominantly parafalcine. This location is less common in direct, unintentional head injury; however, "any subdural hematoma without an adequate explanation strongly suggests physical abuse."[59,70] Other common signs include abnormal vital signs, a bulging fontanelle, and increased head size. Associated physical findings include bruising or fractures where the child was grasped.[62,63,71] Subarachnoid hemorrhage, cerebral edema, and brain parenchyma injuries also occur.

A variation of the shaken infant is the *tin ear syndrome*, in which ecchymosis of an ear, retinal hemorrhages, ipsilateral subdural hematoma, and possibly ipsilateral vitreous hemorrhage are seen. It is postulated to result from a blow to the ear, with consequent rotational stress to the cranial contents.[72]

Cervical spine injury, although considerably less frequent than head injury, does occur in child abuse.[73] It appears that shaking alone is sufficient to produce spinal cord trauma.[74] Significant morbidity can be expected with this injury. Spinal cord injury is identifiable with a thorough neurologic examination. Because children can have spinal cord trauma without fracture or other bony injury, normal radiographs do not exclude injury.

Ophthalmologic Injuries. Ocular trauma from abuse produces many of the same lesions seen in accidental injury, including retinal detachment, dislocated lens, hyphema, corneal abrasion, and periorbital ecchymosis. Glaucoma and diminished vision are among the sequelae.[75,76] The lesions can appear identical to their inadvertent counterparts. If child abuse is suspected, eye injuries should suggest potentially serious head injuries.

Retinal hemorrhages are the most frequent ocular manifestation of child abuse. They are common in newborns as a result of birth trauma, but should be resolved by several weeks of age.[75] In abuse, they are most often the result of head injury, either from blunt trauma or from the shaken-impact syndrome, and are strongly associated with subdural hematoma and cerebral edema.[77,78] The severity of hemorrhages correlates with the severity of neurologic damage.[79] Purtscher retinopathy, retinal hemorrhages resulting from a sudden increase in thoracic pressure, have resulted from intentional chest injury.[80] Several authors suggest that retinal hemorrhage outside the neonatal period is pathognomonic of child abuse, but Goetting and Sowa dispute this.[77,81,82] In this author's opinion, retinal hemorrhage should be considered a result of child abuse until that possibility is excluded.

Oral Injuries. A variety of injuries to the mouth and associated structures may be caused by abuse. Burns transpire from excessively hot food or fluids placed into the child's mouth. Lacerations of the buccal mucosa, particularly the labial frenulum can be caused by blows to the mouth or from jamming an object, such as a bottle, into the child's mouth. Injuries to the tongue, including the lingual frenulum, also occur in this way. Dental injuries result from blows to the mouth or chin.[32,83]

If a long object is jabbed into the child's mouth, severe penetrating injuries to the hypopharynx may occur.[84] Similar injuries have been attributed to sexual abuse (fellatio).[85]

Abdominal and Thoracic Visceral Injuries. Abdominal injuries in child abuse are infrequent, but when present have a high mortality.[35,86,87] The mortality appears to be related both to the severity of initial injury, and to delay in seeking treatment. The latter may result in prehospital demise.[86] Reports of nonaccidental abdominal injury have invariably found it to be the result of blunt trauma with resulting crush/compression injuries to the viscera or shearing forces disrupting vasculature. Hepatic, splenic and renal contusions, pancreatic and duodenal-jejunal hematoma, mesenteric hematoma or laceration, and duodenal-jejunal rupture have been reported most commonly, but the entire spectrum of injuries from abdominal trauma can occur.[86-90] Grosfeld reported the bizarre case of a boy with necrosis of his colon due to a lye enema.[91] Children usually present with bilious vomiting, signs of peritonitis, shock, or localized tenderness. The majority of patients with abdominal injury from abuse will have injuries to the head or skin, but Kleinman et al reported three children with abusive abdominal injury with isolated abdominal findings.[92] Abuse should be considered when a child presents with unexplained shock or peritonitis, particularly associated with anemia.[86,92]

Thoracic visceral injuries are less common than abdominal injuries, but tracheal and esophageal disruption and pulmonary contusion have been described as a result of penetrating oral and blunt chest and neck injury.[85,89,92]

Skeletal Injuries. Fractures were a part of the original description of abused children by Caffey, and skeletal injury, although occurring in no more than half of cases, can provide important evidence of abuse.[1] The physical signs of skeletal trauma (swelling, tenderness, deformity, and diminished range of motion) are not universally present in cases of inflicted fracture.[93] In many cases, healing of the fracture has already begun, and signs of acute injury have resolved. In other cases, the nature of the injuries determines the lack of physical evidence. The most important consideration is whether the injury is consistent with history. The type of fracture (e.g., spiral, transverse, comminuted), as well as its location, should be compared to the history. A four-month-old infant will not suffer a fracture from rolling onto her arm, and a three-year-old child will not have a transverse fracture of the metatarsals slipping on the hall rug.

Fractures in children younger than 1 year of age should arouse suspicion unless clearly explained, and fractures of certain bones are unusual in accidental injury.[94] These bones include the sternum, spinous processes, and scapula.[95-97] Fractures of the femur in children younger than three years of age are often a result of abuse, and spiral fractures of the humerus are worrisome.[98-100] Rib fractures, uncommon in childhood, are common in abused children.[99,101,102] Rib fractures are frequently multiple and bilateral, probably reflecting a squeezing injury to the chest.[93,102] Posterior fractures are the most common, but lateral, anterior, and costochondral injuries do occur. Costovertebral junction injuries are quite difficult to detect on plain radiographs.[102] Vigorous pulmonary resuscitation has not been found to fracture ribs in children.[103] Multiple fractures of varying ages are a clear indication of abuse in the absence of bone disease.[96,101]

Fractures of the epiphyseal-metaphyseal junction are virtually pathognomic of child abuse.[93,95,101,104] Most often seen in long bones, these have been described as "corner" fractures resulting from a planar fracture through the junction of metaphysis and epiphysis, caused by shearing forces when an extremity is violently pulled or twisted. Plain radiographs of these fractures may show only a triangular "chip" from the metaphyseal region, a loop or "bucket-handle" lesion, or metaphyseal lucency, depending on the view, age, and severity of injury. Humeral injuries may have normal radiographs in infancy due to lack of ossification of growth centers.[105] Histologic examination reveals microfractures extending through the metaphysis, a finding which may be useful in unexplained deaths.[104] Fragmentation of the distal end of the clavicle or scapula are similar injuries with identical implications.[93]

Other Manifestations. Concern about toxicologic abuse of children has increased in recent years.[106] These children can present as "accidental" ingestions or with signs/symptoms of ingestion without explanation. Münchausen syndrome by proxy must also be considered (see following section). Virtually any product may be involved, from medications to common household products such as salt.[106,107] The potential presentations are as varied as the chemicals that cause them, but the clinician should consider the possibility of intentional injury in any ingestion.

Abuse may be involved in a significant number of bathtub submersion injuries.[108] The history should be carefully reviewed and a diligent search for injuries conducted. Home investigation may also be warranted, particularly in cases not involving seizures or developmental delay.[109]

Death. The number of unexpected childhood deaths resulting from abuse and neglect is unknown, but almost certainly vastly underreported.[110] Whereas some jurisdictions have established child death evaluation panels, they

TABLE 45-2. Child Abuse Skeletal Survey

Potential skeletal injury	Suggested view(s)
Skull	AP + lateral (include cervical spine)
Chest	Supine AP + lateral (bone technique)
Pelvis	AP
Humeri and forearms	AP
Hands	PA
Femurs, tibias, and feet	AP
Lumbar spine	Lateral

AP, Anteroposterior; *PA,* posteroanterior.

are by no means universal.[111] Recognition of these cases in the acute setting can be difficult, and clinicians want to avoid unwarranted intrusion into the grief of the innocent family. Evaluation by social work service for possible abuse is warranted for unexpected death in children younger than 1 year of age and scene investigation, complete autopsy (including toxicologic studies), and postmortem skeletal survey are indicated in all unexpected childhood deaths.[112-114]

Ancillary Data

Laboratory. A bleeding screen consisting of platelet count, bleeding time, prothrombin time, and partial thromboplastin time should be obtained at the time of examination in cases in which contusions or hematomas are present. This prevents the accused or his lawyers from claiming the child has a chronic bleeding disorder or had a transient one at the time of examination.

Other laboratory tests should be ordered based on the clinical situation, history, and physical findings.

Radiographic Studies. Diagnostic radiology provides additional evidence of abuse in some cases. Radiographic screening is indicated in a child younger than 2 years of age with evidence of abuse, or younger than 1 year of age with evidence of significant neglect or deprivation. Screening should be selective in children from 2 to 5 years of age, and is unlikely to be beneficial for those over that age.[93,97,115,116] In most centers, the screening procedure of choice will be the skeletal survey. The radiographs listed in Table 45-2 should be considered the minimum necessary.[102,117] The single-view "babygram" is inadequate and unacceptable. Meticulous technique and high-detail systems are required for optimal injury detection.[117] Skeletal scintigraphy has been suggested as an alternative to the skeletal survey for routine screening of suspected abuse victims, and may be the procedure of choice in some centers.[93] Plain radiographs are readily available, less expensive, and more easily interpreted. Radionuclide imaging produces less radiation load, requires intravenous access, requires the child to be still for a significant period, and interpretation is technically demanding. The studies are complementary when evaluating lesions, as scintigraphy is more sensitive (except for metaphyseal lesions), whereas the clinical significance of a lesion is better defined by plain films. Any identified injury should have appropriate plain film studies (at least two views).[102] The choice of one over the other depends on the clinical situation, radiologist's experience, and availability of the nuclear medicine study.[97,118-122]

Suspected abuse in a child with head injuries or abnormal neurologic findings is an indication for computed tomography (CT).[123-126] The results may have both clinical and legal implications, and serial examinations have proved useful.[127] CT may be indicated in infants with injuries consistent with shaken-impact syndrome (such as rib fractures), even in the face of a normal neurologic examination. CT is capable of detecting focal lesions, cerebral edema, and evidence of hypoxic-ischemic injury.[128]

Magnetic resonance imaging (MRI) is more sensitive than CT and may better define lesions, but is more expensive and not always available on an acute basis. It is most useful as a supplement to CT or in follow-up.[129-132]

Radiologic imaging of visceral injuries, whether present or suspected, should be individualized.[117,133]

Differential Considerations

Differential diagnosis in child abuse is primarily a matter of deciding whether injuries suffered were inflicted (intentionally or not), unintentionally as a result of neglect, or unintentionally despite reasonable care. The distinction between inflicted and accidental injury is largely presented in the section on diagnostic findings; however there are several conditions which can be misinterpreted as traumatic injury, resulting in misdiagnosis. Keep in mind that the child with a medical problem that can resemble abuse may actually be abused as well.[24]

Several conditions may produce skin lesions resembling abusive injuries. Mongolian spots and other areas of altered pigmentation can be confused with contusions by the uninitiated.[134,135] Lesions of eczema, erythema multiforme, hypersensitivity vasculitis and phytophotodermatitis, and ink or paint have all been reported as resulting from abuse.[136-140] Bruising as a result of hemophilia, Ehlers-Danlos syndrome, idiopathic thrombocytopenic purpura, and other bleeding disorders may also trigger misdiagnosis of abuse.[24,140-142] Burns from a child coming in contact with a car seat which was left exposed to sunlight in a car have been described, as well as ecchymoses, abrasions, and lacerations from an improperly worn seat belt.[143,144] Impetigo may superficially resemble cigarette burns, but the variation in size of the lesions in the former should differentiate the two.[26] Diaper dermatitis has been confused with perineal burns.[140] Comprehensive listings of other conditions mistaken for abuse can be found elsewhere.[145]

Folk medicine practices can provoke confusion. Cao Gió, or coin-rubbing, is a nonabusive folk practice seen among Vietnamese immigrants. It produces linear ecchymoses, usually on the back, but potentially anywhere on the skin.[146] Cupping is similar, except that the circular lesions are produced by placing a heated hemispheric object on the skin. As it cools, the vacuum produced may lead to ecchymosis. This practice seems most common among Eastern European immigrants.[147] Folk medicine can be innocent, as with the examples above, or abusive. The latter is demonstrated in the use of shaking in some Hispanic societies to treat caida de molera ("fallen fontanelle").[70] The burning of the skin with smoldering yarn, a

TABLE 45-3. Differential Diagnosis of Radiologic Findings in Abuse

Condition	Fractures present	Confused with bone injury	Pain or swelling
Obstetric trauma	+	−	+
Metabolic defects			
Scurvy	−	+	+
Rickets	−	+	−
Secondary hyperparathyroidism	+	+	*
Menkes' (kinky-hair) syndrome	−	+	−
Mucolipidosis II	+	+	*
Neuromuscular disease			
Cerebral palsy	+	−	*
Congenital indifference to pain	+	−	−
Myelodysplasia	+	−	−
Skeletal disorders			
Osteogenesis imperfecta	+	−	+
Caffey disease	−	+	+
Drug toxicity			
Methotrexate osteopathy	+	+	*
Prostaglandin E	−	+	−
Hypervitaminosis A	−	+	+
Infection			
Congenital syphilis	+	+	*
Osteomyelitis	−	+	+
Neoplasm			
Leukemia	−	+	+
Metastatic tumors	+	+	+
Primary bone tumors	+	+	+
Poor technique	−	+	−

Adapted from Brill PW, Winchester P: Differential diagnosis of child abuse. In Kleinman PK, editor: *Diagnostic imaging of child abuse*, Baltimore, 1987, Williams & Wilkins; Radkowski MA: *Pediatr Ann* 12:894, 1983.
*Pain if fractures are present.

variant on moxabustion which can resemble cigarette burns, appears to fall somewhere in between.[148]

A number of medical conditions can produce radiological and skeletal findings capable of being misinterpreted as abuse, and some conditions predispose the child to fractures and other bony trauma.[96,145,149] Table 45-3 lists some of these disorders, whether fractures (either pathologic or traumatic) or bony changes occur, and whether pain or tenderness can be present.

MUNCHAUSEN SYNDROME BY PROXY

Munchausen syndrome by proxy is a form of child abuse in which the mother either simulates or produces illness in her child, then presents the child for medical care.[150] Recent reports suggest that fathers and other caregivers may also be the perpetrators of this abuse.[151,152]

Diagnostic Findings

The syndrome affects males and females in equal proportions. Although the mean age of onset is reported as fifteen months of age, children up to 6 years of age are commonly seen.[153,154] About 25% of cases involve simulated illness, in which the child is not directly harmed. In the remainder, the child is actually injured when an artificial illness is produced. The mortality rate in published cases is 9%.[154] The length of time between onset of symptoms and diagnosis generally exceeds 6 months of age, and may be much longer.[155] Cases that go undetected frequently result in increasingly severe symptoms, and serial Munchausen syndrome by proxy has been reported, associated with multiple deaths.[156,157]

The symptoms, signs, or findings in Munchausen syndrome by proxy are legion. The most common in published reports are bleeding, seizures, altered mental status, apnea, diarrhea, vomiting, fever, and rash.[154,158-160] Elaborate histories, including family history, are given, and there may be reports attributed to "witnesses" at school or day care facilities, or of dramatic changes in the home or lifestyles of the family.[161] The mothers frequently request tests, either specific or not, and the factitious illness often results in extensive medical evaluation, with multiple and lengthy hospital admissions, a wide variety of tests (often painful for the child), and consultation with different physicians and centers.

Illness can be produced by a wide variety of actions. Bleeding, for example, has been caused by administration of anticoagulants and exsanguination, and simulated with exogenous blood, phenolphthalein, and lying.[162] Seizures are caused by intoxication, suffocation, or falsely reported. Apnea or altered mental status may result from intoxication, suffocation, or shaking.[163] Administration of ipecac leads to vomiting (and cardiomyopathy in some cases).[164,165] Fever has been triggered by injection of contaminants into intravenous lines.[166-168] The production of illness can continue even though the child is hospitalized unless stringent precautions are taken. Older children may eventually aid in the simulation or production of illness in a "folie a deux." Ultimately, entire families can be involved.[169]

The mothers appear to thrive in the hospital setting, and are often described as very knowledgeable and helpful by the medical staff. Some are nurses or have other medical backgrounds. They will usually insist on staying with their child at all times and may become involved in nursing care. Up to 25% of these perpetrators will themselves have features suggestive of Munchausen syndrome, whereas others may manifest depression, hysteria, or other personality disorders.[154]

In addition to death, long-term physical morbidity may occur, and severe psychologic trauma to the child is likely in this syndrome.[170,171]

NEGLECT AND EMOTIONAL ABUSE

Neglect comprises failure to meet a child's needs in at least one of the areas of medical care, nutrition, supervision, cognitive stimulation, emotional nurture, and physical caregiving.[172] It is usually inadvert and unintentional.[173] Neglect and abuse are thought of as a unit, but neglect encompasses a wide range of problems that parents and other caregivers have little or no control over.[174] The problems of hunger, homelessness, poverty, lack of access to medical care and education are all societal forms of child neglect. These latter may certainly be seen in the emergency department, and may also interact synergistically with intrafamilial problems.

Neglect results from a number of factors, and its etiology is similar to physical abuse in some ways.[175] As discussed in the earlier section on child abuse, the child may be devalued. More important are parental factors. The emotionally ill or socially isolated parent may simply have no emotional energy to spare for the child. The parent may lack the basic knowledge or skills of child care. The parent with unrealistic expectations of the child may not see the necessity of providing care. Support for the family, which could overcome these problems, may be deficient or nonexistent. The final result is child neglect.[8,176-179]

"Emotional abuse refers to the habitual verbal harassment of a child by disparagement, criticism, threat and ridicule, and the inversion of love; by verbal and nonverbal means rejection and withdrawal are substituted."[172] Emotional abuse also occurs with failure to provide a nurturing environment, one aspect of neglect. All other forms of child abuse also cause emotional abuse.

The result of emotional abuse is loss of self-esteem and feelings of worthlessness. As the child grows older, the result may be school failure, depression, crime, and a disregard for others.[180]

Diagnostic Findings

Neglectful caregivers often fail to realize they are causing damage, and may readily provide history if questioned. Some will be unable to provide information because of their lack of involvement with the child, and this negative information is in itself helpful in establishing neglect. Others will unknowingly provide false information. Although this is frequently obvious to the clinician (Physician: "Does your baby roll over?" Parent: "No," after the child was left unattended and fell off a bed), other cases, such as inappropriate feeding, are more obscure. The latter may require detailed questioning to determine, for example, how much formula was consumed, how it was prepared, and whether it was retained in the stomach. A few caregivers will provide elaborately false information to deceive the physician, particularly in cases of medical neglect or lack of safety supervision.

Observation of the caregiver's reactions and emotions during the history can provide clues about attachment to the child, knowledge of child care and development, and understanding of the child's needs. If uncertainty exists, additional information should be elicited.

Common physical findings in neglected infants are developmental delay, grossly poor hygiene, severe diaper dermatitis, alopecia or friction burns from prolonged contact with crib sheets, and failure to thrive (FTT).[181] The latter, in which the child does not grow at an appropriate rate for age, most commonly results from neglect (and is often euphemistically referred to as environmental FTT). Other medical conditions cause FTT, and a complete discussion of the subject may be found in Chapter 50. Lack of attachment is common in these infants, and affection-seeking behavior may occur in preschoolers.[182]

Neglect of safety supervision leads not only to serious injuries, but also to an increased number of minor ones.

Poisonings, falls, burns, and firearms injuries are examples. Any injury should prompt the question "Could this have been prevented by a reasonable caregiver?" Unfortunately in neglect, the answer is yes.

Medical neglect causes or leads to a worsening of a medical or surgical condition. The findings will be those of the condition or its complications, and the only specificity for neglect is whether any reasonable person would fail to seek care before the present time. Burns, asthma, ulcerative colitis (leading to death), and dental caries are only a few among a host of conditions reported as worsening secondary to neglect.[49,177,183-186] Failure to obtain appropriate immunizations is perhaps the most common form of medical neglect. A very difficult situation arises when a parent refuses an indicated medical procedure or treatment on religious grounds. If the indication is clear, and no agreement can be reached, a court order may be required.[173]

Truancy and running away may not be caused directly by neglect, but are a result of it. In the case of neglected runaways, the child is not so much running away from neglect, as running to a perceived or hoped-for caring environment.[187]

Laboratory and radiographic procedures should be ordered as indicated. Virtually any condition or physical or psychological finding may occur as the result of neglect.

SEXUAL ABUSE

Sexual abuse of children (also termed *sexual exploitation*) includes a wide range of activities, and no one definition is universally accepted. A clinically useful definition of child sexual abuse is "the involvement of dependent, developmentally immature children in sexual activities that they do not fully comprehend and therefore to which they are unable to give informed consent and/or which violate the taboos of society."[188] This definition includes but is not restricted to incest, rape, fondling, voyeurism, and the use of a child in pornography. It is apparent that what is abuse in one society or family may not constitute abuse in another.[189-192] Definitions using specific age criteria or specific acts are less useful, as they do not address developmental status or ability to consent.[193] Definitions dependent on physical findings are of virtually no value, as findings are frequently absent.

Incest is sexual activity between relatives, and is a subcategory of sexual abuse. The definition varies from one locale to another, and may be restricted to those closely related by blood or interpreted as including relation by marriage (as in stepchildren).

Sexual abuse of children is now accepted as a widespread problem, but the actual incidence is unknown. In published studies, a history of abuse was reported by 7% to 62% of adult women respondents. For men, the numbers are 6% to 15%.[193] The disparity of incidence may represent differences in sampling or in definition. Undoubtedly, many cases go unreported in childhood because of fear of retribution, ridicule, or separation.

Predisposing Factors

Four preconditions must be met for sexual abuse to occur.[194] The perpetrator must have a motivation to abuse,

his own internal inhibitions must be removed, external inhibitions must be defeated, and the child victim's resistance must be overcome. These preconditions must still be satisfied whether the perpetrator is inside or outside the home; however, they may be more easily met within a family (incest).

The "motivation to abuse" includes any or all of the following: emotional congruence (interest in interacting with children in a sexual fashion); arousal; and blockage (lack of a suitable sexual outlet). Internal inhibitions are sufficient in most adults to prevent acting upon any desires to become sexually involved with children, but these inhibitions may be absent or diminished for several reasons, including drugs and alcohol. External inhibitions include parents primarily, but also teachers, police, and possibly peers. A child who is isolated from others is thus at greater risk. Finally, the child's own resistance must be defeated. This may occur through a lack of understanding on the part of the child, bribery, threats, or lies. Sexual abuse education programs act on this fourth factor, by increasing the child's resistance.[188]

Prior sexual abuse increases the risk for further abuse in both the abuser and the victim. The abused victim may later have an increased interest in sexual relations with children, a poor self-image leading to blockage, and diminished internal inhibitions. A child victim, for similar reasons, may have little or no resistance to future advances, and some sexually abused children may act out sexually by themselves abusing other children. Sexual abuse then becomes a vicious cycle, passed down from generation to generation. Recognition and treatment can be looked upon as helping not only the patient, but potential future victims.

Diagnostic Findings

The emergency physician may encounter victims of sexual abuse under several circumstances. A child may be brought to the emergency department for care of a condition or symptom which includes sexual abuse in its differential diagnosis, for evaluation because the parent is concerned about the possibility of sexual abuse, or by social or law enforcement officials as part of their evaluation.[195] The first of these requires the physician to suspect sexual abuse, for these cases will otherwise be missed. All of these presentations require a physician knowledgeable in the signs and symptoms of child sexual abuse.

Disclosure (revelation of the abusive episode) may occur long after the event itself. The child may feel frightened of the perpetrator, embarrassed, afraid of parental response, or simply uncertain.[196] Younger children may not perceive the experience as unpleasant or wrong until they are older. Many children will "test the waters" by making nonspecific comments to those around them, seeking a response to encourage them to disclose.[188] Parents may also "test the waters," particularly when they feel uncertain about what is best for the child. The alert physician should encourage disclosure in either instance, and arrange for appropriate evaluation.

Sexual abuse occurring within 72 hours of presentation deserves immediate evaluation and should be treated as a medical emergency. Similarly, if recent disclosure has created significant anxiety for parent or child, immediate evaluation should occur. Those cases presenting longer than 72 hours out, without severe anxiety, may be evaluated at a time and place convenient for the family and investigative team.[195] The evaluation is preferably performed by a multidisciplinary team with experience in child sexual abuse, but this may not be practical in many cases because of time constraints or distance from a center. All physicians working in emergency departments should familiarize themselves with the evaluation of these patients.

Clinical Findings. Confirmation of suspicions or allegations of sexual abuse may be made by obtaining a confirming history, specific findings on physical examination, or by specific laboratory findings. These may occur singly or all together. A diagnosis of sexual abuse is usually made on the basis of history, possibly with supportive physical findings. Laboratory results can produce supportive information as well, and certain results may be considered diagnostic.

History. Specific information regarding the alleged sexual abuse should be obtained, from the child if possible. If the child is verbal and comfortable discussing the events with the examiner, the task is easy. In many cases, the child is either too young to provide a meaningful history, or uncomfortable talking about the abuse. However, if the physician is willing to take the time and effort, even very young or distressed children may provide adequate or useful history.[188,193,195,197-199]

The interview is ideally conducted in a quiet area, free from interruptions, and away from the usual bustle in the emergency department. A conference or play room is preferable to an examining room for this purpose. The examiner should be experienced and comfortable dealing with children, and free from other clinical responsibility during this period.[200] Younger children may prefer to have the parents present during the questioning, and they should stay unless they are the alleged abusers. Older children may be quite uncomfortable discussing sexual matters in front of their parents. Other health, legal, and social workers may wish to be present during the history. Their presence may reduce the need for further and repetitive interviews, but may cause embarrassment and anxiety for the patient. The establishment of an interdisciplinary team and plan for obtaining history often provides the best solution.[201] Clinical judgment and the child's wishes are the best guides as to whom should be present. If the child and family provide consent, video and audio recording may prove valuable in reviewing and preparing the medical record of the visit, as well as in future legal proceedings.[197]

A general discussion of the child's life usually provides the best opening for establishing rapport with younger, more anxious, patients. Older children, particularly those who have been interviewed by social or law enforcement services, are invariably aware of the reason for the interview. Depending on the degree of anxiety, a more direct approach may be used. Once rapport is established, a gentle and supportive questioning should ensue in all cases. Tell patients that you have seen children who had bad things happen to them, even by having someone they trusted treat them in a wrong way. Stress that this is never the child's fault and that you want to help. If disclosure was made, tell the child this was a courageous and good act.

Most children will know what you are talking about, and will at this point provide some information to you if they are ever going to do so. Refrain from making promises that cannot be kept (e.g., "this won't happen again"); do not lie; do not threaten; and do not attempt to bribe the child into giving information. If the child is unwilling to provide a history, express that you understand how difficult this is, and that you will still try to help. Avoid showing frustration or anger with the victim. This will add to the trauma already suffered, and will increase the difficulty during physical examination.

Specific information to be obtained includes, but is not restricted to the alleged perpetrator(s), the time(s) of occurrence, the specific acts, whether physical or psychological force was used, any threats if disclosure was made, and witnesses to the event. The child's reactions at the time of the event and presently should also be sought. The child's affect, behavior, and apparent emotional response during the history, as well as the choice of words and descriptions, should be noted. This last aspect is important in deciding on the veracity of the history.[199,202-205]

If necessary, play may be used to help the child relax. Some children will use play as a means of expressing themselves in areas they are unwilling or unable to speak about, so careful observation during play may be illuminating. Children (or the examiner) may also use play activities as an opening for discussion. The use of anatomically correct dolls remains controversial, as no standards have been established for their use. They are particularly useful for identifying the words a child uses for genitalia and as a means for the child to demonstrate actions they cannot or will not verbalize.[206-209] Evidence gained through anatomical doll play is sometimes not admissible in court.[197]

Detailed allegations of sexual abuse are usually true.[210] If the child uses adult terminology or phrasing, "checks" with an accompanying adult before answering questions, or seems emotionally undisturbed by the account, the likelihood of a "coached" history increases, particularly in cases where child custody is disputed. Even with a coached history, there may be some underlying truth.[199,202-204]

Parents and other caregivers should be interviewed individually as well.[197,199,211] This may be done before interviewing the child, allowing a groundwork of vocabulary and environment to be established; or afterwards, to avoid preconceptions during the child's interview. In cases involving very young or nonverbal children, this may be the only history available. In addition to obtaining the specific information noted above, obtain a past medical history and family history (particularly of abuse), changes in the child's behavior and a review of systems.[198,205,212-216] The box on p. 611 lists some behaviors that have been associated with sexual abuse. Observation and inquiry regarding the parent's attitudes and reactions to the alleged events are important in formulating a treatment plan and deciding on the veracity of their history. Depending on the situation, history from siblings may be warranted.

Social and law enforcement workers can also be interviewed. They may provide the only history in some cases, and may augment it in others. As with parents, these workers may have already formed opinions as to what occurred, but the clinician should maintain an open mind.

Behaviors Associated with Prior Sexual Abuse

Refusal to go to place where abuse occurred (e.g., school phobia)
Diminished school performance
Encopresis (especially with anal sodomy)
Enuresis
Abdominal pain
Sleep disturbances
Sexually provocative behavior and promiscuity
Substance abuse
Anxiety
Depression and suicide attempts
Aggression

Physical Examination. A general physical examination serves to identify physical injury and illness. As the examination proceeds, the physician should comment on normal findings. This reassures the child as to his or her normalcy, and helps avoid a narrow focus on the genitalia. The genital examination should follow as a natural part of the overall physical. Techniques for gynecologic examination of children and adolescents may be found in Chapter 53 and in review articles.[217-220] Strictly avoid further trauma (either physical or psychologic) during the examination.[221] Patient and careful explanations, and an unhurried manner, are helpful. Younger patients may wish to participate in the process by holding instruments, retracting their own labia, and positioning themselves. Preschool and toddler age patients are often more comfortable being examined in their parent's lap. Older children may prefer a physician and chaperone to having a parent present. Very agitated patients requiring examination (e.g., vaginal bleeding or forensic evidence collection) may need sedation or evaluation under general anesthesia. There is often a correspondence between history and physical findings, but absence of physical findings rarely confirms the absence of sexual abuse.[222,223]

Magnifying instruments, including the colposcope, can be beneficial during examination, but are not essential.[224] Colposcopy may be helpful in detecting small genital lesions and distinguishing abusive from nonabusive injuries.[225-228] Some experience with the device is needed to obtain these benefits. Documentary photographs are also easy with this device.[229]

Examination should include assessment of growth, development, behavior, and affect. The degree of sexual maturity (Tanner staging) should also be noted. Particular attention should be paid to the mouth, breasts, perineum, buttocks, and anus, as well as the genitals.

Knowledge of normal female genitalia along with normal variants and common abnormalities is essential before examination. Previous examination experience (especially with a seasoned instructor) is most helpful, but atlases of genital anatomy are also useful, particularly for uncommon findings.[230-232]

Examination of the female genitalia begins with inspection of the thighs and labia majora. The labia minora, clitoris and prepuce, urethra and periurethral tissue, fossa navicularis, and posterior fourchette should then be similarly inspected. Bruising, abrasions, erythema, lacerations, foreign material (including hairs and semen), and scarring in any of these areas should be noted. The presence of vaginal discharge should be documented, and appropriate laboratory studies performed.[193,198,219,220,233] Many conditions may produce findings confusing to the examiner including congenital anomalies, hemangiomas, lichen sclerosus, Crohn disease, and accidental trauma.[144,234-240] Vulvovaginitis may have a benign etiology or result from abuse.[241] Comparing the history to the findings can prove critical in distinguishing these cases.

Much attention has been focused on hymenal findings as proof of sexual abuse.[242] The hymen should be examined with particular attention to the morphology and dimensions of the vaginal opening. Various techniques have been described, including supine with labial traction, supine with labial separation, and knee-chest. The length of time allowed for patient relaxation is also variable. The examiner should use whichever technique provides the best patient cooperation and visualization, and note the one(s) used on the chart. Hymenal findings should be interpreted with caution and compared to the history given. Hymenal scarring, tearing, and loss or absence of tissue are "consistent with, but not diagnostic of, sexual abuse."[195] A vaginal opening of greater than 4 to 5 mm has been claimed to suggest abuse; however, the size appears to be related to the technique used for examination, and there is inadequate information on normal sizes.[243-249] Hymenal morphology is quite variable, with mounds, tags, projections, irregular vascularity, notches, and clefts being described in nonabused subjects.[247,250,251] Accurate descriptions (and ideally documentary photographs) of findings allow later review and assessment.

Examination of the male genitalia should include the thighs, penis, and scrotum. Bruising, abrasions, erythema, lacerations, foreign material (including hairs and semen), and scarring in any of these areas should be noted.[33,252] Penile discharge should be noted and cultured.

The anus and perianal structures should be examined in both sexes.[253-257] The majority of sexual abuse directed at males is toward this region.[252] Bruises, scars, and tears should be noted, and anal dilatation (anal "wink") should be assessed.[258,259] Anal sphincter tone should be noted if laxity is present, but digital rectal examination is performed selectively.[195]

Ancillary Data

Laboratory testing is guided by history and physical findings. Nonperinatally acquired gonorrhea is diagnostic of sexual abuse and *Chlamydia, Trichomonas vaginalis,* herpes simplex type 2, and condyloma acuminatum make the diagnosis probable.[195,198] Syphilis is quite suggestive of abuse but is a rare finding.[231,260] It is best to culture children (for gonorrhea and chlamydia) who are unwilling or unable to provide a history, even if no physical findings are present.[200,261-268] Tests other than those noted below can be individualized based on medical and surgical needs.

Obtain cultures for *Neisseria gonorrhoeae* from the oropharynx, rectum, and vagina/cervix in girls, and from the first two plus urethra in boys.* Gram staining may be done, but *must* be confirmed by culture.[273] *Chlamydia* cultures are obtained from the vagina/cervix or urethra. Antigen testing is unreliable and should not be substituted.[274,275]

With the rising incidence of syphilis and its diagnostic value, a Venereal Disease Research Laboratory (VDRL) test or rapid plasmin reagin (RPR) test should be obtained on most victims.[260,272,276,277] Follow-up testing may be necessary. Human immunodeficiency virus (HIV) testing should be done if the assailant is known to be in a high-risk population, claims to have HIV infection, or if the parent or patient requests testing. In most cases, follow-up HIV testing will be necessary.[278]

A vaginal wet mount for sperm and *Trichomonas* is indicated in cases of vaginal discharge, if history is unavailable, or if suggested by history or physical findings. Vaginal secretions may also be tested for acid phosphatase to confirm the presence of spermatozoa. Sperm may also be noted on urinalysis, but should be confirmed by one of the methods above if possible.

Wood Lamp (ultraviolet light) examination of the skin may cause a dark green fluorescence of sperm in dried or moist semen.[279,280] Although not diagnostic, it is a useful screening tool. Semen on the skin, even if dried, may be removed using a saline-moistened swab and tested for acid phosphatase. Moist semen may also be examined for motile sperm.

Condyloma acuminata (venereal warts) may require biopsy for diagnosis, but are recognizable in most cases. Determination of their etiology (whether perinatally acquired or not) is made difficult by the long incubation period of up to 20 months. However their presence should at least raise concern about the possibility of sexual abuse, even in infants.[281-287]

If a forensic evidence collection is being performed, hair combings, clippings, and cuttings of the patient's pubic hair may be requested. In addition, any foreign material should be preserved with a notation of the location from which it was taken. The patient should disrobe over a clean sheet, and the clothing should be saved. Document the patient's activities, including bathing, urinating, defecating, douching, and sexual activity since the time of the assault. Also note menarchal status and previous sexual experience. All materials collected from the patient should be placed in a sealed container and chain of custody scrupulously maintained.

MANAGEMENT

Emergency physicians should be aware of the state and local laws governing child abuse and reporting; support services available within the hospital and local, county, and state governments; medical, social, and surgical consultants available, particularly those with pediatric expertise; and methods for contacting each of these groups. Knowledge of these services will go far toward making evaluations more rapid and effective and less stressful.

If a multidisciplinary management team is available, they should be consulted early during the emergency department stay in cases of suspected abuse. These teams can provide assistance and expertise in a variety of areas, and help reduce the anxiety emergency department personnel feel when dealing with abuse cases.

Careful and complete documentation is essential in these cases. The physician should carefully record, in specific detail, all information obtained by history, examination, laboratory, and radiologic procedures.[288] Times and measurements must be documented specifically if available. Forms with prompts for information are a valuable resource to ensure thorough and appropriate documentation. The physician's assessment should be plainly stated. If other emergency personnel are involved, their records should also be scrupulously complete. After recording, the emergency record should be carefully reviewed by all involved personnel. The physician should sign the record and print his name. Always assume that the record will be seen again in court!

If the child is transferred to another facility or physician, direct communication with the receiving physician is essential. That physician needs to be aware of concerns regarding abuse, whether suspected or confirmed. Transferring a patient does not relieve a physician of the responsibility for reporting (see following section).

Medical-Surgical Treatment

Management of abused children begins with appropriate treatment of injuries and medical problems. Consultation with specialty services is encouraged, as their expertise is helpful clinically, and their experience may prove useful from a diagnostic and legal standpoint.

Sexually transmitted diseases identified before or during evaluation should be treated according to guidelines outlined in Chapter 53. Prophylaxis is probably indicated in victims of sexual assault if an infection is present in the perpetrator or if the patient or parent requests it.[289] Patients with venereal warts should be referred for treatment and follow-up.[281,284,290-292]

If coitus has occurred during sexual abuse, postmenarchal girls with a negative pregnancy test should be offered pregnancy prophylaxis. Hormonal therapy using Ovral (0.05 mg of ethinyl estradiol and 0.5 mg of norgestrel), two tablets within 72 hours of the assault, and two more tablets 12 hours later is effective in preventing pregnancy. A repeat pregnancy test 2 weeks later is recommended.[193,198]

Protection of the Abuse Victim

The second priority in management is protection of the child from further harm, whether it be emotional or physical. Access of the child to the parents must be individualized, as the child may find even abusive parents comforting, whereas in other cases the fear or threat of further harm will only cause more damage to the child. In either case, the child should be observed by medical, law enforcement, or social service workers, particularly when with the caregivers. Reassurance is important to the abuse victim, and medical personnel should remain as calm and nonthreatening as possible. Emotional reaction to the physical findings should be kept under control, as it will agitate

---

* References 200, 231, 259, 266, 269-272.

both parent and child. Whenever possible, time should be taken to explain necessary examinations and testing to the abused child, as they can be perceived as punishment or further abuse. Strictly avoid unnecessary evaluation.

Victims of sexual assault are particularly vulnerable to emotional trauma because of the stigma society attaches to these events. Additional support and counseling may be required both immediately and over the long-term. These patients are also the most likely to perceive medical evaluation as a further assault, and benefit most from a calm, experienced medical team.[293]

Evaluation of Siblings

Siblings of any child suspected of being abused deserve the same level of protection as the proband. Arrange for social and medical evaluation of siblings as quickly as possible. Other children being cared for by the suspected abuser are also at risk, and require rapid identification. Child abusers are not infrequently spouse abusers as well. If suspected, the spouse should be encouraged to seek medical attention and provided with assistance in securing safe shelter.

Family Support and Assistance

Regardless of circumstances, the entire family becomes a victim of child abuse. Nonabusive parents react with guilt, grief, and anger; the abused child suffers emotional and physical trauma; siblings may be abused themselves, or feel "left out" by upset parents. The abuser, if a member of the family, may be mentally ill or guilt stricken because of the abuse; angry at the child for "causing" the abuse and medical personnel for identifying it; and facing censure by society and the family. Emotional support for the family should begin as soon as abuse is identified and continued from that point forward. The emergency physician should avoid being judgmental toward the family or abuser, while remaining an advocate for the victim.

Education is critical for the abusive family. Teaching should begin in the emergency department and should include appropriate child care, coping with stress and aggression and obtaining supporting services. Education is particularly important in the neglectful family. Many of these parents lack rudimentary knowledge and skills of child care, and education may be very beneficial.

Disposition

Notification of Appropriate Agencies. All 50 states now have laws that require a report be filed with the county or state child protective services agency if a health-care worker suspects child abuse or neglect. Reporting should be accomplished as soon as possible after identification of possible abuse. The report will set into motion a procedure to evaluate the child, family, and home; aid in treatment; and provide follow-up. Physicians often fail to report, despite the potential for legal action against the physician. Failure to recognize abuse and its seriousness, desire to avoid legal or bureaucratic involvement, fear of angering the parents, and similar excuses are simply not valid.[294,295] The physician must be knowledgeable and responsible regarding this problem. Good-faith reporters are not liable in cases in which the report turns out to be unproven.

The physician must tell the parents or caregiver about the report. He can explain that the report is required by law, and that the interests of the child and aiding the family are the prime concerns. A helpful, rather than vindictive approach should be taken toward these families, and other personnel should be encouraged to do the same.

Admission vs. Home vs. Protective Care. The abused child must be protected from further injury. Admission is straightforward if required by medical or surgical conditions. Children may be sent home if the abuser will not have access to the child and the parent(s) are comfortable with this decision. If there is doubt about the home situation, the threshold for admission should be low. An alternative is to arrange for a safe home placement with other relatives or through child protective services.

If Munchausen syndrome by proxy is suspected, closely monitor the child, especially when the mother is present. Because of the high mortality associated with this syndrome, the child should be admitted or placed in foster care in almost every case. Proof of the artificial nature of the illness will depend on the presenting signs and symptoms. Perform specific tests if applicable, and interview alleged witnesses and the spouse, as well as the child if verbal. Review medical records of the child and family, and document all information obtained carefully and completely.

In neglect cases, the disposition will depend on an assessment of the safety of the home environment, capacity of the parent to provide adequate care, and in the case of emotional battery, whether the abuse is likely to escalate to the physical level.

If the child is discharged, close follow-up, including social evaluation and medical care must be arranged. This is best provided by a multidisciplinary clinic. Psychiatric, psychologic, and developmental assessment will be necessary in some cases. When possible, the emergency physician should personally contact the physician or clinic seeing the child for follow-up visits.

In sexual assault cases a specific individual should be identified who will obtain culture results and arrange appropriate further evaluation and ongoing treatment if needed.

References

1. Caffey J: Multiple fractures of long bones of children suffering from subdural hematoma, Am J Roentgenol 56:163, 1946.
2. Kempe CH, Silverman FN, Steele BF et al: The battered-child syndrome, JAMA 181:pp 17-24, 1962.
3. U.S. Advisory Board on Child Abuse and Neglect: *Child abuse and neglect: critical first steps in response to a national emergency,* Washington, DC. 1990, U.S. Government Printing Office.
4. Schmitt BD and Clemmens MR: Battered child syndrome. In Touloukian RJ: editor, *Pediatric trauma,* St Louis, 1990, Mosby, pp 161-187.

Physical Abuse

5. American Medical Association: AMA diagnostic and treatment guidelines concerning child abuse and neglect, JAMA 254:796-800, 1985.
6. Steele B: Psychodynamic factors in child abuse. In Helfer RE, Kempe RS: editor, *The battered child.* Chicago, 1987, Univ of Chicago Press, pp 81-114.
7. Ammerman RT: Predisposing child factors. In Ammerman RT, Hersen M, editors: *Children at risk: an evaluation of factors contributing to child abuse and neglect,* New York, 1990, Plenum Press, pp 199-221.

8. Korbin JE: Child abuse and neglect: the cultural context. In Helfer RE, Kempe RS, editors: *The battered child*, Univ of Chicago Press, Chicago 1987, pp 23-41.

9. Boyce WT: The vulnerable child: new evidence, new approaches, *Adv Pediatr* 39:1-33, 1992.

10. Altemeier WA, O'Connor S, Vietze PM et al: Antecedents of child abuse, *J Pediatr* 100:823-829, 1982.

11. Gelles RJ: Child abuse and violence in single-parent families: parent absence and economic deprivation, *Am J Orthopsychiatry* 59:492-501, 1989.

12. Leventhal JM, Garber RB, Brady CA: Identification during the post-partum period of infants who are at high risk of child maltreatment, *J Pediatr* 114:481-7, 1989.

13. Oliver JE: Successive generations of child maltreatment. The children, *Br J Psychiatry* 153:543-53, 1988.

14. Factor DC and Wolfe DA: Parental psychopathology and high-risk children. In Ammerman RT, Hersen M, editors: *Children at risk: an evaluation of factors contributing to child abuse and neglect*, Plenum Press, 1990, New York, pp 171-198.

15. Christian CW: Etiology and prevention of abuse: family and individual factors. In Ludwig S, Kornberg AE, editors: Child abuse: a medical reference, Churchill Livingstone, 1992, New York. pp 39-47.

16. Straus MA and Kantor GK: Stress and child abuse. In Helfer RE, Kempe RS, editors: The battered child, Univ of Chicago Press, Chicago, 1987, pp 42-59.

17. Christian CW: Etiology and prevention of abuse: societal factors. In Ludwig S, Kornberg AE, editors: *Child abuse: a medical reference*, Churchill Livingstone, 1992, New York, pp 25-37.

18. Burrell B, Thompson B, Sexton D: Predicting child abuse potential across family types, *Child Abuse Negl* 18:1039-49, 1994.

19. Marshall WN, Puls T, Davidson C: New child abuse spectrum in an era of increased awareness, *Am J Dis Child* 142:664-7, 1988.

20. Bergman AB, Larsen RM, Mueller BA: Changing spectrum of serious child abuse, *Pediatrics* 77:113-116, 1986.

21. Starling SP, Holden JR, Jenny C: Abusive head trauma: the relationship of perpetrators to their victims, *Pediatrics* 95:259-62, 1995.

22. Kornberg AE: Recognizing and reporting child abuse. In Ludwig S, Kornberg AE, editors: *Child abuse: a medical reference*, Churchill Livingstone, 1992, New York, pp 13-24.

23. Schmitt BD: The child with non-accidental trauma. In Helfer RE, Kempe RS, editors: *The battered child*, Univ of Chicago Press, 1987, Chicago, pp 178-196.

24. Johnson CF and Coury DL: Bruising and hemophilia: accident or child abuse? *Child Abuse Negl* 12:409-15, 1988.

25. Kornberg AE: Skin and soft tissue injuries. In Ludwig S, Kornberg AE, editors: *Child abuse: a medical reference*, Churchill Livingstone, 1992, New York, pp 91-104.

26. Ellerstein NS: The cutaneous manifestations of child abuse and neglect, *Am J Dis Child* 133:906-909, 1979.

27. Richardson AC: Cutaneous manifestations of abuse. In Reece RM, editor: Child abuse: medical diagnosis and management, Lea & Febiger, 1994, Philadelphia, pp 167-184.

28. Wilson EF: Estimation of the age of cutaneous contusions in child abuse, *Pediatrics* 60:750-752, 1977.

29. Johnson CF: Inflicted injury versus accidental injury, *Pediatr Clin North Am* 37:791-814, 1990.

30. Speight N: ABC of child abuse, non-accidental injury, *BMJ* 298:879-81, 1989.

31. Levine LJ: The solution of a battered child homicide by dental evidence, *J Am Dent Assoc* 87:1234-1236, 1973.

32. Bernat JE: Dental trauma and bite mark evaluation. In Ludwig S, Kornberg AE, editors: Child abuse: a medical reference, Churchill Livingstone, 1992, New York, pp 175-190.

33. Slosberg EJ, Ludwig S, Duckett J et al: Penile trauma as a sign of child abuse, *Am J Dis Child* 132:719-721, 1978.

34. Pascoe JM, Hildebrandt HM, Tarrier A et al: Patterns of skin injury in nonaccidental and accidental injury, *Pediatrics* 64:245-247, 1979.

35. Johnson CF and Showers J: Injury variables in child abuse, *Child Abuse Negl* 9:207-215, 1985.

36. Kottmeier PK: The battered child, *Pediatr Ann* 16:343-351, 1987.

37. Laing SA and Buchan AR: Bilateral injuries in childhood: an alerting sign? *BMJ* 2:940-941, 1976.

38. Showers J and Bandman RL: Scarring for life: abuse with electric cords, *Child Abuse Negl* 10:25-31, 1986.

39. Showers J and Garrison KM: Burn abuse: a four-year study, *J Trauma* 28:1581-1583, 1988.

40. Showers J and Apolo J, Thomas J et al: Fatal child abuse: a two-decade review, *Pediatr Emerg Care* 1:66-70, 1985.

41. Rosenberg NM and Marino D: Frequency of suspected abuse/neglect in burn patients, *Pediatr Emerg Care* 5:219-21, 1989.

42. Hight DW, Bakalar HR, Lloyd JR: Inflicted burns in children, Recognition and treatment, *JAMA* 242:517-520, 1979.

43. Hobbs CJ: When are burns not accidental? *Arch Dis Chi* 61:357-361, 1986.

44. Lenoski EF and Hunter KA: Specific patterns of inflicted burn injuries, *J Trauma* 17:842-846, 1977.

45. Purdue GF, Hunt JL, Prescott PR: Child abuse by burning—an index of suspicion, *J Trauma* 28:221-4, 1988.

46. Purdue GF and Hunt JL: Burn injuries. In Ludwig S, Kornberg AE, editors: *Child abuse: a medical reference*, Churchill Livingstone, 1992, New York, pp 105-116.

47. Keen JH, Lendrum J, Wolman B: Inflicted burns and scalds in children, *BMJ* 4:268-269, 1975.

48. Feldman KW, Schaller RT, Feldman JA et al: Tap water scald burns in children, *Pediatrics* 62:1-7, 1978.

49. Ayoub C and Pfeifer D: Burns as a manifestation of child abuse and neglect, *Am J Dis Child* 133:910-914, 1979.

50. Hobbs CJ: ABC of child abuse. Burns and scalds, *BMJ* 298:1302-1305, 1989.

51. Scalzo AJ: Burns and child maltreatment. In Monteleone JA, Brodeur AE, editors: *Child maltreatment: a clinical guide and reference*, St Louis, 1994, GW Medical, pp 89-111.

52. Jewett TC and Ellerstein NS: Burns as a manifestation of child abuse. In Ellerstein NS, editors: *Child abuse and neglect. A medical reference*, New York, 1981, John Wiley & Sons, pp 185-196.

53. Alexander RC, Surrell JA, Cohle SD: Microwave oven burns to children: an unusual manifestation of child abuse, *Pediatrics* 79:255-260, 1987.

54. Billmire ME and Myers PA: Serious head injury in infants: accident or abuse? *Pediatrics* 75:340-342, 1985.

55. Rivara FP, Kamitsuka MD, Quan L: Injuries to children younger than 1 year of age, *Pediatrics* 81:93-97, 1988.

56. Duhaime AC, Alario AJ, Lewander WJ et al: Head injury in very young children: mechanisms, injury types, and ophthalmologic findings in 100 hospitalized patients younger than 2 years of age, *Pediatrics* 90:179-185, 1992.

57. Goldstein B, Kelly MM, Bruton D et al: Inflicted versus accidental head injury in critically injured children, *Crit Care Med* 21:1328-1332, 1993.

58. Helfer RE, Slovis TL, Black M: Injuries resulting when small children fall out of bed, *Pediatrics* 60:533, 1977.

59. Hobbs CJ: ABC of child abuse. Head injuries, *BMJ* 298:1169-1170, 1989.

60. Caniano DA, Beaver BL, Boles ET: Child abuse: an update on surgical management in 256 cases, *Ann Surg* 203:219-224, 1986.

61. Caffey J: On the theory and practice of shaking infants, *Am J Dis Child* 124:161-169, 1972.

62. Caffey J: The whiplash shaken infant syndrome: manual shaking by the extremities with whiplash-induced intracranial and intraocular bleedings, linked with residual permanent brain damage and mental retardation, *Pediatrics* 54:396-403, 1974.

63. Ludwig S and Warman M: Shaken baby syndrome: a review of 20 cases, *Ann Emerg Med* 13:104-107, 1984.

64. Bruce DA: Neurosurgical aspects of child abuse. In Ludwig S, Kornberg AE, editors. *Child abuse: a medical reference*, 1992, Churchill Livingstone, New York, pp 117-129.

65. Hobbs CJ: Skull fractures and the diagnosis of abuse, *Arch Dis Chi* 59:246-252, 1984.

66. Bruce DA and Zimmerman RA: Shaken impact syndrome, *Pediatr Ann* 18:482-484, 1989.

67. Duhaime A-C, Gennarelli TA, Thibault LE et al: The shaken baby syndrome, *J Neurosurg* 66:409-415, 1987.

68. Alexander R, Sato Y, Smith W et al: Incidence of impact trauma with cranial injuries ascribed to shaking, *Am J Dis Child* 144:724-726, 1990.

69. Ommaya AK, Faas F, Yarnell P: Whiplash injury and brain damage, *JAMA* 204:285-289, 1968.

70. Klein DM: Central nervous system injuries. In Ellerstein NS, editors: *Child abuse and neglect. A medical reference*, John Wiley & Sons, 1981:73-93, New York.

71. Dykes LJ: The whiplash shaken infant syndrome: what has been learned? *Child Abuse Negl* 10:211-221, 1986.

72. Hanigan WC, Peterson RA, Njus G: Tin ear syndrome: rotational acceleration in pediatric head injuries, *Pediatrics* 80:618-622, 1987.

73. Case MES: Head injury in child abuse. In Monteleone JA, Brodeur AE, editors: *Child maltreatment: a clinical guide and reference*, GW Medical, 1994, St Louis, pp 75-87.

74. Swischuk LE: Spine and spinal cord trauma in the battered child syndrome, *Radiology* 92:733-738, 1969.

75. Levin AV: Ophthalmologic manifestations. In Ludwig S, Kornberg AE, editors: *Child abuse: a medical reference*, Churchill Livingstone, 1992, New York, pp 191-212.

76. Annable WL: Ocular manifestations of child abuse. In Reece RM, editors: child abuse: medical diagnosis and management, Lea & Febiger, 1994, Philadelphia, pp 138-149.

77. Giangiacomo J and Barkett KJ: Ophthalmoscopic findings in occult child abuse, *J Pediatr Ophthalmol Strabismus* 22:234-237, 1985.

78. Harley RD: Ocular manifestations of child abuse, *J Pediatr Ophthalmol Strabismus* 17:5-13, 1980.

79. Wilkinson WS, Han DP, Rappley MD et al: Retinal hemorrhage predicts neurologic injury in the shaken baby syndrome, *Arch Ophthalmol* 107:1472-1474, 1989.

80. Tomasi LG and Rosman NP: Purtscher retinopathy in the battered child syndrome, *Am J Dis Child* 129:1335-1337, 1975.

81. Kanter RK: Retinal hemorrhage after cardiopulmonary resuscitation or child abuse, *J Pediatr* 108:430-432, 1986.

82. Goetting MG and Sowa B: Retinal hemorrhage after cardiopulmonary resuscitation in children: an etiologic reevaluation, *Pediatrics* 85:585-588, 1990.

83. Donly KJ and Nowak AJ: Maxillofacial, neck, and dental lesions of child abuse. In Reece RM, editor: Child abuse: medical diagnosis and management, Lea & Febiger, 1994, Philadelphia, pp 150-166.

84. McDowell HP and Fielding DW: Traumatic perforation of the hypopharynx—an unusual form of abuse, *Arch Dis Chi* 59:888-889, 1984.

85. Ablin DS and Reinhart MA: Esophageal perforation with mediastinal abscess in child abuse, *Pediatr Radiol* 20:524-525, 1990.

86. Cooper A, Floyd T, Barlow B et al: Major blunt abdominal trauma due to child abuse, *J Trauma* 28:1483-1487, 1988.

87. Chadwick DL, Merten DF, Reece RM: Thoracic and abdominal injuries associated with child abuse. In Reece RM: editor: *Child abuse: medical diagnosis and management*, Lea & Febiger, 1994, Philadelphia, pp 54-68.

88. Kleinman PK, Brill PW, Winchester P: Resolving duodenal-jejunal hematoma in abused children, *Radiology* 160:747-750, 1986.

89. Sivit CJ, Taylor GA, Eichelberger MR: Visceral injury in battered children: a changing perspective, *Radiology* 173:659-61, 1989.

90. Cooper A: Thoracoabdominal trauma. In Ludwig S, Kornberg AE, editor. *Child abuse: a medical reference*, Churchill Livingstone, 1992, New York, pp 131-150.

91. Grosfeld JL and Ballantine TVN: Surgical aspects of child abuse (Trauma-X), *Pediatr Ann* 5:107-120, 1976.

92. Kleinman PK, Raptopoulos VD, Brill PW: Occult nonskeletal trauma in the battered-child syndrome, *Radiology* 141:393-396, 1981.

93. Swischuk LE: Radiographic Signs of Skeletal Trauma, In Ludwig S, Kornberg AE, editors. *Child abuse: a medical reference*, Churchill Livingstone, 1992, New York, pp 151-174.

94. Kogutt MS, Swischuk LE, Fagan CJ: Patterns of injury and significance of uncommon fractures in the battered child syndrome, *Am J Roentgenol Radium Ther Nucl Med* 121:143, 1974.

95. Kleinman PK: Skeletal trauma: general considerations. In Kleinman PK, editors: Diagnostic imaging of child abuse, Williams & Wilkins, 1987, Baltimore, pp 5-28.

96. Radkowski MA: The battered child syndrome: pitfalls in radiological diagnosis, *Pediatr Ann* 12:894-903, 1983.

97. Merten DF, Cooperman DR, Thompson GH: Skeletal manifestations of child abuse. In Reece RM, editor: Child abuse: medical diagnosis and management, Lea & Febiger, 1994, Philadelphia, 23-53.

98. Dalton HJ, Slovis T, Helfer RE et al: Undiagnosed abuse in children younger than 3 years with femoral fracture, *Am J Dis Child* 144:875-878, 1990.

99. Worlock P, Stower M, Barbor P: Patterns of fractures in accidental and non-accidental injury in children: a comparative study, *BMJ* 293:100-102, 1986.

100. Leventhal JM, Thomas SA, Rosenfield NS et al: Fractures in young children, Distinguishing child abuse from unintentional injuries, *Am J Dis Child* 147:87-92, 1993.

101. Leonidas JC: Skeletal trauma in the child abuse syndrome, *Pediatr Ann* 12:875-881, 1983.

102. Merten DF and Carpenter BLM: Radiologic imaging of inflicted injury in the child abuse syndrome, *Pediatr Clin North Am* 37:815-837, 1990.

103. Feldman KW and Brewer DK: Child abuse, cardiopulmonary resuscitation, and rib fractures, *Pediatrics* 73:339-342, 1984.

104. Kleinman PK, Marks SC, Blackbourne B: The metaphyseal lesion in abused infants: a radiologic-histopathologic study, *Am J Roentgenol* 146:895-905, 1986.

105. Merten DF, Kirks DR, Ruderman RJ: Occult humeral epiphyseal fracture in battered infants, *Pediatr Radiol* 10:151-154, 1981.

106. Bays J: Child abuse by poisoning. In Reece RM: editor. *Child abuse: medical diagnosis and management*. Lea & Febiger, 1994, Philadelphia. pp 69-106.

107. Meadow R: Non-accidental salt poisoning, *Arch Dis Child* 68:448-452, 1993.

108. Lavelle JM, Shaw KN, Seidl T et al: Ten-year review of pediatric bathtub near-drownings: evaluation for child abuse and neglect, *Ann Emerg Med* 25:344-348, 1995.

109. Kemp AM, Mott AM, Sibert JR: Accidents and child abuse in bathtub submersions, *Arch Dis Child* 70:435-438, 1994.

110. McClain PW, Sacks JJ, Froehlke RG et al: Estimates of fatal child abuse and neglect, United States, 1979 through 1988, *Pediatrics* 91:338-343, 1993.

111. Ewigman B, Kivlahan C, Land G: The Missouri child fatality study: underreporting of maltreatment fatalities among children younger than five years of age, 1983 through 1986, *Pediatrics* 91:330-337, 1993.

112. Bass M, Kravath RE, Glass L: Death-scene investigation in sudden infant death, *N Engl J Med* 315:100-105, 1986.

113. Christoffel KK, Zierserl EJ, Chiaramonte J: Should child abuse and neglect be considered when a child dies unexpectedly? *Am J Dis Child* 139:876-880, 1985.

114. American Academy of Pediatrics: Committee on Child Abuse and Neglect: Distinguishing sudden infant death syndrome from child abuse fatalities, *Pediatrics* 94:124-126, 1994.

115. Ellerstein NS and Norris KJ: Value of radiologic skeletal survey in assessment of abused children, *Pediatrics* 74:1075-1078, 1984.

116. American Academy of Pediatrics: Section on Radiology: Diagnostic imaging of child abuse, *Pediatrics* 87:262-264, 1991.

117. Kleinman PK: Diagnostic imaging in infant abuse, *J Roentgenol* 155:703-712, 1990.

118. Diament MJ: Should the radionuclide skeletal survey be used as a screening procedure in suspected child abuse victims? *Radiology* 148:573-576, 1983, (letter and response).

119. Haase GM, Ortiz VN, Sfakianakis GN et al: The value of radionuclide bone scanning in the early recognition of deliberate child abuse, *J Trauma* 20:873-875, 1980.

120. Jaudes PK: Comparison of radiography and radionuclide bone scanning in the detection of child abuse, *Pediatrics* 73:166-168, 1984.

121. Merten DF, Radkowski MA, Leonidas JC: The abused child: a radiological reappraisal, *Radiology* 146:377-381, 1983.

122. Sty JR and Starshak RJ: The role of bone scintigraphy in the evaluation of the suspected abused child, *Radiology* 146:369-375, 1983.

123. Cohen RA, Kaufman RA, Myers PA et al: Cranial computed tomography in the abused child with head injury, *Am J Roentgenol* 146:97-102, 1986.

124. Merten DF and Osborne DRS: Craniocerebral trauma in the child abuse syndrome, *Pediatr Ann* 12:882-887, 1983.

125. Merten DF, Osborne DRS, Radkowski MA et al: Craniocerebral trauma in the child abuse syndrome: radiological observations, *Pediatr Radiol* 14:272-277, 1984.

126. Zimmerman RA, Bilaniuk LT, Bruce D et al: Computed tomography of craniocerebral injury in the abused child, *Radiology* 130:687-690, 1979.

127. Sinal SH and Ball MR: Head trauma due to child abuse: serial computerized tomography in diagnosis and management, *South Med J* 80:1505-1512, 1987.

128. Han BK, Towbin RB, De Courten-Myers G et al: Reversal sign on CT: anoxic/ischemic cerebral injury in children, *Am J Roentgenology* 154:361-368, 1990.

129. Alexander RC, Schor DP, Smith WL: Magnetic resonance imaging of intracranial injuries from child abuse, *J Pediatr* 109:975-979, 1986.

130. Ball WS: Nonaccidental craniocerebral trauma (child abuse): MR imaging, *Radiology* 173:609-610, 1989.

131. Levin AV, Magnusson MR, Rafto SE et al: Shaken baby syndrome diagnosed by magnetic resonance imaging, *Pediatr Emerg Care* 5:181-186, 1989.

132. Levitt CJ, Smith WL, Alexander RC: Abusive head trauma. In Reece RM, editor. *Child abuse: medical diagnosis and management.* Lea & Febiger, 1994, Philadelphia, pp 1-22.

133. Kirks DR: Radiological evaluation of visceral injuries in the battered child syndrome, *Pediatr Ann* 12:888-893, 1983.

134. Asnes RS: Buttock bruises = Mongolian spot *Pediatrics* 74:321, 1984, (letter).

135. Dungy CI: Mongolian spots, day care centers, and child abuse, *Pediatrics* 69:672, 1982.

136. Adler R and Kane-Nussen B: Erythema multiforme: confusion with child battering syndrome, *Pediatrics* 72:718-720, 1983.

137. Coffman K, Boyce WT, Hansen RC: Phytophotodermatitis simulating child abuse, *Am J Dis Child* 139:239-240, 1985.

138. Dannaker CJ, Glover RA, Goltz RW: Phytophotodermatitis. A mystery case report, *Clin Pediatr* 27:289-290, 1988.

139. Waskerwitz S, Christoffel KK, Hauger S: Hypersensitivity vasculitis presenting as suspected child abuse: case report and literature review, *Pediatrics* 67:283-284, 1981.

140. Wheeler DM and Hobbs CJ: Mistakes in diagnosing non-accidental injury: 10 years' experience, *BMJ* [Clin Res] 296:1233-1236, 1988.

141. Kirschner RH and Stein RJ: The mistaken diagnosis of child abuse. A form of medical abuse? *Am J Dis Child* 139:873-875, 1985.

142. McNamara JJ, Baler R, Lynch E: Ehlers-Danlos syndrome reported as child abuse, *Clin Pediatr* 24:317, 1985.

143. Schmitt BD, Gray JD, Britton HL: Car seat burns in infants: avoiding confusion with inflicted burns, *Pediatrics* 62:607-609, 1978.

144. Baker RB: Seat belt injury masquerading as sexual abuse *Pediatrics* 77:435, 1986, (letter).

145. Bays J: Conditions mistaken for child abuse. In Reece RM: editor: *Child abuse: medical diagnosis and management,* Lea & Febiger, 1994, Philadelphia, pp 358-385.

146. Yeatman GW, Shaw C, Barlow MJ et al: Pseudobattering in Vietnamese children, *Pediatrics* 58:616-618, 1976.

147. Asnes RS and Wisotsky DH: Cupping lesions simulating child abuse, *J Pediatr* 99:267-268, 1981.

148. Feldman KW: Pseudoabusive burns in Asian refugees, *Am J Dis Child* 138:768-769, 1984.

149. Brill PW and Winchester P: Differential diagnosis of child abuse. In Kleinman PK, editor: *Diagnostic imaging of child abuse.* 1987, Baltimore, Williams & Wilkins.

Munchausen Syndrome by Proxy

150. Meadow R: Munchausen syndrome by proxy: the hinterland of child abuse, *Lancet* 2:343-345, 1977.

151. Makar AF and Squier PJ: Munchausen syndrome by proxy: father as perpetrator, *Pediatrics* 85:370-373, 1990.

152. Jones VF, Badgett JT, Minella JL et al: The role of the male caretaker in Munchausen syndrome by proxy, *Clin Pediatr (Phila)* 32:245-247, 1993.

153. Meadow R: Munchausen syndrome by proxy, *Arch Dis Child* 57:92-98, 1982.

154. Rosenberg DA: Web of deceit: a literature review of Munchausen syndrome by proxy, *Child Abuse Negl* 11:547-563, 1987.

155. Schreier HA and Libow JA: Munchausen by proxy syndrome: a modern pediatric challenge, *J Pediatr* 125:S110-5, 1994.

156. Alexander R, Smith W, Stevenson R: Serial Munchausen syndrome by proxy, *Pediatrics* 86:581-585, 1990.

157. Bools CN, Neale BA, Meadow SR: Co-morbidity associated with fabricated illness (Munchausen syndrome by proxy), *Arch Dis Child* 67:77-79, 1992.

158. Lacey SR, Cooper C, Runyan DK et al: Munchausen syndrome by proxy: patterns of presentation to pediatric surgeons, *J Pediatr Surg* 28:827-832, 1993.

159. Mitchell I, Brummitt J, DeForest J et al: Apnea and factitious illness (Munchausen syndrome) by proxy, *Pediatrics* 92:810-814, 1993.

160. Baron HI, Beck DC, Vargas JH et al: Overinterpretation of gastroduodenal motility studies: two cases involving Munchausen syndrome by proxy, *J Pediatr* 126:397-400, 1995.

161. Warner JO and Hathaway MJ: Allergic form of Meadow's syndrome (Munchausen by proxy), *Arch Dis Child* 59:151-156, 1984.

162. Kurlandsky L, Lukoff JY, Zinkham WH et al: Munchausen syndrome by proxy: definition of factitious bleeding in an infant by ^{51}Cr labeling of erythrocytes, *Pediatrics* 63:228-231, 1979.

163. Berger D: Child abuse simulating "near-miss" sudden infant death syndrome, *J Pediatr* 95:554-556, 1979.

164. Feldman KW, Christopher DM, Opheim KB: Munchausen syndrome/bulimia by proxy: ipecac as a toxin in child abuse. *Child Abuse Negl* 13:257-261, 1989.

165. Goebel J, Gremse DA, Artman M: Cardiomyopathy from ipecac administration in Munchausen syndrome by proxy, *Pediatrics* 92:601-3, 1993.

166. Hodge D, Schwartz W, Sargent J et al: The bacteriologically battered baby: another case of Munchausen by proxy, *Ann Emerg Med* 11:205-207, 1982.

167. Liston TE, Levine PL, Anderson C: Polymicrobial bacteremia due to Polle syndrome: the child abuse variant of Munchausen syndrome by proxy, *Pediatrics* 72:211-213, 1983.

168. Malatack JJ, Wiener ES, Gartner JC et al: Munchausen syndrome by proxy: a new complication of central venous catheterization, *Pediatrics* 75:523-525, 1985;

169. Mehl AL, Coble L, Johnson S: Munchausen syndrome by proxy: a family affair, *Child Abuse Negl* 14:577-585, 1990.

170. McGuire TL and Feldman KW: Psychologic morbidity of children subjected to Munchausen syndrome by proxy, *Pediatrics* 83:289-92, 1989.

171. Eminson DM and Postlethwaite RJ: Factitious illness: recognition and management, *Arch Dis Child* 67:1510-6, 1992.

Neglect and Emotional Abuse

172. Skuse DH: ABC of child abuse. Emotional abuse and neglect, *BMJ* 298:1692-4, 1989.

173. Schmitt BD: Child neglect. In Ellerstein NS, editor: *Child abuse and neglect. A medical reference,* John Wiley & Sons, 1981, pp 297-306, New York.

174. Helfer RE: The neglect of our children, *Pediatr Clin North Am* 37:923-42, 1990.

175. Brayden RM, Altemeier WA, Tucker DD et al: Antecedents of child neglect in the first two years of life, *J Pediatr* 120:426-9, 1992.

176. Helfer RE: The developmental basis of child abuse and neglect: an epidemiological approach. In Helfer RE, Kempe RS, editors: *The battered child,* Univ of Chicago Press, 1987, Chicago, pp 60-80.

177. Jaudes PK and Diamond LJ: Neglect of chronically ill children, *Am J Dis Child* 140:655-658, 1986.

178. Lally JR: Three views of child neglect: expanding visions of preventive intervention, *Child Abuse Negl* 8:243-254, 1984.

179. Polansky NA, Gaudin JM, Ammons PW et al: The psychological ecology of the neglectful mother, *Child Abuse Negl* 9:265-275, 1985.

180. Seagull EA: Childhood depression, *Curr Probl Pediatr* 20:707-755, 1990.

181. Helfer RE: The litany of the smoldering neglect of children. In Helfer RE, Kempe RS: editors: *The battered child,* Univ of Chicago Press, 1987, Chicago, pp 301-311.

182. Ludwig S: Failure-to-thrive/starvation. In Ludwig S, Kornberg AE, editors: *Child abuse: a medical reference,* Churchill Livingstone, 1992, New York, pp 303-319.

183. Ambrose JB: Orofacial signs of child abuse and neglect: a dental perspective, *Pediatrician* 16:188-92. 1989.

184. Boxer GH, Carson J, Miller BD: Neglect contributing to tertiary hospitalization in childhood asthma, *Child Abuse Negl* 12:491-501, 1988.

185. Jackson DL, Korbin J, Youngner S et al: Fatal outcome in untreated adolescent ulcerative colitis: an unusual case of child neglect, *Crit Care Med* 11:832-833, 1983.

186. Johnson CF and Coury DL: Child neglect: general concepts and medical neglect. In Ludwig S, Kornberg AE, editors: *Child abuse: a medical reference,* Churchill Livingstone, 1992, New York, pp 321-331.

187. Kufeldt K and Nimmo M: Youth on the street: abuse and neglect in the eighties, *Child Abuse Negl* 11:531-543, 1987.

Sexual Abuse

188. Krugman R and Jones DPH: Incest and other forms of sexual abuse, In Helfer RE, Kempe RS, editors: *The battered child*, Univ of Chicago Press, 1987, Chicago, pp 286-300.

189. Canavan JW: Sexual child abuse. In Ellerstein NS, editors: *Child abuse and neglect. A medical reference.* New York, 1981, John Wiley & Sons, pp 233-251.

190. De Jong AR: Sexual interactions among siblings and cousins: experimentation or exploitation? *Child Abuse Negl* 13:271-9, 1989.

191. Rosenfeld AA, Wenegrat AOR, Haavik DK et al: Sleeping patterns in upper-middle-class families when the child awakens ill or frightened, *Arch Gen Psychiatry* 39:943-947, 1982.

192. Rosenfeld A, Bailey R, Siegel B et al: Determining incestuous contact between parent and child: frequency of children touching parent's genitals in a nonclinical population, *J Am Acad Child Psychiatry* 25:481-484, 1986.

193. De Jong AR and Finkel MA: Sexual abuse of children, *Curr Probl Pediatr* 20:491-567, 1990.

194. Finkelhor D: *Child sexual abuse. New theory and research,* The Free Press, 1984, New York,

195. American Academy of Pediatrics: Committee on Child Abuse and Neglect: Guidelines for the evaluation of sexual abuse of children, *Pediatrics* 87:254-260, 1991.

196. Sauzier M: Disclosure of child sexual abuse. For better or for worse, *Psychiatr Clin North Am* 12:455-69, 1989.

197. American Academy of Child and Adolescent Psychiatry: Guidelines for the clinical evaluation of child and adolescent sexual abuse, *J Am Acad Child Adolesc Psychiatry* 27:655-657, 1988.

198. Berkowitz CD: Sexual abuse of children and adolescents, *Adv Pediatr* 34:275-312, 1987.

199. Newberger EH: Pediatric interview assessment of child abuse, *Pediatr Clin North Am* 37:943-954, 1990.

200. Paradise JE: The medical evaluation of the sexually abused child, *Pediatr Clin North Am* 37:839-62, 1990.

201. Jaudes PK and Martone M: Interdisciplinary evaluations of alleged sexual abuse cases, *Pediatrics* 89:1164-1168, 1992.

202. Klajner-Diamond H, Wehrspann W, Steinhauer P: Assessing the credibility of young children's allegations of sexual abuse: clinical issues, *Can J Psychiatry* 32:610-614, 1987.

203. Nurcombe B: The child as witness: competency and credibility, *J Am Acad Child Psychiatry* 25:473-480, 1986.

204. Wehrspann WH, Steinhauer PD, Klajner-Diamond H: Criteria and methodology for assessing credibility of sexual abuse allegation, *Can J Psychiatry* 32:615-623, 1987.

205. Friedrich WN: Sexual victimization and sexual behavior in children: a review of recent literature, *Child Abuse Negl* 17:59-66, 1993.

206. Boat BW and Everson MD: Use of anatomical dolls among professionals in sexual abuse evaluations, *Child Abuse Negl* 12:171-179, 1988.

207. Goldberg CC and Yates A: The use of anatomically correct dolls in the evaluation of sexually abused children, *Am J Dis Child* 144:1334-1336, 1990.

208. Schor DP and Sivan AB: Interpreting children's labels for sex-related body parts of anatomically explicit dolls, *Child Abuse Negl* 13:523-31, 1989.

209. Everson MD and Boat BW: Putting the anatomical doll controversy in perspective: an examination of the major uses and criticisms of the dolls in child sexual abuse evaluations, *Child Abuse Negl* 18:113-129, 1994.

210. Keary K and Fitzpatrick C: Children's disclosure of sexual abuse during formal investigation, *Child Abuse Negl* 18:543-548, 1994.

211. Hibbard RA and Hartman GL: Components of child and parent interviews in cases of alleged sexual abuse, *Child Abuse Negl* 17:495-500, 1993.

212. Goldston DB, Turnquist DC, Knutson JF: Presenting problems of sexually abused girls receiving psychiatric services, *J Abnorm Psychol* 98:314-317, 1989.

213. Kolko DJ, Moser JT, Weldy SR: Behavioral/emotional indicators of sexual abuse in child psychiatric inpatients: a controlled comparison with physical abuse, *Child Abuse Negl* 12:529-41, 1988.

214. Mannarino AP and Cohen JA: A clinical-demographic study of sexually abused children, *Child Abuse Negl* 10:17-23, 1986.

215. Reinhart MA and Adelman R: Urinary symptoms in child sexual abuse, *Pediatr Nephrol* 3:381-385, 1989.

216. Yates A: Children eroticized by incest, *Am J Psychiatry* 139:482-485, 1982.

217. Emans SJ: Physical examination of the child and adolescent. In Heger A, Emans SJ, editors: *Evaluation of the sexually abused child: a medical textbook and photographic atlas*, Oxford Univ Press, 1992, New York, pp 39-50.

218. Enos WF, Conrath TB, Byer JC: Forensic evaluation of the sexually abused child, *Pediatrics* 78:385-398, 1986.

219. Seidel JS, Elvik SL, Berkowitz CD et al: Presentation and evaluation of sexual misuse in the emergency department, *Pediatr Emerg Care* 2:157-164, 1986.

220. Tipton AC: Child sexual abuse: physical examination techniques and interpretation of findings, *Adolesc Pediatr Gynecol* 2:10-25, 1989.

221. Lazebnik R, Zimet GD, Ebert J et al: How children perceive the medical evaluation for suspected sexual abuse, *Child Abuse Negl* 18:739-745, 1994.

222. Muram D: Child sexual abuse: relationship between sexual acts and genital findings, *Child Abuse Negl* 13:211-216, 1989.

223. Adams JA, Harper K, Knudson S et al: Examination findings in legally confirmed child sexual abuse: it's normal to be normal, *Pediatrics* 94:310-317, 1994.

224. Muram D and Elias S: Child sexual abuse—genital tract findings in prepubertal girls. II. Comparison of colposcopic and unaided examinations, *Am J Obstet Gynecol* 160:333-335, 1989.

225. Gonçalves-Teixeira WR: Hymenal colposcopic examination in sexual offenses, *Am J Forensic Med Pathol* 2:209-215, 1981.

226. McCann J: Use of the colposcope in childhood sexual abuse examinations, *Pediatr Clin North Am* 37:863-80, 1990.

227. Norvell MK, Benrubi GI, Thompson RJ: Investigation of microtrauma after sexual intercourse, *J Reprod Med* 29:269-271, 1984.

228. Woodling BA and Heger A: The use of the colposcope in the diagnosis of sexual abuse in the pediatric age group, *Child Abuse Negl* 10:111-114, 1986.

229. Ricci LR: Medical forensic photography of the sexually abused child, *Child Abuse Negl* 12:305-310, 1988.

230. Photographic Atlas. In Heger A, Emans SJ, editors: *Evaluation of the Sexually abused child: a medical textbook and photographic atlas*, Oxford Univ Press, 1992, New York.

231. Finkel MA and DeJong AR: Medical findings in child sexual abuse. In Reece RM, editor: *Child abuse: medical diagnosis and management*, Lea & Febiger, 1994, Philadelphia.

232. Berenson AB, Heger AH, Hayes JM et al: Appearance of the hymen in prepubertal girls, *Pediatrics* 89:387-394, 1992.

233. Emans SJ: Evaluation of sexually abused child and adolescent, *Adolesc Pediatr Gynecol* 1:157-163, 1988.

234. Adams JA and Horton M: Is it sexual abuse? *Clin Pediatr* 28:146-148, 1989.

235. Bays J and Jenny C: Genital and anal conditions confused with child sexual abuse trauma, *Am J Dis Child* 144:1319-1322, 1990.

236. Handfield-Jones SE, Hinde FRJ, Kennedy CTC: Lichen sclerosus et atrophicus in children misdiagnosed as sexual abuse, *BMJ* 294:1404-1405, 1987.

237. Hey F, Buchan PC, Littlewood JM, Hall RI: Differential diagnosis in child sexual abuse, *Lancet* 1:283, 1987.

238. Levin AV and Selbst SM: Vulvar hemangioma simulating child abuse, *Clin Pediatr* 27:213-215, 1988.

239. Mor N, Merlob P, Reisner SH: Tags and bands of the female external genitalia in the newborn infant, *Clin Pediatr* 22:122-124, 1983.

240. Bays J: Conditions mistaken for child sexual abuse. In Reece RM, editor: *Child abuse: medical diagnosis and management*, 1994, Philadelphia, Lea & Febiger.

241. Paradise JE, Campos JM, Friedman HM et al: Vulvovaginitis in premenarcheal girls: clinical features and diagnostic evaluation, *Pediatrics* 70:193-198, 1982.

242. Paradise JE: Predictive accuracy and the diagnosis of sexual abuse: the big issue about a little tissue, *Child Abuse Negl* 13:169-176, 1989.

243. Cantwell HB: Vaginal inspection as it relates to child sexual abuse in girls under thirteen, *Child Abuse Negl* 7:171-176, 1983.

244. Cantwell HB: Update on vaginal inspection as it relates to child sexual abuse in girls under thirteen, *Child Abuse Negl* 11:545-546, 1987.

245. Goff CW, Burke KR, Rickenback C et al: Vaginal opening measurement in prepubertal girls, *Am J Dis Child* 143:1366-1368, 1989.

246. Herman-Giddens ME and Frothingham TE: Prepubertal female genitalia: examination for evidence of sexual abuse, *Pediatrics* 80:203-208, 1987.

247. McCann J, Wells R, Simon M et al: Genital findings in prepubertal girls selected for nonabuse: a descriptive study, *Pediatrics* 86:428-39, 1990.

248. McCann J, Voris J, Simon M et al: Comparison of genital examination techniques in prepubertal girls, *Pediatrics* 85:182-187, 1990.

249. Heger A and Emans SJ: Introital diameter as the criterion for sexual abuse, *Pediatrics* 85:222-223, 1990.

250. Adams JA and Wells R: Normal versus abnormal genital findings in children: how well do examiners agree? *Child Abuse Negl* 17:663-675, 1993. (see comments)

251. Bays J and Chadwick D: Medical diagnosis of the sexually abused child, *Child Abuse Negl* 17:91-110, 1993.

252. Spencer MJ and Dunklee P: Sexual abuse of boys, *Pediatrics* 78:133-138, 1986.

253. Finkel MA: Anogenital trauma in sexually abused children, *Pediatrics* 84:317-322. 1989.

254. Hobbs CJ and Wynne JM: Buggery in childhood: a common syndrome of child abuse, *Lancet* II:792-796, 1986.

255. Hobbs CJ and Wynne JM: Sexual abuse of English boys and girls: the importance of anal examination, *Child Abuse Negl* 13:195-210, 1989.

256. McCann J, Voris J, Simon M et al: Perianal findings in prepubertal children selected for nonabuse: a descriptive study, *Child Abuse Negl* 13:179-193, 1989.

257. Muram D: Anal and perianal abnormalities in prepubertal victims of sexual abuse, *Am J Obstet Gynecol* 161:278-281, 1989.

258. McCann J and Voris J: Pereianal injuries resulting from sexual abuse: a longitudinal study, *Pediatrics* 91:390-397, 1993.

259. Berkowitz CD: Child sexual abuse, *Pediatr Rev* 13:443-452, 1992.

260. Lande MB, Richardson AC, White KC: The role of syphilis serology in the evaluation of suspected sexual abuse, *Pediatr Infect Dis J* 11:125-127, 1992.

261. Dattel BJ, Landers DV, Coulter K et al: Isolation of *Chlamydia trachomatis* and *Neisseria gonorrhoeae* from the genital tracts of sexually abused prepubertal females, *Adolesc Pediatr Gynecol* 2:217-220, 1989.

262. Fuster CD and Neinstein LS: Vaginal *Chlamydia trachomatis* prevalence in sexually abused prepubertal girls, *Pediatrics* 79:235-238, 1987.

263. Ingram DL, Runyan DK, Collins AD et al: Vaginal *Chlamydia trachomatis* infection in children with sexual contact, *Pediatr Infect Dis* 3:97-99, 1984.

264. Hammerschlag MR, Doraiswamy B, Alexander ER et al: Are rectogenital chlamydial infections a marker of sexual abuse in children? *Pediatr Infect Dis* 3:100-104, 1984.

265. Hammerschlag MR: Sexually transmitted diseases in sexually abused children, *Adv Pediatr Infect Dis* 3:1-18, 1988.

266. McClure EM, Stack MR, Tanner T et al: Pharyngeal culturing and reporting of pediatric gonorrhea in Connecticut, *Pediatrics* 78:509-510, 1986.

267. Rettig PJ: Pediatric genital infection with *Chlamydia trachomatis*: statistically nonsignificant, but clinically important, *Pediatr Infect Dis* 3:95-96, 1984.

268. Sgroi SM: Pediatric gonorrhea and child sexual abuse: the venereal disease connection, *Sex Transm Dis* 9:154-156, 1983.

269. De Jong AR: Sexually transmitted diseases in sexually abused children, *Sex Transm Dis* 13:123-126, 1986.

270. Kramer DG and Jason J: Sexually abused children and sexually transmitted diseases, *Rev Infect Dis* 4:S883-S890, 1982.

271. Walker FE, Doherty JA, Jessamine AG: STD testing of suspected sexually abused children at a pediatric hospital, *Can Dis Wkly Rep* 14:201-204, 1988.

272. White ST, Loda FA, Ingram DL et al: Sexually transmitted diseases in sexually abused children, *Pediatrics* 72:16-21. 1983.

273. Whittington WL, Rice RJ, Biddle JW et al: Incorrect identification of *Neisseria gonorrhoeae* from infants and children, *Pediatr Infect Dis J* 7:3-10, 1988.

274. Alexander ER: Misidentification of sexually transmitted organisms in children: medicolegal implications, *Pediatr Infect Dis J* 7:1-2, 1988.

275. Hammerschlag MR, Rettig PJ, Shields ME: False positive results with the use of chlamydial antigen detection tests in the evaluation of suspected sexual abuse in children, *Pediatr Infect Dis J* 7:11-14, 1988.

276. Ginsburg CM: Acquired syphilis in prepubertal children, *Pediatr Infect Dis* 2:232-234, 1983.

277. Horowitz S and Chadwick DL: Syphilis as a sole indicator of sexual abuse: two cases with no intervention, *Child Abuse Negl* 14:129-132, 1990.

278. Gellert GA, Durfee MJ, Berkowitz CD: Developing guidelines for HIV antibody testing among victims of pediatric sexual abuse, *Child Abuse Negl* 14:9-17, 1990.

279. Horowitz DA: Physical examination of sexually abused children and adolescents, *Pediatr Rev* 9:25-29, 1987.

280. Koop CE: *The surgeon general's letter on child sexual abuse,* United States Public Health Service, Washington, DC, 1989.

281. Davis AJ and Emans SJ: Human papilloma virus infection in the pediatric and adolescent population, *J Pediatr* 115:1-9, 1989.

282. De Jong AR, Weiss JC, Brent RL: Condyloma acuminata in children, *Am J Dis Child* 136:704-706, 1982.

283. Herman-Giddens ME, Gutman LT et al: Association of coexisting vaginal infections and multiple abusers in female children with genital warts, *Sex Transm Dis* 15:63-67. 1988.

284. McCoy CR, Applebaum H, Besser AS: Condyloma acuminata: an unusual presentation of child abuse, *J Pediatr Surg* 17:505-507, 1982.

285. Rock B, Naghashfar Z, Barnett N et al: Genital tract papillomavirus infection in children, *Arch Dermatol* 122:1129-1132, 1986.

286. Seidel J, Zonana J, Totten E: Condyloma acuminata as a sign of sexual abuse in children, *J Pediatr* 95:553-554, 1979.

287. Gutman LT, St. Claire K, Herman-Giddens ME et al: Evaluation of sexually abused and nonabused young girls for intravaginal human papillomavirus infection, *Am J Dis Child* 146:694-699, 1992.

Management

288. Dubowitz H and Bross DC: The pediatrician's documentation of child maltreatment, *Am J Dis Child* 146:596-599, 1992.

289. Centers for Disease Control: 1993 sexually transmitted diseases treatment guidelines, *MMWR* 42:1-102, 1993.

290. Boyd AS: Condylomata acuminata in the pediatric population, *Am J Dis Child* 144:817-824, 1990.

291. Hanson RM, Glasson M, McCrossin I et al: Anogenital warts in childhood, *Child Abuse Negl* 13:225-233. 1989.

292. Stringel G, Mercer S, Corsini L: Condyloma acuminata in children. *J Pediatr Surg* 20:499-501, 1985.

293. Berson NL, Herman-Giddens ME, Frothingham TE: Children's perceptions of genital examinations during sexual abuse evaluations, *Child Welfare* 72:41-49. 1993.

294. Chang A, Oglesby AC, Wallace HM et al: Child abuse and neglect: physician's knowledge, attitudes, and experiences, *Am J Public Health* 66:1199-1201, 1976.

295. Saulsbury FT and Campbell RE: Evaluation of child abuse reporting by physicians, *Am J Dis Child* 139:393-395, 1985.

Allergic and Immunologic Disorders

Kimberly H. Edwards • *Carden Johnston*

ANAPHYLAXIS

Anaphylaxis is a syndrome whose manifestations are elicited in a hypersensitive subject upon reexposure to a sensitizing antigen.[1] It is a multisystem syndrome involving the cutaneous, respiratory, cardiovascular, and gastrointestinal (GI) systems; two or more systems must be involved for a diagnosis of anaphylaxis.[2] The necessary components of the anaphylactic response are (1) a sensitizing antigen, usually administered parenterally; (2) an immunoglobulin E (IgE)-class antibody response resulting in systemic sensitization of mast cells and basophils; (3) reintroduction of the sensitizing antigen, usually systemically; (4) mast cell degranulation with mediator release, generation, or both; and (5) production of several pathologic responses by the mast cell-derived mediators and manifested as anaphylaxis.[3] Table 46-1 lists the major chemical mediators of anaphylaxis and their effects.[4]

Historically, this term was first used by Richet in 1902 to describe a fatal reaction in dogs upon the reintroduction of minute amounts of antigen to which they had previously been sensitized.[5] The Greek derivation of the word anaphylaxis gives its literal meaning: the opposite (ana) of protection (phylaxis). In contrast to anaphylaxis, anaphylactoid reaction usually refers to non–IgE-mediated responses. Mast cells can be stimulated to degranulate by chemical agents such as opiates, food extracts, radiographic dyes, vancomycin, tubocurarine, and other muscle relaxants.[6]

According to the oversimplified but useful classification of hypersensitivity disorders developed in 1963 by Gell and Coombs, anaphylaxis is a type I hypersensitivity reaction. Type I reactions are caused by IgE antibodies that upon activation by a specific antigen trigger release chemical mediators from the mast cells or circulating basophils to which they are bound. The chemical mediators are responsible for the clinical manifestations of anaphylaxis through their interaction with blood vessels, bronchi, or mucus glands. Type I reactions are usually rapidly manifested following exposure to the offending antigen.

Type II cytotoxic reactions involve an IgG or IgM antibody directed towards a component of a cell or an antigen fixed to a cell. Cell damage results from the complement activation focused onto the cell surface by the antibody, such as occurs with a drug-induced hemolytic anemia.

The most common clinical example of a type III hypersensitivity reaction is serum sickness, discussed later in this chapter. In this type, IgG and IgM antibodies are produced in response to the offending antigen; antigen-antibody complexes circulate in soluble form. Complexes of intermediate size may be deposited in tissues and blood vessel walls where damage to the cells is initiated by the activation of complement, granulocytes, platelets, and possibly basophils.

Type IV reactions, such as the contact dermatitis associated with exposure to poison ivy, and tuberculin skin tests, are caused by T-lymphocytes with specific receptor sites for a certain antigen. Subsequent exposure to the antigen results in proliferation of these cells or may recruit other cytolytic cells.

Pathophysiology

Anaphylaxis involves the release of chemical mediators and their effect on the tissues of the systems involved. Mast cells are central to these reactions and are found in large numbers beneath mucosal and cutaneous surfaces, in close association with blood vessels.[7] Studies have shown that histamine injected subcutaneously induces increased permeability of the postcapillary venules, causing gaps in the lining of the endothelial cell vasculature.[8] Histamine therefore is capable in itself of producing all the recognizable findings of anaphylaxis.

Pathologic findings in cases of fatal systemic anaphylaxis in humans consist of acute pulmonary hyperinflation and edema of the larynx as well as the upper respiratory tract; the edema is noninflammatory in nature. Diffuse microscopic changes in the bronchi, including increased secretions, submucosal edema, vascular congestion, the presence of an eosinophilic infiltrate, and congested viscera are found at autopsy.[7,9]

Etiology

Etiologically, there are many diverse agents and triggers involved in the induction of an anaphylactic event. Anaphylaxis is commonly an iatrogenic disorder related to drug therapy.[9] The majority of the agents involved are protein-based substances.

Since the 1950s penicillin has been the most common cause of anaphylaxis.[9] Approximately 75% of fatal anaphylactic reactions are the result of penicillin administration.[10]

TABLE 46-1. Chemical Mediators of Anaphylaxis

Mediators	Effect
Preformed	
Histamine	Vasodilation, ↑ capillary permeability, chemokinesis, bronchoconstriction
Heparin	Anticoagulation
Enzymes	
Tryptase	Proteolytic C3 convertase
β-glucosaminidase	Cleaves glucosaminidase residues
ECF-A	Chemotaxis of eosinophils
NCF	Chemotaxis of neutrophils
Newly formed	
SRS-A	Vasoactive, bronchoconstrictive,
Chemotactic leukotrienes	chemotactic, or chemokinetic
Prostaglandins	Bronchial muscle constriction
Thromboxanes	
Platelet chemotactic and activating factors	Mediator release from platelets, increased vascular permeability, smooth muscle contraction, neutrophil activation

Adapted from Roitt I, Brostoff J, Male D: *Immunology,* ed 4, London, 1995, Mosby-Wolfe Limited, London, U.K.
ECF-A, Eosinophil chemotactic factor of anaphylaxis; *NCF,* neutrophil chemotactic factor; *SRS-A,* slow-reacting substance of anaphylaxis.

Foods Causing Anaphylaxis

Most Common

Shellfish	Legumes
Crustaceans	Peanuts
Mollusks	Peas
Fish	Beans
Nuts	Milk
Brazil	Egg White
Cashew	Seeds
Walnut	Cottonseed
Pistachio	Flaxseed
Almond	Poppy
Hazelnut	Sesame
Pecan	Sunflower

Less Common

Potato	Bananas
Mango	Melons
Chamomile tea	Citrus fruits
Corn	Other
Grains	
Buckwheat	
Rice	

From Saryan J and O'Loughlin J: *Pediatr Ann* 21(9), 1992.

Serious reactions are about two times as likely after parenteral administration; however, oral penicillin administration may also cause anaphylaxis and death.[3] Other antibiotics that often induce anaphylaxis primarily include cephalosporins (3% to 7% of patients have a cross-sensitivity between penicillins and cephalosporins), sulfamethoxazole-trimethoprim combinations, and vancomycin; virtually all other antibiotics have also been documented as causes of anaphylaxis.[11] Additional medications that cause anaphylaxis include general and local anesthetics, nonsteroidal antiinflammatory drugs, steroids, narcotics and mannitol. Some colloid solutions, contrast media, vaccines, foreign serum, gamma globulin and allergen extracts for desensitization therapy are other etiologic agents of this disorder. Of these agents, general anesthetics, steroids, allergen extracts, vaccines and gamma globulin are IgE-dependent causes of anaphylaxis. In contrast, aspirin, local anesthetics and nonsteroidal antiinflammatory drugs are non-IgE mediated, therefore causing anaphylactoid reactions. Radiocontrast media, opiates, dextran and depolarizing agents cause anaphylactoid reactions via direct nonimmunologic mast cell activation.[3] Clinically, anaphylactic and anaphylactoid reactions are the same; the mechanisms by which the mast cell is activated differ.

Nonpharmacologic agents involved in producing anaphylaxis include preservatives, such as monosodium glutamate, certain dyes and foodstuffs. The most common foods causing anaphylaxis are peanuts (legumes), milk products, eggs, nuts, fish, and shellfish. The frequency of fatal and near-fatal food-induced anaphylactic reactions has risen over the past several years and is likely to continue to rise with increasing use of protein additives in commercially prepared foods.[12] The box above lists foods causing anaphylaxis.

The venom of *Hymenoptera* spp. (wasps, bees, hornets, and yellow jackets) cause allergic reactions at a frequency ranging from 0.8% in children to 3.3% in adults.[13] Solenopsis species (imported fire ants) are estimated to cause anaphylactic reactions in 1% of their victims.[14] Reptile venom has also been reported to produce anaphylaxis.[10] Hormones such as insulin and ACTH may also be responsible for anaphylaxis.[9]

Inhaled antigens may also be implicated in the etiology of anaphylaxis, although they are more often responsible for a single system allergic reaction such as allergic rhinitis or asthma. Administration of any of these agents via oral, parenteral, or inhalation routes may cause anaphylaxis.

A syndrome of exercise-induced anaphylaxis has been described that is clinically separate from exercise-induced asthma and cholinergic urticaria.[15,16] The syndrome often necessitates both exercise and ingestion of particular foods. Most individuals are not aware of concomitant food sensitivity because ingestion of the implicated food does not cause symptoms unless exercise occurs within 2 to 6 hours.[3]

Susceptible persons who develop cold urticaria can develop anaphylactic reactions in response to sudden cold exposure, such as occurs upon diving into a swimming pool.

Idiopathic anaphylaxis describes episodes that occur in the absence of any identifiable inciting antigen, exercise, or other stimulus known to cause anaphylaxis.[17] This particular entity was first reported by Bacal et al in 1978, with several cases having since been identified.[18]

TABLE 46-2. Etiologic Agents Involved in Anaphylaxis

Agent involved	Mechanism
Antigen extracts used for desensitization or skin testing	IgE mediated
Antibiotics, particularly penicillin	IgE mediated
Insect stings (*Hymenoptera*) Hornet, bee, wasp, yellow jacket, fire ants	IgE mediated
Foods Shellfish, eggs, nuts, milk, legumes	IgE mediated
Radiologic contrast media	non-IgE mediated (anaphylactoid)
Local anesthetics	non-IgE mediated (anaphylactoid)
Aspirin	non-IgE mediated (anaphylactoid)
Narcotics	non-IgE mediated (anaphylactoid)
Insulin and ACTH	IgE mediated
Biologic agents, including foreign serum, (usually horse) gamma globulin, and vaccines	IgE mediated
Inhaled allergens, such as dust, dander, and pollen	IgE mediated

Adapted from Barkin RM and Rosen P: *Emergency pediatrics*, ed 4, St Louis, 1994, Mosby.
IgE, Immunoglobulin E; *ACTH*, adrenocorticotropic hormone.

Table 46-2 lists some of the major etiologic agents for anaphylaxis.

Diagnostic Findings

The clinical manifestations of anaphylaxis tend to occur, by history, within 30 minutes of contact with the responsible agent.[7] It is this immediate onset of symptoms that helps establish the diagnosis. The most rapidly evolving reactions tend to be the most severe.

Because of its explosive onset and potentially life-threatening nature, anaphylaxis is the most urgent of all allergic/immunologic events.[19] To make the diagnosis of anaphylaxis, the involvement of two or more systems must be demonstrated.

Clinically, attacks often begin with generalized flushing, and sensations of warmth, tingling, and pruritus in the skin. Many patients will also manifest a feeling of impending doom.

Physical examination is extremely variable because of the varying severity of episodes and the systems that may be involved. Life-threatening signs of cardiovascular collapse, shock, or airway obstruction may be evident. Some patients, however, may only have mild pruritus and urticaria when initially examined; it is important to realize that these patients may progress rapidly to anaphylactic shock.

Anaphylaxis may involve both upper and lower respiratory tracts. Upper respiratory tract involvement may be evidenced by hoarseness of the voice, stridor, or a subjective sensation of throat tightness, itching, or tingling. Lower respiratory tract involvement may be manifest by chest tightness, shortness of breath, coughing, or wheezing. Bronchospasm usually occurs in patients with preexisting asthma.

Cardiovascular symptoms and signs commonly include tachycardia and hypotension, ranging from mild decreases in blood pressure to shock with syncope. Occasionally, conduction defects or dysrhythmias are seen, but these are thought more likely to be secondary to the systemic hypotension or a side effect of the pharmacologic agents used to treat the anaphylaxis, rather than being directly caused by the chemical mediators released. Patients may also complain of chest pain consistent with myocardial ischemia.

GI symptoms are particularly prominent in children. Dysphagia, nausea and vomiting, cramps, tenesmus, and diarrhea may all occur.

Integumentary manifestations, in addition to those already mentioned, include urticaria and angioedema. Table 46-3 summarizes the major signs and symptoms that are commonly noted.

Ancillary Data. There are no specific laboratory tests for anaphylaxis. Ancillary laboratory data helpful in evaluating these patients could include arterial blood gas monitoring, oximetry, and cardiac monitoring to assess for any evidence of hypoxias, dysrhythmias, conduction defects, or ischemia.

Differential Considerations

Usually the temporal relationship between exposure to the offending antigen/agent and the onset of the patient's symptoms helps to establish the diagnosis. The main differential of anaphylaxis is single-organ allergic reactions, where only one system is involved.

Vasovagal syncope is often confused with anaphylaxis. Important points of differentiation include the bradycardia and pallor usually seen with vagal reactions, which is different from the tachycardia and generalized flushing seen in many cases of anaphylaxis. Cutaneous findings and respiratory obstruction are not usually associated with vagal reactions.

Other causes of shock such as sepsis or cardiogenic shock must be differentiated from anaphylactic shock. Upper airway obstruction from croup, epiglottitis, foreign bodies, or congenital malformations is also part of the differential. Hereditary angioedema may also be confused with anaphylaxis at its presentation, but it is not associated with pruritus, flushing, asthma, or urticaria and is of slower onset than anaphylaxis.[3]

Management

As in the treatment of any emergency condition, initial focus must be on the ABCs of resuscitation, both in the prehospital setting and upon arrival in the emergency department. This includes maintaining adequate control over the airway, assisting breathing as necessary, and ensuring adequate tissue perfusion. If cardiopulmonary arrest occurs begin resuscitation (CPR) immediately and continue throughout all other treatment modalities until the patient has effective cardiac output. An organized approach that begins with the ABCs and is tailored to the specific needs and presentation of the patient is the mainstay of therapy.

In anaphylaxis, aqueous epinephrine 1:1,000 in a dose of 0.01 ml/kg SC (with a minimum dose of 0.1 ml and a

TABLE 46-3. Signs and Symptoms of Anaphylaxis

Organ system	Symptoms	Signs
Cutaneous	Pruritus Warmth/flushing	Erythema, urticaria, angioedema
Respiratory	Itching of mouth/throat, dysphagia, swelling of throat, nasal congestions, chest pain and tightness, dyspnea	Wheezing, stridor, hoarseness, cough, sneezing, rhinorrhea, swollen nasal turbinates, mucous secretion, intercostal and suprasternal retractions
Cardiovascular	Faintness, palpitations, sense of impending doom	Tachycardia, hypotension, dysrhythmia
Gastrointestinal	Nausea, cramps, diarrhea, tenesmus	Vomiting, diarrhea
Miscellaneous		
Eye	Itching, watering	Injection, chemosis, lacrimation
Uterus	Cramping	
Urinary bladder	Urgency	

From Guill MF: *Immunol Allerg Clin North Am* 7:3, 1987.

maximum dose of 0.5 to 1.0 ml) is a simultaneous adjunct to standard resuscitation measures. In all cases of anaphylaxis, epinephrine is the drug of choice for first line therapy. Epinephrine relaxes bronchial smooth muscle, supports blood pressure, and reduces subsequent release of mediators from mast cells and basophils. The signs and symptoms of anaphylaxis will generally abate within a few minutes after a single injection. A second epinephrine injection could be given into the site of an insect sting, drug injection, or allergen injection to retard systemic absorption via the vasoconstriction produced.[13] A loosely applied tourniquet may also be placed proximal to the sting or injection site, which decreases systemic absorption by occluding venous and lymphatic return.[20]

In moderate to severe cases of anaphylaxis, symptoms can persist or worsen despite epinephrine, especially if there is delay in administration of the first dose. In such cases airway patency is a major problem because laryngeal edema and laryngospasm may cause upper airway obstruction and necessitate intubation. If intubation is not readily achieved in the patient with an airway obstruction, a cricothyrotomy is indicated as a means of achieving adequate control over the airway. Oxygen (100%) should be given to all patients requiring an artificial airway. In patients whose airway is not compromised, supplemental oxygen should be administered via mask or nasal cannulae at rates of 4 to 10 L/minute. Oximetry can be useful as a guide to the concentrations of oxygen required.

Patients with severe respiratory distress may require assisted ventilation. Bronchospasm is treated aggressively (see Chapter 59).

Cardiovascular support is required in many cases of anaphylaxis. In addition to administering subcutaneous epinephrine, ensure that the patient is supine, in the Trendelenburg position, and obtain intravenous access as quickly as possible. Subcutaneous epinephrine may be repeated every 10 to 15 minutes if needed to a total of 3 doses.[13] In severe cases of hypotension additional support with volume expansion and pressors is indicated. Normal saline can be given in boluses of 20 ml/kg with repeat boluses as required if the patient's cardiovascular system remains compromised. In-travenous fluids may be run at rates of 1.5 to 2 times that of maintenance doses. Addition of vasopressors such as epinephrine, infused at 0.1 to 1.5 ug/kg/min or dopamine (200 mg in 250 ml, infused at 2 to 25 ug/kg/min), may be needed. Except in cases of complete cardiac arrest, intravenous injection of 1:10,000 epinephrine is not indicated because of the vastly increased incidence of dysrhythmia when given via this route. Ongoing monitoring of heart rate, blood pressure, and oxygenation status of patients with severe reactions is required in a pediatric intensive care unit (PICU) setting once they have been initially stabilized.

In patients with less severe disease and no evidence of cardiovascular collapse or upper airway obstruction, treatment must also be initiated and the patient observed for the progression of signs and symptoms. Vital signs must be closely monitored. Diphenhydramine 1 to 2 mg/kg may be given IV, IM, or PO, followed by q 4 to 6 hr administration to treat urticaria, itching, and angioedema. Subcutaneous epinephrine in the dose and concentration noted previously is also of benefit in patients who do not present with a full-blown picture of anaphylactic shock, but in whom two systems are involved.

Steroids may be used, even though they have a slower onset of benefit. Hydrocortisone, 4 to 8 mg/kg IV q 6hr, is useful in preventing or ameliorating late-phase responses.

Cimetidine, an H₂-blocker, has been found to be useful in cases of refractory anaphylaxis in doses of 5 to 10 mg/kg/ IV q 6 hr.

Although beta-blockers are infrequently used in children and adolescents, their presence may counteract the effectiveness of epinephrine, making an anaphylactic reaction more severe, prolonged, and refractory to treatment. Useful agents to consider in the treatment of patients on beta-blockers are nebulized atropine sulfate (0.05 to 0.075 mg/kg q 4 hr) or glucagon (1-5 mg IV) because of its positive inotropic and chronotropic effects.[3,13] The box on p. 623 summarizes the management of anaphylaxis.

Prevention

Prevention is the key in the management of anaphylaxis. The first reaction is, of course, not anticipated and thus

---

Management of Acute Anaphylaxis

1. Administer epinephrine 1:1,000, 0.01 ml/kg (minimum 0.1 ml and maximum 0.5 to 1.0 ml) SC q 10 to 15 minutes up to 3 total doses.

2. Secure and maintain adequate airway. Give 100% oxygen as needed.

3. Administer nebulized beta-agonist for patients with bronchospasm (see Chapter 59).

4. For persistent bronchospasm, consider Aminophylline 5 to 6 mg/kg IV over 20 minutes as a loading dose; then a continuous infusion at 0.7 to 0.9 mg/kg/hr (monitor theophylline levels).

5. Treat hypotension with colloids or normal saline infusion.

6. If needed, administer epinephrine infusion at 0.1 to 1.5 ug/kg/min or dopamine 200 mg in 250 ml, infused at 2 to 25 ug/kg/min.

7. Monitor vital signs frequently.

8. Treat urticaria and angioedema with diphenhydramine 1 to 2 mg/kg IV, IM, or PO q 4 to 6 hr.

9. Hydrocortisone 4 to 8 mg/kg IV q 6 hr for ameliorating late-phase response.

10. Cimetidine 5 to 10 mg/kg IV q 6 hr in refractory cases.

11. Consider nebulized atropine sulfate (0.05 to 0.075 mg/kg q 4 hr) or glucagon 1 to 5 mg IV if patient is on beta-blocking drugs.

12. Observe patient 4 to 8 hours or longer in the emergency department or pediatric intensive care unit for potential delayed reactions.

Adapted from Saryan J and O'Loughlin J: *Pediatr Ann* 21(9), 1992.

---

difficult to circumvent. Although there is generally a higher incidence of atopy, other allergies, and asthma in patients who experience an anaphylactic reaction, the incidence of anaphylaxis is so low that only a history of a previous anaphylactic episode indicates that precautions should be taken. Results of skin tests may be helpful indicators, but only if they are positive; approximately 40% of reactors will have positive results.[10]

The most effective preventive measure is the avoidance of the agent known to have caused anaphylaxis in the past. This also includes such common-sense measures as not walking barefoot in open fields, smelling like a flower, or wearing brightly colored clothing if one has had anaphylactic reactions to bee stings in the past. Patients with known allergies should wear some sort of identifying material, such as a Medic-Alert bracelet, at all times. Patients who have a history of multisystem reactions to insect stings or foods, or those who have documented idiopathic anaphylaxis should be instructed in the use of an emergency anaphylaxis kit. These kits contain epinephrine 1:1,000, and an antihistamine. Patients or their parents should be made aware of how to administer epinephrine subcutaneously if the onset of the symptoms is rapid, or to administer

H_2-blockers in the case of slower evolving reactions. Commercially available kits (Epipen, Epipen Jr, and Ana-kit) are available and these patients should be instructed to carry one at all times. Children whose reaction to insect stings is limited to the skin have less than a 10% chance of having a further reaction. In one study, no follow-up reaction was more severe than the original.[21] Based on these data, the epinephrine kits are not routinely recommended for children whose reactions are limited to the skin.

There is some evidence that metered-dose, aerosolized epinephrine, available as Primatene mist and Medihaler-epi Aerosol, may be as effective as that subcutaneously administered for the population at risk. Mucosal absorption is very rapid and the drug gets directly to one of the systems of major importance: specifically, the upper airway.[22]

Emergency supplies and persons trained and experienced in their use must be available in any setting where parenteral medications are given, including doctors' offices where vaccinations or allergy shots are administered.

Patients at risk for a subsequent reaction to a radiocontrast material, in whom other dyes have been considered and may not be used, and in whom the benefit of reexposure to the dye outweighs the risk, must be pretreated to prevent anaphylaxis. If the radiologic procedure is required on an emergent basis, appropriate measures include use of a nonionic dye or selecting another procedure that could give similar information without the use of a dye. Pretreatment with oral or parent steroids and diphenhydramine is recommended.

Disposition

Disposition of the patient after treatment of an episode of anaphylaxis depends largely on the severity of the event as well as on the caregivers' ability to monitor for resurgence of symptoms and the management of these should they occur. Patients who have experienced mild disease can be observed for 2 to 4 hours and discharged with diphenhydramine and appropriate instructions for returning immediately to the emergency department should symptoms recur. In the case of recurrent symptoms, antihistamines may be all that is indicated, but the patient should be medically evaluated; this decision should not be left up to the caregiver. Because recurrent anaphylactic reactions may occur 12 to 24 hours after the initial episode, patients with severe reactions must be admitted and closely observed for a period of 24 hours after the initial event.[9] The importance of using this time to educate the family on prevention by avoidance of the antigen responsible and on the use of early self-administered medications cannot be overstressed.

Desensitization for Hymenoptera sensitivity may be successful in preventing anaphylaxis in 98% or more of patients.[13] Whether or not to use venom immunotherapy is based on factors such as age, the interval since the sting reaction, and the nature of the anaphylactic symptoms. Patients who have had venom anaphylaxis with more severe symptoms (respiratory distress, hypotension, upper airway edema, or serum sickness-type reactions) and who have positive venom skin tests are candidates for immunotherapy.[23] Patients with penicillin or insulin allergies who need to use these agents can also be desensitized.

JRA: Diagnostic Criteria and Ancillary Manifestations

Diagnostic criteria

Onset at less than 16 years of age

Arthritis in one or more joints defined as swelling or effusion, or by the presence of two or more of the following signs: limitation of range of motion, tenderness or pain on motion, and increased heat

Duration of disease 6 weeks to 3 months

Type of onset of disease during the first 4 to 6 months classified as:

Polyarthritis—five joints or more

Oligoarthritis—four joints or less

Systemic disease

Intermittent fever

Rheumatoid rash

Arthritis

Visceral disease (hepatosplenomegaly, lymphadenopathy, etc.)

Exclusion of other rheumatic diseases

Ancillary manifestations

Morning stiffness

Rheumatoid rash

Intermittent fever

Pericarditis

Chronic uveitis

Cervical spondylitis

Rheumatoid nodules

Tenosynovitis

Antinuclear antibodies

Rheumatoid factors

Adapted from Cassidy JT: *Textbook of pediatric rheumatology,* New York, 1982, John Wiley & Sons.

JUVENILE RHEUMATOID ARTHRITIS

Juvenile rheumatoid arthritis (JRA) is the most common rheumatic disease of childhood.[24] It is one of the more frequent chronic illnesses of children, occurring in about 0.1% of children, with an annual incidence of approximately 10/10,000.[25] Girls are affected twice as often as boys, with the exception of the systemic onset subtype (Still's disease) in which the sex ratio is approximately 1:1. Although the mortality rate in the United States is only about 1%, JRA is an important cause of disability.[25] Some children have prolonged mild joint tenderness; whereas others are confined to wheelchairs or suffer significant morbidity from extraarticular manifestations such as uveitis.

Because of the many organ systems involved as well as the differing modes of presentation, JRA is difficult to define. American College of Rheumatology criteria define arthritis, set an age limit and duration of illness required for diagnosis, specify the different types of onset and indicate the need to exclude other diseases (see box above).[24] The presence of a persistent objective arthritis for at least 6 weeks may be sufficient for a diagnosis; however, duration of at least 6 months is required before the onset type can be defined, unless characteristic systemic features are present.

Pathophysiology

JRA is characterized by chronic synovial inflammation and infiltration by lymphocytes and plasma cells. On biopsy, villous hypertrophy and hyperplasia of the synovial tissues can be seen. Edema is seen in the subsynovial tissues. Fibrin deposits may be incorporated onto the superficial surface of the synovium or within it. Vascular endothelial hyperplasia is also commonly seen.[24,26] Effusions are often present within the joint space. This exuberant inflammatory process leads over a period of time to progressive erosion and destruction of the joints. End-stage disease is characterized by deformity, subluxation, and fibrous or bony ankylosis.

Etiology

The etiology of JRA is as yet unknown. Possible associations with JRA include infection, autoimmunity, trauma, stress, individual immunogenetic predisposition, and possible hereditary predisposition.

Diagnostic Findings

There are three major types of JRA: systemic, polyarticular, and pauciarticular. Systemic JRA is characterized by a high, spiking fever that occurs daily or twice daily, and a classic, although nondiagnostic, salmon-pink evanescent rash.[25] Fever can occur any time but is characteristically present in the late afternoon to evening and is almost always accompanied by the rash.[24] This type of JRA is often accompanied by adenopathy, hepatosplenomegaly, and pleuropericarditis. These systemic symptoms may precede the development of overt arthritis by weeks, months, or, rarely years. Leukocytosis, nonhemolytic anemia, elevated erythrocyte sedimentation rate (ESR), negative ANA, and negative rheumatoid factor are common.[25]

The other two types of JRA are categorized by the total number of joints affected by arthritis in the first 6 months of the patient's illness. The affected joint is warm, tender, and swollen with a diminished range of motion. *Polyarticular* JRA involves five or more joints, whereas pauciarticular JRA involves four or fewer joints.

Children with polyarticular JRA are diagnostically and prognostically divided on the basis of a positive or negative serum rheumatoid factor.[25] Polyarticular JRA is most commonly characterized by an insidious onset with progressive involvement of additional joints. The arthritis may be remittent or indolent, tends to be symmetrical and generally involves the large joints of the knees, wrists, elbows, and ankles. Early or late in the disease there may also be small joint involvement of the hands or feet, and the cervical spine and TMJs are frequently involved. Children who have a positive rheumatoid factor generally have onset of disease late in childhood or adolescence and have a disease characterized by a chronic destructive polyarthritis, sometimes with rheumatic nodules and vasculitis.[25] In contrast, polyarticular JRA with a negative rheumatoid factor, typically affects younger girls, tends to involve fewer joints, with less symmetric involvement, and is less likely to involve the

TABLE 46-4. Modes of Onset of Juvenile Rheumatoid Arthritis

	Systemic	Polyarticular		Pauciarticular	
Presentation	Extraarticular manifestations (fever, rash, organomegaly, serositis, myalgia, hematologic changes); and arthritis	Symmetric arthritis involving large and small joints Five or more joints affected		Asymmetric arthritis involving few joints, usually large Less than five joints affected, frequently only one joint	
Percentage of patients	20%	RF negative 25%-30%	RF positive 10%	Type 1 25%	Type 2 15%-20%
Age at onset (median)	5 years	3 years	> 8 years	2 years	10 years
Sex distribution	M ≃ F	F > M	F > M	F > M	M > F
Rheumatoid factor	Generally negative	Negative	Positive	Generally negative	Generally negative
Antinuclear antibodies	Generally negative	Positive in 25%	Positive in 75%	Positive in 50%	Generally negative
Course	Systemic manifestations are self-limited; arthritis may become chronic, with 25% of patients developing severe destructive arthritis	Majority do well, 10% develop severe sequelae, particularly hip and temporomandibular joint problems	Resembles adult rheumatoid disease; severe destructive arthritis in 50% of cases	Arthritis mild; morbidity associated with ocular problems (e.g., iridocyclitis)	Course variable; patients may develop ankylosing spondylitis pattern

From Jay S, Helm S, Wray BB: *Am Fam Physician* 2692:139-147, 1982.

small joints of the hands or feet. It is also less likely to be associated with rheumatic nodules, and generally tends to improve significantly with therapy. Systemic manifestations may accompany polyarticular JRA but usually are not as acute or persistent as those in systemic onset JRA.

Pauciarticular or oligoarticular JRA accounts for 50% of patients with JRA and is divided nearly evenly between type I and type II. Type I patients generally are young girls who rarely have severe joint destruction but have morbidity associated with the chronic uveitis that eventually affects up to 20% of these children. Type II patients are older, generally male patients, and typically have a lower extremity arthritis. These patients have a variable course and may develop an ankylosing spondylitis pattern. Pauciarticular JRA patients are not systemically ill, and except for chronic uveitis, extraarticular manifestations are distinctly unusual.[24] Table 46-4 summarizes the different types of JRA.

One of the most common presenting symptoms in JRA is that of prolonged fever. Intercurrent fevers in a patient with known JRA must be investigated to rule out infectious causes before the symptom is attributed to an acute flare-up of the chronic disease. One helpful differential point is the spiking nature of the fever and the fact that it is often accompanied by an evanescent macular rash. The fever spikes usually in the morning, early evening, or both rather than simply in a random pattern. When a patient presents to the emergency department with a fever of 1 or more weeks' duration without an obvious source, the diag-

---

Symptoms of JRA Likely to Result in Visits to the Emergency Department

Acute manifestations of chronic disease
  Fever
  Joint pain
  Rash

Pericarditis

C-spine pain or injury
  Neurologic complaints

Injury to an involved joint

---

nosis of JRA should be considered and appropriate follow-up assured. Having the parent record the temperature three or four times a day will be helpful to the consultant. The box above summarizes findings that are likely to present to the emergency department.

Acute Emergent Complications

When the cardiovascular system is involved in JRA, it is often in the form of pericarditis. Myocarditis and endocarditis are relatively rare. The majority of pericardial effusions are subclinical, but clinical pericarditis may

TABLE 46-5. Factors Determining the Risk of Uveitis in Children with JRA

Factor	Low risk	High risk
Sex	Male	Female
Age at onset of arthritis	>6 years	<6 years
Type of onset of arthritis	Systemic	Oligoarticular
Duration of arthritis	>4 years	<4 years
ANA	Absent	Present
RF	Present	Absent
HLA-DR4	Present	Absent
HLA-DR5	Absent	Present

From Cassidy JT and Petty R: *Textbook of pediatric rheumatology,* ed 3, Philadelphia, 1995, WB Saunders.

present as the initial symptom or occurs at any time during the course of the disease, often accompanying a systemic exacerbation. Silent pericarditis may only be evident on chest x-ray examination, electrocardiogram (ECG), or echocardiography. Symptoms of pericardial involvement include chest pain, tachycardia, and dyspnea; physical examination may reveal friction rubs and cardiomegaly.

Myocarditis may occur and progress to congestive cardiac failure. Pneumonitis and pleural effusions may develop and occur in conjunction with carditis. They may also be silent, presenting only on a routine chest x-ray examination, or symptomatic, requiring high inspired concentrations of oxygen and thoracentesis with chest tube placement. Diffuse interstitial fibrosis occurs rarely, but must be considered in a child with JRA who presents with respiratory distress.

Treatment for the cardiac and pulmonary complications is with high-dose systemic steroids, as well as management of the ABCs and supportive therapy.

Involvement of the eyes in children with JRA is usually chronic in nature rather than acute. The outcome can, however, be devastating. The inflammatory process involves the entire uveal tract, predominately affecting the anterior portion of the eye. The frequency of uveitis varies with JRA onset type, patient age at onset, ANA positivity, HLA type, and time since diagnosis. The prevalence of uveitis is lowest in children with systemic JRA and highest in children with type I pauciarticular disease with positive antinuclear antibodies.[25] Table 46-5 summarizes the risk factors for uveitis in JRA.

Occasionally, uveitis presents acutely, usually in older males with pauciarticular JRA, as a red, painful eye, with or without visual disturbances. The more usual scenario is, however, that of an insidious asymptomatic onset. Because of this, ophthalmologic consultation and regular follow-up are mandatory to assess for inflammatory cells in the anterior chamber, punctate keratitis, development of posterior synechiae, and pupillary irregularities. Band keratopathy is pathognomonic of JRA and is a late sign of ocular involvement.

Involvement of the cervical spine, such as atlantoaxial subluxation, is seen less often in children than in adults.

Special consideration should be given to the child with JRA who presents to the emergency department after a traumatic incident because such children are at risk for atlantoaxial instability. Involvement of the C-spine may present merely with pain and stiffness of the neck, torticollis, or paresthesias and other neurologic manifestations. Neurosurgical consultation is mandatory in cases with neurologic compromise.

Airway involvement with cricoarytenoid arthritis is also far less common in the pediatric population than in adults. A presentation of acute airway obstruction, stridor, hoarseness, and dysphagia in a patient with JRA should prompt one to consider involvement of the cricoarytenoids. Treatment is directed at supporting the airway, in conjunction with the parenteral administration of large doses of corticosteroids.

An acutely inflamed joint must be differentiated from bacteremia, tuberculosis, and acute rheumatic fever must be considered because prolonged fever is such a persistent finding in JRA. Evaluation for evidence of previous streptococcal infection is important. Of course, the investigations are geared towards the symptoms and signs that the patient manifests. In sexually active patients, sexually transmitted diseases, including gonococcal arthritis, Reiter syndrome, and syphilis, must be ruled out.

Examination of the joint fluid is of prime importance in these cases (see Chapter 57). As discussed, septic arthritis must be excluded. An acutely inflamed joint must be differentiated from septic arthritis. A septic joint often has no range of motion, rather than merely limited range of motion, and has accompanying erythema. Joint fluid must be examined in any acute joint; treatment for septic arthritis is mandatory if there is evidence that infection is etiologic of the joint complaints (see Chapter 57). Splinting and rest are of prime importance in the treatment of an acutely inflamed arthritic joint; systemic and intraarticular steroids are of benefit once septic arthritis has been excluded.

Ancillary Data. Laboratory investigations useful in diagnosing and following patients with JRA include complete blood count (CBC) with differential and an erythrocyte sedimentation rate, as well as other acute-phase reactants such as C-reactive protein and serum ferritin as nonspecific indicators of inflammation.[27] Other studies include rheumatoid factor (RF) and antinuclear antibodies (ANA), which may or may not be positive depending upon the subtype of the disease. Complement levels, which are frequently elevated, and HLA typing may be useful in determining the subtype of the disease and thus the prognosis. Renal function studies may assist in monitoring extraarticular manifestations of the disease. In patients with fever or acute joint involvement, cultures of blood and appropriate joint fluid must be done. The joint fluid may be examined for crystals and mucin as well as for protein, glucose, Gram's stain, and cell count.

Other ancillary data may include x-ray radiographs of affected joints to exclude evidence of malignancy or trauma in early presentations, and assess for erosions in established JRA. Radiographs of the chest (to assess heart size and pleural involvement), ECGs and echocardiography (if there are symptoms of or laboratory data on screening tests of cardiac involvement) may also be of benefit.

Systemic Onset Juvenile Rheumatoid Arthritis: Differential Diagnosis of Fever of Unknown Origin

Infection
Inflammatory bowel disease
Malignancy
Connective tissue diseases
    Systemic lupus erythematosus
    Juvenile dermatomyositis
    Vasculitis (polyarteritis nodosa)
Castleman disease
Familial Mediterranean fever

From Cassidy JT and Petty RE: *Textbook of pediatric rheumatology,* ed 3, 1995, WB Saunders.

Polyarticular Juvenile Rheumatoid Arthritis: Differential Diagnosis

Seronegative spondyloarthropathy
    Juvenile ankylosing spondylitis
    Juvenile psoriatic arthritis
    Arthritides of inflammatory bowel disease
Systemic lupus erythematosus
Polyarthritis related to infection
    Lyme disease
    Reactive arthritis
Other
    Sarcoidosis
    Familial hypertrophic synovitis syndromes
    Mucopolysaccharidoses

From Cassidy JT and Petty RE: *Textbook of pediatric rheumatology,* ed 3, 1995, WB Saunders.

Differential Considerations

As previously mentioned, JRA is a diagnosis of exclusion; other disorders must be ruled out. The mode of presentation will have some effect on the other entities under consideration.

Infectious disease is the major differential. Infectious causes of fever such as otitis, pneumonia, urinary tract infections, meningitis, bacteremia, tuberculosis, and acute rheumatic fever must be considered because prolonged fever is such a persistent finding in JRA. Evaluation for evidence of previous streptococcal infection is important. Of course, the investigations are geared towards the symptoms and signs that the patient manifests. In sexually active patients, sexually transmitted disease, including gonococcal arthritis, Reiter syndrome, and syphilis, must be ruled out.

A special consideration is the diagnosis of a ruptured popliteal cyst, which presents with pain and swelling of the affected popliteal area and the calf. An important differential in this situation is that of deep venous thrombosis. Examination in either case may reveal a swollen, tender calf, ankle edema, and possibly a positive Homan sign. Once deep venous thrombosis has been excluded, treatment consists of intraarticular steroids and excision of the cyst.

Malignancy is another important differential in any patient with fever of undetermined origin. A careful search must be made to rule out neoplastic disorders, and this may include special imaging studies, bone marrow examination, and hematologic and blood chemistry evaluations (see Chapter 54).

Other connective tissue disorders are also included in the differential diagnosis of JRA. Serum sickness may present with fever, rash, and joint pain. Ankylosing spondylitis may present in a similar fashion to one of the subtype of pauciarticular JRA. The boxes above list the differential diagnosis for each type of JRA.

Management

The treatment of JRA has many facets with both immediate and long-term goals. Acutely, JRA management is

---

Monarticular JRA: Differential Diagnosis

Acute monarthritis
Early rheumatic disease
    Oligoarticular JRA
    Seronegative spondyloarthropathy
Arthritis related to infection
    Septic arthritis
    Reactive arthritis
Malignancy
    Leukemia
    Neuroblastoma
Hemophilia

Chronic monarthritis
Oligoarticular JRA
Juvenile ankylosing spondylitis
Juvenile psoriatic arthritis
Villonodular synovitis
Sarcoidosis

From Cassidy JT and Petty RE: *Textbook of pediatric rheumatology,* ed 3, 1995, WB Saunders.

---

aimed at controlling pain, preserving function, preventing deformities, and controlling the systemic manifestations. Long-term, the treatment regimen should minimize side effects of the disease and its treatment, as well as facilitate normal nutrition, growth and overall development, and well-being.

JRA medication programs have changed significantly in the last few years. The newer nonsteroidal antiinflammatory drugs (NSAIDs) are replacing aspirin as the mainstay of initial treatment. The NSAIDs do not have superior efficacy to aspirin, but rather offer more convenient administration as well as relative freedom from side effects. Some rheumatologists, despite the association with Reye syndrome, continue to use aspirin as first-line therapy since it remains the least expensive choice and has a long history of success. See Chapter 7 for NSAID dosing.

The major change in the treatment of JRA has been the efficacy of subsequent therapy if the first line options are only partially useful. Previously considered experimental or advanced therapies, such as intraarticular glucocorticoids and methotrexate, have proved effective in treating limited joint disease and polyarticular JRA, respectively.[24] Another area of change is in the group of drugs classified as slow-acting antirheumatic drugs which consists of antimalarials, gold salts, penicillamine, and sulfasalazine. Previously considered the mainstay of second-line therapy, these drugs are now falling out of favor and being replaced by low-dose methotrexate, secondary to its efficacy, rapid onset of effect, and acceptable toxicity.

Systemic corticosteroids are seldom used, and only in patients with more severe, refractory disease. The side effects of systemically administered steroids must be weighed against the benefits of their use. They are indicated for any potential life-threatening complications, such as pericarditis, and are also frequently used topically as ophthalmologic preparations for uveitis and via the intraarticular route to treat an acutely inflamed joint.

In order to preserve function, physical and occupational therapy are of prime importance and orthopedic surgery is often undertaken, both preventatively and for reconstructive purposes.

Disposition

Referral to a rheumatologist is mandatory in the management of these patients, particularly because of the chronicity of the illness and the need for good continuity of care. Long-term follow-up is necessary to assess progression of the disease, patient compliance with treatment regimens, and the response of the disease to therapy. Only in this way can modifications be made as required in the treatment plan. The psychosocial aspects of a chronic disease as a stressor to the patient and the family also need to be addressed. A multidisciplinary approach involving physicians, nurses, therapists, social workers, and psychologists needs to be developed and adhered to for each individual patient.

SERUM SICKNESS

Serum sickness, as alluded to previously, is a systemic type III hypersensitivity reaction that usually follows the administration of foreign proteins or chemicals.[28] It is characterized by fever, skin rash, arthritis, and lymphadenopathy.

Serum sickness was first associated with necrotizing vasculitis in man by Clark and Kaplan in 1937. Animal models were developed by various investigators in the 1940s and 1950s in which horse serum or a large dose of a heterologous serum protein was injected into rabbits.[29]

In the preantibiotic era, serum sickness was usually a complication of "serum therapy." Large doses of horse serum were injected for diseases such as diphtheria, and certain individuals would develop antibodies against the foreign protein.[30] Penicillin is now thought to be the most frequent cause of a syndrome that is indistinguishable from true serum sickness.[31]

Pathophysiology

Serum sickness occurs classically with the introduction of a foreign protein into the circulation. The foreign material may be introduced by the oral or parenteral route. Serum sickness can also be seen secondary to the administration of nonprotein drugs.[32] Indeed, some authors state that nearly any foreign substance can cause this syndrome; the immunogenicity of the substance, the route of administration, and the amount of the substance given all have an effect on the development of serum sickness.[33]

Extensive animal studies have defined the pathophysiology and pathogenesis of this disorder. Initial administration of the antigen results in an antigen excess. Antibody against the antigen (IgG and IgM) develops after 4 to 10 days. Immune complexes are formed when the antibody combines with the antigen, and these soluble complexes circulate throughout the vascular tree. If the exposure to the antigen is primary, it may take 7 to 14 days for the antibodies to reach levels that are high enough to cause the formation of immune complexes. If it is a secondary exposure, the antibody-antigen complex formation may occur after 1 to 4 days. These complexes are slowly removed by the mononuclear phagocyte system. The immune complexes, possibly facilitated by IgE-mediated release of vasoactive amines, diffuse into the blood vessel walls where they fixate and activate complement. The chemotactic effect of this causes an influx of polymorphonuclear white blood cells; the release of proteolytic enzymes from the granules can cause tissue damage.

The immune complex deposition and subsequent inflammatory response are the basis for the widespread vasculitic lesions and the symptomatology of serum sickness.[30]

The resolution of the syndrome occurs when the production of antibody rises to a level exceeding the level of antigen. The immune complexes begin to be cleared and the syndrome resolves.

Etiology

As previously mentioned, penicillin is the most frequent cause of reactions similar to serum sickness at the present time.[30] Many of the agents implicated are similar to the agents that are responsible for the development of type I hypersensitivity reactions. Radiocontrast media, cephalosporins (notably cefaclor), sulfonamides, thiouracils, streptomycin, paraamino salicylic acid, hydantoins, dextrans, hydralazine, propranolol, metronidazole, and phenylbutazone have all been implicated.[30]

Equine antitoxins, (e.g., that for botulism) and antivenins are still responsible for serum sickness. Use of more than six vials of horse serum is consistently followed by serum sickness. Antilymphocyte serum is potentially a cause of serum sickness as is Hymenoptera venom; intraarterial streptokinase therapy also has been associated with the development of this disease.[34] Infectious agents such as the Epstein-Barr virus and the hepatitis B virus can also cause reactions similar to serum sickness.

Diagnostic Findings

Because one of the major symptoms of serum sickness is a pruritic rash and the illness is often associated with the use of an antibiotic, serum sickness is often misdiagnosed initially as a type I urticarial reaction. A careful history and physical examination will elicit the important differentiating points, including the length of time that the drug has been taken and other associated physical findings. A particularly important historical point is that the onset of serum sickness is often associated with pain, itching, swelling, and redness at the site of injection if the medication was given via the parenteral route.[29]

The rash is usually urticarial or maculopapular in nature; erythema multiforme and palpable purpuric lesions have also been described. Cutaneous manifestations are found in approximately 95% of cases of serum sickness.[35]

Polyarticular arthritis or arthralgia develops in at least one half of patients.[29] The involved joints are usually the large joints, with knees, elbows, ankles, and wrists being affected most often.

Abdominal pain, nausea, vomiting, and generalized malaise are frequent complaints.

Clinically detectable glomerulonephritis is common in animal models but rare in humans with serum sickness.[29] If present, it is manifested by proteinuria and microscopic hematuria. Low-grade fever is often present. Tender lymphadenopathy may occur and is initially present in nodes that are part of the drainage distribution of the site of administration, if the agent causing the serum sickness was administered intramuscularly. Lymphadenopathy may become generalized and other reticuloendothelial organs such as the spleen and the liver may be involved. Angioedema and other life-threatening allergic reactions such as laryngeal edema, severe asthma, and anaphylactic shock more commonly occur in individuals with a history of atopy.

Cardiovascular involvement is manifested by myocarditis or pericarditis; fortunately, these are not common. The neurologic system is infrequently involved, manifested by peripheral neuritis, classically of the brachial plexus. Cranial nerves are usually spared. A syndrome that is similar in nature to Guillain-Barré syndrome has been described.[29,31] Neurologic involvement is a poor prognostic sign.

Ancillary Data. Laboratory tests are believed to be of limited usefulness in serum sickness. CBC and differential may disclose leukocytosis or leukopenia, and eosinophilia may or may not be present. The erythrocyte sedimentation rate may be increased and complement levels may be decreased or normal. Circulating plasma cells may be found; this is one of the few entities in which this occurs. Electrolytes, blood urea nitrogen (BUN), and creatinine levels are usually normal. A urinalysis may reveal hyaline casts, slight proteinuria, and microscopic hematuria. Nerve conduction studies may be useful in cases with neurologic complaints; a chest radiograph and ECG may be useful in evaluating the possibility of cardiovascular involvement.

Differential Considerations

The differential diagnosis of serum sickness includes a wide variety of infectious and inflammatory disease, especially other connective tissue disorders (see box above). It

---

Differential Diagnosis of Serum Sickness

Erythema multiforme
Stevens-Johnson syndrome
Toxic shock syndrome
Anaphylaxis and anaphylactoid reactions
Urticaria
Juvenile rheumatoid arthritis
Septic arthritis
Viral illnesses
  Rubella
  Rubeola
  Enterovirus
Collagen-vascular disorders
Acute rheumatic fever

---

is important to document a history of exposure to a sensitizing substance at an appropriate preceding time. The differential varies considerably, depending on which systems are involved. Serum sickness usually lasts for only a short period of time; if symptoms persist for more than 1 month, one must either suspect repeated exposure to the responsible antigen or reconsider the diagnosis.

Management

As in any hypersensitivity disorder, the inciting agent must be identified and removed as quickly as possible. Prophylactic treatment with antihistamines has been shown to be of benefit in decreasing the incidence of serum sickness-like reactions. It is believed that negating the action of vasoactive amines and consequently preventing the increased vascular permeability that they induce minimizes or prevents the deposition of circulating immune complexes.[30]

Definitive treatment depends on the nature and severity of the illness. In cases with cardiorespiratory compromise, the basics are first attended to and the disorder is managed in much the same fashion as anaphylaxis, which has been discussed at length earlier in this chapter. However, the majority of serum sickness-like reactions are mild and will resolve spontaneously within a few days or weeks of removal of the inciting agent. Symptomatic and supportive treatment are indicated. Antihistamines, such as diphenhydramine 1 to 2 mg/kg 4 to 6 hours, are useful in controlling urticaria and pruritus and these agents may be administered enterally or parenterally. Ephedrine has been used for these symptoms and antiinflammatory medications may also be indicated. Corticosteroids may help control the manifestations of more severe cases, such as those with severe joint complaints, renal involvement, or cardiovascular involvement. Nonsteroidal antiinflammatory agents may also be of benefit in controlling less significant joint symptoms.

Disposition

Serum sickness is usually limited to a few days to a few weeks in duration. The prognosis is generally good, with full recovery expected after 2 to 4 weeks. In a patient who is only mildly ill, outpatient therapy with close follow-up to monitor symptoms and assess the response to therapy is sufficient. Patients who appear to be more systemically ill with severe joint symptoms, high fevers, or significant involvement of the cardiovascular, neurologic, or renal systems should be treated in hospital and observed more closely. Parenteral treatment is indicated in these patients. In either case, follow-up is important, particularly to ensure that the disease manifestations do not remain present for a prolonged period.

References

Anaphlaxis

1. Kaliner MA: Anaphylaxis, *New Engl Reg Allergy Proc* 5(4):324, 1984.
2. Guill MF: Allergy emergencies, *Immunol Allergy Clin North Am* 7(30):485, 1987.
3. Atkinson TP and Kaliner MA: Anaphylaxis, *Med Clin North Am* 76(4):841,1992.
4. Austen KF: Systemic anaphylaxis in the human being, *New Engl J Med* 291(3):661, 1974.
5. Richet C: Des effects anaphylactique de l'actinotxine sur la pression arterielle, *Comptes Rend Scan Soc Biol* 54:837, 1902.
6. Schatz M and Fung DL: Anaphylactic and anaphylactoid reactions due to anesthetic agents, *Clin Rev Allergy* 4(2):215, 1986.
7. Bonner JR: Anaphylaxis: etiology and pathogenesis, *Ala J Med Sci* 25(3):283, 1988.
8. Majno G and Palad GE: Studies on inflammation. I. The effect of histamine and serotonin on vascular permeability: an electron microscopic study, *J Biophys Biochem Cytol* 11:57, 1961.
9. Sheffer AL: Anaphylaxis, *J Allergy Clin Immunol* 75(2):227, 1985.
10. Parker CW: Allergic drug responses: mechanisms and unsolved problems, *CRC Crit Rev Toxicol* 1:261, 1972.
11. Fisher M: Anaphylaxis, *Dis Mon* Aug:438, 1987.
12. Sampson HA, Mendelson L, Rosen JP: Fatal and near-fatal anaphylactic reactions to food in children and adolescents, *New Engl J Med* 327(6):384,1992.
13. Saryan JA and O'Loughlin JM: Anaphylaxis in children, *Ped Annals* 21(9):592,1992.
14. deShazo RD, Butcher BT, Banks WA: Reactions to the stings of the imported fire ant, *N Engl J Med* 323(7):462, 1990.
15. Sheffer AL and Austen KF: Exercise-induced anaphylaxis, *J Allergy Clin Immunol* 66:106, 1980.
16. Casale TB, Keahey TN, Kaliner M: Exercise-induced anaphylactic syndrome, *JAMA* 255:2049, 1986.
17. Wiggins CA, Dykwicz MS, Patterson R: Idiopathic anaphylaxis: a review, *Ann Allergy* 62:1, 1989.
18. Bacal E, Paterson R, Zeiss CR: Evaluation of severe (anaphylactic) reactions, *Clin Allergy* 8:295, 1978.
19. Sheffer AL: Anaphylaxis, *Insights in Allergy* 5:3, 1990.
20. Bonner JR: Anaphylaxis: prevention and treatment, *Ala J Med Sci* 25(4):408, 1988.
21. Valentine MD, Schuberth KC, Kagey-Sobotka A et al: The value of immunotherapy with venom in children with allergy to insect stings, *N Engl J Med* 323(23):1601, 1990.
22. Heilborn H, Hjemdahl P, Daleskog M et al: Comparison of subcutaneous injection and high-dose inhalation of epinephrine—implications for self-treatment to prevent anaphylaxis, *J Allergy Clin Immunol* 78:1174, 1986.
23. Reisman RE: Stinging insect allergy, *Med Clin North Am* 76(4):889,1992.

Juvenile Rheumatoid Arthritis

24. Cassidy JT and Petty RE: *Textbook of pediatric rheumatology,* ed 3, Philadelphia, 1995, WB Saunders.
25. Warren RW, Perez MD, Wilkings AP et al: Pediatric rheumatic diseases, *Ped Clin North Am* 41(4):788, 1994.
26. Simmons BP and Nutting JT: Juvenile rheumatoid arthritis, *Hand Clin* 5:2, 1989.
27. Petty RE, Cassidy JR, Sullivan DB: Serologic studies in juvenile rheumatoid arthritis: a review, *Arthritis Rheum* 20 (suppl 2):260, 1977.

Serum Sickness

28. Heckbert SR, Stryker WS, Coltin KL et al: Serum sickness in children after antibiotic exposure: estimates of occurrence and morbidity in a health maintenance organization population, *Am J Epidemiol* 132(2):336, 1990.
29. Savage COS and Ng YC: The aetiology and pathogenesis of major systemic vasculitides, *Postgrad Med J* 62:627, 1986.
30. Roitt IM, Brostoff J, Male DK: *Immunology,* ed 4, London, UK, 1995, Mosby-Wolfe Limited.
31. Alanis A and Weinstein AJ: Adverse reactions associated with the use of oral penicillins and cephalosporins, *Med Clin North Am* 67(1):113, 1983.
32. Erffmeyer JE: Serum sickness, *Ann Allergy* 56:105, 1986.
33. Stiehm ER and Fulginetti VA: *Immunologic disorders in infants and children,* ed 3, Philadelphia, 1989, WB Saunders.
34. Totty WG, Romano J, Benian GM et al: Serum sickness following streptokinase therapy, *AJR* 138:143, 1982.
35. Fauci AS: Vasculitis. In Parker CW, editor: *Clinical immunology,* Philadelphia, 1980, WB Saunders.

47

Cardiovascular Disorders

Marilyn M. Li • Terry P. Klassen • Lise K. Watters

Primary cardiovascular problems are infrequent among children who come to emergency departments. However, because of the potentially life-threatening nature of many of these conditions, it is important that they be recognized quickly and managed appropriately. Signs and symptoms that are caused by disorders of the cardiovascular system and that may present to an emergency department include chest pain and heart murmurs, both of which are discussed in detail. Cyanosis, hypertension, and dysrhythmias are covered in Chapters 14, 59, and 60. The specific diagnostic findings considered here include common congenital heart defects, congestive heart failure, endocarditis, myocarditis, pericarditis, acute rheumatic fever, and deep vein thrombosis.

Signs and Symptoms

CHEST PAIN

Chest pain in children is relatively uncommon, comprising about 0.6% of the primary or secondary complaints that present to the emergency department.[1,2] It occurs throughout the pediatric age range of 2 to 18 years with a median age of about 12 years.[1,3-5] Infants cannot indicate specifically if they have chest pain, but toddlers younger than 2 years have been reported to complain of it. Of pediatric patients who have had the complaint for less than 6 months, 65% have a definable etiology.[3] In contrast to adults, chest pain in children and adolescents generally has a benign connotation. In the absence of other physical signs or significant history, the causes are not life threatening and little diagnostic work-up is required.

Pathophysiology

Pain may be derived from any of the structures within the thorax or may be referred from other adjacent visceral organs. The location of the pain, its severity, recurrence, and duration may provide some clues in determining the cause.

In the chest, somatic and visceral structures share sensory pathways. Visceral pathology may have somatic manifestations at the level of T1 through T6. Abdominal pathology may cause chest pain because the posterior and lateral portions of the diaphragm are innervated by intercostal nerves and may be referred to the lower thorax and abdomen. The central and anterior portions of the diaphragm are referred to the neck and shoulders.

A description of the character of the pain is not particularly helpful in providing information about its source or significance. Terms like *crushing*, *squeezing*, or *knifelike* are not well understood, especially by younger children, and are not characteristic of any single condition.

Diagnostic Considerations. A simple classification of diagnostic categories together with the frequency of occurrence provides a focus for the myriad causes of chest pain[6] (Table 47-1).

Chest Wall. Chest wall or musculoskeletal pain is the most common diagnosis; most often, trauma or overuse is the cause of the pain. Costochondritis (Tietze syndrome) is a disease of unknown etiology causing nonsuppurative inflammation of the costochondral junction. It typically occurs in adolescents and young adults and is more frequent in females.[7] The costochondral area is swollen and tender but not erythematous. Although the disease is eventually self-limiting, it may last for months.

In boys and, less frequently, in girls entering puberty, unilateral breast tenderness and swelling is common. A nodule of breast tissue is palpable and may be slightly sore. As long as there is no discharge, changes in the overlying skin, or lymphadenopathy, this is a benign condition that becomes less pronounced as puberty progresses.

Another, less frequent cause of left-sided chest pain in adolescents is what has been termed the *precordial catch syndrome* or *Texidor's twinge*. This is a nonradiating pain that is severe, sudden, and brief (usually <1 min), occurring in the left periapical area of the chest wall. The pain is intensified by inspiration, but its onset is usually spontaneous. It can be recurrent over weeks to years.[8] The etiology is unknown. Physical examination, ECGs, chest x-rays, and echocardiograms are normal.

TABLE 47-1. Diagnostic Categories for Pediatric Chest Pain

Category	Conditions	Percent
Chest wall	Costochondritis, musculoskeletal, breast development	28
Pulmonary	Asthma, pleurisy, pulmonary embolism, pneumothorax	19
Traumatic	Bruise, abrasion, soft-tissue injury, overuse	15
Psychogenic	Hyperventilation, anxiety, depression, conversion disorder	5
Miscellaneous	Cardiac, esophagitis, gastritis, upper respiratory infection, tonsillitis	21
Unknown	Pain of unclear origin	12

Adapted from Rowe BH, et al: *Can Med Assoc J* 143(5):388, 1990.

TABLE 47-2. Causes of Myocardial Infarction in Children

Category	Specific condition
Congenital cardiac disease	Stenosis or atresia of any of the valves, supravalvular aortic stenosis, atrioventricular canal, truncus arteriosus, patent ductus arteriosus, transposition of the great vessels, tetralogy of Fallot, coarctation of the aorta
Coronary artery anomalies	Anomalous origin of coronary arteries, single right or left coronary artery, aneurysm of the coronary arteries (Kawasaki disease)
Primary endocardial or myocardial disease	Endocardial fibroelastosis, cardiomyopathy
Collagen disorders	Rheumatic fever, systemic lupus erythematosus, Kawasaki disease, rheumatoid arthritis
Hematologic/oncologic	Polycythemia, hemoglobinopathy (S-C, SS, H types), anemia, leukemia
Neuromuscular disease	Friedreich's ataxia, muscular dystrophy
Primary cardiac tumors	Myxoma, rhabdomyosarcoma, teratoma, fibroma, lipoma, hamartoma
Miscellaneous	Cocaine use

Adapted from Perry LW: *Contemp Pediatr* 27(Nov-Dec):1985.

Pulmonary. Conditions in the lungs will almost always have associated physical signs or symptoms such as fever, wheezing, rales, dyspnea, or tachypnea. Children with moderate to severe asthma may complain of chest pain, which is more often caused by the physical work of breathing rather than by a pneumothorax. Pneumonia can cause a pleuritic type of pain that is usually unilateral, but more often the pain is muscular and is caused by frequent coughing. A friction rub may be audible near the site of pain; pleural effusions are uncommon. Pleurodynia (Bornholm disease or "the devil's grip") is commonly associated with coxsackievirus type B infections. It is characterized by severe, paroxysmal chest pain accompanied by systemic symptoms such as fever, myalgia, and headache. Pulmonary embolism is rare in children but must be suspected in adolescent girls who have had an abortion, who are on oral contraceptives, or who smoke.

Psychogenic. The diagnosis of depression or anxiety as a cause of chest pain is difficult to establish, and is primarily one of exclusion. The pain is typically recurrent, chronic, and may be quite severe. The physical examination will be negative. A history of a recent heart attack or lung cancer in a parent or relative is common. School performance may be deteriorating or the child may exhibit signs of depression such as abnormal sleep or eating patterns or behavior changes. In a busy emergency department, thorough psychologic evaluation is difficult to do and is time-consuming. If this cause is suspected and other emergent conditions have been ruled out, these patients should be referred to their primary physician for further evaluation and follow-up.

Chest pain associated with hyperventilation may be caused by muscular exertion or by the resultant hypocapneic alkalosis and coronary artery vasoconstriction. Patients often have associated weakness, tingling, and dyspnea responding to rebreathing. It is difficult to assess how much of a role anxiety plays, although when the hyperventilation stops, the symptoms usually cease.

Cardiac. Although cardiac causes of chest pain are rare, they are clinically the most important because of their potentially life-threatening nature. A thorough history and physical examination, including vital signs, should indicate whether or not the likely cause of chest pain is cardiac. As well, a number of important predisposing factors should alert one to the diagnosis of cardiac pain: congenital heart disease, Marfan syndrome (mitral valve prolapse, dissecting aneurysm), Kawasaki disease (coronary artery aneurysm), or a family history of early coronary heart disease or hypercholesterolemia (infarction or ischemia). Myocardial ischemia or infarction is rarely seen in infants and children but should be specifically considered if a predisposing condition is present (Table 47-2).

The diagnosis and management of myocardial infarction in children is similar to that in adults. Pericarditis and myocardial infarction can present with pain of similar type and location. However, the pain in pericarditis is typically aggravated by movement, deep breathing, or coughing. Auscultation reveals a typical pericardial friction rub and the diagnosis is confirmed by echocardiography (see Pericarditis section). Cocaine use in children can cause chest pain from forceful repetitive coughing, pneumomediastinum, cardiac dysrhythmias, or coronary artery vasospasm and myocardial infarction.[9,10] A careful drug history should be taken and toxicologic screening performed when indicated. Regardless of the age of the child, a high index of suspicion should be maintained for this diagnosis. Pain has also been described in children who have mitral valve prolapse.[11] It is thought to be caused by myocardial ischemia or the dysrhythmias that occur with it. However, a

---

Indications for Laboratory Studies

WORRISOME HISTORY

Acute onset of pain

Pain on exertion

History of heart disease

Associated medical problems: diabetes mellitus, asthma, Marfan syndrome, Kawasaki disease, anemia, lupus erythematosus

Drugs: cocaine, oral contraceptives, tobacco

Significant trauma

Associated fever, syncope, palpitations, dizziness

Foreign body aspiration

ABNORMAL PHYSICAL EXAMINATION

Respiratory distress

Subcutaneous emphysema

Decreased breath sounds

Cardiac findings (murmurs, rubs, clicks, dysrhythmias)

Fever

Abnormal vital signs

Large contusions, lacerations, abrasions, or signs of penetrating trauma

Adapted from Selbst S: *Ped Rev* 8(2):56, 1986.

---

recent study has found that children with mitral valve prolapse and chest pain often respond to antacid therapy, which brings the cardiac origin for the pain into question.[12] A trial of antacid therapy is worthwhile.

Miscellaneous. Referred chest pain usually originates in the upper gastrointestinal tract. Esophagitis or gastritis are the most frequent conditions associated with chest pain and may be suspected from the history. Definitive diagnosis may be made by referral to a pediatric gastroenterologist for esophageal manometry, esophagogastroscopy, and esophageal pH monitoring. Pain caused by infections of the upper respiratory tract and tonsils may be described as being from the chest; this is probably not referred pain but simply a reflection of the inability of a young child to localize the source.

Diagnostic Work-Up

Any child who presents to an emergency department with chest pain must have a complete and detailed history and physical examination. Vital signs must be accurately noted. If these are entirely normal and none of the special conditions outlined above are present, then no further investigations are indicated. The accompanying box above describes some indications for laboratory studies.[13] Although chest x-ray studies and ECGs are the most common investigations done, in the presence of a normal respiratory and pulse rate, temperature, blood pressure, and physical examination, these investigations will have a very low yield.[1] If fever, tachypnea, or tachycardia is present or if the history is significant, investigations should be done as necessary.

Prehospital Considerations. Unless the patient is in shock or impending shock, no intervention in the prehospital phase is indicated. If the patient is in respiratory distress, then 100% oxygen by mask should be given. More aggressive airway management may be performed as indicated. Hyperventilating patients may be asked to rebreathe into a bag. However, the majority of children with chest pain are "walk-ins" to the emergency department and will not require care in the prehospital phase.

Therapeutic Trial

Reassurance is the mainstay of therapy in most cases of pediatric chest pain. It is important to discuss the treatment rationale with both the parent and the child and to emphasize the benign nature of the condition. The specific concern that prompted the visit, such as fear of a heart attack or lung cancer, must be acknowledged and directly addressed with the family. In many cases, reassurance causes diminution or complete alleviation of the pain.

Trials of antacids may be used if esophagitis or gastritis is suspected. Heat, rest, and analgesics may be useful if a musculoskeletal origin is likely. A mild analgesic such as acetaminophen (10 to 15 mg/kg/dose q 4 to 6 hr PO/PR PRN) or in children older than 12 years, a nonsteroidal antiinflammatory agent such as ibuprofen (200 to 400 mg/dose q 4 to 6 hr PO PRN) may be prescribed. In cases of more intense pain such as that which occurs with pleurodynia, a narcotic such as codeine (1 mg/kg/dose q 6 hr) may be necessary. However, one should be extremely cautious about prescribing narcotics unless the diagnosis is fairly certain.

Good follow-up with a primary care physician is essential. If the pain does not improve over 24 hours, gets suddenly worse, or if other symptoms develop, the patient should be advised to return to the emergency department immediately.

HEART MURMURS

Murmurs are commonly heard in children who present to emergency departments. When a heart murmur is heard, it is most important to decide whether the murmur is pathologic and if so, whether it is a significant contributor to the presenting complaint.

Pathophysiology

Cardiac murmurs are caused by unusual turbulence of blood flowing through the heart or its main vessels. Abnormal turbulence occurs because of increased flow over normal structures or normal flow over abnormal structures. Examples of the former include the pulmonary flow murmur accentuated by fever or anemia; the latter include the murmurs heard in congenital heart disease or the cervical venous hum.

Diagnostic Considerations

Murmurs are either nonpathologic (functional or innocent) or pathologic. Functional or nonpathologic murmurs are commonly heard in children and adolescents, particularly in the emergency department when fever or anxiety accentuate them. In the initial examination, it is more important to distinguish between pathologic and nonpatho-

TABLE 47-3. Characteristics of Nonpathologic and Pathologic Murmurs

Nonpathologic	Pathologic
Systolic	Systolic or diastolic
Ejection	Holosystolic
Soft or vibratory	Continuous
≤ 3/6	> 3/6
S2 physiologically split	S2 fixed, single
No extra sound or click	Click
Normal precordium	Thrills or heaves
No features associated with cardiac disease (e.g., Down syndrome)	Dysmorphic features

Adapted from Smythe JF: *Can J Pediatr* 2(2):276-278, 1995.

logic murmurs than to determine exactly what type of structural lesion, if any, is present. A careful history and physical examination are usually enough to differentiate them. The main differences between the characteristics of nonpathologic and pathologic murmurs are outlined in Table 47-3.

The classic functional or nonpathologic murmurs heard in childhood are the vibratory systolic murmur (Still's murmur), the pulmonary ejection murmur, the cervical venous hum and in infants, the physiological peripheral, pulmonic stenosis murmur.[14] All of these murmurs can be intensified with anxiety, anemia or fever. The characteristics of each of these are outline in Table 47-4. Still's murmur and pulmonary flow murmurs are best heard with the patient supine and may diminish when the patient stands. The cervical venous hum is the most common murmur of childhood and is best heard in the sitting position, often disappearing when lying down. It is produced by blood flowing around the sharp angle made by the subclavian vein entering the superior vena cava. The murmur of physiologic peripheral pulmonary stenosis is best heard in the supine position and is caused by the blood flow from the large main pulmonary artery to its relatively smaller branches at a sharp take-off angle. As the infant grows, the angle becomes less acute and right and left pulmonary arteries increase in size so the murmur disappears.

The pathologic murmurs, clicks and heart sounds, heard in many types of congenital and acquired cardiac disease are described later in this chapter. If a murmur is heard that is possibly pathologic, then it must be decided whether it is part of the complaint that brings the patient to the emergency department. Once more, a complete history and physical examination should help in the decision making. In the history, symptoms such as shortness of breath, feeding difficulties, fatigue, vomiting, failure to thrive, or episodes of cyanosis or pallor may indicate the presence of cardiac disease. In addition to the murmur heard on auscultation, abnormal vital signs (tachycardia, tachypnea, high or low blood pressure), the quality of the pulses, and signs of congestive heart failure, such as clubbing or cyanosis are signals of cardiac problems. The presence of dysmorphic features associated with particular syndromes

(Down, Turner, Williams) may also be clues to the diagnosis of congenital heart disease.

Diagnostic Work-Up. The definitive examination to determine the cause of the murmur and exclude cardiac disease remains the echocardiogram. Other examinations such as ECGs or chest radiographs may be initially helpful to determine general heart size, chamber size, or axis but are simply not as sensitive or specific as the echocardiogram.

Prehospital Considerations. Murmurs must be managed in the context of the entire clinical picture. The principals of basic life support and advanced life support must be followed in all cases, regardless of what type of murmur is heard.

Therapeutic Trial

Treatment must be directed at correcting the underlying cause of the murmur rather than the murmur itself. If cardiac disease is suspected, then urgent referral to a cardiologist is recommended.

If it is determined that the murmur is pathologic but is of no significance to the presenting complaint, then the patient should be referred to a cardiologist or back to his or her primary care physician for further investigation on a less-urgent basis. Innocent murmurs should be noted but no action need be taken except a reassuring word to the parents.

Diagnostic Entities

CONGENITAL HEART DISEASE

Congenital heart disease refers to structural or functional heart defects that are present at birth. It has been estimated that the incidence of congenital heart disease is 4 to 10/1,000 live births.[15] The underdetection of cardiac defects that are associated with relatively minor physical findings and the overrepresentation of lesions that cause more severe cardiac dysfunction are among the inherent difficulties of the population studies from which these data have been derived (see Chapter 18).

Three common pediatric entities are often not included in population studies of congenital heart disease. These include mitral valve prolapse, which is estimated to occur in 6% to 10% of children, and congenital bicuspid aortic valve, which is the most common congenital heart defect. Regarded as a functional lesion, the patent ductus arteriosus (PDA) of prematurity is often excluded from these studies.[15]

Most forms of congenital heart disease seem to be caused by the interaction among genetic, environmental (e.g., chemical toxins or viral agents), and random factors. In 5% to 8% of patients with congenital heart disease, there is an associated chromosomal defect, with trisomy 21 being the most common. Classic Mendelian single-gene defects are probably responsible for about 3% of cases.[15]

The development of m-mode, two-dimensional, Doppler, and color-flow Doppler echocardiographic techniques represents a very significant advance in pediatric cardiac imaging. Currently, the diagnosis and management of many

TABLE 47-4. Common Nonpathologic Heart Murmurs Heard in Infants and Children

Murmurs	Timing	Location	Quality	Age
Stills	Systole	LLSB—medial to apex	Vibratory, low pitched	>2 years
Pulmonary flow	Systole	LUSB	Blowing, high pitched	All ages
Venous hum	Continuous	Neck (R > L) to base	Humming	All ages
Physiologic peripheral pulmonic stenosis	Systole	LUSB, axilla, back	Blowing, high pitched	<6 months

Adapted from Smythe JF: *Can J Pediatr* 2(2):277, 1995.
LLSB, Left lower sternal border; *LUSB,* left upper sternal border.

cardiac lesions may be based on the information derived from echocardiography, without the need for cardiac catheterization and angiocardiographic studies.[16] Transesophageal echocardiography study tends to be reserved for specific indications, such as the assessment of children in the postoperative period, and the real-time monitoring of selected procedures during cardiac catheterization.[17] Numerous new cardiovascular surgical techniques account for the increase in the length and quality of the lives of many children with congenital heart disease. Several noteworthy examples include the success of heart transplantation for hypoplastic left heart syndrome (among other indications), arterial switch repair of transposition of the great arteries, and balloon valvuloplasty for some cases of pulmonic and aortic stenosis.

Pathophysiology

An appreciation of the normal physiologic and anatomic changes that occur during the transition from fetal to neonatal circulation is helpful in understanding the nature of many of the congenital heart defects. In the fetus, blood with a low oxygen content is delivered via the umbilical arteries from the descending aorta to the placenta where it is oxygenated. Blood with a relatively high oxygen content flows from the placenta into the umbilical vein, which divides into the ductus venosus and the hepatic-portal venous system. Within the inferior vena cava, well-oxygenated blood from the ductus venosus preferentially flows across the foramen ovale into the left atrium and, via the aorta, supplies the myocardium and the brain.

The blood returning from the head and neck is diverted around the inferior vena cava flow within the right atrium to the right ventricle and the pulmonary artery. Because pulmonary artery pressure is high in utero, little of the combined ventricular output goes to the pulmonary circulation and about 60% flows across the patent ductus arteriosus from the pulmonary artery into the descending aorta.

With the newborn's first breath after delivery, the pulmonary vascular resistance falls and blood flow to the lungs increases. Clamping of the umbilical cord leads to an increase in the systemic vascular resistance and left ventricular afterload. Left atrial pressure rises and tends to close the foramen ovale.

Postnatal closure of the ductus occurs in two stages. Functional closure usually takes place within 10 to 15 hours in the full-term infant. The smooth muscle in the wall of the ductus contracts following a change in the balance of factors favoring ductal patency. An increase in Po_2 and the release of vasoactive substances tend to constrict the ductus, which in utero had remained open, due in part to the relaxing effects of endogenous PGE_1 and PGI_2 on local muscle. Within 2 to 3 weeks, the ductus becomes fibrosed and forms the ligamentum arteriosum.[18]

Pulmonary vascular resistance continues to decline over the first week of life, during which time the small muscular pulmonary arteries become widened with thin walls. Right-ventricle pressure reaches adult levels by about 10 days.[19]

Closure of the ductus arteriosus may fail to occur in the neonate who becomes hypoxic or acidotic. With constriction of the pulmonary arterioles in response to these stimuli, pulmonary vascular resistance remains high and the foramen ovale and the ductus remain patent. Right-to-left shunting occurs as a result and the hypoxemia is perpetuated. The cyanotic neonate with persistent pulmonary hypertension (or persistent fetal circulation) may be distinguishable from one with a cyanotic congenital heart defect through the use of the hyperoxic test. Administration of 100% oxygen in the first instance will usually effect an improvement in oxygen saturation but remain low in the latter.[20]

Patients with certain congenital heart lesions are dependent on blood flow through a patent ductus for their survival. These include patients with hypoplastic left heart syndrome, pulmonary or aortic atresia, and transposition of the great vessels with intact ventricular septum. Patients with coarctation of the aorta or interrupted aortic arch require a patent ductus for their initial stability.

Although many congenital heart diseases are associated with variable or nonspecific symptomatology, some cardiac defects may be divided into those that produce cyanosis and those that lead to congestive heart failure (Tables 47-5 and 46-6).[21,22] The age at which most children present with these signs is reasonably predictable for many of the cardiac lesions. In general, lesions that cause severe cyanosis rarely result in congestive heart failure, with the exception of transposition of the great arteries with a ventricular septal defect. Lesions that produce cyanosis may be further divided on the basis of either decreased or increased associated pulmonary blood flow. Acyanotic lesions are accompanied by normal or increased blood flow to the lungs (Table 47-7).[23]

TABLE 47-5. Congenital Heart Diseases Usually Associated With Cyanosis[21,22]

Lesion	Usual time of onset of cyanosis
Transposition of the great arteries	Birth to first week
Total anomalous pulmonary venous return (obstructed)	First week
Tricuspid atresia	Weeks 1-4
Ebstein's anomaly of the tricuspid valve	First week
Tetralogy of Fallot	Weeks 1-12
Severe pulmonary stenosis with intact ventricular septum or ventricular septal defect	Weeks 1-4

TABLE 47-6. Congenital Heart Diseases Usually Presenting With Heart Failure[21,22]

Lesion	Usual time of onset of heart failure
Hypoplastic left heart syndrome	First week
Coarctation of the aorta syndrome	First week
Complete atrioventricular canal	First 2-3 weeks
Ventricular septal defect	Weeks 2-12
Patent ductus arteriosus	Weeks 1-4 (earlier in premature infants)
Complex lesions	Weeks 1-12

TABLE 47-7. Acyanotic vs. Cyanotic Forms of Congenital Heart Disease

Acyanotic	Cyanotic
Normal pulmonary blood flow	**Decreased pulmonary blood flow**
Pulmonary valve stenosis	Severe pulmonary stenosis
Mitral stenosis	Pulmonary atresia
Mitral regurgitation	Tetralogy of Fallot
Aortic stenosis	Transposition of the great arteries with pulmonary stenosis
Coarctation of the aorta	Tricuspid atresia
	Ebstein's anomaly of the tricuspid valve with right-to-left shunt
	Eisenmenger's complex
Increased pulmonary blood flow	**Increased pulmonary blood flow**
Atrial septal defect	Total anomalous pulmonary venous return
Ventricular septal defect	Hypoplastic left heart syndrome
Patent ductus arteriosus	Transposition of the great arteries with or without ventricular septal defect
All left-to-right shunts with pulmonary hypertension	Truncus arteriosus
Atrioventricular canal	

Adapted from Morgan BC: *Pediatr Clin North Am* 25(4):721, 1978.

Tetralogy of Fallot

Tetralogy of Fallot represents the most common type of cyanotic congenital heart disease, and accounts for about 10% of all forms.[24] The tetrad consists of right ventricular outflow tract obstruction, dextroposition and overriding of the aorta, ventricular septal defect, and right ventricular hypertrophy. The nature and severity of cardiac dysfunction is determined primarily by the degree of obstruction of the right ventricular outflow tract. Abnormalities of the pulmonary valve vary from mild changes to complete atresia and hypoplasia of the pulmonary arteries. The ventricular septal defect is usually large.

Pathophysiology. Because of the nature of the anatomic defects, there is a right-to-left shunt that may be mild or severe. Right ventricular hypertrophy occurs as a consequence of the right outflow tract obstruction and the systemic vascular resistance against which blood is pumped across the ventricular septal defect. Eventually, the left ventricle may enlarge and hypertrophy.

Diagnostic Findings

Clinical Findings. The child with tetralogy of Fallot may present in a variety of ways, depending on the degree of pulmonary valve stenosis. Although the patient with tetralogy of Fallot may present with respiratory distress and cyanosis in the newborn period, more commonly the cyanosis appears later with crying or feeding. The occasional infant with a large ventricular septal defect and left-to-right shunt will present much later with signs of heart failure.

Children with tetralogy of Fallot may become dyspneic and assume a squatting position when exerting themselves. The squatting maneuver is accompanied by an increase in oxygen saturation and is in fact therapeutic in the child with tetralogy of Fallot who develops a hypercyanotic spell (see Chest Pain).

On physical examination the patient is cyanotic. Clubbing of the nail beds may be present if the cyanosis is severe. Auscultation of the heart reveals an active precordium. The first heart sound is normal and the second is single and loud. Most individuals have a harsh systolic ejection murmur that is heard maximally in the pulmonic area and radiates to the anterior chest and back. With more severe pulmonic stenosis, the murmur is softer and may disappear during a hypercyanotic spell. The murmur of the ventricular septal defect is not heard.

Complications. Polycythemia places these children at risk for cerebrovascular accidents.[25] They are also at risk for infectious endocarditis and sudden death. Tables 47-8 and 47-9 summarize the surgical procedures of selected congenital heart defects and the potential postoperative complications.

Ancillary Data. Polycythemia is present in patients with tetralogy of Fallot and cyanosis. Arterial blood gases usually show a normal pH and Pco_2 at rest, with a variable Po_2. During a hypercyanotic spell, there is evidence of metabolic acidosis and hypoxemia.

TABLE 47-8. Surgical Procedures for Selected Congenital Heart Defects

Lesion	Procedure
Aortic stenosis	Valvulotomy, prosthetic valve insertion (tissue or mechanical)
Pulmonary stenosis	Valvulotomy
Coarctation of aorta	Resection and end-to-end anastomosis, patch angioplasty, subclavian flap angioplasty
Endocardial cushion defect	Patch closure of ASD and VSD, division of common AV valve and construction of mitral and tricuspid valves
Tetralogy of Fallot	Blalock-Taussig shunt (anastomosis of subclavian artery to pulmonary artery) or Waterston shunt (anastomosis of ascending aorta to right pulmonary artery) for palliation; patch closure of VSD, relief of right ventricular outflow obstruction with valvulotomy and outflow patch, with or without resection of infundibular muscle
Transposition of great arteries	Mustard or Senning repairs (atrial baffle and venous return diversion); arterial switch with transplantation of coronary arteries
Tricuspid atresia	Fontan procedure (anastomosis of right atrium to pulmonary artery either directly or via valved or nonvalved conduits)
Pulmonary atresia with associated lesions	Various shunt procedures for palliation; Rastelli procedure (valved or nonvalved conduit from right ventricular outflow tract to pulmonary artery)

Adapted from Moskowitz WB, Clark BJ III: *Cardiology in principles and practice of clinical pediatrics*, Chicago, 1987, Year Book.

TABLE 47-9. Postoperative Residua and Sequelae of Late Complications Following Repair of Selected Congenital Heart Defects

Lesion	Residua, sequelae, and complications
Aortic stenosis	Residual or recurrent stenosis; aortic insufficiency, prosthetic valve dysfunction or stenosis; thrombosis; life-long anticoagulation
Ventricular septal defect (VSD)	Residual VSD with congestive heart failure; poor ventricular function; AV block; pulmonary vascular disease
Endocardial cushion defect	Mitral, tricuspid regurgitation/stenosis; pulmonary vascular disease; atrial dysrhythmias, residual left-to-right shunt; AV block
Transposition of great arteries	Atrial repair: atrial dysrhythmias and conduction disturbances, ventricular dysfunction, caval or pulmonary venous obstruction, pulmonary stenosis, tricuspid regurgitation; arterial switch: semilunar valve insufficiency, coronary artery ostia or great vessel stenosis at anastomosis site
Rastelli repair	Conduit stenosis; valve stenosis or insufficiency
Fontan repair	Elevated right atrial pressures at rest and with exercise; abnormal cardiac response to exercise
Coarctation of the aorta	Systemic hypertension, recoarctation
Tetralogy of Fallot	Residual VSD or pulmonary stenosis; ventricular dysrhythmias, AV block; pulmonary, tricuspid insufficiency; ventricular dysfunction

Adapted from Moskowitz WB and Clark BJ III: *Cardiology in principles and practice of clinical pediatrics*, Chicago, 1987, Year Book.

There is usually evidence of right axis deviation and right ventricular hypertrophy on the ECG. Evidence of right atrial enlargement and ventricular ectopy are rare findings in infants and young children.

The classic chest x-ray film reveals a boot-shaped heart with an upturned cardiac apex and a reduced main pulmonary artery segment. The pulmonary vascular markings are normal or decreased. A right aortic arch may be seen in about 20% of cases.

Two-dimensional and Doppler echocardiographic demonstration of the anatomic and flow abnormalities in tetralogy of Fallot has in some centers obviated the need for routine preoperative cardiac catheterization and angiocardiography in these patients.

Differential Considerations. The differential considerations include tricuspid atresia, double-outlet right ventricle, single ventricle, critical pulmonic stenosis, pulmonary atresia with intact ventricular septum, and truncus arteriosus.[26] The acyanotic child with mild tetralogy of Fallot may be mistakenly diagnosed as having an isolated ventricular septal defect or isolated pulmonic stenosis.

Management. The patient who presents with cyanosis should receive a therapeutic trial of oxygen. Early consultation with a cardiologist is advised. Some authors recommend starting an infusion of prostaglandin E_1 in the cyanotic newborn with tetralogy of Fallot.[24,25]

Definitive treatment consists of surgical repair of the lesions. Patients with the classic tetralogy and favorable pulmonary arterial anatomy generally undergo primary complete repair. Children who are symptomatic but are not good candidates for repair are usually treated with one of several palliative shunts (see Table 47-8) first. Prophylactic treatment for bacterial endocarditis should be administered when indicated.

Transposition of the Great Arteries

Transposition of the great arteries accounts for 5% to 7% of all forms of congenital heart disease. Simple complete transposition is associated with an aorta arising from the right ventricle and the pulmonary artery coming from the left ventricle.[27] There may be a concurrent ventricular septal defect (30%), patent ductus arteriosus (50%), patent foramen ovale, and less commonly, left ventricular outflow tract obstruction secondary to pulmonic stenosis.

Pathophysiology. The systemic and pulmonary circulations of transposition of the great arteries run in parallel instead of in series, as occurs normally. For gas exchange to occur in this situation, connections between the circuits must exist, i.e., ventricular septal defect, atrial septal defect, patent foramen ovale, patent ductus arteriosus, or bronchopulmonary collateral circulations. Neonates with an intact ventricular septum and a closed ductus will be hypoxic because of the inadequate mixing at the level of the foramen ovale. On the other hand, with adequate interatrial or interventricular shunting, a relatively high oxygen saturation may be attained if the left ventricle can maintain a high-output state. In the presence of left ventricular outflow tract obstruction, arterial oxygen saturation will be decreased even if the size of the anatomic shunts is otherwise adequate.

In transposition of the great arteries, the direction and amount of shunted blood vary throughout the cardiac cycle as determined by local pressure gradients. In the neonate with transposition of the great arteries and intact ventricular septum, right atrial pressure increases after birth secondary to the normal rise in systemic vascular resistance and the foramen ovale tends to remain open with bidirectional shunting across it. The ductus arteriosus in this setting is often patent and for a short time may permit bidirectional shunting. As the ductus arteriosus closes, hypoxemia develops.

Generally, right ventricular function is impaired and hypertrophy occurs secondary to the exercise workload to which it is subjected as the "systemic" ventricle. On the other hand, left ventricular function, at or near birth in patients with transposition of the great arteries and intact ventricular septum, is similar to that in the normal situation and may remain so for a period of about 2 to 3 weeks. With the subsequent fall in pulmonary vascular resistance and left ventricular workload, left ventricular myocardial mass does not usually increase as it does in the normal heart.

In patients with transposition of the great arteries, the early development of pulmonary vascular disease is more frequent than in other forms of congenital heart disease. Those with a ventricular septal defect and high pulmonary blood flow are at particularly great risk.

Diagnostic Findings

Clinical Findings. It is helpful to divide patients with transposition of the great arteries according to anatomic and physiologic factors because the clinical manifestations follow directly from these.[27] Newborns with an intact ventricular septum (group 1) usually have early (within the first day) and rapidly progressive cyanosis, which in the presence of a large patent ductus arteriosus may be more pronounced in the upper body. The neonate may appear otherwise well or be mildly tachypneic and tachycardic. Auscultation of the heart may be normal or reveal a loud first heart sound, a single second heart sound, and a soft systolic ejection murmur (grade 2/6 or less) at the middle to upper left sternal border. The infant with transposition of the great arteries and increased pulmonary blood flow may

undergo "hypoxic" spells, during which the patient is irritable and cyanotic with labored breathing. The patient's mental status is not usually altered as it may be during the hypercyanotic spells associated with tetralogy of Fallot.

The neonate with transposition of the great arteries and a large ventricular septal defect (group 2) often presents with mild cyanosis in the first week. At age 2 to 6 weeks, the patient may develop left heart failure with tachypnea, tachycardia, and cyanosis. Auscultation of the failing heart reveals a grade 3-4/6 pansystolic murmur, a third heart sound, gallop rhythm, and a loud pulmonic component of the second heart sound.

Newborns with transposition of the great arteries, a ventricular septal defect, left ventricular outflow tract obstruction, and diminished pulmonary blood flow (group 3) are severely cyanotic from birth and present in a similar way to patients with tetralogy of Fallot and severe pulmonic stenosis (see section on Tetralogy of Fallot).

Pulmonary vascular disease that occurs in infants with palliated transposition of the great arteries and ventricular septal defects may be manifested by an increase in cyanosis. In late childhood or adolescence, the murmurs of pulmonary or mitral valve insufficiency may be apparent as a result of gross dilation of the left heart.

Complications. Individuals with transposition of the great arteries are at risk for thromboses secondary to polycythemia, notably of the central nervous system, lung, and kidneys. Spontaneous cerebrovascular accidents may occur, particularly in children under the age of 2 years. Brain abscess formation may infrequently complicate the clinical course of children over the age of 2 years with uncorrected transposition of the great arteries.[27] See Table 47-9 for the postoperative complications of this disease.

Ancillary Data. Cyanotic patients with transposition of the great arteries develop polycythemia. Infants over 9 months of age and children with cyanosis may have thrombocytopenia and decreased platelet survival times. Systemic arterial Po_2 levels are infrequently more than 35 mmHg in room air and usually remain below 35 mm Hg during the administration of 100% oxygen. The Pco_2 is usually normal or slightly elevated (less than 45 mm Hg).

The ECG usually shows evidence of right-axis deviation with right (with intact ventricular septum) or combined (with ventricular septal defect) ventricular hypertrophy. The ECG tracing may be normal in the first few days of life.

Chest x-ray studies are very useful in making the diagnosis of transposition of the great arteries. The classic findings include: (1) egg-shaped heart tilted on its side with a narrow mediastinum, (2) increased pulmonary vascular markings, and (3) cardiomegaly. The last two signs are particularly prominent when a ventricular septal defect is present. The chest x-ray film may be normal in the patient with transposition of the great arteries with intact ventricular septum in the first few days to weeks of life.

Two-dimensional and Doppler echocardiography are excellent tools to establish the diagnosis of transposition of the great arteries. Many centers continue to use cardiac catheterization and angiocardiography, particularly in the newborn who is being considered for a balloon atrial septostomy.

Differential Considerations. The differential considerations include pulmonary causes of cyanosis, such as persistent fetal circulation or respiratory distress syndrome, as well as truncus arteriosus, severe tetralogy of Fallot, pulmonary atresia and ventricular septal defect, total anomalous pulmonary venous return, Ebstein's anomaly of the tricuspid valve, or hypoplastic left heart syndrome.

Management. The patient who presents with cyanosis should receive a therapeutic trial of oxygen. The infant who shows signs of heart failure should receive oxygen and appropriate reduction of preload (see section on Congestive Heart Failure). Early consultation with a cardiologist is advised. An IV infusion of prostaglandin PGE_1 should be started before emergency atrial septostomy or arterial switch in the hypoxemic neonate.

Two surgical options exist for the repair of transposition of the great arteries, the first of which is balloon atrial septostomy followed by atrial switch (see Table 47-8). Functional dysrhythmias commonly occur after this procedure and may account for some of the sudden late deaths.[28,29] The second option, arterial switch repair, is best accomplished in the first few weeks of life because delay beyond this time usually requires pulmonary artery banding to prepare the left ventricle for a systemic workload. The distinct advantages of this procedure include good left ventricular function and persistence of normal sinus rhythm in the follow-up studies done to date (8 years vs. 20 years follow-up of patients who had an atrial switch repair).[27,28] Prophylactic treatment for bacterial endocarditis should be given when indicated.

Ventricular Septal Defect

Between 20% and 40% of patients with congenital heart disease have isolated ventricular septal defect (VSD).[15] As such, it is one of the most common forms of congenital heart disease. About 80% of ventricular septal defects are perimembranous. The next largest group, muscular defects, are common in infancy and at least 60% close spontaneously in the first year of life.[18]

Pathophysiology. The normal maturational process of a decrease in pulmonary vascular resistance over the first 2 weeks of life may be delayed in the presence of a large ventricular septal defect. The lungs are thus relatively protected from increased blood flow. During the following few months, as the pulmonary vascular resistance declines, there is an increase in blood return to the left heart and a rise in left atrial and left ventricular pressures. Consequently, the infant's compensatory mechanisms of increased cardiac sympathetic stimulation, myocardial hypertrophy, and increased contractility become inadequate; congestive heart failure develops in the first to third months.

Small ventricular defects provide high resistance to blood flow because of the small area of the defect and a small left-to-right shunt occurs. Moderate-sized defects are usually associated with a moderate left-to-right shunt, volume overload of the left atrium and ventricle, and left ventricular hypertrophy. There is no impedance to blood flow across large defects and both ventricles generate systemic pressures. The term *Eisenmenger complex* applies to patients with a ventricular septal defect in whom the shunt is predominantly right-to-left and pulmonary vascular resistance is very high.

Diagnostic Findings

Clinical Findings. Infants with small defects are usually asymptomatic and diagnosed with a harsh grade 4/6 holosystolic murmur that is best heard at the left lower sternal border and may radiate along the left and right sternal borders. The precordium is quiet. Heart sounds are usually normal and a third heart sound may be present.

Between the ages of 2 weeks and 12 months, infants with moderate or large defects become symptomatic. Typically they are tachypneic (due to pulmonary edema) and they become sweaty (with increased sympathetic tone) and fatigued during feeds. The physical examination of infants with moderate shunts is similar to that of infants with small ventricular septal defects. Infants with large ventricular septal defects have a very active precordium and a decrescendo murmur that is heard best over the lower left sternal border. A third heart sound is present and the second heart sound has a loud pulmonic component.

Children identified with a ventricular septal defect after the age of 2 years may either appear well or, less commonly, show signs of heart failure. Cyanosis may appear in early childhood but is more common in adolescence or early adulthood. The precordium is quiet and there may be a short pulmonic ejection murmur at the upper left sternal border or none at all. A third heart sound may be present and the pulmonic component of the second sound is increased.

Complications. Patients with large ventricular septal defects may develop the Eisenmenger complex with pulmonary vascular obstructive disease and early death from pulmonary hemorrhage, dysrhythmias, cerebral thrombosis, or brain abscess. The risk of infective endocarditis is considered to be negligible when surgical repair of the ventricular septal defect has been effected at least 6 months earlier without residua. Table 47-9 presents the postoperative complications.

Ancillary Data. The ECG is normal in children with small ventricular septal defects. There is evidence of right biventricular hypertrophy and usually left ventricular hypertrophy in patients with moderate defects. With large defects, the ECG tracing shows evidence of biventricular hypertrophy and left atrial hypertrophy in patients with increased pulmonary flow.

The chest x-ray film is normal in patients with small ventricular defects. With moderate defects, there is evidence of cardiomegaly and normal or increased pulmonary vascular markings. The chest x-ray study appearance of patients with large defects is similar; the pulmonary vascular markings are consistently increased.

While two-dimensional with Doppler echocardiographic examination is an excellent method for the diagnosis of moderate and large ventricular septal defects, small defects (<2 mm) and multiple defects are best detected by color-flow mapping studies. The indications for cardiac catheterization in the setting of ventricular septal defect vary according to the experience of the physician.

Differential Considerations. These include endocardial cushion defects, double-outlet right ventricle, infundibular pulmonary stenosis, left ventricle to right atrial communications, double-chambered right ventricle, subaortic steno-sis, truncus arteriosus, and transposition of the great arter-ies with ventricular septal defect.

Management. A cardiology consultation should be ob-tained. Small ventricular septal defects require follow-up only, with prophylactic treatment for bacterial endocarditis where indicated (as for ventricular septal defects of any size). Moderate-sized defects with left-to-right shunts and evidence of heart failure require treatment with digoxin and, in some cases, diuretics[19] (see section on Congestive Heart Failure). Pulmonary infections should be treated aggressively. Definitive treatment consists of patch closure of the defect if a large left-to-right shunt is still present at the age of 4 or 5 years. Patients with large shunts that are not responsive to medical therapy usually require patch closure in the first year of life. Patients who are identified as having severe pulmonary disease and right-to-left shunt-ing are not considered candidates for operation and should restrict their physical activity; their hematocrit level should be monitored.

Secundum Atrial Septal Defect

Secundum atrial septal defect (ASD) is relatively com-mon and accounts for about 7% of all congenital heart disease. Although usually an isolated defect, one of the most common associated lesions is mitral valve prolapse with or without mitral regurgitation.[30]

Pathophysiology. In most cases, the direction and amount of blood flow across the defect is determined by the relative filling resistances in the right and left ven-tricles. There is minimal left-to-right shunting during in-fancy when the right and left ventricular thicknesses are about equal. Pulmonary artery pressure is usually normal even though pulmonary blood flow is often greatly in-creased.

Diagnostic Findings

Clinical Findings. Infants are frequently asymptomatic, and the diagnosis is made when a heart murmur is de-tected in the school-age child. The occasional infant will show poor growth, heart failure, and have frequent respi-ratory infections. The older child is often asymptomatic but may complain of fatigue or dyspnea if there is a moderate to large left-to-right shunt.

The physical examination of the child reveals a systolic impulse along the left lower sternal border and a loud first heart sound. The second heart sound characteristically has fixed splitting. The ejection type murmur is heard maxi-mally at the upper left sternal border with transmission to the upper lung fields. A mid-diastolic murmur may be heard along the lower left sternal border.

Patients with atrial septal defect usually remain asymp-tomatic into childhood. The rare child may develop pulmo-nary vascular disease.

Complications. Atrial dysrhythmias such as junctional rhythms or supraventricular tachydysrhythmias may occur. The risk of developing bacterial endocarditis is considered negligible in patients with isolated secundum atrial septal defect.

Ancillary Data. Although the ECG tracings of most pa-tients show normal sinus rhythms, a small number may have junctional rhythms or supraventricular tachydys-

rhythmias such as atrial flutter.[30,31] There may be evidence of first-degree heart block or of right atrial enlargement.

Usually there is evidence of cardiomegaly and increased pulmonary vascular markings on chest radiograph. Some patients with a large left-to-right shunt have a heart that is normal in size.

The availability of two-dimensional and Doppler echo-cardiographic examinations has obviated the need for car-diac catheterization in most centers.

Differential Considerations. These include ostium pri-mum-type atrial defect, partial atrioventricular canal, ven-tricular septal defect, and mild pulmonic stenosis.

Management. A cardiologist should be consulted. Usu-ally elective surgical repair for large defects is carried out when the patient is 4 or 5 years old, and earlier in infants and children with signs of heart failure or pulmonary hy-pertension. Prophylactic treatment for bacterial endocardi-tis should be given when indicated.

Complete Atrioventricular Canal

A complete atrioventricular canal may require treatment with antidysrhythmic medications and a cardiologist must be consulted. There is a wide variety of atrioventricular canal defects that appear to be caused by maldevelopment of the endocardial cushions and the atrioventricular sep-tum.[32] In almost all instances the mitral valve is improperly formed, as is the anteroseptal commissure of the tricuspid valve on occasion. The main features are a large atrio-ventricular septal defect, a common atrioventricular valve that arises from both atria, and a defective ventricular septum. Complete atrioventricular canal is more often as-sociated with Down syndrome than are other forms of this defect.

Pathophysiology. Pulmonary blood flow is greatly in-creased, as is pulmonary arterial pressure in infants with this lesion. Systemic arterial oxygen desaturation may oc-cur if pulmonary vascular disease is severe. Often the common atrioventricular valve is regurgitant.

Diagnostic Findings

Clinical Findings. Infants usually present by the age of 1 year with heart failure, failure to thrive, and frequent respiratory infections. Physical examination reveals an ac-tive precordium and a loud first heart sound. The second heart sound is usually split in inspiration only, and the pulmonic component is loud. The holosystolic murmur of mitral insufficiency is heard at the left lower sternal border and the apex. A systolic ejection murmur at the upper left sternal border and a mid-diastolic murmur along the lower left sternal border and at the apex can also be heard.

Complications. Infants with this defect are at risk for developing pneumonia, congestive heart failure, pulmonary vascular disease, and infective endocarditis. See Table 47-9 with regard to the postoperative complications.

Ancillary Data. The ECG usually shows a normal sinus rhythm with 1:1 atrioventricular conduction. Most patients have a prolonged P-R interval, and many have evidence of right atrial, left atrial, or biatrial enlargement. Evidence of right ventricular hypertrophy is usually present.

There is evidence of cardiomegaly and increased pulmo-nary markings on the chest x-ray film. Two-dimensional and Doppler echocardiography are very useful in making the diagnosis. Cardiac catheterization is indicated if the diagnosis is uncertain.

Differential Considerations. These include partial atrioventricular canal, large secundum atrial septal defect, common atrium, anomalous pulmonary venous return, and ventricular septal defect. Patients with Down syndrome may have tetralogy of Fallot or a complete atrioventricular canal.

Management. A cardiologist should be consulted. A patient in heart failure may require digoxin and diuretic therapy. Definitive surgical repair is usually done on an elective basis before the age of 2 years and ideally between 6 and 12 months of age. Palliation may be achieved with pulmonary artery banding before complete repair is effected. Prophylactic treatment for bacterial endocarditis should be given when indicated.

Patent Ductus Arteriosus

The incidence of patent ductus arteriosus (PDA) in low-birth-weight premature infants has increased concomitant with the improvement in their rates of survival.[15,33] In one institution, the incidence of patent ductus arteriosus is 8/1,000 total live births. This defect occurs in 1/2,000 full-term live births.

Pathophysiology. The role of the ductus arteriosus in fetal circulation and its normal closure in the postnatal period have been discussed in the introduction to this section. In the postnatal period the degree of left-to-right shunting across the patent ductus arteriosus is regulated by the relatively high pulmonary vascular resistance. Left ventricular and atrial volumes will increase because of this shunt. Left ventricular dilation with increased left ventricular end-diastolic pressure will lead to raised left atrial pressure and will result in left heart failure. Compensatory mechanisms are poorly developed in all newborns, particularly those born prematurely. Right ventricular failure may also occur if the patent ductus arteriosus is large and pulmonary vascular resistance remains elevated.

Aortic diastolic pressure is reduced in the presence of a large PDA and thus myocardial perfusion may be impaired. Anemia and the normal presence of large amounts of fetal hemoglobin may contribute to poor oxygen delivery to the myocardium.

Diagnostic Findings

Clinical Findings. Premature infants without lung disease are generally diagnosed with a heart murmur at 2 to 5 days of age. The murmur is best heard at the second or third left intercostal space, and may extend beyond systole into diastole. However, the classical machinery-type murmur heard in older children with PDA is not usually present. With progression of the left-to-right shunt, an apical third heart sound may appear, the precordium becomes hyperactive, and the peripheral pulses become bounding. Those who develop left ventricular failure will be tachycardiac, tachypneic, and may develop severe bradycardic and apneic spells. Hepatomegaly is a late sign.

The full-term infant with a small PDA is often asymptomatic and the diagnosis is made when a murmur is detected. Those with a moderate left-to-right shunt often show progressive symptomatology with poor feeding and weight gain, irritability, and tachypnea over the first 2 to 3 months of life.

Some infants who have a moderate patent ductus arteriosus compensate with myocardial hypertrophy and do not develop left heart failure. As older children, they may complain of fatigue upon exertion. The physical examination reveals a harsh, continuous machinery-type murmur that radiates to the back. The precordium is active and a thrill may be felt at the upper sternal border. An apical third heart sound is often present.

Complications. Aneurysm formation of the patent ductus arteriosus may occur. The risk of bacterial endocarditis is considered to be negligible when surgical repair of the PDA has been effected at least 6 months earlier without residua. Older infants and children are at risk for failure to thrive, recurrent respiratory infections, congestive heart failure, lobar emphysema or collapse, and pulmonary vascular disease.

Ancillary Data. The ECG is not usually very helpful in making the diagnosis of patent ductus arteriosus in the premature infant. The full-term infant with a small lesion usually has a normal ECG whereas evidence of left ventricular hypertrophy may be seen with large shunts.

Commonly the chest roentgenogram reveals a normal-sized heart with increased pulmonary vascular markings. With a large shunt, the heart may be enlarged. Changes associated with underlying lung pathology may be present.

Two-dimensional and Doppler echocardiographic examinations are usually adequate to make the diagnosis of patent ductus arteriosus. Occasionally, confirmation of the diagnosis requires cardiac catheterization.

Differential Considerations. These include total anomalous pulmonary venous return, ruptured sinus of Valsalva, atrioventricular communication, anomalous origin of the left subclavian artery from the pulmonary artery, absent pulmonic valve, aortic insufficiency and ventricular septal defect, peripheral pulmonary artery stenosis, truncus arteriosus, aortopulmonary fenestration, and pulmonary atresia. In the older child, the findings of a venous hum may resemble those of a patent ductus arteriosus.

Management. A consultation with a cardiologist should be obtained. The very small premature infant does not usually respond to digoxin therapy. Generally, premature newborns require treatment with indomethacin to effect closure of the patent ductus arteriosus. Surgical ligation is indicated if there is persistent left heart failure in the 48 to 72 hours following the administration of indomethacin. The full-term infant does not usually respond to indomethacin. These patients and older children should have surgical ligation of the patent ductus arteriosus.[33] Prophylactic treatment for bacterial endocarditis should be given when indicated.

Coarctation of the Aorta

Coarctation of the aorta accounts for 3% to 7% of congenital heart disease in live-born infants. Among patients with Turner syndrome, coarctation of the aorta represents the most common cardiovascular anomaly. It also occurs in patients with neurofibromatosis.

Pathophysiology. Coarctation of the aorta refers to a constriction of the aorta, which is almost always located at the junction of the ductus arteriosus and the aortic arch, just distal to the left subclavian artery.[34] In one form, there is a segment of severe aortic isthmus narrowing of variable length, and blood flow to the lower trunk occurs across the patent ductus arteriosus from the right heart and main pulmonary artery. In the second form, the obstruction is discrete, with blood flow to the lower trunk supplied by left heart flow into the ascending aorta. In the latter case, the shunt across the patent ductus arteriosus is from left to right. Both isthmic narrowing and discrete obstruction may be present in an individual. Either form of coarctation may be found in infants. The vast majority of patients with coarctation of the aorta who present in the first few months of life have an associated cardiac anomaly. Of these, patent ductus arteriosus, ventricular septal defect, and bicuspid aortic valve are the most common, followed by aortic stenosis, aortic insufficiency, and mitral valve abnormalities. Coarctation of the aorta may also occur with transposition of the great arteries and double-outlet right ventricle.

It is the coarctation itself in most infants with complex coarctation syndrome that is responsible for cardiac decompensation. Both the left and right ventricles face increases in afterload directly caused by the coarctation. In the presence of intracardiac communications, there is also an increase in the preload of each ventricle.

Diagnostic Findings

Clinical Findings. Babies with coarctation of the aorta who present in infancy usually show signs of heart failure, failure to thrive, and, occasionally, low cardiac output. Often the patient is irritable, tachypneic, and tachycardic. Cardiac examination reveals an active precordium and a systolic murmur at the left upper sternal border that may radiate to the back. If there is an associated ventricular septal defect, a harsh pansystolic murmur may be heard at the lower left sternal border. Hepatomegaly is common.

The cardinal features of coarctation of the aorta include weak or absent femoral and pedal pulses, systolic hypertension in the upper limbs, and, usually, decreased blood pressure in the lower limbs. In the severely ill baby, there may be no murmur heard, the upper and lower pulses may be weak or absent, and the blood pressure may be diminished in all four limbs. Following vigorous resuscitation of the infant with low cardiac output, it is essential that the pulses and blood pressure be reassessed in order to detect their characteristic discrepancies and make the diagnosis of coarctation of the aorta.[34]

Generally, patients with coarctation of the aorta who present beyond infancy are asymptomatic, but the child may complain of weakness or pain in the legs after exercise. Physical examination reveals differential blood pressure measurements and pulses, as described for the infant with coarctation of the aorta. Usually it is the right arm pressure that is elevated because of the fact that the right subclavian artery most often arises proximal to the coarctation. A short systolic murmur may be heard in the third and fourth left intercostal spaces, with radiation to the neck and interscapular area of the back. The murmur of mild aortic stenosis may be heard in the third intercostal space and an apical systolic ejection click may be present. The presence of collateral blood flow may be detected by auscultation of a systolic murmur over the left and right chest posteriorly and laterally.

Complications. Children with coarctation of the aorta are at risk for congestive heart failure and infective endocarditis. Patients with associated cerebral aneurysms are at risk for cerebral hemorrhage. Aneurysms may form in the descending aorta or the collateral vessels. Hypertension may develop in the immediate postoperative period or late in the clinical course (see Table 47-9).

The postcoarctectomy syndrome usually occurs in the first week after surgical repair, primarily in children less than 5 years of age. The elevated levels of renin and catecholamines in the postoperative period are believed to cause spasm of the superior mesenteric artery and result in bowel ischemia.[34]

Ancillary Data. The ECG may show evidence of right ventricular hypertrophy and strain in the infant with coarctation of the aorta, with evidence of left ventricular hypertrophy in the first days of life. Usually the ECG tracing is normal in the older child.

The chest x-ray film of the infant with coarctation of the aorta shows evidence of cardiomegaly and increased pulmonary vascular makings. Rib notching secondary to collateral circulation is a characteristic finding in the older child. An area of poststenotic dilation of the aorta may be identifiable on plain radiograph and is best appreciated on barium swallow as displacement of the esophagus and discontinuity of the lateral margin of the aorta below the arch.

Although it is possible to identify discrete coarctation and isthmic narrowing of the aorta with two-dimensional and Doppler echocardiography, cardiac catheterization and angiocardiography remain important parts of the assessment of this lesion, particularly in the young patient.

Differential Considerations. Coarctation of the abdominal aorta may be congenital or it may be acquired in patients with an inflammatory type of aortitis similar to Takayashu arteritis. Abdominal coarctation also occurs in patients with neurofibromatosis. This entity must be considered when typical physical findings and radiographic evidence of coarctation of the aorta are not present.[34]

Management. A cardiology consultation should be obtained. Patients who present with signs of congestive heart failure should receive diuretics, digoxin, and inotropic support. The symptomatic infant requires surgical repair (see Table 47-8).

Ideally, children with coarctation will be identified on routine physical examination before the age of 5 years.[35,36] Optimal timing of elective surgical repair is believed to be between the ages of 3 to 5 years, in order to reduce the risk of complications mentioned earlier (with the exception of infective endocarditis).[34] Balloon dilation of coarctation of the aorta in infancy is associated with a high incidence of recoarctation. However, recoarctation of the aorta is usually treated in this manner, as are older patients with coarctation in some centers.[34,37,38] Prophylactic treatment for bacterial endocarditis should be given when indicated.

Pulmonary Stenosis

Right ventricular outflow tract obstructive lesions occur in 25% to 30% of all patients with congenital heart disease. These lesions include valvular and subvalvular stenosis, supravalvular stenosis, and supravalvular pulmonary artery stenosis of the main pulmonary trunk (seen in children with William syndrome) or the peripheral pulmonary arterial branches (particularly with congenital rubella syndrome). The incidence of isolated valvular pulmonary stenosis is between 8% and 10%.[39]

Pathophysiology. Valvular pulmonary stenosis consists of fused and usually thickened valve leaflets. In patients with Noonan syndrome, the pulmonary valves are often dysplastic. The right ventricle is hypertrophied, particularly in the infundibular area. There may be thickening of the tricuspid valve with right atrial dilation. Usually the foramen ovale is patent and there may be an atrial septal defect. Poststenotic dilation of the pulmonary artery trunk is nearly always present. In some infantile cases, changes associated with a hypertrophic cardiomyopathy may be present.

Right ventricular pressure increases in proportion to the degree of pulmonary valve obstruction. In the fetus with mild-to-moderate pulmonary stenosis, right ventricular output remains relatively normal because of hypertrophy and hyperplasia of the myocardial muscle cells. The infant is initially able to compensate with right ventricular hypertrophy, but over time will develop heart failure if the pulmonary stenosis remains fixed. Because of the diminished pulmonary blood flow at this stage, the patient may become peripherally cyanosed on exertion. Central cyanosis, on the other hand, is the result of right-to-left shunting across the foramen ovale or an atrial septal defect.

Diagnostic Findings

Clinical Findings. Infants with mild-to-moderate valvular pulmonary stenosis are typically asymptomatic. Although dyspnea with effort and mild cyanosis may develop in the older child, some individuals remain symptom-free into adulthood.

Patients with moderate-to-severe stenosis whose capacity to increase right ventricular output during exercise is no longer adequate are at risk for syncope and sudden death. Right ventricular failure may occur in infancy or early childhood in patients with severe stenosis.

Cardiac auscultatory findings in valvular stenosis are usually quite characteristic. A systolic thrill is palpable at the second and third left intercostal spaces and there is a prominent right ventricular systolic impulse. The first heart sound is normal, and the second is split in accordance with the severity of the stenosis. A pulmonary click precedes the systolic ejection-type murmur of pulmonary stenosis, which is best heard at the upper left sternal border and radiates to the precordium, back, and neck. The intensity of the murmur varies with the degree of obstruction. The murmur is usually longer with severe stenosis. With right heart failure there may be a fourth heart sound and the holosystolic murmur of tricuspid regurgitation may be present.

Complications. Complications include the development of congestive heart failure and susceptibility to infective endocarditis.

Ancillary Data. Polycythemia is present in cases with severe cyanosis.

The ECG is normal in up to one half of the cases of mild pulmonary stenosis and in the remainder may show evidence of right ventricular hypertrophy. With moderate-to-severe pulmonary stenosis, there is evidence of right ventricular and sometimes right atrial hypertrophy.

On chest x-ray examination the main pulmonary artery is prominent, and usually the pulmonary vascular markings are normal. Heart size is usually normal unless the stenosis is severe and heart failure is present.

Information from two-dimensional and Doppler echocardiographic examinations is usually sufficient to diagnose valvular pulmonary stenosis.

Differential Considerations. Mild valvular pulmonary stenosis must be differentiated from atrial septal defect, peripheral pulmonary artery stenosis, mitral valve prolapse, aortic stenosis, large arteriovenous malformations of the brain or liver (extracardiac shunt), and innocent murmurs because of potential changing flow patterns. The findings in moderate and severe pulmonary stenosis without cyanosis may resemble those of ventricular septal defect and pulmonary stenosis with right-to-left shunt. Moderate and severe stenosis with cyanosis should be differentiated from tetralogy of Fallot or other lesions with a ventricular septal defect and pulmonary stenosis. Newborns with transposition of the great arteries, pulmonary atresia and intact ventricular septum, and Ebstein's anomaly of the tricuspid valve may present similarly to those with valvular pulmonic stenosis.

Management. Congestive heart failure in neonates with critical pulmonary stenosis rarely responds to digitalis and these babies are best treated with an infusion of PGE$_1$ before balloon valvuloplasty.[39] A consultation with a cardiologist should be obtained. Pulmonary stenosis in the asymptomatic patient who is between the ages of 2 and 4 years is corrected by valvuloplasty.[38,39] Pulmonary stenosis secondary to a dysplastic valve is usually repaired surgically. Prophylactic treatment for bacterial endocarditis should be given when indicated.

Aortic Stenosis

Left ventricular outflow tract obstruction may be secondary to valvular aortic stenosis, subaortic stenosis, narrowing of the supravalvular ascending aorta, and certain forms of hypertrophic obstructive cardiomyopathy. Congenital bicuspid aortic valve probably represents the most common form of congenital heart disease. The incidence of valvular aortic stenosis is 3% to 6%. Not infrequently it is accompanied by other cardiac abnormalities, including patent ductus arteriosus, coarctation of the aorta, ventricular septal defect, and pulmonary stenosis.[40]

Pathophysiology. The aortic valve is thickened and often bicuspid. In severe cases there may be hypoplasia of the aortic valve ring. The pressure gradient across the valve is determined by the size of the aortic opening and the transvalvular flow rate. Critical obstruction is said to exist with a peak systolic pressure gradient over 75 mm Hg.[40] Most children have upper normal left ventricular end-diastolic pressures and normal mean left atrial pressures. An elevation of the former reflects impairment of left ventricle function or decreased left ventricle compliance. Usually cardiac output is normal at rest. Some children with severe stenosis may be unable to increase their cardiac output during exercise.

Left ventricular pressure overload leads to several problems in patients with aortic stenosis and compensatory left ventricular hypertrophy. Diastolic filling may be adversely affected by the left ventricular hypertrophy. With high left ventricular end-diastolic pressure, coronary blood flow is restricted to diastole, coronary driving pressure is reduced, and oxygenation of the myocardium may be impaired under some circumstances.[40]

Aortic insufficiency, which is present in about 25% of patients with valvular aortic stenosis, is not usually clinically significant. Aortic regurgitation secondary to valvular damage from infectious endocarditis is an exception.

Diagnostic Findings

Clinical Findings. Though usually asymptomatic, infants with valvular aortic stenosis may present with severe heart failure. These infants are irritable, pale, tachycardic, tachypneic, hypotensive, and sometimes cyanotic. Cardiac auscultation reveals a systolic murmur at the apex or the lower left sternal border.

Most children with aortic stenosis are asymptomatic, but those with moderate stenosis may complain of fatigue and dyspnea on exertion, abdominal pain, or sweating. Exertional syncope is indicative of critical stenosis.

Physical examination reveals a left ventricular lift and a precordial systolic thrill with moderate or severe stenosis. A systolic aortic click may be heard at the apex and is more common in mild or moderate stenosis. The second heart sound is single and occasionally is paradoxically split. A third heart sound is common and a fourth heart sound is indicative of severe stenosis. A harsh systolic murmur is best heard at the base of the heart and radiates to the apex and the neck.

Complications. The child with aortic stenosis is at risk for infectious endocarditis (risk unchanged after repair) and left ventricular failure. Sclerosis and calcification of the aortic valve may occur in adulthood. Sudden death (often during exercise) may occur in as many as 1% of patients with aortic stenosis per year; dysrhythmias are the suspected cause of death. The subset of patients felt to be at greatest risk of sudden death have severe aortic stenosis with left ventricular hypertrophy and left heart strain, or have a history of chest pain and syncope.[29] Serial echo-Doppler ultrasound assessments are generally recommended at one-to-two year intervals in asymptomatic children.[40]

Ancillary Data. The ECG usually shows evidence of left ventricular hypertrophy or strain. With pulmonary hypertension, there may be evidence of right atrial and right ventricular hypertrophy.

The heart size is usually normal on chest x-ray film. With more severe stenosis, the left atrium may be enlarged and the pulmonary vascular markings increased. Evidence of stenotic dilation of the ascending aorta is commonly seen.

Two-dimensional and Doppler flow echocardiographic studies are currently used to define the lesion. Cardiac catheterization tends to be reserved for use at the time of balloon valvuloplasty.[40]

Differential Considerations.
The diagnosis of patent ductus arteriosus, endocardial fibroelastosis, ventricular septal defect, other forms of aortic stenosis, pulmonary stenosis, peripheral pulmonary arterial stenosis, and rheumatic aortic stenosis should be considered. In the very ill infant, the diagnosis of hypoplastic left heart syndrome or severe coarctation of the aorta should be ruled out.

Management.
Strenuous physical activity should be avoided in patients with severe stenosis. Prophylactic treatment for endocarditis should be given when indicated.

Digitalis therapy is recommended for patients with diminished cardiac reserve, and for patients with left ventricular hypertrophy.[40] Balloon valvuloplasty appears to produce results which are comparable to those of surgical valvotomy. Some authors caution, however, that longer term follow-up is necessary to evaluate the valvuloplasty option.[38]

CONGESTIVE HEART FAILURE

Congestive heart failure (CHF) is defined as cardiac output that is not adequate to meet the metabolic demands of the patient. This manifests itself clinically by symptoms of pulmonary and systemic venous congestion, as well as various adaptive mechanisms that compensate for this failure of the heart.

In the pediatric age group, heart failure usually results from congenital defects in the structure of the heart, with acquired causes playing a minor role. With the predominance of congenital causes, presentation at an early age is the rule. Ninety percent of cases present in the first year of life, most in the first few months.[41] The younger the age of the infant at initial presentation, the worse the prognosis if the condition is left untreated.

The recognition and treatment of heart failure in children presenting to the emergency department will be emphasized.[42-44]

Pathophysiology

Determinants of Cardiac Output. To understand the functional basis of heart failure it is important to review the determinants of cardiac performance. This also helps understand therapeutic strategies in approaching heart failure, especially some of the newer advances that are aimed at altering the loading conditions of the heart.[45,46]

At all ages, cardiac output is determined by four main factors: (1) preload or the diastolic loading of the ventricles, (2) the afterload or systolic loading of the ventricles, (3) cardiac contractility or myocardial function, and (4) heart rate. Alterations in one or more of these factors may result in decreased cardiac output and consequently in congestive heart failure. Conversely, treatment that optimizes one or more of these determinants of cardiac output may alleviate the signs and symptoms of heart failure.

The ventricular preload is determined by the venous return to the heart and by the ventricular compliance. Clinically, atrial pressure is presumed to reflect the ventricular end-diastolic pressure or preload. In practice, right atrial pressure is estimated by measuring the central venous pressure (CVP), and left atrial pressure is estimated by measuring the pulmonary capillary wedge pressure (PCWP).

Increasing the preload results in a compensatory increase in cardiac output as illustrated by the Frank-Starling relationship.[46] However, beyond a certain limit, which is determined in part by the contractile state of myocardium, a further increase in preload will overwhelm the compensatory mechanisms and cause congestive symptoms. Examples of preload causing increased end-diastolic volumes and subsequent heart failure include large volume left-to-right shunts, valvular regurgitation, and volume overload from massive fluid infusions.[47]

There is an inverse relationship between afterload and cardiac output whereby an increasing afterload results in a decreasing cardiac output. This relationship is effected through decreased stroke volume. Conversely, decreasing afterload may result in an augmentation of cardiac output, a factor that has given impetus to the increased use of vasodilators in the treatment of heart failure. Afterload has been difficult to define in an intact heart and in clinical practice usually refers to the aortic pressure alone, although this is an approximation.[46] Examples of outflow tract obstruction that may cause increased afterload include coarctation of the aorta, aortic stenosis, and pulmonic stenosis.

Myocardial contractility refers to that performance of the heart that is independent of either preload or afterload. A decrease in the inotropic state of the heart may result from inflammatory disease such as seen secondary to viral myocarditis or Kawasaki disease. Disturbances of myocardial contractility may be caused by abnormalities in the metabolic milieu of the heart, resulting from electrolyte imbalances, hypoxemia, or hormonal changes (e.g., hypothyroidism).[47] When seen in combination with abnormalities in other determinants of cardiac output, the heart is less able to compensate and hence results in heart failure at an earlier phase than would have occurred with normal pump function.

Cardiac output is usually a product of stroke volume multiplied by heart rate. Hence, an increase in heart rate is used frequently by the body as a compensatory mechanism to maintain normal cardiac output. However, when very fast heart rates are caused by tachydysrhythmias, a fall in cardiac output will actually occur because of a decreased ventricular filling time. Infants seem particularly vulnerable to this; because of their limited cardiac reserve, they tolerate extremely fast heart rates less well than their older counterparts.[46] Extremely slow heart rates, such as those seen from complete heart block, may also result in heart failure.

Adaptive Mechanisms. In response to a cardiac output that is inadequate to meet its needs, the body responds with a variety of adaptive mechanisms. Sometimes, however, these mechanisms, such as increased adrenergic activity and peripheral vasoconstriction, may place the failing heart under increased loading conditions and paradoxically worsen the heart failure.

The ventricle responds to abnormal loading conditions by chamber dilation and hypertrophy. Ventricular dilation causes an increase in end-diastolic ventricular volume, which results in an increased stroke volume and an improvement of cardiac output. Another compensatory mechanism is hypertrophy of the myocardium, which attempts to maintain wall stress within the normal range.[42] However, both these mechanisms increase oxygen requirements and may make the heart more susceptible to ischemia. Fluid retention may develop as an adaptive measure, initially improving contractility along the Starling curve; decompensation may ultimately occur.

Once systemic cardiac output is compromised, the adrenergic system is activated as a homeostatic response, enabling the heart to maintain normal perfusion of the vital organs. Stimulation of the beta-adrenergic function will cause an increase in both cardiac contractility and heart rate, with a resultant increase in cardiac output. The role of the alpha-adrenergic stimulation is redistribution of blood flow. Perfusion of the brain and heart is maintained at the expense of blood flow to the kidneys, gastrointestinal tract, and skin. The reduced blood flow to these organs ensues from vasoconstriction of circulation as alpha-receptors are activated in these regions. This latter response of vasoconstriction can exacerbate cardiac failure because of an increase in the afterload.

Another response to the failing heart is a compensatory mechanism aimed at enhancing oxygen delivery to the tissues. This is accomplished within the red blood cell through increased production of 2,3-diphosphoglycerate, which then shifts the oxyhemoglobin curve to the right and improves the oxygen unloading capacity.[42]

Etiology. The more common causes of congestive failure are listed in the box on p. 646. Further discussion exists in the section on congenital heart disease and exhaustive reviews cover other etiologies in greater detail.[41,43,44] The importance of age at presentation is stressed. The age of presentation depends on the anatomic abnormality, the degree of pulmonary vascular resistance, the patency of the ductus arteriosus, and the limited cardiac reserve of the very young infant heart. About 25% of children with congenital heart disease have an associated extracardiac anomaly.

Birth. Heart failure in the first day of life is usually caused by nenoatal heart muscle dysfunction resulting from asphyxia, sepsis, hypoglycemia, hypocalcemia, or myocarditis.[43] Structural abnormalities that may play a role at this early age include tricuspid or pulmonary regurgitation, or systemic arteriovenous fistula.[41] Contributing neonatal heart rate abnormalities that may cause failure include paroxysmal supraventricular tachycardia or congenital complete heart block.

First Week of Life. A common cause of heart failure in the first week of life is the hypoplastic left heart syndrome.[41,43] These infants present with a sudden onset of a "shock-like" state when the patent ductus arteriosus closes. Other entities that present this early include aortic stenosis, total anomalous pulmonary venous return, and pulmonary stenosis.[43] Heart rate abnormalities and heart muscle dysfunction discussed above remain possibilities.

One to Six Weeks. The coarctation syndrome may present during this time period (7 to 14 days) with sudden onset of severe congestive heart failure.[41,43] This usually occurs when the patent ductus arteriosus constricts. The progressive fall of pulmonary vascular resistance during the first month of life results in worsening of left-to-right shunts. Examples include large ventricular septal defects and atrioventricular canal anomalies.

Later in Infancy. Most of the conditions noted above may present in this age group, but generally the symptoms will appear before the infant is 6 weeks old. Exceptions include patients with myocarditis, endocardial fibroelastosis, and those for whom heart failure is secondary to systemic hypertension or endocrine abnormalities (hypothyroidism or adrenal insufficiency).[43] Although endocardial

---

Causes of Congestive Heart Failure

Volume overload (increased preload)
1. Vascular-congenital heart disease
   Left to right shunt: ventricular septal defect (VSD)
   Anomalous pulmonary venous return
   Valvular regurgitation (aortic insufficiency)
   Patent ductus arteriosus (PDA)
   Arteriovenous fistula
2. Anemia
3. Hypervolemia (malnutrition, iatrogenic)

Pressure overload (increased afterload)
1. Vascular-congenital heart disease
   Ventricular outflow obstruction (aortic stenosis, coarctation)
   Left ventricular inflow obstruction (cor triatriatum)
2. Hypertension

Myocardial dysfunction
1. Vascular
   Pulmonary embolism
   Endocardial fibroelastosis (endocardial fibrosis)
   Anomalous coronary artery
   Pulmonary hypertension (obesity, pickwickian)
2. Dysrhythmia
   Vascular
   Atrial or ventricular: ectopic pacemaker or reentry pathway
   Conduction defect
   Metabolic: electrolyte, Ca^{++}, Mg^{++} abnormalities
   Intoxication: digitalis, tricyclic antidepressants, etc.

3. Infection/inflammation
   Cardiomyopathy
   Viral: coxsackie, influenza
   Bacterial: diphtheria, meningococcemia, sepsis, toxic shock syndrome
   Miscellaneous: toxoplasmosis, spirochetes, parasites
   Bacterial endocarditis
   Pericarditis: viral, bacterial, mycobacterial
   Pulmonary disease: chronic infection, aspiration, cystic fibrosis
4. Endocrine/metabolic
   Newborn: infant of diabetic mother, hypocalcemia, hypomagnesemia
   Hypothyroidism or hyperthyroidism
   Hypoglycemia: glycogen storage disease, etc.
   Pheochromocytoma
   Alpha$_1$-antitrypsin deficiency
5. Trauma/environment
   Cardiac tamponade, contusion or rupture secondary to blunt or penetrating trauma
   Hyperthermia
6. Autoimmune/allergy
   Asthma
   Acute rheumatic fever (ARF)
   Systemic lupus erythematosus (SLE)
7. Deficiency/degeneration
   Anemia
   CNS disease: progressive or degenerative
   Malnutrition: kwashiorkor, beri beri (thiamine), etc.
8. Intoxication: alcohol abuse, heavy metals, cardiac toxins (digitalis, beta blockers)
9. Neoplasm: metastatic or infiltration, atrial myxoma
10. Postsurgical condition

---

fibroelastosis has been decreasing in frequency, a form of familial cardiomyopathy secondary to carnitine deficiency has recently been described.[42,48,49] One acquired condition that must be kept in mind is Kawasaki disease, which may cause coronary arteritis and aneurysm. If sufficient myocardial dysfunction results from these insults, infants may develop heart failure.

Childhood and Adolescence. Congestive heart failure in childhood or adolescence is not common. Older children who have congenital heart disease may develop congestive heart failure because of the onset of valvular regurgitation or tachydysrythmias.[44] An example of this would be the patient with a ventricular septal defect who develops progressive aortic regurgitation with symptoms of heart failure in late childhood or adolescence. Patients with congenital heart disease who have undergone surgery may develop either left- or right-sided heart failure as a postoperative complication.[44]

Acquired heart disease causing heart failure is relatively more common at this age. Myocarditis and endocardial fibroelastosis may cause heart muscle dysfunction in this group. In addition, diseases that cause valvular regurgitation such as rheumatic fever or bacterial endocarditis may also cause heart failure.

Diagnostic Findings

Clinical Findings. In infancy, poor feeding is one of the important symptoms of congestive heart failure. Infants with heart failure may take very long to feed, with a noticeable increase in respiratory effort; hence they frequently consume less than their required caloric intake. Because of this inadequate caloric intake and an increased metabolic rate, weight gain is slow. Caregivers may also notice an increase in sweating, which is a consequence of increased adrenergic activity. These infants are prone to have recurrent lower respiratory infections.[43]

Older children may have a reduced level of exercise tolerance; careful questioning about the degree of physical activity is important. Paroxysmal nocturnal dyspnea may also be a symptom in older children. If there has been a significant degree of fluid retention from congestive heart failure, a recent increase in weight may be elicited. However, if children have been systemically unwell from their disease and have experienced anorexia or nausea, this may result in a documented weight loss.[44]

The classic presentation of congestive heart failure in infants is a pale and sweaty child with an increased respiratory rate. Other common clinical findings are tachycardia, a gallop rhythm, cardiomegaly, tachypnea, and hepatomegaly.

An increase in heart rate is frequently seen as a sign of the failing heart. Tachycardia is secondary to increased adrenergic activity as the body attempts to compensate for inadequate systemic perfusion.

A gallop rhythm is present when, upon auscultation, an S_3 sound is heard in addition to the usual S_1 and S_2 heart sounds. This S_3 gallop sound is believed to result from the rapid filling of a stiff, noncompliant ventricle, a condition seen in heart failure from large left-to-right shunts.[42] As therapy ameliorates the heart failure, this gallop rhythm will disappear.

Cardiomegaly may be difficult to diagnose clinically in infants because of their small thorax. However, the diagnosis would be supported by lateral displacement of the point of maximum impulse and a sternal heave. The definitive way of confirming cardiomegaly is the presence of an enlarged cardiac shadow on a chest x-ray film.

With systemic vasoconstriction, caused by the alpha-adrenergic adaptive response to heart failure, peripheral pulses will be diminished in intensity as compared to central arterial pulsations. In addition, the extremities will be cool and mottled with a prolonged capillary refill (>3 seconds). However, in the case of high-output cardiac failure secondary to a large aortic runoff from a patent ductus arteriosus, one may palpate bounding pulses. Pulsus paradoxus may be noted with large left-to-right shunts, primary myocardial disease, or pericardial tamponade.[42]

Most of the signs of left-sided failure result from pulmonary congestion. Tachypnea is an important early sign reflecting pulmonary venous congestion. As this congestion worsens, breathing becomes more labored, as noted with intercostal retractions, nasal flaring, grunting, and use of accessory muscles.

Adventitial lung sounds are usually not diagnostic of heart failure. Wheezing has been associated with pulmonary congestion.[50] This wheezing may be caused by airway edema ensuing from an accumulation of lung water, or by airway compression from the enlarged left atrium, and may cause the diagnosis to be confused with viral bronchiolitis in infants. Rales are not heard frequently during congestive heart failure in infants; hence their absence does not preclude the diagnosis of pulmonary congestion. Rales heard in a localized region of the lungs may be caused by a pulmonary infection (see section on Pulmonary Edema in Chapter 59).

Enlargement of the liver reflects systemic venous congestion, and usually results from defects producing left-sided heart failure. However, hepatomegaly may also be seen with purely right-sided heart failure, such as defects producing pulmonary hypertension or isolated pulmonary stenosis. In older children, distension of the external jugular vein is evidence of systemic venous congestion. Peripheral edema is rarely seen in children as a consequence of congestive heart failure.

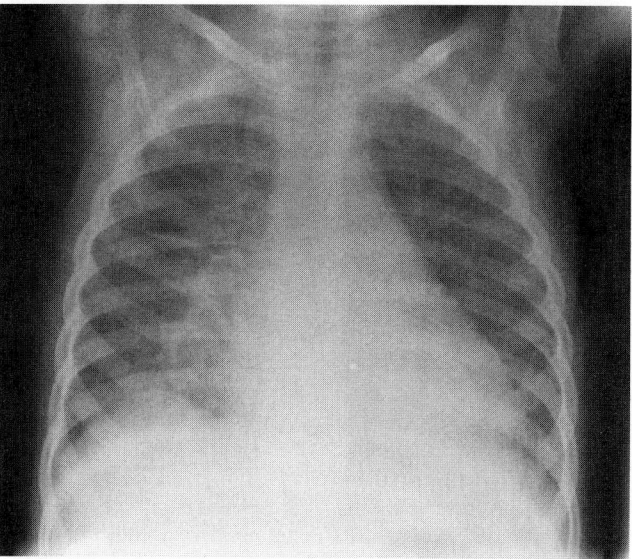

FIG. 47-1. Chest x-ray film of a 1-year-old girl with congestive heart failure due to viral myocarditis. The x-ray film demonstrates cardiomegaly and increased pulmonary vasculature.

Ancillary Data. The plain chest x-ray film is extremely important in assessing whether a child has cardiomegaly or increased pulmonary vascularity. Cardiomegaly is defined as a cardiothoracic ratio greater than 0.55 for infants younger than 1 year of age, and greater than 0.50 for children older than 1 year of age.[43,44] An example of congestive heart failure demonstrating the characteristic features of cardiomegaly and increased pulmonary vascularity is shown in Fig. 47-1. In the case of younger children, the thymus may still be enlarged and simulate cardiomegaly. This must be kept in mind when interpreting the chest radiograph. Although an increased heart shadow usually represents cardiomegaly, it can be seen if a pericardial effusion is present. In this case, the pulmonary vasculature is usually normal. Pulmonary edema is evidenced by the presence of fluffy infiltrates with perihilar haziness, Kerley A and B lines, or pleural effusions.

The ECG is usually not very useful in making the diagnosis of congestive heart failure. It may indicate cardiac chamber enlargement with nonspecific T-wave changes. In myocarditis, one may note low voltages with T-wave abnormalities. Electrocardiography is of course quite useful in determining whether or not the heart failure has indeed been precipitated by a dysrhythmia. Evidence of metabolic abnormalities may also be noted.

Ultrasound of the heart is an extremely useful test in making an etiologic diagnosis of congestive heart failure. For the child who is in severe congestive heart failure, urgent ultrasound of the heart can lead to an early diagnosis and can help to guide therapeutic efforts more specifically. Echocardiography is particularly valuable in assessing cardiac function, pericardial thickening or effusion, cardiac valve vegetations, and atrial myxoma and in monitoring the response to therapy. Nuclear scans may be useful in assessing ventricular contractility, myocardial perfusion, and cellular viability. The ejection fracture is a measure of function representing the percentage of endi-astolic volume that is ejected per stroke using ^{99m}TC radio-isotope.

Assessment of oxygenation may be done through arterial blood gas or pulse oximetry. Mild hypoxemia may be a result of ventilation-perfusion abnormalities caused by pulmonary venous congestion and alveolar edema. Obstruction of pulmonary blood flow or limited mixing from transposition of the great vessels may lead to more severe hypoxemia.[47]

Early in interstitial pulmonary edema one may measure a mild respiratory alkalosis, which is the result of an increased respiratory rate as the stretch receptors in the lungs are activated. As the pulmonary edema worsens and becomes alveolar, ventilation may become inadequate, leading to respiratory acidosis.

Metabolic acidosis may result from an inadequate delivery of oxygen to the tissues, which then causes a secondary lactic acidosis. This inadequate oxygen delivery may be caused by a severe compromise in systemic circulation (e.g., hypoplastic left heart syndrome) or from severe hypoxemia.

Hyponatremia may result from free water retention and reflects the infant's limited ability to handle a water load. Hypoglycemia has been observed in infants with severe congestive heart failure and this may be caused by the depletion of hepatic glycogen stores.[51] In neonates, calcium may be low and restoration to normal levels can improve cardiac function. Electrolytes and a complete blood count should be obtained. Cardiac enzymes including CPK-MB, SGOT, and LDH should be obtained if ischemia or an inflammatory response is suspected.

Differential Considerations. The difficulty lies in diagnosing infants, and the problem is trying to differentiate pulmonary from cardiac disease.[50] Respiratory distress as manifested by an increased respiratory rate or work of breathing is nonspecific. A noisy chest may preclude the adequate assessment of heart sounds and, in addition, heart murmurs may not always be present in cardiac disease. Whereas rales or wheezing are more commonly heard in conjunction with primary lung disease, they may occasionally occur in association with cardiac disease.

True hepatosplenomegaly occurs with congestive heart failure. However, in diseases that produce lung hyperinflation (e.g., bronchiolitis), the diaphragm will depress the liver and spleen into the abdominal cavity, giving a false sense of organ enlargement on palpation. This may be discerned by percussion of the liver, which will reveal a normal span in the case of lung hyperinflation.

An enlarged heart on x-ray study is one of the more important features that supports a cardiac etiology for respiratory distress in an infant. Although primary lung disease may produce mild-to-moderate hypoxemia, extreme hypoxemia usually indicates cardiac disease. Noncardiogenic pulmonary edema must be considered.

Differentiation between cardiac and pulmonary conditions is usually accomplished on a clinical and radiologic basis. However, there may be a few select cases for which this is impossible without echocardiography.

Management. The box above outlines the components of approaching a child who presents with possible conges-

---

General Approach to a Patient with Congestive Heart Failure

1. ABCs

Airway: Oxygenation

Breathing: If patient is in respiratory failure, assist ventilation

Circulation: IV access may be necessary for drug therapy

2. Supportive measures

Monitor blood pressure, pulse, respiratory rate, oxygen saturation

Temperature control

Rest: sedation occasionally required

Position: Semi-Fowler positioning

Diet: NPO if patient is in severe congestive heart failure; otherwise salt restriction

Monitor I and O

3. Specific drug therapy (as determined by patient's condition)

Inotropic support

Diuretics

Vasodilators

PGE_1

---

tive heart failure. The priorities of patient management will depend on the status of the patient, which is established via assessment of the patient's airway, breathing, and circulation (ABCs). Following stabilization, the therapeutic goals must be to improve cardiac performance, augment peripheral perfusion, and decrease systemic and pulmonary venous congestion. Close monitoring of cardiac and respiratory rates, blood pressure, oximetry, and urine output is important.

If the patient is very unstable and in impending respiratory failure or cardiogenic shock, efforts must be directed towards securing the airway, oxygenating the patient, and assisting ventilation as needed. In addition, IV access should be obtained and specific drug treatment administered as required.

If the patient is stable, the first priority after ensuring adequate oxygenation and assessment of the ABCs is to confirm that the diagnosis is indeed congestive heart failure and to identify its underlying pathology. As stated previously, this can usually be established through clinical assessment and ancillary investigations such as chest roentgenograms. If uncertainty still persists, echocardiography may clarify the situation.

Having confirmed that the patient is in congestive heart failure, therapy can be initiated. Basic measures include oxygenation, controlling the temperature, semi-Fowler positioning (patient inclined by raising head of bed), and rest (occasionally, sedation may be helpful).

Specific Drug Therapy. Specific drug therapy aimed at treating heart failure would include inotropic support, diuresis, and drugs that alter the loading conditions of the

TABLE 47-10. Recommended Oral Digoxin Dosage for Congestive Heart Failure

Age	Total loading digitalizing dose (μg/kg)	Maintenance oral dose (μg/kg/day)*
Full-term newborns (≤2 mo)	30	8-10
Infants (<2 yr)	30-50	10-12
Children (>2 yr)	30-40	8-10

Adapted from Park MK: *J Pediatr* 108:871-877, 1986.
*Divided BID; IV dosage is generally 75% of the oral dose for initial digitalization.

heart. At times a prostaglandin E_1 infusion may be lifesaving if a patent ductus arteriosus closes in a patient with a ductal dependent lesion.

Digoxin. If the patient is stable, then in most cases of congestive heart failure digoxin is the agent used for inotropic support (Table 47-10).[52] The inotropic response is determined by pharmacokinetic variables including bioavailability, absorption, volume of distribution, metabolism, and plasma protein binding. End-organ response is affected by the sensitivity of the myocardium and myocardial uptake. Infants often require a relatively larger dose than adults because of the infant's higher body clearance and larger volume of distribution; children require similar or lower doses than adults.

Recent evidence has questioned whether digoxin is in fact effective in all cases of congestive heart failure secondary to left-to-right shunts.[53,54] However, until this question is further clarified, a therapeutic trial of digoxin remains the recommended approach.

The onset of action is usually 5 to 30 minutes when administered intravenously, with renal excretion occurring in 48 to 72 hours. Oral absorption is equivalent to about three quarters of the IV route. In digitalizing emergently ill children, approximately one half of the total digitalizing dose (TDD) is given intravenously initially, one quarter of the TDD is administered in 6 to 8 hours, and the last one quarter of the TDD being administered 6 to 12 hours later, depending on the severity of the CHF. Relatively stable patients may be digitalized by beginning the maintenance dose of digoxin; therapeutic levels are achieved in 5 to 7 days.

Therapeutic levels are in the range of 1 to 2 ng/ml; most infants and children do not show toxicity until levels of 4 ng/ml are reached in the absence of electrolyte abnormalities or myocarditis. Levels should be monitored after initial digitalization, usually 4 hours after IV administration or 8 hours following an oral dose. Normal ECG findings associated with therapeutic digoxin include T-wave depression, ST segment depression (scooped), and prolongation of the P-R interval.

Digoxin is generally contraindicated in patients with idiopathic hypertrophic subaortic stenosis (IHSS) and tetralogy of Fallot and should be used with caution in patients with myocarditis or electrolyte abnormalities. The dose should be reduced in the presence of myocarditis,

pulmonary hypertension, decreased renal function, electrolyte abnormalities, hypoxia, and acidosis.

The therapeutic range between optimal therapeutic dose and toxicity is relatively narrow. Factors that predispose to toxicity caused by high serum levels include decreased renal excretion (premature infant or renal disease), hypothyroidism, high doses, and drug interaction (quinidine or verapamil). Increased sensitivity of the myocardium may be caused by altered myocardium (ischemia or myocarditis), hypokalemia, hypercalcemia, hypoxemia, alkalosis, sympathomimetic drugs, and following cardiac surgery.

Dysrhythmias are a sign of digoxin toxicity. These include bradycardia (infants <80 to 90 beats/min, child <60 to 70 beats/min, and adults <50 to 60 beats/min), atrioventricular dissociation and second- or third-degree block, premature ventricular contractions, ventricular bigeminy, and paroxysmal atrial tachycardia with block. Other evidence may include nausea and vomiting or blurring of vision.

Treatment of digoxin toxicity includes discontinuing the agent and beginning an IV fluid infusion of D5W with 40 to 80 mEq KCl/L at a rate of 0.3 mEq KCl/kg/hr with close monitoring, assuming that block is not present. Atropine may be used for bradycardia. If ventricular dysrhythmias are present, phenytoin 1 mg/kg/dose may be given intravenously over 1 to 2 minutes, and repeated every 5 minutes as needed up to a total dose of 5 mg/kg. Lidocaine and propranolol may sometimes be useful. Digoxin-specific FAB antibody fragments are useful in life-threatening conditions although there is only limited experience in children.

Adrenergic Inotropic Agents. If the patient is in cardiogenic shock, use of adrenergic inotropic agents becomes important.[55] If one is certain of this diagnosis, fluids should be used with caution. If preload is assessed to be low, an initial fluid bolus may improve cardiac output by increasing filling pressure, particularly if the pulmonary capillary wedge pressure (PCWP) is ≤15 to 20 mm Hg. Normal saline at 5 ml/kg over 30 minutes may be administered with careful monitoring.

Dopamine provides inotropic support to the heart, and lower doses will also improve renal perfusion. Dobutamine exerts selective inotropic support without the chronotropic effects but does not selectively improve renal perfusion. Low dosages of dopamine (0.5 to 3 μg/kg/min) may often be combined with dobutamine to maintain renal flow. Isoproterenol has the disadvantage of potentially decreasing coronary perfusion. Epinephrine and norepinephrine are reserved for children who remain in severe cardiogenic shock despite the use of dopamine or dobutamine (Table 47-11).

Diuretics. In pulmonary edema, airway and ventilation require immediate attention. Oxygen should be administered at 3 to 6 L/min by mask or nasal cannula. The need for intubation and mechanical ventilation should be assessed. Diuretics such as furosemide are frequently used to reduce preload and to improve the congestive symptoms present. This may be given orally or intravenously, depending on the severity of congestive heart failure, with 1 to 2 mg/kg used as a starting dose to be given every 8 hours. With large and repeated doses, fluid depletion or electro-

TABLE 47-11. Recommended Dosage of Inotropic Agents

Drug	Dose	Comments
Dopamine	2-5 μg/kg/min IV	Increased renal perfusion
	5-20 μg/kg/min IV	Inotropic effect
	>20 μg/kg/min IV	Vasoconstriction
Dobutamine	2-15 μg/kg/min IV	Mainly inotropic effect
Epinephrine	0.05-0.15 μg/kg/min IV and titrate	Side effects: hypertension and cardiac dysrhythmias
Isoproterenol	0.05-1.5 μg/kg/min IV	May decrease coronary perfusion
Norepinephrine	0.05-0.1 μg/kg/min IV and titrate	Intense vasoconstriction

lyte abnormalities are possible. Thiazide diuretics and spironolactone are usually reserved for ongoing management and rarely have a role to play in the emergency department (Table 47-12).

Vasodilators. In recent years, there has been a greater recognition of the importance of vasodilators in the treatment of congestive heart failure.[45,46,56] These drugs do not augment cardiac performance through direct inotropic support, but rather counteract some of the adaptive mechanisms that cause increased afterload. By lowering this increased load on the heart, cardiac output is improved.

In the emergency department, only rarely would acute use of load-altering agents be necessary. If the assessment showed that markedly increased vasoconstriction was seriously compromising cardiac output, load-altering agents may be considered. In addition, it is imperative that close hemodynamic monitoring be used when administering these drugs; hence this therapy is often reserved for the intensive care setting. Nitroprusside has the advantage of being continuously infused; hence the dose can be titrated according to the response of the patient (Table 47-13). If nitroprusside is unavailable, hydralazine may be a useful alternative. Prazosin has the disadvantage of potentially invoking hypotension. Captopril is used for the treatment of patients with chronic congestive heart failure.

Other Pharmacologic Agents. Morphine sulfate may be used to lower the PCWP and reduce anxiety. In severe pulmonary edema with CHF, 0.1 to 0.2 mg/kg should be administered intravenously slowly in patients with stable vital signs. It should be avoided in patients with intracranial hemorrhage, chronic pulmonary disease, asthma, or narcotic withdrawal. An important side effect is respiratory depression. An alternative for sedation may include chloral hydrate.

Bronchodilator agents may be indicated if there is evidence of bronchoconstriction as a cause for the respiratory distress rather than pulmonary venous congestion (see Chapter 59).

Anemia should be treated if significant (hematocrit <20%) to improve oxygen delivery; 5 to 10 ml/kg of

packed RBCs over 4 to 8 hours with careful monitoring may be administered.

For some infants, systemic perfusion may be dependent on the patency of the ductus arteriosus (e.g., interrupted aortic arch, hypoplastic left heart syndrome, and severe coarctation of the aorta). In such cases, infants may present with a shocklike syndrome when the patent ductus arteriosus closes. These infants may benefit from a continuous IV PGE$_1$ infusion (0.05 μg/kg/min).[57] A positive response is evidenced by a clinical improvement in systemic perfusion and an increase in the arterial pH. Although ideally one should ensure a definite diagnosis before starting an infusion, starting an empiric infusion of PGE$_1$ is warranted in cases in which one of the above syndromes is clinically suspected and the patient is in severe shock.[57]

It is important to emphasize that young infants who present with congestive heart failure may have a potentially life-threatening lesion that may require urgent referral to a cardiologist. At times, early surgical intervention may be critical.

Patients unresponsive to these therapeutic modalities should have other considerations evaluated in consultation with a cardiologist, including reactivation of rheumatic heart disease or concurrent infection such as endocarditis or pericarditis. Electrolyte abnormalities should be excluded, digoxin level measured, dysrhythmias treated aggressively, and pulmonary embolism considered.

Disposition. Factors dictating the disposition of the patient are availability of pediatric cardiac expertise as well as pediatric intensive care facilities. If patients are in mild congestive heart failure, they may be admitted to the pediatric ward where they may be monitored during treatment and further investigated. For patients who are extremely young (<3 months of age) or for older patients who are unstable, admission to a facility that provides very close cardiopulmonary monitoring is recommended.

Patients who may be discharged from the emergency department include those who have been previously diagnosed with cardiac disease, are already on established treatment, and have but a minimal change in their condition.

ENDOCARDITIS, ACUTE AND SUBACUTE

Infectious endocarditis is defined as an infection of the endocardial surface of the heart. It most commonly involves the valves, but may also affect the mural endocardium, septal defects, and vascular endothelium. Although infectious endocarditis may be classified as acute or subacute, the disease tends to be described in terms of the causative agent.[58] *Staphylococcus aureus* and *Streptococcus pneumoniae,* for example, typically cause a fulminant form of infectious endocarditis. Viridans streptococci and enterococci, on the other hand, usually produce a more indolent type of endocarditis.

Many reviews describe an increase in the incidence of infectious endocarditis in the pediatric population over the last two to three decades. Most authors have expressed their data as a proportion, with the total number of admissions to hospital as their denominator. Two large series report the incidence of infectious endocarditis prior to 1970 as 1:4,500 pediatric admissions, whereas the inci-

TABLE 47-12. Diuretics

Drug	Availability	Dosage				Onset of action	Comments/ site of action
		Route	Frequency	Initial	Maximum		
Chlorothiazide (Diuril)	Solution: 50 mg/ml Tablet: 250, 500 mg	PO	q 8-12 hr	10 mg/kg/ 24 hr	20 mg/kg/24 hr (2,000 mg/24 hr)	1-2 hr	↓ K$^+$, ↓ Na$^+$, alkalosis, hyper-glycemia; distal tubule
Hydrochlorothi-azide (HydroDiuril)	Tablet: 25, 50, 100 mg	PO	q 8-12 hr	1 mg/kg/ 24 hr	2 mg/kg/24 hr (200 mg/24 hr)	1-2 hr	↓ K$^+$, ↓ Na$^+$, alkalosis, hyper-glycemia; distal tubule
Furosemide (Lasix)	Ampule: 10 mg/ml	IV, IM	q 6-12 hr	1 mg/kg/ dose	6 mg/kg/dose	5-15 min	↓ K$^+$, ↓ Na$^+$, alkalosis, deaf-ness; may give more often; as-cending loop of Henle
	Solution: 10 mg/ml Tablet: 20, 40 mg	PO	q 6-12 hr	1-3 mg/kg/ dose	6 mg/kg/24 hr	30-60 min	
Spironolactone (Aldactone)	Tablet: 25 mg	PO	q 8-12 hr	1 mg/kg/ 24 hr	3 mg/kg/24 hr (200 mg/24 hr)	3-5 days	↑ K$^+$, ↓ Na$^+$; useful as adjunct, not alone; aldo-sterone antag-onist; collecting tubule
Mannitol	Vial: (250 mg/ml) 25%	IV (slow)		0.5 gm/kg/ dose	2.0 gm/kg/dose	10-30 min	Reduces intracra-nial pressure
Acetazolamide (Diamox)	Vial: 500 mg Tablet: 125, 250 mg	IV PO	q 6-24 hr	5 mg/kg/ 24 hr	8 mg/kg/24 hr	1-6 hr	Carbonic anhy-drase inhibitor; hyperchloremic acidosis
Metolazone (Zaroxolyn)	Tablet: 2.5, 5, 10 mg	PO	q 24 hr	0.2-0.4 mg/kg/24 hr	10 mg/24 hr (adult)	1-2 hr	Useful when marked ↓ glo-merular filtration rate; no experi-ence in children; renal tubule
Bumetanide (Bumex)	Tablet: 0.5, 1, 2 mg	PO	q 12-24 hr	0.015-0.1 mg/kg/dose	0.5-2 mg dose Max: 10 mg/ 24 hr		Little experience in children; side effects: cramps, dizziness; ↓ K$^+$, ↓ Ca^{++}, ↓ Na$^+$, enceph-alopathy. 40 mg furosemide com-parable to 1 mg bumetanide; cross-allergenicity to sulfonamides
	Vial: 0.25 mg/ml	IV	q 8-12 hr	0.1 mg/kg/ dose	0.5-1 mg/dose over 1-2 min Max: 10 mg/ 24 hr		

From Barkin RM and Rosen P: *Emergency pediatrics*, ed 4, St Louis, 1994, Mosby.

dence in the last two decades has been quoted in the range of 1:1,000 to 7:1,000 pediatric admissions.[59-62] In a study involving 30 North American centers, more than 20% of the patients with infectious endocarditis were less than 20 years old.[63] Most children who develop infectious en-docarditis are over the age of 2 years.

The increase in the number of pediatric cases of infec-tious endocarditis may be due to several factors. First,

advances in cardiovascular surgery in the last 30 years have contributed to the greater life expectancy of many children with congenital heart disease.[58] Patients in whom repair of their cardiac defect involves a prosthetic valve or construc-tion of a systemic-pulmonary shunt are at particularly high risk for infectious endocarditis. Second, many critically ill children undergo invasive procedures, such as the place-ment of intravascular lines (e.g., for cardiac pressure moni-

TABLE 47-13. Recommended Dosage for Vasodilators

Drug	Dose and route of administration	Comments
Hydralazine	0.75-3.0 mg/kg/24 hr PO q 6-12 hr up to 200-300 mg/day 0.1-0.2 mg/kg/dose IV q 6 hr	May cause tachycardia, GI symptoms, neutropenia, lupus-like syndrome
Captopril	Infants, 0.5-6.0 mg/kg/24 hr PO q 6-12 hr Children, 12.5 mg/dose PO q 12 hr	May cause neutropenia, proteinuria
Nitroprusside	0.5-8 µg/kg/min IV	May cause thiocyanate or cyanide toxicity
Prazosin	First dose 5 µg/kg PO Up to 25 µg/kg/dose q 6 hr	Initial dose used to evaluate hypotensive effects

Adapted from Friedman WF and George BL: *J Pediatr* 106:697-706, 1985.

toring or the delivery of hyperalimentation) and transvenous pacemaker wires, which may predispose them to the development of infectious endocarditis. Additional risk factors include the presence of a ventriculoatrial shunt for hydrocephalus or a dialysis fistula, abuse of drugs, and immunodeficiency states.[64]

In several large series, an underlying heart defect was identified in 25% to 90% of the cases of childhood infectious endocarditis.[59,60,65,66] With the decline in the incidence of rheumatic heart disease in North America, the vast majority of the cardiac abnormalities associated with infectious endocarditis are of congenital origin.[59-61] The two most common of these defects are tetralogy of Fallot and ventricular septal defect (usually small defects), followed in frequency by aortic stenosis, bicuspid aortic valve, aortic insufficiency, patent ductus arteriosus, coarctation of the aorta, transposition of the great vessels, pulmonic atresia, and pulmonic stenosis.[59,60,67-69] Unlike the older child, the majority of newborns who develop infectious endocarditis have normal hearts.[70]

Although it is recognized that the risk of infectious endocarditis is increased in the subset of patients with mitral valve prolapse who have mitral insufficiency, some authors also consider those patients with isolated mitral valve prolapse (such as some children with Marfan syndrome) to be at risk.[60,70] The subset of patients with a hemodynamically severe form of idiopathic hypertrophic subaortic stenosis appears to be at risk for infectious endocarditis.[71]

The patient with a simple ventricular septal defect has a lifetime risk for infectious endocarditis of 12% to 13%, which is reduced following surgical repair.[72] The patient with aortic stenosis carries a similar risk, which remains the same postoperatively. Infectious endocarditis occurs very rarely in association with an isolated secundum atrial septal defect.[73]

Although infectious endocarditis is no longer a uniformly fatal disease, it is associated with significant morbidity and mortality. The reported mortality rates for children with *Viridans streptococcal* infectious endocarditis and *S. aureus* infectious endocarditis are 9% to 14% and 33% to 47%, respectively.[59,68] Infectious endocarditis may occur in children under the age of 2 years.[60,74-76] The mortality rates for patients who develop infectious endocarditis within 60 days of either the insertion of a prosthetic valve or open

heart surgery are as high as 41% and 50%, respectively.[77,78] Survival of neonates with infectious endocarditis may now be more common.[60,69]

Pathophysiology. For infectious endocarditis to develop, an infective agent must be present in the bloodstream. Transient bacteremia may occur under many circumstances, including invasive surgical (e.g., insertion of central catheters, endotracheal suctioning in the neonate) and dental procedures. Up to 85% of patients will have positive blood cultures following either the extraction of abscessed teeth or periodontal surgery.[64] Although spontaneous bacteremia occurs in humans, it is usually low grade and thereby unlikely to result in the implantation of bacteria on heart defects.

The presumed sequence of events leading to infectious endocarditis in humans begins with the formation of a thrombus composed of platelet and fibrin deposits on the damaged endothelial surface of the valve. This initial phase is referred to as *nonbacterial thrombotic endocarditis*. Subsequently, bacteria or other microorganisms colonize the thrombus and multiply to form a vegetation, which may embolize to other organs.

Injury to the endothelial surface of a heart valve, a great vessel, or the mural endocardium may occur as a result of turbulent blood flow across a pressure gradient. Indeed, vegetations almost always occur distal to the pressure gradient and are found on the atrial surface of the mitral valve and the ventricular surface of the aortic valve when there is accompanying valvular insufficiency. The high degree of turbulence associated with small ventricular septal defects places patients with this congenital abnormality at risk of developing infectious endocarditis.[58]

In addition to hemodynamic factors, the induction of thrombus formation may be associated with stress, exposure to cold, disseminated intravascular coagulation, respiratory distress syndrome of prematurity, and hypoxia.[69]

A crucial step in the colonization of fibrin-platelet deposits on valve surfaces is the ability of certain organisms to adhere to the thrombus. Following endothelial damage, a number of normal components (e.g., fibronectin, fibrinogen) may become exposed to and permit adherence of circulating bacteria (and certain yeasts).[64] In the case of oral streptococci, some strains produce a complex extracellular polysaccharide (dextran), which increases the organism's adherence to valve tissue in vitro.

Following colonization of the valve, very large numbers of bacteria become surrounded by a thick mass of fibrin that essentially protects them from antimicrobials and host defense mechanisms. Growth of the vegetation may be promoted in several ways: (1) the phagocytosis of organisms by monocytes may produce tissue thromboplastin, which induces fibrin deposition; and (2) some organisms themselves may stimulate the production of tissue factor, which causes thrombus formation.[64] There may be little vegetation formation with some of the more virulent bacteria (e.g., *S. aureus*), which may rapidly destroy the valve.

Although immune factors are well described in infectious endocarditis, their role in the pathogenesis is unclear. It is postulated that rheumatoid factor interferes with IgG opsonic activity and may stimulate phagocytosis.[64] Circulating immune complexes have been implicated in the diffuse glomerulonephritis that develops in certain cases of infectious endocarditis, and in some of the peripheral manifestations, such as Osler nodes.

The pathologic changes in infectious endocarditis involve multiple organs. On gross inspection, the vegetations of infectious endocarditis may be single or multiple, measure several millimeters to centimeters, and are usually found along the line of closure of a valve leaflet. There may be destruction of the underlying valve. In addition, there may be evidence of any of the cardiac complications of infectious endocarditis. On microscopy, the vegetations consist of fibrin, platelets, and bacteria.

Emboli from the heart may involve any organ system. At autopsy, the renal, splenic, coronary, and cerebral vasculature are the most frequently involved. The kidney may show evidence of abscess, infarction, or glomerulonephritis (focal segmental glomerulonephritis, diffuse proliferative glomerulonephritis, or, less commonly, membranoproliferative glomerulonephritis). In 10% to 15% of patients, there is evidence of immune complex deposition in the kidney.[79] The immunoglobulin deposits are seen in a subepithelial distribution on electron microscopy in diffuse glomerulonephritis.

The middle cerebral artery of the brain and its branches are the most common sites of cerebral emboli. A wide variety of pathologic processes may be seen, including cerebral infarction, abscess, arteritis, cerebritis, mycotic aneurysm, intracerebral or subarachnoid hemorrhage, meningitis, and encephalomalacia.

Mycotic or infective aneurysms may be found on post mortem examination. They usually arise at the bifurcation points in vessels, which include the cerebral vessels, abdominal aorta, sinus of Valsalva, and the splenic, coronary, pulmonary, and superior mesenteric arteries.[75]

Infarctions of the spleen have been reported at autopsy, as have abscess formations and ruptures. Usually the spleen is enlarged with evidence of lymphoid hyperplasia.

Examination of the lung in the presence of right-sided infectious endocarditis may reveal pulmonary emboli, or evidence of pulmonary infarction, pneumonia, pleural effusion, or empyema.

The peripheral manifestations of infectious endocarditis may be seen at autopsy, including petechiae, Osler's nodes, and Janeway's lesions.

Examination of the retina may reveal hemorrhages with white centers (Roth spots). Rarely, the central retinal artery may be occluded by an embolus.

Etiology. A host of infectious agents may cause infectious endocarditis, the most common of which are streptococci, staphylococci, and gram-negative aerobic bacilli.

One collaborative study from 1979 reported that similar types of bacteria were isolated in patients with and without underlying heart disease.[64]

Streptococci and staphylococci are responsible for up to 80% of the pediatric cases of infectious endocarditis in which an organism is identified.[60,65,80] Among the streptococci that are most commonly isolated in infectious endocarditis are the viridans streptococci, *S. mitior* and *S. sanguis;* the nonhemolytic, non-*group D streptococci (S. mutans);* and the group D streptococci (*S. bovis*).[81]

Staphylococci are responsible for 20% to 39% of cases of infectious endocarditis.[60,65,80] Some authors have found an increase in the incidence of staphylococcal infectious endocarditis over the last decade.[60,82]

Neonatal infectious endocarditis is frequently caused by *S. aureus*, and by *S. epidermidis* when associated with an umbilical venous catheter. *S. epidermidis* is often responsible for the early (< 60 days from surgery) form of prosthetic valve endocarditis. The pathogenesis of late (> 60 days postoperatively) prosthetic valve endocarditis resembles that of endocarditis in patients with native valves.[77]

Gram-negative organisms were isolated in 2.5% of cases of infectious endocarditis in one series of children.[65] Although *Salmonella* species are the most common enterobacteriaceae isolated in infectious endocarditis, *Klebsiella-Enterobacter, E. coli, Pseudomonas,* and other species have also been implicated.

Candida and *Aspergillus* species are most frequently isolated in fungal infectious endocarditis. Neonates, drug abusers, patients who have undergone reconstructive cardiovascular surgery, and those who have received prolonged IV antibiotic therapy are at greatest risk of fungal infectious endocarditis.

Various series report between 8% and 16% of pediatric cases of infectious endocarditis with sterile blood cultures.[83] The multiple reasons for "apparent" culture-negative endocarditis are given in the box on p. 654.

Diagnostic Findings

Clinical Findings. The child with infectious endocarditis may present with a myriad of symptoms and signs, given the variability in the virulence of the infecting organisms and their propensity to cause local cardiac complications and extracardiac organ damage. The diagnosis should be suspected in any child with congenital heart disease and fever, any seriously ill neonate with unexplained septicemia, immunodeficient children with fever, and any child who develops fever postcardiac repair. The latter may not show the classic signs of infectious endocarditis.

Two broad clinical pictures of infectious endocarditis, acute and subacute, have been described. The latter group of patients generally presents with nonspecific symptoms such as malaise, poor appetite, fatigue, weakness, chills, night sweats, nausea, dyspnea, cough, chest pain, delirium, hemoptysis, back pain, vomiting, myalgia/arthralgia, and

Categories of Apparent Culture-Negative Infectious Endocarditis

1. Noninfective endocarditis or incorrect diagnosis
2. Prior antimicrobial treatment
3. "Fastidious" bacteria
4. *Coxiella burnetti*
5. Fungi
6. Acid-fast bacteria
7. *Chlamydia*
8. Forms of bacteria*
9. Virus*
10. Right-sided endocarditis
11. Uremia
12. Mural endocarditis
13. Cultures drawn at end of chronic course (> 3 mos)

Adapted from VanScoy RE: *Mayo Clin Proc* 57:150, 1982.
*Role uncertain.

TABLE 47-14. Clinical Manifestations of Infective Endocarditis

Symptoms	Percentage	Physical findings	Percentage
Fever	80	Fever	90
Chills	40	Heart murmur	85
Weakness	40	Changing murmur	5-10
Dyspnea	40	New murmur	3-5
Sweats	25	Embolic phenomenon	>50
Anorexia	25	Skin manifestations	18-50
Weight loss	25	Osler nodes	10-23
Malaise	25	Splinter hemorrhages	15
Cough	25	Petechiae	20-40
Nausea/ vomiting	20	Janeway's lesion	<10
Headache	15	Splenomegaly	20-57
Myalgia/ arthralgia	15	Septic complications (pneumonia, meningitis, etc.)	20
Chest pain	15	Mycotic aneurysms	20
Abdominal pain	10-15	Clubbing	12-52
Delirium	10	Retinal lesion	2-10
Hemoptysis	10	Signs of renal failure	10-15
Back pain	10		

Adapted from Scheld MW and Sande MA: Endocarditis and intravascular infections. In Mandell GL, Bennett JE, Dolin R, editors: *Principles and practice of infectious diseases*, ed 4, New York, 1995, Churchill Livingstone.

sometimes weight loss, over a period of weeks (6 weeks to 3 months). These patients are often infected with *Streptococcus viridans*, enterococci, nutritionally deficient streptococci, *S. epidermidis*, and anaerobes.

The acute form of infectious endocarditis typically follows a stormy course, with high fever and systemic toxicity developing over days to weeks (6 weeks or less). The organisms responsible for this form, among others, are *S. aureus*, *S. pneumoniae*, other nonviridans, nonenterococcal streptococci, and some of the gram-negative rods.

Fever is a very common finding at the time of diagnosis. A heart murmur occurs in 85% of cases but may be absent in right-sided and mural infectious endocarditis.[65] The "changing" murmur and the new murmur (usually of aortic insufficiency) are relatively uncommon.[84]

Other classical peripheral signs of infectious endocarditis are embolic phenomenon, splinter hemorrhages, and petechiae. Notably, Janeway's lesions and Osler nodes are very unusual findings in children (Table 47-14).

Patients with infectious endocarditis of prolonged duration frequently have splenomegaly. Arthritis may be present. In one series, signs and symptoms related to the musculoskeletal system were the only source of complaint at presentation.[85]

The physical findings that accompany intracardiac and extracardiac complications (due to emboli and circulating immune complexes) are numerous. *S. aureus*, among others, frequently causes cardiac complications secondary to local tissue invasion. Signs of aortic or mitral regurgitation may be present, as may those of valvular stenosis caused by large vegetations. The classic findings of aortic insufficiency, i.e., bounding pulses and wide pulse pressure, may be absent in patients with infectious endocarditis. A decrease in the intensity of an aortic stenosis murmur may reflect valvular destruction, whereas a reduction in the murmur of aortic insufficiency may be indicative, e.g., of an interventricular fistula. Over 90% of patients with a new regurgitant murmur will develop CHF.[64]

Infectious endocarditis in the drug addict typically involves the right side of the heart. These patients may present with signs of tricuspid insufficiency such as a gallop rhythm, systolic regurgitant murmur, and a pulsatile liver. Pulmonary findings compatible with pneumonia, pleural effusions, empyema, or pulmonary infarction may be prominent in patients with right-sided infectious endocarditis.

The clinical picture may be dominated by abnormalities of the central nervous system examination. Signs of stroke with hemiplegia, ataxia, aphasia, or altered mental status may be found. Patients may present with signs of intracranial mycotic aneurysms, such as severe headaches, seizures, visual changes, and cranial nerve palsies. Subarachnoid hemorrhage may occur.

The signs of extracranial mycotic aneurysms may be detected during the acute phase of infectious endocarditis or months to years later.[86] Physical findings may include loss or change in peripheral pulses, local limb pain, or abdominal pain. Occasionally there are no symptoms associated with these aneurysms.

Although the kidney may be affected, it is rare to see hypertension or edema in infectious endocarditis. Signs of uremia may be present in some patients.

Splenic infarction may cause left upper quadrant pain with or without left shoulder pain. Evidence of retinal artery emboli should be sought if the patient complains of sudden complete loss of vision. With pneumococcal endocarditis, a panophthalmitis has been reported to occur.

The neonate with infectious endocarditis typically presents with poor feeding, respiratory distress, and tachycardia. There may be a new or "changing" murmur, signs of congestive heart failure, or hypotension. The classic peripheral manifestations of infectious endocarditis are rarely seen in the neonate.[69]

Complications. Children under the age of 2 years are at high risk for complications.[74-76] *S. aureus* and, to a lesser extent, *S. pneumoniae* and other organisms show a great propensity to cause the following cardiac complications: perforation of valve leaflets; ruptured chordae tendinae, interventricular septum, or papillary muscle; valve ring abscess; pericardial or myocardial fistulae formation; and aneurysm formation of the valve leaflets or sinus of Valsalva. Myocardial abscess with or without conduction disturbances, pericarditis, and myocardial infarction may also develop during the course of acute infectious endocarditis. Uncontrollable congestive heart failure is the leading cause of death from infectious endocarditis.

Emboli to virtually any organ may occur, with the kidney, spleen, lung, and central nervous system among the most frequently affected. Fungal infectious endocarditis is often associated with emboli to major vessels. Some authors have concluded from a retrospective analysis that the risk of embolism is increased in patients with vegetations over 10 mm in size; others have found no correlation between the presence of valvular vegetations and the rate of complications.[87-89]

Mycotic aneurysms may occur in the cerebral vessels, aorta, sinus of Valsalva, and the pulmonary, coronary, splenic, and superior mesenteric arteries. They occur more frequently with *Streptococcus viridans* infectious endocarditis.

The risk of recurrence of infectious endocarditis is particularly high in drug addicts. Patients with prosthetic valves who undergo surgical removal of the valve are at risk for recurrent infectious endocarditis also.

Ancillary Data. The blood culture is the laboratory test that is most critical in making the diagnosis of infectious endocarditis. The bacteremia is usually constant and low grade. According to one review, the first two blood cultures will be positive over 90% of the time.[90] Another study suggests the yield may increase to almost 100% when three blood cultures are drawn.[91]

It is recommended that at least three sets of blood cultures be drawn in the first 24 hours.[92] It may be necessary to draw more blood cultures if there is a history of recent antibiotic administration. In children the volume of blood for culture should equal about 10% of the total volume of the blood culture medium.[58] There is no advantage to drawing arterial rather than venous blood with respect to the yield of positive cultures. As the bacteremia is continuous, it is not necessary to restrict the procurement of blood cultures to those periods of high temperature. Cultures should be held in the laboratory for at least 3 weeks.

Normocytic-normochromic anemia is almost always present. Thrombocytopenia is common in neonatal infectious endocarditis. The peripheral white blood cell count may be elevated. The erythrocyte sedimentation rate is nearly always elevated and may increase with progression of the disease. Serum C-reactive protein levels are usually elevated and may be of use in the follow-up of the patient. In up to 50% of cases of greater than 6 weeks' duration, the rheumatoid factor is positive.[64] The titers fall with therapy. High levels of circulating immune complexes may be found in infectious endocarditis and may be of particular use in the diagnosis of right-sided or culture-negative cases. These levels also fall with therapy.

With renal dysfunction, urea and serum creatinine may be elevated and serum complement levels depressed. The urinalysis is very frequently abnormal, showing microscopic hematuria and proteinuria, as well as red blood cell casts, pyuria, bacteriuria, and, occasionally, white blood cell casts.

Electrocardiographic findings vary with the presence or absence of cardiac structural or functional abnormalities and are not diagnostic of infectious endocarditis.

Although not diagnostic of infectious endocarditis, chest x-ray studies may reveal evidence of cardiac or pulmonary complications such as pulmonary edema, pneumonia, empyema, pleural effusions, pulmonary infarction, or mycotic aneurysms of the pulmonary or cardiac vasculature. The heart shadow may be abnormal if the patient has an underlying cardiac defect.

Echocardiography (two-dimensional and Doppler in particular) is a very important and sensitive diagnostic technique. It has primarily been used to identify the presence and specific location of valvular vegetations and perivalvular abscesses, and the presence of aortic or mitral regurgitation. A recent review showed that the following factors were predictive of a positive echocardiogram: a new or changing murmur, embolic phenomena, congestive heart failure, mechanical ventilation, and persistently positive blood cultures.[93]

The resolution around a prosthetic device tends to be poor and identification of vegetations less than 2 mm in size is not usually possible.[87,88] Despite these limitations, which to some extent, have been overcome with spectral Doppler echocardiography and transesophageal modes, sensitivity has been calculated as high as 90%, with rare false-positive results.[64] A negative study in no way excludes the diagnosis of infectious endocarditis.[69]

The assessment of the severity of aortic regurgitation is readily accomplished with the echocardiogram. If mitral valve preclosure occurs before the Q wave on the ECG, this is indicative of elevation of the left ventricular end-diastolic pressure. Rapid surgical intervention may be needed.

When surgery is being contemplated, cardiac catheterization and cineangiography may be indicated. Radiologic assessment of the various extracardiac complications requiring operative repair may include angiography, CT scan, (e.g., head, abdomen), and lung scan.

Differential Considerations. Several noninfective endocardial disease entities should be considered in children

---

Noninfective Endocardial Diseases

1. Myxoma
2. Rheumatic fever
3. Lupus nonbacterial verrucous endocarditis
4. Marantic endocarditis
5. Endocardial fibroelastosis
6. Fibroplastic endocarditis (Loeffler's)
7. Carcinoid

From Van Scoy RE: *Mayo Clin Proc* 57:150, 1982.

---

with signs and symptoms that are similar to those seen in infectious endocarditis (see box above). When a child presents with predominantly neurologic manifestations, the diagnosis of infectious endocarditis may be confused with that of thrombocytopenic thrombotic purpura. Children with malignancies such as leukemia or connective tissue diseases such as systemic lupus erythematosus, Kawasaki disease, or acute rheumatic fever may present in a similar fashion to patients with complicated infectious endocarditis.

Management. The patient should first be assessed with regard to his or her oxygenation and circulatory status. Patients presenting with signs of congestive heart failure, myocardial dysfunction, pulmonary infarction, or neurologic impairment will require treatment as outlined in the relevant sections.

Once the diagnosis of infectious endocarditis is suspected, the patient should be hospitalized. Admission to the intensive care unit may be necessary if the patient shows signs of cardiac, pulmonary, or central nervous system decompensation. Early consultation with cardiology, cardiovascular surgery, and infectious diseases services is recommended. The patient should be confined to bed in the acute phase and examined frequently with regard to the development of complications. Particular attention should be paid to cardiac auscultation, which is critical in the assessment of changes in valvular function.

General principles in the treatment of infectious endocarditis with antibiotics include the initiation of intravenous antibiotics and the need for lengthy treatment of prosthetic valve infectious endocarditis. In all cases, the minimum inhibitory concentration and the minimum bactericidal concentration must be measured for the antibiotics to be used. Although some controversy exists over the usefulness of the serum bactericidal titer in predicting clinical outcome, most authorities agree that a peak titer of 1:8 or greater is desirable.[94] Standard regimens include two or more antibiotics in order to produce bactericidal synergy.[95]

Guidelines for antibiotic therapy of staphylococcal and streptococcal infectious endocarditis have been developed by several groups, including the recommendations of the American Heart Association.[58,64,94] In all cases, it is imperative that an infectious diseases expert guide the patient's antibiotic regimen from the beginning. It is beyond the scope of this chapter to provide treatment recommendations for all the possible clinical scenarios of infectious endocarditis.

Infectious endocarditis caused by *S. viridans* or *S. bovis* should be treated with penicillin G 200 to 400,000 units/kg/24 hr q 4 to 6 hr (maximum daily dose 20 million units) IV for 4 weeks; *and* gentamicin 7.5 mg/kg/24 hr q 8 hr (maximum dose 80 mg) IV *or* streptomycin 30 mg/kg/24 hr q 12 hr (maximum dose 500 mg) IM for the first 2 weeks. If the patient is allergic to penicillin, vancomycin 40 mg/kg/24 hr q 6 hr (maximum daily dose 2 to 4 gm) IV for 4 weeks may be used. Modifications of these antibiotic regimens will be necessary if the streptococcal organism proves not to be highly susceptible to penicillin.

Enterococcal infectious endocarditis should be treated with penicillin G 250-400,000 units/kg/24 hr q 4 to 6 hr IV for 4 to 6 weeks; *and* gentamicin 7.5 mg/kg/24 hr q 8 hr *or* streptomycin 30 mg/kg/24 hr q 12 hr IM for 4 to 6 weeks.

About 40% of enterococci are resistant to streptomycin and, for this reason, some authorities recommend using gentamicin in combination with penicillin G initially. IV ampicillin in combination with either gentamicin or streptomycin is an alternative. In either case, most authors favor a 6-week therapy regimen. Patients who are penicillin-allergic should be treated with IV vancomycin and gentamicin or streptomycin in doses given for *S. viridans* infectious endocarditis.

Patients with nonprosthetic valve staphylococcal infectious endocarditis should be treated with the following: nafcillin (or oxacillin or cloxacillin) 200 mg/kg/24 hr q 4 hr (maximum daily dose 10 to 12 gm) IV for 4 to 6 weeks, with optional gentamicin 7.5 mg/kg/24 hr q 8 hr (maximum dose 80 mg) IV for 3 to 5 days. If the staphylococcal organism is resistant to methicillin or the patient is allergic to penicillin, the treatment should consist of 4 to 6 weeks of IV vancomycin.

Patients with staphylococcal prosthetic valve infectious endocarditis should always initially be presumed to be infected with a methicillin-resistant strain. The recommended regimen consists of vancomycin 40 mg/kg/24 hr q 6 hr IV and rifampin 20 mg/kg/24 hr q 8 hr (maximum daily dose 600 mg) PO for at least 6 weeks and gentamicin 6 to 7.5 mg/kg/24 hr q 8 hr IV for the initial 2 weeks.

Gram-negative bacillary infectious endocarditis is generally treated with a combination of a penicillin and an aminoglycoside for at least six weeks.[64]

Fungal infectious endocarditis usually requires prolonged treatment with amphotericin B, consideration of 5-fluoroconazole or other antifungal agents for certain fungal species, and, often, surgical intervention.[64]

When no organism is identified in the blood stream of the child with infectious endocarditis, several authorities recommend treatment with IV cloxacillin and penicillin G or ampicillin, *and* gentamicin (or streptomycin).[68] Treatment of neonatal infectious endocarditis should at least consist of a semisynthetic penicillinase-resistant penicillin with the addition of rifampin or an aminoglycoside if the patient is not improving. The duration of treatment should be at least 6 weeks.[69]

There are a number of indications for surgery in the patient with infectious endocarditis. These are as follows: (1) congestive heart failure that is refractory to medical therapy, (2) uncontrolled infection, (3) valve dysfunction, (4) ineffective available antimicrobial therapy (e.g., fungal), (5)

Prophylaxis Recommendations for Cardiac Conditions*

ENDOCARDITIS PROPHYLAXIS RECOMMENDED

Prosthetic cardiac valves, including bioprosthetic and homograft valves

Previous bacterial endocarditis, even in the absence of heart disease

Most congenital cardiac malformations

Rheumatic and other acquired valvular dysfunction, even after valvular surgery

Hypertrophic cardiomyopathy

Mitral valve prolapse with valvular regurgitation

ENDOCARDITIS PROPHYLAXIS NOT RECOMMENDED

Isolated secundum atrial septal defect

Surgical repair without residua beyond 6 months of secundum atrial septal defect, ventricular septal defect, or patent ductus arteriosus

Previous coronary artery bypass graft surgery

Mitral valve prolapse without valvular regurgitation†

Physiologic, functional, or innocent heart murmurs

Previous Kawasaki disease without valvular dysfunction

Previous rheumatic fever without valvular dysfunction

Cardiac pacemakers and implanted defibrillators

From Committee on Rheumatic Fever, Endocarditis, and Kawasaki Disease of the Council on Cardiovascular Disease in the Young of the American Heart Association; *JAMA* 264:2920, 1990.

*This box lists selected conditions but is not meant to be all inclusive.

†Individuals who have a mitral valve prolapse associated with thickening or redundancy of the valve leaflets, particularly men who are 45 years of age or older, may be at increased risk for bacterial endocarditis.

Prophylaxis Recommendations for Dental or Surgical Procedures*

ENDOCARDITIS PROPHYLAXIS RECOMMENDED

Dental procedures known to induce gingival or mucosal bleeding, including professional cleaning

Tonsillectomy and/or adenoidectomy

Surgical operations that involve intestinal or respiratory mucosa

Bronchoscopy with a rigid bronchoscope

Sclerotherapy for esophageal varices

Esophageal dilation

Gallbladder surgery

Cystoscopy

Urethral dilatation

Urethral catheterization if urinary tract infection is present†

Urinary tract surgery if urinary tract infection is present

Prostatic surgery

Incision and drainage of infected tissue†

Vaginal hysterectomy

Vaginal delivery in the presence of infection†

ENDOCARDITIS PROPHYLAXIS NOT RECOMMENDED‡

Dental procedures not likely to induce gingival bleeding, such as simple adjustment of orthodontic appliances or fillings above the gum line

Injection of local intraoral anesthetic (except intraligamentary injections)

Shedding of primary teeth

Tympanostomy tube insertion

Endotracheal intubation

Bronchoscopy with a flexible bronchoscope, with or without biopsy

Cardiac catheterization

Endoscopy with or without gastrointestinal biopsy

Cesarean section

In the absence of infection for urethral catheterization, dilation and curettage, uncomplicated vaginal delivery, therapeutic abortion, sterilization procedures, or insertion or removal of intrauterine devices

From Committee on Rheumatic Fever, Endocarditis, and Kawasaki Disease of the Council on Cardiovascular Disease in the Young of the American Heart Association: *JAMA* 264:2920, 1990.

*This table lists selected procedures but is not meant to be all inclusive.

†In addition to prophylactic regimen for genitourinary procedures, antibiotic therapy should be directed against the most likely bacterial pathogen.

‡In patients who have prosthetic heart valves, a previous history of endocarditis, or surgically constructed systemic-pulmonary shunts or conduits, physicians may choose to administer prophylactic antibiotics even for low-risk procedures that involve the lower respiratory, genitourinary, or gastrointestinal tracts.

mycotic aneurysm that requires resection, (6) most cases of prosthetic valve infectious endocarditis, (7) local cardiac complications (e.g., abscess and heart block, dysrhythmias), and (8) more than one systemic embolus.[58,64,96] Valvular surgery may be indicated after a single embolic episode outside the central nervous system, given that children remain at risk for a cerebral event following the initial embolism.[97] Patients with aortic insufficiency who develop congestive heart failure require prompt surgical attention. In both staphylococcal and prosthetic valve endocarditis, early surgical intervention seems to have improved clinical outcome.[77,82] Patients with right-sided infectious endocarditis often require a tricuspid valvulectomy in addition to their medical therapy.

Prophylaxis. The most recent recommendations by the American Heart Association for the prevention of bacterial endocarditis were published in 1990[98] (see box above). The standard prophylactic regimen for dental, oral, and upper respiratory tract procedures in at-risk patients is oral amoxicillin; oral erythromycin or clindamycin are administered to penicillin-allergic patients (see boxes above right and on p. 658).

An alternative prophylactic regimen for dental, oral, or upper-respiratory tract procedures may be used in patients who are at high risk of infectious endocarditis, e.g., patients with a history of previous infectious endocarditis or those with surgically constructed systemic-pulmonary shunts, or prosthetic valves, although the committee states that the standard prophylactic regimen is adequate. This regimen

Recommended Standard Prophylactic Regimen for Dental, Oral, or Upper Respiratory Tract Procedures in Patients Who Are at Risk*

Drug	Dosage regimen†
	Standard regimen
Amoxicillin	3 gm orally 1 hr before procedure; then 1.5 gm 6 hr after initial dose
	Amoxicillin/penicillin-allergic patients
Erythromycin	Erythromycin ethylsuccinate 800 mg, or erythromycin stearate 1 gm, orally 2 hr before procedure; then half the dose 6 hr after initial dose
or	
Clindamycin	300 mg PO 1 hr before procedure and 150 mg 6 hr after initial dose

From Committee on Rheumatic Fever, Endocarditis, and Kawasaki Disease of the Council on Cardiovascular Disease in the Young of the American Heart Association: *JAMA* 264:2920, 1990.
*Includes those with prosthetic heart valves and other high-risk patients.
†Initial pediatric doses are as follows: amoxicillin, 50 mg/kg; erythromycin ethylsuccinate or erythromycin stearate, 20 mg/kg; and clindamycin, 10 mg/kg. Follow-up doses should be one half the initial dose. *Total pediatric dose should not exceed total adult dose.* The following weight ranges may also be used for the initial pediatric dose of amoxicillin:
< 15 kg, 750 mg; 15 to 30 kg, 1500 mg; and > 30 kg, 3000 mg (full adult dose).

TABLE 47-15. Regimens for Genitourinary/Gastrointestinal Procedures

Drug	Dosage regimen*
Standard regimen	
Ampicillin, gentamicin, and amoxicillin	Intravenous or intramuscular administration of ampicillin 2 gm, plus gentamicin, 1.5 mg/kg (not to exceed 80 mg), 30 min before procedure; followed by amoxicillin, 1.5 gm, orally 6 hr after initial dose; alternatively, the parenteral regimen may be repeated once, 8 hr after initial dose.
Ampicillin/amoxicillin/ penicillin-allergic patient regimen	
Vancomycin and gentamicin	Intravenous administration of vancomycin, 1 gm, over 1 hr plus IV or IM administration of gentamicin, 1.5 mg/kg (not to exceed 80 mg), 1 hr before procedure; may be repeated once 8 hr after initial dose
Alternate low-risk patient regimen	
Amoxicillin	3 gm orally 1 hr before procedure; then 1.5 gm 6 hr after initial dose.

From Committee on Rheumatic Fever, Endocarditis, and Kawasaki Disease of the Council on Cardiovascular Disease in the Young of the American Heart Association: *JAMA* 264:2921, 1990.
*Initial pediatric doses are as follows: ampicillin, 50 mg/kg; amoxicillin, 50 mg/kg, gentamicin 2 mg/kg; and vancomycin, 20 mg/kg. Follow-up doses should be half the initial dose. *Total pediatric dose should not exceed total adult dose.*

consists of ampicillin, 50 mg/kg IV or IM, plus gentamicin, 2 mg/kg (not to exceed 80 mg) IV, 30 minutes before procedure, followed by amoxicillin (25 mg/kg) orally 6 hours after initial dose; alternatively the parenteral regimen may be repeated 8 hours after the initial dose. In the case of genitourinary or gastrointestinal procedures, however, the committee continues to recommend parenteral antibiotics, especially in high-risk patients (Table 47-15).

Erythromycin or an alternative regimen should be used as prophylaxis in patients with rheumatic fever who are taking oral penicillin for secondary prevention of rheumatic fever.

MYOCARDITIS

Myocarditis, a relatively common inflammatory disease of the heart, often accompanies pericarditis or may occur in isolation. Patients with this condition may present with few symptoms or may progress rapidly to cardiogenic shock. The reported mortality rates for children with myocarditis vary widely from 3% to 57%.[99,100] Most children recover completely without complications.[101]

The numerous infectious and noninfectious causes of myocarditis are well documented. Many other features of

this disease, however, remain incompletely defined. The incidence of myocarditis is difficult to establish given the wide spectrum of symptomatology and signs with which children may present. Most estimates of the incidence of myocarditis are based on postmortem examinations. In one series of 90 pediatric cases of sudden and unexpected deaths, 15 (17%) had evidence of myocarditis at autopsy.[102] Others have reported detection rates of 7%, based on autopsies of young adolescents who died unexpectedly in a nonviolent manner.[103]

The lack of consensus regarding the histopathologic diagnosis and staging (acute, subacute, and chronic) of myocarditis precludes a consistent approach to the classification of its causes. It is unclear, for example, whether dilated cardiomyopathy represents the end stage of active persistent myocarditis or is a separate entity.[99]

Pathophysiology. There are a number of possible cardiac findings at autopsy commensurate with the many causes of myocarditis. On gross inspection the heart may appear normal or there may be diffuse dilation with little or no hypertrophy. At the other end of the spectrum, left ventricular hypertrophy and endocardial thickening may accompany dilation of the heart. In the cases of bacterial and tuberculous myocarditis, there may be abscesses and caseous nodules present, respectively.

Myocarditis is generally defined in terms of the microscopic findings, which include the presence of inflammatory cells (usually lymphocytic and mononuclear cells) in the myocardium, with evidence of damaged adjacent myocytes. Evidence of sequential fiber necrosis, as is seen in coronary artery disease and ischemia, must by definition be absent. Although the infiltrates are often located in the perivascular area, they may involve the conduction system and the autonomic nerves. Their distribution in the myocardium may be either focal or diffuse. In an effort to standardize the classification of myocarditis, certain criteria were developed.[104] Accordingly, biopsy material may show evidence of active myocarditis at the onset of the illness, and ongoing, resolving, or resolved myocarditis subsequently. It should be evident from the foregoing that the location and extent of the lesion in the myocardium will determine the nature and severity of the cardiac dysfunction. These factors also influence the chances of obtaining affected tissue on endomyocardial biopsy.[99]

Infectious agents may cause myocardial cytotoxicity directly or by means of a circulating toxin or an immune reaction to the infection. Damage to myocytes may also occur in a nonspecific manner from the inflammatory process itself.[105]

Etiology. A host of infectious agents may cause myocarditis and are listed in the box at right.

In North America, myocarditis is most commonly caused by a virus, with coxsackievirus B and other enteroviruses accounting for a large proportion of these cases.[99] Absolute identification of an infectious agent is not always possible. Not infrequently, circumstantial serologic evidence of a viral infection is all that is available.

Immunocompromised hosts are at particular risk for myocardial infection with many organisms, including cytomegalovirus, Epstein-Barr virus, hepatitis B virus, candida, aspergillus, toxoplasma, and cryptococcus. The effect of human immunodeficiency virus (HIV) on myocytes is not clear.

Bacterial myocarditis is most often one component of a serious multisystem infection. Myocarditis occurs in up to 25% of cases of diphtheria and is the most frequent cause of death in that disease.

Many noninfectious processes may affect the myocardium (see box on p. 660).

Drugs may damage the myocardium by direct toxicity or hypersensitivity reaction. The interval between exposure to the drug and the development of myocarditis may vary from hours to months.[106] Heavy metals such as excessive iron or copper may cause a cardiomyopathy.

In the clinical setting, the cardiomyopathies are generally classified in one of three categories: (1) dilated or congestive, (2) hypertrophic, and (3) restrictive, based on the type of abnormal structure and dysfunction present. If a cause cannot be identified, the term primary is applied to the cardiomyopathy.[107] Although the dilated form is considered by many authors to be primary, others cite the findings of inflammation on some endomyocardial biopsies of cases of dilated cardiomyopathy as evidence of a link to myocarditis.[99]

Infectious Causes of Myocarditis

VIRUSES

Coxsackieviruses A and B
Echoviruses
Polio
Mumps
Rubeola
Varicella-Zoster
Epstein-Barr
Influenza A and B
Adenovirus
Cytomegalovirus
Hepatitis B
Others

BACTERIA AND RICKETTSIA

Corynebacterium diphtheriae
Streptococcus pyogenes
Neisseria meningitidis
Salmonella
Staphylococcus aureus
Mycoplasma pneumoniae
Borrelia burgdorferi
Mycobacterium tuberculosis
Chlamydia psittaci
Others

FUNGI

Aspergillus
Candida
Cryptococcus

PARASITES

Trypanosoma cruzi
Toxoplasma gondii
Others

Adapted from Savoia MC and Oxman MN: Myocarditis and pericarditis. In Mandell GL, Bennett JE, Dolin R, editors: *Principles and practice of infectious diseases*, ed 4, New York, 1995, Churchill Livingstone.

Diagnostic Findings

Clinical Findings. Myocarditis should be suspected in anyone with unexplained heart failure or dysrhythmias in the course of a systemic infection. Depending on the etiology, the stage of the disease, and the age of the patient, myocarditis may present in a number of ways.

Children may in many cases be asymptomatic and the disease may go undiagnosed. With infectious myocarditis children present with a febrile illness, the systemic manifestations of which may overshadow the less obvious signs of cardiac dysfunction. In these cases, the tachycardia is disproportionate to the degree of fever and should alert the physician to the diagnosis.

In other instances, the child may present with myopericarditis and minimal systemic involvement, sudden or recent onset of congestive heart failure, or with a dys-

Noninfectious Causes of Myocarditis[105,106]

COLLAGEN VASCULAR DISEASES
Systemic lupus erythematosus
Rheumatoid arthritis
Still disease
Polyarteritis nodosa
Sarcoidosis
Dermatomyositis
Scleroderma
Inflammatory bowel disease
Kawasaki disease

ENDOCRINE
Hyperthyroidism
Pheochromocytoma

RADIATION-INDUCED

DRUG-INDUCED (DIRECT TOXIC)
Cocaine
Alcohol
Catecholamines
Cyclophosphamide
Adriamycin
Daunorubicin
Arsenic

DRUG-INDUCED (HYPERSENSITIVITY)
Sulfonamides
Penicillin and its derivatives
Chloramphenicol
Streptomycin
Methyldopa
Amphotericin B
Phenytoin
Carbamazepine
Lithium
Emetine
Isoniazid
Hydrochlorothiazide
Indomethacin
Acetazolamide
Others

rhythmia and sudden death. More unusual childhood presentations include the clinical picture of a myocardial infarction (with viral focal myocarditis) and that of pulmonary or systemic embolism.[99]

The older child commonly complains of flu-like symptoms, with weakness and fatigue. He may feel short of breath, and have either chest or abdominal pain if there is a pericardial component. Myalgias are reportedly predominant in myocarditis due to *Mycoplasma pneumoniae*.

On physical examination, the child is tachypneic, tachycardic (may have an irregular rhythm), may or may not have fever, and is usually euvolemic. The first heart sound may be soft, and there may be a systolic murmur of mitral insufficiency (or less commonly, tricuspid insufficiency). In the absence of failure, the lungs are clear to auscultation. With heart failure, there may be cyanosis, a third heart sound, a widely split pulmonic component of the second heart sound, and hepatomegaly. A friction rub may be heard in the case of pericarditis. Hypotension may be present if the child is in cardiogenic shock.

The newborn and the older infant with myocarditis often present with severe respiratory distress and may progress quickly to cardiac collapse.[101] The newborn typically presents in the first 8 to 9 days of life with the sudden appearance of lethargy, pallor or greyness, and poor feeding. Occasionally, there may be a prodrome of poor feeding or diarrhea that is of several hours or days in duration. Commonly the physical examination of the newborn or infant with myocarditis reveals tachypnea, grunting, retractions, clear lungs on auscultation, tachycardia, and hepatomegaly. Fever may or may not be present.

Complications. The short-term complications of myocarditis include sudden death, dysrhythmias, congestive heart failure, and ventricular aneurysm formation. Over the days to years following the onset of myocarditis, a number of sequelae may be seen: persistent dysrhythmias secondary to conduction defects, a decrease in cardiac performance, recurrent inflammation, and chronic dilated cardiomyopathy with mitral insufficiency.[99]

Ancillary Data. The total WBC count and ESR are usually elevated and should be measured. A blood culture and viral serology should be drawn, as well as blood work pertinent to noninfectious causes of myocarditis if these are suspected.

Should the patient's condition warrant it, an arterial blood gas should be drawn. The levels of aspartate transaminase (AST), lactic dehydrogenase (LDH with LD isoenzyme), and creatinine phosphokinase (CPK with MB fraction) may be elevated, and provide supportive evidence of myocarditis.

Throat, stool, urine, and, when appropriate, cerebrospinal fluid specimens should be sent for identification of a viral infection. If tuberculosis is suspected, a purified protein derivative (PPD) should be placed on the skin.

ECG findings are nonspecific and may include diffuse S-T segment abnormalities, evolving T-wave inversion, and atrial and ventricular dysrhythmias with variable degrees of heart block. Occasionally the tracing may be normal.[99]

Chest x-ray studies will in many cases demonstrate evidence of cardiomegaly or pericardial effusion. Evidence of pulmonary edema may be seen when heart failure is present.

Echocardiography is a valuable and sensitive technique in the assessment of left ventricular function and the detection of pericardial effusions.[101] In patients with heart failure, the left ventricular end-diastolic and end-systolic diameters are increased and the shortening fraction is decreased. Very often there is widespread left ventricle free wall asynergistic motion. With mild myocarditis, regional wall motion abnormalities may be detected and the left ventricle size may be normal.

Regional wall motion abnormalities may also be demonstrated with gated blood pool studies.[108] Scintigraphy with gallium 67 (^{67}Ga) citrate is a sensitive but nonspecific method for the identification of myocardial inflammation.[99] Scanning with technetium pyrophosphate may be used to identify patients with focal or diffuse myocardial necrosis.[109]

Endomyocardial biopsy remains the gold standard for the diagnosis of myocarditis, despite the lack of uniform criteria for interpretation of the histologic findings. The diagnostic sensitivity of the endomyocardial biopsy may be enhanced by polymerase chain reaction (PCR) analysis of the tissue. Both adenoviral and enteroviral genomes have been detected by PCR in myocardial specimens from children with suspected acute viral myocarditis.[110] Coronary angiography may occasionally be indicated in the patient with myocarditis who presents with the findings of an acute myocardial infarction.

Differential Considerations. Numerous conditions may cause similar signs and symptoms to those seen in myocarditis. Some authors consider hypertrophic cardiomyopathy to be a primary disorder; others include secondary causes in this category. Among the conditions in which left ventricular hypertrophy may occur are Friedreich ataxia, tuberous sclerosis, Pompe disease, Hurler disease, neurofibromatosis, lentiginosis, certain muscular dystrophies, Turner and Noonan syndromes, and the transient cardiomyopathy of infants of diabetic mothers. Restrictive cardiomyopathy is rare in infants and children. Systemic arteriovenous malformations and anemias may lead to secondary cardiac dilation. Mitral valve prolapse may, in a subset of children, be associated with cardiomyopathy and dysrhythmias.

Management. The patient should first be assessed with regard to oxygenation and circulatory status. Oxygen should be administered and the patient's response to this maneuver should be monitored by oximetry or serial arterial blood gas sampling. Intravenous access should be obtained. Early consultation with a cardiologist is advisable.

If the patient is in cardiogenic shock, the physician should proceed to endotracheal intubation, central venous access, and inotropic support (see Chapter 13).

All patients should be admitted to the intensive care unit for close cardiorespiratory monitoring. Ideally a cardiovascular surgery service should be available. Particular attention should be paid to the development of signs of ventricular failure, which include hypoxia, pleural effusions, and pulmonary edema. Cardiac contractility may be improved with the use of agents that reduce the workload of the heart. However, digoxin must be given with extreme caution because the inflamed myocardium is sensitive. In acute situations, pressor agents may be required. If the preload is adequate and pressor and inotropic agents are not effective, vasodilators may be considered in the patient whose cardiac pressures can be appropriately monitored. Several reports describe successful treatment of young children with acute myocarditis and severe cardiac dysfunction with extracorporeal membrane oxygenation.[111,112]

The patient who develops congestive heart failure may require intravenous furosemide (1 mg/kg/dose). Cardiac pacing is indicated to treat complete heart block, should it develop. Dysrhythmias should be treated with caution, as most antidysrhythmic medications depress the myocardium.[107] Beta-blocker agents should not be used.

Intravenous antibiotics may be started empirically in the infant who presents with myocarditis.[107] Bed rest and adequate oxygenation must be ensured in the acute phase of myocarditis (usually 10 to 14 days in the case of viral myocarditis).

There is preliminary evidence to suggest that treatment of children with acute myocarditis with high-dose intravenous gamma globulin may be associated with improved recovery of left ventricular function. The rate of survival during the year following onset of acute myocarditis appears to be greater among patients who receive this treatment.[113]

Whether or not immunosuppressive agents are indicated in the management of myocarditis is still being debated.[99,101,107] Both beneficial and noxious effects of immunosuppressants have been reported in children with myocarditis.[101,113,114] Certainly there is ample laboratory evidence of a deleterious effect of steroids and of cyclosporine on murine myocardium in the acute phase of coxsackievirus infection.[115] Viral replication and myocardial necrosis were enhanced and the mortality rate increased in these animal models. Similar adverse effects have been documented in animals with viral myocarditis that received early treatment with nonsteroidal antiinflammatory agents.[116] Until the beneficial effect of immunosuppressive therapy is demonstrated in controlled clinical trials, steroid therapy should probably be withheld in acute viral myocarditis.[101,105]

Kawasaki disease may present with symptomatic myocarditis. The reader is referred to the section on infectious disorders for a discussion of the treatment of Kawasaki disease (see Chapter 55).

Throughout the early convalescent phase of viral myocarditis, strenuous physical activity should be avoided. Ambulatory ECG monitoring and exercise testing may provide useful information during the recovery phase of myocarditis, with respect to the identification of residual dysrhythmias and the need for subsequent treatment.[99]

PERICARDIAL DISEASES

Pericarditis is defined as an inflammatory condition of the pericardium that is caused by a number of infectious and noninfectious diseases. Not infrequently, there is an accompanying component of myocarditis. Fluid may accumulate in the pericardial sac as a result of the inflammatory process and may in some instances lead to cardiac tamponade and diminished cardiac output. This life-threatening situation requires immediate recognition and intervention.

The exact incidence of pericarditis is not known. In one large review of purulent pericarditis, more than half of the patients were less than 20 years of age.[117] Although viral pericarditis appears to be a relatively benign and common form of the disease, tuberculous and bacterial pericarditis may cause significant morbidity and mortality.

Pathophysiology. The pathophysiology of pericarditis is best appreciated by examining the anatomy of the pericardium. The pericardial sac consists of two layers, the visceral and the parietal pericardium, between which lie 10 to 15 ml of clear fluid in a healthy child. The pericardium surrounds the heart and the base of the great arteries and is in direct contact with the pleura, the mediastinum and its structures, and the sternum.

When there is an acute build-up of pericardial fluid, cardiac output falls. Several mechanisms explain this fall.[118] The normal pressure gradient between the pulmonary veins and the left atrium falls, as does that across the AV valves. The latter is caused by an increase in end-diastolic filling pressure in the ventricles. As a result, cardiac output and coronary perfusion decrease and a vicious cycle ensues. The reflex vasoconstriction and tachycardia that follow these events during cardiac tamponade are of limited effectiveness in maintaining cardiac output and the blood pressure will eventually fall.

A significant pulsus paradoxus occurs during cardiac tamponade. It is measurable as a fall in pulse pressure during inspiration of more than 10 mm Hg and reflects an exaggeration of the normal decrease in systemic output during inspiration, caused by a reduction of blood return to the left heart.

Etiology. Viruses, particularly the coxsackieviruses, are frequently implicated in the development of myopericarditis. Although viral agents have been isolated from pericardial fluid, more often the evidence of a viral cause has been circumstantial, based on serology or isolation of a virus from another body site.[119] A host of agents have been implicated (see box at right). The entity of acute "benign" pericarditis is usually classified as idiopathic, although a viral etiology is suspected in many of these cases.[119]

The bacteria that account for most of the cases of pyogenic pericarditis include *S. aureus, Haemophilus influenzae, Neisseria meningitidis,* and *Streptococcus pneumoniae,* and are listed in the box at right. In children, *S. aureus* has been reported as the etiologic agent in 43% to 100% of cases in several series.[118,120-122] The bacteria usually reach the pericardium by hematogenous spread from remote foci of infection, which include bone and less commonly lung and skin.[118]

H. influenzae is the second most common infectious cause of pericarditis in children and is associated with a respiratory infection in over 90% of cases.[118,123] In more than 90% of cases caused by *Neisseria meningitides,* meningitis occurs concomitantly.[118] Streptococci other than pneumococcus, which may cause pericarditis, are usually beta-hemolytic streptococci.

Fungal pericarditis may be a rare complication of cardiothoracic surgery. Immunocompromised hosts are at risk for this type of infection.

Pericarditis may occur in association with many noninfectious conditions, which are listed in the box on p. 663. There are reports of pericarditis occurring with inflammatory bowel disease.[124]

The postpericardiotomy syndrome may occur in up to 15% of patients, 1 to 2 weeks postoperatively, at which time the patient generally presents with fever, chest pain, pleural and pericardial effusions, and fluid retention.[118] The fluid accumulation in the pericardial sac appears to be the result of a hypersensitivity reaction to the trauma sustained by the pericardial and epicardial surfaces of the heart.

Diagnostic Findings

Clinical Findings. Typically, the child has respiratory difficulty at the time of presentation, with a history of an upper respiratory tract infection, including fever and cough. The older child may complain of abdominal or chest

---

Infectious Causes of Pericarditis

VIRUSES
Coxsackieviruses A and B
Echovirus
Mumps
Influenza
Epstein-Barr
Varicella-zoster
Cytomegalovirus
Herpes simplex
Hepatitis B

BACTERIA
Streptococcus pneumoniae
Staphylococcus aureus
Neisseria meningitidis
Haemophilus influenzae
Salmonella
Mycoplasma pneumoniae
Mycobacterium tuberculosis
Borrelia burgdorferi
Others

FUNGI
Histoplasma capsulatum
Coccidioides immitis
Blastomyces dermatidis
Cryptococcus neoformans
Candida species
Aspergillus species

PARASITES
Toxoplasma gondii
Entamoeba histolytica
Schistosomes

Adapted from Savoia MC and Oxman MN: Myocarditis and pericarditis. In Mandell GL, Bennett JE, Dolin R, editors: *Principles and practice of infectious diseases,* ed 4, New York, 1995, Churchill Livingstone.

---

pain, which may radiate to the shoulder. The pain is usually described as sharp and may be exacerbated by lying down and relieved by sitting forward. The child may be restless.

Like the symptoms, some of the physical findings will vary according to the rate and degree of pericardial fluid accumulation. The child is in respiratory distress, with tachypnea and tachycardia. He or she may be febrile. The lungs are usually clear upon auscultation. Signs of cardiac tamponade include distension of the neck veins, hepatomegaly, a quiet precordium with distant heart sounds, and a pulsus paradoxus of greater than 10 mm Hg. There may or may not be a friction rub heard over the precordium. Rarely, there may be hypotension.

Complications. Often pericarditis is accompanied by a component of myocarditis.[118,119] Congestive heart failure,

Noninfectious Causes of Pericarditis

COLLAGEN VASCULAR DISEASE
Systemic lupus erythematosus
Rheumatoid arthritis
Polyarteritis nodosa
Sarcoidosis
Scleroderma
Acute rheumatic fever
Kawasaki disease
Inflammatory bowel disease

UREMIA

NEOPLASM
Primary
Metastatic

POSTIRRADIATION

POSTTRAUMA

POSTPERICARDIOTOMY SYNDROME

DRUG-INDUCED
Procainamide
Practolol
Hydralazine
Isoniazid

MYXEDEMA

GOUT

CHRONIC ANEMIAS
Sickle cell disease
Thalassemia
Others

Adapted from Savoia MC and Oxman MN: Myocarditis and pericarditis. In Mandell GL, Bennett JE, Dolin R, editors: *Principles and practice of infectious diseases*, ed 4, New York, 1995, Churchill Livingstone.

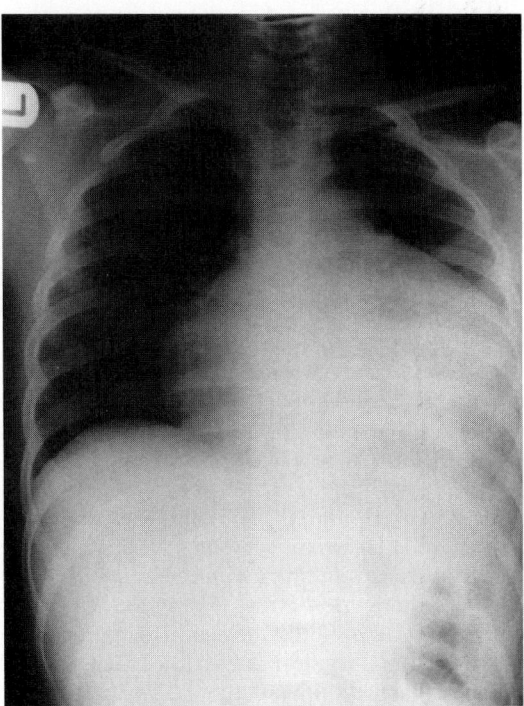

FIG. 47-2. Chest x-ray film shows pericardial effusion. Note "water-bottle" shaped heart.

shock, dysrhythmias, and death number among the immediate complications. Constrictive pericarditis is thought by some to be a late sequela of tuberculous or purulent pericarditis, occurring days to months later.[118] However, in more than 50% of cases of constrictive pericarditis, the etiology is not clear. Recurrences of viral or idiopathic pericarditis may occur.

Ancillary Data. The peripheral WBC count is usually elevated in the case of purulent pericarditis and may be normal in the viral form. Blood cultures should be drawn before antibiotic therapy is begun. Blood urea nitrogen (BUN), creatinine, and arterial blood gases should be measured.

Appropriate diagnostic blood tests may be performed if a noninfectious cause of pericarditis is suspected. Some of these tests are the erythrocyte sedimentation rate, anti-nuclear antibodies, rheumatoid factor, electrolytes, BUN, creatinine, uric acid, and thyroid functions. In addition, viral serology and urine, stool, and throat cultures for isolation of a virus should be sent for analysis. When indicated, a purified protein derivative (PPD) should be placed on the skin.

The ECG may reveal S-T segment elevation and generalized T-wave inversion on the tracing. According to one source, 90% of tracings show these nonspecific abnormalities in the setting of pericarditis.[125]

If a major pericardial effusion is present, the heart shadow will be enlarged in the form of a "water-bottle" (Fig. 47-2) on the chest x-ray film. Generally, the lung fields are clear. There may be evidence of empyema or pleural effusions. Fluoroscopy may be useful in defining the variations in heart size during the cardiac cycle.

The echocardiogram is a very sensitive technique for the detection of a pericardial effusion, which is demonstrable as an echo-free space between the epicardium and the pericardium.

Technetium pertechnetate angiocardiography nuclear scans may be used to confirm the presence of pericardial effusion.[118]

Although it is not necessary in all cases to perform a pericardiocentesis (e.g., in acute benign pericarditis), the examination and culture of pericardial fluid remain the sine qua non in the establishment of the diagnosis of pericarditis.[118] The pericardial fluid should be directly inoculated into bacterial culture medium and sent for gram stain, fungal and mycobacterial culture and stain, cell count and differential, protein, glucose, LDH, and cell cytology. In purulent pericarditis there is usually a marked leucocytosis with a variable protein level and low glucose level. The fluid is usually serous in viral pericarditis, with polymorphonuclear or mononuclear cells. In the case of tuberculosis, the fluid is sanguinous and the cells are primarily lymphocytic.

The procedure is generally performed with the patient supine, leaning backward at a 45-degree angle and supported by the bed or pillows in a reverse Trendelenburg position. After preparing, cleaning, and draping the left subxiphoid area, an 18- or 20-gauge metal 3-inch spinal needle is aimed cephalad and backward toward the tip of the left scapula. The needle is attached to a three-way stopcock and a 20-ml syringe. One end of an alligator clip is attached to the needle's base and the other end to the V lead on an ECG.

The needle is advanced under negative pressure and as the pericardium is entered, generally a distinct "pop" is heard. If there is an injury current with ST-T changes on the ECG, the epicardium has been entered and the needle should be withdrawn slightly. Aspiration is performed. Removal of as little as 50 ml may temporarily relieve tamponade and improve cardiac output. Complications to be monitored include pneumothorax, coronary artery injury, myocardial, liver or aorta laceration, dysrhythmias, and bleeding.[118]

Differential Considerations. Differential diagnoses include sepsis with or without pneumonia, myocarditis, constrictive pericarditis, and congestive or restrictive cardiomyopathy.

Management. Supportive therapy should include delivering oxygen and ensuring an adequate airway. If available, an oximeter is one way of assessing the patient's oxygenation status in an ongoing manner. Intravenous access should be established. Vital signs, including blood pressure, should be monitored closely. Early consultation with a cardiologist is critical.

Decompression of the pericardium should be accomplished by pericardiocentesis if there is evidence of cardiac tamponade (see above) and should be done in an urgent fashion by an experienced physician. Intravenous fluids should be given if hypotension occurs during the procedure. Open surgical drainage is usually necessary if purulent pericarditis is suspected after needle drainage because the fluid is typically thick and loculated in the pericardial sac.[118]

In a well-compensated patient in whom the removal of pericardial fluid is for diagnostic purposes, pericardiocentesis is ideally and most safely accomplished under fluoroscopy or ultrasound guidance in a controlled setting (the intensive care unit or the cardiac catheterization laboratory).[118] This procedure is associated with morbidity and even mortality.

Dysrhythmias should be treated as necessary. Caution should be exercised in the administration of cardiac glycosides if myocarditis or tamponade is present.

Broad-spectrum antibiotic treatment should be started because a bacterial etiology cannot initially be eliminated. Nafcillin (or its equivalent) 150 mg/kg/24 hr q 4 to 6 hr IV and cefotaxime 100 to 150 mg/kg/24 hr q 6 hr IV (or chloramphenicol 100 mg/kg/24 hr IV q 6 hr) should be

started. The maximum daily IV dose for either cefotaxime or nafcillin is 10 to 12 gm. Once the culture and sensitivity results are available, therapy may be directed more specifically at the causative agent. Therapy appropriate for fungi, protozoa, or tuberculosis should be started when one of these agents is identified.

Dialysis is indicated for uremic pericarditis. Specific therapy for Kawasaki disease is discussed in Chapter 55.

In the acute phase of pericarditis, bed rest is essential, usually for a period of several weeks. Salicylates may be useful for the relief of fever and pain in viral or idiopathic pericarditis or in the postpericardiotomy syndrome (50 to 75 mg/kg/24 hr divided into 4 or 6 daily doses).[118] Indomethacin has also been used to treat older patients with recurrent viral pericarditis and the postpericardiotomy syndrome at a dose of 1.5 to 2.5 mg/kg/24 hr q 6 to 8 hr PO (up to 100 mg/24 hr).[119]

Although there may be a role for the use of steroids in certain autoimmune forms of pericarditis (e.g., SLE), most authors recommend avoiding steroids in acute viral pericarditis.[126] It is debatable whether or not steroids may be indicated in recurrent, protracted, or severe viral pericarditis.

Disposition. All patients with pericarditis should be hospitalized. Those with evidence of cardiac tamponade or those who will not be able to receive close monitoring on the ward should be transferred to the intensive care unit where a cardiovascular surgery service is available.

RHEUMATIC FEVER, ACUTE

This is an inflammatory disease that affects the connective tissue of the heart, joints, central nervous system, and subcutaneous tissues. Typically, it presents in school-aged children (5 to 17 years) although it has been described in younger children as well as adults. There is a strong association with the preceding Group A streptococcal infection in the nasopharynx. Since the 1940s when the incidence was 65 per 100,000 population, the incidence of acute rheumatic fever in developed countries has fallen steadily to 9/100,000 in 1978.[127] However, beginning in 1984, new outbreaks of rheumatic fever were reported in several areas of the United States, including Salt Lake City, Pittsburgh, and New York. These cases were not typical in that carditis was more common and severe and the children were from predominantly white, middle class environments, rather than overcrowded, poor socioeconomic conditions previously described.[128] A follow-up study from the Salt Lake City area shows that the incidence has since declined but not to the nadir observed in the late 1970s.[129] In developing countries, acute rheumatic fever is still a major health problem with significant morbidity and mortality.

Pathophysiology. The pathophysiology of this complex disease is unclear. It is thought to be an immune reaction on the part of the host to antigens of certain strains (mucoid types 3, 5, and 18) of Group A streptococcus.[130] The streptococcal cell wall has five layers: the hyaluronic acid capsule, the cell wall containing M-proteins, the group-specific carbohydrate layer, the mucopeptide layer, and the innermost protoplast membrane. The M-proteins are important because of their antigenicity and because they are determinants of the virulence of the organism, likely due to their antiphagocytic properties. The M-protein is believed to be the trigger for antibody production against the myocardium, whereas the capsular protein stimulates antibody production against the joints.[131] Involvement of the heart produces endomyocarditis and valvulitis with typical involvement of the mitral and aortic valves. The joint pathology is completely reversible and involves edema of the synovium and periarticular tissues of the affected joint with effusion.

Etiology. It is clear that a preceding streptococcal infection triggers the disease as well as its recurrences. Treatment of streptococcal pharyngitis will completely prevent the occurrence of the disease. Additionally, prophylactic treatment for streptococcal disease after an attack of rheumatic fever will prevent recurrences. The recent resurgence of the disease is thought to be due to an increased prevalence of strains of Group A streptococci containing M-proteins, which are specific for rheumatic fever—"rheumatogenic" strains.[132] What is still uncertain is the role of other factors such as genetic predisposition of the host, low socioeconomic status, or overcrowded housing conditions.

Diagnostic Findings

Clinical Findings. These patients typically present 2 to 6 weeks after a streptococcal pharyngitis with nonspecific symptoms such as low-grade fever, malaise, joint and abdominal pains, and weight loss. Physical examination may reveal any combination of arthritis, carditis, subcutaneous nodules, chorea, or erythema marginatum. The Jones' criteria were updated in 1992 (see box above right), and form the basis for making the diagnosis of the initial attack of rheumatic fever. They emphasize the use of clinical judgment and caution about overdiagnosis.[133] If there is evidence of a prior Group A streptococcal infection, the presence of two major manifestations or one major and two minor manifestations make the diagnosis highly likely.

Arthritis is the most common symptom, occurring in 60% to 80% of all first attacks. It is polyarticular, migratory, and fleeting and primarily involves large joints (ankle, knee, wrist, or elbow). Usually two or more joints are involved with marked tenderness.

Carditis occurs in 35% to 40% of new cases and can be variable, ranging from a mild myocarditis to severe pancarditis. As a clinical sign, carditis is the most important in the acute phase because of its potentially serious complications. It is manifest by any combination of new cardiac murmurs (typically the apical systolic murmur of mitral regurgitation), a hyperactive precordium, tachycardia, a gallop rhythm, a friction rub, or congestive heart failure.

Chorea (Sydenham chorea or St. Vitus dance) is seen in about 10% of cases. It is defined as a series of sudden purposeless movements that are involuntary, often involving the facial muscles, as well as the extremities. The patient is unable to write, has uncontrollable grimacing, and may complain of weakness. There may be some emotional lability and, as such, it is easy to misdiagnose this condition as a behavior disorder. The child may be brought for medical attention because of problems at school. Chorea may appear months after the streptococcal infection and may be a solitary finding. Its appearance, even without

---

Guidelines for the Diagnosis of Initial Attack of Rheumatic Fever (Jones Criteria, 1992 Update)

MAJOR MANIFESTATIONS

Carditis
Polyarthritis
Chorea
Erythema marginatum
Subcutaneous nodules

MINOR MANIFESTATIONS

Clinical findings
    Arthralgia
    Fever
Laboratory findings
    Elevated acute phase reactants (ESR, C-reactive protein)
    Prolonged PR interval

SUPPORTING EVIDENCE OF ANTECEDENT GROUP A STREPTOCOCCAL INFECTION

    Positive throat culture or rapid streptococcal antigen test
    Elevated or rising streptococcal antibody titer

Adapted from *JAMA:* 268(15):2070, 1992.

---

evidence of an antecedent streptococcal infection, indicates acute rheumatic fever till proven otherwise.

The characteristic erythema marginatum is a serpiginous eruption that appears on the limbs and trunk and lasts only a few days. It is often closely associated with the presence of carditis.

Subcutaneous nodules are rare and are found as small, firm, nontender nodules on the extensor surfaces of the wrists, elbows, and knees.

Minor criteria that may be present include a previous history of rheumatic fever, polyarthralgia, fever, elevated acute-phase reactions (ESR or C-reactive protein), and prolonged PR interval.

Complications. Carditis is potentially the most serious problem because it can cause severe congestive heart failure, myocarditis, pancarditis, valvulitis, dysrhythmias, renal disease, and death.

Ancillary Data. The ECG frequently shows first-degree heart block (prolonged PR interval) and voltage criteria for left ventricular hypertrophy.[134] Doppler echocardiography is an extremely useful diagnostic tool in making this diagnosis because not only will it show valvulitis and flow abnormalities associated with rheumatic fever, but it will also help to rule out congenital aortic or mitral valve abnormalities or other diagnostic considerations. The diagnosis of carditis in acute rheumatic fever, however, should not be made solely on the basis of a positive Doppler examination *without* accompanying auscultatory findings, since abnormal Doppler examinations have been recorded in asymptomatic, healthy children. A chest x-ray film may show cardiomegaly or pulmonary edema. A throat swab positive for Group A streptococcus, an elevated ESR and C-reactive protein as well as high or rising antistreptolysin (ASO) or streptozyme titers will help to confirm the diagnosis. The streptozyme test measures antistreptolysin titers, antihyaluronidase (AH), antistreptokinase (ASK), and antideoxyribonuclease (ADNase), and antinicotinamide-adenine dinucleotidase (ANA-Dase).

Differential Considerations. It is important to differentiate acute rheumatic fever from the many other diseases that may initially present in this nonspecific fashion. This is especially significant because, apart from the small outbreaks mentioned earlier, the disease is relatively rare in North America at present.[135] The updated Jones' criteria are used to make the definitive diagnosis.

The list of differential diagnoses is large and includes juvenile rheumatoid arthritis, septic arthritis, leukemia, myocarditis or cardiomyopathy, Kawasaki disease, viral pericarditis, drug reactions, tumors, cerebral vasculitis, and Huntington chorea.

Management. The initial emergency department management must focus on treating significant complications of shock (see Chapter 13), congestive heart failure, and dysrhythmias. If the patient shows acute decompensation in the emergency department in spite of medical treatment, emergency surgical valve replacement may be indicated. Most often, however, the presentation is more subtle and the patients do not present in an acutely unstable condition.

The mainstays of treatment for the arthritis and carditis are bed rest and antiinflammatory agents. Aspirin (ASA) is prescribed in high doses of 75 to 100 mg/kg/24 hr divided into four daily doses to produce a serum salicylate level in the range of 20 to 30 mg/dl. After a week, the dose may be decreased to 50 mg/kg/24 hr divided into four daily doses for an additional 4 to 6 weeks.

If carditis or congestive heart failure is present, the recommended therapy is the addition of steroids: prednisone or its equivalent in immunosuppressive doses of 1 to 2 mg/kg/day should be given. Treatment is usually continued for 2 weeks after the symptoms have improved and the ESR has returned to normal. The doses of steroids should be tapered over 4 to 6 weeks.

The treatment of chorea, if necessary, is haloperidol 0.01 to 0.03 mg/kg/24 hr divided into 4 doses. Adults receive a maximum dose of 2 to 5 mg/24 hr.

Once the diagnosis of acute rheumatic fever has been confirmed, the patient should be treated with a course of penicillin, even in the absence of cultures positive for Group A streptococcus. The recommended regimen is benzathine penicillin G in a single injection of 1.2 million U or 600,000 U of procaine penicillin G daily for 10 days. Both are administered intramuscularly. If an oral regimen is preferred, penicillin V 25,000 to 50,000 U/kg/24 hr divided into four doses is effective. For patients who are allergic to penicillin, erythromycin may be substituted in a dose of 1 gm orally for 10 days.

Prophylactic therapy should be started as soon as treatment for the acute phase has been completed: benzathine penicillin G in a dose of 1.2 million U should be given monthly by intramuscular injection. Other options include 200,000 U of penicillin orally, administered twice each day, or 1 gm of oral sulphadiazine daily. Recommendations for duration of therapy are variable, the safest being to continue prophylaxis indefinitely. Five years of prophylactic therapy for those without cardiac involvement is the minimum recommendation, whereas a minimum of 10 years is suggested in patients with a residual lesion following carditis.[136]

Disposition. If the diagnosis of acute rheumatic fever is being entertained, early consultation with a cardiologist is advisable, even if the patient does not appear to be acutely ill. Admission to hospital is advised, at least until the diagnosis is confirmed, because clinical deterioration may occur quite rapidly. Given the considerable length of time needed to organize the investigative procedures, it is inappropriate to have these performed in the emergency department.

THROMBOSIS, DEEP VEIN

The true incidence of deep vein thrombosis (DVT) in children and adolescents is not known precisely, but retrospective series have shown clinically diagnosed idiopathic DVT to be 1.2/10,000 hospital admissions[137] and for pulmonary embolus to be 7.8/10,000 hospital admissions for adolescents and young adults.[138] The median age for presentation of DVT and pulmonary embolism has been reported as 13 years (with a range from 3 months to 18 years) with an equal distribution between males and females.[139] DVT is an important clinical problem because of its potential for progressing to a pulmonary embolus, which is a potentially life-threatening condition.[137,140,141] Early recognition and treatment of DVT may prevent this progression. It may occur anywhere in the deep venous system; some examples are venous sinus thrombosis of the central nervous system, which causes neurologic symptoms, and renal vein thrombosis. DVT of the extremities is most common.

Etiology. Table 47-16 shows the predisposing causes in children and adolescents with venous thrombosis of the extremity or pulmonary embolism.[138] The most common causes are an indwelling catheter and surgery.

Endothelial Factors. Disruption of the endothelium may increase the risk of venous thrombosis. This disruption may result from trauma or from the introduction of indwelling catheters.[142]

Venous Stasis. Low venous flow rates also predispose a child to venous thrombosis. Reduced limb movement, one of the causes of venous stasis, has been associated with deep vein thrombosis in the following situations: prolonged bed rest, extremity casting, or extremity paralysis from myelomeningocele.[137,140,143] Low venous flow may also be caused by increased blood viscosity from polycythemia (e.g., secondary to cyanotic heart disease) or by increased venous pressure resulting from congestive heart failure. Severe dehydration has also been associated with an increased risk of venous thrombosis, presumably caused by low flow rates associated with depleted intravascular volume.

Hypercoagulable States. Hypercoagulability may be secondary to increased estrogen levels as seen in pregnancy or with the use of birth control pills. Some patients have a deficiency in antithrombin III, protein C or S, or

TABLE 47-16. Underlying Disorders or Other Predisposing Factors in Children and Adolescents with Venous Thrombosis in the Extremities or Pulmonary Embolism or Both ($N = 308$)

Disorder or other factor	Subjects	
	No.	%
Indwelling catheter	65	21.1
Surgery	40	13.0
Trauma	27	8.8
Systemic lupus erythematosus	23	7.5
Infection	19	6.2
Tumor	18	5.8
None or unknown	17	5.5
Total parenteral nutrition	17	5.5
Disorder of hemostasis causing predisposition to thrombosis	12	3.9
Athletic activity	11	3.6
Leukemia	9	2.9
Nephrotic syndrome	9	2.9
Estrogen use	7	2.3
Obesity	6	2.0
Ulcerative colitis; other enteropathy	6	2.0
Paralysis	5	1.6
Immobilization	4	1.3
Abortion	2	0.7
Homocystinuria	2	0.7
Pregnancy	2	0.7
Ventriculoatrial shunt	2	0.7
Hemolytic anemia	1	0.3
Hughes-Stovin syndrome	1	0.3
Hydrocephalus	1	0.3
Sickle cell anemia	1	0.3
Vascular malformation	1	0.3

From David M and Andrew M: *J Pediatr* 123:337-346, 1993.

plasminogen, which predisposes them to venous thrombosis.[144] Systemic lupus erythematosus is a disease that may rarely cause thrombosis because of the presence of a lupus anticoagulant. Nephrotic syndrome in relapse has also been known to predispose to a deep vein thrombosis.

Diagnostic Findings. The classical clinical findings of a deep vein thrombosis are redness, warmth, swelling, and pain. Pain in the calf region on dorsiflexion of the foot (Homans sign) is commonly seen in this condition but is not always present. However, all these clinical findings are nonspecific; therefore if deep vein thrombosis is suspected, objective diagnostic tests must be done.

The most worrisome complication of a deep vein thrombosis is pulmonary embolism. The symptoms of pulmonary embolism are dyspnea (58% to 81% of patients), pleuritic pain (72% to 84%), cough (50%), hemoptysis (30%), and anxiety. The signs of pulmonary embolism are tachycardia, tachypnea, rales, pleural rub, and an increased S_2 (pulmonic component). The classic triad of hemoptysis, pleuritic chest pain, and dyspnea occur in only 28% of patients.

Ancillary Data. Studies used in determining the presence of a pulmonary embolus include an arterial blood gas, an ECG, and a chest roentgenogram. However, the difficulty of making a definitive diagnosis using only these results lies in the fact that they may at times be normal despite the presence of a pulmonary embolus. Hypoxemia is the expected ABG finding in the presence of pulmonary embolus.

An ECG may show nonspecific changes, but most useful for supporting the diagnosis of pulmonary embolus is the characteristic pattern that occurs with acute cor pulmonale (the S_1-Q_3-T_3 pattern).[143] A normal chest x-ray film is the most common finding, but a pulmonary infiltrate with elevation of the ipsilateral hemidiaphragm suggests a pulmonary infarction.

If there is any clinical concern about the possibility of a pulmonary embolus, a ventilation-perfusion (V-Q) scan should be performed as soon as possible. If uncertainty still persists after a V-Q scan, pulmonary angiography may be necessary.

If a deep vein thrombosis is suspected, definitive diagnostic testing is indicated. In adults, impedance plethysmography has replaced contrast venography as the diagnostic test of choice for initial work-up of a suspected deep vein thrombosis.[145] Because of the differences in anatomy and size between children and adults, it is unlikely that results of studies examining diagnostic tests in adult DVT can be extrapolated to children. Therefore, angiographic studies are still recommended when a thrombotic complication is suspected in children.[138] Early diagnosis is critical, but if there is any anticipated delay in performing diagnostic tests, then heparin therapy until diagnostic confirmation should be done. Other tests that have been used on adults but require more study on children are Doppler ultrasound and I^{139}-fibrinogen leg scanning.

Baseline complete blood count and PT and PTT should be drawn in the event that the diagnosis of deep vein thrombosis is confirmed and therapy needs to be commenced. In addition, any child with a deep vein thrombosis should have underlying thrombotic disorder ruled out by the drawing of blood for levels of antithrombin III, protein C and S, and plasminogen. An antinuclear antibody (ANA) test may be helpful for ruling out systemic lupus erythematosus as the cause for the thrombotic tendency.

Differential Considerations. Because the symptoms of cellulitis overlap with those of deep vein thrombosis, it may be difficult to differentiate between these two entities. Although fever, toxicity, and leukocytosis would make the diagnosis of cellulitis more likely, these findings are not consistently present. If on a clinical basis one is uncertain about the diagnosis, objective diagnostic testing is needed to rule out a deep vein thrombosis.

The patient's history is important in delineating the cause of extremity pain and swelling in this situation. If symptoms occur immediately after an injury, traumatic swelling of the soft tissues is the likely cause. The possibility of venous thrombosis becomes more likely if the pain and swelling begin a day or two after the injury. If uncertainty still exists, objective diagnostic testing should be done.

A Baker's cyst is a synovial fluid cyst located in the popliteal fossa in communication with the knee joint. It is usually seen on patients with underlying rheumatologic conditions, but may also be seen in people with normal knees. If this cyst ruptures, it produces symptoms of calf tenderness with ankle edema, symptoms that are also characteristic of a deep vein thrombosis. The only reliable way to differentiate between these entities is to perform contrast arthrography or venography.[145]

Management. The patient with deep vein thrombosis should be admitted to hospital for bed rest. The involved extremity should be elevated and heat packs applied if appropriate.

Heparin should be started with a loading dose of 75U/kg IV over 10 minutes, followed by a continuous infusion at 22U/kg/hr.[137] The PTT should be tested 4 to 6 hours after starting heparin and the dose of heparin should then be titrated to keep the PTT at about twice control values. The duration of therapy should be 5 to 7 days unless the thrombosis is extensive or the pulmonary embolus is massive.

Hemorrhage is the major side effect of treatment, occurring in 5% to 10% of treated patients.[143] If at any point the patient experiences hemorrhagic complications from heparin therapy, 1 mg of protamine can be given for every 100 U of heparin given concurrently. Contraindications to the use of heparin are existence of an underlying bleeding disorder, central nervous system bleeding, and surgery of the eye, brain, or spinal cord.[143]

Warfarin therapy should be started 48 hours after heparin is instituted. Warfarin is started at 0.2 mg/kg/day PO (maximum dose 10 mg) and is adjusted to keep the INR at 2 to 3.[137] Warfarin should be discontinued after 3 months unless the DVT is recurrent or there is still an underlying cause for the DVT.

The duration of effect is 4 to 5 days. The antidote is vitamin K. The duration of therapy varies from 6 weeks for calf vein thrombosis and from 2 to 3 months for a more proximal thrombosis. The duration will depend on whether or not an underlying clotting disorder is discovered.

Vitamin K can be used as an antidote for hemorrhagic complications while the patient is taking warfarin (infants: 1 to 2 mg/kg/dose IV; children: 5 to 10 mg/kg/dose IV). If the patient is experiencing a serious bleeding problem, fresh frozen plasma (10 to 15 ml/kg body weight) may be given in addition to vitamin K.

Contraindications to warfarin usage are the same as those for heparin (see previous section). However, warfarin should not be used on pregnant patients because it crosses the placenta. Warfarin interacts with many drugs, so if the patient is taking any other medication, it is imperative to check a pharmacology reference source for possible drug interactions. Patients with active bleeding, blood dyscrasia, or cerebral vascular hemorrhage should be monitored closely.

Systemic Thrombolytic Therapy. Systemic thrombolytic therapy may be helpful for massive pulmonary embolus that does not respond to heparin, or for those patients who have an acute, very extensive DVT.[137] However, such therapy should be considered in consultation with a hematologist.

References

Chest Pain

1. Rowe BH, Dulberg CS, Peterson RG, et al: Characteristics of children presenting with chest pain to a pediatric emergency department, *Can Med Assoc J* 143(5):388, 1990.
2. Selbst S: Evaluation of chest pain in children, *Ped Rev* 8(2):56, 1986.
3. Selbst SM, Ruddy RM, Clark BJ, et al: Pediatric chest pain: a prospective study, *Pediatrics* 82:319, 1988.
4. Fukushige J, Tsuchihashi K, Harada T, et al: Chest pain in pediatric patients, *Acta Paediatr Jpn* 30:604, 1988.
5. Rowland TW and Richards MM: The natural history of idiopathic chest pain in children. *Clin Pediatr* 25:612, 1986.
6. Perry LW: Pinpointing the cause of pediatric chest pain, *Contemp Pediatr* Nov/Dec:27, 1985.
7. Brown RT: The adolescent with costochondritis, *Compr Ther* 14(12):27, 1988.
8. Perry LW: Pinpointing the cause of pediatric chest pain, *Contemp Paediatr* Nov/Dec:27, 1985.
9. Woodward GA and Selbst SN: Chest pain secondary to cocaine use, *Pediatr Emerg Care* 3:153, 1987.
10. Schwartz RH: Chest pain in an adolescent: think of cocaine! *Pediatrics* 83(suppl):639, 1989.
11. Bisset GS, Schwartz DC, Meyer RA, et al: Clinical spectrum and long-term follow-up of isolated mitral valve prolapse in 119 children, *Circulation* 62:423, 1980.
12. Woolf PK, Gewitz MH, Stewart JM, et al: Noncardiac chest pain in adolescents and children with mitral valve prolapse, *J Adolesc Health* 12:247, 1991.
13. Selbst SM: Chest pain in children, *AFP* 41(1):179, 1990.

Heart Murmurs

14. Smythe JF: Does every childhood heart murmur need an echocardiogram? *Can J Pediatr* 2(2):275-279, 1995.

Congenital Heart Disease

15. Hoffman JIE: Congenital heart disease, *Pediatr Clin North Am* 37(1):25, 1990.
16. Wiles HG: Imaging congenital heart disease, *Pediatr Clin North Am* 37(1):115, 1990.
17. Sutherland, GR and Stumper OFW: Transthoracic versus transesophageal echocardiography in the pediatric patient, *Curr Opinion Pediatr* 5:598, 1993.
18. Heymann MA: Fetal and postnatal circulations. In Emmanouilides CG, Riemenschneider TA, Allen HD, et al, editors: *Heart disease in infants, children, and adolescents*, ed 5, Baltimore, 1995, Williams & Wilkins.
19. Graham TP Jr, Bender HW, Spach MS: Ventricular septal defects. In Emmanouilides GC, Riemenschneider TA, Allen HD, et al, editors: *Heart disease in infants, children, and adolescents*, ed 5, Baltimore, 1995, Williams & Wilkins.
20. Barkin RM: Cyanosis. In Barkin RM and Rosen P, editors: *Emergency pediatrics*, St Louis, 1990, Mosby.
21. Jordan SC and Scott O, editors: Heart disease in the newborn infant. In *Heart disease in pediatrics*, ed 3, Boston, 1987, Year Book.
22. Rowe RD and Izukawa T: The distressed newborn. In Keith JD, Rowe RD, Vlad P, editors: *Heart disease in infancy and childhood*, ed 3, New York, 1978, Macmillan.
23. Morgan BC: Incidence, etiology, and classification of congenital heart disease, *Pediatr Clin North Am* 25(4):721, 1978.
24. Pinsky WN and Arciniegas E: Tetralogy of Fallot, *Pediatr Clin North Am* 37(1):179, 1990.
25. Zuberbuhler JR: Tetralogy of Fallot. In Emmanouilides GC, Riemenschneider TA, Allen HD, et al, editors: *Heart disease in infants, children, and adolescents*, ed 5, Baltimore, 1995, Williams & Wilkins.
26. Driscoll DJ: Evaluation of the cyanotic newborn, *Pediatr Clin North Am* 37(1):1, 1990.
27. Paul MH: Transposition of the great arteries. In Emmanouilides GC, Riemenschneider TA, Allen HD, et al, editors: *Heart disease in infants, children, and adolescents*, ed 5, Baltimore, 1995, Williams & Wilkins.
28. Kirklin JKW, Colvin EV, McConnell ME, et al: Complete transposition of the great arteries: treatment in the current era, *Pediatr Clin North Am* 37(1):171, 1990.
29. Garson A Jr and Denfield SW: Sudden death in children and young adults, *Pediatr Clin North Am* 37(1):215, 1990.
30. Porter Cj, Feldt RH, Edwards WD, et al: Atrial septal defects. In Emmanouilides GC, Riemenschneider TA, Allen HD, et al, editors: *Heart disease in infants, children, and adolescents*, ed 5, Baltimore, 1995, Williams & Wilkins.

31. Garson A Jr, Bink-Boelkens M, Hesslein PS, et al: Atrial flutter in the young: a collaborative study of 380 cases, *J Am Coll Cardiol* 6:871, 1985.

32. Feldt RH, Porter CJ, Edwards WD, et al: Atrioventricular septal defects. In Emmanouilides GC, Riemenschneider TA, Allen HD, et al, editors: *Heart disease in infants, children, and adolescents,* ed 5, Baltimore, 1995, Williams & Wilkins.

33. Brook MM, Heymann MA: Patent ductus arteriosus. In Emmanouilides GC, Riemenschneider TA, Allen HD, et al, editors: *Heart disease in infants, children, and adolescents,* ed 5, Baltimore, 1995, Williams & Wilkins.

34. Beekman RH: Coarctation of the aorta. In Emmanouilides GC, Riemenschneider TA, Allen HD, et al, editors: *Heart disease in infants, children, and adolescents,* ed 5, Baltimore, 1995, Williams & Wilkins.

35. Strafford MA, Griffiths SP, Gersony WM: Coarctation of the aorta: a study in delayed detection, *Pediatrics* 69:159, 1982.

36. Thoele DG, Muster AJ, Paul MH: Recognition of coarctation of the aorta: a continuing challenge for the primary care physician, *Am J Dis Child* 141(11):1201, 1987.

37. Lock J and Radtke W: Balloon dilation, *Pediatr Clin North Am* 37(1):193, 1990.

38. Rocchini AP: Comparison of risks and short-and long-term results of balloon dilatation versus surgical treatment for pulmonary and aortic valve stenosis and restenosis and coarctation and recoarctation of the aorta, *Curr Opinion Pediatr* 5:611, 1993.

39. Rocchini AP and Emmanouilides GC: In Emmanouilides GC, Riemenschneider TA, Allen HD, et al, editors: *Heart disease in infants, children, and adolescents,* ed 5, Baltimore, 1995, Williams & Wilkins.

40. Friedman WF: Aortic stenosis. In Emmanouilides GC, Riemenschneider TA, Allen HD, et al, editors: *Heart disease in infants, children, and adolescents,* ed 5, Baltimore, 1995, Williams & Wilkins.

Congestive Heart Failure

41. Keith JD: Congestive heart failure. In Keith JD, Rowe RD, Vlad P, editors: *Heart disease in infancy and childhood,* ed 13, New York, 1978, Macmillan.

42. Talner NS: Heart failure. In Emmanouilides GC, Riemenschneider TA, Allen HD, et al, editors: *Heart disease in infants, children, and adolescents,* ed 5, Baltimore, 1995, Williams & Wilkins.

43. Artman M and Graham TP: Congestive heart failure in infancy: recognition and management, *Am Heart J* 203:1040-1055, 1982.

44. Artman M, Parrish MD, Graham TP: Congestive heart failure in childhood and adolescence: recognition and management, *Am Heart J* 204:471-480, 1983.

45. Friedman WF and George BL: Treatment of congestive heart failure by altering loading conditions of the heart, *J Pediatr* 106:697-706, 1985.

46. Friedman WF and George BL: New concepts and drugs in the treatment of congestive heart failure, *Pediatr Clin North Am* 31:1197-1227, 1984.

47. Talner NS: Congestive heart failure in the infant, *Pediatr Clin North Am* 18:1011-1029, 1971.

48. Tripp ME, Katcher ML, Peters HA, et al: Systemic carnitine deficiency presenting as familial endocardial fibroelastosis, *N Engl J Med* 305:385-390, 1981.

49. Waber LJ, Valle D, Neil C, et al: Carnitine deficiency presenting as familial cardiomyopathy: a treatable defect in carnitine transport, *J Pediatr* 101:700-705, 1982.

50. Rudolph AM: Diagnosis and treatment: respiratory distress and cardiac disease in infancy, *Pediatrics* 35:999-1002, 1965.

51. Benzing G, Schubert W, Hug G, et al: Simultaneous hypoglycemia and acute heart failure, *Circulation* 40:209-216, 1969.

52. Park MK: Use of digoxin in infants and children, with specific emphasis on dosage, *J Pediatr* 108:871-877, 1986.

53. Alpert BS, Barfield JA, Taylor WJ: Reappraisal of digitalis in infants with left-to-right shunts and heart failure, *J Pediatr* 106:66-68, 1985.

54. Berman W, Yabek SM, Dillon T, et al: Effects of digoxin in infants with a congested circulatory state due to a ventricular septal defect, *N Engl J Med* 308:363-366, 1983.

55. Perkin RM and Levin DL: Shock in the pediatric patient. II. Therapy, *J Pediatr* 101:319-332, 1982.

56. Rheuban KS, Carpenter MA, Ayers CA, et al: Acute hemodynamic effects of converting enzyme inhibition in infants with congestive heart failure, *J Pediatr* 117:668-670, 1990.

57. Heymann MA: Pharmacologic use of prostaglandin E_1 in infants with congenital heart disease, *Am Heart J* 101:837-843, 1981.

Endocarditis, Acute and Subacute

58. Dajani AS, Taubert KA, Infective endocarditis. In Emmanouilides GC, Riemenschneider TA, Allen HD, et al, editors: *Heart disease in infants, children, and adolescents,* ed 5, Baltimore, 1995, Williams & Wilkins.

59. Johnson DH, Rosenthal A, Nadas AS: A forty-year review of bacterial endocarditis in infancy and childhood, *Circulation* 51:581-588, 1975.

60. Saiman L, Prince A, Gersony WM: Pediatric infective endocarditis in the modern era, *J Pediatr* 122:847, 1993.

61. Kramer H, Bourgeois M, Liersh R, et al: Current clinical aspects of bacterial endocarditis in infancy, childhood, and adolescence, *Eur J Pediatr* 140:253-258, 1983.

62. VanHare GF, Ben-Shachar G, Liebman J, et al: Infective endocarditis in infants and children during the past 10 years: a decade of change, *Am Heart J* 107:1235, 1984.

63. Kaplan EL, Rich H, Gersony W, et al: A collaborative study of infective endocarditis in the 1970s: emphasis on infections in patients who have undergone cardiovascular surgery, *Circulation* 59:327, 1979.

64. Scheld MW and Sande MA: Endocarditis and intravascular infections. In Mandell GL, Bennett JE, Dolin R, editors: *Principles and practice of infectious diseases,* ed 4, New York, 1995, Churchill Livingstone.

65. Kaplan EL: Infective endocarditis in the pediatric age group: an overview. In Kaplan EL and Taranta AV, editors: *Infective endocarditis: an American Heart Association symposium,* Dallas, 1976, American Heart Association.

66. Blumenthal S, Griffiths SP, Morgan BC: Bacterial endocarditis in children with heart disease: a review based on the literature and experience with 58 cases, *Pediatrics* 26:993-1017, 1960.

67. Coutlée F, Carceller AM, and Deschamps L: The evolving pattern of pediatric endocarditis from 1960 to 1985, *Can J Cardiol* 6(4):164-170, 1990.

68. Johnson CM and Rhodes KH: Pediatric endocarditis, *Mayo Clin Proc* 57:86-94, 1982.

69. Millard DD and Shulman ST: The changing spectrum of neonatal endocarditis, *Clin Perinatol* 15(3):587-608, 1988.

70. Clemens JD, Horwitz RI, Jaffe CC, et al: A controlled evaluation of the risk of bacterial endocarditis in persons with mitral-valve prolapse, *N Engl J Med* 307:776, 1982.

71. Chagnac A, Rudniki C, Loebel H, et al: Infectious endocarditis in idiopathic hypertrophic subaortic stenosis: report of three cases and review of the literature, *Chest* 81:346, 1982.

72. Shah P, Singh WSA, Rose V, et al: Incidence of bacterial endocarditis in ventricular septal defects, *Circulation* 34:127-131, 1966.

73. Gersony WM and Hayes CJ: Bacterial endocarditis in patients with pulmonary stenosis, aortic stenosis, or ventricular septal defect, *Circulation* 56(suppl 1):84-87, 1977.

74. Sholler GF, Hawker RE, Celermajer JM: Infective endocarditis in childhood, *Pediatr Cardiol* 6:183, 1986.

75. Parras F, Bouza E, Romero J, et al: Infectious endocarditis in children, *Pediatr Cardiol* 11:77-81, 1990.

76. Johnson DH, Rosenthal A, Nadas A: Bacterial endocarditis in children under 2 years of age, *Am J Dis Child* 129:183-186, 1975.

77. Threlkeld MG and Cobbs CG: Infectious disorders of prosthetic valves and intravascular devices. In Mandell GL, Bennett JE, Dolin R, editors: *Principles and practice of infectious diseases,* ed 4, New York, 1995, Churchill Livingstone.

78. Karl T, Wensley D, Stark J, et al: Infective endocarditis in children with congenital heart disease: comparison of selected features in patients with surgical correction or palliation and those without, *Br Heart J* 58:57, 1987.

79. Levy RL and Hong R: The immune nature of subacute bacterial endocarditis (SBE) nephritis, *Am J Med* 54:645, 1973

80. Wilson WR, Giuliani ER, Danielson GK, et al: General considerations in the diagnosis and treatment of infective endocarditis, *Mayo Clin Proc* 57:81, 1982.

81. Parker MT and Ball LC: Streptococci and aerococci associated with systemic infection in man, *Arch Oral Biol* 13:1249, 1968.

82. Sanabria TJ, Alpert JS, Goldberg R, et al: Increasing frequency of staphylococcal infective endocarditis: experience at a university hospital, 1981 through 1988, *Arch Int Med* 150:1305, 1990.

83. Walterspiel J and Kaplan S: Incidence and clinical characteristics of "culture-negative" infective endocarditis in a pediatric population, *Pediatr Infect Dis J* 5:328, 1986.

84. Danilowicz D: Infective endocarditis, *Pediatr Rev* 16 (4):148, 1995.

85. Churchill MA, Geraci JE, Hunder GG: Musculoskeletal manifestations of bacterial endocarditis, *Ann Intern Med* 87:754, 1977.

86. Mansur AJ, Grinbert M, Leao PP, et al: Extracranial mycotic aneurysms in infective endocarditis, *Clin Cardiol* 9:65, 1986.

87. Jaffe WM, Morgan DE, Pearlman AS, et al: Infective endocarditis, 1983-1988: echocardiographic findings and factors influencing morbidity and mortality, *J Am Coll Cardiol* 15(6):1227, 1990.

88. Martin RP: Editorial comment: the diagnostic and prognostic role of cardiovascular ultrasound in endocarditis: bigger is not better, *J Am Coll Cardiol* 15(6):1234, 1990.

89. Lutas E, Roberts RB, Devereux RB, et al: Relation between the presence of echocardiographic vegetations and the complication rate in infective endocarditis, *Am Heart J* 112:107, 1986.

90. Pelletier LL and Petersdorf RG: Infective endocarditis: a review of 125 cases from the University of Washington hospitals, 1963-72, *Medicine* (Baltimore) 56:287, 1977.

91. Siegal JD: Bacterial endocarditis in infants and children: incidence and pathogenesis, *Pediatr Infect Dis* 3:541, 1983.

92. Werner AS, Cobbs CG, Kaye D, et al: Studies on the bacteremia of bacterial endocarditis, *JAMA* 202:199, 1967.

93. Sable C et al: Indications for echocardiography in the diagnosis of infective endocarditis in children, *Am J Cardiol* 75:801, 1995.

94. Bisno AL, Dismukes WE, Durack DT, et al: Antimicrobial treatment of infective endocarditis due to viridans streptococci, enterococci, and staphylococci, *JAMA* 261:1471, 1989.

95. Behrman RE, Vaughan VC, Nelson WE: Infective endocarditis. In *Textbook of pediatrics*, ed 13, Philadelphia, 1987, WB Saunders.

96. Tolan RW Jr. et al: Operative intervention in active endocarditis in children: report of a series of cases and review, *Clin Infect Dis* 14:852, 1992.

97. Nakayama DK et al: Management of vascular complications of bacterial endocarditis, *J Pediatr Surg* 21:636, 1986.

98. Dajani AS et al: Prevention of bacterial endocarditis. Recommendations by the American Heart Association, *JAMA* 264:2919, 1990.

Myocarditis

99. Kopecky SL and Gersh BJ: Dilated cardiomyopathy and myocarditis: natural history, etiology, clinical manifestations, and management, *Curr Probl Cardiol* 12(10):610, 1987.

100. Press S and Lipkind R: Acute myocarditis in infants, *Clin Pediatr* 29:73, 1990.

101. Lewis AB: Myocarditis. In Emmanouilides GC, Riemenschneider TA, Allen HD, et al, editors: *Heart disease in infants, children, and adolescents*, ed 5, Baltimore, 1995, Williams & Wilkins.

102. Noren GR, Staley NA, Bandt CH, et al: Occurrence of myocarditis in sudden death in children, *J Forensic Sci* 22:188, 1977.

103. Neuspiel DR and Kullen LH: Sudden and unexpected death in childhood and adolescence, *JAMA* 254:1321, 1985.

104. Aretz HT: Diagnosis of myocarditis by endomyocardial biopsy, *Med Clin North Am* 70:1215, 1986.

105. Savoia MC and Oxman MN: Myocarditis and pericarditis. In Mandell GL, Bennett JE, Dolin R, editors: *Principles and practice of infectious diseases*, ed 4, New York, 1995, Churchill Livingston Inc.

106. Taliercio CP, Olney BA, Lie JT, et al: Myocarditis related to drug hypersensitivity, *Mayo Clin Proc* 60:468, 1985.

107. Hohn AR and Stanton RE: Myocarditis in children, *Pediatr Rev* 9(3):83, 1987.

108. Mizlozek CL, Parker JA, Royal HD, et al: Radionuclide ventriculography in viral myopericarditis patients, *Circulation* 62(suppl 3):318, 1980.

109. DesA'neto A, Bullington JB, Dresser KB, et al: Coxsackie B$_5$ heart disease: demonstration of inferolateral wall myocardial necrosis, *Am J Med* 68:295, 1980.

110. Martin AB, et al: Acute myocarditis. Rapid diagnosis by PCR in children, *Circulation* 90:330, 1994.

111. Grundl PD, et al: Successful treatment of acute myocarditis using extracorporeal membrane oxygenation, *Crit Care Med* 21:302, 1993.

112. Stallion A, et al: Myocardial calcification: A predictor of poor outcome of myocarditis treated with extracorporeal life support, *J Pediatr Surg* 29:492, 1994.

113. Drucker NA et al: γ-globulin treatment of acute myocarditis in the pediatric population, *Circulation* 89:252, 1994.

114. Balaji S et al: Immunosuppressive treatment for myocarditis and borderline myocarditis in children with ventricular ectopic rhythm, *Br Heart J* 72:354, 1994.

115. Monrad ES, Matsumori A, Murphy JC, et al: Therapy with cyclosporine in experimental murine myocarditis with encephalomyocarditis virus, *Circulation* 73:1058, 1986.

116. Rezkalla S, Khatib G, and Khatib R: Coxsackievirus B$_3$ murine myocarditis: deleterious effects of nonsteroidal antiinflammatory agents, *J Lab Clin Med* 107:393, 1986.

Pericardial Diseases

117. Boyle JD, Pearce ML, Guze LB: Purulent pericarditis: review of literature and report of eleven cases, *Medicine* 40:119, 1961.

118. Rheuban, KS: Diseases of the pericardium. In Emmanouilides GC, Riemenschneider TA, Allen HD, et al, editors: *Heart disease in infants, children, and adolescents*, ed 5, Baltimore, 1995, Williams & Wilkins.

119. Savoia MC and Oxman MN: Myocarditis and pericarditis. In Mandell GL, Bennett JE, Dolin R, editors: *Principles and practice of infectious diseases*, ed 4, New York, 1995, Churchill Livingstone.

120. Fowler N and Manitsas G: Infectious pericarditis, *Prog Cardiovasc Dis* 16:323, 1973.

121. Van Reken D, Strauss A, Hernandez A, et al: Infectious pericarditis in children, *J Pediatr* 85:165, 1974.

122. Feldman WE: Bacterial etiology and mortality of purulent pericarditis in pediatric patients: review of 1672 cases, *Am J Dis Child* 133:641, 1979.

123. Fyle DA, Hagler DJ, Puga FJ, et al: Clinical and therapeutic aspects of Hemophilus influenzae pericarditis in pediatric patients, *Mayo Clin Proc* 59:415, 1984.

124. Farley JD, Thomson ABR, Dasgupta MK: Pericarditis and ulcerative colitis, *J Clin Gastroenterol* 8(5):567, 1986.

125. Lorell BH and Braunwald E: Pericardial disease. In Braunwald E, editor: *A textbook of cardiovascular medicine*, Philadelphia, 1988, WB Saunders.

126. Bulkey BH and Roberts WC: The heart in systemic lupus erythematosus and the changes induced in it by corticosteroid therapy, *Am J Med* 58:243, 1975.

Rheumatic Fever, Acute

127. Gordis L: The virtual disappearance of rheumatic fever in the United States: lessons in the rise and fall of the disease, *Circulation* 72:1155, 1985.

128. Ferrieri P: Acute rheumatic fever: the comeback of a disappearing disease (editorial), *AJDC* 141:725, 1987.

129. Veasey LG, Tani LY, Hill HR: Persistence of acute rheumatic fever in the intermountain area of the United States, *J Pediatr* 1994;124:9-16.

130. Veasey LG, Wiedmeier SE, Orsmond GS, et al: Resurgence of acute rheumatic fever in the intermountain area of the United States, *N Engl J Med* 316:421, 1987.

131. Ruttenberg HD: Acute rheumatic fever in the 1980s, *Pediatrician* 13:180, 1986.

132. Wald ER: Acute rheumatic fever, *Curr Prob Pediatr* August:264-270, 1993.

133. Special Writing Group: Guidelines for the diagnosis of rheumatic fever, *JAMA* 268(15)2069-2073, 1992.

134. Ruttenberg HD: Acute rheumatic fever in the 1980s, *Pediatrician* 13:180, 1986.

135. Allen UD, Braudo M, Read SE: Acute rheumatic fever: findings of a hospital-based study and an overview of reported outbreaks, *Can J Infect Dis* 1(3):77, 1990.

136. Dajani A, Tauben K, Ferrier P, et al: Treatment of acute streptococcal pharyngitis and prevention of rheumatic fever, *Pediatrics* 96:758, 1995.

Thrombosis, Deep Vein

137. Wise RC and Todd JK: Spontaneous lower-extremity venous thrombosis in children, *Am J Dis Child* 126:766-769, 1973.

138. David M and Andrew M: Venous thromboembolic complications in children, *J Pediatr* 123:337-346, 1993.

139. Bernstein D, Coupey S, Schonberg SK: Pulmonary embolism in adolescents, *Am J Dis Child* 140:667-71, 1986.

140. Jones DRB and MacIntyre IMC: Venous thromboembolism in infancy and childhood, *Arch Dis Child* 50:153-155, 1975.

141. Nguyen LT, Laberge JM, Guttman FM, et al: Spontaneous deep vein thrombosis in childhood and adolescence, *J Pediatr Surg* 21:640-643, 1986.

142. Marcinski A, Barral V, Sauvegrain J: Acquired deep vein thrombosis in children, *Pediatr Radiol* 15:300-306, 1985.

143. Bernstein ML, Esseltine D, Azouz EM, et al: Deep vein thrombosis complicating myelomeningocele: report of three cases, *Pediatrics* 84:856-859, 1989.

144. Corrigan JJ: *Hemorrhagic and thrombotic diseases in childhood and adolescence*, New York, 1985, Churchill Livingstone.

145. Hull RD, Hirsh J, Carter CJ, et al: Diagnostic efficacy of impedance plethysmography for clinically suspected deep-vein thrombosis, *Ann Intern Med* 102:21-28, 1985.

146. Brady HR, Quigley C, Stafford FJ, et al: Popliteal cyst rupture and the pseudothrombophlebitis syndrome, *Ann Emerg Med* 16:1151-1154, 1987.

Dermatologic Disorders

Julia A. Rosekrans

Signs and Symptoms

SKIN LESIONS

The emergency physician caring for children must be able to recognize skin conditions that are true emergencies and others that can cause parental anxiety. The skin problems seen in the emergency department are usually acute, causing symptomatic discomfort or cosmetic disturbances. Defining the underlying condition, alleviating symptoms, and providing appropriate therapy and education about common dermatologic problems is essential.

Dermatology seems daunting because it has developed a unique complex language. When one realizes that the Latinate descriptions of skin lesions are simple descriptive terms, and that skin problems fall into categories on the basis of history, pattern of distribution, and description of the lesion, diagnosis and management of common skin problems is no longer intimidating. A systematic approach to diagnosis allows an emergency practitioner to initiate therapy for most common problems.

Diagnostic Findings

The patient's history should be obtained and include the duration of the problem, location at which the rash started, changes that occurred, exposures, medications, and treatments that were tried, and the presence of any underlying medical problems such as arthritis or pregnancy.

The patient should be examined, and regional distribution of the rash should be noted. Areas of skin that are usually exposed (face, ears, and hands) will be common sites of photosensitivity, insect bites, or contact dermatitis from plants. Intertriginous distribution in axillae, neck folds, and the groin may be indicative of candidiasis.

Note the configuration or shape of lesions because this will also narrow the differential considerations. Annular lesions are ring-shaped, with sharp margins and clear centers, and are often caused by tinea corporis or granuloma annular. Serpiginous lesions are snakelike and have twisty margins as seen in cutaneous larva migrans or urticaria. Dermatomal distribution following a segment of a cutaneous nerve is usually herpes zoster. Target lesions are typically seen in erythema multiforme. Linear lesions may be due to scratching or contact with a linear irritant such as the edge of a plant leaf.

The primary skin lesion usually has the most useful diagnostic features; secondary changes develop as a result of partial treatment, scratching, or infection. Identifying the primary and secondary characteristics of skin lesions is the final step in evaluating a rash (Table 48-1). When the history, distribution, configuration, and type of lesion are identified, a reasonably limited number of diagnostic possibilities is established. Some skin problems require long-term follow-up; however, the emergency physician can be instrumental in recognizing the problem and initiating treatment of the condition, and educating the family.

Entire texts are devoted to the differential diagnosis of skin problems. A color atlas and dermatology text that describe lesions in depth are important reference books for an emergency department library.[1-8]

Diagnostic Entities

ACNE

Although very few people come to an emergency department with a chief complaint of acne, for many adolescents, being seen in an emergency department for an unrelated problem represents their only routine health care contact. Acne is often thought of as a normal burden of the teenage years and not as a condition warranting treatment. However, effective methods of intervention can dramatically change acne lesions. Advising adolescents that their problem is treatable, and initiating a treatment plan can help some patients understand acne, and can prevent physical and emotional scars (Fig. 48-1).

Acne is seen in as many as 85% of American teenagers[9] and ranges from a scattering of facial pimples to severe cystic lesions of the face and trunk. Although some infants have acne lesions, the majority of patients develop acne during the early stages of puberty.

Pathophysiology

Acne is a chronic skin disorder characterized by the presence of inflammatory lesions within hair follicles, which results in the formation of pustules, nodules, and papules. Sebaceous glands become blocked and hair follicles become plugged with desquamative skin cells and sebum.

Obstruction of the follicle leads to a wide, patulous opening filled with stratum corneum cells known as open comedones or "blackheads." Obstruction beneath the opening of the neck of the sebaceous follicles produces cystic lesions, known as closed comedones or "whiteheads," which can progress to inflammatory acne with pap-ules, pustules, cysts, and draining sinus tracts that result in permanent scarring.

Etiology

The bacterium *Propionibacterium acnes* is found in sebaceous follicles and appears to be a major catalyst of inflammatory acne. There is no evidence to support that the composition of chocolate, nuts, milk, or caffeine influences sebum secretion.[10] Stress does appear to influence acne through increased androgen production following altered adrenal-pituitary balance. Increased sweating, high humidity, and microtrauma to acne-prone areas may exacerbate the disease process. Exacerbations of acne have been noted in teenagers working in fast-food restaurants where their skin is exposed to vaporized oils. Heavy makeup to disguise acne blemishes may actually increase the problem. Although it is clear that acne is more severe in men than women and that adrenal conditions associated with increased androgen production are associated with an increased incidence of acne, there is no correlation between measured circulating androgen levels and extent of acne.[11] In addition, acne can develop when exogenous androgens are used.

Diagnostic Findings

Acne can present as a very mild problem of blackheads and whiteheads or it can be a severe problem with the development of deep nodules and cysts. It is located primarily on the face, chest, and back because these are the areas of the body with the greatest concentration of large sebaceous glands.

The acute lesions may be unsightly and uncomfortable, but the long-term complication of permanent scarring is an additional important reason to initiate therapy for acne. Postinflammatory hyperpigmentation is a temporary problem that commonly follows acute lesions. Permanent scars result from cicatricial fibrous contraction of the inflamed follicles. The severity of scarring depends both on the intensity and depth of inflammation and on the individual's susceptibility to form scars.

Differential Considerations

There are several drugs that can cause acne when used systemically. These include androgens, glucocorticoids, isoniazid, and hydantoin. Rosacea in children may result from long-term topical steroid therapy, which also results in erythema and thinning of skin with telangiectasia and formation of papules and pustules.

Infants frequently have a form of acne that can persist for several weeks but does not require treatment to prevent scarring. Newborns also often have miliaria, which are tiny vesicles or papules caused by occluded sweat glands. This heat rash lasts for only a day or two; the infant should be kept cool to reduce sweating.

Flat warts and molluscum contagiosum are sometimes confused with acne, although both lack the red inflammatory component of acne lesions, and both have their own typical appearance.

Angiomas of tuberous sclerosis are found on the face in a distribution typical of acne. In addition, they develop in early adolescence. However, patients do not have black-

TABLE 48-1. Dermatology Differential Diagnosis

MACULE: Flat, not palpable, circumscribed

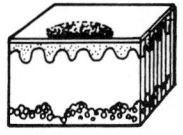

Questions: Color, blanch with pressure, single or multiple, circumscribed or diffuse, sun-exposed areas, length of time present.

Brown	Freckles	*Blue*	Mongolian spot
	Café-au-lait spot		Tattoo
	Postinflammatory hyperpigmentation	*Red*	Urticaria
	Nevi		Erythema marginatum
			Exanthem
White	Tinea versicolor		Telangiectasia
	Pityriasis alba		Burn
	Vitiligo		Fixed drug eruption
	Tuberous sclerosis		

PAPULE: Raised above the skin, < 1 cm in diameter.

Questions: Number, color, presence of scaling, density, length of time present.

Flesh-colored	Acne	*Red, abrupt onset*	Burns	Folliculitis
	Molluscum contagiosum		Goose bumps	Miliaria
	Milia		Urticaria	Viral exanthems
	Flat warts		Drug eruptions	
	Granuloma annular		Erythema multiforme	
	Nevi		Pityriasis rosea	
	Corns, calluses		Polymorphous light eruption	
			Contact dermatitis	
			Insect bites	

VESICLES AND BULLAE: Elevated and contain clear fluid, develop secondary changes rapidly.

Questions: Associated with papules, distribution over body, umbilication.

Associated with red papules	Contact dermatitis	*No associated lesions*	Miliaria
	Erythema multiforme		Dyshidrosis
	Insect bites		Bites
	Scabies		Burns
	Dermatophyte infection		Bullous impetigo
Umbilicated	Herpes simplex		
	Herpes zoster		
	Varicella		

NODULES: Deep in the skin, epidermis can be moved over top.

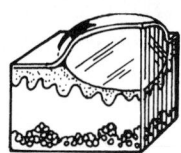

Questions: Color, tenderness.

Subcutaneous fat necrosis	Erythema nodosum
Foreign body	Lymphadenitis
Lipoma	Thrombophlebitis
Hemangioma	Carbuncle
Rheumatoid nodules	Epidermal cysts

PUSTULES: Localized accumulations of inflammatory cells

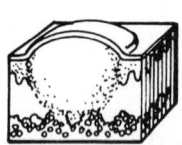

Questions: Distribution on body, abscess formation.

Dermatophyte infection
Folliculitis
Impetigo
Candidiasis
Acne
Dyshidrosis

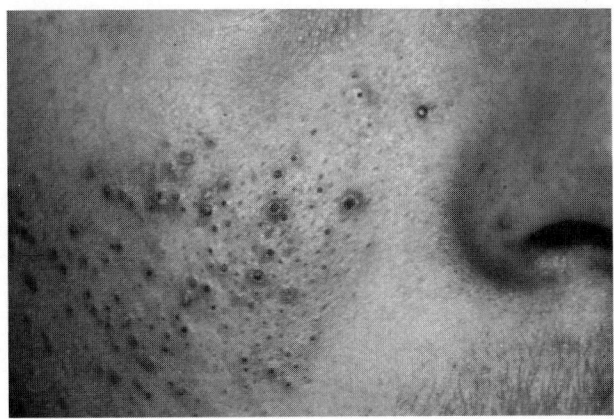

FIG. 48-1. Moderately severe acne deserves recognition as a treatable condition and not just a routine scourge of adolescents. *(Courtesy Mayo Medical Center, Department of Dermatology, Rochester, Minn.)*

TABLE 48-2. Guide to Initial Acne Therapy

Appearance	Treatment
Comedone only	Retinoic acid or benzoyl peroxide once a day
Red papules, few pustules	Retinoic acid cream in evening; benzoyl peroxide gel in morning
Red papules, many pustules	Same as above plus oral antibiotics
Cysts and nodules	Same as above plus oral antibiotics

Adapted from Weston WL and Lane AT: *Color textbook of pediatric dermatology,* St. Louis, 1991, Mosby.

heads present and are rarely without the other neurologic manifestations of this disease.

Management

Initiation of treatment for acne depends on understanding the action and the side effects of various medications. Current therapy focuses on reducing *P. acnes* in sebaceous follicles and unplugging follicles. Mild acne should be treated with simple topical measures and may not need any specific medical follow-up. If the presence of inflammatory papules or pustules warrants prescription medication, therapy such as topical antibiotics or topical retinoid acid can be initiated in the emergency department with a follow-up referral to assess progress and the need for continued treatment. Severe inflammatory or cystic acne should only be treated by a physician familiar with the side effects of the systemic medication needed (Table 48-2).

Benzoyl peroxide is the most widely used medication for acne treatment because it is the active ingredient in most over-the-counter treatments.[12] It acts both as a peeling agent to stop formation of new acne lesions and as an oxidizer of bacterial proteins, thus decreasing the amount of *P. acnes* on the skin. The primary side effect of benzoyl peroxide is an irritant dermatitis because it is very drying and can cause contact sensitization. Although not commonly recognized as a side effect, benzoyl peroxide has the ability to bleach clothing or pillow cases, which is distressing to some users and certainly should be mentioned before initiating treatment.

Topical antibiotics have fewer side effects than systemic preparations. Topical erythromycin is most commonly used. Its main side effect is drying caused by the alcoholic nature of its solvent. A 1.5% or 2% solution applied twice a day is a simple medication for beginning therapy.

Retinoid acid (0.025% cream) applied at bedtime actually decreases the initial formation of acne lesions and is the most effective topical medication. When therapy is initiated, acne may flare up as abnormal follicles already present are irritated. It is very drying and thins the skin, which may result in increased sun sensitivity. This excellent medication

should be used in patients who will continue close follow-up with a dermatologist or primary physician.

Patients with mild acne should be informed that washing with gentle soap once or twice a day is usually enough. Excessive scrubbing with abrasives may actually aggravate acne by causing microtrauma. If makeup is used, it should be water based and used sparingly.

Other medications such as systemic antibiotics and intralesional steroids can be used by patients with good follow-up habits, but are not generally part of the initial therapeutic approach. In the presence of marked disease with marked inflammation, oral antibiotics should be initiated. Tetracycline (0.5 to 1 gm/24 hr PO) is initiated for 2 to 3 months until lesions are suppressed. This should not be used in children under the age of 9 or if there is any pregnancy potential. Minocin may be substituted.

Severe cystic disease may additionally need oral retinoids. Isotretinoin or 13-Cis-retinoid acid (Accutane) may be started at an initial dose of 40 mg once or twice daily PO. It should not be used in women of childbearing age, and requires vigilant monitoring of the patient's liver function and lipid profile. All patients with cystic acne should be informed that treatment is available, and should be referred to a specialist for ongoing therapy with this agent and intralesional steroids.[13]

ATOPIC DERMATITIS

Atopic dermatitis is a chronic relapsing condition with a variable clinical presentation. It appears primarily in people who have a tendency to produce specific IgE when exposed to environmental antigens. There is a familial association with other atopic conditions including allergic rhinitis and asthma (Fig. 48-2, *A*).

Although the term *eczema* is sometimes used synonymously with atopic dermatitis, eczema (which means "boiling over") describes the eruption of erythema, scaling skin, and weeping vesicles. Atopic dermatitis may present with an eczematoid reaction, but other problems such as contact dermatitis and scabies may also be eczematoid (Fig. 48-2, *B*).

Two thirds of patients with atopic dermatitis develop the condition in the first year of life. Many children improve over time, but those with severe infantile dermatitis are likely to continue to have problems as adults. The exact pathogenesis is unknown, although reactions to food allergies and exposure to allergens, such as house mites, have been suggested.[14-16]

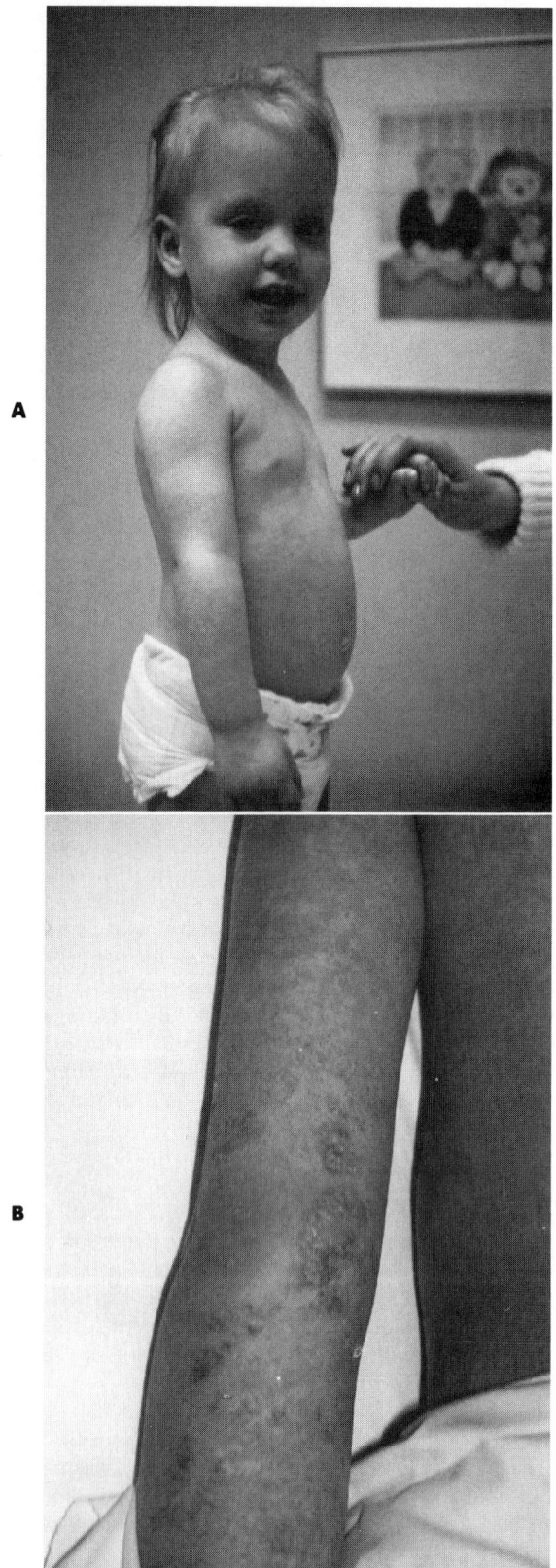

FIG. 48-2. Atopic dermatitis. **A,** Dennie's lines on the lower eyelid and allergic shiners are common findings in toddlers with atopic dermatitis. **B,** Eczematous lesions in the popliteal fossa are commonly seen in childhood atopic dermatitis.

Diagnostic Findings

The symptom most specific to atopic dermatitis is itching. The problem has been described as an "itch that rashes, not a rash that itches."[17] The distribution of the eruption typically varies with the age of the patient. In infancy, the cheeks and the extensor surfaces of the legs are most commonly involved. Later in childhood, the antecubital and popliteal fossae are most affected, whereas an adult usually develops a more diffuse pattern of involved skin.

The rash ranges in severity from dry skin or hypopigmented areas to severe disruption of the skin surface with weeping and open fissures. The physical appearance of atopic dermatitis must be considered in the context of its distribution, the family history of allergic problems, and its chronic nature.

Other findings in patients with this problem include shiny buffed nails from constant rubbing against the skin while scratching. Dennie's sign, which is a double fold in the lower eyelid, and allergic shiners are common associated signs of an atopic individual. These may be enhanced by repeated rubbing of the soft tissue of the lower eyelid, and hyperpigmentation of the skin below the eyelid may result. Very dry skin, which is often worse in the winter, causes hyperkeratotic follicles to develop on the arms and legs. Pityriasis alba or hypopigmented patches are often seen on the face, and may be quite pronounced in children who are tanned or have dark complexions. In addition, patients with atopic dermatitis have unusual reactions to changes in temperature. They show excessive vasoconstriction when their hands or feet are exposed to cold and warm more slowly than those with normal skin.

An important associated problem found with this skin disease is cataract formation.[18] The precise incidence of this complication is unknown, but it has been described in up to 13% of patients with severe atopic dermatitis. There is some suggestion that cataract development may be related to corticosteroid use. Keratoconus, an abnormally shaped cornea, and retinal detachment have also been described in atopic patients.[19]

The most important complication that the emergency physician must recognize is that children with atopic dermatitis tend to develop bacterial skin infections. They have high rates of colonization with *Staphylococcus aureus* and easily develop abscesses, cellulitis, and lymphangitis in eczematoid areas.

Differential Considerations

Atopic dermatitis is most commonly confused with other scaly or papulovesicular disorders such as seborrheic dermatitis, scabies, contact dermatitis, or tinea corporis. In addition, the hypopigmented patches can be mistaken for tinea versicolor. Some metabolic problems such as Hurler syndrome and phenylketonuria may be accompanied by eczematoid rashes.

Management

There is no cure for atopic dermatitis, and education of the patient and family in the care of this chronic problem takes time and patience. Palliative therapy is aimed toward reducing dryness, inflammation, and itching.[20]

Dryness should be treated with moisturizers and preparations that hold water in the skin. Baths should be limited, and soaps that are mild and nonperfumed such as Dove, Basis, Neutrogena, or Aveeno are suggested. Cetaphil cleanser may be substituted. Topical moisturizers such as Eucerin or Vaseline can be very soothing when applied after a bath and before the child is dried. Adding an emollient, such as an oil (Alpha Keri oil) to the bath may be helpful.

For significant weeping and crusting, more aggressive hydration may be essential. Compresses (gauze or soft dishtowels) should be dampened with Burow's solution or tepid water and applied for 2 to 3 days. The wet compresses should be removed every 5 minutes, and damp ones should be reapplied for a total of 15 minutes of treatment. This should be repeated three to five times/day. At night, the child should be bathed and then dressed in cotton pajamas that are wet (but not soaked) with warm water. A pair of dry pajamas are put on over the wet ones to allow slow drying of the lesions following the initial hydration phase.

Inflammation is treated with topical corticosteroids.[21] Because these children will need treatment for years, it is important to use therapy that will cause as few side effects as possible. Topical steroids may be absorbed through the skin and can cause systemic effects when used for long periods of time or when very strong steroid preparations are used (Table 48-3).

An ointment-based corticosteroid will be more effective as a moisturizer than a cream. Fluorinated steroids may cause permanent thinning of the skin and should never be used on the face. Although stronger steroids may be used to initiate therapy, patients should be advised to use milder preparations as soon as the dermatitis begins to resolve. High-potency preparations are rarely needed in children (Table 48-4).

Treatment with H_1 antihistamines such as hydroxyzine hydrochloride (2 to 4 mg/kg/24 hr divided into two or three doses) or diphenhydramine hydrochloride (4 to 6 mg/kg/24 hr, not to exceed 300 mg, divided into three to four doses daily) can be used to relieve itching. New antihistamines, including terfenadine and astemizole, have been tried because they cause less drowsiness. The H_2 antihistamines do not appear to add any advantage and are quite expensive.

Lesions that are secondarily infected need treatment with antistaphylococcal medications. Mupirocin ointment applied in a small amount three times a day is helpful for superficial infections; deep infections require systemic antibiotics such as dicloxacillin 12 to 25 mg/kg/24 hr q 6 hr or cefadroxil 30 mg/kg/24 hr divided into two doses. Antibacterial scrubs are irritating and should be avoided. Topical antibiotics are usually not helpful in this situation. Bacterial infection of atopic dermatitis may require inpatient treatment with parenteral antibiotics and intensive skin care.

On an ongoing basis, hydration should be maximized with daily baths and application of Eucerin and lubricating creams. Routine use of soaps should be avoided because they are drying. Fingernails should be kept short to minimize scratching. Children with severe disease require

TABLE 48-3. Side Effects of Topical Steroids

Local	Systemic
Burning	Suppression of hypothalamic-pituitary axis
Itching	
Irritation	Stunted growth
Folliculitis	Cataracts, glaucoma
Hypertrichosis	Glycosuria
Acneform eruption	Cushing syndrome
Hypopigmentation	
Allergic contact dermatitis	
Maceration of skin	
Skin atrophy	
Striae	
Miliaria	
Rosacea	

long-term follow-up by a physician who can provide the emotional support these children and their families need and who will be able to monitor the child for the potential long-term complications of the disease.

BACTERIAL SKIN INFECTIONS

Although newborn infants are born with skin that is bacteria free, they rapidly become colonized as they are exposed to bacteria either from the birth canal or from normal contact with other people. From the newborn period onward, the skin remains colonized with a small number of residual bacterial species. Pathogenic bacteria are not usually present on the skin although they may be found persistently if skin is damaged or if there is frequent exposure to a source of contamination.

The skin is a good barrier against bacterial infection because it is dry and is shed continuously, which are conditions that do not favor bacterial growth. The presence of established normal bacterial flora contributes to the host-defense system.

Children are prone to developing skin infections because they frequently suffer minor traumatic injuries such as scratched bug bites, abrasions, and lacerations. The most common pathogenic bacteria in children are *S. aureus* and *Streptococcus pyogenes*.[22]

Cellulitis

Cellulitis is a spreading bacterial infection in the loose connective tissue layer of the skin. Although it is not the most common bacterial skin infection, it is significant because there is a risk of mortality in untreated cases.

Pathophysiology. Cellulitis usually spreads from a break in the skin, and lymphangitis may appear as the infection spreads.[23] Regional lymphadenopathy is usually present, although systemic symptoms may not occur in the early stages. Extensive bruising of the skin, lymphedema, immunocompromise, and skin conditions, such as chronic ulcers or atopic dermatitis in which the integrity of the skin is broken, are predisposing factors for developing cellulitis. The disease affects all racial groups equally and can be seen at any age. Cellulitis is most commonly found on the

TABLE 48-4. Potency Guide for Selected Topical Steroids

Dose/form	Generic name	Product name
Lowest potency (antiinflammatory activity = 1)		
0.25%, 0.5%, 1.0%, and 2.5% cream; 1.0% ointment	Hydrocortisone	Synacort, Nutracort, Cort-Dome
0.05% cream and ointment	Desonide	Tridesilon, Desowen
0.1% cream	Dexamethasone*	Decaderm
1.0% cream	Methylprednisolone	Medrol
Moderate potency (antiinflammatory activity = 10-99)		
0.1% and 0.2% cream	Fluocinolone acetonide*	Synalar, Fluonid
0.025% ointment		
0.01% cream, 0.25% lotion	Triamcinolone acetonide*	Kenalog, Aristocort
0.05% ointment	Flurandrenolide*	Cordran
0.05% cream	Desoximetasone*	Topicort L.P.
0.2% cream	Hydrocortisone valerate	Westcort
High potency (antiinflammatory activity = 100-499)		
0.05% cream, solution and ointment	Fluocinonide*	Lidex
0.05% cream and ointment	Bethamethasone Diproprionate*	Diprosone
0.1% cream and ointment	Halcinonide*	Halog
0.1% ointment	Amcinonide*	Cyclocort
0.25% cream and ointment	Desoximetasone*	Tropicort
0.5% cream and ointment	Triamcinolone acetonide*	Kenalog, Aristocort
Highest potency (antiinflammatory activity >500)		
0.05% cream	Clobetasol propionate*	Temovate, Dermovate
0.05% ointment	Betamethasone Dipropionate*	Diprolene

*Fluorinated steroids.

extremities but was found on facial skin in 16% of cases in one survey by a pediatric hospital.[24]

Etiology. There are some clinical patterns of cellulitis that help to distinguish the bacterial cause. It usually appears as a red, tender, swollen induration with indistinct borders that extend outward from a break in the skin. This induration grows over the course of a day, and tends most often to be caused by *S. aureus*[25,26] (Table 48-5).

Certain strains of group A beta-hemolytic streptococci (GABHS) are able to produce a rapidly spreading cellulitis known as erysipelas,[27] which is characterized by a distinct elevated border. The onset of this infection may be quite abrupt, with rapid onset of chills and fever. The inflamed area spreads over a few hours with streaking lymphangitis and bacteremia frequently present. Although erysipelas is most common on the face in adults, it is found on any part of the body in children. It frequently begins at an area of traumatized skin and sometimes complicates surgical wounds. It is more common in children with lymphedema or immunosuppression.

Diagnostic Findings. Common sites of involvement include the extremities, face, and periorbital region. The lesions are generally erythematous, tender, swollen, and edematous. Lymphangitis appears as red lines spread in the direction of regional lymph nodes and is commonly caused by Group A streptococcus.

For children who have no underlying medical conditions that interfere with normal immunity, it may not be neces-

sary to define the specific etiologic agent. When an accurate culture is essential, either a blood culture or a culture obtained by aspirating the infected skin can be attempted. A needle aspiration should be performed using a 24- or 25-gauge needle on a tuberculin syringe containing 0.2 ml of nonbacteriostatic saline. The needle is introduced into the subcutaneous skin at the area of greatest inflammation, and suction is applied. The aspirate should then be plated onto appropriate culture media, determined by the microbiology laboratory responsible for the culture results. Unfortunately, aspirates and blood cultures are only positive about 50% of the time. If an open primary wound is present, cultures taken from the wound correlate well with blood cultures or aspirates. Punch biopsy cultures are also helpful in isolating the causative organism in chronic infectious lesions.

Differential Considerations. Any tender erythematous diffuse swelling may resemble cellulitis. The most common conditions that are confused with cellulitis are reactions to insect bites, the swelling overlying a bad sprain or fracture, and giant urticaria. Swelling and erythema over a joint may be caused by the more serious process of a septic joint or arthritis rather than cellulitis.

Management. Although many early cases of cellulitis will respond to outpatient antibiotic therapy, inpatient parenteral therapy must be seriously considered in every case. If outpatient management is attempted, close observation is required. The patient must be clearly instructed that IV

TABLE 48-5. Cellulitis: Etiologic Characteristics and Treatment

Etiology	Special clinical characteristics	Antibiotics
Haemophilus influenzae	Facial; periorbital; purplish swelling; <9 yr	Cefotaxime 50-150mg/kg/24 hr q 6 hr *or* ceftriaxone 50-75 mg/kg/24 hr q 12 hr IV (*or* cefuroxime 50-100 mg/kg/24 hr q 6-8 hr IV)
Streptococcus pneumoniae	Facial	Penicillin G 25,000-50,000 units/kg/24 hr q 4 hr IV; *if PO:* penicillin V 25,000 units (40 mg)/kg/24 hr q 6 hr PO
Staphylococcus aureus	Often preexisting break in skin	Nafcillin 100-150 mg/kg/24 hr q 4-6 hr IV; *if PO:* dicloxacillin 50-100 mg/kg/24 hr q 6 hr PO; (*or* cephalosporin: cephradine/cephalexin 25-50 mg/kg/24 hr q 6 hr PO; cefadroxil 30 mg/kg/24 hr q 12 hr PO)
Group A streptococci	Often preexisting break in skin; rapidly spreading erythema, induration, pain, lymphadenitis	Penicillin G, as above
Anaerobes (*Clostridium perfringens*)	Possible preexisting injury with necrotic tissue; dirty, foul-smelling, seropurulent discharge	Penicillin G, as above

From Barkin RM and Rosen P: *Emergency pediatrics*, ed 4, St. Louis, 1994, Mosby.

antibiotics may be needed if signs and symptoms worsen or if rapid improvement does not occur. Outpatient therapy can be attempted for cellulitis of the extremities in a child who is not toxic (i.e., does not have high fever and vomiting). Outpatient therapy should not be used for most cases of facial cellulitis, for children with underlying diseases such as nephrotic syndrome or immune compromise, or in children with signs of systemic toxicity such as fever or vomiting. Treatment should be aimed at treating both GABHS and *S. aureus*. Dicloxacillin (50 to 100 mg/kg/24 hr q 6 hr) or cefadroxil (30 mg/kg/24 hr divided into two doses) can be given for outpatient therapy (see Table 48-5). In addition, warm soaks and elevation of the affected area seem to help resolution of cellulitis.

If the infection continues to progress or the child becomes toxic, parenteral antibiotic therapy should be used. Although treatment with penicillin will eradicate GABHS, broad-spectrum antibiotics that will also cover penicillinase-producing staphylococci and *Haemophilus influenzae* are usually used until the bacteriologic agent can be identified by culture, because infections with any of these organisms may have a similar clinical appearance.

Facial Cellulitis

Facial cellulitis is an infection of the soft tissues of the cheek. It may be caused by *H. influenzae* type B, and usually occurs in infants and toddlers under the age of 3.[28]

The incidence of invasive *H. influenzae* disease has declined dramatically in the United States since the introduction of immunizing toddlers with conjugate vaccine, and therefore facial cellulitis in an immunized child will now often be caused by staphylococci and GABHS.

Diagnostic Findings. Swelling and a bluish-hued erythema may develop rapidly on the face of a child who has previously had symptoms of a simple upper respiratory infection. Children with this infection usually have fever, irritability, and vomiting. Two thirds of children have an associated otitis media.

Leukocytosis is usually present, and blood cultures are positive in 80% of patients. There is a significant rate of clinically inapparent meningitis that may accompany the cellulitis; lumbar puncture may be indicated.

Children with a blue discoloration of the cheek, who are afebrile and do not seem ill, often have cold panniculitis (see later section). Trauma and insect bites can cause a red bruised area on the cheek but are not associated with fever or toxic symptoms.

Management. Facial cellulitis is a serious infection that requires inpatient management. Cephalosporins such as cefotaxime (100 to 200 mg/kg/24 hr divided q 6 hr IV) are usually the initial choice while awaiting the results of culture and sensitivity tests.

Periorbital Cellulitis

Cellulitis around the eyelids has great potential for serious complications (see Chapter 51). Periorbital cellulitis may develop following a break in the skin from trauma, insect bites, or chicken pox, in which case it is usually caused by GABHS or *S. aureus*.[29] It may also spread from sinusitis, especially from the ethmoid sinuses. *H. influenzae* type B causes a periorbital cellulitis in unimmunized young children that is similar to facial cellulitis, and can be associated with other focal infections such as meningitis. Children who have received immunization against *H. influenzae* type B and who develop periorbital cellulitis are likely to have infections caused by either staphylococci or GABHS.

Diagnostic Findings. A cellulitis limited to the skin anterior to the orbital septum will not affect the orbital contents. Therefore a child with this infection will have lid swelling and erythema, normal eye movements, and no proptosis, whereas infection within the orbit will cause swelling and pain that restricts eye movement. In some cases, preseptal swelling may be so severe that orbital involvement is difficult to judge, and a CT scan of the orbit may be necessary to determine the extent of infection. It is important to differentiate periorbital or preseptal cellulitis from deep orbital cellulitis because a true orbital cellulitis is a much more difficult infection to manage and often requires surgical drainage.

Many children with swelling of an eyelid have simple conjunctivitis or insect bites on this delicate skin. Children with true cellulitis will have warmth, tenderness, and erythema in addition to swelling; are usually febrile; and may have other systemic symptoms such as vomiting.

Management. Children with a periorbital cellulitis who appear ill or have high fevers should be admitted to the hospital and treated with parenteral antibiotics such as cefotaxime 100 to 200 mg/kg/24 hr q 6 hr IV. If there is a break in the skin, which increases the risk of *S. aureus*, nafcillin (or the equivalent) should be used in addition to the cephalosporin treatment delineated. Some older children with very early infections, no signs of toxicity, and compliant families can be managed on oral antibiotics such as amoxacillin/clavulanate 40 mg/kg/24 hr q 8 hr with very close follow-up.

Folliculitis

Folliculitis is a superficial infection of a hair follicle usually caused by *S. aureus*. In children, it commonly occurs on the scalp and may be associated with trauma to the follicle from traction, which may occur from tight hair braiding, for example.

Simple infections may resolve with topical agents, such as keratolytic shampoos; however, systemic antistaphylococcal antibiotics are often required.

Furuncles may develop in deep layers of the skin following a superficial folliculitis. These lesions are indurated and tender to touch. They often develop fluctuance that requires drainage. Treating with warm compresses and antistaphylococcal antibiotics may speed resolution.

Impetigo

Impetigo is the most common skin infection in children. It occurs more commonly during warm seasons and in tropical climates.

In many cases the normal protective barrier of the skin is interrupted by abrasions or cuts that are then colonized by bacteria. Crops develop on an individual and spread rapidly from child to child. Although single lesions may heal spontaneously, an episode may last for many weeks without spontaneous remission (Fig. 48-3, *A*).

Impetigo is often a secondary problem complicating scabies, head lice, poison ivy, atopic dermatitis, or other pruritic problems (Fig. 48-3, *B*).

Diagnostic Findings. There are two clinically distinguishable types of impetigo: bullous impetigo caused by *S. aureus*, and nonbullous impetigo that has an unclear etiology. In the past it was thought that nonbullous impetigo resulted from infection by GABHS alone; however, *S. aureus* has been implicated as a concurrent pathogen in this form of impetigo.[30]

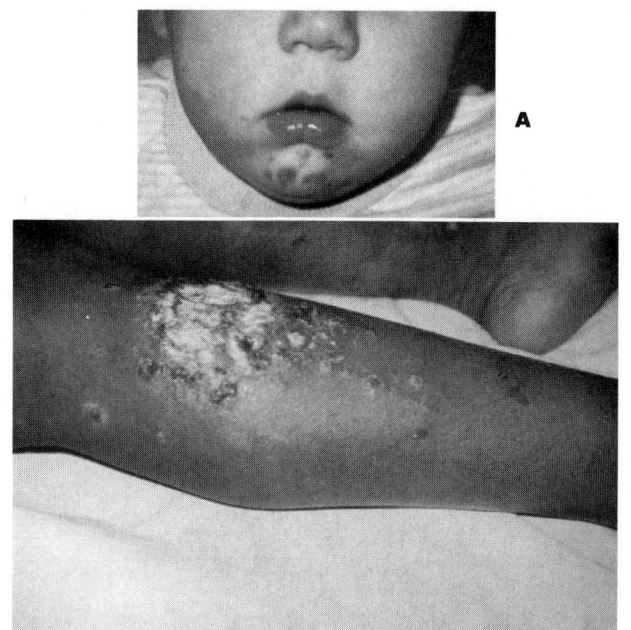

FIG. 48-3. Impetigo. **A,** Blistered lesions on the chin may develop from *Staphylococcal aureus* colonization of the nares. **B,** Icthyma. Impetigo is often a secondary problem complicating other skin conditions such as insect bites.

Bullous impetigo is characterized by clear, very thin-walled blisters that are frequently broken, leaving shiny, round erosions known as "coin" lesions. There is little surrounding erythema, and regional lymph nodes are not usually involved. Blisters frequently begin on normal intact skin and spread rapidly. Bullous impetigo in the neonate is of special concern because infants colonized with staphylococci may develop disseminated infection including pneumonia, septic arthritis, or osteomyelitis. In addition, because it usually develops when the infant is 7 to 14 days old, it raises suspicion of nursery-acquired infection.

Nonbullous impetigo begins as a tiny papule, which may be transiently vesicular, but rapidly develops into a pustule with characteristic golden crusts. Although there is usually little erythema, regional lymph nodes are often involved. As the lesions enlarge, they may develop central clearing.

Differential Considerations. The differential diagnosis of impetigo varies with its stage of development. Herpes simplex, varicella, tinea corporis, and contact dermatitis are easily confused with impetigo lesions. The history of development and distribution of the lesions usually differentiate these conditions.

Management. Impetigo usually heals without any scarring because the lesions are quite superficial, although temporary pigmentation changes may occur. There have been no reports of rheumatic fever or carditis following GABHS impetigo; however, acute glomerulonephritis may follow impetigo that is caused by certain strains of GABHS.[31] Treatment of impetigo may not decrease the incidence of nephritis in an individual, but it will interrupt spread throughout a community. Scarlet fever may be associated with streptococcal species causing impetigo.

Erythromycin in doses of 30 to 50 mg/kg/24 hr divided into 3 doses has been very effective against impetigo in regions where *S. aureus* is sensitive to the medication. When the bacteria are resistant, dicloxacillin 20 to 50 mg/kg/24 hr divided into 4 doses, or cefadroxil 30 mg/kg/24 hr in 2 doses has been suggested. Oral penicillin and injectable bicillin have been mainstays of impetigo treatment in the past, but they are commonly ineffective in our current bacteriologic climate.

Treatment of impetigo with topical antibiotics has traditionally been less effective than treatment with systemic antibiotics.[32] However, topical antibiotic, 2% mupirocin (Bactroban), has proved to be as effective as systemic therapy in many situations.[33] It is very useful in eradicating nasal colonization of *S. aureus* and can be used as an adjunct to systemic therapy. Many practitioners suggest using this topical agent for the initial treatment of impetigo and reserving systemic antibiotics for treatment failures or outbreaks that cover an extensive area of skin.

Scrubbing the crusts and soaking with warm compresses to remove the crusts is often advised; whether this is a necessary adjunct to antibiotic therapy has never been evaluated.[34] Scrubbing with hexachlorophene can actually delay healing, and other antistaphylococcal cleansing agents lack any residual activity. However, it would seem prudent to clean lesions before applying topical antibiotics. Occasionally, home remedies have been used that have increased spread of the infection. Mild topical steroids or ointments have been typically tried with poor results.

Paronychia

Acute paronychia are superficial infections found at the base of the nail bed, usually following trauma such as nail biting, injury to cuticles, or sliver punctures. Maceration of the skin by immersion in water may contribute to development of this infection. Swelling and tenderness around the base of a nail often precede the appearance of an abscess.

S. aureus and anaerobes typical of mouth flora are the most common organisms cultured from paronychia.[35] Treatment includes draining the abscess, which can sometimes be done simply by incising the nail fold, and administering antistaphylococcal antibiotics (see Chapter 32).

Perianal Streptococcus

Infection by group A beta-hemolytic streptococcus of the skin in the perianal region has been recognized since at least 1966.[36,37] This is a superficial process rather than a cellulitis and should be suspected with the appearance of a well-marginated erythematous ring of irritated skin extending evenly from the anus. There is usually no induration, regional lymphadenopathy, or fever. Many children with this problem complain of pain on defecation or perianal itching and may have these complaints before the rash develops.

The majority of cases occur in children under 10 years of age, and it is more common in boys than in girls. The patient frequently has a positive throat culture or has had a recent GABHS pharyngitis. The diagnosis is made by obtaining a culture that is positive for GABHS.

Treatment with oral penicillin will cure most cases; however, treatment failure or recurrence is not uncommon.

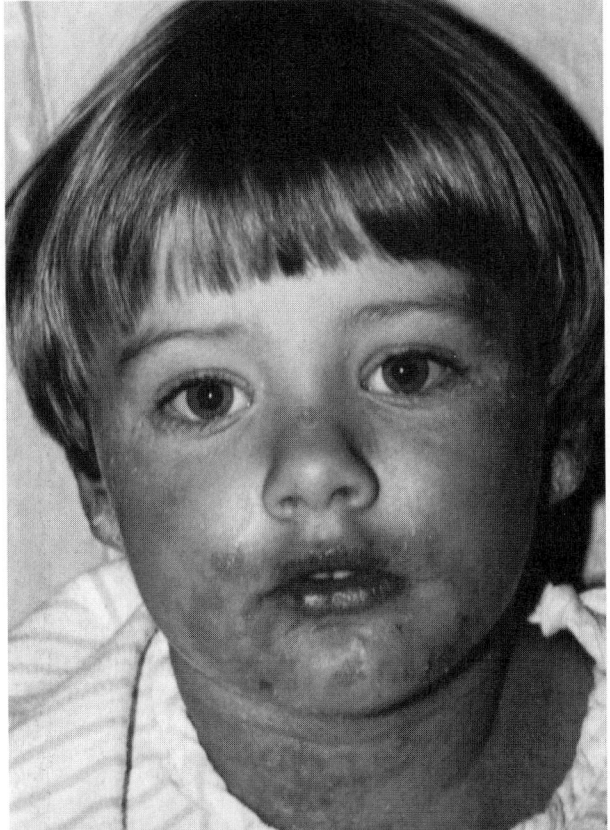

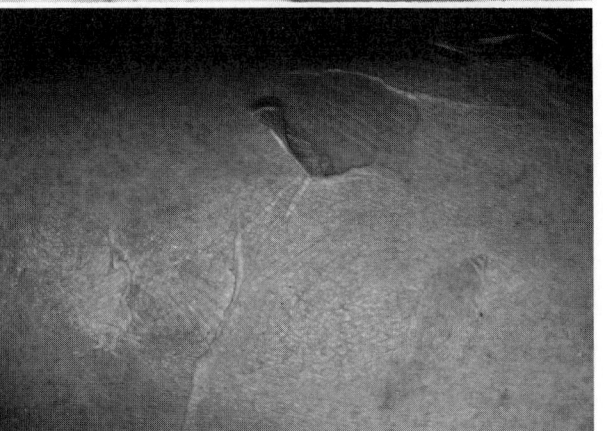

FIG. 48-4. Staphylococcal scalded skin syndrome. **A,** An exfoliative toxin elaborated by certain strains of staphylococcus produces bullous lesions. **B,** Nikolsky's sign. *(Courtesy Mayo Medical Center, Department of Dermatology, Rochester, Minn.)*

Staphylococcal Scalded Skin Syndrome

Among superficial skin infections, staphylococcal scalded skin syndrome (SSSS) has the most serious risk of mortality. It is usually seen in a child under the age of 5 (Fig. 48-4, *A*).

Diagnostic Findings. The initial symptoms are irritability when the child's skin is touched and fever.[38] Generalized erythema is quickly followed by formation of bullae and desquamation of large sheets of skin that split high in the epidermis. The skin can often be rubbed off in thin layers (Nikolsky's sign) (Fig. 48-4, *B*). The clinical presentation ranges from a localized form in which a few large bullae are seen over the lower abdomen or extremities of an infant, to the more severe generalized form. Serous crusting around the mouth and nose is characteristic; however, mucous membranes are not involved.

The peeling skin is produced by an exfoliative toxin elaborated by certain strains of staphylococcus. The same toxin produces bullous impetigo lesions in its localized form. The actual staphylococcal infection site may not involve the skin, but can induce pharyngitis, conjunctivitis, or an umbilical stump infection.[39,40]

Differential Considerations. The initial appearance is similar to scarlet fever, Kawasaki syndrome, toxic shock syndrome, severe forms of erythema multiforme, and even sunburn (see Chapter 55). A similar exfoliating rash in adults called toxic epidermal necrolysis is caused by a systemic drug reaction. A skin biopsy can readily differentiate these conditions if the history of clinical features are unclear.

Management. Because of the loss of skin, fluid and electrolyte imbalance and heat loss are common problems and must receive specific attention as outlined in the section on burn management. Deficits and ongoing fluid loss must be replaced to ensure euvolemia.

Newborns should be treated with IV antibiotics that will eradicate staphylococcus, such as cefazolin 100 mg/kg/24 hr divided into three doses or nafcillin (or equivalent) 100 to 200 mg/kg/24 hr divided into four doses.

Older children should also receive in-hospital parenteral treatment. Rarely, older children with only mild involvement and no toxicity can be treated as outpatients with dicloxacillin 25 to 50 mg/kg/24 hr in four equal doses, if close follow-up can be arranged. Topical antibiotics are not effective. With systemic antistaphylococcal antibiotics and attention to fluid management, most children recover very well without any scarring.

Invasive Group A Beta-Hemolytic Streptococcus

A toxic shock syndrome associated with GABHS has been described in several geographic areas of the United States in recent years. This infection has serious consequences because multiorgan failure and shock occur early in the course of the illness.[41-43] This toxic shock syndrome is thought to be due to an exotoxin produced by a few strains of GABHS.

Diagnostic Findings. In addition to an erythematous rash, children with this severe infection may have a variety of primary infection sites. Pneumonia, osteomyelitis, septic arthritis, pyomyositis, epiglottitis, and sepsis without a focus have all been described. Many of these cases have followed an initial infection with chickenpox. Pharyngitis may be present but is not always seen. Blood cultures are frequently positive.

Local tissue destruction can be severe, and fatality may occur in approximately 30% of cases.

Management. In addition to measures needed to treat hypovolemia and hypoxemia, high dose parenteral antibiotics are necessary to treat the GABS. The course of treatment may be prolonged depending on the underlying in-

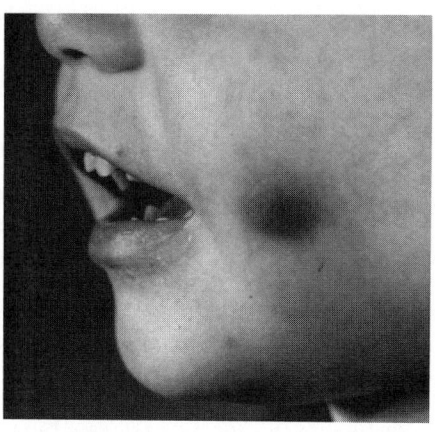

FIG. 48-5. Cold panniculitis. Fat necrosis occurs in toddlers when the skin is exposed to a very cold substance such as a snowbank. *(Courtesy Mayo Medical Center, Department of Dermatology, Rochester, Minn.)*

fection site. Penicillin G is recommended after the organism is identified; however, broad-spectrum coverage to treat other possible organisms is warranted initially.

COLD PANNICULITIS

An infant's skin that is exposed to direct contact with cold may develop nodules that often may not be recognized as being benign. Skin exposed to cold will react differently in people of different ages. The dermal fat in an infant is more highly saturated than the fat in an adult's skin; and highly saturated fat solidifies at colder temperatures than less saturated fat. Therefore an adult exposed to the same level of cold will have no alteration in subcutaneous fat, whereas an infant's fat will harden (Fig. 48-5).

Cold nodules can be produced in all newborns, 50% of 6-month-old children, and an occasional 9-month-old child when they were directly exposed to ice for 50 seconds. The nodules are described as deep, firm, mobile, slightly raised areas that are noticed about 24 hours after direct exposure of the skin to a very cold substance. Although they are minimally erythematous initially, the nodules often develop desquamation and hyperpigmentation, but gradually resolve leaving unblemished skin.

This condition is seen typically in northern climates when unprotected skin is exposed to snow or ice; however, it has also been described in a child who ate a popsicle.[44] It is important to recognize cold panniculitis because it resembles buccal cellulitis, which requires a very different approach to treatment. Children with cold panniculitis are not ill, and the lesion is hard and not usually warm to touch. It is important to avoid biopsy of the lesion because benign neglect is the treatment of choice.[45]

CONTACT DERMATITIS

Contact irritant dermatitis results from skin contact with an exogenous substance. Some irritants will cause a reaction in any person exposed; however, in allergic contact dermatitis only a person sensitized to a particular allergen will have this lymphocyte-mediated reaction. In either of these two reactions, the skin response will be similar and appears as a weepy, vesicular rash or even as an urticarial reaction.[46]

Infants react to many substances that do not trouble older children whose skin is thicker. Common substances that can cause irritant dermatitis in children include detergents, alkalis, acids, solvents, and fiberglass particles.[47] Variations in the extent of the eruption caused by these substances are due to differences in the amount of exposure, the strength of the irritant, and the location of the exposure.

Allergic contact dermatitis is unusual in children less than 8 years of age because they have not had multiple previous exposures to allergens. Allergic dermatitis can develop within 10 days of an initial exposure; however, it is most common to have numerous exposures before a reaction occurs. Parents frequently do not suspect a particular agent if the child has been exposed previously without any problems.

Airborne irritants will typically result in an eruption on skin that is unprotected by clothing. Infants sometimes develop an irritation around the mouth due to an allergic reaction caused by direct contact of food with the skin. Such foods include tomatoes, spinach, or citrus fruits. Ear lobes frequently develop allergic dermatitis to the nickel contained in earrings.[48] Rubber-containing materials, (e.g., waistbands, goggles, or adhesive tape) can cause a contact reaction and should be considered in any eruption that follows the path of the elastic contact on the skin. Feet are often involved in contact reactions. These reactions usually occur in response to the components of shoes that involve chemicals for processing or dyeing fabric and leather, and adhesion.

Cosmetics can commonly cause contact dermatitis. Certain offenders are antiperspirants, eye makeup, lipsticks, and nail care products.[49] Sometimes a person wearing nail polish will rub her eyes and will develop dermatitis of the delicate skin of the eyelids even though her fingers do not react.

The most common cause of significant allergic contact dermatitis in the United States is the rhus group of plants. These include poison ivy, poison oak, and poison sumac (Fig. 48-6). In addition, there are related plants that can cause reactions in sensitive individuals; these plants include mango rind and oil from the cashew nut. Furniture coated with a lacquer made from the Japanese lacquer tree, and a type of ink made from an Indian nut, which is used to mark clothing, can also cause reactions.

Diagnostic Findings

Because the physical appearance of contact dermatitis resembles other skin conditions, reaching a diagnosis of allergic contact dermatitis depends on identifying a responsible agent. Tracking down the exposure history sometimes requires challenging detective work. Distribution of the rash can be an important aid to diagnosis, although spread of the initial irritant through scratching or self-treatment may confuse the picture. Contact dermatitis usually develops abruptly. Typically erythema and a papulovesicular eruption appears in lines if the contact is from a leaf or stem; in geometric shapes if the contact is from metal,

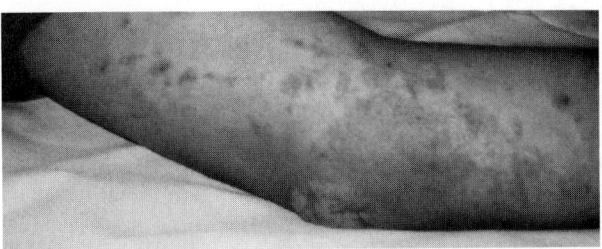

FIG. 48-6. Contact dermatitis. Linear blisters on areas of skin that are not covered by clothing are suggestive of contact with leaves or stems such as poison ivy.

such as a wrist watch; or just on the exposed skin from contact with many environmental irritants.[50]

Management

When a diagnosis is apparent, the first step in treatment is to preserve the skin from further contact. Poison ivy sap can remain on clothing or shoes for long periods of time, so it is advisable to wash everything that could reexpose the child to the irritant. The oleoresin responsible can be spread to areas of the body not originally involved so it is worthwhile to wash exposed skin as quickly as possible, even though this will not prevent the rash on areas already exposed.

Pets who go outdoors where poison ivy weeds grow can carry the oleoresin home on their fur so that the child may develop contact dermatitis from petting the animal.

The fluid in the blisters that develop does not contain the irritant and does not cause the eruption to spread to other areas on the body or to other people. There may be some time lag between different areas of the body developing the rash; this reflects the thickness of the skin and the extent of initial exposure. However, if poison ivy rash continues to develop over several days, the patient is probably being reexposed either by playing in the same areas or by wearing unwashed clothing.

Topical corticosteroids may relieve some of the itch but they do little to hasten resolution of the rash, which may take as long as 2 weeks.[51] In severe cases, a short-term course of systemic steroids, such as prednisone in a dose of 1 to 2 mg/kg/24 hr over 7 to 10 days, can be very helpful. The medication should be tapered gradually because the reaction can rebound if steroids are stopped abruptly or too soon. If this occurs, prednisone should be restarted.

H_1 antihistamines, such as hydroxyzine 2 mg/kg/24 hr divided into four doses, can be used to help relieve itching. Cool compresses with either tap water or Burow's solution are also important measures in relieving discomfort. Calamine lotion may be useful in drying blisters, but it should be emphasized that topical antihistamines or benzocaine are not useful and may cause sensitization.

DIAPER DERMATITIS

Diaper dermatitis refers to many different skin problems that occur in the diaper area. About 10% of infants wearing diapers will develop a significant problem with diaper rash; however, hardly any infant who wears diapers escapes without some diaper dermatitis.[52,53]

Pathophysiology

Diapers are used to contain urine and feces to prevent contaminating the infant's environment. The ideal diaper would also protect the infant's skin from those materials. Many diapers attempt to do this by using absorbent material to draw moisture into deeper layers of the diaper. Whether cloth diapers with or without plastic pants or disposable diapers do a better job of preventing diaper rash has not been conclusively demonstrated.

Ammonia has often been regarded as an agent in the development of diaper rash. The levels of ammonia in infant urine, although easy to smell, are not high enough to cause burns or irritation in normal skin even in the presence of occlusive dressings. Current evidence suggests that urine creates a wet environment and is not a significant source of ammonia.[54]

Feces have not been used experimentally to create dermatitis. It is possible that irritants such as proteolytic enzymes may induce a dermatitis. Some dermatologists suggest that lipase and protease alter the pH of the diaper area, which results in irritation. Water content in infant stool will add to the hydration of infant skin.[55]

Hydrated skin is more vulnerable to friction than dry skin. The injury to the epidermis caused by rubbing makes the skin susceptible to irritation and infection. A skin condition that interrupts normal barrier functions will be made worse by friction in the overhydrated diaper area. The most important variable in developing diaper rash appears to be the length of time a baby's skin is wet.

Bacteria do not play an important initial role in diaper rash. Although bacteria present on the skin do cause the breakdown of urea to ammonia, the level of ammonia produced is not enough to cause dermatitis. *Candida albicans* is recognized as a secondary infection commonly found in diaper dermatitis, but its role as a possible primary cause is not clear. It has been recovered in up to 70% of patients with diaper dermatitis.

Diagnostic Findings

There are several recognizable patterns of diaper rash.[56] The first and most common is dermatitis due to chafing. The skin is mildly reddened, dry, and somewhat thickened on the thighs, buttocks, and around the waist where skin surfaces are rubbed. Papules are sometimes present. This rash tends to appear and resolve quickly. The second, irritant dermatitis, spares intertriginous folds. The skin may be reddened with papules, vesicles, and scaly lesions with most lesions on the lower abdomen, buttocks, and inner thighs.

Candidal diaper dermatitis causes brawny erythema with clearly defined margins; tiny pustules and vesicles are sometimes seen at the periphery of the eruption. Probably over 80% of diaper rashes lasting over 4 days are colonized with *Candida*, even before the classic appearance is manifest. Finally, infants with underlying skin disorders, including atopic or seborrheic dermatitis, commonly have difficulty with diaper rash. Psoriasis may localize to the diaper area and should be considered when there is a family history of psoriasis or typical plaques on other areas of the skin.

Management

Treatment should focus on keeping the skin as dry as possible. Few families are willing to allow infants to be continuously bare-bottomed, but changing diapers frequently is the mainstay of diaper rash therapy. Many young mothers view diaper rash as a sign of inadequacy in caring for an infant and need reassurance that this condition is an expected side effect of diapering.

When the baby is changed, the skin should be rinsed with warm water. If the rash is quite sore, this may need to be done in a sink of warm water to avoid rubbing the skin with a wash cloth or chemical wipe. The baby should gently be patted dry and dusted with a cornstarch powder that will help to reduce friction and rubbing on the skin. It has been shown that cornstarch does not promote candidal growth as it was believed to do in the past. Medicated powders seem to have a helpful antimonilial effect. Zinc oxide emollients provide a barrier that protects the skin from wetness and also decreases friction injury to the skin.

Hydrocortisone (1%) cream applied in a thin coat four times a day at diaper changes will reduce inflammation; often therapy for a few days is all that is needed. If *Candida* is suspected, topical imidazole or nystatin can be used in combination with the hydrocortisone. There is no advantage to using commercially available preparations that combine a steroid and an antifungal agent; some combinations include very strong fluorinated steroids that can cause thinning of the skin when used under occlusion. If candida/diaper dermatitis does not respond to topical therapy, oral nystatin 200,000 U (1 ml in each side of mouth) four times a day for 7 days may be needed to eradicate *Candida* from the gastrointestinal tract. Secondarily infected diaper rash should be treated with appropriate antibiotics.

It is extremely rare for diaper rash to fail to respond to outpatient care. Infants who have not improved within 5 to 7 days will need follow-up evaluation. Rarely, inpatient care may be needed for infants who develop severe bacterial superinfection or in cases where there has been extreme neglect of the child's skin.

ERYTHEMA MULTIFORME

Erythema multiforme (EM) is a hypersensitivity reaction with a controversial definition. The eruption of this disorder is sometimes confused with simple urticaria; however, the papules are duskier in color and tend to evolve in fixed locations over a period of days rather than hours. The characteristic target lesion often has a blister in the center that may develop into an area of tissue necrosis[57,58] (Fig. 48-7).

Erythema multiforme is divided into two categories: erythema multiforme minor, in which lesions are found primarily on the skin, and erythema multiforme major, in which there are prodromal symptoms of fever and malaise, and severe involvement of the mucous membranes. The skin biopsy in both types shows evidence of epidermal damage with perivascular lymphocytic infiltration and edema below the epidermis, thus producing the urticarial lesions. The reaction appears to result from an immune response to a foreign antigen.

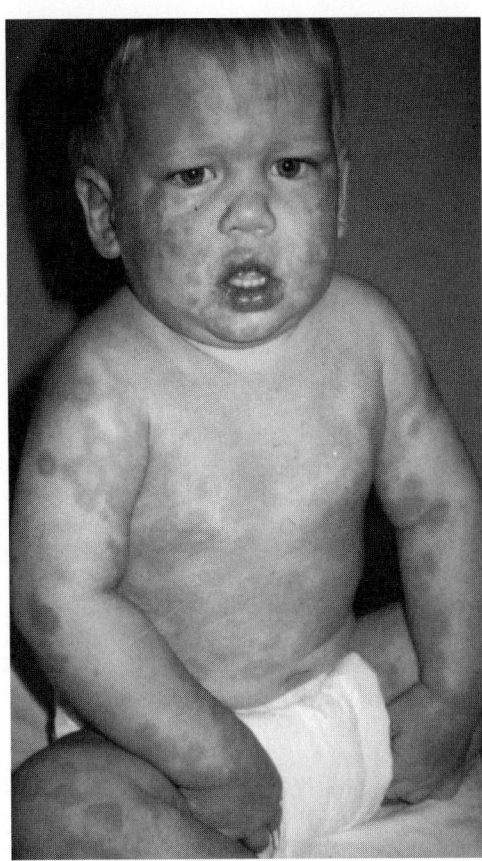

FIG. 48-7. Erythema multiforme. Diagnostic characteristics include target lesions, blistering of the mucous membranes, and a fixed eruption that does not clear with epinephrine.

Infections and drug exposure are the most common etiologic agents. Recurrent herpes simplex infections occur frequently about 10 days before the development of EM. The mechanism for this association is not clear. A clear association between EM and *Mycoplasma pneumoniae* infections is also well known, and frequently develops into Stevens-Johnson syndrome, requiring hospitalization. Drug hypersensitivities may develop after 7 to 14 days of drug therapy or within hours in individuals who have prior sensitization to a drug. Common drugs implicated in EM include sulfa-related antibiotics, penicillins, cephalosporins, phenytoin, and phenylbutazone.

Diagnostic Findings

Simple EM does not involve blistering of mucous membrane surfaces and resolves spontaneously over 10 to 14 days. In approximately one half of EM patients, there is a history of a herpes infection or an upper respiratory infection 1 week before the abrupt onset of the rash. The target-like lesions are distributed symmetrically over elbows, knees, and extensor surfaces.

Differential Considerations

The differential diagnosis of EM includes urticarial reactions. Urticaria may have a similar target lesion appearance; however, the lesions are transient and last for a few hours rather than for several days. Urticarial reactions will clear with subcutaneous epinephrine but erythema multiforme will not. Varicella and other bullous skin diseases may be considered in the initial differential but will be distinguished by their clinical course.

Management

Because simple EM is a benign disorder, it should be managed conservatively by removing any possible offending agent, and initiating symptomatic therapy, such as with oral antihistamines. Patients with any mucous membrane involvement may require inpatient care because they are frequently unable to eat or drink. Local or systemic steroids are not useful in this condition.[59,60]

STEVENS-JOHNSON SYNDROME/TOXIC EPIDERMAL NECROLYSIS

Stevens-Johnson syndrome (SJS) is a polymorphous mucocutaneous eruption characterized by a prodrome of 1 to 14 days of fever, headache, malaise, occasional vomiting, and diarrhea; target lesions of the skin; and blistering of mucous membranes.[61] Toxic epidermal necrolysis (TEN) is a severe exfoliative form of SJS that is frequently drug-induced, in which large areas of skin may be denuded. Although there is considerable overlap in clinical symptoms and etiologic agents, EM and SJS are probably distinct entities.[62] Mild erythema multiforme does not progress to SJS.

Diagnostic Findings

In addition to the cutaneous lesions, at least two mucosal surfaces are involved, and conjunctivitis, rhinitis, proctitis, balanitis, and vulvovaginitis may be identified on physical examination. Iritis and renal involvement are sometimes found, thus indicating internal organ involvement. Some observers have attempted to describe the skin lesions of SJS as flat targets or purpuric macules rather than the raised targets typical of EM.[63]

An association between SJS/TEN and antecedent medication uses has been noticed, particularly with the increased use of cephalosporin antibiotics. Vancomycin, amoxacillin, allopurinol, nonsteroidal antiinflammatory drugs, and phenytoin are among the other drugs implicated in this syndrome. *Mycoplasma pneumoniae* and various viral illnesses may also be involved in the etiology. TEN is usually seen in adults and older children; this is thought to be due to lack of previous exposure to sensitizing drugs in younger children.

Differential Considerations

Severe reactions may be confused with staphylococcal scalded skin syndrome (SSSS) because patients with both diseases have fever and a toxic appearance. When it is necessary to be sure of a diagnosis, the biopsy in SJS or TEN will show a lymphocytic infiltrate with full-thickness necrosis of the epidermis rather than a vasculitis or the intraepidermal cleavage of SSSS. Separation of the skin layers in SJS/TEN occurs at deeper levels below the basement membrane of the upper dermis, whereas skin separation in SSSS occurs at a superficial level.

Management

Patients with SJS or TEN should be treated in-hospital because they may require intravenous hydration, hyperalimentation, and intensive skin care.[64] Patients are best managed in burn units if skin involvement is extensive. The use of systemic corticosteroids for these situations remains highly controversial. Although steroids may help to reduce inflammation very early in the course of a severe reaction, they should not be started without extensive consultation and discussion.

The disorder usually starts abruptly and can last for several weeks. Some studies have suggested a mortality rate of about 15% for SJS, whereas higher mortality rates are seen with TEN because of the severe loss of skin integrity. Dehydration, electrolyte imbalance, inability to regulate body temperature, and secondary infection all contribute to the morbidity of this condition.

FUNGAL INFECTIONS

Fungi are simple plants that lack chlorophyll and obtain nourishment from other living or dead organic material. Fungal infections occur in animals and humans and may be superficial, deep, or systemic. Superficial fungal infections include dermatophytoses, tinea versicolor, and candidiasis. The dermatophytes are a group of fungi that cause infections of skin, hair, and nails commonly referred to as tinea or ringworm. These infections are common and increase in frequency with increased age, hot, humid climate, and crowded living conditions. Infection of the hands, feet, or nails is uncommon before puberty.[65]

Diagnostic Findings

The diagnosis of fungal infections can be confirmed rapidly with a microscopic examination using potassium hydroxide.[66] Skin scales scraped from the most inflammatory edge of a body lesion or hairs from a scalp lesion can be placed on a slide and covered with a drop of 10% potassium hydroxide and 40% dimethyl sulfoxide (DMSO). This solution will dissolve cornified skin cells so that fungal hyphae are easily seen when scanned at X 100 magnification. The reliability of this test depends on the examiner's experience in both gathering the specimen and searching the slide.

A Wood's lamp emits ultraviolet light at 365 nm, which causes a few pathogenic fungi to fluoresce. Unfortunately, the results of the examination are most often negative. Although a Wood's lamp is helpful to examine hair, it is sometimes misused to examine skin scales, which usually appear to fluoresce whatever their cause. Definitive diagnosis of fungal infections is best done by culture on selective media. Although this is not necessary on all superficial fungal infections, cultures should be performed in cases of tinea capitis and tinea of the nails because long-term systemic therapy is usually needed.

Tinea Capitis

Fungal infections of the scalp are most commonly seen in children between 2 and 10 years of age. They occur infrequently after puberty, perhaps because of a change in the fatty acid content of sebum[67] (Fig. 48-8, A).

Etiology. Most cases in the United States are now caused by *Trichophyton tonsurans*, which does not fluoresce under Wood's lamp examination. *Microsporum audouinii*, which does fluoresce, is now seen in less than 10% of cases. Occasionally *M. canis* can be transmitted to a child, but it is usually associated with exposure to an infected cat rather than a dog. Diagnosis of tinea capitis should be confirmed with a fungal culture because clinical diagnostic methods are not foolproof and the treatment is complex.

Diagnostic Findings. There are four patterns of scalp lesions that can be seen with tinea capitis. The most obvious pattern is characterized by round or oval areas of alopecia, about 1 to 5 cm in diameter, which on close inspection show stubby remains of hairs that have broken off a few millimeters above the scalp. The hair stubs produce the "black-dot" appearance. Although this pattern of infection is easy to recognize, it is seen in only 5% of cases.

Kerion formation develops in about one third of cases of tinea capitis. This inflammatory complication resembles a severe bacterial infection with boggy, purulent, crusted lesions and regional lymphadenopathy. Children with this hyperreactive condition often develop generalized scaly papules or plaques (called *id reaction*) on other areas of the body that have no direct fungal involvement; this is probably the result of systemic sensitization to fungal products.

A common presentation of fungal scalp infection, which is often not recognized, resembles diffuse flaky dandruff with little, if any, alopecia. Close examination will show black dots; potassium hydroxide preparation and cultures will be positive.

In some cases, individual discrete pustules resembling folliculitis will actually be tinea capitis. This pattern may also show no alopecia, and lymphadenopathy may be present.

Differential Considerations. The conditions that cause patches of hair loss, such as alopecia areata and trichotillomania, are the major differential considerations. Hair can be broken by repetitive twirling, tight braiding, or yanking (Fig. 48-8, B). In any of these situations, hairs will be broken at different lengths in the affected area. Alopecia areata shows complete hair loss without inflammatory scalp changes (Fig. 48-8, C). Kerion formation is most commonly confused with a bacterial pyoderma; however, the pustules in kerions are sterile. Seborrheic dermatitis, dandruff, and psoriasis should also be considered when evaluating scaly scalp lesions.

Management. Initial therapy for tinea capitis is oral griseofulvin, 15 mg/kg/day in a single dose or divided doses. The medication must be taken for at least 6 weeks. It is reasonable to begin treatment at an acute visit if the diagnosis is certain. Close follow-up to monitor side effects of the medication, such as hepatotoxicity and leukopenia, and to assess the effect of therapy is essential. Ketoconazole is used as a second line of therapy if griseofulvin cannot be tolerated.

Many physicians believe that scarring from kerions can be reduced if oral prednisone, 1 to 2 mg/kg/24 hr, is given. Shampoos containing 2.5% selenium sulfide (Selsun) decrease the amount of shedding of spores when used twice a week and may decrease further spread of infection. Topical antifungal medications have no role in tinea capitis.

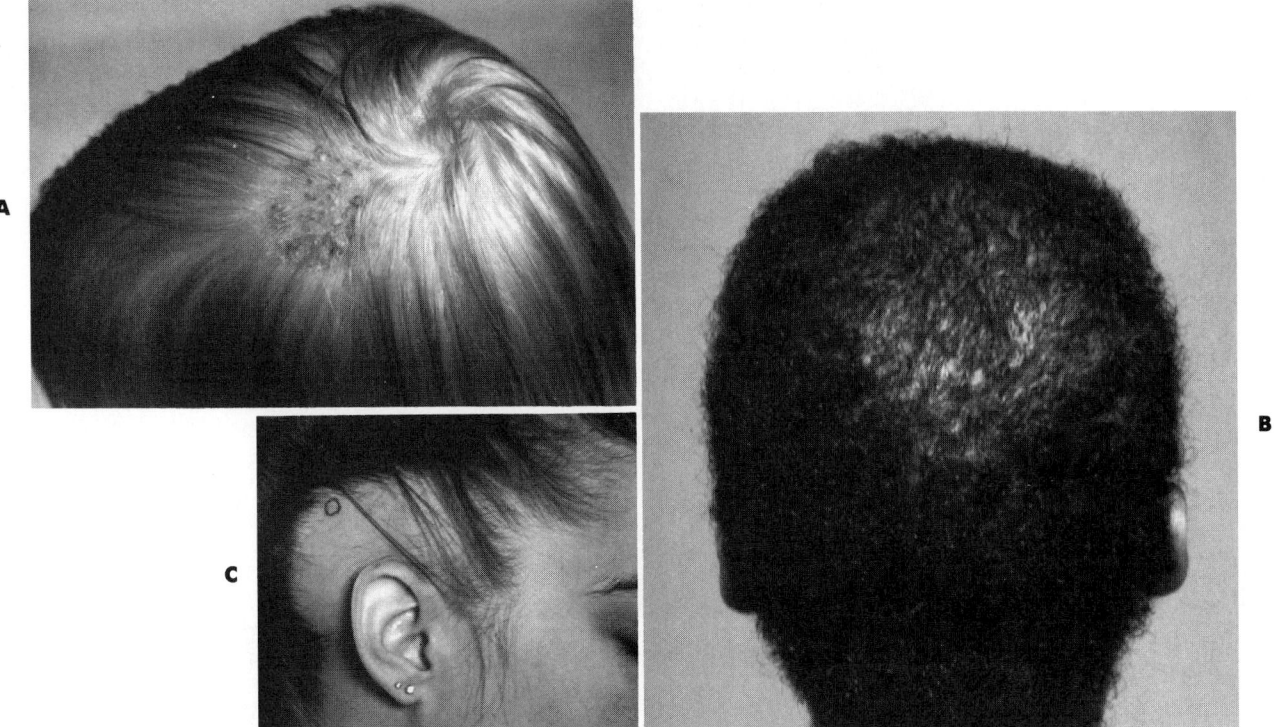

FIG. 48-8. Fungal infections. **A,** Tinea capitis—kerion formation develops in about one third of cases. **B,** Traction alopecia—hair may be broken off at short lengths because of tight braiding. **C,** Alopecia areata—complete loss of hair without inflammatory scalp changes. (*Courtesy Mayo Medical Center, Department of Dermatology, Rochester, Minn.*)   *Continued.*

Fungal spores stay viable in the environment for long periods of time, so barettes, combs, and brushes should be washed frequently in warm soapy water and should not be shared. When an infection is found in one family member, all other children and adults should also be examined. One week after griseofulvin therapy has started, a child can usually return to school. A follow-up visit should be scheduled 2 weeks after beginning therapy to review the culture and assess treatment.

Tinea Corporis

Superficial fungal infections of the skin are most commonly seen in warm climates (Fig. 48-8, *D*). They can be found in infants and adults but are most common in young children. Infected domestic and farm animals are a frequent source of infection. *M. canis* and *T. mentagrophytes* are the dermatophytes that most commonly cause tinea corporis.

Diagnostic Findings. The classic ringworm shape of an expanding oval or round inflammatory border with a clear center is the most recognizable form of tinea corporis. Lesions may also appear as vesicles, papules, pustules, and eczematous patches. Itching is a common problem. Topical corticosteroids are often tried before the diagnosis is reached and may reduce inflammation, making skin lesions difficult to recognize. Regional lymph nodes are usually not enlarged unless impetigo complicates the situation.

Any red scaly rash should be suspected of fungal infection and examined with a KOH prep. A Wood's lamp examination is not helpful. Topical treatment is usually very effective, so many people do not obtain cultures unless there is no response to therapy.

Differential Considerations. Pityriasis rosea, granuloma annulare, and atopic dermatitis are sometimes confused with tinea corporis. Erythrasma, a superficial colonization of the skin with *Corynebacterium minutissimum*, may look like tinea cruris but will have a negative KOH and coral red fluorescence on Wood's lamp examination. Erythrasma requires oral antibiotic treatment.

Management. Treatment of tinea corporis usually results in relief of itching within the first week. It is important to continue treatment for a minimum of 2 to 3 weeks after initial clearing to prevent recurrence. There are several effective topical antifungal agents available to treat tinea corporis: tolnaftate (Tinactin), miconazole (Micatin), haloprogin (Halotex), and clotrimazole (Lotrimin). All are used by rubbing into the affected area twice a day. If there is no improvement in 3 weeks, the patient should be referred for further evaluation.

Tinea Versicolor

A change in skin pigmentation is the most common complaint caused by tinea versicolor (Fig. 48-8, *E*.) The problem results when a yeast called *Malassezia furfur*, which colonizes normal skin, changes to its mycelial form. This change is found more commonly in tropical climates but may also be related to hyperhidrosis, malnutrition, and immunosuppression. Although the yeast is found on the

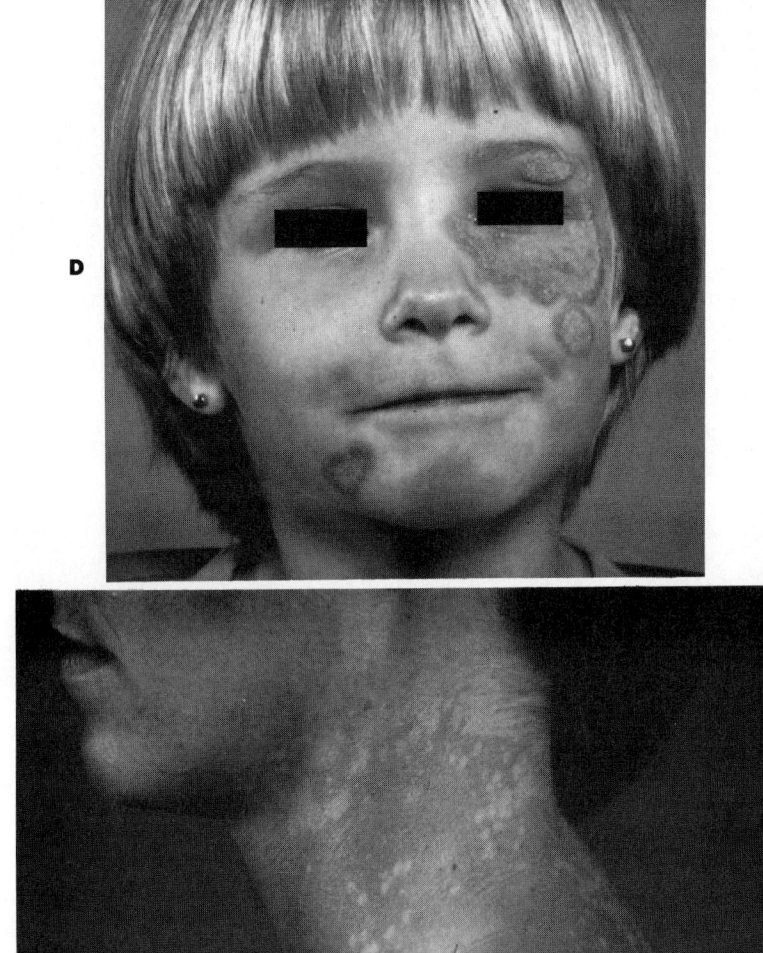

FIG. 48-8, cont'd. Fungal infections. **D**, Tinea corporis — raised, inflamed borders with scales that gradually clear in the center are characteristic. **E**, Tinea versicolor — round scaly patches become prominent in the summer by causing irregular tanning. (*Courtesy Mayo Medical Center, Department of Dermatology, Rochester, Minn.*)

skin of young children, tinea versicolor is rare before puberty.[68]

Diagnostic Findings. Tinea versicolor commonly involves the upper trunk and arms, although it can be more widespread. Many small oval or round scaly patches with no inflammation are seen. It is frequently more prominent in the summer when the patches are accentuated by the irregular tanning that they cause. The patches are usually hypopigmented, although hyperpigmentation can also occur. KOH preparation will demonstrate a "spaghetti-and-meatballs" appearance of clumps of intertwined hyphae and circular spores. A Wood's lamp examination may show

orange fluorescence. It is not possible to culture the organism on usual fungal media; however, the clinical appearance is usually diagnostic.

Differential Considerations. Tinea versicolor can be confused with pityriasis rosea, atopic dermatitis, contact dermatitis, and tinea corporis. Hypopigmented lesions such as vitiligo and pityriasis alba should be considered.

Management. Treatment consists of keratolytics, such as selenium sulfide shampoos, to remove the superficial skin scales in which the mycelium grow, and topical antifungal agents such as clotrimazole, tolnaftate, and miconazole applied once a day. There is a very high rate of recurrence of this problem, and treatment should be aimed toward control, not cure. Abnormal pigmentation will resolve over several months if the infection can be controlled.

Candidiasis

Candida albicans is not found on normal skin; however, it is commonly present in the oral cavity, gastrointestinal tract, and vagina. It occurs as a skin pathogen when host defense mechanisms are impaired either because of a local or a systemic problem.

Oral Candidiasis. Thrush causes painful inflammation of the tongue, palates, and buccal mucosa. The white plaques can be differentiated from curds of milk because they cannot be wiped off the mucous membrane. Most infants with thrush are otherwise entirely healthy. There is not a clear relationship between antibiotic use and thrush, and there is no difference in incidence between bottlefed or breastfed infants. Thrush is rarely seen in newborns and seems to be more common in infants over 2 months of age, probably in relation to decreasing protection from maternal antibodies.[40]

Treatment with oral nystatin suspension, 2 ml (1 ml in each side of mouth) of 100,000 U/ml four times a day, will result in improvement in 85% of infants, usually within 24 hours. The suspension should be used after feedings so that it sits in the mouth for as long as possible. Infants who continue to have thrush after a week of treatment should be seen in a follow-up visit.

Cutaneous Candidiasis. Monilial infections of the skin erupt in the moist warm areas of skin folds such as the axillae, neck folds, and the diaper area. This common problem, known as intertrigo, may complicate seborrheic dermatitis. It is seen in obese children whose skin folds are redundant. In any of the areas affected, the eruption has an appearance similar to glistening red raw skin and may be edematous or oozing. Tiny satellite lesions often appear along the sharp edge of the eruption.

Treatment with topical antifungal agents is very effective. Many preparations are available in powder form, which helps to decrease the moisture in the skin folds. Clotrimazole, miconazole, or nystatin are all quite effective. Combination preparations should be avoided because topical antibiotics can cause sensitization in inflamed areas; corticosteroids can cause thinning of the skin and are absorbed systemically through the skin, but may on occasion be helpful when used cautiously.

HENOCH-SCHÖNLEIN PURPURA

The syndrome of acute purpura and arthritis in children was described in 1837 by Schönlein, and the symptoms of colicky abdominal pain and nephritis were added by Henoch in 1874. This syndrome is seen in children usually between the ages of 2 and 10 years, with a seasonal incidence that peaks in winter. There is no clear etiologic agent, although it has been associated with group A beta-hemolytic streptococcal pharyngitis and viral infections in some cases.[69]

Diagnostic Findings

Palpable purpuras are the usual signs of Henoch-Schönlein purpura. Skin changes develop before other

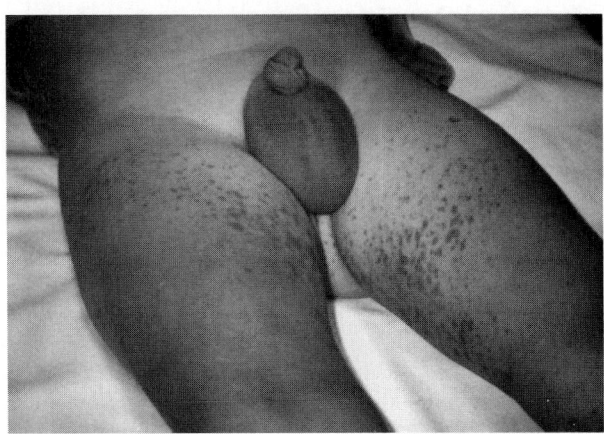

FIG. 48-9. Henoch-Schönlein purpura—purpura over the buttocks, lower extremities, and genitalia.

clinical manifestations in most children. The rash is usually distributed symmetrically over the buttocks and lower extremities with relatively less involvement of the trunk and upper extremities (Fig. 48-9). This distribution is relatively pathognomonic.[70,71] There may be marked swelling and bruising of the scrotum.[72] The rash may begin with urticarial lesions, which then progress to papules that become purpuric within 1 to 2 days. Hemorrhagic vesicles and ulcers can develop in severe cases. The first papules fade after about a week, leaving hyperpigmented areas, but crops of new lesions may continue to develop. Pathology of skin specimens demonstrates an acute vasculitis with IgA deposits in arteriole walls. In some cases arthritis or abdominal pain may develop before the rash appears, and appendicitis has been suspected as an initial diagnosis. Intussusception may occur. Melena or hematest-positive stools are quite common, and are usually unassociated with intussusception.[73]

Arthritis is usually transient and occurs in approximately two thirds of cases, but the pain and disability often seems out of proportion to the signs of inflammation. Large joints, especially the knees and ankles, are usually affected.

Renal involvement is usually mild, with proteinuria or hematuria occurring in about 40% of cases. Hypertension may be present. Pathologic findings on kidney biopsy range from mild focal glomerulitis to proliferative glomerulonephritis. There have been reports of progression of renal disease in up to 10% of older children despite full resolution of the other disease manifestations (see Chapter 60).

Children with Henoch-Schönlein purpura usually recover completely, but they may have relapses of purpura, abdominal pain, and arthritis for 1 or 2 months after the initial occurrence. In general, recurrences are more common in older children.[74]

An elevated white blood cell (WBC) count is often seen along with a mild anemia that may be related to gastrointestinal blood loss. Most importantly, however, platelet count and coagulation studies are normal. Serum IgA levels are frequently elevated, especially in the early stage of the disease. Blood cultures may be necessary to rule out septic causes of purpura.

Differential Considerations

The differential diagnosis includes problems that acutely cause purpura such as meningococcemia, disseminated intravascular coagulation (DIC), and viral illness. Patients often have an acute abdominal pain that begins before the rash is evident; acute appendicitis may be mimicked by Henoch-Schönlein purpura. Child abuse is sometimes considered because the pattern of bruising may resemble paddled buttocks.

Management

After life-threatening conditions are excluded, treatment is generally limited to supportive care with antiinflammatory medications for the arthritis, and intravenous fluids if the child is unable to eat. If severe abdominal pain is present, evaluation to exclude intussusception is essential.

Prednisolone in a dose of 1 to 2 mg/kg/24 hr has been used to control gastrointestinal pain and bleeding.[75] It should not be used if intussusception is a clinical consideration. The efficacy of steroids in relation to treating nephritis has not yet been adequately determined.

The majority of children with Henoch-Schönlein purpura can be treated as outpatients with careful follow-up including urinalysis and blood pressure monitoring. Children require inpatient care when their arthritis cannot be managed at home, when their abdominal pain causes anorexia and dehydration or concern over an acute abdomen, or when observation is needed to distinguish Henoch-Schönlein purpura from serious differential considerations.

HERPES VIRUS INFECTIONS

Skin infections caused by both herpes simplex and herpes zoster are associated with recurrent vesicular eruptions that can occur years after the original infection (Fig. 48-10, A). The mechanism for development of a latent period and for reactivation of the virus is unknown. Both types of herpes virus can be maintained in spinal nerve root ganglia and appear to travel down the nerve to the epidermis when the infection recurs.[76]

Herpes Simplex

Herpes simplex infections are caused by two types of herpes virus, type one (HSV-1) and type two (HSV-2).[77] Although the clinical syndromes produced by these viruses are not entirely distinct, HSV-1 is more common and tends to be found in oral infections, and HSV-2 is usually associated with genital infections. Both types of infections are frequently subclinical; however, once the infection has been acquired, it is present for life.

Diagnostic Findings. Primary infections with herpes simplex occur in an individual with no circulating antibody against the virus. The most common presentation of primary HSV-1 is gingivostomatitis. The peak incidence of this infection is found in children less than 5 years of age. Children frequently have high fever, irritability, and vesicles on the tongue, gingivae, and buccal mucosa. They frequently drool and refuse to eat because of the soreness. Regional lymphadenopathy is usually present. The fever may last for 5 to 7 days, and the mouth sores may last for as long as 2 weeks. Decreased oral intake with the possibility of dehydration, particularly in very young children, is the

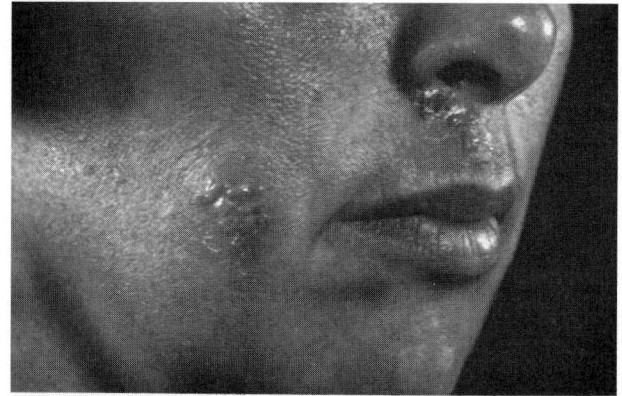

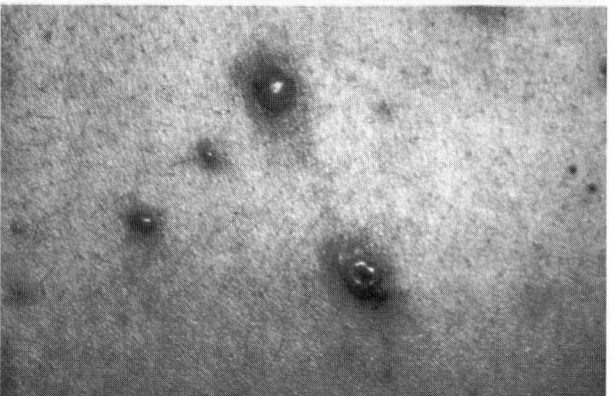

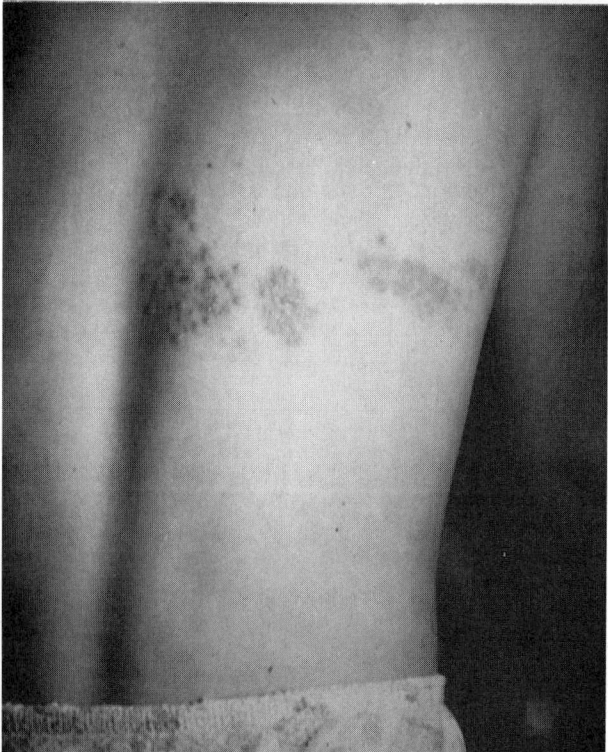

FIG. 48-10. Herpes virus infections. **A,** Herpes simplex—herpes labialis may be a recurrent vesticular eruption. **B,** Varicella—dew-drop-on-a-rose-petal lesions can be seen in different stages of development. **C,** Herpes zoster—vesicles appear along the distribution of a single dermatome. (*Courtesy Mayo Medical Center, Department of Dermatology, Rochester, Minn.*)

major complication. The diagnosis can be confirmed with the discovery of multinucleated giant cells on a Tzanck smear or by viral culture.

Herpetic whitlow is a term describing the presence of grouped vesicles on one or more fingers. Inoculation of the skin on the fingers can occur in children with herpes stomatitis who suck their fingers. A primary herpes infection with fever, lymphadenopathy, and general malaise can occur with local inoculation of the virus through traumatized skin. The herpes virus can be transmitted with a needle stick; this happens most often when physicians, nurses, and dentists are directly exposed to patients with the disease.

HSV-2 is usually acquired through sexual contact, and antibodies against HSV-2 are rarely found in preadolescents.[78] The primary infection is asymptomatic in 75% of cases; however, a primary reaction with fever, regional lymphadenopathy, headache, malaise, and vesicles in the genital region can develop.

Some but not all individuals will develop recurrent infections following a primary herpes infection. About 90% of primary infections are subclinical so most people with recurrent herpes labialis have no history of gingivostomatitis. Lesions occur most often on the vermilion border of the lips, and on the chin or the cheek. A sensation of itching or burning frequently precedes the eruption, which can last for only a few hours or up to 10 days. There is usually no lymphadenopathy. Viral shedding is present initially but rapidly diminishes. There are many examples of triggers for a recurrence, including sunlight, colds, trauma, spicy foods, and stress. Often no trigger can be determined.

After a primary HSV-2 infection, recurrent genital herpes attacks of variable frequency and severity may develop. Some people shed the virus without developing apparent vesicles. It is usually helpful to obtain viral cultures in cases suspected to be genital herpes because this is a very emotionally charged problem, and because antiviral treatment is available.

Differential Considerations. Other vesicular viral infections may be confused with primary herpes infections. Hand, foot, and mouth disease and herpangina resemble herpes gingivostomatitis. Viral cultures can be used to distinguish these diseases if necessary. Aphthous ulcers occur in children who usually do not have systemic symptoms of illness and will have negative Tzanck tests. Although the mouth lesions of erythema multiforme may resemble a herpes infection, the typical target skin lesions should differentiate the problem.

Impetigo and herpes labialis both have yellow serous crusts with erythematous surrounding skin. Gram stain and bacterial culture or Tzanck smear can be used to distinguish these lesions.

Herpetic whitlow is often confused with bacterial cellulitis. A history of exposure to a herpetic infection and a Tzanck smear are very helpful in diagnosing herpes.

Herpes progenitalis may mimic other venereal problems. It is important to be aware that this condition may coexist with gonorrhea or syphilis; smears, cultures and serologic tests are useful diagnostic tools for identification of these problems.

Management. Acyclovir inhibits viral DNA synthesis and will shorten the course of a primary herpes infection if it is started within the first week. For localized skin infections with herpes, 5% acyclovir ointment, applied in a small amount six times a day, may provide some relief of symptoms and shorten the duration of viral shedding.[79]

Primary genital herpes in adults is treated with 200 mg oral acyclovir every 4 hours for five doses throughout the day for 10 days. Local symptomatic treatment includes tepid baths, cool compresses, ice packs, and forcing fluids to maintain dilute urine. Topical anesthetics, such as 2% lidocaine jelly, may provide some relief of pain.

Neither topical nor systemic acyclovir prevents recurrence of herpes simplex infections. Acyclovir may help to shorten the course of viral shedding, thus preventing spread to other skin areas or other people.

Oral herpes simplex infections are very common in children. Because the majority of "cold sores" are asymptomatic, it is not necessary to attempt to isolate children with these infections from school or daycare.[80] However, children with primary gingivostomatitis who are unable to control secretions, should not be in daycare during the period when they have fever, mouth pain, and drooling.

Patients with genital herpes should be counseled to avoid intercourse when they have visible lesions. They should also be made aware that the infection can spread during the latent phase.

Varicella (Chickenpox)

Primary infection with the varicella zoster virus results in chickenpox, a common, highly contagious, usually mild illness of childhood. The incubation period ranges from 14 to 21 days, and most cases occur in people under 14 years of age, with the highest rates occurring in children ages 3 to 6 years. In studies documenting incidence before use of the vaccine, about 20% of children over 8 years of age remained susceptible to varicella.[81] The disease appears to be spread by direct contact, but airborne spread has been documented.[82]

Diagnostic Findings. The illness begins with a mild 1- or 2-day prodrome of respiratory symptoms, malaise, and low-grade fever. The rash usually starts on the trunk with small red macules or papules that progress to tiny vesicles giving the "dew-drop-on-a-rose-petal" appearance (Fig. 48-10, *B*). Crops of vesicles continue to develop for 3 to 5 days, so that all stages of the rash can be found at the same time on any part of the body. When the lesions begin to crust they are thought to no longer be infectious.

Subclinical infections with varicella have been recognized. Children within the same family can develop illness of quite variable severity. Although varicella usually confers lasting immunity after the first infection, second attacks can happen.

The most common complications are bacterial superinfection of the skin lesions and otitis media. Varicella pneumonia, nephritis, meningoencephalitis, orchitis, and appendicitis have been described. Necrotizing fasciitis due to streptococcal infections has been recognized as a complication of chickenpox, and may be increasing in frequency.[83] Inpatient care may be needed for children with cellulitis, pneumonia with respiratory distress, or changes in mental status.[84,85] Varicella infections in an immunocompromised person are often progressive and potentially fatal.

Management. For children who have uncomplicated chickenpox, treatment is symptomatic and supportive. Antihistamines such as diphenhydramine 4 to 6 mg/kg/day, not to exceed 300 mg divided into three or four doses can be given, and oatmeal baths may help relieve itching. Aspirin should be avoided because an association with Reye syndrome has been suggested. Acetaminophen may be used to control fever and discomfort; however, a report showed that lesions erupted for a longer period of time in children given acetaminophen compared to those untreated, suggesting that less treatment may be better.[86] Acyclovir, in a dose of 20 mg/kg/dose (maximum 800 mg/dose) QID PO for 5 days, has been recommended to decrease the severity of illness. However, this treatment is controversial because it must be initiated within the first 24 hours of illness to produce significant effects, and this window of opportunity often occurs before the diagnostic skin lesions appear. It seems most reasonable to use acyclovir for children at risk for severe illness in whom an exact exposure has been documented such as a nonimmune older child with a household exposure, a child with a chronic skin disorder, or a child on corticosteroids or with another immune-compromised state.

Children who are at high risk for severe chickenpox can be treated with varicella-zoster immune globulin (VZIG) to prevent development of disease; however, VZIG must be given within 96 hours of exposure (preferably within 48 hours). The recommended dose of VZIG is 125 U/10 kg IM with a minimum dose of 125 U and a maximum of 625 U. Children with uncomplicated chickenpox should not return to daycare or school until every lesion has a crust. This may take as long as a week after the onset of the rash or may be shorter in children with mild cases.[80,87]

Scars from chickenpox develop most often in lesions that have become superinfected. Chickenpox scars may cause keloid formation in susceptible individuals; however, scars improve in appearance for many months after the initial infection.

Fatal varicella has been seen in apparently healthy children who are on chronic corticosteroid therapy, including children with asthma. Administration of VZIG to attenuate the illness should be considered for children on steroids who have been exposed to chickenpox.[88]

Live attenuated varicella vaccine is now available in the United States for children.[89,90] Current recommendations are for one dose of vaccine for all children under age 13 years who do not have a good history of previous varicella disease. Special attention will be focused on infants between 12 and 18 months in an attempt to provide a high rate of herd immunity. After 13 years of age, two doses of the vaccine are needed to be effective. The most common side effects of the vaccine are pain at the injection site, fever, vesicular rash at the injection site within 2 days of vaccination, and a generalized chickenpox-like rash about 1 to 3 weeks later. The length of sustained immunity into adulthood is not known.

Herpes Zoster

Herpes zoster eruptions are a late complication of chickenpox infections. Varicella zoster virus can persist in latent form in spinal sensory nerve root ganglia and erupt many years after the original infection. Zoster attacks usually are not recurrent. Although they can happen at any age, the attack rate in children under 5 years of age is only about 1 in 100. The rate of zoster is higher in children with underlying immune abnormalities.

Diagnostic Findings. Development of zoster is usually preceded by radicular pain with vesicles appearing along the distribution of a single dermatome, although adjacent dermatomes may be involved (Fig. 48-10, C). Lesions similar in appearance to chickenpox erupt for 1 to 4 days and then crust over. Herpes virus can be cultured from the lesions, and a susceptible person can develop varicella if exposed to someone with zoster. Thoracic and trigeminal nerve dermatomes are most commonly involved. The possibility of ophthalmic complications if the cornea becomes involved, should be suspected if the eyelids or tip of the nose is involved. Postherpetic pain in the region of involvement is very rare in children. Dissemination of the disease, as a consequence of hematogenous viral spread, occurs in immunosuppressed patients and may be seen as a complication of high-dose corticosteroid therapy.

Management. Treatment should be limited to relieving local symptoms with analgesics and drying agents such as Burow's solution and wet compresses. Acyclovir has been used to prevent dissemination in the immunocompromised host. Children with zoster need to be isolated, like children with chickenpox, until there is a crust on every vesicle.

INFECTIOUS EXANTHEMS

Childhood exanthems have become more difficult to recognize because physicians and parents see fewer examples of children with these illnesses, and because these classic infectious exanthems have become modified by vaccine and antibiotic therapy.

In recent years, epidemics of measles have resurfaced, underscoring the need to be able to recognize the classic childhood exanthems. Emergency departments have become a source of care for many children and adults with acute illnesses.[91] They have also been implicated as sources of epidemics because patients waiting to be seen are exposed to other contagious patients. Physicians working in acute care settings must be able to diagnose the infectious exanthem syndromes in order to treat patients accurately and to intervene in community epidemics.

An exanthem is an eruption on the skin associated with a systemic illness.[92-95] The rash is only one manifestation of the total disease. Although the rash may be the chief complaint, it may not be specific enough that a diagnosis can be made without obtaining a history of other symptoms. Diagnosing exanthems depends upon recognition of a set of signs and symptoms.

Most exanthems are part of benign, self-limited viral diseases, but there are situations in which recognition of the syndrome can be important to individuals other than the patient. Both rubella and fifth disease have implications for pregnant women exposed to a patient. In cases such as varicella, parents and physicians need to recognize the complications particular to that disease. A child whose course is benign does not need examination in a setting where other people at risk will be exposed; a child with a complication of chickenpox should not be kept at home

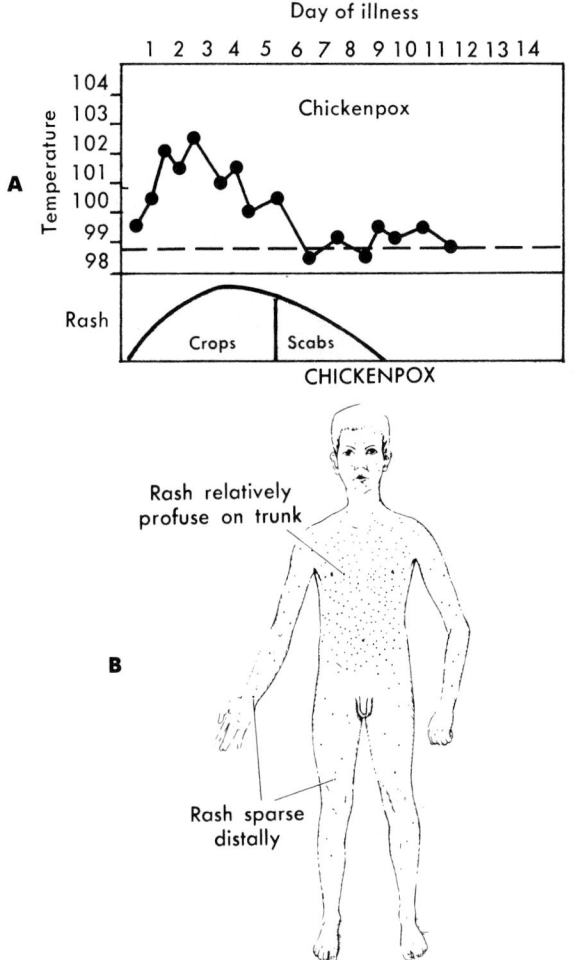

FIG. 48-11. Herpes zoster. **A,** Schematic diagram illustrating clinical course of typical case of chickenpox. Crops of lesions appear with rapid progression from macules to papules to vesicles to scabs. **B,** Schematic drawing illustrating typical distribution of rash of chickenpox. *(From Krugman S et al: Infectious diseases of children, ed 9, St. Louis, 1992, Mosby.)*

without being evaluated. The physician must be ready to assess the rash that appears on a child with an infectious disease who is also taking an antibiotic, so as to determine whether the rash is caused by the illness or the medication.

Early in this century, exanthems were classified and referred to by number with rubeola as first disease, scarlet fever as second disease, and rubella as third disease.[96] Fourth disease does not correspond to any presently known illness. Fifth disease or erythema infectiosum is still referred to by its number but is now known to be caused by a specific viral agent. Roseola infantum is the sixth disease. The majority of viral rashes seen today, however, are caused by enteroviruses and were not part of this numbering system (Figs. 48-11 and 48-12). Viral exanthems are also discussed in Chapter 55.

Rubeola (Measles)

Live attenuated measles virus vaccine was introduced in 1963. Before the vaccine was available, measles was re-

sponsible for at least 600,000 illnesses per year in the United States. Before immunization, the disease was endemic worldwide, and 90% of the population had the disease before reaching adulthood. By 1983 an all-time low of 1,497 cases were reported to the Centers for Disease Control (CDC). Epidemic outbreaks have occurred both in previously immunized college-aged children and in groups of unimmunized younger children.[97] An initial immunization with live attenuated measles virus is suggested at the age of 15 months with a second dose on entry to junior high school.

The measles virus is a single-stranded RNA virus belonging to the paramyxovirus group. It is transmitted by respiratory droplet spread and is highly contagious. The incubation period is 9 to 12 days from the time of exposure to the onset of symptoms. A patient with the disease is thought to be contagious from 3 days prior to the onset of rash until the rash desquamates and is most contagious during the prodromal period. As fewer clinicians are familiar with clinical measles, the clinical diagnosis has become less reliable, and serologic testing should be done to confirm cases when public health concerns require accurate diagnosis.[98]

Diagnostic Findings. Typical measles begins with a prodrome of upper respiratory symptoms that last for 2 to 4 days with gradually increasing fever. Cough, conjunctivitis, and coryza (nasal congestion) are usually present. Koplik spots, which are tiny white spots on erythematous buccal mucosa opposite the lower molars, are diagnostic of measles. They appear during the prodrome and are usually still present when the rash begins.

The exanthem appears 14 days after exposure, classically beginning behind the ears at the hairline and spreading from the head to the feet over a 3-day period. It is erythematous and maculopapular with initial discrete lesions that become confluent as the rash spreads. As the rash fades, skin may appear hyperpigmented, and fine scaling may develop. The patient looks most ill on the second or third day of the rash with high fever, photophobia, and a distressing brassy cough. If no complications of the disease develop, the illness gradually abates, lasting a total of about 7 days. The prognosis is much worse in children who are malnourished or immunosuppressed.

Otitis media is the most common complication of measles. Croup and laryngitis may also occur. Pneumonia is the most common reason for hospitalization, and infiltrates can be found on chest x-rays of most children with measles even without clinical signs of pneumonia. Encephalitis occurs in about 1 in 1,000 cases and may cause permanent neurologic impairment. Hepatitis, thrombocytopenia, Stevens-Johnson syndrome, appendicitis, and colitis have also been associated with this disease.

Modified measles may develop in a partially immune host, such as a child who has received gamma globulin prior to developing the disease, or an infant who has some transplacental antibodies. In this situation, the incubation period may be prolonged and the prodrome shortened. Koplik spots and the exanthem may be present briefly, and the child is usually less ill. It is often difficult to diagnose measles in this setting, although the child is still contagious to others. Atypical measles were seen in children immunized with a killed-type of vaccine (used between 1963 and

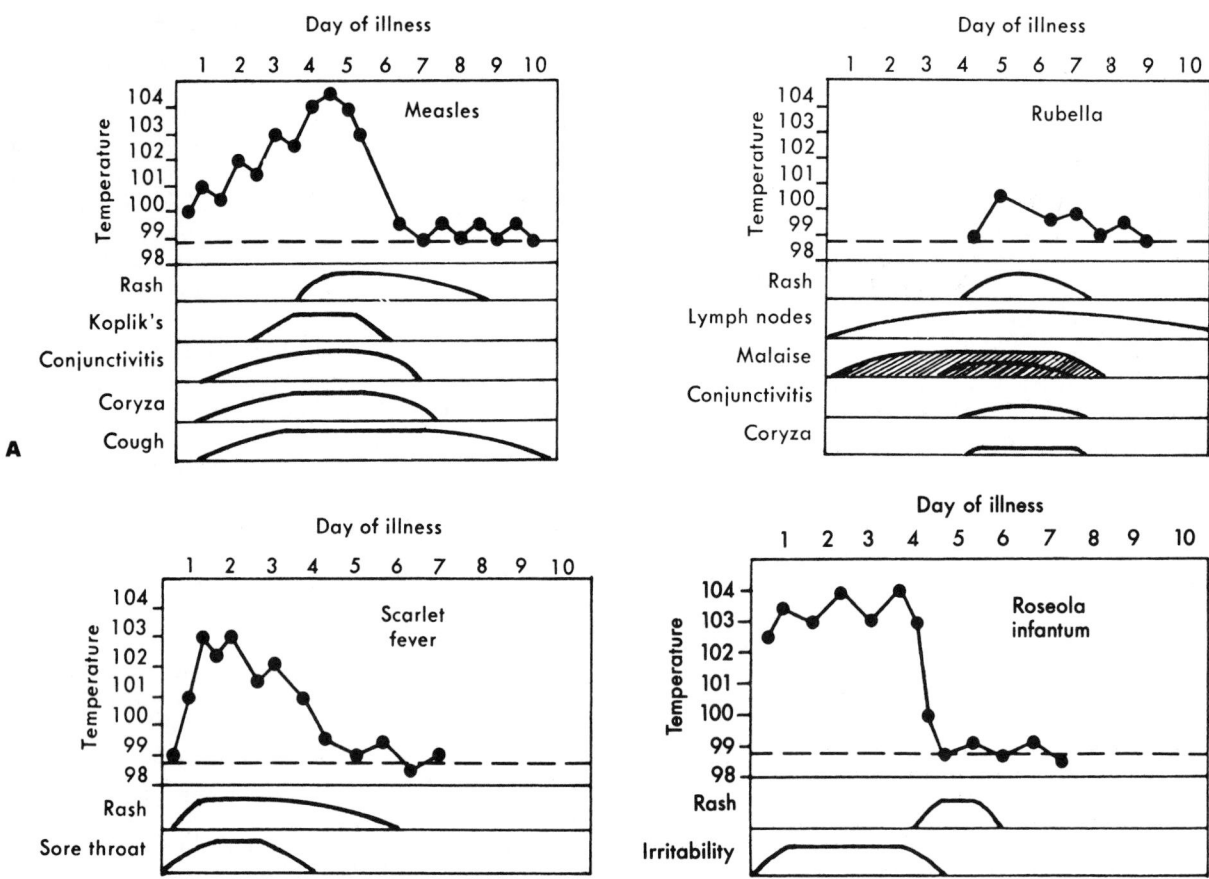

FIG. 48-12. Infectious exanthems. **A,** Schematic diagrams illustrating differences between four acute exanthems characterized by maculopapular eruptions. *(From Krugman S et al: Infectious diseases of children, ed 9, St. Louis, 1992, Mosby.)*   *Continued.*

1967) who were later exposed to wild measles virus. This is no longer seen in children. Serologic confirmation of measles infection may be helpful for documentation.

An exanthem resulting from administration of the measles vaccine can be seen about 7 to 10 days after immunization. Although thrombocytopenic purpura and toxic epidermal necrolysis have been reported as vaccine complications, the majority of people do not develop any systemic illness.

Management. There is no treatment for measles other than symptomatic support. Most children need only antipyretics and bed rest. Secondary infections such as otitis media should be treated with appropriate antibiotics.

The two complications of measles that require inpatient care are meningoencephalitis and respiratory compromise. Mild croup may be managed at home; significant laryngotracheobronchitis and pneumonia both require careful observation because they can progress rapidly.

Measles can be prevented or attenuated in children who have been exposed and are susceptible.[80] Live measles vaccine given within 72 hours of exposure can provide protection. Immune serum globulin 0.25 ml/kg IM, maximum 15 ml, will prevent or modify measles disease if given within 6 days after exposure. This may be helpful for children younger than 1 year of age or for children who are

immunocompromised, because these children are at most risk for developing complications of measles. Children with measles should not attend school or daycare during the 4 days following the rash because this is the period when they will still be contagious after the illness is recognized. Current vaccination recommendations provide for one dose of live attenuated vaccine between 12 and 15 months of age, and a second dose at entry to junior high school. Although vaccine programs have reduced the incidence of measles to 1% of prevaccine levels, the disease has not been eradicated.[99,100]

Whenever a case of measles is documented, it should be reported to local public health authorities who can institute epidemic control measures. All emergency department personnel should have documentation of either measles disease or current immunization to prevent epidemics among hospital personnel.[91]

Scarlet Fever

Although scarlet fever results from a reaction to an erythrogenic toxin produced by several strains of Group A beta-hemolytic streptococci rather than a virus, the appearance of the rash may be difficult to differentiate from viral exanthems. It is commonly associated with GABHS pharyngitis, although it can also develop with impetigo or cellulitis.

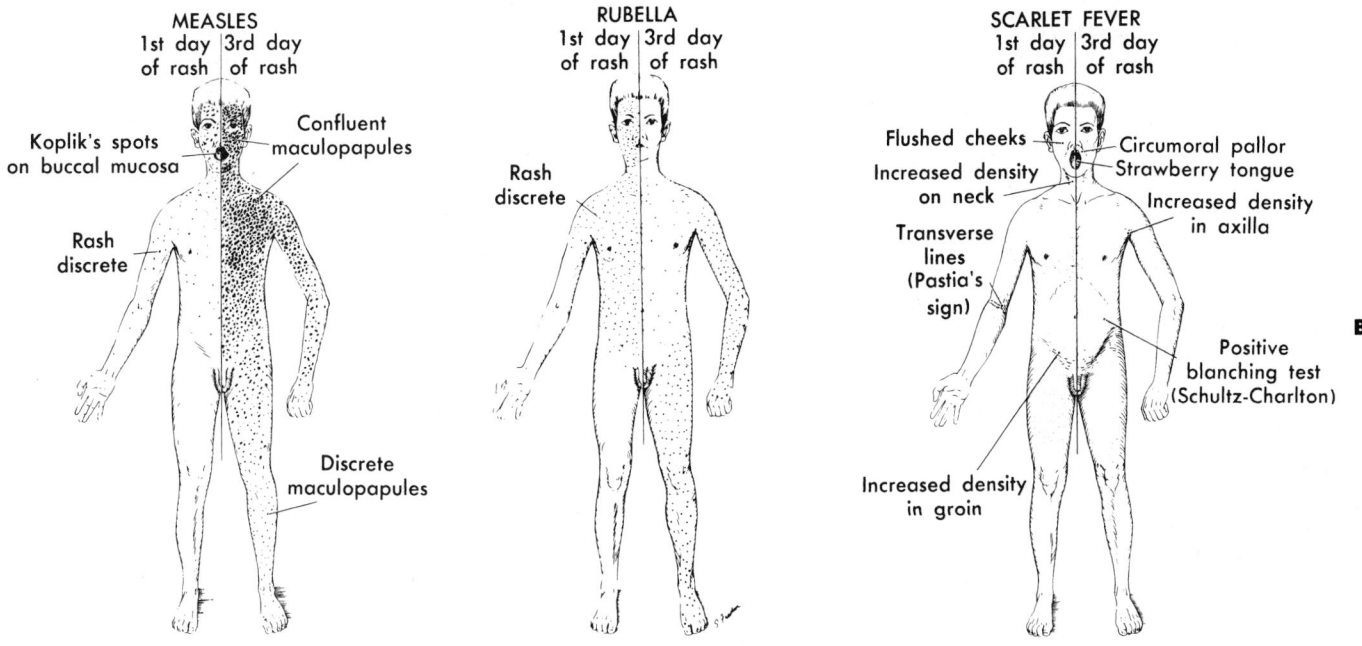

FIG. 48-12, cont'd. Infectious exanthems. **B,** Schematic drawings illustrating differences in appearance, distribution, and progression of rashes of measles, rubella, and scarlet fever. *(From Krugman S et al: Infectious diseases of children, ed 9, St. Louis, 1992, Mosby.)*

Diagnostic Findings. The scarlatiniform rash, which is often described as being rough to touch, like sandpaper, is first noticed in areas of skin folds such as the groin, axilla, and antecubital areas. The area around the mouth and nose is usually not erythematous and has the appearance of circumoral pallor. In a typical case of pharyngitis, the rash usually develops within 12 to 48 hours after the onset of fever, chills, and sore throat. The rash may be accentuated if the patient is wrapped in heavy blankets. Diagnosis of scarlet fever depends on documentation of the GABHS infection because a number of viral infections can also produce a scarlatiniform rash.

Management. When antibiotic treatment of the GABHS infection is started, the rash will be attenuated. Treatment with oral penicillin V 25 to 50 mg (40 to 80,000 U)/kg/24 hr in 4 divided doses or erythromycin 20 to 50 mg/kg/24 hr in 3 to 4 divided doses is adequate, and the risk of complications such as rheumatic fever is no greater than the risk from strep throat without the rash. Without treatment, the rash usually lasts 4 to 5 days, with peeling of the skin noticed, especially on the hands and feet, over the next 2 weeks. Because more than one strain of GABHS is able to produce the toxin, it is possible to have scarlet fever more than once. To control disease spread, children should not return to school until 24 hours after starting antibiotics.[81]

Rubella (German Measles)

The illness of rubella is generally very mild, and the importance of recognizing the syndrome lies in the severe teratogenic effects of the virus. It is caused by an RNA virus that is found worldwide. Man is the only known host. It is transmitted through droplet spread with the period of greatest communicability lasting from a few days before to about 7 days after the onset of the rash. The incubation period after exposure is 14 to 21 days.

Congenital rubella syndrome can develop in infants whose mothers develop rubella infection during the first or early second trimester of pregnancy. These children are frequently growth retarded with microcephaly, cataracts, cardiac defects, sensory neural deafness, and hepatosplenomegaly. They may continue to shed virus in the urine and respiratory secretions for over a year after birth.

Diagnostic Findings. Although the virus is very contagious during epidemics, there is a very high rate of subclinical infection so that many cases are not recognizable. In a typical case, there is a prodrome of upper respiratory symptoms with widespread lymphadenopathy. Postoccipital and postauricular lymphadenopathy are the most notable clinical features that distinguish the rash from other exanthems. The rash appears as small discrete pink maculopapules that coalesce on the trunk on the second day and usually fade on the third day. There is usually mild fever. Because the syndrome is not very distinct, it is difficult to make the diagnosis clinically.

The most common complication of rubella is the development of arthritis or arthralgia, which can begin during the prodrome or several days after the onset of rash. This complication may be useful in distinguishing this exanthem from other infectious ones and does not appear to predispose the patient to arthritis later in life. Serologic confirmation of rubella may be helpful when a nonimmune pregnant woman is exposed to a child with an exanthem.

Management. Rubella is a very mild illness that needs only supportive treatment. Contact isolation is recommended for 7 days after the onset of the rash. Unfortunately the diagnosis is not often made clinically.

Children with congenital rubella syndrome should be considered contagious until they have nasopharyngeal and urine cultures that are negative for rubella virus. This may not happen before 1 year of age.[80]

Erythema Infectiosum (Fifth Disease)

This mild disease is seen in children from about 3 to 12 years of age. It is caused by human parvovirus B19. The illness itself does not produce serious complications in most children, but infection during pregnancy is known to be associated with fatal aplastic anemia and an increased risk of fetal death and miscarriage.

Because the clinical syndrome is so benign and subclinical infections are probably common, the epidemiology of the disease has only been investigated since isolation of the virus in 1975. The infection can be recognized worldwide, and humans are the only known hosts. A significant proportion of adults are immune to the virus. The incubation period from exposure to development of a recognizable syndrome can be from 4 days to several weeks. Transmission of the virus is primarily through respiratory droplet spread. In school epidemics, attack rates from 30% to 60% have been described; infection with this virus can be an occupational hazard for school and daycare personnel.

Diagnostic Findings. The prodrome of the illness is nonspecific and usually ignored. The characteristic rash develops abruptly with bright red cheeks, giving the "slapped" cheek appearance. On the second day a maculopapular, faintly pink rash develops on the trunk and extremities; it clears in a lacy pattern. The child usually appears well and may not have any fever or other symptoms. The rash fades over several days, but it can reappear over several weeks, particularly when the skin is exposed to sun or a warm bath.[101]

Complications are very rare, although arthralgia and arthritis may develop.

There is a transient arrest of red cell production during the infection that is not noticeable in most people but can be significant in people with underlying hemolytic problems. Aplastic crisis in children with sickle cell disease has been related to infection with parvovirus. Immunosuppressed patients, who are unable to clear the virus, may have prolonged anemia. There are no commercially available serologic tests for parvovirus B19 at the present time.

Management. There is no vaccine to prevent the infection, and no specific treatment is needed for the rash. By the time the clinical illness is recognized, the period of greatest contagiousness has passed and exclusion from school or daycare is not necessary. A pregnant woman who has been exposed to children with this illness should be advised to inform her obstetrician.

Human Herpes Virus 6 (Roseola)

Roseola is one of the most common exanthems appearing in young infants.[102] In the 1980s human herpes virus 6 was uncovered as the etiologic agent for this syndrome. Since the discovery of the virus, infection producing rising antibody titers has been found in the absence of rash or fever.[103-105] Passive antibody is common in newborns, indicating a high level of immunity in adults.

Cases are rarely seen before 6 months of age, when maternal antibodies wane, and are not commonly seen after the age of 3 years. The infection is spread by droplets and has an incubation period of between 5 and 15 days.

Diagnostic Findings. The most recognized feature of the illness is the sudden onset of high fever in a surprisingly well-looking child. Some observers have described mild conjunctivitis and periorbital puffiness. Occasionally an infant will have a bulging fontanelle despite lack of evidence of meningeal irritation. These nonspecific findings last for 3 to 4 days, then as the child becomes afebrile, the rash develops. A faint pink, maculopapular, sometimes itchy rash develops mainly over the trunk and resolves within 48 hours.

Febrile seizures sometimes occur with this illness. It is often a child's first febrile illness so parental anxiety may be high despite the benign nature of the disease. There are no significant known complications, no diagnostic laboratory tests, and no vaccines to prevent the illness. Because of the young age of the child, diagnostic tests such as complete blood count, urinalysis, or spinal fluid examination may be necessary to eliminate possible serious treatable illness. These infants are often reexamined several times before the diagnostic rash appears.

Management. Treatment is symptomatic—primarily antipyretics for fever control—and recovery is complete. No special isolation precautions are recommended.

Enteroviruses

At least 30 types of viral exanthems have been associated with coxsackie and ECHO viruses. The most common rashes are maculopapular, but they may also be scarlatiniform, vesicular, and urticarial. Because of the large number of enteroviruses that produce exanthems, the wide variety of clinical presentations, and the number of rare complications, differentiating between different syndromes is usually not possible or necessary.

Diagnostic Findings. Hand, foot, and mouth disease is a distinct exanthem caused by coxsackie A16 and occasionally by A5 and A10.[106] It is seen most commonly in the late summer and fall. The illness develops after an incubation period of 3 to 6 days with a brief prodrome of low fever, malaise, and sometimes abdominal pain. Children may complain of a sore mouth or may refuse to eat. Some infants refuse to walk or complain of sore hands. Vesicles measuring about 5 mm in diameter are found on the palms, soles, buttocks, and sometimes on the extremities and trunk. The oral lesions usually appear later as small red macules and vesicles on the palate, gingivae, buccal mucosa, and tongue. The illness lasts for 3 to 6 days and usually resolves without incident.

Some cases reoccur for several months before completely clearing. Occasional cases of myocarditis, pneumonia, and meningoencephalitis have been reported.

Herpangina, a characteristic exanthem of tiny vesicles on the soft palate, uvula, and tonsillar pillars, can be produced by several enteroviruses and also by herpes simplex. Sore throat and pain with eating are the most common complaints, although fever, headache, vomiting, and myalgia may be present. The ulcers may last for up to a week, but systemic symptoms do not usually persist for more than 1 or 2 days.[107]

Management. Spread of these viruses occurs by the fecal-oral route and possibly by respiratory means. Good hand washing may be the best way to prevent spread.

However, there are many subclinical infections, and isolation in daycare or school settings is impractical. Treatment is symptomatic and no vaccines are available.

Pityriasis Rosea

Pityriasis rosea is an acute self-limited disorder seen most commonly in adolescents and young adults. It is rarely seen in children less than 4 years of age, although it has been reported in infants. Most cases are seen in the winter months, although this may not be true in climates where there is little temperature variation.[108]

The etiology is unknown. An infectious etiology has been suggested because the rash tends to appear in epidemic clusters, and because it only rarely reoccurs. Occasionally a patient may report a prodrome of lymphadenopathy, pharyngitis, and malaise; many patients come for treatment because the rash is not going away rather than because they are feeling ill. It is seen more often in people with a family history of atopic problems.

Diagnostic Findings. The distribution of the rash is pathognomonic. The majority of cases begin with a single oval scaly patch about 2 to 5 cm in diameter. This "herald patch" is often unnoticed until the secondary eruption develops. Crops of small oval scaly patches appear on the trunk parallel to skin cleavage lines creating a "Christmas tree" pattern. The face and extremities are usually spared. In younger children the patches may be urticarial, papular, or even purpuric. Young children may also develop lesions on mucous membranes. The herald patch fades before the smaller scales, which can take up to 12 weeks to resolve. Most patients have some itching, but this is often not serious. Recurrences have been reported in less than 3% of cases.

Laboratory tests and biopsy of the lesion are not helpful in making the diagnosis.

Differential Considerations. The differential diagnosis includes other scaly lesions. The herald patch is sometimes mistaken for tinea corporis. The diagnosis can be confusing if the herald patch has already resolved when the patient is first seen. The most important differential not to be missed is secondary syphilis, and a serologic test should be obtained in all sexually active teenagers. Drug eruptions, nummular eczema, and psoriasis may resemble this disorder; however, it can usually be distinguished by the distribution on the body.

Management. Most patients require no treatment other than reassurance and education about the course of the illness. Exposure to sunlight seems to stop itching and hasten disappearance of the rash.[109] Topical lubricants and colloid baths will help relieve itching, and some patients require systemic antihistamines for severe itching. Topical corticosteroids do not seem to shorten the course of the rash. Whether treated or not, the rash resolves with no sequelae.

MOLLUSCUM CONTAGIOSUM

Molluscum contagiosum is a common viral skin infection caused by a pox virus[110] (Fig. 48-13). Although it can be seen at any age, it is most common in children under 5 years of age, and has even been reported in a 1-week-old infant.[111]

Papules can spread on a child by autoinoculation, and they can be passed to other people by direct contact. The

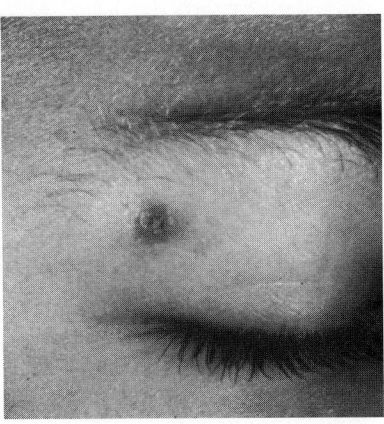

FIG. 48-13. Molluscum contagiosum forms soft flesh-colored papule with a dimpled top. *(Courtesy Mayo Medical Center, Department of Dermatology, Rochester, Minn.)*

infection is more common in children who frequent swimming pools. Papules have been noted in wrestlers in areas of direct body contact. When the infection has been induced experimentally, the papules develop after an incubation period of 2 weeks to several months. They resolve spontaneously in most cases, although this can take from a few weeks to several years.

In adults, molluscum have clearly been shown to spread with sexual contact. Because the chance of autoinoculation is high in children with this viral infection, a genital lesion should not be used as an absolute indicator of sexual abuse. However, the genital area is not a commonly reported site for molluscum in children, and the problem of abuse ought to be considered if a child has only anogenital lesions.

Diagnostic Findings

Lesions can be either solitary or in groups. They are soft, flesh-colored, round papules that have dimpled tops. They can be found on any part of the body but are most frequent on the face, neck, trunk, and axillae. When molluscum occur on the eyelids, the child may have a mild watery conjunctivitis. Most children are asymptomatic, although some complain of itching or soreness around the papules. Occasionally a child can develop an eczematous reaction around a lesion.

Differential Considerations

Small warts, papular urticaria with a central puncture, tiny epidermal cysts, and comedones all resemble molluscum. Careful inspection with a magnifying glass will usually differentiate these umbilicated papules from other bumps.

Management

Treatment may shorten the duration of individual lesions, which will decrease the chance for spread of new lesions. Because of the high rate of spontaneous remission, treatment should be undertaken only if it is relatively painless and does not cause scarring. Because the most popular treatments involve curettage, cryotherapy with liquid nitrogen, or application of vesicants, and will require frequent

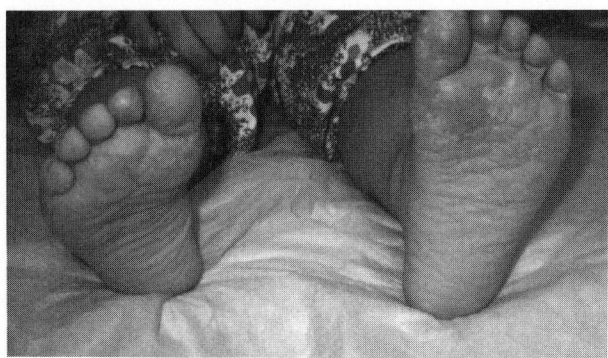

FIG. 48-14. Tinea pedis is extremely uncommon before adolescence.

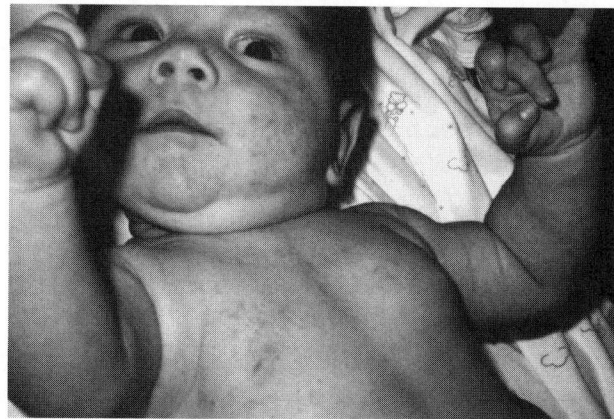

FIG. 48-15. The crusting eruption of the scalp and face of seborrheic dermatitis is common in early infancy.

follow-up examinations, molluscum should usually be referred to a dermatologist.

SCALY FEET

A syndrome named juvenile plantar dermatosis (JPD) accounts for the majority of cases of foot dermatitis in children.[112] Children with this problem have erythema, usually of the forefoot, which can become vesicular or lichenified and fissured. The sole of the foot often appears red and shiny. The problem has commonly been present for several weeks by the time parents notice that the child has difficulty walking because of foot pain.

Diagnostic Findings

Examination of scaly feet shows two patterns that help determine an etiology.

Children whose dermatitis involves the top of the foot frequently have positive patch testing to common contact allergens such as rubber antioxidants and potassium dichromate leather tanning agents. These are both irritants found in shoes. This problem is best treated with topical corticosteroids and a change of footwear.

Children whose dermatitis is found only on the plantar surface of the feet fit the syndrome of JPD. These children do not have an allergic or contact irritant reaction to their shoes, and do not appear to have a higher incidence of atopic problems than the general population. The exact etiology of the problem has not been established; "chapping" of wet feet has been suggested, although scaly feet is not a problem of excessive sweating.

Differential Considerations

Dermatitis of the feet in children is often misdiagnosed as tinea pedis or athlete's foot (Fig. 48-14). Although this is a common condition in adults, it is quite rare in prepubertal children. When children with scaly feet have had KOH testing and fungal cultures performed, the diagnosis of fungal infection has been confirmed in variable frequency from 0% to 50% of cases.[113]

Management

Attempts to dry the feet may increase discomfort; instead emollients and moisturizing agents yield the best results. Topical steroids may be used when inflammation is

severe. The problem resolves by puberty but usually requires attempts at chronic control rather than cure.

SEBORRHEIC DERMATITIS

Seborrheic dermatitis is a scaly crusting eruption that occurs in areas with high concentrations of sebaceous glands, especially the scalp, face, and intertriginous areas (Fig. 48-15). There are two age groups in which seborrhea is prevalent. It is very common in infancy, usually appearing before 6 weeks of age and resolving by 6 months.[114,115] It is then very uncommon until adolescence.

The etiology of this problem is not known; however, it seems to appear most commonly in the spring and summer. There does not seem to be a genetic disposition to developing seborrhea.

Diagnostic Findings

Greasy, yellow scales on the scalp and eyebrows or weeping areas behind the ears are characteristic. Infants are susceptible to diaper rash. Blepharitis with scaling of the eyelids may also occur. Unlike atopic dermatitis, it does not seem to be itchy.

Histologic findings are nonspecific, commonly showing a low-grade inflammatory process. Various theories including allergy to foods, autoimmunity to the epidermis or to *Candida albicans*, as well as infection with other fungal agents have been proposed as etiologic bases for the disease; however, none has been established.

Differential Considerations

The differential diagnosis includes minor problems such as noninflammatory dandruff and serious problems. Letterer-Siwe disease is a lymphoproliferative disorder in which an infant will have purpura, lymphadenopathy, and hepatosplenomegaly as well as a seborrheic rash. Leiner disease, which is caused by complement dysfunction, causes diarrhea and recurrent infections in addition to intractable seborrhea. Psoriasis, yeast infections, and atopic dermatitis share similarities in appearance to seborrhea.

Management

The treatment of infantile seborrhea varies with the severity of the eruption. Low-potency topical corticosteroids

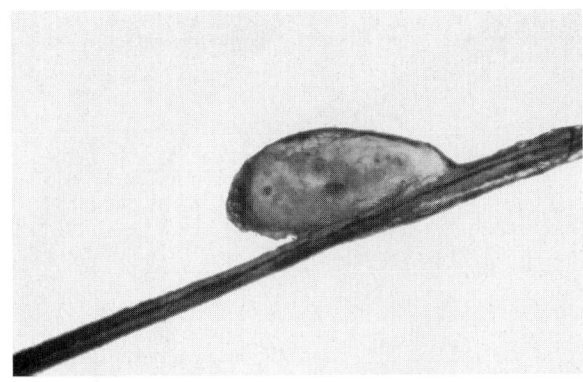

FIG. 48-16. In pediculosis, nits are attached to the hair shaft close to the scalp.

can be used to treat inflamed weepy areas. Scales on the scalp can often be softened with mineral oil and washed off with a keratolytic shampoo such as Sebulex or Selsun. Similar measures should be used for adolescents with seborrhea.

The diaper dermatitis frequently becomes superinfected with monilia and may also develop bacterial infection. Although this can usually be managed with appropriate topical agents, systemic antibiotics are sometimes required. The prognosis for seborrhea is excellent, and most infants are free of the problem before their first birthday. When it occurs in adolescents, seborrhea often follows a relapsing course that responds well to intermittent topical steroids and Selsun shampoo used three times a week.

SKIN PARASITES

Pediculosis

Head lice are frequently diagnosed by school nurses or teachers. Feelings of disgust produced by the thought of insects crawling, biting, and living in a child's scalp may lead to anxious overreaction and requests for treatment of this problem at any hour of the day.

The head louse, *Pediculus humanus capitis*, is a tiny wingless insect about 2 to 4 mm long that exists by feeding on human blood (Fig. 48-16). The condition is usually diagnosed when the egg cases or nits are seen on the scalp hair of a child with an itchy head.[116,117]

Head lice seem to prefer fine straight hair and are seen more commonly in girls than in boys. Caucasians have lice more commonly than blacks in the United States. The prevalence in American primary school children has been estimated as high as 40%. Poor hygiene is not responsible for head lice, which are seen most often in perfectly clean, healthy children. The life cycle of the head louse begins when the egg case is attached to hair close to the scalp. The nymph emerges from the egg case after about a week and then takes another week to mature to the adult insect. An adult can then live for about a month depositing approximately four eggs per day. Lice are quite temperature sensitive and tend to stay in warm areas of hair behind the ears and at the nape of the neck. The nits will be seen on the hair shaft farther from the scalp as the hair grows out if the infestation has been untreated for a long period of time.

Diagnostic Findings. The usual symptom that causes an adult to examine a child for lice is an itchy scalp. Often parents will suspect that nits are present, which upon examination are actually flakes of dandruff or casts of sebum and stratum corneum from the hair follicle. These can be distinguished from nits by their easy movability. Nits are attached to hair with cementlike "nit glue" and are very difficult to dislodge from the hair shaft.

Head lice spread from child to child by direct contact and by sharing clothing or hair utensils. Adult lice will survive for brief periods away from their human host but they will starve if away from the body for more than 10 days. Both eggs and adult lice are very temperature sensitive and are adapted to human body temperature. Hatching of eggs is prevented by exposure to temperatures over 100° F and below 75° F.

Differential Considerations. Neurotic excoriation of the scalp, seborrhea, and dandruff can all be confused with symptoms of infestation with head lice. Hair roots sometimes remain attached to the hair shaft, resembling nits; however, retained roots slide down the hair shaft easily. Head lice anxiety may lead to searches for nits and lice and requests for treatment even in the absence of any symptoms.[118]

Management. Treatment involves prevention of reinfection as well as eradication of adult lice and eggs. Lindane (Kwell) has been used successfully for many years to successfully kill both adults and eggs. One ounce is used as a shampoo that is lathered into the hair, left in place for 10 minutes, and then rinsed out. Because 30% of nits remain viable, the treatment should be repeated in 7 to 10 days. Lindane is also available as a lotion that is applied and left on overnight. Some dermatologists have suggested the lotion for head lice although this has not been studied in a controlled fashion. There has been some concern about possible central nervous system toxicity from absorption of lindane because, if absorbed, this compound could accumulate in fatty tissue such as the brain.[119] Although this possibility exists, it seems to be related to ingestion of the product or frequent repeated applications leading to an accumulation of the toxic substance. The likelihood of toxicity following one or two treatments with lindane is extremely remote if a child has normal skin, is well nourished, is not premature, and does not have an underlying seizure disorder.

Permethrin 1% cream rinse (Nix) has also been successfully used to eradicate head lice.[120] After washing with the child's usual shampoo, the lotion is applied to the hair in an amount that will saturate the hair—about 1 ounce is usually sufficient. It is left on the hair for 10 minutes and then rinsed out. A second treatment is required about 1 week later. It is more pleasant to use than lindane because it has a better smell and leaves hair easier to comb. The potential toxicity of permethrin has not been completely delineated because it has not been used as extensively as lindane.

When a child has head lice, all family members and school contacts should be examined for possible infestation. Clothing and bed linen should be washed in hot water and dried in a hot-air dryer or else dry-cleaned. Combs, brushes, and barrettes should also be washed in hot water. There is no clear evidence that aerosol insecticides for furniture are of any use in killing ambient lice; however, good vacuuming should remove loose lice. Any material that cannot be cleaned can be made noninfectious by sealing it in a plastic bag for about 10 days; any adult lice will have starved in this time.

It is important for parents to know that the child's scalp may remain itchy for several weeks after successful treatment. Some people are so concerned about the infestation that they overtreat the child with multiple courses of insecticide or other disinfectants such as Lysol. This can lead to continued itchiness and further lice phobia. Topical hydrocortisone creams may help to alleviate itching.

Some schools will not allow children to return until all nits are removed from the hair even though the eggs have been killed by insecticide treatment. The egg cases can be very difficult to dislodge and rinsing hair with a solution of equal parts of water and white vinegar seems to soften nit cement. Some people suggest leaving this rinse on the hair for up to an hour. A fine-toothed nit comb may help in nit removal, and sometimes combing the hair backward toward the scalp seems to be more effective in nit removal.

Scabies

Scabies is a very itchy infestation of the skin caused by the microscopic mite, *Sarcoptes scabiei*. It is quite contagious and spreads easily when people live under crowded conditions. It is a common endemic disorder with periodic epidemic outbreaks.[121,122]

The mites are white, transparent creatures with four pairs of legs, and are less than half a millimeter long. The mite is host specific, and normally humans cannot be infected by mites from animals. The gravid female lays two to three eggs per day in a small burrow at the base of the stratum corneum. Larvae emerge after 2 to 3 days and crawl off to make new burrows. It is at this stage that the infestation can be transferred to another person. It takes the mite approximately 30 minutes to burrow into human skin. During the next 10 to 17 days, the insect undergoes three molts before reaching maturity. The adult lives for about 30 to 60 days. The mite secretes a solution that dissolves tissue and then creates a burrow as it digests this material.

Mites are very sensitive to drying and will not survive long periods of time away from the host, particularly in low humidity. Adult mites may be able to survive for 2 days at room temperature, and there is some evidence that eggs can survive for up to 10 days in conditions of low temperature and high humidity.

There are usually very few mites on an infested person. In one series there were an average of 12.3 mites per person. It is more difficult to infect a person who has had scabies before, implying the existence of a mechanism of immunity. Reinfected people will have about the same number of mites as they had on an initial infestation.

Diagnostic Findings. The clinical signs of scabies are quite variable. The lesions usually begin as erythematous papules that then develop an eczematous reaction. Secondary bacterial superinfection is quite common, and epidemics of poststreptococcal glomerulonephritis have been associated with scabies. In older children and adults, scabies papules are found most often on the hands and wrists with typical burrows in the web spaces of fingers. Infants and

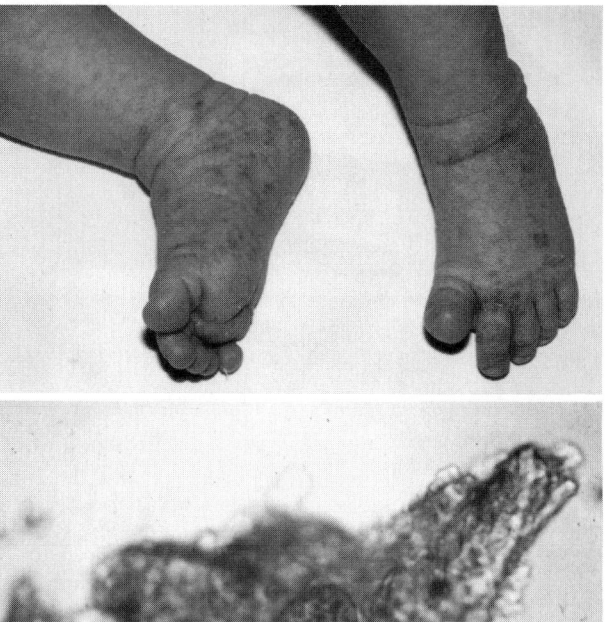

FIG. 48-17. Scabies. **A,** Infants and young children frequently have vesicles on their palms and soles. **B,** Diagnosis of scabies is made by finding mites in a superficial skin scraping. (*Courtesy Mayo Medical Center, Department of Dermatology, Rochester, Minn.*)

young children frequently have vesicles on their palms and soles (Fig. 48-17, *A*). They also develop scabies on their faces and scalps; these areas are very rarely affected in older children. The burrow may be very difficult to find in an infant.[123]

Severe itching is the most common presenting complaint and is believed to be caused by sensitization to mite antigens. In a primary infection, itching usually begins about a month after infection; however, in a reinfection the itch begins early.

Diagnosis of scabies is made by finding the mite or its fecal pellets in a superficial skin scraping (Fig. 48-17, *B*). Fresh lesions that have not yet been scratched are most likely to yield the mite. A drop of mineral oil can be placed on a fresh papule or burrow. The area is then scraped open with a No. 11 scalpel blade, and the oil and scraped material is transferred to a glass slide. A coverslip should be placed over the oil drop, and the specimen should be examined by a microscope with low power. The diagnosis is often difficult in children and may depend on diagnosing the condition in contact cases.

Differential Considerations. Atopic dermatitis, papular urticaria, and simple insect bites are itchy skin reactions of acute onset that are often confused with scabies. Because scabies is so contagious, it is unusual to find only one member of a household affected. A history of itchy bumps should be sought in the rest of the family to confirm the diagnosis of scabies. If no one else in the family has a similar problem, scabies is less likely than another cause of itchy papules.

Management. All close personal contacts and the infested child must be treated with an effective insecticide.[124,125] Lindane lotion (Kwell) has been used effectively for many years. One to two ounces of lotion will cover the entire body in a single application and should be left on for 12 hours. Directions are often written to apply the cream from the neck down, but in infants all affected areas should be covered. If the lotion is washed off during the 12-hour period, it should be reapplied. This often happens when a child's palms and soles are washed at mealtimes.

The use of lindane in infants, pregnant women, and children with severe dermatitis is controversial because it has been associated with possible neurologic toxicity; the potential risks of using lindane in these situations must be weighed against the need to treat the infestation.

Permethrin topical cream (Elimite) is a newer form of scabies treatment that appears to be very effective and safe. It has been used to successfully treat some cases in which lindane did not work. One or two ounces of permethrin lotion should be applied to the entire body. The lotion should remain on the skin for 12 hours and then be rinsed off. A second treatment 7 to 10 days later is suggested to kill any newly hatched larvae.

A third treatment that can be used is crotamiton (Eurax) cream or lotion. One ounce is applied to the entire body at bedtime for two 24-hour intervals and then washed off on the third night. Although this treatment has been considered safer than lindane for infants, it is also much less effective, with a cure rate as low as 60%.

Itching may persist for several days after initial treatment, and parents should be cautioned not to overuse the insecticide. Antihistamines or mild topical steroids have been tried as treatment for itching.

Bed linens and clothing should be washed with ordinary soap and at the usual water temperatures. Because mites do not spread easily through environmental fomites, simple cleaning measures such as vacuuming are sufficient to stop household infestations.

Cutaneous Larva Migrans

Cutaneous larva migrans is a self-limited problem caused when the larval form of a dog hookworm, *Ancylostoma braziliensis*, burrows into the skin of a human host.[126] It is seen most commonly in warmer climates in the southeastern United States. The parasite must spend part of its life cycle in the soil, and it does not survive cold temperatures. Children pick up the parasite when they play in dirt or sand that has been contaminated by feces from infested dogs.

Diagnostic Findings. The larva, which is species specific, is unable to completely invade the skin when it is in the wrong host (Fig. 48-18). It burrows along a wandering path through the epidermis at a rate of about 1 cm a day. The larva causes severe itching, and a child frequently has a large impetiginized area on a foot or lower extremity. The underlying creeping eruption may not be recognized until the superficial bacterial infection is treated.

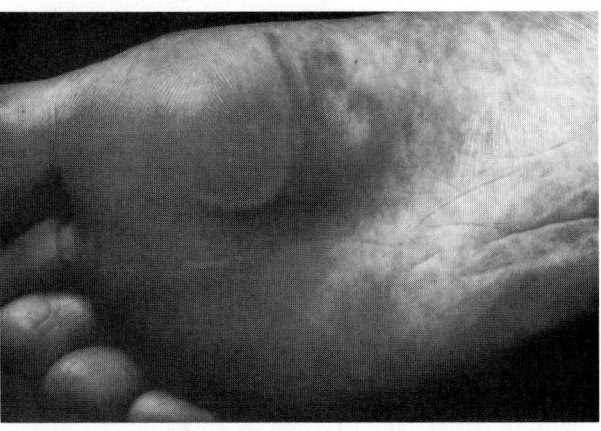

FIG. 48-18. Cutaneous larva migrans is a larval form of a dog hookworm that wanders through the epidermis when it is in the wrong host. *(Courtesy Mayo Medical Center, Department of Dermatology, Rochester, Minn.)*

Differential Considerations. Cutaneous larva migrans can be distinguished by its rapid forward progression and its pruritic nature from granuloma annulare, tinea infections, and urticaria. Secondary superinfection may cause the eruption to look like cellulitis.

Management. The larva eventually dies in the skin, and the eruption will usually last no more than 4 weeks. When symptoms are severe, topical treatment can be used to kill the larva.[127] Thiabendazole 10% suspension should be applied with a cotton ball to the area of skin ahead of the leading point of the tract four times a day for 7 days. Oral thiabendazole, 25 mg/kg/dose, twice a day for 2 days, can also be used; however, this causes gastrointestinal upset with anorexia, nausea, and vomiting, so topical therapy is preferred. Antihistamines by mouth or mild topical steroids may help the itch.

Pinworms

The most common human roundworm is the pinworm *Enterobiasis vermicularis*. It is found in all socioeconomic classes and can affect all ages but is most often diagnosed in children.[128] The usual reason for seeking medical attention is anal itching, which can be quite severe, especially at night.

Children become infected by ingesting eggs that are picked up on fingers when they scratch their bottom. The eggs can also float through the air and be inhaled and ingested when bedclothing is shaken.

The pinworm hatches in the duodenum and matures as it travels through the intestine. The worm migrates out of the rectum to lay its eggs on the perirectal skin. Eggs are not laid inside the intestine so stool samples are usually not helpful in identifying the worm's presence. Eggs mature very quickly, and within a few hours, are ready to start the cycle again.

Diagnostic Findings. Signs and symptoms of pinworm infestation can develop from mechanical irritation, allergic reaction, and movement of the parasite to places where they may become pathogenic.[129] The most common symptom is perianal itching, which may be associated with restless sleep or insomnia. Vaginitis can develop if worms migrate into the vaginal area. Some patients with urticaria show allergic sensitivity to pinworms. There is a slight suggestion that patients with pinworms have increased eosinophil counts. There is no conclusive evidence that pinworms are responsible for abdominal pain, anemia, bed wetting, constipation, nail biting, thumb sucking, nose picking, or tooth grinding. Although pinworms have been found in some inflamed appendices, there is no clear causative relationship.

The diagnosis of pinworms is made by observing a worm or by examining the anal region for eggs using the "scotch tape" test. Transparent sticky tape is touched to perianal skin, then placed on a microscope slide and examined under low power. The eggs are oval, slightly asymmetric, transparent shells. Sometimes the larva can be seen with the egg.

The worm itself is a tiny white roundworm about 1 cm long. In Britain they are called thread worms, which is an excellent description of the worm's appearance. There are no other human parasites that look like this so a parent's description of a pinworm can be used to initiate treatment without further testing.

Management. The infestation is difficult to eradicate because pinworms are highly contagious and reinfection is very likely. The most commonly used medication is mebendazole (Vermox), in the form of 100 mg chewable tablets.[130] The dose for adults and children is a single tablet, although some people recommend a repeat dose in 10 to 14 days. The drug is not absorbed from the gastrointestinal tract and has no major side effects. Since this treatment has become available, many physicians treat rectal itching in children empirically without any diagnostic testing. With a first infection it may be useful to treat the entire family.

Pyrantel pamoate (Antiminth) 11 mg/kg in a single dose, maximum 1 gm, is available as a liquid preparation (50 mg/ml) for children who are too young to chew tablets.

Vaginitis caused by pinworms is self-limited and requires no special treatment beyond medication to eliminate the gastrointestinal infestation.

Attempts to control reexposure to pinworm eggs include vacuuming bedrooms, washing bed linen in warm soapy water, and keeping the child's fingernails short so that eggs will not accumulate under the nails when the child scratches.

Control of pinworms is very difficult, and parents need to be assured that the presence of pinworms does not imply poor hygiene or bad habits on the part of the child. They also need to be told that other than rectal itching, pinworms do not cause serious disease.

SUN REACTIONS

Radiant energy from the sun contains a small spectrum of light that has the property of causing photobiologic reactions. Photochemical reactions occur within the skin that is exposed to ultraviolet light. Melanin, keratin, and many other chemical substances, including DNA and RNA, are capable of absorbing and reacting to ultraviolet energy. The body's entire blood supply is exposed to sunlight because it circulates through the skin several times/minute. Photochemical changes in blood components may ex-

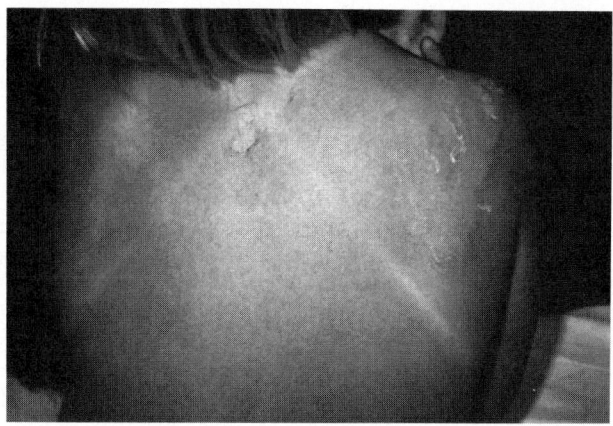

FIG. 48-19. Peeling sunburns are related to development of skin cancer as an adult.

plain some systemic reactions to excessive light exposure (Fig. 48-19).

Ultraviolet light has been divided into three major wavelengths: ultraviolet A (UVA) rays have a length between 320 and 400 nanometers (nm), ultraviolet B (UVB) rays have a length between 290 and 320 nm, and ultraviolet C (UVC) ranges from 200 to 290 nm. UVB is the most powerful spectrum for producing sunburn and tanning. Although much higher doses of UVA are required to produce the same amount of tanning as UVB, these longer wavelengths have better penetrating ability. UVA probably has more affect on collagen breakdown in the skin's dermal layer than UVB. UVC is entirely absorbed in the upper layers of the atmosphere. Although UVC can be shown to cause erythema of skin experimentally, it is not known to be clinically important.[131]

Sunburn

Sunburn is most common sun reaction seen for emergency care. The mechanism of injury involves vasodilation and increased permeability of blood vessels, and migration of leukocytes into the affected area. These reactions may result from direct damage to the vascular epithelium, or may be explained by diffusion of vasoactive material from the epidermis to the vascular bed. Mast cells may release inflammatory substances when damaged by ultraviolet light.

The vulnerability to sunburn varies both with a person's type of skin and the conditions of the exposure. During the midday hours, during the summertime, and at tropical latitudes, the sun's rays are more direct. There is a 4% increase in ultraviolet light for every 1,000 feet of altitude. Ultraviolet light is reflected from surfaces such as white snow and sand, thus increasing potential exposure. Many people are not aware that ultraviolet light can penetrate clear water, and at 50 cm below the water surface, light is still 40% effective. Infants and young children are thought to be at higher risk for sunburn than adults because their epidermis is especially thin.

Diagnostic Findings. Visible erythema does not usually develop until several hours after exposure. Edema and pain of an acute sunburn typically follow development of erythema, peak at 14 to 20 hours after exposure, and last for 24 to 48 hours. Severe sunburns with blister formation and epidermal sloughing resemble second-degree thermal burns.

Management. Symptomatic treatment of sunburn includes application of cool wet compresses of water or Burow's solution and oral antiinflammatory agents such as aspirin or ibuprofen. Topical corticosteroids have not been shown to be useful, although in severe edematous reactions, systemic steroids, such as prednisone 1 to 2 mg/kg/24 hr for 5 days, probably shorten the duration of some of the discomfort. Topical anesthetics such as benzocaine, although commonly available over the counter, should be avoided because they have the potential to cause sensitivity reactions when applied to damaged inflamed skin.

Prevention is the most effective treatment of sunburn. Because it is known that sun exposure causes cumulative damage and that development of skin cancer as an adult is related to both severe sunburn and to prolonged sun exposure in childhood, all children with sunburns should receive information about the importance of sunscreens and skin protection.[132] There are three types of topical sun-blocking preparations currently available. Higher levels of sun protection factor (SPF) provide greater protection. Physical barrier protection is provided by a thick material such as zinc oxide, which reflects UVB. Paraaminobenzoic acid (PABA) and its esters padimate O and padimate A absorb UVB, whereas UVA absorbers include benzophenones and anthranilates. In addition, protective clothing designed to provide sun protection without using chemicals is now available with a skin protective factor of 36.[133]

PABA has been a widely accepted sunscreen because it is generally reasonably priced, cosmetically acceptable, and comes in forms that are water resistant. Unfortunately, it can cause some staining of clothing, and there are people who develop topical sensitivity, particularly when they have had a previous sensitivity to benzocaine or sulfonamide. The PABA esters are less sensitizing, but also can cause photodermatitis or contact irritation. Because of a potential risk of absorption through the skin, the FDA suggests that sunscreens not be used in children under 6 months of age.[134]

Sun exposure should be avoided during the midday hours. Children should wear protective clothing, including hats. Parents should be made aware that wet clothing does not protect against UVB penetration. Parents also should be encouraged to use sun protection for themselves, because setting a good example is the best way to teach children.[135,136] Unfortunately several studies have found that parents are still unaware of the dangers of sun exposure, and children continue to have inadequate sun protection.[137,138]

URTICARIA

Urticaria is probably the most common skin rash for which acute care is sought (Fig. 48-20). Fortunately, this is usually a very benign self-limited condition that causes more alarm than harm. Although an underlying etiology may be discovered, the majority of cases remain diagnostic puzzles. The therapeutic approach consists of a search for possible causes, which is rarely fruitful, and provision of symptomatic relief regardless of the cause.[139,140]

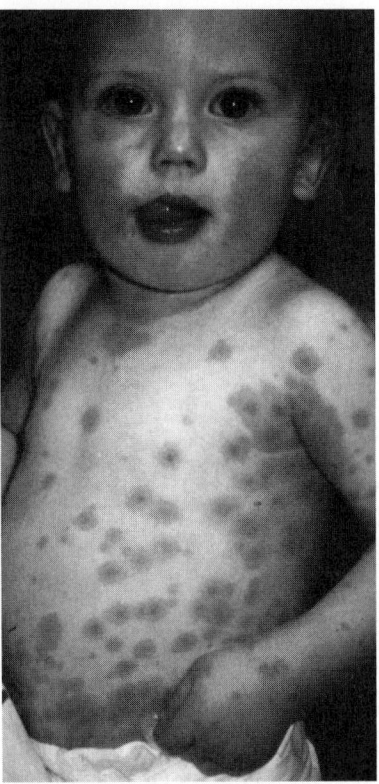

FIG. 48-20. Urticaria is the most common skin rash for which acute care is sought.

Pathophysiology

Mast cell degranulation with release of histamine and other inflammatory mediators is the mechanism by which hives are formed. These chemicals cause vasodilatation and enhance vascular permeability in response to both immunologic and physical agents. Immunologic reactions occur when specific IgE antibody is bound to mast cell membranes, as well as through C3a-mediated reactions. Other complement abnormalities have been found in a small number of patients with urticaria; however, these problems are so rare that they should not be investigated as part of a workup for acute urticaria.

Etiology

The most commonly recognized causes of urticaria include infections, medications, foods, autoimmune diseases, and malignancies. Respiratory infections are thought to be responsible for hives in many children, and acute viral infections including influenza, enterovirus, adenovirus, and infectious mononucleosis and hepatitis viruses have been implicated. Hives may be seen in association with Group A beta-hemolytic streptococcal infection. They have also been attributed to silent focal infections such as dental abscesses, urinary tract infections, and sinus disease.

Medications are frequently implicated in urticarial reactions: penicillins, cephalosporins, sulfa-derived antibiotics, phenytoin, and barbiturates are the most common agents in children. Aspirin and other nonsteroidal antiinflammatory agents that affect prostaglandin synthesis are important causes of urticaria and may increase urticarial reactions from other sources. It should be noted that many children who develop hives while taking these medications are likely to have an urticarial-inducing underlying infection. If there is any need to determine that a medication such as antibiotic is indeed the source of urticaria, a referral for allergy testing would be in order.

There are some foods that are well-recognized causes of urticaria. Many children who have urticarial reactions to eggs and milk lose this sensitivity over time. Reactions to peanuts and seafood do not diminish with age and may actually be quite severe, with respiratory and cutaneous symptoms.

Urticarial reactions to insect stings are fairly common. They should be regarded as the mildest form of an anaphylactic reaction.

Diagnostic Findings

Urticarial lesions occur on all parts of the body and have characteristic raised, erythematous borders with serpiginous edges and blanched centers. They may be very small with a diameter of a few ml or as large as 30 cm. They are characteristically itchy and evanescent. Individual lesions may last for a few minutes or several hours. They typically emerge in areas where there is pressure on the skin, so they are often seen under a waistband. They may also be brought out by temperature changes and may develop during a bath or when a child is wrapped in warm clothing.

Chronic urticaria, defined as hives recurring for over 6 weeks, is rarely seen in children. It is often helpful for parents to know that urticaria lasting for less than this period of time is rarely associated with any systemic problems. Even when urticaria lasts for more than 6 weeks, an etiology is found in fewer than 25% of patients.[141]

There are no routine laboratory tests used in the evaluation of acute urticaria. Simple, inexpensive procedures such as a throat culture for streptococcal screening may be helpful.[142] If an etiologic agent is suggested by the history, that material should be avoided. Otherwise, symptomatic treatment should be given with a referral for a follow-up visit if the hives have not improved within approximately 2 weeks.

Autoimmune diseases such as lupus erythematosus and juvenile rheumatoid arthritis should be considered in the evaluation of chronic urticaria. Childhood malignancies in which urticaria have been described include lymphomas and leukemias. However, investigating these problems should not be part of the standard work-up for acute urticaria.

Differential Considerations

Urticaria and erythema multiforme are frequently confused. Urticaria rarely lasts more than 3 hours; erythema multiforme lesions are fixed and remain for several days. Erythema multiforme does not change with subcutaneous epinephrine whereas urticaria may clear.

Management

If urticaria are severe or if angioedema is present, many patients will improve with subcutaneous epinephrine (1:1,000) at a dose of 0.01 mg/kg; however, this has a short duration. Epinephrine 1:200 (Sus-Phrine) at a dose of 0.05 ml/kg is sometimes helpful for symptomatic relief over a longer number of hours. These medications are not reasonable for use in chronic urticaria.

Antihistamines of the H_1 class are the long-term pharmacologic choice. Over-the-counter products such as diphenhydramine (Benadryl) are inexpensive and effective for most children. Hydroxyzine (Atarax or Vistaril) appear to be the most effective antihistamines. In general, it is best to start with a dose that is in the upper range suggested by the manufacturer and then increase it until the child becomes sedated or until a dose twice the suggested dose is reached. Some clinicians administer H_2 blockers in addition to H_1 blockers. Anticholinergic reactions should not occur at this dose range. The dose should be gradually tapered as the urticaria is controlled (see Chapter 46).

Topical steroids and topical antihistamines are not useful in controlling urticaria. Emollient lotions and baths sometimes provide some symptomatic relief. Systemic corticosteroids have been used in cases that are unresponsive to initial therapy but should be reserved for rare, severe cases.

Children who have urticaria in response to nuts, seafood, or bee stings should be warned about the possibility of anaphylactic reactions in future exposures. An epinephrine administration kit should be provided to the family, and a follow-up visit with an allergist should be arranged.

WARTS

Warts, which are intradermal tumors caused by an infection with a papillomavirus, are among the most common skin problems in children. There are about 40 different types of human papillomaviruses, and each one acts on a specific area of the body[143-145] (Fig. 48-21, A).

The greatest incidence of warts occurs in children 10 to 19 years of age. Transmission through direct contact causes many warts to develop in patterns, which suggests that there has been autoinoculation. Warts can occur in lines as if they are following a scratch, and they are seen as "kissing" lesions on touching surfaces of fingers (Fig. 48-21, B). The incubation period is long and variable so that it is often difficult to identify the source of an infection. Local trauma promotes development of warts, so they are most common at pressure points or in areas that undergo frequent minor trauma such as elbows, fingers, and soles of the feet.

Cellular immunity appears to play an important role in resolution of warts. They develop easily in people who have congenital or acquired immune deficiency. Warts also seem to be among those problems that people outgrow with time, probably by developing immunity with exposure to the virus.

Diagnostic Findings

Common warts appear predominantly on the hands but can be found on other parts of the body. They are skin-colored firm papules found as single lesions or in groups. Facial and scalp warts often develop fingerlike projections that have a hard horny surface.

Flat warts typically develop on the face and extremities. They are tiny smooth-topped flesh-colored papules that are only minimally elevated. They are often spread by the trauma of shaving and are seen more often in adults than in

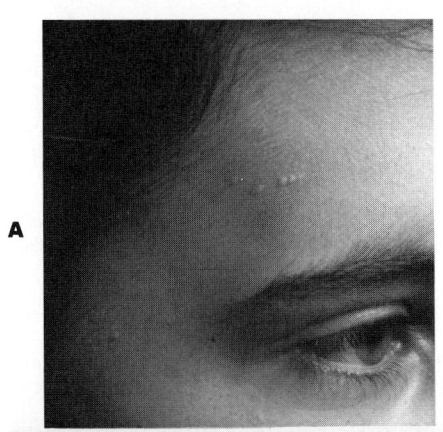

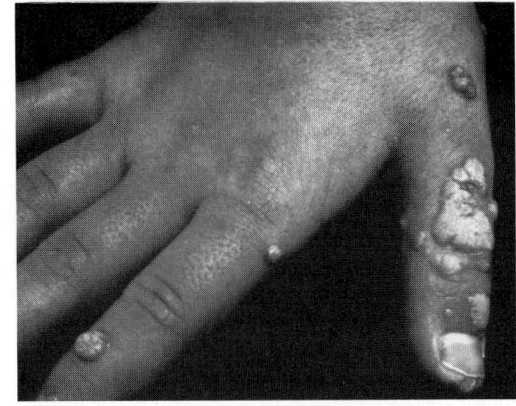

FIG. 48-21. Warts. **A,** Flat warts or verruca planae often develop along a linear scratch. **B,** Verruca vulgaris. *(Courtesy Mayo Medical Center, Department of Dermatology, Rochester, Minn.)*

children. Because it is important to avoid therapies that might cause scarring or changes in skin pigmentation, these warts usually require referral to a specialist.

Children and adolescents with plantar warts are frequently brought to the emergency department for care because the wart causes pain with walking. Because warts develop on pressure points on the feet, a layer of callous-like superficial thickened skin grows over the top of the wart. When the callous is removed, tiny black spots, which are thrombosed superficial capillaries, can be seen in the center of the lesion. These dots help to identify a calloused area as a plantar wart. The prevalence of plantar warts is higher in children who use public swimming pools and gyms.

Anogenital warts and condyloma acuminata are a cause for concern in children because of the risk that the particular papillomavirus that causes these warts may have been transmitted sexually.[144] The possibility of sexual abuse must always be considered when warts are found on a child's perineum. A child with genital warts should be examined for other signs of abuse, and a report should be made to the responsible investigative agency if abuse is suspected. In children who do not have competent immune systems, these warts can grow into fungating lesions that can cause difficulty because of their size. Because these warts are difficult to treat and are located in an anatomic area in which scarring is a serious hazard, treatment should be initiated by a dermatologist.

Management

Treatment of common warts and plantar warts can frequently be managed by families without consulting a specialist; in fact, most warts resolve spontaneously. It is not necessary to initiate treatment for an isolated wart found during a physical examination if it is not causing any problem to the patient. Preschool-aged children are rarely bothered by warts, although most of us can remember the social stigma of a wart for a school-aged child.[146,147]

Patients who come to an emergency department with a wart as their primary problem have usually tried over-the-counter preparations without success or have developed a superficial skin infection after attempting to cut the wart.

Preparations available without prescription usually contain mild keratolytics. Stronger agents, which are quite effective for most patients, contain a combination of salicylic and lactic acids. Preparations in a collodion base (Duofilm, Occlusal) are easily applied directly to the wart. The patient should be warned not to allow the material to touch normal skin. After the medication dries, it should be covered with occlusive tape for 12 to 24 hours. When the tape is removed, the affected area should be soaked in warm water and any loosened skin should be rubbed off with a pumice stone or a rough towel. The treatment is repeated either daily or every other day until the epidermal layer containing the wart peels away. If this treatment has not been effective within 3 months or if the warts are quite widespread, referral to a dermatologist is appropriate.

Most children can be encouraged to treat their problem themselves. Parents may need to apply the medication, but if the child takes care of soaking and rubbing away the loosened skin, not only will their sense of autonomy be encouraged, but the pain that could result from having another person attempt to remove peeling skin will also be avoided. Parents and patients should be cautioned against using a razor blade to shave or cut away at the wart because cellulitis and lymphangitis are potential complications.

Plantar warts are more difficult to treat on very sweaty feet. Efforts to absorb sweat such as wearing thick cotton socks, using absorbent powders, and in some cases, using Burow's solution, can aid resolution of these warts. A tiny doughnut-shaped cushion, such as the type premade for corns, can be positioned over the wart to reduce pressure and pain when walking. Although treatment involving keratolytics will usually take several weeks, it will result in removal of the wart without a scar. It is particularly important to avoid scars on the soles of the feet because they can cause permanent pain.

References

Skin Lesions

1. Callen JP et al: *Color atlas of dermatology,* Philadelphia, 1993, WB Saunders.
2. Cohen B: *Atlas of pediatric dermatology,* St Louis, 1994, Mosby.
3. Fitzpatrick TB et al: *Color atlas and synopsis of clinical dermatology,* New York, 1993, McGraw-Hill.
4. Habif TP: *Clinical dermatology: a color guide to diagnosis and therapy,* St Louis, 1996, Mosby.

5. Hurwitz S: *Clinical pediatric dermatology,* ed 2, Philadelphia, 1993, WB Saunders.
6. Krusinski PA and Flowers FP: *Handbook of pediatric dermatology,* Chicago, 1990, Year book.
7. Schachner LA and Hansen RC: *Pediatric dermatology,* ed 2, New York, 1995, Churchill Livingstone.
8. Weston WL, Lane AT, and Morelli JG: *Color textbook of pediatric dermatology,* St. Louis, 1996, Mosby.

Acne

9. Schachner L: The treatment of acne: a contemporary review, *Pediatr Clin North Am* 30:501-510, 1983.
10. Wilson BB: Acne vulgaris, *Prim Care* 16:695-713, 1989.
11. Lucky A: Endocrine aspects of acne, *Pediatr Clin North Am* 30:495-500, 1983.
12. Yonkosky DM and Pochi PE: Acne vulgaris in childhood pathogenesis and management, *Dermatol Clin* 4:127-136, 1986.
13. Nguyen QH, Kim YA, Schwartz RA: Management of acne vulgaris, *Am Fam Physician* 50:89-96, 99-100, 1994.

Atopic Dermatitis

14. Paller AS: Clinical features of atopic dermatitis, *Clin Rev Allergy* 11:419-426, 1993.
15. Beck HI and Korsgaard J: Atopic dermatitis and house dust mites, *Br J Dermatol* 120:245-251, 1989.
16. Burks AW et al: Atopic dermatitis: clinical relevance of food hypersensitivity reactions, *J Pediatr* 113:447-451, 1988.
17. Krafchik BR: Atopic dermatitis, *Pediatr Clin North Am* 30:669-685, 1983.
18. Roth HL and Kierland RR: The natural history of atopic dermatitis, *Arch Dermatol* 89:209-214, 1964.
19. Brunsting L, Reed WB, Bair HL: Occurrence of cataracts and keratoconus with atopic dermatitis, *Arch Dermatol* 72:237-241, 1955.
20. Charlesworth EN: Practical approaches to the treatment of atopic dermatitis, *Allergy Proc* 15:269-274, 1994.
21. Lester RS: Topical formulary for the pediatrician, *Pediatr Clin North Am* 30:749-764, 1983.

Bacterial Skin Infections

22. Kahn RM and Goldstein EJ: Common bacterial skin infections. Diagnostic clues and therapeutic options, *Postgrad Med* 93:175-182, 1993.
23. Tunnessen WW: Cutaneous infections, *Pediatr Clin North Am* 30:515-532, 1983.
24. Fleisher G, Ludwig S, Campos J: Cellulitis: bacterial etiology, clinical features, and laboratory findings, *J Pediatr* 97:591-593, 1980.
25. Howe PM, Fajardo JE, Orcutt MA: Etiologic diagnosis of cellulitis: comparison of the aspirates obtained from the leading edge and the point of maximal inflammation, *Pediatr Infect Dis J* 6:685-686, 1987.
26. Goldgeier MH: The microbiologic evaluation of acute cellulitis, *Cutis* 31:649-650; 653-654; 656; 1983.
27. Bratton RL and Nesse RE: St. Anthony's Fire: diagnosis and management of erysipelas, *Am Fam Physician* 51:401-404, 1995.
28. Ginsburg CM: Management of selected skin and soft tissue infections, *Pediatr Infect Dis J* 5:735-740, 1986.
29. Powell KR, Kaplan SB, Hall CB, et al: Periorbital cellulitis, *Am J Dis Child* 142:853-857, 1988.
30. Friedman AD: Superficial bacterial and fungal infections of the skin, *Adv Pediatr Infect Dis* 5:205-219, 1990.
31. Dillon HC: The treatment of streptococcal skin infections, *J Pediatr* 76:676-684, 1970.
32. Esterly NB and Markowitz M: The treatment of pyoderma in children, *JAMA* 212:1667-1670, 1970.
33. Hirschmann JV: Topical antibiotics in dermatology, *Arch Dermatol* 124:1691-1700, 1988.
34. Carruthers R: Prescribing antibiotics for impetigo, *Drugs* 36:364-369, 1988.
35. Brook I: Bacteriologic study of paronychia in children, *Am J Surg* 141:703-705, 1981.
36. Kokx NP, Comstock JA, Facklam RR: Streptococcal perianal disease in children, *Pediatrics* 80:659-663, 1987.
37. Krol AL: Perianal streptococcal dermatitis, *Pediatr Dermatol* 7:97-100, 1990.
38. Wikas SM and Tomecki KJ: Staphylococcal scalded-skin syndrome: the Cleveland Clinic experience, *Cleve Clin J Med* 50:141-143, 1983.
39. Hansen RC: Staphylococcal scalded-skin syndrome, toxic shock syndrome, and Kawasaki disease, *Pediatr Clin North Am* 30:533-544, 1983.
40. Hebert A and Esterly WB: Bacterial and candidal cutaneous infections in the neonate, *Dermatol Clin* 4:3-21, 1986.
41. Belani K et al: Association of exotoxin-producing group A streptococci and severe disease in children, *Pediatr Infect Dis J* 10:351-354, 1991.
42. Novotny W, Faden H, Mosovich L: Emergence of invasive group A streptococcal disease among young children, *Clin Pediatr (Phila)* 31:596-601, 1992.
43. Cowan MR et al: Serious group A beta-hemolytic streptococcal infections complicating varicella, *Ann Emerg Med* 23:818-822, 1994.

Cold Panniculitis

44. Epstein EH and Oren ME: Popsicle panniculitis, *N Engl J Med* 282:966-967, 1970.
45. Aronson IK, Zeitz HJ, Variakojis D: Panniculitis in childhood, *Pediatr Dermatol* 5:216-230, 1988.

Contact Dermatitis

46. McAlvany JP and Sherertz EF: Contact dermatitis in infants, children, and adolescents, *Adv Dermatol* 9:205-223, 1994.
47. Weston WL and Weston JA: Allergic contact dermatitis in children, *Am J Dis Control* 138:932-936, 1984.
48. Christensen OB: Nickel dermatitis, *Dermatol Clin* 8:37-40, 1990.
49. deGroot AC et al: The allergens in cosmetics, *Arch Dermatol* 124:1525-1529, 1988.
50. Whittington C: Clinical aspects of contact dermatitis, *Prim Care* 16:729-738, 1989.
51. Zugerman C: Contact dermatitis in children, *Compr Ther* 10:29-36, 1984.

Diaper Dermatitis

52. Janniger CK and Thomas I: Diaper dermatitis: an approach to prevention employing effective diaper care, *Cutis* 52:153-155, 1993.
53. Jordan WE et al: Diaper dermatitis: frequency and severity among a general infant population, *Pediatr Dermatol* 3:198-207, 1986.
54. Berg RW et al: Etiologic factors in diaper dermatitis: the role of urine, *Pediatr Dermatol* 3:102-106, 1986.
55. Buckingham KW and Berg RW: Etiologic factors in diaper dermatitis: the role of feces, *Pediatr Dermatol* 3:107-112, 1986.
56. Rasmussen JE: Classification of diaper dermatitis: an overview, *Pediatrician* 14:6-10, 1986.

Erythema Multiforme

57. Edmond BJ, Huff JC, Weston WL: Erythema multiforme, *Pediatr Clin North Am* 30:631-640, 1983.
58. Brice SL, Huff JC, Weston WL: Erythema multiforme minor in children, *Pediatrician* 18:188-194, 1991.
59. Renfro L et al: Controversy: are systemic steroids indicated in the treatment of erythema multiforme? *Pediatr Dermatol* 6:43-50, 1989.
60. Special symposium: corticosteroids for erythema multiforme? *Pediatr Dermatol* 6:229-250, 1989.

Stevens-Johnson Syndrome/Toxic Epidermal Necrolysis

61. Nethercott JR and Choi BCK: Erythema multiforme (Stevens-Johnson Syndrome)—Chart review of 123 hospitalized patients, *Dermatologica* 171:383-396, 1985.
62. Assier H et al: Erythema multiforme with mucous membrane involvement and Stevens-Johnson syndrome are clinically different disorders with distinct causes, *Arch Dermatol* 131:539-543, 1995.
63. Stewart MG et al: Head and neck manifestations of erythema multiforme in children, *Otolaryngol Head Neck Surg* 111:236-242, 1994.
64. Prendiville JS et al: Management of Stevens-Johnson syndrome and toxic epidermal necrolysis in children, *J Pediatr* 115:881-887, 1989.

Fungal Infections

65. Rasmussen JE: Cutaneous fungus infections in children, *Pediatr Rev* 13:152-156, 1992.
66. Stein DH: Superficial fungal infections, *Pediatr Clin North Am* 30:545-561, 1983.
67. Special symposia: tinea capitis: current concepts, *Pediatr Dermatol* 2:224-237, 1985.

68. Nanda A et al: Pityriasis (tinea) versicolor in infancy, *Pediatr Dermatol* 5:260-262, 1988.

Henoch-Schönlein Purpura

69. Farley TA et al: Epidemiology of a cluster of Henoch-Schönlein purpura, *AJDC* 143:798-803, 1989.
70. Robson WL, Leung AK: Henoch-Schönlein purpura, *Adv Pediatr* 41:163-194, 1994.
71. Causey AL et al: Henoch-Schönlein purpura: four cases and a review, *J Emerg Med* 12:331-341, 1994.
72. Chamberlain RS, Greenberg LW: Scrotal involvement in Henoch-Schönlein purpura: a case report and review of the literature, *Pediatr Emerg Care* 8:213-215, 1992.
73. Saulsburg FT: Henoch-Schönlein purpura, *Pediatr Dermatol* 1:195-201, 1984.
74. Koskimies O et al: Henoch-Schönlein nephritis: long-term prognosis of unselected patients, *Arch Dis Child* 56:482-484, 1981.
75. Rosenblum ND and Winter HS: Steroid effects on the course of abdominal pain in children with Henoch-Schönlein purpura, *Pediatrics* 79:1018-1021, 1987.

Herpes Virus Infections

76. Galasso GJ and Myers MW: The five human herpesviruses: infection, prevention and treatment, *Adv Intern Med* 29:25-28, 1984.
77. Fiumara NJ: Herpes simplex, *Clin Dermatol* 7:23-36, 1989.
78. Raab B and Lorincz AL: Genital herpes simplex: concepts and treatment, *J Am Acad Dermatol* 5:249-263, 1982.
79. Chadwick EG, et al: Advances in antiviral therapy: acyclovir, *Pediatr Dermatol* 2:64-70, 1984.
80. Report of the Committee on Infectious Diseases, *Am Acad Pediatr*, 1994.
81. Finger R et al: Age-specific incidence of chickenpox, *Public Health Rep* 109:750-755, 1994.
82. Wilson GJ et al: Group A streptococcal necrotizing fasciitis following varicella in children: case reports and review, *Clin Infect Dis* 20:1333-1338, 1995.
83. Weller TH: Varicella and herpes zoster: changing concepts of the natural history, control, and importance of a not-so benign virus, *N Engl J Med* 309:1362-1368, 1434-1440, 1983.
84. Fleisher G et al: Life-threatening complications of varicella, *Am J Dis Child* 135:896-899, 1981.
85. Preblud S: Age-specific risks of varicella complications, *Pediatrics* 68:14-17, 1981.
86. Doran T et al: Acetaminophen: more harm than good for chickenpox? *J Pediatr* 114:1045-1048, 1989.
87. Balfour HH Jr: Current management of varicella zoster virus infections, *J Med Virol* 1(suppl):74-81, 1993.
88. Burnett I: Severe chickenpox during treatment with corticosteroids. Immunoglobulin should be given if steroid dosage was (or = 0.5 mg/kg/day) in preceding three months, *BMJ* 310:327, 1995.
89. Krause PR and Klinman DM: Efficacy, immunogenicity, safety, and use of live attenuated chickenpox vaccine, *J Pediatr* 127:518-525, 1995.
90. Anonymous: Recommendations for the use of live attenuated varicella vaccine. AAP Committee on Infectious Diseases, *Pediatrics* 95:791-796, 1995.

Infectious Exanthems

91. Farizo KM et al: Pediatric emergency room visits: a risk factor for acquiring measles, *Pediatrics* 87:74-79, 1991.
92. Hartley AH and Rasmussen JE: Infectious exanthems, *Pediatr Rev* 9:321-329, 1988.
93. Cherry JD: *Viral exanthems: current problems in pediatrics*, Chicago, 1983, Year Book.
94. Cherry JD: Contemporary infectious exanthems, *Clin Infec Dis* 16:199-205, 1993.
95. Frieden IJ and Resnick SD: Childhood exanthems. Old and new, *Pediatr Clin North Am* 38:859-887, 1991.
96. Bialecki C, Feder HM, Grant-Kels JM: The six classic childhood exanthems: a review and update, *J Am Acad Dermatol* 21:891-903, 1989.
97. Markowitz LE et al: Patterns of transmission in measles outbreaks in the United States, 1985-1986, *N Engl J Med* 320:75-81, 1986.
98. Ferson MJ et al: Difficulties in clinical diagnosis of measles: proposal for modified clinical case definition, *Med J Aust* 163:364-366, 1995.
99. Atkinson WL: Epidemiology and prevention of measles, *Dermatol Clin* 13:553-559, 1995.
100. Wood DL and Brunell PA: Measles control in the United States: problems of the past and challenges for the future, *Clin Microbiol Rev* 8:260-267, 1995.
101. Committee on Infectious Diseases: Parvovirus, erythema infectiosum and pregnancy, *Pediatrics* 85:131-133, 1990.
102. Hall CB: The rash of roses, *Arch Dermatol* 125:196-198, 1989.
103. Asano Y et al: Clinical features of infants with primary human herpesvirus 6 infection (exanthem subitum roseola infantum), *Pediatrics* 93:104-108, 1994.
104. Suga S et al: Human herpesvirus-G infection (exanthem subitum) without rash, *Pediatrics* 83:1003-1006, 1989.
105. Asano Y et al: Human herpesvirus-G infection (exanthem subitum) without fever, *J Pediatr* 115:264-265, 1989.
106. Tindall JP and Callaway JL: Hand, foot, and mouth disease: it's more common than you think, *Am J Dis Child* 124:372-375, 1972.
107. Cherry JD and Jahn CL: Herpangina: the etiologic spectrum, *Pediatrics* 36:632-634, 1965.
108. Bjornberg A and Hellgren L: Pityriasis rosea: a statistical, clinical and laboratory investigation of 826 patients and matched healthy controls, *Acta Derm Venereol Suppl (Stockh)* 42:1-68, 1962.
109. Baden H: Sunlight and pityriasis rosea, *Arch Dermatol* 113:377, 1977.

Molluscum Contagiosum

110. Janniger CK, Schwartz RA: Molluscum contagiosum in children, *Cutis* 52:194-196, 1993.
111. Brown ST, Nalley JF, Kraus SJ: Molluscum contagiosum, *Sex Transm Dis* 8:227-234, 1981.

Scaly Feet

112. Weston JA and Weston WL: Foot dermatitis in children, *Pediatrics* 72:824-827, 1983.
113. Broberg A and Faergemann J: Scaly lesions on the feet in children—tinea or eczema? *Acta Paediatr* 79:349-351, 1990.

Seborrheic Dermatitis

114. Yates VM, et al: Early diagnosis of infantile seborrheic dermatitis and atopic dermatitis: clinical features, *Br J Dermatol* 108:633-638, 1983.
115. Janniger CK: Infantile seborrheic dermatitis: an approach to cradle cap, *Cutis* 51:233-235, 1993.

Skin Parasites

116. Elgart M: Pediculosis, *Dermatol Clin* 8:219-228, 1990.
117. Hogan DJ, Schachner L, Tanglertsampan C: Diagnosis and treatment of childhood scabies and pediculosis, *Pediatr Clin North Am* 38:941-957, 1991.
118. Scott JJ and Scott MJ: Nits or not: pseudonits—simple office diagnosis, *JAMA* 243:2325-2326, 1980.
119. Rasmussen JE: The problem of lindane, *J Am Acad Dermatol* 5:507-516, 1981.
120. Bowerman JG et al: Comparative study of permethrin 1% creme rinse and lindane shampoo for the treatment of head lice, *Pediatr Infect Dis J* 6:252-255, 1988.
121. Brown S, Becher J, Brady W: Treatment of ectoparasitic infections: review of the English-language literature, 1982-1992, *Clin Infect Dis* 20(suppl) 1:S104-109, 1995.
122. Meinking TL and Taplin D: Advances in pediatrics, scabies, and other mite infestations, *Adv Dermatol* 5:131-152, 1990.
123. Hurwitz S: Scabies in babies, *Am J Dis Child* 126:226-228, 1973.
124. Rasmussen JE: Scabies, *Pediatr Rev* 15:110-114, 1994.
125. Taplin D et al: A comparative trial of three treatment schedules for the eradication of scabies, *J Am Acad Dermatol* 9:550-554, 1983.
126. Kata R et al: The natural course of creeping eruption and treatment with thiabendazole, *Arch Dermatol* 91:420-424, 1965.
127. Davis CM and Israel RM: Treatment of creeping eruption with thiabendazole, *Arch Dermatol* 97:325-326, 1968.
128. Crawford F and Vermand SH: Parasitic infections in day-care centers, *Pediatr Infect Dis J* 6:744-749, 1987.
129. Brady FJ and Wright WH: Studies on oxyuriasis: the symptomatology of oxyuriasis as based on physical examination and case histories on 200 patients, *Am J Med Sci* 198:367-372, 1939.
130. Drugs for parasitic infections, *Med Lett Drugs Ther* 30:15-24, 1988.

Sun Reactions

131. Kohn G: Photosensitivity and photodermatitis in childhood, *Dermatol Clin* 4:107-116, 1986.
132. Williams M and Sagebiel R: Sunburns, melanoma and the pediatrician, *Pediatrics* 84:381-382, 1989.
133. Federal Register: Sunscreen drug products for over-the-counter human use, II:38206-38369, 1985.
134. Hebert AA: Photoprotection in children, *Adv Dermatol* 8:309-324, 1993.
135. Hurwitz S: The sun and sunscreen protection: recommendations for children, *J Dermatol Surg Oncol* 14:657-660, 1988.
136. Janniger CK: Solar exposure in children, *Dermatology* 189:55-57, 1994.
137. Whiteman DC et al: A survey of sunscreen use and sun-protection practices in Darwin, *Aust J Public Health* 18:47-50, 1994.
138. Bourke JF and Graham-Brown RA: Protection of children against sunburn: a survey of parental practice in Leicester, *Br J Dermatol* 133:264-266, 1995.

Urticaria

139. Twarog FS: Urticaria in childhood: pathogenesis and management, *Pediatr Clin North Am* 30:887-897, 1983.

140. Mahmood T and Janniger CK: Childhood urticaria, *Cutis* 52:78-80, 1993.
141. Halpern SR: Chronic hives in children: an analysis of 75 cases, *Ann Allergy* 23:589-599, 1965.
142. Schuller DE and Elvey SM: Urticaria with streptococcal infection, *Pediatrics* 65:592-596, 1980.

Warts

143. Gellis S: Warts and molluscum contagiosum in children, *Pediatr Ann* 16:69-76, 1987.
144. Shackner L and Hankin DE: Assessing child abuse in childhood condyloma acuminatum, *J Am Acad Dermatol* 12:157-160, 1985.
145. Beutner KR: Cutaneous viral infections, *Pediatr Ann* 22:247-252, 1993.
146. Janniger CK: Childhood warts, *Cutis* 50:15-16, 1992.
147. Special Symposium: Management of warts in children, *Pediatr Dermatol* 4:36-54, 1987.

Ear, Nose, and Throat Disorders

John P. Santamaria • Thomas J. Abrunzo

Signs and Symptoms

DROOLING AND DYSPHONIA

Dysphonia is any impairment of voice; hoarseness is a type of dysphonia that imparts a rough quality to the voice. Drooling or sialorrhea is the excessive flow of saliva from the mouth, and dysphagia or difficulty in swallowing may be an accompanying symptom.

Pathophysiology

Excess salivation occurs from either overproduction of secretions, or more commonly, from inability to effectively swallow salivary secretions. Most normal babies drool secondary to teething, mouth-breathing, and a lack of control of flow of saliva until about 12 months of age.[1]

Hoarseness is indicative of a problem in the larynx and true vocal cords. It can be caused by inflammation (infec-

tions, allergy, chemical, or thermal), obstruction, trauma, or neurologic disease.[2]

Dysphagia may result from anatomic obstruction or compression of the pharynx, or from a physiologic dysfunction of the neuromuscular process of swallowing. Swallowing requires coordination with sucking and breathing. Dysphagia can be caused by congenital and acute processes that may range from mild to life-threatening in nature.

Diagnostic Considerations

The emergent pharyngeal infectious conditions that occur with drooling, dysphonia, or dysphagia include retropharyngeal abscess, peritonsillar abscess, tracheitis, and epiglottitis.

In the infant and toddler, less emergent infectious processes are also known to cause drooling and dysphagia, including the various causes of stomatitis, pharyngitis, and esophagitis. Peritonsillar abscess is more common in children over the age of 12 years.

Chemical agents cause drooling either by direct irritation or by pharmacologic stimulation. Caustics such as drain cleaners and alkalies, hypochlorites, and acids are the common chemical causes of mucosal injury and drooling. Oral burns from hot liquids or objects can also cause injuries. Systemic poisons that cause drooling include organophosphates, mercury, anticholinesterase eye drops, and iodides. Clonazepam and nitrazepam are reported to cause excessive lacrimation and salivation.

Hoarseness may be caused by inflammation secondary to infectious, allergic, chemical, and thermal injuries. Hoarseness in immunocompromised children may be an early indicator of invasive fungal infection.[3]

Foreign body injury can cause drooling or dysphagia by contusion, laceration, perforation, or impaction of the oropharynx and esophagus.

Anterior neck trauma (clothesline or dashboard injury) can fracture thyroid or cricoid cartilage, resulting in dysphonia and dysphagia.

Diagnostic Work-Up

A history of fever, sore throat, drooling, dysphagia, dysphonia with or without stridor, croupy cough, or other sounds of respiratory obstruction, requires immediate steps to diagnose and treat imminent upper airway obstruction. Less toxic-appearing, older children with past history of recurrent tonsillitis, drooling, dysphagia, sore throat, and fever are more likely to have peritonsillar abscess. A history of oral sores or vesicles suggests stomatitis. Caustic, toxic, thermal, and traumatic (foreign body) incidents should be documented.

An acute onset of dysphonia should indicate a foreign body in the airway until proven otherwise.[4]

If respiratory compromise is present, no further invasive physical examination should be done until the airway can be definitively managed. In the absence of significant airway compromise, thorough exam of the aerodigestive anatomy should be undertaken. Oral vesicles and ulcers are signs of stomatitis and gingivitis. Large areas of ulceration and epithelial denudation suggests chemical or thermal burn. Tonsillar infection should be excluded; abscess causes deviation of the uvula, fluctuant swelling, and "hot potato" voice. Ecchymosis, swelling, laceration, and bleeding should be documented. The membranous pharyngitis of diphtheria or other systemic findings should be identified.

Ancillary Data. Soft tissue technique x-ray examination of the upper airway and routine chest x-ray film should be done in the stable patient. A barium swallow may document esophageal injury or the presence of a foreign body. In acute or equivocal cases, stabilization and endoscopy in the operating suite may be necessary.

Prehospital Considerations

With upper airway compromise, follow the protocol recommended for epiglottitis.

Therapeutic Trial

Ensuring airway patency is the first priority. Subsequent therapy is directed by etiology and symptomatology.

EAR DISCHARGE

Ear discharge, or otorrhea, and the underlying causative process may affect hearing or balance.

Pathophysiology

Discharge from the ear is most frequently a manifestation of external or middle ear disease. It may represent an inner ear process or basilar skull fracture. The quality of ear discharge is a clue to the cause.

Ceruminous Discharge. The external ear canal normally contains a thin layer of cerumen produced by glands on its cartilaginous portion. In normal amounts, cerumen can prevent damage to the overlying skin by retained water.[5] Increased cerumen production or impaired clearing may occlude the ear canal and soften enough to create a discharge. Cerumen can cause a conductive hearing loss.

Purulent Discharge. Pus is a product of inflammation, containing leukocytes and the debris of dead cells and tissue elements that have been liquified by leukocytic enzymes. Although the discharge is noted in the external ear canal, the middle ear is often the site of the pathologic process. The pus can rupture through the tympanic membrane or through patent tympanostomy tubes.

Cerebrospinal Fluid Discharge. Fracture of the skull is by far the most common cause of cerebrospinal fluid drainage from the ear. The temporal bone is most frequently involved. Cerebrospinal fluid otorrhea may also result from rupture of the round window, also called *perilymph fistula*. When the window ruptures inward, ambient pressure

---

Ear Discharge by Location and Character

External auditory canal
Impaction (cerumen)
Local trauma (blood)
Foreign bodies (blood)
Otitis externa (pus, blood)
Tumor (blood)

Middle ear
Penetrating injury of the tympanic membrane and middle ear (blood)—curetting wax, myringotomy, tympanostomy
Bullous myringitis (blood, pus)
Acute otitis media (pus, blood)
Tumors/anomalous vessels (blood)
Barotrauma (blood)

Inner ear/intracranial
Round window barotrauma (CSF)
Head trauma (blood, CSF)

---

change in the middle ear space is the culprit, often caused by barotrauma. When the window ruptures outward, excessive physical exertion causes a rise in cerebrospinal fluid pressure.[6]

Bloody Discharge. There are many vascularized structures of the external auditory canal, middle ear, and cranium that can become inflamed or traumatized, resulting in a bloody aural discharge. The skin of the external canal is subject to traumatic tears and inflammatory processes. The tympanic membrane itself can bleed from penetrating trauma, inflammation, or stretching injury. Vascular tumors are seen in the external auditory canal and the middle ear. Congenital vascular anomalies in the middle ear can cause significant bleeding, especially after inadvertent trauma during surgical instrumentation of the canal and eardrum. When fractured, the temporal bone and its soft tissue attachments can cause bleeding into the external ear canal.

Diagnostic Considerations

The box above presents the major differential diagnoses classified by anatomic location.

Diagnostic Work-Up

Historic clues can aid the differential diagnosis of otorrhea. Information regarding the duration of symptoms, change in the character of the discharge, and presence of pain should be noted. Temporal association with surgical procedures, trauma, or foreign body insertion should be determined. Related symptoms of fever, neck pain or swelling, and headache may herald more serious disease.

The physical examination involves a thorough inspection of the ear, cranium, neck, and neurologic system. In inflammatory processes of the external ear, the pinna may be swollen, protruded, erythematous, and tender to palpation or traction. The external auditory canal may be difficult to examine fully because of the presence of discharge or a foreign body. Edema resulting from inflammatory disease may further preclude an adequate view of the canal and tympanic membrane. Removal of the discharge and foreign body will enhance the examination and quicken resolution of the inflammatory process (see section on Foreign Body in the Ear and Nose).

Inspection of the tympanic membrane may reveal changes of color, lucency, light reflex, landmarks, and mobility. Inflammatory conditions of the external and middle ear are often associated with cervical lymphadenitis (see section on Lymphadenitis).

Cerebrospinal fluid otorrhea requires a search for apparent trauma to the head. Presence of periorbital ecchymosis (raccoon eyes) or postauricular ecchymosis (Battle's sign) is suggestive of basilar skull fracture. When significant trauma to the tympanic membrane, middle ear, or round window occurs, the results of a screening hearing examination may be abnormal. Rubbing two fingers together at the external meatus bilaterally can be used as a screening device to detect gross hearing loss or asymmetry.

Ancillary Data. Inspection of the ear discharge often aids in the localization of the disease process (see the box on p. 710). If cerebrospinal fluid otorrhea is suspected but not certain, the fluid can be tested with glucose oxidase paper for confirmation of its normally high glucose content (see the section on Nasal Discharge).

With cerebrospinal fluid otorrhea, the main concern is the status of the intracranial contents. CT scan with bone windows offers the advantage of detailing soft tissue injury and bleeding in addition to evaluating for the presence of fracture.

Prehospital Considerations

When a child has blood or cerebrospinal fluid coming from the ear, the most significant injuries must be considered. Discharge from the ear resembling cerebrospinal fluid always signifies an intracranial injury in the prehospital setting. Unless there is a clear history of local trauma to the external auditory canal, blood from the canal should also initiate head injury precautions until definitive diagnosis is made. Rapid, uninterrupted transport to an appropriate facility should be a high priority.

Therapeutic Trial

Children and parents should be taught not to place anything into the ear canal: "Put nothing smaller than your elbow in your ear."[7] Parents often are not aware that the use of cotton swabs in the ear canal pushes cerumen farther toward the tympanic membrane and can cause an impaction to develop. The ear should be thoroughly dried after swimming and bathing. Fingernails should be kept trimmed and clean. Dermatoses of the external ear canal that may predispose to otitis externa, such as eczema, should be treated.[7] Children should wear helmets when riding bicycles and use age-appropriate restraints when riding in automobiles.

Most external ear disease can be treated topically (see section on Otitis Media). Removal of foreign bodies from the external auditory canal requires careful positioning of the child. Use of an ear curette, suction, or small forceps may facilitate removal. If ear disease is suspected, exami-

nation of the ear should not be compromised by the presence of cerumen, despite the uncooperativeness of most young children for its removal. Bullous myringitis and acute otitis media are usually manageable by using oral antibiotic therapy (see section on Otitis Media).

The diagnosis of skull fracture requires an exhaustive search for associated intracranial injury. If there is a suggestion of intracranial injury by clinical examination, the patient should be observed in an intensive care setting with airway and other resuscitative equipment within reach (see Chapter 21). Round window rupture (perilymph fistula) should be managed by an otolaryngologist.

EAR PAIN

Ear pain or otalgia is the sensation of discomfort at any part of the ear and does not always reflect ear disease. Whether the pain originates from the ear itself or from a distant site may not be discernible by the patient. The severity of the pain may not correlate with the seriousness of underlying pathology.

Pathophysiology

Ear pain reflects the anatomic part that is diseased. The pathology may be intrinsic to the ear or referred by neural pathways from extrinsic disease.

Primary Ear Disease. Pain from the external ear arises from the skin of the pinna or external canal, or the dense connective tissue overlying the cartilage. Inflammatory conditions of the external auditory canal are painful because the skin in the canal is closely adherent to, and stretched tightly over the cartilaginous and bony structures. Middle ear structures that are pain sensitive include the tympanic membrane and the linings of the middle ear cavity and mastoid.

Referred Pain. The fifth, seventh, ninth, and tenth (CN V, VII, IX, and X) cranial nerves and the upper cervical nerves can transmit pain sensation to external and middle ear structures (see box on p. 712). As described by Kreisberg and Turner, "the ear is unique in that no structure in the body of comparable size is supplied by sensory nerves from so many neural segments."[8]

Diagnostic Considerations

Most otalgia seen in the emergency setting is caused by external or middle ear disease. Acute purulent otitis media is the most common middle ear disease presenting as otalgia in childhood (see section on Otitis Media). Otitis externa and foreign bodies in the external ear canal are the most common causes of external ear disease. Otitis externa is usually of bacterial or fungal etiology, readily diagnosed by physical examination, and generally treatable with topical medication (see section on Otitis Externa).

Traumatic injuries to the pinna are frequent and should be treated as indicated. An auricular hematoma may require drainage and close follow-up to prevent formation of a "cauliflower" ear. Localized cellulitis at the site of a recent ear piercing, with swelling and retention of the earring subcutaneously, is common.

Environmental injuries such as frostbite of the pinna may be exacerbated by the contributing factors of unprotected location, lack of subcutaneous insulating fat, and

---

Differential Diagnosis of Referred Ear Pain [9-11]

Trigeminal [V] nerve

Oral cavity: stomatitis, gingivitis, trauma, or infection of tongue

Dental: impacted, traumatized, carious, or abscessed teeth

Temporomandibular joint: malocclusions, bruxism

Other: sinusitis, mastoiditis, parotitis, intracranial process

Facial [VII] nerve

Bell's palsy

Herpes zoster infection (Ramsay-Hunt syndrome)

Glossopharyngeal [IX] nerve

Oropharynx: tonsillitis, posttonsillectomy, retropharyngeal abscess

Nasopharynx: inflammation/infection, foreign body

Vagus [X] nerve

Larynx: trauma, foreign body

Esophagus: foreign body, burn

Thyroiditis

Upper cervical nerves

Lymphadenitis

Infected branchial cleft cysts

Cervical spine injuries or muscle pain

---

terminal blood supply. The appearance of the pinna may vary from erythematous in mild cases to black and necrotic in severe ones (see section on Frostbite). Thermal burns to the pinna occur in a majority of facial burns. Because of the relative absence of subcutaneous tissue, relatively minor burns can cause significant structural and cosmetic disturbance (see Chapter 37).

Perichondritis may complicate many other diseases of the external ear and cause significant pain and swelling. Hematoma, surgery, burns, frostbite, other trauma, and even accupuncture have been associated with the development of this potentially debilitating disease. Commonly caused by *Pseudomonas* or *Staphylococcus* species, the disease progresses with tissue destruction. The resulting cosmetic defect can be significant.[12]

Diseases extrinsic to the ear that can cause otalgia are quite diverse. The box above includes many of these possibilities, grouped according to the proposed neural pathway of pain. Although none of these diseases are frequent causes of childhood otalgia, some are distinct enough to warrant further discussion.

Bell's palsy, caused by peripheral seventh (VII) cranial nerve dysfunction, can cause otalgia and facial paralysis. It can only be diagnosed with certainty after exclusion of otitis media, cholesteatoma, temporal bone fracture, herpes zoster oticus, and tumor. Peripheral (VII) nerve disease causes unilateral upper and lower facial nerve dysfunction. Complete recovery of nerve function occurs in 84% of patients and can be predicted by observing progression and completeness of paralysis during the first 3 weeks of illness.[13] A lesion proximal to the facial nucleus (central VII palsy) spares function of muscles for eye closure and forehead wrinkling because they are controlled by an area in the pons that has input from both cerebral cortices.[14]

Ramsay-Hunt syndrome is an inflammation of the facial nerve (VII) secondary to herpes zoster; other cranial nerves may be involved. Its classic form includes facial paralysis, vesicles on the pinna or in the external canal, and associated pain.[10] Otalgia may be severe and may occur weeks after resolution of the external canal vesicles, which are seen early in the disease process.

Diagnostic Work-Up

The history should determine the child's response to otalgia. From parents of a very young child it is particularly important to establish a change from the usual pattern of behavior. Minor variations in feeding, sleeping, and waking behavior patterns may be all that is present in the young infant. As a child becomes older and more articulate, it becomes possible to elicit a specific history beyond the presence of nonspecific otalgia. Whenever possible, the quality of the pain should be described (e.g., sharp vs. dull); details of its intensity, location, radiation, exacerbating factors (e.g., worsening with chewing may suggest intraoral or temporomandibular joint pathology), and palliative factors should also be elicited.

The primary goal of the physical examination of the patient with otalgia is to determine if primary ear disease is present. The ear examination must be done in a systematic manner. The auricle should be inspected for evidence of swelling, redness, warmth, and tenderness to palpation or traction. The external ear canal should be examined for edema, mass, and discharge. The tympanic membrane must be evaluated for color, lucency, landmarks, light reflex, and mobility.

If the ear examination does not reveal the cause of otalgia, consider referred ear pain. Thorough evaluation of the head, neck, mouth, and neurologic systems may be required to pinpoint the problem (see the box above left). Otalgia has even precipitated unnecessary surgical procedures in a teenager with Munchausen syndrome.[15] Consultation from specialists in otolaryngology, dentistry, neurology, and psychiatry may be necessary.

Ancillary Data. If an exhaustive history and physical examination do not reveal the cause of otalgia, consider radiologic studies. Plain films of the sinuses, mastoid bones, or cervical spine as well as soft tissue techniques of the neck may prove helpful. CT scans, and more recently, MRI scan can detail intracranial processes and assist in visualization of foreign bodies, tumors, or abscesses of the neck and retropharyngeal space.

Prehospital Considerations

Prehospital considerations in the care of the patient with otalgia should follow the same priorities as for any ill or injured patient. Because airway problems can be a cause of referred ear pain, these should be addressed first, followed by stabilization of the cardiopulmonary system. Attention can then be directed to the symptom of pain.

Therapeutic Trial

Treatment of ear pain reflects the etiology. Topical anesthetic otic drops may be useful in differentiating primary pathology from referred pain (see sections on Otitis Externa and Otitis Media).

EPISTAXIS

Epistaxis, or nosebleeding, can be a frightening event for both child and parent. The amount and duration of bleeding are usually overestimated.

Pathophysiology

Most childhood nosebleeds occur before the age of 10 years and are anterior in location, usually from Little's area or the nasal vestibule.[16] Little's area, which contains Kiesselbach's plexus, is an arterial and venous network on the anterior inferior portion of the nasal septum. It is formed from the sphenopalatine branch of the maxillary artery and the septal branches of the superior labial artery, derived from the facial artery. Of small caliber, these vessels lie below a thin mucous membrane. The nasal vestibule is the slightly dilated area just inside the naris that is lined with skin.[17,18] Posterior bleeds are unusual in children. Blood in the nose may also originate from the gastrointestinal or respiratory tract.[19]

Diagnostic Considerations

Trauma is the most frequent cause of nosebleeds in children. The patient's own finger is the most common weapon (epistaxis digitorum). Repeated local trauma causes an inflammatory response and subsequent granulation tissue that can be "picked off," causing bleeding.[19] Nasal foreign bodies can traumatize the nasal mucosa (see section on Foreign Bodies of the Nose and Ear). Following significant nasal trauma, a septal hematoma may develop; the septal vessels bleed and the overlying mucous membrane remains intact. If not recognized and drained, the possibility of abscess formation and septal perforation exists.[18]

Breathing dry air is a major predisposing factor to nosebleeds.[19] A deviated nasal septum may cause the nasal cavity on one side to be relatively narrowed; air passes through the narrowed side at a greater velocity, predisposing that side to nosebleeds.

Given the frequency of infectious and allergic rhinitis in childhood, it is not surprising that they are commonly associated with nosebleeds. Repetitive, forceful nose blowing can rupture the septal venous vessels because of increased intraluminal pressure. During viral or bacterial rhinitis, the child typically has increased vascularity of the inflamed nasal septum (see section on Rhinitis).

Bleeding and other systemic disorders such as ITP, TTP, and leukemia may be associated with epistaxis. Although some authors have suggested that bleeding disorders are only rarely associated with epistaxis, others have demonstrated that success in diagnosing one of these disorders is related to the diligence of the pursuit.[20] Coumadin and aspirin-related drugs are examples of drugs and toxins that must be considered. The Rendu-Osler-Weber syndrome (hereditary hemorrhagic telangiectasia) is autosomal dominant, presenting after puberty with pathologically dilated

---

Equipment for Examination/Treatment of Epistaxis

Light source, preferably head lamp
Nasal speculum
Suction apparatus, including Fraser tips no. 5 to no. 8
Silver nitrate sticks
Vasoconstrictors/anesthetics
    Topical epinephrine 1:1,000
    Topical cocaine 4%
    Topical phenylephrine 0.125%-0.5%
    Injectable lidocaine with epinephrine 1:100,000
Cotton
Topical thrombin or other topical coagulant
Expandable nasal sponges
Forceps
Petrolatum gauze packing
Pneumatic nasal catheters or Foley, various sizes

Modified from Perretta LJ, Denslow BL, Brown CG: *Emerg Med Clin North Am* 5(2):265, 1987.

---

small blood vessels. Epistaxis is common. Sinus barotrauma, tumors, postsurgical changes, and exposure of the nasal mucosa to chemicals are unusual causes in children. It is unclear whether hypertension and epistaxis are associated.[19]

Diagnostic Work-Up

The history will help to determine the etiology of the nosebleed in many cases. Questions regarding recent trauma, upper respiratory illnesses, allergies, and exposure to dry air relate to the most frequently seen etiologies. Easy bruisability, hematoma formation, or prolonged bleeding in the patient or family members should be sought. It may be necessary to ask specifically about circumcision or immunizations to jog the historian's memory. When the nosebleed is bilateral it is helpful to ask on which side the bleeding began; this is usually the side on which the bleeding point is found. Although patients and families frequently overestimate the volume of blood loss, this is still worth asking about. A history of dizziness upon standing, pallor, or change in behavior may be clues that significant hypovolemia has occurred.

The first goal of the physical examination is recognition of hypovolemia. Altered mental status and delayed capillary refill may be the only clinical findings. Frequently, associated sustained tachycardia and tachypnea will be noted. Hypotension is a late sign of hypovolemia in young children.

Once hypovolemia has been excluded or treated, attention should be directed to locating the bleeding site. In the uncooperative child, supplies should be readied before attempting evaluation of the bleeding nose, so that treatment can swiftly follow examination (see box above). Ideally the child will be positioned so that the head is facing slightly downward, preventing blood from running down the nasopharynx and into the stomach. Children who swallow significant amounts of blood tend to have emesis, which can potentially lead to aspiration. In addition to Fraser-tip suction for removal of blood from the nose, a Yankaur tip should be readied to suction particulate matter.

With a careful physical examination, the bleeding point is usually visible. In the cooperative child whose significant nosebleed has stopped, noseblowing on each side will clear away fresh clot. In the uncooperative child, suction will serve this same purpose. Proper restraint is necessary in small children. Fig. 49-1 provides suggestions for restraining and positioning a child for examination and treatment of a nosebleed. Illumination of the nasal cavity by head lamp leaves both hands free for examination. The nasal speculum should be placed into the naris and opened in a rostrocaudal direction. A Fraser suction tip can then be used to clear away fresh blood and pinpoint the bleeding site.

The general examination may provide information regarding the etiology of nosebleed. The posterior pharynx should be checked for evidence of blood dripping down from the posterior nasal cavity. The skin examination may suggest easy bruisability by the presence of petechiae, ecchymoses, or purpura. Telangiectasia is occasionally seen. Lymphadenopathy or splenomegaly may be a clue to the presence of leukemia.

Ancillary Data. In the hypovolemic child, hemoglobin should be determined and the blood should be sent for type and cross. It is the unusual child who has an underlying bleeding diathesis that precipitates nosebleed, yet these children do exist. Katsanis and colleagues developed a clinical scoring system to predict a relatively high risk of bleeding abnormality. Patients rated "severe" by this scoring system had approximately a one in seven chance of having von Willebrand disease. Nosebleeds of high-risk children had frequency: > 25/year, duration: > 10 minutes, volume of blood lost per episode: > 30 ml, presence: > 67% of their lifetime, and bilaterally. Even when these clinical criteria were met, basic clotting profiles (PT, PTT, platelet count, and bleeding time) did not reveal the hemostatic defect. More sophisticated coagulation studies were necessary.[20] Evaluation for a coagulation defect on the basis of epistaxis alone, even if severe, is rarely indicated.

Prehospital Considerations

The danger to the child in the prehospital setting is hypovolemic shock from excessive blood loss. Although rare, appropriate volume resuscitation is indicated in such patient. Ongoing losses should be prevented by squeezing the anterior part of the nose between the thumb and index fingers with continued firm pressure. The other dangers are the potential aspiration of blood or problems maintaining a clear, open airway. Suction and positioning of the child in an upright position is protective.

Therapeutic Trial

Nosebleeds that resolve spontaneously or with prolonged digital pressure generally require no further treatment. Patients whose bleeding has resolved by the time of presentation to the emergency department experience no benefit from treatment.[21] The obvious concern with not treating the cause of the bleeding is that recurrence may occur. History and physical examination will further elucidate the number of recurrences, general health of the patient, and hydration status. All of these factors should be considered when deciding whether or not to treat a nosebleed. Fig. 49-2 provides a protocol that can be used to guide treatment.

Many references recommend identification of the bleeding point and cauterization with silver nitrate sticks. Preparation includes anticipation of untoward events; equipment should be readied before immobilizing the child. Adequate suction equipment for particulate matter should be at the bedside in case of emesis (see box). Successful cautery is more likely in a dry field; Fraser suction tips have fine points and can keep the bleeding site relatively dry while silver nitrate cautery is being performed. Septal perforation has been reported with excessively vigorous application of cautery. Although rare, angiofibroma, a gray mass in the nose, may present with epistaxis; cauterization will worsen the bleeding.[19] The use of a head lamp, although not necessary, affords a well-directed light source while leaving both of the physician's hands free to use the nasal speculum, suction apparatus, cautery sticks, and other equipment. Even with the best-intentioned efforts to prepare well and execute the procedure carefully, cauterization is at best difficult and at worst impossible in children. A child's thin nasal septum is also more prone to perforation by cautery.

Packing the nose with topical thrombin followed by 10 minutes of firm, constant pressure by squeezing the anterior cartilaginous nose between the thumb and index fingers is safer and technically simpler than using of silver nitrate sticks. It is also better tolerated, safer, and very effective. It is helpful to remove as much fresh blood and clot as possible before attempting this procedure.

If bleeding is not controlled in these ways, several other measures may be attempted. Cautery of the area immediately around the bleeding site may slow down the flow. Topical application of a vasoconstrictor such as neosynephrine (0.125% to 0.5%), epinephrine (1:100,000) or cocaine (4%) with a cotton pledget for 5 to 10 minutes is often effective. Although only minimal volumes of drug are necessary in this application, care should be taken to anticipate and treat any untoward effects from systemic absorption, especially with cocaine. In more refractory cases, injection of the site with 1 to 2 ml of lidocaine with epinephrine (1:100,000) is often successful owing to the combination of tamponading and vasoconstrictive effects.[19]

When the above measures are ineffective, nasal packing should be considered. Nasal sponges are now available for this purpose. They are inserted dry and expand upon getting wet. These can be cut to fit any child and offer adequate hemostasis in most cases. Traditional packing with Vaseline-impregnated gauze is an extremely uncomfortable procedure that is often not well tolerated, especially by small children. The need for packing in children is very unusual and should be done in consultation with an otolaryngologist. Sedation with an agent such as chloral hydrate may be necessary. Other complications of nasal packing include syncope during packing, local infection, sinusitis, bacteremia, toxic shock syndrome, and even iatrogenic sleep apnea if bilateral packs are placed.[18,22] To

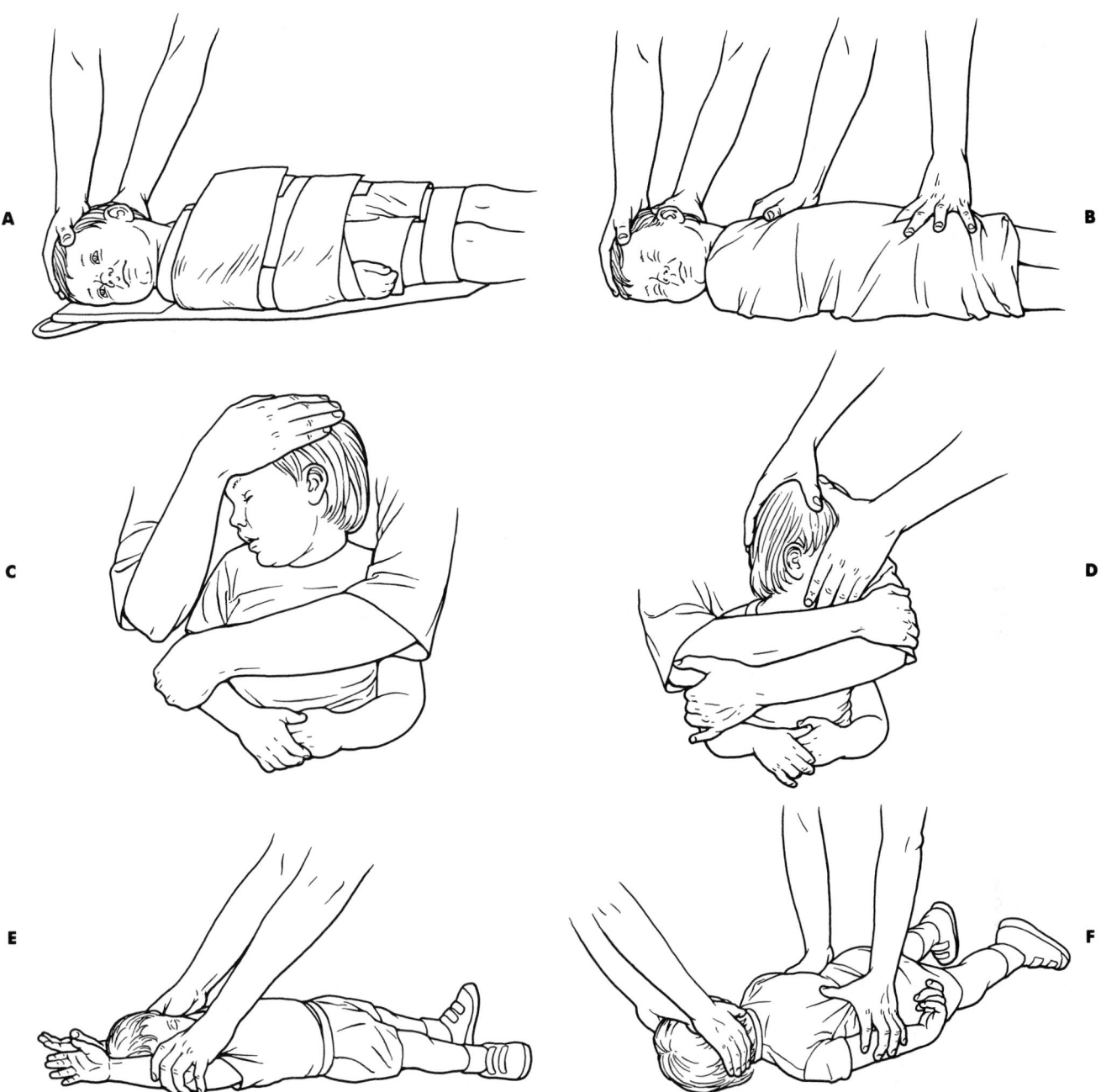

FIG. 49-1. Restraining positions. **A,** Child properly restrained in papoose board. **B,** Child restrained in sheets. **C,** Child restrained while sitting in parent's lap with child's legs between parent's legs, child's back against parent's chest, one of parent's arms encircling the child's upper torso and arms, and the parent's other arm holding the child's head in position to approach the ear or nose. **D,** Child restrained while sitting in parent's lap with child's legs between parent's legs, child's back against parent's chest, both of parent's arms encircling the child's upper torso and arms, and a second adult holding the head with two hands while avoiding the more delicate facial area. **E,** Child restrained while lying supine on examining table. A single assistant is holding both of the child's arms over the head while holding the head motionless between the arms. The examiner's body is draped over the child's torso to minimize wiggling. It should be emphasized that although this method is convenient because only one assistant is needed, it is only practical in very young children. **F,** Child restrained while lying prone on examining table. Two assistants are employed. One assistant holds each of the child's arms at the sides, grasping each arm both above and below the elbow to prevent flexion of the arms and to prevent child's attempts at pushing up from the table. The first assistant's body is draped over the child's buttocks and lower legs (held together) with specific intent of preventing flexion at the waist and hips, each of which can propel the child up from the table. The second assistant's sole duty is to control the head with both hands, being careful to avoid grasping the delicate facial area.

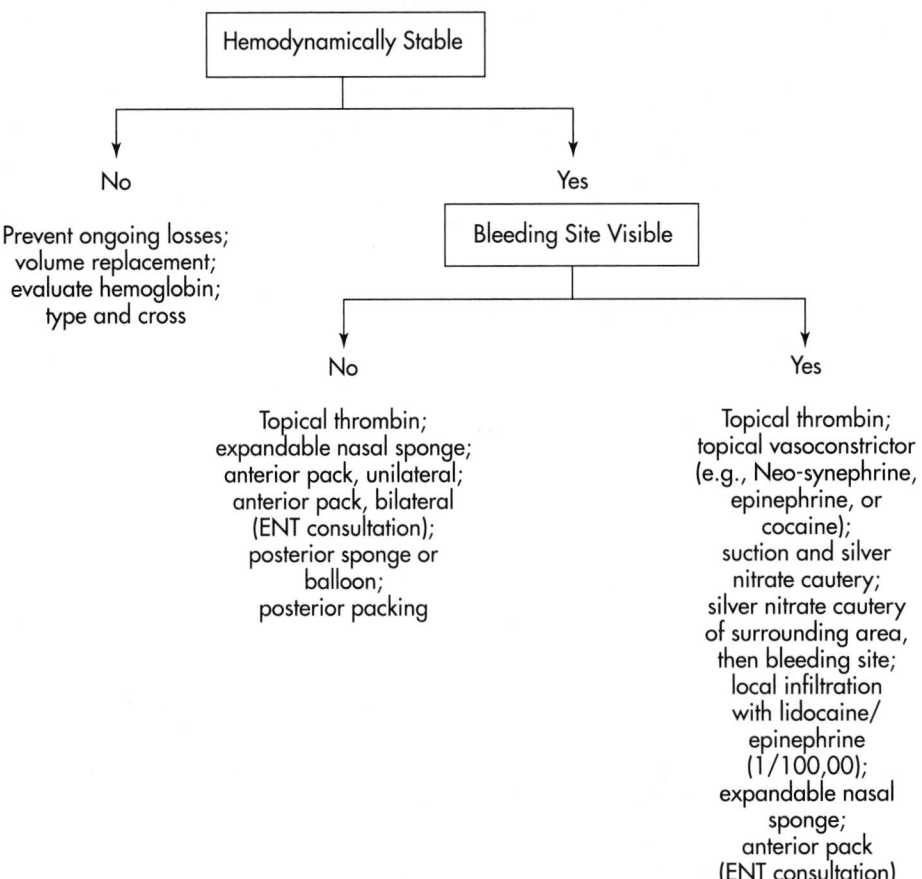

FIG. 49-2. Protocol for treating epistaxis.

lessen these risks, packing should be removed within 48 hours and antibiotic coverage provided while the packing is in place. Antibiotics of choice reflect the fact that most associated infections are from bacteria that inhabit the upper respiratory tract of the child. In young children, amoxicillin is still recommended, but there are more alternatives that provide additional coverage in the extremely rare event of a staphylococcal infection: cefaclor (20 to 40 mg/kg/24 hr q 8 hr PO); erythromycin (20 to 50 mg/kg/24 hr q 6 hr PO), and amoxicillin with clavulanate potassium (20 to 40 mg/kg/24 hr of the amoxicillin component). In the older child, erythromycin is a good choice.

Posterior bleeds are unusual in children and are suspected when a bleeding site cannot be visualized and an anterior pack fails to control bleeding. They should be managed by an otolaryngologist in the hospital. Foley catheters and specially marketed pneumatic nasal catheters have been used successfully. Such catheters have been found to be effective and much better tolerated by patients than petrolatum gauze nasal packs; they may be useful in anterior bleeds as well. Pressure necrosis of the nasal septum and mucosa may occur; removal of the catheter within 24 hours of placement may reduce this complication.[23] When inflated in the posterior aspect of the nose, there is potential for obstruction of the eustachian tube, and subsequent iatrogenic otitis media. The need for a posteriorly

placed pack, arterial ligation, pterygopalatine fossa block, or embolization is rare in a child.[18,19,24]

Because most pediatric epistaxis is a result of local trauma and dry nasal mucosa, it is likely to recur. There are several preventive measures that can be attempted. Humidifiers or vaporizers should be used in the home. In addition, petroleum jelly can be rubbed onto the anterior nasal septum and the skin of the nasal orifice. Fingernails of habitual nosepickers should be kept short. It may become necessary to cover the child's hands with socks.

HALITOSIS

Halitosis or fetor oris is offensive or bad-smelling breath.[25]

Pathophysiology

Fetor oris is usually associated with an acute oral infection or retained nasal foreign body. However, the more common cause is the typical odor of morning breath results from the breakdown of cellular proteins and amino acids to odorous, volatile, sulfur-containing compounds such as methylmercaptan (CH_3SH) and hydrogen sulfide (H_2S). Normal dietary intake such as garlic, onions, and certain spices are absorbed from the intestine, metabolized in the liver, released into the bloodstream, and excreted by the lungs as well as other routes. Poor oral hygiene, inflamma-

TABLE 49-1. Extraoral Sources of Breath Odor

Odor*	Product
Acrid (pearlike)	Paraldehyde
Alcohol	Fruitlike
Bitter almonds	Cyanide
Coal gas	Carbon monoxide
Disinfectants	Phenol, creosotes
Garlic	Phosphorus, tellurium, arsenic, parathion, malathion
Halitosis	Acute illness, poor oral hygiene
Musty fish (raw liver)	Hepatic failure
Pungent, aromatic	Ethchlorvynol
Rotten eggs	Hydrogen sulfide mercaptans
Shoe polish	Nitrobenzenes
Sweet acetone (russet apples)	Lacquer, alcohol, ketoacidosis, chloroform
Stale tobacco	Nicotine
Violets	Turpentine
Wintergreen	Methylsalicylate

Odor*	Disease
Acetone on breath	Diabetes mellitus
Ammoniacal	Uremia
Musty, mousy, horsey	Phenylketonuria
Maple syrup	Maple syrup urine disease
Yeast-like, dried celery-like	Oasthouse urine disease
Sweaty feet	Odor of sweaty feet
Cat's urine	Odor of cat syndrome

*Some odors are generalized and not only on breath.

tion, and bleeding can encourage colonization and growth of putrefactive gram-negative and anaerobic organisms, imparting a foul, metallic odor to the breath.

Diagnostic Considerations

Halitosis can result from oral, paraoral, or extraoral sites. Oropharyngeal infections, nasal foreign bodies, poor hygiene, and specific dietary intake are the most common causes of severe foul breath odor in childhood. Paraoral causes of halitosis include sinusitis, retained foreign bodies (usually nasal), tonsillar infections, bronchiectasis, and lung abscess.[26]

Extraoral sources of breath odor have both physiologic and pathologic bases (Table 49-1). Certain odors have systemic medical significance such as the ammoniacal odor of uremia and the acetone odor of diabetic ketoacidosis.[27] The breath odor of hepatic failure, *fetor hepaticus,* is musty or mousy, like a mixture of rotten eggs and garlic.

Diagnostic Work-Up. Dietary intake should be assessed, as well as symptoms referable to oral and dental pain or a foreign body (foam rubber, paper, and beads). Headache, congestion, nasal discharge, fever, facial swelling, and tenderness may implicate sinusitis. Chest pain, productive cough, wheezing, fever, or dyspnea may be suggestive of pulmonary disease. Vomiting, regurgitating, or choking

may suggest a nasopharyngeal, hypopharyngeal, laryngeal pouch, or esophageal diverticulum that may harbor retained debris.

Examination of the oral cavity should appraise dental, gingival, and lingual hygiene. All teeth should be visualized and palpated for pockets of retained food or pus, tenderness, and instability. Infection of the tonsils should be checked. The nose should be checked for foreign body and drainage. Auscultation and percussion of the chest may reveal signs of bronchopulmonary infection.

Ancillary Data. CBC and specific cultures may be useful in evaluating potential infections. Sinus, chest x-ray, and esophageal studies may be selectively useful.

Therapeutic Trial

Specific etiology may dictate specific approaches. An initial focus on good oral hygiene may be useful in children without a specific etiology.

HEARING LOSS AND TINNITUS, ACUTE

The causes of acute hearing loss range from trivial to life-threatening: hearing loss may be the presentation of a simple cerumen impaction or a subtle, secondary finding in the diagnosis of acute head trauma or meningitis.[28]

Decreased auditory acuity can be characterized by history and physical exam as conductive, sensorineural, or both.[29] The anatomic site of involvement can then be specified and appropriate confirmatory testing, therapy, and referral can be completed.

Tinnitus is a perception of noise in the ear for which there is no source outside the patient. Tinnitus can be characterized as peripheral or central; the peripheral category can be divided into conductive, sensorineural, or mixed. Isolated tinnitus in children is rare; the severity of the symptom is related to the magnitude of the pure-tone hearing loss.[30,31]

Vertigo is a hallucination consisting of an illusion of motion, which is usually rotatory but may be linear, with a sensation of disorientation in space. It suggests a lesion in the labyrinth or along the eighth nerve.[32]

Pathophysiology

The lesion may be in the external, middle, or inner ear, internal auditory meatus, cerebellopontine angle, brainstem, or brain (Table 49-2). Abnormalities of hearing derive from illness or injury affecting any part of the auditory anatomy including its vascular supply. Both the cochlea and vestibular systems derive their blood supply from the basilar artery.

Diagnostic Considerations

External ear problems, such as otitis externa, cerumen impaction, and foreign bodies, account for the most obvious causes of conductive hearing loss. Middle ear pathology including acute otitis media, chronic otitis with or without perforation, cholesteatoma, and trauma to the drum, ossicles, or temporal bone can cause hearing loss and tinnitus. Fracture of the temporal bone can cause sensorineural, conductive, or mixed deficits depending on the site and orientation of the fracture. Inner ear infection, vasculitis, and trauma can result in decreased sensorineural auditory acuity.

TABLE 49-2. Hearing Loss: Diagnostic Considerations

By anatomic site of abnormality[33]					
External canal	Middle ear	Inner ear	Internal auditory canal	Brainstem	Brain
Foreign body	Otitis media	Infection	Tumor	Vascular	Cortical
Cerumen	Trauma	Cochleitis	Neuroma	Tumor	Psychologic
Otitis externa	Barotrauma	Labyrinthitis	Meningioma	Multiple sclerosis	
	Temporal bone	Meningitis			
	Basilar skull fracture	Neuritis			
		Vascular			
		Collagen			
		Hemorrhage			
		Leukemia			
		Sickle cell disease			
		Cochlea			
		Head trauma			
		Barotrauma			

By conductive defect[34]	By neurosensory defect[34]
External canal obstruction	Inner ear malformation
External otitis	Syphilis
Serous otitis	Meniere syndrome
Suppurative otitis	Trauma to temporal bone
Otosclerosis	Rupture of inner ear
Middle ear tumor	Ototoxicity
	Acoustic neuroma
	Idiopathic

Perilymphatic fistula (PF) is a subtle cause of hearing loss, tinnitus, vertigo, and dizziness, which often can only be demonstrated (and repaired) surgically. Salvage of hearing depends on a high index of suspicion. PF is usually traumatic, but may be congenital or idiopathic.[35]

Congenital infections, such as cytomegalovirus (CMV), may produce deafness of delayed onset and gradual progression. Salicylates, quinine, "loop" diuretics, aminoglycosides, and some metals (arsenic and mercury) may be ototoxic.

Acoustic neuroma in the internal auditory canal, at the cerebellopontine angle, or at the brainstem, can cause acute sensorineural hearing loss. This is found almost always in association with neurofibromatosis. The search for other cranial nerve involvement can assist in localizing the source of sensorineural loss. The eighth nerve's location in the brain stem is sufficiently close to the fifth, seventh, ninth, and tenth nerves that these latter nerves may also be affected by brainstem pathology.

Tinnitus may occur alone or in combination with hearing loss. It is usually attributable to middle or inner ear disease, but may also be of central or vascular origin. Objective tinnitus is usually vascular and may represent arteriovenous malformation, inflammatory hyperemia of the ear, aneurysm, transmitted cardiac murmur, hemangioma of the head and neck, or stenosis of the cerebral arteries.[30,31]

Vertigo and dizziness often accompany hearing loss. Vertigo, in association with hearing loss, localizes the lesion to the labyrinth, eighth nerve, or eighth nerve nucleus. Nystagmus, nausea, and vomiting may also be present. Nonvertiginous, nonataxic dizziness is a less specific and less useful sign of auditory disease.

Diagnostic Work-Up

The history of the pattern of onset can be useful. An abrupt onset suggests the acute obstruction of a foreign body, trauma, or a vascular (ischemic) phenomenon. Chronic, recurrent symptoms may indicate migraine or migraine equivalent. Slow progression suggests a tumor or degenerative process. Multiple sclerosis can produce variable occurrences with remissions.[32]

A history of tinnitus, vertigo, or dizziness in the child with hearing loss should be elicited. Some children may not report such symptoms if there is no associated pain; others may be unable to differentiate tinnitus from normal function if there has been a gradual progression.

Specific questioning about facial sensation, nystagmus, and difficulty chewing or swallowing may suggest cranial nerve involvement. A history of ataxia may help localize the lesion to the cerebellum.

Any history of trauma should be thoroughly explored, including minor, mechanical, otic trauma (insertion of foreign objects), and barotrauma from air travel or diving. A family history of hearing loss, past history of congenital infections (syphilis, CMV, etc.), anomalies of the external ear or kidneys, prematurity, neonatal asphyxia, jaundice, meningitis, or ototoxic drug administration may be suggestive of an etiology.

Approximately half of all congenital deafness discovered during childhood is caused by genetic factors. Pendred syndrome consists of congenitally defective thyroid binding of iodine associated with sensorineural hearing loss. Usher syndrome includes retinitis pigmentosa, mental retardation, vestibulocerebellar ataxia, and sensorineural hearing loss. Jervell and Lange-Nielsen syndrome involves a prolonged QT interval, syncope, and sensorineural hearing loss.

Determine gross auditory acuity with a ticking wristwatch or whispered commands. Test for lateralization of sound to one ear (Weber's test), and for air versus bone conduction (Rinne's test).

Weber's test is performed by placing an activated tuning fork firmly on the middle of the forehead or apical scalp. With normal hearing, both ears will hear equally well. With conductive loss, the diseased side will hear best. With sensorineural loss, the diseased side will have decreased sensation.

Rinne's test may be done by holding a vibrating tuning fork firmly on the mastoid process till the patient no longer perceives sound. The fork is then placed next to the ear. With normal hearing, air conduction is better than bone conduction (the sound is heard twice as long in the air). In conductive hearing loss, bone conduction is better than air conduction: the patient will not sense the tone next to the ear. With sensorineural loss, vibration will be heard for a shorter time on the diseased side.

Examine the external canal and drum for trauma, infection, or presence of a foreign body; the neck and head for adenopathy and periauricular swelling; and vessels of the head and ear for bruits. The fistula test (application of positive and negative pressure to the external auditory canal via pneumatic otoscopy produces nystagmus, dizziness, or a sensation of motion) is a sign of perilymphatic fistula.[36]

Anomalies of development should be noted, including those of the first and second branchial arch (microtia, auricular dysplasia, micrognathia) and the neural crest (widely spaced eyes and pigmentary defects). Visible syndromes commonly associated with hearing loss include Waardenburg syndrome (widely spaced eyes, white forelock, iridial heterochromia), Turner syndrome, neurofibromatosis, Treacher-Collins syndrome (malformed auricles, malar and mandibular hypoplasia, antimongoloid slant to eyes), and hypomelanosis of Ito (hypopigmented macules, mental retardation, and seizures).[28,35]

Neurologic examination should specifically evaluate the cranial nerves and cerebellum (i.e., search for nystagmus, ataxia, dizziness, and dysequilibrium).

Ancillary Data. Important data include CT scan and plain-film tomography, especially in cases of trauma and suspected neoplasm. Specific additional studies may include audiometry, acoustic impedance, brainstem auditory evoked response (BAER) testing, electronystagmography, cerebral angiography, and tests confirming specific disease associations.

Prehospital Considerations

Specific causes, such as head trauma, may require specific management.

Major Causes of Nasal Discharge

Allergic
Infectious (viral, bacterial)
Toxic exposures
   Topical/inhaled: decongestants, cocaine, pollutants
   Systemic: estrogens, aspirin
Traumatic (blunt, sharp, retained foreign bodies)

NASAL DISCHARGE AND RHINITIS

Nasal discharge, or rhinorrhea, is most commonly from the nasal mucous membrane and watery in nature. Blood, mucus, pus, and cerebrospinal fluid can be present. The discharge can be stimulated by physiologic, allergic, infectious, and traumatic causes.

Pathophysiology

The mucous membrane of the nose has ciliated and mucous-producing cells. Vascular tone is maintained by the balance of sympathetic and parasympathetic innervation—the latter causes vasodilation and secretion of nasal mucus. The membrane is well vascularized; the venous drainage has direct communication with the cavernous sinus without intervening valves. The ciliated epithelium of the nasal mucosa promotes movement of mucus toward the nasopharynx; impaired ciliary function, or excessive mucus production may overwhelm this mechanism.

Cerebrospinal fluid may enter the nose through a fracture of the cribriform plate or the middle ear via the eustachian tube. Bleeding of the nasal vessels or communicating structures may cause epistaxis. Purulent discharge can be from a primary infection or secondary to a retained foreign body or mucus. Watery, mucoid discharge occurs as a parasympathetic response to a variety of stimuli.

Diagnostic Considerations

The box above outlines the major causes of nasal discharge. Infectious and allergic diseases predominate. Viral rhinitis or the 'common cold' is the single most frequent cause of nasal discharge and is a major cause of school absenteeism and missed parental work days. Although the exact incidence reflects the age of the child, contact with other children at home or in daycare/school, and general state of health, estimates have ranged between 6 and 21 episodes per year.[1] Etiologically, there are over 200 antigenically different viruses including rhinoviruses, influenza, parainfluenza, respiratory syncytial virus (RSV), and adenovirus. The multiple viral serotypes and incomplete immunity account for frequent episodes.[37,38]

Bacterial rhinitis is usually a complication of viral rhinitis heralded by persistence of symptoms and a purulent discharge. Sinusitis may be contributory. *Streptococcus pneumoniae, Haemophilus influenzae, Branhamella catarrhalis,* and staphylococcal species are pathogens. In school-age children *S. pyogenes* most commonly occurs as acute pharyngitis or tonsillitis. In children less than 3 years of age, infection with *S. pyogenes* generally causes streptococcosis, a less acute condition that is characterized by low-grade fever, adenopathy, and rhinitis lasting weeks to months. Sore throat and signs of pharyngitis are not commonly associated with streptococcosis.[39] Furunculosis of a nasal hair follicle is most commonly caused by *S. aureus*. Pertussis, diphtheria, and congenital syphilis are less commonly seen.[1] In children under 2 or 3 months old, a prodrome of nasal congestion, discharge, and sneezing may represent the early stage of a pneumonic process caused by *Chlamydia trachomatis, Ureaplasma urealyticum, Pneumocystis carinii*, or cytomegalovirus.[40]

Allergic rhinitis is an IgE-mediated response to a variety of stimuli, peaking in late adolescence. There are suggestions that the incidence of allergic rhinitis is increasing, possibly secondary to a greater concentration of environmental pollutants and dust mites in the home.[41] In infants and young children, allergens tend to be those to which the patient is exposed earliest and most consistently; allergic rhinitis in these children is generally perennial rather than seasonal. Nonallergic rhinitis with eosinophilia syndrome (NARES) is much less common in children; the response to antihistamines and immunotherapy is poor compared to that of allergic rhinitis.[42,43]

Toxins can cause rhinitis through topical exposures to the nasal mucous membrane (e.g., vasoconstrictor drops, cocaine) or by systemic absorption (e.g., aspirin, estrogens). Rhinitis medicamentosa is a state of chronic nasal congestion and inflammation associated with prolonged use of topical vasoconstrictors, probably due to reactive vasodilation after fatigue of the vasoconstrictive effect on the submucosal vessels. Use of vasoconstrictive nosedrops should be limited to 5 days to avoid this complication. Osguthorpe and Shirley report the case of a neonate (obligate nose breather) with respiratory distress from prolonged use of vasoconstrictive nosedrops.[44]

Trauma may cause the discharge of cerebrospinal fluid (CSF) or blood (epistaxis) from the nose. CSF typically enters the nasal cavity through a fracture of the cribriform plate or temporal bone (see Chapter 21). Epistaxis is discussed elsewhere in this text.

Diagnostic Work-Up

The present illness should be thoroughly investigated by *history*. Precipitants, time and tempo of discharge, exacerbating/relieving factors, and associated symptoms should be ascertained. Previous episodes of nasal discharge, known sensitivities, medications, and response to prior therapy are potentially important. Specific questions about previous use of topical decongestants may be necessary to implicate a rebound phenomenon from these drugs.

Unless the child is in distress, a general *physical examination* should precede a detailed examination of the entire head and neck. A characteristic transverse crease at the junction of the nasal bone and cartilage occurs as a result of the child's repeated rubbing of the nose (*allergic salute*), especially in children with longstanding perennial allergic rhinitis. *Allergic shiners* are dark infraorbital colorings from venous congestion. The child's mouth may be held partially open if chronic nasal congestion is present (*adenoidal facies*).

After inspection of the external nasal surface for asymmetry, trauma, and other abnormalities, the mucous membrane should be visualized using a good light source and nasal speculum or large-caliber otoscope speculum. Proper immobilization of the uncooperative child is essential. Inflammation may be evidenced by swelling, erythema, and secretions of different types. Clear, watery secretions of allergic rhinitis are typically associated with pale, boggy, bluish mucosa and swollen turbinates. Foreign bodies in the anterior segment of the nose can be visualized. With adequate suction to clear away fresh blood, bleeding points of the anterior nose are usually visualized on the anterior inferior nasal septum. Nasal polyps are unusual, raising suspicion of cystic fibrosis or asthma.

Ancillary Data. When the clinical picture is unclear, the laboratory may provide assistance. Lans, Alfano, and Rocklin reported good specificity but poor sensitivity of nasal smear for eosinophils in distinguishing allergic from nonallergic rhinitis.[45] Antigenic skin tests and RAST (radioallergosorbent test) testing are not helpful in directing treatment in the emergency setting. In unusual or persistent cases, gram stain and culture of the discharge may be helpful. However, specimen contamination with normal nonpathogenic flora makes interpretation difficult.

The detection of cerebrospinal fluid rhinorrhea can be important and at times difficult. In the absence of a suggestive history and physical examination (e.g., raccoon eyes, Battle's sign), the associated clear rhinorrhea is easily misinterpreted as allergic or infectious in origin, particularly in a young child. Testing with glucose oxidase-impregnated sticks is useful if precaution is used in interpretation. The basis of a positive test is a high glucose concentration in the nasal drainage that should be confirmed by biochemical analysis for electrolytes, glucose, and protein. This can be falsely elevated by the presence of lacrimal secretions or blood.[46] A negative test is helpful in ruling out CSF rhinorrhea. Basilar skull tomograms and computerized tomography may be diagnostic.[38]

Prehospital Considerations

It is unusual for nasal discharge to be life-threatening. However, nasal discharge may exacerbate nasal obstruction. If a child has concurrent obstruction of the oropharynx from a foreign body, opposed tonsils, trauma, or is an obligate nose breather for any reason (e.g., neonate), nasal discharge may cause respiratory obstruction.

In the prehospital setting, epistaxis is controlled by direct pressure on the cartilaginous anterior nose by firmly compressing the nares between the thumb and index finger.

Therapeutic Trial

Therapy for nasal discharge is disease specific, although empirical management is often appropriate. The management of traumatic injuries and epistaxis is detailed elsewhere. Guidelines for initial therapy of the patient with allergic and infectious rhinitis are outlined in the box on p. 721. Decongestants (vasoconstrictors) may be used orally or topically. Use of topical decongestants is limited to no more than 5 days to avoid rebound vasodilation and worsening rhinorrhea.

Rhinitis medicamentosa, a persistent inflammatory reaction, impedes nasal air flow, further encouraging the use of decongestant nosedrops. Unpublished clinical experience suggests that a single injection of dexamethasone and use of an oral decongestant for a few days may facilitate withdrawal of topical therapy. Nasal decongestant spray may be used on one side only. In approximately 3 days the unsprayed side will open and allow good air flow.

Antihistamines inhibit release of histamine from mast cells. They are more effective in controlling capillary leakage than vasodilation, which explains the successful use of antihistamine/decongestant combinations.[47] Efficacy may be related to the individual child and class of drug. When an antihistamine of one chemical class does not work or has unacceptable side effects, another drug class should be prescribed (see Table 49-3). Although not currently approved in children under 12 years of age, the recent development of newer antihistamines (e.g., terfenadine, astemizole, and loratidine) with long half-lives and low incidences of drowsiness is a major advance.[49,50]

Antibiotics are indicated when evidence of bacterial infection is present. In uncomplicated cases, antibiotics effective against *S. pneumoniae* and *H. influenzae* are adequate initial therapy (e.g., amoxicillin, trimethoprim-sulfamethaxazole, cefaclor). When furunculosis is present, coverage for *S. aureus* is desirable (dicloxacillin, cephalexin, erythromycin).

Agents effective against respiratory syncytial virus and influenza are available and useful in selected cases. Steroids, cromolyn sodium, and immunotherapy are used by the continuing-care physician in the treatment of allergic rhinitis when avoidance, decongestants, and antihistamines fail.

Inhaled steroids are preferred to oral preparations for their low systemic absorption and lack of adrenal suppression. Hynes used rhinometry to demonstrate improved nasal patency after beclomethasone intranasal spray was used in 6- to 13-year-old children with nonpurulent rhinitis.[51] Although onset of action is somewhat delayed, local effects prevent capillary leakage and vasodilation. When environmental allergens precipitate nasal discharge, environmental control is more effective than pharmacologic therapy[52] (see the box on p. 722).

NECK MASS

A neck mass exists in the region between the inferior aspect of the mandible and the level of the clavicles. Once

---

Response to Treatment of Infectious and Allergic Rhinitis

	Infectious	Allergic
Decongestants	Fair	Fair
Antihistamines	Poor	Good
Steroids	None	Excellent
Immunotherapy	None	Variable
Cromolyn	None	Fair
Antibiotics/antivirals	Disease specific	None

TABLE 49-3. Antihistamines[36,48]

Antihistamine	Trade name	Available preparation	Usual dose	Comments
Astemizole	*Hismanal*	Tablets 10 mg	10 mg QD	Nonsedating; little experience under age of 11 yr
Terfenadine	*Seldane*	Tablets 60 mg	60 mg BID	Nonsedating; little experience under age of 11 yr
Alkylamines				
Chlorpheniramine	*Chlor-Trimeton*	Tablets 4 mg; timed-release tablets 8 and 12 mg; syrup 2 mg/5 ml	4 mg q 6 hr (0.35 mg/kg/24 hr)	Least sedating
Brompheniramine	*Dimetane*	Tablets 4 mg; timed-release tablets 8 and 12 mg; syrup 2 mg/5 ml	4 mg q 6 hr (0.5 mg/kg/24 hr)	Least sedating
Ethylenediamines				
Tripelennamine	*Pyribenzamine*	Tablets 25 and 50 mg; elixir 37.5 mg/5 ml	25-50 mg q 6 hr (5 mg/kg/24 hr)	Moderate sedation
Ethanolamines				
Diphenhydramine	*Benadryl*	Capsules 25 and 50 mg; elixir 12.5 mg/5 ml	25-50 mg q 6 hr (5 mg/kg/24 hr)	Most sedating
Piperazines				
Hydroxyzine	*Atarax, Vistaril*	Tablets 10, 25, 50, 100 mg; syrup 10 mg/5 ml	25-50 mg q 6 hr (2 mg/kg/24 hr)	Moderate sedation

From McNamara RM: *Emerg Med Clin North Am* 5(2):279, 1987.

Standard Environmental Control Measures

The patient's **bedroom** is most important, since a significant portion of the day is spent there. Follow these suggestions:

1. The bedroom should contain no stuffed chairs, rugs, or drapes; linoleum or wood floors, wood or metal furniture, and washable cotton curtains or curtains made of plastic or Plexiglas are preferable. Everything in the room should be washable.
2. Avoid storing blankets, woolens, felt hats, or other dust catchers in bedroom closets. Keep the doors closed.
3. If there is a furnace vent in the room, cover it with three layers of cheesecloth. (Exercise caution with flammable material in contact with metal.)
4. Doors and windows in the room must fit tightly. Close windows during major pollen seasons or during pollution alerts.
5. Once or twice a week, clean the room with a damp dustcloth (the patient should avoid the room during and for 3-4 hours after cleaning).
6. Use Dacron or foam pillows and wash monthly.
7. Vacuum mattresses and springs and completely encase in plastic with a zipper closing.
8. Wash blankets; use fuzz-free cotton or Dacron sheets next to patient's body.
9. Have only wooden, plastic, or nonallergenic (not fuzzy) toys.
10. Keep pets out of the bedroom.

In the rest of the house, follow these instructions:

1. **No smoking** should be allowed.
2. The allergic patient should not sit on overstuffed furniture or on rugs. Cotton or nylon rugs backed only with rubber are best.
3. No pets should be kept indoors.
4. Eliminate all house plants (dust and molds).
5. Do not use room deodorizers, mothballs, or bug sprays (strong odors).
6. Have regular furnace cleaning, and provide covers for furnace vents if needed.
7. The allergic patient should not be in the house while the house is being cleaned.
8. Keep humidifiers and air conditioners clean; replace or, if possible, wash filters monthly during heavy use.
9. Masks are helpful during periods of unavoidable allergen exposure. (Flex-a-Lite all-purpose mask with replaceable microfoam filters can be obtained from Flexo Products, Inc., 24864 Detroit Road, Westabe, OH, 44145.)
10. *Consumer Reports* and *Consumer Bulletin* are excellent sources for techniques to modify the environment.

From Lawler G and Fischer T: *Manual of allergy and immunology: diagnosis and therapy,* ed 2, Boston, 1988, Little, Brown.

---

determination is made that the mass does not represent a variant of normal, the pathophysiology and etiology of neck masses should be considered, after which accurate diagnosis and appropriate management are possible.

Pathophysiology

Although neck masses may represent a diverse group of disorders, in the emergency setting the large majority of cases are related to inflammation or infection of lymph nodes. Specific areas of the head and neck drain to anatomically distinct collections of lymph tissue[53] (Table 49-4). Infection or other antigenic stimulation in the head and neck can cause a local reaction and, via afferent lymphatic channels, stimulate lymphocyte production in the lymph node.

Diagnostic Considerations

Malignant tumors are a relatively uncommon cause of childhood neck masses. Less than 2% of suspicious head and neck masses are malignant.[53] The vast majority of neck masses are caused by lymph node swelling or congenital lesions.

Lymph Node. Benign hyperplasia and lymphadenitis are the most common causes of neck masses in children. The many stimuli that can precipitate node enlargement and inflammation include viral, bacterial, mycobacterial, para-

sitic, and fungal infections. Cat-scratch disease, Kawasaki disease, Kikuchi lymphadenitis, sarcoidosis, and antigenic stimulation by drugs, bites, or stings are also potential causes (see section on Lymphadenitis).

Trauma. Soft-tissue swellings of the neck are usually associated with subcutaneous bleeding and edema. Isolated hematoma formation without associated structural damage is rare. When this occurs, a bleeding disorder should be considered. Foreign bodies may cause neck swelling because of the presence of inflammation, abscess formation, hematoma, or the object itself.

Developmental Anomaly. Congenital muscular torticollis is usually seen during the first 2 weeks of life, presenting as a firm, nontender, nonenlarging mass in the sternocleidomastoid muscle. Unilateral fibrosis and contracture of the sternocleidomastoid muscle causes tilting of the head toward the affected side and rotation of the chin toward the opposite side. Venous obstruction has been implicated as the cause of this fibrosis.[54]

Branchial cleft cysts are most commonly seen in children under 10 years of age. They typically occur as the persistence of the second branchial groove, which forms a space lined by squamous epithelium. A thyroglossal duct cyst is caused by persistence of a fetal structure that is usually gone by the eighth week of development. The embryonic thyroid gland migrates from the floor of the pharynx to its

TABLE 49-4. Lymph Nodes of the Head and Neck

Lymph node groups	Areas drained
Occipital	Posterior scalp
Postauricular	Temporal and parietal scalp
Preauricular	Skin anterior to ear, entire pinna
Preparotid-intraparotid	Root of nose, eyelids, temporal scalp, external auditory meatus
Retropharyngeal (Ruvier)	Posterior nose, nasopharynx, paranasal sinuses
Facial	Eyelids, conjunctiva, skin of nose, nasal mucosa, cheek
Submandibular	Cheek, nose, upper lip, lower lip
Submental	Central lower lip, floor of mouth
Superficial cervical	Ear and parotid
Superficial deep cervical	Posterior scalp, posterior neck, tonsil, tongue, larynx, thyroid, palate, nose, esophagus, paranasal sinuses
Inferior deep cervical	Dorsal scalp and neck, superficial pectoral region of arm, superior deep cervical nodes

From Stanievich J: Cervical adenopathy. In Bluestone CD, Stool WC, Scheetz MD, editors: *Pediatric otolaryngology*, Philadelphia, 1990, WB Saunders.

final position in the neck, leaving the thyroglossal duct as a connection to the base of the tongue. Infection of a branchial cleft cyst or thyroglossal duct cyst often precipitates their recognition.

Cystic hygromas and lymphangiomas can be considered together. As lymphatic channels develop in the embryo, they form branches that ultimately drain into the central venous circulation. If a lymphatic space becomes walled off and isolated, an enlarging cystic mass can occur. These cystic hygromas or lymphangiomas can achieve tremendous sizes and cause respiratory compromise and significant cosmetic problems. Dermoid cysts, cervical thymic rests, laryngoceles, and heterotropic salivary gland tissue are rare.[53]

Vascular abnormalities may be recognized in the neonate as a developmental anomaly or, at a later age, subsequent to dilation, trauma, or spontaneous rupture. They may be arterial, venous, or fistulous in nature. Teratomas or hamartoma masses may contain vascular elements.

Neoplasm. Although less than 2% of biopsied head and neck tumors in a large series were malignant, 25% of childhood malignancies will at some time involve the head or neck; this is the primary site in 5% of cases.[55,56] Hodgkin disease and other malignant lymphoid tumors are most common, accounting for more than half of the neoplasms in the head and neck. Addition of rhabdomyosarcomas, other sarcomas, thyroid malignancies, and neuroblastomas account for over 90% of cases.[53] Skin cancer, although possible, is rare in children.

Caffey-Silverman syndrome, or infantile cortical hyperplasia, is a benign condition. There is subperiosteal bone formation over many bones, often noticed over the clavicles and mandible. It usually occurs in children under 6 months of age, after a febrile illness.

Diagnostic Work-Up

A history of the age at onset of symptoms and clinical progression should be clearly established. A history of trauma may be difficult to elicit. The presence of associated ear pain, ear or nose discharge, headache, fever, sore throat, congestion, or sores on the scalp may suggest an inflammatory etiology. Difficulty breathing or swallowing, voice change, and bloody emesis are more ominous symptoms. Children at increased risk of malignancy include those with a prior diagnosis of cancer, prior treatment with carcinogenic drugs or radiation, and those with a family history of childhood malignancy. Although somewhat variable, age at onset can also help differentiate among neoplastic processes; neuroblastomas cluster in the very young, rhabdomyosarcomas in preschool-aged children, non-Hodgkin lymphomas in school-aged children, and Hodgkin disease in adolescence.

The most useful differentiation in the physical examination of a neck mass is the presence or absence of inflammation. A warm, tender, erythematous mass is most likely to be infectious or inflammatory in nature. In such cases, a careful examination of the head and neck should ensue, to search for possible primary disease sites that may have precipitated lymphadenitis. Some developmental anomalies are only detected after the child becomes secondarily infected. Retained foreign bodies and other traumatic injuries, particularly those with violation of the skin barrier or subcutaneous collections of blood, are also prone to infection.

When trauma is suspected, the general examination should be done to observe for evidence of other recent or past injury. The presence of other significant trauma, even if not temporally related to the presenting mass, may be an important clue to the detection of nonaccidental injury. A pulsating mass is suggestive of vascular involvement.

Developmental anomalies may be suspected by features of the physical examination. Branchial cleft cysts usually occur as unilateral, nonpulsatile cystic masses that retract with deglutition and are positioned high in the lateral aspect of the neck. A fistula located along the anterior border of the sternocleidomastoid muscle is pathognomonic of a branchial cleft. Thyroglossal duct cysts are usually midline in position, and although their rostrocaudal position is somewhat variable, are usually just inferior to the hyoid bone. Because of their attachment to underlying structures, thyroglossal duct cysts will move with deglutition and tongue protrusion. Dermoid cysts are also midline, but do not transilluminate; because of their attachments, they move with the skin. Cystic hygromas are compressible and diffuse, enlarge with straining, and transilluminate.[53,57]

A painless, firm neck mass should be considered malignant unless proved otherwise. In Hodgkin and non-Hodgkin lymphoma, cervical adenopathy may be bilateral in over 20% of patients. Upper cervical and submaxillary nodes are most commonly affected. When lower cervical nodes are involved, mediastinal disease is often present.[58] Every child with a suspected malignancy should have a thorough otolaryngologic and systemic examination. Detailed evaluation should be made of all known collections of lymph tissue, especially in the groin and axilla. In addition, a complete abdominal examination should be done.

Ancillary Data. If there is any suggestion of airway compromise and the child is clinically stable, plain x-ray films of the airway should be done. The air column should be well visualized and the adjacent soft tissue examined for presence of foreign body, mixed density, and irregular contour. If the neck mass is noninflammatory, a PA and lateral chest radiograph may reveal mediastinal adenopathy.

When evaluating an inflammatory neck mass, laboratory aids are useful. Culture of abscess material can confirm an infectious etiology. Antigenic skin testing may suggest mycobacterial or fungal disease. CBC and erythrocyte sedimentation rates, although not diagnostic, may be helpful in certain cases.

Histopathologic examination of biopsied tissue is the gold standard for differentiation of malignant processes. In the emergency setting, computerized tomography can delineate size, local extension, proximity to the airway, and presence of cystic components. MRI may provide significantly more soft tissue detail. Although generally not helpful in the emergency setting, arteriography will aid the surgeon in planning a surgical approach by demonstrating the relationship of the mass to vascular structures.

In rare cases, a thyroglossal duct cyst contains the only functioning thyroid tissue in the body. For this reason, convention has advocated the evaluation of a thyroglossal duct cyst by radionucleotide scan or ultrasonography before surgical removal.[59]

Prehospital Considerations

Any mass in the neck, particularly one whose extent and etiology are unclear, has the potential to cause rapid respiratory or cardiovascular compromise. If trauma is suspected, careful management of the cervical spine is a prime concern. Preparations for administration of high-flow oxygen and definitive airway management should be made in anticipation of possible deterioration. A neck mass that is new, enlarging, or has developed clinical evidence of infection should be evaluated on an emergency basis. During transport, the mass should be observed for changes in appearance, effect on pulmonary and cardiovascular system function, and position change with respiration, deglutition, and tongue movements.

Therapeutic Trial

After identifying and treating any life-threatening respiratory and cardiovascular compromise, the next priority is the treatment of infection, if present. The suspected etiology will determine whether antibiotics, antifungals, or antiparasitic drugs will be needed alone or in combination.

Most developmentally-derived masses will require surgical evaluation and ultimate excision. An exception is congenital muscular torticollis, which usually responds to passive stretching exercises done every 4 hours when the child is awake.

The knowledge or suspicion of trauma-related neck mass necessitates the taking of cervical spine precautions (see

Chapter 22). Ice should immediately be applied to acute traumatic soft tissue swellings. The presence of subcutaneous emphysema demands thorough evaluation for concomitant pneumothorax, the latter requiring observation on 100% oxygen and possible thoracostomy tube.

Neoplasms of the neck should have timely otolaryngologic or pediatric surgical evaluation. Portions of the physical examination that are important in these cases are not easily accessible to the emergency physician. The posterior part of the nose, nasopharynx, base of tongue, and larynx should all be visualized. Jaffe and Jaffe reported that one out of six malignant neck masses had an associated nasopharyngeal tumor.[58]

NECK PAIN AND TORTICOLLIS

Torticollis occurs with cervical muscle spasm, often causing twisting of the neck in an unnatural position, involving the sternocleidomastoid and trapezius muscles.

Diagnostic Considerations

The mechanisms of neck trauma are discussed in Chapter 22. Malposition of the neck associated with discomfort can occur from congenital abnormalities of the cervical spine or cervical musculature, lesions of the spine (osteomyelitis, subluxation), and muscles (spasm from primary muscle disease or from paramuscular inflammation), acquired or congenital cervical skin contractures, and from vestibular, cerebellar, toxic (dystonic), and idiopathic causes. Torticollis at birth is usually caused by congenital muscular torticollis (injury to and shortening of the sternocleidomastoid muscle secondary to birth trauma).[60] Contiguous inflammatory disease (cervical adenitis, pharyngitis, cervical Pott disease, retropharyngeal abscess, and apical pneumonitis) may refer pain to the neck and inhibit movement. Phenothiazine-induced dystonia may produce oral, facial, and neck posturing (see box on p. 725).

Diagnostic Work-Up

The history will uncover information about onset, duration, and associated factors, which will pinpoint etiology in most cases. Congenital muscular torticollis and Klippel-Feil syndrome (congenital fusion of cervical vertebra) are present at birth and remain static. Inflammatory causes will be accompanied by fever, swelling and tenderness, depending on the site.[61] Oropharyngeal inflammation is accompanied by a history of pain, dysphagia, stridor, drooling, or hoarseness. Disconjugate gaze is often noted by parents in children with ocular torticollis.

Fever, tachycardia, and respiratory distress (stridor, rales, hoarseness) on physical examination accompany inflammatory upper airway conditions. Thorough inspection and palpation of the neck and airways for range of motion, inflammation, muscular spasm, masses, and tenderness is essential. CNS lesions and extraocular muscle movement abnormalities may reveal vestibular pathology, strabismus, or CNS lesions. Dysarthria and generalized posturing may suggest phenothiazine exposure.

Ancillary Data. Cervical spine, plain and soft tissue x-ray films, and CT scans can evaluate bone or soft tissue (including spinal cord) abnormalities.[62] Other studies should be done as indicated by specific findings.

Differential Diagnosis of Torticollis in Children

I. Congenital
   A. Muscular
      1. Congenital muscular or postural torticollis
      2. Anomalies of the cervical muscles
   B. Branchial cleft anomalies
   C. Osseous
      1. C1-C2 articular lesions
      2. Anomalies of vertebrae
         a. Klippel-Feil syndrome
         b. Sprengel's deformity
         c. Spina bifida, Arnold-Chiari malformation
      3. Anomalies of the skull base
   D. Absence of the transverse ligament of the atlas
II. Acquired
   A. Traumatic
      1. Osseous
         a. Subluxation Cl-C2
         b. Fractures—cervical vertebrae, clavicle, scapula
      2. Muscular
      3. Ligamentous
   B. Nontraumatic
      1. Osseous
         a. C1-C2 articular lesions
         b. Osteoid osteoma
         c. Eosinophilic granuloma
      2. Inflammatory and infectious processes
         a. Grisel syndrome
            i. Upper respiratory tract infection
            ii. Postsurgical inflammation
         b. Cervical adenitis
         c. Postsurgical inflammation
         d. Soft tissue
            i. Nodular fasciitis
            ii. Polymyositis
      3. Ocular
         a. Strabismus and paresis of extraocular muscles
         b. Cranial nerve palsies
         c. Nystagmus
         d. Refractive errors
      4. Neoplastic
      5. Neurologic
         a. Posterior fossa lesions
         b. Dystonic syndromes
         c. Myasthenia gravis
         d. Syringomyelia
         e. Postencephalitis
      6. Miscellaneous
         a. Sandifer syndrome
         b. Paroxysmal torticollis of infancy
         c. Postural
         d. Fibromatosis
         e. Myositis ossificans
         f. Drug-induced: phenothiazines
         g. Injection-induced: steroids
         h. Functional

Prehospital Considerations

Cervical spine immobilization is indicated for potential neck trauma. Primary attention to airway integrity, respiratory effort, and circulatory status is mandatory before any other manipulation or therapy.

Therapeutic Trial

Supportive care is essential. Intravenous diphenhydramine or benzotropine mesylate should be administered if phenothiazine-induced dystonia is suspected. If trauma is the cause, spinal immobilization is to be considered. Pain relief with acetaminophen, or choosing an analgesic and antiinflammatory agent such as ibuprofen is indicated. The patient's condition should be closely followed, especially for persisting symptoms or worsening of pain.

ORAL MASS

Oral masses include growths of the tongue, floor of the mouth, palate, buccal mucosa, gingiva, and bony structures. Benign lesions account for more than 90% of the tumors in this area. Mesenchymal derivatives outnumber cases of epithelial origin by more than five to one. Malignant lesions of the oral cavity, although rare, are most often rhabdomyosarcomas.

Diagnostic Considerations

A large number of diagnostic possibilities provide a framework to evaluate the patient (see the box on p. 726). In about two out of three cases, the mass will originate from soft tissue, including the lips, buccal mucosa, floor of the mouth, and tongue. Next most common are masses derived from the gingiva and jaws, either of odontogenic or nonodontogenic origin. Salivary gland tumors are less frequently seen in children.

Hemangioma, and to a lesser extent lymphangioma, comprise almost one third of all pediatric oral masses. The lip, cheek, and tongue are the most frequent sites. Oral hemangiomas are usually noted at birth in contrast to other highly vascular inflammatory masses, which become apparent as the child gets older. The most common superficial small hemangioma is easily compressible and has a bluish hue. Lymphangiomas are generally soft in texture, pale pink in color, and superficial in location.

Obstruction of a salivary gland duct can cause formation of a retention cyst or ranula. These are located on one side of the floor of the mouth and can get quite large. A ranula is translucent, covered with mucosa, and pale blue in color, having a "frog belly" appearance.[63] Lingual thyroid tissue presents at any age as a midline mass at the base of the

---

Common Masses of the Mouth and Pharynx

A. Oral soft tissues
1. Benign: hemangioma, lymphangioma, fibrous, epithelial, cystic (ranula, thyroglossal duct, branchial cleft)
2. Malignant: rhabdomyosarcoma, epidermoid carcinoma
B. Gingiva and jaws
1. Benign:
a. Gingiva: congenital epulis, melanotic neuroectodermal tumor, giant cell reparative granuloma, pyogenic granuloma, gingival hypertrophy
b. Odontogenic: cysts, cementoma, ameloblastoma, central fibroma
c. Nonodontogenic: hemorrhagic cyst, aneurysmal bone cyst, fibrous dysplasia, cherubism
2. Malignant: Burkitt lymphoma, fibrosarcoma, osteogenic sarcoma, Ewing sarcoma

From Gonzalez C: Tumors of the mouth and pharynx. In Bluestone CD, Stool WC, Scheetz MD, editors: *Pediatric otolaryngology*, Philadelphia, 1990, WB Saunders.

---

tongue and may contain the only functioning thyroid tissue. Thyroglossal duct cyst and branchial cleft cyst may present as a mass (see section on Neck Mass). Epstein's pearls are epithelial inclusion cysts usually found in the midline of the hard palate in newborn infants. These common lesions are small, pearly white, and often multiple. They usually resolve spontaneously in the first month of life.

In a 20-year review of 241 cases by Cunningham, sarcoma, particularly rhabdomyosarcoma, was second only to lymphoma as a cause of malignant tumor of the head and neck.[64] Rhabdomyosarcoma presents in the head and neck in more than one third of cases with bleeding, ulceration, and rapid enlargement. The odontoma is frequently undetected, despite the fact that it is the most common odontogenic tumor of the head and neck. Growing slowly, it is often noted during routine dental radiographs in teenagers and young adults. Enamel, dentin, cementum, and pulp elements occur together. When symptomatic, it presents in association with a retained primary tooth or an impacted permanent tooth. Prompt detection and excision allow for normal tooth eruption.[65]

Epulis results from a persistent inflammatory hyperplasia of the gingiva.[66] Congenital epulis is a benign tumor that primarily affects females. Less than a centimeter in diameter, it presents as a mucosa-covered, round, pink mass. In almost three fourths of cases it is located on the anterior upper gingiva. Pyogenic granuloma is somewhat of a misnomer, resembling a capillary hemangioma more than a granuloma. In the mouth, it projects from the gingival surface on a pink or red stalk and is soft to touch, with a propensity for hemorrhage.

A torus, often seen at puberty in the midline of the hard palate, is a benign overgrowth of bone. It is found in approximately 20% of the general population and sometimes is lobulated.[63]

Diagnostic Work-Up

There are many features of the history that can help to distinguish between benign and malignant masses; in many cases a specific diagnosis can be made. The age at which the mass was first noted, subsequent changes in its size and character, associated pain, bleeding, fluctuance, inflammation, and other masses should be noted. Past medical history should focus on the presence of similar lesions in relatives. Systemic symptoms such as bleeding, fever, malaise, and generalized lymphadenopathy are particularly alarming.[63]

The child's breathing pattern should be evaluated as a clue to intraoral airflow obstruction. The highly vascularized vermilion portion of the lip should be observed for evidence of asymmetry, pallor, cyanosis, or mass. Examination of the teeth and gingiva are important.[67] A significant number of oral masses are of odontogenic origin. Symmetry of the smile (facial-VII), ability to raise the soft palate by saying "ah" (glossopharyngeal-IX and vagus-X), and protrusion of the tongue (hypoglossal-XII) assist in evaluating cranial nerves.

To see the oropharynx and tonsillar areas, it is helpful to have the child raise the soft palate and depress the tongue. In a cooperative patient this can often be accomplished by asking the child to show you how big his or her mouth is while saying "ah," panting like a dog, or singing a note. The child is more likely to understand and cooperate if the examiner also performs this maneuver, particularly if it is done as if in play to see whose mouth opens the widest. If the child is trying but not able to provide enough visualization, singing successively higher notes will often help. Depressing the tongue will allow an adequate view in the uncooperative child. Care should be taken to avoid touching the posterior pharyngeal wall and the posterior tongue because this may precipitate the gag reflex.

The oral mass should be examined carefully to determine its size, color, firmness, attachments, and position. Evidence of bleeding, tenderness, inflammation, and fluctuance should be sought. If the mass appears to be cystic, transillumination should be attempted. Movement with swallowing, speech, breathing, or tongue movement should also be noted. The physical examination requires evaluation of the oral cavity. For palpation of structures in the posterior areas of the oral cavity, such as an attempt to clinically distinguish peritonsillar cellulitis from a peritonsillar abscess, pretreatment with a topical anesthetic may be helpful (see section on Peritonsillar Abscess).

Ancillary Data. Plain radiographs of the airway are indicated if airway compromise is suspected. CT and MRI scans are generally not necessary for emergency management, but may provide invaluable anatomic data. Ultrasound has been used with varied degrees of success in determining the cystic nature of an oral mass. In suspicious lesions, pathologic examination at the time of biopsy or excision will provide a definitive diagnosis.

Prehospital Considerations

Most oral masses are subacute in presentation and do not require specific therapeutic measures before the patient is evaluated in the emergency department.

Therapeutic Trial

The therapy of an oral mass depends largely on its tissue type. Hemangiomas are most frequently encountered; they generally enlarge during the first year of life and then get smaller, often becoming unnoticeable by the time the child is of school age. Aggressive treatment of oral hemangiomas has included surgical removal, cryosurgery, radiation, sclerosing agents, corticosteroids, and carbon dioxide laser surgery. Because all these modalities carry some risk, the preferred management is observation unless unusual complications occur. Significant bleeding, thrombocytopenia, infection, and intractable pain are indications for prompt surgical consultation. Surgical referral can usually be made on an elective basis. Rapid enlargement, interference with normal function, intractable pain, and impingement on vital structures are indications for more timely surgical consultation. Adjuvant chemotherapy, cryosurgery, and radiation therapy are often important in the treatment of malignant processes.[63,64]

SORE THROAT

Sore throat is a common complaint in childhood and generally refers to symptoms caused by pharyngotonsillitis and is further discussed in the section on streptococcal tonsillopharyngitis. Oral ulceration, gingivitis, or uvulitis may appear as sore throat.

Pathophysiology

Inflammatory (infectious, allergic) or traumatic (mechanical, chemical) processes in the oropharynx or neck can occur as a sore throat. Ulcers appear as circumscribed loss of epithelium and local tissue necrosis.

Diagnostic Considerations

Viral infections are the most common infectious cause of sore throat. Group A streptococcus is the most common bacterial cause, but one must also consider *Neisseria gonorrhea* and *Corynebacterium diphtheriae*.[68-70] Rhinovirus and coronavirus, enteroviruses, adenoviruses, and Epstein-Barr (EB) virus are among the most common viral causes of pharyngitis.[71] Type A-3 adenovirus causes pharyngoconjunctival fever. *Chlamydia trachomatis* and *Mycoplasma pneumoniae* are occasionally responsible for pharyngitis in adolescence. Epiglottitis often presents as a severe sore throat in adults and adolescents.

Agranulocytosis, lymphoma, and lymphocytic leukemia, although rare, must be considered in the ill patient with persistent pharyngeal inflammation. A "scratchy" throat may be caused by sinusitis, posterior nasal drip, or respiratory irritants such as smoking.[72]

Childhood oral ulcers can be traumatic, radiation induced (cancer therapy), chemical (antineoplastic agents), bacterial (syphilis, trench mouth), viral (picornaviralcoxsackie A), fungal (*Candida*), autoimmune (Crohn, SLE, Reiter, Behçet), malignant (leukemia), stress related, or idiopathic[73] (see the box above).

Poor oral hygiene and neutropenia may predispose to gingivitis.[74] Mouth breathing from large adenoids, tonsils, nasal blockage or poor lip muscle tone often demonstrate red, inflamed labial gingival tissues about the maxillary incisors. Gingivitis may accompany prepubertal and pubertal maturation. Phenytoin therapy causes gingivitis, yield-

---

Oral Ulcers – Diagnostic Considerations

Aphthous stomatitis
Acute necrotizing gingivostomatitis (trench mouth, Vincent's angina)
Candidiasis (oral thrush)
Chemical
EB virus
Erythema multiforme; Stevens-Johnson syndrome
Hand, foot, and mouth disease
Herpangina
Herpes simplex
Herpetic gingivostomatitis
Radiation-induced
Syphilis (primary and secondary)
Traumatic
Varicella-Zoster

---

ing a painless, extensive, firm, lobulated, gingival hypertrophy.[75] Hypovitaminosis C (scurvy) may cause gingivitis, bone pain, irritability, petechial hemorrhage, poor wound healing, and the sicca syndrome of Sjögren. Primary dental disease, such as pulpitis, periapical abscess, and pericoronitis may cause localized gingival inflammation. Histiocytosis X, a pathologic increase in the monocyte/macrophage line, may cause gingivitis, swelling of the palate, and loss of teeth associated with dermatitis, proctitis, vaginitis, and hepatosplenomegaly.

Uvular inflammation results from bacterial infection, trauma (usually medical instrumentation), and allergy; thermal and chemical injury are less common. Uvulitis is most serious when associated with epiglottitis or angioneurotic edema, which are potentially life-threatening conditions. Bacterial pathogens are Group A hemolytic streptococcus, *H. influenzae* type B, and *S. pneumoniae*.[76-78]

Diagnostic Work-Up

History of sore throat can present subjectively or objectively. Infants and toddlers may have nonspecific irritability, poor feeding, teething, anorexia, drooling, or oral lesions. Older children who can verbalize will localize pain to the throat. Streptococcal pharyngitis typically has an acute onset with fever, dysphagia, and headache. Abdominal pain and vomiting are common. Other respiratory symptoms such as clear rhinorrhea, cough, and hoarseness commonly accompany a viral etiology. In older patients, epiglottitis presents as the "worst" sore throat.

Exposure to the tissue or secretions of infected small animals may suggest tularemia. Tuberculosis and gonorrhea may also be considered.

Tonsillar erythema is nonspecific on physical examination. Exudative pharyngitis may occur in several different kinds of tonsillar infections. A typical fine, erythematous, sandpaper rash of scarlet fever supports the diagnosis of streptococcal infection. The presence of posterior pharyngeal ulcers is likely to represent coxsackie virus. Epstein-Barr (EB) virus causes a diffuse red pharynx with exudate, generalized lymphadenopathy, membranous or ulcerative tonsillitis, and hepatosplenomegaly. Pharyngoconjunctival fever is characterized by low-grade fever, follicular conjunctivitis, sore throat, and cervical lymphadenopathy. A pharyngotonsillar membrane extending to the uvula is highly suspicious for diphtheria. Syphilis may appear in its primary stage as oral, lingual, and tonsillar chancres, and in its secondary stage as "mucous patches": superficial, excoriated, weeping, exudative lesions anywhere in the oropharynx.

With uvular inflammation, fever, stridor, dysphagia, and drooling are suggestive of associated epiglottitis. Urticaria, wheezing, or stridor may suggest an allergic etiology.

Ancillary Data. Routine streptococcal culture, rapid latex agglutination, or enzyme immunoassay should be done in suspected streptococcal infections. Negative rapid streptococcal studies should be followed by routine cultures. A CBC, EB virus titers ("monospot"), RPR, and cultures for *N. gonorrhea* are indicated in complicated cases. The presence of a sexually transmitted disease in childhood is a marker for sexual abuse and must be reported to the appropriate social services investigators.

Prehospital Considerations

No specific management is generally indicated. A severe sore throat or an accompanying airway compromise suggesting epiglottitis or obstruction requires specific attention. The patient should receive oxygen, rest in a position of comfort, and be monitored closely during transport.

Therapeutic Trial

Significant controversy has developed relative to the evaluation and management of the patient with a sore throat. The traditional approach is to perform a throat culture for group A streptococcus and treat only those patients with positive results. A continuing diagnostic problem is the absence of specific signs and symptoms that are sensitive and specific.

Alternatively a rapid strep test can be done, and if positive, antibiotics begun. If negative a routine culture can then be performed. Others emphasize the cost efficiency of treating children with presumptive group A streptococcal tonsillitis without culture documentation. Each clinical setting must evaluate the risks and benefits of specific approaches.

Streptococcal disease and Vincent's angina are treated with penicillin VK 25 to 50 mg/kg/24 hr divided into four doses. Other bacterial diseases require specific and supportive management. Allergic entities frequently require epinephrine, 1:1000 aqueous, 0.01 ml/kg/dose subcutaneously; antihistamine (e.g., diphenhydramine 1.25 to 2.0 mg/kg/dose IM or PO); and corticosteroids (e.g., prednisone 2 mg/kg/dose PO; see section on Anaphylaxis). Gingivitis can usually be significantly improved with good oral hygiene (tooth brushing and washes). Children with stomatitis, ulcers, or severe sore throat may benefit symptomatically from gargling or careful oral administration of a mixture of kaopectate, diphenhydramine, and viscous xylocaine.

TOOTHACHE

Dental pain is usually caused by an abnormality of the tooth, or is referred to the tooth from disease in contiguous structures. Caries, one of the more common causes of dental pain, is caused by bacteria-facilitated disintegration of enamel, dentin, and cementum.

Odontogenic infections include periapical or alveolar abscess and pericoronitis. Infections originate in either the periodontium (the tissue investing and supporting the teeth) or the dental pulp (the soft tissue of the core of the tooth), the latter being the most common. Pericoronitis is an acute localized infection caused by food particles and microorganisms becoming trapped under the gum flaps of partially erupted or impacted teeth. In children it occurs from erupting permanent teeth, and in adolescents occurs from wisdom teeth.[79]

Pathophysiology

Infection of the pulp can be caused by a defect in (1) the enamel and dentin secondary to caries or fracture, (2) the apical foramen or lateral canals because of periapical abscess or pericoronitis, or (3) bacterial hematogenous seeding of pulp that has been mechanically irritated (see Fig. 21-10). Once infected, pus may exit the pulp canal apically, forming a periapical or alveolar abscess, or it may track laterally through the alveolar bone and gingiva to form a parulis (gum boil). Dental infections can extend locally to involve deep fascial spaces causing Ludwig's angina. *Bacteroides*, *Peptostreptococcus*, *Actinomyces*, and *Streptococcus* species are common pathogens of orofacial infections arising from odontogenic sources.[80]

Diagnostic Considerations

Nearly 40% of patients with dental pain presenting to a children's hospital have caries as the cause. Another 30% have pain caused by trauma and its sequelae. A variety of local traumatic, infectious, thermal, and chemical stimuli can be responsible for dental pain. Dry socket is pain caused by either failure of clot formation or dislodgement of a clot postextraction. The incidence is 1% to 3% after routine tooth extraction and 25% to 30% after extraction of impacted wisdom teeth.[81]

Nondental referred pain may occur via the trigeminal nerve because of the close proximity of a large number of anatomic structures and interconnection of nerve pathways. The trigeminal nerve is extensively distributed in the head and neck and is directly responsible for pain conduction from the mandible, maxilla, and teeth. It is also responsible for referred dental pain of facial and aural origin (otitis, temporomandibular joint [TMJ] syndrome, maxillary sinusitis)[82] (see section on Ear Pain). The vagus nerve may cause referred dental pain from cardiac pathology, thyroiditis, and pneumonia; the facial and glossopharyngeal nerves may refer pain to the teeth from the tongue, nasopharynx, and posterior oropharynx.

Diagnostic Work-Up

A history of recent restoration or extraction, tactile (lingual) sensation of a change in restoration surface, and thermal, percussion, or chemical sensitivity suggests failed dental therapy, dental fracture, or new caries as a cause of pain. A dry socket typically occurs 2 to 4 days postextraction in molar teeth. Pain, fever, gingival swelling, and purulent gingival discharge suggest periodontal abscess, periapical abscess, pulpitis, pericoronitis, or gingivitis.[83] Dental caries are heralded by the sudden or gradual onset of sharp or dull throbbing pain in a specific area of the mouth and aggravated by changes in temperature or pressure.

Extradental sources of tooth pain are diverse. Herpes zoster of the mandibular or maxillary branch of the trigeminal nerve may present with tooth pain before the eruption of intraoral vesicles and ulcers. Tic douleroux in its prodromal phase, TMJ syndrome, and posttraumatic neuralgia can also be sources of dental pain. The problem may also be psychogenic or functional in origin.

Dental examination must determine discoloration and fractures, swelling, fluctuance, and percussion tenderness. Complete intraoral, mandibular, sinus, neck, chest, heart, and neurologic examinations will usually demonstrate the etiology of referred pain.

Ancillary Data. Radiographs may be useful when the results of the physical examination are negative. The panoramic x-ray examination of the dentition and mandible is the most useful. A CT scan of the orofacial area may be required if deep fascial space infection is suspected. A complete blood count and site and blood cultures may be useful in the toxic patient. Further work-up is dictated by the postulated source of referred pain.

Therapeutic Trial

Caries require analgesics and dental referral. Pulpitis and periapical abscess also require analgesia, with warm compresses, elevation, and systemic antibiotics (penicillin or erythromycin). Incision and drainage may be necessary. Pericoronitis is treated similarly; irrigation and gentle debridement of operculum may obviate the need for incision and drainage. Dry socket is treated with gauze impregnated with oil of clove, oral analgesics (especially nonsteroidal antiinflammatory agents) and referral to a dentist. Uncomplicated dental infection can be treated on an outpatient basis; deep fascial space infections usually require hospitalization.[84]

Diagnostic Entities

FOREIGN BODY IN THE EAR AND NOSE

The presence of foreign bodies in the ear and nose is one of the problems encountered in the emergency department that can be very rewarding or terribly frustrating. In the best case, a clear history is present, the physical examination is confirmatory, and removal is uneventful. However, there may be no clear history of foreign body insertion, the child may be difficult to restrain, and the foreign body may not be visualized. Attempted removal under suboptimal situations may precipitate reactive edema, bleeding, and displacement of the foreign body to a less accessible location (see Chapter 26).

Anatomy

There are many anatomic characteristics of the external accoustic meatus that predispose to foreign body retention. For example, the external accoustic meatus is oval in trans-

verse section, with one constriction near the medial end of the cartilaginous part and another in the osseus portion[85] (see section on Otitis Externa).

These anatomic relations change considerably during childhood development. The infant's external acoustic meatus is completely cartilaginous except for the osseous tympanic ring. Also, the spatial orientation of the tympanic membrane is horizontal in the upright infant as opposed to vertical in the adult. The result is a short cartilaginous canal with a horizontally oriented tympanic membrane whose superior portion is very close to the lateral meatal opening. The primary clinical importance of this is the relative ease with which an infant's tympanic membrane can be damaged, especially with instrumentation.[86]

A mucous membrane covers the nasal cavity in its entirety except at the vestibules. Contiguous structures that are lined by a continuation of the same mucous membrane include the nasopharynx, conjunctiva, and the paranasal sinuses. It is through the posterior nasal apertures, nasolacrimal duct, lacrimal canaliculi, and the sinus ostia that communication and spread of infection can occur between these parts. Visualization and removal of foreign bodies may be impeded by the three anatomic elevations of the lateral nasal wall, the superior, middle, and inferior conchae.[85]

Pathophysiology

Although a foreign body can become lodged in the nose or ear in a variety of ways, self-insertion is the most common. Often placed in play, it may also be a response to an itch or irritation. Trauma is another frequent mechanism for foreign body retention. Animals, most commonly insects, worms, and larvae, can enter as mobile adults or be deposited as eggs. In unusual cases nasal foreign bodies have been associated with dental procedures and endotracheal intubation.[87-89]

The extent of tissue reaction and bleeding that ensues is largely a function of the size, position, movement, and antigenicity of the foreign body. The only limits on the size and shape of nasal and aural foreign bodies are the physical limits of the cavities into which they are placed. The fact that these normal spaces can be expanded, especially in the nose, is evidenced by numerous case reports of large retained foreign bodies. Even in children of apparently normal intelligence these can go unnoticed for long periods of time. A rhinolith is a nasal foreign body that has become mineralized. A rhinolith will continue to increase in size as mineral salts are deposited onto its surface. The outer surface is usually composed of calcium phosphate, water, and organic material.[90] It is usually an incidental finding on plain x-ray radiograph.

Etiology

Only one's imagination limits the variety of possible retained foreign bodies in the nose and ear.[87-99] At approximately 9 months of age a child develops the pincer grasp mechanism and the ability to pick up small objects. From this time until late school age when the child understands the consequences of placing foreign bodies in a nose or ear, they remain at high risk for self-insertion. Older children are at greater risk for accidental traumatic insertion. Malhotra et al described the case of a teenager who, as a result of a motor vehicle accident, had a broken door handle over 7 cm long lodged in his nose for 24 days before diagnosis.[89] Forrest reported the case of a teenage boy who had an 8.5-cm wood fragment lodged in his nose as a result of a bicycle accident for 5 months before diagnosis.[91]

Retained foreign bodies can be classified as animal, vegetable, or mineral. The primary reason for making these distinctions is for the somewhat different approach to their removal. Insects and other animate objects are usually easier to remove and cause less trauma when they are not flapping their wings or wriggling their bodies. For this reason, it is generally recommended that they be killed before removal is attempted. Vegetable matter such as wood fragments tends to swell if moistened and should be removed in as dry an environment as possible. Mineral-based foreign bodies, especially if round, and plastic can be difficult to grasp.

Excessive cerumen is so common as to be called the "bread and butter" of pediatric emergency medicine. Clinical manifestations of this problem can be quite variable, including a painful, itchy, or draining ear, headache, and hearing loss. Ethnic, familial, and individual factors may predispose to particular types and amount of cerumen. Children with trisomy 21 often have dry cerumen and are more prone to impaction because they have tortuous canals of small caliber. Attempts at home cleaning, particularly with cotton swabs, may further pack the cerumen into the canal, sometimes adding cotton fibers to the impaction. For this reason the patient is advised "not to put anything smaller than an elbow into the ear canal." Even if the cerumen itself is asymptomatic, removal is often necessary to get a full view of the tympanic membrane, especially if otitis media is suspected.

Diagnostic Findings

The patient's history often reveals insertion of one or more foreign bodies by the child or older sibling, but may be completely devoid of such clues. The child may instead have a history of recurrent epistaxis, foul smell (odor), painful nose or ear, fever, alteration in hearing or olfaction, lump in the neck, discharge, or may be completely asymptomatic.

Findings on physical examination follow these same patterns. In cases of both nasal and aural foreign bodies, bleeding and purulent discharge can impede visualization. It is important to carefully examine both sides of the nose and ear, even when only a single foreign body is suspected. The same stimulus to insert one foreign body may provoke several; in fact, it is not uncommon for children's noses and ears to be filled to capacity.

Cerumen is the most common obstructive material seen in children's ears. Although it cannot properly be termed a "foreign body," the cerumen will occasionally be symptomatic and often will significantly impede an adequate physical examination of the tympanic membrane.

Complications. Complications can occur as a result of the foreign body itself, examination, or removal. Intranasal button batteries, for example, can release chemicals that release low-voltage current on contact, causing chemical burns, tissue necrosis, and septal perforation.[100] Physical obstruction of the external auditory canal or nares can interfere with normal hearing or olfaction. Infection can closely follow the presence of a foreign body in both the ear and the nose. The sinus ostia in the anterior section and the eustachian tube in the posterior section of the nose can become blocked, predisposing the patient to sinusitis and otitis media.

Previously undetected nasal foreign bodies may present with recurrent epistaxis because of local irritation and mucosal erosion. Formation of a rhinolith may be considered a complication because its size gradually increases. Subsequent violation of contiguous structures may complicate removal or predispose the patient to serious infection. In a review of 495 cases by Polson in 1943, one death from meningitis as a complication of rhinolithiasis was reported.[92]

Examination of a struggling child and removal of the foreign body are also fraught with potential complications. The best way to prevent these problems is with secure restraint of the child and judicious use of conscious sedation before attempting instrumentation (see Chapter 7 and Fig. 49-1). Vigorous or overzealous restraint can cause vascular compromise or ecchymosis. Perforation of the tympanic membrane has occurred. Pushing a foreign body into the nasopharynx can lead to esophageal impaction or aspiration.

Ancillary Data. Plain radiographs may be helpful in cases of suspected nasal foreign bodies, but there are many nonradioopaque objects that will give false-negative results. Although rarely necessary, CT scans can demonstrate the presence of a foreign body in the posterior portion of the nose that cannot be readily seen on examination. In traumatic cases prior to removal, radiographic x-ray studies can demonstrate the size of a retained foreign body and involvement of adjacent structures.

Differential Considerations

Nasal or aural foreign bodies have masqueraded as tumors, chronic infections, recurrent epistaxis, and even generalized body odor (bromhidrosis).[96-99] However, these distinctions are usually obvious after taking the patient's history and a physical examination.

Management

First do no harm. Removal of a nasal or aural foreign body should only be attempted if success is expected. Cases that appear to be too difficult for emergency department removal should be referred to an otolaryngologic consultant. It is true that the first attempt at removal is the most likely to be successful. Anatomic considerations reinforce clinical experience that unsuccessful manipulation may stimulate mucosal edema, bleeding, and displacement of the object to a less accessible area. Although many cases will not require all the recommended supplies, it is prudent to have those that are potentially useful at hand before attempting removal (see the box on p. 731).

Before proceeding with immobilization, the entire procedure should be explained to the family and child as age and maturity permit. If removal can be accomplished without violating the child's trust, everyone will fare better. Sedation should be considered if the child is still flailing to prevent immobilization. Adequate personnel should be employed so that the child is quickly and completely overpowered. This

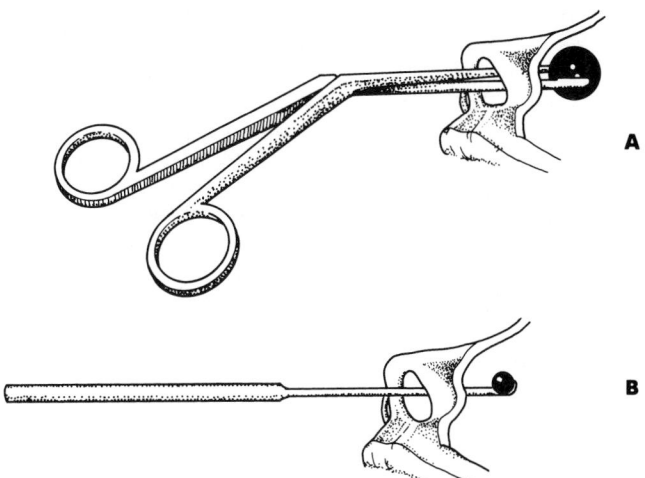

Equipment for Examination or Removal of a Nasal or Aural Foreign Body

Immobilization device (e.g., sheet or papoose board)

Sedative medications (see Chapter 7)

Otoscope that allows for instrumentation under direct visualization

Nasal speculum and headlight (optional)

Topical vasoconstrictor (e.g., phenylephrine 0.125%-0.5%)
  cocaine 4%
  epinephrine 1:1,000

Alligator or Hartmann forceps

Wire loop or curette

Suction apparatus including catheters of various sizes

Foley or Fogarty catheter no. 8 (optional)

FIG. 49-3. Removal of foreign body. **A,** Object grasped with a Hartmann forceps. **B,** Wire loop passed behind foreign body before withdrawing. (*From Shapiro RS: Foreign bodies of the nose. In Bluestone CD, Stool WE, Scheetz MD:* Pediatric otolaryngology, *ed 2, Baltimore, 1990, WB Saunders.*)

will lessen the chance of injury to the child and emergency department staff. In older children this may require one person assigned to each limb and a fifth to control the head. Use of a papoose board or immobilization device fashioned from sheets is less labor intensive and often safer than completely manual restraint (see Fig. 49-1).

A good light source is mandatory. An otoscope with provision for instrument placement under direct visualization is adequate for most foreign bodies of the nose and ear. For nasal foreign bodies, a headlight and nasal speculum are preferable. The nasal speculum should be opened vertically to avoid septal damage. Removal of nasal foreign bodies that are associated with significant tissue edema may be facilitated by topical vasoconstriction before instrumentation[101] (see box above).

The choice of technique or instrument for removal of a specific foreign body is largely related to its exact location, shape, composition, and physician preference. A widely used method that is adaptable to a variety of situations is physically grasping the foreign body with forceps (Fig. 49-3, A). Insect removal from the ear is facilitated by killing the insect with prior instillation of alcohol. Objects that are round or may break when grasped may be more easily removed with a curette or wire loop (Fig. 49-3, B). In cases of impaction with hard wax, softening may be attempted with a variety of otic drops. The curette is often particularly useful in removal of excess cerumen deposits. Disposable cerumen loops and spoons are available. It is helpful to use a curette that has a familiar feel, preferably one with a small loop with rounded, smooth edges that is slightly bent at the junction of the handle, and a curette ring to lift out the cerumen. Preparations should be made and removal completed as for other foreign bodies. The canal should then be checked for trauma, which could predispose the patient to infection. If the canal is abraded or otherwise traumatized, treatment is begun for acute otitis externa as detailed in the section on Otitis Externa.

The potential for damage to the ear canal or tympanic membrane with an otoscope or curette is real, especially when examining a struggling child. When holding an otoscope, curette, or other instrument near the ear canal, part

of that hand should be anchored against the child's head. Then, if the child moves suddenly, the head, examining hand, and instrument will move together (see Fig. 49-7).

Irrigation may be particularly useful in removal of small aural foreign bodies close to the tympanic membrane. The presence of vegetable matter is a relative contraindication to this procedure because swelling of the foreign body and further obstruction may result. Many different irrigation solutions are recommended, but body temperature tap water is acceptable as long as no perforation exists. The ideal irrigating equipment will deliver an adequate volume of water with a brisk flow to a well-defined area. These parameters are satisfied by a 30- to 60-ml syringe attached to a plastic infusion catheter (e.g., an Angiocath) or preferably a butterfly needle tubing cut off about 3 cm from the hub. The flexibility and softness of the butterfly tubing allow it to be inserted into the lateral margin of the external accoustic meatus and then directed so that the water can flow around a partial obstruction, thus allowing the foreign body to be removed with the lateral water outflow.

Henry and Chamberlain published a method of nasal foreign body removal using a No. 8 Foley catheter in which the catheter was passed beneath and past the object, filled with 2 to 3 ml of saline and slowly withdrawn.[102] Others have endorsed the use of suction apparatus when foreign bodies are round and difficult to grasp.

Several methods of foreign body removal from the nose without instrumentation have been developed. Messervy recommended that in cooperative children the unobstructed nostril be occluded, the mouth closed, and forceful exhalation be attempted at least 15 times. He suggested that uncooperative children be stimulated to sneeze by inhaling pepper while the unobstructed nostril and mouth are briefly occluded.[103]

After removal, the child should be reexamined for evidence of other retained foreign bodies. It is not unusual for a child to pack an ear or nose with several objects at once.

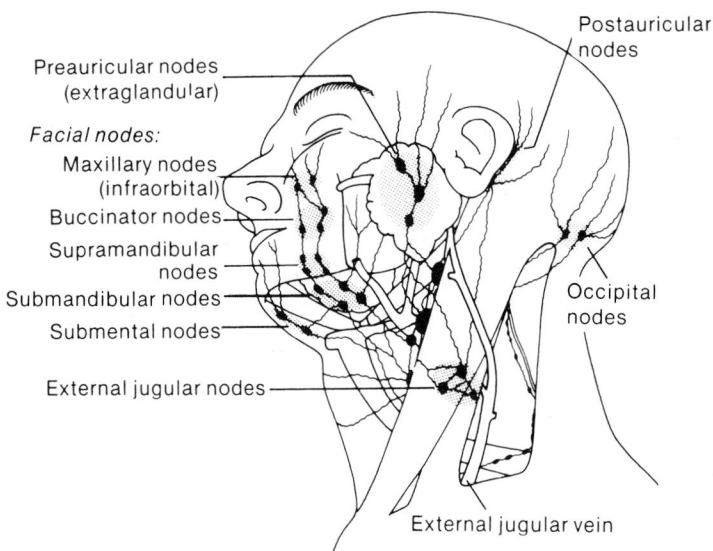

FIG. 49-4. Superficial cervical and facial nodal drainage patterns. (*From Cummings CW: Otolaryngology-head and neck surgery, ed 2, St Louis, 1992, Mosby.*)

Disposition

The child can be discharged from the emergency department after removal of the foreign body and control of hemorrhage. If emergency department removal is not possible, an outpatient otolaryngology referral is desirable unless the clinical situation warrants immediate removal. Children who are discharged with retained foreign bodies should be started on oral antibiotics to avoid infection of the obstructed orifice with normal upper respiratory flora.

LYMPHADENITIS

The high incidence of neck masses in children is usually secondary to lymphadenitis. Lymphadenitis is inflammation of one or more lymph nodes.[104] There are often clinical clues that can help narrow the differential possibilities to a manageable number.

Anatomy

Lymph nodes are encapsulated, soft, ovoid, discrete collections of lymph tissue that are generally between a few and 20 mm in diameter.[105] The lymph tissue of the neck is the final common pathway for lymph to drain from the entire head and neck before draining into the thoracic duct and the central venous circulation. All the lymph channels of the head and neck drain into the deep cervical lymph nodes, sometimes after passing through neighboring collections of lymph tissue. In the neck, the most prominent regional groups of lymph nodes are the submandibular, submental, anterior cervical, and superficial cervical groups. These drain into the upper and then the lower deep cervical nodes and ultimately into the thoracic duct and the central venous circulation.[106] Fig. 49-4 details the lymph node groups of the head and neck, illustrating the areas drained by each group.

Pathophysiology

Palpable lymph nodes in children can be normal. It is impossible to place absolute limits on normal-sized nodes in every age child and anatomic location. Palpable head and neck nodes are detected in 25% of normal children and 34% of neonates. Younger children most commonly have nodes in the occipital and postauricular areas. Older children have them predominantly in the cervical and submandibular regions. However, a lymph node that has changed in size or is asymmetric should be carefully evaluated. The pathophysiology of lymphadenitis is somewhat dependent upon the etiology. Even without exogenous stimulation, lymph nodes are constantly changing. Trivial injuries and subclinical infections can effect changes in the cervical lymph nodes. Any antigenic material, infectious or otherwise, can cause inflammation and enlargement of local or regional lymph nodes. This can occur by the presence of antigenic material itself or by stimulation of lymphocyte production. Particularly virulent infections can cause dramatic lymphatic enlargement and can sometimes result in permanent scarring.[105]

Etiology

By far, *S. aureus* and Group A streptococcus are the prominent microbiologic causes of primary cervical lymphadenitis in childhood. Several large clinical series have estimated the combined incidence of these two bacteria to be between 60% and 85% of cases. A majority of the staphylococcal species isolated are resistant to penicillin. There are many other possible although rare etiologic agents: mycobacteria tuberculosis, nontuberculous mycobacteria (e.g., *M. scrofulaceum*), and anaerobic bacteria.[107-110]

When the cause is unusual, the possibilities are so vast as to frustrate the most earnest attempts at discovery. *Francisella tularensis* (tularemia), *Yersinia pestis* (plague), *Brucella melitensis* (brucellosis), *Chlamydia* genus, *Mycoplasma pneumoniae*, *Treponema pallidum* (syphilis), *Actinomyces israelii* (actinomycosis), Group B streptococcus, *H. influenzae*, *Pseudomonas aeruginosa*, and *Toxoplasma gondii* (toxoplasmosis) have been associated with cervical lymphadenitis in children.[111-113] These facts highlight the importance of having a systematic approach to aid further diagnostic and therapeutic efforts.

Systemic viral diseases are frequently associated with inflamed cervical lymph nodes. Most commonly, a viral pharyngitis or tonsillitis caused by rhinovirus, adenovirus, or enterovirus will cause lymphadenitis that is transient and resolves without specific therapy in less than 2 weeks. Identifiable clinical syndromes such as mumps, rubella, rubeola, chickenpox, and herpes simplex can also cause cervical lymphadenitis.

Because of their distinctive features, several illnesses deserve special mention. Mononucleosis is caused by the Epstein-Barr virus and its presentation may include tonsillitis with an overlying necrotic greyish membrane, fever, hepatosplenomegaly, malaise, and generalized lymphadenopathy (see section on Neck Mass).

Mucocutaneous lymph node syndrome (Kawasaki disease) is important to diagnose because of the potential for aneurysmal dilatation of the coronary vessels. Early recognition and treatment can reduce mortality from this complication. The child who presents with a temperature over 101° F for several days with cervical adenitis should be examined carefully for other clinical findings of this syndrome: stomatitis, conjunctivitis, polymorphous exanthem, peripheral edema, or desquamation of the hands and feet can all be clues to this diagnosis.

Kikuchi disease (necrotizing lymphadenitis) is a benign condition of unknown cause. It primarily affects young Oriental females as tender swelling of the cervical lymph nodes, variably associated with fever and leukopenia. First described in the Japanese literature in 1972, all cases have resolved completely within 4 months of onset. The main concern with this disorder is its possible confusion with lymphoma. In questionable cases, lymph node biopsy will resolve this issue.

Cat-scratch disease is frequently suspected on the basis of a cat scratch within 10 days from the onset of a nonpruritic erythematous papule and subsequent regional lymphadenitis. A specific antigenic skin test (Hanger-Rose test) now exists for this disorder and a "cat-scratch bacillus" can be demonstrated on biopsy material that also reveals noncaseating granuloma.[114,115]

Diagnostic Findings

The history and physical examination of the patient with cervical lymphadenitis will not generally reveal a specific microbiologic diagnosis. However, they may provide important information that will direct further evaluation and initial treatment measures. History should include information about concurrent sore throat, skin lesions of the scalp or face, associated fever, dental problems, exposure to farm animals, pets in the home, family history or known exposure to tuberculosis and other infectious diseases, duration of symptoms, and prior upper respiratory infection.

Although inflammation is present in all cases of cervical lymphadenitis, there is wide variation in physical findings. The most acute presentation is that of a "hot" node, which is erythematous, warm, tender, and sometimes fluctuant. A thorough examination of the head and neck often reveals a primary infection that has caused reactive lymphadenitis. The scalp, dentition, ears, and tonsillar areas are particularly rewarding places to examine.

Some nodes are only minimally inflamed, or "cold." These can be quite challenging to diagnose and require an even more thorough search for associated disease than the "hot" node. Care should be taken in basing diagnostic and therapeutic decisions on the clinical appearance of the node. For example, cat-scratch disease, tuberculosis, and nontuberculous mycobacterial infections are known to present as subacute "cold" cervical lymphadenitis. However, in a series of 19 cases of nontuberculous mycobacterial lymphadenitis, White found 28% of cases to have "hot" nodes, which are typical of bacterial disease. Needle aspiration and incision/drainage in these cases led to a high incidence of prolonged sinus formation.[116]

Complications. Serious complications of cervical lymphadenitis are unusual and primarily related to airway compromise. It is possible to misdiagnose an infected branchial cleft cyst or other developmentally-derived neck mass as cervical lymphadenitis.

Abscess formation is most likely with bacterial etiology. Although uncommon, systemic toxicity and sepsis can occur. Neonates and children with altered immunity are at particular risk for this complication.

Ancillary Data. Laboratory evaluation is of limited assistance in the evaluation of cervical lymphadenitis in the acute care setting. In unusual cases, the laboratory may be of some assistance. In children with suspected sepsis, a white blood count with differential may be of benefit in evaluating the response to infection. The child with a viral etiology may demonstrate a preponderance of lymphocytes on the peripheral smear; infectious mononucleosis may have a disproportionate number of atypical lymphocytes along with a positive "monospot" test. When lymphadenopathy of malignancy such as lymphoma or leukemia mimics lymphadenitis, the child may exhibit markedly depressed or elevated white blood counts with immature forms noted on the peripheral smear.

Antigenic skin testing may be helpful with prolonged lymphadenitis. If living in an endemic area for tuberculosis, if a known exposure has occurred, or if there is suspicion on clinical grounds, a 5 TU PPD skin test should be placed intradermally on the volar aspect of the forearm. A control skin test on the contralateral volar forearm is useful when properly identified both on the patient and the chart so that a negative PPD cannot be attributed to anergy. Nontuberculous mycobacteria sometimes reacts weakly to PPD, but this is not a consistent finding. If such infection is suspected, specific organism-derived skin tests may be placed. Even these specific nontuberculous antigens for skin testing are unreliable, and their usefulness is limited.

Needle aspiration or incision/drainage of cervical nodes, although tempting, should be deferred by the emergency physician if possible. However, there will be cases that present with draining nodes and provide an excellent opportunity to get a microbiologic diagnosis upon follow-up. In neonates, immunocompromised patients, or in cases that have failed initial antibiotic therapy, the abscess material should be cultured for aerobic and anaerobic bacteria, mycobacteria, and fungus. If mycobacteria is the suspected etiology, aspiration should be considered carefully since chronic drainage may occur. Aspiration of a fluctuant node can be performed using providone iodine (Betadine) skin preps, a 20-ml syringe, and a large bore (e.g., 18-gauge) needle. The Betadine should be wiped off the skin surface before aspiration to avoid inadvertent sterilization of the sample.

In cervical lymphadenitis, a throat culture is most useful in the documentation of a streptococcal infection. However, because the suggested empiric antibiotic therapy will include excellent coverage for this organism, the throat culture is often of academic interest only.

X-ray studies are generally not needed in the evaluation and management of cervical lymphadenitis in the acute setting. Plain films of the airway and soft tissue lateral neck may be helpful in unusual cases of airway compromise and to exclude deep neck infections. When doubt exists as to the presence of an embryologically-derived mass with superimposed infection, computerized tomography or magnetic resonance imaging can provide additional information. These modalities can also help the surgeon to assess proximity to vital structures, including vessels that should be avoided during excisional surgery.

Differential Considerations

The diagnosis of cervical lymphadenitis suggests the prior elimination of other causes of neck masses in children (see section on Neck Mass). Once the presence of lymphadenitis has been established, there are three major diagnostic groups to consider.

Regional lymph node enlargement can be a response to antigenic stimulation, usually infectious, elsewhere in the head and neck. Tonsillitis, peritonsillar abscess, dental pathology, scalp trauma or infection, and ear disease are common causes of regional lymph node enlargement.

Secondly, cervical lymphadenitis can be a local manifestation of a systemic disease. Frequently mononucleosis, less commonly sarcoidosis, tuberculosis, or Kawasaki disease, and rarely toxoplasmosis, syphilis, neoplasm, and other systemic diseases can cause inflammatory changes in the cervical lymph nodes.

If another site of inflammation cannot be detected and there is no evidence of systemic disease, primary lymph node infection is likely.

Management

In most cases, oral antibiotic therapy for S. aureus and S. pyogenes is all that is necessary. However, because of the extensive differential diagnosis, a series of questions should be answered before embarking on this course (Fig. 49-5). Is there evidence of another primary inflammatory process of the head or neck? If there is, treatment must be directed toward the primary process. Is there evidence of a primary systemic disease? If there is evidence of such a process, e.g., in a patient with mononucleosis who is noted to have associated exudative pharyngitis, general malaise, and splenomegaly, treatment efforts should be directed toward relieving symptoms of the primary process.

If the answers to these two questions are "No," then primary lymph node infection is likely. If the child has been in an endemic area or has had a known exposure to tuberculosis, a 5 TU PPD and a suitable control to exclude anergy should be placed on the opposite forearm. If there

are historical or clinical clues to an unusual microbiologic etiology, these should be pursued. As previously mentioned, there are specific antigenic skin tests available for some of the nontuberculous mycobacteria. Culture is the only reliable means of pinning down this diagnosis. Differentiation of tuberculous from nontuberculous mycobacterial disease is important because the treatment is different. Tuberculosis is treated by medical means, whereas nontuberculous mycobacterial infections usually require complete node excision to effect a cure.[116,117]

Once these preliminary measures have been taken, treatment to cover the common bacterial causes of lymphadenitis should begin. As discussed previously, "hot" or suppurative nodes are most commonly caused by beta-hemolytic Group A streptococci (S. pyogenes) and penicillin-resistant S. aureus. Although microbiologic considerations would suggest that a semisynthetic penicillin such as dicloxacillin (25 to 50 mg/kg/24 hr divided into 4 doses) is the drug of choice, the practical consideration of palatability makes cephalexin (25 to 50 mg/kg/24 hr divided into 4 doses) and amoxicillin-clavulanic acid (20 to 40 mg/kg/24 hr divided into 3 doses) superior choices. Although not as consistently effective against S. aureus, erythromycin (30 to 50 mg/kg/24 hr divided into 4 doses) should also be considered, particularly when cost is a significant concern. Patients should be advised to take each dose with food to prevent gastrointestinal irritation. The use of second- and third-generation cephalosporins is unnecessary and inferior to more narrow-spectrum first-generation drugs such as cephalexin. Trimethoprim-sulphamethoxazole combinations have reasonably good activity against S. aureus but are not very effective against S. pyogenes.

Advanced disease, unreliable follow-up, toxic appearance, young age, immunocompromised host, unresponsiveness to oral therapy, or inability to tolerate oral medications are indications for inpatient IV therapy. A semisynthetic penicillin such as nafcillin (50 to 100 mg/kg/24 hr divided into 4 to 6 doses) is the drug of choice. Quite often the considerations that make inpatient management preferable initially are resolved before the full course of IV antibiotics is given. In these cases, a change to oral antibiotics is a reasonable way to complete the therapy.[118]

Disposition

Before discharge, parents should be advised to return at once if the condition worsens while the child is on antibiotics. In particular, children should be observed for dyspnea, voice change, or inability to tolerate fluids or antibiotics. Follow-up visits in 2 or 3 days are helpful to assess the progress of therapy. Also, this is a good time to read skin tests if placed, and to observe for signs of abscess formation. Inpatient therapy is indicated in the very young, immunocompromised, or toxic-appearing child. Advanced disease, inability to tolerate oral therapy, or disease progression on oral antibiotics should also prompt hospital admission.

Surgical consultation should be requested if cervical lymphadenitis is unresponsive to optimal medical management. Incision and drainage of the nodes by the emergency physician should be avoided because a persistent draining sinus can result, especially when the infection is caused by nontuberculous mycobacteria. As emphasized previously,

APPROACH TO LYMPHADENITIS

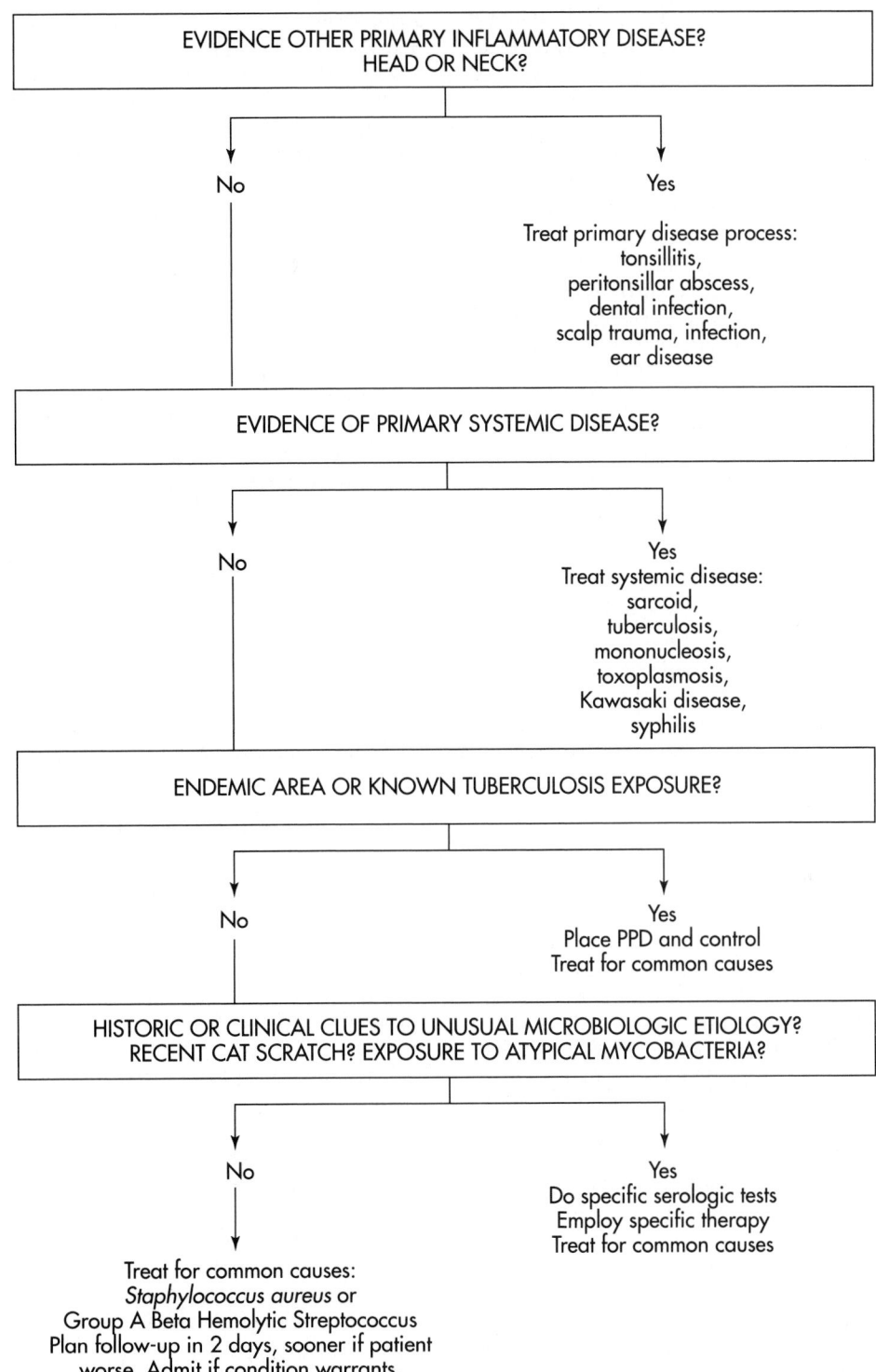

FIG. 49-5. Evidence of other primary inflammatory processes of the head and neck.

distinguishing bacterial from mycobacterial disease is frequently not possible from physical examination. Total surgical excision of the node can cure the patient, prevent this complication, and allow a clear etiologic diagnosis in the vast majority of cases.

MASTOIDITIS

Although less common since the early, aggressive use of antibiotics, mastoiditis remains an important sequela of otitis media. The best chance of recovery without complication requires early recognition and aggressive treatment.[119]

Anatomy

The mastoid is the posterior part of the temporal bone. At birth the mastoid antrum is well developed, achieving almost adult size. It communicates with the tympanic cavity via the aditus. The mastoid air cells are well formed by age 2 years, but continue to enlarge through puberty. The size, number, and position of these air cells vary greatly from person to person. The mucous membrane that lines the mastoid air cells is continuous with that of the mastoid antrum, aditus, and tympanic cavity, which facilitates the easy movement of air, fluid, and microorganisms among these structures. However, it is the anatomic relationships of the mastoid antrum and air cells to surrounding structures that provides a clear understanding of the potential complications of mastoiditis. In addition to the aditus and mastoid air cells, the antrum is bordered by the semicircular canals, the middle cranial fossa, the temporal lobe of the brain, and the path of the facial nerve. The air cells vary more in location and are sometimes found beyond the confines of the mastoid bone. Other anatomic neighbors may include the superior jugular bulb, the auditory tube, the carotid canal, the labyrinth, and the abducent nerve.[120] Fig. 49-6 depicts the relationships between the tympanic cavity, aditus, antrum, and air cells.

Pathophysiology

Most cases of suppurative otitis media have associated mastoid inflammation; clinical mastoiditis is infrequently seen.[121] In the early stages of mastoiditis, before periostitis or coalescence of air cells occurs, there are no specific signs. For these reasons, the preclinical form of mastoiditis probably occurs frequently. Elucidation of mastoiditis has been hampered by its infrequent occurrence and inconsistent diagnostic criteria, which make interstudy comparisons difficult.

In most cases, mastoiditis is a complication of acute purulent otitis media. The mucous membrane, which is continuous between the tympanic and the mastoid cavities, becomes hyperemic and edematous. If the process is not reversed, the infection may spread to the periosteum of the mastoid bone, potentially causing a subperiosteal abscess. Extensive suppuration can occur, filling the air cells and causing an osteitis that destroys the bony network separating the communicating air cells. Because of the resultant coalescence of the air cells, this process has been descriptively termed *acute coalescent mastoiditis.*[122] In some cases, acute mastoiditis is a primary osteitis of the middle ear cleft.[123]

Etiology

The successful identification of a bacteriologic etiology varies greatly from series to series. Isolation rates are far better from mastoid mucosa and subperiosteal aspirates than blood culture and culture of middle ear exudate. Most commonly, acute mastoiditis is caused by the same bacteria that are associated with acute purulent otitis media. *S. pneumoniae* and *H. influenzae* are frequent isolates. Also seen are infections with *S. epidermidis, S. aureus, S. pyogenes, Escherichia coli, Proteus* species, *P. aeruginosa,* and anaerobes.[124]

Diagnostic Findings

The child with mastoiditis may have a history of fever, prior diagnosis of otitis media, and antibiotic treatment. Ear pain, discharge, and nonspecific symptoms of headache, malaise, and upper respiratory congestion are also common. Physical findings of acute purulent otitis media are often seen, but mastoiditis may progress slowly and occur in the absence of any demonstrable middle ear disease. In a study of 98 children with mastoiditis over a 5-year period in an economically-deprived South African population, Pfaltz noted a peak in mastoiditis between the ages of 3 and 6 months after the onset of otitis media.[125] When present, fever, otorrhea, abnormal tympanic membrane examination, and regional lymph node swelling may be helpful for diagnostic purposes. In advanced cases, there is more likely to be erythema and swelling over the mastoid bone. Unilateral outward and downward protrusion of the pinna and sagging of the posterior external auditory canal are highly suggestive of subperiosteal abscess.

Complications. Although more properly considered to be the later stages of disease rather than complications, subperiosteal abscess and osteitis should be considered because they can significantly affect management and prognosis. True complications are caused by local bacterial extension. Fig. 49-6 shows the relationship of the mastoid aditus, antrum, and air cells to surrounding structures. Soon after the first clinical signs of mastoiditis intracranial complications such as labyrinthitis, encephalitis, intracranial abscess, meningitis, and cranial nerve inflammation can occur.[123]

Ancillary Data. There is no specific diagnostic laboratory test for mastoiditis. An elevated erythrocyte sedimentation rate and leukocytosis are often noted but are of no consequence in diagnosis or management. Blood cultures should be done with a low expectation of bacterial recovery. Aspiration of subperiosteal abscess cavity and culture of mastoid mucosa are the best sources of bacterial confirmation. Tympanic cavity aspiration is of intermediate value. When purulent material is cultured from the external acoustic meatus, every attempt should be made to first remove debris and collect the specimen just as it passes through the tympanic membrane. Anaerobic cultures should also be done.[126]

CT scans of the temporal bone may provide further detailed information about the mastoid cavity and are preferred to plain x-ray films. Acute mastoiditis initially may show only clouding. As the disease progresses, coalescence of the air cells and abscess formation can be seen. CT scans can also help to identify complications of mastoiditis such as bone resorption, intracranial abscess, and facial nerve involvement.

Differential Considerations

As described previously, the early stages of acute mastoiditis are characterized by nonspecific symptoms. Even in the later stages, diagnosis may be difficult. Widely disparate disease processes such as cervical adenopathy, parotitis, mastoid trauma, basilar skull fracture, and various cysts and tumors can have presentations similar to mas-

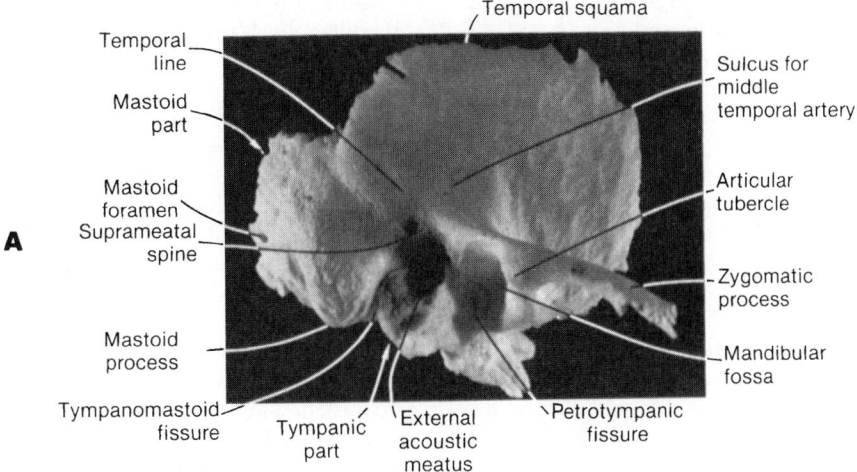

Temporal squama

Temporal line

Mastoid part

Mastoid foramen

Suprameatal spine

Mastoid process

Tympanomastoid fissure

Tympanic part

External acoustic meatus

Petrotympanic fissure

Sulcus for middle temporal artery

Articular tubercle

Zygomatic process

Mandibular fossa

A

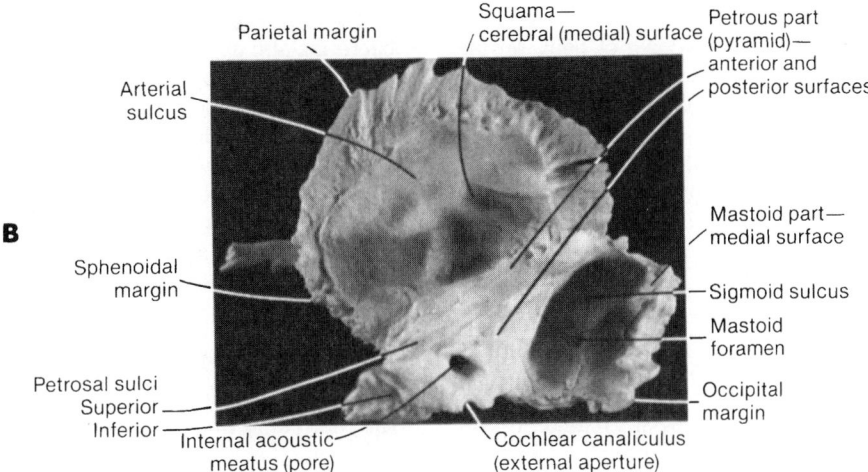

Parietal margin

Squama— cerebral (medial) surface

Petrous part (pyramid)— anterior and posterior surfaces

Arterial sulcus

Sphenoidal margin

Petrosal sulci
Superior
Inferior

Internal acoustic meatus (pore)

Cochlear canaliculus (external aperture)

Mastoid part— medial surface

Sigmoid sulcus

Mastoid foramen

Occipital margin

B

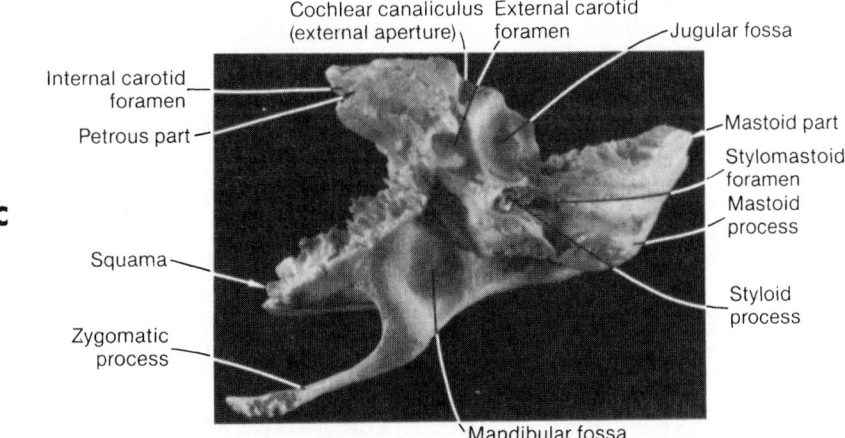

Cochlear canaliculus (external aperture)

External carotid foramen

Jugular fossa

Internal carotid foramen

Petrous part

Squama

Zygomatic process

Mandibular fossa

Mastoid part

Stylomastoid foramen

Mastoid process

Styloid process

C

FIG. 49-6. Right temporal bone. **A,** Lateral view. **B,** Medial view. **C,** Inferior view. Note the narrow connection between the middle ear and the mastoid inhibiting drainage from the mastoid into the middle ear. (*From Cummings CW: Otolaryngology-head and neck surgery, ed 2, St Louis, 1992, Mosby.*)

toiditis. Puczynski, Stankiewicz, and Ow described the case of a 3-year-old who had fever, otitis media, swelling and tenderness over the right mastoid, and clouding of the right mastoid antrum on CT scans. Within 2 days the child met diagnostic criteria for mucocutaneous lymph node syndrome (Kawasaki syndrome), and the mastoid swelling resolved.[127]

Management

The diagnosis of mastoiditis should prompt otolaryngologic consultation. In children, many cures can be effected with IV antibiotics. A broad-spectrum cephalosporin (e.g., ceftriaxone, 50 to 75 mg/kg/24 hr q 12 hr IV); or combination therapy with a penicillinase-resistant penicillin (e.g., oxacillin, 200 mg/kg/24 hr q 4 to 6 hr IV) and aminoglycoside (e.g., gentamicin, 5 to 7.5 mg/kg/24 hr q 8 hr IV) are both acceptable until bacterial confirmation is made.[128,129] The patient should be afebrile for at least 72 hours before IV antibiotics are discontinued. After that time, a 2-week course of oral antibiotics is usually given. Adjunctive therapy with a narcotic analgesic such as meperidine or codeine is often helpful.[130]

Presence of mastoid osteitis (breakdown of bony septae between air cells) or subperiosteal abscess is an indication for immediate mastoidectomy. A less absolute but widely accepted additional criterion for mastoidectomy is unresponsiveness to 48 hours of IV antibiotics. When otitis media with effusion is present, tympanostomy tubes are placed at the time of mastoidectomy.

Disposition

All children with mastoiditis should be admitted to the hospital with otolaryngologic consultation. Prognosis is largely dependent on the occurrence of suppurative complications. Although largely dependent on the personal experience of the individual otolaryngologist, treatment with oral antibiotics will often be considered after the child has been clinically stable and afebrile for at least 3 days.

OTITIS EXTERNA, ACUTE

Acute otitis externa refers to any inflammatory condition of the external ear and is a frequent problem in children. Eczema, seborrhea, and furunculosis of the ear canal, as well as diseases of the pinna have been discussed in Chapter 48.

Anatomy

The external acoustic meatus (ear canal) is a cul-de-sac extending from the pinna to the tympanic membrane. Stratified squamous epithelium covers the cartilaginous and bony portions, which change as the child develops. In infancy, the meatus is completely cartilaginous except for the osseous tympanic ring. The adult external acoustic meatus is approximately 2.5 cm long, 5 mm wide, and S-shaped. The lateral one third, or cartilaginous meatus, has ceruminous glands, hair follicles, and tightly applied skin. It is in part the tissue tension that causes inflammatory conditions in this area to be so painful. The medial two thirds, or osseous meatus, is generally more painful to touch.[131,132]

Protruding from the lateral surfaces of the head, the pinnae are prone to physical insult, both traumatic and thermal. The cartilage of the pinna and external acoustic meatus is not well vascularized and therefore less able to mobilize host resources in wound healing and infection control.

Pathophysiology

Acute otitis externa is dependent upon the presence of microorganisms and an environment that is moist and warm. The cartilaginous portion of the canal is relatively resistant to infection, due in part to the presence of glands that produce bacteriostatic cerumen. The bony canal at the blind end of the cul-de-sac is a prime target for bacterial growth. It lacks ceruminous glands, traps moisture, and approximates body temperature. Moisture retention can be caused by anatomic factors such as a narrow, tortuous canal or obstruction. Acute otitis externa has been called *swimmer's ear* because increased exposure of the ear canal to water is a major predisposing factor. A study of 100 patients and 150 matched controls found that regular swimming, hair washing, and showering were significantly more common in patients with acute otitis externa.[133] The normal acid pH of the external acoustic canal is a physiologic bacteriostatic mechanism. Inadequate cerumen from washout or production deficit adversely affects this protection. Presence of alkaline substances such as soap can also raise the pH of the canal. Trauma and dermatitis can interrupt the integrity of the epithelial lining and predispose the ear canal to infection. Eczema, seborrhea, psoriasis, systemic lupus erythematosus, neurodermatitis, contact dermatitis, and draining otitis media can all affect the ear canal in this way.[132] Table 49-5 summarizes the predisposing factors to acute otitis externa and outlines appropriate preventative measures.

In the early stage, itching is present, which promotes scratching and instrumentation of the canal. Interruption of the epithelial lining provides microorganisms easy access into the traumatized, macerated skin. With ensuing growth, degradation byproducts alter the normal pH and a moist exudate fills the canal, which further promotes moisture retention and microorganism proliferation. If this process is not promptly recognized and adequately treated, perichondritis and other complications can develop.[131]

Etiology

Although almost any microorganism can grow in the external acoustic meatus, *Pseudomonas* species are responsible for a majority of cases of acute otitis externa. Other bacteria, including gram-negative organisms, *Staphylococcus* species, *Streptococcus* species, and diphtheroids are less frequently implicated. Otomycosis, or acute external otitis of fungal etiology, is caused by *Aspergillus* in approximately 90% of cases. It is more common in patients who are immunosuppressed or have uncontrolled hyperglycemia.[131]

Diagnostic Findings

As inflammation is developing in the external acoustic meatus, local itch and pain are common. Bacteria invade the epithelial and perichondral surfaces, with progressive edema and increased tissue tensions. At this stage pain can be quite severe, and is exacerbated by pressing on the

TABLE 49-5. Acute Otitis Externa: Predisposition and Prevention

Predisposing factors	Prevention
Moisture retention	
Anatomic factors	Dry ear canals (e.g., with blow
Tortuous, narrow canal	dryer); position head to pro-
Obstructive cerumen,	mote drainage
foreign body	
Exposure	
Swimming, bathing	
Loss of acidic environment	
Inadequate cerumen	Do not use soap in ears; mini-
Decreased production	mize irrigation
Lavage	
Alkaline exposure	
Soap	
Bacterial degradation by-	
products	
Interruption of epithelial lining integrity	
Trauma	Avoid manipulation of ear
	canal with cotton swabs or
	other nonessential maneuvers
Dermatitis	Treat dermatitis

tragus, applying traction to the pinna, or moving the jaw from side to side.[132] Exudate and swelling of the ear canal are common. Acute otitis externa is characterized by local symptoms. Systemic toxicity suggests another diagnosis.

In children with disease of a fungal etiology, hyphae may be seen in the external acoustic meatus as white, yellow-green, or dark pigmented masses.[131,134] In children with occluded ear canals secondary to cerumen, diagnosing acute otitis media may be particularly difficult.

Complications. Otitis externa in children generally does not progress beyond the stage of moderate local inflammation. Complications are unusual. Although possible, extension to other cranial nerves, the meninges, and the brain does not occur in children as it does in adults.[131]

Malignant otitis externa is a severe form of infection that is characterized by a progressive course that is refractory to conventional treatment. It typically occurs in adults with diabetes mellitus and has a high mortality rate. In contrast, malignant otitis externa in children is rare, and sequelae are generally limited to facial nerve paresis, stenosis of the external canal, and hearing loss. Susceptible children include diabetic adolescents and the immunosuppressed.[135,136] *P. aeruginosa* is essentially always involved and invades the deeper tissue of the external acoustic meatus causing local thrombosis, vasculitis, and necrosis. Bone, cartilage, the mastoid air spaces, parotid gland, facial nerve, lymph glands, and other contiguous structures can become involved.

Ancillary Data. Laboratory evaluation is not necessary in uncomplicated cases of otitis externa. When disease is unresponsive to usual treatment or when unusual microor-

ganisms are suspected, stains and cultures of ear discharge for bacteria and fungi may be helpful.

Radiographic studies have no role in the evaluation or management of uncomplicated otitis externa. In malignant otitis externa, CT scans can help the otolaryngologist detect involvement of contiguous structures.

Differential Considerations

Acute otitis externa is usually easily recognizable by its clinical picture. Inflammation and exudate of the ear canal in a patient with a painful ear, particularly with traction on the pinna, is a classic presentation. However, there are other conditions that can mimic otitis externa and make diagnosis more difficult.

A retained foreign body can, by several of the same pathophysiologic mechanisms, promote bacterial growth in the external acoustic meatus. It may be only after thorough cleansing of exudate from the canal that a foreign body is noted.

Furuncles can originate in a hair follicle of the external acoustic meatus. A localized pyogenic infection is most frequently caused by *S. aureus*; the furuncle is treated with warm compresses and systemic antibiotics such as dicloxacillin, amoxicillin with clavulanic acid, a first-generation cephalosporin, or erythromycin, with consideration given to local bacterial susceptibilities. The patient should be followed closely and advised that this, as any early abscess, has the potential to become fluctuant and require surgical drainage.

Eczema frequently occurs on the pinna, especially along the posterior sulcus, but can also affect the external acoustic canal. The skin is noted to be erythematous and weeping with microvesicle formation in the epidermis. Histologically, the characteristic finding is intraepidermal edema. Typical causes are atopy, seborrheic or contact dermatitis, or dyshidrosis. Eczematous changes of other dermatoses can occur from scratching and irritation. If possible, treatment should be tailored to the specific cause[137] (see Chapter 48).

Moderately inflamed ear canals can make visualization of the tympanic membrane difficult or impossible. In such cases, the patient may have concurrent otitis media and externa. Alternately, there may be otitis media with perforation, which causes inflammation and exudate in the canal.

Management

Appropriate therapy begins with cleansing of the ear canal. This can be accomplished by suction, dry mopping, curetting, or irrigation. Care must be taken not to abrade or otherwise further damage the epithelial surface. Cleansing removes exudate, which promotes the inflammatory response; it also allows topical therapeutic agents to contact the diseased epithelium. Foreign bodies, if present, should be removed. Topical agents may be directly instilled into the external acoustic canal or applied to a wick. Enough medication should be instilled to fill the entire canal. In teenagers, a minimum of 4 to 6 drops are necessary; smaller children will require proportionally fewer drops.[138] Use of a Merocel wick (Pope Otowick) provides some advantages over direct instillation of drops and traditional packing with cotton gauze. The wick places and maintains medication in direct contact with the epithelium of the ear

---

Recommended Initial Treatment for Uncomplicated Otitis Externa

Itchy, mildly erythematous canal	Acetic acid otic solution (e.g., VoSol)
As above, with associated edema	Acetic acid otic with hydrocortisone solution (e.g., VoSol HC)
As above, with associated discharge	Polymyxin B sulfate-neomycin sulfate-hydrocortisone suspension (e.g., cortisporin otic suspension or equivalent such as Lidosporin otic suspension)

All drops should be used 4 times a day in adequate amounts to fill the ear canal.

If Polymixin B sulfate-neomycin sulfate-hydrocortisone suspension causes a hypersensitivity reaction, the patient should be changed to acetic acid with hydrocortisone.

In patients with edematous canals and significant discharge, the suspension is preferred to the solution in the event that an undetected tympanic perforation exists. The suspension is thought to be less toxic to the middle ear structures.

---

canal, absorbs moisture from the canal, and is relatively painless to insert. Precautions to its use are those associated with leaving any foreign material in an infected area. A wick is most helpful when edema of the canal is present, and should optimally be removed 1 or 2 days after placement.

Commonly used, effective topical preparations contain polymyxin B, neomycin, cortisporin, lidosporin, and hydrocortisone. Polymyxin B is effective against *Pseudomonas*; neomycin is effective against other gram-negative bacteria and staphylococci, although it may cause contact dermatitis. Both are acidifying and help the ear canal regain its physiologic pH. Hydrocortisone has antiinflammatory and antipruritic effects. In consideration of cost, risk of allergic reaction, and development of bacterial resistance, several authors have compared the efficacy of antiseptic drops (e.g., acetic acid, boric acid, or aluminum acetate) to that of commonly used antibiotic-steroid preparations, and have demonstrated relative comparable results.[139,140] Other authors are reporting success with topical steroids alone and a spray formulation of neomycin/dexamethasone.[141,142] A suspension should be used if the eardrum is perforated. Fungal otitis externa can require prolonged treatment. Several weeks of topical tolnaftate therapy is usually effective, but because of the possibility of therapeutic failure and suspicion of underlying disease, an otolaryngologist should be consulted.[3] See the box above for specific therapeutic recommendations.

The treatment of malignant otitis externa requires prolonged IV antibiotic therapy and sometimes surgical debridement. This necessitates admission and consultation with an otolaryngologist.

Disposition

In children who live in warm humid environments or are active in aquatic activities, preventive measures may be necessary to avoid recurrent disease. Drying the external canal after water exposure can be accomplished by jumping with the head tilted to one side, fanning, and drying with a hair blowdryer. The use of topical agents that promote drying and acidification of the ear canal (e.g., aluminum acetate) is also a good preventive measure.[132]

Children with uncomplicated cases of acute otitis externa should be followed on an outpatient basis after an appropriate therapeutic trial. Children with disease refractory to usual measures should be seen by an otolaryngologist. If systemic toxicity occurs or there is suspicion of malignant externa otitis, hospital admission and immediate otolaryngologic consultation are indicated.

OTITIS MEDIA

Otitis media is a very common diagnosis in febrile children presenting to the emergency department. Peaking between the ages of 6 and 13 months, otitis media accounts for more than 30 million oral antibiotic prescriptions each year in the United States. Myringotomy with placement of tympanostomy tubes is the most common surgical procedure performed on children.[143] Accurate diagnosis and proper treatment are important to relieve and prevent untoward sequelae. The term *otitis media* encompasses the clinical syndromes of acute suppurative/purulent otitis media and otitis media with effusion. Although pathologically different in their pure forms, these clinical syndromes have overlapped significantly in their pathology, pathophysiology, microbiology, clinical findings, and treatment.

Anatomy

The middle ear is an air-filled cavity within the temporal bone. It is bordered laterally by the tympanic membrane and medially by the inner ear. The tegmen tympani bone lies superior to the middle ear space, separating it from the cranial contents. The superior bulb of the internal jugular vein lies adjacent to the floor of the middle ear cavity, separated only by a thin bony structure that is not consistently present. The posterior wall of the middle ear communicates with the mastoid antrum and air cells via the aditus.[144-146]

The osseous part of the eustachian tube originates in the anterior wall of the middle ear space and connects to the cartilaginous portion, communicating with the nasopharynx. The osseous eustachian tube originates from a point 4 mm above the floor of the middle ear cavity, affecting the clearance of middle ear fluids.[144] The osseous eustachian tube normally remains open while the cartilaginous portion is closed at rest, opening during contraction of the tensor veli palatini muscle during swallowing, Valsalva, and other maneuvers.[145] The eustachian tube doubles in length from birth to adulthood. This, and the fact that it is much closer to the horizontal plane during infancy, partially explains the greater susceptibility of infants to inadequate middle ear drainage, middle ear effusions, and subsequent infections.[144,145]

Pathophysiology

Although many factors have been implicated in the pathogenesis of otitis media, eustachian tube dysfunction appears to be the most important. The eustachian tube has three major functions: equilibration of middle ear and atmospheric air pressures, protection from secretions and sound pressures of the nasopharynx, and clearance of middle ear secretions into the nasopharynx.[144]

Typically, the eustachian tube becomes congested as a result of an upper respiratory infection, allergy, or anatomic predisposition. Most significantly affected is the narrowed isthmus where the bony and cartilaginous portions meet. The mucosa of the middle ear continues to produce its secretions, which have no way to exit. As middle ear secretions accumulate, they serve as a good culture medium for bacterial pathogens. Suppuration, filling of the middle ear cavity, and bulging or rupture of the tympanic membrane may result.[144]

Infection can also occur from reflux or insufflation of nasopharyngeal pathogens into the middle ear via the eustachian tube. The supine position and shorter eustachian tube in infants enhances flow of nasopharyngeal contents into the middle ear, thus predisposing to otitis media. Hematogenous spread of bacteria into the middle ear is thought to occur in some newborns but is probably uncommon.[144]

Etiology

Bacterial infection, although not uniformly demonstrable, is a contributing factor in most cases of otitis media. *S. pneumoniae* and *H. influenzae* are major pathogens, accounting for more than half of the cases in most series.[147] Contrary to prior notions that *H. influenzae* infection was only significant in the preschool-age child, it is now known that its relative importance in otitis media remains approximately constant throughout childhood and adulthood.[144] *Moraxella catarrhalis,* an infrequent isolate in middle ear disease before the early 1980s, is now markedly increased in importance.[148] Group A streptococcus and *S. aureus* are significant but are much less frequently isolated in otitis media.

The bacteriology of otitis media in the newborn deserves special mention. During the first 2 weeks of life, even otherwise healthy full-term infants with otitis media are at increased risk of infection with Group B streptococcus, *S. aureus,* and gram-negative enteric bacteria. After 2 weeks of age, the bacteriologic spectrum of disease is the same as for older children.[144]

Chlamydia trachomatis is known to cause otitis media in infants less than 6 months old, and its role may be underestimated. Because it is an obligate intracellular organism, it is not likely to be recovered in middle ear effusions. *Mycoplasma pneumoniae* is not frequently isolated but should be considered in cases unresponsive to initial therapy, especially if bullous myringitis is noted on examination. The role of viruses in the etiology of otitis media is still poorly understood.[147]

Diagnostic Findings

Historic findings in the child with otitis media commonly include fever, pain, hearing loss, and ear discharge. Systemic symptoms such as abdominal pain, emesis, diarrhea, lethargy, irritability, and anorexia may also be present.[144] Earache in children having upper respiratory tract infection is predictive of acute otitis media; however, the converse is not true.[149]

Physical examination of the ear should begin with an overall assessment reflecting activity, toxicity, and underlying conditions. The postauricular area, pinna, and external auditory canal should be examined for evidence of inflammation. Using a pneumatic otoscope with a well-fitting speculum, the tympanic membrane should be evaluated, and a description recorded of the color, lucency, light reflex, ossicular landmarks, and mobility. The classic picture of otitis media is that of a tympanic membrane that is erythematous, opaque, and devoid of bony landmarks, with a splaying or absence of the light reflex, and abnormal mobility. However, otitis media may be present without all of these findings. More importantly, the crying child without otitis media may demonstrate abnormalities of the tympanic membrane color, lucency, light reflex, and ossicular landmarks. The only reliable sign of otitis media in the crying child is tympanic membrane mobility.[150]

Schwartz has published an entertaining and compelling argument for the routine use of pneumatic otoscopy. "The clinician afflicted with educational inertia believes that the pneumatic otoscope is cumbersome, complicated, and unnecessary. If you use the pneumatic otoscope correctly, you will be able to read in detail the tympanic membrane—the 'Rosetta stone' of the middle ear. Without pneumatoscopy, a 'best-guess' approach to the diagnosis of middle ear problems may lead to underdiagnosing or overdiagnosing middle ear diseases"[150] (Fig. 49-7 and the box on p. 742).

Examination of the ear should not be compromised by the presence of cerumen, despite the uncooperativeness of most children during its removal. Positioning of the uncooperative child for ear examination and cerumen removal is illustrated in Fig. 49-1. The choice of instrument will be largely determined by the characteristics of the cerumen (e.g., hard, wet, flaky) and prior experience of the examiner. Several methods should be mastered (e.g., curette, suction, irrigation) so that a variety of clinical situations can be successfully managed. If available, suction is optimal for liquid wax that is not adherent to the ear canal. Wax that is present in small hard chunks may be particularly amenable to irrigation. The procedure and apparatus for aural irrigation is described in the section on Foreign Body. In experienced hands, a curette is valuable for removing wax that is sticky or adherent to the walls of the ear canal. This should be attempted under direct visualization through an otoscope. Disposable cerumen loops are available; however, it is helpful to use an instrument with a familiar feel, preferably one with a small loop and rounded, smooth edges that is slightly bent at the juncture of the handle and curette ring to facilitate the lifting out of cerumen. When curetting a large piece of hard adherent wax, it is helpful to loosen its attachments to the canal by gently lifting up the visible edges of the cerumen, getting behind the impaction,

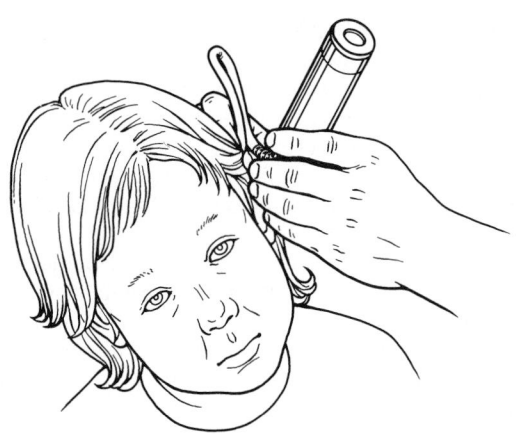

FIG. 49-7. The speculum of the otoscope is inserted into the ear canal. The seal between the speculum and the cartilaginous part of the canal must be airtight; an elastic band cut from tourniquet tubing may be placed around the speculum tip to effect a good seal. The handle of the otoscope should be pointing toward the ceiling, and the side of the little finger of that hand should rest against the side of the child's head to prevent any sudden movement from forcing the speculum deeper into the ear canal. A tube is attached to the otoscope for pneumatic otoscopy.

and lifting it out in one piece. The operating hand of the examiner should be firmly anchored against the child's head so that perforation of the tympanic membrane will not occur if the child moves during the procedure. Again, the need for adequate immobilization cannot be overemphasized. If during the procedure the ear canal is abraded or otherwise traumatized, treatment for otitis externa is begun as detailed in the section on Otitis Externa.

Complications. Although all complications and sequelae of otitis media are relatively rare because of early recognition and the aggressive use of antibiotics, those that are localized within the temporal bone are more common than intracranial complications. Some degree of hearing loss occurs in most children and is often associated with chronic serous otitis media with effusion. Less frequent intratemporal complications and sequelae include perforation of the tympanic membrane, chronicity, cholesteatoma, mastoiditis, labyrinthitis, facial paralysis, and infectious eczemoid dermatitis.[144,151,152]

The incidence of intracranial suppurative complications of acute otitis media has declined and is now more likely to be associated with chronic otitis media and mastoiditis. Suppuration in the middle ear or mastoid may spread to contiguous structures, causing meningitis, encephalitis, brain abscess, or lateral sinus thrombosis. Any child with known otitis media and associated irritability, intractable headache or vomiting, lethargy, or worsening ear pain on antibiotics should be suspected of having an intracranial complication, such as concurrent meningitis. The presence of stiff neck, visual changes, papilledema, focal seizure, or other focal neurologic abnormality should further heighten one's level of suspicion.[144]

**Essential Components to Examination
of the Middle Ear**[150]

Well-designed, functioning otoscope and insufflator without air leaks
Ear canal free of cerumen or foreign body
Cooperative or adequately immobilized child
Routine use of pneumatic otoscopy
Validation of otoscopic skills by tympanometry or expert otoscopist

---

Ancillary Data. The white blood count, C-reactive protein, and erythrocyte sedimentation rate have been shown to be elevated in children with otitis media that is caused by a bacterial pathogen; these differences are not generally of practical value in the emergency setting.[144]

Tympanocentesis and culture of middle ear fluid may relieve extreme pain and provide a microbiologic diagnosis in the toxic-appearing child. It may also be indicated in the presence of intracranial complications, otitis media in the newborn or immunologically compromised child, and impending tympanic membrane rupture.[144,153] Tympanocentesis should only be performed by those trained and experienced in the proper technique. Important considerations include adequate immobilization, sterilization of the canal by prior instillation and removal of 70% alcohol, and entrance at the posterior inferior portion of the tympanic membrane. A 3.5-inch, 22-gauge spinal needle bent to an angle of 30 degrees to enhance visualization through the otoscope is ideally suited to this use. Potential complications may outweigh diagnostic or therapeutic usefulness in the emergency department.

Plain film radiographs of the paranasal sinuses may be helpful in identifying concurrent or preexisting sinusitis in the child who presents with recurrent or persisting otitis media. CT scans will give more information at a higher cost and should be considered in difficult cases. When suspicion of mastoiditis or other intratemporal/intracranial complication occurs, CT scans are preferred to plain x-ray radiographs.[144]

Tympanometry can provide an objective measurement of tympanic membrane mobility and middle ear pressure, thus enabling the clinician to identify a variety of abnormal middle ear conditions.[143] This data is not routinely used in the emergency department setting and much of the same information can be obtained by careful examination with a pneumatic otoscope. However, because many clinicians are not entirely confident of their ability to assess tympanic membrane mobility accurately, common discrepancies in clinical findings among experienced observers and the relative ease in using a tympanometer should give tympanometry further consideration. Such testing must only be used as a supplement to a complete ear examination, including insufflation.[154] Although not generally available in the emergency department, audiology is an important part of the follow-up evaluation of children with otitis media, especially in chronic or recurrent cases.

Differential Considerations

Otalgia can be caused by primary ear disease or be referred from another site (see section on Ear Pain). The emergency physician must be particularly careful not to overdiagnose otitis media in the young febrile child. By treating a child with occult meningitis or other serious bacterial illness with oral antibiotics, the illness may smolder and go unrecognized for extended periods, presenting at a future time in an advanced state of illness. Whenever the diagnosis of otitis media is entertained, other coexisting bacterial illnesses must be carefully considered.

The febrile, crying, struggling child can have tympanic membranes that appear red, opaque, or lack a light reflex and bony landmarks. Presence of tympanic membrane mobility with insufflation will help differentiate this as a normal variant associated with crying. Myringitis, typically associated with bullae, is an infection of the tympanic membrane caused by *Mycoplasma pneumoniae*, bacteria, or viruses.

Trauma to the tympanic membrane or dysbaric injury (diving, ascent to high altitudes, or slap to ear) can cause physical findings similar to otitis media. Careful history and assessment for tympanic membrane mobility can help differentiate these conditions.

The presence of cerumen or pus in the ear canal precludes an adequate examination of the tympanic membrane. In such cases, cerumen should be removed. One can only make a presumptive diagnosis of otitis media when purulent material has ruptured through the tympanic membrane or passed through a tympanostomy tube. Otitis externa can be clinically indistinguishable unless the external canal is cleansed (see section on Otitis Externa).

Management

Erythromycin, first-generation cephalosporins (e.g., cephalexin and cephradrine), sulfonamides, and penicillin should not be used alone to treat otitis media.[155] There are many antibiotics that are appropriate for the outpatient management of otitis media; however, considerable debate rages over the relative merits of these drugs. Although significantly different antibacterial activity exists among antibiotics used to treat acute otitis media, they are similarly efficacious ("Pollyanna phenomenon").[156] Issues such as antibiotic distribution into the middle ear and spontaneous resolution of acute otitis media are being studied to explain this phenomenon.

Rational use should take into account the local microbiologic spectrum of disease, efficacy, patterns of drug resistance, palatability, dosing frequency, cost, need for refrigeration, and untoward effects[157-165] (Table 49-6). Based on these criteria, amoxicillin or trimethoprim-sulfamethoxazole is recommended as a first-line agent.[144,166]

When faced with a therapeutic failure with one of these drugs, patient characteristics and knowledge of local microbiologic trends can help guide subsequent therapy. In a patient with gastrointestinal symptoms, amoxicillin-clavulanate and erythromycin-sulfisoxazole may exacerbate

symptoms. Children with cervical lymphadenitis or exudative tonsillitis should not be given trimethoprim-sulfamethoxazole due to the high incidence of Group A streptococcus infection and this agent's ineffectiveness in management of this organism. When purulent conjunctivitis and acute otitis media co-exist, there is a significant chance of *H. influenzae* infection; when pneumonia or sinusitis is associated with acute otitis media, concerns about *H. influenzae* and *S. aureus* producing beta-lactamase also exist. An antibiotic resistant to beta-lactamase such as amoxicillin-clavulanate or cefixime is a reasonable choice. Erythromycin-sulfisoxazole is a good choice if pneumonia is present when the child is less than 6 months old (*C. trachomatis*) or school age (*M. pneumonia*). Sulfa drugs are not recommended for use in children less than 8 weeks old due to the theoretic risk of kernicterus.[167] If noncompliance demands a convenient dosing schedule, cefixime should be considered even though *S. aureus* is likely to be resistant.[144] Efficacy of ceftriaxone in a single IM dose of 50 mg/kg has also been suggested.[168]

The resistance of penicillin to *S. pneumoniae* is becoming a worldwide problem of increasing importance. These organisms that are resistant to beta-lactam can also be resistant to trimethoprim-sulfamethoxazole, tetracycline, and erythromycin. Beta-lactam antibiotic concentrations in middle ear fluid are generally inadequate to control even some intermediately-resistant pneumonococci; ceftriaxone or clindamycin therapy has been suggested. Although any recommendations in this area must be considered preliminary at best, there is also a suggestion that increasing the dose of amoxicillin increases middle ear concentrations of the drug to a therapeutic level, even for resistant organisms.[169]

Owing to the increasing emergence of beta-lactamase strains of *H. influenzae* and *M. catarrhalis* in certain areas, it has been suggested that for some families the initial use of a more expensive and broad-spectrum antibiotic may save significant time and money in the long term.[170] As new information concerning microbiologic patterns of resistance become available, choices of antibiotics should be reevaluated.

Of children with otitis media, 3% have co-existing bacteremia, and this incidence increases with higher fevers. Blood culture collection should be considered when treating acute otitis media in children with very high temperatures or toxic appearances.[171]

Treatment of neonates with otitis media is controversial. Traditionally otitis media in the newborn has been significantly associated with hematogenously spread disease, including disease from gram-negative bacilli or *S. aureus*. This association therefore mandates that newborns receive a complete evaluation for sepsis and be admitted for IV administration of broad-spectrum antibiotics pending culture results. Others suggest that in the otherwise well neonate over 2 weeks old, otitis media without systemic toxicity can be treated as in older infants and children.[144] Until this issue is further elucidated, a cautious approach should be taken concerning the neonate with otitis media, especially if associated with fever (Table 49-7).

Decongestants, antihistamines, and topical adrenocorticosteroids have no demonstrated efficacy in the treatment

TABLE 49-6. Comparative Frequency of Bacterial Isolates and Antibiotic Sensitivities in Otitis Media[157-165]

Frequency of bacterial isolates	Amoxicillin (Amoxil) (20-50 mg/kg/ 24 hr q 8 hr)	Trimethoprim-sulfamethoxazole (Septra, Bactrim) (8-10 mg trimetho-prim/kg/24 hr = 1 ml/kg/24 hr q 12 hr)	Amoxicillin-clavulanate (Augmentin) (20-40 mg/kg/ 24 hr q 8 hr)	Cefaclor (Ceclor) (20-40 mg/kg/ 24 hr q 8 hr)	Erythromycin-sulfisoxazole (Pediazole) (30-50 mg erythromycin/kg/ 24 hr q 6 hr)	Cefixime[162] (Suprax) (8 mg/kg/ 24 hr q 24 hr)
S. pneumoniae (27%-52% [39%])*	Sensitive	Sensitive	Sensitive	Sensitive	Sensitive	Variable
H. influenzae (16%-52% [27%])*	<10% resistant	Sensitive	Sensitive	Sensitive	Sensitive	Sensitive
M. catarrhalis (2%-15% [10%])*	Variable	Sensitive	Sensitive	Variable	Sensitive	Sensitive
Group A streptococci (0%-11% [3%])*	Sensitive	Resistant	Sensitive	Sensitive	Sensitive	Sensitive
S. aureus (0%-16% [12%])	Resistant	Resistant	Sensitive	Sensitive	Sensitive	Resistant

*Percentage of children with pathogen (range [mean]).

TABLE 49-7. Acute Otitis Media: Common Pathogens and Treatment

Age-group/ condition	Common pathogens	Antibiotics*	Dosage† (mg/kg/24 hr)	Frequency/ route	Minimum duration	Comments
<2 mo	S. pneumoniae, H. influenzae, group A streptococci, S. aureus, gram-negative enteric	Ampicillin; and gentamicin or cefotaxime	100-200 5.0-7.5 50-100	q 4 hr IV q 8 hr IV q 8 hr IV	3-7 days, then appropriate PO	Appropriate if signs of systemic illness; tympano-centesis indicated; hospitalize; if no signs or symptoms, use 2 mo-8 yr regimen
>2 mo	S. pneumoniae, H. influenzae, M. catarrhalis, group A streptococci	Amoxicillin; or erythromycin and sulfisoxazole‡; or erythromycin and trimethoprim-sulfamethoxazole; or augmentin; or cefaclor; or cefixime	30-50 30-50 100-150 30-50 8.0/40 20-40 (amox) 20-40 8	q 8 hr PO q 6 hr PO q 6 hr PO q 6 hr PO q 12 hr PO q 8 hr PO q 8 hr PO q 24 hr PO	10-14 days 10-14 days 10-14 days 10-14 days 10-14 days 10-14 days 10-14 days 10-14 days	
Persistent		Sulfisoxazole; or trimethoprim-sulfamethoxazole; or amoxicillin	100-150 8.0/40 20	q 6 hr PO q 12 hr PO q 8 hr PO	14 days 14 days 14 days	Use after initial course; if no resolution, consider tympano-centesis
Recurrent		Sulfisoxazole; or trimethoprim-sulfamethoxazole	50-75 8.0/40 4.0/20	q 12 hr PO q 24 hr PO	2-4 mo 2-4 mo	Should be done in conjunction with otolaryngologist

Modified from Barkin RM and Rosen P: *Emergency pediatrics*, ed 4, St Louis, 1994, Mosby.
*Additional acceptable antibiotics are available but are either broader in spectrum or more costly.
†See Appendix C for adult (maximum) doses.
‡Available as a single combination (Pediazole).

of otitis media.[144] In light of the inconclusive evidence of beneficial effect and potential for adverse effects, systemic adrenocorticosteroids are not recommended for treatment of otitis media.[144]

Disposition

Some improvement is expected within 3 days of starting antibiotics.[172] The child should be seen for follow-up examination immediately if clinical worsening occurs, and 3 days after onset of antibiotic therapy if symptoms are not improving. The importance of a follow-up examination in approximately 2 weeks, even if the child is completely asymptomatic, should be strongly emphasized. It should be explained that the primary purpose of this follow-up visit is to assess for persistence of middle ear fluid. The child who is toxic-appearing or has a suspected concomitant systemic infection should be admitted to the hospital for IV administration of antibiotics as the clinical condition warrants. The nontoxic-appearing child with persistent hearing loss, poor response to treatment with multiple appropriate courses of antibiotics, or frequently recurring otitis media, should be referred to an otolaryngologist.

PAROTITIS AND SALIVARY GLAND INFECTIONS

Salivary gland secretions have mechanical and protective functions. They protect oral mucosa from trauma and drying, and are important in normal deglutition and dental hygiene.[173] The parotid and submandibular glands are predominantly involved.[174] Inflammation of the submandibular and sublingual spaces may lead to Ludwig's angina, a potentially life-threatening submandibular cellulitis.

Anatomy

The parotid gland is situated in the space formed by the deep cervical fascia as the fascia splits to enclose the parotid gland. The space is separated from the submandibular (or submaxillary) space inferiorly by the stylomandibular ligament. The medial aspect of the parotid capsule is incomplete, allowing direct communication of the parotid space with the parapharyngeal (also called the pterygopharyngeal or lateral pharyngeal) space, thus potentially leading to peritonsillar abscess.[175]

The mylohyoid muscle horizontally separates the floor of the mouth into the sublingual and submandibular spaces. The sublingual space, located above the mylohyoid muscle, contains the sublingual gland, hypoglossal nerve, part of the submandibular gland, and loose connective tissue. The sublingual gland is limited superiorly by the mucosa of the floor of the mouth, anteriorly and laterally by the mandible, medially by the septum of the tongue, and posteriorly by the hyoid bone. The submandibular space contains the submandibular gland and lymph nodes. There is direct communication between the two spaces at the posterior aspect of the mylohyoid muscle; infection spreads bilaterally with ease.[175]

Ludwig's angina most commonly follows infection of the second or third mandibular molars or develops after extraction of impacted or diseased teeth. The submandibular space is primarily involved because the roots of the teeth are located below the attachment of the mylohyoid muscle to the mandible. Primary bacterial sialoadenitis can also lead to Ludwig's angina.[176]

Pathophysiology

Decreased salivary flow (dehydration, drugs) may facilitate retrograde infection. Primary or secondary infection and hematogenous seeding may also result in parotid infection.

Etiology

Mumps is the most common viral cause of parotitis, but a host of other viruses (and mycoplasma) have been implicated, including coxsackie, Epstein-Barr, influenza A, parainfluenza type 1 and 3, and herpes simplex.[177]

Primary or secondary infection caused by obstruction and acute suppurative sialoadenitis is caused by coagulase-positive *S. aureus* and *S. viridans*. Less commonly, *S. pneumoniae*, *E. coli*, *Bacteroides melaningelicus* and *S. micros* are the causative agents. Granulomatous parotitis is caused by mycobacteria, mycotic infections, cat-scratch fever, *Treponema pallidum*, *Franciscella tularensis*, and *Brucella abortus*.[178] Other causes include autoimmune and vasculitic diseases (SLE, Sjögren, Mickulicz, sarcoid), liver disease, diabetes, malnutrition, iodine and lead exposure, hypothyroidism, hyperuricemia, cystic fibrosis, and allergic/hypersensitivity conditions.[177]

Trauma, stones, cysts (first branchial arch and dermoid), and tumors can also result in parotid or submandibular disease. Stones are most common in the submandibular duct because of its "uphill" course, viscous alkaline secretion, and high concentration of calcium and phosphorus.[173]

Diagnostic Findings

Suppurative parotitis usually presents with sudden onset of swelling, pain, heat, erythema, cervical adenitis, trismus, and purulent drainage from Stenson's duct; clear definition of the angle of the mandible is lost. Fever and malaise are frequently present.

Viral parotitis, typified by mumps, begins with fever, anorexia, and malaise; usually within 24 hours, earache and parotid tenderness are present along with clear drainage from Stenson's duct. Pain may be severe during the period of rapid swelling, which becomes maximal within 2 to 3 days and usually disappears after 6 days of illness. Mumps may be accompanied by submandibular adenitis, epididymitis, orchitis, oophoritis, pancreatitis, and meningoencephalitis. Paralysis or weakness of the facial nerve with parotid swelling usually indicates malignancy. The relationship of the lingual and hypoglossal nerves to the submandibular glands is less intimate, so neuropathy is less predictive.

Ludwig's angina occurs with tender, symmetric, indurated swelling in the submandibular area, which often has a "bull-neck" appearance. The tongue may enlarge two or three times its normal size. Patients may have upper airway obstruction requiring urgent intervention; fever, drooling, and trismus are common.

Complications. Parotid suppuration may become complicated by fulminant glandular necrosis, contiguous osteomyelitis, septicemia, and facial nerve palsy. Complications of viral parotitis are specific to the pathogenic virus; EB virus and CMV may cause hepatitis whereas meningoencephalitis is associated with herpes, CMV, and coxsackie virus. Ludwig's angina can evolve rapidly to obstruct the airway.

Ancillary Data. The WBC count is frequently elevated in suppurative disease; eosinophilia is present in allergic parotitis. The serum amylase will be elevated with salivary gland inflammation. Specific bacteriologic data may be obtained by gram stain of Stenson's duct secretions. Specific serologies, skin tests, etc., may be useful to exclude uncommon etiologies.

Plain x-ray studies may reveal a stone in the gland's main duct. Contrast sialography or CT scanning will delineate stones, duct abnormalities, trauma, abscess, and tumor, but is rarely indicated.

Differential Considerations

Primary suppurative lymphadenitis, recurrent parotitis, odontogenic infection, neoplasm, and trauma must be considered and can usually be excluded by physical examination.

Management

Treat suppurative parotitis with systemic antibiotics, local heat, massage, hydration, sialogogues (lemon juice, sour candy), and surgical drainage if unresponsive. For nontoxic children, initiate dicloxicillin 50 mg/kg/24 hr q 6 hr PO or a cephalosporin. Systemically ill children should receive nafcillin (or equivalent) 100 mg/kg/24 hr q 6 hr IV on an inpatient basis.

Viral parotitis is managed supportively with rest, hydration, analgesics, and antipyretics.

Ludwig's angina requires immediate airway stabilization, often with intubation, surgical drainage as indicated, and broadspectrum antibiotics including nafcillin (100 mg/kg/24 hr q 6 hr IV) and a third-generation cephalosporin (cefotaxime 150 mg/kg/24 hr q 6 hr IV or ceftriaxone 100 mg/kg/24 hr q 12 hr IV).

Disposition

Uncomplicated salivary gland infections can be treated on an outpatient basis with support unless the child appears unusually toxic or there is potential for airway compromise, in which case hospitalization may be indicated. All patients with persistent abnormal parotid and submandibular tissue must be referred for reevaluation by an otolaryngologist.

PERITONSILLAR ABSCESS

Peritonsillar abscess is the most common deep infection of the head and neck. Usually a complication of bacterial tonsillitis, it can occur simultaneously with EB virus infection and is rare in children under 12 years of age, but has been reported in children as young as 4 months.[179]

Anatomy

The peritonsillar space contains loose connective tissue and is bordered by the capsule of the tonsil medially, the superior constrictor muscle laterally, and the anterior and posterior pillars. Infections in this space may extend to the peripharyngeal space and tissues (e.g., the parotid gland).[180]

Pathophysiology

An infection in the tonsil breaks through the tonsillar capsule and lies between the capsule and the muscle of the superior constrictor.

Etiology

Most peritonsillar abscesses are polymicrobial infections. Group A streptococci are predominant; peptostreptococcus, peptococcus, fusobacterium, and other normal mouth flora including anaerobes may also be detected.[181] Uncommonly *H. influenzae*, *S. pneumoniae*, and *S. aureus* are cultured.

Diagnostic Findings

The history is usually of gradually increasing pharyngeal discomfort and ipsilateral otalgia, followed by trismus, dysarthria, dysphagia, and odynophagia. Drooling is not unusual and is usually secondary to swelling and odynophagia. The voice has a muffled, "hot potato" quality. Patients often have symptoms of toxicity.

Examination of the oropharynx may fail to distinguish the stages of inflammation in the continuum from peritonsillar cellulitis to abscess. Cellulitis is commonly associated with a diffuse swelling in the peritonsillar region. The abscess causes varying degrees of trismus. There is a peritonsillar mass effect, which displaces the soft palate medially. Fluctuance can frequently be palpated. The uvula is pushed contralaterally and there is usually edema of the soft palate and uvula. Ipsilateral cervical adenopathy and mild elevation of temperature are frequently present.[181-183]

Extension beyond the peritonsillar space produces complications, which may become evident after the pharyngitis has resolved. Peripharyngeal extension may be heralded by spiking fevers, chills, neck stiffness and pain, torticollis toward the opposite side (from sternocleidomastoid spasm), and swelling around the parotid gland. Necrotizing fasciitis has been reported as a lethal complication. Airway obstruction, aspiration pneumonia, mediastinitis, lung abscess, thrombophlebitis, and sepsis have been reported.

Ancillary Data. The WBC count may be elevated, and the throat culture will often document a streptococcal infection. Rapid latex agglutination and routine cultures should be done. Blood and tonsillar aspirate cultures are useful for directing antibiotic therapy.[184] Tonsillar aspiration is usually left to an experienced consultant otolaryngologist. This procedure can be both diagnostic and curative.[185] The technique may need to be performed promptly if there is airway obstruction. A needle placed in the fluctuant area can be lifesaving. Although not yet widely available, intraoral ultrasonography has recently been demonstrated as useful in the diagnosis and evaluation of peritonsillar abscess.[186]

A CT scan of the head and neck is vital for delineating the extent of involvement if extension from the peritonsillar space is suspected and the patient is not responding to traditional antibiotics.

Differential Considerations

Peritonsillar cellulitis can be mimicked by infectious mononucleosis and diphtheria. It is not uncommon for streptococcal infections to co-exist with infectious mononucleosis. Peritonsillar abscess may be confused with peripharyngeal space infections, cervical adenitis and abscess, foreign bodies, dental infections, tetanus, salivary gland infections, and tumors.

Management

Generally, patients will require hospitalization for hydration, IV antibiotics, analgesia, and surgical drainage, if indicated. Antibiotics usually include a third-generation cephalosporin such as ceftriaxone (100 mg/kg/24 hr q 12 hr IV) or cefotaxime (150 mg/kg/24 hr q 6 hr IV). Many clinicians add penicillin G, 25 to 50 mg (40,000 to 80,000 U)/kg/24 hr q 4 hr IV, initially if the child is toxic. If resolution is slow, nafcillin (or equivalent) 100 to 150 mg/kg/24 hr q 4 to 6 hr IV is started.

Needle aspiration is sometimes used diagnostically to differentiate between cellulitis and abscess. Some otolaryngologists use needle aspiration therapeutically to replace incision and drainage in cooperative patients. Tonsillectomy after the acute episode is advocated by many but is rarely necessary in childhood except for recurrent problems or slow resolution of symptoms.[184]

Disposition

As noted above, only the earliest and mildest cases of peritonsillar abscess will be treated on an outpatient basis. These patients must have an immunologically-intact host without underlying disease, the ability to tolerate oral intake of medication, and a follow-up visit within 24 hours. Hospitalization is otherwise appropriate.

RETROPHARYNGEAL ABSCESS

Retropharyngeal abscess can be a life-threatening infection, because of possible airway compromise, invasion of contiguous structures, or sepsis.

Anatomy

The retropharyngeal space is a pocket of connective tissue that extends from the base of the skull approximately to the tracheal carina. It harbors two paramedian chains of lymphoid tissue—nodes of Ruvier—that drain the nasopharynx, the adenoids, and the posterior paranasal sinuses. These lymphatic chains begin to atrophy around the third or fourth year of life. Retropharyngeal abscess occurs in 50% of children between the ages 6 and 12 months; 96% of cases occur in children under the age of 6 years.[187-190]

Pathophysiology

Bacterial infections of the areas drained by the retropharyngeal nodes may result in suppuration of the nodes and abscess formation. Otitis media and nasopharyngeal infection may lead to the suppuration of nodes of the small lymph chains between the buccopharyngeal and prevertebral fascia. Less commonly, extension of infection from penetrating injuries or vertebral osteomyelitis may cause retropharyngeal abscess.[191]

Etiology

S. aureus and Group A hemolytic streptococci are the most common pathogens. *H. influenzae* and anaerobes such as *Bacteroides*, *Peptostreptococcus*, and *Fusobacterium* spe-

cies are also pathogenic. Recently, a variety of anaerobes have also been recovered.[192]

Diagnostic Findings

Retropharyngeal abscess is usually characterized by a prodromal nasopharyngitis or pharyngitis that progresses to an abrupt onset of high fever, dysphagia, refusal to eat, severe throat pain, hyperextension of head, and noisy respirations. Previous trauma or evidence of associated infectious conditions should be sought. In addition, the patient has labored respirations, drooling, and possible stridor. Frequently, a bulge in the retropharynx is visible. Swelling of the neck, deviation, crepitus, and trauma should be defined. Meningismus may result from irritation of the paravertebral ligaments. Pain in the back of the neck or shoulder may be precipitated by swallowing.

Complications. The most serious acute complications are airway obstruction and aspiration. The abscess may rupture into the esophagus, mediastinum, or lungs. Empyema and pneumonia can result. Blood vessels may be eroded and hemorrhage can occur. Inadequate drainage can allow re-formation of the abscess.

Ancillary Data. The WBC count may be elevated with a shift to the left. This is generally not helpful in decision making. The discovery of neutropenia, however, especially in the immunocompromised host, may reflect decompensation and the need for more aggressive therapy. Cultures and gram stain of purulent material obtained from incision and drainage is essential.

A lateral view x-ray radiograph of the soft tissue of the neck is frequently helpful in making the diagnosis of retropharyngeal abscess.

A soft tissue lateral neck x-ray study will usually demonstrate the retropharyngeal mass in the stable patient. Normal prevertebral spaces are as follows: anterior to C2: ≤7 mm in children and adults; anterior to C3 and C4: ≤5 mm in children and adults; or <40% of the AP diameter of the C3 and C4 vertebral bodies. Adequate hyperextension of the head and neck is necessary to properly interpret the film if there is no history of trauma.

Differential Considerations

Airway obstruction by retropharyngeal abscess may mimic epiglottitis, croup, and other infectious processess such as peritonsillar abscess and infectious mononucleosis. Other considerations include cystic hygroma, hemangioma, and primary neurogenic neoplasm. Trauma to the retropharynx from foreign body ingestion, instrumentation, and cervical spine injury can cause localized swelling.[188]

Management

Using the standard, primary orientation to airway maintenance is vital because airway obstruction and aspiration can occur at any time. Patients will require hospitalization for hydration, IV antibiotics, analgesia, and surgical drainage. Antibiotics usually include penicillin G 25 to 50 mg (40,000 to 80,000 U)/kg/24 hr q 4 hr IV, or nafcillin (or equivalent) 100 to 150 mg/kg/24 hr q 4 to 6 hr IV. A third-generation cephalosporin such as ceftriaxone (100 mg/kg/24 hr q 12 hr IV) or cefotaxime (150 mg/kg/24 hr q 6 hr IV) may also be added. Clindamycin 15 to 40 mg/

kg/24 hr q 6 to 8 hr IV may be considered for anaerobic coverage.

Emergent surgical intervention and drainage is necessary, with particular attention paid to airway patency and ventilation.

Disposition

Hospitalization and immediate otolaryngologic intervention is essential.

SINUSITIS

Sinusitis is an inflammation of the lining of the paranasal sinuses caused by infection, allergy, or both.[193-195] The diagnosis is considered in two clinical settings: persistent or severe upper respiratory inflammation and headache (see also section on Mastoiditis).

Anatomy

The paranasal sinuses consist of four paired structures: maxillary, ethmoidal, sphenoidal, and frontal. Maxillary and ethmoidal sinuses are aerated soon after birth; the frontal and sphenoidal sinus are visible radiographically by the seventh and ninth years, respectively. The presence of functioning sinuses at birth means that sinusitis can occur at any age, with the maxillary and ethmoidal sinuses being involved most frequently.

The sinuses drain beneath two of the three shelflike turbinates of the lateral nasal wall. The sphenoidal and posterior ethmoidals drain into the ostium of the superior meatus; the maxillary, frontal, and anterior ethmoidals drain into the middle meatus.

Pathophysiology

Normal function of the paranasal sinuses depends on patency of the sinus ostia, function of the ciliary apparatus, and the nature of sinus secretions. Abnormality of any of the latter factors will predispose to bacterial infection.[193]

Etiology

Predisposing clinical problems include allergies, rhinitis, foreign bodies, choanal atresia, cleft palate, neoplasm, septal deviation, adenoidal hypertrophy, polyps (allergic, cystic fibrosis), dental infection, immunodeficiency, and immotile cilia syndromes (Kartagener syndrome). Swimming, trauma, and rhinitis medicamentosa may also cause mucosal swelling and sinus ostium obstruction. Cystic fibrosis patients have thick, tenacious mucus that may obstruct the ostia because the mucus-secreting cells have a defect in ion transport.

In acute sinusitis (<30 days duration), common bacteria isolated from positive aerobic cultures include *H. influenzae* (19% to 32%), *S. pneumoniae* (9% to 28%), Group A streptococcus (17% to 27%), *S. aureus* (6% to 21%), *B. catarrhalis* and nontypable *H. influenzae*.[194] Staphylococci and anaerobes are more important pathogens in chronic sinusitis (more than 30 days duration). Chronic or refractory sinusitis requires specific diagnostic and therapeutic maneuvers[196] (see below).

Diagnostic Findings

The key to differentiating an uncomplicated upper respiratory infection (URI) from sinusitis is the unusual severity or protraction of symptoms found in the latter. Measures of severity may include fever >39° C, purulent nasal discharge, and periorbital swelling. Protracted (>10 days) findings are common, including nasal discharge (clear or purulent), cough that is frequently worse at night, bad breath, facial pain, and periorbital edema that is worse in the morning. Fatigue, malaise, decreased appetite, and weight loss are sometimes noted. Headache, dental pain and facial tenderness are less common complaints in children than adults.

The physical examination should seek purulent drainage from the middle meatus. There may also be boggy nasal mucosa, postnasal drip, and cobblestoning of the posterior pharynx. Only 8% of patients have tenderness overlying the frontal, ethmoid, or maxillary sinuses, whereas 76% have unequal or poor transillumination. Transillumination is of limited value in children because of the variable development of sinuses before the age of 8 to 10 years.

Sphenoidal sinusitis is uniquely associated with occipital pain, which may be the only symptom. It is rare in children. Because isolated sphenoid sinusitis can result in severe intracranial complications (extension to brain) in the absence of the typical respiratory prodrome, it is an important consideration in the differential diagnosis of headache.[197]

Complications. Sinusitis can seed the systemic circulation, resulting in septicemia. Local extension can result in facial cellulitis, facial abscess, periorbital and orbital cellulitis, osteomyelitis of the skull (Pott's puffy tumor), cavernous sinus thrombosis, epidural abscess, subdural empyema, meningitis, and brain abscess.

Ancillary Data. The WBC count may be useful in assessing the patients response to infection. Blood cultures may occasionally be useful in patients with signs of toxicity. If a sinus puncture is done, a gram stain should be performed and cultured aerobically and anaerobically.

An initial, uncomplicated episode of sinusitis can be treated on the basis of clinical findings. Radiographic studies can be reserved for persistent or recurrent problems after appropriate therapy.

Radiologic plain film examination of children has variable reliability. Normal sinus films are helpful. Abnormal sinus films are difficult to interpret, although in children over the age of 6 years the interpretation can be more definitive. Sinusitis appears as clouding, mucosal thickening, or air-fluid levels within the sinuses, the latter being most helpful in defining acute infection. Preferred plain views and the corresponding sinus studied include:

View	Sinus
Occipitomental (Water's)	Maxillary sinuses
Anteroposterior (Caldwell)	Frontal and ethmoidal sinuses
Submentovertex	Sphenoidal sinus
Lateral	Sphenoidal sinus

For most small children in whom maxillary sinusitis is suspected, a single Water's view will suffice. Mucosal thickening >4 mm is a less specific though suggestive sign of disease.

With equivocal results from plain x-ray studies, CT scan is indicated as the definitive evaluation of acute or chronic infection. It is usually indicated if the child is seriously ill, has had recurrent episodes, or has chronic disease or suspected suppurative complications.[193]

Differential Considerations

In evaluating the patient with suspected sinusitis, other entities that cause comparable presentations must be excluded. An acute upper respiratory tract infection or allergy may initially have similar symptoms, whereas a foreign body, neoplasm, or polyp commonly causes unilateral drainage and obstruction, possibly as a predisposing factor in the development of sinusitis. Functional and organic causes of headache should also be excluded.

Management

Although sinusitis may occasionally resolve spontaneously, antibiotic therapy is indicated to hasten resolution of symptoms and to prevent complications. For the nontoxic patient, a course of 2 to 3 weeks with one of the following agents is appropriate:

Amoxicillin 50 mg/kg/24 hr q 8 hr PO
Amoxicillin with clavulanic acid 50 mg/kg/24 hr q 8 hr PO
Cefaclor 40 mg/kg/24 hr q 8 hr PO
Trimethoprim-sulfamethoxazole (TMP-SMX) 10 mg TMP/50 mg SMX/kg/24 hr q 12 hr PO

Failure to respond justifies the addition of specific coverage for *S. aureus* (dicloxacillin 50 mg/kg/24 hr q 6 hr PO) and anaerobic organisms. In toxic children and those with evidence of sphenoid sinusitis, inpatient admission and parenteral administration of antibiotics are indicated initially. The emergence and increasing prevalence of penicillin-resistant streptococcus pneumoniae in specific geographic areas may dictate the choice of antibiotic in those areas. Knowledge of public health department and local hospital bacteriology lab data can be extremely helpful in antibiotic choice.

The use of standard doses of antihistamines, decongestants, steroids, and cromolyn sodium are controversial regarding their efficacy in the treatment of sinusitis. Input from the consultant pediatrician or otolaryngologist is useful in developing a specific, personalized therapeutic regimen.

Needle or surgical drainage is necessary in those patients who are unresponsive to antibiotics. Antral puncture by an otolaryngologist is indicated if there is severe pain that is unresponsive to medical management, sinusitis in a seriously ill toxic child, an unsatisfactory response, suppurative complications, or if the patient is immunocompromised.

Recurrent or refractory sinusitis is sometimes further evaluated by antral lavage to establish a definitive bacteriologic diagnosis. Persistent infection that is unresponsive to multiple antibiotics is treated surgically by the creation of an antral window[196] or functional endoscopal sinus surgery.

Disposition

Degree of toxicity, ability to tolerate oral fluids, complicated or serious disease, age of the patient, and reliability of follow-up will dictate whether inpatient management is necessary. Immunocompromised patients with diabetes will frequently require inpatient therapy.

STREPTOCOCCAL TONSILLOPHARYNGITIS

Group A streptococcus is the most common bacterial cause of pharyngitis in children greater than 3 years of age.[198] In children under 3 years, purulent rhinitis is the predominant presentation of streptococcal upper respiratory infection.

Anatomy

Streptococcal infections commonly involve Waldeyer's ring, which is the ring of posterior pharyngeal lymphoid tissue that consists of the tonsils and adenoids, and the surrounding lymphoid tissue; distant lymphatic tissue (Peyer's patches of the intestines) may also be affected.

Pathophysiology

Streptococcal disease is transmitted by close contact. It is present in saliva and nasal secretions. Food and water-borne outbreaks have been documented.

Etiology

Group A beta-hemolytic streptococci are responsible for the pharyngitis as well as the suppurative and nonsuppurative complications. Groups B, C, and G also cause pharyngitis but do not cause the nonsuppurative findings.

Diagnostic Findings

Pharyngeal pain, dysphagia, fever, exudate over the tonsils and posterior pharyngeal wall, and tender, swollen anterior cervical adenopathy are common presentations in school-age children and adults. Headache, vomiting, abdominal pain, and a scarlatiniform (fine, erythematous, sandpaper-like) rash are also noted. Infants commonly have excoriated nares. Streptococcal pharyngitis most often occurs in late winter and early spring. A scarlatiniform rash is diagnostic of streptococcal infections (Table 49-8) (see Chapter 48).

Suppuration can spread to contiguous tissue, causing peritonsillar abscess (Quinsy) and life-threatening "post-anginal sepsis" (aerobic or anaerobic bacteremia from septic thrombophlebitis of the tonsillar vein). Streptococcal infection may exist simultaneously with infectious mononucleosis, increasing the incidence of relative airway obstruction. Streptococcal pharyngitis may progress to peritonsillar cellulitis and abscess, retropharyngeal abscess, otitis media, cervical adenitis, or sinusitis. Hematologic spread may result in mesenteric adenitis, meningitis, brain abscess, cavernous sinus thrombosis, suppurative arthritis, endocarditis, osteomyelitis, sepsis, and septic embolization to the lung.

Recurrent pharyngitis may occur, which may make management a difficult problem. Often the histories for such episodes are unreliable. Culture documentation is essential.

Nonsuppurative syndromes include scarlet fever or scarlatiniform rash, acute rheumatic fever, and glomerulonephritis.

Ancillary Data. The WBC count may be elevated, more so in patients who develop complications, but is a nonspecific response. Additional studies may be useful to exclude complications in complex cases; these include evaluation of the urinalysis, immunologic response to the infection, and renal function.

Rapid streptococcal detection by latex agglutination or enzyme immunoassay are useful when positive on throat cultures. False positives with this test are uncommon (high

TABLE 49-8. Tonsillopharyngitis: Diagnostic Signs and Symptoms

| | Group A streptococci | | | |
	Infant	School-age	Adult	Viral
Onset	Gradual	Sudden	Sudden	Gradual
Chief complaint	Anorexia, rhinitis, listlessness	Sore throat	Sore throat	Sore throat, cough, rhinitis, conjunctivitis
Diagnostic findings				
Sore throat	+	+ + +	+ + +	+ + +
Tonsillary erythema	+	+ + +	+ + +	+ +
Tonsillar exudate	+	+ +	+ + +	+
Palatal petechiae	+	+ + +	+ + +	+
Adenitis	+ + +	+ + +	+ + +	+ +
Excoriated nares	+ + +	+	+	+
Conjunctivitis	+	+	+	+ + +
Cough	+	+	+	+ + +
Congestion	+	+	+	+ + +
Hoarseness	+	+	+	+ + +
Fever	Minimal	High	High	Minimal
Abdominal pain	+	+ +	+	+
Headache	+	+ +	+ +	+
Vomiting	+	+ +	+ +	+
Scarlatiniform rash	+	+ + +	+ + +	+
Streptococcal contact	+ + +	+ + +	+ + +	+
Ancillary data				
Positive streptococcal culture	+ + +	+ +	+ + +	+
Elevated WBC	+ +	+ +	+ + +	+

From Barkin RM and Rosen P: *Emergency pediatrics*, ed 4, St Louis, 1994, Mosby.

specificity: 88% to 100%), but false negatives occur frequently (lower sensitivity: 72% to 95%). A negative rapid streptococcal test should be confirmed by a routine streptococcal culture using an aerobic culture on sheep blood medium with bacitracin disk.[199] Infants should have their noses cultured rather than their throats. Local suppurative complications manifested by symptoms such as severe dysphagia, stridor, dysphonia, and odynophagia may require more aggressive diagnostic testing such as soft tissue x-ray studies of the lateral neck and CT scan of the neck.

Children with recurrent positive streptococcal cultures may be carriers. To investigate this possibility, a streptozyme (including ASO titer) should be ordered. Low titers are consistent with the chronic carrier state.

Differential Considerations

An exudative pharyngitis is commonly associated with Group A streptococci, EB virus (infectious mononucleosis), *Corynebacterium diphtheriae*, and adenovirus. Exudative pharyngitis in children is commonly caused by a virus in children under 3 years of age and more frequently caused by Group A streptococci in those over 6 years of age. Soft palate petechiae are found with Group A streptococcal and EB virus infections, vesicles or ulcers on the posterior tonsillar pillars with enterovirus infection, and ulcers on the anterior palate with adenopathy in herpes infection (Table 49-8).

Management

Symptomatic therapy may be achieved by gargling with warm water, sucking hard candy, and taking acetaminophen or aspirin.

Antibiotics should generally be administered for a total of 10 days. Penicillin V, 25 to 50 mg (40,000 to 80,000 U)/kg/24 hr q 6 to 8 hr PO or benzathine penicillin, 25,000 U/kg IM (up to 1.2 million U) as a single dose are therapeutic.[200] Alternatives include erythromycin 40 mg/kg/24 hr q 8 hr, a first-generation cephalosporin 50 mg/kg/24 hr, or clindamycin 20 to 30 mg/kg/24 hr q 6 hr PO for penicillin-allergic children and in those with recurrent disease. Do not use sulfa or tetracycline.[201]

Problematic children with streptococcal carriage may be treated with benzathine penicillin in combination with rifampin 10 mg/kg/dose q 12 hr PO for 8 doses (4 days).[202,203] Indications for tonsillectomy for recurrent sore throats are controversial and remain undefined.

Disposition

Uncomplicated pharyngitis can be treated with antibiotics, analgesics, antipyretics, and fluids. Children should improve rapidly following diagnosis and may return to school or daycare in 24 hours. Complicated infections should be admitted for IV hydration, antibiotics, and medical/surgical observation. Patients with a history of endocarditis, or those at risk for endocarditis should be on antibiotic prophylaxis against streptococcal infection.

References

Drooling and Dysphonia

1. Illingsworth RS: *Common symptoms of disease in children*, Oxford, 1975, Blackwell Scientific Publications.
2. Hess GP: An approach to throat complaints, foreign body sensation, difficulty swallowing, and hoarseness, *Emerg Med Clin North Am* 5:313, 1987.
3. Hass A, Hyatt AC, Kattan M, et al: Hoarseness in immunocompromised children, *J Pediatr* 111:731, 1987.
4. Phillips DE and Childs D: Hoarse cry with fatal outcome, *BMJ* 299:847, 1989.

Ear Discharge

5. Williams PL, editor: *Gray's anatomy*, Philadelphia, 1989, WB Saunders.
6. Schloss MD: Otorrhea. In Bluestone CD, Stool WE, Scheetz MD, editors: *Pediatric otolaryngology*, Philadelphia, 1990, WB Saunders.
7. Burke P: The diagnosis and management of the discharging ear, *Practitioner* 233:742 May, 1989.

Ear Pain

8. Kreisberg MK and Turner J: Dental causes of referred otalgia, *Ear Nose Throat J* 66:30, 1987.
9. Chasin WD: Otalgia. In Bluestone CD, Stool WE, Scheetz MD, editors: *Pediatric otolaryngology*, Philadelphia, 1990, WB Saunders.
10. Wazen JJ: Referred otalgia, *Otolaryngol Clin North Am* 22(6):1205, 1989.
11. Williams PL, editor: *Gray's anatomy*, Philadelphia, 1989, WB Saunders.
12. Martin R, Yonkers AJ, Yarington CT: Perichondritis of the ear, *Laryngoscope* 86:664, 1976.
13. May M: Facial paralysis in children. In Bluestone CD, Stool WE, Scheetz MD, editors: *Pediatric otolaryngology*, Philadelphia, 1990, WB Saunders.
14. Sundsten JW: The peripheral nerves, spinal cord, and brainstem. In Patten HD et al, editors: *Introduction to basic neurology*, Philadelphia, 1976, WB Saunders.
15. Gilbert RW, Pierse PM, Mitchell DP: Cryptic otalgia: a case of Munchausen syndrome in a pediatric patient, *J Otolaryngol* 16(4):231, 1987.

Epistaxis

16. Padgam N: Epistaxis: anatomical and clinical correlates, *J Laryngol Otol* 104:308, 1990.
17. Williams PL, editor: *Gray's anatomy*, Philadelphia, 1989, WB Saunders.
18. Culbertson MC and Manning SC: Epistaxis. In Bluestone CD, Stool WE, Scheetz MD, editors: *Pediatric otolaryngology*, Philadelphia, WB Saunders.
19. Perretta LJ, Denslow BL, Brown CG: Emergency evaluation and management of epistaxis, *Emerg Med Clin North Am* 5(2):265, 1987.
20. Katsanis E, Luke KH, Hsu E, et al: Prevalence and significance of mild bleeding disorders in children with recurrent epistaxis, *J Pediatr* 113(1):73, 1988.
21. John DG, Alison AI, Scott DJA, et al: Who should treat epistaxis? *J Laryngol Otol* 101:139, 1987.
22. Fairbanks DNF: Complications of nasal packing, *Otolaryngol Head Neck Surg* 94(3):412, 1986.
23. Elwany S, Kamel T, Mekhamer A: Pneumatic nasal catheters: advantages and drawbacks, *J Laryngol Otol* 100:641, 1986.
24. Votey S and Dudley JP: Emergency ear, nose, and throat procedures, *Emerg Med Clin North Am* 7(1):117, 1989.

Halitosis

25. Bogdasarian RS: Halitosis, *Otolaryngol Clin North Am* 19:111, 1986.
26. Claycomb CK and Shearer TR: Malodors of the mouth, *J Ohio Dent Assoc*, Summer, 1986.
27. McMillan JA, Nieburg PI, Oski FA: *The whole pediatrician catalogue: a compendium of clues to diagnosis and management*, Philadelphia, 1977, WB Saunders.

Hearing Loss and Tinnitus, Acute

28. Grundfast KM: Hearing loss. In Bluestone CD, Stool SE, Scheetz MD, editors: *Pediatric otolaryngology*, ed 2, Philadelphia, 1990, WB Saunders.
29. Lawerence LJ and Brown CG: Approach to decreased hearing, *Emerg Med Clin North Am* 5:193, 1987.
30. Black FO and Lilly DJ: Tinnitus. In Bluestone CD, Stool SE, Scheetz MD, editors: *Pediatric otolaryngology*, ed 2, Philadelphia, 1990, WB Saunders.
31. Viani LG: Tinnitis in children with hearing loss, *J Laryngol Otol* 103:1142, 1989.
32. Busis SM: Vertigo. In Bluestone CD, Stool SE, Scheetz MD, editors: *Pediatric otolaryngology*, ed 2, Philadelphia, 1990, WB Saunders.
33. Bellman SC: Hearing disorders in children, *Br Med Bull* 43:966, 1987.
34. Bredenkamp JK and Shelton C: Sudden hearing loss, *Postgrad Med* 86:125, 1989.
35. Coplan J: Deafness: ever heard of it? Delayed recognition of permanent hearing loss, *Pediatrics* 79:206, 1987.
36. Parnes LS and McCabe BF: Perilymph fistula: an important cause of deafness and dizziness in children, *Pediatrics* 80:524, 1987.

Nasal Discharge and Rhinitis

37. Belensky WM: Nasal obstruction and rhinorrhea. In Bluestone CD, Stool WE, Scheetz MD, editors: *Pediatric otolaryngology*, Philadelphia, 1990, WB Saunders.
38. McNamara RM: Approach to rhinitis, *Emerg Med Clin North Am* 5(2):279, 1987.
39. Wald ER: Purulent nasal discharge, *Pediatr Infect Dis J* 10:329, 1991.
40. Stagno S, Brasfield DM, Brown MB, et al: Infant pneumonitis associated with cytomegalovirus, chlamydia, pneumocystis, and ureaplasma: a prospective study, *Pediatrics* 68:322, 1981.
41. Lee TH: Asthma and allergic rhinitis, *Curr Opin Immunol* 1:654, 1989.
42. Perlman DS: Chronic rhinitis in children, *J Allergy Clin Immunol* 81(5):962, 1988.
43. Fireman P: Allergic rhinitis. In Bluestone CD, Stool E, Scheetz MD, editors: *Pediatric otolaryngology*, Philadelphia, 1990, WB Saunders.
44. Osguthorpe JD and Shirley R: Neonatal respiratory distress from rhinitis medicamentosa, *Laryngoscope* 97:829, 1987.
45. Lans DM, Alfani N, Rocklin R: Nasal eosinophilia in allergic and nonallergic rhinitis: usefulness of the nasal smear in the diagnosis of allergic rhinitis, *Allergy Proc* 10:275, 1989.
46. Steedman DJ and Gordon M: CSF rhinorrhoea: significance of the glucose oxidase strip test, *Injury* 18:327, 1987.
47. Curley FJ, Irwin RS, Pratter MR, et al: Cough and the common cold, *Am Rev Respir Dis* 138:305, 1988.
48. Barnhart ER, publisher: *Physicians' desk reference*, Oradell, NJ, 1991, Medical Economics.
49. Berkowitz RB, Connell JT, Dietz AJ, et al: The effectiveness of the nonsedating antihistamine loratadine plus pseudoephedrine in the symptomatic management of the common cold, *Ann Allergy* 63:336, 1989.
50. Nuutinen J, Holopainen E, Malmberg H, et al: Terfenadine with or without phenylpropanolamine in the treatment of seasonal allergic rhinitis, *Clin Exp Allergy* 19:603, 1989.
51. Hynes B, Cole P, Forte V, et al: The evaluation of intranasal topical beclomethasone spray in the treatment of children with nonpurulent rhinitis using rhinometric, cytologic, and symptomatologic assessment, *J Otolaryngol* 18(4):151, 1989.
52. Lawler G and Fischer T, editors: *Manual of allergy and immunology: diagnosis and therapy*, Boston, 1981, Little, Brown.

Neck Mass

53. Stanievich J: Cervical adenopathy. In Bluestone CD, Stool WE, Scheetz MD, editors: *Pediatric otolaryngology*, Philadelphia, 1990, WB Saunders.
54. Lidge RT, Bechol RC, Lambert CN: Congenital muscular torticollis: etiology and pathology, *J Bone Joint Surg* 39A:1165, 1957.
55. Bleyer WA: The impact of childhood cancer on the United States and the world, *CA* 40:355, 1990.
56. Sutow W and Montaugue E: Pediatric tumors. In MacComb W and Fletcher G, editors: *Cancer of the head and neck*, Baltimore, 1967, Williams & Wilkins.
57. May M: Neck masses in children: diagnosis and treatment, *Ear Nose Throat J* 57:12, 1978.
58. Jaffe B and Jaffe N: Head and neck tumors in children, *Pediatrics* 51:731, 1973.

59. Sherman NH, Rosenberg HK, Heyman S, et al: Ultrasound evaluation of neck masses in children, *J Ultrasound Med* 4:127, 1985.

Neck Pain and Torticollis

60. Green M: *Pediatric diagnosis: interpretation of symptoms and signs in different age periods*, Philadelphia, 1980, WB Saunders.
61. Bredenkamp JK and Maceri DR: Inflammatory torticollis in children, *Arch Otolaryngol Head Neck Surg* 116:310, 1990.
62. Kiwak KJ, Deray MJ, Shields J: Torticollis in three children with syringomyelia and spinal cord tumor, *Neurology* 33:946, 1983.

Oral Mass

63. Gonzalez C: Tumors of the mouth and pharynx. In Bluestone CD, Stool WE, Scheetz MD, editors: *Pediatric otolaryngology*, Philadelphia, 1990, WB Saunders.
64. Cunningham MJ, Myers EN, Bluestone CD: Malignant tumors of the head and neck in children: a twenty-year review, *International J Pediatr Otorhinolaryngol* 13:279, 1987.
65. Thwaites MS and Camacho JL: Complex odontoma: report of case, *ASDC J Dent Child* 54(4):286, 1987.
66. *Stedman's medical dictionary*, Baltimore, 1990, Williams & Wilkins.
67. Kramer S: Dangers stemming from superficial examination and diagnosis, *NY State Dent J* 55(9):58, 1989.

Sore Throat

68. Klein MD: Streptococcal pharyngitis in children, *Pediatr Emerg Care* 5:259, 1989.
69. Kenna MA: Sore throat in children: diagnosis and management. In Bluestone CD, Stool WE, and Scheetz MD, editors: *Pediatric otolaryngology*, Philadelphia, 1990, WB Saunders.
70. Gluckman JL: Inflammatory disease of the mouth and pharynx. In Bluestone CD, Stool WE, Scheetz MD, editors: *Pediatric otolaryngology*, ed 2, Philadelphia, 1990, WB Saunders.
71. Amren DP, Green JL, Roe TLW: Acute pharyngitis, American Board of Pediatrics Program for Renewal of Certification in Pediatrics, 1990.
72. Illingsworth RS: *Common symptoms of disease in children*, Cambridge, Mass, 1974, Blackwell Scientific Publications.
73. Nelson JD: *Pocketbook of pediatric antimicrobial therapy*, ed 9, Baltimore, 1991, Williams & Wilkins.
74. Rapp R: Dental and gingival disorders. In Bluestone CD, Stool WE, Scheetz MD: *Pediatric otolaryngology*, ed 2, Philadelphia, 1990, WB Saunders.
75. Massler M: Epidemiology of gingivitis in childhood, *J Am Dent Assoc* 45:319, 1952.
76. Behrman RE, Vaughan VC, Nelson WE: *Nelson textbook of pediatrics*, Philadelphia, 1987, WB Saunders.
77. Megran DW, Scheifele DW, Chow AW: Odontogenic infections, *Pediatr Infect Dis J* 3:257, 1984.
78. Wynder SG, Lampe RM, Shoemaker ME, et al: Uvulitis and *Hemophilus influenzae* β-bacteremia, *Pediatr Emerg Care* 2:23-25, 1986.

Toothache

79. Megran DW, Scheifele DW, Chow AW: Odontogenic infections, *Pediatr Infect Dis J* 3:257, 1984.
80. Rapp R: Dental and gingival disorders. In Bluestone CD, Stool WE, Scheetz MD: *Pediatric otolaryngology*, ed 2, Philadelphia, 1990, WB Saunders.
81. Kahn CS: "Dry socket": etiology and management, *Compendium* 10:48, 1989.
82. Solberg WK and Graff-Radford SB: Orodental considerations in facial pain, *Semin Neurol* 8:318, 1988.
83. Kureishi A and Chow AW: The tender tooth: dentoalveolar, pericoronal and periodontal infections, *Infect Dis Clin North Am* 2:163, 1988.
84. Thaller SR and Thaller JL: Handling dental emergencies when the dentist's away, *Emerg Med* Feb 28, 1990.

Foreign Body in the Ear and Nose

85. Williams PL, editor: *Gray's anatomy*, Philadelphia, 1989, WB Saunders.
86. Bergstrom L: Diseases of the external ear. In Bluestone CD, Stool WE, Scheetz MD, editors: *Pediatric otolaryngology*, Philadelphia, 1990, WB Saunders.

87. Marrone MP, Goodwin M, Genovese M: A unique foreign body in the nose: case report, *Ann Dent* 27:156, 1968.
88. McAndrew PG: The lost tooth, *J Dent* 4:144, 1976.
89. Malhotra C, Arora MML, Mehua YN: An unusual foreign body in the nose, *J Laryngol Otol* 84:539, 1970.
90. Appleton SS, Kimbrough RE, Engstrom HIM: Rhinolithiasis: a review, *Oral Surg Oral Med Oral Pathol* 65(6):693, 1988.
91. Forrest AW: A large foreign body in the nose, *J Laryngol Otol* 101:1280, 1987.
92. Polson CJ: On rhinoliths, *J Laryngol Otol* 58:79, 1943.
93. Jones DC, O'Bree WD, Macintyre DDR: Intranasal foreign body: an incidental radiographic finding, *Dental Update* 14:408, 1987.
94. Nazif M: A rubber dam clamp in the nasal cavity: report of case, *J Am Dent Assoc* 82:1099, 1971.
95. Shapiro RS: Foreign bodies of the nose. In Bluestone CD, Stool WE, Scheetz MD, editors: *Pediatric otolaryngology*, Philadelphia, 1990, WB Saunders.
96. Golding IM: An unusual cause of bromidrosis, *Pediatrics* 36:791, 1965.
97. Katz HP, Katz JR, Bernstein M, et al: Unusual presentation of foreign bodies in children, *JAMA* 241:1496, 1979.
98. Feinstein RJ: Nasal foreign bodies and bromidrosis, *JAMA* 242:1031, 1979 (letter).
99. Stegman JC: Unusual presentation of nasal foreign bodies, *Am J Dis Child* 141:239, 1987 (letter).
100. Palmer O et al: Button battery in the nose-an unusual foreign body, *J Laryngol Otol* 108:871-872, 1994.
101. Brownstein DR and Hodge D III: Foreign bodies of the eye, ear, and nose, *Pediatr Emerg Care* 4:215, 1988.
102. Henry LN and Chamberlain JW: Removal of foreign bodies from esophagus and nose with the use of a Foley catheter, *Surgery* 71:918, 1972.
103. Messervy M: Forced expiration in treatment of nasal foreign bodies, *Practitioner* 210:242, 1973.

Lymphadenitis

104. *Stedman's medical dictionary*, Baltimore, 1990, Williams & Wilkins.
105. Robbins S: *Pathologic basis of disease*, Philadelphia, 1974, WB Saunders.
106. Williams PL, editor: *Gray's anatomy*, Philadelphia, 1989, WB Saunders.
107. Barton LL and Feigen RD: Childhood cervical lymphadenitis: a reappraisal, *J Pediatr* 84:846, 1974.
108. Dajani AS, Garcia RE, Wolinsky E: Etiology of cervical lymphadenitis in children, *N Engl J Med* 268:1329, 1963.
109. Scobie WG: Acute suppurative adenitis in children: a review of 964 cases, *Scott Med J* 14:352, 1969.
110. Yamauchi T, Ferrieri P, Anthony BF: The aetiology of acute cervical adenitis in children: serological and bacteriological studies, *J Med Microbiol* 13:37, 1980.
111. Stanievich J: Cervical adenopathy. In Bluestone CD, Stool WE, Scheetz MD, editors: *Pediatric otolaryngology*, Philadelphia, 1990, WB Saunders.
112. Rathore MH: Group B streptococcal cellulitis and adenitis concurrent with meningitis, *Clin Pediatr (Phila)* 28:411, 1989.
113. Crandall JP and Shah BR: Group B streptococcal lymphadenitis in a child with AIDS, *Clin Pediatr (Phila)* 27:404, 1988.
114. Aburajab A: Necrotizing lymphadenitis: case report and review of the literature, *Trop Geogr Med* 40:64, 1988.
115. Hoyt DJ and Fisher SR: Kikuchi's disease causing cervical lymphadenopathy, *Otolaryngol Head Neck Surg* 102:755, 1990.
116. White MP, Bangash H, Goel KM, et al: Nontuberculous mycobacterial lymphadenitis, *Arch Dis Child* 61:368, 1986.
117. Schaad UB, Votteler TP, McCracken GH, et al: Management of atypical mycobacterial lymphadenitis in childhood: a review based on 380 cases, *J Pediatr* 95:356, 1979.
118. Wright JE: Cervical lymphadenitis in childhood: which antibiotic agent? *Med J Aust* 150:150, February, 1989.

Mastoiditis

119. Zoller H: Acute mastoiditis and its complications, *South Med J* 65(4):477, 1972.
120. Williams PL, editor: *Gray's anatomy*, Philadelphia, 1989, WB Saunders Co.

121. Nadal D, Hermann P, Baumann A, et al: Acute mastoiditis: clinical, microbiological, and therapeutic aspects, *Eur J Pediatr* 149:560, 1990.

122. Rogers SM, Wedro BC, Overholt SL: Emergency presentation of coalescent mastoiditis, *Am J Emerg Med* 7(4):413, 1989.

123. Luntz M, et al: Acute mastoiditis-revisited, *Ear Nose Throat J* 73:9, 1994.

124. Scott TA and Jackler RK: Acute mastoiditis in infancy: a sequela of unrecognized acute otitis media, *Otolaryngol Head Neck Surg* 101(6):683, 1989.

125. Pfaltz CR: Complications of acute otitis media in children, *Adv Otorhinolaryngol* 40:70, 1988.

126. Ogle JW and Lauer BA: Acute mastoiditis, *Am J Dis Child* 140:1178, November 1986.

127. Puczynski MS, Stankiewicz JA, Ow PE: Mucocutaneous lymph node syndrome mimicking acute coalescent mastoiditis, *Am J Otol* 7(1):71, 1986.

128. Bluestone CD and Klein JO: Otitis media, atelectasis, and eustachian tube dysfunction. In Bluestone CD, Stool WE, Scheetz MD, editors: *Pediatric otolaryngology*, Philadelphia, 1990, WB Saunders.

129. Bluestone CD and Klein JO: Intratemporal complications and sequelae of otitis media. In Bluestone CD, Stool WE, Scheetz MD, editors: *Pediatric otolaryngology*, Philadelphia, 1990, WB Saunders.

130. Scheibel WR and Urtes MA: Mastoiditis, *AFP* 35(6):123, 1987.

Otitis Externa, Acute

131. Bergstrom L: Diseases of the external ear. In Bluestone CD, Stool WE, Scheetz MD, editors: *Pediatric otolaryngology*, Philadelphia, 1990, WB Saunders.

132. Strauss MB and Dierker RL: Otitis externa associated with aquatic activities (swimmer's ear), *Clin Dermatol* 5(3):103, 1987.

133. Russell JD, et al: What causes acute otitis externa? *J Larnygol Otol* 107:898-901, 1993.

134. Liston SL and Siegel LG: Tinactin in the treatment of fungal otitis externa, *Laryngoscope* 96:699, June, 1986.

135. Nir D, Nir T, Danino J, et al: Malignant external otitis in an infant, *J Laryngol Otol* 104:488, June, 1990.

136. Wolff LJ: Necrotizing otitis externa during induction therapy for acute lymphoblastic leukemia, *Pediatrics* 84(5):882, 1989.

137. Esterly NB: Eczema. In Behrman RE and Vaughn VC, editors: *Nelson's textbook of pediatrics*, Philadelphia, 1987, WB Saunders.

138. Stewart IA, Guy AM, Sherwen PJ: Topical antibiotics in otitis externa, *N Z Med J* 99(812):816, 1986.

139. Clayton MI, Osborne JE, Rutherford D, et al: A double-blind, randomized, prospective trial of a topical antiseptic versus a topical antibiotic in the treatment of otorrhoea, *Clin Otolaryngol* 15:7, 1990.

140. Slack RWT: A study of three preparations in the treatment of otitis externa, *J Laryngol Otol* 101:533, 1987.

141. Smith RB and Moodle J: A general practice study to compare the efficacy and tolerability of a spray ('Otomize') versus a standard drop formulation ('Sofradex') in the treatment of patients with otitis externa, *Curr Med Res Opin* 12(1):12, 1990.

142. Ruth M, Ekstrom T, Aberg B, et al: A clinical comparison of hydrocortisone butyrate with oxytetracycline/hydrocortisone acetate-polymyxin B in the local treatment of acute external otitis, *Eur Arch Otorhinolaryngol* 247:77, 1990.

Otitis Media

143. Bluestone CD: Modern management of otitis media, *Pediatr Clin North Am* 36(6):1371, 1989.

144. Bluestone CD and Klein JO: Otitis media, atelectasis, and eustachian tube function. In Bluestone CD, Stool SE, Scheetz MD, editors: *Pediatric Otolaryngology*, Philadelphia, 1990, WB Saunders.

145. Lisby-Sutch SM, Nemec-Dwyer MA, Deeter RG, et al: Therapy of otitis media, *Clin Pharm* 9:15, 1990.

146. Williams PL, editor: *Gray's anatomy*, Philadelphia, 1989, WB Saunders.

147. Kemp ED: Otitis media, *Prim Care* 17(2):267, 1990.

148. Van Hare GF et al: Acute otitis media caused by *Branhamella catarrhalis*: biology and therapy, *Rev Infect Dis* 9(1):16, 1987.

149. Heikkinen T and Ruuskanen O: Signs and symptoms predicting acute otitis media, *Arch Pediatr Adolesc Med* 149:26-29, 1995.

150. Schwartz RH: Pneumatic otoscopy: getting the most out of the ear exam, *J Resp Dis* 4(5):82, 1983.

151. Jacobsson M, Nylen O, Tjellstrom A: Acute otitis media and facial palsy in children, *Acta Paediatr* 79:118, 1990.

152. Farrior J: Complications of otitis media in children, *South Med J* 83(6):645, 1990.

153. Koltai PJ, Maisel BO, Seskin F, et al: Otitis media in the immunosuppressed child, *Ear Nose Throat J* 67:88, 1988.

154. Jehle D and Cottington E: Acoustic otoscopy in the diagnosis of otitis media, *Ann Emerg Med* 18(4):396, 1989.

155. Kempthorne J and Giebink GS: Pediatric approach to the diagnosis and management of otitis media, *Otolaryngol Clin N Am* 24:4, 1991.

156. Marchant CD, et al: Measuring the comparative efficacy of antibacterial agents for acute otitis media: the "Pollyanna phenomenon," *J Pediatr* 120:1, 1992.

157. Bergeron MG, Ahronheim G, Richard JE, et al: Comparative efficacy of erythromycin-sulfisoxazole and cefaclor in acute otitis media: a double blind randomized trial, *Pediatr Infect Dis J* 6:654, 1987.

158. Carlin SA, Marchant CD, Shurin PA, et al: Early recurrences of otitis media: reinfection or relapse? *J Pediatr* 110:20, 1987.

159. Harrison CJ, Marks MI, Welch DF: Microbiology of recently treated acute otitis media compared with previously untreated acute otitis media, *Pediatr Infect Dis J* 4:641, 1985.

160. Kaleida PH, Bluestone CD, Blatter MM, et al: Sultamicillin (ampicillin-sulbactam) in the treatment of acute otitis media in children, *Pediatr Infect Dis J* 5:33, 1986.

161. Kaleida PH, Bluestone CD, Rockette HE, et al: Amoxicillin-clavulanate potassium compared with cefaclor for acute otitis media in infants and children, *Pediatr Infect Dis J* 6:265, 1987.

162. Kenna MA, Bluestone CD, Fall P, et al: Cefixime vs. cefaclor in the treatment of acute otitis media in infants and children, *Pediatr Infect Dis J* 6:992, 1987.

163. Marchant CD, Shurin PA, Johnson CE, et al: A randomized controlled trial of amoxicillin plus clavulanate compared with cefaclor for treatment of acute otitis media, *J Pediatr* 109:891, 1986.

164. Odio CM, Kusmiesz H, Shelton S, et al: Comparative treatment trial of augmentin versus cefaclor for acute otitis media with effusion, *Pediatrics* 75:819, 1985.

165. Rodriguez WJ, Schwartz RH, Sait T, et al: Erythromycin-sulfisoxazole vs. amoxicillin in treatment of acute otitis media in children, *Am J Dis Child* 139:766, 1985.

166. Feldman W, Momy J, Dulberg C: Trimethoprim-sulfamethoxazole v. amoxicillin in the treatment of acute otitis media, *Can Med Assoc J* 139:961, 1988.

167. Canafax DM and Grebiak GS: Antimicrobial treatment of acute otitis media, *Ann Otol Rhinol Laryngol* 103:11-14, 1994.

168. Green SM, Rothrock SG: Single dose intramuscular ceftriaxone for acute otitis media in children, *Pediatrics* 91:23-30, 1993.

169. McCracken GH: Emergence of resistant streptococcus pneumonia: a problem in pediatrics, *Pediatr Infect Dis J* 14:424-428, 1995.

170. Weiss JC and Melman ST: Cost effectiveness in the choice of antibiotics for the initial treatment of otitis media in children: a decision analysis approach, *Pediatr Infect Dis J* 7:23, 1988.

171. Schutzman SA, et al: Bacteremia with otitis media. *Pediatrics* 87:1, 1991.

172. Pelton SI and Klein JO: The draining ear—otitis media and externa, *Infect Dis Clin North Am* 2(1):117, 1988.

Parotitis and Salivary Gland Infections

173. Seibert RW: Diseases of the salivary glands. In Bluestone CD, Stool SE, Scheetz MD, editors: *Pediatric otolaryngology*, ed 2, Philadelphia, 1990, WB Saunders.

174. Meyer C and Cotton RT: Salivary gland disease in children: a review, *Clin Pediatr* 26:314, 1986.

175. Richardson MA: The neck: embryology and anatomy. In Bluestone CD, Stool SE, Scheets MD, editors: *Pediatric otolaryngology*, ed 2, Philadelphia, 1990, WB Saunders.

176. Megran DW, Scheifele DW, Chow AW: Odontogenic infections, *Pediatr Infect Dis J* 3:257, 1984.

177. Loughran DH and Smith LG: Infectious disorders of the parotid gland, *N J Med* 4:311, 1988.

178. Jacobs RF, Condrey YM, Yamauchi T: Tularemia in adults and children: a changing presentation, *Pediatrics* 76:818-822, 1985.

Peritonsillar Abscess

179. Shenoy P and David VC: A case of quinsy in a fifteen month old child, *J Laryngol Otol* 107:354, 1993.
180. Baker AS and Montgomery WW: Oropharyngeal space infections, *Curr Clin Top Infect Dis* 8:227, 1987.
181. Hardingham M: Peritonsillar infections, *Otolaryngol Clin North Am* 20:273, 1987.
182. Brodsky L, Sobie SR, Korwin D, et al: A clinical prospective study of peritonsillar abscess in children, *Laryngoscope* 98:780, 1987.
183. Shoemaker M, Lampe RM, Weir MR: Peritonsillitis: abscess or cellulitis? *Pediatr Infect Dis J* 5:435, 1986.
184. Votey S and Dudley JP: Emergency ear, nose, and throat procedures, *Emer Med Clin North Am* 7:149-151, 1989.
185. Weinberg HD: Treatment of otitis media twice daily for five days, *Clin Pediatr* 30:6, 1991.
186. Haeggstrom A, Gustafsson O, Engquist S, et al: Intraoral ultrasonography in the diagnosis of peritonsillar abscess, *Otolaryngol Head Neck Surg* 108:243, 1993.

Retropharyngeal Abscess

187. Thompson JW, Cohen SR, Reddix P: Retropharyngeal abscess in children: a retrospective and historical analysis, *Laryngoscope* 98:589, 1988.
188. McCook TA and Felman AH: Retropharyngeal masses in infants and children, *Am J Dis Child* 133:41, 1979.
189. Berhman RE, Vaughan VC, Nelson WE: *Nelson textbook of pediatrics*, ed 2, Philadelphia, 1987, WB Saunders.
190. Morrison JE and Pashley NRT: Retropharyngeal abscesses in children: a 10-year review, *Pediatr Emerg Care* 4:9, 1988.
191. Grosso J and Myer CM: Radiological cases of the month, *Am J Dis Child* 144:1349, 1990.
192. Asmar BI: Bacteriology of retropharyngeal abscess in children, *Pediatr Infect Dis J* 9:595, 1990.

Sinusitis

193. Wald ER: Rhinitis and acute and chronic sinusitis. In Bluestone CD, Stool SE, Scheetz MD, editors: *Pediatric Otolaryngology*, ed 2, Philadelphia, 1990, WB Saunders.
194. Seigle JD: Diagnosis and management of acute sinusitis in children, *Pediatr Infect Dis J* 6:95-99, 1987.
195. Wald ER: Sinusitis in children, *Pediatr Infect Dis J* 7:S150-S153, 1988.
196. Rachelefsky GS: Chronic sinusitis: the disease of all ages, *Am J Dis Child* 143:886-888, 1989.
197. Turkewitz D and Keller R: Acute headache in childhood: a case of sphenoid sinusitis, *Pediatr Emerg Care* 3:155-157, 1987.

Streptococcal Tonsillopharyngitis

198. Kenna MA: Sore throat in children: diagnosis and management. In Bluestone CD, Stool SE, Scheetz MD, editors: *Pediatric otolaryngology*, ed 2, Philadelphia, 1990, WB Saunders.
199. Medical Letter: Rapid diagnostic test for group A streptococcal pharyngitis, 33:40-41, May 3, 1991.
200. Nelson JD: The effect of penicillin therapy on the symptoms and signs of streptococcal pharyngitis, *Pediatr Infect Dis J* 3:10-13, 1984.
201. Nelson JD: *Pocketbook of pediatric antimicrobial therapy*, ed 9, Baltimore, 1991, Williams & Wilkins.
202. Krober MS, Bass JW, Michels GN: Streptococcal pharyngitis: placebo-controlled double-blind evaluation of clinical response to penicillin therapy, *JAMA* 253:1271-1274, 1985.
203. Randolph MF, Gerber MA, DeMeo KK, et al: The effect of antibiotic therapy on the clinical course of streptococcal pharyngitis, *J Pediatr* 106:870-875, 1985.

Endocrine and Metabolic Disorders

Richard A. Saladino

Signs and Symptoms

FAILURE TO THRIVE/GROWTH DEFICIENCY

Definition

Failure to thrive/growth deficiency (FTT/GD) refers to an infant or child with growth failure. Traditionally, FTT/GD was considered failure to gain weight consistent with peers of the same age.[1] In particular, FTT/GD has been defined as weight below the fifth or third percentile on a weight and height chart or as weight 20% or more below the ideal weight for an infant's height.[2,3] More important than a single measurement, though, is detection of a slowing of the velocity of growth or a falloff from a previously appropriate growth curve. Failure to grow or gain weight appropriately occurs in the presence of organic and nonorganic illness, but these causes are not mutually exclusive. Given these considerations, *growth deficiency* more accurately describes this disorder.[4]

Pathophysiology

Poor caloric intake results in poor weight gain and growth, but FTT/GD is often complex in pathogenesis and etiology. Many congenital or acquired organic illnesses may result in a child's failure to grow because of the inherent pathophysiologic condition. Furthermore, children with chronic illness may have a psychosocial component to the poor growth. Purely nonorganic failure to grow has long been described as a specific entity; careful investigation has shown that psychosocial difficulties compound diminished growth in one fourth to one half of patients with organic illnesses and failure to grow.[5,6]

Differential Considerations

Although nonorganic causes are most common, one third to one half of patients with FTT/GD have underlying organic disease, but up to half of these patients also have psychosocial problems.[3,6] Common causes of FTT/GD are outlined in the box on p. 756. FTT/GD may not be caused by only one disease and should not be approached as a diagnosis by exclusion. Rather, an investigation for positive organic and nonorganic findings should proceed when evaluating a child who has not grown appropriately.

Failure to gain weight when the child has normal height and head circumference is due to inadequate caloric intake or absorption, or to organic causes of increased caloric requirements (e.g., hyperthyroidism or chronic infection). Normal head circumference with depressed weight and linear growth are manifestations of intrauterine growth retardation or endocrine disease. Abnormally small head circumference is usually due to congenital defects or central nervous system (CNS) disease.

Diagnostic Work-Up

History. The most important component in the evaluation of the child who fails to grow appropriately is a detailed history, including psychosocial data (e.g., family makeup, living arrangements, socioeconomic status, and stressors in the home and at work); see the box on p. 756. Growth records should be obtained and examined. Weight, height, and head circumference measurements should be plotted on standard growth curves (see Appendix A) to determine the patterns of growth failure. Physical, environmental, or social changes that are temporally related to a growth fall off should be noted. Finally, constitutional growth delay may be identified by obtaining growth records of parents and siblings.

Physical Examination. A careful examination is imperative to identify congenital causes of FTT/GD and to detect physical findings of systemic disease (see box on p. 756). Observation in the emergency department and during hospitalization may provide clues to feeding and emotional difficulties, or situations of neglect or abuse. Signs of neglect may include poor hygiene, severe diaper rash, impe-

Common Causes of Failure to Grow

ORGANIC CAUSES

Congenital

Genetic syndromes (e.g., Turner, Noonan, Williams, Russell-Silver)
Inborn errors of metabolism

Gastrointestinal

Malabsorption syndromes, including cystic fibrosis
Inflammatory bowel disease
Liver disease
Obstructive disease (e.g., pyloric stenosis, Hirschsprung disease)

Cardiopulmonary

Congenital heart disease
Cystic fibrosis
Chronic lung disease (e.g., bronchopulmonary dysplasia, severe asthma)

Renal

Anatomic abnormalities with renal failure
Chronic infection
Renal tubular acidosis

Immunologic

Severe combined immunodeficiency
DiGeorge syndrome
Acquired immunodeficiency syndrome

Endocrinologic

Hypopituitarism
Thyroid disease
Diabetes mellitus (DM)

NONORGANIC CAUSES

Parent-child dysfunction

Perinatal factors (e.g., insufficient family and emotional support systems)
Neonatal factors (e.g., bonding and feeding problems)
"Difficult child"
Developmental delay
Attentional disorders
Care requirements for chronic disease

Family psychosocial dysfunction

Socioeconomic factors
Family discord
Child abuse or neglect

Historic Considerations for FTT/GD

Pregnancy	Intrauterine growth retardation Medicine/drug exposures
Perinatal	Complications during the immediate postnatal period
Nutritional	Feeding: formulas, feeding patterns, problems
Medical	Review of systems, illnesses
Growth	Obtain records to track growth: weight, length, head circumference
Development	Motor, language and behavioral developmental milestones
Family history	Parental heights, growth patterns, inherited diseases
Psychosocial	Family stress, parental interpretation of growth deficit

tigo, and inappropriate parent-infant behaviors (e.g., lack of eye contact, smiling, or cuddling). Feeding patterns and parental bonding are observed as well.

Ancillary Data. Laboratory and radiologic testing does not usually help in the evaluation of infants and children with FTT/GD.[5,6] However, judiciously applied testing may yield different diagnoses. Screening studies include urinalysis, electrolyte and glucose determinations (renal dis-

ease and diabetes mellitus), peripheral WBC count, erythrocyte sedimentation rate and urine culture (infection), hematologic indices (anemia), and radiologic evaluation of bone age. Investigation of many of the organic causes may require additional studies.[7]

Therapeutic Trial

Initial therapy for infants and children with FTT/GD includes correction of any fluid and electrolyte abnormalities. Identifiable underlying organic disorders may also require treatment. Initiation of appropriate and specific alimentation should begin only after the child is physiologically stable. Involvement of medical and psychosocial personnel should accompany parental observation and involvement, and careful follow-up visits must always be arranged.

Disposition

In the case of severe undernutrition, hospitalization is mandatory to carefully correct altered fluid and electrolyte status, and to monitor response to therapy. Outpatient management of children with less severe growth deficiency requires close and frequent contact with the primary health-care providers. The entire health-care team (e.g., physicians, social services personnel, nutritional support staff, and visiting nurses) must guide and monitor the progress of the patient. Growth and psychomotor development must be observed and recorded regularly. Attention to the child and the family provides a supportive environment that optimizes growth potential.

HYPOGLYCEMIA

Definition

Hypoglycemia in infants and children is defined by a serum glucose concentration less than 40 mg/dl in a child and less than 30 mg/dl in full-term and preterm neonates.[8] These definitions are practical, although somewhat controversial.[9,10] Some authors suggest that hypoglycemia is defined by a blood glucose concentration less than 45 mg/dl, regardless of age.[10,11] This is a chemical diagnosis, and hypoglycemia in childhood should be interpreted in the context of age, precipitating factors, and symptoms.

Pathophysiology

An optimum blood glucose level is maintained via exogenous substrate supply (i.e., oral intake of carbohydrates, protein, and fats), and appropriate gluconeogenesis and glycogenolysis. In turn, mobilization and use of glucose is hormonally mediated by insulin, epinephrine, glucagon, cortisol, and growth hormone.

In the fasting state, glucose is the product of hepatic glycogenolysis and gluconeogenesis. Muscle stores of glycogen are not available as free glucose, but as liberated amino acids—in particular, alanine and glycine—that are used in gluconeogenic pathways. Lactate, which is generated in various tissues, is an important precursor for gluconeogenesis through the Krebs cycle. Finally, lipolysis occurs during fasting, generating free fatty acids and glycerol, which are useful fuel sources.[10,12]

The balance of glycogenolysis and gluconeogenesis with glycogen synthesis and peripheral use of glucose is primarily a function of the secretion of insulin. Insulin stimulates glucose uptake in skeletal and cardiac muscle and adipose tissue and affects various anabolic conversions, including glycogen synthesis. The result is a lowering of blood glucose concentrations. Hormones that oppose the effect of insulin—glucagon, cortisol, catecholamines, and growth hormone—inhibit glucose uptake into muscle, activate lipolysis, mobilize amino acids for gluconeogenesis, and hence raise blood glucose concentrations.[10,13]

Hypoglycemia occurs when any of these mechanisms are altered. Exogenous sources must be present because fasting is not tolerated by the body for prolonged periods, especially in a small or ill child. Defects in the enzymes necessary for endogenous glucose supply result in less effective glucose homeostasis and leave the child at higher risk for hypoglycemia. Finally, abnormalities of the hormonal control of glucose metabolism can result in hypoglycemia.

Differential Considerations

The causes of hypoglycemia in infancy and childhood, based on the preceding discussion of pathophysiologic conditions, are outlined in the box above. Insufficient exogenous substrate is common in childhood because decreased intake or absorption often accompanies many infectious illnesses. Chronic malnutrition or malabsorption syndromes predispose the child to hypoglycemia because of resultant inadequate body energy stores.

Inborn errors of metabolism include disorders of hepatic gluconeogenesis, glycogenolysis, glycogen storage diseases, and enzyme defects of amino acid mobilization. In particular, *glycogen storage diseases* usually are accompanied by hepatomegaly and hypoglycemia. Characteristic features vary with the type of disease but may include poor feeding, vomiting, diarrhea, growth failure, jaundice, protuberant abdomen, acidemia, hyperlipidemia, hyperuricemia, and bleeding diathesis. The most common form of galactose metabolism is classic galactosemia. Normal at birth, infants

---

Pathogenesis of Hypoglycemia in Childhood

Diminished substrate

Exogenous sources

Decreased intake
  Fasting
  Anorexia: illness-related or psychiatric
  Chronic malnutrition
Decreased absorption
  Infection: diarrheal illness
  Malabsorption syndromes

Endogenous sources (inborn errors of metabolism)

Gluconeogenic enzyme deficiencies
Glycogenolytic enzyme deficiencies
Inadequate glycogen storage diseases
Amino acid metabolism defects

Abnormal hormonal mediation

Hypopituitarism
Hypothyroidism
Adrenal insufficiency (congenital adrenal hyperplasia)

Inappropriate insulin

Endogenous causes: nesidioblastosis and islet cell adenoma
Exogenous causes: insulin therapy and oral hypoglycemic agents

Associated disorders

Sepsis
Reye syndrome
Poisonings (e.g., salicylates, ethanol, and propranolol)

---

with galactosemia experience vomiting, diarrhea, jaundice, and FTT/GD in the first month of life. Hepatomegaly, ascites, peripheral edema, and cataracts may be noted. Renal tubular dysfunction manifests as galactosuria, proteinuria, and aminoaciduria. Liver failure and sepsis are life-threatening complications of galactosemia. Hereditary fructose intolerance produces symptoms with the ingestion of fructose. Hypoglycemia may then manifest as vomiting, pallor, diaphoresis, lethargy, and seizures. In addition, FTT/GD, hepatosplenomegaly, acidemia, fructosuria, and liver and renal failure (with related findings) may be noted.

Children with growth hormone deficiency, hypothyroidism, and cortisol deficiency (e.g., congenital adrenal hyperplasia) are prone to hypoglycemia because they lack some degree of insulin-opposing effect.[13,14] Conversely, excess insulin, whether endogenous or exogenous in origin, is a cause of hypoglycemia. In particular, hypoglycemia as a complication of the insulin therapy of diabetes mellitus is common in children.

A number of syndromes are associated with hypoglycemia resulting from high blood insulin concentration.[14] Nesidioblastosis is the most common cause of hypoglycemia in the neonate and is due to pancreatic beta-cell dysfunction with abnormal islet cells budding from the ductile elements. Neonates with Beckwith-Wiedemann (macroglossia-microcephaly-gigantism) syndrome may have hypoglycemia due to beta-cell hyperplasia. In the first 24 hours of life, the neonate with islet cell adenoma experiences hypoglycemia and seizures.

Hypoglycemia from other causes must not be overlooked. Low blood sugar is often present in the infected infant or young child. Reye syndrome after influenza or varicella infection often occurs with hypoglycemia, especially in younger patients.[8,15] Finally, toxic ingestions frequently are complicated by hypoglycemia, especially with aspirin, ethanol, insulin, oral hypoglycemic agents, and propranolol.[8]

Diagnostic Work-Up

History. Historic data are extremely important in the evaluation of a patient with hypoglycemia. Dietary intake must be considered, especially in the context of infection; most children have poor oral intake during acute illnesses and may predispose themselves to hypoglycemia. The possibility of a toxic ingestion must always be investigated. Family history may reveal a hereditary pattern.

Physical Examination. Signs and symptoms of hypoglycemia may be absent or few and subtle. Infants especially manifest nonspecific symptoms, including irritability, lethargy, vomiting, pallor or cyanosis, tachycardia, and tachypnea; these symptoms are also present in sepsis and must be evaluated and treated as indicated. Hypoglycemic children can manifest the adrenergic symptoms of low blood glucose (i.e., nervousness, diaphoresis, tremor, and altered mental status), which may progress to seizures or coma.

Ancillary Data. Any acutely ill child should be evaluated for hypoglycemia. Prompt diagnosis is imperative and is made by serum glucose measurement, although rapid assessment should be made using a glucose-specific coated strip (e.g., Chemstrip bG).* Urine should be analyzed for glucose, ketone bodies, and non–glucose-reducing substances. Further studies should be guided by historical data and contextual information. Serum and urine should be obtained for indicated studies such as plasma insulin, plasma glucagon, and serum lactate liver function tests, and a comprehensive screen for toxins should be sent if there is a suspicion that a toxic substance has been ingested.

Therapeutic Trial

Rapidly delivered IV glucose 0.25 to 0.50 gm/kg is the treatment for hypoglycemia. It can be given as 25% dextrose in water 1 to 2 ml/kg. Appropriate serum glucose levels can then be maintained by continuous infusion of dextrose-containing IV fluids, 4 to 6 mg/kg/min.[13,16] Glucagon 0.1 to 0.2 mg/kg IM can be used if excess insulin is known to be present. Underlying illness should be expeditiously evaluated and treated.

Patients who have less severe hypoglycemia may be treated with oral sources of glucose when appropriate. Approximately 20 gm of glucose is present in milk (13 oz), orange or apple juice (12 oz), Coca-cola (13 oz), ginger ale (15 oz), or a Hershey's milk chocolate bar (2 oz).

*Available from Boehringer Mannheim, Inc, Indianapolis, IN.

Diagnostic Entities

ADRENAL HYPERPLASIA, CONGENITAL

Congenital adrenal hyperplasia (CAH) is a group of disorders that result from enzymatic defects in adrenocortical synthesis of cortisol, and are inherited as autosomal traits.[17] Impaired cortisol production, resulting from a specific enzyme defect, results in chronic elevation of plasma corticotropin levels via negative feedback at the anterior pituitary. Corticotropin excess results histologically in hyperplasia of the adrenal cortex. Steroidogenic enzyme deficiencies manifest differently, depending on their place in the synthetic pathway. Nearly 95% of cases of CAH are a result of 21-hydroxylase deficiency, a relatively common inborn error of metabolism with an incidence as high as one in 10,000 births in a Caucasian population.[18,19] The salt-wasting form of "classic" 21-hydroxylase often leads to acute adrenal insufficiency in the first weeks of life of an infant with CAH; the acute condition necessitates prompt evaluation and treatment.[11,16,20]

Pathophysiology

CAH results from an enzymatic defect at any one of the five steps of cortisol synthesis from cholesterol (Fig. 50-1).[18,19] The biochemical result of such a blockade in synthesis is accumulation of the steroid precursors proximal to the defect; these precursors are then shunted toward the androgen biosynthetic pathway. Enzyme deficiencies may be incomplete or total, so clinical expression of CAH is variable.[17,21]

A 21-hydroxylase deficiency occurs in 90% to 95% of CAH cases. There are two variants of 21-hydroxylase deficiency: simple virilizing and salt-wasting. One third of patients with 21-hydroxylase deficiency manifest virilization.[21] Diminished cortisol production leads to hypersecretion of corticotropin, in turn resulting in an accumulation of pregnenolone and subsequent overproduction of virilizing androgens. Two thirds of patients with 21-hydroxylase deficiency also have a deficiency in aldosterone synthesis, and their bodies less efficiently conserve sodium and excrete potassium.[18,19] Clinical and biochemical evidence of classic CAH is often present at birth or in the first weeks of life. Patients with "nonclassic" 21–hydroxylase-deficient CAH are born without clinical or biochemical abnormalities but develop signs of androgen overproduction at any age and to varying degrees.[18,22] For this reason, nonclassic 21-hydroxylase deficiency is referred to as *late-onset* or *attenuated CAH*.

Although infrequently seen, 11 beta-hydroxylase deficiency accounts for approximately 3% of CAH cases. In addition to virilization like that seen in 21-hydroxylase deficiency, patients with 11 beta-hydroxylase deficiency can have significant hypertension.[20,23] Accumulation of 11-desoxycorticosterone occurs, and its mineralocorticoid effect results in sodium and water retention and varying degrees of hypertension.[21,22]

Etiology

The diminished enzymatic activity in CAH may involve any step of steroid synthesis; defects have been described

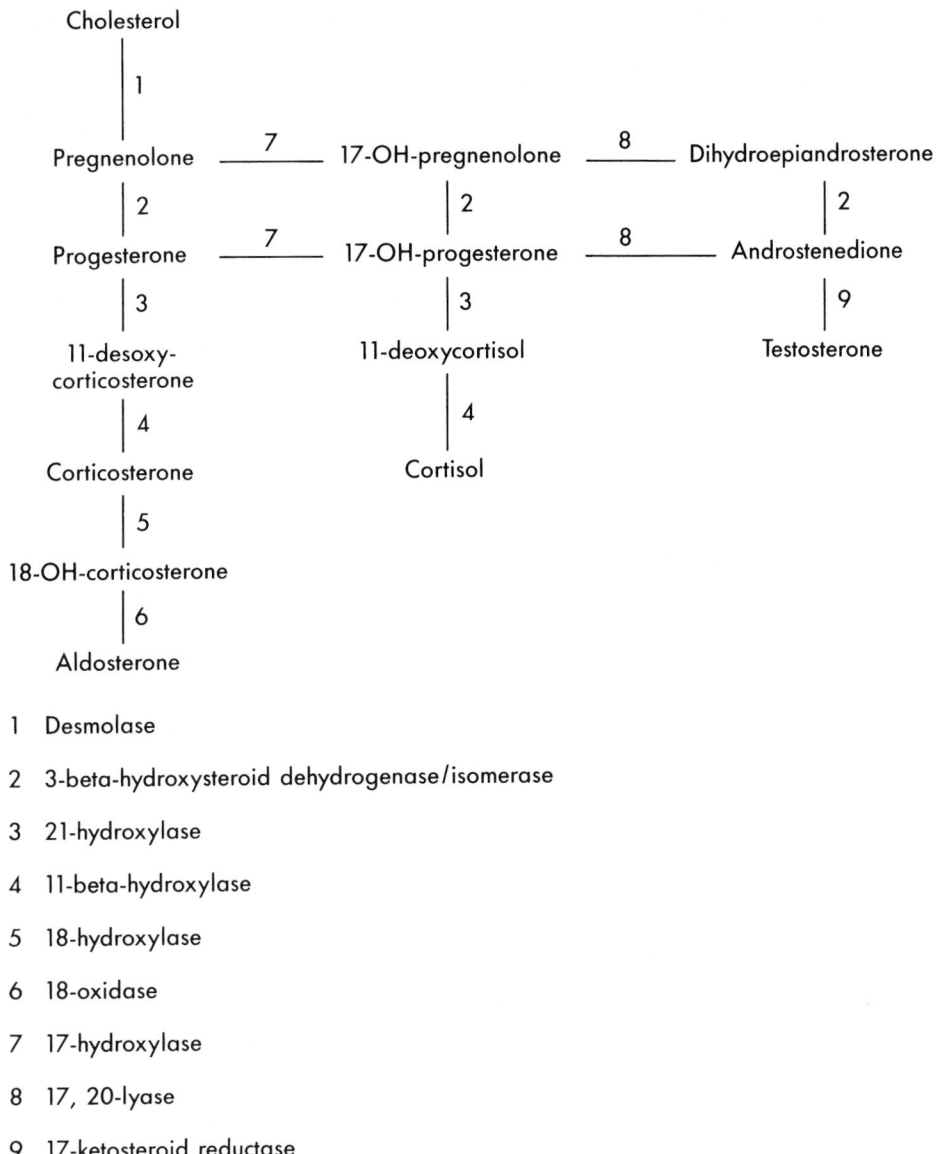

FIG. 50-1. Adrenocorticosteroid synthetic pathways.

for 21-hydroxylase, 11 beta-hydroxylase, 3 beta-hydroxysteroid dehydrogenase, 17-hydroxylase and 17,20 lyase. All have well-described biochemical profiles.[3] In addition, human leukocyte antigen (HLA) linkage and genetic mapping have located the genes for these inherited disorders, allowing earlier detection and definitive diagnosis of the different forms of CAH.[17-22]

Diagnostic Findings

Clinical Findings and Complications. These findings follow from the biochemical derangements of specific enzyme deficiencies. Classic virilizing CAH is unlikely to necessitate emergent care. Often the diagnosis is suspected at birth in a girl because of virilized ambiguous genitalia whereas male infants are at higher risk for a missed diagnosis. Patients with classic salt-wasting CAH are more likely to need emergent intervention, usually in the first few weeks of life.[24,25] Signs of adrenal crisis (insufficiency) may be present and include lethargy, vomiting, and dehydration (see box on p. 760). Cardiovascular instability may manifest as tachycardia, poor peripheral perfusion, and hypotension. Vascular collapse may lead to death. In both forms, virilization may be obvious or undetectable. Classic simple virilizing and, more so, nonclassic CAH often occur later in childhood or puberty. Virilization may be present at birth as mild-to-prominent clitoromegaly or complete labial fusion in a girl. Later signs of virilization in either sex include precocious appearance of pubic hair, accelerated somatic growth, and early fusion of epiphyses.[22,23,25] Hyperpigmentation may be present in the axillae and groin, especially at the scrotum and labia; this results from the presence of the corticotropin precursor, proopiomelanocortin.[18]

Ancillary Data. Laboratory findings in CAH result from the enzyme deficiencies and subsequent altered steroidogenesis.[26,27] Hyponatremia and hyperkalemia may be apparent in classic salt-wasting CAH because of diminished mineralocorticoid (aldosterone) levels. Hypoglycemia may

---

Acute Adrenal Insufficiency (Addisonian Crisis)

Historic findings:	Fatigue, weakness
	Anorexia
	Abdominal pain
	Vomiting
Physical examination findings:	Unexplained fever
	Hypotension or shock
	Confusion or coma
	Abdominal pain
Laboratory findings:	Unexplained hypoglycemia
	Hyponatremia
	Hyperkalemia
	Acidosis
	Decreased serum cortisol

Initial Management of Acute Adrenal Insufficiency

Immediate intervention

Patent airway

Supplemental oxygen if altered mental status or shock occurs

Restoration of intravascular volume: intravenous normal saline, 10 to 20 ml/kg

Correction of hypoglycemia: IV 25% dextrose in water, 2 ml/kg

Treatment with glucocorticoid*

First dose (stress dose): IV hydrocortisone, 36 to 60 mg/m^2

Maintenance doses: IV or oral hydrocortisone, 15 mg/m^2 day in two or three divided doses

Treatment with mineralocorticoids

Oral fludrocortisone (Florinef), 0.1 to 0.2 mg/24 hr

*Basal secretion rate of cortisol is 12 to 15 mg/m^2/day.[13] Stress dose of glucocorticoid is considered 3 to 5 times the maintenance dose.

---

be present, resulting from low levels of cortisol and complicated by poor feeding or vomiting. Hence, blood should be drawn for electrolyte and glucose measurements, and an electrocardiogram should be performed to evaluate for hyperkalemia with peaked T waves. Arterial blood gas determination should be done if evidence of cardiovascular instability or significant dehydration is present. Furthermore, blood and urine samples should be obtained to measure cortisol precursors and adrenal androgens, and plasma cortisol, aldosterone, and renin levels. Consultation with a pediatric endocrinologist is essential.

Differential Considerations

Any infant with lethargy, vomiting, and dehydration may have overwhelming sepsis. Evaluation for and treatment of sepsis should precede or coincide with the evaluation and treatment of CAH. Other inborn errors of metabolism should be considered. Abdominal problems, including malrotation with volvulus and necrotizing enterocolitis, should be excluded because they often occur with lethargy, poor feeding, vomiting, hypoglycemia, and cardiovascular instability. Finally, hypertrophic pyloric stenosis should be considered because vomiting and dehydration often occur during the first several weeks of life but infants with these problems commonly have characteristically different electrolyte abnormalities.

Management

Prehospital considerations should address management of airway compromise and shock. If an infant or child is known to have adrenal insufficiency, intramuscular hydrocortisone or cortisone acetate can be given by the caretakers at home or by transport personnel before arriving at the emergency department.[28]

Upon arrival to the emergency department, the infant with salt-losing crisis must be immediately assessed for adequacy of a patent airway, especially if the patient is in a depressed mental status or coma. Oxygen should be ad-ministered to any infant who has altered consciousness or evidence of shock. Intravascular volume should be rapidly restored with intravenous saline (see box above). Sodium and fluid deficits can be calculated and repleted over 24 to 36 hours.

Glucocorticoid therapy should be initiated with fluid therapy when cardiovascular collapse is present (Table 50-1). When the diagnosis is suspected and the infant is otherwise stable, blood should be obtained for steroid analysis before glucocorticoid administration.[27] Hydrocortisone is a physiologically active glucocorticoid and should be given as a stress dose for adrenal crisis, which is three to four times the physiologic dose. Subsequent doses are physiologic, 12 to 15 mg/m^2/day in two to three divided doses.[16,21,25] After IV fluid and salt repletion has been provided and the infant has resumed feeding, oral mineralocorticoid replacement can begin; usually fludrocortisone (Florinef) is the agent of choice.[16]

Disposition

All infants with adrenal crisis should be hospitalized and carefully monitored. Blood pressure, cardiac rhythm, and changes in electrolyte levels must be tracked. Consultation with an endocrinologist is essential for diagnosis and short- and long-term management. The expression of virilization may require surgical intervention in affected girls. Normal growth and pubertal development depends on appropriate mineralocorticoid use. Finally, mineralocorticoid therapy is guided not by normal serum electrolyte composition but by age-appropriate plasma renin levels.[25]

ADRENAL INSUFFICIENCY, ACUTE

Adrenal insufficiency due to any cause is rare in childhood, but the associated morbidity and mortality require

TABLE 50-1. Adrenal Corticosteroids

Drug	Availability	Dose*	Frequency (hr)	Glucocorticoid effect†	Mineralocorticoid effect†
Glucocorticoids					
Cortisone	IM: 25, 50 mg/ml	0.25 mg/kg/24 hr	q 12-24	100 mg	100 mg
	PO: 5, 25 mg	0.5-0.75 mg/kg/24 hr	q 6-8		
Hydrocortisone	PO: 5, 10, 20 mg	0.5 mg/kg/24 hr	q 8		
(Solu-Cortef)	IV/IM: 100, 250,	Shock‡: 50 mg/kg/dose		80 mg	80 mg
	500 mg	(maximum: 500 mg)			
		Asthma§: 4-5 mg/kg/dose	q 6		
Prednisone	PO: 1, 5, 10, 20 mg,	0.1-0.15 mg/kg/24 hr	q 12	20 mg	Little effect
	5 mg/5 ml	Asthma: 1-2 mg/kg/24 hr	q 6		
Methylprednisolone	IV: 40, 125, 500,	Shock‡: 30-50 mg/kg/dose		16 mg	No effect
(Solu-Medrol)	1000 mg	Asthma: 1-2 mg/kg/dose	q 6		
Dexamethasone	IV/IM: 4, 24 mg/ml	Shock‡: 3 mg/kg/dose		2 mg	No effect
(Decadron)		Cerebral edema‖: 0.25-	q 6		
		0.5 mg/kg/dose			
		Croup: 0.25 mg/kg/dose	q 6		
Mineralocorticoids					
Fludrocortisone	PO: 0.1 mg	0.05-0.1 mg/24 hr	q 24	5 mg	0.2 mg
(Florinef)					
Desoxycorticosterone	IM: 5 mg/ml (in oil)	1-5 mg/24-48 hr	q 24-48	No effect	2 mg
(DOCA)					

From Barkin RM and Rosen P: *Emergency pediatrics*, ed 4, St Louis, 1994, Mosby.
With long-term therapy, dose requires adjustment. Attempt QOD dosing when employing pharmacologic doses. Long-acting preparations for physiologic replacement are available with monthly (or longer) activity.
*Physiologic replacement unless otherwise indicated.
†Equivalent doses required for same clinical effect.
‡Use of steroids for septic shock is controversial and may be detrimental.
§Asthma, status asthmaticus.
‖Remains controversial.

appropriate inclusion of adrenal crisis as a potential etiology of acute illness or decompensation of clinical status in a child.

Pathophysiology

Acute adrenal insufficiency may be primary (Addison disease), secondary (pituitary), or tertiary (hypothalamic). Pathology at any level results in insufficient production of corticosteroids by the adrenal cortex.

Primary adrenal insufficiency results from destruction of adrenal cortical tissue; therefore deficiencies of both mineralocorticoids and glucocorticoids are apparent. The striking features of adrenal crisis are manifest as a lack of the normal glucocorticoid response to stress (infection, trauma, burns, surgery). Aldosterone deficiency is the primary cause of electrolyte disturbances seen in acute adrenal insufficiency.

Secondary and tertiary adrenal insufficiency are primarily pure glucocorticoid deficiency states because mineralocorticoid secretion usually remains normal under the control of the renin-angiotensin system.

Etiology

Primary adrenal insufficiency is rare in childhood; 80% of cases are due to autoimmune destruction of adrenal cortical tissue (see box at right). Acute adrenal crisis associated with bilateral hemorrhage in the adrenal gland is

---

Causes of Acute Adrenal Insufficiency

Primary adrenal insufficiency:
Congenital adrenal hyperplasia
Adrenoleukodystrophy
Autoimmune destruction
Adrenal hemorrhage
Tuberculosis

Secondary and tertiary adrenal insufficiency:
Congenital hypopituitarism
CNS tumors
CNS surgery or irradiation
Suppression of hypothalamic-pituitary-adrenal function by glucocorticoid administration

---

rarely described in the context of sepsis,[29,30] particularly in overwhelming meningococcemia.[31] Congenital adrenal hyperplasia is discussed earlier in this chapter.

Secondary and tertiary adrenal insufficiency are more common, and of late, most cases are due to either CNS tumors and related treatment, or exogenous administration of glucocorticoids for a number of chronic diseases (e.g., nephrotic syndrome, asthma).[32-34]

Diagnostic Findings

Clinical Findings and Complications. Although clinical manifestations of adrenal insufficiency may be gradual in onset, acute symptoms may occur as "Addisonian crisis" (see box on p. 760). Insidious signs and symptoms that are present in nearly all cases include anorexia and weight loss, fatigability and malaise, nausea and vomiting, and hyperpigmentation. Salt craving and dizziness (postural hypotension) are reported in 10% to 20% of cases.[31,35]

Ancillary Data. The primary pathophysiology of acute adrenal insufficiency results from mineralocorticoid deficiency[20,35]; hence hyponatremia and hyperkalemia are laboratory clues to the diagnosis (see box on p. 760). Peaked T waves and a widened QRS complex due to elevated serum potassium may be present on electrocardiogram. Glucocorticoid deficiency is manifested as hypoglycemia and contributes to hypotension.[26] This is common in acute adrenal hemorrhage that accompanies overwhelming sepsis, in particular, fulminant meningococcemia (Waterhouse-Friderichsen syndrome).[29-31]

Differential Considerations

Any infant or child with altered mental status and shock may have overwhelming sepsis. Evaluation for and treatment of sepsis should precede or be concomitant with evaluation and therapy of adrenal insufficiency. The differential diagnosis of vomiting and abdominal pain should be considered, including pneumonia, gastroenteritis, abdominal obstruction, urinary tract infection, and DKA. Finally, polyglandular endocrine disease should be considered when the diagnosis of adrenal insufficiency is made.

Management

Management of the patient with known adrenal insufficiency should be prompt. Intramuscular hydrocortisone or cortisone acetate can be given by the caretakers at home or by transport personnel before arriving at the emergency department.[28]

The child with adrenal crisis should be assessed for patency of the airway, and oxygen should be administered if altered mental status or shock is present. Intravenous access should be rapidly obtained, and intravascular volume replacement begun immediately (see box on p. 760). Blood should be sent for electrolyte and glucose determination, and if possible, cortisol and corticotropin measurements.[27]

The immediate goal is to reverse hypotension and hypoglycemia, and replete intravascular volume. Stress-dose glucocorticoid replacement is intravenous hydrocortisone, 50 mg/m², which is 3 to 5 times the physiologic secretion rate. Subsequent maintenance therapy is 12 to 15 mg/m²/day, in two to three divided doses.[16,28,32,35] As fluid and electrolyte correction is attained, mineralocorticoid replacement is begun (see box on p. 760).

Disposition

Any child with suspected or known adrenal crisis should be hospitalized and carefully monitored. Cardiac rhythm, blood pressure, intravascular volume status, and electrolytes should be evaluated at regular intervals, in consultation with an endocrinologist.

ANTIDIURETIC HORMONE DISORDERS

Diabetes Insipidus

Children with the syndrome of diabetes insipidus (DI) experience failure of antidiuresis because of serum hyperosmolality and hypoosmolar urine. DI is characterized by one of two abnormalities: antidiuretic hormone (ADH or vasopressin) deficiency or impaired renal response to ADH.[36] ADH deficiency causes central DI (neurogenic, ADH-sensitive), whereas impaired renal response to ADH causes nephrogenic DI (ADH-resistant). DI is uncommon in childhood but has many causes (see box below).

Pathophysiology. Normal body water balance is briefly discussed in the section concerning the syndrome of inappropriate secretion of ADH. The biologic action of ADH depends on its synthesis in the hypothalamus and secretion from the posterior pituitary and appropriate response to its binding at the basolateral plasma membrane of the collecting duct.[20] A defect in the secretion or renal response to ADH results in an inability to produce maximally concentrated urine and, if normal thirst mechanisms are intact, results in large volumes of hypotonic urine.

Causes of the Syndrome of DI in Childhood

Central (ADH-deficient)

Idiopathic
Familial (congenital; autosomal dominant)
Sporadic

Secondary
Head injury
Infection: meningitis, encephalitis, Guillain-Barré syndrome
Neoplasm (suprasellar or intrasellar)
Septooptic dysplasia
Granulomas: histiocytosis X, sarcoid
Vascular: sickle-cell disease, cerebral hemorrhage, or thrombosis
Iatrogenic: postintracranial surgery

Nephrogenic (ADH-resistent)

Idiopathic
Familial (congenital; x-linked)
Sporadic

Secondary
Renal disease: polycystic kidney disease, ureteral obstruction, and pyelonephritis
Electrolyte abnormalities: hypokalemia, hypercalcemia
Toxins: alcohol, phenytoin, lithium, demeclocycline, and angiography dyes
Granulomas: histiocytosis X, sarcoid
Vascular: sickle-cell disease

Data from Alberti K: *Arch Intern Med* 137:1367, 1977; Fisher J, Shahshahani M, Kitabachi A: *N Engl J Med* 297(5):238, 1977; and Dillon E, Riggs H, Dyer W: *Am J Med Sci* 192:360, 1965.

Etiology. Central DI is idiopathic in approximately half of cases. Of the remainder, the majority of patients have DI with head injury or neoplasm or after intracranial surgery. Plasma levels of ADH are low or absent, although DI is often transient in the instances of head injury or intracranial surgery.

Idiopathic nephrogenic DI is a rare but severe disorder; infants with this disease continue to excrete hypoosmolar urine even with significant hypernatremic dehydration. More common, nephrogenic DI is acquired and rarely severe.[36] Maximal renal concentrating ability is impaired, but affected individuals can usually produce a hypertonic urine.

Diagnostic Findings

Clinical Findings. Polyuria, usually with large urine volumes (including nocturia), characterizes DI. If the thirst mechanism is intact and fluids are accessible, polydipsia can be marked. The onset of polyuria is usually sudden in central DI, whereas it may be less so in patients with nephrogenic DI. In addition, urine volumes may be more moderate in acquired DI. In all cases, though, clinical signs and symptoms may be few or vague, such as with enuresis and poor school performance. If thirst mechanisms are compromised or access to fluids is not ad libitum, hypertonic dehydration may develop quickly, manifesting as irritability or further depression of mental status, including coma. Physical examination may be normal or reveal signs of dehydration, including weight loss, dry mucous membranes, and decreased skin turgor.

Ancillary Data. Laboratory findings of DI are low urinary osmolality and increasingly hypertonic serum with brief water deprivation.[36,37] Serum osmolality greater than 290 mOsm/L and serum sodium levels greater than 145 mEq/L with urine osmolality less than 150 mOsm/L support the diagnosis. Radioimmunoassay for plasma ADH is available but not helpful in the acute setting. Diagnosis is confirmed with a formal water deprivation test and through the use of exogenous ADH.[36,38]

Differential Considerations. A lethargic infant or child with signs of dehydration may indicate a septic condition; evaluation and treatment must consider infection. Hypernatremia from other causes must also be considered. Free water loss in excess of sodium loss results in states of low total body sodium such as in diarrheal illnesses and osmotic diuresis. Free water loss with a normal total body sodium level may occur with diarrheal illnesses and states of increased insensible losses (e.g., fever or respiratory disease). Finally, hypernatremia associated with increased total body sodium levels results from hyperaldosteronism, Cushing syndrome, and exogenous salt poisoning. In nearly all cases, urine is isotonic or hypertonic. Individuals who compulsively drink water (psychogenic polydipsia) also manifest polyuria with hypotonic urine but have no concentrating defect; these patients are polyuric because of their polydipsia.

Management. Any infant or child with depressed mental status requires careful maintenance of a patent airway and provision of supplemental oxygen. Naloxone should be administered if narcotic poisoning is suspected, and hypoglycemia should be treated promptly if noted. Immediate management of hypernatremic dehydration may require repletion of intravascular volume if tachycardia or hypotension are present or if signs of dehydration are severe. Rapid volume replacement is achieved with isotonic saline 10 to 20 ml/kg IV over 30 to 60 minutes.

Fluid replacement in DI produces normal levels of total body sodium. Free water deficit can be calculated and replaced carefully over 24 to 48 hours.

$$\text{Total body water} = 10 \text{ kg} \times 0.60 = 6.0 \text{ L}$$

Free water necessary to correct serum sodium to 140 mEq/L in a 10 kg child with a serum sodium of 155 mEq/L can be calculated as:

$$\frac{155 \text{ mEq/L}}{140 \text{ mEq/L}} \times 6 \text{ L} = 6.6 \text{ L}$$

thus $\qquad 6.6 \text{ L} - 6.0 \text{ L} = 0.6 \text{ L}$ free water deficit.

Maintenance fluids are delivered concomitantly, and urinary losses are replaced. Because large volumes of fluids may be necessary, the dextrose concentration of IV fluids may need to be reduced from 5% to 2.5% to avoid osmotic diuresis.

ADH or its analogs may be used during the treatment of DI but almost never are appropriate in the emergency department setting.[39-43] Routes of administration, duration of effect, and individual response vary for different forms of ADH (Table 50-2), and use of ADH requires careful monitoring of response and fluid and electrolyte balance.

Disposition. The underlying cause for DI should be investigated and treated as indicated. The child with significant dehydration or hypernatremia must be closely monitored during therapy. Fluid and electrolyte input and output should be carefully measured. Hospitalization is required, and endocrinologic consultation should be sought, especially for ADH therapy.

Syndrome of Inappropriate Secretion of ADH

Inappropriate or excess secretion of ADH results in hyponatremia and low serum osmolality. In this context, and

TABLE 50-2. Hormonal Treatment of Diabetes Insipidus

Agent	Dosage	Duration of effect (hr)
Aqueous ADH	5 units IM, SC or 0.5-1.0 μU/ kg/hr IV	3-6
ADH tannate in oil	5 units IM	24-72
1-desamino-8-d-arginine (dDAVP)	0.5-2 μg/kg IN or 1.25, 2.5, or 5 μg IN every 12-24 hr	12-24

Data from Berl T and Schrier R: Disorders of water metabolism. In Schrier R, editor: *Renal and electrolyte disorders*, Boston, 1986, Little, Brown; Fjellestad-Paulsen A, Tubiana-Rufi N, Harris A, et al: *Acta Endocrinol (Copenh)* 115:307, 1987; Giacoia G, Watson S, Karathanos A: *South Med J* 77(1):75, 1984; Beclier D and Foley T: *J Pediatr* 92(6):1011, 1978; Robinson A: *N Engl J Med* 294(10):507, 1976; and Weigle C: Metabolic and endocrine diseases in pediatric intensive care. In Rogers M, editor: *Textbook of pediatric intensive care*, Philadelphia, 1982, Williams & Wilkins.

ADH, Antidiuretic hormone; *IM,* intramuscular; *IN,* intranasal; *IV,* intravenous; *SC,* subcutaneous.

in the presence of normal renal and adrenal function, urine concentration is high with extracellular free water excess.[36,44,45]

Etiology. In childhood, numerous disorders have been associated with a syndrome of inappropriate secretion of ADH (SIADH). These are outlined in the box below.

Disorders Associated with SIADH

CNS DISORDERS

Infection
    Meningitis (bacterial, viral, or fungal)
    Encephalitis
    Brain abscess
    Guillain-Barré syndrome

Brain trauma
    Subarachnoid hemorrhage
    Subdural hematoma

Brain tumor

Hypoxic or ischemic insult

Vascular process
    Cerebral thrombosis
    Cavernous sinus thrombosis
    Rocky Mountain spotted fever

Increased intracranial pressure or hydrocephalus

Acute intermittent porphyria

INTRATHORACIC DISORDERS

Infection
    Pneumonia (bacterial, viral, or fungal) or tuberculosis
    Abscess or empyema

Positive-pressure ventilation

Lung tumor
    Decreased left atrial pressure: pneumothorax, asthma, cystic fibrosis, mitral valve commissurotomy, or ligation of patent ductus arteriosus

MEDICATIONS

Increased ADH secretion
    Vincristine
    Cyclophosphamide
    Carbamazepine
    Morphine sulfate
    Phenothiazine
    Vidarabine (Ara-A, adenine arabinoside)

Potentiation of ADH renal effects
    Acetaminophen
    Indomethacin

MISCELLANEOUS DISORDERS

Bacterial infection
    Lymphadenitis
    Arthritis
    Sepsis

Diabetic ketoacidosis

Pathophysiology. Normal body water balance is maintained by regulation of plasma osmolality within a relatively narrow range. This osmoregulation occurs in the anterior hypothalamus. Osmoreceptors control the extracellular tonicity via thirst and the effects of ADH, which are synthesized in the supraoptic and paraventricular nuclei of the hypothalamus and secreted by the posterior pituitary. Plasma ADH levels are low or undetectable when plasma osmolality falls below 280 mOsm/L, whereas ADH secretion is maximal when plasma osmolality exceeds 290 to 295 mOsm/L.[37,45] Inappropriate secretion of ADH implies that (1) secretion of ADH is independent from osmoreceptor control, (2) the threshold plasma osmolality is "reset" and ADH is suppressed only at abnormally low osmolality, or (3) there is a "leak" of ADH with hypotonicity and hyponatremia.[36,37]

The physiologic consequence of ADH in the kidney is a reduction of free water excretion resulting from increased reabsorption in the collecting tubule. Free water excess results in dilutional hyponatremia and depressed serum osmolality.[46]

In most cases, peripheral edema is not present because of urinary sodium losses. This natriuresis partially corrects the expansion of body fluids and has two likely mechanisms. Expansion of plasma volume results in an increase in the filtered load of sodium and a decrease in sodium reabsorption by the proximal tubule. In addition, atrial natriuretic peptide effects an increased urinary sodium excretion in this high-volume state.[37,45,47] In summary, the inappropriate presence of ADH results in dilutional hyponatremia, hypotonicity, and urine that is usually hypertonic. Urine volume may increase with natriuresis.

Diagnostic Findings

Clinical Findings and Complications. The clinical findings in SIADH are usually not manifested until the serum sodium level is depressed below 120 mEq/L. Nonspecific signs and symptoms of hyponatremia may be present and include lethargy, listlessness, headache, disorientation, anorexia, nausea, and vomiting. More severe signs include seizures and coma.[46] Signs of increased intracranial pressure may be evident.[37,47]

Ancillary Data. The classic laboratory findings of SIADH are hyponatremia, hypoosmolality of plasma, inappropriately hypertonic urine relative to concomitant plasma osmolality, inappropriately high urinary sodium concentration relative to concomitant serum hyponatremia, and weight gain that occurs despite natriuretic compensation.[46] To establish the diagnosis of SIADH, evidence of volume depletion must not be present and renal, adrenal, and thyroid function must be normal.[48]

Differential Considerations. Hyponatremia of different causes must be excluded before making the diagnosis of SIADH. Hypervolemic hyponatremia is present in congestive heart failure, nephrotic syndrome, and cirrhosis of the liver. Hypovolemic hyponatremia occurs with diarrheal losses, significant hemorrhage, adrenal insufficiency, hypothyroidism, and loop diuretic use.[37] Factitious hyponatremia occurs with hyperglycemia, hyperlipidemia, and hyperproteinemia. Most importantly, cerebral salt wasting, although rare, should be ruled out as a cause of hyponatremia and natriuresis.[49]

Management. The overt symptoms of SIADH are not frequently severe, but the vital signs and neurologic status of any child with obtundation or coma should be vigilantly monitored, and a patent airway carefully maintained. Pursuit of the underlying cause of the SIADH should take place, and appropriate therapy instituted.

The hyponatremia and hypotonicity of SIADH responds to carefully monitored fluid restriction of two thirds to three fourths of maintenance volumes. It is important to individualize this therapy and closely follow serum sodium and osmolality values, concomitant urine and sodium concentrations, and body weight.

The treatment of symptomatic hyponatremia (seizures and coma) must be aggressive. Hypertonic saline (3% saline = 0.513 mEq/ml of sodium) is used to correct serum sodium to a conservative level of 125 mEq/L. For example, to calculate for sodium replacement in hyponatremia[50] (correct to 125 mEq/L):

$$mEq \, Na^+{}_{(needed)} = 0.6 \times body \, weight \, (kg) \times (125 - Na^+{}_{(measured)})$$

The infusion volume of 3% saline is calculated and given carefully over 15 minutes, with attention directed to the IV site because the solution is hyperosmolar and consequently an irritant to veins and tissues. The remainder of the sodium deficit can be replaced over the next 24 hours. Furosemide 1 mg/kg will enhance free water loss, but diuretic use requires electrolyte and urinary fluid loss replacement.[50]

Disposition. The underlying cause for SIADH in a child must be appropriately investigated and treated. Symptomatic hyponatremia must be treated aggressively in an intensive care setting; moderate hyponatremia can be slowly corrected in a hospital ward. Mild hyponatremia and chronic therapy for SIADH may not require hospitalization.

DIABETIC KETOACIDOSIS

Despite advances in the management of insulin-dependent DM in children, the incidence of diabetic ketoacidosis (DKA) has remained essentially unchanged over the last 20 years. Ketoacidosis is not an uncommon complication of diabetes in children; it accounts for approximately 15% of hospitalizations for diabetes and is the most common cause of death in diabetic children, with a case fatality rate of 2% to 3%.[51-54] Hence, DKA is a serious and commonly seen illness in emergency departments.

Pathophysiology

Definition. Hyperglycemic ketoacidosis (DKA) is defined as follows[55]:

1. Hyperglycemia with a serum glucose concentration greater than 250 mg/dl
2. Ketonemia measured quantitatively in the serum, or ketonuria measured qualitatively in the urine with a nitroprusside reaction (e.g., Chemstrip uGK* or Acetest†)

*Boehringer Mannheim Inc., Indianapolis, IN.
†Miles Inc, Elkhart, IN.

3. Acidemia with a blood pH less than 7.30 or serum bicarbonate level less than 15 mEq/L

Ketoacidosis is generated with insulin deficiency and elevated levels of hormones that oppose the action of insulin ("counter-regulatory" hormones).[56,57] These catabolic counter-regulatory hormones—epinephrine, glucagon, cortisol, and growth hormone—are secreted in response to stress and, in the diabetic child with an absolute or relative lack of insulin, more fully express their actions. Epinephrine raises blood glucose and free fatty acid levels via increased gluconeogenesis, glycogenolysis, and lipolysis; hepatic ketogenesis is activated. Glucagon exacerbates the hyperglycemia by stimulating gluconeogenesis and glycogenolysis, and further prompts hepatic ketone production. Cortisol decreases peripheral glucose use. Growth hormone secretion has less immediate effects but causes increased hepatic gluconeogenesis and lipolysis with resultant hepatic ketogenesis.[53,58,59] In concert and unopposed by insulin, these hormones drive blood glucose concentrations higher by increasing glucose production in the liver and inhibiting peripheral glucose use by tissues. Therefore ketone body production is elevated and peripheral use is likewise depressed. The result is hyperglycemia and acidosis secondary to ketosis.

Etiology

For basic understanding of the causes of DKA, a discussion of the multifactorial cause of insulin-dependent DM (IDDM) is necessary. IDDM seems to be genetic. Individuals who develop it have associated chromosome 6 HLA two times more often than the normal population; in particular, they have HLA B8/DR3 or HLA B15/DR4.[60] Infectious or otherwise, a toxic insult to the pancreatic beta-islet cell occurs, leading to a chronic autoimmune destruction of beta-cells and a consequent decline in insulin production. This is supported by the circulating antiislet cell antibodies that are found in the serum of 85% of newly diagnosed patients with IDDM.[60]

In this setting a child with undiagnosed diabetes or, more exactly, insulin deficiency is at risk of developing ketoacidosis. Nearly any stress and counter-regulatory hormone response may initiate the pathogenetic cascade to hyperglycemia and ketoacidosis. Similarly, the child with known IDDM may develop a "relative" insulin deficiency resulting from a counter-regulatory hormone response to stress. In either case, an absolute or relative insulin deficiency and an increase in the level of counter-regulatory hormones are necessary for the progression to DKA.[55,61] Underlying causes that may trigger ketoacidosis are numerous and are outlined in the box on p. 766. In the undiagnosed diabetic who has DKA and in the known insulin-dependent patient, the cause or underlying stress must be sought.

Diagnostic Findings

The hyperglycemia and ketosis of DKA produce several clinical findings. Patients not previously diagnosed may report polyphagia or poor appetite, weight loss, polyuria, and polydipsia, and have some degree of dehydration. In patients who have been diagnosed with IDDM, it is im-

Common Underlying Causes of Ketoacidosis

Infection

Sepsis

Upper respiratory infection, including otitis media

Pharyngitis, including group A streptococcus

Pneumonia

Genitourinary infections

Gastroenteritis

Noninfectious causes

Trauma

Metabolic or endocrine derangements (e.g., hyperthyroidism, adrenal insufficiency, and pregnancy)

Poisonings (accidental and nonaccidental)

Surgery

Psychiatric conditions (emotional problems and environmental stress)

TABLE 50-3. Range of Metabolic and Electrolyte Abnormalities in Patients with DKA

	DKA	Normal
Glucose (mg/dl)	300-1200	80-120
Sodium (mEq/L)	120-135	135-145
Potassium (mEq/L)	2.0-6.0	3.5-5.0
Bicarbonate (mEq/L)	3.0-15.0	20.0-24.0
Arterial pH	6.90-7.30	7.35-7.45
Osmolality (mOsm/L)	300-325	280-300

Data from Holman R, Herrar C, Sinnock P: *Am J Public Health* 73(10):1169, 1985; and Foster D and McGarry J: *N Engl J Med* 309(3):159, 1983.

TABLE 50-4. Fluid and Electrolyte Daily Losses and Maintenance Requirements in DKA

	Daily loss (range)	Maintenance
Water	100 ml/kg	1500 ml/m²
Sodium	6 mEq/kg (5-13)	45 mEq/m²
Potassium	5 mEq/kg (4-6)	35 mEq/m²
Chloride	4 mEq/kg (3-9)	30 mEq/m²
Phosphate	3 mEq/kg (2-5)	10 mEq/m²

From Sperling MA. In Lebovitz HD, editor: *Therapy for diabetes mellitus and related disorders*, American Diabetes Association, 1991.

portant to document the duration of insulin therapy, usual insulin dosage and regimen, presenting symptoms, and possible precipitating factors.

The child with DKA is usually quite alert and, although the patient appears ill, behavior is appropriate. In addition, the progression of ketoacidosis produces tachypnea and Kussmaul's (deep, rapid) respirations, tachycardia, orthostatic changes in blood pressure, acetone breath, and vomiting. Abdominal pain is common and may mimic an acute surgical condition, although this resolves with treatment of the acidosis. Severe dehydration or acidosis may depress the level of consciousness, and coma is infrequently seen.

Complications. Dehydration with metabolic acidosis is common. Hyperglycemia invokes an osmotic diuresis that is manifested by polyuria as the renal threshold for glucose is exceeded. Electrolyte losses accompany this diuresis, and volume contraction progresses, resulting in greater hyperglycemia and hypertonicity (Table 50-3). Measured serum osmolality is elevated. Fluid losses accelerate with increasing glucose concentration; dehydration may rapidly progress in the child who does not respond well to thirst mechanisms, especially with vomiting or a depressed mental status. However, because of the osmotic gradient created by hyperglycemia and resultant fluid shift from the intracellular to extracellular compartment, the severity of clinical dehydration may be underestimated.[62] Net free water losses may be as high as 100 to 150 ml/kg.[53,62] Clinical signs of this dehydration are apparent; almost without exception, patients with DKA have very dry mucous membranes and some degree of tachycardia. Tissue perfusion is usually diminished, as evidenced by delayed capillary refill time. Less frequently, hypotension is present.

The acidosis of DKA may be moderate or severe and has two sources. Osmotic diuresis, dehydration, and volume contraction lead to diminished tissue perfusion and lactic acidosis. In addition, the excessive ketone body formation in DKA favors the production of the strong organic acids,

beta-hydroxybutyric acid and acetoacetic acid.[53,62,63] These acids produce a positive urine nitroprusside reaction, which can be measured using a diagnostic test strip (Chemstrip uGK).

As renal perfusion declines, all of these acids are less readily cleared, and acidemia worsens; pH is reduced below 7.30. The clinical signs of acidosis are usually overt; patients with DKA are nearly always tachypneic, or if acidosis is severe, Kussmaul's respirations are evident.

Hyperosmolar nonketotic coma with glucose measurements from 800 to 1,200 mg/dl, is rare in children. Such patients may not be acidotic with hyperglycemia, hyperosmolality, and dehydration.

Ancillary Data. Electrolyte losses that accompany the metabolic derangements and osmotic diuresis of DKA can be quite significant and are summarized in Table 50-4. Urinary sodium loss and osmotic dilution of the extracellular fluid space usually result in mild-to-moderate hyponatremia. A spurious component of hyponatremia results from the lipemic nature of the plasma; sodium is distributed in water only, but the concentration calculation also includes the volume contribution of lipids.[56,62] "Actual" or corrected sodium concentration may be calculated as follows:

$$Sodium_{corrected} = Sodium_{measured} + 1.6 \times (glucose - 100)/100$$

Measured potassium concentration may be high, normal, or low, but total body potassium stores are often markedly depleted. During acidosis, intracellular potassium shifts to the extracellular compartment, only to be lost with diuresis; this loss is also due to the heightened aldosterone effect during dehydration.[53,59,64] Measured serum potassium rises 0.5 mEq/L with each 0.1 decrease in blood pH. Elevated serum potassium levels may be evident on an electrocardiogram as heightened T waves.

Phosphate is also lost in the urine with the intracellular to extracellular shifts that accompany ketosis. Phosphate deficits may result in diminished 2,3-diphosphoglycerate levels, effecting a shift of the oxygen dissociation curve to the left and diminished oxygen release at the tissues.[59,65] The serum bicarbonate level is depressed because ketoacids and lactic acid consume the serum's buffering capacity. Other laboratory findings in DKA include leukocytosis, which may be an indication of a coexistent infection.[53]

Initial diagnostic investigation for DKA includes arterial blood gas determination and serum glucose, sodium, potassium, chloride, bicarbonate, urea nitrogen, calcium, phosphate osmolality, and triglycerides measurement. An electrocardiogram should be obtained. Glycosylated hemoglobin (HbA_{1c}) should be measured. At many centers, blood is analyzed for antiislet-cell and antiinsulin antibodies in patients who have been newly diagnosed with diabetes. Appropriate cultures should be obtained.

Differential Considerations

The diagnosis of DKA can be relatively obvious and straightforward. However, especially in the young child who has not been diagnosed with DM, infection or sepsis is often initially thought to be the cause of dehydration, lethargy, and acidosis. In addition, diagnoses that manifest acidemia must be considered; these include lactic acidosis (as a result of hypovolemia and shock), toxic ingestions (commonly salicylates, alcohols, and glycols), congenital metabolic derangements (inborn errors of metabolism), and renal failure.

Management

As with any acutely ill child, careful attention must be paid to maintenance of a patent airway. Compromise of a child's level of consciousness may impair air exchange. Oxygen should be administered to the patient who is not fully conscious. Cardiorespiratory monitoring should be continuous.

The most important principle in the management of DKA is individualization of therapy. Careful monitoring of mental status, cardiovascular status, and fluid and electrolyte balance must be a priority.

Fluids and Electrolytes. Intravascular volume and tissue perfusion are restored with an isotonic IV solution (normal saline or Ringer's lactate solution); this is done over the first hour of therapy as outlined in the box above. Fluid and electrolyte deficits are calculated and carefully replaced over 48 hours. Use the corrected serum sodium concentration to guide this replacement. Potassium is also replaced based on serum concentration; half is replaced as potassium chloride and the other half as potassium phosphate to replete phosphate losses. Potassium repletion should begin immediately after initial intravascular volume restoration.

The use of IV bicarbonate in the management of DKA remains controversial.[66,67] Bicarbonate is used in two in-

---

Treatment Guidelines for DKA

Repletion of intravascular volume
Give 10 to 20 ml/kg IV normal saline.

Fluid and electrolyte replacement
Give crystalloid infusion of 0.45% normal saline with potassium salts (as determined below)
If corrected sodium ≤ 140 mEq/L; replace half of the deficit over first 16 hours and restore total deficit over 36 hours.
If corrected sodium ≥ 140 mEq/L, restore total deficit evenly over 48 hours.

Replace potassium and phosphate
Potassium should be given half as potassium chloride and half as potassium phosphate as follows:

Serum potassium (mEq/L)	Potassium in infusate (mEq/L)
<3	40-60
3-4	30
4-5	20
5-6	10

Bicarbonate therapy
Bicarbonate therapy is indicated only with shock or severe acidemia (pH <7.0); give sodium bicarbonate, 1 to 2 mEq/kg, IV over 1 to 2 hours.

Dextrose administration
As glucose falls below 300 mg/dl, add 5% dextrose to IV fluids.

Insulin therapy
Begin low-dose insulin therapy with regular insulin after the diagnosis of ketoacidosis is confirmed.
Give initial dose of 0.1 units/kg pushed IV.
Give continuous infusion of 0.1 units/kg/hr IV.
Monitor serum glucose levels hourly.

---

stances, severe acidemia (i.e., pH less than 7.0) and cardiovascular instability. The physician administers 1 to 2 mEq/kg IV over 1 to 2 hours and monitors blood gas values. Correction to pH 7.1 is usually sufficient and avoids overcorrection.

Insulin. Insulin replacement is also initiated after ketoacidosis is confirmed. Restoration of intravascular volume with an isotonic fluid will improve renal perfusion and result in a significant reduction in blood glucose concentration via diuresis. Insulin will "turn off" ketosis and reverse acidosis. Low-dose continuous infusion of insulin is well documented as effective and does not have the adverse side effects of high-dose insulin regimens such as with hypoglycemia and hypokalemia.[68,69] The optimum fall in measured glucose is 100 mg/dl/hr. The alternative to a continuous infusion of insulin is hourly IM injections of 0.1 mg/kg/hr of regular insulin.

Dextrose should be added to the IV fluids as measured serum glucose levels fall below 300 mg/dl. The hourly insulin dose may be adjusted but never discontinued because insulin is required for halting ketosis and reversal of acidosis. After acidosis resolves (pH >7.30), continuous insulin can be discontinued 30 to 60 minutes after the first SC dose.

Further insulin therapy does not usually take place in the emergency department, but an endocrinologist should be involved in management. Long-acting insulin is typically given SC in a total daily dose of 0.6 to 0.8 units/kg/24 hr; two thirds of this dose is usually given before breakfast and one third before dinner. At each time, the dose is commonly delivered as neutral protamine Hagedom (NPH) and regular insulin in a ratio of 2:1. Newly diagnosed diabetic patients are often very sensitive to exogenous insulin and therefore have lower initial insulin requirements (the "honeymoon phase").

Brain Swelling. The risk for the development of subclinically or clinically apparent brain swelling, during or as a result of the course of treatment of DKA, remains controversial.[70-75] Cerebral edema is unpredictable in onset and without warning signs, although it usually occurs 8 to 12 hours after initiation of treatment[76] (see box above). Two recent reports describe alarmingly early onset of cerebral edema in DKA, one before treatment and one about 2 hours after treatment had begun.[76,77] Abrupt changes in mental status, pupillary changes, and posturing progressed to coma, with a mortality rate of 90%.[74] Unfortunately, it is difficult to identify specific treatment variables that predispose a patient to the development of cerebral edema.[78] Prompt use of IV mannitol may help to reverse cerebral edema in these instances.[79] Therefore the goal of therapy is careful, individualized fluid and electrolyte replacement delivered to minimize osmotic changes. Rapid rates of fluid administration and a total fluid dose greater than 4 L/m²/ day have correlated with an increased risk for cerebral edema.[69,72,73] A slower repletion regimen may lower the risk for brain swelling and intracerebral crises, but further studies are required.[80]

Disposition

All patients with ketoacidosis should be hospitalized. Criteria for admission to an intensive care unit (ICU) vary in different institutions, but any child with abnormal mental status or evidence of shock or cardiac dysrhythmia requires the close observation and invasive monitoring possible in an ICU. In addition, admission to an ICU should be considered for patients with DKA who are younger than 12 to 24 months of age or for those patients with an initial glucose measurement greater than 1,000 mg/dl or pH less than 7.0. Less severely ill patients may be cared for on a pediatric ward, provided that frequent clinical and chemical monitoring can be performed. Finally, patients with newly diagnosed DM need intensive education initiated early in the illness.

PHEOCHROMOCYTOMA

Catecholamine-secreting pheochromocytoma is an uncommon cause of systemic hypertension, hence diagnosis requires a high degree of suspicion by the clinician. Pheo-

---

> ### Signs and Symptoms of Cerebral Edema in DKA
>
> Headache
> Agitation, disorientation
> Abnormal pupillary findings (sluggish or nonreactive, asymmetric)
> Papilledema
> Ophthalmoplegia
> Depressed level of consciousness
> Abnormal vital signs (tachycardia or bradycardia, hypertension or hypotension)
> Seizures
> Posturing

---

chromocytoma is a rare entity; only 5% to 20% of all pheochromocytomas are found in the pediatric population.[81,82] Even in adult populations incidence is less than 2/100,000/ year.[83]

Etiology

Pheochromocytoma is a catecholamine-secreting tumor that arises from the chromaffin cells of the adrenal medulla, and in 30% of children, it arises from the extraadrenal sympathetic ganglia chains.[84] Pheochromocytoma can be associated with a number of syndromes and diseases including neuroectodermal conditions (neurofibromatosis, von Hippel-Lindau disease, Sturge-Weber syndrome, and tuberous sclerosis), multiple endocrine neoplasia (MEN) type II, and tumors of the amine precursor uptake and decarboxylation (APUD) system.[81]

Pathophysiology

About 70% of pheochromocytoma in children arise from the chromaffin cells of the adrenal medulla, whereas the remainder are extraadrenal, (usually intraabdominal), arising from the sympathetic chains. Tumors found in the pediatric population occur bilaterally in 20% of cases and are multiple in 30%. Malignant pheochromocytoma occurs in as many as 10% of cases.[84]

The chromaffin cells of the pheochromocytoma are the source of the excess catecholamines. Dopamine, norepinephrine, and epinephrine are synthesized form tyrosine, and these products are excreted unchanged. Further metabolism yields normetanephrine, metanephrine, and finally vanillylmandelic acid (VMA), which is secreted in even greater quantities.[85] All of these metabolites are responsible for the symptoms found in patients with pheochromocytoma.

Diagnostic Findings

Clinical Findings and Complications. The clinical manifestations of pheochromocytoma are attributed to sustained or episodic release of catecholamines. The classic triad of headache, palpitations and diaphoresis is highly sensitive and specific.[86,87] Hypertension is the most common finding in children and is a sustained reaction rather than episodic or paroxysmal in 90% of cases.[84,88] Hypertension tends to be more severe in children than in adults and may lead to congestive heart failure, retinopathy, and hypertensive crisis, including encephalopathic conditions and death.[81] Common associated findings, especially during a paroxysm of hypertension, include headache, visual blurring, palpitations, diaphoresis, and tremors. Flushing or pallor has also been described.[81,84] Pheochromocytoma should be considered in any child with hypertension and in any child who manifests blood pressure instability or a hypertensive response to the induction of anesthesia.[85] An abdominal mass is palpable in only 10% of patients.[84]

Ancillary Data. Laboratory findings on initial examination are few. Electrocardiographic evidence of a tachydysrhythmia may be present.[85] The diagnosis of pheochromocytoma is made by measurement of urinary catecholamines, metanephrines, and VMA. One or more of these metabolites is increased in 95% of cases, but urinary metanephrine and plasma catecholamine measurements are the most sensitive indicators of pheochromocytoma. Furthermore, when plasma catecholamines, urinary VWA, and metanephrine are increased, specificity is quite high.[89,90] Pharmacologic provocation and suppression tests are also available but rarely used because urinary and plasma catecholamine measurements are sufficient in nearly all cases.

Tumor localization is important for subsequent management and is almost always accomplished by CT or MRI scan. More than 90% of tumors can be detected by one of these modalities.[85,89,90] Because tumors may be multiple and may be found at any site in the sympathetic chain, scintigraphy is sometimes used for localization of pheochromocytoma. Selective angiography can be useful when information regarding tumor blood supply is needed.[81]

Differential Considerations

Hypertension in children has many causes, including renal disease, hyperthyroidism, coarctation of the aorta, and CNS problems (infection and tumors). Renal diseases include glomerulonephritis associated with streptococcal disease, Henoch-Schönlein purpura, systemic lupus erythematosus, hemolytic-uremic syndrome, chronic pyelonephritis, and renal vascular stenosis. Headache and visual blurring may be present in migraine syndromes. Anxiety states can produce the symptoms of pheochromocytoma.

Management

Definitive therapy for pheochromocytoma is surgical excision.[85] Symptomatic and preparative treatment must be given before surgery after localizing the tumor by imaging studies. Phenoxybenzamine is a long-acting noncompetitive alpha-adrenergic blocking agent that is given orally in a starting dose of 1 to 2 mg/kg/24 hr in four divided doses.[81,85,90] Beta-adrenergic blockade is rarely necessary in children because norepinephrine is the predominant catecholamine secreted.[81]

Disposition

Children who have hypertensive crisis need immediate therapeutic intervention and hospitalization. In cases of less severe symptoms hospitalization may not be necessary, but full investigation must proceed expediently. After a diagnosis of pheochromocytoma is made, the tumors must be localized for future surgical removal.

THYROID DISORDERS

Hyperthyroidism

Hyperthyroidism in children is nearly always due to Graves disease (also called *diffuse toxic goiter*), and accounts for 10% to 25% of all childhood thyroid disorders.[91,92] Girls are much more likely to be affected than boys (4:1 to 7:1).[91,93] Onset depends on age. Approximately 15% of children have hyperthyroidism from birth to 5 years of age, 25% of children are 6 to 10 years old when affected, and 60% are older than 10 years.[91]

Pathophysiology. Graves disease is an autoimmune thyroid disorder associated with thyroid-stimulating immunoglobulins (TSIs): most notably, antithyroglobulin antibodies (ATAs), antimicrosomal antibodies (AMAs), and thyroid-stimulating hormone (TSH) receptor antibodies. The immunopathogenesis of a hyperthyroid state involves these antibodies stimulating the thyroid follicular cells responsible for the production and secretion of thyroid hormone. This process occurs independently from the pituitary-thyroid axis of feedback control.[94,95] Unchecked synthesis and release of triiodothyronine (T_3) and thyroxine (T_4) results in the clinical and laboratory abnormalities of Graves hyperthyroidism.

Etiology. The autoimmune process from which childhood hyperthyroidism arises may be stimulated by any number of unknown etiologies. In particular, antibodies to plasmid-encoded capsular proteins of *Yersinia enterocolitica* and other similar microorganisms may cross-react with the TSH receptor.[96] Antithyroid antibodies have also been detected in the presence of viral thyroiditis, which is also caused by stimulation of the TSH receptor.[97]

Diagnostic Findings

Clinical Findings. The most common clinical manifestations of childhood hyperthyroidism are goiter (97% to 100% of cases), nervousness (60% to 92%), tachycardia (65% to 91%), exophthalmos (55% to 78%), and tremor (40% to 76%). Weight loss has been reported in 50% to 67% of cases, but weight gain occurred in 12%. Bone age may be advanced and height may be greater than average for age. Parents may report declining school performance, labile behaviors, and increased irritability. Heat intolerance, diaphoresis, palpitations, diarrhea, and amenorrhea have also been reported. Symptoms and signs usually appear gradually over 6 weeks to several months but may occur more abruptly.[91,92,94,95]

Thyroid storm or thyrotoxic crisis is a life-threatening complication of severe hyperthyroidism; it is almost always abrupt in onset. A precipitating factor is usually present such as infection, trauma, surgery, acute cardiopulmonary disease; and metabolic derangements (diabetic ketoacidosis and dehydration) have been associated with thyroid storm. Fever heralds the onset of crisis and can be high. Cardiovascular symptoms include marked tachycardia and progression to congestive heart failure or cardiogenic shock. CNS manifestations of tremor, restlessness, and agitation

TABLE 50-5. Thyroid Function Tests

Disease	T_4	T_3-resin uptake	TSH
Hyperthyroidism	↑	↑	↓
Chronic lymphocytic thyroiditis			
Euthyroidism	nl	nl/↑	nl/↑
Hyperthyroidism	↑	↑	↓
Hypothyroidism	↓	nl/↓	↑
Congenital hypothyroidism	↓	↓	↑

Modified from Fisher D: *J Pediatr* 82:187, 1973.
nl, Normal; *TSH*, thyroid stimulating hormone.

may progress to confusion, mania, psychosis, or coma. In addition, gastrointestinal symptoms are common; abdominal pain, nausea, vomiting, and diarrhea have all been described.[98,99]

Ancillary Data. The laboratory diagnosis of hyperthyroidism includes radioimmunoassay measurement of serum T_3 and T_4. The serum concentration of T_3 and T_4 should be compared with age-matched controls; thyroid hormone levels are significantly higher at birth than in adults, and they decline with age.[91] Elevation of T_4 is almost always found, although marked elevation of T_3 is invariable.[91,92,95] TSH measurement and the T_3-resin uptake test are confirmatory (Table 50-5). Therefore childhood hyperthyroidism is a clinical diagnosis that cannot really be confirmed. Electrocardiography should be performed to evaluate associated dysrhythmias, and a radiograph of the chest may alert the physician to cardiomegaly or congestive heart failure.

Differential Considerations. Goiters can be found in approximately 5% of school-age children.[100] The differential diagnosis of goiter can be narrowed by evaluating the physical characteristics of the thyroid gland. Nodular goiters may indicate adenoma, cyst, colloid nodule, or cancer, and may account for less than 20% of goiters in children. A diffusely enlarged thyroid is likely to be lymphocytic as in thyroiditis (33%), especially Hashimoto's thyroiditis, or Graves disease (25%).[100]

Not all children with hyperthyroidism have goiter. In addition, any child with symptoms consistent with hyperthyroidism or thyrotoxic crisis should be rapidly evaluated for infection, cardiovascular disease or dysrhythmias, metabolic derangements, and ingestion of poisons. Finally, pheochromocytoma has many symptoms in common with patients with hyperthyroidism.

Management. Treatment options of childhood hyperthyroidism exist but are not without controversy.[91-93,101,102] They are: total or subtotal surgical thyroidectomy, radioiodine treatment (I^{131}), and antithyroid drug therapy. Only the treatment for severe hyperthyroidism or thyroid storm will be discussed here.

Therapy for the child in thyroid storm is directed at the precipitating factor, cardiovascular complications, and the thyroid gland itself. Any child with a depressed mental status or coma requires maintenance of a patent airway. Oxygen should be administered if signs of shock or congestive heart failure are present. Hyperpyrexia can be treated with acetaminophen and cooling blankets.

IV access is necessary for treatment of shock or dysrhythmias. Beta-adrenergic blockade blunts the heightened peripheral response to catecholamines in patients with thyrotoxicosis.[91,98,103] Propranolol may improve many of the signs of hyperthyroidism, reducing tachycardia and ameliorating symptoms of nervousness, agitation, and tremor. Propranolol is titrated to clinical effect (reduction of tachycardia) in doses of 0.1 mg/kg. Antithyroid drugs, commonly propylthiouracil (PTU), inhibit thyroid hormone synthesis and peripheral conversion of T_4 to T_3. PTU is given 5 to 10 mg/kg/24 hr PO in 3 divided doses.[91,97-104] In addition, a single daily dose of methimazole (0.5 to 0.7 mg/kg) may be used.[95]

Iodide inhibits the release of thyroid hormone. Potassium iodide as a saturated solution of potassium iodide (saturated solution of potassium iodide [SSKI], and Lugol's solution [5% iodine and 10% potassium iodide]) is usually begun 1 hour after PTU to avoid increasing thyroid gland stores before the antithyroid effect occurs. Lugol's solution is given 5 drops/q 8 hr PO.[98]

Disposition. Children who have a history and signs consistent with hyperthyroidism should be fully evaluated by an endocrinologist before initiation of treatment. Patients who show evidence of thyroid storm should be promptly treated, admitted to the hospital, and closely monitored, preferably in an ICU. Response to therapy must also be monitored carefully.

Hypothyroidism, Acquired

Acquired hypothyroidism does not occur with emergent signs or symptoms. The most common cause of acquired hypothyroidism in childhood is chronic lymphocytic thyroiditis, and one third to half of these patients will have goiter, which may prompt a visit to the emergency department.[94,100,105] Of these cases with chronic lymphocytic thyroiditis, 70% will be euthyroid and 10% will evidence hyperthyroidism, but 20% will manifest hypothyroidism.[94,100,106,107]

Pathophysiology. Lymphocytic thyroiditis is an autoimmune disease of the thyroid and is associated with circulating antithyroid antibodies (ATA), antimicrosomal antibodies (AMA), and in 40% to 60% of cases, thyroid stimulating immunoglobulin (TSI).[106] In cases that proceed to hypothyroidism, these immunoglobulins attack and render the host thyroid tissue inadequate for thyroid hormone synthesis and secretion.

Etiology. The majority of acquired hypothyroidism in childhood is associated with antithyroid antibodies. Other causes of acquired hypothyroidism include thyroid dysgenesis, decreased response to thyroid hormones, hypothalamic-pituitary hypothyroidism (TSH deficiency), and iodine deficiency (endemic hypothyroidism).[99]

Diagnostic Findings

Clinical Findings and Complications. The clinical findings of hypothyroidism are insidious in onset and often very subtle. Historic data include failure to gain weight or decreased growth velocity, lethargy, poor appetite, constipation, cold intolerance, and precocious or delayed puberty. Findings on examination may include flattened affect, puffiness, goiter, mild bradycardia, and slow return of deep tendon reflexes.[105]

Ancillary Data. Radioimmunoassay for serum T_4 is low, and the T_3 resin-uptake test is reduced. Serum TSH level is high, and bone age is delayed on radiography.[94,105]

Differential Considerations. The nonspecific and sometimes scant number of symptoms of hypothyroidism makes this a difficult diagnosis. The differential diagnosis of goiter depends on physical characteristics. About 40% of diffusely enlarged goiters are due to chronic lymphocytic thyroiditis, whereas nearly one third are due to Graves hyperthyroidism.[100] Acute or chronic toxic drug ingestion should be considered in children and adolescents with altered mental status or significant lethargy.

Management. Treatment for hypothyroidism is thyroxine replacement. The dose of levothyroxine decreases with age, from 10 to 15 mg/kg/24 hr for the neonate, to 2 to 3 mg/kg/24 hr for the adolescent and young adult.[108] Replacement therapy should be guided by an endocrinologist. Response to treatment and growth and developmental advancement must be monitored.

Disposition. The child with hypothyroidism rarely needs hospitalization but absolutely requires close monitoring of therapeutic measures and drug effects.

Hypothyroidism, Congenital

Routine screening for inborn errors of metabolism has revealed the occurrence of abnormal thyroid function in 1 in 3,750 to 4,400 live births and much more frequently in premature infants.[105,109,110] Despite screening programs, failure of notification occasionally occurs, and an infant may be brought to the emergency department with subtle signs of hypothyroidism. In addition, parental anxiety concerning the diagnosis may prompt a visit.

Pathophysiology. Thyroid dysgenesis (aplastic, hypoplastic, and ectopic gland) is responsible for up to 80% of cases of permanent congenital hypothyroidism. The second most frequent cause of primary congenital hypothyroidism is an inborn error of thyroid hormone synthesis, usually an organification defect.[105,110] Secondary causes of congenital hypothyroidism include hypopituitarism and septooptic dysplasia. Hyposecretion of thyroid hormone leads to the clinical manifestations of hypothyroidism, however subtle.

Diagnostic Findings
Clinical Findings. Clinical manifestations of congenital hypothyroidism may be vague or absent. The classic appearance of a child with this disease is only infrequently seen and includes puffy facies, depressed nasal bridge, macroglossia with protrusion of the tongue, large fontanelles with widened sutures, abdominal distension with umbilical hernia, hypotonia, and delayed deep tendon reflex return. More commonly, the infant with hypothyroidism has nonspecific findings such as lethargy, poor feeding, constipation, and prolonged jaundice.[105,110]

Ancillary Data. Radioimmunoassay for serum T_4 is usually markedly low compared with age-matched normals, and serum TSH level is elevated. Other laboratory findings include a low T_3 resin-uptake test and usually a normal or minimally lowered serum T_3 level. Thyroid-binding globulin (TBG) is measured as part of a complete evaluation. Furthermore, serum glucose levels should be measured in any lethargic infant, and an evaluation for sepsis should be performed as indicated.

Differential Considerations. Any infant who is lethargic should be evaluated for hypoglycemia and sepsis; consideration of adrenal crisis (congenital adrenal hyperplasia) is imperative.

Management. A patent airway must be maintained in the lethargic infant. Oxygen and IV fluids should be administered if signs of shock are present, although these are exceedingly unlikely in an infant with only hypothyroidism.

The infant with congenital hypothyroidism should be started on levothyroxine immediately after confirmatory blood studies are obtained. The usual dosage is 10 to 15 mg/kg/24 hr.[99,110]

Disposition. The child with hypothyroidism should be followed closely by an endocrinologist to avoid undertreatment or overtreatment and to monitor growth and development.

Thyrotoxicosis, Neonatal

Neonatal thyrotoxicosis is a transient hyperthyroidism acquired by transplacental passage of TSIs from mother to fetus. Although infants with thyrotoxicosis are almost always born to mothers who are or who have been hyperthyroid, this disease has been reported in infants of mothers without known thyroid disease or lymphocytic thyroiditis.[91,98] The signs of hyperthyroidism in the neonate are usually noticed in the newborn nursery, especially when the mother has had thyroid disease. Unsuspected or delayed onset of hyperthyroidism in the neonate may not present until after 10 or more days of life.[98,111] Neonatal thyrotoxicosis is a life-threatening disorder with a mortality rate of 16%.[91]

Pathophysiology. Transplacental transfer of a maternal TSH–receptor-stimulating antibody has been implicated in the pathogenesis of neonatal thyrotoxicosis.[106] The half-life of immunoglobulin G (IgG) is 10 to 14 days; however, these TSIs have been reported to effect infants 12 weeks of age.[112] As in childhood hyperthyroidism, thyroid hormone is synthesized and secreted in excess independent from the pituitary-thyroid gland axis.

Diagnostic Findings
Clinical Findings. The clinical findings of neonatal thyrotoxicosis may be noticed before birth by a fetal heart rate greater than 160 beats/minute.[91] Affected infants are commonly born before term and may be microcephalic with craniosynostosis.[91,94] Clinical manifestations of excess thyroid hormones include restlessness, hyperthermia, respiratory distress, and tachycardia that may rapidly produce congestive heart failure. Goiter and exophthalmos may not be present. Advanced bone age is common.[91,94,98]

Ancillary Data. Radioimmunoassay measurement of T_4 and T_3 reveals elevated serum levels compared with age-matched controls. Measurement of TSHs and a T_3-resin uptake test are helpful in the diagnosis. Electrocardiography is an important evaluation for dysrhythmias. Chest radiography is likewise important in the neonate as part of the investigation for congestive heart failure and respiratory distress.

Differential Considerations. Prematurity in an infant warrants investigation of possible causes such as infection and metabolic disease. In addition, any neonate with temperature instability, respiratory distress, or tachycardia may be manifesting signs of sepsis, hypoglycemia, inborn error of metabolism, congenital heart disease, or drug withdrawal.

Management. Treatment of neonatal thyrotoxicosis parallels the treatment of thyroid storm in the child. Propranolol is used to ameliorate the cardiovascular symptoms in a dosage of 1 to 2 mg/kg/24 hr in three divided doses.[94,98] Propylthiouracil, 5 to 10 mg/kg/24 hr or methimazole, 0.5 to 0.7 mg/kg in divided doses, is given to inhibit the hypersecretion of thyroid hormone.[91,94,95,98,112] Iodide is then given as a supersaturated potassium iodide solution (Lugol's solution), 1 drop orally every 8 hours.[94,98,112]

Disposition. Neonatal thyrotoxicosis is transient but can be severe and life-threatening. Treatment and monitoring, and consultation with an endocrinologist should be done. The ICU is the appropriate setting for continuous monitoring and attention to the therapeutic regimens and response.

References

Failure to Thrive/Growth Deficiency

1. Wilcox W, Nieburg P, Miller D: Failure to thrive: a continuing problem of definition, *Clin Pediatr (Phila)* 28(9):391, 1989.
2. Failure to thrive revisited, *Lancet* 336:662, 1990.
3. Schmitt B and Mauro R: Nonorganic failure to thrive: an outpatient approach, *Child Abuse Negl* 13:235, 1989.
4. Bithoney WG, Dubowitz H, Egan H: Failure to thrive/growth deficiency, *Pediatr Rev* 13:453-460, 1992.
5. Goldbloom R: Failure to thrive, *Pediatr Clin North Am* 29(1):151, 1982.
6. Ludwig S and Homer C: Categorization of failure to thrive, *Am J Dis Child* 135:848, 1981.
7. Nazarian LF: Special records for special conditions—failure to thrive, *Pediatr Rev* 15:69-71, 1994.

Hypoglycemia

8. Haymond M: Hypoglycemia in infants and children, *Endocrinol Metab Clin North Am* 18(1):211, 1989.
9. Koh THHG, Eyre JA, Anysley-Green A: Neural dysfunction during hypoglycaemia, *Arch Dis Child* 63:1353-1358, 1988.
10. Bonham JR: The investigation of hypoglycaemia during childhood, *Ann Clin Biochem* 30:238-247, 1993.
11. Fernandes J and Berger R: Hypoglycaemia: principles of diagnosis and treatment in children, *Baillieres Clin Endocrinol Metab* 591-609, 1993.
12. Pagliara A, Karl I, Haymond M, et al: Hypoglycemia in infancy and childhood, *I J Pediatr* 82(3):365, 1973.
13. Cornblath M and Poth M: Hypoglycemia. In Kaplan S, editor: *Clinical pediatric and adolescent endocrinology*, Philadelphia, 1982, WB Saunders.
14. Haywood N, Forsman P, Kenny F, et al: Hypoglycemia in hypopituitary children, *Am J Dis Child* 129:918, 1975.
15. Reye R, Morgan G, Barel J: Encephalopathy and fatty acid degradation of the viscera: a disease entity of childhood, *Lancet* 2:749, 1963.
16. Czernichow P and Sizonenko PC: Paediatric endocrine and metabolic emergencies. *Baillieres Clin Endocrinol Metab* 193-216, 1992.

Adrenal Hyperplasia, Congenital

17. New M: Molecular genetics and the characterization of steroid 21-hydroxylase deficiency, *Endocr Res* 12(4):505, 1986.
18. White P and New M: Congenital adrenal hyperplasia, *N Engl J Med* 316(24):1519, 1987.
19. New M and Josso N: Disorders of gonadal differentiation and congenital adrenal hyperplasia, *Endocrinol Metab Clin North Am* 17(2):339, 1988.
20. Rosler A: The natural history of salt-wasting disorders of adrenal and renal origin. *J Clin Endocrinol Metab* Oct;59(4):689-700, 1984.
21. Miller W and Levine L: Molecular and clinical advances in congenital adrenal hyperplasia, *J Pediatr* 111(1):1, 1987.
22. New M: Congenital adrenal hyperplasia, *Biochem Soc Trans* 16:691, 1988.
23. Zachman M, Tassinari D, Prader A: Clinical and biochemical variabil-

ity of congenital adrenal hyperplasia due to 11-hydroxylase deficiency: a study of 25 patients, *J Clin Endocrinol Metab* 56:222, 1983.
24. Drucker S and New M: Disorders of adrenal steroidogenesis, *Pediatr Clin North Am* 34(4):1055, 1987.
25. Hughes I: Management of congenital adrenal hyperplasia, *Arch Dis Child* 63:1399, 1988.
26. Artavia-Loria E, Chaussain JL, Bourgneres PF, et al. Frequency of hypoglycemia in children with adrenal insufficiency, *Acta Endocrinol* 279 (suppl):275-278, 1986.
27. Snow K, Jiang NS, Kao PC, et al: Biochemical evaluation of adrenal dysfunction: the laboratory perspective, *Mayo Clin Proc* 67:1055-1065, 1992.
28. Aoki BY and McCloskey K, editors: Renal, metabolic and endocrine disorders. In *Evaluation, stabilization, and transport of the critically ill child*, St. Louis, 1992, Mosby.

Adrenal Insufficiency, Acute

29. Ryan CA, Wenman W, Henningsen C, et al: Fatal childhood pneumococcal Waterhouse-Friderichsen syndrome, *Pediatr Infect Dis J* 12:250-251, 1993.
30. Gertner M, Rodriguez L, Barnett SH, et al: Group A beta-hemolytic streptococcus and Waterhouse-Friderichsen syndrome, *Pediatr Infect Dis J* 11:595-596, 1992.
31. Duffy TP: Clinical problem solving. The sooner the better, *N Eng J Med* 329:710-713, 1993.
32. Urban MD and Kogut MD: Adrenocortical insufficiency in the child, *Curr Ther Endocrinol Metab* 5:131-135, 1994.
33. Zwann CM, Odink RJH, Delemarre-van de Wall, et al: Acute adrenal insufficiency after discontinuation of inhaled corticosteroid therapy, *Lancet* 340:1289-1290, 1992.
34. Philip M, Aviram M, Leiberman A, et al: Integrated plasma cortisol concentration in children with asthma receiving long-term inhaled corticosteroids, *Pediatr Pulmonol* 12:84-89, 1992.
35. Girard FO, Raux-Demay MC: Adrenal insufficiency. In *Pediatric endocrinology: physiology, pathophysiology and clinical aspects*, ed 2, Philadelphia, 1993, Williams & Wilkins.

Antidiuretic Hormone Disorders

36. Berl T and Schrier R: Disorders of water metabolism. In Schrier R, editor: *Renal and electrolyte disorders*, Boston, 1986, Little, Brown.
37. Vokes T and Robertson G: Disorders of antidiuretic hormone, *Endocrinol Metab Clin North Am* 17(2):281, 1988.
38. Hendricks S, Lippe B, Kaplan S, et al: Differential diagnosis of diabetes insipidus: use of dDAVP to terminate the seven-hour water deprivation test, *J Pediatr* 98(2):224, 1981.
39. Seif S, Zenser T, Ciarochi F, et al: dDAVP (1-desamino-8-d-arginine vasopressin) treatment of central diabetes insipidus: mechanism of prolonged antidiuresis, *J Clin Endocrinol Metab* 46(3):381, 1978.
40. Fjellestad-Paulsen A, Tubiana-Rufi N, Harris A, et al: Central diabetes insipidus in children: antidiuretic effect and pharmacokinetics of intranasal and per oral 1-desamino-8-d-arginine vasopressin, *Acta Endocrinol (Copenh)* 115:307, 1987.
41. Giacoia G, Watson S, Karathanos A: Treatment of neonatal diabetes insipidus with desmopresin, *South Med J* 77(1):75, 1984.
42. Beclier D and Foley T: 1-Desamino-8-d-arginine vasopressin in the treatment of central DI in childhood, *J Pediatr* 92(6):1011, 1978.
43. Robinson A: dDAVP in the treatment of central diabetes insipidus, *N Engl J Med* 294(10):507, 1976.
44. Bartter FC, Schwartz WB: The syndrome of inappropriate secretion of antidiuretic hormone, *Adv Pediatr* 27:247-274, 1980.
45. Kaplan S and Feigin R: Syndromes of inappropriate secretion of antidiuretic hormone in children, *Adv Pediatr* 27:247, 1980.
46. Arieff A, Llach F, Massry S: Neurologic manifestations and morbidity of hyponatremia: correlation with brain water and electrolytes, *Medicine (Baltimore)* 55(2):121, 1976.
47. Sakamoto H, Inove K, Marumo F: High plasma atrial natriuretic peptide independent of sodium balance in SIADH, *JAMA* 256:1293, 1986 (letter).
48. Brown LW and Feigin RD: Bacterial meningitis: fluid balance and therapy, Pediatr Ann 23:93-98, 1994.
49. Ganong CA and Kappy MS: Cerebral salt-wasting in children. The need for recognition and treatment, *AJDC* 147:167-169, 1993.
50. Weigle C: Metabolic and endocrine diseases in pediatric intensive

care. In Rogers M, editor: *Textbook of pediatric intensive care*, Philadelphia, 1982, Williams & Wilkins.

Diabetic Ketoacidosis

51. Connell F and Couden J: Diabetes mortality in persons under 45 years of age, *Am J Public Health* 3(10):1174, 1983.
52. Holman R, Herrar C, Sinnock P: Epidemic characteristics of mortality from diabetes with acidosis or coma, United States, 1970-1978, *Am J Public Health* 73(10):1169, 1983.
53. Foster D and Mcgarry J: The metabolic derangements and treatment of diabetic ketoacidosis, *N Engl J Med* 309(3):159, 1983.
54. Rosenbloom AL and Schatz DA: Diabetic ketoacidosis in childhood, *Pediatr Ann* 23:284-288, 1994.
55. Sperling MA: Diabetes mellitus. In *Clinical pediatric endocrinology*, ed 2, Philadelphia, 1990, WB Saunders.
56. Cryer P: Glucose counterregulation in man, *Diabetes* 30:261, 1981.
57. Shamoon H, Hendler R, Sherwin R: Synergistic interaction among anti-insulin hormones in the pathogenesis of stress hyperglycemia in humans, *J Clin Endocrinol Metab* 52:1235, 1981.
58. Miles J, Rizza R, Haymond M, et al: Effects of acute insulin deficiency on glucose and ketone body turnover in man, *Diabetes* 29:295, 1980.
59. Kreisberg R: Diabetic ketoacidosis: new concepts and trends in pathogenesis and treatment, *Ann Intern Med* 88(5):681, 1978.
60. Lebovitz H: Etiology and pathogenesis of diabetes mellitus, *Pediatr Clin North Am* 31(3):521, 1984.
61. Barnes A, Kohmer E, Bloom S, et al: Importance of pituitary hormones in the etiology of diabetic ketoacidosis, *Lancet* 1:1171, 1978.
62. Krane E: Diabetic ketoacidosis, *Pediatr Clin North Am* 34(4):935, 1987.
63. Adrogue H, Wilson H, Boyd A, et al: Plasma acid-base patterns in diabetic ketoacidosis, *N Engl J Med* 307:1603, 1982.
64. Fulop M: Serum potassium in lactic acidosis and ketoacidosis, *N Engl J Med* 300:1087, 1979.
65. Kanter Y, Gerson J, Begman A: 2,3-diphosphoglycerate, nucleotide phosphate, and organic and inorganic phosphate levels during the early phases of diabetic ketoacidosis, *Diabetes* 26:429, 1977.
66. Kaye R: Diabetic ketoacidosis—the bicarbonate controversy, *J Pediatr* 87(1):156, 1975.
67. Ellis E: Concepts of fluid therapy, *Pediatr Clin North Am* 37(2):313, 1990.
68. Alberti K: Low-dose insulin in the treatment of diabetic ketoacidosis, *Arch Intern Med* 137:1367, 1977.
69. Fisher J, Shahshahani M, Kitabachi A: Diabetic ketoacidosis: low-dose insulin therapy by various routes, *N Engl J Med* 297(5):238, 1977.
70. Dillon E, Riggs H, Dyer W: Cerebral lesions in uncomplicated fatal diabetic acidosis, *Am J Med Sci* 192:360, 1965.
71. Speirs A, Stewart D, Adams H, et al: Fatal increase of intracranial pressure during management of diabetic ketosis, *Lancet* 2:879, 1971.
72. Duck S, Weldon V, Pagliara A, et al: Cerebral edema complicating therapy for diabetic ketoacidosis, *Diabetes* 25:111, 1977.
73. Duck S and Kohler E: Cerebral edema in diabetic ketoacidosis, *J Pediatr* 98(4):674, 1981.
74. Krane E, Rockoff M, Waldman J, et al: Subclinical brain swelling in children during treatment of diabetic ketoacidosis, *N Engl J Med* 312(18):1147, 1985.
75. Rosenbloom A: Intracerebral crisis during treatment of diabetic ketoacidosis, *Diabetes Care* 13(1):22, 1990.
76. Mel JM, Werther GA: Incidence and outcome of diabetic cerebral oedema in childhood: are there predictors? *J Paediatr Child Health* 31:17-20, 1995.
77. Glasgow A: Devastating cerebral edema in diabetic ketoacidosis before therapy, *Diabetes Care* 14(1):77, 1991 (letter).
78. Couch R, Acott P, Wong G: Early onset fatal cerebral edema in diabetic ketoacidosis, *Diabetes Care* 14(1):78, 1991 (letter).
79. Franklin B, Liu J, Ginsburg-Fellner F: Cerebral edema and ophthalmoplegia reversed by mannitol in a new case of insulin-dependent diabetes mellitus, *Pediatrics* 69(1):87, 1987.
80. Harris G, Fiordalisi I, Harris W, et al: Minimizing the risk of brain herniation during treatment of diabetic ketoacidosis: a retrospective and prospective study, *J Pediatr* 117(1):22, 1990.

Pheochromocytoma

81. Stringel G, Ein S, Creighton R, et al: Pheochromocytoma in children: an update, *J Pediatr Surg* 15(4):496, 1980.

82. Farrelly C, Daneman A, Martin D, et al: Pheochromocytoma in childhood: the important role of computed tomography in tumour localization, *Pediatr Radiol* 14:210, 1984.
83. Beard C, Sheps S, Kurland L, et al: Occurrence of pheochromocytoma in Rochester, Minnesota, 1950 through 1979, *Mayo Clin Proc* 58:802, 1983.
84. Samaan N and Hickey R: Pheochromocytoma, *Semin Oncol* 14(3):297, 1987.
85. Sheps S, Jiang N, Klee G: Diagnostic evaluation of pheochromocytoma, *Endocrinol Metab Clin North Am* 17(2):397, 1988.
86. Aguilo F, Tamayo N, Vazquez-Quintana E, et al: Pheochromocytoma: a twenty-year experience at the University Hospital, *P R Health Sci J* 10:135-142, 1991.
87. Huddle KR, Mannell A, James MF, et al: Phaoechromocytoma. A report of 10 patients, *S Afr Med J* 79:217-220, 1991.
88. Daneman A: Adrenal neoplasms in children, *Semin Roentgenol* 23(3):205, 1988.
89. Fonesca V and Bouloux PM: Phaeochromocytoma and paraganglioma, *Ballieres Clin Endocrinol Metab* 7:509-544, 1993.
90. Bravo EL and Gifford RW: Phaeochromocytoma: diagnosis, localization, and management, *N Engl J Med* 11:1298-1303, 1984.

Thyroid Disorders

91. Levy W, Schumacher P, Gupta M: Treatment of childhood Graves' disease, *Cleve Clin J Med* 55(4):373, 1988.
92. Barnes H and Blizzard R: Antithyroid drug therapy for toxic diffuse goiter (Graves' disease): 30 years experience in children and adolescents, *J Pediatr* 91(2):313, 1977.
93. Maanpaa J and Kuusi A: Childhood hyperthyroidism, *Acta Paediatr* 69:137, 1980.
94. Lee W: Thyroiditis, hyperthyroidism and tumors, *Pediatr Clin North Am* 26(1):53, 1979.
95. Zimmerman D, Gan-Gaisano M: Hyperthyroidism in children and adolescents, *Pediatr Clin North Am* 37:1273-1295, 1990.
96. Wenzel BE, Heesemann J, Wenzel KW, et al: Patients with autoimmune diseases have antibodies to plasmid-encoded proteins of enteropathogenic *Yersinia*, *J Endocrinol Invest* 11:139-140, 1988.
97. Volpe R, Row VV, Ezrin C: Circulating viral and thyroid antibodies in subacute thyroiditis, *J Clin Endocrinol Metab* 27:1275-1284, 1967.
98. Hoffenberg R: Thyroid emergencies, *Clin Endocrinol Metab* 9(3):503, 1980.
99. Fisher DA: The thyroid. In: *Clinical pediatric endocrinology*, ed 2, Philadelphia, 1990, WB Saunders.
100. Mahoney C: Differential diagnosis of goiter, *Pediatr Clin North Am* 34(4):891, 1987.
101. Hamburger J: Management of hyperthyroidism in children and adolescents, *J Clin Endocrinol Metab* 60(5):1019, 1985.
102. MacDougal I: Which therapy for Graves' hyperthyroidism in children? *Nucl Med Commun* 10:885, 1989.
103. Ingbar S: Management of emergencies: thyrotoxic storm, *N Engl J Med* 274(2):1252, 1966.
104. Gorton C, Sedeghi-Nejad A, Senior B: Remission in children with hyperthyroidism treated with propylthiouracil: long-term results, *Am J Dis Child* 141:1084, 1987.
105. LaFranchi S: Hypothyroidism: congenital and acquired. In Kaplan S, editor: *Clinical pediatric and adolescent endocrinology*, Philadelphia, 1982, WB Saunders.
106. Fisher D, Pandian M, Carlton E: Autoimmune thyroid disease: an expanding spectrum, *Pediatr Clin North Am* 39(4):907, 1987.
107. Foley T: Acute, subacute and chronic thyroiditis. In Kaplan S, editor: *Clinical pediatric and adolescent endocrinology*, Philadelphia, 1982, WB Saunders.
108. Lafranchi S: Thyroiditis and acquired hypothyroidism, *Pediatr Ann* 21:29-39, 1992.
109. January 1, 1990 Report: *New England Regional Newborn Screening Program*, Boston, 1990, (booklet).
110. Fisher D and Klein A: Thyroid development and disorders of thyroid function in the newborn, *N Engl J Med* 304(12):702, 1981.
111. Zakarija M and McKenzie M: Pregnancy associated changes in the thyroid-stimulating antibody of Graves' disease and the relationship to neonatal hyperthyroidism, *J Clin Endocrinol Metab* 57:1036, 1983.
112. Clayton G: Thyrotoxicosis in children. In Kaplan S, editor: *Clinical pediatric and adolescent endocrinology*, 1982, WB Saunders.

51

Eye Disorders

Jacalyn S. Maller

The emergency department is often the first place that eye disorders are brought to medical attention. Problems encountered can range from those that can be adequately diagnosed and treated by the emergency physician (e.g., conjunctivitis and periorbital cellulitis) with ophthalmologic follow-up if symptoms do not improve, to those considered ophthalmologic emergencies (e.g., acid/alkali burns and ruptured globe), when prompt intervention or immediate consultation with an ophthalmologist can improve visual outcome. Unfortunately, in the setting of a busy emergency department, eye disorders may be overlooked when present with other serious injuries (e.g., in the patient with multiple trauma), when the physician fails to perform a thorough eye examination (patient with a swollen eye), or when the examiner is not comfortable examining infants and children.

DIAGNOSTIC FINDINGS

Patient history can guide the examiner in assessing the seriousness of the problem. If a history of acid or alkali exposure is obtained, the patient should receive immediate irrigation with saline before further evaluation is attempted. If the history or physical examination suggests a penetrating ocular injury or ruptured globe, the eye should be immediately patched with a nonpressured protective shield. No further manipulation or examination should be attempted until an ophthalmologist is present (see Chapter 21).

If neither a chemical burn nor penetrating ocular injury is present, a more detailed history can be obtained. Important questions include the nature of the pain or complaint, duration of symptoms, location, exacerbating and relieving factors, occurrence of trauma, and the presence of fever or other systemic symptoms. A complete history may not be given if a child was hurt while engaging in a forbidden activity (e.g., playing with fireworks or BB guns) or if a parent intentionally injured a child. Important points in the past medical history include history of eye problems, prematurity, in utero exposures (e.g., drugs or rubella) that may result in congenital eye abnormalities, birth trauma, prior visual acuity, and previous eye injury (e.g., hyphema) that may result in subsequent eye problems months to years later (e.g., glaucoma or cataracts).

Using toys to elicit attention and making the practitioner seem less threatening facilitates the examination. Doing as much of the examination as possible without touching the patient and examining the unaffected eye first is helpful.

The assessment of visual acuity is the most important part of the eye examination in children. Although normal visual acuity does not exclude eye pathology, it is rare to have a serious injury requiring immediate ophthalmologic intervention with normal acuity. In the infant, the ability to fixate and follow a target is the most reliable test of visual acuity in the emergency department setting. This ability is usually obvious by 6 weeks of age. The object used for fixation can include a brightly colored toy, a human face, or a sound-producing object (even though the latter may not be visually pure, it will more readily engage the infant).[1] Subjective testing of vision is usually not possible until a child is 2½ to 3 years old.[2] The Allen picture card examination, which tests each eye separately, is the best test at this age. The "E" test can usually be performed on children by age 4; after a pretest practice session to teach the child, the test is then taken. The adult type of Snellen acuity chart may be used with the 5 to 6 year old who knows numbers and letters.[1] The definition of normal visual acuity varies by age and is discussed in a subsequent section.

In the uncooperative patient, objective testing is not possible. A gross estimation of visual abilities can be obtained by checking for light perception (manifested by blinking or light aversion) recognizing hand motion, and object movement (fix and follow), distinguishing faces (recognize a parent), or counting fingers (recorded at best distance).[3]

Before touching the patient, observe the child for evidence of trauma or facial asymmetry. Marked blepharospasm or blinking suggests light sensitivity and possible corneal inflammation or, in rare cases, glaucoma. A child who is constantly scratching the eyes may have an allergic

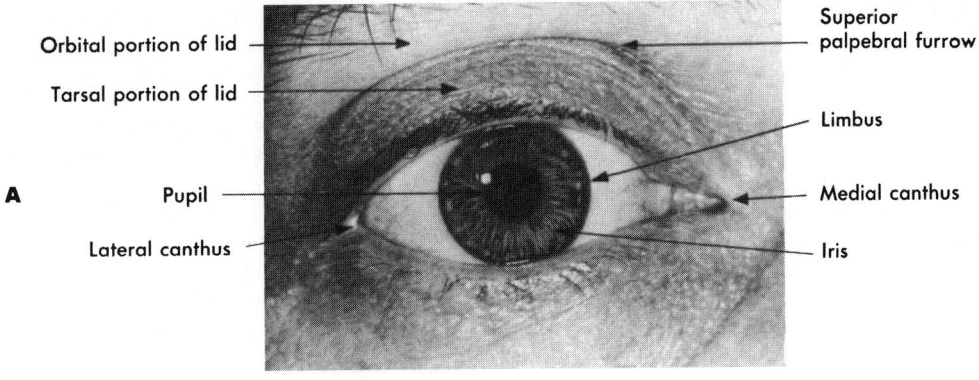

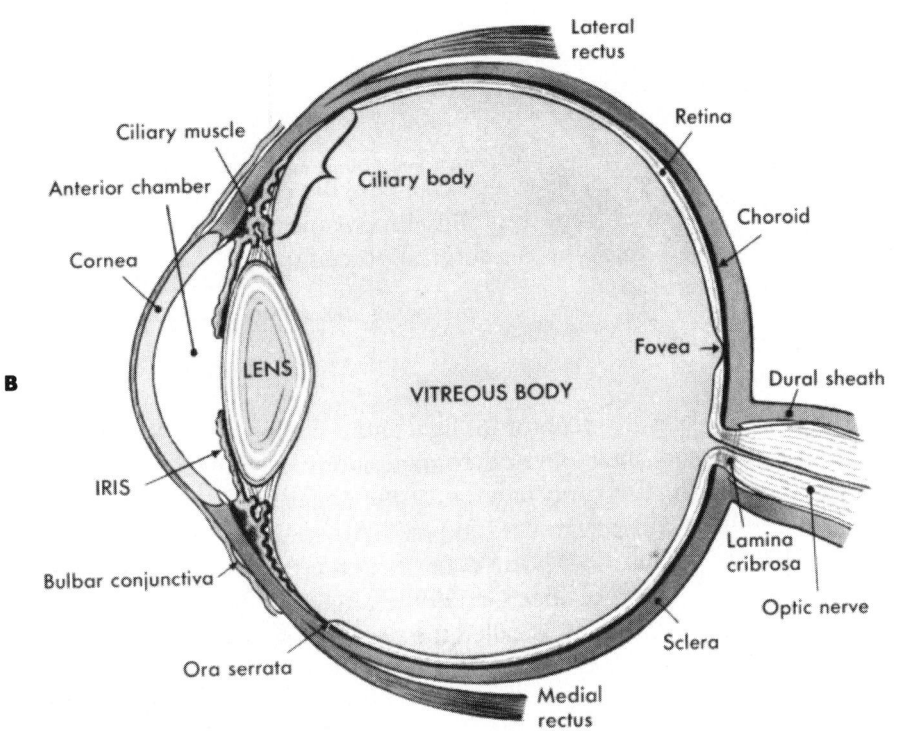

FIG. 51-1. A, Surface anatomy of the eye. **B,** The eye cut in horizontal section. (*From Stein HA, Slatt BJ, Stein RM: Ophthalmic terminology, ed 2, St Louis, 1987, Mosby.*)

conjunctivitis or a new corneal abrasion. In the young child, somnolence or lethargy may be the first manifestation of a globe perforation.

The external structures of the eye—including the face, brow, lids, and lashes—are examined next (Fig. 51-1). A complete examination of the upper lid and palpebral conjunctiva requires lid eversion. This involves pulling the upper lid lashes outward with one hand and using a cotton swab to act as a fulcrum against the upper skinfold to evert the upper lid.[1] Lid eversion is particularly important to evaluate the possibility of a foreign body. Any laceration of the lid margin in the area of the medial canthus may involve the lacrimal duct system and require suturing by an ophthalmologist. In the event that marked lid swelling is present and examination of the internal structures is difficult, the use of lid retractors is indicated. The orbital bones are palpated while looking for a step-off, localized tenderness, or the presence of subcutaneous emphysema, which indicates a sinus or nasal fracture. Decreased sensation in the distribution of the infraorbital nerve suggests an orbital floor fracture.

The conjunctiva should be examined for evidence of inflammation, hemorrhage, or laceration. The cornea is examined for any evidence of opacification. If a corneal abrasion is suggested by history or abnormal reflection of light, the instillation of fluorescein is necessary to outline the defect. For this procedure, fluorescein-impregnated sterile paper strips should be used rather than the bottled solution, which can readily become contaminated with *Pseudomonas aeruginosa*. After anesthetizing the eye with a topical anesthetic, saline may be used to drip the fluorescein over the conjunctival surface. Fluorescein is taken up by subepithelial corneal tissue because of a more acidic pH and appears dark green when viewed under a Wood's lamp or other fluorescent light.

The anterior chamber, although usually examined with a slit lamp, may be grossly inspected with a penlight and magnifying glass for the presence of blood (hyphema) or pus (hypopyon).

The pupils are assessed for size, symmetry, shape, and reactivity. Although in most cases the size is equal, anisocoria may be present in approximately 25% of healthy individuals.[1] Pupillary reactivity indicates functioning afferent and efferent pathways. In the neonate the resting pupil size is small, and reactivity is slightly more sluggish than in the older child. Although absence of a pupillary reaction to light indicates an abnormality of the retina or optic nerve, the presence of a reactive pupil is not synonymous with normal visual acuity.[1] Pupillary irregularity may suggest a prolapsed iris. In the comatose or uncooperative patient, evidence of a Marcus-Gunn pupil (i.e., dilation instead of constriction of the contralateral pupil on light stimulation of an injured eye) suggests a visual defect. A white pupillary reflex, leukokoria, is the most common sign of retinoblastoma.[1]

Ocular alignment and extraocular motility are assessed for limitations of gaze or eliciting diplopia. This is particularly important in the patient with suspected orbital cellulitis and in the patient with a possible orbital fracture with extraocular muscle entrapment.

Internal examination of the eye with a direct ophthalmoscope is done to assess for papilledema and evidence of retinal hemorrhages (shaken baby syndrome). Direct ophthalmoscopy is not helpful in examining the periphery of the retina and may overlook a retinal detachment. Therefore any time visual acuity is reduced, direct ophthalmoscopy by the emergency department physician must be supplemented by indirect ophthalmoscopy to adequately visualize the retinal periphery.

In the patient with constricted pupils a combination of a short-acting mydriatic and cycloplegic agent may be used, provided contraindications (e.g., head trauma or suspected globe perforation) do not exist. For young children a combination of 1% cyclopentolate hydrochloride (Cyclogyl) and 2.5% phenylephrine hydrochloride (Mydfrin) may be used for pupillary dilatation and cycloplegia.[1] Cycloplegia is usually achieved 45 minutes after instillation. In children with darker skin pigmentation a second drop of these medications 5 to 10 minutes after the first may be necessary.

Visual field examination by confrontation is appropriate whenever there is decreased visual acuity or the possibility of a visual field cut. Abnormal findings may indicate a retinal detachment or intracranial pathology.

The slit lamp demonstrates a magnified view of the external eye and anterior segment. It may help detect a small foreign body or hyphema and is essential in evaluating the eye with suspected uveitis.

Tonometry is indicated whenever increased intraocular pressure is suspected. This procedure is difficult to perform accurately in the infant or uncooperative young child. Therefore these cases should be referred to an ophthalmologist when the diagnosis of glaucoma is an absolute contraindication, whereas the presence of corneal infections or ulcers are relative contraindications to the procedure.[4] Suspected globe perforation is suggested by the emergency department evaluation.

In the next section, specific eye complaints, including evaluation of visual impairment, paralysis and movement disorders, and the approach to red eye are discussed in greater detail.

Signs and Symptoms

IMPAIRED VISION

Most children who come to the emergency department with acute complaints of impaired vision have a readily definable cause. Trauma and infection are by far the most common causes of visual disturbances in children.[1] The two most emergent conditions for the emergency department physician to diagnose and treat are chemical burns, particularly those caused by alkali, and central retinal artery occlusion.[1] Unfortunately, in the pediatric population, many children with impaired vision may be preverbal and unable to complain, or may have subtle visual abnormalities that can only be tested by careful assessment of visual acuity and a complete ophthalmologic examination. Therefore the emergency department physician must assess visual acuity in all pediatric patients with visual complaints or eye pathology on physical examination.

The definition of normal visual acuity in the preschool population, when most quantitative testing can be determined, differs by age. An acuity of 20/40 is considered normal for a 3-year-old child, whereas 20/30 is the accepted norm for a 4-year-old child. The normal adult vision of 20/20 is not usually evident until age 5 or 6 years.[5] Whenever possible, it is best to use a full chart of symbols rather than single symbols, since the latter will yield better visual acuity results, particularly in the amblyopic eye.[2] It is also preferable to use a patch rather than a handheld occluder when testing each eye's acuity to avoid the possibility of peeking.[2] When using an eye chart, a difference of greater than one line between the two eyes is considered abnormal and requires further ophthalmologic evaluation.

Pathophysiology

Visual impairment may be due to a variety of causes. Anything that physically obstructs the passage of light through the eye (e.g., a swollen lid and corneal or lens opacities) impairs normal visual acuity. Refractive abnormalities that distort image formation (e.g., myopia, hyperopia, and astigmatism) cause visual disturbance on a more chronic basis and are not discussed. Neuroretinal deficits that prevent retinal perception of light or preclude its transmission to the visual cortex (e.g., tumors, drugs, retinal detachment, or head trauma) cause visual difficulties.[6]

Differential Considerations

Conjunctivitis, which is due to excessive mucopurulent discharge or, when viral, corneal involvement, may cause mild visual impairment. Recurrent herpes simplex keratoconjunctivitis is the most common cause of corneal scarring and infectious blindness in the United States.[7] When conjunctivitis occurs within the first 2 to 4 weeks of life, the possibility of *Neisseria gonorrhoeae* infection must be considered, since if left untreated, the disease may progress to corneal ulceration with perforation and subsequent septicemia and blindness.

Periorbital or orbital cellulitis may cause visual impairment. In periorbital cellulitis, any decrease in visual acuity usually is due to eyelid swelling and tenderness, but the eye itself should be normal, unless there has been a history of trauma to the globe. The presence of decreased vision, ophthalmoplegia, proptosis, or pain on eye movement indicates orbital cellulitis. In the latter case, ophthalmoscopy may demonstrate retinal vein congestion or optic disc edema.

Uveitis occurs with symptoms of blurred vision, unilateral eye pain, headache, and photophobia. The degree of visual impairment increases with posterior uveal tract involvement. More severe visual loss is found with endophthalmitis, which may follow eye surgery or penetrating injury. A unilateral, painful, visually impaired eye with a hypopyon suggests endophthalmitis.[8]

Trauma may cause impaired vision by interference with light perception or transmission. Blunt trauma that produces an eyelid hematoma or edema obstructs the ability of the eye to receive an image. Orbital trauma may increase the probability of ocular complications because of the close proximity of the nerves, blood vessels, and extraocular muscles to the orbital bones. Severe visual loss may result from damage to the optic nerve or compromise of its blood supply, especially when a lateral wall fracture is present.[1] A blowout fracture, resulting from blunt trauma to the orbital rim, most commonly damages the medial wall and orbital floor (i.e., the weakest orbital bones). Visual impairment, most specifically double vision, may be related to incarceration of the inferior rectus or inferior oblique muscle, causing restriction of upward gaze.[9] An intramuscular hematoma of the extraocular muscles may also prevent normal motility and result in impaired vision.

Traumatic injury to the cornea may cause epithelial defects or abrasions, resulting in severe lacrimation, photophobia, and blurring of vision. Fluorescein staining and lid eversion delineate the defects and reveal foreign bodies on the upper lid. Corneal and scleral lacerations may result from blunt or penetrating trauma and cause subsequent visual impairment. A hyphema is usually the result of trauma that causes rupture of blood vessels of the iris or ciliary body. The degree of visual impairment depends on the extent of filling of the anterior chamber. Complications of hyphemas include rebleeding, elevated intraocular pressure with resultant glaucoma, and corneal bloodstaining, which may cause amblyopia and may require surgery. Glaucoma may also occur as a late complication of blunt trauma to the eye (see Chapter 21).

Trauma to the lens may result in a cataract, which may ultimately decrease visual outcome, depending on the extent of involvement. More acutely, ocular trauma may result in lens subluxation, with diplopia and iridodonesis (trembling of the iris).

Trauma to the posterior segment of the eye may result in vitreous hemorrhage and occurs with sudden, profound loss of vision.[9] Other nontraumatic causes of vitreous hemorrhage include diabetes mellitus, hypertension, sickle cell disease, and leukemia.[8]

Berlin's edema, or commotio retinae, is contusion edema of the retina from blunt trauma. Visual acuity may be decreased and a "milky white haze" of the retina with retinal hemorrhage may be evident on funduscopic examination.[1] Visual prognosis depends on the degree of retinal damage. Retinal detachment in children is most commonly secondary to trauma. Often the tear is in the retinal periphery, and therefore few ocular symptoms are noted. Diagnosis may be delayed by several months or even years, since symptoms may not be evident until the macula is involved. Involvement of the macula is suggested by symptoms of flashing lights or a "curtain" in the visual field.

Chemical burns, particularly those caused by alkali, may result in significant visual impairment and are the most common vision-threatening emergencies in children. Alkali quickly penetrates the cornea by reacting with fats to form soaps, whereas acid quenches its own ability to cause more extensive damage by precipitating tissue proteins. Immediate copious irrigation with careful testing of eye pH is necessary to minimize the extent of visual impairment (see Chapter 43).

Ultraviolet and infrared light can cause corneal damage within 24 hours of exposure. Patients may have a red, swollen eye and complaints of photophobia, decreased vision, lacrimation, and severe blepharospasm. Symptoms should gradually abate over the next few days without treatment.

Blunt head trauma may result in transient cortical blindness. The patient may seem unaware and unconcerned about the lack of vision. There are no pupillary or retinal abnormalities found on physical examination and often the diagnosis of "hysterical" blindness is made. Recovery occurs over several hours to several weeks, beginning peripherally and moving centrally.[8]

The remaining causes of visual impairment are neither traumatic nor infectious. Errors in refraction (e.g., myopia, hyperopia, and astigmatism) usually will not be presented as an acute emergency. Strabismus, paralytic or nonparalytic, may present as diplopia, squinting, or with various head tilts that the child adopts to eliminate double vision. Amblyopia, abnormal visual acuity in one eye without abnormalities of the retina, is often the result of strabismus or unequal refractive errors of the two eyes. It reflects the ability of the cortex to ignore all visual input when the image is distorted or misaligned. Glaucoma may be congenital or result from trauma. Visual acuity is decreased, and immediate ophthalmologic consultation is indicated.

Retinal vein or artery occlusion is rare in pediatric patients but is a true ophthalmologic emergency. Both cause a sudden painless loss of vision in one eye, generally more complete with artery occlusion. With retinal artery occlusion, funduscopic examination reveals a cherry red spot of the fovea, a pale optic disc and narrowed arteries, along with a Marcus-Gunn pupil. Causes include trauma or embolic obstruction, which may occur in sickle cell disease or systemic lupus erythematosus. The funduscopic examination of a patient with retinal vein occlusion may reveal retinal hemorrhages with a blurred optic disc, engorged, tortuous veins, and narrowed arteries. Causes of retinal vein occlusion include trauma, leukemia, and cystic fibrosis.[4,8]

Optic neuritis occurs with acute, unilateral loss of vision. In children with papillitis or intraocular optic neuritis, symptoms are usually bilateral and part of a systemic disease such as meningitis, varicella, or a nonspecific febrile illness. Various toxins such as lead or high-dose chloramphenicol can also cause papillitis. Funduscopic examination reveals disc swelling with hemorrhages, exudates, and a Marcus-Gunn pupillary defect.[1]

Toxins may impair vision through effects on the retina or optic nerve and include methanol, mercury, salicylates, quinidine, naphthalene, and the halogenated hydrocarbons. Diagnosis may be made by a history of ingestion or the associated symptoms of the ingestion.

Migraine headaches may cause bilateral field loss or total blindness, most commonly in the adolescent population. The symptoms usually last from 10 to 15 minutes and may be followed by nausea, vomiting, or headache.

Diagnostic Work-Up

Information useful in defining the cause of visual impairment includes the degree of impairment, rapidity of onset and progression of the symptoms, and presence of pain, trauma, fever, or other systemic symptoms. A history of blunt trauma requires evaluation for hyphema, cataract, or lens dislocation; with complete loss of vision, a retinal detachment or retinal vessel occlusion may be present. Foreign-body sensation with photophobia may result from the presence of a foreign body, corneal abrasion, or thermal or ultraviolet burn. A history of blunt head trauma with complete loss of vision and no apparent physical findings on examination suggests cortical blindness. A past medical history of cystic fibrosis, lupus, or sickle cell disease will lead one to consider a retinal vessel occlusion as the cause for painless loss of vision. Exposure to various toxins such as lead, methanol, or drugs such as chloramphenicol, salicylates, and quinidine should be elicited. A history of migraine headaches may aid the physician in defining the cause of bilateral visual field loss.

Physical examination of the patient with impaired vision should include visual acuity testing if some degree of vision is present. External examination may reveal evidence of trauma (ecchymoses) or infection (periorbital swelling and erythema). The anterior chamber should be checked for a hyphema or hypopyon. Examination of the cornea with fluorescein may reveal a foreign body, corneal abrasion, or diffuse uptake found in viral conjunctivitis. Extraocular muscle testing may reveal abnormalities resulting from muscle entrapment from orbital fractures or hematomas. Pupillary reactivity may be abnormal with retinal artery occlusion. Abnormal visual-field testing may indicate a retinal detachment. Funduscopic examination with evidence of disc swelling and hemorrhages may suggest a papillitis. When abnormal vessels are present, the diagnosis of retinal vessel occlusion also may be considered. Fluorescein testing helps delineate a foreign body, corneal abrasion, or infectious keratitis.

Ancillary Data. Conjunctivitis in the neonatal period requires a gram stain and culture of the eye discharge to rule out gonococcal or chlamydial conjunctivitis. With periorbital or orbital cellulitis, a complete blood count (CBC) and differential and blood culture are indicated, particularly in children under 5 years of age when *Haemophilus influenzae* is a potential hematogenous pathogen. When the history and physical examination suggest an orbital cellulitis, a head CT scan is indicated to rule out an orbital or subperiosteal abscess and look for evidence of sinusitis. In patients with extraocular muscle entrapment after blunt trauma or with a physical examination suggestive of an orbital fracture, an orbital CT scan should be obtained to look for a fracture; fluid in the sinuses, which indirectly indicates a fracture; or evidence of a foreign body. Ophthalmology should be consulted whenever the diagnosis of gonococcal or herpes simplex conjunctivitis, orbital cellulitis, endophthalmitis, or hyphema is made or anytime vision is impaired acutely, regardless of whether trauma has occurred. If a toxic ingestion is suspected, a drug screen and quantitative levels of the suspected drug should be sent.

Prehospital Considerations

Immediate irrigation of the eye for all acid or alkali exposures has been described previously. Patching the eye with suspected globe perforation has also been described.

Therapeutic Trial

All patients with acute onset of impaired vision should be seen by an ophthalmologist. After irrigation and ophthalmologic assessment of a chemical burn, a cycloplegic agent (atropine 1%) is instilled to decrease ciliary spasm and formation of adhesions. Topical antibiotics and steroids are recommended to prevent infection and decrease inflammation, respectively.[9] The presence of hyphema usually necessitates admission to the hospital because of the risk of rebleeding and permanent visual sequelae. A unilateral painless loss of vision may be the result of a retinal vein or artery occlusion and is considered an ophthalmologic emergency requiring immediate oxygenation of the ischemic retina with a mixture of 95% oxygen and 5% carbon dioxide and ophthalmologic consultation.[4] The treatment of conjunctivitis and periorbital and orbital cellulitis is discussed in a subsequent section.

PARALYSIS AND MOVEMENT DISORDERS

Complaints of double vision or the presence of abnormal eye movements may be the initial manifestation of serious neurologic, infectious, or oncologic disease. A history of the complaint, including age of onset, length of symptoms, presence of systemic symptoms, and whether trauma occurred helps the emergency department physician differentiate between the more benign entities and those requiring immediate diagnosis and management.

Disorders of eye movements may occur as the following:

1. Extraocular muscle palsies.
2. Abnormal head positions (e.g., head tilt, face turn, and torticollis).
3. Disorders of conjugate (paired eye movements) gaze.
4. Abnormal eye movements (nystagmus, opsoclonus, and ocular bobbing).[10]

Strabismus refers to a muscle imbalance that causes improper eye alignment. Paralytic strabismus refers to paralysis of an extraocular muscle with a deviation varying according to the direction of gaze and is primarily neurologic in origin. In nonparalytic or concomitant strabismus, there is no muscle or nerve palsy and the amount of deviation is constant in all fields of gaze. The latter is primarily an ophthalmologic problem that may be related to visual defects such as cataracts, high refractive error, or retinal lesions (retinoblastoma).[1] Esotropia is persistent inward deviation of the eyes, whereas exotropia is divergent or outward eye deviation. Esophoria and exophoria relate to an eye that tends to deviate inward or outward, respectively. Nystagmus refers to involuntary rhythmic oscillations of the eyes and may be physiologic or pathologic depending on the age of onset, direction (vertical or horizontal), and other clinical symptomatology.

Pathophysiology

The pathophysiology of eye movement disorders is complex and is not described in detail. In simple terms, however, problems with abnormal eye movements or paralysis can be ascribed to the following lesions that are most likely to appear acutely in the emergency department:

1. Lesions of the afferent visual pathway (e.g., cataracts, optic nerve tumors, or retinal lesions), causing visual sensory deprivation and subsequent esotropia, exotropia, or nystagmus.
2. Lesions of cranial nerve nuclei III, IV, and VI or their pathways that control motor innervation of the six extraocular muscles. Cranial nerve (CN) III supplies all of the extrinsic ocular muscles except for the superior oblique (innervated by CN IV) and the lateral rectus (innervated by CN VI). The paths of these nerves are long and may be affected anywhere in their course by infections or inflammatory processes, vascular disease, trauma with resultant rise in intracranial pressure, tumor, toxins, and degenerative or demyelinating disease.
3. Lesions of the neuromuscular junction (e.g., myasthenia gravis) prevent nerve-to-muscular transmission of impulses.

4. Lesions of the midbrain centers (medial longitudinal fasciculus) that control convergence and divergence.
5. Primary muscle disorders.[10]

Differential Considerations

Muscle. The most common primary extraocular muscle abnormality seen in the emergency department results from an orbital fracture with localized hemorrhage and muscle entrapment.

Most commonly, the eye cannot move in the direction opposite the fracture. Thyroid disease causes inflamed extraocular muscles with restricted eye movements (Table 51-1).

Neuromuscular System. Myasthenia gravis may present initially with external ophthalmoplegia and ptosis. The symptoms fluctuate in severity, worsening with fatigue and improving with rest and anticholinesterase medication.

Cranial Nerves. The majority of extraocular muscle palsies are due to cranial nerve abnormalities and neurologic disease.[10] Cranial nerve palsies are rare in children, but when the onset is acute, may indicate life-threatening central nervous system (CNS) disease, including meningitis, tumor, and an epidural or subdural hemorrhage.

TABLE 51-1. Differential Diagnosis of Diplopia

Common etiologies	Physical findings
Neurogenic palsy cranial nerves	
VI: Head trauma	Loss of lateral eye movement
↑ ICP	Horizontal diplopia
Tumor	If chronic, face turns *toward*
Meningitis/encephalitis	side of paretic muscle
Postviral (benign)	
Gradenigo syndrome	
III: Head trauma	Eye deviated down and
Tumor	outward
Infection	Ptosis
Migraine	Pupil dilation
IV: Head trauma	Vertical diplopia
Tumor	Head tilt to side opposite
	palsied muscle
Muscle	
Orbital floor fracture	Entrapment of inferior rectus muscle
	Restricted upgaze
	Enophthalmus
	Proptosis secondary orbital hemorrhage
Thyroid ophthalmopathy	Restricted eye movements secondary inflamed extraocular muscles
Neuromuscular	
Myasthenia gravis	Bilateral ptosis
	Oculomotor impairment
	Worse with fatigue
Botulism	Oculomotor palsies
	Bilateral ptosis
	Poor suck and gag
	Hypotonia

Oculomotor (CN III) palsies are more frequently congenital than acquired, resulting from developmental abnormalities or birth trauma. They present with exotropia and downward deviation of the eye, ptosis, pupillary dilation and impaired adduction, depression, and elevation. Most acute oculomotor palsies in children are caused by increased intracranial pressure (tumor) or trauma. Less common acute causes include infection and ophthalmoplegic migraine.

A trochlear (CN IV) palsy is also more commonly congenital rather than acquired. If congenital, it will present at approximately 1 month of age with a head tilt to the side opposite the palsied superior oblique muscle. Most commonly, acquired fourth nerve palsies are due to head trauma or a midbrain tumor such as a pinealoma.[11]

In contrast, most sixth nerve palsies are acquired, with trauma being the most common cause. Patients may have lateral rectus weakness or paralysis, convergent strabismus, horizontal diplopia that worsens on gaze toward the involved side and, if longstanding, a compensatory face turn toward the side of the paretic muscle. The palsied abducens (CN VI) nerve is a nonspecific, nonlocalizing sign of increased intracranial pressure secondary to hydrocephalus, tumor, an intracranial hemorrhage, or cerebral edema. Other acute causes include meningitis, cavernous sinus thrombosis, vascular disease, and neurotoxins (e.g., lead).[10]

A benign acquired sixth nerve palsy that is painless and resolves spontaneously may occur in children after a viral illness. The child with accommodative esotropia will have a more gradual onset of symptoms with greater diplopia for near than far objects.[11] In contrast, Gradenigo syndrome is an acquired painful sixth nerve palsy. Pain occurs in the distribution of the homolateral trigeminal nerve along with photophobia, diplopia, and lacrimation. It is due to disease involving the petrous portion of the sixth nerve; otitis media and mastoiditis with inflammation of the petrous bone are the most likely causes.[10] Meningitis, extradural or brain abscesses, and tumor are less common but more potentially life-threatening causes of Gradenigo syndrome.

A congenital syndrome often confused with a sixth nerve palsy is Duane congenital retraction syndrome in which the lateral rectus is innervated by an anomalous third nerve. Patients have deficiency of abduction with retraction of the globe and palpebral fissure narrowing on adduction.

Multiple cranial nerve palsies affecting eye movement (specifically CN III, IV, V, and VI) may be seen in cavernous sinus syndromes with ophthalmoplegia, ptosis, lack of accommodation, venous engorgement and edema of the lids, conjunctiva, and ptosis. The most common conditions in children are related to sepsis, but tumor, inflammatory disorders, and vascular etiologies are also causes.

Conjugate Gaze. Conjugate gaze disorders, or defects in paired movements of the two eyes in any direction, signify supranuclear or higher cortical lesions. Vertical gaze palsies (e.g., Parinaud syndrome) may occur with hydrocephalus, third ventricle or midbrain tumors, aqueductal stenosis, and after trauma. Patients with hydrocephalus and ventriculoperitoneal shunts may develop Parinaud syndrome when their shunt is malfunctioning.

Internuclear ophthalmoplegia, characterized by failure of adduction on conjugate gaze with associated nystagmus of the abducting eye, signifies a lesion of the medial longitudinal fasciculus. If unilateral, a brainstem tumor or vascular process should be suspected. Bilateral disease is associated with demyelination (e.g., multiple sclerosis).

Nystagmus and Other Abnormal Eye Movements. Nystagmus may be physiologic, induced by various stimuli, or pathologic. To differentiate the various causes, one must be aware of symptom duration, variation by direction of gaze, as well as whether the oscillations are pendular (equal speed in both directions) or jerky (slow in one direction and rapid in opposite direction).

Physiologic forms of nystagmus includes end-gaze nystagmus, which commonly occurs in extreme lateral gaze when the object being watched is beyond the binocular field of vision. The jerk is always in the direction of gaze and is usually symmetric but may be greater in the abducting eye. Nystagmus should not occur on vertical gaze.

Nystagmus may be evoked in healthy individuals by irrigation of the ear with cold or warm water (the basis of caloric testing in comatose individuals when cranial nerve integrity is in question) or by acceleration and deceleration of the head. Both processes produce nystagmus by displacing endolymph in the semicircular canals. The mnemonic COWS (cold opposite, warm same) describes the direction of the rapid jerk with caloric testing. Optokinetic nystagmus is similarly a physiologic nystagmus that occurs by watching a series of objects move across the field of vision.

Spontaneous and pathologic nystagmus may be ocular (attributable to a defect in afferent visual pathways) or neurologic (attributable to a lesion in the posterior fossa or motor pathways). Ocular nystagmus may be due to poor central vision, either congenital or lost within the first 2 years of life. This form of nystagmus is horizontal and pendular and may be seen in association with optic atrophy, chorioretinitis, macula colobomas, high refractive errors, and cataracts.

Spasmus mutans is an acquired form of nystagmus presenting in the first year of life with a characteristic triad of rapid, horizontal pendular nystagmus, head nodding, and torticollis. The nystagmus may be variable in different directions of gaze and may be asymmetric or unilateral. The cause is unclear and usually disappears by age 3.[11]

Posterior fossa disease may cause nystagmus that is horizontal or jerky in both the horizontal and vertical directions. Generally vertical nystagmus is a more ominous sign of pathology. Brainstem or cerebellar disease may cause nystagmus with the rapid component toward the side of the lesion.

Various drugs, in particular phenytoin and barbiturates, can evoke nystagmus in the horizontal or vertical plane.

Nystagmus may indicate peripheral or central vestibular dysfunction. Peripheral labyrinth disease or viral labyrinthitis may be associated with vertigo, tinnitus, difficulty hearing, and nausea or vomiting. Symptoms are associated with an upper respiratory infection or otitis media and begin to resolve within 2 weeks. Central vestibular nystagmus may be caused by tumor, encephalitis, or demyelinating disease. The nystagmus is a horizontal rotary jerk nystagmus that changes direction with gaze and may become vertical on upward and downward gaze. Tinnitus, deafness, and vertigo are not prominent features and the nystagmus remains until the underlying cause is eliminated. There may be evidence of multiple cranial nerve abnormalities. Trauma to the vestibular system may elicit spontaneous nystagmus with nausea, vomiting, and vertigo as prominent symptoms.[10]

Opsoclonus, which may be confused with nystagmus, denotes spontaneous, nonrhythmic chaotic eye movements. There may also be associated myoclonic jerks of the face, trunk, and extremities. Causes include an occult neuroblastoma and encephalitis.[11]

Diagnostic Work-Up

Diplopia is the most common subjective manifestation of ocular muscle paralysis. It is important to elicit whether the onset is acute or chronic, whether trauma has occurred, and whether the patient is systemically ill. Sudden onset of diplopia with associated physical examination findings consistent with ocular palsies are indicative of serious CNS pathology such as meningitis, encephalitis, or tumor. A history of trauma suggests the possibility of an epidural or subdural hemorrhage or cerebral edema. A history of fever, stiff neck, vomiting, and mental status changes suggest meningitis or encephalitis. A longer history of headache with new onset diplopia may point to a CNS tumor, or in a patient with known migraines, an ophthalmoplegic migraine. A patient with otitis media or mastoiditis may develop Gradenigo syndrome. Similarly, a patient with sinusitis and pain with extraocular movements or ophthalmoplegia may have orbital cellulitis, abscess, or cavernous sinus thrombosis.

Important past medical history includes a history of previous chronic illnesses such as myasthenia gravis, collagen vascular disease, diabetes, Lyme disease, and cyanotic congenital heart disease, or a tick bite. Exposure to drugs such as phenytoin, barbiturates, and antihistamines should be elicited in the patient with nystagmus. Endogenous toxins such as diphtheria, tetanus, and botulism can give rise to ophthalmoplegia. Similarly, exogenous toxic exposures such as lead and snake or wasp venom may give rise to ocular motor palsies.

Although diplopia is a common complaint in patients with extraocular muscle abnormalities, young children cannot verbalize it and may squint, cover one eye with their hand, or assume compensatory head positions to avoid double vision. These head positions may be confused with idiopathic torticollis if specific extraocular muscle palsies are not considered. The general appearance of the patient, including presence of fever, stiff neck, hydration status, mental status, and toxicity should be assessed. External evidence of trauma must be sought, even if no history of trauma is forthcoming. Ophthalmologic examination should assess pupil size, reactivity, accommodation, whether ptosis or proptosis is present, and visual acuity. A thorough examination of the actions of the six extraocular muscles should be performed, with close attention to the positions of the two eyes in primary gaze and movement. Abnormal eye movements, including nystagmus, should be assessed, with vertical nystagmus being a more worrisome indicator of CNS disease. Evidence of conjunctivitis with periorbital swelling and proptosis points to orbital cellulitis or cavernous sinus syndrome as causes of ophthalmoplegia. Fundi should be examined for evidence of papilledema, optic atrophy, or retinal hemorrhages. Evidence of otitis media or mastoiditis would lead one to consider Gradenigo syndrome as a cause of a sixth nerve palsy. The neurologic examination needs to determine whether a focal lesion exists, suggesting a brain tumor or abscess, and whether multiple cranial nerve involvement is present. Look for evidence of rash or arthritis, with collagen vascular disease or Lyme disease as possible causes.

Ancillary Data. In a trauma setting, focal neurologic findings, suspected orbital cellulitis, or evidence of increased intracranial pressure (ICP) indicate a head CT scan. Patients who are systemically ill, with suspected meningitis or encephalitis, require a lumbar puncture, unless evidence of increased ICP is present. A child with risk factors for a brain abscess (right-to-left shunting) and new onset focal neurologic symptoms and fever should not have a lumbar puncture, unless a head CT scan has ruled out an abscess. Orbital CT scans with coronal and axial views are indicated after blunt trauma with impaired extraocular motility for a suspected fracture. If opsoclonus/myoclonus is present, an abdominal ultrasound or CT scan and a urine test for catecholamine metabolites can help diagnose an occult neuroblastoma.

Therapeutic Trial

Patients who have extraocular muscle abnormalities related to head trauma and increased intracranial pressure should be intubated and hyperventilated and should receive mannitol 0.25 to 0.5 gm/kg if evidence of acute herniation is present. Neurosurgical involvement is mandatory and a head CT scan should be obtained to look for hemorrhage, cerebral edema, hydrocephalus, or tumor. If the patient's blood pressure is adequate, fluids should be restricted.

If meningitis or encephalitis is suspected, a sepsis work-up should be done and the appropriate antibiotics for age given parenterally either before or after the lumbar puncture, depending on the degree of toxicity of the patient.

Patients with a mass lesion seen on a head CT scan, which is suggestive of an abscess or tumor, require neurosurgical consultation and broad spectrum antibiotics if infection is likely.

When the physical examination is suggestive of orbital cellulitis, ophthalmologic consultation is indicated and antibiotics (nafcillin sodium 150 mg/kg/24 hr q 4 to 6 hr IV and ceftriaxone 100 mg/kg/24 hr q 12 hr IV) are given. A head CT scan showing an orbital or subperiosteal abscess or sinusitis indicates the need for surgical drainage and otolaryngologic involvement.

Patients with ventriculoperitoneal shunts who have vomiting, lethargy, or difficulty with upgaze (Parinaud syndrome) require neurosurgical involvement, a head CT scan, and possibly a shunt tap to evaluate opening pressure and evidence of infection.

If drug intoxication is suspected as a cause of nystagmus, levels should be sent and appropriate treatment measures undertaken to eliminate the toxin.

For patients with long-standing strabismus or nystagmus or a gradual onset head tilt with no evidence of increased intracranial pressure on examination and an otherwise normal neurologic examination, an ophthalmology referral can be made. Patients with a sixth nerve palsy with pain and evidence of otitis media or mastoiditis, should be evaluated by an otorhinolaryngologist.

RED EYE

Red eye, or conjunctival hyperemia, usually refers to reactivity of conjunctival vascular tissue to a variety of infectious, inflammatory, traumatic, or allergic insults.[7] In most cases the cause will be infection or allergy or related to trauma (corneal abrasion or foreign body); however, more serious vision-threatening causes (e.g., glaucoma, uveitis, or recurrent herpes simplex infection) and ocular manifestations of systemic illness (e.g., Stevens-Johnson, Kawasaki, or toxic shock syndrome) may also occur as a red eye. A thorough history and physical examination is mandatory to exclude these latter causes.

Pathophysiology

The conjunctiva, which lines the posterior surface of the lids and the eyeball, is a highly reactive vascular tissue that responds to noxious stimuli with vasodilation, migration of inflammatory cells to the site of injury, pain, and reflex tear secretion.[7]

Differential Considerations

The most common causes of red eye are related to trauma, infection, or allergies. Uveitis and glaucoma, although rare, should be considered and diagnosed to avoid permanent damage to vision.

The most common traumatic causes of red eye are foreign bodies and corneal abrasions. Foreign bodies may present with pain on blinking, injected conjunctiva, and watery discharge. Fluorescein examination often delineates corneal abrasions or the foreign body itself. The foreign body often lodges in the conjunctival cul de sac and may be removed by eversion of the lid. Intraocular foreign bodies may occur when a high speed, small caliber object (e.g., BB pellets) lacerates the globe. Complications include infection, tissue reactions to metallic particles, and chronic inflammation.[12]

Corneal abrasions are extremely common in children. Whenever a corneal abrasion is present, a foreign body must be sought, although a fingernail or a scratch from a toy may be the source. The exposure of sensory nerve endings make corneal abrasions extremely painful. One should consider the diagnosis of a corneal abrasion in the colicky infant with no obvious cause for crying. Symptoms include tearing, photophobia, blepharospasm, and occasionally, visual blurring. The diagnosis is easily made by fluorescein examination.

Ultraviolet keratitis, resulting from the selective absorption of ultraviolet light by corneal epithelium, may result from exposure to direct or reflected sunlight (i.e., snow blindness) or artificial sunlight. Symptoms are similar to those found with corneal abrasions and include foreign-body sensation, photophobia, and occasional decreased vision; bilateral involvement is most commonly present. Diagnosis is made by fluorescein staining in which fine central corneal stippling may be appreciated. The patient

with contact lens overuse with corneal anoxia presents in a similar fashion with comparable findings on fluorescein examination.[12]

Chemical burns are ocular emergencies, requiring immediate action to limit damage to the eye. The mechanism of toxicity, treatment, and severe consequences of alkali burns have already been discussed. A white eye after an alkali burn is an ominous sign, indicating necrosis of perilimbal vessels and the probability of cataract formation, secondary glaucoma, or visual loss.

Of the infectious causes of red eye in children, conjunctivitis is the most common. Conjunctivitis may be bacterial, viral, or allergic. It usually presents with unilateral or bilateral conjunctival injection with purulent discharge and occasionally with lid edema. Pain and foreign-body sensation are uncommon, and vision should be normal (Table 51-2).

Viral conjunctivitis may clinically resemble bacterial conjunctivitis except for the presence of a watery discharge and preauricular adenopathy. The presence of pharyngitis, fever, or other systemic symptoms is more consistent with a viral cause. Corneal involvement may account for decreased visual acuity.

Herpes simplex may cause a keratoconjunctivitis. Corneal involvement is rare in primary disease but is almost inevitable with recurrent infection. Fluorescein staining of the cornea may reveal the characteristic dendritic pattern with recurrent disease. Steroids must never be used before ophthalmologic consultation if herpes infection is suspected.

Allergic conjunctivitis often accompanies hay fever or other environmental allergens. Patients have itchy, watery eyes, injected conjunctiva, and eyelid swelling, which is usually bilateral.

Chemical conjunctivitis is a common cause of red eye in the early newborn period because of silver nitrate prophylaxis given to prevent *N. gonorrhaeae* infection. The onset is several hours after the administration of medication, and it usually lasts 24 to 48 hours. Neonatal conjunctivitis caused by *N. gonorrhaeae* and *Chlamydia trachomatis* usually present in the first 2 weeks of life. Early diagnosis and treatment may prevent serious sequelae.

Glaucoma is an uncommon cause of red eye in children but if not diagnosed and treated promptly, may decrease visual potential. Symptoms include photophobia, tearing, and severe blepharospasm attributable to irritation of the cornea from increased intraocular pressure. Corneal diameter is often increased, and corneal haziness from epithelial edema may be present. Funduscopic examination may reveal an increased cup-size-to-disc ratio. Immediate ophthalmologic consultation is indicated.[1]

Inflammation of the uveal tract, which includes the iris, ciliary body, and choroid, may cause red eye. This may be a result of trauma, juvenile rheumatoid arthritis (JRA), or various infections such as rubella, CMV, toxoplasmosis, syphilis, or tuberculosis (TB).[1]

Iritis may be the result of direct blunt injury to the eye. Patients may have photophobia, hazy vision, and red eye. Findings on physical examination may include a miotic pupil, circumlimbal injection, fine punctate keratopathy on fluorescein examination, and aqueous flare and cells under slit lamp magnification.

TABLE 51-2. Infective Conjunctivitis: Etiology and Management

Etiology	Epidemiology	Diagnostic findings						
		Vision	Pain	Photo-phobia	Discharge/microscopic	Cornea	Conjunctiva	Management*
Bacteria†								
S. pneumoniae H. influenzae	Bilateral, history of exposure	WNL	None	None	Purulent; PMN on smear	WNL	Injected papillary	Topical antibiotics
Viral‡								
Adenovirus§ types 8, 19, 3, and 7	Incubation: 5-14 days; history of exposure; systemic symptoms; preauricular node	Often decreased	FBS	±	Mucoid; mononuclear on smear	Punctate keratopathy	Injected follicles	Cool compresses; artificial tears
Herpes‖	Unilateral; often secondary	±	FBS	+	Mucoid; mononuclear on smear	Dendrite	Injected follicles	Refer to ophthalmologist
Varicella (chickenpox)	"Pox" may involve lid, rarely cornea	WNL	±	±	Mucoid; mononuclear on smear	±	Injected follicles	Follow, refer
Chlamydia	May be recurrent if inadequately treated	WNL	±	±	Inclusion bodies (Giemsa): fluorescent antibody	WNL	Injected follicles (except in newborn period)	Erythromycin for 2-3 wk

*Do not prescribe topical analgesics for prn use.
†"Bacterial" conjunctivitis unresponsive to topical antibiotics more often results from viral agents or iritis than from insensitivity to antibiotics.
‡Prolonged treatment with neomycin-containing antibiotics can cause local sensitivity.
§Adenoviral conjunctivitis also is known as epidemic keratoconjunctivitis. Children should be kept out of school until resolution.
‖Herpes simplex can be difficult to diagnose. Since steroids dramatically worsen herpes keratitis, they should not be prescribed without clear indications.
FBS, Foreign body sensation; *PMN*, polymorphonuclear cells; *WNL*, within normal limits.

Patients with JRA have chronic uveitis in which classic symptoms of uveitis (i.e., pain, photophobia, lacrimation, and decreased vision) are absent. Slit lamp examination may reveal band-shaped keratopathy attributable to calcium deposition in the superficial cornea. In the acute state, conjunctival inflammation with a small pupil and watery discharge is present. Slit lamp examination reveals anterior chamber flare attributable to leakage of protein and leukocyte migration into the aqueous humor.

Many other systemic diseases may present with red eyes and will usually be differentiated by the accompanying symptoms. Kawasaki disease presents with bilateral, non-exudative conjunctival injection within the first week after the onset of fever. Conjunctival involvement is more prominent in the bulbar portion, and anterior uveitis without complaints of photophobia or eye pain may be diagnosed by slit lamp examination. Stevens-Johnson syndrome is an allergic vasculitis with anterior segment involvement, exudative discharge, and occasional conjunctival epithelial sloughing. The differential diagnosis of red eye with fever and rash is extensive and includes streptococcal and staphylococcal toxin-mediated diseases (e.g., scarlet fever and toxic shock syndrome), adenovirus, enterovirus, measles, and multiple collagen vascular diseases (e.g., systemic lupus erythematosus, inflammatory bowel disease, and postinfectious immune complex disease).[13]

Diagnostic Work-Up

The history should focus on the age of the patient, length of symptoms, presence of discharge, whether trauma or other damaging exposures preceded the symptoms, unilateral or bilateral involvement, and whether visual changes are present. Red eye with discharge in the neonate requires a more thorough diagnostic approach and search for a causative organism than would similar symptoms in an older child. A history of trauma may point to the presence of a corneal abrasion or a foreign body. Similarly, a history of radiation or sunlamp exposure may lead one to look for ultraviolet keratitis. If any other family members or personal contacts have similar symptoms, an infectious cause is likely. A purulent discharge may favor the diagnosis of bacterial conjunctivitis, although adenovirus can also present with a purulent conjunctivitis.[14] In a unilateral conjunctivitis, one must inquire whether the patient has ever had a previous herpes infection, since recurrent herpes keratitis can produce extensive corneal scarring and visual loss if untreated. A history of allergies or hay fever with watery, itchy eyes favors an allergic cause. The presence of visual changes suggests corneal involvement, resulting from a keratitis secondary to herpes, adenovirus, a corneal abrasion, or the multiple systemic diseases with uveitis as a component. Recurrent tearing or discharge in the newborn, without the appearance of conjunctival hyperemia, most commonly is due to a lacrimal duct obstruction. However, glaucoma must always be considered if symptoms persist and the physical examination is abnormal.

As with all eye disorders, visual acuity testing should always be performed. Acuity should be normal with bacterial conjunctivitis but may be decreased with adenovirus, herpes simplex keratoconjunctivitis, uveitis, corneal abrasions, or foreign-body invasion. Acuity almost always is abnormal with glaucoma. External examination may suggest the occurrence of trauma and the possibility of a corneal abrasion or intraocular trauma. Examination of the cornea is unremarkable in bacterial conjunctivitis but is cloudy in glaucoma with a shallow anterior chamber. In addition, asymmetry of corneal diameter and a palpable hard lid suggests glaucoma in the tearing, photophobic infant. A small pupil, resulting from spasm of the ciliary sphincter muscle, and circumlimbal flush, may suggest iritis, uveitis, or a corneal abrasion. Eversion of the lid may reveal the presence of a foreign body. Examination of the cornea with fluorescein may reveal diffuse punctate or focal epithelial uptake with a corneal abrasion or ulcer or diffuse punctate keratopathy with adenovirus. Fine bilateral central corneal stippling may be seen on fluorescein staining with an ultraviolet keratitis. The presence of fever and a rash suggests the possibility of systemic viral, bacterial, or collagen vascular disease.

Ancillary Data. Evaluation of red eye begins with fluorescein staining. In the neonate with red eye and discharge, cultures and gram stain of the discharge are indicated to rule out gonococcal or chlamydial conjunctivitis. Similarly, cultures of eye discharge may be indicated if the symptoms are chronic (i.e., lasting more than 2 weeks) or if more virulent organisms are suspected, as with contact lens use or with a preceding history of penetrating eye trauma. If the presence of a metallic foreign body is suggested by history or physical examination, a radiograph may be indicated. Slit lamp examination is indicated for the patient with impaired vision or trauma. When the diagnosis of glaucoma is considered, tonometry measurements of intraocular pressure, consultation with an ophthalmologist, and examination under anesthesia is indicated.

Prehospital Considerations

Prehospital management of chemical burns has already been discussed.

Therapeutic Trial

If a foreign body is found, a topical anesthetic agent may be applied. A cotton-tipped applicator or irrigation with saline is all that is needed for its removal. Occasionally, the foreign body, when embedded in the cornea, may require removal in the operating suite by an ophthalmologist. This may occur after drilling or sawing when a "rust ring" surrounding the foreign body is found on examination. The risk of fungal infections is increased if a plant- or vegetable-matter source is involved.[12]

Treatment of a corneal abrasion requires a short-acting cycloplegic agent such as cyclopentolate (Cyclogyl, 1%) or tropicamide (Mydriacyl, 1%) to decrease pain from ciliary spasm, and a broad-spectrum antibiotic ointment such as polymyxin B sulfate (Polysporin) or sulfacetamide sodium

(Sulamyd) to prevent bacterial superinfection. A semipressure patch is applied to the eye to relieve the discomfort from photophobia, decrease lid movement, and allow the epithelial defect to heal. Topical anesthetic agents should never be prescribed, since they may retard epithelial healing and worsen the keratitis. Similarly, topical steroids impair epithelialization and promote corneal infection and should never be used under these circumstances. The patient with ultraviolet keratitis or contact lens overuse is treated the same as for corneal abrasions (see Chapter 21).

Traumatic iritis is treated, in consultation with an ophthalmologist, with cycloplegics to reduce ciliary spasm and topical steroids to reduce inflammation.

The treatment of infectious and allergic conjunctivitis is discussed in a later section.

Diagnostic Entities

CHALAZION AND HORDEOLUM

Eyelid infections, or blepharitis, in children are often localized to the sebaceous glands lining the lid. An external hordeolum or stye is an acute suppurative infection of the glands of Zeis, which are sebaceous glands attached to the hair follicles. An internal hordeolum is an acute infection of a meibomian gland, which produces an abscess within the tarsal plate.[7] A chalazion is a localized painless swelling of the lid, located in the tarsus, which occurs as a chronic lipogranulomatous reaction to retained secretions and is due to obstruction of the meibomian gland.[1,7]

Commonly, blepharitis is due to *Staphylococcus aureus*, although *S. epidermidis* may also be involved. These organisms are part of the normal flora but may increase in number because of poor hygiene or contamination. The incidence is increased in children with seborrhea, atopy, tear deficiency, and immunodeficiency. One theory speculates that mites may block gland ductules leading to the creation of hordeola. Hordeola are frequently associated with staphylococcal blepharitis.[7]

Diagnostic Findings

Hordeola begin with diffuse eyelid edema and hyperemia, which is painful and eventually localizes to the lid margin (Fig. 51-2). The lesion often points and drains spontaneously. Internal hordeola similarly but are only seen on lid eversion. With time they may develop into a chalazion. A chalazion is characteristically painless, causing mainly cosmetic difficulties (Fig. 51-3).[7]

Differential Considerations

The differential diagnosis of external hordeolum includes contact dermatitis and allergic conjunctivitis. The latter two conditions are associated with itching, erythema, and periorbital swelling but should not have a focal indurated area associated with a hordeolum.[7]

The differential diagnosis of an internal hordeolum or chalazion includes eyelid tumors, cysts, or lymphoma. Differentiation is made by lack of clinical response to medical therapy and eventual biopsy of the lesion.[7]

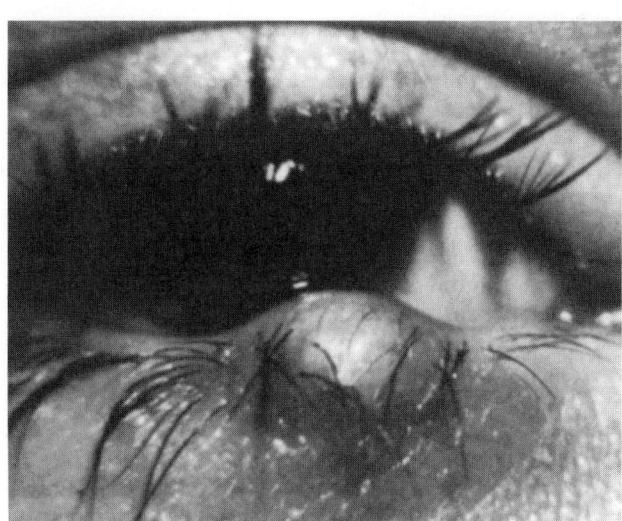

FIG. 51-2. Acute hordeolum of the lower eyelid. (*From Newell FW: Ophthalmology: principles and concepts, ed 7, St Louis, 1992, Mosby.*)

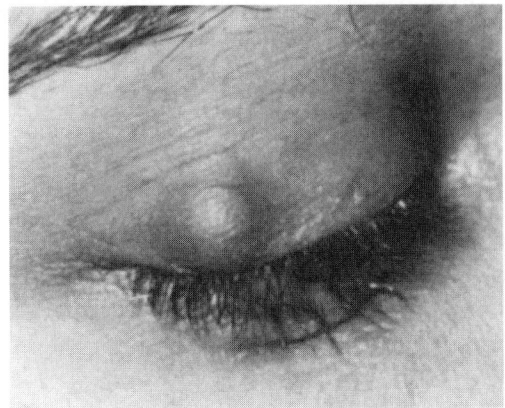

FIG. 51-3. Chronic chalazion (lipogranuloma) of meibomian gland of the upper eyelid. (*From Newell FW: Ophthalmology: principles and concepts, ed 7, St Louis, 1992, Mosby.*)

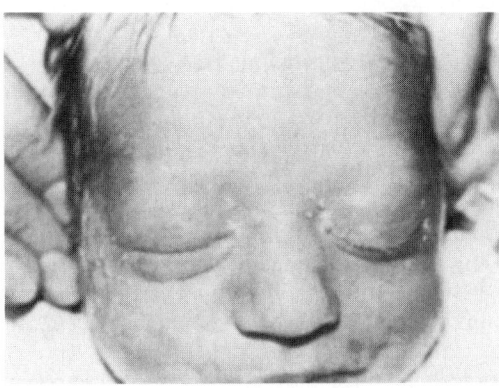

FIG. 51-4. Ophthalmia neonatorum. (*From Helveston EM: Pediatric ophthalmology practice, ed 2, St Louis, 1984, Mosby.*)

Management

External and internal hordeola are treated with warm compresses several times a day and eyelash scrubs with baby shampoo on a washcloth. The *S. aureus* should be treated with antibiotic ointment such as polymyxin B sulfate (Polysporin) or erythromycin (Ilotycin) twice a day, particularly when conjunctivitis is present. These measures should aid in spontaneous drainage and resolution of the lesion.

Chalazia are treated similarly for 2 weeks. Occasionally these measures are inadequate, and incision and curretage or steroid injections are necessary to resolve the lesion. Indications for surgical intervention include ptosis or the development of astigmatism.[7]

Both hordeola and chalazia frequently recur. Tear deficiency and lid scarring may result from multiple excisions of chalazia.[7] Rarely hordeola progresses to periorbital cellulitis, usually because of *S. aureus*. Under these conditions, oral antistaphylococcal medication is sufficient to treat the cellulitis if the symptoms are mild.[15]

CONJUNCTIVITIS

Conjunctivitis is the most common cause of red eye in children.[15] It may occur alone or as a manifestation of a systemic process.[16] In most cases the process is benign and self-limited; however, certain causes of conjunctivitis may pose a greater threat to visual integrity than others, especially in the newborn period. The emergency department physician must know the various causes and required treatments of conjunctivitis and must also be able to differentiate conjunctivitis from other causes of red eye.

The conjunctiva is a transparent mucous membrane that covers the eye; the palpebral portion lines the posterior surface of the lids, and the bulbar portion lines the entire eyeball except for the cornea.[1]

The conjunctiva is protected from most noxious or infectious insults by a variety of mechanisms, including the flushing mechanism of tears, the mechanical barrier provided by the eyelid blink and an intact conjunctiva, and the immunologic components of tears (i.e., the enzyme lysozyme, IgA specific antibodies, and complement).[1,17] Local irritation from cosmetics, contact lenses, or other foreign bodies, or effects of air pollution on tear lysozyme may be factors that affect the host's ability to contain disease.[7]

When infection does occur, the conjunctiva responds with vasodilation and mobilization of inflammatory cells to the site of injury, producing pain and tear secretion.[7]

Conjunctivitis can be subdivided by age of occurrence (e.g., neonatal or childhood); by type of infecting organism (bacterial, viral, or other); or by length of symptomatic course (acute: less than 2 weeks' duration vs. chronic).

Ophthalmia Neonatorum

Ophthalmia neonatorum, or conjunctivitis during the first month of life, is common (Fig. 51-4).[16] The cause may be infectious or related to silver nitrate prophylaxis. Accurate diagnosis of the infecting organism is crucial to avoid long-term visual damage from gonococcal conjunctivitis.

TABLE 51-3. Ophthalmia Neonatorum: Etiology

Etiology	Incubation period	Diagnostic findings	Management
Chemical Silver nitrate	24 hr	Diffuse injection; culture: negative	Wait and watch
Gonococcal *N. gonorrhoeae*	24-72 hr	Hyperpurulent discharge; history of infected birth canal or infected contact; smear: typical gonococcus	Systemic and topical antibiotics; hospitalize
***Chlamydia* organism** (inclusion conjunctivitis) *C. trachomatis*	7-10 days	Indolent, although often purulent; history of infected birth canal; may have had partial response to topical antibiotics; no follicles in infant; smear: cytoplasmic inclusion; culture: negative	Systemic erythromycin or sulfonamides; exclude systemic disease
Other bacteria	2-5 days	Purulent or hyperpurulent discharge	Topical antibiotics

Pathophysiology. Bacteria from the maternal genital tract during the birth process or from the environment can be inoculated onto the conjunctiva. When membranes are prematurely ruptured, transmission of maternal genital organisms can occur before birth.

Diagnostic Findings. Chemical conjunctivitis occurs in approximately 10% of newborns who receive silver nitrate prophylaxis, which is used to prevent eye infections from *N. gonorrhoeae*. [16] Silver nitrate works by sloughing superficial cells. Bilateral conjunctival injection and discharge are evident several hours after instillation of silver nitrate, and symptoms should resolve spontaneously in 24 to 48 hours.

C. trachomatis is the most common infectious agent causing ophthalmia neonatorum, accounting for 20% to 40% of neonatal conjunctivitis.[1,17,18] It occurs 5 to 14 days postpartum as a mucopurulent conjunctivitis with lid edema, chemosis, and lid erythema.[1] The conjunctiva may be red and friable,[17] and generally palpebral involvement is greater than bulbar involvement.[16] Diagnosis can be made by looking for cytoplasmic inclusions on smears of the conjunctival discharge when stained with Wright or Giemsa stain and by culture. The baby is inoculated at multiple sites during birth, including the eye and nasopharynx. Ocular complications such as scars and pannus formation are rare.[19] However, nasopharyngeal carriage is associated with the development of pneumonia at 3 to 19 weeks of age, characterized by staccato cough, congestion, tachypnea, and rales, usually without fever.[18,19] Chest radiograph may show hyperinflation with interstitial infiltrates.

The incidence of conjunctival infection with *N. gonorrhoeae* is low; however, the potential for destruction and permanent visual disabilities remains high if the diagnosis is delayed. The organism is acquired by passage through an infected birth canal. Symptoms typically appear 2 to 4 days after birth and include a bilateral, hyperpurulent discharge, conjunctival hyperemia, chemosis, and lid edema. There is a wide variability to the symptoms, and therefore the diagnosis should be suspected in all patients with conjunctivitis in the first month of life; most cases, however, should appear by 2 weeks of age. Both ocular complications, which

may include corneal ulceration, perforation, and endophthalmitis, and systemic toxicity are possible.[1] Diagnosis may be suspected by a gram stain of the discharge, which shows intracellular gram-negative diplococci and is confirmed by culture of the discharge on Thayer-Martin plates. A blood culture and cerebrospinal fluid culture may be taken before starting systemic therapy in the hospital (Table 51-3).

Neonatal herpes simplex can be disseminated or localized within the eye, CNS, or skin. The infection is acquired during passage through the birth canal or occasionally by ascending infection if maternal membranes are ruptured prematurely. Symptoms occur between 2 days and 2 weeks after birth. The characteristics of the conjunctivitis are not clinically distinctive and may result in keratitis, cataracts, chorioretinitis, and optic neuritis.[7] Fluorescein examination may reveal dendritic formation. A Tzanck preparation from the eye or skin lesions may reveal multinucleated giant cells or intranuclear inclusions.[16] Cultures will be positive within 48 hours.

Neonatal conjunctivitis may also be caused by other bacteria, including *S. aureus, Haemophilus* species, *S. pneumoniae,* gram-negative enteric rods, and enterococci. Most cases occur in the first 2 weeks of life. The conjunctiva is red with a purulent discharge. Gram stain of the discharge may reveal WBC and an organism; the correlation between gram stain and culture results are variable. Gonococcal disease should be sought in neonates.

Differential Considerations. In addition to chemical conjunctivitis and the infectious causes listed previously, a variety of noninfectious conditions may cause red eye in the neonatal period. Trauma to the eye during birth, a fingernail scratch, or rubbing the eyes can cause injected conjunctiva and corneal abrasion. Neonatal glaucoma may occur with red eye but may also reveal an enlarged and cloudy cornea. Congenital nasolacrimal duct obstruction may occur with recurrent tearing and bacterial blepharoconjunctivitis. The key to this diagnosis is its recurrence and the persistence of tearing between bouts of conjunctivitis.[7]

Management. All patients with conjunctivitis in the first month of life should have the discharge sent for gram and

Giemsa stain and gonococcal and chlamydial cultures. Fluorescein testing should be performed to rule out the presence of a foreign body or a corneal abrasion. A careful eye examination should be performed to locate corneal abnormalities or cataracts, which may be seen in neonatal intrauterine viral infections or neonatal glaucoma.[16]

If the gram stain is suggestive of gonococcal conjunctivitis, the patient should be hospitalized for IV antibiotics after an appropriate sepsis evaluation and should be seen by an ophthalmologist. Recommended initial therapy used to be penicillin G (50,000 units/kg/24 hr); however, with the increasing prevalence of penicillin-resistant gonococci, ceftriaxone sodium 50 mg/kg IV or IM once a day for 7 days may be a better first-line agent. The risk of inadequate coverage could result in permanent visual sequelae.[20] Ophthalmology should be consulted, and the eye should be irrigated with saline frequently until the discharge is eliminated.[19] Topical erythromycin is also started pending results of chlamydial cultures. Parents should be referred for treatment of gonorrhea.

If the Giemsa stain is suggestive of chlamydia, the child can be treated as an outpatient. Topical therapy alone has not been shown to be adequate at eradicating nasopharyngeal carriage and preventing pneumonia.[21,22] Therefore when there is a high index of suspicion for chlamydial infection, erythromycin 50 mg/kg/24 hr PO is the treatment of choice for 14 days.[19] The parents should also be treated when the diagnosis is confirmed.

If the diagnosis of herpes simplex is suggested by history or physical examination, the child should be seen by an ophthalmologist and hospitalized for topical and parenteral viral therapy.

Most cases of bacterial conjunctivitis can be treated topically with erythromycin (Ilotycin) or polymixin B (Polysporin) ophthalmic ointment and discharged with appropriate follow-up in a few days.

Childhood Conjunctivitis

Conjunctivitis beyond the neonatal period is also extremely common.[16] The majority of children with acute conjunctivitis have a bacterial cause. Viral infections begin to play a larger role in the older patients. In most cases the disease is self-limited and benign and can be treated without knowing the specific organisms involved.

Etiology. Bacterial conjunctivitis is responsible for over 50% of cases of infectious conjunctivitis.[14,23] Recent studies using age and season-matched controls show that nontypable *H. influenzae* is the most common bacterial isolate in over 40% of the cases, occurring most frequently in the winter.[14,23] *S. pneumoniae* was the second most commonly isolated bacterial pathogen followed by *M. catarrhalis*.[24] *S. aureus* has been found in both control and diseased patients and is not believed to be an important cause of acute conjunctivitis in the absence of trauma or disruption of skin integrity.[14,17] *S. aureus* may be important in patients with a primary eyelid infection, allergic eye disease, immunodeficiency syndrome, and with toxin-producing strains of *S. aureus* with toxic shock or staphylococcal scalded skin syndrome.

Gonococcal conjunctivitis may occur in sexually active adolescents and in children who have been sexually abused.[16] Clinical symptoms can mimic orbital cellulitis with severe chemosis, and restricted and painful ocular motility.[24]

Viral conjunctivitis is most commonly caused by adenovirus, which accounts for approximately 20% of cases of infectious conjunctivitis.[14] Enterovirus may cause an acute hemorrhagic conjunctivitis with characteristic bulbar conjunctival hemorrhages, fever, and malaise.[7] Herpes simplex may cause a unilateral acute conjunctivitis, which causes corneal scarring and visual disturbance when it is recurrent (see Table 51-2).

Fungal infection of the conjunctiva is uncommon, except in cases of ocular trauma or in children who wear contact lenses.[16]

Conjunctivitis may occur in other systemic infections, including measles, rubella, Epstein-Barr virus, varicella, Rocky Mountain spotted fever, and Kawasaki disease. Parinaud syndrome may be an ocular presentation of cat-scratch disease with conjunctivitis and preauricular adenopathy.[16]

Allergic conjunctivitis is common in children, usually related to hay fever or another environmental allergen. Vernal conjunctivitis is a distinct form of allergic conjunctivitis, which occurs most often in males with a family history of atopy. It appears as a recurrent, bilateral conjunctivitis and is worse in the spring and summer.[1]

Toxic conjunctivitis can occur as a reaction to various drugs, including miotics, neomycin, and cosmetics. Scarring may result from severe reactions.[7]

Diagnostic Findings. Bacterial conjunctivitis is characterized by conjunctival injection, mucopurulent discharge, and occasional lid edema. Early bilateral involvement within 1 to 2 days is more typical than with viral disease.[14] Pain is uncommon, and vision should be normal. Physical examination reveals hyperemic palpebral and bulbar conjunctiva with a purulent exudate revealing polymorphonuclear cells on gram stain. Corneal involvement is rare unless a corneal abrasion has occurred from frequent rubbing of the eyes. The mean age of patients with bacterial conjunctivitis is less than the mean age for adenovirus, but the age range is comparable.[14]

Patients with concurrent otitis media and conjunctivitis may have the "conjunctivitis-otitis media syndrome," which is most often caused by nontypable *H. influenzae*, and rarely by *S. pneumoniae*. The incidence of concurrent otitis media and conjunctivitis has ranged from 20% to 75% of all patients with purulent conjunctivitis.[14,25-27] Younger patients, below the age of 4 years, and those patients with greater than three episodes of acute otitis media the previous year were more likely to develop conjunctivitis-otitis syndrome than conjunctivitis alone.[27]

Clinically, viral conjunctivitis may resemble bacterial conjunctivitis. The discharge is described as watery or mucoid rather than purulent, but adenovirus may also have with a purulent exudate.[14] Follicular hypertrophy of the conjunctiva occurs in response to viral disease in patients over 3 months of age.[7]

Pharyngoconjunctival fever is most commonly attributable to adenovirus, which is characterized by fever, pharyngitis, and conjunctivitis.[1] Early bilateral disease is less common than with bacterial conjunctivitis, and preauricular adenopathy is usually present on the involved side.[14] Symptoms may last from 4 days to 2 weeks.[1]

Epidemic keratoconjunctivitis, also caused by adenovirus, is similar but without significant fever or respiratory symptoms. Tearing and chemosis are common, and subconjunctival hemorrhage and eyelid ecchymoses may occur.[7] Corneal involvement with punctate keratopathy is more likely with resultant decreased visual acuity. Symptoms and infectious potential may last up to 2 weeks; corneal changes may persist for years but gradually resolve without scarring.[1]

Herpes keratoconjunctivitis occurs initially as a unilateral acute conjunctivitis with lymphadenitis in the first decade of life. Pain and foreign-body sensation are common complaints. Skin lesions, typically grouped vesicles or crusted ulcers, may be obvious or hidden in the nose or beneath the lashes. Recurrent disease with corneal involvement may cause scarring and visual loss. The discharge is mucoid and may reveal mononuclear cells on gram stain. Fluorescein examination should be performed to look for the characteristic dendritic ulcer, which is most common with recurrent disease.[1,7]

Allergic conjunctivitis is characterized by itchy eyes with a watery discharge. Bilateral involvement, eyelid swelling, and chemosis are common. Hayfever and other environmental allergens may cause seasonal conjunctivitis. Atopic keratoconjunctivitis, occurring in children with eczema, is nonseasonal and has similar symptoms. Vernal conjunctivitis is marked by severe itching, tearing, redness, and photophobia. The discharge is thick and yellow, and "cobblestone" papillae may be seen with lid eversion of the upper lid. In severe cases, papillary hypertrophy may cause drooping of the upper eyelid.[1,7]

Differential Considerations. When evaluating patients with conjunctivitis, important points include age, onset of symptoms, known exposure to conjunctivitis, type of discharge if present, presence of pain or decreased visual acuity, preceding trauma or toxin exposure, and presence of systemic signs of illness. The presence of bilateral disease, a purulent discharge, or concurrent otitis media is more consistent with a bacterial cause. A watery discharge with preauricular adenopathy, accompanied by fever and sore throat is consistent with a viral cause, particularly adenovirus. A history of herpes conjunctivitis or a unilateral conjunctivitis with skin lesions and corneal involvement is consistent with herpes keratoconjunctivitis. Conjunctivitis in the first 24 to 48 hours of life is primarily chemical and is due to instillation of silver nitrate prophylaxis. Anytime after the first 2 days of the neonatal period, cultures and gram or Giemsa stain of eye discharge are necessary to make a specific diagnosis. A history of eczema or allergies with bilateral, watery, itchy eyes or follicular hypertrophy is consistent with an allergic conjunctivitis. Finally, contact lenses predispose wearers to keratitis and fungal conjunctivitis.

Other conditions that may cause red eye and have been discussed previously include foreign bodies, corneal abrasion, trauma, chemical, toxic or ultraviolet exposure, and glaucoma. Fluorescein examination, careful review of patient history, and physical examination help differentiate these conditions from the infectious and allergic causes of conjunctivitis.

Management. Although most forms of acute bacterial conjunctivitis are believed to be self-limited, the use of topical antibiotic therapy has been demonstrated to shorten the clinical course and more quickly eradicate the organism from the conjunctiva, thereby shortening the period of contagion.[28] With the exception of ophthalmia neonatorum, the routine use of gram stain and culture for acute bacterial conjunctivitis is not indicated, since they are not predictive of the infecting organism when compared with culture results.[14]

Bacterial conjunctivitis is treated empirically with topical ophthalmic ointments or drops. The advantage of ointments is their lower frequency of administration (four times a day). Drops require administration every 2 to 4 hours to be effective, and compliance is generally lower.[17] Ointment, however, can blur vision, which may be more disconcerting for the older child. At bedtime, ointment is indicated for its longer-lasting effect. Specific drugs include polymyxin B sulfate (Polysporin) ointment, which has a broad spectrum of action and good *H. influenzae* coverage; sulfacetamide sodium (10%) ointment or drops (Sulamyd); and the newest medication for conjunctivitis, trimethoprim-polymyxin B (Polytrim). Polytrim has been found to be more effective than sulfacetamide or gentamicin at eliminating *H. influenzae*, and has a broad spectrum of activity against gram-positive and gram-negative bacilli, including *Pseudomonas aeruginosa*.[29] Sulfacetamide may cause burning and stinging and has a low risk of causing Stevens-Johnson syndrome.[17] Erythromycin (Ilotycin) ointment is effective against most *H. influenzae* and *Streptococcus pneumoniae*, although resistant strains of *H. influenzae* are emerging, and gram-negative enterics, which may be cultured from children with poor hygiene, are resistant to erythromycin. Gentamicin and tobramycin cover gram-negative organisms well but will not affect *S. pneumoniae*, which is a more common cause of conjunctivitis in children; therefore they are not indicated as first-line therapy. Neosporin may cause a hypersensitivity reaction in up to 10% of patients. Chloramphenicol drops have been associated with aplastic anemia in rare idiosyncratic reactions.[17]

Children with conjunctivitis-otitis media syndrome require systemic antibiotics. This form of therapy has been shown to be equally effective in achieving clinical and microbiologic cure, regardless of whether topical therapy is included.[28] Patients with purulent conjunctivitis who were treated with systemic antibiotics appeared to develop a lower incidence of subsequent otitis media than those treated topically.[27] Despite these studies, most ophthalmologists prefer to treat conjunctivitis topically to get the highest concentration of antibiotics into the affected tissue and reserve systemic antibiotics for conjunctivitis with systemic involvement.[17]

Patients with persistent or recurrent conjunctivitis should be evaluated by an ophthalmologist and have cultures sent to help revise therapy.

Treatment of viral conjunctivitis is primarily supportive, with cool compresses and artificial tears to relieve the discomfort. Broad-spectrum topical therapy has been used to prevent bacterial superinfection, but the value of this is unproved and generally not indicated in the immunocompetent host.[1]

Allergic conjunctivitis should be treated with cool compresses, elimination of the offending allergen, and systemic antihistamines such as diphenhydramine (Benadryl) 5 mg/kg/24 hr q 4 to 6 hr PO or hydroxyzine (Atarax or Vistaril) 2 mg/kg/24 hr QID PO. Treatment of vernal conjunctivitis may require a topical vasoconstrictor such as Naphazoine HCl (Vasocon-A). Advanced cases may require topical steroids, given under the direction of an ophthalmologist.

Herpes keratoconjunctivitis should always be seen by an ophthalmologist and treated parenterally and topically with antiviral therapy, a cycloplegic agent, and occasionally topical steroids for deeper corneal involvement.

Disposition. Most patients with conjunctivitis that are no longer neonates can be treated as outpatients. Topical therapy should be continued until the discharge is gone for two consecutive mornings.[15] The high level of contagion of infectious conjunctivitis should be stressed, and good handwashing and separate towels should be used. Patients should be reexamined in 72 hours if the symptoms have not resolved. Referral to an ophthalmologist is indicated for an infection lasting longer than 1 to 2 weeks, whenever vision is decreased, or when pain is present.

PERIORBITAL AND ORBITAL CELLULITIS

Periorbital swelling is a common complaint in the emergency department. When the onset is sudden and erythema is present, the differential diagnosis may include allergic reactions, insect bites, trauma, and more serious infections such as periorbital and orbital cellulitis. Prompt diagnosis and management is essential to avoid the visual or potentially life-threatening, infectious complications of periorbital and orbital cellulitis.

The mechanism of periorbital swelling can be best understood by reviewing the relevant anatomy. The orbit is a fixed bony cavity surrounded by the sinuses; superiorly lies the frontal sinus, inferiorly lies the maxillary sinus, and medially lies the ethmoid sinus which is separated by the paper-thin lamina papyracea. The orbital septum is a layer of fibrous tissue that extends from the orbital walls to the tarsal plate as an extension of the periosteum of the orbit.[30] The preseptal space lies between the orbital septum and the eyelid skin. The connective tissue in this space is elastic, and therefore large amounts of fluid or inflammatory cells may accumulate in response to an infectious or inflammatory insult. The venous drainage system of the orbit and sinuses lacks valves and lymphatic drainage and empties into the cavernous sinus. The spread of infection from the sinuses to the orbital or periorbital area is facilitated by these freely communicating valveless vessels, and the thin lamina papyracea. In addition, reactive periorbital edema without evidence of infection may occur because of pressure on sinus vessels from sinusitis causing impedence of blood flow.[7,31]

Periorbital Cellulitis

Periorbital or preseptal cellulitis is an infection occurring in the superficial tissue space surrounding the eye anterior to the orbital septum.[32] Although symptoms can occur at any age, the majority of patients are under the age of 6 years, with a peak incidence between 2 and 4 years.[33] Infections of the preseptal area are much more common in

children than are orbital infections.[34] Since the pathogenesis, bacteriology, treatment, and complications of these two entities are distinct, it is crucial for the clinician to differentiate between them.

Etiology. Predisposing conditions may be found in as many as 75% of patients with periorbital cellulitis. A history of skin or lid infections (e.g., impetigo, or hordeolum), insect bites, or trauma may precede periorbital cellulitis in 25% of these cases, most often in patients over the age of 3 years.[32,34] Most commonly, infection in this case is due to *S. aureus, S. pyogenes,* and anaerobes. Human and animal bites to the periorbital area may produce polymicrobial infections.[7]

In those patients without preceding trauma or skin lesion a history of an upper respiratory tract infection, otitis media, or pharyngitis may be found, which may extend to involve the conjunctiva and periorbital tissues.[35] *H. influenzae* type B and *S. pneumoniae* are the most common causes for preseptal cellulitis in these patients, who are usually under age 3.[7] The incidence of *H. influenzae* type B has decreased with widespread HB immunization. Cellulitis is believed to be due to bacteremia and seeding of the preseptal space.

Periorbital cellulitis may also be associated with sinusitis, especially with ethmoid involvement attributable to the extremely thin barrier between the ethmoid sinus and preseptal tissues. It is unclear whether the sinusitis precedes the cellulitis or is a complication of the cellulitis. In any case, the organisms involved are those associated with acute sinusitis, including *H. influenzae, S. pneumoniae,* and occasionally anaerobic bacteria.[32]

Other predisposing conditions to periorbital cellulitis include dental abscesses, herpes, varicella, adenovirus, osteomyelitis of the maxillae, and nasolacrimal duct obstruction.[32,36] Periorbital cellulitis also has been found to be the primary complaint of a brain abscess and ethmoid sinusitis in a 2-month-old infant.[37]

Diagnostic Findings. Periorbital cellulitis occurs with acute unilateral lid swelling, erythema, tenderness, and warmth. The absence of proptosis, ophthalmoplegia, or changes in visual acuity distinguish it from the more serious orbital involvement. Fever is present in two thirds to three fourths of patients.[33,34] The absence of fever does not rule out a cellulitis in patients with a suggestive physical examination. There is unilateral involvement in the vast majority of patients with the left side predominating approximately two thirds of the time.[33] Lymphedema can cause swelling of the contralateral lid, which may account for the 4% incidence of bilateral involvement.[38] A violaceous color has been described in association with both *H. influenzae* and *S. pneumoniae* periorbital disease.[39] Chemosis and conjunctival injection, with or without a purulent discharge, may be present in approximately one fourth of the patients.[7,40] Clinical symptoms suggestive of sinusitis, including nasal discharge, pain, or localized tenderness may also be present, although sinusitis as a cause in periorbital disease remains controversial.[40]

Although proptosis, abnormalities in extraocular muscle testing, pain on eye movement, or visual acuity changes should not occur with periorbital cellulitis, they may be present if trauma preceded the cellulitis and additional eye pathology is present. It may be difficult to assess visual acuity and extraocular movement testing because of large amounts of eyelid swelling or tenderness. If this occurs, testing of the afferent visual pathway may still be done by noting the consensual pupillary light response in the uninvolved eye.[7] Further ophthalmologic evaluation and a head CT scan may be needed to exclude orbital involvement.

Complications. Complications of periorbital cellulitis most commonly occur in the CNS. When cellulitis occurs in the absence of a history of trauma or disruption of skin integrity in the child under age 5, *H. influenzae*, or *S. pneumoniae* are likely pathogens. Bacterial seeding of the meninges, joints, and other sites are potential complications. Meningitis has been reported in children under 2 years of age with periorbital cellulitis and with no signs of meningeal irritation on examination other than mild irritability; cerebrospinal fluid (CSF) cell counts were normal, but CSF and blood cultures grew either *H. influenzae* or *S. pneumoniae*.[41] Although meningitis is the most common complication, subdural and epidural empyemas, lid abscess,[34] and brain abscess complicating ethmoid sinusitis, have been reported.[37]

Ancillary Data. A complete blood count with differential may help define those patients with periorbital cellulitis who are more likely to be bacteremic. Mean WBC counts tend to run higher in patients who are bacteremic than those who are not, although there is still a significant percentage of false positives, as well as false negatives.[39,40] A CBC may be more helpful in differentiating a bacterial from a noninfectious cause of periorbital swelling.

For patients with preceding trauma or skin lesions, a culture of the wound or skin lesions and a blood culture should be taken to help isolate the organism responsible.[32] In most cases the blood culture will be negative, and wound or skin cultures are often positive for gram-positive skin flora, including *S. aureus* and *S. pyogenes*.[7,32,34,38] When there is no history of preceding trauma or disruption in skin integrity, blood cultures should be done and will be positive in approximately 25% of cases. Before the advent of the *H. influenzae* type B vaccine for young infants in 1990, *H. influenzae* was the most common organism isolated in the blood followed by *S. pneumoniae*, which is currently the leading blood culture isolate. In general, nasopharyngeal and conjunctival cultures and gram stain are not believed to correlate well with the isolated causative organism from blood, wound, or sinus aspirates.[32]

A history of trauma or skin lesions may occur in patients with documented *H. influenzae* type B cellulitis and therefore should not exclude the possibility of systemic bacterial disease.[39] The age of the patient, degree of fever, toxicity, and WBC must be taken into account when deciding on the appropriate antibiotic therapy.

A lumbar puncture should be considered in all patients with possible *H. influenzae* disease, especially those under 2 years of age.[41] A positive CSF culture prolongs the length of treatment with parenteral antibiotics.

Patients unlikely to have meningitis are afebrile, appear well, or have cellulitis associated with a nonbacteremic etiology.[42] *H. influenzae* immunization status must also be considered.

Countercurrent immunoelectrophoresis (CIE) may be helpful in identifying a cause when the patient has been pretreated with antibiotics. Samples taken from blood, urine, CSF, or tears have a sensitivity of 50% and a specificity of 93% in detecting *H. influenzae*, using positive blood cultures as a gold standard. These methods are not as helpful in identifying patients with *S. pneumoniae* infections.[39]

The value of radiographs in evaluating patients with periorbital cellulitis is controversial and generally not indicated. Abnormal sinus films are often found when periorbital swelling is present without true cellulitis or may indicate a concurrent upper respiratory infection without sinusitis in the young child.[30]

CT scan of the orbit is indicated when the diagnosis of orbital cellulitis is suspected to look for evidence of subperiosteal or orbital abscess or whenever eyelid swelling and tenderness precludes adequate examination of the globe[43] (Fig. 51-5).

Differential Considerations. The differential diagnosis of periorbital swelling may be due to a large variety of infectious and noninfectious causes. The most common noninfectious causes include reactions to insect bites, allergic reactions, contact dermatitis, reactive edema, and trauma. The patient with an insect bite may have a red, swollen eye, but should not have clinical evidence of cellulitis. A puncture should be sought but may not always be found. The patient with allergies may have nasal discharge, watery, injected eyes, or urticaria.[38] To differentiate between infectious and allergic causes, one can observe the child for several hours and give the patient epinephrine 0.01 ml/kg/dose SC or diphenhydramine HCI (Benadryl) 2 mg/kg/dose PO. Allergic swelling may recede with these measures, but cellulitis should continue to progress.[31] Reactive periorbital edema may be due to underlying sinusitis. The onset is less acute, fever may be present, and swelling often decreases as the day progresses. Swelling related to trauma may have a history indicating that trauma occurred and usually will appear reddish-blue. Fever should not be present. Contact dermatitis, especially from poison ivy, may be confused with periorbital cellulitis. Differentiating features include absence of fever, history of recent outdoor play, the presence of vesicles and linear streaks, and pruritus. Superinfection is always possible, especially in the case of an insect bite or poison ivy exposure. Therefore signs of cellulitis should always be assessed even when the history suggests a noninfectious cause.

Other infectious causes of periorbital erythema and lid swelling include conjunctivitis, hordeolum, dacrocystitis, and dacroadenitis.[38] A hordeolum or localized infection of a hair follicle or sebaceous gland will be present along the eyelid, either externally or internally. Dacrocystitis, attributable to lacrimal duct obstruction, may cause periorbital swelling, erythema, and tenderness, often marked medial and inferior to the eye. These patients are generally less than 4 months old, and diagnosis often can be made by expressing purulent drainage from the lacrimal duct, the so-called toothpaste sign. Dacroadenitis is a rare infection of the lacrimal gland. Conjunctivitis, especially when severe, may present with periorbital swelling. Both *N. gonorrhoeae* and adenovirus conjunctivitis have been reported in association with periorbital swelling or cellulitis.[24,36]

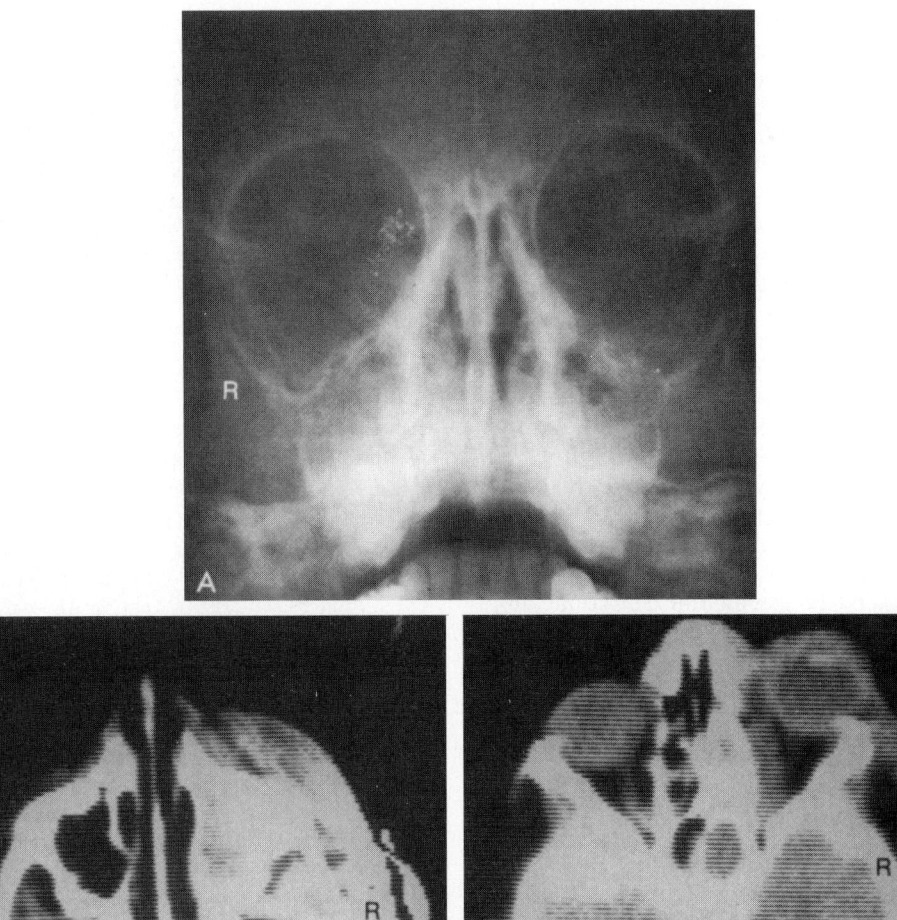

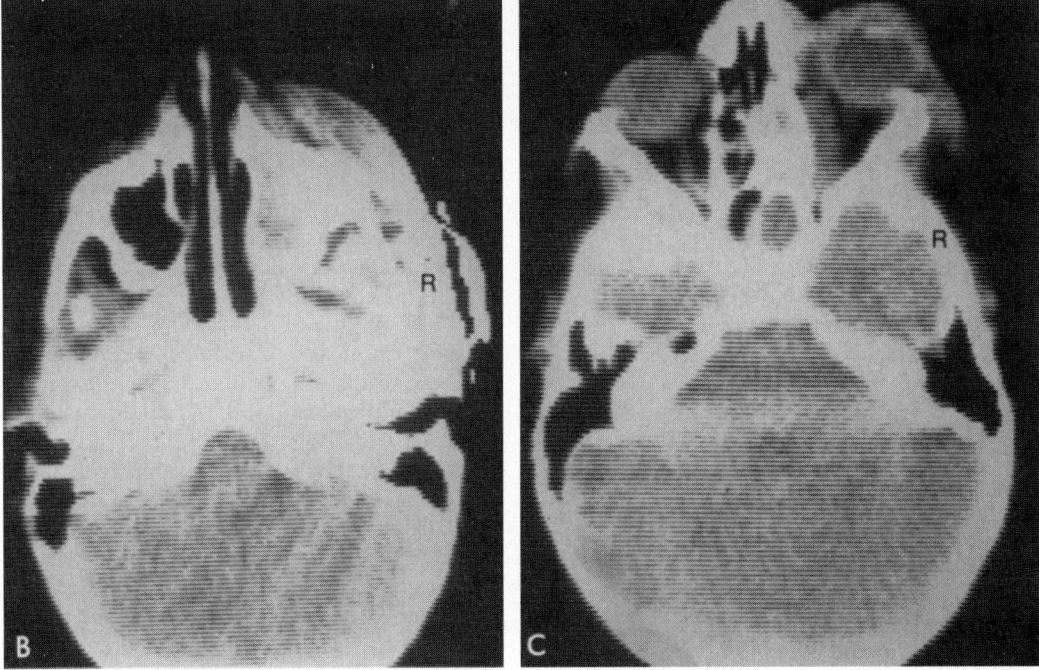

FIG. 51-5. Periorbital cellulitis. **A,** Water's view of orbits showing opaque right *(R)* maxillary and ethmoid sinuses and generalized soft tissue swelling over the right *(R)* orbit. **B,** CT scan through the level of the maxillary sinus showing superficial soft tissue edema and fluid within the right (R) maxillary sinus. **C,** CT scan through the mid-plane of the orbit showing proptosis of the right *(R)* globe and edema along the medial wall of the orbit behind the globe. The right *(R)* ethmoid sinus is filled with fluid, but there is no evidence of bone destruction. *(From Harley RD: Pediatric ophthalmology, ed 2, Philadelphia, 1983, WB Saunders.)*

Rare causes of periorbital swelling, which may be of rapid onset, include malignancies such as retinoblastoma or rhabdomyosarcoma, trichinosis infection, and renal disease.

Management. Antibiotic therapy for periorbital cellulitis should be selected based on the age of the patient and predisposing conditions. For patients under the age of 5 years with no preceding history of trauma or insect bites, *H. influenzae* or *S. pneumoniae* must be considered. IV antibiotics should be given to cover *H. influenzae* and gram-positive cocci. Regimens could include a penicillinase-resistant antistaphylococcal agent (nafcillin 150 mg/kg/24 hr) and a beta-lactamase resistant agent to cover *H. influenzae* such as cefuroxime 75-100 mg/kg/24 hr or ceftriaxone 100 mg/kg/24 hr). For patients older than 5 years old, or when the cellulitis is clearly related to a trauma or skin lesion, oxacillin sodium or nafcillin sodium 150 mg/

kg/24 hr IV will cover the most likely organisms, *S. aureus* and group A beta-hemolytic streptococci. For the child under age 5 with a history of trauma but with fevers and an elevated WBC count, coverage with both a penicillinase-resistant penicillin and cephalosporin for beta-lactam resistant *H. influenzae* is indicated until an agent is identified by culture.[34] The emergence of strains of *S. pneumoniae* that are resistant to penicillin and cephalosporins mandates use of vancomycin 40 mg/kg/24 hr q 6 hr IV if meningitis is suspected or clinical improvement does not occur as anticipated.

An alternative outpatient regimen or daily ceftriaxone sodium IM has been studied in patients with periorbital and buccal cellulitis. Complications included *H. influenzae* meningitis in a 4-month-old with buccal cellulitis, and a second episode of periorbital cellulitis in a 15-month-old.[44] The remainder of the patients did well with five daily injections of ceftriaxone 50 to 75 mg/kg/24 hr IM.

For the patient under age 5 with clinical cellulitis and a history of trauma or bite who is afebrile and who has a normal CBC, an intermediate regimen of ceftriaxone IM after a blood culture is obtained, followed by an oral cephalosporin with good staphylococcal coverage such as cephalexin (Keflex) 25 to 50 mg/kg/24 hr QID PO may be used in addition to a 24-hour follow-up visit.

Extremely mild cases of periorbital cellulitis attributable to bacterial conjunctivitis, hordeolum, or mild trauma, in which the incidence of bacteremia is rare, could be treated with oral penicillinase-resistant penicillins (cephalexin) as long as follow-up and compliance are likely.

Disposition. Patients who are admitted to the hospital are treated intravenously until fever and symptoms resolve, which usually occurs within 3 to 5 days, followed by subsequent discharge on oral antibiotics, which are chosen based on cultures and sensitivity testing. Evidence of meningitis or a positive CSF culture necessitates a longer course of parenteral therapy.

Orbital Cellulitis

Orbital cellulitis is an infection of the orbital tissues posterior to the orbital septum, characterized by periorbital swelling, erythema, and evidence of proptosis, ophthalmoplegia, or loss of visual acuity (Fig. 51-6). In children, it is most commonly found as a complication of sinusitis, although it may also follow trauma or intraorbital surgery.[43] The majority of patients with orbital disease are older than the population with periorbital cellulitis, although the age of patients afflicted ranges from newborns to adults.[34] Extension of orbital cellulitis may result in subperiosteal, orbital abscess, or cavernous sinus thrombosis.

Pathophysiology. About 75% of the time, orbital cellulitis occurs as a result of a sinus infection.[34] Anatomically, this can be explained by the proximity between the sinuses and the orbit, as well as the common venous and lymphatic system, which is devoid of valves. The pathophysiology of this process is related to the buildup of pressure within the sinus, which obstructs venous and lymphatic drainage, resulting in periorbital swelling. The orbit becomes more edematous, and inflammatory cells and bacteria infiltrate the orbit by direct spread from the sinuses or by venous connections. The buildup of orbital pressure causes pro-

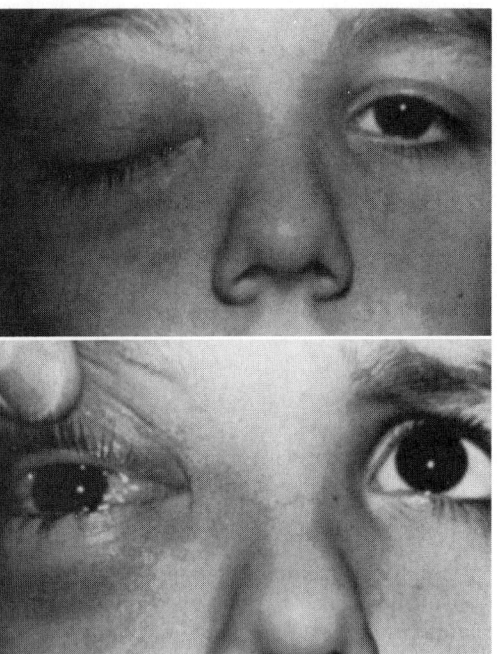

FIG. 51-6. Orbital cellulitis. (*From Helveston EM:* Pediatric ophthalmology practice, *ed 2, St Louis, 1984, Mosby.*)

gressive tenderness, pain with extraocular movements, chemosis, proptosis, and ophthalmoplegia. Subperiosteal and orbital abscesses may form, displacing the orbital contents and globe. Visual acuity may be hindered by the buildup of pressure on the optic nerve when an orbital abscess is present. The infectious process can extend via the valveless veins of the orbit into the cavernous sinus, thus resulting in thrombosis, bilateral symptoms, and further impairment of vision.[43]

The remaining cases of orbital cellulitis are the result of trauma, particularly penetrating ocular injury, skin infection, or intraorbital surgery.[43]

Etiology. Orbital cellulitis is most commonly caused by *S. aureus*, especially when trauma or surgery is the predisposing event[7] and in the newborn period.[34] *S. pneumoniae*, group A beta-hemolytic streptococci and nontypable *H. influenzae* are common organisms when the cellulitis is due to a sinus infection or dental abscess. Anaerobic organisms and *Branhamella catarrhalis* may be isolated from infected sinuses or dental abscesses, causing an orbital cellulitis.[7]

Less common causes of orbital cellulitis include tuberculosis, fungal disease, syphilis, and parasitic disease.[33,34]

Diagnostic Findings. Patients with orbital cellulitis may have a history of sinusitis, preceding trauma, or eye surgery. The onset of lid edema and erythema is acute and proceeds rapidly. As with periorbital cellulitis, fever is present approximately 75% of the time[34,38] and unilateral involvement is characteristic. The patient often appears systemically ill. On physical examination the eyelid is red or purple and markedly swollen. There may be injection of the conjunctiva, moderate-to-marked chemosis, proptosis, pain on eye movement, and decreased ocular mobility. Visual acuity may be decreased. If sinusitis is the cause of the cellulitis, the patient may have headache, rhinorrhea, and boggy nasal mucosa. With subperiosteal or orbital abscess formation, the globe will be further displaced. Examination of the fundus may reveal retinal vein congestion or swelling of the optic disc.

Complications. Complications of orbital cellulitis are far more devastating than with periorbital disease. Before the advent of antibiotic therapy, 17% of patients with orbital cellulitis died from meningitis, and 20% of survivors had permanent visual loss.[33] The case fatality rate for orbital cellulitis is 2%, which is tenfold greater than with periorbital disease. The fatality rate in newborns, however, remains high at 11%.[34]

CNS infections are the most common complications attributable to direct spread from infected abscesses or bone or through hematogenous dissemination. Meningitis and intracranial or parenchymal abscesses are the most common cause of morbidity and mortality, followed by septicemia.[34] Orbital and subperiosteal abscesses are the most common eye complications. With further venous extension of an orbital infection, cavernous sinus thrombosis may occur, characterized by abnormalities of cranial nerves III, IV, V, and VI. Symptoms may include ptosis, ophthalmoplegia, pupillary rigidity, loss of accommodation, marked edema, and venous engorgement of the lids and orbital tissues.[10]

Less common but potential complications when diagnosis is delayed include partial or total visual loss, optic atrophy, enucleation of the eye, keratitis, and osteomyelitis of the orbit.[34]

Ancillary Data. Laboratory evaluation is not extremely helpful in differentiating orbital from periorbital disease. A CBC with differential and blood culture are usually obtained to look for evidence of an increased WBC count or leftward shift and for a causative organism. A normal CBC would not affect management when the diagnosis of orbital cellulitis is made clinically. Cultures of any external wounds that may have preceded the cellulitis, or of an abscess or sinus obtained in the operating room may help isolate the causative agent.

In the newborn with orbital cellulitis a lumbar puncture should be performed, since bacterial seeding is the most likely mechanism of spreading of the infection.

Sinus films often show evidence of ethmoid or maxillary involvement. A head CT scan is the preferred radiologic study when the diagnosis of orbital cellulitis is suspected, to look for evidence of an abscess, which would need to be drained, or to identify sinusitis. The degree of proptosis, ophthalmoplegia, or impaired visual acuity does not clinically correlate with the presence or absence of an abscess. Other indications for a head CT scan in the setting of periorbital swelling have been discussed previously.[31,43]

Differential Considerations. The differential diagnosis of orbital cellulitis is similar to the entities described for periorbital cellulitis. Allergic, reactive edema, and contact dermatitis are less likely to be confused with orbital cellulitis because of the absence of globe involvement with these processes. Retinoblastoma and rhabdomyosarcoma may mimic orbital cellulitis by their acute onset of lid edema, conjunctival injection, chemosis, proptosis, and decreased extraocular motility. Fever is generally absent and

WBC count is normal. Examination by an ophthalmologist should help make these diagnoses. Neonatal conjunctivitis and dacrocystitis may have large amounts or eyelid swelling, but there is no evidence of globe involvement. Aseptic cavernous sinus thrombosis may occur after trauma or surgery. The classic symptoms of cavernous sinus thrombosis include bilateral involvement and cranial nerve palsies, but the lack of pain with extraocular movements differentiate aseptic cavernous sinus thrombosis from orbital cellulitis with extension to the cavernous sinus. Finally, idiopathic inflammatory orbital pseudotumor may present with the acute onset of pain, periorbital swelling, conjunctival injection, chemosis, proptosis, and abnormal extraocular motility. This condition may be differentiated from orbital cellulitis by the absence of fever or visual complaints, even though vision is decreased, and the amount of swelling decreases as the day progresses. Eosinophilia and elevated erythrocyte sedimentation rate may be found on laboratory evaluation.[7]

It is most important to differentiate periorbital cellulitis from orbital cellulitis. Although lid edema, erythema, fever, and even mild chemosis may be found in both conditions, the presence of ophthalmoplegia, proptosis, pain with eye movement, or abnormal visual acuity indicates orbital involvement.[34]

Management. Patients with orbital cellulitis must be admitted to the hospital and treated intravenously for organisms associated with sinusitis: *H. influenzae, S. pneumoniae, S. aureus,* and anaerobes (e.g., ceftriaxone 50-100 mg/kg/24 hr q 12 hr IV and clindamycin 15-40 mg/kg/24 hr q 6-8 hr IV).[45] An ophthalmologist and otolaryngologist should be consulted if the course of the illness is unusual. Surgical intervention is required for drainage of an abscess. Sinus drainage may be attempted if medical therapy alone is ineffective. Other indications for surgery include persistence of fever, evidence of optic nerve compression with decreased vision or color perception, worsening proptosis or globe displacement, or isolated muscle weakness.[7,43] Once a cause is identified from cultures, antibiotic therapy can be narrowed.

Disposition. Most patients with orbital cellulitis require a more prolonged hospitalization than those with periorbital disease, especially when complicating abscesses form. Defervescence alone is not a reliable sign, since abscesses have been noted to progress in the absence of fever.[43] Given the serious nature and risk of long-term complications with orbital cellulitis, a prolonged IV course of therapy is recommended.

References

Diagnostic Findings

1. Nelson LB: *Pediatric ophthalmology,* Philadelphia, 1984, WB Saunders.
2. Robb RM: *Ophthalmology for the pediatric practitioner,* Boston, 1981, Little, Brown.
3. Shingleton BJ: Eye injuries, *N Engl J Med* 325(6):408, 1991.
4. Clark R: Common ophthalmologic problems. In Rosen P et al, editors: *Emergency medicine concepts and clinical practice,* St Louis, 1988, Mosby.

Impaired Vision

5. Allen HF: Testing of visual acuity in preschool children, *Pediatrics* 19:1093, 1957.

6. Beauchamp GR: Causes of visual impairment in children, *Pediatr Ann* 9:414, 1980.
7. Gans LA and Shackelford PG: Ocular infections. In Feigin RD and Cherry JD, editors: *Textbook of pediatric infectious diseases,* ed 2, Philadelphia, 1987, WB Saunders.
8. Felter RA and Burnstine RA: Visual disturbance. In Fleisher GR, et al, editors: *Textbook of pediatric emergency medicine,* ed 2, Baltimore, 1988, Williams & Wilkins.
9. Ervin-Mulvey LD, et al: Pediatric eye trauma. *Pediatr Clin North Am* 30(6):1167, 1983.

Paralysis and Movement Disorders

10. Martyn LJ: Ophthalmic manifestations of central nervous system disorders in children. In RD Harley, editor: *Pediatric ophthalmology,* ed 2, Philadelphia, 1983, WB Saunders.
11. Keltner JL: Neuro-ophthalmology for the pediatrician, *Pediatr Ann* 6:78, 1977.

Red Eye

12. Oglesby R: Eye trauma in children, *Pediatr Ann* 6:11, 1977.
13. Smith LBH et al: Kawasaki syndrome and the eye, *Pediatr Infect Dis J* 8:116, 1989.
14. Gigliotti F et al: Etiology of acute conjunctivitis in children, *J Pediatr* 98(4):531, 1981.

Chalazion and Hordeolum

15. Sprague J: Eye disorders. In Barkin RM and Rosen P, editors: *Emergency Pediatrics,* ed 3, St Louis, 1990, Mosby.

Conjunctivitis

16. Fisher MC: Conjunctivitis in children, *Pediatr Clin North Am* 34:1446, 1987.
17. Brunell PA, moderator: *Pediatric ocular infections.* Supplement to Infectious Diseases in Children, April 1991.
18. Friendly DS: Ophthalmia neonatorum, *Pediatr Clin North Am* 30(6):1033, 1983.
19. Chlamydial Infections. In G Peter: *Report of the Committee on Infectious Diseases,* 22nd ed, Elk Grove Village, 1991, American Academy of Pediatrics.
20. Laga M et al: Single dose therapy of gonococcal ophthalmia neonatorum with ceftriaxone, *N Engl J Med* 315:1382, 1986.
21. Patamasucon P et al: Oral vs. topical erythromycin therapies for chlamydial conjunctivitis. *Am J Dis Child* 136:817, 1982.
22. Heggie AD et al: Topical sulfacetamide vs. oral erythromycin for neonatal chlamydial conjunctivitis, *Am J Dis Child* 139:564, 1985.
23. Weiss A et al: Acute conjunctivitis in childhood, *J Pediatr* 122:10-14, 1993.
24. Legido A and Joffe M: Gonococcal conjunctivitis mimicking orbital cellulitis in a young adolescent, *Am J Dis Child* 143:443, 1989.
25. Bodor FF: Conjunctivitis-otitis syndrome, *Pediatrics* 69(6):695, 1982.
26. Bodor FF et al: Bacterial etiology of conjunctivitis-otitis media syndrome, *Pediatrics* 76(1):26, 1985.
27. Harrison CJ et al: Relation of the outcome of conjunctivitis and the conjunctivitis-otitis syndrome to identifiable risk factors and oral antimicrobial therapy, *Pediatr Infect Dis J* 6:536, 1987.
28. Gigliotti F et al: Efficacy of topical antibiotic therapy in acute conjunctivitis in children, *J Pediatr* 104:623, 1984.
29. Lohr JA et al: Comparison of three topical antimicrobials for acute bacterial conjunctivitis, *Pediatr Infect Dis J* 7:626, 1988.

Periorbital and Orbital Cellulitis

30. Shapiro ED et al: Periorbital cellulitis and orbital cellulitis a reappraisal, *Pediatr Infect Dis* 1:91, 1982.
31. Luten RC: Evaluation of periorbital swelling. In Barkin RM, editor: *The emergently ill child,* Rockville, Md, 1987, Aspen Publishers.
32. Lucht RG and Hamilton GC: Periorbital cellulitis. In Barkin RM, editor: *The emergently ill child,* Rockville, Md, 1987, Aspen Publishers.
33. Gellady AM et al: Periorbital and orbital cellulitis in children, *Pediatrics* 61:272, 1978.
34. Israele V and Nelson JD: Periorbital and orbital cellulitis, *Pediatr Infect Dis J* 6:404, 1987.
35. Smith TF et al: Clinical implications of preseptal (periorbital) cellulitis in childhood, *Pediatrics* 62:1006, 1978.
36. Herman J and Katzuni E: Periorbital cellulitis complicating adenovirus infection, *Am J Dis Child* 140:745, 1986.
37. Zellers TM and Donowitz LG: Brain abscess and ethmoid sinusitis presenting as periorbital cellulitis in a two month old infant, *Pediatr Infect Dis J* 6(2):213, 1987.
38. Teele DW: Management of the child with a red and swollen eye, *Pediatr Infect Dis J* 2:258-62, 1983.
39. Powell KR et al: Periorbital cellulitis: clinical and laboratory findings in 146 episodes, including tear countercurrent immunoelectrophoresis in 89 episodes, *Am J Dis Child* 142:853, 1988.
40. Barkin RM et al: Periorbital cellulitis in children, *Pediatrics* 62:390, 1978.
41. Sankrithi UM and Lipuma JJ: Clinically inapparent meningitis complicating periorbital cellulitis, *Pediatr Emerg Care* 7:28, 1991.
42. Ciarallo LR and Rowe PC: Lumbar puncture in children with periorbital and orbital cellulitis, *J Pediatr* 122:355-359, 1993.
43. Goldberg F et al: Differentiation of orbital cellulitis from preseptal cellulitis by computed tomography, *Pediatrics* 62:1000, 1978.
44. Dagan R et al: Outpatient treatment of serious community-acquired pediatric infections using once daily intramuscular ceftriaxone, *Pediatr Infect Dis J* 6:1080, 1987.
45. Powell KR: Orbital and periorbital cellulitis, *Pediatr Rev* 16(5): 163–164, 1995.

CHAPTER

◆ **52** ◆

Gastrointestinal Disorders

DOUGLAS A. BOENNING • *BRUCE L. KLEIN*
Evaline A. Alessandrini • *Robert A. Belfer* • *James M. Chamberlain* • *Marc H. Gorelick*
• *Lisa Sinclair Hart* • *Kathleen A. Lillis* • *Julian B. Orenstein* • *Daniel W. Ochsenschlager*
• *Mary D. Patterson* • *Yeheskel Waisman* • *Joseph L. Wright*

Signs and Symptoms

ABDOMINAL MASS

MARC H. GORELICK

Abdominal masses are commonly palpated in children. Some produce symptoms or signs, whereas others remain silent even when large. They are usually discovered by a parent or caretaker or as an incidental finding during routine physical examination. Prompt diagnosis is necessary because of the frequency of malignancy: 15% in neonates and up to 50% in older infants and children.

Differential Considerations

The majority of abdominal masses are caused by hepatosplenomegaly, which is discussed in a later section. Other masses originate in the peritoneum, retroperitoneum, or pelvis. The frequency with which such masses arise from a specific organ system is related to age; however, in all age groups the urinary tract is the most common site of origin (Tables 52-1 and 52-2).[1] In addition, it is important to note that mass lesions of a congenital nature may first be detected in older children.[2]

Diagnostic Work-Up

Important points to delineate include the age of the child, type and duration of symptoms, and any change in size of the mass. In newborns, delayed passage of meconium is consistent with Hirschsprung disease or cystic fibrosis. Neonatal umbilical vessel catheterization is suggestive of portal vein thrombosis. At all ages, a family history of polycystic kidney disease or other anomalies should be elicited. A menstrual and sexual history is important in postpubescent girls. Finally, a history of trauma suggests a perinephric hematoma or pancreatic pseudocyst.

TABLE 52-1. Site of Origin of Abdominal Masses*

	Renal	Other retroperitoneal	GI	Genital
Neonates	55%	10%	20%	15%
Infants and children	55%	23%	18%	4%

*Excluding hepatosplenomegaly.

Symptoms indicative of gastrointestinal obstruction (abdominal pain and tenderness, vomiting, and constipation) or urinary tract obstruction (oliguria, dribbling, increased urinary frequency, and recurrent urinary tract infection) should be sought. If there is abdominal pain, its location, character, and pattern can be helpful in making the diagnosis. For example, colicky abdominal pain associated with vomiting and currant-jelly stools is classic for intussusception, whereas persistent localized pain with tenderness and high spiking fevers is more likely to be caused by an abscess.

Careful attention to technique is essential to a successful abdominal examination. The child should be as relaxed as possible; distracting older children is helpful, as are warm hands and a stethoscope. The infant may need to be examined initially on the parent's lap. The examination should start with visual inspection, followed by auscultation. Percussion may differentiate solid from cystic masses and define their extent. Finally, the mass should be palpated, with position, size, consistency, texture, mobility, and tenderness all noted. Other abdominal organs should also be palpated. A useful maneuver in young children is to flex the legs with one hand while palpating with the other. One should palpate gently, because the mass may have bled internally and could easily rupture. Occasionally, if an infant's stomach is distended with swallowed air, evacuation with a nasogastric tube is necessary to allow an adequate examination. Rectal examination is essential in the evaluation of a child with an abdominal mass. This allows better palpation of pelvic or anterior spinal masses and detection of occult fecal blood.[3]

The remainder of the examination may also provide clues. Nonspecific findings such as fever or weight loss are seen with infectious or neoplastic masses. Tumors of endocrine origin may lead to hormonal manifestations such as precocious puberty or hypertension. Some genetic disorders are associated with renal anomalies. Rashes may be indicative of Henoch-Schönlein therapy with intussusception. Finally, a pelvic examination should be performed on adolescent girls; in boys, the scrotum should be examined for tumors or hydroceles, both of which can be associated with abdominal masses.

Ancillary Data. Flat and upright abdominal x-ray studies are usually the first imaging studies obtained in the emergency department. These help to confirm the location of the mass and determine the presence or absence of intestinal obstruction or calcification (see box on p. 797). If intussusception is suspected on clinical grounds, a barium enema may be diagnostic as well as therapeutic.

TABLE 52-2. Classification of Abdominal Masses by Age at Presentation*

Most commonly detected in neonates	Most commonly detected in older infants, children, and adolescents
Urinary tract masses	
Hydronephrosis	Wilms' tumor
Multicystic or polycystic kidney	Perinephric hematoma
Distended bladder	
Renal vein thrombosis	
Ectopic or horseshoe kidney	
Urachal cyst	
Mesoblastic nephroma	
Gastrointestinal masses	
Pyloric stenosis	Constipation
Bowel duplication	Intussusception
Intestinal obstruction	Appendiceal abscess
Imperforate anus	Pancreatic pseudocyst
Hirschsprung disease	Mesenteric or omental cyst
Meconium ileus	
Genital tract masses	
Hydrometrocolpos	Intrauterine or ectopic pregnancy
Follicular ovarian cyst	Ovarian teratoma
	Ovarian tumor
	Ovarian cyst
	Tuboovarian abscess
	Hematocolpos
	Ovarian torsion
Hepatobiliary	
Choledochal cyst	Hepatoblastoma
Hepatic cyst	Choledochal cyst
Hemangioma	Hydrops of the gallbladder
Hydrops of the gallbladder	
Other	
Adrenal hematoma	Neuroblastoma
Sacrococcygeal teratoma	Lymphoma
Anterior meningomyelocele	Rhabdomyosarcoma
	Wandering spleen

*Some causes of hepatosplenomegaly excluded.

An abdominal ultrasound is a particularly useful test, providing information regarding the size, morphology (i.e., cystic vs. solid), and organ of origin of the mass. The advantages of ultrasound are its low cost and the fact that there is no exposure to ionizing radiation or contrast media. Computed tomography, which has those drawbacks, is less operator dependent, shows better anatomic detail of the mass and associated structures, and provides information regarding function. These two imaging modalities have largely supplanted IV pyelography, which was formerly the study of choice. However, because the majority of pediatric abdominal masses are of renal or perirenal origin, IV pyelography may be a useful tool when ultrasound and CT scanning are unavailable.[1]

Abdominal Masses Commonly Associated with Calcification

Neuroblastoma
Teratoma
   Ovarian
   Sacrococcygeal
Adrenal hematoma
Hepatic hemangioma
Meconium peritonitis

Laboratory evaluation has a limited role in the diagnosis of abdominal masses. Urinalysis, serum blood urea nitrogen and creatinine are useful when the mass is suspected to be renal in origin. Serum amylase and liver function tests are helpful on occasion. A complete blood count should be done if there is evidence of bleeding or if infectious or neoplastic causes are being considered. Increased urinary excretion of catecholamines and VMA suggest neuroblastoma. A urine pregnancy test should be obtained in sexually active females, especially before radiologic studies are performed.

Therapeutic Trial

The most important consideration in the emergency department evaluation of a child with an abdominal mass is determining which patient requires immediate intervention. Potential causes of intestinal gangrene (e.g., volvulus) or peritonitis and sepsis (e.g., appendiceal abscess) must be diagnosed and treated expeditiously. So too must conditions that can result in a loss of function (e.g., tuboovarian abscess) or those that may be caused by overwhelming disease (e.g., renal vein thrombosis). Once emergent and urgent conditions have been excluded, further studies as outlined above may be performed. If on the basis of the initial evaluation a malignancy is suspected or cannot be ruled out, the patient should be admitted for further diagnostic work-up.

ABDOMINAL PAIN

KATHLEEN A. LILLIS

Abdominal pain is a very common complaint in children and making an accurate diagnosis is often difficult. Nearly one third of the children who presented to an emergency department with abdominal pain did not receive a specific diagnosis.[4] However, it is necessary to recognize the signs and symptoms of the serious causes of abdominal pain so treatment can be instituted without delay, and the incidence of morbidity and mortality reduced. Because of the significance of abdominal pain, diagnostic entities are discussed in detail in sections focusing on the specific condition later in this chapter.

Pathophysiology

Visceral Pain. Visceral or splanchnic pain originates in the intraabdominal organs with visceral peritoneum. Im-

pulses are conducted to the spinal cord via visceral afferent nerve fibers. Stimuli for visceral pain arise from pathologic conditions of the viscera, including increased hollow viscus wall tension, solid viscus capsular stretching, and ischemia. Visceral pain tends to be midline, diffuse, and difficult to localize. It is often described as a "deep" pain. Severe visceral pain can cause autonomic reflexes such as sweating, tachycardia or bradycardia, hypotension, cutaneous hyperalgesia, hyperesthesia, and involuntary spastic contractions of the abdominal musculature.[5,6]

Somatic Pain. Somatic or parietal pain originates from the abdominal wall, the root of the mesenteries, or the diaphragm. It is mediated by somatic afferent nerve fibers in segmental spinal nerves. Somatic pain is usually sharper and more distinct than visceral pain, and is well localized to the site of stimulation.[5,6]

Referred Pain. Pain arising from a site distant to the pathology is called referred pain. The distant site is often along a dermatome from the pathologic site. Diaphragmatic irritation is associated with shoulder pain through C4 distribution; biliary tract disease often produces pain in the back from T9 distribution.[5,6]

Differential Considerations

The diagnostic alternatives are broad, requiring specific evaluation. Generally, conditions diagnosed or considered in a younger age group may require exclusion and consideration in older children, although these divisions by age are somewhat arbitrary.

Infancy. Abdominal pain is seen in patients of all ages. There are some diseases that are most prevalent in infancy. However, these are not unique to that group and may be seen in children of different ages (Table 52-3).

Intussusception is a telescoping of a proximal section of bowel into the more distal segment. It is the most common cause of intestinal obstruction in children less than 2 years of age.[7] It occurs most commonly in infants between 5 and 12 months of life, with a male predominance.[8,9] The most frequent site is the ileocecal valve. In older children, there is frequently a lead point, which includes polyp, Meckel's diverticulum, foreign body, hypertrophied Peyer's patch, or hematoma. An increased incidence is associated with cystic fibrosis, Henoch-Schönlein purpura, and idiopathic thrombocytopenic purpura.[7,8] When the upper portion of the intestine invaginates into the lower, there is constriction of the mesentery, which obstructs venous return and produces edema and inflammation of the bowel wall.[10]

Volvulus results from a congenital abnormality in the fixation of the mesentery and normal bowel migration. A malrotation predisposes the bowel to twist on itself, producing intestinal obstruction and vascular compromise. Complete volvulus can lead to bowel necrosis in 1 to 2 hours.[7,9]

Incarcerated hernias may develop in children with inguinal, femoral, and umbilical hernias. Inguinal hernias are the most common indication for surgery in children less than 2 years of age. Forty percent of inguinal hernias are apparent by 6 months of age. These are usually unilateral and have a 9:1 male to female ratio.[7,9,10]

Hirschsprung disease or aganglionic megacolon is a congenital disorder of the peristaltic activity of the large bowel

TABLE 52-3. Abdominal Pain by Ages

Infancy	Childhood	Adolescence
Intussusception	Gastroenteritis	Ectopic pregnancy
Volvulus	Appendicitis	Pelvic inflammatory disease
Incarcerated hernia	Pancreatitis	Testicular torsion
Hirschsprung disease	Henoch-Schönlein purpura	Inflammatory bowel disease
Necrotizing enterocolitis	Hemolytic uremic syndrome	Biliary disease
Colic	Ulcers	
Perforation	Constipation	
	Urinary tract infection	
	Functional causes of abdominal pain	

produced by an absence of ganglionic cells in the submucosal and myenteric plexuses. Involvement of the colon may range from a small segment at the rectum to the entire colon. This is the most common cause of intestinal obstruction in the neonate, accounting for 33% of all neonatal obstructions. The incidence is 1 in 1,500 to 3,000 live births. There is an increased incidence in male infants and in those with Down syndrome.[8,10]

Necrotizing enterocolitis (NEC) is the most common serious abdominal emergency in neonates. The etiology is unknown. NEC is characterized by varying degrees of mucosal or transmural necrosis of the intestines. The disease occurs primarily in premature infants, although it can occur in term infants as well. Perinatal stress may predispose the infant to the disease, including asphyxia, hypothermia, birth trauma, early feeding, or umbilical vessel catheterization.[8,9,11]

Colic refers to paroxysmal abdominal pain associated with severe crying. It occurs most commonly in infants under 3 months of age. The attacks begin suddenly, and the crying may last for hours. The etiology of these attacks is not known, but colic may be associated with swallowed air passed into the intestines or may be related to hunger. Certain foods may be responsible for excessive fermentation in the intestines, but a change in diet only rarely reduces attacks. Attempts should be made to improve feeding techniques including frequent burping, identifying possible allergenic foods in the diet, and avoiding overfeeding or underfeeding. Careful physical examination is essential to rule out the possibility of intussusception, strangulated hernia, otitis, pyelonephritis, and a hair or scratch in the eye. Support and reassurance are important in dealing with the family of a child with colic.[12]

Perforation should be considered in children who present with abdominal pain. Seventy-five percent of gastrointestinal perforation in children occurs in patients less than 2 years of age. Aside from NEC, ulcers are the most common cause of perforations, followed by complications of Hirschsprung disease, atresias, meconium ileus, and volvulus. Trauma and child abuse have also been associated with perforation.

There is a sudden onset of abdominal distension and peritonitis. The child will progress to shock without early intervention. Diagnosis can be confirmed by evidence of free air on radiographs.

Treatment involves supportive care with fluid management and surgical repair.[13]

Childhood. *Gastroenteritis* is the most common cause of abdominal pain in children. Viral agents account for 70% to 80% of cases of acute gastroenteritis. The most common viruses that produce gastroenteritis in children are rotavirus, Norwalk virus, and enteric adenovirus. Bacteria produce 10% to 20% of gastroenteritis in children, with the most common causes including *Escherichia coli*, *Salmonella*, and *Shigella*. Less common bacteria include *Campylobacter*, *Clostridium*, *Staphylococcus aureus*, *Vibrio*, and *Yersinia*. Parasites responsible for producing acute gastroenteritis in children are *Entamoeba histolytica*, *Giardia lamblia*, *Cryptosporidium*, and *Strongyloides stercoralis*.[14]

Appendicitis is the most common nontraumatic surgical emergency in children.[7] Peak incidence of appendicitis is from 9 to 12 years of age; approximately 1 out of every 15 individuals will develop appendicitis sometime during their lifetime.[7,8,13] There is a male predominance.[8,15,16] In appendicitis there is obstruction of the lumen, followed by distension and compromise to the blood supply. The appendix develops ischemia and infarction. As bacteria invade the wall of the appendix, the appendix becomes necrotic and gangrenous; perforation may occur.[15-17]

Pancreatitis is becoming more commonly recognized as a cause of acute abdominal pain in children. The pancreas is particularly susceptible to inflammation because its glands contain potentially destructive proenzymes that can rapidly destroy pancreatic tissue when activated. Most of the cases of pancreatitis in childhood occur after the age of 10 years and are related to drugs, toxins, trauma, or viral illnesses.[19,20]

The child with pancreatitis presents a constant epigastric pain that sometimes radiates to the back. Nausea, vomiting, and abdominal distension are also present. In more advanced cases, jaundice, acolic stools, ascites, and pleural effusions may be seen.

Henoch-Schönlein purpura (HSP) or anaphylactoid purpura is a systemic vasculitis. An acute inflammatory reaction occurs in the skin, and involves the polymorphonuclear cells, eosinophils, red cells, and IgA. An erythematous maculopapular rash progresses to petechiae or purpuric lesions and then ecchymoses. Abdominal pain is seen in two thirds of the children; this is usually colicky pain and is often associated with vomiting. Stools are grossly bloody or positive for occult blood in greater than half the patients; hematemesis may be present. In rare cases the renal manifestations of hematuria, proteinuria, azotemia, hypertension, and oliguria can result in chronic renal failure. Central nervous system involvement is a rare but serious manifestation that can produce seizures, paresis, and coma. Hepatosplenomegaly and lymphadenopathy may also occur.[8,13,21] (also see Chapter 60).

Hemolytic uremic syndrome (HUS) has been associated with bacterial and viral infections. This disease is characterized by a microangiopathic hemolytic anemia, acute renal failure, and thrombocytopenia.

The syndrome is most common in children under the age of 5 years and is usually preceded by gastroenteritis or an upper respiratory tract infection. Five to ten days after the initial illness, the child usually develops pallor, irritability, weakness, and lethargy. Of these children, 25% to 50% have crampy abdominal pain and diarrhea. Anemia, hypertension, and oliguria may develop over the next 2 weeks. Physical examination may be significant for dehydration, petechiae, edema, hepatosplenomegaly, and irritability. Intussusception, toxic megacolon, and perforation have been associated with HUS. More than 90% of the patients with acute renal failure survive the acute phase, and the majority recover normal renal function. Treatment involves peritoneal dialysis and supportive care[13,22] as delineated in Chapter 60.

Ulcer disease occurs much less commonly in children than in adults. During the first and second year of life, duodenal and gastric ulcers occur with similar frequency; however, after the sixth year, duodenal ulcers are much more common.

The clinical presentation includes dull or achy abdominal pain, acute or chronic blood loss, and vomiting in young children. An upper GI series is helpful in making the diagnosis. Gastroduodenoscopy is indicated when radiographs are unable to confirm the diagnosis.

Treatment consists of antacids. Cimetidine and ranitidine have been successful in the treatment of ulcers in children, although neither of these drugs have been approved for this age group.[23]

Constipation is one of the most common causes of abdominal pain in children. Children often withhold stool because they associate its passage with pain or are resisting toilet training. Colonic spasm may produce vague, recurrent, and severe abdominal pain. The child may also have nausea, vomiting, and abdominal distension. Hard stools will be palpated on the abdominal examination and the rectal exam. The diagnosis should be made by history and physical examination, and radiographs are unnecessary.

Treatment may include digital disimpaction followed by enemas. Caution must be exercised not to produce electrolyte imbalances secondary to absorption of the enemas. The child's parents should be counseled on dietary changes; mineral oil should be prescribed to prevent further complications with hard stools.[8,13]

A *urinary tract infection (UTI)* may be responsible for abdominal pain at any age. A history of urinary frequency, dysuria, dribbling, nocturnal enuresis, and daytime incontinence are important clues to the diagnosis, and can be elicited through a complete history in an older child. Ab-

dominal pain may also be present. Infants and young children may have a urinary tract infection even when abdominal pain is the only symptom elicited. Vomiting may also be a frequent symptom of a UTI in infants. On physical examination, tenderness may be noted in the flank region. Fever and an elevated white blood cell count may be present.

Urinalysis is necessary for the diagnosis. A catheterized specimen or a suprapubic tap may be required if the child is unable to provide a clean-catch midstream urine specimen. Bacteriuria indicates a UTI; pyuria alone does not. Pyuria may be caused by an adjacent inflamed appendix.[13]

The treatment for a UTI is antibiotics. After resolution, further investigations should exclude structural abnormalities that would predispose the child to urinary tract infections, as discussed in Chapter 60.

Functional causes of abdominal pain are common. Children who have abdominal pain and no organic cause can be classified into three categories: somatization disorders, hypochondriasis, and factitious abdominal pain. In somatization disorders, children have multiple, recurrent episodes of vague abdominal pain, abnormal vomiting, and bowel difficulties. The child is rarely free of symptoms, and has a history of multiple diagnostic tests without a diagnosis. One study reports that 95% of intermittent abdominal pain lasting greater than 3 months in a child over the age of 5 is on a functional basis. Hypochondriasis is a consequence of the interpretation of normal bodily functions and sensations as abnormal and indicative of disease. Factitious abdominal pain involves the conscious fabrication of signs and symptoms of disease for various purposes. These include children with Munchausen syndrome and the malingering patient.[24] The diagnosis of functional abdominal pain can not be made in the emergency department because ongoing evaluation and follow-up visits are required.

Adolescence. *Ectopic pregnancy* must be considered in every postmenarchal female who complains of lower abdominal pain. Approximately 95% of ectopic pregnancies are in the fallopian tube; rarely are they ovarian, abdominal, or cervical. Most ectopic pregnancies occur at 6 to 12 weeks of gestation. Risk factors include a history of pelvic inflammatory disease, previous ectopic pregnancy or tubal ligation, infertility, previous abortions, or an intrauterine device (IUD) in place or recently removed.

Abdominal pain is present in 97% of cases. The pain may be sharp or dull, intermittent or constant, and diffuse or localized. Some form of abnormal vaginal bleeding is seen in most cases including amenorrhea, delayed menses, abnormal period, or noncyclic bleeding. Nausea, vomiting, symptoms of pregnancy or urinary tract infection, and rectal complaints may be noted. Fever is rare; peritoneal signs are not seen in an unruptured ectopic pregnancy. The classic presentation of a ruptured ectopic pregnancy consists of sudden onset of severe pelvic and abdominal pain, shoulder pain, an urge to defecate, and syncope in the absence of hypovolemia; 10% to 20% of patients are in shock. The remaining patients have abdominal, adnexal, or cervical tenderness. Adnexal fullness and uterine enlargement may be evident at 6 to 8 weeks of gestation.

The diagnosis is made by a positive pregnancy test and ultrasound, as discussed in Chapter 53. Because the placenta produces less human chorionic gonadotropin (HCG) in an ectopic pregnancy, a false-negative test result can occur. Serum HCG testing is very reliable and should be performed on any girl in whom an ectopic pregnancy is suspected. Ultrasounds are 70% to 90% accurate and may determine whether the pregnancy is intrauterine or extrauterine. Culdocentesis and laparoscopy are alternative techniques for diagnosis.

Conservative surgical management may include manual expression of the ectopic pregnancy, linear salpingostomy, midsegment tubal resection with reanastomosis, or tubal reimplantation. These methods have been successful in preserving fertility although there is a 15% to 18% incidence of recurrence. Resuscitation is necessary before surgical management.[8,13]

Pelvic inflammatory disease (PID) develops in one out of every eight sexually active female adolescents. It is more prevalent in females with multiple sexual partners. It is the leading cause of infertility and is associated with an increased incidence of ectopic pregnancies. Infectious organisms responsible for this disease include *Neisseria gonorrhoeae, Chlamydia trachomatis,* and *Mycoplasma hominis* (see Chapter 53).

Lower abdominal pain is the most common symptom. Vaginal discharge, followed by vaginal bleeding, dysuria, and gastrointestinal complaints are frequently seen. Physical examination reveals significant lower abdominal and adnexal tenderness. Up to 30% of patients have right upper quadrant tenderness. Cervical tenderness and vaginal discharge are found in the majority of cases of pelvic examination. Diagnosis is made by history and physical examination. A positive cervical gram stain helps to support the diagnosis.[8,13]

Testicular torsion may occur with abdominal pain originating from the testicles. Examination of the external genitalia is essential in any male who has abdominal pain. Torsion of the testicle should be considered an emergency, and efforts should be made to correct the situation as soon as possible to avoid loss of the testicle. Compromise to the vascular supply of the testicle can result in death to the testicle within hours. Torsion most commonly occurs during or shortly after puberty when the testicle is increasing in size and weight. A congenital lack of testicular attachment to the scrotum also creates an additional increased risk.

The boy experiences scrotal or lower abdominal pain that may be sudden or insidious in onset. Physical examination usually reveals a swollen, tender, erythematous hemiscrotum with a high-riding testicle. Other findings that may be present are lack of a cremasteric reflex on the affected side and lack of relief of pain with elevation of the testicle. Assessing blood flow to the testicle by Doppler effect may be useful, but is associated with false negatives and positives; however, it has been found to be helpful in confirming the diagnosis. False negatives have been found late in the course. Epididymitis and torsion of the appendix testis may mimic testicular torsion. Testicular blood flow scans have been successful in demonstrating decreased blood flow on the ipsilateral side in torsion and increased blood flow in epididymitis. Torsion of the appendix testis usually occurs in prepubertal children and shows more localized pain. A "blue dot" may be seen over the torsed appendix testicle. The pain in epididymitis is usually more insidious in onset and initially localizes to the epididymis.

Inflammatory bowel disease (IBD) including Crohn disease and ulcerative colitis should be considered in the adolescent with abdominal pain. Although both diseases classically consist of a variety of other gastrointestinal and systemic symptoms, abdominal pain may be the predominant clinical manifestation. A significant history of bloody, mucous diarrhea, fecal urgency, tenesmus, fever, anorexia, chronic malaise, and joint symptoms may be indicative of IBD. Typically, there will be a more chronic change in bowel habits. Radiographic studies or colonoscopy may be necessary to confirm the diagnosis.[9,25]

Biliary tract disorders are less common causes of acute abdominal pain in children than adults. Abdominal pain is the most frequent complaint in children with biliary disease. Often, children are unable to locate the pain well, which contributes to the difficulty of diagnosis. The pain is generally constant, of sudden onset, and gradual resolution. Hemolytic disorders such as sickle cell anemia, hereditary spherocytosis, and thalassemia are commonly associated with biliary disease. Other predisposing factors appear to be chronic use of parenteral nutrition, abdominal sepsis, dehydration, ileal resection, obesity, and pregnancy.[9,13,19,20]

Other Extraabdominal Causes. *Sickle cell anemia* often causes abdominal pain secondary to vasoocclusive crisis. This event is frequently precipitated by infection, exertion, dehydration, hypovolemia, cold exposure, hypoxemia, acidosis, or depression. The pain is severe and continuous, but may be throbbing in nature. The abdomen is involved approximately one third of the time. Symptoms associated with vasoocclusive crisis include fever, nausea, vomiting, and diarrhea. Bone or joint pain is usually also present. Physical examination may reveal tachycardia, jaundice, ileus, and in some cases, a tender, rigid abdomen resembling a surgical abdomen. A marked elevation in liver enzymes may be seen.

Treatment consists of narcotic analgesics, nonsteroidal antiinflammatory medications, hydration, and close observation. Surgical consultation may be necessary to rule out concurrent intraabdominal pathology.[8,24]

Pneumonia in the right lower lobe may produce irritation of the lower intercostal nerve and pain in any quadrant of the abdomen. Usually the child has a history of upper respiratory symptoms, with cough and fever. Physical examination is significant for tachypnea, shallow breathing, splinting, and pleuritic pain. Chest auscultation demonstrates rales, dullness, and decreased breath sounds. Some abdominal guarding may be found, but rigidity and peritoneal signs are absent. Although the chest radiograph will confirm the diagnosis, radiographs may lag behind the clinical symptoms by 24 hours.[13,24]

Diabetic ketoacidosis may cause abdominal pain and vomiting. Typically, there is a history of polyuria, polydipsia, and weight loss. Depending on the degree of dehydration, the child may be lethargic or somnolent, and frequently ketones are detected on the breath. Laboratory studies reveal hyperglycemia and a metabolic acidosis. Urinalysis is positive for glucose and ketones.[13] A bedside glucose test should be performed on any child who has abdominal pain and decreased level of consciousness.

Lead intoxication may occur in children who ingest lead-based paint. It is most common in children between 1 and 6 years of age. Symptoms include anorexia, intermittent colicky abdominal pain, constipation, and hyperirritability. On physical examination, some abdominal tenderness may be seen. Flecks of opaque material may be found on abdominal radiographs. Broad bands of increased density on the metaphyses of the long bones support the diagnosis.[13] The diagnosis is confirmed by elevated serum lead levels. Treatment consists of chelation.

Porphyria may occur initially with abdominal pain. The porphyrias are characterized by errors in pyrrole metabolism. Symptoms rarely develop before puberty and are usually insidious in onset. The abdominal pain is usually colicky in nature and is localized in the epigastric region or right lower quadrant. At times the pain is severe and is usually associated with vomiting and constipation. On physical examination, mild, diffuse abdominal tenderness and photodermatitis are present. Hypertension also may be seen. The classic burgundy-red urine may or may not be present. The diagnosis is confirmed with a positive Hoesch test for porphobilinogen.[13]

Poisoning and foreign body ingestions should also be considered in the diagnosis of a child with abdominal pain. Drugs and other toxins produce abdominal pain through a variety of different mechanisms. Ingestion of substances such as aspirin, iron, mercury, and acidic or alkali agents produce abdominal pain through corrosive injury. Ingestion of activated charcoal, anticholinergic drugs, narcotics, and drug-filled packets used by "body packers" can produce obstruction and an ileus. Abdominal pain manifested as a sign of systemic toxicity is seen with a black widow spider bite and ingestion of heavy metals. Ergotamines and sympathomimetic drugs can produce intestinal ischemia.[20] Foreign bodies in the gastrointestinal tract usually cause little or no problems, whereas large objects and long objects with sharp points (such as sewing needles) may cause perforation.[7]

Diagnostic Work-Up

Important information that should be obtained in a diagnostic work-up of a child with abdominal pain is outlined in the box at right.

A careful history is essential in evaluating a child with abdominal pain. It is also important to determine if this is an acute or chronic problem. Chronic abdominal pain is less likely to be life-threatening, although complications may evolve. Determine if the pain is as usual or different.[7]

The onset of the pain can provide clues to the diagnosis (Table 52-4). Sudden onset of pain is more likely to be associated with perforation, intussusception, ectopic pregnancy, and torsion. Slow onset is associated with an inflammatory process such as appendicitis, pancreatitis, and cholecystitis. Colicky pain that is severe, crampy, and intermittent usually originates from a hollow, muscular viscus such as the intestine, biliary tree, pancreatic duct, uterus, or fallopian tube. Severe chronic pain may be seen in children with sickle cell anemia, inflammatory bowel disease, or cystic fibrosis. If a patient is brought to the emergency department within 24 hours after the onset of the

---

Diagnostic Work-Up for Abdominal Pain

History

Characteristic of pain: type of pain at onset, presentation, aggravating factors, relieving factors, previous episodes

Location of pain: site at onset and presentation, radiation

Associated symptoms: vomiting—hematemesis; diarrhea—hematochezia, melena; urinary symptoms—frequency, dysuria, fever, anorexia

Past medical history: menstrual history, sexual history, medications, and allergies

Review of system: coughing, gastrointestinal bleeding, vaginal bleeding, discharge

Physical examination

Observation: interactions, different positions

Vital signs: tachycardia, tachypnea, fever, hypotension

Skin: rashes, petechiae, purpura

Complete physical examination: otitis media, pneumonia

Abdominal examination:

    Observation: scaphoid, distended, evidence of trauma, discolored hernia

    Auscultation: bowel sounds

    Percussion: tympany, organ size

    Palpation: masses, guarding, rebound tenderness, peritoneal signs

External genitalia: cryptorchism, high-riding testicle, penile discharge, vaginal atresia

Rectal examination: tenderness, masses, stool, sphincter tone

Ancillary data

Laboratory studies: CBC, electrolytes, BUN, creatinine, liver function tests, amylase, HCG if indicated; urinalysis

Imaging studies: Radiographs: two abdominal views, chest (if indicated); sonography (if indicated); CT scans (if indicated)

---

pain, the underlying condition is more likely to be of a surgical nature.[8,13]

The location of the pain may also provide information regarding its underlying etiology (Fig. 52-1). Periumbical pain is associated with the small bowel and proximal colon. Hypogastric pain is associated with the distal colon, bladder, ovary, and fallopian tubes; pain in the epigastric region is related to the esophagus, stomach, duodenum, biliary tree, and pancreas. Shoulder pain may result from diaphragmatic involvement, whereas back pain may reflect pathology of the pancreas, retroperineum, or sacrum. Right scapular pain may occur with gallbladder pathology. Sacral pain is related to gynecologic pathology or rectal etiology.[8,13]

Associated symptoms are helpful in the diagnostic process. Low-grade fever is commonly seen in gastroenteritis, appendicitis, perforation, and peritonitis.[8] The level of elevation of the body temperature is of little help diagnostically. Vomiting that occurs with the onset of pain is usually associated with gastroenteritis, intussusception, or ureteral

TABLE 52-4. Characteristics of Abdominal Pain

Pain	Characteristic
Sudden onset	Perforation, intussusception, ectopic pregnancy, torsion
Slow onset	Appendicitis, pancreatitis, cholecystitis
Colicky pain	From intestines, biliary tree, pancreatic duct, uterus, fallopian tube
Severe chronic pain	Sickle cell disease, inflammatory bowel disease, cystic fibrosis

colic. Delayed vomiting is suggestive of peritoneal inflammation or obstruction. Bilious emesis indicates mechanical obstruction.[8,13] Diarrhea may be seen in gastroenteritis, Hirschsprung disease, and inflammatory bowel disease.

Past medical history is important and may reveal such illnesses as nephrotic syndrome, ascites, or immune deficiency, which might suggest peritonitis. A history of abdominal trauma or use of steroids might lead to the investigation of pancreatitis. A positive family history of sickle cell disease, cystic fibrosis, or hemophilia may be suggestive of the etiology of the pain.[13]

A thorough review of systems is essential and often aids in the diagnosis. A history of gastrointestinal bleeding associated with the abdominal pain is seen with intussusception, HSP, and Meckel's diverticulum. Coughing with pleuritic chest pain suggests pneumonia. Hematuria may be present with sickle cell disease, HUS, and HSP. Polyuria and polydipsia are suggestive of diabetes. Premenarchal pelvic pain suggests a follicular cyst rupture, ovarian torsion, or pelvic appendicitis. Postmenarchal patients may experience abdominal pain secondary to ectopic pregnancy, torsion of tumors, or hemorrhagic cysts. Vaginal bleeding, a history of unprotected sexual intercourse, and a missed period suggest an ectopic pregnancy. A history of multiple sex partners and the use of an IUD suggests PID.[8,13] The history should also contain information regarding medications, allergies, and recent hospitalizations.

The examination of a child should be done with patience and gentleness. Gaining the child's trust is important. The child should be observed interacting with his parents and nurse. The physician should obtain a sense of the severity of the illness. A sick or toxic-appearing child will be lethargic and withdrawn. A child with peritoneal irritation will tend to be quiet, lying with knees flexed and drawn up. A child with colicky pain frequently moans with discomfort, often rocking back and forth.[8] Have the child stand erect and jump up and down; this exercise can provide useful information.

A complete physical examination should be performed to look for extraabdominal causes of the abdominal pain. Vital signs provide essential information. If a postmenarchal female is in shock from blood loss, an ectopic pregnancy should be suspected. Hypertension may be associated with Henoch-Schönlein purpura or hemolytic uremic syndrome.[13] Evidence of tachycardia or orthostatic findings might suggest compensated shock and be indicative of

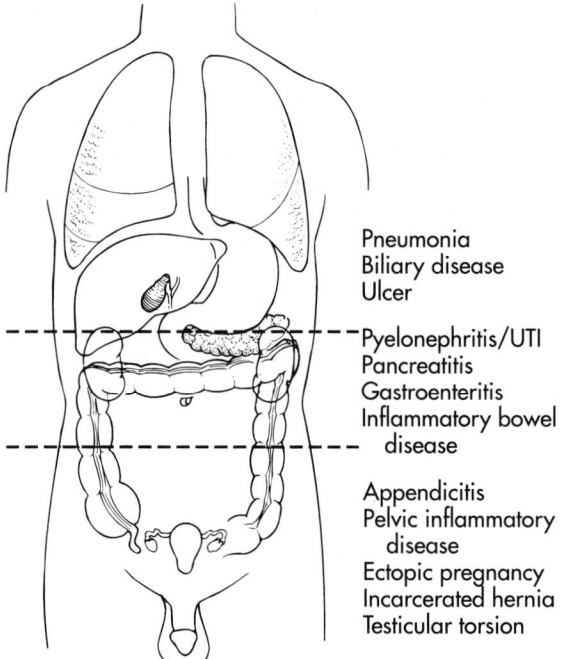

Pneumonia
Biliary disease
Ulcer

Pyelonephritis/UTI
Pancreatitis
Gastroenteritis
Inflammatory bowel
  disease

Appendicitis
Pelvic inflammatory
  disease
Ectopic pregnancy
Incarcerated hernia
Testicular torsion

FIG. 52-1. Location of abdominal pain.

sepsis or hypovolemia. The pattern of respiration should be noted. Rapid shallow respirations along with abdominal pain suggests peritonitis or lower lobe pneumonia. Kussmaul respirations points to diabetic ketoacidosis.[7] Examination of the skin may reveal a maculopapular rash on the lower extremities, which is suggestive of HSP. Erythema nodosum and pyoderma granulosum may suggest inflammatory bowel disease.

The abdominal examination should be performed only after completing the rest of the examination. The examination of the abdomen should begin with observation. What is the shape of the abdomen? Is it flat, distended, or scaphoid? Can peristaltic waves be seen? Is there any evidence of trauma or child abuse? Is there a high-riding torsed testicle or discolored hernia? Auscultation should be done by lightly placing the stethoscope upon the abdomen and listening in all quadrants. High-pitched, crescendo sounds interspersed with periods of silence suggest an obstruction. Hypoactive bowel sounds in the presence of peritoneal irritation suggest peritonitis. Bowel sounds that are absent for 5 minutes may indicate an ileus.[8] Before placing one's hands upon a child's abdomen, the child should be asked to point to the area that hurts the most and the physician should avoid examining that region initially. If possible, the child should be distracted with conversation about school or home. The child's facial expressions should help the physician to evaluate the effect of the interaction.[8] Percussion should be the next step in the abdominal examination. The gentle jarring produced by percussion can be enough to elicit rebound tenderness. Percussion is useful in estimating organ sizes. Tympany may be seen with bowel obstruction or perforation.[5]

Palpation is the fourth and most informative part of the abdominal examination. Gentle, systematic palpation can be done with the stethoscope on an anxious child. If palpation of the abdomen reveals rigidity, perforation should be suspected. Guarding and rebound tenderness suggest a surgical disease.[5] Palpation during the deep breaths between sobs will allow the physician to check for masses or guarding. It is often better to use an alternative method of determining rebound tenderness in a child such as rocking the child's pelvis, tapping the child's soles, or asking the child to cough. The child should sit up for the back examination to determine evidence of costovertebral angle tenderness and for palpation of the spine.[8]

Examination of the external genitalia should be performed for evidence of penile and scrotal findings. Balanitis and urethritis may produce abdominal pain. Evidence of cryptorchidism should raise the suspicion of an intraabdominal torsed testicle.[8] In female patients, the external genitalia should be examined for evidence of vaginal atresia and imperforate hymen, which can present as an abdominal mass or an acute abdomen.[9] A pelvic examination with consent is important in an adolescent even if she denies sexual activity.[8] Prepubescent girls rarely require a formal pelvic examination. Pelvic masses can be palpated during the rectal examination. The rectal examination should be the last part of the examination because it may be somewhat distressing for some children. The rectal examination provides useful information regarding tenderness, presence of masses and stool, melena, and sphincter tone. The rectal examination should be explained to the child before the procedure begins. Generous amounts of lubricant should be used, and the procedure should be done slowly and as gently as possible.[8]

Ancillary Data. Laboratory evaluation can provide some helpful clues into the diagnosis of the abdominal pain.

A CBC provides essential information regarding infection and blood loss. Leukocytosis is seen in most cases of acute appendicitis, in somewhat fewer cases of cholecystitis, and in approximately half of the cases of intestinal obstruction. Gastroenteritis and abdominal pain of unknown etiology are associated with leukocytosis in 43% and 31% of the cases respectively.[7] The CBC detects anemia, suggesting blood loss or underlying hematologic abnormalities such as sickle cell disease.[8] The peripheral smear should be examined for evidence of red cell destruction and thrombocytopenia, which may be indicative of hemolytic-uremic syndrome.[8,13] Serum electrolytes are helpful in children with pronounced vomiting or diarrhea. A nonanionic gap metabolic acidosis may be present in children with prolonged or severe diarrhea. The finding of an anion gap metabolic acidosis in the setting of abdominal pain suggests sepsis, hypovolemic shock, ingestion, diabetic ketoacidosis (DKA), or renal failure. An arterial blood gas should be performed in the presence of an anion gap metabolic acidosis and abdominal pain, and abdominal pain associated with tachypnea or shortness of breath. Serum glucose to exclude DKA or other causes of hyperglycemia should be entertained. Blood nitrogen urea (BUN) and creatinine are useful in evaluating hydration and kidney status.[5] Other serum blood chemistries such as amylase and liver function tests (LFT) should be obtained on those children who may have pancreatitis, biliary tract disease, or hepatitis.[13]

A urinalysis is essential in the work-up of a child with abdominal pain. Bacteriuria and pyuria are consistent with a UTI. An inflamed appendix lying adjacent to a urethra or bladder may cause pyuria (increased white cells present on urinalysis). Hematuria is present with passage of a urethral stone or may be seen with a urinary tract infection.[13] If the hematuria is present with proteinuria, HSP and HUS should be considered.[8,13] Glycosuria is seen in diabetes or sepsis.[13] Ketonuria, which is present in diabetes mellitus, may also be seen in children with poor oral fluid intake.[8] Burgundy-colored urine suggests porphyria.[13]

An HCG test, or pregnancy test, whether on serum or urine, is necessary in adolescent girls who are sexually active. This test is essential to rule out intrauterine pregnancy or ectopic pregnancy as a cause of abdominal pain.[8] A pregnancy test should be performed on all sexually active females before obtaining any radiographs. Gram stains and other studies of cervical and vaginal specimens obtained during the pelvic examination are helpful in diagnosing pelvic inflammatory disease.[13]

If there is a high suspicion of intraabdominal pathology, radiographs should be performed. At least two views should be obtained: a supine film and an erect or upright film. Because many children are too young or too uncomfortable to stand erect, a left lateral decubitus is an excellent alternative to the erect film. If there are any signs or symptoms that might suggest pneumonia such as cough, tachypnea, or shortness of breath, a chest radiograph should also be obtained.[7,8,13] The radiographs should be examined for evidence of air-fluid levels, free air, bowel obstruction, calcifications or foreign bodies, and masses. Air-fluid levels, sentinel loops, and a gasless abdomen suggest an obstruction. Free air is suggestive of perforation. Soft tissue masses may be represented by displacement of adjacent loops of bowel that contain gas. Radiopaque foreign bodies and calcifications can be consistent with a fecalith of a Meckel's diverticulum or appendix, right upper quadrant gallstones, renal stones, and flecks of calcification suggesting lead-containing paint.[13]

Obstruction of the lower intestinal tract often requires further investigation to distinguish small bowel obstruction from large bowel obstruction. A small bowel obstruction may be seen in diseases such as ileal stenosis or atresia, meconium ileus, midgut volvulus, or total colonic aganglionosis. A large bowel obstruction can be seen with Hirschsprung disease and a meconium plug. A barium enema may help to identify a distended large bowel, an abnormally positioned colon, and possibly a patent appendix.[8]

If the abdominal radiographs are equivocal, sonography may be useful. Ultrasound is ideal for children. Little preparation is required and it is painless. It emits no radiation, requires no contrast, and allows the examiner to image multiple systems simultaneously. Ultrasound is very helpful in determining the etiology of lower abdominal pain in a female adolescent and in establishing the diagnosis of pancreatitis, cholecystitis, intraabdominal and appendiceal abscesses, and hydronephrosis.[25] The presence of a gestational sac can determine if the pregnancy is intrauterine or ectopic.[13]

Other imaging studies that may be helpful in the work-up of a child with abdominal pain include CT scans and Doppler ultrasound. CT scanning is a useful adjunct in the work-up of a child with abdominal pain. Its major role is in diagnosing abdominal trauma and masses. Testicular blood flow scan is very successful in the evaluation of acute scrotum. Decreased blood flow is demonstrated on the ipsilateral side in torsion and increased blood flow is demonstrated in epididymitis.[8]

Prehospital Considerations

Children present a unique challenge to emergency medical personnel who transport them. Special considerations that should be given to transporting a child who has abdominal pain involve the basics of life support. Children who have severe abdominal pain of unknown etiology should be treated as if a major intraabdominal process is evolving. Establishing airway, breathing, and circulation should always be a priority. Precautions should be taken for early recognition and treatment of shock. Vital signs should be closely monitored and an IV line should be established. In patients with significant concern that some abdominal trauma may have occurred, IV lines should be established in the upper extremities to avoid pooling in the intraabdominal cavity if there has been a disruption of the inferior vena cava. Supporting ABCs and proper treatment of shock is the most important management of a child with abdominal pain who is being transported. Until a definitive diagnosis can be made, the child should not be allowed to take anything by mouth during the transport.

Therapeutic Trials

Therapeutic trials should be specific to the diagnosis responsible for producing the abdominal pain. Nonspecific therapeutic intervention should not be used in a child in the absence of a diagnosis. If no diagnosis is made and the abdominal pain is severe, the child should be hospitalized for further work-up or observation.

CONSTIPATION

JULIAN B. ORENSTEIN

Constipation is a symptom of a variety of conditions; pathologic and functional disorders frequently overlap. Evaluation of this symptom differs for infants and older children. In either case the concern is in distinguishing a medical or surgical emergency from a functional disorder of long or short duration.

Pathophysiology

Normal bowel continence requires intact mechanisms of fluid and electrolyte transport, sensory and motor functions, and behavioral/psychologic components.

Large-bowel mucosa absorbs sodium and water as long as it remains in contact with feces. The prolonged transit time of chronic stool retention results in hardening of the stool by continuous water reabsorption.

Sensation of stool in the rectum occurs as a threshold volume (TV); a larger critical volume (CV) is required to initiate normal internal anal sphincter (IAS) relaxation. When this involuntary (smooth muscle) reflex occurs, the external anal sphincter (EAS) voluntarily constricts (stri-

ated muscle) to permit timely defecation in older, toilet-trained children. In infancy and before toilet training, however, the EAS relaxes when the IAS relaxes.

Manometric studies in chronically constipated children have demonstrated that both the TV and CV rise in a parallel fashion. In encopretics, newly arrived liquid stool seeps around the older harder stool and leaks out before the child is conscious of rectal distension and before the rectum is able to relax and accommodate it. Such children often claim that they do not know they are going to stool until after the event has occurred. Recognition has also grown in the past few years of intestinal neuronal dysplasia, which causes dysfunctional colonic motility. Manometric examination distinguishes this disorder from normal innervation and true functional disorders.[26]

Finally, a child's conscious control of defecation is a combination of behavioral and psychologic factors. The child must have the patience to sit on a toilet and consciously attempt to defecate, the process must be a pain-free one, the child must have some sense of reward either pleasing himself or his parents, and it should be a part of the daily routine, such as dressing or brushing one's teeth. Any part of this constellation can be disrupted, and children can easily overcome the normal continence mechanisms and withhold stool until it becomes an abnormal, painful, and punishing experience. Such children can maintain abnormally high EAS tone and demonstrate paradoxic contraction of the EAS upon defecation, thereby defeating what otherwise might be a normal attempt to defecate.

Differential Considerations

When evaluating a "constipated" child, it is important to understand normal bowel habits. In the first 2 or 3 months, anything from one bowel movement per feeding to one every other day may be noted. From 2 months to 1 year, two to three per day is normal, and from 1 to 5 years, one or two per day is typical.[27] The approach to constipated infants is different from the approach to older children who are constipated.

Infants. Infants with a complaint of constipation may not be "constipated," and if they are, they may be asymptomatic, colicky, or just straining at stools. Often the parent needs reassurance and education as well as recommendations for management. Causes for constipation in the first 2 months of life are listed in the box on p. 805. Diet is a consideration: breastfed infants have fewer stools than formula-fed babies. Iron-fortified formulas do not cause constipation although there is some evidence that cow milk protein allergy may produce constipation in some infants.[28] In infants who are acutely ill with a viral syndrome or gastroenteritis, infrequent stooling may be related to poor intake, recovery from diarrhea, or pain from fissures or perianal dermatitis. Infant botulism is an unusual but life-threatening cause of constipation.

History and Physical. The history should pay attention to the number of stools beginning from the neonatal period. Stool consistency and color, diet, and presence of systemic signs (e.g., vomiting, fever, and lethargy) should be defined. On physical examination note abdominal girth, presence of bowel sounds, and masses. The rectal exam

Constipation in Newborns and Infants

I. General
   A. Sepsis
   B. Respiratory distress syndrome
   C. Maternal drugs
      1. Opiates
      2. MgSO$_4$
   D. Hypothyroidism
   E. Infant botulism
   F. Breastfed
II. Stomach/duodenum
   A. Antral web
   B. Pyloric stenosis
   C. Duodenal atresia
   D. Anular pancreas
III. Small intestine
   A. Meconium ileus/meconium plug
   B. Volvulus
IV. Large intestine
   A. Hirschsprung disease
V. Anus
   A. Anteriorly displaced anus
   B. Anal fissure
   C. Perianal dermatitis

Constipation in Older Children

I. Gastrointestinal
   A. Hirschsprung disease
   B. Status post (S/P) repair of Hirschsprung disease
   C. Anterior displacement of anus
II. Diet
   A. Low fiber
   B. Anorexia
III. Neurogenic
   A. Cerebral palsy
   B. Mental retardation
   C. Spina bifida
   D. Neuronal intestinal dysplasia
   E. Neurofibromatosis (colonic neurofibromas)
   F. Myotonia/muscular dystrophy
   G. Infantile botulism
   H. Chagas disease
IV. Endocrine/Metabolism
   A. Dehydration
      1. Fever
      2. Heat
      3. Poor oral intake
   B. Diabetes
      1. Neuropathy
      2. Dehydration
   C. Hypercalcemia
   D. Hypokalemia
   E. Lead poisoning
   F. Hypothyroidism
V. Drugs
   A. Opiates
   B. Diuretics
   C. Anticholinergics
   D. Antihistamines
   E. Phenothiazines
   F. Antacids
   G. Chemotherapy (vincristine)
VI. Psychogenic (voluntary)
   A. Encopresis
   B. Sexual abuse
   C. Pain
   D. Depression
   E. Parental conflict

should note presence of an anal fissure, tone, and whether or not there is a "shelf" (anteriorly-displaced anus) or "sleeve" (Hirschsprung disease). In the well-appearing infant with a history of infrequent, nonbloody, formed stools who is not surgically obstructed, an extensive evaluation (i.e., radiologic and manometric studies) can be reserved until symptoms are recurrent or nonresponsive to therapy. If an obstruction is suspected, the evaluation starts with an abdominal radiograph and proceeds with contrast studies or ultrasonography.

Treatment. Therapy in infants for whom there is significant discomfort in passing a bowel movement should start with the addition of Karo syrup or other mild stool-softeners to the diet. The parents of infants who have infrequent stools should be reassured that their baby is normal; rectal manipulation to increase the frequency of stools should be discouraged. It is important to avoid laying the groundwork for future behavioral problems surrounding bowel movements. In the emergency department an important intervention is to refer such problems back to the family physician.

Older Children. Constipation in the older child presents a far more difficult problem because of the high frequency of functional problems and children who are chronically constipated; however, surgical problems can occur in these children, too. Constipation is seen frequently in neurologically disabled children either because of a primary neurologic deficit (spina bifida, muscular dystrophy) or secondary problems related to lack of coordination of defecation (cerebral palsy, mental retardation). In children with recent viral illness, poor appetite and dehydration may cause acute, uncomplicated "constipation." Chronically ill children may be predisposed to constipation, particularly children who are receiving chemotherapy or those with metabolic disorders. Children receiving over-the-counter cold medications may get enough anticholinergic medication to cause constipation (see box above).

The possibility of sexual abuse is also a consideration. In a series of children who were sexually abused, 17% had initial complaints not related to the abuse, and of these 9% had constipation and rectal bleeding.[29]

History and Physical. The child with a complaint of constipation may initially give only a history of abdominal

TABLE 52-5. Treatment of Constipation*

Method	Amount	Advantage	Disadvantage	Onset
Enema				
Fleet	2.5 oz	Rapid, direct	Rectal irritation	Immediate
Normal saline	150 ml		Na^+ changes	
Bulk-forming laxatives				
Bran	0.5-1 tsp	Increases bulk, softness	Delayed onset	1-3 days
Psyllium (Metamucil)		Shortens transit time		
Osmotic laxatives				
Sorbitol	1 tsp-2 tbsp	Shortens transit time	Possible fluid/electrolyte shifts	1-3 hours
Lactulose			Avoid Mg^{++} salts in renal failure	
Mg^{++} phos salts (Milk of Magnesia)				
Polyethylene glycol (Golytely)	150 ml/kg	Immediate effect; useful for neurologically impaired patients	May require NG tube and admission	Immediate
Irritant laxatives				
Bisacodyl (Dulcolax)	5-10 mg	Increases mucosal secretion; can be used with bulk-forming laxatives	Abdominal cramping	6-8 hours
Senna (Senokot)	0.5-1 tsp			
Cascara	2-8 ml		Melanosis coli	
Lubricant laxatives				
Mineral oil	1-2 tbsp		May absorb fat-soluble vitamins; slight risk of aspiration pneumonitis	1-3 days

*1 tsp = 5 ml; 1 tbsp = 15 ml.

pain. The initial evaluation then must be directed to the presence of fever, vomiting, onset of pain, and characteristics of the pain. If the diagnosis of chronic constipation is suggested by lack of fever and vomiting, obtain a history for frequency, duration, and character of stools. Stools passed every 2 or 3 days or less; large, hard stools that may block a toilet occurring on a weekly basis, alternating with more frequent small soft or pebbly stools; and soiling episodes with a prior history of such events all suggest chronic constipation. Even if such a diagnosis is suspected, an acute, surgical condition must be ruled out if there is a history of progressive pain, fever, or vomiting because the two can occur together. If the child does not have a history of chronic symptoms, it is important to obtain a history of prior surgery or evaluations of the GI tract, recent viral symptoms, nonprescription medication, or narcotics for pain.

The physical examination usually is not helpful if the patient has chronic or acute constipation. A palpable abdominal mass is occasionally present; it is usually soft, mobile and nontender or minimally tender without guarding or rebound tenderness, and located in the left lower quadrant or suprapubic area. If the abdomen is distended or tympanitic, a small or large bowel obstruction should be suspected, and a surgeon consulted. A rectal examination should look for fissures, tone, masses, and occult blood. The absence of a rectal mass does not rule out constipation as the child may have evacuated a small amount of stool from the rectal vault; however, a large amount of rock-hard stool

(positive "scraped knuckle" sign) is evidence of longstanding constipation.

Work-up. If the child is suspected of having chronic or uncomplicated acute constipation, an abdominal radiograph may be obtained. However, when history and physical examination are considered with chronic constipation, radiographic evaluation rarely adds useful diagnostic information and may be omitted. A large amount of stool or gas in the colon corresponds with but does not prove the diagnosis. A normal abdominal radiograph rules out longstanding constipation. Further radiologic diagnosis is not necessary.

Therapeutic Trial. Management of the acutely constipated child is generally easier than treatment of chronic constipation. Improving oral hydration and softening stool orally is generally sufficient, and treatment should almost never require enemas or suppositories. Once the acute episode has been resolved, the child's natural toilet training and diet should allow a return to normal stooling. In the chronically constipated child, there are three separate steps that must be taken, all of which can be discussed in the emergency department, but must be followed through by the primary physician: cleanout, maintenance, and behavior modification (Table 52-5).

Cleanout can be accomplished "from above and below" and should be limited to 10 to 14 days. Use of once-a-day enemas, suppositories, and laxatives can be given as a 3-day cycle during which time the patient or parent should keep a record of how much stool is produced per intervention to monitor progress of the cleanout. *Maintenance* begins after the cleanout period ends, and involves keeping the stool soft and the child defecating on a regular basis. This is done with stool softeners or laxatives, which are gradually withdrawn.

Behavior modification occurs during both phases. A reward system that motivates the child to comply with treatment is implemented. During this time the threshold volume (TV) and critical volume (CV) are returning to normal, so that at the end of the cleanout period, the child is able to sense a smaller and more normal bolus of stool. Also the child can be taught to relax the external anal sphincter (EAS) normally during defecation by sitting on the toilet at regular intervals after meals in order to take advantage of the gastrocolic reflex. Although diet changes are not strictly a form of behavior modification, encouraging a higher intake of fiber promotes the easier passage of stools. The emergency department physician should establish at the beginning of treatment that behavior modification is a long process, and that frequent, regular visits to the primary physician will be needed. Success depends on a variety of factors, such as frequency of soiling episodes, severity of the constipation, and particularly the absence of a paradoxical EAS contraction during defecation.[30]

Criteria for admission are difficult to quantify; the severely constipated child who is experiencing severe and frequent abdominal pain or the neurologically impaired child who may be difficult to clean out may need to be admitted for polyethylene glycol (Golytely) treatment. The outcome of chronic constipation is variable. Follow-up studies of 3 to 12 years have shown that chronic constipation persists in a large number of children; follow-up remains an important mainstay of treatment. Complications are exceedingly rare but may occur as urinary retention,[31] respiratory distress due to pressure on the diaphragm,[32] or even aspiration pneumonia with shock during treatment with mineral oil.[33]

DIARRHEA

DOUGLAS A. BOENNING

Diarrhea is an increased number of watery loose stools per day. This definition must take into account the tremendous age-related range for normal. The young infant often stools after each feeding; up to 24 stools per day may be normal in the newborn. Gastroenteritis implies both vomiting and diarrhea but is often used interchangeably with acute diarrhea alone. Dysentery is a febrile illness characterized by bloody, mucousy stools associated with abdominal pain and tenesmus.

Diarrhea is the leading cause of childhood morbidity and mortality worldwide. In developing nations, dehydrating diarrhea is often fatal in children less than 2 years of age, particularly when superimposed upon malnutrition. Global estimates are that 4 to 10 million children die annually as a result of diarrheal disease. In the United States, diarrhea is a leading cause of hospital admission in the first years of life, responsible for over 210,000 hospitalizations per year. The millions of diarrhea episodes that children experience are a frequent reason for seeking care in an emergency facility.[34]

Pathophysiology

In the normal preschool-age child, approximately 5 L of fluid pass into the upper small intestine each day, of which 1 L originates from ingested material and 4 L represents endogenous secretion. Most of this fluid (85% to 90%) is absorbed before reaching the large intestine where again approximately 90% of water is absorbed; this leaves about 100 ml of water that comprises normal stool volume (see Chapter 15).

There are three major mechanisms that contribute to the production of diarrhea in children. These mechanisms of disease are linked and may overlap in the individual child. The first is *osmotic slowing of water absorption*. When movement of water into the gut lumen exceeds its absorptive capacity, watery diarrhea results. This state can result from overloading the gut with compounds like sorbitol or from malabsorption of ingested substances such as carbohydrates. Unabsorbed carbohydrates undergo fermentation to organic acids, further increasing the osmotic load and eventual water content in the gut lumen. The second mechanism of diarrhea involves *transit disorders*. A hypomotile bowel allows for bacterial overgrowth in the small intestine leading to absorptive defects. Conversely, a hypermotile bowel resulting from an acute infection, laxatives, thyrotoxicosis, or secreting tumor increases the transit time and sends more unabsorbed fluid into the colon. *Impaired electrolyte and water transport* is the third major mechanism of diarrhea in children. This impairment results from direct mucosal injury or effects of intraluminal compounds and bacterial toxins. Direct mucosal injury typically occurs with viral infections such as rotavirus and Norwalk virus. Mucosal cells of the small intestinal villi are lysed, causing the villi to shorten and effectively decrease the total surface area available for absorption in the intestine. Intraluminal or circulating factors that impair water and electrolyte transport include deconjugated bile salts secondary to bacterial overgrowth of the small bowel and hydroxylated acids produced by the action of colonic flora on unabsorbed fats. Some secreting tumors such as neuroblastoma produce humoral agents that stimulate electrolyte and water secretion. Toxins from enteropathogens stimulate fluid secretion from mucosalcrypt cells in the small intestine and may also block the absorption of electrolytes and water by the villus cells. Infectious causes of secretory diarrhea with toxin production include species of *Vibrio* and *E. coli.*[34-36]

Differential Considerations

Most children with diarrhea will have an acute self-limited episode secondary to a primary infection of the gastrointestinal tract or as an associated symptom of another illness—the "parenteral" diarrhea that accompanies such illnesses as urinary tract infections or otitis media. The most common agents of acute gastroenteritis in the United States are viral (specifically, rotavirus, Norwalk virus, enteric adenovirus, astrovirus, and calicivirus). These viruses predominate in the winter months in contrast to bacterial agents that predominate in the summer and fall months. The most prevalent bacterial pathogens are species of *Campylobacter, Shigella, Salmonella,* and *Yersinia.* Bacterial gastroenteritis is more likely to occur in children

TABLE 52-6. Common Diagnostic Considerations: Diarrhea

Sick	Not sick
Acute onset	
Fever common, ± vomiting/ dehydration	*Usually afebrile, hydrated*
Acute infectious gastroen- teritis	Transient malabsorption
Viral (rotavirus, Norwalk	High fat intake
virus, enteric adenovirus)	Food intolerance/adverse
Bacteria or toxin (*Campylo-	reaction to food
bacter, Shigella, Salmonella,*	Protozoal gastroenteritis
Staphylococcus toxin)	(*Giardia, Entamoeba,*
"Parenteral" diarrhea (sec-	*Cryptosporidium*)
ondary to otitis, UTI)	Psychogenic—anxiety/stress
Medication related	
Antibiotic-associated diar-	
rhea	
Pseudomembranous colitis	
Chronic course	
Failing to thrive, ± dehydra- tion	*Thriving, afebrile, hydrated*
Postinfectious diarrhea	Age-specific variant of normal
Starvation stools (pro-	Breast-feeding stools (0-2
longed liquid diet)	mo old infant)
Lactose intolerance posten-	Chronic nonspecific diar-
teritis	rhea of infancy/childhood
Inflammatory bowel disease	(up to age 3 yr)
Hirschsprung disease	Medication related
Chronic malabsorption	Laxative abuse in adoles-
Protein (celiac disease)	cents
Fat (cystic fibrosis, pancre-	Sorbitol content of cough
atic diseases)	syrups/bronchodilators
Carbohydrates (acquired	Encopresis—overflow in-
lactase deficiency)	continence
Protozoal diarrhea (also cause	
of acute process)	

with a history of blood in the stool in combination with either a fever over 38° C or at least 10 stools in the previous 24 hours.

Protozoal agents are present year-round and seem to have become more common over the last decade with the rise in daycare center attendance. Common protozoal agents are *G. lamblia, E. histolytica,* and *Cryptosporidium.* In all of these cases, the major question facing the emergency physician is whether the child can be managed as an outpatient or requires admission to the hospital. The clinician must also distinguish *acute* from *chronic* causes of diarrhea; the latter are defined as loose stools lasting for more than 2 weeks (Table 52-6).[34,37]

Diagnostic Work-Up

Ascertain the normal diet of the child and how intake and output has varied in the previous 24 to 48 hours. Determine the usual stool and urine output of the child and how that has changed during the illness. Is the illness characterized by fever or vomiting? Historical points that suggest dehydration include dry diapers (reduced urine volume and frequency), minimal intake of fluids, weight loss, and lethargy. Has the caretaker noted blood or mucus in the stool? What home remedies, including fluids and medications, have been used? Inquire about the child's past hospitalizations or chronic medical problems, if any. Additional points in the history should include source of drinking water, recent travel, and ill contacts at home or daycare center.

A complete physical examination should be conducted, with particular attention to signs that indicate dehydration. For clinical assessment, dehydration is characterized as mild, moderate, or severe—corresponding to approximately <5%, 5% to 10%, and ≥15% dehydration, respectively. The precise percentage of dehydration can be calculated by comparing current weight to a recent preillness weight. The mildly dehydrated child has slightly dry, tacky mucous membranes, dry skin without loss of turgor, and a normal fontanelle in the young child. The moderately dehydrated child exhibits dry mucous membranes, decreased skin turgor, a sunken anterior fontanelle, sunken eyes, and some lethargy. The severely dehydrated child appears quite ill, with parched mucous membranes, decreased skin turgor with tenting of the skin, sunken anterior fontanelle in the young child, sunken eyes, and absent tears. Mental status is abnormal with all or some of the following: lethargy, unresponsiveness to verbal stimuli, or decreased responsiveness to pain. Signs of shock include tachycardia with weak distal pulses and delayed capillary refill (>2 seconds)[39] (see Chapters 13 and 15).

Ancillary Data. Laboratory data are obtained based on the severity of the dehydration and chronicity of the diarrhea. In acute diarrhea with mild dehydration, no laboratory tests may be necessary. Any child who is moderately or severely dehydrated requires laboratory investigation including, at a minimum, electrolytes, BUN, and CBC with differential. The severely dehydrated child also requires the determination of an arterial or venous pH, blood glucose, and a complete evaluation for sepsis, including cultures of blood, urine, and CSF in the febrile child under 2 years of age.

The presence of bloody diarrhea necessitates a stool culture. Cultures are useful in determining the bacterial etiology of an acute diarrheal illness, but should be reserved for those patients in whom the results will have a therapeutic or epidemiologic impact. Rectal swabs handled expeditiously provide a good culture source if stool is unavailable. Cultures should be routinely done in children under 1 year of age who are febrile or toxic on arrival with diarrhea and who have polymorphonuclear (PMN) leukocytes in their stool. Cultures are also important if multiple members of the same family are ill, if any member of the family is a food handler, if the patient has recently traveled, or if symptomatic children are immunosuppressed or have a hemoglobinopathy. Children with diarrhea who are enrolled in daycare centers usually merit a stool culture in light of their infectious potential for other children.

Methylene blue smears for PMN leukocytes are particularly useful in excluding a number of bacterial causes; bacterial gastroenteritis is commonly associated with the presence of PMN cells in the smear. Over 90% of diarrhea resulting from *Salmonella* or *Shigella* organisms has PMN leukocytes in the stool. Fecal leukocytes are often found in patients with *Campylobacter* organisms, *Y. enterocolitica*, invasive *E. coli*, and *V. parahaemolyticus*.[40]

To perform this study, a small amount of mucus is placed on a clear glass slide and mixed with two drops of methylene blue. A cover glass is placed on the slide and nuclear staining occurs over 2 minutes. Microscopic examination for PMN leukocytes is performed and is considered positive if there are more than 5 WBC per high powered field (HPF).

During endemic periods, stool can be sent for rapid enzyme-linked immunosorbent assays for rotavirus and other infectious agents.

The CBC may be helpful. When the ratio of band forms over total neutrophils (segmented plus bands) is >0.10, *Shigella*, *Salmonella*, or *Campylobacter* organisms should be suspected. The WBC is usually <10,000 WBC/mm³, with a marked shift to the left in patients with *Shigella* infection. In *Salmonella* infection (except typhoid fever), the WBC is increased with a mild shift to the left. A high WBC count may also be found in patients with *Campylobacter* and *Yersinia*.

Prehospital Considerations

Paramedics should exercise enteric precautions, washing their hands after transporting a child with diarrhea. All severely dehydrated and some moderately dehydrated children require prompt IV access and fluid resuscitation with normal saline. This maneuver should be started before reaching the emergency department for any child who appears sick enough to require hospital admission.

Therapeutic Trial

Regardless of the etiology, a child with acute diarrhea and dehydration requires fluid and electrolyte replacement. The patient with chronic diarrhea who is not dehydrated needs further work-up on a scheduled basis from a primary care provider or gastroenterologist. The acute management should be based on the degree of dehydration present. The mildly dehydrated child may be managed with oral fluid therapy alone with a commercial electrolyte solution. The moderately dehydrated child with 5% to 10% weight loss also may be treated with oral rehydration therapy. That child should demonstrate adequate interest in drinking and the ability to consume and retain an electrolyte-containing solution in the emergency department.[41] The moderately dehydrated child who either refuses to drink or is unable to retain fluids will require IV rehydration. Severely dehydrated children require IV or intraosseous fluid resuscitation. Normal saline boluses of 20 ml/kg body weight should be given every 30 minutes until spontaneous urine output is established. Many severely dehydrated children will require up to 60 to 100 ml/kg fluid replacement for the first phase of rehydration. Following stabilization and rehydration, dextrose-containing IV fluids should be continued with lesser sodium concentrations and oral rehydration therapy may be started under the supervision of health-care providers. The severely dehydrated child requires hospital admission. Remember to avoid using potassium in any IV solution until it is clear that the child is not experiencing acute or chronic renal failure.

DYSPHAGIA

JOSEPH L. WRIGHT

Swallowing represents a complex series of neuromuscular events. Dysphagia, or difficulty in swallowing, is defined as any defect in the transport of food or endogenous secretions to the stomach. A systematic approach to the child with dysfunctional swallowing includes an awareness of the normal physiology of deglutition.

Pathophysiology

The act of deglutition proceeds through three distinct stages: the oral, pharyngeal, and esophageal stages. Dysfunction during any of these stages can result in dysphagia.

Oral Stage. The manipulation of food within the oral cavity is mediated by the fifth, seventh, ninth, tenth, and twelfth cranial nerves and is dependent on the anatomic integrity of intraoral structures. Hence, any abnormality of the lips, palate, or tongue can produce a poor suck. Additionally, global neurologic deficits from central nervous system hypoxic insults or specific bulbar palsies can result in failure to propel food into the pharynx.

Pharyngeal Stage. Entry of food into the pharynx stimulates a rapid sequence of reflex actions that are designed primarily to protect the airway. The glossal, soft palatal, and pharyngeal mucosa are rich with afferent nerve fibers essential to the coordination of these actions. This renders the pharyngeal stage particularly vulnerable to conditions that affect sensory receptors, such as acute infections or inappropriate use of topical anesthetizing agents. Problems during this stage can lead to aspiration and pneumonia, the most serious potential consequence of dysfunctional swallowing.

Esophageal Stage. The esophageal stage is initiated by relaxation of the cricopharyngeus muscle, or upper esophageal sphincter (UES), and is partially governed by vagus nerve innervation. Peristalsis through the lower two thirds of the esophagus is achieved by the autonomic action of the myenteric nerve plexus. Problems here may occur secondary to incoordination of the intrinsic esophageal musculature (achalasia) or from extrinsic pressure.[42-46]

Etiology

The causes of dysfunctional swallowing in children are myriad and diverse. Potential etiologic disorders cross broad physiologic and anatomic boundaries. For the emergency physician, the differential diagnosis is best categorized in terms of the three functional stages of deglutition. The history and physical examination can then be directed at each of the stages in a sequential fashion. Conditions that include dysphagia as part of a global neurologic or systemic process are considered separately[47-50] (see box on p. 810).

Diagnostic Work-Up

In the young child, signs and symptoms of dysphagia can be elusive. Such a patient is unlikely to actually complain

---

Conditions Associated with Dysphagia

Oral stage

A. Anatomic/congenital
 1. Choanal atresia (nasal obstruction)
 2. Cleft lip/cleft palate
 3. Craniofacial syndromes with micrognathia
  a. Pierre-Robin
  b. Treacher-Collins
  c. Crouzon
  d. Goldenhar
 4. Macroglossia
B. Constitutional
 1. Normal variation
 2. Prematurity
 3. Hypoxic-ischemic CNS injury
C. Infections
 1. Oral thrush
 2. Gingivostomatitis
D. Acquired
 1. Mucosal scald injury (e.g., microwave-heated infant formula)
 2. Trauma
  a. Temporomandibular joint dislocation
  b. Mandibular fracture

Pharyngeal stage

A. Infections
 1. Febrile dysphagia
  a. Epiglottitis
  b. Tonsillopharyngitis
  c. Peritonsillar abscess
  d. Retropharyngeal abscess
 2. Miscellaneous
  a. Botulism
  b. Poliomyelitis
  c. Diphtheria
B. Anatomic
 1. Pharyngeal diverticulum
 2. Laryngeal cyst
C. Acquired
 1. Trauma
  a. Instrumentation
  b. Impalement injury (e.g., from pencil in mouth)
 2. Foreign body
 3. Topical anesthesia
  a. Over-the-counter teething preparations (benzocaine 7.5%)
  b. Viscous lidocaine 2%
 4. Extrapyramidal effects of antipsychotic medications
  a. Dystonic reaction
  b. Neuroleptic malignant syndrome

Esophageal stage

A. Anatomic/obstructive
 1. Intrinsic
  a. Tracheoesophageal fistula/esophageal atresia
  b. Esophageal diverticulum
  c. Esophageal duplication
  d. Esophageal web
 2. Extrinsic
  a. Vascular ring (e.g., double aortic arch)
  b. Mediastinal mass
  c. Diaphragmatic hernia
  d. Thyroiditis
  e. Cystic hygroma
  f. Neoplasm
B. Acquired
 1. Stricture caused by corrosive ingestion
 2. Foreign body
 3. Trauma
  a. Instrumentation
  b. Blunt (i.e., esophageal disruption)
C. Disordered motility
 1. Gastroesophageal reflux
 2. Achalasia
 3. Cricopharyngeal incoordination
D. Inflammatory bowel disease
 1. Crohn disease
 2. Ulcerative colitis
E. Infections
 1. Candidiasis (immunocompromised host)
 2. Chronic trypanosomiasis (Chagas disease)
F. Psychogenic—globus hystericus

Neuromuscular diseases and syndromes

A. Myotonic muscular dystrophy
B. Werdnig-Hoffman syndrome (spinal muscular atrophy)
C. Myasthenia gravis
D. Mobius syndrome
E. Riley-Day syndrome (familial dysautonomia)
F. Prader-Willi syndrome

Systemic diseases with prominent esophageal involvement

A. Collagen-vascular
 1. Scleroderma
 2. Dermatomyositis/polymyositis
 3. Sjögren syndrome
 4. Mixed connective tissue disease
B. Postinfectious—Guillain-Barré syndrome
C. Miscellaneous
 1. Angioneurotic edema
 2. Stevens-Johnson syndrome

---

of odynophagia (painful swallowing), and symptoms often masquerade as upper respiratory problems. Therefore, a detailed history and thorough physical examination, including observation of the feeding pattern, are paramount to the evaluation. Imaging and endoscopic studies may be definitive but are not always immediately available in the acute care setting.

The history must include details of the prenatal course and a review of the family and developmental histories. The pregnancy may reveal evidence of maternal infections, bleeding, toxemia, drug or medication use.[51] Antihypertensives are known to cross the placenta and cause nasal obstruction in the neonate. First trimester exposure to diazepam is associated with cleft lip and palate. Polyhydramnios frequently occurs from oral, pharyngeal, or esophageal dysfunction. Details of the labor and delivery may reveal prolonged hypoxia or the need for resuscitation; direct laryngoscopy, deep suction, nasogastric tube placement, and endotracheal intubation can all damage the delicate aerodigestive anatomy. Prematurity predisposes the infant to early feeding fatigue with poor suck and swallow coordination. Human immunodeficiency virus exposure raises the possibility of opportunistic infection and odynophagia related to herpetic gingivostomatitis, mucocutaneous candidiasis, or cytomegalovirus esophagitis.

Family history of neurologic disease such as myotonic dystrophy, or anatomic problems like cleft palate can alert the physician to the possibility of similar conditions in the infant. Developmental history should focus on the presence or absence of primitive reflexes and the attainment of early milestones, looking for evidence of retardation.

History of the present illness should ascertain whether symptoms are acute or chronic, intermittent or constant. For example, sudden onset of dysphagia suggests a recent foreign body ingestion, whereas more indolent symptoms might represent stricture development from an unsuspected corrosive substance ingestion or reflux esophagitis. Obstructive symptoms of a progressive nature could occur from an impinging mediastinal mass or tumor. For this reason, it is important to document dietary tolerance with particular attention to any transition from solid to liquid food preference. In addition, the nature of associated upper respiratory symptoms, such as cough or stridor, ought to be characterized as to onset and temporal relationship to food intake.[52]

Finally, a history of trauma should be elicited. A blow to the chin can produce an occult mandibular fracture or dislocation producing acute dysphagia. Children undergoing repair of a chin laceration should be carefully examined for signs of mandibular injury.[53,54] Esophageal disruption from blunt trauma is a rare but lethal injury if unrecognized. A linear tear in the ampulla region is caused by forceful injection of gastric contents into the esophagus from a severe abdominal blow. Such an injury should be suspected if there is severe odynophagia and mediastinal air on chest radiograph. Potential complications are mediastinitis and pleural empyema. Primary surgical repair is the definitive therapy.

Assessment of airway patency must be the task first undertaken on physical examination. Any child with fever, drooling, and air hunger must be considered to have a threatened airway until proven otherwise. Invasive examination and excessive manipulation should be deferred until the airway has been appropriately secured. Other than in such a scenario, the examination is best conducted in an oral, pharyngeal, esophageal progression that includes observation of the feeding pattern.

Plotting of the growth parameters and an assessment of the child's nutritional status may yield clues about the chronicity of symptoms. The facies should be scrutinized for craniofacial or mandibulofacial disproportion, misshapen or low set ears, and micrognathia. Intraoral inspection should reveal any obvious cleft lip or palate defects, but the examiner must also palpate the soft palate to exclude a submucosal cleft. Patency of the choanae can be ascertained by passage of a catheter through each naris into the nasopharynx. This is important because infants, as obligate nose breathers, are unable to feed and breathe effectively when nasal obstruction is present. Finally, the tongue should be observed for fasciculations characteristic of spinal muscular atrophy (Werdnig-Hoffman syndrome).

Upon visualization of the pharynx, the examiner should note the symmetry and anatomic integrity of the pharyngeal vault, as well as any inflamed, infected, or denuded mucosa. Voice quality and the presence or absence of a gag reflex should be checked. Reflex sensation in this area can be blunted by overzealous use of topical anesthetics, like the teething agent benzocaine 7.5% (Ora-Jel, Anbesol).

The esophageal phase is best evaluated during actual observation of deglutition. Both liquid and solid matter should be swallowed and attention given to the precise point at which pain, gasping, gagging, or vomiting occurs. For instance, a patient with a tracheoesophageal fistula may begin coughing and choking after only a few seconds of feeding, whereas an obstructive lesion like an esophageal web does not manifest symptoms until overflow of the proximal esophagus occurs. In the infant, coordination of the suck, swallow, and breathe sequence should be observed to look for nasal regurgitation or stridor, which are signs of cricopharyngeal incoordination. Such a patient is at increased risk for aspiration and requires expedient therapeutic intervention.

The necessity of a complete neurologic examination with special attention to the cranial nerves cannot be overemphasized. The infant with underlying neurologic problems usually demonstrates a decreased level of alertness and can exhibit generalized hypotonia, as with the Prader-Willi syndrome.

Ancillary Data. Plain radiographs sometimes are helpful in the diagnostic evaluation of dysphagia. Lateral airway films may reveal obstructive lesions or foreign bodies, whereas chest radiograph may show evidence of aspiration. Contrast study, however, is the technique of choice for defining specific lesions in the aerodigestive tract. Esophagogram and cine-esophagogram should be performed with introduction of the radiopaque medium at the most proximal point possible. Nipple or intranasal instillation of contrast allows for study of both anatomy and function. Computed tomography (CT) and magnetic resonance imaging (MRI) can be useful for lesions that are difficult to define.[55,56]

Endoscopic procedures, including laryngoscopy, bronchoscopy, and esophagoscopy, can be both diagnostic and therapeutic, but in most instances ought to be performed by the subspecialist in an operating room or endoscopy suite.

Therapeutic Trial

The child with sudden onset of dysphagia is likely to have ingested a foreign body or be suffering from an acute infectious process. The goal of prehospital management, regardless of etiology, is maintenance of airway patency.

This is best achieved by allowing the child to assume a position of comfort and delivering 100% oxygen in a non-threatening manner, preferably via a parent or caretaker.

Treatment is directed at correction of the underlying cause and often requires a multidisciplinary team approach. In the emergency department, the immediate goals of therapy are to minimize the risk of aspiration and ensure airway patency. Appropriate positioning and nasogastric suction are generally sufficient, but in extreme instances endotracheal intubation may be required. Foreign bodies and some intrinsic esophageal lesions are amenable to endoscopic repair but the majority of obstructive lesions require surgical intervention. Most of the conditions associated with disordered esophageal motility are successfully managed conservatively with tube feedings and high-calorie, high-density formulas. More severely affected children may require hyperalimentation and gastrostomy tube placement.

When counseling new parents in the emergency department or primary care setting, it is important to provide anticipatory information about normal physiologic variation in the development of the swallowing mechanism. Periodic sputtering, disorganized sucking, and regurgitation without cyanosis are acceptable in the neonate. Reassurance, anticipatory guidance, and expectant management with close follow-up should be provided in this situation. However, when dysphagia occurs in malnourished or immunocompromised patients, or in association with cyanosis, dyspnea, pain or fever, hospital admission is warranted.[57]

GASTROINTESTINAL BLEEDING

DANIEL W. OCHSENSCHLAGER

The causes of bleeding from the gastrointestinal tract in children are almost limitless; the more common etiologies will be the focus here. GI bleeding may be manifested by vomiting (hematemesis) or rectal bleeding (melena).

Pathophysiology

Lesions proximal to the ligament of Treitz will usually result in nasogastric aspirates that are positive for blood. Bright red hematemesis indicates that there is little or no contact with gastric juices; it results from an active bleeding site at or above the cardia. In children it is usually caused by varices or esophagitis. Occasionally, brisk duodenal or gastric bleeding may be bright red. Coffee-ground aspirates indicate that there has been an alteration of blood by gastric acid.

Rectal bleeding reflects the amount and site of blood loss. Hemorrhage proximal to the ileocecal valve produces black, tarry stools caused by alteration of blood by intestinal enzymes (melena). Gross blood is generally associated with lower intestinal bleeding; rapid-transit upper GI hemorrhage may cause similar appearing stools (hematochezia).

Hemoptysis must be differentiated from hematemesis, the former usually appearing with a red, frothy material mixed with sputum.[58]

Differential Considerations

Massive uncontrolled bleeding is rare and usually stops early in the course of disease. In fact, most GI bleeding is

TABLE 52-7. Causes of Upper and Lower Gastrointestinal Bleeding by Age

Age	Upper GI	Lower GI
0–1 month	Idiopathic	Anal fissure
	Gastritis	Upper gastrointestinal bleeding
	Stress ulcers	
	Esophagitis	Volvulus
	Swallowed maternal blood	Necrotizing enterocolitis
	Congenital blood dyscrasia	Swallowed maternal blood
	Vascular malformation	Infectious colitis
		Milk allergy
		Blood dyscrasia
		Duplication
1 month–1 year	Gastritis	Anal fissure
	Esophagitis	Intussusception
	Stress ulcer	Meckel's diverticulum
	Mallory-Weiss tear	
	Vascular malformation	Infectious diarrhea
		Milk allergy
	Duplication	Duplication
		Pseudomembranous colitis
1 year–12 years	Esophageal varices	Polyps
	Peptic ulcer disease	Anal fissure
	Stress ulcer	Meckel's diverticulum
	Gastritis	
	Mallory-Weiss tear	Infectious diarrhea
	Foreign body	HSP
	Esophagitis	HUS
		Intussusception
		Pseudomembranous colitis
Adolescent	Esophageal varices	Polyps
	Peptic ulcer disease	Hemorrhoids
	Gastritis	Inflammatory bowel disease
	Mallory-Weiss tear	
	Esophagitis	Infectious diarrhea
	Stress ulcer	

minor in nature and is often mucosal bleeding from vomiting or irritation. Therefore, making the precise diagnosis in the emergency department is generally unnecessary. Emergency surgery is rarely indicated unless there is evidence of bowel ischemia (e.g., volvulus, nonreducible intussusception) or massive bleeding. Diagnostic evaluation should proceed in a logical and orderly progression based upon the clinical presentation. The location of bleeding can be determined in about 95% of patients. Radiologic techniques have been largely supplanted by newer endoscopic procedures.

Unlike adults, children seldom have a malignancy as a cause of bleeding. The most common causes of gastrointestinal bleeding in the pediatric age group tend to be age-specific[59] (Table 52-7).

Neonate (Birth to 1 Month). The most common cause of upper GI bleeding during the first month of life is idiopathic (i.e., no specific source can be identified). This bleeding typically occurs within the first 48 hours of life, and although the blood loss may be significant, it tends to stop spontaneously within 24 hours. Other causes include gastritis, esophagitis, and peptic ulcer disease. Ulcers in neonates are commonly stress related secondary to sepsis, intracranial pathology, or heart disease. Primary ulcers are distinctly uncommon in neonates.

Swallowed maternal blood either at delivery or from bleeding nipples also can occur as hematemesis. Maternal adult hemoglobin can be differentiated from fetal hemoglobin by the Apt test. Fetal hemoglobin resists alkaline reduction whereas adult hemoglobin becomes brown when mixed with alkali. It is important that only red blood and not partially denatured blood (i.e., melena or coffee-ground material) be used because denatured hemoglobin has already been reduced to hematin and will falsely look like "adult" hemoglobin when tested.

Congenital bleeding disorders can occur in the neonatal period. It is important to ask about family history and look for bleeding from other sites such as circumcisions and venipunctures. Abnormal coagulation studies are diagnostic. Vitamin K deficiency can result from failure to administer it at birth or from compromised fetal production secondary to transplacental passage of maternal drugs such as phenytoin or promethazine. Vitamin K (1 mg IM) should be given if a vitamin K deficiency is suspected and should be repeated daily for 5 days.

Lower GI bleeding in the neonatal period is most frequently caused by a benign anal or rectal lesions such as fissures or local trauma. Necrotizing enterocolitis is relatively common in the premature infant but can also occur in the full-term child up to 1 month of age with birth asphyxia or cyanotic congenital heart disease. Necrotizing enterocolitis begins with abdominal distension, bilious vomiting, and lower gastrointestinal bleeding. Abdominal radiographs are helpful when they demonstrate pneumatosis intestinalis. Most of these patients can be treated medically with hospitalization, bowel rest, IV antibiotics, and hyperalimentation, but surgery is indicated for cases of suspected or definite perforation.

The true surgical emergency in this age group is midgut volvulus, which occurs as abdominal pain, bilious vomiting, and melena (see volvulus).

Infant (30 Days to 1 Yr). Upper GI bleeding in infancy is most commonly caused by esophagitis, gastritis, or peptic ulcer. Anorectal lesions remain the most frequent source of lower GI bleeding, but there are other common causes.

Infectious diarrhea can produce bright red blood in the stool. Although many bacteria have been associated with hematochezia, species of *Campylobacter, Salmonella, Shigella,* and *Yersinia* are the most common. Viral agents causing bloody diarrhea include rotavirus and Norwalk virus.

Milk allergy is rare but does exist and can be associated with GI bleeding. Changing the formula results in a cessation of symptoms; a subsequent challenge feeding of cow's milk reproduces the symptoms.[60]

Intussusception is most frequently diagnosed in this age group. Presenting symptoms include intermittent abdomi-

nal pain, vomiting, and sometimes lethargy. Stools are usually positive for blood and can look like currant jelly (see section on Intussusception).

Few immunocompromised infants have presented with gastrointestinal bleeding. However, the number of pediatric AIDS patients is increasing and GI bleeding will be a serious consideration in this group of children. Bleeding is usually secondary to various opportunistic infections that cause lesions anywhere in the GI tract. GI tumors are a much rarer source of bleeding in these patients.

Child (1 to 12 Yrs). Massive hematemesis may be the initial presentation of esophageal varices. Varices are secondary to extrahepatic portal hypertension the majority of the time; intrahepatic obstruction from biliary cirrhosis, Alpha 1 antitrypsin deficiency, hepatitis, and cystic fibrosis are less common. Initial hemorrhage occurs before 8 years of age in 85% of these patients and before 5 years of age in two thirds of this group. On physical examination, other signs of portal hypertension or liver disease can be found: splenomegaly, hepatomegaly, or dilated abdominal veins. The diagnosis is confirmed by endoscopy. Most variceal bleeding will stop spontaneously. Treatment of uncontrolled bleeding is controversial. Some institutions favor IV administration of vasopressin, whereas others prefer emergency endosclerosis, which can be up to 40% effective in controlling the acute hemorrhage. Rarely, balloon tamponade by Sengstaken-Blakemore tube or a related variant is necessary. Serious complications, which include upper airway obstruction and esophageal perforation, can occur with these types of devices in 20% of patients. Maintaining proper position and traction are absolutely necessary and can be best managed by physicians who are familiar with such devices.

Another cause of upper GI bleeding in this age group is drug use. Salicylates, NSAIDs, and anticoagulants are the most common etiologic agents. A careful history of drug usage or unintentional ingestion of warfarin-containing rodenticides is necessary in all children with GI bleeding.

Juvenile polyps are the most frequent cause of lower GI bleeding in children, with a peak incidence at 3 to 7 years of age. These are nonmalignant lesions and in one third of cases there is only a solitary lesion. Up to 75% can be reached by digital examination and 85% are within the reach of the sigmoidoscope. Initial symptoms are intermittent, painless, bright red rectal bleeding. These patients should be referred for further evaluation and polyp removal. It is important to obtain a histologic diagnosis to ensure that the lesion is not premalignant in nature such as adenomatous polyps (familial polyposis coli, Gardner syndrome, Turcot syndrome) or hamartomatous polyps (Peutz-Jeghers syndrome).

Meckel's diverticulum can cause massive blood loss in this age group and is discussed in detail in another section.

Infectious diarrhea is common in this age group. Considerably less common are two syndromes that can cause bloody stools in children. One is Henoch-Schönlein purpura (HSP), anaphylactoid purpura, which is usually diagnosed by its characteristic rash on the lower extremities. However, GI bleeding may be the first sign of this disorder. Bleeding results from the generalized vasculitis or from an associated intussusception. The other syndrome is hemolytic uremic syndrome (HUS). The bleeding is secondary to thrombosis of small vessels and ischemia to the mucosa. Hemolytic anemia, nephritis, and mental status changes are also parts of this disorder.

Adolescent (13 to 19 Yrs). Esophagitis and peptic ulcer disease are the most common sources of upper GI bleeding in this age group. Juvenile polyps and anal fissure are the most common cause of lower GI bleeding. However, it is during adolescence that inflammatory bowel disease usually appears, although it can appear much earlier. This diagnosis is made by contrast radiography or endoscopy. Unless there is obstruction or massive bleeding, which is rare, emergency surgery is not necessary.

Diagnostic Work-Up

The diagnostic evaluation must initially focus on the potential for hemodynamic instability and the site and etiology of the hemorrhage.

The history should assess the onset, progression, character, frequency, and quality of bleeding, as well as the degree of the vomiting, diarrhea, and abdominal pain. A personal or family history of bleeding problems should be noted. History of ingestion of irritants such as aspirin, alcohol, caustic agents, and other toxins may be contributory.

Hemodynamic stability should be assessed on physical examination. Abdominal examination should evaluate masses, bowel sounds, tenderness, rebound, guarding, and rectal disease.

Several questions should be asked during the evaluation:

1. Is the bleeding actually from the GI tract? Epistaxis, bleeding from oral lesions, and hemoptysis can be easily mistaken for hematemesis. Similarly, hematuria, menstrual bleeding, and bleeding caused by urethral prolapse or from perianal skin excoriation may appear as hematochezia.
2. Is the colored material actually blood? Tomato and cranberry juice, red food coloring, and drugs such as amoxicillin and rifampin can look like blood. Ingestion of iron, bismuth, spinach, or dark chocolate can produce a melanotic-like stool. In order to prevent unnecessary and costly evaluation, the suspected material should be tested with one of the rapid chemical screening tests. These tests are usually sensitive (i.e., 1 mg hemoglobin/ml fluid can be detected). Because an acidic pH can diminish the sensitivity of the oxidation-reduction reaction, only the screening test designed for gastric contents should be used to detect blood in stomach contents (Gastroccult). Several substances may decrease the accuracy of these screens: activated charcoal, vitamin C, N-acetylcysteine, rifampin, some antacids, bismuth subsalicylate, and foods such as red chili, pepper, and spaghetti sauce. False positive results may be caused by iodine, supplemental iron, and ingestion of red meat.
3. Where is the source of the bleeding? Hematemesis implies bleeding proximal to the ligament of Treitz, melena implies bleeding proximal to the ileocecal valve or ascending colon, and hematochezia implies bleeding from the descending colon. Bright red blood

on the toilet tissue and only on the outside of the stool suggest that the source of bleeding is in the lower rectum or anus. The color of the stool is related to metabolism of hemoglobin in the GI tract and this rate of conversion is proportional to the amount of time the blood remains in contact with intestinal bacteria and enzymes. Stool transit time varies a great deal in children. Because blood can be a potent cathartic, bleeding from the stomach or duodenum can occur as hematochezia if the transit time is rapid. Similarly, bleeding in the lower colon can occur as melena if the transit time is delayed. A small amount of blood in vomitus or stool is relatively common in acute gastroenteritis.

4. How much blood has been lost? Often this is difficult to determine clinically and the history can be inaccurate. A few milliliters of blood may seem like a huge blood loss to an anxious parent; hypotension only develops after an acute loss of greater than 20% of total blood volume. Chronic blood loss, unless severe, does not result in hypotension. Fortunately, massive blood loss is rare in children.

If significant upper GI bleeding is suspected, aspiration of the stomach through an oral or NG tube should be performed. If the gastric aspirate is positive, the tube should be left in place to monitor blood loss. Lavage with saline (10 ml/kg) until active bleeding stops. Iced saline and other therapeutic agents do not have any advantage over room-temperature saline as an irrigation fluid and may actually exacerbate the bleeding. Unstable patients may require intubation to prevent aspiration during NG lavage. Bleeding from the duodenum may not be detected in the aspirate. Esophageal varices are not a contraindication to placement of an NG tube.

Ancillary Data. Initial laboratory studies should include a CBC, platelet count, PT, PTT, BUN, electrolytes, liver enzymes, and type and crossmatch. It should be noted that a relatively normal hemogram can be seen initially with a large amount of acute blood loss. Frequently it takes several hours for the hematocrit to equilibrate.

Blood can be confirmed by the various screening card tests. Positive results are usually indicated by a blue color. False positives and negatives can occur.

Swallowed maternal blood in the neonate may be identified by performing the Apt test. One part of gastric contents or stool is mixed with five parts of water and centrifuged. Add 0.1 ml of 0.2 N sodium hydroxide to the supernatant fluid. A pink color that develops in 2 to 5 minutes indicates fetal hemoglobin and a brown color signifies adult hemoglobin.

Specific evaluation of the stool should include fecal leukocytes, bacterial culture, and examination for ova and parasites when appropriate.

Endoscopic examination (gastroduodenoscopy for upper GI bleeding and proctosigmoidoscopy for lower GI bleeding) identifies the location of bleeding in about 90% of patients. Radiological studies are usually less helpful than endoscopy but include an upper gastrointestinal tract study or barium enema for specific presentations.[61] Nuclear scans may be helpful, especially for Meckel's diverticulum.

An abdominal AP and upright can be helpful in diagnosing some causes of GI bleeding, especially obstructive lesions, masses, enterocolits, and perforations. However, by no means does a normal abdominal film eliminate a serious etiology.

Prehospital Considerations

Obviously, the hemodynamic stability of the patient should be reflected in resuscitation efforts in the prehospital setting. Intravenous crystalloid fluids and oxygen should be initiated if there is any evidence of abnormal vital signs including orthostatic signs, delayed capillary refill, or significant past or ongoing bleeding.

Therapeutic Trial

If there is evidence of hypovolemia (i.e., anxiety, tachycardia, tachypnea, thready pulses, increased capillary refill time, or hypotension), immediate intervention is necessary. Two large-bore peripheral IV lines should be inserted and 20 ml/kg of 0.9% NS or LR infused rapidly. Additional fluid boluses, warmed if possible, should be given as indicated by frequent reevaluations. An NG tube should be placed in the stomach, and lavage with saline should be performed. Oxygen should be administered. Blood should be administered for massive bleeding or if electrolyte solution boluses are ineffective. Completely crossed packed red cells are preferred. But type O non-crossmatched blood may be utilized if blood is needed immediately.

Unstable patients should be admitted to the Intensive Care Unit and be carefully monitored including central venous pressure. Gastroenterologists and surgeons should be consulted as soon as possible for complicated or unstable patients. An antacid, 1 ml/kg, or cimetidine, 20 to 30 mg/kg/day QID PO, can be administered if gastritis is suspected.

HEPATOSPLENOMEGALY

JAMES M. CHAMBERLAIN

The causes of hepatosplenomegaly are legion and often require a systematic diagnostic approach beyond the scope of the emergency department. Nevertheless, patients may present with hepatomegaly or splenomegaly. As with all illness, the emergency department physician must classify the patient's condition as follows:

1. Immediately life-threatening disorder requiring emergent therapy
2. Illness for which immediate treatment is beneficial
3. Illness that must be referred to another provider for diagnosis or definitive care

Many cases of hepatosplenomegaly in children fall into the last category, representing chronic or subacute illness. This section focuses on the first two categories and addresses only briefly those conditions for which referral is made electively for treatment or more extensive work-up.

The clinician uses the physical examination to screen for enlargement of the liver and spleen; however, this estimation of enlargement may be inaccurate if the distance below the costal margin is used as the sole criterion for enlargement.[62] Ultrasonography is the best method to evaluate liver and spleen volume and may provide useful information as to the cause of enlargement but is impractical for every patient.[63]

Physical examination of the spleen should be done with the patient in the supine and left lateral decubitus positions. Gentle palpation starting from the lower quadrants and moving superiorly is necessary in order to avoid missing a massively enlarged organ. Palpation of a 1 to 2 cm spleen tip is normal in infants, and a 1 cm spleen tip is palpable in 1% of normal children and adolescents and 3% of college freshmen.[64-66] Palpation of a larger spleen or a spleen that is firm or tender is abnormal. Percussion of the spleen with the patient in the right lateral decubitus position is recommended in adults and may be useful in adolescent patients. Dullness beyond intercostal spaces 9 to 11 suggests splenomegaly.[63]

Estimation of liver size is best performed by percussion of the vertical span in the right midclavicular line. Extension below the costal margin is affected by inflation of the lungs and body habitus and may be inaccurate. Reiff and Osborn measured a mean liver span of 5.9 + 0.8 cm in 100 healthy newborns.[67] Similar measurements of 5.65 + 0.68 cm were obtained by Weisman et al.[68] In contrast, Lawson determined liver spans for infants and toddlers and found much smaller mean values.[69]

Data are available providing 95% confidence intervals for liver span as a function of body weight and age in older children.[70]

Based on these data, hepatomegaly is present if the span in the midclavicular line is greater than 9.5 cm at age 5 years (or weight 20 kg), 10.5 cm at age 9 (30 kg), or 11.5 cm at age 13 (55 kg). Fig. 52-2 depicts mean liver span and upper limits of normal for newborns and older children. The data for infants and toddlers are estimated by extrapolation.

Pathophysiology

The spleen is the largest lymphatic organ in the body. It is the only effective site for the clearance of encapsulated bacteria when antibodies are absent. In addition, it functions as a reservoir for platelets and as a filter for abnormal blood cells.[71]

Enlargement of the spleen occurs because of hyperplasia of the monocyte-phagocyte system (previously called the reticuloendothelial system), vascular congestion, infiltration with neoplastic cells or abnormal storage products, space-occupying lesions such as hematomas, or extramedullary hematopoiesis. Hyperplasia of the monocyte-phagocyte system is most common and results from excessive antigenic stimulation caused by infections, excessive destruction of blood cells as in hemolytic diseases, and disorders of immunoregulation (e.g., juvenile rheumatoid arthritis, systemic lupus erythematosus, serum sickness). Infections, particularly viral infections, are the most common etiology.[65] The most common infectious etiology worldwide is malaria.

Hepatomegaly occurs for many of the same reasons, including Kupffer cell hyperplasia caused by infections, vascular congestion, and infiltration by neoplastic cells or storage of abnormal products of metabolism. Because of

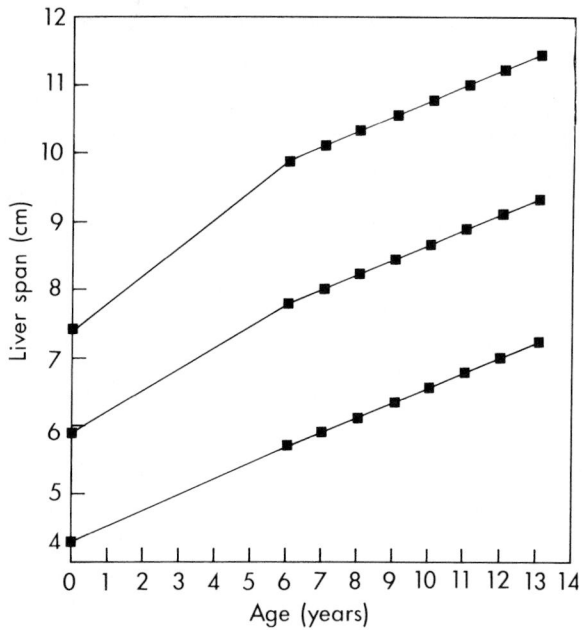

FIG. 52-2. Liver span as a function of age. The mean liver span and 95% confidence intervals are depicted. Estimated measurements for 1 year to 5 years are extrapolated. (*Newborn data from Reiff MI and Osborn LM: Pediatrics 71:46, 1983; older children data from Younoszai MK and Mueller S: Clin Pediatr 14:378, 1975.*)

the liver's role in detoxification, fatty infiltration from toxins may occur. In addition, inflammation (i.e., hepatitis) and bile duct obstruction can cause hepatomegaly.[72]

Diagnostic Considerations

Table 52-8 depicts most of the causes of hepatosplenomegaly classified according to urgency.

Immediately Life-Threatening Etiologies. The immediately life-threatening causes of hepatosplenomegaly include hypersplenism, severe hemolytic anemias, trauma, and sepsis. Hypersplenism results in sequestration of peripheral blood cells. Sickle cell hemoglobinopathy is the most common life-threatening cause of this syndrome in children. Extrahepatic or intrahepatic obstruction can also cause hypersplenism. Extrahepatic venous obstruction (e.g., thrombosis caused by omphalitis, shock, or umbilical venous catheterization) causes portal hypertension and resultant hypersplenism. Intrahepatic obstruction (e.g., cirrhosis caused by hepatitis, alpha-1-antitrypsin deficiency, cystic fibrosis, or parasitic infections) is less common in children.[65]

Hemolytic anemias may be life-threatening if the rate of hemolysis exceeds the rate of production. Immune hemolytic anemias, in particular, often present de novo and anemia may be severe. Trauma causing splenic or hepatic laceration can be fatal if fluid resuscitation is not instituted. Sepsis may result in hepatosplenomegaly and urgent therapy is required. Reye syndrome is life-threatening and causes a soft, enlarged liver.

TABLE 52-8. Etiology of Hepatosplenomegaly Classified by Emergency Department Triage Criteria

Emergent therapy	Immediate therapy	Referral
Trauma	Congestive heart failure	Infectious mononucleosis
Hypersplenism	Neoplasm	Immunodeficiencies
Sequestration crisis	Hematopoietic	AIDS
Immune hemolytic anemia	Metastatic	Severe combined immunodeficiency
Sepsis	Infections	Chronic granulomatous disease
Reye syndrome	Congenital syphilis	Congenital infections
	Rickettsiae	Toxoplasmosis
	Malaria	Cytomegalovirus
	Hepatitis	Other infections
	Viral	Parasites
	Toxin-induced	Fungi
	Hemolytic anemia	Protozoa
	Hypersplenism	Tuberculosis
	Extrahepatic obstruction	Brucellosis
	Intrahepatic obstruction	Leptospirosis
		Tularemia
		Typhoid fever
		Mycobacteria
		Disorders of immunoregulation
		Juvenile rheumatoid arthritis
		Systemic lupus erythematosus
		Serum sickness
		Storage disease

Etiologies for Which Immediate Therapy is Indicated. Diseases for which immediate therapy is helpful include congestive heart failure, neoplasias, congenital syphilis, certain infections, and toxic liver injury. Congestive heart failure is not usually imminently life-threatening unless associated with complications, but should be diagnosed and treated in the emergency department. If neoplastic disease is suspected, the child should be admitted. Viral hepatitis is a common cause of hepatomegaly and may require inpatient care for complications. Congenital syphilis is increasing in incidence and should be suspected in any infant with hepatosplenomegaly.[73] Malaria should be considered if exposure has occurred. Rickettsial and parasitic infections benefit from specific therapy but definitive diagnosis is often delayed. When rickettsial disease is likely, presumptive therapy should be started pending confirmation of the diagnosis. Hepatomegaly may be caused by an acute toxin (e.g., acetaminophen, phenytoin, valproate, corticosteroids).

Etiologies for Which Referral is Necessary for Diagnosis or Treatment. AIDS is an increasingly common cause of splenomegaly. Other immunodeficiency disorders (e.g., severe combined immunodeficiency) may appear similarly. Storage diseases (e.g., Gaucher) affect both organs and generally result in massive enlargement. Less common infectious causes of an enlarged liver or spleen are listed in Table 52-8.

Diagnostic Work-Up

The history assists in the classification of the disease as acute, subacute, or chronic. Truly acute hepatosplenomegaly is uncommon. Possible causes include trauma, sepsis, dehydration and shock, and splenic sequestration crisis. Subacute causes include infections, congestive heart failure, portal hypertension other than that caused by sepsis and shock, hemolysis, autoimmune (rheumatologic) diseases, and neoplasias. Chronic causes include the storage disorders, cirrhosis, chronic anemias with extramedullary hematopoiesis, immunodeficiency states, and assorted rare diseases.

A history of travel to an endemic area may be helpful in diagnosing many of the infectious causes of hepatosplenomegaly, including parasitic or rickettsial infections. Contact with animals or soil known to harbor leptospirosis or histoplasmosis, for example, suggests the presence of these infections.

Systemic symptoms such as weight loss or persistent fever should prompt consideration of neoplasia or chronic infection. Bruising or bleeding suggests dysfunction of the bone marrow, as in neoplastic infiltration, or severe liver disease. Poor feeding in an infant may suggest anemia or congestive heart failure. Fatigue in the older child may be caused by anemia or heart failure or may be a manifestation of the infectious mononucleosis syndrome, which is caused by Epstein-Barr (EB) and other viruses. The symptoms of hepatitis or biliary tract disease include anorexia, nausea and vomiting, abdominal pain, jaundice, dark urine, and alcholic stools. Hepatitis is likely to be preceded by a prodrome of fatigue, anorexia, and nausea, possibly followed by urticaria or arthritis. Inquire about trauma to the abdomen, and hematemesis should be explored. Hemorrhoids suggest portal venous hypertension with collateral circulation. Immunodeficiencies should be considered in an infant with a history of failure to thrive and recurrent opportunistic infections. Denial of high-risk behaviors for AIDS and other sexually transmitted diseases is common among adolescents. A history of recent exposure to medication raises the possibility of serum sickness. Finally, a family history of autoimmune disorders is frequently present with such entities as juvenile rheumatoid arthritis and systemic lupus erythematosus.

The physical examination of the patient with hepatosplenomegaly should include an accurate estimation of liver and spleen size. Drawing lines on the abdomen to mark the span of the liver and spleen is useful for future reference. Massive enlargement of the spleen is characteristic of infiltration with storage materials or malignant cells or splenic sequestration.

The child's general appearance should be noted, and particular attention should be paid to signs of weight loss or systemic disease. A cushingoid appearance may suggest hepatomegaly caused by the use of exogenous steroids. Vital signs should be examined for tachycardia or low blood pressure suggestive of shock, tachypnea associated with heart failure, and fever. The skin may be jaundiced with liver or biliary tract disease, pale with anemia, or mottled with congestive heart failure. Sepsis may cause the skin to appear either warm and pink with bounding pulses or gray and poorly perfused. Rickettsial infections, congenital syphilis, and the rheumatologic diseases may exhibit characteristic rashes. The storage disorders may manifest as a thick, doughy skin.

Lymphadenopathy is suggestive of infection or malignancy. Generalized lymphadenopathy in an infant with failure to thrive and recurrent candidal infections may be indicative of AIDS or other immunodeficiency disorder. A gallop rhythm is usually present with congestive heart failure. Children may have prominent superficial abdominal blood vessels or hemorrhoids or, more commonly, splenomegaly as the sole manifestation of portal venous hypertension. Pain in the upper quadrant(s) with a tender liver or spleen is indicative of capsular distension and is common with trauma and infections. An abdominal mass may represent a primary tumor such as neuroblastoma or Wilms' tumor, which causes hepatomegaly or splenomegaly because of metastasis. Encephalopathy may be seen with severe systemic disturbances such as sepsis or shock, or it may be a manifestation of liver dysfunction as in Reye syndrome or cirrhotic liver disease.

Ancillary Data. The purpose of the initial laboratory work-up for the patient with hepatosplenomegaly is to test the function of the spleen, the liver, and the bone marrow. The single most important test is examination of the peripheral blood smear for CBC, differential, and reticulocyte count. Cytopenias can be classified as resulting from either decreased production or increased destruction based on the presence or absence of immature forms (i.e., reticulocytes). Decreased production of one or more cell lines is suspicious for neoplastic or storage product infiltration of the bone marrow, but marrow suppression can result from viral infections. Aspiration of the bone marrow is generally required to make a definitive diagnosis. Increased destruction of more than one cell line generally indicates hypersplenism whereas increased destruction of red blood cells only may indicate an immune-based hemolytic anemia or chronic hemolysis. The peripheral smear and a Coombs' antibody test help to distinguish between these causes. Anemia alone, with a history of trauma to the abdomen, suggests splenic or hepatic laceration. Child abuse must be considered in the differential diagnosis. Leukocytosis may indicate infection but examination of the marrow for leukemic infiltration is necessary if splenomegaly is a prominent finding. Eosinophilia suggests parasitic infection. Lymphocytosis and atypical lymphocytosis are common with infectious mononucleosis caused by EB virus, even in young children.[74] The combination of anemia, monocytosis, and thrombocytopenia suggests congenital syphilis.

Initial tests of liver function include glucose, coagulation times, and serum and urine bilirubin. Bilirubin may be elevated with hepatitis or biliary tract disease. Disturbances of glucose and coagulation profiles indicate global hepatic dysfunction of a severe degree. Elevated transaminase levels indicate injury to liver cells and may be seen with trauma, infectious hepatitis, biliary tract disease, toxin-induced hepatitis, liver abscess, parasitic infection, and Reye syndrome.

Further laboratory studies are indicated by the history and physical examination. Because infection with EB virus is a common cause of splenomegaly, serologic tests for this infection should be performed. The heterophil antibody response may be negative in children less than 4 years of age; EB virus-specific immunoglobulin titers should be performed.[75] The heterophil antibody also may be negative in the first week of illness and become positive in the second week. Further serologic testing (e.g., for syphilis, Rocky Mountain spotted fever, toxoplasmosis, cytomegalovirus, etc.) is indicated by history or physical findings. Peripheral adenopathy may require biopsy or serologic testing for AIDS. Bone marrow aspiration has already been discussed and is indicated whenever peripheral blood smear testing suggests marrow failure. Tests for antinuclear antibody or rheumatoid factor may be indicated if rash or arthritis is present.

Electrocardiography and echocardiography are indicated if congestive heart failure is the cause of hepatosplenomegaly. A plain roentgenogram of the chest and abdomen may provide the diagnosis of tuberculosis or neuroblastoma, for example, and will assist in accurately assessing organ size. CT scan of the abdomen is the radiographic study of choice if splenic or hepatic trauma is suspected. Ultrasonography may be useful in other situations to provide reliable measurements of liver and spleen size and to identify cysts, infarcts, accessory organs, and biliary stones. Radionuclide scanning can test hepatic and splenic functioning. More invasive tests, such as angiography or biopsy, are indicated in rare cases in childhood.

JAUNDICE

LISA SINCLAIR HART

Jaundice is defined as "a syndrome characterized by hyperbilirubinemia and deposition of bile pigment in the skin, mucous membranes and sclera with resulting yellow appearance of the patient."* Its clinical appearance can be confused with carotenemia; however, in the latter disorder the jaundiced appearance is accompanied by a normal serum bilirubin level.

Jaundice or hyperbilirubinemia is divided into two types—conjugated and unconjugated. In conjugated hyperbilirubinemia the direct reacting component of the serum bilirubin exceeds 30% of the total. In unconjugated hyperbilirubinemia the direct reacting component is less than 15% of the total. A direct reacting fraction of 15% to 30% is inconclusive, and the patient cannot be placed clearly in either category.

Pathophysiology

Bilirubin is the final product formed from the breakdown of heme. Heme proteins are present not only in hemoglobin but also in myoglobin and certain heme-containing enzymes. The majority of heme breakdown occurs in the reticuloendothelial system. Heme is converted into biliverdin by the action of the enzyme heme oxygenase. Biliverdin is subsequently converted into bilirubin by the enzyme biliverdin reductase. Bilirubin is a yellow, toxic metabolite that is not soluble in water. When it is released in the plasma it binds to albumin and is transported to the liver for conjugation.

The uptake of bilirubin into the liver is thought to involve the action of two proteins—the "y" protein or ligandin and the "z" protein. Once in the hepatocyte, glucuronyl transferase converts the bilirubin into its monoglucuronide or diglucuronide conjugated form. The conjugated bilirubin is then excreted into the bile canaliculus and transported through the biliary system into the intestine.

Prenatally unconjugated bilirubin is excreted via the placenta. At birth the fetal liver must quickly adapt to metabolize the circulating unconjugated bilirubin. Physiologic hyperbilirubinemia of the newborn occurs due to the inability of the immature neonatal liver to handle this bilirubin load. In the newborn's liver there is a transient deficiency of the y protein, which leads to impaired uptake into the hepatocyte. In addition a deficiency of glucuronyl transferase leads to impairment of the ability to conjugate bilirubin. Finally, there is defective excretion of bilirubin into the bile canaliculus. This immaturity of the neonatal liver is accompanied by a high bilirubin load (6 to 8 mg/kg/24 hr in the neonate vs. 3 to 4 mg/kg/24 hr in adults).[76] The neonatal liver quickly adapts and physiologic hyperbilirubinemia resolves during the first 1 to 2 weeks of life.

Unconjugated Hyperbilirubinemia

Infants

Differential Considerations. The differential diagnosis of unconjugated hyperbilirubinemia in infancy is relatively long (see box on p. 819). The most common cause of unconjugated hyperbilirubinemia in neonates is physiologic jaundice of the newborn. Approximately 60% of newborns

---

* *Dorland's Illustrated Medical Dictionary*, ed 28, Philadelphia, 1994, WB Saunders.

become visibly jaundiced during their first week of life due to this entity. The pathophysiology has been previously discussed. The emergency department physician evaluating a jaundiced neonate must be able to quickly differentiate infants with true pathology from this large number of physiologically jaundiced infants. The classic pattern of physiologic jaundice is described as an absence of jaundice on the first day of life followed by a steady rise in bilirubin to approximately 6 mg/dl on the third day of life followed by a decline to normal levels by the tenth to twelfth day of life. This pattern is classically followed by most formula-fed infants and does not merit further diagnostic work-up unless the level of hyperbilirubinemia becomes marked or is particularly prolonged. The American Academy of Pediatrics has published guidelines to assist the clinician in diagnosing and managing hyperbilirubinemia in newborns.[77] The new revisions propose a less aggressive approach in evaluation of infants with suspected physiologic jaundice by giving con-

crete guidelines for when to pursue a full diagnostic work-up and raising the threshold for when to consider phototherapy and exchange transfusion (Table 52-9).

The second most common cause of neonatal jaundice is breast milk jaundice. The exact cause of breast milk jaundice is not completely understood. In the first few days of life the bilirubin level generally increases at the same rate as formula-fed infants; however, in most of these babies the level continues to rise. The bilirubin level generally reaches a peak between days 10 and 27 of life and then persists for 3 to 10 weeks with the bilirubin remaining at a lower level. The American Academy of Pediatrics suggests five possible approaches to management of the newborn with severe breast milk jaundice (see box on p. 820).[77]

Jaundice that is visible in the first 24 hours of life or a rise in serum bilirubin greater than 0.5 mg/dl/hour is always considered abnormal and merits further diagnostic work-up. Specifically the clinician should consider the possibility of severe hemolytic disease, congenital TORCHS infections (toxoplasmosis, rubella, cytomegalovirus, herpes, and syphilis), and sepsis.

Unconjugated hyperbilirubinemia that occurs or persists after the first week of life and is not caused by breastfeeding should be considered pathologic and evaluated further. Hemolytic anemias such as spherocytosis, elliptocytosis, and pyruvate kinase deficiency can occur as persisting jaundice. In addition, genetic disorders such as Crigler-Najjar and Gilbert syndrome may become manifest at this time. Sepsis, UTI, upper GI tract obstruction, and congenital hypothyroidism should also be considered in these infants.

Diagnostic Work-Up. In evaluating the jaundiced infant certain risk factors should be elicited from the history. A family history of other children with hyperbilirubemia or severe hemolytic disease should be sought. Parents should also be questioned about genetic and metobolic disorders or unexplained infant deaths. A history of infection during pregnancy would suggest congenital TORCHS infection. Fever in the mother just before delivery should lead the clinician to suspect sepsis.

The abnormal skin color of the child is generally the most noteworthy finding during the physical examination

---

Differential Diagnosis of Unconjugated Hyperbilirubinemia in Infants

1. Physiologic jaundice of the newborn
2. Breast milk jaundice
3. Hemolysis
   a. ABO or Rh incompatibility
   b. Membrane defects (i.e., spherocytosis)
   c. Enzyme deficiencies (i.e., pyruvate kinase deficiency)
   d. Breakdown of hematomas formed from birth trauma (i.e., cephalohematomas)
4. Infections
   a. TORCHS (see Chapter 18)
   b. Sepsis/UTI
5. Crigler-Najjar syndrome
6. Gilbert syndrome
7. Congenital hypothyroidism
8. Upper GI tract obstruction

TABLE 52-9. Management of Hyperbilirubinemia in the Healthy Term Newborn

Age, hours	TSB* level, mg/dl (µmol/L)			
	Consider phototherapy†	Phototherapy	Exchange transfusion if intensive phototherapy fails‡	Exchange transfusion and intensive phototherapy
≤24§	—	—	—	—
25-48	≥ 12 (170)	≥ 15 (260)	≥ 20 (340)	≥ 25 (430)
49-72	≥ 15 (260)	≥ 18 (310)	≥ 25 (430)	≥ 30 (510)
>72	≥ 17 (290)	≥ 20 (340)	≥ 25 (430)	≥ 30 (510)

From *Pediatrics* 94:558, 1994.
*TSB indicates total serum bilirubin.
†Phototherapy at these TSB levels is a clinical option, meaning that the intervention is available and may be used *on the basis of individual clinical judgment.*
‡Intensive phototherapy should produce a decline of TSB of 1 to 2 mg/dl within 4 to 6 hours and the TSB level should continue to fall and remain below the threshold level for exchange transfusion. If this does not occur, it is considered a failure of phototherapy.
§Term infants who are clinically jaundiced at ≤24 hours old are not considered healthy and require further evaluation (see text).

Treatment Options for Jaundiced Breastfed Infants

Observe

Continue breastfeeding; administer phototherapy

Supplement breastfeeding with formula, with or without phototherapy

Interrupt breastfeeding; substitute formula

Interrupt breastfeeding; substitute formula; administer phototherapy

From *Pediatrics* 94:558, 1994.

---

of the jaundiced infant. Jaundice becomes clinically apparent when the bilirubin level is greater than 5 mg/dl. The abnormal color is due to the accumulation of unconjugated and conjugated bilirubin in the skin. Indirect hyperbilirubinemia tends to give the skin a bright yellow or orange color whereas direct hyperbilirubinemia usually leads to a muddy yellow or greenish color. Jaundice appears first in the face and progresses caudally as the serum bilirubin level rises. However, it is impossible to tell with certainty the level or type of hyperbilirubinemia based only on skin color; therefore serum levels must be checked.

The physical examination should look for signs that might indicate the cause of the jaundice. For example, microcephaly would suggest congenital TORCHS infection. Cephalohematomas or extensive bruising might suggest hemolysis due to birth trauma. Poor feeding and lethargy could increase the suspicion of sepsis although this is often present in severe hyperbilirubinemia without sepsis.

The clinician should also look for findings that may be suggestive of bilirubin encephalopathy or kernicterus. Kernicterus is caused by bilirubin deposition in the CNS, especially the basal ganglia, which leads to permanent neurologic deficits and occasionally death. In the 1990s, severe kernicterus is distinctly unusual because of the aggressive treatment of hyperbilirubinemia in newborns. From historical cases we know that it usually manifests early by subtle signs such as lethargy and poor feeding. As it progresses, the infant appears acutely ill and has a bulging fontanel, opisthotonus, diminished reflexes, twitching, and a shrill cry. In its severe state there can be muscular rigidity, convulsions, and death. Infants who survive may have severe permanent neurologic deficits. In milder cases, more appropriately called bilirubin encephalopathy, they may be uncoordinated, partially deaf, and have learning disabilities.[78,79]

The laboratory work-up of unconjugated hyperbilirubinemia can be extensive. The history and physical examination will help to dictate what studies are needed. Because the majority of newborn infants develop physiologic jaundice, standards are needed to determine which infants merit a jaundice work-up. The following criteria have been suggested.[76,80,81]

1. Jaundice appearing at less than 24 hours of age.
2. Serum bilirubin rise of greater than 5 mg/dl/day or greater than 0.5 mg/dl/hr.
3. Serum bilirubin level greater than 12 mg/dl in a full-term infant or greater than 14 mg/dl in a premature infant.
4. Jaundice persisting for more than 1 week in a full-term infant or for more than 2 weeks in a premature infant.
5. All conjugated hyperbilirubinemia.

The jaundice work-up generally consists of measurement of the total serum bilirubin level with direct and indirect fractions. Maternal prenatal testing should have included ABO and Rh(D) typing and a serum screen for unusual isoimmune antibodies. When the mother has not had a prenatal screen the infant should have a blood type, Coombs' status, and CBC checked. In addition the peripheral smear should be reviewed for signs of hemolysis. Generally these preliminary tests will lead to a diagnosis. A screening test for G6PD deficiency, TORCHS screen, liver and thyroid functions tests, sepsis work-up, and further metabolic work-up may be needed if the clinical picture suggests.

Therapeutic Trial. The treatment of unconjugated hyperbilirubinemia in the newborn is designed to slow the rise in serum bilirubin and thus prevent kernicterus. Phototherapy and exchange transfusion remain the cornerstones of therapy in the 1990s. Hydration should be assessed and assured.

The revised guidelines for initiation of phototherapy or exchange transfusion are given in Table 52-9. For premature and sick infants the exchange level and "light" level are lower.[76] The reader should refer to standard neonatology texts to determine appropriate levels in these infants. Phototherapy converts bilirubin into unconjugated isomers that can be excreted in the bile. Intensive phototherapy often combined with hydration should result in a decline in serum bilirubin by 1 to 2 mg/dl within 4 to 6 hours. Side effects include diarrhea, skin rashes, and dehydration. There is also potential for bronze baby syndrome and ocular damage.

Exchange transfusion is used when bilirubin levels are nearing a toxic range or if there are any clinical signs of kernicterus. The treatment of jaundice also includes prevention of risk factors for kernicterus. Hypoxemia, hypercarbia, acidosis, hypoglycemia, hypoalbuminemia, hypothermia, and dehydration should be corrected. If possible oral feeds should be continued because this will stimulate the enterohepatic circulation, which may help to decrease the bilirubin level.

Older Children and Adults. There are very few diagnostic considerations in determining the cause of unconjugated hyperbilirubinemia in older children and adults (see box on p. 821). One of the most common causes is hemolysis due to sickle cell disease or other congenital hemolytic anemias. Certain drugs (chloramphenicol and pregnanediol) may also induce transient elevations of unconjugated bilirubin levels. If the patient appears healthy and has no signs of anemia, hepatocellular damage, or exposure to hepatotoxic drugs, Gilbert disease and Crigler-Najjar syndrome should be considered. Treatment will depend on the underlying cause of the hyperbilirubinemia.

Differential Diagnosis of Unconjugated Hyperbilirubinemia in Older Children and Adults

1. Hemolytic anemia (i.e., sickle cell disease)
2. Genetic defect
   a. Gilbert syndrome
   b. Crigler-Najjar syndrome
3. Hepatotoxic drugs (i.e., chloramphenicol, pregnanediol)
4. Prolonged fasting

Conjugated Hyperbilirubinemia

Infants

Differential Considerations. Conjugated hyperbilirubinemia is *always* pathologic. The differential diagnosis in infancy is particularly extensive and complex. A quick review of the diagnostic considerations listed in the box at right reveals that most of these disorders are life-threatening. For this reason the clinician must pursue a diagnostic work-up expeditiously. Certain disorders require further clarification.

Extrahepatic biliary atresia is a pathologic process in which there is absence or atresia of some portion of the extrahepatic biliary system. Landing proposed that extrahepatic biliary atresia, choledochal cysts, some cases of intrahepatic biliary atresia, and neonatal hepatitis were all manifestations of a single basic disease process in which there is inflammation at different points in the biliary system that leads to functional obstruction.[82] The exact cause of this inflammatory process is unknown but may be related to reovirus 3.[83]

Infectious agents are sometimes implicated as the cause of conjugated hyperbilirubinemia in infancy. In particular gram-negative sepsis is commonly identified. It appears there is an endotoxin present in the cell wall of gram-negative bacteria that impairs the ability of the hepatocyte to excrete conjugated bilirubin.

Diagnostic Work-Up. The history should aid the diagnostic evaluation by attempting to identify known causes of neonatal cholestasis. The infant's medical history should be reviewed for exposure to hepatoxic drugs or total parenteral nutrition. A family history should focus on stillbirths or infant deaths to elucidate risk factors for genetic or metabolic defects. A history suggestive of infection in the mother would increase suspicion for sepsis or TORCHS infection in the infant.

The physical examination should initially focus on ruling out obvious genetic syndromes. From that point, the examination should attempt to differentiate extrahepatic from intrahepatic causes of cholestasis. It has been stated often that infants with extrahepatic atresia are generally full-term infants of normal weight who clinically appear well except for the jaundice, obvious hepatomegaly, and acholic stools. In contrast, infants with intrahepatic cholestasis are often preterm, small for gestational age, ill-

---

Differential Diagnosis of Conjugated Hyperbilirubinemia in Infants

I. Obstructive causes
   A. Extrahepatic
      1. Extrahepatic biliary atresia/hypoplasia
      2. Choledochal cyst
      3. Bile duct strictures
      4. Mass (neoplasia, stone)
      5. Inspissated bile syndrome
      6. Spontaneous bile duct perforation
   B. Intrahepatic
      1. Intrahepatic biliary atresia/hypoplasia
      2. "Neonatal hepatitis"
      3. Alagille syndrome
      4. Byler disease
      5. Congenital hepatic fibrosis
II. Infectious causes
   A. Bacterial
      1. Gram-negative sepsis
      2. UTIs
      3. Congenital infections (i.e., toxoplasmosis, syphilis)
      4. Listeriosis
      5. Tuberculosis
   B. Viral
      1. CMV
      2. Hepatitis B
      3. Rubella
      4. Varicella
      5. Herpes
      6. Coxsackie
      7. Echovirus
      8. HIV
III. Drugs/toxins (i.e., total parenteral nutrition)
IV. Metabolic/genetic causes
   A. Errors of amino acid metabolism—tyrosinemia
   B. Errors of carbohydrate metabolism
      1. Galactosemia
      2. Hereditary fructose intolerance
      3. Glycogen storage disease type IV
   C. Errors of lipid metabolism
      1. Niemann-Pick
      2. Wolman disease
      3. Gaucher disease
      4. Cholesterol ester storage disease
   D. Chromosomal disorders
      1. Down syndrome
      2. Turner syndrome
      3. Trisomy 18
   E. Miscellaneous
      1. Alpha-1-antitrypsin deficiency
      2. Cystic fibrosis
      3. Dubin-Johnson syndrome
      4. Neonatal hypopituitarism
      5. Zellweger syndrome
      6. Donohue syndrome—leprechaunism
      7. Rotor syndrome

appearing infants who have both hepatomegaly and spleno-megaly.

An extensive laboratory work-up is indicated in each case of conjugated hyperbilirubinemia because examination findings are nonspecific. All infants with cholestasis need certain baseline tests. These include a CBC, differential, platelet count, bilirubin (total and direct), SGOT, SGPT, alkaline phosphatase, GGT, PT/PTT, total protein, albumin, cholesterol, and ammonia level. In addition, all infants should have a urinalysis and urine test for reducing substances. As previously stated, a sepsis work-up should be strongly considered. Most of these preliminary tests can be initiated in the emergency department and the child can then be admitted for further evaluation. Other diagnostic studies to consider after admission includes thyroid function tests, urine metabolic screen, serum amino acids, TORCHS titers, hepatitis B serology, ophthalmologic evaluation, sweat test, and long bone films.

An ultrasound can determine the presence of a chole-dochal cyst or obvious stones or stenosis leading to dilation of the biliary tree. If the ultrasound does not reveal a cyst or obvious extrahepatic obstruction, a Disida scan is done. If the scan shows biliary excretion into the intestine, extrahepatic biliary atresia is effectively ruled out. If excretion is absent, a percutaneous liver biopsy should be performed. If the liver biopsy suggests biliary atresia (bile duct proliferation and portal perilobular fibrosis), an intraoperative cholangiogram is indicated. If extrahepatic bile ducts are not patent on this study a diagnosis of extrahepatic biliary atresia is made and a Kasai procedure is performed.

Therapeutic Trial. The treatment of conjugated hyperbilirubinemia depends entirely on its cause. Initial management of these patients in the emergency department focuses on the prompt identification of the etiology of the cholestasis. In particular the clinician must quickly identify potentially devastating disorders that depend on early identification and treatment (i.e., sepsis, metabolic disorders). There are certain general principles that can be applied to the management of cholestasis in infancy; however, most of these are not relevant in the emergency department and are largely issues for inpatient management. For example, the child's diet should be adjusted to account for the malabsorptive difficulties that are apparent in children with hepatic dysfunction.[84,85] Maintaining adequate nutritional intake is particularly important in patients who are surgical candidates. Aside from diet, further management focuses on stimulating bile flow and reducing pruritus. Phenobarbital is a drug that is commonly used for this purpose. The surgical treatment of biliary atresia is discussed in detail in the section on biliary atresia.

Older Children and Adults
Differential Considerations. The diagnosis, evaluation, and management of direct hyperbilirubinemia in older children and adults vary markedly from infantile cholestasis. The diagnosis and evaluation are made somewhat simpler by the fact that fewer diseases occur with cholestasis in older children. The differential diagnosis of cholestasis in older children is presented in the box above. By far the most common cause of conjugated hyperbilirubinemia in childhood is viral hepatitis.

Differential Diagnosis of Congenital Hyperbilirubinemia in Older Children and Adults

1. Extrahepatic obstruction
   a. Tumor
   b. Stone
   c. Bile duct stricture (i.e., chronic pancreatitis)
2. Infections
   a. Sepsis
   b. Hepatitis/mononucleosis
3. Hepatotoxins (i.e., estrogens, acetaminophen, etc.)
4. Metabolic/genetic
   a. Dubin-Johnson syndrome
   b. Rotor syndrome
   c. Wilson disease
   d. Cystic fibrosis
   e. Alpha-1-antitrypsin deficiency
5. Inflammatory bowel disease
6. Hepatic crisis in sickle cell disease
7. Cholestatic jaundice of pregnancy
8. Cirrhosis
9. Sclerosing cholangitis

Diagnostic Work-Up. The initial history taken in the emergency department should focus on excluding easily identifiable causes of jaundice. A recent history of fevers, malaise, nausea, and vomiting would suggest possible viral hepatitis. In considering this diagnosis the clinician should inquire about risk factors for hepatitis such as recent transfusions or a history of IV drug abuse. In addition, a recent travel history or exposure to foods known to carry hepatitis A (i.e., seafood) should be elicited. Exposure to known hepatoxic agents (e.g., estrogens, tetracycline, alcohols, and certain types of mushrooms) should also be determined. The history should identify any similar episodes of jaundice in the patient or his or her family. The clinician should also attempt to identify any recurring symptoms present over the preceding months that might suggest a more chronic disorder. For example, a history of recurrent arthralgias, rash, or GI complaints might suggest inflammatory bowel disease. A history of failure to thrive with or without respiratory symptoms would be suggestive of cystic fibrosis or alpha-1-antitrypsin deficiency.

The physical examination may also aid in narrowing the diagnostic considerations. One of the most useful findings will be the presence or absence of hepatomegaly and hepatic tenderness. Tenderness over the liver is nearly universal in viral hepatitis; hepatomegaly is inconsistently found. Hepatomegaly is more commonly seen in infiltrative processes (i.e., storage disorder, malignancies) and congestive heart failure. Hepatic tenderness, when present, must be differentiated from tenderness caused by inflammation of the gall bladder (cholecystitis, cholelithiasis). Choledochal cyst presenting with the classic triad of right upper quadrant mass, tenderness, and jaundice must also be considered.

Other physical findings suggestive of systemic disease should be sought. A chronically wasted appearance would lend support to a diagnosis of an ongoing systemic disorder. The presence of pulmonary findings such as tachypnea or rales suggests further testing for cystic fibrosis or alpha-1-antitrypsin deficiency is needed. Abnormal joint findings or skin rashes suggest inflammatory bowel disease. The presence of Kayser-Fleischer rings on ophthalmologic examination suggests Wilson disease, particularly when neurologic abnormalities are also present.

Laboratory work-up will be directed by the findings of the history and physical examination. A CBC, differential, electrolytes, BUN, creatinine, glucose, SGOT, SGPT, alkaline phosphatase, total protein, albumin, and PT/PTT are essential. Titers for viral hepatitis should be sent. Serum total and direct bilirubin levels should be measured but the clinician should remember that all cases of conjugated hyperbilirubinemia are accompanied by some rise in unconjugated bilirubin level. To reiterate, conjugated hyperbilirubinemia is defined as an elevated serum bilirubin level with greater than 30% in the conjugated form.

Other laboratory tests should be considered depending on the initial findings. Urine and blood culture should be considered if sepsis is suspected. A toxicologic screen should be sent if the child has acute hepatic failure without a clear etiology. A chest x-ray film may be helpful in the child with pulmonary findings. Further diagnostic studies such as the sweat test, ceruloplasmin levels, ammonia, abdominal ultrasound, and abdominal CT scan should be considered as part of the inpatient evaluation.

Therapeutic Trial. Many patients with conjugated hyperbilirubinemia will require inpatient evaluation and treatment unless the cause of the jaundice can be clearly identified in the emergency department. In the latter case outpatient management may be considered if the etiology is not life-threatening and close outpatient follow-up can be maintained. Treatment in the hospital will be dictated by the initial findings; often the inpatient treatment consists of further diagnostic studies to identify the cause of the hyperbilirubinemia.

VOMITING

MARY D. PATTERSON

Vomiting may be the chief complaint or it may be a symptom associated with a multitude of diagnostic entities. Illnesses as common as otitis media and as unusual as a posterior fossa tumor may appear with vomiting.

Vomiting is the "violent expulsion of gastric contents through the mouth."[86] True vomiting can be characterized by three stages: nausea, retching, and emesis.[87]

Nausea is evoked by "emotional, labyrinthine, and visceral stimuli."[87] It is marked by a strong desire to vomit and may be associated with such autonomic symptoms as salivation, pallor, sweating, and tachycardia.[87] Nausea is associated with relaxation of the body and fundus of the stomach, as well as frequent contractions of the gastric antrum. Retrograde peristalsis may occur.[87,88]

Retching is the result of "spasmodic and abortive respiratory movements with the glottis closed."[88] Inspiratory

TABLE 52-10. Diagnostic Vomitus Characteristics

Characteristic	Comment
Undigested food	Esophageal lesion at or above cardia
Nonbilious vomiting	Lesion proximal to pylorus
Bilious vomiting	Obstruction beyond the ampulla of Vater (second portion duodenum) or adynamic ileus
Fecal odor	Peritonitis or lower obstruction
Bloody	Lesion proximal to ligament of Treitz
Bright red	Vomitus has little or no contact with gastric juices; active bleeding site at or above cardia
Coffee grounds	Bloody vomitus altered by gastric juices

movements of the chest and diaphragm occur simultaneously with expiratory contractions of the abdominal musculature.[87,88] The fundus relaxes while the antrum and pylorus contract.[87,88]

The actual act of vomiting occurs as the gastric contents are forcefully expelled through the open mouth. This is the result of a forceful sustained contraction of the abdominal muscles and diaphragm; at the same time, the pylorus and antrum contract. Vomiting is accompanied by a temporary elevation of the gastroesophageal junction above the diaphragm. This results in decreased pressure on the lower esophageal sphincter and allows the expulsion of gastric contents.[87,89]

Pathophysiology

Two central nervous system centers serve as the basis for vomiting, both located in the medulla. The vomiting center is found in the lateral reticular formation and responds to afferent stimuli from the pharynx, pleura, heart, urogenital tract, gastrointestinal tract, and biliary tree.[87,89] The chemoreceptor trigger zone (CTZ) is located in the floor of the fourth ventricle. The CTZ is sensitive to metabolic disturbances (i.e., uremia, electrolyte abnormalities, ketones, adrenaline, estrogen) and various drugs (i.e., morphine, cardiac glycosides, antimetabolites, and ipecac).

Differential Considerations

Because a wide variety of afferent stimuli may produce vomiting, there are many diagnoses to consider. The vast majority of children with emesis will have a self-limited viral gastroenteritis; however, consideration of more serious illnesses is essential and the characteristics of the vomitus may be useful in distinguishing the anatomic pathology (Table 52-10). The specific nature of the vomited material may provide early clues about the location of the pathology leading to emesis. Differential considerations vary greatly by age and many etiologies are more prevalent in specific age groups (Table 52-11).

Diagnostic Work-Up

The evaluation of the patient should initially focus on the history related to the nature of the vomiting and the child's

TABLE 52-11. Causes of Vomiting

Birth to 3 mo	3 mo to 2 yr	2 yr to 12 yr	Adolescents
Infectious	**Infectious**	**Infectious**	**Infectious**
Viral gastroenteritis	Viral gastroenteritis	Viral gastroenteritis	Viral gastroenteritis
Meningitis/encephalitis	Meningitis/encephalitis	Meningitis/encephalitis	Meningitis/encephalitis
Pneumonia/pertussis	Pneumonia/bronchiolitis	Pneumonia	Pneumonia
Sepsis	Sepsis	UTI/pyelonephritis	Sinusitis
UTI	UTI/pyelonephritis	Otitis media/pharyngitis	Pyelonephritis
	Hepatitis	Sinusitis	Pharyngitis
Anatomic/congenital	Otitis media	Hepatitis	Hepatitis
Tracheoesophageal fistula	Pharyngitis	Peptic ulcer disease	PID
Duodenal/jejunal stenosis			Peptic ulcer disease
Esophageal web	**Anatomic/congenital**	**Anatomic**	
Hernia	Incarcerated hernia	Appendicitis	**Anatomic**
Pyloric stenosis	Intussusception	Pancreatitis	Appendicitis
Annular pancreas	Abdominal neoplasm		Testicular torsion
Gastroesophageal reflux	Malrotation with volvulus	**Metabolic**	Renal colic
		Diabetic ketoacidosis	
Metabolic	**Metabolic**	Thyrotoxicosis	**Metabolic**
Congenital adrenal hyperplasia	Uremia	Uremia	Diabetic ketoacidosis
Urea cycle defects	Diabetic ketoacidosis		Thyrotoxicosis
Organic acidemias		**CNS**	Uremia
Amino acid metabolism defect	**CNS**	Head trauma	
Hereditary fructose intolerance	Intracranial tumor	Seizure disorder	**CNS**
	Head trauma	Intracranial tumor	Migraine headache
CNS		Pseudotumor cerebri	Intracranial tumor
Hydrocephalus	**Other**		Head trauma
Intracranial tumor	Reactive airway disease	**Other**	
	Appendicitis	Ingestion/drug	**Other**
Other	Ingestion/drug	Reactive airway disease	Pregnancy
Milk allergy	Bezoars	Cyclic vomiting	Ingestion/ethanol
Bezoars	Reye syndrome		Drugs
			Bulimia
			Reactive airway disease

age. Physical and laboratory considerations may provide further diagnostic data. An age-related discussion may be particularly helpful.

Birth to 3 Months. Congenital anomalies and acquired illness are common entities. The prenatal and neonatal history are relevant; congenital anomalies should be considered. The nature of onset and the vomitus may be diagnostic.

Vital signs may reveal fever as an indication of infection or tachypnea and tachycardia associated with volume depletion. The abdominal examination is more easily accomplished if the hips are flexed, thus relaxing the abdominal musculature.

In the well-appearing infant with emesis as the sole complaint, gastroesophageal reflux or chalasia is extremely common and results from a relaxed lower esophageal sphincter. The majority of infants experience reflux at some time, although it is seen more often in premature infants.[87] These children are often described as "spitting up" or regurgitating after every feeding since birth or shortly thereafter. Because the majority of these children thrive and remain well hydrated, they can be managed with conservative measures such as thickened feedings and antireflux positioning (prone with the head elevated at an angle

of 30 degrees) and careful slow feeding. Typically, infants outgrow reflux by 6 to 9 months of age as the lower esophageal sphincter muscles mature. A small percentage of infants experience such severe reflux that they fail to gain weight; aspiration pneumonia or esophagitis may develop. These patients require more extensive investigation including a focused barium swallow, esophageal pH monitoring, or radionuclide milk scans. Anticholinergic agents such as bethanecol (0.4 mg/kg/24 hr QID PO) may be helpful. A Nissen fundoplication is reserved to reduce the reflux and aspiration in severe cases.

Children with hypertrophic pyloric stenosis typically experience no emesis until 2 to 3 weeks of age or later. Vomiting usually increases gradually in volume and frequency and often becomes projectile. Affected males outnumber females by a ratio of 5:1; first-born infants are commonly affected.[90] Approximately 1 of 150 males and 1 of 750 females develop pyloric stenosis.[91]

Duodenal and jejunal atresia may present in the nursery; partial or stenotic lesions may evolve later.[90] Approximately 95% of children with malrotation develop problems early.[90] Intestinal obstruction is associated with bilious vomiting, requiring rapid evaluation, stabilization, and surgery. Volvulus with or without malrotation accompanied with vascular compromise of the midgut requires surgical intervention, often following confirmation by a barium study.[91]

Emesis can be the presenting symptom of metabolic abnormalities. Organic acidemias, urea cycle defects, congenital adrenal hyperplasia, disorders of amino acid metabolism, and hereditary fructose intolerance can occur in the first few weeks of life.[92,93] Lethargy, seizures, and coma may accompany vomiting. Dysmorphic features, unusual urine odors, organomegaly, and ambiguous genitalia should be noted if present.

Infectious viral gastroenteritis is a common cause of vomiting. Vomiting may be a nonspecific symptom of other infections including meningitis, pneumonia, and urinary tract infection, all of which require diagnostic work-up and often empirical antibiotic management.

Three Months to 2 Years. Viral gastroenteritis accounts for the vast majority of emesis in this age group. During the winter, rotavirus is epidemic in many regions and is frequently associated with familial or daycare exposure. These children develop fever, vomiting, and diarrhea. The physical examination and laboratory evaluation reflect the hydration status. Oral or IV fluids are usually curative, the exact management being determined by hydration, response, and ongoing losses.

Fever and vomiting without diarrhea should lead to consideration of meningitis, pneumonia, urinary tract infection, otitis media, and pharyngitis. The child in this age group may also have vomiting that is associated with respiratory disease. Children with bronchiolitis or reactive airway disease often vomit during acute episodes, presumably because of tachypnea and coughing (posttussive emesis).[94,95]

As in the neonate, the determination that an acute surgical abdomen exists is more important than the exact diagnosis.[96] Conditions to consider include intussusception, volvulus, and incarcerated inguinal hernia. Fever is usually not present early in the course of illness unless frank peritonitis occurs. The most common obstructive lesion in this age group is intussusception with telescoping of the bowel into itself, which results in ischemia and eventual infarction; this most often involves the ileocolic junction.[87]

Unrecognized esophageal foreign bodies or caustic ingestions (e.g., button batteries) may result in obstruction or stricture of the esophagus. This can lead to chronic emesis and inability to swallow solids, and sometimes liquids as well.

Ingestion of drugs or toxins may be associated with vomiting. Unintentional administration or the ongoing use of agents such as theophylline or erythromycin may cause vomiting. Several cases have actually been reported in which syrup of ipecac was administered to small children on a chronic basis.[97]

Anatomic or metabolic abnormalities often noted in infants may cause vomiting in this age group.

Two to 12 Years. The majority of children with vomiting will have an infectious cause with viral gastroenteritis being the most common. Other considerations must include meningitis, pneumonia, otitis media, pharyngitis, and urinary tract infection. Staphylococcal food poisoning or other ingested toxic may also be contributory.

In the last several years it has been recognized that peptic ulcer disease is associated with *Helicobacter pylori* infection or colonization. A wide variety of symptoms have been described, but one study demonstrated that hematemesis was more likely in patients subsequently proven to have *H. pylori* infection.[98] Effective therapy seems to require a combination of antibiotics, bismuth salicylate, and H_2 antagonists.[99]

Cyclic vomiting is a rare cause of severe recurrent emesis. Although the pathophysiology of this syndrome is not well understood, erythromycin has been shown to be effective in the management of these symptoms in one pediatric series.[100]

An acute appendicitis should also be considered. The presentation in the young child is often atypical, with nonspecific severe abdominal pain making perforation more likely before diagnosis.[101]

Metabolic disorders may be contributory. New-onset diabetes mellitus may occur with vomiting and dehydration, requiring an assessment of glucose metabolism for confirmation. An unfortunate scenario is the young child who has vomiting and abdominal pain and is diagnosed as having viral gastroenteritis, only to return later with severe ketoacidosis.

A central nervous system etiology of vomiting is a common cause of concern; trauma and tumor producing increased intracranial pressure are associated with vomiting. In the child who has experienced a closed head injury, vomiting is common. One study reported that posttraumatic emesis is more common in children over 2 years of age and in children who had eaten within 1 hour of the injury. The presence of skull fracture was not associated with an increased incidence of emesis; vomiting was more likely following minor head injury.[102]

Vomiting secondary to intracranial tumor is often prolonged over several weeks, usually occurring in the early morning or evening.[103] Patients may be well between episodes and usually have a weight loss. Obviously, meticulous examination and intracranial imaging studies are indicated.

Adolescents. The history in the adolescent is usually more useful once trust is established. The evaluation and diagnostic considerations can often be rapidly narrowed down. Acute infectious and surgical illnesses are common in this age group.

In the female, pregnancy and pelvic inflammatory disease must be considered. A thorough pelvic examination and pregnancy testing are indicated.

Vomiting may also be self-induced. Bulimia (binge-purge syndrome) is common, but frequently unrecognized as a cause of chronic vomiting. It may be associated with anorexia nervosa. In one study, 13% of teenagers reported purging behavior on a regular or occasional basis.[104] Eighty-seven percent of patients with binge-purge cycle behavior are female.[105] It is commonly seen in those attempting to control or lose weight. Unusual findings on physical examination include dental abnormalities secondary to deterioration of enamel, parotid enlargement, and even callous formation on the dorsum of the hand related to gagging oneself.[105] Laboratory evaluation may reveal hypokalemia and metabolic alkalosis.

Diagnostic Entities

ANORECTAL DISEASE

EVALINE A. ALESSANDRINI

Anal Fissure

Anal fissure is the most common proctologic disease of infants and children and the most frequent cause of rectal bleeding in the first year of life. One study found that 17% of all children with GI bleeding had an anal fissure as the cause.

Etiology. Anal fissures are usually associated with constipation. Tearing of the sensitive squamous anal mucosa occurs after passage of a hard stool. Subsequently, the child withholds stools to avoid pain, thus worsening the constipation and creating a vicious cycle. Anal fissures may also be seen after a bout of severe diarrhea with ensuing anal irritation.

Diagnostic Findings. A history of constipation is usually elicited from the parent. There may be blood streaks on the surface of the stools and defecation may be painful. Older children sometimes complain only of nonspecific abdominal pain.[106,107]

The diagnosis is made on physical examination. Direct inspection of the anus is facilitated by having the patient lie on his side with legs flexed and drawn towards the chest. The anal canal can be averted by gently spreading the skin of the perineum. Fissures appear as ½ to 1 cm longitudinal splits in the anal mucosa. In older children they are found mostly on the posterior aspect, whereas in infants they are often multiple and involve the anterior and lateral aspects of the anal canal as well. Some physicians find that inserting a clear test tube with lubricant into the anal opening facilitates visualization of deep fissures.

Differential Considerations. Because constipation often accompanies fissures, it is important to consider disease processes that cause constipation, such as congenital hypothyroidism, diabetes insipidus, or functional bowel obstruction. An anal fissure may be the first sign of Crohn disease in an older patient. Importantly, sexual abuse must be considered when evaluating an anal fissure, and an appropriate social history obtained and a careful examination of the genitalia performed.

Management. Management of acute, superficial anal fissures is conservative and consists primarily of improved anal hygiene and stool softening. Softening of stools can be achieved by increasing free water intake. Additionally, stool softeners, such as Karo syrup in infants or Maltsupex in older children, are effective (see Table 52-5). Twice-daily Sitz baths may be helpful. Application of emollient ointments (e.g., petroleum jelly) around the anus at each diaper change is also recommended. Occasionally, the fissure may cause such severe pain as to warrant application of topical anesthetics, but one must use these cautiously in order to avoid desensitization. Fissures that are not responsive to routine medical management may be superinfected with Group A beta-hemolytic streptococci, which can be treated with oral penicillin.

Very rarely, anal fissures become chronic and require fissurectomy with sphincterotomy or dilatation to eliminate scars and granulation tissue.[108] This procedure is not recommended for patients who are immunosuppressed because healing will be poor.

Perianal Abscess

A perianal abscess is an infection of the perianal glands and ducts. The latter originate from the bottom of the crypts of Morgagni (anal sinuses) near the distal rectum. There is often no clear etiology for these abscesses. However, chronic constipation or acute gastroenteritis can produce anal fissures that become superinfected and form abscesses in poorly draining perianal ducts.

Etiology. The majority of perianal abscesses are found in healthy boys less than 3 years of age. Immunosuppressed children are particularly likely to develop them. Cultures yield *S. aureus* and enteric organisms such as *E. coli*.

Diagnostic Findings. There is a history of anal redness and swelling, and the older child may complain of painful defecation. Intermittently, purulent discharge may be found in the diaper or underpants.

Physical examination may reveal fever, perianal edema, erythema, and induration that is 1 to 2 cm in size. Fluctuance evolves if the abscess is left untreated. Digital examination may demonstrate spread into the perirectal area.

Fistulae in ano, which is an extension of the abscess to the skin and to the inside of the anal canal, complicates 25% to 30% of perianal abscesses. In children, as opposed to adults, the fistulous tract is generally very straight. Symptoms of fistulae in ano include drainage of mucus and pus. Frequent exacerbations and remissions are the rule.[109]

Perianal abscesses may extend into deeper tissues and form ischiorectal abscesses. These are detectable by rectal palpation.

Differential Considerations. Perianal cellulitis due to Group A beta-hemolytic streptococcus may be confused with a perianal abscess. This type of cellulitis also includes symptoms of perianal erythema, edema, and tenderness. Often there is a history of a preceding streptococcal pharyngitis; perianal cultures are positive for streptococci. Perianal cellulitis can be treated orally with penicillin VK (25 to 50 mg/kg/24 hr QID PO).

Condyloma acuminatum, which is caused by the human papillomavirus, is often found in the perianal region. Although transmission from infected mothers at delivery does occur, this infection can result from sexual abuse, and an appropriate history, physical examination, and laboratory evaluation should be performed. Condyloma acuminatum in children can be attributed to maternal transmission when it is detected within the first 2 years of life in a child born vaginally.

Management. The abscess should be incised and drained and antibiotic therapy prescribed. Amoxicillin/clavulanate potassium (30 to 50 mg AMX/kg/24 hr TID PO) or cephalexin (25 to 50 mg/kg/24 hr QID PO) are good initial choices; subsequently, the antibiotic can be chosen based on culture results. Sitz baths and good perianal hygiene, in conjunction with stool softeners, are useful. Recurrences are rare unless the patient is immunocompromised.

Juvenile Polyps

Juvenile polyps should be considered in the differential diagnosis of lower gastrointestinal bleeding, particularly in school-aged children. These are pedunculated hamartomas and account for 90% of all gastrointestinal polyps in children. They can be single or multiple and are always benign. The peak incidence is in children 3 to 4 years of age. They are rare before 1 year of age, and, because most juvenile polyps autoamputate, they are also rare after the age of 15 years. Males are afflicted twice as often as females.

Diagnostic Findings. A history of bright red blood on the surface of the stool is the most common complaint. Usually the amount of bleeding is small, but occasionally it can be profuse. Juvenile polyps can also cause occult bleeding, resulting in anemia. Crampy abdominal pain may be reported due to traction on the polyp; occasionally, a colicocolic intussusception may result, with the polyp acting as the lead point. In other situations, the parent may even bring the polyp, found in the stool, to the physician.

The rectal examination is particularly important as 70% of juvenile polyps are found in the rectum and nearly half of these are palpable on digital examination.

Laboratory values may reveal anemia. Proctosigmoidoscopy is the method of choice for diagnosing suspected rectal juvenile polyps. Barium enema is useful if the history is less suggestive of polyps.

Differential Considerations. The various polyposis syndromes, such as Gardner and Peutz-Jeghers, should be considered in the case of multiple polyps because these have malignant potential. Some rectal juvenile polyps may prolapse from the anus and be misdiagnosed as hemorrhoids.

Management. Many juvenile polyps, especially the ones located distally in the GI tract, autoamputate as traction is placed upon them from formed stools. However, as soon as a polyp is found, the treatment indicated is polypectomy via colonoscopy after appropriate bowel preparation. The entire colon is visualized to rule out multiple polyps. In good hands, complications are rare and the prognosis is excellent because these polyps are benign.

Hemorrhoids

Hemorrhoids are varicosities of the rectal veins. They are unusual in children but somewhat more common in adolescents. Nearly all those found are external hemorrhoids, which are varicosities of the inferior rectal veins covered by skin. Internal hemorrhoids, which are varicosities of the superior rectal veins covered by mucosa, are part of the portal-caval system and are extremely rare in children.

Etiology. External hemorrhoids may occur with chronic constipation or be secondary to anal infections that spread to the inferior rectal veins. They also may be found with anorectal disease in Crohn disease.

Internal hemorrhoids occur in approximately one third of pediatric patients with portal hypertension. Extrahepatic causes of portal hypertension (e.g., portal vein occlusion) are more likely to result in hemorrhoids than intrahepatic etiologies (e.g., cirrhosis).[110]

Diagnostic Findings. Bleeding, anal pain, and hemorrhoidal prolapse are the most common symptoms. Hemorrhoids may be found on direct inspection or by anoscopy. They appear as small purple varicosities around the anus and may be single or multiple. Internal hemorrhoids are accompanied by other signs of portal hypertension such as angiomata of the skin and hepatosplenomegaly.

Differential Considerations. A perianal abscess, prolapsed rectal polyp, or rectal prolapse is often mistaken for a hemorrhoid and is more likely to be the correct diagnosis, at least in a young child.

Management. Conservative management is usually effective and includes stool softeners and sitz baths. Topical anesthetic ointments may be helpful on occasion. To decrease the spread of the buttocks, which can exacerbate the hemorrhoids, a child should use a child-sized toilet seat. Surgery is sometimes recommended for evacuation of painful thrombosed external hemorrhoids.

Rectal Prolapse

Rectal prolapse is an abnormal protrusion of the rectum through the anus. Partial prolapse involves the mucosa and submucosa and is most common in children who are less than 3 years of age.[111] Prolapse of the entire rectal wall is termed *procidentia* and occurs more frequently in older children, especially those with an underlying disease.

Etiology. In most cases of mucosal prolapse, the etiology is unknown. Diarrhea and straining with bowel movements are provoking factors.[112] *Clostridium difficile* infection has recently been described as an etiology of rectal prolapse.[112] It is hypothesized that rectal prolapse occurs more often in young children because they have recently assumed the erect position and their rectal musculature is still weak. Similarly, children with meningomyelocele, prune-belly syndrome, and exstrophy of the bladder are predisposed to rectal prolapse. Procidentia in an older child warrants an investigation for diseases associated with this condition, such as cystic fibrosis, rectal polyps, or illnesses associated with ascites or sustained cough.[109,114]

Diagnostic Findings. Rectal prolapse is diagnosed by history and physical examination. The parent reports a 1 to 2 cm protrusion from the anus during defecation. The prolapse is painless and may resolve spontaneously with relaxation. Stools may contain much mucus and small amounts of blood. On physical examination, mucosal prolapse appears as radial folds of mucosa protruding through the anus. True rectal procidentia is usually longer than an inch and exhibits circular rugal folds caused by contraction of the muscle fibers of the rectum. Severe or prolonged prolapse may result in edema and congestion of the involved segment of bowel, and although uncommon, ischemia of the involved segment.

Laboratory studies are generally not helpful, but a sweat chloride test can diagnose cystic fibrosis. Performing a barium enema to exclude polyps or other rectal lesions may disclose a precipitating cause.

Management. Most rectal prolapses resolve spontaneously, and these respond to simple measures and time.

Stool softeners such as mineral oil help avoid straining. A child toilet seat is recommended, as with hemorrhoids, to reduce spread of the gluteal folds. Some prolapses require manual reduction, which is achieved best with sedation, elevation of the buttocks, and bimanual reduction using gauze for better grip of the mucosa.

If there is no response to conservative measures, surgery is warranted. Phenol and glycerin or 30% saline injections around the rectal wall cause fibrosis of the perirectal tissues, and many authors report an excellent success rate. Alternatively, sutures may be used subcutaneously around the perianal area. Major surgical procedures as performed on adults are rarely necessary in children.[114]

BILIARY TRACT DISEASE

JAMES M. CHAMBERLAIN

The biliary tract consists of the intrahepatic bile canaliculi and bile ducts, and the extrahepatic duct system. The extrahepatic system starts with the right and left hepatic ducts, which join to form the common hepatic duct. The common hepatic duct then meets the cystic duct from the gallbladder to form the common bile duct, which ends at the sphincter of Oddi in the duodenum. The precise location of the union of this system with the pancreatic duct is variable.

The gallbladder is a hollow pear-shaped organ with walls of smooth muscle and fibrous tissue. The lumen is lined with epithelium containing cholesterol and fat globules. Mucus is formed and secreted by the alveolar glands lining the infundibulum.

Motor nerve supply is via the vagus nerve and postganglionic fibers from the celiac ganglion. Sensory fibers course with the sympathetic nerves through the celiac plexus to T_8 and T_9 spinal roots on the right. As with the other hollow viscera, pain may be caused by distension or ischemia. Acute distension of the common bile duct causes colicky abdominal pain, whereas gradual distension with identical pressures causes a vague feeling of distress without colic.[115] Inflammation contributes to pain by causing dysfunctional peristalsis, by lowering the pain threshold, and by causing congestion, which worsens the ischemia. Pain originating in the biliary tract may be referred to the back in the T_6 to T_{10} distribution.[116]

Pathophysiology. The gallbladder secretes, stores, and concentrates bile. Bile is the main vehicle in which bilirubin cholesterol and the metabolic products of several hormones are excreted. The secretion of bile is controlled by complex humoral and neurogenic mechanisms. The gallbladder concentrates bile tenfold; mucus production protects the mucosa from the irritant effects of the concentrated bile. The main stimulus to empty the gallbladder is cholecystokinin, which is produced in response to food in the duodenum. Emptying of the gallbladder requires coordination of contractions of the gallbladder with relaxation of the sphincter of Oddi.[117]

Bilirubin, the breakdown product of heme, is conjugated by glucuronyl transferase in the liver. Excretion of this conjugated (direct) bilirubin is the rate-limiting step in elimination. Interference with excretion of conjugated bilirubin causes it to back up, leaking into the serum. Thus liver diseases in general and biliary tract diseases usually lead to an elevation of predominantly conjugated rather than unconjugated (indirect) bilirubin. Only with massive hepatic damage will hepatocyte dysfunction cause a predominant rise in unconjugated bilirubin. Differentiation of hepatic vs. biliary tract disease, therefore, is marked elevation of liver transaminases (signifying hepatocyte damage) in the former.

Cholelithiasis and Acute Cholecystitis

Complications of gallstones represent a common cause of abdominal pain in adult patients who come to emergency departments. In contrast, the pediatrician is far less likely to encounter patients with this disorder. Cholelithiasis is defined as gallstones in the gallbladder or cystic duct; choledocholithiasis is defined as stones in the common duct. Cholecystitis is inflammation of the gallbladder and is usually caused by stones impacting in the cystic duct. Acalculous cholecystitis, or inflammation without gallstones, will be discussed below.

Pathophysiology. There are two types of gallstones commonly seen in the United States: cholesterol stones and bile pigment stones. Both types contain calcium, cholesterol, and bile pigments in varying proportions. The suspension of cholesterol in bile depends on the formation of micelles and is effected by a fine balance between the concentrations of bile acid, cholesterol, and lecithin.[118] If bile acids or lecithin are too low or the cholesterol is too high, cholesterol will crystallize out of solution, predisposing the patient to stone formation. Low bile acids are important in the formation of stones associated with cystic fibrosis and regional enteritis, whereas high cholesterol is the primary cause in obese patients.[119,120] Mechanical or functional stasis from previous stones or from neurogenic causes (e.g., autonomic neuropathy in diabetes mellitus) contributes to the formation of gallstones. Other factors that may be involved include genetic predisposition, infection, and reflux of pancreatic juices into the gallbladder.[115] Bile pigment stones occur in the presence of increased red blood cell destruction and bilirubin metabolism.

The association of cholelithiasis with pregnancy is controversial but cholestasis occurs in some women during the third trimester, and several studies have identified recent pregnancy as the most frequent predisposing factor for cholecystitis in adolescents.[115,121-124] There is an increased risk of gallstones in women taking oral contraceptives.[125]

The etiology of gallstones in children can be divided into three groups on the basis of age. Adolescents form gallstones chiefly because of pregnancy, obesity, and hemolytic disease. Younger children most commonly have gallstones on the basis of hemolytic disease. Gallstones in infants occur predominantly in intensive care–nursery patients or graduates and are associated with total parenteral nutrition, abdominal surgery, sepsis, and necrotizing enterocolitis.[126]

Diagnostic Findings. The clinical findings in patients with gallstones are variable. Many patients are asymptomatic for long periods.[127] Patients with cholecystitis complain of abdominal pain as the most frequent symptom, followed by nausea or vomiting. The pain is epigastric or in the right upper quadrant in most children and radiates to the back in about one third.[121-124,128,129] Young patients, however, may be unable to localize the pain to the right upper quadrant.[130] Occasional patients will have atypical locations such as the right lower quadrant.[121]

Patients with gallstones may have recurring episodes of colicky pain associated with fatty foods or may seek medical attention after their first episode. Acute inflammation, which is present with cholecystitis, adds a persistent nature to the pain, so that patients may have a mixed picture of colic and persistent severe pain. In uncomplicated cases, inflammation subsides with gradual resolution of pain over 12 to 18 hours.[120]

Nausea and vomiting are frequent symptoms in patients with cholecystitis.[121,122,124,128,129] Abdominal pain generally precedes vomiting.[118] A history of fatty food intolerance and dyspepsia is present in many cases.[122,124,128,131-133] Low-grade fever is common.

The physical examination with acute cholecystitis usually demonstrates tenderness in the right upper quadrant. Guarding may be present. A palpable mass is present in 25% to 50% of cases.[124,133,134] Jaundice, either on presentation or by history, occurs in up to a third of patients.[122,124,132] In older children, one may attempt to elicit Murphy's sign: ask the patient to inspire while placing the fingers under the liver border. Inspiration is arrested by painful contact of the descending gallbladder with the examiner's fingers.

Complications. Dehydration and electrolyte abnormalities can occur if vomiting is severe. Atelectasis and pneumonia may result from splinting respirations or intraoperative manipulation. Pancreatitis occurs when stones lodge in the common duct and obstruct pancreatic outflow. The most serious risk of acute cholecystitis is necrosis with perforation, but this is rare in children. Diagnosis of perforation will be made at laparotomy in most instances; the diagnosis should be considered if the patient develops signs of peritonitis or if pain, tenderness, and fever fail to subside with conservative medical management. Blood loss and wound infection are possible complications of surgery.

Ancillary Data. Patients with acute cholecystitis often have leukocytosis, and a predominance of neutrophil, mild elevations in alkaline phosphatase or transaminases, and hyperbilirubinemia occur in up to one third of patients.[122,124,132,134] The degree of hyperbilirubinemia does not correlate with the presence of common duct stones.[128] Serum or urinary amylase may also be elevated in some children.

Plain abdominal roentgenograms will show calcified gallstones in approximately 15% of symptomatic adults.[120] The frequency may be as high as 40% to 56% in young children because of higher proportions of calcium bilirubinate in the stones.[121,126,129,132,135] Adolescent females are like adults in this regard because their stones are predominantly made up of cholesterol.[124,133]

Ultrasonography is currently the best emergent modality to support the diagnosis of acute cholecystitis caused by gallstones.[136] In adults, sonography has a sensitivity of 90% to 98% for detecting gallstones or evidence of inflammation (e.g., wall thickening, enlargement, round shape). The specificity varies from 70% to 98% because stones may be visualized that may not be causing acute symptoms and

TABLE 52-12. Features Distinguishing Acute Cholecystitis from Other Diseases

Differential consideration	Distinguishing features
Right lower lobe pneumonia	Abnormal chest roentgenogram
Hepatitis	Markedly elevated transaminases
Peptic ulcer disease	Anemia, positive stool guiac
Pancreatitis	Elevated amylase and lipase, hypocalcemia
Fitz-Hugh-Curtis syndrome	Abnormal pelvic examination
Nephrolithiasis	Hematuria, abnormal roentgenogram
Pyelonephritis	Pyuria, bacteriuria

sonography cannot demonstrate cystic duct obstruction, which is the sine qua non of acute calculous cholecystitis.[136,137] Nevertheless, ultrasound provides rapid indirect evidence supporting the diagnosis of cholecystitis; it is safe, noninvasive, and can be performed on most patients. Cholescintigraphy with ^{99m}Tc-IDA is the procedure of choice for definitively demonstrating cystic duct obstruction but cannot be performed rapidly in the emergency department.[136,138,139]

Differential Considerations. In patients with sickle cell hemoglobinopathies, acute cholecystitis must be differentiated from abdominal pain crisis. The localization of the pain and tenderness of cholecystitis to the right upper quadrant should be helpful, although the differentiation from hepatic crisis may be difficult without sonography.[140] Hepatic crisis generally causes greater rises in serum transaminases. A history of intermittent colicky pain in the past suggests cholelithiasis.

In atypical cases, the differentiation from appendicitis may be difficult, but DeDombal demonstrated that movement aggravated pain in only 6% of adults with acute cholecystitis as opposed to 57% of those with appendicitis.[141] Appendicitis also has a more progressive course in general.[142]

Other disorders in the differential diagnosis include renal stones, pyelonephritis, right lower lobe pneumonia, hepatitis, Fitz-Hugh-Curtis syndrome (associated with pelvic inflammatory disease), pancreatitis, and peptic ulcer disease. In addition to differences in the history and physical examination, some of the distinguishing characteristics of these diseases are presented in Table 52-12. Admission and further testing are often necessary to differentiate cholecystitis from pancreatitis and peptic ulcer disease.

Management. Patients with cholecystitis should be admitted for observation, pain control, and fluid resaturation and management. After acute inflammation has subsided in 48 to 72 hours, cholecystectomy can be performed more safely.[120] An exciting new treatment is the use of percutaneously applied shock waves (lithotripsy) to fragment gallstones; this technique may preclude the need for surgery. This technology is still in its infancy and is undergoing clinical trials.[143] No data are available in children.

Children with cholecystitis generally do well. Perforation is rare and surgery is well tolerated. Even patients with sickle cell hemoglobinopathies will tolerate cholecystectomy with few complications if adequate preparations are made before surgery.[144]

Acalculous Cholecystitis

The clinical presentation of children with acalculous cholecystitis is similar to children with cholecystitis caused by gallstones; however, the predisposing factors are different. Acalculous disease is usually associated with acute systemic disturbances such as burns, sepsis, or dehydration. Infections with *Salmonella typhi*, *Shigella*, or intestinal parasites such as *Ascaris* are also associated.[127] Physical examination and results of diagnostic tests are similar to calculus cholecystitis except that sonography will demonstrate signs of inflammation in the absence of calculi. In addition, the differential diagnosis includes gallbladder hydrops (see next section).

Treatment is similar to that of acute calculous cholecystitis, with specific attention to the underlying etiology.

Hydrops of the Gallbladder

Acute noncalculous distension of the gallbladder without inflammation occurs rarely and almost exclusively in children.[127]

Frequently there is an underlying or predisposing illness such as an upper respiratory infection or gastroenteritis. In addition, hydrops is associated with leptospirosis and Kawasaki disease.[145] The etiology of hydrops is unclear but it may be caused by mesenteric adenitis in some cases.[146] A review of 46 cases associated with Kawasaki disease revealed that the clinical findings of gallbladder hydrops were similar to those of acute cholecystitis except that more (40%) had jaundice with hydrops.[147] In addition, a right upper quadrant mass is more frequent and occurs in 75% to 100% of cases.[146-148]

Sonography reveals a markedly enlarged gallbladder without calculi. The differentiation of this disorder from acute acalculous cholecystitis can be difficult if the results of sonography and scintigraphy are at all equivocal.[149] The use of CT scan may be helpful in this situation.[150]

Treatment is conservative in most cases but laparotomy may be necessary for impending or actual perforation or when the diagnosis is unclear.[146,147,151]

Acute Cholangitis

Acute cholangitis is an infection within the biliary tree and is largely a disease of the elderly. However, it may be seen in children following biliary surgery.

FOREIGN BODY INGESTIONS

ROBERT A. BELFER

Children commonly ingest foreign bodies. Fortunately, most pass through the gastrointestinal tract and infrequently cause problems.

The majority of foreign body ingestions occur in children between the ages of 6 months and 6 years. Young children are especially prone because:

1. They tend to mouth objects while exploring their environment
2. They lack the proper dentition to crush small hard foods
3. Their protective oral reflexes are less developed, allowing objects in their mouths to slip into the esophagus more easily[152]

Because toddlers do not report such incidents, they are particularly likely to have symptoms of unknown etiology, and the possibility of a foreign body should always be kept in mind.

Pathophysiology

The majority of foreign bodies in the gastrointestinal tract lodge in the esophagus, the narrowest region except for the appendix.[153] There are three areas of physiologic narrowing in the esophagus: the upper esophageal sphincter (cricopharyngeus), the midportion at the level of the aortic arch, and the lower esophageal sphincter at the diaphragmatic inlet. The most common location for an esophageal foreign body is at the cricopharyngeus. Foreign bodies tend to lodge at the cricopharyngeus because strong propulsive pharyngeal muscles force the object to this point, and weaker esophageal muscles cannot propel it further. The alignment is typically coronal. Preexisting abnormalities of the esophagus and extrinsic esophageal compression from vascular rings can cause ingested material that would normally pass through the esophagus to become lodged in the esophagus. Approximately 60% of all ingested foreign bodies pass through the esophagus to the stomach. Once a foreign body has reached the stomach, it has an 80% to 90% chance of traversing the gut without problems, usually within 7 to 10 days. Past the stomach, potential sites of impediment include the pylorus, the duodenal sweep, the ileocecal valve, and the anus. Less than 1% perforate the gut; the ileocecal valve is the most common site of perforation.[154]

The pathophysiology of gastrointestinal foreign body ingestion is dependent upon the age of the child, the type and size of the foreign body, the length of time it has been in place, and the exact anatomic location. The risk of impaction in the esophagus increases with a younger patient age and a larger object, especially with button batteries. In general, the longer a foreign body has been lodged in the gastrointestinal tract the greater the tissue reaction. When it remains for some period of time, it is harder to extract and complications arise more frequently. Smooth, slippery objects pose little problem and tend to travel through the gastrointestinal tract without incident. Foreign bodies that are sharp or pointed are especially worrisome because of the risk of perforation.

Etiology

Coins are the most common esophageal foreign bodies in the United States (Fig. 52-3).[155,156] Food, a common esophageal foreign body in adults, is uncommon in children if the esophagus is otherwise normal. The incidence of ingestion of safety pins has decreased with the rise in popularity of disposable diapers. The dramatic rise in plastics manufacturing has led to increasing ingestions of materials that pose diagnostic challenges due to their radiolucency and

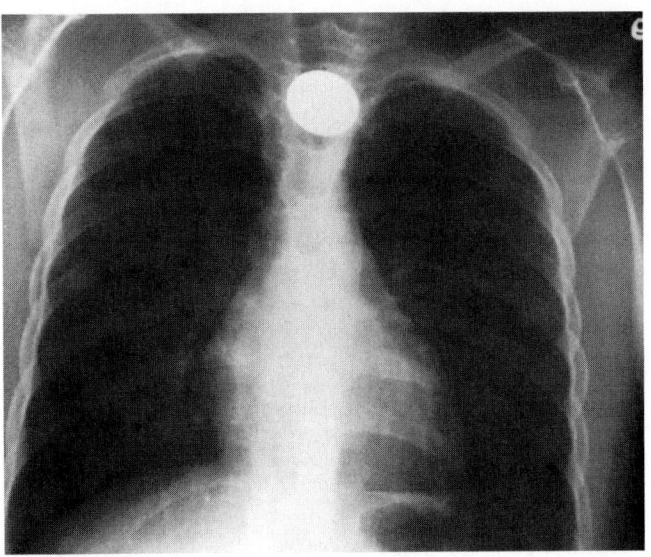

FIG. 52-3. Coin lodged in the proximal esophagus in the coronal position.

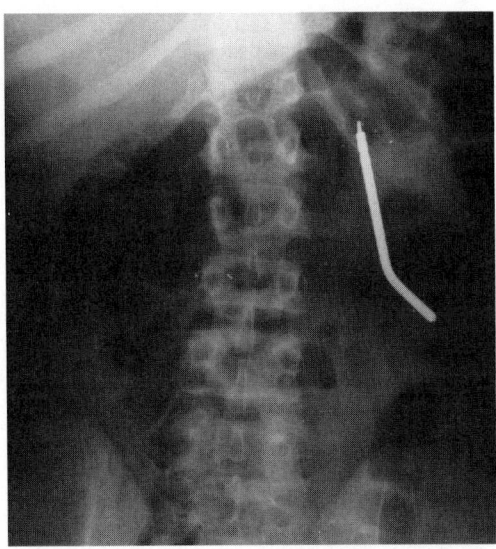

FIG. 52-4. Dental instrument, accidentally swallowed, located in the small intestine.

inertness. The incidence of button battery ingestions from hearing aids, watches, and games has also increased in recent years.

Diagnostic Findings

Clinical Findings. Specific manifestations depend on the type of foreign body, its location, and the length of time that has elapsed since ingestion. Most ingestions are unwitnessed; thus the history may be negative or misleading in over half of all cases.[155] The most common symptoms of an esophageal foreign body include refusal to feed, increased salivation, vomiting, and pain or discomfort with swallowing. These initial symptoms may subside and be followed by a relatively asymptomatic period. The predominately liquid and soft diets of children sometimes allow them to go months before obstruction becomes manifest. In 1950, Jackson and Jackson reviewed 1400 cases of aerodigestive foreign bodies and found that a significant number had been overlooked for periods of 1 month to 4 years.[157] The primary reason for this delay in diagnosis was failure of the clinician to consider the possibility of a foreign body.

The majority of foreign bodies in the stomach are asymptomatic. Pain, fever, bleeding, or vomiting suggests pyloric obstruction or mucosal disruption. In the intestine, angulations at the duodenal sweep, ligament of Treitz, terminal ileum, ileocecal valve, and sigmoid colon are potential sites of obstruction. Fortunately, this rarely occurs; once in the intestine nearly all foreign bodies pass without problem (Fig. 52-4).

Complications. Esophageal foreign bodies can cause signs and symptoms that simulate respiratory disorders such as asthma, croup, bronchitis, or pneumonia.[158] If the foreign body is large and compresses the trachea, the child may have symptoms referable to both the airway (e.g., cough, stridor, wheeze) and esophagus (e.g., drooling, food refusal, weight loss). In addition to direct compression of the trachea, symptoms may be due to periesophageal in-

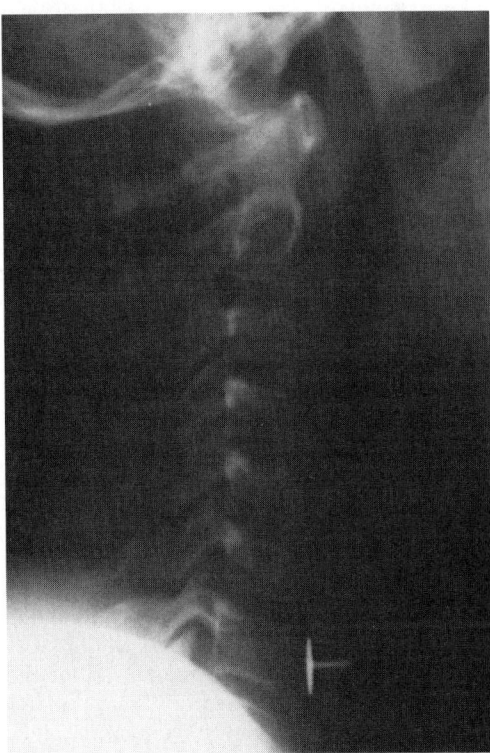

FIG. 52-5. Thumb tack located in upper esophagus.

flammation from the retained foreign body. Furthermore, recurrent aspiration secondary to esophageal obstruction may lead to pneumonia, bronchiectasis, or lung abscess.

Most esophageal perforations are caused by sharp objects although pressure erosion by smooth objects can produce perforation (Fig. 52-5). The majority of perforations are rapidly symptomatic, producing fever, pain, and dysphagia.

Long-standing esophageal foreign bodies may result in secondary infection with erosion, leading to perforation, stricture formation, or rarely, tracheoesophageal fistula.[159] Other less frequent complications of esophageal foreign bodies include mediastinitis, cardiac tamponade, and aortic aneurysm. Rarely, intestinal foreign bodies cause obstruction, hemorrhage, or perforation.

Button batteries may cause esophageal mucosal injury due to liquefaction necrosis from the leakage of alkali and via the production of an electrochemical burn by direct current from the battery. The incidence of complications is less than 1%, yet morbidity from strictures or perforations is significant. Button batteries in the stomach are usually asymptomatic, although endoscopy has shown evidence of superficial ulcers even in asymptomatic patients.[160]

Radiologic Studies. Radiologic evaluation can be extremely useful and help locate many foreign bodies. All patients suspected of harboring an esophageal foreign body should undergo posteroanterior and lateral neck radiographs and a chest radiograph. Neck films will rule-out any radiopaque object in the hypopharynx, whereas the chest x-ray will detect the presence of coins, batteries, and other radiopaque objects and will locate their position. These films can also evaluate the presence of mediastinal or subcutaneous air.[161] If endoscopy is delayed, films should be repeated just prior to attempted retrieval in order to demonstrate any distal migration of the object. Diagnosing a radiolucent foreign body is much more difficult. The chest and lateral soft tissue neck radiographs are often normal, and careful fluoroscopic studies including barium examination of the esophagus may be necessary for diagnosis. Esophagrams can demonstrate radiolucent foreign bodies through persistent filling defects.

Button batteries have a distinctive appearance on radiography with a "double-density" on PA view and a "step-off" at the junction of the cathode and anode on lateral view.[160]

Metal detectors have been shown to be viable alternatives to radiography in the clinical detection and localization of metallic foreign body ingestions. Metal detectors represent a simple and safe method of eliminating ionizing radiation exposure and reducing the patient expense associated with coin ingestions. In addition, metal detectors may be an effective alternative to repeat radiographs in patients requiring reevaluation of coin location before therapeutic interventions.[162-164]

CT scanning, although not routinely used for the evaluation of an esophageal foreign body, may be helpful in delineating adjacent soft tissue inflammation and abscess formation. MRI, with its superb soft tissue resolution, may play an increasing role in demonstrating periesophageal pathology. The clinician must keep in mind that negative imaging procedures do not rule out a foreign body.

Serial plain films of the abdomen are useful in locating and monitoring the progress of foreign bodies in the stomach and intestines. When suspicious of perforation, water-soluble contrast studies can be done to rule out a leak.

Management

Several methods are used for the removal of blunt esophageal foreign bodies including esophagoscopy in the operating room, flexible esophagoscopy in the outpatient setting, and the fluoroscopic foley catheter technique. A major concern during removal of an esophageal foreign body is protection of the airway. Some believe that the safest method for retrieval of an esophageal foreign body is under general anesthesia with a protected airway.[156] Esophagoscopy in the operating room has traditionally been the technique of choice for removal of impacted esophageal foreign bodies.

Fluoroscopic foley catheter techniques avoid the risks and costs of general anesthesia, operating room esophagoscopy, and hospitalization. Controversy regarding this technique stems from its safety. Risks include lack of control when the object passes through the hypopharynx and aspiration when done without airway control.[165,166] Schunk's review of an 11-year experience with this technique showed success rates of 96% when blunt objects were impacted in the esophagus for less than 3 days.[167] The magnitude of the risks associated with this technique has been debated in the literature and appears to depend on the expertise available at a given institution.[161]

If lodged in the upper or middle third of the esophagus, esophageal foreign bodies require immediate removal because of the risk of aspiration and the unlikelihood of passing them into the stomach. A possible exception to the need for immediate removal is when a small rounded object is swallowed and is in the distal third of the esophagus. In asymptomatic patients, an observation period of 12 to 24 hours may be warranted; there is a high likelihood that the object will spontaneously pass into the stomach without problems.[154,168]

The major indications for removal of foreign bodies in the stomach and proximal duodenum are failure of progression and risk of perforation. Since most pass through the remainder of the gastrointestinal tract without any problem, stomach foreign bodies can be managed conservatively. If an object remains in the stomach for several days, it may become embedded in the gastric wall. It is advisable to remove the object if no progress is made after 3 to 7 days. A conservative approach is also recommended in all cases of foreign bodies lodged in the intestine except when complications develop.

Management recommendations for sharp object ingestions distal to the gastroesophageal junction vary considerably. Asymptomatic ingestions can be managed on an individual basis.[169] If symptomatic, surgical or gastrointestinal consultation for endoscopy or laparotomy is indicated. Surgical removal is recommended for perforations or if the foreign body does not progress in the lower gastrointestinal tract.

The lodging of button batteries in the esophagus may lead to mucosal damage and full-thickness mucosal necrosis necessitating immediate removal. Endoscopic removal of the battery in the operating room permits evaluation of the extent of mucosal injury. Steroids and antibiotics have no role in the treatment of esophageal mucosal burns from a button battery.[170] Although exposure to gastric acid is associated with a remote risk of leakage, virtually all button batteries that reach the stomach pass spontaneously without any complications.[171] Daily abdominal x-rays are recommended to demonstrate progression from the stomach.

The majority of batteries that have passed the pylorus pass through the gut without problem.[171] Indications for endoscopy or surgery include esophageal location, fixation to the stomach or gut mucosa for a prolonged period, and signs of peritonitis.[170]

Cathartics, stool softeners, whole bowel irrigation, and special diets are of no proven benefit in the management of most foreign bodies.[172]

GASTROENTERITIS, ACUTE INFECTIOUS

DOUGLAS A. BOENNING

Acute infectious diarrhea is second only to cardiovascular disease worldwide as a cause of death. In many parts of the world, it is the leading cause of childhood mortality. Public health officials estimate that more than 12,000 children die each day from diarrheal disease in Asia, Africa, and Latin America. The United States averages 1.5 to 1.9 diarrheal illnesses/person annually, with young children experiencing 2 to 3.2 diarrheal episodes/year, and up to 5 illnesses if attending daycare centers.

The management and disposition of children with acute infectious gastroenteritis can be distilled into a few issues. Acute management is based upon the relative severity of dehydration and toxicity of the child. The other central question is whether antimicrobial or antiparasitic agents will be useful given the particular etiology of the diarrhea. Rarely are radiologic studies indicated, except when the possibility exists of a surgical abdomen (e.g., obstruction, appendicitis, volvulus, or intussusception) (also see section on Diarrhea).

Pathophysiology

The intestine is designed for absorption of digestive material. Visible redundant folds in the lumen and microscopic outpouchings (villi) vastly increase the surface area available for absorption and secretion. The lumen of the adult intestine has a surface area of 400 m^2.

Infectious agents produce diarrhea by interfering with intestinal absorption and secretion of fluids and electrolytes. Surface area is decreased by viral destruction of mucosal cells. This results in a loss of digestive enzymes located on cell surfaces. Many bacterial pathogens produce toxins that promote fluid secretion into the gut lumen, blocking some absorptive functions. Increased osmolality of luminal fluid and altered transit time also lead to production of frequent watery stools.

Stool characteristics have been reported to be pathognomonic for specific etiologies. However, many symptoms of viral, bacterial, and protozoal diarrhea overlap and are indistinguishable. The gold standard in diagnosis is culture for bacterial pathogens, immunoassays for viral agents, or direct microscopy for identification of parasites. Immunoassays are under development for rapid diagnosis of some bacterial and protozoal agents. A few clues may aid in the presumptive diagnosis; knowledge of local epidemiology is invaluable (i.e., geographic predilection of organisms, seasonal influences, reported outbreaks, and relative presence of pathogen isolation).[173,174] Characteristics of the host are important including age, immunocompetence, personal hygiene, travel, and exposure to ill contacts at home or in a daycare center. Gastric acidity provides an important barrier because most pathogens are killed at a normal gastric pH (<4); achlorhydric stomachs do not have a similar effect. Normal intestinal motility is essential for the absorptive process and to maintain distribution of enteric flora.[175-177]

Specific Diagnostic Patterns

Viral Agents. Viral diarrhea accounts for 30% to 40% of all infectious diarrhea in the United States and 80% in children. Viral diarrhea is second only to the common cold in episodic illnesses affecting families.[178]

Rotavirus. Rotavirus accounts for 30% to 60% of all episodes of severe diarrhea in young children. The peak incidence of the disease is between 3 and 15 months of life, and older children and adults can have a milder form of disease after close contact with an infected infant. The virus attacks mature enterocytes on the tips of the small intestinal villi. Pancreatic trypsin cleaves a viral surface protein VP-4 in the lumen of the small intestine, which allows the virus to enter intestinal cells. Cells are lysed, causing villi to shorten and crypt cells to enlarge. The infection spreads from the proximal small bowel to the ileum over 1 to 2 days. Carbohydrate malabsorption occurs within the gut lumen, leading to osmotic diarrhea during rotaviral infection. Rotavirus is spread by the fecal-oral route and usually occurs in the winter months in temperature climates, which is commonly from October to May in the United States.

The typical illness lasts for 5 to 7 days with fever and vomiting preceding the onset of diarrhea as hallmarks of illness. Bloody diarrhea is uncommon; stools are commonly loose and relatively frequent (>5 stools/day). In the young infant, fluid losses from vomiting and diarrhea often necessitate hospitalization to correct dehydration and treat ongoing losses. Respiratory symptoms may be noted.

Toxic children should have a baseline CBC and electrolytes. A rapid immunoassay is available for the rotavirus antibody. Diagnosis may be confirmed by electron microscopy.

A vaccine for rotavirus is under development, with some attenuated animal strains conferring immunity in children.[179]

Norwalk Virus. The Norwalk virus and Norwalk-like agents (named for the sites of an outbreak) are small, round-structured viruses that may belong to the calicivirus family. These viruses are responsible for 40% of gastroenteritis outbreaks that affect older children or adults in schools, camps, institutions, or cruise ships. The viruses are isolated year round and cause low levels of "background" infection in individuals until the infected patient contaminates a common source and an epidemic occurs. Transmission occurs via person-to-person spread, airborne droplets, contaminated swimming water, and contaminated food (undercooked food, shellfish, salads, and cake frosting).

After a 12 to 48 hour incubation period, the illness is characterized by nonbloody, mild diarrhea, vomiting, abdominal cramps, and marked nausea secondary to delayed gastric emptying. One quarter of patients report fever, chills, headache, and myalgias. The illness lasts 12 to 60 hours but the patient remains infective for up to 2 days following resolution of symptoms. Malabsorption of lactose and fat can occur for up to 2 weeks.

Adenovirus. After rotavirus, enteric adenovirus is the next most common cause of viral gastroenteritis in young children and is responsible for 4% to 10% of inpatient and outpatient cases. Serotypes 40, 41, and 31 cause enteric disease predominantly in children who are under the age of 2 years. Transmission is person-to-person without seasonality. Incubation ranges from 3 to 10 days, and the illness lasts an average of 5 to 12 days, both of longer duration than other viral diarrheas. Symptoms include watery diarrhea followed by mild vomiting for 1 to 2 days. Fever is low grade, averaging 38° C and lasts for 2 to 3 days. Respiratory symptoms are rarely part of the infection. Asymptomatic shedding occurs in only 2% of cases. The presumptive diagnosis is made with electron microscopy and confirmed with DNA analysis or specific monoclonal antibody immunoassays. Treatment is supportive.[180]

Calicivirus. Calicivirus causes a self-limited illness similar to rotavirus A infection: diarrhea, vomiting, abdominal pain, possible fever, and upper respiratory symptoms. Like rotavirus A, most people develop antibody to calicivirus in early childhood. Two strains of calicivirus share immunologic properties with Norwalk virus. Three to five serologically distinct strains of calicivirus exist. Diagnosis is made by electron microscopy or immunoassay.

Children between the ages of 3 months and 6 years are primarily affected. The illness lasts an average of 4 days after a 1 to 3 days incubation. Person-to-person transmission is presumed in institutional outbreaks with a 50% to 70% attack rate, although drinking water, cold food, and shellfish have been implicated as vehicles of transmission. Calicivirus comprises 3% of cases of daycare center diarrhea and hospitalized children with gastroenteritis. No seasonal peaks are reported, and some infections may be asymptomatic. Supportive management is essential.

Astrovirus. Five serotypes of astrovirus cause a short illness less severe than rotavirus that is characterized by watery diarrhea, vomiting, fever, and abdominal pain. Children from infancy to 7 years of age are predominantly affected. This organism comprised 4% of hospitalized cases of gastroenteritis in the United Kingdom. Over two thirds of British children have antibody to this virus by the age of 4. A winter peak of infectivity is likely. Transmission is from person-to-person and contaminated water and shellfish have been reported vehicles. A kindergarten outbreak affected 50% of children, and one third of their families had members who became infected. Incubation is short (24 to 36 hours) with the illness lasting only 1 to 4 days. Asymptomatic shedding has been reported.[181]

Bacterial Agents

Campylobacter. Campylobacter infections are caused by *C. jejuni* or *C. coli*. Campylobacter is the leading cause of bacterial gastroenteritis in the United States. It was known primarily as a veterinary pathogen for many years until the advent of selective culture medium in the 1970s leading to the recognition of its important role in human disease. Newborn puppies and food sources such as chicken and turkeys are important reservoirs for the organ-

ism. The virus is transmitted person-to-person or pet-to-person. The incubation period is 2 to 5 days.

The illness is characterized by fever and severe abdominal cramping. Bloody diarrhea is a frequent component of the illness. Although the patient may be asymptomatic, the onset of illness can be marked by high fever, myalgia, headaches, abdominal cramps, and vomiting. Diarrhea is profusely watery, mucousy, and bloody. Leukocytes are common in the stool.

Symptoms often resolve spontaneously over 3 to 4 days; treatment should be based on the need to eradicate the organism from the feces. Children attending daycare centers deserve treatment that has been shown to be effective in eliminating the organism from the stools. Treatment with erythromycin during the illness has been generally found to have no significant effect on the severity or duration of the diarrhea or the abdominal pain. The usefulness of erythromycin may be confined to patients with the dysenteric form of the illness. No accurate, rapid diagnostic test exists for diagnosing *Campylobacter* infections. Some laboratories have touted the ability of a microscopic examination to identify motile, comma-shaped gram-negative organisms but this test is of questionable sensitivity.[182]

Salmonella. Salmonella gastroenteritis is caused by two species of *Salmonella*: *S. enteritidis* (over 1700 biotypes) and *S. choleraesuis* (one biotype). This infection is an important cause of bacterial diarrhea in infants, especially in urban areas of the United States. The reservoirs for the organisms are animals, contaminated food or water, and humans. Animals that are frequently incriminated include poultry, pet turtles, and livestock, which may develop multiply resistant organisms from antibiotics in their feeds. Foods such as chicken, eggs, unpasteurized milk, and cantaloupes (presumably grown on contaminated soil) have all been linked to outbreaks. Transmission occurs by ingestion or via the fecal-oral route in person-to-person transmission. The incubation period is usually less than 24 hours but ranges from 6 to 72 hours. The minimum infective dose is 10^6 to 10^8 organisms. The highest attack rate occurs in children who are under 1 year old. Many children will have a prolonged carrier state causing particular problems if they are enrolled in a daycare center. In contrast to some other enteropathogens, *Salmonella* has a predilection for developed countries.

The illness is characterized by fever, watery diarrhea, and stools that may show streaks of blood or test positive for occult blood. It primarily affects children under 5 years of age. Symptoms of fever, vomiting, and diarrhea begin 24 to 48 hours after exposure, diminishing over 3 to 5 days. Young children appear to be prone to developing extraintestinal complications with penetration of the lamina propria; bacteremia, osteomyelitis, septic arthritis, endocarditis, pneumonia, urinary tract infection, and meningitis have been reported. Children under 1 year of age and those who have sickle cell disease or other hemoglobinopathies or immunoincompetence are at increased risk of developing septicemia. Older children may have abdominal pain, which is often confused with acute appendicitis.

Suspected *Salmonella* infections occurring in infants 3 months and younger or those with significant toxicity, deserve hospital admission and treatment with IV antibiotics.

Older infants and children with fever and bloody diarrhea who appear to be candidates for outpatient management, merit a blood culture in addition to stool culture. Beyond infancy, treatment with antibiotics, either IV or oral, may prolong the carrier state of the organism or lead to development of antibiotic resistance by the *Salmonella*.

S. typhi causes severe, prolonged disease with gastroenteritis associated with fever, malaise, headache, and myalgias. Hepatosplenomegaly and rose spots (2 mm maculopapular lesions) may appear.

Shigella. *Shigella* gastroenteritis is caused by four species of the organism: *S. sonnei, S. flexneri, S. dysenteriae,* and *S. boydii.* The first two species cause most infections in developed countries. Epidemics of dysentery in developing countries are frequently caused by the *S. dysenteriae* serotype. In warmer regions of the United States such as the Southwest, *Shigella* is the leading cause of bacterial gastroenteritis. The reservoir for the organism is infected patients, which helps to explain the high intrafamilial attack rate. As few as 100 organisms can cause disease. The incubation period ranges from 1 to 5 days. *Shigella* invades the colonic epithelium causing an inflammatory colitis, killing the epithelial cells, and invading adjacent cells with resultant focal ulcers and mucosal inflammation. Ultimately, bloody mucoid exudate forms in the gut lumen.

The illness occurs most frequently in children under 5 years of age and is characterized by fever and malaise initially with the subsequent development of watery and often bloody diarrhea, averaging 10 to 25 stools per day. Abdominal cramps are a common feature. Tenesmus secondary to proctitis leads to rectal prolapse in younger patients.

Seizures occur frequently, sometimes before the onset of diarrhea. The seizures are nonfocal, often occur only once, and are associated with a rapidly-rising fever. Other associated findings include a relatively low WBC (under 10,000 cells/mm³) with a marked shift to the left, hyponatremia from *S. dysenteriae* type 1 infection, and occasionally toxic megacolon. Anorexia can persist for weeks into the convalescent period, and a protein-losing enteropathy can push the marginally fit child into a state of protein-calorie malnutrition.[183]

The treatment for *Shigella* is antibiotics. Antibiotic therapy helps to control symptoms and stops organism excretion within 1 to 2 days. The drug of choice is trimethoprim-sulfamethoxazole but ampicillin is an alternative for susceptible strains. Antibiotics should be prescribed for 5 days. Single-dose therapy in children older than 2 years of age has been effective in eradicating symptoms but is not as capable of eliminating the organism from stool.

Yersinia. Although *Yersinia enterocolitica* causes a gastroenteritis often indistinguishable from other bacterial causes in infants and young children, school-aged children may develop symptoms that mimic appendicitis. The reservoir for the organism is swine, and transmission occurs by ingestion of contaminated food (particularly uncooked pork products), unpasteurized milk, or person-to-person spread by the fecal-oral route. One notable outbreak in upstate New York affected over 200 schoolchildren who drank contaminated chocolate milk. The incubation period averages 4 to 6 days, ranging from 1 to 14 days. The organism initially appeared to predominate in colder climates but now has been reported in all parts of the United States.

The illness in infants and young children is characterized by fever, vomiting, bloody diarrhea, and often toxicity reflecting a bacteremic state. The older child develops gastroenteritis with associated symptoms of headache, pharyngitis, and often right lower quadrant pain secondary to mesenteric adenitis or terminal ileitis. The latter symptoms of "pseudoappendicitis" have led many physicians to take such children to the operating room. Skin manifestations may include maculopapular or erythema multiforme findings. Reactive arthritis may occur weeks after acute infection. Children with excess iron in their tissues (either chronically from conditions such as thalassemia or acutely from iron overdosage) are at increased risk of developing *Yersinia* infections.

The organism is susceptible to aminoglycosides, cefotaxime, trimethoprim-sulfamethoxazole, and tetracycline in children who are older than 9 years old. Bacteremic infants require hospital admission and IV antibiotics. Treatment of outpatient children with oral antibiotics reduces the time of excretion but may not have a notable effect on the other clinical symptoms.

Enterotoxigenic and Invasive Escherichia Coli. Diarrhea due to *E. coli* is categorized according to the mechanism of microbial action and resultant symptoms. *E. coli* strains include enterotoxigenic (ETEC), enteroinvasive (EIEC), enterohemorrhagic (EHEC), enteropathogenic (EPEC), and enteroadherent (EAEC) varieties.

The microbiologic diagnosis of an *E. coli* syndrome may have to be performed by a reference laboratory with selective media and specific antisera to identify toxins. The illnesses are usually self-limited and for practical purposes the time and expense of identifying specific strains may not aid in managing the individual patient.

Enterotoxigenic *E. coli* (ETEC) is associated with *traveler's diarrhea* and diarrhea in children under the age of 3 in developing countries. Symptomatically, patients have abdominal cramps, tenesmus, vomiting, nausea, chills, anorexia, and watery diarrhea. Prophylactic treatment and support are essential.

Enterohemorrhagic *E. coli* (EHEC) strains have been implicated in foodborne outbreaks (undercooked hamburger). Specifically the O157:H7 serotype has been associated with the development of hemolytic uremic syndrome.[184]

Food Poisoning. Several bacterial agents may result in an acute diarrheal illness following a specific dietary ingestion. Staphylococcal food poisoning results from a common-source food that has been poorly refrigerated. Vomiting, marked prostration, and diarrhea occur within 12 to 16 hours of ingestion.

Clostridium perfringens. Abdominal pain and diarrhea are common within 12 to 24 hours after the ingestion of contaminated food. Fever, nausea, and vomiting are rare. Resolution occurs within 24 to 48 hours.

C. botulinum. Although not directly causative of diarrheal illness, *C. botulinum* may produce clinical symptoms within 12 to 36 hours after the ingestion of contaminated foods: usually home-preserved vegetables, fruit, or fish. Honey may cause infantile botulism in children under 1 year of age. Patients develop nausea, vomiting, diplopia, dysphagia, dysarthria, and dry mouth. Ptosis, mydriasis, nystagmus, and paresis of extraocular muscles may be noted. Treatment includes support and antitoxin (see Chapter 55).

Clostridium Difficile. *Clostridium difficile* was identified in the 1970s as the major cause of pseudomembranous colitis. Many infants and children are colonized with this organism in balance with the normal flora of their bowel. Antibiotic usage changes the normal flora leading to overgrowth with *C. difficile.* A spectrum of illness ranging from antibiotic-associated diarrhea to full-blown pseudomembranous colitis with friable mucosal plaque formations may evolve.

The organism or its spores are hardy and have been known to have survived for long periods on inanimate objects such as bed rails, call buttons, and floors in the rooms of infected hospital patients. The attack rate in daycare centers is reported to be 32%; as a nosocomial infection the attack rate is probably even higher. Hospital roommates of culture-positive patients become colonized in an average of 3.2 days.

Almost all antibiotics have been reported to cause pseudomembranous colitis. The most frequently cited drugs are clindamycin, lincomycin, broad-spectrum antibiotics (including third-generation cephalosporins), and anticancer drugs.

If *C. difficile* and its cytotoxin are isolated from the stool, treatment with the nonabsorbable antibiotic vancomycin (50 mg/kg/24 hr QID PO for 7 days; adults: 150 to 500 mg QID PO) is effective in most cases. Metronidazole is an alternative drug for treatment.

Cholera. A heat-labile enterotoxin of *Vibrio cholerae* (primarily the El Tor biotype) causes a diarrheal disease that can lead to severe dehydration, hypokalemia, shock, and death. The Gulf regions of Texas and Louisiana are endemic areas in the United States. Man is the only natural host; contaminated water can affect raw or undercooked crabs and other shellfish.

The minimum infective dose is 10^5 to 10^8 organisms; some mild and asymptomatic infections occur. The incubation period averages 2 to 3 days, ranging from a few hours to 5 days. The organisms adhere to small bowel mucosa and multiply there, producing a protein enterotoxin. First, the B subunit of the toxin binds to receptors on the brush border of mucosal cells. Then an A_1 subunit crosses the cell membrane to stimulate cyclic AMP production, pumping out chloride ions while inhibiting sodium chloride absorption. Profuse watery diarrhea results, classically described as *rice water stools*—colorless and with small flecks of mucus. The patient is usually febrile without abdominal pain or tenesmus. Stool electrolyte losses can produce hypokalemia, muscle cramps, severe acidosis, and seizures. Hypovolemia can be severe enough to reduce renal blood flow and produce acute tubular necrosis. Treatment involves massive and vigorous fluid and electrolyte replacement. Antibiotics reduce fluid losses. First choices for antibiotics are trimethoprim-sulfamethoxazole or tetracycline for children older than 9 years of age.

Aeromonas. A prospective study in Australia first called clinical attention to this organism when 6.5% of children with diarrhea yielded *A. hydrophilia* on stool culture. In prevalence studies that followed, it was found in 1.1% to 18% of patients with bacterial stool cultures and occurred more commonly in the warmer months. *Aeromonas* is found in fresh and brackish water, particularly water contaminated by nonfecal organic matter such as decaying leaves or plant matter.

Symptoms of infection include low-grade fever and mild to moderate watery diarrhea lasting greater than 10 days in half of patients. One fourth of patients have bloody stools and vomiting whereas one third report abdominal cramps or pain. Most patients do not require antibiotic treatment.

Plesiomonas shigelloides. Closely related to *A. hydrophilia,* *P. shigelloides* produces a similar illness. If these organisms are suspected, the clinician should alert the microbiology laboratory to culture specifically for these pathogens.

Parasitic Agents

Cryptosporidium. First recognized in 1907 as a veterinary pathogen, this acid-fast staining, coccidian protozoan has been identified as the cause of watery diarrhea in patients with AIDS and in daycare attendees where the attack rate ranges from 30% to 65%. Hosts for the organism are birds, reptiles, and mammals. The disease is transmitted by person-to-person contact. The parasite is not killed by chlorine and may escape filtration, thus explaining why some waterborne outbreaks have been reported. In 1993 over 400,000 people were infected in Milwaukee, Wisconsin when the city water supply became contaminated.[185] The organism superficially invades the mucosal epithelial cells in the small intestine causing mild villus atrophy. After an incubation period that ranges from 2 to 14 days, a noninflammatory diarrhea results, lasting an average of 10 days (range 5 to 20 days). A more prolonged course exists in malnourished or immunocompromised patients. In developing countries, cryptosporidium may be one of the top four agents of acute diarrhea in infants and young children. In Costa Rica, it is reported to cause 4% of all cases of childhood diarrhea.

Associated symptoms include nausea, vomiting, and low-grade fever. Treatment with the macrolide antibiotic spiramycin shortened the duration of diarrhea by 2.1 days and shortened the excretion of oocysts by 1.4 days.[186]

Supportive care is the treatment of the immunocompetent host. Up to 25% have been reported to be asymptomatic carriers in some daycare centers.

Giardia Lamblia. Protozoa are typically considered causes of chronic diarrhea in children. *G. lamblia* is a flagellate protozoan that causes acute and chronic diarrhea. It is the most common parasitic enteropathogen in the United States. Children in daycare centers serve as a major reservoir of infection. Prevalence rates in those centers range from 17% to 90% where infection often may be asymptomatic and may last for up to 6 months. Animals such as beavers and possibly muskrats contaminate rural streams and water supplies with the parasite. Treatment of drinking water must include adequate filtration because chlorination alone is ineffective in killing *Giardia* cysts. Patients with cystic fibrosis or secretory IgA deficiency are especially susceptible to this protozoa.

One reason the attack rate is so high in daycare centers is that the minimum infective dose is as low as 10 to 100 cysts. The incubation period ranges from 1 to 4 weeks and averages 6 to 15 days in adult volunteer studies. Most infected patients have symptoms within 10 days but may not excrete cysts until later. The common symptoms are nausea, anorexia, and malodorous stools that appear pale, watery, and greasy. Abdominal distention, cramps, belching, and flatulence are also frequent.[187]

In children over the age of 5 years constipation may alternate with intermittent diarrhea. Chronic malabsorption of fats, carbohydrates, vitamin A, vitamin B_{12}, and folate leads to weight loss and failure to thrive. The illness may resolve spontaneously in 4 to 6 weeks.

Diagnosis of *Giardia* infection can be established in a few ways. Traditionally, stools have been microscopically examined for cysts on 3 consecutive days. This method proved highly sensitive in well-nourished Danish children. However, malnourished children in other studies failed to excrete trophozoites that were firmly attached to the duodenal or proximal jejunum. In those cases, duodenal fluid was obtained for microscopy by aspiration or swallowed string that was removed with duodenal secretions. Newer ELISA and counterimmune electrophoresis assays are now available for detecting *Giardia* antigens. Three agents have proven effective for treatment of symptomatic infection: quinacrine hydrochloride, furazolidone, and metronidazole.

Ancillary Data. A CBC and electrolytes should be obtained in toxic or dehydrated children. When the ratio of band forms over total neutrophils (segmented and bands) is over 0.10, *Shigella*, *Salmonella*, or *Campylobacter* organisms should be suspected. The WBC is usually under 10,000/mm³ with a marked shift to the left in children with *Shigella*, whereas in those with *Salmonella* the WBC count is often increased. *Campylobacter* and *Yersinia* have a high WBC as well. A blood culture is indicated for infants and young children who have high fever and significant toxicity.

Cultures of the stool are useful in determining the bacterial etiology when the results will have a therapeutic or epidemiologic impact. Cultures should be done in febrile or toxic children under 1 year of age, in those with PMNs in the stool, or if a member of the family is a food handler. Such studies should also be done if the patient has traveled extensively, or if the child is immunosuppressed or has a hemoglobinopathy.

Fecal leukocytes are a reliable test to determine the etiologic agent because over 90% of patients with diarrhea caused by *Salmonella* or *Shigella* have PMNs in the stool. Other etiologies associated with >5 WBC/high-power field include *Campylobacter*, *Y. enterocolitica*, invasive *E. coli*, and *V. parahemolyticus*. A small amount of mucus is placed on a glass slide and mixed with two drops of methylene blue. A cover slip is placed on the slide and nuclear staining indicates a PMN.[188]

Rotavirus may be identified by electron microscopy, radioimmunoassay, or the easier ELISA test.

Ova and parasite examination is important when parasitic pathogens are suspected. With *Giardia* organisms, cysts are present in formed stools and trophozoites are present in watery stools or duodenal aspirates.

Management

The initial assessment must focus on toxicity and hydration status. If dehydration is present, basic and advanced support should be initiated as outlined in Chapter 15.

Antibiotics are used only after the specific pathogen has been identified. In general, they are not useful in most diarrheal disease. Specific pathogens as outlined in Table 52-13 may benefit from pharmacologic management. Antibiotic therapy in children with documented *Salmonella* is controversial; the carrier state may be prolonged but the bacteremia must be treated if it is suspected or proven. Ceftriaxone is more effective than ampicillin in the treatment of shigellosis. *Campylobacter* responds to erythromycin (see Table 52-13). Vancomycin may be indicated for the treatment of *C. difficile* pseudomembranous colitis.[189,190]

Antidiarrheal agents include kaolin and pectin and have no beneficial therapeutic value. Diphenoxylate (Lomotil) may enhance abdominal cramping, particularly in children with *Shigella*, and is generally not used. Loperamide (Imodium) is occasionally recommended for a short period by some clinicians.

Bile acid may cause gastrointestinal irritation, usually in those children in whom clear liquids or NPO status has not resolved the diarrhea. A short course of aluminum hydroxide (Amphojel) 2.5 to 5 ml QID PO or cholestyramine (1 gm/24 hr in children under 1 year of age, up to 4 gm/24 hr in older children) may be useful in recalcitrant diarrhea. Nonsteroidal antiinflammatory agents may be indicated empirically.

Traveler's diarrhea prophylaxis is useful. Acute management must involve fluid resuscitation. Guidelines regarding administration must be individualized. Severe diarrhea (>3 stools in 8 hours with nausea, vomiting, or fever) is treated with doxycycline (children over 8 years) or trimethoprim-sulfamethoxazole. Reduction in diarrhea may be achieved by bismuth subsalicylate 2 tablets QID PO or 30 ml q 30 min for 3 hours. Loperamide 4 mg (adult) initially and then a 2-mg capsule after each unformed stool for 2 days (maximum: 8 capsules/day) may be effective.[191,192]

Disposition

Children who are moderately or severely dehydrated are generally admitted to hospital, particularly if they are not taking fluids well. Toxicity and fever should also be considered criteria for admission. Other reasons for admission include severe acidosis, abnormal serum sodium, and elevated BUN.

The parents of patients who are discharged should receive specific instructions regarding dietary restrictions of clear liquids, and a slow and deliberate progression of additional fluids and foods.

VIRAL HEPATITIS

MARY D. PATTERSON

Hepatitis can be diagnosed clinically in the emergency department. However, the exact diagnosis will require serologic testing, the results of which are often not available for several days. A focused clinical diagnosis will require

TABLE 52-13. Antibiotic Indications in Infectious Diarrhea

Etiologic agent	Drug of choice	Dose: mg/kg/24 hr (adult dose)	Route/frequency	Comments
Salmonella	Ampicillin **and** chloramphenicol*	200-400 (1 gm) 75-100 (1 gm)	IV q 4-6 hr IV q 6 hr	Only in toxic patient when bacteremia is a concern; prolongs carrier status
Shigella	Trimethoprim-sulfamethoxazole, **or**	8-10/40-50 (double strength)	PO q 12 hr	Preferred, depending on sensitivity; treat 5 days
	Ampicillin; **or**	50-100 (0.5 gm)	PO q 6-8 hr	Do not use amoxicillin; may give parenterally for very toxic patients
	Ceftriaxone	50	IM q 24 hr	Treat for 5 days; more effective than ampicillin
Campylobacter	Erythromycin	30-50 (0.5 gm)	PO q 6-8 hr	Effectiveness unproved; reduces length of excretion
Yersinia enterocolitica	Trimethoprim-sulfamethoxazole	8-10/40-50	PO q 12 hr	With severe toxicity, may use tetracycline (>8 yr old) and aminoglycoside
Giardia	Furazolidone; **or**	6-8 (0.1 gm)	PO q 6 hr	7-10 days; suspension available
	Quinacrine; **or**	6 (0.1 gm)	PO q 8 hr	5 days; poorly tolerated if <5 yr old
	Metronidazole	15 (0.25 gm)	PO q 8 hr	5 days

*Controversial. Other approaches include ampicillin and gentamicin; trimethoprim-sulfamethoxazole (IV). Drug must reflect local sensitivity patterns and treatment approaches.

historical information such as previous transfusions, travel history, diet (i.e., ingestion of raw shellfish), and high-risk behaviors such as parenteral drug use and multiple sexual partners. In the case of small children, ethnic background, daycare exposure, and information regarding the parents' risks are important.

Pathophysiology

The classic pathologic lesion of viral hepatitis is acute inflammation of the liver.[192] Hepatic cell necrosis is accompanied by leukocytic and histiocytic reaction and infiltration. Lymphadenopathy and splenomegaly are often associated with viral hepatitis.[193]

Etiology

A number of viruses and toxins can produce a hepatitis-like picture. Typically, infectious hepatitis A (HAV), hepatitis B (HBV), delta hepatitis (HDV), hepatitis C (HCV), and hepatitis E (HEV) are the primary etiologic considerations in the patient who has acute hepatitis. Less commonly, the following viruses are implicated: cytomegalovirus, herpes, varicella zoster, EB virus, rubella, and coxsackie B virus.[194] The differential diagnosis of hepatitis includes other infectious causes of hepatitis such as leptospirosis, secondary syphilis, brucellosis, and Q fever.[195]

Drugs have also been implicated, including acetaminophen, carbon tetrachloride, isoniazid, heavy metals, and vitamin A overdose, all of which can mimic viral hepatitis. Wilson disease may also present as an acute hepatitis associated with a hemolytic anemia.[196]

Diagnostic Findings

Most acute cases of viral hepatitis will have a self-limited course following an episode of variable symptomatology. Abdominal discomfort, jaundice, nausea, and vomiting are typical symptoms, combined with laboratory abnormalities reflecting severity and type of hepatitis (Table 52-14).

On occasion, viral hepatitis may be associated with acute pancreatitis or myocarditis. Both aplastic anemia and Guillain-Barré syndrome may be seen as late sequelae of viral hepatitis.[193]

An important complication of viral hepatitis is fulminant hepatitis, which occurs in 1% to 2% of all cases.[194] These patients have acute liver failure and encephalopathy within days to weeks of the onset of disease. The longer the interval between the onset of disease and development of symptomatology, the poorer the prognosis.[193] These patients develop vomiting, fever, and confusion. In contrast to patients with acute hepatitis, they have small, shrunken livers.[193]

Ancillary Data. Laboratory examination demonstrates leukocytosis and an elevated prothrombin time. The degree of elevation of transaminases is not prognostic; however, prolongation of the PT screen that does not respond to vitamin K administration is indicative of a poor response. Sixty to ninety percent of children with fulminant hepatitis will die.[194]

Management

The initial treatment of viral hepatitis consists only of supportive care; steroids are not helpful.[194] Hospitalized

TABLE 52-14. Acute Viral Hepatitis

	Hepatitis A	Hepatitis B	Hepatitis C
Epidemiologic features			
Incubation (weeks)	2-7	6-27	2-22
Onset	Acute	Insidious	Insidious with relapses
Cluster	Epidemic	Sporadic	Sporadic
Transmission	Fecal-oral, common source; rarely parenteral	Parenteral; rarely nonparenteral	Transfusions, rarely nonparenteral
Age distribution	Children	Adolescents, adults	Adolescents, adults
Duration	Weeks	Weeks to months	Often chronic
Diagnostic findings			
Fever	High	Moderate	Minimal
Nausea, vomiting	Common	Rare	Rare
Serum sickness (arthralgia, rash)	Rare	Common	Variable
Severity	Mild	Severe	Moderate
Carrier state	No	Yes	Yes
Ancillary data			
Transaminase elevation	1-3 wk	Months	Months to years
Bilirubin elevation	Weeks	Months	Often chronic
Prophylaxis	IG	HBIG	Not effective

IG, Immune serum globulin; *HBIG*, hepatitis B immunoglobulin.

patients should be isolated, and good universal precautions should be observed. Enteric precautions can be observed once the type of hepatitis is specified.

Alpha-interferon has shown some promise in adults but not yet in children.[197] years is not improved significantly but has not been demonstrated to show clinical improvement.[197]

Hepatitis A

Hepatitis A accounts for 20% to 25% of cases of clinical hepatitis in developed countries. In the United States, it is estimated that one third of hepatitis A cases occur in children. However, this number is probably underestimated because most children are only mildly symptomatic.[194] HAV is endemic in certain areas, particularly in tropical regions. In developing countries, 90% of children have antibodies to hepatitis A by 10 years of age.

The hepatitis A virus (HAV) is an RNA virus that is spread from person-to-person by the fecal-oral route.[194] Spread of this disease is exacerbated by poor hygiene and overcrowding. In this country, daycare centers frequently serve as reservoirs for this illness. This finding is particularly true in those centers where food preparation and diaper changing occur in the same area. Institutionalized children are also at high risk.[194]

Consumption of uncooked shellfish is another risk factor. No known carrier state exists. Interestingly, the patient is most contagious in the preicteric phase of the illness; once the patient becomes icteric, the viral shedding in stools decreases.[194] The incubation period is 15 to 45 days with a mean of approximately 30 days.

Diagnostic Findings. The patient typically complains of fever, headache, anorexia, vomiting, and diarrhea. Painful hepatomegaly is a common finding.[194] Dark urine and light stools may appear within the first week of the illness, followed by jaundice.[198] However more than half of children under 4 years of age who acquire HAV will be anicteric.[199] The illness may last 4 to 6 weeks, but over 95% of children will recover with supportive care alone.

Ancillary Data. A rise in aminotransferases occurs 1 week after infection and these may be normal 1 to 2 weeks later; the average incubation period is 25 to 30 days. The specific diagnosis of hepatitis A is made by the detection of antibody to HAV. Detection of anti-HAV IgM may be possible only transiently, peaking 1 week after the onset of infection, even before the jaundice occurs, and indicating recent infection. Anti-HAV IgG peaks at 1 to 2 months and persists for years.[194]

Management. Children require supportive care. No specific diet, medication, or treatment regimen is required. After stabilization, specific attention must be directed to intravascular volume. CNS management must be specific if encephalopathy is present including insertion of an NG tube, dietary manipulation, and treatment of cerebral edema (mannitol, steroids, and hyperventilation). Nutrition, bleeding, isolation, and fluid balance must be watched closely.

Prevention of hepatitis A requires attention to hygiene and good handwashing. Once an index case has been identified, prevention of further spread involves passive immunization of all household and daycare contacts with standard immune globulin (IG) at a dose of 0.02 ml/kg.[194] This is 80% to 90% effective if administered within 2 weeks of exposure.[198]

Administration of IG is indicated in the following specific epidemiologic circumstances:

1. Daycare facility with all children being over 2 years of age or toilet trained. When a case is identified in an employee or enrolled child, administer IG to those in contact with employee or in same room as index case.
2. Daycare facility with children not toilet trained. Following identification of a case in an employee, child, or household contacts of two of the enrolled children, IG should be given to all employees and enrolled children.
3. If the recognition of the outbreak is delayed at which time three or more families are involved, IG should be considered for all employees, children, and household contacts of all enrolled children in diapers.

Children and adults with hepatitis should be excluded from daycare or school for 1 week after the onset of the illness or until jaundice, if present, has disappeared.

Schoolroom exposures do not generally pose a significant risk unless there is close personal contact with the infected person. In institutions and hospitals, residents and staff with close personal contact with the index patient should be immunized if there is an outbreak.

Preexposure prophylaxis for travelers to endemic areas with poor hygiene may be done by administering IG right before departure, 0.02 ml/kg for children (2 ml in adult) for stays under 3 months and 0.06 ml/kg for longer stays (5 ml in adult). An inactivated hepatitis A vaccine has been developed, which has been demonstrated in several studies to induce good antibody levels within 1 month of immunization. This vaccine is not yet routinely available in the United States.[200,201]

Hepatitis B

Hepatitis B virus (HBV) is a DNA virus that is usually transmitted parenterally. Typically this virus is spread by blood or blood products, needles shared among IV drug users, sexual contact, and vertical transmission between mother and newborn. Health-care providers who have a high exposure to blood products and unintentional needle puncture, and institutionalized children are at high risk of contracting hepatitis B. In addition there are a number of areas where HBV is endemic. For example, 45% of Alaskan Eskimos and 85% of Australian aborigines are positive for hepatitis B surface antigen (HBsAG). In the Taiwanese population, 15% to 20% are HBV carriers, and 80% have antibodies to HBV.[194] Offspring of mothers who are carriers are at high risk of contracting the infection themselves. Moreover, 90% of those children who become infected with HBV as infants will become chronic carriers with an increased chance of developing hepatocellular carcinoma.[194]

Diagnostic Findings. The incubation period is 50 to 180 days with an average of 120 days. Patients with acute HBV infection may have symptoms somewhat more severe than those associated with hepatitis A and these can include urticaria, arthralgia, and arthritis.[194] Hepatitis B may also be associated with an illness similar to serum sickness, membranous and membranoproliferative glomerulonephritis, nephrotic syndrome, and polyarteritis nodosa.[194] Approximately 60% to 70% of acute hepatitis B infections are subclinical.[202]

Although HBsAg may be detected 3 to 6 days after exposure (Table 52-15), it is typically not found until 1 to 3

TABLE 52-15. HBV Diagnostic Tests

Hepatitis B antigen/antibody	Interpretation
Surface antigen (HBsAg)	Carrier or acutely infected
Antibody to surface antigen (Anti-HBs)	Prior infection with HBV; immunity following vaccine
e Antigen (HBeAg)	Carrier with high risk of transmitting HbsAg
Antibody to e antigen (Anti-HBe)	HBsAg carrier with low risk of infectiousness
Antibody to core antigen (Anti-HBc)	Prior HBV infection
IgM antibody to core antigen (IgM Anti-HBc)	Acute or recent HBV infection

TABLE 52-16. Dosage Schedule for Hepatitis B Vaccines*

| Group | Vaccine μg (ml) | | |
	Heptavax B	Recombivax	Energix-B
Infants of HBV mother	10 (0.5)	5 (0.5)	10 (0.5)
Children (<11 yrs)	10 (0.5)	2.5 (0.25)	10 (0.5)
Adolescents (11-19 yrs)	20 (1.0)	5 (0.5)	20 (1.0)
Adults	20 (1.0)	10 (1.0)	20 (1.0)

*Immunization is typically given IM at 0, 1, and 6 months.

months after exposure. This is followed by the appearance of hepatitis Be antigen (HBeAg) and antibody to the core antigen (anti-HBc-IgM).[198] Elevation of aminotransferases is seen 14 to 60 days after appearance of HBsAg.[194] This is followed by the rise of hepatitis B surface antibody (HBsAb) and anti-HBc-IgG, which may persist for years.[198]

Those patients who become chronic carriers typically demonstrate the persistence of HBsAg for 6 months or more. Presence of HBeAg is associated with a high degree of infectivity. Over 90% of infants and 20% of children infected will become carriers of the virus.[198]

Management. Treatment of hepatitis B is mainly supportive; mortality of the acute infection is 1%.[203] Prevention of the disease is possible.

Preexposure prophylaxis for high-risk individuals is available from a recombinant vaccine containing 10 to 40 μg HBsAg protein/ml. A series of three doses induces a response in 90% of healthy patients when given at intervals of 0, 1, and 6 months (Table 52-16). Children in this group include those from families with HBV infection, chronic carriers, those in institutions for the mentally retarded, and those receiving large amounts of blood and blood products.

Postexposure prophylaxis must reflect the type of exposure (blood or percutaneous needlestick or mucosal membrane) and the HBsAg status of the donor. Exposed infants under the age of 12 months should receive both hepatitis B immunoglobulin (HBIG) (0.06 ml/kg or 5 ml for adults) and vaccine. Children over the age of 12 months living in a home with acute HBV infection should be followed serologically to determine if the index case becomes a carrier, and if so, household contacts should be immunized. For those who are unvaccinated and have a percutaneous or transmucosal exposure to blood known to be HBsAg positive, a dose of hepatitis B vaccine is recommended and the hepatitis B vaccine given as soon as possible and 1 and 6 months after exposure. Generally, such exposed persons should receive the first dose of hepatitis B vaccine within 7 days of exposure, and the series should be completed as recommended. Obviously, the blood of both the donor and the exposed individual should be tested for HBsAg and HIV.[199]

Sexual contacts of persons with hepatitis B infections are at increased risk of acquiring the disease. All susceptible persons whose sexual partners have acute hepatitis B should receive a single dose of HBIG if it can be given within 14 days of the last sexual contact or if sexual contact is ongoing. A series of hepatitis B vaccines should also be given.[204]

Infants of mothers known to be positive for HBsAg should receive hepatitis B IG (0.5 ml/dose) within 12 hours of delivery; the hepatitis B vaccine series should be begun at birth and administered at 1 and 6 months. HBsAg testing should be done at 6 months to monitor status. Universal immunization for hepatitis B is now recommended for all infants in the United States; implementation has been sporadic. In addition, adolescents should be immunized before they become sexually active.[205]

Hepatitis D

Hepatitis D virus (HDV) or delta agent is caused by an RNA-containing viral particle. This delta agent is unique because it can only infect patients who are also positive for the HBsAg. This can occur either in the midst of an acute HBV infection or in a HBV carrier. The mortality ranges from 2% to 20%.[203]

Patients who develop simultaneous infections with HBV and HDV are characterized as having a coinfection. Coinfections are usually self-limited, with only 5% of patients developing chronic hepatitis.[203] However, chronic carriers of HBsAg who then become infected with HDV develop what is known as a superinfection. As many as 80% of these patients will develop chronic hepatitis.[203]

Diagnosis of HDV is made by detection of anti-HDV antibody. Coinfection may be distinguished from superinfection by the presence of anti-HBc-IgM, which is the marker of acute HBV infection.[203]

HDV infection can occur in epidemic form among chronic carriers of HBsAg. In South America, there have been a number of outbreaks of severe fulminant hepatitis that have been attributed to the delta agent. This disease mainly strikes children and may be rapidly fatal with mortality ranging from 10% to 20%.[203]

The best hope for the prevention of this disease lies in the prevention of hepatitis B. Supportive care is the mainstay of therapy, though alpha-interferon and liver transplantation have shown some promise for those with chronic hepatitis.[203]

Hepatitis C

Hepatitis C (HCV, formerly known as non-A, non-B hepatitis) is a parenterally transmitted RNA virus that is believed to account for the vast majority of cases of posttransfusion hepatitis in this country.[199] Diagnosis is made by anti-HCV assay; however, this is limited in that the antibody may not be detected for a number of months after infection.[206]

This virus is transmitted parenterally and not only by transfusion. In 1987, only 5% of patients with this type of hepatitis had a history of transfusion, whereas 42% had a history of IV drug use. Approximately 10% had a history of sexual contact with someone who had hepatitis or had multiple sexual partners.[207] Nevertheless, in the pediatric population, children who have received multiple transfusions, required cardiac surgery, or hemodialysis represent the majority of patients.[209] Perinatal transmission is a much less important causative factor.[209] The average incubation period is 7 to 9 weeks, with a range of 2 to 12 weeks. Sixty percent of patients will develop chronic hepatitis, and 10% to 20% of those will develop cirrhosis.[207]

Treatment is mainly supportive. There is a small series of children with hepatitis C in whom alpha-interferon therapy resulted in normalization of liver function tests.[210]

Hepatitis E

Hepatitis E (HEV) is an enterically transmitted non-A, non-B hepatitis. It was originally confined to the Indian subcontinent, but has now been reported in Asia, Africa, and Mexico.[199] HEV is remarkable in that it causes a 10% to 20% mortality rate among pregnant women who contract it.[207] In certain developing countries, hepatitis E is believed to be a common cause of acute hepatitis.[211,212]

The incubation period ranges from 15 to 60 days. Although no diagnostic test is widely available, certain laboratories have developed fluorescent antibody assays and polymerase chain reaction tools that identify this RNA virus.[205]

Immunoglobulin prepared in the United States is not considered effective prophylaxis for hepatitis E.[205]

INFLAMMATORY BOWEL DISEASE

ROBERT A. BELFER

Inflammatory bowel disease (IBD) is being recognized in children with increasing frequency. Ulcerative colitis and Crohn disease constitute the major entities. Although the initial diagnosis of inflammatory bowel disease is infrequently made in the ED, patients with IBD are seen because of exacerbations, relapses, and complications of their existing disease.

Pathophysiology

Ulcerative colitis is an idiopathic recurrent inflammatory disease of the colon. Histologically the inflammation is confined to the mucosa and submucosa. It typically begins in the rectum and spreads proximally. In most patients only the rectum and left colon are affected, but in severe cases the entire colon is diseased.[213]

Crohn disease is a subacute idiopathic inflammatory disease. It can affect any part of the gastrointestinal tract in a segmental manner. In approximately one third of patients, only the terminal ileum is involved; in one fifth of patients, only the colon is involved; and in half the patients, both the small and large intestines are involved.[213] Crohn disease may involve one or all layers of the bowel. Pathologically, it consists of granulomas and giant cells; occasionally, there also may be bowel wall fistulas and abscesses.

Etiology

The etiology of ulcerative colitis and Crohn disease remains obscure and is most likely multifactorial. Inflammatory bowel disease occurs more commonly among the Jewish populations in North America and Europe. Multiple familial occurrences are documented in 15% to 40% of patients with inflammatory bowel disease.[214] Males and females are equally affected. Ulcerative colitis affects 15% of patients before the age of 20, usually in adolescence.[215] Crohn disease is diagnosed in 18% to 30% of patients before the age of 20.[215] Although rare, both ulcerative colitis and Crohn disease have been reported in children under the age of 1 year.[216]

Diagnostic Findings

Clinical Findings. Over 90% of pediatric patients with ulcerative colitis have moderate to severe disease.[214] Bloody diarrhea is the most common feature. Other signs and symptoms include rectal bleeding, abdominal pain, weakness, weight loss, and fever. In the ED, 50% of patients have had an insidious onset of diarrhea, and 33% have had a dramatic onset with a sudden acute appearance of bloody stools. Ten percent of patients develop a fulminating course, characterized by fever, bloody diarrhea, abdominal pain, and distention, and, possibly, toxic megacolon. Werlin and Grand's[217] characteristics of severe colitis include either toxic megacolon or meeting four of the following five criteria: (1) five or more grossly bloody stools a day; (2) oral temperature > 100° F; (3) tachycardia > 90; (4) hematocrit < 30%; and (5) serum albumin < 3 gm/dl.

Crohn disease often has an insidious onset. The most common symptoms are abdominal pain and diarrhea (usually watery, not bloody). Less frequent signs and symptoms are rectal bleeding, fever, anorexia, and weight loss. At times, patients may have appendicitis-like symptoms, and only at laparotomy is the diagnosis of Crohn disease evident.[218]

Extraintestinal manifestations seen in both forms of inflammatory bowel disease include growth failure (10% to 40%), polyarthritis and ankylosing spondylitis (10% to 15%), skin manifestations (erythema nodosum and pyoderma gangrenosum) (10%), hepatobiliary dysfunction (8%), and uveitis (3%). These may precede the gastrointestinal symptoms, particularly in children.[216] Additionally, calcium oxalate nephrolithiasis may occur.

Complications. Both ulcerative colitis and Crohn disease are associated with a variety of complications. Massive hemorrhage may occur during fulminant episodes, which is more common in ulcerative colitis. Intestinal obstruction occurs in about 8% of children with Crohn disease. It may occur secondary to severe inflammation, abscess formation,

or chronic inflammation with stricture formation. The most common site of obstruction is the ileocecal region. Crohn disease may be complicated by formation of fistulas, leading to pathologic connections between different sites in the gastrointestinal tract as well as between bowel and other sites (e.g., bladder, skin). Perianal skin tags, fissures, fistulas, and abscesses occur frequently.[219]

Toxic megacolon, a medical and surgical emergency, occurs in 5% of patients with inflammatory bowel disease.[217] It usually involves the transverse colon in addition to other regions of the colon. The course is one of progressive deterioration with a mortality rate of up to 25%. Antidiarrheal agents (anticholinergic agents), opiates, and an antecedent barium enema have been implicated in this complication. Toxic megacolon occurs in the presence of severe pancolitis. Clinically, the child is toxic-appearing, with an acutely distended and tender abdomen. Fever, dehydration, elevated WBC count, and abdominal films showing dilation of the transverse colon are seen. Hemorrhage, gram-negative sepsis, and perforation are life-threatening complications of toxic megacolon. The presenting symptoms of perforation are those of classic peritonitis, although these features may be masked by high-dose corticosteroid therapy.

Patients with inflammatory bowel disease have an increased risk of developing carcinoma. In ulcerative colitis, the risk is 3% in the first decade and 20%/decade after that.[214] Patients with Crohn disease also have an increased risk of carcinoma over that of the general population, although this risk is less than that of patients with ulcerative colitis.

Ancillary Data. In moderate to severe ulcerative colitis, abdominal radiographs may reveal "thumb printing" indicative of edematous bowel mucosa. In Crohn disease, abdominal films can demonstrate incomplete small bowel obstruction, distended loops of bowel, and air fluid levels. In toxic megacolon, the transverse colon is grossly dilated, usually greater than 5 to 7 centimeters, and x-rays may also show signs of perforation. In mild inflammatory bowel disease, however, the films are usually normal.

Barium x-ray studies in acute ulcerative colitis show mucosal irregularity, effaced haustrations, and a shortened narrowed colon due to muscular rigidity. Barium examination in Crohn disease demonstrates irregular or cobblestone-like mucosa and enteric fistulas. The lesion's segmental distribution is diagnostic. Cautiously perform contrast studies in patients with Crohn disease because it is not uncommon for a flare-up in disease activity or even toxic megacolon to follow a barium enema.

Laboratory findings include an elevated white blood cell count with a left shift, anemia, and elevated sedimentation rate. Stool cultures to exclude bacterial etiologies and analysis of the stool for the presence of red and white blood cells should be performed. After the initial evaluation, if the clinician is still suspicious of inflammatory bowel disease, a gastroenterologist should be consulted. Sigmoidoscopy and colonoscopy are procedures used by the specialist to confirm the diagnosis and also help in the ongoing management of these patients. In ulcerative colitis, colonoscopy demonstrates an inflamed and friable mucosa, and biopsy of these lesions demonstrates polymorphonuclear infiltrates with crypt abscesses. In Crohn disease, biopsy of the mucosa reveals granulomas with chronic inflammation to all layers of bowel.

Differential Considerations

Infectious colitis can occur with diarrhea, at times bloody; stool cultures for ova and parasites and bacterial pathogens are likely to distinguish this entity. Allergic colitis usually occurs in infancy and responds to removal of the offending agent. Patients with hemolytic uremic syndrome have a prodrome of abdominal pain and bloody diarrhea and go on to develop acute renal failure, hemolytic anemia, and thrombocytopenia. Radiation enteritis should be considered in a child with cancer and pseudomembranous colitis in a child taking antibiotics. HIV infection can result in chronic diarrhea, low grade fever, and cachexia. Acute appendicitis can mimic an exacerbation of inflammatory bowel disease. The extraintestinal manifestations of inflammatory bowel disease may mimic the initial presentations of juvenile rheumatoid arthritis, rheumatic fever, or other collagen vascular diseases.

Management

When caring for patients with inflammatory bowel disease in the emergency department, it is prudent to involve a gastroenterologist in the decision-making process. The management of a patient with ulcerative colitis depends on the severity of the attack. A mild attack characterized by diarrhea, abdominal pain, and minimal rectal bleeding without systemic signs can be treated as an out-patient with sulfasalazine, which is a drug used to induce and maintain remission of disease. Moderate attacks of ulcerative colitis in which there is bloody diarrhea (more than six times a day), abdominal pain, and systemic signs such as low-grade fever, anorexia, leukocytosis and mild anemia, generally require a short hospitalization. Corticosteroids are the most effective drugs and may be given either orally, rectally, or intravenously. Clinical improvement is seen within 1 to 2 weeks. For fulminant colitis unresponsive to conventional treatment, cyclosporine A has been shown to be efficacious in children to induce remission and avoid precipitous colectomy.[220] Indications for surgery include failed medical management, profuse hemorrhage, perforation, and sometimes toxic megacolon and obstruction.[221]

A variety of agents are useful in the management of Crohn disease. Steroids induce remission in a majority of patients. Immunosuppressive agents (azathioprine and 6-mercaptopurine) have been used to maintain remissions and are frequently used in children refractory to corticosteroids. Metronidazole also has recently been shown to be an effective therapeutic agent for perianal disease. Sulfasalazine has been shown to be a useful adjunct to prednisone in the treatment of colonic disease.

Management of toxic megacolon is a medical emergency. Treatment includes making the patient NPO, inserting a nasogastric tube, administering parenteral fluids, and correcting fluid and electrolyte abnormalities. Erect and supine abdominal films must be obtained to rule out viscous perforation. Opiates should be avoided since they can precipitate or worsen toxic megacolon. Parenteral steroids and broad-spectrum antibiotics should be administered. Most

patients require colloid and blood transfusions. Early consultation with both a gastroenterologist and a surgeon is necessary.

PANCREATITIS, ACUTE

YEHESKEL WAISMAN

Acute pancreatitis is considered relatively rare in childhood but more recent reports suggest that it might be more common than previously suspected.[222-225] The incidence of pancreatitis in children is estimated to be 1 in 50,000.[226] Because of its relative rarity and frequently atypical presentation, pancreatitis may be overlooked. It should be considered in children with abdominal trauma, epigastric pain associated with nausea or vomiting, ascites or pleural effusion of unknown origin, or unexplained shock. Pancreatitis can result in a fulminant or even fatal course. Compilation of mortality data from the literature suggests that the mortality rate in childhood pancreatitis is 14%; unfortunately, some of these cases were diagnosed only at autopsy.[223-227] Early treatment may improve the outcome.

Pathophysiology

The pancreas contains many destructive enzymes which, when activated, initiate a process of pancreatic autodigestion. The morphologic appearance of acute pancreatitis gives no clue to its cause. Early stages of pancreatitis are characterized by peripancreatic fat necrosis and interstitial edema; the parenchyma remains intact in general. Acinar cells may be fused, depleted of zymogen granules, and loaded with autophagic vacuoles containing various cell elements. These changes are consistent with the initial release of enzymes across the wall of acinar cell, a stage known as *acute edematous pancreatitis.* Acute edematous pancreatitis is most common in children. The process may progress to coagulation necrosis of the pancreatic tissue and surrounding fat, a stage called *necrotizing pancreatitis.* Finally, there may be hemorrhage from rupture of blood vessels within the necrotizing gland or its surroundings, a stage known as *hemorrhagic pancreatitis.*[228]

Complications can be significant and may manifest early or late. Tissue debris, pancreatic juice, blood and fat droplets accumulating in areas of necrosis can form a pseudocyst. Inflammation of peritoneal surfaces by activated pancreatic enzymes and leukocytes can produce pancreatic ascites, and propagation of this process through the diaphragmatic lymphatics to the pleural space may cause a sterile pleural effusion and occasionally a pneumonitis. Pancreatic abscesses may result from secondary infection of necrotic tissue by enteric bacteria.[225] Activation of kallikrein, a potent vasoactive peptide, can induce vasodilatation and increase vascular permeability, leading to hypotension and shock. Whereas acute edematous pancreatitis is associated with a self-limited course and complete recovery, acute hemorrhagic pancreatitis has a 40% to 80% mortality.

Etiology

Children over the age of 10 years are most commonly affected. In contrast to adults in whom alcoholism and

Etiology of Pancreatitis in Children and Adolescents

Trauma:

Blunt, penetrating, surgical

Drugs/toxins:

Steroids, thiazides, azathioprine, L-asparaginase, alcohol, valproic acid, tetracycline, oral contraceptives, furosemide, ethacrynic acid, sulfasalazine, rifampin, pentamidine, metronidazole

Infection:

Mumps, hepatitis A and B, coxsackievirus B, influenza A, Epstein-Barr, cytomegalovirus, rubella, rubeola, *Mycoplasma pneumoniae*, *Salmonella*, leptospirosis, *Ascaris*, sepsis

Biliary tract disease:

Congenital—Choledochal cyst, duplication cyst, anomalous bile duct, duodenal stenosis, pancreas divisum
Acquired—Cholelithiasis, tumors

Systemic:

Systemic lupus erythematosus, periarteritis nodosa, Kawasaki disease, hemolytic-uremic syndrome, Reye syndrome, cystic fibrosis, Henoch-Schönlein purpura, Crohn disease, sickle cell disease, glycogen storage disease Type I, alpha-1-antitrypsin deficiency, hyperlipidemia, hypercalcemia, hyperparathyroidism, end-stage renal failure, diabetes mellitus ketoacidosis, and organ transplantation

Miscellaneous:

Perforated duodenal ulcer

Hereditary:

Hereditary pancreatitis

Idiopathic

cholelithiasis are the most common causes, the etiologies of childhood pancreatitis are more diverse and are listed in the box above. Accumulated data from 304 cases show that trauma (22%), structural (15%), drugs/toxins (13%), systemic illness (13%), and infection (11%) share a fairly even distribution.[223] Mechanisms of trauma include motor vehicle accidents and falls from bicycles, typically onto the handlebars. However, the pancreas may also be contused or ruptured by what might have seemed to be an insignificant trauma, because it is a soft, parenchymatous, and extremely vascular structure.[227] Mumps is the most common cause of viral pancreatitis but accounts for only 10% to 15% of all cases.[223,225,227] It rarely occurs in children under the age of 5 years, is seldom severe, and parotitis may or may not be present. Despite the long and growing list of etiologies, idiopathic causes still account for up to 30% of the cases.[223,225]

Diagnostic Findings

Abdominal pain associated with nausea and vomiting is the dominant symptom of acute pancreatitis and occurs in more than 75% of cases.[222,224] It begins insidiously over several hours, localizes to the epigastric or periumbilical areas, and is described as knifelike and constant in nature. It may have a more acute onset, radiating to the back or to upper quadrants. Its severity can vary from tolerable to incapacitating. Patients usually prefer a sitting position or lay still on their sides in a knee-chest position in an attempt to obtain some relief. Vomiting may be severe and protracted, is aggravated by food, and does not relieve the pain. Slight fever is common; high temperatures are usually associated with extensive pancreatic necrosis or abscess formation.

On physical examination, the abdomen tends to be distended and tender. Mild to moderate voluntary guarding and rebound tenderness may be present over the epigastric area. Bowel sounds may be normal, hypoactive, or absent depending on the severity of peritoneal inflammation and fluid and electrolyte abnormalities. The finding of an abdominal mass suggests the presence of a pseudocyst. Ascites or pleural effusion are rare but may be found in severe cases. Bluish discoloration over the periumbilical area (Cullen's sign) or flanks (Grey Turner's sign) suggests the diagnosis of hemorrhagic pancreatitis. This is usually associated with severe abdominal pain, rigidity, and increased vascular permeability, which can result in ascites, pleural effusion, and hypotension. Hemorrhagic pancreatitis is associated with a poor prognosis and is not diagnosed until postmortem examination in 25% of cases. Because pancreatitis can be part of a systemic disease, associated findings may include parotitis, jaundice, hepatosplenomegaly, skin rashes, petechiae, or clinical signs of hypocalcemia.

Ancillary Data. Blood should be sent for amylase, CBC, glucose, electrolytes, calcium, BUN, creatinine, liver function tests, and coagulation screen. Urinalysis and urine amylase and creatinine should be obtained. An arterial blood gas may be useful.

Confirming the diagnosis of pancreatitis can be difficult since there is no pathognomonic test for pancreatitis. Symptoms and signs of pancreatitis are nonspecific; suggestive biochemical or radiological abnormalities may be absent (in 10% of cases of proven pancreatitis).[222,229-230] The most useful diagnostic tests are the serum amylase, urine amylase, and amylase/creatinine clearance ratio. In uncomplicated cases, serum amylase levels begin to rise within hours of onset of symptoms, peak during the first day, and return to normal within 2 to 3 days.[222,230] A threefold increase in serum amylase in the appropriate clinical context is diagnostic for pancreatitis, but children with pancreatitis may have normal levels. Furthermore, because hyperamylasemia is observed in other diseases, conditions such as parotitis, renal failure, common bile duct obstruction, hepatic trauma, acute salpingitis, ectopic pregnancy, opiate administration, and intestinal infarction must be excluded before the diagnosis of acute pancreatitis can be made.[229] Analysis of amylase isoenzymes may help to determine whether an elevated value is of pancreatic origin; however, it cannot determine whether patients with a normal amylase have pancreatitis. The amylase/creatinine clearance ratio (AM/CCR) is more accurate than the amylase level alone. It is calculated from the formula:

$$\text{Cam/Ccr \%} = \frac{\text{urine amylase}}{\text{serum amylase}} \times \frac{\text{serum creatinine}}{\text{urine creatinine}} \times 100$$

This ratio reflects defective tubular reabsorption of amylase and a ratio greater than 5% has been considered indicative for pancreatitis in the past. However, the more recent literature questions its diagnostic validity.[231-233] Other conditions such as diabetic ketoacidosis and thermal burns may elevate the ratio and must be excluded. When further confirmation is needed, serum lipase level or trypsinogen should be obtained. An elevated lipase value correlates well with pancreatitis and remains elevated after the amylase level has returned to normal.[234]

Hyperglycemia may result from damage to beta cells. Unexplained hypocalcemia frequently occurs in severe cases and is a poor prognostic sign if it occurs in presentation, at least in adults.[225]

Radiographic studies can also help to diagnose pancreatitis and its complications. Abdominal roentgenograms may reveal a distended segment of small intestine near the pancreas (sentinel loop), generalized paralytic ileus, or spasm in the transverse colon with absent colonic gas beyond this point (colon cut-off sign).[7] Pancreatic calcifications are specific for chronic pancreatitis but rare in children, except in hereditary pancreatitis. Chest radiographs should exclude pleural effusion, pulmonary infiltrate, and atelectasis. Ultrasonography may demonstrate an enlarged pancreas with reduced echodensity and is particularly helpful in detecting pseudocysts. Abdominal CT scans (Fig. 52-6) may also show pancreatic enlargement and identify complications such as pseudocysts, abscesses, hemorrhage, or biliary obstruction. In comparative studies it has been found to be more accurate than ultrasonography; therefore it is considered the imaging method of choice for any pancreatic disease, especially when complications are suspected.[228,230,234,235] Endoscopic retrogade cholangiopancreatography is of value in defining the ductal anatomy when investigating relapsing pancreatitis but is contraindicated during the acute illness.[236]

Differential Considerations

Acute cholecystitis, biliary colic, gastritis, intestinal obstruction, appendicitis, and penetrating peptic ulcer may have a similar symptomatology and should be considered in the differential diagnosis.

Management

In the emergency department a combined diagnostic and therapeutic approach should be initiated simultaneously. The objectives of therapy are to rest the pancreas, treat shock and electrolyte abnormalities, and relieve pain. Oral intake should be discontinued and IV fluid resuscitation should be begun. Type, volume, and rate of fluids depend on the state of hydration and circulation. For a clinically stable patient, 1.5 times the maintenance dose of a crystalloid solution is recommended. In shock or circulatory failure, however, repeated boluses of a crystalloid (20

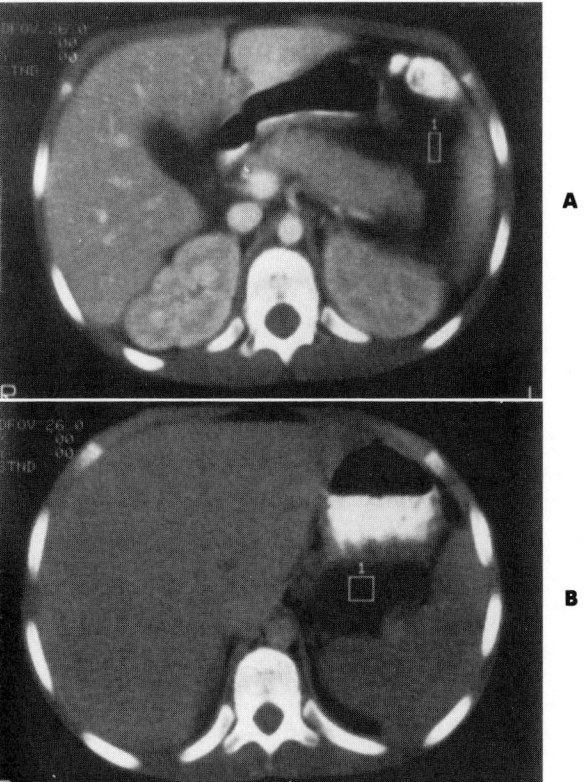

FIG. 52-6. A, Axial cross-section abdominal CT scan with contrast of a 10-year-old girl with abdominal trauma showing swelling of the pancreas and inflammation of the tail 7 days after the event. **B,** Pseudocyst formation 2 weeks later.

ml/kg 0.9% NS or LR), or colloid (10 ml/kg 5% albumin) should be administered. The latter is preferable due to the increased capillary leak. Frequent assessment of response to treatment (vital signs, tissue perfusion, and urinary output every 5 to 10 minutes) is the key to appropriate and successful fluid resuscitation in severe cases. A nasogastric tube should be placed and connected to suction. Aspiration of gastric contents reduces pancreatic hormonal stimulation, relieves pain, and prevents ileus. The use of anticholinergics to reduce pancreatic secretions is controversial and is not generally recommended. Meperidine (1 mg/kg) can be used to control pain; morphine should not be used because it causes spasm at the sphincter of Oddi. Hypocalcemia must be corrected with calcium gluconate infusions. Antibiotics are not indicated unless an abscess is suspected. Steroids are of no use.

New patients with acute pancreatitis should be hospitalized. Emergency surgery is rarely necessary and should be reserved for selected cases of traumatic pancreatitis.

REYE SYNDROME

DOUGLAS A. BOENNING

First described in 1963, Reye syndrome is an encephalopathy associated with fatty infiltration of the liver and

TABLE 52-17. Clinical Staging of Reye Syndrome (CDC)

Stage	Level of consciousness
0	Alert, wakeful
I	Sleepy, lethargic
II	Delirious, combative
III	Unarousable, decorticate
IV	Unarousable, decerebrate
V	Unarousable, flaccid paralysis
	Areflexia, unresponsive pupils

mitochondrial injury. The exact etiology is not known but a clear epidemiologic link has been established with salicylate exposure during viral infections. Public awareness of this association has lead to a reduction in the use of aspirin in children and a similar decline in the cases of Reye syndrome. Now, only approximately 20 confirmed cases are reported annually in the United States.

Epidemiologically, Reye syndrome in the United States arose as a disease of suburban white children in the Midwest. Reported cases rose during the 1970s, peaking at 555 cases in 1980 for a calculated incidence of 0.88 cases/100,000 population under the age of 18. From 1974 to 1985 the mean case fatality rate was 32%.

During the 1980s, the incidence of Reye syndrome began to decline as evidence accumulated that aspirin was linked to its development. In 1982, the Surgeon General recommended that parents avoid using aspirin for treatment of acute febrile illnesses in their children. In 1984, a well-designed case control study by the United States Public Health Service found 93% of identified cases of Reye syndrome had salicylate exposure as compared with 28% of emergency room controls and 55% of community children. Aspirin manufacturers placed a warning label on their products in 1986. In the late 1980s, cases of confirmed Reye syndrome declined to fewer than 50 per year.[237-240]

In 1989, the Centers for Disease Control (CDC) issued the following case definition for Reye syndrome:

1. Acute noninflammatory encephalopathy documented by alteration in the level of consciousness and either: (a) a record, if available, of cerebrospinal fluid (CSF) containing < 8 leukocytes/mm^3; or (b) histologic sections of the brain demonstrating cerebral edema without perivascular or meningeal inflammation.
2. Hepatopathy documented either by biopsy or autopsy considered to be diagnostic of Reye syndrome or by threefold or greater rise in the levels of either serum aspartate aminotransferase (AST), serum alanine aminotransferase (ALT), or serum ammonia.
3. No more reasonable explanation for the cerebral or hepatic abnormalities.

The clinical staging of Reye syndrome has been useful in describing the progression and prognosis of the disorder.

The stages reflect deepening levels of stupor and coma (Table 52-17).

In recent years, the term *Reye-like syndrome* has been increasingly used to describe a variety of pathologic conditions resulting from defects in urea and fatty acid metabolism, toxicologic injury, and impaired gluconeogenesis.

Pathophysiology

Whereas the etiology of the disorder is unknown, widespread mitochondrial damage is found in all parts of the body with pathognomonic changes seen under electron microscopy. Mitochondrial enzyme disruption produces derangements in urea synthesis, gluconeogenesis, and the Krebs cycle, leading to elevated ammonia levels, hypoglycemia, cellular lipid accumulation, and lactic acidosis.

Diagnostic Findings

The child with altered mental status and liver dysfunction is immediately suspected of having Reye syndrome. The classic history is one of a viral illness such as an upper respiratory infection, influenza, or varicella. Within 3 to 5 days persistent vomiting develops that is intractable to the usual interventions at home. The child then becomes listless or drowsy with a change in personality. Disorientation may lead to delirium and convulsions. The child may become confused, disinterested, lethargic, or may experience hallucinations (stage I). The subtle signs of encephalopathy give way to more overt manifestations—combativeness and delirium (stage II). Most children are brought to the ED for care at stage II. Rapid deterioration may follow with hyperventilation, coma, and decorticate posturing (stage III), followed by deeper coma and decerebrate posturing (stage IV). Physiologically the brain is swelling and the liver is enlarging; the latter is often clinically detectable within the first 2 days of presentation.[241]

An important point to elicit in the history is medication usage. Salicylate exposure is common and may occur through over-the-counter medicines with "hidden" salicylates such as bismuth subsalicylate. The adolescent patient tends to self-medicate and parents may not know about salicylate usage. Antiemetics such as promethazine or prochlorperazine suppositories may contribute to patient lethargy and cloud the issue of Reye syndrome.[242]

Laboratory data includes elevated aminotransferase and ammonia, decreased serum glucose, and prolonged PT. The CSF is normal and the EEG is of no predictive value.

Differential Considerations

There are five major diagnoses to consider in the patient with suspected Reye syndrome:

1. The first and most common is viral syndrome with dehydration. Most children suffering from this entity improve rapidly with vigorous hydration—they also have normal hepatic function.
2. A child with sepsis or meningitis who has lethargy, seizure, and coagulopathy often has laboratory evidence of focal infection such as pyuria or CSF pleocytosis. Serum ammonia remains normal. Toxic shock

syndrome may include hepatic dysfunction and elevated prothrombin time, but is notable for pathognomonic skin and mucous membrane changes.

3. Acute liver failure presents with hepatic dysfunction, hepatomegaly, and altered mental status but is distinguished from Reye syndrome by the presence of hyperbilirubinemia.

4. A toxin or drug exposure characterized by vomiting, lethargy, coma, and hepatic dysfunction can be distinguished from Reye syndrome by obtaining a history of illicit drug use, massive salicylate ingestion, or overuse of phenothiazine antiemetics. Regardless of history, suspected cases should undergo toxicology screening of urine and blood.

5. Inborn errors of metabolism with overlapping features such as acidosis, hyperammonemia, hypoglycemia, and hepatomegaly are difficult to distinguish from Reye syndrome. Many purported cases of Reye syndrome diagnosed in the 1970s and 1980s were probably inherited metabolic abnormalities. Their distinguishing features are an age less than 2 years, history of delayed growth and development, recurrent attacks, a family history of metabolic disorder, and an abnormal serum aminogram or abnormal serum organic acids. Major metabolic disturbances that can be confused with Reye syndrome are defects in ureagenesis such as ornithine transcarbamylase deficiency, carbamoyl phosphate synthetase deficiency, and citrullinemia; amino acid degradation defects (e.g., types I and II glutaric acidemia and isovaleric acidemia); and fatty acid oxidation disorders (e.g., carnitine deficiency and medium- and long-chain acyl coenzyme A dehydrogenase deficiency).[243]

Management

The child with suspected Reye syndrome deserves immediate attention. Conduct a focused neurologic examination and administer IV fluids containing dextrose to prevent hypoglycemia. Perform routine laboratory evaluations including complete blood count, electrolytes, serum glucose, lumbar puncture with complete analysis, and toxicology screens. If lethargy persists after adequate fluid resuscitation and both CNS infection and toxic exposure have been ruled out, then Reye syndrome is a more likely possibility. Limit fluid administration to prevent complications of cerebral swelling. Expand the laboratory evaluation to include liver enzymes, serum ammonia, and PT/PTT. A urine and serum metabolic screen should be obtained because some inborn errors of metabolism occur in a Reye-like manner. Consult with intensivist and gastroenterology colleagues to maximize supportive care.

A liver biopsy should be considered if a child is in stage II (delirious, combative) or worse. If the patient progresses from CDC stage II to III, intubation and placement of an intracranial pressure monitor are indicated. Intracranial pressure should be controlled with hyperventilation and osmotic and diuretic agents.[244] Suspected cases of Reye syndrome should be reported to the national registry based at the CDC.

CONDITIONS REQUIRING SURGERY
Appendicitis

LISA SINCLAIR HART

Appendicitis is the most common acute surgical condition of the abdomen. Approximately 6% of the population will develop appendicitis during their lifetime. The disease can present at any age but is most common in the second and third decades. Males outnumber females by a ratio of 2 to 1. Appendicitis is more common in developed countries than in primitive societies although the reason for this is unclear.[245] The mortality rate in the United States for unruptured appendicitis is 0.1%, whereas if ruptured the rate climbs to 3% to 5%.[246,247]

Accurately diagnosing appendicitis is a challenge. Approximately 25% of patients undergoing laparotomy for suspected appendicitis have a normal appendix removed. However, attempts to decrease the number of "negative appendectomies" has resulted in a higher rate of perforated appendicitis. Thus early surgery for suspected appendicitis has remained the cornerstone of treatment. Clinicians must consider appendicitis in any child with fever and abdominal pain since many patients do not present with "classic" signs and symptoms. The adage remains "when in doubt, take it out."

Pathophysiology. At birth the cecum is shaped like an inverted pyramind with the appendix forming a small diverticulum off the inferior border. The primitive shape of the appendix and the paucity of lymphatic tissue during infancy make it unlikely to become obstructed.[246] Hence, acute appendicitis is rare in this age group. As the child grows the appendix assumes its adult configuration and there is an increase in lymphatic tissue. The amount of lymphatic tissue in the appendix correlates with the incidence of acute appendicitis; both peak during the adolescent years.

Acute appendicitis occurs when the lumen of the organ becomes obstructed. This initial obstruction may be caused by fecaliths, lymphatic hyperplasia, fruit or vegetable matter, worms, inspissated barium, or tumors. Obstruction by hypertrophied lymphatic tissue appears to be a major factor in children because appendicitis often occurs following gastroenteritis, an upper respiratory infection, measles, or infectious mononucleosis.

Obstruction of the appendiceal lumen triggers a sequence of events. The mucosa of the appendix continues to secrete its normal fluid leading to distension of the appendix. This stimulates visceral afferent autonomic nerves that enter the spinal cord at T_8 to T_{10}. The patient develops referred pain at these dermatomes, which is perceived as epigastric or periumbilical pain. As the appendix distends further, veins become engorged and inflammation spreads to the serosa and parietal peritoneum. This inflammation triggers local somatic pain fibers, causing the pain to move to the right lower quadrant. The distension eventually cuts off the arterial supply to the appendix, and its walls infarct and subsequently perforate. In adults, inflammatory cells and a well-developed omentum wall off the infection and prevent its diffuse spread. However, in young children the omentum is less well-developed and rupture of the appendix quickly leads to diffuse peritonitis. This complication may be a contributing factor to the higher mortality of young children with appendicitis.

Diagnostic Findings

Clinical Findings. Patients with acute appendicitis often have "classic" signs and symptoms that clearly point the physician toward the correct diagnosis. However, appendicitis is equally likely to occur with misleading symptoms by history and atypical findings on physical examination. For these reasons, appendicitis should be considered in the differential diagnosis of every child with acute abdominal pain.

Generally, the patient first notices a diffuse, periumbilical, continuous abdominal pain. Anorexia develops early in the course of the illness, followed by a cramping feeling as local inflammation triggers peristalsis. This is often followed by nausea and vomiting; diarrhea is unusual. There may be mild elevation of the temperature (approximately 1° C), but high spiking fever is unusual in nonruptured appendicitis. After 1 to 12 hours (average 4 to 6 hours), inflammation spreads to involve the peritoneum, and local pain receptors trigger a severe right lower quadrant pain. At this point patients usually seek medical attention if they have not done so already. Clearly in young children the symptoms vary considerably from the typical adult symptoms. O'Shea found that vomiting and fever were the most reliable findings in children with appendicitis.[248]

Physical examination of the patient with appendicitis typically reveals the patient lying supine with legs drawn up close to the abdomen. Pain occurs with movement. Vital signs are usually normal with the exception of a low-grade fever. The patient usually can localize the pain to a single point in the right lower quadrant, classically called *McBurney's point* (originally described as 1 to 2 inches from the anterior superior iliac spine on a line drawn between it and the umbilicus). The patient usually has rebound tenderness that often can be elicited simply with light percussion. There may be pain referred to the right lower quadrant with percussion of the left lower quadrant (Rovsing's sign). Involuntary guarding of the right lower quadrant and cutaneous hyperesthesia in this area are common. As inflammation of the appendix worsens the organ may rupture, leading to higher fever and tachycardia accompanied by worsening peritoneal signs. Occasionally an abscess will form and it may be palpable as a diffuse fluctuant mass in the right lower quadrant.

The tip of the appendix occasionally lies in unusual positions, leading to variations in the examination. For example, if the appendix lies in a retrocecal position, the patient will complain of pain in the flank or back and may not have the classic peritoneal findings. An appendix that lies near the psoas muscle will produce pain with extension of the right hip (positive psoas sign). If the tip of the appendix lies in the left lower quadrant, the patient will have pain in that location. Finally, when the appendix lies in the pelvis the patient will complain of more diffuse abdominal or suprapubic pain. The inflamed appendix lying near the rectum may provoke diarrhea. A rectal examination will reveal localized tenderness and occasionally a fluctuant mass. The patient with a pelvic appendix will also generally have pain with internal rotation of the flexed right hip (positive obturator sign).

Complications. As a result of earlier diagnosis and improvements in surgical and anesthetic techniques, the mortality from nonruptured acute appendicitis has fallen to 0.1%.[247] In gangrenous appendicitis, the mortality rate is 0.6%. Once perforation occurs, the mortality increases markedly to 5%. Obviously the main goal in acute appendicitis is to diagnose the condition before perforation and its attendant complications.

The pathophysiology leading to rupture and its clinical manifestations were described previously. After the appendix ruptures a phlegmon is produced, consisting of a mass of matted intestines and omentum with little pus. (When the appendix ruptures, generally less than 0.1 ml of pus is extruded because of its small luminal capacity.) As the infection progresses, an expanding collection of pus is produced that is walled off to form an abscess. If this walling off is incomplete, there will be a diffuse peritonitis rather than a focal abscess. Occasionally the patient can develop pylephlebitis, which is a septic phlebitis of the portal veins. Clinically the symptoms of this condition are high fever, chills, jaundice, and a toxic appearance. This complication has a high morbidity and mortality.[246]

Approximately 30% of patients with acute appendicitis have a perforated appendix at the time of surgery; a review of reported series reveals that this ranges from 18.6% to 41%.[249-251] Harberg reports that acute appendicitis progresses to perforation in 10% of patients by 24 hours and in nearly 50% by 48 hours.[253]

Preschool-age children have a much higher rate of perforation, variably reported as 50% to 85%.[246,252] The higher perforation rate is most likely due to delay in diagnosis because of the nonspecific nature of the symptoms in this age group. Young children also are more likely to develop a diffuse peritonitis because they have more difficulty "walling-off" the infection in the periappendiceal region. For this reason, surgical colleagues should be consulted quickly when a diagnosis of appendicitis is being considered in any preschool-age child.

Because of the high morbidity and mortality associated with appendiceal rupture, surgeons often will err on the side of removing the appendix in questionable cases. This conservative approach leads to a higher rate of laparotomies with removal of a normal appendix, as many as 20% to 25% of cases.[253,254] Surgeons must weigh the morbidity and mortality of ruptured appendicitis against the morbidity and mortality of a negative laparotomy. Other complications that can occur from appendectomy include wound infection,[251,254,255] small bowel obstruction, and prolonged ileus.[249,251]

Ancillary Data. No laboratory test is diagnostic for appendicitis. For this reason an extensive laboratory evaluation is unnecessary. However, each patient should have a CBC with differential and a urinalysis. A type and crossmatch should be considered. Further tests are indicated only as dictated by unusual findings on history and physical examination.

The CBC will be most remarkable for a moderate leukocytosis with a predominance of PMN cells. Over 80% of patients with acute appendicitis have a WBC count greater than 10,000/mm.[256-259] A similar percentage will have a left-shifted differential with more than 75% neutrophils.[9,13,15] When considered together, only 4% of patients with acute appendicitis have a normal WBC and neutrophil count.[256-258] The WBC count in acute appendicitis is generally in the range of 10,000 to 15,000 cells/mm^3. If it exceeds 15,000 cells/mm^3, the patient is more likely to have a perforated appendix.[249] Perhaps the greatest value of the WBC count is if it is normal. In that case, if the examination is equivocal, the surgeon may decide to watch the patient for a few hours rather than immediately proceeding to the operating room.[256-259]

The urinalysis in a patient with appendicitis is usually normal with the exception of findings consistent with dehydration.[246] Many patients with appendicitis will have mildly abnormal microscopic findings with small numbers of white or red cells in the urine secondary to ureteral inflammation. However, any patient with more than 30 RBCs/HPF or 20 WBCs/HPF, especially with clumps of cells or casts in the urine, should be evaluated carefully for a urinary tract infection.

Radiologic Studies. An extensive radiologic evaluation is not necessary in classic appendicitis because it only delays definitive treatment and is costly for the patient. Radiologic evaluation should be saved for patients with equivocal physical findings or for women in their childbearing years who usually need to have a sonographic evaluation of their uterus and ovaries. However, radiologic evaluation of patients with appendicitis remains an active focus of research and controversy.

Plain x-ray films of the abdomen, although commonly ordered, are generally not helpful. Several "classic" radiographic findings are suggestive of appendicitis but are not pathognomonic for the disease. Examples of common findings include loss of the psoas shadow on the right, localized air-fluid collections in the cecum and terminal ileum, scoliosis of the lumbar spine, fecalith, gas in the appendix, haziness over the right sacroiliac joint, obliteration of the right properitoneal fat line, and free air.[246,255,260] Fecaliths, though classically described in appendicitis, were only present in 1.14% of 570 patients studied by Lewis et al.[254]

Graded compression ultrasonography is a promising technique that is receiving increasing attention in the literature. There is a characteristic appearance of an inflamed appendix on ultrasound. In adults this has been described as a noncompressible appendix with a diameter of 7 mm or greater in anterior-posterior diameter.[261,262] However, no specific size criterion has been developed for acute appendicitis in children. Identification of a noncompressible appendix is strongly suggestive of appendicitis as is the presence of fecaliths, free fluid in the region of the cecum, increased echogenicity of the periappendiceal fat, and loss of the submucosal layer of the appendix.[263] One study of graded compression ultrasonography in 98 children less than 13 years old reported a sensitivity of 85%, specificity of 94%, and overall diagnostic accuracy of 91.8%.[263] This has been comparable to the clinical validity in adult studies.[261,264] The low sensitivity reflects false negative ultrasounds that are particularly concerning. Several authors have mentioned that perforated appendicitis is harder to visualize on ultrasound and may lead to a false negative.[265,266]

A barium enema may be helpful in some equivocal cases. An examination in which the appendix fails to fill with barium is suggestive of appendicitis. Still it should be noted that in approximately 10% of patients without appendicitis, the appendix does not fill.[250,267-270] The sensitivity of barium enema has been reported as 90% to 100%, with a specificity of 75% to 98%.[250,261,269]

The accuracy of CT scan, nuclear medicine scans, and laparoscopy and their exact role in diagnosing appendicitis need further study.[271,272]

Differential Considerations. Other disease entities can simulate appendicitis with symptoms of right lower quadrant pain and peritoneal findings. The disease most commonly confused with appendicitis in children is mesenteric lymphadenitis. Usually the associated pain is less pronounced and less sharply localized. Acute gastroenteritis in young children can also appear with right lower quadrant pain. (*Yersinia enterocolitica* infection is a classic example.) Women of childbearing age present a diagnostic challenge because several gynecologic disorders can mimic appendicitis, including pelvic inflammatory disease, ovarian torsion, ruptured ovarian cyst, and ruptured ectopic pregnancy. Women in this age group have a negative laparotomy for appendicitis in 30% to 50% of cases.[255] Other conditions that have been confused with appendicitis in the past include Meckel's diverticulitis, regional enteritis, intussusception, urinary tract infection, perforated peptic ulcer, nephrolithiasis, HSP, acute intermittent porphyria, child abuse, testicular torsion, epididymitis, and right lower lobe pneumonia[254,273,274] (see section on Abdominal Pain).

Putnam and Emmens reported a series of pediatric patients with a negative laparotomy rate of only 1.5%.[251] They maintain that such accuracy in diagnosis resulted from admitting and observing all children with equivocal findings on examination. Their perforation rate at the time of surgery was 30%, which is well within acceptable limits for the pediatric age group.

Management. The emergency physician must stabilize the patient and consider the etiology of an acute abdomen, if present. Coordination of surgical consultation, fluid resuscitation, and preparation for surgery are important components of management. Minimally invasive surgical techniques have significantly reduced the morbidity and length of stay associated with surgical management.

Fluid resuscitation and correction of electrolyte disturbances is essential following evaluation and stabilization of the airway and breathing. Oxygen may often be appropriate. Some patients, particularly young children, may have symptoms of shock because of sepsis or hypovolemia. Hypovolemia is often secondary to vomiting, diarrhea, anorexia, and third-space losses into the inflamed bowel. Patients should be resuscitated with a minimum of 20 ml/kg of crystalloid consisting of 0.9% NS or LR. Surgical consultation should be sought concurrent with efforts to stabilize the patient.

If there is evidence of peritonitis, antibiotic therapy should be administered preoperatively and continued after surgery to cover the most common offending organisms including *Bacteroides fragilis, E. coli,* and enteric streptococcal species.[246,249,251] Many authors recommend triple antibiotics consisting of ampicillin (100 to 200 mg/kg/24 hr q 4 hr IV), clindamycin (30 to 40 mg/kg/24 hr q 6 hr IV), and gentamicin (5 to 7.5 mg/kg/24 hr q 8 hr IV).[251,252,275]

NG tube suction may be useful in cases of small bowel obstruction, peritonitis, or abdominal distension.

If there is any difficulty in making the diagnosis, a period of observation may be warranted. This should provide an increased data base and reduce the high rate of perforation, particularly in young children.

Hirschsprung Disease

JULIAN B. ORENSTEIN

Hirschsprung disease is defined as the absence of intramural ganglion cells from the rectum to the sigmoid or proximal colon. In the Emergency Department, patients present with enterocolitis or chronic constipation.

Pathophysiology. Arrest of migration of ganglion cells results in aganglionosis in the rectosigmoid in 77% of patients and in the entire colon in 15%. The genetic defect responsible for this altered migration recently has been localized to chromosome 10.[277] Rarely, there is involvement of the entire intestinal tract or "ultrashort" disease affecting only the distal rectum. Skip segments within the colon do not occur. While the transition zone to ganglionized bowel is usually well-demarcated histologically, it often appears as a conical segment at surgery or radiographically. In the aganglionic segment, normal colonic relaxation does not occur, and dysmotility and spasm result in constipation or acute obstruction.

Etiology. The incidence of Hirschsprung disease is 1 in 5,000 births. It occurs equally in African-Americans and whites and four times more commonly in males than in females. Hirschsprung disease has been associated with Down syndrome and, less frequently, with deafness (Waardenburg syndrome) and genitourinary anomalies.[276]

Diagnostic Findings. The diagnosis is usually made in the newborn nursery and should be suspected if there has been no passage of meconium for 24 to 48 hours. Vomiting, abdominal distension, and tenderness, and other signs of obstruction may occur.

Beyond the newborn period, children with Hirschsprung disease have moderate to severe constipation associated with abdominal discomfort and bloating. They also can have toxic megacolon, which is an acute enterocolitis characterized by fever, explosive bloody diarrhea, vomiting, abdominal distension, and tenderness. There is erosion and ulceration of the mucosa above the aganglionic segment, and perforation, pneumoperitoneum, severe electrolyte derangements, shock, and death can ensue. The length of the aganglionic segment does not help to predict either the development of enterocolitis or the clinical course. Postoperative enterocolitis also occurs in a significant number of patients and is thought to develop from chronic residual damage to the colonic mucosa. The frequency of postoperative enterocolitis has decreased in recent years because of earlier diagnosis and improved surgical management.[278]

Ancillary Data. An abdominal x-ray series and a barium enema should be performed initially. The cone-shaped transition zone and dilated segment of proximal colon may be seen, particularly on the lateral view at the rectum. The transition zone is usually evident in older children but it may not be as obvious in infants, with the rectosigmoid having a "sawtooth" appearance. In cases of total aganglionosis, the colon may appear entirely normal or short with rounding of the hepatic and splenic flexures. In such cases, the diagnosis should still be suspected if there is delayed passage of barium over the next 2 to 3 days. Ultrashort segment Hirschsprung disease is characterized by presence of ganglion cells on biopsy but with abnormal manometry studies typical of Hirschsprung disease. Internal anal sphincter myomectomy is curative in these patients.[279]

In most children, rectal manometry demonstrates paradoxical contraction of the internal anal sphincter. A definitive diagnosis of Hirschsprung disease is made surgically by rectal biopsy, which demonstrates an absence of ganglion cells in the rectal submucosa. The colonic mucosa is biopsied proximally until ganglion cells are demonstrated at some level.

Differential Considerations. In newborns, the main diagnosis to exclude is meconium plug syndrome due to cystic fibrosis. Barium enema is both diagnostic and therapeutic, and the diagnosis can be confirmed by a sweat chloride test. In older children, differentiation from functional or other causes of constipation can be difficult (see section on Constipation). An acquired form of this disease can be found in trypanosomiasis (Chagas disease), in which there is destruction of ganglion cells in the heart and distal rectum.[280]

Management. The chronically constipated infant or child in whom Hirschsprung disease is suspected should be referred for radiographic and manometric studies. The acutely ill child with enterocolitis requires fluid resuscitation and stabilization. The standard surgical approach includes a decompressing colostomy at the time of diagnosis followed by a definitive repair and colostomy closure at about 1 year of age. Older patients may tolerate a single stage repair, which also has been performed in infants under 3 months of age with no increase in morbidity.[281] Almost all children regain full continence within 1 year after surgery.

Early complications of surgery include stenosis and anastomotic leak with perineal abscess formation. Late complications include constipation and enterocolitis in up to 9% of patients. Enterocolitis is characterized by abdominal distension, bloody diarrheal stools, fever, and an elevated WBC. Plain films of the abdomen will show signs of obstruction with dilated loops of bowel and air-fluid levels. Hospital admission is required for a rectal tube or dilation, colonic irrigations every 6 to 8 hours, antibiotics, fluid support, and possible emergency colostomy. Blood and stool cultures are usually negative, although many patients develop high titers of *C. difficile* toxin. Vancomycin is the treatment of choice in this situation.

Patients with total aganglionosis may have a different postoperative course and develop chronic liquid diarrhea, presenting to the emergency department with rectal distension and liquid feces. This complication can be relieved with a rectal tube, and admission should be considered for further monitoring and fluid management.

Inguinal Hernia

DANIEL W. OCHSENSCHLAGER

Inguinal hernias in infants and children are a frequent reason for seeking medical evaluation in an emergency department. Representing approximately 37% of all surgical procedures, inguinal herniorrhaphy is the most commonly performed surgical procedure in the pediatric age group.

Pathophysiology. To understand the pathogenesis of inguinal hernias, it is necessary to review the embryology of gonadal descent. At about the third month of gestation, a protrusion of the ventral abdominal wall, the processus vaginalis, appears. In males, this sac evaginates through the internal inguinal ring, and the testicle begins its descent, reaching the distal scrotum between the seventh and ninth months of gestation. Shortly before or at birth, the processus vaginalis looses its communication with the peritoneum, becomes atretic, and forms a fibrous cord between the internal inguinal ring and the upper portion of the scrotal sac. Failure of the processus vaginalis to obliterate increases the likelihood of both indirect inguinal hernias and hydroceles.

In females, normally, there is no external migration of gonads; however, a diverticulum of the peritoneum, the canal of Nuck, corresponds to the processus vaginalis in males. Failure of closure of the canal of Nuck predisposes to the development of inguinal hernias. The fallopian tube with or without the ovary is found in the hernia sacs of 21% of females with inguinal hernias[282] (see Chapter 60).

Only a small percentage of patients with a patent processus vaginalis or canal of Nuck actually develop inguinal hernias. Approximately 60% of infants less than 1 year of age, 40% of children less than 2 years of age, and 20% of adults have a patent processus vaginalis, but few have clinically apparent inguinal hernias.[282]

Etiology. Among 1,000 live births approximately 10 to 20 will have inguinal hernias. Virtually all inguinal hernias in the pediatric age group are indirect. They are largely a phenomenon of infancy. Inguinal hernias occur in 30% of premature infants, and approximately one third of all inguinal hernias are diagnosed by 6 months of age.[282] Right-sided hernias occur more commonly than left-sided ones (60% vs. 30%), and they occur bilaterally in about 10% of cases.[283] Boys are approximately six times more likely than girls to have inguinal hernias.[283-285]

Entities associated with an increased incidence of inguinal hernias are listed in the box above. Excess peritoneal fluid causes increased intraabdominal pressure, forcing open the processus vaginalis. Patients with cystic fibrosis are more likely to develop hernias because of poor nutrition, increased intraabdominal pressure due to coughing, or generalized muscle or tissue wasting. Infants with intersex syndromes, especially phenotypic females, frequently have hernias containing a gonad. In testicular feminization syndrome this gonad is really a testis, and in hermaphroditism an ova-testes.

Diagnostic Findings

Clinical Findings. Parents usually report a bulge or mass in the groin that becomes larger with crying or other

---

Entities Associated with an Increased Incidence of Inguinal Hernias

Increases in volume of peritoneal fluid
  Ventricular-peritoneal shunt
  Peritoneal dialysis
  Ascites
Increases in abdominal pressure
  Tumors
Connective tissue disorders
  Ehlers-Danlos syndrome
  Marfan syndrome
Mucopolysaccharidoses
  Hunter syndrome
  Hurler syndrome
Cystic fibrosis
Genitourinary abnormalities
  Exstrophy of the bladder
  Hypospadias
  Epispadias
Intersex syndromes
  Testicular feminization syndrome
  Hermaphroditism

---

forms of the Valsalva maneuver and disappears when the infant is quiet. The infant may seem fussy or in pain. An older child may complain of vague groin pain especially during exercise. Parents should be asked about signs and symptoms of intestinal obstruction such as vomiting and abdominal distension. It is also important to determine how long the hernia has been noted; generally, the longer a hernia has protruded, the more difficult it is to reduce.

On physical examination, a smooth, firm, sausage-shaped, nontender or slightly tender mass can be seen and palpated in the groin. This structure seems to originate proximally at the external inguinal ring and may extend completely into the scrotum. A definitive diagnosis can be made during reduction, which usually occurs with a gurgling sound and a "swoosh." Because the hernia often reduces before the patient is examined by a physician, it helps to have a cooperative child perform the Valsalva maneuver (e.g., cry, cough, strain, or blow up a balloon). Detecting the "silk glove" sign can also be useful. This is accomplished by rubbing one's index finger over the spermatic cord at the pubic tubercle. A slippery feel similar to two layers of silk rubbing together is considered positive. This silky sensation results from the movement of the two layers of the hernia sac against each other. Finally, one must remember to evaluate for signs of intestinal obstruction.

Ancillary Data. X-ray studies should not be needed for diagnosis. Occasionally, however, they can help to demonstrate intestinal obstruction. Also visualization of bowel gas in the scrotum will confirm the presence of a hernia. Ocassionally translumination may be positive especially if the bowel is filled with fluid.

Differential Considerations. Hydroceles are commonly mistaken for hernias, and the differentiation can be difficult. A hydrocele is also formed by an outpocketing of the peritoneum and a lack of complete obliteration of the processus vaginalis. Rarely, there can be a hydrocele of the canal of Nuck. A hydrocele usually becomes apparent during the first few months of life and disappears spontaneously by 1 year of age. It is asymptomatic, although it may cause considerable anxiety to the parents. The fluid-filled mass can form anywhere along the course of the spermatic cord from the testicle to the abdomen. A slightly soft to firm spherical, freely movable, nontender mass is palpable in the scrotum, separate from the testicle. Translumination is positive, revealing a brilliant fluid-filled structure. Unless the hydrocele communicates with the peritoneal cavity, its size does not change when a Valsalva maneuver is performed or upon recumbency; however, communicating hydroceles can be made smaller by squeezing. A hydrocele "reduces" much more slowly than an inguinal hernia and, unlike a hernia, never completely disappears. It usually resolves spontaneously by 1 year of age; if it does not resolve by the age of 2, it is unlikely to resolve at all and most surgeons recommend operating at this time.[286]

Inguinal lymphadenopathy can be confused with inguinal hernias; however, enlarged lymph nodes generally do not involve the inguinal canal and usually are smaller, finer, and multiple. In lymphadenopathy, the spermatic cord should be palpated easily. There may be an associated adjacent skin infection or an infection of the ipsilateral extremity.

An undescended or high-riding testicle in the inguinal canal or upper scrotum may seem like a hernia. When diagnosing a hernia, it is important that a testicle be felt in the scrotum. Undescended or high-riding testicles are usually smaller and more discrete than hernias, and sometimes they can be retracted into the scrotum.

Certain urologic problems (e.g., torsion of a testicle, torsion of an appendix testes, and epididymitis) result in a tender, enlarged scrotum. Except for torsion of a testicle, which sometimes occurs in the neonatal period, these are more common in prepubertal and pubertal boys. Furthermore, they are associated with considerable pain upon palpation. Finally, these masses, which at times seem to occupy the entire scrotum, do not extend into the inguinal canal.

Management. First, the clinician needs to determine whether there are signs or symptoms of intestinal obstruction or perforation such as abdominal distention, intensifying pain, rebound tenderness, bilious vomiting, bloody stools, absent bowel sounds, decreased mental status, or shock. If intestinal obstruction or perforation is suspected, blood studies should be obtained, IV line inserted and fluids administered, nasogastric tube placed, and emergency surgery consultation sought.

If there is no evidence of a surgical emergency and the hernia does not reduce spontaneously (i.e., it is incarcerated), an attempt should be made to reduce it. Ninety-five percent of all inguinal hernias can be reduced without surgery by applying gentle persistent pressure on the hernia sac.[284] Afterwards, it is important to confirm that the sac is completely reduced and that the inguinal canal is entirely empty.

If simple pressure does not reduce the hernia, more aggressive means can be attempted. It sometimes helps to have the patient in a Trendelenburg position with ice or cold compresses placed over the inguinal area to reduce edema. Many surgeons try various muscle relaxants, sedatives, or analgesics to promote reduction. In case immediate surgery is necessary, these drugs should not be given by mouth.

If the hernia still cannot be reduced, surgical consultation should be requested. The hernia may be strangulated, implying ischemic damage to the intestine. Applying greater pressure to the hernia sac is not likely to be successful. Although it is supposedly axiomatic that infarcted bowel cannot be reduced, this is not always the case.

An ovary can be difficult to reduce. Compared to incarcerated bowel, the likelihood of strangulation is less, therefore some surgeons believe that surgery can be delayed if the ovary appears normal (i.e., nontender and neither red nor enlarged). If there are signs suggesting vascular compromise, however, emergency surgery is necessary.

All patients with hernias need surgery at some date, and arrangements for surgical follow-up should be made. If the hernia reduces spontaneously or is easily reduced, the patient can be discharged and surgery performed at a later date although some surgeons prefer to observe all patients for several hours as inpatients. Before discharge, the parents should be instructed to immediately seek medical care if the hernia cannot be easily reduced by gentle pressure at home. If the hernia was reduced with some difficulty, the patient should be admitted for observation and early surgery. Surgery should be planned as early as possible because up to 35% of children with an inguinal hernia will have an episode of incarceration before the time of elective surgery.[287]

Intussusception

YEHESKEL WAISMAN

Intussusception is one of the most common abdominal emergencies of infancy and early childhood. It is defined as a prolapse of one part of the intestine into the lumen of an immediately adjoining part. Complications of intussusception include intestinal hemorrhage, necrosis and bowel perforation, and shock. Spontaneous reduction of an intussusception rarely occurs; therefore, if left undiagnosed and untreated, it can result in death. Administration of timely treatment, however, ensures a 99% survival.

Pathophysiology. The intussusception usually starts with a lead point just proximal to the ileocecal valve causing an ileocolic invagination. The prolapse can continue through the colon for a variable distance, occasionally as far as the rectum. Ileoileal and colocolic forms may also occur but these are far less common. During invagination, the mesentery is dragged along with the intussusceptum (invaginating portion) into the intussuscipiens (recipient portion), obstructing the venous return. Engorgement of the intussusceptum eventually occurs, resulting in edema and bleeding from the mucosa and the development of bloody mucousy stools ("current-jelly" stools). If entrapment of the bowel and mesentery continues, mounting pressure causes obstruction to the arterial blood supply, which leads to intestinal gangrene and perforation. Most intussusceptions do not result in strangulation of the bowel within the first 24 hours.

Etiology. Male infants (male-to-female ratio = 2:1) 3 to 12 months of age are most commonly affected, and there is a seasonal prevalence with peaks in the spring and autumn. In children younger than 2 years of age, a pathologic lead point for the intussusception is found in less than 10% of cases, and hypertrophied Peyer's patches secondary to a viral infection are believed to be the cause. However, in children over the age of 5 years, an underlying lesion such as a polyp, ileal duplication, lymphoma, inverted Meckel's diverticulum, or Henoch-Schönlein intramural hematoma is found in over 75% of the cases.

Diagnostic Findings. The classic triad of symptoms includes intermittent colicky abdominal pain, vomiting, and passage of stool mixed with blood and mucus. Although characteristic, the full triad is infrequently encountered (21% of cases), and in 70% of the cases only two symptoms are present.[288] Typically, the colicky pain appears first (70% to 80% of cases) and dominates the clinical picture. It is episodic and persists for about 4 to 5 minutes, during which the infant may pull his knees up in distress. Between attacks there is 10 to 20 minutes of complete relief. Gradually, the child becomes more irritable, anorectic, and begins to vomit (90% of cases). Later, the vomitus may become bilious because of intestinal obstruction. Currant-jelly stools may appear either spontaneously or after a rectal examination but usually not before 12 hours after the onset of pain. Because these stools occur in only 50% of the cases, their absence does not exclude the diagnosis of intussusception. On the other hand, stools with occult blood in children with nonspecific signs and symptoms is supportive of intussusception.[289] Prostration and fever can ensue as symptoms progress. Occasionally, lethargy, pallor, and unresponsiveness mimicking a postictal state dominate the clinical picture.[290]

On physical examination, the finding of an elongated mass in the right upper quadrant with absence of bowel in the right lower quadrant (Dance's sign) is pathognomonic. The abdomen may be distended and tender and show signs of peritoneal irritation when necrosis or perforation occurs. Rarely, the intussusception can be palpated in the rectum or seen protruding through it.

Ancillary Data. Blood for a CBC, electrolytes, glucose, and type and crossmatch should be obtained. Urine output should be monitored. Plain abdominal films can be normal early in the disease, but if symptoms persist for longer than 8 to 12 hours, they may show signs of intestinal obstruction with distended loops and air-fluid levels proximal to the obstruction and paucity of gas distally. Occasionally, the soft tissue mass of the intussusception can be seen radiographically. Free air can be seen in cases complicated by perforation. Currently, barium enema is the "gold standard" for both diagnosis and therapy. Classic signs are a "cervix-like" mass as the barium reaches the intussusception (Fig. 52-7, A) and a coiled-spring appearance on the evacuation film (Fig. 52-7, B).

There is emerging literature regarding the use of ultrasonography in the diagnosis of intussusception. It has been reported that in experienced hands ultrasonography can reach a 98% sensitivity and a 100% specificity in the diag-

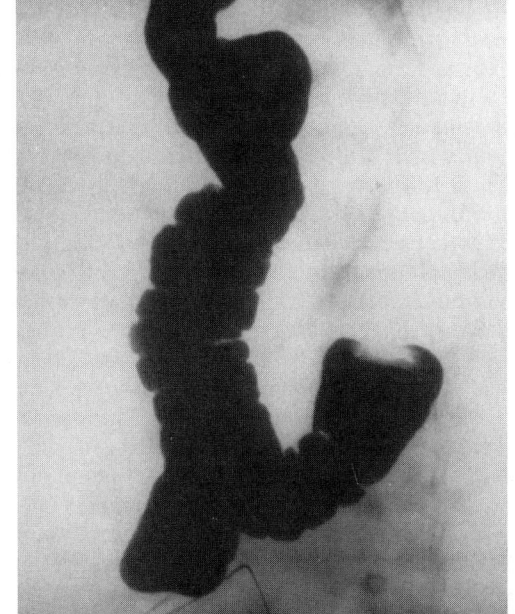

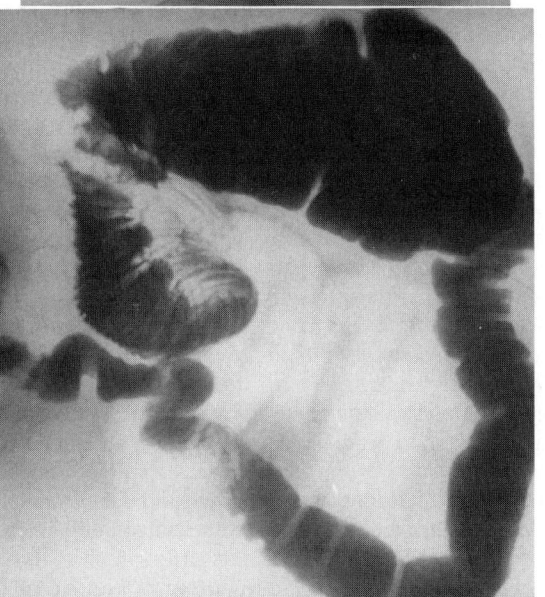

FIG. 52-7. A, Barium enema of a 12-month-old boy showing a "cervix-like" mass as the barium reaches the intussusception. **B,** An evacuation film during a barium enema demonstrating a coiled-spring appearance in the distal ileum confirming reduction of an intussusception.

nosis of intussusception.[291,292] This modality might be particularly helpful in the diagnosis when contrast studies are contraindicated.[289]

Differential Considerations. Although intussusception following gastroenteritis can be difficult to diagnose, in gastroenteritis the pain is generally milder, less regular, and not completely relieved between bouts of cramps. The bloody stools from Meckel's diverticulum are usually painless. In HSP there are additional findings such as skin rash or involvement of joints; because the two conditions may co-exist, however, a barium enema cannot be avoided. Other causes of intestinal obstruction such as Hirschsprung disease, incarcerated inguinal hernia, or malrotation should also be considered.

Management. An IV line should be inserted and IV fluids administered to correct volume deficits. Hypovolemia can be further exacerbated by fluid drawn from the intravascular compartment into the bowel lumen by the hyperosmotic barium. A nasogastric tube should be placed to decompress the obstructed bowel and reduce the risk of vomiting and aspiration. Surgical consultation should be sought.

Hydrostatic reduction by barium enema is successful in 50% to 90% of cases; however, certain contraindications exist. It is absolutely contraindicated if there is perforation, peritonitis, or profound hypovolemic shock, and the patient should be taken to surgery. Prolonged symptomatology (greater than 5 days), radiologic signs of severe intestinal obstruction, and fever associated with leukocytosis and toxicity are considered by some to be relative contraindications because of the risk of causing perforation or reducing unsuspected nonviable bowel.[288,293] Furthermore, because of its low success rate and the possibility of missing a pathologic lead point, barium enema is relatively contraindicated in older patients or patients with recurrent intussusceptions. Relative contraindications vary and must be decided upon on an individual basis.

Potential complications of hydrostatic reduction include bowel perforation, reduction of necrotic bowel, incomplete reduction with a delay in surgery, and overlooking a pathologic lead point.[293,294] To minimize these risks the patient must be well hydrated parenterally before the procedure, which should be performed by a radiologist skilled in the procedure, because results improve with experience. A surgeon should be involved in the evaluation and management and be available for any complications that may require immediate transfer of the patient to the operating room.

The "rule of threes" should be adhered to. The barium column should not exceed a height of 3 feet above the patient, no more than 3 attempts at reduction should be performed, with only 3 minutes/attempt. Manual manipulation of the abdomen during the procedure has been considered contraindicated for many years, but a recent re-evaluation of this historical technique has been found potentially useful.[294] Full reduction must be confirmed by normal reflux of barium into the ileum; otherwise, an ileo-ileal component of intussusception might be left unreduced.

An IV analgesic should be administered to any agitated child because crying, straining, or performing Valsalva maneuvers can increase intraabdominal pressure, decreasing the success rate and increasing the risk of perforation. Fentanyl citrate, morphine, or midazolam have been advocated. Glucagon, a smooth-muscle relaxant, was initially reported to increase the success rate but has not proven beneficial in controlled studies. The child should be closely monitored throughout the procedure. If hydrostatic reduction fails, the patient must be taken to the operating room. Broad-spectrum antibiotics should be administered before surgery in consultation with a surgical colleague.

Reduction of intussusception by air insufflation has been the standard treatment in the Far East for the last decades,[295,296] but was reintroduced to the West only in the mid-1980s.[297,298] This technique is gaining acceptance and popularity in North America. In experienced hands, success rates of pneumatic reduction are comparable to barium enema reductions with fewer complications.[297,299]

Intussusception recurs in 7% to 10% of radiologic and 2% to 5% of surgical reductions, respectively. Recurrence usually occurs within the first 24 hours after reduction, so hospitalization and a follow-up film is recommended.

Meckel's Diverticulum

BRUCE L. KLEIN

Meckel's diverticulum occurs in approximately 2% of the population.[300] It is the most frequent congenital abnormality of the small intestine.[300,301] Symptomatic patients are more likely to be male, whereas there is no sexual predominance when diverticula are discovered incidentally at surgery.[302] Symptomatic patients also tend to be younger.[301,303,304] Forty-five percent of patients who have symptoms are less than 2 years old.[300]

Meckel's diverticulum was first described by Fabricius Hildanus in 1598.[303] Johann Friedrich Meckel unraveled its embryologic origins in the early 1800s.

Pathophysiology. Meckel's diverticulum is a vestige of the omphalomesenteric (vitelline) duct. The latter connects the embryo's gut to its yolk sac and should disappear completely by the seventh week of gestation. When it fails to do so, a variety of anomalies ensue. Meckel's diverticulum is by far the most common and is reported in 97% of vitelline duct remnants.[305] The tip of the diverticulum is free in 76%.[305] It is attached to the body wall or another structure in the remainder, usually by a fibrous band.[305] Omphaloileal fistulas, enterocystomas, and umbilical sinuses are other anomalies that result from incomplete obliteration of the omphalomesenteric duct that sometimes co-exist with a Meckel's diverticulum.[305,306]

Its blood supply is derived from the right vitelline artery. This usually terminates in the diverticulum itself but can continue to the abdominal wall.[300] In addition, fibrous vestiges of the vitelline vessels may persist and extend between the abdominal wall, Meckel's diverticulum, ileum, or small intestine mesentery.[300,307]

Meckel's diverticulum arises from the antimesenteric border of the ileum. It is typically located 40 to 100 cm proximal to the ileocecal valve, but lies even closer in children who are less than 2 years old.[300,308] In one study comprised mostly of asymptomatic adults, its average length was 2.99 cm and width was 1.92 cm (range: 1 cm $\times$ 0.3 cm to 11 cm $\times$ 3.5 cm).[302] It is smaller in young children. The mouth tends to be wide and is often equal in diameter to the lumen of the small intestine itself (Fig. 52-8).[301]

Meckel's diverticulum is a true diverticulum, consisting of all layers of the bowel wall.[300] Up to 60% of cases contain heterotopic tissue.[309] Some authors note a much lower incidence, however.[304,308] The frequency seems to depend upon the complaints of the patients from whom the specimens were obtained and the thoroughness of the his-

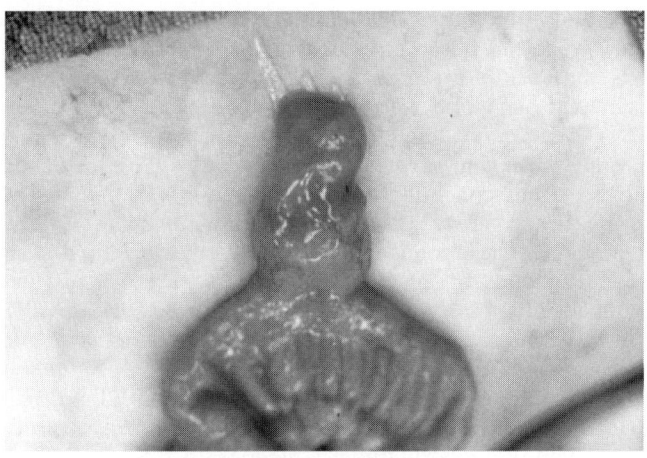

FIG. 52-8. Meckel's diverticulum.

tologic examinations. Isolated gastric mucosa is the most common finding overall, although pancreatic, duodenal, jejunal, colonic, rectal, and endometrial tissue have also been reported.[300,301,303,310] Patients who hemorrhage are particularly prone to have ectopic gastric mucosa.[306,311]

Diagnostic Findings. Only 4% of people with Meckel's diverticula will actually develop complications during their lifetimes, and the majority will do so by the age of 20.[301,304,308,312] From 6 series that totalled 830 cases of all ages, Amoury found the incidence of complications to be as follows: intestinal obstruction including intussusception (35%); bleeding (32%), diverticulitias with or without perforation (22%); umbilical fistula (10%); and other umbilical lesions, hernias, and tumors (1%).[300] These frequencies might differ if only infants and pediatric patients were studied.[313]

Intestinal obstruction can result from a variety of mechanisms. The diverticulum may act as a lead point for an ileoileal or ileocolic intussusception, or there may be herniation through or volvulus around a persistent remnant of the vitelline duct or vessels.[300,303,307,314] None of the symptoms or signs are pathognomonic for Meckel's diverticulum so the diagnosis is rarely made preoperatively.[300,304] Typical findings include abdominal pain, tenderness and distension, hyperactive bowel sounds, and vomiting. A mass may be palpated in a case of intussusception. The process can progress to bowel ischemia or infarction and produce rectal bleeding and peritoneal signs.

Isolated rectal bleeding is a particularly common mode of presentation in children under 5 years of age.[300,301] Most have ectopic gastric mucosa and the bleeding originates from a peptic ulcer within the diverticulum itself or the adjacent ileum.[300,302,304,308] Although classically described as being painless, some children experience pain.[307] Hemorrhage tends to be acute and episodic; Meckel's diverticulum is rarely a cause of chronic blood loss.[300,303] Bleeding may be massive and result in shock.[300,303,310] The stools appear brick red or like currant-jelly when the bleeding is brisk, and tarry if bleeding is minor.[300,301,303]

In contrast, diverticulitis occurs more frequently in older patients.[302,303,307] Ectopic mucosa is often found but this is not invariably so.[309] The presentation mimics appendicitis,

and the correct diagnosis is virtually never made before laparotomy.[300-302] Findings include vomiting and abdominal pain and tenderness. The pain originates in the periumbilical area before moving to the lower abdomen. About ⅓ of cases are complicated by perforation, which results in diffuse peritonitis or a localized abscess.[300]

Other rare entities that have been reported include perforation of a diverticulum by a sewing needle and incarceration of diverticula in femoral, inguinal, or umbilical hernias.[302-304] Neoplasms, which can be benign or malignant, are also uncommon; these usually affect the elderly.[302,303]

Ancillary Data. Routine tests are nonspecific but should initially include a CBC, electrolytes, BUN, glucose, bleeding screen, and type and crossmatch. Abdominal x-ray studies may demonstrate obstruction or perforation. The hemoglobin and hematocrit will be low when blood loss is significant.

The Meckel's scan is the most widely employed specific diagnostic study. Tc[99]-pertechnetate is injected intravenously, and the abdomen is scanned continuously by gamma camera for 30 to 45 minutes. Because the test depends upon the affinity of the radionucleotide for gastric mucosa, only diverticula having ectopic mucosa will be detected. It is therefore particularly useful in young children who have bleeding. The Meckel's scan is about 95% accurate for detection of gastric mucosa.[315] Administration of pentagastrin or cimetidine may increase this yield.[300,301,315,316] Although both false-negative and false-positive scans have been reported in the past, these are less common using modern techniques.[315] False negatives can result when there is only a small amount of ectopic gastric mucosa present.

Other studies can help occasionally. A large-volume barium meal or a small bowel barium enema may localize a diverticulum.[311,317] Active bleeding may be demonstrated by arteriography or by scintigraphy using ^{99m}Tc-sulfur colloid, ^{99m}Tc-human serum albumin, or ^{99m}Tc-red blood cells.[315] These are not specific for bleeding from a Meckel's diverticulum, however. Laparoscopy can also diagnose a Meckel's diverticulum.[318]

Differential Considerations. Many diseases produce abdominal pain, rectal bleeding, or symptoms of obstruction so there is a long list of differential diagnoses. These are mentioned in previous sections on gastrointestinal bleeding, which most commonly results from intestinal polyps, intussusception, anal fissures, and volvulus. A definitive diagnosis of Meckel's diverticulum is rarely made before surgery.

Management. Emergency department evaluation and treatment will vary with the mode of presentation. The patient should have a large-bore IV catheter inserted, and oral intake should be restricted. Crystalloid fluid resuscitation is generally sufficient; red blood cell transfusions are required when there is significant hemorrhage. A nasogastric tube should be placed in a patient who is obstructed and this can be connected to low suction. Surgical consultation should be obtained. Antibiotics should be administered when there is suspected strangulation. As stated previously, the Meckel's scan is most helpful in the case of a child who has bleeding and remains stable. If the child is unstable or has peritoneal signs, necessary surgery should not be delayed. A barium enema should be performed if intussusception is suspected; hydrostatic reduction often fails when a Meckel's diverticulum is the lead point.

Symptomatic diverticula must be treated surgically. For the majority of cases that present to the emergency department, the surgery should be done expeditiously. A simple diverticulectomy may suffice in some cases, whereas a more extensive resection is needed in others. The exact technique depends upon the pathology discovered at laparotomy.[300] Postoperative morbidity tends to be low. Laparoscopic diverticulectomy has recently been reported to be successful in selected cases.[318,319]

Pyloric Stenosis, Infantile Hypertrophic

BRUCE L. KLEIN

Harald Hirschsprung, a Danish pediatrician, reported two cases of pyloric stenosis in 1888.[320,321] Pyloric stenosis had been recognized more than a century earlier, but Hirschsprung described its characteristic features and is credited with establishing it as a unique disease.

Pathophysiology. The pyloric hypertrophy most likely develops postnatally. Pyloric stenosis is uncommon in the first few days of life and is almost never found in stillbirths.[321-323] Rollins performed abdominal ultrasound examinations on 1,400 consecutive newborns shortly after birth. All nine babies who ultimately developed pyloric stenosis had normal initial ultrasounds.[322] This parallels the classic history of vomiting that begins at 3 weeks of age.

Macroscopically, the pylorus is elongated and thickened, averaging 3 cm in length and 1.5 cm in diameter.[320] Microscopically, there is marked hypertrophy and hyperplasia of the circular muscle layer, which can be four times wider than normal.[320,324] There is also mucosal edema, lymphocytic infiltration of the submucosal muscle layers, and an increase in connective tissue. Changes in autonomic nerve fibers and nerve-supporting cells have been reported by some, but the significance of these changes remains uncertain.[320,324,326,327]

Etiology. Pyloric stenosis is the most common disorder requiring abdominal surgery in infancy, occurring in approximately 1 in 250 births.[325] The incidence is increasing, and there appears to be regional variations.[320,321,324,328] Whites are afflicted more often than African-Americans, and the disease is rare in Asians.[321,323,324] Males are affected four times as frequently as females.[324,325] Jedd confirmed that firstborn boys are particularly prone to developing pyloric stenosis.[329] A child of an affected parent has a nearly 7% incidence of disease; the incidence is even higher if the mother had it.[321,325] The relationship of pyloric stenosis to breast or bottlefeeding is still being debated.[329,330] Despite these interesting associations, its cause still remains unknown.

Diagnostic Findings. Vomiting is the initial complaint. It typically begins at around 3 weeks of age but can occur earlier or later.[320,321,324,325] The vomitus contains partially digested milk and mucus. It is never bile stained, although it may be blood streaked if there is an associated mucosal tear.[320,321,324,325] It occurs just after or near the end of a feeding. Afterwards, the infant will refeed hungrily unless he or she has become so malnourished that he or she has lost interest in drinking.[325] The vomiting progresses gradually and eventually becomes projectile and quite forceful. Constipation is common because the baby does not retain enough milk and may get dehydrated.[320,324,325]

Physical examination demonstrates a hungry infant who has failed to gain weight sufficiently or has even lost weight. Although emaciation is rare nowadays, signs of dehydration are frequently found. These include absence of tears, dry mucous membranes, and poor skin turgor. Jaundice is seen in 1% to 2% of cases,[321] secondary to an immature liver and starvation; it resolves rapidly after surgery.[320,321,325]

Peristaltic waves can be seen passing from left to right across the upper abdomen just before the baby vomits. Palpation of a pyloric tumor ("olive") is pathognomonic. If it is present, one can be sure of the diagnosis. This lump is usually felt near the lateral margin of the right rectus muscle below the liver edge, although it is sometimes more medial or a little lower. Although it has been reported to be palpable in 85% of patients, others have not had quite as much success.[331] Because a distended antrum can obscure the olive, it is best to feel for it right after the child has vomited or after the gastric contents have been emptied with a nasogastric tube.

Ancillary Data. Gastric secretions contain large amounts of hydrogen and chloride ions and smaller quantities of sodium and potassium ions. Moreover, the kidneys compensate by conserving sodium and wasting potassium and hydrogen. Consequently, as the vomiting progresses, a hypokalemic, hypochloremic metabolic alkalosis develops.[320,332,333] Electrolytes, glucose, BUN, and CBC should be obtained. The sodium tends to be normal, but it may be particularly low if the baby has been fed water or dilute formula.[332,333] Urine specific gravity, blood urea nitrogen, and hematocrit are elevated, reflecting volume deficit. An indirect hyperbilirubinemia is occasionally noted.[320,321,325]

If the olive can be palpated, further studies are unnecessary. If not, sonography is recommended.[325,334] Abdominal ultrasound demonstrates an increased pyloric diameter, a thickened muscle wall, and an elongated pyloric canal. Although it is reported to be at least 95% accurate, this reflects the experiences of the sonographer using a high-resolution machine.[335] False positives tend to be rare, whereas false negatives occur in up to 19% of cases.[324,336,337] The latter may result from bowel gas overlying and obscuring the tumor.[338] When sonography is negative, an upper GI series should be performed.[325,334] This reveals delayed gastric emptying, indentation of the antrum by the olive, and elongation and narrowing of the pyloric channel (the "string sign"). It too is at least 95% accurate, but its drawbacks include exposure to radiation and a risk of aspiration.[324,334] Endoscopy may prove diagnostic in younger infants but is rarely necessary.[339]

Differential Considerations. Although many disorders produce vomiting, gastroesophageal reflux is the one that is most often confused with pyloric stenosis. In contrast, it occurs even earlier, is usually not as severe, and does not tend to be as characteristically progressive. If an olive cannot be palpated, an ultrasound or upper gastrointestinal series should distinguish the two.

Management. The infant should have a parenteral fluid initiated and oral intake restricted. Any dehydration or electrolyte abnormalities should be corrected before surgery, even if this delays the definitive procedure.[320,321,324,325] Much of the reduced morbidity and mortality that has been seen recently can be attributed to meticulous monitoring of fluid and electrolyte levels.

Surgery is the treatment of choice. There is no role for medical management. The Ramstedt pyloromyotomy was first described in 1912, and the operation has changed little since then.[320,321,324] A longitudinal incision is made along the anterosuperior surface of the pylorus through the serosa and the circular muscle layer. The circular muscle layer is then spread bluntly until the gastric submucosa bulges through.[321,324] The main complication encountered during surgery is perforation of the duodenum but this is uncommon.[320,321,324] Recently, laparoscopic pyloromyotomy has been reported to be both safe and successful.[340]

Mortality is rare.[321] Approximately 6 to 8 hours postoperatively, oral feedings are begun.[321,341] Although vomiting may occur during this period, most babies can be discharged within 36 to 72 hours of the surgery if good follow-up and compliance can be ensured.[321,325,341]

Malrotation And Midgut Volvulus

JOSEPH L. WRIGHT

Volvulus refers to a complete twisting of a loop of bowel about its mesenteric base of attachment. It can occur at several points along the alimentary tract including the sigmoid colon, cecum, and small bowel. This section focuses on midgut volvulus around the superior mesenteric artery, which is the most common and dangerous complication of malrotation in infants.

Pathophysiology. At 6 weeks gestation, the rapidly elongating intestine leaves the embryonic abdominal cavity, prolapsing into the yolk sac. Upon reentry at 10 weeks, the midgut (i.e., duodenum, small intestine, and colon up to its midtransverse portion) undergoes a 270° counterclockwise turn around the superior mesenteric artery. Additionally, the third portion of the duodenum is fixed in the retroperitoneum by the ligament of Treitz, the cecum in the right lower quadrant by peritoneal bands, and the small intestine in the peritoneum by a broad mesenteric attachment along its base.[342]

Abnormal rotation and inadequate fixation can occur at any stage in this reentry process.[343,344] Incomplete rotation or malrotation leaves the cecum high in the midabdomen with its peritoneal attachments (Ladd's bands) straddling the duodenum in an obstructing manner. Furthermore, the duodenum becomes narrowed and kinked near the duodenal-jejunal junction due to abnormal fixation by the ligament of Treitz. Finally, the mesentery fails to fan out, remaining bunched in the epigastrium. These anatomic relationships suspend the midgut and its entire vascular supply by a narrow pedicle, rendering it susceptible to twisting and infarction. Complete obstruction is mostly related to duodenal kinking and volvulus rather than the effects of transduodenal bands.[343] However, bands may contribute to the recurrent abdominal symptoms seen in older children with unrecognized malrotation and incomplete volvulus.

Epidemiology. The incidence of malrotation of the midgut is approximately 1 in 500 live births with a rare familial predilection. In the newborn period, there is a 2:1 male predominance that disappears after 1 year of age.[345,346] Midgut volvulus, as a complicating feature of malrotation, occurs in 45% to 80% of cases with a mortality rate of 3% to 15%.[345-351] Associated congenital anomalies, primarily involving the gastrointestinal tract, are found in 46% to 62% of laparotomy-confirmed cases of malrotation.[346,348,349]

Diagnostic Findings. Malrotation with midgut volvulus can present in a number of ways. The most dramatic is the sudden onset of an acute abdomen and shock in a newborn infant. A rigid, discolored abdomen associated with bilious or bloody vomiting and bloody stools indicates the presence of gangrenous bowel. These infants are extremely volume depleted and require vigorous fluid resuscitation before surgery. Alternatively, the abrupt onset of obstructive symptoms in an infant with a history of feeding intolerance and episodic vomiting represents an advancing volvulus until proven otherwise. Even if only transient, green or yellow emesis is never normal in a neonate.

There is an inverse relationship between age at the onset of symptoms and the probability of midgut volvulus. Seventy-five percent of cases occur within the first month of life.[342,343,352] Bilious emesis is the hallmark of presentation evident 77% to 100% of the time.[346,347,349,351] Malrotation without volvulus can go unrecognized until late childhood or even adulthood. These individuals often have a history of recurrent abdominal pain and other vague gastrointestinal symptoms, and their symptoms are frequently ascribed to psychogenic or emotional problems. The frequency of midgut volvulus complicating malrotation in this age group is lower than in the neonatal period, ranging from 14% to 65% in several series.[346-349] However, older children, like newborns, still have a propensity to have symptoms of sudden abdominal pain, shock, and unsalvageable bowel.[349,352]

On examination, malrotation is typically accompanied by few, if any, abnormal physical findings. Even in early volvulus, patients may appear well with few signs of serious underlying pathology.[347,351] A high index of suspicion must be exercised in order to recognize the evolving condition in progress. When the diagnosis is delayed, patients may appear pale and have grunting respirations. The abdomen is diffusely and persistently tender, ranging from mild to rebound. A dilated loop of bowel is sometimes palpated, but abdominal distension is minimal because the intestinal obstruction is high and decompressed by vomiting. Blood from the rectum is ominous, indicating significant vascular compromise. As ischemia progresses, bowel necrosis with perforation, pneumoperitoneum, peritonitis, severe fluid and electrolyte derangements, and hypovolemic and septic shock ensue.

Ancillary Data. A complete blood count, electrolytes, BUN, and urinalysis should be components of the initial examination. A type and crossmatch should also be done.

Upright, flat plate, and cross-table lateral abdominal x-ray examinations may demonstrate evidence of small bowel obstruction, including air-fluid levels, a paucity of

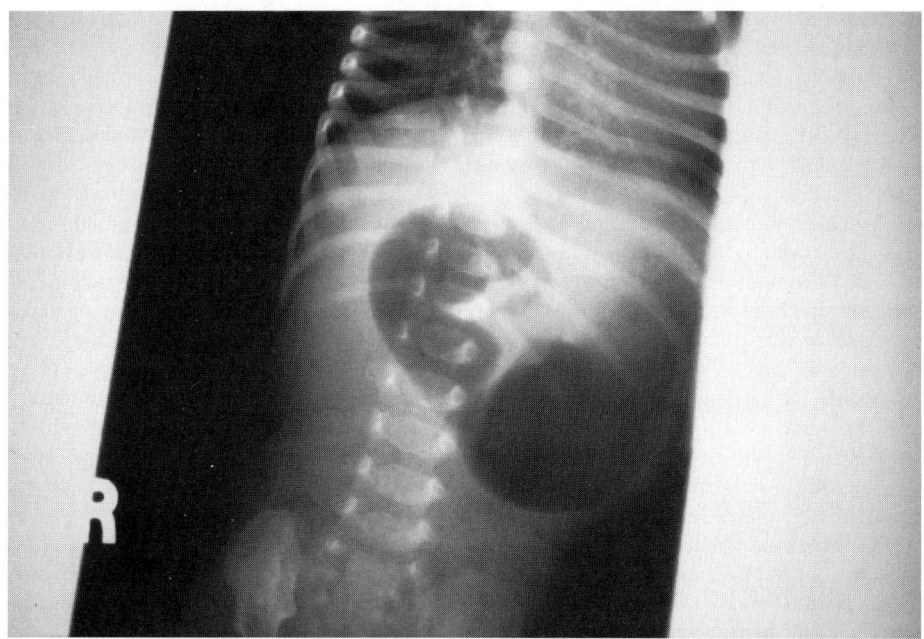

FIG. 52-9. Double-bubble sign on air-contrast study associated with malrotation and midgut volvulus.

bowel gas distally, dilated loops overlying the liver shadow, and a markedly dilated duodenum and stomach.[353,354] However, sometimes the abdomen is gasless or the bowel gas pattern appears relatively normal and contrast studies are warranted.

A simple air contrast study may reveal the "double-bubble" sign, signifying gastric and duodenal dilatation (Fig. 52-9). An upper gastrointestinal series using barium is preferable to a barium enema; the latter study is only likely to demonstrate a high cecum, which can be a normal variant in some infants.[353,354] The upper gastrointestinal series reveals narrowing at the site of obstruction, spiraling of the small bowel about the superior mesenteric artery, and malrotated small intestine occupying the right side of the abdomen. Using this technique, malrotation can only be excluded if the duodenal-jejunal junction (ligament of Treitz) is located to the left of the spine at the same level as the duodenal bulb.[351]

An ultrasound study can be a useful adjunct by showing duodenal distension, intraluminal fluid, and bowel wall edema. In equivocal cases, computed tomography and magnetic resonance imaging have been used to demonstrate the abnormal orientation of the mesenteric vessels inside the twisted pedicle.[351,353,355-357]

Differential Considerations. Intrinsic anatomic lesions, including duodenal webs, duodenal stenosis, and duodenal atresia, can produce a clinical picture similar to midgut volvulus. More distal obstructions also produce bilious vomiting but are more likely to present with distention. Occasionally, a septic child with an adynamic ileus vomits bile as well.

Management. Prompt diagnosis, repair of fluid and electrolyte deficits, and surgery are crucial to the emergency department management of malrotation and midgut volvulus. The patient should be made NPO, an intravenous

line inserted, and 20 ml/kg of 0.9% NS or LR solution administered rapidly. Further boluses may be necessary. A nasogastric tube should be placed and connected to low suction. If vascular compromise is suspected, antibiotic coverage for enteric pathogens should be initiated with ampicillin (100 to 200 mg/kg/24 hr q 4 hr IV), clindamycin (30 to 40 mg/kg/24 hr q 6 hr IV), and an aminoglycoside (gentamicin 5 to 7.5 mg/kg/24 hr q 8 hr IV). The diagnosis can be supported with contrast studies in a stable patient but surgery should not be delayed in an unstable child.

Primary surgical intervention should occur within 1 hour if bowel ischemia is to be reversed. At laparotomy, the volvulized pedicle is identified and untwisted in a counterclockwise fashion, and the obstructing Ladd's bands are divided. The mesentery and the superior mesenteric artery branches are then splayed out, identifying and dividing any further abnormal peritoneal bands and assessing the viability of the bowel. Fixation of the bowel is not generally advocated. [343,352,358] In cases of questionably viable bowel, relief of the volvulus can be followed by abdominal skin closure and a second-look procedure within 24 hours.[343,352,358] This technique may save some bowel from being removed, but even in the best of hands, delayed recognition can lead to death and significant morbidity characterized by the short gut syndrome and the need for hyperalimentation.

References
Abdominal Mass
1. Merten DF and Kirks DR: Diagnostic imaging of pediatric abdominal masses, *Pediatr Clin North Am* 32:1397, 1985.
2. Koop CE: *Visible and palpable lesions in children,* New York, 1976, Grune & Stratton.
3. Hutson JM and Beasley SW: *The surgical examination of children,* Oxford, 1988, Heinemann Medical Books.

Abdominal Pain

4. Reynolds SL and Jaffe DM: Children with abdominal pain: evaluation in the pediatric emergency department, *Pediatr Emerg Care* 6:8-12, 1990.
5. Hickey MS, Kiernan GJ, Weaver KE: Evaluation of abdominal pain, *Emerg Med Clin North Am* 7:437-452, 1989.
6. Adams RD and Martin JB: Pain. In Petersdorf RG, Adams RD, Braunwald E et al, editors: *Harrison's principles of internal medicine,* ed 10, New York, 1983, McGraw-Hill.
7. Felter RA: Nontraumatic surgical emergencies in children, *Emerg Med Clin North Am* 9:589-610, 1991.
8. Buchert GS: Abdominal pain in children: an emergency practitioner's guide, *Emerg Med Clin North Am* 7:497-517, 1989.
9. Neblett WW, Pietsch JB, Holcomb GW: Acute abdominal condition in children and adolescents, *Surg Clin North Am* 68:415-430, 1988.
10. Shandling B: Congenital and perinatal anomalies of the gastrointestinal tract and intestinal obstruction. In Behrman RE and Vaughan VC, editors: *Nelson textbook of pediatrics,* ed 13, Philadelphia, 1987, WB Saunders.
11. Kliegman RM and Behrman RE: Diseases of the newborn infant: premature and full-term. In Behrman RE and Vaughan VC, editors: *Nelson textbook of pediatrics,* ed 13, Philadelphia, 1987, WB Saunders.
12. Barness LA: Nutrition and nutritional disorders. In Behrman RE and Vaughan VC, editors: *Nelson textbook of pediatrics,* ed 13, Philadelphia, 1987, WB Saunders.
13. Stevenson RJ: Abdominal pain unrelated to trauma, *Surg Clin North Am* 65:1181-1215, 1985.
14. Grisanti KA and Jaffe DM: Dehydration syndromes: oral rehydration and fluid replacement, *Emerg Med Clin North Am* 9:565-588, 1991.
15. Shandling B and Fallis JC: Acute appendicitis. In Behrman RE and Vaughan VC, editors: *Nelson textbook of pediatrics,* ed 13, Philadelphia, 1987, WB Saunders.
16. Doherty GM and Lewis FR: Appendicitis: continuing diagnostic challenge, *Emerg Med Clin North Am* 7:667-681, 1989.
17. Hatch EI: The acute abdomen in children, *Pediatr Clin North Am* 32:1151-1164, 1985.
18. Forstner G: The exocrine pancreas. In Behrman RE and Vaughan VC, WB Saunders: *Nelson textbook of pediatrics,* ed 13, Philadelphia, 1987, WB Saunders.
19. Young M: Acute diseases of the pancreas and biliary tract: management in the emergency department, *Emerg Med Clin North Am* 7:555-573, 1989.
20. Mueller PD and Benowitz NL: Toxicologic causes of acute abdominal disorders, *Emerg Med Clin North Am* 7:667-681, 1989.
21. Schaller JG and Wedgwood RJ: Rheumatic diseases of childhood. In Behrman RE and Vaughan VC, editors: *Nelson textbook of pediatrics,* ed 13, Philadelphia, 1987, WB Saunders.
22. Bergstein JM and Michael AF: Glomerular diseases. In Behrman RE and Vaughan VC, editors: *Nelson textbook of pediatrics,* ed 13, Philadelphia, 1987, WB Saunders.
23. Herbst JJ: Noninfective inflammatory gastrointestinal diseases. In Behrman RE and Vaughan VC, editors: *Nelson textbook of pediatrics,* ed 13, Philadelphia, 1987, WB Saunders.
24. Purcell TB: Nonsurgical and extraperitoneal causes of abdominal pain, *Emerg Med Clin North Am* 7:721-739, 1989.
25. Preger L, Gronner AT, Glazer H et al: Imaging of the nontraumatic acute abdomen, *Emerg Med North Am* 7:453-496, 1989.

Constipation

26. Di Lorenzo C, Flores AF, Reddy SN et al: Use of colonic manometry to differentiate causes of intractable constipation in children, *J Pediatr* 120:690-695, 1992.
27. Weaver LT and Steiner H: The bowel habit of young children, *Arch Dis Child* 59:649-652, 1984.
28. Iacono G, Carroccio A, Cavataio F et al: Chronic constipation as a symptom of cow milk allergy, *J Pediatr* 126:34-39, 1995.
29. Seidel JS, Berkowitz CD, Day C: Presentation and evaluation of sexual/misuse in the emergency department, *Pediatr Emerg Care* 2:157-164, 1986.
30. Loening-Baucke V: Factors determining outcome in children with chronic constipation and faecal soiling, *Gut* 30:999-1006, 1989.
31. Kaneti J and Bar-Ziv J: Case profile: urinary retention due to fecal impaction in a child, *Urology* 23:307, 1984.

32. Milanese A, Schechter NL, Ganeshananthan M: Constipation presenting as respiratory distress, *J Adol Health* 7:255-258, 1986.
33. McGuire T, Rothenberg MB, Tyler DC: Profound shock following intervention for chronic untreated stool retention, *Clin Pediatr (Phila)* 23:459-461, 1983.

Diarrhea

34. Guerrant RL, Lohr JA, Williams EK: Acute infectious diarrhea. I. Epidemiology, etiology and pathogenesis, *Pediatr Infect Dis J* 5:353, 1986.
35. Williams EK, Lohr JA, Guerrant RL: Acute infectious diarrhea. II. Diagnosis, treatment and prevention, *Pediatr Infect Dis J* 5:455, 1986.
36. Barkin RM: Acute infectious diarrheal disease in children, *J Emerg Med* 3:1, 1985.
37. Kapikian AZ, Whakin H, Whatt RG et al: Human reovirus-like agent as the major pathogen associated with "winter" gastroenteritis in hospitalized infants and young children, *N Engl J Med* 294:965, 1976.
38. DeWitt TJ, Humphrey KF, McCarthy P: Clinical predictors of acute bacterial diarrhea in young children, *Pediatrics* 76:551, 1985.
39. Finkelstein JA, Schwartz JS, Torrey S et al: Common clinical features as predictors of bacterial diarrhea in infants, *Ann J Emerg Med* 7:469, 1989.
40. Harris JC, Dupont HL, Hopnick RB: Fecal leukocytes in diarrheal illness, *Ann Intern Med* 76:699, 1972.
41. Avery ME and Snyder JD: Oral therapy for acute diarrhea, *N Engl J Med* 323:891, 1990.

Dysphagia

42. Weiss MH: Dysphagia in infants and children, *Otolaryngol Clin North Am* 21:4, 1988.
43. Shapiro J and Healy GB: Dysphagia in infants, *Otolaryngol Clin North Am* 21:4, 1988.
44. Christensen JP: Gastrointestinal Motility. In West JB, editor: *Best and Taylor's physiological basis of medical practice,* Baltimore, 1991, Williams and Wilkins.
45. Stevenson RD and Allaire JH: The development of normal feeding and swallowing, *Pediatr Clin North Am* 38:6, 1991.
46. Kahrilas PJ: Anatomy, physiology and pathophysiology of dysphagia, *Acta Otorhinolaryngol Belg* 48:2, 1994.
47. Illingworth RS: Sucking and swallowing difficulties in infancy: diagnostic problem of dysphagia, *Arch Dis Child* 44:6, 1969.
48. Deron P: Dysphagia with systemic diseases, *Acta Otorhinolaryngol Belg* 48:2, 1994.
49. Cohen SR: Difficulty with swallowing. In Bluestone C and Stool S, editors: *Pediatric otolaryngology,* Philadelphia, 1990, WB Saunders.
50. Vandenplas Y: Dysphagia in infants and children, *Acta Otorhinolaryngol Belg* 48:2, 1994.
51. Stoschus B and Allescher HD: Drug-induced dysphagia, *Dysphagia* 8:2, 1993.
52. Castell DO and Donner MW: Evaluation of dysphagia: a careful history is crucial, *Dysphagia* 2:2, 1987.
53. Meldon SW and Bonadio WA: An unusual cause of acute dysphagia and trismus in a child, *Pediatr Emerg Care* 10:3, 1994.
54. Hubbard KA, Klein BL, Hernandez M et al: Mandibular fractures in children with chin lacerations, *Pediatr Emerg Care* 11:2, 1995.
55. Swischuk LE: Stridor and occult dysphagia, *Pediatr Emerg Care* 2:4, 1986.
56. Tuchman DN: Dysfunctional swallowing in the pediatric patient: clinical considerations, *Dysphagia* 2:4, 1988.
57. Pressman H and Morrison SH: Dysphagia in the pediatric AIDS population, *Dysphagia* 2:3, 1988.

Gastrointestinal Bleeding

58. Cox K and Ament MR: Upper gastrointestinal bleeding in children and adolescents, *Pediatrics* 63:408, 1979.
59. Hyams JS, Leichtner AM, Schwartz AN: Recent advances in diagnosis and treatment of gastrointestinal hemorrhage in infants and children, *J Pediatr* 106:1, 1985.
60. Jenkins HR, Pincott JR, Soothill JF et al: Food allergy: the major cause of infantile colitis, *Arch Dis Child* 59:326, 1984.
61. Steer ML and Silen W: Diagnostic procedures in gastrointestinal hemorrhage, *N Engl J Med* 309:646, 1983.

Hepatosplenomegaly

62. Dommerby H, Stangerup SE, Stangerup M et al: Hepatosplenomegaly in infectious mononucleosis assessed by ultrasonic scanning, *J Laryngol Otol* 100:573, 1986.

63. Haynes BF: Enlargement of lymph nodes and spleen. In Wilson JD et al, editors: *Harrison's principles of internal medicine*, New York, 1991, McGraw-Hill.

64. Mimouni F, Merlob P, Ashkenazi S et al: Palpable spleens in newborn term infants, *Clin Pediatr (Phila)* 24:197, 1985.

65. Sills RH: The spleen and lymph nodes. In Oski FA et al, editors: *Principles and practice of pediatrics*, Philadelphia, 1990, JB Lippincott.

66. McIntyre OR and Ebaugh FG: Palpable spleens in college freshmen, *Ann Intern Med* 66:301, 1967.

67. Reiff MI and Osborn LM: Clinical estimation of liver span in newborn infants, *Pediatrics* 71:46, 1983.

68. Weisman LE, Cagle N, Mathis R et al: Clinical estimation of liver size in the normal neonate, *Clin Pediatr (Phila)* 21:596, 1982.

69. Lawson EE, Grand RJ, Neff RK et al: Clinical estimation of liver span in infants and children, *Am J Dis Child* 132:474, 1978.

70. Younoszai MK and Mueller S: Clinical assessment of liver size in normal children, *Clin Pediatr (Phila)* 14:378, 1975.

71. Hess CE: Diseases of the spleen. In Conn RB, editor: *Current diagnosis*, Philadelphia, 1985, WB Saunders.

72. Walker WA and Mathis RK: Hepatomegaly: an approach to differential diagnosis, *Pediatr Clin North Am* 22:929, 1975.

73. Dorfman DH and Glaser JH: Congenital syphilis presenting in infants after the newborn period, *N Engl J Med* 323:1299, 1990.

74. Fleisher GR, Paradise JE, Lennette ET: Leukocyte response in childhood infectious mononucleosis caused by Epstein-Barr virus, *Am J Dis Child* 135:699, 1981.

75. Sumaya CV and Ench Y: Epstein-Barr virus infectious mononucleosis in children: heterophil antibody response and viral-specific responses, *Pediatrics* 75:1011, 1985.

Jaundice

76. Polin RA and Burg FD: *Workbook in practical neonatology*, Philadelphia, 1983, WB Saunders.

77. American Academy of Pediatrics: Practice parameter: management of hyperbilirubinemia in the healthy term newborn, *Pediatrics* 94:558, 1994.

78. Behrman RE and Kliegman RM: Non-infectious diseases of the newborn. In Behrman RE and Vaughn VC, editors: *Nelson's textbook of pediatrics*, 1983, WB Saunders.

79. Perlman M and Frank JW: Bilirubin beyond the blood-brain barrier, *Pediatrics* 81:304-313, 1988.

80. Rosenthal P and Sinatra F: Jaundice in infancy, *Pediatr Rev* 11:79-85, 1989.

81. Maisels MJ: Jaundice in the newborn, *Pediatr Rev* 3:305-319, 1982.

82. Landing BH: Considerations on the pathogenesis of neonatal hepatitis, biliary atresia and choledochal cyst: the concept of infantile obstructive cholangiopathy, *Prog Pediatr Surg* 6:113-139, 1974.

83. Glaser JH and Morecki R: Reovirus type 3 and neonatal cholestasis, *Semin Liver Dis* 7:100, 1987.

84. Sokol RJ: Medical management of the infant or child with chronic liver disease, *Semin Liver Dis* 7:155, 1987.

85. Fitzgerald JF: Cholestatic disorders of infancy, *Pediatr Clin North Am* 35:357-373, 1988.

Vomiting

86. Toccalino H, LiCastro R, Quastavino E et al: Vomiting and regurgitation, *Clin Gastroenterol* 6:267, 1977.

87. Dodge JA: Vomiting and regurgitation. In Walker WA, editor: *Pediatric gastrointestinal disease*, Philadelphia, 1991, BC Decker.

88. Feldman M: Nausea and vomiting. In Sleisenger MH and Fordtran JS, editors: *Gastrointestinal disease: pathophysiology, diagnosis and management*, Philadelphia, 1989, WB Saunders.

89. Dodge JA: The stomach. In Anderson CM, Burke V, Gracey M, editors: *Pediatric gastroenterology*, Chicago, 1987, Blackwell Scientific Publications.

90. Jewett TC and Karp MP: Congenital lesions of the gastrointestinal tract. In Lebenthal E, editor: *Textbook of gastroenterology and nutrition in infancy*, New York, 1989, Raven Press.

91. Below ME: One-month-old infant with vomiting, *Indiana Med* 83:258, 1990.

92. Edstrom CS: Hereditary fructose intolerance in the vomiting infant, *Pediatrics* 85:600, 1990.

93. Burton BK: Inborn errors of metabolism: the clinical diagnosis in early infancy, *Pediatrics* 79:359, 1987.

94. Schreier L, Cutler RM, Saigal V: Vomiting as a dominant symptom of asthma, *Ann Allergy* 58:118, 1987.

95. Osundwa VM and Dawod ST: Vomiting as the main presenting symptom of acute asthma, *Acta Pediatr* 78:968, 1989.

96. Swischuk LE: Acute vomiting and abdominal pain in an infant, *Pediatr Emerg Care* 2:201, 1986.

97. McClung HJ, Murray R, Braden NJ et al: Intentional ipecac poisoning in children, *Am J Dis Child* 142:637, 1988.

98. Reifen R, Rasooly I, Drumm B et al: *Helicobacter pylori* infection in children. Is there specific symptomatology? *Dig Dis Sci* 39: 1488, 1994.

99. Rosioru C, Glassman MS, Halata MS et al: Esophagitis and *Helicobacter pylori* in children: incidence and therapeutic implications, *Am J Gastroenterol* 88:510, 1993.

100. Vanderhoof JA, Young R, Kaufman SS et al: Treatment of cyclic vomiting of childhood with erythromycin, *J Pediatr Gastroenterol Nutr* 17:387, 1993.

101. McHardy G: The appendix. In Berk JE, editor: *Bockus gastroenterology*, Philadelphia, 1985, WB Saunders.

102. Hugenholtz H, Izukawa D, Shear P et al: Vomiting in children following head injury, *Childs Nerv Syst* 3:266, 1987.

103. Squires RH: Intracranial tumors: vomiting as a presenting sign, *Clin Pediatr (Phila)* 28:351, 1989.

104. Killen JD, Taylor CB, Telch MJ: Self-induced vomiting and laxative and diuretic use among teenagers, *JAMA* 255:1447, 1986.

105. Oster JR: The binge-purge syndrome, *South Med J* 80:58, 1987.

Anorectal Disease

106. Silber G: Lower gastrointestinal bleeding, *Pediatr Rev* 12:85, 1990.

107. Hillemeir C: Rectal bleeding in childhood, *Pediatr Rev* 5:35, 1983.

108. Oh C, Divino CM, Steinhagen RM: Anal fissure 20 year experience, *Dis Colon Rectum* 38(4):378-382, 1995.

109. Leape L: Other disorders of the rectum and anus. In Welch KJ et al, editors: *Pediatric surgery*, Chicago, 1986, Mosby.

110. Heaton ND, Davenport M, Howard ER: Incidence of haemorrhoids and anorectal varices in children with portal hypertension, *Br J Surg* 80(5): 616-618, 1993.

111. Corman ML: Rectal prolapse in children, *Dis Colon Rectum* 28: 535-539, 1985.

112. Zempsky WT, Rosenstein BJ: The course of rectal prolapse in children, *Am J Dis Child* 142: 338-339, 1988.

113. Harris PR and Figueroa-Colon R: Rectal prolapse in children associated with *Clostridium difficile* infection, *Pediatr Infect Dis J* 14(1): 78-80, 1995.

114. Kay NRM and Zachary RB: The treatment of rectal prolapse in children with injections of 30% saline solutions, *J Pediatr Surg* 5:334, 1970.

Biliary Tract Disease

115. Schwartz SI: Gallbladder and extrahepatic biliary system. In Schwartz SI et al, editors: *Principles of surgery*, New York, 1989, McGraw Hill.

116. Hickey MS and Weaver KE: Evaluation of abdominal pain, *Emerg Clin North Am* 7:437, 1989.

117. Grace PA, Poston GJ, Williamson RCN: Biliary motility, *Gut* 31:571, 1990.

118. Small DM: Gallstones, *N Engl J Med* 279:588, 1968.

119. Shwachman H: Gastrointestinal manifestations of cystic fibrosis, *Pediatr Clin North Am* 22:787, 1975.

120. Knauer CM and Silverman S: Alimentary tract and liver. In Schroeder SA et al, editors: *Current medical diagnosis and treatment*, East Norwalk, Conn, 1990, Appleton & Lange.

121. Holcomb GW, O'Neill J, Holcomb GW: Cholecystitis, cholelithiasis and common duct stenosis in children and adolescents, *Ann Surg* 191:626, 1980.

122. Sears HF, Golden GT, Horsley S: Cholecystitis in childhood and adolescence, *Arch Surg* 106:651, 1973.

123. Buiumsohn A, Albu E, Gerst PH et al: Cholelithiasis and teenage mothers, *J Adolesc Health Care* 11:339, 1990.

124. Odom FC, Oliver BB, Kline M et al: Gallbladder disease in patients 20 years of age and under, *South Med J* 69:1299, 1976.

125. Boston Collaborative Drug Surveillance Program: Oral contraceptives and venous thromboembolic disease, surgically confirmed gallbladder disease, and breast tumours, *Lancet* 1:1399, 1973.

126. Friesen CA and Roberts CC: Cholelithiasis: clinical characteristics in children, *Clin Pediatr (Phila)* 28:294, 1989.

127. Kamath KR: Abnormalities of the biliary tree, *Clin Gastroenterol* 15:157, 1986.

128. Andrassy RJ, Treadwell TA, Ratner RA, et al: Gallbladder disease in children and adolescents, *Am J Surg* 132:19, 1976.

129. Hanson BA, Mahour GH, Woolley MM: Diseases of the gallbladder in infancy and childhood, *J Pediatr Surg* 6:277, 1971.

130. Brewer RJ, Golden GT, Hitch DC et al: Abdominal pain: an analysis of 1000 consecutive cases in a university hospital emergency room, *Am J Surg* 131:219, 1976.

131. Pokorny WJ et al: Cholelithiasis and cholecystitis in childhood, *Am J Surg* 148:742, 1984.

132. MacMillan RW, Schullinger JN, Santulli TV: Cholelithiasis in childhood, *Am J Surg* 127:689, 1974.

133. Grace N and Rodgers B: Cholecystitis in childhood: clinical observations based on 30 surgically treated cases, *Clin Pediatr* (Phila) 16:179, 1977.

134. Pieretti R, Auldist AW, Stephens CA: Acute cholecystitis in children, *Surg Gynecol Obstet* 140:16, 1975.

135. Takiff H and Fonkalsrud EW: Gallbladder disease in childhood, *Am J Dis Child* 138:565, 1984.

136. American College of Physicians Health and Policy Statement: How to study the gallbladder, *Ann Intern Med* 109:752, 1975.

137. Krishnamurthy GT: Diagnosing gallbladder disease, *Ann Intern Med* 110:493, 1989 (letter).

138. Preger L, Gronner AT, Glazer H et al: Imaging of the nontraumatic acute abdomen, *Emerg Med Clin North Am* 7:453, 1989.

139. Tweedie JH: Management of acute biliary disease, *Br J Hosp Med* 53, 1987.

140. Karayalcin G, Hassani N, Abrams M et al: Cholelithiasis in children with sickle cell disease, *Am J Dis Child* 133:306, 1979.

141. DeDombal FT: Analysis of symptoms in the acute abdomen, *Clin Gastroenterol* 14:531, 1985.

142. Young M: Acute diseases of the pancreas and biliary tract: management in the emergency department, *Emerg Clin North Am* 7:555, 1989.

143. Ferrucci JT, Freeny PC, Stark DD et al: Advances in hepatobiliary radiology, *Radiology* 168:319, 1988.

144. Ariyan S, Shessel FS, Pickett LK: Cholecystitis and cholelithiasis masking as abdominal crises in sickle cell disease, *Pediatrics* 58:252, 1976.

145. Bell MJ, Ternberg JL, Feigin RD: Surgical complications of leptospirosis in children, *J Pediatr Surg* 13:325, 1978.

146. Chamberlain JW and Hight DW: Acute hydrops of the gallbladder in childhood, *Surgery* 68:899, 1970.

147. Choi CYS and Sharma B: Gallbladder hydrops in mucocutaneous lymph node syndrome, *South Med J* 82:397, 1989.

148. Bradford BF, Reid BS, Weinstein BJ et al: Ultrasonographic evaluation of the gallbladder in mucocutaneous lymph node syndrome, *Radiology* 142:381, 1982.

149. Hyams JS, Baker E, Schwartz AN et al: Acalculous cholecystitis in Crohn's disease, *J Adolesc Health* 10:151, 1988.

150. Mirvis SE, Vainwright JR, Nelson AW et al: The diagnosis of acute acalculous cholecystitis: a comparison of sonography, scintigraphy, and CT, *Am J Radiol* 147:1171, 1986.

151. Slovis TL, Hight DW, Philippart AI et al: Sonography in the diagnosis and management of hydrops of the gallbladder in children with mucocutaneous lymph node syndrome, *Pediatrics* 65:789, 1980.

Foreign Body Ingestions

152. Kenna MA and Bluestone CD: Foreign bodies in the air and food passages, *PIR* 10:25, 1988.

153. Suita S et al: Management of pediatric patients who have swallowed foreign objects, *The American Surgeon* 55:585, 1989.

154. Hacker J and Cattau E: Management of gastrointestinal foreign bodies, *AFP* 34:101, 1981.

155. Stool S and Manning S: Foreign bodies of the pharynx and esophagus. In Bluestone and Stool, editors: *Pediatric otolaryngology,* Philadelphia, 1990, WB Saunders, 1009.

156. Friedman E: Caustic ingestions and foreign bodies in the aerodigestive tract of children, *Pediatr Clin North Am* 36:1403, 1989.

157. Jackson C and Jackson CL: *Bronchoesophagology,* Philadelphia, 1936, WB Saunders.

158. Smith PC et al: An elusive and often unsuspected cause of stridor or pneumonia: the esophageal foreign body, *Am J Roetgenol* 122:80, 1974.

159. Obiako MN: Tracheo-esophageal fistula: a complication of foreign body, *Ann Otol Rhinol Laryngol* 91:325, 1982.

160. Sheikh A: Button battery ingestions in children, *Pediatr Emerg Care* 9:224, 1993.

161. Quinn PG and Connors PJ: The role of upper gastrointestinal endoscopy in foreign body removal, *Gastrointest Endosc Clin N Am* 4:571, 1994.

162. Sacchetti A, Carraccio C, Lichenstein R: Hand-held metal detector identification of ingested foreign bodies, *Pediatr Emerg Care* 10:204, 1994.

163. Biehler JL, Tuggle D, Stacy T: Use of the transmitter-receiver metal detector in the evaluation of pediatric coin ingestions, *Pediatr Emerg Care* 9:208, 1993.

164. Ros SP and Cetta F: Detection of ingested foreign bodies with a metal detector, *J Pediatr* 121:837, 1992.

165. Campbell JB et al: Foley catheter removal of blunt esophageal foreign bodies, *Pediatr Radiol* 13:116, 1983.

166. Carlson D: Removal of coins in the esophagus using a Foley catheter, *Pediatrics* 50:475, 1972.

167. Schunk JE, Harrison M, Corneli HM et al: Fluoroscopic foley catheter removal of esophageal foreign bodies in children: experience with 415 episodes, *Pediatrics* 94:709, 1994.

168. Connors GP, Chamberlain JM, Oschsenschlager DW: Symptoms and spontaneous passage of esophageal coins, *Arch Pediatr Adolesc Med* 149:36, 1995.

169. Paul R and Jaffe D: Sharp object ingestion in children: illustrative cases and literature review, *Pediatr Emerg Care* 4:245, 1988.

170. David TJ and Ferguson AP: Management of children who have swallowed button batteries, *Arch Dis Child* 61:321, 1986.

171. Litovitz TL: Battery ingestions: product accessibility and clinical course, *Pediatrics* 75:469, 1985.

172. Henderson C et al: Foreign body ingestion: review and successful guidelines for management, *Endoscopy* 19:68, 1987.

Gastroenteritis, Acute Infectious

173. DeWitt TG, Humphrey KF, McCarthy P: Clinical predictors of acute bacterial diarrhea in young children, *Pediatrics* 76:551, 1985.

174. Finkelstein JA, Schwartz JS, Torrey S et al: Common clinical features as predictors of bacterial diarrhea in infants, *Am J Emerg Med* 7:469, 1989.

175. Guerrant RL, Lohr JA, Williams EK: Acute infectious diarrhea. I Epidemiology, etiology, and pathogenesis, *Pediatr Infect Dis J* 5:353, 1986.

176. Williams EK, Lohr JA, Guerrant RL: Acute infectious diarrhea. II Diagnosis, treatment, and prevention, *Pediatr Infect Dis J* 5:455, 1986.

177. Higgens JA, Code CF, Orvis AL: The influence of motility on the rate of absorption of sodium and water from the small intestine of healthy persons, *Gastroenterology* 31:708, 1956.

178. Northrup RS and Flanigan TP: Gastroenteritis, *Pediatr Rev* 15:461, 1994.

179. Kapikian AZ, Whakin H, Wyatt RG et al: Human reovirus-like agent as the major pathogen associated with "winter" gastroenteritis in hospitalized infants and young children, *N Engl J Med* 294:965, 1976.

180. Kotloff KL, Losonsky GA, Morris JG Jr et al: Enteric adenovirus infection and childhood diarrhea: an epidemiologic study in three clinical settings, *Pediatrics* 84:219, 1989.

181. Herrmann JE, Taylor DN, Echeverria P et al: Astroviruses as a cause of gastroenteritis in children, *N Engl J Med* 324:1757, 1991.

182. Karmali MA and Fleming PC: *Campylobacter* enteritis in children, *J Pediatr* 94:527, 1979.

183. Ashkanazi S, Dinari G, Zegulknov A et al: Convulsions in childhood shigellosis, *Am J Dis Child* 141:208, 1983.

184. Singh-Naz N and Rodriquez WJ: Acute enteritis in pediatric infectious disease. In Jenson HB and Baltimore RS, editors: *Pediatric infectious diseases: principles and practice,* Norwalk, Conn, 1995, Appleton and Lange, pp 1081-1138.

185. Vakil NB, Schwartz SM, Buggy BP et al: Biliary cryptosporidiosis in HIV-infected people after the waterborne outbreak of cryptosporidiosis in Milwaukee, *N Engl J Med* 334:19-23, 1996.

186. Current WL, Reese NC, Ernst JV et al: Human cryptosporidiosis in immunocompetent and immunodeficient persons, *N Engl J Med* 308:1252, 1983.
187. Dupont HL and Sullivan PS: Giardiasis: the clinical spectrum, diagnosis, and therapy, *Pediatr Infect Dis* 5:131, 1986.
188. Pickering LK, DuPont HL, Olarte J et al: Fecal leukocytes in enteric infections, *Am J Clin Pathol* 68:562, 1977.
189. Varsano I, Eidlitz-Marcus T, Nussinovitch M et al: Comparative efficacy of ceftriaxone and ampicillin for the treatment of severe shigellosis in children, *J Pediatr* 118:627, 1991.
190. St Geme JW III, Hodes HL, Marcy SM et al: Consensus: management of *Salmonella* infection in the first year of life, *Pediatr Infect Dis J* 7:615, 1988.
191. DuPont HL, Ericcson CD, Johnson DC et al: Prevention of traveler's diarrhea by the tablet formulation of bismuth subsalicylate, *JAMA* 257:1347, 1987.
192. Diarrheal Disease Study Group: Loperamide in acute diarrhea in childhood: results of a double-blind, placebo-controlled multicentre clinical trial, *Lancet* 289:1263, 1984.

Viral Hepatitis

193. Sherlock S: *Viral hepatitis in diseases of the liver and biliary system*, ed 8, Oxford, 1989, Blackwell Scientific Publications.
194. Balistreri WF: Viral hepatitis, *Pediatr Clin North Am* 35:375-407, 1988.
195. Schroeder SA, Krupp MA, Tierney LM Jr et al, editors: *Current medical diagnosis and treatment*, East Norwalk, Conn, 1991, Appleton & Lange.
196. Gur H, Aderka D, Finkelstein A: Fulminant Wilsonian hepatitis: difficulties in diagnosis and treatment, *Am J Gastroenterol* 83:679-681, 1988.
197. Levin S, Liebowitz E, Torten J et al: Interferon treatment in acute progressive and fulminant hepatitis, *Isr J Med Sci* 25:364-372, 1989.
198. Friedman LS: Viral hepatitis: current status, *Del Med J* 62:933-941, 1990.
199. Walker WA, Durie JB, Hamilton RS et al: *Pediatric gastrointestinal disease: pathophysiology, diagnosis, and management*, Philadelphia, 1991, BC Decker.
200. Clemens R, Safary A, Hepburn A et al.: Clinical experience with an inactivated hepatitis A vaccine, *J Infect Dis* 171(S1): S44, 1995.
201. Balcarek KB, Bagley MR, Pass RF et al.: Safety and immunogenicity of an inactivated hepatitis A vaccine in preschool children, *J Infect Dis* 171(S1):S70, 1995.
202. Hoofnagle JH, Shafritz DA, Popper H: Chronic type B hepatitis and the healthy HBsAg carrier state, *Hepatology* 7:758-763, 1987.
203. Hoofnagle JH: Type D (Delta) hepatitis, *JAMA* 261:1321-1325, 1989.
204. Georges P, editor: *Report of the Committee on Infectious Diseases*, ed 22, 1991, American Academy of Pediatrics.
205. Kuo G, Choo QL, Alter HJ et al: An assay for circulating antibodies to a major etiologic virus of human non-A, non-B hepatitis, *Science* 244:362-364, 1989.
206. Alter MJ: Non-A, non-B hepatitis: sorting through a diagnosis of exclusion, *Ann Intern Med* 110:583-585, 1989.
207. Georges P, editor: *Report of the Committee on Infectious Diseases*, ed 23, 1994, American Academy of Pediatrics.
208. Chang MH, Ni YH, Hwang LH et al.: Long term clinical and virologic outcome of primary hepatitis C virus infection in children: a prospective study, *Pediatr Infect Dis J* 13:769, 1994.
209. Napoli N, Fiore G, Vella F et al.: Prevalence of antibodies to hepatitis C virus among family members of patients with chronic hepatitis C, *Eur J Epidemiol* 9:629, 1993.
210. Ruiz-Moreno M, Rua MJ, Castillo I et al.: Treatment of children with chronic hepatitis C with recombinant interferon-alpha: a pilot study, *Hepatology* 16:882, 1992.
211. Hyams KC, McCarthy MC, Kaur M et al.: Acute sporadic hepatitis in children living in Cairo, Egypt, *J Med Virol* 37:274, 1992.
212. Arankalle VA, Tsarev SA, Chadha MS et al.: Age-specific prevalence of antibodies to hepatitis A and E viruses in Pune, India, 1982 and 1992, *J Infect Dis* 171:447, 1995.

Inflammatory Bowel Disease

213. Werman HA: Inflammatory bowel disease. In Harwood-Nuss A et al, editors: *The clinical practice of emergency medicine*, Philadelphia, 1991, JB Lippincott p 962.

214. Ament ME et al: Advances in ulcerative colitis, *Pediatrician* 15:45, 1988.
215. Grand RJ and Homer DR: Approaches to inflammatory bowel disease in childhood and adolescence, *Pediatr Clin North Am* 22:835, 1975.
216. Miller RC and Larsen E: Regional enteritis in early infancy, *Am J Dis Child* 122:301, 1971.
217. Werlin SL and Grand RJ: Severe colitis in children and adolescents: diagnosis, course and treatment, *Gastroenterology* 73:828, 1977.
218. Justinich CJ and Hyams JS: Inflammatory bowel disease in children and adolescents, *Gastrointest Endosc Clin N Am* 4:39, 1994.
219. Hofley PM and Piccoli DA: Inflammatory bowel disease in children, *Med Clin North Am* 78:1281, 1994.
220. Treem WR, Davis PM, Hyams JS: Cyclosporine treatment of severe ulcerative colitis in children, *J Pediatr* 119:994, 1991.
221. Motil KJ and Grand RJ: Ulcerative colitis and Crohn disease in children, *Pediatr Rev* 9:109, 1987.

Pancreatitis, Acute

222. Warner Jr RL, Othersen Jr HB, Smith CD: Traumatic pancreatitis and pseudocyst in children: current management, *J Trauma* 29(5):597-601, 1989.
223. Mader TJ and McHugh TP: Acute pancreatitis in children, *Pediatr Emerg Care* 8:157-161, 1992.
224. Haddock G, Coupar G, Youngson GG et al: Acute pancreatitis in children: a 15-year review, *J Pediatr Surg* 29:719-722, 1994.
225. Weizman Z and Durie PR: Acute pancreatitis in childhood, *J Pediatr* 113:24-29, 1988.
226. Cox KL: *Pancreatitis in children. Pediatric case reports in gastrointestinal disease*, vol 6, No 3, Newten, PA, 1986, Associates in Medical Marketing, pp 1-7.
227. Jordan SC and Ament ME: Pancreatitis in children and adolescents; *J Pediatr* 91(2):211-216, 1977.
228. Soergel KS: Acute Pancreatitis. In Sleisenger MS and Fordtran JS (4th eds): *Gastrointestinal disease: pathophysiology, diagnosis, management*, ed 4, vol 2, Philadelphia, 1989, WB Saunders, pp 1814-1841.
229. Fonkalsrud EW: Pancreatitis in children. In Howard JM, Jordan JL, Howard R: *Surgical diseases of the pancreas*, Philadelphia, 1987, Lea & Febiger pp 342-347.
230. Cox KL, Ament ME, Sample WF et al: The ultrasonic and biochemical diagnosis of pancreatitis in children, *J Pediatr* 96:407-411, 1980.
231. Levitt MD: Clinical use of amylase clearance and isoamylase measurements, *Mayo Clin Proc* 54:428-431, 1979.
232. Clavien PA, Burgan S, Mossa AR: Serum enzymes and other laboratory tests in acute pancreatitis, *Br J Surg* 76:1234-1243, 1989.
233. Steinberg WM, Goldstein SS, Davis ND et al: Diagnostic assays in acute pancreatitis, *Ann Intern Med* 102:576-580, 1985.
234. Silverstein W, Isikoff MB, Hill MC et al: Diagnostic imaging of acute pancreatitis: prospective study using CT and sonography, *AJR* 137:597-602, 1981.
235. Williford ME, Foster WL, Halvorsen RA et al: Pancreatic pseudocyst: comparative evaluation by sonography and computed tomography, *AJR* 140:53-57, 1983.
236. Bluestein PK, Gaskin K, Filler R et al: Endoscopic retrograde cholangiopancreatography in pancreatitis in children and adolescents, *Pediatrics* 68:387-393, 1981.

Reye Syndrome

237. Barrett MJ, Hurwitz ES, Schonberger LB et al: Changing epidemiology of Reye syndrome in the United States, *Pediatrics* 77:598, 1986.
238. Waldman RJ, Hall WN, McGee H et al: Aspirin as a risk factor in Reye's syndrome, *JAMA* 247:3089, 1982.
239. Arrowsmith JB, Kennedy DL, Kuritsky JN et al: National patterns of aspirin use and Reye syndrome reporting, United States, 1980-1985, *Pediatrics* 77:598, 1986.
240. Forsyth BW, Horwitz RI, Acampora D et al: New epidemiologic evidence confirming that bias does not explain the aspirin/Reye syndrome association, *JAMA* 261:2517, 1989.
241. Lovejoy FH, Smith AL, Bresnan MJ et al: Clinical staging of Reye's syndrome, *Am J Dis Child* 128:36, 1974.
242. Glasgow JFT: Clinical features and prognosis of Reye's syndrome, *Arch Dis Child* 59:230, 1984.

243. Rowe PC, Valle D, Brusilow SW: Inborn errors of metabolism in children referred with Reye's syndrome, *JAMA* 260:3167, 1988.

244. Trauner DA: What is the best treatment for Reye's syndrome? *Arch Neurol* 43:729, 1986.

Appendicitis

245. Walker AR and Segal I: What causes appendicitis? *J Clin Gastroenterol* 12:127, 1990(editorial).

246. Schwartz SI: Appendix. In Schwartz SI, editor: *Principles of surgery,* New York, 1989, McGraw-Hill.

247. A sound approach to the diagnosis of acute appendicitis, *Lancet* 1:198, 1987.

248. O'Shea TS, Bishop HE, Alermo AJ et al: Diagnosing appendicitis in children with acute abdominal pain, *Pediatr Emerg Care* 4:172, 1988.

249. Stringel G: Appendicitis in children: a symptomatic approach for a low incidence of complications, *Am J Surg* 154:631, 1987.

250. Schey WL: Use of barium in the diagnosis of appendicitis in children, *Am J Roentgenol Radium Ther Nucl Med* 118:95, 1973.

251. Putnam TC and Emmens RW: Appendicitis in children, *Surg Gyn Obstet* 170:527, 1990.

252. Harberg FJ: The acute abdomen in childhood, *Pediatr Ann* 18:169, 1989.

253. Bolton JP, Craven ER, Croft RJ et al: An assessment of the value of the white cell count in the management of suspected acute appendicitis, *Br J Surg* 62:906, 1975.

254. Lewis FR, Holcroft JW, Boey J et al: Appendicitis: a critical review of diagnosis and treatment in 1000 cases, *Arch Surg* 110:677, 1975.

255. Hoffman J and Rasmussen AB: Aids in the diagnosis of acute appendicitis, *Br J Surg* 76:774, 1989.

256. Sasso RD, Hanna EA, Moore DL: Leukocytic and neutrophil counts in acute appendicitis, *Am J Surg* 120:563, 1970.

257. Lee PWR: The leukocyte count in acute appendicitis, *Br J Surg* 60:618, 1973.

258. Raflery AT: The value of the leukocyte count in the diagnosis of acute appendicitis, *Br J Surg* 63:143, 1976.

259. English DC, Allen W, Coppola ED et al: Excessive dependence of the leukocytosis and in diagnosing appendicitis, *Am Surg* 43:399, 1977.

260. Swichuk LE: Abdominal pain and distention, *Pediatr Emerg Care* 4:45, 1988.

261. Puylaert JB: Acute appendicitis: ultrasound evaluation using graded compression, *Radiology* 158:355, 1986.

262. Jeffrey RB Jr, Laing FC, Lewis FR: Acute appendicitis: high-resolution real-time findings, *Radiology* 163:11, 1987.

263. Yacoe ME and Jeffrey RB: Sonography of appendicitis and diverticulitis, *Radiol Clin North Am* 32:899, 1994.

264. Ooms IIW, Koumans RK, Ho Kang You PJ et al: Ultrasonography in the diagnosis of acute appendicitis, *Br J Surg* 78:315, 1991.

265. Crady SK, Jones JS, Wyn T et al: Clinical validity of ultrasound in children with suspected appendicitis, *Ann Emerg Med* 22:1125, 1993.

266. Quillin SP, Siegel MJ, Coffin CM: Acute appendicitis in children: value of sonography in detecting perforation, *AJR* 159:1265, 1992.

267. Sakover RP and del Fava RL: Frequency of visualization of the normal appendix with the barium enema examination, *Am J Roentgenol Radium Ther Nucl Med* 121:312, 1974.

268. Jona JL, Belin RP, Selke AC: Barium enema as a diagnosis and in children with abdominal pain, *Surg Gynecol Obstet* 144:351, 1977.

269. Rajugopulan AE, Mason JH, Kennedy M et al: The value of the barium enema in the diagnosis of acute appendicitis, *Arch Surg* 112:531, 1977.

270. Smith DE, Kirchner NA, Stewart DR: Use of the barium enema in the diagnosis of acute appendicitis and its complications, *Am J Surg* 138:829, 1979.

271. Balthazar EJ and Gordon RB: CT of appendicitis: seminar in ultrasound, *Semin Ultrasound CT MR* 10:326, 1989.

272. Henneman PL, Marcus CS, Inkelis SH et al: Evaluation of children with possible appendicitis using technetium 99m leukocyte scan, *Pediatrics* 85:838, 1990.

273. Doherty CM and Lewis FR: Appendicitis: continuing diagnostic challenge, *Emerg Clin N Am* 7:537, 1989.

274. Blalock JB: Improving diagnostic accuracy in appendicitis, *Ala Med* 1989.

275. Rosser SB and Nazem A: Appendicitis in the pediatric age group, *J Natl Med Assoc* 80:401, 1988.

Hirschsprung Disease

276. Qualman SJ and Murray R: Aganglionosis and related disorders, *Hum Pathol* 25:1141-1149, 1994.

277. Rudolph C and Benaroch L: Hirschsrung disease, *Pediatr Rev* 16:5-11, 1995.

278. Loening-Baucke V: Constipation in children, *Curr Opin Pediatr* 6:556-561, 1994.

279. Neilson IR and Yazbeck S: Ultrashort Hirschsprung's disease: myth or reality, *J Pediatr Surg* 25:1135-1138, 1990.

280. Koberlle F: Enteromegaly and cardiomegaly in Chagas' disease, *Gut* 4:399, 1963.

281. Carcassone M et al: Management of Hirschsprung's disease: curative surgery before 3 months of age, *J Pediatr Surg* 24:1032, 1989.

Inguinal Hernia

282. Rowe MI and Lloyd DA: Inguinal hernia. In Welch KJ et al, editors: *Pediatric surgery,* Chicago, 1986, Mosby.

283. Rowe MI, Copelson LW, Clatworthy HW: The patent processus vaginalis and the inguinal hernia, *J Pediatr Surg* 4:102, 1969.

284. Sparnon AL, Kiely EM, Spitz L: Incarcerated inguinal hernia in infants, *BMJ* 293:376, 1986.

Intussusception

285. Scherer LR and Grosfeld JL: Inguinal hernia and umbilical anomalies, *Pediatr Clin North Am* 40:1121, 1993.

286. Skoog SJ and Conlin MJ: Pediatric hernias and hydroceles—the urologist's perspective, *Urol Clin North Am* 22:119, 1995.

287. Stylianos S, Jacir NN, Harris BH: Incarceration of inguinal hernia in infants prior to elective repair, *J Pediatr Surg* 28:582, 1993.

288. Bruce J, Huh YS, Cooney DR et al: Intussusception: evolution of current management, *J Pediatr Gastroenterol Nutr* 6:663, 1987.

289. Rachmel A, Rosenbach Y, Amir J et al: Apathy as an early manifestation of intussusception, *Am J Dis Child* 137:701, 1983.

290. Losek JD and Fiete RL: Intussusception and the diagnostic value of testing stool for occult blood, *Am J Emerg Med* 9:1-3, 1991.

291. Lee HC, Yeh HJ, Leu YJ: Intussusception: the sonographic diagnosis and its clinical value, *J Pediatr Gastroenterol Nutr* 8:343, 1989.

292. Shanbhogue RL, Hussain SM, Meradji M et al: Ultrasonography is accurate enough for the diagnosis of intussusception, *J Pediatr Surg* 29:324-327, 1994.

293. Weast KW, Stephens B, Vane DW et al: Intussusception: current management in infants and children, *Surgery* 102:704, 1987.

294. Grasso SN, Katz ME, Presberg HJ et al: Transabdominal manually assisted reduction of pediatric intussusception: reappraisal of this historical technique, *Radiology* 191:777-779, 1994.

295. Guo J, Ma X, Zhou Q: Results of air pressure enema reduction of intussusception: 6396 cases in 13 years, *J Pediatr Surg* 21:1201-1203, 1986.

296. Jinzhe Z, Yenzia W, Linchi W: Rectal inflation of intussusception in infants, *J Pediatr Surg* 21:30-32, 1986.

297. McDermott VG, Taylor T, Mackenzie S et al: Pneumatic reduction of intussusception: clinical experience and factors affecting outcome, *Clin Radiol* 49:30-34, 1994.

298. Meyer JS: The current radiologic management of intussusception: a survey and review, *Pediatr Radiol* 22:323-325, 1992.

299. Palder SB, Ein SH, Stringer DA et al: Intussusception: barium or air? *J Pediatr Surg* 26:271-274, 1991.

Meckel's Diverticulum

300. Amoury RA: Meckel's diverticulum. In Welch KJ et al, editors: *Pediatric surgery,* Chicago, 1986, Mosby.

301. Trier JS and Winter HS: Anatomy, embryology and developmental abnormalities of the small intestine and colon. In Sleisenger MH and Fordtran JS, editors: *Gastrointestinal disease: pathophysiology, diagnosis, management,* Philadelphia, 1989, WB Saunders.

302. Weinstein EC, Cain JC, ReMine WH: Meckel's diverticulum: 55 years of clinical and surgical experience, *JAMA* 182:251, 1962.

303. Brown CK and Olshaker JS: Meckel's diverticulum, *Am J Emerg Med* 6:157, 1988.

304. Ludtk F, Mende V, Kohler H et al: Incidence and frequency of complications and management of Meckel's diverticulum, *Surg Gynecol Obstet* 169:537, 1989.

305. Soderlund S: Meckel's diverticulum, a clinical and histologic study, *Acta Chir Scand Suppl* 248:13, 1959.

306. Michas CA, Cohen SE, Wolfman EF: Meckel's diverticulum: should it be excised incidentally at operation? *Am J Surg* 129:682, 1975.

307. Brophy C and Seashore J: Meckel's diverticulum in the pediatric surgical population, *Conn Med* 53:203, 1989.

308. Yamaguchi M, Takeuchi S, Awazu S: Meckel's diverticulum: investigation of 600 patients in Japanese literature, *Am J Surg* 136:247, 1978.

309. Murali VP, Divaker D, Thachil MV et al: Meckel's diverticulum in adults, *J Indian Med Assoc* 87:116, 1989.

310. DeBartolo HM and vanHeerden JA: Meckel's diverticulum, *Ann Surg* 183:30, 1976.

311. Dixon PM and Nolan DJ: The diagnosis of Meckel's diverticulum: a continuing challenge, *Clin Radiol* 38:615, 1987.

312. Soltero MJ and Bill AH: The natural history of Meckel's diverticulum and its relation to incidental removal, *Am J Surg* 132:168, 1976.

313. Kusumoto H, Yoshida M, Takahashi I et al: Complications and diagnosis of Meckel's diverticulum in 776 patients, *Am J Surg* 164:382, 1992.

314. Pfalzgraf RR, Zumwalt RE, Kenny MR: Mesodiverticular band and sudden death in children, *Arch Pathol Lab Med* 112:182, 1988.

315. Majd M: Nuclear medicine. In Franken EA and Smith WL, editors: *Gastrointestinal imaging in pediatrics*, Philadelphia, 1982, Harper and Row.

316. Treves S, Grand RJ, Eraklis AJ: Pentagastrin stimulation of technetium-99m uptake by ectopic gastric mucosa in a Meckel's diverticulum, *Radiology* 128:711, 1978.

317. Lachaux AG, Descos BP, Bret P et al: Meckel's diverticulum in children: a radiological challenge? *J Pediatr Gastroenterol Nutr* 7:939, 1988.

318. Teitelbaum DH, Polley TZ, Obeid F: Laparoscopic diagnosis and excision of Meckel's diverticulum, *J Pediatr Surg* 29:495, 1994.

319. Huang CS and Lin LH: Laparoscopic Meckel's diverticulectomy in infants: report of three cases, *J Pediatr Surg* 28:1486, 1993.

Pyloric Stenosis, Infantile Hypertrophic

320. Spicer RD: Infantile hypertrophic pyloric stenosis: a review, *Br J Surg* 69:128, 1982.

321. Benson CD: Infantile hypertrophic pyloric stenosis. In Welch KJ et al, editors: *Pediatric surgery*, Chicago, 1986, Mosby.

322. Rollins MD, Shields MD, Quinn RJ et al: Pyloric stenosis: congenital or acquired? *Arch Dis Child* 64:138, 1989.

323. Zenn MR and Redo SF: Hypertrophic pyloric stenosis in the newborn, *J Pediatr Surg* 28:1577, 1993.

324. Stringer MD and Brereton RJ: Current management of infantile hypertrophic pyloric stenosis, *Br J Hosp Med* 43:266, 1990.

325. McGuigan JE and Ament ME: Anatomy, embryology, and developmental anomalies. In Sleisenger MH and Fordtran JS, editors: *Gastrointestinal disease: pathophysiology, diagnosis, management*, Philadelphia, 1989, WB Saunders.

326. Kobayashi H, O'Brian S, Puri P: Selective reduction in intramuscular nerve supporting cells in infantile hypertrophic pyloric stenosis, *J Pediatr Surg* 29:651, 1994.

327. Okazaki T, Yamataka A, Fujiwara T et al: Abnormal distribution of nerve terminals in infantile hypertrophic pyloric stenosis, *J Pediatr Surg* 29:655, 1994.

328. Incidence of infantile hypertrophic pyloric stenosis, *Lancet* 1:888, 1984 (editorial).

329. Jedd MB, Melton LJ, Griffin M et al: Factors associated with infantile hypertrophic pyloric stenosis, *Am J Dis Child* 142:334, 1988.

330. Webb AR, Lari J, Dodge JA: Infantile hypertrophic pyloric stenosis in South Glamorgan 1970-1979, *Arch Dis Child* 58:586, 1983.

331. Zeidan B, Wyatt J, Mackensie A et al: Recent results of treatment of infantile hypertrophic pyloric stenosis, *Arch Dis Child* 63:1060, 1988.

332. Touloukian RJ and Higgins E: The spectrum of serum electrolytes in hypertrophic pyloric stenosis, *J Pediatr Surg* 18:394, 1983.

333. Breaux CW Jr, Hood JS, Georgeson KE: The significance of alkalosis and hypochloremia in hypertrophic pyloric stenosis, *J Pediatr Surg* 24:1250, 1989.

334. Breaux CW Jr, Georgeson KE, Royal SA et al: Changing patterns in the diagnosis of hypertrophic pyloric stenosis, *Pediatrics* 81:213, 1988.

335. Allen AE: Ultrasound investigation of pyloric stenosis, *Radiogr Today* 54:49, 1988.

336. Blumhagen JD: Ultrasonography in diagnosis of hypertrophic pyloric stenosis, *J Pediatr* 103:496, 1983.

337. Reilly DT and Hershman MJ: Diagnosis of infantile hypertrophic pyloric stenosis by ultrasound, *BJCP* 43:339, 1989.

338. Khamapirad T and Athey PA: Ultrasound diagnosis of hypertrophic pyloric stenosis, *J Pediatr* 102:23, 1983.

339. DeBacker A, Bove T, Vandenplas Y, et al: Contribution of endoscopy to early diagnosis of hypertrophic pyloric stenosis, *J Pediatr Gastroenterol Nutr* 18:78, 1994.

340. Najmaldin A and Tan HL: Early experience with laparoscopic pyloromyotomy for infantile hypertrophic pyloric stenosis, *J Pediatr Surg* 30:37, 1995.

341. Georgeson KE, Corbin TJ, Griffen JW et al: An analysis of feeding regimens after pyloromyotomy for hypertrophic pyloric stenosis, *J Pediatr Surg* 28:1478, 1993.

Malrotation and Midgut Volvulus

342. Snyder WH and Chaffin L: Embryology and pathology of the intestinal tract: presentation of 40 cases of malrotation, *Ann Surg* 140:368, 1954.

343. Raffensperger JG: Malrotation. In Raffensperger JG, editor: *Swenson's pediatric surgery*, New York, 1990, Appleton and Lange.

344. Ladd WE: Congenital obstructions of the duodenum in children, *N Engl J Med* 206:277, 1932.

345. Stewart DR, Colodny AL, Daggett WC: Malrotation of the bowel in infants and children: a fifteen year review, *Surgery* 79:716, 1976.

346. Torres AM and Ziegler MM: Malrotation of the intestine, *World J Surg* 17:326, 1993.

347. Seashore JH and Touloukian RJ: Midgut volvulus: an ever-present threat, *Arch Pediatr Adolesc Med* 148:43, 1994.

348. Powell DM, Othersen HB, Smith CD: Malrotation of the intestine: the effect of age on presentation and therapy, *J Pediatr Surg* 24:777, 1989.

349. Spigland N, Brandt ML, Yarbeck S: Malrotation presenting beyond the neonatal period, *J Pediatr Surg* 25:1139, 1990.

350. Messineo A, MacMillan JH, Palder SB et al: Clinical factors affecting mortality in children with malrotation of the intestine, *J Pediatr Surg* 27:1343, 1992.

351. Bonadio WA, Clarkson T, Naus J: The clinical features of children with malrotation of the intestine, *Pediatr Emerg Care* 7:348, 1991.

352. Smith EI: Malrotation of the intestine. In Welch KJ et al, editors: *Pediatric surgery*, Chicago, 1986, Mosby.

353. Swischuk LE: Volvulus. In Swischuk LE, editor: *Emergency radiology of the acutely ill or injured child*, Baltimore, 1994, Williams and Wilkins.

354. Berdon WE, Baker DH, Bull S et al: Midgut malrotation and volvulus: which films are most helpful, *Radiology* 96:375, 1970.

355. Dufour D, Delaet MH, Dassonville M et al: Midgut malrotation, the reliability of sonographic diagnosis, *Pediatr Radiol* 22:21, 1992.

356. Leonidas JC, Magid N, Soberman N et al: Midgut volvulus in infants: diagnosis with ultrasound, *Radiology* 179:491, 1991.

357. Shatzkes D, Gordon DH, Haller JO et al: Malrotation of the bowel: malalignment of the superior mesenteric artery-vein complex shown by CT and MR, *J Comput Assist Tomogr* 14:93, 1990.

358. Guzzetta PC, Anderson KD, Altman RP et al: Malrotation and midgut volvulus. In Schwartz SI et al, editors: *Principles of surgery*, New York, 1994, McGraw-Hill.

53

Gynecologic and Obstetric Disorders

Angela Sirnick • Marlene D. Melzer-Lange

APPROACHING THE GYNECOLOGIC EXAMINATION

The pediatric gynecologic examination may seem daunting, but technically, particularly in the young child, it is much simpler than in the adult. The greatest barriers are parental anxiety, adolescent embarrassment, and physician apprehension. Young children are primarily afraid of pain. In most cases a simple explanation of the procedure reassures the parents and the child and facilitates the examination. The physician's approach should be one of gentleness, sensitivity, and patience.

Under no circumstances should a child be forced to have a gynecologic examination; such an act may constitute sexual assault, depending on state or provincial laws. When the examination is necessary for medical reasons (e.g., vaginal foreign body or traumatic vaginal bleeding) and the child remains uncooperative, examination by a gynecologist with the child under anesthesia is indicated. In less urgent cases, examination under sedation may be considered if the examination is medically necessary. The pediatric gynecologic examination may need to be deferred to the child's pediatrician or family doctor if it is medically nonurgent and the child will not cooperate.[1]

Position

Prepubertal. A comfortable position for most children is supine in the frog-leg position, with the hips flexed and the soles of the feet touching. The knee-chest position has been recommended for better visualization of the vagina, since the tissues fall forward because of gravity. However, this position may be more threatening, particularly in a child who has suffered sexual abuse.

Very anxious children may need to be examined in their mother's lap or between their mother's legs on the examining table. Whereas draping is necessary for the adolescent, young children often want to see what is happening. Having the child assist the examiner by separating the labia may be reassuring to the child. With the examiner depressing the perineum downward and laterally, on either side of the introitus, the hymenal ring and vagina may be visualized (Fig. 53-1, *A*).

Asking the patient to cough or take a big breath sometimes results in relaxation of the vaginal walls and further aids in visualization. If this method is not successful, the labia may be gently held between index finger and thumb and pulled upward and outward (Fig. 53-1, *B*). In the vast majority of young children, no further examination or instrumentation is necessary.

Pubertal. The adolescent may be examined in the traditional lithotomy position. For the first pelvic examination, it may be reassuring for the patient to be examined in a semisitting position, without the use of stirrups so that she can see what is happening.[2] Before examination, rapport should be established. This is usually easily accomplished by obtaining a general medical history, including information about school and hobbies. Questions about sexual activities should be straightforward and nonjudgmental and preferably asked without the parent in the room. At the same time, the adolescent should be asked whether she would like a family member or friend present during the examination. With increasing age, most adolescents prefer to be accompanied by a female nurse. For medicolegal

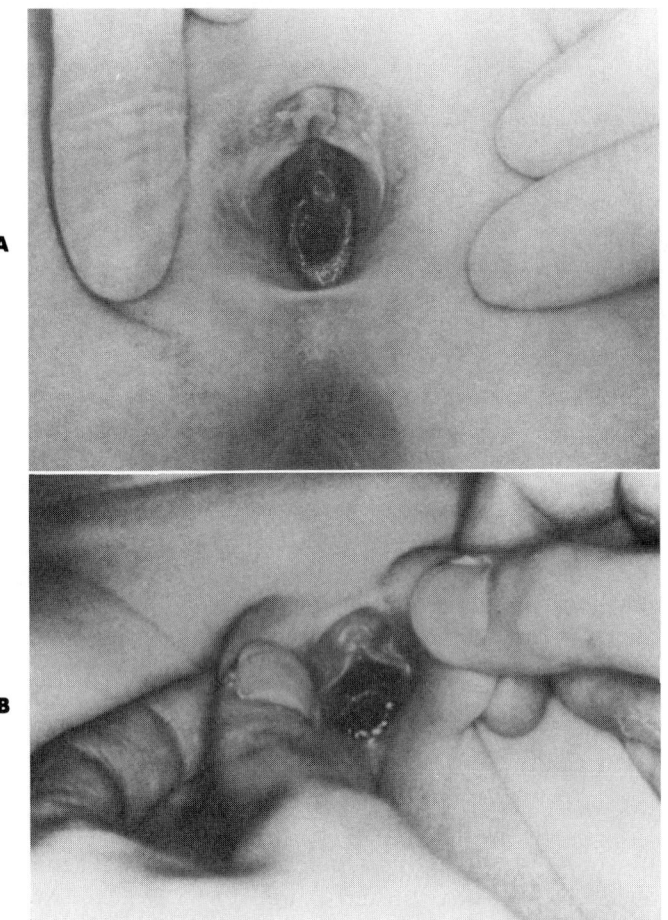

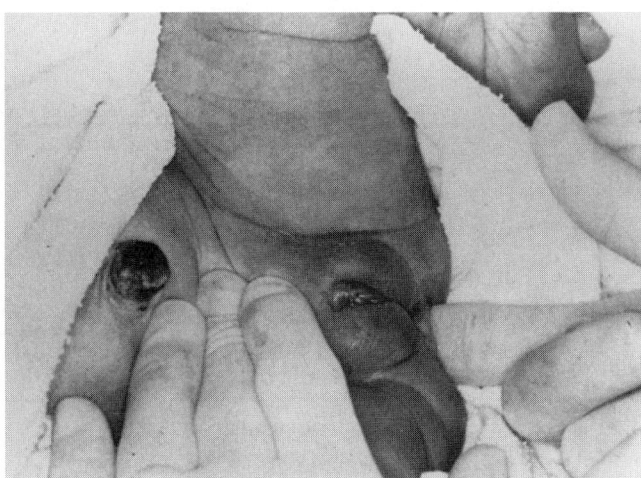

FIG. 53-2. The gynecologic examination of infants, children, and young adolescents. (*From Cowell CA:* Pediatr Clin North Am *28(2):259, 1981.*)

FIG. 53-1. A, Visualization of hymenal ring and vagina. **B,** Holding labia gently while pulling upward and outward. (*From Emans JS, Goldstein DP:* Pediatric and adolescent gynecology, *Boston, 1990, Little, Brown.*)

reasons and support, some suggest that a female assistant be present during examination by a male physician.

Equipment

In prepubertal children, neither the speculum examination nor the traditional bimanual vaginal examination is a routine part of the pelvic examination. If bimanual examination is required, inserting the index or little finger into the rectum and palpating the abdomen may provide information about the presence of a vaginal foreign body or an ovarian tumor (Fig. 53-2).

The only equipment used routinely are those required to obtain specimens (e.g., cotton-tipped swabs, eye dropper, and light source). If further visualization is necessary to remove a foreign body or to exclude internal lacerations caused by straddle injuries, instrumentation may be required. An ordinary otoscope without a speculum may provide adequate visualization of the vagina in a cooperative child. Alternatively a vaginoscope, cytoscope, or nasal speculum may be used. These later examinations are usually performed by a gynecologist on an anesthetized patient.

In adolescents the bimanual vaginal examination and use of the speculum is routine, as it is in adults. Special con-

sideration is needed when examining the young adolescent who has never been sexually active. Insertion of one finger for palpation and use of a small speculum may be necessary. The Huffman speculum is appropriate. For most adolescents who are sexually active the Pederson speculum, which is narrower than the "adult" Graves speculum, is optimal. The infant speculum is rarely used (Fig. 53-3).

Specimens

Specimens may be obtained for culture Gram stain, wet mount, potassium-hydroxide preparation, cytology (Papanicolaou smear), and seminal-fluid analysis.

In prepubertal children a cotton-tipped applicator or Q-tip may be used. Care must be taken to moisten the applicator before insertion because a dry cotton applicator may cause discomfort and pain to the unestrogenized vagina. Preferred techniques include the use of a calcium alginate swab, urethral swab, eye dropper, or catheter. A thin nasopharyngeal Caligeswab moistened with nonbacteriostatic saline can be inserted into the vagina without pain if the hymenal edges are avoided. Similarly a cotton-tipped urethral swab may be inserted and gently scraped along the lateral vaginal wall to obtain a specimen for *Chlamydia* culture. Cultures for *Chlamydia trachomatis* are recommended rather than indirect tests in prepubertal children because of the possibility of false-positive results and the association of this organism with sexual abuse. Culture for *Neisseria gonorrhoeae* should be plated on modified Thayer-Martin-Jembec media at the time of examination. Vaginal washings for seminal fluid are obtained by injecting 2 to 3 ml of nonbacteriostatic saline into the vagina with a sterile eye dropper or catheter and then aspirating the fluid. In the adolescent, specimens are usually obtained during the speculum examination. For the Pap smear, an Ayer spatula is rotated around the cervix and the material obtained is applied to a slide. An endocervical specimen should also be obtained, preferably by cytobrush. Wet preparations are collected with a cotton-tipped applicator inserted into the posterior vagina. Cultures for *N. gonorrhoeae* and *C. trachomatis* require endocervical swabs.

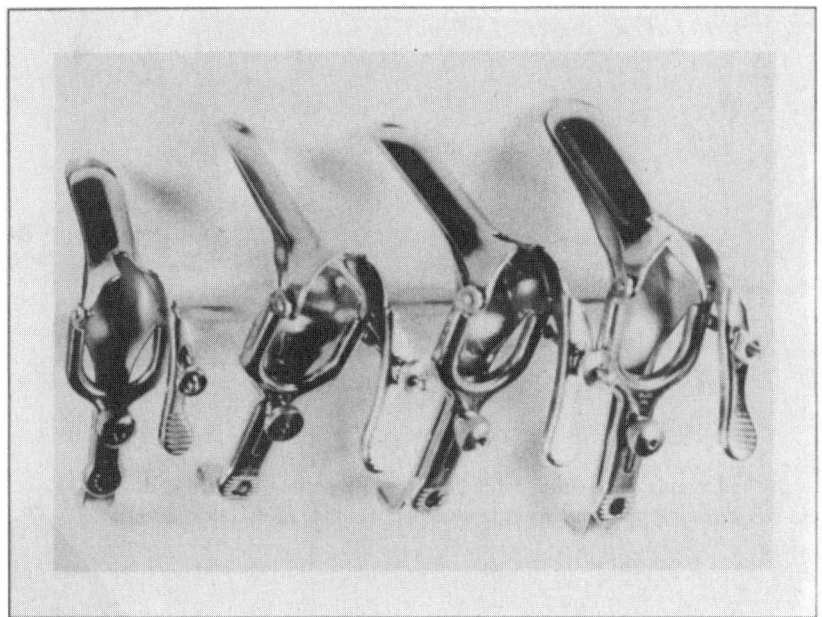

FIG. 53-3. Types of specula (from left to right): infant, Huffman, Pederson, and Graves. (*From Emans JS, Goldstein DP: Pediatric and adolescent gynecology, Boston, 1990, Little, Brown.*)

Gynecologic Examination

The gynecologic examination of a prepubertal child usually involves direct visualization of the external genitalia. A recent study reported that the majority of physicians have very poor knowledge of the normal findings in a prepubertal child. An outline of the normal anatomy is depicted in Fig. 53-4. Hymenal shapes are varied. Most common are the fimbriated, circumferential, and posterior rim shapes.

The size and shape of the hymen has assumed importance because of the increase in allegations of child sexual abuse; thus knowledge of normal findings is essential (Figs. 53-5 and 53-6). Numerous authors have documented the hymenal diameter in prepubertal children. White and colleagues concluded that a "vaginal introital diameter less than 4 mm is highly associated with a history of sexual contact."[3] Paradise cautioned against the use of the hymenal orifice diameter as a sole confirmatory test for sexual abuse but agreed with White in stating that "an introital diameter less than 4 mm does not negate a history of fondling or penetration."[4] As a guideline, the upper limit of normal in a prepubertal child is 1 mm for each year of age (e.g., 7 mm for a 7-year-old child). For the emergency physician, accurate documentation of all findings is key and allows for further interpretation by experts in the field (see Chapter 45).

Signs and Symptoms

ANGELA SIRNICK

VAGINAL BLEEDING

Vaginal bleeding may be a normal physiologic event in the neonate because of maternal estrogen withdrawal or in the prepubertal child because of serious disease such as

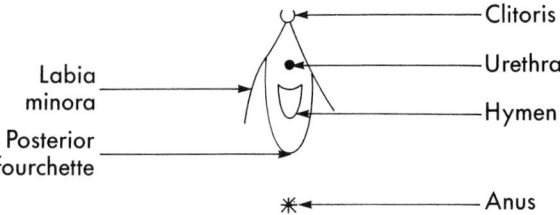

FIG. 53-4. Outline of normal anatomy.

vulvovaginitis, vaginal foreign body, precocious puberty, blood dyscrasias, or genital tumor. It is rarely functional. In the infant a blood-stained diaper may be hematuria or rectal bleeding rather than vaginal blood. In the postpubertal child (adolescent) the most frequent causes of abnormal vaginal bleeding are related to disorders of menstruation (e.g., dysfunctional uterine bleeding or complications of pregnancy). Other causes include local infections, complications of medications, bleeding dyscrasias, endocrine disorders, and chronic illnesses.

Prepubertal

Before birth, newborn infants are exposed to high levels of maternal estrogen, which stimulates the uterine endometrium and breast tissue. In the first 2 to 3 weeks of life, hormonal withdrawal results in endometrial sloughing and a few days of vaginal bleeding. On examination of the infant, breast enlargement may be noted. These changes are part of the normal physiology of the newborn period and do not require any treatment. Parents usually require a simple reassuring explanation.

Vulvovaginitis. Vulvovaginitis is a common cause of bleeding in the prepubertal child. It may occur as a result of pruritus and scratching because of pinworm infection. Excoriations are usually present in the anal area as well.

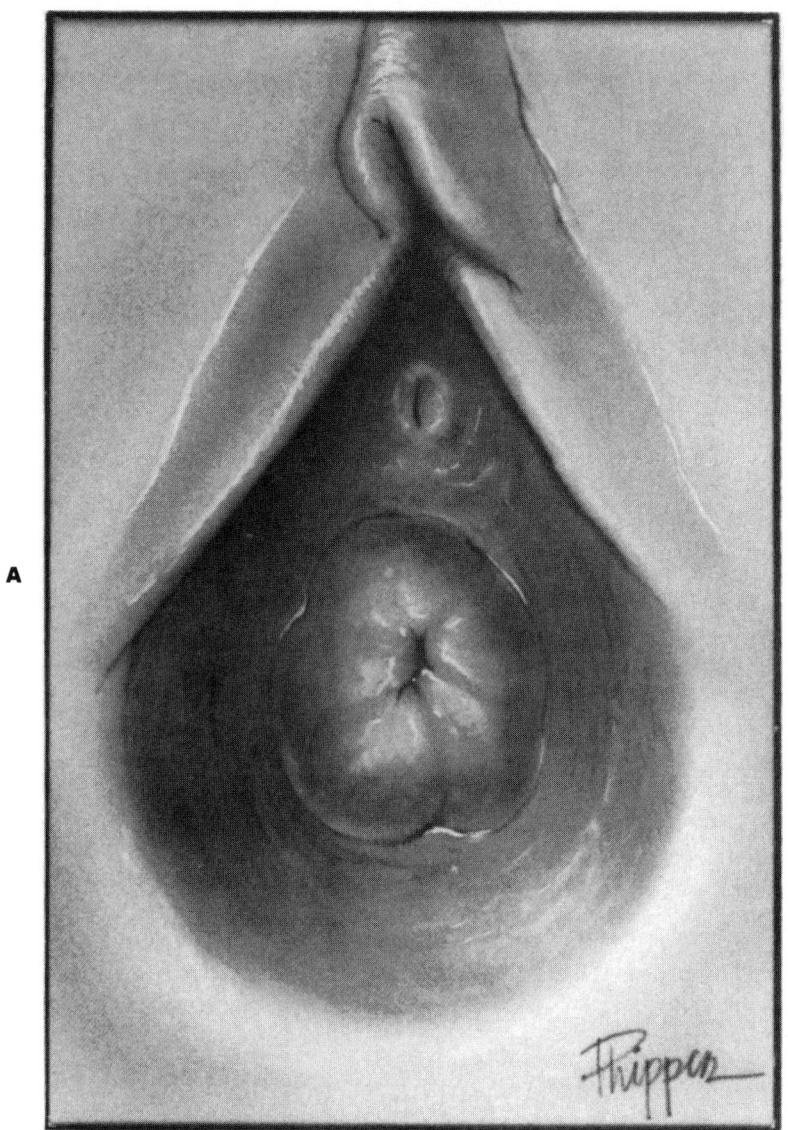

FIG. 53-5. Hymenal shapes. **A,** Fimbriated. (*A, B,* and *C from Pokorny SF:* Am J Obstet Gynecol *157(4):951-953, 1987.*)   *Continued.*

Organisms especially associated with vaginal bleeding include group A β-hemolytic streptocci and *Shigella.* Other signs of infection are usually present (e.g., vulvar inflammation and vaginal discharge). There may be a recent history of diarrhea.

Diagnostic work-up includes a Scotch-tape test for pinworms and cultures for group A β-hemolytic streptococci and enteric organisms.

Management initially should be symptomatic with local creams and sitz baths. If pinworms are suspected, treat with a single dose of pyrantel pamoate 11 mg/kg or mebendazole 100 mg PO. Local measures alone have not been effective for *Shigella* and group A β-hemolytic streptococci. Appropriate oral antibiotics should be prescribed, depending on the culture and sensitivity of the organism.

Trauma. Straddle injuries commonly result in bruising or hematomas in the vulva and periclitoral folds. Superficial lacerations of the labia minora, periurethral tissue, and posterior fourchette may be seen. Tears of the hymen are very uncommon unless a penetrating injury has occurred. In the absence of an appropriate history consistent with the physical findings, sexual abuse should be considered. Children with straddle injuries may be difficult to examine because of their anxiety and pain. Reassurance, a simple explanation of the procedure, and a supportive parent often allay the problem. Sitting in a lukewarm bath may ease the pain and allow examination. For better visualization of a vulvar laceration with bleeding, 2% lidocaine jelly may be applied with a gauze, followed by irrigation of the area with warm water. With minor abrasions, Gelfoam or Surgigel may be applied to the area. If sutures are deemed necessary, sedation or anesthesia are often required. Most children with straddle injuries can be managed with supportive care (e.g., sitz baths and local hygiene).

Trauma caused by penetrating objects such as broom handles can cause life-threatening injuries and may ini-

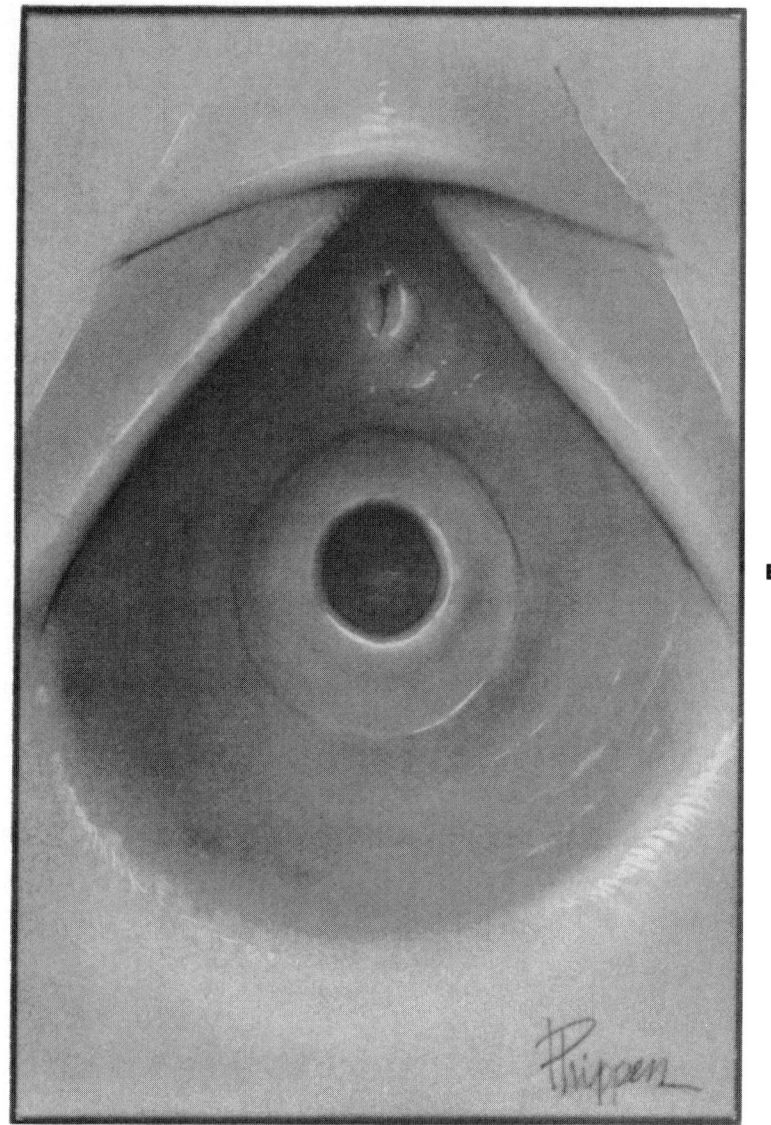

FIG. 53-5, cont'd. Hymenal shapes. **B,** Annular or circumferential. *Continued.*

tially present with no physical findings other than vaginal bleeding. Damage to the bowel, bladder, and rectum may occur. Careful examination should be performed to look for any signs of abdominal tenderness or rectal lacerations. However minor the genital injury may seem initially (e.g., hymenal tear with minimal bleeding), a careful vaginal examination should be performed. This often requires gynecologic consultation and administration of general anesthesia. Initial management includes assessment for signs of shock, intravenous fluids when appropriate, baseline hemoglobin, and urinalysis.

Foreign Body. The presence of vaginal bleeding should alert the examining physician to the possibility of a foreign body. In most prepubertal children a foul-smelling discharge does not accompany the bleeding.[5] Objects commonly found include bits of tissue or toilet paper, crayons, beads, or pins. When strongly suspected on the basis of history, and if the foreign body cannot be visualized in the knee-chest position, gentle irrigation of the vagina with

normal saline using a 25-ml syringe and small urethral catheter may be considered. If unable to visualize, examination under anesthesia is warranted.

Rectal examination can sometimes be helpful in confirming the presence of large objects such as crayons. X-ray studies are useful only if the object is radiopaque.

Lichen Sclerosus. Lichen sclerosus is a rare disorder of the vulvovaginal and perianal skin, presenting with ecchymoses, excoriations, and bleeding, which may lead parents or physicians to suspect sexual abuse. Characteristically white papules and atrophic plaques are present; superinfection may occur. Referral to a dermatologist or gynecologist usually confirms the diagnosis. Treatment may include steroid emollients or antifungal creams.

Genital Tumors. Genital tumors are an uncommon cause of vaginal bleeding. The most frequent malignant tumor is sarcoma botryoides or embryonal rhabdomyosarcoma. Along with bleeding it may present with vaginal discharge, abdominal pain or mass, and the passage of

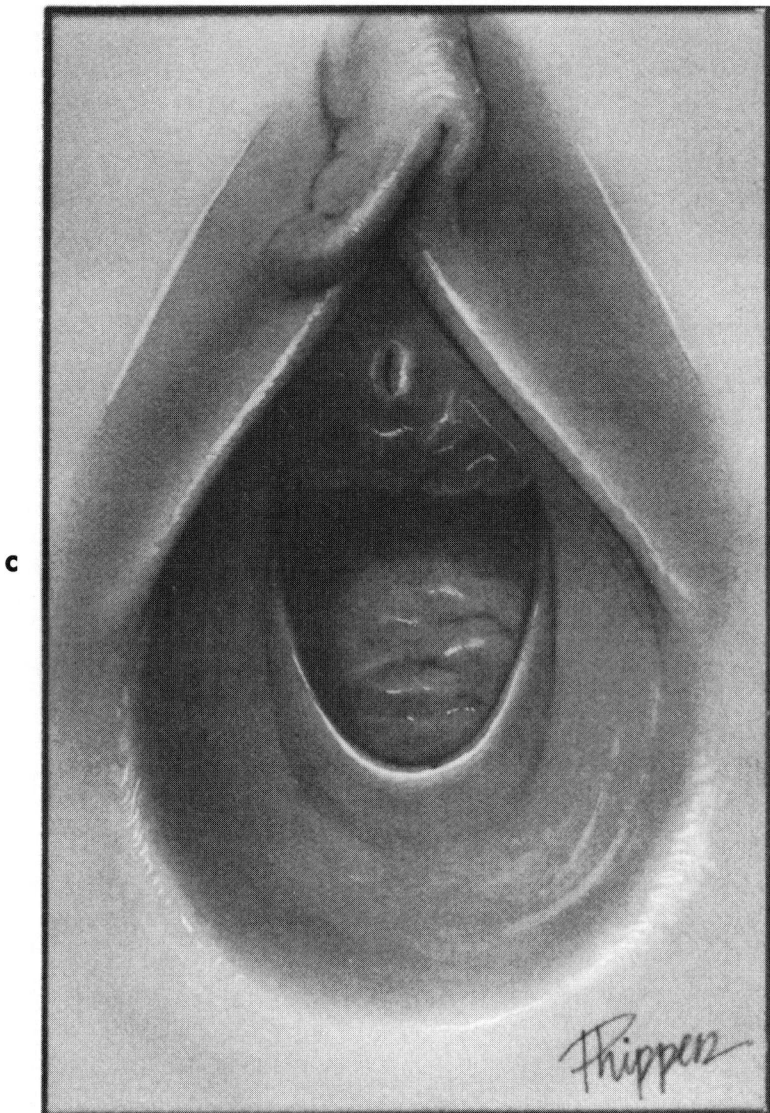

FIG. 53-5, cont'd. Hymenal shapes. C, Posterior rim or crescentic. Configuration of the prepubertal hymen.

grapelike lesions. Treatment consists of chemotherapy and aggressive surgery.

Clear-cell adenocarcinoma of the vagina or cervix occurs in about 0.2% of girls who were exposed to diethylstilbestrol or other estrogen-containing drugs in utero. Treatment consists of radiotherapy.

Urethral Prolapse. Urethral prolapse frequently presents with bleeding that is often thought to be vaginal in origin. Other symptoms may include dysuria and urinary frequency. Diagnosis is made by the characteristic appearance of the doughnut-shaped friable red-blue mass that at times obscures the vaginal introitus. In mild cases the prolapse resolves with use of sitz baths and emollient creams. If the tissue appears necrotic, surgical excision will be required.

Precocious Puberty. Cyclic vaginal bleeding associated with the onset of other signs of puberty (e.g., breast development and pubic hair growth) before the age of 8 signifies precocious puberty and requires investigation (see box on p. 871). Although the majority of cases are idiopathic or constitutional, the differential diagnosis includes ovarian and central nervous system (CNS) tumors and neurocutaneous disorders (McCune-Albright syndrome). The examining physician should check specifically for abdominal masses and café au lait spots. Referral to a pediatric endocrinologist on an outpatient basis is suggested.

Postpubertal

Recognition of abnormal vaginal bleeding requires an understanding of the patient's normal menstrual patterns. Normal variation in flow and cycle length is discussed later in this chapter in the section on dysfunctional uterine bleeding. For the physician, recognition of disorders that are potentially dangerous and may require urgent treatment is a priority. Other than dysfunctional uterine bleeding, vaginal bleeding is most often related to complications

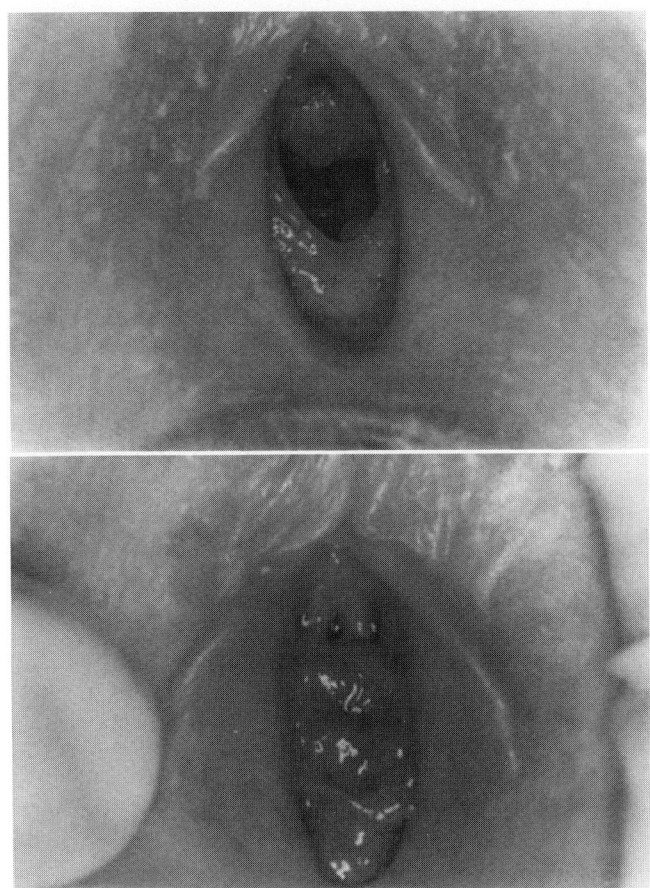

FIG. 53-6. A, Annular hymen. **B,** Fimbriated hymen. (*From Chadwick D et al: Color atlas of child sexual abuse, Chicago, 1989, Year Book Medical.*)

of pregnancy (e.g., ectopic pregnancy, placenta previa, and bleeding dyscrasias).

Dysfunctional Uterine Bleeding. Dysfunctional uterine bleeding refers to irregular and often excessive painless bleeding caused by the immaturity of the pituitary-ovarian axis and results in anovulatory cycles and withdrawal bleeding.

Initial history should include the amount and acuity of blood loss to evaluate and determine the need for fluid resuscitation, details of menstrual pattern, possibility of pregnancy or pelvic infection, use of contraceptives or other medications, and history of bleeding diathesis.

Physical examination should initially assess hemodynamic stability. An acute abdomen suggests causes other than dysfunctional uterine bleeding. A pelvic examination provides information about source and amount of bleeding and excludes other causes of vaginal bleeding. Laboratory data should include a hemoglobin test to assess the degree of anemia, a platelet count to rule out thrombocytopenia, and a pregnancy test.

Management depends on the severity of bleeding and the resultant hemoglobin level, assuming the patient was not previously anemic. For mild bleeding (Hgb >11 gm/dl) only reassurance may be required. For moderate bleed-

ing (Hgb 9 to 11 gm/dl) oral contraceptives and iron supplements are sufficient. With severe bleeding (Hgb <9 gm/dl) acute management consists of fluid resuscitation and transfusion as necessary, as well as intravenous estrogen. If blood products are required, blood samples should be taken for a coagulation profile because transfusion will obscure the results (see also section on Dysfunctional Uterine Bleeding).

Complications of Pregnancy. The possible complications of pregnancy include spontaneous abortion (incomplete, complete, or threatened), ectopic pregnancy, molar pregnancy, abruptio placenta, and placenta previa. Because of the increase in teenage pregnancies, particularly in adolescents younger than 15 years of age, a careful history about sexual activity should be sought. Since teenagers are often reluctant to convey this information, a pregnancy test should be performed routinely in the investigation of vaginal bleeding. Spontaneous abortion presents with varying amounts of bleeding and uterine cramps. A pelvic examination assists in determining whether the abortion is threatened or incomplete. Septic abortion presents with signs of infection and bleeding. In all cases an obstetrician should be consulted.

In any patient with vaginal bleeding who presents in shock with an unknown or first-trimester pregnancy, ruptured ectopic pregnancy must be considered. Immediate stabilization is necessary, followed by appropriate investigations. Culdocentesis, laparoscopy, or laparectomy may be necessary to confirm the diagnosis.

In the second or third trimester of pregnancy, placenta previa and abruptio should be considered. Pelvic examination may trigger sudden hemorrhage and thus should be avoided until the patient has been stabilized with an intravenous line, the fetal heart rate is monitored, baseline blood work has been obtained (hemoglobin or hematocrit, platelet count, prothrombin time, and partial thromboplastin time), and an obstetrician has been consulted (see also section on Complications of Pregnancy).

Complications of Contraceptives. Breakthrough bleeding may occur in adolescents on oral contraceptives and unless the patient is specifically asked about the use of the pill, the diagnosis may be missed.

Intrauterine devices are often associated with regular heavy bleeding at the time of each menstrual cycle.

Medications. History should be asked regarding use of medications. Anticoagulants, platelet inhibitors, gonadal and adrenal steroids, monoamine oxidase inhibitors, morphine, and anticholinergics have been associated with vaginal bleeding.[6]

Pelvic Inflammatory Disease. Salpingitis and endometritis caused by *N. gonorrhoeae* and *C. trachomatis* frequently cause heavy or irregular bleeding. Appropriate cultures should be taken. An elevated ESR may aid in diagnosis as discussed later in this chapter.

Endometriosis. Endometriosis has been associated with irregular menses because of anovulatory cycles and with brown spotting before menstruation. Other symptoms reported include abdominal pain, vaginal discharge, and dyspareunia.

Bleeding Dyscrasias. A bleeding disorder may present with an unusually heavy first menstrual period or excessive bleeding at the time of delivery in a pregnant patient. Most common disorders presenting in this manner are qualitative and quantitative platelet disorders, including hereditary or acquired thrombocytopenia, von Willebrand disease, and factor VIII or IX deficiencies.

Trauma. Trauma may be accidental, caused by falls and straddle injuries, or it may be inflicted by sexual assault. In adolescents the most frequent foreign body causing vaginal bleeding is a retained tampon. If the tampon has been left in for several days to weeks, there is usually an associated foul-smelling discharge.

Systemic Illnesses. Any systemic illness that interferes with the hypothalamic-pituitary-gonadal axis may cause irregular bleeding. Renal dialysis has been associated with both amenorrhea and heavy menses. Similarly stress, excessive exercise, and eating disorders have been associated with irregular menses and, more commonly, with amenorrhea. Systemic diseases may also directly interfere with coagulation resulting in heavy bleeding (e.g., viral-induced thrombocytopenia and idiopathic thrombocytopenic purpura [ITP]).

Endocrine Disorders. Both hypothyroidism and hyperthyroidism may result in menstrual irregularities. Polycystic ovary syndrome and prolactinomas classically present with amenorrhea but initially may be indistinguishable from dysfunctional uterine bleeding. Clinical characteristics determine the need for measuring prolactin, follicle-stimulating hormone (FSH), and luteinizing hormone (LH) levels. Anovulation may also be caused by adrenal disorders such as Cushing and Addison disease.

Tumors. Tumors of the genital tract are uncommon but must be considered in the differential diagnosis of vaginal bleeding. Vaginal adenocarcinoma caused by maternal intake of diethylstilbestrol has already been mentioned. Cervical polyps and hemangiomas rarely may present with vaginal bleeding. Cervical cancer should be considered, particularly in the sexually active adolescent who has been exposed to the human papillomavirus. Uterine abnormalities such as congenital anomalies and submucous myomas may present with irregular bleeding (see box above).

VAGINAL DISCHARGE

Vaginal discharge may be normal or physiologic in the first 2 to 3 weeks of life and just before menarche. In the newborn, stimulation of the vaginal mucosa and cervical epithelium by maternal estrogen before birth results in a physiologic discharge that consists of thick mucoid material

---

Postpubertal Vaginal Bleeding
Dysfunctional uterine bleeding
Complications of pregnancy
Complications of contraceptives
Other medications
Pelvic inflammatory disease
Endometriosis
Trauma
Foreign body
Systemic illnesses
Bleeding dyscrasias
Endocrine disorders
Tumors

and superficial squamous epithelial cells. It may be blood-tinged or grossly bloody secondary to withdrawal from in utero estrogen stimulation of the endometrium. The physiologic discharge of the newborn usually wanes within 7 to 10 days. Similarly, just before menarche there may be a sudden increase in vaginal discharge that is copious, gray-white and non-foul-smelling, resulting from increasing ovarian estrogen activity. Physiologic leukorrhea requires only reassurance and local hygiene measures.

Abnormal vaginal discharge results from specific infections including sexually transmitted organisms, nonspecific infections, physical agents (e.g., vaginal foreign body, sand, soap, and deodorant spray), structural defects (e.g., ectopic ureter and congenital fistula), systemic illnesses, vulvar skin disease, and psychosomatic causes (see box on p. 873).

Prepubertal

Vulvovaginal problems in the prepubertal child are common. Predisposing factors include an underdeveloped labia minora and the absence of pubic hair for protection, atrophic vulvovaginal mucosa, an alkaline vaginal pH that is ideal for bacterial growth, and poor perineal hygiene.

Nonspecific vulvovaginitis results from mixed bacterial infections for which no specific cause can be identified. Symptoms consist of dysuria, vulvar discomfort, and inflammation. Poor hygiene and local irritation by clothing or physical agents have been implicated. Treatment consists of attention to hygiene, education about wiping from front to back, sitz baths, avoidance of irritating substances and tight clothing, and frequent changes of white cotton underpants. In severe cases topical measures such as 1% hydrocortisone cream may be used for 2 to 3 days. With persistent or recurrent nonspecific vulvovaginitis a 10- to 14-day course of oral amoxicillin or cephalosporin or application of estrogen-containing creams to the vulva for 2 weeks may be helpful.

Specific infections may be bacterial, viral, or protozoal caused by respiratory, enteric, or sexually transmitted organisms. After an upper respiratory tract infection, vaginal infection with group A β-hemolytic streptococcus, *Streptococcus pneumoniae*, *Haemophilus influenzae* type B, and *Neisseria meningitidis* may occur. Treatment is specific for the organism. *Shigella* and group A β-hemolytic streptococci may present with bleeding or a bloody discharge.

Causes of Vulvovaginitis in Childhood and Adolescence

Bacterial

Nonspecific: mixed flora

Specific: *Neisseria gonorrhoeae*, Group A β-*hemolytic streptococci*, *Gardnerella vaginalis*, *Neisseria meningitidis*, *Streptococcus pneumoniae*, *Shigella flexneri*, and *Chlamydia trachomatis*

Protozoal

Trichomoniasis, amoebiasis, and schistosomiasis (in endemic areas)

Candida albicans

Pinworms

Viral

Varicella, smallpox, vaccinia, rubeola, herpes, and *condylomata acuminata*

Physical agents

Vaginal foreign body, sand, soap, fabric softener, deodorant spray, bubble bath, diapers, leotards, and medications

Structural defects

Prolapsed urethra, ectopic ureter, congenital fistula, inflammatory bowel disease with fistulae, and labial adhesions

Vulvar skin problems

Seborrhea, atopic dermatitis, tinea, *molluscum contagiosum*, scabies, and pediculosis

Syphilis

Neuropsychiatric problems

The presence of sexually transmitted diseases (STDs) should alert the physician to the possibility of sexual abuse and appropriate questions should be asked and referral made to social services. Gonorrhea tends to present with a purulent discharge. Chlamydia is frequently asymptomatic. *Trichomonas vaginalis* in the first few months of life may have been acquired during delivery.

Skin infections caused by *Staphylococcus aureus* and β-hemolytic streptococci and *Proteus mirabilis* may also cause vulvitis. Candidal vulvovaginitis is less common in prepubertal children than in adolescents and adults because of its preferential growth on estrogenized tissues. In young children, there frequently is a history of a prior course of antibiotics. With frequent or severe candidal infections, diabetes mellitus and immunodeficiency status should be considered. *Enterobius vermicularis* (pin-worms) frequently causes intense perianal and vaginal pruritus. Discharge may not be present.

Retained foreign bodies may present with vaginal bleeding and discharge. In young children tissue or toilet paper, beads, and pins are frequently found.

Systemic illnesses with vaginal manifestations include chickenpox, measles, scarlet fever, and diphtheria. Chronic granulomatous disease may present with a draining vaginal fistula.

Structural defects include prolapsed urethra, labial adhesions, ectopic ureter, and congenital fistula. An ectopic ureter presents with persistent watery discharge. The ureter may exit from the trigone urethra, just below the urethra or vagina. Congenital fistulas from the rectum to the posterior vagina or posterior fourchette present with recurrent and persistent infections. There may be an associated imperforate anus. Agglutination of the labia minora results from subclinical vulvitis; treatment consists of application of estrogenic cream. Although usually benign, urinary tract infections may result from partial obstruction of the urinary stream and formation of an artificial urogenital sinus.

Vulvar skin problems may be caused by generalized skin diseases such as seborrheic dermatitis, psoriasis, atopic dermatitis, and, rarely, lichen sclerosus. Vulvovaginitis occurs from secondary infection.

Recurrent genital complaints without obvious findings may be the presentation of a child who has been sexually abused. Appropriate questions should be asked.

Postpubertal

In adolescents with vaginal discharge the most frequent causes are infection and foreign bodies. Candidal vaginitis presents with an itchy, white discharge. Predisposing factors include antibiotics, oral contraceptives, diabetes, and pregnancy. Clinical associations included pruritus, caseous discharge, perineal edema, or erythema. A watery discharge and urine odor were good predictors of an alternate diagnosis. Gram stain showing yeast was the most accurate laboratory test; saline microscopy, potassium hydroxide, and methylene blue were moderately accurate.[8]

Treatment consists of local antifungal creams and suppositories. *Gardnerella vaginalis* presents with a fishy odor. Clue cells are evident on wet mount. *Trichomonas vaginalis* is often seen in sexually active adolescents. Presenting complaints may include pruritus and a frothy discharge that is more frequent after menses. Wet mount reveals motile trichomonads.[9] Gonorrhea and chlamydial infection may cause vaginitis, cervicitis, salpingitis, and systemic complications.[10,11]

The most frequent foreign body in an adolescent is a retained tampon. This usually presents with a foul-smelling discharge. Symptoms usually resolve with removal of the foreign body.

Diagnostic Entities

MARLENE MELZER-LANGE

BREAST DISORDERS

Neonatal

Because of intense maternal hormonal stimulation of the neonatal breast, engorgement is frequently seen 2 to 3 weeks after birth. The engorgement is usually bilateral and can occur in both boys and girls. Occasionally, drops of blood or milk may be seen; expressing this milk may lead to excoriation of the breast and subsequent mastitis. Parents should be reassured that neonatal breast hyperplasia is normal and that manipulation of the infant nipple should be avoided.

Erythema, increased warmth, and induration of the infant breast indicates mastitis. Mastitis may be associated with neonatal sepsis; infants should have a septic work-up and should be treated empirically for sepsis until their condition improves and cultures are negative. Broad antibiotic coverage should be used initially, including a penicillinase-resistant penicillin such as nafcillin 100 to 150 mg/kg/24 hr q 4-6 hr IV combined with gentamicin 7.5 mg/kg/24 hr q 8 hr IV or an equivalent agent.

Prepubertal

Premature thelarche (i.e., growth of breasts before the age of 8), is a common complaint in the prepubertal child. Breast development may occur on one side initially, with the other breast developing later. Examination of the genitalia will reveal normal, prepubertal development without estrogen effect of the vulva. The breasts may initially be tender. No further evaluation is necessary in these girls, unless hormonal changes of the genitalia are present. The patient and her parents should be reassured; routine follow-up should be done with her primary physician.

Adolescence

Normal Breast Development. Most girls begin to develop breast tissue sometime after the age of 8. Initially one nipple develops a palpable, usually tender "breast bud." The other breast may develop concurrently but frequently may lag weeks to months behind. Asymmetric breast development is a frequent concern to the young adolescent; she should be reassured that this asymmetry is normal. In the past physicians have mistakenly performed biopsies in cases of early normal breast development because they were concerned that the breast bud represented an abnormal malignancy. Patients and their parents should be reassured that asymmetric breast development is common and normal.

Gynecomastia. Enlargement of one or both breasts occurs frequently in boys during adolescence. The teen may notice tenderness and a small subareolar nodule. Enlargement up to 3 cm in diameter is considered normal and occurs in approximately two thirds of adolescent boys, usually at 14 to 15 years of age.[12] The teen should be reassured that this minimal breast development is a normal part of male puberty and very common. In teens with breast enlargement of greater proportions, counseling and occasional surgical reduction of the enlarged breast(s) may be necessary to improve male body image.[13]

Nipple Irritation. Scaliness, redness, or tenderness of nipples may occasionally occur. Sports, including jogging and biking, have been implicated.[14] Lubrication of the nipples in conjunction with the use of soft, smooth "sports bras" will prevent further maceration. In girls with hair growth on the nipples, plucking may cause irritation and folliculitis of areola; patients should be cautioned to avoid removal of these hairs.[15]

Breast Infections. Lactational mastitis is the most common problem among adolescents.[16] Usually postpartum, the blockage of milk in the ducts of the breast causes stasis and subsequent infection. Fever, marked tenderness of the breast, erythema of the skin, and a firm or fluctuant mass are signs and symptoms of mastitis. Trauma from prolonged nursing may play a part in the pathophysiology. *S. aureus*, group A streptococcus, *Escherichia coli*, and other organisms are usually the cause.[17]

Treatment should include an oral antibiotic such as ampicillin 30 to 50 mg/kg/24 hr (adult: 250 to 500 mg/dose) PO QID or erythromycin 30 mg/kg/24 hr (adult: 250 mg/dose) PO QID, warm compresses, and rest. Occasionally drainage may be required; careful drainage with a circumareolar incision and gentle dissection of the abscess helps minimize damage to the breast tissue.[18]

Nonlactational mastitis may also occur. Trauma caused by foreplay, sports, needle or open biopsies, local skin infections, and epidermal cysts may predispose the nonlactating breast to mastitis. Treatment is the same as for lactating breast infections.

Breast Masses. Adolescents may present to the emergency department after detection of a breast mass. The anxiety produced by such masses may be considerable; patient, parent, and physician all can be involved. Because discovery of a breast mass in adulthood mandates careful investigation to eliminate breast cancer as a diagnosis, a mass in adolescence frequently precipitates a similar response. Although breast cancer does occur in adolescents, it is far less common than after the age of 35. History of tenderness, timing, size change, and relationship to the menstrual cycle should be noted. Size, distribution, and texture should be evaluated in the affected breast and in the contralateral side. Drainage from the nipple should be noted.

Fibroadenoma. Fibroadenoma is the most common breast tumor in adolescents, particularly black youngsters; 95% of lesions biopsied were found to be fibroadenomas in one series.[19] Their consistency may be from firm to rubbery and the mass tends to be smooth, movable, and well-demarcated within the breast tissue. Although most are 3 to 4 cm at presentation, they may enlarge to 15 cm. They may enlarge significantly and may occasionally regress spontaneously. Fibroadenomas may be multiple or bilateral, most commonly in the upper outer quadrant of the breast. Management should be with close, repeated physical examinations. Slow growth of a characteristic lesion may be followed clinically; needle or open biopsy should be considered if rapid growth or patient anxiety ensues.[20] Large or rapidly expanding lesions should be surgically excised to prevent asymmetry and distortion of the breast.

Trauma. Injury to the breast during sports may cause contusions, hematomas, and subsequent fat necrosis that may present as a breast mass. Conversely, trauma to the breast may precipitate a breast examination, during which a preexisting lump may be discovered. Breast masses discovered immediately after trauma are most likely to be preexisting masses that are unrelated to the trauma.[21] Management of acute injuries includes cool compresses, support with a comfortable bra, and analgesics.

Other breast masses include giant or juvenile fibroadenoma, cystosarcoma phylloides, intraductal breast papilloma, breast carcinoma, and others. Masses that are firm and nonmovable, indiscrete from the remaining breast tissue, very rapidly enlarging, or associated with breast discharge should be closely evaluated by a surgeon or breast specialist.[22] Needle or excisional biopsy may be indicated.[23]

EXTERNAL GENITALIA

Bartholin Gland Abscess

In adolescents, acute onset of swelling and pain in the vulvar area may be the initial signs of a Bartholin gland abscess. Although *N. gonorrhoeae* and *Chlamydia* are frequently the cause in adolescents, other organisms have been cultured from these abscesses.[24,25] Clinical findings include an erythematous, unilateral, indurated, or fluctuant mass in the posterior portion of the vulva. Due to the tenderness of these abscesses, a speculum examination at the initial presentation is usually impossible. Treatment includes incision and drainage of the abscess with appropriate cultures; placement of a Word catheter in the abscess cavity should be considered in the case of large abscesses. The patient should be treated with antibiotics to cover *N. gonorrhoeae* and *Chlamydia*.

Imperforate Hymen and Hematoculpos

In rare instances, the hymen may be imperforate. Clinically, the young girl will be asymptomatic until the time of menarche. At that time, collection of the menstrual flow behind the imperforate hymen may result in distension of the uterus and tubes and subsequent hematoculpos.

Physical examination reveals a bulging hymen that is occasionally blue-purple or yellow in color. An opening in the hymen is not visible. Abdominal pain and possibly distension may also occur. Surgical incision of the imperforate hymen relieves blockage.

Labial Adhesions

Labial adhesions, the fusion of the labia minora, is also called *labial agglutination, labial synechiae,* and *labial fusion.* Labial adhesions are believed to be an acquired problem. After denuding of the labial epithelium by either trauma, dermatitis, or infection, a thin bridge of connective tissue is formed, fusing the labia minorae partially or completely.[26] Low estrogen levels have also been thought to contribute to the formation of labial adhesions.[27] Labial adhesions have been described in childhood sexual abuse but are not pathognomonic.[28,29] Their peak incidence is between 1 and 6 years of age[30]; they occur equally among all races.

Diagnostic Findings. Many labial adhesions are asymptomatic and may present only on routine examination or be noted by parents. Dysuria and frequency are common complaints; some labial adhesions are associated with urinary tract infections.[30] Examination reveals either partial or complete fusion of the labia minora by a "thin, translucent central line of fusion (raphe) extending from the posterior fourchette toward the clitoris"[31] (Fig. 53-7). Inquiry regarding sexual abuse should be considered, particularly if the fusion appears irregular or thick.[29] Urinary tract infection should be excluded.

Management. Treatment of labial adhesions is conservative. Good hygiene and the application of an estrogen

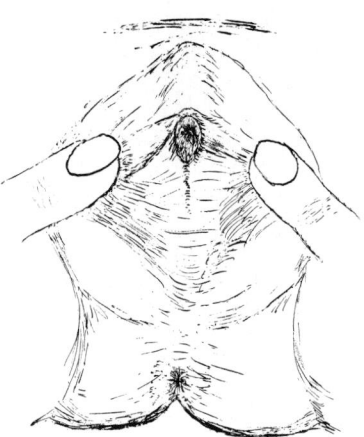

FIG. 53-7. Labial adhesions. Note the adherence of the labia obscuring the introitus. (*Courtesy RM Hanson, MD.*)

cream such as Premarin to the raphe at bedtime for up to a month usually results in separation of the adhesions. Estrogen cream should be used sparingly over a short period of time because breast tenderness and vulvar pigmentation frequently occur after treatment. These changes are reversible once treatment is discontinued. After separation of the adhesions, good hygiene and lubrication of the vulva with petroleum jelly prevent further recurrences.

Lichen Sclerosus

Although uncommon, cases of lichen sclerosus of the vulvovaginal and perianal skin may present to the emergency department; fear that the characteristic rash may represent infection or sexual abuse prompts caregivers to seek emergency care. Lichen sclerosus is believed to be an autoimmune phenomenon; heredity may also play a part.[32]

Complaints include burning, pruritus, nocturia, dysuria, and bleeding. The vulva appears to have areas of "fine wrinkling" and pallor, occasionally with white papules[33] (Fig. 53-8). Involvement of the perianal skin may also occur. Blistering, bleeding, excoriations, and, occasionally, superinfection may also be seen. The diagnosis may be made clinically by an experienced dermatologist. Occasionally skin biopsy may be required to confirm the diagnosis.

Because of the marked irritation and bleeding that may accompany lichen sclerosus, it is understandable that sexual abuse may be considered. There is, however, no evidence that sexual abuse has any relationship to lichen sclerosus.[34]

Treatment may include steroid, emollient, or antifungal creams, particularly if there is superinfection. In many girls, lichen sclerosus disappears spontaneously, usually by puberty.

Urethral Prolapse

In urethral prolapse the mucosa of the distal urethra protrudes out through the urethral meatus. Because of the constricting forces of the urethral meatus, the portion of prolapsing urethra becomes engorged and edematous. In severe cases the prolapsed tissue may become necrotic.

Prolapse occurs at two ages: in prepubertal children, usually between 2 and 12 years, and in postmenopausal

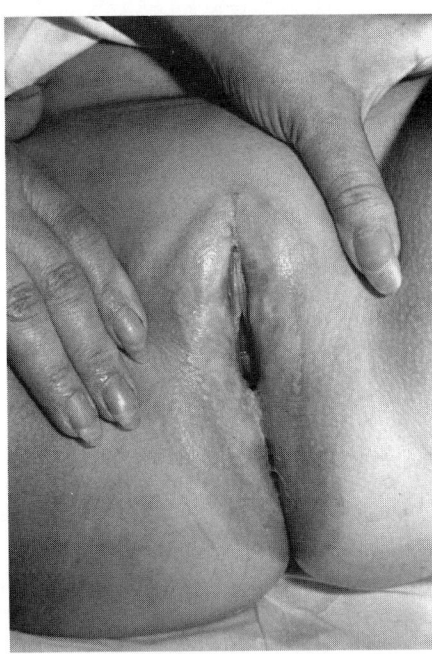

FIG. 53-8. Lichen sclerosis. (*Courtesy N Esterly, MD.*)

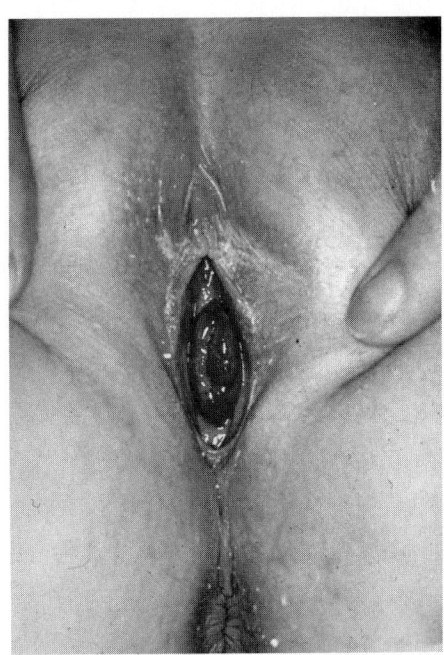

FIG. 53-9. Urethral prolapse. Note doughnut-shaped mass completely obscuring vaginal opening. (*Courtesy E Shapiro, MD.*)

women. Approximately 95% of pediatric cases have been reported in black girls.[35] The causes are controversial; an episodic increase in intraabdominal pressure may precede the prolapse in girls who may have poorly developed smooth muscle supports of the urethra.[36] Seizures, prolonged spasmodic coughing, sexual abuse, burns, straddle injury, or urinary tract infection were associated with the onset of prolapse in two thirds of the children.

Diagnostic Findings. Girls present with vaginal bleeding or spotting if significant urethral prolapse is present. Dysuria, urinary frequency, and occasionally urinary retention may also be symptoms. In some patients the bleeding may be confused with menstruation, hematuria, or rectal bleeding. Most children will not complain of genital pain in association with urethral prolapse.

Physical examination reveals a doughnut-shaped mass at the site of the urethral meatus (Fig. 53-9). The mass is usually hyperemic and friable; occasionally a scant bloody drainage can be observed on the surface of the prolapsed area. A punctum present in the center of the mass represents the urethral meatus. If the examiner is unable to identify the meatus, a urinary catheter may be introduced to locate the urethra. The examiner should perform a careful examination of the genitalia with an attempt to identify the vaginal introitus as a separate structure posterior to the prolapsed urethra. On occasion it may be difficult to visualize the vaginal area because the prolapse may actually be large enough to conceal the introitus.

Urinalysis should be performed. Red blood cells (RBCs) may be present because of the external irritation of the urethral meatus. Urine cultures are generally negative. X-ray studies are not helpful.

Differential Considerations. Differential diagnoses include urethral polyps, papilloma, caruncle, prolapsed ec-

topic ureterocele, condylomata acuminata, sarcoma botryoides, and periurethral prolapse.[36] All these entities are rare; the symmetry of the mass of urethral prolapse distinguishes it from these other conditions.

Management. Management in mild cases without necrosis includes reassurance, warm sitz baths, and emollient creams to the area. Betadine, estrogen cream, vaseline, and zinc oxide have all been used with some success in the girl with a small viable-appearing prolapse.[37] Most mild prolapses resolve in a week or two. Parents should be cautioned that prolapses may recur weeks to months after initial resolution. Follow-up should be arranged with either the child's primary physician or a urologist.

In the patient with necrotic or purple mucosa, urologic consultation should be obtained. Various surgical procedures have been described for these patients; most involve excision of the necrotic, prolapsed areas and repair of the remaining viable tissue.[38] The procedure should be performed under general anesthesia within days of presentation; ambulatory surgery is usually recommended. Recurrence is uncommon after surgical intervention.[39]

SEXUALLY TRANSMITTED DISEASES

Chlamydial Infection

C. trachomatis is the most common STD in adolescence; its prevalence is underestimated because many cases are asymptomatic in both males and females.[40] Although more common in urban, minority teens, suburban teens are frequently infected; rates in sexually active teens range from 10% to 30%.[41,42] Increased number of sexual partners is a risk factor. *C. trachomatis* is an obligate intracellular parasite; frequently it accompanies gonorrheal infection.[43] In the emergency department the following three clinical syndromes occur: (1) mucopurulent cervicitis, (2) pelvic inflammatory disease, and (3) asymptomatic disease. Younger adolescent girls and girls using oral contraceptives appear to be at higher risk of cervicitis.[44]

Diagnostic Findings. Clinical symptoms, if present, may include discharge, dysuria, urinary frequency, and pelvic pain. Cervical erythema and friability may be visualized. Complications of chlamydial infections include conjunctivitis, pelvic inflammatory disease (PID), urethritis, bartholinitis, and perihepatitis (Fitz-Hugh-Curtis syndrome).[45]

Diagnosis may be made by McCoy cell culture, monoclonal antibodies (Microtrak), or by enzyme-linked immunosorbent assay (ELISA) (Chlamydiazyme) analysis of the endocervical secretions. All laboratory evaluations have limitations; ELISA and monoclonal antibody tests yield much quicker results and are more commonly used in clinical practice.[46-49] Cultures should be taken for gonorrhea; serologic tests for syphilis should be drawn. Pathogens that must be excluded include gonorrhea, trichomonas, and candida.

Management. Uncomplicated *C. trachomatis* should be treated with azithromycin 1 gm once[50] or with doxycycline 100 mg BID PO for 7 days in nonpregnant, nonallergic patients. Compliance may be improved with the one-time azithromycin regimen in adolescents, especially if the drug is administered in the emergency department. Erythromycin base or stearate 500 mg QID PO for 7 days should be used in pregnancy or for patients who are allergic to doxycycline. Treating the patient for gonorrhea as well should be seriously considered.

To enhance compliance in treating the patient's sexual partner(s), written instructions including the diagnosis *chlamydia* and treatment protocol may be handed to the patient; she may have her partner take this note to a health-care provider to expedite his treatment. Because many adolescents may find it difficult to locate inexpensive, confidential health care, a list of available clinics in the area should be given to the patient, both for her care and for her partner's treatment. Patients and their partners should be encouraged to use condoms to protect themselves from future sexually transmitted infections, including AIDS.

Gonococcal Infection

Gonorrhea is a gram-negative, intracellular diplococcus. In sexually active adolescent girls, gonococcal infections are relatively common. In family planning and adolescent clinics, routine screening of patients yields rates of 7% to 10%.[51,52] Patients presenting with genital symptoms in an emergency department probably have a higher infection rate. Patients with new sexual partners or those who use oral contraceptives are at increased risk.[53]

Diagnostic Findings. Three clinical syndromes may be seen in the emergency department: vaginal discharge secondary to a mucopurulent cervicitis, pelvic pain secondary to gonococcal PID, or asymptomatic. Each is equally common. PID is discussed in the next section.

Symptoms of cervicitis may include copious purulent vaginal discharge, vulvar irritation, urinary frequency, and dysuria. Symptoms may occur as early as 3 to 8 days after intercourse with an infected person. A yellow exudate may be seen at the introitus; exudate may be expressed from the urethra, Skene gland, or Bartholin gland. The cervix may appear normal or may have purulent drainage from the cervical os. Occasionally the cervix may bleed readily on manipulation. Complications include PID, tuboovarian abscess, abscess of Bartholin gland, pharyngitis, rectal infection, or disseminated gonococcal arthritis.[54]

Differential Considerations. Differential diagnosis includes chlamydial infection, *Trichomonas vaginitis,* urinary tract infection, and bacterial vaginosis. The cervical os should be freshly cultured for gonorrhea on Thayer-Martin media; Gram stain of the cervical exudate may show gram-negative intracellular diplococci but is not as reliable as culture. Many public health laboratories prefer to monitor sensitivity to the antibiotic; resistance to penicillin occurs not infrequently.

Management. Because strains of *N. gonorrhoeae* have shown antibiotic-resistance to penicillin, tetracycline, and other multiple antibiotics and because chlamydial infections are frequently associated with gonorrheal infection, treatment of uncomplicated gonorrhea in adolescents is with cefiximine 400 mg PO or ceftriaxone 250 mg IM followed by azithromycin 1 gm PO once or doxycycline 100 mg BID PO for 7 days.[55-58] For patients who are allergic to penicillin, spectinomycin 2 gm IM may be used in place of ceftriaxone. In pregnant adolescents, erythromycin 500 mg QID PO should be administered for 7 days in place of doxycycline.

Patients should be tested for syphilis and offered HIV testing. Sexual partners should be seen, tested for STDs, and treated presumptively. Patients should be encouraged to use "safe-sex" practices (e.g., abstinence and condoms) in the future. Currently, test of cure is not recommended because the above regimen rarely fails. Cultures and reexamination should be performed 1 to 2 months after the initial infection to screen for reinfection. Compliance to follow-up for venereal disease has been shown to be poor among adolescents, particularly males.[59]

Herpes Genitalis

Herpes genitalis is caused by the herpes simplex virus (HSV). HSV-1, more commonly found in the mouth as cold sores, may cause genital infection in the young child either by autoinoculation from mouth-hand-genitals, or by contact with another infected person. Infection from another may be transmitted by hand, oral, or sexual contact. HSV-2 infections are transmitted by sexual contact, and are more common in adolescence. HSV-1 infections of the genitalia have become more common in adolescents, perhaps because of changing sexual practices.[60] History of contact with an infected person may not be obtained because carriers may be asymptomatic.

Diagnostic Findings. Symptoms of an HSV infection include painful urination, vulvar pruritus and burning, discomfort when walking, and occasionally fever. Inability to urinate or defecate may occur because of severe pain. Primary lesions usually occur within a week of contact. They appear as erythematous macular areas that progress to papules and then to vesicles on an erythematous base. As the vesicles break, crusting and ulcerations appear. Lesions are usually limited to the vulvar and perianal skin in prepubertal children (Fig. 53-10). In adolescents, vaginal and cervical mucosa may also be involved.

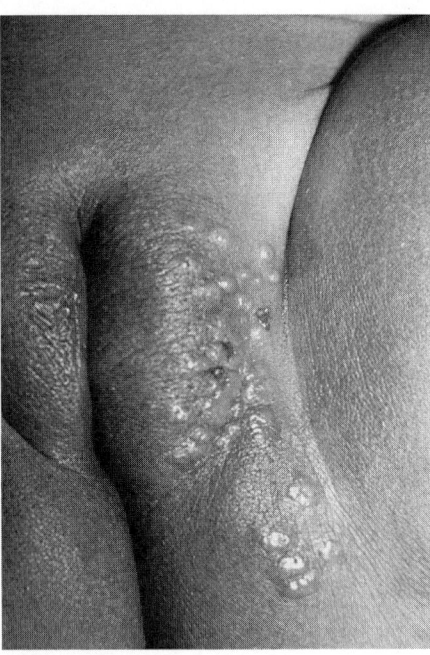

FIG. 53-10. Herpes genitalis in a prepubertal girl. (*Courtesy N Esterly, MD.*)

Stained smears of lesions show characteristic multinucleated giant cells. Viral cultures should be taken, particularly in prepubertal children, because HSV-2 infections are more commonly associated with sexual contact. Serologic tests for HSV-1 and HSV-2 may also be helpful.

Differential diagnosis includes varicella and inflicted burns. In varicella, other extragenital lesions should be present.

Management. Treatment of HSV infections in the prepubertal child is limited to local hygiene, antipruritic agents, and pain medications. In cases of urinary retention, sitz baths, and allowing the child to void in the bath water may be helpful. Since HSV-2 infections are frequently associated with sexual contact, a social service referral should be sought to evaluate the child for sexual abuse.

In adolescents with primary genital herpes, acyclovir 400 mg PO three times a day for 7 to 10 days is recommended. For recurrent episodes, acyclovir 400 mg PO three times a day for 5 days may offer some benefit. Patients with frequent recurrent episodes may improve with daily suppressive therapy over months or years.[61] Acyclovir is contraindicated in pregnancy. Although lesions disappear, shedding of the HSV virus from the cervix and vagina continues for weeks to months after an infection. Sexual partners should be made aware of HSV infection. Use of condoms should be encouraged. The patient should also be cultured for other STDs.

In young children, secondary bacterial infection of lesions may occur. In the adolescent, complications may include serious systemic involvement, risk of perinatal transmission in the case of pregnant teens, and long-term increased risk of genital malignancies. Follow-up with a gynecologist should be established for the patient with genital infections that are caused by the herpes simplex virus.

Pelvic Inflammatory Disease

Of the many complications of the early initiation of sexual activity in adolescence, pelvic inflammatory disease (PID) is one of the most serious. Infertility, pelvic pain, and ectopic pregnancy have all been associated with a past history of PID. Risk factors that increase the incidence of PID include use of intrauterine devices, nonwhite racial background, multiple sexual partners, young age, prior history of PID, and biologic immaturity of the adolescent cervix.[62] Approximately one in eight 15-year-old females have suffered from PID, as compared with one in eighty 24 year olds.[63] Contraceptive barriers, such as condoms, diaphragms, and spermicides, decrease the risk of PID. The immature adolescent cervix frequently has columnar endothelial cells exposed at the os, which appear to increase the chance of PID. Patients frequently present in the days after completion of their menses with PID.[64]

The pathogenesis of PID is complex; many suspect that the existence of certain organisms in some hosts with a vulnerable genital tract leads to the clinical syndrome. *N. gonorrhoeae* and *C. trachomatis*, as well as facultative anaerobes and aerobes, have all been cultured from patients with PID; usually more than one organism is recovered in culture. Many other bacteria, such as *G. vaginalis* and *Mycoplasma hominis*, may also play a role.[65] The disease is believed to be an ascending problem; organisms are forced through the cervix, into the endometrium of the uterus, up into the tubal mucosa, and potentially into the abdominal cavity. Acute and chronic changes surrounding the pelvic organs may occur.

Diagnostic Findings. It is very difficult to correlate the clinical signs and symptoms with laparoscopy-proven findings of PID. Only 65% of women with clinical evidence of PID were found to have signs via laparoscopy.[66] Because of the serious long-term problems if PID goes undetected, a clinician must remain vigilant for potential cases. Fever, vaginal discharge, irregular vaginal bleeding, and abdominal pain are all symptoms of PID. Presentation in the days after cessation of menses is also suggestive. Clinically, lower abdominal tenderness, cervical motion tenderness, and adnexal tenderness should all be present to make the diagnosis of PID. Fever, an increased peripheral white blood cell (WBC) count, an ESR that is greater than 15, purulent material on culdocentesis, mass on bimanual pelvic examination or ultrasound, more than five WBC on Gram stain of the endocervix, or infection with *N. gonorrhoeae* or *C. trachomatis* may also be present. Although laparoscopy is the only definitive way to diagnose PID, it is not a practical method given its risks, cost, patient discomfort, and time.[67,68] By methodically piecing together the constellation of symptoms with clinical signs on pelvic examination (see box on p. 879) and aggressively treating suggestive cases, the clinician can help to prevent the complications of PID.

Complications include recurrent PID, infertility,[69] ectopic pregnancy, chronic abdominal pain, tuboovarian abscess, perihepatitis (Fitz-Hugh-Curtis syndrome), and sacroiliitis. The emergency physician should be aware that both ectopic pregnancy and tuboovarian abscess are life-threatening problems requiring immediate gynecologic intervention.

Clinical Findings Diagnostic of Pelvic Inflammatory Disease

All of the following must be present:
1. Lower abdominal pain by history or physical examination
2. Cervical motion tenderness on pelvic examination
3. Adnexal tenderness

One of the following must be present:
1. Fever greater than 38° C
2. WBC count greater than 10,500/mm^3
3. Pelvic abscess on bimanual examination or sonography
4. Purulent material from peritoneal cavity on culdocentesis or laparoscopy
5. ESR >15 mm/hr
6. Positive monoclonal antibody for *C. trachomatis* from endocervix
7. Gram stain with gram-negative diplococci from cervix
8. WBC per oil immersion field on gram stain of endocervical discharge

Data from Jacobson L and Westrom L: *Am J Obstet Gynecol* 105(7):1088-1098, 1969.

Possible Reasons for Failure in Treatment of Pelvic Inflammatory Disease

Illness not recognized by adolescent or her physician

Physician insistence on strict criteria before diagnosing PID

Treatment of gonococcus only

Lack of careful early follow-up to assess clinical response

Inability of adolescent to obtain outpatient prescriptions for PID because of lack of funds, insurance, or understanding

Fear of breach of confidentiality in follow-up or in obtaining prescriptions

Failure to treat sexual partners for gonorrhea and chlamydia

Treatment Regimens for Acute PID

Inpatient treatment (strongly consider for all adolescents)

Treatment A

Cefoxitin 2 gm q 6 hr IV or cefotetan 2 gm q 12 hr IV; PLUS doxycycline 100 mg q 12 hr PO/IV given for 48 hr after patient improves clinically. Doxycycline 100 mg BID PO for a total of 10 to 14 days.

Treatment B

Clindamycin 900 mg q 8 hr IV; plus Gentamicin loading dose (2 mg/kg) IV/IM followed by a maintenance dose 1.5 mg/kg q 8 hr given for 48 hr after patient improves clinically. Doxycycline 100 mg BID PO for 10 to 14 days or clindamycin 450 mg orally 4 times a day for 14 days total

Ambulatory management of PID (reserve for less toxic, very compliant adolescents)

Cefoxitin 2 gm IM plus probenecid 1 gm PO concurrently or ceftriaxone 250 mg IM; PLUS Doxycycline 100 mg BID PO for 14 days, **or** tetracycline 500 mg QID PO for 10 to 14 days **or** erythromycin 500 mg QID PO for 10 to 14 days (only if patient is sensitive to tetracyclines). If no improvement as outpatient, patient should be hospitalized

NOTE: Tetracycline and doxycycline should not be given to children 8 years of age and younger.
Centers for Disease Control: *MMWR* 42:RR14, 75-81, September 1993

Evaluation should include endocervical cultures for *N. gonorrhoeae* and *C. trachomatis,* a potassium hydroxide (KOH) preparation for Candida, and a wet mount for Trichomonas. A urinalysis and a urinary β-human chorionic gonadotropin (HCG) pregnancy test should be obtained. A Venereal Disease Research Laboratory (VDRL) should be performed on teens presenting with signs of PID. Ultrasonography of the pelvis is quite helpful in many patients, particularly if ectopic pregnancy, tuboovarian abscess, or inflammatory bowel involvement is suspected.[70,71] Golden, Neuhoff, and Cohen found that 85% of adolescents with suspected PID admitted to the hospital had either adnexal enlargement or tuboovarian abscesses on pelvic ultrasound.[72]

Differential diagnosis includes appendicitis, cholecystitis, urinary tract infection, ectopic pregnancy, inflammatory bowel disease, ovarian cyst with torsion, and spontaneous or septic abortion.[73]

Management. Treatment early in the course of acute PID has been shown to preserve tubal patency.[74] Several factors have been cited as reasons for failure in the treatment of PID (see box, top right).

Treatment is based on antibiotic sensitivities of the various bacteria implicated in PID rather than on carefully tested clinical trials; the Centers for Disease Control (CDC) recommends a polymicrobial coverage for gonorrhea, chlamydia, and anaerobes. Some small clinical trials have shown that alternative drugs have been promising in the treatment of PID.[75-77] Various regimens currently recommended are shown in the box at right.

Hospital admission should be strongly considered for many adolescents to prevent the long-term complications of infertility and the increased risk of future ectopic pregnancy; in many cases hospitalization may be the only

way to ensure administration of medication and clinical improvement while minimizing long-term sequelae. Adolescents who are discharged from the emergency department should be seen by their pediatrician or gynecologist in 24 to 48 hours to assess their clinical improvement. If follow-up cannot be assured, hospitalization is indicated if the patient (1) has a pelvic or tuboovarian abscess, (2) has peritonitis, (3) is pregnant, (4) has an intrauterine device (IUD), (5) is unable to comply with regimen, or (6) is not responding clinically.[78]

Patients should be encouraged to return immediately if symptoms of fever or pain increase; patients failing outpatient management should be admitted to the hospital without delay.

Abstinence from sexual intercourse should be encouraged for 2 to 3 weeks after beginning treatment for PID treatment. Test of cure should be done at the end of this time.

Sexual partners should be treated as soon as possible. Condom and contraceptive use should be encouraged in these patients, not only to prevent STDs, including AIDS, but also to prevent adolescent pregnancy. To ensure compliance, the emergency physician should take the time to discuss the diagnosis, the seriousness of the illness, and possible complications with the adolescent in a caring and confidential matter. The physician should also make sure that the adolescent and her partner have access to the follow-up visit and the ability to fill any prescriptions.

Syphilis

A thin, motile spirochete, *Treponema pallidum*, causes syphilis. Outside of congenitally acquired cases, syphilis is transmitted by sexual contact. It is more common in urban areas, among drug addicts, prostitutes, and in HIV-positive patients, probably because of "drugs-for-sex" transactions. A recent increase of syphilis has been reported in the United States and among adolescents.[79]

Diagnostic Findings. Primary syphilis presents with open, nontender, ulcerative lesions, usually on the genitals, 10 to 90 days after inoculation. These lesions or chancres usually heal in one week. Inguinal adenopathy may ensue in the following weeks. VDRL or rapid plasma reagin (RPR) serology may be negative at the time of the chancre, but dark-field microscope examination of scrapings of the lesion or fluid from the nodes usually will demonstrate the spirochete.[80]

Secondary syphilis occurs 6 to 20 weeks after exposure as a maculopapular, symmetric rash that involves the palms and soles. Fever, splenomegaly, generalized lymphadenopathy, and condylomata lata (Fig. 53-11) may be present. Serology is usually positive.

Management. Treatment should be initiated by the emergency physician for all known or suspected cases of early, primary, or secondary syphilis because follow-up may be difficult. Current treatment for early syphilis (< 1 year's duration) or for syphilis contacts is 2.4 million units of benzathine penicillin G administered intramuscularly in one dose. In penicillin-allergic, nonpregnant patients, doxycycline 100 mg BID PO for 2 weeks or tetracycline 500 mg QID PO for 2 weeks is the treatment of choice. The patient should be evaluated for other STDs; conversely, patients presenting with other STDs should undergo a serologic test for syphilis.

Follow-up of patients treated for either presumptive or known syphilis should be at 3 and 6 months, when a serologic test should be redrawn. HIV testing should be

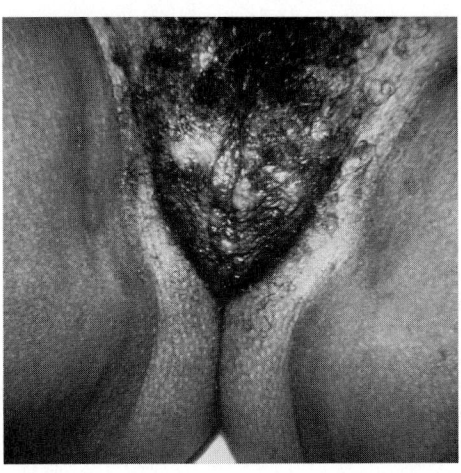

FIG. 53-11. Condylomata in an adolescent. (*Courtesy N Esterly, MD.*)

strongly advised because of the close association between the two diseases. Persons known to be positive for HIV and syphilis should have more frequent follow-up serology according to CDC guidelines; a cerebrospinal fluid (CSF) examination is not indicated in patients with early syphilis unless neurologic problems such as optic, auditory, cranial nerve, or meningeal symptoms occur.

Viral Vulvovaginitis

Condylomata Acuminata. Human papillomavirus is a slow-growing virus that causes condylomata acuminata or veneral warts. In the prepubescent girl the virus is believed to be transmitted by exposure during delivery to an infected mother, close contact with an infected person, sharing baths or towels with an infected person, or by being sexually abused by an infected perpetrator.[81] Cases of condylomata acuminata have been found in several siblings in a single family; bathing together is believed to be the source of infection.[82] In adolescent girls, transmission of the virus is believed to be only by sexual contact. Common warts on hands and feet are in the papillomavirus family and recently have been found by viral typing to be associated with condylomata acuminata on the genitalia.[83,84]

Diagnostic Findings. In prepubescent girls, condylomata appear as small, soft, nontender, cauliflowerlike, nonulcerative lesions. Early lesions are small, discrete papules. The mucosa of the periurethral, vaginal, inner labia minora, or perirectal area is most frequently involved in girls (Fig. 53-12). Boys may exhibit lesions on the penis, particularly at the urethral opening, and perirectally. In teenagers, condylomata rapidly proliferate causing large masses of greyish sessile warts with redundant folds. Most appear at the introitus although warts may be present in the vagina and on the cervix. In adolescents the lesions may be itchy or painful. A discharge may be visible on the surface on the condylomata. Perirectal lesions may also be present.

Differential diagnosis includes the condyloma latum of secondary syphilis and perineal tumors. Diagnosis of condyloma acuminata is usually a clinical one; biopsy of the

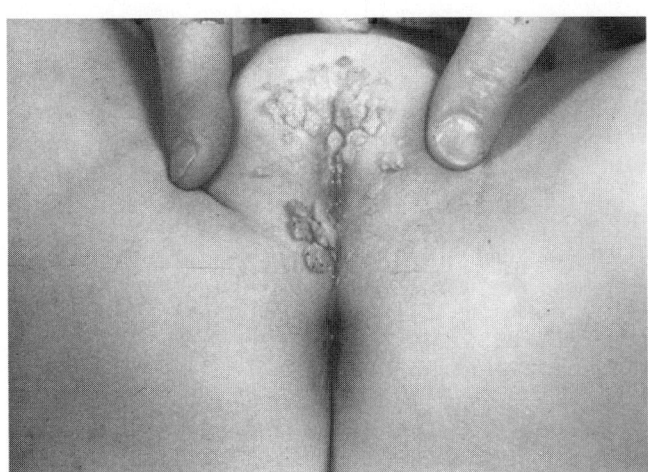

FIG. 53-12. Condyloma acuminata in a prepubertal girl. (*Courtesy N Esterly, MD.*)

lesion or testing by polymerase chain reaction may be needed in atypical cases.[85]

Management. Treatment of condyloma acuminata should be performed by a gynecologist, dermatologist, or pediatric surgeon familiar with venereal warts. In the prepubertal girl, cryotherapy under general anesthesia with either solid carbon dioxide or liquid nitrogen usually eradicates the warts. In teenagers, podophyllin ointment applied only to the warts may resolve the problem. Cautery and cryotherapy are other alternatives. Although warts may be recurrent, most disappear with the initial treatment. In young girls with condylomata a thorough investigation looking for sexual abuse should be done by a trained social worker. Sexual abuse is less likely to be the cause if the child's mother had genital warts at the time of delivery, if the child has cutaneous warts, if the parent has cutaneous warts, or if the child is younger than 3 years of age. Close follow-up and reexamination should be encouraged, both to ensure resolution of the warts and to monitor the social situation carefully.

Acquired Immunodeficiency Syndrome

Human immunodeficiency virus (HIV), which causes acquired immunodeficiency syndrome (AIDS), is a special threat to the sexually active adolescent, whether heterosexual or homosexual.[86] Because the virus remains asymptomatic for many years, adolescents do not realize the threat of infection nor the risk that they take when engaging in sexual activities.[87] The emergency physician plays a special role in the education of adolescents who may be presenting with STDs or complaints referable to the genitalia. Because of the heightened awareness of the adolescent who presents with a sexual complaint, counseling regarding safe sex or abstinence may prove more pertinent and useful to that patient than in a primary care setting.

HIV testing is controversial.[88] The emotional and social repercussions of positive test results should be considered before testing is carried out. Some promiscuous adolescents who receive negative test results may believe that "risk-taking" sex is "OK"; this may encourage an even more careless attitude. Adolescents who present to the emergency department with STDs should be encouraged to practice safe sex[89]; those with syphilis should be encouraged to consider HIV testing after counseling. Anonymous testing sites that ensure confidentiality may be helpful to the adolescent.

VULVOVAGINITIS

Prepubertal Vulvovaginitis

The gynecologic examination of the prepubertal patient requires sensitivity and patience. Careful explanations and reassurance should accompany the examination. This may present the necessity to anesthetize the patient. The most shy children are often 11- to 13-year olds who are just experiencing puberty.

Younger girls are best examined in the presence of their mothers. The external genitalia can be inspected with the child on the mother's lap. If appropriate, have the child assist by separating the labia and simultaneously depress the perineum. Particular attention should be focused on observing for trauma, foreign bodies, lacerations, discharges, vesicles, ulcers, and adenopathy.

The child may then be placed in the knee-chest position with her buttocks held up in the air and apart by an assistant. The girl is asked to lie on her abdomen with her bottom up and to let her stomach and back sag. Instrumentation is rarely necessary, the short vagina of the prepubertal girl allows enough visualization to rule out a foreign body or other lesion. Samples of secretions, discharges, and seminal fluid for culture, cell cytology, or forensic examination may be obtained by using a moistened cotton-tipped applicator or an eye dropper. A small vaginoscope or nasal speculum should be used if direct visualization is necessary.

Physiologic Vaginal Discharge. In the newborn period, many infant girls may have what appears to be excess vaginal discharge.[90] The tenacious grey drainage is visible on the vulva and in the introitus and is a result of the stimulation of the infant vagina and cervix by maternal hormones. The vagina and hymen show hypertrophy that is also caused by this hormonal stimulation. Occasionally, a scant bloody drainage also occurs for a few days in the infant girl, caused by diminishing levels of maternal hormones.[91] Nonpurulent vaginal discharge of the infant girl is physiologic and requires no intervention.

Girls just entering puberty frequently have a profuse, clear or white vaginal discharge as well.[92] This drainage is caused by the hormonal stimulation of the genitalia by the start of endocrine ovarian function and is frequently noted by the patient in the few months before menarche. Physical examination will show a patient with an estrogenized hymen and vulva and copious vaginal fluid. The patient should have secondary sex characteristics such as breast development and pubic and axillary hair. A speculum examination or cultures of the discharge are not necessary unless the drainage is purulent. Girls and their parents need to be reassured that this is a normal occurrence and that simple cleansing of the vulvar folds and frequent changes of underwear may prevent vulvar irritation.

Nonspecific Vulvovaginitis. In the prepubertal child, nonspecific vulvovaginitis refers to inflammation of the genitalia in which bacterial cultures yield mixed flora; none of the bacterial cultures may be positive for gonorrhea. The majority of prepubertal children presenting with vaginal discharge suffer from nonspecific vulvovaginitis.

The vaginal mucosa is relatively thin and alkalotic in the prepubertal girl; both these factors cause her to be more vulnerable to infections. The introitus and labia minora are not yet covered by the larger outer labia majora in the young girl. Infection because of poor toilet hygiene, scratching with dirty hands, and pinworms frequently can be a problem. Vaginal foreign bodies may precipitate nonspecific vulvovaginitis. Girls with high posterior commissures may be at higher risk for recurrent vulvovaginitis because the vagina is less likely to drain completely.

Diagnostic Findings. History should include duration of discharge, amount of discharge based on child's history, and soiling of underpants. The physician should inquire about vulvar or perianal scratching. Questions about the child's toileting habits, use of soaps or bubble baths, and family history of genital infections are all important. Family social living conditions and history of child sexual abuse should be considered in the evaluation of a child with genital discharge. A review of old records may reveal prior histories of vaginal infection.

The physical examination should include a general pediatric examination in conjunction with examination of the genitalia and perineum. The vulvar skin should be inspected for excoriations and fecal soiling; inflammation, pinworms, and fecal soiling of the perianal skin should be noted. The vaginal opening should be examined for the presence of erythema, discharge, and foreign bodies. The vaginal discharge associated with nonspecific vulvovaginitis is usually thin, grey, and mucoid.

Vaginal discharge should be cultured for general bacteria and for *N. gonorrhoeae* and *C. trachomatis* isolation. In many young girls, bacterial culture may yield *E. coli* or multiple organisms.[93] Pinworms or pinworm ova may be identified by touching the perianal area with Scotch tape and affixing the tape to a slide to examine under a microscope.

Management. Treatment of nonspecific vulvovaginitis includes frequent sitz baths in plain tap water, good toilet hygiene, daily underwear changes, and removal of the precipitating problem. Foreign-body removal usually results in subsequent disappearance of an offending vaginal discharge. If pinworms are identified, the child and all her family should be treated with a single dose of either pyrantel pamoate 11 mg/kg or mebendazole 100 mg PO. Avoidance of soaps, perfumes, or fabric softeners may also reduce the discharge.

Rarely topical creams may be helpful. Sultrin cream, aminoacridine hydrochloride suppositories, and Premarin estrogen cream have all been advocated as useful in resistant cases of nonspecific vaginitis.[94] Cream may be applied with an eyedropper; cutting suppositories in half lengthwise may make them small enough for use in the prepubertal girl.

Parenteral or oral antibiotics are generally not helpful in the treatment of vulvovaginitis and may cause *Candida albicans* overgrowth of the perineum.

Specific Bacterial Vulvovaginitis

Candidal Vulvovaginitis. Mycotic infections in the prepubescent child are usually the result of systemic antibiotic use or underlying diabetes; they are not sexually transmitted.

Dysuria, vaginal discharge, and pruritus of the vulva are usually noted by the patient. Examination of the vulva reveals erythema of both the skin and mucosa; white plaques of the vaginal area may also be seen. A vaginal discharge with white curds may also be noted. A wet mount of the discharge reveals hyphae and spores.

Treatment is to apply nystatin cream to the vulva. In stubborn cases, nystatin suspension may be instilled into the vaginal orifice with a soft catheter that is attached to a syringe.[95]

Chlamydia Vulvovaginitis. In the prepubescent girl, *C. trachomatis* is a rare pathogen for vulvovaginitis. In young infants the infection may occur after birth to an infected mother; these infants, however, are usually asymptomatic.[96] Infection in the prepubertal girl with *C. trachomatis* has been associated with sexual abuse in several series.[97-99] Many of these children were concurrently infected with *N. gonorrhoeae*.

Mucopurulent vaginitis and serosanguinous discharge may be present in infected prepubertal children. Some children are asymptomatic. Cultures for chlamydia by McCoy cell tissue culture are the best diagnostic tool but can delay treatment. Testing for serum chlamydia antibodies or by immunofluorescence of vaginal secretions is less reliable but facilitates clinical management. The discharge should be cultured for *N. gonorrhoeae* as well. Treatment is with erythromycin base, 40 mg/kg/24 hr (adult: 250 to 500 mg) PO QID for a period of 10 days. An evaluation for sexual abuse should be made in children with culture-proven chlamydial infections.

Gonorrheal Vulvovaginitis. Vulvovaginitis may be caused by *N. gonorrhoeae* in the prepubertal child. It is caused by contact of the genitalia with infected material.[100] Because a history of sexual contact is difficult to obtain in the young child, the epidemiology of gonorrhea is problematic. Direct genital contact by infected adults or children has resulted in infection with *N. gonorrhoeae* in case studies.[101] Noncoital contact with the genitals of infected males may result in infection. Sexual abuse must be suspected in all cases of gonorrhea presenting in prepubertal girls.[102-104]

Diagnostic Findings. Children with gonorrhea vulvovaginitis may complain of genital pain, dysuria, urinary frequency, and discharge on underwear. Fever is not a problem. Vaginal infection with *N. gonorrhoeae* is rarely asymptomatic. A careful history should be taken for genital discharges in other family members.

When possible, the child should be interviewed for the possibility of sexual abuse; interviews without care givers or parents present may yield a more frank history of sexual abuse. A social worker skilled in interviewing children for sexual abuse may be helpful to the physician.

Infection with *N. gonorrhoeae* causes a copious purulent vaginal discharge in prepubertal girls because the vaginal mucosa is thin, friable, and susceptible to infection. Prepubertal children, however, do not manifest signs of cervicitis or PID. Examination of the genitalia yields hyperemia of the vulvar and vaginal mucosa and a thick purulent discharge. Excoriations of the vulvar area may also be present. The Bartholin glands are not involved in gonorrheal infections of prepubertal children. The genitalia should be examined for signs of sexual abuse.

Cultures of the vaginal discharge should be taken at the vaginal introitus for *N. gonorrhoeae* and for general bacterial culture and chlamydia. Although Gram stain of the discharge may exhibit gram-negative diplococci, the diagnosis of *N. gonorrhoeae* should not be made until the culture is diagnostic. The social and legal implications of the diagnosis of *N. gonorrhoeae* in a prepubertal child force the physician to base the diagnosis on reliable culture results.[105] Because other strains of the organism may grow on gonococcal-selective media, the clinical laboratory must verify with a standardized laboratory that an organism is specifically *N. gonorrhoeae*.

Management. Treatment of gonorrhea vulvovaginitis includes antibiotics and a complete social-work investigation. The child should be interviewed for a history of sexual abuse and the family should be cultured for gonorrhea, particularly if they are symptomatic. Siblings of the index case should be examined and cultured.

The decision to treat for gonorrhea at the time of the initial emergency department visit may be based on the preliminary gram stain exhibiting gram-negative intracellular diplococci because future follow-up may be delayed. The decision to initiate investigation by a social worker and particularly protective service notification should be based on substantial laboratory evidence of *N. gonorrhoeae*. Discussion with the family regarding gonorrhea infection should only be made if definitive laboratory evidence is established.

The increasing incidence of penicillinase-producing *N. gonorrhoeae* (PPNG) demands the use of ceftriaxone. In one series of 33 children with gonorrheal infection in New York City, 26% of the episodes were caused by penicillinase-producing *N. gonorrhoeae*.[106] These children were treated with ceftriaxone 125 mg IM if they weighed less than 45 kg and with ceftriaxone 250 mg if they weighed more than 45 kg; the ceftriaxone was administered as a one-time dose. All patients had clinical responses with repeat cultures being negative. No side effects were noted.

To cover additional potential pathogens including *C. trachomatis*, combined therapy is often recommended. The single-dose management is appropriate if there is no infection. However, because this is often difficult to determine, gonorrhea treatment is usually followed in children over 8 years of age with tetracycline 500 mg QID PO or doxycycline 100 mg BID PO for 7 days.

Shigella Vulvovaginitis. Shigella species may cause vulvovaginitis in young girls. The direct contact of infected loose stools to the vagina, particularly in infants wearing diapers, may predispose the young girl to shigella vaginitis. History of diarrhea may occasionally be present. The vulvovaginitis may present weeks to months after the diarrheal illness and may persist for weeks to months if untreated. In a series by Murphy and Nelson, 38 children were identified with shigella vulvovaginitis; *S. flexneri* was isolated in 87% of the cases, *S. sonnei* in 10% of cases, and *S. boydii* in 2% of the cases.[107] About half the patients had bloody discharge; most others had a mucopurulent discharge. Younger children were more likely to have diarrhea preceding the episode of vulvovaginitis.

The vaginal discharge should be cultured for enteric pathogens in cases of bloody vaginal discharge or in cases of vulvovaginitis after a diarrheal episode. *S. vaginitis* should be considered in children who do not respond to the usual treatment for vaginitis. Treatment with oral antibiotics based on sensitivity of the organism usually cures the vulvovaginitis. Local creams and sitz baths alone have not been effective.[108]

Streptococcal Vulvovaginitis. Vaginitis caused by group A β-hemolytic streptococcus is fairly common, especially in the fall and winter months; it may be associated with a pharyngeal, upper respiratory, or skin infection. It may frequently be associated with scarlet fever.[109,110]

Symptoms include vaginal discharge, pruritus, and dysuria, and are usually abrupt in onset. Inspection of the genitalia reveals hyperemia of the vulva and a seropurulent discharge. Cultures specifically for group A streptococcus using blood agar should be performed because cultures placed on Thayer-Martin media do not yield this organism. Urine cultures are negative.

Treatment is with penicillin V 40 mg/kg/24 hr QID PO; symptoms usually resolve quickly once treatment is begun.[111] Local measures are not helpful in the treatment of streptococcal vulvovaginitis.

Postpubertal Vulvovaginitis

Bacterial vaginosis. *G. vaginalis* is a pleomorphic, gram-variable, anaerobic, fastidious coccobacillus that is believed to contribute to the syndrome currently known as *bacterial vaginosis* and previously known as *nonspecific vaginitis*. In this syndrome, anaerobic bacteria and *G. vaginalis* replace the normal lactobacillus flora of the vaginal vault. It is unclear whether *G. vaginalis* or the accompanying anaerobic bacteria is the cause of the vaginal discharge; both are present in affected patients. *G. vaginalis* has been found in the sexual partners of infected girls, and is currently believed to be an STD.[112,113]

Diagnostic Findings. Patients complain primarily of a malodorous, thin discharge. The odor of the vaginal discharge has been described as "fishy"; occasionally pruritus, dyspareunia, and dysuria may occur. Physical examination reveals a thin, grey discharge that tends to adhere to the vaginal walls. The pH is usually above normal, in the 5.0 or greater range. Laboratory evaluation of bacterial vaginosis relies on evidence of an homogeneous discharge, the fishy odor when KOH is added to vaginal fluid ("whiff test"), a vaginal pH greater than 4.5, and clue cells on wet mount. Clue cells are cells surrounded by coccobacillary bacteria adhering to the cell walls. Recently the coccobacillary bacteria have been identified as *G. vaginalis*.[114] Other laboratory efforts to identify *G. vaginalis* in a more efficient way include rehydrated wet mounts, rapid identification method (RIM) immunofluorescence, and improved culture media.[115-118]

Differential diagnosis includes candidal, gonorrheal, and chlamydial vaginitis; differentiation can be made by clinical findings of a grey discharge and laboratory cultures and serologic tests.

Management. Treatment for bacterial vaginosis is metronidazole 500 mg BID PO for 7 days. Treatment is believed to be successful because metronidazole is effective against both anaerobes and *G. vaginalis*. A more convenient dosage scheme of 2 gm on day 1 may be effective.[119] In pregnancy, metronidazole is contraindicated during the first trimester; clindamycin cream may be used if the diagnosis is well established. During the second and third trimester, oral metronidazole or metronidazole cream may be used. Currently, no treatment is recommended for sexual partners or asymptomatic women. Patients undergoing treatment, however, are advised to practice abstinence or to use condoms.

Candidiasis. Fungal infections of the vulva and vagina are much more common in adolescent girls than in children and are usually caused by *C. albicans*. Although colonization of the vagina with yeast is fairly common, only some girls become symptomatic.[120] As the pH rises after the onset of menstruation, the vagina becomes more susceptible to yeast infections. Estrogen and progesterone have also been shown to stimulate the growth of yeast.[121] This may explain why yeast infections are more common during pregnancy and in patients using oral contraceptives. Although *Candida* may be sexually transmitted, it frequently occurs in girls who are not sexually active. Tight clothing, obesity, menstruation, poor hygiene, infected toiletries, oral antibiotic use, and chronic diseases such as diabetes are all predisposing factors for yeast infections. Many yeast infections, however, occur in healthy young teens.

Diagnostic Findings. Symptoms include burning, pruritus, erythema of the vulva, and a whitish discharge. Many adolescents present with complaints in the week after completion of menses. Physical examination reveals an erythematous vulva, occasionally with shiny fissures or a maculopapular rash. The rash may extend to the perianal area or down onto the thighs. The vaginal wall may be reddened; only in about 20% of cases will there be the classic white plaques on the wall of the vagina. There may be a white cheesy vaginal discharge; the discharge may have a yeasty odor.

Recurrences are common. Occasionally, patients may exhibit the generalized rash of an id reaction. Other complications are rare in healthy adolescents.

Laboratory evidence of yeast infections may be made by using a KOH preparation of the cotton-applicator scraping of the vaginal wall. Under the microscope, yeast buds or hyphae in filamentous forms may be seen. Cultures using Nikerson's or Sabouraud's medium may be used if clinical findings or the KOH preparation are inconclusive.

Differential Considerations. Differential diagnosis includes allergic dermatitis, trichomonal vaginitis, and *G. vaginitis*.[122] *Vaginitis associated with foreign bodies can be differentiated by the malodorous vaginal discharge.*

Management. Recommended treatments for *Candida vulvovaginitis* include clotrimazole cream or vaginal suppositories, 100 mg intravaginally every night for 7 days or miconazole cream or vaginal suppositories, 100 mg intravaginally every night for 7 to 14 days. A newer antifungal agent, terconazole, has been shown to be effective in 90% of cases when used topically as an 80-mg vaginal suppository or a 5-gm vaginal cream for 3 to 7 days.[123] Recurrences of vaginal candidiasis may be prevented by postmenstrual application of a 500-mg clotrimazole vaginal

tablet.[124] Oral therapy may be indicated.[125,126] Fluconazole (Diflucan) 150 mg orally has been noted to be equivalent to 7 days of topical medications. Patients who remain symptomatic after their course of treatment should be advised to see their physician. Treatment of sexual partners is usually not required unless the vulvovaginitis remains resistant to treatment.

Foreign Body. In adolescence the presence of a foreign body can cause a copious malodorous discharge; tampons, diaphragms, condoms, and masturbation items may be found. Removal of the foreign body relieves the symptoms of vaginitis. If removal is not possible via the use of a forceps vaginally, occasionally a rectal examination with pressure exerted through the rectovaginal septum may disengage the foreign body.

Trichomonas Vaginalis. *Trichomonas vaginalis* is an anaerobic, flagellated protozoan that is a fairly common pathogen causing vulvovaginitis. Because it is an STD in almost all circumstances, *Trichomonas* is seen quite often in the sexually active adolescent girl.[127] Number of sexual partners and amount of sexual activity are both associated with risk for the disease.[128] Other STDs such as *C. trachomatis* and *N. gonorrhoeae* are frequently isolated from patients with *Trichomonas*. *Trichomonas* has been known to be viable away from the body: towels have been implicated as the vector for spread. *Trichomonas* has been isolated from a chlorinated swimming pool.[129]

Diagnostic Findings. Clinical complaints include severe pruritus, dysuria, frequency, a profuse, frothy yellow-green vaginal discharge with a musty odor, and dyspareunia. Between 10% and 50% of girls may be initially asymptomatic.[130] Symptoms tend to occur after menses. Incubation is from 4 to 30 days. The vulva and vaginal walls are usually bright red and inflamed, occasionally with excoriations. The pH of the fluid is usually between 5 and 7.

A fresh saline wet mount of vaginal secretions reveals the ovoid, motile trichomonads and an increase in leukocytes. A monoclonal immunofluorescence technique has also been developed that may be helpful in detecting *Trichomonas* in dried and fresh specimens.[131,132] Differential diagnosis includes candidiasis, bacterial vaginosis, and vaginal foreign body; concurrent gonorrheal and chlamydial infections should be considered.

Management. Treatment for trichomoniasis is metronidazole 2 gm PO in a single dose or metronidazole 250 mg BID PO for 7 days. Although the 1-week course of medication has a slightly better cure rate (95% vs. 88%), the single dose is more likely to be accepted by the adolescent girl; administration of metronidazole 2 gm PO in the emergency department ensures patient compliance. Sexual partners should be treated in like manner to prevent reinfection. Metronidazole may cause nausea and a metallic taste in the mouth. Urticaria and reversible leukopenia are occasionally seen. Seizures and peripheral neuropathy are rare.[133] Alcoholic beverages should not be imbibed during and immediately after metronidazole therapy because the drug blocks the metabolism of ethinyl 2-aldehyde intermediaries. Treatment of *Trichomonas* with metronidazole is contraindicated in pregnancy and nursing mothers because it may have mutagenic and carcinogenic effects.[134] The use of 100-mg vaginal suppositories of clotrimazole at bedtime for a week may have some symptomatic benefit in pregnant adolescents.[135] Follow-up should include treatment of sexual partners; patients with recurrent infections should be treated for a week.

MENSTRUAL PROBLEMS

Normal Menstruation

The release of gonadotropic-releasing hormone triggers the secretion of FSH and LH from the anterior pituitary gland. Breast budding typically occurs at the age of 11 years, ranging from 8 to 13 years of age. Pubic hair develops next, although it may be the first external evidence in 15% of girls.

Estrogen leads to uterine growth and maturation, associated with physiologic leukorrhea.

The age range of menarche is 12 to 16 years, commonly after the mother's pattern. Initial periods are anovulatory and irregular, often for up to 24 months.

Although the typical cycle interval is 28 days, the actual range is 21 to 45 days. The average blood loss per cycle is 30 to 40 ml or about 10 to 15 tampons or pads. Flow is generally heaviest on days 1 through 3, with decreased loss thereafter.

Dysfunctional Uterine Bleeding

Dysfunctional uterine bleeding is a clinical syndrome of irregular and occasionally excessive menstrual bleeding. In most cases, no cause is identifiable for this problem that is distressing, particularly to the adolescent girl. The bleeding is usually painless and without a particular pattern.[136] Anemia may be one of the presenting symptoms of dysfunctional uterine bleeding.

Normal menstruation occurs approximately every 28 days, with a range of 21 to 35 days. The duration of flow is usually about 5 days with heavy bleeding only on the first few days. Bleeding is considered heavy if the girl reports soaking of six or more pads per day.[137] Girls with short cycles and heavy flow during their periods may easily become anemic.

Cycles during the first 2 years after menarche are often irregular. Widholm reported that 43% of adolescents in their first year of menstruation had irregular periods; after 5 years, 20% still had irregular periods.[138] Many of these girls do not present to medical attention with complaints because their mothers may recognize that irregular periods are common in early adolescence.

In girls with heavy bleeding who do seek medical attention, approximately 95% have dysfunctional bleeding.[139] In a study of teens hospitalized for heavy, uncontrollable menstrual bleeding, Claessens and Cowell noted that 74% had dysfunctional uterine bleeding, 19% had a coagulation disorder, and 7% had other problems.[140]

Anovulatory cycles in adolescence are the cause of dysfunctional uterine bleeding. In the first years after menarche the pituitary-ovarian axis is immature; approximately 50% of cycles are anovulatory in the first years after menarche.

In an ovulatory cycle, FSH stimulates the ovary to produce estrogen; estrogen stimulates the endometrium to proliferate. LH surges, causing the release of an ovum. The corpus luteum produces progesterone and subsequently estrogen. As the unfertilized corpus luteum involutes, estrogen and progesterone fall and the endometrium is shed as menses.

In an anovulatory cycle, FSH surges and the ovarian follicle produces estrogen, thus stimulating proliferation of the uterine endometrium. LH, however, does not surge at midcycle and so no ovum is released; thus, no progesterone-producing corpus luteum is formed. Without progesterone, the endometrium remains proliferative as estrogen remains elevated. As the follicle finally involutes, estrogen falls and a withdrawal bleed occurs. Withdrawal bleeds, however, result in less organized shedding of the endometrium; menses may be irregular or prolonged. Dysfunctional bleeding is generally painless because of the anovulatory quality of the cycles.

Diagnostic Findings. A careful gynecologic history should be taken; age at menarche, bleeding length and quality during menstruation, and frequency of vaginal bleeding should all be noted. It is frequently difficult to assess the amount of bleeding; questions regarding number and type of sanitary pads or tampons may help the physician to approximate the extent of blood loss. History of sexual activity, contraceptive use, and prior STDs should be taken in a confidential manner when parents are absent from the examination room. Possibility of pregnancy or history of induced abortion should be considered and discussed with the teen in a nonjudgmental fashion. Symptoms of breast tenderness, mittelschmerz, or cramping with bleeding are more suggestive of pregnancy or ovulation. Bleeding during dental or operative procedures or easy bruisability should suggest a bleeding diathesis. Questions regarding aspirin use should also be asked.

The physical examination should be directed to first maintaining hemodynamic stability and then to ascertaining the cause of the bleeding. Vital signs including orthostatic blood pressures should be followed. Signs of pallor, petechiae, shock, or decreased mental status should be noted. The abdomen should be palpated for tenderness, guarding, and masses.

Pelvic examination is indicated in most patients even when bleeding is active. The examination should attempt to visualize the source and quantity of bleeding. The examiner should remember that bleeding may occur from the urinary bladder and rectum, as well as the genital tract. Cultures and smears of cervical secretions should be taken. A bimanual exam should focus on discovery of masses and tenderness within either the uterus or adnexa. A rectovaginal exam may replace a bimanual examination in virginal girls. Patients who are not sexually active, who have recent onset of menarche (less than 2 years), and who experience short periods of bleeding without excessive blood loss may be followed initially without a pelvic examination.

Laboratory examination should include a hemoglobin or hematocrit. In cases of anemia, a reticulocyte count, iron level, and hemostasis panel should be considered. Pregnancy tests should be performed in all sexually active girls. Cervical discharge should be cultured for sexually transmitted diseases.

Differential Considerations. Besides dysfunctional uterine bleeding, extensive vaginal bleeding may also be caused by other entities.

TABLE 53-1. Management of Dysfunctional Uterine Bleeding

Mild	Moderate	Severe
Characteristics		
Hgb >11 gm/dl	Hgb 9-11 gm/dl	Hgb <9 gm/dl
Acute treatment		
Reassure	OCP 4 pills/day tapering to 1 pill/day over 21 days	Transfusion as needed
		Estrogen 25 mg IV q 4 hr for 4 doses
		Enovid 5 mg 4 pills/day tapering to 1 pill/day over 21 days
Long-term treatment		
Reexamine in 2 mo	OCP daily for 4 mo thereafter	OCP daily for 4 mo
	Iron supplements	Iron supplements
	Follow-up in 2 weeks	Daily reevaluation until stable

OCP, Oral contraceptive pills.
Adapted from Coupey SM, Ahlstrom P: *Pediatr Clin North Am* 36(3):558, 1989.

Prolonged vaginal bleeding may be the first symptom of coagulation disorders, particularly von Willebrand disease and idiopathic thrombocytopenic purpura. Endocrine abnormalities such as hypothyroidism, hyperthyroidism, or polycystic ovary syndrome may present with heavy vaginal bleeding. Pregnancies complicated by a septic induced abortion, threatened abortion, or ectopic implantation may present with irregular vaginal bleeding. Unusual vaginal bleeding may also occur in PID.

Management. Management of the young woman with dysfunctional uterine bleeding is practically always medical rather than surgical (Table 53-1). Therapy should be guided by the extent of bleeding and anemia present in the patient. Since immature hormonal physiology of the adolescent is the frequent cause of anovulatory cycles and dysfunctional uterine bleeding, therapy is aimed at controlling menstrual cycles with exogenous hormones, specifically estrogen and progestin.

In the girl with mild dysfunctional uterine bleeding, cycles may be more frequent or irregular; anemia is not present. Reassurance, close follow-up, and repeat hematocrit should be planned.

The girl with moderate dysfunctional bleeding has anemia, with a hematocrit that ranges between 25% and 35%. The girl is hemodynamically stable. A combination of estrogen and synthetic progestin given in 21-day cycles separated by 7 days without therapy usually regulates the menstrual cycle. Oral contraceptives offer the convenience of the hormonal combination in a package designed to ease daily use. Active bleeding may be controlled by administering up to four tablets of the combination oral contraceptive at the time of the emergency visit, and then prescribing tapering doses over the next few days down to one tablet per day during a 21-day cycle. (Two oral contraceptive packages will need to be partially used because packages contain only 21 tablets each.) Parents should be reassured that hormonal therapy in adolescent girls is safe; if parents object to the use of oral contraceptives, ethinyl estradiol 50 to 100 µg can be prescribed in combination with norethindrone 5 to 20 mg. Iron supplementation and close, possibly even daily follow-up is indicated in these patients. Because withdrawal bleeding may occur if tablets are stopped suddenly, patients and their parents should be counseled to follow medication schedules closely. Diaries kept by the patient and her parent may be helpful to her physician in follow-up. Hormonal therapy is usually continued for about 6 months.

Severe dysfunctional bleeding causes massive bleeding, hemodynamic compromise, and hematocrits of less than 25%. The girl with severe dysfunctional bleeding should be treated as an emergent patient; initial stabilization should include establishing large-bore intravenous lines, isotonic fluid resuscitation, and type and crossmatch for blood. Coagulation studies should be drawn, especially before transfusion. Occasionally blood transfusions are indicated in these patients. Bleeding should be controlled with the intravenous administration of water-soluble conjugated equine estrogen (Premarin) 25 mg q 4 to 6 hr. Hospitalization with close monitoring is mandatory for the patient who presents with hemodynamic compromise. Curettage is rarely necessary to control bleeding.

Close follow-up is especially important for the patient with moderate or severe dysfunctional bleeding because recurrent bleeding and subsequent anemia may occur.[141]

Dysmenorrhea

Dysmenorrhea is the crampy abdominal or back pain noted in conjunction with a menstrual period. Occasionally nausea, vomiting, diarrhea, or headache may also occur. In a survey of young American girls, 39% of 12 year olds and 72% of 17 year olds reported cramping pain with their menstrual periods.[142]

Primary dysmenorrhea exists when there is no identifiable pathologic cause for the pain. Primary dysmenorrhea is associated with ovulatory cycles; therefore, periods during the first year or two after menarche are usually not associated with dysmenorrhea.

Researchers have found increased levels of prostaglandins E-2 and F-2 α in women with dysmenorrhea.[143] These prostaglandins increase the tone and contractions of the uterus and lead to pain. Prostaglandin F-2 α has also been shown to cause headache, flushing, nausea, and diarrhea when infused.[144]

Secondary dysmenorrhea exists when there is an underlying pathologic condition causing the painful menstruation. PID, endometriosis, congenital malformations, and occasionally, psychosocial factors may cause dysmenorrhea. PID may precipitate pain in a girl who had previously painless menstrual periods. Dysmenorrhea associated with endometriosis usually worsens as the teen gets older, because of the extension of the disease.[145] Congenital malformations such as bicornuate uterus usually present with painful menstruation at menarche because of the obstruction caused by the malformation. Although most girls who complain of dysmenorrhea do not have underlying psychologic problems, an occasional girl may present with complaints of excessive pain with menstruation.[146] Sexual abuse, rape, school problems, or family unrest may affect a girl's perception of pain related to periods.

Diagnostic Findings. History should include the age at menarche, duration of periods, quantity of flow, cycle length, and associated pain. The physician should note whether pain was always associated with menses, or whether it is a new complaint. Crampy abdominal pain in the lower-to-middle abdomen and radiating to the back and thighs is associated with menses, often beginning 6 to 18 months after menarche. The discomfort normally begins within 1 to 4 hours of menstruation, continuing for as long as 24 hours. It may vary from month to month in severity.

A history of vaginal discharge and sexual activity should be noted. Emotional problems should be sought if the pain occurs at menarche or on anticipation of menses. Bloating and irritability with edema may be noted. A family history of pain with menses should also be noted. The physician should ask about the impact that the pain has on the patient's daily activities and school participation.

Physical examination should include examination of the external genitalia in virginal girls. In girls with prolonged or severe pain a pelvic examination should be considered with special attention to pelvic masses on a rectovaginal or bimanual vaginal examination. In adolescents who are sexually active a complete pelvic examination including cultures for STDs is indicated.

Pregnancy testing, cultures for STDs, and, occasionally, ultrasonography or laparoscopy may be indicated in the adolescent girl. One author suggests the use of nifedipine to differentiate primary from secondary dysmenorrhea.[147]

Differential Considerations. A number of entities should be considered, including complications of pregnancy such as threatened abortion, ectopic pregnancy, or a septic induced abortion; any of these should be suspected when a patient presents with an isolated episode of dysmenorrhea.

Mittelschmerz is associated with a typical dull and aching pain, occurring midcycle and predominantly in one lower quadrant. It is caused by ovulatory bleeding into the peritoneal cavity. Mittelschmerz may last for 6 to 8 hours but may be severe and last for several days. Differentiation from appendicitis, torsion or rupture of an ovarian cyst, and ectopic pregnancy may be difficult.

Management. Management of primary dysmenorrhea focuses on blocking the production of the prostaglandins in the uterine wall. NSAIDs such as aspirin, ibuprofen, naproxen sodium, and mefenamic acid are effective, especially if taken at the first sign of cramping (Table 53-2). Patients find that using these drugs on the first 3 days of a menstrual period usually controls pain. In sexually active adolescents with dysmenorrhea, low-dose oral contraceptives are an alternative therapy. Because oral contraceptives block ovulation, they also block the prostaglandin release that is responsible for dysmenorrhea. However, oral contraceptives should not be used in pregnant women or in those who have a history of thromboembolic disease, coronary artery disease, myocardial ischemia, neoplasm, hepatic dysfunction, or hypertension. Narcotics should never be prescribed for dysmenorrhea. Close follow-up is essential.

TABLE 53-2. Nonsteroidal Antiinflammatory Drugs for Primary Dysmenorrhea

Generic name	Brand name	Dosage
Aspirin		650 mg q 6 hr
Ibuprofen	Motrin Advil	400 mg q 6 hr
Naproxen sodium	Anaprox	550 mg then 275 mg q 12 hr
Mefenamic acid	Ponstel	500 mg then 250 mg q 6 hr

PREGNANCY

Adolescent pregnancy has become a major problem,[148] particularly among girls who are between 15 to 18 years old. Approximately 43% of all girls will become pregnant before their twentieth birthday.[149] Many will seek an initial diagnosis in the emergency department setting. Fear of breach of confidentiality between their primary physician and parents may be one reason; lack of a primary physician or health-care funding may be another. Finally, many adolescents do not understand how to access the health-care system and they view the emergency department as their only resource. In some cases, other acute problems such as bleeding, vomiting, abdominal pain, or attempted suicide may precipitate a visit to the emergency department. Teens may not suspect or admit pregnancy. Denial of pregnancy is a frequent issue in the sexually active teen.

Hormonal changes underline the basis for clinical diagnosis. About 14 days before the next expected menstruation, ovulation is triggered by a surge of LH. Approximately 9 days later (1 to 2 days after implantation), HCG becomes detectable; HCG maintains the corpus luteum of pregnancy, supporting the secretion of estrogen and progesterone.

HCG is a sialoglycoprotein with α and β subunits secreted by the fertilized ovum from the time of implantation, approximately 8 to 9 days after ovulation. The β-subunits are immunologically specific. HCG initially increases about twofold every day during the first 30 days of pregnancy.

Diagnostic Findings

History of breast tenderness, nausea, vomiting, fatigue, weight gain, urinary frequency, and amenorrhea are all suggestive of pregnancy. These questions are best asked in the absence of a parent or family member. The teen should be reassured that the visit is confidential; questions regarding sexual activity and contraception will usually then be answered candidly by the adolescent. Questions like, "Do you feel that you may be pregnant?" or "Are you worried about anything?" may reveal concerns.

Setting the tone of the visit by asking about the girl's school life, her friends, and the existence of a boy friend will make it easier for her to answer more sensitive questions. The physician should observe cues such as eye contact, giggling, and other body language; reassuring the patient that some questions may make her uncomfortable usually results in a more rewarding history.

By sitting down in the examination room to take a history, the physician shows concern and courtesy to the patient.

The physical examination should include a breast, abdominal, and pelvic examination. Seeing or feeling fetal movement or hearing fetal heart sounds is diagnostic. Doppler techniques can detect fetal heart tones at 10 weeks of gestation; a fetoscope can detect sounds at 17 to 19 weeks. Fetal movement is generally felt by the mother at 16 to 20 weeks and the abdomen and uterus are enlarged. The uterus is about the size of an orange at 6 to 8 weeks of gestation. It can be palpated at the level of the symphysis pubis by 12 weeks and at 16 to 20 weeks it is noted at the level of the umbilicus. Uterine size measured from the symphysis pubis to the fundus is the quickest means of estimating gestational age. The distance in centimeters equals the gestational age in weeks. For a rough guide, when the dome of the uterus extends beyond the umbilicus, the fetus is potentially viable. Softness or blueness of the cervix may be present.

Early vaginal bleeding in pregnancy may be mistaken for menstrual bleeding and delay the diagnosis of pregnancy.[150]

Ancillary Data. After the assessment of the patient, the physician should decide if a pregnancy test is needed. In cases where the adolescent denies emphatically the possibility of pregnancy, urine pregnancy testing should be presented as a "routine" part of the evaluation of her symptoms. Occasionally the physician may choose to order pregnancy testing without discussing it with the adolescent. To set the stage for counseling, the physician may encourage the teen to consider what she will do if her pregnancy test is positive.[151]

Qualitative pregnancy tests should be correlated with the results of the clinical examination and ultrasound, the latter demonstrating intrauterine pregnancy at β-HCG levels of 750 to 1000 mIU/ml when the vaginal probe is used. Conventional ultrasound can identify intrauterine pregnancy at a β-HCG level of about 1800 mIU/ml. Traditional hemagglutination and latex agglutination inhibition as available in home pregnancy tests detect HCG in material urine at levels of 150 to 4,000 mIU/ml. Enzyme-linked or solid-phase immunoassays are sensitive to a level of 25 to 50 mIU/ml. These assays for HCG are accurate within 2 days of implantation or 4 to 5 days after the missed menses.[152] Qualitative serum pregnancy tests having a threshold from 10 to 50 mIU/ml may actually be positive before a missed menses. Because these tests detect very early stages of pregnancy, they may detect pregnancies that may terminate spontaneously. These tests may yield positive results for up to 4 weeks after a therapeutic abortion as well. Very rarely, urinary β-HCG may be positive in malignant tumors.[153]

Counseling

The diagnosis of pregnancy should be made by using the signs and symptoms of the patient in conjunction with a positive urinary pregnancy test. In discussing the newly diagnosed pregnancy with the adolescent the physician should take time and show concern. The discussion should be done in a confidential manner, without the presence of parents or others. The physician should be nonjudgmental in his or her approach. In a busy emergency department the physician should ensure that confidentiality is maintained among other personnel and that family members be told only if the teen agrees and in the presence of the patient.

The physician should be prepared to face the adolescent's feelings of fear, anger, guilt, sadness, or panic. By being caring, the physician can help the adolescent to begin the decision-making process; the teen must be enabled to explore her options and the resources in her family and community. In young adolescents, particularly those younger than 15 years of age, it is important to include family members in the discussion. Younger teens, in particular, appreciate a family member being notified of the pregnancy; this notification, however, must be done with the permission of the teen and is best done in the examination room in the presence of the patient. Encouraging discussion between the patient and her family members or partner at the time of the emergency department visit frequently defuses questions and concerns. The possibility of rape or incest should be considered, particularly in younger pregnant adolescents. In some hospitals, social workers may prove to be invaluable resources for the immediate counseling of the pregnant teen and her family.

Well-planned follow-up must be arranged for the pregnant teen. Community resources for counseling and specialized prenatal care should be offered to the patient. Early prenatal care helps to prevent the complications of teen pregnancies, including low birth weight and poor nutrition.[154,155] If the teen chooses to continue her pregnancy, she should be encouraged to initiate prenatal care as soon as possible. Written information, including the date of the positive pregnancy test, the "due date," and the phone numbers of community resources help the adolescent to face the reality of her pregnancy and to initiate follow-up medical care.

COMPLICATIONS OF PREGNANCY

Miscarriage

Spontaneous miscarriage refers to the cessation of pregnancy before 20 weeks of gestation. Fetal abnormalities and uterine infections or structural abnormalities may be the cause of spontaneous abortion. Approximately 15% of all pregnancies terminate in spontaneous abortion.

Vaginal bleeding occurring two or more weeks after a missed period should raise consideration of a spontaneous abortion. Cramping and abdominal pain during the first trimester of pregnancy are other symptoms. Since the patient may not give adequate history of sexual activity or of menstrual dates, the physician needs to maintain a high index of suspicion for pregnancy and its complications.

A *threatened miscarriage* refers to bleeding during the first half of pregnancy, without immediate expulsion of the fetus. Approximately 20% to 25% of clinically pregnant women experience some bleeding and about one half of these women miscarry. Examination reveals a closed cervix. Ultrasound and quantitative serial HCG measurements may be helpful in establishing the viability of the pregnancy. Other than reassurance, no treatment other than

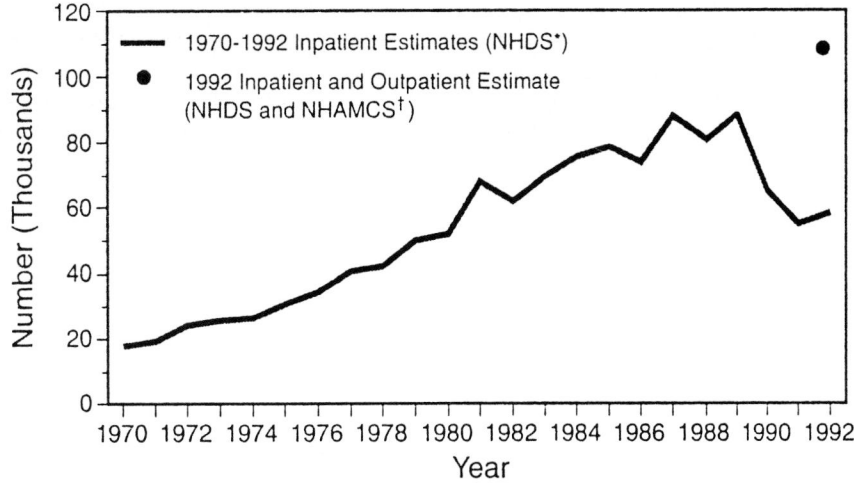

*National Hospital Discharge Survey.
†National Hospital Ambulatory Medical Care Survey.

FIG. 53-13. Number of ectopic pregnancies — United States, 1970–1992.

watchful waiting is needed. A miscarriage is inevitable when the cervix is open. If products of conception are present at the open cervical os or in the vaginal canal, permitting only partial expulsion of the products of conception, the miscarriage is considered incomplete.

A *complete miscarriage* refers to the complete emptying of the uterus of the products of conception in a spontaneous fashion. The cervix closes, and the uterus contracts. Cramping and bleeding resolve; no further treatment is necessary.

An *incomplete miscarriage* refers to partial expulsion of the products of conception. Cramping and bleeding continues until the uterus is completely emptied. Examination reveals an open cervix with clots or tissue. Curettage provided by a gynecologic specialist is indicated. Fluids or blood may be needed in cases of severe bleeding.

A *missed abortion* refers to the situation in which the fetus dies but remains in the uterus without any accompanying uterine growth. Patients may note some brief vaginal bleeding or abdominal pain; missed abortion frequently occurs during the second trimester. Sonography and serial hormonal assessment confirms this event. Because a maternal coagulopathy may occur, curettage should be performed in a timely manner.

A *septic abortion* occurs usually after a nonsterile attempt to effect a therapeutic abortion. Clinically, the patient appears quite toxic and uncomfortable. Pelvic examination may reveal pus from the cervix and vagina. Fever and shock may be present. Intravenous antibiotics and complete evacuation of the uterus is necessary.

In all cases of suspected spontaneous abortion the emergency physician must be careful to consider ectopic pregnancy in the differential diagnosis. Because symptoms of cramping and nonmenstrual bleeding, as well as detectable levels of HCG, may be present in both situations, a careful assessment of the patient is necessary. Treatment should focus on the gynecologic and hemodynamic consequences of the pregnancy complication. Ergonovine or methergonovine (0.2 mg BID PO) may be useful to stimulate uterine involution. Administration of anti-D immunoglobulin should be

considered if the woman is Rh negative — 50 mg is administered in women miscarrying during the first trimester, whereas 300 mg is given following later miscarriages.

Ectopic Pregnancy

Implantation of a fertilized ovum into any site other than the uterine endometrium is called *ectopic pregnancy.* Most implantations occur in the fallopian tubal lining; occasionally they may occur in the intraperitoneal space.

Ectopic pregnancies have increased each year to 110,000 ectopic pregnancies in 1992[156] (Fig. 53-13). Ectopic pregnancy represented 1.7% of all pregnancies in 1987, but 12% of maternal deaths in 1987.[156] Fortunately, mortality rates for ectopic pregnancy have declined, probably because of more sensitive urinary pregnancy tests and increased physician awareness. Adolescents, however, have the highest case-fatality rate of any age group.

Predisposing Factors. PID, IUD, prior pelvic surgery, and congenital abnormalities of the fallopian tube are all believed to be risk factors for the development of ectopic pregnancy. Bobrow and Bell found that approximately 95% of tubes removed surgically for ectopic pregnancy had evidence of prior tubal infection.[157] Young women exposed to diethylstilbestrol had tubes with poor peristalsis and an increased risk of ectopic pregnancy.[158]

When the fertilized egg implants in the fallopian tube, it begins to secrete HCG. At 4 to 6 weeks after implantation the embryo penetrates the tube wall and causes distension and usually abdominal pain. Because the uterine decidua is not supported by the defective trophoblast, withdrawal vaginal bleeding may occur that a patient may misconstrue as a menstrual period. At 6 to 10 weeks, tubal distension continues and the tube eventually ruptures releasing blood and conceptual products into the peritoneal cavity.

Diagnostic Findings. Symptoms may include early pregnancy signs such as nausea, breast tenderness, amenorrhea or a "light" period, and weight gain. When taking the history, the physician should try to compare the most recent period in quantity and duration with prior "normal" periods. Abdominal pain, particularly in the pelvic area, is usually but not always present in ectopic pregnancy. Pain in the shoulder or chest, the sensation of the need to defecate, or pelvic pain may occur because of the intraperitoneal bleeding. Weakness or syncope may occasionally be a complaint if intraperitoneal bleeding is significant. Because the symptomatology can be vague and frequently suggestive of other problems, ectopic pregnancy must be considered in patients with amenorrhea, abdominal pain, and vaginal bleeding accompanying symptoms of pregnancy. However, it must be recognized that the triad of abdominal pain, abnormal vaginal bleeding, and mass are present in only 45% of patients with ectopic pregnancy.

Responses to questions regarding sexual activity may not be accurate in the adolescent girl; accuracy is somewhat improved if the girl's parents are not present in the examining room. Prior episodes of PID, therapeutic abortions, ectopic pregnancy, or pelvic surgery should be noted and should increase the emergency physician's suspicion for ectopic pregnancy. Obviously, these questions are best asked in a confidential manner.

The physical findings of ectopic pregnancy can also be quite elusive, and depend on the amount of fallopian tube distension and on the presence of rupture and intraperitoneal bleeding. Patient cooperation and physician skill are particularly important in detecting signs of ectopic pregnancy. Abdominal tenderness is usually present; rebound, guarding, localized tenderness to one side, and decreased bowel sounds may occur if rupture has ensued.

Pelvic examination usually reveals a somewhat enlarged, soft uterus because of hormonal stimulation; size will not necessarily correspond to week of gestation based on duration of amenorrhea, if known. About half the time, an adnexal mass may be appreciated.[159] Occasionally, this mass may be bilateral or on the contralateral side because of intraperitoneal blood or a corpus luteum cyst.[160] Cul-de-sac fullness on rectovaginal examination is occasionally noted as well. Hypovolemic shock, tachycardia, orthostatic hypotension, and narrow pulse pressure should be sought but generally are absent findings in early ectopic pregnancy because the tube has not yet ruptured. Frequent and occasional physical findings are presented in the box above. The clinician must realize that many of these findings are not present in most cases of ectopic pregnancy presenting to the emergency department. Because an ectopic pregnancy can result in hypovolemic shock and death, it is important to assess at-risk patients carefully.

Ancillary Data. Laboratory evaluation begins with a urinary or serum pregnancy test, developed with sensitivity and specificity for the β-HCG hormone. Studies have shown that these tests approach 100% reliability in detecting pregnancies if the specific gravity of urine is greater than 1.015.[161] Although levels of β-HCG are lower in ectopic pregnancy than in normal pregnancy for the same duration of gestation, the new urinary pregnancy tests have been found to be sensitive enough to detect levels as low as 30 to 50 mIU HCG/ml. Most ectopic pregnancies yield positive urinary pregnancy tests when sensitive tests are used.

Pelvic transabdominal ultrasound is useful in the ectopic pregnancy dilemma. By detecting an intrauterine pregnancy complete with fetal heart movement on ultrasound,

---

Ectopic Pregnancy: Frequent and Occasional Findings

Symptoms

Abdominal pain
Amenorrhea/"light" period
Syncope
Previous PID
Vaginal bleeding
Prior induced abortion

Signs

Abdominal tenderness
Adnexal mass: unilateral/bilateral
Adnexal tenderness/fullness
Cul-de-sac fullness
Diminished bowel sounds
Shock

Data from Webster HD, et al: *Am J Obstet Gynecol* 92:23, 1965; Weckstein LN, Boucher AR, Tucher H, et al: *Obstet Gynecol* 65:393, 1985; and Helvacloglu A, Long M, Yang S: *J Reprod Med* 22(2):87, 1979.

---

the physician is able to rule out ectopic pregnancy. Only in the unusual case of an intrauterine pregnancy concurrent with an ectopic pregnancy would the physician err. Ultrasound can pick up an intrauterine pregnancy by 7 to 8 weeks of gestation, which is usually about the time that an ectopic pregnancy begins to present.[162] Lack of an intrauterine pregnancy on ultrasound in the face of a positive pregnancy test, however, does not absolutely indicate an ectopic pregnancy. Because of its sensitivity, the pregnancy test may be positive before the intrauterine pregnancy is mature enough to be detected on ultrasound. Visualizing the ectopic pregnancy itself on ultrasound may be difficult because fetal heart movement may be too small to be detected directly. Transvaginal ultrasound detects pregnancies as early as 2½ weeks after conception.[163-166] In the hands of an experienced ultrasonographer the transvaginal approach appears to be more sensitive in picking up both early ectopic and intrauterine pregnancies. Intrauterine pregnancies normally have evidence of an intrauterine gestational sac and double ring sign. Pelvic ultrasound, then, is useful to rule out ectopic pregnancy if an intrauterine pregnancy is detected. Culdocentesis is now considered obsolete.[167]

Differential Considerations. Differential diagnosis includes PID, gastroenteritis, dysfunctional uterine bleeding, appendicitis, threatened abortion, tuboovarian abscess, and ruptured corpus luteum cyst (see the box on p. 891). Pregnancy testing is helpful and should be performed in all patients in whom PID is suspected. Because adolescents frequently have poor recall of their menstrual history and irregular menses, pregnancy testing should be performed in all girls presenting with abdominal pain, regardless of menstrual or sexual histories.

Management. Fluid resuscitation through two large-bore intravenous lines, administration of type-specific blood if

Differential Considerations of Ectopic Pregnancies

Diagnosis	Distinguishing features
Acute or chronic salpingitis	Menses usually normal; fever often present; bilateral pain and tenderness usual
Spontaneous abortion of intrauterine pregnancy	Increased bleeding; decreased pain
Ovarian cyst; twisted/ torsioned/ruptured	Signs of pregnancy lacking; discrete mass palpable
Appendicitis	Signs of pregnancy lacking; great "mimicker" of salpingitis and ectopic pregnancy
Intrauterine device	Positive history; crampy abdominal pain common; bleeding present
Acute gastroenteritis	Nausea, vomiting, diarrhea, abdominal pain may all be present; other family members may be affected

From Ammerman S et al: *J Pediatr* 117(5):683, 1990.

appropriate, administration of oxygen, immediate urinary pregnancy testing, measurement of hematocrit, and notification of the gynecologist should be performed in the hemodynamically unstable patient suspected of having an ectopic pregnancy. Delay in consulting the gynecologist and in aggressive management for shock are two serious mistakes the emergency physician should avoid.

In the stable patient presenting with symptoms of ectopic pregnancy a careful approach should be taken in conjunction with obstetric colleagues. If the pregnancy test is positive, ultrasonography should be obtained.

A full bladder enhances the use of ultrasonography and may be accomplished by a bolus of IV fluids. Transvaginal ultrasonography eliminates this requirement and facilitates examination. If ultrasonography shows an intrauterine pregnancy, the physician should consider other diagnoses. If ultrasonography shows a tubal pregnancy or no clear intrauterine pregnancy, gynecologic consultation for surgery is indicated. If the patient is in a very early stage of pregnancy, tubal or intrauterine pregnancy may not be visible by ultrasonography. If the patient is certain of having had a normal menstrual period 6 weeks before presentation, a quantitative serum HCG may be helpful. If the β-HCG is less than 6,500 mIU/ml, the patient is most likely to have an early intrauterine pregnancy and may be carefully followed clinically. If the quantitative serum β-HCG is greater than 6,500 mIU/ml, more aggressive evaluation is indicated. Laparoscopy may be used in

equivocal cases in some centers.[168,169] A management algorithm is shown in Fig. 53-14.[170]

Close, continuous monitoring of the patient with suspected ectopic pregnancy is mandatory. Vital signs, abdominal pain, and mental status should be followed both in the emergency department and the radiology suite. Adolescents in whom the diagnosis is equivocal and in whom watchful waiting is prescribed should be admitted to the hospital in a monitored unit for observation.

Abbott and colleagues have reported several pitfalls in diagnosis in a review of ectopic pregnancies[171] (see the box on p. 893). They found that some ectopic pregnancies presented without pain, that adnexal masses were rarely palpable by emergency physicians, and that transabdominal ultrasound was frequently not helpful. Further, a patient's history of "passing tissue" was interpreted as a complete abortion when it actually represented a withdrawal bleed. Scrutiny of vital signs to detect early hypovolemia was also encouraged.

Treatment of ectopic pregnancy is generally surgical. Current procedures include salpingectomy, fimbrial expression, and partial salpingectomy, among others.[172,173] Early aggressive treatment of ectopic pregnancy is important not only to prevent maternal morbidity and mortality, but also to ensure future fertility. Sherman and colleagues found that surgery before rupture of the ectopic pregnancy significantly improved fertility compared with surgery after rupture.[174]

Less surgical approaches to ectopic pregnancy have included the use of methotrexate as well as observation of the stable patient without intervention.[175]

Ectopic pregnancy may be an elusive diagnosis for the emergency physician caring for the adolescent girl. A high index of suspicion, coupled with careful interpretation of diagnostic modalities, and consideration of differential entities allows the physician to initiate early treatment to prevent mortality and future infertility.

Complications of the Third Trimester

Abruptio Placentae and Placenta Previa. About 4% of pregnancies have bleeding during the second half of pregnancy. Abruptio placentae is the premature separation of a normally implanted placenta with a peak incidence between 20 and 29 weeks of gestation and again at 38 weeks. It accounts for about 30% of bleeding episodes. Spontaneous hemorrhage into the decidua basalis causes separation and compression of the adjacent placenta. Separation may be associated with blunt trauma to the abdomen.

Patients with *abruptio placentae* classically have vaginal bleeding and abdominal pain. The extent of pain reflects the degree of disruption of the myometrial fibers and intravasation of blood at the site of bleeding. Vaginal bleeding is variable and may be concealed. The uterus is uniformly tender. Hypotension, fetal distress, and death may result with significant separation.

Placenta previa occurs with implantation of the placenta over the cervical os. Marginal placental vessels are torn as the uterine wall elongates or with cervical dilatation. Painless, fresh vaginal bleeding is common. Digital or instrumental probing of the cervical os may produce hemorrhage.

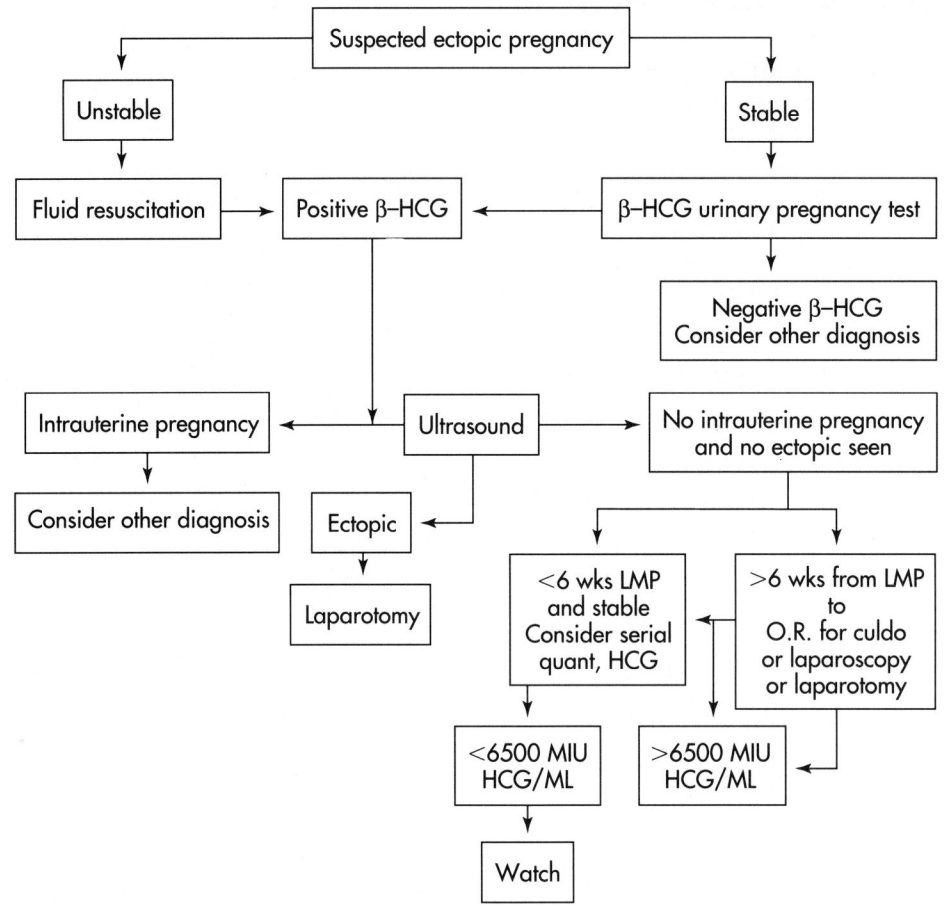

FIG. 53-14. Management of the patient with suspected ectopic pregnancy. (*Adapted from Hockberger RS: Ectopic pregnancy, Emerg Clin North Am 5(3):481-493, 1987.*) *LMP,* Last menstrual period.

Ultrasonography may identify the location and condition of the placenta.

Management involves the localization of the placenta on ultrasonography while hemodynamic stability is achieved. Obstetric consultation is required in the emergency department. Special attention must be given to monitoring for disseminated intravascular coagulation and acute tubular necrosis. Examination during stabilization should be done expeditiously, using an expectant approach. The initial pelvic examination is normally done in an operating (or obstetric) room with a double set-up procedure.

Infants under 2,500 gm born after third trimester bleeding may be adversely affected. After abruptio placentae, infants had lower Apgar scores at 1 minute and higher rates of acidosis. Infants with placenta previa had a higher incidence of respiratory distress syndrome. Third trimester bleeding is a risk factor for neurodevelopmental impairment in low-birth-weight infants.[176]

Other Complications. Preeclampsia is accompanied by pregnancy-induced hypertension and complicates about 2.6% of births. Patients with mild findings have proteinuria and mild systolic or diastolic blood pressure elevation. In severe preeclampsia, diastolic blood pressure may exceed 110 mm Hg, proteinuria is severe, and vasospastic end-organ damage presents with central nervous system (CNS) effects (headache or visual disturbances), liver function ab-

normalities, thrombocytopenia, and renal dysfunction. Eclampsia may develop, accompanied by seizures or coma, hyperactive reflexes, and renal dysfunction.

Management focuses on initial evaluation of end-organ effects and close monitoring. Specific treatment includes control of hypertension, treatment of seizures, and monitoring and maintenance of urine output.

Rh (anti-D) immunization occurs when a Rh-negative woman is exposed to Rh-positive blood during pregnancy or delivery. Sensitization may occur at the time of delivery or during uterine manipulation. Transplacental hemorrhage should also be considered during miscarriage, during surgery for ectopic pregnancy, and during amniocentesis. Anti-D immunoglobulin (Rhogam) should be administered according to the following schedule in consultation with an obstetric consultant when these events occur: 50 mg of Rhogam: < 12 weeks—ectopic pregnancy, threatened or complete abortion; 300 mg of Rhogam: ≥ 12 weeks—ectopic pregnancy, threatened or complete abortion; and amniocentesis.

Rhogam is not required if the father or fetus (from cord blood) is known to be Rh negative. Treatment is also indicated if fetomaternal transfusions is suspected after trauma.

Urinary tract infections tend to be more commonly symptomatic during pregnancy. Symptomatic infections occur in 1% to 3% of pregnant women and acute pyelone-

Pitfalls in Diagnosis of Ectopic Pregnancies

	No. of patients (%)	95% confidence intervals
Clinical		
Atypical or absent pain	26 (92%)	(76%, 99%)
Absence of adnexal mass	25 (89%)	(72%, 98%)
Failure to recognize signs of blood loss	9 (32%)	(16%, 52%)
Failure to recognize risk factors	7 (25%)	(11%, 45%)
Passage of uterine tissue	4 (14%)	(4%, 33%)
Ancillary study interpretation		
Nondiagnostic ultrasound ($n = 41$)	19 (46%)	(31%, 63%)
Ultrasound misinterpretation ($n = 41$)	11 (27%)	(14%, 43%)
Quantitative HCG interpretation ($n = 20$)	5 (20%)	(9%, 49%)
Ultrasound correlation with HCG levels	2 (7%)	(1%, 32%)
Dry or serous culdocentesis ($n = 28$)	16 (57%)	(37%, 76%)

HCG, Human chorionic gonadotropin.
From Abbott J, Emmans LS, Lowenstein SR: Am J Emerg Med 8:515, 1990.
$n = 28$ patients with delayed diagnosis of ectopic pregnancy.

phritis develops in 1% to 2% of women. Dysuria, urinary frequency, urinary urgency, as well as upper tract symptoms of fever, malaise, and back pain may be noted.

Differential considerations must include vaginitis, herpes genitalis, or chlamydial infection of the urethra. Appendicitis, cholecystitis, pancreatitis, and liver disease must be considered. As many as 20% of patients with appendicitis have pyuria without bacteriuria.

Outpatient management for 7 to 10 days is appropriate for asymptomatic patients and those with lower tract signs and symptoms. Intravenous management in a hospital is desirable for patients who present with acute pyelonephritis. Referral and close follow-up are essential.

Gastrointestinal presentations not uncommonly accompany pregnancy. Appendicitis, gallbladder disease, acute fatty liver, and cholestasis may present clinically to the emergency department, requiring evaluation and management in coordination with an obstetric consultant.

References

Vaginal Bleeding

1. Baldwin DD and Landa HM: Common problems in pediatric gynecology, *Urol Clinics North Am* 22:161-176, 1995.
2. Rimsza ME: An illustrated guide to adolescent gynecology, *Pediatr Clin North Am* 36(3):640, 1989.
3. White ST, Ingram DL, Lyra PR: Vaginal introital diameter in the evaluation of sexual abuse, *Child Abuse Negl* 13:217-224, 1989.
4. Paradise JE: Predictive accuracy and the diagnosis of sexual abuse: a big issue about a little tissue, *Child Abuse Negl* 13:169-176, 1989.
5. Paradise JE and Willis ED: Probability of vaginal foreign body in girls with genital complaints, *Am J Dis Child* 139:472, 1985.
6. Anderson M, Irwin CE, Sayder DL: Abnormal vaginal bleeding in adolescents, *Pediatr Ann* 15(10):696-707, 1986.

Vaginal Discharge

7. Aruda MM: Vulvovaginitis in the prepubertal child, *Nurse Pract Forum* 3:149-151, 1992.
8. Abbott J: Clinical and microscopic diagnosis of vaginal yeast infection: a prospective analysis, *Ann Emerg Med* 25:587-91, 1995.
9. Krieger JN, Tam MR, Stevens CE: Diagnosis of trichomoniasis, *JAMA* 259:1223, 1988.
10. Abromowicz M: Treatment of sexually transmitted diseases, *Med Lett Drugs Ther* 30:5, 1988.
11. Hammerschlag MR: Chlamydial infections, *J Pediatr* 114:727, 1989.

Breast Disorders

12. Nydick M, Bustos J, Dale JH et al: Gynecomastia in adolescent boys, *JAMA* 178:449-451, 1961.
13. Schonfield WA: Gynecomastia in adolescence: effects on body image and personality adaptation, *Psychosom Med* 24:379, 1962.
14. Levit F: Jogger's nipples, *N Engl J Med* 297:1127, 1977.
15. Beach RK: Routine breast exams: a chance to reassure, guide, and protect, *Contemp Pediatr* 4:70-100, 1987.
16. Sandison AT and Walker JC: Diseases of the adolescent female breast: a clinicopathological study, *Br J Surg* 55:443-448, 1968.
17. Greydanus DE and Hoffman AD: The thorax. In Hoffman AD, Greydanus DE, editors: *Adolescent medicine*, Norwalk, Conn, 1989, Appleton and Lange.
18. Gogas J, Sechas M, Skalkeas G: Surgical management of diseases of the adolescent breast, *Am J Surg* 137:634-637, 1979.
19. Daniel WA Jr and Mathews MD: Tumors of the breast in adolescent females, *Pediatrics* 41:743-749, 1968.
20. Wile AG and Killin M: Office management of the breast mass, *Postgrad Med* 81:137-143, 1987.
21. Farrow JH and Ashikari H: Breast lesions in young girls, *Surg Clin North Am* 49:261, 1969.
22. Bauer BS, Jones KM, Talbot CW: Mammary masses in the adolescent female, *Surg Gynecol Obstet* 165:63-65, 1987.
23. Goldstein DP and Miller V: Breast masses in adolescent females, *Clin Pediatr* 21:17-19, 1982.

External Genitalia

24. Aghajanian A et al: Bartholin's duct abscess and cyst: a case-control study, *Southern Med J* 87:26-29, 1994.
25. Lee YH, et al: Microbiological investigation of Bartholin gland abscesses and cysts, *Am J Obstet Gynecol* 129:150-153, 1977.
26. Rimsza ME and Feingold M: Picture of the month, *Am J Dis Child* 143:381-382, 1989.
27. Bowles HE and Childs LS: Synechias of vulva in small children, *Am J Dis Child* 66:258-263, 1953.
28. Berkowitz CD, Elvik SL, Logan MK: Labial fusion in prepubescent girls: a marker for sexual abuse? *Am J Obstet Gynecol* 156:16, 1987.
29. McCann M, Voris J, Simon M: Labial adhesions and posterior fourchette injuries in childhood sexual abuse, *Am J Dis Child* 142:659-663, 1988.
30. Capraro VJ and Greenberg H: Adhesions of the labia minora: a study of 50 patients, *Obstet Gynecol* 39:65, 1972.
31. Clair DL and Caldamone AA: Pediatric office procedures, *Urol Clin North Am* 15(4):716, 1988.
32. Shirer JA and Ray MC: Familial occurence of lichen sclerosus et atrophicus, *Arch Dermatol* 123:485-488, 1987.
33. Berth-Jones J, Graham-Brown RAC, Burns DA: Lichen sclerosus, *Arch Dis Child* 64:1204-1206, 1989.
34. Handfield-Jones SE, Hinde FRJ, Kennedy CTC: Lichen sclerosus et atrophicus in children misdiagnosed as sexual abuse, *BMJ* 294:1404-1405, 1987.
35. Capraro VJ, Boyonet-Rivera NP, Magoss I: Vulvar tumor in children due to prolapse of urethral mucosa, *Am J Obstet Gynecol* 108:572, 1970.
36. Lowe FC, Hill GS, Jeffs RD, et al: Urethral prolapse in children: insights into etiology and management, *J Urol* 135:100, 1986.
37. Richardson DA, Jaijj SN, Herbst AL: Medical treatment of urethral prolapse in children, *Obstet Gynecol* 59:69, 1982.

38. Jerkins GR, Verheeck K, Noe HN: Treatment of girls with urethral prolapse, *J Urol* 132:732, 1984.

39. Anveden-Hertzberg L et al: Urethral prolapse: an often misdiagnosed cause of urogenital bleeding in girls, *Ped Emerg Care* 11:212-214, 1995.

Sexually Transmitted Diseases

40. Brady M, Baker C, Neinstein L: Asymptomatic *Chlamydia trachomatis* infections in teenage males, *J Adol Health Care* 9:72-75, 1988.

41. Smith PB, Phillips LE, Faro S et al: Predominant sexually transmitted diseases among different age and ethnic groups of indigent sexually active adolescents attending a family planning clinic, *J Adolesc Health Care* 9:291-295, 1988.

42. Fisher M, Swenson PD, Risucci D et al: *Chlamydia trachomatis* in suburban adolescents, *J Pediatr* 111:617-620, 1987.

43. Fraser JJ Jr, Rettig PJ, Kaplan DW: Prevalence of cervical *Chlamydia trachomatis* and *Neisseria gonorrheae* in female adolescents, *Pediatrics* 72:333-336, 1983.

44. Chacko MR, Lovchik JC: *Chlamydia trachomatis* infection in sexually active adolescents: prevalence and risk factors, *Pediatrics* 73:836-840, 1984.

45. Stamm WE, Holmes KK: *Chlamydia trachomatis* infections of the adult. In Holmes KK, Mardh PA, Sparling F et al, editors: *Sexually transmitted diseases,* New York, 1984, McGraw-Hill.

46. Krowchuck DP, Anglin TM, Lembo RM et al: Use of enzyme immunoassay for the rapid diagnosis of *Chlamydia trachomatis* endocervical infection in female adolescents, *J Adolesc Health Care* 9:296-300, 1988.

47. Shafer MA, Vaughan E, Lipkin ES et al: Evaluation of fluorescein-conjugated monoclonal antibody test to detect *Chlamydia trachomatis* in adolescent girls, *J Pediatr* 108:779-783, 1986.

48. Yang LI et al: Detection of *Chlamydia trachomatis* endocervical infection in asymptomatic and symptomatic women: a comparison of deoxyribonucleic acid probe test with tissue culture, *Am J Obstet Gynecol* 165 (5 Part 1):1444-1453, 1991.

49. Ferris DG, Martin WH: A comparison of three rapid chlamydial tests in pregnant and nonpregnant women, *J Fam Pract* 34:593-597, 1992.

50. Martin DH et al: A controlled trial of a single dose of azythromycin for the treatment of chlamydial urethritis and cervicitis, *N Engl J Med* 327:921-925, 1992.

51. Oh MK, Feinstein R, Pass RF: Sexually transmitted diseases and sexual behavior in urban adolescent females attending a family planning clinic, *J Adolesc Health Care* 9:67-71, 1988.

52. Smith PB, Phillips LE, Faro S et al: Predominant sexually transmitted diseases among different age and ethnic groups of indigent sexually active adolescents attending a family planning clinic, *J Adolesc Health Care* 9:291-295, 1988.

53. Louv WC, Austin H, Perlman J et al: Oral contraceptive use and the risk of chlamydial and gonococcal infections, *Am J Obstet Gynecol* 160:396-402, 1989.

54. Dallabetta G, Hook EW: Gonococcal infections, *Infect Dis Clin North Am* 1:25-54, 1987.

55. Schwarcz SK, Zenilman JM, Schnell D et al: National surveillance of antimicrobial resistance in *Neisseria gonorrhea,* *JAMA* 254(11):1413-1417, 1990.

56. Seigel WM et al: Hyperendemic penicillinase producing *Neisseria gonorrhoeae* genital infections in an inner city population, *J of Adolesc Health* 16:41, 1995.

57. CDC: 1993 Sexually transmitted diseases treatment guidelines, *MMWR* 42:47-52, 1993.

58. Handsfield HH et al: Oral cefixime for gonorrhea, *N Engl J Med* 325:1337, 1991.

59. Chacko MR, Wells RD, Phillips SA: Test of cure for gonorrhea in teenagers, *J Adolesc Health Care* 8:261-265, 1987.

60. Chang T: Genital herpes, the source of infection, *Int J Dermatol* 14:201-202, 1975.

61. Stone KM, Whittington WL: Treatment of genital herpes, *Rev Infect Dis* 12(suppl 16):S609-S610, 1990.

62. McCormack WM: Pelvic inflammatory disease (review), *N Engl J Med* 330:115-119, 1994.

63. Westrom L: Incidence, prevalence, and trends of acute pelvic inflammatory disease and its consequences in industrialized countries, *Am J Obstet Gynecol* 138:880-892, 1980.

64. Sweet RL, Blankfort-Doyle M, Robbie MO et al: The occurrence of chlamydia and gonococcal salpingitis during the menstrual cycle, *JAMA* 255:2062-2064, 1986.

65. Moeller BR: The role of mycoplasmas in the upper genital tract of women, *Sex Transm Dis* 10:281-284, 1983.

66. Jacobson L and Westrom L: Objectivized diagnosis of acute pelvic inflammatory disease, *Am J Obstet Gynecol* 105(7):1088-1098, 1969.

67. Sellors J et al: The accuracy of clinical findings and laparoscopy in pelvic inflammatory disease, *Am J Obstet Gynecol* 164:113-120, 1991.

68. Kahn JG et al: Diagnosing pelvic inflammatory disease: a comprehensive analysis and considerations for developing a new model, *JAMA* 226:2594-2604, 1991.

69. Sweet RC: Pelvic inflammatory disease and infertility in women, *Infect Dis Clin North Am* 1:199-215, 1987.

70. Jehle D, Davis E, Evans T et al: Emergency department sonography by emergency physicians, *Am J Emerg Med* 7:605-611, 1989.

71. Eschenbach DA: Acute pelvic inflammatory disease, *Urol Clin North Am* 11(1):65-81, 1984.

72. Golden N, Neuhoff S, Cohen H: Pelvic inflammatory disease in adolescents, *J Pediatr* 114(1):138-143, 1989.

73. Jacobson L: Differential diagnosis of acute pelvic inflammatory disease, *Am J Obstet Gynecol* 138:905-1008, 1980.

74. Viberg L: Acute inflammatory conditions of the uterine adnexa, *Acta Obstet Gynecol Scand* 43(54):1-86, 1964.

75. Martens MG, Faro Sebastian, Hammill H et al: Comparison of cefotaxime, cefoxitin and clindamycin plus gentamicin in the treatment of uncomplicated and complicated pelvic inflammatory disease, *J Antimicrob Chemother* 26(A):37-43, 1990.

76. Wolner-Hanssen PW, Paavonen J, Kiviat N et al: Ambulatory treatment of suspected pelvic inflammatory disease with Augmentin, with or without doxycycline, *Am J Obstet Gynecol* 158:577-579, 1988.

77. CDC: 2993 Sexually transmitted diseases treatment guidelines, *MMWR* 42, RR-14, 38-39, 1993.

78. American Academy of Pediatrics: *1994 Red Book of the Report of the Committee on Infectious Diseases,* 1994, Elk Grove Village, Ill.

79. Centers for Disease Control: Increases in primary and secondary syphilis—United States, *MMWR* 36(25):393-397, 1987.

80. US Public Health Service: Criteria and techniques for the diagnosis of early syphilis, *Bulletin* 98-376, 1974.

81. De Jong AR, Weiss JC, Brent RL: *Condyloma acuminata* in children, *Am J Dis Child* 136:704-706, 1982.

82. Patel R and Groff DB: *Condyloma acuminata* in childhood, *Pediatrics* 112:1329, 1972.

83. Obalek S, Jablonska S, Favre M, et al: *Condylomata acuminata* in children: frequent association with human papillomaviruses responsible for cutaneous warts, *J Am Acad Dermatol* 23:205-213, 1990.

84. Cohen B, Honig P, Androphy E: Anogenital warts in children: clinical and virologic evaluation for sexual abuse, *Arch Dermatol* 126:1575-1580, 1990.

85. Bauer HM, Ting Y, Greer CE et al: Genital human papillomavirus infection in female university students as determined by a PCR-based method, *JAMA* 265:472-477, 1991.

86. Hein K: Acquired immunodeficiency syndrome in adolescents: a rationale for concern, *NY State J Med* 87:290-295, 1987.

87. Strunin L and Hingson R: Acquired immunodeficiency syndrome and adolescents: knowledge, beliefs, attitudes, and behaviors, *Pediatrics* 79:825-828, 1987.

88. Remafedi GJ: Preventing the sexual transmission of AIDS during adolescence, *J Adolesc Health Care* 9:139-145, 1988.

89. Centers for Disease Control: Condoms for prevention of sexually transmitted diseases, *MMWR* 37(9):133-137, 1988.

Vulvovaginitis

90. Rey-Stocker I: Vulvitis and vaginitis in the infant, *Gynaecologia* 168:413, 1969.

91. Huber A and Kalkschmid W: L'hemorragie physiologique du nouveaune', *Gynecol Prat* 23:69, 1972.

92. Huffman JW, Dewhurst CJ, Capraro VJ: *The gynecology of childhood and adolescence,* ed 2, Philadelphia, 1981, WB Saunders.

93. Hammerschlag MR, Alpert S, Rosner I et al: Microbiology of the vagina in children: normal and potentially pathogenic organisms, *Pediatrics* 62:57-62, 1978.

94. Gardner H: The vulvovaginitides. In Traymor M and Green T Jr, editors: *Progress in gynecology,* vol 6, New York, 1975, Grune & Stratton.

95. Huffman JW: Premenarchal vulvovaginitis, *Clin Obstet Gynecol* 20:581-593, 1977.

96. Schachter J, Grossman M, Holt J et al: Infection with *Chlamydia trachomatis:* involvement of multiple anatomic sites in neonates, *J Infect Dis* 129:232-234, 1979.

97. Rettig PJ and Nelson JD: Genital tract infection with *Chlamydia trachomatis* in prepubertal children, *J Pediatr* 99:206-210, 1981.

98. Bump RC: *Chlamydia trachomatis* as a cause of prepubertal vaginitis, *Obstet Gynecol* 65:384-388, 1985.

99. Hammerschlag MR, Doraiswamy B, Alexander ER et al: Are rectogenital chlamydial infections a marker of sexual abuse in children? *Pediatr Infect Dis* 3:100-104, 1984.

100. Srivastava AC: Survival of gonococci in urethral secretions with reference to the nonsexual transmission of gonococcal infection, *J Med Microbiol* 13:593-595, 1980.

101. Odugbemi T and Onile BA: Pediatric gonorrhea: is it receiving adequate attention? *Am J Reprod Immunol Microbiol* 18:32-34, 1988.

102. Ingram DL: The gonococcus and the toilet seat revisited, *Pediatr Infect Dis J* 8:191, 1989.

103. Ingram DL, White ST, Durfee MF et al: Sexual contact in children with gonorrhea, *Am J Dis Child* 136:994-996, 1982.

104. Branch G and Paxton P: A study of gonococcal infections among infants and children, *Public Health Rep* 80:347-352, 1965.

105. Whittington WL, Rice RJ, Biddle JW et al: Incorrect identification of *Neisseria gonorrhea* from infants and children, *Pediatr Infect Dis J* 7:3-10, 1988.

106. Rawstron SA, Hammerschlag MR, Gullans C et al: Ceftriaxone treatment of penicillinase-producing *Neisseria gonorrhea* infections in children, *Pediatr Infect Dis J* 8:445-448, 1989.

107. Murphy TV and Nelson JD: Shigella vaginitis: report of 38 patients and review of the literature, *Pediatrics* 63:511-516, 1979.

108. Davis TC: Chronic vulvovaginitis in children due to *Shigella flexneri, Pediatrics* 56:41, 1975.

109. Heller RH, Joseph HM, Davis HJ: Vulvovaginitis in the premenarcheal child, *J Pediatr* 74:370-377, 1969.

110. Hedlund P: Acute vulvovaginitis in streptococcal infections, *Acta Paediatr* 42:388-389, 1953.

111. Straumanis JP and Bocchini JA: Group A beta-hemolytic Streptococcal vulvovaginitis in prepubertal girls: a case report and review of the past twenty years, *Pediatr Infect Dis J* 9:345-348, 1990.

112. Pheifer TA, Forsyth PS, Durfee MA, et al: Nonspecific vaginitis: Role of *Haemophilus vaginalis* and treatment with metronidazole, *N Engl J Med* 298:1429-1434, 1978.

113. Elsner P and Hartman AA: *Gardnerella vaginalis* in the male upper genital tract: a possible source of reinfection of the female partner, *Sex Transm Dis* 14:122-123, 1987.

114. Cook RL, Reid G, Pond DG, et al: Clue cells in bacterial vaginosis: immunofluorescent identification of the adherent gram-negative bacteria as *Gardnerella vaginalis, J Infect Dis* 160:490-496, 1989.

115. Larsson PG, Platz-Christensen JJ: Enumeration of clue cells in rehydrated air-dried vaginal wet smears for the diagnosis of bacterial vaginosis, *Obstet Gynecol* 76:727-730, 1990.

116. Lien EA and Hillier SL: Evaluation of the enhanced rapid identification method for *Gardnerella vaginalis, J Clin Microbiol* 27:566-567, 1989.

117. Hansen W, Vray B, Miller K, et al: Detection of *Gardnerella vaginalis* in vaginal specimens by direct immunofluorescence, *J Clin Microbiol* 25:1934-1937, 1987.

118. Chowdhury A, Bhujuwala RA, Shriniwas: *Gardnerella vaginalis:* isolation and identification, *Indian J Pathol Microbiol* 33:151-156, 1990.

119. Jerve F, Berdol TB, Bohman P, et al: Metronidazole in the treatment of nonspecific vaginitis (NSV), *Br J Vener Dis* 60:171-174, 1984.

120. Connell EB and Tatum HJ: *Sexually transmitted diseases: diagnosis and treatment,* Durant, Okla, 1985, Creative Informatics.

121. Paavonen J and Stamm WE: Lower genital tract infections in women, *Infect Dis Clin North Am* 1(I):179-198, 1987.

122. Reed BD, Huck W, Zazove P: Differentiation of *Gardnerella vaginalis, Candida albicans,* and *Trichomonas vaginalis* infections of the vagina, *J Fam Pract* 28:673-680, 1989.

123. Weisberg M: Terconazole—a new antifungal agent for vulvovaginal candidiasis, *Clin Ther* 11(5):659-668, 1989.

124. Roth AC, Milsom I, Forssman L: Intermittent prophylactic treatment of recurrent vaginal candidiasis by postmenstrual application of a 500-mg clotrimazole vaginal tablet, *Genitourin Med* 66:357-360, 1990.

125. Merkus JM: Treatment of vaginal candidiasis: orally or vaginally? *J Am Acad Dermatol* 23:568-572, 1990.

126. Sobel JD: Individualizing treatment of vaginal candidiasis, *J Am Acad Dermatol* 23:572-576, 1990.

127. Oh MK, Feinstein RA, Pass RF: Sexually transmitted diseases and sexual behavior in urban adolescent females attending a family planning clinic, *J Adolesc Health Care* 9:67-71, 1988.

128. Paavonen J and Stamm WE: Lower genital tract infections in women, *Infect Dis Clin North Am* 1(I):179-198, 1987.

129. Friedrich E: *Vulvar disease,* Philadelphia, 1976, WB Saunders.

130. Fouts AC and Kraus SJ: *Trichomonas vaginalis:* reevaluation of its clinical presentation and laboratory diagnosis, *J Infect Dis* 141:137-143, 1980.

131. Paavonen J and Stamm WE: Lower genital tract infections in women, *Infect Dis Clin North Am* 1(I):179-198, 1987.

132. Krieger JN, Tam MR, Stevens CE et al: Diagnosis of trichomoniasis: comparison of conventional wet-mount examination with cytologic studies, cultures, and monoclonal antibody staining of direct specimens, *JAMA* 259(8):1223-1227, 1988.

133. Martien K and Emans SJ: Treatment of common genital infections in adolescents, *J Adolesc Health Care* 8:1129-1136, 1987.

134. Godman P: Metronidazole, *N Engl J Med* 303:1212-1218, 1980.

135. Schnell JD: The incidence of vaginal candida and trichomonas infections and treatment of *Trichomonas vaginitis* with clotrimazole, *Postgrad Med J* 50:S79, 1974.

Menstrual Problems

136. Goldfarb JM and Little BA: Abnormal vaginal bleeding, *N Engl J Med* 302(12):660, 1980.

137. Coupey SM and Ahlstrom P: Common menstrual disorders, *Pediatr Clin North Am* 36(3):558, 1989.

138. Widholm O and Kantero RL: Menstrual patterns of adolescent girls according to chronological and gynecological ages, *Acta Obstet Gynecol Scand* (Suppl) 14:19, 1974.

139. Huffman JW, Dewhurst CJ, Capraro VJ, editors: *The gynecology of childhood and adolescence,* Philadelphia, 1981, WB Saunders.

140. Claessens EA and Cowell CA: Acute adolescent menorrhagia, *Am J Obstet Gynecol* 139:277, 1981.

141. Wathen PI, Henderson MC, Witz CA: Abnormal uterine bleeding. *Med Clin North Am* 79:329-344, 1995.

142. Klein JR and Litt IF: Epidemiology of adolescent dysmenorrhea, *Pediatrics* 68(5):661, 1981.

143. Alvin PE and Litt IF: Current status of the etiology and management of dysmenorrhea in adolescence, *Pediatrics* 70(4):516, 1982.

144. Jones GS and Wentz AC: The effect of prostaglandin F2 alpha infusion on the corpus luteum function, *Am J Obstet Gynecol* 114:393, 1972.

145. Goldstein DP and DeCholnoky C: Adolescent endometriosis, *J Adolesc Health Care* 1:37-41, 1980.

146. Lawlor CL and Davis AM: Primary dysmenorrhea: relationship to personality and attitudes in adolescent females. *J Adolesc Health Care* 1:208, 1981.

147. Ulmsten U: Calcium blockade as a rapid pharmacological test to evaluate primary dysmenorrhea, *Gynecol Obstet Invest* 20:78-83, 1985.

Pregnancy

148. Fraser AM, Brockert JE, Ward RH: Association of young maternal age with adverse reproductive outcomes. *New Engl J Med* 332:1113-1117, 1995.

149. Forrest JD: Proportion of U.S. women pregnant before age 20: a research note, Unpublished paper, New York, Alan Guttmacher Institute.

150. Stevens-Simon C, Roghmann KJ, McAnarney ER: Early vaginal bleeding, late prenatal care, and misdating in adolescent pregnancies, *Pediatrics* 87:838-840, 1991.

151. Stephenson JN: Pregnancy testing and counseling, *Pediatr Clin North Am* 36(3):681-696, 1986.

152. Gelletlie R and Nielsen JB: Evaluation and comparison of commercially available pregnancy tests based on monoclonal antibodies to human choriogonadotropin, *Clin Chem* 32(12):2166-2170, 1986.

153. Fletcher JL: Update on pregnancy testing, *Prim Care* 13:667-677, 1986.

154. Friede A, Baldwin W, Rhodes PH, et al: Young maternal age and infant mortality: the role of low birth weight, *Public Health Rep* 102:192-199, March 1987.

155. Clark JFJ, Westney LS, Laawyer CJ: Adolescent pregnancy: a 25-year review, *JAMA* 79(4):377-380, 1987.

Complications of Pregnancy

156. CDC: Ectopic pregnancy—United States, 1990-1992, *MMWR* 44:46-49, 1995.

157. Bobrow ML and Bell HG: Ectopic pregnancy: a 26 year survey of 905 cases, *Obstet Gynecol* 16:51, 1960.

158. De Cherney AH: Structure and function of the fallopian tubes following exposure to DES during gestation, *Fertil Steril* 36:741, 1982.

159. Webster HD et al: Ectopic pregnancy, *Am J Obstet Gynecol* 92:23, 1965.

160. Weckstein LN, Boucher AR, Tucher H et al: Accurate diagnosis of early ectopic pregnancy, *Obstet Gynecol* 65:393, 1985.

161. Helvacioglu A, Long EM, Yang S: Ectopic pregnancy: an eight-year review, *J Reprod Med* 22(2):87-92, 1979.

162. Cartwright PS, Victory DF, Moore RA et al: Performance of a new-enzyme-linked immunoassay urine pregnancy test for the detection of ectopic pregnancy, *Ann Emerg Med* 15:1198, 1986.

163. Kelly MT, Santos-Ramos R, Duehoelter JH: The value of sonography in suspected ectopic pregnancy, *Obstet Gynecol* 58:703, 1979.

164. Barnhart K et al: Prompt diagnosis of ectopic pregnancy in an emergency setting, *Obstet Gynecol* 84:1010-1015, 1994.

165. Carson SA and Buster JE: Ectopic pregnancy (review). *New Engl J Med* 329:1174-1181, 1993.

166. Brown DL and Doubilet PM: Transvaginal sonography for diagnosing ectopic pregnancy, *J Ultrasound Med* 13:259-266, 1994.

167. Braffman BH, et al: Emergency department screening for ectopic pregnancy: a prospective U.S. study, *Radiology* 190:797-802, 1994.

168. Glezerman M, Press F, Carpman M: Culdocentesis is an obsolete diagnostic tool in suspected ectopic pregnancy, *Arch Gynecol Obstet* 252:5-9, 1992.

169. Weckstin LN, Boucher AR, Tucher H et al: Accurate diagnosis of early ectopic pregnancy, *Obstet Gynecol* 65:393, 1985.

170. Hockberger RS: Ectopic pregnancy, *Emerg Clin North Am* 5(3):481-493, 1987.

171. Abbot J, Emmans LS, Lowenstein SR: Ectopic pregnancy: ten common pitfalls in diagnosis, *Am J Emerg Med* 8:515-522, 1990.

172. Stromme WB, McKelvey JL, Adkins CD: Conservative surgery for ectopic pregnancy, *Obstet Gynecol* 19:249, 1962.

173. Timonen S and Nieminen U: Tubal pregnancy, choice of operative method of treatment, *Acta Obstet Gynecol Scand* 46:327, 1967.

174. Sherman D, Langer R, Sadovsky G et al: Improved fertility following ectopic pregnancy, *Fertil Steril* 37:497, 1982.

175. Miller JF, Williamson E, Blue J, et al: Fetal loss after implantation: a prospective study, *Lancet* 2:554, 1980.

176. Wolf GC et al: Completely nonsurgical management of ectopic pregnancies, *Gynecol Obstet Invest* 37:232-235, 1994.

177. Spinillo A, Fazzi E, Stronati M, et al: Early morbidity and neurodevelopmental outcome in low-birthweight infants born after third trimester bleeding, *Ann J Perinatology* 11:85-90, 1994.

## 54

Hematologic and Oncologic Disorders

David T. Bachman • Roger M. Barkin • Sharon A. Brennan • Michael Recht

Pediatric patients with hematologic and oncologic disorders frequently seek care in the emergency department. Even for the physician well-versed in the care of children their management can prove challenging.

Signs and Symptoms

ANEMIA

Children with a red cell volume or hemoglobin concentration that is below the third percentile for the patient's age group are anemic. In general, a hemoglobin level below 11 gm/dl is consistent with anemia, although there is marked age-specific variability (Fig. 54-1). Although nutritional deficiencies account for many cases of anemia in childhood, a variety of congenital and acquired forms are quite common in the pediatric population. In fact, in the United States it has been observed that the overall prevalence of iron deficiency is declining because of changes in nutrition, and that the number of children with inherited hemoglobin disorders is increasing as the result of the influx of families of Asian and African backgrounds.[1]

Pathophysiology

Maintenance of a normal hemoglobin requires an ongoing balance between red cell production and destruction. Anemia and chronic hypoxia serve as stimuli to red cell production, which is regulated by erythropoietin, a glycoprotein made by the kidneys. Inadequate erythropoiesis can result from impaired red cell production, maturation, or release from the bone marrow. Red blood cells normally have a life span of 100 to 120 days, which may be shortened by hemolysis or acute sequestration. Chronic blood loss, as can occur with peptic ulcer disease, can also lead to anemia, generally with a component of iron deficiency. That acute hemorrhage can produce anemia is self-evident; the focus in this chapter will be on other causes of anemia.

Differential Considerations

Diagnostic evaluation of the patient with anemia requires a careful review of the complete blood count with particular attention to the red blood cell indices and morphology. The peripheral smear is invaluable in evaluating the size, color, shape, and morphology of the cells (Fig. 54-2). It must be first determined using age-specific norms whether or not the child is truly anemic. A relative anemia occurs during infancy with typical hemoglobins of 10.5 gm/dl at 2 months and 11 gm/dl at 3 months. This "physiologic" anemia does not require any particular treatment or investigation. Premature infants often have a further exaggeration of anemia, with the hemoglobin falling in the normal preterm infant to as low as 8 gm/dl at 2 to 3 months of age.

Nutritional iron deficiency is the most common cause of anemia between the ages of 9 months and 2 years. Typically, it results from excessive intake of cow's milk, which may induce occult gastrointestinal blood loss, and from inadequate consumption of iron-rich foods. Iron-deficiency anemia in children over 2 years of age should be investigated for the possibility of chronic blood loss.[2] In women of childbearing age, it is typically menstrual blood loss that leads to iron depletion and anemia. When uncomplicated by the co-existence of an inherited hemoglobin disorder (e.g., thalassemia trait), iron deficiency produces a hypochromic microcytic anemia with the mean corpuscular volume (MCV) in the range of 65 to 70 fL. To establish the diagnosis, additional studies including the free erythrocyte protoporphyrin (FEP) and serum ferritin may be obtained. An FEP greater than 30 μg/dl of whole blood and a serum ferritin of less than 10 ng/ml are typical of iron deficiency. An iron saturation (serum iron/total iron-binding capac-

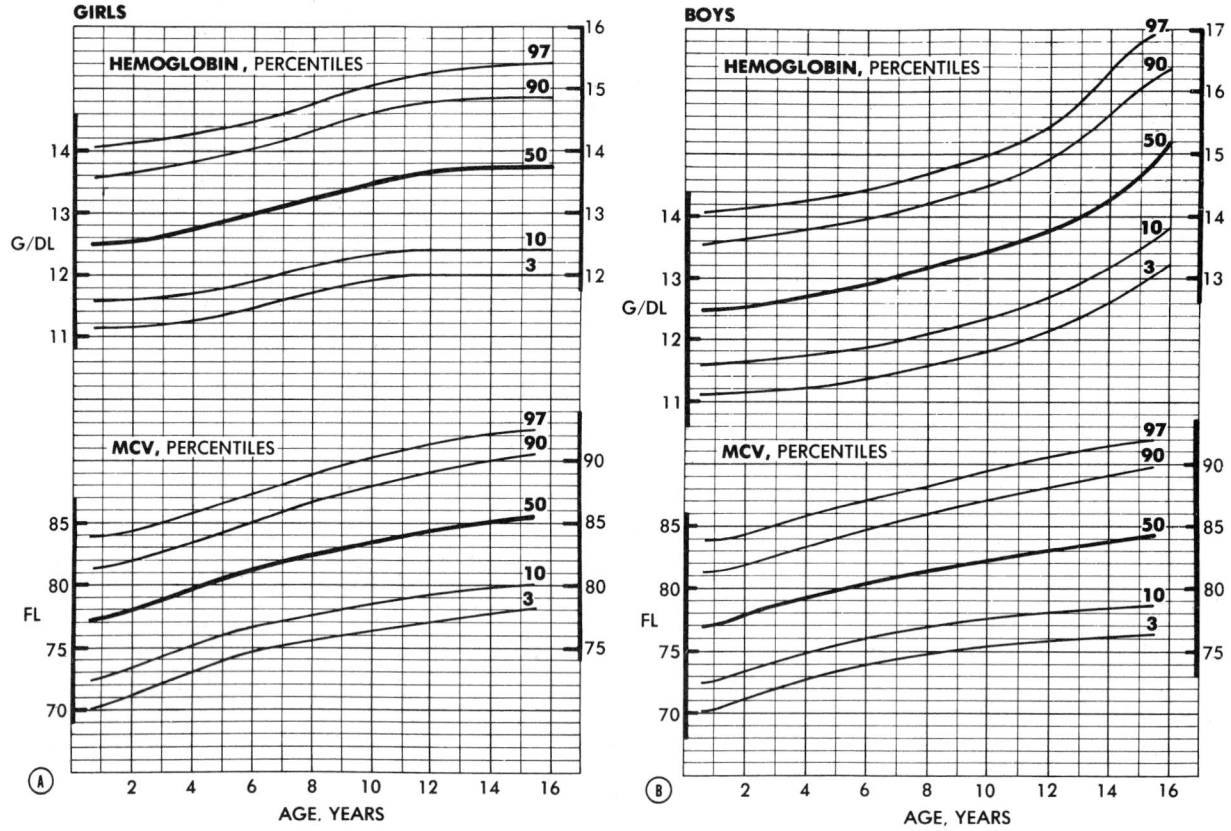

FIG. 54-1. Normal hemoglobin values by age. **A,** Hemoglobin and MCV percentile curves for girls. **B,** Hemoglobin and MCV percentile curves for boys. (*From Dallman PR and Siimes MA: J Pediatr 94:26, 1979.*)

ity × 100) of less than 20% is indicative of iron deficiency, but is subject to greater error because of the diurnal and acute dietary fluctuations in serum iron. An FEP greater than 50 to 60 µg/dl of whole blood strongly suggests lead poisoning, either alone or in combination with iron deficiency.

In asymptomatic patients with apparent iron-deficiency anemia a number of alternatives exist. The clinician may elect to do a complete diagnostic evaluation as noted above before beginning treatment. In clear-cut cases, it is acceptable to begin empiric treatment with 3 to 6 mg/kg/24 hr TID PO of *elemental iron.* The reticulocyte count should increase within 3 to 5 days, and the hemoglobin should rise after 1 week. Such a response can generally be viewed as confirmatory of the diagnosis of iron deficiency. Therapy is then continued for at least 2 to 3 months. Iron-rich foods should be encouraged, as should juices containing vitamin C, which increases iron absorption. Cow's milk should be limited to 24 ounces/day. The increasing evidence linking iron-deficiency with delays in psychomotor development in children under age 2 years strengthens the argument that iron deficiency, although rarely a problem demanding emergency department care, should be treated in a timely manner even when incidentally discovered in that setting.

Although iron deficiency ranks as the leading cause of microcytic anemia, it is hardly the only cause. Of particular importance are the thalassemias, autosomally recessive disorders marked by defective synthesis of one or more of the globin chains (see later discussion). In fact alpha-thalassemia ranks as the most common genetic disorder worldwide.[3] Thalassemia major results from a homozygous defect in globin chain production and is primarily found in Mediterranean and southeast Asian populations. Affected individuals have severe anemia, hepatosplenomegaly, jaundice, growth retardation, and abnormal development in infancy. Microcytosis and mild anemia with target cells are seen with heterozygous beta-thalassemia (thalassemia minor or thalassemia trait). A patient who is homozygous for beta-globin deficiency but produces enough hemoglobin to survive without chronic transfusions is said to have thalassemia intermedia.

Although most alpha-thalassemia syndromes are not of clinical importance, the more severe forms may result in significant pathology. There are normally 2 alpha-globin genes on each chromosome 16 (for a total of 4 alpha genes). The alpha-thalassemia syndromes result from deletions of one or more of these genes, with disease severity dependent on the number of deletions. A deletion of one gene is silent. Deletion of two genes causes alpha-thalassemia trait, which is also asymptomatic. (Of note is that in African-Americans with alpha-thalassemia trait there is usually one gene deletion on each chromosome, while in southeast Asian populations both deletions occur on the same chromosome.) Three gene deletion results in hemoglobin H disease, whereas a deletion of four genes is associated with hydrops fetalis and fetal death.[4] Deletions of

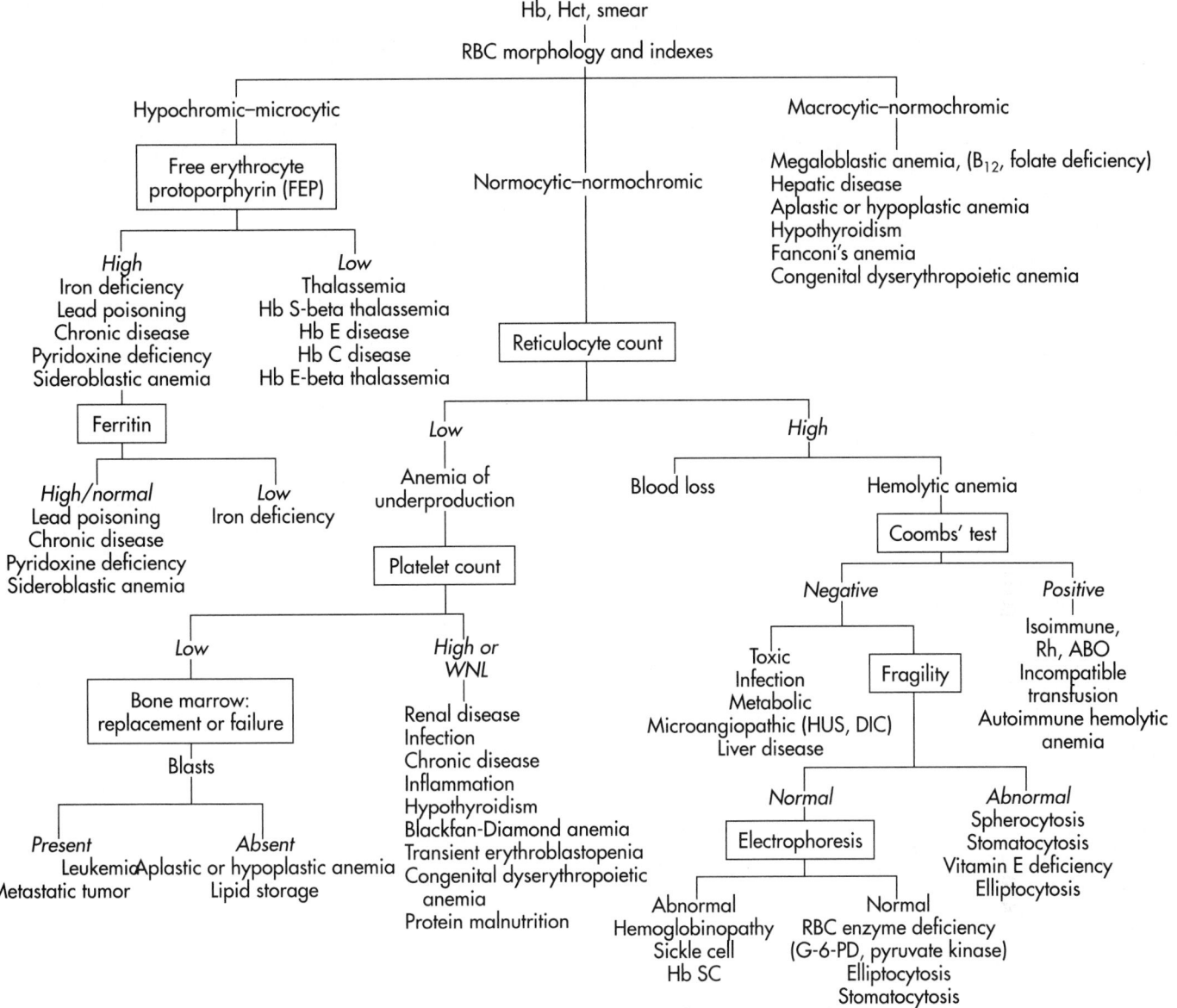

FIG. 54-2. Evaluation of anemia. (*From Barkin RM and Rosen P: Emergency pediatrics, ed 4, St Louis, 1994, Mosby.*)

three or more genes requires inheritance of at least one chromosome with deletions of both alpha genes. These disorders thus occur primarily in southeast Asian and not African-American populations. Patients with hemoglobin H disease have anemia, reticulocytosis, and splenomegaly; acute drops in hemoglobin with reticulocytopenia can occur in the setting of infection.[1]

No doubt the hemoglobinopathy of greatest clinical concern in the emergency department setting is sickle cell disease, which is discussed in detail later in this chapter. Other than when associated with beta-thalassemia trait, the red blood cells in hemoglobin SS are normocytic. Review of the smear, however, will reveal red blood cells of various sizes and shapes including sickle and target cells. Howell-Jolly bodies appear in children with nonfunctioning spleens; reticulocytosis reflective of chronic hemolytic anemia is evident as early as 3 months of age. Neonatal screen-

ing (now done in 40 states) detects most individuals with sickle cell disease. Unfortunately, sometimes the diagnosis becomes evident only in the setting of an acute complication when recognition may not always be straightforward.

Accurate diagnosis of sickle cell anemia and other hemoglobinopathies requires a hemoglobin electrophoresis, the results of which are not immediately available to the emergency physician. Clinical features including growth retardation, hepatosplenomegaly, and jaundice should suggest the possibility of a hemoglobin disorder. Review of the peripheral blood smear can help distinguish iron deficiency from the major hemoglobinopathies. The MCV/RBC ratio, termed the *Mentzer index*, can be used to distinguish iron deficiency from thalassemia minor. A ratio greater than 13.5 suggests iron deficiency; values less than 11.5 occur with thalassemia minor. The advent of automated tests for RBC indices allows calculation of the red cell distribution width (RDW), a statistical description of the heterogeneity of RBC size (calculated by dividing the standard deviation of the red cell volume by the MCV and then multiplying by 100). Normal values are less than 14. Higher values occur with iron deficiency and the more severe hemoglobinopathies, particularly with a significant reticulocytosis. With thalassemia traits, the RDW is normal, unless there is co-existing iron deficiency.[1,5]

Hematologic changes suggestive of sickle cell disease occur as early as 10 weeks of age, with mean hemoglobins of 9.3 gm/dl in one large cohort study.[6] A persistent and rising reticulocytosis also becomes evident in infancy, with mean percentages ranging from 4.0% to 6.7% in the first year of life. In one study, the sensitivity of a reticulocyte count >2% for the detection of sickle cell anemia was 93%. A high reticulocyte count combined with anemia and abnormal RBC morphology was 99% sensitive.[7]

Normocytic, normochromic anemia occurs in a number of different settings in childhood, including recent blood loss without iron deficiency, transient erythroblastopenia of childhood (TEC), and anemia of chronic disease. The role of even relatively mild infections in producing transient anemia has been increasingly apparent in recent years.[1,8] It is thought that the inflammatory response accompanying febrile illnesses of more than 3 days duration can significantly alter iron metabolism and thus affect erythropoiesis. The resultant anemia can persist for a month or more. It is preferred, then, that a child be screened for anemia when well. More severe and prolonged anemia is seen with TEC, now recognized as a common cause of normocytic, normochromic anemia in otherwise healthy children aged 6 months to 6 years.[9,10] In TEC there is a temporary failure of erythropoiesis, most likely on an autoimmune basis, which results in the slow development of anemia. The manifestations include pallor and symptoms of anemia. Only rarely will the child have hypovolemic shock.[11] The CBC is notable for a normocytic anemia, often profound, with reticulocytopenia, a normal leukocyte count, and a normal or occasionally elevated platelet count. Bone marrow examination, which may be necessary for diagnosis, is normal except for a paucity of erythroid precursors. Differential considerations include the Blackfan-Diamond syndrome, acute hemolysis, and acute leukemia. Treatment is limited to RBC transfusions in severe cases. Recovery usually occurs spontaneously within a few weeks.

Anemia of chronic disease, another form of normocytic normochromic anemia, accompanies a number of pediatric infectious and inflammatory disorders (e.g., osteomyelitis and autoimmune diseases). Normocytic normochromic anemia also occurs with renal disease and endocrinopathies. Bone marrow infiltration from malignancy or storage disease impairs production of red blood cells; a normocytic anemia with the characteristic form of a teardrop is observed.

Hemolytic anemias, both congenital and acquired, are relatively commonplace in the pediatric population. Abnormalities of the erythrocyte membrane result in chronic hemolysis in individuals with hereditary spherocytosis, in which transmission occurs in an autosomal dominant pattern in 80% of cases. Clinical features may include splenomegaly, pigmentary gallstones, anemia with hemoglobin

levels of 6 to 10 gm/dl, reticulocytosis, and hyperbilirubinemia. Some patients are well-compensated with higher hemoglobin levels. Examination of the blood smear and review of the family history are important diagnostic features; osmotic fragility studies are confirmatory. Unlike acquired autoimmune hemolytic anemias, in which spherocytes can also be evident on the peripheral smear, the direct Coombs' test is negative in hereditary spherocytosis. Serious complications are relatively infrequent; aplastic crises (generally associated with parvovirus infections) rank as the most serious. Splenectomy is curative, but is generally delayed until the child has reached age 5 or 6 with the hope of minimizing the risk of overwhelming postsplenectomy sepsis.[9] Hereditary elliptocytosis is another autosomal dominant erythrocyte membrane defect. It is of less clinical importance in that significant hemolysis occurs in only 10% of affected individuals.

Inherited abnormalities of erythrocyte enzymes can also result in hemolytic anemias. Of importance is glucose-6-phosphate dehydrogenase (G6PD) deficiency, which for the most part comes to clinical attention only when infections or certain drugs precipitate acute hemolysis. (For further discussion see Specific Anemias.) Other inherited enzyme disorders do occur (e.g., pyruvate kinase deficiency), but only infrequently come to the attention of the emergency physician.

Acquired autoimmune hemolytic anemia is rare during infancy but is a common cause of acquired anemia after the first year of life. Some cases occur in the setting of clinically distinct entities (e.g., infectious mononucleosis); others follow less well-defined infections. On occasion, drugs, including commonly used antimicrobials (penicillins, cephalosporins, sulfonamides), can trigger hemolysis via immune-complex formation.[12] Secondary cases of autoimmune hemolytic anemia may accompany diseases such as systemic lupus erythematosus and malignancies (e.g., Hodgkin disease and leukemia). The onset of anemia can be quite precipitous, with pallor, jaundice, and hemoglobinuria. The red blood cell indices are usually normal to macrocytic due to a prominent reticulocytosis. Spherocytes and nucleated red blood cells are seen on the peripheral smear. The direct Coombs' test is positive, indicative of the role of antibodies on the red blood cells in the hemolytic process. In idiopathic cases, the prognosis is generally favorable, with corticosteroids being of greatest initial benefit (starting dose: prednisone, 2 to 4 mg/kg per day).

Microangiopathic hemolytic anemia occurs in the setting of disseminated intravascular coagulation (DIC), vascular anomalies, cardiac defects, or platelet activation as seen in the hemolytic uremic syndrome (HUS) and thrombotic thrombocytopenia purpura (TTP). In addition to manifestations of hemolysis, the clinical features will include those of the underlying disorder (e.g., thrombocytopenia and renal dysfunction in HUS and TTP). Schistocytes and other fragmented erythrocyte forms are prominent on the peripheral smear.

Another cause of anemia of increasing importance in childhood is HIV infection.[13] Nearly all HIV-infected children are anemic to some degree right from the onset of their disease. The anemia can result both from a direct effect of the HIV virus on stem cells and from the production of autoantibodies leading to peripheral hemolysis. Pancytopenia is common. It is worthwhile, then, to consider the possibility of HIV infection when evaluating an anemic child and to inquire about the recognized risk factors.

Megaloblastic anemia results from defective DNA synthesis because of a lack of the coenzyme forms of vitamin B_{12} and folic acid. The cells are macrocytic, with the MCV greater than 100 fL. Macrocytosis can result from extreme reticulocytosis or may be an early sign of congenital hypoplastic anemia (Blackfan-Diamond syndrome) or congenital aplastic anemia (Fanconi syndrome). Overall, these forms of anemia are of less importance to the emergency physician.

Finally, brief mention should be made of the sideroblastic anemias, in which various defects in porphyrin synthesis result in hypochromic anemia. The disorders are typified by the presence of ringed sideroblasts, abnormal erythroid precursors, which are evident on bone marrow examination. Of the sideroblastic anemias, the one resulting from lead toxicity is of greatest importance in the pediatric age group. In addition to hypochromia, microcytosis and basophilic stippling of the erythrocytes are generally evident on the peripheral smear.[14] The FEP will be markedly elevated. Direct measurements of the serum lead level are confirmatory.

Diagnostic Work-Up and Initial Management

When evaluating a child with anemia, the physician must determine whether or not anemia is acute or chronic, diagnostic studies are indicated, and if immediate transfusion is necessary (see Fig. 54-2). Consultation with a hematologist is strongly encouraged in problematic cases. The history should take into account the child's age, ethnic background, family history, and diet. Constitutional symptoms such as pallor, fatigue, and dizziness should be noted. With rapid onset of anemia, evidence of intravascular deficit may include headache, dizziness, postural hypotension, tachycardia, and high-output cardiac failure. Details regarding antecedent illnesses and growth and development are also of importance. If HIV infection is a consideration, risk factors should be assessed.

On physical examination, evidence of cardiovascular instability should be sought, paying particular attention to the vital signs, orthostatic changes, capillary refill, cardiac function, and mental status. Pallor, petechiae, purpura, and ecchymoses must be noted, as should lymphadenopathy, splenomegaly, hepatomegaly, and blood in the stool. Evidence of systemic or underlying disease must be documented.

Ancillary Data. The initial laboratory data should include a CBC with hemoglobin, hematocrit, and RBC indices. The white blood cell and platelet counts, peripheral smear, and reticulocyte count should be obtained. Indices (mean corpuscular volume and mean corpuscular hemoglobin) are particularly useful in defining the differential considerations. The RDW can also be of value, as was discussed previously.

In many instances, additional studies will be needed for accurate diagnosis. The actual studies needed will be dictated by the clinical scenario. Studies to consider include stool for occult blood, iron studies, free erythrocyte protoporphyrin, serum lead, a Coombs' test (direct and indirect), screens for hemolysis (serum bilirubin, LDH, and haptoglobin), folate or B_{12} levels, osmotic fragility studies, and hemoglobin electrophoresis. On occasion, screens for autoimmune disease will be needed. In the febrile or immunocompromised child, blood and urine cultures and chest radiographs will also be indicated. A bone marrow examination will be necessary in certain acute cases when the risk of systemic or invasive disease is high.

Blood Transfusions. When caring for an anemic child, the emergency physician is obligated to determine if immediate transfusion is necessary. Obviously, care must always be taken first to obtain all required diagnostic blood studies unless the urgency of the situation dictates otherwise. It is well-recognized that hemoglobin levels of less than 3 gm/dl may lead to high-output cardiac failure and death, especially if anemia develops rapidly; transfusion is essentially mandated for all such extremely anemic patients.[15] Above that level there is no absolute hemoglobin value that can be considered as an automatic indication for transfusion—although it is accepted that many patients with a hemoglobin of less than 7 gm/dl will require transfusion (the need for transfusion is less imperative in those patients with chronic anemia of that level). In deciding when to transfuse, it is necessary to take into account both the nature of the anemia (acute or chronic, stable or progressive) and the condition of the patient. When there is evidence of cardiopulmonary compromise or tissue hypoxia, transfusion must be strongly considered even with hemoglobin levels of greater than 7 gm/dl.

Of equal importance as the decision to transfuse an anemic child is the actual rate of transfusion, particularly in the severely anemic child (Hgb <5 gm/dl). Overzealous transfusion can lead to circulatory overload and outright cardiac failure. One accepted approach is to administer multiple transfusions of 3 to 5 ml/kg of packed red blood cells (PRBC), with each transfusion occurring over 3 to 4 hours and separated from the next by several hours. An alternative approach suggested by one study is to transfuse PRBC at a rate of 2 ml/kg/hr continuously until the desired volume has been administered.[16] The latter protocol was used successfully with 22 children with severe anemia of varying etiologies (but not sickle cell anemia with sequestration, which requires more rapid correction). As a group, they were transfused from an initial mean hemoglobin of 3.5 gm/dl to a mean posttransfusion level of 11.2 gm/dl; no patient developed evidence of congestive heart failure. For the patient with evidence of severe anemia and heart failure, concomitant diuretic administration or partial exchange transfusion rather than either of the approaches described before will be necessary.

NEUTROPENIA

Most often while pursuing a fever evaluation, but occasionally while treating a noninfectious condition, the emergency physician may discover that a child is leukopenic (total WBC <5000/mm³). Generally, neutropenia will be the issue (defined as an absolute neutrophil count [ANC] <1500/mm³, with the ANC = WBC × [% bands + % neutrophils] × 0.01). Of importance is recognizing when the neutropenia is of immediate clinical significance, that is, when further investigation is needed and when antibiotic treatment is warranted.

Pathophysiology

Neutropenia, like anemia, can result from an abnormality in either the production or destruction of white blood cells. The degree of neutropenia can be stratified as mild (ANC of 1000 to 1500/mm³), moderate (ANC 500 to 1000/mm³), or severe (ANC <500/mm³). Such a stratification is most useful in defining risk of infection, particularly in immunocompromised patients. In this group of patients, it is recognized that the likelihood of infection correlates inversely with the ANC, with the greatest susceptibility being to infections caused by gram-negative organisms and *Staphylococcus aureus*. It is important in caring for the pediatric patient to distinguish the intrinsic (congenital) forms of neutropenia from the acquired ones.[17,18]

Differential Considerations

Most congenital neutropenias are diagnosed in early infancy, either as the result of phenotypic abnormalities (e.g., dwarfism in Schwachman-Diamond syndrome) or because of repeated infections (e.g., severe congenital neutropenia or combined immune deficiencies). When febrile, such patients will generally require hospitalization for broad-spectrum antibiotic coverage. There is a form of congenital neutropenia with a lower risk of infection, so-called chronic benign neutropenia. In addition, an alloimmune neutropenia mediated by maternal IgG can occur in newborns; resolution by the age of 2 months is the rule.

Of greater importance to the emergency physician are the acquired forms of neutropenia. It is important to attempt to distinguish those neutropenic children who have an obvious underlying disease from those who do not. Is there evidence of sepsis as the cause of the neutropenia? Does the physical examination or CBC suggest an aplastic anemia or the possibility of a malignancy involving the bone marrow, either primarily or via metastases? Or has the child become neutropenic as the result of chemotherapy for a known malignancy? Are there risk factors suggestive of HIV infection, the hematologic manifestations of which can include leukopenia, neutropenia, and lymphopenia?[13,19] Are there features suggestive of a systemic autoimmune disorder, such as systemic lupus erythematosus or rheumatoid arthritis? Or is there evidence of any of a number of the other childhood infections associated with neutropenia? The latter include mononucleosis, influenza, measles, varicella, hepatitis A and B, and RSV as well as bacterial infections such as typhoid and tuberculosis.

When there is no evidence of an underlying disease, consideration must be given to the possibility of neutropenia occurring either on an immune basis, from exposure to a drug, or, by default, idiopathically. Cases of autoimmune neutropenia are well-described; circulating antineutrophil antibodies have been identified. The prognosis is favorable with infectious complications limited to skin infections, otitis media, and upper respiratory processes responsive to routine antibiotic therapy. Drugs, including commonly prescribed antiinflammatories, antibiotics, and anticonvulsants (phenytoin), can induce neutropenia via imprecisely de-

fined, idiosyncratic mechanisms. The rate of recovery is variable, ranging from days to months to years.

Ancillary Data

Often, a CBC with differential will be the only study needed on the immediate basis unless symptoms or signs suggestive of an underlying disorder are present. If the neutropenia is felt to have resulted from a viral process, reexamination and a repeat CBC in 2 to 3 days are warranted. Resolution of the neutropenia may already be evident by that time. Of note is that the presence of significant monocytosis suggests chronic neutropenia. More complicated cases require hematologic consultation for consideration of bone marrow examination or more specialized testing of immune function.

Management

For many children with neutropenia, management will be dictated by the nature of the congenital or underlying process. Management is also straightforward for the otherwise healthy, afebrile child with isolated neutropenia. Such patients require no emergent interventions; close outpatient follow-up with weekly CBCs is adequate. All nonessential drugs should be discontinued. A bit more problematic is the well-appearing, previously healthy child who is found to be neutropenic during an acute febrile illness. Current evidence suggests that the risks of serious infectious complications in such a child are minimal, and that outpatient management is adequate.[20-22] Neither extensive laboratory studies nor empiric antibiotic therapy is indicated. This low risk of infectious complications apparently even extends to febrile infants under 8 weeks of age. In one study, 7% (70/1000) of febrile infants were found to be neutropenic. Only one had a bacterial process identified (*Salmonella enteris*). The remainder had either aseptic meningitis (6 cases) or a presumed or proven viral syndrome (63 cases).[23] These findings suggest that considerations other than the presence of neutropenia alone should guide management of the febrile infant.

THROMBOCYTOPENIA

Thrombocytopenia is not uncommon in pediatric emergency department patients, and its causes are many.[24,25] Mechanisms of thrombocytopenia include increased platelet destruction, decreased platelet production, and platelet sequestration (see box on p. 903). The practitioner must obviously rely on features of the history and physical examination and the results of the complete blood count so as to narrow an otherwise broad differential diagnosis. One common cause, idiopathic thrombocytopenia purpura, is discussed at length later in this chapter.

BLEEDING DISORDERS

Bleeding occurs in children as the result of trauma and numerous congenital or acquired conditions.

Pathophysiology

Physiologic hemostasis involves a fine balance between coagulation and fibrinolysis. This balance depends on the normal function of multiple interrelated systems, notably the vascular endothelium, platelets, coagulation factors, the

Causes of Thrombocytopenia

Sequestration
Splenomegaly

Increased destruction of platelets
Immune
Idiopathic thrombocytopenia purpura
HIV associated
Systemic lupus erythematosus
Evans syndrome
Alloimmune thrombocytopenia

Microangiopathy
Sepsis
Disseminated intravascular coagulation
Necrotizing enterocolitis
Giant hemangiomas (Kasabach-Merritt syndrome)

Drug associated
Heparin
Quinidine
Valproic acid
Others

Platelet activation
Hemolytic uremic syndrome
Thrombotic thrombocytopenia purpura

Decreased production of platelets
Marrow infiltration
Leukemia, lymphoma, certain solid tumors
Granulomas
Storage diseases
Myelofibrosis

Marrow dysfunction—congenital
Wiskott-Aldrich syndrome
TAR (thrombocytopenia, absent radii) syndrome
Amegakaryocytic thrombocytopenia
Congenital giant platelet syndromes

Infections - viral, such as HIV

Drugs
Cytotoxic (chemotherapeutic agents)
Antibiotics (sulfa, rifampin, chloramphenicol)
Others

Aplastic anemia
Idiopathic
Posthepatitis
Toxin induced
Congenital: Fanconi syndrome, dyskeratosis
    congenita, etc.

From Goebel RA: Thrombocytopenia, *Emerg Med Clin North Am*
11:445-463, 1993.

fibrinolytic system, and anticlotting mechanisms.[26,27] The endothelial cells lining the vessels are an important barrier to macromolecules. Platelets serve to stop bleeding initially; fibrin clot formation follows as a result of activation of the plasma protein coagulation pathways (Fig. 54-3). The intrinsic, extrinsic, and common pathways are modulated by control proteins and anticoagulants, thus preventing generalized thrombosis.

Differential Considerations

When a patient has a bleeding disorder, the nature of the bleeding relative to preceding injury will hold clues to the underlying pathophysiology (Table 54-1).[28] Abnormalities of primary hemostasis (platelet plug formation) typically cause petechiae, ecchymoses, mucous membrane bleeding, and immediate perioperative hemorrhage. When secondary hemostasis (fibrin polymerization) is abnormal, delayed bleeding after injury or surgery is characteristic.

Diagnostic Work-Up

A careful patient and family history is essential. A history of excessive bleeding after procedures such as circumcision, tonsillectomy, or tooth extraction may be helpful. Patients may also report a history of menorrhagia or epistaxis. In addition, recent use of drugs or foods that interfere with platelet function should be determined (the most common of these being aspirin and nonsteroidal antiinflammatory agents). The patient's hemodynamic status should be assessed and resuscitation initiated if the patient is unstable. The site, extent, and nature of the bleed should be determined. If bruises or bleeding are unexplained or inconsistent with the history and examination, the possibility of child abuse should be considered.[29,30]

Ancillary Data. Initial laboratory studies should include a CBC with differential and review of the peripheral smear, a platelet count, and other assays as clinically indicated by the patient's history and physical. These labs may include a bleeding time, PT, PTT, fibrinogen, fibrin split/degradation products (FDP), and D-dimers, as well as specific factor and cofactor levels. Clinical conditions and the laboratory abnormalities associated with them are presented in Table 54-2.

The CBC provides an assessment of the degree of blood loss although the actual loss may not be reflected immediately in a decrease in hematocrit. Patients with platelet counts below 20,000/mm³ are at higher risk of significant spontaneous bleeding. The actual level of risk varies somewhat with the underlying condition and the age of the platelets. For example, the risk of hemorrhage is usually greater in a leukemia patient with a platelet count of 20,000/mm³ than in a child with idiopathic thrombocytopenic purpura (ITP) with the same platelet count. In ITP the circulating platelets are younger and thus more physiologically active; the risk of hemorrhage is relatively low even when the count is as low as 3,000 to 4,000 platelets/mm³. Obviously, the platelet count does not reflect function.[28]

Evaluation of the coagulation pathways includes several specific assays. Assessment of the extrinsic and common pathway requires measurement of the prothrombin time (PT), whereas the intrinsic and common pathways are evaluated using the partial thromboplastin time (PTT). Hemophilia A and B cause elevation of only the PTT.[30] The

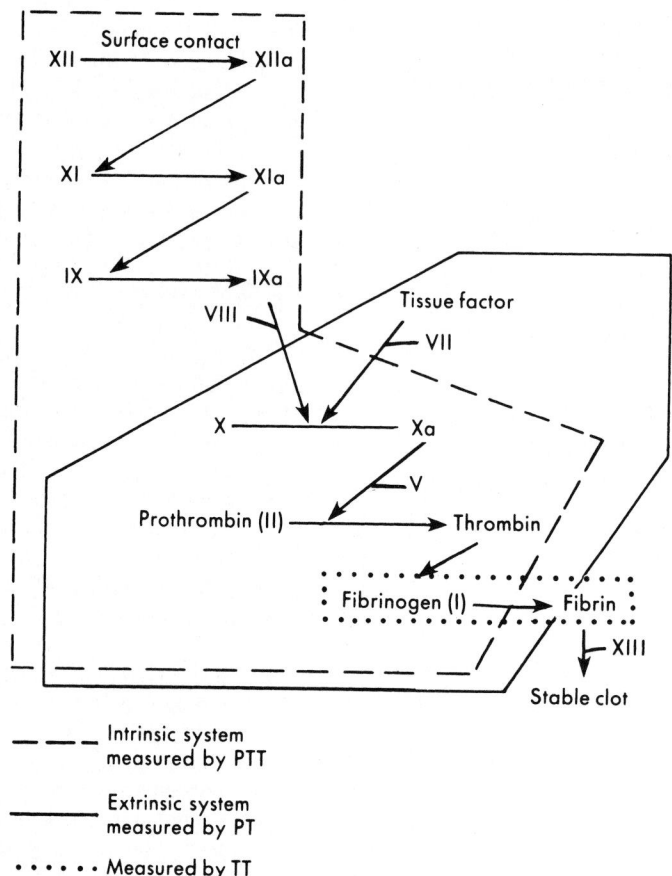

FIG. 54-3. Blood coagulation scheme. (*From Barkin RM and Rosen P:* Emergency pediatrics, *ed 4, St Louis, 1994, Mosby.*)

TABLE 54-1. Patterns of Bleeding

Diagnostic findings	Small vessel hemostasis defect (platelet or capillary)	Intravascular defect (coagulation)
Bleeding pattern		
Spontaneous	Small, superficial, diffuse bleeding involving mucous membranes (epistaxis, GI, menorrhagia)	Major bleeding (musculoskeletal, CNS)
Superficial cut or abrasion	Profuse, prolonged	Minimal
Deep cut or tooth extraction	Immediate; good response to pressure	Delayed; poor response to pressure
Hemarthrosis	Rare	Common
Petechiae	Common	Rare
Ancillary data	Prolonged BT Abnormal platelets	Prolonged PTT, PT

bleeding time assesses vascular integrity and platelet function. It is a standardized test requiring an incision of 1 mm deep × 1 cm long on the volar aspect of the forearm; during this time the arm is held by a blood pressure cuff at 40 mm Hg. The time is measured until the blood from the wound is no longer absorbed by a filter paper. The normal time is less than 9 minutes; a bleeding time longer than 10 minutes is abnormal.[31] The plasma fibrinogen level reflects a balance of production and consumption of fibrinogen and may be decreased by impaired production, liver dysfunc-

tion, or overconsumption. Fibrinogen production is increased in inflammatory diseases and during pregnancy. Specific factor levels may be measured by coagulation based or chromogenic assays. Inhibitor screening tests may be useful in hemophilic patients in whom antibodies may prolong the normal plasma clotting process.

Therapeutic Trial

If the patient is hemodynamically stable, a trial of direct pressure at the site of bleeding should be attempted. If the

TABLE 54-2. Screening of the Bleeding Patient

Condition	Screening tests					Comments
	Platelet count	BT	PTT	PT	TT	
Normal (WNL) (varies with lab)	150-400,000/mm^3	4-9 min	25-35 sec	12-13 sec	8-10 sec	Fibrinogen 190-400 mg/dl
Hereditary disorders Hemophilia						
Factor VIII (Classic: A)	WNL	WNL	↑	WNL	WNL	Factor assay
Factor IX (Christmas: B)	WNL	WNL	↑	WNL	WNL	Factor assay
Factor XI	WNL	WNL	↑	WNL	WNL	Factor assay
Factor XII	WNL	WNL	↑	WNL	WNL	Factor assay
Factor II, V, X	WNL	WNL	↑	↑	WNL	Factor assay
Factor VII	WNL	WNL	WNL	↑	WNL	Factor assay
von Willebrand (many variants)	WNL	↑	WNL/↑	WNL	WNL	vWF antigen, vWF activity, ristocetin cofactor
Platelet dysfunction	WNL/↓	↑	WNL	WNL	WNL	Platelet aggregation studies
Acquired disorders						
DIC	↓	↑	↑	↑	↑	↓ fibrinogen, ↑ fibrin split products, ↑ D-dimer
ITP	↓	↑	WNL	WNL	WNL	
HSP	WNL	WNL	WNL	WNL	WNL	
HUS, TTP	↓	Varies with platelet count	WNL	WNL	WNL	Microangiopathic hemolytic anemia; renal failure
Liver failure (severe)	WNL/↓	WNL/↑	↑	↑	WNL/↑	↓ fibrinogen, ↑ fibrin split products
Uremia	WNL	↑	WNL	WNL	WNL/↑	
Anticoagulants						
Heparin	WNL	WNL	↑	WNL/↑	↑ ↑	
Coumadin	WNL	WNL	WNL/↑	↑	WNL	
Aspirin, other NSAID	WNL	↑	WNL	WNL	WNL	

HSP, Henoch-Schönlein purpura; *HUS,* hemolytic uremic syndrome; *TTP,* thrombotic thrombocytopenia purpura.

bleeding is minor, further therapy may not be needed. If bleeding persists or is significant, additional therapy will be necessary, with the choice of components dependent on the underlying process.

MANIFESTATIONS OF COMMON CHILDHOOD MALIGNANCIES

Childhood malignancies are uncommon with an estimated incidence of only 10 to 12 cases per 100,000 children per year. On the other hand, cancer ranks only behind injury as a cause of death in children aged 1 to 14 years. For the most part, visits of the pediatric patient to the emergency department derive from complications of the primary disease or treatment (see discussion later in this chapter). Only infrequently will the emergency department physician have the opportunity to make the initial diagnosis of a malignancy in a child or adolescent.

In a retrospective study, only 16 of 220 (7.3%) children with newly diagnosed malignancies first sought medical attention in the emergency department.[32] Overall, these children represented only 1 out of every 4,500 emergency department visits in this particular facility. In keeping with relative frequency of various malignancies in childhood, 7 of the 16 patients were diagnosed with leukemia, 4 with CNS tumors, and 5 with non-CNS solid tumors. Leukemia most commonly occurred with pallor and lassitude as well as hepatomegaly, petechiae or ecchymoses, fever, tachycardia, or an abnormal CBC. Children with CNS tumors were noted to have headache, vomiting, fever, or balance problems. A delay in diagnosing brain tumors occurred. Children with non-CNS solid tumors had symptoms related to the location of their neoplasm.

Common appearance of symptoms may be nonspecific initially (Table 54-3).[33] For example, although musculoskeletal injuries are common in adolescents, persistent bone or joint pain should prompt consideration of leukemia, neuroblastoma, and bone tumors as alternative diagnoses. Similarly, lymphomas often occur as cervical masses;

TABLE 54-3. Manifestations of Common Childhood Malignancies[33]

Malignancy	Common manifestations
Leukemia	Anorexia, lethargy, fever (25%)
	Bruising, epistaxis, gingival bleeding
	Pallor
	Splenomegaly (67%), diffuse lymphadenopathy
	Bone, joint, back pain, joint swelling
	CBC abnormalities
Lymphoma	Lymphadenopathy (cervical, supraclavicular, axillary)
	Night sweats, fever, weight loss, anorexia, fatigue
	Anterior mediastinal mass with tracheal shift or compression (stridor, orthopnea, dyspnea), superior vena cava obstruction
	Abdominal pain, swelling, ascites
CNS tumor	Diffuse or occipital headache, worse in morning, may awaken patient from sleep, often with vomiting
	Neurologic findings (up to 95%): may include pupil abnormalities, changes in acuity and visual fields, papilledema, nystagmus, motor or sensory abnormalities, polydipsia, ataxia, tremors
	Seizures
	Macrocephaly (infants)
Neuroblastoma	Nodular abdominal mass
	Posterior mediastinal mass +/− spinal cord compression (may present with torticollis, scoliosis)
	Pallor, irritability, weight loss
	Chronic diarrhea, flushing, hypertension, tachycardia (from increased catecholamines)
	Periorbital ecchymosis, proptosis (orbital)
	Opsoclonus-myoclonus (may be initial symptom)
	Bone pain
Nephroblastoma (Wilms' tumor)	Abdominal mass, +/− vomiting, pain
	Gross hematuria, hypertension
Bone tumors	Painful limp, bone pain (worse at night)
	Pleural effusion, pneumothorax (pulmonary metastases)
	Weight loss, anorexia, malaise, fever (especially with Ewing tumor)
Retinoblastoma	Leukoria (60%), strabismus, decreased acuity, dilated pupil
Rhabdomyosarcoma (Head and neck)	Periorbital edema, proptosis, ptosis, cranial nerve abnormalities
	Chronic nasal congestion, recurrent epistaxis
	Ear pain, chronic otorrhea
	Neck mass, stridor

close follow-up and consideration of biopsy are suggested whenever apparent lymphadenitis fails to respond to conventional antibiotic therapy. Children with persistent headaches, especially when associated with vomiting, merit a thorough neurologic examination and, in many instances, CT (or MRI) studies must be performed so as to exclude a CNS tumor as the cause.

Diagnostic Entities

SPECIFIC ANEMIAS

Glucose-6-Phosphate Dehydrogenase Deficiency

Oxidative damage to circulating RBCs is principally prevented by the actions of four reducing enzymes, of which G6PD is the most important clinically. The gene for G6PD is x-linked and is polymorphic; more than 400 variants have been described. G6PD deficiency affects an estimated 200 to 400 million people worldwide. The prevalence rates among individuals of Mediterranean, Middle Eastern, and tropical African and Asian background vary from 5% to 25%. Deficiency due to the presence of an unstable isoenzyme called G6PDA$^-$ occurs in 11% of African-Americans. Despite these high prevalence rates, the likelihood of an affected individual suffering any clinical consequences is quite low.[12,34-36]

Although the enzyme is found in all cells, it is anemia that is the most frequent manifestation of G6PD deficiency. Deficiency of the enzyme increases the susceptibility of the RBC to oxidative stress and hemolysis. It is the older erythrocytes that are most subject to hemolysis as the activity of the enzyme declines with the increasing age of the RBC. Hemolysis occurs only in certain circumstances, notably following infection, after exposure to certain drugs, and after ingestion of fava beans. Severe hyperbilirubinemia requiring exchange transfusion can occur during the neonatal period (generally observed only in certain parts of the world, notably Greece).

Although it was drug-induced hemolysis (by primaquine) that first brought G6PD deficiency to clinical attention, infections are now thought to be the leading cause of hemolysis in affected individuals. Viral infections, including upper respiratory and gastrointestinal illnesses, appear to be particularly important in children. Pneumonia, infectious hepatitis, and typhoid fever are frequent precipitants; numerous other bacterial, viral, and rickettsial processes have been implicated.

The role of drugs as precipitants of acute anemia in G6PD deficient individuals is well-recognized, although there has often been confusion about which drugs are actually capable of inducing hemolysis. For an exhaustive listing, the reader is referred to Beutler's review.[35] Among the drugs to be avoided in G6PD deficiency are the following: ciprofloxacin, furazolidone (Furoxone), methylene blue, nalidixic acid, naphthalene (mothballs), nitrofurantoin, phenazopyridine (Pyridium), primaquine, sulfacetamide, and sulfamethoxazole. (Susceptibility to sulfamethoxazole, a component of Bactrim and Septra, is limited to the Asian variant of G6PD and does not occur in African-Americans with more common G6PDA⁻ variant.) Drugs that can be safely administered in the setting of G6PD deficiency include acetaminophen, aspirin, diphenhydramine, phenytoin, quinidine, sulfisoxazole, and trimethoprim among many others. Many of these agents had previously been implicated as precipitants. As a general rule, reference to standard drug references is recommended before prescribing any drug to an individual with known G6PD deficiency.

Another important precipitant is the fava bean, a staple in many Mediterranean diets. Not all individuals with G6PD deficiency will develop hemolysis following ingestion of uncooked fava beans, but hemolysis, when it does occur, can be quite severe and even fatal. It can occur even in breastfed infants whose mothers have eaten the beans.

The clinical manifestations are essentially those of the other hemolytic anemias, with onset of pallor, jaundice, and hemoglobinuria within 24 to 48 hours of exposure to a precipitant. Examination of the peripheral smear will reveal reticulocytosis and bite cells. Heinz bodies (denatured protein particles adherent to the RBC membrane) can be seen with special staining. Quantitative assays of G6PD are necessary to confirm the diagnosis. False-negative results can be obtained following hemolytic episodes because the surviving erythrocytes are disproportionately younger cells higher in enzyme activity. Treatment consists of removing the inciting agent and transfusing packed RBCs. In most instances, the latter are not necessary as the hemolytic process is self-limited. Folate supplementation for several weeks after an acute hemolytic episode is recommended.

Sickle Cell Disease

Sickle cell disease is an inherited disease of hemoglobin synthesis resulting from a single amino acid substitution (valine for glutamate) in the beta-globin chain of the hemoglobin molecule. Gene carriage is approximately 8% in African-Americans, with homozygous (SS) disease occurring in 0.15% of African-American newborns. On occasion sickle syndromes may be seen in individuals from the

TABLE 54-4. Hematologic Values in Sickle Cell Anemia

	Normal values	Sickle cell (SS) disease	
		Average	Range
Hemoglobin (gm/dl)	12	7.5	5.5-9.5
Hematocrit (%)	36	22	17-29
Reticulocytes (%)	1.5	12	5-30
WBC count (/mm³)	7,500	20,000	12,000-35,000

From Pearson HA and Diamond LK: In Smith CA, editor: *The critically ill child*, Philadelphia, 1985, WB Saunders.

Mediterranean, Middle East, and India. Antenatal detection is now possible, and newborn screening is routinely done in many states. Important heterozygote variants include the sickle-beta thalassemia and hemoglobin SC, conditions of variable severity. Sickle trait (heterozygous hemoglobin SA) is rarely of clinical consequence other than under conditions of severe hypoxia.[37-39]

Baseline hematologic values for individual patients with sickle cell disease vary and are particularly important in the evaluation of acute problems (Table 54-4). The anemia is normocytic with multiple target and sickle cells and abnormal shapes. The number of sickle forms seen on the peripheral blood smear does not reflect the degree of in vivo sickling, which depends upon oxygenation and hydration. Nucleated red blood cells may be present. The hemoglobin is usually between 7 and 10 gm/dl and may drop as low as 3 gm/dl during aplastic crises. The reticulocyte count is elevated.[39]

The sickling process occurs with local tissue hypoxia, dehydration, acidosis, and hypertonicity. The abnormal sickled cells are less deformable and produce thromboses and obstruction of small vessels with subsequent infarcts. Painful crises and functional asplenia result. Because high levels of fetal hemoglobin are present following delivery and the beta-hemoglobin chain is not usually predominant until after 3 months of age, symptoms are usually delayed until 6 to 12 months of life. Hematologic changes indicative of the disorder become evident as early as 10 weeks of age (see discussion under Anemia earlier in this chapter).

The clinical course is one of chronic illness with acute exacerbations ("crises") that threaten the life and comfort of the patient (Table 54-5).[40,41] Life expectancy has dramatically increased in the last 30 years, with 50% of patients surviving beyond the fifth decade. Of note is that one third of deaths occur during acute crisis in individuals clinically free of organ failure. Specifically, deaths result from painful crises, the acute chest syndrome, and cerebrovascular events.[42,43] Infection remains the leading cause of death in early childhood, with a peak incidence in children aged 1 to 3 years. For children aged 10 to 20 years, cerebrovascular accidents and trauma rank as the leading causes of death. Deaths in children also continue to occur as the result of acute chest syndrome as well as aplastic and splenic sequestration crises.[44]

Diagnostic Findings. In general, when evaluating a patient with sickle cell disease, it is obviously crucial to consider the pattern of past events, the current status of the

TABLE 54-5. Sickle Cell Disease: Diagnostic Findings

Category	Infant (5 mo-5 yr)	Child (5-12 yr)	Adolescent (13-18 yr)	Management
Vasoocclusive	Dactylitis			Pain control, hydrate
		Painful crisis	→	Pain control, hydrate
		Stroke	→	Hospitalize, hydrate, and replace sickle cells with normal RBC (partial exchange transfusion)
		Hematuria	→	Observe
		Hyposthenuria	→	Observe
		Autosplenectomy		Observe for infection
			Aseptic necrosis of bone	Conservative treatment; arthroplasty
			Acute pulmonary syndrome	Hospitalize; hydrate, O_2; possibly replace sickle cells with normal RBC (simple or partial exchange transfusion)
Increased red cell destruction	Aplastic crisis	→		Hospitalize, transfuse to restore RBC mass
		Impaired growth	→	Observe
			Delayed puberty	Observe
			Psychosocial problems	Counseling
Sequestration and stasis	Splenomegaly			Observe
	Splenic sequestration crisis			Hospitalize, hydrate, support intravascular volume, transfuse to replace sequestered RBC
		Hepatomegaly	→	Observe
		Priapism	→	If severe, hospitalize; hydrate; possibly replace sickle cells with normal RBC (simple or partial exchange transfusion); pain control
Functional asplenia	Sepsis Pneumonia Meningitis Osteomyelitis	→		Hospitalize Give antibiotics

disease, baseline hemoglobin and reticulocyte count values, prior treatment, and patient/parental expectations.

Fever is one of the more common chief complaints among sickle cell patients seeking emergency department care. It is well-recognized that functional asplenia from autoinfarction leads to an increased risk of bacterial infection, particularly caused by *Streptococcus pneumoniae, Haemophilus influenzae, Neisseria meningitidis, Salmonella* species, *Escherichia coli, Mycoplasma pneumoniae,* and *S. aureus.* Bacteremia, meningitis, pneumonia, urinary tract infection, and osteomyelitis are common. Overwhelming, fulminant infections with *S. pneumoniae* are of particular importance, with rates 30 to 100 times greater in children with sickle cell anemia under the age of 5 years than in healthy children.[45] The dramatic efficacy of penicillin prophylaxis in preventing pneumococcal septicemia in sickle cell patients under the age of 5 years has been demonstrated; unfortunately parental compliance is far from universal.[46,47] The benefits of current pneumococcal vaccines, although uniformly recommended for children over age 2 years, are not quite as clear-cut.[45] *H. influenzae* type B vaccines have been shown to be immunogenic in sickle cell patients and are also recommended.[48] For patients with hemoglobin SC or sickle beta-thalassemia, antibiotic prophylaxis is also recommended when there is evidence of splenic dysfunction. Fatal septicemia, although much less common than with SS disease, is well-described in SC disease. In sickle SC, functional asplenia, which can be

TABLE 54-6. Sickle Cell Disease: Infections and Antibiotic Therapy

Infection	Common organisms	Initial antibiotic therapy

Fever (no focus)	S. pneumoniae*
	 H. influenzae
	 N. meningitidis
		Low risk: outpatient (see text for criteria):
		     Ceftriaxone 50 mg/kg/24 hr (max: 2 gm) IV/IM q 24 hr
		 High risk: inpatient-cefotaxime 150 mg/kg/24 hr (max: 6-12 gm) IV q 6 hr or
		     ceftriaxone 50-75 mg/kg/24 hr (max: 2-4 gm) IV q 24 hr

Sepsis	S. pneumoniae* H. influenzae N. meningitidis	Same as for high risk fever above

Meningitis	S. pneumoniae*
	 H. influenzae
	 N. meningitidis
		Cefotaxime 200 mg/kg/24 hr (max: 12 gm) IV q 6 hr or ceftriaxone 100 mg/
		     kg/24 hr (max: 4 gm) IV q 12 hr; *plus* vancomycin 45-60 mg/kg/24 hr (max: 2
		     gm) IV q 6 hr

Pneumonia	S. pneumoniae* H. influenzae M. pneumoniae	Cefuroxime 150 mg/kg/24 hr (max: 4.5 gm) IV q 8 hr If *Mycoplasma* add erythromycin 30-50 mg/kg/24 hr PO q 6 hr for 10 days

Osteomyelitis	Salmonella
	 S. aureus
	 S. pneumoniae*
		Oxacillin 200 mg/kg/24 hr (max: 12 gm) IV q 4-6 hr; *plus* cefotaxime 150 mg/
		     kg/24 hr (max: 6-12 gm) IV q 6 hr or ceftriaxone 50-75 mg/kg/24 hr (max: 2-4
		     gm) IV q 24 hr

Data from Jenson HG and Baltimore RS: *Pediatric infectious diseases,* Norwalk, Conn, 1995, Appleton & Lange.

NOTE: Whenever possible, samples for microbiologic studies should be collected before antibiotic therapy. Therapy should be adjusted when culture and susceptibility data become available.

*In critically ill children, consider addition of vancomycin 45-60 mg/kg/day (max: 2 gm) IV q 6 hr for resistant *S. pneumoniae.*

assessed using erythrocyte pit counts, is uncommon prior to age 3. Some have suggested, then, that penicillin prophylaxis be considered for patients with SC disease[49]; all febrile illnesses in SC patients should be investigated promptly.

Ancillary Data. The long-standing recommendation has been that all children under the age of 5 with sickle cell anemia should be promptly evaluated whenever febrile to over 38.5° C. Laboratory studies should include a CBC, differential, reticulocyte count, urinalysis, and blood, urine, and throat cultures. When reviewing the CBC and differential, attention should be paid to the absolute band count (= % bands × total WBC). With bacterial infection (and to a lesser extent during painful crises), elevations of the absolute band count over 1000/mm^3 are common.[50] When well, children with sickle cell disease typically have elevations of the total WBC but not of the total band count. Cough, chest pain, or other pulmonary symptoms should prompt a chest radiograph, just as the presence of meningeal signs or an altered mental status should prompt consideration of a lumbar puncture. Antibiotic therapy should be instituted as soon as specimens are obtained (that is, even before any laboratory results are known). Recommended agents include those providing adequate coverage for *S. pneumoniae, H. influenzae,* and other encapsulated organisms; common choices include cefuroxime, cefotaxime, and ceftriaxone (Table 54-6). It should be noted that cefuroxime is inadequate for CSF penetration. The emergence of pneumococcal strains resistant to penicillin and third generation cephalosporins means that the addition of vancomycin with or without rifampin must be considered, particularly in cases of meningitis and overwhelming sepsis.[51]

The traditional approach has been for young children with sickle cell disease and fever to be hospitalized until

culture results become available. The low rate of positive blood cultures in such patients has lead to the suggestion that outpatient management could be adequate in selected cases.[52] Further support for outpatient care has emerged from a randomized study comparing hospitalization with outpatient treatment with ceftriaxone for children aged 6 months to 12 years.[53] Specifically excluded were patients judged to be at higher risk for sepsis on the basis of an ill-appearance, hypotension, poor perfusion, a temperature above 40.0° C, a WBC >30,000 or <5,000/mm^3, a platelet count <100,000/mm^3, or a history of pneumococcal sepsis. Also excluded were children with dehydration, a segmental or larger pulmonary infiltrate, severe pain, or a Hgb <5.0 gm/dl. All children promptly received 50 mg/kg of ceftriaxone and were observed until initial laboratory results became available. No episodes of bacteremia occurred among those children who were discharged; follow-up with administration of a second dose of ceftriaxone occurred within 20 to 30 hours. For children fulfilling **all** of the criteria outlined above, consideration of outpatient management can be viewed as a safe, cost-effective option provided that close follow-up can be guaranteed. The pharmacokinetics of ceftriaxone is such that intramuscular administration is acceptable.

Complications. The diagnosis of osteomyelitis in sickle cell patients can be particularly problematic, if simply because the clinical findings are similar to those occurring with bony infarction. Patients with osteomyelitis are more likely to have high fevers (>39° C), elevated erythrocyte sedimentation rates (>20 mm/hr), and prominent local findings than those with bony infarction, but considerable overlap occurs. When there is involvement of multiple sites, bony infarction is more likely.[54] Radiographic studies may prove useful in some cases. Typical pathogens causing osteomyelitis in sickle cell patients include *Salmonella* species and *S. aureus.* Incision and drainage or needle aspiration is recommended whenever possible before instituting antibiotic therapy.[55]

Another potentially fatal complication of sickle cell disease in younger children is that of splenic sequestration—at times it may be the first manifestation of the disorder. With sequestration, there is rapid pooling of a large portion of peripheral blood volume in the spleen. A common symptom is syncope. Profound anemia and hypovolemic shock rapidly ensue. Death can occur within hours. Children ages 5 months to 2 years are most at risk; autoinfarction of the spleen makes sequestration unusual in children over age 6 with SS disease. Splenic autoinfarction and dysfunction occur later in patients with SC disease or sickle beta[+]-thalassemia, making them subject to sequestration at older ages. Prompt recognition and transfusion are necessary to avoid irreversible circulatory collapse. Splenectomy is often recommended as a preventative measure following the first episode of severe sequestration. The value of parental education regarding this complication has been demonstrated; parents can be taught to palpate the spleen and seek prompt medical attention whenever enlargement is noted.[56]

Aplastic crisis is another complication of sickle cell disease more common in pediatric than adult patients. With an aplastic crisis, there is impairment of red cell production in the bone marrow, exacerbating the chronic hemolytic anemia. High-output congestive heart failure may result. Patients generally complain of dyspnea and increased fatigue. The CBC will reveal a more marked anemia than the patient's baseline, with few or no reticulocytes. Folate deficiency is an occasional contributor, but most cases are precipitated by infection. In recent years parvovirus B19 has been recognized as an important cause of aplastic crises, on occasion in near epidemic outbreaks.[57,58] Spontaneous resolution within 5 to 10 days generally occurs; transfusions may sometimes be necessary.

Painful crises, which affect sickle cell patients of all ages, are no doubt the most problematic complication of the disease for the emergency physician. Despite perceptions to the contrary, not all patients with sickle cell disease experience painful crises. In one study, 39% of patients had no episodes of pain, and only 1% had more than 6 episodes per year. Approximately one third of all painful episodes occurred in just over 5% of the patients.[59] The reasons underlying this disproportionate distribution of painful crises are not well understood, although there is some correlation of painful crises with higher hematocrits and lower fetal hemoglobin levels.

Musculoskeletal and abdominal pain are particularly common forms of crisis, with abdominal pain being particularly prevalent during adolescence. Often the patient has experienced comparable discomfort in the past. In infancy, the hand-foot syndrome (dactylitis) with painful swelling of the hands and feet may be the first manifestation of the disorder. Precipitants of painful crises include dehydration, infection, hypoxia, fatigue, exposure to cold, and psychological stress.[60-62] Abdominal pain is caused by small infarcts of the mesentery and viscera, usually without peritoneal signs or decreased bowel sounds. When evaluating a child with an apparent painful abdominal crisis, the exam-

iner must also consider the possibility of an acute surgical condition and other processes associated with abdominal pain including urinary tract and pulmonary infections.

The acute chest syndrome is characterized by chest pain, dyspnea, fever, leukocytosis, pulmonary infiltrates, and pleural effusions. Pulmonary infarction is difficult to differentiate from pneumonia, although in children under 12 years of age infection is a more common cause of acute chest syndrome.[63,64] It is not unusual for acute chest syndrome to occur *after* 24 to 48 hours of hospitalization; debate continues as to whether narcotic analgesic therapy and fluid administration contribute to its development.[65,66] In one prospective, randomized study, incentive spirometry proved markedly effective in preventing pulmonary complications in patients with chest or back pain. The results prompted the investigators to suggest that chest splinting from pain leads to the development of atelectasis or infiltrates and thus the acute chest syndrome itself.[67] In addition, investigation continues into the role of pulmonary fat embolism[68] and *Chlamydia pneumoniae*[69] in the development of the chest syndrome. There is no disagreement, however, about the contribution of the acute chest syndrome to overall mortality in sickle cell disease.[70]

Management. When treating a suspected painful crisis, the emergency physician must make an effort to identify possible precipitants, particularly infection. Low-grade fever is common; temperatures over 38.5° C should raise clinical suspicions. A CBC and reticulocyte count are generally indicated. Suspicions regarding infection should heighten further when the WBC is >20,000/mm³. A below normal reticulocyte count should prompt the examiner to consider an aplastic crisis. A blood culture is suggested whenever there is fever or leukocytosis. Routine performance of a urinalysis, urine culture, and chest radiograph should be considered, even when there are no specific symptoms or signs.[41,71] Oxygen saturation should be measured as well.

Hydration and analgesia comprise the mainstay of treatment for painful crises. Although the benefit of oxygen administration has never been convincingly demonstrated, it remains in widespread use. Supplemental oxygen should be provided when there is evidence of hypoxia. In many instances, patients can maintain adequate oral hydration. For those who cannot, intravenous hydration at a rate of 1½ to 2 times maintenance is suggested. The choice of analgesic agent will depend upon the severity of the pain and the prior at-home treatment. For individuals in mild pain who have had no therapy before the emergency department visit, oral nonsteroidal agents or codeine may suffice. Patients with more severe episodes and those who have already tried oral opiates will require parenteral therapy.

Presently, morphine administration is generally favored for patients with painful crises. Pharmacokinetic considerations, particularly the accumulation of a metabolite thought to provoke seizures, have caused meperidine to fall out of favor. Continuous intravenous infusions of morphine are frequently used; an initial bolus of 0.15 mg/kg is followed by an infusion of 0.07 to 0.10 mg/kg/hr.[72] Marked variations in patient tolerance and pharmacokinetics make individual titration necessary.[73] Such infusions are not without risks—at least one death has been attributed to excessive dosing and improper monitoring.[74] Patient-controlled analgesia has been advocated as a safer, more effective approach.[75]

Several new pain management options have come to attention in recent years. Ketorolac, an injectable nonsteroidal agent, has been used with variable success. One study demonstrated a narcotic-sparing effect[76] while another did not.[77] The efficacy of epidural analgesia in managing pain refractory to conventional therapy was demonstrated in one case series of nine children.[78] But perhaps the most promising new therapy for pain in pediatric patients is high-dose intravenous methylprednisolone.[79] When children and adolescents with pain received high-dose methylprednisolone (15 mg/kg over 30 minutes upon admission with a second dose 24 hours later), the duration of inpatient analgesia therapy decreased to 41 hours compared with 71 hours in a control group. The steroid group did, however, have a greater rate of rebound attacks upon discontinuation of therapy. There are ongoing efforts to define methods of preventing painful crises. Hypertransfusion protocols have been used with some success, but pose the risk of iron overload. Hydroxyurea has been shown to be beneficial in adult patients[80]; combination therapy with erythropoietin may offer additional benefits.[81] Uncertainties about the long-term side effects of hydroxyurea administration preclude its use in children at present.

When the acute chest syndrome develops, consideration must be given to antibiotic therapy and transfusion. Although disagreement exists regarding the overall role of infection in producing the syndrome, most advocate antibiotic coverage when it develops. An agent that covers the typical pulmonary pathogens is usually adequate (e.g., cefuroxime). Some advocate coverage of atypical organisms with a drug such as erythromycin. Closely monitored oxygen therapy is essential. The results of one small case series suggest that nebulized albuterol may be of some adjunctive benefit, even in the absence of overt bronchospasm.[82] With progressive anemia or respiratory deterioration, exchange transfusion must be considered. It has been suggested that careful measurement of the room air alveolar-arterial oxygen gradient ($[A-a]Po_2$) can guide decision making about transfusion. An $(A-a)Po_2$ greater than 30 mm Hg was the best predictor of the need for transfusion in one study.[83] Using the following formula, obtain an arterial blood gas with the patient breathing room air:

$$(FIo_2 = 0.21), \text{ the } (A-a)Po_2 = \\ (713 \times FIo_2) - (Pco_2 \times 1.2) - Po_2$$

Intubation and positive pressure ventilation are required when respiratory failure develops. Despite such intensive support, refractory respiratory distress leading to death will occur in some cases. Hypoxic stroke is another potential complication of the acute chest syndrome.

Thrombotic and hemorrhagic strokes, at times fatal, occur in 6% to 12% of patients with sickle cell disease. Clinical manifestations include headache, transient ischemic attacks, seizures, motor deficits, aphasia, and coma. Hemiparesis is particularly common in children.[84,85] Diagnosis is based on clinical features, with CT scan providing additional data. Therapy will vary with the clinical scenario. Close monitoring for the development of increased intracranial pressure is necessary, instituting hyperventilation and other measures when it develops. Anticonvulsants are recommended for seizure activity. Exchange transfusion must be considered with hemorrhagic infarcts and when acute coma occurs in the setting of a normal CT study. In the latter situation, acute, potentially reversible, sickling of erythrocytes in the cerebral arterioles is thought to take place. Transfusion therapy offers some benefits as a strategy to prevent recurrent stroke.[85]

Other complications of sickle cell disease are of lesser importance to the emergency physician and will be mentioned only briefly here. Children generally have impaired growth and delayed puberty. High-output congestive heart failure may be noted; cardiomegaly and flow murmurs occur in most. Retinopathy secondary to sequestration of the blood in the conjunctival vessels is marked by dilated and tortuous retinal vessels, microaneurysms, and retinal hemorrhage. Gastrointestinal tract involvement may include cholelithiasis caused by chronic hemolysis, particularly after 6 years of age. Acute cholecystitis can ensue. Irreversible renal damage causing hyposthenuria is present in almost all patients by 3 years of age. This may progress to renal failure requiring transplantation. Hematuria as the result of sickling in the vasa recta or renal papillary necrosis is commonplace. Refractory hematuria may require hospitalization for bedrest, hydration, and a trial of epsilon aminocaproic acid (2 to 8 gm/day orally). Patients with sickle cell trait may also develop hyposthenuria or hematuria but at a later age. Priapism can occur as the result of obstruction of the venous drainage of the corpus cavernosum. Management can be very problematic.[86] Osteonecrosis of the femoral head occurs in about 10% of patients: hip arthroplasty may be necessary.[87] As with many chronic diseases, psychosocial problems are common.

Hospitalization is indicated for children with splenic sequestration, aplastic crisis with severe anemia, stroke, pulmonary infarction, suspected bacterial infection, severe or prolonged priapism, and severe vasoocclusive pain crisis in which parenteral analgesia, fluids, or antibiotics are required. Patients not responding in the first 2 hours of appropriate ambulatory management should generally be admitted to the hospital. Long-term follow-up is essential. Prophylactic antibiotics should be administered to patients 6 years old and younger, vaccines and chronic transfusion therapy should be arranged as indicated. Genetic counseling, periodic ophthalmologic examination for retinopathy, and psychosocial counseling should also be considered.[88]

Thalassemia

Microcytic hemolytic anemia is the hallmark of the thalassemias, a diverse group of disorders characterized by defective synthesis of the globin chains. Gene frequencies range from 5% to 20% in people of Mediterranean, Middle Eastern, and southeast Asian backgrounds. Individuals with thalassemia minor (heterozygous beta-thalassemia) are generally asymptomatic, although splenomegaly, cholelithiasis, and leg ulcers may rarely be observed. It may be at times difficult to distinguish thalassemia minor from iron deficiency and lead poisoning (see discussion on Anemia earlier in this chapter). The severity of disease is variable in individuals with thalassemia intermedia; aplastic crises requiring transfusion do occur. It is patients with beta-thalassemia major, in which there is absent (beta°) or decreased (beta⁺) synthesis of the beta-globin chain, who are most likely to come to the attention of the emergency physician. Thalassemia intermedia refers to the clinical variant of homozygous beta-thalassemia in which patients are not absolutely dependent upon transfusion for survival.

Thalassemia major, also known as Cooley or Mediterranean anemia, is marked by ineffective erythropoiesis, chronic hemolysis, and thus severe anemia. Most cases are detected during infancy, although in isolated instances, the diagnosis does not manifest itself until age 3 to 4 years.[89,90] Without transfusions, affected infants demonstrate severe anemia (see earlier discussion), physical stigmata of extramedullary hematopoiesis, and growth retardation. Death from infection or congestive heart failure follows within 1 to 2 years of life. With a program of regular transfusion, splenectomy, and iron chelation, the prognosis is altered dramatically, with median survival of 31 years. Complications are frequent, both as the result of the underlying disease and the therapeutic regimen.

With the institution of a program of regular transfusions during infancy, patients with thalassemia major can achieve normal growth and development. Transfusion reactions can occur, although they can be minimized by use of washed or leukocyte poor RBCs. With multiple transfusions, the risk of transmission of CMV and hepatitis increase. Once again, the risks can be decreased with careful screening and white cell filtration of donor units and hepatitis B immunization. Aplastic and hemolytic crises are an ongoing concern, as with any hemoglobinopathy. In addition, alterations in immune function lead to an increased susceptibility to infection.

Despite a program of regular transfusion, patients with thalassemia major may still develop hypersplenism. Splenectomy is generally required by the time affected children reach age 6 to 8 years. Following splenectomy, the risk of overwhelming sepsis increases significantly despite penicillin prophylaxis and vaccinations against pneumococcus and *H. influenzae*. An aggressive approach to fever (>38.5° C) is thus essential in all patients who have undergone splenectomy. Empiric antibiotic therapy until results of blood, urine, and throat cultures are known is generally indicated.

Transfusion therapy inevitably leads to iron overload and its complications, most importantly cardiac dysfunction, which are the leading cause of death in thalassemia major. Even with routine chelation beginning at age 4 to 5 years, iron accumulation cannot be avoided. Multiple organ systems are affected. Manifestations that may demand acute attention include pericarditis, diabetes mellitus, hypothyroidism, hypoparathyroidism, and coagulation disorders (with platelet dysfunction and prolongation of the prothrombin time). The greatest risks are posed by cardiac hemosiderosis, signs of which include dysrhythmias and refractory congestive heart failure. Clearly then, given the broad range of pathology possible, consultation with a hematologist and other subspecialists should be considered whenever the emergency physician encounters a patient with thalassemia major.

TABLE 54-7. Clinical Manifestations of DIC

Organ system	Thrombotic	Hemorrhagic
Skin	Peripheral cyanosis Purpura fulminans Gangrene	Petechiae, ecchymoses, oozing from venipunctures
CNS	Coma/delirium	Intracranial hemorrhage
Renal	Azotemia/oliguria Cortical necrosis	Hematuria
Lungs	Pulmonary infarction Hypoxemia	Pulmonary hemorrhage
Gastrointestinal	Infarction Ulceration	Hemorrhage/melena

BLEEDING DISORDERS

Disseminated Intravascular Coagulation

Disseminated intravascular coagulation (DIC) is an acquired condition that occurs in multiple different clinical settings. DIC is considered both a thrombohemorrhagic disorder and a consumptive coagulopathy.

Pathophysiology. In DIC, activation of both the coagulation and fibrinolytic systems results in microthrombi formation and subsequent tissue ischemia in addition to bleeding secondary to consumption of clotting factors, thrombocytopenia, and fibrinolysis. Given that the mortality rate from DIC is extremely high, it is important to recognize this entity and to treat both the underlying pathology and the DIC as rapidly as possible.[91]

Etiology. There are numerous conditions associated with DIC. Infection is one of the most common triggers. DIC can occur in the setting of gram-negative sepsis (especially meningococcemia), gram-positive sepsis (including *S. pneumoniae* and *S. aureus*), viral infections (herpes, cytomegalovirus, measles, influenza, varicella, and hepatitis), rickettsial infections (including Rocky Mountain spotted fever), and chlamydial, fungal, mycobacterial, and protozoal infections (including *Plasmodium falciparum* malaria). Other causes of DIC include trauma, crush injuries, burns, extensive surgery, pregnancy, malignancy, acute hemolytic transfusion reactions, vascular malformations, snake bites, heat stroke, hypothermia, hyperthermia, anoxia, acidosis, and anaphylaxis.[92]

Diagnostic Findings. The clinical and laboratory findings associated with DIC are diverse, in keeping with the pathophysiology and the range of associated underlying conditions. A number of specific signs and symptoms relate directly to thrombosis and hemorrhage as summarized in Table 54-7.

Ancillary Data. Multiple laboratory tests are helpful in the diagnosis and management of DIC. The peripheral smear may show thrombocytopenia and microangiopathic hemolytic anemia with schistocytes. Subtle signs of fibrin damage to red blood cells may precede quantitative manifestations of DIC. The PT and PTT are prolonged in the majority of patients with DIC because there is consumption of all the clotting factors. Decreased levels of fibrino-

TABLE 54-8. Differential Diagnosis: DIC

Disease	Similarities	Differences
Vitamin K deficiency	Increased PT	Normal fibrinogen
	Increased PTT	Normal FDP
Liver disease	Increased PT	Worsening
	Increased PTT	Coagulopathy will be seen with DIC—
	Thrombocytopenia	serial measurements needed
Lupus (SLE)	Increased PT, PTT, anemia, thrombocytopenia	Normal fibrinogen
Thrombotic thrombocytopenia purpura	Thrombocytopenia, microangiopathy	Normal clotting factors
Renal failure	Increased FDP anemia	Clinically different
Dysfibrinogenemia	Increased FDP	Clinically different

DIC, Disseminated intravascular coagulation; *FDP,* fibrin split/degradation products; *PT,* prothrombin time; *PTT,* partial thromboplastin time; *SLE,* systemic lupus erythematosus.

gen are often seen in DIC, although an elevated fibrinogen level may occur early in DIC as part of an acute phase reaction. The measurements of fibrinogen and fibrin split/degradation products (FDP) are important in the diagnosis and management of DIC. Fibrinogen levels of less than 50 mg/dl place the patient at high risk for serious hemorrhage. The level of FDP, although a sensitive measure of fibrinolytic activity, is not a specific test for DIC. The D-dimer, a breakdown product of polymerized fibrin but not fibrinogen, is specific for DIC, as it verifies the production of both thrombin and plasmin. Control proteins of the coagulation system are also depleted in DIC.

Differential Considerations. Several conditions can appear similar to DIC, and they should be considered in the differential diagnosis. Their similarities and differences are outlined in Table 54-8.

Management. The management of DIC remains controversial. The most important objective of treatment is to diagnose and treat the underlying disease while stabilizing the patient hemodynamically. Specific therapy for DIC may not be required if the precipitating event is quickly reversed. Once treatment of the underlying process has begun, there are three categories of treatment that may be considered. These include the replacement of clotting factors, controlling proteins and platelets, using anticoagulants and fibrinolytic therapy. Laboratory values may reveal a low fibrinogen level, low clotting factor levels, and thrombocytopenia. If the patient is actively bleeding, replacement of depleted coagulation factors is usually appropriate. Replacement with fresh frozen plasma (FFP), cryoprecipitate, or platelets may be indicated. Antithrombin III concentrate replacement is being evaluated as another therapeutic modality for DIC.

FFP is the usual first line therapy for DIC. FFP contains all factors and is usually given in a dose of 10 to 15 ml/kg (which also provides volume replacement). Cryoprecipitate contains primarily factor VIII and fibrinogen in a concentrated form. When a patient is severely deficient in fibrinogen (<50 mg/dl), use of cryoprecipitate may allow effective fibrinogen replacement without volume overload. The initial dose of cryoprecipitate is 1 unit IV for every 5 kilograms of body weight. Severe thrombocytopenia (<20,000/ml³) and thrombocytopenia with ongoing bleeding are indications for platelet transfusion. Platelet concentrates are given at a rate of 1 pack per 5 to 6 kg of body weight to a maximum of 6 units. For infants, one unit of platelet concentrate can be given as long as the transfused volume is not excessive.[93]

The use of heparin in DIC remains controversial. Heparin is most commonly used in the management of those illnesses that are thought to have a strong thrombotic component (e.g., meningococcemia with purpura fulminans and acute promyelocytic leukemia). Heparin therapy may be considered for the patient with active bleeding who has not been controlled with FFP, platelets, and treatment of the underlying disorder. The initial dose of heparin for DIC is 50 units/kg IV followed by a continuous infusion of 10 to 15 units/kg/hr. Replacement therapy with FFP and platelets should continue during the heparin infusion to minimize bleeding. Close monitoring of coagulation studies, fibrinogen levels, and platelet counts is essential. Future therapy of DIC may include the use of low molecular weight heparin, antithrombin III concentrates, and protein C concentrates. Management of DIC will be temporizing at best unless the underlying disorder is treated aggressively at the same time.

Hemophilia

Hemophilia A (classical hemophilia) is an X-linked recessive disorder of blood coagulation resulting from a lack of factor VIII activity. The incidence of hemophilia A is approximately 1 in 7,500 live male births. Occurring less frequently (1:30,000 males), hemophilia B (Christmas disease) results from a decrease in factor IX activity. Hemophilia A and B are clinically indistinguishable.[94,95] The severity of the bleeding tendency is dependent upon the degree of clotting factor deficiency as follows: severe (<1%), moderate (1% to 5%), and mild (>5%).

Pathophysiology. Patients with hemophilia have a defect in the intrinsic cascade of secondary hemostasis—the formation of fibrin. Primary hemostasis (platelet plug formation) is not affected by factor VIII or IX deficiency; this process, however, is not adequate to control hemorrhaging beyond superficial skin abrasions. In hemophilia, the failure to form a firm fibrin clot leads to a cycle of rebleeding.

Because factor VIII or IX deficiency results in incomplete hemostasis, life-threatening bleeding can occur even with trivial trauma to the airway, central nervous system, or internal organs.[96]

The hallmark of hemophilia is hemorrhage into the joints (hemarthrosis). The accumulated blood and resulting hemosiderin eventually are cleared from the joint space by phagocytosis and proteolytic degradation. Prolonged and recurrent hemarthroses cause progressive joint damage and can lead to disabling hemophilic arthropathy.

Diagnostic Findings. Typical manifestations of bleeding in hemophilia vary with the severity of the factor deficiency and the age of the child. Prolonged bleeding after circumcision may be the first indication that an infant has a bleeding disorder but this does not occur in all cases. Instances of significant bleeding are rare during the first year of life. Easy bruising is apparent in most affected infants and toddlers; the pattern of bruising is different from that seen in child abuse. Typical sites include the knees, shins, and buttocks as the child learns to crawl and walk. Specific injuries may be caused by points of pressure related to toys or furniture. Mucous membrane hemorrhaging secondary to minor trauma is common in this age group. Eruption of primary teeth rarely causes bleeding since the gingival tissues become devascularized as the tooth emerges. Later in life, as the tooth's root is reabsorbed before loss, the sharp base of the primary tooth may cause gingival hemorrhage.

Hemarthrosis and soft tissue bleeding are the most common manifestations of hemophilia during childhood. Early signs and symptoms of both joint and soft tissue bleeding are pain or difficulty in the use of a limb. Later findings of warmth, swelling, decreased range of motion, and erythema occur only after a significant quantity of blood has collected. The joints most frequently affected are the knees, ankles, and elbows; bleeding into the shoulder and hip occur less often. Bleeding in the forearm or calf may compress a muscle compartment and cause neurovascular compromise with pain, paresthesia, anesthesia, or decreased blood flow.

Individuals with mild hemophilia may not experience any of these early childhood bleeding manifestations. The first episode may not occur until adolescence or even adulthood. Patients with mild hemophilia generally do not experience spontaneous bleeding but may be brought to the emergency department with excessive hemorrhage after trauma. A common history would be a patient with prolonged or excessive clinical findings out of proportion to the type of injury.

Complications. Approximately 15% of patients with severe hemophilia A develop factor VIII inhibitors, which are IgG antibodies that inactivate transfused factor concentrates. Inhibitor antibodies to factor IX occur in only 1% of patients with severe hemophilia B.[97] The number of treatments before inhibitor formation varies but most patients who develop inhibitors will do so before the age of 20 years. Not all inhibitors that can be detected in the laboratory, however, interfere with the ability to treat the patient with factor replacement. Acquired hemophilia, which is caused by autoantibodies to one of the clotting factors, is extremely uncommon in the pediatric age group.

Patients with low titer–low responder inhibitors can often be treated with the usual factor replacement therapy by increasing the dose. Patients with high titer–high responder inhibitors have an anamnestic rise in antibody titer after exposure to factor. These patients are treated with hemostatic preparations such as prothrombin complex concentrate (PCC) or activated PCC, which attempt to activate coagulation by an alternative mechanism (Table 54-9). This approach to therapy is not as effective as correction of the specific factor deficiency; thus, these patients are at greater risk for serious hemorrhage. Most patients with inhibitors have a lower inhibitor titer against porcine factor VIII than human factor VIII (average 1:5 ratio of inhibitor titers). Factor VIII replacement with Hyate C (porcine factor VIII) may be possible in this situation.

When pooled factor concentrates came into general use for the treatment of hemophilia, transmission of viral infections (specifically HIV and hepatitis) became a major problem.[98] Fortunately, viral inactivation procedures for factor concentrates instituted during the past decade have eliminated the transmission of HIV and markedly decreased risk of hepatitis transmission[97] (see Table 54-9). Hepatitis A and B vaccines are recommended for all patients with hemophilia. Clinical studies of recombinant, pasteurized, and immunoaffinity purified (monoclonal) concentrates have demonstrated these products to be free of hepatitis and HIV contamination. Solvent detergent concentrates may carry a small risk for hepatitis A transmission.

Ancillary Data. The goal of therapy is to correct the hemorrhagic diathesis promptly—even before any signs of hemorrhage are present on clinical examination. Older children and adults are usually managed by home infusion of factor for joint and soft tissue hemorrhage. Young children with hemophilia will come to the emergency department primarily for assistance with intravenous infusion of factor concentrates. In these cases, no laboratory studies are needed. Measurement of the PTT is of no value for a patient whose hemophilia has been previously diagnosed. In cases of life- or limb-threatening hemorrhage, imaging studies and factor assays *are* important. Appropriate management for these cases will be discussed in the following section.

Management. When patients with hemophilia come to the emergency department, they should be assessed and stabilized, and appropriate factor replacement should be administered as soon as possible. Infusion of factor concentrates will temporarily correct the bleeding disorder. For patients with a history of a documented or suspected inhibitor, a citrated plasma sample for inhibitor titers against both human and porcine factor VIII should be obtained before the infusion of factor concentrates. Subsequent replacement therapy may depend upon the patient's inhibitor titers. Titers cannot be measured once exogenous factor has been administered. It may also be necessary to document the response to factor therapy by comparing preinfusion and postinfusion levels for an appropriate rise in the factor level.

In the absence of an inhibitor, the circulating factor VIII level will be increased by 2% after the infusion of one unit/kg of body weight of factor VIII concentrate. The half-life of factor VIII is approximately 12 hours. For factor

TABLE 54-9. Hemophilia Therapies Used in the United States

Therapeutic product	Clinical indication	Brand name (manufacturer)	Additional information
Recombinant factor VIII	Factor VIII replacement	Kogenate (Miles) Recombinate (Hyland) Bioclate (Armour) Helixate (Armour)	Pasteurized human albumin added as stabilizer
Ultrapure, plasma-derived factor VIII	Factor VIII replacement	Monoclate-P (Armour) Hemofil M (Hyland) AHF-Method M (Baxter)	Pasteurized human albumin added as stabilizer
Intermediate and high purity, plasma–derived factor VIII	Factor VIII replacement	Humate-P (Armour) Alphanate (Alpha)* Prolifate OSD (Alpha)* Koate HP (Miles)*	See note below regarding solvent-detergent method
Affinity purified factor IX	Factor IX replacement	Alphanine SD (Alpha) Mononine (Armour)	
Prothrombin complex concentrate	Factor IX replacement or mild/moderate bleeding when inhibitors present	Konyne-80 (Cutter) Proplex T (Hyland) Profilnine SD (Alpha)* Bebulin VH (Immuno)	Risk for thrombotic complications, hepatitis a potential risk (HIV inactivated by all methods)
Activated prothrombin complex concentrate	Only used for patients with inhibitors	Autoplex T (Hyland) Feiba VH Immuno (Immuno)	Risk for thrombotic complications, hepatitis a potential risk (HIV inactivated by all methods)
Desmopressin	Mild hemophilia Type I von Willebrand	Nasal spray: Stimate (Armour) Injectable: DDAVP (Rhone-Poulenc Rorer)	DDAVP nasal spray (Rhone-Poulenc Rorer) should not be used because concentration is too low
Products under investigation Recombinant Factor VIIa Recombinant Factor IX	Patients with inhibitors Factor IX replacement	Novoseven (NovoNordisk) Genetics Institute	

*These products are prepared using a solvent-detergent method that does not inactivate nonlipid enveloped viruses (hepatitis A, parvovirus).

TABLE 54-10. Initial Management of Bleeding in Hemophilia*

Degree of hemorrhage	Desired factor level	Initial dosage Factor VIII*	Initial dosage Factor IX*	Typical follow-up
Moderate				
Hemarthrosis	40%-50%	25 units/kg	50 units/kg	Rest, application of ice; telephone follow-up next day
Muscle/soft tissue	30%-50%			
Laceration requiring sutures	40%-50%	25 units/kg	50 units/kg	Factor correction for 1-10 days depending on severity
Mouth, tongue	40%-50% (aminocaproic or tranexamic acid alone if minor)	25 units/kg	50 units/kg	Oral aminocaproic or tranexamic acid therapy for several days; close telephone follow-up
Life- or limb-threatening				
Airway	100%	50 units/kg	100 units/kg	Hospitalization; maintain normal hemostasis
CNS, spinal cord				Surgical intervention as appropriate
Eye				
Gastrointestinal				
Retroperitoneal				
Compartment syndrome (forearm, calf)	100%	50 units/kg	100 units/kg	Hospitalization; maintain normal hemostasis Surgical intervention generally not needed
Other				
Head injury—no evidence of CNS hemorrhage	50%	25 units/kg	50 units/kg	Monitor for head injury; CT scan if delay between injury and factor treatment
Hematuria	0%	0	0	Rest and fluids for 48 hr; if no improvement, prednisone 2 mg/kg/day for 4 days

*For patients without inhibitors.

IX concentrates, however, the infusion of one unit/kg of body weight increases the factor IX level by only 1% and the half-life is approximately 24 hours. The various clotting factor preparations are listed in Table 54-9.

Dosages of factor VIII and factor IX concentrates will vary in number of units and intervals between doses according to the nature of the hemorrhage. For life- or limb-threatening hemorrhages, the initial goal of therapy is to achieve a factor VIII or factor IX level of 100%, and normal hemostasis must be maintained for at least 10 days. Transient correction to 50% is adequate for minor bleeding episodes. Typical therapeutic goals for various types of hemorrhaging are found in Table 54-10.

Adequate factor coverage should be administered before invasive procedures such as lumbar puncture, venous cutdown, joint aspiration, incision and drainage of an abscess, and suturing of a deep laceration. The need for and timing of follow-up doses will vary according to the nature of the procedure. Factor replacement for 7 days may be justified after lumbar puncture.

Bleeding from the oral mucosa is a common occurrence in young patients with hemophilia. Therapy, which can be initiated at home, generally consists of oral aminocaproic acid, 100 mg/kg/dose q 6 hr, and may also include the application of topical thrombin. For bleeding uncontrolled by these medications, a dose of factor concentrate followed by several days of oral aminocaproic acid (or tranexamic acid) may be required.

Hematuria in the absence of abdominal trauma should be managed initially without factor replacement. Upper tract blood clots can lead to renal colic. If there is no pain associated with the hematuria, the patient should be instructed to rest and to increase fluid intake for 24 to 48 hours. For persistent or progressive symptoms, a short course of oral prednisone is indicated. Symptoms generally resolve within a few days.

Diagnostic imaging studies are indicated for episodes of significant bleeding and in instances of trauma, particularly when the site of injury involves the head, neck, chest, abdomen, or groin. However, factor therapy should not be withheld to wait for an imaging study or its results. A head CT scan (without contrast) should be performed to assess for intracranial hemorrhage on any patient presenting to the ED with hemophilia and significant head trauma or positive neurological signs/symptoms. Imaging may also be warranted for the patient with a history of mild head trauma who did not receive prompt factor coverage.

For the patient with airway trauma or difficulty in breathing or swallowing, lateral neck films are useful in determining the threat of the hemorrhage to the airway. A CT scan of the neck may be indicated to further define the extent of bleeding.

If the hemophilic patient comes to the ED with complaints of abdominal or groin pain, with or without a history of significant trauma, these complaints are likely due to intraabdominal hemorrhage. Bowel wall or abdominal hematomas may mimic acute appendicitis or gastritis. Retroperitoneal bleeding may occur as pain in the knee or hip in addition to findings directly related to the groin or abdomen. Prompt clinical response to factor infusion suggests that the problem is acute hemorrhage; and these patients should have diagnostic imaging in an attempt to define the source of bleeding. An ultrasound of the abdomen may be able to detect large hematomas, whereas a CT scan would be most helpful in characterizing a retroperitoneal iliopsoas hematoma. In cases of scrotal or testicular trauma or swelling, an ultrasound to eliminate torsion or epididymitis should be considered.

Hemophilic hemarthrosis nearly always responds to factor infusion alone without surgical intervention. If compartment syndrome is suspected, however, an ultrasound of the affected forearm or calf should be considered. Doppler studies can also be use to evaluate blood flow. Evaluation should include orthopedic consultation but initial therapy should be limited to factor replacement, elevation, and positioning.

Patients with mild classical hemophilia can be treated with desmopressin acetate (injectable or intranasal).[97] Desmopressin is an analog of the pituitary hormone 8-arginine vasopressin. It increases plasma factor VIII and von Willebrand factor concentrations to two to four times baseline values and is therefore useful in patients with factor VIII levels of >5%. The exact mechanism of action remains unknown, but it is thought to be the release of endothelial storage site proteins. The injectable form of desmopressin (DDAVP 4 μg/ml) is infused at a dose of 0.3 μg/kg over 15 to 30 minutes. The intranasal preparation (Stimate) contains 1.5 mg/ml of desmopressin; one metered spray dose delivers 0.1 ml or 150 μg. Patients under 50 kg should receive one spray; heavier patients require two sprays (300 μg). Note: The intranasal DDAVP solution used to treat enuresis and diabetes insipidus contains only 0.1 mg/ml and has no effect on factor levels.

In the emergency department, a patient who has had a previously effective therapeutic trial of desmopressin can be assumed to respond similarly as long as 7 to 10 days have elapsed between treatments. Maximal factor levels are seen 15 to 30 minutes after administration of desmopressin. Patients may experience facial flushing or headache after infusion; blood pressure and heart rate should be monitored. Hyponatremia has been reported in children under 4 years of age; thus careful monitoring of patients in this age group is needed. Desmopressin administration can be repeated every 12 hours but tachyphylaxis usually develops with significant loss of clinical response after the second or third dose. Full response to DDAVP will recover in 7 to 10 days if therapy is suspended.

Special Cases. Patients treated before 1985 may have contracted HIV from contaminated blood products. In most instances, the management of their infections or opportunistic infections would be the same as for other HIV-positive patients. It would be prudent, however, to remember that soft tissue bleeding and hemarthroses may serve as actual or potential reservoirs for infection. The patient's clotting disorder should be corrected to provide adequate hemostasis during invasive procedures. For those HIV-positive patients who are also thrombocytopenic, additional doses of factor concentrates may be required to prevent postprocedural bleeding.

Consultations with other specialties should be considered in the following instances:

1. Neurosurgery: suspected/documented CNS bleeding, spinal cord trauma
2. Orthopedics: persistent joint swelling/pain despite appropriate management, patient's first hemarthrosis into a joint, suspected compartment syndrome
3. Dentistry: loose primary tooth "rocking" against the gumline (may require removal)
4. Surgery: abdominal pain not responsive to factor infusion

Consultation with a hematologist in a comprehensive hemophilia center is often helpful when a patient with hemophilia seeks care for a problem potentially related to the disease.[99]

Immune Thrombocytopenic Purpura (ITP)

ITP results from increased destruction of platelets on an autoimmune basis. In children, ITP often occurs 2 to 3 weeks after an immunization or a viral illness (e.g., measles, rubella, mumps, varicella, infectious mononucleosis, and the common cold.) Most cases in children are self-limited with 90% resolving within 6 months.

Diagnostic Findings. Patients are generally healthy, aged 2 to 10 years, and have sudden onset of bruising and petechiae. Mucosal bleeding including epistaxis, buccal mucosal hemorrhage, or menorrhagia occasionally occurs. Patients with such "wet purpura" are at greatest risk for serious hemorrhage. There is usually no history of fatigue, recurrent fevers, decreased appetite, bone pain, or weight loss. These patients typically have no adenopathy or hepatosplenomegaly when physically examined.

The rare death from acute ITP is almost always secondary to intracranial hemorrhage, which occurs in <1% of patients with ITP. Most patients who suffer these hemorrhages have platelet counts of less than 20,000/mm³. Gastrointestinal hemorrhage and hematuria, although infrequent, can also be life-threatening.

Ancillary Data. The CBC with platelet count and peripheral smear should be reviewed. A patient with ITP will have a normal hemoglobin hematocrit (unless there has been extensive hemorrhage), white cell count, and differential. The peripheral blood smear should reveal normal blood cell morphology. Microangiopathy points towards TTP, HUS, or DIC as a diagnosis. Giant platelets may indicate a congenital giant platelet disorder. Teardrop and nucleated red cells are suggestive of infiltrative bone marrow disease, and polychromasia or microspherocytes may signal hemolytic anemia. The platelet count is usually less than 50,000/mm³ in children with ITP. Patients with platelet counts of less than 10,000 to 20,000/mm³ are at higher risk for spontaneous hemorrhage.

If there is any history of bone pain, weight loss, recurrent fever, or any evidence of hepatosplenomegaly, adenopathy, anemia, leukopenia, or leukocytosis to suggest an alternate diagnosis, an examination of the bone marrow is necessary. If the patient is to be treated with steroids, many hematologists recommend the performance of a bone marrow aspirate because using only steroids in the treatment of a child with acute leukemia may adversely affect long-term prognosis. A patient with "atypical" findings on physical examination or laboratory studies must have a bone marrow aspiration.[100,101] The marrow of a patient with ITP will reveal a normal or increased number of megakaryocytes but will otherwise be normal, thus confirming the destruction of platelets in the peripheral blood.

ITP may be the first manifestation of HIV infection (10% of cases). A careful history of HIV risk factors should be obtained, and HIV serologic testing should be considered.

Differential Considerations. Possible mechanisms for thrombocytopenia include increased platelet destruction, decreased platelet production, and platelet sequestration. Common causes of thrombocytopenia are listed in the box on p. 903.

Management. There has been great controversy in the literature about therapy for pediatric patients with acute ITP. Possible therapeutic approaches include expectant waiting, intravenous gamma globulin or immune globulin (IVIG), and corticosteroids. Since there is increasing risk of spontaneous hemorrhage with counts less than 20,000/mm^3, the goal of therapy is to raise the platelet count as quickly as possible to prevent CNS bleeding. If the decision is made to treat the patient pharmacologically, initial therapy is usually either IVIG or steroids.[102,103] IVIG is administered in doses of 0.8 to 1.0 gm/kg daily for 1 to 2 days.[104] Corticosteroids may be given parenterally (30 mg/kg of IV methylprednisolone daily for 3 days) or orally (4 mg/kg of oral prednisone daily for 2 to 4 days, followed by 2 mg/kg/day for 10 to 14 days, and then tapered over the next 2 weeks). Neither IVIG nor steroids have altered the long-term prognosis of patients. However, both have increased the platelet count more rapidly than expectant observation in the majority of patients.

Patients with signs or symptoms of intracranial hemorrhage (vomiting, headache, or neurologic symptoms) should be promptly evaluated with a head CT scan. Multimodality therapy is indicated in this instance, including IVIG, steroids, and possibly splenectomy. Patients with ITP have destructive antiplatelet antibodies and platelets; therefore platelet transfusions are usually ineffective. In patients with life-threatening bleeding, however, intermittent or continuous platelet transfusions are recommended to help control hemorrhage.

In 80% to 90% of children, ITP resolves within 6 months whether therapy is instituted or not. Patients with persistent ITP 6 months after diagnosis are considered to have chronic ITP, although there is a small chance that they may recover as long as 10 years after diagnosis.[105] Chronic ITP is more common in females and in patients older than 10 years of age. These patients may have HIV, or autoimmune or collagen vascular disease. Therapy for chronic ITP may include anti-Rh(D), splenectomy, vinca alkaloids, danazol, azathioprine, and cyclophosphamide.

Disposition. The decision whether or not to admit the patient to the hospital depends on several important

factors: the platelet count and age (a toddler vs. school-age child). Since patients with platelet counts of less than 10,000 to 20,000/mm^3 are at risk for spontaneous hemorrhage, many hematologists will admit these patients for observation and therapy. It is also generally easier to limit the activity of a toddler in the hospital. Close observation and activity restrictions are most important for children with mucous membrane bleeding because these children are thought to be at highest risk for intracranial hemorrhage. Contact sports should be avoided for all patients with ITP. No intramuscular injections should be given, and aspirin and other anticoagulants should be withheld. Platelet counts should be monitored, with the frequency dependent on the severity of thrombocytopenia and the presence of bleeding.

von Willebrand Disease

von Willebrand disease results from quantitative or qualitative congenital abnormality of von Willebrand factor, which is a protein facilitating the adherence of platelets to damaged endothelium. von Willebrand disease (vWD) is thought to be present in 2% or more of the population, but because of its often mild clinical manifestations, the true incidence of the disease is not known. The disease is usually inherited in an autosomal dominant pattern; thus males and females are equally affected.[106]

Pathophysiology. von Willebrand factor (vWF) is a larger multimeric protein (MW up 20×10^6) that facilitates platelet adhesion to exposed subendothelium at a site of vascular injury. vWF also serves as the necessary carrier protein for factor VIII; thus a decrease in the amount of vWF results in a decrease in plasma factor VIII. Patients with Type III vWD (severe) have defective primary and secondary hemostasis. A number of different genetic defects are known to cause vWD, and these produce a number of clinical variants (Table 54-11). vWD results from one of three processes: a reduction in the amount of vWF—types I and III; production of abnormal vWF—types IIA, IIB; and an abnormal interaction of vWF with platelets—platelet type vWD. Typical clinical manifestations of vWD include ecchymoses, epistaxis, postoperative bleeding, and menorrhagia.

Diagnostic Findings. The patient with vWD may first be recognized by the astute emergency physician. Hemorrhage out of proportion to the severity of an injury should alert the examiner to the possibility of a bleeding disorder. Referral for hemostasis evaluation should be based upon clinical judgment.

Of all the variants, Type I vWD is the most common (70% to 80% of vWD patients). Patients with Type I vWD have a decrease in both von Willebrand antigen and von Willebrand activity as measured by the ristocetin cofactor assay. Factor VIII coagulant activity is also mildly depressed (see Table 54-11). The next most common variant is Type IIA disease, which accounts for another 10% to 12% of patients. Patients with type IIA disease will have a significant reduction of ristocetin cofactor, and a mild reduction of von Willebrand antigen. Type IIB vWD accounts for 3% to 5% of von Willebrand patients, and approximately 1% of patients have platelet-type vWD. These two groups of patients will demonstrate a hyperresponsiveness of von Willebrand fac-

TABLE 54-11. Diagnosis and Management of von Willebrand Disease

Diagnosis	vWF antigen	vWF activity	Factor VIII activity	RIPA (LD)	Usual therapy
Type I vWD	↓	↓	↓	Absent	Desmopressin
Type IIA vWD	Nl to ↓	↓ ↓ ↓	Nl to ↓	Absent	Humate-P unless known response to desmopressin
Type IIB vWD	Nl to ↓	Nl to ↓	Nl to ↓	Increased	Humate-P (desmopressin contraindicated)
Type III vWD	↓ ↓ ↓	↓ ↓ ↓	↓ ↓ ↓	Absent	Humate-P
Platelet type vWD	Nl to ↓	Nl to ↓	Nl to ↓	Increased	Platelet transfusion (desmopressin contraindicated)

Nl, Normal; *vWD*, von Willebrand disease; *vWF*, von Willebrand factor; *RIPA (LD)*, ristocetin-induced platelet aggregation (low dose).

tor (vWF) to platelets on ristocetin-induced platelet aggregation, low dose (RIPA-LD).

Approximately 1% to 3% of patients have type III disease. These patients have either an autosomal recessive or double heterozygous inheritance of their defect and, as a result, they will display an absence of von Willebrand factor and ristocetin cofactor. It is important to identify patients with type IIB and platelet type vWD because desmopressin therapy causes platelet agglutination and thrombocytopenia in these patients and is therefore contraindicated.

Management. Over 90% of patients with Type I disease will respond to intravenous desmopressin (DDAVP) with a twofold to fourfold increase of their von Willebrand factor levels (see Table 54-11). Patients with type I disease should have a trial of intravenous DDAVP at diagnosis to determine their responsiveness. The dose is 0.3 μg/kg IV in 30 to 50 ml of saline, delivered over 30 minutes. Intranasal desmopressin (Stimate 1.5 mg/ml) has also been used at a dose of 150 μg/nostril in adults. The intranasal delivery has varied efficacy possibly due to the variable absorption. (Note: There are two concentrations of intranasal desmopressin available. The 0.1 mg/ml strength (DDAVP) is used for the treatment of diabetes insipidus and is ineffective in treating vWD.)

For patients with type IIA vWD, intravenous DDAVP may work transiently but most patients will require vWD replacement. There are some intermediate purity, plasma-derived factor VIII concentrates that contain factor VIII complexed to vWF (see Table 54-9). Humate-P is one of these pasteurized preparations, and has been documented to be efficacious in the treatment of vWD and poses no risk in the transmission of hepatitis or HIV. Cryoprecipitate is no longer recommended since it cannot be rendered free of virus.

Patients with type IIB disease have abnormal von Willebrand molecules that bind spontaneously to platelets, causing agglutination and subsequent thrombocytopenia. As a result, stress (including pregnancy and surgery) and desmopressin therapy can release increased amounts of abnormal von Willebrand factor, thus worsening the thrombocytopenia. These patients must be treated with factor VIII and vWF complex (Humate-P).

Since patients with type III disease usually have unmeasurable levels of von Willebrand factor, desmopressin therapy is usually not effective. On the other hand, some patients who have extremely low plasma vWF levels may have higher platelet vWF levels; thus a therapeutic trial with desmopressin is worthwhile. If there is an inadequate rise in the vWF level, an antihemophilic factor must be given (Humate-P).

In platelet type vWD, the primary defect is in the platelet receptor GPIb, with a secondary loss in vWF. Although results of assays are similar to patients with type IIB vWD, platelet type should be treated with platelet transfusion. Once the patient is treated with platelets, the vWF levels will increase.

Rarely, a patient will have vWD of an unknown type. If there is severe hemorrhage, these patients should have blood drawn for typing followed by treatment with vWF. This will adequately treat all patients except those with platelet-type disease. Since administration of desmopressin might worsen thrombocytopenia in patients with type IIB disease or be ineffective in patients with type IIA disease, it is risky to use desmopressin during acute hemorrhage for the initial treatment of a patient with poorly characterized vWD.

COMPLICATIONS OF COMMON CHILDHOOD MALIGNANCIES

Fever and Neutropenia

Fever, a single oral temperature elevation of 38.3° C or three oral temperature elevations of 38° C in 24 hours is a common occurrence in children with cancer. Although fever in cancer patients is frequently due to infection, noninfectious causes must also be considered. Pyrogenic medications (particularly cytotoxic agents such as bleomycin and cytosine arabinoside), blood products, allergic reactions, and the malignant process itself are potential causes of fever.

In a neutropenic child, fever may the first and only sign of infection. Other signs and symptoms indicative of an infectious process may be blunted. Infections in the setting of severe neutropenia may progress very rapidly and result in overwhelming sepsis. Therefore fever and neutropenia demand careful and rapid attention.

Although the definition of neutropenia is somewhat arbitrary, most pediatric cancer centers consider patients with an absolute neutrophil (ANC) count of less than 500/mm³ to be severely neutropenic. Children whose ANC is between 500/mm^3 and 1000/mm^3 but falling due to antineoplastic therapy should also be in the same category.

The initial evaluation of the febrile neutropenic child necessitates an expeditious and meticulous physical examination, with particular attention to those sites that are commonly the source of infection in neutropenic patients such as the skin (particularly sites of intravenous access), lungs, and the perioral and perirectal areas. This initial evaluation of the neutropenic patient yields a clinically or microbiologically defined site of infection in less than half of those who become febrile.[107] Even subtle indications of inflammation must be considered presumptive signs of infection in the presence of neutropenia because the neutrophil-mediated signs are likely to be diminished. After the initial history and physical examination, all febrile, neutropenic children should have cultures from all lumens of indwelling venous catheters. A routine urinalysis and urine culture should be obtained. In young children, catheterization of the bladder is to be avoided. Children with diarrhea should have a stool culture for bacterial, viral, and protozoal agents; and an assay for *Clostridium difficile* toxin. Although the yield of routine chest radiographs in asymptomatic neutropenic patients is small, the study should be performed because it provides an important baseline for comparison with later films (if required).[108]

The management of fever and neutropenia is somewhat controversial, and actual practice varies widely. There is no uniformly agreed upon specific regimen. The following approach is used at many centers.

After the initial evaluation, all febrile neutropenic patients should be promptly placed on broad-spectrum antibiotics. In the absence of definitive microbiologic data, the initial goal of empiric antibiotic therapy is to provide broad-spectrum bactericidal coverage. The most common pathogens are gram-positive organisms, especially staphylococci (both coagulase-positive and coagulase-negative) and streptococci. The most common gram-negative bacteria are *E. coli*, followed by *Klebsiella pneumoniae*, *Pseudomonas* species, and *Enterobacter* species.

Appropriate empiric antibiotic regimens must ultimately be individualized at each institution. Oncology centers have different patterns of microbial isolates and antibiotic resistance. Nevertheless, there is good evidence that the initial empiric management of a febrile, neutropenic cancer patient may be accomplished with a single antibiotic such as ceftazidime. The efficacy of ceftazidime as a monotherapeutic regimen has been supported by the results of a prospective, randomized trial at the National Cancer Institute where ceftazidime monotherapy was compared to a combination of cephalothin, carbenicillin, and gentamicin for the initial empiric management of 550 episodes of febrile neutropenia.[109] Overall, the results demonstrated equivalent rates of success (i.e., survival of the patient through neutropenia, with or without antibiotic modifications of the initial regimen) between ceftazidime and the combination regimen.

There are concerns regarding the use of monotherapy.

1. The relative lack of activity of third-generation cephalosporins against gram-positive cocci has prompted some to advocate the inclusion of vancomycin in the primary regimen.[110]

2. Some have argued for the inclusion of an aminoglycoside in the initial regimen to maximize the activity against gram-negative pathogens and to decrease the emergence of resistant organisms.

Analysis of the data from the National Cancer Institute trial demonstrated that vancomycin was ultimately required in 26 of the 53 primary infections, but was added only after the identification of a resistant isolate in 14 of 17 cases. There were no deaths or significant morbidity associated with the addition of vancomycin after the identification of an organism resistant to the initial regimen. The routine inclusion of vancomycin in the initial empiric therapy would have overtreated most patients, needlessly exposing them to a potentially toxic compound and increasing the cost of care without improving the overall clinical response.

Most patients never required an aminoglycoside, and the inclusion of one of these drugs as part of the initial empiric therapy would have unnecessarily exposed the patients to potential ototoxicity and nephrotoxicity.

How long to continue empiric antibiotics is the most controversial aspect of fever and neutropenia management. A conservative approach is to continue therapy until the absolute neutrophil count returns to over 1500/mm^3.

Varicella Prophylaxis. An important objective in the care of children with cancer is the prevention of infection. Primary varicella is a significant concern for the child with cancer, because the mortality rate in untreated children ranges from 7% to 20%. If a seronegative child is exposed to varicella (continuous household contact, a playmate contact, or a hospital contact) varicella-zoster immune globulin (VZIG), 1 vial/10 kg, should be administered no later than 96 hours after exposure. Children who have received ablative therapy associated with bone marrow transplantation should receive VZIG regardless of their immune status.[111]

Genitourinary Emergencies

Hemorrhagic Cystitis. Hemorrhagic cystitis consists of painful urination with leukocytes, erythrocytes, or clots in the urine because of bleeding and inflammation of the bladder. Cyclophosphamide and ifosfamide are the most common causes of hemorrhagic cystitis.[112] Damage is caused by acrolein, a by-product of cyclophosphamide metabolism.

The diagnosis is made by history and urinalysis. Immediate treatment consists of hydration, transfusion, correction of thrombocytopenia and coagulation abnormalities, and removal of clots by a catheter or cystoscopically. Hemorrhagic cystitis can be prevented by vigorous hydration during and after treatment, and by the use of intravenous or oral sodium-2-mercaptoethanesulfonate (Mesna).[113]

Urinary Flow Obstruction. Lesions of the spinal cord and bulky pelvic tumors may cause acute urinary retention. These lesions include retroperitoneal sarcomas and lymphomas, ovarian tumors, bladder wall rhabdomyosarcomas, and "drop" metastases from brain tumors. All have characteristic radiographic and sonographic appearances. The initial management of the obstruction consists of catheterization or nephrostomy.

Hyperleukocytosis

Hyperleukocytosis is defined as a peripheral leukocyte count exceeding 100,000/μl, and can lead to death from CNS hemorrhage or thrombosis, pulmonary leukostasis, or tumor lysis–associated metabolic derangements. Hyperleukocytosis may occur in lymphoblastic leukemias, particularly those of T-cell lineage. The most severe problems occur, however, when the cells are of myeloid origin in acute myelogenous leukemia. The difference apparently lies in the higher capacity of the latter type of cells for aggregation and adherence to the vascular endothelium.

Many children will have no particular signs or symptoms, but some show signs of hypoxia and acidosis with dyspnea, blurred vision, agitation, confusion, delirium, and stupor. Management of hyperleukocytosis has not been investigated in controlled studies. Hydration, alkalinization, and allopurinol administration should start immediately. The use of exchange transfusion, leukophoresis, and cranial radiation is controversial. At best these modalities are temporizing measures, and definitive treatment must include chemotherapy to ablate production of the abnormal cells in the bone marrow.

Metabolic Emergencies

Tumor Lysis Syndrome. The tumor lysis syndrome consists of the metabolic triad of hyperuricemia, hyperkalemia, and hyperphosphatemia. Secondary renal failure and symptomatic hypocalcemia are common complications. Tumor lysis syndrome occurs before therapy or 1 to 5 days after the start of specific cytotoxic therapy for tumors with a high growth fraction and sensitivity to chemotherapy. It is seen most commonly in Burkitt's lymphoma and in T-cell leukemia/lymphoma.[114] The syndrome generally does not occur in acute nonlymphocytic leukemia or in nonlymphomatous solid tumors.

The tumor lysis syndrome is a direct result of the degradation of malignant cells and of inadequate renal function. All three metabolites involved—uric acid, phosphorus, and potassium—are excreted by the kidney. Elevated uric acid comes from breakdown of nucleic acids. Phosphates are released when tumor cells lyse. Lymphoblasts are especially rich in phosphate, having four times the content of normal lymphocytes.[115] When the calcium:phosphorus product exceeds 60, calcium phosphate precipitates in the microvasculature, leading to renal failure. The second major consequence of hyperphosphatemia is hypocalcemia and seizures.[116] Potassium, the principal intracellular cation, is released with tumor cell lysis. Hyperkalemia can also result from secondary renal failure, and can lead to ventricular arrhythmias and death.

Prevention of renal failure entails hydration, alkalinization, and allopurinol. Hydration is probably the most critical factor. Patients should receive two to four times the maintenance fluid volume as 5% glucose in 0.25 normal saline with 50 to 100 mEq of sodium bicarbonate/L, to produce a urine pH of 7.0 to 7.5 with a specific gravity of no more than 1.010. (Alkalinization of the urine to a pH greater than 7.5 can contribute to the precipitation of calcium stones.) Hydration and alkalinization promote uric acid and phosphate excretion. Allopurinol inhibits xanthine oxidase, which is the enzyme that forms uric acid from the

purine degradation products, hypoxanthine and xanthine. Generally, potassium should not be added to the intravenous solution.

Frank or impending renal failure requires additional therapeutic measures. Hyperkalemia usually presents the most immediate threat to life. All potassium intake should be stopped. Sodium polystyrene sulfonate (Kayexalate), a potassium-binding resin, (1 gm/kg orally with 50% sorbitol) should be started. Calcium gluconate (100 to 200 mg/kg/dose) can induce shift of potassium intracellulary and stabilize myocardial conduction. Insulin with glucose also induces the intracellular flux of potassium. If hyperkalemia and renal failure cannot be controlled, dialysis should be started.

Hypercalcemia. Hypercalcemia refers to a serum calcium greater than 10.5 mg/dl. Normally, serum calcium must be maintained between 9.0 and 10.5 mg/dl. Levels above 12.0 mg/dl disturb virtually every organ system. Hypercalcemia is an infrequent complication of pediatric cancer. The childhood tumors associated with hypercalcemia are acute lymphoblastic leukemia, non-Hodgkin lymphoma, neuroblastoma, and Ewing sarcoma.[117]

Most malignant hypercalcemia results from excessive bone resorption. Normal calcium homeostasis is maintained by a balance between bone deposition and bone resorption. The hypercalcemia of cancer patients is mediated by the same factors that lead to normal bone resorption: parathyroid hormone, prostaglandin E_2, polypeptide growth factors, osteoclast-activating factor, and osteoclasts that are derived from mononuclear phagocytes. A tumor can often be the source of these factors.

Gastrointestinal, renal, neuromuscular, and cardiovascular symptoms dominate the clinical picture of malignant hypercalcemia. The diagnosis is made on the basis of the serum calcium level and the presence of cancer. Other factors that may co-exist in cancer patients to cause hypercalcemia or exacerbate tumor-mediated hypercalcemia include use of thiazide diuretics, oral contraceptives, antacids with calcium carbonate, hypervitaminosis A or D, adrenal insufficiency, fractures, and immobilization.

Treatment of hypercalcemia involves close monitoring of intravascular status. For a serum calcium level less than 14 mg/dl, saline repletion with standard furosemide diuresis is usually sufficient. With higher serum calcium levels, a more vigorous diuresis can be forced with saline levels three times the maintenance dose, and furosemide every 2 hours.[118] Oral phosphorus is effective in controlling chronic but not acute elevations of serum calcium.

Neurologic Emergencies

Acute Change in Mental Status. Changes in mental status often occur in the child with cancer who is medically unstable because of systemic illness or primary CNS dysfunction. These changes consist of lethargy, stupor, and coma, and can be caused by intracranial hemorrhage, cerebrovascular accident, metastatic disease, primary CNS fungal or bacterial infection, viral encephalitis, sepsis/DIC, metabolic abnormality, or leukoencephalopathy.

The emergency evaluation of coma begins with the assessment of vital signs, followed by examination for evidence of cerebral herniation, increased intracranial pressure, and focal neurologic deficits. Special attention should be give to breathing patterns, pupillary size and reactivity, extraocular movements, spontaneous motor function, and the response of the patient to verbal or physical stimuli.

Evaluation in the emergency department should include a complete blood count, serum glucose and electrolytes, hepatic and renal function tests, a coagulation profile, and a toxin screen. If the vital signs of the child are abnormal, life-threatening respiratory and circulatory disturbances must be corrected. Symptoms or signs of increased intra-cranial pressure should be managed with measures to de-crease that pressure, including hyperventilation, intrave-nous dexamethasone (1 to 2 mg/kg) and possibly infusion of mannitol in a 20% solution at 0.5 to 1.0 gm/kg.

Spinal Cord Compression. Of children with cancer who develop spinal cord dysfunction, 4% usually have a tumor-related compression. Sarcomas account for 50% of meta-static spinal cord disease in childhood, with neuroblastoma, lymphomas, and leukemias causing most of the rest.[119] The spinal cord and cauda equina may be compressed by tumor in the epidural or subarachnoid space or by metastatic spread to the cord parenchyma. Epidural compression is the most common.

Any child with cancer and back pain should be consid-ered to have spinal cord compression until proved other-wise. Detailed neurologic examination with attention to extremity strength, reflexes, anal tone, and determination of a sensory level is mandatory. The diagnosis is usually established by MRI studies. If the history suggests rapidly progressive spinal cord dysfunction, or physical examina-tion documents an anatomic level of dysfunction, the treat-ment of choice is immediate dexamethasone in a dose of 1 to 2 mg/kg q 6 hr for 96 hr. For the child with back pain and possible cord compression but without loss of function, the situation is subacute and a lower dose of dexametha-sone (0.25 to 0.5 mg/kg q 6 hr) may be given. Treatment options include surgery, radiation, or chemotherapy.

Syndrome of Inappropriate ADH Secretion. The syn-drome of inappropriate ADH secretion (SIADH) is charac-terized by continuous release of antidiuretic hormone (ADH) without any relation to plasma osmolality. ADH causes the kidneys to conserve water and to concentrate urine. The clinical consequences are hyponatremia and water intoxication. The symptoms of SIADH include fa-tigue, weight gain, lethargy, confusion, seizures, and coma. To make the diagnosis of SIADH, it is necessary to docu-ment a urine osmolality and to exclude renal, adrenal, or thyroid disease and simple hypotonic dehydration.

Fluid restriction is the mainstay of therapy of chronic SIADH or of acute SIADH if the sodium is above 120 mEq/dl and the patient is asymptomatic.[120] If fluid restric-tion is not possible when the patient is having seizures, furosemide and 3% saline to replace sodium losses can correct the situation in 6 hours. There has been some concern that too rapid a correction of sodium can cause further neurologic deterioration and death; a rate of correc-tion of 2 mEq/dl/hr is recommended.[121]

Thoracic Emergencies

Superior Vena Cava Syndrome. Superior vena cava syndrome (SVCS) results from compression, infiltration, or thrombosis of the superior vena cava. Signs of obstruction dominate the clinical presentation in adults, whereas in children, tracheal compression and respiratory distress may also occur.

The superior vena cava (SVC) is a thin-walled vessel with low intraluminal pressure that is surrounded by lymph nodes, which drain the right side and lower left side of the chest, and by the thymus in the anterior superior mediastinum. When the thymus or nodes become involved with tumor, they may compress the SVC. The trachea and right main-stem bronchus are relatively rigid compared with the SVC, but in children these structures also may be compressed by tumor. The relatively small intraluminal diameter of the infant's trachea and bronchi can accommo-date little edema before obstructive symptoms occur. Com-pression, clotting, and edema reduce air flow and blood return from the head, neck, and upper thorax. Collateral vessels enlarge to compensate, but fail to do so adequately.

Common symptoms of SVCS are cough, hoarseness, dys-pnea, orthopnea, and chest pain. Less frequent, but more sinister, are anxiety, confusion, lethargy, distorted vision, and a sense of fullness in the ears. Syncope is a particularly worrisome symptom. Symptoms may be aggravated when the patient is supine or flexed (as for a lumbar puncture).

Signs of SVCS include swelling, plethora, and cyanosis of the face, neck, and upper extremities, edema of the conjunctiva, diaphoresis, and wheezing or stridor. The veins of the chest wall may be engorged. If the right arm is raised above the patient's head, the brachial veins remain full. In children and adolescents, the symptoms often progress rapidly over days. Chest radiographs show a mass in the anterior superior mediastinum. Pleural and pericar-dial effusions may be apparent.

When SVCS is caused by a malignant mass, the situation is a true medical emergency. Establishing a histologic di-agnosis, usually of primary importance, may become sec-ondary to relieving the obstruction. The traditional therapy in such situations has been irradiation. T-cell leukemia and non-Hodgkin lymphoma are the most common causes of SVCS in childhood. These causes of SVCS are usually exquisitely radiosensitive, and many patients improve within 12 hours after the first dose of radiation therapy. In the rare case when symptoms become life-threatening be-cause of postirradiation airway edema a course of pred-nisone 40 mg/m²/day in divided doses q 6 hr may be nec-essary.

Empiric chemotherapy consisting of steroids, cyclophos-phamide, or both in combination with an anthracycline is a reasonable alternative to radiation. Like irradiation, em-piric chemotherapy may confound the diagnosis. Consulta-tion with a pediatric oncologist is recommended to deter-mine the choice of initial therapy and the appropriateness of diagnostic tests before initiating therapy.

Although most chemotherapy- and radiotherapy-sen-sitive anterior mediastinal tumors in children are lympho-mas, dysgerminomas and seminomas may also respond. Alpha-fetoprotein and human chorionic gonadotropin as-says may help to differentiate these from lymphomas.

If the tumor fails to respond to either irradiation or chemotherapy, the differential should include a number of benign lesions including complications from congenital cardiac defect repairs, ventriculoatrial shunts, histoplasmosis, granuloma, and thrombosis of the SVC.[122]

Pleural and Pericardial Effusions. Effusions are classified as either transudates or exudates. Transudates are caused by a sympathetic response to a tumor in the chest or abdomen, fluid overload, heart failure, or hypoproteinemia. Exudates may be caused by local invasion or metastatic spread of tumor or infection. Exudates have protein concentrations exceeding 2.5 gm/dl, a specific gravity greater than 1.015, and a high cell count. Transudates have low protein concentrations, low specific gravity, and low cell counts.

Small, clinically silent pleural and pericardial effusions are often detected on radiographs as part of the evaluation of the extent of disease in patients with a number of childhood tumors. Thoracentesis is indicated when fluid is needed to exclude infection, to establish the stage or diagnosis, to relieve respiratory or cardiac distress, or to eliminate a potential reservoir for drugs such as methotrexate.

Cardiac Tamponade. Cardiac tamponade is the inability of the left ventricle to maintain output, usually because of extrinsic pressure or, rarely, because of an intrinsic mass. Tamponade is caused by compression with pericardial fluid, constrictive fibrosis from previous irradiation, and primary tumors of the cardiac muscle or pericardium.

Symptoms of impending tamponade resemble those of heart failure: cough, chest pain, dyspnea, hiccups, and nonspecific abdominal pain. Signs may include cyanosis and a pulsus paradoxus of more than 10 mm Hg. Patients with constrictive pericarditis may have friction rubs, diastolic murmurs, and atrial dysrhythmia. Radiographs show a typical "waterbag" cardiac shadow. The electrocardiogram may show low-voltage QRS complexes, have flattened or inverted T waves, and electrical atrial and ventricular alterans. Echocardiography of the posterior wall will show two echoes—one from the cardiac muscle and one from the pericardium. Tamponade must be differentiated from congestive heart failure, infections, myocarditis, and therapy-induced myocardiopathy.

Supportive care for malignant pericardial effusion consists of hydration, oxygen, and positioning the patient to maximize cardiac output. Diuretics are usually contraindicated. The specific treatment of tamponade is immediate removal of fluid under echocardiographic guidance.

References

Anemia

1. Graham EA: The changing face of anemia in infancy, *Pediatr Rev* 15:175-183, 1994.
2. Oski FA and Stockman JA III: Anemia due to inadequate iron stores or poor iron utilization, *Pediatr Clin North Am* 27:237, 1980.
3. Bayless PA: Selected red cell disorders, *Emerg Med Clin North Am* 11:481-493, 1993.
4. Orkin SH and Nathan DG: The thalassemias, *N Engl J Med* 295:710, 1976.
5. Evans TC and Jehl D: The red blood cell distribution width, *J Emerg Med* 9(Suppl):71-74, 1991.
6. Brown AK et al.: Reference values and hematologic changes from birth to 5 years in patients with sickle cell disease, *Arch Pediatr Adolesc Med* 148:796-804, 1994.
7. Losek JD et al.: Diagnostic value of anemia, red blood cell morphology, and reticulocyte count for sickle cell disease, *Ann Emerg Med* 21:915-918, 1992.
8. Haschke F and Javaid N: Nutritional anemias, *Acta Paediatr Suppl* 374:38-44, 1991.

9. Martin PL and Pearson HA: The hemolytic anemias. In Oski FA, et al: *Principles and practice of pediatrics*, ed 2, Philadelphia, 1994, JB Lippincott.
10. Skeppner G and Wranne L: Transient erythroblastopenia of childhood in Sweden: incidence and findings at the time of diagnosis, *Acta Paediatr* 82:574-578, 1993.
11. Chabali R: Transient erythroblastopenia of childhood presenting with shock and metabolic acidosis, *Pediatr Emerg Care* 10:278-280, 1994.
12. Berkowitz FE: Hemolysis and infection: categories and mechanisms of their interrelationship, *Rev Infect Dis* 13:1151-1162, 1991.
13. Hilgartner M: Hematological manifestations in HIV-infect children, *J Pediatr* 119:S47-49, 1991.
14. Brown RG: Determining the cause of anemia. General approach with emphasis on microcytic hypochromic anemias, *Postgrad Med* 89:167-170, 1991.
15. Simon TL: Evolution in indications for blood component transfusion, *Clin Lab Med* 12:655-667, 1992.
16. Jayabose S et al: Transfusion therapy for acute anemia, *Amer J Pediatr Hem Onc* 15:324-327, 1993.

Neutropenia

17. Gin-Shaw S and Moore GP: Selected white cell disorders, *Emerg Med Clin North Am* 11:495-516, 1993.
18. Roskos RR and Boxer LA: Clinical disorders of neutropenia, *Pediatr Rev* 12:208-12, 1991.
19. Suarez AD et al.: Prevalence of lymphopenia in children with AIDS, *Clin Pediatr (Phila)* 33:204-208, 1994.
20. Alario AJ and O'Shea J: Risk of infectious complications in well-appearing children with transient neutropenia, *Am J Dis Child* 143:973-976, 1989.
21. Alario AJ: Management of the febrile, otherwise healthy child with neutropenia, *Pediatr Infect Dis J* 13:169-170, 1994.
22. Valiaveedan R et al.: Transient neutropenia of childhood, *Clin Pediatr (Phila)* 26:639-642, 1987.
23. Bonadio WA et al: Clinical significance of newly documented neutropenia in febrile young infants evaluated for sepsis, *Pediatr Infect Dis J* 10:407-408, 1991.

Thrombocytopenia

24. Beardsley DS: Platelet abnormalities in infancy and childhood. In Nathan DG and Oski FA: *Hematology of infancy and childhood*, ed 4, Philadelphia, 1994, WB Saunders.
25. Bussel JB: Thrombocytopenia in newborns, infants, and children, *Pediatr Ann* 19:181-193.

Bleeding Disorders

26. Bleyer WA, Hakami N, Shepard TH: The development of hemostasis in the human fetus and newborn infant, *J Pediatr* 79:838, 1971.
27. Clouse LH and Comp PC: The regulation of hemostasis: the protein C system, *N Engl J Med* 314:1298, 1986.
28. Montgomery RR and Hathaway WF: Acute bleeding emergencies, *Pediatr Clin North Am* 27:327, 1980.
29. Bennett JS: Blood coagulation and coagulation tests, *Med Clin North Am* 68:557, 1985.
30. Buchanan G: Hemophilia, *Pediatr Clin North Am* 27:309, 1980.
31. Harker LA and Slichte AJ: The bleeding time as a screening test for evaluation of platelet function, *N Engl J Med* 287:155, 1972.

Manifestations of Common Childhood Malignancies

32. Jaffe D et al: Detection of cancer in the pediatric emergency department, *Pediatr Emerg Care* 1:11-15, 1985.
33. Pollack ES: Emergency department presentation of childhood malignancies, *Emerg Med Clin North Am* 11:517-529, 1993.

Glucose-6-Phosphate Dehydrogenase Deficiency

34. Beutler E: Glucose-6-phosphate dehydrogenase deficiency, *N Engl J Med* 324:169-174, 1991.
35. Beutler E: G6PD deficiency, *Blood* 84:3613-3636, 1994.
36. Mehta AB: Glucose-6-phosphate dehydrogenase deficiency, *Postgrad Med J* 70:871-877, 1994.

Sickle Cell Disease

37. Kark JA, Posey DM, Schumacher HR, et al: Sickle-cell trait as a risk for sudden death in physical training, *N Engl J Med* 317:781, 1987.

38. Mentzer WC: Is sickle cell trait harmless? *Resid Staff Phys* 38:15-18, 1992.

39. Buchanan GR and Glader BE: Leukocyte counts in children with sickle cell disease, *Am J Dis Child* 132:398, 1978.

40. Davies SC and Wonke B: The management of haemoglobinopathies, *Baillieres Clin Haematol* 4:361-389, 1991.

41. Pollack CV, Jr: Emergencies in sickle cell disease, *Emerg Med Clin North Am* 11:365-378, 1993.

42. Platt OS et al: Mortality in sickle cell disease. Life expectancy and risk factors for early death, *N Engl J Med* 330:1639-1644, 1994.

43. Gray A et al: Patterns of mortality in sickle cell disease in the United Kingdom, *J Clin Pathol* 44:459-463, 1991.

44. Leikin SL et al: Mortality in children and adolescents with sickle cell disease, *Pediatrics* 84:500-508, 1989.

45. Wong WY, et al: Infection caused by *Streptococcus pneumoniae* in children with sickle cell disease: epidemiology, immunologic mechanisms, prophylaxis, and vaccination, *Clin Infect Dis* 14:1124-1136, 1992.

46. Gaston MH et al: Prophylaxis with oral penicillin in children with sickle cell anemia, *N Engl J Med* 314:1593-1599, 1986.

47. Pegelow CH et al: Experience with the use of prophylactic penicillin in children with sickle cell anemia, *J Pediatr* 118:736-738, 1991.

48. Kaplan SK et al: Immunogenicity of *Haemophilus influenzae* type b polysaccharide vaccine in children with sickle hemoglobinopathy or malignancies, and after systemic *Haemophilus influenzae* type b infection, *J Pediatr* 120:367-370, 1992.

49. Lane PA et al: Fatal pneumococcal septicemia in hemoglobin SC disease, *J Pediatr* 124:859-862, 1994.

50. Buchanan GR and Glader BE: Leukocyte counts in children with sickle cell disease, *Am J Dis Child* 132:396-398, 1978.

51. Wong WY et al: Multi-drug resistance to *Streptococcus pneumoniae* in sickle cell anemia, *Am J Hematol* 48:278-279, 1995.

52. West TB et al: The presentation, frequency, and outcome of bacteremia among children with sickle cell disease and fever, *Pediatr Emerg Care* 10:141-143, 1994.

53. Wilimas JA et al: A randomized study of outpatient treatment with ceftriaxone for selected febrile children with sickle cell disease, *N Engl J Med* 329:472-476, 1993.

54. Syrogiannopoulos GA, et al: Osteoarticular infections in children with sickle cell disease, *Pediatrics* 78:1090-1096, 1986.

55. Epps CH Jr et al: Osteomyelitis in patient who have sickle-cell disease. Diagnosis and management, *J Bone Joint Surg* 73:1281-1294, 1991.

56. Powell RW et al: Acute splenic sequestration crisis in sickle cell disease: early detection and treatment, *J Pediatr Surg* 27:215-219, 1992.

57. Rao SP et al: Transient aplastic crisis in patients with sickle cell disease. B19 parvovirus studies during a 7-year period, *Am J Dis Child* 146:1328-1330, 1992.

58. Mallouh AA and Qudah A: An epidemic of aplastic crisis caused by human parvovirus B19, *Pediatr Infect Dis J* 14:31-34, 1995.

59. Platt OS et al: Pain in sickle cell disease, *N Engl J Med* 325:11-16, 1991.

60. Resar LM and Oski FA: Cold water exposure and vaso-occlusive crises in sickle cell anemia, *J Pediatr* 118:407-409, 1991.

61. Serjeant GR et al: The painful crisis of homozygous sickle cell disease: clinical features, *Br J Haematol* 87:586-591, 1994.

62. Shapiro BS: Pain management in sickle cell disease, *Pediatr Clin North Am* 36:1029-1045, 1989.

63. Mills ML: Life-threatening complications of sickle cell disease in children, *JAMA* 254:1487, 1985.

64. Poncz M, Kane E, Gill FM: Acute chest syndrome in sickle cell disease: etiology and clinical correlates, *J Pediatr* 107:861, 1985.

65. Sprinkle RH et al: Acute chest syndrome in children with sickle cell disease, *Am J Pediatr Hem Onc* 8:105-110, 1986.

66. Weil JV et al: Pathogenesis of lung disease in sickle hemoglobinopathies, *Am Rev Resp Dis* 148:249-256, 1993.

67. Bellett PS et al: Incentive spirometry to prevent acute pulmonary complications in sickle cell diseases, *N Engl J Med* 333:699-703.

68. Vichinsky E et al: Pulmonary fat embolism: a distinct cause of severe acute chest syndrome in sickle cell anemia, *Blood* 83:3107-3112, 1994.

69. Miller ST et al: Role of *Chlamydia pneumoniae* in acute chest syndrome of sickle cell disease, *J Pediatr* 118:30-33, 1991.

70. Castro O et al: The acute chest syndrome in sickle cell disease: incidence and risk factors. The Cooperative Study of Sickle Cell Disease, *Blood* 84:643-649, 1994.

71. Pollack CV, Jr, et al: Usefulness of empiric chest radiography and urinalysis testing in adults with acute sickle cell pain crisis, *Ann Emerg Med* 20:1210-1214, 1991.

72. Cole TB, et al: Intravenous narcotic therapy for children with severe sickle cell pain crisis, *Am J Dis Child* 140:1255-1259, 1986.

73. Dampier CD, et al: Intravenous morphine pharmacokinetics in pediatric patients with sickle cell disease, *J Pediatr* 126:461-467, 1995.

74. Gerber N and Apseloff G: Death from a morphine infusion during a sickle cell crisis, *J Pediatr* 123:322-325, 1993.

75. Gonzalez ER, et al: Intermittent injection vs patient-controlled analgesia for sickle cell crisis pain. Comparison in patients in the emergency department, *Arch Intern Med* 151:1373-1378, 1991.

76. Perlin E, et al: Enhancement of pain control with ketorolac tromethamine in patients with sickle cell vaso-occlusive crisis, *Am J Hematol* 46:43-47, 1994.

77. Wright SW, et al: Ketorolac for sickle cell vaso-occlusive crisis pain in the emergency department: lack of a narcotic sparing effect, *Ann Emerg Med* 21:925-928, 1992.

78. Yaster M, et al: Epidural analgesia in the management of severe vaso-occlusive sickle cell crisis, *Pediatrics* 93:310-315, 1994.

79. Griffin TC, et al: High-dose intravenous methylprednisolone therapy for pain in children and adolescents with sickle cell disease, *N Engl J Med* 330:733-737, 1994.

80. Charache S, et al: Effect of hydroxyurea on the frequency of painful crises in sickle cell anemia. Investigators of the Multicenter Study of Hydroyurea in Sickle Cell Anemia, *N Engl J Med* 332:1317-1322, 1995.

81. Rodgers GP, et al: Augmentation of erythropoietin of the fetal-hemoglobin response to hydroxyurea in sickle cell disease, *N Engl J Med* 328:73-80, 1993.

82. Handelsman E and Voulalas D: Albuterol inhalations in acute chest syndrome (letter), *Am J Dis Child* 145:603-604, 1991.

83. Emre U, et al: Alveolar-arterial oxygen gradient in acute chest syndrome of sickle cell disease, *J Pediatr* 123:272-275, 1993.

84. Balkaran B, et al: Stroke in a cohort of patients with homozygous sickle cell disease, *J Pediatr* 120:360-366, 1992.

85. Ohene-Frempong K: Stroke in sickle cell disease: demographic, clinical, and therapeutic considerations, *Semin Hematol* 28:213-219, 1991.

86. Hamre MR, et al: Priapism as a complication of sickle cell disease, *J Urol* 145:1-5, 1991.

87. Milner PF, et al: Sickle cell disease as a cause of osteonecrosis of the femoral head, *N Engl J Med* 325:1476-1481, 1991.

88. Galloway SJ and Harwood-Nuss AL: Sickle cell anemia: a review, *J Emerg Med* 6:213, 1988.

Thalassemia

89. Davies SC and Wonke B: The management of haemoglobinopathies, *Baillieres Clin Haematol* 4:361-389, 1991.

90. Giardina PJ and Hilgartner MW: Update on thalassemia, *Pediatr Rev* 13:55-62, 1992.

Disseminated Intravascular Coagulation

91. Corrigan JJ Jr: Disseminated intravascular coagulation, *Pediatrics* 64:37, 1979.

92. Feinstein DI: Diagnosis and management of disseminated intravascular coagulation: the role of heparin therapy, *Blood* 60:284, 1982.

93. Gill JC and Montgomery RP. Principles of therapy for coagulation factor deficiency. In Nathan DG and Oski FA, *Hematology of infancy and childhood*, ed 4, Philadelphia, 1994, WB Saunders.

Hemophilia

94. Bell B, et al: Hemophilia: an updated review, *Pediatr Rev* 16:290-298, 1995.

95. Ingram GIC: The history of hemophilia, *J Clin Pathol* 29:469, 1976.

96. Gill FH: Congenital bleeding disorders: hemophilia and von Willebrand's disease, *Med Clin North Am* 68:601, 1984.

97. Hoyer LW: Hemophilia A, *N Engl J Med* 330:38-45, 1994.

98. Eyster ME, Goedert JJ, Sarngadharan MG, et al: Development and early natural history of HTLV-III antibodies in persons with hemophilia, *JAMA* 253:2219, 1985.

99. Kasper et al: Hemophilia in the 1990s: principles of management and improved access to care, *Semin Thromb Hemost* 18:1-10, 1992.

Immune Thrombocytopenic Purpura

100. Halperin DA and Doyle JJ: Is bone marrow examination justified in idiopathic thrombocytopenic purpura? *Am J Dis Child* 142:508, 1988.
101. Dubansky AS et al: Isolated thrombocytopenia in children with acute lymphoblastic leukemia: a rare event in a pediatric oncology group study, *Pediatrics* 84:1068-1071, 1989.
102. Sartorius JA: Steroid treatment of idiopathic thrombocytopenic purpura in children: preliminary results of a randomized cooperative study, *Am J Pediatr Hematol Oncol* 6:165, 1984.
103. Bussel JF, Goldman A, Imbach P, et al: Treatment of acute idiopathic thrombocytopenia of childhood with intravenous infusions of gammaglobulin, *Pediatrics* 106:886, 1985.
104. Blanchette V et al: Randomised trial of intravenous immunoglobulin G, intravenous anti-D, and oral prednisone in childhood acute immune thrombocytopenic purpura, *Lancet* 344:703-707, 1994.
105. Water AH: Autoimmune thrombocytopenia: clinical aspects, *Semin Hematol* 29:18-25, 1992.

von Willebrand Disease

106. Casella JF: Disorders of Coagulation. In Nathan DG and Oski FA: *Hematology of infancy and childhood*, ed 4, Philadelphia, 1994, WB Saunders.

Complications of Common Childhood Malignancies

107. Pizzo PA, et al: Fever in the pediatric and young adult patient with cancer: a prospective study of 1001 episodes, *Medicine (Baltimore)* 61:153-165, 1982.
108. Pizzo PA: Management of fever in patients with cancer and treatment-induced neutropenia, *N Engl J Med* 328:1323-1332, 1993.
109. Pizzo PA et al: A randomized trial comparing ceftazidime alone with combination antibiotic therapy in cancer patients with fever and neutropenia, *N Engl J Med* 315:552-558, 1986.
110. Karp JE et al: Empiric use of vancomycin during prolonged treatment-induced granulocytopenia: randomized double-blind, placebo-controlled clinical trial in patients with acute leukemia, *Am J Med* 81:237-242, 1986.
111. Committee on Infectious Diseases and Peter G, editor: *1994 Redbook: report of the Committee on Infectious Diseases*, Elk Grove, IL, 1994, American Academy of Pediatrics.
112. Droller MJ et al: Prevention of cyclophosphamide induced hemorrhagic cystitis, *Urology* 20:256-258, 1982.
113. Shepard JD et al: Mesna versus hyperhydration for the prevention of cyclophosphamide induced hemorrhagic cystitis in bone marrow transplantation, *J Clin Oncol* 9:2016-2020, 1991.
114. Cohen LF et al: Acute tumor lysis syndrome, *Am J Med* 68:486-491, 1980.
115. Rigas DA et al: The nucleic acids and other phosphorus compounds of human leukemic leucocytes: relation to cell maturity, *J Lab Clin Med* 48:356-378, 1956.
116. Zusman J et al: Hyperphosphatemia, hyperphosphaturia and hypocalcemia in acute lymphoblast leukemia, *N Engl J Med* 289:1335-1340, 1973.
117. Harguindey S et al: Hypercalcemia complicating childhood malignancies, *Cancer* 44:2280-2290, 1979.
118. Suki WN et al: Acute treatment of hypercalcemia with furosemide, *N Engl J Med* 326:1196-1203, 1992.
119. Lewis DW et al: Incidence, presentation, and outcome of spinal cord diseases in children with systemic cancer, *Pediatrics* 78:438-443, 1986.
120. Narins RG: Therapy of hyponatremia: does haste make waste? *N Engl J Med* 314:1573-1574, 1986.
121. Wezman Z et al: Combined treatment of severe hyponatremia due to inappropriate antidiuretic hormone secretion, *Pediatrics* 69:610-612, 1982.
122. Issa PY et al: Superior vena cava syndrome in childhood, *Pediatrics* 71:337-341, 1983.

CHAPTER

55

Infectious Disorders

Robert A. Felter • John R. Bower

Signs and Symptoms

FEBRILE CHILD

Fever has been recognized as a symptom of disease since Hippocrates. However, it was only during the sixteenth century that fever was thought to be caused by an irritating or invading agent. Galileo invented the first thermometer in 1592; in the early 18th century Andus Celsius used thermometry in clinical practice. By the nineteenth century Karl Wunderlich established that fever was a symptom and not a disease itself.

Fever has remained an important symptom of illness and is a frequent complaint in children, accounting for up to 20% of emergency department visits. Although the vast majority of children seeking medical care for evaluation of a fever can be easily diagnosed and have minor illnesses, there remains an important group of patients who present one of the greatest clinical challenges to the emergency physician.

Fever as a symptom in children has been a concern to the medical profession as well as parents. Myths often imply that fever in and of itself is damaging and should be treated aggressively, perhaps stemming from Bernard's animal studies in the mid-nineteenth century. However, it is generally the underlying condition that impacts the outcome rather than the fever itself.[1]

Physiologic mechanisms to control body temperature include sweating and hyperventilation to lower temperature and vasoconstriction and shivering to raise temperature. Circulating interleukins, prostaglandins, and prostacyclins mediate the febrile response.

A child is generally considered febrile when the rectal temperature is $\geq 38.0°$ C ($100.4°$ F). The reliability of other methods of temperature measurement is variable. There is a normal diurnal variation in children of up to $1.1°$ C; this is less pronounced in younger children. Seriously ill infants may be euthermic or hypothermic.[2-5]

The *site* for temperature measurement must reflect proximity to major arteries, absence of inflammation, degree of precision required, safety, and insulation from external factors (e.g., drinking). *Rectal* temperature provides precision and should be the technique used in infants, especially those younger than 90 days of age. A risk of rectal perforation and emotional trauma exists. *Axillary* temperatures are appropriate in thermostable environments or when absolute precision is not mandatory, neither of which exists in

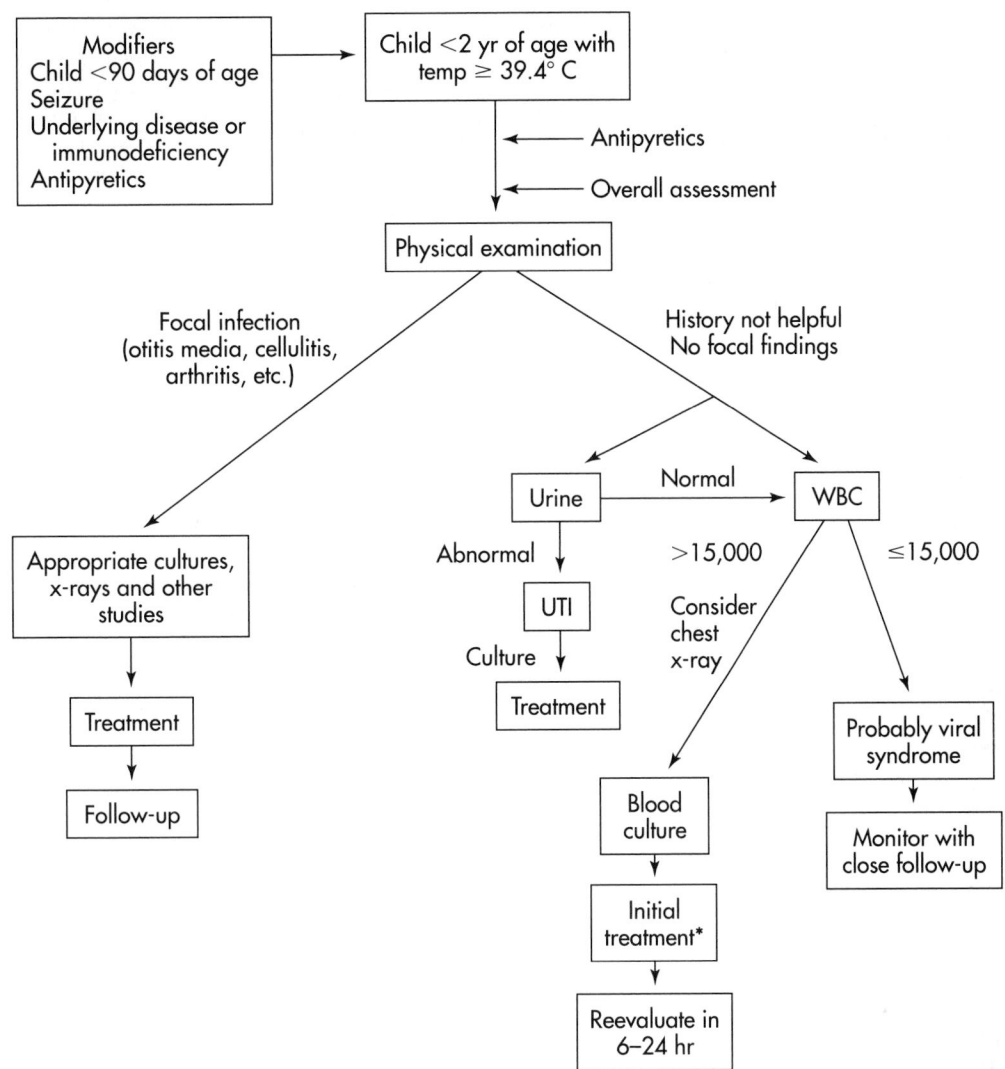

FIG. 55-1. Evaluation of the febrile child younger than 2 years of age (see text). *Ceftriaxone 50 mg/kg/dose IM/IV; ampicillin 50 to 75 mg/kg/dose IM/IV; or amoxicillin 50 mg/kg/24 hr q 8 hr PO. (*From Barkin RM and Rosen P: Emergency pediatrics, ed 4, St. Louis, 1994, Mosby.*)

the emergency department setting. The *oral* or *sublingual* site is useful in a cooperative older child who does not have a rapid respiratory rate. The *tympanic membrane* has been employed with great reproducibility but appears to be less accurate in infants younger than 6 months of age, yielding falsely low values; children younger than 90 days of age should have the temperature taken rectally. It measures the infrared radiation emitted by the tympanic membrane. Speed of measurement must be balanced by the relative inaccuracy of the method. When the tympanic membrane approach is used, an ear "hug" done by pulling posteriorly and superiorly on the external ear at the midpoint between the apex of the helix and the inferior border of the lobule may improve the accuracy.[6-8]

Although the vast majority of underlying illness is infectious in origin, the obligation is to assure that children with significant and potentially life-threatening conditions are distinguished from those with self-limited problems. The nonspecific nature of presentation in neonates and infants and their impaired immunocompetency require aggressive evaluation and treatment in children younger than 90 days of age, but recent patterns of management have introduced greater support for individualizing treatment beyond 30 days.[9-13]

Diagnostic Findings (Fig. 55-1)

Parents usually report nonspecific observations of behavior. The history is important in defining the nature of the illness; the height and duration of fever; dosage, frequency, and response to antipyretics; and past medical problems. A measured or reported elevated temperature within the previous 6 hours is usually considered significant. Associated symptoms and behavioral patterns should be reviewed; particularly look for irritability, response to the environment, respiratory or gastrointestinal findings, limp, and other localizing findings. Exposures to other ill children or adults, immunizations, travel, and source of water may be useful. Preexisting medical conditions (e.g., sickle cell disease, immunodeficiency, respiratory, cardiac, renal disease) should be delineated. Prematurity and associated problems may affect the assessment, particularly during the first 6 months of life.

The physical examination should be systematic and thorough. Specific findings may suggest the source of infection and appropriate therapy.

To assess responsiveness, focus on careful observation of the child at play and encourage the youngster to follow lights and bring objects to parents. Components of this overall assessment as parts of the Yale Observation Scale include:

1. Child looks and focuses on the clinician and spontaneously explores the room.
2. Child spontaneously makes sounds or talks in a playful manner.
3. Child plays and reaches for objects.
4. Child smiles and interacts with parent or practitioner.
5. Child quiets easily when held by parents.[14-16]

While the child is distracted with play objects, obvious physical abnormalities such as limitations of limb movement, rashes, and points of tenderness should be defined. The chest, heart, and abdomen require a gentle hand and patience. Tachypnea disproportionate to fever (>59/min in child <6 months, >52/min in those 6-11 months, and >42 in children 1 to 2 years of age) must be carefully evaluated.[17]

Early antipyretic therapy is imperative in facilitating observation. Many children who are irritable and uninterested in their environment improve markedly with antipyretic management. Acetaminophen (15 mg/kg q 4 to 6 hr PO or PR) should be administered to children with temperatures >38.5° to 39° C on arrival in the emergency department to ensure optimal observation by reducing temperature and permitting a more accurate assessment of the child. Ibuprofen (5 to 10 mg/kg q 6 to 8 hr PO) may be useful as an ancillary agent. Children who are particularly uncomfortable may additionally benefit from a lukewarm water sponge bath. Studies have documented that the clinical response to antipyretics is not predictive of the nature of the illness; the response may facilitate evaluation.[18,19]

As a general rule, infants have less specific findings. In the first few months of life, studies have suggested that febrile children are far more likely to have serious illness. Fever may be the only early symptom; few signs and symptoms may exist. Children with serious disease, as mentioned, may be normothermic. The absence of specific findings mandates complete laboratory evaluation, admission, and antibiotics in this age group.

The older the patient, the more reliable findings are noted. Meningitis in youngsters may merely present with irritability or lethargy, whereas in the teenager, meningismus, pain on extension of the knee with the leg positioned in flexion at the hip (Kernig's sign), and reflex flexion at the knee and hip when the neck is flexed (Brudzinski's sign) are noted.

Specific Entities

Occult Bacteremia. Although bacteremia occurs in association with a host of clinical entities, including meningitis, septic arthritis, epiglottitis, cellulitis, pneumonia, and kidney infection, about 6% of febrile patients without a defined focus have positive blood cloture results. The most common pathogen is *Streptococcus pneumoniae*, accounting for nearly 85% of positive cultures. The majority of the remaining cultures are *Haemophilis influenzae* infections, although this is decreasing with widespread immunization. *Neisseria meningitidis, Salmonella* spp. and other pathogens may also be found.

The highest risk group are those 24 months of age or younger with a fever ≥39.4° C and a white blood cell (WBC) count of 15,000/mm³ or greater. An erythrocyte sedimentation rate (ESR) >30 mm/hr may also be predictive.

Each degree of elevation >39° C increases the risk; children with a temperature of 39.5° to 39.9° C had approximately a 3% incidence of bacteremia, 40° to 40.9° C a 4% risk, and >41° C a 10% risk.

It is essential to evaluate such children carefully to be certain no underlying disease exists. If pneumococcal bacteremia is suspected, consideration should be given to initiating prophylactic antibiotics, but the benefit is controversial. Retrospective review of *H. influenzae* and *Neisseria meningitidis* bacteremia suggested that children sent home on oral antibiotics do better when compared with those sent home without therapy. Another study demonstrated enhanced defervescence when oral amoxicillin was started but did not prevent major morbid events. In general, children younger than 60 to 90 days of age with suspected occult bacteremia in whom empiric antibiotics are initiated should have a full sepsis evaluation including a lumbar puncture.

Hyperpyrexia. True hyperpyrexia, defined as a temperature >41° C (105.8° F), is uncommon but more commonly associated with serious infections. Approximately 20% of children with fevers >41° C will have convulsions. Ten percent of children with temperatures >41.1° C have bacterial meningitis, whereas an additional 7% have bacteremia without meningitis. Press noted that eight of fifteen (53%) children with temperatures >41.1° C had serious disease (two had bacterial meningitis, two bacteremia, two pneumonia, one pericarditis, and one Kawasaki disease).[20,21]

Temperatures >42° C often have noninfectious etiologies such as hyperthermia, head injury, ingestion of psychotropic drugs, and malignant hyperthermia during anesthesia.

Antipyretic management is appropriate and patients should receive a minimum of a complete blood count (CBC), urinalysis, and blood culture. Lumbar puncture (LP) should be considered and a chest-x-ray obtained if there is any suggestion of respiratory findings.

Immunocompromise. Children with a history of recurrent serious bacterial infection should be evaluated for immunodeficiency. Children undergoing cancer chemotherapy or having a history of asplenia (e.g., congenital, trauma) are obviously at risk. Those with sickle cell disease have a 400-fold increased risk of pneumococcal septicemia if younger than 5 years of age and a fourfold risk of *H. influenzae* septicemia if younger than 9 years of age.[22,23]

Such children require aggressive and anticipatory evaluation and treatment as described in Chapter 54.[24,25]

Fever and Petechiae. Children with fever and petechiae may have a viral illness, Rocky Mountain spotted fever, or invasive bacterial disease. Rapid intervention is required. In one study of 190 patients with fever and petechiae, 15 had bacterial disease, half of which was meningitis. The most common pathogen was *N. meningitidis*, accounting for 13 of the 15 patients with invasive disease. Group A streptococcus and respiratory syncytial virus were the most common causes of noninvasive bacterial disease.

Children with fever and petechiae who have a normal lumbar puncture, a WBC count that is neither elevated or decreased, a normal absolute neutrophil and band count, and a temperature <40° C are less likely to have a bacterial infection.[26]

Fever of Unknown Origin. A fever of unknown origin (FUO) is commonly used to refer to a febrile illness of unknown etiology lasting 14 days or more. Most children have actually had two or more febrile illnesses within a short period. When the prolonged fever is continuous, etiologies to consider include inflammatory bowel disease, Hodgkin disease, other neoplasm, juvenile rheumatoid arthritis, systemic lupus erythematosus, infectious mononucleosis, Kawasaki disease and tropical infections such as malaria (see box at right). In a study of 100 children, 52 had an infectious origin, 20 collagen-inflammatory disease, 6 malignancy, and 12 were undiagnosed. A systematic approach to evaluation and referral for ongoing management is appropriate.[27]

Ancillary Data. Following the initial assessment, laboratory studies may be useful in delineating the nature of the underlying illness. No laboratory or historical factors may definitively exclude serious underlying bacterial disease. The peripheral WBC count >15,000 cells/mm³ or below 5,000 cells/mm³ may indicate a serious infection. Meningococcemia, disseminated intravascular coagulation (DIC), or septic shock classically have low counts. Guidelines have suggested that a febrile, non-toxic-appearing child younger than 12 weeks of age has an 8.6% probability of having a serious bacterial infection. Studies have suggested that a band to neutrophil ratio of 0.2 is associated with bacterial infections.[9]

The ESR is a nonspecific test for infection, inflammatory bowel disease, and collagen vascular disease. Its utility is limited by the length of time required for the study.

Cultures are appropriate for specific indications as discussed in the section on Management. Blood cultures for aerobic and anaerobic organisms should be obtained in patients suspected of having bacteremia.[28]

Urinalysis is important in children with fever and no source. In the neonate, the urinalyses may be unremarkable in up to 80% of children with a documented positive culture. Twenty percent of older children with urinary tract infections have a normal urine with negative leukocyte, esterase, or nitrite. A gram stain of the spun urine sediment is the most sensitive screening test. The only reliable methods to obtain a urine sample are straight catheterization or suprapubic bladder aspiration. Table 55-1 provides an interpretation of culture results. Bagged urines are useful to document the degree of hydration or the presence of hematuria, proteinuria, or glucosuria. Urine cultures should be processed promptly.[29-31]

Etiology of Pediatric Prolonged Fever of Unknown Origin

Infection
Bacterial
    Sinusitis
    Pyelonephritis
    Mastoiditis
    Endocarditis
    Adenitis
Viral
    Infectious mononucleosis
    Hepatitis A, B, or C
    Cytomegalovirus
Chlamydial
Mycoplasma
Fungal
    Cysticercosis, blastomycosis, histoplasmosis
Rickettsial
    Q fever
    Rocky Mountain spotted fever
Parasitic
    Malaria
    Toxoplasmosis

Collagen vascular
Juvenile rheumatoid arthritis
Lupus erythematosus
Vasculitis, postinfectious
Acute rheumatic fever
Ulcerative colitis/regional enteritis

Malignancy
Leukemia, lymphoma, neuroblastoma, Wilms tumor

Drug-induced
Antineoplastic, anticonvulsants, antituberculosis agents
Quinidine, procainamide
Serum sickness

Other
Kawasaki disease
AIDS
Hypothalamic dysfunction
Factitious

Lumbar punctures are appropriate to exclude meningitis when this diagnosis is considered as discussed in Chapter 56. The fluid should be cultured and studies should include cell count, gram stain, protein, and glucose (with concurrent blood glucose).[32] There is no conclusive evidence that performing a lumbar puncture on a bacteremic child significantly increases the risk of developing meningitis. Stool smear examination for polymorphonuclear (PMN) leukocyte cells is useful in children with diarrhea, since 90% of infections with salmonella or shigella have accompanying cells; *Campylobacter*, toxigenic *Escherichia coli*, and *Yersinia* sp. may also have PMN leukocytes.

TABLE 55-1. Criteria for Diagnosis of UTI

Collection method	Probability of infection (based on colony forming units/ml*)		
	Unlikely	Probable	Likely
Suprapubic	$< 10^3$		$\geq 10^3$
Catheterization	$< 10^3$	10^3-10^4	$\geq 10^4$
CCMS			
Male	$< 10^3$	10^3-10^4	$\geq 10^4$
Female	$< 10^3$	10^4-10^5	$\geq 10^5$
Bag	$< 10^3$	10^4-10^5	$\geq 10^5$

Adapted from Dubin WA: *Pediatr Infect Dis* 3:564, 1984, and from Barkin RM and Rosen P: *Emergency pediatrics*, ed 4, St Louis, 1994, Mosby.
*Pure culture.
CCMS, Clean catch midstream.

Chest x-ray studies are recommended in young febrile children with evidence of lower respiratory tract disease such as coughing, wheezing, tachypnea, dyspnea, retractions, grunting, nasal flaring, or focally decreased breath sounds. Tachypnea disproportionate to the child's age as noted previously may be an additional risk factor. An abnormal radiograph result in the absence of respiratory findings of cough, rales, or wheezing is unusual in children younger than 8 weeks of age.[33-35]

Management

As no consensus exists regarding the evaluation and management of young febrile children, a conservative yet responsible approach appears mandatory, while recognizing the need to individualize assessment and care.[9]

Children Younger Than 90 Days of Age. A rational and conservative approach is essential in infants. This history is rarely more specific than the triad of fever, irritability, and poor feeding. The physical examination may fail to reveal specific focal findings, despite the presence of systemic infections, which may be enteric, as well as the more common organisms infecting older children. Children younger than 3 months of age with a temperature above 38.5° C have more than a twentyfold greater risk of having a serious infection than do older children with similar temperatures. High fever has some correlation with serious illness but the absence of this finding does not exclude bacterial infections.

Prospective studies have demonstrated that clinical judgment alone is not adequate in the assessment of febrile infant. There are no clear factors that are sensitive or specific enough to be relied on in decision making. However, factors that have been most consistently associated with bacterial disease include age younger than one month, breast feeding, history of lethargy, no contact with an ill person, PMN neutrophil count above 10,000 cells/mm³, and band count greater than 500 cells/mm³. No laboratory or historic factors should be used to exclude underlying bacterial infection.

During the first 30 days of life, infants undergo tremendous developmental and immunological change and are difficult to assess. In one study, one in nine neonates with

The Rochester Criteria

1) Infant appears generally well
2) Infant has been previously healthy
   - Born at term (≥ 37 weeks gestation)
   - Did not receive perinatal antimicrobial therapy
   - Was not treated for unexplained hyperbilirubinemia
   - Had not received and was not receiving antimicrobial agents
   - Had not been previously hospitalized
   - Had no chronic or underlying illness
   - Was not hospitalized longer than mother
3) No evidence of skin, soft tissue, bone, joint, or ear infection
4) Laboratory values:
   - Peripheral blood WBC count 5.0 to 15.0 × 10⁹ cells/L (5,000 to 15,000/mm³)
   - Absolute band form count $\leq 1.5 \times 10^9$ cells/L ($\leq 1,500$/mm³)
   - ≤ 10 WBC per high power field (×40) on microscopic examination of a spun urine sediment
   - ≤ 5 WBC per high power field (×40) on microscopic examination of a stool smear (only for infants with diarrhea)

WBC, White blood cell.
From Jackiewicz JA, McCarthy CA, Richardson AC et al: Febrile infants at low risk for serious bacterial infection. An appraisal of the Rochester Criteria and implications for management, *Pediatrics* 94:390-396, 1994.

serious bacterial infection appeared clinically well. Furthermore, the etiologic agents evolve from vaginal flora (*E. coli,* group B streptococcus, *Listeria monocytogenes,* herpes, and chlamydia) to more traditional community acquired disease. Children in this age group require admission after a full sepsis work-up for administration of parenteral antibiotics and monitoring until culture results are negative at 48 to 72 hours. These children should have blood, urine, and cerebrospinal fluid (CSF) cultures as well as consideration for other studies as indicated. Antibiotics should be initiated including ampicillin 100 to 200 mg/kg/24 hr q 4-6 hrs IV and cefotaxime 50 to 100 mg/kg/24 hr q 8 hr IV. Gentamicin 5 to 7.5 mg/kg/24 hr q 8 hr IV or ceftriaxone 50 to 100 mg/kg/24 hr q 12 hr IV may substitute for cefotaxime, the latter in children older than 30 days of age.

From 30 to 60 days of age, the assessment has greater validity because of the enhanced developmental skills of the child and maturing immune system. Blood and urine cultures, complete blood count (CBC), and LP should be done in febrile children in this age group. An LP is indicated in those children who have an abnormal examination or evaluation or in whom antibiotics are prescribed. Admission is indicated in children with systemic findings toxic appearance, or any abnormal laboratory findings and those who do not meet the low risk Rochester criteria delineated in the box above. Children requiring treatment should be treated with antibiotics identical to those for children younger than 30 days of age.

Children 60 to 90 days of age should have a CBC, urinalysis and urine culture done. If any of these are abnormal, a blood culture should be done. An LP is appropriate if indicated by the examination of the child or if antibiotics are to be started. Admission is appropriate if low risk criteria (see box on p. 930) are not present, the child appears toxic, or the physical or laboratory evaluation is abnormal in any aspect. Additional studies should be considered as indicated by the examination.[36-38]

Children 90 Days to 36 Months. From 90 days to 36 months, the evaluation is more specific and the examination may provide information about a specific diagnostic direction. Studies have shown that the majority of children with serious infections can be identified by the initial evaluation. Furthermore, beyond the greater reliability of the examination, the mature immune status provides reassurance regarding the nature of infection. Clearly, toxic-appearing children need extensive evaluations, whereas children without specific findings who appear nontoxic can generally be managed by ambulatory observation. When the temperature is >39.4° C or 103° F, a CBC is indicated and when the WBC is >15,000/mm^3, a blood culture to exclude occult bacteremia is appropriate. For those who are to receive antibiotics, males younger than 6 months of age, and girls a urinalysis and culture should be obtained as well.

If blood cultures are obtained, many suggest presumptive treatment with antibiotics, although this is controversial and may not reduce the incidence of significant complications. Follow-up observation is essential, usually in 12 to 24 hours, depending on clinical and logistical constraints. This is particularly important in children at high risk for bacteremia.[39]

Disposition

Obviously, close follow-up is essential in all children presenting with a febrile illness, usually within 24 hours either by phone or return visit to the emergency department or primary care physician. Changing clinical status, evolving foci, or other parameters should be evaluated, and cultures obtained initially should be checked for culture results.

If the blood culture remains negative, follow-up on an outpatient basis is appropriate if the patient remains without focal findings. Antibiotics, if started, should be stopped after 48 hours and the patient followed until the illness resolves.

If the blood culture is positive, thereby documenting bacteremia, reexamination of the patient is essential. If the patient is totally normal and the culture contains a gram-positive organisms, close follow-up and continuing antibiotics may be continued for a total 10-day course. If the child is febrile or toxic, has an evolving focus, or the organism is a gram-negative one, admission and intravenous antibiotics are indicated.

Diagnostic Entities

ACQUIRED IMMUNODEFICIENCY SYNDROME

Acquired immunodeficiency syndrome (AIDS) is a persistent and progressively debilitating viral infection affecting multiple systems, particularly the immune and nervous systems.[40] The impact of AIDS in the emergency department includes early diagnosis, management of acute disease complications, and implementation of universal precautions in the care of all patients. AIDS was first recognized as a disease entity in 1981. The etiologic agent, a retrovirus now known as the human immunodeficiency virus (HIV), was first identified in 1984.[41] Screening of the U.S. blood supply for HIV began in 1985. The incidence of pediatric AIDS has risen steadily since the first pediatric case was reported in 1982 and is now the seventh most common cause of death in children 1 to 5 years of age.[42]

Today, over 90% of pediatric HIV infections are the result of vertical transmission from the mother to the infant. Other routes for HIV infection in children include transfusion with contaminated blood or blood products, and sexual abuse. Infants born to HIV-infected mothers have approximately a 25% risk of acquiring infection.[42] Recent studies, however, have shown that the risk of vertical transmission is significantly reduced following maternal zidovudine therapy.[43] HIV-infected mothers acquire the virus primarily through intravenous drug use or sexual contact with an HIV-infected male and are often asymptomatic at the time their child is diagnosed.[44] A family history is often unavailable in the emergency department, as in the case of foster children.

The pathogenesis of AIDS stems from the ability of the virus to specifically recognize and infect CD4 T-helper cells. The CD4 T-cells play a pivotal role in the immune response, interacting with multiple components of the immune system. A depletion in the number of CD4 T-cells, therefore, results in widespread immune dysfunction.[45] Other tissues, such as nervous tissue, may express a receptor similar to that on CD4 T-cells and are targets for primary infection.

Diagnostic Findings

Children infected with HIV present with a diverse array of clinical manifestations ranging from asymptomatic infection to AIDS.[41,46-49]

The disease course in children is often more rapid and has a shorter incubation period than in adults. This makes early diagnosis vital; however, only 35% to 55% of HIV-exposed children are identified before becoming symptomatic.[50] The median age at diagnosis of perinatally acquired AIDS is about 12 months and the majority of cases present by 2 years of age. A small number of children have been diagnosed as late as 13 years of age.[51]

Many of the presenting signs and symptoms of HIV infection are nonspecific. These include recurrent fever, generalized lymphadenopathy, failure to thrive, recurrent oral candidiasis, chronic diarrhea, hepatomegaly, or splenomegaly.[41,46]

Serious or recurrent bacterial infections are a frequent occurrence in HIV-infected children and may present in a variety of forms including bacteremia, otitis media, sinusitis, pneumonia, urinary tract infection, gastroenteritis and meningitis. The most commonly occurring bacterial pathogens isolated from the blood are *S. pneumoniae*, *Salmonella*, *Enterococcus*, *Staphylococcus aureus*, *H. influenzae*, *Pseudomonas*, and *E. coli* (see box on p. 932). An increased

---

Frequent Bacterial Isolates from HIV Patients with Bacteremia

Streptococcus pneumoniae
Haemophilus influenzae
Salmonella
Staphylococcus aureus
Coagulase negative staphylococcus
Other streptococci
Enterococcus
Other enterobacteriaceae
Pseudomonas

Modified from Bernstein et al: *Pediatr Infect Dis J* 4:472-475, 1985; Krasinski et al: *Pediatr Infect Dis J* 7:323-328, 1988; and Spector et al: *N Engl J Med* 331:1181-1187, 1994. Massachusetts Medical Society.

---

incidence of tuberculosis and syphilis has also been observed. Patients presenting to the emergency department with serious or recurrent bacterial infections should be assessed for possible HIV risk factors.[51-54]

Neurologic manifestations are common in HIV-infected children. A static or progressive encephalopathy is the most frequent presentation and is characterized by developmental delay, deterioration in motor skills or intellectual performance, muscle weakness, pyramidal tract signs, ataxia, acquired microcephaly, or seizures. CSF findings are usually normal although there may be mild pleocytosis or an increase in protein concentration.[55] The computed tomography (CT) scan may demonstrate varying degrees of cortical atrophy and basal ganglia calcifications. Central nervous system (CNS) infections occur less frequently in children than in adults. Common causes include *Toxoplasma gondii*, *Cryptococcus neoformans*, bacterial meningitis, syphilis, *Mycobacterium tuberculosis*, and various viruses.[56]

Opportunistic infections develop in patients with significantly depressed cell-mediated immunity. *Pneumocystis carinii* pneumonia (PCP) is the most common opportunistic infection in children with AIDS. The incidence of PCP is highest in children younger than 12 months of age, peaking between 3 to 6 months of age.[50] Infants with PCP characteristically present with acute onset of fever, cough, tachypnea, and retractions. The chest x-ray reveals diffuse bilateral alveolar infiltrates but may show minimal changes early in the disease. The diagnosis of PCP is by bronchoalveolar lavage or lung biopsy. Lymphocytic interstitial pneumonitis (LIP) may resemble PCP. LIP is an idiopathic pneumonitis that occurs in approximately 20% of children with AIDS.[57] The chest x-ray typically reveals fine reticular or reticulonodular infiltrates. Children with LIP develop cough, tachypnea, and hypoxia. There may also be evidence of bronchospasm. Definitive diagnosis of LIP requires biopsy. *Mycobacterium avium-intracellulare* complex (MAC) is an opportunistic infection that typically presents as a multisystem disease with recurrent fever, pneumonia, abdominal pain, and diarrhea. Organisms can be isolated from the blood

and infected tissues.[58] Disseminated CMV may present similarly to MAC with pneumonia, hepatitis, colitis, meningitis, or retinitis.[40,58] Candidial infections that extend beyond the oral mucosa are considered opportunistic. Candidal esophagitis should be suspected in patients with oral candidiasis, dysphagia, or decreased appetite. The diagnosis requires endoscopy. Chronic herpes simplex virus infections present as frequently recurring lesions that persist for longer than one month. Other opportunistic infections include *Cryptosporidium, Cryptococcus, Toxoplasma,* and *M. tuberculosis.*[40,46]

Ancillary Data. Routine laboratory studies generally reveal nonspecific abnormalities. Anemia, thrombocytopenia, neutropenia, and lymphopenia are common findings.[59] Liver function studies may be elevated, suggesting a primary or secondary hepatitis. The urinalysis is often abnormal. As many as 30% to 55% of HIV-infected patients may develop renal disease with findings of azotemia and proteinuria.[60] Studies of the immune system generally show an elevation in quantitative immunoglobulins and a decrease in the CD4 T-cell count.

The diagnosis of HIV in children older than 18 months is by enzyme immunoassay (EIA). Any positive EIA must be repeated and confirmed by western blot analysis to establish a serologic diagnosis. In children younger than 18 months a positive EIA may be due to the presence of maternal antibody. In these children the diagnosis of HIV infection is accomplished using either HIV viral culture or HIV polymerase chain reaction (PCR) and detection of p24 antigen (acid dissociated). HIV culture and PCR are highly sensitive and specific in detecting HIV by the time a child is 6 months of age. However, any positive result must be confirmed with a second test performed on a separate blood sample.[61-63]

Management

Preventive health care and careful monitoring constitutes the long-term management of HIV-infected children. Zidovudine (AZT) and Didanosine (DDI) are antiretroviral agents approved for use in HIV-infected children with evidence of immune dysfunction or symptoms of HIV.[64] Acute illness in the HIV-infected child ranges from common childhood illnesses to serious manifestations of opportunistic infections. Aggressive and sensitive medical and emotional support is essential.

A common management consideration is the febrile HIV-infected child. Evaluation of an HIV-infected patient with fever requires a thorough history, physical examination, and assessment of the patient's general condition. In addition, a CBC and blood culture should be obtained because of the increased risk for bacterial infection. Apart from the well-appearing child with an obvious focus of infection, such as middle ear or upper respiratory infection, the evaluation should also include urinalysis, stool culture (in the presence of diarrhea), and chest x-ray (even in the absence of respiratory symptoms). Febrile patients who appear toxic should be hospitalized and evaluated for serious bacterial or opportunistic infection.[65-67]

Pneumonia in any HIV-infected child is a potentially serious complication and presents an extensive differential diagnosis including bacterial, mycobacterial, fungal, viral,

Universal Precautions for Exposure to Blood and Body Fluids of All Patients

Handwashing is necessary after physical contact with all patients and after removing gloves.

I. Body fluids and procedures for which gloves are recommended (barrier eye protection should be used whenever spattering is likely):

Blood

Body fluids: semen, vaginal secretions, and tissue, cerebrospinal, synovial, pericardial, pleural, and amniotic fluids

Blood-contaminated fluids

Intubation

Endoscopy

Dental procedures

Wound irrigation

Phlebotomy

Arterial puncture

Vascular catheter placement

Tracheostomy suctioning

Rinsing of used instruments

Lumbar puncture

Puncture of other cavities (e.g., pleural, peritoneal)

II. Body fluids for which only handwashing is recommended:

Urine

Stool

Vomitus

Tears

Nasal secretions

Oral secretions

Diaper contents

Management of Occupational Exposure to HIV-Contaminated Blood or Body Fluids

Definition:

Occupational exposure is defined as a percutaneous injury (e.g., a needlestick or cut with a sharp object), contact of mucous membranes, or contact of skin (especially when the exposed skin is chapped, abraded, or afflicted with dermatitis or the contact is prolonged or involves an extensive area) with blood, tissues, or other body fluids to which universal precautions apply, including: (1) semen, vaginal secretions, or other body fluids contaminated with visible blood, because these substances have been implicated in the transmission of HIV infection; (2) cerebrospinal fluid, synovial fluid, pleural fluid, peritoneal fluid, pericardial fluid, and amniotic fluid, because the risk of transmission of HIV from these fluids has not yet been determined; and (3) laboratory specimens that contain HIV.

Management of workers with percutaneous or permucosal exposure:

Test both source patient and exposed worker for HIV and hepatitis B virus. Testing must be performed in compliance with hospital and state regulations for maintaining confidentiality.

1. If the source patient is HIV-negative, no further testing is required unless there is reason to suspect that the source patient has only recently been infected.

2. If the source patient is positive or is suspected to be positive because of significant risk factors, the exposed worker should be counseled regarding risk of infection and the role of zidovudine (AZT) prophylaxis. The role of zidovudine in preventing HIV infection has not been established. The CDC or health department should be contacted for the most current treatment regimen.

3. Workers exposed to hepatitis B–contaminated blood should be managed as described in Appendix 55B.

HIV, Human immunodeficiency virus; *CDC,* Centers for Disease Control and Prevention.

Adapted from Public Health Service: *MMWR* 39 (RR-1): 1-14, 1990.

and idiopathic etiologies. Because of the multiple etiologies and the risk for rapid deterioration, HIV-infected children with clinical or radiographic evidence of pneumonia should be hospitalized for further evaluation and management.[66,68]

Prevention. The rising incidence of HIV infection makes compliance with "universal precautions" an important aspect of patient management, particularly in the emergency department where exposure to contaminated fluids is common and where knowledge of a patient's HIV status is unlikely. Therefore, all patients should be considered as infectious for HIV and other bloodborne pathogens.[69] Universal precautions are designed to prevent parenteral, mucous membrane, and nonintact skin exposures to bloodborne pathogens by the appropriate use of barriers including gloves, eyewear, gowns, and masks (see box above).

Gloves should be worn on both hands whenever there is potential contact with blood, body fluids, or any fluid containing visible blood. Gloves should never be washed and reused. Long-sleeved, fluid-resistant gowns should be worn whenever there may be splattering of contaminated fluids over clothing. Eye protection, preferably goggles and

masks, should be worn whenever splattering of infective material is likely.[70]

Hands and other skin surfaces should be washed immediately and thoroughly following contact with blood or other body fluids included under universal precautions. Hands should be washed after removing gloves, even if the gloves appear intact.[70]

Occupational exposure to blood or body fluids is a frequent concern in the emergency department and requires immediate evaluation for risk of HIV and hepatitis B infection (see box above). Both the worker and the source patient should be tested for HIV and hepatitis B. HIV testing must be performed in compliance with hospital and state guidelines to maintain patient confidentiality. All occupational exposures should be referred to the hospital occupational health officer or to a local health department.

The risk of HIV infection following percutaneous exposure to known HIV-infected blood is approximately 0.4%. The risk following perimucosal exposure is probably even less. Workers who have been exposed to HIV-positive blood or body fluids should be counseled regarding AZT prophylaxis. The prophylactic efficacy of AZT has not yet been established. Short-term side effects are primarily a reversible anemia/neutrepenia. Long-term effects such as teratogenicity are unknown.[71]

At present, there is no established AZT prophylaxis regimen although many hospitals have instituted protocols. Current treatment regimens should be obtained by contacting the hospital occupational health officer, local health department, or the Centers for Disease Control and Prevention (CDC).

BOTULISM

Botulism is a toxin-mediated neuromuscular disease having three clinical forms; classical, infant, and wound botulism. Infant botulism is the most common form of the disease in the United States with 60 to 70 cases reported each year, affecting mostly infants younger than 6 months of age.[72] Classical or foodborne botulism typically occurs in outbreaks and is most commonly associated with home-prepared foods. Wound botulism is quite rare.[73]

The etiologic agent, *Clostridium botulinum*, is an anaerobic gram-positive bacillus capable of producing one of three exotoxins (A, B, or E). These extremely powerful neurotoxins bind irreversibly to the synaptic membrane of the neuromuscular junction, preventing acetylcholine release. The organism is capable of growth in a wide pH range and is inactivated only by boiling for at least 5 minutes. The toxin may accumulate in a food source, as in classical botulism, or be produced following growth of the bacillus in the patient, as in infant and wound botulism.[74] Honey may be a source of the bacillus in children younger than 12 months.

Diagnostic Findings

The clinical features of classical botulism develop 12 to 72 hours after ingestion of the toxin and involve generalized weakness and autonomic dysfunction. Weakness proceeds in a symmetrical, descending fashion beginning with the cranial nerves. Blurred vision, dilated or fixed pupils, diplopia, and dysphagia are followed by muscular weakness. Postural hypotension, constipation, and urinary retention are common. Respiratory muscles are frequently involved and patients often require ventilatory support.[75] Slurred speech, dysphagia, and sore throat are reported. Nausea, vomiting, and dry mouth may also occur. The sensorium and sensory examination are normal.

The clinical manifestations of infant botulism are often more subtle and gradual in onset than classical botulism. A history of recent honey or corn syrup consumption may be suggestive, but absent in most cases.[76,77] The most common signs and symptoms of infant botulism include generalized weakness, poor feeding, constipation, decreased activity, and poor cry; the term "floppy infant" with hypotonia may be applied (Table 55-2).

TABLE 55-2. Presenting Signs of Infant Botulism

Sign	Percentage of infants (N = 57)
Floppiness or generalized weakness	88
Poor feeding	79
Constipation	65
Lethargy or decreased activity	60
Poor cry	18
Irritability	18
Respiratory difficulties	11
Seizures	2

Adapted from Schreiner M, Field E, Ruddy R: *Pediatrics* 87:159, 1991.

Complications of botulism include respiratory failure, malnutrition, pneumonia, syndrome of inappropriate antidiuretic hormone (SIADH), seizures, apnea, urinary retention, and autonomic instability.[77-79]

Routine laboratory findings are not revealing in botulism. Specific diagnosis of botulism requires identification of either the toxin or organism. In foodborne botulism a food sample or blood specimen (obtained before administration of antitoxin) should be submitted for botulinum toxin analysis.[72] CSF may have increased protein.

Definitive diagnosis of infant botulism requires identification of toxin or organisms in the stool. However, the amount of stool required for toxin identification (50 to 60 gm) in a patient that typically has severe constipation makes this a difficult test. EMG has been used to establish a preliminary diagnosis of infant botulism[64]; however, the sensitivity and specificity of electrodiagnosis has been questioned.[80]

Differential Considerations

The differential diagnosis of infant botulism includes hypotonia, sepsis, metabolic disorders, endocrine abnormalities, subdural hematoma, and Wernig-Hoffman syndrome. Entities that may present similarly to classical botulism include myasthenia gravis, chemical intoxication, Guillain-Barré syndrome, tick paralysis, and Eaton-Lambert syndrome.[78,79]

Management

The most vital aspect of management is supportive care. Patients should be evaluated for evidence of respiratory compromise and managed accordingly. All patients require intensive monitoring. A study of 57 children with infant botulism revealed that 77% required intubation and mechanical ventilation.[78] Patients with classical botulism who are suspected of ingesting toxin should be treated with trivalent (ABE) antitoxin. Individuals exposed to the same contaminated source should also receive antitoxin. Trivalent antitoxin can be obtained by contacting the state health department or, failing that, by calling the CDC (404) 639-3670 in the daytime or (404) 639-2888 at night.

Patients with suspected infant botulism do not benefit from antitoxin, as there is very little circulating toxin in the blood stream. These patients should be managed with supportive care.[76]

Botulism may be prevented by boiling all foods adequately (over 10 minutes). Children younger than one year of age should not eat honey.

DIPHTHERIA

Diphtheria is a rare disease in most developed countries, but the continued presence of the causative organism producing sporadic outbreaks and deaths requires the clinician to be familiar with the disease process. High levels of immunization affect the frequency and severity of cases, and in developing countries where < 10% of children are immunized, diphtheria accounts for up to one million deaths per year.[81] Outbreaks in Scandinavia, where this disease was considered to be eradicated, clearly point to the distinct danger of diphtheria even in highly immunized populations and the need for continued immunizations of adults against this disease.[82]

The causative organism for diphtheria, *Corynebacterium diphtheriae*, was first isolated by Loeffler in 1895 and is a clubshaped gram-positive pleomorphic bacillus. Diphtheria was the subject of great interest around the turn of the century and was a leading cause of death among children, with a case fatality rate from 50% to 80%. The advances in medical knowledge from this intensive investigation were considerable and led to many now widely accepted theories from the germ theory to the carrier state theory.[83]

Diagnostic Findings

The clinical manifestations of diphtheria depend on the location of the infection, the host's immune status, and the virulence of the infecting bacterium. The incubation period is 2 to 5 days. In the acute phase, infections can be broadly classified into cutaneous and pharyngeal, the latter being the most common. The pharyngeal form presents with fever, sore throat, cervical lymphadenopathy, thick gray-white membrane, and tachycardia. The cervical adenopathy may be so pronounced that historically it has been called bull neck. Early in the disease, before the membrane is pronounced, the patient is often diagnosed as having streptococcal pharyngitis or infectious mononucleosis. There is a characteristic odor to the breath of patients with pharyngeal diphtheria but, because of its rarity, is not generally recognized by clinicians.[84]

The laryngeal form is less common, initially presenting with hoarseness or loss of voice, and may extend into the pharynx. Nasal disease presents with a serosanguinous discharge that may persist for weeks. Cutaneous diphtheria presents with a sharply demarcated ulcer with a membranous base.

In addition to the local infection, the bacterium elaborates a toxin that predominantly affects the cardiac and nervous systems. The complications of the toxin are seen several days to several weeks after the acute infection.

Early morbidity is usually caused by respiratory embarrassment from the spreading membrane and upper airway obstructions. The fact that most children with diphtheria die of suffocation led to the development of intubation as a therapeutic modality by O'Dwyer in 1886. With intubation and tracheostomy well established, early deaths now are usually due to the hemorrhagic complications, although the exact etiology of the bleeding diathesis associated with this form of diphtheria remains unclear.

Later complications causing morbidity and mortality are the toxin-mediated myocarditis, endocarditis, dysrhythmias, thrombocytopenia, and paralysis. Vocal cord paralysis and an ascending paralysis similar to Guillain-Barré syndrome may occur. As the antitoxin only neutralizes circulating toxin, the rapid elimination of the causative organism as well as antitoxin administration is essential. Delay in diagnosis leads to irreversible damage to tissues on which the toxin is already fixed.[85] Because of this, suspected cases should be treated before definitive diagnosis by culture is made.

Specimens for culture should be obtained from the nose, throat, and any lesions. Material from beneath the membrane or a portion of the membrane should be cultured. The laboratory should culture material on Loeffler medium and tellurite agar. The CBC is variable, often with decreased platelets. Cardiac enzymes, electrocardiogram (ECG), and arterial blood gas (ABG) are usually appropriate.

Management

Treatment of pharyngeal diphtheria begins with suspicion of its presence with suggestive clinical findings rather than an absolute diagnosis, especially in nonimmunized or incompletely immunized children. Immediate administration of intravenous equine antitoxin after appropriate sensitization testing is recommended. Intradermal and conjunctival tests for horse-serum sensitivity should be done using 0.1 ml after 1:10 dilution for conjunctival testing or 1:100 dilution for intradermal testing. Desensitization may be necessary. The dose is based on the estimated degree of toxicity and duration of illness.[86] If the membrane is pharyngeal or laryngeal and of less than 48 hours' duration, 20,000 to 40,000 U should be administered. Nasopharyngeal lesions require 40,000 to 60,000 U; extensive prolonged (>3 days) disease may need 80,000 to 100,000 U.

Antibiotic therapy consists of erythromycin (40 to 50 mg/kg/24 hr) for 2 weeks or penicillin G (aqueous crystalline, 100,000 to 150,000 U/kg/24 hr q 6 hr) or procaine (25,000 to 50,000 U/kg/24 hr q 12 hr IM) for 2 weeks.[86]

It is also imperative to test and treat potential carriers and those exposed to active cases, including health-care professionals. Close contacts, regardless of their immunization status, should be cultured and treated with oral erythromycin or intramuscular penicillin G. Previously immunized contacts should receive a booster dose if they have not received one in more than 5 years. In unimmunized persons or those with uncertain immunization status, active immunization is begun based on age. Contacts who cannot be kept under surveillance should be given erythromycin or penicillin G for 7 days, or benzathine penicillin G (600,000 U for those over 30 kg and 1.2 million U for others) and appropriate immunization.[86]

Since the introduction of diphtheria toxoid, diphtheria has become a rare disorder and therefore is more difficult to recognize. Although children still make up a majority of cases, they are a much smaller percentage than historically. This probably is because of the decreased levels of immunity among adults. Immunization decreases the likelihood and severity of illness but is protective only against the phage-mediated toxin and not against infection by *C. diphtheriae*.[81] Widespread immunization leads to a "herd immunity" but recent outbreaks demonstrate that there are still carriers and susceptible individuals. In North America cases most commonly occur in nonimmunized children or adults from lower socioeconomic groups.

Cutaneous diphtheria, once considered to be a strictly tropical disease, is making up a larger percentage of cases. The cutaneous form is considered more infectious than the nose or throat carrier forms and several recent cases of pharyngeal diphtheria have been traced to an individual with the cutaneous form.[87] Because the skin lesions are often confused with impetigo or an infected wound or ulcer and the incubation period may be up to 1 week long, the index case may be difficult to detect.[88,89]

As morbidity and mortality of infected patients has not changed in recent years, efforts must be directed at early detection, as well as initial and continued immunization. The emergency physician has a unique opportunity to aid in this process by administering the combined diphtheria and tetanus toxoid to older patients and those who have not received such immunization in more than 10 years, and to ensure the initial immunization of children.

EMPORIATRICS

The emergency physician is presented daily with a wide spectrum of diseases. Making a definitive diagnosis is not always possible on a single visit to the emergency department, yet this is often expected. Diseases related to international travel and those that occur rarely, if ever, in the United States may not be considered initially in a given patient. But it is often the emergency physician who is faced with the problems of (1) recommending prophylactic treatment for international travelers, (2) treating foreign visitors who become ill while in the United States, and (3) treating patients who return or become ill soon after international travel.

Emporiatrics, or the study of travel medicine, is a new field brought about by the incredible numbers of people who travel around the world every year. Because not every city has a specialist in emporiatrics, the emergency physician must often fill that role.

Even though practitioners of emergency medicine in large metropolitan areas, especially where large populations of immigrants live, are more aware of tropical diseases, most may never see any of these "exotic" diseases. As the entire spectrum of tropical medicine cannot be discussed here, a few diseases that are more likely to be seen are discussed. In addition to having the name of a local specialist for the identification of mushrooms, having a tropical medicine consultant available is advisable for any emergency department, especially in large urban areas.

Recommendations for prophylaxis for would-be travelers are presented in the CDC's *Health Information for International Travel*. This is updated annually and provides the best information regarding immunization, prophylaxis, and general advice according to country and risk of disease. In addition, the CDC publishes a biweekly "blue sheet" updating specific diseases occurring in specific countries at that time (e.g., cholera).

Treating the foreign visitor who becomes ill is a more difficult problem. As if the frequent language barrier were not bad enough, lack of information on immunization status, unfamiliarity with drugs used in other countries, and the wide array of foreign as well as domestic disease possibilities make diagnosis incredibly difficult.

First, any recent travel must be established. This is not a typical question to ask when confronted with a febrile child but the emergency physician must always keep this in mind, especially when the presenting complaints are complex or unusual.

Once travel to specific areas is determined, a detailed history must be elicited. In the young child this may be difficult, especially if the child was not accompanied by an adult to the emergency department. A detailed itinerary, including season, place of residence (rural vs. urban, 5-star hotel vs. tent), what foods were eaten, what precautions were taken (including sexual history), insect bites, and skin lesions, should be obtained. In addition, any prophylactic measures, either prescribed or self-medicated, must be documented. Then a detailed history of the illness should be elicited; remember that some diseases appear within days after or during travel (traveler's diarrhea), whereas others develop weeks or months after exposure (some forms of malaria). Illness in other members of a traveling group and a thorough physical examination are also necessary. Laboratory evaluation must be directed at likely illnesses as well as those that are important to exclude. The physician must remember that in addition to diseases endemic to the tropics, familiar but rare diseases (e.g., measles) can be contracted in countries with less prevention.

The chief complaints of patients returning from travel abroad include diarrhea (30% to 35%), upper respiratory symptoms (15%), fever with or without rash (10%), and abdominal pain or malaise (5%).[90] Of the acute febrile illnesses most fall into one of the following categories: typhoid or one of the enteric fevers, infectious diarrhea or dysentery, tuberculosis, viral hepatitis, or malaria.[91]

Of the diarrheal diseases, the most common cause of "traveler's diarrhea" is *E. coli*, although many other agents may be responsible. The clinical course may suggest a particular diagnosis. Examination of stool specimen for WBCs and blood, as well as ova and parasites, and stool culture may establish the diagnosis. Treatment is based on the infecting organism and the child's clinical condition.

Of the febrile illnesses associated with travel, malaria, typhoid fever, and dengue are briefly discussed (see following). Table 55-3 summarizes the pharmacologic management of commonly encountered parasitic diseases.

Malaria

Although once endemic in the United States, malaria is seldom encountered except in those who travel to foreign countries. Before World War II, it was estimated that one third of the world's population had had malaria. Currently, malaria is probably the leading infectious disease worldwide, causing up to three million deaths per year, with one third of the patients younger than 5 years of age.[90]

Malaria is not uncommonly seen in this country because of large numbers of civilian and government personnel

TABLE 55-3. Antiparasitic Drugs

Parasitic diseases	Management
Amebiasis (*Entamoeba histolytica*)	
Asymptomatic carrier	Iodoquinol (previously diiodohydroxyquin) 40 mg/kg/24 hr q 8 hr PO (adult: 650 mg/dose) × 20 days; **or** diloxanide furoate (Furamide) (CDC) 20 mg/kg/24 hr q 8 hr PO (adult: 500 mg/dose) × 10 days
Mild to moderate colitis	Metronidazole (Flagyl) 35 mg/kg/24 hr q 8 hr PO (adult: 750 mg/dose) × 10 days; **plus** iodoquinol, as above
Severe colitis	Metronidazole, as above × 10 days; **plus** iodoquinol, as above
Extraintestinal	Metronidazole, as above × 10 days; **plus** iodoquinol, as above
Ascariasis (*Ascaris lumbricoides*)	Mebendazole (Vermox) 100 mg q 12 hr PO × 3 days (children >2 yr); **or** pyrantel pamoate (Antiminth) 11 mg/kg/dose (maximum: 1 gm) PO × 1 (one dose only)
Balantidiasis (*Balantidium coli*)	Tetracycline 40 mg/kg/24 hr q 6 hr PO (children >8 yr only) (adult: 500 mg/dose) × 10 days; **or** iodoquinol 40 mg/kg 24 hr q 8 hr PO (adult: 650 mg/dose) × 20 days
Cutaneous larva migrans or creeping eruption (cutaneous hookworm)	Thiabendazole (Mintezol) 50 mg/kg/24 hr (maximum: 1.5 gm/dose) q 12 hr PO × 2-5 days
Cysticercosis (*Taenia solium*)	Surgical excision most satisfactory; Praziquantel (Biltricide) 50 mg/kg/24 hr q 8 hr PO × 14 days (± steroids)
Dientamoebiasis (*Dientamoeba fragilis*)	Iodoquinol 40 mg/kg/24 hr q 8 hr PO (adult: 650 mg/dose) × 20 days
Filiariasis	
Onchocerciasis (*Onchocerca volvulus*)	Ivermectin 150 μg/kg once and repeated every 6-12 mo; **or** diethylcarbamazine (Hetrazan) 1.5 mg/kg/24 hr q 8 hr PO (maximum: 25 mg/24 hr) × 3 days, then 3 mg/kg/24 hr q 8 hr PO (maximum: 50 mg/24 hr) × 3-4 days, then 4.5 mg/kg/24 hr q 8 hr PO (maximum: 100 mg/24 hr) 3-4 days, then 6 mg/kg/24 hr q 8 hr PO (maximum: 150 mg/24 hr) × 14-21 days, *followed by* suramin 10-20 mg (test dose) IV, then 20 mg/kg IV at weekly intervals × 5 wk (adult: 100-200 mg [test dose] IV, then 1 gm IV at weekly intervals × 5 wk)
Other forms (Loa loa, tropical eosinophilia) (*Wuchereria bancrofti, Brugia malayi*)	Diethylcarbamazine (Hetrazan) 25-50 mg/24 hr q 24 hr PO (maximum: 50 mg/24 hr) × 1 day; then 75-150 mg/24 hr q 8 hr PO (maximum: 150 mg/24 hr) × 1 day; then 150-300 mg/24 hr q 8 hr PO (maximum: 300 mg/24 hr) × 1 day; then 6 mg/kg/24 hr q 8 hr PO × 17 days; surgical excision of subcutaneous nodules; allergic reactions may require steroids or antihistamines
Flukes Liver (*Opisthorchis viverrini*) Lung (*Paragonimus westermani*) Chinese liver (*Clonorchis sinensis*)	Praziquantel (Biltricide) 25 mg/kg/dose PO × 3 doses (doses to be taken in 1 day)
Giardiasis (*Giardia lamblia*)	Furazolidone (Furoxone) 6-8 mg/kg/24 hr (adult: 100 mg/dose) q 6 hr PO × 7-10 days; **or** quinacrine (Atabrine) 6 mg/kg/24 hr (adult: 100 mg) q 8 hr PO × 5 days; **or** metronidazole (Flagyl) 15 mg/kg/24 hr (adult: 250 mg) q 8 hr PO × 5 days
Hookworm *Necator americanus* *Ancylostoma duodenale*	Mebendazole (Vermox) 100 mg q 12 hr PO (children >2 yr) × 3 days; **or** pyrantel pamoate (Antiminth) 11 mg/kg/24 hr q 24 hr (maximum: 1 gm/24 hr) PO × 3 days
Leishmaniasis *Leishmania donovani* (kala azar) *L. braziliensis* (American mucocutaneous leishmaniasis) *L. mexicana, L. tropica*	Stibogluconate sodium (Pentostam, Tricostam) (CDC) 20 mg/kg/24 hr (maximum: 800 mg/24 hr) q 24 hr IM, IV × 20 days; may need to repeat

Continued.

living in endemic areas, as well as frequent travel by tourists. Also, there was outbreak of *Plasmodium vivax* malaria in San Diego County in 1985; the disease exhibited sustained transmission through several generations.[92] One author (RF) personally saw three children in a 3-year period at a busy urban pediatric emergency department who presented with fever and were diagnosed as having malaria by the finding of infected red cells on a peripheral smear. That same medical facility recently reported 64 children diagnosed with malaria from 1983 to 1992. This reflects a

TABLE 55-3. Antiparasitic Drugs—cont'd

Parasitic diseases	Management
Malaria	
Prophylaxis	
For areas without chloroquine-resistant *Plasmodium falciparum*	Chloroquine 5 mg base/kg (adult: 300 mg) base q wk PO, beginning 1 wk before potential exposure and continuing for 6 wk after last exposure; **plus,** primaquine phosphate 0.3 mg base/kg (adult: 15 mg base) q 24 hr PO × 14 days after departure from endemic area
For areas with chloroquine-resistant *P. falciparum*	For **short-term** (<3 wk) travel: chloroquine 5 mg base/kg (adult: 300 mg base) q wk PO, beginning 1 wk before potential exposure and continuing for 6 wk after last exposure; **plus,** patient should be given single-treatment dose of pyrimethamine-sulfadoxine (Fansidar)* and advised to take promptly if febrile illness develops, no medical care is available, and there is no known intolerance (2-11 mo: ¼ tab/wk; 1-3 yr: ½ tab/wk; 4-8 yr: 1 tab/wk; 9-14 yr: 2 tab/wk; >14 yr [adult]: 3 tab/wk PO) For **long-term** travel to high-risk area: chloroquine, as above; **plus** consider pyrimethamine-sulfadoxine, as above. Proguanil is suggested in Africa south of the Sahara.
Treatment	
P. vivax, P. ovale	Chloroquine phosphate (Aralen, Nivaquine) 10 mg base/kg then 5 mg/base/kg at 6 hr, 24 hr, and 48 hr after initial dose (adult: 600 mg base, then 300 mg base at 6 hr, 24 hr, and 48 hr **plus** primaquine 0.3 mg base/kg (adult: 15 mg base) q 24 hr PO × 14 days; parenteral chloroquine (CDC) is available for central nervous system (CNS) disease
P. malariae	Chloroquine, as above
P. falciparum (non-chloroquine-resistant)	Chloroquine, as above
P. falciparum (chloroquine-resistant)	Quinine 25 mg/kg/24 hr (adult: 650 mg/dose) q 8 hr PO × 3 days; **plus** pyrimethamine 1 mg/kg/24 hr (adult: 25 mg/dose) q 12 hr PO × 3 days; **plus** sulfadiazine 120-150 mg/kg/24 hr (adult: 500 mg/dose) q 6 hr PO × 5 days; parenteral therapy (CDC) is administered for severe disease
Pinworms (*Enterobius vermicularis*)	Mebendazole (Vermox) 100 mg PO once (children >2 yr) (repeat in 1 wk) **or** pyrantel (Antiminth) 11 mg/kg/dose (maximum: 1 gm) PO once (repeat in 1 wk)
Pneumocystis pneumonia (*Pneumocystis carinii*)	Trimethoprim (TMP)-sulfamethoxazole (SMX) (Bactrim, Septra) 20 mg TMP, 100 mg SMX/kg/24 hr q 6-8 hr PO, IV × 10-14 days. (Also trimetrexate with leucovorin [NIAID])
Schistosomiasis *Schistosoma haematobium* *S. japonicum* *S. mansoni*	Praziquantel (Biltricide) 20 mg/kg PO × 3 doses in 1 day
Tapeworms *Taenia saginata* *Taenia solium* (see Cysticercosis) *Hymenolepis nana* *Diphyllobothrium latum*	Niclosamide (Niclocide, Cesticide) 11-34 kg: single dose 1 gm (2 tab) PO; >34 kg: single dose 1.5 gm (3 tab) PO (adult: 2 gm or 4 tab PO) For *H. nana,* treat with 11-34 kg: single dose 1 gm (2 tab) PO, then 0.5 gm (1 tab)/24 hr PO × 6 days; >34 kg: single dose 1.5 gm (3 tab) PO, then 1 gm (2 tab)/24 hr PO × 6 days (adult: 2 gm or 4 tab/24 hr PO × 7 days)
Toxoplasmosis (*Toxoplasma gondii*)	Pyrimethamine (Daraprim) 2 mg/kg/24 hr (adult: 25 mg/24 hr) q 12 PO × 3 days, then 1 mg/kg/24 hr q 12 hr PO × 4 wk (supplement with folinic acid 5-10 mg/24 hr); **plus** trisulfapyrimidines or sulfadiazine 120-150 mg/kg/24 hr (adult: 4-6 gm/24 hr) q 6 hr PO × 28 days
Trichinosis (*Trichinella spiralis*)	Thiabendazole (Mintezol) 50 mg/kg/24 hr q 12 PO (maximum: 3 gm/24 hr); **or** mebendazole (Vermox) 200-400 mg (children >2 yr) q 8 hr PO × 5-10 days
Trypanosomiasis Chagas disease (*Trypanosoma cruzi*)	Nifurtimox (Bayer 2502) (CDC) 6-10 yr: 15-20 mg/kg/24 hr q 6 hr PO × 90 days; 11-16 yr: 12.5-15 mg/kg/24 hr q 6 hr PO × 90 days; adult: 8-10 mg/kg/24 hr q 6 hr PO × 120 days
Visceral larva migrans (*Toxocara canis*)	Thiabendazole (Mintezol) 50 mg/kg/24 hr q 12 hr PO (maximum: 3 gm/24 hr) × 5 days or longer
Whipworm (*Trichuris trichiura*)	Mebendazole (Vermox) 100 mg q 12 hr PO × 3 days

CDC, Available from the Centers for Disease Control and Prevention Parasitic Drug Service, Atlanta; call: (404) 639-3670. For emergencies on nights, weekends, and holidays, call: (404) 639-2888.

*Associated with serious adverse reactions, including erythema multiforme, Stevens-Johnson syndrome, toxic epidermal necrolysis, and serum sickness. Discontinue if any mucocutaneous lesions develop. Presumptive treatment with pyrimethamine-sulfadoxine (Fansidar): 2-11 mo: ¼ tab; 1-3 yr: ½ tab; 4-8 yr: 1 tab; 9-14 yr: 2 tab; >14 yr (adult): 3 tab as single dose PO.

NIAID, Available from the National Institute of Allergy and Infectious Diseases, call 1-800-537-9978.

national trend in urban emergency departments as well as community hospitals to see increasing numbers of patients with malaria.[93] In general, half of the children are recent immigrants and half have had recent travel to endemic areas, especially, West Africa. Most children have been seen for the same illness and misdiagnosed.[93] Thus malaria must remain in the differential of the febrile child without obvious source.

Of the 100 species of the protozoan *Plasmodium*, only four are associated with human disease: *P. falciparum, P. vivax, P. ovale,* and *P. malariae.* They vary in distribution, clinical course, severity of illness, and resistance to prevention and therapeutic medications. Plasmodium is transmitted by the Anopheles mosquito, as well as by needle sharing, blood transfusion, and congenitally.

Diagnostic Findings. The sporozoite form is injected into the host and settles in the liver. During a variable incubation phase, from 8 to 28 days depending on the species, the sporozoites mature and multiply asexually. When released from the hepatocytes, the mature merozoites invade red blood cells (RBCs), initiating the early clinical stage of the disease, which is characterized by malaise, headache, vomiting, and anorexia. In the RBCs the merozoites change into trophozoites and then into the sexually mature form, the schizont. The schizonts may reproduce, produce more merozoites, rupture the host cells, and invade new red blood cells. This occurs in a periodic fashion, which leads to the characteristic pattern of intermittent fever, chills, and hypotension. These occur every several days, depending on the species involved. Children may have nonspecific complaints and physical findings including nausea, vomiting, malaise, abdominal pain, and headache. Fever is the most consistent finding although the characteristic patterns are often absent. Splenomegaly and hepatomegaly are common and care during examination is necessary because of the possibility of splenic rupture.

The most severe complications, cerebral malaria and anemia, are the most frequent causes of death, usually due to *P. falciparum,* and may occur in young children. Cerebral malaria should be suspected in a febrile child who has a seizure and prolonged postictal phase or decreasing level of consciousness.[94] A recent study has shown that the physician cannot reliably distinguish between meningitis and cerebral malaria based on duration of fever, presence or absence of nuchal rigidity, fontanelle fullness, or physical blood malaria smear.[95] Thus, an examination of the CSF fluid is required in children with suggestive historic or physical findings. The LP may be delayed in children who exhibit signs of increased intracranial pressure, thus necessitating treatment for both meningitis and cerebral malaria. Although *P. falciparum* malaria kills more children worldwide, in the United States, children have the lowest mortality from this species.[96] As the infected RBCs have a tendency to sludge, in addition to hemolysis, clinical illness can show signs of multiorgan tissue ischemia, including coma, pulmonary edema, renal failure, and anemia.[97]

Diagnosis is made by finding the parasites in the peripheral blood smear, thick or thin preparation. Because an individual specimen may be negative, repeated specimens should be obtained for several days in suspected cases.

Because most emergency departments use automated equipment for CBCs, children with normal white blood cell, red blood cell, and platelet counts will not have their peripheral smears reviewed. This can occur in up to half of children with malaria.[93] In addition, there is usually a normochromic, normocytic anemia, with a relative monocytosis, and thrombocytopenia. Liver enzymes may be elevated as well as bilirubin and there may be hypoglycemia, especially in children who have had limited oral intake. New methods for rapid detection of the *P. falciparium* HRP-2 antigen have been described.[98,99]

Management/Prevention. Priorities include stabilization of the critically ill patient and determination of which form of malaria is present. *P. falciparium* is the most serious and has the highest rate of chloroquine resistance. Admission to hospital is advisable for children, especially if *P. falciparum* is suspected or the child appears ill. Although chloroquine is the drug of choice, for *P. falciparum* infections or in children with cerebral symptoms, severe anemia, and renal failure, quinidine hydrochloride administered intravenously in a monitored setting is recommended in addition to general and specific supportive measures (see Table 55-3).

Despite the ability to prevent most cases of malaria, studies have shown that most travelers to endemic areas do not take prophylactic medicines or personal precautions (see Table 55-3). The emergency physician can be instrumental in stressing the need for these precautions. Malaria should be considered in all febrile children who have lived abroad in an endemic area within the last 12 months.

Dengue Fever

Dengue fever is caused by an arbovirus, more specifically a flavivirus, and was once prevalent in the United States. The infection can be caused by dengue virus 1-4. There is no cross protection between these viruses and repeat infection increases the likelihood of more severe disease.[100] It remains prevalent throughout the world, but its presence in Puerto Rico, the United States' Virgin Islands, and other neighboring countries increases the likelihood of its presence in the United States. The virus is transmitted by the *Aedes aegyptii* mosquito, which prefers to breed in small collections of water around dwellings. A second vector, *Aedes albopictus,* has recently been proposed.[97]

Diagnostic Findings. Dengue has a 2- to 8-day incubation period and has two possible presentations. Classic dengue fever presents with acute onset of fever, headache, retroorbital pain, and myalgia. The latter may be very severe and is why dengue is commonly called *breakbone fever.*[90,97] The acute phase may last for several days. The patient improves only to have a "relapse" several days later with predominately gastrointestinal symptoms, nausea, vomiting, abdominal pain, as well as fever and rash.[97] There is a prolonged convalescence, often accompanied by fatigue and depression.[90,97]

A second presentation is called *dengue hemorrhagic fever* or *dengue shock syndrome,* a more severe disease thought to have both an infectious, as well as an immunologic, basis. Thus it more frequently occurs in patients who have had classic dengue fever. These patients are severely ill and if untreated may have a 50% mortality.[90] An epidemic of dengue fever in the Lao Peoples Democratic Republic in 1994 had 375 cases with 3 deaths. Ninety eight percent of cases were children younger than age 16 years.[100]

These patients show a bleeding diathesis, with hemoconcentration, vasodilatation, pulmonary edema, and shock; hydrothorax and ascites may be present.[90,97] The virus can be isolated from whole blood or the buffy coat obtained during the acute phase of the illness but this technique is performed by a limited number of laboratories.

Management. Diagnosis is clinical and treatment is supportive in the hospital.

Typhoid Fever

Typhoid fever is caused by the ingestion of a large amount (10^6 to 10^9) of organisms of Salmonella typhi from food or water that is contaminated by human fecal material. It is one of the most common causes of bacteremia in endemic areas.[97] Typhoid vaccine provides 50% to 70% protection, depending on the size of the innoculum.

Diagnostic Findings. Typhoid fever has a wide spectrum of clinical presentations beginning 10 to 14 days after exposure. Initially, fever with a temperature/pulse disassociation (relative bradycardia), headache, and abdominal pain occur. This progresses over the next week to an ill-appearing patient, often with a characteristic rash (rose spots), abdominal pain and distension, hepatomegaly, and watery diarrhea. During this phase delirium and prostration may occur. Improvement occurs by the fourth week.[90,97]

Complications include myocarditis, encephalitis, and hepatitis; however, the most common severe complication is intestinal perforation and hemorrhage, occurring in 2% to 3% of patients.[97]

Diagnosis is suspected clinically; blood cultures are positive in 80% of patients in the first week and stool cultures are frequently positive in the second and third weeks (see Chapter 52).

Management. Treatment involves hospitalization, stabilization of fluid status, close monitoring, and antibiotic therapy when cultures are positive. Useful antibiotics include chloramphenicol, ampicillin, amoxicillin, or trimethoprim-sulfamethoxazole. Multiple drug-resistant S. typhi (MDRST) reports are increasing, and a study from India in 1993 showed a 66.6% MDRST in children younger than age 2 years of age diagnosed with typhoid fever.[101] For MDRST, a recent study has shown oral cefixime (8 mg/kg/24 hr q 12 to 24 hr PO) to be as effective as parenteral ceftriaxone.[102] Children infected with MDRST have a higher incidence of severe complications (shock, encepholophathy, myocarditis and gastric hemorrhage).[103] Precautions for health-care personnel and evaluation of family members are warranted. Intestinal perforation obviously requires surgical consultation.

HERPES VIRUS INFECTION
Perinatal Herpes Simplex

One of the most serious infections for the neonate is herpes simplex virus (HSV) infection. Acquired at a time when host immunity is restricted, HSV infection can disseminate widely or remain localized to the CNS. The in-

fection is rapidly progressive and, even in treated cases, the morbidity and mortality is high. The disease incidence in the United States is low, occurring in 1:3,000 to 1:5,000 live births; however, reports indicate that the incidence is rising in certain populations and regions of the country.[104]

The principal route of transmission is by intrapartum exposure to genital HSV infection. Not surprisingly, therefore, HSV type 2 is responsible for 70% to 80% of perinatally acquired HSV infections. Postpartum transmission of HSV occurs much less frequently and usually results from exposure to orolabial, hand, or breast lesions. The absence of a maternal history of genital herpes does not exclude the possibility of neonatal HSV infection because there is a high rate of asymptomatic maternal infection.[105]

Diagnostic Findings. Clinical manifestations of HSV infection in the newborn include skin, eye, and mouth (SEM) manifestations, encephalitis, and disseminated disease. Symptoms occur as early as a few days or as late as 4 to 6 weeks after birth.[104,106-108]

SEM manifestations usually present during the first or second week of life. Skin lesions often appear over the area that was the presenting surface during birth. Breaks in the skin such as result from fetal scalp monitors may also become sites of local infection. Eye infection manifests itself as keratoconjunctivitis and has potential for causing significant injury to the eye. Oropharyngeal involvement consists of the characteristic ulcers of the buccal mucosa and tongue. Newborns developing encephalitis or disseminated infection often first develop SEM manifestations.[104,106-108]

Encephalitis occurs in about 34% of HSV-infected newborns. It may present with or without SEM findings and be the result of infection localized to the CNS or disseminated to other organ systems. Seizures (either focal or generalized), irritability, poor feeding, and bulging fontanels are common findings.[104,106,109]

Disseminated HSV infection most often presents during the first 2 weeks of life and most commonly affects the skin, liver, adrenals, and central nervous system. The lungs, kidneys, and heart are less frequently involved. Newborns commonly present with skin lesions, encephalitis, shock, jaundice, and hepatomegaly. Newborns with disseminated disease may also have symptoms that are very similar to those of bacterial sepsis.[104,106-108]

The differential diagnosis includes (1) causes of vesicular skin rashes such as Varicella zoster, enteroviruses, and cytomegalovirus; (2) viral or bacterial etiologies of meningoencephalitis; and (3) causes of shock such as bacterial sepsis and metabolic or cardiac diseases.[104]

Diagnosis of neonatal HSV infection is by viral culture. Cultures should be obtained from skin lesions, mouth or nasopharynx, CSF, eyes, urine, blood, and stool. Newborns with CNS involvement will grow virus from the CSF in 20% to 40% of cases. Rapid diagnostic studies, such as direct fluorescent antibody (DFA), are helpful in evaluating suspicious vesicular lesions (see Chapter 18).

Management. Treatment for all neonatal HSV infections is with intravenous acyclovir.[110] Acyclovir 30 mg/kg/24 hr divided q 8 hr IV is indicated in the following situations: (1) newborns with skin, eye, or mouth manifestations of HSV; (2) newborns with viral meningitis or encephalitis in whom no other etiology can be identified; (3) newborns with a septic appearance and no identifiable cause or etiologic agent (especially in cases involving pneumonitis or hepatitis) in whom HSV is a consideration; and (4) newborns with evidence of meningitis or sepsis and a mother with HSV genital lesions or excretion at the time of birth.[111]

Herpes Simplex Encephalitis (HSE)

Herpes simplex virus is a frequent cause of severe focal encephalitis and accounts for 2% of all cases of encephalitis. HSE occurs in all ages with a third of cases occurring in individuals younger than 20 years of age and 10% occurring in children from 6 months to 10 years of age. The great majority of cases are caused by either primary or recurrent HSV type 1 infections.[112]

HSE presents acutely with fever, headache, alteration in consciousness, personality changes, vomiting, and focal neurologic findings. Neurologic findings include dysphasia, autonomic dysfunction, ataxia, hemiparesis, and seizures (focal or generalized).[112]

Examination of the CSF fluid reveals WBC counts ranging from 5 to 2,000 cells/mm^3; however, the majority of patients have counts of 50 to 500/mm^3. Early in the disease, neutrophils may predominate. RBCs of varying number are a common finding. The CSF protein is frequently elevated and the glucose is decreased in only a small number of patients.[112]

The CT scan is frequently normal in the early stages of HSV encephalitis. Magnetic resonance imaging (MRI) scan has shown much greater sensitivity than CT in identifying the characteristic fronto-temporal lesions early in the disease course.[113]

The electroencephalogram (EEG) is another sensitive tool early in the disease and classically displays paroxysmal lateral epileptiform discharges (PLEDS).[114] Definitive diagnosis requires brain biopsy[115,116]; however, newer diagnostic approaches such as the PCR assay may prove equally sensitive and specific.[113]

CSF for PCR should be sent only to laboratories with demonstrated expertise in PCR; samples should be carefully handled to avoid contamination. Prompt treatment with acyclovir is indicated in those children with suspected disease until the diagnosis can be excluded.

Herpetic Gingivostomatitis

After the neonatal period gingivostomatitis is the most frequent form of HSV infection in children. Affected children present with fever, irritability, and inflammation of the gingiva and mucous membranes of the mouth. Although most children tolerate this infection well, some may have significant enough involvement that they refuse feeding and become dehydrated, thus requiring admission to hospital.

In those less severely affected, supportive care is all that is required. Analgesics, such as acetaminophen with codeine elixir, may be required for pain relief. Use of topical lidocaine should be discouraged, unless used with great caution, especially in the younger child, because there have been cases of lidocaine toxicity secondary to its use for this purpose. A mixture of Kaopectate, diphenhydramine, and viscous xylocaine may be useful (see Chapter 49).

Herpetic Whitlow

HSV infection may present as a painful, red distal phalanx that eventually shows a herpetic vesicle, called a whitlow.

Before the appearance of the vesicle, it may be confused with a felon. Treatment is analgesics as needed.

Recurrent HSV

In some patients, HSV infection will show repetitive outbreaks of vesicles, usually in the same location. Presence of a vesicle typical of a herpetic lesion should prompt the emergency physician to ask if this has occurred before.

Treatment is supportive although referral to a dermatologist may be helpful. Antiviral therapy has minimal effect on recurrent genital herpes. Oral acyclovir initiated within 2 days of onset of symptoms shortens the mean clinical course by 1 day. Viral excretion may be diminished. The dose in adults is 200 mg five times per day or 800 mg twice a day for 5 days.

Oral acyclovir administered on a daily basis for suppressive therapy has been effective in decreasing the frequency of recurrences of active disease in persons with frequent recurrences (six or more episodes per year) of genital infection.

Herpes Zoster

Although more frequent in adults, herpes zoster or shingles may occur in children. There is usually a history of varicella in the past (see Chapter 48). Initial symptoms may be pain, followed by vesicles in a dermatome distribution; except in the immunocompromised patient or when the trigeminal distribution is involved, treatment is symptomatic. The former may require admission and referral to the ophthalmology department.

INFLUENZA

Influenza remains a major cause of illness for mankind. Occurring in epidemics and pandemics, it has been responsible for innumerable deaths. The pandemic of influenza following World War I took more lives than the war itself. Outbreaks continue to occur yearly with frequent pandemics. The influenza virus is an orthomyxovirus. Although four types (A through D) are known, only A and B are frequent causes of illness. Type A infects man as well as many animals. Type B and C are only known to occur in humans; type C influenza is rare, causes mild disease, and is rarely diagnosed.[117] Although both A and B are indistinguishable clinically, type A is responsible for the massive outbreaks.

Outbreaks usually occur in the winter months and generally begin in school-aged children. They usually last 1 to 2 months in a given community. The virus is spread by respiratory droplets and patients are most contagious from the day before to several days into the disease.[118]

Diagnostic Findings

The clinical picture varies with the virulence of the infecting organism, general health of the patient, and patient's immune status, especially previous influenza exposure. The presentation is more variable in children. Very young children often present a picture similar to bacterial sepsis.[119] Older children may present with the more typical sudden onset of fever, chills, headache, diffuse myalgia, and dry cough. Respiratory symptoms, sore throat, nasal congestion, and cough usually predominate.[118] Younger children have a higher incidence of rhinorrhea and abdominal symptoms. A recent survey of children hospitalized with influenza B infection showed a 38% occurrence of vomiting and diarrhea although abdominal pain was not as prevalent in previous reports.[120] Because of the variable and nonspecific presentation of influenza infections in younger children, physicians must suspect this diagnosis, especially in children hospitalized during an influenza outbreak. The inability to diagnose influenza quickly has shown to lead to nosocomial infections, increased morbidity and prolonged hospitalizations.[121] Several tests are available for the rapid detection of influenza A infections.[122]

Complications of influenza include primary viral or secondary bacterial pneumonia, which is probably responsible for the majority of deaths from the disease.[117] Children particularly at risk are asthmatics and those with chronic lung conditions, as well as children with any chronic debilitating disease. Although the myalgias of influenza are often severe, rhabdomyolysis is a rare complication. Other complications include Reye syndrome, especially with the use of aspirin, and other central nervous system diseases such as Guillain-Barré syndrome. Influenza has been known to cause croup.

Diagnosis is made clinically, especially during an outbreak. Viral cultures are accurate from nasopharyngeal swabs taken during the first 3 days of illness. These tests are rarely useful to the emergency physician.

Management

Although recent studies have shown some benefit in using aerosolized ribavirin, children with either influenza A and B respond to supportive care.[123] Aspirin should be strictly avoided in patients with potential influenza. Very ill patients or those with underlying diseases or complications may require admission to hospital and treatment. Amantadine has been used successfully against influenza A. Dosage is 4.4 mg/kg/day given orally twice a day. For children younger than the age of 9 years of age and those weighing <45 kg, the maximum daily dose should not exceed 150 mg per day. Older children and those weighing >45 kg should receive 100 mg twice a day. Therapy should begin as soon after diagnosis is suspected. The treatment course varies with response but may be from 2 to 7 days. In 1993, rimantadine was approved for prevention and treatment of influenza in adults and prevention of influenza in children. For children 1 to 10 years of age, the oral dose is 5 mg/kg with a maximum single daily dose of 150 mg; the adult dose is 100 mg BID PO.[124] Prophylaxis may be considered after exposure, the treatment continuing for 10 days.

The influenza virus has the property of constant change in antigenicity; thus the vaccine for influenza is the only one in widespread use that must be updated to be useful against new variants.[102] The efficacy of the vaccine is difficult to assess, especially in children. Recommendations for use in high-risk children change somewhat on an annual basis. High-risk children include those with chronic pulmonary disease (severe asthma, bronchopulmonary dysplasia, cystic fibrosis), severe cardiac disease, immunosuppressed patients, and those with sickle cell and other hemoglobinopathies. Children with other chronic diseases such as diabetes mellitus and renal disease should also be considered for immunization. Health-care workers who are likely to be exposed to influenza (emergency personnel) should consider use of the vaccine. Emergency departments can play a vital role in the control of influenza. They should be able to offer information regarding why, where, and how to obtain the vaccine.[125]

KAWASAKI DISEASE

Kawasaki disease (KD) or mucocutaneous lymph node syndrome is an acute, self-limiting, multisystem disease of unknown etiology. The disease affects mostly young children and results in serious cardiac sequelae in 20% of untreated patients. Major advances in its management have significantly reduced this high rate of complications; however, early diagnosis is vital. The diagnosis of KD is based on a characteristic group of nonspecific clinical features and requires familiarity with both the clinical presentation and course of the disease.[126,127]

KD was first recognized in Japan by Kawasaki in 1967, and in the United States by Melish in 1976.[127] The disease is now recognized worldwide. In the United States an estimated 2,000 to 4,000 cases occur annually.[63]

The peak incidence is 18 to 24 months of age with 80% of cases occurring in children younger than 4 years of age and 95% of cases occurring in children younger than 10 years of age.[128] Males are affected more often (1.5:1) and children of Asian descent are at increased risk.[128] The disease appears year round with the incidence increasing during late winter and early spring. Reported outbreaks appear to occur in 2- to 3-year cycles.[128] Person-to-person transmission of the disease has not been demonstrated; however, studies suggest that the general incidence of the disease is slightly higher among family members.[128,129] Recurrent KD has been reported in a small number of patients.[130]

Clinically and epidemiologically KD behaves as an infectious agent. A number of viral, bacterial, and environmental associations have been made but the causative factor remains unknown.[131]

Diagnostic Findings

The principal pathologic feature of this disease is a systemic vasculitis that affects the microvessels (arterioles, venules, and capillaries) and arteries.[128,132] Nearly every organ system is involved, particularly the heart, where the vasculitic process results in coronary aneurysm formation in 20% of untreated patients. Autopsy studies have described the sequence of pathologic changes in the heart.[132] These changes begin with a perivasculitis of the microvessels and small arteries. This early inflammation usually peaks by day 10 of the illness and is responsible for the myocarditis, pericarditis, and endocarditis that develop early in the disease. Following inflammation of the small vessels, perivasculitis and panvasculitis of the major coronary arteries develop, resulting in variable degrees of inflammation and necrosis. Necrosis of the musculoelastic layers may create sufficient weakness in the vessel wall to form an aneurysm. Thrombus or scar formation within the aneurysm may result in severe stenosis or obstruction.[128,132] Aneurysm formation in other large arteries such as the brachial, renal, femoral, and iliac arteries, and the aorta are known to occur. Circulating immune complexes have been identified in patients with KD and may play a role in aneurysm pathogenesis.[133]

The diagnosis is based entirely on clinical findings. The diagnostic guidelines, outlined in the box above, require fever over 38° C of 5 days or more and at least four of five clinical features in order to establish the diagnosis of KD.[134] Use of the diagnostic guidelines, however, is subject to two important qualifications. First, all symptoms need not be present simultaneously and may vary in severity, time of onset, and duration.[126,128] Secondly, cases of atypical or incomplete KD are being increasingly reported.[135,136] In patients with atypical KD, one or more of the necessary diagnostic clinical features is absent. Patients, therefore, presenting with fever of more than 5 days should have atypical Kawasaki disease included in their differential diagnosis.

The clinical manifestations, complications, and laboratory findings of KD appear at characteristic times in the clinical course. The course of the illness has therefore been divided into several clinical phases: acute, subacute, and convalescent.[127,128] The acute or febrile phase lasts 7 to 15 days and is the period when most diagnostic clinical features occur. After resolution of the fever, the subacute phase begins and continues for 10 to 25 days. During the subacute phase, the remaining acute symptoms resolve or improve. It is in the subacute phase that coronary artery aneurysms as well as hydrops of the gallbladder begin to appear. Other important features of the subacute phase include desquamation of the fingers and toes and thrombocytosis. The convalescent phase begins following complete resolution of all clinical manifestations and continues until all laboratory findings have normalized, often by 6 to 10 weeks.

Fever is commonly the first symptom of the acute phase. The fever lasts from 7 to 15 days (mean 12 days), often exceeding 40° C and is erratic. Cervical adenopathy is another early symptom. The nodes are usually unilateral, nonsuppurative, and measure > 1.5 cm in size. Bulbar conjunctivitis is bilateral, nonexudative, and usually quite prominent, although on occasion it may be mild. Changes involving the oropharynx include erythema and cracking of the lips and erythema of the buccal mucosa and posterior pharynx. Lingual papillae may become prominent giving the tongue a strawberry appearance. The rash is quite variable and may appear morbilliform, maculopapular, or scarlatiniform. Vesicular rashes are rare. In infants the rash may be most apparent in the perineum. Changes in the peripheral extremities occur as induration of the dorsum of the hands and feet with erythema over the palms and soles. Induration and erythema are followed by desquamation of the fingers and toes, usually in the subacute phase.[126-128,132,137,138]

Other clinical findings that may occur are listed in the box on p. 944. Although not diagnostic criteria, these other clinical findings are often useful in supporting the diagnosis. Gastrointestinal manifestations include vomiting, abdominal pain, diarrhea, mild jaundice, and hepatitis. Arthritis and arthralgia occur in as many as 30% of patients. The majority of patients with joint involvement have onset during the subacute phase, although it may appear earlier in the acute phase. Both large and small joints may be involved, especially weight-bearing joints like the hips, knees, and ankles.[127]

Joint aspirates may have WBC counts from 90,000 to 300,000 cells/mm³. Central nervous system involvement often presents as extreme irritability or occasionally as aseptic meningitis. Examination of the CSF may reveal a mild pleocytosis (10 to 50 WBC/mm³) with predominantly mononuclear cells. CSF glucose and protein are normal.[126]

Cardiovascular manifestations of the disease comprise the major complications of KD (see box on p. 944). Patients with KD have approximately a 20% risk of developing coronary aneurysms without treatment. Patients younger than 1 year of age have an even greater risk.[139] Following treatment the risk of coronary aneurysm is reduced to 4% to 5%. Most aneurysms develop after the acute phase between days 15 to 45 of the illness. Myocardial infarction and dysrhythmia are the most common causes of sudden death and occur in 1% to 2% of patients, usually in the third to fourth week.[140]

Hydrops of the gallbladder is a self-limiting complication that occurs in 3% of patients and is a functional rather than obstructive distension.[127] Iridocyclitis or anterior uveitis develops in about 80% of patients.[141] Sensorineural hearing loss may range from mild to severe.[142]

Ancillary Data. Laboratory findings are nonspecific in patients with KD. The CBC often shows an elevated WBC count with a left shift. A mild nonhemolytic anemia may be present. Thrombocytosis is an important finding in KD; however, platelets are usually normal in the acute phase

---

Other Significant Clinical and Laboratory Findings of Kawasaki Disease

Cardiovascular
  Gallop rhythm
  Dysrhythmias
  Electrocardiogram changes
  Pericardial effusion
  Valvular insufficiency
  Coronary aneurysm
Central Nervous System
  Irritability
  Meningitis
  Photophobia, uveitis, iritis
  Cerebrospinal pleocytosis
Hematologic
  Anemia
  Thrombocytosis (after 10 or more days)
Genitourinary
  Urethritis
  Sterile pyuria
  Proteinuria
Respiratory
  Cough
  Rhinorrhea
  Pulmonary infiltrate
Gastrointestinal
  Diarrhea
  Nausea and vomiting
  Abdominal pain
  Gallbladder hydrops
  Elevated transaminases
  Mild jaundice

Complications of Kawasaki Disease

Cardiovascular
  Coronary aneurysms
  Valvular insufficiency
  Congestive heart failure
  Myocardial infarction
  Dysrhythmias
  Rupture of aneurysm
  Pericardial effusion
Hydrops of the gallbladder

---

and become elevated only in the subacute phase. At this time the platelet count is generally greater than 650,000/ mm[3] and may exceed one million. Acute-phase reactants such as the ESR and the CRP are markedly elevated. Serum transaminases may be mildly elevated and serum chemistries occasionally show hyponatremia and hypoalbuminemia. Urinalysis often demonstrates pyuria, which probably results from urethritis. Bilirubinuria may be an early sign of hydrops of the gallbladder.[143]

Pulmonary infiltrates or cardiomegaly may be noted on chest radiographs. The ECG may reveal a variety of changes including dysrhythmias, prolonged PR or QT intervals, and nonspecific ST-T wave changes. Two-dimensional echocardiography may demonstrate coronary artery dilatation or aneurysm as well as pericardial effusion or decreased contractility and mitral and aortic valve function and is generally followed serially.[138]

Differential Considerations

The differential diagnosis is extensive because of the nonspecific nature of its clinical features (see box on p. 945). Other infectious agents may present with a similar erythroderma. Most viral exanthems can be eliminated based on the clinical course, absence of sufficient diagnostic features, and by epidemiologic considerations such as age and immunization status. Group A beta-hemolytic streptococcal or staphylococcal infections can usually be excluded by the differences in the clinical appearance and isolation of the organism. Toxic shock syndrome occurs in mostly older children and adolescents who present with fever, erythroderma, hypotension, thrombocytopenia, and multisystem organ involvement. Leptospirosis may present with sudden onset and multisystem involvement and is diagnosed by culture and serology. Arthritis can be mistaken for juvenile rheumatoid arthritis and these patients often require rheumatologic evaluation. Drug reactions, especially secondary to sulfisoxazole, sulfamethoxazole, and nitrofurantoin may present with parallel findings.

Management

All patients diagnosed with KD should be hospitalized immediately for administration of IV gamma globulin (IVGG), aspirin therapy, and cardiac evaluation (see box on p. 945). Patients with severe disease should be monitored closely for cardiac complications such as CHF.[137]

IVGG is administered as a single dose of 2 gm/kg infused over 8 to 12 hours with specific protocols to monitor the patient. Single-dose IVGG has been shown to be as effective as divided doses, has fewer complications, and may reduce the duration of hospitalization.[144] Patients receiving IVGG require cardiorespiratory monitoring during the infusion; however, severe adverse reactions to IVGG are rare. Mild reactions include flushing, chills, headache, nausea, and vomiting; these can be managed by slowing the infusion rate.[108]

Aspirin therapy is started at 100 mg/kg/24 hr QID PO and continued until the fever has resolved. Low-dose aspirin at 3 to 5 mg/kg/24 hr QD PO (maximum, 40 to 80 mg/24 hr) is then continued for 2 to 3 months or until the platelet count has normalized. Salicylate levels should be monitored during high-dose aspirin therapy.[108,132] Echocardiography should be performed on all patients at the time of presentation, especially in seriously ill patients. A cardiologist should be involved in the evaluation and follow-up of any patient with Kawasaki disease. Repeat echocardiograms are usually performed 14 days and 6 to 8 weeks after onset of the illness, or more frequently if there is evidence of cardiac involvement.[138,145]

The prognosis for patients receiving treatment within the first 10 days of the illness is good. The majority of aneurysms resolve within the first year with no apparent sequelae; however, sudden death occurs in 1% to 2% of

---

Other Illnesses Sharing Features Common with Kawasaki Disease

Viral
Rubeola
Rubella
Epstein-Barr virus
Adenovirus
Enteroviruses

Bacterial
Staphylococcal
    Scalded skin syndrome
    Toxic shock syndrome
Streptococcal
    Scarlet fever

Spirochete
Leptospirosis

Rickettsial
Rocky Mountain spotted fever

Rheumatologic
Juvenile rheumatoid arthritis
Behçet disease
Reiter syndrome (affects older individuals)

Other
Stevens-Johnson syndrome
Drug reaction

Management and Treatment of Kawasaki Disease

Evaluation
Routine laboratory (CBC, UA, electrolytes)
Liver profile
Chest x-ray
Electrocardiogram, echocardiogram
Studies to exclude other diagnoses

Treatment
IVGG dose: 2 gm/kg IV infused over 8-12 hours as a
    single one-time dose
Aspirin
High dose: 100 mg/kg/day divided into 4 doses; monitor
    salicylate levels
                        followed by
Low dose: 3-5 mg/kg/day as a single daily dose; continue
    until the platelet count has normalized

---

patients and the long-term morbidity caused by small lesions is unknown.[138]

MENINGOCOCCEMIA

N. meningitidis, a gram-negative diplococcus, can cause a meningitis or a rapidly fatal sepsis. At the turn of the century the mortality rate in children approached 80%. With the use of antibiotics and supportive measures the fatality rate is around 10%.[146] A recent study showed an overall mortality of 6.6%, but over one-third of the patients with septic shock died.[147] Most cases occur in young children with the peak attack being in the 6- to 12-month age group.[148] The study just mentioned showed the highest incidence in the 0- to 4-year and 15- to 19-year age groups.[147] Along with *H. influenzae* and *S. pneumoniae*, *N. meningitidis* is the most frequent bacterial pathogen causing meningitis after the age of 2 months. The signs and symptoms of *N. meningitidis* meningitis are indistinguishable from other causes of bacterial meningitis. Diagnosis can be made by finding gram-negative diplococci on gram stain of the CSF or a positive latex agglutination test.

Meningococcemia is usually characterized by rapid onset of fever, chills, malaise, and a rash. The onset is variable, ranging from insidious to fulminant. Two patterns of skin eruption are noted. A pink maculopapular and generalized petechial rash may develop, including involvement of the palms and soles. Purpuric and ecchymotic lesions may be associated with a very high mortality.

As this disease can be rapidly fatal within hours, early recognition and prompt intervention are essential. Patients may develop meningitis or meningoencephalitis, pericarditis, cervicitis, hypotension, and DIC. It is important to realize that in fulminant cases, death can occur within hours despite adequate medical therapy.[149] Survival is usually determined in the first 12 hours after treatment has begun. Prognostically, unfavorable factors include the presence of petechiae for less than 12 hours before hospitalization, shock, absence of meningitis (≤ 20 WBC/mm^3 in CSF), and a normal or low WBC count and ESR. A recent study noted that the development of purpura fulminans (extensive purpuric rash with cardiovascular collapse) was the major risk factor for death. Additional risk factors from that study included infection with serogroup A and age of less than 1 year or over 10 years.[150]

All patients with consideration of meningococcemia should have a WBC count, platelet count, and bleeding screen. Cultures of blood, spinal fluid, nasopharynx, and other involved organs should be obtained. Skin scraping of the purpuric lesion may have a positive culture.

Approximately 20% of children with fever and petechiae have bacterial infections. Of these, 50% are caused by *N. meningitidis*, 30% by *H. influenzae*, and the remaining by a variety of agents. Management requires immediate resuscitation and support. Penicillin 250,000 U/kg/24 hr q 4 hr IV with a maximum of 20 million U/24 hours should be given for 7 to 10 days. Chloramphenicol is an alternative in allergic patients. Use of penicillin alone should be reserved until the isolate has been determined to be a penicillin-sensitive strain. Isolates have been recovered recently which have reduced sensitivity to penicillin. Prophylaxis of exposed persons is essential (see Appendix 55A).

MONONUCLEOSIS, INFECTIOUS

Infectious mononucleosis (IM) is a common, usually self-limited disease caused by the Epstein-Barr virus (EBV) a member of the herpes family. This virus is known to be the cause of Burkitt lymphoma, which occurs endemically in equatorial Africa. There is a wide range of clinical severity from asymptomatic to fatal. Worldwide testing for evidence of EBV infection shows that over 90% to 95% of people over the age of 30 years are seropositive.[151] In developing countries and lower socioeconomic environments seroconversion occurs at an earlier age.[152] In the developed countries, IM is diagnosed most frequently in adolescence. Up to 50% of children will show evidence of EBV infection by the age of 5, even with no clinical history.[151] In several studies in college students, of those who were EBV negative on college admission, almost half converted during the succeeding 4 years; nearly one third did not demonstrate clinical symptoms.[153]

IM was first named in 1920 by Sprunt and Evans although a similar disease called *glandular fever,* described several decades earlier, may have represented the same infection. The ubiquitous nature of the infection and the high rate of subclinical disease made determination of the etiologic agent and laboratory confirmation difficult. Serendipity played a role several times in the history of IM and led to the discovery of EBV as the causative agent and the heterophil antibody as a useful means of diagnosis. In addition, Downey in 1923 described the atypical lymphocytes that bear his name and remain key in the diagnosis of the illness.[154] Studies have also shown that clinical and laboratory presentations identical to IM, with the exception of absence of the heterophil antibody, occur in 10% to 20% of cases of parallel illness caused by cytomegalovirus infection, *Toxoplasma gondii,* hepatitis virus, or rubella virus and have led to the term *heterophil-negative infectious mononucleosis.* More recently, HIV infection has been added to this list.[155]

Diagnostic Findings

As EB virus is ubiquitous and sheds after acute infection from several months to a lifetime with a reservoir in the salivary glands, determination of the transmitting person is often difficult. Because of its predilection for the salivary glands, IM has been called the kissing disease, but transmission can also occur from less intimate interaction. After exposure, susceptible individuals have an incubation period of approximately 6 weeks.

The prodromal phase consists of up to a week of malaise, anorexia, headaches, fatigue, and night sweats. The acute phase consists of the classical triad of fever, exudative tonsillitis, and generalized lymphadenopathy. The posterior cervical lymph nodes are most often affected. Other symptoms associated with the acute phase include splenomegaly, palatal petechiae, periorbital edema (Hoagland signs), hepatomegaly, conjunctival injection, and exanthems. Although these are the most common clinical findings, virtually every organ system can be affected by the infection and occasionally some of the unusual complications may be the only presenting symptoms. An erythematous, maculopapular rash may develop, often associated with the use of ampicillin. It is most prominent on the trunk and proximal extremities.

As mentioned before, many cases of IM are subclinical. At the other extreme is a rare x-linked lymphoproliferative syndrome in which the EBV infection may be lethal sec-

ondary to fulminant hepatitis, lymphoma, or agammaglobulinemia. Fatal complications show a median age of 10.7 years in sporadic IM vs. 2.4 years in the x-linked lymphoproliferative syndrome.[156] There is a suggested increase in risk of Hodgkin disease in persons who have had IM, but the widespread nature of this infection raises some doubt as to its significance.

Complication rates vary, probably based on the definition of a complication and the age of the patients studied, ranging from 1% to over 20%.[151,152,157] The most common complications include splenic enlargement and rupture, the risk being greatest between the first 14 and 28 days of illness. Upper airway obstruction from marked tonsillar hypertrophy occurs. Peritonsillar abscess, meningitis, encephalitis, peripheral neuropathy (Bell palsy), ataxia, Guillain-Barré pneumonia, thrombocytopenia and autoimmune hemolytic anemia, pericarditis, myocarditis, hepatitis, proteinuria, microsporic hematuria and pyuria, and erythema multiforme are reported.[151,157-159]

Peritonsillar abscess must be considered with persistent or worsening pharyngeal complaints and breathing difficulty.[160] Concurrent group A streptococcal infection is common and should be considered in all patients with significant pharyngitis.

Deaths from IM are fortunately rare; 200 were reported to the CDC in a 10-year period.[158] Fatalities involve airway compromise, CNS involvement, and involvement of heart, liver, or spleen. These areas must be monitored closely during the clinical course.

Initially the EB virus infection starts in the salivary gland or adenotonsillar tissue and after about 2 weeks circulates in the B lymphocytes to the entire body. This viremia may last for several weeks.[154] Clinically after the acute phase the convalescent phase may last 2 to 8 weeks longer, with resolution of symptoms in a gradual or waxing and waning progression.[155] Fatigability is often prominent, especially in older patients, and is the basis for the recommended gradual return to full activity.

The clinical course is similar in patients of all ages with few exceptions. Children tend to have more abdominal pain and rashes; children under the age of 4 have increased frequency of hepatosplenomegaly and upper respiratory infections, including otitis media. In very young children, presentation may be similar to a failure-to-thrive picture.[157] Children younger than 2 years of age have a higher incidence of asymptomatic disease.[155]

Ancillary Data. Criteria for diagnosis of IM were published by Hoagland in 1973.[161] These include the clinical features noted above, relative and absolute lymphocytosis with more than 20% atypical lymphocytes, and positive Paul-Bunnell-Davidsohn (PBD) test or rapid slide test. In the emergency department, a CBC ordered on a patient with a typical history and physical, with blood held for a rapid slide test, is appropriate in initial evaluation. Younger children show a higher total WBC count but the relative percentage of lymphocytes remains similar in all ages. A lymphocyte count of 50% or more is usually present in all ages, but older children have a greater percentage of atypical lymphocytes.[155] In older patients the percentage of atypical lymphocytes has been used to determine if further testing is indicated.

If over 40% atypical lymphocytes are present, the diagnosis is considered firm; if 20% to 40% are present, the rapid slide test is indicated; if less than 20% are present, wait and repeat the evaluation.[153] This process may not be appropriate in younger children as many with confirmed IM will have a low percentage of atypical lymphocytes.

There are several rapid slide tests available with differing sensitivity and specificity.[151] These tests aim at detecting the presence of the heterophil antibody. The antibody may be absent early in the disease; 40% will be positive in the first week and 80% will be positive within 3 weeks.[162] Positive heterophil tests using horse and RBCs may remain positive for over a year. This pseudo-false-positives test must be considered when using these tests.[155] There is a much lower frequency of detectable heterophil antibodies in children younger than 4 years of age[163]; in the under-1-year age group only about one fourth will be positive.[152] In children in whom a diagnosis is required, especially early in the course, the detection of the IgM antibody to EBV-capsid antigen is the single most valuable specific serologic test of acute EBVM, when accompanied by compatible clinical and hematologic findings, and should be done in all patients younger than 4 years of age in whom the rapid test is negative.[163]

A routine throat culture for group A beta-hemolytic streptococci is recommended as well as liver function tests.

Management

Early diagnosis in the emergency department, especially in young children, presents challenges in both clinical and laboratory diagnosis. Because of its routinely benign course and the lack of isolation precautions, ambulatory management in confirmed or suspicious cases is often appropriate. Discharge instructions should be given and follow-up is recommended to monitor the patient and fully establish the diagnosis.

Treatment of IM is mainly supportive, as most cases are benign and self-limited. The use of steroids, except in cases with upper airway compromise, has been shown to be ineffective in altering the course of the disease. With the possibility of airway compromise, patients should be admitted to the hospital and placed on steroids: 1 to 2 mg/kg/day of prednisone can be used and tapered when adequate response is noted. Intubation may be required in rare cases.[164] Oral prednisone (1 to 2 mg/kg/24 hr PO) or hydrocortisone (Solu-Cortef 16 to 20 mg/kg/24 hr q 6 hr IV) may be used.

Because of the prolonged course of the disease a gradual resumption of normal activities is recommended. Relapses have occurred in patients who attempted to resume normal activities too early. Splenic enlargement presents a significant problem, especially in the athlete. No athletic activity should be allowed for at least 1 month; those patients involved with contact sports should have documentation of normal splenic size before resuming activity. Because splenic rupture can occur spontaneously or with minimal trauma, abdominal pain, especially left upper quadrant pain, should be evaluated carefully in a child with IM.

It has been suggested that use of aspirin prolongs the symptomatic period so its use should be discouraged. Initial reports showed an apparent high incidence of associated group A beta-hemolytic streptococcal throat infection with IM, but more recent studies have refuted this.[163,164] The routine prescribing of antibiotics is therefore not recommended, especially as there is a higher percentage of skin reaction with antibiotic usage in IM (almost 100% with ampicillin/amoxicillin and 40% with penicillin vs. 3% to 4% in those persons not treated).[165] A throat culture should be obtained in patients with pharyngitis or tonsillitis and antibiotics initiated if the culture is positive.[166]

MUMPS

Mumps is a systemic disease caused by the mumps virus, which belongs to the family of paramyxoviruses. Although infection and swelling of the parotid gland is generally considered the hallmark of this disease, central nervous system infection and testicular involvement occur frequently. Other complications include renal involvement, arthritis, thyroiditis, mastitis, and hearing impairment.[108]

Mumps was once considered a normal childhood illness; however, there has been a dramatic decrease in reported cases since the introduction of the mumps vaccine in 1967. Sporadic outbreaks have occurred in North America, usually in adolescents and young adults, with a peak in 1986 and 1987. These were thought to be secondary to the lack of emphasis on the need for mumps vaccination, which left a group of children unimmunized in a milieu of decreasing disease prevalence. Most cases occurred in states where mumps vaccination was not required.[167,168] Although mumps is more common in older patients in the United States and Canada, a recent report from England shows a trend toward a resurgence in preschool-aged children.[169] In the years before vaccination, 50% of children contracted mumps before starting school.[170] Other viral agents cause parotitis, which is clinically similar to mumps.

Diagnostic Findings

Humans are the only known reservoir of the mumps virus. After exposure of a susceptible individual, there is an incubation period of an average of 16 to 18 days, which ranges from 12 to 25 days.[108] Contagion is considered to occur for 7 days before and 9 days after onset of parotid swelling.[171] Although the hallmark of mumps is parotid swelling, up to one third of cases may not show this or any other sign of infection. For several days before parotid swelling there may be fever, malaise, and headache. Earache often precedes the parotid swelling. Although one parotid gland may be affected first, both are affected in the majority of cases.

Complications. Other organ systems are frequently affected by the mumps virus. Meningitis and encephalitis are the most serious complications. Before the vaccine era, mumps virus was the leading cause of meningoencephalitis in North American children.[170] Some reports state it still is.[170] Up to half the patients with mumps will show a CSF pleocytosis; approximately one in 10 persons with parotitis will develop clinical meningitis.[171] Males predominate in the development of meningitis.[170] A recent outbreak reported 17% of patients with meningeal involvement.[168] Symptoms of mumps meningitis are similar to those of other aseptic meningitides, and it should be considered in the differential diagnosis of aseptic meningitis because up to 50% of the cases do not show parotid swelling.[172] Mumps encephalitis has a higher morbidity and mortality with up to one in four cases showing neurologic sequelae.[170] Presenting symptoms include headache, vomiting, nuchal rigidity, delirium, hemiplegia, and seizures.[171] The encephalitis that occurs late in the clinical course may have long-term sequelae. Other nervous system complications include transverse myelitis, ataxia, Guillain-Barré syndrome, and deafness.[172] In fact, mumps has historically been considered the most common cause of acquired deafness in children and may remain so.[173]

Orchitis is a frequent complication in postpubertal males with a 19% occurrence cited in a recent outbreak.[168] Although debilitating, the orchitis rarely leads to fertility problems. A recent report of a fatality secondary to mumps myocarditis suggests that although death is rare, myocardial involvement is common.[174]

With the complications mentioned above, mumps is seen not as a benign childhood illness, but as a disease with significant morbidity, especially in older patients.

Diagnosis of mumps is usually made clinically. Serum amylase is often elevated and can indicate parotid or pancreatic involvement. Viral studies are usually of little use to the emergency physician.

Differential Considerations

Differential diagnosis of parotid swelling includes supporative parotitis, which is usually caused by *Staphylococcus aureus* or *Streptococcus pyogenes*. This is rare in children and usually secondary to salivary stasis due to obstructions.[175] The child presents with a swollen, markedly tender parotid gland. Stensen duct is often inflamed and purulent material can be expressed. Treatment includes antibiotics directed against the above organisms until cultures return; probing and relief of the obstruction may be indicated. Many other viruses and fungi can cause a parotitis and must be considered, particularly in children who are immunized.[176]

In addition, there is a condition that is associated with recurrent, noninfectious swelling of the parotid gland. In these patients the gland is usually not tender, the child does not appear ill, and pus cannot be expressed from Stensen duct.

Management

Treatment of mumps is supportive and depends on the severity of the illness. In the usual case, antipyretics, analgesics, and warm or cool compresses to the affected parotid are adequate. Similar recommendations can be made for mumps orchitis. More seriously ill children may require admission to hospital for supportive care.

PERTUSSIS

Pertussis, or whooping cough, is an acute bacterial respiratory infection that may have life-threatening complications, particularly in children younger than 6 months of age. Despite high immunization rates pertussis continues to be an important part of the differential diagnosis of acute respiratory disease.[177]

The causative agent, *Bordetella pertussis,* is a small gram-negative bacterium transmitted by contact with respiratory droplets from infected individuals. Attack rates of susceptible household contacts often approach greater than 90%.[178] In 1993 approximately 6,500 cases of pertussis were reported. The great majority of cases, however, go unrecognized or unreported. Over 40% of reported cases occur in children younger than 1 year of age and nearly 65% of cases occur in children younger than 4 years of age.[179] Most of these children lack a complete immunization series. Children should not be considered immune until they have completed the primary immunization series. Older children and adults may contract the disease and serve as reservoirs because of waning immunity.[180]

Multiple virulence factors allow *Bordetella* to establish and maintain infection in the human. Upon entering the respiratory tract the fimbriae of the bacterium attach to the surface of respiratory epithelial cells. After attachment the bacterium rapidly proliferates, producing a number of toxins. Among these toxins are pertussis toxin, adenylate cyclase toxin, and tracheal cytotoxin. The combined effect of these toxins on the respiratory tract is loss of ciliary function, accumulation of cellular debris, increased mucus production, and lymphocytic and granulocytic infiltration. The accumulated mucus and debris result in bronchiolar congestion, obstruction, and necrosis, which create conditions for secondary bronchopneumonia, atelectasis, and bronchiectasis.[181]

Diagnostic Findings

The incubation period for *Bordetella* is 6 to 20 days, with most symptoms beginning 7 days after exposure. The symptoms of pertussis typically occur in three stages (Table 55-4). The first stage, or the catarrhal stage, lasts for 1 to 2 weeks and consists of rhinorrhea, lacrimation, and mild cough. Fever is low grade throughout the disease and rarely exceeds 101° F.

Following the catarrhal stage the patient enters the paroxysmal stage, which may last from 2 to 4 weeks and is the period during which most morbidity and mortality occurs. The prominent feature is paroxysmal cough characterized by as many as 5 to 10 expulsions before inspiration. The patient often appears cyanotic, plethoric, anxious, or diaphoretic, with protrusion of the tongue and bulging of the eyes. Immediately following the cough the patient may

TABLE 55-4. Clinical Stages of Pertussis

Stage	Duration	Clinical features
Catarrhal	1-2 weeks	Rhinorrhea, lacrimation, mild cough, fever (usually low grade)
Paroxysmal	2-4 weeks	Paroxysmal cough, neurologic and respiratory complications
Convalescent	1-4 weeks	Gradual improvement in symptoms. Paroxysmal cough may persist for up to 6 months

produce an inspiratory "whoop," appear limp and exhausted, and begin vomiting.[181] There are two important considerations when evaluating patients for pertussis. First, all patients do not whoop. Second, younger infants, especially those younger than 6 months of age, may lack the paroxysmal cough and may present with choking episodes, apnea, cyanotic episodes, or failure to thrive.[182]

The convalescent stage begins following a gradual improvement in symptoms and lasts 1 to 4 weeks. Spontaneous paroxysms may continue to appear for 6 months. Bronchopneumonia is the most common complication of pertussis and is reported to occur in 14% of hospitalized patients.[183] Neurologic complications occur in 2% to 4% of patients in the form of seizures and encephalopathy and probably result from both repeated episodes of hypoxia and toxin-mediated effects.[183,184] Other complications include rectal prolapse, pneumothorax, hernia, and hemorrhagic events such as petechiae, subconjunctival hemorrhages, and subdural hematomas.

Ancillary Data. The most striking laboratory finding in pertussis is leukocytosis and lymphocytosis. A WBC count of >15,000 cells/mm^3 with an absolute lymphocytosis may be helpful in establishing a diagnosis of pertussis; however, the absence of this finding does not discount the possibility of pertussis, especially in the child younger than 6 months of age.[185] Eosinophilia, although not common, may occur and its presence should suggest the possibility of pertussis.[181]

Hypoglycemia may develop in some patients with no other blood chemistry abnormalities. The ESR is typically normal and an elevation should suggest secondary infection.[185] Chest x-ray radiographs may reveal atelectasis or pneumonia often accompanied by peribronchial thickening, infiltrates, and a "shaggy" heart border.

Early diagnosis is important in reducing disease morbidity and spread.[186] A presumptive diagnosis can be quickly made when a paroxysmal cough and inspiratory whoop is present. However, patients with mild symptoms, or small infants with atypical presentations require specific identification of Bordetella.[182] Differential considerations should include other causes of pneumonia.

Culture of the organism remains the gold standard of diagnosis; however, success is dependent on the experience of the laboratory as well as the quality and handling of the specimen. Nasopharyngeal swabs should be rapidly inoculated onto prewarmed culture plates, using a selective medium such as Bordet-Gengou. Cough plates are not recommended. Fluorescent antibody staining of nasopharyngeal swabs offers a more rapid approach to diagnosis; however, specificity and sensitivity is unpredictable. All fluorescent antibody assays should be accompanied by culture.[63,185]

Management

Antibiotic therapy does not hasten clinical improvement during the paroxysmal stage of disease. It does, however, eradicate the organism from the respiratory tract, which is crucial in containing the spread of disease.

The drug of choice is erythromycin estolate (50 mg/kg/24 hr in 4 divided doses) for 14 days. The higher serum levels of erythromycin achieved with the estolate form afford a theoretical advantage over other forms of erythromycin.[187,188] Patients should be instructed to repeat vomited doses. Trimethoprim/sulfamethoxazole (TMP/SMX) (8 mg TMP/kg/24 hr BID PO) is an alternative for patients who do not tolerate erythromycin, although its efficacy has not been thoroughly studied. Patients treated with TMP/SMX should be closely observed and require a longer period of isolation.[63]

Several reports have suggested that corticosteroids and albuterol may reduce the frequency and severity of symptoms but further studies are needed to establish their efficacy and safety.[189,190]

All household contacts and other close contacts should receive prophylactic treatment with erythromycin estolate (50 mg/kg/24 hr QID PO) for 14 days. TMP/SMX (8 mg TMP/kg/24 hr BID PO) can be used when erythromycin is not tolerated. Its efficacy, however, has not been established.[63]

All close contacts younger than 7 years of age and children who are unimmunized or have received less than four diphtheria-pertussis-tetanus doses [DPTs] should receive immunizations according to the routine immunization schedule.

All patients younger than 6 months of age with clinical evidence of pertussis should be hospitalized for evaluation because of the high rate of complications in this age group.

All patients should be isolated for 5 days after beginning erythromycin therapy or until 3 weeks after the onset of paroxysms if appropriate antimicrobial therapy is not given.

Prophylaxis of household and other close contacts of pertussis cases should be considered. All household or other close contacts younger than 1 year of age (regardless of DTP immunization status) should receive a 14-day course of oral erythromycin (40 mg/kg/24 hr QID PO). Household and other close contacts 1 to 7 years of age who have had less than four DTP doses or whose last DTP was more than 3 years ago should receive 14 days of oral erythromycin as above, and many physicians recommend receiving another DTP immunization.

Asymptomatic household or other close contacts need not be excluded from school if they are taking antibiotics. Persons who have a positive laboratory test for pertussis should be excluded from school or work until they have taken antibiotics for 14 days. All household contacts older than 7 years of age should receive antibiotics if the last DTP immunization was given 3 years ago or longer.

RABIES

Human rabies is an acute viral infection with predominantly CNS manifestations that almost invariably results in death. The decline of rabies in domestic pets over the last 40 years has made human rabies extremely rare.[191] The frequency of animal bites and the rising incidence of rabies in wild animals makes evaluation for postexposure prophylaxis a major consideration in the emergency department. Tremendous geographic variability exists and local disease patterns should be explored.

Transmission of the rabies virus occurs following penetration of the skin, as occurs with bites or scratches, or by contamination of an open wound or mucous membrane.

TABLE 55-5. Rabies Postexposure Prophylaxis

Animal type	Evaluation and disposition of animal	Postexposure prophylaxis recommendations
Dogs and cats	Healthy and available for 10 days observation*	Do not begin prophylaxis unless animal develops symptoms of rabies
	Rabies or suspected rabies	Begin vaccination immediately
	Unknown (escaped)	Consult public health officials
Skunks, raccoons, bats, foxes, and other carnivores; woodchucks	Regarded as rabid unless geographic area is known to be free of rabies or animal is proven negative by laboratory tests†	Begin vaccination immediately
Livestock, rodents, and lagomorphs (rabbits and hares)	Considered individually	Consult public health officials. Bites of squirrels, hamsters, guinea pigs, chipmunks, rats, mice, and other lagomorphs almost never require antirabies prophylaxis

From the Advisory Committee on Immunization Practices: *MMWR* 40(RR-3):1-19, 1991.
*During 10-day holding period treatment with HRIG and rabies vaccine should begin at first sign of rabies. The symptomatic animal should be killed immediately and tested.
†The animal should be killed and tested as soon as possible. Holding for observation is not recommended. Treatment should be discontinued if laboratory testing is negative.

The etiologic agent is the rabies virus, a neurotrophic ribonucleic acid (RNA) virus that rapidly ascends peripheral nerves to the CNS.[192]

Human rabies is characterized by agitation, bizarre behavior, pharyngeal and laryngeal spasm, flaccid paralysis, and coma. Death generally results from cardiac or respiratory failure.[193]

Sources of rabies in the United States include wild and domestic animals. The occurrence of rabies in domestic animals may vary with the region of the United States; however, in most regions the incidence is very low. Fully vaccinated dogs and cats are rarely infected with the virus.[191]

Wild animals represent the most significant source of rabies in the United States. The highest incidence is among carnivores (especially skunks, raccoons, and foxes) and bats. Rodents such as squirrels, hamsters, guinea pigs, chipmunks, gerbils, rats, and mice are rarely infected. The major exception is the woodchuck, which constitutes 70% of the rabies reported in rodents.[191]

The diagnosis of an animal infected with rabies is by immunofluorescent examination of the brain tissue for virus. Animals to be tested for rabies should be killed in a manner that preserves the brain intact. The reference laboratory should be consulted for the proper method of obtaining and transporting the specimen.[191]

Diagnostic Findings

Management is outlined in Table 55-5. Wounds inflicted by dogs and cats that appear healthy represent the lowest risk and should be managed by observing the animal for 10 days. If the animal appears rabid or becomes ill during the period of observation, the contact patient should be started on postexposure prophylaxis immediately pending laboratory testing. Other considerations should include the circumstances of the biting incident, the type of exposure (bite or nonbite), and epizootic conditions in the area. Treatment should be discontinued upon receiving a nega-

tive result. Unprovoked attacks or behavioral changes in the animal, such as agitation or malaise, should be interpreted as possible signs of rabies. Unwanted or stray animals should be killed and tested. Patients injured by dogs or cats that escaped should be managed after consultation with public health officials.[191]

All carnivores (especially skunks, raccoons, and foxes), bats, and woodchucks should be regarded as rabid and contacts should be administered postexposure prophylaxis unless the animal is confirmed to be negative by laboratory testing.[191]

The risks from livestock, rodents, and rabbits is low and public health officials should be consulted before administering postexposure prophylaxis.[191]

Management

Management of patients with wounds inflicted by animals should begin with thorough cleaning of the wound and administration of tetanus prophylaxis when indicated. Postexposure prophylaxis consists of the concurrent administration of human rabies immune globulin (HRIG) and human rabies vaccine (Table 55-6).

HRIG (150 IU/ml) is administered as a single dose of 20 IU/kg, with up to one half the dose infiltrated around the wound, when possible, and the remainder given intramuscularly in the gluteal area. Human rabies vaccine (1 ml) is given intramuscularly in the deltoid area at days 0, 3, 7, 14, and 28. Two rabies vaccines are available in the United States—the human diploid cell rabies vaccine (HDCV) and the rabies vaccine adsorbed (RVA). Administration is the same for either vaccine.[191,194] If vaccine or immune globulin is not readily available, call the Centers for Disease Control ([404] 639-3670 during working hours or [404] 639-2888 on nights, weekends, and holidays).

Preexposure HDCV (1 Movax Rabies) may be administered to at-risk individuals. In adults, give 1 ml IM in 3 doses at 0, 7, and 29 days with a booster every 2 years; 0.1 ml intradermally may also be given according to this schedule.

TABLE 55-6. Rabies Postexposure Prophylaxis Regimen

Vaccination status	Treatment	Regimen
Not previously vaccinated	Local wound cleansing	Thorough cleansing with soap and water
	HRIG	20 IU/kg; if anatomy permits, half dose is infiltrated around wounds and remainder given IM in gluteal area
	Vaccine	HDCV or RVA 1 ml IM in deltoid.* One each on days 0, 3, 7, 14, and 28.
Previously vaccinated†	Local wound cleansing	Thorough cleansing with soap and water
	HRIG	HRIG should not be administered
	Vaccine	HDCV or RVA 1 ml, IM in deltoid.* One each on days 0 and 3.

From the Advisory Committee on Immunization Practices: *MMWR* 40(RR-3):1-19, 1991.
*The deltoid is the only acceptable site of vaccination for adults and older children. For younger children, the outer aspect of the thigh may be used. Vaccine should never be administered in the gluteal area.
†Any person with a history of preexposure vaccination with HDCV or RVA, prior postexposure prophylaxis with HDCV or RVA, or previous vaccination with any other type of rabies vaccine and a documented history of antibody response to the prior vaccination.

STAPHYLOCOCCAL AND STREPTOCOCCAL SYSTEMIC DISEASE

Toxic Shock Syndrome

Toxic shock syndrome (TSS) was first described by Todd in 1978 in seven children.[195] It is possible that this was not a new disease but a rediscovered one, as reports of a similar complex appeared as early as 1927.[196] Although Todd reported the syndrome in seven children, it soon became a disease associated with menstruation and tampon use.[197] Menstrual cases still predominate; TSS has been associated with staphylococcal infections in a wide variety of other clinical settings including staphylococcal pneumonia complicating influenza A and B, superficial skin infections, major and minor burns, ear piercing, nasal packing, poison oak dermatitis, sinusitis, and bacterial tracheitis.[198-208] As more reports appear, it is apparent that a staphylococcal infection, either primary or secondary, caused by the appropriate strain in a susceptible individual may lead to TSS. The CDC have developed a list of criteria for diagnosis of TSS (see box at right). Although suggested modifications have been published, these remain the standard.

For undetermined reasons the number of reported cases of TSS peaked in 1980 and has declined since. Because of the high morbidity associated with TSS, especially the nonmenstrual form, as well as an often subtle initial presentation, it is imperative that clinicians remain alert for this disease.

As mentioned earlier, the majority of cases of TSS have occurred in menstruating females, but cases have been reported in children of all ages. Investigation into risk factors other than menstruation and tampon use has met with limited results and it appears that multiple bacterial and host factors are involved.[209] The disease complex is secondary to a toxin elaborated by certain strains of staphylococcus. This toxin has been called various names but most commonly *toxic shock syndrome toxin 1 (TSST-1)*. Although most menstrual cases are caused by strains producing TSST-1, nonmenstrual cases are much more variable. Also, the fatality rate for cases of TSS with non–TSST-1-producing strains is much higher than for strains that do produce TSST-1.[209] Thus there is a great likelihood that other toxins are involved.

Toxic Shock Syndrome Case Definition*

1. Fever (temperature $\geq 39.2°$ C [102° F])
2. Rash (diffuse macular erythroderma)
3. Desquamation, 1-2 weeks after onset of illness, particularly of palms and soles
4. Hypotension (systolic blood pressure ≤ 90 mm Hg for adults or less than the 5th percentile by age for children < 16 years of age, or orthostatic syncope)
5. Involvement of three or more of the following organ systems:
   A. Gastrointestinal (vomiting or diarrhea at onset of illness)
   B. Muscular (severe myalgia or creatinine phosphokinase level $\geq 2 \times$ ULN)
   C. Mucous membrane (vaginal, oropharyngeal, or conjunctival hyperemia)
   D. Renal (BUN or Cr $\geq 2 \times$ ULN or ≥ 5 WBCs per high power field—in the absence of a urinary tract infection)
   E. Hepatic (total bilirubin, SGOT [AST], or SGPT [APT] $\geq 2 \times$ ULN)
   F. Hematologic (low platelet count)
   G. Central nervous system (disorientation or alterations in consciousness without focal neurologic signs when fever and hypotension are absent)
6. Negative results on the following tests, if obtained:
   A. Blood throat or cerebrospinal fluid cultures
   B. Serologic tests for Rocky Mountain spotted fever, leptospirosis, or measles

*Criteria from the Centers for Disease Control and Prevention, 1980. *ULN*, Upper limit of normal range; *BUN*, blood urea nitrogen; *Cr*, serum creatinine; *WBCs*, white blood cells; *SGOT*, serum glutamate oxaloacetate transaminase (aspartate aminotransferase); *SGPT*, serum glutamate pyruvate transaminase (alanine aminotransferase).

Although children have a higher incidence of minor staphylococcal infections than adults, the incidence of TSS in children is lower. This may point to the fact that the focus of infection plays a greater role in the elaboration of the toxin than is generally believed.

These toxins are produced by particular strains of staphylococcus when in appropriate local conditions, such as aerobic conditions, neutral pH, 6% carbon dioxide, and presence of protein—conditions that are often found in infectious foci.[210] In addition, studies have shown that patients with TSS do not develop a significant antibody response to TSST-1.[211] This may explain why there is a significant recurrence rate for TSS.

Diagnostic Findings

Because of the rapid progression and low incidence of TSS in children, it is important to suspect this disorder in any unusual illness that presents with consistent symptoms. There is often a sudden onset of high fever associated with vomiting, myalgia, dizziness, hypotension, and rash. Additional symptoms include headache, arthralgia, sore throat, abdominal pain, diarrhea, and stiff neck. The skin findings may be dramatic and present as a severe, diffuse erythroderma or may be evanescent if localized.

Desquamation, which is a key factor, occurs later in the disease. Obviously, if there is a primary disease (e.g., bacterial tracheitis, influenza), those symptoms may initially predominate.

Physical examination may be deceptively benign but a thorough search for the source of infection is mandatory. The actual infected site may not be impressive, with minimal purulence. Identification and elimination of this focus is necessary.

The toxin(s) in TSS affect multiple organs and many laboratory abnormalities are possible. No specific laboratory test can make the diagnosis but there are several frequently found abnormalities. A CBC may show a normal total count, but there is frequently a large percentage of band and immature forms, often with toxic granulations. Platelet counts may be low. Clotting studies are usually normal except in the rare patient who develops DIC. Evaluation of renal function frequently shows elevated blood urea nitrogen (BUN) and creatinine as well as WBCs and RBCs in the urine. Liver function tests frequently show some elevation of liver enzymes and bilirubin. Electrolyte abnormalities are variable and often reflect the degree of gastrointestinal involvement. Calcium may be decreased. With severe hypotension, the patients are often acidotic. Some patients may develop adult respiratory distress with associated blood gas and chest x-ray film abnormalities. Cultures of the blood, throat, and CSF fluid, skin lesions and localized infections are useful. Vaginal cultures may be appropriate in menstruating females.

Although cardiac abnormalities are not common in children, ECG may reveal nonspecific ST segment and T-wave abnormalities and decrease in QRS voltage; one case of complete heart block has been recorded.[212,213] Thus the toxins cause some myocardial damage as well.

Management

Management of TSS depends on its prompt recognition as well as on identification of the infectious focus. This focus must be drained and foreign material (e.g., nasal packing) must be removed. Antibiotics directed against Staphylococcus such as nafcillin or cefazolin (150 mg/kg/24

> **Differential Diagnosis of Toxic Shock Syndrome**
>
> Kawasaki disease
> Staphylococcal scalded skin syndrome
> Scarlet fever
> Rocky Mountain spotted fever
> Leptospirosis
> Erythema multiforme major
> Drug reaction
> Gram-negative septic shock

---

hr q 4-6 hr IV) are recommended but their effect on the morbidity and mortality is uncertain. Corticosteroids (methylprednisolone [Solu-Medrol]) are recommended within 2 to 3 days of illness but also have not been shown to conclusively affect eventual outcome. Because of the difficulty in distinguishing KS from TSS, especially in younger children, IVGG may be considered if this distinction is difficult (see box on p. 945).[214]

The remainder of therapy depends on the severity and extent of symptoms. Hypotension is initially treated with fluids and pressors are used if fluids are unsuccessful. Renal failure may necessitate dialysis. Children have a higher incidence of respiratory problems and need ventilatory assistance more frequently than adults.[210] This may be associated with the frequent association of TSS with bacterial tracheitis in children. Correction of electrolyte, calcium, and hematologic abnormalities is directed by the patient's condition. Hospitalization is required.

Group A Streptococcal Sepsis

Although there are many diseases on the list of differential diagnoses of TSS (see box above), recently a very similar syndrome associated with group A streptococcal infection has been described.[215,216] Unlike TSS, the site of infection is often an obvious cellulitis or necrotizing fasciitis, or secondary to infected varicella; there is a frequent positive blood culture in the streptococcal disease.[217] Like TSS, this syndrome appears to be mediated by a toxin elaborated by the streptococcus, specifically pyrogenic exotoxin A. This toxin has rarely been found in isolates since the earlier part of this century, so this syndrome may represent a reemergence of a previous strain that is capable of producing this toxin. Indeed, scarlet fever was a virulent disease that reached its peak at the turn of the century but has recently been considered a minor illness. This may now change.[218] This latter toxin has similar properties to staphylococcal enterotoxin B, which may play a role in nonmenstrual TSS.[219]

Diagnostic Findings. Clinical presentation in addition to the primary source of infection includes erythroderma, hypotension, renal dysfunction, hypoalbuminemia, hypocalcemia, and respiratory failure. Pain is often severe and abrupt in onset.[205] Other symptoms are nonspecific and include fever, chills, myalgia, and diarrhea. Desquamation often occurs within 2 weeks. A recent population based study suggested that there are distinct groups of invasive group A streptococcal disease: (1) those with organ system involvement; (2) those with skin and mucus membrane involvement; and (3) those with necrotizing fasciitis. The development of shock is associated with the first two groups.[220]

Diagnosis can be suspected by culturing the streptococcus or serologic evidence of infection. Laboratory evaluations resemble TSS with normal WBC count but elevated immature forms, evidence of renal failure, hematuria, as well as those mentioned previously. Again, blood cultures are frequently positive.

Management. Management includes antibiotics against group A streptococcus such as penicillin (100,000 to 150,000 U/kg/24 hr q 4 hr IV) and supportive measures depending on the severity of symptoms. A recent report suggests that IVGG may be useful.[221] Because this is a recently "rediscovered" disease, more information on prevalence, risk factors, and therapy should be forthcoming. The child should be admitted.

TETANUS

Tetanus is a toxin-mediated disease resulting in either generalized or localized muscular spasm. The incidence of pediatric tetanus in the United States has diminished significantly over the last 30 years because of effective immunization practices. Despite the rarity of the disease the physician is frequently required to evaluate patients for tetanus prophylaxis.[222]

The causative organism, *Clostridium tetani*, is an anaerobic, spore-forming, gram-positive bacillus commonly present in the environment. The organism is usually introduced into the wound as a spore. Conditions in the wound may allow the spore to develop into the toxin-producing vegetative form. The exotoxin produced by *C. tetani* is a neurotoxin, *tetanospasmin*, which acts on the CNS and skeletal muscle motor endplates. Toxin produced at the site of the wound may remain in the vicinity, affecting only adjacent muscle groups, or it may be absorbed and hematogenously distributed throughout the body. The wounds most commonly associated with tetanus are puncture wounds, lacerations, and abrasions. Up to a third of tetanus cases result from injuries that went unnoticed or were considered trivial.[223]

Diagnostic Findings

Generalized tetanus is the most common form of the disease and presents with severe muscular spasms involving the jaw, face, neck, and back, giving rise to the classic features of trismus and opisthotonos.[223] Localized tetanus arises in the muscle group closest in proximity to the site of contamination and is characterized by isolated muscular spasm.[224] Localized tetanus often progresses into generalized tetanus. Cephalic tetanus is a form of localized tetanus that involves the head and neck muscles.[223]

Complications include musculoskeletal injuries, especially vertebral fractures and respiratory compromise. Case fatality rates average 20%.[223]

TABLE 55-7. Tetanus Prophylaxis in Routine Wound Management

History of tetanus immunizations	Clean minor wound		All other wounds*	
	Td[†]	TIG	Td	TIG
Unknown or less than 3 doses	Yes	No	Yes	Yes
3 or more doses[‡]	No[§]	No	No[‖]	No

From *MMWR* 39(3):37-41, 1990; Committee on Infectious Diseases: *AAP* 409-414, 1994.
*Such as, but not limited to, wounds contaminated with dirt, feces, soil, and saliva; puncture wounds; avulsions; and wounds resulting from missiles, crushing, burns, and frostbite.
[†]For children younger than 7 years of age give DTP (or DT if pertussis is contraindicated).
[‡]If only 3 doses of *fluid* toxoid have been received, a fourth dose of absorbed toxoid should be given.
[§]Yes, if more than 10 years since the last dose.
[‖]Yes, if more than 5 years since the last dose.

Routine laboratory findings are not helpful in diagnosing tetanus. WBC counts and blood chemistries are generally normal. LP results are normal except for an occasional elevation in the protein. Wounds should be cultured anaerobically for *C. tetani*.[223]

The differential diagnosis of tetanus includes drug or chemical ingestion, drug reactions, metabolic or endocrine causes, and hysteria or conversion reactions.

Management

Management of tetanus involves administration of tetanus immune globulin (TIG) to neutralize circulating antibody, surgical debridement of wounds, antibiotic therapy (penicillin G 100,000 U/kg/6 hr IV for 10 days) and control of muscle spasms with diazepam or lorazepam.[63,225,226]

TIG should be administered as a single dose of 3,000 to 6,000 U IM with a portion of the dose infiltrated around the wound. If TIG is not available, equine tetanus antitoxin (TAT) may be given after appropriate testing for sensitivity. TAT is administered as a single dose of 50,000 to 100,000 U. Approximately 20,000 U of this dose should be given intravenously.[108] IVGG may be considered for treatment if TIG is not available. However, this is not an approved use of IVGG and the dosage is not established.[63]

All patients with tetanus should receive supportive care and management in an intensive care unit.

Prevention. The management of all patients presenting to the emergency room with even trivial wounds requires evaluation for tetanus prophylaxis, which is outlined in Table 55-7. Minor wounds are considered clean, superficial lacerations or abrasions. Wounds contaminated with soil, feces, saliva, or other potentially contaminated material represents a higher risk for infection as do puncture wounds, avulsions, and wounds resulting in areas of devitalized tissue.[227] Management of persons exposed to tetanus lacking sufficient immunity requires the administration of tetanus toxoid vaccine and TIG for all but clean minor wounds.

Tetanus toxoid is available as either a fluid preparation (which requires four doses for primary immunity) or an absorbed preparation (which requires only three doses for primary immunity). Absorbed tetanus toxoid is the preferred preparation.

Diphtheria and tetanus toxoid mixtures all contain the same amount of tetanus toxoid and are available as DTP, DT, and Td. DTP, which contains the pertussis component, is the preferred vaccine for all children younger than 7 years of age requiring tetanus prophylaxis and not having a contraindication for the pertussis component. DT is recommended for all other children younger than 7 years of age. Td is indicated for all children 7 years of age or older and contains a small-dose diphtheria toxin to provide a diphtheria booster.[228]

TICK-BORNE INFECTIOUS DISEASES

Ticks are widely distributed throughout the world and serve as major vectors of human disease. In the United States, the rising incidence of tick-borne disease has heightened public awareness of the tick as a disease vector.[229,230]

The most common tick habitats are rural and wilderness areas but may also include city parks, golf courses, and vacant lots.[231] Ticks serve as reservoirs for a variety of pathogens that are efficiently transmitted during the blood meal. Individual pathogens are generally restricted to a particular species of tick.[229]

The most common tick-borne infectious diseases include Lyme disease, Rocky Mountain spotted fever, and tularemia. Less common diseases include ehrlichiosis, relapsing fever, and Colorado tick fever. Several of these illnesses are potentially life threatening and require prompt diagnosis and treatment (Table 55-8).

Colorado Tick Fever

Colorado tick fever is an acute febrile illness that typically occurs in the Rocky Mountains, northwestern United States, and western Canada during the warm-weather months. The etiologic agent is a reovirus that is transmitted by the tick, *Dermacentor andersoni*. The incubation period is from 3 to 6 days.

The common clinical manifestations include fever, headache, myalgia, and malaise. Less common manifestations include nonexudative pharyngitis, conjunctivitis, stiff neck, abdominal pain, vomiting, and diarrhea. Symptoms may persist for up to 8 weeks, resulting in a prolonged or biphasic clinical course. Leukopenia ($>4500/mm^3$) occurs in the majority of patients and is usually the only laboratory abnormality. Treatment is supportive.[232]

Ehrlichiosis

Human ehrlichiosis was first described in the United States in 1987 and is caused by the rickettsia, *Ehrlichia chaffeensis*. The infection appears to be transmitted by ticks, although little is known regarding which tick species serve as reservoirs.[233] Over 90% of cases present between the months of April and September and occur predominantly in the southcentral and southeastern United States (especially Oklahoma, Missouri, and Arkansas). Most cases

have been reported in adults and the disease has a fatality rate of approximately 1% to 2%.

Clinically, ehrlichiosis is similar to Rocky Mountain spotted fever, although rash is less common and leukopenia more common. The most frequent signs and symptoms include fever, malaise, headache, myalgia, arthralgia, anorexia, nausea, vomiting, and diaphoresis. Mental confusion, diarrhea, and abdominal pain occur less frequently. Rash occurs in only about 30% of patients in the first week and may be maculopapular or petechial. Common laboratory findings include leukopenia, elevated alanine aminotransferase (ALT) and aspartate aminotransferase (AST), and thrombocytopenia.[233,234]

Doxycycline appears to be the drug of choice in the treatment of ehrlichiosis. Children younger than 9 years of age should be treated with chloramphenicol (50 to 75 mg/kg/24 hr QID PO). However, because tetracyclines appear superior to chloramphenicol in the treatment of rickettsial infections, some clinicians have compared the benefits and risks of tetracycline in children younger than 9 years of age, and prefer to use a tetracycline; parental consent is appropriate.[63,233,234]

Lyme Disease

Lyme disease (LD) is a systemic infection causing predominantly dermatologic, neurologic, cardiac, and musculoskeletal symptoms and is the most common tick-borne disease in the United States. The sharp rise in the incidence of LD as well as the broad range of symptoms has made this illness a frequent concern for the parent and a diagnostic dilemma for the physician.

LD was first described by Steere in 1977, following the outbreak of a juvenile rheumatoid arthritis-like illness in Lyme, Conn.[235] Evidence, however, suggests that the disease dates back many years.[236]

The etiologic agent, *Borrelia burgdorferi*, was a previously unknown spirochete until its discovery by Burgdorfer in 1981. Before the etiologic agent was correctly identified the deer tick was thought to be the disease vector based on epidemiologic data. The deer tick, *Ixodes dammini*, is the most common vector of LD in the United States, except in the Pacific region where *I. pacificus* is the predominant vector.[237]

Approximately 13,000 cases were reported in the United States in 1994; this is 58% more than the number of cases reported in 1993.[238] Nearly every state in the United States has reported cases of LD with the northeastern, mid-Atlantic, northcentral, and Pacific coastal states reporting the highest incidence.[239]

LD is most common in warm-weather months with the peak incidence occurring in June and July. The age range from LD is from 2 to 88 years; however, the peak age incidence is in 9- to 12-year-olds.[239]

The spirochete enters the wound during the tick's blood meal and establishes an area of localized infection in the skin that results in the erythema migrans rash. The organism then invades adjacent blood or lymph vessels with lymphohematogenous dissemination to the various organ systems. The spirochete has been isolated from a variety of tissues and fluids including skin, blood, heart, CSF, and

TABLE 55-8. Tick-Transmitted Diseases

	Tularemia	Relapsing fever	Rocky Mountain spotted fever (RMSF)	Colorado tick fever	Ehrlichiosis	Lyme disease
Etiology	*Francisella tularemia*	*Borrelia recurrentis*	*Rickettsia rickettsii*	Colorado tick fever virus	*Ehrlichia chaffeensis*	*Borrelia burgdorferi*
Tick vector	*Dermacentor*	*Orinthodoros*	*Dermacentor*	*Dermacentor*		*Ixodes scapularis* *I. pacificus*
Incubation	1-14 days	5-9 days	2-14 days	3-6 days	7-21 days	3-32 days
Diagnostic findings	Headache, persistent fever, malaise, anorexia, lymphadenopathy, conjunctivitis	Relapsing fever, headache, malaise, myalgia, cough, meningismus, lymphadenopathy, leukocytosis	Resistant fever, headache, malaise, arthralgia, periorbital edema, conjunctivitis, meningismus, coma, centrifugal hemorrhagic rash, petechiae	Sudden onset of fever, retro-orbital headache, myalgia, anorexia, meningismus, rash, conjunctivitis, leukopenia	Fever, headache, malaise, arthralgia, myalgia, nausea, vomiting, rash (30% of cases)	Erythema chronicum migrans (ECM) (macular/papular becoming annular), flu-like symptoms (headache, anorexia, chills) with later neurologic complications (encephalopathy, cranial neuropathy, peripheral radiculoneuropathy) or joint complications (arthralgia); remissions; ELISA
Antibiotics	Gentamicin	Tetracycline,* penicillin, chloramphenicol	Tetracycline,* chloramphenicol	None (support)	Tetracycline,* chloramphenicol	Doxycycline,* amoxicillin

ELISA, Enzyme-linked immunosorbent assay.
Adapted from Barkin RM and Rosen P: *Emergency pediatrics,* ed 4, St Louis, 1994, Mosby.
*Do not use in children <9 yr.

synovium.[240] The clinical features of LD are caused both by the direct effects of the live spirochete and by the formation of immune complexes.[241,242] An unusual feature of the spirochete is the capacity to alter its own surface antigens, allowing it to evade host immune defenses and establish persistent or relapsing infection.[243]

Diagnostic Findings. The clinical manifestations of LD occur in three stages: early localized, early disseminated, and late persistent.[237,238,242] (Table 55-9) Early localized LD (stage I) manifestations include erythema chronicum migrans (ECM), fever, and flu-like symptoms. Erythema migrans, the most common and important feature of LD, is found in about 60% to 80% of cases and usually appears 4

to 20 days after a tick bite. Up to half of patients developing erythema migrans will have no history of tick bite. The rash begins as a small macule with a rapidly expanding annular border. Erythema migrans appears singly (50% of cases) or as a group of 2 or 3 macules. The lesion may appear flat or raised and the size varies from less than 1 cm to over 60 cm. Erythema migrans usually resolves within 3 weeks; however, chronic recurrences may continue for up to a year in untreated or inadequately treated patients. Fever is usually low grade but may be as high as 40° C. Malaise, myalgia, arthralgia, headache, and sore throat occur frequently.[244] Early LD presenting as a flu-like illness without erythema migrans has been reported.[245]

TABLE 55-9. Principal Clinical Manifestations of Lyme Disease

System	Stage 1	Stage 2	Stage 3
Skin	Erythema chronicum migrans (ECM)	Recurrent ECM	Acrodermatitis chronica atrophican
Central nervous system	Headache	Neurologic Aseptic meningitis Mild encephalitis Cranial nerve palsy Radiculoneuropathy Cerebellar ataxia Chorea	Persistent central and peripheral nervous system involvement
Musculoskeletal	Arthralgia	Arthritis	Intermittent or chronic arthritis
Cardiac		Cardiac manifestations Atrioventricular block Myopericarditis Left ventricular dysfunction	
Constitutional symptoms	Fever, malaise, myalgia	Malaise	Malaise

Early disseminated (stage II) LD presents primarily with neurologic and cardiac manifestations. Arthralgia, myalgia, hepatitis, recurrent erythema migrans, and fatigue may also be observed. Neurologic symptoms generally appear within 4 weeks (range 2 to 11 weeks) of the tick bite and occur in 15% to 20% of patients.[246] Aseptic meningitis is the most common neurologic finding, presenting with typical signs of headache, stiff neck, irritability, photophobia, nausea, and vomiting. CSF findings are similar to those of viral meningitis. Other frequently occurring clinical findings include seventh cranial nerve palsy and meningoencephalitis. Chorea, cerebellar ataxia, radiculopathy, myelitis, and pseudotumor cerebri may also occur. Cardiac manifestations are found in 8% to 10% of patients and usually present within 5 weeks of the tick bite (range 3 to 21 weeks).[247] The most common abnormality is atrioventricular block of varying degrees. Complete heart block has been reported in children but is more common in young adult men. Other cardiac abnormalities include myopericarditis and left ventricular dysfunction. Cardiac abnormalities are generally transient, resolving 1 to 6 weeks after onset.

Late persistent (stage III) LD manifestations include chronic or relapsing arthritis, ongoing neurologic syndromes, and acrodermatitis chronica atrophicans, a chronic skin lesion. Arthritis is the second most common finding in LD, after erythema migrans, and is present in up to 50% of patients.[248] Although arthralgia and transient arthritis may be seen with early LD, arthritis usually does not appear until 3 to 4 weeks after the tick bite. The knee is the most commonly involved joint (70% of patients with arthritis), followed by the ankle, shoulder, wrist, spine, temporomandibular joint, and hip. Smaller joints are infrequently involved. Arthritis may present without a history of erythema migrans in up to 50% of patients.

The diagnosis of LD is based on clinical findings. Epidemiologic factors, such as season, tick exposure and outdoor activity in an endemic area, are also important. Serologic testing may be of value in confirming suspect cases of LD but results should be interpreted cautiously.[249] The two most commonly available serologic assays are the indirect fluorescent antibody assays (IFA) and the enzyme immunoassay (EIA). The EIA is generally more sensitive and specific; however, both assays have a high rate of false-positive and false-negative results (especially when performed by nonreference laboratories). Western blot analysis is both sensitive and specific and may be useful in confirming serologic results.[63,250] Patients with characteristic erythema migrans should be treated regardless of serology. Similarly, treatment should not be withheld from patients, with clinical and epidemiologic features suggestive of disease, because of negative serology. Serology should not routinely be obtained in patients with vague, nonspecific complaints because of the high false-positive rate.[249]

Differential Considerations. The differential diagnosis of LD is extensive and includes causes of rapidly expanding rashes such as cellulitis, insect bite, erythema multiforme, and erythema marginatum. Aseptic meningitis of LD appears similar to viral meningitis and, in cases of persistent or chronic aseptic meningitis, should be differentiated from tuberculous meningitis. Cranial nerve palsies may present as a Bell palsy or intracranial lesion. The associated arthritis may have features similar to juvenile rheumatoid arthritis, acute rheumatic fever, Kawasaki disease, or serum sickness.

Management. Patients presenting with only a tick bite and no evidence of disease should not routinely be treated because of the low risk of infection even in endemic regions.[251]

Mild LD may be treated with oral antibiotics. Doxycycline (100 mg PO BID) is the drug of choice in the treatment of children older than 9 years of age. For children younger than 9 years of age, penicillin V 50 mg/kg/24 hr TID PO (up to 2 gm/24 hr) or amoxicillin 25 to 50 mg/kg/24 hr TID PO (up to 2 gm/24 hr) is preferred.

Penicillin-allergic patients may be treated with erythromycin 30 mg/kg/24 hr. Clarithromycin and azithromycin have in vitro activity against *B. burgdorferi*; the clinical efficacy of these newer macrolides remains to be shown and they will only be useful in older children.[63,252] Treatment should be for 10 to 30 days. Patients who are toxic or who have manifestations of late disease should be treated with ceftriaxone 75 to 100 mg/kg IV or IM as a single daily dose or with penicillin G 300,000 U/kg/24 hr q 4 hr IV. Parenteral therapy should be continued for 14 to 21 days. Studies suggest that ceftriaxone may be more effective in treating the persistent arthritis and neurologic manifestations of LD.[63,253]

Patients with LD having evidence of severe or advanced disease should be hospitalized for evaluation, observation, and parenteral therapy. Hospitalized patients require no isolation because person-to-person spread has not been documented.

Relapsing Fever

Relapsing fever, or borreliosis, is an uncommon recurrent febrile illness that occurs in the western states (particularly mountainous regions). Outbreaks often involve tourists visiting national parks or other wilderness areas and exposed tourists may return home before the onset of symptoms. The incubation period is from 4 to 18 days. Patients presenting in nonendemic areas with a recurrent febrile illness should be questioned regarding travel over the preceding 1 to 3 weeks. In the United States, the disease is caused by one of several different species of the spirochete *Borrelia recurrentis* and is transmitted by ticks of the genus *Orinthodoros*.

The predominant clinical features of relapsing fever are recurrent, 3- to 6-day periods of fever, headache, and myalgia with intervening afebrile periods of varying duration. Hepatosplenomegaly is common. Pleomorphic rash may occur in up to 30% of patients.[254,255]

Diagnosis requires identification of the spirochetes in dark field preparations or in Wright- or Giemsa-stained thick and thin smears of peripheral blood. Relapsing fever has been successfully treated using tetracycline, penicillin, erythromycin and chloramphenical. Treatment for children older than 9 years of age is tetracycline or erythromycin for 10 days. For children younger than 9 years of age penicillin or erythromycin is indicated. Treatment of relapsing fever may induce a Jarisch-Herxheimer reaction in a significant percentage of patients. To modify or prevent this reaction the initial antibiotic dose should be reduced and the patient observed for 8 hours following antibiotic administration. For a febrile child, oral penicillin V 7.5 mg/kg as a single oral dose (or penicillin G 10,000 U/kg IV given over 30 minutes) is given initially, followed by a conventional 10-day course.

Rocky Mountain Spotted Fever

Rocky Mountain spotted fever (RMSF) is a serious systemic illness and the most common rickettsial infection in the United States. Once thought to be confined to remote, discrete areas, RMSF is now reported from nearly every state in the United States, with a predominance in the East and Midwest. Despite the availability of antibiotic therapy the mortality rate is 3% to 5%. Early diagnosis is important in reducing both morbidity and mortality and requires familiarity with the wide range of clinical presentations.

The etiologic agent of RMSF is *Rickettsia rickettsii*, a small coccobacillus that grows and multiplies intracellularly but is also capable of a cell-free existence in blood or tissue. Ticks serve as the natural hosts for *R. rickettsii* and provide a persistent reservoir of infection by transovarially passing the organism on to succeeding generations. Common tick vectors include the dog tick, *Dermacentor variabilis*, in the East; the wood tick, *D. andersoni*, in the West; and the Lone Star tick, *Amblyomma americanum*, in Texas.[256]

The incidence of RMSF varies widely, with some areas being notorious "hotspots" of disease. Primarily a warm-weather disease, about 80% of cases of RMSF occur between May and August. Over half the cases of RMSF have been reported in individuals who are younger than 20 years old.[257]

Infection by *R. rickettsii* begins with the blood meal of the tick. Organisms from the tick's saliva enter the wound and are hematogenously disseminated. The rickettsia infect and replicate within the endothelial cells of the small blood vessels, resulting in cell injury, both directly and by the host's inflammatory response. The principal pathologic feature of RMSF is a widespread vasculitis involving the small blood vessels. The result is endothelial proliferation, a loss of vascular integrity, thrombus formation, and vascular occlusion of the small blood vessels.[258]

Diagnostic Findings. The incubation period for *Rickettsia* is from 1 to 14 days, clinical manifestations appearing in the first 7 days of the illness. The disease course varies widely from a mild self-limited course to prolonged severe life-threatening disease. The most common clinical features of RMSF are fever, rash, headache, and myalgia. A history of either tick exposure or bite may be obtained in up to 50% of children. A presumptive diagnosis of RMSF is readily made when patients present with all these findings. Many patients, however, lack one or more of the characteristic findings early in the course, making diagnosis difficult and often delaying diagnosis.[256,259]

Rash is the most characteristic feature of RMSF and is present in about 90% of patients. Only 50% of patients, however, will exhibit rash during the first few days of illness. The rash commonly appears first on the extremities and then extends to the trunk. The rash may appear macular, maculopapular, or as a fine erythema, and then progress to a petechial appearance. Involvement of the palms and soles is an important feature in suggesting the diagnosis. Fever is present in almost all cases; however, up to 30% of patients may have no fever early in the disease. Headache and myalgia range from mild to severe.[256,259]

Other presenting signs and symptoms include nausea, vomiting, diarrhea, abdominal pain, conjunctivitis, lymphadenopathy, edema, ataxia, meningoencephalitis, hepatosplenomegaly, seizures, dysrhythmias, and myocarditis.[259,260]

Complications of RMSF include hypovolemic shock, renal failure, seizures, skin necrosis, congestive heart failure, and complications caused by hemostasis.

Ancillary Data. Laboratory data may be useful in diagnosing suspicious or atypical cases. A normal or near-normal total WBC count with a significant left shift is a suggestive feature.[259] Thrombocytopenia of varying degrees is common.[259] Studies suggest as many as 30% of patients have platelet counts less than 150,000/mm[3].[261] Hyponatremia (< 130 mEq/L) has been reported in 20% to 50% of patients and may result from vascular leakage or inappropriate ADH secretion.[262] Elevation in the serum enzymes serum glutamate oxaloacetate transaminase (SGOT), creatinine phosphokinase (CPK), and lactate dehydrogenase (LDH) occurs in up to 40% of patients.[259] DIC, as demonstrated by prolonged prothrombin time (PT) and partial thromboplastin time (PTT) studies, may develop in severe cases.[259]

Abnormal chest x-ray findings occur in 10% to 40% of patients and include localized or diffuse infiltrates and cardiomegaly.[263] Myocarditis or dysrhythmia may be evident on ECG.[264]

Specific laboratory diagnosis of RMSF can be performed by immunostaining skin biopsies or serology. Immunostaining biopsies of skin lesions for organisms is a rapid means of diagnosis; however, it has a low sensitivity and is not widely available.[256]

Serologic tests include the Weil-Felix test, the indirect fluorescent antibody assay, and the indirect hemagglutination assay. The Weil-Felix test has low specificity and sensitivity but is widely available. The Weil-Felix test relies on antigenic similarities between *Rickettsia* and *Proteus* (strains OX19 and OX2) and is usually positive by day 10 to 14 of the illness. A fourfold rise in titer or an initial titer $> 1:160$ is suggestive of RMSF.

The indirect fluorescent antibody and indirect hemagglutination assays both have high sensitivity and specificity and detect antibody usually by day 7 to 10 of the illness. All serologic tests should be performed by using acute and convalescent paired sera.[108,256] Culturing of *Rickettsia* is not practical because of the risk to laboratory personnel.

Differential Considerations. The differential diagnosis of RMSF includes viral infections such as measles, EBV, coxsackievirus, and adenovirus. Bacterial agents presenting with similar complaints include *N. meningitidis*, *Borrelia*, and *Leptospira*.

Management. The drug of choice for children ≥ 9 years of age is tetracycline (30 to 40 mg/kg/24 hr q 6 hr PO *or* 20 mg/kg/24 hr q 8 to 12 hr IV infused over 2 hours). Children younger than 9 years of age should be treated with chloramphenicol (50 to 75 mg/kg/24 hr QID PO). Some clinicians, having compared the benefits and risks of tetracycline in children younger than 9 years of age, prefer to use tetracycline.[63] Therapy is continued until the patient is afebrile for at least 2 to 3 days. A usual course is 6 to 10 days.

Tularemia

Tularemia is an acute bacterial illness with six clinically recognized syndromes: ulceroglandular, glandular, pneumonic, oculoglandular, oropharyngeal, and typhoidal. The disease is often severe, with mortality rates as high as 5% to 7% in untreated cases.[265] Milder forms of the disease, however, are being recognized with increasing frequency.[266] Tularemia occurs in most regions of the United States and is capable of being transmitted by a variety of animal and arthropod vectors.

The infecting organism (*Francisella tularensis*) is an intracellular gram-negative coccobacillus. Transmission may occur following the bite of bloodsucking insects such as ticks, deerflies, or mosquitoes; or by exposure to contaminated animals such as rabbits, squirrels, and muskrats. The most common vectors in the United States are ticks and rabbits. Most cases occur in the warm weather months and during the rabbit hunting season. The West Central states (especially Missouri, Arkansas, and Oklahoma) report the highest incidence; however, scattered cases are reported throughout the country each year.[267]

Diagnostic Findings. The organism may be introduced in a wound during the blood meal of an arthropod, or by contact with mucous membrane surfaces such as the conjunctiva, oropharynx, or respiratory tract. Upon entry, organisms invade local and regional lymph nodes. Necrotic and granulomatous lesions develop. Superficial lymph nodes may suppurate, forming cutaneous ulcers. Hematogenous dissemination is a frequent occurrence and can result in lesions forming in the spleen, liver, and other organs, and is the major cause of septicemia.[268]

The incubation period for *F. tularensis* is 1 to 21 days, with most symptoms appearing by days 2 to 5. Symptoms common to all forms of tularemia include fever, influenza-like symptoms, and lymphadenopathy. Fever is present in 87% of patients; it may be high- or low-grade and lasts an average of 20 days (range of 3 to 60 days). The influenza-like symptoms include headache, chills, myalgia, and sometimes pharyngitis. Lymphadenopathy is the most frequent finding in tularemia, present in 96% of patients, and develops shortly after the onset of fever and constitutional symptoms. A history of contact with ticks or other known vectors is present in about 80% of cases.[265,266,268-270]

Ulceroglandular and glandular tularemia are the most common forms of the disease in children, representing 48% and 25% of cases respectively. Following cutaneous infection, regional lymph nodes become swollen and painful. In ulceroglandular tularemia a papule develops over the affected node, which ruptures to leave an ulcerated lesion that may persist for weeks. Glandular tularemia usually lacks ulcerations and is characterized by a milder clinical course.[265,266,268,270]

Pneumonic tularemia occurs in up to 14% of infected children and represents either primary infection or dissemination from another site of infection. Pneumonic tularemia is associated with a high mortality rate.[269]

Oculoglandular tularemia is an uncommon manifestation of the disease; it follows conjunctival inoculation with infected material. Conjunctivitis is followed by the appearance of multiple small papules and ulcerations over the palpebral conjunctiva. Regional lymph nodes of the head and neck are commonly involved.[268]

Rare manifestations of tularemia include pharyngeal tularemia and typhoidal tularemia, which typically presents as sepsis.[269]

Ancillary Data. Routine laboratory data contribute little to the diagnosis. Gram stain of material from draining lesions typically does not reveal organisms and culture of the material is not recommended because of the potential danger to laboratory personnel.

A suspicion of tularemia, based on history and clinical findings, requires specific laboratory confirmation. The serum agglutination assay is the most widely used and available test. A fourfold or greater rise in antibody titer or a single titer of greater than 1:160 is considered diagnostic. Antibody is typically absent in the initial stages of the disease and does not appear until the second week or later.[108,271]

Differential Considerations. The differential diagnosis of tularemia includes most causes of lymphadenitis such as bacterial, mycobacterial, viral, and cat-scratch disease. Pneumonic disease must be distinguished from the other causes of atypical pneumonia such as mycoplasma, legionnaires disease, and tuberculosis.

Management. The drug of choice for *F. tularensis* is gentamicin (6 mg/kg/24 hr q 8 hr IM, IV).[63,272] Tetracycline (25 to 50 mg/kg/24 hr q 6 hr PO) and chloramphenicol (50 to 75 mg/kg/24 hr q 6 hr PO) have been used successfully but are associated with a higher incidence of relapse. Tetracycline should not be administered to children younger than 9 years of age.[108] Suppurative lymph nodes may need to be incised and drained. Caution should be exercised with the highly infectious drainage.

Patients who appear toxic or have evidence of pulmonary involvement should be hospitalized. Strict drainage precautions should be used to prevent nosocomial infections from occurring.

TUBERCULOSIS

Despite major therapeutic advances, tuberculosis remains a major public health concern throughout the world, including the United States. The majority of children with tuberculosis are asymptomatic and have self-limited infections; however, early identification and treatment of tuberculosis is vital in preventing serious sequelae and reducing the reservoir of infection.[273]

In 1993 over 25,000 cases of tuberculosis were reported in the United States; approximately 2,300 of these cases involved children and adolescents.[274] Children of minority groups are especially at risk, with nearly 70% of cases occurring in blacks, Hispanics, Asian/Pacific Islanders, and Native Americans. Living in crowded or urban settings presents an additional risk factor. Tuberculosis is found throughout the United States; half of all cases are reported from California, New York, Florida, Texas, and Illinois.[274]

The etiologic agent, *M. tuberculosis,* is primarily spread by inhalation of small droplets produced by adults with reactivated pulmonary disease. Children themselves rarely transmit the disease because of insufficient inoculum in their respiratory tract.[275] Upon entering the alveolus the organism establishes a foci of infection with spread to regional lymph nodes. Lymphohematogenous spread occurs in nearly all cases of primary tuberculous infection.[276]

Diagnostic Findings

The period from exposure until a positive tuberculin skin test is usually 2 to 10 weeks, although a delay as long as 3 months may be seen. Most tuberculous infections resolve without clinical evidence of disease. Manifestations of tuberculous disease often appear within the first 6 months, although some infections may remain latent for 1 or more years. Clinical presentations of tuberculosis are classified as either pulmonary or extrapulmonary. Pulmonary disease is the most common form of tuberculous disease and comprises 80% of cases. Extrapulmonary disease manifestations include miliary tuberculosis, tuberculous meningitis, superficial tuberculous lymphadentitis, renal tuberculosis, and bone/joint infections.[276]

The great majority of children infected with *Mycobacterium* have asymptomatic infections and are identified by routine tuberculin skin testing or following an index case investigation. The chest x-ray of asymptomatic children is generally normal; however, all individuals with a positive tuberculin skin test should have a chest x-ray performed to identify early pulmonary tuberculous disease.

Most patients with pulmonary tuberculosis have few clinical findings. Low-grade fever may be present and cough is usually mild or absent. The most frequent manifestation of pulmonary tuberculosis is hilar and mediastinal adenopathy. Pulmonary lesions are characteristically subpleural and are located slightly more often in the right upper lobe. Patients with pleural involvement present more acutely with fever, chest pain, shortness of breath, and evidence of pleural effusion. Bronchial compression from enlarging lymph nodes may result in segmental atelectasis. This is particularly common in infants.[277] Patients with bronchial compression often present with a more severe cough or pneumonia. All patients with pleural effusion or pneumonia unresponsive to antibiotics should be evaluated for tuberculosis.

Complications. The most serious extrapulmonary manifestations of tuberculous disease are miliary tuberculosis and tuberculous meningitis. Children with tuberculous meningitis usually present with a gradual onset of symptoms over 2 to 3 weeks. Early nonspecific symptoms, such as irritability, are followed by findings of meningeal irritation and eventually by evidence of increased intracranial pressure. CSF findings include an increased opening pressure, increased protein, low glucose, and a pleocytosis that rarely exceeds 1,200 WBC/mm^3 and is predominantly lymphocytic. Acid-fast staining of the CSF for organisms is frequently positive. Most children with tuberculous meningitis have evidence of pulmonary disease on chest x-ray.[278]

Miliary tuberculosis results from the evacuation of a caseous node into the blood stream with seeding of multiple organs. Clinical findings include persistent fever, hepatosplenomegaly, and abnormal auscultatory findings on lung examination. The chest radiograph reveals characteristic diffuse mottling, usually after several weeks.[275]

Ancillary Data. The tuberculin skin test is the major diagnostic test for tuberculous infection. A positive skin test is defined as (1) >15 mm of induration in healthy individuals 4 years of age or older with no risk factors; (2) >10 mm in individuals younger than 4 years of age or with risk factors; and (3) >5 mm in patients with HIV infection, documented exposure, or with radiographic evidence of disease (see box on p. 960).

All patients suspected of having tuberculosis should have tuberculin skin testing and a chest x-ray film. The tuberculin skin testing should be performed using purified protein derivative (PPD) by the method of Mantoux in

---

Definition of a Positive Mantoux Skin Test (5TU-PPD) in Children*

Reaction ≥5 mm

Children in close contact with known or suspected infectious cases of tuberculosis:
- Households with active or previously active cases if:
  - Treatment not verified as adequate before exposure
  - Treatment initiated after period of child's contact
  - Reactivation suspected

Children suspected to have tuberculosis:
- Chest roentgenogram consistent with active or previously active tuberculosis
- Clinical evidence of tuberculosis

Children with immunosuppressive conditions† or HIV infection

Reaction ≥10 mm

Children at increased risk of dissemination from:
- Young age (younger than 4 years of age)
- Other medical risk factors, including Hodgkin disease, lymphoma, diabetes mellitus, chronic renal failure, and malnutrition

Children with increased environmental exposure:
- Born, or whose parents were born, in regions of the world where tuberculosis is highly prevalent
- Frequently exposed to adults who are HIV infected, homeless, users of intravenous and other street drugs, poor and medically indigent city dwellers, residents of nursing homes, incarcerated or institutionalized persons, and migrant farm workers

Reaction ≥15 mm

Children ≥4 years of age without any risk factors

From Committee on Infectious Diseases: *Pediatr* 93:131-134, 1994.
*These recommendations should apply regardless of whether BCG has been previously administered.
†Including immunosuppressive doses of corticosteroids.

---

which five tuberculin units (0.1 ml) of PPD are injected intracutaneously onto the volar aspect of the forearm, often with a skin test control such as candida. Multiple puncture tests are unpredictable and should not be used to diagnose patients with suspected tuberculosis. The Mantoux test is read at 48 and 72 hours for size of induration. All patients with a positive multiple puncture skin test should be retested using the Mantoux method. False-positive PPD skin tests may occur and are commonly due to cross reactivity with nontuberculous mycobacteria. Skin-test reactivity in patients previously immunized with BCG is variable. Reactions due to BCG are usually less than 10 mm of induration and reactivity wanes several years after vaccination. A skin test with greater than 10-mm induration should be considered suspicious in a BCG recipient.[63,279,280]

Cultures for *M. tuberculosis* should be obtained from all infected children or their source case due to the increasing incidence of drug resistance. Obtaining cultures from small children in cases of pulmonary tuberculosis is difficult. Gastric washings are positive in only 40% of cases.[279] Sputum cultures should be obtained from older children and adolescents. Identification of *Mycobacterium* by culture may require up to 6 to 10 weeks.

Management

Patients with a positive skin test who are asymptomatic should be started on preventive therapy with isoniazid (INH) 10 mg/kg/24 hr (300 mg maximum) as a daily dose for 9 months. In select cases twice-a-week therapy may be administered by the health department.[63]

Treatment for uncomplicated pulmonary tuberculosis is a 6-month course consisting of single daily doses of INH (10 mg/kg/24 hr [300 mg maximum]), rifampin (10 to 15 mg/kg/24 hr [600 mg maximum]), and pyrazinamide (20 to 30 mg/kg/24 hr [2 gm maximum]) for the first 2 months, followed by twice-weekly doses of INH (20 to 40 mg/kg/dose [900 mg maximum]) and rifampin (10 to 20 mg/kg/dose [600 mg maximum]) for the remaining 4 months. Tuberculous meningitis, miliary disease, or bone-joint infections should be treated for 12 months with INH, rifampin, pyrazinamide, and streptomycin for the first 2 months, followed by INH and rifampin for the remaining 10 months.[63]

The treatment of drug-resistant strains of *M. tuberculosis* requires familiarity with local drug resistance patterns. In addition, foreign-born persons, the homeless, and patients previously treated for tuberculosis are at increased risk for harboring drug-resistant strains. Outbreaks of multiply resistant strains of *M. tuberculosis* have been reported, especially in the homeless and HIV-infected patients.[281] Consultation with a specialist in tuberculosis is important in managing patients with drug-resistant disease.[63,279]

Asymptomatic individuals or patients with mild pulmonary disease may be managed as outpatients. In many areas directly observed therapy is utilized to ensure compliance and reduce the incidence of drug resistance.[282] Because of the increased incidence of tuberculosis in HIV-infected individuals, patients with tuberculosis should be offered HIV testing.

EXANTHEMS

Around the turn of the century, the common childhood diseases associated with exanthems were ordered:

1. Measles, rubeola
2. Scarlet fever
3. German measles (rubella)
4. Filatov-Dukes disease or fourth disease
5. Erythema infectiosum or fifth disease
6. Roseola

Since that time, several changes have occurred in naming these diseases. The term *fourth disease* was dropped because the disease was thought not to be a distinct clinical entity but possibly a staphylococcal or streptococcal infection. The remainder of the numeric categorization has fallen into disuse with the exception of the term *fifth disease*, which is still used often. There is some overlap in the clinical presentation, but most of these disorders can be clinically diagnosed by history and physical examination, although this takes more than one visit (Table 55-10). However, the emergency physician does not always have the luxury of several examinations to determine the precise diagnosis. Each of these disorders will be discussed in this chapter (see also Chapter 48) with emphasis on characteristic physical and historical information, because, with rare exceptions, laboratory evaluation is of little help in the emergency department. The relative frequency and expression of the disease has been greatly effected by vaccines. Varicella is also discussed in Chapter 48.

Erythema Infectiosum or Fifth Disease

Erythema infectiosum is an acute viral illness caused by a parvovirus B-19.[283] The disease predominantly affects school-aged children and frequently occurs in epidemic fashion,[284-286] often in winter and spring months. The virus is spread by respiratory droplets and has an incubation period of about a week. This is followed by a viremia that may last several days, during which time the patient is contagious. During this time the child may have nonspecific signs of mild fever, pruritus, malaise, headache, and occasional arthralgias.[287] Older patients often have more severe symptoms.

Diagnostic Findings. The hallmark of the disease is an erythematous, erysipeloid rash on the cheeks, which gives this disease its common name of *slapped-cheek disease.* The patient is not contagious when the rash presents.[288] The rash then spreads to the upper arms and legs and then to the trunk with a maculopapular erythematous form; it gradually fades into a reticular or "lace-like" pattern.[289] The rash may fade only to reappear with skin irritation from warm baths, sunlight, or trauma. There are no characteristic laboratory findings.

Management. Treatment is symptomatic. There is a known risk of spontaneous abortion in mothers with parvovirus infection, but because the child is not contagious at the time of appearance of the rash, prevention of transmission to susceptible persons is difficult. Women exposed during the first 20 weeks of gestation may be referred to their physicians. Further recommendations for pregnancy have been published by the American Academy of Pediatrics.[288] Patients with chronic hemolytic anemias are prone to aplastic crises with this infection and may continue to shed the virus for a longer period.[288]

Hand-Foot-and-Mouth Disease

Although not listed as one of the five exanthems of childhood, hand-foot-and-mouth disease is a common infection seen in children. It is caused by the coxsackievirus. The children are usually not ill appearing and have nonspecific symptoms with low-grade fever and malaise. The chief complaint may be the rash, which causes characteristic lesions in the mouth, hands, and feet, although it may appear on other areas of the body.

The lesions begin as bright red, blanching macules, which develop into flattened vesicles, often showing the underlying skin creases. This gives them the characteristic "flame-shaped" appearance. The lesions in the mouth may be more vesicular.

The children usually tolerate this infection well; however, the mouth lesions may be painful.

Management is with antipyretics and analgesics. The infection is contagious and may spread to other family members. Although usually a disease of children, it may spread to adults as well.

Roseola (Exanthem Subitum)

Roseola is one of the more common, least serious, but often most problematic of diseases for the emergency physician. Roseola infantum and exanthem subitum refer to an illness that was recently discovered to be caused by human herpes virus 6 (HHV-6).[290-292] The disease occurs in young children, with 95% of cases occurring in children between 6 months and 3 years of age.[293] It is a common disorder and will develop in up to 30% of children by the age of 2 years.

It is mildly contagious and presents with a sudden onset of high fever, which lasts around 3 days. With defervescence there is an appearance of a macular (occasionally papular) rose-pink rash that begins on the trunk and spreads to the proximal extremities. Except for the fever, the child has no physical findings and appears well. With the onset of the fever, there may be a febrile seizure in up to 6% of cases.[294] A careful history, physical examination, appropriate evaluation, and close follow-up are essential.

Although the diagnosis is rarely made by the emergency physician unless the child is brought in for the rash, this can be mentioned as a possible cause of the child's fever and the parents can be prepared for its appearance. If the child presents with the typical rash, is afebrile, and has had several days of fever, the diagnosis can be made with some confidence. No other laboratory tests are indicated. Therapy should focus on support and symptomatic improvement. Rarely there are complications, such as meningoencephalitis, requiring specific evaluation and treatment.[295] Therapy should generally focus on support and symptomatic improvement.

Rubella

Rubella, also called "three-day measles" or German measles, is caused by a togavirus. Before the introduction of the rubella vaccine this illness was commonly seen, but today is rarely seen except in older adolescents and young adults.[280] Spread is by respiratory droplets with a 2- to 3-week incubation period. In older patients there is a prodrome marked by malaise and enlarged tender postauricular nodes. Within 24 hours of the fever the rash begins on the scalp and face and rapidly moves down the body. It may be accompanied by myalgias, arthralgias, and headaches, although younger children may look clinically well.

The rash appears as multiple, small, discrete macules and papules that coalesce and fade rapidly.[289] In up to 20% of patients, Forchheimer sign (petechiae on the soft palate) may be seen early in the disease.

No diagnostic studies are indicated. This is a generally benign disease with the greatest risk to the fetus, especially during the first trimester.

Rubeola

Rubeola or measles is the most common cause of death among children worldwide that is preventable by use of a vaccine.[296] Although greatly reduced in frequency in coun-

TABLE 55-10. Common Exanthems

	Measles (rubeola)	Rubella (German, 3-day measles)
Incubation	10-14 days	14-21 days
Prodrome	3 days high fever, cough, conjunctivitis, and coryza; child appears toxic, lethargic	May be none; lymphadenopathy (especially postauricular, suboccipital), malaise, variable low-grade fever
Exanthem	Reddish-brown; begins on face and progresses downward; generalized by third day; confluent on face, neck, upper trunk; lasts 7-10 days; desquamates; atypical measles: maculopapular, purpuric, petechial, or vesicular rash	Pink; begins on face and progresses rapidly downward; generalized by second day; discrete; lasts 2-3 days, fades in order of appearance
Enanthem	Koplik spots (2 days before rash, on buccal mucosa opposite molars)	None
Complication	Pneumonia Encephalitis Otitis media Thrombocytopenia Hemorrhagic measles Pneumothorax Hepatitis Exacerbation of TB	Arthritis (common in women) beginning after 2-3 days' illness; knee, wrist, finger Congenital rubella syndrome Encephalitis Thrombocytopenia
Management	Supportive; may require hospitalization; active immunization of contacts; immune serum globulin (0.05 ml/kg) for children <1 yr; reportable	Supportive; isolate from pregnant women; active immunization of contacts; reportable
Comments	Rare with immunization	Rare with immunization; serologic diagnosis

tries with high immunization rates, rubeola remains a serious illness. In the United States, although outbreaks among college students are reported, it still most commonly occurs in preschool-aged children.[287] Populations at risk remain children younger than 15 months of age, which is the recommended age for immunization; unimmunized patients; and those who received killed-virus vaccine or vaccines that have been improperly handled. The latter are susceptible to a variation of the disease called *atypical measles*. Rubeola is caused by a paromyxovirus and is spread by respiratory droplets.

There is a 10- to 14-day incubation period, followed by a prodrome of fever, malaise, cough, coryza, and conjunctivitis.

Diagnostic Findings. The earliest skin findings are exanthems on the buccal mucosa called Koplik spots. These look like white grains of sand on an erythematous base. This is the only pathognomonic finding of rubeola. The rash, which begins 3 to 4 days into the illness, begins on the scalp, face, and neck and often follows the hairline. The rash spreads downward to affect most of the body, the older areas coalescing into raised macular areas that are deep red in color. The rash leaves in the same direction in which it came, often leaving a brownish discoloration to the skin.[271]

Rubeola has a number of complications, the most frequent being secondary bacterial infections, especially pneumonia and otitis media. Rubeola can cause a primary viral pneumonia, encephalitis, and postinfectious encephalomyelitis. A rare form of rubeola, hemorrhagic measles, is complicated by disseminated intravascular coagulation.

Atypical measles can occur in patients who received the killed vaccine, which was used from 1963 to 1967; thus it should no longer appear in pediatric patients. This disease has a variable presentation of fever, headache, myalgia, and a rash that begins on the extremities. Most patients have infiltrates on x-ray radiographs. This disease was most often confused with Rocky Mountain spotted fever.

There is no specific laboratory test useful to the emergency physician. A CBC will usually show a leukopenia. Serologic testing can be obtained on those patients in whom a diagnosis is required.

Management. Rubeola is not a benign disease because the children are often ill during its course and it has significant complications. Treatment is supportive but bacterial superinfection must be carefully sought and treated; follow-up is essential.

Roseola (exanthema subitum)	Fifth disease (erythema infectiosum)	Enterovirus	Scarlet fever
10-14 days	7-14 days	Variable (short)	2-4 days
3-4 days high fever in otherwise well child, preceding rash	None	Variable; fever, malaise, vomiting, sore throat, rhinorrhea	1-2 days fever, vomiting, sore throat; often toxic
Appears after defervescence; rose, discrete; initially on chest, spreads to involve face and extremities; fades quickly	Erupts in 3 stages: (1) red-flushed cheeks with circumoral pallor (slapped cheek), (2) maculopapular eruption on extremities (lacelike), (3) may recur secondary to heat, sunlight, trauma	Maculopapular, discrete, nonpruritic, generalized; rubella-like; hand, foot, and mouth distribution	Erythematous, punctate, sandpaper texture; appears first in flexor areas, then generalized; most intense on neck, axilla, inguinal, popliteal skin fold; circumoral pallor; lasts 7 days, then desquamates
None	Variable	Variable	Red pharynx, tonsils; palatal petechiae; strawberry tongue
Febrile seizure	Transient arthritis	Aseptic meningitis Myocarditis Hepatitis	Rheumatic fever Acute glomerulonephritis
Supportive; good fever control	Rarely need care	Supportive	Penicillin
Usually 1-4 yr olds	May be caused by human parvovirus	Concurrent family illness, gastroenteritis, herpangina	Group A streptococci

From Barkin RM and Rosen P: *Emergency pediatrics*, ed 4, St Louis, 1994, Mosby.
TB, Tuberculosis.

Scarlet Fever

Scarlet fever, also called *scarlatina*, is currently a relatively benign disease caused by toxin-producing strains of group A beta-hemolytic streptococci. It occurs throughout the year but more often in winter and early spring. The peak incidence is in 4- to 8-year-olds.

The primary infection is usually in the tonsils and begins with sore throat, fever, headache, and several episodes of vomiting. The characteristic rash spreads quickly from the head and chest to the remainder of the body. There is a generalized erythema with multiple small papules that give the skin a rough or sandpaper-like texture. The area around the mouth is often spared (circumoral pallor), the skin creases are often reddened (Pastia lines), and the tongue may be coated white with red or bright-red splotches (strawberry tongue).

In addition to the typical rash, examination will show a pustular tonsillitis with anterior cervical lymph node enlargement. Desquamation is typical after one week. Diagnosis can be made by rapid latex agglutination or standard throat culture tests as discussed in Chapter 49.

Treatment is similar to that of streptococcal pharyngitis. Penicillin VK 25 to 50 mg (40,000 to 80,000 U)/kg/24 hr QID PO or erythromycin 30 to 50 mg/kg/24 hr TID PO may be used.

Infections located elsewhere in the body, such as wounds secondarily infected by beta-hemolytic streptococcus, can cause a similar clinical picture with the absence of tonsillitis and the involvement of regional lymph nodes. This is often called *surgical scarlet fever*. One must look carefully for the site of infection as it may be subtle.

Scarlet fever today is considered a relatively benign disease, although this has not always been the case. A recurrence of a severe streptococcal infection is reminiscent of the severity of scarlet fever at the turn of the century (see section on Toxic Shock Syndrome).

References

1. Baker D, Fosarelli P, Carpenter R: Childhood fever: correlation of diagnosis with temperature response to acetaminophen, *Pediatrics* 80:315-318, 1987.
2. McCarthy P: Acute infectious illness in children, *Compr Ther* 14:51-57, 1988.
3. Gehlback S: Fever in children younger than three months of age, *J Fam Pract* 27:305-312, 1988.
4. Kruse J: Fever in children, *Am Fam Physician* 37:127-135, 1988.

5. Bonadio W: Incidence of serious infection in afebrile neonates with a history of fever, *Pediatr Infect Dis J* 6:911-914, 1987.

6. Ogren JM: The inaccuracy of axillary temperatures measured with an electronic thermometer, *Am J Dis Child* 144:109-111, 1990.

7. Muma BK, Treloar DJ, Wurmlinger K et al: Comparison of rectal, axillary and tympanic membrane temperatures in infants and young children, *Ann Emerg Med* 20:41-44, 1991.

8. Stewart JV and Webster D: Reevaluation of tympanic thermometer in the emergency department, *Ann Emerg Med* 21:158-161, 1992.

9. Baraff LJ, Bass JW, Fleisher GR et al: Practice guidelines for the management of infants and children 0 to 36 months of age with fever without source, *Ann Emerg Med* 22:1198-1210, 1993.

10. Jaskiewicz JA, McCarthy CA, Richardson AC et al: Febrile infants at low risk for serious bacterial infection. An appraisal of the Rochester criteria and implications for management, *Pediatrics* 94:390-396, 1994.

11. Baker MD, Bell LM, Avner JR: Outpatient management without antibiotics of fever in selected infants *N Engl J Med* 329:1437-1441, 1993.

12. Lieu TA, Baskin MN, Schwartz JS, et al: *Pediatrics* 89:1135-1144, 1992.

13. Baraff LJ, Oslund SA, Schriger DL, et al: Probability of bacterial infections in febrile infants less than three months of age: a meta analysis, *Pediatr Infect Dis J* 11:257-265, 1992.

14. McCarthy P, Sharpe M, Spisel S et al: Observation scales to identify serious illness in febrile children, *Pediatrics* 70:802-809, 1982.

15. Baker D, Avner J, Bell J: Failure of infant observation scales in detecting serious illness in febrile four to eight-week-old infants, *Pediatrics* 85:1040-1043, 1990.

16. McCarthy PL, Sznajerman SD, Lustman-Findling K et al: *J Pediatr* 116:200-206, 1990.

17. Graves G and Rhoedes P: Tachycardia as a sign of early onset neonatal sepsis, *Pediatr Infect Dis J* 3:404-406, 1984.

18. Walson PD, Galletta G, Chomilo F et al: Comparison of multidose ibuprofen and acetaminophen therapy in febrile children, *Am J Dis Child* 146:626-632, 1992.

19. Baker RC, Tiller T, Bausher JC et al: Severity of disease correlated with fever reduction in febrile infants, *Pediatrics* 83:1016-1019, 1989.

20. Press S and Fawcett NP: Association of temperature greater than 41.1 degrees C (106 degrees F) with serious illness, *Clin Pediatr* 24:21-25, 1985.

21. McCarthy PL and Dolman TO: Hyperpyrexia in children, *Am J Dis Child* 130:849-851, 1976.

22. Vichinsky E, Lubin BH: Suggested guidelines for the treatment of children with sickle cell anemia, *Hematol Oncol Clin North Am* a:483-501, 1987.

23. Williams JA, Flynn PM, Harris S et al: A randomized study of outpatient treatment with ceftriaxone for selected febrile children with sickle cell disease, *N Engl J Med* 329:472-476, 1993.

24. Langley J, Gold R: Sepsis in febrile neutropenic children with cancer, *Pediatr Infect Dis* 7:34-37, 1988.

25. Pizzo PA, Rubin M, Freifeld A et al: The child with cancer and infection. I. Empiric therapy for fever and neutropenia and preventive strategies, *J Pediatr* 119:679-694, 1991.

26. Baker RC, Sequin JH, Leslie N et al: Fever and petechiae in children, *Pediatrics* 84:1051-1055, 1989.

27. Pizzo PA, Lovejoy FH, Smith DH: Prolonged fever in children: review of 100 cases, *Pediatrics* 55:468-473, 1975.

28. Kramer M, Lane D, Mills E: Should blood cultures be obtained in the evaluation of young febrile children without evident focus of bacterial infections? A decision analysis of diagnostic management strategies, *Pediatrics* 84:18-27, 1989.

29. Crain E and Gershel J: Urinary tract infections in febrile infants younger than 8 weeks of age, *Pediatrics* 86:363-367, 1990.

30. Goldsmith B and Campo J: Comparison of urine dipstick, microscopy and culture for the detection of bacteriuria in children, *Clin Pediatr* 29:214-218, 1990.

31. Pollack CV, Pollack ES, Andrew ME: Suprapubic bladder aspiration versus urethral catheterization in ill infants: success, efficiency, and complication rates, *Ann Emerg Med* 23:225-230, 1994.

32. Joffe A, McCormick M, De Angelis C: Which children with febrile seizures need lumbar puncture, *Am J Dis Child* 60:1045-1049, 1983.

33. Zukin DD, Hoffman JR, Cleveland RH et al: Correlation of pulmonary signs and symptoms with chest, *Ann Emerg Med* 15:792, 1986.

34. Crain EF, Bulas D, Bijur PE et al: Is a chest radiograph necessary in the evaluation of every febrile infant less than 8 weeks of age? *Pediatrics* 88:821-824, 1991.

35. Patterson R, Bissett G, Kirks D et al: Chest radiographs in the evaluation of the febrile infant, *Am J Radiol* 155:833-835, 1990.

36. Bonadio WA, Webster H, Wolfe A et al: Correlating infectious outcome with clinical parameters of 1130 consecutive febrile infants aged zero to eight weeks, *Pediatr Emerg Care* 9:84-86, 1993.

37. Baskin MN, O'Rourke EJ, Fleisher GR: Outpatient treatment of febrile infants 28 to 89 days of age with intramuscular administration of ceftriaxone, *J Pediatr* 120:22-27, 1992.

38. Klassen TP and Rowe PC: Selecting diagnostic tests to identify febrile infant less than 3 months of age as being at low risk for serious bacterial infection: a scientific overview, *J Pediatr* 121:671, 1992.

39. Fleisher GR, Rosenberg N, Vinci R et al: Intramuscular versus oral antibiotic therapy for the prevention of meningitis and other bacterial sequelae in young febrile children at risk for occult bacteremia.

Acquired Immunodeficiency Syndrome

40. Falloon J, Eddy J, Wiener L et al: Human immunodeficiency virus infection in children, *J Pediatr* 114(1):1-30, 1989.

41. The HIV/AIDS epidemic: the first 10 years, *MMWR* 40(22):357-369, 1991.

42. Rogers M, Caldwell M, Gwinn M et al: Epidemiology of pediatric human immunodeficiency virus infection in the United States, *Acta Paediatr Suppl* 400:5-7, 1994.

43. Connor E, Sperling R, Gelber R et al: Reduction of maternal-infant transmission of human immunodeficiency virus type 1 with zidovudine treatment, *N Engl J Med* 331:1173-1180, 1994.

44. Update: AIDS among women—United States, 1994, *MMWR* 44(5):81-84, 1995.

45. Epstein F: The immunopathogenesis of human immunodeficiency virus infection, *N Engl J Med* 328:327-335.

46. Barrett D: The clinician's guide to pediatric AIDS, *Contemp Pediatr* 5:24-47, 1988.

47. Pahwa S, Kaplan M, Fikrig S et al: Spectrum of human T-cell lymphotropic virus type III infection in children, *JAMA* 225(17):2299-2305, 1986.

48. Rogers M, Thomas P, Starcher E et al: Acquired immunodeficiency syndrome in children: report of the Centers for Disease Control national surveillance, 1982 to 1985, *Pediatrics* 79(6):1008-1014, 1985.

49. Crain E and Bernstein L: Pediatric HIV infection for the emergency physician: epidemiology and overview, *Pediatr Emerg Care* 6(3):214-218, 1990.

50. 1995 Revised guidelines for prophylaxis against *Pneumocystis carinii* pneumonia for children infected with or perinatally exposed to human immunodeficiency virus, *MMWR* 44(RR-4), 1995.

51. Pizzo P, Wilfert C: *Pediatric aids*, ed 2, Baltimore, 1994, Williams and Wilkins, p 14.

52. Krasinski K, Borkowsky W, Bonk S et al: Bacterial infections in human immunodeficiency virus-infected children, *Pediatr Infect Dis J* 7:323-328, 1988.

53. Bernstein L, Krieger BZ, Novick B et al: Bacterial infection in the acquired immunodeficiency syndrome of children, *Pediatr Infect Dis J* 4(5):472-475, 1985.

54. Nicholas SW: The opportunistic and bacterial infections associated with pediatric human immunodeficiency virus disease, *Acta Paediatr Suppl* 400:46-50, 1994.

55. Belman A, Diamond G, Dickson D et al: Pediatric acquired immunodeficiency syndrome, *Am J Dis Child* 142:29-35, 1988.

56. Butler C, Hittleman J, Hauger S: Approach to neurodevelopmental and neurologic complications in pediatric HIV infection, *J Pediatr* 119(1):S41-S46, 1991.

57. Pizzo P, Wilfert C: *Pediatric aids*, ed 2, Baltimore, 1994, Williams and Wilkins, p 477.

58. Burroughs M, Edelson P: Medical care of the HIV-infected child, *Pediatr Clin North Am* 38(1):45-68, 1991.

59. Hilgartner M: Hematologic manifestations in HIV-infected children, *J Pediatr* 119(1):S47-S49, 1991.

60. Tarshish P: Approach to the diagnosis and management of HIV-associated nephropathy, *J Pediatr* 119(1):550-552, 1991.

61. Kline M, Lewis D, Hollinger F et al: A comparative study of human immunodeficiency virus culture, polymerase chain reaction and anti-

human immunodeficiency virus immunoglobulin A antibody detection in the diagnosis during early infancy of vertically acquired human immunodeficiency virus infection, *Pediatr Infect Dis J* 13:90-94, 1994.

62. Miles S, Balden E, Magpantay L et al: Rapid serologic testing with immune-complex-dissociated HIV p24 antigen for early detection of HIV infection in neonates, *N Engl J Med* 328:297-302, 1993.

63. Peter G, Halsey N, Marcuse E et al: Report of the committee on infectious diseases, ed 23, Elk Grove Village, Ill, 1994, American Academy of Pediatrics.

64. Krasinski K: Antiretroviral therapy for children, *Acta Paediatr Suppl* 400:63-69, 1994.

65. Nicholas S: Management of the HIV-positive child with fever, *J Pediatr* 119(1):S21-S24, 1991.

66. Dorfman D, Crain E, Bernstein L: Care of the febrile child with HIV infection in the emergency department, *Pediatr Emerg Care* 6(4):305-310, 1990.

67. Pinkert H, Harper M, Cooper T et al: HIV-infected children in the pediatric emergency department, *Pediatr Emerg Care* 9(5):265-269, 1993.

68. Rubinstein A, Morecki R, Silverman B et al: Pulmonary disease in children with acquired immune deficiency syndrome and AIDS-related complex, *J Pediatr* 108:498-503, 1986.

69. Gershon R, Karkashian C, Felknor S: Universal precautions: An update. *Heart Lung* 23:352-358, 1994.

70. Guidelines for prevention of transmission of human immunodeficiency virus and hepatitis B virus to healthcare and public safety workers, US Dept of Health and Human Services, 1989.

71. Public Health Service statement on management of occupational exposure to human immunodeficiency virus, including considerations regarding zidovudine postexposure use, *MMWR* 39(RR-1):1-14, 1990.

Botulism

72. Dowell VR: Botulism and tetanus: selected epidemiologic and microbiologic aspects, *Rev Infect Dis* 6(1):S202-S207, 1984.

73. Burningham M, Walter F, Mechem C et al: Wound botulism, *Ann Emerg Med* 24:1184-1187, 1994.

74. Feigin R and Cherry J: *Textbook of pediatric infectious diseases*, ed 2, New York, 1987, WB Saunders.

75. Hughes J, Blumenthal J, Merson M et al: Clinical features of types A and B food-borne botulism, *Ann Emerg Med* 95:442-445, 1981.

76. Arnon S: Infant botulism: anticipating the second decade, *J Infect Dis* 154(2):201-205, 1986.

77. Long S, Gajewski J, Brown L et al: Clinical, laboratory, and environmental features of infant botulism in southeastern Pennsylvania, *Pediatrics* 75(5):935-941, 1985.

78. Johnson R, Clay S, Arnon S: Diagnosis and management of infant botulism, *Am J Dis Child* 133:586-593, 1979.

79. Schriener M, Field E, Ruddy R: Infant botulism: a review of 12 years' experience at the Children's Hospital of Philadelphia, *Pediatrics* 87(2):159-165, 1991.

80. Graf W, Hays R, Astley S et al: Electrodiagnosis reliability in the diagnosis of infant botulism, *J Pediatr* 120:747-749, 1992.

Diphtheria

81. Chen R, Broome C, Weinstein R et al: Diphtheria in the United States, 1971-1981, *Am J Public Health* 75(12):1393-1397, 1985.

82. Karzon D and Edwards K: Diphtheria outbreaks in immunized populations, *N Engl J Med* 318(1):41-43, 1988.

83. English P: Diphtheria and theories of infectious disease: centennial appreciation of the critical role of diphtheria in the history of medicine, *Pediatrics* 76(1):1-9, 1985.

84. Kwantes W: Diphtheria in Europe, *J Hyg Camb* 93:433-437, 1984.

85. Singh M, Azizullah S, Bakhtiar A et al: Diphtheria in Afghanistan—a review of 155 cases, *J Trop Med Hyg* 88:373-376, 1985.

86. Peter G, Lepow M, McCracken G et al: *Diphtheria—report of the committee on infectious disease*, ed 22, Elk Grove Village, Ill, 1991, American Academy of Pediatrics.

87. Bowler IC, Mandal BK, Schlecht B et al: Diphtheria—the continuing hazard, *Arch Dis Child* 63:194-210, 1988.

88. Dixon J: Diphtheria in North America, *J Nyg Camb* 93:419-432, 1984.

89. Ringham SRN: An outbreak of diphtheria, *Nursing Times*, Aug 1983.

Emporiatrics

90. Shepherd S and Talbot-Stern J: Evaluation of the traveler: an introduction to emporiatrics for the emergency physician, *Emerg Med Clin North Am* 9(2):273-303, 1991.

91. Cunha B: Case studies in infectious disease. 1. Fever in returning travelers, *Emerg Med* 15:27-31, 1988.

92. Maldonaldo Y, Nahlen L, Roberto R et al: Transmission of *Plasmodium vivax* malaria in San Diego county, California, 1986, *Am J Trop Med Hyg* 42(1):3-9, 1990.

93. McCaslin R, Pikis A, Rodriguez W: Pediatric *Plasmodium falciparum* malaria: a ten-year experience from Washington, DC, *Pediatr Infect Dis J* 13(8):709-715, August 1994.

94. Jotte RS, and Scott J, Malaria: Review of features pertinent to the emergency physician, *J Emerg Med* 11:729-736, 1993.

95. Wright PW, Avery WG, Aprill WD, and McLarty JW: Initial clinical assessment of the comatose patient: cerebral malaria vs meningitis *Pediatr Infect Dis J* 12(1):37-41, Jan 1993.

96. Greenberg A and Lobel H: Mortality from *Plasmodium falciparum* malaria in travelers from the United States, 1959-1987, *Ann Intern Med* 113(4):326-327, 1990.

97. Panosian C: Emporiatrics in the emergency department, *Top Emerg Med* 10(4):53-65, 1989.

98. Beadle C, Long GW, Weiss WR et al: Diagnoses of malaria by detection of *Plasmodium falciparum* HRP-2 antigen with a rapid dipstick antigen-capture assay, *Lancet*, 343:564-568, March 5, 1994.

99. Dietze R, Perkins M, Boulos M et al: The diagnosis of *Plasmodium falciparum* infection using a new antigen detection system, *Am J Trop Med Hyg* 52(1):45-49, 1995.

100. *Weekly Epidemiological Record*, Sept 9, 1994, pp 265-266.

101. Garg RA and Krashak R: Typhoid fever before two years of age *Indian Pediatr* 30:805-808, June 1993.

102. Bhutta ZA, Khan IA, Molla AM: Therapy of multi-drug resistant typhoid fever with oral cefixime vs intravenous ceftriaxone *Pediatr Infect Dis J* 13(11):990-994, Nov 1994.

103. Sharma A and Gathwala, G: Clinical profile and outcome in enteric fever *Indian Pediatr Vol* 30(1):47-50, Jan 1993.

Herpes Virus Infection

104. Whitley R: Neonatal herpes simplex virus, *Clin Perinatol* 15(4):903-916, 1988.

105. Prober C, Hensleigh P, Boucher F et al: Use of routine viral cultures at delivery to identify neonates exposed to herpes simplex virus, *N Engl J Med* 318(15):887-891, 1988.

106. Sullivan J, Hull H, Wilson C et al: Presentation of neonatal herpes simplex virus infections: implications for a change in therapeutic strategy, *Pediatr Infect Dis* 5(3):309-314, 1986.

107. Whitley R, Corey L, Arvin A et al: Changing presentation of herpes simplex virus infection in neonates, *J Infect Dis* 158(1):109-116, 1988.

108. Peter G, Lepow M, McCracken G: Report of the committee on infectious diseases, ed 22, Elk Grove Village, Ill, 1991, American Academy of Pediatrics.

109. Whitley R, Arvin A, Prober C et al: Predictors of morbidity and mortality in neonates with herpes simplex virus infections, *N Engl J Med* 324:450-454, 1991.

110. Whitley R, Arvin A, Prober C et al: A controlled trial comparing vidarabine with acyclovir in neonatal herpes simplex virus infection, *N Engl J Med* 324:444-449, 1991.

111. Overall JC: Empiric therapy with acyclovir for suspected neonatal herpes simplex infection, *Pediatr Infect Dis J* 8(11):808-809, 1989.

112. Whitley R, Soong S-J, Linneman C et al: Herpes simplex encephalitis, *JAMA* 247(3):317-320, 1982.

113. Lakeman FD and Whitley RJ: Diagnosis of Herpes simplex encephalitis: application of polymerase chain reaction to cerebrospinal fluid from brain-biopsied patients and correlation with disease, National Institute of Allergy and Infectious Disease Collaborative Antiviral Study Group, *J Infect Dis* 171:857-863, 1995.

114. Nahmias AJ, Whitley RJ, Visintine AN et al: Herpes simplex virus encephalitis: laboratory evaluations and their diagnostic significance, *J Infect Dis* 145(6):829-836, 1982.

115. Whitley R, Cobbs G, Alford C et al: Diseases that mimic herpes simplex encephalitis, *JAMA* 262(2):234-239, 1989.

116. Fishman M: Herpes simplex encephalitis: the brain biopsy controversy, *J Pediatr* 113(3):575-578, 1988.

Influenza

117. Heilman C and Montagne J: Influenza: status and prospects for its prevention, therapy, and control, *Pediatr Clin North Am* 37(3):669-688, 1990.
118. Peter G, Leopow M, McCracken G, et al: Report of the committee on infectious diseases: influenza, ed 22, Elk Grove Village, Ill, 1991, American Academy of Pediatrics.
119. Dagan R and Hall C: Influenza A virus infection imitating bacterial sepsis in early infancy, *Pediatr Infec Dis J* 3(3):218-221, 1984.
120. Liou Y, Barbour S, Bell L et al: Children hospitalized with influenza B infection, *Pediatr Infect Dis J* 6(6):541-543, 1987.
121. Serwint JR, Miller RM: Why diagnose influenza infections in hospitalized pediatric patients, *Pediatr Infect Dis J* 12(3):200-204, March 1993.
122. Dominguez EA, Taber LH, and Couch RB: Comparison of rapid diagnostic techniques for respiratory syncytial and influenza A virus respiratory infections in young children, *J Clin Microbiol* 31(9):2286-2290, Sept 1993.
123. Rodriguez W, Hall C, Welliver R, Simoes, E, et al: Efficacy and safety of aerosolized ribavirim in young children hospitalized with influenza: a double-blind multicenter, placebo-controlled trial. *J Pediatr* 125(1):129-135, July 1994.
124. Rimantadine for influenza A prevention and treatment. *Drug News* 19(9):22-23, Sept 1994.
125. Prevention and control of influenza: part I, vaccines. Recommendations of the advisory committee on immunization practices, *MMWR* 43(RR-9):1-13, May 27, 1994.

Kawasaki Disease

126. Yanagihara R and Todd J: Acute febrile mucocutaneous lymph node syndrome, *Am J Dis Child* 134:603-614, 1980.
127. Hicks R, Melish M: Kawasaki syndrome, *Pediatr Clin North Am* 33(5):1151-1175, 1986.
128. Rowley A, Gonzalez-Crussi F, Shulman S: Kawasaki syndrome: reviews of infectious diseases, *Rev Infect Dis* 10(1):1-15, 1988.
129. Fujita Y, Fujita N, Yosikazu S et al: Kawasaki disease in families, *Pediatrics* 84(4):666-669, 1989.
130. Vargo T, Huhta J, Moore W: Recurrent Kawasaki disease, *Pediatr Cardiol* 6:199-202, 1986.
131. Ichida F, Fatica N, O'Loughlin J et al: Epidemiological aspects of Kawasaki disease in a Manhattan hospital, *Pediatrics* 84(2):235-241, 1989.
132. Fujiwara H, Hamashima Y: Pathology of the heart in Kawasaki disease, *Pediatrics* 61:100-107, 1978.
133. Mason W, Jordan S, Sakai R et al: Circulating immune complexes in Kawasaki syndrome, *Pediatr Infect Dis* 4(1):48-51, 1955.
134. American Heart Association committee on rheumatic fever, endocarditis, and Kawasaki disease: diagnostic guidelines for Kawasaki disease, *Am J Dis Child* 144:1220-1222, 1990.
135. Levy M Koren G: Atypical Kawasaki disease: analysis of clinical presentation and diagnostic clues, *Pediatr Infect Dis* 9:122-126, 1990.
136. Fukushige F, Takahashi N, Ueda Y et al: Incidence and clinical features of incomplete Kawasaki disease, *Acta Paediatr* 83:1057-1060, 1994.
137. Shulman S, Bass J, Bierman F et al: Management of Kawasaki syndrome: a consensus statement prepared by North American participants of the third international Kawasaki disease symposium, Tokyo, Japan, December 1988, *Pediatr Infect Dis* 8:663-665, 1989.
138. Gersony W: Diagnosis and management of Kawasaki disease, *JAMA* 265(20):2699-2703, 1991.
139. Rosenfeld EA, Corydon KE, Shulman ST: Kawasaki disease in infants less than one year of age, *J Pediatr* 126:524-529, 1995.
140. Kohr R: Progressive asymptomatic coronary artery disease as a late fatal sequela of Kawasaki disease, *J Pediatr* 108(2):256-259, 1986.
141. Smith L, Newburger J, Burns J: Kawasaki syndrome and the eye, *Pediatr Infect Dis* 8:116-118, 1989.
142. Sundel R, Newburger J, McGill T: Sensorineural hearing loss associated with Kawasaki disease, *J Pediatr* 117:371-377, 1990.
143. Friesen C, Gamis A, Riddell L et al: Bilirubinuria: an early indicator of gallbladder hydrops associated with Kawasaki disease, *J Pediatr Gastroenterol Nutr* 8:384-386, 1989.
144. Barron K, Murphy D, Silverman E et al: Treatment of Kawasaki syndrome: a comparison of two dose regimens of intravenously administered immune globulin, *J Pediatr* 117:638-644, 1990.
145. Dajani A, Taubert K, Takahashi M et al: Guidelines for long-term management of patients with Kawasaki disease, *Circulation* 89:916-922, 1994.

Meningococcemia

146. Havens P, Garland J, Brook M et al: Trends in mortality in children hospitalized with meningococcal infections 1957 to 1987, *Pediatr Infect Dis J* 8(1):8-11, 1989.
147. Berg S, Trollfors B, Alestig K, and Jodal U: Incidence, serogroups and case-fatality rate of invasive meningococcal infections in a Swedish region 1975-1989, *Scan J Infect Dis* 24:333-338, 1992.
148. Peter G, Lepow M, McCracken G et al: *Meningococcal infections, report of the committee on infectious diseases*, ed 22, Elk Grove Village, Ill, 1991, American Academy of Pediatrics.
149. Peter G, Halsey N, Marcuse E, Pickering L editors: *Redbook report of the committee on infectious disease: meningococccocal infections*, ed 23, 1994, American Academy of Pediatrics pp 323-324.
150. Olivares R, Bouyer J, Hubert B: Risk factors for death in meningococcal disease, *Path Biol* 41:164-168, 1993.

Mononucleosis, Infectious

151. Papadakis M: Infectious mononucleosis, *West J Med* 137:141-144, 1982.
152. White L and Karofsky P: Review of the clinical manifestations, laboratory findings and complications of infectious mononucleosis, *Wisc Med J* 84:19-25, 1985.
153. McSherry JA: Diagnosing infectious mononucleosis, *Am Fam Physician* 32(4):129-132, 1985.
154. Pochedly C: Etiology of infectious mononucleosis: solving the riddle, *NY State J Med* June:352-355, 1987.
155. Cheeseman S: Infectious mononucleosis, *Semin Hematol* 25(3):261-268, 1988.
156. Markin R, Linder J, Zuerlein K et al: Hepatitis in fatal infectious mononucleosis, *Gastroenterology* 93:1210-1217, 1987.
157. Sumaya C and Ench Y: Epstein-Barr virus infectious mononucleosis in children. I. Clinical and general laboratory findings, *Pediatrics* 75(6):1003-1010, 1985.
158. Murray B: Medical complications of infectious mononucleosis, *Am Fam Physician* 30(5):195-199, 1984.
159. Erzurum S, Kalavsky S, Watanakunakorn C: Acute cerebellar ataxia and hearing loss as initial symptoms of infectious mononucleosis, *Arch Neurol* 40:760-762, 1983.
160. Portman M, Ingall D, Westenfelder G et al: Peritonsilar abscess complicating infectious mononucleosis, *J Pediatr* 104(5):742-744, 1984.
161. Hoagland RJ: General features of infectious mononucleosis. In Glade PR, editor: *Proceedings of symposium on infectious mononucleosis, New York, April 7, 1972*, Philadelphia, 1975, JB Lippincott.
162. Cook L, Midgett J, Willis D et al: Evaluation of latex-based heterophile antibody assay for diagnosis of acute infectious mononucleosis, *J Clin Microbiol* 25(12):2391-2394, 1987.
163. Sumaya C and Ench Y: Epstein-Barr virus infectious mononucleosis in children. II. Heterophil antibody and viral-specific responses, *Pediatrics* 75(6):1011-1019, 1985.
164. Zwaveling J, Ruding P, Nortter H et al: Airway obstruction: an unusual complication of infectious mononucleosis, *J Crit Care Med* 15(4):333, 1987.
165. Collins M, Fleisher G, Fager S: Incidence of beta-hemolytic streptococcal pharyngitis in adolescent with infectious mononucleosis, *J Adolesc Health Care* 5:96-100, 1984.
166. Merriam S and Keeling R: Beta-hemolytic streptococcal pharyngitis: uncommon in infectious mononucleosis, *South Med J* 76(5):575-576, 1983.

Mumps

167. Wharton M, Cochi S, Hutcheson R et al: A large outbreak of mumps in the postvaccine era, *J Infect Dis* 158(6):1253-1260, 1988.
168. Sosin D, Cochi S, Gunn R et al: Changing epidemiology of mumps and its impact on university campuses, *Pediatrics* 84(5):779-784, 1989.
169. Palmer SR and Biffin A: Incidence of mumps, *J R Coll Gen Pract* Jan:34, 1989.
170. McDonald J, Moore D, Quennec P: Clinical and epidemiologic features of mumps meningoencephalitis and possible vaccine-related disease, *Pediatr Infect Dis J* 8(11):751-755, 1989.

171. McCarthy C: Mumps: a 1990 update, *Pediatr Virol* 5(4):1990.
172. Ichiba N, Miyake Y, Sato K et al: Mumps induced opsoclonus-myoclonus and ataxia, *Pediatr Neurol* 4(4):224-227, 1988.
173. Garty B, Danon Y, Nitzan M: Hearing loss due to mumps? *Arch Dis Child* 63:105, 1988.
174. Ozkutlu S, Soylemezoglu O, Calikoglu A et al: Fatal mumps myocarditis, *Jpn Heart J* 30(1):109-114, 1989.
175. Myer C and Cotton R: Salivary gland disease in children: a review, *Clin Pediatr* 25(6):314-322, 1986.
176. Krilov L and Swenson P: Acute parotitis associated with influenza A infection, *J Infect Dis* 152(4):853, 1985.

Pertussis

177. Bass J and Stephenson S: The return of pertussis, *Pediatr Infect Dis J* 6:141-144, 1987.
178. Long S, Welkon C, Clark J: Widespread silent transmission of pertussis in families: antibody correlates of infection and symptomatology, *J Infect Dis* 161:480-486, 1990.
179. Pertussis surveillance: United States: 1986-1988, *MMWR* 39:5766, 1990.
180. Mortimer E: Pertussis and its prevention: a family affair, *J Infect Dis* 161:473-479, 1990.
181. Olson L: Pertussis, *Medicine* 54(6):427-469, 1975.
182. Sotomayor J, Weiner L, McMillan J: Inaccurate diagnosis in infants with pertussis: an eight-year experience, *Am J Dis Child* 139:724-727, 1985.
183. Romanus V, Jonsell R, Bergquist S-O: Pertussis in Sweden after the cessation of general immunization in 1979, *Pediatr Infect Dis J* 6(4):364-371, 1987.
184. Davis L, Burstyn D, Manclark C: Pertussis encephalopathy with a normal brain biopsy and elevated lymphocytosis-promoting factor antibodies, *Pediatr Infect Dis J* 3(5):448-451, 1984.
185. Onorato I, Wassilak S: Laboratory diagnosis of pertussis: the state of the art, *Pediatr Infect Dis J* 6(2):145-149, 1987.
186. Bass J: Pertussis: current status of prevention and treatment, *Pediatr Infect Dis J* 4(6):614-619, 1985.
187. Bergquist SO, Bernander S, Dahnsjo H et al: Erythromycin in the treatment of pertussis: a study of bacteriologic and clinical effects, *Pediatr Infect Dis J* 6(5):458-461, 1987.
188. Bass J: Erythromycin for treatment and prevention of pertussis, *Pediatr Infect Dis J* 5(1):154-157, 1986.
189. Krantz I, Norrby SR, Trollfors B: Salbutamol vs placebo for treatment of pertussis, *Pediatr Infect Dis J* 4(6):638-640, 1985.
190. Zoumboulakis D, Anagnostakis D, Albanis V et al: Steroids in treatment of pertussis: a controlled clinical trial, *Arch Dis Child* 48:51-54, 1973.

Rabies

191. Rabies prevention—United States, 1991, Recommendations of the immunization practices advisory committee (ACIP), *MMWR* 40(RR-3):1-19.
192. Plotkin S, Clark F: Rabies. In Feigin RD and Cherry JD, *Textbook of pediatric infectious diseases*, ed 2, Philadelphia, 1987, WB Saunders.
193. Bhatt D, Hattwick M, Gerdsen R et al: Human rabies, *Am J Dis Child* 127:862-869, 1974.
194. Bernard AW, Parham GL, Winler WG et al: Rabies: Report of the committee on infectious diseases, ed 22, Elk Grove Village, Ill, 1991, American Academy of Pediatrics.

Staphylococcal and Streptococcal Systemic Disease

195. Todd J, Fishaut M, Kapral F et al: Toxic shock syndrome associated with phage-group-I Staphylococci, *Lancet* 2:1116-1118, 1978.
196. Stevens FA: The occurrence of staphylococcal infection with a scarlatiniform rash, *JAMA* 119:1491-1495, 1927.
197. Shands KN, Schmid BP, Dan BB: Toxic shock syndrome in menstruating women: its association with tampon use and *Staphylococcus aureus* and the clinical features in 52 cases, *N Engl J Med* 303:1436-1442, 1980.
198. Sperber S, Francis JB: Toxic shock syndrome during an influenza outbreak, *JAMA* 257(8):1086-1087, 1987.
199. Conway E, Haber R, Gumprecht J et al: Toxic shock syndrome following influenza A in a child, *Crit Care Med* 19(1):123-125, 1991.
200. MacDonald K, Osterholm M, Hedberg C et al: Toxic shock syndrome: a newly recognized complication of influenza and influenza-like illness, *JAMA* 257(8):1053-1058, 1987.

201. Kniffin W, Smith R, Stashwick C: Toxic shock syndrome in three adolescent males, *J Adolesc Health Care* 10(2):166-169, 1990.
202. Heywood AJ, Al-Essa S: Toxic shock syndrome in child with only 2% burn, *Lancet* 335:867, 1990.
203. Farmer B, Bradley J, Smiley P: Toxic shock syndrome in a scald burn victim, *J Trauma* 25(10):1004-1006, 1985.
204. McCarthy V, Peoples W: Toxic shock syndrome after ear piercing, *Pediatr Infect Dis J* 7(10):741-742, 1988.
205. Mansfield C, Peterson M: Toxic shock syndrome: associated with nasal packing, *Clin Pediatr* 28(10):443-445, 1989.
206. Kishaba RG, Losek J: Toxic shock syndrome associated with poison oak dermatitis, *Pediatr Emerg Care* 5(1):40-42, 1989.
207. Ferguson M, Todd J: Toxic shock syndrome associated with *Staphylococcus aureus* sinusitis in children, *J Infect Dis* 161:953-955, 1990.
208. Chenaud M, Leclerc F, Martinot A: Bacterial croup and toxic shock syndrome, *Eur J Pediatr* 145:306-307, 1986.
209. Resnick S: Toxic shock syndrome: recent developments in pathogenesis, *J Pediatr* 116(3):321-328, 1990.
210. Todd JK, Todd BH, Franco-Buff A et al: Influence of local growth conditions on the pathogenesis of toxic shock syndrome, *J Infect Dis* 155:673-681, 1987.
211. Crass B, Bergdoll M: Toxin involvement in toxic shock syndrome, *J Infect Dis* 153(5):918-926, 1986.
212. McMahon W, Patrenos E, McConnell M et al: Complete heart block in toxic shock syndrome, *Am J Dis Child* 144:748-750, 1990.
213. Rolston R, Yabek S, Florman A et al: Severe cardiac conduction abnormalities associated with atypical toxic shock syndrome, *J Pediatr* 117(1):89-92, 1990.
214. Gamillscheg A, Zobel G, Karpf EF, Dacar D et al: Atypical presentation of Kawasaki disease in an Infant, *Pediatr Cardiol* 14(4):223-226, 1993.
215. Stevens D, Tanner M, Winship J et al: Severe group A streptococcal infections associated with a toxic shock-like syndrome and scarlet fever toxin A, *N Engl J Med* 321(1):1-7, 1989.
216. Cone L, Woodard D, Schlivert P et al: Clinical and bacteriologic observations of a toxic shock-like syndrome due to Streptococcus pyogenes, *N Engl J Med* 317(3):146-149, 1987.
217. Begovac J, Marton E, Lisic M et al: Group A gb-hemolytic streptococcal toxic shock-like syndrome, *Pediatr Infect Dis J* 9(5):369-370, 1990.
218. Stollerman G: Changing group A streptococci: the reappearance of streptococcal "toxic shock," *Arch Intern Med* 148:1268-1270, 1988.
219. Barter T, Dascal A, Carroll K et al: Toxic strep syndrome: a manifestation of group A streptococcal infection, *Arch Intern Med* 148:1421-1424, 1988.
220. Hoge CW, Schwartz KB, Talkington DF, Breiman RF et al: The changing epidemiology of invasive group A streptococcal infections and the emergence of streptococcal toxic shock-like syndrome. A retrospective population-based study, *JAMA* 269:(3)384-389, Jan 20, 1993.
221. Nadal D, Lavener R, Braegger C, Kaufhold A et al: T cell activation and cytokine release in streptococcal toxic shock-like syndrome, *J Pediatr* 122(5)Pt 1:727-729, 1993.

Tetanus

222. Brand D, Acampora D, Gottlieb L et al: Adequacy of antitetanus prophylaxis in six hospital emergency rooms, *N Engl J Med* 309(11):636-640, 1983.
223. Weinstein L: Medical intelligence current concepts tetanus, *N Engl J Med* 289(24):1293-1296, 1973.
224. Millard H, Wales MB, Lond MB: Local tetanus, *Lancet* October 23:S44-S46, 1954.
225. Richardson J, Knight A: The management and prevention of tetanus, *J Emerg Med* 11:737-742, 1993.
226. McCarthy P, Lembo R, Fink H et al: Observation, history and physical examination in diagnosis of serious illnesses in febrile children less than 24 months *J Pediatr* 110(1):26-30, 1987.
227. Tetanus: United States, 1987 and 1988, *MMWR* 39(3):138-141, 1990.
228. Plotkin S, Mortimer E: *Tetanus*, Philadelphia, 1988, WB Saunders.

Tick-Borne Infectious Diseases

229. Doan-Wiggins L: Tick-borne diseases, *Emerg Med Clin North Am* 9(2):303-325, 1991.

230. Wright S, Trott A: North American tick-borne diseases, *Ann Emerg Med* 17:964-972, 1988.

231. Salgo MP, Telzak EE, Currie B et al: A focus of Rocky Mountain spotted fever within New York City, *N Engl J Med* 318:1345, 1988.

232. Goodpasture H, Poland J, Francy B et al: Colorado tick fever: clinical, epidemiologic, and laboratory aspects of 228 cases in Colorado in 1973-1974, *Ann Intern Med* 88:303-310, 1978.

233. Fishbein D, Dawson J, Robinson L: Human ehrlichiosis in the United States, 1985 to 1990. *Ann Int Med* 120:736-743, 1994.

234. Standaert S, Dawson J, Schaffner W et al: Ehrlichiosis in a golf-oriented retirement community, *N Engl J Med* 333:420-425, 1995.

235. Steere A, Malawista S, Snydman D et al: Lyme arthritis, arthritis, and rheumatism, *Arthritis Rheum* 20(1):7-17, 1977.

236. Persing D, Telford S, Rys P et al: Detection of *Borrelia burgdorferi* DNA in museum specimens of *Ixodes dammini* ticks, *Science* 249:1420-1423, 1990.

237. Balani K, Regelmann W: Lyme disease in children, *Rheum Dis Clin North Am* 15(4):679-691, 1989.

238. Lyme disease surveillance—United States, 1994, *MMWR* 44(24): 459-462.

239. Andiman W: Lyme disease: epidemiology, etiology, clinical spectrum, diagnosis, and treatment, *Adv Pediatr Infect Dis* 1:163-186, 1986.

240. Steere A, Grodzicki R, Kornblatt A et al: The spirochetal etiology of Lyme disease, *N Engl J Med* 308(13):733-739, 1983.

241. Hardin J, Steere A, Malawista S: Immune complexes and the evolution of Lyme arthritis, dissemination and localization of abnormal C1q binding activity, *N Engl J Med* 301(25):1358-1363, 1979.

242. Steere A: Lyme disease, *N Engl J Med* 321(9):586-596, 1989.

243. Duffy J: Lyme disease, *Ann Allergy* 65:1-13, 1990.

244. Williams C, Strobino B, Lee A et al: Lyme disease in childhood: clinical and epidemiologic features of ninety cases, *Pediatr Infect Dis J* 9:10-14, 1990.

245. Feder H, Gerber M, Krause P et al: Early Lyme disease: A flu-like illness without erythema migrans, *Pediatrics* 91:456-459, 1993.

246. Pachner A and Steere A: The triad of neurologic manifestations of Lyme disease: meningitis, cranial neuritis, and radiculoneuritis, *Neurology* 35:47-53, 1985.

247. Steere A, Batsford W, Weinberg M et al: Lyme carditis: cardiac abnormalities of Lyme disease, *Ann Intern Med* 93:8-16, 1980.

248. Eichenfeld A, Goldsmith D, Benach J et al: Childhood lyme arthritis: experience in an endemic area, *J Pediatr* 109:753, 1986.

249. Gerber M, Shapiro E: Current literature and clinical issues; Diagnosis of Lyme disease in children, *J Pediatr* 121:157-161, 1992.

250. Dressler F, Whalen J, Reinhardt B et al: Western blotting in the serodiagnosis of Lyme disease, *J Infect Dis* 167:392-400, 1993.

251. Shapiro E, Gerber M, Holabird N et al: A controlled trial of antimicrobial prophylaxis for Lyme disease after deer tick bites, *N Engl J Med* 327:1769-1773, 1992.

252. Denver L, Jorgensen J, Barbour A: Comparitive in vitro activities of clarithromycin, azithromycin, and erythromycin against *Borrelia burgdorferi*, *Antimicr Agents Chemo* 37:1704-1706, 1993.

253. Pfister HW, Preac-Mursic V, Wilske B et al: Randomized comparison of ceftriaxone and cefotaxime in Lyme neuroborreliosis, *J Infect Dis* 163:311-318, 1991.

254. Burgdorfer W: The enlarging spectrum of tick-borne spirochetoses (RR Parker memorial address) *Rev Infect Dis* 8(6):932-940, 1986.

255. Outbreak of relapsing fever—Grand Canyon National Park, Arizona, *MMWR* 40(8):296-303, 1990.

256. Fischer J: Rocky Mountain spotted fever: when and why to consider the diagnosis, *Postgrad Med* 87(4):109-118, 1990.

257. Wilfert C, MacCormack N, Kleeman K et al: Epidemiology of Rocky Mountain spotted fever as determined by active surveillance, *J Infect Dis* 150(4):468-479, 1984.

258. Feigin R, O'Neil J: Rickettsial diseases. In *Textbook of pediatric infectious diseases,* Philadelphia, 1987, WB Saunders.

259. Helmick C, Bernard K, D'Angelo L: Rocky Mountain spotted fever: clinical, laboratory and epidemiological features of 262 cases, *J Infect Dis* 150(4):480-496, 1984.

260. Middleton R: Rocky Mountain spotted fever: gastrointestinal and laboratory manifestations, *South Med J* 71(6):629-632, 1978.

261. Rubio T, Riley D, Nida J: Thrombocytopenia in Rocky Mountain spotted fever, *Am J Dis Child* 116:88-96, 1968.

262. Kaplowitz L, Robertson G: Hyponatremia in Rocky Mountain spotted fever: role of antidiuretic hormone, *Ann Intern Med* 98(3):334-335, 1983.

263. Wells M III, Choplin R, Shertzer M: The chest radiograph in Rocky Mountain spotted fever, *Am J Radiol* 139:889-893, 1982.

264. Marin-Garcia J, Gooch WM, Coury D: Cardiac manifestations of Rocky Mountain spotted fever, *Pediatrics* 67(3):358-361, 1981.

265. Markowitz L, Hynes N, de la Cruz P et al: Tick-borne tularemia, *JAMA* 254:2922-2925, 1985.

266. Schmidt GP, Kornblatt AN, Connors CA et al: Clinically mild tularemia associated with tick-borne *Francisella tularensis, J Infect Dis* 148(1):63-67, 1983.

267. Summary of notifiable diseases—United States, *MMWR* 38(54):1990.

268. Yow M: Tularemia. In *Textbook of pediatric infectious diseases,* ed 2, Philadelphia, 1987, WB Saunders.

269. Jacobs R, Condrey Y, Yamauchi T: Tularemia in adults and children: a changing presentation, *Pediatrics* 76(5):818-822, 1985.

270. Uhari M, Syrjala H, Salminen A: Tularemia in children caused by *Francisella tularensis biovar palaeartica, Pediatr Infect Dis J* 9:80-83, 1990.

271. Doan-Wiggins L: Tick-borne diseases, *Emerg Med Clin North Am* 9(2):303-325, 1991.

272. Nelson J: *Pocketbook of pediatric antimicrobial therapy,* Baltimore, 1991-1992, Williams & Wilkins.

Tuberculosis

273. Dowling P: Return of tuberculosis: screening and preventive therapy, *Am Fam Physician* 43(2):457-467, 1991.

274. Summary of notifiable diseases, United States, 1993, *MMWR* 42(53), 1994.

275. Smith M: Tuberculosis in children and adolescents, *Clin Chest Med* 10(3):381-395, 1989.

276. Jacobs R, Eisenach K: Childhood tuberculosis, *Adv Pediatr Infect Dis* 8:23-51, 1993.

277. Vallejo J, Ong L, Starke J: Clinical features, diagnosis, and treatment of tuberculosis in infants, *Pediatrics* 9:1-7, 1994.

278. Molavi A, LeFrock J: Tuberculosis meningitis, *Med Clin North Am* 69(2):315-331, 1985.

279. Starke J, Jacobs R, Jereb J: Medical progress: Resurgence of tuberculosis in children, *J Pediatr* 120:839-855, 1992.

280. Huebner R, Schein M, Bass J: The tuberculin test, *Clin Infect Dis* 17:968-975, 1993.

281. Frieden T, Sterling T, Pablos-Mendez et al: The emergence of drug resistant tuberculosis in New York City, *N Engl J Med* 328:521-526, 1993.

282. Weis S, Slocum P, Blais F et al: The effect of directly observed therapy on the rates of drug resistance and relapse in tuberculosis, *N Engl J Med* 330:1179-1184, 1994.

Exanthems

283. Anderson M, Lewis E, Kidd I et al: An outbreak of erythema infectiosum associated with human parvovirus infection, *J Hyg (Camb)* 93:85-93, 1984.

284. Mynott MJ: An epidemic of *erythema infectiosum* in a school, *Practitioner* 229:767-768, 1985.

285. Mansfield F: *Erythema infectiosum,* slapped face disease, *Austr Fam Physician* 17(9):737-738, 1988.

286. Tuckerman J, Brown T, Cohen B: *Erythema infectiosum* in a village primary school: clinical and virological studies, *J R Coll Gen Pract* June:267-270, 1986.

287. Bialecki C, Feder H, Grant-Kels J: The six classic childhood exanthems: a review and update, *J Am Acad Dermatol* 21(5):891-903, 1989.

288. Plotkin S: Committee on infectious disease, American Academy of Pediatrics, parvovirus, erythema infectiosum, and pregnancy, *Pediatrics* 85(1):131-133, 1990.

289. Bligard C and Millikan L: Acute exanthems in children, *Postgrad Med* 79(5):150-167, 1986.

290. Hall CB: Herpes and the rash of the roses: a new virus, HHV-6, as a cause of an old childhood disease, Roseola, *Pediatr Ann* 19(9):517-521, 1990.

291. Irving WL, Change J, Raymond D et al: Roseola infantum and other syndromes associated with acute HHV-6 infection, *Arch Dis Child* 65:1297-1300, 1990.

292. Yamanishi K, Okuno T, Shiraki K et al: Identification of human herpesvirus-6 as a causal agent for exanthem subitum, *Lancet* 1:1065-1067, 1988.

293. Yoshiyama H, Suzuki E, Yoshida T et al: Role of human herpesvirus infection in infants with exanthem subitum, *Pediatr Infect Dis J* 9:71-74, 1990.
294. Meade R: Exanthem subitum (roseola infantum), *Clin Dermatol* 7(1):92-96, 1989.
295. Ishiguro N, Yamada S, Takashashi T et al: Meningoencephalitis associated with HHV-6 related exanthem subitum, *Acta Paediatr Scand* 79:987-989, 1990.
296. Markowitz L, Orenstein W: Measles vaccine, *Pediatr Clin North Am* 37(3):603-625, 1990.

Appendix 55A: Postexposure Prophylaxis for Common Viral and Bacterial Pathogens

Children and adults may require prophylaxis following exposure to a variety of specific viral or bacterial pathogens. The decision to administer prophylaxis following a documented exposure is based on several considerations including (1) the pathogen involved, (2) the individual's risk for disease and disease complications, and (3) the nature of the exposure. Household contacts are among the most frequently evaluated exposures and are defined as those individuals living in the same house as the index case or who have spent 4 or more hours with the index case for at least 5 of the 7 days before the index case becomes ill. Prophylaxis is accomplished using either immunization or antimicrobial agents.[1]

IMMUNE PROPHYLAXIS

Immune prophylaxis may be indicated following exposure to hepatitis A and B, varicella zoster, measles, rabies, and tetanus. Protective antibody is provided either passively, actively, or in combination. Passive immunization employs immune globulin products that are prepared either from the plasma of pooled donors (immune globulin: IG) or from donors having high titers of a specific antibody (hyperimmune immune globulin: HBIG, HRIG, TIG, or VZIG). Immune globulin products are not known to transmit infectious agents such as HIV and hepatitis.[1,2]

Immune globulin preparations are administered by deep intramuscular injection. The injected volume for a single site should not exceed 1 to 3 ml in infants and small children and 5 ml in large children and adults. The most common side effect is pain. Serious reactions such as anaphylaxis are rare.[2,3]

1. *Hepatitis B Virus:* Postexposure management involves administration of HBIG, the hepatitis B vaccine, either singly or in combination. The dose for HGIG is 0.5 ml IM for newborns and infants younger than 12 months of age and 0.06 ml/kg for children and adults (maximum: 5 ml). Vaccine is administered as a series of three doses at 0, 1, and 6 months. The vaccine dose for newborns and infants younger than 12 months of age is 0.5 ml IM and for children and adults is 1 ml IM.[3] Indications for hepatitis B prophylaxis include:
   a. *Newborns of Hepatitis B surface antigen (HBsAg)-positive mothers:* All newborns born to HBsAg-positive mothers should receive HBIG and hepatitis B vaccine within 12 hours of birth. HBIG may be administered as late as 48 hours but with a significant loss in efficacy. Hepatitis B vaccine is efficacious if administered within 7 days of birth.[1,3]
   b. *Household contacts:* Children younger than 12 months of age whose primary caregiver has acute hepatitis B are more likely to become chronic carriers if infected and therefore should receive HBIG and hepatitis vaccine. If the index case is a chronic carrier, all susceptible household contacts, regardless of age, should be vaccinated.[1,3]
   c. *Sexual contacts:* Sexual contacts of HBsAg-positive individuals should receive HBIG and hepatitis B vaccine within 14 days of the last sexual contact.[1,3]
   d. *Percutaneous and permucosal contacts:* Risk assessment following percutaneous or permucosal exposure to blood involves testing the source patient for HBsAg and determining the immune status of the exposed person. Exposed persons previously vaccinated should be tested for anti-HBs response. Management is outlined in Table 55A-1.[1,3]
2. *Hepatitis A:* Postexposure prophylaxis should not be administered until there is serologic confirmation of the index case (IgM anti-Hepatitis A virus [HAV]). Prophylaxis should not be administered if more than 2 weeks have passed since the exposure. IG is administered as a single dose of 0.02 ml/kg IM. Indications for postexposure immune globulin prophylaxis include:
   a. *Household and sexual contacts:* All household and sexual contacts should receive immune globulin.[1,3]
   b. *Day care centers and schools:* All staff and attendees of day care centers in which diapered children are enrolled must be immunized if: (1) HAV is diagnosed in one or more employees or attendees or (2) if two or more households of attendees have cases of HAV. In day care centers in which no diapered children are enrolled, only the classroom contacts need to receive prophylaxis. Contacts within elementary and secondary schools represent a low risk and do not require prophylaxis, unless there is evidence of an outbreak.[1,3]
   c. *Institutions and hospitals:* Institutions providing custodial care, such as chronic care facilities, are at increased risk for the spread of HAV. All staff and residents in close contact with an index case should receive prophylaxis. Hospital employees do not routinely require prophylaxis.[1,3]
   d. *Common source outbreaks:* Individuals exposed to common source outbreaks usually are not identified early enough following the exposure to warrant prophylaxis. Individuals whose exposure to a known HAV-contaminated food or water source of less than 2 weeks should receive prophylaxis.[1,3]
3. *Varicella zoster:* Prophylaxis against varicella is indicated for high-risk individuals at increased risk for disease complications. Those at increased risk include immunocompromised children, susceptible adolescents (≥ 15 years of age) and adults, pregnant women, and newborns, if the mother develops chickenpox within 5 days before or 2 days after delivery.[1] All candidates for VZIG 15 years of age or older should, if possible, be tested for immunity because the majority of these individuals will have serologic evidence of prior infection.

TABLE 55A-1. Recommendations for Hepatitis B Prophylaxis Following Percutaneous or Permucosal Exposure

Exposed person	Treatment when source is found to be		
	HBsAg-positive	HBsAg-negative	Source not tested or unknown
Unvaccinated	HBIG × 1 (0.06 ml/kg), begin HB vaccine	Initiate HB vaccine	Initiate HB vaccine
Previously vaccinated; known responder	Test exposed person for anti-HBs — if adequate, no treatment; if inadequate, HB vaccine booster dose	No treatment	No treatment
Known nonresponder	HBIG × 2 or HBIG × 1 plus 1 dose of HB vaccine	No treatment	If known high-risk source, may treat as if source is HBsAg-positive
Response unknown	Test exposed person for anti-HBs — if inadequate, HBIG × 1 plus HB vaccine booster dose; if adequate, no treatment	No treatment	Test exposed person for anti-HBs — if inadequate, HBIG × 1 plus HB vaccine booster dose; if adequate, no treatment

From Advisory Committee on Immunization Practices recommendations for protection against viral hepatitis, *MMWR*, 39(S-2):1-26, 1990.

The dose of VZIG is one vial (125 U) for each 10 kg of body weight. The maximum dose is 5 vials (625 U). VZIG should be administered within 48 hours, but no later than 96 hours, after exposure.[1]

4. *Measles:* Susceptible individuals exposed to a physician-documented case should receive postexposure prophylaxis using measles vaccine or IG. Susceptible persons include all unvaccinated persons born after 1957 and those receiving the vaccine before their first birthday. The vaccine should be administered within 72 hours of exposure to all susceptible individuals 6 months of age or older unless there is a contraindication to the vaccine. Contraindications for measles vaccine include immunocompromised patients (excluding HIV), pregnant women, administration of IG within the previous 3 months, and anaphylactic hypersensitivity to eggs or neomycin. The vaccine of choice is the measles, mumps, rubella (MMR). IG may be effective in preventing or modifying disease if given within 6 days of exposure. IG should be used for individuals having a vaccine contraindication and in exposures occurring within the previous 3 to 6 days. IG may also be considered in infants younger than 12 months of age because of the risk for severe disease. The IG dose is 0.5 ml/kg for immunocompromised individuals and 0.25 ml/kg for all others. Maximum dose is 15 ml.[1,2,4,5]

ANTIMICROBIAL PROPHYLAXIS

Common pathogens for which antimicrobial prophylaxis is indicated include *N. menigitidis, H. influenzae,* pertussis, tuberculosis, and sexually transmitted pathogens. The postexposure management of *N. menigitidis* and *H. influenzae* type B will be discussed here. The prophylaxis of the remaining pathogens is considered in their respective sections (see sections on Pertussis, Tuberculosis, and Chapter 53 on Sexually Transmitted Diseases).

Rifampin is the drug of choice for prophylaxis of both *N. meningitidis* and *H. influenzae* exposures. Rifampin is available as 150 mg and 300 mg capsules. For small children a liquid preparation can be formulated or the contents of a capsule can be mixed with applesauce.[1] Common side effects of rifampin include nausea, vomiting, gastric irrita-tion, and diarrhea. Rifampin is excreted in most body fluids and secretions, giving them a characteristic orange color. Individuals with soft contact lenses should be advised not to wear them during treatment.

Management

H. Influenzae Type B. Antibiotic prophylaxis is indicated for all household contacts (regardless of age or immunization status), if any one contact is younger than 48 months of age. Prophylaxis of household contacts should be administered as soon as possible following diagnosis and should include the index case.[1]

The risk to exposed day care and nursery school children has been the subject of considerable debate and no specific guidelines exist.[1,6,7] Studies suggest that following day care center exposures to invasive *H. influenzae* disease, children younger than 2 years of age not receiving rifampin prophylaxis have a higher rate of secondary disease.[6,7] Rifampin prophylaxis should be considered for day care center contacts if children younger than 2 years of age are enrolled. Day care centers having two or more cases of invasive disease within a 6-month period should have rifampin prophylaxis administered to all staff and attendees.[1]

Rifampin is administered at a dose of 20 mg/kg/dose (maximum dose: 600 mg) once a day for 4 days. The dose for infants younger than 1 month of age should be decreased to 10 mg/kg/dose.[1]

N. Meningitidis. All household, day care center, and nursery school contacts should receive antibiotic prophylaxis within 24 hours of the index case being diagnosed. Prophylaxis for older children and adults is not indicated unless contact included kissing or sharing of food and drink. Medical personnel do not routinely require prophylaxis unless in close contact with secretions as may occur with suctioning and endotracheal intubation. Any exposed individual who subsequently develops a febrile illness should be medically evaluated.[1]

Rifampin is administered at a dose of 10 mg/kg/24 hr/q 12 hr (maximum dose: 600 mg) for a total of four doses. Sulfasoxizole may be used if the organism is shown to be sensitive to sulfa drugs.[1]

Appendix 55B: Acute Exposure to Blood That May Contain HBsAg

For accidental percutaneous (needlestick, laceration, or bite) or permucosal (ocular mucous membrane) exposure to blood, the decision to provide prophylaxis must include consideration of several factors: (1) whether the source of the blood is available, (2) the HBsAg status of the source, and (3) the hepatitis B vaccination and vaccine-response status of the exposed person. Such exposures usually affect persons for whom hepatitis B vaccine is recommended. For any exposure of a person not previously vaccinated, hepatitis B vaccination is recommended.

Following any such exposure, a blood sample should be obtained from the person who was the source of the exposure and should be tested for HBsAg. The hepatitis B vaccination status and anti-HBs response status of the exposed person (if known) should be reviewed. The outline below and Table 55A-1 summarize prophylaxis for percutaneous or permucosal exposure to blood according to the HBsAG status of the source of exposure and the vaccination status and vaccine response of the exposed person.

For greatest effectiveness, passive prophylaxis with HBIG, when indicated, should be given as soon as possible after exposure. (Its value beyond 7 days after exposure is unclear.)

Source of Exposure HBsAg-Positive

Exposed person has not been vaccinated or has not completed vaccination. Hepatitis B vaccination should be initiated. A single dose of HBIG (0.06 ml/kg) should be given as soon as possible after exposure and within 24 hours, if possible. The first dose of hepatitis B vaccine (see Table 55A-1) should be given intramuscularly at a separate site (deltoid for adults) and can be given simultaneously with HBIG or within 7 days of exposure. Subsequent doses should be given as recommended for the specific vaccine. If the exposed person has begun but not completed vaccination, one dose of HBIG should be given immediately, and vaccination should be completed as scheduled.

Exposed person has already been vaccinated against hepatitis B, and anti-HBs response status is known.

a. If the exposed person is known to have had adequate response in the past, the anti-HBs level should be tested unless an adequate level has been demonstrated within the last 24 months. Although current data show that vaccine-induced protection does not decrease as antibody level wanes, most experts consider the following approach to be prudent.
   (1) If anti-HBs level is adequate, no treatment is necessary.
   (2) If anti-HBs level is inadequate, a booster dose of hepatitis B vaccine should be given.
b. If the exposed person is known not to have responded to the primary vaccine series, the exposed person should be given either a single dose of HBIG and a dose of hepatitis B vaccine as soon as possible after exposure, or two doses of HBIG (0.06 ml/kg), one given as soon as possible after exposure and the second 1 month later. The latter treatment is preferred

for those who have failed to respond to at least four doses of vaccine.

Exposed person has already been vaccinated against hepatitis B, and the anti-HBs response is unknown. The exposed person should be tested for anti-HBs.

a. If the exposed person has adequate antibody, no additional treatment is necessary.
b. Source of exposure known and HBsAg-negative.
   (1) Exposed person has not been vaccinated or has not completed vaccination. If unvaccinated, the exposed person should be given the first dose of hepatitis B vaccine within 7 days of exposure, and vaccination should be completed as recommended. If the exposed person has not completed vaccination, vaccination should be completed as scheduled.
   (2) Exposed person has already been vaccinated against hepatitis B. No treatment is necessary.

Source of Exposure Unknown or Unavailable

Exposed person has not been vaccinated or has not completed vaccination. If unvaccinated, the exposed person should be given the first dose of the hepatitis B vaccine within 7 days of exposure and vaccination completed as recommended. If the exposed person has not completed vaccination, vaccination should be completed as scheduled.

Exposed person has already been vaccinated against hepatitis B, and anti-HBs response status is known.

a. If the exposed person is known to have had adequate response in the past, no treatment is necessary.
b. If the exposed person is known to have responded to the vaccine, prophylaxis as described previously in section on Source of Exposure HBsAg-Positive may be considered if the source of the exposure is known to be at high risk of HBV infection.

Exposed person has already been vaccinated against hepatitis B, and the anti-HBs response is unknown. The exposed person should be tested for anti-HBs.

a. If the exposed person has adequate anti-HBs, no treatment is necessary.
b. If the exposed person has inadequate anti-HBs, a standard booster dose of vaccine should be given.

References

1. Peter G, Lepow M, McCracken G: *Report of the committee on infectious diseases*, ed 22, 1991, American Academy of Pediatrics.
2. Weintrub PS: Uses of immune globulins in the prophylaxis and treatment of viral infections, *Clin Lab Med* 7(4):897-910, 1987.
3. Protection against viral hepatitis, Recommendations of the immunization practices advisory committee (ACIP), *MMWR* 39(S-2):26, 1990.
4. Measles prevention: recommendations of the immunization practices advisory committee (ACIP), *MMWR* 38(S-9):1-17, 1989.
5. Markowitz L and Orenstein W: Measles vaccines, *Pediatr Clin North Am* 37(3):603-625, 1990.
6. Osterhold M, Pierson L, White K et al: The risk of subsequent transmission of Hemophilus influenzae type B disease among children in daycare, *N Engl J Med* 316(1):1-5, 1987.
7. Makintubee S, Istre G, Ward J: Transmission of invasive Haemophilus influenzae type B disease in day care settings, *J Pediatr* 111:180-186, 1987.

CHAPTER

56

Neurologic Disorders

SUSAN M. FUCHS

• *Roger M. Barkin* • *Mananda S. Bhende* • *Javier A. Gonzalez del Rey* • *Douglas Holtzman*
Daniel J. Isaacman • *Raymond B. Karasic* • *Ronald I. Paul*

Signs and Symptoms

ATAXIA

MANANDA S. BHENDE

Ataxia is incoordination of movement with intact muscle strength, which may or may not be associated with disturbance of balance.[1,2]

Pathophysiology

The cerebellum coordinates movement by modifying muscle tone and contraction, resulting in smooth movements.[3,4] Dysfunction of the cerebellum causes ataxia, referred to as cerebellar ataxia. The cerebellum is connected to the brain by three large paired peduncles: the superior, middle, and inferior peduncles through which pass the afferent and efferent connections to and from the cerebellum and the rest of the nervous system. The inferior peduncle carries important sensory fibers via the dorsal spinocerebellar tract and also afferent fibers from the vestibular apparatus. The middle peduncle carries afferent fibers from the central cortex; efferent fibers from the cerebellum are mainly located in the superior peduncle.[3,4-6]

The cerebellum consists of a midline structure called the vermis and two lateral hemispheres. There are two distinct cerebellar ataxic syndromes, depending upon which of the cerebellar regions are affected. The vermis and the flocculonodular lobes of the hemispheres control equilibrium. Dysfunction of this area leads to axial (truncal) ataxia (i.e., swaying of the trunk and titubation when sitting, standing, and walking). The lateral cerebellar hemispheres control ipsilateral limb movements. Dysfunction in the cerebellar hemisphere leads to ataxia in the respective limb, depending upon the location of the lesion. Because the cerebellum also forms the roof of the fourth ventricle, an expanding lesion can obstruct cerebrospinal fluid (CSF) flow and result in hydrocephalus and cause truncal ataxia.[3,4-6]

Ataxia can also be caused by dysfunction in structures other than the cerebellum, such as cerebral cortex (frontal ataxia), peripheral sensory nerves and spinal cord (sensory ataxia), and the vestibular labyrinthine system (labyrinthine ataxia).[3] Besides structural pathology, ataxia can also be caused by metabolic and pharmacologic processes such as drugs, toxins, hypoglycemia, and rarely by a psychiatric disorder, such as a conversion reaction.[7]

Differential Considerations

Although many conditions may cause ataxia, the most commonly occurring are drug intoxication, postinfectious acute cerebellar ataxia, and a posterior fossa tumor (see box on p. 973). Ataxia can be divided according to the modes of presentation: acute, acute remitting, and chronic.[3] Acute ataxia refers to an acute onset of ataxia in a previously healthy child; acute remitting ataxia occurs when bouts of ataxia are interspersed with illness-free periods; chronic ataxia is persistent ataxia. The most common type of ataxia seen by the emergency physician is acute ataxia.

Acute cerebellar ataxia occurs after an antecedent nonspecific viral illness. It occurs after influenza, poliomyelitis, coxsackie B, echovirus type 6, herpes simplex virus, mononucleosis, mycoplasma, and most commonly after varicella.[8-14] Patients usually present with severe ataxia. Most have dysarthria; half have nystagmus. The computed tomography (CT) scan is normal and the CSF usually has mild pleocytosis. The course of illness is usually benign, the ataxia resolving within a few weeks to a few months. Residual symptoms, such as persistent gait disturbances, truncal tremor, abnormal eye movements, and impaired

Causes of Acute Ataxia in Childhood

Postinfectious: acute cerebellar ataxia
Drug ingestion/intoxication
Posterior fossa tumor
Head trauma
Occult neuroblastoma
Guillain-Barré syndrome
Stroke
Vasculitis

speech may persist for up to 6 years after the initial episode in about one third of patients.[15]

Drug ingestion is one of the most common causes of acute ataxia.[16] Patients taking anticonvulsants, especially phenytoin, may have toxic levels and present with ataxia. Other drugs and toxins producing ataxia are alcohol, tricyclic antidepressants, hypnotics, sedatives, benzodiazepines, heavy metals (lead), insecticides, and drugs of abuse (PCP).[16]

Posterior fossa tumors such as medulloblastoma, astrocytoma, and ependymoma or a brain stem glioma can present as acute ataxia due to cerebellar dysfunction or hydrocephalus. The patient usually has a history of headaches, vomiting, and, in frontal lobe tumors, behavioral changes. Papilledema may occur.

Head trauma is commonly encountered in the emergency department. Ataxia may occur as a part of postconcussion syndrome.[1] A CT scan is necessary to rule out a hemorrhage, edema, or contusion. A rapidly increasing cerebellar hematoma is a neurosurgical emergency and immediate intervention can be lifesaving. Basilar skull fractures can also damage the vestibular system with resultant ataxia.

A triad of acute ataxia, opsoclonus (jerky, random eye movements), and myoclonus is associated with occult neuroblastoma.[17,18] Weakness may be mistaken for acute ataxia. Thus patients with Guillain-Barré syndrome, transverse myelitis, tick paralysis, or myasthenia gravis can all present with an ataxic gait.[19] Acute infections such as meningitis, encephalitis, or labyrinthitis can all present with acute ataxia. Some patients with stroke or vasculitis as in systemic lupus erythematosus may have ataxia as a presenting complaint.

Inherited metabolic conditions such as Hartnup disease, maple syrup urine disease, argininosuccinicaciduria, ornithine transcarbamoylase deficiency, multiple carboxylase deficiencies, and hypothyroidism can all present with multiple acute ataxic symptoms.[20] Metabolic conditions including hypoglycemia, hyponatremia, and hyperammonemia must also be kept in mind.

Chronic ataxias are associated with tumors; hydrocephalus; hereditary ataxias such as Friedreich and Leigh syndromes; congenital disorders such as Arnold-Chiari and Dandy-Walker malformations, ataxia telangiectasia, and Wilson and Refsum disease; and acquired diseases such as multiple sclerosis, vitamin B_{12}, Vitamin E, or folate deficiency.[21,22]

Diagnostic Work-Up

An accurate history and detailed physical examination are essential for arriving at a diagnosis and for choosing the appropriate laboratory tests.

Some important *historic questions* to ask include the following: Is the ataxia of acute onset? Has the patient had ataxia previously, which resolved completely, or is this ataxia chronic? Does the ataxia involve only the trunk, or are the limbs also involved? An antecedent history of a viral illness such as influenza, varicella, or mononucleosis may suggest postinfectious acute cerebellar ataxia.[1,2] A history of fever, sore throat, rash, lymphadenitis, or pneumonia should be elicited. Headaches, blurred vision, nausea, vomiting, and mental status changes suggest the possibility of a tumor. A patient could present with ataxia after head injury.[3,23] One should also inquire about drug ingestion and the presence or absence of associated neurologic symptoms such as sensory paresthesias.

A thorough general physical examination should be performed. Critically ill children may have meningitis, shock, increased intracranial pressure, or hypoglycemia, which requires immediate therapeutic intervention.[23] The head should be examined for any evidence of injury. The eyes should be examined for cranial nerve palsies, papilledema, nystagmus, or opsoclonus. The presence of opsoclonus associated with myoclonus and ataxia is associated with occult neuroblastoma. The throat and neck should be examined for pharyngitis and lymphadenitis, and the ears for chronic otitis. Chest examination may reveal heart murmurs, which may account for embolic phenomena giving rise to ataxia, or lungs may have evidence of mycoplasma pneumonia. The abdomen should be checked for masses and the skin for rashes.

A detailed neurologic examination is essential. Testing of the cranial nerves; motor system for tone, power, and deep tendon reflexes, which are absent in Guillain-Barré and Fisher syndrome; sensory system; and gait is important. Mild gait impairments can be elicited if the child walks in a tandem fashion. Tests of cerebellar function (i.e., finger-to-object, toe-to-object, heel-to-shin-to-knee) should be conducted to detect asynergy and dysmetria, and rapid alternating movements should be checked for dysdiadochokinesia. The Romberg test (standing with toes and heels together, arms at sides, and eyes closed) should be positive (falling) in sensory ataxia. In a younger child, much information can be obtained by watching the child at play with the parents.

Ancillary Data. Blood and urine toxicology screens should be obtained to rule out drug overdose as a cause of ataxia. Serum electrolytes, glucose, and ammonia are obtained to rule out hyponatremia, hypoglycemia, or hyperammonemia.[22] A complete blood count may reveal the presence of atypical lymphocytes of infectious mononucleosis. A CT scan or magnetic resonance imaging (MRI) scan of the brain is indicated in most cases to detect a space-occupying lesion or hydrocephalus. A lumbar puncture is usually performed after obtaining a head CT scan. If the patient presents with a triad of ataxia, opsoclonus, and myoclonus, radiographic or ultrasound studies of the abdomen and chest and 24-hour urine for homovanillic acid (HVA) and vanillylmandelic acid (VMA) are indicated to rule out occult neuroblastoma.[17,18] An electroencephalogram (EEG), electromyogram (EMG), nerve conduction studies, and vestibular function tests may be indicated in certain cases.[3]

Prehospital Considerations

Routine monitoring should be performed on all patients who are being transported. If an ataxic patient becomes increasingly obtunded, stabilizing the airway and breathing is essential. If there are signs of increased intracranial pressure, such as unresponsiveness with pupillary inequality, bradycardia, and hypertension, hyperventilation and rapid transport for definitive therapy are of utmost importance.

Therapeutic Trial

Because no specific therapy is available for most ataxia, therapy is usually symptomatic. The physician should be able to diagnose treatable conditions and those that need quick intervention, such as hypoglycemia. Neurosurgical consults are indicated in patients with tumors, abscesses, and trauma. Drug screen should guide therapy in case of toxic ingestions, and acute cerebellar ataxia is a diagnosis of exclusion even if a prior antecedent history of a viral illness is present. Psychiatric consultations are indicated in suicide attempts with drug overdose and conversion reaction. Increased intracranial pressure is treated with hyperventilation and mannitol; an immediate neurosurgical consultation should be obtained. Most patients are admitted for diagnostic evaluation. Very close follow-up of the discharged patient should be maintained. Wearing helmets to prevent head injury and physiotherapy may be indicated. Avoid prescribing sedatives, since these can cause an exacerbation of the symptoms.

COMA AND ALTERED MENTAL STATUS

DANIEL J. ISAACMAN

As defined in the superb treatise by Plum and Posner, coma is "the absence of awareness of one's self and one's environment."[24] Because this definition is descriptive, determining that someone is in a coma is generally a function of both their appearance at rest and response to stimulation. A spectrum of alterations in consciousness exists, with a wide variety of terms used to describe the various states. Lethargy is a term describing a reduced wakefulness in which the primary defect is one of attention. Confusion is a state of reduced awareness in which the patient often misrepresents oncoming stimuli, particularly visual ones. Delirium is a more floridly abnormal state characterized by disorientation, fear, irritability, misrepresentation of sensory stimuli, and often visual hallucinations. Obtundation is literally defined as mental blunting, manifested by slow responses to stimuli and often an increase in time asleep. Stupor is a condition of deep sleep from which the patient can be aroused only by vigorous and repeated stimuli. As soon as the stimulus ceases, most stuporous subjects return to an unresponsive state.

Although these terms aid somewhat in the description of a patient's clinical status, several objective scales have been developed that aid in standardizing patient classification. The most widely used scale is the Glasgow Coma Scale (GCS), developed by Jeanette and Teasdale and used internationally since 1976 (see Table 20-1 in Chapter 20). Several advantages make this a useful scale in the emergency setting: (1) It is a practical scale, which can be administered quickly at the bedside; (2) it has good interrater reliability among medical personnel; and (3) it is a reliable barometer of neurologic impairment and an accurate indicator of eventual outcome of head trauma patients. It is important to note that the scale was initially tested on patients seen some 6 hours after head injury and that application of the GCS earlier than that time may be less useful.[25] Application of the GCS in the prehospital setting has not shown the same accuracy as when applied in the emergency department.[26] Although developed for head trauma patients, the GCS is also useful for the classification of nontrauma patients.

Because the GCS requires evaluation of verbal responses, it is not applicable to preverbal children. Several pediatric coma scores have been proposed, but none have gained the widespread acceptance of the GCS.[27-29] Multimodality-evoked potential recordings may serve as a useful adjunct to clinical examinations and other diagnostic aids in predicting outcome.[30]

Pathophysiology

Human consciousness requires neurologic communication between the cerebral cortex and subcortical structures in the diencephalon, midbrain, and upper pons. Superimposed on the higher integrative functions of the cerebral cortex is a physiologic arousal system located in the ascending reticular activating system (ARAS) that maintains behavioral alertness. Transection of the ARAS leads to prolonged unresponsiveness.

Coma is caused by extensive damage either to both cerebral cortices or to the ARAS. Nontraumatic pathways leading to coma include inadequate delivery of a necessary substrate, inadequate removal of a waste product, or production of an exogenous toxin. Nontraumatic categories include anoxic damage, metabolic derangement, hormonal or electrolyte abnormalities, or exogenous toxins.

Both traumatic and nontraumatic causes of coma can cause herniation—displacement or compression of the brain tissue against the dural folds that support it. There are three major loci of herniation. When forces shift supratentorial structures laterally, herniation of the cingulate gyrus may occur under the falx cerebri from one side of the brain to another. Clinical signs, although not uniformly present, include the loss of leg function as a result of compression of one or both anterior cerebral arteries.

The second area of cerebral herniation is at the foramen magnum. In transtentorial or central herniation, the diencephalon (thalamus and hypothalamus) is displaced through the foramen magnum into the posterior fossa with resultant compression and ischemia of the brain stem. Central herniation usually results from increases in intracranial pressure that involve both hemispheres equally. Examples include diffuse cerebral edema or hydrocephalus with third ventricular or aqueductal stenosis. Mass lesions confined to a single hemisphere can also lead to central herniation as

TABLE 56-1. Clinical Signs in Transtentorial (Central) Herniation

Stage	Respiratory pattern	Pupillary size reactivity	Eye movements	Motor changes
Diencephalic	Cheyne-Stokes	Small, reactive	Full doll's eyes Normal caloric testing	Normal
Midbrain/Pontine	Central hyperventilation	Midposition, fixed	Dysconjugate or absent	Decerebrate
Medullary	Slow, irregular/apnea	Midposition/dilated, fixed	Absent	Flaccid

TABLE 56-2. Differentiating Characteristics of Structural and Metabolic Coma

Supratentorial lesions	Infratentorial lesions	Toxic, metabolic, or infectious processes
Initial focal signs	Brain stem abnormalities are often initial signs	Confusion/stupor often precede motor signs
Rostrocaudal progression seen	Sudden onset of coma	Symmetrical examination
Asymmetric examination often present early	Cranial nerve abnormalities often seen	Pupillary reactions preserved
	Respiratory pattern often altered	Respiratory rate often altered

forces initially directed laterally become translated in a downward direction. Early symptoms may include headache, vomiting, stiff neck, or head tilt. As herniation progresses, neurologic deterioration becomes pronounced and follows an orderly progression affecting progressively lower brain stem centers. Neurologic deterioration is monitored by following respiratory pattern, pupillary changes, eye movements, and motor changes and is categorized into stages corresponding to the level of brain stem involvement (Table 56-1).

The third and most frequent location for cerebral herniation is at the tentorial edge from the supratentorial to the infratentorial compartment. This type of herniation, commonly referred to as uncal herniation, often occurs as a result of an expanding mass lesion that occupies the middle cranial fossa or parenchyma of the temporal lobe. Medial displacement of the uncus and hippocampal gyrus occurs with encroachment initially on the oculomotor nerve and later on the diencephalon. Clinical signs of uncal herniation include headache and decreased level of consciousness followed by unilateral pupillary dilation, usually on the same side of the expanding lesion. Progression of herniation is heralded by motor impairment of the oculomotor nerve with resultant ptosis and loss of adduction of the ipsilateral eye. Decerebrate posturing or hemiparesis of the contralateral extremities may then occur. Ultimately, uncal herniation syndrome is converted into transtentorial herniation. Dilation of the opposite pupil ensues followed by motor impairment of the ipsilateral side. Terminal events resulting from brain stem compression include altered respirations, bradycardia, systemic hypertension, and respiratory arrest.

Differential Considerations

Although many of the etiologies of coma in the infant and child are similar to that of adults, the relative frequency is somewhat different and a few etiologies are

---

Coma Mnemonic "TIPS from the Vowels (AEIOU)"

Trauma/tumor	Alcohol/Abuse
Insulin and hypoglycemia	Epilepsy/Encephalopathy
Intussusception	Infection/Inborn errors
Poisoning/psychogenic	Opiates
Shock	Uremia

---

unique to this age group. Few authors have attempted to provide data on the frequency of various diagnoses as causes for coma presenting as traumatic or nontraumatic conditions. Reviews show intracranial infection was the most frequent nontraumatic cause of coma, followed by anoxic encephalopathy, status epilepticus, metabolic derangement, and vascular lesions[31,32] (Table 56-2).

To some extent one can still use the adult mnemonic "TIPS from the Vowels" when remembering diagnostic possibilities (see box above). The following purely pediatric diagnoses must be added to this list.

Ingestion, although included in the adult mnemonic, should always be suspected in the young child with an unexplained alteration in consciousness. A complete history of medications in the household should be obtained early in the evaluation of these patients.

Lead encephalopathy continues to be a concern in the pediatric age group, particularly in children living in older buildings where leaded paint may still be present. Children can have rapid rises in blood lead levels by ingesting loose paint chips or by sucking items contaminated with lead paint, dust, and soil. An antecedent history of fatigue, vomiting, or abdominal pain in a child living in an older dwelling should alert the clinician to the possibility of this diagnosis. Occasionally, radiopaque lead chips will be found on abdominal X-ray film. Diagnostic tests include blood lead, free erythrocyte protoporphyrin, and complete blood count. Treatment includes chelation therapy and depends upon lead level and clinical status.

Child abuse must be considered in any child presenting in coma, particularly when there are discrepancies between elements of the history and physical examination. The clinician must thoroughly look for subtle physical signs of trauma including bruising, cranial tenderness or swelling, and retinal hemorrhages.

Reye disease, although decreasing in incidence, is a consideration in any child presenting with a history of pernicious vomiting leading to altered mental status, particularly when there is a history of an antecedent varicella, flulike illness, or aspirin use.[33]

Inborn errors of metabolism should be suspected, particularly when the onset of symptoms are early in life and are characterized by vomiting, seizures, or metabolic acidosis. Urine screens for organic and amino acids are often diagnostic.

Intussusception has been known to present with mental status changes prior to the presentation of abdominal findings.[34,35] If the child is less than 3 years of age with a decreased level of consciousness, this diagnosis should be considered.

Finally, ketotic hypoglycemia, probably the most common cause of hypoglycemia in childhood, is typically overlooked in the differential diagnosis. These children are often young (18 months to 5 years of age), and low birth weight is a common characteristic of affected children. Attacks are episodic, most apt to occur in the morning (after an overnight fast), and frequently are associated with ketonuria. Hypoglycemic episodes respond promptly to the administration of glucose.

The differential diagnosis of altered mental status changes with age. The common diagnostic considerations by age are listed in Table 56-3.

Diagnostic Work-Up

The child with altered mental status arrives at the emergency department at one point of what may be a rapidly evolving process. Although a complete history and physical examination should eventually be performed, the urgency of the situation demands a rapid, organized approach to determine the severity of the situation and to identify rapidly treatable conditions.

Immediate Considerations. The initial approach to the child in coma should be to ensure that the brain is receiving adequate substrate to maintain viability. As with any critically ill patient, the emergency physician must first address the status of the airway, breathing, and circulation (ABCs). Vital signs including temperature, heart rate, blood pressure, respiratory rate, Dextrostix, and Chemstrip should be immediately assessed. If head trauma is suspected, immobilize the cervical spine. The physician must look for signs of increased intracranial pressure or cerebral herniation. Any asymmetry to the examination suggests focal rather than diffuse neurologic disease.

An abbreviated, targeted history is often indicated at this point. The physician should ascertain whether the child

TABLE 56-3. Common Considerations of Altered Mental Status at Various Ages

Infant	Child	Adolescent
Infection	Ingestion	Ingestion,
Inborn error of	Infection	intentional
metabolism	Intussusception	Trauma
Metabolic	Seizure	Drug/alcohol overdose
Abuse	Abuse	

has had any chronic or recent illness, antecedent fever, vomiting, or trauma. An assessment of the rapidity of onset of the change is often helpful. A history of all medications in the household should be obtained.

Secondary Considerations. After initial assessment and stabilization, a more complete history and physical examination should be performed. Four pathophysiologic variables ascertain the nature of the lesion that affects the brain, the functional level of involvement, and the rate and extent of progression of the disease process: the pattern of respiration, the size and reactivity of the pupils, spontaneous and induced eye movements, and motor responses.

Respiratory Pattern. Control of ventilation is governed by centers located in the lower pons and medulla and modulated by cortical centers located mainly in the forebrain. Respiratory abnormalities signify either metabolic derangement or neurologic insult. Several characteristic patterns exist. Posthyperventilation apnea is generally characterized by brief periods of apnea lasting 10 to 30 seconds after voluntary deep breathing. It is generally representative of forebrain lesions.

Cheyne-Stokes respiration is a pattern of breathing in which phases of hyperpnea regularly alternate with apnea. The depth of breathing waxes in a smooth crescendo and wanes in an equally smooth decrescendo after a peak. Cheyne-Stokes respiration usually implies dysfunction of structures deep within both cerebral hemispheres or in the diencephalon. It commonly occurs in metabolic encephalopathy.

Central neurogenic hyperventilation is manifested by sustained regular and rapid respirations in the face of a normal Po_2 and a low Pco_2. This finding is both rare and serious and suggests midbrain dysfunction.

Apneustic breathing is characterized by brief inspiratory pauses lasting 2 to 3 seconds, often alternating with end expiratory pauses. Clinically, this pattern is characteristic of pontine infarction but occasionally can be seen in anoxic encephalopathy or severe meningitis. With lesions lower in the pons or high in the medulla, disorganized clusters of breaths are noted with irregular pauses between them.

Eye Examination. Specific eye findings can define much about the level of the lesion and prognosis. Pupillary size and responsiveness, spontaneous and induced eye movements, and results of funduscopic examination should be noted.

The pupillary reactions, constriction and dilation, are controlled by the sympathetic and parasympathetic nervous system. Because brain stem areas that control con-

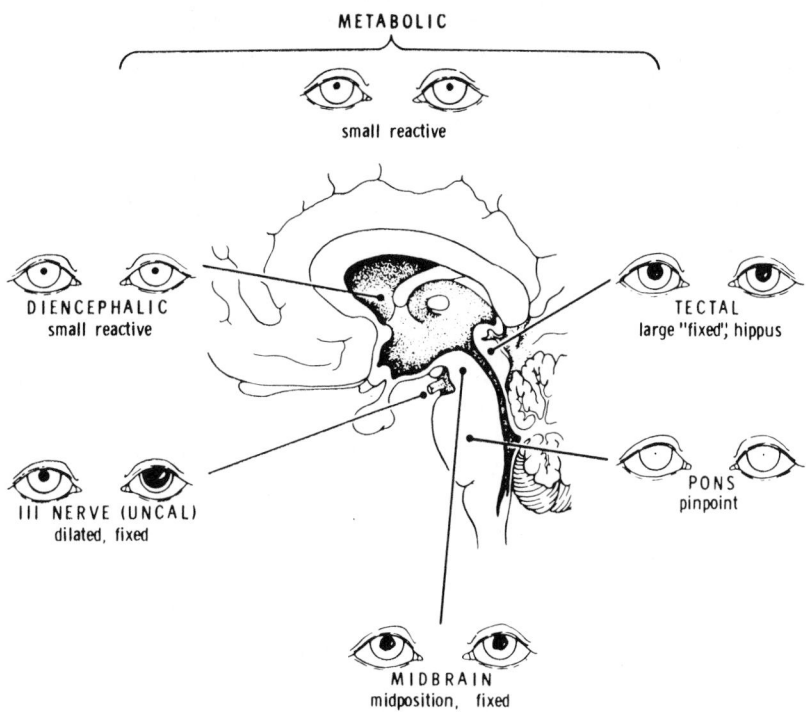

FIG. 56-1. Pupillary abnormalities in the patient with coma. (*From Plum F and Posner J:* The diagnosis of stupor and coma, *Philadelphia, 1980, FA Davis.*)

sciousness are adjacent to those that control the pupils, pupillary changes are often informative. In addition, because pupillary pathways are relatively resistant to metabolic insult, the presence or absence of a light reflex is the single most important physical finding that distinguishes structural from metabolic disease. Most metabolic conditions affecting the central nervous system (CNS) lead to pupils that are constricted but that remain reactive to light. At times the pupils are so small that they appear light fixed, but reactivity is readily apparent when a bright light is used and when the pupils are visualized with a magnifying glass. Pupillary findings are invalid if eye-altering medications have been accidentally ingested or therapeutically administered.

Pupillary responses to structural lesions depend on the site of the primary disturbance and on secondary effects of increased intracranial pressure. Hypothalamic damage usually produces ipsilateral pupillary constriction associated with ptosis and anhidrosis (Horner syndrome). Pupillary function is usually preserved. Horner syndrome is often the first clear sign of impending transtentorial herniation. Uncal herniation is usually heralded by a unilaterally fixed and dilated pupil caused by compression of the oculomotor nerve by the medially displaced uncus of the temporal lobe. Midbrain lesions produce clear cut pupillary findings. Classically, these lesions result in midposition round regular pupils that are light fixed but may spontaneously fluctuate in size (due to sparing of the response to accommodation). Pontine lesions interrupt both the sympathetic and parasympathetic pathways producing small pupils with a preserved response to light that may be difficult to appre-

ciate. Selected pupillary abnormalities are presented in Fig. 56-1.

Funduscopic Examination. A brief funduscopic examination should be performed to assess the presence of papilledema or retinal hemorrhages. Although not generally an early finding, papilledema is suggestive of increased intracranial pressure and merits efforts aimed at its control. Retinal hemorrhages are often the result of shearing forces exerted when young infants are shaken (shaken baby syndrome). Although initially felt to be pathognomonic of child abuse, retinal hemorrhages have also been postulated to result from aggressive resuscitative efforts or extraordinary force.[36-38]

Induced Eye Movements. Two specific eye maneuvers are helpful in evaluating the comatose child. The oculocephalic, or doll's eye reflex, is performed by holding the eyelids open and briskly rotating the head from side to side. This test is contraindicated in any child in whom cervical spine injury is a possibility. The normal, or positive, doll's eye response is conjugate deviation of the eyes contrary to the direction in which the head is turned. The stimulus for this reflex involves either the vestibular system, the proprioceptive afferents in the neck, or possibly both. Various abnormal oculocephalic reflexes are illustrated in Fig. 56-2.

The oculovestibular reflex, better known as caloric testing, is performed by flexing the patient's head to 30 degrees and slowly injecting 50 ml of ice water through a catheter placed in the external auditory canal. This technique causes vestibular stimulation. In the normal awake patient, the response to ice water testing is nystagmus with

CONDITION: OCULAR REFLEXES IN UNCONSCIOUS PATIENTS

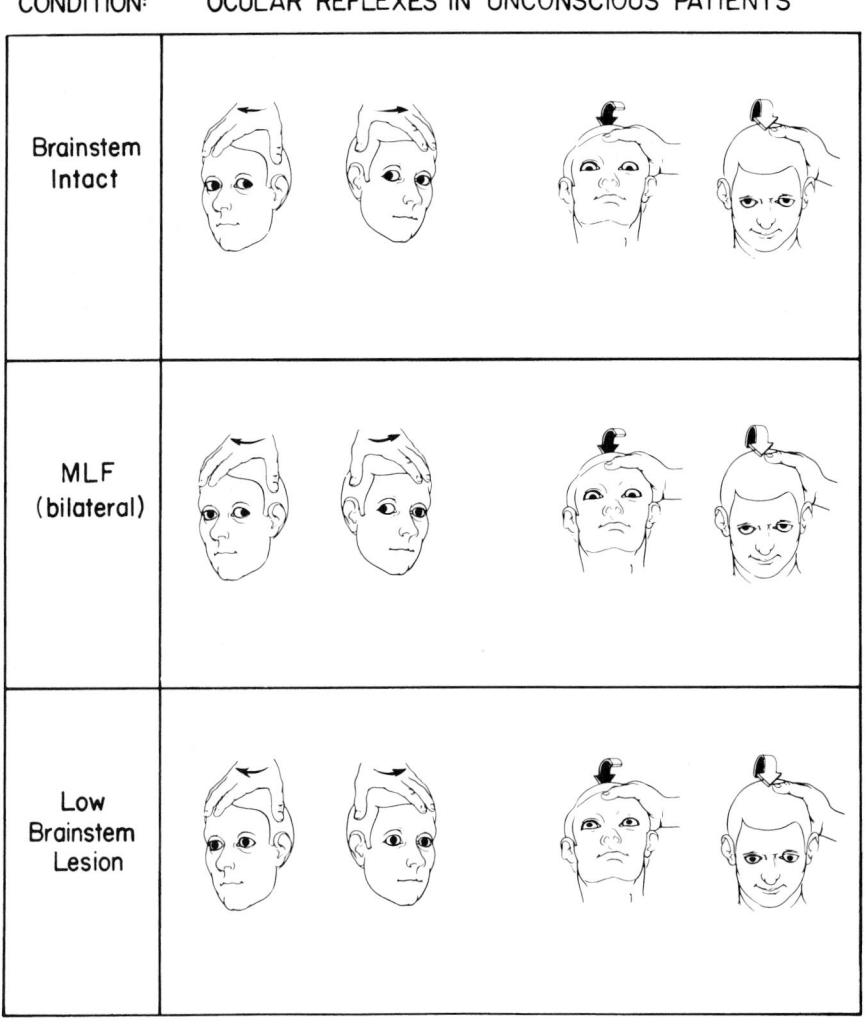

FIG. 56-2. Oculocephalic (doll's eyes) reflexes. (*Adapted from Plum F and Posner J:* The diagnosis of stupor and coma, *Philadelphia, 1980, FA Davis.*)

the slow component toward the irrigated ear and the fast nystagmus away from the irrigated ear. In the unconscious patient whose brain stem is intact, the fast nystagmus is abolished; the eyes move toward the stimulus and remain tonically deviated for a minute or more before slowly returning to the midline. The integrity of this reflex is dependent on the function of the labyrinths, the vestibular nerves and nuclei, the oculomotor nerve, and their connection, the medial longitudinal fasciculus. Because these structures encompass a large portion of the medulla, pons, and midbrain, a normal response indicates that much of the brain stem is intact. Abnormal oculovestibular responses are illustrated in Fig. 56-3.

Conjugate deviation of the eyes at rest is also of great diagnostic significance. With cerebral lesions, conjugate deviation is noted toward the side of the lesion, whereas with brain stem lesions, conjugate deviation is away from the lesion. The setting sun sign, characterized by downward deviation of the eyes, is associated with upper midbrain lesions. Third nerve paralysis generally causes the eyes to point down and out.

Motor Examination. The comatose patient should be evaluated to elicit responses to stimuli, either auditory or physical. Muscle strength, tone, and deep tendon reflexes should be assessed for normality and symmetry. The ability of the patient to localize, as well as the presence or absence of abnormal posturing, also helps in characterizing the severity of involvement. Decorticate posturing (flexion of the upper extremities with extension of the lower extremities) suggests involvement of the cerebral cortex and subcortical white matter with preservation of brain stem function. Decerebrate posturing (rigid extension of the arms and legs) generally represents added brain stem involvement, usually at the level of the pons. Finally the flaccid patient with no response to painful stimuli carries the gravest prognosis and generally has suffered injury deep into the brain stem (Fig. 56-4).

Ancillary Data. Laboratory evaluation of the patient with altered mental status can be divided into the routine and the specific. Patients with altered mental status should undergo blood testing for complete blood count, electrolytes, blood urea nitrogen (BUN), creatinine, and glucose.

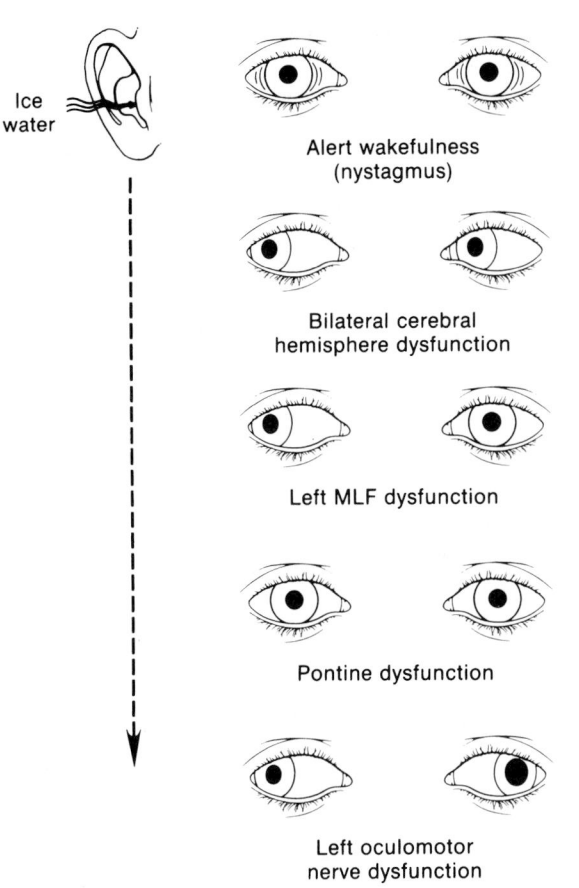

FIG. 56-3. Caloric responses in the unconscious patient. (*Adapted from Plum F and Posner J: The diagnosis of stupor and coma, Philadelphia, 1980, FA Davis.*)

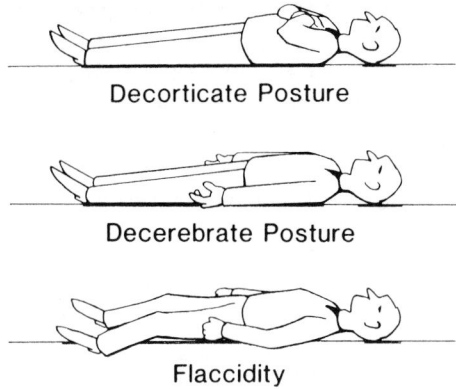

FIG. 56-4. Motor responses in the unconscious patient. (*From Pellock and Meyer: Neurologic emergencies in infancy and childhood, Philadelphia, 1984, Harper and Row.*)

When a metabolic cause for coma is suspected, liver enzymes, ammonia, and toxicology screens should be strongly considered in addition to those routinely done. Arterial blood gases are useful in monitoring the adequacy of ventilation and oxygenation. In the patient who remains an enigma, a stat EEG should be considered because status epilepticus is at times not clinically obvious. Lumbar puncture should confirm clinical suspicion of meningitis provided no signs of increased intracranial pressure are present. Additional laboratory tests to consider when clinically indicated include blood alcohol level, thyroid function tests, free erythrocyte protoporphyrin (FEP), blood lead level, blood culture, skeletal survey, and barium enema (to rule out intussusception).

Prehospital Concerns

Prehospital management of the patient with altered mental status should be directed at assuring adequate delivery of substrate to the brain, providing C-spine immobilization when appropriate, and initiating treatment for suspected increased intracranial pressure.

On arrival at the scene, a quick history should be taken as to rapidity of onset, underlying medical problems, history of fever, ingestion, trauma, or pernicious vomiting. An assessment of the ABCs is made, and C-spine immobilization is provided for patients with suspected traumatic in-

jury. A Dextrostix or Chemstrip should be obtained while IV access is obtained.

Accurate communication with base stations is important in describing the clinical status of the patient. An objective scale such as the GCS or AVPU system (Alert, responds to Verbal stimuli, responds to Painful stimuli, or Unresponsive) should be used to communicate the status of the patient. All too frequently, clinical descriptions such as "comatose, but combative" or "intermittently comatose" are ineffective in transmitting useful information to the base station (see Chapters 19 and 20).

For those patients with suspected metabolic causes for coma, trials of glucose and naloxone can be attempted while en route to the hospital. Glucose (50% dextrose) should be given at the dose of 1 gm/kg, and naloxone should be administered at an initial dose of 0.1 mg/kg up to 2 mg IV. Flumazenil, a benzodiazepine antagonist, is indicated in the patient with a known or suspected ingestion of benzodiazepines. It should not be administered indiscriminately to all patients with altered mental status because it is known to produce refractory seizures in those with a preexisting seizure disorder.[39] Patients whose mental status improves and subsequently deteriorates may require repeated doses or a continuous maintenance infusion. Patients suspected of having increased intracranial pressure should be hyperventilated gently to achieve Pco_2 lower than 35 mm Hg while en route to the hospital. If transport time will be greater than 15 minutes and physician back-up is available, consideration should be given to measures to decrease intracranial pressure, such as mannitol and positioning.

Therapeutic Trial

Guided by results of the initial history and physical examination, the emergency physician must first address life-threatening concerns while pursuing a definitive diagnosis. After assessment of the ABCs, dextrostix, chemstrip, and C-spine immobilization, the physician must turn attention to assessment and treatment of possible increased intracranial pressure or cerebral herniation. Suspected increased intracranial pressure should be managed with oxygenation and hyperventilation to a target Pco_2 of 30 to 35

Management of the Child with Altered Mental Status

1. Stabilize airway, breathing, and circulatory status. Cardiorespiratory and oximetry monitors.
2. Draw baseline laboratories and Dextrostix.
3. Assess for evidence of herniation.
4. Assess/treat evidence of increased intracranial pressure.
   a. Hyperventilation (target P_{CO_2} 30-35 mm Hg)
   b. IV mannitol (0.5-1 gm/kg)
   c. +/− Dexamethasone (0.5-1.0 gm/kg)
   d. Consider need for intracranial monitoring.
5. Evaluate for signs of meningitis. Lumbar puncture indicated for suspected infection without signs of increased intracranial pressure. If any evidence of increased intracranial pressure, perform CT scan to document safety of procedure.
6. Evaluate for focal deficit. If focal deficit present, CT scan is indicated.
7. Administer trials of glucose (1 gm/kg) and naloxone (0.1 mg/kg) sequentially.
8. Evaluate and treat for possible toxic ingestion.
9. Consider stat EEG for undiagnosed patients.
10. Place indwelling catheter.
11. Transfer to intensive care unit.

---

mm Hg. Although hyperventilation is rapidly effective in lowering intracranial pressure, experimental data suggest that its effects are transient. Often an osmotic diuretic such as mannitol (0.5 g to 1.0 g/kg) is indicated for brain swelling. When osmotic diuretics are used, one must monitor urine output, serum osmolarity, and serum electrolytes. Corticosteroids, although controversial, are an additional adjunct. Dexamethasone at a dose of 0.5 to 1 mg/kg is most effective in controlling intracranial pressure related to CNS tumors. Its effects are generally not seen for 24 hours and its efficacy in the setting of head injuries is controversial.[40-43] If dexamethasone is used, care must be taken to monitor potential deleterious side effects such as the development of gastric ulceration (see box above).

After concerns about intracranial pressure are addressed, other rapidly remediable diagnoses must be considered. A review of all possible toxic exposures should be undertaken, and consideration given to administration of appropriate antidotes. Concerns about intracranial infection should then be addressed. A search for unsuspected traumatic injury should also be performed. Focal abnormalities or signs of increased intracranial pressure generally mandate a CT scan once the patient is stabilized.

A recent retrospective review by Davis suggested no intracranial injuries in 49 children with GCS of 15 who had normal neurologic examinations and no evidence for basilar or depressed skull fractures.[44] In a study of children with coagulopathies who experienced head trauma, Dietrich found no CT scan abnormalities in the absence of alterations in mental status or focal neurologic deficit.[45] Further studies are indicated to define the clinical significance of these findings.

Patients with suspected increased intracranial pressure and intracranial infection should be treated presumptively for infection before lumbar puncture is performed and after a blood culture is obtained, rather than risk precipitating herniation.

When increased intracranial pressure is a concern, it should be monitored. Insertion of an intracranial pressure monitor provides a guide to therapeutic decisions.[46,47] If intracranial pressure remains elevated despite these measures, patients should be sedated and paralyzed for optimal control. In addition, the induction of barbiturate coma may be necessary.[48-50] This mode of therapy should only be implemented in an intensive care setting where central venous pressure monitoring is available.

Prognosis

In general, the prognosis of the pediatric coma patient is much better than adult counterparts. Particularly in relation to traumatic etiologies, age appears to be a major independent factor affecting both mortality and morbidity.[51-53] Bruce[54] suggested that the child's brain shows a different pathophysiologic response to injury than the adult as evidenced by the differences in the vascular response to brain injury.

At this time, no scale has been developed that can successfully separate children destined to a uniformly good prognosis from those destined to severe morbidity. Predictors suggestive of poor outcome from traumatic coma include the GCS < 9, age less than 2, and the presence of skull fracture.[55]

The best early predictors appear to be the postresuscitation GCS as well as the findings on CT scan. Bilateral swelling with or without midline shift appears to be related to poor outcome as does the presence of a mass lesion.[56]

Choi documented that a significant proportion of children continuously improve during the first 6 months after head injury. Outcomes tend to stabilize at this point, suggesting that the 6-month response may be a good predictor of ultimate disability and the appropriate end point for clinical trials in severe head injury.[57]

The long-term outcome for children discharged from the hospital in a persistently vegetative state is poor. Forty percent of such patients die, and at best, children show only minimal awareness after an average of 4½ years.[58]

Predictors found by Margolis and Shaywitz to be suggestive of a less than normal outcome in nontraumatic cases include anoxia as a cause of coma, elevated intracranial pressure of greater than 2 days duration, and deep coma of greater than 2 weeks duration.[59]

Guidelines for determination of brain death in children outlined by the American Academy of Pediatrics Task Force involve an observation period of a minimum of 24 hours for children less than 1 year and 12 hours for children older than 1 year.[60] Thus the diagnosis of brain death is not appropriate in the emergency setting. The emergency physician must gather a complete history to ensure the absence of remediable or reversible conditions, which may influence physical examination findings. Especially important are detections of toxic and metabolic disorders, sedative-hypnotic drugs, paralytic agents, hypothermia, hypotension, and surgically remediable conditions.

Until better predictive models are developed, one needs to be cautiously optimistic about the potential for recovery in most children presenting with altered mental status.

HEADACHE

RAYMOND B. KARASIC

Headache is defined as pain involving the scalp, skull, or intracranial contents. It is a common pediatric symptom with a wide spectrum of severity and clinical significance. Because children less than 5 years rarely have headaches, an organic etiology is highly likely. Although headaches in children, as in adults, are often mild and self-limited, on occasion the symptom can be a harbinger of a serious underlying condition. Fortunately, a carefully performed history and physical examination are the only tools needed to make an accurate diagnosis.

Pathophysiology

Headache can arise from any of the pain-sensitive structures of the head or neck. Intracranial structures that are sensitive to pain include large arteries and veins; the dura at the base of the skull; cranial nerves V, VII, and X; and the upper cervical nerves. Pain-sensitive extracranial structures include the eyes and orbits, ears and mastoid air cells, nose and paranasal sinuses, teeth and oropharynx, scalp, neck, and cervical spine. The brain, skull, most of the dura, and the ependymal lining of the ventricles are insensitive to pain. Pain originating from intracranial structures above the tentorium is referred to the front of the head, whereas pain arising from the posterior fossa is referred to the back of the head or neck.[61,62]

Diagnostic Considerations

A useful way of classifying headaches is by their pathophysiologic mechanism and diagnostic considerations (see box at right).[62,63]

Inflammatory Headache. The most serious inflammatory processes causing headache are meningitis and encephalitis, which require prompt diagnosis and rapid initiation of antimicrobial therapy if a bacterial etiology is suspected or cannot be ruled out. Patients with CNS infection typically have fever and an altered level of consciousness (lethargy or irritability); nuchal rigidity and other signs of meningeal irritation may be present, although these signs are less reliable in infants. The diagnosis of meningitis must be confirmed by examination of the CSF (see p. 1000).

Fever is a common cause of headache. The headaches associated with fever tend to be frontal or bitemporal and have a throbbing, vascular quality.

Infection of the paranasal sinuses is a recognized cause of headache, the location of which usually relates to the specific sinus involved. Maxillary sinusitis typically causes facial pain rather than headache, whereas sphenoid sinusitis classically produces occipital pain and ethmoid sinusitis results in eyeball pain.[64] In the absence of fever or prolonged respiratory symptoms, frontal headache in young

---

Headache Diagnostic Considerations

Infection/inflammation
Meningitis/encephalitis
Sinusitis
Abscess, cerebral
Dental abscess

Vascular
Migraine
Cluster
Subarachnoid or cerebral bleed
Hypertensive encephalopathy

Functional
Tension
Conversion reaction
Depression

Trauma
Postconcussive
Subdural
Fracture

Intoxication
Carbon monoxide
Lead

Neoplasm
Cerebral
Cerebellar
Pseudotumor cerebri

Autoimmune
Temporal arteritis
Trigeminal neuralgia

Miscellaneous
Eye: glaucoma, refractive error
Epilepsy
High altitude
Temporomandibular joint (TMJ) disease
Status-post lumbar puncture

---

children (whose frontal sinuses have not pneumatized) should not be attributed to sinusitis. Sinus x-ray studies and occasionally CT scans are required for definitive diagnosis (see Chapter 49).

Dental infections are often accompanied by headache. In most cases the headache is accompanied by localized symptoms (tooth pain and temperature sensitivity) and signs of dental disease.

Vascular Headaches. Vascular headaches result from dilation of pain-sensitive blood vessels. The hallmark of such headaches is their pulsatile, throbbing quality. Vascular headaches can represent a primary derangement (e.g., migraine) or may be secondary to an underlying pathologic process (e.g., hypertension or hypoxia).

Migraine headaches are relatively common in children. The most distinctive, although not the most common, presentation is the classic migraine, characterized by an aura, transient neurologic symptoms, unilateral throbbing headache, nausea, vomiting, and usually a family history of migraine. The most prevalent type of migraine in children is the common migraine, which lacks an aura and tends to cause bilateral head pain, often associated with nausea and vomiting.[65] Other forms of migraine (confusional, hemiplegic, ophthalmoplegic, vertebrobasilar) can also occur; these entities are discussed in more detail in a later section.

Cluster headaches, although rare in children, are paroxysmal and unilateral in presentation. The headache tends to be retroorbital, periorbital, or frontal. Unilateral autonomic symptoms may develop including nasal stuffiness, lacrimation, or Horner syndrome. The headaches tend to cluster in short periods of time separated by long pain-free intervals; discomfort lasts for 30 to 120 minutes but may occur several times in a 24-hour period, and is not associated with an aura.[62,64]

Traction Headache. Traction on pain-sensitive structures can be produced directly by mass lesions or indirectly by any process causing increased intracranial pressure. These headaches tend to be daily and progressive, occur most often in the morning, and are exacerbated by coughing or straining (Valsalva maneuver).[63] The major categories of mass lesions in children include neoplasm, hematoma, arteriovenous malformation, and brain abscess. In addition to mass lesions, the principal causes of increased intracranial pressure are hemorrhage, hydrocephalus and cerebral edema (including pseudotumor cerebri).[62,63] Because of the nature of the underlying disease processes, traction headaches represent true emergencies that demand prompt diagnosis and institution of treatment.

Tension or Muscle Contraction Headache. "Tension" headaches are common in children and result from sustained contraction of scalp or neck muscles. The pain, which is located in the back of the head or neck, is constant and generally has a squeezing, bandlike quality. In many patients the symptom can be attributed to fatigue, a chronically stressful environment, or a particular life event. Psychiatric problems such as conversion reaction and depression may also be causative.[62,63,65]

Trauma. After head trauma, some patients experience headaches or other vague symptoms for variable periods of time. Such postconcussive headaches are often described as "dull" and "achy" but sometimes have a throbbing, vascular quality. Posttraumatic headaches must be distinguished from true intracranial complications of head trauma (e.g., subdural hematoma).[64]

Intoxication/Toxins. Carbon monoxide intoxication may cause headache, weakness, and dizziness. The poisoning may progress to seizures and coma. A carboxyhemoglobin level should be measured, since these symptoms may occur even with mild elevations. Lead intoxication often caused by pica may lead to a diffuse and persistent headache. Headaches can also occur secondary to drugs and food additives. Among the most commonly implicated are alcohol, nitrites (in cured meat), and monosodium glutamate (MSG).[64]

Miscellaneous. Eye strain and other ocular disturbances may be an infrequent cause of headache in children. Clinicians should consider this diagnosis in patients who have an identifiable ophthalmologic problem (e.g., refractive error) and whose headaches are relieved by correction of the underlying abnormality. Epilepsy may cause paroxysmal headaches with an abrupt termination. Temporal arteritis and trigeminal neuralgia may also be associated with headaches. High altitude sickness may cause a diffuse headache with increasing altitude; relief usually occurs with return to lower altitudes. Temporomandibular joint (TMJ) disease discomfort and headache are usually exacerbated by chewing or teeth clenching.[62-64,66]

Diagnostic Work-Up

The key to making an accurate diagnosis of headache is a detailed history. The child's headache should be characterized in terms of its quality, location, chronology, change in symptoms or severity, progression, associated symptoms, and factors that relieve or worsen the headache. The quality or character of the headache (pounding, squeezing, aching) is best determined by questioning the child directly, using understandable terms and providing appropriate examples. A pulsatile or throbbing headache generally indicates a vascular etiology, whereas a constant, squeezing headache suggests muscle contraction as the mechanism.

The location of the headache and the pattern of radiation can provide clues to the diagnosis, but are generally not as discriminating as other aspects of the history. For example, frontal headache can result from a variety of mechanisms, including inflammatory processes, vascular events (e.g., migraine), traction from a mass lesion, or muscle contraction. Additional information from the history or physical examination is needed to refine the list of diagnostic possibilities (Table 56-4).

The chronologic features of the headache (onset, frequency, duration, pattern) are extremely important in determining its etiology. Headaches associated with mass lesions tend to be most prominent upon wakening, tension headaches typically occur later in the day (and more often on weekdays than on weekends), and migraines frequently have an identifiable "trigger" event (e.g., head trauma, fatigue). Chronic headaches that occur with increasing frequency and intensity over time suggest the presence of a progressive intracranial process, such as a mass lesion or hydrocephalus. In contrast, acute, recurrent headaches are more likely to represent migraine or some other paroxysmal disorder.

Most headache syndromes have associated symptoms that can help pinpoint the diagnosis. The child or parent should be queried about fever and other symptoms indicating the presence of a specific inflammatory process. Information should be sought about visual or other neurologic symptoms; transient symptoms are most compatible with a migrainous disorder, whereas a fixed or progressive neurologic deficit, such as a gait disturbance, suggests a mass lesion or other intracranial pathology. Vomiting associated with headache should always be taken seriously; although this combination can be seen with migraine disorders and a variety of minor illnesses (e.g., viral gastritis, streptococcal pharyngitis), the possibility of increased intracranial pressure must also be considered.

Additional information that should be elicited from the history includes precipitating factors (e.g., coughing, stress,

TABLE 56-4. Differentiation of Headache Type by Signs and Symptoms

	Type of headache
Associated events	
Abrupt onset	Convulsive
Afternoon	Muscle contraction
Present on arising	Convulsive (following nocturnal seizure), emotional depression, traction (tumor), vascular
Preceded by aura	Convulsive, vascular (migraine)
Exacerbated by coughing	Paranasal sinus, traction (tumor, increased intracranial pressure), vascular
Followed by lethargy	Convulsive, vascular
Followed by focal CNS deficit	Convulsive (Todd's paresis), traction (tumor), vascular (hemiplegic migraine)
Related to posture	Posttraumatic, traction (tumor and following lumbar puncture)
Related to stress	Muscle contraction, vascular (migraine)
Nausea and vomiting	Migraine, convulsive, traction (tumor)
Character of pain	
Steady	Emotional depression, muscle contraction, sinus, traction (tumor, increased intracranial pressure)
Throbbing	Convulsive, posttraumatic, traction (tumor, increased intracranial pressure), vascular (migraine, vasculitis, inflammatory)
Location	
Frontal	Traction (supratentorial tumor), vascular
Occipital and neck	Muscle contraction, sinus (ethmoid), traction (posterior fossa tumor)
Unilateral	Traction (lateralized supratentorial tumor), vascular (migraine)

From Kriel RL: Headache. In Swaiman KF and Wright FS, editors: *The practice of pediatric neurology,* ed 2, vol 1, St. Louis, 1982, Mosby.

medications, foods, sleep deprivation, menses), antecedent trauma, medications used (and which ones relieve the headache), environmental exposures (e.g., carbon monoxide), underlying medical problems (e.g., hypertension), recognized stressors, and family history of headaches.

The initial goal of the physical examination in patients with headache is to identify or rule out serious conditions requiring immediate treatment, such as infections of the CNS, severe hypertension, mass lesions, or increased intracranial pressure. Accordingly a complete set of vital signs, including temperature and blood pressure, must be obtained. Patients should be evaluated for signs of meningeal irritation, as evidenced by nuchal rigidity or a positive Brudzinski's or Kernig's sign. A careful ophthalmologic examination, including measurement of visual acuity, should be performed; retinal hemorrhages are a clue to the diagnosis of a subarachnoid hemorrhage, whereas papilledema generally indicates the presence of increased intracranial pressure. The cornerstone of the physical examination is a thorough neurologic examination, including evaluation of the cranial nerves, muscle strength and tone, deep tendon reflexes, plantar responses, gait, cerebellar and posterior column function, and sensation.

Once life-threatening processes have been ruled out, the remainder of the physical examination should focus on identifying specific illnesses (e.g., dental infection) that may be responsible for the patient's headache. It is essential to consider organic etiologies in children under 5 years who present with headaches.[62,66,67]

Ancillary Data. In many patients with headache, the diagnosis is apparent from the history and physical examination alone and laboratory studies are unnecessary. In other individuals, specific tests (e.g., lumbar puncture, dental x-ray films, throat culture) may be useful for confirming the diagnosis of an underlying condition.

A CT scan should be performed in any patient who has evidence of a mass lesion, hydrocephalus, hemorrhage, or other intracranial pathology or has a history of recent significant trauma. MRI scan is an alternative technique that appears to be more sensitive than the CT scan for detecting intracranial lesions in the temporal lobe and posterior fossa. Despite the enormous value of these imaging techniques, they should be used selectively and not routinely.

Prehospital Considerations

Because the diagnosis of headache is generally not apparent before medical evaluation, the prehospital management of patients with headache is primarily supportive. Careful administration of intravenous fluids may be indicated for the treatment of vomiting; analgesics should be considered in patients with severe pain.

Therapeutic Trial

When headache is caused by an identifiable underlying process, therapy should be directed at that condition. For example, headaches resulting from hypertension are treated primarily with antihypertensive medication, whereas headaches caused by sinusitis require antimicrobial therapy. The treatment of migraine headaches is discussed in a later section.

Rest and analgesics, including acetaminophen and nonsteroidal antiinflammatory drugs (NSAIDs), are useful for the symptomatic relief of headache. The choice, route, and dose should be appropriate for the patient's age and degree of pain.[63,64] Medication for migraine headaches is discussed in a later section.

MOVEMENT DISORDERS

SUSAN M. FUCHS

A variety of disorders cause abnormal muscular movements on an involuntary basis. Clinically and emotionally these require definition and evaluation (see section on Paralysis and Hemiplegia).

Chorea is a quick, random jerk of a part of the body. Any body part can be included, but the limbs are most commonly affected.[68,69] Sydenham chorea, which may occur months after streptococcal pharyngitis, is one of the major Jones' criteria for the diagnosis of rheumatic fever (see box on p. 665). Huntington chorea is an autosomal-dominant disease that usually manifests in later years of life and is associated with dementia.[69] However, the juvenile form, characterized by rigidity, occurs in 10% of patients and begins in childhood.[70] Chorea may be a presenting or prominent symptom in many other genetic disorders. Chorea can be induced by drugs (anticonvulsants, oral contraceptives, psychotropic agents, stimulants, and antiemetics) and has been seen in thyrotoxicosis and lupus erythematosus.[68,69]

Athetosis is a slow, irregular writhing movement of the extremities.[68,69] It is associated with perinatal injury including hypoxia, ischemia, and kernicterus. Choreoathetosis may be due to infectious diseases including meningitis and viral encephalitis or metabolic disorders such as phenylketonuria, porphyria, and Wilson disease.[68,69]

Ballismus is an irregular, violent hurling or flailing of one limb (monoballismus); ipsilateral upper and lower extremity (hemiballismus); or both limbs (biballismus).[71] This disorder is associated with infectious etiologies including viral encephalitis or a stroke involving the subthalamic nucleus.[69,71]

Dystonia is a disorder of the basal ganglia characterized by an abnormal posture of the body with or without a facial grimace, the result of the simultaneous contraction of agonist and antagonist muscles, which can affect the limbs, trunk, or face. The involvement of a single body part is called focal dystonia; a single limb and adjacent trunk, segmental dystonia; and limbs and face, generalized dystonia.[68] These movements tend to be exacerbated by stress and disappear during sleep.[70] Focal dystonias include blepharospasm and writer's cramp. Dystonia musculorum deformans (primary torsion dystonia) is a genetically based focal dystonia that progresses to a generalized dystonia without intellectual deterioration. Progressive dystonia with seizures and coma may be an indication of several metabolic disorders including aminoacidopathies, such as phenylketonuria, and organicacidopathies.[70] Acquired dystonias can result from trauma, infections, intoxication (carbon monoxide), hypoxic-ischemic encephalopathy, tumors, and hydrocephalus.[68-70] Focal or generalized dystonia can be induced by haloperidol, phenothiazines, and metoclopramide (Reglan).[68-70]

Torticollis is an abnormal tilt of the head and neck. In a fixed torticollis, the neck cannot be moved back to the neutral position and should prompt investigation of the cervical spine. Nonfixed torticollis usually occurs with benign paroxysmal torticollis or familial paroxysmal choreoathetosis.[68] Paroxysmal infantile torticollis consists of intermittent episodes of torticollis that last for minutes to hours and may recur for weeks or months. This should not be confused with Sandifer syndrome, which is associated with gastroesophageal reflux. Infants and children with this disorder have intermittent or persistent torticollis, retrocollis, or even opisthotonus, behavioral irritability often associated with feeding, which may result in failure to thrive.[70]

Myoclonus involves involuntary, rapid jerks of any body part due to muscle contractions. They can be symmetric or asymmetric, rhythmic, focal, or generalized. They can be activated by visual or tactile stimuli (reflex myoclonus) or purposeful movements (action myoclonus). Physiologic (benign) myoclonus may occur during sleep (nocturnal or sleep myoclonus) and consists of jerking of the legs. This may be difficult to distinguish from juvenile myoclonic epilepsy (of Janz), which consists of myoclonic movements upon awakening that may occur before the onset of seizures.[70] Essential myoclonus may be familial (autosomal dominant), which involves movements of the face, trunk, and proximal muscles, and begins in childhood. Symptomatic myoclonus is usually a symptom of an underlying neurologic disease such as a lysosomal storage disease, aminoacidopathy, metabolic encephalopathy, or degenerative diseases. It can be toxin-, anoxia-, or trauma-induced; infection-mediated (viral encephalopathy); or due to a brain stem or spinal cord lesion.[68,69] Myoclonic encephalopathy of infancy (myoclonus-opsoclonus) consists of severe jerking of the head and trunk with rapid fluttering eye movement in all directions. This may be a form of encephalitis, from which most infants recover; however, some have persistent ataxia and recurrence during subsequent illnesses.[70] Another important cause of myoclonus-opsoclonus in infants and children is an occult neuroblastoma or ganglioneuroblastoma.[70]

Tics or habit spasms are stereotyped, quick, and purposeless movements or utterances not associated with an impairment of consciousness. Face, neck, and shoulders are commonly involved.[68,69,71] Tics increase in frequency when the patient is under stress or excited. A simple motor tic occurs in 10% of children and may last for up to 1 year. Complex tics are a combination of verbal and motor tics that tend to be chronic. Tourette syndrome is an inherited (autosomal dominant) complex tic, which includes movements of the facial muscles, hopping, truncal or pelvic gyrations, and vocalizations including grunts, snorts, barks, and occasionally obscenities.[69,71]

Tremors are involuntary, rhythmic oscillations that usually affect the hands. Essential (familial) tremor is inherited as an autosomal-dominant trait, which occurs only in a limb being used (action tremor). Its onset is usually in adulthood. A postural tremor (physiologic tremor) occurs when the patient extends the arms forward and can be enhanced by exercise, fatigue, stress, or drugs (xanthines, methylprednisone, nicotine, thyroid hormone); it often occurs with hyperthyroidism.[68,69]

Spasmus nutans is episodic abnormal head posturing and nodding associated with nystagmus, which occurs in infants 4 to 12 months of age and then resolves spontaneously.[71]

Parkinsonism consists of tremor, rigidity, bradykinesia, and abnormal posture. Although uncommon in children, it may be a component of other inherited neurologic disorders or may be idiopathic.[70]

Pathophysiology

All of the involuntary movement disorders mentioned here are thought to originate in the basal ganglia. The basal ganglia include the caudate, putamen, subthalamic nucleus, globus pallidus, and substantia nigra. These structures are also known as the extrapyramidal system. They connect with each other as well as with the cerebral cortex, thalamus, and cerebellum through numerous pathways. Excitatory and inhibitory effects are associated with neurotransmitters including acetylcholine, serotonin, dopamine, gamma-aminobutyric acid (GABA), glutamate, substance P, and enkephalins.[69] Recent advances in the treatment of some movement disorders are due to pharmacologic agents that affect the actions and concentration of these neurotransmitters.

Diagnostic Considerations

One of the most difficult decisions is whether the abnormal movement represents a movement disorder or a focal seizure. Some helpful clues include the following: (1) involuntary movements usually disappear during sleep, seizures do not; (2) movement disorders do not produce a loss of consciousness; (3) movement disorders are more stereotyped than seizures; and (4) an EEG performed during an abnormal movement will be normal.[69]

Diagnostic Work-Up

Observing a patient is the best way to classify a movement disorder. Since these movements are paroxysmal, a videotape may be necessary.

A movement disorder may be acute or insidious. Sometimes the disorder is mistaken for clumsiness or is masked by the child's attempt to hide it. The age at onset is important, since movement disorders can be due to birth trauma, progressive degenerative diseases, infections, or drugs.

Most movement disorders will worsen or become more prominent during stressful or anxiety-provoking situations. Because many of these disorders are inherited, they may be the initial manifestation of the disease or may progress with the underlying disease.

An antecedent history of a sore throat (even months prior to the episode) in a child with chorea can suggest the diagnosis of Sydenham chorea. Although a documented history of streptococcal pharyngitis would confirm the diagnosis, one must consider rheumatic fever if other symptoms and laboratory findings (Jones' criteria) are present. Because many of the movement disorders may be manifestations of viral encephalitides, an antecedent history of a viral illness is also important to elicit. Underlying disorders (e.g., liver or renal disease), vitamin deficiencies, lupus erythematosus, and pregnancy may manifest as movement disorders.

Many inherited metabolic disorders (e.g., phenylketonuria, Wilson disease) may present with a movement disorder. Chorea can be due to many acquired metabolic disorders including hypocalcemia, hypoglycemia, hypomagnesemia, and hypernatremia. Endocrinologic disorders such as thyrotoxicosis, hypoparathyroidism, and Addison disease can also cause chorea or tremors.[69,71]

Both toxic exposure as well as therapeutic use of medications (i.e., phenothiazines, haloperidol, and metoclopramide) can cause drug-induced movement disorders.

Inquire about the birth history, since athetosis is associated with hypoxia, ischemia, and kernicterus, which can occur in the perinatal period; choreiform or dystonic movements of children with cerebral palsy may be related to perinatal problems.

A normal developmental history followed by a gradual loss of milestones should prompt investigation for a genetic/metabolic disorder. Failure to thrive with recurrent torticollis and behavioral irritability with or without vomiting can provide clues to the presence of Sandifer syndrome.

Emotional lability may be a manifestation of Sydenham and Huntington chorea. In some cases, a tremor is the first manifestation of hysteria.[71]

It is extremely important to ask about other family members who may have movement disorders, since many of these disorders are inherited.

The key to diagnosis is to witness the movement disorder and describe it specifically. The finding of an injected pharynx, enlarged thyroid gland or Kayser-Fleischer rings (Wilson disease), or optic atrophy (Hallervorden-Spatz syndrome) may provide clues as to the underlying disorder. A stiff neck or meningismus should prompt evaluation for viral encephalitis. The presence of hypertrophied muscles, especially of the lower limbs, may be found in torsion dystonia.[70]

Since chorea can be a manifestation of rheumatic fever, the heart should be examined for evidence of murmurs, clicks, or rubs. The presence of jaundice, hepatomegaly, or other evidence of hepatic failure should suggest Wilson disease.

It is important to look for other specific neurologic manifestations of the underlying process including dysarthria, incoordination, weakness, hypotonia (chorea), or oculogyric crisis (drug-induced dystonia). It is imperative to make a distinction between ataxia and incoordination of gait due to a movement disorder, since ataxia implies a very different list of potential diagnoses.

Specific tests to elicit the presence of chorea include the milkmaid sign (the patient is unable to maintain a tight grip on the examiner's fingers), the pronator test (the patient's palms face outward when the hands are held over the head), and "spooning" (wrist flexion and hyperextension of the metacarpophalangeal joints when the arms and hands are extended).[69]

Ancillary Data. Laboratory studies performed should be based upon the specific movement disorder. Appropriate studies include electrolytes, glucose, BUN, creatinine, calcium, magnesium, liver functions, thyroid functions, copper, ceruloplasmin levels, toxicology screens, and urine for amino and organic acids.

Documentation of a streptococcal infection should include a throat culture, antistreptolysin O (ASO), titer, and sedimentation rate. Since an elevated ASO titer can also occur in lupus erythematosus, other antibody tests such as anti-DNase B and antinuclear antibody (ANA) should be ordered.

If an infectious etiology is considered, appropriate blood cultures or viral titers should be ordered. If viral encephalitis is a possibility, a lumbar puncture should be performed assuming there is no evidence of increased intracranial pressure.

Imaging studies should be directed by the differential diagnosis. A child with torticollis may warrant a radiograph of the cervical spine, whereas if a tumor, arteriovenous malformation, or stroke is suspected, a CT scan or MRI scan of the head should be obtained. Further imaging of the paraspinal region or abdomen is appropriate for an infant with myoclonus-opsoclonus. If the movement disorder may potentially be a seizure, an EEG should be obtained. An esophageal pH probe and esophagram to document gastroesophageal reflux are diagnostic for infants with Sandifer syndrome.[70]

Prehospital Considerations

Since the diagnosis of a movement disorder involves a long differential, attention should be directed toward the ABCs. If there is a history of trauma in a child with torticollis, the child should be immobilized on a backboard, with the head and neck in the position favored by the child.

Therapeutic Trial

Since movement disorders encompass a wide variety of diseases, therapeutic trials should be based on the specific diagnosis and consultation with a neurologist. However, specific emergency therapy for dystonia due to phenothiazines includes the use of diphenhydramine (Benadryl) 1 mg/kg/dose given IV, IM, or PO or benztropine (Cogentin) 1 to 2 mg IM.

PARALYSIS AND HEMIPLEGIA

SUSAN M. FUCHS

Paralysis implies a loss of function, whereas paresis is a partial or complete weakness. The areas affected are differentiated as paraplegia, affecting the lower half of the body; hemiplegia, affecting one side; and quadriplegia, affecting all limbs.

Pathophysiology

Acute onset of any of these neurologic deficits is a true emergency. Quadriplegia or paraplegia of an acute onset usually indicates a spinal cord lesion, whereas hemiplegia indicates brain involvement.[72] Peripheral nerve involvement can also result in paraplegia; however, the course as well as findings on neurologic examination will help identify spinal origin. Because neuromuscular disorders can cause weakness in both patterns, it is important to localize the level of involvement. The neuromuscular system has two parts: the upper motor neuron, which arises in the cerebral cortex and traverses the brain stem and spinal cord, and the lower motor unit, which includes the lower motor neuron (anterior horn cells), the neuromuscular junction, and the skeletal muscle[72] (Table 56-5).

TABLE 56-5. Upper Motor Neuron vs. Motor Unit Differences

Finding	Upper motor neuron	Motor unit (lower motor neuron, neuromuscular junction, and muscle)
Muscles affected	Muscle groups	Individual muscles or groups
Reflexes	Increased	Decreased or absent
Tone	Increased	Decreased
Fasciculations	Absent	Present
Atrophy	Absent or minimal	Present

Modified from Rodenberg M, Gratton M, Bennett J, et al: *Ann Emerg Med* 20:672, 1991.

Etiology of Paraplegia in Childhood

Trauma: spinal cord fracture, dislocation
Vascular: occlusion—anterior spinal artery anomaly—arteriovenous malformation
Tumor: ependymoma, astrocytoma, neuroblastoma
Infection: epidural abscess, osteomyelitis, diskitis
Miscellaneous: transverse myelitis, poliomyelitis, Guillain-Barré syndrome, botulism, tick paralysis, heavy metals, myasthenia gravis, dyskalemic paralysis
Congenital malformations: meningomyelocele, aplasia of odontoid

---

Paraplegia

Diagnostic Work-Up. Acute onset or rapid progression (minutes to hours) of paraplegia is generally due to trauma resulting in spinal cord compression or a vascular event involving the spinal cord (anterior spinal artery occlusion). A subacute presentation (hours to days) is usually due to a tumor, infection, or inflammation (myelitis). Slowly progressive symptoms are characteristic of chronic disorders[73] (see box above).

Refusal to walk or stand is often the first symptom of a subacute process and is often interpreted by the child or parent as leg weakness or pain. Progression should be noted, such as initial refusal to run or climb steps advancing to an inability to go from sitting to standing without help. Clumsiness of gait usually indicates a slowly progressive, chronic disorder. Disturbances in bowel or bladder control should be determined, since this will often assist in determining the progression of the disease.

The presence of other associated symptoms such as fever, back pain or tenderness, headache, neck pain or stiffness, the pattern of paresthesias, or weakness (distal, proximal, symmetric, ascending) before the onset of paraplegia should be determined, as should a history of recent illness.

A mass lesion such as a tumor or abscess will often result in localized back pain. The common spinal cord tumors of childhood include ependymoma, astrocytoma, and neuroblastoma. Because astrocytomas are often long, they can extend from the lower brain stem to the cord, resulting in neck pain as well as paraplegia. Neuroblastomas can produce neurologic dysfunction by direct invasion or metastasis. Other spinal cord tumors of childhood include sarcoma, neurinoma, dermoid, teratoma, and epidermoids.[74]

Arteriovenous malformations of the spinal cord, although rare in childhood, should also be considered. Symptoms such as back or abdominal pain and weakness may progress slowly or seem to improve; a subarachnoid hemorrhage is often the initial manifestation.

An infectious cause of paraplegia is epidural abscess; however, initial symptoms can be similar to those for diskitis and osteomyelitis. Most epidural abscesses are due to hematogenous spread of bacteria, especially *Staphylococcus aureus*, rather than extension from osteomyelitis; therefore, it is important to elicit a history of a preceding infection or trauma to the back. Symptoms in addition to back pain include fever, headache, vomiting, and stiff neck. Vertebral osteomyelitis is also due to hematogenous spread and therefore results in more systemic symptoms such as fever, anorexia, and back pain. Bacterial etiologies include *Salmonella* (especially in children with sickle cell disease) and tuberculosis. Diskitis (inflammation of a disk space) usually presents with walking difficulty in children less than 3 years of age and back pain in those older than 3 years. A low-grade fever and abnormal posture may also be present.

Transverse myelitis is an acute demyelinating disorder of the spinal cord, which is inflammatory in origin, but can be difficult to distinguish from (the aforementioned) infectious disorders and is often preceded by a viral illness, including infectious mononucleosis, mumps, rubella, and varicella.[75] Symptoms include severe back or radicular pain followed by fever, generalized muscle aches, and a stiff neck. The combination of optic neuritis and transverse myelitis is called Devic disease.

Poliomyelitis is a disorder of the anterior horn cells characterized by an asymmetric motor weakness. The course of the disease can be gradual or fulminant. Bulbar involvement can result in disturbances of respiratory function.[75]

Some of the causes of peripheral neuropathy, especially motor polyneuropathies, can cause gradual weakness and paralysis. Guillain-Barré syndrome, characterized by a gradually ascending symmetric weakness, can also follow viral illnesses or immunizations. Cranial nerves may be affected, with oculomotor involvement in the Fisher syndrome. Tick paralysis is a toxin-mediated ascending paralysis that presents similar to Guillain-Barré syndrome and is thought to involve the neuromuscular junction. Botulism, caused by the endotoxin of *Clostridium botulinum*, can cause nausea, vomiting, abdominal pain, and cranial nerve dysfunction, which can progress to paralysis. Infant botulism can present with flaccid paralysis, although constipation is usually the first symptom.[76] Other toxins such as organophosphates, chemotherapeutic agents, and heavy metals (lead, arsenic, mercury) should also be considered in the differential diagnosis. Myasthenia gravis is an autoimmune disorder that also causes muscle fatigability, which results in cranial nerve and limb weakness.[77]

Dyskalemic paralysis, including familial periodic paralysis (hypokalemic, hyperkalemic, and normokalemic forms), and acquired hypokalemic paralysis (usually secondary to drugs such as diuretics, amphotericin B, albuterol, laxatives, or licorice) result in muscle weakness and even paralysis. This is actually a myopathy which ascends from the lower extremities, usually affecting proximal muscles first. Respiratory muscles and cranial nerves are usually spared.[78]

A detailed trauma history should be obtained, as motor-vehicle accidents and sports-related injuries account for many cases of acute paraplegia. Although injuries such as fractures, dislocations, or spinal cord concussion will present acutely, a spinal epidural hematoma, which results from vertebral trauma, may result in progressive cord compression, and back trauma may be an antecedent event in the development of an epidural abscess.

Obvious causes of paraplegia at birth include congenital malformations such as a meningomyelocele. However, birth trauma should be considered, especially congenital aplasia of the odontoid process leading to atlantoaxial dislocation. Other disorders associated with an increased risk of atlantooccipital dislocation include Down syndrome, Morquio syndrome (mucopolysaccharidosis IV), and Klippel-Feil syndrome.[74] The presence of a dermal sinus, tuft of hair, or port wine stain in a child with a slowly progressive disorder should prompt one to think of spina bifida occulta, which may be associated with a tethered spinal cord (anchoring of the conus medullaris to the base of the spine, which results in stretching of the spinal cord and neurologic deficits of the lower extremities as a child grows).[74]

Cerebral palsy is another disorder thought to have its etiology in the prenatal and perinatal periods. Although the degree of impairment is variable, motor symptoms predominate and can affect all limbs.[74] Family history is important to elicit, as some genetic disorders cause progressive spastic paraplegia.[74]

A complete and detailed physical examination is essential not only for determining the level and degree of paralysis, but also for use as a baseline by which to document progression or improvement of the disease process.

Vital signs including temperature, pulse, respirations, and blood pressure should be obtained. Pay special attention to the respiratory rate, as well as the depth of respirations and ability to handle secretions. The ophthalmologic examination should include assessment of pupil size, reactivity, range of motion (cranial nerves III, IV, and VI), vision, and funduscopy. Pain, discomfort, or neck swelling should be noted. The abdomen should be assessed for masses (neuroblastoma). Rectal tone, as well as the presence or absence of an anal wink, must be evaluated. The presence of back tenderness—generalized or localized, swelling or erythema—or the presence of a sacral dimple should be noted.

The neurologic examination must be comprehensive. Motor strength should be assessed on a 5-point scale, and all muscle groups should be evaluated: 0, lack of muscle contraction; 1, trace contraction; 2, active movement without gravity; 3, active movement against gravity; 4, active movement against resistance (and gravity); and 5, normal strength.[72] Symmetric weakness/paraplegia suggests a lesion in the spinal cord or conus medullaris, whereas asymmetric weakness or weakness in one (lower) limb suggests a nerve root or peripheral nerve disorder.[72] If limb weakness is found, distal weakness implies a nerve disorder, whereas proximal weakness is more suggestive of a myopathy.[72]

Reflexes should be assessed not only for their presence or absence, but also for symmetry. Hyperreflexia or sustained clonus implies an upper motor neuron disorder and decreased or absent reflexes a lower motor unit problem[72] (see Table 56-5). An acute spinal cord lesion may cause loss of reflexes at and below the lesion, whereas slowly progressive disorders may cause hyperreflexia below the lesion. The loss of a single reflex can be due to a nerve root disorder such as a disk problem or tumor pressing on a nerve. A symmetric decrease in reflexes may be the result of a peripheral nerve disorder.[73]

Evaluation of touch, pain, temperature, and position (or vibration) sense should be performed as part of the sensory examination. Because pain and temperature cross in the spinal cord and touch and vibration do not, a cord lesion will be suggested by the loss of pain and temperature on one side and touch and position on the other. The loss of all sensations on one side suggests a brain lesion. Rectal tone and anal wink are extremely important to assess, since intrinsic cord lesions spare this area, whereas extrinsic lesions do not. An absent anal wink suggests spinal cord or conus involvement.[73] Polyneuropathies may cause decreased or a total loss of sensation, but in a pattern different from that caused by a spinal cord lesion. The distribution may be in a stocking and glove pattern or limited to the areas supplied by one or several nerves.

Ancillary Data. Blood work should include a complete blood count with differential. Other laboratory studies should be directed towards the differential diagnosis, but can often include sedimentation rate, electrolytes, glucose, BUN, creatinine, calcium, creatinine phosphokinase, and toxicology screening (urine and blood). If the child is febrile, blood cultures should be obtained.

Radiographs of the spine at the suspected level of the lesion should be obtained. Look for fracture, collapse or narrowing of vertebral body height, widening of the spinal canal, or bony erosion. ECG may be helpful in the rapid detection of electrolyte abnormalities.

A lumbar puncture will be necessary for the diagnosis of some causes of paraplegia; however, if a mass lesion is suspected, CT scan of the head and spine should be performed beforehand. If a mass lesion is present and a lumbar puncture performed, the patient may decompensate acutely due to blockage of CSF. Therefore if a mass is suspected, it is important to involve neurologic or neurosurgical specialists before this test because specific CSF studies (CSF protein, glucose, viral studies, protein patterns) or a myelogram (to determine the exact location of the lesion) may be required.

A CT scan should be performed to delineate bony lesions, erosions, or fractures, whereas an MRI scan is useful to evaluate the spinal cord or paraspinal lesions. A myelogram is useful to define the degree of spinal cord compression and blockage but should be performed by or under the supervision of a neurosurgeon. Other studies such as electromyography, nerve conduction studies, nerve or muscle

---

Etiology of Hemiplegia in Childhood

Trauma: neck—carotid artery injury
      head—epidural or subdural hematoma
      birth—carotid artery injury
Vascular: cerebral infarction, moyamoya disease, arteriovenous malformations
Seizure: epilepsia partialis continua
Infections: meningitis, thrombosis of cavernous sinus secondary to otitis, mastoiditis, sinusitis
Metabolic: homocystinuria
Underlying illnesses: sickle cell anemia; congenital heart disease; vasculopathies (SLE); protein S, protein C, or antithrombin III deficiency; cancer; IDDM; migraine headaches; neurocutaneous syndromes

---

biopsies, or edrophonium (Tensilon) test can be ordered later, as determined by the results of the previous studies and the patient's condition.

Prehospital Considerations. For any child with paraplegia, with or without a history of trauma, the entire spine should be immobilized before transport.

Therapeutic Trial. Therapy depends upon the diagnosis. Mass lesions may require rapid laminectomy, spine fractures require immobilization and may require surgical stabilization, and infections require antibiotic therapy. Supportive therapy is needed for Guillain-Barré syndrome and transverse myelitis.

Hemiplegia

Diagnostic Work-Up. The onset of hemiplegia can be divided into acute, which has its onset over a period of hours, to chronic, which evolves over days, weeks, or months (see box above). The sudden onset of hemiplegia implies a vascular disorder or epilepsy. The major vascular disorder is a cerebral infarction (stroke), with or without hemorrhage. If hemiplegia is preceded by focal and intractable seizures (epilepsia partialis continua), the probability of a permanent motor deficit is twice as high as when a seizure does not precede the hemiplegia.[79]

Forewarning signs may be present in some of the more slowly progressive disorders such as moyamoya disease (stenosis or occlusion of the carotid artery with the development of collaterals), where recurrent headaches or transient ischemic attacks may occur. Headaches, focal seizures, or neurologic deficits may also be the warning signs of an arteriovenous malformation or cerebral aneurysms.[80]

Infections can predispose to stroke through various mechanisms including thrombosis of the cavernous sinus by infections of the ears, mastoids, or sinuses. Meningitis (bacterial, viral, tuberculous, or fungal) can cause vasculitis or thrombophlebitis leading to arterial occlusion.[80] Unilateral cerebral infarction may also result from cat-scratch disease and *Mycoplasma pneumoniae* thought to be secondary to arteritis of the carotid artery adjacent to an infected lymph node.[79]

Head trauma resulting in epidural or subdural hematoma or intracerebral hemorrhage can cause hemiplegia. Trauma to the neck during exercise or sports can injure the carotid artery, leading to thrombosis and the gradual development of hemiparesis. Falling with an object in one's mouth can lead to injury and occlusion of carotid artery.[79,80]

Neonatal strokes can occur secondary to polycythemia, disseminated intravascular coagulation, or birth trauma to the carotid artery. The usual presentation is the development of seizures.[79]

Some of the predisposing illnesses associated with cerebrovascular disease include sickle cell disease secondary to a thrombotic vasoocclusive crisis; congenital heart disease (especially cyanotic) due to venous thrombosis associated with dehydration and polycythemia; arterial embolization of a thrombus or vegetation; and vasculopathies including systemic lupus erythematosus secondary to cerebral infarction or hemorrhage, Takayasu arteritis, and periarteritis nodosa. Cancer can result in infarction secondary to thrombosis due to disseminated intravascular coagulation, metastasis (neuroblastoma), homocystinuria, or chemotherapy-induced problems. Other inherited coagulation disorders such as protein S, protein C, and antithrombin III deficiency predispose to arterial or venous thrombosis.[81] Children with insulin-dependent diabetes mellitus (IDDM) may also develop acute transient hemiparesis. The attack often occurs with a respiratory illness and is characterized by a headache in conjunction with hemiparesis, which tends to affect the face and arm more than the leg. Children with neurocutaneous syndromes such as neurofibromatosis, Sturge-Weber syndrome, and tuberous sclerosis are also at risk for vascular occlusive disease, especially involving the carotid artery.[80] A child with a seizure disorder may develop transient hemiparesis (Todd paralysis) following a generalized or focal seizure. The degree and distribution of weakness is variable and may last for minutes or days.[79]

It is especially important to inquire about a family history of migraines, since they tend to be familial. There are two types of migraines that can cause hemiplegia. A complicated migraine is a headache with a transient, usually reversible focal motor deficit including hemiplegia. The hemiplegia is often followed by a contralateral headache, nausea, and vomiting.[79,80] In familial hemiplegic migraines, all family members with migraines have at least one hemiplegic attack, which is precipitated by trivial head trauma.[79]

The key finding on examination will be hemiplegia, but some clues to etiology may be found on physical examination. Hydration status should be assessed because dehydration can contribute to thrombosis. The presence of central cyanosis should suggest underlying congenital heart disease, and jaundice may be a clue to sickle cell or liver disease.

The neck should be evaluated for stiffness, bruises, or swelling and auscultated for bruits. The cardiac examination should include assessment of heart rate, rhythm, murmurs, clicks, and comparison of peripheral and central pulses. Evidence of petechiae or purpura may be a clue to disseminated intravascular coagulation (DIC), whereas a malar rash may indicate systemic lupus erythematosus. The skin should be checked for the presence of neurofibromas, cafe-au-lait spots, hemangiomas, or adenoma sebaceum. A complete neurologic examination (as outlined in the previous section) is essential.

Ancillary Data. Laboratory studies should include a complete blood count with a differential, platelet count, and sedimentation rate. If sickle cell disease is suspected, a sickle prep should be obtained, and if positive, a hemoglobin electrophoresis should be performed. If the patient is known to have sickle cell disease, a reticulocyte count should be obtained. If a bleeding disorder is suspected, partial thromboplastin time (PTT) and prothrombin time (PT), as well as other studies looking for disseminated intravascular coagulation disorders, are needed.

Baseline electrolytes, glucose, BUN, creatinine, calcium, phosphorus, and liver function tests should be obtained. Depending upon the etiology of the hemiparesis, other laboratory studies can be ordered, including ANA if a vasculitic origin is suspected; protein S, protein C, antithrombin III, or fibrinogen levels (for these deficiencies); lipid profile (for lipoprotein disorders); and lactic acid, for *mitochondrial encephalopathy, lactic acidosis, and stroke-like syndrome* (MELAS). A urinalysis should be obtained, paying special attention to the presence of protein or blood.

An ECG and echocardiogram should be obtained in order to look for dysrhythmias, underlying heart disease, mitral valve prolapse, bacterial endocarditis, or rheumatic heart disease.

Imaging studies such as a CT scan or MRI scan of the head can identify an infarction, bleeding, or structural shifts. The decision about which study should be performed is based upon the likely diagnosis and availability of such studies. A CT scan without contrast is useful for an acute hemorrhage (<12 hours). However an MRI scan is better for infarction, small aneurysms, arteriovenous malformations, venous sinus and central vein thrombosis, and moyamoya. Contrast-enhanced CT scans are used to identify abscesses or tumors.[80,81] Cerebral angiography is often necessary to determine the exact site of vessel occlusion, unusual vessel patterns, and small aneurysms.[80] Electroencephalogram may be useful if there are focal findings or if a seizure disorder remains in the differential diagnosis. Newer imaging modalities, such as positron emission tomography (PET) scans, and single photon emission computed tomography (SPECT) scans are useful later in the course of an illness, not in the acute diagnostic phase.[80]

Prehospital Considerations. If there is a history of trauma, the entire spine should be immobilized. All children with hemiplegia should be given oxygen during hospital transport.

Therapeutic Trial. Treatment is dependent upon the etiology of hemiplegia; however, as warranted, treatment may include seizure control (see section on Seizures), correction of dehydration, control of intracranial pressure, exchange transfusion, and antibiotic therapy.

SYNCOPE

SUSAN M. FUCHS

Syncope is a sudden, transient loss of consciousness caused by inadequate blood, oxygen, or substrate delivery to the brain.[82,83] It is usually brief and may be precipitated by intercurrent illness, hypovolemia, anemia, vasodilation, drug use, prolonged bed rest, or inactivity. Warning signs are common and include nausea, a feeling of warmth, perspiration, lightheadedness or dizziness, blurred vision, and pallor.[83] The period of unconsciousness is usually brief, during which the patient will be limp; however, clonic movements of the limbs and face may occur. On awakening, the patient may be tired and weak but is aware of his or her surroundings.[84]

Syncope is often referred to as a fainting spell or simple faint. However, due to the many forms of syncope, including some that result from a serious underlying illness or disorder, a thorough evaluation is required. If these causes of syncope are eliminated, then the episode can be referred to as a simple faint.[85]

Pathophysiology (see box at right)

Reduced Peripheral Vascular Resistance/Abnormalities of Circulatory Control/Reflex. When one goes from sitting to an upright position, blood pools in the lower extremities, resulting in decreased blood flow to the heart. To maintain normal blood pressure, there is a reflex increase in peripheral vascular resistance and increase in heart rate and contractility. If this sequence of events is disturbed, syncope can result.[86]

Orthostatic Hypotension. If there is volume depletion or hypovolemia (as could result from bleeding, gastrointestinal [GI] losses, or dehydration) or if drugs that interfere with the normal orthostatic reflex (i.e., phenothiazines, antihypertensives, nitrates, calcium channel blockers, and diuretics) are prescribed or ingested, the reflex can be overwhelmed. The usual compensatory mechanism is an increase in heart rate.[84,86]

Vasodepressor (Vasovagal, Neurally Mediated) Syncope. The most common cause of the simple faint and one of the most common causes of syncope, vasodepressor syncope may be precipitated by stress, anxiety, fear, pain, a shocking incident, or a prolonged period in a warm, crowded environment. Patients are usually sitting or standing and often report a prodrome of nausea, diaphoresis, blurred vision, or weakness. Vasodilation and decreased peripheral vascular resistance result in a decrease in venous return to the heart, which results in increased ventricular contraction. Sympathetic activity decreases (a paradoxical reaction) and further vasodilation and a slower heart rate result. This response can cause hypotension, bradycardia, decreased cerebral perfusion, and a loss of consciousness.[87] Placing the patient in a supine position with the head down usually results in a return of consciousness.[82,84,86]

Cough Syncope. Cough syncope refers to a brief loss of consciousness that occurs after paroxysms of coughing. It is thought to be due to an increase in intrathoracic pressure that causes decreased venous return to the heart.[84,88]

Micturition Syncope. Micturition syncope is a loss of consciousness following voiding. Bladder emptying may stimulate a reflex decrease in peripheral vascular resistance, leading to syncope.[88]

Autonomic System Dysfunction. Because the usual reflex response to hypotension is tachycardia and is autonomic-mediated, if a patient has a blunted or abnormal response, syncope can result. Autonomic dysfunction can be primary as in primary dysautonomia (Riley-Day) and

Causes of Syncope in Children

Vascular/Reflex
  Orthostatic hypotension
  Vasodepressor (vasovagal)
  Cough
  Micturition
  Carotid sinus syndrome
Low volume
  Anemia, dehydration
Cardiovascular
  Obstruction
    Aortic stenosis, pulmonic stenosis, hypertrophic cardiomyopathy, anomalous origin of left coronary, tetralogy of Fallot, coarctation of aorta
  Acquired
    Myocarditis, dilated cardiomyopathy, pulmonary hypertension, tumor
  Dysrhythmias
    Heart block, prolonged QT (familial, idiopathic, and drug-induced), supraventricular tachycardia (SVT), ventricular tachycardia (VT), Wolff-Parkinson-White syndrome
Metabolic
  Hypoglycemia
  Hypocalcemia
  Hypomagnesemia
Neurologic
  Epilepsy
  Vertigo
  Autonomic dysfunction
Psychologic
  Hyperventilation
  Hysterical
Drugs
  Diuretics
  Antihypertensives
  Phenothiazines
  Beta-blockers
  Alcohol
  Cocaine

Shy-Drager syndrome or secondary to spinal cord injury or diabetes mellitus.[82,86,89] Two methods of testing the autonomic nervous system are the cold pressor test and the Valsalva maneuver. The cold pressor test is performed by submerging a hand in ice water for several minutes; the normal response is an increase in blood pressure.[89] The normal response to a Valsalva maneuver is an initial increase in blood pressure, followed by a mild decrease and then an even more profound increase, while the heart rate slows.[89]

Carotid Sinus Syndrome. This is a rare cause of syncope in children, which results from an exaggerated cardioinhibitory response to carotid sinus massage.[84,85]

Cardiovascular Syncope. The major factor in cardiac syncope is a decrease in cardiac output, which then decreases cerebral perfusion.[84] Because cardiac output depends upon stroke volume and heart rate, if stroke volume decreases without an appropriate increase in heart rate, syncope can result.[89] Cardiovascular syncope can be due to congenital heart disease such as aortic stenosis, pulmonic stenosis, hypertrophic cardiomyopathy (all forms of outflow obstruction), anomalous origin of the left coronary artery, tetralogy of Fallot, or coarctation of the aorta.[83] It can also be acquired secondary to myocarditis, dilated cardiomyopathy, pulmonary hypertension, or a tumor. On the other hand, if the heart rate is too slow and stroke volume cannot be increased, or if the heart rate is too fast to allow adequate filling of the heart, syncope can result. This can occur with dysrhythmias, including heart block, prolonged QT syndrome and Wolff-Parkinson-White syndrome; supraventricular, ventricular, or atrial tachycardia; atrial flutter; or ventricular fibrillation.[89] The long QT syndrome can be familial, Romano-Ward syndrome or Jervell and Lange-Nielsen syndrome where deafness is also an association, idiopathic, or drug-induced.[90] QT prolongation, ventricular dysrhythmias, and torsades de pointes have resulted from overdoses of antidysrhythmic drugs such as procainamide and quinidine, as well as normal use of tricyclic antidepressants, phenothiazines, and nonsedating antihistamines; terfenadine (Seldane); and astemizole (Hismanal), especially if used with erythromycin, troleandomycin, or ketoconazole.[90,91]

Patients who have had surgical correction of congenital heart disease are at greater risk of complete heart block. Risk factors include first degree AV block and right or left bundle branch blocks.[90] Children who have undergone a Mustard or Senning procedure for repair of transposition of the great vessels may develop bradycardia or the tachycardia-bradycardia syndrome (also called the "sick-sinus" syndrome), in which atrial tachycardia or flutter is followed by brief asystole and syncope.[90,91]

Some of the most important clues to cardiac syncope are a family history of syncope or sudden death, exercise-induced syncope, and even syncope while sitting.[83]

Metabolic Disorders. The main metabolic disorder that can cause syncope is hypoglycemia.[82] It is often preceded by confusion, an altered level of consciousness, and weakness. Occurrence of syncope before breakfast in normal individuals or in diabetics who have received too much insulin is suggestive of this etiology. There is a rapid reversal of symptoms with the administration of glucose or other sugar-containing foods or beverages. Hypocalcemia and hypomagnesemia can also cause syncope secondary to dysrhythmias from electrolyte disturbances.[89]

Neurologic. Both epilepsy and vertigo can be confused with syncope, although they are not true causes of syncope. Seizures cause a sudden but transient loss of consciousness, and atonic seizures cause a sudden loss of muscle tone, resulting in a child falling to the floor from a standing or sitting position. Depending on the type of seizure, a child may have an aura, tonic clonic-movements of the extremities, incontinence, and confusion after the seizure. This is not present in syncopal attacks.[84,92]

Vertigo can also be confused with syncope, since the child will lose balance and fall, although consciousness is never lost. The prominent symptom before the attack is

dizziness or a feeling of the room spinning, although nausea, sweating, and pallor may also occur beforehand.[92]

Psychologic. Hypocapnia (reduction in Pco_2 that occurs with hyperventilation) causes cerebral vasoconstriction and therefore decreased cerebral perfusion, which results in syncope. The patient may complain of numb extremities or have an altered level of consciousness before the syncopal episode.[82,89]

Hysterical syncopal episodes occur when the patient falls to the ground without injury and without a true loss of consciousness.[84] Although organic etiologies must be considered initially, clues such as a precipitating, often anxiety-producing event; witnesses; and awareness by the patient of the surroundings during the event are suggestive of hysterical syncope.[84,86]

Drugs. Many prescription drugs can cause syncope due to their effects on blood pressure (diuretics, antihypertensives, phenothiazines, nitrates, and barbiturates) or due to their effects on heart rate (beta-blockers, digitalis). Drugs of abuse, such as cocaine, as well as alcohol can also result in syncope.[84,89]

Diagnostic Considerations

Although most cases of syncope in children, in contrast to adults, reflect a benign condition, the possibility of serious underlying pathology, especially cardiovascular, must be excluded. Other factors may predispose a patient to have a syncopal event, where syncope itself is a result of the body's reaction to the underlying problem (e.g., hypotension and syncope secondary to anemia, hypovolemia, or drugs). Metabolic disorders may present with syncope, and the distinction between seizures and syncope can affect a patient's long-term diagnosis and treatment.

Diagnostic Work-Up

An accurate history of the event may be the most important part of the work-up. Obtain information about events preceding the episode, including any prodromal symptoms and prior activity. Inciting events such as exertion, a change in posture, trauma, pain, fear, micturition, an aura, or hyperventilation can assist in determining the possible etiology of the syncopal event. The presence of palpitations, a "funny feeling in the chest," or chest pain point to a cardiac etiology. A report of the duration of the event, the presence of any focal neurologic activity, tongue-biting, eye position, incontinence, or postictal state may suggest a neurologic problem. Because the patient may not be able to provide some of this information, any information from witnesses or prehospital care providers may be beneficial. Information about the patient's level of consciousness or impaired memory after the episode, any postsyncopal symptoms, or a history about previous similar or dissimilar events should also be obtained. The physician should also ask about a family history of sudden death, cardiac problems, syncope, or deafness, as these can provide a clue to the presence of a prolonged QT syndrome.

Obtain a complete medication or drug use history. Many prescribed medications can cause syncope as a side effect of normal use, but especially when overused or in combination with other drugs or used inappropriately. Drugs of abuse, especially cocaine, can have direct toxic effects on both the cardiovascular and neurologic systems and can cause seizures, tachycardia, myocardial infarction, and sudden death.

The patient's vital signs, including orthostatic vital signs, should be measured (i.e., pulse and blood pressure measurement in the supine and sitting [legs dependent] or standing positions). A positive test would be the increase in heart rate by 20 beats/minute, the development of bradycardia, a decrease in systolic blood pressure by 20 mm Hg, or feelings of dizziness when going from supine to any other position.[93-95] A thorough examination should include looking for signs of head trauma; a complete eye examination (including pupil size, reactivity, and funduscopic examination); identification of masses in the ears, nose, or throat; hearing; inspection of the mouth for bite marks; and palpation of the cervical vertebrae for pain, tenderness, or step-offs. Abdominal examination should include evaluation for masses, including the possibility of pregnancy.

Cardiac evaluation includes assessment of the heart rhythm (whether it is fast or slow, regular, or irregular); the presence of any murmurs or extra sounds such as gallops, rubs, thrills, or bruits; and the strength and quality of all pulses. A child with structural heart disease usually has a murmur. Some murmurs indicate specific pathology. A harsh mid-to-late systolic murmur, with an ejection click, is indicative of aortic stenosis. The murmur of hypertrophic cardiomyopathy can be varied, but may include a palpable S_4 at the apex and a late systolic murmur, which increases in intensity during a Valsalva maneuver.[82] A mid-systolic click or late systolic murmur can occur in mitral valve prolapse; a loud P_2 and right ventricular heave can suggest pulmonary hypertension.[82] A child with coarctation of the aorta may not have a murmur but will have diminished or absent femoral pulses, upper extremity hypertension, and low blood pressure in the legs.[85] The presence of a rub can suggest pericardial effusion or pericarditis.[96] A child who has undergone repair for congenital heart disease can have various findings including murmurs and thrills, although the absence of a murmur may also be a concern.

Neurologic examination must include an assessment of the patient's level of consciousness and age-appropriate mental status, memory for events preceding the syncopal episode, the episode itself, and events afterwards. The presence of any focal abnormalities or defects must be clearly elicited and documented.

Ancillary Data. Certain basic tests should be performed in any child with syncope: a hemoglobin, hematocrit, and complete blood cell count; electrolytes with bicarbonate; glucose; calcium; and magnesium. As mentioned previously, anemia and hypoglycemia can cause syncope. Electrolyte abnormalities, especially potassium, calcium, and magnesium, can cause dysrhythmias. The presence of an elevated bicarbonate may provide a clue to hyperventilation, whereas a low bicarbonate level may result from hypoxia after a seizure.[82,89] Other laboratory tests, including serum pregnancy test, toxicology/drug screens, or arterial blood gas, should be ordered based on clinical impressions or suspicions.

A patient who is being evaluated for a syncopal episode should be monitored; a recorded 12-lead ECG is essential. The ECG will provide information on heart rate and rhythm and the presence of ectopy and conduction abnormalities, including prolonged PR and QT intervals and AV blocks.[89] (Correction of the QT interval [QTc] is the QT interval divided by the square root of the RR interval in seconds, with normal QTc being <0.44 sec).[90] An abnormal QRS axis or ventricular hypertrophy may suggest a structural problem. The presence of ischemic changes, such as Q-waves, T-wave abnormalities, or ST segment depressions, should be noted.

Tilt testing is a method used to study and replicate the changes in heart rate and blood pressure that occur upon standing, and is therefore used to diagnose vasodepressor syncope. Several protocols exist, but the main features are the use of a mechanical tilting table (with safety restraints), a 15-minute period in the supine position with baseline vital signs, followed by tilting the table to 60 degrees (maximum 80 degrees) for 15 to 60 minutes, with continuous vital signs. The test is terminated (and positive) if the patient develops symptoms such as pallor, lightheadedness, nausea, a feeling of malaise or being hot, a change in mental status, or the heart rate increases by more than 20 beats/min or there is a sudden drop in blood pressure without a change in heart rate.[87,90,91] If the initial test is negative, it can be repeated during an increasing infusion of isoproterenol, which has been found to increase the sensitivity of the test.[87,90]

Although the information obtained from a careful history, physical examination, and ECG can point to the etiology of syncope in most cases, if a cardiac etiology is suspected, further evaluation will be warranted.

Two-dimensional echocardiography is a noninvasive way to identify structural heart disease. It can identify hypertrophic cardiomyopathy, aortic stenosis, mitral valve prolapse, depressed myocardial contractility, ventricular enlargement, and pericardial effusions, which can occur in myocarditis. Recent additions of pulsed and continuous wave Doppler can also allow quantification of the severity of some of these defects.[85] Echocardiography may not show anomalous coronary arteries or small tumors; therefore a normal echo does not necessarily exclude a cardiac etiology for syncope.[85]

Ambulatory ECG recording (Holter monitor) is a tape-recording device that allows continuous recording of all heartbeats. It is very useful in detecting transient dysrhythmias, periods of tachycardia or bradycardia, blocks, and Wolff-Parkinson-White syndrome. The patient or parent can document a time period when syncope or syncopal symptoms occur, and this can be matched to the ECG.[85] Holter monitoring is useful to evaluate a child with recurrent syncope or suspected heart disease, the athlete, and children who have undergone surgical correction of congenital heart defects.[89,90] Unfortunately, a normal Holter reading may not be definitive because the dysrhythmia/syncopal episode is so transient and does not occur in every 24-hour period. In such cases, specific telemetry studies or event recorders, which can be used for periods longer than 24 hours, may be necessary.[90]

Stress testing is important in evaluating patients with exercise-induced syncope, occult coronary artery disease, or anomalies. Transient dysrhythmias or ST segment depression may be detected before, during, or after exercise.[89,96]

Cardiac catheterization and electrophysiology studies may be required for a few children with cardiac syncope (i.e., those in whom the previous studies have not determined an etiology or in whom further study is necessary to determine appropriate therapy).[85]

All children who undergo a cardiac evaluation of syncope should undergo chest radiography.

If there is strong suspicion of a seizure disorder, an EEG should be performed. This test can be negative in 50% of patients; however, specific provocative tests, including sleep deprivation, may increase diagnostic accuracy. In addition, a video EEG can prove useful in children with hysterical seizures and syncopal attacks. Further neurologic studies, such as a CT scan, MRI scan; or lumbar puncture, should be performed only when neurologic findings are present on physical examination.[92]

Prehospital Considerations

A child with a syncopal event can be found by prehospital care providers to be awake and alert, as opposed to a child who is seizing or in cardiac arrest. The keys to prehospital care should still involve assessment of the ABCs. Vital signs, including blood pressure, should be performed. (It is not necessary to do orthostatic vital signs in the field). The child should be given oxygen and attached to a cardiac monitor. Depending upon the history of the event, the patient's condition, findings on quick patient assessment, and the providers' capabilities, further diagnostic and therapeutic modalities can be performed: Chemstrip or Dextrostix to check for serum glucose, with administration of PO or IV glucose (D50W 0.5 to 1.0 gm/kg: dilute 1:1 with sterile water and give 2 to 4 ml/kg in children <2 yrs) or IM, IV, or SC glucagon (0.1 mg/kg for children <10 kg and 1 mg/dose for children >10 kg) as needed; initiation of IV access and fluid therapy (D5W if hypoglycemic, otherwise normal saline) for a child with low blood pressure or evidence of hypovolemia or dehydration; or administration of antiseizure medication.

In most cases, transporting the child to the hospital in a recumbent position may be all that is required after the patient's initial assessment.

Therapeutic Trial

Once the child is determined to be hemodynamically stable and the level of consciousness has returned to normal, the next decision involves treatment. Depending on the history, physical examination, and basic laboratory studies, a likely etiology for the syncope can be determined. Children with hypovolemia will benefit from fluid, and those with hypoglycemia from glucose. In cases where a cardiovascular cause is suspected, if studies can be performed immediately or within a short time frame, outpatient studies may be appropriate. For those patients with initial symptomatology of great severity of either a cardiac or neurologic etiology, inpatient evaluation may be warranted. Most syncopal episodes in children are due to vasovagal syncope or other reflex phenomena. Therefore most are benign and the children generally have a good outcome. Reassurance and avoidance of the precipitating event are often all that is needed to prevent a recurrence.

Those children who have recurrent episodes of syncope

Causes of Vertigo in Children

Infectious: meningitis, otitis media, labyrinthitis, vestibular neuritis, encephalitis, epidural abscess
Migraine headaches: benign paroxysmal vertigo
Drugs
Epilepsy
Meniere disease
Motion sickness
Multiple sclerosis
Psychogenic (hyperventilation)
Trauma
Tumor: posterior fossa

---

require good follow-up care to determine the etiology. Those found to have a cardiac or neurologic cause should have follow-up with their respective specialists.

VERTIGO

SUSAN M. FUCHS

Vertigo is the sensation of motion, which can be described as spinning, rotation, or even linear movement. This feeling is often accompanied by nystagmus, and is produced by a disturbance in the vestibular system.[97,98]

Dizziness, on the other hand, has been described as a disturbance in balance or a feeling of lightheadedness and faintness accompanied by nausea. It is produced by an alteration in the interaction of the eyes, proprioception system, labyrinth, cerebellum, or cerebrum.[97]

Pathophysiology

The semicircular canals, the vestibule within the labyrinth, and the vestibular portion of cranial nerve VII are the peripheral components of the sensory pathway that can result in vertigo. The stimulus for excitation of the semicircular canals is rotary motion of the head, whereas for the vestibule it is gravity. This information is transmitted by the vestibular nuclei in the brain stem and cerebellum, through connections in the medial longitudinal fasciculus to the superior temporal gyrus and frontal lobe (central components).[97]

Differential Considerations

Because children do not often complain about vertigo, further questioning of those with a complaint of dizziness involving a sensation of motion is warranted. The sensation of rotation of the subject or the environment separates vertigo from dizziness, syncope, or ataxia (see box above).

Infectious. Otitis media and meningitis are the leading causes of vertigo in children. Acute suppurative labyrinthitis secondary to otitis media is uncommon; however, serous labyrinthitis can cause vertigo due to inflammation and is accompanied by a hearing loss.[99] A cholesteatoma secondary to chronic otitis media may cause labyrinthine damage.[97]

Vestibular neuritis (or neuronitis) is a viral infection of the labyrinth or vestibular nerve, characterized by vertigo, vomiting, and ataxia.[99] It can be secondary to mumps, measles, or infectious mononucleosis. Encephalitis and an epidural abscess can also cause vertigo.

Epilepsy. Many people with vertiginous seizures experience an aura, which consists of a feeling of vertigo. The occurrence of a seizure after a feeling of vertigo will make diagnosis of the primary problem easy. However, some people with complex partial seizures have vertigo as the only manifestation of the seizure. Vestibulogenic seizures are triggered by a stimulus to an abnormal labyrinth system.[99]

Migraine. Many individuals who suffer from basilar artery migraine headaches experience vertigo before the headache. Other symptoms include visual symptoms such as scotoma, blurred vision; paresthesias; loss of consciousness; and drop attacks.[99] Benign paroxysmal vertigo is a specific syndrome in children ages 1 to 4, which is characterized by (1) multiple, brief, sporadic episodes of disequilibrium, anxiety, and often nystagmus, pallor, sweating, and vomiting; (2) no loss of consciousness and a normal neurologic examination; (3) normal EEG; and (4) abnormal response to caloric stimulation of the ears (abnormal labyrinthine function).[97,100,101] These brief, recurrent episodes of vertigo in infants and children are now recognized as migraine equivalents.[99,101,102]

Drugs and Toxins. Aminoglycoside antibiotics are known to disturb vestibular function. Streptomycin and gentamicin are known to cause vestibular damage when given in high doses. Minocycline causes nausea, vomiting, dizziness, and ataxia at therapeutic doses.[97]

Anticonvulsants such as diphenylhydantoin and carbamazepine can cause ataxia and incoordination at toxic doses, but vertigo is not usually the major complaint.

Meniere Disease. Although uncommon in children, Meniere disease is thought to be a rupture of the labyrinth due to an overaccumulation of endolymph causing the clinical features of hearing impairment, tinnitus, and vertigo. An attack consists of vertigo (often preceded by tinnitus), ear fullness, or loss of hearing. Nystagmus is present during the attack, with the fast component initially toward the abnormal ear. As the attack subsides, the fast component of nystagmus is away from the abnormal ear. The attacks last for 1 to 3 hours and occur at sporadic intervals for years and then decrease in frequency or even stop; however, the patient is then left with permanent hearing loss.[97]

Motion Sickness. Motion sickness occurs when the body senses some acceleration or movement, but the visual input is stationary. Symptoms include pallor followed by nausea and vomiting.

Multiple Sclerosis. Although ataxia and blindness are the most common presenting signs of this disease, vertigo may occur during an attack.[1]

Psychogenic (Hyperventilation). Psychogenic vertigo, or hyperventilation, should be a diagnosis of exclusion. The patient often has episodes of vertigo during hyperventilation, but this is probably more a feeling of lightheadedness than true vertigo. To differentiate this entity, the patient can be made to hyperventilate; if the patient complains of vertigo, but nystagmus is absent, true vertigo does not exist.[103]

Trauma

Head Injury. After a closed head injury, many children complain of dizziness, headache, and nausea for a few days. Because some also have vertigo, it is important to determine whether there has been trauma to the labyrinth (vestibular or labyrinthine concussion).

Vestibular or Labyrinthine Concussion. Injury to this structure can follow trauma to the parietooccipital or temporal region of the head. The child usually complains of vertigo immediately after the injury and will have an unsteady balance for a few days. Symptoms resolve, but the child will have recurrent episodes of vertigo and nausea lasting for 5 to 10 seconds, precipitated by specific movements of the head.[99,100]

Tympanic Membrane Perforation. Rupture of the round or oval window secondary to trauma or sudden changes in barometric pressure (decompression) can create a perilymphatic fistula. This results in the sudden onset of vertigo and a hearing loss.[99]

Whiplash Injury. After a whiplash or whiplash-type injury, vertigo and tinnitus may occur. The etiology is thought to be basilar artery spasm.[97]

Tumor. The presence of unremitting vertigo and neurologic findings such as cranial nerve defects, ataxia, or pyramidal signs are suggestive of a tumor in the posterior fossa, brain stem, or cerebellopontine angle.[99]

Diagnostic Work-Up

When eliciting a history, ask the patient to describe the feelings of the attack without suggestions (e.g., without using the word *dizzy* or asking if the room was spinning or moving). Words spoken, such as *spinning* or *rotating*, help distinguish vertigo from lightheadedness or presyncope. The patient should be asked about the concomitant occurrence of hearing loss, impairment, or tinnitus. The course of the illness, duration and frequency of attacks (whether acute, recurrent, or chronic), and the severity of symptoms with each subsequent attack should be determined. Because some of the causes of vertigo are precipitated by infections (otitis), trauma (head injury), or positional changes, these items should be included in the history. Medications being used at the present time or in the past, including antibiotics, over-the-counter, or recreational drugs, should be identified. A family history of seizures or migraines may assist in narrowing the differential diagnosis.[97,103]

A physical examination should include a thorough otoscopic examination including the external auditory canal (looking for trauma, infection, or cerumen) and the tympanic membrane (for evidence of perforation, infection, cholesteatoma, or hemotympanum). Ophthalmologic examination should note nystagmus (both spontaneous and induced), extraocular muscle movements, and visual acuity.

Neurologic testing should include all cranial nerves, gait, past pointing, and Romberg tests. Since an infant cannot perform these tests, the vertical acceleration test can be used to test vestibular function. For this test, the infant is held at arm's length in the supine position; then the examiner suddenly descends to a semicrouched position. The normal response is abduction and extension of the arms, then an embrace.[99] For young children, the Romberg test may be possible, with the patient falling toward the side of a unilateral labyrinthine problem. A more sensitive test for older children is the tandem Romberg test. The child stands with one foot in front of the other and closes his or her eyes; a normal (negative test) is maintenance of posture for 6 to 7 seconds, a positive test is falling toward one (the affected) side.[99]

Ancillary Data

Caloric Test. The canal must be inspected to determine that the external auditory canal is clear and the tympanic membrane is intact. The patient should lie supine with the head raised on a pillow to approximately 30 degrees. Cool water (30° C) is instilled into the external canal and the eyes are observed for nystagmus. Warm water (44° C) is then instilled and the direction of nystagmus noted. A normal response in the fast component of nystagmus is to the opposite side with cold water and to the same side with warm water (Fast *cows: c*old *o*pposite, *w*arm *s*ame). If cool water does not elicit a response, the test can be repeated with ice water, but severe nausea can result. Absence of nystagmus indicates peripheral vestibular nerve disease, whereas a hyperactive response indicates irritation. Directional preponderance is a symmetric response caused by partial dysfunction.[97,99,104]

Nylen-Hallpike Technique. From the sitting position, the patient is moved to the supine position so that the head hangs below the level of the examining table. The head is then turned 45 degrees to the right and the eyes are observed for nystagmus. The patient should be returned to the sitting position and the test repeated, with the head being turned 45 degrees to the left and then tilted 45 degrees backwards.[97,99]

Fistula Test. The patient should be positioned with the head looking 60 degrees to the ceiling, and positive air pressure with a pneumatic otoscope is applied to the external canal. The eyes should be checked for nystagmus and the patient asked if this reproduces the symptoms. Also, test to see if the patient is vertiginous. A positive test (vertigo and nystagmus) most commonly occurs with labyrinthitis, perilymph fistula, or cholesteatoma, but the test can also be positive with a perforated tympanic membrane.[99,101]

Weber Test. Hold the tuning fork in midline and check for lateralization of sound. Sound travels toward the affected ear with conductive hearing loss and away from the affected ear with sensorineural hearing loss.[105]

Rinne Test. Hold the tuning fork to the mastoid and then the ear. Normally air conduction is greater than bone conduction by a 2:1 ratio.[105]

Audiometric Testing. True audiometric testing can determine the degree of hearing loss, specific tone loss, or threshold fluctuation. Brain stem auditory evoked potentials (BAEPs) are more useful for infants and young children, who may not cooperate for formal hearing tests.[99]

Laboratory Testing. Unless an infection is suspected, blood tests do not usually help in the differential diagnosis of vertigo.

Electronystagmography (ENG). ENG records eye movements and therefore allows better assessment of caloric and positional testing. The primary tests are performed as described above, and the duration and velocity of nystagmus is recorded.

Lumbar Puncture. Because meningitis or encephalitis can cause vertigo, the presence of meningismus along with vertigo is reason to perform a lumbar puncture. However, if there are signs of increased intracranial pressure or an epidural abscess is suspected, a CT scan should be performed before the lumbar puncture, preceded by the administration of antibiotics. If multiple sclerosis is in the differential, this can be confirmed by elevation of oligoclonal bands and gamma globulin in the CSF.[99]

EEG. Because vertigo may be a component of epilepsy, an EEG may be warranted.

Radiographs/CT Scan/MRI Scan. The history of head trauma or the presence of mastoid tenderness should prompt radiologic investigation. Although appropriate x-ray studies may prove or disprove the diagnosis, a CT scan is often needed to visualize the problem fully. In mastoiditis, clouding of the mastoid air cells will secure the diagnosis but will not allow for visualization of bone erosion. Skull radiographs will demonstrate skull fractures, but special views of the petrous bone are needed to determine vestibular concussion. An MRI scan is helpful to detect small tumors or inflammatory conditions.[99]

Prehospital Considerations

Because the differential diagnosis of vertigo is complex, the most beneficial function of prehospital transport is to allow the patient to ride in a position of comfort.

Therapeutic Trial

The key to management is to treat the underlying cause before initiating therapeutic trials. Because vertigo and the symptoms of vertigo can be disabling, certain medications may help alleviate symptoms. During the acute phase of an attack, bed rest, sedation, and antiemetics may be beneficial. Diazepam (0.1 mg/kg/24 hr) given orally; scopolamine PO given as Donnatal with dosage based on weight, or transdermally as a 0.5 mg patch (except in young children); promethazine (Phenergan 0.5 mg/kg/dose q 12 hr PO or per rectum); dimenhydrinate (Dramamine 5 mg/kg/24 hr); or in children older than 12 years old meclizine (Antivert 12.5 to 25 mg BID) can be used.

Diagnostic Entities

BREATH-HOLDING SPELLS

SUSAN M. FUCHS

There are two clinical types of breath-holding spells that refer to the child's color during the episode.

The *cyanotic breath-holding spell*, often referred to as the classic spell, is the result of cerebral hypoxia. It is more common than the pallid breath-holding spell. The child usually begins to cry due to anger, frustration, or fear. Shortly thereafter, the child stops breathing in expiration and cyanosis ensues rapidly, followed by limpness and loss of consciousness. The loss of consciousness allows the autonomic respiratory mechanism to resume; thus the hypoxia that develops is never severe. If the attacks are of short duration, the child may resume normal behavior or continue crying after awakening.[106-108] For longer attacks, there may be posturing and tonic-clonic movements of the body, similar to those that occur with a seizure (although these episodes are not indicative of an underlying seizure disorder or epilepsy). After such a spell, the child may have a prolonged period of sleep after initial arousal.[109]

A *pallid breath-holding spell* is actually a form of vasovagal or cardiac syncope characterized by vagally mediated bradycardia or asystole. It is thought to be due to increased vagal discharge or increased sensitivity to vagal stimulation. A positive response is asystole longer than 2 seconds after vagal stimulation.[110] The sequence of events usually begins with a sudden, unexpected, painful event such as bumping one's head. The child will then stop, may cry or gasp, turn pale and limp, and fall to the floor. The body may stiffen after the period of limpness, and there may be arching of the back and, occasionally, tonic-clonic movements.[106,107] The spell is brief, although it may seem like hours for a parent or observer. Afterward, the child is normal but may be sleepy.

Diagnostic Findings

The age of onset for both pallid and cyanotic breath-holding spells is the same—less than 5 years. They often begin between 6 and 18 months of age and cease by 4 to 8 years. Differentiation between pallid and cyanotic spells is based on the history of the spell: the precipitating event and the presence or absence of cyanosis. Often there is a family history of spells, especially pallid spells.[108,109,111]

Ancillary Data. A provocative test for pallid breath-holding spells—ocular compression, which involves applying pressure over both eyeballs—has been positive in 61% to 78% of children with pallid breath-holding spells, but only 25% to 33% of children with cyanotic breath-holding spells.[110,111] A positive test is characterized by (1) a prompt and sustained bradycardia of 50% or less than resting heart rate during 10 seconds of compression, (2) cardiac asystole for 2 seconds or longer, or (3) the precipitation of a spell.[110-112] Obviously, a child should be monitored closely during this type of study. An EEG during a pallid or cyanotic spell shows nonspecific slowing, but between attacks it is normal.[107]

Differential Considerations

It is sometimes difficult to distinguish between a breath-holding spell and a seizure. The history of a precipitating event is the key differentiating factor for the diagnosis of a spell. Because both spells may result in tonic-clonic movement, information about the actual event may not be helpful. After most spells, however, the child is normal, whereas, after a tonic-clonic or akinetic seizure, the child's level of consciousness is impaired.[108] In addition, with a seizure the change in muscle tone develops before the color change.[112]

The differentiation between a spell and syncope (simple faint) can be based on a prodrome of pallor and sweating before a loss of consciousness.[106] Although syncope usually occurs in an older child or adolescent, there does seem to be an increased incidence of syncope in children who had breath-holding spells when younger.[111]

A recent study reported several children with recurrent cyanotic episodes and sudden death. Investigation revealed severe arterial and cerebral hypoxemia due to an intrapulmonary shunt and prolonged expiratory apnea, which may be related to the mechanism for sudden infant death.[113]

Management

For pallid breath-holding spells, reassurance is the best therapy. Atropine 0.01 mg/kg/dose BID to TID PO has been recommended if the spells recur very frequently, or affect the parent-child relationship or child rearing.[111,112] This regimen is thought to result in a parasympathetic block to the vagal stimulation that results in the bradycardia or asystole.[109]

For cyanotic breath-holding spells, the most important management strategy is parental reassurance and behavior modification. Explain to the parent that although the child is cyanotic, it does not harm the child. For a child who has a seizure-like episode as part of the breath-holding spell, the parents should be instructed to ensure that the child is not injured by nearby objects. They should not attempt to place anything in the child's mouth, but should position the child on the left side.

Once spells begin, the frequency may increase initially and then decline before stopping spontaneously. Parents should be told not to pay special attention to the spells, since the child can use them for secondary gain. If parents find it difficult to reduce the episodes by focusing on behavioral modification, counseling may be helpful.[106,108]

MENINGITIS, BACTERIAL

ROGER M. BARKIN

Meningitis is an inflammatory process of the meninges surrounding the brain. It is life threatening if not treated expeditiously and has a relatively high incidence of sequelae. The increasingly widespread use of *Haemophilus influenzae* conjugate vaccine has produced a marked decrease in the incidence of meningitis and other systemic disease resulting from this pathogen. The incidence of bacterial meningitis in the United States is estimated to be about 4.6 to 10 cases/100,000 per year, occurring most commonly between 3 and 8 months of age. Nearly 90% of pediatric bacterial meningitis occurs in the first 5 years of life.[115] The incidence of *H. influenzae* declined from 59 cases/100,000 children in 1986 to 6 cases/100,000 children in 1991.[114] Mortality rates have decreased from *H. influenzae* from 1.71 deaths/100,000 children in 1980 to 0.11 deaths/100,000 children in 1991.[116,117]

Pathophysiology

The inflammatory response caused by the bacterial infection in the subarachnoid space leads to liberation of the bacterial cell wall constituents. Host inflammatory mediators and cytokines, including interleukin-1, tumor necrosis factor, arachidonic acid metabolites, and platelet-activating factor are produced and secreted by central nervous system macrophages and endothelial cells.[118] Antibiotics produce bacterial lysis. The activation of leukocytes, endothelial injury, altered vascular permeability, and thrombosis produce brain swelling, edema, and decreased cerebral perfusion; tissue injury occurs.

A variety of modes of infection are possible. The upper respiratory tract is the major reservoir of pathogens, often being colonized by *Streptococcus pneumoniae, H. influenzae,* and *Neisseria meningitidis.* Hematogenous transmission is common, bacteremia often preceding the onset of meningitis. Up to one third of children have a distant focus of infection.[119] Meningitis may follow bacterial invasion from a local focus of infection such as the mastoids, paranasal sinuses, or osteomyelitis of the skull. Bacterial meningitis associated with otitis media generally follows bacteremia, although direct invasion has occurred.

Host factors influence susceptibility to meningitis. Males and young children are affected more frequently than females and older children.[120,121] Children with a compromised immunologic response are at enhanced risk. Congenital or acquired dysgammaglobulinemia, sickle cell disease, recent irradiation or immunosuppressive agents, and malnutrition predispose to bacterial meningitis. Cole et al[122] reported recurrent infection in normal children less than 2 years of age, probably on the basis of immature immunologic and inflammatory responses. After splenectomy, there is greater incidence of infection; the frequency depends on the age at the time of splenectomy, number of years since the procedure, and indications for removal. An increased frequency of infection is noted in children with diabetes mellitus, renal or adrenal insufficiency, hypoparathyroidism, and cystic fibrosis, probably associated with defective chemotaxis and phagocytosis.[123]

Mechanical factors, including recent neurosurgical procedure or skull fracture associated with a persistent fluid leak, increase risk. Infection is usually seen within two weeks of the initial trauma, although it may be delayed for years.[124] Congenital dermoid sinus tracts or meningomyeloceles provide communication between the skin and meninges, predisposing to infection, often on a recurrent basis.

Meningitis in the newborn occurs largely through colonization of the newborn by pathogens through vertical transmission from maternal intestinal or genital tract or from horizontal transmission from nursery personnel or caregivers in the home setting.[125] After colonization, bacteremia probably develops, although the role of the immunologic incompetency of this age group remains unclear.

After bacterial invasion of the meninges, a purulent exudate accumulates around the veins, venous sinuses, and the brain. Ventriculitis is a common finding. Vascular and parenchymal changes occur with microthrombi and vasculitis, producing impaired blood flow and potentially leading to cerebral edema.[126] Inflammation of the pain-sensitive spinal nerves and roots probably account for the meningeal signs seen during an acute illness; residual sensory or motor deficits stem from injury to peripheral nerves.

Meningeal inflammation associated with increased vascular permeability and loss of albumin fluid into the subdural space may produce subdural effusion.[127] Hydrocephalus is usually communicating, resulting from adhesive thickening of the arachnoid about the cisterns at the base of the brain.

TABLE 56-6. Etiology of Bacterial Meningitis by Age Group

Age group	Predominant organism
<2 mon	*E. coli,* group B streptococci, *L. monocytogenes, N. meningitidis, S. pneumoniae*
2 mon-9 yrs	*H. influenzae, N. meningitidis, S. pneumoniae*
>9 yrs	*N. meningitidis, S. pneumoniae*

Etiology

S. pneumoniae is most common, followed by *H. influenzae* type B, and *N. meningitidis,* accounting for 90% to 95% of the organisms causing meningitis in children older than 2 months of age. *Staphylococcus aureus, Staphylococcus epidermidis,* and *Listeria monocytogenes* are cultured as well, typically associated with a ventriculoperitoneal shunt, abnormal anatomy, or immunosuppressed host. *Escherichia coli* and other coliforms account for one fourth of cases, and group B streptococcus are responsible for one half of cases of neonatal meningitis (Table 56-6).

Diagnostic Findings

The history and physical examination are often nonspecific early in the course of bacterial meningitis. The findings reflect the age of the child and progression of illness. Historically, the course of the illness, associated signs and symptoms, exposures, and underlying health problems are important. Often the condition has developed over a matter of hours, whereas in other children it may be insidious.

In some children, health care may have been sought and antibiotics initiated before diagnosis is confirmed, leading to partial treatment of the meningitis. Partially treated children less commonly have temperatures over 38.3° C and altered mental status. Their clinical progression is usually less rapid.

Children are reported to have altered responsiveness ranging from lethargy to irritability, often resisting handling. Decreased appetite or interest in eating and nonprojectile vomiting may be noted. Respiratory pattern changes and apnea may be manifestations of seizure activity or central dysfunction (see Chapter 59). Tachypnea with or without respiratory distress is not uncommon and is usually without pulmonary findings.

Fever is common, although not universally present. One half of neonates have a normal or depressed temperature.[127] About 10% of children under 2 years of age with temperatures of 41.1° C have meningitis. Petechiae and fever may be associated with *N. meningitidis.*

In neonates and those under 3 months of age, the initial presentation is nonspecific, including fever, hypothermia, dehydration, bulging fontanelle, lethargy, irritability, anorexia, vomiting seizures, respiratory distress, or cyanosis. The absence of nuchal rigidity in children under one year of age does not preclude an intracranial infection. The diagnosis therefore is often difficult to confirm clinically; a lumbar puncture remains the definitive test.[127]

Older patients may have the signs and symptoms found in younger children, as well as the more classic findings of

TABLE 56-7. Bacterial Meningitis: Presentation by Age

Diagnostic findings	< 2-3 mo	2-3 mo-2 yr	> 2 yr
Apnea/cyanosis	Common	Rare	Rare
Fever	Common	Common	Common
Hypothermia	Common	Rare	Rare
Altered mental status	Common	Common	Common
Headache	Rare	Rare	Common
Seizures	Early finding	Early finding	Late finding
Ataxia	Rare	Variable	Early finding
Jitteriness	Common	Common	Rare
Vomiting	Common	Common	Variable
Stiff neck	Rare	Late finding	Common
Bulging fontanelle	Common	Common	Closed

nuchal rigidity, Kernig's sign (pain on extension of legs), Brudzinski's sign (flexion of the neck producing flexion at the knees and hips), and headaches. Alternatively, a child may be asked to touch the knees as an active motion. If this movement can only be performed with rapid flexion of the knees or if it cannot be completed, meningeal inflammation is possible. It is only in children over 2 years of age that patients commonly have headache, photophobia, and stiff neck. Focal findings of hemiparesis, facial palsy and visual field defects are noted in 15% of patients (Table 56-7).[128]

Patients with a ventriculoperitoneal (VP) shunt may have a somewhat different presentation associated with a low-grade ventriculitis that includes headache, nausea, minimal fever, and malaise. The shunting device consists of three parts. The ventricular catheter is passed into the anterior horns of the lateral ventricles through a right occipital or frontal burr hole. The catheter is attached subcutaneously to a reservoir that may be percutaneously tapped to obtain ventricular fluid. A distal catheter containing a pump and one-way valve to regulate pressure and flow in the system is attached to the reservoir. This distal catheter commonly passes into the peritoneum.

To assess shunt function, the reservoir is pumped and if it cannot be depressed, a distal block is present; if it pumps but does not refill, it is blocked proximally at the ventricular end. If it pumps poorly, there may be a relative dysfunction. Withdrawing fluid from the shunt for analysis or because of abnormal pumping requires consultation with a neurosurgeon.[129]

Aseptic meningoencephalitis from viral, fungal, or mycobacterial agents is usually less toxic and more insidious in presentation.

Complications. Manifestations of meningitis are varied, with a high potential for significant complications. Five percent to 10% of children initially present with circulatory collapse marked by poor perfusion, mottling, delayed capillary refill, and altered mental status, all of which are usually due to vasoconstriction, redistribution, and increased venous pooling. Tachypnea and tachycardia may be present. With progression, evidence of septic shock, end organ damage, and metabolic acidosis may develop.[129] Patients may develop disseminated intravascular coagulation as a component of septic shock. The mortality rate in neo-

---

Complications of Bacterial Meningitis

Acute	**Long-term**
General	Seizure disorder
Shock	Hydrocephalus
Bacteremia	Paresis
Neurologic	Sensorineural hearing loss
Seizure	Cranial nerve palsy
Herniation	Blindness
Subdural effusion	Hearing, speech, or behavioral disorders
Cerebral edema and infarction	
Inappropriate ADH (SIDH)	
Other	
Anemia	
Disseminated intravascular coagulation	
Myocarditis	
Septic joint	

---

nates remains high. Beyond the neonatal age, this rate is about 5% (see box above).[130]

Bacteremia with associated hematogenous involvement of joints, particularly the hip, may occur. The pericardium and myocardium may also be involved.

Anemia, especially with *H. influenzae,* is common, probably as a result of a low-grade hemolytic process.

Seizures occur in as many as one third of patients.[131] The distinction between a simple febrile seizure and a seizure complicating meningitis is often difficult in younger children and made only by performing a lumbar puncture. Focal seizures have a significant poor prognostic significance, potentially representing focal intracranial pathology. The presence of persistent neurologic deficits is the only long-term predictor of subsequent afebrile seizures.[132,133]

Increased intracranial pressure may develop secondary to cerebral edema on a vasogenic or cytotoxic basis. Headache and vomiting may occur. Inappropriate secretion of antidiuretic hormone (SIADH) may further exacerbate this condition (see Chapter 50). Bradycardia, hypertension, and respiratory compromise often precede herniation. Ultimately, such patients demonstrate uncal herniation marked by hyperventilation, hypertension, impaired mental status, and abnormal pupillary response. Lateral rectus muscle abnormality, facial paralysis, vertigo, and deafness may accompany altered mental status as evidence of increased intracranial pressure.[134,135] Bulging fontanelle, widening of skull sutures, and decerebrate or decorticate posturing also may be present.

Subdural effusions are reported in 39% of patients with bacterial meningitis in children aged 1 to 18 months. The associated risk factors include young age, rapid onset of illness, low peripheral WBC count, and high CSF protein. Patients with a subdural effusion are more likely to have seizures, although there is no greater ongoing incidence of patients to have seizure, hearing loss, neurologic deficits, or developmental delay.[136] Long-term follow-up of children with *H. influenzae* meningitis indicates that the sequelae after 10 years includes about 4% of children with serious neurologic abnormalities and about 10% with residual sensorineural hearing loss.[137]

Of those patients with meningococcal or pneumococcal meningitis, 90% are afebrile by the sixth day in contrast to only 72% of those with *H. influenzae* as the etiologic agent. The early introduction of dexamethasone in management may alter the temperature pattern. Conditions associated with this persistent fever include untreated or partially treated disease, subdural effusion, nosocomial infection, phlebitis, and drug fever.

Ancillary Data. A number of studies should be conducted concurrent with the lumbar puncture. A CBC may be elevated after a spinal tap.[124]

Electrolytes should be measured to provide baseline data to exclude SIADH, as well as to evaluate for abnormal fluid intake or output. Serial monitoring is essential. A blood culture is essential and is generally positive in 90% of patients with *N. meningitidis* or *H. influenzae* and 80% of those with *S. pneumoniae*. Cultures of focally infected sites such as purpuric lesions, joints, and abscesses should be obtained. Coagulation studies should be performed in patients suspected of having DIC.

Counterimmunoelectrophoresis (CIE) is a particularly useful rapid diagnostic test to detect the capsular antigen to *H. influenzae*, *S. pneumoniae*, *N. meningitidis*, and group B streptococci. However, studies have shown that the gram stain of the CSF is faster and just as sensitive as bacterial antigen tests.[138] Other studies have suggested a false positive rate of 54% and a true positive rate of 38%. The greatest yield was on CSF specimens with a cell count over 50 white cells/mm^3 and a negative culture at 48 hours. Specimens from children recently vaccinated with HIB conjugate may have a positive urine and CSF for the rapid test.

Urinalyses should be considered a component of the routine evaluation of such children.

Lumbar puncture and analysis of CSF are the basis for evaluation of the patient with suggestive clinical signs of meningitis. Clinical circumstances in which a lumbar puncture is indicated in children are summarized in the box above.

Common Indications to Consider Performing Lumbar Puncture in Children[110,111]

Suspected meningitis

Suspected neonatal sepsis

Toxic febrile child without source of infection, particularly if under 1 year of age and altered mental status

Focal infection and altered mental status associated with intracranial infection (otitis media, orbital/periorbital/facial cellulitis, septic arthritis, pneumonia, etc.)

Increasingly toxic child with previously negative lumbar puncture

Documented bacteremia in child with altered mental status, especially *H. influenzae*

Febrile illness after intimate contact with child with *N. meningitidis* or *H. influenzae*

Febrile seizure in child <18 months of age

Nuchal rigidity with no obvious etiology

Petechial rash and fever

Sepsis suspected in immunocompromised child

Penetration of dura and subsequent CNS or traumatic findings

It is important to exclude the potential of significantly increased intracranial pressure on the basis of history and physical examination before performing the procedure. If there is any question, a CT scan should be obtained before the lumbar puncture is performed, but increased intracranial pressure is unusual unless there is a history of trauma or major alteration in mental status.

The key to performing a lumbar puncture is to properly position and immobilize the child. The patient should be placed at the edge of a firm examination table and maintained in a position, with the neck flexed and the knee drawn upward into the fetal position. The shoulders should be perpendicular to the table. An alternative position for the small infant is to hold the patient sitting, flexing the thighs up to the abdomen. Cardiac respiratory arrest may result from the child being held too tightly with subsequent impairment in venous return; careful monitoring is essential.

The back is cleansed with povidone-iodine and alcohol and draped. Meticulous sterile technique is required. Local anesthesia should be used for comfort and to enhance cooperation. The puncture is at the intersection of the line joining the superior portion of the iliac crest with the spine. This point is the spinous process of L4 (Fig. 56-5). A 22-gauge, 1.5-inch needle is inserted at L3-L4, but may be inserted one space above or below. A 20-gauge, 3-inch needle may be used with adolescents and adults.

The needle is inserted perpendicular to the back, aiming at the umbilicus. In younger children it is advisable to puncture the skin and allow the child to calm down and then reassess the position before proceeding. A "pop" may not be felt in younger children, and it is advisable to remove the stylet frequently and examine the needle hub for fluid as the needle with stylet is advanced. Intraspinal

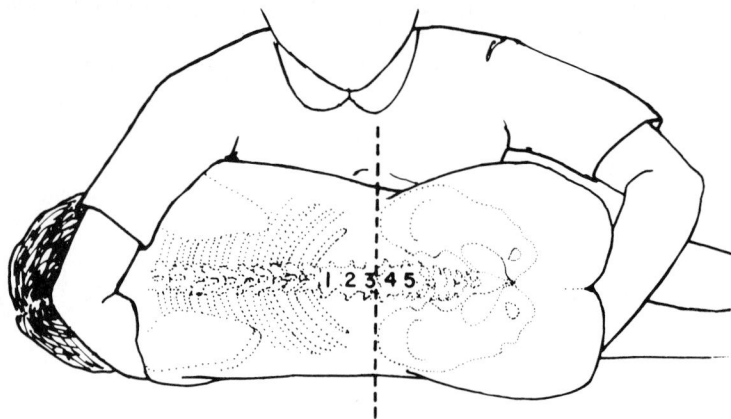

FIG. 56-5. Position for lumbar puncture.

dermoids are avoided by using only needles with stylets. Penetration of a nerve causes pain. In this case, the needle is withdrawn and redirected.

Manometry may be performed in cooperative children, particularly those over 5 years of age. Normal relaxed pressure is 5 to 15 cm H_2O. If increased pressure is noted at the time of the procedure, only a small amount of fluid should be withdrawn and the needle quickly removed. The patient obviously requires immediate evaluation and treatment. Optimally a lumbar puncture is avoided in such patients.

Complications associated with the procedure are rare but may include local problems including pain or hematoma, persistent CSF leak, radiculopathy and nerve injury (cauda equina), and an epidermoid cyst. Systemic conditions may include a post-lumbar puncture headache, infection, herniation syndrome, spinal subarachnoid hemorrhage, and respiratory or circulatory compromise due to impaired venous return or reduced ventilatory capacity.

Partial treatment with antibiotics before lumbar puncture will rarely alter the CSF enough to interfere with appropriate interpretation.[139] If it is difficult to distinguish between bacterial and viral meningitis on the basis of the initial CSF test, a repeat lumbar puncture in 6 to 8 hours may be helpful. The second lumbar puncture may demonstrate a marked decrease in the percentage of polymorphonuclear (PMN) leukocytes and an increase in lymphocytes in untreated viral meningitis.[140] Although there is conflicting evidence that a lumbar puncture can potentially seed the meninges in bacteremic patients, this consideration is theoretical and should not delay obtaining spinal fluid. One author has suggested that a ratio of immature-neutrophils to total neutrophils on peripheral WBC count over 0.12 is associated with, and is more sensitive for, bacterial meningitis than the total peripheral WBC count, but under no circumstances should peripheral studies be used to avoid performing a spinal tap.[114]

A lumbar puncture may be delayed if the patient is hemodynamically unstable, the airway is unprotected, or there is generalized seizure activity. If increased intracranial pressure is suspected secondary to a subdural or epidural fluid collection, cavernous sinus thrombosis, lateral sinus thrombosis, cerebral hemorrhage, brain tumor, cord tumor, or brain abscess, further evaluation by CT should be considered before a lumbar puncture is performed. The removal of the CSF enhances the risk of cerebral herniation and specific intervention may be required.[142] Children with special deformities may require fluoroscopic direction of the needle. Those with lumbosacral cutaneous infection such as abscess, cellulitis, or varicella lesions present a unique risk. In such circumstances in which clinical or logistical issues suggest delaying the procedure, antibiotics should be administered empirically after a blood culture is obtained.

Analysis of the CSF is essential (Table 56-8). Classically, the CSF is cloudy or turbid when meningitis is present. Two to three percent of patients with culture-proven bacterial meningitis have an otherwise normal analysis.[143] In very low birth–weight infants, the findings may be different (Table 56-9). The *gram stain* will often identify the causative organism. If the gram stain is negative, a methylene blue stain may distinguish intracellular bacteria from nuclear material.

The CSF glucose usually is low in patients with bacterial meningitis. The normal CSF/serum glucose ratio is approximately 0.6, although some consider a ratio of 0.4 as normal. A greater specificity for bacterial meningitis is a CSF/glucose ratio of 0.30.[144] The lumbar puncture procedure may actually increase the peripheral glucose as well as WBC.[145] The *protein* is elevated in an inflammatory response, bleed, endocrinopathy, or degenerative disorder. CSF lactic acid may have some discriminatory function.

The cell count should have less than eight leukocytes. The absolute number of white cells and the predominance of PMN leukocytes vs. lymphocytes help to distinguish viral from bacterial disease.

Bloody spinal punctures create a diagnostic dilemma. Hemorrhage into the subarachnoid space due to a bleed results in an equal number of red blood cells (RBC) in the first and last samples. The fluid is usually xanthochromic. Although the appraisal may be inexact and fraught with errors, the number of WBC in spinal fluid obtained after a traumatic tap may be estimated. One thousand RBC/mm^3 in the CSF contribute 1 to 2 WBC/mm^3 in the CSF,

TABLE 56-8. Cerebrospinal Fluid Analysis

	Normal			Bacterial	Viral
	Preterm	Term	>6 mo		
Cell count (WBC/mm³)*					
Mean	9	8	0	>500	<500
Range	0-25	0-22	0-4		
Predominant cell type	Lymph	Lymph	Lymph	80% PMN leukocyte	PMN leukocyte initially; lymphocyte later
Glucose (mg/dl)					
Mean	50	52	>40	<40	>40
Range	24-63	34-119			
Protein (mg/dl)					
Mean	115	90	<40	>100	<100
Range	65-150	20-170			
CSF/blood glucose (%)					
Mean	74	81	50	<40	>40
Range	55-150	44-248	40-60		
Gram stain	Negative	Negative	Negative	Positive†	Negative
Bacterial culture	Negative	Negative	Negative	Positive‡	Negative

Modified from Sarff LD, Platt LH, McCracken GH Jr: *J Pediatr* 88:473, 1976; Portnoy JM and Olson LC: *Pediatric* 75:484, 1985.
*Total WBC/mm³ by age in the normal child can be further delineated as follows (mean ± 2 SD): <6 wk: 3.7 ± 6.8; 6 wk-3 mo: 2.9 ± 5.7; 3 mo-6 mo: 1.9 ± 4.0; 6-12 mo: 2.6 ± 4.9; >12 mo: 1.9 ± 5.4.
†If gram stain is negative, a methylene blue stain may distinguish intracellular bacteria from nuclear material.
‡85% of partially treated patients will have a positive gram stain and >95% have positive cultures. (CIE may be helpful if the culture is negative.)

TABLE 56-9. CSF Findings in Very Low Birthweight Infants

Finding	Group 1 (<1,000 gm)		Group 2 (1,001-1,500 gm)	
	Mean ± SD	Range	Mean ± SD	Range
Birthweight (gm)	763 ± 115	550-980	1,270 ± 152	1,020-1,500
Gestational age (wks)	26 ± 1.3	24-28	29 ± 1.4	27-33
Leukocyte count (cells/mm³)	4 ± 3	0-14	6 ± 9	0-44
Erythrocytes (mm³)	1,027 ± 3,270	0-19,050	786 ± 1,879	0-9,750
Polymorphonuclear cells (%)	6 ± 15	0-66	9 ± 17	0-60
Mononuclear cells (%)	86 ± 30	34-100	85 ± 28	13-100
Glucose (mg/dl)	61 ± 34	29-217	59 ± 21	31-109
Protein (mg/dl)	150 ± 56	95-370	132 ± 43	5-227

From Rodriguez AF, Kaplan SL, Mason EO: *J Pediatr* 116:971, 1990.
*All infants in study had birthweights appropriate for gestational age, negative CSF bacterial cultures, and no evidence of intracranial bleed.

whereas 1,000 RBC/mm³ in the CSF raises the protein to about 1.5 mg/dl. The calculation is as follows:

$$\text{Number of WBC introduced/mm}^3 = \frac{(\text{peripheral WBC}) \times (\text{RBC in CSF})}{\text{peripheral RBC count}}$$

The result of this calculation is then compared with the actual number of cells counted in the CSF.[146]

Approximately 90% of children with ventriculoperitoneal shunts with CSF WBC count over 100 cells/mm³ will be infected. The CSF glucose is usually normal and the organisms are less pathogenic.[147]

Radiographic studies may be helpful in evaluating the chest if consideration is given to pleural, pericardial, or parenchymal disease. If there is any evidence of an intracranial process or concern about cerebral edema and increased intracranial pressure, a CT should be performed.[148]

Differential Considerations

A number of presenting complaints must be considered when evaluating the patient with suspected bacterial meningitis. Stiff neck is a common presentation and diagnoses to be excluded include meningitis, cervical adenitis, osteomyelitis, trauma with secondary fracture, hematoma or muscle injury, tumor, hysteria, and oculogyric crisis from drugs such as phenothiazines.

Altered mental status associated with fever or systemic toxicity may result from a number of diagnostic entities.

TABLE 56-10. Infectious Causes of Aseptic Meningitis

Bacteria	Partially treated meningitis
Virus	Enterovirus, mumps, Epstein-Barr, arbovirus (eastern, western, and St. Louis equine), cytomegalovirus, lymphocytic choriomeningitis, varicella-zoster, herpes simplex, HIV
Mycoplasma	*M. pneumoniae, M. hominis*
Spirochete	Syphilis, leptospirosis, Lyme disease
Fungi	*Candida albicans, Crytococcus, neoformons, Coccidioides*
Rickettsiae	Rocky Mountain spotted fever
Protozoa	*Toxoplasma gondii*, malaria
Other	Parameningeal, brain, or epidural abscess, bacterial endocarditis

Because of the nonspecific nature of the signs and symptoms, particularly in younger children, it is often difficult without a lumbar puncture to distinguish meningitis from a number of other infections including pneumonia, acute gastroenteritis with dehydration, and an acute illness associated with a febrile seizure. Less often, brain abscess, subdural empyema, and acute obstruction of a VP shunt should be considered.

Children with aseptic meningitis or meningoencephalitis are usually less toxic than children with a low-grade fever. Enterovirus accounts for approximately 85% of all cases of aseptic meningitis. Retroorbital, global, or bifrontal headaches occur in the vast majority of patients; and vomiting is noted in over half. Anorexia, malaise, myalgia, photophobia, and seizures may be present. Meningism is present in about 75% of patients but is persistent and severe in only about 15%. Focal neurologic abnormalities are usually absent.[149,150] Herpes simplex infection may require specific treatment with acyclovir (see Chapters 18 and 55). Usual management of other causes is supportive, often including pain management.

Encephalitis and meningoencephalitis are an inflammatory illness of the brain and meninges. Etiologic agents include viruses spread person to person (e.g., adenovirus, herpes, varicella, EB virus, enterovirus) and from mosquitoes (arbovirus) or warm-blooded mammals (rabies, lymphocytic choriomeningitis). Bacterial pathogens, as well as rickettsial disease, mycoplasma, fungi, protozoan, and cat scratch disease, have also been demonstrated to be causative (Table 56-10). Children typically have diffuse disease with behavioral and personality changes, decreased consciousness, generalized or localized seizures, hemiparesis, movement disorders, cranial nerve defects, and ataxia. The initial findings are usually fever with headache.[151,152]

Vascular disorders may also cause a rapid deterioration. Subarachnoid bleeding or a cerebrovascular accident may develop acutely and may be associated with a systemic infection.

The stress of an acute infection may lead some individuals to overdoses, either purposeful or accidental. Infection may change the kinetics of drugs such as theophylline.

Head trauma producing a subdural or epidural hematoma may be difficult to distinguish, sometimes necessitating a CT scan before the lumbar puncture. Heatstroke may cause fever, dehydration, meningism, and marked changes in mentation.

Management

The initial management of the child with suspected bacterial meningitis must focus on stabilizing the patient. Assessment of vital signs with concomitant evaluation for hypoxia, adequacy of ventilation, dehydration, increased intracranial pressure, acidosis, electrolyte abnormalities, and DIC should be performed as appropriate. Intravenous access should be ensured once adequate airway and ventilation are assured.

After stabilization is achieved, a lumbar puncture should be performed and analyzed. Concomitant additional laboratory studies are performed as indicated. A variety of specific pharmacologic agents should be initiated rapidly once bacterial meningitis is confirmed or suspected on the basis of the CSF analysis.

Antibiotics should be initiated parenterally using the gram stain, patient's age, underlying disease, immunologic status, and allergy history as guides to selection. Although chloramphenicol has been a mainstay of therapy, it has largely been replaced by third generation cephalosporins. If the spinal tap cannot be performed for any one of the reasons discussed earlier, antibiotics should be initiated after obtaining a blood culture with the anticipation that the lumbar puncture will be completed in the next few hours. If bacterial meningitis is diagnosed or suspected and venous access cannot be achieved, intramuscular administration should be considered. If the child is in shock, intraosseous administration of antibiotics and fluids may be appropriate. Antibiotics should be altered once culture and sensitivity data are available. Ceftriaxone has been reported to cause biliary pseudolithiasis in children and displaces bilirubin from albumin in neonates (see box on p. 1003).[150-157]

Penicillin- and cephalosporin-resistant *S. pneumoniae* isolates have been reported. Vancomycin has been recommended when resistance is prevalent in a specific area or is documented by sensitivity testing. It should also be considered in children who respond poorly to therapy. However, its CSF penetration is reflective of the degree of inflammation that may be reduced by dexamethasone.[158,159] The dose is typically 40 to 60 mg/kg/24 hr q 6 hr IV with somewhat lower doses in neonates. Vancomycin therapeutic ranges are a trough of 4 to 10 μg/ml while the peak is 20-40 μg/ml, depending on the laboratory.

Fluid therapy should be conservative, reflecting hydration and vital signs. After stabilization is achieved, fluids should be continued at 80% to 100% of maintenance re-

---

Antibiotic Management of Bacterial Meningitis

< 2 mo

Unknown etiology	Ampicillin 100-200 mg/kg/24 hr q 4-6 hr IV *and* cefotaxime (or equivalent) 100-150 mg/kg/24 hr q 8-12 hr IV; or ampicillin *and* gentamicin 5-7.5 mg/kg/24 hr q 8-12 hr IV (or tobramycin 4-6 mg/kg/24 hr q 8-12 hr IV)
E. coli	Chloramphenicol 50-100 mg/kg/24 hr q 6 hr IV or cefotaxime, as above; treat 21 days or longer
Group B streptococci	Penicillin G 150,000-250,000 units/kg/24 hr q 4-6 hr IV *and* gentamicin, as above; treat 14 days or longer
L. monocytogenes	Ampicillin, as above; treat 14 days or longer

2 mo-9 yr

Unknown etiology	Cefotaxime 200 mg/kg/24 hr q 6 hr IV (or ceftriaxone 100 mg/kg/24 hr q 12 hr IV or cefuroxime 200 mg/kg/24 hr q 6 hr IV); or ampicillin 200-400 mg/kg/24 hr q 4 hr IV *and* chloramphenicol 100 mg/kg/24 hr q 6 hr IV (rarely used)
H. influenzae	Cefotaxime 200 mg/kg/24 hr q 6 hr IV (or ceftriaxone 100 mg/kg/24 hr q 12 hr IV or cefuroxime 200 mg/kg/24 hr q 6 hr IV or ceftizoxime 200 mg/kg/24 hr q 6-8 hr IV); or ampicillin 200-400 mg/kg/24 hr q 4 hr IV *and* chloramphenicol 100 mg/kg/24 hr q 6 hr IV (rarely used); treat 10 days
S. pneumoniae†	Penicillin G 250,000 units/kg/24 hr q 4 hr IV; treat 10 days
N. meningitidis	Penicillin G 250,000 units/kg/24 hr q 4 hr IV; treat 7-10 days

>9 yr

Unknown etiology	Penicillin G 250,000 units/kg/24 hr q 4 hr IV*
S. pneumoniae†	Penicillin G 250,000 units/kg/24 hr q 4 hr IV*; treat 10 days
N. meningitidis	Penicillin G 250,000 units/kg/24 hr q 4 hr IV*; treat 7-10 days

Serum concentration of chloramphenicol should be maintained at 10-25 μg/ml.

Duration of therapy in uncomplicated cases in children <2 mo of age is generally 14-21 days or longer. Older children may generally be treated for 10 days, depending on the response to therapy and the pathogen. Patients with complicated cases require longer duration.

*Adult: 10 million-20 million units/24 hr q 4 hr IV.

†If resistance suspected, initiate vancomycin 40-60 mg/kg/24 hr q 6 hr IV.

---

quirements during the first 24 hours. Serum sodium should be monitored and if decreased, spot urine and serum sodium potassium and osmolality should be measured. If hyponatremia secondary to inappropriate ADH secretion occurs, fluid should be restricted.

Administration of steroids during the treatment of bacterial meningitis reduces the incidence of subsequent sensorineural hearing loss. A selective approach is indicated, suggesting that when meningitis is microscopically confirmed or the CSF profile is suggestive, dexamethasone 0.15 mg/kg/dose IV should be administered every 6 hours for four days or a total of 16 doses. The initial dose of antibiotics should be given concomitant or 10 to 15 minutes after the initial dose of dexamethasone.[160-163]

Serial physical examinations, including a head circumference, should occur daily. Particular attention should be given to secondary complications such as septic arthritis or subdural effusion in performing daily examinations. Fluid status must be concurrently monitored.

Seizures should be treated with diazepam (Valium) 0.2 to 0.3 mg/kg/dose q 5 to 10 minutes IV (maximum: 10 mg) or lorazepam (Ativan) 0.05 to 0.10 mg/kg/dose IV. Obviously, metabolic and anatomic abnormalities should be excluded. Phenobarbital or phenytoin may be initiated, thereafter.

Cerebral edema is an infrequent complication but may develop with focal neurologic signs or evidence of hernia-

tion. If the patient is intubated, hyperventilate to maintain the P_{CO_2} at about 25 mm Hg. Mannitol (20% solution) 0.5 to 1.0 gm/kg/dose q 4 to 6 hr IV may also be given if the patient is hemodynamically stable.

Disposition

All patients require hospitalization. Those at highest risk include those who are less than 1 year or demonstrate shock, coma, seizures, petechiae for less than 12 hours, low CSF glucose, or a very high protein; close monitoring is required.

If the patient is seen initially in a setting without facilities to perform a lumbar puncture and has signs and symptoms suggestive of bacterial meningitis, blood cultures should be obtained and parenteral antibiotics (preferably IV) administered before transport.

Chemoprophylaxis is indicated in specific children and is discussed in the Appendix to Chapter 55. Individuals who have had intimate contact with a parent with meningitis due to *N. meningitidis* should receive prophylaxis or rifampin 10 mg/kg/dose q 12 hr PO for 4 doses (adult: 600 mg/dose q 12 hr PO for 4 doses; children <1 month: 5 mg/kg/dose q 12 hr PO for 4 doses).

Prophylaxis for exposure to systemic disease is generally indicated. It is recommended for all household contacts, regardless of age, in those households with at least one contact younger than 48 months. Day care facilities with children under 2 years of age with 25 or more hours of contact per week should usually initiate prophylaxis. Those with older children need to begin therapy. In settings with multiple cases within 60 days, treatment should be initiated. The dosage of rifampin is 20 mg/kg/dose (max: 600 mg/dose) q 24 hr PO for 4 doses. In neonates, the dose is 10 mg/kg/dose q 24 hr PO although some recommend reducing the dose to 10 mg/kg/dose in infants less than 1 month old. Rifampin can be administered to children by having a liquid formulation prepared or crushing the tablets. Do not give the medication to patients with liver disease or pregnant females.

Exposed children who develop a febrile illness should receive prompt medical evaluation, with treatment initiated if indicated. Parents must be informed of the increased risk of children under 1 year of age developing secondary cases of *H. influenzae* meningitis. In epidemic *N. meningitidis*, immunization of potential contacts is appropriate.[156]

All children should undergo audiologic evaluation after acute management.[164]

Immunization with *H. influenzae* vaccine is now routinely available to children at 2, 4, 6, and 15 months. Generally, children less than 2 years of age who have recovered from *H. influenzae* meningitis should be immunized, since the disease does not provide long-term protection.[156]

MIGRAINE HEADACHES

MANANDA S. BHENDE

Headaches are common complaints in childhood and adolescence.[165] Migraine is an episodic headache that is unilateral or bilateral, pulsating, of moderate to severe intensity, and exacerbated by physical activity.[166] Associated symptoms include nausea, vomiting, photophobia, and phonophobia. Migraines are one of the most common cause of headaches in children.[167]

Migraines may be classified *migraine with aura* (previously called classic migraine) and *migraine without aura* (previously called common migraine) according to the presence or absence of premonitory neurologic symptoms.[168] Between the episodes of headache, the patient is essentially symptom free.

Migraines are more common in adolescent girls. The largest study of headaches in school children between the ages of 7 to 15 was reported by Bille in 1962.[169] He found that about 4% of school children had vascular headaches. By 7 years of age 2.5% and by about 15 years 5% of children will have experienced a migraine attack. About half of all individuals who develop migraines have their first attack prior to age 20. In early childhood boys are affected more than girls, but after puberty girls have more migraines than boys.[165,170] Other studies have confirmed Bille's original findings that headache frequently increases with age.[165] A history of motion sickness and sleep disorders has been found to be associated with migraines.[165,171] There is also an association between migraine and epilepsy. Migraneurs have an epilepsy incidence of 2% to 8%, which is higher than the general population and about 15%

of epileptics will develop migraine. EEG changes in migraine are variable and may be only transitory during the attack.[172]

Pathophysiology

The exact pathophysiology of migraine has not been elucidated, but there are many hypotheses about the pathogenesis. The vascular theory of migraine, popular until the 1980s, emphasized that vasoconstriction causes the aura while vasodilation produces the headache.[173] It is now believed that the primary event is neuronal, which in turn initiates biochemical and vascular changes. The aura is caused by spreading depression of neuronal activity, first described by Leao, from the occiput forward at the rate of 2 to 3 mm/minute because of a spreading decrease in cerebral blood flow.[173-176] Positive emission tomography (PET) scans of cerebral blood flow supports a hypoxic model of ischemia leading to calcium excesses and cerebral dysfunction.[177] A PET scan recorded during a spontaneous migraine headache has demonstrated the bilateral spread of cerebral hypoperfusion.[178] This hypothesis best explains the gradual evolution of a migraine (rather than a sudden onset); the march of symptoms suggest a progressive involvement of the cortical areas.

Involvement of serotonin (5-HT) in the pathogenesis of migraine has been documented repeatedly.[166,168,173,176,179] Probably 5-HT is released from platelets at the onset of an attack, which is associated with an increase of free 5-HT in the plasma. Later stages are characterized by lower levels of 5-HT. 5-HT acts in many different receptors and may induce vasodilation or vasoconstriction depending on the type of receptor dominant in a particular blood vessel. On this basis, Humphries et al developed the 5-HT agonist sumatriptan to treat migraines.[176]

Other neurotransmitters implicated include prostaglandins, prolactin, gamma-aminobutyric acid (GABA), dopamine, substance P, neuropeptide 7, and vasoactive intestinal peptide.[173] Increased platelet aggregation, endorphin deficiencies, excessive epinephrine release, and lipoprotein abnormalities are also implicated in the pathophysiology.[180] Disparate 5 hydroxytryptamine (5-HT) and norepinephrine (NE) metabolisms have been shown in classic and common migraines.[181] It was thought that the vasodilation caused the headache; now it is thought that dilated vessels are hyperpermeable to polypeptides, resulting in sterile perivascular inflammation and activation of the perivascular trigeminal nocioceptive receptors.[174,176] Fluctuating levels of monoamines in the peripheral circulation probably reflect changes in central neurotransmitter substances, causing the vascular changes found in migraines.[175]

There is also evidence that the brain is not the only organ affected by migraine: alterations in renal function, especially polyuria and increased histidine excretion, have been demonstrated. Thus although many theories have been postulated, the exact mechanism remains unknown.[182]

Etiology

Migraine headaches are probably a genetically transmitted disease, as there is a positive family history in 70% to 90% of cases.[170,171] The mode of transmission is unclear but seems to be autosomal dominant with variable penetrance, which is greater in females.[171] Offspring of female migraine patients have a 25% chance of developing migraines.[173] The child with a genetic predisposition to migraines may suffer from these headaches, depending on numerous precipitating events.[167]

Diagnostic Criteria

Prensky and Sommers[183] described certain diagnostic criteria for both common and classic migraine. Migraines are periodic headaches that are separated by symptom-free intervals and associated with at least three of the following:

1. Abdominal pain with nausea or vomiting
2. Unilateral headache (hemicrania)
3. Throbbing, pulsating quality
4. Aura: visual, sensory, or motor preceding the headache
5. Positive family history
6. Relief by sleep

Criteria 1, 5, and 6 occur most frequently in childhood migraines. Common migraine in which no aura precedes the headache is the usual type seen in childhood: the headache is usually bilateral so these criteria may be too restrictive.[173] Nausea, vomiting, abdominal pain, and relief after sleep are found in 90% of the patients; 69% have a positive family history. Throbbing pulsatile headache is found in about 58% of patients, hemicrania in 36%, and aura in 17% of the patients.[173]

Description of a Typical Migraine Attack.[168] The migraine attack has been divided into the following five phases:

1. *Prodrome* occurs hours or days before the headache
2. *Aura* comes immediately before the headache
3. *Headache*
4. *Headache termination*
5. *Postdrome*

No one particular phase is required for the diagnosis. The prodrome can occur in up to 60% of migraines and can occur hours to days prior to the onset of the headache. It includes psychologic, neurologic, constitutional and autonomic features. Psychologic features can include depression, euphoria, irritability, restlessness, mental slowness, hyperactivity, fatigue, and drowsiness. Neurologic symptoms include photophobia and phonophobia; constitutional symptoms like stiff neck, sluggishness, increased thirst or urination, anorexia, diarrhea, or constipation may occur. Some patients report a poorly characterized feeling that a migraine is coming.

The aura develops over the course of 5 to 20 minutes, usually lasts less than 60 minutes, and can be characterized by visual, sensory or motor phenomena. Visual aura is the most common, including scintillations, fortification spectra, photopsia, or negative visual features like scotomas. This can be accompanied by tingling, numbness, hemiparesis, dysphasia, or aphasia if the dominant hemisphere is involved.

The headache is typically unilateral and throbbing, moderate to marked in severity and aggravated by physical activity. It lasts 4 to 72 hours in adults and 2 to 4 hours in children.

Classification of Migraine

Migraine without aura (common migraine)

A. At least 5 attacks filling criteria B to D
B. Headache lasting 4 to 72 hours (untreated or unsuccessfully treated)
C. Headache has at least 2 of the following:
   1. Unilateral
   2. Pulsating
   3. Moderate or severe intensity
   4. Aggravation by physical activity
D. During the headache, at least one of the following occurs:
   1. Nausea or vomiting
   2. Photophobia and phonophobia
E. At least one of the following is present:
   1. History and physical/neurologic examination rules out organic disorder
   2. Investigation rules out organic disorder
   3. Organic disorder is present but migraine attacks do not occur for the first time in close temporal relation to the disorder.

Migraine with aura (classic migraine)

A. At least 2 attacks fulfilling criteria B
B. At least 3 of the following 4 are present:
   1. One or more fully reversible aura symptoms occur indicating brain dysfunction
   2. At least 1 aura symptom develops gradually over more than 4 minutes or 2 or more symptoms in succession
   3. No single aura, symptoms last >60 minutes
   4. Headache follows the aura with a free interval of <60 minutes (it may also begin simultaneously or before the aura)
C. History/physical examination and diagnostic tests where appropriate exclude a secondary cause

---

As the headache terminates, the pain wanes and the patient has a washed out, tired feeling. Some may become irritable, listless and have impaired consciousness. They may complain of scalp tenderness and mood changes—some may feel unusually refreshed or euphoric after an attack.

Classification

The International Headache Society established diagnostic criteria and classification of headaches, which were published in 1988.[168] This has been the singular advance in headache research and provides the best diagnostic gold standard for both the clinician and the investigator.

Migraine has been classified into migraine without aura (common), migraine with aura (classic), complicated, and variant (see box above).

Complicated migraines are associated with transient neurologic disturbances. These neurologic abnormalities are assumed to be secondary to intracranial vasoconstriction and resultant ischemia and edema of the affected cerebral areas.[1] Classically, the deficit precedes the headache but may follow it. The pattern for any individual may be constant except for laterality. If this occurs on only one side, intracranial pathology must be ruled out. Any patient with complicated migraine must have diagnostic studies to exclude intracranial pathology.

Hemiplegic or *hemisensory migraine* is more common in children than adults. In recurrent attacks, alternate sides can be affected and are usually associated with aphasia and paresthesias. When it occurs posttrauma, hemiplegic or hemisensory migraines can present a diagnostic dilemma. After the onset of hemiparesis, contralateral headache and motor or sensory deficits follow and can last for days. Most resolve without sequelae, but permanent deficits have been reported. Similar disorders have been observed in patients with cardiogenic emboli, thrombotic disorders in sickle cell disease, moyamoya disease, postictal Todds paralysis, and intracranial hemorrhage, as well as in patients taking oral contraceptives. Angiography should be avoided because it worsens the attack.

Ophthalmoplegic migraine is accompanied by third nerve palsy and the headache may precede, accompany, or follow the ophthalmoplegia. Third nerve dysfunction consists of strabismus, ptosis, diplopia, and mydriasis. Age of onset is usually under 10 years, but patients as young as 1 year have been reported. It is more common in males. The possibility of vascular anomalies should be excluded.

Basilar artery migraine was initially described by Bicherdoff in 1961 and consists of a combination of visual symptoms (transient bilateral blindness, blurred vision, scotoma) along with vertigo, ataxia, loss of consciousness, and drop attacks. These symptoms are thought to be produced by vertebro-basilar insufficiency. Many patients go on to develop classic or common migraine and a few develop neurologic symptoms.[173,182]

Acute confusional state is an unusual form of migraine in which patients are restless, combative, and hyperactive or have altered consciousness and reduced response to painful stimuli. Attacks may last up to several hours, and it is important to distinguish from acute encephalopathy secondary to toxic or metabolic causes, psychotic states, and non-convulsive status epilepticus. Prognosis is usually good.

Alice in Wonderland syndrome is unusual because it causes distortion of body image, spatial relations, and time sense. Micropsia metamorphopsia, olfactory, auditory, and gustatory hallucinations have been reported.[165,171,172] Symptoms may vary before, during, or after the headache. It is more common in adults and is thought to be caused by ischemia of the parietal lobe.[170,172]

Migraine variants are syndromes that are thought to be a symptomatic equivalent of migraine in young children and include abdominal migraine, cyclic vomiting, and benign paroxysmal vertigo.[165,170] In abdominal migraine, children present with recurrent acute severe abdominal pain, nausea, and often an associated headache. Cyclic vomiting occurs with recurrent bouts of nausea and vomiting. *Migraine sine hemicrania* is a variant in which ophthalmologic manifestations are present without the headache and is more common in adolescent girls.[171]

Posttraumatic migraine occurs in children after mild head injury.[171,183,184] The migraine may present within a few minutes or hours after the trauma and may recur later in the absence of trauma. It is seen more frequently in children with a strong family history of migraine. Usually one has to obtain diagnostic studies to rule out intracranial pathology.

Diagnostic Findings

A detailed *history* about the headache is of utmost importance. The physician should obtain the details of aura, GI symptoms, location, type of headache, and any associated signs and symptoms. Anorexia and photobia are concomitant symptoms.

Triggering factors should be elicited. Stress, missed meals, excitement, post-excitement letdown, anxiety, fatigue, exercise, any intercurrent illness, menstrual periods, too much or too little sleep, and life events have all been known to trigger migraine attacks.[182] Certain foods, such as chocolate, cheese, citrus fruits, bananas, nuts, food additives, Chinese food with monosodium glutamate, alcohol (especially red wine), and processed meats that contain nitrites (hot dogs), have been known to trigger migraines in some individuals. These foods contain oxalates, nitrites, histamine, dopamine, tyrosine, and phenylalanine, which are the alleged precipitants for migraine attacks.[182] Delayed allergy to certain foods may be associated with migraines in children.[180] Birth control pills and mild head trauma may also cause migraine headaches.

Trying to pinpoint the cause of a migraine attack is beneficial in preventing or reducing further attacks. The history should include symptoms, intracranial pathology, family history, and psychosocial history. Children with migraines often show a characteristic meticulous, compulsive personality, strive to excel, and have difficulty in expressing rage or anger.[185]

The physical examination should include vital signs, especially blood pressure to check for hypertension; examination of head to detect sinusitis; temporomandibular joint dysfunction; tooth abscess; and skin to exclude any neurocutaneous syndromes.[180] The fundus should be examined for signs of papilledema. A thorough neck examination should include auscultation to elicit bruits, which may indicate the presence of vascular anomalies.[165] The presence of neck stiffness suggests subarachnoid hemorrhage or CNS infections such as meningitis, and head tilt may be found in some posterior fossa tumors. The neurologic examination should be very thorough to pinpoint any deviations from normal.

Ancillary Data. If the physical examination is normal and the history classic, no further laboratory data are necessary. In complicated migraine, the presence of any neurologic deficit or signs and symptoms of increased intracranial pressure or subarachnoid hemorrhage mandate diagnostic studies such as CT scans, with and without contrast, or MRI scans. Sometimes an EEG or LP may be indicated when seizures and intracranial infection are under consideration. A lumbar puncture should generally be preceded by a CT scan of the brain to avoid brain herniation. Diagnostic studies should be obtained in all children less than 6 years, as well as those having large head circumferences, exhibiting new neurologic signs, failing to return to a normal state of health between headaches, experiencing an increase in headache frequency or severity, or demonstrating personality changes.[186]

Differential Considerations

Included in the differential diagnosis of migraine headaches are intracranial pathology of any etiology, intracranial vascular malformation, Arnold-Chiari malformation, syndrome of postconcussion headache, benign muscle contraction, tension headaches, and seizures.[182] Because the child with migraines should be healthy between migraine attacks, the diagnosis of migraine is made by exclusion and longitudinal observation.[186]

Management

Most patients with migraines can be treated by the pediatrician or family practitioner but should be referred to the neurologist if there is any question. The steps in treatment include the following:

1. Reassurance—patients and parents want to be reassured that there is no brain tumor. Once this has been confirmed, they are usually less anxious and the child is more relaxed, which in itself may decrease the headache frequency.
2. Education of both the patient and parents
3. General nonpharmacologic treatment
4. Specific pharmacologic therapy, which includes therapy for the acute attack and prophylactic therapy to prevent/reduce further attack
5. Specific nonpharmacologic therapy such as biofeedback, if appropriate[165]

Both parents and patient should understand that migraine is a life-long condition, and relief but not cure is possible.[165] Parents should also be taught not to be overprotective, which inadvertently cause their children to be overdependent, and avoid allowing any secondary gains to the child because of the condition.

General nonpharmacologic therapy should focus on removing the trigger factors. Reducing stress, exertion, avoiding certain foods, eating meals on time, sleeping and waking at regular times, and avoiding oral contraceptives all help to reduce the incidence. Special nonpharmacologic therapy, including biofeedback techniques, relaxation therapy, psychotherapy, and hypnotherapy, should be provided by experts.[172,180,187,188] Children are more amenable than adults to these techniques.

Pharmacologic therapy has two purposes: to treat the acute attack and to use prophylactic therapy to prevent further attacks.

Treatment of Acute Attack

Medications used in acute headache treatment include analgesics, antiemetics, anxiolytics, nonsteroidal antiinflammatory drugs (NSAIDS), ergots, steroids, major tranquillizers, narcotics and more recently 5-HT (serotonin) agonists.[166,168,179] The choice of acute treatment depends on severity, frequency of headaches, and the patient's re-

sponse profile. The symptomatic treatment begins with the use of either nonprescription or prescription analgesics.

Simple analgesics, such as salicylates and acetaminophen, and rest in a quiet, dark room are sufficient to treat mild attacks. Fiornal (butalbital, aspirin, and caffeine) may be used if the preceding measures are not effective, in the dose of one-half tablet in a child less than 5 years, 1 tablet for a child between 5 and 11 years and 1 to 2 tablets for older children. Fiornal should be used with caution, since it can be habit forming.

Neuroleptic agents such as chlorpromazine or prochlorperazine when given IV or IM are useful not only for nausea and vomiting, but also for migraine pain.[189,190] Metoclopramide (Reglan) in a dose of 10 mg IV has been shown to be useful in adults with migraines for both reducing the nausea and vomiting and also the headache.[191] Very few studies have been reproduced in children. Smaller doses in adolescent patients may be helpful in select patients with migraine.

More potent narcotic analgesics such as propoxyphene, meperidine (Demerol), morphine, hydromorphone, and oxycodone are available, which may be used for infrequent severe attacks. Medication overuse poses a threat for rebound headache and should be avoided; narcotics should be administered with caution to prevent addiction. These are usually administered with an antiemetic such as hydroxyzine (Vistaril).

NSAIDS inhibit the enzyme cyclo-oxygenase to prevent the synthesis of prostaglandins, which account for their antiinflammatory, analgesic, and antipyretic properties. Ketorolac has been studied in adults and shown to help migraines.[192] It is the first NSAID that can be given parenterally but has not been studied in children with migraine. Older adolescents require the full dose of 60 mg, while 10- to 12-year-olds with migraine respond to one half the dose, 30 mg IM.

If simple analgesics do not provide satisfactory headache relief, then dihydroergotamine (DHE) or ergotamine can be used.[193] The bioavailability of ergot depends on the route of administration. Ergotamine can be given orally, sublingually, per rectum, and DHE can be given via the IV or SC route. Patients who cannot tolerate the accompanying nausea should be pretreated with metoclopramide, prochlorperazine, or promethazine. With oral ergot, the dosage is 1 to 2 tabs initially, followed by 2 additional tabs at half-hour intervals. No more than 4 tabs should be given for one attack and no more than 8 tabs should be taken in one week. When DHE is administered, the dose in adults is 1 mg IV/IM and repeated in one hour up to a total dose of 3 mg. When this is occasionally used in the adolescent, we give 0.5 mg IV, usually admitting to the hospital for repeated dosing. Contraindications to DHE are hypertension, sepsis, renal or hepatic failure, and coronary, cerebral, or peripheral vascular disease. Phenergan or other antiemetics may be needed.

Sumatriptan is a relatively new acute treatment for migraine. It is a selective $5HT_1$ receptor agonist and has been studied extensively in adults with success.[194,195] The studies in children are yet to be done. Neurologists have occasionally used it in a patient under close supervision. The adult dose is 6 mg SC and repeated in one hour if not responding. Side effects include pain at injection site, tingling, flushing, burning, dizziness, heaviness, neck pain and dysphoria, and rarely chest pressure.

Prophylaxis. Various agents have been tried for prophylaxis for frequent headaches, when a child has more than 4 headaches per month, or if the headaches are severe enough to disrupt work or school. The advantages and disadvantages of the medication must be considered, and the patient should be followed closely. Many drugs have been tried, including serotonin agonists and antagonists, tranquilizers, antidepressants, antihistamines, anticonvulsants, calcium channel blocking agents, vasoconstrictors, and vasodilators.[171]

Propranolol, the most commonly used drug for prophylaxis, has consistently shown greater efficacy than placebo.[171] The dose is 2 mg/kg/24 hr in 3 divided doses PO with a gradual increase until therapeutic efficacy or bradycardia is reached. Side effects include nausea, fatigue, bradycardia, hypotension, hypoglycemia, and depression. If the drug is stopped abruptly, patients can experience rebound headaches.[171] Propranolol is contraindicated in patients with asthma, with congestive heart failure, or suffering from depression.

Anticonvulsants such as phenobarbital and phenytoin (Dilantin) have been used successfully in younger patients in doses similar to those used for seizures (3 to 5 mg/kg/24 hr). Side effects include drowsiness, impaired learning, idiosyncratic hypersensitive responses, gingival hyperplasia, hirsutism, and ataxia. Amitriptyline (Elavil), 0.2 to 0.5 mg/kg as a single dose at night, can be given to older children with a depressive component. The side effects are dry mouth, dizziness, fatigue, urinary retention, constipation, and weight gain. Methysergide (Sansert) was one of the first agents used but is seldom used now because of its serious side effect, retroperitoneal fibrosis. Calcium channel blockers are currently being tested for migraine prophylaxis in children. They seem to work via their effect on smooth muscle and prevent vasoconstriction. Flunarizine and verapamil have been shown to be beneficial in adults, and cyproheptadine and nifedipine have been studied in children. Cyproheptadine (Periactin) is also an antihistamine and has antiserotonin activity but can cause weight gain and sedation.[171] The dose is 0.2 to 0.4 mg/kg/24 hr q 6-8 hr PO (max: 32 mg/24 hr). In adults, low dose aspirin prophylaxis has been shown to decrease the incidence of migraine,[196] and it may have beneficial effects in some children.[167]

Disposition

The vast majority of patients respond to therapy. Patient and family education enhance any treatment protocol, and education may help decrease triggering factors. The patient must be followed for prolonged periods. There is little correlation between migraine type, frequency, or severity of attacks and the ultimate prognosis; however, age of onset of migraines is a prognostic factor. Patients with onset after puberty usually continue to have migraines into adult life.[170] Bille reported that more than half his patients were migraine-free and one third improved after 4 to 6 years.[169,173] He followed some patients into adult life and found that about one fourth of them continued to have attacks as adults, and many were intermittently headache-free for prolonged periods of time.

IDIOPATHIC INTRACRANIAL HYPERTENSION (PSEUDOTUMOR CEREBRI)

RONALD I. PAUL • DOUGLAS HOLTZMAN

Idiopathic intracranial hypertension (IIH), also known as pseudotumor cerebri, is a syndrome characterized by the clinical manifestations of increased intracranial pressure with normal CSF constituents and a normal brain with normal or small ventricles on imaging studies. First described by Heinrich Quincke in 1893, the syndrome still has an elusive pathophysiology and etiology. Although called benign, the clinical course is not always harmless (with occasional severe complications).

Pathophysiology

Over the years, multiple theories have evolved to explain the mechanism behind the raised intracranial pressure. It is still not known why the ventricles fail to dilate under increased CSF pressure and volume. Recent studies have revealed an increase in the volume of free brain water (vasogenic brain edema) and may explain why the ventricles remain normal in size.[197] Studies also support the idea that absorption of cerebral spinal fluid through the arachnoid villi is decreased.[195] Other proposed mechanisms include the following: (1) overproduction of CSF, (2) increased intracranial blood volume, (3) increased venous pressure, (4) cerebral edema, (5) immune response, and (6) toxins.[199]

Etiology

Despite the lack of definitive knowledge of the pathophysiology, multiple conditions have been found in association with IIH (see box on p. 1009). In studies of childhood and adolescent IIH, an etiology was found in 33% to 75% of cases.[200-202] Those found most often included otitis media, corticosteroid use, obesity, and mild head trauma.

Diagnostic Findings

Although the peak incidence of IIH occurs in patients in their thirties, cases have been described in infants as young as 4 months. The most common adult patient is young, female, and obese; in contrast, no sex predilection has been found in the pediatric population. Headache is the most common presenting symptom, occurring in 50% to 75% of cases. It is typically generalized, episodic, throbbing, and worse in the morning. Other common symptoms include double or blurred vision, tinnitus, nausea and vomiting, and dizziness. Infants often initially present with somnolence, apathy, or irritability.[203] Occurrences have been documented in asymptomatic children in which papilledema was found on routine eye examination.

Physical findings include papilledema in almost all cases, retinal hemorrhages, unilateral or bilateral rectus muscles palsy, and slight ataxia. Younger children may have a bulging fontanelle, irritability, or listlessness. Most children initially do not have impairment of visual acuity.

Pseudotumor Cerebri — Underlying Conditions

Infectious
Otitis media
Roseola infantum
Sinusitis

Metabolic/endocrinologic
Corticosteroids (withdrawal or systemic therapy)
Hyperthyroidism
Obesity
Menstrual irregularities
Oral contraceptives
Addison disease
Hypoparathyroidism
Empty-sella syndrome
Pregnancy

Toxins
Tetracycline
Vitamin A
Nitrofurantoin
Nalidixic acid

Miscellaneous
Allergy
Minor head trauma
Immune complex disorder
Anemia
Sarcoidosis

Complications. In most children with IIH, the course is self-limited and results in no unfavorable sequelae. However, permanent visual loss secondary to papilledema does occur and is the major long-term complication. Studies of children have revealed a loss of visual acuity in 0% to 17% of patients. Unfortunately, ophthalmologic follow-up is not well documented. In adult series, loss of visual function was more likely to occur in patients with high grade or atrophic papilledema or subretinal hemorrhages.

Ancillary Data. The diagnosis of IIH must be clearly established. Symptoms and physical signs are suggestive of an intracranial mass lesion and hence frequently require CT scan. Findings on CT scan include small ventricles, empty sella, enlarged cisterna magna, and dilated optic nerve sheaths.

MRI scanning has been performed in several patients with IIH and has revealed no white matter signal abnormalities. The clinical use of both CT and MRI scans is primarily in the exclusion of other diseases that may present with similar clinical symptoms and signs.

After eliminating the possibility of an intracranial mass, a lumbar puncture should usually be performed to exclude infection, preferably in a relaxed patient whose head and legs are extended (a position difficult to achieve in an uncooperative child). Opening pressure greater than 20 cm H_2O, a normal or low CSF protein level, and a normal glucose and cell count confirm the diagnosis.

Management

No prospective randomized controlled clinical studies comparing treatment modalities have been performed on patients with IIH. Treatment successes and failures are also skewed by a large group of generalists and specialists who treat and provide follow-up, including pediatricians, internists, neurologists, neurosurgeons, and ophthalmologists. Most investigators agree that management should be dictated by the extent and the rapidity of the patient's visual deterioration. Medical management should be started initially, with surgical treatment reserved for refractory cases in which visual derangements worsen or if vision is severely affected at time of diagnosis.[203]

Treatment of any underlying condition should be concurrent with medical management of IIH, which begins with a short course of serial lumbar punctures, each removing enough CSF to reduce the manometric pressure to less than 20 cm H_2O. Repeated spinal taps are painful and may become progressively more difficult to perform. They also may produce persistent CSF leaks. Frequently after the first spinal tap, symptoms including headaches abate, at least temporarily. Adjunctive therapy may include the use of acetazolamide (Diamox), a carbonic anhydrase inhibitor of CSF production, in a dose of 5 mg/kg/dose (adult 250 to 375 mg/dose) given orally every 24 to 48 hours. This drug should be administered if symptoms such as visual defects worsen or if repeated lumbar punctures are ineffective or impossible to perform. If corticosteroids have recently been withdrawn (i.e., asthma), a course of prednisone or dexamethasone has been shown to be effective in selected patients. If prominent, obesity should be addressed, but in itself diet control will not provide a rapid enough resolution of symptoms. Surgical techniques including subtemporal decompression, lumbar peritoneal shunt, and optic nerve sheath fenestrations have been effective in cases unresponsive to medical management to limit or prevent visual field and acuity loss. Studies now show optic nerve sheath fenestrations to be the procedure of choice in adults.[203]

After the diagnosis is ascertained and treatment initiated with the first lumbar puncture, further treatment usually may be performed as an outpatient. If available, an ophthalmologist should evaluate the patient before discharge because it is important to document visual field acuity and field defects. Due to the seriousness of potential complications, careful follow-up needs to be established, even if mild symptoms abate. A neurologist and ophthalmologist should provide a team approach for further treatment and decide when surgical intervention is necessary. A neurosurgeon may be needed as well for refractory cases.

SEIZURES

SUSAN M. FUCHS

A *seizure* is a sudden, paroxysmal, excessive electrical discharge of neurons within the cerebral cortex.[202] The clinical manifestations of the seizure depend on the part or parts of the cortex involved, the rate, direction of spread of the discharge within the brain, and the age of the child.[204,205] Because of cortical immaturity, a seizure in a newborn infant is often fragmentary and subtle, manifesting as eye deviation, chewing movements, or apnea.[205-207] As a child matures so does the cortex; therefore generalized tonic-clonic movements occur in childhood, and specific sensations that occur with partial complex seizures can be expressed in an older child.[204]

Epilepsy is a disorder characterized by recurrent (two or more) seizures that occur in the absence of provoking factors.[204,208] The incidence of epilepsy in children (less than 14 years) is between 45 and 83/100,000.[208]

An *epileptic syndrome* is an epileptic disorder characterized by specific signs and symptoms that occur together, which can be defined by history, seizure type, recurrence, and findings on neurologic examination and ancillary studies (EEG) (i.e., febrile seizures, neonatal seizures).[208]

Classification of Seizures and Epilepsies

The Commission on Classification and Terminology of the International League Against Epilepsy classified seizures in 1981.[204,209] The seizure classification was based on a clinical description of the seizure and ictal and interictal EEGs.[210] In 1989, a system was developed based on generalization, localization, undetermined (focal or generalized), and special syndromes.[205,210,211]

There are two categories of seizures: *partial* (old terms: focal or local) seizures, which arise in one part of the brain and have focal abnormalities on an EEG, and *generalized* seizures, which involve all or large parts of the cerebral cortex.[205]

Partial Seizures. Partial seizures are further classified into simple (i.e., no loss of consciousness) and complex (i.e., an impairment of consciousness).[205,209,210] Included in these categories are simple partial seizures with motor symptoms (jacksonian epilepsy), somatosensory or special sensory symptoms (e.g., metallic taste, headache, "pins and needles"), autonomic symptoms (e.g., flushing, sweating), or psychic symptoms (déjà vu, déjà entendu).[205,209,210,212]

Complex partial (psychomotor) seizures are further subdivided into those involving impairment of consciousness only (temporal lobe seizures) and those that generalize secondarily to tonic-clonic seizures.[205,209,210] An aura often occurs before the impairment of consciousness in complex partial seizures, with symptoms such as automatisms, alterations in perception (micropsia and macropsia), hallucinations, and other symptoms similar to those in simple partial seizures.[212,213]

Generalized Seizures. Generalized seizures are subclassified into specific movement patterns, including absence (petit mal), atypical absence, tonic, clonic, myoclonic (minor motor), atonic or astatic (akinetic, drop attacks), and tonic-clonic (grand mal).[205,209,210]

Absence seizures are characterized by brief lapses in awareness, which may or may not be accompanied by minor motor manifestations (staring, rhythmic eye blinking or head drooping) without postictal impairment.[212,213]

Tonic movements (and seizures) refer to sustained muscle contraction that results in limb and trunk rigidity. This rigidity can result in inhibition of respiration, leading to cyanosis.[213,214] *Clonic* movements (and seizures) are the rhythmic jerking and flexor spasms of the extremi-

ties.[213,214] *Tonic-clonic* seizures are generalized seizures, involving both tonic and clonic movements. Myoclonic seizures are brief muscle contractions that occur unilaterally or bilaterally.[213] Atonic seizures are characterized by an abrupt loss of muscle tone, causing the child to collapse (or drop) to the floor.[213,215]

Epileptic Syndromes. The epilepsy classification system encompasses several of the childhood epilepsy syndromes. Localization-related (focal) epilepsies have a proven site of origin of the seizure, generalized epileptic syndromes involve both hemispheres, and undetermined epilepsies have focal and generalized seizures with no specific site of onset.[211,216] These are further subclassified:

- Idiopathic (or primary epilepsy)—no underlying cause except for a possible genetic component
- Symptomatic—due to a suspected or known CNS disorder
- Cryptogenic—unknown, but presumed symptomatic origin.[216]

Benign childhood epilepsy with centrotemporal spikes, also known as benign rolandic epilepsy, is an example of an idiopathic, localization-related epilepsy. Its onset is between age 3 and 13 years, and the seizures consist of facial movements, grimacing, and vocalizations, which often wake the child from sleep. These symptoms may be confused with night terrors. The diagnosis is based on the finding of centrotemporal spikes on an interictal EEG. It has a good prognosis, with spontaneous remission by age 20.[216-218]

West syndrome (infantile spasms) is a generalized, symptomatic, or cryptogenic epileptic syndrome characterized by infantile spasms, sudden tonic contractions of the extremities, head, and trunk that occur in clusters; an EEG pattern known as hypsarrhythmia; and mental retardation.[216-218] The onset is between 4 and 18 months. Some of the infants with this disorder have evidence of previous CNS damage such as prenatal ischemia-hypoxia, cerebral dysgenesis (tuberous sclerosis), brain malformations, intrauterine infections (TORCHS—*t*oxoplasmosis, *r*ubella, *c*ytomegalovirus, *h*erpes, *s*yphilis), and inborn metabolic disorders (phenylketonuria, nonketotic hyperglycinemia). Therapy has consisted of ACTH (corticotropin) or prednisone.[216,218]

Lennox-Gastaut syndrome is another cryptogenic or symptomatic generalized epileptic syndrome characterized by an age of onset of 1 to 8 years, multiple types of seizures (atonic, atypical absence, myoclonic or tonic), diffuse spikes and slow waves on the interictal EEG, and mental retardation.[215-217]

Juvenile myoclonic epilepsy of Janz is an idiopathic, generalized seizure syndrome with onset between 12 and 18 years of age. Although myoclonic seizures, especially on awakening, are the hallmark, tonic, tonic-clonic, and absence seizures also occur. Often precipitated by stress, lack of sleep, or excessive alcohol consumption, it has a diagnosis confirmed by a unique EEG pattern of fast spike-and-wave discharges, with a multiple spike-and-wave pattern when aroused from sleep. Valproic acid is the treatment of choice and is often needed for life.[217]

Neonatal seizures are considered epilepsies and syndromes of undetermined origin.[211,216] The seizures are fragmentary and not well sustained, but have been described as (1) subtle seizures characterized by eye deviation or fluttering, sucking, changes in respirations, and apnea; (2) focal clonic seizures; (3) multifocal clonic seizures; (4) tonic seizures; and (5) myoclonic seizures.[206,207] Another classification method takes into account that not all of these behaviors are correlated with EEG changes. Electroclinical seizures have clinical findings and EEG correlates; clinical seizures involve some observed seizure or change in activity that may be correlated with a change in EEG; and electrographic seizures occur when seizure activity is recorded on the EEG but no clinical seizure is observed.[219,220]

Febrile seizures are classified under the heading of special syndromes.[211] It is the most common seizure disorder of childhood, characterized by onset between age 3 months and 5 years, and is associated with a fever but without evidence of intracranial infection or defined cause.[214]

Status epilepticus, also classified under the special syndrome category, is defined by an epileptic seizure that is so prolonged or so frequently repeated that a fixed epileptic condition exists.[221] A practical definition is any tonic-clonic (or convulsive) seizure that lasts more than 30 minutes or any series of seizures (including nonconvulsive) in which the patient does not regain consciousness between seizures.[221-223]

Etiology

Although the most common etiology of seizures in children is a fever, the diagnosis of a febrile seizure must exclude other causes. The specific etiologies of a febrile seizure, as well as diagnostic work-up and treatment, will be discussed in the section on Febrile Seizures. Specific etiologies of seizures by age of onset are listed in Table 56-11.

The onset of seizures in the neonatal period should prompt a thorough evaluation. Within the first 48 to 72 hours of life, the most common etiology is perinatal anoxia or hypoxia, often intrauterine hypoxia.[206,207,219,220] In full-term and premature infants, 50% to 65% of newborn seizures are due to hypoxic-ischemic encephalopathy.[207,219] Birth trauma, including subarachnoid and subdural hemorrhage in full-term infants, and intraventricular hemorrhage in preterm infants cause 15% of neonatal seizures, and another 5% to 10% are caused by infection, cerebral malformations, inborn errors of metabolism, or toxins.[206,207,219]

Metabolic disorders, especially hypoglycemia, hypocalcemia, and hypomagnesemia, can be primary or secondary disorders (e.g., small-for-age, perinatal asphyxia, hemorrhage, or infection) in a newborn infant that result in early-onset seizures. Although primary hypocalcemic seizures occur at 7 to 14 days, it is important to remember that when treating primary or secondary hypocalcemia, hypomagnesemia may be concurrent or may be made worse by the administration of calcium.[207,220] Pyridoxine (vitamin B_6) deficiency, although rare, is another cause of repeated neonatal seizures.[206] Inborn errors of metabolism such as aminoacidurias (maple syrup urine disease, phenylketonuria), urea cycle defects (ornithine carbamoyltransferase deficiency, citrullinemia), and organic acidurias (propionic acidemia) should be considered if seizures begin on days 4 to 14 of life.[206,207,219]

TABLE 56-11. Seizures: Cause by Age of Onset

First month of life
First day

Hypoxia	Hyperglycemia
Drugs	Hypoglycemia
Trauma	Pyridoxine deficiency
Infection	

Day 2-3

Infection	Developmental malformation
Drug withdrawal	Intracranial hemorrhage
Hypoglycemia	Inborn error of metabolism
Hypocalcemia	Hyponatremia/hypernatremia

Day >4

Infection	Developmental malformation
Hypocalcemia	Drug withdrawal
Hyperphosphatemia	Inborn error of metabolism
Hyponatremia	

1-6 mo
As above

6 mo-3 yr

Febrile seizures	Trauma
Birth injury	Metabolic disorder
Infection	Cerebral degenerative disease
Toxin	

>3 yr

Idiopathic	Trauma
Infection	Cerebral degenerative disease

Although infections such as meningitis (group B-streptococci, *E. coli*) and meningoencephalitis (TORCHS) are causes of neonatal seizures (usually days 3 to 7), one must not forget that meningitis and encephalitis, especially herpes, can cause seizures throughout childhood.[206,207]

Major CNS structural anomalies (lissencephaly) or neurocutaneous disorders (neurofibromatosis, Sturge-Weber disease, tuberous sclerosis) may be manifest during the newborn period or result in seizures later in infancy or childhood.[207,219]

Two types of neonatal seizures have no apparent etiology, a favorable prognosis, and are considered benign. Benign familial neonatal convulsions (BFNC) begin in the first 3 days of life, and there is a strong family history of neonatal seizures or epilepsy. Benign idiopathic neonatal convulsions (BINC), also called "fifth day fits," occur on the fifth day of life.[219,220]

Toxins can cause seizures in all age groups. In the newborn, toxic substances have passed from the mother and may include narcotics, especially cocaine. Some of the substances to be considered in young children include lead, prescribed medications such as theophylline, tricyclic antidepressants, and over-the-counter medications such as diphenhydramine; in older children and adolescents alcohol, narcotics, or other illicit drugs must be considered.[207,214] On the other hand, a child with a known seizure disorder who stops taking prescribed anticonvulsant medication is at risk for a seizure.

Head trauma may precipitate a seizure immediately following the injury or several hours to days later.[206,214] Although the immediate posttraumatic seizure is in response to the blow, the later forms are often due to the underlying brain injury.[206,214] Tumors and vascular problems, more common etiologies of new-onset seizures in adults, can also cause seizures in children.[210]

Diagnostic Findings

The most important aspect of the evaluation of a seizure is a careful history, including potential precipitating factors such as fever, trauma, ingestion, or underlying medical illness (hypertension, renal disease, metabolic disorders such as diabetes mellitus).[224,225] A description of the seizure, including presence of an aura, eye findings, movements, cyanosis, incontinence, and duration; loss of consciousness during the seizure; and level of consciousness after the seizure are important in classifying the seizure. If there have been recurrent seizures, a pattern or time of recurrence may be evident (e.g., on awakening, during sleep, hyperventilation).[213]

A complete physical and neurologic examination should be performed to detect previously unsuspected disorders or disease manifestations such as hypertension, skin findings (adenoma sebaceum, café au lait spots), eye findings (chorioretinitis, papilledema), and physical findings such as a stiff neck or focal deficits.[214,225]

Complications. After a first nonfebrile, unprovoked seizure, the risk of recurrence depends on several factors and ranges from 27% to 61%.[224] Definite risk factors include an abnormal EEG and underlying neurologic abnormality.[214,224,226] Factors that increase the likelihood of recurrence include the type of seizure (partial seizure), a family history of epilepsy, and a history of prior febrile seizures.[224,227] Factors that do not affect recurrence include duration of seizure, age at first seizure, status epilepticus, or treatment after first seizure.[224-226]

If a child experiences a recurrent seizure, the risk of another seizure also increases to 50% to 75%, usually within 6 to 12 months of the first seizure, regardless of risk factors outlined previously.[227]

There is no way to predict the occurrence of status epilepticus, nor does its initial occurrence predict its recurrence. Only drug withdrawal in individuals with known seizure disorders is a major precipitant of status.[227] Adverse outcomes after status epilepticus are often the result of the underlying disorder (meningitis), not the seizure itself.[224] The morbidity of aggressively treated status epilepticus in the absence of an acute neurologic insult or progressive neurologic disorder is low.

A single, brief (<30 minutes) seizure causes no permanent brain damage.[227] Injuries such as falls, cuts, bruises, or loss of teeth can occur during a seizure; however, these are due to the loss of consciousness of the child at the time of the seizure.[224,227]

Ancillary Data. There is no routine work-up for a child with a new-onset seizure; the evaluation should be based on clinical information supplied by the history and physical examination, seizure type, and likelihood of an underlying disorder.

A fingerstick Chemstrip or Dextrostix should be performed to rule out hypoglycemia. Confirmatory serum glucose, electrolytes, calcium, and magnesium levels should be obtained based on suspicion of a metabolic disturbance. BUN and creatinine are helpful only if renal disease is suspected. A white blood cell count may be beneficial for an infectious etiology; however, the seizure itself may cause an elevation as a result of the adrenergic-mediated leukocyte demargination.[228] Liver enzymes and platelet count, although not beneficial in the work-up of seizures, may be helpful as a baseline if antiepileptic drug therapy is initiated. Other laboratory studies, such as serum ammonia, drug levels or toxicology screens (urine and blood), or urine for amino or organic acids, should be based on clinical suspicion.

If meningitis or encephalitis is suspected, a lumbar puncture should be performed; however, if a mass-occupying lesion is also in the differential, a CT scan should be performed prior to the spinal tap, with consideration of initiating antibiotic or antiviral therapy before the definitive evaluation.

A head CT scan, often with and without contrast, should be reserved for the evaluation of children with focal seizures, focal findings on physical examination, suspicion of a CNS abnormality (e.g., intracranial lesion or bleed, tumor, vascular or congenital abnormality), a change or worsening of preexisting seizures, or a focal abnormality on EEG.[205,213,225] An MRI scan may be superior to CT scan in the diagnosis of certain tumors and vascular malformations, but it is often not available or practical in the acute work-up of seizures in children.[205,214]

The study of choice in the evaluation of childhood seizures is an EEG. The most beneficial EEG is one recorded during a seizure (ictal EEG); however, since this is not always possible, when an EEG is performed it should include recordings during sleep and wake, as well as during photic stimulation and hyperventilation.[205,213,214] Because EEGs recorded just after a seizure often show slowing, an EEG should be performed (or repeated) several days to several weeks after a seizure.[225] Unfortunately, an EEG performed between seizures (interictal) often shows diffuse slowing and is not diagnostic of epilepsy, nor does a normal EEG rule out a seizure disorder.[205,214] However, the finding of focal slowing at any time indicates a focal disturbance and warrants further diagnostic evaluation, whereas specific spike-and-wave patterns are characteristic of absence seizures and juvenile myoclonic epilepsy of Janz.[218,225]

Differential Considerations

A good history is important to differentiate among seizurelike episodes such as breath-holding spells, syncope, and cataplexy, which are often precipitated by events such as anger, fright, or injury.[214,215,225] Hysterical seizures or pseudoseizures usually occur in teenage girls and can be associated with a variety of movements, but rarely with incontinence or bodily injury.[214] Other clinical entities simulating seizures are outlined in the box on p. 1013.

Management

Acute—Tonic-Clonic Status Epilepticus

Stabilization (ABCs). Airway, breathing, and circulation are the first priority. The patient should be positioned to assure an open airway and, if needed, an airway adjunct such as a nasopharyngeal or oral airway should be inserted. Oxygen should be administered by nasal cannula, blow-by, or face mask; suction equipment should be available. Because bag-valve-mask ventilation may be required to oxygenate the patient and intubation may be needed to minimize the risk of aspiration, this equipment should also be available. Prophylactic intubation is rarely indicated unless the seizures do not abate or the patient has a compromised airway or cannot be ventilated by bag-valve-mask.

Pulse, respirations, blood pressure, and oxygen saturation should be monitored frequently.[221,222,229] Rectal temperature should be checked and, if elevated, treated. The patient should be protected against inflicting self-injury.

An intravenous catheter should be placed and blood drawn for appropriate studies, with a drop left for a bedside Dextrostix/Chemstrip. An infusion of normal saline should be started. If intravenous access cannot be achieved, intraosseous infusion is an alternative for children younger than 6 years.

If the glucose is less than 60 mg/dl or a bedside glucose evaluation not performed, glucose should be infused by giving 50% glucose in a dosage of 1 gm/kg IV. In children less than 2 years, this should be diluted to 25% dextrose by mixing 1:1 with sterile water and giving 4 ml/kg. In neonates, 10% dextrose should be given at 10 ml/kg (dilute 50% dextrose 5:1 with sterile water, if needed) over 10 to 20 minutes.

If there is any suspicion of drug exposure, administer naloxone (Narcan) 0.1 mg/kg/dose IV up to 2 mg/dose. Very large doses may be required for propoxyphene (Darvon) or pentazocine (Talwin) overdoses. Thiamine 100 mg/dose IV or IM initially (then BID orally for maintenance) may be considered if alcoholism or malnutrition is suspected.

Anticonvulsants. Pharmacologic management should be initiated during stabilization, although the appropriate drug and order of administration are controversial. A sequential approach to seizure management is preferred. Lorazepam or diazepam are preferred for acute termination of the seizure, but a second drug is required for long-term management. Since this protocol increases the risk of respiratory depression, oxygen and a bag-valve-mask should be available before any medication is administered.

If the patient has been taking anticonvulsants, it is essential to measure drug levels. If the levels are subtherapeutic, the maintenance dose should be increased with full or partial loading at the time of the acute seizure. If poor compliance is the basis for low levels, education and close follow-up are essential.

Lorazepam (Ativan) 0.05 to 0.10 mg/kg, administered IV at a rate of 2 mg/min, is preferred because it has a longer half-life than diazepam (3 to 24 hrs vs. 20 min).[223,229,230] A repeat dose is rarely beneficial, but may be considered up to a total of 0.15 mg/kg in children (the adult dose is 2.5 to 10 mg). Intramuscular administration is not recommended due to erratic absorption.

If lorazepam is not available, diazepam (Valium) 0.2 to 0.3 mg/kg (up to 10 mg) at a rate of 1 mg/min can be administered. Seizure control may require a repeat of the dose in 5 to 10 minutes up to a maximum dose of 10 mg in children and 30 mg in adults.[222,229,230] Because one of the side effects of diazepam and, to a lesser extent, lorazepam is respiratory depression, the patient may require breathing assistance for a short time with a bag-valve-mask.

If IV access is not available, diazepam can be administered rectally: the IV solution is placed in a 1 ml TB syringe, 14 G plastic angiocatheter, or feeding tube and given initially at a dose of 0.5 mg/kg (the second dose if needed is 0.25 mg/kg).[231] The intraosseous route may be effective as an alternate route at the IV dose. Intramuscular administration of diazepam is unreliable, and endotracheal use may cause pneumonitis.

If the foregoing medications are not effective in aborting the seizure, phenytoin (Dilantin), 15 to 20 mg/kg, should be given at a rate no faster than 40 mg/min or 0.5 mg/kg/min (max total dose 1,250 mg).[222,229] Because phenytoin precipitates in dextrose solutions, it must be given in saline.[229] Because the peak effect occurs in 15 to 20 minutes, phenytoin should be administered to prevent seizure recurrence, even if diazepam or lorazepam does stop the initial seizure.[221,222,229] Side effects of phenytoin include bradycardia, cardiac dysrhythmias, and hypotension; therefore the patient must be closely monitored during slow administration.

Phenobarbital (Luminal) given in a loading dose of 20 mg/kg, at a rate of 30 mg/min or 1 mg/kg/min IV, is the third drug of choice if seizures persist or as an alternative to ongoing control with phenytoin. Although not preferred, IM administration is possible. Because diazepam has a synergistic effect on respirations and vascular tone, respirations and blood pressure must be carefully monitored; many patients will require assisted ventilation or even intubation.[221,223,229]

Another alternative to phenytoin or phenobarbital is an intravenous diazepam drip in a concentration of 100 mg of diazepam diluted in 500 ml 5% dextrose. The adult infusion rate is 40 ml/hr or <1 mg/kg/hr.[222]

If seizures continue, paraldehyde rectal solution can be administered (the IV formulation is no longer available in the United States). Paraldehyde is mixed 2:1 with oil (peanut, olive, cottonseed) and given at 0.3 ml/kg/dose, which can be repeated in 2 to 4 hours. Glass syringes must be used with paraldehyde, since the agent dissolves plastic.[221,223,229]

Pentobarbital (pentobarbital coma) can also be used for refractory seizures. A loading dose of 20 mg/kg is followed by a continuous infusion at 1 to 2 mg/kg/hr. Although serum levels (usually kept between 20 to 40 µg/ml) can be followed, the best method of gauging success is by electrographic suppression on an EEG.[223]

If the seizures continue or persist for more than 1 hour, general anesthesia with halothane and neuromuscular blockade and continuous EEG recording should be considered.[221,222,229]

All metabolic abnormalities must be corrected. Rarely will anticonvulsants be totally effective in the presence of significant metabolic abnormalities. Hypoglycemia is managed as noted above. Hyponatremia can be partially corrected (up to a sodium of 125 mEq/L) by administering 3% saline (0.5 mEq Na$^+$/ml) at a rate of 4 ml/kg IV over 10 to 30 minutes. Further correction up to a sodium of 140 mEq/L should be achieved over 16 hours. Hypernatremia is corrected over 24 to 48 hours. Hypocalcemia may be treated initially with an infusion of 0.5 to 1.0 ml/kg of 10% calcium gluconate over 5 minutes. Ongoing management combines IV (5 to 8 ml/kg/24 hr of 10% calcium gluconate given in four to six doses) and oral calcium gluconate (200 to 500 mg/kg/dose every 6 hours) as needed. Magnesium sulfate can be given in a dose of 25 to 50 mg/kg/dose IV slowly every 4 to 6 hours for three to four doses to correct hypomagnesemia.

For neonatal seizures, phenobarbital, 18 to 20 mg/kg IV slowly, is the drug of choice. Additional boluses of phenobarbital, 5 to 10 mg/kg every 5 to 10 minutes up to a total of 50 to 60 mg/kg, may be required. Lorazepam 0.05 to 0.1 mg/kg is another option, but phenobarbital will be required for maintenance. If seizures continue, phenytoin, 15 to 20 mg/kg IV slowly (1 mg/kg/min), is the next option. If seizures remain unresponsive, therapy at this point should include pyridoxine, 50 to 100 mg IV.[206,207,219,232] If seizures are not abated, diazepam (0.3 mg/kg followed by a continuous infusion at 0.3 to 0.8 mg/kg/hr), paraldehyde (0.3 mg/kg per rectum), lidocaine (2 mg/kg IV load, followed by infusion at 4 to 6 mg/kg/hr), acetazolamide (10 to 30 mg/kg/24 hrs divided BID or TID), or primidone (15 to 25 mg/kg) remains as a therapeutic modality.[219,232]

Acute and Nonconvulsive Status Epilepticus. Although not usually life-threatening emergencies, these forms of status epilepticus are often difficult to diagnose.[221] Typical absence status is characterized by mental confusion but no motor activity. A benzodiazepine such as diazepam or lorazepam are the drugs of choice for this rare disorder, followed by ethosuximide, valproic acid, or clonazepam.[223,229]

Atypical absence status also presents with mental confusion but may have associated myoclonic or atonic seizures. These seizures are difficult to treat; valproic acid (20 mg/kg) orally, via nasogastric tube, or rectally is the drug of choice followed by diazepam or lorazepam.[223,229]

TABLE 56-12. Antiepileptic Therapy of Seizure Disorders of Childhood

Seizure type	Drugs of choice	Alternative
Generalized tonic-clonic	Carbamazepine Phenytoin	Phenobarbital Primidone Valproate
Absence	Ethosuximide	Valproate Clonazepam Felbamate
Myoclonic	Valproate Clonazepam	Lamotrigine
Atonic	Valproate Clonazepam	Ethosuximide Lamotrigine
Partial; simple and complex	Carbamazepine Phenytoin	Valproate Phenobarbital Primidone Gabapentin Lamotrigine
Infantile spasms	ACTH (corticotropin)	Prednisone

Modified from references 205 and 233-240.

Simple partial status is a prolonged focal seizure or recurrent focal seizures with no loss of consciousness. The medications used are the same as outlined for tonic-clonic status.[229]

Complex partial status may be found in a patient with a prolonged period of mental confusion, potentially associated with psychomotor or sensory symptoms. Treatment is the same as for tonic-clonic status.[229]

Long-term Prevention. The decision to initiate treatment is based on an appraisal of many factors, not just the seizure itself. Included in this assessment are the patient's age, predisposing factors, time of seizure occurrence, type of seizure, and risk of recurrence, as well as the potential psychologic, emotional, vocational, and social consequences of further seizures.[205,214,233]

Recommendations for the treatment of seizures with medication include recurrent generalized tonic-clonic seizures, absence seizures, and partial complex seizures (Tables 56-12 and 56-13).[233]

Drug Therapy and Monitoring. Drug therapy offers many options. Some principles to follow include the following:

1. Choose a drug effective for the particular type of seizure. If several are available, use the least toxic drug.
2. Initiate therapy with a single drug, calculated based on body weight. If a range of dosage is available, use the lower end.
3. The drug used must be given for a long enough time to reach a steady state, which is approximately five times the half-life of the drug (7 to 10 days for many antiepileptic drugs). Blood levels may be useful at this time if seizure control has not been achieved (before increasing the dose or adding a new medication).

TABLE 56-13. Common Anticonvulsants

Drug/availability	Primary indications	Maintenance dosage (mg/kg/ 24 hr PO)	Loading dose (mg/kg)	Serum half-life (hr)	Serum therapeutic range (μg/ml)
Phenobarbital Elix: 20 mg/5 ml Tab: 15, 30, 60, 90, 100 mg Vial: 65, 130 mg/ml	Grand mal	3-8	15-20 IV or IM (<1 mg/kg/min IV)	48-72	10-35 (may be higher)
Phenytoin (Dilantin) Susp: 30,125 mg/ 5 ml Tab (chew): 50 mg Cap: 30, 100 mg Amp: 50 mg/ml	Grand mal, partial, psychomotor	5-10	15-20 IV (<40 mg/min or 0.5 mg/kg/min)	6-30	10-20
Diazepam (Valium) Vial: 5 mg/ml	Status epilepticus	NA	0.2-0.3 IV (<1 mg/min)	.33	
Lorazepam (Ativan) Vial: 2, 4 mg/ml	Status epilepticus	NA	0.05-0.10 IV	16	
Carbamazepine (Tegretol)* Tab: 100 (chew), 200 mg	Grand mal, partial, psychomotor	15-30		12	4-14 (varies with laboratory)
Ethosuximide (Zarontin) Syr: 250 mg/5 ml Cap: 250 mg	Petit mal (absence)	20-40		30	40-100
Valproic acid (Depakene) Syr: 250 mg/5 ml Cap: 250 mg	Petit mal (absence) myoclonic, atonic; grand mal	15-60		6-18	50-100
Primidone (Mysoline) Susp: 250 mg/5 ml Tab: 50, 250 mg	Partial, psychomotor generalized	10-25		12	6-12 (or pheno-barbital level)
Clonazepam (Klonopin) Tab: 0.5, 1, 2 mg	Myoclonic, atonic	0.05-0.2		18-50	0.020-0.080 (20-80 ng/ml)
Felbamate (Felbatol)	Lennox-Gastaut	15-45			
Gabapentin (Neuron-tin)	Partial	20-70			
Lamotrigine (Lamictal)	Myoclonic, atonic, Lennox-Gastaut	5-15†			
Vigabatrin (Sabril)	Partial, infantile spasms	75-100			

*Patients with atypical absence seizures as well as other types of seizures may be predisposed to exacerbation of seizures when carbamazepine (Tegretol) is used.
†Depends on other concurrent antiepileptic medication.
NOTE: Generic carbamazepine and primidone may have variable bioavailability. Erythromycin decreases clearance of carbamazepine.

4. Once seizure control is achieved, periodic blood tests should be performed to monitor blood levels as well as any adverse side effects.[213] When monitoring serum levels of anticonvulsants, it should be remembered that the reported blood level is a combination of the free and protein-bound drug. The "free" or unbound drug accounts for the therapeutic effect as well as dose-related toxicity (protein-bound drug does not cross the blood-brain barrier), so free drug assays may be needed. This is especially true for phenytoin (90% protein-bound), or when the patient requires a higher than expected dose to achieve seizure control or is demonstrating signs of toxicity with a therapeutic drug level.[213]

5. Although therapeutic ranges for most drugs exist, some children may have adequate seizure control

with lower drug levels. In other patients, it may be necessary to exceed this range if seizures are not controlled and the patient is not experiencing the toxic side effects.[218]

Phenytoin (Dilantin). Phenytoin is useful for generalized tonic-clonic, partial seizures; simple and complex seizures; and status epilepticus. The dose is 5 to 10 mg/kg/24 hr given BID (once a day may be used in older children). Major side effects include gum hyperplasia (90%) and hirsutism. It can cause drowsiness, nystagmus, drug rashes (Stevens-Johnson syndrome), and occasional liver or hematologic side effects.[225,233,235] If the liquid form is used, it should be shaken vigorously before use to ensure adequate mixing of the drug.[211] If this drug is used, it should be remembered that generic forms are effective in controlling seizures, but due to varying rates of absorption and bioavailability, the blood level may change when switching from Dilantin to generic forms or vice versa.[225,229] Therapeutic serum levels are 10 to 20 μg/ml.[233,235,237] When using phenytoin in combination with other antiepileptic drugs, it is important to monitor drug levels (both drugs), since phenytoin can decrease the effectiveness of carbamazepine, clonazepam, and primidone but increase the effectiveness of phenobarbital.[235] Antacids (cimetidine), isoniazid, chloramphenicol, chlorpromazine, anticoagulants, and estrogens may increase phenytoin levels.[213,235]

Phenobarbital. Phenobarbital is useful for generalized tonic-clonic, partial seizures; simple and complex, neonatal seizures; as well as status epilepticus; however, its side effects can be problematic. The dose is 3 to 8 mg/kg/24 hr given once a day or BID. There is a 30% to 40% incidence of hyperactivity, lethargy, sleep disorders, and behavioral disorders.[213,224,225,235] Recent studies have shown that children taking phenobarbital have scored lower on performance and IQ tests.[224,241]

Therapeutic serum levels of phenobarbital are 10 to 35 μg/ml, although higher levels may be required and tolerated. The combination of phenobarbital and clonazepam may result in decreased effectiveness of clonazepam.[235]

Carbamazepine (Tegretol). Carbamazepine is effective against generalized tonic-clonic seizures, as well as partial seizures: simple, complex, and secondarily generalized. The usual dose is 15 to 30 mg/kg/24 hr given BID to QID. It should be started at 10 mg/kg/24 hr and increased every 3 to 4 days by 5 mg/kg/24 hr, until an effective maintenance dose is reached.[234,235] Dose-related side effects, including drowsiness, blurred vision, or diplopia, occur 1 hour after a dose.[225,233,234] Other side effects include allergic and idiosyncratic reactions, rashes (5%), and dose-related leukopenia (10%).[234] Rare, but potentially serious side effects include blood dyscrasias (agranulocytosis and aplastic anemia) and cardiac and hepatic toxicity.[234,235]

Therapeutic serum levels range from 4 to 14 μg/ml.[233-235] Toxic carbamazepine levels can result if a patient is on macrolide antibiotics (erythromycin), isoniazid, cimetidine (Tagamet), verapamil, diltiazem, and propoxyphene (Darvon).[234,235] In addition, the effectiveness of oral contraceptives is reduced by carbamazepine.[234,235]

Valproate, Valproic Acid (Depakote, Depakene). Valproate and valproic acid have been most useful for the treatment of absence and myoclonic seizures although they can be used for generalized tonic-clonic and partial seizures—simple and complex.[233,234] The dose is 15 to 60 mg/kg/24 hr BID to QID, to be started at 10 mg/kg/24 hr and increased weekly by 10 mg/kg.[233,234] Side effects include GI distress (especially with the syrup), drowsiness, weight gain, and hair loss. Idiosyncratic reactions include neutropenia, thrombocytopenia, and hepatotoxicity (increased risk in children <2 years on other drugs as well as valproate).[233-235]

Therapeutic serum concentration should be 50 to 100 μg/ml, depending on the laboratory.[233-235] Valproate causes increased serum levels of phenobarbital, phenytoin, carbamazepine, diazepam, clonazepam, and ethosuximide; therefore serum levels of these drugs should be monitored carefully.[234,235]

Ethosuximide (Zarontin). Ethosuximide is used for management of absence seizures. The dose is 20 to 40 mg/kg/day BID.[218,233,234] Side effects include nausea, vomiting, hiccups, and headache. Erythema multiforme, Stevens-Johnson syndrome, and a lupus-like syndrome have been reported as rare occurrences.[233,234] Serum levels should be kept between 40 and 100 μg/ml.[233-235]

Primidone (Mysoline). Since one of the metabolites of primidone is phenobarbital, it is effective for the same types of seizures and causes similar side effects. The dose is 10 to 25 mg/kg/24 hr BID to QID; however, nausea, sedation, and ataxia occur unless the drug is started at a very low dose.[233,235] Therapeutic serum levels are in the range 6 to 12 μg/ml.[233,235]

Clonazepam (Klonopin). Clonazepam is an alternative for the treatment of myoclonic and atonic seizures, although it can also be used for absence seizures. The dose is 0.05 to 0.2 mg/kg/24 hr BID to QID. Side effects include drowsiness, ataxia, and drooling.[233,235] Therapeutic drug levels are in the .020 to .080 μg/ml (20 to 80 nanogram/ml) range.[235]

New Drugs. In the last 3 years, several new medications have been introduced for the control of seizures. Although most of the original studies involved adults, several have involved children. Some are currently available in the United States, while others remain under study.

FELBAMATE (FELBATOL). Felbamate was initially approved for monotherapy (single drug use) for adults with partial and generalized seizures and for children with Lennox-Gastaut syndrome because when used with other medications there were more side effects. The dose in children is 15 to 45 mg/kg/24 hr, given 3 to 4 times a day. The lowest dose should be started initially, and if tolerated for 1 to 2 weeks can be increased.[236-238] When given concomitantly, it raises the drug levels of phenytoin and valproic acid and decreases those of carbamazepine. Side effects include insomnia, anorexia, vomiting, and somnolence. To minimize these side effects it should be taken after meals, with the last dose after dinner rather than at bedtime if insomnia is a problem.[236,238] Since Felbamate's release, additional major side effects have been reported and include aplastic anemia and acute hepatic failure. For these reasons, use has drastically decreased, but if the child continues taking this drug, frequent blood tests to include complete blood counts and liver enzymes are needed.[235]

GABAPENTIN (NEURONTIN). Gabapentin was approved for adjunctive therapy for patients with refractory partial and secondarily tonic-clonic seizures, but its use in children has been limited to those over 12 years.[235,236] The adult dose is 300 mg/day, to be increased to 600 to 1800 mg/kg over 2 to 3 days, with 20 to 70 mg/kg the dose for children.[218,238] It has no effect on the concentration of other antiepileptic drugs.[236,239] Side effects include somnolence, ataxia, and dizziness.[238]

LAMOTRIGINE (LAMICTAL). Lamotrigine is approved for adults as adjunctive treatment for partial seizures. Studies are underway for the indications for use in children. At this point, it appears best for myoclonic, tonic, and atonic seizures and Lennox-Gastaut syndrome.[236,240] Since it can alter drug levels of other antiepileptic medications, the dose is based on what other medications the child is taking. For those taking valproic acid, the dose is 5 mg/kg/24 hr, and for those on phenytoin, carbamazepine, phenobarbital, or primidone, the dose is 15 mg/kg/24 hr, taken once or twice a day, which should be achieved over a 1 month period.[236,238,240] Side effects include rash, sedation, and ataxia.[236-238]

VIGABATRIN (SABRIL). Although not currently available in the United States, vigabatrin has been used in Europe since 1979; studies are underway in the United States. It is most effective for partial seizures and infantile spasms.[238] The starting dose is 50 mg/kg/24 hr and is increased to 75 to 100 mg/kg/24 hr (given once or twice a day) if there has been a partial response with the initial dose.[236,238] If seizures do not improve, or become worse, the child is considered resistant to vigabatrin.[236,240] Of note, in a subgroup of infants with infantile spasms and tuberous sclerosis, infantile spasms were replaced by partial seizures, which was considered an improvement.[240,241] Side effects include hyperactivity, agitation, and insomnia.[236,237]

Disposition. Parents should understand that the treatment of seizures is a balancing act. One must weigh the risks of seizures—their recurrence, risk of injury, and psychosocial stigmata—against drug therapy—their effects on behavior, intelligence, idiosyncratic reactions, toxicity, and expense.[224,225] Although complete seizure control is the goal of treatment, if side effects of medication impair the child's functioning, drug therapy should be reevaluated. Parental anxiety must be addressed so that overprotection or undue restriction of activity does not result. Appropriate educational or vocational training and support services can be arranged to assist both patient and family.[205,241]

Most children with a seizure disorder can be managed by a primary care physician, but this can take time. For most children with generalized tonic-clonic seizures, if seizures continue despite adequate drug levels, consultation with a neurologist is recommended. For those children with evidence of focal slowing on EEG, acquired changing, or progressive developmental or neurologic deficit, neurologic consultation should be obtained.[242]

FEBRILE SEIZURES

JAVIER A. GONZALEZ DEL REY

Febrile seizures are best defined as convulsions that occur in early childhood in association with a febrile illness with no evidence of intracranial infection or other defined CNS pathology or previous afebrile seizures. They account for 30% of all childhood seizures and usually occur in infants and children between 3 months and 5 years of age.[243] Approximately 3% to 5% of all children will have experienced at least one febrile seizure between the age of 6 months and 6 years.[244] Although most episodes are benign and self-limited, requiring only supportive intervention, they are very dramatic events that create immense anxiety in parents and challenge in management for emergency physicians.

Febrile seizures have been classified into two major categories. *Simple* or *typical* convulsions usually occur in otherwise normal children. They are self-limited, generally not lasting more than 15 minutes and are generalized, tonic-clonic with one convulsive episode during the first 24 hours of the febrile illness. Simple febrile convulsions represent the vast majority of cases (97%).[245] The term *complex* or *atypical* febrile convulsion is used if the seizure lasts more than 15 minutes, there is more than one episode within the first 24 hours, or the convulsion has a focal component.

Pathophysiology

The peak incidence for febrile convulsions is between 9 to 30 months of age, with an average age of 23 months for the first episode.[246] Most series report a higher incidence in boys than girls (2:1) and slightly higher prevalence in black versus white children (4.2% vs. 3.4%).[246,247]

Although the cause of febrile seizures is still unknown, fever, infections, and the age of the child all seem to play an important role. Millichap[243] has suggested that the fever lowers the convulsive threshold, causing the seizure in susceptible children. It is unclear whether the seizures are related to the rate of rise of temperature or to the peak value attained. Some studies suggest that a high sustained fever is of more importance than a rapid rise in temperature.[248]

Only 11% of children with febrile seizures convulse at temperatures <37.9° C, 14% to 40% at temperatures between 38° and 38.9° C, and 40% to 56% at temperatures between 39° and 39.9° C. Temperatures of 40° C or greater are reported in 20% of children with febrile seizures.[249]

Viral infections are associated with 80% of cases in which an etiology has been determined. Upper respiratory tract infections represent 38% to 40% of cases. Others include otitis media (15% to 23%), pneumonia (15%), acute gastroenteritis (7% to 9%), roseola infantum (5%) and "flu" (1.4%).[243,247]

There appears to be a strong genetic predisposition. The mode of transmission has not been established but an autosomal dominant or a polygenic transmission appears to be most likely.[250] A family history (siblings or parents) of febrile seizures can be elicited in 25% to 40% of children with febrile seizures.[251,252] The offspring of parents who convulsed when febrile during childhood have a risk of febrile seizures over four times that of the general population. The siblings of a patient with febrile convulsions have a 3.5 times greater risk than that of the general population with an actual prevalence of 8%.[253]

Natural History

In general, children who experience a simple febrile seizure will have no complications. The chance of having further febrile seizures will depend primarily on age of presentation of the first convulsion and associated risk factors. One third of children will have one or more recurrences and 50% of these episodes occur in children who experienced a febrile seizure during the first year of life.[254] For children having their first seizure after the first year of life, only a 28% recurrence rate has been documented. Fifty percent of recurrences occurred within 6 months of the initial febrile seizure, 73% within one year, and 90% within two years. Although the classification of simple vs. complex is useful in approach and management, recurrence rates are not known to differ between these two groups.

A very small percentage of children with febrile seizures will develop epilepsy (afebrile seizures). In a collaborative study conducted by the National Institutes of Health, significant risk factors were found to identify children at high risk of nonfebrile seizures: abnormal neurologic or developmental examination prior to the febrile convulsion and atypical or complex febrile seizure.[255] If a child has two of these factors (only 6% of patients), the chances of developing epilepsy is 9.6% to 13%.[246] With only one risk factor, only 2% to 3% will develop epilepsy. In the absence of risk factors, the overall incidence of developing epilepsy after a febrile convulsion is 0.9%, compared to 0.5% incidence in the general population with no history of febrile seizures. These data do not represent a statistically significant difference, indicating that the majority of children with febrile convulsions have minimal or no chance of subsequent epilepsy.

Patients with normal neurologic and developmental examination prior to the first febrile convulsion showed no deficits in IQ scores when compared with asymptomatic siblings. These observations were confirmed in a British cohort study that evaluated children with febrile convulsions and a normal neurologic examination prior to the seizure. No significant difference was found at age 5 with peers who were free of febrile convulsions.[256]

Diagnostic Findings

Controversy exists as to the approach and extent of laboratory tests in the evaluation of a child with the first febrile convulsion. Usually a complete history and physical examination will provide the practitioner with all the necessary information for management decisions. The medical history should emphasize the type and length of the febrile illness and the type and length of convulsion. Past medical history should focus on the presence of abnormal neurologic or developmental examinations prior to the seizure. The physical examination should be complete, with detailed documentation of the patient's general status, neurologic findings, and when discoverable, the source of fever.

Ancillary Data. The most controversial aspect of the laboratory evaluation is the value and indications for a lumbar puncture. Some 13% to 18% of children with meningitis may initially present with a febrile convulsion and 40% of them may have no clinical signs of meningeal irritation.[257] In these series, the majority of children were younger than 2 years of age, and a careful differentiation of simple vs. complex febrile convulsions was not made. Combining data from several series, less than 1% of all patients who present with a febrile convulsion had meningitis and most were viral in origin.[258-260] Only one had a bacterial etiology and the seizure was described as complex.

Several recommendations can be made regarding lumbar puncture. It is clear that children with evidence of meningitis either by history or physical examination must have a lumbar puncture to confirm the diagnosis. On the other hand, the approach to the patient with a simple febrile convulsion and no meningeal findings or suspicious history is very controversial. Some authors recommend performing the procedure in all children with their first febrile convulsion; others will order a lumbar puncture if the child is younger than 16 or 18 months of age regardless of the history or presentation.[257,260-263] Another factor that frequently clouds the decision in these young children is the inability to adequately assess neurologic status during the postictal period. When the practitioner is presented with these conflicting recommendations, the elaboration of a practical and uniform approach may be difficult and, in most instances, is the origin of anxiety because of the chances of missing meningitis. Keeping in mind that the incidence of meningitis in children who experience simple febrile convulsions is low, the physician should individualize each case. The decision regarding the need for a lumbar puncture should be based on presentation, clinical findings, individual judgment, and experience, always with consideration to err on the safe side.

Blood glucose, serum calcium, serum electrolytes, BUN, and serum creatinine should be reserved for patients in which there is a suggestion of an underlying disorder, for patients who are not clinically normal at the time of evaluation, or for those who have significant risk factors for developing epilepsy.[264] The use of blood and urine cultures as well as CBC and urinalysis should be limited to the investigation of the source of fever. Children with simple febrile seizures are at approximately the same risk for bacteremia as children with fever alone.[265]

Other diagnostic tests including skull radiographs and head CT scans are seldom helpful in the evaluation of a simple febrile convulsion. Usually the history or abnormal findings on physical examination will be the major indication for these tests. The EEG is abnormal in 95% of patients shortly after a febrile convulsion. Approximately 30% of patients will have occipital slowing that resolves in 7 to 10 days following a febrile seizure.[251] Again, the EEG may be useful only in patients with a possible underlying brain disorder. Complex febrile seizures may warrant a more detailed evaluation and extensive laboratory evaluation, often including a CT scan and perhaps a lumbar puncture.

Management

Acute Management. In most cases, by the time the patient is brought to the emergency department, the child is either in a postictal state or fully recovered from the convulsion. In the event of prolonged seizures, immediate supportive measures should be taken. An adequate, clear, and secure airway must be kept at all times. Afterward, emphasis should focus on ventilation and oxygenation. Many patients with prolonged seizures may develop laryngospasm requiring assisted ventilation with positive pressure. Cardiorespiratory monitor, pulse oximeter, and IV access are the next priorities in acute management.

Once the initial phase is completed, seizure control and temperature regulation should be addressed, as discussed in the previous section on Seizures. For the latter, reduction of body temperature may be achieved by conductive or evaporative cooling and by the administration of antipyretics such as acetaminophen (15 mg/kg) or ibuprofen (10 mg/kg).

If the seizure continues, diazepam (0.1 mg/kg/dose) or lorazepam (0.05 to 0.10 mg/kg/dose) should be given IV. Both have a rapid onset of action (2 to 3 minutes); lorazepam has a longer antiepileptic duration of action than diazepam (24 hours vs. 1 hour).[266,267] If peripheral perfusion is compromised due to a prolonged seizure, the underlying problem causing the fever and in some instances hypoventilation, it may be difficult to establish IV access. In such cases, the use of the intraosseous route for drug administration should be considered, but a more commonly used alternative is diazepam (IV solution) given per rectum (0.5 mg/kg for the first dose, 0.25 mg/kg on subsequent doses), administered by inserting a TB syringe or 14 G plastic catheter into the rectum. Rectal Valium has been successful in treating febrile seizures, since therapeutic levels are reached 3 to 5 minutes after administration.[268] Diazepam given as suppositories or IM is not suitable for the treatment of seizures in progress. If seizure control is not established in 5 to 10 minutes, a second dose of the drug may be given. It is important constantly to reevaluate the airway and respiratory status because of the continuing possibility of respiratory depression, especially with the use of benzodiazepines.

Phenytoin, at a dose of 10 to 15 mg/kg, is the second line of therapy for a prolonged febrile convulsion. Although it does not cause respiratory depression, if given in a fast infusion, it can cause cardiac dysrhythmias and hypotension.

Phenobarbital, 10 mg/kg given over 2 to 3 minutes IV, may be used as an alternative and provides a peak brain concentration within 30 minutes. Respiratory depression may occur if given shortly after a dose of benzodiazepine. Protection of the airway and ventilatory support may become necessary (see Chapter 11).

Long-Term Management. Controversy continues regarding the long-term management of children with febrile convulsions. Current consensus is that in view of the benign nature and low risk of complications in most simple febrile seizures, there is no need for long-term medication.[255] Prophylaxis with anticonvulsants should be individually considered and reserved for patients with either an abnormal neurologic examination, a prolonged or focal seizure, a seizure associated with a transient or permanent neurologic deficit, or a family history of nonfebrile seizures. It is important to consider that even when two risk factors are present, 87% of those patients will not develop epilepsy.

Studies have demonstrated that antipyretic therapy with aspirin or acetaminophen, although effective in reducing fever, is not effective in reducing the frequency of febrile convulsions.[269,270]

Phenobarbital is the traditional drug used in prophylaxis and long-term management of febrile convulsions. It is not effective when used intermittently at the onset of fever.[271] Even its effectiveness in long-term prophylaxis is debatable. Although some studies suggest that the rate of recur-

rence is decreased by continuous dosing (serum levels of 15 µg/ml), others have shown contradictory results.[272-277] Side effects due to daily use of phenobarbital include behavioral changes (hyperactivity, irritability, somnolence) and changes in sleep patterns, which often result in discontinuation of therapy. The IQ in children receiving phenobarbital on a long-term basis is lower than controls of the same age.[271]

Other anticonvulsants such as carbamazepine and phenytoin have been found to be ineffective in the prevention of seizure recurrence.[277,278] Although valproic acid has been shown to be effective as a prophylactic agent, the severity of its side effects (toxic hepatitis, hepatic failure, and pancreatitis) makes it an unacceptable alternative.[271,272,279]

Rectal diazepam suppositories (0.5 mg/kg/24 hr), given every 12 hours beginning with the onset of fever, is as effective as continuous phenobarbital.[280-283] Most failures were related to inadequate recognition of a fever by the parents at the time of onset of febrile illness. Oral diazepam (0.5 mg/kg/24 hr) and clonazepam (0.1 mg/kg/24 hr) divided in 3 doses have also been effective in decreasing the recurrence rate.[284,285] Rosman et al conducted a randomized, double-blind, placebo-controlled trial comparing oral diazepam to placebo. A dose of 0.33 mg/kg was administered at the onset of a febrile illness to prevent febrile seizures. The authors concluded that oral diazepam is safe and reduces the risk of recurrent seizures. It is important to mention that 39% of the 153 children in this study who took at least one dose of diazepam experienced a reversible side effect including ataxia, lethargy, and irritability.[286] These side effects could make the evaluation of a febrile child more difficult.

In summary, the use of prophylactic anticonvulsant therapy is still controversial. Each case should be carefully evaluated. Long-term therapy should be considered only in those patients presenting with one or more of the aforementioned risk factors. If treatment is necessary, the preferred drug is phenobarbital for 2 years after the most recent febrile seizure. If parents are able to recognize a fever early, rectal or oral diazepam or oral clonazepam may be considered as alternatives.

References

Ataxia

1. Fenichel GM: Ataxia. In Fenichel GM, editor: *Clinical pediatric neurology: a signs and symptoms approach*, Philadelphia, 1988, WB Saunders.
2. Chutorian AM and Pavlakis SG: Acute ataxia. In Pellock JM and Meyer EC, editor: *Neurologic emergencies in infancy and childhood*, ed 2, Boston, 1993, Butterworth-Heinemann.
3. Berman PH and Packer RJ: Ataxia. In Fleisher G, editor: *Textbook of pediatric emergency medicine*, ed 3, Baltimore, 1993, Williams & Wilkins.
4. Guyton AC: The cerebellum, the basal ganglia, and overall motor control. In Guyton AC, editor: *Textbook of medical physiology*, ed 8, Philadelphia, 1991, WB Saunders.
5. Brown JR: Localizing cerebellar syndromes, *JAMA* 141:518,1949.
6. Brazis PW, Masdeu JC, Biller J: *Localization in clinical neurology*, Boston, 1985, Little, Brown.
7. Bell WE: Ataxia in childhood, *Lancet* 85(1):2, 1965.
8. Curnen EC and Chamberlin HR: Acute cerebellar ataxia associated with poliovirus infection, *Yale J Biol Med* 34:219, 1962.

9. Berg R and Jelke H: Acute cerebellar ataxia in children associated with coxsackie viruses group B, *Acta Paediatr Scand* 54:497, Sept 1965.

10. Marzetti G and Midulla M: Acute cerebellar ataxia associated with echo type 6 infection in two children, *Acta Paedietr Scand* 56:547, 1967.

11. Dano G: Acute cerebellar ataxia associated with herpes simplex virus infection, *Acta Paediatr Scand* 57:151, 1968.

12. Cleary TG, Henle W, Pickering LK: Acute cerebellar ataxia associated with Epstein-Barr virus infection, *JAMA* 243(2):148, 1980.

13. Steele JC, Gladstone RM, Thanasophon S, et al: Acute cerebellar ataxia and concomitant infection with Mycoplasma pneumoniae, *J Pediatr* 80(3):467, 1972.

14. Peters ACB, Versteeg J, Lindeman J, et al: Varicella and acute cerebellar ataxia, *Arch Neurol* 35:769, 1978.

15. Weiss S and Carter S: Course and prognosis of acute cerebellar ataxia in children, *Neurology* 9(11):711, 1959.

16. Garretton LK: Poisoning. In Pellock JM and Meyer EC, editors: *Neurologic emergencies in infancy and childhood*, ed 2, Boston, 1993, Butterworth-Heinemann.

17. Solomon GE and Chutorian AM: Opsoclonus and occult neuroblastoma, *N Engl J Med* 279:475, 1968.

18. Korobkin M, Clark RE, Palubinskas AJ: Occult neuroblastoma and acute cerebellar ataxia in childhood, *Pediatr Radiol* 102:151, 1972.

19. Schwartz JF: Acute ataxia. In Gellison SS and Kagan BM, editors: *Current Pediatric Therapy*, ed 13, Philadelphia, 1990, WB Saunders.

20. Gordon N: Intermittent ataxia and biochemical disorders, *Dev Med Child Neurol* 15:208, 1973.

21. Stumpf DA: Friedreich's ataxia and other hereditary ataxias. In Tyler HR and Dawson DM, editors: *Current neurology,* Boston, 1978, Houghton-Mifflin.

22. Stumpf DA: Ataxic syndromes. In Rudolph AM, Hoffman JIE, Rudolph CD, editors: *Rudolph's pediatrics*, ed 19, Norwalk, CT, 1991, Appleton & Lange.

23. Stumpf DA: Acute ataxia, *Pediatr Rev* 8(10):303, 1987.

Coma and Altered Mental Status

24. Plum F and Posner J: *The diagnosis of stupor and coma*, Philadelphia, 1980, FA Davis.

25. Jennet B and Teasdale G.: Aspects of coma after severe head injury, *Lancet* 1:878, 1977.

26. Winkler JV, Rosen P, Alfry E: Prehospital use of the Glasgow Coma Scale in severe head injury, *J Emerg Med* 2:1, 1984.

27. Morray J, Tyler D, Jones T: Coma scale for use in brain-injured children, *Crit Care Med* 12:1018, 1984.

28. Raimondi A and Hirshauer J: Head injury in the infant and toddler. Coma scoring and outcome scale, *Child's Brain* 11:12, 1984.

29. Simpson D and Reilly P: Pediatric coma scale, *Lancet* 2:450, 1982.

30. Goodwin SR, Friedman WA, Bellefleur M: Is it time to use evoked potentials to predict outcome in comatose children and adults, *Crit Care Med* 19:518, 1991.

31. Seshia S and Seshia M: Coma in childhood, *Dev Med Child Neurol* 19:614, 1977.

32. Vannucci RC and Wasiewski WW: Diagnosis and management of coma in children. In Pellock JM and Myer EC, editors: *Neurologic emergencies in infancy and childhood*, ed 2, Boston, 1993, Butterworth-Heinemann.

33. Barret, Michael J, et al: Changing epidemiology of Reye syndrome in the United States, *Pediatrics* 77:598, 1986.

34. McCabe JB, Singer JI, Love T, et al: Intussusception: a supplement to the mnemonic for coma, *Pediatr Emerg Care* 2:118, 1987.

35. Singer JI: Altered consciousness as an early manifestation of intussusception, *Pediatrics* 64:93, 1979.

36. Kanter RK: Retinal hemorrhage after cardiopulmonary resuscitation or child abuse, *J Pediatr* 108:430, 1986.

37. Johnson DL, Braun D, Friendly D: Accidental head trauma and retinal hemorrhage *Neurosurgery* 33:231, 1993.

38. Goetting MG and Sowa B: Retinal hemorrhage after cardiopulmonary resuscitation in children: an etiologic reevaluation, *Pediatrics* 85:585, 1990.

39. Winkler E, Almog S, Kriger D, et al: Use of flumazenil in the diagnosis and treatment of patients with coma of unknown etiology, *Crit Care Med* 21:538, 1993.

40. Molofsky WJ: Steroids and head trauma, *Neurosurgery* 15:424, 1984.

41. Dearden NM, Gibson JS, McDowall DG, et al: Effect of high-dose dexamethasone on outcome from severe head injury, *J Neurosurg* 64:81, 1986.

42. Braughler JM and Hall ED: Current application of "high dose" steroid therapy for CNS injury. A pharmacologic perspective, *J Neurosurg* 62:806, 1985.

43. Jooma R: Dexamethasone and the serious head injury, *Br J Neurosurg* 1:400, 1987.

44. Davis RL, Mullen N, Makela M, et al: Cranial computed tomography scans in children after minimal head injury with loss of consciousness, *Ann Emerg Med* 24:640, 1994.

45. Dietrich AM, James CD, King DR, et al: Head trauma in children with congenital coagulation disorders, *J Pediatr Surg* 29:28, 1994.

46. Tasker RC, Matthew DJ, Dinwiddie R, et al: Monitoring in nontraumatic coma. Part 1: invasive intracranial measurements, *Arch Dis Child* 63:888, 1988.

47. Nussbaum E, Maggi C: Intracranial pressure monitoring by subarachnoid bolt in comatose children, *Clin Pediatr* 24:329, 1985.

48. Eisenberg HM, Frankowski RF, Conant CF, et al: High-dose barbiturate control of elevated intracranial pressure in patients with severe head injury, *J Neurosurg* 69:15, 1988.

49. Rea GL and Rockswold GL: Barbiturate therapy in uncontrolled intracranial hypertension, *Neurosurgery* 12:401, 1983.

50. Rockoff MA, Marshall LF, Shapiro M: High-dose barbiturate therapy in humans: a clinical review of 60 patients, *Ann Neurol* 56:498, 1979.

51. Seshia S, Johnston B, Kasian G: Non-traumatic coma in childhood: clinical variables in prediction of outcome, *Dev Med Child Neurol* 25:493, 1983.

52. Leurssen T, Klauber M, Marshall L: Outcome from head injury related to patient's age, *J Neurosurg* 68:409, 1988.

53. Mahoney W, D'Souza B, et al: Long term outcome of children with severe outcome and prolonged coma, *Pediatrics* 71:756, 1983.

54. Bruce D, Schut L, et al: Outcome following severe head injury in children, *J Neurosurg* 48:679, 1978.

55. Kraus J, Fife D, Conroy C: Pediatric brain injuries: the nature, clinical course, and early outcomes in a defined United States population, *Pediatrics* 79:501, 1987.

56. Levin HS, Aldrich EF, Saydjari C, et al: Severe head injury in children: experience of the Traumatic Coma Data Bank, *Neurosurgery* 31:435, 1992.

57. Choi SC, Barnes TY, Bullock R, et al: Temporal profile of outcomes in severe head injury, *J Neurosurg* 81:169, 1994.

58. Fields AI, Coble DH, Pollack MM, et al: Outcomes of children in a persistent vegetative state, *Crit Care Med* 21:1890, 1993.

59. Margolis L and Shaywitz B: The outcome of prolonged coma in childhood, *Pediatrics* 65:477, 1980.

60. Special Task Force of the American Academy of Pediatrics: Guidelines for the determination of brain death in children, *Pediatrics* 80:298, 1987.

Headache

61. Lance JW: Headache, *Ann Neurol* 10:1, 1981.

62. Rothner AD: Headache. In Swaiman KF, editor: *Pediatric neurology: principles and practice*, ed 2, St. Louis, 1994, Mosby.

63. Singer HS and Rowe S: Chronic recurrent headaches in children, *Pediatr Ann* 21:369, 1992.

64. Caeser R, Kramer DA, Gavin LJ: Acute headache management: the challenge of deciphering etiologies to guide assessment and treatment, *Emerg Med Reports* June 1995.

65. Rothner AD: A practical approach to headaches in adolescents, *Pediatr Ann* 20:200, 1991.

66. Shinnar S and D'Souza BJ: Diagnosis and management of headaches in children, *Pediatr Clin North Am* 29:79, 1981.

67. Kriel RL: Headache. In Swaiman KF and Wright FS, editors: *The practice of pediatric neurology,* ed 2, St. Louis, 1982, Mosby.

Movement Disorders

68. Fenichel GM: Movement disorders. In Fenichel GM, editor: *Clinical pediatric neurology: a signs and symptoms approach,* Philadelphia, 1988, WB Saunders.

69. Swaiman KF: Movement disorders. In Swaiman KF, editor: *Pediatric neurology: principles and practice,* St. Louis, 1994, Mosby.

70. Butler IJ: Movement disorders of children, *Pediatr Clin North Am* 39:727, 1992.

71. Berg BO: Movement disorders. In Berg BO, editor: *Child neurology: a clinical manual*, Greenbrae, CA, 1984, Jones Medical Publications.

Paralysis and Hemiplegia

72. Rodenberg H, Gratton M, Bennett J, et al: Left upper extremity weakness in an 18-year-old man, *Ann Emerg Med* 20:672, 1991.

73. Freeman JM: Diagnosis and evaluation of acute paraplegia, *Pediatr Rev* 4:327, 1983.

74. Fenichel GM: Paraplegia and quadriplegia. In Fenichel GM, editor: *Clinical pediatric neurology: a signs and symptoms approach*, Philadelphia, 1988, WB Saunders.

75. Swaiman KF: Anterior horn cell and cranial motor neuron disease. In Swaiman KF, editor: *Pediatric neurology: principles and practice*, ed 2, St. Louis, 1994, Mosby.

76. Avner JR, Cunningham S, Dorfman D, et al: Office management of neurologic emergencies, *Pediatr Ann* 19:649, 1990.

77. Swaiman KF: Diseases of the neuromuscular junction. In Swaiman KF, editor: *Pediatric neurology: principles and practice*, ed 2, St. Louis, 1994, Mosby.

78. Leshner RT and Teasley JE: Pediatric neuromuscular emergencies. In Pellock JM and Myer EC, editors: *Neurologic emergencies in infancy and childhood*, ed 2, Boston, 1993, Butterworth-Heinemann.

79. Fenichel GM: Hemiplegia. In Fenichel GM, editor: *Clinical pediatric neurology: a signs and symptoms approach*. Philadelphia, 1988, WB Saunders.

80. Solomon GE: Acute therapy of childhood stroke. In Pellock JM and Myer EC, editors: *Neurologic emergencies in infancy and childhood*, ed 2, Boston, 1993, Butterworth-Heinemann.

81. Trescher WH: Ischemic stroke syndromes in childhood, *Pediatr Ann* 21:1374, 1992.

Syncope

82. Linzer M, Osborn HH, Gabelman M, et al: Syncope: how to evaluate, when to admit, *Hosp Phys* 8, Nov 1983.

83. Farmer TW and Greenwood RS: Paroxysmal disorders. In Farmer TW, editor: *Pediatric neurology*, ed 3, Philadelphia, 1983, Harper & Row.

84. Fineman JR and Soifer SJ: Syncope. In Grossman M and Dieckman RA, editors: *Pediatric emergency medicine: a clinician's reference*, Philadelphia, 1991, JB Lippincott.

85. Gillette PC and Ross BA: Cardiovascular Syncope, *Pediatr Emerg Casebook* 4:3, 1986.

86. Kienzle MG: Syncope: Mechanisms and manifestations, *Hosp Pract* 77, Dec 1990.

87. Samoil D, Grubb BP, Kip K, et al: Head-upright tilt table testing in children with unexplained syncope, *Pediatrics* 92:426, 1993.

88. Kapoor WN, Karpf M, Wieand S, et al: A prospective evaluation and follow-up of patients with syncope, *N Engl J Med* 309:197, 1983.

89. Ruckman RN: Cardiac causes of syncope, *Pediatr Rev* 9:101, 1987.

90. Hannon DW and Knilans TK: Syncope in children and adolescents, *Curr Probl Pediatr* 23:358, 1993.

91. Scott WA: Evaluating the child with syncope, *Pediatr Ann* 20:350, 1991.

92. Duchowny MS: Atonic seizures, *Pediatr Rev* 9:43, 1987.

93. Pratt JL, Fleisher GR: Syncope in children and adolescents, *Pediatr Emerg Care* 5:80, 1989.

94. Lerman-Sagie T, Rechavia E, Strasberg B, et al: Head-up tilt for the evaluation of syncope of unknown origin in children, *J Pediatr* 118:676, 1991.

95. Fuchs SM and Jaffe DM: Evaluation of the "tilt test" in children, *Ann Emerg Med* 16:386, 1987.

96. Hardy CE: Syncope and chest pain: to worry, or not? *Contemp Peds* 11:19, 1994.

Vertigo

97. Fenichel GM: Lower brainstem and cranial nerve dysfunction. In Fenichel GM, editor: *Clinical pediatric neurology: a signs and symptoms approach*, Philadelphia, 1988, WB Saunders.

98. Busis SN: Diagnostic evaluation of the patient presenting with vertigo, *Otolaryngol Clin North Am* 6:3, 1973.

99. Eviatar L: Vertigo. In Swaiman KF, editor: *Pediatric neurology: principles and practice*, St. Louis, 1995, Mosby.

100. Lockman LA: Nonepileptic paroxysmal disorders. In Swaiman KF, editor: *Pediatric neurology: principles and practice*, St. Louis, 1995, Mosby.

101. Berg BO: Convulsive disorders. In Berg BO, editor: *Child neurology: a clinical manual*, Greenbrae, CA, 1984, Jones Medical Publications.

102. Fenichel GM: Migraine as a cause of benign paroxysmal vertigo of childhood, *J Pediatr* 71:114, 1968.

103. Dunn DW and Synder CH: Benign paroxysmal vertigo of childhood, *Am J Dis Child* 130:1099, 1976.

104. Jongkees LBW: The caloric test and the patient with vertigo, *Otolaryngol Clin North Am* 6:73, 1973.

105. DeGowin EL, DeGowin RL: *DeGowin's diagnostic examination*, ed 6, New York, 1993, McGraw-Hill, Health Professions Division.

Breath-Holding Spells

106. Vining EPG and Freeman JM: Paroxysmal events which are not seizures, *Pediatr Ann* 14:726, 1985.

107. Fenichel GM: Paroxysmal disorders. In Fenichel GM, editor: *Clinical pediatric neurology: a signs and symptoms approach*, Philadelphia, 1988, WB Saunders.

108. Gordon N: Breath-holding spells, *Dev Med Child Neurol* 29:805, 1987.

109. Lockman LA: Nonepileptic paroxysmal disorders. In Swaiman KF, editor: *Pediatric neurology: principles and practice*, ed 2, St. Louis, 1994, Mosby.

110. DiMario FJ, Chee CM, Berman PH: Pallid breath-holding spells: evaluation of the autonomic nervous system, *Clin Pediatr* 9:17, 1990.

111. Lombroso CT and Lerman P: Breathholding spells (cyanotic and pallid infantile syncope), *Pediatrics* 39:563, 1967.

112. DiMario FJ: Breath-holding spells in childhood, *Am J Dis Child* 146:125, 1992.

113. Southall DP, Samuels MP, Talbert DG: Recurrent cyanotic episodes with severe arterial hypoxaemia and intrapulmonary shunting: a mechanism for sudden death, *Arch Dis Child* 65:953, 1990.

Meningitis (Bacterial)

114. Erickson RL and Kelley DW: Decreases in invasive *Haemophilus influenzae* diseases in US army children, 1984-1991, *JAMA* 269:227, 1993.

115. Claesson B, Trollfors B, Joda U, et al: Incidence and prognosis of *Haemophilus influenzae* meningitis in children in a Swedish region, *Pediatr Infect Dis* 3:35, 1984.

116. Schoendorf KC, Adams WG, Kiely JL, et al: National trends in *Haemophilus influenzae* meningitis mortality and hospitalization among children, 1980-1991, *Pediatrics* 93:663, 1994.

117. Control: Progress toward elimination of *Haemophilus influenzae* type B disease among infants and children—United States, 1993-1994, *MMWR* 44:545, 1995.

118. Mustafa MM, Ramilo O, Saez-Llorens X, et al: Cerebrospinal fluid prostaglandins, interleukin-1B, and tumor necrosis factor in bacterial meningitis: clinical and laboratory correlations in placebo and dexamethasone treated patients, *Am J Dis Child* 144:883, 1990.

119. Smith AL: Pathogenesis of *Haemophilus influenzae* meningitis, *Pediatr Infect Dis* 7:83, 1987.

120. Yogev R: Suppurative intracranial complications of upper respiratory tract infections, *Pediatr Infect Dis J* 6:324, 1987.

121. Smith DH: The challenge of bacterial meningitis, *Hosp Pract* 11:71, 1976.

122. Cole FS, Saryan JA, Smith AL: The risk of additional systemic bacterial illness in infants with systemic *Streptococcus pneumoniae* disease, *J Pediatr* 99:91, 1981.

123. Eraklis AJ, Kevy SV, Diamond LK, et al: Hazard of overwhelming infection after splenectomy in childhood, *N Engl J Med* 276:1225, 1967.

124. Garvey JC and Trott A: Recurrent meningitis: a case report, *J Emerg Med* 5:185, 1987.

125. Baker CJ and Barrett FF: Transmission of group B streptococci among parturient women and their neonates, *J Pediatr* 83:919, 1973.

126. Sande MA, Scheld WM, McCracken GH: Pathophysiology of bacterial meningitis: implications for new management strategies, *Pediatr Infect Dis* 6:1167, 1987.

127. Groover RV, Sutherland JM, Landing BH: Purulent meningitis of newborn infants, *N Engl J Med* 264:1115, 1961.

128. Lipton JD and Schafermeyer RQ: Evolving concepts in pediatric bacterial meningitis. *Ann Emerg Med* 22:1602, 1993.

129. Pryor RW, Kline MW, Matson JR, et al: Septic shock: principles of management in the emergency department, *Pediatr Emerg Care* 5:193, 1989.

130. Oliver LG and Harwood-Nuss AL: Bacterial meningitis in infants and children: a review, *J Emerg Med* 11:555, 1993.

131. Green SM, Rothrock SG, Clem KJ: Can seizures be the sole manifestation of meningitis in febrile children? *Pediatrics* 92:527, 1993.

132. Pomeroy SL, Holmes SJ, Dodge PR et al: Seizures and other neurologic sequelae of bacterial meningitis in children, *N Engl J Med* 323:1651, 1990.

133. Floret D: Cerebellar infarction as a complication of pneumococcal meningitis, *Pediatr Infect Dis J* 8:57, 1989.

134. Dodge PR and Swartz MN: Bacterial meningitis. A review of selected aspects. II. Special neurologic problems, postmeningitic complications and clinicopathological correlations, *N Engl J Med* 272:1003, 1965.

135. Bonadio WA: Cerebral herniation syndrome as the presenting sign of *Haemophilus influenzae* meningitis, *Pediatr Emerg Care* 3:253, 1987.

136. Snedeker JB, Kaplan SL, Dodge PR, et al: Subdural effusion and its relationship with neurologic sequelae of bacterial meningitis in infancy: a prospective study, *Pediatrics* 86:163, 1990.

137. Pomeroy SC, Holmes SJ, Dodge PR, et al: Seizures and other neurologic sequelae of bacterial meningitis in children, *N Engl J Med* 323:1651, 1990.

138. Ballard TL, et al: Comparison of three latex agglutination kits and counterimmunoelectrophoresis for the detection of bacterial antigens in a pediatric population, *Pediatr Infect Dis* 6:30, 1987

139. David SD, Hill SR, Feigl P, et al: Partial antibiotic therapy in *Haemophilus influenzae* meningitis: its effect on cerebrospinal fluid abnormalities, *Am J Dis Child* 129:802, 1975.

140. Hamson SA and Risser W: Repeat lumbar puncture in the differential diagnosis of meningitis, *Pediatr Infect Dis J* 7:143, 1988.

141. Lembo RM, Rubin DH, Krowchuk DP, et al: Peripheral white blood cell counts and bacterial meningitis, implications regarding diagnostic efficacy in febrile children, *Pediatr Emerg Care* 7:4, 1991.

142. Crosby RM: Risk of diagnostic lumbar puncture in acute bacterial meningitis, *Pediatr Emerg Care* 2:180, 1986.

143. Polk DB and Steele RW: Bacterial meningitis presenting with normal cerebrospinal fluid, *Pediatr Infect Dis* 3:239, 1984.

144. Donald PR, Malan C, Van Der Walt A: Simultaneous determination of cerebrospinal fluid glucose and blood glucose concentrations in the diagnosis of bacterial meningitis, *J Pediatr* 103:413, 1983.

145. Shohat M, Goodman Z, Ragovin H, et al: The effect of lumbar puncture procedure on blood glucose level and leukocyte count in infants, *Clin Pediatr* 26:477, 1987.

146. Rubenstein JS and Yogev R: What represents pleocytosis in blood contaminated ("traumatic tap") cerebrospinal fluid in children, *J Pediatr* 107:249, 1985.

147. Odio C, McCracken GH, Nelson JD: CSF shunt infections in pediatrics, *Am J Dis Child* 138:249, 1984.

148. Heyderman RS, Robb SA, Kendall BE, et al: Does computed tomography have a role in the evaluation of complicated acute bacterial meningitis in childhood? *Dev Med Child Neurol* 34:870, 1992.

149. Lepow ML, Coyne N, Thompson LB, et al: A clinical and epidemiologic and laboratory investigation of aseptic meningitis during the four year period 1955-1958. II. The clinical disease and its sequelae, *N Engl J Med* 266:1188, 1962.

150. Deibel R, Flanagan TD, Smith V: Central nervous system infections in New York State: etiologic and epidemiologic observations, 1974, *New York State J Med* 75:2337, 1975.

151. Moore M: Enteroviral disease in the United States, 1970-1979, *J Infect Dis* 146:103, 1982.

152. Koskiniemi M, Manninen V, Vaheri A, et al: Acute encephalitis: a survey of epidemiological, clinical and microbiological features covering a twelve-year period, *Acta Med Scand* 209:115, 1981.

153. Schaad UB, Suter S, Gianella-Borradori A, et al: A comparison of ceftriaxone and cefuroxime for the treatment of bacterial meningitis in children, *N Engl J Med* 322:141, 1990.

154. Schaad UB, Wedawoof-Krucko J, Tschaepoeler H: Reversible ceftriaxone associated biliary pseudo-lithiasis in children, *Lancet* 2:1411, 1988.

155. Arditi M, Herold BC, Yogev R: Cefuroxime treatment failure and *Haemophilus influenzae* meningitis: case report and review of literature, *Pediatrics* 84:132, 1989.

156. Committee on Infectious Diseases: report, 1991, Elk Grove Village, Ill, American Academy of Pediatrics.

157. Jacobs RF, Well TG, Steele RW, et al: A prospective randomized comparison of cefotaxime vs ampicillin and chloramphenicol for bacterial meningitis in children, *J Pediatr* 107:129, 1985.

158. Briemán R, Butler J, Tenover F, et al: Emergence of drug resistant pneumococcal infections in the United States, *JAMA* 271:1831, 1994.

159. Viladrich P, Guidol F, Linares J, et al: Evaluation of vancomycin for therapy of adult pneumococcal meningitis, *Antimicrob Agents Chemother* 35:2467, 1991.

160. Lebel MH, Freis B, Syroglannopoulos GA, et al: Dexamethasone therapy for bacterial meningitis, *N Engl J Med* 319:964, 1988.

161. Feigin RD, McCracken GH Jr, Klein JO: Diagnosis and management of meningitis, *Pediatr Infect Dis J* 11:785, 1992.

162. Wald E, Kaplan S, Mason E, et al: Dexamethasone therapy for children with bacterial meningitis, *Pediatrics* 95:21, 1995.

163. American Academy of Pediatrics: Report of the Committee on Infectious Diseases, Elk Grove Village, 1994, AAP.

164. Kotagel S, Rosenberg C, Ruddet US: Auditory evoked potentials in bacterial meningitis, *Arch Neurol* 38:693, 1981.

Migraine Headaches

165. Gascon GG: Chronic and recurrent headaches in children and adolescents, *Pediatr Clin North Am* 31:1027, 1984.

166. Welch KMA: Drug therapy of migraine, *N Engl J Med* 329:1476, 1993.

167. Chutorian AM: Paroxysmal disorders of childhood. In Rudolph AM, Hoffman JI, Rudolph CD, editors: *Rudolph's pediatrics*, ed 19, Norwalk, CT, 1991, Appleton & Lange.

168. Silberstein SD and Lipton RB: Overview of diagnosis and treatment of migraine, *Neurology* 44(7 suppl):S6, 1994.

169. Bille B: Migraine in school children. *Acta Pediatr Scand* 136(51 suppl):14, 1962.

170. Shinnar S: An approach to the child with headaches, *Int Pediatr* 6:140, 1991

171. Fenichel GM: Headache. In Fenichel GM, editor: *Clinical pediatric neurology: a signs and symptoms approach*, Philadelphia, 1985, WB Saunders.

172. Shinnar S and D'Souza B: Migraine in children and adolescents, *Pediatr Rev* 3:257, 1982.

173. Rothner AD: Migraine headaches. In Swaiman KF, editor: *Pediatric neurology: principles and practice*, St. Louis, 1989, Mosby.

174. Solomon S: Migraine: current approaches to diagnosis and management. *Hosp Pract* 26:95, 1991.

175. Lance JW: The pharmacotherapy of migraine, *Med J Aust* 144:85, 1986.

176. Olesen J: Understanding the biologic basis of migraine, *N Engl J Med* 331:1713, 1994.

177. Schuler ME, Goldman MP, Munger MA. The role of calcium channel blocking agents in the prevention of migraine, *Drug Intell Clin Pharm* 22:187, 1988.

178. Woods RP, Iacoboni M, Mazziotta JC: Bilateral spreading cerebral hypoperfusion during spontaneous migraine headache, *N Engl J Med* 331:1689, 1994.

179. Raskin NH: Acute and prophylactic treatment of migraine: practical approaches and pharmacologic rationale, *Neurology* 43(3 suppl):S39, 1993.

180. Olness KN and MacDonald JT: Recurrent headaches in children: diagnosis and treatment, *Pediatr Rev* 8:307, 1987.

181. D'Andrea G, Welch KM, Grunfeld S, et al: Platelet norepinephrine and serotonin balance in migraine, *Headache* 29:657, 1989.

182. Fernandez F: Migraine headaches in children. In Fishman MA, editor: *Pediatric neurology*, Orlando, 1986, Grune & Stratton.

183. Prensky AL and Sommers D: Diagnosis and management of migraine in children, *Neurology* 29:506, 1979.

184. Haas DC and Lourie H: Trauma triggered migraine: an explanation for common neurological attacks after mild head injury. Review of the literature. *J Neurosurg* 68:181, 1988.

185. Menkes JH: Paroxysmal disorders. In Menkes JH, editor: *Textbook of child neurology*, ed 4, Philadelphia, 1990, Lea & Febiger.

186. Hockaday JM: Management of migraine, *Arch Dis Child* 65:1174, 1990.

187. Hodes RL: The biofeedback treatment of neurologic and neuropsychological diseases of childhood and adolescence. In Reynolds CR and Janzen EH, editors: *Handbook of clinical child neuropsychology*, New York, 1989, Plenum Press.

188. Olness K: Hypnotherapy: a cyberphysiologic strategy in pain management, *Pediatr Clin North Am* 36:873, 1989.

189. Jones EB, Gonzalez ER, Boggs JG, et al: Safety and efficacy of rectal prochlorperazine for the treatment of migraine in the emergency department, *Ann Emerg Med* 24:237, 1994.

190. Jones J, Sklar D, Dougherty J, et al: Randomized double-blind trial of intravenous prochlorperazine for the treatment of acute headache, *JAMA* 261:1174, 1989.

191. Ellis GL, Delaney J, DeHart DA, et al: The efficacy of metoclopramide in the treatment of migraine headache, *Ann Emerg Med* 22:191, 1993.

192. Larkin GL and Prescott JE: A randomized, double-blind, comparative study of the efficacy of ketorolac tromethamine versus meperidine in the treatment of severe migraine, *Ann Emerg Med* 21:919, 1992.

193. Saadah HA: Abortive headache therapy in the office with intravenous dihydroergotamine plus prochlorperazine, *Headache* 32:143, 1992.

194. Ferrari MD, et al: The Subcutaneous Sumatriptan International Study Group. Treatment of migraine attacks with sumatriptan. *N Engl J Med* 325:316, 1991.

195. Akpunonu BE, Mutgi AB, Federman DJ, et al: Subcutaneous sumatriptan for treatment of acute migraine in patients admitted to the emergency department: a multicenter study, *Ann Emerg Med* 25:464, 1995.

196. Buring JE, Peto R, Hennekens CH: Low-dose aspirin for migraine prophylaxis, *JAMA* 264:1711, 1990.

Idiopathic Intracranial Hypertension (Pseudotumor Cerebri)

197. Radhakrishnan K, Ahlskog JE, Garrity JA, et al: Idiopathic intracranial hypertension, *Mayo Clin Proc* 69:169, 1994.

198. Johnston I and Paterson A: Benign intracranial hypertension II. CSF pressure and circulation, *Brain* 97:301, 1974.

199. Lehman LB: Pseudotumor cerebri: an enigmatic process, *Hosp Pract* 23(12):127, 1988.

200. Weisberg LA and Chutorian AM: Pseudotumor cerebri of childhood, *Am J Dis Child* 131:1243, 1977.

201. Grant DN: Benign intracranial hypertension; a review of 79 cases in infancy and childhood, *Arch Dis Child* 46:651, 1971.

202. Amacher AL and Spence JD: Spectrum of benign intracranial hypertension in children and adolescents, *Childs Nerv Syst* 1:81, 1985.

203. Lessell S: Pediatric pseudotumor cerebri (idiopathic intracranial hypertension), *Surv Ophthalmol* 37:155, 1992.

Seizures

204. Vining EPG and Freeman JM: Introduction: epilepsy in children, *Pediatr Ann* 14(11):705, 1985.

205. Scheuer ML and Pedley TA: The evaluation and treatment of seizures, *N Engl J Med* 323:1468, 1990.

206. Vining EPG and Freeman JM: Seizures which are not epilepsy, *Pediatr Ann* 14(11):711, 1985.

207. Glaze DG: Neonatal seizures. In Fishman MA, editor: *Pediatric neurology,* Orlando, 1986, Grune & Stratton.

208. Holmes GL: Introduction and commentary, *Pediatr Ann* 20(1):13, 1991.

209. Commission on Classification and Terminology of the International League Against Epilepsy: Proposal for revised clinical and electroencephalographic classification of epileptic seizures, *Epilepsia* 22:489, 1981.

210. Vining EPG and Freeman JM: Classification and evaluation of seizures, *Pediatr Ann* 14(11):730, 1985.

211. Commission on Classification and Terminology of the International League Against Epilepsy: Proposal for revised classification of epilepsies and epileptic syndromes, *Epilepsia* 30:389, 1989.

212. Holmes GL: Partial seizures in children, *Pediatrics* 77:725, 1986.

213. Zion TE: Diagnosis and pharmacologic therapy of epilepsy. In Fishman MA, editor: *Pediatric neurology.* Orlando, 1986, Grune & Stratton.

214. Hirtz DG: Generalized tonic-clonic and febrile seizures, *Pediatr Clin North Am* 36:365, 1989.

215. Duchowny MS: Atonic seizures, *Pediatr Rev* 9(2):43, 1987.

216. Papazian O: Common epileptic syndromes of children, *Pediatr Ann* 20(1):15, 1991.

217. Vining EPG and Freeman JM: Special types of seizures, *Pediatr Ann* 14(11):757, 1985.

218. Vining EPG: Pediatric seizures, *Emerg Med Clin North Am* 12:973, 1994.

219. Stafstrom CE: Neonatal seizures, *Pediatr Rev* 16:248, 1995.

220. Horton EJ and Snead OC: Diagnosis of neonatal seizures, *Semin Neurol* 13:48, 1993.

221. Vining EPG and Freeman JM: Status epilepticus, *Pediatr Ann* 14(11):764, 1985.

222. Delgado-Escueta AV, Wasterlain C, Treiman DM, et al: Management of status epilepticus, *N Engl J Med* 306:1137, 1982.

223. Pellock JM: Status epilepticus in children: Update and review, *J Child Neurol* 9(Suppl):2S27, 1994.

224. Shinnar S and Ballaban-Gil K: An approach to the child with a first unprovoked seizure, *Pediatr Ann* 20(1):29, 1991.

225. Vining EPG and Freeman JM: Management of nonfebrile seizures, *Pediatr Rev* 8(6):185, 1986.

226. Shinnar S, Berg AT, Moshe SL, et al: Risk of seizure recurrence following a first unprovoked seizure in childhood: a prospective study, *Pediatrics* 85:1076, 1990.

227. Freeman JM, Tibbles J, Camfield C, et al: Benign epilepsy of childhood: a speculation and its ramifications, *Pediatrics* 79:864, 1987.

228. Turnbull TL, Vanden Hoek TL, Howes DS, et al: Utility of laboratory studies in the emergency department patient with a new-onset seizure, *Ann Emerg Med* 19:373, 1990.

229. Shields WD: Status epilepticus, *Pediatr Clin North Am* 36(2):383, 1989.

230. Lacey DJ, Singer WD, Horwitz SJ, et al: Lorazepam therapy of status epilepticus in children and adolescents, *J Pediatr* 108:771, 1986.

231. Albano A, Reisdorff EJ, Wiegenstein JG: Rectal diazepam in pediatric status epilepticus, *Am J Emerg Med* 7:168, 1989.

232. Snead OC and Horton EJ: Treatment of neonatal seizures, *Semin Neurol* 13:53, 1993.

233. Vining EPG and Freeman JM: Where, why, and what type of therapy, *Pediatr Ann* 14(11):741, 1985.

234. Mikati M: The newer antiepileptic drugs: carbamazepine and valproic acid, *Pediatr Ann* 20(1):34, 1991.

235. The Medical Letter: Drugs for epilepsy. In Abramowicz M, editor: *Drugs of choice from the medical letter,* New Rochelle, NY, 1995, Medical Letter.

236. Leppik IE, Graves N, Devinsky O: New antiepileptic medications, *Neurol Clin* 11:923, 1993.

237. Dodson E and Bourgeois BFD: Pharmacology and therapeutic aspects of antiepileptic drugs in pediatrics, *J Child Neurol* 9(suppl): 2S1, 1994.

238. Devinsky O, Vazquez B, Luciano D: New antiepileptic drugs for children: Felbamate, gabapentin, lamotrigene, and vigabatrin, *J Child Neurol* 9(suppl):S33, 1994.

239. The Medical Letter: Gabapentin—a new anticonvulsant. In Abramowicz M, editor: *The Medical Letter.* New Rochelle, NY, 1995, Medical Letter.

240. The Medical Letter: Lamotrigene for epilepsy. In Abramowicz M, editor: *Medical Letter.* New Rochelle, NY, 1995, Medical Letter.

241. Lortie A, Chiron C, Mumford J, et al: The potential for increasing frequency, relapse, and appearance of new seizure types with vigabatrin, *Neurology* 43(Suppl 5):S25, 1993.

242. Vining EPG and Freeman JM: Monitoring: the most important role of the pediatrician. *Pediatr Ann* 14(11):747, 1985.

Febrile Seizures

243. Millichap JG: *Febrile convulsions,* New York, 1968, Macmillan.

244. Van den Berg BJ and Yerushalemy J: Studies on convulsive disorders in children: I. Incidence of febrile and non-febrile convulsions by age and other factors, *Pediatr Res* 3:289, 1968.

245. Livingston S: *Comprehensive management of epilepsy in infancy, childhood and adolescence,* Springfield, 1972, Charles C. Thomas.

246. Nelson KB and Ellenberg JH: Prognosis in children with febrile seizures, *Pediatrics* 61:720, 1978.

247. Gururaj VJ: Febrile seizures, *Clin Pediatr* 19:731, 1980.

248. Minchom PE and Wallace SJ: Febrile convulsions: electroencephalographic changes related to rectal temperature, *Arch Dis Child* 59:371, 1970.

249. Friderichsen C and Melchoir JC: Febrile convulsions in children: frequency and prognosis. *Acta Paediatr Scand Suppl* 43:307, 1954.

250. Wallace SJ: *The child with febrile seizures,* London, 1988, John Wright.
251. Frantzen E, Lennox-Buchtal M, Nygaard A: Longitudinal EEG and clinical study of children with febrile convulsions. *Electroencephalogr Clin Neurophysiol* 24:197, 1968.
252. Hauser WA and Kurland LT: The epidemiology of epilepsy in New Rochester, Minnesota, 1935 through 1967. *Epilepsia* 16:1, 1975.
253. Hauser WA, Annegers JF, Anderson E, et al: The risk of seizure disorders among relatives of children with febrile seizures, *Neurology* 35:1268, 1985.
254. Ellenberg JH and Nelson KB: Febrile seizures and later intellectual performance, *Arch Neurol* 35:17, 1978.
255. National Institutes of Health: Consensus development conference on febrile seizures, *Pediatrics* 66:1009, 1980.
256. Blennow G, Brierley JB, Meldrum BS, et al: Epileptic brain damage: the role of systemic factors that modify cerebral energy metabolism, *Brain* 101:687, 1978.
257. Samson JH, Apthrop J, Finley A: Febrile seizures and purulent meningitis, *JAMA* 210:1918, 1969.
258. Wolf SM: Laboratory evaluation of the child with a febrile convulsion. *Pediatrics* 62:1074, 1978.
259. Frantzen E: Spinal findings in children with febrile convulsions, *Epilepsia* 12:192, 1972.
260. Rutter N and Smales ORC: Role of routine investigations in children presenting with their first febrile convulsion, *Arch Dis Child* 52:188, 1977.
261. Asnes RS, Novick LF, Nealis J, et al: The first febrile seizure: a study of current paediatric practice, *J Pediatr* 87:485, 1975.
262. Oullette EM: The child who convulses with fever. *Pediatr Clin North AM* 21:467, 1974.
263. Ratcliffe JC and Wolf SM: Febrile convulsions caused by meningitis in young children, *Ann Neurol* 1:285, 1977.
264. Gerber MA and Berliner BC: The child with a "simple" febrile seizure, *Am J Dis Child* 135:431, 1981.
265. Chamberlain JM and Gorman RL: Occult bacteremia in children with simple febrile seizures, *Am J Dis Child* 142:1073, 1988.
266. Homam RW and Unwin DH: Benzodiazepines: lorazepam. In Levy RH, Dreyfuss FE, Mattson RH, et al, editors: *Antiepileptic drugs,* ed 3, New York, 1989, Raven Press.
267. Treiman DM: General principles of treatment: responsive and intractable status epilepticus in adults. In Delgado-Escueta AV, Wasterlain CG, Treiman DM, et al, editors: *Advances in neurology, Vol 34: Status epilepticus,* New York, 1883, Raven Press.
268. Knudsen FU: Plasma diazepam in infants after rectal administration in solution and by suppository, *Acta Paediatr Scand* 66:563, 1977.
269. Camfield PR, Camfield CS, Shapiro SH, et al: The first febrile seizure—antipyretic instruction plus either phenobarbital or placebo to prevent recurrence, *J Pediatr* 97:16, 1980.
270. Camfield PR: Effects of anticonvulsants on developing systems: section discussion. In Nelson KB and Ellenberg JH, editors: *Febrile seizures,* New York, 1981, Raven Press.
271. Farwell JR, et al: Phenobarbital for febrile seizures—effects on intelligence and on seizure recurrence, *N Engl J Med* 322:364, 1990.
272. Wallace SJ and Aldridge-Smith J: Successful prophylaxis against febrile convulsions with valproic acid or phenobarbitone, *Brit J Med* 280:353, 1980.
273. Wolf SM, Carr A, Daves DC, et al: The value of phenobarbital in the child who has had a single febrile seizure: a controlled prospective study, *Pediatrics* 59:378, 1977.
274. Faero L, Kastrup KW, Lykkegaard-Nielsen E, et al: Successful prophylaxis of febrile convulsions with phenobarbital, *Epilepsia* 13:279, 1972.
275. Livingston S, Paul LL, Pruce I, et al: Febrile convulsions: diagnosis, treatment, and prognosis, *Pediatr Ann* 8:133, 1979.
276. Millichap JG, Hernandez P, Zalez MR, et al: Studies in febrile seizures. IV. Evaluation of drug effects and development of potential new therapy (Pyrictal), *Neurology* 10:575, 1960.
277. Hirtz DG, et al: Survey on the management of febrile seizures, *Am J Dis Child* 140:909, 1986.
278. Campfield PR, Campfield CS, Tibbles AR: Carbamazepine does not prevent febrile seizures in phenobarbital failures, *Neurology* 32:388, 1982.
279. Mamelle N, et al: Prevention of recurrent febrile convulsions—a randomized therapeutic assay: sodium valproate, phenobarbital and placebo, *Neuropediatrics* 35:37, 1984.
280. Knudsen FU and Vestermark S: Prophylactic diazepam or phenobarbitone in febrile convulsions: a prospective, controlled study, *Arch Dis Child* 53:660, 1978.
281. Wilensky AJ, et al: Chlorazepate and phenobarbital as antiepileptic drugs: a double-blind study, *Neurology* 31:1271, 1981.
282. Franzoni E, Carboni C, Lambertini A: Rectal diazepam: a clinical and EEG study after a single dose in children, *Epilepsia* 24:35, 1981.
283. Knudsen FU: Recurrence risk after first febrile seizure and effect of short term diazepam prophylaxis, *Arch Dis Child* 60:1045, 1985.
284. Dianese G: Prophylactic diazepam in febrile convulsions, *Arch Dis Child* 54:244, 1979.
285. Lalande J and De Paillerets F: Prevention of hyperthermic convulsions: utility of discontinuous treatment with clonazepam. In Meinardi H and Rowan AJ, editors: *Advances in epileptology 1977. Psychology, pharmacotherapy and new diagnostic approaches,* Amsterdam, 1978, Swets and Zeitlinger.
286. Rosman NP, Colton T, Labazzo J, et al: A controlled trial of diazepam administered during febrile illnesses to prevent recurrence of febrile seizures, *N Engl J Med* 329:79, 1993.

## 57

Orthopedic Disorders

Paula C. Fink • James E. Dufort • Deborah L. Smith-Wright

Signs and Symptoms

PAULA C. FINK

ARTHRALGIA AND JOINT PAIN

Arthralgia is joint pain with or without signs or symptoms of inflammation. When arthritis accompanies joint pain, inflammation of the synovium, with redness, warmth, swelling, and pain are usually present.

Pathophysiology

The three major sources of arthralgias in children include inflammation of the joint, muscular pain, or bone pain. Arthritis can result from infection, autoimmune response, or trauma. The synovium reacts to these insults with an increase of synovial fluid and thickening of the tissues, which results in pain and a loss of mobility.[1] Injury to muscles that stabilize joints can result in arthralgia by putting stress on the joints when the injured muscles are in spasm. Bone pain resulting from a fracture, osteomyelitis, or malignancy may present as joint pain.

Differential Considerations

Many differential considerations of arthralgia can be grouped according to medical etiology (Table 57-1). A categorical discussion of possible diagnoses follows.

Traumatic. Traumatic injury is one of the most common causes of arthralgia. In the nonverbal child the injury is often unwitnessed and the precise site of the injury is unknown. However, the joint will usually be swollen, red, and tender to manipulation. The injury can be as benign as a contusion or muscle strain or as serious as a fracture or ruptured tendon.[2] A foreign body in the joint space can be a nidus for infection and is an emergent situation; if not removed it can result in a septic arthritis.

When the description of the mechanism of injury does not fit the severity of the injury, child abuse should be considered. Nonaccidental injury or child abuse should be investigated when epiphyseal or "bucket-handle" fractures of the tibia and fibula are found on x-ray examination (Fig. 57-1).[3] These fractures are usually caused by a twisting motion of the limb.

Chronic overuse of a limb can put low constant amounts of stress on a joint and result in acute and chronic disorders of that joint. Little League elbow and swimmer's knee are examples of the overuse syndromes that can cause joint pain.[4]

Inflammation/Infection. Osteomyelitis and septic arthritis are the two major infectious causes of arthralgia and are often misdiagnosed. The infection can occur in any joint or growing bone, and the site is usually swollen and red. The usual pathogen is bacterial, primarily *Staphylococcus aureus*. Mycobacterium, fungi, rubella, hepatitis, and varicella-zoster viral infections have also caused septic arthritis.[5] Hematogenous spread, usually from a distant site, is the common route of infection. Direct trauma to the site with a penetrating injury causing injection of a foreign body into a joint can result in infection. A child who is immunosuppressed or has sickle cell disease has an increased risk of septic arthritis.

Delay in treatment of osteomyelitis and septic arthritis can be catastrophic (see following sections on Osteomyelitis and Septic Arthritis). When suspected, the joint or bone should be aspirated for a gram stain and culture. Treatment should be delayed until samples are obtained.[6]

Toxic synovitis of the hip is a common benign cause of hip pain in children.[7] It is thought to be secondary to nonspecific inflammation and hypertrophy of the synovial membrane; it can be seen in children until skeletal maturity, with a peak age between 1 and 7 years of age. The pain may not localize in the hip but may be referred to the groin, trochanter region, or anterolateral thigh.[8] The misdiagnosis of a septic arthritis as toxic synovitis can result in the delay of treatment and possible joint damage. Therefore, toxic synovitis is a diagnosis of exclusion.

Chronic inflammation of the synovium is the pathologic description of juvenile rheumatoid arthritis (JRA). The disease is divided into distinct subgroups as shown in Table 57-2. The systemic onset of JRA includes symptoms of fever, rash, and organomegaly, as well as arthritic symp-

TABLE 57-1. Differential Diagnosis of Arthralgia

Condition	Joints involved	Diagnostic findings
Traumatic		History of injuries; swelling, tenderness, reduced movement, x-ray findings
Sprain	Monoarticular	
Fracture		
Overuse injuries		
Inflammation/infection		
Septic arthritis	Monoarticular	Fever, local findings of infection (warm, tender, swollen, red), x-ray evidence of effusion, joint aspiration
Osteomyelitis	Monoarticular	Fever, local findings of infection (warm, tender, swollen, red), x-ray possible lytic lesion; bone scan—increased uptake; aspiration of bone
Toxic synovitis	Hip	History of viral illness and limp; aspiration to rule out infection
Juvenile rheumatoid arthritis	Variable joints	(See Table 57-2)
Henoch-Schönlein purpura	Migratory polyarthritis	Swollen, red, tender joints with limited motion; purpuric rash over legs and trunk
Kawasaki disease	Migratory polyarthritis	History of fever, rash, conjunctivitis, stomatitis, lymphadenopathy, vasculitis of coronary arteries
Neoplasm	Variable joints	X-ray findings of bone involvement; abnormal CBC
Degenerative		
Slipped capital femoral epiphysis	Unilateral or bilateral hips	Limited range of hip motion, x-ray findings, obese child
Legg-Calvé-Perthes disease	Hip	Limited range of motion, x-ray findings, age 4-10 yr
Osgood-Schlatter disease	Knee	Pain over insertion of quadriceps tendon, x-ray findings
Congenital		
Hemophilia	Monoarticular	History of bleeding or trauma; swollen and tender joint
Functional		
Growing pains	Polyarticular	Tender but no edema or erythema

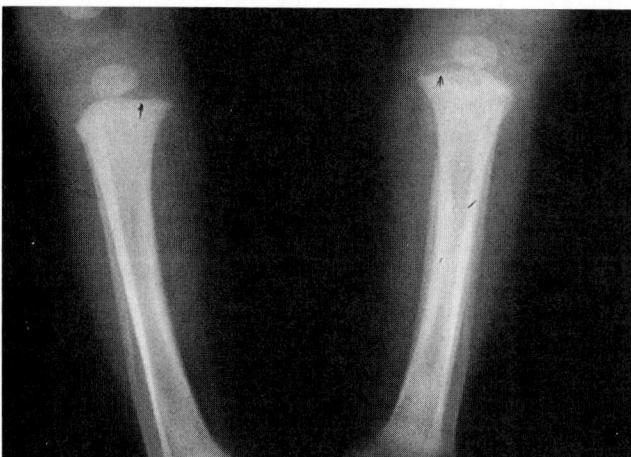

FIG. 57-1. Epiphyseal "bucket-handle" separation of fibia often associated with child abuse.

toms. Polyarticular and pauciarticular JRA have fewer systemic symptoms, but the arthritis is more severe. Polyarticular JRA involves smaller joints and can destroy the joints. Pauciarticular JRA usually involves larger joints and can be associated with iridocyclitis (see Chapter 51). Ar-

thritides, such as ankylosing spondylitis and spondyloarthropathy, can affect the sacroiliac joints and joints of the spine.

Other autoimmune disorders can result in inflammation of the joints. Inflammatory bowel disease can include transient bouts of arthritis that are usually easily controlled.[9] Uncommon in children, but worth noting, are Reiter syndrome and psoriatic arthritis. Reiter syndrome is typified by the triad of arthritis, conjunctivitis, and urethritis. Psoriatic arthritis may be difficult to control and is associated with psoriasis. Systemic lupus erythematosus (SLE) is a multisystem autoimmune disease that can include arthritis. The clinical picture of nephritis, anemia, polyserositis, and central nervous system involvement combined with abnormal laboratory results usually confirms the diagnosis of SLE. Poststreptococcal rheumatic fever includes symptoms of large joint arthritis, rash, carditis, and subcutaneous nodules as the major manifestations. Minor manifestations include fever, previous rheumatic fever, and arthralgia combined with positive laboratory levels of C-reactive protein (CRP) and a high erythrocyte sedimentation rate (ESR).[10]

Another group of autoimmune diseases can include arthralgia/arthritis as the major presenting symptom. This group includes the vasculitides of Henoch-Schönlein purpura (HSP), Kawasaki disease, and serum sickness. Ana-

TABLE 57-2. Classification of JRA

Type	Percent of all JRA	Clinical findings	Laboratory findings
Systemic	30	Rash, fever, polyarticular, involvement of liver, heart, spleen, and lymph nodes	Anemia, ESR elevated, leukocytosis, −rheumatoid factor, ±ANA
Pauciarticular	45	Usually lower extremity arthritis, less than five joints	+ANA, ESR elevated, + some HLA-B27
Polyarticular	25	Greater than four joints, resembles adult rheumatoid arthritis	ESR elevated, ±rheumatoid factor

phylactoid purpura or HSP can exhibit polyarticular arthritis a few days before the characteristic rash appears. The arthritis is never chronic and resolves spontaneously, whereas the associated nephritis, can become a chronic problem. Kawasaki disease is described as a vasculitic syndrome that includes fever, conjunctivitis, stomatitis, rash, lymphadenopathy, coronary artery vasculitis, desquamation of hands and feet, and arthritis.[11] The arthritis is self-limiting; however, coronary artery vasculitis may be chronic or fatal. Serum sickness, an immune complex reaction developing 6 to 21 days after exposure to a drug, can also include polyarthritis with joint effusions and pain (see Chapter 46).

Neoplasm. Osteogenic sarcoma, caused by the infiltration of malignant cells into the periosteum of the bones around the joint, may present as joint pain. The peak incidence is in rapidly growing children, usually in their teenage years. The most common sites are the distal femur and proximal tibia. Vague migratory musculoskeletal pain may be the first sign of leukemia so the working diagnosis of rheumatoid arthritis may mistakenly be given to a child with leukemia. Osteochondrosis dissecans and osteoid osteoma are benign disorders of the bone that may become symptomatic with joint pain.

Degenerative. Slipped capital femoral epiphysis (SCFE), a displacement of the femoral head from the femoral neck through the growth plate, can present as knee or hip pain. This may be an acute slip secondary to severe trauma or a gradual slip from a large shear force exerted over an extended period of time. The majority of these cases are chronic, gradual displacements and most are due to the chronic stress of excess weight on the hip joint. Eighty-eight percent of patients with SCFE are obese.[11]

Knee pain originating at the anterior tibial tuberosity can be caused by Osgood-Schlatter disease. This disease, the result of strenuous physical activity, can result in microtrauma to the insertion of the quadriceps tendon. It is commonly found in boys during the rapid growth of adolescence. Chondromalacia of the patella, damage to the knee's articular cartilage by abnormal mechanical forces on the knee, may be another cause of knee pain. The pain is usually worse after the knee has been resting and is suddenly flexed; it then lessens after the patient has walked for a short distance. Chondromalacia is most commonly found in teenage girls.[12]

Congenital. Hemophilia, sickle cell disease, and Gaucher disease are a few congenital diseases that can cause

joint pain. Trauma to the joints of a hemophiliac can result in hemarthroses. Pain crises with sickle cell disease may produce joint pain. Gaucher disease can cause bone pain and produce weak bones, allowing fractures at the neck of the femur. Limb length discrepancy and undetected scoliosis may cause hip pain during late adolescence.

Vascular. Legg-Calvé-Perthes disease (LCPD), avascular necrosis of the femoral head, can present as knee or hip pain. Although there is no known cause of LCPD, it has been noted that children with LCPD have a delayed bone age and are primarily boys.[13] Avascular necrosis can also result from sickle cell disease.

Functional. Growing pains, an annoying ache in the muscles of the thighs and legs, may present with knee or hip pain. The pain sometimes localizes to the area behind the knees. Multiple etiologies have been proposed ranging from environmental to psychological factors; however, it is the clinician's duty to rule out all treatable diagnoses.[14] Adolescents are prone to hysterical transference of pain and may come to the emergency department with acute pain.[15] Psychogenic pain is very real and must be dealt with by finding the inciting cause.

Iatrogenic. Chronic cortisone treatment for JRA or asthma may produce osteoporosis and vertebral compression fractures that can cause hip pain. Cortisone-induced necrosis of the femoral head can result in an identical presentation as LCPD. Intraarticular injections of cortisone for joint pain (usually in athletes) can produce a severe arthropathy.

Diagnostic Work-Up

A complete medical history is necessary to determine the general well-being of the child and is the primary diagnostic tool of the physician. The history of the joint pain can be determined, using the following questions:

- How long has the patient had the pain?
- When did it start?
- Was trauma thought to be the cause of the pain and, if so, what was the exact nature of the trauma?
- How many joints are involved and is the pain migratory, affecting multiple joints?
- Is the pain intermittent or continuous; is it localized or generalized?
- Is the character of the pain sharp, dull, or burning?
- Does the child refuse to use the joint or is it only mildly painful?

• How does the pain relate to the strength of the child; is it worse when the child is fatigued or does it subside when the child has been active?

The child's medical history should be carefully examined for trauma or changes in activity. The family history must also be examined for any congenital diseases that may present with joint pain.

The physical examination should be complete with special attention to the tender joint but general enough to prevent missing symptoms of systemic illnesses. If the hip, knee, or ankle is the joint involved, the gait should be observed carefully concentrating on the function of the problem joint.

The joint examination should include range of motion, laxity, stiffness, and guarding. The passive joint motion angle and length of the limb with the pain should be measured and compared with the normal side. Signs of fluid in the knee joint should be sought. The patella should track smoothly during the full range of motion of the knee. Crepitus of the knee may represent chondromalacia.[12,13] Contiguous joints should be examined; hip disease may present with knee pain. The circumference of the muscle masses of the limbs should be measured around involved joints, looking for atrophy of the muscles. A full neurologic examination of muscle function and strength should be done, comparing the normal and abnormal side.

Ancillary Data

Laboratory and x-ray studies should reflect the medical history and physical examination to support the diagnosis of joint pain. A CBC, differential, and ESR are usually necessary but may not be diagnostic in defining the etiology of the arthralgia. The ESR can often be used to follow the resolution of the inflammation of an arthritis. Laboratory studies specific to JRA, such as antinuclear antibodies and rheumatoid factors, are not easily determined in the acute setting but may aid in the diagnosis of the arthralgia. A urinalysis may be useful in the evaluation of possible SLE or HSP. When there is a concern of a septic arthritis, aspiration of the joint is necessary to obtain the cell count, differential, protein, and glucose levels, and bacterial and viral cultures of the synovial fluid. Specific laboratory tests, such as a factor VII level or liver function test, should be obtained if indicated by the presenting symptoms.

Radiologic studies are almost always indicated in the evaluation of joint pain. In the evaluation of hip pain, attention to the space between the femoral head and the acetabulum should be made; it may show asymmetry indicative of fluid in the joint space and infection. Plain x-ray films of the limb in question can also show radiolucencies or cortical changes that can be caused by neoplasm. The bone scan has been helpful in identifying inflammation when routine x-ray films are normal. It shows increased or decreased metabolic activity that can help in the diagnosis of neoplasm, infection, and avascular disorders.[16] Magnetic resonance imaging (MRI) scanning is especially helpful in the knee examination. Both the computed tomography (CT) and MRI scanning are usually not easily available in the emergency department but can be helpful in a follow-up evaluation.[17]

Therapeutic Trial

Many specific etiologies and treatments of arthralgia are discussed in other sections of this chapter. Toxic synovitis of the hip and JRA are treated with rest and analgesics for severe discomfort. The clinical response to aspirin may be useful in confirming the diagnosis of JRA. Referral to a pediatric rheumatologist is appropriate for a child with suspected JRA or unresolving arthralgia.

BACK PAIN

Back pain is a common complaint in the general population with up to 70% to 80% of adults complaining of low back pain at some time in their lives.[18] However, in children this accounts for less than 2% of all referrals to pediatric orthopedic surgeons.[19] Back pain in children may be indicative of a significant illness or injury. The emergency physician should not be fooled by the commonality of back pain in adults and assume that overuse or strain is the cause of a child's complaint of back pain. Minimal back pain in children may be the result of a major illness.

Pathophysiology

Back pain can originate from injury or inflammation of muscle, nerve, or bony tissue. Inflammation of the kidney as in pyelonephritis may present as back pain. Direct trauma to the back muscles can result in contusions and hematomas causing acute back pain. Rarely, a child complains of postexercise pain, but in this era of competitive sports starting at an early age, overuse injuries can result from the chronic stress of sports practice.[20] Nerve injury or compression is often the cause of severe pain. Back pain associated with neurologic findings can be the result of a herniated or ruptured disk.[21] Nerve impingement from spondylolysis (fracture of the pars interarticularis) or spondylolisthesis (the forward slipping of a vertebra on the one below) can cause lower back pain.[22] Inflammation of the spine, as found in diskitis or vertebral osteomyelitis, can cause irritation of the nerves and back pain.

Differential Considerations (Table 57-3)

Neurologic. Herniation of the nucleus pulposus and rupture of the intervertebral disk are rare but not unknown in children. There is usually an underlying malformation of the vertebral column in the lumbar sacral region, like spina bifida, allowing for herniation in children.[23] When back pain is accompanied by sciatica, decreased spine mobility, or scoliosis, then a herniated intervertebral disk is a possible diagnosis. Because this is so rare, more common causes of back pain with neurological findings like infection, spondylolysis, and tumor should be considered first.

Traumatic. Only large forces can injure the back (see Chapter 22). Chronic stress and injury to the back resulting in back pain is less frequent in children than in adults. Children are very active and usually never experience muscle pain from overexertion. However, with the recent focus on competitive sports and intense training, more children are presenting with back pain that results from overuse.[20] Gymnastics, with frequent flexion and extension stunts, and football, with increased pressure loads on the shoulders and back, can produce back pain. Modifying the level of activity will allow the pain to resolve.

TABLE 57-3. Differential Diagnosis of Back Pain

Condition	Diagnostic findings	Ancillary data
Neurologic		
Ruptured/herniated disk	Severe back pain, motor deficit, weakness, foot drop, sensory deficit	X-ray studies: disk space asymmetries; CT/MRI scans: showing ruptured/ herniation
Traumatic		
Vertebral fracture	Severe point tenderness, sensory or motor deficit dependent on area injured	X-ray studies: disk space asymmetries and fracture visualized; motor deficits; CT/MRI scans: showing fracture
Overuse injuries	Muscle tenderness, pain relieved with rest	X-ray studies: usually normal
Spondylolysis/spondylolisthesis	Gait abnormalities, lumbar lordosis, pain relieved with rest	X-ray studies: often a slip of L5 over S1, congenital sacral deficit; bone scan to show acute uptake
Infection/inflammation		
Intervertebral diskitis	Fever, irritability, back and hip pain, change in gait, pain with straight-leg raising	Elevated ESR; x-ray studies: narrowing of disk space
Vertebral osteomyelitis	Fever, irritability for weeks, point tenderness	Elevated ESR and WBC; x-ray studies: narrowing of disk space or collapse of vertebrae
Collagen vascular diseases (ankylosing spondylitis)	Usually adolescence, limited range of motion	+ HLA B27; + RF; elevated ESR and WBC; x-ray studies: nonspecific
Neoplasm		
Variety of primary benign and malignant and secondary metastatic tumors	Initially diffuse complaints over a few weeks escalating to severe pain and neurologic findings	Positive blood tests dependent on the type of neoplasm; x-ray studies: may show lytic lesions or masses; MRI/CT scans: helpful
Degenerative		
Scheuermann disease	Back pain, thoracic kyphosis, lumbar lordosis	X-ray studies: lateral spine, vertebral end plate irregularities, wedging of vertebral bodies
Scoliosis	Back pain, neurologic findings	X-ray studies: scoliosis

A stress fracture of the pars interarticularis, spondylolysis is a cause of back pain in active children from 10 years of age to adolescence. This is often accompanied by spondylolisthesis, the forward slipping of a vertebra on the one below it. Severe spondylolisthesis with listhesis of >30% may require surgical fusion to prevent future back pain and limitation of activities (Fig. 57-2).[24] The pain is usually found in the lumbosacral spine without neurologic findings. As with overuse injuries, aggressive training for gymnastics, football, rowing, and dance can result in these injuries. The diagnosis can be made with radiographic studies of the spine.[22]

Infection/Inflammation. Intervertebral diskitis, both sterile and infectious, is an etiology of back pain in children younger than 10 years of age. It is usually bacterial and caused by hematogenous spread. Children's symptoms include complaints of back pain and pain with walking, weeks of irritability, intermittent fever, and malaise. Cultures from biopsies are positive 25% of the time with *Staphylococcus aureus*.[25]

Presenting with a similar set of symptoms, vertebral osteomyelitis usually occurs in children over 8 years of age. Caused by hematogenous spread of bacteria, vertebral osteomyelitis produces complaints of a dull, constant back pain and a history of 3 to 4 months of fevers and lethargy. Eighty percent of these cases are caused by *S. aureus*, confirmed by culture of a bone specimen.[26]

Paravertebral abscesses, though rare, usually present as back pain and are often caused by *S. aureus*. They may be difficult to diagnosis and delay in surgical drainage and antibiotics can result in bone damage and subsequent nerve root damage.[27]

Inflammatory disorders of the collagen vascular diseases may present as back or neck pain. Children with JRA often complain of cervical pain from inflammation of the cervical vertebral joints. Ankylosing spondylitis can include lower back pain in the adolescent age.[28]

Pyelonephritis can cause inflammation of the kidney and costovertebral angle pain that may not be accompanied by the other symptoms of fever, nausea, or dysuria. Checking

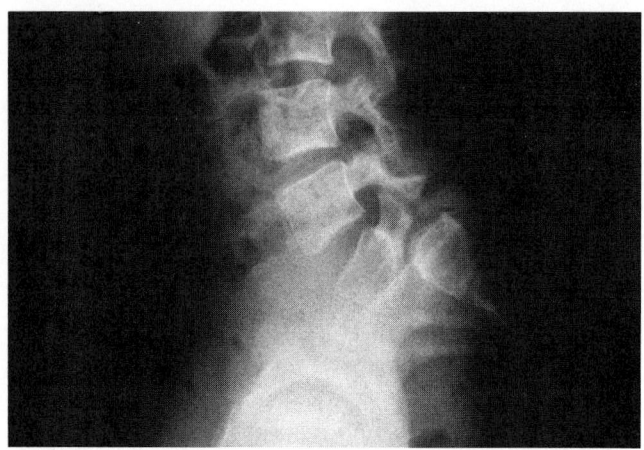

FIG. 57-2. Spondylolysis associated with a fracture of the pars interarticularis.

a urinalysis will rule out this common cause of back pain.

Neoplasm. Neoplasm is rare as a cause of back pain. Tumors can be either primary or, more commonly, metastatic. Not all tumors causing back pain are malignant. Lipomas, neurofibromas, teratomas, and hemangiomas are a few benign tumors that may be excised. Malignant spinal cord tumors are rare in children and may be the direct extension of paravertebral tumors, like gliomas; or astrocytomas. Ependymomas can originate in the cauda equina and cause lower back pain.[23]

Back pain localized to a specific vertebra may be the result of neoplasms of the vertebral column. These can be either benign or malignant, primary or metastatic. Primary lesions include giant cell tumor, aneurysmal bone cyst, osteoid osteoma, or eosinophilic granuloma. Any of the neoplasms that metastasize to the bone can involve the vertebral column and cause back pain. Back pain is a common symptom of leukemia.

Degenerative. Degenerative disorders of the vertebral column, like osteoarthritis, are major causes of back pain in adults but rare in young children. Studies have shown that about 30% of adolescents, ages 11 to 17, have complained of low back pain, and approximately 7% of those seek medical attention.[18] Early signs of disk degeneration have been found with MRI in adolescents with low back pain and many of those were associated with Scheuermann-type changes.[29] Scheuermann disease, juvenile kyphosis, is one of the few degenerative causes of back pain in children. Described by Scheuermann in 1964, it is the epiphyseal aseptic necrosis of the vertebral bodies producing a thoracic kyphosis. Currently, there is no known cause of necrosis[28] but half of affected children complain of thoracic pain, and the majority of children are girls in the teenage years.[23]

Idiopathic scoliosis in the adolescent years should never be painful, and other etiologies of the pain should be sought. However, scoliosis, resulting in a mechanical derangement of the spine, can cause degenerative changes of the vertebral bodies and the ribs. Nerve impingement and muscle spasm may produce disabling pain. Childhood scoliosis may also be the cause of future back pain or decreased pulmonary function.[30]

Functional. It is unusual for a child to exhibit stress with physical complaints; back pain without a physiologic etiology should not be ignored.[28] Children do observe their adult role models and often see the reaction that back pain elicits. The diagnosis of conversion reaction should be one of exclusion for a child with back pain, but it may be the correct diagnosis.[31]

Iatrogenic. Chronic steroid treatment for illness, such as in JRA or severe asthma, may produce osteoporosis and vertebral body compression fractures. A child with a chronic disease complaining of back pain should be closely evaluated.

Diagnostic Work-Up

A complete medical history of the child is necessary to determine the general health of the child, as well as the history of the back pain. Timing and mode of onset should be determined by the following questions:

- How long has the child had the back pain and when did it start?
- Was trauma thought to be the cause of the pain and, if so, what was the exact nature of the trauma?
- Has there been a change in activity or has the child started a new sport?
- Is the pain migratory, affecting the back and other joints of the body?
- Is the pain radiating to the arms and legs?
- Is the pain intermittent or continuous, is it localized or generalized?
- What is the character of the pain: sharp, dull, or burning?
- Does the child refuse to walk or is walking only mildly painful?
- How does the pain relate to the strength of the child: is it worse when the child is fatigued, or does it subside when the child has been active?
- Is the discomfort relieved with pain relievers like aspirin?

The child's medical history should be carefully examined, as well as the family history, for any congenital diseases that may present with back pain (e.g., are there any relatives with chronic back pain and when did their pain manifest itself?).

The physical examination should be complete with special attention to the back but general enough to prevent missing the symptoms of systemic illnesses. The gait should be observed carefully concentrating on the different phases, swing and stance (see following section on Limp). Special attention should be given to the hips, looking for a tilt or lurch of the pelvis. The child should be asked to squat and stand on the toes to exhibit leg and back strength.

The back examination should begin with an overview of the back from top to bottom. The child's general posture should be evaluated. The cervical region should be noted for torticollis, tilt, or list. Lumbar lordosis, thoracic kyphosis, list, and scoliosis should be excluded. The skin should be observed for a sacral dimple or hair patch that may indicate spina bifida occulta. The café-au-lait spots of neurofibromatosis should be noted if present. The child should be asked to bend over to check for the asymmetries of scoliosis and to observe the fluidity of motion. Direct palpation of the spine is necessary to determine point tenderness and search for masses.[19]

A full neurologic examination should be done, looking for any denervation of muscle groups, asymmetry of reflexes, or sensory loss. Joint-motion angle and leg length should be measured on each side. Limb circumference should be measured, looking for atrophy of the muscles.

Ancillary Data. Laboratory and x-ray studies should be obtained based on the medical history and physical examination in an effort to support the possible diagnoses of back pain. CBC, differential, and ESR are usually necessary. Often the ESR can be used to follow the resolution of the inflammation of arthritis or osteomyelitis. Laboratory studies specific to collagen vascular diseases, such as antinuclear antibodies (ANA), HLA B27, and rheumatoid factors, are not easily determined in the acute setting but may aid in diagnosis.[32] When there is any concern of a vertebral osteomyelitis or diskitis, an aspiration or biopsy of the area in question is necessary to obtain white blood cell count, differential, protein, glucose levels, and cultures for bacterial and viral pathogens.[33]

X-ray studies are almost always indicated in the evaluation of back pain. Anteroposterior and lateral views of the back can show disk-space abnormalities, asymmetry of the vertebra, and spondylolysis. The bone scan is helpful in showing inflammation secondary to neoplasm, infection, or spondylolithesis.[34] It will show increased or decreased metabolic activity that can help in the diagnosis of neoplasm, infection, and avascular disorders.

The MRI scan is helpful as the definitive back examination tool.[35]

Therapeutic Trial

Specific etiologies of back pain are covered elsewhere (see Chapter 22). Local treatment, such as heat, cold, and the response to antiinflammatories, may be diagnostic. Collagen vascular diseases are not covered in detail; treatment is usually rest, analgesics for pain, and often antiinflammatory drugs.

LIMP

Limp is defined as an abnormality of gait. A limp is never normal. A child with acute onset of a limp will often be brought into the emergency department for evaluation, providing a diagnostic challenge for the physician. The range of etiologies of a limp can run from a benign contusion, a malfitted shoe, or a malignant neoplasm.

Pathophysiology

Normal gait is the coordinated action of the entire lower extremity. It can be divided into two phases, the swing and the stance. When one segment of the leg is dysfunctional because of pain, weakness, congenital malformation, or denervated muscle, a limp results.[36]

Trunk and Pelvis. Irritation to the abdominal musculature secondary to appendicitis or pelvic inflammatory disease can cause an irregular gait. This stooped gait abnormality easily indicates that its etiology is in the abdomen. Most gait disorders are not so easily identified.

The antalgic limp is caused by a child trying to avoid weight bearing on a painful limb by shortening the stance phase on the painful extremity.[37] Any cause of lower extremity pain (contusion to the ankle, fractured tibia, or osteogenic sarcoma) can result in an antalgic limp. Children with diskitis or vertebral osteomyelitis can have an antalgic gait to avoid jarring the spine.

Weakness in the gluteus medius muscle may result in a lurching Trendelenburg gait. In this limp, the gluteus medius, which usually stabilizes the hip, is weak and the child's trunk dips to the weak side during the swing phase to minimize the work of that extremity. The child then shifts the weight back to the strong side during the stance phase to minimize the pain producing a dip to the opposite side. A test for this can be performed by having the child stand on one leg and then the other. The test is positive for gluteal weakness if the pelvis tilts to the contralateral side of the weight bearing leg. Children with LCPD or SCFE can have a Trendelenburg gait resulting from gluteus medius pain. A waddling gait will result in a child with bilateral congenital hip dislocation because of weak bilateral gluteus medius muscles.[37]

Weakness in the gluteus maximus secondary to Duchenne muscular dystrophy or spinal vascular atrophy produces a unique gait. The child hyperextends the trunk and pelvis to maintain the center of gravity behind the pelvis and remain erect, producing a gait with the back held in lordotic extension.[36]

Knee. Limitation of the knee's normal 70 degrees of flexion can result in a limp. A child with limited flexion will usually elevate the pelvis and swing the leg around the opposite foot. A weak quadriceps femoralis will inhibit proper lifting of the knee despite a near normal gait. However, the knee will hyperextend and lock at the end of the stance phase of the gait and the child will vault over the extremity.[36]

Foot and Ankle. The push off from the stance phase of the gait depends on the 20 degrees of plantar flexion and 10 degrees of dorsiflexion. Lack of dorsiflexion secondary to neurologic illness, such as Charcot-Marie-Tooth disease or Friedreich ataxia, produces a foot drop and a steppage gait.[36] The lack of dorsiflexion prevents the normal deceleration before heel strike, and foot-slap develops. Spastic contraction of the gastrocnemius muscle because of cerebral palsy can result in a toe-walking gait.

Differential Considerations

Many differential considerations can be grouped according to the age of common occurrence, while others occur throughout childhood (Table 57-4). A categoric discussion of possible diagnoses follows (Table 57-5).

Traumatic. In the nonverbal child, traumatic injury is one of the most common causes of limp. The injury was often unwitnessed, and the precise site of the injury is unknown. If witnessed, the force of the accident is thought to be too trivial to have caused any significant damage. Toddler's fractures are an example of this phenomenon (Fig. 57-3). They occur with mild trauma and are usually a nondisplaced fracture of the diaphysis of the tibia.[38] It is

TABLE 57-4. Differential Diagnosis of Limp by Age

1-3 yr	4-10 yr	10-16 yr	Not age-specific
Congenital hip dislocation	Toxic synovitis	Spondylolysis	Septic arthritis
Muscular dystrophy	Legg-Calvé-Perthes disease	Slipped capital femoral epiphysis	Neoplasms
Congenital scoliosis	Leg length discrepancies	Osgood-Schlatter disease	Osteomyelitis
Juvenile rheumatoid arthritis	Rickets	Chondromalacia	
Cerebral palsy			
Toddler's fracture			
Osteomyelitis			
Diskitis			

thought that this fracture is common because the bone is still a woven matrix and has not yet ossified.

Less serious causes of limping in the nonverbal child include splinters and foreign bodies in the foot. Poorly fitted shoes can also cause a limp, especially if the child's feet are different sizes.[37]

In verbal children and adolescents, the history of traumatic injury is more easily ascertained. Nondisplaced fractures or avulsion fractures may be minimally painful and allow the child to walk with a limp. Stress fractures may also be seen in children participating in sports where there is repetitive loading and use of their legs. Other traumatic causes of limp in young children include contusions or muscle strains. Ankle sprains, in general, do not occur in children; avulsion fracture of the preosseous cartilage is the probable injury. Possible sprains of the ankle should be closely evaluated with x-ray studies. Knee injuries and strains are common in adolescence and may cause a limp.

Infection/Inflammation. Osteomyelitis and septic arthritis are two major causes of limp that are often misdiagnosed; delay in treatment can result in permanent damage. When the site is swollen and red, there is little problem in the correct diagnosis of septic arthritis or osteomyelitis, but often a limp is the only clue. The site of infection may be any joint or growing bone. The spine and pelvis should be evaluated for possible septic diskitis and sacroiliac septic arthritis. Tuberculosis of the bone and joint is uncommon in the United States; however, the disease has not been eradicated, and it should be considered in the case of osteomyelitis or septic arthritis without a bacterial etiology.[39]

Toxic synovitis of the hip is a common benign cause of limp and hip pain in children. Thought to be secondary to nonspecific inflammation and hypertrophy of the synovial membrane, it can be seen in children before skeletal maturity. The pain may not localize in the hip but may be referred to the groin, trochanter region, or the anterolateral thigh. The misdiagnosis of an infectious arthritis as toxic synovitis can result in delay of treatment and possible joint damage. Therefore, toxic synovitis is a diagnosis of exclusion and the treatment is observation and pain relief.[40]

The primary autoimmune cause of inflammation that can produce a limp in a child is rheumatologic. New onset of JRA, especially pauciarticular arthritis, can present with a single knee or ankle affected. Careful visual examination looking for iridocyclitis, which is associated with JRA, can assist in the diagnosis of JRA (see Chapter 46).[41]

Other causes to consider in a child with a limp include appendicitis, pelvic inflammatory disease, and Guillain-Barré syndrome. In these cases, the limp would usually not be an isolated symptom but part of a constellation of symptoms.

Neoplasm. Osteogenic sarcoma can present as a new onset limp or as limb pain. The peak incidence is in rapidly growing children, usually in their teenage years. The most common sites are the distal femur and proximal tibia. There is often a history of trauma before the diagnosis; however, it is thought that this is coincidence.[42] Ewing sarcoma presents usually at the same age of osteogenic sarcoma and can start in the long bones of the leg. Vague migratory bone and joint pain may be the first signs of leukemia. It may manifest in a limp or refusal to walk. Malignancies that have spread to the bone marrow can produce bone pain.

Neuroblastoma of the sympathetic paraspinus chain can produce a limp that may progress into nerve impingement and paraplegia.[43] Osteochondromas and osteoid osteoma are benign tumors of the bone and may become symptomatic with limb pain or a limp.

Degenerative. SCFE is a displacement of the femoral head from the femoral neck through the growth plate (Fig. 57-4). This may be an acute slip secondary to severe trauma or a gradual slip from a large shear force exerted over an extended period of time. The majority of these cases are chronic, gradual displacements. Since 88% of the patients with SCFE are obese, it is thought that the chronic stress of excess weight on the hip results in this displacement.[40] The hip pain that accompanies SCFE is usually localized to the anterior or lateral groin or the knee.[44]

Limp resulting from pain at the anterior tibial tuberosity could be caused by Osgood-Schlatter disease because microtrauma to the insertion of the quadriceps tendon occurs. Usually found in boys during rapid adolescent growth, it is aggravated by strenuous physical activity.[45]

Chondromalacia patella may be another cause of knee pain in the region of the patella, resulting in a limp. Damage to the knee's articular cartilage by abnormal mechanical forces on the knee produces chondromalacia. The pain usually is worse after the knee has been resting and is suddenly flexed; the pain lessens after the patient has walked for a short distance.[46]

TABLE 57-5. Differential Diagnosis of Limp

Condition	Diagnostic findings	Ancillary data
Traumatic		
Sprains/strains	History of trauma, tenderness, erythema, restricted range of motion	X-ray studies: no fracture, soft tissue injury
Fracture	History of trauma, tenderness, erythema, edema, restricted range of motion	X-ray studies: positive/negative for fracture; if negative, then serial x-ray films, bone scan, or CT/MRI scans
Foreign body/splinter in foot	Acute onset, site of injury	X-ray studies: needed at times to localize foreign body
Infection/inflammation		
Osteomyelitis	Fever, local tenderness, edema, monoarticular	ESR/WBC elevated; x-ray studies: increased fluid or lytic lesion in bone scan positive; bone/joint aspirate positive for bacteria
Arthritis, bacterial	Febrile, monoarticular, local edema and erythema	X-ray studies: effusion; elevated WBC and ESR, positive bacteria on joint aspiration, positive bone scan
Toxic synovitis of hip	Preceding viral illness, limited range of motion	WBC positive, ESR variable; x-ray studies: positive/negative effusion; aspirate if necessary
Juvenile rheumatoid arthritis	See Table 57-2	WBC elevated
Appendicitis	Abdominal symptoms, stooped over gait, fever	
Pelvic inflammatory disease	Abdominal, pelvic symptoms	
Neoplasm		
Osteogenic or Ewing sarcoma	Painful limb	X-ray studies: lytic or cortical lesions
Metastatic involvement of bone marrow	Migratory pain	X-ray studies: lytic lesions, abnormal blood tests
Degenerative		
Slipped capital femoral epiphysis	Acute or chronic pain, obese child, pain in anterior groin	X-ray studies: slipped femoral head
Osgood-Schlatter disease	Tender over anterior tibia, active child	X-ray studies: usually normal may show elevation of tibial tuberosity
Chondromalacia of patella	Tender over knee, resolves with rest	X-ray studies: normal
Congenital		
Hemophilia	Variable history of trauma, history of bleeding and bruising	Blood factor tests
Sickle cell anemia	Bone pain diffuse	Sickle screen
Scoliosis	Limp in adolescents after exercise	X-ray studies: scoliosis
Leg length discrepancy	Chronic limp	Physical findings
Vascular		
Legg-Calvé-Perthes disease	Tender hip, chronic pain	X-ray studies: bulging capsule, bone scan positive uptake

Congenital. Hemophilia, sickle cell disease, and Gaucher disease are a few of the congenital diseases that can cause leg pain, resulting in a limp. Trauma to the legs of a hemophiliac can result in hemarthrosis or severe contusions. Pain crises of sickle cell disease also cause leg pain. Gaucher disease can cause bone pain and produce weak bones, allowing fractures at the neck of the femur. Congenital hip dislocation left untreated can produce a Trendelenburg limping gait.[35] Limb length discrepancy may cause a limp, but usually this is not a painful limp until adolescence, when it is associated with back pain. Undetected scoliosis may result in a limp during late adolescence.

Vascular. Avascular necrosis of the femoral head, Legg-Calvé-Perthes disease (LCPD), can present as knee pain or a limp (Fig. 57-5). The patient will have an antalgic gait with limited hip motion. Although it has been noted that patients with LCPD have a delayed bone age and are

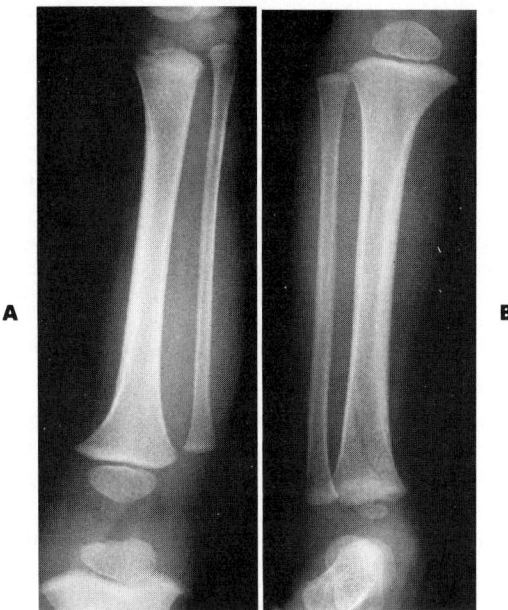

FIG. 57-3. Toddler's fracture. Nondisplaced fracture of the diaphysis of the tibia. Often this is only seen on an x-ray view of the extremity.

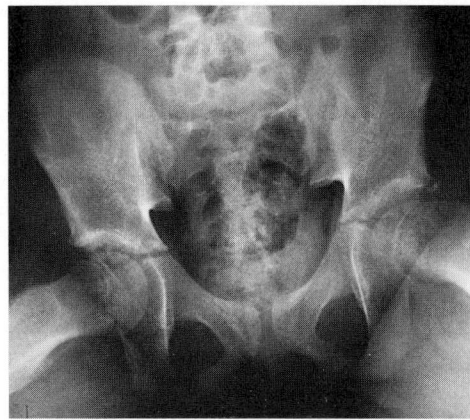

FIG. 57-4. Slipped capital femoral epiphysis. Femoral head is displaced from the femoral neck through the growth plate.

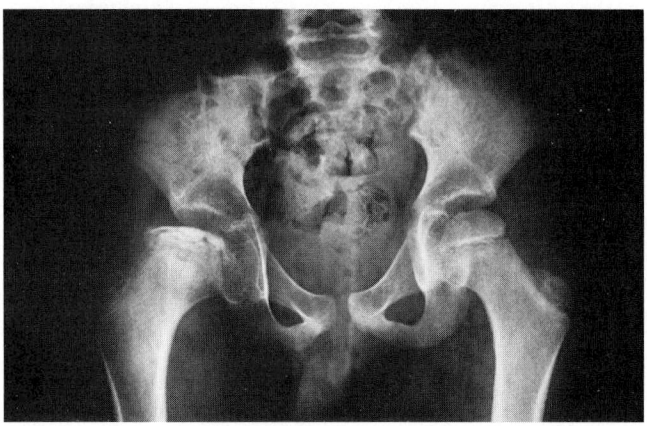

FIG. 57-5. Legg-Calvé-Perthes disease. Avascular necrosis of the femoral head.

primarily boys, there is no known cause. Avascular necrosis can also result from sickle cell disease[40] (Table 57-6).

Nutritional. Limp and leg pain may be the presenting symptoms of children with rickets secondary to vitamin D deficiency. These children will also have the concomitant symptoms of bowing of the legs and a large head.[47] Scurvy, vitamin C deficiency, and hypervitaminosis A have also presented with limp.

Functional. A limp may not be the result of a physical problem but of a psychologic problem, especially in adolescents. Psychogenic pain can cause a limp and must be dealt with by finding the inciting cause.[48,49] Young children may exhibit limps for attention, especially if they have an adult role model with a limp.

Iatrogenic. Cortisone-induced necrosis of the femoral head can result in a case similar to LCPD. Injections of vaccines can produce aseptic abscess in muscle tissue and leg pain leading to a limp in a toddler.

Diagnostic Work-Up

A complete medical history of the child is necessary to determine the general health status of the child and if there have been any recent illnesses. The history of the limp should be determined by the following questions:

- How long has the patient had it? When did it start?
- Was there recent trauma and, if so, what was the exact nature of that trauma?
- Is pain associated with the limp? If so, is the pain intermittent or continuous, is it localized or generalized?
- Is the character of the pain sharp, dull, or burning?
- Does the child refuse to walk or is the pain a mild nuisance?
- How does the limp relate to the strength of the child? Is it worse when the child is fatigued or is it better after use?

The child's medical history should be carefully examined. The family history must be closely examined for any congenital diseases that may produce a limp as a primary symptom.

The physical examination is the next most important phase of the evaluation. A full set of vital signs should be obtained. The gait should be observed carefully, concentrating on the separate phases of stance and swing. Then the components of the leg, trunk, pelvis, knees, and feet should be observed separately during the full gait. Particular attention to the smoothness of motion or the lack of flowing motion should be made. Listening to the foot strike may be helpful: the slapping foot of a foot drop; the uneven sound of a heavy, nonpainful foot strike; or the soft strike of the painful leg in an atalgic gait. The child should be observed both barefoot and wearing shoes. The shoes the child has been wearing should be closely examined for worn areas and scrapes, indicating the initial foot strike and if the foot is being dragged across the floor during the stride. The shoes should be examined on the child to check the fit.[37]

A complete systematic physical examination should follow. The examination should be generalized to prevent

TABLE 57-6. Differential Diagnosis of Painful Hip

	Toxic synovitis	Legg-Calvé-Perthes disease	Septic arthritis	Slipped capital femoral epiphysis
Age	2-12 yr	4-10 yr	Any age	8-16 yr
Sex	3:2	5:1	1:1	2:1
Trauma	+/−	+/−	+/−	+/−
Weight	Normal	Low	Normal	High
Fever	Normal	Normal	+	+
X-ray studies	−	+	+	+
WBC	Normal	Normal	Elevated	Normal
ESR	Normal	Normal	Elevated	Normal
Bone scan	+	+	+	+

+, Present/positive; −, absent/normal.

missing symptoms of systemic illness. The joint examination should check the range of motion, laxity, stiffness, and guarding. Joint angle and leg length of the abnormal limb should be measured and compared with the normal side. Crepitus of the knee should be noted; it could represent chondromalacia. The knee should be palpated for signs of fluid; the track of the patella normally moves smoothly during full range of motion of the knee.[46] Hip disease may present as knee pain. The circumference of the thigh and calf should determine if atrophy is present. A full neurologic examination of muscle function and strength should compare the normal with the abnormal side.

Ancillary Data

Laboratory and x-ray studies should only supplement the medical history and physical examination in the diagnosis of the limp. A CBC, differential, and ESR are usually necessary but do not provide a definitive diagnosis. When there is a concern of a septic joint, aspiration is necessary obtaining the cell count, differential, protein, and glucose levels, and cultures for bacterial and viral pathogens. Specific laboratory tests, like factor VIII level or liver function tests, can be indicated by the symptoms presented. If Guillain-Barré syndrome is suspected, evaluation of the cerebrospinal fluid (CSF) is essential.

X-ray studies are almost always indicated in the evaluation of limp, but rarely are they helpful. Only when the limp is obviously caused by malfitted shoes or a splinter in the foot, are x-rays not used. The area to examine by x-ray study requires careful thought, since the pain of the limp may be referred to an unaffected site. Routine examination of a large area will prevent missing the injured area. Close attention to the space between the femoral head and the acetabulum can show fluid suggestive of an infection. Plain x-ray films of the limb with the limp can also show radiolucencies or cortical changes that could be caused by neoplasm. The bone scan has been helpful in locating the source of pain. It will show increased or decreased metabolic activity that can help in the diagnosis of neoplasm, infection, and avascular disorders. CT scans with specific bone windows may aid in the diagnosis. MRI scans are being used with increased frequency in diagnosis of nervous system disorders, but it may also be useful in ortho-

pedic disorders. It is especially helpful in the knee and back examination. Both the CT and MRI scans are not easily used in the emergency department but can be used in a follow-up evaluation.[50]

Therapeutic Trial

Limp should be treated according to its specific etiology. The acute treatment for toxic synovitis and JRA is analgesics for pain and rest. The response to antiinflammatory drugs may be useful in diagnosis.

Diagnostic Entities

JAMES E. DUFORT ● DEBORAH L. SMITH-WRIGHT

OSTEOMYELITIS

Osteomyelitis is an infection of the bone. Before the antibiotic era, osteomyelitis and septic arthritis in infancy and childhood resulted in a 50% mortality rate. Substantial morbidity from chronic infection and bony destruction with growth and functional disturbance is still noted, usually because of delays in diagnosis and inadequate treatment.[51-54]

The true incidence of osteomyelitis in the pediatric patient is unknown. Bremmer and Negliman estimated that 1 in 5,000 children younger than 13 years of age develop osteomyelitis.[55] During a 28-year period (1959-1986), 365 children with osteomyelitis were hospitalized at the Children's Medical Center in Dallas.[54]

Pathophysiology

Osteomyelitis can result from bacteria entering the bone via hematogenous spread, direct inoculation, or contiguous extension. Hematogenous spread is thought to be the most common mode of infection.

As early as 1921, Hobo hypothesized that bacteria entered the bone via the bloodstream.[56] Bacteria lodged in the medullary cavity of the bone rarely lead to infection because of the massive phagocytic activity in this region. However, bacteria lodged in the end arterial loops beneath the epiphyseal plate are not subject to such massive phagocyte attack; osteomyelitis primarily develops at these rapidly growing ends of bone. However, the actual mechanism of infection is not clearly understood.[53] Simply inoculating the bloodstream with bacteria in multiple in vitro studies has failed to produce osteomyelitis. Also, in children the long bones are infected more often than other bones.

One mechanism of infection is preceding trauma. In a large series of osteomyelitis, a prior traumatic event occurred in 30% to 40% of all cases.[52,54,57-60] In the laboratory, it has been shown that osteomyelitis can be produced if a small crack is made in the epiphyseal plate with subclinical bacteremia. Baxter and Finnegan reviewed 26 cases of neonatal Group B streptococcal skeletal infections associated with trauma.[57] Fifteen had complicated obstetric histories; eleven of these had traumatic deliveries. Seventeen of the 26 cases involved the proximal humerus. The common proximal humeral site may be secondary to trauma to the shoulder as it came through the maternal pelvic rim.[57,59] Other predisposing factors may include drug abuse, systemic bacterial disease, sickle cell disease, and impaired immunologic status.

Contiguous extension or direct inoculation may also be causative. Brook reviewed 26 cases of anaerobic osteomyelitis in children, most secondary to a continuous focus of a mucous membrane.[61] Faden reviewed 135 children with acute osteomyelitis; eight (6%) had infection with *Pseudomonas aeruginosa*, confirming the association with a penetrating wound of the foot through a rubber soled shoe.[60,62] *Pseudomonas osteomyelitis* is also seen in drug abusers.[63,64]

Infection usually begins at the end of a rapidly growing long bone, spreading to the subperiosteal space in the metaphyseal area. The cortex in this area is porous. Once in the subperiosteal space, the infection and inflammation lift the loosely attached periosteum along with the blood supply of the cortex, forming dead bone. The periosteum that maintains its blood supply will begin the formation of new bone. If the metaphysis where the infection begins lies within the joint capsule, infection can spread to the joint itself; septic arthritis may ensue. This is true in anatomic locations, such as the proximal femur (hip), the proximal humerus (shoulder), the distal tibia (ankle), and the proximal radius (elbow). In infants and neonates, the metaphysis where infection occurs may be next to a ligamentous attachment that may preclude infection of the joint. In infants, where no epiphyseal plate is present or ossification site has appeared, the cartilage model at the growth end of a bone is often infected.

Etiology

Multiple organisms may cause osteomyelitis. Historically, *S. aureus* has been most frequently implicated in osteomyelitis regardless of age, accounting for 52% of cases in one study.[52] In the review by Faden of 135 children, it was identified as the causative agent for 47% of these cases. No organism is identified in 20% to 25% of cases.[52,53,58,60]

Haemophilus influenzae type B was the second most frequent identifiable cause of osteomyelitis, ranging from 4.4% to 12%, but will probably decrease in frequency with widespread immunization.[52,60] *H. influenzae* has not been reported in a child over the age of 5. It accounted for 13%

to 33% of osteomyelitis in children between the ages of 1 to 24 months. The pathogen is associated with a preceding or concurrent upper respiratory infection, frequent joint effusions, and concurrent joint disease. It is the second leading cause of osteomyelitis in pediatric patients with sickle cell disease.[65]

Salmonella organism is the most commonly reported pathogen when osteomyelitis occurs in children with sickle cell disease. It accounts for 50% of the cases in the series reported by Syrogiannopoulos.[65] Gram-negative bacteria may be causative in children with sickle cell anemia, as well as in newborns.

Streptococcus pneumoniae has been reported as a cause of osteomyelitis in normal children. Jacobs reported that *S. pneumoniae* is more common in children under 24 months of age.[66] Group A streptococcus has been cited in 4% to 9% of children, and coagulase-negative staphylococcus has been reported in 2% to 4% of pediatric patients.[58,60] Group B streptococcus and *S. aureus* are the two predominant organisms responsible for neonatel osteomyelitis.[67,68] Other organisms include gram-negative bacilli, coagulase negative staphylococcus, *S. pneumoniae*, and *Candida albicans*. Invasive procedures and technological advancements such as fetal monitoring, umbilical and central line placement, total parental nutrition, and heelsticks are related to the increased incidence of neonatal osteomyelitis.

In children with immunologic disorders including HIV, unusual pathogens may be found as the causative agent of osteomyelitis.

Diagnostic Findings

Clinical Findings. Osteomyelitis has been called the great mimicker; diagnosis may be difficult. Morrissey and Shore have broken the diagnosis down into three steps: suspect the diagnosis, localize the area, and isolate the organism.[53]

Evaluation requires a thorough medical history and physical examination. From the medical history the physician wants to know answers to the following questions:

- What symptoms are present?
- How long have symptoms been present?
- Has there been a concurrent or antecedent infection or wound?
- Has there been a history of trauma?
- Does the child have a chronic or underlying medical condition?
- Has the child been on antibiotic therapy?
- Has there been previous skeletal joint disorders?
- Is there familial history of skeletal disorders?

Pain is the most common presenting characteristic and is manifested according to age and the site of involvement. The verbal child will localize and communicate pain to caregiver and physician.

The physical examination will reveal pain, tenderness, warmth, and erythema over the involved bone. Decreased range of motion, limping, and refusal to bear weight or walk may become manifest.

Orthopedic examination attempts to localize the pain and assess joint involvement. A single bone is involved in over 90% of the cases.[53,58] Fifty percent of patients have lower extremity, primarily femur and tibia, involvement. Upper extremities account for 25% of the cases. In the neonate the proximal femur is the most common site of infection. Forty percent have multiple sites.[68-70] In a follow-up study of nonhip neonatal osteomyelitis, six patients had destruction of growth plates. Four of the six patients had multiple sites of infection. Growth plate disruptions in these patients were found at an average age of 9 years. Vertebral osteomyelitis can masquerade as back pain, neck pain, and torticollis. Mandibular osteomyelitis can be depicted as painful or difficult mastication.

In a series of children with pelvic osteomyelitis, an admitting diagnosis of pelvic osteomyelitis was made in only 16% to 25% of patients.[54,71] Acute abdomen, nephrolithiasis, rhabdomyosarcoma, toxic synovitis, septic hip, and buttock cellulitis were a few of the admitting diagnoses of these patients with pelvic osteomyelitis.

Fever >38.5° C has been found in 70% to 85% of children with osteomyelitis.[52,53,60] Infants and nonverbal children with osteomyelitis may only present with irritability, decreased feedings, and lethargy with little systemic toxicity. Neonates are commonly afebrile. Swelling and pseudoparalysis of the involved site are common focal signs.[67,70]

Complications may include septic arthritis, chronic osteomyelitis, and growth disturbance of the extremity with disruption of the epiphyseal growth plate. The latter can lead to limb length discrepancy, limb deformity, and permanent disability.

Ancillary Data. If osteomyelitis is suspected, plain radiographs may localize the area of involvement. X-ray films are often normal early in the course of the disease. However, soft tissue changes may be detectable in the first 3 to 10 days. Initially deep soft tissue swelling can be seen as a shift of the lucent deep muscle plane away from the bone. Eventually this lucent plane will be obliterated altogether. At 10 to 12 days into the disease process, bone lytic destruction and periosteal elevation are apparent on x-ray films.

Further attempts to localize osteomyelitis can be made with other imaging techniques. Radionuclide technetium (TC) 99m scanning may be useful in a child with suspected osteomyelitis and normal plain radiographs. This is particularly true in the toddler age group as shown by Aronson.[72] A normal TC 99m scan with a negative screening examination (history, physical, temperature, WBC count, ESR) allowed the children to be observed as outpatients. Thus unnecessary hospitalizations and expenses were avoided. Radionuclear scanning will show abnormal areas of skeletal physiology. The scan often becomes abnormal 1 to 2 days after the onset of symptoms with increased uptake in the inflammation area. It will not differentiate between the diagnosis of osteomyelitis, cellulitis, septic arthritis, tumor, or trauma. The scan often is normal in the early stages of disease and may need to be repeated.[51,72]

Ultrasound, CT, and MRI scans have been shown to be useful in evaluating patients with clinically suspected osteomyelitis but may have limited availability.[72-76] These scans can help differentiate between osteomyelitis and soft tissue abscesses, localize the specific site for aspiration or surgical drainage, and detect the recurrence of infection.

Because of their ability to evaluate soft tissues, CT and MRI scans have been helpful in achieving the diagnosis of pelvic, vertebral, and mandibular osteomyelitis.

Both ESR and CRP have been shown to be elevated in osteomyelitis.[52,53,60,77] The ESR mean value in these cases was 60 to 70 mm/hr, whereas CRP was 65 mg/L. However, 4.5% to 11% of patients had normal values. ESR and CRP when elevated, are useful in monitoring therapy. White blood cell (WBC) count has not been helpful diagnostically; only 31% of children have an elevated count.[60,77]

Attempting to isolate the organism, a blood culture is obtained at the time of venipuncture. In 50% of children with osteomyelitis, an organism can be isolated on blood cultures. Aspiration of the bone may provide definitive identification in 50% to 69% of children with osteomyelitis.[52,58,60] Aspiration of bone yields important information. First, recovery of pus confirms infection. Secondly, a gram stain of the aspirate may help to initially direct specific antibiotic therapy. Finally, aspiration may help determine the need for specific surgical therapy. If pus is obtained, drainage and curettage may be needed.

Management

All children suspected or known to have osteomyelitis require admission to the hospital for intravenous antibiotic therapy. The antibiotic therapy chosen will depend on the age of the child, the site involved, the organism suspected, community patterns of antibiotic resistance, and any underlying medical conditions. Guidelines are provided in the box on p. 1038. Intravenous antibiotic therapy should generally be initiated in consultation with orthopedic consultation, often following bone aspiration. The duration and route of administration of antibiotic therapy is controversial. In the routine care of osteomyelitis caused by *S. aureus*, patients are normally treated parenterally for 5 to 7 days, assuming decreasing local inflammation and normalization of the ESR/CRP. Following this period, patients may often be switched to oral therapy for 3 to 6 weeks. Symptomatology, degree of bone involvement, skeletal maturation, and compliance may modify this approach.

Compliance must be assured during the oral phase of treatment. Serum bactericidal levels or serum antibiotic levels are monitored. A trough bactericidal titer of 1:8 or greater is acceptable.

Immobilization, if the site of osteomyelitis is an extremity, using a simple sling or splint minimizes pain in the initial treatment stages.

Prognosis. Most children with osteomyelitis have a favorable outcome without sequela. Delay in diagnosis and inadequate treatment are the most important factors determining prognosis. Chronic infection and bony destruction with growth disturbance, residual deformity, and functional disability can result if diagnosis and treatment are not instituted promptly. Long-term follow-up is mandatory after appropriate therapy particularly in the neonate.

SEPTIC ARTHRITIS

Septic arthritis (also bacterial, suppurative, or infectious arthritis) refers to the presence of organisms inducing purulent material within the joint space, leading to inflammation of the joint. The importance of recognition and man-

---

**Antibiotic Management of Osteomyelitis
and Septic Arthritis**

Nafcillin 100-200 mg/kg/24 hr q 4 hr IV (or equivalent
semisynthetic penicillin); followed by dicloxicillin 75-
100 mg/kg/24 hr QID PO

Alternative: if penicillin allergic, cefazolin or cephalothin
100 mg/kg/24 hr q 4-6 hr IV; followed by cephalexin
50-100 mg/kg/24 hr q 6 hr PO **or** if penicillin and
cephalosporin allergic, (1) clindamycin 15-25 mg/kg/
24 hr QID PO **or** (2) vancomycin 40 mg/kg/24 hr QID
PO

Special situations

1. Newborn (child <1 mo) or sickle cell patient *ADD* cefotaxime 100-150 mg/kg/24 hr q 8 hr IV **or** gentamicin
5 to 7.5 mg/kg/24 hr q 8-12 hr IV and ampicillin 200
mg/kg/24 hr q 4 hr IV
2. Child <5 years consider *ADDING* cefuroxime 150
mg/kg/24 hr q 6-8 hr IV
3. Puncture wound or drug abuser (may require surgical
drainage)
   Carbenicillin 400 to 600 mg/kg/24 hr q 4 hr IV and
   Gentamicin, as above; **or**
   Ceftazidime 100 to 150 mg/kg/24 hr q 8 hr IV
4. Immunosuppressed child
   Vancomycin 30-40 mg/kg/24 hr q 6-8 hr IV and
   ceftazidime 100 mg to 150 mg/kg/24 hr q 8 hr
   IV; **or** ticarcillin/clavulanate 200-300 mg/kg/24
   hr q 4-6 hr IV and tobramycin 6-7.5 mg/kg/24 hr
   q 8 hr IV

Antibiotic should be adjusted to reflect identification and
sensitivity of known pathogen.

---

agement of this condition cannot be overemphasized.
Delay in diagnosis and treatment increases the risk of
serious complications, which include joint destruction and
long-term disability.

Septic arthritis is more common in children than in
adults. Although the disease can occur at any age, most
cases occur in infants to children up to 5 years of age, with
the highest incidence in infants 6 to 24 months old.[78-82]

A number of factors predispose to infection. Significant
trauma occurs in approximately 30% to 45% of cases. There
may be preceding upper respiratory infection or otitis media. Skin and soft tissue infections have been associated
with septic arthritis, especially when *S. aureus* is the causative agent. In addition, intravenous drug abuse, traumatic
puncture wounds, and femoral venipuncture in neonates
can lead to direct penetration and inoculation arthritis.[78,80,82-84]

Pathophysiology

Bacteria can enter the joint space through three
mechanisms: hematogenous spread, direct inoculation, or
contiguous extension. Of these, hematogenous spread is
the most common mode of infection in the pediatric population.[82,83]

In patients with bacteremia and hematogenous spread, a
large number of bacteria are delivered in the synovial
membranes of diarthrodial joints, which have a high effective blood flow. If infection occurs, PMN leukocyte infiltration, vascular congestion, and lining cell proliferation
ensue. In some cases, this initial joint infection may be
eradicated by host defense mechanisms. This phase may be
represented by the transient arthritis and arthralgias associated with some septicemic and viremic illnesses. If this
stage progresses and bacterial proliferation occurs, a persistent purulent effusion develops, accompanied by the
clinical findings of a swollen, tender joint. Eventually proteolytic enzymes released by PMN leukocyte, as well as
direct pressure, lead to cartilage and bone destruction.

Direct inoculation usually occurs following trauma or
surgical manipulation. Cellulitis or osteomyelitis may lead
to septic arthritis of the contiguous joint.

Etiology

Historically, *S. aureus* has been the organism most frequently implicated in septic arthritis, accounting for
greater than 50% of those cases with known pathogens.[83]
Recent reviews have documented an increased incidence
of *H. influenzae* infections, the latter being responsible for
19% to 46% of all cases, although this may change with
increasing immunization of infants. The bacterial etiology
varies with age.[78,80,82,84] In neonates, group B Streptococcus and *S. aureus* predominate; gram-negative enteric organisms are another important source of infection. In children beyond the neonatal period up to 24 months of age, *H.
influenzae* is most prevalent and *S. aureus* remains an important causative agent. From age 2 to 5 years, *H. influenzae*, *S. aureus*, and Streptococcal species (group A and
pneumococcal) are most common, while *S. aureus* is the
pathogen most often identified in children older than 5
years old. Other important organisms include *Neisseria
gonorrhoeae* in sexually active adolescents, and *P. aeruginosa* in puncture wounds.[83,84] It should be noted that in
large series, no organism is recovered in approximately
30% of patients with diagnosed septic arthritis.[78,80,82-84]
Dagan[85] suspected that fastidious organisms may be responsible for a considerable number of culture negative
cases. They isolated *Kingella kingae* after innoculating synovial fluid into blood culture bottles.

Children with hemophilia have an increased risk of septic arthritis.[86] Studies by Gregg-Smith[87] and Merchan[88]
suggest the incidence may be increasing because of the
increasing frequency of HIV in these patients. *S. pneumoniae* has been the most common pathogen isolated.

Diagnostic Findings

Children with septic arthritis are frequently misdiagnosed on their initial visit to the physician; in one study, 10
out of 32 patients were originally given an incorrect diagnosis despite presenting with complaints of musculoskeletal pain.[84] Because there is often a history of trauma, a
diagnosis of posttraumatic arthritis may be confused on the
first evaluation. Delay in diagnosis is one of the major
causes of complications.

Morrissy and Shore[89] have identified the following three
steps in diagnosis:

- Suspect the infection.
- Localize the area.
- Isolate the organism.

Children with septic arthritis typically have complaints of pain in an extremity, a limp, or decreased active motion about the involved joint. Seventy-five percent have fever greater than 38.3° C.[78,81,89] Constitutional signs of systemic illness are usually present within the first few days of infection. In neonates, the disease may not produce fever or toxic appearance; rather, nonspecific signs of septicemia may be present, such as poor feeding, irritability, or lethargy.

Joints involved in order of frequency are the knee, hip, and ankle; the elbow, shoulder, and wrist are less commonly involved. Six percent to eleven percent of patients will have involvement of more than one joint.[78,80,82,83]

On physical examination, the manifestations are those of any localized infection (i.e., erythema, swelling, tenderness, and pain). There is a noticeable lack of active motion of the affected limb. Because pain fibers are located only in the joint capsule, anything that increases intracapsular pressure will also produce pain. Therefore joints are held in a position of minimum hydrostatic pressure. For the hip, this includes moderate flexion (70 degrees to 80 degrees), slight abduction (15 degrees to 20 degrees), and slight external rotation (15 degrees). The knee is held in 25 degrees to 50 degrees of flexion, the ankle in 15 degrees of plantar flexion, the elbow in 20 degrees to 30 degrees of flexion, and the shoulder in slight abduction and lateral rotation. Passive range of motion is limited, and even gentle manipulation produces pain. There may be considerable muscle spasms about the joint.

Assessing range of motion is not difficult when the joint involved moves in only one plane (i.e., the knee or elbow). The hip joint presents a special problem, but an adequate evaluation can be accomplished by performance of radiographs, ESR, CRP, CBC, and, often, a bone scan.

Ancillary Data. Plain film radiographs should be obtained but are of limited use early in the course of infection. Widening of the joint space and bone destruction are late findings. Fat lines are displaced early in septic arthritis because of capsular distension. Views of the contralateral side may be useful for comparison.

Ultrasonography can be a useful adjuvant. It documents the presence of a joint effusion and aids needle aspiration. However, it cannot differentiate between septic and nonseptic effusions.[90] CT and MRI scans because of their improved soft tissue resolution can aid diagnosis. The availability and interpretation of these scans can be limited in the emergency department.

In cases of suspected septic arthritis, laboratory studies should be obtained, including a CBC, differential, ESR, CRP, and blood and throat cultures; joint fluid should be collected for analysis (cell count, Gram stain, glucose) and culture. The total CBC will be mildly elevated in most patients; however, this test lacks sensitivity, since approximately 50% of patients will have counts of less than 15,000 cells/mm[3]; ESR and CRP values are highly sensitive tests for the presence of septic arthritis.[78,91] The ESR is high in greater than 90% of cases and is typically evaluated with mean values ranging from 68 to 82 mm/hr.[78,84] Although

sensitive, the ESR is relatively nonspecific and may be elevated in the presence of other infectious or immunologic conditions. The CRP value may be the most useful laboratory test for primary diagnosis of children with septic arthritis. In one study, CRP values greater than 20 mg/L had a sensitivity of 94%, a specificity of 92%, and high predictive values in identifying children with septic arthritis.[81] The CRP value was more accurate than the WBC or ESR in distinguishing septic arthritis from other forms of acute arthritis.

Analysis of joint fluid is essential. The primary criterion for the diagnosis of septic arthritis is the isolation of an organism from the joint fluid. Gram-stained specimens must be examined carefully; joint fluid may exert a bacteriostatic effect on microorganisms, and those that can be seen on the smear may not grow in culture.

Joint fluid should also be analyzed for total WBC count and differential, and glucose concentration. The fluid should be collected in a heparinized syringe; large clot formation does not interfere with WBC count determination. Total WBC count is usually greater than 50,000 cells/mm[3] with 90% PMN leukocytes; the range is generally from 50,000 to 200,000 cells/mm[3], but counts as low as 5000 cells/mm[3] have been found in patients with septic arthritis.[89] Glucose concentration is typically < 40 mg/dl or < 30% of the serum concentration (Table 57-7).[83]

A specific pathogen is not identified in about 30% of cases. The organism is most often recovered from the joint fluid, accounting for up to 80% of positive cultures.[78,80,82,84] When obtained, 40% of blood cultures are positive; they are the only source from which the causative agent is isolated in up to 11% of cases.[78,80,82,84]

Other potential sites have been reported to have concurrent infection and may serve as an additional mechanism of defining the pathogen: urine (gram-negative bacilli), CSF (*H. influenzae*), skin/wound (*S. aureus*), and urethra, cervix, rectum, and pharynx (*N. gonorrhoeae*). The decision to obtain cultures from these sites will be dictated by the age of the child and the clinical circumstances. Latex agglutination tests may be useful in children at risk for infection with *H. influenzae*. Welkon noted that 11% of septic arthritis resulting from *H. influenzae* had a bacterial pathogen defined by latex agglutination only.[78]

Differential Considerations

The differential considerations of septic arthritis include viral arthritis, traumatic arthritis, toxic synovitis, periarticular cellulitis, osteomyelitis with reactive arthritis, Henoch-Schönlein purpura, JRA, acute rheumatic fever, Lyme disease, postinfectious reactive arthritis, leukemia, and diskitis.

Toxic synovitis is particularly difficult to differentiate in younger children. This self-limited condition is common in children from 1 to 7 years of age. Children often have a preceding viral-like illness and are nontoxic. The hip joint may have some limited range of motion. The CBC and ESR are generally normal, whereas the hip x-ray study shows a variable effusion.

Management

The management of children with septic arthritis involves a team approach. Medical therapy includes prompt

TABLE 57-7. Common Synovial Fluid Findings

Category	Etiology	Appearance	Leukocytes (cells/mm^3)	Percentage of neutrophils	Percentage of glucose $\left[\dfrac{\text{synovial}}{\text{blood}}\right]$	Mucin* clot
Normal		Clear	< 100	25	> 50	Good
Bacterial	Septic arthritis	Turbid, purulent	> 50,000	> 75	< 50	Poor
Inflammatory	JRA Rheumatic fever Mycobacterial, viral, and fungal arthritis	Clear or turbid	500-75,000	50	> 50	Poor
Traumatic		Clear or bloody	< 5,000†	< 50	> 50	Good

*For mucin clot: add 4 ml of water to 1 ml of synovial fluid supernatant. Mix in 2 drops of 5% glacial acetic acid. If normal, a tight rope of mucin will form. If infection or inflammation is present, clot will flake and shred.
†May have red cells.

initiation of parenteral antibiotics. The selection of specific antimicrobial agents should be guided by the age of the child, the suspected organism, community pattern of antimicrobial resistance, and any underlying medical condition of the child (see box).[80,91-93] Specific clinical situations may dictate further alterations in the selection of antibiotics. Traditionally, parenteral antibiotics are continued for a minimum of 2 (S. pneumoniae and H. influenzae) to 3 (S. aureus and gram-negative enterics) weeks. For infections from P. aeruginosa and N. gonorrhoeae 1 week of therapy is indicated. Duration of antibiotic therapy should be dictated by clinical findings. Some clinicians prefer to begin oral therapy after 1 week of parenteral agents, while carefully monitoring serum bactericidal levels. For oral therapy to be successful, compliance must be ensured and bactericidal level must be maintained at 1:8 or greater.

Surgical management includes obtaining specimens for microbiological diagnosis, evaluating the need for surgery and performing surgery when indicated. Indications for surgery in the child with septic arthritis are arthritis of the hip or shoulder joint, the presence of large amounts of fibrotic debris within the joint space, and arthritis not improving after 3 days of medical management.

Most children with septic arthritis have a favorable outcome without orthopedic sequelae. Delay in diagnosis and treatment is the most important factor affecting prognosis.[78,84,94] Welkon demonstrated a significant association between delay of therapy of 4 or more days duration and the development of orthopedic complications. Infants and patients with infections involving the hip also tend to have less favorable outcomes. Sequelae can result in long-term disability and include avascular necrosis, limb length discrepancy, residual deformity, and decreased range of motion. Long-term follow-up is indicated.

References

Arthralgia and Joint Pain

1. Schaller JG: Arthritis in children, *Pediatr Clin North Am* 33(5):1565, 1986.
2. Lane SE: Severe ankle sprains, *Physician Sports Med* 18(11):43, 1990.
3. Merten DF and Carpenter BL: Radiologic imaging of inflicted injury in the child abuse syndrome, *Pediatr Clin North Am* 37(4):815, 1990.
4. Garrick JG: Sports medicine, *Pediatr Clin North Am* 33(6):1541, 1986.
5. Morrissy RT and Shore SL: Bone and joint sepsis, *Pediatr Clin North Am* 33(6):1551, 1986.
6. Waldvogel FA and Vasey H: Osteomyelitis, the past decade, *N Engl J Med* 303(7):360, 1980.
7. Swischuk LE: Limp in young child, *Pediatr Emerg Care* 6(1):65, 1990.
8. Renshaw TS: *Pediatric orthopedics*, Philadelphia, 1986, WB Saunders.
9. Lindsley CB and Schaller JG: Arthritis associated with inflammatory bowel disease in children, *J Pediatr* 84(1):16, 1974.
10. Stollerman GH (chairman): Committee report: Jones criteria (revised) for guidance in the diagnosis of rheumatic fever, *Circulation* 32:664, 1965.
11. Chung SMK: Disease of the developing hip joint, *Pediatr Clin North Am* 33(6):1457, 1986.
12. Gruber MA: The conservative treatment of chondramalacia patellae, *Orthop Clin North Am* 10(1):105, 1989.
13. Smith JB: Knee problems in children, *Pediatr Clin North Am* 33(6):1439, 1986.
14. Peterson H: Growing pains, *Pediatr Clin North Am* 33(6):1365, 1986.
15. Maloney MJ: Diagnosing hysterical conversion reactions in children, *J Pediatr* 97(6):1016, 1980.
16. Conway JJ: Radionuclide bone scintigraphy in pediatric orthopedics, *Pediatr Clin North Am* 33(6):1313, 1986.
17. Wilkinson R: Imaging, *Pediatr Clin North Am* 33(6):1299, 1986.

Back Pain

18. Olson TL et al: The epidemiology of low back pain in an adolescent population, *Am J of Public Health* 82(4):606, 1992.
19. Turner PG, Green JH, Galasko CSB: Back pain in childhood, *Spine* 14(8):8, 1989.
20. King HA: Back pain in children, *Pediatr Clin North Am* 31(5):1083, 1984.
21. Smith RF and Taylor TKF: Inflammatory lesions of intervertebral discs in children, *J Bone Joint Surg* 49-A(8):1507, 1967.
22. Hensinger RN: Spondylolysis and spondylolisthesis in children and adolescents, *J Bone Joint Surg* 71-A(7):1098, 1989.
23. Menkes JH: *The textbook of child neurology*, ed 2, Philadelphia, 1980, Lea and Febiger.
24. Comstock CP, Carragee EJ, O'Sullivan GS: Spondylolisthesis in the young athlete, *Physician Sports Med* 22(18):39, 1994.
25. Boston HC, Bianco AJ, Rhodes KH: Disk space infections in children, *Orthop Clin North Am* 6(4):953, 1975.
26. Syriopoulou VP and Smith AL: Osteomyelitis and septic arthritis. In Feigin RD, Cherry JD, editors: *Textbook of pediatric infectious diseases*, Philadelphia, 1987, WB Saunders.
27. Bernini PM, Gorczyca JT, Modlin JF: Cat-scratch disease presenting as a paravertebral abscess. A case report, *J Bone Joint Surg* 76(12):1858, 1994.
28. Bunnell WP: Back pain in children, *Pediatr Clin North Am* 13(3):587, 1982.
29. Tertti MO et al: Low-back pain and disk degeneration in children: a case-control MR imaging study, *Radiology* 180(2):503, 1991

30. Bunnell WP: Spinal deformity, *Pediatr Clin North Am* 33(6):1475, 1986.
31. Maloney MJ: Diagnosing hysterical conversion reactions in children, *J Pediatr* 97(6):1016, 1980.
32. Cassidy JT: *Textbook of pediatric rheumatology,* New York, 1986, John Wiley & Sons.
33. Collert S: Osteomyelitis of the spine, *Acta Orthop Scand* 18:283, 1977.
34. Conway JJ: Radionuclide bone scintigraphy in pediatric orthopedics, *Pediatr Clin North Am* 33(6):1313, 1986.
35. Wilkinson R: Imaging, *Pediatr Clin North Am* 33(6):1299, 1986.

Limp

36. Hensinger RN: Limp, *Pediatr Clin North Am* 33(6):1355, 1986.
37. Phillips WA: The child with a limp, *Orthop Clin North Am* 18(4):489, 1987.
38. Rang M and Wright J: Pitfalls on fractures, *Pediatr Ann* 18(1):53, 1989.
39. Morrissy RT and Shore SL: Bone and joint sepsis, *Pediatr Clin North Am* 33(6):1551, 1986.
40. Chung SM: Diseases of developing hip joint, *Pediatr Clin North Am* 33(6):1457, 1986.
41. Cassidy JT: *Textbook of pediatric rheumatology,* New York, 1982, John Wiley & Sons.
42. Rosen G: Spindle cell scarcoma-osteogenic scarcoma. In Sutow WW, Fernbach DJ, Vietti TJ, editors, *Clinical pediatric oncology,* ed 3, St. Louis, 1984, Mosby.
43. Menkes JH: *The textbook of child neurology,* ed 2, Philadelphia, 1980, Lea & Febiger.
44. Renshaw TS: *Pediatric orthopedics,* Philadelphia, 1986, WB Saunders.
45. Smith JB: Knee problems in children, *Pediatr Clin North Am* 33(6):1439, 1986.
46. Gruber MA: The conservative treatment of chondramalacia patellae, *Orthop Clin North Am* 10(1):105, 1979.
47. Edidin DV et al: Resurgence of nurtritional rickets associated with breast-feeding and special dietary practices, *Pediatr* 65(2):232, 1980.
48. Maloney MJ: Diagnosing hysterical conversion reactions in children, *J Pediatr* 97(6):1016, 1980.
49. Conway JJ: Radionuclide bone scintigraphy in pediatric orthopedics, *Pediatr Clin North Am* 33(6):1313, 1986.
50. Wilkinson R: Imaging, *Pediatr Clin North Am* 33(6):1299, 1986.

Osteomyelitis

51. Fleisher GR, Paradise JE, Plotkin SA et al. Falsely normal radionuclide scans for osteomyelitis, *Am J Dis Child* 134:499, 1980.
52. Lebel MH and Nelson JD: *Haemophilus influenzae* type b osteomyelitis in infants and children, *Pediatr Infect Dis J* 7:250, 1988.
53. Morrissy RT and Shore LS: Bone and joint sepsis, *Pediatr Clin North Am* 33(6):1551, 1986.
54. Mustafa MM, Saez-Llorens X, McCracken GH et al: Acute hematogenous pelvic osteomyelitis in infant and children, *Pediatr Infect Dis J* 9:416, 1990.
55. Bremmer A and Neligman G: Pyogenic osteitis, *Recent Adv Pediatr* 2:354, 1958.11.
56. Hobo T: Fur Pathogenese du Akuten-hematogenen Osteomyelitis, mit Berucksichtigung du Vital Farbungslehre, *Acta Scholae Med Imp Kioto* 4:1, 1921.
57. Baxter MD and Finnegan MA: Skeletal infection by group B beta haemolytic streptococci in neonates, *J Bone Joint Surg* 70B:812, 1988.
58. Dich VQ, Nelson JD, Hallalin KC: Osteomyuelitis in infants and children, *Am J Dis Child* 129:1273, 1975.
59. Edwards MS, Baker CJ, Wagner ML et al: An etiologic shift in infantile osteomyelitis: the emergence of the group B streptococcus, *J Pediatr* 93:578, 1978.
60. Faden H and Grossi M: Acute osteomyelitis in children, *Am J Dis Child* 145:65, 1991.
61. Brook I: Anaerobic osteomyelitis in children. *Pediatr Infect Dis J* 5:550, 1986.
62. Fisher MC, Goldsmith JF, Gilligan PH: Sneakers as a source of *Pseudomonas aeruginosa* in children with osteomyelitis following puncture wound, *J Pediatr* 107:161, 1985.
63. Roca RP and Yoshikawa TT: Primary skeletal infections in heroin users: a clinical characterization, diagnosis and therapy, *Clin Orthop* 144:238, 1979.
64. Sequeira W, Jones E, Siegel ME: Pyogenic infections of the pubic symphysis, *Ann Intern Med* 96:604, 1982.
65. Syrogiannopoulos GA, McCracken GH, Nelson JD: Osteoarticular infections in children with sickle cell disease, *Pediatrics* 78:1090, 1986.
66. Jacobs NM: Pneumococcal osteomyhelitis and arthritis in children, *Am J Dis Child* 145:70, 1991.
67. Dormans JP: Pediatric hematogenous osteomyelitis: New trends in presentation, diagnosis and treatment, *J Am Acad Orthop* 2(6):333, 1994.
68. Knudsen CJM: Neonatal osteomyelitis, *J Bone Joint Surg Br* 72(5): 846, 1990.
69. Green NE: Bone and joint infections in children, *Orthop Clin North Am* 18(4):555, 1987.
70. Peters W: Long-term effects of neonatal bone and joint infection on adjacent growth plates, *J Pediatr Orthop* 12:806, 1992.
71. Highland TR: Osteomyelitis of the pelvis in children, *J Bone Joint Surg* 65A:230, 1983.
72. Aronson J: Efficiency of the bone scan for occult limping toddlers, *J Pediatr Orthop* 12:38, 1992.
73. Nath AK: Use of ultrasound in Osteomyelitis, *Br J Radiol* 65:649, 1992.
74. Mah ET: Ultrasonic Features of acute osteomyelitis in children, *J Bone Joint Surg Br* 76-B:969, 1994.
75. Azouz EM: CT evaluation of primary epiphyseal bone abscesses, *Skeletal Radiol* 22:17, 1993.
76. Erdman WA: Osteomyelitis: Characteristics and pitfalls of diagnosis with MR imaging, *Radiology* 180:533, 1991.
77. Unkila-Kallio L: Serum c-reative protein, erythrocyte sedimentation rate and white blood cell count in acute hematogenous osteomelitis of children, *Pediatrics,* 93:59, 1994.

Septic Arthritis

78. Welkon CH, Long SS, Fisher MC et al: Pyogenic arthritis in infants and children: a review of 95 cases, *Pediatr Infect Dis J* 5:669, 1986.
79. Peterson S, Knudsen FU, Anderson EA et al: Acute hematogenous osteomyelitis and septic arthritis in childhood, *Acta Orthop Scand* 51:451, 1980.
80. Barton LL, Dunkle LM, Habib FH: Septic arthritis in childhood, *Am J Dis Child* 141:898, 1987.
81. Kunnamo I, Kallio P, Pelkonen P et al: Clinical signs and laboratory tests in the differential diagnosis of arthritis in children, *Am J Dis Child* 141:34, 1987.
82. Nelson JD and Koontz WC: Septic arthritis in infants and children: a review of 117 cases, *Pediatrics* 38:966, 1966.
83. Syriopoulou VPH and Smith AL: Osteomyelitis and septic arthritis in Feigin RD and Cherry JD, editors: *Textbook of pediatric infectious diseases,* ed 2, Philadelphia, 1987, WB Saunders.
84. Morrey BF, Bianco AJ, Rhodes KH: Septic arthritis in children, *Orthop Clin North Am* 6:923, 1975.
85. Dagan R: Management of acute hematogenous osteomyelitis and septic arthritis in the pediatric patient, *Pediatr Infect Dis J* 12:88, 1993.
86. Fajardo JE: Suppurative arthritis and hemophilia, *Pediatr Infect Dis J* 5:593, 1986.
87. Gregg-Smith SJ: Septic arthritis in haemophilia *J Bone Joint Surg* 75-B:368, 1993.
88. Merchan ECR: Septic arthritis in HIV positive haemophiliacs, *International Orthop* 16:302, 1992.
89. Morrissey RT and Shore SL: Bone and joint sepsis, *Pediatr Clin North Am* 33:1551, 1986.
90. Zawin JK: Joint effusion in children with an irritable hip: US diagnosis and aspiration, *Radiology* 187:459, 1993.
91. Molteni RA: The differential diagnosis of benign and septic joint disease in children, *Clin Pediatr* 17:19, 1978.
92. Scoles PV and Aronoff SC: Antimicrobial therapy of childhood skeletal infections, *J Bone Joint Surg* 66-A:1487, 1984.
93. Nelson JD: Evaluation of new anti-infective drugs for the treatment of acute suppurative arthritis in children, *Clin Infect Dis* 15:5172, 1992.
94. Lunseth PA and Heiple KG: Prognosis in septic arthritis of the hip in children, *Clin Orthop* 139:81, 1979.

Psychiatric and Behavioral Disorders

Theodore M. Barnett

EVALUATION OF THE DISTURBED CHILD

As the pattern of health care in the United States changes, more and more children are receiving their primary medical care through the emergency department. Many of these children will have emotional, psychiatric, or behavioral disturbances, and a significant number (5%-15% of school age children) will have functional impairment as a result.[1]

These children may present with a chief complaint specific to an emotional or behavioral problem, and thus be easily recognized. More commonly, when children are seen for a physical or unrelated complaints, the underlying psychiatric, social, behavioral, or emotional problems remain hidden. This latter group may go undiagnosed and untreated without an appropriate focus on these areas.[2] Being alert to inappropriate interaction between parent, child, and medical staff and willing to ask specific questions of the parent and child regarding potential problems will allow identification of these patients.

Unlike adults, evaluation of the child requires evaluation of the family. The child with a psychiatric, emotional, or behavioral disorder is brought for medical care as a result of failed family coping mechanisms. The family believes (whether true or not) that they can no longer care for the child's problems in a family setting. The family may have exhausted their normal coping mechanisms or be unable or unwilling to use the supports that exist. The child may also present as a result of dysfunction in another family member or the family as a whole. The clinician is not taking care of a single patient, but the family as a unit. All must be assessed and treated.

Signs and Symptoms

ENURESIS

Enuresis, the involuntary voiding of urine, is commonly divided into primary and secondary and diurnal and nocturnal categories. Primary enuresis refers to involuntary voiding in a child who has never had voluntary control ("not toilet trained"). Secondary enuresis occurs in children who were previously continent for a period of 1 year, and is less common.

Girls normally have bladder control after 5 years of age; boys may not have control until 6.[3] Diurnal (daytime) enuresis usually disappears first and accounts for 20% of enuretics.[4] Nocturnal (night-time) voiding exists in approximately 15% of 5-year-old children, 7% of 8-year old children, and 3% of 12-year-old children.

Pathophysiology. Continent voiding of urine requires that the bladder have sufficient capacity for the urine produced, that voluntary sphincter tone remain adequate until voiding is desired, and that the bladder not contract and overcome the urinary sphincter.[5] Several factors can interfere with this physiology. Structural abnormalities, such as ectopic ureter, may cause incontinence, though a careful history will often show that continence was never fully achieved. Increased volume of urine resulting from polydipsia or diuretic effect (from medication, hyperosmolar effect, or hormonal effect as in diabetes insipidus) can result in enuresis with an otherwise normal urologic system. Loss of renal medullary gradient, as in sickle cell disease, leads to larger urine volumes.[6,7] Urinary tract infection can lead to bladder contraction and poor sphincter control. Central and (less often) peripheral nervous system lesions can affect both bladder and sphincter control. Inappropriate voiding habits, such as repeatedly "holding urine" until the child can no longer wait, results in diurnal enuresis.[4] These habits are often associated with resistance to toilet training. Finally, psychogenic causes, particularly sexual abuse, depression, and anxiety may provoke either diurnal or nocturnal enuresis.[8]

History for Children with Enuresis

· Presence of fever, pain, or discomfort in abdomen-back
· Quality of urinary stream; color and odor of urine
· Pattern of enuresis and voiding; previous episode(s)
· Toilet training experience
· Personality or behavioral changes and recent stress
· Associated medical conditions, dietary changes, and medication
· Family history of renal or voiding problems

Primary enuresis represents a variation in maturation of bladder control. Many of these children will have a family history of late attainment of continence and most will have spontaneous improvement and resolution.[9]

Differential Considerations. Constitutional delay in neuromuscular maturation or a small functional bladder capacity often underlie primary enuresis. Anatomic abnormalities of the genitourinary tract, such as ectopic ureters, or of the central nervous system (CNS), such as meningomyelocele, may be present.[5] Abnormal bladder function from a variety of causes and urinary tract infection (UTI) may be contributory. Constipation, pinworms, vulvovaginitis, vaginal foreign bodies, and neurologic lesions such as spinal cord tumors have been implicated in enuresis.[3,10,11]

Diagnostic Findings. The history should begin with the general health of the child. Specific questioning should include the items in the box above. Items one through five are often positive in UTI. Items six and seven may point to a direct cause of enuresis (i.e., diuretic effect or polydipsia) or indirect cause (i.e., diabetes). A child, particularly a girl, who voids infrequently (only two or three times a day) is exhibiting "holding on" behavior. So is the child with diurnal enuresis who has a history of squatting, pressing her thighs together, pressing her hands against her perineum, or squirming. Questioning about previous episodes and continence training may indicate that the problem is actually primary enuresis. Previous episodes in association with other symptoms may also suggest recurrent UTI. A history of personality changes concurrent with the onset of enuresis may be a result of abuse or stress. Specific questioning of both the child and the parents about unpleasant events or stress may identify the problem. Family history of renal or voiding problems is particularly useful in primary enuresis.

A thorough physical examination, including the genitalia, should be performed, particularly looking for signs of maltreatment, genitourinary abnormalities, abdominal masses, and irritation of the urethral meatus or surrounding structures. Blood pressure should be measured.

Ancillary Data. A urinalysis, including specific gravity, chemistry, and microscopic examination, is necessary in the evaluation of all children with secondary enuresis. The urinalysis, history, or examination may suggest the need for other laboratory tests such as electrolytes, creatinine, blood urea nitrogen, serum glucose, and urine culture. If structural abnormalities of the urinary tract are suspected, an ultrasound is often useful as a screening examination.

Management. Management will depend on the diagnosis. Primary enuretics should be referred to a physician who can provide evaluation, longitudinal care, and support.[3,12-14] Patients with inappropriate voiding patterns should be encouraged to void every 1½ hours while awake, take time to void completely, and increase fluid intake.[4] A system of support and positive reinforcement should be implemented by the family, providing consistency and appropriate expectations. Pharmacologic agents are rarely necessary. These patients also require longitudinal follow-up. Victims of abuse and those with urinary tract infections are discussed in Chapters 45 and 60, respectively.

ENCOPRESIS

The term *encopresis* was derived from the word enuresis and originally referred only to psychogenic passage of bowel movements in inappropriate places.[15] Encopresis is defined as "repeated, involuntary defecation into clothing, occurring in children 4 years of age and older, of at least 1 month's duration."[16] Boys are affected about three times as often as girls.

Pathophysiology. Virtually all children with encopresis have stool retention, at least intermittently. The pattern of retention may begin in early infancy, and is usually well established by the age of 4. Some of these patients will have had simple constipation, anorectal disorders, or anorectal manipulation (e.g., with enemas, suppositories) during the first 2 years of life. Due to pain, fear, or anxiety, the child begins delaying or withholding defecation. The retention is often increased during the toilet-training period because of parental attitudes and reactions, fear of the toilet itself, and stresses during the struggle for autonomy in early childhood development.[17] Once the child goes to school, the more scheduled environment may lead to incomplete defecation. Some children delay defecation to avoid the lack of privacy or verbal abuse they suffer in the school bathroom.

Encopresis may also result from organic disorders of rectal motility or sphincter control.[16] These problems may then be exacerbated by the factors listed previously. In either case, when stool is retained, the colon and rectum must enlarge to accommodate the increased volume. As time passes, this interferes with the bowel's sensory feedback; the stretched rectum loses some of its contractility. Large, painful stools may be passed, leading the child to try further to withhold stool.[18] Stool may be passed (often without sensation) around the impaction and overflow diarrhea (with or without water loss) may occur. The result is a vicious cycle of gradually increasing retention and loss of normal function. Eventually, the patient is unable to sense the need to defecate, nor is able to control the passage of stool. Indeed, the child with encopresis may not be able to smell his own feces, due to accommodation to the omnipresent odor.

Encopresis carries a severe social stigma. A child suffering from encopresis will often become socially isolated, depressed, and display behavior problems.[19] These are usually the result of the child's shame, reinforced by the reaction of parents, siblings, and peers. The child is often blamed for the problem or accused of being lazy. Eventually, a feeling of hopelessness pervades the child, making treatment quite difficult.[18,20]

Diagnostic Considerations. Defecation into clothing may occur occasionally when the child is under stress or as an "accident" if play results in a delay in reaching the bathroom. Persistent encopretic stooling suggests a more difficult problem to solve. Toilet training issues may become a battleground between parent and child. In older children, school-related stresses may contribute.

The child with an anteriorly placed anus may have an anatomic and correctable obstruction and deserves further evaluation by a pediatric surgeon or gastroenterologist. The possibility of Hirschsprung disease should always be considered, although it is not common in the school-aged child. Stool retention from birth, abdominal pain, failure to thrive, and large stool size should increase the suspicion of Hirschsprung disease.[15] Mental retardation or CNS disorders may result in delay in achieving adequate stool control.

Diagnostic Findings. The physician should obtain a thorough stooling history on the encopretic child, looking for evidence of the retention problems described previously. This should include the stooling pattern in infancy and its progression as the child got older; problems with and results of toilet training; medical problems related to the gastrointestinal tract; and the current frequency, circumstances, and volume of the incontinence. Assessment of the school environment, parental and peer attitudes, and the child's psychosocial reactions may also helpful when counseling the family.[16]

Children with encopresis and chronic constipation typically appear physically healthy, but may appear depressed or anxious. The examination may be normal or have a palpable abdominal or rectal stool mass. The anus is anatomically normal; tone is variable.

In the child who is suspected of having stool retention by history, but whose examination is unrevealing, a flat-plate x-ray film of the abdomen may show the full extent of retained stool.

Management. The child and parents should be counseled that although this problem is not uncommon, the treatment may be lengthy and patience will be necessary. The child will require long-term follow-up.[16,21] Immediate management involves emptying the bowel to allow reestablishment of sensory feedback. The aggressive regimen for the constipated child described in Chapter 52 is appropriate. The child should eat a diet with increased bran cereals, fruits, and vegetables. A regular toilet time should be established twice a day during which the child will sit on the toilet for 10 minutes. Mineral oil or Sennecot may be added to the regimen if desired.[15] Fecal disimpaction by manual removal or by administration of hypertonic phosphate enema (Fleet pediatric: 30-60 ml/10 kg, or adolescent: 120 ml, may be used after overnight mineral oil. Add 100 mg docusate (colace) to each enema. Other approaches include mineral oil at 1 to 2 ml/kg up to 120 ml BID PO for 2 to 7 days until the rectal effluent is clear. The dose may gradually be increased to 300 ml BID PO as a maximum. Senokot may also be used as an alternative (<5 yr: 1-2 tsp syrup; >5 yr: 2-3 tsp syrup).

The parents and child should be given an explanation of the problem and the child's blamelessness. Encourage the parents to support and guide the child during treatment, and avoid recriminations. Stress the importance of compli-

ance with the prescribed regimen, despite the time required. Most importantly, provide hope and reassurance for the child. Treatment without hope is doomed to failure.

SLEEP DISTURBANCES

Many children suffer from a variety of sleep disorders and disturbances.[22] Sleep problems seen in the emergency department include nighttime awakenings, night terrors, sleep walking and sleep talking, and nightmares. Despite genuine parental concern regarding the child's health, sleep problems are usually brought to the physician's attention based on the accompanying disturbance of parental sleep patterns.[23] This disturbance may trigger significant intrafamilial tension, with anger directed at the child, frustration between marital partners, and guilt felt by everyone.

Pathophysiology. The sleep patterns of the newborn infant show little day-night differentiation. By 3 to 6 months of age, most infants have a more organized sleep pattern, with the bulk of sleep occurring at night, and a total of 14 to 15 hours of sleep a day. Two or three naps a day are common. A one-year-old child requires about 11.5 hours of sleep a day. By 5 years of age, this amount is usually 11 hours; the nine-year-old child requires 10 hours. Naps are gradually consolidated, as the sleep pattern matures. They are usually eliminated by age 3, but may persist to age 5.[24]

Night awakenings are not truly a problem of awakening, which occurs in all children, but a problem of inability to fall back to sleep without parental intervention. The parents may inadvertently reinforce this problem in their attempts to comfort the child upon normal nighttime awakening; thus, the child never learns to fall asleep on his or her own.[23]

Night terrors (pavor nocturnus), *sleepwalking* (somnambulism), and *nightmares* (dream anxiety attacks) all belong to a group of disorders known as *parasomnias.* In adults and older adolescents, these disorders may be a signal of underlying psychopathology; however, in children, they appear to be a normal variant of sleep maturation and associated psychopathology is uncommon.[25]

Diagnostic Considerations. Sleep terrors and nightmares can usually be distinguished by the difference in time of occurrence, recall, ease of awakening, and physical activity. Psychomotor epilepsy may initially appear similar to sleepwalking, but there is a more pronounced postictal phase with the former, and patients are not as likely to return to bed. Epileptic seizures may also mimic sleep terrors, but no past or family history of seizures makes this diagnosis much less likely. An electroencephalogram during an episode will distinguish them.[22,25,26]

Pain, itching, and cough may trigger nonnormal night awakenings. A careful history and physical examination should detect causes of these symptoms.[24]

Diagnostic Findings

Night Awakenings. These usually present as a result of parental sleep disruption. The parents will complain that the child awakens a number of times at night, cries, and will not return to sleep until the parents comfort him. This comforting may be prolonged and involve a ritual. The child may have no other problems, or show other signs of separation difficulties.

Disorders of Arousal. *Sleep terrors* occur in the first third of sleep. The child sits up, screams, and appears frightened and agitated. Further screams or speech may occur, usually incoherent. The child may have movement of arms and legs, including ambulation. Signs of autonomic discharge (fight or flight) are present. Arousal during the episode is quite difficult. The episode typically lasts about 15 minutes, after which the child will again return to normal sleep. There is amnesia for the event in the morning.[22,23,25]

Sleepwalking is characterized by subconscious motor behavior during the first third of sleep, and often within the first hour. The behaviors are commonly simple, such as walking or opening doors, but complex behaviors have been described. The child responds to the environment in a limited fashion, avoiding running into furniture, but not responding to conversation. Violent activity is rare, but injuries due to limited response to the environment may occur. The child is difficult to arouse. The event usually lasts seconds to a few minutes before returning to sleep. Amnesia for the event may be partial or total.[22,25]

Nightmares are distinguished from sleepwalking and sleep terrors by being a rapid eye movement (REM) sleep disturbance. They occur in the latter third of sleep, and are usually recalled well. The nightmare usually contains a threat to the dreamer's physical safety or self-respect. Awakening is relatively easy. Physical activity on the part of the sufferer is rare owing to REM sleep paralysis. Like other parasomnias in children, nightmares do not appear to be associated with psychopathology.[26]

Management. Medical causes of abnormal awakening should be treated as appropriate. Parents should set firm bedtimes that are consistent with the child's age and sleep requirements. For example, a nine-year-old child who has a set bedtime of 9 PM can be expected to awaken at 7 AM. If the child awakens during the night, the parent should wait to see if the child will fall back to sleep. If not, a brief visit to comfort the child is appropriate. The parent should then leave while the child is awake. If the child cries again, the parent may again go to bring comfort, but after a longer delay, and again leave before the child falls asleep. This is continued progressively until the child is able to fall asleep without the parent entering the room. The entire training process may require as long as several weeks if the parents are compliant with the regimen.[24,27]

Sleep terrors and sleep walking are normal variants, and the parents should be assured that this is not a sign of a psychiatric disorder or epilepsy. No medical treatment is needed. Nightmares are also normal variants; parental comforting of the child is reassuring. The parent should not remain in the room until the child has fallen asleep again to avoid creating problems with future sleep transition.[22]

After counseling and reassurance, most of these children can be discharged into their parents' care and have routine follow-up with their regular physician. Families with a great deal of anxiety, anger, or dysfunction due to sleep disruption require close follow-up, and even admission to defuse the situation may be warranted.

IRRITABILITY

Irritability is a relative term—parental expectations and the child's previous behavior provide the best definition. Irritability may result from or be a cause of parental anxi-

---

Etiologies of Irritability

Ear-nose-throat and ophthalmologic
  Otitis media and externa
  Foreign bodies in ear or airway
  Teething
  Pharyngitis
  Corneal abrasion and foreign bodies
Cardiopulmonary
  Hypoxia
  Congestive heart failure
  Tachydysrhythmias
  Pulmonary infections
Abdominal and pelvic
  Abdominal and pelvic pain (variety of etiologies)
  Urinary tract infection
  Gastritis and esophagitis
Musculoskeletal and cutaneous
  Fractures
  Contusions
  Tourniquet syndromes (penis, clitoris, or digit)
  Dermatitis
Neurologic
  Intracranial hematomas
  Meningitis and encephalitis
Endocrine and metabolic
  Electrolyte disturbances (particularly sodium, calcium, and magnesium)
  Hypoglycemia
  Intoxications with a variety of agents
  In utero cocaine exposure
Psychosocial
  Emotional or physical neglect or abuse
  Depression or anxiety in parent

---

ety, and precipitates a significant number of emergency visits. Changes in personality are probably best gauged by parents and are often a reflection of illness or stress in the child or family. Most children have some period of the day when they are most irritable, usually near evening; however, acute onset of irritability requires specific attention.

Differential Considerations. Specific findings will depend on the etiology, and the causes of irritability are legion. The box above lists some of the more frequent ones. Further discussion of causes can be found in other chapters. An etiology that has dramatically increased in recent years is in utero exposure to toxic agents, particularly crack cocaine.[28]

Diagnostic Findings. The one invariable finding in all cases is an alteration in the child's normal personality. Unfortunately for the clinician, the alteration may be transitory, and only the parent's report will provide a clue. These reports should be taken seriously, and a careful evaluation performed.

Colic is episodes of irritability, fussiness, or crying in an infant less than three months old. It occurs in as many as 10% of infants. Carey recommends a definition of over three hours a day, for four or more days a week, and that the crying must be full force.[29] However, if the parents are distressed by the crying, some intervention is usually required.[30] These infants are otherwise healthy, with normal growth. There are no specific findings in colic, and the diagnosis is one of exclusion.

Management. Establishing a diagnosis will direct the physician to appropriate treatment. It will also provide some relief for the parents, who are often very anxious about their child. If no cause can be found, support and reassurance for the parents may be more important. They may blame themselves for the problem, and the guilt they feel may worsen the child's symptoms. Regardless of the therapy or diagnosis, a specific follow-up plan should be developed to provide an outlet for parental anxiety.

Most infants with colic will have spontaneous resolution of their symptoms by 4 months of age. Many treatments have been suggested, but reduction of parental anxiety, and either a reduction in holding or increase in holding the baby may be helpful.[29,30] Changing formulas (with elimination of cow's milk) may improve some cases.[31] This author has found a warm, soothing environment, with a small amount of motion to be effective.

"Crack babies" may be particularly difficult for the emergency physician. The natural parents have (or have had) inherent problems of their own, and foster families may be unfamiliar with the child. These infants tend toward overstimulation and are difficult to comfort and console. Much effort and patience on the part of the family will be required to determine how best to handle each of these children.

Diagnostic Entities

Many, if not most children presenting to the emergency department have some psychosocial problem. This may be anxiety (fear) of pain, strange people, or separation from parents. It may be an adjustment disorder brought on by school change, parental divorce, loss of a sibling, or some other life stress. It may be inappropriate behavior from a variety of etiologies. It may be a major depression or psychosis, with risk of self-harm. The emergency physician must recognize that psychiatric problems not only occur in children, but that they are common. Unless the physician is willing to accept their existence, these problems will go untreated and possibly worsen. The physician must also recognize that organic disorders may mimic many of these conditions and must be excluded before a psychiatric diagnosis is made. Finally, the physician must decide whether the problem can be managed in an outpatient setting or if admission is required, and whether psychiatric consultation is needed.

PSYCHIATRIC ASSESSMENT OF CHILDREN

The goals of the psychiatric assessment are to obtain information in order to make a diagnosis, to make a decision regarding the need for immediate intervention or referral, and to begin the therapeutic process for the family. The psychiatric assessment should ideally take place in a calm, quiet atmosphere and the physician should minimize interruptions and allow adequate time.[32] Reassurance of the patient and parents is a critical part of the evaluation. By diminishing anxiety, more information can usually be gathered and coping mechanisms can be identified and brought into play. The emergency department is often a less-than-ideal environment, but an effort should be made to find a quiet location in which to talk with the family and perform the assessment. The physician must ensure that he or she, the patient, and other individuals in the emergency department are safe. This may require physical or chemical restraint of the patient or the presence of others during the interview. Only when the physician feels secure should interviewing begin.[33]

Authorities differ on who should be to interviewed initially: the child, parent, or both. Interviewing the child or adolescent first allows an assessment unbiased by the parent's report, but may be difficult without some guiding information from the parents. Interviewing the parents first can be useful in talking to the preschool or school aged child, but may increase suspicion in the adolescent that the physician is merely an agent of the parents.[34] The advantage to the last is in observing the interaction of the family members, and obtaining a broad view of the perceived problem. If the child cannot separate from the parents without great difficulty, it is usually best not to force the issue. Otherwise, the choice must be individualized based on the age of the child and the physician's sense of family interaction.

Most children who are brought to a physician with psychiatric or behavioral complaints are not coming of their own free will. Some are unaware of the reason for the visit. Others are well aware of the cause. The former group is often unable or unwilling to provide information to the examiner. The latter group includes children who cannot control their actions, as well as children who use their actions as a cry for help or expression of anger. These children may be psychologically or physically abused, and may come from financially, socially, or emotionally deprived environments. The interviewer must be a sympathetic and interested listener to identify these problems and obtain information from this group. Unless the situation is emergent, do not force or press the patient to answer questions.[32]

Respect should be shown to all patients, but particularly adolescents. They are often suspicious of adults and especially self-conscious. Body language and tone of voice of the examiner are as important as the specific questions asked. False attempts to be "one of the guys" are likely to engender contempt and should be avoided.[34]

During the interview process, both the patient and family members should be queried. School and social workers can also provide valuable information.[35] The interviewer should inquire into the patient's recent and past medical history, social situation, family history, and psychiatric history. Specific questioning should include family tensions and arguments, other personal problems, and activities of daily life (hobbies, friends, pets, school performance, and enjoyment).[32] Particularly important is the perception of each family member (including the patient) regarding the problem. Family members often have very different ideas regarding the problem and varying expectations about treatment and outcome. Past and present stressors are also an important area to address. An acute event usually has precipitated the emergency visit, but the problem will more often have caused and be a result of chronic stress. Actual and potential efforts to harm others or the patient himself must be detected, and the degree of risk established. A physical exam, including neurological, should be completed.

The information obtained may not allow a specific diagnosis to be made, or even whether the problem is organic or functional; however, it should allow an assessment of whether the patient should be admitted or discharged, and whether psychiatric consultation is required immediately or at a later time. When assessment is felt to be inadequate, specialty consultation should be obtained, or the patient admitted until the situation is clarified.

MOOD DISORDERS

Mood disorders are characterized by an alteration in *mood,* "a prolonged emotion that colors the perception of the world."[36] This alteration may be upward (elation), also termed *manic,* or downward (depression). The alteration in mood must extend across a range of situations, and is distinguished from reaction to events such as death of a parent or sibling (although these may contribute to the development of depression).[37] These disorders can appear for brief single episodes, in multiple episodes, or for prolonged periods.

The etiology of mood disorders appears to be multifactorial. A family history of mood disorders increases the chance of their occurrence, even when controlling for environmental influences. Environmental factors such as other mental illness in parents, separation from family, child abuse, medical illness, and many others may play a role in the development of depressive disorders.[37-39] Several biologic factors have been studied, but to date, no one factor has been implicated as the cause of mood disorders.

Depression

Diagnostic Findings. Depression is characterized by a depressed mood (which in children and adolescents may be flattened, sad, or irritable), or a loss of interest or pleasure in most daily activities. The above may be accompanied by significant alteration in weight or appetite; lack of energy; altered sleep pattern; agitation or lethargy; feelings of worthlessness; inability to concentrate; and preoccupation, thoughts, or plans of death. Any four of these, combined with one of the former two, and lasting for two weeks fulfill the DSM-IV criteria for major depressive episode. *Major depressive disorder* consists of one or more major depressive episodes.[36]

The diagnosis of *dysthymic disorder* requires a depressed mood, associated with any two of the following: change in appetite, change in sleep habits, fatigue, diminished self-esteem, hopelessness, and poor concentration. These must be present for a majority of the time for 1 year without major depression.[36]

Depressed mood may be the chief complaint for some patients. More commonly, the child's mood will be demonstrated by the choice of words used, tone, body language, and interaction with the examiner. The clinician will also rely on the parent's report of behavior and emotional state.

Findings displayed by individual patients vary with age. In addition to depressed mood, infants will demonstrate no interest in interaction, and may withdraw from it. Lethargy, poor weight gain, and developmental delay are common. Lack of a nurturing environment, whether due to parental loss or illness or neglect, is the proximate cause in this age group. Preschool aged children may describe themselves as "bad" or "worthless," be overly active or lethargic, and complain of somatic symptoms, notably abdominal pain.[37]

Older children and adolescents have presentation more similar to adults. They are more likely to verbalize cognitive changes such as feelings of hopelessness, guilt, or preoccupation with death. Diminished school performance and withdrawal from friends frequently occur.[40] Suicide plans or thoughts are most common in this age group, but may be seen even in very young children.

Differential Considerations. Organic causes of altered mood to be considered and excluded include brain tumors, drug abuse, and accidental ingestions. Abuse and neglect are causes of depression in young children and may produce similar symptoms in this and other age groups. Conduct disorder, separation anxiety, and schizophrenia may also be confused with depression. Mild mood disturbance secondary to acute psychological stress should be classified as adjustment disorder. Bereavement is likewise excluded from this diagnostic category.

Management. Identification of major depressive disorder or dysthymia, or symptoms suggestive of either, should prompt a psychiatric consultation. This allows treatment to begin as early as possible in the illness. Assessment of the patient's risk of self-injury will lead to the decision to admit or discharge in most cases. When in doubt about the need for inpatient treatment, emergency consultation is advisable or admit the patient until the consultant is available.

Bipolar Disorders

Diagnostic Findings. Bipolar disorders include all conditions in which manic or hypomanic episodes occur. A *manic episode* is defined by a "period of abnormally and persistently elevated, expansive, or irritable mood," markedly impairing function, lasting at least 1 week, and associated with at least three of the following: increased self-esteem, decreased sleep requirements, garrulousness, flight of ideas, easy distractibility, agitation, and risk-taking behavior. A *hypomanic episode* is differentiated by mood being different but not necessarily abnormal, and by change in (not markedly impaired) function.[36]

In addition to the symptoms noted above, patients suffering from mania may act inappropriately, as a result of diminished impulse control and egotism. Recklessness may lead to physical injury. Delusions and hallucinations, often of a grandiose sort, may occur.

Bipolar disorders are divided into *bipolar I disorder,* in which at least one manic episode has occurred usually accompanied by major depressive episodes; *bipolar II disorder,* in which at least one hypomanic episode accompanies a major depressive episode; and *cyclothymic disorder,* in which hypomanic episodes alternate with periods of depressed mood.[36]

Differential Considerations. Bipolar disorders are quite rare in children, but underdiagnosed in adolescents. The latter is due in part to confusion with attention-deficit hyperactivity disorder and conduct disorders. Delusions and hallucinations frequently lead to the (incorrect) diagnosis of schizophrenia. Depending on when the patient is seen, bipolar disorders may be confused with each other and depressive disorders.[38]

Management. Identification of a mood disorder should prompt a psychiatric consultation. Consultation in fairly mild behavioral or emotional symptoms suggestive of a mood disorder can be beneficial by preventing progression to a more serious problem, and allowing treatment to begin as early as possible in the illness. Waiting to see if the disorder will "go away on its own" is inappropriate.[37] Psychotherapy, involving both patient and parents, is usually required. Pharmacologic therapy may be needed as an adjunct, but should be avoided without consultation.

Assessment of the patient's risk of self-injury will lead to the decision to admit or discharge in most cases. When in doubt about the need for inpatient treatment, emergency consultation is advisable, or the patient can be admitted until the consultant is available.

ANXIETY DISORDERS

Disorders in this category are those in which there is an abnormally high level of anxiety. This may occur as a result of excessive reaction to an outside stress, but in some cases, no stress can be identified as the inciting agent. *Anxiety* itself is a sense of fear, uneasiness, or apprehension that keeps the individual at a heightened level of vigilance. Physiologic changes associated with these feelings include tachycardia and tachypnea. Panic attacks, in which the patient has intense fear or discomfort associated with severe somatic symptoms, have been described in children.[41]

Anxiety disorders are more common in certain families. Whether this represents genetic or environmental effects (or both) remains unclear.[42]

Separation Anxiety Disorder

Separation anxiety disorder includes what was previously called *school phobia.* Children with school phobia have a reluctance to attend school associated with anxiety and, particularly in adolescents, symptoms of depression.

Diagnostic Findings. School phobia most commonly occurs with initial entrance into school or with change to a new school. Physical symptoms, including abdominal pain, headache, nausea, and vomiting are common, especially in the morning. These patients often have difficulty in coping with other stresses in daily life. The families tend to be either chaotic and unsupportive, or clinging and encouraging of the behavior.[42,43]

Differential Considerations. School refusal may appear as a symptom of separation anxiety disorder. Generalized anxiety in many different situations is characteristic of overanxiety disorder.[42] School refusal may also represent one aspect of depression. In truancy, there is voluntary avoidance of school, rather than excessive anxiety. If physical complaints predominate, organic etiologies should be considered.

Management. School phobia is best treated with firm insistence that the child attend school. Simultaneously, parents should discuss the child's fears and provide reassurance, as well as encouraging peer relationships. School officials should be alerted to the problem to assist the parents and support the child. The child should see a physician on any day of absence.[44]

Phobias

Fears in children are ubiquitous, but usually transient, and rarely present to the emergency department. *Specific phobias* are more persistent, interfere with normal routines, produce intense anxiety, and lead to avoidance of the phobic stimulus. If the child is afraid of the scrutiny of others or of acting in an embarrassing or humiliating fashion, the term *social phobia* is applied. Pharmacologic management is not appropriate for these problems. Parents should be instructed to be reassuring and supportive; however, follow-up with a longitudinal care provider is often necessary.[45]

SOMATOFORM DISORDERS

The somatoform disorders are a heterogeneous group of conditions in which symptoms (not under the conscious control of the patient) suggesting a physical illness are predominant. Malingering and factitious illness are excluded. Somatization disorder, in which patients have many physical complaints over a long period of time, will not be discussed in detail here. These patients require longitudinal care and should be referred to a pediatrician or psychiatrist for follow-up.[46]

Conversion Disorder

Conversion disorder is the somatic expression of a problem with no organic basis. It represents an attempt to communicate discomfort felt by the patient, a sort of coded message that the patient is unable (for whatever reason) to communicate in words. The trigger may be virtually anything uncomfortable for the patient, and any bodily process that can be perceived may become the focus of the complaint. Conversion reaction is distinguished from malingering in that the former is not a voluntary act.[47]

Diagnostic Findings. Conversion reaction may occur as early as 7 years of age but is more common in adolescence. Girls are affected about twice as often as boys. Education level and socioeconomic status have no correlation with the frequency of occurrence; however, less sophisticated patients tend to produce more "physiologically believable" symptoms. Conversion reaction may present as a group phenomenon (epidemic hysteria).[48]

Any body system can be involved. Common presentations include alteration or loss of sensation, tremors or paralysis, inability to walk or stand, limb pain, headache, abdominal pain, hyperventilation, vomiting, and visual symptoms.[48,49] The presentation can be quite elaborate, with nearly exact duplication of an organic process, or bizarre and easily recognizable as not resulting from an organic cause.

Differential Considerations. Recognition of conversion reaction depends on considering it in the differential diagnosis of somatic complaints. Patients with this disorder are often less willing to talk about stresses in their lives, display emotional lability, and may have a history of multiple unexplained somatic complaints, psychiatric illnesses, and be indifferent to their symptoms. Another family member who has or had similar symptoms, recent stress, or obvious secondary gain from the "illness" should also alert the examiner.[48-50] The symptom invariably serves a purpose (albeit an unconscious one) for the patient. Careful history may elucidate this purpose.

Management. Evaluation of the patient with a possible or suspected conversion reaction must proceed along both functional and organic paths. Demonstration of nonorganic etiology is difficult, if not impossible. The clinician must use judgment in deciding how far to work up organic causes of the patient's symptoms, bearing in mind that both conversion reaction and organic disease may occur simultaneously. Schecker recommends "at the minimum, the normal history, physical, and laboratory examinations undertaken in the emergency department to resolve the differential diagnosis."[50]

If the diagnosis can be established, mild disturbances may be treated with reassurance, and suggestions to decrease attention to and secondary gain from the symptoms. More severe or persistent problems usually require multiple visits, and should be referred to a pediatrician or psychiatrist for follow-up.[50,51] If the diagnosis is uncertain, the need for admission is determined by the possible organic causes. Follow-up should be both medical and psychosocial in nature.

DISRUPTIVE BEHAVIOR DISORDERS

The term *disruptive behavior disorders* encompasses attention-deficit hyperactivity disorder (ADHD), conduct disorder, and oppositional-defiant disorder. There is much overlap in the symptoms seen in all three, and some patients may progress from one to another (e.g., ADHD to conduct disorder). They are characterized by behaviors that intrude, injure, or annoy others and that, at the extreme, are dangerous and destructive. It may be difficult to distinguish between normal behavior and disruptive behavior disorder in less severe cases.

The etiology of these disorders remains unclear. The cause is probably multifactorial; a combination of biochemical, environmental, genetic, and traumatic. They are a particular concern in the long-term care of the brain-injured patient.[52]

Attention-Deficit/Hyperactivity Disorder

Inattention, hyperactivity, and impulsivity (in various combinations) are the hallmarks of ADHD. Currently, children are grouped into three types: predominantly inattentive, predominantly hyperactive-impulsive, and combined.[36] Due to their activity and impulsivity, children in the latter two groups tend to be frequent visitors to the emergency department. Estimates of the frequency of this disorder are 2% to 5% of school-aged children.[53]

Diagnostic Findings. Children suffering from ADHD with hyperactive-impulsive symptoms have difficulty remaining in one place. Even when seated, they tend to squirm and fidget. They are easily distracted by outside stimuli, and have difficulty maintaining attention on the job at hand. They tend to not wait their turn, talk excessively, blurt out answers to uncompleted questions, and interrupt others. They often engage in dangerous activities without considering the consequences.[54] The difference between the above and age-appropriate overactivity is that the latter is organized and the former is not.

Hyperactive-impulsive patients may be seen for injuries resulting from errors in judgment or lack of self-control, or be brought in for their disruptive actions. Children with primarily inattentive symptoms are less likely to come to the emergency department, but may be brought by parents frustrated by poor school performance.

Differential Considerations. Establishing the diagnosis of ADHD requires a significant time investment in observing the child and obtaining thorough history. Due to the emergency department environment, this is usually best accomplished in follow-up. The symptoms of ADHD overlap with other disruptive behavior disorders, as well as personality, anxiety, and mood disorders. Comorbidity of ADHD and other disorders also occurs. Mental retardation, autism, deafness, seizure disorder, Tourette syndrome, substance abuse, and child abuse must all be considered in the differential. As several of these are remediable and the treatment differs widely, the importance lies in assuring appropriate follow-up, and communicating findings and concerns to that person.

Management. The emergency physician should avoid beginning pharmacotherapy for ADHD in the emergency department. Some patients will not require it, and necessary monitoring cannot be assured in the emergency department. An exhaustive evaluation is warranted before initiating drug therapy. In addition to referral to a pediatrician or child psychiatrist, helping the parents to set limits and specify rules represents a good first step in treatment. They should focus on good behaviors, catching the child "being good." From there, a program designed to alter one behavior at a time may begin. Whereas the parents may be able to carry out behavior modification on their own, medical supervision is often needed, and school personnel involvement is almost always necessary.[53,55]

Children may present to the emergency department already on medication for ADHD. These children also deserve careful evaluation and follow-up as noted above. The primary agents used to treat ADHD are the CNS stimulants, including methylphenidate (Ritalin), dextroamphetamine (Dexedrine), and pemoline (Cylert). By enhancing certain neurotransmitters, these drugs may improve behavioral, cognitive, and academic function in some children with ADHD.[56,57] Withdrawal or decreasing the dosage of these medications may unmask ADHD symptoms or lead to depression, whereas increasing the dosage may lead to undesirable side effects such as decreased appetite, insomnia, somatic complaints, or tic disorders. Dosage or medication changes should only be done in consultation with a physician who can provide close follow-up.

The child may be discharged into the parents' care following appropriate counseling and arrangement of follow-up unless the child's behavior is dangerous, or the parents are unable to deal with the situation. In the latter circumstances, admission or immediate psychiatric consultation should be sought.

Conduct Disorder

Conduct disorder is "characterized by a persistent and repetitive pattern of aggressive, noncompliant, intrusive, and poorly self-controlled behaviors that violate either the rights of others or age-appropriate societal norms."[58] Because violent acts and substance abuse can occur in this disorder, it is of special concern for the emergency physician.

Diagnostic Findings. Criteria for diagnosis include intimidation of others, physical threats, assaults (with and without weapons), cruelty, theft, destruction of property, lying, and serious rule/law violations. These must be associated with significant impairment of function in an academic or social setting. The disorder can be classified as mild, moderate, or severe based on both the number of problems and the degree to which others are harmed.[36]

Differential Considerations. Within the above guidelines are virtually endless combinations of symptoms of varying severity. As in ADHD, a thorough evaluation requires a substantial time investment usually not possible in the emergency department. Behaviors resulting from conduct disorder tend to be pervasive, frequent, and severe when compared to usual childhood mischief. Conduct disorder must also be differentiated from lying or disobedience in preschoolers, which is not uncommon.[58,59] *Oppositional defiant disorder* also has elements of hostility and negativity, but is less severe and "does not violate societal norms."[58] This latter diagnosis should be used with caution in ages 18 to 36 months of age as oppositional behavior is normal at that age.

Management. The management of these disorders can be lengthy and frustrating. Protection of health-care workers, the community, and the patient are primary goals. Admission or incarceration may be required depending on the severity of symptoms; clinical judgment combined with input from social, law enforcement, and psychiatric services will facilitate this determination. Longitudinal follow-up is a requirement regardless of the disposition, and should be arranged (personally, when possible) before the patient leaves the emergency department.[52,58,59]

EATING DISORDERS

The disorders in this category are all characterized by "severe disturbances in eating behavior."[36] *Pica* and *rumination disorder* occur primarily in young children, whereas *bulimia nervosa* and *anorexia nervosa* occur almost exclusively in adolescents and may be unrelated to the former two.

Nutritional deficiency (notably iron) can lead to pica, but the condition can also occur without another organic or psychiatric cause.[60] Mental retardation, autism, and schizophrenia are other disorders in which pica appears. Rumination is thought to result from a disordered mother-infant relationship, and may be a form of self-stimulation.[61,62]

The etiology of anorexia and bulimia nervosa is probably multifactorial. Many risk factors for the development of these disorders have been identified, but no single factor appears to be responsible. Increased incidence of concordance in monozygotic twins suggests a genetic factor, but environmental factors, including cultural ideals of beauty and parental expectations are also important. Self-perception (body image), medical illness, and difficulties in autonomy are personal factors associated with these disorders.[63-65]

Diagnostic Findings. Ingestion of nonnutritive substances is the essential feature of pica.[36] Pulling and eating of hair (trichotillomania), paint chips, dirt, and paper, as well as other items is seen. The child may eat a regular diet in addition to the above. Toxicity from the ingestion, such as lead from paint chips, must be considered. Most cases resolve by school age, but the condition may persist into adulthood.

Rumination is regurgitation of food with rechewing and subsequent reswallowing or ejection from the mouth.[36] Rumination usually starts between 3 and 12 months of age, but may begin later in those with mental retardation. This activity is not accompanied by nausea, retching, or other signs of distress, and in fact may seem pleasurable to the infant. Infants with this disorder often are irritable and hungry between rumination episodes, and inadequate weight gain is the rule. Without intervention, life-threatening weight loss can occur.

Anorexia nervosa is characterized by inability to maintain a body weight more than 15% below that predicted by height and age, accompanied by fear of gaining weight or becoming fat, and a distorted body self-image (i.e., perception of being fat even when quite thin). Females account for 95% of the cases, and often have amenorrhea as well. Onset is typically in adolescence, but may occur earlier or later. Although the majority of cases will only have a single episode, other patients will suffer persistent or recurrent episodes, with males at particular risk. Mortality rates from 5% to 18% have been reported.[65,66]

Patients with bulimia nervosa suffer from recurrent attacks of binge eating in which large volumes of food will be consumed. This activity is associated with a feeling of loss of control over eating habits. The bulimic also practices some act to prevent weight gain such as forced vomiting, purging with laxatives, or fasting. Bulimics have an "overconcern with body shape and weight," and must have an average of two episodes per week for 3 months to fulfill DSM-IV criteria. Bulimia is more likely to occur in females, and to start in adolescence or early adulthood.[36,65,67] Body weight may be normal or above normal, and activities of daily living are often unaffected.

Differential Considerations. Pica as a primary disorder must be distinguished from pica resulting from nutritional deficiency. This relatively straightforward determination can be made by excluding iron-deficiency anemia. Observation and history should exclude other psychiatric causes. If rumination itself is observed, the diagnosis is assured. If only vomiting is seen, then organic causes of vomiting (e.g., bowel obstruction) must be ruled out.

Anorexia can be differentiated from bulimia by body weight below normal minimums. In the emaciated patient, organic causes and other psychiatric illness should usually be excluded by lack of historical or physical findings. If doubt exists, further evaluation can be performed as indicated.[68]

Management. Management of eating disorders in the emergency department involves exclusion of organic disease, assessment of the severity of illness and need for admission, and arrangement of follow-up. Treatment of pica should also involve removing potential ingestants from the reach of the child and careful observation. Increased stimulation and careful feeding with increased parental involvement have been suggested as helpful in rumination syndrome.[62,69] Patients with anorexia, and especially bulimia, may have severe electrolyte disturbances or dehydration and require immediate fluid therapy. In anorexia, bulimia, and rumination, early restoration of adequate nutrition is the primary goal.[65,66]

Longitudinal follow-up of all eating disorder patients is mandatory. Careful monitoring of weight and physical condition, in addition to behavioral and psychiatric treatment is needed. Patients whose weight loss or physical condition has deteriorated substantially usually require admission to stabilize the situation. Similarly, those in which follow-up is uncertain should be admitted. If the decision to discharge is made, follow-up with a specific physician (whether pediatrician or psychiatrist) or facility should be arranged.

TIC DISORDERS

Tics are a common problem in childhood, occurring in 4% to 10% of children. The vast majority are simple tics of brief duration and spontaneous duration; some children will have complex or persistent symptoms with significant social impairment.

Tourette syndrome is manifested by multiple motor and vocal tics, changing with time, occurring many times a day, persisting for over a year. If only motor or vocal tics occur, the disorder is termed *chronic motor disorder* or *vocal tic disorder. Transient tic disorder* refers to those cases in which single or multiple tics occur many times a day for a period of at least 2 weeks, but not greater than a year.[36] Many children will have tics that do not meet the criteria above because of low frequency of occurrence or brief duration.[70]

Studies suggest that Tourette syndrome is inherited in an autosomal dominant fashion with variable penetrance. The etiology appears to lie in dysfunction of dopaminergic, as well as adrenergic, serotonergic, and cholinergic neurotransmitter systems, but the exact problem remains elusive.[71] Environmental factors also seem to be involved. Other tic disorders, and even the transient simple tics may represent a continuum, with Tourette being the worst case scenario.

Diagnostic Findings. Tics range from simple acts such as eye blinking, head nodding, grunting, or sighing to more complex tasks, such as posturing, smelling an object, echokinesis (imitation of another's movements), coprolalia (use of scatology), echolalia (repeating a speaker's words), or palilalia (repeating one's own words). Tics are involuntary, but usually disappear or lessen during sleep or with intense concentration such as reading or studying. They often worsen with stress. Social discomfort, depression, and shame may be present as a result of the tics, and can significantly impair the patient's ability to function. Tics may have their onset as early as 2 years of age, and rarely later than early adolescence. Depending on their frequency, the clinician may have to rely on the parent's observations to arrive at a tentative diagnosis.[70]

Differential Considerations. The diagnosis is often obvious after observation of the patient for a time, but tic disorder must be distinguished from myoclonus (more shocklike and less complex), chorea (less stereotyped), athetosis (slower and writhing), and hemiballismus (sudden flinging of an extremity).[70]

Head banging, body rocking, bruxism, breath holding, and nose-picking are "intentional and repetitive behaviors that are nonfunctional." If they cause physical injury or "markedly interfere with normal activities," these are included in the *stereotypic movement disorder* in DSM-IV, and are not tic disorders; otherwise, they are considered a normal variant.

Management. Transient tics should be treated with parental reassurance and benign neglect. If the tic disorder is very disturbing to the patient or family, referral to a pediatrician or psychiatrist is indicated. Pharmacotherapy is not indicated in the emergency department. Tic disorders rarely require admission unless the patient is so distressed by the symptoms as to consider harm to himself or herself.

DISORDERS WITH PSYCHOTIC FEATURES

Psychosis is an altered contact with reality. The disorders discussed in this section all have psychosis in common. Functional psychotic disorders are uncommon in childhood, and a child presenting with psychosis in the emergency department deserves a thorough search for an organic etiology.

Pervasive developmental disorders include the subtypes of *autistic disorder, Rett disorder, Asperger disorder, childhood disintegrative disorder,* and pervasive developmental disorder not otherwise specified (PDDNOS). In these disorders, there is a marked impairment in reciprocal social interaction, communication skills, or a limited variety of behaviors, interests, and activities. Onset is in infancy or childhood, and delusions, hallucinations, and loosening of associations are not present.[36]

Schizophrenia is defined by the presence of any two of the following: (1) hallucinations, delusions, catatonia, inappropriate or flat affect, and loosening of associations; (2) bizarre delusions; or (3) prominent hallucinations involving a voice or voices discussing the person's actions or thoughts. Functional impairment must be present, other disorders must be excluded, and the duration of symptoms must be longer than 6 months' duration.[36]

The many causes of psychosis will be discussed in the following section on Differential Considerations. Psychotic disorders appear to have a multifactorial etiology in which genetic predisposition plays an important role.[72]

Diagnostic Findings

Pervasive Developmental Disorders. Autistic disorder has an onset before the age of 36 months. Many parents note abnormal interaction in infants as young as 2 months. This is marked not only by delays in development, but in aberrant development. Communication skills are usually severely impaired, and this may be detectable in the preverbal stages. Both receptive and expressive communication can be impaired. Social skills are similarly impaired, often with avoidance of interaction with others. Other findings include unusual and erratic reactions to external stimuli, repetitive and self-stimulating behaviors, stereotyped body movements, and preoccupation with details (particularly parts of objects). It is usually quite obvious to the clinician that these children have some disorder, due to the gross impairment in interaction.[72-74]

Whereas children with autistic disorder will suffer problems in all the areas mentioned above and are frequently noted to be abnormal in early infancy, those with Asperger disorder have normal language and cognitive development. Rett disorder occurs only in females and is characterized by normal development until at least 5 months of age, followed by deceleration of head growth and severe psychomotor retardation with loss of previously acquired skills. Childhood disintegrative disorder victims may have abnormalities in all areas mentioned, but have at least 2 years of normal development before onset.[36,74]

Childhood Schizophrenia. Whether this entity exists before 5 years of age is a matter of debate. The symptoms are difficult to recognize in younger children, primarily due to lack of verbal skills. Children with schizophrenia present similarly to adults. Delusions, especially of outside forces controlling the patient are common. Hallucinations, most frequently auditory, may be present.[75] Emotional reactions are blunted (flat affect) or inappropriate, and patients relate a disinterest in normal activities. Bizarre movements, social isolation, impulsiveness, and loss of identity are also seen. Paranoid schizophrenia is rare in childhood, but may occur in adolescents. These patients may present with almost any behavior, including violence and sexual acting out, or be withdrawn and quiet.

Differential Considerations. As noted above, psychosis in childhood is more likely to be a result of organic causes than a purely psychiatric disorder. Toxic, metabolic, traumatic, and infectious etiologies must be excluded in the emergency department evaluation of childhood psychosis. A list of organic etiologies of psychosis is presented in Table 58-1, with mechanisms to differentiate them. In general, organic psychoses tend to have abrupt onset, with no past or family history of similar problems. Physical examination, vital signs, and level of consciousness are more frequently altered than with functional causes.[76]

In addition to excluding organic causes, other psychiatric causes of psychosis must be considered. Mood disorders, particularly bipolar disorders, can produce psychosis. It is important to distinguish these, as the therapy is quite different. If psychosis is of brief duration (less than 1 month) and occurs within a short time of a severe stress (e.g., loss of a loved one), a diagnosis of *brief reactive psychosis* is likely. Symptoms of schizophrenia for a period less than 6 months are consistent with *schizophreniform disorder.* *Schizoaffective disorder* is a grab-bag including those cases with both a schizophrenic and mood disturbance that do not meet the criteria for either.[36]

Finally, the clinician should be wary of false-positive responses to questions regarding delusions and hallucinations with younger children, because they lack understanding of such questions.[77]

Management. Management of these disorders in the emergency department centers on excluding organic causes of psychosis and obtaining prompt psychiatric consultation. Patients who are out of control may require acute administration of psychopharmacologic agents.[78] Table 58-2 lists several of these agents with dosages and potential

TABLE 58-1. Organic Etiologies of Childhood Psychosis

Etiology	Diagnostic test
Toxic	
Drugs of abuse	Toxicologic screens, physical examination
Alcohol, cocaine, PCP, LSD, amphetamines, marijuana	
Prescription drugs	Toxicologic screens, physical examination
Tricyclic antidepressants, phenobarbital, phenytoin, isoniazid, benzodiazepines, captopril, digitalis, corticosteroids	
OTC drugs	Toxicologic screens, physical examination
Antihistamines, decongestants, antitussives	
Metabolic	
Electrolyte alterations	Blood chemistry
Hypothyroidism and hyperthyroidism	Examination, thyroid function tests
Cushing and Addison diseases	Examination, cortisol levels
Vitamin deficiencies	Examination, history of inadequate diet
Hepatic dysfunction	Liver function tests, ammonia
Renal dysfunction	Urinalysis, creatinine, BUN
Diabetic ketoacidosis	Blood chemistry, glucose, history
Hypoglycemia	Blood glucose, history of diabetes
Traumatic	
Subdural hematoma	History, examination, CT scan
Cerebral contusion	History, examination, CT scan
Infectious	
Meningitis, encephalitis	Examination, CSF examination
Pneumonia	Examination, chest x-ray film
Typhoid fever	History, examination, stool culture
Rocky Mountain spotted fever	History, examination, serology
Syphilis	Serology, CSF examination
Malaria	History, blood smear
Sepsis	Examination, cultures
Other	
Hypoxia	Examination, blood gas, oximetry
Anemia	Examination, hemoglobin, hematocrit
Shock	Examination
Collagen vascular disease	History, examination, serology

side effects. Physical restraint may also be needed. Due to their lack of touch with reality, these patients should always be treated with caution, even when docile. Regardless of the etiology, all children with acute psychosis should be admitted for observation and treatment.

TABLE 58-2. Emergency Psychopharmacologics

Drug	Dose (maximum)	Route	Important side effects
Diphenhydramine	1 mg/kg (100 mg)	PO, IM, IV	Sedation, (hypotension with IV)
Lorazepam	0.05 mg/kg (4 mg)	IM	Sedation, respiratory embarrassment
	0.04 mg/kg (2 mg)	IV	
Chlorpromazine	0.5 mg/kg (25 mg)	IM	Dystonia, hypotension, autonomic symptoms, sedation
	1.0 mg/kg (100 mg)	PR	
Thioridazine	0.5 mg/kg (100 mg)	PO	Dystonia, autonomic symptoms, sedation

PO, By mouth; *IM,* intramuscular; *IV,* intravenous; *PR,* per rectum.

SUICIDE

A *suicide attempt* is any act of non-fatal self-injury with intention to harm or call attention to oneself.[79] *Suicide* (completed suicide) occurs if the attempt results in death. Despite efforts to reduce it, suicide continues to increase in the 15-19 year age group, and has *more than doubled in the 10-14 year age group* in the latest available figures.[80] Younger children are also affected, although suicide is only rarely reported in the five to nine age group. All of these figures undoubtedly understate the problem.[81,82]

In addition to the completed suicides and attempts, a third group of "unintentional" attempters has been described. These patients had self-inflicted injuries, but denied suicidal intent. Unfortunately, these patients had as high a rate of previous suicide attempts as the intentional group, but a much lower rate of psychiatric intervention.[79]

Diagnostic Findings. A number of factors are associated with an increased risk of suicidal behavior. These are listed in the box at right. Caucasians and Native Americans are more likely to engage in suicidal behavior. Suicide and suicide attempts become more frequent with advancing age. Girls attempt suicide at least three times as frequently as boys, but boys outnumber girls in completing suicides by about 4:1 because they tend to use more effective means such as firearms and hanging.[83] Second attempts are most common within 3 months of the initial event.[84]

Any child who presents with evidence of self-injury deserves consideration of suicidal intent. The alert clinician will also suspect suicidal behavior in patients with less obvious injuries, particularly those with several of the characteristics noted above. Although the evaluation of suicidal intent is ideally performed by a psychiatrist, this may not be possible in every case. The emergency physician should not be afraid to bring up the subject and discuss it with children, regardless of age.

Interviewing should include a discussion of the events preceding the injury-attempt. The patient's reactions and emotions to these events, as well as the facts themselves should be noted.[85,86] Following this, the patient's past and family medical history, including psychiatric illnesses, previous suicide attempts, and any previous self-inflicted injuries should be reviewed. Social history, including family discord, absences, or loss, can be analyzed.

The suicide attempt itself must be evaluated for lethality, chance of discovery, planning, and patient intent. Lethality is usually determined by method. Shooting oneself in the head is clearly more lethal than taking 10 aspirin. A lower

---

Risk Factors for Suicidal Behavior

Psychiatric illness
    Mood disorders
    Psychosis
    Conduct disorders
    Family history of mood disorders and suicide
Substance abuse
Past suicide attempts
Personality
    Hopeless
    Hostile
    Impulsive
    Perfectionism
    Poor social skills
Environmental
    Abused or neglected
    Parental absence or discord
    Exposure to suicide
    Stress (especially multiple)
Seizure disorder

---

chance of discovery also suggests a higher level of lethality. Well-planned attempts may be more lethal, but also suggest a lengthier problem, with greater potential for future attempts. Patient intent is extremely important. The patient taking 10 aspirin in the belief they were truly deadly is at greater risk than the patient taking 100 acetaminophen thinking they were just like candy.

Family members should be interviewed to determine their interest in the patient, perception of the seriousness of the incident, and ability to observe the patient, as well as confirm details of the attempt.

Finally, an assessment of the patient's risk of recurrence, based on continuing suicidal ideation and ability to carry out a plan must be performed.[82-84,87]

Management. Medical management of suicide attempts depends on the method chosen and resulting injuries. Psychiatric management will depend on the results of the evaluation described previously. In the emergency department it is imperative that the patient be prevented from further harming himself. This may require physical restraint, and at the least, close observation.

Most of these patients will need admission. Only those with no medical need for observation or treatment, *and* with virtually no risk for recurrence, *and* with family members available and competent to watch and assure follow-up should be discharged from the emergency department. Psychiatric consultation should be obtained before discharge. If admission is required, the assessment of further suicide potential should be communicated to the inpatient staff, and appropriate precautions taken.

Many patients at risk for suicide present to the emergency department for other reasons than a suicide attempt. The emergency physician should evaluate a child or adolescent with depression, psychosis, or any of the risk factors noted above in a similar fashion, and obtain psychiatric consultation if the risk of suicidal behavior appears significant. Even if psychiatric consultation is not needed, the presence of risk factors indicates a need for medical follow-up.[79,83,84]

SUBSTANCE ABUSE

Despite an overall decline in the prevalence of substance abuse among Americans of high-school age in the 1980s, abuse of alcohol, illicit, and prescription drugs remains a major problem. Abuse of marijuana, LSD, and amphetamines has been on the rise in the 90s. Usage of alcohol and tobacco products remained high during the 1980s, and is even higher in the 1990s. Worse yet, we are seeing younger children abusing these drugs, often on a regular basis.[88] Substance abuse is a significant risk factor in suicide, and is associated with other psychiatric disorders, notably depression.[89,90] When it occurs in conjunction with other psychiatric disorders, substance abuse may result from the disorder, exacerbate the disorder, or uncover a latent disorder. *Substance abuse must be considered in any patient presenting with psychiatric complaints or symptoms.* Appropriate evaluation to exclude drug effects should be completed and any necessary treatment begun in the emergency department before making a disposition of these patients.

A detailed discussion of substance abuse is beyond the scope of this chapter, and comprehensive emergency department management can be found in other sources.[91,92]

References

Evaluation of the Disturbed Child

1. Rutter M, Tizard J, Whitmore K: *Education, Health, and Behavior*, London, 1970, Longman.
2. Costello EJ: Primary care pediatrics and child psychopathology: a review of diagnostic, treatment, and referral practices, *Pediatrics* 78:1044-1051, 1986.

Enuresis

3. Novello AC & Novello JR: Enuresis, *Pediatr Clin North Am* 34:719-733, 1987.
4. Hurley RM: Enuresis: the difference between day and night, *Pediatr Rev* 12:167-170, 1990.
5. Maizels M, Gandhi K, Keating B, et al: Diagnosis and treatment for children who cannot control urination, *Curr Probl Pediatr* 23:402-50, 1993.
6. Readett DRJ, Morris J, Serjeant GR: Determinants of nocturnal enuresis in homozygous sickle cell disease, *Arch Dis Chi* 65:615-618, 1990.
7. Readett DRJ, Morris JS, Serjeant GR: Nocturnal enuresis in sickle cell haemoglobinopathies, *Arch Dis Chi* 65:290-293, 1990.

8. Klevan JL & De Jong AR: Urinary tract symptoms and urinary tract infection following sexual abuse, *Am J Dis Child* 144:242-244, 1990.
9. Alon US: Nocturnal enuresis, *Pediatr Nephrol* 9:94-103, 1995.
10. O'Regan S, Yazbeck S, Hamberger B, et al: Constipation a commonly unrecognized cause of enuresis, *Am J Dis Child* 140:260-261, 1986.
11. Scharf MB, Pravda MF, Jennings SW, et al: Childhood enuresis. A comprehensive treatment program, *Pediatr Clin North Am* 10:655-665, 1987.
12. Fergusson DM, Horwood LJ, Shannon FT: Factors related to the age of attainment of nocturnal bladder control: an 8-year longitudinal study, *Pediatrics* 78:884-890, 1986.
13. Foxman B, Valdez RB, Brook RH: Childhood enuresis: prevalence, perceived impact, and prescribed treatments, *Pediatrics* 77:482-487, 1986.
14. Howe AC & Walker CE: Behavioral management of toilet training, enuresis, and encopresis. *Pediatr Clin North Am* 39:413-32, 1992.

Encopresis

15. Hatch TF: Encopresis and constipation in children, *Pediatr Clin North Am* 35:257-280, 1988.
16. Nolan T and Oberklaid F: New concepts in the management of encopresis, *Pediatr Rev* 14:447-51, 1993.
17. Amsterdam B: Chronic encopresis: a system based psychodynamic approach, *Child Psychiatry Hum Dev* 9:137-44, 1979.
18. Rappaport LA, Levine MD: The prevention of constipation and encopresis: a developmental model and approach, *Pediatr Clin North Am* 33:859-869, 1986.
19. Gabel S, Chandra R, Shindledecker R: Behavioral ratings and outcome of medical treatment for encopresis, *J Dev Behav Pediatr* 9:129-133, 1988.
20. Levine MD: Encopresis: its potentiation, evaluation, and alleviation, *Pediatr Clin North Am* 29:315-330, 1982.
21. Seth R & Heyman MB: Management of constipation and encopresis in infants and children, *Gastroenterol Clin North Am* 23:621-36, 1994.

Sleep Disturbances

22. Lozoff B, Zuckerman B: Sleep problems in children, *Pediatr Rev* 10:17-24, 1988.
23. Ferber RA: Behavioral "insomnia" in the child, *Psychiatr Clin North Am* 10:641-653, 1987.
24. Ferber R: Sleeplessness, night awakening, and night crying in the infant and toddler, *Pediatr Rev* 9:69-82, 1987.
25. Thorpy MJ & Glovinsky PB: Parasomnias, *Psychiatr Clin North Am* 10:623-639, 1987.
26. Erman MK: Dream anxiety attacks (nightmares), *Psychiatr Clin North Am* 10:667-674, 1987.
27. Schmitt BD: The "two-step" approach to infant sleep problems, *Contemp Pediatr* 9:37-38, 1992.

Irritability

28. Hawley TL: New developments: the development of cocaine-exposed children, *Curr Probl Pediatr* 24:259-266, 1994.
29. Carey WB: Colic—Primary excessive crying as an infant-environment interaction, *Pediatr Clin North Am* 31:993-1005, 1984.
30. Schmitt BD: The prevention of sleep problems and colic, *Pediatr Clin North Am* 33:763-774, 1986.
31. Forsyth BWC: Colic and the effect of changing formulas: a double-blind, multiple crossover study, *J Pediatr* 115:521-526, 1989.

Psychiatric Assessment of Children

32. Jellinek MS: Interviewing in pediatric outpatient practice, *Curr Probl Pediatr* 20:575-588, 1990.
33. Sugar J: Emergency ward triage. In Jellinek MS, Herzog DB, editors: Massachusetts General Hospital Psychiatric Aspects of General Hospital Pediatrics, Chicago, 1990, Year Book.
34. Lucas SE, Spear B, Daniel WA: Interviewing the adolescent, *Pediatr Ann* 15:811-814, 1986.
35. Brent DA: Psychiatric assessment of the school age child, *Pediatr Ann* 14:371-375, 1985.

Mood Disorders

36. American Psychiatric Association: Diagnostic and statistical manual of mental disorders, Washington, DC, American Psychiatric Association, 1994.

37. Seagull EA: Childhood depression, *Curr Probl Pediatr* 20:707-755, 1990.
38. Carlson GA: Bipolar disorders in children and adolescents. In Garfinkel BD & Carlson GA, Weller EB, editors: *Psychiatric disorders in children and adolescents*, Philadelphia, 1990, WB Saunders.
39. Weller EB & Weller RA: Depressive disorders in children and adolescents, In Garfinkel BD, Carlson GA, Weller EB, editors: Psychiatric disorders in children and adolescents, Philadelphia, 1990, WB Saunders.
40. Schowalter JE: Depression in children and adolescents, *Pediatr Rev* 3:51-55, 1981.

Anxiety Disorders

41. Swedo SE, Leonard HL, Allen AJ: New developments in childhood affective and anxiety disorders, *Curr Probl Pediatr* 24:12-38, 1994.
42. Bernstein GA: Anxiety disorders, In Garfinkel BD, Carlson GA, Weller EB, editors: Psychiatric disorders in children and adolescents, Philadelphia, 1990, WB Saunders.
43. Mattison RE: Pediatric management of anxiety disorders, *Pediatr Ann* 18:114-118, 1989.
44. Schmitt BD: When your child has school phobia, *Contemp Pediatr* 7:41-42, 1990.
45. Schowalter JE: Fears and phobias, *Pediatr Rev* 15:384-388, 1994.

Somatoform Disorders

46. Rickert VI & Jay MS: Psychosomatic disorders: the approach, *Pediatr Rev* 15:448-454, 1994.
47. Purcell TB: The somatic patient, *Emerg Med Clin North Am* 9:137-159, 1991.
48. Prazar G: Conversion reactions in adolescents, *Pediatr Rev* 8:279-286, 1987.
49. Schecker N: Childhood conversion reactions in the emergency department: part 2—general and specific features, *Pediatr Emerg Care* 6:46-51, 1990.
50. Schecker NH: Childhood conversion reactions in the emergency department: part 1—diagnostic and management approaches within a biopsychosocial framework, *Pediatr Emerg Care* 3:202-208, 1987.
51. Hodgman CH: Conversion and somatization in pediatrics, *Pediatr Rev* 16:29-36, 1995.

Disruptive Behavior Disorders

52. Gerring JP: Psychiatric sequelae of severe closed head injury, *Pediatr Rev* 8:115-121, 1986.
53. Rostain AL: Attention deficit disorders in children and adolescents, *Pediatr Clin North Am* 38:607-635, 1991.
54. Coleman WL & Levine MD: Attention deficits in adolescence: description, evaluation, and management, *Pediatr Rev* 9:287-298, 1988.
55. Baren M: Managing ADHD, *Contemp Pediatr* 11:29-48, 1994.
56. Barkley RA & Murphy JV: Treating attention-deficit hyperactivity disorder: medication and behavior management training, *Pediatr Ann* 20:256-266, 1991.
57. Culbert TP, Banez GA, Reiff MI: Children who have attentional disorders: interventions, *Pediatr Rev* 1994; 15:5-14.
58. Gottlieb SE & Friedman SB: Conduct disorders in children and adolescents, *Pediatr Rev* 12:218-223, 1991.
59. Lewis DO: Conduct disorders. In Garfinkel BD, Carlson GA, Weller EB, editors: *Psychiatric disorders in children and adolescents*, Philadelphia, 1990, WB Saunders.

Eating Disorders

60. Pearson HA: The nutritional anemias. In Oski FA, DeAngelis CD, Feigin RD et al, editors: Principles and practice of pediatrics, Philadelphia, 1990, JB Lippincott.
61. Richmond JB, Eddy E, Green M: Rumination: a psychosomatic syndrome of infancy, *Pediatrics* 1958; 22:49-55.
62. Sheagren TG, Mangurten HH, Brea F, et al: Rumination—a new complication of neonatal intensive care, *Pediatrics* 66:551-555, 1980.
63. Comerci GD & Williams RL: Eating disorders in the young. Part 1: anorexia nervosa and bulimia, *Curr Probl Pediatr* 15:1-57, 1985.
64. Goldbloom DS & Garfinkel PE: Eating disorders: anorexia nervosa and bulimia nervosa. In Garfinkel BD, Carlson GA, Weller EB, editors: Psychiatric disorders in children and adolescents, Philadelphia, WB Saunders, 1990.
65. Harper G: Eating disorders in adolescence, *Pediatr Rev* 15:72-77, 1994.

66. Comerci GD: Eating disorders in adolescents, *Pediatr Rev* 10:37-47, 1988.
67. Woodside DB: A review of anorexia nervosa and bulimia nervosa, *Curr Probl Pediatr* 25:67-89, 1995.
68. Wright K, Smith MS, Mitchell J: Organic diseases mimicking atypical eating disorders, *Clin Pediatr* 29:325-328, 1990.
69. Fleisher DR: Infant rumination syndrome, *Am J Dis Child* 133:266-269, 1979.

Tic Disorders

70. Golden GS: Tic disorders in childhood, *Pediatr Rev* 8:229-233, 1987.
71. Barabas G: Tourette's syndrome: an overview, *Pediatr Ann* 17:391-393, 1988.

Disorders with Psychotic Features

72. Pomeroy JC: Infantile autism and childhood psychosis, In Garfinkel BD, Carlson GA, Weller EB, editors: Psychiatric disorders in children and adolescents, Philadelphia, 1990, WB Saunders.
73. Stone WL, Lemanek KL, Fishel PT et al: Play and imitation skills in the diagnosis of autism in young children, *Pediatrics* 86:267-272, 1990.
74. Bauer S: Autism and the pervasive developmental disorders: part 1. *Pediatr Rev* 16:130-136, 1995.
75. Kemph JP: Hallucinations in psychotic children, *J Am Acad Child Adolesc Psychiatry* 26:556-559, 1987.
76. Frame DS, Kercher EE: Acute psychosis. Functional versus organic, *Emerg Med Clin North Am* 9:123-136, 1991.
77. Breslau N: Inquiring about the bizarre: false positives in diagnostic interview schedule for children (DISC) ascertainment of obsessions, compulsions, and psychotic symptoms, *J Am Acad Child Adolesc Psychiatry* 26:639-644, 1987.
78. Biederman J, Steingard R: Psychopharmacology for children and adolescents, In Jellinek MS, Herzog DB, editors: Massachusetts General Hospital Psychiatric Aspects of General Hospital Pediatrics, Chicago, 1990, Year Book.

Suicide

79. Trautman PD, Shaffer D: Pediatric management of suicidal behavior. *Pediatr Ann* 18:134-143, 1989.
80. CDC: Suicide among children, adolescents, and young adults—United States, 1980-1992, *MMWR* 44:289-291, 1995.
81. Holinger PC: The causes, impact, and preventability of childhood injuries in the United States. Childhood suicide in the United States, *Am J Dis Child* 144:670-676, 1990.
82. Shaw KR, Sheehan KH, Fernandez RC: Suicide in children and adolescents, *Adv Pediatr* 34:313-334, 1987.
83. Brent DA, Kolko DJ: Suicide and suicidal behavior in children and adolescents, In Garfinkel BD, Carlson GA, Weller EB, editors: *Psychiatric disorders in children and adolescents*, Philadelphia, 1990, WB Saunders.
84. Brent DA: Suicide and suicidal behavior in children and adolescents, *Pediatr Rev* 10:269-275, 1989.
85. Pearce CM, Martin G: Predicting suicide attempts among adolescents, *Acta Psychiatr Scand* 90:324-8, 1994.
86. Cappelli M, Clulow MK, Goodman JT et al: Identifying depressed and suicidal adolescents in a teen health clinic, *J Adolesc Health* 16:64-70, 1995.
87. Pfeffer CR: Assessment of suicidal children and adolescents, *Psychiatr Clin North Am* 12:861-872, 1989.

Substance Abuse

88. O'Malley PM, Johnston LD, Bachman JG: Adolescent substance use: epidemiology and implications for public policy, *Pediatr Clin North Am* 42:241-260, 1995.
89. Berman AL, Schwartz RH: Suicide attempts among adolescent drug users, *Am J Dis Child* 144:310-314, 1990.
90. Armentano ME: Assessment, diagnosis, and treatment of the dually diagnosed adolescent, *Pediatr Clin North Am* 42:479-490, 1995.
91. Savitt DL, Roberts JR, Merigian KS: Psychoactive drug abuse. In Rosen P, Barkin RM, Braen GR et al: editors: *Emergency medicine: concepts and clinical practice*, St Louis, 1992, Mosby.
92. Rogers PD, Speraw SR, Ozbek I: The assessment of the identified substance-abusing adolescent, *Pediatr Clin North Am* 42:351-370, 1995.

Respiratory Disorders

MARY A. LETOURNEAU • *SUZANNE SCHUH*
Marianne Gausche

Signs and Symptoms

APNEA

Apnea is defined as a cessation of breathing for 20 seconds or longer, or a shorter respiratory pause associated with bradycardia, cyanosis, or pallor (see box on p. 1057).[1,2] It must be distinguished from normal sleep breathing patterns, which consist of alternating periods of regular breathing and respiratory pauses of 10 seconds without color change in up to 3% of sleep time.[3] Normal newborns, especially premature infants, may demonstrate periodic breathing, which is a regular recurrence of respiratory pauses of 3 seconds or more, followed by a breathing period of 20 seconds or less, repeated at least three times (see box on p. 1116).[4] There is no evidence that increased amounts of periodic breathing in infants have any adverse prognostic significance if hypoxemia does not occur.[5] The term *apparent life-threatening event* (ALTE) describes an episode characterized by a combination of apnea, color change (usually cyanosis but occasionally erythema or plethora), marked change in muscle tone (usually limp-

ness), and choking or gagging. This condition was previously known as *near-miss SIDS* (Sudden Infant Death Syndrome), and the term ALTE was introduced to eliminate the unclear connection between apnea and SIDS.[6]

Apnea can be either central or obstructive. Central apnea is marked by an absence of respiratory effort that results from the lack of activation of the musculature producing air flow. Obstructive apnea occurs when airflow ceases even though respiratory effort with chest and abdominal breathing continues.[3] Mixed apnea may also exist, with the central type usually occurring after the obstructive type.[7]

The evaluation of apnea can pose problems with diagnosis and subsequent management. The underlying cause of apnea is often difficult to identify. However, the presence of apnea requires immediate diagnostic evaluation and treatment; consequences can include neurologic sequelae, cor pulmonale, and sudden death.[8] Because there is still no reliable method to predict or prevent SIDS, apnea of infancy and ALTE continue to be focused on as possible precursors to SIDS, although the relationship is unclear[5] (see later section in this chapter).

Pathophysiology

Normal respiratory activity is controlled through respiratory centers in the pons and medulla. These centers receive afferent input from peripheral and central chemoreceptors, airway and lung receptors, and the cerebral and reticular activating systems. The peripheral carotid and aortic bodies are primarily sensitive to hypoxemia, whereas the central medullary chemoreceptor is primarily sensitive to hydrogen ion concentration and responds to changes in arterial Pco_2 or pH.[5] The efferent impulses from the respiratory centers travel via the vagus, phrenic, and intercostal nerves to produce muscular contraction and respiratory effort. Ventilation depends on the orderly sequence of muscular contraction.[8] Contraction of the upper airway muscles is necessary to maintain patency of the upper airway. The negative pressure generated by the diaphragm, combined with contraction of the intercostal muscles, allows the normal bellows function of the respiratory cycle.[8]

Normal sleep produces changes in muscular tone and the control of ventilation. During rapid eye movement (REM) sleep, there is a depression of all skeletal muscle tone, including the upper airway and intercostal muscles,

Apnea of Infancy: Differential Considerations

Infection
Lower respiratory tract (RSV and pertussis)
Pneumonia
Sepsis
Meningitis
Encephalitis

Central nervous system
Seizures
Intracranial hemorrhage
Increased intracranial pressure
Central hypoventilation
Encephalopathy

Gastrointestinal system
Gastroesophageal reflux
Swallowing disorders
Tracheoesophageal fistula

Pulmonary system
Respiratory distress syndrome
Pulmonary edema
Pulmonary hemorrhage
Hypoplastic lung

Cardiovascular system
Congenital heart disease
Shock
Dysrhythmias

Metabolic disorders
Hypoglycemia
Hypocalcemia
Hyponatremia
Inborn errors of metabolism

Musculoskeletal system
Infant botulism
Guillain-Barré syndrome
Congenital myopathies (Werdnig-Hoffman)

Other
Severe anemia
Poisoning
Hypothermia
Hyperthermia
Breath-holding spells
Child abuse
Idiopathic

Adapted from Fan LL: *Primary Care* 11(3):443, 1984.

sponse to hypercarbia, hypoxia, and airway stimulation is depressed.[8] Respiratory control during non-REM sleep is similar to that in the awake state.

Newborn and young infants are particularly prone to apneic episodes because the afferent inputs from the chemoreceptors, lung and airway receptors, and central nervous system (CNS) are immature. Maturational changes in the response to hypercarbia and hypoxia are also seen in newborns. A mature response depends on gestational and postnatal age and may reflect changes in neurologic development and in pulmonary mechanics.[5]

The role of hypoxia and hypoxemia is important in the pathophysiology of apnea in infants. In older children and adults, hypoxemia normally produces an increase in respiratory rate. In newborns, however, a brief increase in the respiratory rate is followed by depression of the respiratory drive, hypoventilation, and subsequent apnea.[3] Immature development of elastic fibers in the septae of the alveoli surrounding the conducting airways allows them to collapse and is further aggravated by low lung volumes in infants, which decline even more during REM sleep.[8]

Differential Considerations

Apnea of Infancy. Apnea is a nonspecific response to a variety of clinical conditions as shown in the box. A variety of ventilatory defects present during sleep are most likely responsible for the development of an abnormal respiratory pattern. These ventilatory defects include excessive periodic breathing, decreased ventilatory response to carbon dioxide, and an abnormal arousal response to hypoxia.[5]

Other infants may have an underlying cause of the apnea. Infectious processes can result in apnea of infancy. Infants with lower respiratory tract infections, including bronchiolitis and pneumonia, may present with apnea of infancy, presumably from hypoxia or increased work of breathing. Central apnea also may occur in infants with respiratory syncytial virus (RSV) who have no evidence of lower respiratory tract involvement.[7] Infants with a history of prematurity are particularly vulnerable to apnea of infancy from RSV infections.[9] Pertussis syndrome (see Chapter 55) in early infancy may also present with respiratory symptoms and apnea.[7] Apnea in infants has also clearly been associated with sepsis, meningitis (see Chapter 56), and encephalitis, all of which can occur in an infant without other more specific signs indicating the source of infection.

Apnea of infancy has been associated with a variety of neurologic conditions including seizures, intracranial hemorrhage, increased intracranial pressure, and central loss of ventilatory control. Apnea with or without color change may precede or follow a seizure, but it is often difficult to define the primary disorder in infants.[2] Apnea may be the sole manifestation of seizures, accompany a more generalized primary seizure, or precipitate a seizure from hypoxia.[10] Intracranial hemorrhage in infants can also produce apnea as seen in premature infants who develop intraventricular hemorrhages, in full-term newborns, or in infants secondary to trauma, particularly the shaken baby syndrome. Apnea can also result from increased intracranial pressure, which may develop in infants for various reasons. Infants with congenital central alveolar hypoventilation

which may result in instability of the rib cage, thus decreasing tidal volume. During non-REM sleep, however, the tone of the upper airway and intercostal muscles remains intact.[8] During REM sleep, the ventilatory response to hypercarbia and hypoxia decreases; and the arousal re-

(Ondine's curse) experience apnea secondary to failure of automatic control of ventilation only when they are asleep, perhaps because of defective central chemoreceptors.[11]

Apnea in infants can occur secondary to abnormalities within the gastrointestinal (GI) system. Gastroesophageal reflux may trigger either central apnea or oxygen desaturation with subsequent apnea or ALTE.[12,13] Apnea and reflux in the same patient does not necessarily prove cause and effect.[7] Other swallowing disorders can also produce apnea in infants. Premature infants may experience reflex apnea during feeding, secondary to stimulation of the laryngeal chemoreceptors and pulmonary receptors.[8] A recent study reports airway obstruction at the laryngeal level with the aryepiglottic folds closing over and across the vocal cords in premature infants with ALTEs, which are most likely due to an exaggerated airway protective reflex of the laryngeal chemoreceptors.[14]

Several disorders of the cardiopulmonary systems may also produce apnea in infancy. Premature or newborn infants with respiratory distress syndrome can develop apnea. Apnea has also been associated with pulmonary edema, pulmonary hemorrhage, or hypoplastic lungs, as seen in infants with diaphragmatic hernias. In addition, congenital heart disease such as atrial septal defect, patent ductus arteriosus, or ventricular septal defect may be associated with apnea in infants.[3] It also can result from shock secondary to hypovolemia, sepsis, or cardiogenic abnormalities. Apnea may be the primary symptom in patients with cardiac dysrhythmias, particularly prolonged Q-T syndrome (see Chapter 14). However, the prolongation of the Q-T interval may be seen only during REM sleep.[7]

Apnea may result from metabolic derangements including hypoglycemia, hypocalcemia, hyponatremia, and acidosis resulting from inborn errors of metabolism.[15]

A variety of progressive neuropathies and myopathies will eventually involve the respiratory system, leading to weakened respiratory muscles and ultimately producing apnea. Infant botulism and Guillain-Barré syndrome are usually acute in onset and should be suspected based on the history and physical examination.[16] Chronic, progressive disease processes, including the congenital myopathies, will also eventually produce apnea.

Other processes that can produce apnea in infants include severe anemia, ingestions or poisonings, and environmental abnormalities including hypothermia and extreme hyperthermia.[2,8,17,18] Breath-holding spells, although uncommon in early infancy, can produce apnea in association with severe crying episodes and thus is a diagnosis of exclusion.[2]

Child abuse in the form of recurrent apneic episodes secondary to suffocation has been increasingly reported. It has been recognized as Munchausen syndrome by proxy and is important in the differential diagnosis of apnea or apparently life-threatening events.[19,20]

Obstructive Apnea. Obstructive apnea is more common in older children, although it also can occur in infants. Obstructive apnea, like apnea of infancy, often occurs during sleep. In infants and children, structural abnormalities of the airway can produce fixed or dynamic airway narrowing or instability and thus predispose the child to obstructive sleep apnea or hypoventilation (see box above).[21] Hypertrophy of the tonsils and adenoids is a common cause.[22]

**Obstructive Apnea:
Differential Considerations**

Structural abnormalities
Hypertrophy of tonsils and adenoids
Choanal atresia or stenosis
Nasal septal deviation
Airway hematoma or tumor
Temporomandibular joint dysfunction
Subglottic stenosis
Laryngomalacia
Tracheomalacia

Craniofacial abnormalities
Micrognathia (Pierre Robin syndrome)
Macroglossia (Down and Beckwith-Wiedemann syndromes)
Crouzon disease
Cleft palate

Vascular abnormalities
Double aortic arch
Aberrant arteries

Neuromuscular disorders
Down syndrome
Hypotonic cerebral palsy
Muscular dystrophy
Congenital myopathy (Werdnig-Hoffman disease)

Metabolic disorders
Hypothyroidism
Prader-Willi syndrome
Morbid obesity

Infection
Epiglottitis
Croup
Tonsillitis
Pharyngitis

Other
Airway trauma
Foreign body

Adapted from Mark JD and Brooks JG: *Pediatr Clin North Am* 31(4):907, 1984.

Other structural abnormalities that may predispose the child to the development of obstructive sleep apnea include choanal atresia or stenosis, nasal septal deviation, upper airway hematoma or tumor, temporomandibular joint dysfunction, subglottic stenosis, laryngomalacia, and tracheomalacia,[21] in addition to craniofacial abnormalities such as micrognathia, macroglossia, midface hypoplasias, and cleft palates.[8] Airway obstruction secondary to vascular abnormalities, including double aortic arch and aberrant arteries, may also occur with sleep-associated apnea.[3]

Children with neuromuscular weakness or hypotonia are predisposed to the development of obstructive sleep apnea resulting from collapse of the pharyngeal wall, which allows the tongue to fall back into the airway.[21] Examples of this cause include Down syndrome, hypotonic cerebral palsy, muscular dystrophy, and progressive congenital myopathies such as Werdnig-Hoffman disease.[23] Children with neuromuscular disorders often have chronic pulmonary disease and impaired ability to clear pharyngeal secretions, which further complicates their airway obstruction.

Hypothyroidism, Prader-Willi syndrome, and severe obesity may also produce obstructive sleep apnea in children.[3,24] A number of infectious processes of the upper airway may produce acute upper airway obstruction leading to the development of apnea. These include epiglottitis, and severe croup, tonsillitis, and pharyngitis. These illnesses are usually accompanied by fever and other signs and symptoms of acute upper airway obstruction including stridor. Obstructive apnea may also develop as a result of trauma to the airway or palate or secondary to an airway foreign body.[3]

Diagnostic Work-Up

The patient's history is essential to substantiate the significance of the episode, demonstrate associated problems, and define possible underlying causes.[3] The primary decision is whether the episode can be dismissed as a minor problem of childhood or whether the event is significant enough to require further investigation. Unfortunately, because of the vague history often surrounding such episodes, that decision may not be easy to make.[6]

A careful history about the nature of the episode should include questions about the wake or sleep state of the infant; appearance of the infant with regard to color, tone, and movement; and intervention required, if any, to terminate the episode. Feeding or crying, duration, and condition of the infant immediately after the episode are also important to define.[7] History of associated problems such as vomiting or spitting up with feeding, intercurrent illness (particularly respiratory infections), and mental status before the episode should also be obtained.[3] Previous history of apnea, seizures, or metabolic abnormalities is important to obtain; recurrent episodes of apnea should raise the possibility of life-threatening apnea.[6] The sleeping position and pattern of the child should also be determined including fitfulness, restlessness, snoring, and daytime hypersomnolence.[3,25] Family history of apnea, SIDS, respiratory and cardiac disease, seizure, or metabolic abnormalities should be specifically obtained.

The initial assessment of the patient with apnea should focus on the status and stability of the pulmonary and cardiovascular system while attempting to identify the underlying cause. The emergency physician must be able to identify and treat life-threatening events such as persistent or recurrent apnea, hypoxia, shock, and hypoglycemia. Vital signs, upper airway evaluation, cardiopulmonary assessment, and neurologic evaluation (including mental status) are essential components. At times, findings on physical examination suggest the underlying cause of the apnea, although the examination is usually entirely normal.[8]

Ancillary Data. If the clinical presentation of the patient points to a specific diagnosis, a general evaluation may not be necessary. If the clinical presentation is nonspecific,

however, a general diagnostic evaluation should be performed to assess for several common causes.[7] Pulse oximetry and cardiorespiratory monitoring should be instituted at the initial evaluation and continued during hospitalization. Routine screening tests should include a complete blood count (CBC), serum glucose, electrolytes, calcium, magnesium, chest radiograph, and electrocardiogram (ECG).[5] Further tests should be obtained as directed by the history, physical examination, and screening tests. An electroencephalogram (EEG) should be obtained if there is any question of seizure activity, nystagmus or eye deviation associated with the episode, or altered mental status on physical examination.[3] Studies for RSV and pertussis should also be considered in infants even if there is no evidence of respiratory disease.[7] An arterial blood gas should be obtained if apnea persists, other respiratory symptoms are present, or the pulse oximetry monitoring indicates hypoxemia. In febrile patients or in afebrile infants less than 1 month of age, appropriate cultures including blood, urine, and cerebrospinal fluid by lumbar puncture should be obtained. A barium swallow may be necessary to evaluate a possible gastroesophageal reflux (GER) in infants with a history of feeding difficulties or vomiting. Studies such as esophageal pH monitoring or esophageal manometry may be indicated to confirm a diagnosis of GER if the barium swallow is abnormal.[12] Further evaluations including cranial ultrasound or CT scan of the head, echocardiogram, and Holter monitoring should be obtained as directed by the history, physical examination, and routine screening tests.[5]

If obstructive apnea is suspected, investigations to identify the underlying cause should include lateral neck radiographs, transnasal fiberoptic endoscopy, and direct observation of patient's sleep.[26] Sleep studies, in which nasal and oral airflow, arterial oxygen saturation, chest wall motion, ECG, EEG, and sleep stages are measured, can be helpful in identifying the type and significance of apnea and quantifying the apneic events.[27] However, this evaluation technique is available only in major sleep laboratories, and referral to such a center may be necessary if the significance or cause of the apnea remains unclear and in-depth evaluation is indicated.

Prehospital Considerations

The appropriate care of children with apnea begins in the field if that is the first contact by the health-care system. Emergency medical service (EMS) personnel should be properly trained in the assessment and management of airway and cardiopulmonary problems in children. The primary responsibility in prehospital care is evaluation and stabilization of airway, breathing, and circulation. Supplementary humidified oxygen should be administered as this initial assessment occurs. Respiratory and cardiac monitoring should be instituted along with pulse oximetry, if available. Maneuvers to assure airway patency including chin lift/jaw thrust positioning, or placement of nasal or oropharyngeal airways may be necessary if evidence of decreased pharyngeal tone causing airway obstruction is present, particularly in patients with altered mental status or neuromuscular disease. If apnea recurs or persists, artificial respirations will need to be maintained by bag-valve-mask ventilation or an artificial airway with tracheal intubation and supportive ventilation may need to be placed.

Therapeutic Trial

Therapeutic trials may include a variety of diagnostic and therapeutic approaches. Any infant or child with a significant apneic episode or ALTE requires hospitalization with monitoring and further evaluation on an inpatient basis. If a demonstrable abnormality is detected on screening, treatment of the specific problem often results in the resolution of apnea. Apnea associated with seizures commonly diminishes with institution of anticonvulsant therapy. Episodes resulting from gastroesophageal reflux usually decrease if the reflux is treated adequately.[12]

If no underlying cause is identified for the apnea or ALTE after a complete evaluation, home cardiorespiratory monitoring may be appropriate.[6] The use of home cardiorespiratory monitoring remains controversial, however, and the benefits vs. risks have not yet been established. Families who have a child on a home monitor require substantial medical and emotional support, and one should not undertake this form of therapy unless such support can be provided on a 24-hour basis.[6] This support is usually only available at major sleep centers.

COUGH

A cough helps clear debris and secretions from the respiratory tract and aids the expulsion of foreign matter that may be inhaled accidentally.[28,29]

Pathophysiology

To cough effectively, the patient must have an intact irritant-receptor reflex, laryngeal function, and effective chest musculature and diaphragm. The cough reflex consists of five primary components:

1. Cough receptors in the various parts of the respiratory tree including the nose, pharynx, pleura, pericardium, and diaphragm, which are very sensitive to touch, inflammation, pressure, and chemical irritation.
2. Afferent nerve pathways, which include primarily the vagus nerve fibrils around and in the larynx, trachea, and large bronchi, as well as cranial nerves V and IX (from the nose and pharynx) and the phrenic nerve (from the diaphragm).[29-31]
3. Central cough center in the medulla.
4. Efferent pathway including the vagus and phrenic nerve, and the various motor nerves.
5. Relevant musculature of the chest, abdominal muscles, and diaphragm.

The cough itself is initiated by a deep inspiration followed by a glottis closure. Contraction of the laryngeal smooth muscle and the respiratory muscles follows, resulting in the opening of the glottis and a rapid, forceful expulsion of the intrathoracic air. At the same time, the airways are compressed, and the alveolar and bronchial secretions are propelled proximally. In addition, there appears to be a relationship between the cough reflex and bronchoconstriction.[30]

Failure of an adequate cough mechanism may result from abnormalities at any level in the cough reflex pathway. Those affected include children with chronic repetitive as-

---

Causes of Cough

Infection
Pharyngitis
Laryngitis, laryngotracheobronchitis
Sinusitis
Pneumonia
Bronchiolitis
Pertussis
Bronchiectasis
Tuberculosis

Inflammatory
Asthma
Allergy

Traumatic/toxic
Foreign body aspiration
Trauma to the neck/chest
Smoke inhalation
Hydrocarbon ingestion

Genetic/metabolic
Cystic fibrosis

Neoplastic and other extrinsic compressions
Mediastinal tumors
Lymphoma
Neuroblastoma
Teratoma
Airway anomalies (e.g., vascular ring)

Aspiration
Tracheoesophageal fistula
Gastroesophageal reflux
Neuromuscular incoordination

Psychogenic

---

piration, laryngeal anatomic or neurologic abnormalities, and those who are comatose, on large doses of narcotics, or have poor intercostal muscle and diaphragmatic function.

Differential Considerations

It is helpful to think of the cough as either relatively acute and of recent onset (usually less than a week) or persistent or chronic (often more than 2 weeks). Most of the conditions listed in the box above fit into either category, depending on the time of presentation. Those with a relatively sudden or recent onset include patients with a viral infection such as pharyngitis, laryngitis, bronchiolitis, and commonly certain types of bacterial pneumonias, foreign body aspiration, toxic inhalation, or ingestion. These conditions usually (though certainly not always) present little diagnostic difficulty (because the history tends to be quite suggestive) and require relatively little investigation. If the cough has been present for a long time, the differential diagnosis tends to be more complex and the investigation and follow-up more involved.

Categorization by age also establishes a helpful approach to cough.

Infants. Infants with persistent cough must be evaluated thoroughly for respiratory disease. Infants between 1 and 4 months of age with staccato cough and mild congestion may have chlamydial pneumonia. Coexistent inclusion conjunctivitis may or may not be present.[32] Other organisms, notably cytomegalovirus, *Ureaplasma*, and pneumocystitis, may cause similar pulmonary symptoms in infants.[33] Bacterial or viral pertussis syndrome, should be considered in an infant who has episodic bouts of severe paroxysmal cough (often without whoop), but is quite well and comfortable the rest of the time. The cough of bronchiolitis may be similar to that of pertussis (usually less severe), but bronchiolitis usually produces some degree of respiratory distress and wheezing at rest. Both illnesses, if sufficiently severe, result in periodic apnea or cyanosis.

In cystic fibrosis the cough is often wet and persistent. Although it may be confused with bronchiolitis or pertussis, most children also develop a chronic wheeze, which poorly responds to treatment, recurrent pneumonia, or abnormal stools with signs of nutritional deficiency. Cough resulting from various congenital anatomic anomalies such as tracheoesophageal fistula (TEF) or laryngeal cleft usually starts at birth or very shortly after and is caused by chronic aspiration of liquids. Infants with congenital developmental problems such as tracheomalacia (barking cough) or swallowing incoordination (cough with feeding) also present very early in life. In infants with a fixed congenital airway problem (e.g., a vascular ring, bronchogenic cyst, or pulmonary sequestration) the cough may be present only during intercurrent viral illness.[34]

Although most infants who have aspirated a foreign body tend to have a very sudden and recent onset of choking cough during play or feeding, there can be a significant diagnostic lag time in many patients.[35,36] Chronic cough, sometimes associated with chronic wheezing, atelectasis, or pneumonia may thus be the presenting picture. The esophageal foreign body can also produce cough due to airway obstruction because the posterior trachea is adjacent to the anterior esophagus.[34]

Preschool. Cough is also common in preschool-aged children. Asthma is probably the most common cause. Cough may be the only manifestation, since some children with reactive airway disease have no wheezing or respiratory distress (cough variant asthma).[37] It is often chronic (lasting many weeks) and dry, getting worse at night, after exercise, an emotional event, or cold weather. Viral upper respiratory infections are common precipitants. Whereas children with postnasal drip cough only for a few days, those with hyperreactive airways tend to cough longer. Many of these children get misdiagnosed as having persistent and frequent colds or pneumonias; multiple courses of antibiotics and antitussives with poor results are common. Relatively recent onset of cough with fever of several days duration may be due to pneumonia (bacterial or viral). Respiratory distress may or may not be present. Many children with pneumonia resulting from *Streptococcus pneumoniae*, beta-hemolytic streptococcus, or *Haemophilus influenzae* tend to be ill and toxic-looking. Auscultatory chest signs may be absent in small children.

A child with a prolonged cough history with severe, protracted (>7 days) nasal symptoms (often with purulent nasal discharge) may have sinusitis. It is worth noting that in preschoolers the complaints may be quite vague, including occasionally, malodorous breath.[38] Preschoolers may, of course, also aspirate a foreign body.

School-aged Children. Asthma remains a common cause of chronic cough. The relevant history often dates back to the infant or preschool years. The child may be unable to keep up with the others or avoid sports altogether. The cough is usually seasonal, associated with a known environmental allergen, or (usually) worsened by one of the many known precipitating factors, especially viral infections and exercise. *Mycoplasma pneumoniae* is also common in this age group, although it may occur in 4 to 5-year-olds as well. These children usually look surprisingly well and nontoxic and have minimal or no chest findings. A week or more may pass before the onset of vague symptoms such as low-grade fever, malaise, sore throat, and a dry cough. A fairly high proportion of these patients demonstrate wheezing.[39] Other etiologies, pneumonia, and sinusitis may also occur. Active or passive smoking are potentially aggravating or precipitating factors. Because of a rising incidence of *Mycobacterium tuberculosis* disease in North America, the agent has to be considered, especially in suspected contacts, recent immigrants, HIV-positive patients or visitors from areas where tuberculosis (TB) prevalence is high in the native population. A mediastinal mass may have to be ruled out in a child with a dry, barking cough associated with weight loss, chronic fever, anorexia, or lymphadenopathy. Psychogenic cough may also occur in the adolescent. Most often, it is due to a habit developed after an airway irritation associated with a viral infection. The cough is dry, barking, honking, and explosive; it is often precipitated by a reference to it and is absent at night during sleep. Associated family tension, school problems, and secondary gains are often present.[29]

Hemoptysis (coughing up blood often mixed with sputum) appears red and frothy and is an unusual pediatric condition. Infection is most common, resulting from pneumonia (group A streptococcus and tuberculosis), pertussis, pulmonary abscess, bronchiectasis, or viral infections. A foreign body, neoplasm, bleeding diathesis, pulmonary hemosiderosis, or acute asthmatic attack may also be underlying conditions. Pulmonary embolism, mitral stenosis, and pulmonary hypertension may be causative. Pseudohemoptysis may result from Munchausen syndrome, epistaxis, gingival bleeding, or gastrointestinal hemorrhage.

Diagnostic Work-Up

A careful history is essential for correct diagnosis and therapy, and to assure appropriate investigations and follow-up.

Historically, it is imperative to determine the duration, frequency, quality, timing, and productivity of the cough. Inciting and ameliorating conditions, and other respiratory findings including shortness of breath, wheezing, exercise tolerance, stridor, and chest pain should be defined.

The onset of the cough is important. Infants with a persistent cough that began at or shortly after birth should be evaluated for congenital malformations (see previous section). Those with tracheomalacia have associated chronic stridor, and the cough has a barking quality. Those with sudden onset of a choking episode may have aspirated a foreign body.

The description and character of the cough may be inaccurate and misleading. For example, a "rattling wet cough" may not represent any lower airway pathology, but rather a congested upper airway. Nevertheless, certain features tend to be helpful. A staccato, dry cough in a small infant may be due to *Chlamydia trachomatis* pneumonia. A dry, barking cough is usually due to tracheal pathology. Although the psychogenic cough is also dry and slightly barking, it has a honking and bizarre quality. In contrast to croup, it never occurs during sleep, and there is no respiratory discomfort. Coughs that worsen at night usually are caused by posterior nasal drips from allergy or infection. When parents report paroxysmal cough, pertussis should be considered, although reactive airway disease, *Mycoplasma*, and *Chlamydia* may also produce paroxysmal coughing.[29] The child with persistent production of purulent sputum may have a form of suppurative lung disease such as bacterial pneumonia, bronchiectasis, cystic fibrosis, or lung abscess. These children are acutely or chronically ill, often febrile, and miserable. Small children may swallow the sputum rather than expectorate; significant hemoptysis is rare. It usually occurs in older children with well-established disease. After a recent epistaxis is excluded (causing hematemesis rather than hemoptysis), the possibilities include a foreign body, cystic fibrosis, bronchiectasis, pulmonary hemosiderosis, and tuberculosis.

The temporal relationship of the cough to activity may be useful. In small infants, aspiration often causes coughing after feeding; in older children, cough associated with exercise, anxiety, or cold weather suggests reactive airway disease. Contrary to most causes of cough, the psychogenic cough is present only in the awake state. Cough caused by airway compression or cardiac disease may worsen with exercise. If the cough starts suddenly, an aspirated piece of food (e.g., peanuts or popcorn) is often causative. A severe chronic cough occurring on most days over many months suggests a persistent lesion such as airway compression, bronchomalacia, or cystic fibrosis.[34]

Systemic complaints should be defined, including fever, headache with facial pain and green nasal discharge (sinusitis), acute dyspnea (pneumonia, asthma, and cardiac disease), acute dysphagia (swallowed foreign body), significant weight loss (malignancy, TB, and cystic fibrosis), abnormal stools or chronic diarrhea (cystic fibrosis), and difficult and slow feeding with diaphoresis (cardiac problem).

In some patients a past history of severe infections may be relevant if immunodeficiency is considered. Immunization status should be determined. A family history of atopy, recent infections, or exposures may be relevant.

A thorough physical examination may occasionally lead to diagnosis. First impressions are often important. For example, does the child look acutely ill and toxic, or is the child short of breath, irritable and anxious? Is there evidence of chronic illness, weight loss, and clubbing? Is the child clearly failing to thrive? Is there muscle wasting and weakness, suggesting neuromuscular disease?

A good head and neck examination should include looking for sinus tenderness, otitis, pharyngitis, nasal polyps, and evidence of allergic features (e.g., boggy nasal mucosa, transverse nasal crease, and allergic shiners). Cyanosis, pathologic heart murmurs, or congestive heart failure point to a significant cardiac lesion.

The chest examination may show tachypnea, hyperinflation, long expiratory phase, poor or unequal air entry, unilateral or bilateral wheezes, or crackles. The adequacy of ventilation needs to be specifically evaluated. Color, respiratory rate, pattern, effort, retractions and flaring should be noted. It is important to mention that a normal chest examination does not eliminate significant respiratory pathology (e.g., hyperreactive airway disease, *M. pneumoniae* or an aspirated foreign body). Although infants with bacterial pneumonia usually look ill, the chest signs may be minimal (and so may the cough!). In many cases, the chest examination will be normal and will yield no clues as to the diagnosis.[40]

Ancillary Data

A careful history and a thorough examination may be all that is required. Many patients require no investigations, especially when the diagnosis is obvious (e.g., typical bronchiolitis) or if the cough is clearly related to a known diagnosis responding to treatment (e.g., croup).

The chest x-ray study is the first and the single most useful method in excluding various pathologies.[32,41] This is especially true of small infants with chronic cough. Unless the child is truly critically ill, posteroanterior and lateral films should be requested. The radiograph should be evaluated for hyperinflation, alveolar or interstitial infiltrates, increased bronchial markings, atelectasis, or localized emphysema. If a diagnosis of a foreign-body aspiration is in question, then inspiratory-expiratory radiographs should be performed. Films taken with the child in the left and right lateral decubitus position may help when the former method is difficult; persistent unilateral hyperinflation, which does not change in a dependent position, may be noted. Abnormal maxillary sinus radiographs in children over 1 year old usually indicate inflammatory disease.[42] If a diagnosis of gastroesophageal reflux or chronic aspiration are likely, a fluoroscopic barium swallow may be indicated. It is also useful in diagnosing external tracheal compression (e.g., a vascular ring) in which a fixed esophageal indentation is seen. Other sophisticated imaging techniques may be necessary in unusual diagnoses (e.g., CT scan for the exact extent of a mediastinal mass or an echocardiogram and angiogram for suspected vascular compression of the airway).

Bronchoscopy is useful for suspected foreign-body aspiration, tracheoesophageal fistula, or bronchiectasis. A child with smoke inhalation and cough or any other respiratory symptoms must undergo laryngoscopy and early intubation in anticipation of airway obstruction.

Any child with cough who is in respiratory distress or is cyanotic should undergo a transcutaneous pulse oximetry, which provides an accurate measurement of arterial oxygen saturation.[43] Children who are 5 or 6 years old or older can usually cooperate with simple spirometry. A reduced baseline forced expiratory volume in 1 second (FEV_1) or peak expiratory flow rate (PEFR) and their improvement after an inhaled bronchodilator suggest reactive airway disease. An arterial blood gas is indicated in children with respiratory distress.

Blood cultures may be useful in toxic-looking children with pneumonia. Other tests depend on specific situations such as the serology for *Chlamydia* or viruses, elevated lymphocyte count in pertussis, or eosinophilia in *C. pneumoniae*. In a child with suspected immunodeficiency or unexplained bronchiectasis, immunoglobulin status examination is indicated.[44]

Nasopharyngeal swabs for fluorescent antibody, *Bordetella pertussis* IgA antibody, and cultures are indicated in those with suspected pertussis.[45,46] Similarly, *C. trachomatis* may be cultured, and its antibody detected in nasopharyngeal or conjunctival secretions.[29] If cystic fibrosis is suspected, a sweat chloride test should be performed. If tuberculosis is a possibility, a tuberculin skin test should be performed, often concomitant with specific cultures.

Prehospital Considerations

Only a minority of children with cough have respiratory distress. Children most likely to have trouble are those with severe asthma, bronchiolitis, or croup; small infants having pertussis with cyanotic or apneic episodes; children with extensive pneumonia; victims of smoke inhalation or tracheal foreign body aspiration; and those with a large mediastinal mass. Careful attention to the airway patency and adequate oxygenation are of prime importance.

Therapeutic Trial

The response to treatment depends on the underlying cause. Therefore whenever possible, a specific diagnosis should be sought and treated accordingly (see the specific sections). Attention to the airway and oxygen saturation at or above 95% are of prime importance. Patients with smoke inhalation or mediastinal masses often look quite healthy initially, yet acutely decompensate with sudden airway obstruction without warning. In relatively healthy-looking children, certain diagnoses are easily missed unless specifically investigated. Mild bronchiolitis in an infant with upper respiratory infection (URI) but persistent tachypnea (often without wheezing), or asthma in a child with persistent dry cough and little else, may often respond to a trial of inhaled bronchodilators, thus providing diagnostic clues. Other easily missed diagnoses include sinusitis and *M. pneumoniae*, both of which respond well to the appropriate antibiotics, (usually cefaclor or amoxicillin-clavulanate and erythromycin, respectively). Although a diagnosis of foreign-body aspiration is often obvious, bronchoscopy should also be strongly considered in a child with a chronic cough and persistent pneumonia or atelectasis on chest x-ray examination.

Antitussive medications have limited use in pediatrics because (1) the cough often responds only to a specific therapy (e.g., bronchodilators in asthma, antibiotics in sinusitis), (2) the suppression of cough is contraindicated in conditions with increased sputum production (e.g., pneumonia), and (3) codeine, the most effective antitussive, is known to reduce mucokinesis.[32] On occasion, children with nonspecific, dry, nonproductive, and sleep-disturbing cough that serves no useful physiologic function, do require antitussive therapy. A short course of codeine 1 mg/kg/24 hr q 4 to 6 hr PO in such situations is often effective and well tolerated. Over-the-counter cough suppressant mixtures usually are not effective; many contain expectorants to increase mucus production, or antihistamines, which cause fatigue or excitability. Their use is not recommended, especially in small children.

Cool high humidity via a humidifier is often beneficial for a child with the dry cough associated with viral URI because of its soothing effect on the nasal, pharyngeal, and tracheal mucosa, and for those with a posterior nasal drip.

CYANOSIS

Cyanosis is a physical sign characterized by a bluish discoloration of the skin and mucous membranes produced by the color of blood within the capillaries of the dermis and mucous membranes. The detection of cyanosis is highly subjective and can be difficult to correlate with the degree of arterial oxygenation.[47,48] However, its presence requires immediate treatment and diagnostic evaluation.

Pathophysiology

Cyanosis is determined by the absolute amount of reduced hemoglobin in the blood; the amount of oxygenated hemoglobin present has little influence.[49] Cyanosis is clinically evident when there are at least 5 gm of reduced hemoglobin in 100 ml of capillary blood.[50] This amount is usually associated with an arterial oxyhemoglobin saturation of 85% or less.[51] The increase in the amount of reduced hemoglobin in the capillary vessels can be due to an increased quantity of venous blood in the skin, dilation of the venules, or a decrease in the oxygen saturation of the capillary blood.[52] The oxygen saturation of the blood depends on the oxygen content of the blood and tissue, and the oxyhemoglobin dissociation curve.

The detection of cyanosis is influenced by different factors including the light conditions present for examination, the cutaneous pigment and thickness of the skin, the rate of blood flow through the capillaries, and the skill of the individual examiner.[47,50] Cyanosis is most evident in areas where the epidermis is thin, the pigment is minimal, and the capillaries are abundant.[53] The mucous membranes and tongue are the most sensitive sites for observing central cyanosis, whereas the tips of fingers and toes, nailbeds, and earlobes are less reliable.[54]

Cyanosis suggests the possibility of tissue hypoxia and requires a thorough clinical evaluation. The absence of cyanosis, however, does not confirm the absence of tissue hypoxia. An infant may have hypoxia without cyanosis secondary to an increased affinity of fetal hemoglobin for oxygen.[53] Cyanosis may not be detected in hypoxic patients with severe anemia; inadequate hemoglobin may be in the reduced state.[47,48]

Central Cyanosis

Central cyanosis is reflected clinically in the tongue, mucous membranes, and peripheral skin.[53] It is seen when arterial blood is desaturated or in the presence of an abnormal hemoglobin. A decrease in arterial oxygen saturation may result from a decrease in atmospheric pressure because of high altitude, impaired pulmonary ventilation, or decreased pulmonary perfusion. Cyanosis secondary to decreased pulmonary and alveolar ventilation or impaired oxygen diffusion usually improves with the administration of 100% oxygen. However, cyanosis seen with decreased pulmonary perfusion resulting from intracardiac shunting of blood, (as in congenital heart disease) shows little response to the administration of 100% oxygen.[53]

Cyanosis from an abnormal hemoglobin is most commonly caused by methemoglobinemia, which may be either congenital or acquired. Another aberrant hemoglobin results from sulfhemoglobinemia, which is usually secondary to sulfonamide drugs. Carboxyhemoglobinemia does not cause cyanosis but may produce a cherry-red flush of the skin, retina, or mucous membranes.

Peripheral Cyanosis

Peripheral cyanosis is a bluish discoloration of the skin resulting from slowing of blood flow to an area and increased extraction of oxygen from normally saturated arterial blood. It commonly has a vascular cause and can be seen in sepsis, shock states, and newborns with temperature changes or metabolic abnormalities secondary to vasomotor instability. Peripheral cyanosis can be caused by venous obstruction, capillary stasis, and conditions such as Raynaud's phenomenon. Hematologic disorders such as polycythemia secondary to congenital heart disease, chronic hypoxia, or maternal-fetal or twin-twin transfusion can also result in peripheral cyanosis.

Differential Considerations

Vascular

Cardiac (See Chapter 47). The diagnostic considerations when approaching a pediatric patient with central cyanosis can be quite broad as seen in the box on p. 1065, although the most common causes of cyanosis in infants and children are abnormalities of the pulmonary and cardiac systems. The primary cardiac cause of cyanosis in the pediatric age group is congenital heart disease. A decrease in arterial oxygen saturation with evidence of cyanosis may result from anomalies with intracardiac shunting secondary to obstruction to right ventricular outflow, leading to a decrease in pulmonary blood flow as in pulmonary atresia, pulmonary stenosis, tetralogy of Fallot, and tricuspid atresia. Congenital heart disease with increased pulmonary blood flow caused by defects that result in admixture of pulmonary and systemic venous return such as transposition of the great vessels, total anomalous pulmonary venous return, truncus arteriosus, and hypoplastic left heart syndrome, can also produce cyanosis.[55] Infants with cyanosis resulting from congenital heart disease usually have some degree of respiratory distress, and the differentiation between cardiac and primary pulmonary disease can be difficult.

Congestive heart failure can lead to cyanosis because of decreased alveolar ventilation and decreased pulmonary perfusion secondary to intrapulmonary shunting. When it develops in the first year of life, it is usually due to congenital heart disease; in older children it is more likely due to an acquired abnormality.[56] Pulmonary edema produces cyanosis by a similar pathophysiology. Any condition that causes cardiac shock can produce cyanosis by decreasing pulmonary perfusion.

Pulmonary. Cyanosis may be caused by vascular abnormalities that directly affect the pulmonary vessels and decrease alveolar perfusion. Pulmonary hemorrhage, pulmonary embolism, and pulmonary hypertension can all lead to the development of cyanosis in children. Besides cyanosis, dyspnea will also be present. However, with pulmonary hemorrhage and embolism, the clinical and radiologic picture often suggests pneumonia, and the diagnosis may be difficult to make. Persistent fetal circulation in newborns presents with cyanosis from birth with varying degrees of respiratory distress. This syndrome results in a true right-to-left shunt; patients show little improvement in arterial oxygen saturation with the administration of 100% oxygen, and can be difficult to distinguish from infants with cyanotic heart disease.

The presence of an anomalous pulmonary vascular abnormality such as a ring can impair ventilation and produce cyanosis secondary to compression of the trachea. Symptoms are usually present from infancy and can include wheezing respirations, cough, and vomiting.

Respiratory

Upper Airway. Diseases of the pulmonary system producing cyanosis can be divided into those involving either the upper or lower airways. Upper airway obstruction produces cyanosis primarily because of impaired ventilation. Pulmonary edema may accompany upper airway obstruction in children, further impairing alveolar ventilation.[57,58] Croup, epiglottitis, bacterial tracheitis, and retropharyngeal abscess are the most common infectious diseases that lead to obstruction of the upper airway in children. Other causes, including foreign bodies and anatomic abnormalities, should also be considered. Signs of respiratory distress seen with upper airway obstruction include stridor, tachypnea, and accessory muscle use with retractions.

Lower Airway. Diseases of the lower airway are particularly common in infants and children and are the most likely cause of cyanosis presenting beyond the neonatal period. The primary mechanism is a decrease in alveolar ventilation; pulmonary perfusion abnormalities may be present as well. Pneumonia, asthma, bronchiolitis, atelectasis, aspiration, or foreign body are common diseases of the lower airway in children that must be considered in the differential diagnosis of cyanosis. These conditions are usually accompanied by signs of respiratory distress including tachypnea, grunting, nasal flaring, retractions, crackles, and wheezing. A chest x-ray study may be helpful in differentiating causes. Other pediatric diseases involving the lower airways include respiratory distress syndrome, bronchopulmonary dysplasia, and cystic fibrosis.

CNS. Vascular abnormalities in the CNS causing intracranial hemorrhage or increased intracranial pressure may lead to cyanosis by depressing the respiratory center and leading to alveolar hypoventilation. This development occurs primarily as a result of trauma in children but can also be seen with congenital disorders.

Infection. Serious systemic infections in children such as meningitis or sepsis can be accompanied by cyanosis caused by abnormalities of ventilation and perfusion. Whenever a child presents cyanosis and evidence of toxic-

Central Cyanosis: Diagnostic Considerations

Vascular

Cardiac

Congenital heart disease:

↓ *pulmonary blood flow*

Pulmonary atresia

Pulmonary stenosis

Tetralogy of Fallot

Triscuspid atresia

Transposition with pulmonary stenosis

↑ *pulmonary blood flow*

Transposition of the great vessels

Total anomalous pulmonary venous return

Truncus arteriosus

Hypoplastic left heart syndrome

Congestive heart failure

Pulmonary edema

Shock

Pulmonary

Pulmonary hemorrhage

Pulmonary embolism

Persistent fetal circulation

Pulmonary hypertension

Vascular ring

Respiratory

Upper airway

Croup

Epiglottitis

Retropharyngeal abscess

Foreign body

Lower airway

Pneumonia

Bronchiolitis

Asthma

Atelectasis

Aspiration/foreign body

Respiratory distress syndrome

Bronchopulmonary dysplasia

Cystic fibrosis

Systemic infection

Meningitis

Sepsis

Trauma

Pneumothorax

Hemothorax

Pulmonary contusion

Drowning

Congenital

Hereditary abnormal hemoglobin

Diaphragmatic hernia

Choanal atresia

Hypoplastic mandible

Tracheolaryngomalacia

Intoxication

Anesthetics (benzocaine, prilocaine)

Nitrates/nitrites

Aniline dyes

Sulfonamides

Neurologic

Intracranial hemorrhage

Breath holding

Seizure

---

ity including fever, respiratory distress, poor perfusion, or altered mental status, systemic infection should be considered and treatment instituted while attempts at diagnosis continue.

Trauma. Cyanosis may result from trauma for many different reasons, depending on the organs and systems of the body involved. Hypoventilation may be due to CNS injury or chest trauma with associated pneumothorax, hemothorax, or pulmonary contusion. Direct myocardial injury secondary to contusion can decrease cardiac output leading to a decrease in pulmonary perfusion. A shock state can result from abdominal, pelvic, or severe extremity injury. The pulmonary system may be primarily involved as in drowning or with the development of adult respiratory distress syndrome (ARDS) after multiple or severe trauma.

Congenital. Newborns presenting with cyanosis may have various congenital anomalies; the most common organ system causing cyanosis in neonates is the cardiovascular system. Airway abnormalities including hypoplastic man-dible, choanal atresia, subglottic stenosis, or tracheolaryn-gomalacia need to be considered in the differential diagnosis. Diaphragmatic hernia will usually present from birth with severe respiratory distress accompanied by cyanosis.

Intoxication. Intoxication or ingestions may produce cyanosis by the development of abnormal hemoglobins, and the most common are methemoglobinemia and sulfhemo-globinemia. Anesthetics including benzocaine and prilo-caine, nitrates and nitrites (e.g., contaminated well water, plant nitrates, food additives), oxidant agents (e.g., disinfectants), aniline dye absorbed from diapers, and furniture polish have all been implicated in the development of methemoglobinemia in children.[59] It has also been described in infants with diarrhea and an associated acidosis.[60] A congenital form of methemoglobinemia affects the enzyme methemoglobin reductase, resulting in structural alterations of the hemoglobin molecule. Methemoglobin-emia produces cyanosis when it exceeds 15% of the total hemoglobin. Because methemoglobin is incapable of binding with oxygen, the symptoms that develop are secondary to hypoxia. Sulfhemoglobinemia usually results from ingestion of an oxidizing drug, the most common being the sulfonamides and phenacetin, which can also cause methemoglobinemia.

Diagnostic Work-Up

A thorough history should be obtained early and focus on potential contributing conditions. The age of the patient is important; the most likely cause of cyanosis differs by age group. In newborns the most common causes of cyanosis are congenital cardiac disease and pulmonary disease. In older children, cyanosis more frequently results from diseases of the upper and lower airways.

The onset and pattern of cyanosis, temporal relationships, and alleviating or exacerbating factors should be obtained. Does it occur with feeding in an infant, after exertion, or does it improve with rest? It is important to obtain information about associated symptoms, particularly respiratory distress, cough, stridor, wheezing, or fever. Any history of congenital heart or pulmonary disease or perinatal problems needs to be elicited. Family history of cardiac or pulmonary disease should also be obtained.

Further history should include any recent traumatic episodes or possibility of foreign-body ingestion or aspiration. History of ingestion of well water, drugs, or inhalation or intoxication with other agents including carbon monoxide should be obtained to assess for methemoglobinemia. It is also important to obtain information about any recent changes in mental status or behavior.

Initial physical assessment of the patient with cyanosis should focus on the status and stability of the pulmonary and cardiovascular systems and attempt to differentiate between central and peripheral cyanosis. Emergency evaluation includes ensuring adequacy of airway, breathing, and circulation. Vital signs should be obtained while this initial assessment occurs. A focused examination of the pulmonary system should include an assessment of the upper airway; adequacy of air exchange including chest expansion; adventitial lungs sounds such as wheezing or crackles; and signs of respiratory distress including grunting, use of accessory muscles, or nasal flaring. In general, cyanotic infants with pulmonary disease are more tachypneic and appear to have greater respiratory distress than infants with cyanotic congenital heart disease.[55]

A complete cardiovascular examination should include evaluation of precordial activity, the regularity of heart sounds, the presence of heart murmurs or gallops, and the presence and quality of pulses, including peripheral perfusion by eliciting capillary refill time. It is important to look for signs of congestive heart failure such as crackles on auscultation of the lungs, hepatomegaly, or an increase in jugular venous distension. Evaluation of the neurologic system, including mental status, should follow as the remainder of the physical examination is completed.

Ancillary Data. Laboratory evaluation of central cyanosis needs to include an assessment for hypoxemia and decreased arterial oxygen saturation. Pulse oximetry monitoring should be instituted immediately; it provides a noninvasive, continuous, and generally valid measure of arterial hemoglobin oxygen saturation and the arterial pulse.[61] A

cardiac monitor should also be placed on the patient. An arterial blood gas (ABG) should be obtained to measure the P_{O_2} and the P_{CO_2}, the latter reflecting ventilation. It should confirm the oxygen saturation readings obtained with the pulse oximeter; if it does not, an abnormal hemoglobin should be suspected. An ABG also provides information about the patient's ventilatory status and acid-base balance; however, this is particularly vulnerable to errors introduced by improper sampling, handling, and storage. Special attention should be paid to the most common sources of error: excessive amounts of heparin, presence of air bubbles, or failure to reduce the temperature of the specimen by placing on ice immediately.[52]

Other laboratory studies should include a hemoglobin and hematocrit to diagnose anemia or polycythemia. A methemoglobin level should be obtained if the blood turns chocolate color when exposed to air or if exposure is suggested by history. A chest radiograph is commonly indicated in all patients as part of the evaluation of the cardiac and pulmonary systems. Attention should be paid to the lung fields, pulmonary vascular markings, and heart size and silhouette. Further evaluation of the cardiac system, including an ECG and echocardiogram, should proceed if heart disease is suspected. Specific studies such as a barium swallow, bronchoscopy, and CT scan should be obtained as indicated to exclude specific entities.

Prehospital Considerations

The appropriate care of patients with cyanosis begins in the field if that is where first contact by the health-care system occurs. EMS personnel should be properly trained in the assessment and management of airway and cardiopulmonary problems in children. Oxygen 100% should be administered as airway, breathing, and circulation are assessed and stabilized. Respiratory and cardiac monitoring should be instituted along with pulse oximetry if available. If symptoms or signs of upper airway obstruction are evident, the patient should be transported with as little distress as possible while being comforted and held by the parent. If wheezing or signs of lower airway obstruction are present, treatment with an inhaled bronchodilating agent should be attempted (see section on Asthma).

Therapeutic Trial

The response to oxygen should be measured by comparing the P_{O_2} from the arterial blood gas or oximetry reading in room air with that obtained during administration of 100% oxygen. This comparison assists in differentiating between primary cardiac disease, which does not respond because of ventilation-perfusion defects, and pulmonary disease, which is primarily due to ventilation deficits and should show improvement with supplemental oxygen.[53] Cyanosis secondary to an abnormal hemoglobin will not be relieved by the administration of oxygen.

RESPIRATORY DISTRESS/DYSPNEA

Dyspnea, or difficult, labored respirations is a symptom described as a subjective feeling of respiratory discomfort.[62] Respiratory distress occurs when the respiratory system has difficulty in maintaining gas exchange at a rate that matches the body's metabolic demands.[63] Respiratory failure results when the pulmonary system fails to meet the body's metabolic demands by providing adequate oxygen and eliminating carbon dioxide, and this impairment becomes a threat to life.[64] Respiratory distress accounts for approximately 10% of all pediatric emergency department visits.[65] Any underlying disorder that presents with respiratory distress may eventually become life-threatening. Respiratory distress accompanied by acute respiratory failure accounts for a large portion of pediatric deaths yearly in the United States. Therefore the presence of respiratory distress in an infant or child requires immediate intervention and evaluation for the underlying cause.

Pathophysiology

The human body coordinates many complex elements into an integrated system to provide normal respiratory activity. The CNS, including the cerebral cortex and the respiratory centers in the pons and medulla of the brainstem, provide outgoing impulses that travel via the spinal cord and peripheral nervous system to the neuromuscular junctions of the muscles of the chest wall, neck, and abdomen.[64] These muscles, in conjunction with the supporting skeletal framework of the body (particularly the spine and ribs), allow the bellows function of the pulmonary system to occur in response to the CNS stimuli.[64] Air traverses the conducting airways to the alveoli where gas exchange occurs. The cardiovascular and lymphatic systems maintain the fluid balance in the lungs, allowing this normal exchange of gases.

Respiratory distress may occur as a result of impairment anywhere along this ventilatory pathway. Term infants, and particularly premature newborns, have an immature central respiratory control center, which is easily affected by environmental or metabolic changes.[64] Infants also have a relatively compliant chest wall with poorly developed intercostal muscles compared to older children and adults, which leads to inward chest wall movement rather than to lung expansion during respirations.[66] In an infant the diaphragm is the primary muscle responsible for most of the work of respiration. All of the muscles involved in respiration, including the diaphragm, can become easily fatigued in an infant. The smaller lung volumes and lower residual capacities of infants provide a minimal reserve of oxygen, making them unable to tolerate any interruption in the supply of oxygen.[64]

The most important factor predisposing infants and younger children to respiratory dysfunction is the smaller diameter of their airways. Because resistance varies inversely with the fourth power of the radius of the airway, a small change in the airway diameter increases resistance to airflow dramatically.[67] This is particularly important in newborns because their tracheas and bronchis are respectively one third and one half the diameter of adult trachea and bronchi.[64] The smaller airways and alveoli of infants are more susceptible to collapse because of a lower elastic recoil.[64]

Differential Considerations

As shown in the box on p. 1068, respiratory distress most commonly occurs in children because of abnormalities within the pulmonary, cardiovascular, or metabolic systems

or secondary to a disruption of the CNS drive. In the presence of respiratory distress, it is important to make an initial differentiation within the pulmonary system between upper and lower airway disease based on the presence or absence of stridor on physical examination[68] (see Stridor).

Upper Airway Disease. Diseases of the upper airway are characterized primarily by inspiratory stridor, because as inspiration begins, the negative pressure (relative to atmospheric pressure) of the pleural space is transmitted to the airways, and the partially obstructed airway produces turbulent air flow.[69] Inspiratory stridor usually indicates a supraglottic obstruction, whereas expiratory and biphasic respiratory stridor generally point to an obstruction below the larynx. Children with inspiratory and expiratory stridor or expiratory stridor alone usually have a more significant obstruction. If stridor is present but the voice remains normal, the lesion is usually subglottic or tracheal. A hoarse voice or muffled cry indicates glottic, pharyngeal, or supraglottic pathology.[68] Diseases of the upper airway primarily result in abnormalities of ventilation; with severe degrees of obstruction, perfusion abnormalities can also result.

Acute upper airway obstruction in childhood is most often caused by infection or aspiration of a foreign body. Croup, epiglottitis, and bacterial tracheitis are the three most common causes of infectious upper airway obstruction.[66] In children with croup the infection is predominantly viral in origin and is often preceded by symptoms of an upper respiratory infection. Symptoms of the illness typically are gradual in onset and include a hoarse "seal-bark" cough and accompanying fever. The child usually does not appear toxic, although the degree of respiratory distress present can be variable.[70]

On the other hand, children with acute epiglottitis, a more serious bacterial infection of the epiglottitis caused primarily by *H. influenzae*, have rapid onset of an illness characterized by stridor, high fever, and signs of toxicity. The child will often appear anxious. Other common symptoms include sore throat, drooling, and a muffled voice.[66] The incidence of invasive disease caused by *H. influenzae*, including epiglottitis, has declined dramatically since the introduction of conjugate vaccination in the United States.[71]

Bacterial tracheitis has some features of both croup and epiglottitis. It is often a secondary infection caused by *Staphylococcus aureus* or *H. influenzae* involving an inflamed trachea from an antecedent viral infection.[68]

Because it is a subglottic lesion, bacterial tracheitis can mimic croup; yet it also has many characteristics of epiglottitis because of the bacterial cause, including the presence of high fever and a toxic appearance. One frequently reported feature is the presence of copious amounts of purulent sputum. Other less common infectious causes of stridor in children include peritonsillar abscess, retropharyngeal abscess (see Chapter 49), and diphtheria, which, although rare, still occurs in the United States.[66,72]

The most common noninfectious cause of acute stridor in the pediatric age group is an aspirated foreign body,[66] which can be seen in all age groups. The aspirated object can cause airway obstruction and stridor by lodging in various places within the upper airway or GI tract includ-

Respiratory Distress: Diagnostic Considerations

Upper airway disease

Infection

Croup (acute laryngotracheobronchitis)
Epiglottitis
Bacterial tracheitis
Peritonsillar abscess
Retropharyngeal abscess
Diphtheria

Trauma

Foreign body
Neck injury
Vocal cord paralysis
Smoke inhalation
Subglottic stenosis

Congenital

Vascular ring
Laryngeal web
Vocal cord paralysis
Laryngomalacia
Tracheomalacia
Micrognathia (Pierre Robin syndrome)
Glossoptosis (Down syndrome, hypothyroidism,
  Beckwith-Wiedemann syndrome)

Allergic

Spasmodic croup
Anaphylaxis
Angioneurotic edema

Neoplasms

Tracheal
Laryngeal
Esophageal
Neck

Lower airway disease

Infection

Pneumonia (bacterial and viral)
Bronchiolitis
Pleural effusions
Empyema
Sepsis

Allergic

Asthma
Anaphylaxis

Cardiovascular

Congestive heart failure
Congenital heart disease
Pulmonary edema
Pleural effusions
Pulmonary embolism

Polycythemia
Severe anemia

Trauma

Foreign body
Pneumothorax
Pulmonary contusion
Diaphragmatic defect
Smoke inhalation
Near drowning
Spinal cord injury

Congenital

Cystic fibrosis
Diaphragmatic defect

Neoplasm

Pulmonary tumors
Mediastinal masses

Other

Sarcoidosis
Pulmonary hemosiderosis
Scoliosis

Nervous system disease

Infection

Meningitis
Encephalitis

Trauma

Increased intracranial pressure
Intracranial hemorrhage

Neuropathy/myopathy

Guillain-Barré syndrome
Infant botulism
Werdnig-Hoffman disease
Muscular dystrophy
Myasthenia gravis

Other

Ingestions
Seizures

Metabolic disease

Metabolic acidosis

Dehydration
Sepsis
Diabetic ketoacidosis
Salicylate intoxication
Other toxins

Increased oxygen demand

Fever
Hyperthyroidism

ing the pharynx, larynx, trachea, or esophagus.[73] There may be an accompanying history of possible foreign-body ingestion or aspiration, but it is not unusual for the diagnosis to be delayed until after a work-up, (including obtaining radiographs) for the respiratory distress has been initiated. Other traumatic causes of upper airway obstruction manifested by stridor include trauma to the neck with subsequent soft-tissue swelling impinging on the airway, vocal cord paralysis, smoke inhalation, or traumatic subglottic stenosis.[62]

Infants less than 6 months of age who present with stridor should be considered to have a possible underlying anatomic abnormality that may now be symptomatic secondary to an accompanying illness. Common congenital anatomic abnormalities that may predispose infants to upper airway obstruction include anomalous vascular rings, laryngeal webs, vocal cord paralysis, laryngomalacia, or tracheomalacia. Micrognathia, seen in Pierre Robin syndrome, and glossoptosis, seen in multiple syndromes including Down syndrome, hypothyroidism, and Beckwith-Wiedemann syndrome, can also produce significant upper airway obstruction with subsequent respiratory distress.[62]

Allergic or immunologic processes may also lead to the development of upper airway obstruction. Spasmodic croup, anaphylaxis, and angioneurotic edema can all lead to respiratory distress with accompanying stridor. Neoplasms involving the larynx or trachea, the upper GI tract, or other structures of the neck may become symptomatic by pressing on the airway and presenting with signs of upper airway obstruction.[62]

Lower Airway Disease. Diseases of the lower airways and lung parenchyma that commonly cause respiratory distress in childhood and can lead to respiratory failure include pneumonia, bronchiolitis, asthma or reactive airway disease, and pulmonary edema secondary to congenital heart disease. The common pathway to respiratory distress and failure in lower airway disease includes alveolar and airway closure causing hypoxemia with the subsequent development of ventilation and perfusion abnormalities.[66]

The most common infectious diseases involving the lower airways in children are pneumonia and bronchiolitis. Pneumonia involves infection of the interstitium or alveoli of the lung. It occurs in every pediatric age group and can have various underlying causes. Children with bacterial pneumonia, commonly caused by *Streptococcus pneumoniae, H. influenzae,* or *S. aureus,* frequently present with cough, fever, crackles, and decreased breath sounds on auscultation of the lungs.[74] Viral pneumonias are characterized by a preceding upper respiratory infection, fever, and variable pulmonary findings. Other atypical pneumonias, such as those caused by *Mycoplasma pneumoniae* and *Chlamydia trachomatis,* may present with findings similar to those seen with viruses.[74]

Bronchiolitis is an important cause of lower airway disease with airway obstruction in infants and young children. It is an acute, small-airway infection, usually caused by RSV, although it has been reported to occur with parainfluenzae infection, often in conjunction with RSV.[75] The presentation of the illness varies from mild wheezing in an otherwise happy-appearing infant to severe respiratory distress with tachypnea, nasal flaring, and intercostal retractions. Other infectious processes that may present with respiratory distress include parapneumonic pleural effusions with empyemas and generalized sepsis, which lead to leaky pulmonary capillaries and subsequent pulmonary edema.

Asthma is one of the most common diseases of the lower airway affecting children and requiring medical intervention in emergency departments. Asthma is defined as recurrent episodes of airway obstruction responsive to bronchodilator therapy.[75] An acute first episode of wheezing should cause the examiner to consider a possible aspirated foreign body.[73] Children with asthma present in varying degrees of respiratory distress, depending on the degree of airway obstruction present. In children with wheezing accompanied by urticaria, mucosal edema, and other signs of histamine release an anaphylactic allergic reaction should be considered.[76]

A variety of cardiovascular conditions in children can occur with respiratory distress. Congestive heart failure, most commonly resulting from congenital heart disease, can lead to the development of pulmonary edema and pleural effusions, both of which can cause impairment in pulmonary ventilation and perfusion. Pulmonary edema and pleural effusions can also result from primary disease processes involving the hepatic or renal systems. Children with congestive heart failure may have complaints of orthopnea or paroxysmal nocturnal dyspnea, although these symptoms are much less commonly reported in children than in adults.[62] Fever is usually absent but may be present if the heart failure has been precipitated by an infectious process. Respiratory distress can also result from a pulmonary embolism. Polycythemia or severe anemia can produce respiratory distress by interfering with oxygen transport or precipitating heart failure.[68]

A number of different traumatic causes can lead to the development of respiratory distress in children. As previously noted, aspirated foreign bodies are a common cause of both upper and lower airway obstruction in children. Unfortunately, the history of a possible aspirated lower airway foreign body is often unavailable, and suspicions should be raised if it is the first wheezing episode in a child or if differential wheezing or air entry is present.[72] Blunt chest trauma, often seen in children involved in motor vehicle accidents or falls, may result in a pneumothorax, hemothorax, or pulmonary contusion. Children who have sustained smoke inhalation, near drowning, or an acute spinal cord injury can also experience respiratory distress secondary to their injuries.[77]

Other disease processes involving the lower airway in children include congenital diaphragmatic defects, cystic fibrosis, pulmonary or mediastinal neoplasms, sarcoidosis, pulmonary hemosiderosis, and musculoskeletal anomalies such as scoliosis.[62]

Nervous System Disease. The central and peripheral nervous systems make up an important part of the ventilatory pathway. Alterations in the CNS control can lead to hyperventilation or hypoventilation, loss of protective airway reflexes, or a decrease in pharyngeal tone with subsequent upper airway obstruction.[64] CNS infections, including meningitis and encephalitis, can interfere with the respiratory pathway at various levels with subsequent respiratory compromise. Increased intracranial pressure, whether resulting from CNS infection, intracranial hemorrhage, or other mass lesions such as a tumor, can disrupt the respiratory center impulses and produce several abnormal respiratory patterns including apnea. Drug ingestions or seizure activity can cause CNS depression with subsequent respiratory suppression.[78] A variety of progressive neuropathies and myopathies will eventually involve the respiratory system, leading to weakened respiratory muscles. These include Guillain-Barré syndrome and infant botulism, which are usually more acute in onset, Werdnig-Hoffman disease, muscular dystrophy, and myasthenia gravis.[62] In the absence of specific signs or symptoms of a CNS disorder, it is important to remember that altered mental status, seizures, coma, or other symptoms may be a consequence of preceding hypoxemia or hypercarbia rather than the primary cause of the respiratory abnormalities.

Metabolic Disease. Metabolic acidosis is a common metabolic abnormality in infants and children in which respiratory stimulation occurs as a compensatory mechanism producing respiratory distress.[68] It can result from a number of underlying disorders but it should be aggressively treated to prevent further respiratory compromise. Dehydration, sepsis, diabetic ketoacidosis, salicylate intoxication, or other toxins may be responsible for the development of the metabolic acidosis. Conditions altering the metabolic state of the body, including fever and hyperthyroidism, can increase the metabolic rate and subsequently lead to an increase in oxygen demand, resulting in tachypnea and signs of respiratory distress.[68]

Diagnostic Work-Up

Acute respiratory distress in a child is an emergency that requires prompt action to identify the underlying cause and to begin appropriate therapeutic measures in a timely fashion. Despite advances in technology that permit precise measurement of physiologic parameters, the patient's history and physical examination remain the basis for evaluating respiratory distress. In general, children with respiratory distress should be approached according to the severity of their signs and symptoms. Alert children should be allowed to remain with their parents in the most comfortable position and approached as gently as possible.

History. A thorough history should be obtained early and focus on the presenting problem and contributing conditions. The most likely causes of respiratory distress, as shown in the box above, often differ by age group. In children under 2 years of age, common causes of respiratory distress include pneumonia, reactive airway disease (RAD) presenting as bronchiolitis or asthma, croup, foreign-body aspiration, congenital heart disease, sepsis, submersion injury, and congenital anomalies of the airway, particularly in infants less than 6 months old. Respiratory distress in older children is more frequently due to asthma, pneumonia, ingestions, submersion injury, trauma, cystic fibrosis, or peripheral neuropathies.[68]

The onset and pattern of the respiratory distress, temporal relationships, and alleviating or exacerbating factors

---

Common Causes of Respiratory Distress

Children < 2 years old
Pneumonia
Bronchiolitis
Asthma/RAD
Croup
Foreign body aspiration
Congenital heart disease
Sepsis
Submersion injury

Children > 2 years old
Asthma/RAD
Pneumonia
Ingestions
Submersion injury
Trauma
Cystic fibrosis
Nervous system disease

---

should be obtained along with information about associated symptoms including stridor, wheezing, fever, cough, snoring, chest pain, or recent changes in mental status or behavior. Any previous history of pulmonary disease such as asthma or cystic fibrosis, congenital heart disease, or perinatal problems, including bronchopulmonary dysplasia, should also be obtained early in the evaluation of the patient. Further history should include any recent traumatic episodes or possibility of foreign-body aspiration. History of ingestion or inhalation of any material, including poisons or smoke, should also be noted. Family history of cardiac, pulmonary, metabolic, and infectious diseases should also be obtained.

Physical Examination. Initial assessment of the patient presenting with respiratory distress should focus on the status and stability of the pulmonary and cardiovascular system while attempting to identify the underlying cause. The initial examination should consist of a rapid evaluation of airway, breathing, and circulation with an assessment of the degree of respiratory distress using the following clinical variables: mental status; color; respiratory rate; presence of signs of respiratory distress including grunting, nasal flaring, and retractions; and the quality of air entry on auscultation of the lungs.[65] The presence of stridor to differentiate between upper and lower airway disease should also be determined early in the examination.[68]

A full set of vital signs should be obtained during this initial assessment. It is important to know the normal respiratory rate, pulse, and blood pressure for children of different ages. A more focused examination of the pulmonary system should include the upper airway to assess the degree and timing of stridor if present, evaluation of the adequacy of air exchange including chest expansion, and auscultation for the presence of any adventitial lung sounds such as wheezes or crackles. It is important to note that the absence of wheezing in a child with asthma may indicate severe airway obstruction with poor air exchange; attention should be paid to the patient's respiratory rate, quality of air exchange, and presence of other signs of respiratory distress. The oropharynx should be examined cautiously by direct visualization only, without instrumentation, until the diagnosis of epiglottitis has been excluded.[70]

A complete cardiovascular examination should include evaluation of precordial activity, the regularity of heart sounds, the presence of heart murmurs or gallops, and the presence and quality of pulses including assessment of peripheral perfusion by eliciting capillary refill time. Signs of congestive heart failure such as crackles on auscultation of the lungs, hepatomegaly, or an increase in jugular venous distension should be specifically noted. A full neurologic examination should follow as the remainder of the physical examination is completed. It is important not to underestimate the degree of respiratory distress nor to leave the child unattended in the emergency or radiology departments until the initial evaluation and stabilization are complete.

Close observation with frequent reassessment is important in all children with respiratory distress. Progression to respiratory failure may be heralded by the clinical findings of decreasing air entry, increasing retractions with accessory muscle use, development of expiratory grunting or cyanosis, a decreasing level of consciousness, including the development of confusion or agitation, decreasing muscle tone, and vital sign changes including progressive tachycardia, increasing tachypnea, or apnea.[66]

Ancillary Data. In children with acute upper respiratory disease with obstruction, laboratory tests are usually ancillary to direct visualization of the upper airway. However, this investigation must proceed with great caution and only in a setting where controlled placement of an airway by experienced personnel is available, preferably in the operating room with the child under general anesthesia.[70]

Further laboratory and radiographic evaluation should be guided by the degree of respiratory distress and assist in identifying the underlying process. The initial laboratory evaluation of respiratory distress should include an assessment for hypoxemia. Pulse oximetry monitoring should be instituted immediately, because it provides a noninvasive, continuous, and generally valid measure of arterial hemoglobin oxygen saturation and the arterial pulse.[79] A cardiac monitor should also be placed on the patient. An ABG would be optimal to assess the patient's oxygenation status, measure the Pco_2, and provide information about the acid-base balance of the patient. It is important, however, to avoid making the patient worse by manipulations, particularly in the child with severe upper respiratory obstruction, until the capability for controlled placement of an airway is available. ABG evidence of respiratory failure in most clinical situations includes a Pco_2 greater than 50 mm Hg or Po_2 less than 50 mm Hg, or both, breathing room air at sea level.[64] A Pco_2 greater than 40 mm Hg in a child with asthma who is exhibiting signs of respiratory distress is an indication of impending respiratory failure.[64] Hematology and chemistry studies should be obtained as appropriate, including a CBC to assess for anemia, polycythemia, or evidence of infection, and electrolytes and glucose if metabolic disease is suspected. A blood culture should be obtained in the febrile patient.

In children with upper respiratory disease, lateral and anteroposterior radiographs of the soft tissues of the neck may be performed to assess airway narrowing if the diagnosis is uncertain, if a foreign body is suspected, or to evaluate the epiglottitis. If epiglottitis is suspected, airway films should be considered, with the patient remaining under observation in the emergency department, although many prefer direct visualization under very controlled conditions. For children with lower airway involvement confirmed by history and physical examination, a chest radiograph should be obtained as part of the evaluation of both the pulmonary and cardiovascular systems. Attention should be paid to the lung fields, pulmonary vascular markings, and heart size and silhouette. If a lower airway foreign body is suspected, inspiratory and expiratory or bilateral decubitus chest radiographs should be obtained. The decubitus x-ray studies are more appropriate for younger children who may not be able to cooperate to obtain films on maximal inspiration and expiration.

If heart disease is suspected, further evaluation of the cardiac system should include an ECG and echocardiogram. In the febrile, toxic-appearing child with respiratory distress without an obvious source of infection, sepsis and meningitis should be considered and a lumbar puncture may be warranted. A toxicology screen of both urine and blood should be obtained in children presenting with respiratory distress combined with an altered level of consciousness, or a respiratory acidosis with an anion gap. If neurologic symptoms predominate or if there is a history of preceding head trauma, a CT scan of the head may be indicated. If the presence of a foreign body in the respiratory or GI tract is confirmed or strongly suspected, the child should proceed to the operating room for laryngoscopy and bronchoscopy under controlled conditions.

Prehospital Considerations

The appropriate care of children presenting with respiratory distress begins with the first contact by health-care workers, which may be paramedical personnel working in the field. EMS personnel should be properly trained in the assessment and management of airway and respiratory problems in children. The primary responsibility in prehospital care is evaluation and stabilization of airway, breathing, and circulation. Supplementary 100% humidified oxygen should be administered as this initial assessment occurs. Respiratory and cardiac monitoring should be instituted along with pulse oximetry if available. If symptoms or signs of upper airway obstruction are present, it is important to transport the patient with as little distress as possible in the parent's arms, allowing the child to find the most comfortable position. Maneuvers to assure airway patency including chin lift/jaw thrust positioning or nasal or oropharyngeal airways may be necessary if evidence of decreased pharyngeal tone causing airway obstruction is present, particularly in patients with altered mental status or neuromuscular disease. Placement of an artificial airway by tracheal intubation may be indicated for airway support or respiratory failure but should be performed only by trained personnel. If wheezing or signs of lower airway obstruction are present, treatment with an inhaled or injected bronchodilating agent should be attempted.

Therapeutic Trials

As initial evaluation of the patient proceeds, attention should be directed to the stabilization of airway, breathing, and circulation. In children with respiratory distress, stabilization of the airway is central to any therapeutic plan and should not be delayed by obtaining excessive ancillary data.[68] One hundred percent or high-flow humidified oxygen should be administered to the patient as the airway is evaluated. Children with symptoms and signs of upper airway obstruction should be manipulated as little as possible until the airway has been stabilized. They should be allowed to be held and comforted by their parents and they should be allowed to find the most comfortable position to maintain their airway. The parent may attempt to blow oxygen by the child's face if it is not too distressing. Airway obstruction may occur secondary to poor pharyngeal muscle tone, particularly in children with an altered level of consciousness, such as the postictal state after a seizure or with neuromuscular disease. Head positioning to optimize the airway with the chin lift–jaw thrust maneuver may be helpful in this situation. A nasal or oropharyngeal airway can also be placed to maintain the airway but may be difficult to keep in place in an alert patient.

Airway intubation with mechanical ventilation may be required to protect the airway in cases of upper airway obstruction including epiglottitis, bacterial tracheitis, and severe croup or if the protective airway reflexes have been lost. Mechanical ventilation may also be indicated for patients with disturbances of respiratory rate or rhythm including apnea, hemodynamic instability including shock states, unresponsive metabolic acidosis, signs of increased intracranial pressure, or for patients progressing to respiratory failure noted by a combination of clinical signs and physiologic parameters.

STRIDOR

Stridor is a crowing, high-pitched sound commonly heard during inspiration. It is usually indicative of obstruction in the larynx or the extrathoracic trachea associated with partial obstruction of the upper airway. It is typically heard during inspiration, but may be present during both inspiration and expiration when the anatomic site of obstruction is more distal. It demands immediate attention and evaluation.

Pathophysiology

Stridor is produced by the turbulence of airflow that develops from a laryngeal or tracheal obstruction.[80] Inspiratory stridor usually indicates obstruction at the laryngeal level or above, whereas expiratory or biphasic stridor points to a lesion in or around the trachea.[81] During inspiration, there is negative intraluminal pressure immediately below the tracheal obstruction, which leads to a dynamic narrowing of the extrathoracic trachea and air turbulence.[81] This dynamic tracheal compression occurs quite readily in children because of the softness of the tracheal tissue. Moreover, the inspiration also creates negative pleural pressure. Because infants have very compliant chest walls, they also have marked suprasternal retractions. In contrast, children with lower airway disease usually do not have stridor. Respiratory distress tends to be greater in the

younger children due to the small size of the infant larynx; the presence of loose, submucous, connective tissue in the supraglottic and subglottic regions; and the tight encirclement of the subglottic area by the cricoid cartilage, which is the narrowest airway point in children under 8 years old. Any edema, inflammation, or excessive mucus results in significant impingement on the airway.

The quality of the stridor may indicate the level of obstruction. Stridor originating in the larynx or subglottic region tends to be high-pitched and associated with hoarseness or aphonia, whereas stridor resulting from lower tracheal or bronchial pathology is often biphasic and associated with expiratory wheeze.

Differential Considerations

When considering different causes of stridor, it is helpful to determine whether the stridor is relatively acute (present from a few hours to a few days) or chronic. The causes of stridor are summarized in the boxes on p. 1073 and Table 59-1. Some children may have an acute stridor superimposed on a chronic cause. For example, infants with a subglottic stenosis or a vascular ring are predisposed to frequent severe acute croup. In babies with acute stridor the diagnosis is usually fairly certain; the main concern is one of management (e.g., croup, retropharyngeal abscess, aspirated or swallowed foreign body, or airway trauma). In patients with a chronic or frequently recurring stridor the urgency with which to search for an anatomic cause depends on the degree of physiologic impairment.[82]

The most common cause of acute stridor in the emergency department is viral laryngotracheobronchitis (croup). This condition is usually accompanied by coryza, a hoarse voice, and a barking cough. The stridor is often very loud, frightening, and abrupt in onset in the middle of the night. Nevertheless, many children arrive somewhat improved after a trip in the cool night air. They tend to be playful, active, and nontoxic looking.

In contrast to croup, children with bacterial tracheitis are toxic. They may have had typical croup for a few days but then deteriorate over several hours.[83] High fever, toxicity, and marked respiratory distress with signs of both upper and lower airway disease are typical. Compared with viral croup, bacterial tracheitis is a rare entity. Stridor associated with epiglottitis tends to be mild or absent; crying is weak or muffled.[84] These children are almost always anxious and tachycardic and tend to sit upright. Immunization has decreased the frequency of epiglottitis. Children with retropharyngeal abscess usually have a longer history and often assume a supine opisthotonic position, with the neck hyperextended to make breathing easier. In contrast to croup, children with either one of these two diagnoses are hesitant to eat or drink because of a profoundly sore throat. It is quite rare for a patient with severe adenoidal enlargement (e.g., infectious mononucleosis) or peritonsillar abscess to have stridor. It develops late in the illness in older children.

Allergic angioedema is likely in preschool- and school-aged children and is associated with facial swelling and an urticarial rash. Foreign-body inhalation must be considered if there is a history of a choking episode and abrupt onset of biphasic stridor. Drooling and dysphagia usually

Causes of Chronic/Frequently Recurrent Stridor

Nasopharynx
Choanal atresia
Macroglossia
Craniofacial anomalies
Thyroglossal duct cyst

Larynx
Laryngomalacia
Laryngeal web and cleft
Laryngocele
Subglottic stenosis

Trachea
Tracheal web and cysts

Vascular
Vascular ring
Large hemangiomas in upper airway

Neoplasm
Benign and malignant in neck and chest

Traumatic
Subglottic stenosis (postintubation)

Neurologic
Poor pharyngeal muscle tone
Laryngeal paralysis (may be sudden in Arnold-Chiari malformation)

Causes of Acute Stridor

Infectious
• Laryngotracheobronchitis (croup)
• Bacterial tracheitis
• Epiglottitis
• Retropharyngeal abscess
• Peritonsillar abscess
• Massive adenotonsillar enlargement (e.g., infectious mononucleosis)
• Diphtheria

Inflammatory
• Angioneurotic edema

Traumatic
• Foreign body in nasopharynx, larynx, trachea, or esophagus
• Laryngeal fracture
• Postintubation
• Ingestion of corrosives

Metabolic
• Hypocalcemia

Psychogenic

accompany an esophageal foreign body. A laryngeal fracture requires significant trauma to the neck. Crepitus and subcutaneous emphysema may be present.

Hypocalcemia is a very rare cause of stridor. Because of associated neuronal excitability, there are often associated seizures, tremor, or carpopedal spasm, and tetanic adduction of the vocal cords.[85] Hyperventilation may induce stridor in chronically hypocalcemic patients because of its attendant respiratory alkalosis and a further drop in the ionized calcium.[86,87] On rare occasions, psychogenic stridor may occur in adolescents, either acutely or intermittently.[88] These patients are able to talk freely and have no other demonstrable organic reason for the symptom; stridor tends to appear within the context of severe psychologic distress.[89] Because misdiagnosis may be life-threatening, organic causes should be ruled out.

Chronic stridor is less frequent and often starts during the newborn period. Causes are numerous, most of them being congenital anomalies.[90] Of these, tracheolaryngomalacia is the most common. It is due to a weakness of the tracheal walls of the supporting cartilage leading to collapse during inspiration.[91] It begins within the first 10 days of life. The stridor is often intermittent, increasing with agitation and decreasing with lying prone. The cry is normal; there are no swallowing or feeding abnormalities and dyspnea is usually absent.[81]

Severe cases of tracheolaryngomalacia may occur, causing respiratory distress and apnea. These children sometimes tolerate viral infections poorly and may decompensate acutely.[92] A neonate with a weak or absent cry, stridor, respiratory distress, and feeding problems may have a vocal cord paralysis. This clinical picture may coexist with other anomalies (e.g., Arnold-Chiari malformation with an elevated cerebrospinal fluid pressure and subsequent pressure on the vagal nuclei).[91]

Children with severe subglottic stenosis present with chronic inspiratory and expiratory stridor and recurrent episodes of severe croup. Mild cases may exhibit stridor with exercise or stress and frequent croup.[80] Although this may be a primary lesion (presenting at birth), many of these babies have a history of prolonged neonatal ventilation and prematurity. Babies who have tracheal compression from a vascular ring tend to have both inspiratory stridor and an expiratory wheeze, swallowing problems because of an esophageal compression, and episodes of severe croup. The underlying chronic symptoms may be quite mild; careful physician's questioning and subsequent parental recollection of the historical details during all acute croup episodes brings the diagnosis to light.

Diagnostic Work-Up

The first priority in the emergency setting is to determine the likelihood of epiglottitis or respiratory failure requiring immediate airway stabilization. Once these two entities are deemed unlikely, an orderly history should be taken. Onset at or very shortly after birth suggests a congenital airway or a vascular anomaly (e.g., tracheomalacia, congenital subglottic stenosis, congenital bilateral vocal

TABLE 59-1. Acute Presentation of Stridor—Common Causes

	Age	Drooling	Fever	Posture	Common etiology	X-Ray findings	Other distinguishing features
Epiglottitis	May happen over wide range, including newborn or adults	+	Usually high; 40% afebrile (may be absent)	Sitting up; leaning forward	*H. influenzae*	Enlarged epiglottis "thumbprint"*	Usually short history; toxic-looking; stridor usually mild
Croup viral, spasmodic	6 months-3 yr	–	Variable; absent	Lying down	Viral; laryngeal spasm	Subglottic narrowing; ballooning hypopharynx variable	Barking cough; hoarse voice
Foreign body	>9 months	+/–	–	Variable	N/A	Depends on radiopacity; air trapping in expiration*	
Peritonsillar abscess	>12 yrs	+/–	High	Upright; painful neck movement	Beta-hemolytic streptococci (group A)	–	Stridor usually mild or absent; visible on exam of oropharynx; severe sore throat
Trauma	Variable	–	–	Variable	N/A	Fractures; soft tissue swelling	History often suggestive; skin exam may reveal diagnosis
Retropharyngeal abscess	<6 yr (50% <12 months)	+	Often high but variable	Hyperextension	Beta-hemolytic streptococci *S. aureus*	Enlarged retropharyngeal space*	History often longer than 12-24 hr
Bacterial tracheitis	1-5 yr	–	High	Variable	*H. influenzae* *S. aureus*	Irregular tracheal wall	Inflammation; tracheal pseudomembrane noted during endotracheal intubation; toxic looking

*Most distinguishing feature.
N/A = Guidelines only. A significant degree of overlap exists in these parameters.

cord paralysis, laryngeal web and cyst, facial skeletal anomaly, or a vascular ring compressing the trachea). However, neither laryngomalacia nor vascular compression may manifest until a few weeks after birth.[90]

If the stridor is acute, look for a history of viral symptoms, fever, barking cough, difficulty in swallowing, sore throat, neck trauma, toxic ingestion, smoke inhalation, or a sudden choking episode. Dysphagia with drooling suggests a foreign body, retropharyngeal abscess or hematoma, or epiglottitis or diphtheria. A chronic or recurrent history may be due to an underlying fixed obstruction (e.g., vascular ring) with superimposed edema resulting from a viral infection.

Other findings that should be sought include associated feeding problems, swallowing difficulties, cyanosis with feeding, cough, hoarseness, and position-dependent symptoms. A perinatal history of hydramnios (laryngeal cleft), birth trauma (vocal cord palsy), prematurity, or neonatal ventilation is useful, as is information about previous pneumonia or recent chest or neck surgery.

A great deal of information can be obtained by initially observing the child during the physical examination. First, the severity of airway obstruction must be assessed and the respiratory distress alleviated. Some of the warning signs are altered consciousness reflected as anxiety, restlessness, undue fatigue, and decreasing level of consciousness; respiratory findings of persistent tachycardia; tachypnea; and suprasternal, intercostal, and subcostal retractions. In babies, head bobbing with each breath is suggestive of severe distress.[93] Decreased air entry and respiratory effort, extreme pallor, and cyanosis require immediate intervention. The examiner should note the preferred position (sitting up vs. lying down); hyperextension or another abnormal position of the neck (abscess, tumor); drooling (epiglottitis, abscess, foreign body in the esophagus); and signs of trauma to the face, neck, or chest.

The quality of stridor is rarely diagnostic on its own but may be important; the nasal and hypopharyngeal stridor (stertor) tends to be low-pitched, whereas the pitch of more distant lesions is usually higher.[82] The presence of an expiratory component of the stridor points toward the subglottic lesion or below. The physician should also note the quality of the voice. Aphonia suggests a vocal cord lesion such as a cyst, web, cord paresis; muffling occurs with supraglottic lesions; and hoarseness is associated with laryngeal pathology. Associated wheezing is also important and may be due to laryngotracheobronchitis (croup) with or without associated asthma, foreign body in the airway or esophagus, mediastinal mass or congenital lesion such as a vascular ring, subglottic hemangioma, and distal tracheal stenosis.[94] Anaphylaxis, smoke inhalation, and psychogenic problems may also cause the combination of these two signs.[92,94-98]

The level of conssciousness is a sensitive barometer of cerebral hypoxia. Restlessness and irritability may reflect pain, sepsis, shock, dehydration, or hypoxia. Seizures or coma can occur as a result of severe hypoxia.

In stable children with chronic stridor, the emergency pediatrician may wish to look for failure to thrive, which is indicative of chronic hypoxia, chronic respiratory distress associated with excessive caloric expenditure, neurologic problems or hydrocephalus (vocal cord palsy due to compression of vagal nuclei),[99] cutaneous hemangiomas (airway hemangiomas may be associated), craniofacial anomalies (e.g., Pierre Robin or Treacher Collins syndrome), or macroglossia.[82,99]

Ancillary Data

In a stridorous child, ensuring an adequate airway must take precedence over diagnostic maneuvers. Moreover, unnecessary intervention may increase the underlying distress, potentially placing the child at significant risk.[91] Some children have a rather obvious diagnosis, require little or no investigation, and need to be stabilized and treated immediately. Examples include epiglottitis, severe croup, bacterial tracheitis, foreign body in the upper airway or trachea, smoke inhalation, anaphylaxis, or airway trauma. Most patients with stridor (acute or chronic) are stable and allow some time for evaluation. Investigations may have to be conducted on an emergent or urgent basis, whereas others are semielective. Respiratory compromise, worsening stridor, craniofacial anomalies with stridor, suspected neck or chest mass, stridor after recent neck or mediastinal surgery, and symptomatic smoke inhalation all require urgent pediatric anesthesia or ENT consultation.[82]

The emergency physician should generally admit children with stridor who are very young and have problems such as failure to thrive, stridor with drinking (tracheoesophageal fistula), apnea with feeding, cutaneous hemangioma, stridor with hydrocephalus, or a history of stridor aggravated by sleep; consultation is appropriate.[82] Babies with chronic or frequent stridor but no respiratory distress may often be evaluated electively.

Chest x-ray studies are indicated in most patients with obscure stridor and in all stridorous newborns.[90] Look for a right-sided aortic arch (associated with a vascular ring or sling), an air leak, mediastinal mass, or tracheal compression. Anteroposterior and lateral neck x-ray radiographs are also indicated in children with undiagnosed cause for stridor. It may be diagnostic of a foreign body, retropharyngeal mass, or epiglottitis, although if epiglottitis is considered,

direct visualization is often preferred. Good positioning of the head and neck are essential to avoid misinterpretation. Personnel skilled in airway management should be in attendance. Most children with croup do not need an x-ray film.

Transcutaneous pulse oximetry is useful for those with respiratory distress. Invasive procedures such as blood gases or blood cultures should be postponed until after the airway has been stabilized.

Flexible indirect endoscopy can be performed by an experienced pediatric surgeon, otolaryngologist, or pulmonologist. One can assess the nasal cavity, the base of the tongue, the supraglottic region, and the larynx, including the vocal cords. It is useful in patients with no respiratory compromise to rule out nasal masses, choanal atresia, congenital lesions at the base of the tongue, and vocal cord palsy. It is also useful in a cooperative, stable patient with possible early epiglottitis. An anesthetist must be present to intubate a patient if decompensation occurs during this procedure.[80] Rigid endoscopy (laryngoscopy, bronchoscopy, and esophagoscopy) must be performed under a general anesthetic in the operating room. This procedure is useful both diagnostically (to define the exact lesion along the airway down to the trachea and bronchi) and therapeutically (e.g., to remove a foreign body or to drain a pharyngeal abscess).

A barium esophagogram is indicated if vascular ring or tracheoesophageal fistula or laryngeal clefts are suspected. A CT scan or MRI are valuable for delineating the extent of a mediastinal or neck mass. Digital subtraction angiography is useful in looking at the great vessel anatomy in vascular tracheal compression. Fluoroscopy and xeroradiography may occasionally be useful in diagnosing obscure foreign bodies in the upper airway. None of these investigations are necessary in the Emergency Department.

Prehospital Considerations

Special attention must be paid to the airway patency, degree of respiratory distress, and oxygenation. The airway must be assessed and stabilized at the nearest hospital. Intervention may include humidified oxygen, racemic epinephrine, and corticosteroids in suspected croup; endotracheal intubation in children with epiglottitis, bacterial tracheitis, smoke inhalation, large mediastinal masses, or certain types of severely obstructed congenital airway lesions may be required expeditiously. Patients with stridor and respiratory compromise requiring an interhospital transfer should not be transported until their airway is secure; physician attendance is appropriate.

Therapeutic Trial

If the stridor is chronic and the patient is stable, fully examine and admit, or discharge the patient with a scheduled pediatric or ENT follow-up visit. Discharging the patient depends on the necessity of knowing the diagnosis right away, parental anxiety, and presence or absence of the "warning signs" (see previous discussion).

If the stridorous child is in respiratory distress, airway assessment and stabilization must take precedence over all other therapeutic steps. This procedure includes minimal disturbance, upright positioning, and humidified oxygen (usually via a hose held next to the infant's face, since masks are usually not well tolerated). Patients with suspected supraglottic pathology, a foreign body in the airway, or imminent respiratory failure evidenced by a decreasing level of consciousness, cyanosis, and respiratory fatigue must undergo emergent endotracheal intubation or foreign-body removal. The endotracheal tube size used in upper airway obstruction should be slightly smaller than normal: preterm, 2.0 mm; neonate, 2.5 mm; <6 months, 3.0 mm; 6 months to 2 years, 3.5 mm; 2 to 5 years, 4.0 mm; >5 years, 4 to 5 mm.[90] Further management of the individual child depends on the condition (see Chapters 11, 12, and 17 and specific sections of this chapter). Certain causes of stridor, such as smoke inhalation or large mediastinal mass, have a propensity for sudden deterioration without warning. The patient should be monitored continuously in the ICU, and consideration should be given to intubation during the early stages of airway obstruction to prevent a sudden, catastrophic deterioration. Cervical spine precautions must be maintained if there is a suspected traumatic etiology for the child's stridor. After the patient has been stabilized, therapeutic trials should reflect diagnostic considerations.

WHEEZING

Wheezing is a hissing, often musical expiratory sound, usually indicative of a medium-sized intrathoracic airway obstruction. Accompanying obstruction of the large bronchi or the upper airway is likely if wheezing is heard during inspiration. In young children, this sound is often harsh and nonmusical.

Pathophysiology

Wheezing is generated by bronchial wall vibrations and air flow turbulance because of an increase in the linear air flow velocity from narrowing of the airway.[100,101] The site of the origin of the wheeze is usually the larger bronchi because only at that level is the air velocity high enough to generate the sound. The primary airway pathology may be either bronchospasm (dynamic) or infection, inflammation, and intrinsic or extrinsic compression of the airway (fixed) involving the bronchi, trachea, or smaller airways (the bronchioles). The associated wheezing, however, is due to the concurrent dynamic narrowing of the larger airways caused by the positive pleural pressure generated during expiration to overcome the resistance.[100] Even in the presence of small airway disease, there is dynamic narrowing of the trachea and larger bronchi. In this situation, the pleural pressure outside the larger airways exceeds the insufficient expiratory pressure inside; the airway partially collapses.[101]

Infants are prone to severe airway obstruction and its accompanying complications such as atelectasis and respiratory failure. Contributing factors include the following:

1. The infantile airway is small in absolute caliber; therefore, resistance to airflow is dramatically increased by any obstructive disease.[102]
2. Peripheral airways may be disproportionately narrow in infancy due to a much higher peripheral airway resistance in small children.[103]
3. Babies have a compliant airway that lacks elasticity, resulting in an early airway closure and lower oxygen

---

> ### Causes of Wheezing
>
> **Reactive airway disease (RAD) asthma**
> Bronchopulmonary dysplasia
> Infection/inflammation
>   Bronchiolitis (RSV)
>   Pneumonia
> Intrinsic
> Allergic/anaphylaxis
>
> **Aspiration and aspiration syndromes**
> Foreign body
> Neuromuscular swallowing abnormality
> Esophageal obstruction
> Tracheoesophageal fistula or other abnormal communication between GI and respiratory tracts
>
> **Metabolic**
> Cystic fibrosis
>
> **Extrinsic compression of airway**
> Vascular anomalies
> Mediastinal masses
> Foreign body in esophagus
>
> **Cardiac disease** (CHF, large left to right shunt, large left atrium)
>
> **Anomalies of the tracheobronchial tree**
> Narrowing or deformity of larynx, trachea, bronchi

---

tension even during normal respiration.[104] This creates a potential for early disturbance in gas exchange.

4. The rib cage of a small child is very compliant. This fact, along with the horizontal insertion of the diaphragm to the rib cage, results in increased work of breathing.[105]

Differential Considerations

Although most children who come to the emergency department with wheezing will have asthma or bronchiolitis as a cause of reactive airway disease (RAD), other important diagnoses must be considered (see box above). On occasion known asthmatics may develop a new cause for wheezing such as myocarditis, foreign body aspiration/ingestion, and others.

First Episode of Wheezing. Most of these children have viral bronchiolitis, especially those who have wheezing during the winter with symptoms of a preceding upper respiratory infection (URI) and developing cough and respiratory distress. Those who present with a second wheezing episode probably have a RAD.

Sudden Onset of Wheezing. If wheezing occurs suddenly, especially when the child is awake, during meals, or play, aspiration of a foreign body should be ruled out even when no definite history of aspiration is obtained. (The history is negative in approximately 15% of cases.[106]) Unilateral wheeze with decreased breath sounds are common but not always obvious. Occasionally, the foreign body is radiolucent and causes a very minor occlusion of the airways; the physical and radiologic signs may be normal.[100] A suspicious history of unexplained sudden onset of wheezing becomes critical in such circumstances. In 17% of cases the diagnosis is not made until a month or more after aspiration.[100] Failure of management may be signaled by persistent wheezing, chronic cough, or the development of pneumonia.[107] Esophageal foreign bodies may on occasion cause wheezing (or stridor) by tracheal compression.[101]

Prolonged Wheezing Over Several Weeks or Frequent Wheezing Relapses. Although most of these patients will turn out to be inadequately managed asthmatics, other diagnoses should be considered, especially in a small child. A history of foreign-body aspiration may be unclear or forgotten. Tiny infants with prolonged wheezing and inadequate response to therapy should have the diagnosis of cystic fibrosis excluded by a formal sweat test; failure to thrive and malabsorption may be absent.[100] Aspiration symptoms, another diagnostic possibility in this situation, consist of swallowing incoordination, esophageal reflux, or a communication between the respiratory and GI tract.

Associated Feeding Difficulties. A history of chronic vomiting soon after feeding (often exaggerated by lying prone or a sudden change in position), or of coughing or choking associated with feeding, must be taken seriously and aspiration syndromes ruled out.

Associated Documented Persistent or Recurrent Pneumonia. A foreign body triggers a local inflammatory response; the atelectasis and trapped secretions become infected.[107] The associated pneumonia responds poorly or incompletely to medical therapy, and bronchoscopy to remove the foreign body is necessary. With repeated inhalations resulting from aspiration syndromes, chronic interstitial pneumonia may occur. Immune deficiency syndromes may occur with persistent wheezing[107]; recurrent severe bacterial pneumonias are common. A nontoxic older child (age 3 years and older) with fever, pneumonia on chest x-ray radiograph, and wheezes in the chest (often first time) may have *M. pneumoniae* infection.[108]

Associated Grunting, Slow Feeding, and Borderline Weight Gain. Undiagnosed cardiac disease may be responsible for these symptoms, especially in the first few months of life. Babies may have signs of heart failure (e.g., tachycardia with gallop rhythm, tachypnea, and hepatomegaly) or pathologic murmurs, usually because of large left-to-right shunts or mitral valve anomalies.[100,109] On occasion, especially in those with cardiomyopathy, murmurs may be absent. Severe grunting is more common in heart failure than in asthma or bronchiolitis.[110] Heart failure should be ruled out in infants with persistent grunting. Associated borderline skin perfusion and marginal blood pressure with tachycardia point to myocarditis.[110]

Accompanying Stridor. Infants with congenital vascular ring such as a double aortic arch, right aortic arch with rudimentary ligamentum aorteriosum, or an anomalous innominate artery, usually have significant tracheal compression. Stridor (constant or recurrent) is usually the rule, but wheezing also frequently occurs.[111] Periodic unexplained apnea or cyanosis with feeding may be noted. Congenital airway anomalies, such as laryngeal webs or stenosis, or subglottic atelectasis (congenital or postintubation), have

stridor as a primary symptom. Those with tracheal webs or bronchial strictures, however, may have only chronic wheeze, which is often both inspiratory and expiratory. Children with croup often have acute onset of mild wheezing, resulting from bronchial involvement; inspiratory stridor, barking cough, and hoarseness predominate. Rare instances of hypocalcemia have been documented in infants with stridor and wheezing.[112]

Associated Systemic Symptoms. Symptoms such as weight loss, excessive fatigue, or chronic low-grade fever may accompany wheezing because of the various mediastinal masses such as lymphoma or neuroblastoma. Sudden airway obstruction may occur with large mediastinal masses.

History of Prematurity and Neonatal Ventilation. Children with bronchopulmonary dysplasia have ongoing bronchial hyperreactivity.[113]

Diagnostic Work-Up

A careful history complements the evaluation discussed under diagnostic considerations. It is essential to determine whether the patient is a known asthmatic and if the exacerbation is typical. Preceding viral symptoms, fever, and atopic history should be sought. Past episodes of vomiting, coughing, or choking with drinks and feeding suggest aspiration, whereas recurrent or chronic pneumonia or persistent bacterial infections may suggest immunodeficiency. The response to previous therapeutic intervention such as inhaled bronchodilators may be useful diagnostically. Associated findings such as weight loss, failure to thrive, feeding problems, chronic grunting, and sudden onset of wheezing suggest underlying illness other than reactive airway disease.

The most important step is to evaluate the degree of respiratory distress by physically analyzing the patient. Examine the patient's level of consciousness. Hypoxic infants usually demonstrate persistent irritability. However, infants calm down amazingly fast when their oxygenation improves. Patients who are somnolent, lethargic, or exhausted may have an elevated Pco_2 or diminished Po_2. Cyanosis usually indicates severe airway obstruction with severe hypoxia and impending respiratory failure. Many cyanotic infants demonstrate perioral and nailbed pallor rather than frank, obvious cyanosis. However, absence of cyanosis does not necessarily exclude severe airway compromise. Patients should be examined for severe intercostal and suprasternal retractions, tachypnea (>60/minute in infants and >30/minute in school-aged children), tachycardia, pulsus paradoxus (≥ 15 mm), poor air entry (unilateral or bilateral), and inability to speak in sentences. A paucity or absence of wheezes, usually accompanied by markedly decreased air exchange, indicates severe respiratory distress. Significant airway compromise or respiratory failure may necessitate immediate intervention.

After airway assessment and stabilization, an in-depth physical examination is needed to confirm or change likely diagnoses and to initiate the proper investigations. Special attention should be paid to height and weight as indications of failure to thrive (cystic fibrosis, immunodeficiency, severe gastroesophageal reflux, or chronic congestive heart failure); evidence of atopy (accompanying asthma); clubbing (chronic hypoxia and cystic fibrosis); associated stridor (croup, foreign body, or airway anomaly); grunting, gallop rhythm, and hepatomegaly (congestive heart failure); and unilateral chest findings (foreign bodies).

Ancillary Data. Many children with minimal wheezing, especially known asthmatics and infants with bronchiolitis responding well to therapy, do not require any investigation. Further testing is usually dictated by the degree of respiratory distress and by the emergency physician's suspicion of certain diagnoses.

Transcutaneous pulse oximetry is useful for children with significant respiratory discomfort. It is well tolerated and provides a reliable, noninvasive measuring of oxygen saturation.[114] Regardless of their therapeutic response, few asthmatics with a initial saturation of 92% or less (sea level) are able to be discharged home without early relapse, whereas those with the initial saturation of 95% or higher usually do well at home.[115]

Arterial gases are necessary to assess ventilation only in children with severe respiratory distress not responding well to therapy. These cases are a distinct minority of wheezing children. Most moderate and many severe asthmatics improve after aggressive inhaled bronchodilator treatment combined with early steroid use. Serum potassium should be evaluated in children who have received many frequent albuterol inhalations (see section on Asthma). Acute and convalescent mycoplasma titers, cold agglutinins, or DNA studies may be fruitful in a preschool-aged child with suspected infection with *M. pneumoniae*.

Measurement of FEV_1 is the best indicator of severity in acute bronchospasm.[116] It can be measured in most cooperative children aged 5 years or older using a battery-operated, handheld portable spirometer, both before and after treatment. Many emergency departments have inexpensive peak flow meters, and there is evidence that the PEFR can be substituted for FEV_1.[117]

Chest x-ray studies are useful in an asthmatic patient that is not responding to treatment to rule out underlying conditions, complications, and in a child with first time wheezing (except in mild bronchiolitis) to exclude other diagnoses such as pneumonia, mediastinal mass, cardiomegaly, or congenital airway problems (e.g., right aortic arch). Physicians should obtain a chest radiograph of first-time wheezing infants under 6 months of age,[118] particularly in babies not responding well to treatment. Heart size is often normal in myocarditis, hence ECG and echocardiogram are necessary to rule out this diagnosis. Inspiratory-expiratory films are useful in a suspected diagnosis of foreign body, usually showing unilateral obstructive emphysema (but ipsilateral atelectasis or pneumonia may also be found, especially later on). Because these studies may be difficult to obtain in small infants, lateral decubitus films may serve the same purpose.

Depending on circumstances, the emergency physician may arrange or refer the child for other selected procedures on emergent, urgent, or semielective basis. Echocardiography is a useful noninvasive method in evaluating congenital cardiac and vascular anomalies that cause wheezing. Barium swallow is indicated for babies with suspected airway compression (e.g., vascular ring, where the esophagus is often indented); in those with gastroesophageal reflux (swallow may be normal in cases of significant reflux and other tests such as esophageal pH monitoring may be needed); or in patients with suspected aspiration syndromes.[100] Angiography may be needed for a precise anatomic diagnosis of a vascular ring. Urgent CT scan is useful for delineating the character, size, and exact location of the mediastinal masses.

An urgent bronchoscopy is necessary for diagnosis and removal of suspected inhaled foreign bodies (even when the initial appropriate x-ray films are normal), and to indicate the precise anatomic location of abnormal GI respiratory communications or congenital airway anomalies.

Regardless of nutritional status, any infant who has chronic wheezing and responds poorly to therapy should undergo a sweat test. Children with biphasic wheezing or stridor may need more complicated diagnostic tests than patients with uniphasic noises. The investigation may include an inspiratory/expiratory chest x-ray and lateral neck film, and on occasion an endoscopy, barium swallow, and serum calcium level test may need to be added.[112,119]

Prehospital Considerations

Particular attention must be paid to the presence of respiratory distress, and signs of hypoxemia, dehydration, and cardiovascular instability. These problems should be resolved; the patient may need to be transferred to a tertiary care facility for a more definitive diagnosis and management. If the child is ill, the airway must be stabilized before transfer.

It is often helpful to give the severe asthmatic patient several doses of continuous inhaled bronchodilators along with corticosteroids when en route to an emergency department. Continue the therapy until the child improves and becomes more stable. Seemingly stable patients with a large mediastinal mass may obstruct suddenly and without warning. Therefore personnel skilled in intubation must accompany the child.

Therapeutic Trial

Most children who have recurrent episodes of wheezing will have hyperreactive airway disease. Inhaled bronchodilators and other drugs (see section on Asthma) are indicated. The same protocol should be followed in a first wheezing episode, especially if other problems such as a foreign body are unlikely. Patients with diagnoses such as pneumonia, cystic fibrosis, or congestive heart failure are unlikely to respond well to bronchodilators. On occasion, these diagnoses may not be obvious initially and only become so after careful reassessment. Therefore the emergency physician needs to ensure that children with suspicious physical findings or history, and chronic or frequent wheezing who respond poorly to bronchodilators should receive appropriate referral and follow-up. Both depend on the suspected diagnosis and degree of distress.

Diagnostic Entities

ASTHMA

Asthma is a chronic pulmonary disease characterized by recurrent and usually reversible airway obstruction.[120]

Epidemiology

Asthma affects 5% to 10% of children[121] and is associated with a recent apparent increase in associated morbidity and mortality.[122] A recent U.S. study suggests that asthma is more prevalent among lower income, inner city, black children, and in those with a history of low birth weight or young mothers.[123]

The most important risk factor for development of asthma is the combination of RSV-related bronchiolitis and a genetic predisposition for atopic disease.[124] Diminished baseline lung function in early infancy (before any lower respiratory tract illness) may be a risk factor for bronchiolitis and subsequent asthma.[125] Allergic inflammatory reaction in the airways is probably an integral part of this disease.[126]

Pathophysiology

Asthma results from widespread obstruction of the airways because of bronchospasm, mucosal edema with inflammation, and aspirated secretions. Both bronchospasm and extensive airway inflammation constitute an integral part of acute exacerbations.[127] Microscopically, there is edema of the epithelium, damage to the ciliated cells, and inflammatory infiltrate involving the entire bronchial wall, including the muscle and mucous glands. The most characteristic finding is inflammatory secretions in the bronchial lumen, the amount of which is further augmented by the abnormalities of mucociliary clearance.[128,129]

The precise pathogenetic mechanism has not been clarified. Enhanced bronchial reactivity appears to be primary. An intrinsic defect in the bronchial smooth muscle or neural control of the airway may contribute[128]; bronchial inflammation is the consistent finding. Bronchoconstriction occurs because of an interaction between the allergen and a specific IgE-sensitized mast cell membrane, leading to release of bronchoconstrictive and inflammatory mediators such as histamine, kallikrein, and neutrophil and eosinophilic chemotactic factors. Polymorphs and eosinophils are capable of generating inflammatory mediators. Disruption of the cell membrane can liberate arachidonic acid from membrane phospholipids, which get metabolized to prostaglandins, thromboxanes, and leukotrienes, many of which are potent bronchoconstrictors.[130] The protein components of the eosinophilic granules are cytotoxic to the respiratory epithelium, which may further enhance bronchial hyperresponsiveness.[131,132] Accompanying microvessel disruption and release of plasma proteins into the airway lumen may worsen the inflammatory response and mucus plugging.[128]

Pharmacologic agents may affect bronchoconstriction. An increase in intracellular cyclic adenosine 3′ to 5′ monophosphate (AMP) secondary to the promotion of its biosynthesis (beta-adrenergic agents) or inhibition of its degradation (theophylline) produces bronchodilation. An increase in cyclic guanosine monophosphate (GMP), which is produced by parasympathetic stimulation caused by cholinergic receptors, causes bronchoconstriction. Parasympathetic agents such as atropine decrease vagal tone and produce relaxation, thereby promoting bronchodilation.

During an asthma attack, the maximum expiratory flow is reduced because of increased airway resistance. The increased respiratory rate leads to gas trapping with incom-

---

Precipitating Factors in Asthma

Infection
Usually viral
Mycoplasma pneumoniae

Allergens/irritants
Fumes, smoke, dust, air pollution, ammonia, chlorine
Pollens, mold, animal dander

Exercise

Weather
Cold exposure and humidity changes

Psychologic factors
Emotional stress and phobias

Drugs
Aspirin and beta-blockers

---

plete expiration via the obstructed bronchi. High lung volumes are required to maintain necessary pressures, and the work of breathing increases. Hyperinflation, airway obstruction, atelectasis, and decreased compliance cause regional decreases and abnormal ventilation perfusion ratios with marked hypoxemia. Carbon dioxide readily diffuses across alveolar capillary membranes and thus is not retained in mild cases in which ventilation is adequate. As the obstruction increases, ventilation-perfusion mismatch progresses and the carbon dioxide level rises.

Another potentially useful sign reflecting the severity of reactive airway disease is pulsus paradoxus. During severe attacks of asthma with large swings in the intrathoracic pressure and elevated right ventricular pressure, there is an increase in interventricular septal movement during inspiration and subsequent impediment to left ventricular function, thus causing pulsus paradoxus.[133]

Although a small drop in systolic blood pressure during inspiration is normal, pulsus paradoxus of 10 mm Hg or more is abnormal. There tends to be a good correlation between a pulsus paradoxus of greater than 20 mm Hg and a P_{CO_2} over 40 mm Hg.[120] However, a low pulsus paradoxus in no way guarantees only mild bronchospasm.

Respiratory decompensation occurs much more readily in asthmatic infants than in older children. Contributing factors include the small diameter of the infantile airway, soft and compliant rib cage, decreased airway recoil, early airway closure, and a high density of mucous glands in the bronchial mucosa.

Numerous precipitating factors may lead to an asthma attack (see box above). Only a minority can be directly attributed to a specific allergen. Viral infections seem to be extremely common triggers in infants and older children alike, and are associated with 19% to 42% of cases. Although their exact mechanism of action is not clear, among the suggested ones are the viral effect on IgE production, inflammatory response, mediator release, and on autonomic nervous system.[134,135] Many children display worsening of their symptoms after exercise. During exercise, water loss occurs from the respiratory tract, leading to mucosal cellular hyperosmolarity and subsequent mast cell mediator release.[134,136] Vagal mechanisms may be responsible for emotion-induced bronchospasm.[128] Aspirin-induced asthma is caused by blockage of the cyclooxygenase pathway of arachidonic acid, favoring production of bronchoconstrictive oxygenase products.[120] Low barometer pressure, cold temperatures, and sudden humidity changes have been associated with increased emergency department visits for asthma.[137-139] Cigarette smoke acts as a nonspecific irritant to sensitive airways. Parental smoking contributes to airway responsiveness at an early age and an increased risk of lower respiratory illness. There is clear evidence that this exposure leads to more severe pulmonary findings. Clearly, polygenic and multifactorial inheritance patterns have been demonstrated.[128]

Diagnostic Findings

Clinical Findings. A child with asthma typically experiences coryza followed by cough, shortness of breath, wheezing, and signs of respiratory distress. Children who experience their first attack after 3 years of age tend to have milder, infrequent episodes with no interval symptoms or signs.[128] Approximately 50% of these patients are symptom-free by early adolescence.[140] Those with first attacks before 3 years of age often have more frequent episodes and occasionally have persistent evidence of airway obstruction despite absent symptoms. The third pattern is that of chronic or persistent asthma. Many of these children have prolonged wheezing in the first 2 years of life.[128] They are chronically ill, adapting to chronic breathlessness, and even accept their limitation of activities as normal.[141] These patients often decompensate with a relatively minor precipitating cause, leading to recurrent pneumonia.

It is essential to focus on the acute episode as well as previous experiences and management. Medications (type, dose, and time of last dose), duration of acute symptoms, associated illness, and history of aspiration must be delineated. Cough, wheezing, chest tightness, sputum production, associated rhinitis, sinusitis, nasal polyposis, and atopic dermatitis may be noted. Patterns related to seasonality, episodic versus continuous, onset, duration, frequency, and progression may be diagnostic and useful in developing a treatment plan.

It is essential to define the extent of previous evaluations, episodes, response to treatment, and ongoing management and evaluation. Prior hospitalizations and ventilatory support should be assessed.

The medical history should include any allergic manifestations, gastrointestinal disturbances, reactions to drugs and food, and early injury to airway (bronchopulmonary dysplasia, pneumonia, intubation, croup, reflux, or passive exposure to smoking). Allergic or asthmatic problems in the family should be outlined. The living environment provides clues such as exposure to dust, pets, smoke, and heating or cooling system problems.

More subtle presentations may occur, including cough variant asthma with a prolonged history of dry cough (often exacerbated by exercise), paroxysmal cough with occasional vomiting, poor exercise tolerance, recurrent "chest infec-

---

Urgent History and Physical Findings
Urgent questions
Duration of the attack. Is it typical?
Precipitating factor (e.g., infection or anaphylaxis)
Previous severe episodes (including ICU admissions)
Current therapy, doses, and frequency
Associated medical conditions
Adverse drug reactions in past
Warning signs
Severe anxiety, persistent irritability, and inability to speak
Decreasing level of consciousness
Tachypnea, tachycardia, and pulsus paradoxus
Poor air entry, severe intercostal and suprasternal retractions (often with minimal wheezing), and nasal flaring

---

tions" with prolonged cough, or recurrent "pneumonia." Although the chest examination may be normal, the FEV_1 is often decreased and symptoms improve with bronchodilators; wheezing may be noted after prolonged and controlled exercise testing.

Certain key questions should be asked and physical signs sought while initiating treatment (see box above). Patients who have had severe attacks or previous respiratory failure tend to have severe recurrences.[142] Knowledge of past adverse reactions to medication (e.g., vomiting or severe abdominal pain while on theophylline) eliminate their use unless absolutely necessary. Patients with a history of recurrent asthma-related medical visits often have insufficient control of their disease or an alternate explanation for their symptoms.

Physical findings must assess respiratory status and distress. Tachypnea, labored respirations with retractions, nasal flaring, tachycardia, and pulsus paradoxus over 15 to 20 mm Hg are all indicators of disease severity.[143-145] Diffuse inspiratory and expiratory wheezing is noted with prolonged expiratory phase. The patient with respiratory distress and without wheezing may not be moving enough air to generate air movement and thus may have a "silent chest." A child with severe bronchospasm may develop wheezing, which was initially absent, after the initiation of therapy and improved aeration. Oxygen requirements may actually increase during this period; rales and rhonchi may be present. Hypoxic infants tend to be persistently irritable. Those who appear exhausted, lethargic, somnolent, or diaphoretic may have an elevated P_{CO_2}. Inability to speak in sentences is an important warning sign.

Pulsus paradoxus may accompany severe asthma, pericardial tamponade, and pneumothorax. Its presence is determined by having the patient breathe quietly while the clinician lowers the blood pressure cuff toward the systolic level. The pressure when the first sound is heard is noted. The pressure is further dropped until sounds can be heard through the respiratory cycle. A difference of 10 mm Hg or greater indicates the presence of pulsus paradoxus.

TABLE 59-2. Estimation of Severity of Acute Exacerbations of Asthma in Children

Sign/symptom	Mild	Moderate	Severe
Peak expiratory flow rate*	70%-90% predicted or personal best	50%-70% predicted or personal best	<50% predicted or personal best
Respiratory rate, resting or sleeping	Normal to 30% increase above the mean	30%-50% increase above the mean	Increase over 50% above the mean
Alertness	Normal	Normal	May be decreased
Dyspnea†	Absent or mild; speaks in complete sentences	Moderate; speaks in phrases or partial sentences; infant cry is softer and shorter; infant has difficulty sucking and feeding	Severe; speaks only in single words or short phrases; infant cry is softer and shorter, infant stops sucking and feeding
Pulsus paradoxus‡	<10 mm Hg	10-20 mm Hg	20-40 mm Hg
Accessory muscle use	No intercostal to mild retractions	Moderate intercostal retraction with tracheosternal retractions; use of sternocleidomastoid muscles; chest hyperinflation	Severe intercostal retractions; tracheosternal retractions with nasal flaring during inspiration, chest hyperinflation
Color	Good	Pale	Possibly cyanotic
Auscultation	End-expiratory wheeze only	Wheeze during entire expiration and inspiration	Breath sounds becoming inaudible
Oxygen saturation	>95%	90%-95%	<90%
P_{CO_2} (mm Hg)	<35	<40	>40

From National Asthma Education Program: *Guidelines for the diagnosis and management of asthma*, Bethesda, MD, 1991, National Institutes of Health, US Department of Health and Human Services, Publication 91-3042/3042A.
NOTE: Within each category, the presence of several parameters (but not necessarily all) indicates the general classification of the exacerbation.
*For children 5 years of age or older.
†Parents' or physicians' impression of degree of child's breathlessness.
‡Pulsus paradoxus does not correlate with phase of respiration in small children.

Pulsus paradoxus may be difficult to measure in small children; the parameters of level of consciousness, degree of tachypnea, retractions and distress, and response to treatment may be more useful. Oximetry is a better predictor of outcome than the presenting signs and symptoms, which underlines the importance of measuring this parameter in patients with any respiratory compromise and repeating this measurement following treatment if intervention is not on a continuous basis. Multiple parameters are useful in estimating the severity of an acute exacerbation (Table 59-2). Status asthmaticus is usually considered to be present in the child with moderate-to-severe asthma if there is no significant response to rapid administration of multiple dose beta-agonist agents.

It is essential to monitor the patient's response to therapy by using serial observations, oximetry, and reevaluations. It is not unusual for the child who is initially "tight" with minimal air movement to develop increased wheezing and oxygen requirements during early management with nebulized bronchodilators. Therefore reassessment is mandatory. Although there are several scoring systems for asthma, they are more useful in describing severity than in predicting outcome.[143,146,147]

Complications. Acute, life-threatening asthma (status asthmaticus) is associated with severe airway obstruction not responding to initial standard beta-agonist bronchodilator treatment. It is more frequent in younger children but also occurs in older asthmatics.[148] Acute respiratory failure associated with a P_{O_2} <50 mm Hg and a P_{CO_2} >50 mm Hg (room air at sea level) may occur as a result of delayed recognition or inadequate therapy. Patients can develop significant retractions, decreased or absent breath sounds, wheezing, impaired mental status and agitation, decreased response to pain, and labored speech.

Atelectasis and segmental collapse may develop. These children often have unexplained tachypnea with little or no wheezing after the initial treatment. This tachypnea often causes deterioration after beginning therapy in children who were initially doing well. With large areas of lung collapse, there is persistent poor air entry to other areas of the lung, which ultimately respond to aggressive bronchodilators and physiotherapy.[128] Mediastinal emphysema and pneumothorax occasionally occurs usually with severe disease.[149] Pneumothorax, a very rare complication, is due to air escaping from a ruptured alveolus. Pneumomediastinum usually develops from air tracking into the mediastinum and subcutaneous tissue of the neck and rarely requires specific treatment. Dehydration may evolve due to poor fluid intake and measured insensible losses. Theophylline may be associated with adverse responses (see Chapter 43). Death is secondary to respiratory failure with cardiac decompensation or dysrhythmias.

Diminished level of consciousness usually signals arterial hypoxemia and hypercarbia. Irritability may also be associated with hypoxemia. The syndrome of inappropriate antidiuretic hormone (SIADH) is rare, except with profound hypoxemia. Seizures are also uncommon, indicating severe hypoxemia, underlying CNS disease, or theophylline toxicity.

Most children with moderate-to-severe asthma have sinus tachycardia, with rates in the sick infant often reaching 160 to 200 bpm. This tachycardia is usually due to the asthma itself and does not necessitate reducing aggressive therapy while the child is in severe respiratory distress. Cardiac dysrhythmias are almost never seen except with severe theophylline toxicity. Dysrhythmias resulting from selective beta-2 agonists are extremely rare.

Ancillary Data. Transcutaneous pulse oximetry is a reliable, noninvasive way to measure oxygen saturation and should be performed on all asthmatics.[150] Oximetry is a guide to the severity of the disease and the response to therapy. Low initial oxygen saturation (below 92% sea level, at room air) has been identified as a predictor of when a child with acute asthma should be hospitalized.[151,152] While a low oxygen saturation usually correlates with severe disease, near-normal saturation ($\geq 95\%$) does not guarantee a mild illness.[153] Arterial blood gas (ABG) is unnecessary in all but severe asthmatics with poor ventilation or inadequate response to therapy in whom ventilation must be specifically assessed. Although P_{CO_2} values above 40 mm Hg correlate with clinical disease severity and may serve as a guide to the need for ventilation, lower P_{CO_2} values may still be present in severe disease and should in no way eliminate the potential need for continuous observation or admission to an intensive care unit. Oximetry should not be viewed as a substitute for ABGs; ventilation must be assessed.

Pulmonary function tests (PFTs) have a definite but limited role in the ED assessment of acute asthmatic children. They are particularly useful when the diagnosis is uncertain, in those patients suspected of having chronic poor asthma control, and in children with borderline therapeutic response, especially those with labile disease history and past ICU admissions. On the other hand, initial PFTs do not appear to correlate well with subsequent need for hospitalization.[154] Studies have demonstrated that both low oxygen saturation and low FEV_1 tend to confirm the clinical impression of severe disease but airway obstruction can occasionally exist in the absence of typical clinical signs.[153] To be reliable, the child should be at least 5 years of age, cooperative, and able to perform the respiratory maneuvers consistently. The measurement of greatest utility is the FEV_1. Measurement of PEFR is a useful substitute. The values are obtained on a handheld spirometer or a peak flowmeter and then compared with the standard values for the same height and sex or with baseline values established by the patient during a healthy period between attacks[155] (Table 59-3).

Chest x-ray studies are usually of little value. They classically demonstrate hyperinflation, sometimes increased bronchial markings, atelectasis, and in rare cases, infiltrate. Children with increasing respiratory distress or who fail to respond as expected to conventional therapy should be studied to exclude an associated process that requires specific therapy or other causes of wheezing. Any patient with signs suggestive of an air leak or foreign-body aspiration should be studied. Radiographs are rarely indicated in children who respond well to initial therapy.

TABLE 59-3. Reference Values for Spirometry

Height (CM)	Female			Male		
	FVC (L)	FEV₁ (L)	PEFR (L/min)	FVC (L)	FEV₁ (L)	PEFR (L/min)
110	1.22	1.12	145	1.11	1.03	—
115	1.38	1.26	157	1.28	1.18	160
120	1.55	1.42	170	1.46	1.34	175
125	1.74	1.58	184	1.67	1.51	191
130	1.94	1.75	199	1.89	1.70	208
135	2.15	1.94	216	2.13	1.90	226
140	2.38	2.14	234	2.39	2.12	247
145	2.62	2.35	253	2.67	2.36	269
150	2.88	2.57	274	2.98	2.61	293
155	3.16	2.81	296	3.30	2.88	319
160	3.45	3.06	321	3.66	3.17	348
165	3.75	3.32	347	4.03	3.48	379
170	4.08	3.60	376	4.43	3.80	414
175	4.42	3.89	407	4.86	4.15	451
180	4.78	4.20	441	5.32	4.51	491

NOTE: Spirometry may be a reflection of patient's level of cooperation and understanding of the procedure and clinical condition at the time of evaluation. Reference standards listed are for white population.
FEV₁, forced expiratory volume in 1 sec; *FVC*, forced vital capacity; *PEFR*, peak expiratory flow rate.

The serum theophylline level is crucial in managing patients with an acute episode who are taking therapeutic doses of theophylline. Therapeutic levels are in the range of 10 to 20 µg/ml. Rapid assays may facilitate this monitoring. Serum potassium levels should be monitored in patients on prolonged, frequent albuterol therapy, whereas other electrolytes are useful in children with inadequate intake. The CBC has little value, particularly if obtained after administration of beta-adrenergic agents.

Differential Considerations

The most common consideration in older children is *M. pneumoniae*. In infants, common considerations include bronchiolitis, pertussis, or an aspirated foreign body (see section on Wheezing). Although most children with wheezing do have asthma, one should pursue other diagnostic entities in those who wheeze for the first time and those with an unusual presentation, very sudden onset, poor response to treatment, or associated suspicious findings such as a pathologic heart murmur, failure to thrive, or other systemic findings. Exposure to toxic gases or hydrocarbons suggest the potential of a chemical pneumonitis.

Inspiratory stridor is usually accompanied by upper airway disease. Suprasternal and supraclavicular retractions are more common than intercostal retractions.

The young infant with tachypnea and wheezing typically has bronchiolitis. The seasonality (winter and early spring), age, and epidemic nature of this illness are helpful diagnostically. Infants with a past history of prematurity or ventilatory support often have a viral illness accompanied by wheezing and tachypnea, which is managed comparable with reactive airway disease. Finger clubbing is suggestive of chronic illness such as cystic fibrosis rather than asthma.

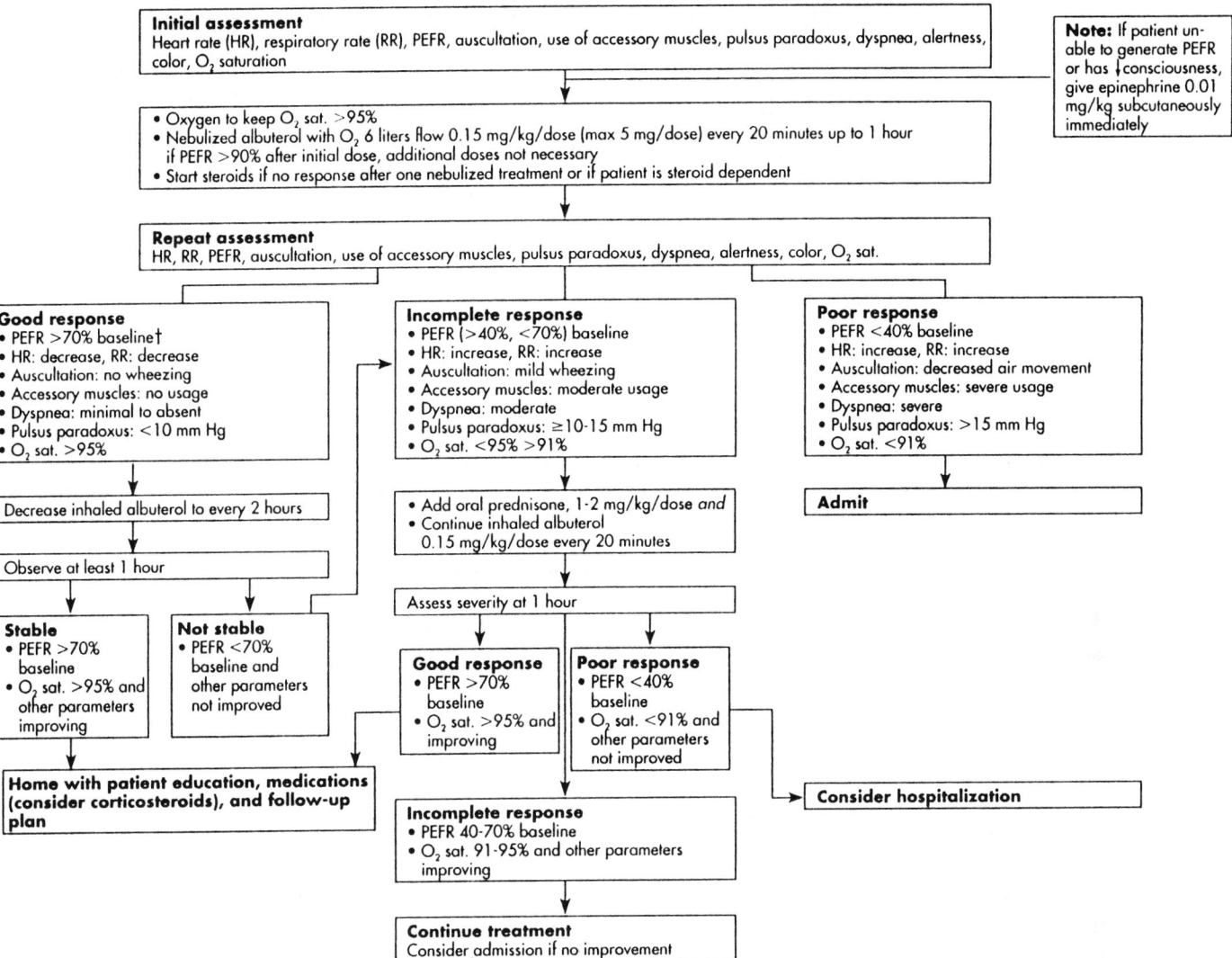

Initial assessment
Heart rate (HR), respiratory rate (RR), PEFR, auscultation, use of accessory muscles, pulsus paradoxus, dyspnea, alertness, color, O_2 saturation

Note: If patient unable to generate PEFR or has ↓consciousness, give epinephrine 0.01 mg/kg subcutaneously immediately

• Oxygen to keep O_2 sat. >95%
• Nebulized albuterol with O_2 6 liters flow 0.15 mg/kg/dose (max 5 mg/dose) every 20 minutes up to 1 hour
  if PEFR >90% after initial dose, additional doses not necessary
• Start steroids if no response after one nebulized treatment or if patient is steroid dependent

Repeat assessment
HR, RR, PEFR, auscultation, use of accessory muscles, pulsus paradoxus, dyspnea, alertness, color, O_2 sat.

Good response
• PEFR >70% baseline†
• HR: decrease, RR: decrease
• Auscultation: no wheezing
• Accessory muscles: no usage
• Dyspnea: minimal to absent
• Pulsus paradoxus: <10 mm Hg
• O_2 sat. >95%

Incomplete response
• PEFR (>40%, <70%) baseline
• HR: increase, RR: increase
• Auscultation: mild wheezing
• Accessory muscles: moderate usage
• Dyspnea: moderate
• Pulsus paradoxus: ≥10-15 mm Hg
• O_2 sat. <95% >91%

Poor response
• PEFR <40% baseline
• HR: increase, RR: increase
• Auscultation: decreased air movement
• Accessory muscles: severe usage
• Dyspnea: severe
• Pulsus paradoxus: >15 mm Hg
• O_2 sat. <91%

Decrease inhaled albuterol to every 2 hours

• Add oral prednisone, 1-2 mg/kg/dose *and*
• Continue inhaled albuterol 0.15 mg/kg/dose every 20 minutes

Admit

Observe at least 1 hour

Assess severity at 1 hour

Stable
• PEFR >70% baseline
• O_2 sat. >95% and other parameters improving

Not stable
• PEFR <70% baseline and other parameters not improved

Good response
• PEFR >70% baseline
• O_2 sat. >95% and improving

Poor response
• PEFR <40% baseline
• O_2 sat. <91% and other parameters not improved

Home with patient education, medications (consider corticosteroids), and follow-up plan

Consider hospitalization

Incomplete response
• PEFR 40-70% baseline
• O_2 sat. 91-95% and other parameters improving

Continue treatment
Consider admission if no improvement

FIG. 59-1. Acute exacerbations of asthma in children: emergency department management. Therapies are often available in a physician's office. However, most acutely severe exacerbations of asthma require a complete course of therapy in an emergency department. †A baseline of PEFR% refers to the norm for the individual, established by the clinician. This may be a percentage predicted on the basis of standardized norms or the patient's personal best. (*From National Asthma Education Program:* Guidelines for the diagnosis and management of asthma, *Bethesda, MD, 1991, National Institutes of Health, US Department of Health and Human Services, Publication 91-3042/3042A.*)

An even more common problem is underdiagnosis. Many physicians are hesitant to diagnose asthma in infants, preferring to wait until several episodes of wheezing have occurred. Similarly, many children with a chronic cough or exercise intolerance have undiagnosed reactive airway disease.

Vocal cord dysfunction because of adduction of the true and false vocal cords throughout the respiratory cycle may mimic asthma but is a form of conversion reaction.

Management

The patient is usually the best source of previous experiences and effective therapeutic regimens. If the history or physical suggests reactive airway disease, appropriate intervention and evaluation are appropriate. For management of acute exacerbations of asthma see Figs. 59-1 and 59-2. When other causes of wheezing are likely, additional studies are indicated. Oxygen should be given to all those with any respiratory discomfort and the transcutaneous oxygen saturation level should be maintained above 95% at sea level. Humidified delivery is preferred. Oxygen may be administered using a mask or cannula. In uncooperative children, blow-by may be the only successful technique. When appropriate, airway, ventilation, and blood pressure should be stabilized and correction of acid-base abnormalities initiated. Cardiac and oximetry monitoring is appropriate.

Pharmacologic Agents. Inhaled bronchodilators should be given concurrently, usually by ultrasonic or jet nebulization. Optimal deposition of drug particles to the lower respiratory tract to assure high aerosol output, small par-

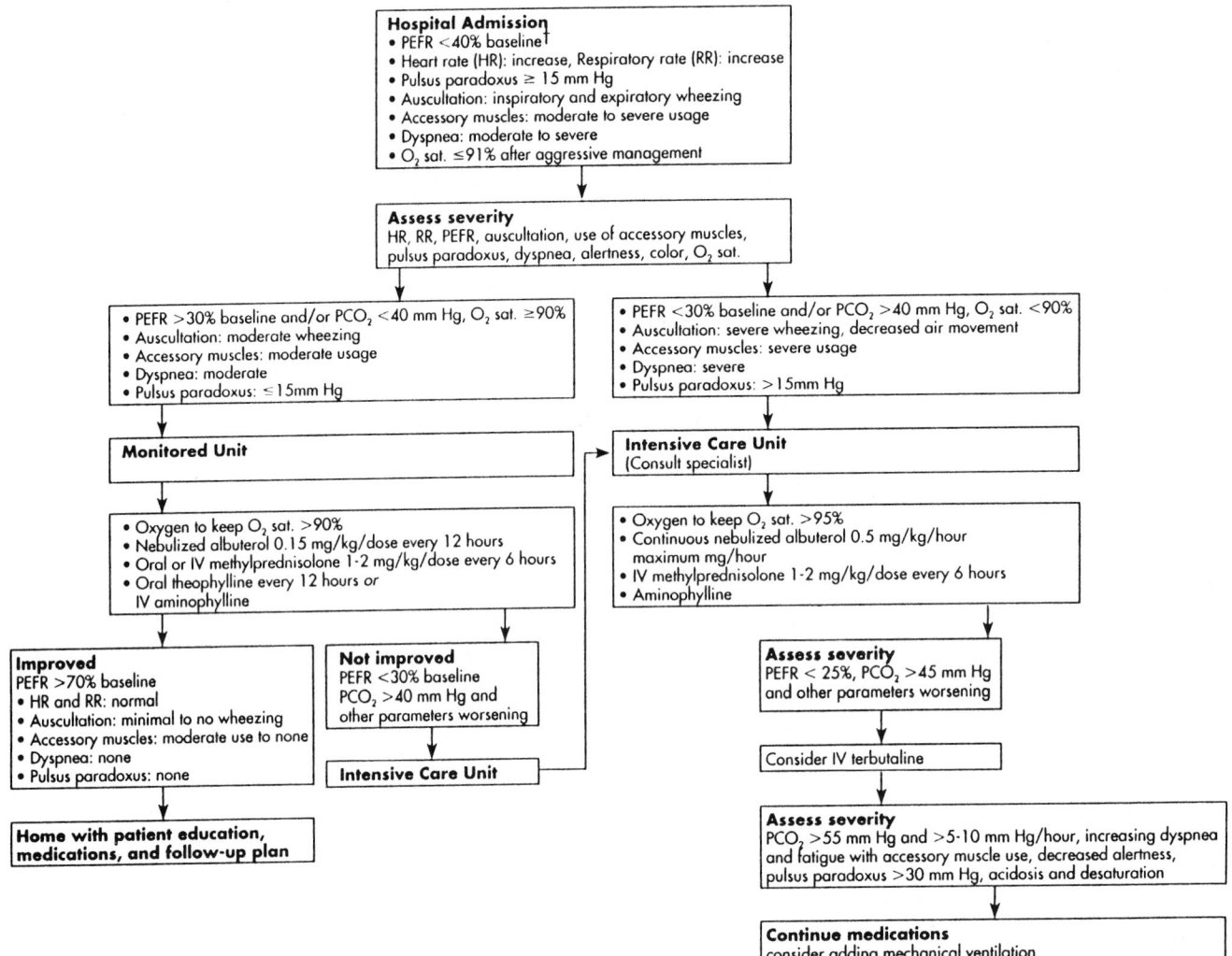

FIG. 59-2. Acute exacerbations of asthma in children: hospital management. †A baseline of PEFR% refers to the norm for the individual, established by the clinician. This may be a percentage predicted on the basis of standardized norms or the patient's personal best. (*From National Asthma Education Program:* Guidelines for the diagnosis and management of asthma, *Bethesda, MD, 1991, National Institutes of Health, US Department of Health and Human Services, Publication 91-3042/3042A.*)

ticle size, and short treatment time is achieved by a flow of 6 to 7 L/min and a nebulization total volume of 4 ml.[156,157] The primary bronchodilator in the management of acute asthma are beta-agonists; ipratropium, where available, is a useful adjunctive measure.

Beta-Agonists. The relatively nonspecific catecholamine derivatives (e.g., epinephrine and isoproterenol) have been largely replaced by more specific beta-2 agonists including albuterol (Proventil and Ventolin), fenoterol, or terbutaline. Metaproterenol and isoetharine have limited use because of their alpha and beta-1 agonist side effects. As noted, these agents work by activation of the beta-2 receptor-dependent adenyl cyclase, with subsequent elevation of cyclic-AMP, reduction of myoplasmic calcium, and bronchodilation.[158]

Nebulized inhalation administration is generally more effective than parenteral therapy and is the ideal route. Such administration is clearly more effective than the oral or parenteral routes. Parenteral administration may have a role in the uncooperative, severely ill patient or when inhalation therapy is logistically impractical (i.e., equipment problem, poor cooperation, etc). The wide therapeutic index of albuterol and terbutaline allow for the safe administration of doses, often exceeding standard recommendations. High doses are needed because only about 10% actually reaches the lung; the decreased airway caliber and altered respiratory pattern decreases the aerosol's penetration.[159-161] The superiority of frequent, high dosing in moderate and severe asthma is well documented.[162] During stabilization of a severe asthmatic, patients may be given several doses in a row as tolerated; however, tolerance has not been a problem. Nebulized inhalation is usually administered by a tight-fitting plastic face mask although other techniques have been effective.

Albuterol (Proventil or Ventolin), 0.5% solution (or 5 mg/ml) is given in a dose of 0.15 mg (0.03 ml)/kg/dose up to a maximum of 5.0 mg (1.0 ml)/dose. It should be diluted in 2 to 3 ml of 0.9% NS and administered by a nebulizer with oxygen flow 6 to 7 L/min. Frequency of administration during the acute phase varies from continuous to hourly, depending on severity and degree of clinical response. With sustained improvement, the intervals are gradually lengthened. Peak of onset is 30 to 60 minutes with a duration of 4 to 6 hours.

Metered dose inhalers (MDIs) are also available. Although popular and useful for home use, the experience with MDI use in the ED management of acute pediatric asthma is very limited. The optimal frequency of administration is unknown as is the efficacy in infants under 6 months of age and in patients with severe disease. Spacers increase aerosol delivery into the lung,[163] and are recommended for children of all ages. Spacers with a plastic face mask are useful in infants and preschool children who are to take five to six normal breaths between puffs.[164,165] Patients over 6 years of age can usually follow the standard deep inhalation technique with each puff, followed by a few normal breaths before the next dose. Tube-shaped spacers are recommended for children over 6 years of age. Care should be taken to shake the MDI before each puff. Although the ideal dose of albuterol via MDI is not known, approximately 0.3 puffs/kg/dose (maximum 10 puffs; 100 μg/puff) are known to have a similar efficacy as the comparable weight-appropriate nebulizer dose already described.

There has been limited experience with fenoterol. The 0.5% solution has been used as 0.1 ml/dose in children ≤2 years; those 2 to 9 years received 0.2 ml/dose; and children over 9 years were given 0.3 ml/dose.

Terbutaline, 0.1% solution or 1 mg/ml for parenteral administration, (Brethine) may also be given by nebulization. Doses of 0.03 mg (0.03 ml)/kg/dose, up to a maximum of 0.5 ml/dose, in 2 to 4 ml of 0.9% NS can be administered by nebulization q 4 hr or as often as tolerated. The peak of onset is 30 minutes with a duration of 3 to 4 hr. Parenteral terbutaline may be given in a dose of 0.01 ml (0.01 mg)/kg/dose, up to a maximum of 0.25 ml/dose, q 15 to 20 minutes subcutaneously as needed, often as an adjunct to nebulization therapy in the critically-ill child. However, nebulization therapy is usually more effective. Use the parenteral solution for nebulization.

Epinephrine (Adrenalin 1:1000), given in a parenteral dose of 0.01 ml (0.01 mg)/kg/dose, to a maximum of 0.35 ml/dose, q 20 minutes subcutaneously (up to three doses), may also be used if tolerated and the heart rate is less than 180 beats/min. Its efficacy, however, is less than inhaled agents and its significant alpha- and beta-agonist side effects limit its usefulness. Epinephrine 1:200 (Sus-Phrine) has a more prolonged effect but can result in inconsistent administration unless a single vial ampule is used for each patient; side effects are similar to epinephrine 1:1000. Inhaled beta-2 agonists have largely replaced this mode of treatment.

Oral agents are occasionally useful for the ongoing treatment after discharge of small infants wheezing for the first time and without significant respiratory problems, for whom the purchase of inhalation equipment may be unnecessary. Oral agents have no role in acute stabilization. Albuterol

(Proventil) 2 mg/5 ml is an excellent option at a dose of 0.1 to 0.15 mg/kg/dose q 6 to 8 hr PO up to a dose of 4 mg/dose. It is also available in 2 and 4 mg tablets. Peak of onset is 1 to 2 hr and the duration is 4 to 6 hr.

Anticholinergics. Decreasing the intracellular production of cyclic GMP (guanosine 3,5-monophosphate) inhibits smooth muscle contraction and may be achieved by using anticholinergics.[166] Ipratropium bromide (Atrovent) acts on both the large and small airways, whereas albuterol only affects the small airways. The rationale for using a combination of atropine or ipratropium and albuterol is that together they are particularly effective because of the different pharmacologic mechanisms by which bronchodilation is achieved. Two pediatric studies have documented this approach,[167,168] however, both used low doses of albuterol. A recent trial demonstrated significantly superior efficacy of multiple ipratropium administrations when added to continuous albuterol therapy in severe disease.[169] Ipratropium should thus be added (adult: 500 μg/dose) to the first several albuterol nebulizations during the ED management of severe asthma. Pediatric nebulization dosages have not been fully determined for children but may be extrapolated. Some suggest an initial dose of 250 μg by nebulization mixed with saline. The systemic absorption of ipratropium is poor and therefore does not cause tachycardia, pupillary dilation, visual problems, or elevated intraocular pressure, even at high doses.[170,171] The maximum response occurs in 30 to 120 minutes after inhalation.[172] Ipratropium has been recently licensed for nebulization in the United States. It is also available as an MDI in which the adult dose is two inhalations (36 μg) QID. If ipratropium bromide is unavailable, atropine may be substituted as 0.02 mg/kg/dose, up to a maximum of 2 mg/dose, in 2 ml of 0.9% NS administered by nebulization q 4 to 6 hr or as tolerated.

Corticosteroids. Corticosteroids block the release of inflammatory substances by indirectly blocking the phospholipase alpha-2 activity.[173] In addition, they may increase the number and affinity of beta-adrenergic receptors.[174] There also appears to be a direct bronchodilator effect, which is supported by a more rapid onset of action (within 1 hour) than previously thought for corticosteroids.[175] Several studies have shown that parenteral corticosteroids can decrease hospitalization rates among patient with acute asthma and reduce the period of hypoxia,[174,176] although this finding is not universal.[177,178] A recent trial demonstrated that oral prednisone reduces the need for hospitalizations among children with severe asthma treated in the ED with frequent beta-2 agonist nebulizations.[179] Patients who have taken steroids within 12 months (including those taking steroids by inhalation), or who have a history of respiratory failure associated with asthma require early administration. Orally administered corticosteroids are as effective as intravenous therapy.[180,181]

Steroids should be initiated as soon as possible after arrival to the ED in all children with moderate to severe disease. Exceptions include patients with mild exacerbations, especially if there is an excellent response to inhaled bronchodilator therapy. Most children can be successfully treated with oral steroid preparations. Indications for intravenous therapy include critically-ill status and repetitive vomiting. Useful regimens include oral prednisone 2 mg/kg/dose after arrival in the ED followed by 1 mg/kg/dose once daily for 5 days. Toxicity is not significant nor is tapering required.[182] Those needing intravenous treatment will benefit from methylprednisolone (Solu-Medrol) 1 to 2 mg/kg/dose q 6 hr IV or hydrocortisone (Solu-Cortef) 5 mg/kg/dose q 6 hr IV.

In preschool-aged children with repeated attacks related to URIs, administration of steroids with the onset of cough and cold may reduce progression of acute exacerbation.[183] If more than four bursts have been given in 1 year, a brief course of glucocorticoids should be initiated for stressful situations such as surgery.

At present there is no evidence to suggest that inhaled steroids benefit patients with acute exacerbations but they are useful for chronic management. Although these preparations may be given continuously along with or after the course of oral steroids, children with acute exacerbations should not be treated with inhaled corticosteroids alone. Beclomethasone (Vanceril or Beclovent) is provided in a metered dose inhaler delivering 42 to 50 µg/puff. The doses used vary widely; most children use 200 to 400 µg/day, although higher doses are sometimes necessary. Duration of treatment needs to be individualized according to the frequency of exacerbations and disease severity. The mouth should be rinsed after each inhalation.

Theophylline. The mechanism of theophylline action includes its influence on intracellular free calcium, prostaglandin antagonism, and as a cyclic-AMP analog.[184] It is a weaker bronchodilator than the beta-2 agonists.[185] Several adult studies have actually failed to show an early additive effect when theophylline is added to beta-agonists for acute asthma exacerbation.[185-187] A pediatric trial also failed to show additional benefit of theophylline in hospitalized children on inhaled beta-agonists.[188] Children may experience nausea, abdominal pain, vomiting, and sleeping and behavioral problems, even with safe, therapeutic levels. There is a trend away from the routine use of theophylline for either acute or chronic therapy. Beta-2 agonists, anticholinergics, and corticosteroids constitute the mainstay of acute asthma therapy. A trial of theophylline may be warranted in critically-ill asthmatics unresponsive to these measures.

If the patient is taking theophylline at the time of the encounter, many clinicians continue the agent. It is imperative to determine the amount and time of the last dose and duration of therapy. Generally, a theophylline level is required. If the patient is taking a subtherapeutic dose or has not had any medication for 6 hours, half of the loading dose may be given pending the determination of the theophylline level; if an adequate dose has been administered within 6 hours, maintenance can be given pending determination of levels. Therapeutic theophylline is 10 to 20 µg/ml and the administration of 1 mg/kg of theophylline raises the theophylline concentration by about 2 µg/ml. The clearance of theophylline is altered by several conditions outlined in the box above, requiring dosage adjustment and close monitoring of levels. The dose is determined on the basis of lean body weight, reflecting measured serum theophylline levels. Aminophylline is approximately 85% theophylline.[189]

Influences on Theophylline Clearance

Increase dose (clearance increased)	Decrease dose (clearance decreased)
Drugs: phenobarbital, phenytoin, rifampin, carbamazepine, and marijuana	Drugs: cimetidine, erythromycin, and oral contraceptives
Smokers	Illness: viral infection, fever, congestive heart failure, abnormal liver or renal function
Diet: high protein, low carbohydrate, and charcoal-broiled meat	Other: infants <3 mo, pregnancy, especially third trimester
Other: hyperthyroidism and cystic fibrosis	

Parenteral therapy of theophylline is indicated for severe obstructive disease that is unresponsive to adrenergic agents (status asthmaticus) and when the child is deteriorating. In children not receiving ongoing theophylline therapy, a loading dose of 5 to 6 mg of theophylline should be given over 20 minutes and may be repeated q 6 hr. Alternatively, a sustained maintenance dose of 0.7 to 0.9 mg/kg/hr in an infusion pump may be initiated after the loading dose. The lower dose is used in children under 1 year of age and in those 10 years and older. There appears to be no advantage to intermittent vs. continuous infusion[128]; however, continuous therapy facilitates adjustment of drug levels.

Maintenance dosing of theophylline in infants less than 1 year requires careful monitoring because of the variability of pharmacokinetics. Guidelines are summarized in the box on p. 1087.

Oral therapy with theophylline is usually reserved for special circumstances requiring ongoing therapy for which beta-agonists, cromolyn, and intermittent steroid management is ineffective alone. Acute episodes of mild-to-moderate disease are ideally managed with beta-2 agonist agents. Short-acting formulations may be used in children who need only sporadic therapy with exacerbations. Stable patients are often treated with an initial loading dose using a short-acting theophylline and initiating a sustained-released drug.

Patients requiring ongoing therapy may receive theophylline, usually beginning at a dose of 16 mg/kg/24 hr and then adjusted to reflect serum and daily maximum levels (see box on p. 1087).

Patients usually do well when maintained at therapeutic levels. Some patients require levels that are either lower or higher than normal therapeutic levels.

Toxicity primarily results from the sympathomimetic effects of theophylline including tachycardia, dysrhythmias (atrial fibrillation and ventricular tachycardia), and hypertension. Patients may be agitated and restless. The mean theophylline level of patients having seizures is probably in the range of 45 µg/dl.

Supportive care following overdose must include monitoring levels, gastric emptying, charcoal, and catharsis. Se-

---

Theophylline Doses in Children < 1 Year

Preterm infants up to 40 weeks postconception (postconception age = gestational age at birth + postnatal age):
1 mg/kg q 12 hr

Term infants either at birth or infants 40 weeks postconception
  Up to 4 weeks postnatal: 1 to 2 mg/kg q 12 hr
  4 to 8 weeks: 1 to 2 mg/kg q 8 hr
  Beyond 8 weeks: 1 to 3 mg/kg q 6 hr

Maximum Theophylline Levels

< 1 yr	Max: 8 mg + 0.3 × age (wk)
1 to 9 yr	Max: 22 to 24 mg/kg/24 hr
9 to 12 yr	Max: 20 mg/kg/24 hr
12 to 16 yr	Max: 18 mg/kg/24 hr
> 16 yr	Max: 12.5 mg/kg/24 hr or 600 to 800 mg/24 hr

---

rial activated charcoal must be given to adults as 10 gm q 1 hr or 20 gm q 2 hr to a total dose of 120 gm; children are given proportionately less. This approach decreases the half-life of elimination. If the level is not decreasing, bowel washout may be appropriate. If the level is >50 μg/dl, dialysis should be considered (see Chapter 60).

Other Measures. Cromolyn (Intal) is sometimes used in conjunction with beta-agonist agents for chronic therapy, especially in those with exercise- or cold-induced problems or in conjunction with other elements of ongoing intervention. It has a stabilizing effect and may decrease reliance on frequent nebulization therapy. The adult dose is 1 ampule or 20 mg/dose. The infant and neonatal dose is proportionately less, usually about 10 mg/dose QID. Its role in acute management is uncertain.

IV albuterol has few side effects but is not generally available in the United States at the present time. It is usually initiated in an intensive care setting. The initial loading dose is 1 μg/kg/min for 10 minutes, followed by a continuous infusion of 0.2 μg/kg/min. This dose can be increased by 0.1 μg/kg q 15 minutes, based on the patient's response.[167]

IV isoproterenol in a dose of 0.1 mg/kg/min by infusion, then increased by 0.1 μg/kg/min q 15 minutes according to response, has been effective but can potentially cause tachycardia and a rebound rise in arterial carbon dioxide during infusion.

Other agents include magnesium sulfate, which was demonstrated to be particularly useful in adults.[190,191] Minimal data are available in children at present although a recent pediatric report showed promising results in occasional asthmatics who were refractory to other treatment measures.[192] The dose is estimated to be 40 mg/kg given IV over 20 min.

Intubation. Patients with severe asthma who are in respiratory failure, patients with persistent hypoxemia and hypercarbia on maximal therapy, and patients fatiguing or failing to respond to aggressive bronchodilation management, may require intubation. The need to intubate an asthmatic is fortunately rare with current medications and usually involves an exhausted, moribund-looking patient. Ketamine, a sedative and bronchodilator, may be a useful agent in children requiring ventilation.

Classification

Mild Asthma. Initial stabilization should obviously include assessment of ventilation and oxygenation, the latter using pulse oximetry. Albuterol should be administered with a maximum effect at least at hourly intervals in a dose of 0.15 mg or 0.03 ml/kg, and can be administered more often as needed. The child receiving albuterol should be reevaluated frequently. The maximum effect is achieved about 10 to 15 minutes after inhalation. Two or three hourly doses are usually sufficient in most mild asthmatics. Even the mild asthmatic should usually be discharged on continued inhaled bronchodilator therapy for 5 to 10 days. Any need for oral steroids needs to be individualized.

Occasionally a child improves initially only to relapse in 30 minutes. These children benefit from two to three additional frequent inhalations, steroids, and 1 to 2 hours of observation and monitoring of oximetry after the last treatment to detect relapse. A persisting need for inhalations at 1- to 2-hour intervals signals the need for hospitalization. Ipratropium may be useful in the management of these children.

Moderate to Severe Asthma. If the response to the first inhalation therapy is suboptimal or the child is in distress at presentation, several frequent, high-dose inhalational administrations of albuterol are indicated. In severe disease, continuous albuterol should be continued until the child improves. Corticosteroids should be initiated early.

Ipratropium is a useful adjunctive agent in these patients, particularly during the early management. A dose of 250 μg or 1 ml should be given for the first few treatments. Ipratropium may be added to the albuterol inhalations, and the dose can be repeated two or three times at 20 minute intervals if necessary.[169]

Drug resistance does not usually account for treatment failures with beta-2 agonist and sympathomimetic agents.[193] Transient tremor, hyperactivity, and tachycardia may be noted. Vomiting may occur but is often due to the illness itself. These problems are usually short lived and well tolerated and only occasionally require postponement of the next dose. Albuterol can cause hypokalemia by interfering with membrane Na-K-ATPase, and thus requires monitoring of potassium.[194]

Theophylline may be considered in critically-ill children with poor response to multiple frequent bronchodilator inhalations and systemic corticoidsteroids. Close monitoring of vital signs, cardiac rhythm, oxygenation, ventilation, and level of consciousness is imperative. Measurement of arterial oxygen and carbon dioxide is necessary to follow severity; noninvasive measurements are increasingly being used. It is often a good idea to watch a tired, severely distressed asthmatic in an intensive care setting, despite acceptable blood-gas results. These patients may deteriorate suddenly and unexpectedly.

Risk Factors for Considering Admission

- Presence of symptoms for over 24 hours
- Marked retraction, hypoxia, or hypercapnia
- Low oxygen saturation on admission to the ED (<90%-93% at sea level)
- Respiratory obstruction (PEFR ≤ 10% of expected)
- Poor response to initial beta-agonist agent (PEFR ≤ 40% of expected). Failure to respond to initial ED management requires admission.
- History of hospitalization or respiratory failure
- Multiple drug therapy; chronic or intermittent steroid use
- Concurrent infection
- Progressive fatigue
- Multiple visits for episode
- Poor parental compliance and follow-up

In the future, IV albuterol and other agents may be useful for patients who have failed aggressive inhaled bronchodilators, as described previously, to attempt to avoid intubation.[195] It is effective and has fewer side effects than parenteral isoproterenol.

Disposition

The indications for hospitalization include either an inadequate response to several frequent doses of inhaled bronchodilators, a relapse while waiting for the next hourly bronchodilator dose, initial oxygen saturation of 92% or less (sea level), progressive fatigue, significant complications, and poor social situation. Risk factors include a prolonged, poorly controlled episode, prior hospitalization for respiratory failure, multiple visits for the episode, and multiple bronchodilator drug therapy. Many children with a history of life-threatening asthma should also be admitted (see box above). Except for mild cases, emergency department observation for at least 1 hour after the last bronchodilator inhalation may prevent unexpected return visits a few hours later.

Most children with acute asthma go home on inhaled beta-2 agonists. Home compressors are useful, especially for younger infants and those with severe disease. MDIs are also valuable and successfully used by most asthmatic children.[196] Standard doses of albuterol given q 4 to 6 hr should be used. The usual dose of albuterol required by MDI administration is approximately one fourth to one fifth of that given by nebulizer.[197] This translates into approximately 0.3 puffs/kg/dose q 4 hr (100 μg/puff, maximum 10 puffs).[198] The patients need to be instructed to return if the prescribed dose does not work or needs to be given more frequently than every 4 hours. Mandatory reassessment within 48 hours is important to reevaluate the clinical state and the ongoing therapy. Oral albuterol may also be used in young infants with first-time wheezing or infrequent attacks. The addition of oral steroids is important as noted previously. They should be used in all acute asthmatics except those with a mild attack who have relapsed on insufficient beta-2

agonist therapy at home and who exhibit an excellent response to inhaled bronchodilators in the ED.

How many medications should the child who is discharged home receive? In general, previous therapy needs to be intensified (i.e., inhaled albuterol given TID should be increased to every 4 hr), the dose optimized, or another drug added. Patients should be released on more intensive therapy than the dose they were taking when they experienced relapse. Regardless of the drugs used, all asthmatics should be reevaluated within 24 to 48 hours, or earlier if necessary.

Sporadic cases of unusually severe or fatal varicella have been reported in immunocompetent children on oral corticosteroids for asthma. Although this event is extremely rare in healthy patients, it is wise to recommend that patients seek medical care if they are exposed to or develop varicella within 2 to 3 weeks of steroid therapy.

Prognosis

Asthma is associated with considerable morbidity. The single most important risk factor for morbidity is failure to diagnose asthma from recurrent wheezing.[128] Many of these children suffer from undiagnosed chronic fatigue, night cough with loss of sleep, recurrent pneumonias, and poor school attendance. Repetitive administration of antibiotics and cough mixtures is predictably ineffective. Moreover, the known adolescent asthmatic often denies the disease. Adolescents are also at the highest risk of death from asthma.[199] Most fatalities occur in outpatients, usually as a result of overreliance on bronchodilators with a delay in seeking medical care.[200] It is likely that most incidents of sudden fatal episodes had a chronic significant obstruction with a poor respiratory reserve.[128] Recognition, aggressive management, and good follow-up of high-risk patients are essential. Deaths from asthma within the hospital are rare. Likewise, it is now known that the beta-2 agonists themselves do not directly cause death when used appropriately.[201]

BRONCHIOLITIS

Bronchiolitis is a viral lower respiratory infection affecting infants under 2 years of age; the highest incidence occurs in infants less than 1 year of age. Bronchiolitis produces inflammatory obstruction of the airways and may also be related to underlying airway hyperactivity.

Pathophysiology

A virus-induced necrosis of the bronchiolar epithelium, peribronchial lymphocytic inflammatory reaction, and proliferation of nonciliated cuboid cells lead to obstruction of the bronchi and bronchioles with cellular debris and fibrin. Respiratory secretions are profuse and handled inefficiently due to a lack of normal airway clearance mechanism.[202] These factors contribute to small airway obstruction, producing patchy areas of hyperinflation or focal atelectasis. Furthermore, increased airway reactivity has been documented in viral-induced respiratory infections.[203] Immediate immunologic hypersensitivity to viral antigens appears to play a contributing role in bronchiolitis, as demonstrated by the production of virus-specific IgE and release of mediators of bronchoconstriction, the quantities of which correlate with the severity of illness.[204] In addition, other mechanisms may lead to viral-induced airway constriction such as increased thromboxane production stimulated by viral antigen-antibody complexes, beta-blockage in granulocytes in prone individuals, and possible subsequent exaggerated IgE response to inhaled antigens because of viral-induced respiratory epithelial damage.[205-207]

Many children manifest evidence of hyperreactive airway disease after the initial bronchiolitis episode. A recent prospective study shows that respiratory syncytial virus (RSV) bronchiolitis appears to be an important risk factor for the development of subsequent asthma, especially in children with heredity for atopy or asthma.[208] Why some infants develop bronchiolitis after RSV exposure whereas others do not is not clear. Genetic predisposition does not appear to be a major factor[209] but preexisting bronchial reactivity may be a factor.[210]

Infants are particularly prone to develop severe manifestations of lower airway obstruction because of the small airway diameter, very high airway resistance, poor airway elastic recoil, and high rib-cage compliance.[211] All these factors lead to increased work when breathing. Air trapping, high resistance, and atelectasis produce ventilation-perfusion defect and almost universal hypoxemia. As the minute ventilation falls, the infant becomes fatigued, and severe airway involvement produces carbon dioxide accumulation.

Etiology

RSV is the major cause of bronchiolitis, especially in epidemics, and accounts for about 90% of isolates.[212,213] Other causative infectious agents include parainfluenza virus, influenza, adenovirus, rhinovirus, and rarely enterovirus, herpes simplex, or *M. pneumoniae*. Bacterial superinfection is uncommon. Bronchiolitis caused by adenovirus is more severe than that resulting from RSV. It frequently involves the alveolar respiratory epithelium causing high morbidity and mortality and chronic respiratory disease.[214,215] Viral secretions continue for up to 3 weeks, and reinfection may occur within months.[216]

Bronchiolitis occurs primarily in winter and early spring, especially if RSV-induced. Most affected infants are under 1 year of age.

Diagnostic Findings

Bronchiolitis is usually preceded by several days of mild-to-moderate upper respiratory tract infection with rhinorrhea, mild cough, and sometimes a low-grade fever. Despite displaying an obvious labored breathing, many children with a moderate disease are remarkably alert, playful, and happy-looking.

With progression, the cough becomes more bothersome in both severity and frequency, occasionally becoming paroxysmal in nature. Vomiting and poor intake may occur. The infant becomes irritable, sleeps and feeds poorly, and ultimately may develop marked respiratory distress. On examination these infants exhibit tachypnea, tachycardia, and intercostal retractions. Wheezing is common, but it may be absent both in mild and moderate disease, and in infants with poor air entry. Crepitations are commonly heard. Respiratory rates tend to be directly related to the severity of the disease and indirectly to arterial oxygenation.

With severe disease, nasal flaring, suprasternal retractions, and grunting are commonplace. Persistent irritability or lethargy must be taken seriously because they often accompany hypoxemia or hypercarbia. Cyanosis tends to occur late in respiratory failure; its absence does not exclude severe disease. Although feeding difficulties are quite common, significant dehydration is rare.

Bronchiolitis has a variable duration. Some infants recover in 7 to 10 days, whereas others remain ill for 3 to 4 weeks or even longer. A rapid deterioration in clinical status may be due to significant atelectasis.

Certain children tend to have a more severe clinical course. Very young infants and those with underlying chronic lung disease, hemodynamically significant congenital heart problems, or immunodeficiency tend to have more severe disease.[217,218]

Complications. Children with severe tachypnea and tachycardia (respiratory rate often approaching 80 breaths/min and heart rates close to 200 bpm) must be watched carefully for impending respiratory failure, especially if accompanied by changes in the level of consciousness and signs of severe respiratory distress. Accompanying alveolar involvement and pulmonary infiltrates are not uncommon, but bacterial infiltration is very rare. Atelectasis may occur, producing rapid deterioration and increased oxygen requirement. Children with underlying cardiac or lung pathology, immunodeficiency, or congenital anomalies are at greatest risk of death associated with respiratory failure.[219] The mortality rate varies but is probably around 0.5%.[220] Apnea may occur, particularly in children under 6 months of age who were born prematurely and have severe disease. Pneumothorax is very rare.

Many children have long-term evidence of airway hyperreactivity and abnormal pulmonary function after bronchiolitis.[221-223] Moreover, patients with bronchiolitis often develop subsequent wheezing episodes. Although it seems likely that bronchiolitis develops in patients with underlying hyperreactive airway predisposition, it is not clear whether viral bronchiolitis actually contributes to the subsequent wheezing.[207]

Bronchiolitis fibrosa obliterans results from progressive fibrotic reaction, and thus obliterates the bronchioles.

Ancillary Data. Transcutaneous oxygen saturation measurement (pulse oximetry) is a useful, noninvasive monitoring tool for the emergency physician. It reliably reflects arterial oxygenation.[224] ABGs are not generally needed. However, in those with severe disease who do not respond to aggressive management or deteriorate while on therapy, ABGs may be useful. In severe disease the blood pH may be low and the Pco_2 is elevated.[225,226]

Other blood tests add little. The WBC count is frequently elevated; there may be a modest left shift.[227] Monitoring electrolyte levels is useful in dehydrated children.

Chest radiographs are probably not necessary in infants with mild disease or those who respond promptly to therapy. It is useful, however, for those who have severe respiratory manifestations, fail to improve with initial therapy, have a prolonged course or recurrent wheezing, or look toxic; it is also useful when the diagnosis is in doubt. Films may be useful to exclude significant complications, such as pneumonia or pneumothorax, and to define the degree of atelectasis or exclude other diagnoses such as congenital lung, cardiac anomalies, or foreign body. Atelectasis occurs with more severe disease.

Radiologic findings in bronchiolitis are variable. Although the majority show prominent bronchial markings and hyperinflation, others have accompanying interstitial infiltrates or segmented atelectasis, which are often confused with pneumonia.[228,229] About 10% of radiographs are normal. Radiographs should be repeated if a child deteriorates; they often document increasing atelectasis.

Although rapid viral detection techniques are available, deep nasopharyngeal swabs or nasal washings are often useful in establishing a specific diagnosis by fluorescent antibody (FA) testing for RSV and viral cultures.[230] This rapid test is useful in providing rapid diagnostic information and cohorting hospitalized patients. A virus can be identified in 60% to 75% of cases.[231]

Differential Considerations

Little diagnostic difficulty arises in congested infants with typical signs and symptoms, particularly during the winter and spring when epidemics occur. Rhinorrhea, tachypnea, and tachycardia are almost universal, whereas wheezing may be absent or intermittent, especially in relatively mild cases (see section on Wheezing). However, other diagnostic entities may need to be considered if the child has a chronic wheezing episode or exhibits unusual findings.

Severe bronchiolitis that responds poorly to therapy often accompanies coexisting viral pneumonia. Bacterial pneumonia and sepsis should be considered in a child with respiratory distress who looks toxic. When wheezing persists for several weeks, a sweat test should be performed to diagnose possible cystic fibrosis. Persistent wheezing may also occur in infants with bronchopulmonary dysplasia (BPD); these patients usually having bronchial hyperactivity.[232] This latter group tends to have more severe infection when infected with RSV.

A second wheezing episode strongly suggests reactive airway disease, especially in families with a positive history of atopic disease. Aspiration should also be considered. Prolonged episodes of grunting, wheezing, and tachypnea over several weeks may be associated with cardiac disease, especially large left-to-right shunts.[233] The dilated pulmonary artery and enlarged left atrium compress the bronchial tree causing atelectasis and emphysema. Pulmonary vascular congestion because of congestive heart failure due to cardiomyopathy, or from pulmonary venous obstruction due to mitral stenosis, cor triatriatum, or anomalous venous drainage, may cause wheezing.[234] Heart murmurs may be poorly audible although they are usually present in large shunts. The heart is usually enlarged except in cor triatriatum. Failure to thrive and poor feeding may be present.

Paroxysmal coughing may be due to pertussis or aspiration. Unlike infants with pertussis, those with bronchiolitis are rarely totally well between coughing spells. Swallowing incoordination, esophageal reflux, esophageal obstruction, or an abnormal communication between the respiratory and GI tract may be present in those with feeding difficulties. An appropriate history of foreign-body aspiration is sometimes absent.[235]

Apnea associated with wheezing and stridor may be a sign of vascular anomalies involving the trachea such as a double aortic arch, right aortic arch with ligamentum arteriosum, anomalous innominate artery, or pulmonary artery sling.[236] Recurrent stridor is common.

Management

The hallmark of therapy is the administration of humidified oxygen by mask, cannula (pediatric or infant size), or hood, because most patients are hypoxemic.[237] (Also see section on Asthma.) Many irritable infants calm down once oxygenation improves. If the baby does not tolerate standard administration routes, a parent can hold the oxygen hose close to the baby's face. Oxygen saturation must be monitored and should be maintained at or above 95% (sea level). Croupettes should be discouraged because they reduce the baby's visibility and the mist does not reach the lower airway.[238]

Although controversial, the use of beta-agonist agents appears to be beneficial. Initially there was little proven therapeutic effect[239-244]; however, these studies were methodologically flawed. A good response to subcutaneous epinephrine in young infants has been demonstrated.[245] Three double-blind, placebo-controlled trials demonstrated a clinically significant beneficial response to nebulized albuterol,[246-248] although this finding is not universal.[249] The usual high doses used are 0.15 mg (0.03 ml)/kg/dose diluted in 3 ml of 0.9% NS administered at least q hr initially to those with moderate disease and q 15 to 20 minutes for those in severe distress. The solution is best administered using an oxygen flow of 6 to 7 L/min. The side effects are mild and well tolerated. Terbutaline may be used by nebulization but is particularly helpful when given parenterally to children in whom nebulization therapy is difficult. Parenteral dosing of 0.01 ml/kg/dose subcutaneously, up to a maximum of 0.25 ml/dose, may be a useful adjunct to albuterol nebulization. Oxygen requirements may actually transiently increase after several nebulization treatments. Many children, following stabilization and tolerance of room air, still require bronchodilation therapy and may ultimately be discharged on nebulization therapy to be administered at home. Some infants with this disease do not appear to respond to inhaled beta-2 agonists. Several frequent doses (three to four) should be given before it is decided the infant is a "nonresponder". If such is the case the beta-2 agonist should be stopped. These babies should get adequate supportive therapy, minimal disturbance, and careful observation.

Ipratropium (Atrovent), which has been found to be synergistic in the management of children with asthma, has not been found useful in those with bronchiolitis who are also receiving albuterol.[250-254] Theophylline has no therapeutic effect.[255] The efficacy of corticosteorids in bronchiolitis is unknown at present. It seems reasonable to add ipratropium and corticosteroids in the management of children with critical disease.

Antibiotics are not routinely indicated. Aerosolized ribavirin is an antiviral drug approved for severe RSV infection that is usually given after documentation of the cause. It is a synthetic guanosine analog that interferes with the expression of messenger RNA and inhibits viral protein synthesis.[256] Several randomized, double-blind trails have shown modest clinical improvement after ribavirin both in previously well children and in those with cardiopulmonary problems; however, the length of hospitalization, oxygen therapy for ventilation, and mortality rate probably remain unaffected.[257-261] Ribavirin should be considered for severe disease especially if there is underlying severe cardiopulmonary pathology or immunosuppression.[257-261] Special precautions are required for children who need mechanical ventilation. Ribavirin reduces the duration of mechanical ventilation, oxygen treatment, and hospital stay in infants requiring respiratory support.[262] However, more recent data show similar RSV-induced mortality in children with and without congenital heart disease.[263] This evidence supports the use of ribavirin in a limited number of highly selected cases.[264] Ribavirin plays no role in the management of bronchiolitis in the ED.

Periodic reassessment is essential. Small infants may deteriorate suddenly and unexpectedly. Therefore constant nursing care or observation in intensive care is a good idea for a tired-looking, distressed baby, even with acceptable blood gases. Although no absolute levels of P_{CO_2} or P_{O_2} dictate the need for ventilatory support, rising oxygen requirements and carbon dioxide levels, along with a worsening clinical status or frequent apneic spells, warrant intubation and ventilation. Continuous positive airway pressure (CPAP) may often be attempted before mechanical ventilation.

Appropriate hydration is essential. Small, frequent feedings are usually offered to children with moderate disease; an IV line is necessary for those in severe distress or if fluid intake is questionable.

Respiratory isolation is required for all patients. Hospital personnel are important reservoirs for nosocomial spread.

Disposition

Patients in significant distress who do not respond to bronchodilators or who do not feed should be admitted. Specific factors that have been associated with more severe disease include the child's ill or toxic appearance, an oxygen saturation less than 95% (sea level), gestational age under 34 weeks, a respiratory rate greater than 70 breaths/min, atelectasis on chest radiograph, and an age less than 3 months. Oxygen saturation is the single best objective predictor.

A low threshold for admission is appropriate for children who were previously ventilated or have residual pulmonary disease (e.g., BPD), cardiac disease, are less than 3 months of age, or have a history suggestive of apnea.

Parents of patients going home should receive detailed instructions regarding observation for signs of worsening respiratory distress (e.g., lethargy or poor feeding). Smaller, frequent feedings are often better tolerated. Home administration of bronchodilators for 7 to 10 days is usually necessary. Therapeutic options include albuterol administration via a metered dose inhaler with a spacer and a mask (2 to 3 puffs, 100 μg per puff/dose q 4 hr); wet nebulizer (0.15 mg/kg/dose q 4 hr) or orally (0.1 to 0.15 mg/kg/dose q 6 hr) for 7 to 10 days. Close follow-up is essential. Prophylactic immune globulin has been studied to reduce the severity of disease in high risk children.

CROUP (LARYNGOTRACHEOBRONCHITIS)

Croup can be defined as an acute viral clinical syndrome characterized by barking cough, hoarse voice, inspiratory stridor, and variable degree of respiratory distress.

Pathophysiology

The initial portal of entry of infection occurs within the nose and nasopharynx, hence the initial symptomatology of nasal stuffiness. Subsequently, the infection spreads to the larynx and trachea. There is erythema and edema of the tracheal walls, and an inflammatory exudate within the tracheal lumen.[265] The vocal cords are swollen and their mobility impaired, which leads to stridor, hoarseness, and barking cough. The associated hypoxemia in severe croup also appears to be the result of impaired alveolar ventilation and ventilation-perfusion imbalance.[266] It should be remembered that the infant's subglottic region is surrounded by a firm cartilaginous ring. Any edema, therefore, results in a significant airway compromise because of the normally narrow infantile airway.

Spasmodic croup occurs at night and is characterized by a sudden onset of dyspnea, barking cough, and stridor in a previously well, afebrile child. The croup quickly disappears with humidity, only to recur in the same pattern for 3 or 4 consecutive nights. There is subglottic, noninflammatory edema. The cause of this entity is unknown, but some authors believe it represents the mild end of the broad spectrum of laryngotracheitis.[267,268]

Etiology

Parainfluenza virus type I is the most common cause of croup, and it is also often responsible for the yearly winter epidemics. Mild sporadic cases may be caused by parainfluenza type III, adenovirus, and respiratory syncytial virus.[269] Influenza A virus is often responsible for very severe cases. Bacterial suprainfection is uncommon, but if it occurs it causes the more serious entity of bacterial tracheitis. The highest attack rate occurs in children between 6 and 36 months of age, usually peaking in late fall and early winter.[270]

Diagnostic Findings

Typically, the child experiences 1 to 2 days of coryzal symptoms followed by hoarse voice and harsh barking cough. The accompanying respiratory stridor often begins at night between 1 AM and 5 AM, awakening the child from sleep. It is often quite loud and very frightening to parents. Fever is common, but toxicity does not occur. The chest is usually clear, although there may be mild wheezing.

In severe cases, the stridor may be both inspiratory and expiratory, and there is both suprasternal and intercostal indrawing during inspiration (as a result of a negative intrapleural pressure), indicating a component of associated lower airway disease. Air entry may be poor. Significant hypoxemia is often present in severe croup, resulting in lethargy or agitation. Progressive tachycardia and tachypnea are other warning signs of severe disease. Tachypnea

Clinical Scoring System for Croup

Level of consciousness

Normal (including sleep)	0
Disoriented	5

Cyanosis

None	0
Cyanosis with agitation	4
Cyanosis at rest	5

Stridor

None	0
When agitated	1
At rest	2

Air entry

Normal	0
Decreased	1
Markedly decreased	2

Retractions

None	0
Mild	1
Moderate	2
Severe	3

From Westley CR, Cotton EK, Brooks JG: Nebulized racemic epinephrine by IPPB for the treatment of croup, *Am J Dis Child* 132 (5): 484-487, 1978.

tends to be the best indicator of low arterial oxygen tension.[266] Cyanosis is a late and ominous sign.

In general, any child with persistent stridor at rest (despite therapeutic measures) must be observed carefully. The presence of resting sternal retractions on admission identifies a high-risk child who sometimes requires more prolonged hospital stay and multiple drug therapy, and may go on to need artificial airway support.[271]

A clinical score modified from Westley and colleagues[272] (see box above) is useful in monitoring the child's response to therapy in the emergency department. Croup usually lasts 4 to 7 days or occasionally longer.

Complications. Complications occur in a small minority of cases. The most common complication is increasing severity of upper airway obstruction. The inflammatory process may extend into the lower airway causing tachypnea and mild wheezing. The inflammation usually responds well to inhaled bronchodilators. Pneumonia is uncommon and usually associated with bacterial tracheitis rather than viral croup. Other extraepiglottic foci may include lymphadermitis and otitis media. Dehydration is also uncommon and, if present, requires specific fluid management. Airway management should always precede an IV line insertion in a child with severe airway compromise.

Ancillary Data. Transcutaneous oximetry is a reliable noninvasive way of monitoring the arterial oxygenation and is generally normal. Hypoxia is an ominous finding. ABGs are usually not necessary. Almost all children respond to standard therapy.

In typical cases, there is little to be gained from a radiologic examination of the neck and chest. The usual signs include narrowing and smudging of subglottic region and bulbous hypopharynx. The classic radiologic sign of a narrowed subglottic region on posteroanterior view of the neck (the steeple sign) is absent in 50% to 60% of cases, and the procedure only aggravates further the already miserable child.[273,274] Cautious direct visualization of the throat may be appropriate in children with suspected croup to exclude epiglottitis.

Differential Considerations

The box on p. 1093 lists some of the entities that rarely may be confused with croup, although the diagnosis of croup is usually straightforward (see section on Stridor).

Croup vs. Epiglottitis. Children with croup are usually noisy; stridor, loud barking cough, and hoarse cry can often be heard behind closed doors. Nevertheless, many are active, appear well, and readily consume fluids. In contrast, patients with epiglottitis are anxious, occasionally toxic children who sit fairly immobile, seemingly afraid to talk or cry; cough is usually absent and stridor minimal. Saliva pools under the tongue and drooling is common. Although this differentiation is easy in most cases, some children do have a somewhat confusing clinical picture, either on arrival or during therapy for "croup" in the emergency department. This picture includes a well-looking croupy infant with an atypical sign for croup such as drooling, refusal to drink, weak voice, undue restlessness, or an older child with stridor and a very sore throat. Epiglottitis needs to be ruled out by visualization in the operating room if there are any of these epiglottitis signs, even in a child with a viral prodrome, cough, or other croup-associated features.[275] In a rare child, croup and epiglottitis may co-exist. These atypical cases do not respond to the usual croup therapy and deteriorate in a few hours, necessitating airway support for supraglottic obstruction.[275,276]

Croup vs. Other Diagnoses. A toxic-looking child with signs of severe croup who does not promptly respond to treatment may have bacterial tracheitis that almost always requires intubation, intensive management, and appropriate antibiotics (see later in this chapter). A lateral x-ray study of the neck may be useful as it may reveal soft tissue densities within the trachea. Immunization history against diphtheria should always be obtained since this disease may mimic croup as well.

Management

An adequate airway and effective ventilation must be assured. Respiratory distress or failure is excluded. Most children with croup but no stridor at rest can be managed as outpatients once the diagnosis is certain. Gentle handling is important because persistent crying increases oxygen demands and respiratory muscle fatigue, and makes the obstruction worse. Medical procedures should be kept at a minimum. Most stable croupy infants welcome small frequent drinks of their favorite juice, and this activity should be encouraged. Careful observation of heart rate, respiratory rate, and respiratory distress are important to detect early hypoxia.

Although the value of high humidity has not been proven, it seems to be beneficial to most children. Humid-

---

Differential Considerations of Croup

Infectious

Croup	Loud stridor and prominent cough
	Not toxic and drinks well
Bacterial tracheitis	"Croup" for 2 to 3 days, then deterioration over hours; toxic
Epiglottitis	Poor response to croup therapy
	Short history (hours)
	Very sore throat and poor fluid intake
	Stridor mild (absent) and cough absent
Retropharyngeal abscess	History of several days dysphagia and drooling
	Stridor minimal; cough and hoarseness absent
	Neck extended
	Stridor and hoarse voice rare
Diphtheria	Check immunizations

Traumatic

Foreign body	Onset at play or feeding
	Stridor often biphasic
Subglottic stenosis	History of prolonged intubation
	Recurrent severe croup
Inhalation burns	Smoke inhalation
Laryngeal fracture	Significant neck trauma

Congenital
(see Stridor)

Vascular ring	Recurrent severe croup
	Feeding problems common
Laryngomalacia	Baseline stridor
	Normal voice
Subglottic stenosis	

---

ity presumably works by moistening the secretions and soothing the inflamed laryngeal mucosa.[277] Humidity also decreases the viscosity of secretions in the trachea, thus facilitating their clearance by coughing.[278] Hypoxemia is uncommon in croup; high-humidity air is useful.[266] Since most infants do not tolerate strange beds, croupettes, or masks very well, it may be best to deliver the mist via a respiratory hose held by a parent a few inches from the child's face while their offspring plays on their lap.

Racemic epinephrine (Vaponefrin) has been found to be effective.[271,279-283] It works primarily by adrenergic-stimulated mucosal vasoconstriction,[273] although its beta-2 activity also leads to bronchial smooth muscle relaxation. Its effect lasts 2 hours or less.[273,279,280] We have found that 0.5 ml of the 2.25% solution in 3 ml saline given via a nebulizer and repeated at 1 to 2 hours if necessary is a useful universal dose. Previously feared rebound phenomenon appears quite uncommon, although some patients do return to their baseline status after the effect of the drug wears off. Some patients sustain their improvement after racemic epinephrine (particularly if steroids are begun early) and may be safely discharged after an appropriate period of observation. A nebulizer is better tolerated than positive pressure breathing.[280] A mandatory period of observation of at least 3 to 4 hours is necessary for all those who have received this drug. Those who were initially severely ill, responded incompletely, relapsed during observation, or required multiple doses must be hospitalized. Racemic epinephrine can be used in moderate and severe croup not responding to humidified oxygen. Tachycardia may occasionally develop[281] but this is uncommon. Two or three consecutive doses are necessary in very severely ill children to provide some relief, to provide time for ENT and anesthesia consultants to make provision for artificial airway placement, and even to avoid the need to intubate some patients who stabilize soon thereafter.

Early use of steroids is beneficial in the emergency department. Several studies have demonstrated clinical benefit of parenteral corticosteroids in hospitalized patients with croup.[281,284-287] A single dose of IM dexamethasone (0.6 mg/kg) is useful in reducing the overall severity starting in the first 4 to 24 hours after injection.[288] The majority of children with this disease tolerate dexamethasone orally (1 mg/kg/dose). Due to a long biologic half-life of dexamethasone (up to 54 hours), only one injection is usually necessary, although many clinicians use several doses over 3 days. Dexamethasone should be given to all children who require racemic epinephrine and to all who need hospitalization. Although the efficacy of dexamethasone has not been evaluated in an outpatient setting, it is useful to administer this drug in the emergency department before discharge, especially in those who still have mild respiratory distress or a bothersome cough after mist therapy, and to those who respond to and remain well after racemic epinephrine. Inhaled corticosteroids may be useful in the acute management of this disease[289] but at the present time there is insufficient evidence to recommend their routine use.

Fluids given intravenously may occasionally be required in dehydrated children. Dexamethasone may also be given intravenously.

It is unusual for a child with viral croup to be unresponsive to this therapy, either in the emergency department or during hospitalization. Patients with severe croup should receive immediate humidified oxygen, two or three doses of frequent nebulized racemic epinephrine, and parenteral steroids. Failure to respond to these measures requires urgent consultation from both ENT and anesthesia consultants with a view to endoscopy, both to provide an artificial airway and to rule out other diagnoses. Nasotracheal intubation compares favorably with tracheostomy, especially because of a shorter period of intubation and avoidance of a tracheostomy wound.[290,291] Special attention should be paid to selecting the tube (size 3.5 for infants 6 months to 3 years, 4.0 for 3- to 5-year-olds, and 4.5 for those over 5 years) to avoid pressure necrosis and subglottic stenosis, yet permit adequate ventilation.[292] These children need to be managed in a pediatric intensive care unit with well-trained staff and good facilities. Endoscopy should be considered in severe cases (before intubation), as well as in atypical or recurrent cases (after recovery).[293]

If a child with severe croup is to be transferred to another hospital, therapy should be given and the airway stabilized, if necessary and appropriate, before transfer.

Disposition

Children with croup often benefit from staying several hours in the observation unit, particularly those children with mild to moderate residual respiratory distress or stridor at rest after mist therapy, and those with excellent response to racemic epinephrine. Patients with persistent stridor at rest and significant respiratory distress, those who need multiple doses or exhibit incomplete response to racemic epinephrine, those in whom alternate diagnosis is entertained, and those with a poor social situation require hospitalization.

Most children can go home if stridor at rest is not present. Parents need to be reassured regarding the usually benign course of this illness. As stridor tends to last for several days, parents should be warned that their offspring may still feel miserable and have some noisy breathing for the next 2 to 3 nights. Letting the child sit and play in a steamy bathroom is often helpful, as is a brief car ride on a cool, humid night (usually on the way to the hospital). It is possible that giving one dose of oral dexamethasone (1 mg/kg) to those with mild distress or mild stridor at rest prior to discharge may be beneficial.

EPIGLOTTITIS

Epiglottitis (supraglottitis) is a life-threatening bacterial infection of the epiglottitis and the surrounding structures.

Pathophysiology

The hallmark of this illness is supraglottic cellulitis involving the epiglottitis, aryepiglottic folds, ventricular bands, and arytenoids. This massive inflammatory edema may lead to ulceration and microabscess formation with mucosal necrosis.[294] Secretions often accumulate in the hypopharynx. The inflammation also may extend to the posterior tongue and the uvula.[295] All of these are responsible for the sore throat, dysphagia, and rapidly increasing upper airway obstruction. The muffled stridor and dysphonia are due to decreased air flow in the upper airway. The vocal cords and the subglottic region are usually not involved; hence loud stridor and significant cough are often lacking. Total airway obstruction may occur as a result of aspiration of secretions in the already narrowed airway.

Etiology

Before the introduction of the *H. influenzae* vaccine, almost all pediatric cases were caused by *H. influenzae* type B and accompanying bacteremia directly invading the supraglottic structures.[296] Other organisms have rarely caused epiglottitis in children; however, isolated cases have been reported with *S. pneumoniae*, *S. aureus*, and group A and group C beta-hemolytic streptococci.[297-303]

Bacteriology of this condition in teenagers includes a varied spectrum of organisms.[303] In addition, *H. influenzae* type B caused a significant percentage of adult epiglottitis cases as well.[304] However, since the introduction of the *H. influenzae* vaccine, acute epiglottitis has considerably diminished in frequency, and in some regions with a fully immunized population, has been nearly eradicated.[305,306] Epiglottitis therefore tends to be caused by organisms other than *H. influenzae* type B.[305] Although the bacteremia tends to be of relatively short duration and of low density, 70% to 90% of the blood cultures yield the responsible organism.[307]

Epiglottitis may occur at any time of the year and in any age group, including (rarely) the newborn.[308,309] Before advent of the *H. influenzae* vaccine, up to 25% of pediatric cases occurred in children under 2 years of age[310]; since the vaccine, patients with this condition tend to be older.[305] Although rare, several cases of thermal epiglottitis have been reported.[311]

Diagnostic Findings

Epiglottitis typically causes several hours of fever, sore throat, and poor fluid intake, and these symptoms progress to respiratory distress. Viral prodrome is usually absent. Upon arrival to the ED the child is usually anxious, toxic, and prefers to sit upright. The voice or crying is weak and muffled, and stridor, if present, tends to be soft.[308] There may be varying degrees of respiratory distress with slight tachypnea and poor air entry or cyanosis. Tachycardia is common. The mouth is often held open, and quick inspection reveals pooling of saliva beneath the tongue and drooling.

However, atypical presentation may occasionally occur and epiglottitis may be missed unless meticulous history is taken and the child is carefully examined and assessed. Some children may initially have no respiratory distress and appear quite comfortable. A history of severe sore throat with dysphagia, therefore, must be taken seriously (especially if the pharynx appears normal or mildly erythematous) and epiglottitis ruled out. The finding of pharyngitis or uvulitis does not always exclude a concurrent supraglottic infection.[295] Up to 40% of epiglottitis patients are afebrile.[312] In adults a severe sore throat is a common initial complaint.

On rare occasions, some children may initially present with crouplike features, and their lack of response to initial therapy or a subsequent subtle deterioration in the emergency department could indicate epiglottitis.[313-315] Rarely, subglottic obstruction may co-exist with epiglottitis.[316,317]

Children with streptococcal epiglottitis tend to be older and have a longer prodrome and a more protracted clinical course.[301] Adolescents and young adults with epiglottitis often have a preceding history of viral infection and a slow clinical evolution over several days.[318] Sudden airway obstruction, however, still occurs. Rarely, epiglottitis may co-exist with concurrent bacterial seeding elsewhere, such as meningitis.[312,315]

Complications. Unrecognized epiglottitis leads to increasing airway obstruction with subsequent respiratory arrest and death. Airway deterioration may occur suddenly because of extreme fatigue from trying to maintain airflow, aspiration of secretions, and subsequent laryngospasm.[319,320] Airway deterioration may occur spontaneously or be precipitated by severe crying, forcibly trying to make the child assume a supine position, or by instrumentation of the pharynx by inexperienced personnel. Other infectious foci may co-exist with epiglottitis: pneumonia (common), meningitis, septic arthritis, or pericarditis (rare).[307,315,321]

Ancillary Data. Laboratory investigations are contraindicated before establishing the airway in a child with a strongly suspected diagnosis of epiglottitis. Blood, throat, and epiglottitis cultures and the IV line are accomplished in the operating room after intubation. The WBC count is almost always elevated, with predominance of polymorphonuclear leukocytes and high numbers of immature neutrophil precursors.[322] Most blood and epiglottis cultures are positive.[323,324]

Similarly, lateral neck x-ray studies are potentially dangerous because of the resultant delays in definitive diagnosis and treatment and usually contribute little to management if the emergency department physician strongly suspects epiglottitis. Careful and continuous clinical monitoring is essential. However, a good quality lateral neck x-ray is often helpful in early or atypical cases. Care must be taken to prevent neck flexion during the imaging to avoid buckling of soft tissues and subsequent difficulty in interpretation. X-ray films are not always accurate.[325] The epiglottitis per se may occasionally be normal even though there is edema of other supraglottic structures. Although a perfectly normal supraglottic radiograph may be reassuring in an infant with very ambiguous presentation, a high quality picture is often difficult to obtain and false-negative examinations have required direct visualization. Direct pharyngoscopy performed in the Emergency Department by an otolaryngologist or an experienced physician is a useful tool to rule out epiglottitis in early or atypical presentations. It should be done in cooperative children when respiratory distress is absent.

Differential Considerations

Any child with crouplike features who has or develops any signs of epiglottitis (especially drooling, dysphagia, and preference for sitting position) must have supraglottic obstruction ruled out by direct visualization, optimally in the operating room.

Those patients with bacterial tracheitis usually have several days of typical croup and subsequently become toxic with worsening stridor that clinically mimics epiglottitis (see section on Stridor). Their upper airway obstruction is severe, does not respond to the croup therapy, and almost always requires intubation. Retropharyngeal abscess usually requires several days to develop. These children are often afebrile, rarely toxic, and hold their neck in a slightly extended position. Epiglottitis and uvulitis may co-exist.

Other diagnoses can usually be excluded. Obtaining a brief history while carefully observing the child helps to eliminate problems such as trauma or burn to the larynx, most cases of foreign-body inhalation, or diphtheria. The diagnosis of peritonsillar abscess is usually quite straightforward, although it is sometimes made by the ENT surgeon when they carefully examine the pharynx after referral for possible epiglottitis. Infectious mononucleosis is usually quite easy to diagnose as well. Most of these children are older (and thus cooperative), and permit examination of the throat. Large, swollen tonsils with exudate, marked cervical lymphadenopathy, and nasal congestion with or without splenomegaly help to establish the diagnosis. Those with respiratory difficulty (usually resulting from marked lymphoid tissue edema) should be admitted, moni-

tored, hydrated, cultured, given IV penicillin (pending culture results), and steroids. Small children with severe pharyngitis often drool and refuse fluids. Respiratory distress is absent, and crying is loud. A gentle examination of the pharynx usually reveals the source of the problem.

Management

Prehospital. Any child suspected of having supraglottic obstruction (at home or in a physician's office) must be urgently transferred by the fastest and safest route (via an aircraft or ambulance—never by a family car) to the nearest emergency facility where an artificial airway support can be provided, antibiotics initiated, and the child transferred elsewhere if necessary. A quick call to the local emergency department is helpful so that the anesthetist and operating room team can be summoned and the equipment assembled before the child's arrival. The physician must accompany the patient (or paramedics if the transfer is from home). The child should remain in the upright position in the parent's arms, and humidified oxygen provided using the best tolerated technique. If a complete airway obstruction occurs en route, jaw-thrust with bag-valve-mask ventilation is the treatment of choice and is usually preferred over an emergency tracheostomy.[326,327] Intubation in epiglottitis is often difficult, even under ideal circumstances, and should generally be deferred if possible until the patient reaches the hospital. When the airway is secure, a transfer should be arranged to the nearest pediatric ICU.

Emergency Department Management. The child with suspected epiglottitis must be seen and assessed immediately and managed according to predetermined protocols (see box on p. 1096). Every effort should be made to keep the patients calm, in the most comfortable position, and not separated from parents. Parents can assist in holding a tube with humidified oxygen a few inches from the face and in placing the probe on the skin for transcutaneous oxygen monitoring. Excellent information can usually be obtained by observing the child from a distance and auscultation of the chest. A brief history can usually be taken during this time. Particular attention should be paid to the rapidity of onset, fluid intake, foreign-body aspiration, trauma to the neck, and immunizations. When epiglottitis is likely, an anesthesia and ENT specialist must be summoned emergently. The rest of the examination should be deferred. The throat examination must be performed by a team skilled in establishing the airway.[328]

The child is taken to the operating room (with the parents assisting in transport) where a nasotracheal intubation is performed under general anesthesia. The nasotracheal tube should be 0.5 to 1.0 mm smaller than that predicted for the patient's age (0 to 6 months, 3 mm; 6 to 36 months, 3.5 mm; 36 months to 5 years, 4 mm; > 5 years, 4 to 5 mm).[327] Nasotracheal intubation is preferred to tracheostomy since it avoids surgery and reduces the duration of intubation and hospital stay.[329] Orotracheal intubation is an alternative. Rigid endoscopy and tracheostomy are also acceptable if personnel skilled in intubation and its aftercare are not available at the facility providing initial or definitive care (Fig. 59-3). Patients remain intubated for 36 ± 14 (1 SD) hours.

Sample Protocol for Management of Upper Airway Obstruction Caused by Infection in Children

Overview

Children with evidence of upper airway obstruction commonly have stridor, most commonly inspiratory if the pathology is supraglottic (extrathoracic), whereas expiratory stridor emanates from the trachea. For children with stridor or any evidence of upper airway obstruction, it is imperative to rapidly evaluate the degree of respiratory distress and intervene in an appropriate fashion, taking into account the degree of compromise, the diagnostic considerations, and the personnel, equipment, and facilities available.

Obviously, management (described below) of the child with severe croup or epiglottitis as the underlying pathology requires a markedly different intervention than does management of the child with a suspected or proved foreign body. Furthermore, mild croup unassociated with significant respiratory distress often can be managed after a careful evaluation with humidification at home and parental education regarding the danger signals indicating progression of disease.

Management

1. When the diagnosis of upper airway obstruction with respiratory compromise is suspected, secondary to an infectious process, a designated senior physician (attending or fellow) experienced in airway management should be called and should remain in constant attendance to coordinate and facilitate the patient's care. The senior physician should be responsible for activating this protocol.

2. The child should be kept in the company of parents, given humidified oxygen by mask, monitored for cardiac and respiratory function, and allowed to remain in the most comfortable position. Keep the child calm, reducing anxiety wherever possible.

3. After rapid assessment of the severity and pattern of progression of the respiratory obstruction, the senior physician should call the pediatric pulmonary and surgery fellows and the attending anesthesiologist.

4. If significant obstruction appears to be present, the operating room personnel should be alerted to prepare for direct laryngoscopy and possible intubation. Preparations also should be made for rigid bronchoscopy and tracheostomy.

5. Should the operating room be unable to accommodate the patient immediately, transfer the patient to the PACU (recovery room). The third line of transfer is the pediatric intensive care unit.

6. For children who probably have severe croup rather than epiglottitis and when there is a delay in achieving definitive visualization, a trial of nebulized racemic epinephrine (dilute 0.25 to 0.50 ml in 2.5 ml sterile water or saline and administer by nebulizer) may be of value. This should be done only in *stable, cooperative* patients under constant supervision who are not progressing rapidly and who have no evidence of impending total obstruction.

7. Do not agitate the child while obtaining blood samples and x-ray studies, starting IVs, or separating the child from the parents. Do not leave the child unattended or send the patient for any diagnostic studies.

8. *Do not* attempt laryngoscopy in the emergency department unless other options do not exist. The cause of progressive airway obstruction is best delineated under optimal conditions in the operating room where the patient can be given inhalation anesthesia and the epiglottis visualized under total control. If the diagnosis of epiglottitis is confirmed, the patient will be intubated with a tube 0.5 to 1.0 mm smaller than would normally be used.

9. In the event of an acute obstructive event in the emergency department, ventilation usually can be achieved using positive pressure ventilation and a self-inflating bag with 100% oxygen until definitive stabilization is achieved with available resources.

10. After satisfactory establishment of the airway, diagnostic studies can be obtained, pharmacologic therapy initiated, and transfer to the pediatric intensive care unit accomplished.

11. Management of croup with stridor at rest in the emergency department. Stridor at rest is an indication for hospital admission. Visualization of the epiglottis should be performed in the emergency department before admission to the ward or ICU if there is *no* evidence of obstruction and epiglottitis is not considered to be the likely diagnosis. The attending emergency department physician should be notified of the presence of such patients and involved with the procedure. At the time of visualization, the child should have been preoxygenated and a nurse and attending physician should be present. Equipment necessary for airway management, including self-inflating bag, appropriate endotracheal tube size (with stylet), oxygen, suction, and laryngoscope, must be immediately available. Frequently, nebulized racemic epinephrine (see management 6) may be administered to the cooperative patient. Steroids often are given to patients who require nebulized racemic epinephrine.

NOTE: This protocol should be modified to reflect the availability of personnel, equipment, and facilities, as well as the service and educational focus in a given situation.

Once intubated, blood and throat cultures are obtained, IV line placed, and antibiotics given. The child is then moved to a pediatric ICU. If this move involves an inter-hospital transfer, it is advisable to have a pediatric ICU transport staff or experienced physician involved. The antibiotics must include coverage for *H. influenzae*. Acceptable parenteral regimen include cefuroxime 75 mg/kg/24 hr q 8 hr, cefotaxime 150 mg/kg/24 hr q 6 hr or ceftriaxone 100 mg/kg/24 hr q 12 hr. Cefuroxime should not be given if concurrent meningitis is present or suspected. Additional

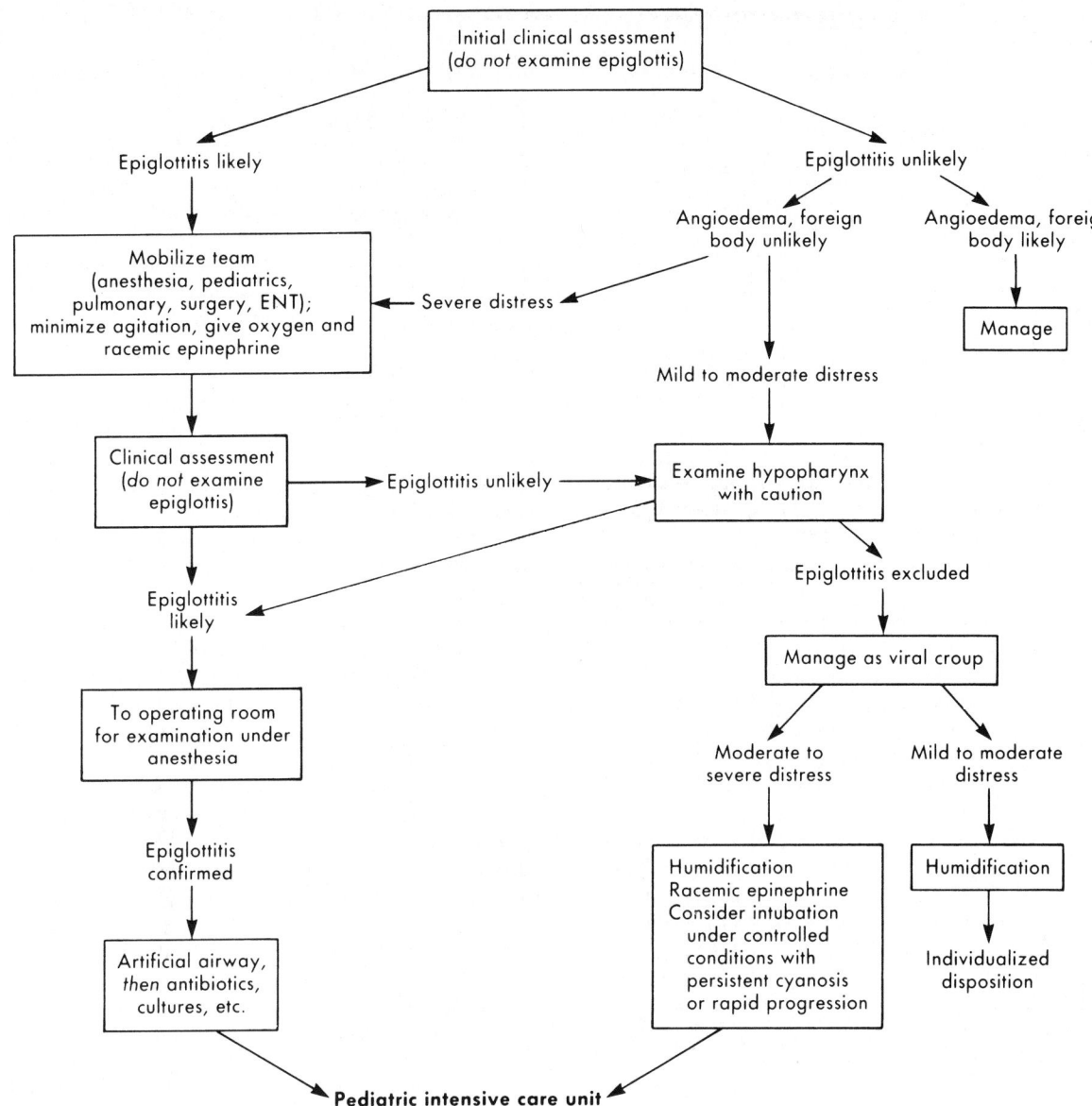

FIG. 59-3. Optimal assessment and management of upper airway obstruction due to epiglottitis or severe croup. Care must be individualized to reflect resources and logistic issues within a given institution. (*From Barkin RM and Rosen P: Emergency pediatrics, ed 4, St Louis, 1994, Mosby.*)

coverage is indicated if *S. aureus* is suspected. Corticosteroids have not been shown to be efficacious in epiglottitis.

Rarely, some intensivists choose to manage carefully selected patients without intubation.[312] This decision must be made in the operating room by the experienced airway consultants and never in the emergency department or in the community hospital. These patients will require round-the-clock observation in the pediatric ICU with skilled intubation personnel immediately available. A child who is to be transferred should be intubated before the journey. Transport must be completed with equipment and personnel to control the airway and ventilation.

Household contacts of patients with *H. influenzae* type B infection are at increased risk for this type of infection.[330] Rifampin prophylaxis 20 mg/kg/24 hr (600 mg/dose maximum) is recommended for all household contacts, espe-

cially if there is a young child (4 years of age or younger) in the contact group (see Appendix to Chapter 55). The emergency physician should also instruct the parents that a prompt visit to the family physician or pediatrician is advised for any febrile illness.

Mild or Unlikely Cases. If other diagnoses are likely, respiratory distress is absent, and the child is cooperative, the mouth and throat may be gently inspected. Pooling of the saliva beneath the tongue (often initially with little or no drooling) may be an early clue to epiglottitis in a child with sore throat and few other symptoms. Severe pharyngitis or peritonsillar or retropharyngeal abscess may also become obvious this way. If the findings are negative and epiglottitis is still a possibility, direct pharyngoscopy is a quick and reliable way to establish the diagnosis, provided the child is reasonably calm and cooperative. Pharyngoscopy can be performed in the emergency department by experienced emergency medicine personnel, or an ENT or anesthesia physician, with intubation equipment at hand. In many cases direct pharyngoscopy is a safer and better procedure than lateral neck x-ray films, especially in older children when performed under controlled conditions. The x-ray study may be helpful in ruling out unlikely cases if it is of a high quality but should not be the primary modality to exclude epiglottitis because of the rate of false-negative results.

TRACHEITIS

Bacterial tracheitis (membranous laryngotracheobronchitis) is a rare but serious subglottic bacterial infection.

Pathophysiology

Bacterial tracheitis is characterized by subglottic edema and inflammation of the larynx, trachea, bronchi, and sometimes the lung. There is usually copious purulent secretions and pseudomembrane formation in the trachea and bronchi.[331] Microscopically, there is mucosal ulceration, microabscess formation, and submucosal edema.[332] Extension of the disease into the bronchi and alveoli is common.

Etiology

Reports of concurrent positive viral isolation suggest the possibility of bacterial superinfection in viral disease.[332-334] *S. aureus* is the most common causative agent, followed by *S. pneumoniae*, group A beta-hemolytic streptococci, and *H. influenzae*.[332,335,336] Most patients with this disease tend to be older than those with uncomplicated viral croup.[333,337]

Diagnostic Findings

Most children have an upper respiratory infection for 1 to 2 weeks and several days of mild to moderately severe croup, followed by a rapid deterioration over several hours.[337] The child is febrile, very toxic, anxious or lethargic, and exhibits signs of severe upper airway obstruction: significant stridor, suprasternal indrawing, and poor air entry. Signs of lower airway disease such as crepitation, wheezing, and tachypnea are commonly associated. Respiratory distress tends to be severe and is unresponsive to therapy for croup. This diagnosis must be kept in mind for any child with crouplike features who appears unusually toxic or who deteriorates during therapy.

Complications. If unrecognized and not promptly treated, these patients are at risk of increasing upper and lower airway obstruction, with its attendant risk of hypoxemia, respiratory arrest, and death. Pneumonia often occurs as well, and its absence may imply a better prognosis.[337-339] A rare association with toxic shock syndrome has been reported.[340]

Ancillary Data

As in severe croup and epiglottitis, laboratory investigations add little to early diagnosis and should be postponed until the airway is secure. Transcutaneous oximetry is useful. Radiographs of the airway often show irregular tracheal densities, subglottic narrowing,[275] and varying degrees of opacification of the airway due to secretions. The whole blood cell count is usually high, suggesting an acute bacterial infection. Interestingly, positive blood cultures are unusual in bacterial tracheitis.[333] The tracheal culture during intubation usually grows the causative organisms.

Differential Considerations

The most common differential diagnosis is that of a severe viral croup and epiglottitis (see sections on Croup, Epiglottitis, and Stridor). Often, children appear clinically to have had croup, and with progression, the condition resembles epiglottitis. Occasionally, the x-ray radiographic reading of the tracheal air column may be falsely interpreted as a foreign body.[341]

Management

Tracheitis is usually suspected in febrile children with moderate croup who deteriorate in respiratory status and fail to respond to the usual croup management. These children need to be managed aggressively because of the high morbidity accompanying this illness. The approach is similar to that with epiglottitis (see previous section). Emergent intubation is usually required. Endoscopy may be beneficial, not only for early diagnosis and cultures, but also for the removal of the copious obstructive secretions by meticulous suction.[342] Frequent suctioning and pulmonary irrigation may be indicated. IV antibiotics for the causative organisms should be initiated as soon as the child's airway is stabilized. Useful initial antibiotic coverage includes nafcillin 100 to 150 mg/kg/24 hr q 6 hr IV with ceftriaxone 100 mg/kg/24 hr q 12 hr IV or another third generation cephalosporin. Gram stain and culture of the tracheal secretions may permit a more selective antibiotic choice. IV hydration must be provided, and the child should be carefully monitored in the ICU.

PLEURAL DISEASE

Pleuritis is defined as inflammation of the pleural membranes. It may occur as either an acute or chronic process. The inflammation may be associated with a pleural effusion, which is an accumulation of fluid into the pleural cavity. Pleural inflammation with effusion is an important cause of pulmonary disability and death in pediatric patients.[343] It may occur as a manifestation of a variety of clinical entities.

Pathophysiology

The serous membrane lining the lungs, visceral pleura, thoracic cavity, and parietal pleura completely enclose a potential space known as the pleural cavity.[344] The pleura is moistened with a serous secretion that facilitates the movements of the lung in the chest. The pleural fluid is created as a filtrate of the parietal pleural capillaries, which are supplied by the systemic circulation.[344] This filtrate is in turn absorbed by low-pressure visceral pleural capillaries. Additional drainage of the pleural fluid and high-molecular-weight proteins occurs by way of the lymphatic system, which drains centrally into the superior mediastinal lymph nodes. Under normal conditions, a dynamic equilibrium is reached in which there is a small amount of pleural fluid, and fluid formation equals fluid absorption.[345]

Various mechanisms may account for abnormal pleural fluid accumulation including alterations in hydrostatic or colloid osmotic pressures, altered capillary permeability secondary to diseases of the pleural surface, and changes in the lymphatic reabsorption of proteins and fluid.[344] Pleural effusions can be divided into transudates or exudates based on the mechanism of abnormal fluid accumulation. Transudates result from an increase in capillary hydrostatic pressure or a decrease in colloid osmotic pressure.[346] The pleura itself is usually not diseased. A transudate is essentially a plasma filtrate, containing relatively low concentrations of proteins and cells.[346]

An exudate is fluid that has escaped from blood vessels, usually as a result of inflammation or disease of the pleura. Exudates contain relatively larger amounts of protein, cells, and cellular debris than transudates contain. The mechanisms leading to production of an exudate include infection or inflammatory processes, which damage the pleural capillary endothelium, allow leakage of protein into the pleural space, and obstruct the lymphatic system (seen primarily with neoplastic diseases in children).[346] An empyema is a purulent parapneumonic effusion that represents true infection of the pleural space.[347]

The identification of pleural fluid as a transudate or exudate can help determine the cause of fluid accumulation. Pleural fluid has been classified as an exudate if the total protein concentration exceeds 3.0 gm/dl.[348,349] However, this level can result in incorrect classification of over 10% of effusions.[348,350] Better classification of pleural fluid into transudates and exudates can be achieved by comparing the concentrations of proteins and lactate dehydrogenase (LDH) found in the serum and pleural fluid. The pleural fluid properties of an exudate include any of the following: (1) ratio of pleural fluid protein to serum protein >0.5, (2) ratio of pleural fluid LDH to serum LDH >0.6, or (3) an absolute value of LDH >200 IU.[346]

Etiology

Transudative Pleural Effusions. A transudate occurs when the systemic factors influencing the formation or absorption of pleural fluid are altered. Various disease states can lead to this abnormal fluid collection as shown in the box on p. 1100. Elevated capillary hydrostatic pressure as a result of elevated left atrial pressure secondary to congestive heart failure or restrictive pericarditis can cause accumulation of pleural fluid.[351]

Transudates secondary to a decrease in plasma colloid osmotic pressure are generally seen in patients with hypoproteinemic conditions, including renal disease with nephrosis, hepatic failure, protein-losing enteropathy, severe malnutrition, or extensive burns.[351] A transudative pleural effusion can also be seen in patients undergoing peritoneal dialysis or with sarcoidosis.[345]

Exudative Pleural Effusions. Pleural fluid exudates primarily result from diseases of the pleural surface. Infectious diseases are the most common cause of pleural inflammation in the pediatric age group, with pneumonia being the most common specific cause producing an exudative pleural effusion.[347] Various bacteria including *S. aureus*, *S. pneumoniae*, group A streptococci, and *H. influenzae* may all produce pneumonia with an associated empyema.[352] Although *S. aureus* has been the most frequently isolated pathogen in adults and children, a significant de-

cline in the proportion of cases resulting from that pathogen and a concomitant rise in those resulting from *H. influenzae* has been noted in children.[353,354] Anaerobic bacteria have also been isolated from empyemas occuring in children and adolescents.[352] *M. pneumoniae* and viral infections caused by coxsackie, Epstein-Barr, and herpes zoster viruses can also cause exudative pleural effusions. Tuberculosis remains an important pathogen to consider in the child presenting with pleural disease.[347] Less common fungal and parasitic infections such as histoplasmosis, coccidiodomycosis, blastomycosis, and amebiasis can also present with a pleural effusion, particularly in the immunocompromised patient.[345,355] Visceral leishmaniasis is increasingly reported in immunocompromised patients, including patients with AIDS, and can present with pleural effusions.[356]

Pneumocystis carinii pneumonia, the most common opportunistic pulmonary infection in patients with AIDS, recently has been reported as occurring as both a primary pleural infection and as a parapneumonic infection complicating underlying *Pneumocystis* pneumonia.[357]

Neoplastic diseases are the second most common cause of pleural effusions in children.[347] Mesothelioma is a primary malignancy of the pleura itself and is very rare in children. Pleural effusions are more commonly seen with metastatic disease in children, with the primary tumor most commonly occurring as leukemia, lymphoma, carcinoma, or sarcoma.[351]

Other underlying causes of an exudative pleural effusion in children include collagen vascular diseases such as systemic lupus erythematosus or juvenile rheumatoid arthritis, GI disorders, pulmonary embolism or infarction, and drug hypersensitivity or reactions.[351,358] A hemothorax or chylothorax can result from accidental or nonaccidental trauma, or it can occur iatrogenically secondary to medical procedures. Other conditions known to be associated with pleural disease with effusion in children include exposure to asbestos, uremia, radiation therapy, and congenital abnormalities of the lymphatics.[345]

Diagnostic Findings

Clinical Findings. Although the signs and symptoms are often related to the underlying disease, a pleural effusion itself will be symptomatic after enough fluid has accumulated in the pleural space. Common symptoms and complaints include dyspnea at rest or on exertion, nonproductive cough, and fever. Pleuritic chest pain, the most characteristic symptom of pleural effusion, usually occurs when infection is the underlying cause.[347] It may be mild but is often severe, and is described as sharp or knifelike, with severity increasing with inspiration. The pain is generally localized to the chest without radiation. Gastrointestinal complaints include anorexia, vomiting, and abdominal distension and may be present due to an associated partial paralytic ileus. Infants and younger children will often have much less specific symptoms of respiratory illness including dyspnea, cough, lethargy, or feeding difficulties.[347]

The findings on physical examination are variable and are often related to the underlying cause of the pleural effusion. The patient is usually tachypneic with short, shal-

Etiology of Pleural Effusions

Transudates

Increased hydrostatic pressure
Congestive heart failure
Constrictive pericarditis

Decreased osmotic pressure
Renal disease with nephrosis
Hepatic failure
Protein-losing enteropathy
Severe malnutrition
Extensive burns

Other
Peritoneal dialysis
Sarcoidosis
Idiopathic

Exudates

Infections
Bacterial: *S. aureus, S. pneumoniae, H. influenzae,* group A
    streptococci, and anaerobes
Viral: Coxsackie, EBV, and herpes zoster
M. pneumoniae
Tuberculosis
Fungal: histoplasmosis, coccidiodomycosis, and blastomycosis
Parasitic: ameba, filaria, visceral leishmaniasis, *Pneumocystis
    carinii*
Hepatitis

Neoplasms
Mesothelioma
Leukemia
Lymphoma

Metastatic carcinoma
Sarcoma
Chest wall tumors

Collagen vascular diseases
Systemic lupus erythematosus
Juvenile rheumatoid arthritis

Gastrointestinal diseases
Pancreatitis
Esophageal rupture
Subphrenic abscess
Hepatic abscess
Diaphragmatic hernia
Peritonitis

Trauma
Hemothorax
Chylothorax
Esophageal rupture

Drug hypersensitivity
Nitrofurantoin
Methotrexate

Other
Pulmonary infarction
Asbestos exposure
Uremia
Postradiation therapy
Drug reactions
Congenital lymphatic abnormalities

Adapted from Light RW: *Med Clin North Am* 61(6):1339, 1977.

---

low respirations. Signs of respiratory distress including grunting, flaring, and accessory muscle use may be present. Attention to the chest findings on physical examination is important, particularly if only a small amount of pleural fluid is present. The pleural effusion itself results in a decrease in breath sounds on the affected side and dullness to percussion over the fluid collection.[343] Tactile fremitus will be decreased over the effusion because the fluid conducts vibrations less well than air.[343] A pleural friction rub may be heard directly over an area of pleural inflammation early in the disease process when little effusion is present. The rub is an audible, low-pitched sound that may be grating in nature. It is heard throughout the respiratory cycle but is maximal on inspiration.[343]

Complications. The primary complication associated with pleural inflammation with effusion is the progression to acute respiratory failure with inadequate oxygenation and ventilation. The patient's course will also be complicated by the nature and extent of the underlying disease process. Empyemic pleural fluid is associated with a more prolonged and complicated hospital course. Bronchopleu-

ral fistula and tension pneumatocele are rare but may delay full recovery.[343] In contrast to adults, infants and children have a remarkable ability to resolve a thickened pleura with little effect on subsequent lung growth and function.[343]

Ancillary Data. Ancillary tests should be used to evaluate the cardiorespiratory status of the patient and to identify the underlying disease process. Hematologic studies should include a CBC to look for evidence of infection or thrombocytopenia, and coagulation studies, particularly if thoracentesis is planned. An erythrocyte sedimentation rate should be obtained, as it may be elevated with malignant or collagen vascular diseases. Laboratory studies including electrolytes, renal function tests, liver enzymes, serum protein, and albumin may reveal underlying abnormalities. A serum LDH should also be obtained to use for comparison with the pleural fluid value. The urine should be checked for both protein and blood. An arterial blood gas assesses both the oxygenation and ventilation status of the patient, as well as the acid-base balance. The development of a respiratory acidosis should raise concerns of respiratory decompensation. Appropriate cultures, including a blood culture, should be obtained in the presence of a fever. An ECG should be obtained if an underlying cardiac abnormality is suspected.

A chest x-ray film is necessary in all patients presenting with signs or symptoms of pleural effusion. On an upright chest film, blunting of the costophrenic angles is the earliest sign of a pleural effusion. As fluid accumulation increases, a concave density develops along the lateral chest wall. The lateral view may show a fluid collection in the posterior costophrenic angle.[359] Decubitus views may reveal small quantities of pleural fluid that are completely invisible on the routine upright radiographs. On a lateral decubitus view, the effusion layers out on the dependent side if it is not loculated.[360] The effusion also shifts in the decubitus position, allowing a view of the underlying lung. Supine films may suggest an effusion by diffuse haziness because the fluid layers posteriorly, although it may be very difficult to identify if effusions are present bilaterally. The radiographic appearance of pleural fluid may be confusing at times, even if the fluid is not loculated. Free fluid within the fissures may simulate a mass, loculated effusion, or focal infiltrate. Large amounts of subpulmonic fluid may simulate an elevated diaphragm or subphrenic abscess.[360] The radiologic findings of any underlying cardiac or pulmonary process may also be present.

Extracardiac chest ultrasonography can also be used as a technique for characterization and localization of pleural disease by an experienced ultrasonographer. In children with evidence of a pleural effusion, opaque hemithorax, or suspected pulmonary or mediastinal masses, chest ultrasonography can be an accurate and useful imaging modality in cases not easily diagnosed from conventional radiographs.[361,362] A CT scan of the chest can be helpful in the differential diagnosis of diffuse pleural disease, particularly in differentiating malignant from benign conditions.[363,364] Interventional radiology with image-guided management of intrathoracic collections by CT scan or ultrasonography is increasingly being used as an alternative to traditional thoracentesis and surgical therapy.[365]

Thoracentesis. Thoracentesis is indicated for diagnostic purposes when a sufficient quantity of pleural fluid effusion or empyema is demonstrated, and for therapeutic purposes when the fluid accumulation is extensive enough to cause dyspnea. With the proper technique, thoracentesis can be performed quickly, safely, and with minimum discomfort to the patient. The intercostal vessels and nerves run below the inferior margin of the rib; therefore, the needle should always be inserted over the superior margin of the rib to avoid the neurovascular bundle.

Technique. The patient is prepared and draped. Mild sedation may be required in the uncooperative child if respiratory distress is not present. The child should be positioned leaning forward against a pillow or embracing the backrest of a chair. Small infants can be held against the chest of an assistant. With the arm on the involved side elevated, the lower tip of the scapula lies just above the seventh intercostal space in the posterior axillary line. The position of the fluid should be confirmed by dullness to percussion on physical examination and by radiograph or ultrasound. Ultrasound localization and monitoring of needle insertion can be particularly useful.

The puncture site is prepped with povidone-iodine solution and draped to permit visualization of the landmarks. Adequate local anesthesia should be achieved by infiltrating 1% lidocaine without epinephrine down to the rib periosteum and pleura. A three-way stopcock, tubing, and 20-ml syringe can be attached to an 18-gauge needle, angiocath, or catheter system. The needle is generally inserted along the posterior axillary line, corresponding to the fluid level, just above the edge of the rib to avoid the intercostal vessels running along the lower edge of the ribs. The sixth to seventh interspace is usually appropriate. Insertion of the needle at other sites may be elected as dictated by the location of the fluid loculations. If pneumothorax rather than fluid is present, the needle is best inserted at the second or third intercostal space at the midclavicular line.

The needle is inserted so that as much of its length is exposed as needed to traverse the chest wall, to maximize control over the needle, and to prevent inadvertent puncture of the underlying lung. The syringe should be attached to the needle, with aspiration occurring as the needle is advanced to ensure that the needle has reached the pleural fluid. To fix the position of the needle on the skin surface, a hemostat can be clamped across the needle barrel. If a catheter is used, it can be advanced after removal of the stylet, in a caudal direction into the thoracic cavity while covering the hub with a finger.

The fluid is slowly aspirated using a T-connection, syringe, and three-way stopcock. Aliquots of 50 to 100 ml can be removed for diagnostic studies or to provide symptomatic relief. Some of the fluid should be collected in test tubes for analysis. After the fluid is removed, the needle or catheter should be removed quickly and a sterile occlusive dressing can be applied.

An upright chest x-ray film should be obtained after the procedure is completed to verify the absence of complications such as pneumothorax, hemothorax, or underlying parenchymal disease. Infection, pulmonary edema, and fluid shifts with intravascular depletion can also complicate this procedure.

Contraindications to the procedure include a significant bleeding diathesis, thrombocytopenia <50,000 platelets/mm³), prolonged partial thromboplastin time (PTT >1.5 normal), chest wall herpes zoster, and insufficient quantity of pleural fluid.

Interpretations. The fluid obtained from thoracentesis can be classified as either a transudate or an exudate, using the previously stated criteria based on the protein and LDH levels in the pleural fluid. In addition to establishing these levels, other laboratory evaluations should be performed on a routine basis, including gross examination of the fluid, RBC and WBC count with differential, glucose and amylase levels, pH, gram stain and cultures, and cytologic analysis.

On gross examination, most transudates appear clear, straw-colored, quite fluid, and odorless. A white milky appearance indicates a chylothorax or pyothorax. The fluid from a frank empyema is viscid, opaque, and often malodorous.[345]

A grossly bloody pleural effusion with a RBC count greater than 100,000/mm[3] is suggestive of trauma, malignancy, or pulmonary embolization.[366] A RBC count between 5,000 and 100,000/mm[3] is much less specific, since over 15% of transudates and 40% of all types of exudates are blood tinged. A Wright stain of the pleural sediment showing hemoglobin inclusion bodies stained pink in the macrophages indicates that the blood has been in the pleural space for a period of time and was not introduced via the thoracentesis.[345]

The pleural fluid WBC count is of limited value. A pleural WBC count of 1,000/mm[3] suggests a transudate rather than an exudate, but not as effectively as the protein and LDH comparisons.[345] Transudates have a protein of <3 gm/dl and relatively low LDH (<200 IU/L), whereas exudates have a higher protein and a high LDH (>200 IU/L) (see earlier discussion as well). Pleural fluid WBC counts greater than 10,000/mm[3] are most common with parapneumonic effusions, but are also seen with pancreatitis, pulmonary infarction, collagen vascular diseases, malignancy, and tuberculosis.[366] Examination of the WBC count differential is important to further define the underlying cause.

The pleural fluid glucose level of transudates and most exudates is similar to the serum level. Low pleural fluid glucose levels of less than 60 mg/dl, however, can be seen with parapneumonic effusions, rheumatoid diseases, tuberculosis, and malignancy.[367] An elevated amylase level helps establish a diagnosis of underlying pancreatitis. The pleural fluid pH can be a useful prognostic index in patients with acute bacterial pneumonia and pleural effusion. An arterial pH should be obtained for comparison with the pleural fluid value. In adult patients, it appears that pleural fluid pH can discriminate free-moving, unloculated effusions (pH >7.30) from loculated exudates and frank empyema (pH <7.30), thus having therapeutic and prognostic importance.[343] In children a pleural fluid pH value of less than 7.20 in parapneumonic effusions correlates with more severe disease evidenced by a prolonged hospital course or failure of treatment of antibiotics alone, and usually requires chest tube drainage.[368,369]

When a diagnostic thoracentesis is performed, a gram stain should be performed, and the fluid should be cultured for aerobic and anaerobic organisms. Mycobacterial and fungal cultures should also be considered. The pleural fluid can also be stained for acid-fast bacteria, but the yield is low even in tuberculous effusions.[345]

Pleural fluid should undergo cytologic analysis because it may lead to the diagnosis of a malignant effusion. When indicated by clinical circumstances, additional parameters such as triglyceride, cholesterol, complement, rheumatoid factor, or lupus erythematosus cells may be determined.

Other. When diagnoses such as tuberculosis or malignancy are suspected, a needle biopsy of the parietal pleura should be considered to complete the analysis of the pleural fluid. It is not an emergency procedure, however, and should be performed only in a well-controlled environment.

Differential Considerations

The differential diagnosis of a patient presenting with the specific symptom of pleuritic chest pain should include rib fractures and costochondritis. It is also important to note that the physical findings of atelectasis of an entire lung and a large pleural effusion can be very similar, except that the trachea deviates away from the involved side when a pleural effusion is present, and toward the involved side with atelectasis.

Management

The treatment of pleural disease should be directed toward specific management of the underlying cause and relief of the associated symptoms. As in all resuscitation efforts, attention should first be directed toward airway, breathing, and circulation. General supportive measures should include initial stabilization of the pulmonary status with the reversal of hypoxemia by the administration of humidified oxygen and mechanical ventilation if necessary. The patient should be kept in a comfortable position with cardiac and pulse oximetry monitoring.

The chest pain associated with pleural inflammation without effusion requires treatment. Analgesics, bed rest, and mild sedation may be indicated. It is important to note, however, that the restlessness and irritability seen in a patient with pleural disease may be due to the chest pain, high fever, or hypoxia. With severe chest pain, lying on the affected side sometimes provides relief by splinting the involved thorax.[343] As a pleural effusion accumulates, the chest pain is usually relieved.

Thoracentesis is indicated as a therapeutic measure when the pleural fluid accumulation is large enough to cause dyspnea. If thoracentesis is performed, it is important to have adequate intravenous access so that hypovolemia secondary to fluid shifts can be rapidly treated with an infusion of an isotonic crystalloid solution (normal saline or lactated Ringer's solution) or a 5% albumin solution. Continuous chest tube drainage may be indicated if rapid reaccumulation of the effusion occurs and the patient remains symptomatic. Further specific management should be directed at the underlying disease process.

Disposition

Nearly all patients presenting with a clinically significant and radiologically identified pleural effusion require admission to the hospital for management and determination of the underlying cause. The rare patient with a known underlying condition and with minimal clinical symptoms and close follow-up available on an outpatient basis, can be discharged from the emergency department.

PNEUMONIA

Pneumonia is an inflammation of the lung parenchyma involving either the interstitium or the alveoli usually secondary to an infectious process.[370] Acute respiratory infections in general are one of the most common illnesses occurring in children in the United States.[371] Most of these infections are mild and refer to the upper respiratory tract. However, lower respiratory tract infections, including pneumonia, remain a leading cause of significant morbidity in infancy and childhood. Pneumonia is the most common discharge diagnosis made in children under 10 years of age who are hospitalized with respiratory disease.[371] This group makes up just a small portion of the total, since the majority of children with pneumonia are managed outside of the hospital.

Pathophysiology

Multiple defense mechanisms protect the respiratory tract from infection. The epiglottal reflex prevents aspiration of infected secretions from the upper respiratory tract. The mucous blanket of the respiratory tract, to which airborne mechanisms adhere, is cleared from the respiratory epithelium by ciliary action. Aspirated foreign material that passes through the glottis is generally propelled out of the lower respiratory tract by the cough reflex. The alveoli are lined by phagocytic cells that act as the first line of attack against invading microorganisms.[372]

The defense mechanisms of the pulmonary system are most often disturbed by a viral infection, which frequently precedes the development of bacterial pneumonia. Different cells within the respiratory epithelium support the replication of these viruses in various ways related to the distinctive patterns of clinical disease and associated with various agents.[373] The virus causes damage directly to the cell it invades, resulting in the response of nonspecific and specific inflammatory and immunocompetent cells to the site of infection. This produces immunologically mediated lysis of the viral infected cells with the subsequent alteration of the capillary and mucous membranes, permeability to serum proteins, alterations of the mucosal handling of water and electrolytes, and mucus hypersecretion.[373]

Bacteria may invade the lower respiratory tract by two routes, primarily facilitated by previous injury secondary to infection with respiratory viruses. The first, but less common route, is via the bloodstream. Inflammation of the nasal mucosa may allow direct seeding into the bloodstream, or it may trap bacteria in the middle ear or paranasal sinuses leading to a purulent infection and the additional possibility of bacteremia. The blood-borne bacteria may be filtered out in the lung or visceral pleura, resulting in pneumonia with or without empyema.[374] The second route allows bacteria in the nasopharynx to invade the lower respiratory tract and produce bacterial pneumonia after a breakdown of normal pulmonary clearance mechanisms has occurred secondary to a viral infection.[374] Understanding the pathogenesis of pneumonia is important because the two classifications of viral and bacterial infection are not mutually exclusive.

Etiology

A variety of different infectious agents can produce pneumonia and lower tract respiratory illness in children as shown in the box at right, including bacteria, viruses, parasites, fungi, and other agents such as *C. trachomatis*, *M. pneumoniae*, and *M. tuberculosis*. Studies of the bacterial flora of the nasopharynx of children with pneumonia have shown that the potential pathogens usually associated with bacterial pneumonia are found with nearly the same frequencies in healthy children as in ill children.[375,376] Clinical signs and symptoms, laboratory data, and radiography can help the clinician determine that pneumonia is present and may be useful in determining cause. Awareness of outbreaks in particular areas may also facilitate determining cause in individual children. However, the

effect of age on the likely pathogens of a child with pneumonia is probably the single most important variable to be considered when determining the probable microorganisms involved.[377]

Neonates. Neonates are at increased risk of pneumonia, and other bacterial and viral infections, primarily because of the trauma of the birthing process itself combined with immature host defenses against infection.[378] Most babies with neonatal pneumonia have congenitally-acquired or hospital-acquired rather than community-acquired infections. Some newborns, however, may have pneumonia that

---

Etiologic Agents in Pneumonia

Bacterial

Common organisms
S. pneumoniae
H. influenzae
S. aureus
Group A streptococci
Group B streptococci

Uncommon organisms
Bordetella pertussis
Pseudomonas aeruginosa
Escherichia coli
Klebsiella pneumoniae
Legionella pneumophila
Listeria monocytogenes
Peptostreptococcus

Viral

Common organisms
Respiratory syncytial virus (RSV)
Parainfluenzae
Influenzae
Adenovirus
Enterovirus
Rhinovirus

Uncommon organisms
Measles
Varicella-zoster
Cytomegalovirus
Herpes simplex

Fungal
Coccidioides immitis
Histoplasma capsulatum

Parasitic
Pneumocystis carinii

Other
M. pneumoniae
C. trachomatis
M. tuberculosis
Coxiella burnetti (Q fever)

TABLE 59-4. Common Etiologic Agents in Pneumonia by Age Group

	Bacterial	Viral	Other
Neonates (< 1 mo)	Group B streptococci *E. coli* *Klebsiella* *Pseudomonas* *Listeria*	RSV Varicella	*Chlamydia*
Young Infants (1 to 3 mo)	Group B streptococci *H. influenzae* *S. pneumoniae* Group A streptococci Pertussis	RSV Parainfluenzae Influenzae Adenovirus	*Chlamydia*
Infants and Young Children (3 mo to 5 yr)	*S. pneumoniae* *H. influenzae* *S. aureus* Group A streptococci Pertussis	RSV Parainfluenzae Influenzae Adenovirus Enterovirus Rhinovirus	*Chlamydia*
Older Children (> 5 yr)	*S. pneumoniae* *H. influenzae* Group A streptococci	Parainfluenzae Influenzae Adenovirus Rhinovirus	*Mycoplasma*

is recognized only after discharge from the hospital. The spectrum of organisms causing pneumonia in neonates is much different from that in older infants and children as shown in Table 59-4. Neonates are protected by transplacental antibodies against the more common causes of pneumonia in older children such as *S. pneumoniae* and *H. influenzae*.[378] Respiratory viral infections are also less common in infants than in older children because of the limited exposure of newborns to large numbers of people. The most common bacterial pathogen in neonatal pneumonia remains group B streptococci. It is characterized by a very fulminating course, with mortality exceeding 50%, particularly in the immediate newborn period.[371] Gram-negative bacteria, such as *Escherichia coli, Klebsiella pneumoniae,* and *Pseudomonas aeruginosa* are also important pathogens, especially in small, premature infants requiring intensive care.[371] These bacteria are generally acquired during delivery through a vaginal tract that is colonized with these organisms. Less frequently, *Listeria monocytogenes*, a bacteria infants can acquire in utero, can produce pneumonia in newborns.[377] Because of their relatively immunocompromised state, neonates may also develop viral pneumonia with RSV, varicella, cytomegalovirus, or herpes simplex virus.[378]

Young Infants. Infants between 1 and 3 months of age pose a difficult diagnostic problem because they are old enough to be colonized with the respiratory pathogens of older children but young enough to have disease because

of agents acquired at birth.[377] For these infants, the immune system is somewhat more mature, protecting them from the more unusual pathogens seen in neonates. However, they are beginning to lose their protective maternal antibodies against *S. pneumoniae* and *H. influenzae* and are becoming more susceptible to these pathogens. Pneumonia caused by *C. trachomatis* has come to be recognized as one of the most common forms of pneumonia during the first 3 months of life.[379] It is considered to be an infection caused by agents acquired at birth. Young infants less than 6 months of age are also at risk for developing respiratory tract infection caused by *B. pertussis*. Infection with this agent persists primarily in large urban areas where children's immunizations may be delayed or not obtained at all. The infection, however, is usually transmitted to children from adult carriers of the organism.[380]

Infants and Young Children. In children between 3 months of age and approximately 5 years, the relative importance of potential causative agents changes significantly. In infants and preschool-aged children, the major causative agents producing pneumonia are viruses, with the highest incidence of infection occurring between 6 and 12 months of age.[381] RSV and parainfluenzae virus types 1, 2, and 3 are the most important causes of lower respiratory tract infections, including pneumonia, in infants and children in this age group. Infection with RSV is the most common, primarily occurring during the winter and spring.[373] Influenza virus, usually occurring in winter epidemics, can also produce pneumonia in this age group. Adenovirus infections vary yearly, but can cause a very severe pneumonia, particularly in young infants. Other viruses such as enteroviruses and rhinoviruses can also be a source of lower respiratory tract infection in children.[373]

Bacteria are far less likely than viruses to cause pneumonia in this age group of children. Those that do produce infection are quite different from the causative agents seen in neonates. The most common bacterial cause of pneumonia in older infants and children is *S. pneumoniae*.[381] Children with sickle cell disease are particularly at risk to develop pneumococcal pneumonia.

Up until recently, *H. influenzae* type B had been one of the most common causes of bacterial pneumonia in infants and young children. However, the routine immunization of young children with *H. influenzae* type B vaccine has significantly decreased the incidence of invasive disease secondary to this organism.[382] However, it is not unusual for this bacteria to cause concomitant infection in other areas of the body such as otitis media, meningitis, epiglottitis, pericarditis, or septic arthritis.[383,384]

Less commonly seen bacterial causes of childhood pneumonia include *S. aureus* and group A streptococci. Pneumonia produced by *S. aureus* is decreasing in frequency among children, but remains a very serious illness often complicated by the development of pneumatoceles, pneumothoraces, and empyema.[385] Infection with group A streptococci usually follows one of the childhood exanthematous illnesses, particularly measles, varicella, or scarlet fever.[372] Infection with *P. aeruginosa* can be seen in debilitated or immunocompromised hosts, particularly children with cystic fibrosis. *L. pneumophilia* can also cause pneumonia, although it is rarely seen in children.

Older Children. As children enter their school years, infection with *M. pneumoniae* becomes increasingly more likely to cause pneumonia than viruses or bacteria. It reaches its peak occurrence in the 10- to 12-year-old age group.[386] Infection with *H. influenzae* drops off sharply after ages 6 or 7 so that by 10 years of age, the nonviral causes of pneumonia are primarily *Mycoplasma* and *S. pneumoniae*.[387]

Although tuberculosis is no longer a common cause of respiratory disease in most areas of the United States, after decades of steady decline it has begun to rise in some vulnerable communities.[388] Those particularly at risk for the development of tuberculosis include recent immigrants, particularly from Southeast Asia and Mexico, who have been previously infected. The homeless, the poor living in crowded areas, and those with underlying immunodeficiencies, including the acquired immunodeficiency syndrome (AIDS), are also susceptible.[388]

Another infectious cause of pneumonia in the pediatric age group is the parasite *Pneumocystis carinii*. It is becoming more frequently diagnosed in children of all ages with primary immune deficiency disorders and in patients receiving immunosuppressive drugs for malignancies or organ transplantation. Fungal agents such as histoplasmosis and coccidiomycosis also rarely produce pneumonia in children. Primary infection of the lung with *Histoplasma capsulatum* occurs primarily in endemic areas, such as in the southeast area and Mississippi Valley of the United States.[372] Infection with *Coccidioides immitis* is common in the arid regions of the southwestern United States, Mexico, and Central America. Almost all cases of this disease heal without treatment. A rickettsial organism, *Coxiella burnetii*, can cause an illness known as Q fever. It is an interstitial pneumonitis, which is endemic in sheep and is frequently transmitted to sheep handlers.[372] The infection is usually self-limited, lasting approximately 3 weeks.

Diagnostic Findings

Clinical Findings. The clinical symptoms associated with the diagnosis of pneumonia are varied and may be rather nonspecific. An older child may have symptoms of cough, fever, pleuritic chest pain, dyspnea, or tachypnea. The presence of a productive cough in adults is a hallmark of pneumonia, but the child with pneumonia usually swallows sputum rather than expectorate it.[371] These typical symptoms may not be present in the young child or infant who may have nonspecific symptoms, including fever, irritability, poor feeding, decreased physical activity, vomiting or diarrhea, or apneic episodes.

Viral pneumonia is typically preceded by an upper respiratory infection with the insidious onset of further symptoms including cough, coryza, myalgias, and low-grade fever. An apneic episode may be the first symptom to occur with RSV infections in young infants less than 3 months old.[373] Bacterial pneumonia, particularly pneumococcal pneumonia, is characterized by a more rapid onset of symptoms and a high degree of toxicity with fever, chills, cough, and often, pleuritic pain. *H. influenzae* produces a pneumonia that may be mild in course, closely resembling a viral pneumonia, or it may be extremely severe with the symptoms similar to infection with *S. pneumonia*.[371] Infection with *Mycoplasma* usually produces a mild illness of insidious onset with a protracted course characterized by a productive cough, malaise, headache, and fever.[387]

Young infants with *Chlamydia* pneumonia have an illness characterized by an afebrile, gradually progressive course with increasing tachypnea. Many infants with this infection exhibit a distinctive staccato-like cough that may be associated with posttussive cyanosis. Approximately half of infected infants have a concurrent or previous conjunctivitis.[379] Infection with *B. pertussis* clinically appears with an initial catarrhal stage followed by the development of a staccato, paroxysmal cough. The classic "whoop" may be heard in between cough paroxysms.[380]

The feeding history of the patient, particularly in young infants, can aid in assessing the severity of the illness. Infants who feed slowly, with evidence of respiratory distress during feeding, or who refuse feedings entirely may be more severely affected than infants who maintain their normal feeding patterns.

It is important to obtain history regarding any underlying diseases. Children with preexisting cardiac or pulmonary disease may be more seriously compromised by an episode of pneumonia. A history of frequent infections, immunosuppressive therapy, or primary immune deficiencies should raise suspicion about the possibility of infection with an opportunistic organism. Children with chronic disease involving other systems such as liver disease, metabolic disease, or chronic renal failure can also have their course complicated by acute pulmonary infections.

The clinical signs present in pneumonia vary according to cause and also from child to child. Tachypnea is a helpful clue to the possibility of pneumonia, particularly in the first year of life.[371] It is important to observe the child quietly at rest before auscultation to note this finding along with the degree of effort required to maintain respirations. Signs of increased respiratory effort include accessory respiratory muscle use with substernal, intercostal, or suprasternal retractions, nasal flaring, or grunting. A prolonged expiratory phase suggests airway obstruction as in asthma or bronchiolitis. Fever is usually present in all children with pneumonia but may not be present in young infants infected with *Chlamydia*.[379]

Auscultation may reveal rales or moist crackles, which are highly specific signs for pneumonia, if present. However, these signs may not be appreciated in the young child who is unable to cooperate with the examination or who may not be ventilating the involved area of the lung.[371] Localized findings of decreased breath sounds and dullness to percussion suggest the possibility of consolidation or a pleural effusion. In young children, careful back-and-forth comparison of both lung fields may help to reveal areas of diminished breath sounds. The presence of wheezing on auscultation suggests a viral infection, particularly RSV.[373] However, it can also be seen in children with *Chlamydia* or *Mycoplasma* pneumonia.[387] Occasionally, in children with lower lobe pneumonias, GI signs including abdominal distension and tenderness may mimic GI pathology.

Complications. The specific complications associated with pneumonia vary depending on the underlying pathogen. As with all pulmonary processes, progression to acute respiratory failure with inadequate oxygenation and ventilation can complicate the course of any type of pneumonia. The most common complication of pneumonia in younger children is dehydration, primarily due to poor oral intake. Pulmonary infections because of *H. influenzae* can be complicated by the development of pleural effusions, pneumatoceles, or bacteremia with concomitant infections such as otitis media, meningitis, epiglottitis, pericarditis, or septic arthritis.[383,384] Pleural effusions, pneumatoceles, and pneumothoraces are also frequently seen with pneumonia caused by *S. aureus.*[372] Significant morbidity resulting from respiratory failure with RSV infection can be seen in children with underlying diseases and those who are very young. Long-term complications from infection with the RSV include a small risk for recurrent apnea but a moderately increased risk for the development of hyperreactive airways later in life.[373]

Ancillary Data. Laboratory studies in the evaluation of pneumonia should be individualized for the specific patient and the presenting clinical complex. An ABG may be obtained on patients with pneumonia who have significant respiratory distress, apnea, or cyanosis.[370] Oximetry should be done on all patients with pneumonia. A WBC count with differential may be helpful in differentiating viral from bacterial disease. Very high peripheral WBC counts greater than 15,000 cells/mm³ with a shift to immature forms of polymorphonuclear cells are suggestive of bacterial infection.[389] However, normal or low WBC counts can occur in infants and children with overwhelming bacterial infection. An elevated WBC count with an associated lymphocytosis can be seen in viral infections or with pertussis. Infections with *Chlamydia* may produce a mild eosinophilia.[386] The use of the erythrocyte sedimentation rate or C-reactive protein, together with the WBC count, may increase the sensitivity for detecting bacterial infection.[389] The combination of these tests, however, have not shown consistently high enough predictive values to add significantly to the clinical impression.[371]

A blood culture should be obtained in all patients who have a suspected bacterial pneumonia and in those children with pneumonia requiring hospitalization. Although they will only be positive in approximately 10% of bacterial pneumonias, the information obtained from a positive culture can be extremely important and helpful with directing therapy.[377] Because the culture result will not be available at the time of the initial emergency department visit, appropriate follow-up should be available so that a positive blood culture result will not be missed.

A blood specimen can be obtained to test for cold agglutinins. Cold agglutinins develop in response to a variety of infectious agents but are present in highest titer in *Mycoplasma* infections. Although they may be positive in adolescents, they are much less consistently positive in younger children.[387]

Nasopharyngeal cultures for bacteria are of little value in identifying the causative agent of pneumonia, since healthy children can be colonized normally by pathogenic organisms. They may be useful if the diagnosis of pertussis is suspected, since this organism can be isolated from a nasopharyngeal specimen.[370] Documentation of nasopharyngeal carriage of *C. trachomatis,* along with its detection in conjunctival scrapings by direct immunoflourescent anti-

gen or culture, can confirm the diagnosis of *Chlamydia* pneumonia.[386] Sputum for culture is usually difficult to obtain from children and is often contaminated with mouth flora.

Antigen-detection techniques for the identification of bacterial polysaccharides in serum and urine have become available. They have appeared promising as an aid in the diagnosis of pneumonia, particularly in the emergency or outpatient department, since the test is noninvasive and test results are available in a few hours. However, a study of various latex agglutination and countercurrent immunoelectrophoresis methods showed both poor sensitivity and specificity in the diagnosis of causative agents in pneumonia.[390] It may be difficult to judge the exact sensitivity and predictive value of these techniques, since no comparison has been made with a definitive standard for diagnosis, such as lung puncture and aspiration.[371]

Further diagnostic procedures may be indicated for patients with severe life-threatening infections, for those failing to respond to appropriate antibiotic therapy, and for immunocompromised patients.[370] Serologic tests can be obtained for viral, fungal, and parasitic infections. Total IgM antibodies may be elevated in congenital viral pneumonias. A skin test for the detection of tuberculosis should be performed in high-risk patients, including indigent urban children and those with a history of exposure to tuberculosis.[391]

More invasive procedures can be used to obtain material directly from the lungs including suctioning the trachea via direct laryngoscopy or through an endotracheal tube, bronchoscopy to obtain bronchial washings, or by direct needle aspiration of the lung. If a pleural effusion is present, thoracentesis (see section on Pleural Disease) can be performed to obtain pleural fluid for examination and culture. Transtracheal aspiration has been used in adults to obtain specimens for culture, but the procedure is difficult to perform in children and should be avoided because of the risk to structures adjacent to the trachea.[370] The risk of these procedures must be weighed against the benefits of diagnosis for each patient on an individual basis. All of these procedures should be performed only by an experienced physician, using the appropriate equipment in a controlled environment. With the exception of thoracentesis, rarely are these procedures necessary on an emergent basis in the emergency department.

Radiographic Studies. Chest radiographs should be obtained on all children appearing in the emergency department with signs and symptoms suggestive of pneumonia. Anteroposterior and lateral views should be obtained on a routine basis. A lateral decubitus radiograph can help to define an associated pleural effusion. If a foreign body of the airway is suspected, inspiratory and expiratory or bilateral decubitus radiographs should be obtained to look for asymmetric hyperexpansion. The pattern of infiltrate noted on x-ray study may be helpful in defining the cause of the infection. Classic radiographic findings consistent with a bacterial process include distinct consolidation localized to one or two lobes, with rapid progression over hours or days. An associated pleural effusion is highly suggestive of a bacterial cause.[392] Chest radiographs in viral infections of the lower respiratory tract most commonly show perihilar or peribronchial infiltrates but can vary from normal appearing to diffusely hazy. Diffuse, patchy, multilobular parenchymal infiltrates are also seen with *Mycoplasma* infections, which can mimic viral infections radiographically.[392] A diffuse, homogeneous pattern can be seen with neonatal group B streptococci, *Pneumocystis*, cytomegalovirus, varicella, or *Chlamydia*. Pulmonary hyperinflation combined with peribronchiolar "cuffing" is characteristic of RSV infections in infants. The results of chest radiographs alone have been shown to be insensitive in differentiating viral and bacterial causes of pneumonia.[393] Therefore radiographic results should be combined with the clinical picture and laboratory values to help in determining the cause of infection. Occasionally, a chest x-ray film in a child with clinical evidence of pneumonia may be clear of infiltrates if the radiograph is obtained early in the course of the illness or if the patient is dehydrated; follow-up radiographs may be useful. In patients with unusual patterns on chest x-ray studies, CT scans may be required to define the nature of the pathology.

Differential Considerations

The differential diagnosis of a patient with the signs and symptoms of pneumonia should include asthma, lower airway foreign body, atelectasis, congestive heart failure with pulmonary edema, hydrocarbon ingestions, near drowning, recurrent aspiration of gastric contents, and primary or metastatic neoplasms.[370] The information obtained from history and physical examination will be the most helpful in differentiating these disease processes from pneumonia.

Management

The majority of patients with pneumonia have only mild disease and require no immediate stabilization or airway support. If respiratory distress is present, however, stabilization of the pulmonary status with the assurance of airway and breathing is the first priority. Humidified oxygen should be initiated if respiratory distress is present to reverse hypoxemia and help reduce the work of breathing. Continuous pulse oximetry and cardiac monitoring should be instituted. Airway intubation with mechanical ventilation may be required for the patient unable to maintain the airway or progressing to respiratory failure. Respiratory failure may be noted by a combination of clinical signs and physiologic parameters including a Pco_2 greater than 50 mm Hg and Po_2 less than 50 mm Hg on an arterial blood gas specimen obtained in room air at sea level.[370] If signs of dehydration or shock are present, circulation should be supported by obtaining IV access and administering parenteral fluids. Inhaled bronchodilators are indicated if wheezing or evidence of lower airway obstruction is present (see section on Asthma).

Antibiotics should be administered to all patients with pneumonia in which bacteria or *Mycoplasma* are the suspected pathogens (Table 59-5). The differentiation of viral and bacterial pneumonias can be difficult, however, and the decision to treat with antibiotics is often empiric. Appropriate specimens for culture should be obtained before antimicrobial therapy is instituted. Results from these cultures may be used to guide subsequent therapy. The majority of patients may be treated with oral medications on

TABLE 59-5. Oral Antibiotics for Bacterial Pneumonia

Drug	Dose (mg/kg/24 hr)	Interval
Amoxillin	25-50	TID
Amoxicillin-clavulanate	20-40 as amoxicillin	TID
Erythromycin-sulfisoxazole	40-50 as erythromycin	QID
Trimethoprim-sulfamethoxazole	6-10 as trimethoprim	BID
Cefaclor	20-40	TID
Cefixime	8	Q/day or BID
Cefuroxime axetil	20-30	BID
Erythromycin ethylsuccinate	40-50	QID
Clarithromycin	20-30	BID

an outpatient basis.[372] Specific antimicrobial agents should be chosen on the basis of the patient's age and likely pathogen, known allergies, and known bacterial sensitivity patterns. Antibiotic failures commonly result from resistant organisms, particularly *H. influenzae*, viral infections, or poor compliance.[370]

Antibiotic choice for the inpatient treatment of pneumonia will differ by age group. In the neonatal period, ampicillin, 100 to 200 mg/kg/24 hr q 4 to 6 hr IV, paired with cefotaxime, 100 mg/kg/24 hr q 8 to 12 hr IV, or with an aminoglycoside antibiotic (often gentamicin 5 to 7.5 mg/kg/24 hr q 8 hr IV) should be initiated. Infants between 1 and 3 months of age may develop pneumonia resulting from neonatal pathogens or bacteria found in older children. A combination of ampicillin plus cefotaxime (100 mg/kg/24 hr q 8 to 12 hr IV) provides broad coverage against the most likely organisms in this age group. In young infants demonstrating the afebrile pneumonia syndrome characteristic of *Chlamydia*, erythromycin or a sulfonamide is the drug of choice.[371]

Children between 3 months and 5 years of age with bacterial pneumonia should be treated with antimicrobial agents effective against the two most frequent pathogens, *S. pneumoniae* and *H. influenzae*. Although approximately 20% to 25% of *Haemophilus* strains are resistant to the penicillins by virtue of beta-lactamase production, the much lower frequency of *Haemophilus* pneumonia as compared with pneumococcal pneumonia still permits amoxicillin therapy initially in most circumstances.[391] Other considerations for outpatient therapy include beta-lactamase-resistant drugs such as amoxicillin-clavulanate, erythromycin-sulfisoxazole, trimethoprim-sulfamethoxazole, and various cephalosporins including cefaclor, cefixime, and cefuroxime axetil. More seriously ill children require treatment with parenteral antibiotics in the hospital. A second-generation cephalosporin such as cefuroxime is effective initial therapy against the most common pathogens in this age group. Other IV antimicrobial drugs that are effective against both *S. pneumoniae* and *H. influenzae* include cefotaxime and ceftriaxone.[391]

In children older than 5 years, erythromycin or clarithromycin is preferred for initial therapy for mild-to-moderate pneumonia, since *M. pneumoniae* emerges as the most likely causative organism and *H. influenzae* becomes less common.[394] Both are also active against *S. pneumoniae*. If the child is ill enough to be admitted to the hospital, treatment should be directed toward *S. pneumoniae* with IV penicillin or ampicillin. If the child fails to respond to this initial therapy, erythromycin or a penicillinase-resistant penicillin should be considered.[370]

In all age groups, additional coverage is necessary for the treatment of staphylococcal pneumonia with a penicillinase-resistant penicillin, such as nafcillin 100 mg/kg/24 hr q 4 to 6 hr IV. All patients with suspected pneumonia produced by *S. aureus* require admission to the hospital and parental antibiotics. Infection with other organisms such as *P. carinii*, tuberculosis, or fungal agents require alternative therapy.

Disposition

The majority of pediatric patients with pneumonia without underlying disease can be treated with oral antibiotics on an outpatient basis. Hospitalization and treatment with parental antibiotics is rarely necessary but is indicated if the child shows signs of significant toxicity including high fever, dyspnea, apnea, cyanosis, fatigue, or evidence of potential respiratory failure. Children who are dehydrated should also be admitted to the hospital for initial antibiotic therapy and appropriate rehydration. Generally, infants less than 2 to 3 months should be admitted to the hospital for parenteral antimicrobial therapy and close observation of respiratory status. Hospitalization with IV antibiotics is also indicated for patients who are immunocompromised because of primary immunodeficiencies, underlying malignancy, treatment with immunosuppressive agents, or sickle cell disease. Any patient requiring thoracentesis for diagnosis or treatment of a complicating pleural effusion should be admitted for observation after the procedure. Those patients with an unreliable home environment or who are unavailable for follow-up care after discharge from the emergency department should also be considered for initial inpatient therapy.[370]

For those patients who are discharged home, follow-up in 24 hours is important to assess the patient's condition and ensure response to therapy. The choice between phone contact and a return visit for the follow-up should be based on the physician's assessment of the degree of illness present and the parents' ability to accurately report the status of the child.[371] If no improvement has occurred at the time of the reassessment in 24 hours, the child may have developed an empyema, bacteria may be resistant to the initial therapy, the patient may not have received the antibiotics, or the infection may have a viral cause.[391] If the follow-up examination reveals a pleural effusion, the child should be admitted to the hospital for treatment with parenteral antibiotics. If there is no evidence of a pleural effusion and there has been good patient compliance with the antibiotics, consideration should be given to switching treatment to a beta-lactamase resistant drug.[391] A follow-up chest radiograph is probably not necessary in normally healthy children who show a prompt response to therapy.

PULMONARY EDEMA

Pulmonary edema is the abnormal extravascular accumulation of fluids in the pulmonary tissues and air spaces due primarily to changes in hydrostatic forces in the capillaries or to increased capillary permeability. It is characterized clinically by intense dyspnea and, in the intraalveolar form, by expectoration of frothy pink serous fluid. Pulmonary edema develops when the outward flow of fluid from the pulmonary circulation exceeds the capacity of the lymphatic system to clear it from the interstitium from either cardiogenic or noncardiogenic causes.[395]

The primary cause of pulmonary edema in the pediatric population is congestive heart failure secondary to underlying cardiac disease.[396] Pulmonary edema is a common pathologic finding in infants who die from an array of cardiorespiratory disorders.[397] Noncardiogenic causes of pulmonary edema may result from a number of different clinical entities. However, acute pulmonary edema in itself is a life-threatening medical emergency that requires immediate diagnosis and treatment.

Pathophysiology

The fluid and protein exchange between the bloodstream and the interstitial spaces of the lung is an ongoing process. That exchange is affected by a number of different factors. Hydrostatic pressure differences and colloid osmotic pressure gradients between the intravascular and interstitial compartments, the permeability of the pulmonary microvascular membranes, lymphatic drainage from the lungs, and changes in transpulmonary pressures can all affect the balance of fluids and proteins in the lungs.[398]

The Starling equation is a formulation that quantitates fluid movement across the pulmonary microvascular membrane in relation to the microvascular hydrostatic and osmotic forces.[398] The equation states:

$$Q_f = K_f [(P_c - P_i) - \delta (\pi_c - \pi_i)]$$

in which Q_f = fluid flow across pulmonary microvascular membrane

K_f = filtration coefficient

P_c, P_i = capillary and interstitial fluid hydrostatic pressures

π_c, π_i = capillary and interstitial fluid osmotic pressures

δ = reflection coefficient represents degree to which the membrane presents a physical barrier to protein molecules

Pulmonary edema develops when there is an imbalance in these forces at work. It is probable that the net pressure of the Starling equation is outward, causing a small lymph flow in humans under normal conditions.[398] As the fluid flow exceeds the capacity of the lymphatics, it leaks into the interstitium of the alveolar walls. This fluid pulls proteins across the normally restrictive alveolar epithelium. As the fluid crosses the alveolar epithelium into the alveolar spaces, the alveoli are unable to be ventilated, and oxygenation of the blood passing through becomes impossible.[398] With increasing pulmonary congestion, lung compliance and vital capacity decrease, and gas exchange is further impaired.[395]

Etiology of Pulmonary Edema

Increased pulmonary capillary pressure

Cardiac

Congestive heart failure
  Coarctation of the aorta
  Severe aortic stenosis
  Myocardial disease (cardiomyopathy and myocarditis)
Congenital heart disease with left-to-right shunts
  Ventricular septal defect
  Patent ductus arteriosus
  Iatrogenic shunts

Noncardiac

Iatrogenic fluid overload
Pulmonary embolism
Fat embolism
Pulmonary venoocclusive disease

Altered membrane permeability

Pneumonia (infectious and aspiration)
Hypersensitivity pneumonitis
Autoimmune disease (SLE)
Near drowning (fresh or seawater)
Adult respiratory distress syndrome (ARDS)
Vasoactive substances
  Asthma
  Anaphylaxis
  Neoplasms
  Endotoxic shock
  Hemorrhagic shock
  Snake and scorpion venom
Inhaled toxins
  Smoke

Carbon monoxide
Sulfur dioxide
Herbicides (paraquat)
Cocaine
Drugs
  Narcotics (heroin and methadone)
  Barbiturates
  Alcohol
  Salicylates
  Amphetamines

Decreased colloid osmotic pressure

Renal disease with nephrosis
Hepatic failure
Protein-losing enteropathy
Severe malnutrition
Extensive burns

Changes in transpulmonary pressures

Upper airway obstruction
  Croup and epiglottitis
  Hypertrophied tonsils/adenoids

Decreased lymphatic drainage

Superior vena cava obstruction
Interstitial emphysema/fibrosis

Mixed or unknown mechanisms

High-altitude pulmonary edema
Neurogenic pulmonary edema
  Cerebral anoxia
  Head trauma
  Seizures

Etiology

As previously noted, fluid and protein exchange in the lung is largely determined by the balance of intravascular and interstitial hydrostatic and colloid osmotic pressures, pulmonary microvascular permeability, transpulmonary pressures, and lymphatic drainage. Pulmonary edema may develop after any of these factors are altered, depending on the disease state involved as shown in the box above. Pathologically, pulmonary edema can generally be classified into cardiogenic and noncardiogenic causes.

Increased Pulmonary Capillary Pressure. Increases in pulmonary capillary pressure can occur as a result of abnormalities in cardiac function with development of elevated left atrial pressures, often secondary to congestive heart failure. Pulmonary edema resulting from congestive heart failure may be seen with severe aortic stenosis, coarctation of the aorta, or myocardial diseases such as myocarditis or cardiomyopathy. Children with congenital heart disease with left-to-right vascular shunting, as in ventricular septal defect and patent ductus arteriosus, often have an increased pulmonary blood flow, which can lead to edema. In other congenital cardiac conditions such as hypoplastic

left heart syndrome and mitral stenosis, pulmonary edema may occur secondary to increased pulmonary capillary hydrostatic pressures.[399] Pulmonary edema has been observed after the creation of systemic-pulmonary-artery shunts, probably on the basis of increased capillary hydrostatic pressures related to increased flow through one lung or a segment of one lung.[400] Generalized accumulation of salt and water with overall expansion of the extracellular space, as in fluid overload, tends to increase the liquid accumulation in the lung. Left-sided pressures may also be elevated in this form of pulmonary edema.[401]

Flow obstruction may involve the pulmonary veins, producing an increase in pulmonary capillary hydrostatic pressure independent of cardiac disease. This effect can be seen in children with pulmonary thromboembolic disease, fat embolism secondary to trauma or fractures, air embolism, or pulmonary venoocclusive disease.[395]

Decreased Colloid Osmotic Pressure. Low intravascular colloid osmotic pressure from a decrease in plasma proteins, primarily albumin, can disturb lung fluid clearance and precipitate pulmonary edema. Hypoalbuminemia can develop in children with nephrosis, liver failure, protein-losing enteropathies, severe malnutrition, or extensive burns.

Altered Membrane Permeability. Alterations in the permeability of the alveolar microvascular membrane can result in direct physical or chemical damage to the alveolar epithelial or capillary endothelial cells.[395] Pulmonary infections such as bacterial or viral pneumonia may be associated with inflammatory edema as a result of alveolar or capillary injury. Inhalation of aspirated liquid into the lungs can result in pulmonary edema, with the amount of edema accumulation depending on inherent toxicity, pH, and osmolarity of the aspirated liquid.[395] Aspiration of hydrochloric acid results in particularly florid edema.[402] Drowning results in filling the lungs with fluid, which is a form of pulmonary edema. In both freshwater and saltwater drowning, the lungs become filled with high-protein edema fluid, suggesting an alteration of pulmonary capillary permeability produced by osmotic damage from the aspirated water.[395] The term adult respiratory distress syndrome (ARDS) is used to describe the pulmonary complications of a wide variety of conditions such as shock, trauma, and postcardiopulmonary bypass. Many different causes are involved in the development of ARDS, and the common abnormality may be alteration of pulmonary capillary permeability.[395]

The liberation of chemical mediators and vasoactive substances such as histamine, serotonin, kinins, and prostaglandins in disorders such as asthma, anaphylaxis, neoplasms, and both endotoxic and hemorrhagic shock can produce pulmonary edema.[403] This is also the mechanism related to the development of pulmonary edema from the circulating toxins of snake and scorpion venom.[404,405] These chemical mediators may also be involved in hypersensitivity pneumonitis and pneumonias associated with connective tissue immune-complex diseases such as systemic lupus erythematous.[406] Changes in permeability and direct injury to pulmonary alveolar or capillary cells can result from the inhalation of noxious agents such as smoke and gases from fires including carbon monoxide, atmospheric pollutants such as sulfur dioxide, certain herbicides (paraquat), and cocaine.[407-410] Pulmonary edema can occur secondary to the use of certain drugs including barbiturates, alcohol, salicylates, and amphetamines and has been well described with the use of narcotics, particularly heroin and methadone.[411,412]

Changes in Transpulmonary Pressures. In patients with upper airway obstruction, exaggeration of the transmural pulmonary vascular hydrostatic pressure gradient is the most likely pathogenic mechanism.[413] The highly negative intrapleural pressures that develop in the face of the tracheal airway obstruction lead to a decrease in pulmonary interstitial hydrostatic pressures with a net movement of fluid and protein out of the pulmonary capillaries and into the interstitial spaces. This is the mechanism involved in the development of pulmonary edema following postoperative laryngospasm.[414,415] With acute obstruction of the upper airway as seen in croup and epiglottitis, however, the development of pulmonary edema usually follows relief of the obstruction after the patient has been intubated or obstructive tonsils/adenoids removed.[413,414] This relief in the obstruction likely results in an abrupt drop in airway pressures with a subsequent increase in venous return and increase in pulmonary microvascular pressures, further changing the hydrostatic pressure gradient leading to extravasation of fluid into the alveoli.[414] Cor pulmonale with development of pulmonary edema can result from chronic upper airway obstruction as seen in children with adenoidal or tonsillar hypertrophy.[416]

Decreased Lymphatic Drainage. Pathologic disturbances in the pulmonary lymphatic system can result in abnormal lung fluid transport. Fluid may accumulate in the lungs if the lymphatics must pump against an exceedingly high central venous pressure as seen with obstruction of the superior vena cava.[399] In patients with interstitial emphysema and fibrosis, the air or scar tissue can block lymphatic flow, leading to fluid accumulation and pulmonary edema.

Mixed or Unknown Mechanisms. High-altitude pulmonary edema (HAPE) is a severe, potentially life-threatening form of noncardiogenic pulmonary edema seen almost exclusively in those who ascend over 9,000 ft (2,740 m) of elevation. The pathophysiology is uncertain but is probably due, at least in part, to hydrostatic and capillary permeability abnormalities of the pulmonary vascular bed in response to hypobaric hypoxia.[417] High-altitude pulmonary edema is associated with rapid ascent, strenuous activity on arrival, cold, respiratory tract infections, sedation, and young age[417] (see Chapter 40).

Injuries to the CNS such as trauma or cerebral anoxia may be associated with the development of pulmonary edema although the mechanism responsible is not completely understood. Evidence suggests an acute sympathetic discharge after head injury or sudden increases in intracranial pressure. This discharge results in a marked generalized vasoconstriction with subsequent increased pulmonary vascular pressures and blood volume producing pulmonary edema.[418] The same mechanism is likely responsible for the pulmonary edema that infrequently follows seizures in children.[419]

Diagnostic Findings

Although there are specific findings with pulmonary edema, the majority of signs and symptoms are related to the underlying cause.[396] The development of symptoms associated with pulmonary edema is variable but may be rapid. Progressive dyspnea, shortness of breath, tachypnea, and chest pain are frequently present. Pink, frothy sputum production as classically reported with pulmonary edema is not always present in children. Infants may have a history of feeding difficulties associated with respiratory difficulty.

On physical examination, the child may appear pale with clammy skin. Vital signs vary, but tachycardia is usually present and the blood pressure may be elevated. Tachypnea is almost uniformly present with pulmonary edema. Further examination of the pulmonary system may show retractions, nasal flaring, and grunting as the child attempts to prevent alveolar collapse. Cyanosis may be present secondary to ventilation/perfusion abnormalities. Decreased breath sounds and moist crackles are the most common auscultatory findings, but they may not be apparent if the volume of intrapulmonary fluid is small. Wheezing may also be heard due to the compression of small airways by tissue fluid. If a pleural effusion accompanies the pulmonary edema, dullness to percussion and decreased breath sounds will be evident over the posterior basilar lung fields. On examination the cardiovascular findings should reflect any underlying pathology. Specific signs of congestive heart failure, including increased heart sounds, a gallop rhythm, and elevated jugular venous distension, may be present. Heart murmurs associated with any underlying defects may also be elicited. CNS examination abnormalities may be present including mental status changes that can progress to coma if the patient's condition deteriorates. Respiratory abnormalities of CNS origin, such as Cheyne-Stokes respiration or apnea, may occur with cerebral hypoxia.

Complications. The primary complication associated with pulmonary edema is the progression to acute respiratory failure marked by inadequate oxygenation and ventilation, progressive disease or fatigue, and respiratory acidosis. Pulmonary edema may also be complicated by cardiac failure with left or right ventricular failure, since this may be the underlying cause producing the excess intrapulmonary fluid. Superimposed pulmonary infection, disseminated intravascular coagulation (DIC), or even cardiopulmonary arrest may also complicate the course of pulmonary edema.

Ancillary Data. Ancillary tests should be used to evaluate pulmonary status and to identify and assess the underlying primary cause. A CBC may show anemia, evidence of infection, or thrombocytopenia suggesting septic shock or DIC. Chemistries including electrolytes, renal function tests, liver enzymes, serum protein, and albumin may reveal underlying abnormalities. An ABG assesses both the oxygenation and ventilation status of the patient, as well as the acid-base balance. Attention should be paid to the development of respiratory acidosis indicating respiratory decompensation. A toxicology screen on both urine and blood should be obtained if poisoning is suspected. Urine should also be dipped for protein. A 12-lead ECG will reflect the abnormalities associated with any underlying heart disease.

A chest x-ray film is necessary in all patients with symptoms or signs of pulmonary edema. It may be difficult, however, to separate pulmonary edema from the findings of underlying pulmonary disease. In addition, the small initial fluid accumulations seen in pulmonary edema may be difficult to detect at all on chest x-ray study. The radiographic findings usually seen with pulmonary edema include diffuse bilateral alveolar infiltrates most marked in the periphery and basilar areas of the lung. Kerley A and B lines representing lymphatic and interstitial fluid accumulation may be visible. Kerley A lines appear as straight nonbranching lines in the upper lung field that run diagonally toward the hilum. Kerley B lines are horizontal nonbranching lines at the periphery of the lower lungs. These represent interlobular septal edema. Pleural effusions may also be present and x-ray findings should indicate any underlying cardiac or pulmonary process. As the intrapulmonary fluid increases and the pulmonary edema worsens, it may be very difficult to radiographically differentiate edema, atelectasis, and pneumonia.[420]

If a pleural effusion is present and is large enough to interfere with respiratory effort or accompany respiratory deterioration, thoracocentesis should be performed (see section on Pleural Effusions). Analysis of the fluid should include protein, glucose, LDH, amylase, cell count, gram stain, and culture. Further studies such as an echocardiogram to evaluate cardiac anatomy and function and to assess for pulmonary hypertension (Swan-Ganz catheter) should be obtained as indicated.

Differential Considerations

The differential diagnosis of a patient with the signs and symptoms of pulmonary edema needs to include pneumonia, asthma or anaphylaxis, and vascular abnormalities such as pulmonary embolism or intrapulmonary hemorrhage. The latter is often accompanied by hemoptysis, chest pain, and an infiltrate on chest x-ray film.[396]

Management

The treatment of pulmonary edema should be directed towards the correction of the underlying cause. The pulmonary status should initially be stabilized with the reversal of hypoxemia with the administration of oxygen and mechanical ventilation if necessary. The patient should be maintained in a semirecumbent position with cardiac and pulse oximetry monitoring.

As in all resuscitation efforts, attention should first be directed toward airway and breathing as shown in the box on p. 1112. Improving oxygenation is the first priority and humidified oxygen, preferably at 100% or 8 to 10 L/min, high flow by mask should be administered. Airway intubation with mechanical ventilation may be required for the patient progressing to respiratory failure (Pco_2 >50 mm Hg and Po_2 <50 mm Hg at room air, sea level) to protect the airway, for a decreased level of consciousness, or to treat an unresponsive metabolic acidosis.[396] Mechanical ventilation should include the use of positive end-expiratory pressure (PEEP) beginning at 5 cm H_2O if the Po_2 remains >50 mm Hg at an Fio_2 of 50%. The PEEP needs to be titrated as necessary in combination with ventilatory assistance in a closely monitored setting in the ICU. Mechanical ventilation with the use of PEEP improves oxygenation by keeping the alveoli from collapsing, reducing the work of breathing by decreasing oxygen consumption, and assists with the reabsorption of intrapulmonary fluid.[399]

Circulation should next be addressed with fluid resuscitation. IV access will be required. Fluids may be necessary to improve cardiac output but must be balanced carefully with the possibility of increased pulmonary flow and edema. Administering fluids may require the placement of a Swan-Ganz catheter and monitoring in the ICU setting,[396] particularly if the underlying cause is not readily reversible. Crystalloid (normal saline or lactated Ringer's solution) is the initial resuscitation fluid of choice and should be used to maintain urine output at 0.5 ml/kg/hr. An indwelling bladder catheter may need to be placed for adequate monitoring of fluid output. If the pulmonary edema is secondary to hypoalbuminemia, 25% albumin administered at a dose of 1 gm/kg over 2 to 4 hr may be administered; it is often used in conjunction with diuretics.

Diuretics are indicated if the pulmonary edema is cardiogenic in origin. If it is noncardiogenic, diuretics may not

---

Treatment of Pulmonary Edema

Airway and breathing

Oxygen 100% by mask

Intubation

Mechanical ventilation with PEEP

Circulation

Crystalloid fluid (0.9% NS, LR)

Maintain urine output >0.5 ml/kg/hr

Albumin 25% if hypoalbuminemic

Diuretics

Furosemide 1 to 2 mg/kg q 6 hr IV

Morphine

0.1 to 0.2 mg/kg IV slowly

Monitor for respiratory suppression and hypotension

Treatment of shock

Dopamine 5-20 µg/kg/min IV continuous infusion

Dobutamine 2-15 µg/kg/min IV continuous infusion

Digitalis

Other considerations

Afterload reduction

Bronchodilator

---

be useful when the underlying pathophysiology is not a fluid overload.[396]

Furosemide at a dose of 1 to 2 mg/kg q 6 hr is the initial choice. It can be repeated up to every 2 hours as indicated but should not be used if the patient is anuric. Furosemide usually produces an abrupt diuresis with a decrease in pulmonary microvascular pressures and an increase in the concentration of plasma proteins, further inhibiting fluid filtration into the lungs.

Morphine sulfate can be an important adjunct in the management of pulmonary edema because it dilates the venous system and decreases the pulmonary wedge pressure. It also relieves patient dyspnea and anxiety. However, it should be used with caution with continuous monitoring for respiratory suppression and hypotension. In severe pulmonary edema, 0.1 to 0.2 mg/kg IV should be administered slowly.[396] The use of morphine is contraindicated in the presence of unstable vital signs, including hypotension, intracranial hemorrhage, asthma, chronic pulmonary disease, or narcotic withdrawal.[396]

Shock may accompany pulmonary edema secondary to low cardiac output and must be treated aggressively. The adrenergic agents of choice in children include dopamine administered by continuous IV infusion at a rate of 5 to 20 µg/kg/min or dobutamine at 2 to 15 µg/kg/min IV infusion. There has been extensive experience with the use of dopamine in children.[396] Digitalis can also be used to increase cardiac contractility. To achieve a more rapid response, however, the use of dopamine or dobutamine is preferable.

Afterload reduction may be useful to diminish pressure overload. If response to initial management of pulmonary edema is inadequate, agents that diminish afterload by decreasing peripheral resistance may improve cardiac output. These drugs should be used only with indwelling arterial monitoring and a Swan-Ganz catheter in place. Sodium nitroprusside is initiated at an infusion of 0.1 µg/kg/min and increased to an infusion of 0.5 to 8.0 µg/kg/min until the desired response is achieved. The clinical response is noted in 1 to 2 minutes. Nitroglycerine has no established dosage in children but may be useful in acute treatment. Sublingual and IV nitroglycerine may be useful in patients with obvious cardiac decompensation. Combination therapy using other agents is still evolving.

Bronchodilators may be useful if wheezing is present and there is evidence of bronchoconstriction. They also act to improve cardiac contractility. Any cardiac dysrhythmia that develops because of hypoxia or multiple drug therapy requires urgent treatment. Patients in renal failure must be observed for possible refractoriness to the usual treatment. Treatment of neurogenic pulmonary edema should focus on reduction of intracranial pressure, when possible, and the pharmacologic reduction of systemic arterial blood pressure.

Disposition

The majority of patients with pulmonary edema require admission to an ICU for appropriate monitoring, intervention, and treatment of the pulmonary edema and for management of the underlying condition. Only the rare patient with a mild, slowly progressive pulmonary edema with a known underlying condition can be discharged to be managed on an outpatient basis if compliance and follow-up can be ensured.[396]

PULMONARY EMBOLISM

A pulmonary embolism develops when a free segment of a thrombus is carried to the pulmonary circulation and causes partial or complete occlusion of a pulmonary artery or one of its branches. It may be associated with infarction of a portion of the lung.

Pulmonary embolism is a leading cause of morbidity and mortality in the adult population, affecting over 650,000 adults per year and accounting for approximately 50,000 fatalities annually.[421,422] The incidence in hospitalized adults has been estimated at between 15% and 30%.[423] Because of the lack of specific clinical and routine laboratory findings, it is probably greatly underdiagnosed.

Despite being a common cause of death in adults, pulmonary embolism is rarely diagnosed in children. In autopsy series the reported incidence of this disorder in children is between 0.5% and 3.7%.[424-426] A recent report from the Canadian Registry of venous thromboembolic complications in children established in 1990 showed an incidence of deep vein thrombosis/pulmonary embolism of 5.3/10,000 hospital admissions of 0.07/10,000 children in Canada.[427] One of the reasons children are much less afflicted than adults is that they are generally healthy, and healthy individuals are at much less risk for this disorder (see Chapter 47). Because it is rare in children, only a very high index of suspicion will lead to early diagnosis and appropriate intervention.

Pathophysiology

Pulmonary emboli are not a primary phenomenon but are the consequence of thrombosis elsewhere in the body. In adults, approximately 70% develop an embolis from a thrombus in the deep venous system of the lower extremities.[421] In children an autopsy series showed the associated venous thromboses to be more commonly located in the chambers of the right heart, mesenteric, and cerebral vessels or the inferior or superior vena cava.[426] The classic triad of factors associated with the development of venous thrombosis include venostasis, hypercoagulability, and altered vascular integrity or inflammation of the vessel wall.[421]

Vascular occlusion of the pulmonary vessel results from fragmentation or loosening of the thrombus with migration through the vena cava, right atrium, and right ventricle to a branch of the pulmonary artery. Obstruction of the vascular flow distal to the embolism develops, creating a ventilation/perfusion mismatch. Infarction of a surrounding portion of the lung may occur but is infrequent due to the fact that the lung normally receives oxygen from three sources: pulmonary arteries, bronchial arteries, and the airways.[424] Resulting hemodynamic effects such as the development of pulmonary hypertension depend on the extent of vascular obstruction and degree of associated hypoxia.[428] The pulmonary vascular bed is so extensive that in patients without preexisting cardiopulmonary disease, as is the case in most children, pulmonary arterial pressures generally do not become significantly elevated.[428]

Besides the mechanical forces in the vessels, the embolus has other important effects on the lung. The embolus contains platelets that degranulate, releasing chemical mediators such as histamine, prostaglandins, and serotonin, which produce both bronchoconstriction and pulmonary vasoconstriction.[421] This leads to the development of both alveolar hypoventilation and intrapulmonary shunting of blood. The decreased perfusion reduces surfactant synthesis contributing to additional atelectasis.[421] The atelectasis can produce further shunting of blood flow and persistent hypoxia for several days after the acute embolic event.[458] The ventilation/perfusion mismatch present will cause hypoxia in approximately 85% of adult patients with acute pulmonary embolism.[429]

Etiology

With pulmonary emboli, the venous thrombosis is the primary process and embolism the complication. Therefore the etiology of the pulmonary embolism can be thought of as the conditions that lead to the factors associated with thrombus formation: stasis, hypercoagulability, and altered vascular integrity, as shown in the box above. It is rare for a pulmonary embolism to develop in the absence of risk factors.

In children, as in adults, stasis appears to be the primary predisposing factor in the development of venous thrombosis.[428] Children at increased risk of thrombosis on this basis include those with spinal cord injury; abdominal, pelvic, and lower extremity trauma; burns; prolonged states of immobilization or unconsciousness; and neuromuscular diseases including Guillain-Barré syndrome.[428,430-432] Stasis may result not only from the immobilization of the

---

Predisposing Conditions for Pulmonary Embolism

Stasis
Spinal cord injury
Trauma: abdominal, pelvic and lower extremity
Burns
Neuromuscular diseases
Congenital heart disease
Prolonged immobilization
Increased blood viscosity
Severe dehydration
Surgery
Obesity

Hypercoagulable states
Oral contraceptive use
Antithrombin III deficiency
Neoplasms
Nephrotic syndrome
Pregnancy
Collagen vascular disease

Altered vascular integrity
Ventriculoatrial shunts
Indwelling central venous catheters

---

patient but also from an increase in viscosity of the blood, as seen in children with severe dehydration, congenital heart disease with polycythemia, and hyperproteinemic states.[428]

Hypercoagulable states also increase the risk for venous thrombosis. This risk can be seen with oral contraceptive use, antithrombin III deficiency, neoplasms, nephrotic syndrome, and collagen vascular diseases.[428,433-435]

Altered vascular integrity in pediatric patients is most commonly due to indwelling venous catheters causing local trauma to the vessel wall. This problem is becoming more common in the pediatric population, since central venous catheters may be placed to provide hyperalimentation, to determine central venous pressure, or to ease administration of long-term chemotherapeutic agents or antibiotics.[436,437] The Canadian Registry on venous thromboembolic complications in children reported that 33% of children with deep vein thrombosis/pulmonary embolism had a central venous line in place.[427] IV drug use by adolescents can also lead to vessel inflammation and predispose to thrombus formation.[433] Hydrocephalic patients with ventriculoatrial shunts are also included in the group considered at higher risk for pulmonary embolism.[428]

Adolescents as a group are at a higher risk for development of pulmonary emboli, since they share a mixture of risk factors present in younger children and adults. These risk factors include oral contraceptive use, abortion, IV drug use, obesity, pregnancy, trauma, infection, malignancy, collagen vascular disease, and surgery, particularly renal transplantation.[433]

Sources of thrombi other than the venous system include formation of fat emboli after long-bone fractures, air embolism introduced iatrogenically, amniotic fluid emboli, septic emboli particularly from bacterial endocarditis, and foreign-body emboli such as catheter fragments.[421,438]

Diagnostic Findings

Clinical Findings. Because pulmonary emboli are somewhat rare in children, the majority of the clinical data are derived from adult studies. In both populations, however, the majority of patients have nonspecific signs and symptoms, and because there are no pathognomonic laboratory abnormalities, the diagnosis is difficult to confirm.

The classic triad of dyspnea, pleuritic chest pain, and hemoptysis is present in only a minority of patients.[439] Dyspnea is the most common symptom and is especially suggestive if it seems disproportionate to the degree of abnormal findings.[439] The pleuritic chest pain results from inflammation of the pleura overlying the area of pulmonary infarction. Occasionally it may be substernal with radiation to the shoulders.[421] Additional symptoms can include nonproductive cough, anxiety or apprehension, fever, and palpitations.

On physical examination, tachypnea and tachycardia are almost uniformly present but are very nonspecific signs.[429] Fever may be present but is also nonspecific. Hypotension, although uncommon, is usually associated with massive embolization and is a poor prognostic sign. Other abnormalities on the physical examination are often lacking. Cyanosis may be present and should suggest a serious underlying respiratory process. Auscultation of the lung fields may reveal decreased or distant breath sounds, rales, or wheezing. A pleural friction rub rarely may be heard if there has been a large associated pulmonary infarction.[421] If pulmonary hypertension is present, a loud P_2 heart sound may be heard on auscultation of the heart.[428]

Complications. The primary complication associated with pulmonary embolism is the progression to acute respiratory failure with inadequate oxygenation and ventilation. In patients with preexisting cardiopulmonary disease, pulmonary hypertension may develop after a significant embolism occurs, causing an increase in pulmonary vascular resistance leading to right ventricular failure.[428] Rarely, a massive pulmonary embolism in a child or adolescent can lead to cardiorespiratory arrest and sudden death.

Ancillary Data. Ancillary tests should be used to evaluate the cardiorespiratory status of the patient and to identify the contributing disease process or risk factors. Hematologic studies should include a CBC with differential and coagulation studies to look for evidence of polycythemia, infection, disseminated intravascular coagulation, or other hypercoagulable states. An erythrocyte sedimentation rate may be elevated in the presence of serious infection, malignancy, or collagen vascular disease. Chemistries including electrolytes, renal function tests, liver enzymes, serum protein, and albumin may help identify the underlying abnormality. An ABG should be obtained on all patients with signs or symptoms of pulmonary embolism. Hypoxemia with a P_{O_2} of less than 85 mm Hg at sea level has been demonstrated in a majority of adult patients with pulmonary emboli.[429] However, a normal P_{O_2} does not exclude embolism. A decrease in P_{CO_2} may be present secondary to the tachypnea. The development of a respiratory acidosis with an elevated P_{CO_2} should raise suspicion of acute respiratory decompensation. An ECG may show nonspecific ST-T wave changes. The appearance of right heart strain manifested by P-pulmonale, right bundle branch block, right axis deviation, or S1 Q3 T3 is suggestive of pulmonary embolism but is infrequent even in the adult population.[440] Although most ECG changes of pulmonary embolism are nonspecific, if present, they help to raise the clinical suspicion.

A chest x-ray film should be obtained, and although it will often be read as normal, it can be helpful in excluding other causes of acute pulmonary disease.[441] In the presence of a pulmonary embolism the chest x-ray study may reveal subtle findings of an elevated hemidiaphragm reflecting the loss of lung volume, a parenchymal infiltrate as a result of atelectasis or infarction, a pleural effusion, or segmental or subsegmental atelectasis. The classic radiographic finding associated with pulmonary embolism is "Hampton's hump," a pleural-based density with an apex pointing toward the hilum.[442]

A ventilation-perfusion lung scan can be used to help establish the diagnosis of pulmonary embolism. Indications for its use include clinical suspicion along with abnormalities present on chest x-ray film, ABG, and ECG. It should also be obtained if the diagnosis is strongly suspected, even if no abnormalities are present on the supportive tests.[441] The perfusion scan alone is a very sensitive but relatively nonspecific test.[443] A scan revealing no perfusion defect excludes the diagnosis of clinically significant pulmonary embolism. A positive scan, however, does not confirm the diagnosis, since perfusion defects on scanning may result from other forms of pulmonary pathology, such as pneumonia, collagen vascular disease, and sickle cell disease.[424] If a perfusion scan reveals a segmental or larger defect, the addition of a ventilation scan increases the specificity if a mismatched defect is found. With a mismatched defect and high degree of clinical suspicion, the diagnosis of pulmonary embolism can be made without further testing.[443]

If the ventilation-perfusion scan is read as low or moderate probability but the clinical suspicion of pulmonary embolism is high, pulmonary angiography may be indicated.[441] Currently, it is considered the "gold standard" test for the diagnosis of pulmonary embolism and the definitive study.[421,444] This examination is very specific because it allows direct visualization of any existing embolus by demonstrating intravascular filling defects or complete pulmonary arterial occlusion. The reliability of this study diminishes with time after the embolism and should be performed within the first 24 to 48 hours.[444] The angiogram is an invasive procedure that carries a significant associated morbidity and mortality, and is rarely used in children for fear of the complications of the procedure.[424] It should be considered in circumstances in which the diagnosis of pulmonary embolism is not certain but is strongly suspected and the risk of anticoagulant therapy is high.[445]

Because of the inexactness of ventilation-perfusion scans and the risks of pulmonary angiography, many new techniques are being evaluated to diagnose pulmonary embolism. Digital subtraction angiography has shown good results in identifying pulmonary emboli with the use of peripheral contrast injection and image enhancement techniques to generate images of the pulmonary vasculature. The technique is simple, fast, and does not require pulmonary artery catheterization.[446] Recently, the use of contrast-enhanced electron-beam CT for the noninvasive evaluation of pulmonary vascular disease including pulmonary emboli in adults showed it to be both more sensitive and specific than ventilation-perfusion scans using pulmonary angiography as the standard of reference.[447] Magnetic resonance imaging is generally useful in evaluating abnormalities of the pulmonary vasculature, and because of this, there are current studies researching its potential use in the diagnosis of pulmonary emboli. As experience grows with MRI, the sensitivity may improve and MRI may establish itself as a useful noninvasive diagnostic modality.[424]

Differential Considerations

The differential diagnosis of a patient with the nonspecific signs and symptoms of pulmonary embolism should include pneumonia, pleural effusion, asthma, ARDS, congestive heart failure, pneumothorax, hyperventilation syndrome, and musculoskeletal chest pain, fractured ribs, or costochondritis.

Management

The initial treatment of a patient with suspected pulmonary embolism should be directed toward stabilization of the cardiopulmonary system with reversal of hypoxemia and maintenance of ventilation and circulation. Further management should then be directed toward preventing deep vein thrombosis or other predisposing conditions. Initial attention should be paid to airway, breathing, and circulation with the administration of humidified oxygen and ventilatory support as indicated for respiratory failure. IV access should be obtained as part of the stabilization process. If hypotension is present after a pulmonary embolism is suspected, it is a poor prognostic sign and the patient will require intensive medical care, including mechanical ventilatory support. Volume loading may be helpful but the pulmonary wedge pressures and cardiac output should be monitored to better assess the patient's intravascular volume status. Inotropic agents such as dopamine or dobutamine may be necessary.[428]

Definitive therapy can then be directed toward prevention of further deep vein thrombosis by the administration of IV heparin.[448] Historically, adults treated with heparin for pulmonary embolism who survived beyond the first 2 hours of symptoms had a survival rate of 92%. Therefore as soon as a diagnosis of pulmonary embolism is strongly suspected and the decision to use thrombolytic therapy is made, intravenous heparin should be started without delay.[449] An initial dose of 50 to 75 units/kg has been advocated to further prevent platelet aggregation and to minimize the effect of thrombin on platelet degranulation. A continuous infusion of 25 units/kg/hr should be initiated within 2 hr after the initial bolus. The efficacy of heparinization can be determined by following the partial thromboplastin time (PTT), which should be maintained at 1.5 to 2 times the control value.[428] A significant morbidity is associated with the use of IV heparin; it is the leading cause of drug-related deaths in hospitalized patients.[421] Surveillance for bleeding complications should be part of the management plan. Heparin is contraindicated in patients at high risk for bleeding such as those with GI or postoperative bleeds. Bleeding after heparin administration can be reversed with protamine sulfate. Each milligram of protamine reverses approximately 100 units of heparin.[421] Heparin therapy should be maintained for 7 to 10 days while the thrombus stabilizes in the vessel wall. Oral warfarin sodium (Coumadin) therapy should be initiated 4 to 5 days after beginning anticoagulation with heparin. In the absence of persistent risk factors for deep venous thrombosis, the existing data suggest that anticoagulant therapy should be continued for 2 to 3 months.[428]

Specific therapy can also be directed toward the existing embolus with the use of thrombolytic enzymes such as streptokinase and urokinase, which convert plasminogen to the fibrinolytic agent plasmin. In studies of adults, the pulmonary emboli resolved more rapidly when treated with these agents than with IV heparin alone. However, these agents were not shown to decrease the mortality secondary to pulmonary embolism.[450] There has been no significant experience in the pediatric population with these agents for this particular diagnosis.

Tissue plasminogen activator (tPA) has recently been used in adult and pediatric patients to treat thromboembolic states after conventional thrombolytic agents have failed.[451-453] In one study involving children, 11 of 12 patients had partial to complete clot lysis. However, 6 of 12 patients had bleeding complications, although all were controlled by clinically available means.[452] Further studies are necessary to determine if tPA offers any advantages over other thrombolytic agents.

Disposition

Children who are evaluated in the emergency department and found to have a low clinical suspicion for a pulmonary embolus along with a normal chest x-ray film, ABG, and ECG can be discharged to home as long as their clinical condition is stable and adequate medical follow-up is available on an outpatient basis. Any patient who is clinically suspected to have a pulmonary embolus and is found to have abnormalities on a chest x-ray study, ABG, or ECG should be admitted to the hospital for further evaluation to include a ventilation-perfusion scan. The same course of action should be followed for the patient suspected of having a pulmonary embolus regardless of the results of the supportive tests. After admission, these patients should also be thoroughly evaluated to identify any predisposing conditions that can be corrected or treated. Any patient who has an unstable cardiopulmonary status, including hypotension after initial stabilization and treatment in the emergency department, should be admitted to an ICU.

SUDDEN INFANT DEATH SYNDROME (SIDS)

MARIANNE GAUSCHE

Sudden infant death syndrome (SIDS) is the sudden death of a young child who is generally between 1 month and 1 year of age, which is unexpected by history and for which a thorough postmortem examination fails to define an adequate cause of death.[454,455] Only 2% of deaths occur in infants over 1 year of age; 88% occur in those less than 5.5 months, with a peak between 2 and 4 months of age.[456]

SIDS is the leading cause of death in infants under 1 year of age; approximately 7,000 to 10,000 infants die annually in the United States. The overall incidence of SIDS in the United States is approximately 1.5/1,000 live births.[456] The incidence varies significantly by racial groups: African-Americans—2.98 to 5.04/1,000 live births; American Indians—3.0 to 5.93/1,000 live births; Inuit—4.95/1,000 live births; whites—1.5/1,000 live births; Hispanics—1.1/1,000 live births; and Asians—0.5 to 1.8/1,000 live births.[457,458]

Multiple maternal, neonatal, and postneonatal factors are associated with SIDS. Maternal cigarette smoking, including passive smoking, and an age less than 20 years at the first pregnancy are the factors with the highest relative risk.[456,459] Other maternal factors including illicit drug use, short interpregnancy interval, illness during pregnancy, and unmarried and low socioeconomic status are particularly prevalent in mothers of SIDS infants.[456,457,460] Prenatal factors include intrauterine growth retardation, preterm birth, and low birth weight. Neonatal risk factors include cyanosis, tachycardia, fever, respiratory distress, and irritability. The National Institute of Child Health and Development (NICHD) Cooperative Epidemiological Study documented similar rates of apnea between SIDS and control infants when the infants were matched for low birth weight and race.[456] In the postneonatal period, symptoms of diarrhea, vomiting, or listlessness were common in the 2 weeks before death.[456,457] Although some investigators have suggested an association between viral syndromes such as RSV infection and apnea, no clear association exists among viral infection, upper respiratory tract infection, and SIDS.[461] Other authors have shown a relationship between overheating and sleeping on a soft surface pillow or polystyrene-filled cushion and SIDS.[462-464]

Children sleeping on their back or side appear to have a reduced incidence of SIDS.[465-469] In June, 1992, the American Academy of Pediatrics Task Force on Infant Positioning and SIDS issued a statement calling for healthy infants to be placed on their back or side when positioned for sleep.[465] This recommendation was based on epidemiologic evidence from several countries showing a greater than 50% decrease in the incidence of SIDS when child-care practices changed to placing the infant in the side or back position for sleeping.[465-469] Although many of these studies showed other child-care and environmental factors (swaddling, lack of central heating, increased incidence of infant sleeping with a parent) that may affect the rate of SIDS in that country, the evidence suggests a correlation (odds ratio 1.3 to 11.7) between the prone position and SIDS.[465-470]

Other factors that may increase risk are male sex, multiple births (triplets have an incidence of 8.3/1,000 live births), and cold weather months.[471,472] Maternal alcohol use, diphtheria-tetanus-pertussis (DTP) vaccine, and being the sibling of an SIDS victim are not epidemiologically related.[472-475]

A number of definitions are commonly used for apnea and periodic breathing that relate to SIDS (see box above).[475]

Definitions for Apnea and Periodic Breathing

Apnea: Cessation of airflow. The respiratory pause may be central or diaphragmatic without respiratory effort, obstructive because of upper airway obstruction, or mixed. Central apnea lasting less than 15 seconds without clinical change may occur in normal children. If this respiratory pause is 20 seconds or longer or accompanied by cyanosis, hypotonia, or bradycardia, it is considered pathologic.

Periodic breathing: A breathing pattern with three or more respiratory pauses lasting longer than 3 seconds, with less than 20 seconds between pauses. This pattern may be normal. If it is associated with apnea in a premature infant, it is considered to be *apnea of prematurity* and will generally resolve by 37 weeks of age but may occasionally persist for several weeks past term. Infants greater than 37 weeks of age suffering a pathologic apnea episode without specific cause are considered to have *apnea of infancy.*

Apparent life-threatening event (ALTE): An episode characterized by a combination of apnea, color change (usually cyanosis but occasionally erythema or plethora), marked change in muscle tone (usually limpness), and choking or gagging. This condition was previously termed *near-miss SIDS.*

From Consensus statement: National Institutes of Health Consensus Development Conference on Infantile Apnea and Home Monitoring, *Pediatrics* 79:292, 1987.

Pathophysiology

The majority of deaths are unexplained. Pathologic data have implicated a role for hypoxia and possibly autonomic dysfunction. Abnormalities in the control of ventilation lead to hypoventilation.[455] The resultant hypoxia may directly or indirectly cause end organ changes. The pulmonary artery vasculature responds to the hypoxia by vasoconstriction ultimately leading to pulmonary muscle wall hyperplasia and enhanced vascular resistance on the right heart. Increased ventricular afterload may cause tachycardia and decreased cardiac output.[476,477]

Astrocyte gliosis has been found in the brainstem at autopsy, reflecting the dysfunction of the respiratory center and autonomic control. Other findings more commonly found in SIDS infants than in those dying of other causes include abnormalities in the carotid body, intrathoracic petechiae, increased periadrenal brown fat, liver hematopoiesis, fetal hemoglobin, and neuroepithelial bodies in the tracheal bronchial tree.[476,478-480]

The role of apnea in SIDS is controversial. Mothers of SIDS infants are more likely to report apneic episodes compared with control mothers. High-risk infants have been shown to exhibit abnormal responses to hypoxemia and hypercarbia. Southall and Talbert have suggested that lung function may be affected during the infant's development by changes in the intrauterine (maternal drug use or smoking) or extrauterine environments.[477] The changes produce an abnormal response to stimuli by the lung or respiratory control centers leading to expiratory apnea. Others have suggested that primary autonomic dysfunction leads to poor respiratory drive or cardiac dysrhythmias.[480]

Diagnostic Findings

A history of an ALTE requires emergent evaluation and intervention as outlined in Chapter 12. The child may look normal at presentation; however, all ALTEs require further evaluation and monitoring. All infants require a complete history of past medical problems, the event, and subsequent findings and response to management. Possible maternal and postnatal factors should be defined.

The physical examination after stabilization and evaluation of the life-threatening event requires attention to bruising, retinal hemorrhages, and other signs of hemorrhage. Rarely, child abuse may be implicated.

Obviously, in patients who cannot be resuscitated, support for the family is a high priority.

Ancillary Data. Evidence of contributing conditions should be sought. Oximetry, electrolytes, glucose, magnesium, calcium, and CBC should be assessed. Infection and metabolic abnormalities should be excluded. Patients who are hospitalized with ALTE should undergo a series of evaluations that may include a pneumogram, polysomnography, continuous ECG recording, barium swallow, EEG, CT scan of the head, and a toxin screen.

An autopsy should be performed on all patients who die of an apparent SIDS death.[481] The coroner, infant's pediatrician, and the emergency physician who was involved in the resusciatiation of the infant may all participate in a postautopsy conference with the parents to answer questions about their infant's death.[481]

Differential Considerations

The differential of ALTE is extensive. Head trauma or child abuse may be difficult to distinguish initially in the absence of a reliable history; however, less than 5% of patients dying of apparent SIDS are later discovered to have died of child abuse.[482] Infection may be causative from overwhelming and acute infection. Encephalopathy or meningitis may be associated with apnea.

Congenital metabolic derangements, particularly those producing hypoglycemia such as glycogen storage disease, may be causative. Intracranial bleeding and cardiac dysrhythmias may occur. Accidental or intentional poisoning can produce coma, with subsequent hyperventilation, arrest, hypoxia, and death.

The initial assessment should be thorough but not necessarily aimed at establishing a definitive diagnosis. In the case of ALTE, admission and monitoring are required; in the case of SIDS, a thorough on-scene investigation is indicated.[480,482,483]

Management

The child with an ALTE needs initial hospitalization and admission. After stabilization and resuscitation, appropriate evaluation is indicated.

Respiratory stimulants such as caffeine or theophylline may be considered. A study of 300 patients with ALTE or increased epidemiologic risk were given theophylline 6 to 7.5 mg/kg/24 hr PO. Theophylline normalized the pneumogram in 94% of infants and improved the study in 100%.[484] Theophylline levels in the range of 10 to 15 gmm/ml are effective and should be monitored periodically.

Home Monitoring. Home monitoring of high-risk infants is another approach, although it is controversial. Groups that may benefit from the use of monitors include (1) symptomatic premature infants who continue to exhibit apnea when they otherwise could be discharged home, (2) infants with tracheostomies or severe bronchopulmonary dysplasia, and (3) infants with a history of ALTE who required vigorous stimulation or resuscitation.[475] Some physicians also monitor infants who are siblings of SIDS victims, although no studies have documented the usefulness of such intervention.[485] Mothers who have a home monitor for their infant experience increased situational anxiety but suffer no untoward health effect.[486]

Home-monitoring devices measure chest wall movement and heart rate. Impedance monitoring is subject to false alarms due to shallow breathing or normal cardiac variability. Parents obviously need training in the use of the monitoring and comprehensive technical and medical support. Home monitoring has not been shown to decrease the mortality of SIDS and is therefore of questionable value in the management of patients with ALTE.[468,469]

Prevention. In 1994, the US Public Health Services joined with the AAP, SIDS Alliance, and the Association of SIDS Program Professionals in launching a national campaign ("Back to Sleep") calling for health professionals to educate parents to place infants on their backs or sides instead of the stomach for sleeping.[487] The supine position appears to be optimal. Emergency physicians can participate in this prevention effort and recognize other opportunities for SIDS prevention such as encouraging parents not to smoke and not to overbundle their infant.[469,487]

Psychosocial Considerations. The death of a child is difficult for parents, relatives, and health professionals (see Chapter 8). Parents, even those who are not responsible in any way for their child's death, universally experience intense guilt feelings for months or years.[488] The immediate reaction of parents may vary from hysteria to complete silence, reflecting cultural background, spiritual beliefs, and previous experiences with death.[489] Parents who initially seem detached or unemotional are actually in a "state of shock." It is essential to allow families to openly express their grief, vocalize their feelings, and clarify any misconceptions. A quiet room for parents to grieve or spend time alone with the infant may be useful. The health-care team including a nurse, social worker, chaplain, emergency department physician, and pediatrician must do their respective parts to provide support for the grieving family. This support may include providing help in funeral arrangements and ultimately reviewing the autopsy results and answering further questions at a later date. Ongoing support must be ensured.[453] Many communities have parent support groups as a component of the National Sudden Infant Death Syndrome Alliance, (800) 221-7437.

The psychosocial effects of SIDS may be profound. Parents may become very accusatory and feel an intense feeling of guilt for months or years.[490] Siblings may also have guilt over the loss of their sibling if, for example, they may have been jealous.[491] Suspicion from neighbors and friends may intensify any problems if there is not an open discussion about what causes SIDS.

Health professionals may have similar feelings and should be allowed to discuss their feelings. Communicating these feelings with one another often does much to relieve stress.

References

Apnea

1. American Academy of Pediatrics: Task force on prolonged apnea, *Pediatrics* 76:129, 1985.
2. Brooks JG: Apnea of infancy and sudden infant death syndrome, *Am J Dis Child* 136:1012, 1982.
3. Barkin RM: Apnea. In Barkin RM and Rosen P, editors: *Emergency pediatrics*, ed 3, St Louis, 1990, Mosby.
4. Barrington K and Finer NN: Periodic breathing and apnea in preterm infants, *Pediatr Res* 27(2):118, 1990.
5. Brooks JG: Abnormalities of control of ventilation. In Rudolph AM, Hoffman JIE, Rudolph CD, editors: *Pediatrics*, ed 20, Stamford, Connecticut, 1996, Appleton and Lange.
6. National Institutes of Health Consensus Development Conference on Infantile Apnea and Home Monitoring: *Pediatrics* 79:292, 1987.
7. Fan LL: Apnea of infancy and childhood, *Prim Care* 11(3):443, 1984.
8. Leistner HL: Apnea in infants and children. In Zimmerman SS and Bilden JH, editors: *Critical care pediatrics*, Philadelphia, 1985, WB Saunders.
9. Henderson FW: Pulmonary infections with respiratory syncytial virus and the parainfluenza virus, *Semin Respir Infect* 2(2):112, 1987.
10. Hewertson J, Poets CF, Samuels MP, et al: Epileptic seizure-induced hypoxemia in infants with apparent life-threatening events, *Pediatrics* 94(2):148, 1994.
11. Green M: Respiratory distress; dyspnea, apnea. In Green M, editor: *Pediatric diagnosis*, ed 5, Philadelphia, 1992, WB Saunders.
12. Friesen CA, Streed CJ, Carney LA: Esophagitis and modified Bernstein tests in infants with apparent life-threatening events, *Pediatrics* 94(4):541, 1994.
13. Wetmore RF: Effects of acid on the larynx of the maturing rabbit and their possible significance to the Sudden Infant Death Syndrome, *Laryngoscope* 103:1242, 1993.
14. Ruggins NR and Milner AD: Site of upper airway obstruction in infants following an acute life-threatening event, *Pediatrics* 91 (3) 595, 1993.
15. Arens R, Gozal D, Williams JC, et al: Recurrent apparent life-threatening events during infancy: a manifestation of inborn errors of metabolism, *J Pediatr* 123 (5):415, 1993.
16. Hurst DL and Marsh WW: Early severe infantile botulism, *J Pediatr* 122 (6):909, 1993.
17. Singer J and Janz T: Apnea and seizures caused by nicotine ingestion, *Pediatr Emerg Care* 6(2):135, 1990.
18. Gozal D, Colin AA, Daskalovic YI, et al: Environmental overheating as a cause of transient respiratory chemoreceptor dysfunction in an infant, *Pediatrics* 82(5):738, 1988.
19. Meadow R: Suffocation, recurrent apnea, and sudden infant death, *J Pediatr* 117(3):351, 1990.
20. Mitchell I, Brummitt J, DeForest J, et al: Apnea and factitious illness (Munchausen Syndrome) by Proxy, *Pediatrics* 92 (6):810, 1993.
21. Mark JD and Brooks JG: Sleep-associated airway problems in children, *Pediatr Clin North Am* 31(4):907, 1984.
22. Gislason T and Benediktsdottir B: Snoring, apneic episodes, and nocturnal hypoxemia among children 6 months to 6 years old: an epidemiologic study of lower limit of prevalence, *Chest* 107(4):963, 1995.
23. Potsic WP: Obstructive sleep apnea, *Pediatr Clin North Am* 36(6):1435, 1989.
24. Mallory GB Jr, Fiser DH, Jackson R: Sleep-associated breathing disorders in morbidly obese children and adolescents, *J Pediatr* 115(6):892, 1989.
25. Chiodini BA and Thach BT: Impaired ventilation in infants sleeping face down: potential significance for sudden infant death syndrome, *J Pediatr* 123(5):686, 1993.
26. Stradling JR, Thomas G, Warley ARH, et al: Effect of adenotonsillectomy on nocturnal hypoxaemia, sleep disturbance, and symptoms in snoring children, *Lancet* 335:249, 1990.
27. Poets CF, Samuels MP, Noyes JP, et al: Home event recordings of oxygenation, breathing movements, and heart rate and rhythm in infants with recurrent life-threatening events, *J Pediatr* 123(5):693, 1993.

Cough

28. Murray JF: *The normal lung*, Philadelphia, 1986, WB Saunders.
29. Phelan PD, Landau LI, Olinsky A: Cough. In Phelan PD, Landau LI, Olinsky A, editors: *Respiratory illness in children*, ed 3, 1990, Cambridge, Mass, Blackwell Scientific Publications.
30. Braman SS and Corrao WM: Cough: differential diagnosis and treatment, *Clin Chest Med* 8:177-188, 1987.
31. Sant Ambrogio G: Afferent pathways for the cough reflex, *Bull Eur Physiopathol Respir* 23:105, 19-24, 1987.
32. Eigen H: The clinical evaluation of chronic cough, *Pediatr Clin North Am* 29:1, 67, 1982.
33. Cloud G, Cassell G, Tiller R, et al: Infant pneumonitis associated with cytomegalovirus, chlamydia, pneumocytis, and ureaplasma, *Pediatrics* 79(1):76-83, 1987.
34. Morgan WJ and Taussig LM: The child with persistent cough, *Pediatr Rev* 8:8, 249-253, 1987.
35. Mok J and Levison H: The wheezing infant. In Tinkelman DG, Fallis CJ, Naspitz CK, editors: *Childhood asthma—pathophysiology and treatment*, New York, 1987, Marcel Dekker.
36. Kim I, Brummitt W, Humphrey A, et al: Foreign body in the airway: a review of 202 cases, *Laryngoscope* 83:347-354, 1973.
37. Cloutier MM and Loughlin GM: Chronic cough in children: a manifestation of airway hyperreactivity, *Pediatrics* 67:6-12, 1981.
38. Wald ER, Pang D, Milmore G, et al: Sinusitis and its complications in the pediatric patient, *Pediatr Clin North Am* 28:4, 777-796, 1981.
39. Sabato AR, Martin AJ, Marmion BP, et al: *Mycoplasma pneumoniae*: acute illness, antibiotics and subsequent pulmonary function, *Arch Dis Child* 59:1034-1037, 1984.
40. Reisman J, Canny GJ, Levison H: The approach to chronic cough in childhood, *Ann Allergy* 61:163-169, 1988.
41. Mellis CM: Evaluation and treatment of chronic cough in children, *Pediatr Clin North Am* 26:553-564, 1979.
42. Kovatch AL, Wald ER, Ledesma-Medina J, et al: Maxillary sinus radiographs in children with non-respiratory complaints, *Pediatrics* 73:306-308, 1984.
43. Fanconi S, Doherty P, Edmonds JF, et al: Pulse oximetry in pediatric intensive care, *J Pediatr* 107:3,362-366, 1985.
44. Umetsun DM, Ambrosino DM, Quinti I, et al: Recurrent pulmonary infection and impaired antibody response to bacterial capsular polysaccharide antigen in children with IgG deficiency, *N Engl J Med* 313:1247-1251, 1985.
45. Whitaker JA, Donaldson P, Nelson JD: Diagnosis of pertussis by the fluorescent antibody method, *N Engl J Med* 263:850-851, 1960.
46. Goodman YE, Wort AJ, Jackson FL: Enzyme-linked immunosorbent assay for detection of pertussis immunoglobulin A in nasopharyngeal secretions as an indication of recent infection, *J Clin Microbiol* 13:286-292, 1981.

Cyanosis

47. Comroe HH Jr and Botelho S: The unreliability of cyanosis in the recognition of arterial anoxemia, *Am J Med Sci* 214:1, 1947.
48. Geraci JE and Wood EH: The relationship of the arterial oxygen saturation to cyanosis, *Med Clin North Am* 35:1185, 1951.
49. Lin YT, Yen LC, Oka Y: Pathophysiology of general cyanosis, *NY State J Med* 77:1393, August 1977.
50. Lundsgaard C and Van Slyke DD: Cyanosis, *Medicine* 2:1, 1923.
51. Martin L and Khalil H: How much reduced hemoglobin is necessary to generate central cyanosis? *Chest* 97(1):182, 1990.
52. Harwood-Nuss AL: Cyanosis. In Tintinalli JE, Krome RL, Ruiz E, editors: *Emergency medicine. A comprehensive study guide*, New York, 1988, McGraw-Hill.
53. Barkin RM: Cyanosis. In Barkin RM and Rosen P, editors: *Emergency pediatrics*, ed 4, St Louis, 1994, Mosby.
54. Blount SG Jr: Cyanosis: pathophysiology and differential diagnosis, *Prog Cardiovasc Dis* 13(6):595, 1971.

55. Driscoll DJ: Evaluation of the cyanotic newborn, *Pediatr Clin North Am* 37(1):1, 1990.
56. Barkin RM: Congestive heart failure in children, *J Emerg Med* 4:378, 1986.
57. Kanter RK and Watchko JR: Pulmonary edema associated with upper airway obstruction, *Am J Dis Child* 138:356, 1984.
58. Sofer S, Weinhouse E, Tal A, et al: Cor pulmonale due to adenoidal or tonsillar hypertrophy or both in children, *Chest* 93(1):119, 1988.
59. Dolan MA and Luban NLC: Methemoglobinemia in two children: disparate etiology and treatment, *Pediatr Emerg Care* 3(3):171, 1987.
60. Yano SS, Danish EH, Hsia YE: Transient methemoglobinemia with acidosis in infants, *J Pediatr* 100(3):415, 1982.
61. Kulick RM: Pulse oximetry, *Pediatr Emerg Care* 3(2):127, 1987.

Respiratory Distress/Dyspnea

62. Green M: Respiratory distress. In Green M, editor: *Pediatric diagnosis*, ed 5, Philadelphia, 1992, WB Saunders.
63. Anas NG and Perkin RM: Resuscitation and stabilization of the child with respiratory disease, *Pediatr Ann* 15(1):43, 1986.
64. Newth CJL: Recognition and management of respiratory failure, *Pediatr Clin North Am* 26(4):614, 1979.
65. McGravey AR: Pediatric respiratory emergencies, *Hosp Physician* 24, 1989.
66. Karlson KH Jr: Acute respiratory distress in children, *Compr Ther* 13(7):9, 1987.
67. West JB: *Respiratory physiology—the essentials*, ed 4, Baltimore, 1990, Williams and Wilkins.
68. Barkin RM: Respiratory distress (dyspnea). In Barkin RM and Rosen P, editors: *Emergency pediatrics*, ed 3, St Louis, 1990, Mosby.
69. Maze A and Block E: Stridor in pediatric patients, *Anesthesiology* 50(2):132, 1979.
70. Hen J: Current management of upper airway obstruction, *Pediatr Ann* 15(4):274, 1986.
71. American Academy of Pediatrics: *Haemophilus influenzae* infections. In Peter G, editor: *1994 Red Book: report of the Committee on Infectious Diseases*, ed 23, Elk Grove Village, IL, 1994, American Academy of Pediatrics.
72. Lichenstein R: Retropharyngeal cellulitis: an unusual case of respiratory distress in infancy, *Pediatr Emerg Care* 6(2):138, 1990.
73. Laks Y and Barzilay Z: Foreign body aspiration in childhood, *Pediatr Emerg Care* 4(2):102, 1988.
74. Grossman LK: Pneumonia in infants and children, *Compr Ther* 12(2):15, 1986.
75. Fireman P: The wheezing infant, *Pediatr Rev* 7(8):247, 1986.
76. Ho AM-H: Food anaphylaxis-an important cause of acute respiratory distress in children, *Anesth Analg* 77:1289, 1993.
77. Scannell G, Waxman K, Tominaga GT: Respiratory distress in traumatized and burned children, *J Pediatr Surg* 30(4):612, 1995.
78. Lindsay CA, Williams GD, Levin DL: Fatal adult respiratory distress syndrome after diphenhydramine toxicity in a child: a case report, *Crit Care Med* 23(4):777, 1995.
79. Kulick RM: Pulse oximetry, *Pediatr Emerg Care* 3(2):127, 1987.

Stridor

80. Phelan PD, Landau LI, Olinsky A: Respiratory noises. In Phelan PD, Landau LI, Olinsky A, editors: *Respiratory illness in children*, Cambridge, Mass, 1990, Blackwell Scientific Publications.
81. Maze A and Bloch E: Stridor in pediatric patients—review, *Anesthesiology* 50:132, 1979.
82. Freidberg J: An approach to stridor in infants and children, *J Otolaryngol* 16:203, 1987.
83. Friedman EM, Jorgensen K, Healy GB, et al: Bacterial tracheitis—two year experience, *Laryngoscope* 95:9, 1985.
84. Barker GA: Current management of croup and epiglottitis, *Pediatr Clin North Am* 26:565, 1979.
85. Gutson AC: *Human physiology and mechanisms of disease*, ed 4, Philadelphia, 1987, WB Saunders.
86. Moore EW: Ionized calcium in normal serum, ultrafiltrates, and whole blood determined by ion-exchange electrodes, *J Clin Invest* 49:318, 1970.
87. Hidalgo HA and Davis SH: Intermittent stridor and hypocalcemia in childhood, *Pediatr Pulmonol* 7:110, 1989.
88. Geist R and Tallett SE: Diagnosis and management of psychogenic stridor caused by a conversion disorder, *Pediatrics* 86:315, 1990.

89. American Psychiatric Association: *Diagnosis and statistical manual of mental disorders*, ed 5, 1987, Washington, DC, The Association.
90. Kilham H, Gillis J, Bengamin B: Severe upper airway obstruction, *Pediatr Clin North Am* 34:1, 1987.
91. Zalzal GH: Stridor and airway compromise, *Pediatr Clin North Am* 36:1389, 1989.
92. Friedman EM, Vastola AP, McGill TJI, et al: Chronic pediatric stridor: etiology and outcome, *Laryngoscope* 100:277, 1990.
93. Santamaria JP and Schafermeyer R: Stridor—a review, *Pediatr Emerg Care* 8:4, 229-234, 1992.
94. Poole SR, Mauro RD, Fan LL, et al: The child with simultaneous stridor and wheezing, *Pediatr Emerg Care* 6:33, 1990.
95. Kolski GB: Allergic and pulmonary emergencies. In Fletcher G and Ludwig S, editors: *Textbook of pediatric emergency medicine*, Baltimore, 1983, Williams and Williams.
96. Cohen MA and Guzzardi LJ: Inhalation of products of combustion, *Ann Emerg Med* 12:628, 1983.
97. Smith MS: Acute psychogenic stridor in an adolescent athlete treated with hypnosis, *Pediatrics* 72:247, 1983.
98. Barnes SD, Grob CS, Lachman BS: Psychogenic upper airway obstruction presenting as refractory wheezing, *J Pediatr* 109:1067, 1986.
99. Bluestone CD, Delerme AN, Samuelson GH: Airway obstruction due to vocal cord paralysis in infants with hydrocephalus and meningomyelocele, *Ann Otol Rhinol Laryngol* 81:778, 1972.

Wheezing

100. Mok J and Levison H: The wheezing infant. In Tinkelman JG, Falliers CJ, Naspitz CK, editors: *Childhood asthma—pathophysiology and treatment*, New York, 1987, Marcel Dekker.
101. Phelan PD: Respiratory noises. In Phelan PD, Landau LI, Olinsky A, editors: *Respiratory illness in children*, ed 3, Cambridge, Mass, 1990, Blackwell Scientific Publications.
102. Fireman P: The wheezing infant, *Pediatr Rev* 7:8, 1986.
103. Hogg JC, Williams J, Richardson JB, et al: Age as a factor in the distribution of lower airway conductance and in the pathologic anatomy of obstructive lung disease, *N Engl J Med* 282:1283, 1970.
104. Bryan AC, Mansel AL, Levison H: Development of mechanical properties of the respiratory system. In Hodson WA, editor: *Development of the lung*, vol 6, New York, 1977, Marcel Dekker.
105. Muller NL and Bryan AC: Chest wall mechanics and respiratory muscles in infants, *Pediatr Clin North Am* 26:503, 1979.
106. Kim GL, Brummitt MW, Humphrey A, et al: Foreign body in the airway: a review of 202 cases, *Laryngoscope* 83(1):347, 1973.
107. Holroyd HJ: Foreign body aspiration: potential case of coughing and wheezing, *Pediatr Rev* 10:59, 1988.
108. Mok JYQ, Ingliss JM, Simpson H: *Mycoplasma pneumoniae* infection: a retrospective review of 103 hospitalized children, *Acta Paediatr* 68:833, 1979.
109. Moss AJ and McDonald LV: Cardiac disease in the wheezing child, *Chest* 71 (suppl 2):187, 1977.
110. Singer JI, Isaacm DJ, Bell LM: The wheezers that wasn't, *Pediatr Emerg Care* 8:2, 107-109, 1992.
111. Keith HH: Vascular rings and tracheobronchial compression in infants, *Pediatr Ann* 6:8, 1977.
112. Abrunzo T: An infant fatality associated with inspiratory and expiratory wheezing, *Pediatr Emerg Care* 11:1 48-51, 1995.
113. Smyth JA, Tabachnik E, Duncan WJ, et al: Pulmonary function and bronchial hyperreactivity in long-term survivors of bronchopulmonary dysplasia, *Pediatrics* 68:336, 1981.
114. Fanconi S, Doherty P, Edmonds JF, et al: Pulse oximetry in pediatric intensive care, *J Pediatr* 107:362, 1985.
115. Geelhoed GC, Landau W, LeSouef PN: Predictive value of oxygen saturation in emergency evaluation of asthmatic children, *BMJ* (Clin Res) 297:395, 1988.
116. Spiegel RL and Twarog FJ: Emergency room therapy of the pediatric patient with status asthmaticus, *J Asthma* 19:47, 1982.
117. Nowak RM, Pensler MI, Sarkar DD, et al: Comparison of peak expiratory flow and FEV_1 admission criteria for acute bronchial asthma, *Ann Emerg Med* 11:64, 1982.
118. Franklin WH, Sietrich Am, Hichey RW, et al: Anomalous left coronary artery masquerading as infantile bronchiolitis, *Pediatr Emerg Care* 8:6, 338-341, 1992.

119. Poole SR, Mauro RD, Fan CC, et al: The child with simultaeous stridor and wheezing, *Pediatr Emerg Care* 6: 33-37, 1990.

Asthma

120. Sly RM: Evolving views of asthma. In Tinkelman DG, Falliers CJ, Naspitz CK, editors: *Childhood asthma*, New York, 1987, Marcel Dekker.
121. Bierman C and Pearlman D: Asthma. In Chernick V, Kendig EL, editors: *Disorders of the respiratory tract in children*, ed. 5, Philadelphia, WB Saunders, 1990.
122. Burney P: Epidemiology, *Br Med Bull* 48:10, 1992.
123. Schwartz J, Gold D, Dockery D, et al: Predictors of asthma and persistent wheeze in a nationale sample of children in the United States, *Am Rev Respir Dis* 142:555, 1990.
124. Sigurs N, Bjarnason R, Sigurbegsson F, et al: Asthma and Immunoglobulin E antibodies after respiratory syncytial virus bronchiolitis, *Pediatrics* 95:4, 500-505, 1995.
125. Martinez F, Morgan W, Wright A, et al: Diminished lung function as a predisposing factor for wheezing respiratory illness in infants, *N Engl J Med* 219:1112, 1988.
126. Morgan WJ and Martinez FD: Risk factors for developing wheezing and asthma in childhood, *Pediatr Clin North Am* 39:6 1185-1203, 1995.
127. Siegel SC: Infantile and childhood asthma. In Nussbaum E and Gallant SP, editors: *Pediatric and respiratory disorders*, Orlando, Fla, 1984, Grune & Stratton.
128. Phelan PD, Landau LI, Olinsky A: Asthma: pathogenesis, pathophysiology and epidemiology. In Phelan PD, Landau LI, Olinsky A, editors: *Respiratory illness in children*, ed 3, Cambridge, Mass, 1990, Blackwell Scientific Publications.
129. Wanner A: The role of mucociliary dysfunction in bronchial asthma, *Am J Med* 67:477, 1979.
130. Goetzel EJ: Oxygenation products of arachidonic acid as mediators of hypersensitivity and inflammation, *Med Clin North Am* 65:809, 1981.
131. Chung KF: Role of inflammation in the hypersensitivity of the airways in asthma, *Thorax* 41:657, 1986.
132. Cuss FM and Barnes PJ: Epithelial mediators, *Am J Respir D Crit Care Med* 136:532, 1987.
133. Scharf S: Mechanical cardiopulmonary interaction with asthma, *Clin Rev Allergy* 3:487, 1985.
134. Busse WW: Respiratory infection: their role in airway responsiveness and the pathogenesis of asthma, *J Allergy Clin Immunol* 85:4, 671, 1990.
135. Eggleston PA, Kagey-Sobotka A, Schleimer RP, et al: Interaction between hyperosmolar and IgE mediated histamine release from basophils and mast cells, *Am J Respir Crit Care Med* 130:86, 1984.
136. Hahn A, Anderson SD, Morton AR, et al: A reinterpretation of the effect of temperature and water content of the inspired air in exercise induced asthma, *Am Rev Respir Dis* 130:575, 1984.
137. Salvagio J, Hasselbad V, Seaburg S, et al: New Orleans Asthma. II. Relationship of climatologic and seasonal factors to outbreaks, *J Allergy* 45:257, 1970.
138. Derrick EH: Childhood asthma in Brisbane. Epidemiological observations, *Austr Paediatr J* 9:135, 1973.
139. Carey MJ and Cordon J: Asthma and climatic conditions, *BMJ* 293:843, 1986.
140. Martin AJ, McLennan LA, Landau LI, et al: The natural history of childhood asthma to adult life, *BMJ* 280:1397, 1980.
141. Gillam GL, McNico K, Williams HE: Chest deformity, residual airways obstruction and hyperinflation and growth in children with asthma II, *Arch Dis Child* 45:789, 1970.
142. Westerman, DE, Benatar SR, Potgieter PD, et al: Identification of the high risk asthmatic patient, *Am J Med* 66:565, 1979.
143. Fisch MA, Pitchenick A, Giander LB: An index predicting relapse and need for hospitalization in patients with acute bronchial asthma, *N Engl J Med* 305:783, 1981.
144. Gallant SP, Groncy CE, Shaw KC: The value of pulsus paradoxus in assessing the child with status asthmaticus, *Pediatrics* 61:46, 1987.
145. Skoner DP, Fisher TJ, Gormley G, et al: Pediatric predictive index for hospitalization in acute asthma, *Ann Emerg Med* 16:25, 1987.
146. Wood DW, Downes JJ, Lecks HI: A clinical screening system for the diagnosis of respiratory failure, *Am J Dis Child* 123:227, 1972.

147. Kerem E, Canny G, Tibshirani R, et al: Clinical-physiological correlations in acute asthma of childhood, *Pediatrics* 87:4, 481, 1991.
148. Simpson H, Mitchell I, Inglis JM, et al: Severe ventilatory failure in asthma in children, *Arch Dis Child* 52:714, 1978.
149. Eggleston PA, Ward BH, Pierson WE, et al: Radiographic abnormalities in acute asthma in children, *Pediatrics* 54:442, 1974.
150. Fanconi S, Doherty P, Edmonds JF, et al: Pulse oximetry in pediatric intensive care, *J Pediatr* 107:3 362, 1985.
151. Kerem E, Tibshirani R, Canny G, et al: Predicting the need for hospitalization in children with acute asthma, *Chest* 98:6 1355, 1990.
152. Geelhoed GC, Landau LI, Le Soeuf GC: Predictive value of oxygen saturation in emergency evaluation of asthmatic children, *BMJ* 297: 395-396, 1988.
153. Kerem E, Canny G, Tibshirani R, et al: Clinical physiological correlations in acute asthma in childhood, *Pediatrics* 87:4 481-486, 1991.
154. Geelhoed GC, Landau LI, Le Soeuf GC: Oximetry and peak expiration flow in assessment of acute childhood asthma, *J Pediatr* 117:6 907-909, 1990.
155. Weng T and Levison H: Standard of pulmonary function in children, *Am J Respir Crit Care Med* 99:879, 1969.
156. Freelander M and van Asperen PP: Nebuhaler versus nebulizer in children with acute asthma, *BMJ* 288:1873, 1984.
157. Newman SP and Clarke SW: Therapeutic aerosols. I. Physical and practical considerations, *Thorax* 58:881, 1983.
158. Lofdahl CG and Barnes PJ: Calcium channel blockage and asthma-the current position, *Eur J Respir Dis* 67:193-203, 1986.
159. Newhouse MT and Dolovich MB: Control of asthma by aerosols, *N Engl J Med* 315:870, 1986.
160. Dolovich M, Sanchis H, Rossman C, et al: Aerosol penetrance: a selection index of peripheral airways obstruction, *J Appl Physiol* 40:468, 1976.
161. Brain JD and Valberg PA: Deposition of aerosol in the respiratory tract, *Am Rev Respir Dis* 120:1325, 1979.
162. Schuh S, Parkin P, Rajan A, et al: High-versus low dose frequent nebulized albuterol in children with severe acute asthma, *Pediatrics* 83:513, 1989.
163. Newman SP, Millar AB, Jones TR, et al: Improvement of pressurized aerosol deposition with nebuhaler spacer device, *Thorax* 39:935-41, 1984.
164. Hickey RW, Gochman RF, Chande V, et al: Albuterol deliveries via metered dose inhaler with spacer for outpatient treatment of young children with wheezing, *Arch Pediatr Adolesc Med* 148:189, 1994.
165. Kerem E, Levison H, Schuh S, et al: Efficacy of albuterol administration by nebulizer versus spacer device in children with acute asthma, *J Pediatr* 123:313, 1993.
166. Mann JS and George CS: Anticholinergic drugs in the treatment of airway disease, *Br J Dis Chest* 79:209, 1985.
167. Beck B R, Robertson CF, Galdes-Sebaldt M, et al: Combined salbutamol and ipratropium bromide by inhalation in the treatment of severe acute asthma, *J Pediatr* 107:605, 1985.
168. Reisman J, Galdes-Sebaldt M, Kazim F, et al: Frequent administration by inhalation of salbutamol and ipratropium bromide in the initial management of severe acute asthma in children, *J Allergy Clin Immunol* 81:1, 16, 1988.
169. Schuh S, Johnson D, Callahan S, et al: Efficacy of frequent nebulized ipratropium bromide added to frequent albuterol therapy in severe childhood asthma, *J Pediatr* 126:4, 639, 1995.
170. Gross NJ and Skorudin MS: State of the art: anticholinergic, antimuscarinic bronchodilators, *Ann Rev Respir Dis* 129:856, 1984.
171. Lichterfeld A: Safety of Atroven, *Scand J Respir Dis* 60:(suppl 103)143, 1979.
172. Karpel JP, Appel D, Breidbart D, et al: A comparison of atropine sulfate and isoproterenol sulfate in the emergency treatment of asthma, *Am J Respir Crit Care Med* 133:727, 1986.
173. Fanci AS, Dale DC, Balow BE: Glucocorticosteroid therapy. Mechanism of action and clinical considerations, *Ann Intern Med* 84:304, 1976.
174. Littenberg B and Gluck EH: A controlled trial of methylprednisolone in the emergency treatment of acute asthma, *N Engl J Med* 314:150, 1986.
175. Ellul-Micallef R and Fenech FF: Effect of intravenous prednisolone in asthmatics with diminished adrenergic responsiveness, *Lancet* 2:1269, 1975.

176. Schneider S, Pipher A, Britton H, et al: High-dose methylprednisolone as initial therapy in patients with acute bronchospasm, *J Asthma* 25:189-193, 1988.

177. Stein L and Cole R: Early administration of corticosteroids in emergency room treatment of acute asthma, *Ann Intern Med* 112:822-827, 1990.

178. Rodrigo C and Rodrigo G: Early administration of hydrocortisone in the emergency room treatment of acute asthma: a controlled clinical trial, *Respir Med* 88:755-761, 1994.

179. Scarfone RJ, Fuchs SM, Nager AL, et al: Controlled trial of oral prednisone in the emergency department treatment of children with acute asthma, *Pediatrics* 92:4, 513-518, 1993.

180. Ratto D, Alfaro C, Sipsey J, et al: Are intravenous corticosteroids required in status asthmaticus? *JAMA* 260:527, 1988.

181. Rowe B., Keller J, Oxman A: Effectiveness of steroid therapy in acute exacerbation of asthma, *Am J Emerg Med* 10:301-310, 1992.

182. Weinberger M: Anti asthmatic therapy in children, *Pediatr Clin North Am* 36:5, 1251, 1989.

183. Harris JB, Weinberger M, Nasif E, et al: Early intervention with short courses of prednisone to prevent progression of asthma in ambulatory patients incompletely responsive to bronchodilators, *J Pediatr* 110:627, 1987.

184. Weinberger M: The pharmacology and therapeutic use of theophylline, *J Allergy Clin Immunol* 73:525, 1984.

185. Rossing TH, Fanta CH, Goldstein DH, et al: Emergency therapy of asthma: comparison of the acute effects of parenteral and inhaled sympathomimetics and infused theophylline, *Am J Respir Crit Care Med* 122:365-371, 1980.

186. Siegel D, Sheppard D, Gelb A, et al: Aminophylline increases the toxicity but not the efficacy of an inhaled beta-adrenergic agonist in the treatment of acute exacerbation of asthma, *Am J Respir Crit Care Med* 132(2):283, 1985.

187. Littenberg B: Aminophylline treatment in severe acute asthma, a meta analysis, *JAMA* 259:1678, 1988.

188. Carter E, Cruz M, Chestown S, et al: Efficacy of intravenously administered theophylline in children hospitalized with severe asthma, *J Pediatr* 122:470, 1993.

189. Barkin RM and Rosen P: Pulmonary disorders. In Barkin RM and Rosen P, editors: *Emergency pediatrics*, ed 4, St Louis, 1994, Mosby.

190. McNamara RM, Spivey WH, Skobeloff E, et al: Intravenous magnesium sulfate in the management of acute respiratory failure complicating asthma, *Ann Emerg Med* 18:2, 197, 1989.

191. Noppen M, Vanmaele L, Impeus N, et al: Bronchodilating effect of intravenous magnesium sulfate in acute severe bronchial asthma, *Chest* 97:2, 373, 1990.

192. Pabon H., Monem G, Kissoon N: Safety and efficacy of magnesium sulfate infusions in children with status asthmaticus, *Pediatr Emerg Care* 10:4, 200-203, 1994.

193. Rossing TH, Fanta CH, McFadden ER: Effect of outpatient treatment of asthma with beta agonists on the response of sympathomimetics in an emergency room, *Am J Med* 75:781, 1983.

194. Whyte KF, Addis GJ, Whitesmith R, et al: The mechanism of salbutamol-induced hypokalemia, *Br J Clin Pharmacol* 23:65, 1987.

195. Bohn DJ, Kalloghlian A, Jenkins J, et al: Intravenous salbutamol in the treatment of status asthmaticus in children, *Crit Care Med* 12:892, 1984.

196. Conner WT, Dolovich MB, Frame RA, et al: Reliable salbutamol administration in 6 to 36 month old children by means of a metered dose inhaler and aerochamber with mask, *Pediatr Pulmonol* 6:263, 1989.

197. Bennton G, Thomas RC, Nickerson BG, et al: Experience with a metered-dose inhaler with a spacer in the pediatric emergency department, *Am J Dis Child*, 143:678, 1989.

198. Kerem E, Levison H, Schuh S, et al: Efficacy of albuterol administered by nebulizer versus spacer device in children with acute asthma, *J Pediatr* 123:2, 313-318, 1993.

199. Kravis LP: An analysis of fifteen childhood asthma fatalities, *J Allergy Clin Immunol* 80:467, 1987.

200. Benatar SR: Fatal asthma, *N Engl J Med* 314:423, 1986.

201. Lanes SF and Walker A: Do pressurized bronchodilator aerosoles cause death among asthmatics? *Am J Epidemiol* 125:755, 1987.

Bronchiolitis

202. Tercier JA: Bronchiolitis: a clinical review, *J Emerg Med* 1:119, 1983.

203. Aquelina AT, Hall WJ, Douglas G, et al: Airway reactivity in subjects with viral upper respiratory tract infections, *Am J Respir Crit Care Med* 122:3, 1980.

204. Welliver RC, Wong DT, Sun M, et al: The development of respiratory syncytial virus-specific IgE and the release of histamine in nasopharyngeal secretions after infection, *N Engl J Med* 305:841, 1981.

205. Faden H, Kaul TN, Ogra PL: Activation of oxidative and arachidonic acid metabolism in neutrophils by RSV antibody complexes, *J Infect Dis* 148:110, 1983.

206. Busse W: Decreased granulocyte response to isoproterenol in asthma during upper respiratory infections, *Am J Respir Crit Care Med* 115-783, 1977.

207. Gershwin LJ, Osebold JW, Zee YC: Immunoglobulin E-containing cells in mouse lung following allergen inhalation and ozone exposure, *Int Arch Allergy Immunol* 65:266, 1981.

208. Sigurs N, Bjarnason R, Sigurbegsson F, et al: Asthma and Immunoglobulin E antibodies after respiratory syncytial virus bronchiolitis, *Pediatrics* 95:4, 500-505, 1995.

209. Murray M, Webb MSC, O'Callaghan C, et al: Respiratory status and allergy after bronchiolitis, *Arch Dis Child* 67:482-487, 1992.

210. Martinez FD, Morgan WJ, Wright AL, et al: Initial airway function is a risk factor for recurrent wheezing respiratory illnesses during the first three years of life, *Am J Respir Crit Care Med* 143:312-316, 1991.

211. Hogg JC, Williams J, Richardson JB, et al: Age as a factor in the distribution of lower-airway conductance and in the pathologic anatomy of obstructive lung disease, *N Engl J Med* 282:1283, 1970.

212. Sandiford BR and Spencer B: Respiratory syncytial virus in epidemic bronchiolitis of infants, *BMJ* 2:881, 1962.

213. Cherry JD: Newer respiratory viruses: their role in respiratory illness of children. In Shulman I, editor *Advances in pediatrics,* vol 20, Chicago, 1973, Year Book.

214. Lang WR, Howden CW, Laws J, et al: Bronchopneumonia with serious sequelae in children with evidence of adenovirus type 21 infection, *BMJ* 1:73, 1969.

215. Chernick V and MacPherson RI: Respiratory syncytial and adenovirus infections of the lower respiratory tract in infancy, *Clin Notes Respir Dis* 10:3, 1971.

216. Hall CB, Walsh EE, Long CE, et al: Immunity to and frequency of reinfection with respiratory syncytial virus, *J Infect Dis* 163:693, 1991.

217. MacDonald WE, Hall CB, Suffrin SC, et al: Respiratory syncytial viral infection in infants with congenital heart disease, *N Engl J Med* 307:397, 1982.

218. Hall CB, Powell KR, MacDonald NE, et al: Respiratory syncytial viral infection in children with compromised immune function, *N Engl J Med* 315:77, 1986.

219. Hall CB and McBride JT: Respiratory syncytial virus, *N Engl J Med* 325:1, 51, 1991.

220. Clarke SKR, Gardner SP, Poole PM, et al: Respiratory syncytial virus infection: admissions to hospital in industrial, urban, and rural areas, *BMJ* 2:796, 1978.

221. Gurwitz D, Mindorff C, Levison H: Increased incidence of bronchial reactivity in children with a history of bronchiolitis, *J Pediatr* 98:551, 1981.

222. Kattan M, Keens TG, Lapierre JG, et al: Pulmonary function abnormalities in symptom-free children after bronchiolitis, *Pediatrics* 59:683, 1977.

223. Stokes GM, Milner AD, Hodges IGC, et al: Lung function abnormalities after acute bronchiolitis, *J Pediatr* 98:871, 1981.

224. Fanconi S, Doherty P, Edmonds JF, et al: Pulse oximetry in pediatric intensive care: comparison with measured saturation and transcutaneous oxygen tension, *J Pediatr* 107:362, 1985.

225. Downes JD, Wood DW, Striker TW, et al: Acute respiratory failure in infants with bronchiolitis, *Anesthesiology* 29:426, 1968.

226. Simpson H, Matthew DJ, Habel AH, et al: Acute respiratory failure in bronchiolitis and pneumonia in infancy, *BMJ* 2:632, 1974.

227. Portnoy B, Hanes B, Salvatore MA, et al: The peripheral white blood count in respirovirus infection, *J Pediatr* 68:181, 1966.

228. Simpson W, Hacking PM, Court SDM, et al: The radiologic findings in respiratory syncytial virus infection in children I and II, *Pediatr Radiol* 2:97, 105, 1974.

229. Rice RP and Loda F: A roentgengraphic analysis of respiratory syncytial virus pneumonia in infants, *Radiology* 87:102, 1966.

230. Krilov LR, Lipson SM, Barone SR, et al: Evaluation of a rapid diagnostic test for respiratory syncytial virus: potential for bedside diagnosis, *Pediatrics* 93:903, 1994.

231. Hall CB and Douglas RG: Clinically useful method for the isolation of respiratory syncytial virus, *J Infect Dis* 131:1, 1975.

232. Smyth JA, Tabachnik E, Duncan WJ, et al: Pulmonary function and bronchial hyper-reactivity in long-term survivors of bronchopulmonary dysplasia, *Pediatrics* 68:336, 1981.

233. Moss AJ and McDonald LV: Cardiac disease in the wheezing child, *Chest* 71(suppl 2):187, 1977.

234. Mok J and Levison H: The wheezing infant. In Tinkelman D, editor: *Childhood asthma-pathophysiology and treatment*, New York, 1987, Marcel Dekker.

235. Kim GI, Brummitt MW, Humphrey A, et al: Foreign body in the airway: a review of 202 cases, *Laryngoscope* 83(1):347, 1973.

236. Keith HH: Vascular rings and tracheobronchial compression in infants, *Pediatr Ann* 6:8, 1977.

237. Simpson H, Mathew DJ, Inglis JM, et al: Virological findings and blood gas tensions in acute lower respiratory tract infections in children, *BMJ* 2:629, 1974.

238. Bau SK, Aspin N, Wood DE, et al: The measurement of fluid deposition in humans following mist tent therapy, *Pediatrics* 48:605, 1971.

239. Lenney W and Milner AA: At what age do bronchodilator drugs work? *Arch Dis Child* 53:532, 1978.

240. Stokes GM, Milner AD, Hodges IGC, et al: Nebulized therapy in acute severe bronchiolitis in infancy, *Arch Dis Child* 58:279, 1980.

241. Hughes DM, Lesonef RN, Landau LI: Effect of salbutamol on respiratory mechanics in bronchiolitis, *Pediatr Res* 22:83, 1987.

242. Rutter N, Milner AD, Hiller EJ: Effects of bronchodilators on respiratory resistance in infants and young children with bronchiolitis and wheezy bronchitis, *Arch Dis Child* 50:719, 1975.

243. Phelan PD and Williams HE: Sympathomimetic drugs in acute viral bronchiolitis, *Pediatrics* 44:493, 1969.

244. Tal A, Bavilski C, Yohai D, et al: Dexamethasone and salbutamol in the treatment of acute wheezing in infants, *Pediatrics* 71:13, 1983.

245. Lowell DE, Lister G, Van Koss H, et al: Wheezing in infants: the response to epinephrine, *Pediatrics* 79:939, 1987.

246. Schuh S, Canny G, Reisman J, et al: Nebutilized albuterol in acute bronchiolitis, *J Pediatr* 117:633, 1990.

247. Klassen TP, Rowe PC, Sutcliffe T, et al: Randomized trial of salbutaneol in acute bronchiolitis, *J Pediatr* 118:5, 807, 1991.

248. Schweich PJ, Hurt TL, Walkley EI, et al: The use of nebulized albuterol in wheezing infants, *Pediatr Emerg Care* 8:4, 184-188, 1992.

249. Gadomski Am, Lichenstein R, Horton L, et al: Efficacy of albuterol in the management of bronchiolitis, *Pediatrics* 93:6, 1994.

250. Hodges IGC, Groggins RC, Milner AD, et al: Bronchodilator effect of inhaled ipratropium bromide in wheezy toddlers, *Arch Dis Child* 56:729, 1981.

251. Stokes GM, Milner AD, Hodges IGC, et al: Nebulized therapy in acute severe bronchiolitis in infancy, *Arch Dis Child* 58:4, 279, 1980.

252. Henry RL, Milner AD, Stokes GM: Ineffectiveness of ipratropium bromide in acute bronchiolitis, *Arch Dis Child* 58:11, 925, 1983.

253. Seidenberg J, Masters IB, Hudson I, et al: Effect of ipratropium bromide on respiratory mechanics in infants with acute bronchiolitis, *Aust Pediatr J* 23:169, 1987.

254. Schuh S, Johnson D, Canny G et al: Efficacy of nebulized ipratropium bromide in acute bronchiolitis, *Pediatrics* 90:920, 1992.

255. Brooks LJ and Cropp GJ: Theophylline therapy in bronchiolitis, *Am J Dis Child* 135:934, 1981.

256. Smith RA, et al: *Background and mechanisms of action of ribavirin in clinical applications of ribavirin*, 1984, Orlando, Fla, Academic Press.

257. Hall CB, McBride JT, Walsh EE, et al: Aerosolized ribavirin in the treatment of infants with respiratory syncytial virus infection, *N Engl J Med* 308:1443, 1983.

258. Rodriquez WJ, Kim HW, Brandt CD, et al: Aerosolized ribavirin in the treatment of patients with respiratory syncytial virus disease, *Pediatr Infect Dis J* 6:159, 1987.

259. Barry W, Cockburn F, Cornall R, et al: Ribavirin aerosol for acute bronchiolitis, *Arch Dis Child* 61:593, 1986.

260. Taylor LH, Knight V, Gilbert BE, et al: Ribavirin aerosol treatment of bronchiolitis associated with respiratory syncytial virus infection in infants, *Pediatrics* 72:5, 613, 1983.

261. Hall CB, McBride JT, Gala CL, et al: Ribavirin treatment of respiratory syncytial virus infection in infants with underlying cardiopulmonary disease, *JAMA* 254:21, 3047, 1985.

262. Smith DW, Frankel LR, Mathers LH, et al: A controlled trial of aerosolized ribavirin in infants receiving mechanical ventilation for severe respiratory syncytial virus infection, *N Engl J Med* 325:1, 24, 1991.

263. Moler FW, Khan AS, Meliones JN, et al: respiratory syncytial virus morbidity and mortality estimates in congenital heart disease patients: a recent experience, *Crit Care Med* 20:1406-1413, 1992.

264. Wald ER and Dashefsky B: Ribavirin Red Book committee recomendations questioned, *Pediatrics* 93:4, 672-673, 1994.

Croup (Laryngotracheobronchitis)

265. Szpumar J, Glowacki J, Laskowski A, et al: Fibrinous laryngotracheobronchitis in children, *Arch Otolaryngol Head Neck Surg* 93:173, 1971.

266. Newth C, Levison H, Bryan AC: The respiratory status of children with croup, *J Pediatr* 81:1068, 1972.

267. Koren G, Frand M, Barzilay Z, et al: Corticosteroid treatment of laryngotracheotitis vs. spasmodic croup in children, *Am J Dis Child* 137:941, 1983.

268. Zach M, Erben A, Olinsky A: Croup, recurrent croup, allergy and airways hyperreactivity, *Arch Dis Child* 56:336, 1981.

269. Cherry JD: Croup. In Feigin RD and Cherry JD, editors: *Textbook of pediatric infectious diseases*, ed 2, Philadelphia, 1987, WB Saunders.

270. Jenny FW, Murphy TR, Clyde WA, et al: Croup: an 11 year study in a pediatric practice, *Pediatrics* 71:871, 1983.

271. Wagner JS, Landan LI, Olinsky A, et al: Management of children hospitalized for laryngotracheobronchitis, *Pediatr Pulmonol* 2:3, 159, 1986.

272. Westey CR, Cotton EK, Brooks JG: Nebulized racemic epinephrine by IPPB for the treatment of croup: a double-blind study, *Am J Dis Child* 132:484, 1978.

273. Baugh F and Gillmore BB: Infectious croup: a critical review, *Otolaryngol Head Neck Surg* 95:40, 1986.

274. Rothrock SG, Pignatiello GA, Howard RM: Radiologic diagnosis of epiglottitis: objective criteria for all ages, *Ann Emerg Med* 19:978, 1990.

275. Schuh S, Huang A, Fallis JC: Atypical epiglottitis, *Ann Emerg Med* 17:2, 168, 1988.

276. Kissoon K and Mitchell I: Adverse effects of racemic epinephrine in epiglottitis, *Pediatr Emerg Care* 1:143, 1985.

277. Skolnik NS: Treatment of croup—a critical review, *Am J Dis Child* 143:1045, 1989.

278. Dulfano MJ, Adler K, Wooten O: Physical properties of sputum. Effects of 100 percent humidity and water mist, *Am Pediatr Respir Dis* 107:130, 1972.

279. Taussig LM, Castro O, Beaudry PH, et al: Treatment of laryngotracheobronchitis (croup), *Am J Dis Child* 129:790, 1975.

280. Fogel JM, Berg IJ, Gerber MA, et al: Racemic epinephrine in the treatment of croup, *J Pediatr* 25:1028, 1982.

281. Kunsela AL and Vesidari T: A randomized double-blind, placebo trial of dexamethasone and racemic epinephrine in the treatment of croup, *Acta Paediatr* 77:99, 1988.

282. Husby S, Agertoft L, Mortensen S, et al: Treatment of croup with nebulized steroids (budesonide), *Arch Dis Child* 68:353, 1993.

283. Remington S and Meakin G: Nebulized adrenaline 1:1000 in the treatment of croup, *Anaesthesia* 41:923, 1986.

284. James JA: Dexamethasone in croup, *Am J Dis Child* 117:511, 1969.

285. Leipzig B, Oski TA, Cummings CW, et al: A prospective randomized study to determine the efficacy of steroids in treatment of croup, *J Pediatr* 94:194, 1979.

286. Muhlendahl KE, Kahn J, Spohr HL, et al: Steroid treatment of pseudo-croup, *Helv Paediatr Acta* 37:431, 1982.

287. Kairys SW, Olmstead BA, O'Connor GT: Steroid treatment of laryngotracheobronchitis: a meta-analysis, *Pediatrics* 83:683, 1989.

288. Super DM, Cartelli NA, Brooks LV, et al: A prospective randomized double-blind study to evaluate the effect of dexamethasone in acute laryngotracheobronchitis, *J Pediatr* 115:2, 323, 1989.

289. Klassen TP, Feldman ME, Waters LK et al: Nebulized budesomide for children with mild-to-moderate croup, *N Engl J Med* 331:285-289, 1994.
290. Barker GA: Current management of croup and epiglottitis, *Pediatr Clin North Am* 26:565, 1979.
291. Zullinger JJ, Schuller DW, Beach TP, et al: Assessment of intubation in croup and epiglottitis, *Am Otol·Rhinol Laryngol* 91:403, 1982.
292. Phelan PD, Landau LI, Olinsky A: Croup. In Phelan PD, Landau LI, Olinsky A, editors: *Respiratory illness in children*, Cambridge, Mass, 1990, Blackwell Scientific Publications.
293. Cressman Wr and Myer CM: Diagnosis and management of croup and epiglottitis: *Pediatr Clin North Am* 41:2, 265-276, 1994.

Epiglottitis

294. Jones HM: Acute epiglottitis: a personal study over twenty years, *Proc Roy Soc Med* 63:706, 1970.
295. Rapkin RH: Simultaneous uvulitis and epiglottitis, *JAMA* 243:1848, 1980.
296. Todd JK: The sore throat—pharyngitis and epiglottitis, *Infect Dis Clin North Am* 2:1, 149, 1988.
297. Faden HS: Treatment of *Haemophilus influenzae* type b epiglottitis, *Pediatrics* 63:402, 1979.
298. Berenberg W and Kelly S: Acute epiglottitis in childhood, *N Engl J Med* 258:870, 1958.
299. Breivik H and Klaastad O: Acute epiglottitis in children, *Br J Anaesth* 50:505, 1978.
300. Lewis JK, Gartner JC, Galvis AG: Protocol for management of acute epiglottitis, *Clin Pediatr (Phila)* 17:494, 1978.
301. Lacroix J, Ahronheim G, Arcand P, et al: Group A streptococcus supraglottitis, *J Pediatr* 109:1, 20, 1986.
302. Schwartz RH, Knerr RJ, Hermansen K, et al: Acute epiglottitis caused by B-hemolytic group C streptococci, *Am J Dis Child* 136:558, 1982.
303. Sarant G: Acute epiglottitis in adults, *Ann Emerg Med* 10:58, 1981.
304. Khilahani U and Khatib R: Acute epiglottitis in adults, *Am J Med Sci* 287:65, 1984.
305. Gorelick MH and Baker MD: Epiglottitis in children, 1979 through 1992, *Arch Pediatr Adolesc Med* 148:47, 1994.
306. Vadheim CM, Greenberg DP, Eriksen E, et al: *Eradication of Hemophilus influenzae* type b disease in Southern California, *Arch Pediatr Adolesc Med* 148:51, 1994.
307. Daum RS and Smith AL: Epiglottitis. In Feigin RD and Cherry JD, editors: *Textbook of pediatric infectious diseases*, ed 2, Philadelphia, 1987, WB Saunders.
308. Barker GA: Current management of croup and epiglottitis, *Pediatr Clin North Am* 26:3, 565, 1979.
309. Baxter JD: Acute epiglottitis in children, *Laryngoscope* 77:1358, 1967.
310. Schuller DE and Birch HG: The safety of intubation in croup and epiglottitis, *Laryngoscope* 85:33, 1975.
311. Harjacek M, Koruberg AE, Yates EW, et al: Thermal epiglottitis after swallowing hot tea, *Pediatr Emerg Care* 8:6, 342-344, 1992.
312. Sendi K and Crysdale WS: Acute epiglottitis—decade of change, *J Otolaryngol* 16:196, 1987.
313. Bass JW, Steele RW, Wiebe RA: Acute epiglottitis: a surgical emergency, *JAMA* 229:671, 1974.
314. Kissoon N and Mitchell I: Adverse effects of racemic epinephrine in epiglottitis, *Pediatr Emerg Care* 3:143, 1985.
315. Schuh S, Huang A, Fallis JC: Atypical epiglottitis, *Ann Emerg Med* 17:2, 168, 1988.
316. Shackelford GD, Siegel MJ, McAllister WH: Subglottic edema in acute epiglottitis in children, *Am J Roentgenol* 131:603, 1978.
317. Gratton-Smith T, Forer M, Kilham H, et al: Viral supraglottitis, *J Pediatr* 110:434, 1987.
318. Warshawski J, Havas TE, McShane D, et al: Adult epiglottitis, *J Otolaryngol* 15(6):362, 1986.
319. Adair JC and Ring WH: Management of epiglottitis in children, *Anaesth Analg* 54:622, 1975.
320. Hannallah R and Rosales JK: Acute epiglottitis: current management and review, *Can J Anaesth* 25(2):84-91, 1978.
321. Costigan DC and Newth CJL: Respiratory studies of children with epiglottitis and without an artificial airway, *Am J Dis Child* 137:139, 1983.
322. Molteni R: Epiglottitis: incidence of epiglottic infection: report of 72 cases and review of the literature, *Pediatrics* 58:526, 1976.

323. Branefors-Holander P and Jeppsson PH: Acute epiglottitis: a clinical, bacteriological and serological study, *Scand J Infect Dis* 7:103, 1975.
324. Margolis CZ, Colletti RB, Grundy G: *Haemophilus influenzae* type b. The etiologic agent in epiglottitis, *J Pediatr* 87:322, 1975.
325. Stankiewicz JA and Bowes AK: Croup and epiglottitis: a radiologic study, *Laryngoscope* 95:1159, 1985.
326. Szold PD and Glicklich M: Children with epiglottitis can be bagged, *Clin Pediatr (Phila)* 15:792, 1976.
327. Diaz JA: Croup and epiglottitis in children: the anaesthesiologist and a diagnostician, *Anesth Analg* 64:621, 1985.
328. Fried MP: Controversies in the management of supraglottitis and croup, *Pediatr Clin North Am* 26:931, 1979.
329. Oh TH and Motoyama ED: Comparisons of nasotracheal intubation and tracheotomy in management of acute epiglottitis, *Anesthesiology* 46:214, 1977.
330. Granoff DM and Daum RS: Spread of *Haemophilus influenzae* type b: recent epidemiologic and therapeutic considerations, *J Pediatr* 97:854, 1980.

Tracheitis

331. Fried MP: Controversies in the management of supraglottitis and croup, *Pediatr Clin North Am* 26:931, 1979.
332. Edwards KM, Dundon MC, Alte WA: Bacterial tracheitis as a complication of viral croup, *Pediatr Infect Dis J* 2:390, 1983.
333. Liston S, Gehrz R, Jarvis C: Bacterial tracheitis, *Arch Otolaryngol Head Neck Surg* 107:561, 1981.
334. Naqui SH and Dunkle LM: Bacterial tracheitis and viral croup, *Pediatr Infect Dis J* 3:282, 1981.
335. Denneny JC and Handler SD: Membranous laryngotracheotrachitis, *Pediatrics* 70:705, 1982.
336. Nelson WE: Bacterial croup: a historical perspective, *J Pediatr* 105:52, 1984.
337. Friedman EM, Jorgensen K, Healy GB, et al: Bacterial tracheitis—two year experience, *Laryngoscope* 95:9, 1985.
338. Jones R, Santos JI, Overall JC: Bacterial tracheitis, *JAMA* 242:721, 1979.
339. Sofer S, Duncan P, Chernick V: Bacterial tracheitis—an old disease rediscovered, *Clin Pediatr (Phila)* 22:6, 407, 1983.
340. Cheseand M, Ledre F, Marsenot A: Bacterial croup and toxic shock syndrome, *Eur J Pediatr* 145:306, 1986.
341. Henry RC, Mellis CM, Benjamin B: Pseudomembranous croup, *Arch Dis Child* 58:3, 180, 1983.
342. Phelan PD, Landau LI, Olinsky A: Tracheitis. In Phelan PD: *Respiratory illness in children*, ed 3, Cambridge, Mass, 1990, Blackwell Scientific Publications.

Pleural Disease

343. Pagtakhan RD and Montgomery MD: Pleurisy and emphysema. In Chernich V, editor: *Kendig's disorders of the respiratory tract in children*, ed 5, Philadelphia, 1990, WB Saunders.
344. Sahebjami H and London RG: Pleural effusion: pathophysiology and clinical features, *Semin Roentgenol* 12(4):269, 1977.
345. Light RW: Pleural effusions, *Med Clin North Am* 61(6):1339, 1977.
346. Light RW, MacGregor MI, Luchsinger DC, et al: Pleural effusions: the diagnostic separation of transudates and exudates, *Ann Intern Med* 77:507, 1972.
347. Wolfe WG, Spock A, Bradford WB: Pleural fluid in infants and children, *Am J Respir Crit Care Med* 98:1027, 1968.
348. Carr DT and Power MH: Clinical values of measurements of concentration of protein in pleural fluid, *N Engl J Med* 259:926, 1958.
349. Paddock FR: The diagnostic significance of serous fluids in disease, *N Engl J Med* 223:1010, 1940.
350. Leuallen E and Carr D: Pleural effusion: a statistical study of 436 patients, *N Engl J Med* 252:79, 1955.
351. Jay SJ: Diagnostic procedures for pleural disease, *Clin Chest Med* 6(1):33, 1985.
352. Brook I: Microbiology of empyema in children and adolescents, *Pediatrics* 85(5):722, 1990.
353. Freif BJ, Kusmiez H, Nelson JD, et al: Parapneumonic effusions and empyema in hospitalized children: a retrospective review of 227 cases, *Pediatr Infect Dis J* 3(6):578, 1984.
354. Fajardo JE and Chang MJ: Pleural empyema in children: a nationwide retrospective study, *South Med J* 80(5):593, 1987.

355. Kinasewitz GT, Penn RL, George RB: The spectrum and significance of pleural disease in blastomycosis, *Chest* 86(4):580, 1984.

356. Chenoweth CE, Singal S, Pearson RD, et al: Acquired Immunodeficiency Syndrome—related visceral leishmaniasis presenting in a pleural effusion, *Chest* 103(2):648, 1993.

357. Horowitz ML, Schiff M, Samuels J: *Pneumocystis carnii* pleural effusion, *Am J Respir Crit Care Med* 148:232, 1993.

358. Rosenow EC III: Drug-induced bronchopulmonary pleural disease, *J Allergy Clin Immunol* 80(6):780, 1987.

359. Swischuk LE: *Emergency imaging of the acutely ill or injured child*, ed 3, Baltimore, 1994, Williams and Wilkins.

360. Henschke CI, Davis SD, Romano DM, et al: The pathogenesis, radiologic evaluation, and therapy of pleural effusions, *Radiol Clin North Am* 27(6):1241, 1989.

361. Glasier CM, Leithisor RE, Williamson SL, et al: Extracardiac chest ultrasonography in infants and children: radiographic and clinical implications, *J Pediatr* 114(4):540, 1989.

362. Rothlin MA, Naf R, Amgwerd M, et al: Ultrasound in blunt abdominal and thoracic trauma, *J Trauma* 34(4):488, 1993.

363. Leung AN, Muller NL, Miller RR: CT in differential diagnosis of diffuse pleural disease, *Am J Radiol* 154:487, 1990.

364. Aquino SL, Webb WR, Gushiken BJ: Pleural exudates and transudates: diagnosis with contrast-enhanced CT, *Radiology* 192:803, 1994.

365. Klein JS, Schultz S, Heffner JE: Interventional radiology of the chest: image-guided percutaneous drainage of pleural effusions, lung abscess, and pneumothorax, *Am J Radiol* 164:581, 1995.

366. Light RW, Erozan YC, Ball WC Jr: Cells in pleural fluid: their value in differential diagnosis, *Arch Intern Med* 132(6):854, 1973.

367. Light RW and Ball WC Jr: Glucose and amylase in pleural effusions, *JAMA* 225(3):257, 1973.

368. Hoff SJ, Neblett WW, Edwards RM, et al: Parapneumonic empyema in children: decortication hastens recovery in patients with severe pleural infections, *Pediatr Infect Dis J* 10(3):194, 1991.

369. Heffner JE, Brown LK, Barbieri C, et al: Pleural fluid chemical analysis in parapneumonic effusions: a meta-analysis, *Am J Respir Crit Care Med* 151:1700, 1995.

Pneumonia

370. Barkin RM: Pneumonia. In Barkin RM and Rosen P, editors: *Emergency pediatrics*, ed 3, St Louis, 1990, Mosby.

371. Grossman LK: Pneumonia in infants and children, *Compr Ther* 12(4):15, 1986.

372. Campbell II PW: Pneumonias. In Rudolph AM, Hoffman JIE, Rudolph CD, editors: *Pediatrics*, ed 20, Stamford, Connecticut, 1996, Appleton and Lange.

373. Henderson FW: Pulmonary infections with respiratory syncytial virus and the parainfluenza viruses, *Semin Respir Infect* 2(2):112, 1987.

374. Khampirad T and Glezen WP: Clinical and radiographic assessment of acute lower respiratory tract disease in infants and children, *Semin Respir Infect* 2(2):130, 1987.

375. Loda FA, Clyde WA Jr, Glezen WP, et al: Studies on the role of viruses, bacteria, and *M. pneumoniae* as causes of lower respiratory tract infections in children, *J Pediatr* 72(2):161, 1968.

376. Glezen WP, Collier AM, Loda FA: Significance of *Diplococcus pneumoniae* and *Haemophilus influenzae* cultured from the nasopharynx of children, *Pediatr Res* 8:425, 1974.

377. Teele D: Pneumonia: antimicrobial therapy for infants and children, *Pediatr Infect Dis J* 4(3):330, 1985.

378. Gilsdorf JR: Community-acquired pneumonia in children, *Semin Respir Infect* 2(2):146, 1987.

379. Rettig PJ: Infections due to *Chlamydia trachomatis* from infancy to adolescence, *Pediatr Infect Dis J* 5(4):449, 1986.

380. Lewis K: Pertussis. In Rudolph AM, Hoffman JIE, Rudolph CD, editors: *Pediatrics*, ed 20, Stamford, Connecticut, 1996, Appleton and Lange.

381. Denny FW and Clyde WA Jr: Acute lower respiratory tract infections in nonhospitalized children, *J Pediatr* 108(5):635, 1986.

382. American Academy of Pediatrics: *Haemophilus influenzae* infections. In Peter G, editor: *1994 Red Book: Report of the Committee on Infectious Diseases*, ed 23, Elk Grove Village, IL, 1994, American Academy of Pediatrics.

383. Asmar BI, Slovis TL, Reed JO, et al: *Haemophilus influenzae* type b pneumonia in 43 children, *J Pediatr* 93(3):389, 1979.

384. Ginsburg CM, Howard JB, Nelson JD: Report of 65 cases of *Haemophilus influenzae* b pneumonia, *Pediatrics* 64(3):283, 1979.

385. Al-Ujayli B, Nafziger DA, Saravolatz L: Pneumonia due to *Staphylococcus aureus* infection, *Clin Chest Med* 16(1):111, 1995.

386. Leigh MW and Clyde WA Jr: Chlamydial and mycoplasmal pneumonias, *Semin Respir Infect* 2(2):146, 1987.

387. Hammerschlag MR: Atypical pneumonias in children. *Adv Pediatr Infect Dis* 10:1, 1995.

388. Inselman LS: Tuberculosis in children: an unsettling forecast, *Contemp Pediatr* 7:10, 1990.

389. McCarthy PL, Frank AL, Ablow RC, et al: Value of the C-reactive protein test in the differentiation of bacterial and viral pneumonia, *J Pediatr* 92(4):454, 1978.

390. Isaacs D: Problems in determining the etiology of community-acquired childhood pneumonia, *Pediatr Infect Dis J* 8(3):143, 1989.

391. Grossman M, Klein JO, McCarthy PL, et al: Consensus and management of presumed bacterial pneumonia in ambulatory children, *Pediatr Infect Dis J* 3(6):497, 1984.

392. Swischuk LE: *Emergency imaging of the acutely ill or injured child*, ed 3, Baltimore, 1994, Williams and Wilkins.

393. Courtoy I, Lande AE, Turner RB: Accuracy of radiographic differentiation of bacterial from nonbacterial pneumonia, *Pediatrics* 28(6):;261, 1989.

394. Sabato AR, Martin AJ, Marmion BP, et al: *Mycoplasma pneumoniae*: acute illness, antibiotics, and subsequent pulmonary function, *Arch Dis Child* 59(11):1034, 1984.

Pulmonary Edema

395. Robin ED, Cross CE, Zelis R: Pulmonary edema, parts 1 and 2, *N Engl J Med* 288(5,6):239, 292, 1973.

396. Barkin RM: Pulmonary edema. In Barkin RM and Rosen P, editors: *Emergency pediatrics*, ed 3, St Louis, 1990, Mosby.

397. Bland RD: Edema formation in newborn lung, *Clin Perinatol* 9:593, 1982.

398. West JB: *Respiratory physiology—the essentials*, ed 4, Baltimore, 1990, Williams and Wilkins.

399. Mellins RB: Pulmonary edema. In Chernick V, editor: *Kendig's disorders of the respiratory tract in children*, ed 5, Philadelphia, 1990, WB Saunders.

400. Albus WH and Nadas AS: Unilateral chronic pulmonary edema and pleural effusion after systemic-pulmonary artery shunts for cyanotic congenital heart disease, *Am J Cardiol* 19:861, 1967.

401. Opdyke DF, Duomarco J, Dillion WH, et al: Study of simultaneous right and left atrial pressure pulses under normal and experimentally altered conditions, *Am J Physiol* 154:258, 1948.

402. Alexander GS: The ultrastructure of the pulmonary alveolar vessels in Mendelson's (acid pulmonary aspiration) syndrome, *Br J Anaesth* 40(6):408, 1968.

403. Brigham KL, Bowers RE, Haynes J: Increased sheep lung vascular permeability caused by *Escherichia coli* endotoxin, *Circ Res* 45(2):292, 1979.

404. Ramsey HW, Synder GK, Taylor WJ: Pulmonary hemodynamics after infusion of *Micrurus f. fulvius* (coral) venom, *Clin Res* 19(2):355, 1971.

405. Amaral CFS, de Rezende NA, Freire-Maia L: Acute pulmonary edema after *Tityus Serrulatus* scorpion sting in children, *Am J Cardiol* 71:242, 1992.

406. Massumi RA and Legier JF: Rheumatic pneumonitis, *Circulation* 33:417, 1966.

407. Peitzman AB, Shires GT, Texidor HS, et al: Smoke inhalation injury: evaluation of radiographic manifestations and pulmonary dysfunction, *J Trauma* 29(9):1232, 1989.

408. Clark DG, McElligott TF, Hurst EW: The toxicity of paraquat, *Br J Ind Med* 23:126, 1966.

409. Efferen L, Palat D, Meisner J: Nonfatal pulmonary edema following cocaine smoking, *NY State J Med* 89(7):415, 1989.

410. Batlle MA and Wilcox WD: Pulmonary edema in an infant following passive inhalation of free-base ("Crack") cocaine, *Clin Pediatr*, Feb 1993:105.

411. Frand UI, Shim CS, Williams MH Jr: Methadone-induced pulmonary edema, *Ann Intern Med* 76(6):975, 1972.

412. Steinberg AD and Karliner JS: The clinical spectrum of heroin pulmonary edema, *Arch Intern Med* 122:122, August 1968.

413. Kanter RK and Watchko JF: Pulmonary edema associated with upper airway obstruction, *Am J Dis Child* 138:356, 1984.

414. Galvis AG: Pulmonary edema complicating relief of upper airway obstruction, *Am J Emerg Med* 5(4):294, 1987.

415. Halow KD and Ford EG: Pulmonary edema following postoperative laryngospasm: a case report and review of the literature, *Am Surg* 59:444, 1993.

416. Sofer S, Weinhouse E, Tal A, et al: Cor pulmonale due to adenoidal or tonsillar hypertrophy or both in children, *Chest* 93(1):119, 1988.

417. Rabold M: High-altitude pulmonary edema: a collective review, *Am J Emerg Med* 7(4):426, 1989.

418. Theodore J and Robin ED: Speculations on neurogenic pulmonary edema (NPE), *Am J Respir Crit Care Med* 113:405, 1976.

419. Mulroy JJ, Michell JJ, Tong TK, et al: Postictal pulmonary edema in children, *Neurology* 35:403, 1985.

420. Swischuk LE: *Emergency radiology of the acutely ill or injured child*, ed 3, Baltimore, 1994, Williams and Wilkins.

Pulmonary Embolism

421. Dunmire SM: Pulmonary embolism, *Emerg Med Clin North Am* 7(2):339, 1989.

422. Goldhaber SZ: Thrombolysis for pulmonary embolism, *Prog Cardiovasc Dis* 34:113, 1991.

423. Freijman DG, Suyemoto J, Wessler S: Frequency of pulmonary thromboembolism in man, *N Engl J Med* 272:1278, 1965.

424. Evans DA and Wilmott RW: Pulmonary embolism in children, *Pediatr Clin North Am* 41(3):569, 1994.

425. Buck JR, Connors RH, Coon WW, et al: Pulmonary embolism in children, *J Pediatr Surg* 16(3):385, 1981.

426. Byard RW and Cuz E: Sudden and unexpected death in infancy and childhood due to pulmonary thromboembolism, *Arch Pathol Lab Med* 114:142, 1990.

427. Andrew M, David M, Adams M, et al: Venous thromboembolic complications (VTE) in children: first analyses of the Canadian registry of VTE, *Blood* 83(5):1251, 1994.

428. Zimmerman SS: Pulmonary embolism. In Zimmerman SS and Gilden JH, editors: *Critical care pediatrics*, Philadelphia, 1985, WB Saunders.

429. Bell WR, Simon TL, Stengle JM, et al: The urokinase-streptokinase pulmonary embolism trial (phase II) results, *Circulation* 50:1070, 1974.

430. Shackford SR and Moser KM: Deep venous thrombosis and pulmonary embolism in trauma patients, *J Intensive Care Med* 3(1):87, 1988.

431. Desai MH, Linares HA, Hemdon DN: Pulmonary embolism in burned children, *Burns* 15(6):376, 1989.

432. McBride WJ, Gadowski GR, Keller MS, et al: Pulmonary embolism in pediatric trauma patients, *J Trauma* 37(6):913, 1994.

433. Berenstein D, Coupy S, Schonberg SK: Pulmonary embolism in adolescents, *Am J Dis Child* 140:667, 1986.

434. Whitlock JA, Janco RL, Phillips JA: Inherited hypercoagulable states in children, *Am J Pediatr Hematol Oncol* 11(2):170, 1989.

435. Mehls O, Andrassy K, Koderisch J, et al: Hemostasis and thromboembolism in children with nephrotic syndrome: differences from adults, *J Pediatr* 110(6):862, 1987.

436. Leiby JM, Purcell H, DeMaria JJ, et al: Pulmonary embolism as a result of Hickman catheter-related thrombosis, *Am J Med* 86:228, 1989.

437. Collery CM, Sullivan ID, Bauraind O, et al: Thrombosis and embolism in long-term central venous access for parenteral nutrition, *Lancet* 344:1043, 1994.

438. Shulman St and Grossman BJ: Fat embolism in childhood, *Am J Dis Child* 120:480, 1970.

439. Barkin RM: Cardiovascular disorders. In Barkin RM and Rosen P, editors: *Emergency pediatrics*, ed 3, St Louis, 1990, Mosby.

440. Kutty K: Pulmonary embolism: how to nail down the diagnosis, *Postgrad Med* 88:72, 1990.

441. The PISA-PED Investigators: invasive and noninvasive diagnosis of pulmonary embolism: preliminary results of the Prospective Investigative Study of Acute Pulmonary Embolism Diagnosis (PISA-PED), *Chest* 107(1):33S, 1995.

442. Greenspan RH, Ravin CE, Polansky SM, et al: Accuracy of the chest radiograph in the diagnosis of pulmonary embolism, *Invest Radiol* 17(6):539, 1982.

443. Hull RD, Hirsh J, Carter CJ, et al: Diagnostic value of ventilation perfusion lung scanning in patients with suspected pulmonary embolism, *Chest* 88(6):819, 1985.

444. Goodman PC: Pulmonary angiography, *Clin Chest Med* 5(3):465, 1984.

445. Henschke CI, Mateescu I, Yankelevitz DF: Changing practice patterns in the workup of pulmonary embolism, *Chest* 107(4):940, 1995.

446. van Rooijh W-JJ, den Heeten GJ, Sluzewski M: Pulmonary embolism: diagnosis in 211 patients with use of selective pulmonary digital subtraction angiography with a flow-directed catheter, *Radiology* 195(3):793, 1995.

447. Teigen CL, Maus TP, Sheedy II PF, et al: Pulmonary embolism: diagnosis with contrast-enhanced electron-beam CT and comparison with pulmonary angiography, *Radiology* 19492):313, 1995.

448. Agnelli G: Anticoagulation in the prevention and treatment of pulmonary embolism, *Chest* 107(1):39S, 1995.

449. Robinson PJ: Lung scintigraphy: doubt and certainty in the diagnosis of pulmonary embolism, *Clin Radiology* 40:557, 1989.

450. The urokinase-streptokinase embolism trial: phase II results, *JAMA* 229(12):1606, 1974.

451. Goldhaber SZ, Marks JE, Meyerwitz MF, et al: Acute pulmonary embolism treated with tissue plasminogen activator, *Lancet* 2:886, 1986.

452. Levy M, Benson LN, Burrows PE, et al: Tissue plasminogen activator for the treatment of thromboembolism in infants and children, *J Pediatr* 118(3):467, 1991.

453. Pyles L, Peirpont MEM, Steiner ME: Fibrinolysis by tissue plasminogen activator in a child with pulmonary embolism, *J Pediatr* 116(5):801, 1990.

Sudden Infant Death Syndrome (SIDS)

454. Merritt TA, Bauer WI, Hasselmeyer EG: Sudden infant death syndrome: the role of the emergency room physician, *Clin Pediatr* 14:1095, 1975.

455. Naeye RL: Sudden infant death, *Sci Am* 242:56, 1980.

456. Hoffman HJ, Damus K, Hillman L, et al: Risk factors for SIDS: results of the National Institute of Child Health and Human Development SIDS cooperative epidemiological study, *Ann NY Acad Sci* 533:13, 1988.

457. Kelly DH and Shannon DC: Sudden infant death syndrome and near sudden infant death syndrome: a review of the literature, 1964-1982, *Pediatr Clin North Am* 29:1241, 1982.

458. Grether JK and Schulman J: Sudden infant death syndrome and birth weight, *J Pediatr* 114:561, 1989.

459. Dwyer T and Ponsonby AL: SIDS epidemiology and incidence, *Pediatr Ann* 24:7:350-356, 1995.

460. Chavez CJ, Ostrea EM, Stryker JC, et al: Sudden infant death syndrome among infants of drug dependent mothers, *J Pediatr* 95:407, 1979.

461. Church NR, Anas NG, Hall CB, et al: Respiratory synctial virus. Related apnea in infants, *Am J Dis Child* 138:247, 1984.

462. Kemp JS and Thach BT: Sudden death in infants sleeping on polystyrene-filled cushions, *N Engl J Med* 324:26:1858-1864, 1991.

463. Miller JM and Redgrave AP: Overheating and cot death, *Lancet* 338:1595, 1991.

464. Ponsonby AL, Dwyer T, Gibbons LE, et al: Factors potentiating the risk of sudden infant death syndrome associated with the prone position, *N Engl J Med* 329:6,378-382, 1993.

465. Kattwinkel J, Brooks J, Myerberg D: Positioning and SIDS: AAP Task Force on Infant Positioning and SIDS, *Pediatrics* 89:6:1120-1126, 1992.

466. Dwyer T, Ponsonby AL, Blizzard L, et al: The contribution of changes in the prevalence of prone sleeping position to the decline of sudden infant death syndrome in Tasmania, *JAMA* 273:10:783-789, 1995.

467. Mitchell EA, Brunt JM, Everard C: Reduction in mortality from sudden infant death syndrome in New Zealand: 1986-92, *Arch Dis Child* 70:291-294, 1994.

468. Freed GE, Steinschneider A, Glassman M, et al: Sudden infant death syndrome prevention and an understanding of selected clinical issues, *Pediatr Clin North Am* 41:5:967-990, 1994.

469. Willinger M: SIDS prevention, *Pediatr Ann* 24:358-364, 1995.

470. Klonoff-Cohen HS, Edelstein SL, Lefkowitz ES, et al: The effect of passive smoking and tobacco exposure through breast milk on sudden infant death syndrome, *JAMA* 273:10:795-798, 1995.

471. Bergman AB, Ray CC, Pomeroy MA et al: Students of sudden infant death syndrome in King County, Washington. III. Epidemiology, *Pediatrics* 49:860, 1972.

472. Peterson DR, Sabotta EE, Daling JR: Infant mortality among subsequent siblings of infants who died of sudden infant syndrome, *J Pediatr* 108:911, 1986.

473. Griffin MR, Ray WA, Livingood JR: Risk of sudden infant death syndrome after immunization with the diphtheria-tetanus-pertussis vaccine, *N Engl J Med* 319:618, 1988.

474. Haidmayer R and Kenner T: Physiological approaches to respiratory control mechanisms in infants: assessing the risk of SIDS, *Ann NY Acad Sci* 533:377, 1988.

475. National Institutes of Health Consensus Development Conference on Infantile Apnea and Home Monitoring: Consensus statement, *Pediatrics* 79:292, 1987.

476. Valdes-Dapena M: Sudden infant death syndrome: overview of recent research developments from a pediatric pathologist's perspective, *Pediatrician* 15:222, 1988.

477. Southall DP and Talbert DG: Mechanisms for abnormal apnea of possible relevance to the sudden infant death syndrome, *Ann NY Acad Sci* 533:329, 1988.

478. Beckwith JB: Intrathoracic petechial hemorrhages. A clue to the mechanisms of sudden infant death syndrome? *Ann NY Acad Sci* 533:37, 1988.

479. Giulian GG, Gilbert EF, Moss RL: Elevated fetal hemoglobin levels in sudden infant death syndrome, *N Engl J Med* 316:1122, 1987.

480. Schwartz PJ: The quest for the mechanisms of sudden infant death syndrome: doubts and progress, *Circulation* 75:53, 1987.

481. Valdes-Dapena M: The postmortem examination, *Pediatri Ann* 24:7:365-372, 1995.

482. Krugman RD, Bays JA, Chadwick DL, et al: Distinguishing sudden infant death syndrome from child abuse fatalities: Committee on Child Abuse and Neglect, *Pediatrics* 94:1:124-126, 1994.

483. Bass M, Kravath RE, Glass L: Death-scene investigation in sudden infant death, *N Engl J Med* 315:100, 1986.

484. Hunt CE and Brouillette RT: Methylxanthine treatment in infants at risk for sudden infant death syndrome, *Ann NY Acad Sci* 533:119, 1988.

485. Kahn A, Blum D, Muller MF, et al: Sudden infant death syndrome in a town: a comparison of sibling histories, *Pediatrics* 78:146, 1986.

486. McElroy E, Steinschneider A, Weinstein S: Emotional and health impact of home monitoring on mothers: a controlled prospective study, *Pediatrics* 78:780, 1986.

487. Elders JM: Reducing the risk of sudden infant death syndrome, *JAMA* 272:21:1646, 1994.

488. Smialek Z: Observations on immediate reactions of families to sudden infant death, *Pediatrics* 63:670, 1978.

489. Limerick S: Family and health-professional interactions, *Ann NY Acad Sci* 533:145, 1988.

490. Schwartz LZ: The origin of maternal feelings of guilt in SIDS: relationship with the normal psychological reactions to maternity, *Ann NY Acad Sci* 533:132, 1988.

491. Mandell F, McClain M, Reece R: The sudden infant death syndrome: siblings and their place in the family, *Ann NY Acad Sci* 533:129, 1988.

Urinary and Renal Disorders

JOSEPH A. WEINBERG

Julio Castillo • Felton E. Combest • Earl R. Dixon • Martin I. Herman • Amy L. Hertz
• Warren L. Hutcheson • John G. Knepper • James A. O'Donnell II • Mary P. Sweeney • David G. Ward

The urinary tract is a common source of problems confronting practitioners who treat ill and injured children. Disorders such as urinary tract infection (UTI) and phimosis are routine, whereas acute renal failure occurs less frequently. Traumatic injuries to the urinary tract are discussed in Chapter 25.

The kidney serves as the primary filter, maintaining internal homeostasis. An endocrine organ, it produces renin, erythropoietin, prostaglandins, and 1,25-hydroxyvitamin D and is a target organ of the hormones aldosterone and vasopressin.

A full complement of nephrons is generally present at birth; nephron induction ceases at approximately 26 weeks of gestation. Newborn nephrons have underdeveloped, heterogeneous proximal tubules. There is an elevenfold difference in length between the longest and shortest proximal tubules in infants compared to a twofold variability in adults. Glomeruli also vary in size and this correlates with their respective tubules.[1] This size variability disappears by the time the child is 12 to 14 months. As individual nephrons grow, there is elongation of the loops of Henle and increased tortuosity of the proximal convoluted tubules.[2]

The remainder of the urinary system develops synchronously with the renal bud. The separation of the urinary system from the rectum occurs at about the sixth week. The urachus normally is a fibrous remnant of the ureteral bud. Lower tract obstruction can inhibit this process resulting in a patent urachus with urine being excreted at the umbilical cord. Fetal urine is excreted into the bladder by 10 to 11 weeks of gestation.

The male genitalia are induced by proteins coded on the Y chromosome starting in the seventh to eighth week of gestation. The primitive gonad develops into a testis and the mesonephric duct into wolffian ducts. The absence of the Y chromosome factors allows differentiation of the ovary and the müllerian duct system. The urogenital sinus and genital tubercle will develop into separate urinary and genital structures of the male and female perineum; the testes ultimately migrate into the scrotal sac.

Because the placenta is the major homeostatic organ in utero, renal blood flow and glomerular filtration rate (GFR) are low before birth and correlate with gestational age at birth. These values are approximately 10% of adult values at term and reach maturation by 12 to 24 months of age. The mean GFR at birth is 38 ml/min/1.73 m^2, at 1 year 77 ml/min/1.73 m^2, and 1.31 ml/min/1.73 m^2 and 117 ml/min/1.73 m^2 in adult males and females, respectively. This maturation increase in GFR with age must be taken into account in calculating dosages of renal excreted drugs, interpreting laboratory values, and calculating fluid requirements (see box on p. 1128).

A normal 1-year-old child would be expected to have a creatinine level of 0.375 mg/dl. A level of 1.0 mg/dl can represent a significant change in GFR in that child (Table 60-1).[5]

Tubular function also continues to mature postnatally.[6] Newborn infants have a limited ability to conserve sodium and excrete a sodium load. They can only concentrate urine to 400 to 600 mOsm/L. These tubular functions mature by 3 months of age. Tubular reabsorption of glucose does not reach maturation until 12 to 24 months of age.

GFR Estimation

GFR can be estimated from plasma creatinine (Pcr) by the formulas

GFR = 0.45 L/Pcr for full-term infants in the first year of life

GFR = 0.55 L/Pcr in older children

where L = length in centimeters.[3] Schwartz has also estimated Pcr for individuals 1 to 20 years of age with the formulas[4]

Pcr (mg/dl) = 0.35 + 0.025 × age (yrs) for males

Pcr (mg/dl) = 0.35 + 0.018 × age (yrs) for females

TABLE 60-1. Plasma Creatinine Levels at Different Ages

Age	Height (cm)	True plasma creatinine (mg/dl) Mean	Range (±2SD)
Cord blood		0.75	0.51-0.99
0-2 weeks	50	0.50	0.34-0.66
2-26 weeks	60	0.39	0.23-0.55
1 year	70	0.32	0.18-0.46
2 years	87	0.32	0.20-0.44
4 years	101	0.37	0.25-0.49
6 years	114	0.43	0.27-0.59
8 years	126	0.48	0.31-0.65
10 years	137	0.52	0.34-0.70
12 years	147	0.59	0.41-0.78
Adult male	174	0.97	0.72-1.22
Adult female	163	0.77	0.53-1.01

Conversion factor µmol/L = mg/dl × 88.4.
From Chantler C and Barratt TM: Laboratory evaluation. In Holliday MA, Barratt TM, Vernier RL, editors: *Pediatric nephrology,* Baltimore, 1987, Williams & Wilkins.

Signs and Symptoms

DYSURIA AND PYURIA

AMY L. HERTZ

Dysuria, marked by painful or difficult urination, may be present throughout or toward the end of micturition, indicating inflammation of the urinary tract. Dysuria may be associated with pelvic or suprapubic pain. These symptoms may be helpful in determining the cause of the dysuria. Occasionally, systemic symptoms such as fever, nausea, and vomiting may also be present.

Pyuria, the presence of white blood cells (WBCs) in the urine, is a sign of inflammation of the genital region or urinary tract. The presence of ≤10 WBC/mm^3 has been associated with a higher incidence of true UTIs compared to <10 WBC/mm^3, which has been associated with sterile urine cultures.[7] Pyuria may also be present with urethritis

---

Etiologies of Dysuria

Infections
Urinary tract infection; cystitis (bacterial or viral) or pyelonephritis
Vaginitis or urethritis
Balanitis
Pinworms

Irritants
Bubble bath
Feminine hygiene products
Soaps and douches containing perfumes and certain chemicals

Trauma
Masturbation
Sexual or physical abuse
Straddle injury
Foreign body causing local trauma or inflammation

Other
Labial adhesions
Hypercalciuria
Stones

---

and vaginitis in adolescent females and urethritis in adolescent males. Balanitis in a young male may also be a cause of pyuria. Because of the many etiologies of pyuria and dysuria, it is imperative to document any infectious cause with the appropriate cultures (e.g., urine, vaginal, or urethral discharge).

Differential Considerations

Although infection is the most common cause of dysuria, many other possible causes must be evaluated (see box above). Certain etiologies vary with patient age. Cystitis causes the classic triad of dysuria, urgency, and frequency of urination. Pyelonephritis generally causes flank pain and fever. Other constitutional symptoms may also be present. In adolescent females, vaginitis can result from a number of organisms, including *Trichomonas vaginalis, Candida albicans, Gardnerella vaginalis,* and bacterial overgrowth from a foreign body. These organisms cause periurethral and perivaginal irritation, inflammation, and resultant dysuria. Urethritis and cervicitis are most commonly caused by *Chlamydia trachomatis* and *Neisseria gonorrhoeae.* Infections with these two organisms account for approximately 10% of dysuria in the adolescent female.[8] Pelvic inflammatory disease should be considered in an adolescent female who presents with lower abdominal pain and fever. A vaginal discharge may or may not be present. Infection with *C. trachomatis* is associated with the presence of endocervical mucopus and the microscopic finding of 10 or more WBCs per high power field in cervical mucus.[9]

Common irritants include bubble bath, shampoo, feminine hygiene products, powders, and soaps. In younger children, pinworms *(Enterobius vermicularis)* may cause dysuria and vaginitis because of the abrasions that result from periurethral and perivaginal itching and subsequent scratching. In young, uncircumcised boys, balanitis can cause dysuria and pyuria.

Trauma to the area, such as a straddle injury may result in abrasions and local inflammation. Foreign bodies in the vagina may cause dysuria and pyuria. There is often an associated vaginal discharge present. One must look carefully for evidence of sexual or physical abuse because the history is often denied. Masturbation may also cause dysuria, although this history is often difficult to obtain. Finally, there have been reports that labial adhesions or fusion can cause dysuria in young, prepubertal girls.[10]

Diagnostic Work-Up

The history is very important when evaluating a child with a chief complaint of dysuria. One must question the patient about use of hygiene products, bubble baths, soaps, and other irritants. Trauma to the area may not always be evident and often the patient does not remember a minor injury. A history of abuse or masturbation is often difficult to obtain and is often denied by the patient.

A physical examination with emphasis on the genitourinary tract should be performed when evaluating a child with dysuria. It is important to rule in or out an infectious cause of the dysuria; this is based on history, physical examination, and subsequent cultures. When no other signs or symptoms are present, it is imperative to carefully examine the genitalia. Abrasions, tears, foreign bodies, erythema, edema, and discharge are all helpful diagnostic signs. A pelvic examination should be performed on all adolescent females with dysuria, pelvic pain, and a vaginal discharge.[11] One must consider a diagnosis of hypercalciuria in some children with persistent dysuria in whom infectious and other causes have been ruled out. These children generally have an increased urinary calcium excretion.[12]

Ancillary Data. It is imperative to document the infectious causes of dysuria with the proper cultures. Urine should be collected using sterile technique and sent immediately for urinalysis and culture. The specimen may be obtained either by clean-catch or bladder catheterization, depending on the age and level of cooperation of the patient. Leukocytes present in the urine usually are indicative of a UTI, although it is possible to have a UTI without pyuria.[13] Conversely, pyuria may be present without an infectious cause, as in a febrile or dehydrated child. One may want to recollect the urine after a child has been adequately hydrated. Chemical irritants may also produce pyuria resulting from the inflammation of the urethral mucosa.

A urethral or vaginal discharge from a female or a urethral discharge from a male suggests an infection of the genitalia. Most often these infections are the result of sexually transmitted diseases such as gonorrhea or chlamydia.[3] A gram stain that shows gram-negative intracellular diplococci is indicative of *N. gonorrhoeae* in a prepubertal female. In this instance one must immediately suspect sexual abuse. Normal vaginal flora from a postpubertal female may have the same appearance as *N. gonorrhoeae*. Therefore it is necessary to culture any vaginal, cervical, or

---

> ### Measures to Prevent Dysuria
>
> Wear cotton undergarments
> Use only warm water, not soap, to clean genital area
> Avoid using feminine hygiene products
> Avoid using bubble baths
> Wipe front to back (females)
> Urinate after intercourse

urethral discharge before beginning treatment on any patient.

Poor personal hygiene is a common cause of dysuria, especially in young girls. Many of these patients present with vulvovaginitis, with or without a vaginal discharge. Most prepubertal girls with either vulvitis or normal appearing genitalia will have relief of their symptoms once their hygiene has improved or a local irritant has been removed.[14]

Therapeutic Trials

In cases of dysuria as a result of chemical urethritis, warm sitz baths are helpful in relieving some of the discomfort. Educating both the patient and parents about proper hygiene is often the key to preventing future episodes of dysuria (see box above). Treatment of associated vaginal pathology may be curative.

HEMATURIA

JOSEPH A. WEINBERG

Hematuria is the presence of blood in the urine. The blood can be visible to the naked eye (macroscopic) and may have clots appearing in the urine. Hematuria may be detected only through the use of chemical reagent strips and microscopic urinalysis (microscopic). The following section discusses nontraumatic hematuria; traumatic hematuria is discussed in Chapter 25.

Up to 1 million red blood cells (RBCs) are excreted in the urine in overnight collections in normal people, using Addis counts or cell counts reporting RBCs/ml. Greater than 100,000 RBCs in a 12-hour urine or 6 RBCs/mm^3 in a counting chamber is abnormal. The most common method of reporting is RBCs/high power field (HPF). Good evidence exists that 8 RBCs/HPF under phase microscopy or 2 to 3 RBCs/HPF by light microscopy should be investigated.[15,16] The incidence of asymptomatic hematuria ranges from 0.15% to 4.1% of school-aged children based on a single specimen and less than 1% on recurrent testing. Experts argue about the definition and significance of asymptomatic hematuria in children.[17]

Pathophysiology

RBCs can enter the urine throughout the urinary tract from the glomerulus to urethra. Infection, inflammation, or anatomic lesions anywhere in the urinary tract can cause bleeding. The glomerular basement membrane is imper-

1156 PART VIII DIAGNOSTIC CATEGORIES

Causes of Red Urine

Hematuria
Hemoglobinuria
Myoglobinuria
Bilirubinuria
Drugs: phenazopyridine, phenothiazines, ibuprofen,
  levodopa, phenolphthalein, methyldopa,
  Adriamycin, deferoxamine-Fe complex, phenytoin,
  aminopyrine, antipyrine, quinine, sulfonamides,
  chloroform, naphthalene, oxalic acid, Fe-sorbitol,
  salicylates, rifampin, nitrofurantoin, metronidazole,
  chloroquine
Foods: Beets, blueberries, rhubarb, fava beans
Dyes: Aniline dyes, food coloring
Red diaper syndrome
Alcaptonuria
Tyrosinosis
Urate crystals

---

meable to RBCs and large proteins such as hemoglobin. Myoglobin is normally freely filtered. Damage to the glomerular endothelium and glomerular basement membrane disrupts the endothelial-epithelial barrier, allowing red cells to enter Bowman's capsule. If the urine is hypotonic, the red cells may lyse, resulting in a reagent strip positive for hemoglobin with a negative microscopic examination.

Exercise, fever, and other hypermetabolic states are known to cause hematuria.[16] Exercise-related hematuria is due to direct trauma to the kidney and bladder, as well as ischemic injury.[18] It is caused by the shifting of blood flow from the renal circulation to the heart, lung, and skeletal muscles during periods of high demand.

Differential Considerations

An evaluation of a child with hematuria involves determining the site and cause of bleeding. In infants, bleeding on the diaper from either the vagina or rectum can be confused with a urinary source. The menstruating female can also confuse vaginal with urinary bleeding. Red urine does not necessarily equate with hematuria (see box above). A positive reagent strip test can be caused by hemoglobinuria (massive hemolysis) or myoglobinuria (rhabdomyolysis). In these cases, no red cells will be seen on microscopic examination. The serum will be pink in the presence of hemoglobin and clear in the presence of myoglobin. Other pigments can cause a red urine with a negative reagent strip.[19] The red diaper syndrome describes a red color on the diaper. This is caused by *Serratia marcescens* in the infant stool, which produces a pigment after incubation in the diaper pail.

Numerous conditions can be the source of hematuria, including those from outside the urinary tract or those from within the urinary tract beyond the glomerulus. Cases of feigned hematuria to gain admission to the hospital or to obtain narcotics have been reported.[20] Causes of hematuria are listed in the box at right.

Causes of Hematuria

Extrarenal
Coagulation disorders: hemophilia, von Willebrand disease, platelet disorders
Anticoagulant therapy
Salicylates
Sickle cell disease/trait
Factitious

Extraglomerular
Urinary tract infection: cystitis, pyelonephritis
Hemorrhagic cystitis (viral, bacterial, drug, schistosomiasis)
Urethritis, urethral, or meatal ulceration, masturbation
Nephrolithiasis
Hypercalciuria
Interstitial nephritis
Hydronephrosis
Polycystic kidney disease
Renal vein thrombosis
Papillary necrosis
Hemangiomas
Tumors: Wilms', bladder sarcoma
Foreign body
Posterior urethral valves
Ureteropelvic junction obstruction
Renal tuberculosis

Glomerular
Idiopathic, acute glomerulonephritis (GN)
Acute poststreptococcal GN/acute postinfectious GN
IgA nephropathy
Membranoproliferative GN
Chronic GN
Alport syndrome
Exercise
Thin basement membrane disease/familial benign hematuria
Focal glomerulosclerosis
Membranous GN
Antiglomerular basement membrane disease
Sporadic benign hematuria

Systemic conditions
Allergic disorders
Hepatitis B antigenemia
Subacute bacterial endocarditis
Shunt nephritis
Artificial heart valves
Systemic lupus erythematosus
Henoch-Schönlein purpura
Hemolytic-uremic syndrome
Polyarteritis
Still disease
Malaria
Infectious mononucleosis

The bleeding may be due to an underlying bleeding disorder. Qualitative and quantitative platelet disorders as well as hemophilia can cause both gross and microscopic bleeding. A history of other bleeding sites, either concurrently or in the past, or a family history of a bleeding disorder is usually present. Hematuria can also be present in sickle cell conditions, especially with sickle cell disease or sickle cell trait.

Hematuria is also associated with a number of systemic conditions. These infections and inflammatory conditions are usually multisystem diseases involving the glomerulus. Hematuria may be the presenting sign.

Extraglomerular renal causes include anatomic abnormalities such as hydronephrosis. Although a palpable mass may also be present, hematuria may be the index sign that triggers an investigation.

Hypercalciuria is now known to be an important cause of hematuria.[21] This is a familial autosomal dominant condition characterized by excessive urinary calcium excretion that can be found in 3% to 6% of asymptomatic children. In a multicenter study, 35% of children with unexplained isolated hematuria had idiopathic hypercalciuria.[22] Hypercalciuria is more common in white males and patients with a positive family history of urolithiasis, gross hematuria, and calcium oxalate crystals in the urine. A 24-hour urine collection will have more than 4 mg Ca^{++}/kg/24 hr. The spot urine Ca^{++}/Cr ratio varies with age: 0-7 months, 0.86; 7-18 months, 0.6; 19 months-6 years, 0.42; and adults, 0.22.[23] Such children are at risk for developing renal calculi. Enuresis, dysuria, polyuria, short stature, or rickets may occur in severe cases. The excess calcium may be due to a renal tubular leak, which can be decreased by thiazide diuretics. Other patients have excess intestinal absorption of calcium. These patients should limit dietary calcium and sodium to 500 to 600 mg/day and maintain a large daily fluid intake. Restricting calcium, at least in adults, can increase stone formation.

Acute interstitial nephritis mimics glomerular disease with proteinuria and red cell casts and is associated with antibiotic administration, such as methicillin and other penicillins. Acute renal failure may develop.

Tumors are uncommon in childhood. Wilms' tumor is the most frequent and, similar to neuroblastoma, usually presents as a mass rather than isolated hematuria.

Glomerular causes include generally benign conditions such as acute poststreptococcal glomerulonephritis (APSGN), as well as those conditions leading to chronic renal failure. APSGN is the most common condition in this group. IgA nephropathy is the most common cause of recurrent macroscopic and microscopic hematuria. Alport syndrome is a familial nephropathy with associated deafness, ocular abnormalities, and renal failure.

Thin basement membrane disease (benign familial hematuria) is usually discovered as an incidental finding of microhematuria with proteinuria. Family members may not be aware of their asymptomatic hematuria without screening urinalyses. There has been some concern about progression to chronic renal disease.[24] Attenuation of the glomerular basement membrane is often seen on microscopy.[25] The relationship between this condition and Alport syndrome remains to be clarified.[26]

Transient hematuria is frequent after strenuous exercise proportional to the amount of exercise and trauma to the urinary tract. Hemoglobinuria and myoglobinuria can occur in the same setting.[18]

Diagnostic Work-Up

History. The patient or family should describe the color, frequency, and timing of the hematuria; presence of clots; and nature of the urinary stream. Gross hematuria may imply a bladder lesion but can be seen in other conditions such as sickle cell trait, IgA nephropathy, or glomerular lesions.[27] The smoky urine of acute glomerulonephritis is characteristic.

Associated symptoms of fever, dysuria, frequency, or urgency may indicate infection.

Abdominal pain is common in Henoch-Schönlein purpura, whereas colic may indicate stones. A history of recent trauma, exercise, associated bleeding sites, or recent throat or skin infections should be sought. Gross hematuria after minimal trauma can indicate a renal abnormality such as ureteropelvic-junction (UPJ) stenosis.

A history of poor growth may indicate chronic renal disease; weight gain, edema, and acute onset may indicate acute renal failure. Joint pain, nausea, vomiting, headache, or rash may indicate systemic disease. Medication usage may be a clue to interstitial nephritis. Furosemide can cause hypercalciuria leading to hematuria. Caution should be used in ascribing bleeding to anticoagulant use; many of these patients will have an underlying urinary lesion.[28] A family history of renal disease, deafness, or hematuria should be elicited.

Physical Examination. The patient should be examined for signs of trauma, bruising, or bleeding. Edema, ascites, hypertension, cardiac murmurs, pulmonary rales, and joint involvement are important findings. The abdomen and back should be examined for masses and tenderness. Deafness or pinna abnormalities may be associated with renal disease. The genitalia should be inspected carefully for local sources of bleeding or inflammation (trauma, meatitis, urethral prolapse). Associated skin rashes, healing impetigo, or petechia are noted.

Ancillary Data. Urinalysis and culture are essential initial tests. A fresh urine should be carefully examined for casts. In the office setting, a morning urine is preferred to obtain a concentrated urine; dilute specimens may miss certain elements. This is not possible in the emergency setting. If the findings are consistent with infection, no further testing is indicated pending culture results. A urine should be appropriately collected and sent for culture, as UTI is a common cause, especially with macroscopic hematuria.[29]

The urinalysis depends on the chemistry reagent strip and microscopic examination of the spun urine sediment to detect hematuria. The sensitivity of the microscopic examination has been questioned. A finding of 1 to 3 RBCs/HPF had a sensitivity of only 63% in detecting greater than 2,000 RBCs/ml. A cytometer count may be more sensitive but has not gained general acceptance.[30]

The common reagent strips are based on the peroxidase-like activity of hemoglobin and detect intact red cells, free hemoglobin, and myoglobin. False-positive tests can occur with UTIs (microbial peroxidases), ascorbic acid concentration greater than 5 mg/ml, and Betadine. Studies of adults have shown that reactions of trace or greater are significant. Another study found that negative dipsticks missed 16% of patients with significant hematuria. Multiple repeat negative examinations did not miss any pathology.[15]

Thus a complaint of hematuria must be evaluated with careful microscopic evaluation and follow-up examinations and not disregarded on the basis of a negative dipstick on a random urine in the emergency setting. Confirmation of a positive dipstick with the presence of the RBCs on microscopic examination is also important. A negative microscopic examination may indicate hemoglobinuria or myoglobinuria.

Evaluation of the RBCs in the urine may localize the site of bleeding. Casts demonstrate a glomerular etiology. In glomerular lesions, red cells exhibit dysmorphic appearance under phase microscopy with findings of doughnut cells, extruded cytoplasm, budding cells, and ruptured cells.[31] The red cell volume reported by cell counts may also differentiate bleeding sites. The modal cell volume from glomerular sites (35 to 50 fl) was significantly lower than bleeding from nonglomerular sources (65 to 148 fl)[32] and is easier to perform and less operator-dependent than phase contrast microscopy.[33]

Coexistent proteinuria is indicative of glomerular disease. Gross hematuria may give proteinuria from the blood itself. Protein greater than 2+ cannot be attributed to the blood. The selectivity of the protein excreted can also be used to localize the bleeding source.

Creatinine and protein excretion using a 24-hour urine collection should be measured in asymptomatic hematuria. Urine and plasma calcium and the calcium-creatinine ratio should be measured. Associated colic or abdominal pain suggests a calculus, necessitating a plain abdominal film and a renal ultrasound. Henoch-Schönlein purpura and hemolytic-uremic syndrome would also be considerations. Coagulation studies and a platelet count are also indicated in the presence of hematuria.

If a glomerular lesion is suspected, a throat culture, serum tests for streptococcal antibodies, erythrocyte sedimentation rate, complement studies (C_3, C_4), an ANA, and a hepatitis B serology test should be considered. The patient's sickle cell status must be determined. Electrolytes, total protein, and albumin are indicated in the presence of proteinuria, edema, or hypertension. In any case, BUN and creatinine should be obtained to assess renal function.

Hematuria rarely requires invasive imaging techniques. Real time ultrasound is capable of detecting most lesions. Intravenous urograms and cystoscopy are rarely needed. A VCUG should be performed based on ultrasound findings (hydronephrosis, dilated ureters, small or scarred kidneys).

Based on laboratory evaluations, physical findings, and follow-up with a nephrologist, a renal biopsy may ultimately need to be performed.

Therapeutic Trials

Hematuria itself requires no specific therapy. Patients with azotemia, edema, or hypertension should be admitted. Patients with a calculus should receive a urologic consultation in the emergency department. UTI should be tested appropriately. Patients with asymptomatic hematuria do not require a definitive evaluation in the emergency department. They should be referred for pediatric evaluation and follow-up. In many cases, the degree of further evaluation will depend on whether the hematuria is transient or persistent.

HYPERTENSION

JOSEPH A. WEINBERG

The true meaning of hypertension in the pediatric population is still unknown. Traditional pediatric concern has been with patients with serious hypertension secondary to an underlying disease and clearly requiring therapy. Renal disease is the most common cause of this hypertension. Thus the pediatric nephrologist may be the emergency physician's best resource in the face of hypertensive crisis. However, the relationship of childhood blood pressure to adult hypertension and the diagnosis of essential hypertension in childhood are coming under increasing scrutiny.[34,35] The prevalence of hypertension in childhood has been reported to be between 0.8% to 5%.[36]

The definition of high blood pressure in children is not precise. The adult definition should be kept in mind with a value of 140/90 mm Hg as an upper limit and a diastolic pressure of 90 to 104 mm Hg as mild, 105 to 114 mm Hg as moderate, greater than 114 mm Hg as severe, and greater than 129 mm Hg as malignant. Hypertensive crisis is defined as severe elevation of blood pressure without end-organ damage. Hypertensive emergencies occur with associated symptoms involving the central nervous system (CNS) (confusion, visual problems, seizures), heart (congestive heart failure), or kidneys. The terms *malignant* and *accelerated* hypertension are often used to imply severe hypertension with progressive end-organ damage. When neurologic findings are prominent, the term *hypertensive encephalopathy* is often used. Headaches, confusions, lethargy, impaired vision, and seizures may occur. In the emergency setting, the blood pressure requiring treatment depends both on the level of pressure and associated symptoms.

The best definition of blood pressure norms in pediatrics comes from the 1987 report of the second Task Force on Blood Pressure Control in Children from the National Heart, Lung, and Blood Institute. These figures do not take into account the effect of physical maturation on blood pressure. Height-age correlations have been done on this data base, and these more refined charts are available.[37] The figures used here are adequate for emergency department purposes[38] (Figs. 60-1 to 60-6).

There are no risk data to stratify levels of hypertension. The task force developed definitions based on experience and consensus. Normal is defined as a systolic and diastolic less than the 90th percentile for age and sex, high normal as between the 90th and 95th percentiles, and hypertension as systolic or diastolic equal to or greater than the 95th percentile (Table 60-2). These measurements should be obtained on at least three occasions. They further define two classes of hypertension: significant, between the 95th and 99th percentile, and severe, at or above the 99th per-

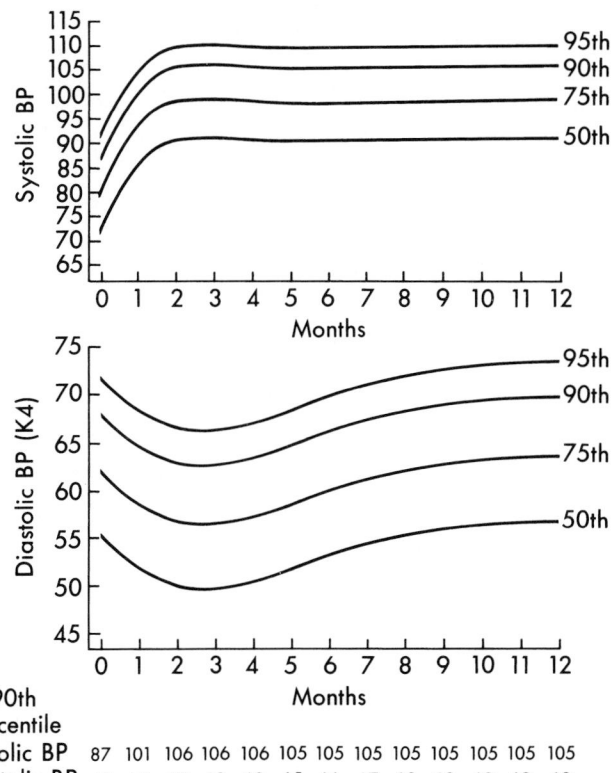

90th
Percentile

Systolic BP	87	101	106	106	106	105	105	105	105	105	105	105	105
Diastolic BP	68	65	63	63	63	65	66	67	68	68	69	69	69
Height cm	51	59	63	66	68	70	72	73	74	76	77	78	80
Weight kg	4	4	5	5	6	7	8	9	9	10	10	11	11

FIG. 60-1. Age-specific percentiles of blood pressure measurements in **boys—birth to 12 months of age;** Korotkoff phase IV (K4) used for diastolic blood pressure. (*From Task Force on Blood Pressure Control in Children: Report of the second task force on blood,* Pediatrics 79:1, 1987.)

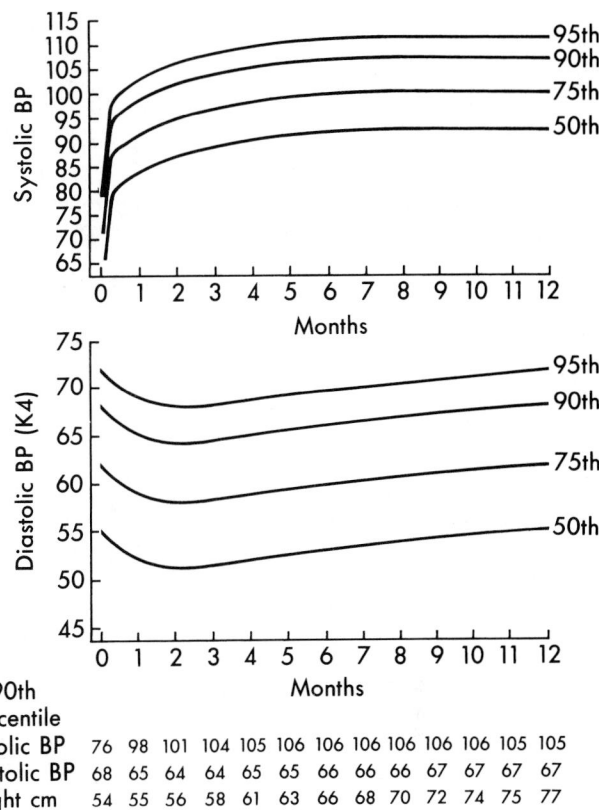

90th
Percentile

Systolic BP	76	98	101	104	105	106	106	106	106	106	106	105	105
Diastolic BP	68	65	64	64	65	65	66	66	66	67	67	67	67
Height cm	54	55	56	58	61	63	66	68	70	72	74	75	77
Weight kg	4	4	4	5	5	6	7	8	9	9	10	10	11

FIG. 60-2. Age-specific percentiles of blood pressure measurements in **girls—birth to 12 months of age;** Korotkoff phase IV (K4) used for diastolic blood pressure. (*From Task Force on Blood Pressure Control in Children: Report of the second task force on blood,* Pediatrics 79:1, 1987.)

centile (Table 60-3). The task force utilized muffling (K4) for children 1 to 13 years of age and disappearance (K5) for children 13 and older to determine diastolic blood pressure. It is now more common to use K5 at all ages.

Pathophysiology

The acute effects of high blood pressure are related to the elevation of perfusion forces. Starling forces cause the transudation of fluid into tissue. Increased intraluminal pressure leads to vascular damage. The resultant edema causes vision disturbances and increased intracranial pressure. Reactive vasoconstriction causes organ ischemia, which further compromises CNS function, and results in pulmonary hypertension and myocardial and renal dysfunction. Unchecked, this can lead to renal failure, cerebral hemorrhage and infarction, coma, and death. The vessels of patients with chronic hypertension adapt by becoming thickened. This protective mechanism does not exist in the sudden onset of hypertension seen in acute glomerulonephritis, leading to encephalopathy at lower pressures.

The physiologic basis of the hypertension depends on the underlying etiology. Renal hypertension depends on decreased perfusion pressure to the afferent arteriole of the glomerulus, resulting in the secretion of renin from the juxtaglomerular apparatus. The resultant aldosterone se-

cretion leads to sodium retention and potassium loss in the kidneys. The sodium retention results in hypervolemia and increased cardiac output. The renin-induced angiotensin production increases peripheral vascular resistance. This combination increases blood pressure. Chronic renal disease also causes sodium retention with resultant hypervolemia and alterations in production of renin and vasodilators such as bradykinin, kallidin, and prostaglandin A₂. The hypertension of coarctation of the aorta depends on pressure load and renal mechanisms. Constricted flow to the kidneys activates the renin angiotensin axis noted previously.[39] Hypertension may develop postcoarctation repair because of a persistent hyperdynamic state, pressure gradients, increased sympathetic tone, or abnormalities in the renin-angiotensin system.[40]

Differential Considerations

It is estimated that in 79% to 98% of cases, hypertension in childhood is usually secondary to an underlying cause,[39] the predominant cause being renal. Londe reported that 80% of secondary hypertension is due to renal causes. The second leading cause was coarctation of the aorta, found in 2% of these patients.[40] Hypertension may persist even after surgical repair. Endocrine causes represent an important but small group of patients. The incidence of renal and

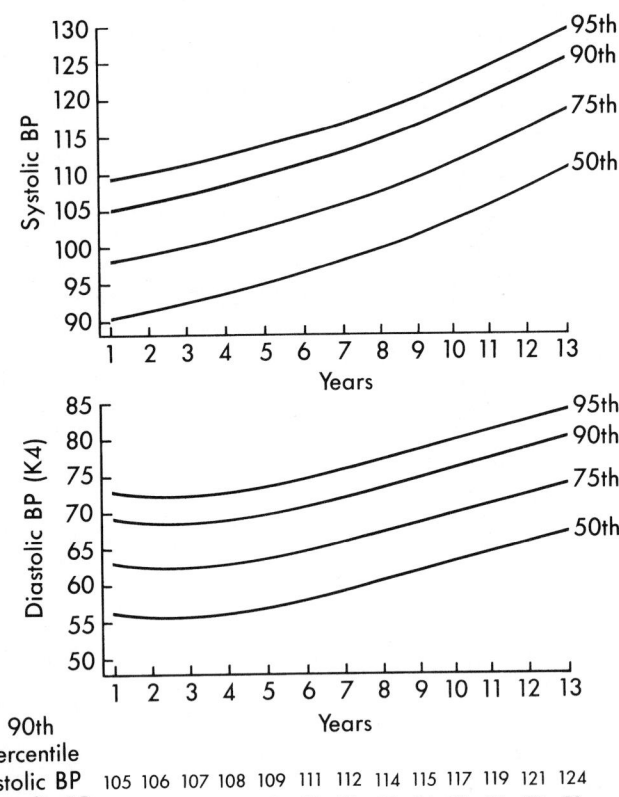

90th
Percentile

Systolic BP	105	106	107	108	109	111	112	114	115	117	119	121	124
Diastolic BP	69	68	68	69	69	70	71	73	74	75	76	77	79
Height cm	80	91	100	108	115	122	129	135	141	147	153	159	165
Weight kg	11	14	16	18	22	25	29	34	39	44	50	55	62

FIG. 60-3. Age-specific percentiles of blood pressure measurements in **boys—1 to 13 years of age;** Korotkoff phase IV (K4) used for diastolic blood pressure. (*From Task Force on Blood Pressure Control in Children: Report of the second task force on blood,* Pediatrics 79:1, 1987.)

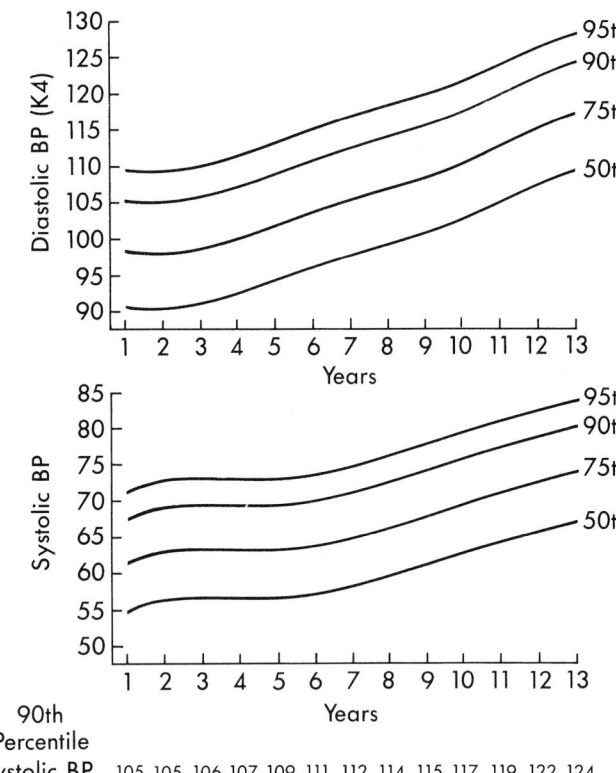

90th
Percentile

Systolic BP	105	105	106	107	109	111	112	114	115	117	119	122	124
Diastolic BP	67	69	69	69	69	70	71	72	74	75	77	78	80
Height cm	77	89	98	107	115	122	129	135	142	148	154	160	165
Weight kg	11	13	15	18	22	25	30	35	40	45	51	58	63

FIG. 60-4. Age-specific percentiles of blood pressure measurements in **girls—1 to 13 years of age;** Korotkoff phase IV (K4) used for diastolic blood pressure. (*From Task Force on Blood Pressure Control in Children: Report of the second task force on blood,* Pediatrics 79:1, 1987.)

secondary hypertension increases in studies from tertiary centers as opposed to primary care settings.[41,42]

Essential or idiopathic hypertension is being increasingly recognized. There is probably an interplay of genetic factor and environmental elements that begins in childhood and leads to adult hypertension.[43] It is still not clear if childhood blood pressure percentiles track into adulthood. Loggie[44] suggests that secondary hypertension is most likely in children under age 10, in white females aged 10 to 20 years, and in adolescents with a diastolic pressure greater than 100 mm Hg. White males and black teenagers are much more likely to have idiopathic hypertension.

Many of the causes of hypertension in children and adolescents are listed in the box on p. 1137. Hypertension may be the presenting sign in cases of renal disease, especially with chronic infection, reflux nephropathy, or some forms of chronic renal disease. Acute poststreptococcal glomerulonephritis, hemolytic-uremic syndrome, and anaphylactic purpura have hypertension as a significant complication of the characteristic disease. Hypertension can also be secondary to acute stress situations such as major burns, CNS infections and tumors, or autonomic dysfunction in dysautonomia.

Ingestions should always be considered in unexplained hypertension. Renovascular hypertension should be espe-

cially considered if there is unexplained severe hypertension, in cases of umbilical artery catheterization, renal trauma, Williams syndrome, neurofibromatosis, systemic arteritis, progeria states, and refractory hypertension.[42]

Diagnostic Work-Up

A previous history of renal, cardiac, or other systemic disease should be elicited. Preeclampsia and toxemia during pregnancy, difficult neonatal course, instrumentation, abnormal growth, headaches, dizziness, epistaxis, joint pain, edema, weakness, abnormal menses, or drug ingestion should be sought. Prior measurements of blood pressure may be helpful.

A family history of hypertension, cardiac disease, or renal disease may be significant. Essential hypertension is rare in childhood and a positive family history should not preclude a search for an underlying cause.

Hypertensive measurements in children may be due to inappropriate measurement techniques. It is essential that the correct size blood pressure cuff be used. Cuff size refers to the air bladder itself and not its cloth covering. Six cuff sizes should be available (Table 60-4). The cuff should be fitted to the extremity part that fits best and should cover three fourths of the extremity part, and the air bladder should be long enough to almost encircle the circum-

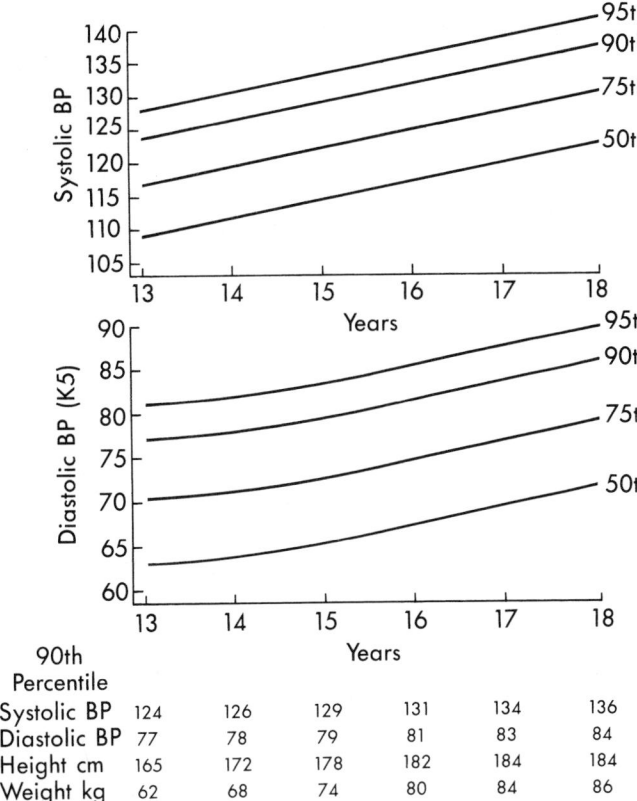

90th Percentile						
Systolic BP	124	126	129	131	134	136
Diastolic BP	77	78	79	81	83	84
Height cm	165	172	178	182	184	184
Weight kg	62	68	74	80	84	86

FIG. 60-5. Age-specific percentiles of blood pressure measurements in **boys—13 to 18 years of age;** Korotkoff phase V (K5) used for diastolic blood pressure. (*From Task Force on Blood Pressure Control in Children: Report of the second task force on blood,* Pediatrics 79:1, 1987.)

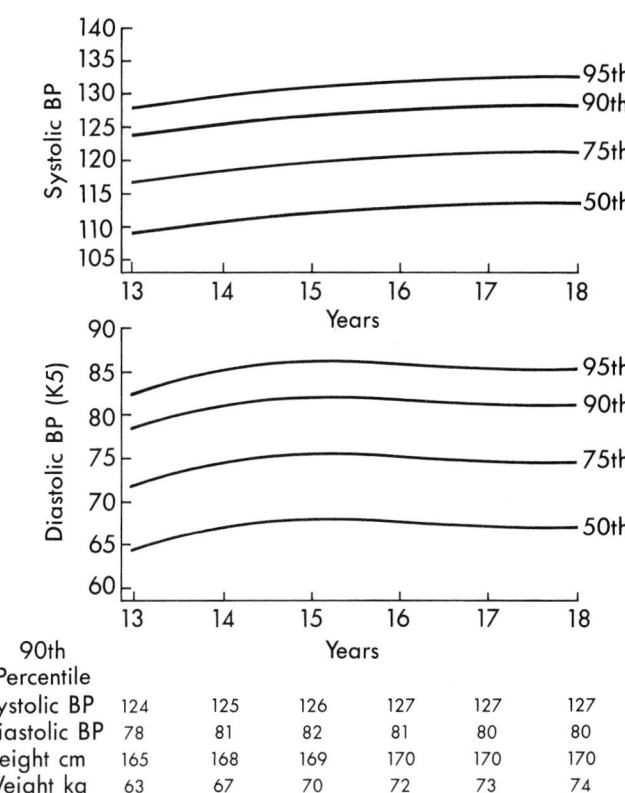

90th Percentile						
Systolic BP	124	125	126	127	127	127
Diastolic BP	78	81	82	81	80	80
Height cm	165	168	169	170	170	170
Weight kg	63	67	70	72	73	74

FIG. 60-6. Age-specific percentiles of blood pressure measurements in **girls—13 to 18 years of age;** Korotkoff phase V (K5) used for diastolic blood pressure. (*From Task Force on Blood Pressure Control in Children: Report of the second task force on blood,* Pediatrics 79:1, 1987.)

ference.[38] The latter is often overlooked, causing the selection of a cuff that only encircles a small part of the extremity. This causes a high blood pressure reading. It is best to err toward too large a cuff; a small cuff causes greater distortion of pressure measurements. The manufacturers' markings for acceptable arm sizes for a given cuff are not always accurate.[45]

If the proper fit can be made on the arm, blood pressure can be taken by the auscultation method. The systolic pressure, pressure at muffling, and pressure at disappearance should be recorded. Disappearance may not be detectable in some children. Londes observed that this is related to too much pressure on the stethoscope chest piece.[46]

The Doppler and oscillometric techniques allow use of the arm, forearm, thigh, or calf. Diastolic pressure is difficult to determine using a hand-held Doppler. Many automatic devices use the oscillometric technique and are useful except in cases of profound shock. It has been suggested that the Dinamap may be more reliable than auscultation.[47] Other investigations have found that the Dinamap readings are 6 to 9 mm Hg lower than auscultation values and caution against using published normative values when pressures are obtained using a Dinamap.[48]

The examiner must also consider the physical factors affecting this measurement. The patient's position (sitting, lying, standing) may affect the measurement. The pressure

TABLE 60-2. Definitions

Term	Definition
Normal BP	Systolic and diastolic BP <90th percentile for age and sex
High normal BP*	Average systolic and/or average diastolic BP between 90th and 95th percentiles for age and sex
High BP (hypertension)	Average systolic and/or average diastolic BPs ≥95th percentile for age and sex with measurements obtained on at least three occasions

From Task Force on Blood Pressure Control in Children: Report of the second task force on blood, *Pediatrics,* 79:1, 1987.
*If the BP reading is high normal for age, but can be accounted for by excess height for age or excess lean body mass for age, such children are considered to have normal BP.

may be increased by 20 to 30 mm Hg if the arm is held down along the trunk rather than at the level of the heart.[49] Several measurements must sometimes be taken to eliminate anxiety. In children, fear, pain, and anxiety can be major factors in the acute medical setting. There are respiratory variations. Blood pressure is low in the morning and peaks in the early evening. Traube-Hering waves resulting

TABLE 60-3. Classification of Hypertension by Age Group

Age group	Significant hypertension (mm Hg)	Severe hypertension (mm Hg)
Newborn		
7 d	Systolic BP ≥ 96	Systolic BP ≥ 106
8-30 d	Systolic BP ≥ 104	Systolic BP ≥ 110
Infant	Systolic BP ≥ 112	Systolic BP ≥ 118
(< 2 yr)	Diastolic BP ≥ 74	Diastolic BP ≥ 82
Children	Systolic BP ≥ 116	Systolic BP ≥ 124
(3-5 yr)	Diastolic BP ≥ 76	Diastolic BP ≥ 84
Children	Systolic BP ≥ 122	Systolic BP ≥ 130
(6-9 yr)	Diastolic BP ≥ 78	Diastolic BP ≥ 86
Children	Systolic BP ≥ 126	Systolic BP ≥ 134
(10-12 yr)	Diastolic BP ≥ 82	Diastolic BP ≥ 90
Adolescents	Systolic BP ≥ 136	Systolic BP ≥ 144
(13-15 yr)	Diastolic BP ≥ 86	Diastolic BP ≥ 92
Adolescents	Systolic BP ≥ 142	Systolic BP ≥ 150
(16-18 yr)	Diastolic BP ≥ 92	Diastolic BP ≥ 98

From Task Force on Blood Pressure Control in Children: Report of the second task force on blood, *Pediatrics*, 79:1, 1987.

from variations in autonomic activity can cause wide swings in pressure. Careful, repeat measurements are important.[39]

Once hypertension is established, a careful examination should be performed for an etiology. Table 60-5 delineates important aspects of the history and physical examination. The most common entities in the differential diagnosis in children with severe hypertension are renal/renovascular disease and pheochromocytoma. Acute hypertensive conditions such as anaphylactoid purpura, hemolytic-uremic syndrome, or acute glomerulonephritis are usually obvious from associated findings such as rash, blood smear findings, or urinalysis.

The retina should be examined for signs of long-standing hypertension (e.g., arteriovenous nicking, copper or silver wire vessels, exudates). Neurologic deficits such as hemiparesis or a Bell palsy may also indicate chronic hypertension, often with acute acceleration.[49] The possibility of drug ingestion should also be considered. The lower extremity pulses and blood pressures should be evaluated to avoid missing coarctation of the aorta.

Hypertensive encephalopathy must be differentiated from primary CNS lesions with secondary hypertension. Intracranial hemorrhage, stroke, encephalitis, and mass lesions must be considered.

Ancillary Data. The patient with stable hypertension requires very little laboratory evaluation in the emergency department. A detailed diagnostic evaluation can generally be performed by the patient's primary physician. A screening urinalysis, hemoglobin, electrolytes, creatinine, BUN, and chest x-ray film can be obtained to detect abnormalities requiring immediate intervention.

If the patient has acutely symptomatic hypertension, a CBC, electrolytes, BUN, creatinine, phosphorus, cholesterol, triglycerides, and uric acid should be measured. Uric acid evaluation may be the only indication of impaired renal function. Urine should be obtained for a urinalysis looking for proteinuria, hematuria, RBC casts, and other abnormalities; urine output is closely monitored. A renin level should be obtained before treatment. Hormonal studies, ECG and chest x-ray study should be obtained but should not delay emergency therapy. An echocardiogram should be obtained to establish baseline left ventricular mass and function to evaluate target organ damage.

Specific studies for nonrenal causes of hypertension are discussed in their respective sections. A chest x-ray film can exclude pulmonary edema and cardiomegaly. If a renal cause is suspected, an ultrasound and disodium monomethanearsonate (DMSA) nuclear scan should be obtained. Special studies will be needed if renovascular hypertension is suspected. Renal radionuclide studies, possibly with a captopril challenge; computed tomography (CT) scans; angiography; scintigraphy for pheochromocytoma localization; and digital imaging may be considerations. The array of available imaging options makes consultation important in planning an appropriate evaluation.

Management

The decision to treat is based on the combination of blood pressure and symptoms. The desired rate of decreasing blood pressure must be considered. In a patient with chronic hypertension, higher pressures may be needed to maintain organ perfusion. A rapid decrease in pressure can compromise end-organ function. CNS status must be carefully monitored. If it deteriorates, treatment should be stopped pending normalization of blood pressure and CNS signs. A child with the rapid onset of hypertension, such as with acute glomerulonephritis, may develop symptoms at a diastolic pressure of 100 mm Hg.[35]

Feld and Springate[42] recommend the urgent treatment of blood pressures that exceed age-related norms or previous blood pressure measurements by 30%. This arbitrary definition must be combined with clinical signs of encephalopathy, heart failure, renal failure, and stroke to determine the need for emergency therapy. Consultations with a specialist are essential in these cases. The goals of treatment should be to reduce pressure within 1 hour to a range of 160 to 170/100 to 110 or by 25% in younger children.

The patient with acute renal failure and hypertension is often fluid overloaded. A dose of furosemide (Lasix), 1 mg/kg intravenously, should be given in that setting and may be sufficient to treat the hypertension. If the patient has pulmonary edema, encephalopathy, acute worsening of renal function, or a diastolic pressure greater than 120 mm Hg, more aggressive treatment is indicated. Diuretics may worsen salt depletion and should be used only in the context of overt fluid overload.

Nifedipine, 0.25 to 0.5 mg/kg, is the pharmacologic agent of choice beyond diuretics. The drug is removed from the capsule by having the patient bite the capsule and then swallow it or by removing the drug and administering it orally by syringe.[50] It can also be given rectally.[51]

Blood pressure will fall within minutes with maximum effect in 30 to 60 minutes. The effect lasts for 3 to 4 hours and is still present 6 hours after the dose. The dose can be repeated in 30 minutes if there is no effect but is usually given every 6 to 8 hours.[52] This calcium-channel blocker has negative inotropic effects and may worsen congestive heart failure. Nicardipine, a potent arterial vasodilator, is

Etiology of Hypertension in Infants and Children

Renal
Acute glomerulonephritis (including poststreptococcal/
    postinfections)
Alport syndrome
Amyloidosis
Acute renal failure
End-stage renal disease
Fabry disease
Hemolytic-uremic syndrome
Henoch-Schönlein purpura
Hypoplastic/dysplastic kidney
Hydronephrosis
Nephrotic syndrome
Periarteritis nodosa
Polycystic kidney/medullary cystic disease
Postrenal transplantation
Pyelonephritis
Renal calculi
Renal vein thrombosis
Renovascular
    Fibromuscular dysplasia
    Neurofibromatosis
    Renal artery stenosis
    Takayasu disease
    Thromboembolus (including postumbilical catheter)
    Williams syndrome
Systemic lupus erythematosus
Trauma
Wilms' tumor

Cardiovascular
Coarctation of the aorta
Atherosclerosis/progeria syndromes
Aortic arteritis

Essential hypertension

Endocrine
Pheochromocytoma
Cushing syndrome
Hyperthyroidism
Hypercalcemia
Hyperaldosteronism
Neuroblastoma
Congenital adrenal hyperplasia
Turner syndrome
Ovarian tumor

Neurologic
Dysautonomia
Increased intracranial pressure
Guillain-Barré syndrome
Stress, including major burns
Orthopedic procedures

Drug ingestion
Amphetamines/sympathomimetic agents
Cocaine
Lead
Licorice
Mercury
Oral contraceptives
Phencyclidine
Reserpine
Steroids

TABLE 60-4. Commonly Available Blood Pressure Cuffs

Cuff name*	Bladder width (cm)	Bladder length (cm)
Newborn	2.5-4.0	5.0-9.0
Infant	4.0-6.0	11.5-18.0
Child	7.5-9.0	17.0-19.0
Adult	11.5-13.0	22.0-26.0
Large arm	14.0-15.0	30.5-33.0
Thigh	18.0-19.0	36.0-38.0

From Task Force on Blood Pressure Control in Children: Report of the second task force on blood, *Pediatrics*, 79:1, 1987.
*Cuff name does not guarantee that the cuff will be appropriate size for a child within that age range.

an intravenous calcium-channel blocker. The calcium-channel blockers, like other vasodilators, can cause tachycardia, but have been reported to cause less side effects than nitroprusside because they have much less effect on preload.[53] Nicardipine does not have the negative inotropic effects of nifedipine. There is limited experience in children, but a dose of 1 μg/kg/min continuous IV resulted in a 10% decrease in blood pressure without affecting heart rate. A loading dose is contraindicated and the dose can be titrated up to 3 μg/kg/min continuous IV.[54] Calcium-channel blockers should not be used in patients on beta-blocker treatment. They are contraindicated in intracranial hemorrhage, since they cause an increase in cerebral blood flow.[55]

Labetalol is a combined alpha- and beta-blocker that is often used for hypertensive crises. An initial loading dose of 0.2 to 1.0 mg/kg can be followed with a continuous infusion of 0.25 to 1.5 mg/kg/hr.[56] Labetatol may be the drug of choice in cocaine and other sympathomimetic agent abuse.[35] It should not be used when beta-blockers are contraindicated such as in patients with bronchospasm, bradycardia, or congestive heart failure.

Diazoxide, a potent vasodilator, can be used to quickly decrease blood pressure. The drug is given as a rapid IV bolus. If given slowly, it is rapidly protein-bound and will be ineffective. The blood pressure fall is unpredictable. Blood pressure must be measured every 5 minutes to monitor for hypotension, which can lead to renal failure, myocardial and

TABLE 60-5. Etiology of Hypertension: Signs and Symptoms

Signs and symptoms	Etiology
Flushing, palpitations, diarrhea, tachycardia	Pheochromocytoma, hyperthyroidism
Poor growth, fevers, UTI, edema, hematuria, trauma, family history of renal disease	Renal
Abdominal mass	Renal, neuroblastoma, Wilms' tumor
Virilization	Congenital adrenal hyperplasia
Striae, moon facies, truncal obesity	Cushing syndrome
Weakness, muscle cramps	Hyperaldosteronism
Heart murmur, decreased femoral pulses or leg blood pressures	Coarctation of the aorta
Butterfly rash	Systemic lupus erythematosus
Abdominal bruit	Renovascular, abdominal coarctation of the aorta
Prematurity, umbilical catheterization	Renal artery thrombosis
Café-au-lait spots, neurofibromas	von Recklinghausen disease
Funduscopic changes, Bell palsy, stroke, CHF, cardiomegaly	Chronic hypertension
Elfin facies	Williams syndrome

cerebral ischemia, and coma. Hypotension will respond to fluid administration. The risk of hypotension will be decreased by giving the drug in a 1 to 3 mg/kg bolus over 5 to 10 seconds. These mini boluses can be repeated every 10 minutes, titrating against the blood pressure.

A less dramatic decline in blood pressure will occur with hydralazine. It is often effective in acute situations, such as APSGN or eclampsia. Hydralazine can be given 0.1 to 0.2 mg/kg/dose IV or IM. The vasodilation may cause reflex tachycardia, which can be blunted with propranolol.

In severe cases, a continuous infusion of nitroprusside can be used. Nitroprusside is both an arteriolar and venous dilator. The patient generally requires continuous blood pressure monitoring with an arterial line. The blood pressure can be titrated against the infusion rate, since onset of effect is within seconds. If hypotension develops, the infusion can be slowed or stopped and pressure will rise in minutes. Cyanide toxicity causes metabolic acidosis and clinical deterioration. Thiocyanate levels must be monitored. The drug is given at a continuous infusion rate of 0.5 to 10 μg/kg/min.

These patients should have ongoing cardiopulmonary monitoring. Intake and output should be meticulously managed. Close monitoring of neurologic status and renal function is imperative. Hydralazine and nitroprusside may cause cerebral vasodilation and worsen encephalopathy.

Prazosin, an alpha-blocker, is used for hypertension secondary to pheochromocytoma at a dose of 50 mcg/kg IV. Phenoxybenzamine and phentolamine can still be used.[57] The dose of phentolamine is 0.1 to 0.2 mg/kg/dose IV.

Captopril, an angiotensin-converting enzyme (ACE) inhibitor, requires slow incremental dose increases, which limits its effectiveness in the acute setting. The ACE inhibitors may precipitate acute renal failure in patients with renal artery stenosis. The drug is given initially orally 0.3 mg/kg/dose. The dose is doubled every 2 hours to a maximum of 2 to 6 mg/kg/24 hr until the desired effect is achieved. Higher doses may be required. It may be particularly useful in infants with renovascular hypertension secondary to the use of umbilical artery catheters.[58] Neonates are very sensitive to the drug and dosage should be started at a dose of 0.01 mg/kg po.[58] Enalapril may have fewer side effects than captopril but has not been well studied in children. The dose is one tenth of the captopril dose.[59]

Disposition

Any patient who requires emergency blood pressure treatment should be admitted to an intensive care unit (ICU) for close monitoring. Stable patients with newly diagnosed hypertension should be referred to their primary care provider for follow-up within 1 to 2 days. If screening tests demonstrate electrolyte abnormalities or impaired renal function, the patient should be admitted for evaluation. Patients with symptoms of headaches, visual disturbances, or other neurologic problems should also be admitted.

It is important to counsel a patient with a blood pressure greater than the 95th percentile before discharge from the emergency department. A single reading in the artificial setting of the emergency department is not sufficient to diagnose hypertension. However, the finding may be highly significant. In the series of Watson,[60] 9 of 17 patients with renovascular hypertension were initially identified during routine office examinations. Thus the emergency physician must emphasize the importance of follow-up in the asymptomatic patient without causing undue alarm to the family.

PROTEINURIA

JOSEPH A. WEINBERG

Protein in the urine is easily detected and commonly found on routine urinalysis. Screening examination in children have demonstrated an incidence of up to 85% if trace protein is included. The incidence peaks during adolescence and hot weather.[61,62] Asymptomatic proteinuria has a varying incidence of from 1.8% to 11.6% in different studies.[63] Trace to two-plus proteinuria is not uncommon in the acute care setting of stressed, febrile, or dehydrated patients.

Pathophysiology

Normally, the glomerulus is virtually impermeable to large-molecular-weight proteins such as albumin. The small amounts that are filtered are almost completely reabsorbed and degraded in the proximal tubule. Low-molecular-weight proteins are freely filtered, with greater than 95% reabsorption in the proximal tubule.[64] Significant proteinuria can reflect glomerular disease with increased filtration or tubular injury with decreased reabsorption. Glomerular disease is marked by excretion of large-molecular-weight proteins. Tubular injury results in the increased excretion of low-molecular-weight proteins such as lysozyme or B_2 microglobulin.

Proteinuria may be benign and asymptomatic,[63] or a marker of underlying disease.[63,65,66] The physiologic impact depends on the amount of protein lost. If hypoproteinemia results (albumin <2.0 gm/dl, protein <4.0 gm/dl), as in the nephrotic syndrome, then edema and ascites may develop. In most cases, the proteinuria is asymptomatic.

Differential Considerations

Proteinuria can be divided conveniently into conditions affecting the glomerulus or the tubule (Table 60-6). Transient proteinuria is due to benign situations such as stress, fever, exercise, and dehydration. Persistent proteinuria may be benign or a sign of underlying disease.[67]

Fortunately, benign conditions are the most common.[62] Orthostatic proteinuria occurs in 2% to 5% of adolescents[68] and may be transient or fixed. The total excretion is usually less than 1 gm/24 hr.[69] Patients should have normal blood pressure, no microscopic hematuria, and normal renal function.[68] The prognosis is excellent. Factitious proteinuria has been reported.[70]

Diagnostic Work-Up

A history suggestive of renal disease should be sought. Important considerations are growth failure, developmental delay, edema or swelling, weight gain, polydipsia, deafness, UTIs, exercise, stress, fever, or fluid loss. A family history of renal disease, diabetes, or hypertension is significant.

Blood pressure should be measured in all patients. A careful examination should be performed for signs of edema, which is classically periorbital in renal disease and may be subtle.

Ancillary Data. A positive initial screen for proteinuria requires a complete urinalysis including a microscopic examination. Associated hematuria, crystalluria, or cyclindruria may indicate underlying disease.

Protein is usually detected by color change on a reagent strip, turning from pale to dark green with increasing protein, reading 0 to 4+ (0 to >2,000 mg/dl). These colorimetric strips are sensitive to about 20 mg/dl of albumin.[71] They will not detect nonalbumin proteinuria. False-positive results can be obtained as a result of highly concentrated urine, sodium bicarbonate ingestion or other highly alkaline urines, macroscopic hematuria, or phenazopyridine.[72]

A more sensitive screening test is sulfasalicylic acid (SSA). Ten drops of SSA are added to 5 ml of urine. The precipitate is graded on a scale of 0 to 4+. False-positive results occur in the presence of macroscopic hematuria, radiocontrast dyes, penicillin, cephalosporins, tolbutamide, tolmetin, and sulfonamides.[73]

Ultimately, quantitation of protein excretion is necessary. A normal adult excretes less than 150 mg/24 hr; the excretion rate can be as high as 300 mg/24 hr in children under

TABLE 60-6. Etiology of Proteinuria

Type	Etiology
Glomerular	
Nephrotic syndrome	Orthostatic
Acute glomerulonephritis	Exercise
IgA nephropathy	Emotional stress
Chronic glomerulonephritis	Cold exposure
Posttransplantation rejection	Fever
Incomplete foot process disease	Dehydration
Sialidosis (mucolipidosis I)	
Tubular	
Acute vasomotor nephropathy	Vesicoureteric reflux
Heavy metal poisoning	Polycystic kidney disease
Acute UTI	Fanconi syndrome
Chronic pyelonephritis	Myeloma
Diabetes mellitus	Hydronephrosis
Asymptomatic low-molecular-weight proteinuria	

18 years of age. Children normally excrete less than 100mg/m²/day. Full-term infants can excrete up to 145mg/m²/day and premature infants up to 185mg/m²/day in the first month of life. Severe proteinuria is defined as greater than 3,500 mg/24 hr/1.73 m² in adults and greater than 40 mg/hr/m² in children.[74] Timed urinary specimens have been required, since protein excretion varies with activity, posture, and time of day.

Single early morning specimens have been advocated to alleviate the problems of timed collections.[75] Creating a ratio with the urinary creatinine has allowed the use of single specimens. The normal ratio is less than 0.15 in children. Severe proteinuria is indicated by a ratio greater than 1.0. A persistent ratio of greater than 2.5 is diagnostic of nephrotic syndrome.[76] Quantitative protein excretion can be established by the formula

$$\text{Total protein (gm/m}^2\text{/24 hr)} = 0.63 \text{ (urine protein/urine creatinine)}^{77}$$

Single specimens obtained in the emergency department to calculate 24-hour protein excretion in this manner may be inaccurate because of the circadian rhythm of protein excretion.[78]

These more detailed analyses are not required in the acute setting. Proteinuria less than 3+ requires no further testing in the emergency department unless the need for a culture is suggested by other findings. Proteinuria, 3+ and 4+, should be evaluated with a urine culture, serum protein and albumin, serum electrolytes, serum urea nitrogen, and creatinine.

Therapeutic Trial

Treatment is aimed at the underlying conditions. Patients with edema and hypoproteinemia should be treated as noted in the section on Nephrotic Syndrome, generally with diuretics and steroids. ACE inhibitors can reduce protein excretion by 60% to 70%.[79]

Patients with less than 3+ proteinuria should have their acute illness treated and referred for follow-up urinalysis.[80] Patients with 3+ and 4+ proteinuria, normal blood pressure, serum proteins, and renal function should undergo a urine culture and be referred to their primary care provider for urgent renal evaluation.

If renal function is impaired in the presence of persistent significant proteinuria, further anatomic evaluation by ultrasound should be considered. Any patient with instability, hypertension, hypoalbuminemia, or markedly evolving impairment of renal function should be admitted for diagnosis and treatment.

SCROTAL PAIN AND SWELLING

MARTIN I. HERMAN

A red, tender, and swollen hemiscrotum can challenge even the most experienced clinician's diagnostic acumen.[81]

Pathophysiology

Within the hemiscrotum the testis rests just under the epididymis, suspended by the spermatic cord and nourished by a testicular artery intimately entwined in the cord apparatus. Normally the testis lies with the long axis in the vertical plane with the epididymis just above the posterior to the gonad. The testis is attached posteriorly and inferiorly by a residual of the gubernaculum. Anterolaterally, the testis is embedded in the tunica vaginalis, an extension of the peritoneum formed during the descent of the testis from its abdominal origins. The processing vaginalis lies above the testis and epididymis. This structure provides the potential site for the formation of hydroceles and indirect inguinal hernias. The spermatic cord is composed of the nutrient arteries, vas deferens, spermatic veins (pampiniform plexus), and nerves, all of which are surrounded by three layers of fascia. These layers include the dartos tunic, a thin muscular layer, which is continuous, with the abdominal and perineal fascias. Under the dartos tunic is the cremaster muscle and the internal and external spermatic fascia.[82]

If the epididymis comes to rest in a more superior position on the gonad (bell clapper deformity), the superior and posterior attachment of the testis allows the entire epididymotesticular complex to rotate freely within the scrotum. The blood supply to the testis is cut off, producing arterial ischemia. The ischemic testis becomes painful and swollen, producing the acute scrotum.[81]

Inflammation of the epididymis with swelling may also produce the clinical picture of an acute scrotum.

Differential Considerations

Torsion of the spermatic cord, one of the more common causes for an acute scrotal presentation, demands timely surgical intervention (see section on Testicular Torsion).[81,83] Other diagnostic entities that must be addressed immediately include incarcerated or strangulated inguinal hernias and ruptured testicles.

Dividing the causes of scrotal swelling into those that are and are not associated with pain may be helpful. The presence or absence of scrotal transillumination, cremasteric reflex or testicular enlargement is also useful in mak-

TABLE 60-7. Causes of Scrotal Swelling

Painful	Painless
Testis enlarged	**Testis enlarged**
Testicular torsion	Testicular tumor
Torsion appendage testis	Testicular leukemia
Trauma	Gumma
Epididymoorchitis	Cysts of testes
Tumor, acute hemorrhage	Tuberculosis
Testis normal	**Testis normal**
Torsion appendage testis	Tumor
Communicating hydrocele	Antenatal testicular torsion
Cellulitis	Incarcerated hernia
Nontraumatic hydrocele	Hydrocele
Trauma	Idiopathic scrotal edema
Hernia	Systemic edema states (Henoch-Schönlein purpura, Kawasaki disease, etc.)
Varicocele	Sarcoidosis
	Fat necrosis
	Hypertriglyceridemia

ing a diagnosis. Differentiating various causes of scrotal swelling can be very difficult; early surgical consultation is often appropriate (Table 60-7).[84]

Some 96% of acute scrotum cases are due to either acute torsions of the spermatic cord, torsions of the appendix testis, or epididymitis, which are discussed in detail in this chapter.[85] The remaining 4% of acute scrotal pathologies include varicoceles, hydroceles, testicular trauma, testicular tumors, and idiopathic scrotal edema (ISE). Extrascrotal disease such as inguinal hernia or ruptured appendices may also appear to involve the scrotum.

Varicocele. This "bag of worms" is found most often in the left hemiscrotum as a result of incompetent spermatic vein valves and is one cause of the painless swollen scrotum. Poor drainage of the pampiniform plexus leads to dilation and elongation of the spermatic veins, which on examination simulate a mass both superior and posterior to the testis. These can be tender at times.[83]

The left spermatic vein empties directly into the left renal vein and the right into the inferior vena cava, explaining the left-sided preponderance of varicoceles. A right-sided varicocele should prompt a search for intraabdominal disease such as a tumor compressing the inferior vena cava or thrombosis of that vein. New onset left varicocele may reflect the development of a renal cell carcinoma obstructing the left renal vein. Intravenous pyelogram (IVP), ultrasound, angiography, and arterial catheterization may be needed to define the underlying pathology.[86]

Uncomplicated varicoceles may resolve spontaneously or remain asymptomatic for years. Diminished spermatogenesis and motility has been ascribed to the presence of a varicocele and occasionally a surgical remedy is sought to improve fertility.

Inguinal Hernia. Indirect inguinal hernia is the invagination of abdominal contents into a peritoneal sac, the processus vaginalis, which then traverses the inguinal canal.[87] These may present as scrotal swelling and may be tender. Differentiation from other causes of scrotal pathology may be difficult, unless one can palpate the testis. Unlike torsions of the spermatic cord, incarcerated inguinal hernias are found more commonly in infant males. Persistent incarceration may result in ischemia of the entrapped bowel and present as an acutely painful inguinoscrotal mass. Using ice packs, analgesia, and steady manual pressure, 80% to 95% of incarcerated hernias can be reduced. Reduction of the inguinal hernia will allow the examiner to adequately check the scrotal contents for other pathology. Testicular compromise has been found in 3% to 5% of cases with incarcerated inguinal hernias.[88]

Hydrocele. When fluid accumulates within the tunica vaginalis of the scrotum, a hydrocele results. Communicating hydroceles occur with failure of the upper processus vaginalis to obliterate, resulting in a conduit between the peritoneum and the scrotum. The upper processus vaginalis is closed with a noncommunicating hydrocele.[88] If only fluid is present, the pathology is a hydrocele, whereas if bowel invaginates into the processus vaginalis, an indirect hernia exists. Hydroceles are more common on the right; most are painless and present at birth, resolving by 18 months of age.

Examination will find scrotal fullness that transilluminates. The size of the scrotum may change with position, straining, or squeezing.[89] Although tempting, aspiration of hydroceles is to be avoided. When the physician cannot differentiate between a scrotal hydrocele and an inguinal hernia, a surgical consultation is warranted.

Occasionally a patient will present with an acute, painful hydrocele. This may represent acute intraabdominal pathology such as ruptured appendix or meconium hydrocele from prenatal rupture of viscus necessitating surgical consultation. Other causes of painful hydrocele include epididymitis, torsions, tumor, or trauma. In these situations the ipsilateral testis will be tender and enlarged, although the examination may be compromised by the size of the hydrocele. Scintigraphy or color Doppler ultrasound may be helpful.

Trauma. Blunt trauma to the scrotum may produce a variety of injuries, from simple contusion of the scrotal skin to rupture of the testicle.[83] Injury limited to minimal swelling, bruising, or tenderness may be managed conservatively with immobilization, ice, and analgesia. Large scrotal hematomas may represent more significant testicular injuries and require surgical evaluation. Blunt trauma may rupture the testicle when it is trapped against the pubic ramus. Be aware that acute torsions have been reported after blunt scrotal trauma.[90] When acute torsion of the spermatic cord cannot be ruled out or rupture of the testis is possible, ultrasound, scintigraphy, or exploration is indicated.[87,91] The time elapsed from insult to treatment may be crucial in these patients, similar to the patient with a torsion, because testicular blood supply may be compromised.

Testicular Tumor. Testicular tumors account for less than 2% of all pediatric solid tumors and have an incidence in boys under 15 years of age of 0.5/100,000.[92] They occur most frequently in 2-year-old males with a second peak in the pubertal years.[88] Patients with solid tumors of the testicle present with painless, heavy and firm, asymmetrical scrotal mass. Ultrasonography can be confirmatory.[89] Testicular tumors may present as acute painful swelling resulting from hemorrhage or necrosis into the tumor. For the nontender, swollen testicle a nonemergent surgical referral is more appropriate.

Idiopathic Scrotal Edema. ISE is seen in prepubertal males, with 77% of the cases occurring before age 10. Etiology of ISE is uncertain but characteristics of allergic disease have been found. Typically patients have sudden onset of swelling without pain. Every patient displays scrotal erythema and edema but has very little tenderness. Occasionally the swelling extends to the phallus. Fever is rare. Scrotal edema from nephrotic syndrome may look similar to ISE but is also present in the lower extremities. A urinalysis should quickly differentiate ISE from nephrosis. Episodes of ISE resolve spontaneously in 1 to 4 days and require little treatment beyond reassurance.[88,89]

Miscellaneous Conditions. There are other conditions that may present as scrotal pain or swelling mimicking the acute scrotum. Inguinal adenopathy is usually associated with physical findings such as penile vesicles or lower extremity lesions. Cysts and angiomas, sarcoidosis, Henoch-Schönlein purpura, and hypertriglyceridemia can all present as scrotal pain or swelling.[84]

Diagnostic Work-Up

The clinician should determine whether the patient has pain, swelling, or both in the scrotal region and should determine the onset and progression of pain and history of previous episodes. As many as 30% of patients with torsions of the spermatic cord or appendix testis will report an earlier experience with similar types of pain.[88]

Age is another factor. Knight and Vassy found that patients with acute spermatic cord torsions averaged 13 ± 3.5 years of age, whereas those with torsion of the appendix testis averaged 9.9 ± 2.9 years.[85] Other discriminating historic facts include the presence of dysuria, history of earlier UTIs, anatomic abnormalities, urinary tract instrumentation, or gradual onset of pain. These features are found in epididymitis and not torsion of the spermatic cord.[85] Trauma may precede a ruptured testicle but may also be associated with spermatic cord torsion.[91]

The physical examination can yield important information. On inspection of the scrotum is there edema of the skin? Are there skin lesions present suggesting insect bites or allergy? Is there ecchymosis, implicating a traumatic injury? The scrotum may have a tense area of swelling with a bluish color to it, typically seen with a hydrocele. This area should transilluminate. Often there are traumatic hydroceles in association with testicular torsions.[83] In torsion the testis will lie transversely and be elevated. The left testicle usually sits lower than the right; when this relationship is reversed, suspect a torsion. Palpate the intrascrotal contents and try to delineate the epididymis from the testicle. In torsions, the epididymis is shifted to the front of the scrotum.[81] Examination of the intrascrotal structures may be impossible because of the extreme degree of discomfort these patients have. Patients with torsions of the appendix testis have a faintly visible blue nodule located on the upper pole of the testes (blue dot sign).[83,88] Also palpate the spermatic cord for the presence of varicoceles, usually painless unless a thrombus has occurred. Hernias may be palpable in the inguinal canal and extend into the scrotum (see Chapter 52). The presence of the cremasteric reflex (retraction of the testicle with stroking of the inner thigh) is a reliable sign eliminating testicular torsion from the differential consideration, whereas Prehn's sign (relief of pain with elevation of the scrotum in epididymitis and no relief or exacerbation of pain with elevation in testicular torsions) is worthless.[89]

When the diagnosis cannot be made on the basis of the history or examination, color Doppler ultrasound or testicular scintigraphy may provide useful information about the presence of blood flow or the anatomy of the scrotum (see section on Testicular Torsion).

Prehospital Considerations

The acute scrotum in an adolescent requires the prehospital providers to assure expeditious evaluation and possible exploration. Delay can be disastrous; the opportunity for saving a torsed testicle lasts only 6 to 10 hours from the onset of pain. Emergency responders should give intravenous fluids if vomiting has occurred. Transport the patient with the scrotum supported and ice packs applied to help relieve the pain and swelling.

Therapeutic Trial

In the case of the acute scrotum, there are two caveats. First, a wait-and-see approach can be disastrous for the patient with a testicular emergency. Secondly, be cautious in assigning the diagnosis of epididymitis to patients because an error here may well mean that a torsion of the spermatic cord has been overlooked.[88]

Diagnostic Entities

CIRCUMCISION COMPLICATIONS

JAMES A. O'DONNELL II

Whether the incidence of circumcision in the newborn in the immediate postdelivery period is declining is open to debate.[93] Circumcision in the immediate postdelivery period is usually performed just prior to discharge. This fact, coupled with the now commonplace shorter postdelivery hospitalization stays, will tend to increase pediatric emergency department visits for the actual and supposed complications of circumcision.

There are generally three methods of circumcision commonly in use. These are the dorsal slit, the use of either Gomco or plastibell clamps, and excision.[94-96] Physicians for children should familiarize themselves with these techniques so as to develop expertise in the normal postoperative course and complications of the infant who has been circumcised.

There are several reasons why circumcision can be advocated in the male including prevention of penile cancer and UTIs[94]; improved hygiene; prevention of phimosis, paraphi-

mosis, posthitis (prepuce inflammation), and balanitis; or inflammation of the glans penis.[93] There is, however, no acceptable reason for females to be circumcised. If such an event comes to the attention of the physician, an investigation for abuse is warranted.[97]

Severe complications including necrosis and complete or partial amputation of the penis are rare and usually due to inappropriate techniques.[98] For the most part circumcision is safe and perhaps one of the most commonly performed surgical procedures in the United States.[93]

Intraoperative complications of circumcision include hemorrhage, localized and systemic infection, Fournier syndrome, necrotizing fasciitis, and excessive penile skin or inadequate prepuce removal as well as meatal problems. Hemorrhage is usually minor and controlled by pressure on the wound. Other methods used to control bleeding include the application of silver nitrate, epinephrine, fibrin and suture placement.[96]

The second most common complication is infection. This can be either localized or generalized with the circumcision site serving as the entry for invading organisms. Organisms that have been implicated in localized infections include *Staphylococcus aureus*, *Klebsiella pneumoniae*, *Staphylococcus epidermidis* (coagulase-negative), *Escherichia coli*, and *Proteus mirabilis*.[99] Additionally, *E. coli* and group D streptococcus have been implicated as the causative agents in Fournier syndrome, the gangrenous infection of the scrotum, penis, and perineum.[100] Group D salmonella has also been identified as the cause of postcircumcision scrotal abscess.[101] Necrotizing fasciitis has also been described. Cultures in these cases yielded mixed flora.[102] Primary penile tuberculosis has been described, presenting with bilateral inguinal lymph node enlargement and a draining sinus.[103]

In addition to localized infection, meningitis and septicemia can follow circumcision. *S. aureus*, group B beta-hemolytic streptococcus, and *Proteus* species have been implicated as causative agents in this setting.[104,105] UTIs have also been reported as a complication of circumcision.[106] Kaplan also reports osteomyelitis, pulmonary abscess, diphtheria, and tetanus as complications of circumcision.[94]

Inherent in the operative procedure of circumcision is the possibility of causing meatal stenosis or ulcers. With circumcision the glans loses the protection afforded by the prepuce to the glans and the urethral meatus and is susceptible to injury from ammonia compounds produced by bacterial action on urine held in place by the infant's diaper.[96] Patients with meatal stenosis present with symptoms of penile pain with micturition, the presence of a high velocity stream, and the need to sit or stand back from the toilet to void.[107] The reported incidence of meatitis is between 8% and 31%.

Excessive skin removal at the time of circumcision from the penile shaft, coupled with an inadequate amount of the inner prepuce epithelium being removed, leads to the concealed penis. The penile shaft is forced into the suprapubic fat and a stenotic preputial ring is formed that lies at or just above the skin level of the abdominal wall.[94,96] This can lead to bladder outflow obstruction. Should such a patient present, the stenotic ring can be dilated using a hemostat to provide temporary relief; if this fails a dorsal slit can be made until definite correction by repeat circumcision is performed.[108] This must be differentiated from a penis hidden by fat deposits in the suprapubic area; retracting the fat deposits makes this distinction.

Laceration of the glans or the penile shaft at the time of circumcision has the potential for excessive scarring, which may lead to chordee formation and angulation of the penis either in the flaccid or erect state. This can cause pain. Likewise, the retention of excessive or asymmetric amounts of the foreskin can lead to scarring, which could result in acquired phimosis or paraphimosis.[94] The urethra can be damaged because of its ventral position on the penis at the time of circumcision. This can also lead to the formation of urethrocutaneous fistulas. Iatrogenic hypospadias and epispadias may result if the glans penis is split during circumcision.[96]

Postoperative complications include pain that generally lasts from 12 to 24 hours, urinary retention, skin bridge and inclusion cyst formation, and problems that are related to either retention of the plastibell or the size of the plastibell used.

Postoperative swelling caused by edema of the glans or the presence of obstructing surgical dressings may cause urinary retention. The urinary retention may be associated with secondary symptoms such as poor feeding, emesis, irritability, and even cyanosis of the lower extremities. One case has been described in which the circumcision dressing led to urinary obstruction of such a degree that gross bladder distension and bilateral hydroureteronephrosis resulted.[109] Usually removal of the offending surgical dressing causes prompt resolution of the urinary retention and secondary symptoms, although at times adjunctive treatment is necessary until all complications resolve.[110]

When the plastibell device is employed, it is imperative to use the proper size "bell." If the bell is too small, the ring can restrict normal venous return from the glans causing edema or can adhere to the glans causing scarring and tissue necrosis. With time this can lead to meatal stenosis, chordee, or sulcus formation. If the plastibell is too large it can become displaced proximally until it encounters the larger penile shaft. The ring can then act like a tourniquet in this position and cause distal edema and even necrosis. Plastibell complications appear to be more common in those patients who retain the device for more than 10 days after circumcision. Parents should be advised to have the circumcision checked if they suspect any problems or if the plastibell is present for more than 10 days after application.[94,95,111,112]

Skin bridges consist of small bands of tissue that bind the glans to the penile shaft because of the incomplete separation of the inner preputial epithelium and the glans at the time of circumcision. Fibrosis fusion of these bands causes chordee formation and, in addition to deformation and pain, can serve as a nidus for infection. Inclusion cysts are formed as the result of retained smegma implanted in the wound or the involution of the epidermis during the circumcision. These present as small cystic bumps along the edge of the circumcision. Like skin bridges they too can later become infected and thus cause problems. The definitive treatment for both conditions is surgical resection.[94,96]

EPIDIDYMITIS

MARTIN I. HERMAN

Infection or inflammation of the epididymis as a cause of scrotal pain and swelling is uncommon in prepubertal males; however, it is the most common cause of the acute scrotum in adults. Differentiating epididymitis from acute testicular torsions may be very difficult. Incorrect diagnosis may result in lower testicular salvage rates.

Epididymitis is an inflammation of the epididymis. The epididymis is the elongated cordlike structure resting along the posterior border of the testicle that acts as a storage site for spermatozoa.

The epididymis, composed of a tortuous duct, is comma-shaped and closely applied to the posterior margin of the testis, overlapping the superior pole and lateral surface. A testicle is attached by 15 to 20 efferent ductules and by a common segment of tunica vaginalis. Turek surveyed the epididymal anatomy in 112 boys: 84% had the typical relationship between epididymis and testicle (type 1), 13% had the epididymis fused along the entire curvature (type 2 on bell clapper deformity), and the remaining 3% had other variants.[113]

Pathophysiology

Retrograde flow of urine induced by straining may be a factor in the development of epididymitis. Urine reflux can induce an inflammatory response in the vas and epididymis. Young patients with acute epididymitis typically have a history of earlier UTIs, anatomic abnormalities, instrumentation, or symptoms referable to the urinary tract, such as dysuria or pyuria.

Etiology

Adolescents presenting with epididymal pain may not have any demonstrable bacterial infection; in these cases a viral or atypical bacterium is suspected. *N. gonorrhoeae* and *C. trachomatis* can cause epididymitis, especially in the sexually active patient. In patients with UTI, *Enterobacteriaceae* or *Pseudomonas* may be causative. Other etiologies have included brucellosis, and in young children, *Haemophilus influenzae.*[114]

Diagnostic Findings

Clinical Findings. Physical examination may find a tender, swollen epididymis in its normal position, posterior and lateral to the testes. The pain may be exquisite, prohibiting an adequate examination. If so, the cord can be blocked with lidocaine to allow for a more comfortable and meaningful examination. A urethral discharge or boggy prostate may be present on examination. The history may reveal gradual onset, fever, nausea, vomiting, urinary complaints, urethral discharge, urinary surgery or instrumentation, abnormal bladder function, or anatomic abnormalities of the genitourinary system. Prehn's sign (relief with elevation) is unreliable.[89] A reactive hydrocele may be present confounding the physical assessment of the scrotal contents. As the infection advances to include the testes, differentiating epididymitis from torsion becomes very difficult because the anatomic landmarks are obscured.

Ancillary Data. Urine cultures can help in selecting antibiotic coverage, especially if sensitivity is tested. A urinalysis will report leukocytes or may be normal. Urethral discharge cultures, chlamydia antigen detection, and gram stain may also be valuable when a discharge is present.

When faced with the challenge of selecting between epididymitis and other causes of an acute scrotum, the clinician may find scintigraphy or ultrasound useful (see section on Testicular Torsion). Complete blood counts are not helpful because both spermatic cord torsions and epididymitis can have elevated white blood cell counts.

Complications

Most cases of epididymitis will resolve with the combination of antibiotics, rest, and scrotal elevation. A few patients will continue to have significant pain, which may represent abscess formation requiring surgical drainage or orchiectomy. A repeat ultrasound may reveal the abscess. Chronic epididymitis can also be caused by an acute infection and long-term epididymal atrophy can result. Infertility is rare after epididymitis unless bilateral involvement was noted.

Differential Considerations
(See Section on Scrotal Pain and Swelling)

Acute epididymitis must be differentiated from acute testicular torsion as well as other less threatening entities (See Table 60-7).

Management

Prehospital management may involve pain relief with ice packs or intravenous analgesia. Place the patient in a position of comfort and elevate the scrotum by propping it on a pillow. Fluids may be needed if there has been significant vomiting.

When a patient presents with acute scrotal pathology the emergency physician should be notified immediately to evaluate differential considerations (see section on Scrotal Pain and Swelling). Urine, blood, and urethral specimens can be obtained and sent off for the appropriate studies.

After the diagnosis of epididymitis is made, therapy is fairly straightforward. Septic- or toxic-appearing patients, as well as those who are immunocompromised, are admitted for intravenous antibiotics, usually ceftriaxone or cefotaxime. Low-risk patients can be treated for their pain and discharged. If there is urethral discharge, therapy for *N. gonorrhoeae* with parenteral ceftriaxone, 125 mg, and a prescription for doxycycline, 200 mg/24 hr BID PO, or tetracycline, 2 gm/24 hr QID PO, should be initiated. Consult the CDC guidelines for alternative treatment strategies in the allergic patient. Children under 9 years should receive erythromycin (50 mg/kg/day [max: 2 gm] QID PO).[114] Other cases of epididymitis without a bacterial source can be treated with ampicillin, trimethoprim-sulfamethoxazole, erythromycin, clarithromycin, azithromycin, cephalexin, or one of the fluoroquinolones. Treat for 10 to 14 days. Note the fluoroquinolones and azithromycin are not approved for use in children. Analgesia should not be overlooked in these patients whether admitted or sent home.

Disposition

Patients undergoing treatment for acute epididymitis will need urologic follow-up care. Persistent pain warrants urgent repeat evaluation. If the inflammation and pain respond to therapy, a recheck in a week would be appropriate. Positive gonorrhea cultures need to be reported and the patient followed up to assess the efficacy of therapy. These patients also need to be screened for other sexually transmitted diseases. Any patient who has not had the urinary tract evaluated prior to infection should also undergo voiding cystourethrography and renal ultrasound.

GLOMERULONEPHRITIS, ACUTE POSTSTREPTOCOCCAL

JOHN G. KNEPPER

Acute glomerulonephritis (AGN) follows infections resulting from strains of group A beta-hemolytic streptococci. These infections can be either pharyngeal or cutaneous (impetigo, pyoderma). The disease most commonly occurs between ages 3 and 7 years and rarely under 2 years.

The pathogenesis is poorly understood but probably results from the deposition of circulating immune complexes in the kidney. These immune complexes are deposited on the glomerular basement membrane and result in a decrease in glomerular filtration.[115,116]

Diagnostic Findings
(See Section on Renal Failure, Acute)

There is usually a preceding streptococcal infection or exposure 1 to 2 weeks before the onset of glomerulonephritis. Patients may develop a sudden onset of oliguria with the production of dark brown or blood urine resulting from hematuria. Fluid retention and edema, hypertension, fever, malaise, and abdominal pain are often noted.

The physical findings vary depending on the length of illness. Initial findings may be only some mild facial and extremity edema with a minimal rise in blood pressure. Some children may present with complications of circulatory congestion and pulmonary edema, malignant hypertension, and cardiac dysrhythmias. Anuria and renal failure occur in 2% of patients.

Ancillary Data. Laboratory findings include an abnormal urinalysis with a large amount of blood and protein, red cell casts on microscopic examination in 60% of patients, and normal urinary concentrating ability. Leukocyturia and hyaline and granular casts are common. The fractional excretion of sodium may be reduced (see section on Renal Failure, Acute).

Total serum complement, and specifically C3 complement, is depressed in 90% to 100% of patients during the first 2 weeks of illness, returning to normal in 3 to 4 weeks. Persistently low levels suggest that an ongoing, chronic process is present.[116]

Antistreptolysin (ASO) is elevated. Immunoglobulin G levels are elevated, often associated with a positive rheumatoid factor titer over 1:32. Anemia may be present. The BUN is elevated disproportionately to the serum creatinine. Hyponatremia and hyperkalemia may be present and are specifically related to the degree of oliguria.

Management

Initial focus must be on fluid and salt restriction to maintain a normal intravascular volume as discussed in the section on Renal Failure, Acute. Diuretics may be required. Blood pressure, weight (fluid retention), and urinalysis should be followed closely on an outpatient basis if the illness is mild. Patients with complications should be monitored to treat the problems associated with acute renal failure. Hypertension should be managed acutely and chronically (see section on Hypertension). Congestive heart failure and azotemia may need specific inpatient management.

The prognosis for complete recovery from acute glomerulonephritis in children is excellent. Approximately 80% to 90% recovery without any measurable renal abnormality is expected. All patients who have evidence of uncontrolled hypertension, congestive heart failure, or azotemia should be hospitalized. Children without any of these problems can be followed at home but must have adequate medical care available, including frequent blood pressure measurements. A nephrologist should be consulted. Follow-up will reflect clinical condition, response to therapy, and normalization of laboratory findings.

HEMOLYTIC-UREMIC SYNDROME

JULIO CASTILLO ● MARY P. SWEENEY

The hemolytic-uremic syndrome (HUS) is a multisystem disorder with diverse etiologies, variable clinical presentations, and multiple pathophysiologies. HUS was described in children by Gasser in 1955. A similar syndrome in adults was described in 1925 by Moschowitz as thrombotic thrombocytopenic purpura (TTP).[117] Both disorders share clinical features (thrombocytopenia, acute nephropathy, hemolytic anemia, CNS symptoms, and fever), as well as arteriolar and capillary microthrombolic pathologic lesions.[118] TTP affects mainly adults who develop a generalized vasculopathy, have a high fatality rate, and respond better to plasmapheresis and fresh-frozen plasma (FFP).

The syndrome occurs most frequently in infants and young children, with a mean age in the United States of 3 years; it rarely occurs after 5 years of age and neonatal cases are uncommon. HUS has no sex predilection and a worldwide distribution; it is rare in blacks and endemic in Argentina, South Africa, and southern California.[119] Seasonal variations with peaks during the summer months have been reported as well as sporadic and epidemic outbreaks, most commonly associated with food contaminated by verotoxin producing *E. coli.*

Pediatric HUS without diarrhea has been described as a subset of cases with a different presentation and outcome from typical HUS.[120] Familial HUS, type 1, occurs in siblings who have a brief period between onsets, good prognosis, and no recurrences. Type 2 occurs in siblings whose onset is more than one year apart and whose prognosis is poor (genetic predisposition, autosomal recessive mode). Type 3, the autosomal dominant mode, has been reported

in adults and has an extremely high mortality rate. The majority of nonfamilial adult cases are associated with pregnancy, essential hypertension, use of oral contraceptives, collagen vascular disease, malignancies, or hyperacute renal homograft rejections.[117,121,122]

Pathophysiology

The probable initial pathogenic event is an injury to the endothelial cells of the renal microvasculature induced either by a viral or bacterial agent or their toxins. The vascular endothelial cell injury is characterized by edema and detachment of the basal membrane followed by local fibrin deposits. A microangiopathic hemolytic anemia develops as a result of mechanical damage to the red cells by the fibrin strands as the erythrocytes pass through the narrowed vessels. The damaged red cells are sequestered by the reticuloendothelial system, resulting in a decrease in the RBC count and associated decrease in the hemoglobin level.[121] There may also be injury directly to the red blood cell membranes, endothelial cells, and platelets, since fragmented erythrocytes have been described in HUS patients without microangiopathic changes.[118]

The platelets aggregate around the damaged vessel walls and liberate the vasoconstrictor agent thromboxane A_2 and the platelet aggregatory stimulating factor, producing microthrombi and secondary hypoxia. Recanalization of occluded vessels is inhibited by decreased fibrinolysis, which appears to be mediated by increased levels of plasminogen activator inhibitor.[123,124] Lack of stimulation of production of prostacyclin, an antiplatelet aggregation agent, may add to the development of microthrombi.

Platelets, fibrin, and complement also deposit in the lumina of the glomeruli resulting in decreased glomerular filtration and ultimately renal failure.[117] Glomerular capillary wall thickening and subendothelial electron-dense deposits of fibrin are characteristic. Focal areas of necrosis leading to permanent damage may evolve.[117,121,125,126]

Etiology

The organism most frequently found in association with the typical cases of HUS is *E. coli* (serotype 0157:H7), which produces a cytotoxin (also referred to as a verotoxin). This cytotoxin is a protein synthesis inhibitor and causes cell death. The organism is spread by both person-to-person contact and contaminated food, typically beef or unpasteurized milk.[126,127] In a large recent outbreak in the northwestern United States, HUS was associated with *E. coli* 0157:H7, traced to a fast food chain, pointing out the need for public health intervention in monitoring food quality.[128] The use of antibiotics in treatment of diarrhea caused by *E. coli* 0157:H7 may increase the risk of developing HUS. An agent may also increase the incidence of HUS.

In underdeveloped countries, *Shigella* and *Salmonella* infections have been associated with HUS. Shigatoxin, produced by *Shigella dysenteriae-1*, is essentially identical to the cytotoxins produced by *E. coli* and thus may have an identical cell receptor, mechanism of action, and pathogenetic significance.[129]

Neuraminidase-producing organisms, such as *Streptococcus pneumoniae* and possibly some viruses, are also associated with HUS. Neuraminidase will cleave the N-acetylneuraminic acid in the T-F antigen region on erythrocytes, platelets, endothelial cells, lymphocytes, and glycosubstances in the brain and will expose this antigen to anti-T-F antigen antibodies (IgM) present in the patient's plasma, leading to polyagglutination with hemolysis. The IgM anti-T-F antigen antibodies may have been induced in a previous exposure to intestinal bacteria or may be present in plasma infusates.[117]

Diagnostic Findings

The prodromal symptoms may include severe cramping abdominal pain, watery diarrhea followed by grossly bloody diarrhea, emesis, and occasionally upper respiratory symptoms. This is followed by acute renal failure, pallor, low-grade fever, hematuria, oliguria, petechiae, prostration, gastrointestinal bleeding, and CNS deterioration that may present as irritability, lethargy, gait disorder, personality disorder, seizures, hemiparesis, cortical blindness, or coma. The absence of a gastrointestinal prodrome is associated with a poor prognosis.

HUS can present as an acute abdominal emergency resulting from bowel perforation, colitis with bowel ischemia, intussusception, colonic stricture, and toxic megacolon. Occasionally, HUS may mimic acute hepatitis, with jaundice seen in up to 30% of the cases. The hemolysis occurs rapidly and the hemoglobin may fall to 4 to 5 gm/dl within a few hours. Thrombocytopenia rarely persists beyond 2 weeks and has no prognostic significance.

Hypertension is present in 40% to 50% of the patients and may contribute to the encephalopathy and cardiac failure. Seizures occur in 40% of cases, especially in patients with hyponatremia or severe azotemia. Electrolyte imbalance, especially hyponatremia and hypocalcemia, is common. The spectrum of renal disease may be very variable, ranging from a mild elevation of BUN to total anuria caused by acute nephropathy.

Pancreatic insufficiency leading to permanent insulin-dependent diabetes mellitus has been reported. Autopsies and CT scans of the head have revealed infarcts and hemorrhages. Cardiac involvement has included cardiomyopathy, cardiac aneurysms, high-output cardiac failure, and myocarditis.[121,125,126]

Recurrences can occur, often without a prodrome and associated with a mortality rate of 30%.

Ancillary Data. Due to the multisystem compromise, close monitoring is essential. Daily weights, record of intake and output, and frequent measurement of the blood pressure are essential. Neurologic examinations will assess the progression of the CNS involvement. The presence of seizure or coma may indicate CNS hemorrhage.

Electrolytes, BUN, creatinine, calcium, phosphate, CBC, platelet count, reticulocyte count, prothrombin time (PT), partial thromboplastin time (PTT), and fibrinogen split products need periodic monitoring. In dehydration without renal involvement, the BUN is often elevated and should decrease by 50% over the first 24 hours of appropriate rehydration. The peripheral blood smear will demonstrate morphologic changes in the erythrocytes (tear drop cells, burr cells, helmet cells, microspherocytes). The WBC may be elevated and platelets may be decreased below 50,000/

mm^3. Low total protein measurement on admission may be an indicator for renal failure and subsequent need for support and potential dialysis.[130] Serologic testing for antibodies to the lipopolysaccharide of E. coli 0157:H7 provides evidence of infection with E. coli 0157:H7 when fecal bacteria or verotoxin cannot be detected.[131]

Differential Considerations

Inflammatory processes may have similar presentation. Ulcerative colitis may be accompanied by bloody diarrhea and anemia. The length of illness may be helpful. Surgical abdominal processes or acute dehydration and acute tubular necroses may have parallel characteristics.

Other causes of acquired hemolytic anemia should be considered (see Chapter 54).

Management

Supportive therapy for patients with mild features of HUS but without anuria has been responsible for the decline in the mortality rate to 5% to 10%. None of the many therapeutic approaches that have been used have proved uniformly successful. The use of heparin (due to the presence of fibrinogen degradation products), immunosuppressive agents (steroids and vincristine), antiplatelet agents (aspirin, dipyridamole), fibrinolytic agents (urokinase, streptokinase), prostacyclin (PGI2) infusions, intravenous IgG infusions (to abolish platelet aggregating activity), or vitamin E (to correct peroxidase damage) has not been consistently beneficial.[118,132,133] The use of FFP and plasma exchange to provide prostacyclin and remove its inhibitors, although still controversial, is a frequently used treatment modality.

The early institution of peritoneal dialysis probably has been most efficient in improving the outcome for patients with HUS and is usually indicated in severely affected patients with anuria for more than 24 hours or the simultaneous presence of hypertension, seizures, and oliguria.

Rehydration therapy should be initiated promptly. In the euvolemic patient, fluids should be limited to 350 to 400 ml/m^2 surface plus ongoing renal and gastrointestinal losses. Inappropriate administration of fluids when oliguria is wrongly suspected to be prerenal may produce edema, hyponatremia, or congestive heart failure. Patients with edema and hyponatremia require a negative salt and water balance.

Hyperkalemia is common and may require emergency management in the presence of cardiotoxicity (sodium bicarbonate, 50% dextrose plus regular insulin, calcium gluconate) (see section on Renal Failure). Emergency dialysis for severe hyperkalemia should be instituted as soon as possible. Hyponatremia and hypocalcemia should be corrected to prevent potentially life-threatening seizures. Hyperphosphatemia is best treated with dialysis.

Packed red blood cells (p-RBC) are recommended if the hematocrit drops to a level less than 15% to 20% or the hemoglobin is less than 5 to 6 gm/ml and the hemolytic process has not ceased or hemodynamic status is not stable. Transfusion should be accomplished in small amounts, slowly (5 ml/kg over 4 hours) to minimize overload. Platelet replacement is indicated only if there is active bleeding with a platelet count consistently below 20,000/mm^3, as further platelet plugging and decreased platelet survival time will occur.[126,133]

Hypertension that persists after control of volume overload should be treated with antihypertensive drugs. Nifedipine is recommended for diastolic readings above 120 to 130 mm Hg. If the hypertension is persistent, labetalol, captopril, or hydralazine may be used (see section on Hypertension).

Seizures not associated with hyponatremia will respond to diazepam and phenytoin. Prophylactic anticonvulsant therapy is controversial in patients with neuromuscular irritability marked by muscle twitching. In the presence of elevated intracranial pressure, aggressive therapy with hyperventilation, mannitol, and fluid restriction is indicated. Total parenteral nutrition or oral administration of carbohydrate-essential amino-acid preparations can help to limit the azotemia.[133]

The management of fluid and electrolyte balance, the control of hypertension and seizures, and the control of anemia and active bleeding secondary to thrombocytopenia have been primarily responsible for the decreased morbidity and mortality rates. Patients should be admitted for treatment. HUS usually resolves 1 to 3 months after presentation, with no residual complications in 80% to 85% of these cases. Long-term follow-up is indicated. Siblings and other household members should be monitored concurrently.

HENOCH-SCHÖNLEIN PURPURA

JOHN G. KNEPPER

Henoch-Schönlein purpura (HSP) is a vasculitis presenting with abdominal pain, arthritis, and purpura. Although the etiology is undefined, HSP is associated with group A streptococci, *Mycoplasma*, and viral (varicella, Epstein-Barr virus [EBV]) infections; drugs (penicillin, tetracycline, aspirin, sulfonamides, and erythromycin); and allergens (insect bites, chocolate, milk, and wheat). It most commonly occurs in winter months and has a male predominance.[134]

Diagnostic Findings

Skin lesions are pathognomonic, beginning on the gravity-dependent areas of the legs and buttocks and the extensor surfaces of the arms. They begin as erythematous, maculopapular lesions that blanch and become petechial and purpuric, at which time they are often palpable. They may be discrete, confluent, clustered, or individual. The entire body may be involved, although the lower extremities usually demonstrate the greatest eruption. A rash is the presenting symptom in 50% of patients and may recur in 40% of patients within 6 weeks, often without systemic signs.[135]

Colicky abdominal pain with diarrhea, often bloody, is common. Approximately 60% to 85% of patients have melena or hematemesis. Intussusception or perforation must be considered. Nephritis may develop, associated with hematuria, proteinuria, and other nephrosis. Renal involvement is almost always the ultimate determinant of outcome and long-term sequelae but cases of intestinal perforation with life-threatening sequelae have been reported.[136] Mi-

gratory polyarthritis, often transient, is present with greatest tenderness of ankles, knees, or wrists. CNS changes may include mental status change, hemiparesis, seizures, and intracranial hemorrhage. Other findings include soft tissue edema of the scalp, ear, face, and dorsum of the hands and feet; testicular pain; and parotitis.

Multisystem involvement occurs primarily in children 2 to 11 years of age with progression of renal disease occurring more commonly in older children and adults (children, 5%; adults, 13%). Children under 3 months commonly have only skin manifestations without gastrointestinal or renal involvement.

Ancillary Data. The WBC is usually elevated and anemia may be present. Bleeding screen and platelet count are normal. The erythrocyte sedimentation rate may be elevated. Urinalysis reflects the degree of renal involvement. Hematuria, proteinuria, leukocytosis, and cylindruria may be noted. If the urinalysis is abnormal, other assessments of renal function are indicated.

Other evaluation that may be indicated include a throat culture for group A streptococci, blood cultures, and serum complement, which should be normal. Renal biopsy is ultimately performed in patients with severe nephropathy after the acute phase of illness.

Radiographic studies to exclude intussusception may be required in patients with severe abdominal pain (see Chapter 52).

Differential Considerations

Diagnoses that should be considered include those presenting with a purpuric rash, such as meningococcemia and Rocky Mountain spotted fever. Thrombocytopenic purpura with a low platelet count and nonthrombocytopenic purpura (Ehlers-Danlos syndrome, scurvy, steroid therapy) may be considered. Intraabdominal pathology such as intussusception, trauma, and appendicitis as well as primary renal pathology should be excluded. A ureteral stone with colic may be considered because of the association of abdominal pain and hematuria.

Management

Supportive care is essential if there is evidence of gastrointestinal hemorrhage or hypovolemia, and fluid resuscitation should be initiated. Abdominal pathology, underlying renal disease, and septicemia should be considered, requiring emergent consultation.

With significant gastrointestinal symptoms and once an acute abdomen is excluded, steroids may be useful in severely affected children (prednisone 1 to 2 mg/kg/24 hr q 12 hr PO for 1 week). Some evidence suggests that steroids may also be beneficial in soft tissue and joint swelling as well as glomerulonephritis, the latter requiring high-dose, pulsed therapy. Therapy with intravenous immunoglobulins (IVIG) has also been recommended in patients with severe renal involvement.[137] IVIG has also been tried in patients with severe abdominal pain secondary to gastrointestinal involvement, with good results.[138]

Specific treatment is required for renal failure or nephrosis in consultation with a nephrologist. Patients should be hospitalized unless skin manifestations are the only problem and good follow-up is possible. A poor prognosis is associated with children less than 6 years old and those with nephrotic syndrome or crescent formation in the glomeruli. Patients with renal involvement may improve and then much later develop progressive renal disease. All patients with HSP with renal involvement should have long-term follow-up.[139]

NEPHROTIC SYNDROME

WARREN L. HUTCHESON

Nephrotic syndrome (NS) is classically defined by proteinuria, hypoproteinemia, hyperlipidemia, and edema. Patients may have variable features of the syndrome during the course of the disease process. Confusion arises with attempts to categorize patients. Primary NS as opposed to secondary NS is that disease state occurring in the absence of glomerulonephritis or in association with a known disease state. Patients may also be categorized by their histologic characteristics from renal biopsy. Patients with NS are probably best categorized into various subgroups based on the pattern of steroid response. This has important diagnostic, therapeutic, and prognostic value for the treating physicians and appears to be the single most important clinical parameter in patients with primary NS as well as secondary NS.[140]

Minimal change NS (MCNS), the most common form of childhood NS, is based on a characteristic histologic pattern. It represents the classic form of primary NS, only rarely having features of nephritis. Most important, 93% of patients with minimal change in NS respond to a course of steroids. In addition, 92% of all children with NS who respond to steroids will have MCNS and thus a good prognosis.[141]

Epidemiology

Boys are affected with primary NS twice as often as girls. The sexes are affected equally in adulthood. The incidence of new cases of NS in children less than 16 years old ranges anywhere from 2 to 7/100,000/year. The prevalence is approximately 15 cases/100,000 in the pediatric population.

Some 90% of children with NS have primary disease. Approximately 85% of primary NS is MCNS, 10% focal sclerosis, and 5% mesangial proliferation. More than 70% of all NS children between the ages of 1 to 7 years of age have MCNS.[141,142] In comparison, only 50% of older children, even fewer adolescents, and only 25% to 30% of adults have MCNS.[141] Congenital NS is known as the Finnish-type NS, commonly presenting in the first 3 minutes of life and associated with a poor prognosis.

Pathophysiology

Generally, all of the abnormalities encountered in the patient with NS result from the presence of proteinuria and subsequent hypoproteinemia. In the normal kidney, the glomerular filter contains negatively charged proteins (sialoglycoproteins) that line the epithelial podocytes. These negatively charged sites are responsible for the transport of both cations and anions across the glomerular basement membrane. Evidence suggests that in NS, there is a loss of the sialoglycoproteins, which in turn results in a loss of the negative charge on the basement membrane by 50%. This increases glomerular permeability to proteins resulting in massive proteinuria.[143,144] The loss of the negative charge is also believed to cause the epithelial foot-process fusion seen in patients with MCNS.[143]

Because of the urinary losses of primarily albumin, hypoalbuminemia is present and is responsible for the decrease in the plasma oncotic pressure. In accordance with the Starling forces, there is a shift of fluid from the vascular to the interstitial spaces causing a shrinking plasma volume and systemic edema. In the presence of a diminished blood volume, the reninangiotensin-aldosterone system is activated and produces an increase in tubular sodium chloride reabsorption.[145] Edema formation is worsened. Hepatic synthesis of albumin may increase, but is unable to compensate for the urinary losses.

The serum cholesterol level is inversely related to the serum albumin level in the nephrotic state, but the mechanism for this hyperlipidemia is poorly understood. An increase in the hepatic synthesis of lipids and lipoproteins is postulated, but the activity of lipoprotein lipase is decreased. The elevated levels of serum cholesterol persist long after the urinary protein losses and serum albumin levels have returned to normal.[146]

Etiology

The etiology of primary NS is unknown and is generally idiopathic. There have been no certain associations with antecedent infections; respiratory infection often precedes the onset. Bacterial, viral (hepatitis, cytomegalovirus, EBV), and protozoan infections and malaria have been implicated. Other causes that have been loosely related to primary NS include insect stings, ingestion of certain drugs (heroin, mercury, probenecid, and silver), allergic reactions (poison ivy or oak, pollens), tumors, and recent immunizations.[143] Current research is investigating an immunologic basis for NS.

Causes of secondary NS include collagen vascular diseases, such as systemic lupus erythematosus and polyarteritis nodosa, vascular diseases (such as HUS and renal vein thrombosis), and certain drugs such as penicillamine. Other associations include HSP and as a complication following hepatitis B and poststreptococcal glomerulonephritis.[145]

Diagnostic Findings

The usual presenting sign in a child with NS is the presence of edema. There may be a prodrome of asymptomatic proteinuria, which allows for early detection of the illness. The edema is usually first noted around the eyes, especially in the morning. It is often attributed to a cold or allergy. As the edema becomes more generalized, parents often believe their child is gaining weight, although the appetite may actually be decreased. In early stages of illness, edema may disappear only to reappear as the disease progresses.

The child generally does not appear ill, unless the degree of fluid retention has progressed and ascites or respiratory distress is present. Ascites is due to the edema of the intestinal mucosa itself and is the cause of abdominal pain, diarrhea, and vomiting in many of these patients. Respiratory distress is a result of pleural effusions or pulmonary edema. Many children have a decreased elasticity of the cartilage of the ear.

Although blood pressure is usually normal or slightly decreased, it is elevated in approximately 5% to 10% of children with MCNS.[147] If the blood pressure remains elevated, a histologic lesion other than MCNS should be sought.[142] Transient hematuria is sometimes present. Occasionally, a child becomes oliguric, but this development is rarely associated with renal failure.

Complications. Acute renal failure is uncommon in primary NS in children and usually thought to be secondary to severe intravascular volume depletion, bilateral renal vein thrombosis, severe hypertension, and a variety of other causes. Reversible idiopathic acute renal failure in children with primary NS has been described.[148]

Many of the complications seen in children with NS are masked by the corticosteroid therapy, especially if a bacterial infection is present. Because these patients are immunocompromised and have an increased susceptibility to infections, one must have an increased degree of suspicion when evaluating the child in the emergency department. Children with NS have decreased levels of IgG and factors B and D (proteins needed in the alternate pathway of complement activation) resulting from urinary losses. Low levels of factor B are believed to lead to impaired opsonization of encapsulated bacteria such as *E. coli* and *S. pneumoniae*.[142,149]

Children are susceptible to all types of infection, most notably cellulitis, peritonitis, and pneumonia. Sepsis and meningitis are not uncommon. Infections are most commonly due to gram-positive organisms, particularly *S. pneumoniae*, but gram-negative organisms also play an important role.

Thrombotic events are among the more serious complications that occur in patients with NS. One study showed 1.8% of nephrotic children to have thromboembolic complications.[150] Many vessels, both arteries and veins, are involved, particularly the renal veins. Renal vein thrombosis is an underdiagnosed problem and occurs more commonly than indicated by the clinical signs and symptoms of flank pain, hematuria, and deterioration of renal function.[142] Causes for the hypercoagulable state include changes in the blood levels of various factors, decreased fibrinolytic activity, platelet tendency to aggregate, venostasis, and increased blood viscosity due to the hyperlipidemia.[143,150] Because of the hypercoagulable state, children should never have any deep venous punctures performed.

Hypovolemia usually occurs in a previously diagnosed patient who is fluid restricted and may be on diuretic therapy. Because of the edema resulting from increased interstitial fluid, there is a relative intravascular depletion, leading to hypovolemia and often shock.

Other complications of NS include pleural effusions, ascites, decreased total thyroxine (T_4) and total triiodothyronine (T_3), and impaired growth, most often caused by corticosteroid therapy. Acute leukoencephalopathy during combined therapy with prednisolone and cyclosporin A was recently reported in a 13 year old who presented with altered mental status and seizure.[143,151]

Ancillary Data. The hallmarks of NS, in addition to edema, include proteinuria, hypoproteinemia, and hyperlipidemia. Proteinuria is heavy and is defined as >3.5 gm protein/1.73 m^2/24 hr or >50 mg/kg/24 hr. These values result in a 3+ to 4+ reading by the "dipstick" methods for qualitative protein excretion. The spot protein/creatinine ratio is 2.5. As a result of the proteinuria, the urine-specific gravity is usually high, exceeding 1.025. Hyaline casts may also be present secondary to the large amounts of protein in the urine. Occasionally, patients may have microscopic hematuria. Gross hematuria is rare in children with MCNS; if present, a different diagnosis should be sought.

Several blood studies should be obtained when evaluating a patient with NS. Hypoproteinemia is common to all of these patients. Total serum protein is reduced and ranges from 4.5 to 5.5 gm/dl. Serum albumin levels fall to less than 2 gm/dl and are often below 1 gm/dl.

Hyperlipidemia results from an increase in serum cholesterol, and levels are usually >400 mg/dl. Plasma cholesterol carriers (low-density lipoprotein [LDL] and very low–density lipoprotein) are increased. Serum electrolytes are most often normal. Serum sodium may be mildly reduced (130 mEq/L) but usually does not require special treatment. BUN and serum creatinine are also within normal range; however, the BUN may be elevated as a result of a reduced clearance of urea. In the event of hemoconcentration, hemoglobin levels and hematocrits may be elevated. Serum C_3 and C_4 levels are usually within normal range.

Radiographic studies include chest and abdominal x-ray studies. The heart is usually normal in size, but may be small due to hypovolemia. Pleural effusions or pulmonary edema may also be present. The abdominal film may show the presence of ascites. Ultrasound should exclude renal anatomic abnormality.

Renal biopsy should be considered if the patient is over 6 years, there is evidence of azotemia, decreased complement, hematuria, or persistent hypertension or if the patient fails to respond to steroids.

Differential Considerations

Renal concerns that cause edema include associated renal failure and glomerulonephritis. Congestive heart failure, vasculitis, and acute thrombosis may be contributory. Newborns may be edematous secondary to hemolytic disease of the newborn. Gastrointestinal conditions produce hypoalbuminemia resulting from cirrhosis, protein-losing enteritis, cystic fibrosis, or lymphangitis.

Management

The goal of the emergency department management of NS is to restore the patient's intravascular volume and to treat the symptomatic edema. Hypovolemic shock is treated with the usual volume resuscitation despite the presence of edema. The risks of hypertension, which develops due either to the disease itself or to the therapy, is increased; prompt recognition and intervention are important. Hydration status may be followed by serial hematocrits, as the hematocrit is often elevated secondary to hemoconcentration (Fig. 60-7).

The mainstay of therapy for NS is corticosteroids in patients without complications including those between 1 and 6 years, and with normal complement, no gross hema-

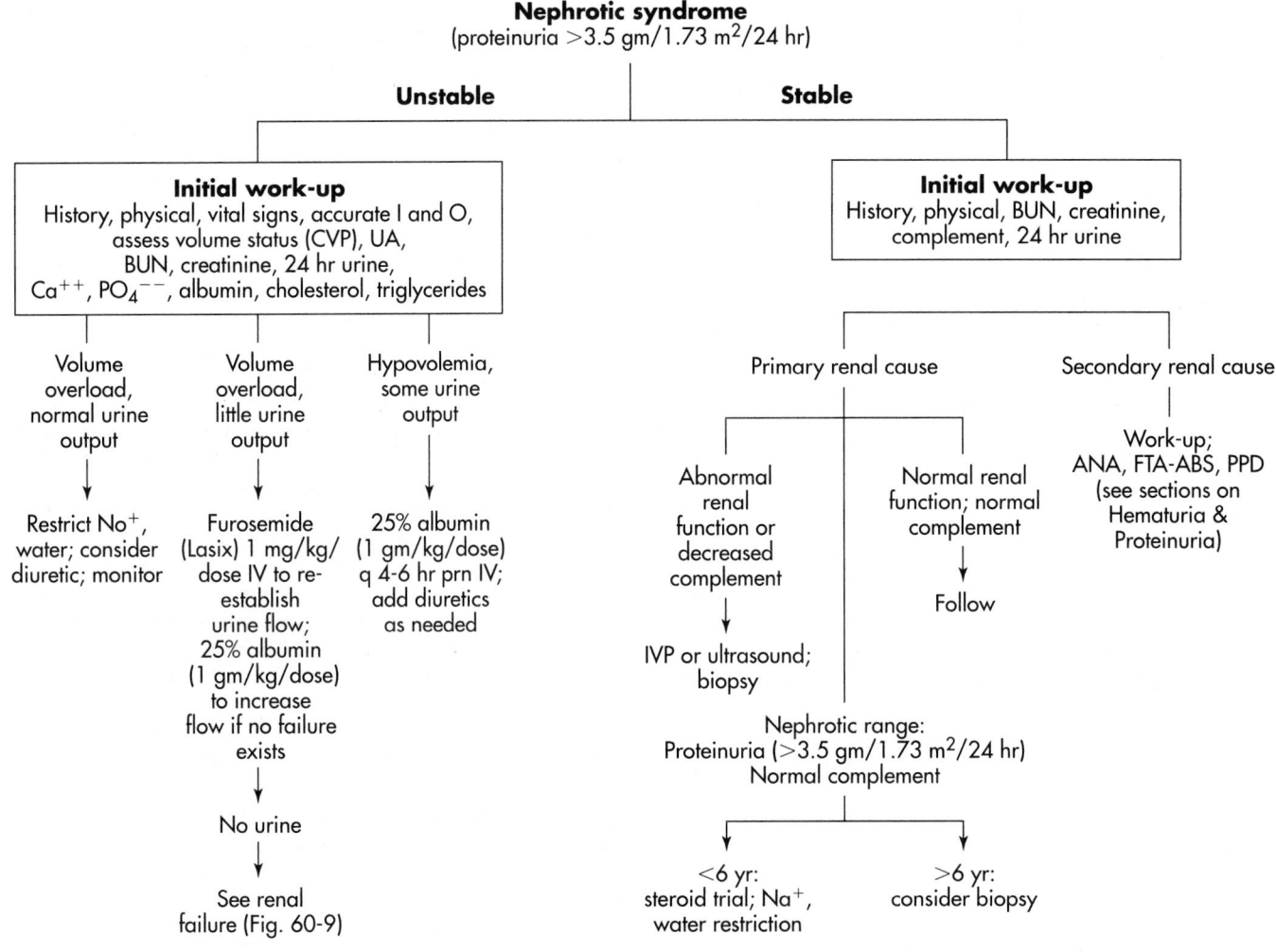

Nephrotic syndrome
(proteinuria >3.5 gm/1.73 m²/24 hr)

Unstable

Stable

Initial work-up
History, physical, vital signs, accurate I and O, assess volume status (CVP), UA, BUN, creatinine, 24 hr urine, Ca⁺⁺, PO₄⁻⁻, albumin, cholesterol, triglycerides

Initial work-up
History, physical, BUN, creatinine, complement, 24 hr urine

Volume overload, normal urine output

Volume overload, little urine output

Hypovolemia, some urine output

Primary renal cause

Secondary renal cause

Restrict No⁺, water; consider diuretic; monitor

Furosemide (Lasix) 1 mg/kg/ dose IV to re-establish urine flow; 25% albumin (1 gm/kg/dose) to increase flow if no failure exists

25% albumin (1 gm/kg/dose) q 4-6 hr prn IV; add diuretics as needed

Abnormal renal function or decreased complement

Normal renal function; normal complement

Work-up; ANA, FTA-ABS, PPD (see sections on Hematuria & Proteinuria)

No urine

IVP or ultrasound; biopsy

Follow

See renal failure (Fig. 60-9)

Nephrotic range: Proteinuria (>3.5 gm/1.73 m²/24 hr) Normal complement

<6 yr: steroid trial; Na⁺, water restriction

>6 yr: consider biopsy

FIG. 60-7. Management of nephrotic syndrome.

turia, or large protein loss. Generally, patients are started on prednisone, 2 mg/kg/24 hr (maximum: 80 mg/24 hr) PO, in 2 to 3 divided doses. This regimen should not be initiated until the initial evaluation (including placement of a tuberculin test) is completed to prevent complications. Approximately 90% of patients with MCNS will respond (urine protein trace or negative over 3 days) by the end of 4 weeks of steroid therapy. Reducing and tapering the dosage is variable. In a recent study comparing four treatment regimens in children with frequently relapsing, steroid-sensitive NS, relapse-free intervals were the longest with long-term daily prednisone therapy.[152] If a child does not respond to daily steroid therapy, referral and a renal biopsy are needed; steroid resistance increases the chance that the renal pathology is not minimal change.

Frequent relapses or steroid resistance may initially require a second steroid course; the use of immunosuppressant therapy such as chlorambucil or cyclophosphamide may be necessary if there are multiple relapses or if the patient is not responsive to steroids. Recently cyclosporine has been used to treat NS.[153,154] Consultation is necessary.

Diuretics may be warranted if edema is severe enough to cause respiratory distress or ascites. Furosemide, 1 to 2 mg/kg/24 hr PO or IV, in divided doses may be used.

Additional diuretics such as hydrochlorothiazide, spironolactone, or metolazone may be added and potentiate the action of the loop diuretics (see Fig. 60-7 and Table 47-12). However, loop diuretics remain most effective. The diuresis associated with diuretics is small compared to that observed when the patient responds to steroid therapy.

Patients should be monitored closely for volume depletion and electrolyte disturbances. Occasionally, severely hypoalbuminemic (<1.5 gm/dl) children fail to respond to diuretics. These children require the administration of salt-poor albumin (0.5 to 1.0 gm/kg intravenously over 2 hours) followed by IV furosemide (1 to 2 mg/kg). This regimen should be used only in the presence of volume contraction and the patient monitored closely for excessive volume expansion.

Salt restriction is required as long as there is evidence of proteinuria and edema. Water intake should be limited only if the edema progresses despite sodium restriction or if there is an impaired ability to excrete normal quantities of water leading to hyponatremia.

Because these patients are immunosuppressed, infection is always a risk. The use of steroids may mask the signs and symptoms of a bacterial infection. All children with a fever or signs of peritonitis in the absence of a fever must be fully evaluated. Appropriate cultures should be obtained and a diagnostic paracentesis performed if peritonitis is a concern. Peritoneal fluid should be sent for gram stain and culture. Antibiotics should not be initiated until the cultures have been obtained. Penicillin has been the drug of choice in the past to treat *S. pneumoniae* infections; however, with the increase in the gram-negative infections, it is prudent to broaden the coverage with a cephalosporin.

Immunization recommendations in patients with NS have been controversial. Studies have contradicted one another on the effectiveness of pneumococcal vaccine in children with NS. The effectiveness of other vaccines has not been well tested. Other issues besides that of efficacy have been raised. The risk of treating NS patients with a live virus (in the new varicella vaccine) and concern that vaccination provides an immunogenic stimulus for relapse of NS are among other reasons why there is not a consensus among nephrologists regarding vaccination.[155]

Disposition

Any patient with respiratory distress or shock must be admitted to the hospital after stabilization has occurred in the emergency department. Other patients with NS who require hospitalization include those with infections, refractory edema, renal insufficiency, and hemoconcentration (HCT >50%). In addition, newly diagnosed patients should be hospitalized, not only to complete the initial evaluation, but also to educate patient and parent about NS and its management.

ORCHITIS

MARTIN I. HERMAN

Usually presenting in adolescence, orchitis can be due to bacterial or viral agents. Bacterial infection is rare and the more typical offending agent is a virus. Orchitis may occur from hematogenous spread of virus or as a result of adjacent epididymitis.[156] Mumps (paramyxovirus) is the most common agent involved in primary orchitis; however, orchitis can be caused by coxsackievirus, adenovirus, and enteroviral infections.[157] Other viral agents shown to be causative include EBV, dengue (arbovirus), and arenavirus (agent of lymphocytic choriomeningitis). Brucellosis and filariasis have also been found in cases of orchitis.[158]

Typically the patient with orchitis will have a gradual onset of scrotal pain and swelling along with the constitutional symptoms concordant for the viral infection. Examination finds a very tender swollen testicle possibly with a reactive hydrocele.[156] Orchitis is most often found in conjunction with epididymitis; acute torsion of the spermatic cord should be excluded. Viral orchitis is self-limiting and therapy is focused on relief of pain and swelling.[156]

About 30% to 38% of postpubertal males with mumps will develop orchitis.[159] Orchitis is generally noted at the end of the first week of the mumps illness. Patients will have testicular pain, swelling, and tenderness. Facial swelling is not always seen. Atrophy may result from the infection. Fertility is maintained because infection is typically unilateral. Infertility has been reported following bilateral orchitis.[156,159]

Pathophysiology

Testicular infection results in diffuse swelling, associated with edema and discoloration of the scrotum. Microscopically, there is infiltration of the gonad by leukocytes, lymphocytes, and other cells. Tubular structures degenerate but the Leydig cells are typically spared, thus preserving androgenic function.[156]

Diagnostic Findings

Clinical Findings. Physical findings of the patient with orchitis may help determine the etiologic agent involved. In mumps severe systemic symptoms are rare. Parotid swelling may be the first sign of illness. Temperatures may elevate, but only moderately.[159] When the orchitis is due to other agents, systemic findings will tend to be consistent with those specific diseases.

The scrotum will be erythematous and swollen. On examination the testis is enlarged and very tender.[156] It may be difficult to delineate the testis from the epididymis, since the adjacent epididymis may also be infected. Bilateral disease does occur and reactive hydroceles may also be noted. Urethral discharge, dysuria, or a tender prostate implicates a concurrent epididymal infection.[160]

Complications. Orchitis is usually a self-limited disease but can be very painful. About 50% of patients with orchitis will experience testicular atrophy (mumps orchitis) and rarely infertility due to bilateral disease.[159] Although bacterial orchitis is rare, abscess formation can result, necessitating surgical drainage or orchiectomy.

Ancillary Data. Serologic testing for paramyxovirus, coxsackievirus, or other causative viral agents should be avoided because it is expensive, time-consuming, and does not impact on therapy. A serum monotest might be worthwhile, since patients with mononucleosis need to be monitored for splenic swelling and hepatitis.

CBC may demonstrate a leftward shift when bacterial infection is present or the white count may be low, suggesting a viral infection. Scintigraphy, MRI scans, or color Doppler ultrasound can be helpful when the diagnosis is in doubt.

In primary orchitis infections the urine is clear, although urinalysis may be abnormal when a concurrent epididymitis exists. Urethral discharges should be cultured for gonococcal or chlamydial organisms and wet mount preparations performed for trichomonads.

Differential Considerations

Isolated orchitis may appear the same clinically as epididymitis, scrotal trauma, scrotal cellulitis, acute torsion of the spermatic cord, torsions of the appendix testis, and most causes of the acute scrotum (see section on Scrotal Pain and Swelling).

Management

Rest, analgesia, and scrotal elevation may ameliorate patient discomfort. Mild analgesics, such as nonsteroidal antiinflammatory agents, may be sufficient for some cases. Combinations of acetaminophen and codeine or hydrocodone should be adequate for all but the most severe patients. Antibiotics are of limited value, except for cases of epididymitis. Fluoroquinolones (ciprofloxacin) in older patients or second and third generation cephalosporins (ceftriaxone, cefprozil) are the drugs of choice in the non-allergic patient with epididymitis or bacterial orchitis. Doxycycline and other tetracyclines have also been helpful. Medical management should be instituted only after carefully eliminating those entities for which surgery is warranted.

PHIMOSIS AND PARAPHIMOSIS

JAMES A. O'DONNELL II

During the third month of gestation the foreskin begins as a fold of skin at the base of the glans. From its origin it grows forward over the base of the glans with more rapid growth occurring dorsally; initially only the dorsum of the glans is covered. As the glanular urethra closes, the ventral prepuce fuses producing the ventral frenulum. Failure of urethral development limits foreskin formation and results in either hypospadias or epispadias depending on the location of the failed development. By the fifth month of gestation fusion occurs between the stratified epithelium of the glans and the prepuce. As gestation progresses, and under the influence of androgens, the stratified epithelium of the fused glans-prepuce begins to degenerate, keratinize, and desquamate. This leads to the formation of squamous epithelium that in turn forms into whorls or cell nests. Shortly before term the cell nests degenerate and, as a result, clefts are formed. As these clefts enlarge, the preputial space is formed. Thus at term this separation of the glans from the prepuce is usually incomplete. In newborn boys only 4% will have a foreskin that is fully retractable. Of the remaining group, the urethral meatus can only be visualized in 54% and the tip of the glans cannot be seen in 42%.

Phimosis

Phimosis is characterized by constriction of the distal prepuce, preventing easy passage of the foreskin over the glans. Depending upon age, this is more likely to be physiologic than pathologic. By 6 months of age the foreskin is retractable in 25% of males. About 50% of 1-year-old males will have a fully retractable foreskin; this can be found in 80% of two-year-old males. By the age of 4 years 90% of males will have a fully retractable prepuce.[161,162]

True phimosis is rare in children. More often the child is brought to the physician because of parental concerns about the inability to retract the foreskin. When true phimosis does occur, it may be the result of circumcision complications, repeated trauma, infections, or chemical irritation.[163] All of these insults lead to scar formation. Collections of smegma can also produce adhesions between the foreskin and the glans. Phimosis may also be seen in combination with infection of the adjacent glans (balanitis) or glans and prepuce (balanoposthitis). In addition local lichen sclerosus et atrophicus can cause phimosis in boys. This can be identified preoperatively by the presence of a whitish ring at the tip of the phimotic prepuce.[164]

Diagnostic Findings. True phimosis with marked constriction of the distal prepuce is suggested by the presence of decreased urinary stream, hematuria, or pain in the area of the prepuce.

Frank urinary outlet obstruction is rare. One case of severe accelerated hypertension in conjunction with phimosis has been described. Relief of this patient's urinary outlet obstruction by circumcision also reversed his hypertension.[165]

Management. Physicians should recognize that the ability to fully retract the foreskin is an age-related process. Reassurance and education constitute the management in younger males. The parents should also be counseled against attempting forceful retractions of the prepuce; adequate hygiene should be stressed. If the child presents with acute urethral outlet obstruction, an attempt at gentle dilation should be made to relieve bladder spasm until a more definitive treatment can be undertaken.

Classically, circumcision was the definitive treatment for all forms of phimosis. Such intervention is indeed indicated for phimosis accompanied by recurrent cases of balanoposthitis and urinary tract obstruction and infection. There are limited cases that respond to topical steroid therapy and balloon dilation.[166,167]

Paraphimosis

Paraphimosis occurs when a relatively tight foreskin becomes retracted over the glans and fixed in position. The tight preputial ring acts like a tourniquet obstructing venous return from the glans. This in turn produces distal edema, inflammation, and engorgement. Ultimately the foreskin cannot be returned to its normal position.

Diagnostic Findings. Typically, the patient is anxious and may complain of bladder spasm. Inspection of the penis will reveal a flaccid proximal penis up to the level of the obstruction unless there is accompanying balanoposthitis or infection of the penis. Pathogens involved in such an infection include spirochetes, bacteria and *Candida albicans*. If there is infection present, instead of a sharply demarcated area of erythema and edema, the proximal phallus will show more diffuse induration.[163] Idiopathic penile edema, usually as a result of insect bites or irritation, can also mimic paraphimosis or an infected penis.

If there is no history of circumcision, the phallus must be searched for a foreign body that has encircled and is causing an obstruction. Hair that has become entwined around the penis to form a tourniquet is a common offender; clothing, metallic objects, and rubber bands have also been found as causative agents. Although hair and clothing can accidentally encircle the penis, any material may have been purposely placed either as experimentation, for excitement, or for punishment. Because of the degree of edema present and the lack of accurate information as to whether the patient has been circumcised, the physician may be unable to exclude the possibility of a foreign body.

Management. The treatment of paraphimosis should be individualized by the diagnostic concerns that accompany each case. The management of swelling and pain are the primary concern. Pain can be managed by either general sedation measures or a local dorsal penile block using 1% lidocaine without epinephrine.[161,168] Cooling the phallus with compresses or wrapping the penis, starting at the glans and moving proximally toward the base with a folded gauze bandage, will begin to control edema.[169] A bandage may need to be adjusted a few times to ensure that proper compression is applied to the phallus.

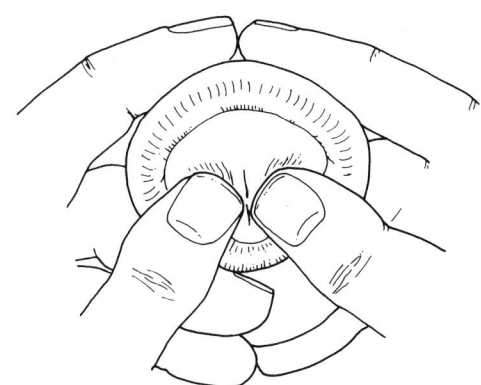

FIG. 60-8. Reduction of paraphimosis by combined traction and compression upon the foreskin with simultaneous counterpressure against the glans penis. (*From Kelalis PP, King LR, Bleman AB: Clinical pediatric urology, vol 2, ed 2, Philadelphia, 1985, WB Saunders.*)

Once edema is controlled, repeat inspection of the penis may disclose constricting foreign bodies. Removal of such an object is mandatory and should provide resolution of phallic edema. If repeat examination discloses only findings consistent with paraphimosis, manual reduction (Fig. 60-8) may be attempted. This is done by pushing gently on the glans through the edematous prepuce tissue while traction is on the prepuce. This has been likened to "turning a sock inside out." Postreduction bleeding, if it occurs, is slight and generally responds to pressure.

An alternative method involves lubricating and anesthetizing the foreskin and glans by applying lidocaine jelly. This is left in place for 2 minutes. The foreskin is then retracted and the glans is placed in ice water. To easily facilitate this, the tip of a latex examination glove is removed after the glove is filled with ice water. The glans is placed in the thumbhole of the glove and the glove is pushed down the shaft of the penis until it rests on the symphysis pubis. The glove is held in place for 5 minutes or until the edema is reduced. The glove is then removed and the prepuce is slipped back over the glans into its normal position.[164] A third method for the reduction of paraphimosis is the "puncture" method.[170] This employs the use of a single 21 gauge needle to puncture the edematous foreskin once sedation or a penile nerve block has been provided. This allows drainage of the edematous fluid with manual compression. Once the edema is resolved, the foreskin is manually returned to its normal position over the glans. The child may be discharged following voiding. Follow-up with a pediatric surgeon or urologist should be encouraged. If the above measures fail, prompt surgical consultation for removal of the foreign body or a dorsal slit procedure or circumcision is mandated.[171]

PRIAPISM

EARL R. DIXON

Priapism is defined as a persistent, usually painful penile erection not necessarily associated with sexual stimulation or desire. During childhood it is primarily hematologic in etiology. Long-standing priapism can result in impotence.

Pathophysiology

The penis contains valves in the arteries, arterioles, and the sinusoidal spaces that are under tonic contraction due to sympathetic input. This causes most of the blood flow to bypass the corpora cavernosa and go directly to the emissary veins that drain the penis during the flaccid state. Similar valves in the venous system remain patent by the same neurogenic stimuli.[172] During an erection, parasympathetic stimuli cause a reversal of events with arteriolar dilation and sinusoidal filling. The valves in the venous system are closed, thus impeding the egress of blood. The corpora cavernosa then becomes distended, elongated, and erect with blood.

In priapism, there is pain and persistent engorgement of the corpora cavernosa. This can be due to a low flow rate of blood into the sinusoids combined with the impediment of egress of blood from the corpora cavernosa. High flow rate has also been described as the cause of priapism in sickle cell patients.[173] This can result in hypoxia, edema, and inflammation and can progress to thrombosis, fibrosis, and ultimately impotence. In sickle cell disease, sludging of sickle red blood cells in the sinusoids causes impairment of normal venous drainage. This promotes local hypoxia and acidosis, and sets up a cycle for more sickling and sludging, resulting in more obstruction of venous drainage.[174] A similar mechanism may occur in hyperviscous states such as polycythemia and leukemia.

Etiology

Sickle cell disease is the most common cause of priapism in the pediatric age group. It accounts for approximately two thirds of all pediatric cases and can occur in all genotypes of sickle cell disease.[175] However, only approximately 2% to 10% of all patients with sickle cell disease develop priapism.[174,176,177]

Leukemia accounts for approximately 11% of cases.[175] A small percentage of cases are also due to idiopathic priapism. Local trauma from a straddle injury can be a rare cause of priapism, as well as excessive sexual stimulation, anticoagulation therapy, and diabetes mellitus.

Diagnostic Findings

A detailed history and physical examination should be done to identify any underlying medical conditions that could precipitate priapism. In cases of sickle cell disease, the focus should also be to identify other coexisting conditions such as infection or painful crisis. Some patients may complain of voiding difficulty, since urinary retention may complicate the condition.

Priapism differs from a normal erection in that only the dorsal paired corpora cavernosa are involved in priapism, and the glans and ventral surface (corpus spongiosum) remain flaccid. Although priapism may arise as a result of sexual stimulation, the tumescence is not associated with continued sexual pleasure, nor is it relieved by ejaculation. Its onset mostly occurs at night or in the early morning.[178] In sickle cell disease, priapism is frequently an isolated finding. Sequestration, infection, and painful vasoocclusive crises should also be considered in these patients. Furthermore, some patients may have a low-grade fever with no source of infection.

Complications. The most acute complication of priapism is urinary retention. This may be due to either hesitancy to void because of pain or mechanical obstruction secondary to the edematous engorged corpora cavernosa that impedes flow through the urethra.[179] Some patients will urinate after the pain is controlled. Careful urethral catheterization should be done if urinary retention persists. In trauma-induced priapism with urinary retention, a urologic consultation should be considered. A retrograde urethrogram should be done to investigate the urethra's integrity. Rarely, infection, ischemia, and gangrene occur due to priapism.

The long-term complication of priapism is impotence. The exact incidence is not well defined. Various studies suggest that the risk of impotence increases with multiple episodes and with increased duration. The younger the age of onset of priapism, the less likely that impotence will develop following a specific episode.[180]

Ancillary Data. No laboratory data or radiographic studies are necessary to confirm priapism, since it is a clinical entity. Serum electrolytes, BUN, creatinine, and a urinalysis may be helpful to establish the patient's hydration status. A CBC can confirm sickle cell anemia or suggest a leukemic or polycythemic process. In a patient with coagulation defect, PT and PTT may help to guide anticoagulation therapy if priapism is secondary to penile vein thrombosis. In most patients, the history will confirm sickle cell disease; a CBC and reticulocyte count may be helpful to guide therapy.

Differential Diagnosis

Priapism has been reported to occur in the newborn.[181] Most infants with sustained erection do not, however, appear to be in pain. Phimosis with erection may produce pain, a result of the stretched preputial tissue over the firm glans. In priapism, the glans is usually flaccid. In paraphimosis, the penis is painful and swollen with an engorged glans resulting from constriction by the foreskin around the base of the glans. This is a distinguishing characteristic from priapism. Urethral foreign body should also be considered, and a careful history will be helpful. In addition, penile pain with erection can be caused by Peyronie disease. This is accompanied by penile curvature caused by plaque formation secondary to tissue fibrosis. Finally, cervical and thoracic spinal cord injury can present with penile erection secondary to the lack of sympathetic input.

Management

Treatment of priapism is aimed at relieving the pain and detumescence and returning penile function to normal while preserving sexual potency. The patient should be hospitalized for pain control and monitoring of urinary retention. Patients with sickle cell disease are most often treated conservatively with narcotic analgesia and hydration. This management most often involves a hematologic consultation. Some patients require red blood cell transfusion or exchange to decrease the sickle cell load, which usually results in detumescence in the majority of patients, and surgical intervention is not required. There is controversy concerning how much hydration and how many units of blood these patients should receive before surgical intervention takes place. Hydration and pain management should be similar to the management of other painful sickle cell crises as discussed in Chapter 54. Case reports of hydralazine relieving priapism in sickle cell patients suggest that vasodilatory therapy may be of some benefit.[182]

The management of patients with concurrent leukemia should focus on treatment of their malignancy. It may take days to weeks before detumescence occurs. In some patients with unresolving priapism, surgical intervention is necessary. A cavernosa-glans shunt will be curative in most of these cases; however, priapism may persist in a small percentage of patients, and a cavernosa-spongiosum shunt should then be required.

PROSTATITIS

FELTON E. COMBEST • DAVID G. WARD

Prostatitis is an acute infection of the prostate. It is rare in the adolescent years and exceedingly unusual in the prepubertal patient.[183,184] Daum has described prostatitis as "a poorly defined clinical syndrome, frequently diagnosed in the absence of objective evidence."[185] This disease more commonly is found in men between the ages of 20 and 40 years.[186]

Pathophysiology

The infection is presumed to develop by direct extension of the organism up the urethra or hematogenous seeding.[187] An animal model has been developed for study and research into several areas, including sex hormone influence on prostate infection, prostatic antibacterial factor, zinc and polypeptide activity in prostatitis, and bacterial surface antibody detection.[185]

Etiology and Epidemiology

Organisms often implicated in acute prostatitis include the usual urinary pathogens such as *E. coli, Klebsiella, Enterobacter, Proteus, Pseudomonas,* and *Staphylococcus* species. *N. gonorrhoeae* and the chlamydial organisms are found in the postpubertal patient and are sexually transmitted, although there is dispute as to the role of chlamydia.[185] *Trichomonas* is reported to be a cause of infection in both the prostate and urethra.[185,188]

Diagnostic Findings

Clinical Findings. Acute prostatitis commonly presents with symptoms similar to those of acute cystitis or urethritis, including cloudy urine, malodorous urine, frequency, dysuria, burning, and urgency. Additional symptoms may include fever, pain in the suprapubic, perineal, or low back region, or referred pained to the testes. Systemic signs of urosepsis such as chills, fever, and prostration may be present.

Examination of the genitourinary system may reveal a urethral discharge. A tender, enlarged, "boggy" prostate gland may be palpated on rectal examination. An enlarged and tender epididymis or testicle is often noted. Because of the possibility of retrograde seeding of the epididymis and possible bacteremia, some feel that prostatic massage should not be performed during the acute infection. A fluctuant mass may be palpable on rectal examination if a prostatic abscess is present.

Complications. Acute obstruction with urinary retention requiring suprapubic diversion of the urinary stream may occur secondary to edema of the gland. Rarely, an abscess occurs requiring surgical intervention.[189] Extension of the infection along the vas deferens to the epididymis and testis may occur resulting in epididymitis or orchitis. Bacteremia may occur if the infection is not diagnosed in time. Systemic gonorrhea, associated coexisting diseases of syphilis, acquired immunodeficiency syndrome (AIDS), and other sexually transmitted diseases may be present but unrecognized.

Ancillary Data. If a urethral discharge is present, samples should be obtained for culture and gram stain. A urinalysis may reveal hematuria, pyuria, and bacteriuria. In the patient with systemic symptoms, leukocytosis ($>20,000$ WBC/mm^3) or other signs of acute inflammation may be present. Blood cultures should be obtained in the patient with signs of urosepsis.

When the site of infection along the genitourinary tract is unclear, the three-glass urinary test may be used to locate the site. To perform the test, the patient voids the first 10 ml of urine into the first container (to wash the anterior urethra of bacteria), voids the majority of the remainder of the urine into a second container, and voids the last few milliliters into a third container. If prostatic massage is to be performed, it is done between the second and third collections and the secretions are expressed or collected with the third specimen. Each urine specimen is specifically labeled by order of collection and sent for urinalysis. If the majority of the blood or pus cells are found in the first container, the infection is localized to the anterior urethra. If the largest number of cells are found in the third specimen, infection is in the prostate, bladder neck, or the posterior urethra. If the number of cells is the same in all three specimens, the site of disease is probably above the bladder neck, and antibiotic therapy is needed before the prostate can be fully evaluated.[190,191]

Evaluation of the anatomy of the genitourinary tract should be performed after the acute phase has subsided. Studies using intravenous pyelogram (IVP), ultrasound, and cystoscopy may be indicated. Instrumentation of the genitourinary tract is usually delayed until after the acute phase, except in the case of urinary retention (requiring percutaneous suprapubic drainage) or prostatic abscess (requiring percutaneous needle aspiration).[187]

Differential Considerations

Signs and symptoms of infection in most of the urinary tract, but especially in the lower portion, are similar. Systemic symptoms such as malaise, fever, nausea, vomiting, and arthralgias may be present. Local symptoms such as frequency, dysuria, burning, and nocturia with referral of pain to areas such as the testicle, lower abdomen, flank, and back are usually present. A nonprostatic UTI may be confused initially with prostatitis, but the rectal examination should be diagnostic. Seminal vesiculitis is usually a complication of prostatic infection but may occasionally occur as a primary infection. It may be differentiated from prostatitis by findings of a normal prostate with tender nodules

in the area above the prostate on rectal examination.[187] Urethritis must be considered, and care must be taken to identify sexually transmitted diseases. Chronic prostatitis may be considered in the patient with recurrent episodes of prostatitis and a lack of systemic symptoms.

Management

Infants and children with prostatitis caused by sepsis should be treated for the sepsis with broad-spectrum antibiotic coverage. After cultures are obtained, empiric parenteral antibiotics should be started until an organism is identified.

Adolescents with prostatitis should be treated for chlamydia and gonorrheal disease with ceftriaxone, 125 mg IM, and doxycycline, 100 mg PO BID, or tetracycline, 500 mg PO QID. Alternative regimens include use of azithromycin instead of doxycycline, or doxycycline and either spectinomycin or ciprofloxacin.[192] If nonsexually transmitted organisms are suspected, antibiotic therapy should be directed toward the likely pathogens until cultures are available and then tailored to the susceptibility results. Trimethoprim/sulfamethoxazole, 160/800 mg PO BID, for up to 12 weeks has been advocated.[193] More recent reports have suggested that fluoroquinolones may be effective, although some agents are age-restricted to older patients.[194]

Symptomatic relief of pain may be obtained by rest, increased oral fluid intake, sitz baths, and analgesics. The currently available antispasmodics and urinary antiseptics may also afford some relief. Urologic consultation should be sought in cases complicated by acute urinary retention or prostatic abscess.

Disposition

A patient who appears acutely ill or septic should be admitted to the hospital for administration of intravenous antibiotics and fluid resuscitation. Referral for evaluation of the prostate after the acute symptoms have subsided may be helpful to delineate the chronic case (the treatment of prostatitis is a long-term engagement that has frequent failures) or an underlying anatomic abnormality.

RENAL FAILURE, ACUTE

JOHN G. KNEPPER

Acute renal failure is a sudden decrease in GFR; the functions of fluid balance, blood pressure control, acid-base balance, and solute excretion are inadequate. Two manifestations are readily apparent in the acutely ill child: a decrease in urine output and an increase in solute retention (BUN, creatinine). Although the actual urine output of the child is rarely known upon arrival in the emergency department, monitoring of the output will frequently yield valuable information. A urinary output of 1 ml/kg/hr is usually considered an adequate output, but in the somewhat dehydrated child, 0.5 ml/kg/hr is probably an appropriate response and may be a sign of acceptable renal function.[195]

Nephrotoxic agents, such as mercury, and some aminoglycosides can initially cause an increase in urine output, a result of renal tubular damage. In these patients, the solute retention is reflected by the rising BUN and creatinine; urinary volume output may be normal or high.[195]

Diagnostic Findings

Acute renal failure can be divided clinically and pathophysiologically into three classes: prerenal (decreased renal perfusion), renal (intrinsic parenchymal damage), and postrenal (obstructive) (see box at right).

Decreased renal perfusion or prerenal causes of acute renal failure fall into three broad groups. The hypovolemic group is caused by dehydration or acute blood loss. Patients often have a history of vomiting, diarrhea, diabetic ketoacidosis, decreased intravascular volume secondary to NS, burns, or shock resulting from hemorrhage, sepsis, cardiac failure, or anaphylaxis. The loss of circulatory volume results in decreased perfusion. Decreased cardiac output, secondary to congestive heart failure may produce prerenal failure. The third group is characterized by decreased intravascular volume with a normal or increased extracellular fluid volume, as seen in cirrhosis, NS, burns, and septic shock.

The renal or parenchymal causes are associated with either glomerular or tubular damage. The glomerular damage is usually inflammatory, resulting in destruction of glomeruli or damage to the glomerular basement membrane. The most common cause is acute poststreptococcal glomerulonephritis, which is usually a self-limited, reversible condition. Patients often have a history of hematuria, proteinuria, edema, or hypertension. HUS, nephrotic exposure, massive crush injuries, and overwhelming sepsis may be contributory. Less common forms of glomerular damage are associated with systemic lupus erythematosus, NS, and other progressive glomerulonephritis, which have a worse prognosis.

Tubular damage, commonly called acute tubular necrosis, can follow a toxic insult, such as heavy metal poisoning, or can result from the presence of myoglobin or hemoglobin in the tubule following a severe burn, crush injury, or hemolytic crisis. Additionally, the most common cause of acute tubular necrosis is renal ischemia, precipitated by hypovolemic shock. In this situation, determining whether decreased urinary output is secondary to hypovolemia or to acute tubular damage is essential in emergency department intervention (see Management).

Postrenal or obstructive failure can be brought about by posterior urethral valves, tumors, or infections resulting in ureteral dilation and pressure on the trigone of the bladder.[195] Usually, unilateral obstructive abnormalities do not result in failure. Abdominal and flank pain may be present.

Finally, in considering the diagnosis of acute renal failure in the individual patient, it is always important to consider the possibility of acute decompensation of underlying chronic renal disease.[196]

Complications. Five life-threatening complications of acute renal failure underscore potential presentations to the emergency department.

1. Severe hyperkalemia
2. Pulmonary edema and fluid overload
3. Hypertension progressing to hypertensive encephalopathy
4. Septic shock (secondary to obstruction and infection)

Common Causes of Acute Renal Failure

Prerenal (decreased perfusion of an intact nephron)
Shock: hypovolemic
  Dehydration
  Hemorrhagic
  Diabetic ketoacidosis
  Burn
Shock: distributive
  Septic
  Anaphylactic
Shock: cardiogenic
Nephrotic syndrome with intravascular volume depletion
  from decreased oncotic pressure
Renal vessel injury with obstruction

Intrarenal (damage of the actual nephron)
Primary glomerular disease
  Acute poststreptococcal nephritis
  Membranoproliferative glomerulonephritis
  Progressive glomerulonephritis
Systemic disease
  Henoch-Schönlein purpura
  Hemolytic-uremic syndrome
  Vasculitides
  Bacterial endocarditis
  Systemic lupus erythematosus
Nephrotoxins
  Antibiotics (aminoglycoside, methicillin)
  Metals (gold, lead)
  Antihypertensives (captopril)
  Anticonvulsant (phenytoin)
  Rhabdomyolysis (pigment damage to nephron)
  Radiocontrast materials
  Organic solvent (carbon tetrachloride, methanol, toluene)
Neoplasm
Vascular
  Renal vein thrombosis
  Renal artery thrombosis or embolism
Acute tubular necrosis (caused by prolonged decreased perfusion)

Postrenal (downstream obstruction with initially intact nephron*)
Posterior urethral valves
Ureteropelvic junction abnormality
Stones
Crystals
  Sulfonamides
  Uric acid
Retroperitoneal fibrosis or tumor
Trauma to collecting system
Ureterocele

*Prolonged obstruction eventually leads to irreversible nephron damage.

TABLE 60-8. Renal Function Studies

Prerenal	Intrarenal	Postrenal
Ultrasound: normal	Ultrasound: can have increased renal density or slight swelling	Ultrasound: dilated bladder or kidney
Serum BUN to creatinine ratio $>15:1$		History and examination may be diagnostic
Urine Na^+ <15 mEq/L	Urine Na^+ >20 mEq/L	Indices not helpful
Urine osmolality >500 mOsm/kg H_2O	Urine osmolality <350 mOsm/kg H_2O	
Urine to plasma creatinine ratio $>40:1$	Urine to plasma creatinine ratio $<20:1$ (often $<5:1$)	
Fractional excretion of Na^+ <1 (<2.5 in neonates)	Fractional excretion of Na^+ >2 (>2.5 in neonates)	

$$\text{Fractional excretion of } Na^+ = \frac{\text{Urine } Na^+ \text{ mEq/L}}{\text{Plasma } Na^+ \text{ mEq/L}} \times \frac{\text{Plasma creatinine mg/dl}}{\text{Urine creatinine mg/dl}} \times 100$$

From Barkin RM and Rosen P: *Emergency pediatrics,* ed 4, St Louis, 1994, Mosby.

5. Seizures (from metabolic derangement or hypertensive encephalopathy)

These medical emergencies will be discussed in detail in the Management section. Azotemia with elevated potassium, BUN, and creatinine are noted. Dysrhythmias, hypocalcemia and hyperphosphatemia, acidosis, and impaired level of consciousness are seen.

Ancillary Data. The routine laboratory determinations that may prove helpful in assessing the patient with renal failure are CBC, BUN, electrolytes, calcium, phosphorus, creatinine, urinalysis (including careful microscopic examination), and urine culture. Additional laboratory determinations that may prove useful in specific cases include an antistreptolysin-O (ASO) titer and C_3 complement (in suspected acute poststreptococcal or lupus nephritis), total serum albumin, albumin/globulin (A/G) ratio, cholesterol (in NS and cirrhosis), and Wright stain of the urinary sediment (in suspected methicillin nephritis). Examination of the urine output and sediment must be performed by someone who is skilled in interpreting the findings because the finding of red cell casts clearly points toward a glomerulonephritis picture; white cell casts are suggestive of an infectious etiology and hyaline casts suggest either dehydration or acute tubular necrosis.

Laboratory differentiation between the classic etiologies of acute renal failure is outlined in Table 60-8. Combining data from serum, urine, and ultrasonography is valuable.

The creatinine clearance is a good measure of GFR and is particularly helpful in monitoring children with renal disease. As discussed earlier, 24-hour urine collection is required:

$$\text{Creatinine clearance (ml/min/1.73 m}^2) = \frac{UV}{P} \times \frac{1.73}{SA}$$

A rapid approximation can be made by using the formula:

$$\text{Creatinine clearance (ml/min/1.73 m}^2) = \frac{0.55 \times \text{Ht (cm)}}{P}$$

where U = urinary concentration of creatinine (mg/dl); V = volume of urine divided by the number of minutes in collection period (24 hr = 1,440 min); P = plasma concentration of creatinine (mg/dl); and SA = surface area (m²).

Normal newborn and premature infants have a mean creatinine clearance of 38 ml/min/1.73 m². Mean creatinine clearance GFR at one year of age has increased to 77 ml/min/1.73 m². Normal children between 4 and 10 years have value of 109 ml (female) and 124 ml (male)/min/1.73 m², and adult values are 117 ml (female) and 131 ml (male)/min/1.73 m² (see Table 60-1).

A single voided urine sample in adults may have some predictive value. In patients with stable renal function, a spot protein/creatinine ratio of >2.5 can represent nephrotic range proteinuria; a ratio of <0.15 is normal.

Renal ultrasound has replaced the intravenous pyelogram (IVP) as the first line test in the search for obstructive causes of renal failure.[197] The ultrasound has two distinct advantages. The first is the lack of a need for dye, and accordingly, the absence of a risk of anaphylactic reactions. Additionally, no urine production is necessary with ultrasound, in contrast to the IVP in which a certain minimal renal function is necessary.[197] The IVP localizes the site of obstruction and is a more readily interpreted test in the absence of a skilled ultrasonographer. In obstructive uropathies, the voiding cystourethrogram identifies posterior urethral valves and demonstrates extrinsic pressure on the bladder neck.[197] A chest x-ray study may exclude congestive heart failure.

Management

A systematic approach to the evaluation and treatment of the patient with acute renal failure is essential based on a full assessment of the patient (Fig. 60-9). Four questions must be considered immediately in the management of suspected acute renal failure:

1. Is there decreased renal perfusion (prerenal)?
2. Are any life-threatening complications present?
   a. Hypertension with encephalopathy
   b. Severe hyperkalemia
   c. Seizures
   d. Septic shock
3. Is there evidence of infection with obstruction?
4. Is there a need for immediate dialysis?

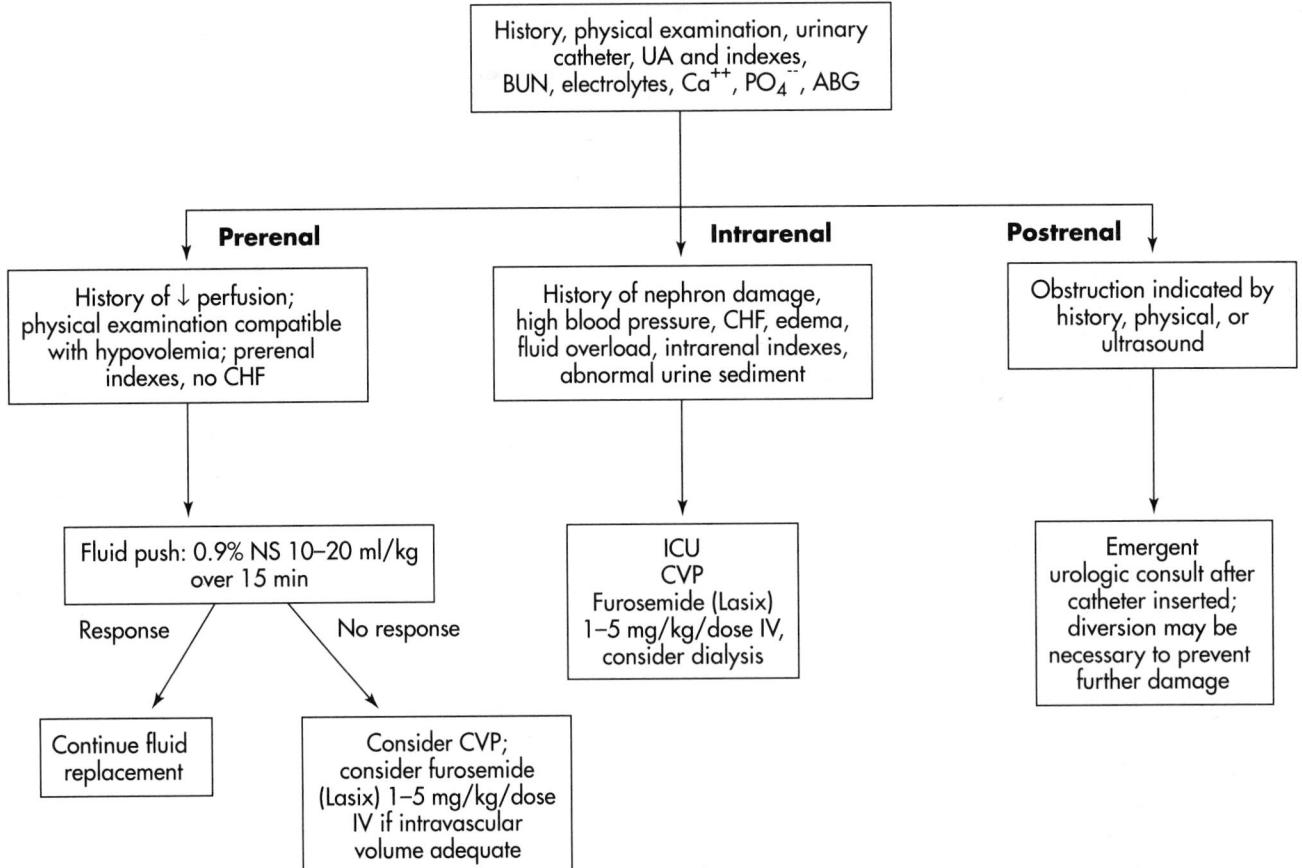

FIG. 60-9. Acute renal failure: initial assessment and treatment.

If *hypovolemia* (dehydration or acute blood loss—shock) is the suspected cause of renal failure, immediate vigorous fluid resuscitation is mandatory to prevent a possible progression to acute tubular necrosis. The goal is to rapidly restore a normal circulating blood volume. Initially, normal saline should be given as a 20 ml/kg IV bolus.[198] If urine output improves with a return of blood pressure to normal, the problem is most likely prerenal. Therapy then is directed at further correction of the fluid deficit. If a single bolus does not achieve a return of adequate urine output, a second bolus should be considered. The placement of a central venous pressure monitor is recommended to prevent overhydration in the patient who may be developing acute tubular necrosis secondary to renal ischemia while ensuring adequate fluid resuscitation to preserve renal failure.

If there is no response to administration of fluids, other modalities should be considered. Diuretics such as furosemide at 1 mg/kg/dose q 2 to 6 hours IV may be useful in the euvolemic patient if there is no evidence of obstruction. Bumetanide (Bumex) in a dose of 0.015 to 0.1 mg/kg/dose q 6 to 24 hr IV up to 10 mg/24 hr can also be tried. Mannitol may be useful if there is no response to furosemide in patients with prerenal failure and if responses can be monitored closely. Some clinicians use mannitol in combination with furosemide. Give mannitol 0.75 gm/kg/dose q 6 hours IV over 3 to 5 minutes. Obviously mannitol raises the potential risk of fluid overload and should not be given if there is evidence of obstruction or acute intrarenal failure.

If the patient remains oliguric or anuric, fluids should be administered to keep the patient intravascularly normal. Replace insensible (350 to 400 ml/m²/24 hr), extraordinary losses and urine output in the previous 24 hours. Maintain normoglycemia and metabolic balance. In patients with nonoliguric renal failure, it is imperative to replace insensible losses with D5W or D10W and urine output (milliliter-for-milliliter replacement with fluid reflecting electrolyte contents of urine).[199]

Low-dose dopamine may be infused (1 to 5 μg/kg/min) to increase renal blood flow, GFR, and sodium excretion. Dialysis may be used to produce euvolemia.

If hypertension with an associated encephalopathy develops, several drugs are useful in controlling hypertension in the anuric or oliguric patient as discussed in an earlier section. Nitroprusside and nifedipine are excellent drugs in this emergency situation.[200] Doses are as follows:

Nitroprusside 0.5 to 10 μg/kg/min IV infusion
Nifedipine (0.25 to 0.5 mg/kg to a maximum of 10 to 20 mg) PO or sublingual or buccal, q 6 to 8 hours[200]
Captopril 0.3 mg/kg up to 25 to 50 mg PO q 6 to 8 hours[201]
Diazoxide 1 to 3 mg/kg maximum 150 mg/dose, rapid IV push[200]

It is important in treating the acute hypertensive crisis to aim at achieving a 15% to 25% reduction in mean arterial pressure, rather than a return to "normal" blood pressure.

Overaggressive therapy can result in complications due to hypoperfusion of end-organs (brain, heart, and kidney).[202]

In addition to the antihypertensive drugs, a trial of furosemide to stimulate renal function is worth considering if intravascular volume is adequate or overloaded. The dose of furosemide should be 1 mg/kg/dose IV with expected maximum effect within 30 minutes.[203] The dose may be increased up to 6 mg/kg.

Hyperkalemia is a potentially serious complication of acute renal failure. It may produce membrane excitability with possible cardiac dysrhythmias. A potassium over 6.5 mEq/L may cause ECG changes associated with peaked T waves and eventually a widened QRS complex. A potassium level over 7.0 mEq/L requires emergent intervention.

In the patient with an abnormal ECG, calcium chloride 10% should be given at a dose of 0.2 to 0.3 ml (20 to 30 mg)/kg/dose (maximum: 5 ml or 500 mg/dose) IV slowly over 10 to 15 minutes, monitoring for bradycardia. The calcium changes the cell action potential, protecting the heart from dysrhythmias; the effect is short-acting and may be repeated in 5 minutes if indicated.[200]

Alkalosis helps to exchange H^+ for K^+, moving potassium intracellularly and normalizing membrane potential. If hyperkalemic dysrhythmias persist, sodium bicarbonate, 1 to 2 mEq/kg/dose IV push q 4 hr or as required by pH, is useful in emergent situations, usually in combination with sodium polystyrene sulfonate (Kayexalate) for hyperkalemia.[204]

If dysrhythmias persist, load the patient with glucose (D50W), giving 0.5 to 1.0 gm/kg initially followed by an infusion of D25W accompanied by 1.0 units/insulin for every 4 gm of glucose infused to keep the glucose between 120 and 300 mg/dl. Potassium is thereby moved intracellularly.

Albuterol can be used in an emergency in an aerosol form. It also causes the shift of extracellular potassium into the cell and can lower the serum K^+ by 1.0 to 1.5 mEq/L over 30 minutes.[200] Dialysis may ultimately be used in rare and unresponsive circumstances.

Kayexalate is an ion exchange resin that may be used in stable patients without ECG changes, often in combination with sodium bicarbonate in patients with a K^+ <5.8 mEq/L. Normally, give 1 gm resin/kg/dose q 2 to 4 hr, often mixed in children over 1 year with 70% sorbitol. It may cause hypocalcemia and hypomagnesemia, gastric irritation, and diarrhea.[200]

Seizures can be caused by either hypertensive encephalopathy or a metabolic disturbance, the most common of which is hyponatremia. Hyponatremia in the acute renal failure patient is almost never caused by sodium depletion. The total body sodium is usually normal and the hyponatremia is purely dilutional. Nevertheless, in the patient with intractable hyponatremic seizures, administration of hypertonic saline may be necessary. In these cases, saline is best accompanied with rigorous water restriction and is often only an intermediate stop to dialysis (see Chapter 56).[205] As in hyperkalemia, hyponatremia may ultimately be best treated by dialysis.

Other metabolic abnormalities include metabolic acidosis, usually managed by infusion of sodium bicarbonate. The goal is to maintain a pH of 7.2 or greater and the serum bicarbonate (HCO_3) above 16 mEq/L. The amount of bicarbonate necessary can be determined using the formula: Base deficit = 0.6 × (body weight in kg) × (the desired bicarbonate level − the observed level), all divided by 2.

Give ½ the replacement in the first 2 to 3 hours and the remainder over the next 24 hours.[199] Patients with congestive heart failure (CHF) will not tolerate the sodium necessary to correct a significant acidosis with sodium bicarbonate. In these cases, the correction can be accomplished using tromethamine (THAM) available in 0.3 M solution. The amount of THAM necessary can be calculated as: ml of 0.3 M THAM + (body weight in kg) × (the base deficit in mEq/L). THAM is given slowly and with careful monitoring and should be reserved for intensive care situations.

Hyperphosphatemia may also occur and is managed by administration of calcium carbonate 300 to 400 mg/kg/day, PO or NG.[199]

Rapid dialysis, either peritoneal or hemodialysis, may be indicated for fluid overload refractory to medical management with congestive heart failure, pulmonary edema or hypertension, severe hyperkalemia, hyponatremia, hypernatremia, unresponsive metabolic acidosis, azotemia, HUS with hemoglobinuria, burns or crush injuries with myoglobinuria, and altered mental status.

Septic shock may also develop. Relief of any obstructive uropathy by catheter or nephrostomy is essential to control infection and shock and to preserve renal function.[206,207]

RENAL FAILURE, CHRONIC

JULIO CASTILLO • MARY P. SWEENEY

Chronic renal failure (CRF) implies an irreversible and progressive reduction in the GFR to below 25% of normal (greater than 30 ml/min/1.73 m²) that is present for at least 3 months. The incidence of CRF is estimated at 3 to 6 children/million.[208] In the emergency setting, it is essential to focus on the presentation of potential complications and work closely with the child's nephrologist.

Chronic renal insufficiency defines the stage in which residual renal function remains between 25% and 50% of normal. End-stage renal disease (ESRD) is associated with a GFR of less than 10 ml/min/1.73 m²; dialysis or transplantation must be considered.[209] Renal and metabolic responses consist of hematuria, proteinuria, anemia, hypertension, osteodystrophy, growth retardation, oliguria, and uremic symptoms. Uremia is characterized early by anorexia, nausea, vomiting, somnolence, and malaise. Convulsions, coma, cardiac failure, and gastrointestinal bleeding may develop if no treatment is instituted.[209,210]

Pathophysiology

The onset of CRF is gradual with mild biochemical changes. The progressive loss of functional nephrons causes an increase in the glomerular capillary blood flow and pressure and single nephron GFR. Hypertrophic response in the glomeruli and proximal tubules has been observed.[209] Endogenous vasoactive substances are believed responsible for the increased glomerular capillary blood flow by constrictive action on the efferent arteriole facilitating an increase in single nephron GFR.

As single nephron GFR increases, solute load per nephron also increases. In general, reabsorption from the proximal loop of Henle balances a single nephron GFR. This hyperperfusion stage produces intraglomerular hypertension, endothelial damage (expansion of mesangial matrix), and finally glomerular sclerosis.[211]

Glomerular sclerosis will induce systemic hypertension and aggravate hyperfusion. Proteinuria and hematuria appear as a result of hyperfiltration and the mesangial injury. Ongoing immunologic injury may also play an important role in the progression of the glomerular sclerosis (intraglomerular coagulation).

Etiology

Congenital renal disease (renal hypoplasia, renal dysplasia, and obstructive uropathy) is the most common cause of CRF in children younger than 5 years. Hereditary, metabolic, or acquired CRF occurs more frequently in older children. Among the hereditary cases, juvenile nephritis, cystic disease, and Alport syndrome are the most frequent diseases encountered. The principal metabolic diseases are cystinosis and oxalosis, and among the acquired etiologies, chronic glomerulonephritis and HUS are most important.

Diagnostic Findings

Clinical Findings. The progressive decline in GFR affects almost all organ systems. The findings are largely a result of complications of renal failure. Hypertension is common in children with acquired gomerulonephritides, perhaps related to salt and water retention and excessive renin secretion. Heart failure, stroke, seizures, headache, blurred vision, and deteriorating renal function may be the initial clinical presentation. The focus of the emergency evaluation must be on establishing baseline status, treating acute exacerbation or complications, and assuring communication with the patient's nephrologist.

Mental retardation, personality changes, cognitive disturbances, encephalopathic seizures, and coma may develop. Paresthesias of the palm and soles (uremic neuropathy) and pericarditis are common with uremia. These CNS alterations have been attributed to hypertension, uremia, acidosis, hypocalcemia, and the effects of aluminum absorption from aluminum containing phosphate-binding agents.

Renal Osteodystrophy. The progressive loss of nephrons decreases the conversion of 1,25-dihydroxyvitamin D_3 from 25-hydroxycholecalciferol formed by the liver leading to poor calcium absorption in the gastrointestinal tract, hypocalcemia, and osteomalacia. Secondary hyperparathyroidism develops, promoting calcium resorption from the bones and later osteitis fibrosa. Inadequate renal phosphate excretion occurs with the reduction of functioning nephrons and hyperphosphatemia develops. The hyperphosphatemia will inhibit the 1,25-dihydroxyvitamin D_3 synthesis and will further stimulate the secretion of parathyroid hormone.[212] Rachitism, pathologic fractures, valgus deformity of lower extremities, slipped capital femoral epiphysis, and other skeletal deformities develop.[208,210]

Excessive intake of aluminum contained in phosphate binders, which are often prescribed, may produce a severe form of renal dystrophy characterized by severe deformities and multiple fractures.

Growth Retardation. Factors associated with growth retardation include poor caloric intake, anorexia, renal osteodystrophy, metabolic acidosis, anemia, and hypertension. Children less than 2 years with CRF will be more affected because of the greater velocity of linear growth and rate of brain development. Growth velocity is decreased and there is progressive bone age retardation before puberty. Serum growth hormone and insulin-like growth factor I (somatomedin C) concentrations can be normal or elevated in children. Exogenous growth hormone therapy may accelerate growth.[213-216]

Electrolyte Disturbances. Impairment of sodium excretion appears as the number of functioning nephrons decreases. This retention produces edema, hypertension, and eventually congestive heart failure. Poor urinary concentrating capacity and the inability to conserve sodium in the patient with congenital renal disease will produce a salt-wasting state with severe extracellular volume contraction and a rapid decline in the CRF.[217]

Hyperkalemia results from the catabolic state, decreased renal excretion, and metabolic acidosis. Chronic metabolic acidosis secondary to inadequate ammonia excretion to buffer hydrogen ion occurs as the number of functioning nephrons decreases. Respiratory alkalosis and bone alkali used to titrate the hydrogen ion are the homeostatic responses, the latter resulting in bone demineralization and increased calciuria that aggravate the renal osteodystrophy. Renal bicarbonate wasting in patients with Fanconi syndrome, type IV renal tubular acidosis, and secondary hyperparathyroidism may aggravate the acidotic state.

Other Findings. *Delayed puberty* is related to insufficient production of gonadal steroids associated with elevated gonadotropin concentrations. Alterations in the pulsatile daily secretions of gonadotropins (luteinizing hormone and growth hormone) in pubertal children undergoing dialysis have been found.[218]

Progressive anemia is caused by the decrease in production of erythropoietin, toxic inhibitors of erythropoiesis, and a shortened half-life of the erythrocytes induced by the uremia. Although there is low serum iron level and elevated iron-binding capacity, the anemia is generally normocytic and normochromic with a low reticulocyte count and normal ferritin level.

Protein intake has been restricted traditionally to the recommended daily allowances for age, ensuring the highest proportion of essential amino acids. The rate of progression of renal insufficiency may be slowed with protein restriction. Reduction of the protein intake to 8% of the total recommended daily allowance is suggested; 100% of daily caloric intake has been recommended in children with creatinine clearance less than 50% who do not have uremic symptoms and are not on dialysis.[219]

Phosphorus and sodium intake limitation is also recommended. Calcium carbonate as a phosphate binder is indicated because the patients with renal failure receive a diet restricted in dairy products due to the high phosphate content. Their diet is also deficient in calcium, requiring calcium and vitamin D supplements.

Multivitamin supplement is indicated to replace water-soluble vitamins. Children undergoing dialysis will suffer from a loss of folate.[209]

Ancillary Data. Regular monitoring of biochemical and hematologic parameters is recommended. Blood count, reticulocytes, electrolytes, glucose, BUN, creatinine, serum osmolality, calcium, phosphorus, serum proteins, triglycerides, cholesterol, alkaline phosphatase, ferritin level, urine osmolality, urine electrolytes, and urine creatinine are indicated. Platelet dysfunction and vasopressin-resistant diabetes insipidus are common.[217] Bone age evaluation of the changes from rachitism or renal osteodystrophy is obtained at regular 3 to 6 month intervals.

Management

Renal transplantation is the treatment of choice for patients with ESRD. Children with CRF require conservative management to protect residual renal function, prevent the acceleration of renal injury and metabolic abnormalities, and treat the complications of CRF.

Fluid restriction is indicated in the presence of edema, hypertension, or congestive heart failure. The use of diuretics may be indicated. Sodium supplementation in children with renal salt-wasting syndrome may prevent hyponatremia, dehydration, and eventually renal hypoperfusion; signs of hyponatremia may be vague consisting of poor weight gain and malaise.[212] Sodium replacement in the salt-wasting condition can be estimated from a 24-hour urinary sodium measurement.

Anemia may be treated with recombinant human erythropoietin and may minimize the need for blood transfusion.[216,220,221]

Specific management of acidosis, hyperkalemia, dysrhythmias, and other metabolic abnormalities are discussed elsewhere in this chapter. Calcium-channel blockers such as nifedipine given sublingually are particularly useful for acute hypertensive crises.

Dialysis. Dialysis therapy is used to regulate solute concentration and fluid volume in the patient with ESRD. Dialysis allows children to wait until conditions for a renal transplant are optimal or is used for patients in whom renal transplantation is not possible.

A GFR of less than 5% of normal or 5 ml/min/1.73 m² is usually an indication for dialysis treatment. In general, the development of uremic encephalopathy, peripheral neuropathy, pericarditis, and bleeding diathesis are absolute indications for dialysis. Congestive heart failure, hyperkalemia, metabolic acidosis, and hypertension uncontrolled by conservative measures are also common indicators.

Even infants and small children can undergo hemodialysis, which is more efficient than peritoneal dialysis, although it is used less frequently. Hemodialysis requires a permanent vascular access shunt or fistula. Patients usually undergo treatment for 4 hours, three times per week, at an outpatient facility.

Peritoneal dialysis requires a catheter insertion for instillation of a dialysis solution into the peritoneal cavity for 4 to 8 hours, four to five times per day. The retained body metabolite will diffuse from the blood to the solution via the peritoneum. Continuous ambulatory peritoneal dialysis (CAPD) and continuous cycling peritoneal dialysis (CCPD) are effective and well tolerated, allowing the recollection of the infused fluid in plastic bags concealed under clothing. In CCPD, overnight cycling of dialysate is performed automatically.

The advantages of peritoneal dialysis in children include decreased transfusion requirements, better blood pressure control, increased serum levels of bicarbonate, increased caloric intake, and no interference with usual daily activities such as school or family traveling.[210] The main complications are mechanical (pain, bleeding, leakage, inadequate drainage, local edema, intestinal perforation), infectious (peritonitis, tunnel infection, exit-site infection), cardiovascular (fluid overload, hypertension, acute pulmonary edema), metabolic (hyperglycemia, hyponatremia, hypoproteinemia) and neurologic (cerebral edema), and psychosis (seizures in new patients).[222]

Peritonitis is the major complication. Children have cloudy peritoneal fluid, fever, and abdominal pain. The fluid will usually contain greater than 100 WBCs per mm³ with 50% neutrophils. Gram stain will show organisms in only 25% of cases. *S. epidermidis* and *S. aureus* are the pathogens in 70% of cases. Antibiotics may be used intravenously or intraperitoneal. Catheter exit-site infection requires aggressive IV antibiotic therapy. Painful dialysis may represent early peritonitis or intolerance to the acid pH of the dialysate. Bloody peritoneal fluid may indicate disseminated intravascular coagulation, trauma, ovulation, or true peritoneal hemorrhage.

Renal Transplantation. Renal transplantation is the principal definitive treatment in ESRD. Successful transplantation is technically feasible in most children, regardless of the underlying renal disease. Controversies in management are diverse: the type of graft (live related donors vs. cadaveric transplants), optimal recipient age for transplant, and the safest immunosuppressive therapy.[223-225]

The North American Pediatric Renal Transplant Cooperative Study has registered 3,438 renal transplants between January 1987 and December 1991. The one-year graft survival has risen steadily each year from 72% in 1987 to 83% in 1991; likewise two-year graft survival increased from 65% in 1987 to 78% in 1991. Reasons for improvement include increasing use of anti-T cell therapy, higher doses of cyclosporine A, and decreased need for transfusions with the availability of erythropoietin.[226]

It is essential to understand potential complications. Immunologic damage to the renal allograft is mediated by cellular and humoral mechanisms leading to humoral, acute cellular, and chronic humoral rejection. Acute humoral rejection occurs in hosts with preformed cytotoxic antibodies against the blood groups ABO- or HLA-associated antigens present in the transplanted organ.

Chronic humoral rejection occurs over time and produces arteriolar and interstitial fibrosis. The patient will present within days of the transplant with fever, graft pain and tenderness, decreased urine output, hypertension, increased BUN and creatinine levels, hematuria, proteinuria, and weight gain. Differential diagnosis includes acute urinary obstruction, cyclosporine nephrotoxicity, urinary extravasation, and persistent acute tubular necrosis. Most acute cellular rejection episodes will respond to corticosteroids or, if persistent, to antithymocyte globulin.

The risk of opportunistic infection is obviously higher as the immunosuppressive regimen becomes more potent. Cytomegalovirus infection occurs in 60% of patients during the first year after transplantation. When this occurs, the dose of steroids must be reduced or the infection will be prolonged and more severe. Hypertension will occur in more than 70% of children after transplantation, accelerating the deterioration of the allograft. Potential etiologies of hypotension include side effects of cyclosporine and corticosteroids, transplant arterial stenosis, acute or chronic rejection, or recurrence of the primary renal disease. Steroid toxicity includes posterior subcapsular cataracts in more than half of the patients 1 year after transplantation and, possibly, aseptic necrosis of bone, especially the femoral head.

Prepubertal recipients experience significant height gain after transplantation; children with a bone age greater than 12 years at the time of renal transplantation grow minimally. Recombinant growth hormone treatment results in accelerated height velocity, especially after the second and third years of treatment.[214] In general, sexual maturation proceeds after renal transplantation. Rehabilitation of children after successful renal transplantation is complicated, as evidenced by low self-esteem, defective social adaptation, noncompliance with immunosuppression, poor school performance, growth retardation, and pubertal delay in many children.

TESTICULAR TORSION

MARTIN I. HERMAN

Testicular torsion, or more correctly torsion of the spermatic cord, is one of the three most common causes of an acutely tender and swollen scrotum. Early relief of the compromised blood flow can result in testicular rescue; failure to act quickly will result in loss of spermatogenesis or testicular atrophy.

Testicular torsions affect 1/4,000 males, usually in their adolescent years, with a peak incidence occurring around age 13. Before 1966, orchiectomy rates were as high as 90%, presumably due to delay in referral and diagnosis. In 1977, as a result of more aggressive surgical intervention, testicular survival approached 50%; testicular survival rates now approach 90%.[227,228]

Testicular survival is dependent on at least two factors: duration of the torsion and the tightness of the twist. In rats, arterial occlusion has been documented within 30 minutes of a surgically produced torsion of 720 degrees.[229] In data that Hastie presented, two turns of the spermatic cord in rats will produce ischemia in 6 hours and four turns will produce zero perfusion in 10 minutes. In humans the data is indirect. Knight and Vassy reported salvage rates of 96%, 93%, 80%, 40%, and less than 10% when surgical intervention occurs at less than 4 hours, between 4 and 8 hours, 8 and 12 hours, 12 and 24 hours, and more than 24 hours, respectively. This data supports modifying the aggressive attitude toward early scrotal exploration when the pain has been present for more than 24 hours.

Pathophysiology

The testis descends from the abdomen and enters the scrotum through the inguinal canal. The peritoneum invaginates into the scrotum to become the tunica vaginalis. This tunica may envelop the testicle and epididymis either partially or completely. The majority of the time the tunica surrounds only part of the testicle and epididymis and attaches to the posterior wall of the hemiscrotum and the superior pole of the testis, resulting in testicular fixation (Fig. 60-10). For a torsion to occur, the tunica has to surround the entire complex and attach higher up on the cord structures (bell clapper deformity), allowing for minimal fixation of the testis (Fig. 60-11). In this situation the testicle may rotate within the tunica vaginalis and thereby impede its arterial blood supply. Extravaginal torsion is seen most commonly in neonates, especially prematures. The torsion occurs outside of the tunica.

Once a twist exists in the spermatic cord the blood supply to the testis is compromised.[228] Venous occlusion occurs, leading to swelling, arterial occlusion, and then testicular infarction.

What precipitates a torsion is still unknown. Speculation has included a relationship with testosterone surges and there is a chronologic relationship to minor trauma, bicycle riding, and strenuous exercise.[230,231]

In addition to having a detrimental effect on spermatogenesis, testicular torsion causes pain and swelling. Following significant torsion, the morphology and number of spermatogonia are decreased. Even after successful derotation and orchiopexy about one third of testis will atrophy and in some, complete resorption of the organ occurs.[232]

Torsion not only affects the ipsilateral testicle; it can have disastrous effects on the contralateral organ, too. After surgically induced torsions for six hours, the contralateral testis in rats displayed decreased spermatogenesis and smaller seminiferous tubular diameter.[233] An immunologic reaction has been proposed. But it is not seen in prepubertal rats, possibly due to the absence of antigens derived from mature spermatozoa.[232] There is human evidence that substantiates the rat experience.

Diagnostic Findings

Clinical Findings. Pathognomonic findings for torsion include an elevated testicle with a palpable twist, abnormal axis of the testicle, abnormal scrotal position of epididymis, absent cremasteric reflex, and an abnormal testicular axis in the contralateral testis. Other findings associated with testicular torsion, but not pathognomonic, include age (13 ± 3.5 years), left testicular pain (78 of 130), duration of pain (< 24 hours [74/130], > 24 hours [56/130]), nausea, vomiting, acute onset of pain, and past episodes of similar pain (30/130). About 10% of patients had painless swelling. Leukocytosis is present in about half the cases and a left shift is seen in about two thirds of cases. Findings of acute UTIs, epididymal tenderness, urethral discharge, past history of imperforate anus, abnormal bladder anatomy, or hypospadias repair are more suggestive of epididymitis.

A cryptorchid testis may be more prone to torsion and may need to be considered in the child with abdominal pain.[234]

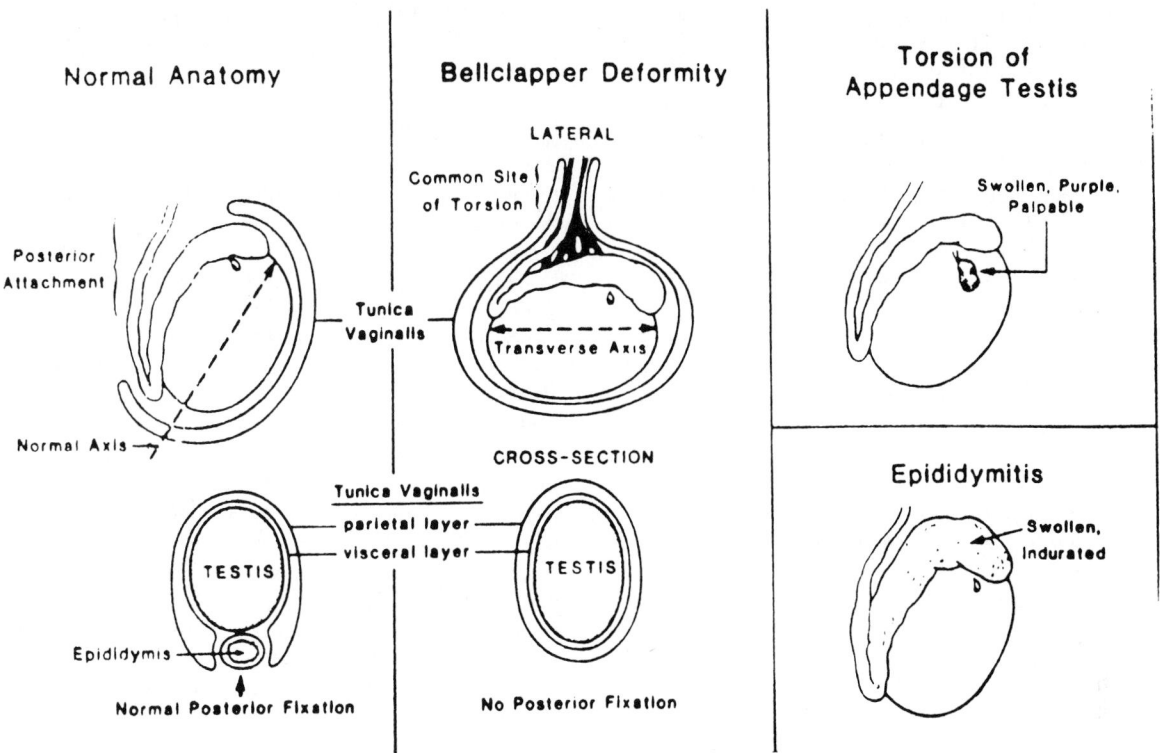

FIG. 60-10. Physical findings in normal boys and in boys with torsion of the spermatic cord, torsion of an appendage, or acute epididymitis. (*From Knight PJ and Vassy LE: The diagnosis and treatment of the acute scrotum in children and adolescents,* Ann Surg 200:664, 1984.)

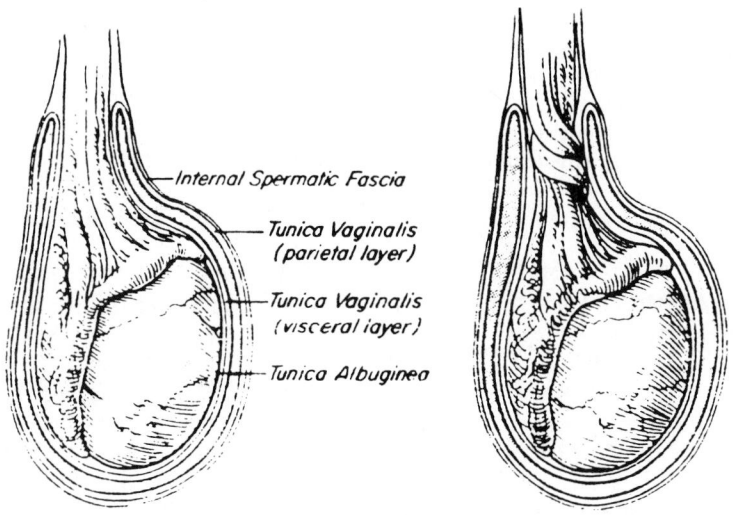

FIG. 60-11. Intravaginal torsion. The testicle twists upon its vasculature within the investing tunica vaginalis. This type occurs primarily during the pubertal age. (*From Cilento BG et al: Cryptorchidism and testicular torsion,* Ped Clin North Am, Pediatric Surgery 40(6):1133, 1993.)

Complications (See section on Scrotal Pain and Swelling). An untreated testicular torsion will lead to hemicastration by infarction. Since the same anatomy that led to the torsion in the first testis may exist in the contralateral scrotum, a contralateral torsion may result if an orchiopexy is not carried out subsequent to the index torsion, resulting in complete castration. Outcome after treatment is dependent on the timeliness of intervention. Spermatogenesis can be impaired after as little as 4 hours of ischemia and atrophy of the organ has been noted after 4 to 6 hours of torsion.

Ancillary Data. Although the history and physical examination are the most important factors in determining the need for detorsion, ancillary testing may help with making management decisions. At least three types of imaging modalities are adjuncts in the evaluation of the acutely swollen scrotum: color Doppler ultrasonography (CDU), technetium pertechnetate scintigraphy, and magnetic resonance imaging (MRI) of the scrotum. MRI has not been evaluated in pediatric patients; however, it appears promising in adult studies. Its utility will depend on whether the study can be performed expeditiously.

CDU, advocated since the late 1980s, is reported to have a sensitivity of 82% to 86% and a specificity approaching 100%. In fact, when compared to scintigraphy, CDU seems to be as sensitive and specific without ionizing radiation exposure.[235] Several reports advocate and confirm the utility of CDU or pulsed Doppler ultrasonography in evaluating the pediatric scrotum.[235-238] There are some questions remaining about the ability of CDU to detect true torsion, intermittent torsions, and spontaneous detorsion just based on the appearance of diminished flow.[239] Nevertheless, CDU is easier to get, has the ability to assess other anatomic relationships, and does not involve exposure to ionizing radiation.

Scintigraphy has been promoted as the imaging study for the acute scrotum, probably based on testicular scanning's reported sensitivities of 80% to 100% and a specificity of 89% to 100% in the detection of spermatic cord torsion.[240] In 1991, Atkinson noted that scintigraphy has an advantage over CDU for imaging flow in children due to the smaller size of the nutrient vessels.[241] Even though scintigraphy was plagued by poor resolution, subjective interpretation, and unavoidable delays in availability, it held a position as the imaging modality to use until CDU was refined.

Imaging does not replace clinical judgment. Surgical exploration has a 100% diagnostic accuracy and is still the treatment of choice for the patient who presents with pain of less than 12 hours duration with a history suggestive of torsion. Imaging is reserved for those cases with a small likelihood of torsion or presented late in the course of their disease.

Differential Considerations
(See Section on Scrotal Pain and Swelling)

Management

"Once the diagnosis is made, treatment is straightforward."[242] Surgical exploration is the only course to take if the patient has had his pain for less than 12 hours. For patients having pain for over 24 hours, the option to wait and observe can be considered.[227,228] If the diagnosis of a torsion is confirmed, the patient should be scheduled for orchiectomy of the nonviable testis. An elective orchiopexy of the contralateral testis is needed; 40% of contralateral testes have the bell clapper deformity and therefore will be at risk for a torsion of their spermatic cord if not fixed. There is some controversy regarding the removal of the infarcted testicle. However, there is mounting evidence that by leaving the ischemic organ in place, the surgeon is risking damage to the contralateral testicle from the previously described immunologic response.[232,233]

Other management modalities include manual detorsion, ultrasound-guided manual detorsion, and pharmaceutical adjuncts. Since the testicle usually twists from lateral to medial, reversal by rotating the testicle in a medial to lateral fashion should bring pain relief. Repeat the procedure if a twist can still be palpated in the cord, since torsions may have rotated more than once. Detorsion can be monitored by ultrasound, documenting the return of blood flow to the testis.[243] Allopurinol prior to detorsion has been advocated to avoid injury caused by the peroxidation of cell membrane lipids after reperfusion; in rats, allopurinol has a protective effect.[242]

Disposition

Patients presenting with acute scrotal pain demand immediate attention. If a twist in the cord can be felt or the testicular axis is abnormal, manual detorsion can be attempted. Surgical consultation to assess the need for scrotal exploration should be obtained immediately because delay may jeopardize testicular salvage. For cases that present late (pain >24 hours) a less urgent approach may be followed. Still surgical consultation is advisable. Make the patient comfortable, give intravenous fluids, and maintain the patient's readiness for surgery. It may be advisable to obtain a CBC, electrolytes, urinalysis, and any other tests needed to clear the patient for anesthesia. If there is going to be a delay in the consultant's arrival and CDU is readily available, proceed with the imaging study. Imaging studies should never delay the surgeon's evaluation or impede the patient's transition to the operating room.

URINARY TRACT INFECTION

AMY L. HERTZ

UTI is a major bacterial disease of childhood. Anywhere from 3% to 5% of all girls and 1% of boys will experience a symptomatic UTI before puberty.[244,245] Girls will often have recurrences of the infection. In infants less than 3 months of age, the incidence of UTI is higher in males than females.[246]

The prevalence of asymptomatic bacteria (significant bacteriuria found during routine screening of asymptomatic children) in the preschool/school-aged girl is approximately 1%.[247,248] Both symptomatic and asymptomatic UTIs can result in serious complications, including hypertension, renal stones, and in rare circumstances, ESRD. The complications are often preventable if adequate treatment and follow-up are obtained.

The definition of UTI is the presence of a significant number of bacteria anywhere in the urinary tract. Cystitis refers to inflammation or infection of the kidney, whereas pyelonephritis involves the renal tissue. The term *significant* or *true bacteriuria* is used to distinguish bacteria multiplying within the urinary tract from bacteria present in the urine specimen resulting from contamination of the specimen from inadequate collection techniques.

Timely evaluation and diagnosis will ultimately require an understanding of relative risk factors, particularly in febrile children. Children under 2 years of age who appear at greatest risk of having a UTI include females, particularly caucasians, with temperatures over 39° C and children with no source delineated.[249]

Pathophysiology

A variety of predisposing factors enable bacteria to enter the urinary system. Poor perineal hygiene, the short urethra of females, infrequent voiding, and sexual activity increase the risk for UTI, possibly resulting from bacteria harbored in the foreskin leading to increased meatal contamination.[250]

The acute, uncomplicated infection is most often confined to the bladder. The inflammatory changes of the bladder and urethral mucosa are responsible for the symptoms of frequency, urgency, and dysuria. Recurrent infections distort the normal bladder-ureter anatomic relationship. This leads to incompetence of the vesicoureteral valve resulting in reflux of the urine into the ureter, especially during voiding. Reflux allows for direct access of the infecting organism to the kidney parenchyma with resultant pyelonephritis and the development of parenchymal scars. Continued infection alters the normal urinary concentrating mechanisms and leads to polyuria.

Etiology

Infection usually occurs by an ascending route from the external genitalia. Females are affected more commonly than males because of the shorter urethra and ease of contamination of the bladder. Bacteremia is generally a consequence and not a cause of the UTI in older children but may be causative in neonates.

E. coli is the most frequently isolated organism responsible for UTI in patients without a complicating disorder of the urinary system. Up to 80% to 90% of all UTIs are due to *E. coli* because of its increased prevalence on the gastrointestinal system and its ability to multiply rapidly once inside the bladder. Other infectious causes of UTI are listed in the box above.

Diagnostic Findings

Signs and symptoms of UTI vary, especially according to patient age. Because neonatal UTI is associated with bacteremia, signs are nonspecific and are more consistent with generalized septicemia, including lethargy, poor appetite, irritability, and tenderness to touch. Many of these patients present with jaundice. Fever may not always be present. Occasionally, a workup for failure to thrive reveals a UTI. When treated appropriately, the neonate promptly begins to gain weight.

Infants and toddlers often have a fever associated with a symptomatic infection. Generalized signs and symptoms such as irritability, abdominal pain, vomiting, and meningismus may be present. In other cases, the only complaint is that a child has smelly diapers and hematuria may be present. Generalized symptoms may be lacking.

Older children present with more localized symptoms including dysuria, frequency, and urgency. Previously toilet-trained children may have accidents. Urine may have a strong odor. Hematuria may be the presenting complaint. *E. coli* is associated with more severe symptoms than bacteria such as *Proteus*, *Staphylococcus*, and *Pseudomonas* species.[251] It is felt that high fever, flank pain (especially

---

Common Causative Agents of UTI in children

Escherichia coli
Proteus species
Klebsiella species
Staphylococcus saprophyticus
Enterococcus species

---

costovertebral angle), and leukocytosis are suggestive of pyelonephritis. Children with chronic infections may be symptom-free.

It is imperative to remember that not all urinary symptoms are secondary to infection. Anything that causes irritation to the urethra may cause dysuria and urgency in children. Bubble baths, soaps, masturbation, vaginitis, and trauma may all be sources of irritation, producing inflammation and resultant bacteria in the urinary tract (see section on Dysuria).

Complications of recurrent UTIs include chronic renal failure, bacteremia, perinephric abscess, and urolithiasis.

Ancillary Data. The urinalysis may provide limited information. A gram-stained smear of the urine sediment is the most sensitive screening test and is often combined with evaluation for WBCs or a positive leukocyte esterase and nitrate. In the neonatal period, the urinalysis may initially be unremarkable and the culture may be positive. About 20% of neonates with UTIs will have a normal urinalysis or negative leukocyte esterase or nitrite or both.[252]

A common error made in the diagnosis of UTI is the reliance on inadequately collected and transported urine specimens. If a urine specimen is not promptly processed, there may be an overgrowth of bacteria, resulting in false-positive tests.[253] The methods of collection include urine bag, clean-catch, catheterization, and suprapubic bladder aspiration.

Collection Techniques. The urine bag collection system is commonly used on infants and small children because of its ease and lack of invasion; however, it has its own inherent problems. There is an increased risk of contamination of the urine with vaginal and fecal flora because of the difficulty in thoroughly cleansing the perineum and this approach should not be used if antibiotics are to be initiated. Although a negative urine culture from a bag specimen is helpful in ruling out a UTI, positive cultures should be confirmed by a more accurate method such as catheterization or suprapubic bladder aspiration.

Clean-catch urine specimens in children also are frequently contaminated by perineal bacteria. The reliability of these specimens increases with the age of the patient. It is sufficient to clean the perineum with soft soap and water, since any antibacterial agent left on the skin may result in a false-negative urine culture.

The most reliable method of urine collection is that which is obtained directly from the bladder, either by urethral catheterization or suprapubic bladder aspiration. Catheterization may be difficult in uncircumcised boys or neonates, and there is a slight risk of urethral trauma or introduction of secondary infection in uninfected children.

Straight in and out catheterization is relatively simple and not associated with a significant risk of nosocomial infection. The patient's anterior urethra should be thoroughly cleansed. A pliable #5 feeding tube should be passed into the bladder until urine flow is seen. It is important not to collect the first amount of the urine flowing out because this allows the urethral organisms to flow out; a later sample should be collected. Larger catheters are not recommended because of the risk of urethral irritation and contamination of the sample with urethral bacteria.[248]

Suprapubic Aspiration. Suprapubic bladder aspiration is a safe method for obtaining urine from the newborn and infants because distended bladder in this age group is primarily intraabdominal. The infant's bladder must be full, which may be partially confirmed by the diaper having been dry for at least 45 minutes. A first morning urine is the optimal specimen.

The child is restrained in the supine position and a site 2 cm or 1 fingerbreadth above the symphysis is identified in the midline. After surgical cleansing with povidone-iodine, the symphysis and point of insertion are identified and a 1.5-inch, 22 gauge needle attached to a 5-ml syringe is inserted. The needle is angled at 10 to 20 degrees cephalad and advanced through the skin under negative pressure.

Entry into the bladder is indicated by return of urine. If no urine is obtained, the needle should be angled more perpendicular to the frontal plane. Avoid excessive probing or manipulation. If no urine is obtained, try again in 15 minutes or use a different technique such as catheterization.

The procedure is generally safe but not entirely without risk. Some hematuria is common after the procedure. Complications include gross hematuria, anterior abdominal wall abscess, and bowel puncture.

After the specimen is obtained, it should be cultured within 30 minutes or placed in a refrigerator to prevent the colony count from being unreliably elevated. Urinalysis is a useful, but not definitive, diagnostic test. Pyuria may not be present in up to 50% of children with culture-proven UTI. Pyuria is generally defined as ≥ 10 WBC/HPF in a centrifuged urinary sediment. A count of < 10 WBC/HPF has been associated with sterile urine cultures, whereas a count of > 10 WBC/HPF has been associated with positive urine cultures.[252] There are many causes of pyuria not associated with a UTI (see section on Pyuria). The presence of leukocyte esterase correlates with the presence of pyuria, whereas a positive nitrite test implies that bacteria capable of fixing the nitrate normally found in urine is present and is used as a screening test for bacteriuria.

Because bladder urine is normally sterile, quantitative urine culture is the "gold standard" for the diagnosis of UTI. There are several methods of culturing urine, including the loop culture method and the dipslide method (a convenient test suited for office use). The standard criterion used to diagnose UTI is to document the growth of 10^5 bacterial colonies of a single type per milliliter of urine from a clean-catch specimen. Any bacterial growth from a suprapubic urine specimen or a specimen obtained by

TABLE 60-9. Diagnostic Significance of Colony Counts in Urinary Specimens

Method of collection	Colony count (pure culture)	Probability of infection
Suprapubic aspiration	Gram-negative bacilli: any number Gram-positive staphylococci: > a few thousand	>99%
Catheterization	$> 10^5$	95%
	10^4 to 10^5	Infection likely
	10^3 to 10^4	Suspicious: repeat
	$< 10^3$	Infection unlikely
Clean-voided (male)	$\geq 10^4$	Infection likely (foreskin retracted or absent and glans penis well cleansed)
	3 specimens: $> 10^5$	95%
	2 specimens: $> 10^5$	90%
	1 specimen: $> 10^5$	80%
Clean-voided (female)	$5 \times 10^4 - 10^5$	Suspicious: repeat symptomatic*
	$10^4 - 5 \times 10^4$	Suspicious: repeat asymptomatic Infection unlikely
	$< 10^4$	Infection unlikely

*The culture should be repeated in the presence of symptoms of upper or lower urinary infection or unexplained fever.
From Hellerstein S: *Urinary tract infections in children*, St. Louis, 1982, Mosby.

straight catheterization suggests infection.[254] Table 60-9 indicates the likelihood that a positive culture reflects a UTI.[244]

Low colony count in a urine culture may indicate that the urine is dilute, the processing is incorrect, or an improper growth medium has been used. Other causes that may be considered include recent ingestion of antibiotics, fastidious organisms, bacteriostatic agents in urine, and complete obstruction of the ureter.

Because one may have bacteriuria without pyuria or pyuria without bacteriuria, a urine culture for diagnosis is imperative. In older children with uncomplicated UTI, other laboratory tests are not required. If there are clinical signs and symptoms of decreasing renal function, such as decreased urine output or hypertension, BUN and serum creatinine should be determined. In neonates, young children, and children with complicated infections, these studies should be part of the initial evaluation. Several tests (C-reactive protein, ESR) have been used to differentiate upper from lower tract infections, but their reliability is poor.

Radiologic Studies. In most patients with a UTI, radiologic imaging of the urinary tract is imperative to detect urologic abnormalities, to identify patients in whom renal scarring has resulted from previous UTI, and to assist in the diagnosis of pyelonephritis. Opinions differ regarding which radiologic tests should be performed.[254,255]

It is generally agreed that neonates, infants, and all males regardless of age should be evaluated with radiologic studies after the first UTI. Others who require imaging studies include female patients with recurrent UTI, patients with pyelonephritis and all children with hypertension, abnormal voiding patterns, or elevated BUN or serum creatinine.[247] There are others who believe that all children under the age of 5 years should have imaging studies performed after their first UTI.[255] Approximately 30% of infants and 50% of older children demonstrate an anatomic abnormality on investigation.[253] The most common finding is vesicoureteral reflux (VUR).

The renal ultrasound is the initial evaluation of a patient with a UTI. Many abnormalities, especially urinary tract obstruction and renal abnormalities can be identified with a renal ultrasound. A voiding cystourethrogram (VCUG) is appropriate 2 to 4 weeks after the diagnosis of UTI is made. The VCUG will diagnose VUR and is helpful in defining urethral and bladder anatomy. The IVP has been considered the "gold standard" when evaluating patients with UTI and should be obtained if the ultrasound is abnormal. Renal scars and other urinary tract abnormalities can easily be detected with IVP. It is not the procedure of choice to evaluate neonates and children with renal failure because of their inability to concentrate and excrete the contrast adequately.[254] More recently studies have shown that renal cortical scintigraphy using technetium-99m (^{99m}Tc)-labeled glucoheptonate or dimercaptosuccinic acid (DMSA) is preferable to the IVP and ultrasound in detecting renal parenchymal involvement. When compared to the IVP, the Tc-99m DMSA scan is more sensitive for the diagnosis of acute pyelonephritis, is better in detecting early renal scars and uses less radiation.[245,256]

Differential Considerations

Causes of pyuria other than UTI include chemical (bubble bath, feminine hygiene products) or physical (masturbation, abuse) irritation, other irritation, dehydration, renal tuberculosis, acute glomerulonephritis, respiratory infections, appendicitis and other abdominal or pelvic infections, gastroenteritis, and administration of oral polio vaccine.

Viral, mycobacterial, and fungal agents may cause dysuria, pyuria, and frequency. Vaginitis, urethritis, and pinworms may also cause local irritation and inflammation with discomfort.

Hemorrhagic cystitis is a benign self-limited disease in school-aged children. Adenovirus types 11 and 21 are implicated as the viral etiology. Gross hematuria, dysuria, and other symptoms may be similar to acute bacterial cystitis, lasting only a few days. Treatment includes vigorous hydration.

Management

Antibiotics should be initiated when a UTI is highly suspected after an adequate urine specimen for culture has been obtained. The antibiotics can be discontinued if the culture is negative. Waiting 1 or 2 days for laboratory

TABLE 60-10. Commonly Used Oral Antibiotics for UTI

Drugs	Dosage (mg/kg/24 hr)
Amoxicillin	20-40
Ampicillin	50-100
Amoxicillin/potassium clavulanate	40-50 (AMX)
Nitrofurantoin	5-7
TMP-SMZ	8-12 TMP
	40-60 SMZ
Cefaclor	20-40
Cephalexin	25-50
Sulfisoxazole	120-150

results may increase the likelihood for renal scarring or VUR. Therefore treatment should be initiated pending culture results if the urinalysis and symptoms support the diagnosis. However, if a child has a small amount of pyuria only, it is feasible to hold antibiotic treatment for 24 to 48 hours until the culture report is known. Treatment for 7 to 10 days is generally sufficient to eliminate bacteria from an otherwise normal urinary tract, assuming the organism is sensitive to the chosen antibiotic and no stone, foreign body, or obstruction is present. Several studies in children have looked at short courses of antibiotic therapy for simple UTI. Although some studies found no difference between the short course and conventional treatment, others have shown that with an abbreviated course of antibiotics the cure rate was lower, the reinfection rate was higher, and there was a higher rate of recurrent UTI.[256-258] When appropriate antibiotics are chosen, sterilization of the urine usually occurs within 24 hours and symptoms resolve dramatically.

It is necessary to repeat a urinalysis and culture 48 hours after treatment is begun. If infection is still present, resistance to the antibiotic, noncompliance, or anatomic defect must all be considered.

The drugs of choice for the simple, uncomplicated UTI include ampicillin or amoxicillin, trimethoprim/sulfamethoxazole (TMP-SMZ), or a sulfonamide. Oral cephalosporins are more expensive. Amoxicillin/potassium clavulanate is also expensive and offers an advantage only in the rare case of an infection due to a beta-lactamase-producing organism. Commonly used antibiotics and their dosages are listed in Table 60-10.

A urinary analgesic such as phenazopyridine (Pyridium) 10 mg/kg/24 hr PO TID for 2 days may be helpful for acute dysuria in children older than 6 years. This may turn the patient's urine orange. Increasing oral fluid intake to dilute the urine is also recommended.

Exceptions to these treatment guidelines include neonates and children who are significantly toxic or vomiting. Both warrant hospital admission and treatment with IV antibiotics. The treatment should include an aminoglycoside (gentamicin 5 to 7.5 mg/kg/24 hr q 8 hr IM or IV) or a cephalosporin, generally third generation, singly or in combination.[248,250] Children with pyelonephritis usually require hospitalization as do individuals who are pregnant or immunocompromised. Hospitalization should also be considered in those with previous renal disease and impaired renal function, foreign bodies (catheter), or stones.

Treatment should be initiated with parenteral antibiotics in these high-risk patients and changed to oral antibiotics pending sensitivity of the organism and the clinical course. Antibiotics should be continued for 14 days with good follow-up. To help prevent recurrent infections, particularly in girls, patients should be instructed to wipe correctly from front to back, not to use bubble bath, to minimize constipation, and to wear cotton underwear. Children should also be encouraged to have a high fluid intake and to void frequently.

Once the first infection is treated, the patient with a UTI requires close follow-up. Because of the risk of recurrence, periodic screens for UTI should be performed at increasing intervals (1 month, 3 months, 6 months, 12 months, and yearly).[248] Most children with a simple UTI can be managed successfully without urologic consultation. Occasionally a child experiences frequent episodes of symptomatic cystitis despite a normal urinary tract. This is an indication for prophylactic antibiotic therapy, which should be continued until the patient is infection-free for 6 to 12 months.[247] For significant abnormalities, the child should be referred to a pediatric urologist. Some clinicians suggest a radiologic evaluation of infant siblings because of the increased risk of abnormalities.

UROLITHIASIS

DAVID G. WARD

Stones in the urinary tract are now an uncommon event in children, occurring at a rate of 0.94 cases per 1,000 hospital admissions compared to 3.3 cases per 1,000 admissions in adults.[259-262]

Pathophysiology

Urinary stones are composed of crystals formed from ionic elements and organic protein compounds in the urine. The initial formation is called nucleation. Complex physiochemical factors are involved in the formation of stones, including crystal supersaturation, growth inhibitors, growth promoters, matrix composition, heterogenous nucleation, infection, urine flow obstruction, urine pH, site of stone formation, retention, and growth. The presence of congenital anomalies may lead to UTI in various ways, which may predispose to infection stones. Injury to the urinary tract lumen may provide a nidus upon which stone formation may occur.[263]

Etiology and Epidemiology

Calcium-containing stones (57.6%) are the most common composition followed, in decreasing frequency, by struvite, uric acid, and cystine stones (see box above).[264]

Calcium-containing stones in children have a male predominance of 1.3:1 and a mean age at diagnosis of 9 years. Approximately one third to one half of patients have a metabolic cause and up to one third have a congenital anomaly of the urinary tract. Infection stones are the second most common cause of stones in children, occurring in approximately 25% of cases. In infection calculi, the mean

---

Composition of Calculi

Calcium lithiasis

Hypercalciuria
    Normocalcemic hypercalciuria
        Idiopathic
        Distal renal tubular acidosis
        Drug-induced
    Hypercalcemic hypercalciuria
        Associated with calcium resorption from bone
            Primary hyperparathyroidism
            Immobilization
            Adrenocorticosteroid excess or insufficiency
            Osteolytic metastases
        Associated with gastrointestinal hyperabsorption
            Hypervitaminosis D
            Sarcoidosis
            Milk alkali syndrome
Hyperoxaluria
    Hereditary
    Enteric hyperoxaluria
Hyperuricosuria
Hypocitraturia
    Distal renal tubular acidosis
    Idiopathic calcium urolithiasis (adults)

Uric acid lithiasis

Struvite (infection) stones

Cystinuria

Other inborn errors of metabolism associated with lithiasis
Hereditary xanthinuria
Orotic aciduria

Modified from Polinsky MS, Kaiser BA, Balvarte LJ: Urolithiasis in childhood, *Pediatr Clin North Am* 34:683, 1987.

---

age of diagnosis is 5 years and the male predominance is 2.2:1. Pediatric stone disease is 3 to 4 times more common in white than nonwhite children.[265]

Metabolic Stones. Idiopathic hypercalciuria (normocalcemic hypercalciuria) is the most prevalent form of urolithiasis, accounting for up to 81% of all unexplained calculi. It may have an autosomal dominant inheritance.[266-270] Factors predisposing to uric acid stones include acidic pH of the urine, hyperuricosuria, and decreased urine flow. Cystinuria is an acute somal recessive disorder with defective transport of the amino acids cystine, lysine, arginine, and arnithine.[264,265,271]

Infection Stones. Urine pH > 7.20 causes precipitation of crystals of magnesium ammonium phosphate or carbonate apatite. Urease from urea-splitting bacteria is responsible for the pH changes and is primarily produced by *Proteus*, although *Klebsiella, Serratia, Pseudomonas,* and *Staphylococcus* species and Enterobacteria and Mycoplasmas are capable of producing urease.[265] *E. coli* does not produce urease. The production and growth of the crystal is rapid and the organism becomes an integral part of the stone. Factors such as neurogenic bladder or instrumentation that increase the risk of infection of the urinary tract predispose to formation of struvite, the composition of infection stones.[265]

Diagnostic findings

Clinical Findings. The most common presenting symptoms are pain, fever, and associated findings of hematuria and UTI.[272] Symptoms in younger children are nonspecific. In children under 5 years the primary complaint is malaise. Older children and adolescents may describe more localized flank pain, but in general most children only complain of abdominal pain.

Abdominal pain is usually "colic" in nature, waxing and waning, or radiating to the groin. Other signs of UTI should be sought, including fever, nausea, vomiting, lethargy, depressed appetite, irritability, frequency, urgency, malodorous urine, hematuria, or passage of gravel or stones in the urine. A history of previous episodes of UTIs, unusual infecting organisms such as *Proteus* species, or a family history of urolithiasis should be noted. Dietary history, fluid intake history, and vitamin use (including over-the-counter and health food products) must be specifically explored.

A thorough physical examination should be performed.

Complications. Obstruction of the collecting system can lead to renal injury or loss from urine stasis with risk of urease producing bacteria and struvite formation complicating the disease further or risk of increased collecting system pressure resulting in papillary necrosis. Untreated infections can lead to deteriorating renal function. Struvite calculi can recur as a result of incomplete removal of stone or failure to adequately clear the UTI.

Ancillary Data. Laboratory testing for patients suspected of urolithiasis may be selectively done but may include serum samples for a CBC, electrolytes, BUN, creatinine, alkaline phosphatase, uric acid, total protein, and albumin. Urine should be examined for routine urinalysis and culture. Urine should be collected using a urine strain and crystal products collected for chemical analysis. An abdominal x-ray film may be useful, with about 90% of calculi being visible.[273] An IVP may be considered to identify the exact location of the stone, presence of obstruction and urine stasis, renal function, and to assist in planning surgical treatment options. A nonopaque-filling defect identified on IVP may represent a calculus, blood clot, tumor, fungus ball, neoplasm, or other entity that may require ultrasound or CT scan to delineate.

Follow-up testing should include serum C-terminal parathyroid hormone, first-morning-fasting urine sample for urine calcium:creatinine ratio, an x-ray film of the hands, and a voiding cystourethrogram. A 24-hour collection of urine should be analyzed for calcium, phosphorus, magnesium, oxalate, uric acid, citrate, cystine, protein, and creatinine. The collection should be obtained while the patient is eating a normal, unrestricted, and unaltered diet.[274]

Differential Considerations

Considerations for patients with the most common constellation of presenting symptoms of urolithiasis include UTIs, appendicitis, pancreatitis, hydronephrosis, tumor, and inflammatory bowel disease. Hematuria as the presenting finding has a wide differential discussed in another section of this chapter. Abdominal pain has a wide group of entities reviewed in Chapter 52.

Cholelithiasis, vascular calcifications, lymph node calcifications, phleboliths, and malignancy with calcification may all present with radiographic calcifications.[273]

Management

Assuming a patient is stable, attention should next be directed to the patient's pain, infection and volume status.

Pain may be severe and generally requires narcotics. If suspected, treatment of infection must be initiated after cultures have been obtained. Antibiotic therapy will not eliminate struvite calculi but should be administered until definitive therapy is completed. UTI can coexist with urolithiasis and not involve struvite stones. In such cases antibiotic therapy is indicated and the infection will clear, provided the cause of the infection is also corrected. (Antibiotic choice and dose is discussed in the section on Urinary Tract Infections in this chapter.) If struvite stones are suspected, coverage must include *Proteus* species until another organism is identified.

In patients that present with fever, anorexia, vomiting, or malaise sufficient to cause volume depletion, attention to the fluid and electrolyte status is important and, in some patients, may reveal renal insufficiency or failure. The goal of fluid therapy should be to maintain fluid and electrolyte homeostasis and sufficient urine flow through the urinary collection system to prevent urinary stasis from contributing to stone formation. Administration of excessive fluid in an attempt to increase urine flow in the affected kidney, "forcing" the stone to dislodge and clear the obstruction, should be discouraged.

The treatment of infection stones is removal. Anatrophic nephrolithotomy, a combination of percutaneous lithotripsy and shock wave lithotripsy25 and extracorporeal shock wave lithotripsy[275], have been reported. Failure of therapy is generally due to the inability to remove all stone elements, thereby allowing a source of stone nidus and bacteria to remain in the collecting system.

Specific medical management of the metabolic abnormalities is usually done in consultation with nephrologists and endocrinologists.[274]

Disposition

Older pediatric patients (those that have the ability and capability to communicate with adults) may be considered for outpatient management in consultation with a pediatric urologist and nephrologist if their pain, fluid, and infection status are easily controlled. All pediatric patients with urolithiasis should be referred for consultation (or follow-up evaluation if seen in the emergency department with a recurrent episode) with a urologist and a nephrologist.

References

1. Fetterman GH, et al: The growth and maturation of human glomeruli and proximal convulations from term to adulthood: studies by microdissection, *Pediatrics* 35:601, 1965.

2. McCrory WW: Renal structure and development. In Holliday MA, Barratt TM, Vernier RL, editors: *Pediatr nephrol*, Baltimore, 1987, Williams & Wilkins.

3. Schwartz GJ, Feld LG, Langford DJ: A simple estimate of glomerular filtration rate in full term infants during the first year of life, *J Pediatr* 104:849, 1984.

4. Schwartz GJ, et al: Plasma creatine and urea concentration in children: normal values for age and sex, *J Pediatr* 88:828, 1976.

5. Chantler C and Barratt TM: Laboratory evaluation. In Holliday MA, Barratt TM, Vernier RL, editors: *Pediatr nephrol*, Baltimore, 1987, Williams & Wilkins.

6. Hogg RJ and Stapleton FB: Renal tubular function. In Holliday MA, Barratt TM, Vernier RL editors: *Pediatr nephrol*, Baltimore, 1987, Williams & Wilkins.

Dysuria and Pyuria

7. Hoberman A, et al: Pyuria and bacteriuria in urine specimens obtained by catheter from young children with fever, *J Pediatr* 124:513, 1994.

8. Goldenring J: Tracking down the cause of dysuria in adolescent girls, *Contemp Pediatr* 3:50, 1986.

9. Brunham RC, et al: Mucopurulent cervicitis—the ignored counterpart in woman of urethritis in men, *N Engl J Med* 311:1, 1984.

10. Baker RB: Dysuria: presenting compliant in labial fusion, *Am J Dis Child* 140:1100, 1986.

11. Rosenfeld WD and Clark J: Vulvovaginitis and cervicitis, *Pediatr Clin North Am* 36:489, 1989.

12. Alon U, et al: Hypercalciuria in the frequency-dysuria syndrome of childhood, *J Pediatr* 116:103, 1990.

13. Pyrles CV and Eliot CR: Pyuria and bacteriuria in infants and children, *Am J Dis Child* 110:628, 1965.

14. Paradise JE, et al: Vulvovaginitis in premenarcheal girls: clinical features and diagnostic evaluation, *Pediatrics* 70:193, 1982.

Hematuria

15. Arm JP, et al: Significance of dipstick haematuria. 1. Correlation with microscopy of the urine, *Br J Urol* 58:211, 1986.

16. Fitzwater DS and Wyatt RJ: Hematuria, *Pediatr Rev* 15:102, 1994.

17. Vehaskari VM: Asymptomatic hematuria—a cause for concern?, *Pediatr Nephrol* 3:240, 1989.

18. Abarbanel J, et al: Sports hematuria, *J Urol* 143:887, 1990.

19. Kallen RJ: What's causing the hematuria, *Contemp Pediatr* 3:55, 1986.

20. Abrol RP, et al: Self-induced hematuria, *J Natl Med Assoc* 82:127, 1990.

21. Stapleton FB: Idiopathic hypercalciuria: association with isolated hematuria and risk for urolithiasis in children, *Kidney Int* 37:807, 1990.

22. Venkat RG, et al: A blind controlled trial of phase contrast microscopy by two observers for evaluating the source of haematuria, *Nephron* 441:304, 1986.

23. Sargent JD, et al: Normal values for random urinary calcium to creatinine ratios in infancy, *J Pediatr* 123:393, 1993.

24. Disch FE, et al: Abnormally thin glomerular basement membranes associated with hematuria, proteinuria or renal failure in adults, *Am J Nephrol* 5:103, 1985.

25. Yoshikawa N, et al: Benign familial hematuria, *Arch Pathol Lab Med* 112:794, 1988.

26. White RHR: The investigation of hematuria, *Arch Dis Child* 64:159, 1989.

27. Ingelfinger JR, et al: Frequency and etiology of gross hematuria in a general pediatric setting, *Pediatrics* 59:557, 1977.

28. Barkin M, et al: Unexplained Hematuria, *Can J Surg* 26:501, 1983.

29. Yadin O: Hematuria in children, *Pediatr Ann* 23:474, 1994.

30. Froom P, et al: Sensitivity of the high-power field method in detecting red blood cells in the urinary sediment, *Isr J Med Sci* 23:1118, 1987.

31. Kitamoto Y, et al: Differentiation of hematuria using a uniquely shaped red cell, *Nephron* 64:32, 1993.

32. de Caestecker MP, et al: Localization of haematuria by red cell analysers and phase contrast microscopy, *Nephron* 52:170, 1989.

33. Lettgen B, Hestermann C, Rascher W: Differentiation of glomerular and nonglomerular hematuria in children by measurement of mean corpuscular volume of urinary red cells using a semi-automated cell counter, *Acta Paediatr* 83:946, 1994.

Hypertension

34. Ingelfinger JR: Pediatric hypertension, *Curr Opin Pediatr* 6:198, 1994.

35. Calhoun DA and Oparil S: Treatment of hypertensive crisis, *N Engl J Med* 323:1177, 1990.

36. Morgenstern BZ: Hypertension in pediatric patients: Current Issues, *Mayo Clin Proc* 69:1089, 1994.

37. Rosner B et al: Blood pressure nomograms for children and adolescents, by heights, sex, and age, in the United States, *J Pediatr* 123:871, 1993.

38. Task Force on Blood Pressure Control in Children: Report of the second task force on blood pressure control in children—1987, *Pediatrics* 79:1, 1987.

39. Moss AJ: Blood pressure in infants, children and adolescents, *West J Med* 134:296, 1981.

40. Kimball TR, et al: Persistent hyperdynamic cardiovascular state at rest and during exercise in children after successful repair of coarctation of the aorta, *J Am Coll Cardiol* 24:194, 1994.

41. Lieberman E: Hypertension in childhood and adolescence. In Kaplan NM, editor: *Clinical hypertension*, ed 5, Baltimore, 1990, Williams & Wilkins.

42. Feld LG and Springate JE: Hypertension in children, *Curr Probl Pediatr* 18:321, 1988.

43. Zinner SH, et al: A longitudinal study of blood pressure in childhood, *Am J Epidemiol* 100:437, 1974.

44. Loggie JMH: Hypertension in children and adolescents, *Hosp Pract* 81, 1975.

45. Abbott D et al: Guidelines for measurement of blood pressure, follow-up, and lifestyle counseling, *Can J Public Health* 85:S29, 1994.

46. Mehta SK: Pediatric hypertension: a challenge for pediatricians, *Am J Dis Child* 141:893, 1987.

47. Park MK and Menard SM: Accuracy of blood pressure measurement by the dinamap monitor in infants and children, *Pediatrics* 79:907, 1987.

48. Weaver MG, Park MK, Lee DH: Differences in blood pressure levels obtained by auscultatory and oscillometric methods, *Am J Dis Child* 144:911, 1990.

49. Jung FF and Ingelfinger JR: Hypertension in childhood and adolescence, *Pediatr Rev* 14:169, 1993.

50. Sinaiko AR: Treatment of hypertension in children, *Pediatr Nephrol* 8:603, 1994.

51. Uchiyama M and Sakai K: Rectal administration of perforated nifedipine capsules in severe hypertension in children, *Br J Clin Pract* 46:100, 1992.

52. Lopez-Herce J, et al: Treatment of hypertensive crisis in children with nifedipine, *Intensive Care Med* 14:519, 1988.

53. Neutel JM, et al: A comparison of intravenous nicardipine and sodium nitroprusside in the immediate treatment of severe hypertension, *Am J Hypertens* 7:623, 1994.

54. Treluyer JM, et al: Intravenous nicardipine in hypertensive children, *Eur J Pediatr* 152:712, 1993.

55. Farine M and Arbus GS: Management of hypertensive emergencies in children, *Pediatr Emerg Care* 5:51, 1989.

56. Bunchman TE, Lynch RE, Wood EG: Intravenously administered labetalol for treatment of hypertension in children, *J Pediatr* 120:140, 1992.

57. Hohn AR: *Guidebook for pediatric hypertension*, Mount Kisco, New York, 1994, Futura Publishing.

58. Mirkin BL, et al: Efficacy and safety of captopril in the treatment of severe childhood hypertension: report of the International Collaborative Study Group, *Pediatrics* 75:1091, 1985.

59. Lieberman E: Pediatric hypertension: Clinical perspective, *Mayo Clin Proc* 69:1098, 1994.

60. Watson AR, Balfe JW, Hardy BE: Renovascular hypertension in childhood: a changing perspective in management, *J Pediatr* 106:366, 1985.

Proteinuria

61. Peggs JF, Reinhardt RW, O'Brien JM: Proteinuria in adolescent sports physical examinations, *J Fam Pract* 22:80, 1986.

62. Maxson WT: Benign proteinuria of childhood and adolescents: a survey, *Clin Pediatr* 2:662, 1963.

63. Feld LG, et al: Evaluation of the child with asymptomatic proteinuria, *Pediatr Rev* 5:248, 1984.

64. Peterson A, Ervin E, Berggard I: Differentiation of glomerular, tubular, and normal proteinuria: determination of urinary excretion of B_2-microglobulin, albumin, and total protein, *J Clin Invest* 48:1189, 1969.

65. Bell FG, Wilkin TJ, Atwell JD: Microproteinuria in children with vesicoureteric reflux, *Br J Urol* 58:605, 1986.

66. Gibb DM, et al: Renal tubular proteinuria and microalbuminuria in diabetic patients, *Arch Dis Child* 64:129, 1989.

67. Glassock RJ: Postural (orthostatic) proteinuria: no cause for concern, *N Engl J Med* 305:639, 1981.

68. Thompson AC, Durrett RR, Robinson RR: Fixed and reproducible orthostatic proteinuria VI: result of a ten-year follow-up, *Ann Intern Med* 73:325, 1970.

69. Dodge WF, et al: Proteinuria and hematuria in children: causes and appropriate diagnostic studies, *J Pediatr* 88:327, 1976.

70. Tojo A, et al: Factitious proteinuria in a young girl, *Clin Nephrol* 33:299, 1990.

71. Chavers BM and Vernier RL: Proteinuria and enzymuria, *Semin Nephrol* 6:371, 1986.

72. Wechsler D, Ibsen L, Fosarelli P: Apparent proteinuria as a consequence of sodium bicarbonate ingestion, *Pediatrics* 86:318, 1990.

73. Striegel J, Michael AF, Chavers BM: Asymptomatic proteinuria benign disorder or harbinger of disease, *Postgrad Med* 83:287, 1988.

74. Wagner MG, et al: Epidemiology of proteinuria: a study of 4807 schoolchildren, *J Pediatr* 73:825, 1968.

75. Elises JS, et al: Simplified quantification of urinary protein excretion in children, *Clin Nephrol* 30:225, 1988.

76. Kelsch RC and Sedman AB: Nephrotic syndrome, *Pediatr Rev*, 14:30, 1993.

77. Abitbol C, et al: Quantitation of proteinuria with urinary protein/creatinine ratios and random testing with dipsticks in nephrotic children, *J Pediatr* 116:243, 1990.

78. Koopman MG, et al: Circadian rhythm of proteinuria: consequences of the use of urinary protein: creatinine ratios, nephrology, dialysis, *Transplantation* 4:9, 1989.

79. Trachtman H and Gauthier B: Effect of angiotensin-converting enzyme inhibitor therapy on proteinuria in children with renal disease, *J Pediatr* 112:295, 1988.

80. Harrison NA, et al: Proteinuria—what value is the dipstick? *Br J Urol* 63:202, 1989.

Scrotal Pain and Swelling

81. Noseworthy J: Testicular torsion. In Ashcraft KW, Holder TM, editor: *Pediatric surgery*, ed 2, Philadelphia, 1993, WB Saunders.

82. Glenister TW: Urogenital system. In Hamilton WJ, editor: *Textbook of human anatomy*, St Louis, 1976, Mosby.

83. Kogan SJ: Acute and chronic scrotal swelling. In Gillwater JY, Grayback JT, Howard S, et al, editors: *Adult and pediatric urology*, ed 2, St Louis, 1991, Mosby.

84. Tunnessen W: Scrotal swelling. In Tunnessen W, editor: *Signs and symptoms in pediatrics*, ed 2, Philadelphia, 1988, JB Lippincott.

85. Knight PJ and Vassy LE: The diagnosis and treatment of the acute scrotum in children and adolescents, *Ann Surg* 200:664, 1984.

86. Govan DE, Kessler R: Urologic problems in the adolescent male, *Pediatr Clin North Am* 27(1):122, 1980.

87. Caldamone AA, Alvo Jr, et al: Acute scrotal swelling in children, *J Pediatr Surg* 19(5):581, 1984.

88. Gilchrist BF, Lobe TE: The acute groin in pediatrics, *Clin Pediatr*, Aug:488, 1992.

89. Schul MW, Keating MA: The acute pediatric scrotum, *J Emerg Med* 11:565, 1993.

90. Soper R: Testicular torsion. In Grosfield JL, editor: *Common problems in pediatric surgery*, St Louis, 1991, Mosby.

91. Zivkovic S and Janjic G: Traumatic rupture of the testis and epididymis, *J Pediatr Surg* 15(3):287, 1980.

92. Snyder CL, Holder TM: Miscellaneous tumors. In Ashcraft KW and Holder TM, editors: *Pediatric surgery*, ed 2, Philadelphia, 1993, WB Saunders.

Circumcision Complications

93. Wiswell TE: Neonatal circumcision: a current appraisal, *Focus & Opinion:Pediatr*, 1:93, 1995.

94. Kaplan GW: Circumcision: an overview, *Curr Probl Pediatr* 7:1, 1977.

95. Anderson GF: Circumcision. In Ashcraft KW and Holder TM, editors: *Pediatric surgery*, ed 2, Philadelphia, 1993, WB Saunders.

96. Niku SD, Stock JA, Kaplan GW: Neonatal circumcision, *Urol Clin North Am* 22:57, Feb. 1995.

97. Schroeder P: Female genital mutilation, *N Engl J Med* 331:739, 1994.

98. Stefan H: Reconstruction of penis after necrosis due to circumcision burn, *Eur J Pediatr Surg* 4:40, 1994.

99. Gee WF and Ansell JS: Neonatal circumcision: a ten year overview: with comparison of the Gomco clamp and plastibell device, *Pediatrics* 58:824, 1976.

100. Sussman SJ, Schiller RP, Shashilumar VL: Fournier's syndrome: report of three cases and review of the literature, *Am J Dis Child* 132:1189, 1978.

101. Uwyyed K and Korman SH: Scrotal abscess with bacteremia caused by salmonella group D after ritual circumcision, *Pediatr Infect Dis J* 9:65, 1990.

102. Woodside JR: Necrotizing fasciitis after neonatal circumcision, *Am J Dis Child* 134:301, 1980.

103. Annobil SH, al-Hilfi A, Kazi T: Primary tuberculosis of the penis in an infant, *Tubercle* 71:229, 1990.

104. Cleary TG and Kohl S: Overwhelming infection with group B beta-hemolytic streptococcus associated with circumcision, *Pediatrics* 64:301, 1979.

105. Kirkpatrick BV and Eitzman DV: Neonatal septicemia after circumcision, *Clin Pediatr* 13:767, 1974.

106. Wiswell TE and Geschke DW: Risks from circumcision during the first month of life compared with those for uncircumcised boys, *Pediatrics* 83:1011, 1989.

107. Persad R, Sharma S, McTavish J, et al: Clinical presentation and pathophysiology of meatal stenosis following circumcision, *Br J Urol* 75:91, 1995.

108. Trier WC and Drach GW: Concealed penis: another complication of circumcision, *Am J Dis Child* 125:276, 1973.

109. Craig JC, Grigor WG, Knight JF: Acute obstructive uropathy—a rare complication of circumcision, *Eur J Pediatr* 153:369, 1994.

110. Fraud M, Berant N, Brand N, et al: Complication of ritual circumcision in Israel, *Pediatrics* 54:521, 1974.

111. Johnsonbaugh RE, Meyer BP, Catalano JD: Complication of circumcision performed with a plastic bell clamp, *Amer J Dis Child* 118:781, 1969.

112. Johnsonbaugh RE: Complication of a circumcision performed with a plastic disposable circumcision device:long term follow-up, *Amer J Dis Child* 133:438, 1979.

Epididymitis

113. Turek PJ, et al: Normal epididymal anatomy in boys, *J Urol* 151:726, 1994.

114. Report of the Committee on Infectious Diseases, *American Academy of Pediatrics*, American Academy of Pediatrics, 1991.

Glomerulonephritis, Acute Poststreptococcal

115. Mezzano S, et al: Incidence of circulating immune complexes in patients with acute post-streptococcal glomerulonephritis and in patients with streptococcal impetigo, *Clin Nephrol* 26:65, 1988.

116. Jordan S and Lemire J: Acute glomerulonephritis—diagnosis and treatment, *Pediatr Clin North Am* 29:857, 1982.

Hemolytic-Uremic Syndrome

117. Levin M, Walters M, Barratt T: Hemolytic uremic syndrome, *Adv Pediatr Infect Dis* 4:51, 1989.

118. Kaplan B and Proesmans W: The hemolytic uremic syndrome of childhood and its variants, *Semin Hematol* 24:148, 1987.

119. Tarr P and Hickman R: Hemolytic uremic syndrome epidemiology: a population-based study in King County, Washington, 1971 to 1980, *Pediatrics* 80:41, 1987.

120. Neuman M and Urizar R: Hemolytic uremic syndrome: current pathophysiology and management, *Anna J* 21:137, 1994.

121. Miller K and Kim Y: Hemolytic uremic syndrome. In Barratt T and Vernier R, editors: *Pediatric nephrology*, ed 2, Baltimore, 1987, Williams & Wilkins.

122. Gottschall JL, et al: Quinine induced immune thrombocytopenia with hemolytic uremic syndrome: clinical and serological findings of nine patients and review of literature, *Am J Hematol* 47:283, 1994.

123. Menzel D, et al: Impaired fibrinolysis in the hemolytic uremic syndrome of childhood, *Ann Hematol* 68:43, 1994.

124. Chant ID, et al: Plasminogen activator inhibitor activity in diarrhea associated hemolytic uremic syndrome, *QJM* 87:736, 1994.

125. Argyle H, et al: A clinicopathological study of 24 children with hemolytic uremic syndrome: a report of the Southwest Pediatric Nephrology Study Group, *Pediatr Nephrol* 4:52, 1990.

126. Salmon R and Baum M: Hemolytic uremic syndrome. In Levin D and Morriss F, editors: *Essentials of pediatric intensive care*, St Louis, 1990, Quality Medical Publishing.

127. Cleary T: Cytotoxin—producing *Escherichia coli* and the hemolytic uremic syndrome, *Pediatr Clin North Am* 35:485, 1988.

128. Brandt JR, et al: *E. coli* 0157:H7-associated hemolytic uremic syndrome after ingestion of contaminated hamburgers, *J Pediatr* 125:1519, 1994.

129. Cleary T and Lopez E: The shiga-like toxin producing *Escherichia coli* and hemolytic uremic syndrome, *Pediatr Infect Dis J* 8:720, 1989.

130. Serebruany VL, et al: Hypoproteinemia in the hemolytic uremic syndrome of childhood, *Pediatr Nephrol* 7:72, 1993.

131. Chart H, et al: Serological identification of *Escherichia coli* 0157:H7 infection in haemolytic uraemic syndrome, *Lancet* 337:138, 1991.

132. Ashkenazi S, et al: Anticytotoxin—neutralizing antibodies in immune globulin preparations: potential use in hemolytic-uremic syndrome, *J Pediatr* 113:1008, 1988.

133. Siegler R: Management of hemolytic-uremic syndrome, *J Pediatr* 112:1014, 1988.

Henoch-Schönlein Purpura

134. Hurley RM and Drummon KN: Anaphylactoid purpura nephritis: clinicopathological correlations, *J Pediatr* 81:904, 1972.

135. Yoshikawa NI, et al: Henoch-Schönlein nephritis and IgA nephropathy in children: a comparison of clinical course, *Clin Nephrol* 27:233, 1987.

136. Okano M, et al: Anaphylactoid purpura with intestinal perforation, *Pathol Int* 44:303, 1994.

137. Rostoker G, et al: High dose immunoglobulin therapy for severe IGA nephropathy and Henoch-Schönlein purpura, *Ann Intern Med* 120:476, 1994.

138. Heldrich F, et al: Intravenous immunoglobulins in Henoch-Schönlein purpura: a case study, *Maryland MD Med J* 42:577, 1993.

139. Robson W and Leung A: Henoch-Schönlein purpura, *Adv Pediatr* 41:163, 1994.

Nephrotic Syndrome

140. Gulak S, et al: Steroid response pattern in Indian children with nephrotic syndrome, *Acta Paediatr* 83:530, 1994.

141. Warshaw BL: Nephrotic syndrome in children, *Pediatr Ann*, 23:495, 1994.

142. Vernier RL: Primary (idiopathic) nephrotic syndrome. In Barratt TM and Vernier RL, editors: *Pediatrics*, ed 2, Baltimore, 1987, Williams & Wilkins.

143. Schnaper HW and Robson AM: Nephrotic syndrome: minimal change disease, focal glomerulosclerosis, and related disorders. In Schrier RW and Gottschalk CW, editors: *Kidney disease*, ed 4, Boston, 1988, Little, Brown.

144. Michael AF, Blao E, Vernier RL: Glomerular polyanion: alterations in aminonucleoside nephrosis, *Lab Invest* 23:649, 1970.

145. Barnett HL, et al: The nephrotic syndrome. In Edelmann EM, editor: *Pediatric kidney disease*, Boston, 1978, Little, Brown.

146. Zillervelo G, et al: Persistence of serum lipid abnormalities in children with idiopathic nephrotic syndrome, *J Pediatr* 104:61, 1984.

147. International study of kidney disease in children, the nephrotic syndrome in children, prediction of histopathology from clinical and laboratory characteristics at the time of diagnosis, *Kidney Int* 13:43, 1978.

148. Abdullah S, et al: Reversible idiopathic acute renal failure in children with primary nephrotic syndrome, *J Pediatr* 125:723, 1994.

149. McLean RH, et al: Decreased serum factor B concentrations associated with decreased opsonization of *Escherichia coli* in the idiopathic nephrotic syndrome, *Pediatr Res* 11:910, 1977.

150. Cameron JS: Coagulation and thromboembolic complications in the nephrotic syndrome. In Bach JF, et al, editors: *Advances in nephrology*, Chicago, 1984, Year Book Medical Publishers.

151. Shimizy C, et al: Acute leukoencephalopathy during cyclosporin A therapy in a patient with nephrotic syndrome, *Pediatr Nephrol* 8:483, 1994.

152. Winger AM, et al: Comparison of different regimens of prednisone therapy in frequently relapsing nephrotic syndrome, *Acta Paediatr Scand* 79:305, 1990.

153. Kitano Y, et al: Cylosporin treatment in children with steroid dependent nephrotic syndrome, *Pediatr Nephrol* 4:474, 1990.

154. Tejani A, et al: Cyclosporine—induced remission of relapsing nephrotic syndrome in children, *J Pediatr* 111:1056, 1987.

155. Schnaper HW: Immunization practices in childhood nephrotics syndrome: a survey of North American pediatric nephrologists, *Pediatr Nephrol* 8:4, 1994.

Orchitis

156. Kogan SJ: Acute and chronic scrotal swelling. In Gillenwater JY, Grayback JT, Howard S, et al, editors: *Adult and pediatric urology*, ed 2, St Louis, 1991, Mosby.

157. Cherry JD: Nonpolio enteroviruses: coxsackieviruses, echoviruses, and enteroviruses. In Feigin RD and Cherry JD, editors: *Textbook of pediatric infectious diseases*, Philadelphia, 1981, WB Saunders.

158. Report of the Committee on Infectious Diseases, *American Academy of Pediatrics*, American Academy of Pediatrics, 1991.

159. Brunell PA: Mumps. In Feigin RD and Cherry JD, editors: *Textbook of pediatric infectious diseases*, Philadelphia, 1981, WB Saunders.

160. Knight PJ and Vassy LE: The diagnosis and treatment of acute scrotum in children and adolescents, *Ann Surg* 200:664, 1984.

Phimosis and Paraphimosis

161. Anderson GF: Circumcision. In Ashcraft KW and Holder TM, editors: *Pediatric surgery*, ed 2, Philadelphia, 1993, WB Saunders.

162. Niku SD, Stock JA, Kaplan GW: Neonatal circumcision, *Urol Clin North Am* 22:57, 1995.

163. Super DM: Phimosis. In Hoekelmann RA et al, editors: *Primary pediatric care*, ed 2, St Louis, 1992, Mosby.

164. Meuli M, Briner T, Hanimann B, et al: Lichen sclerosus et atrophicus causing phimosis in boys: a prospective study with 5 year followup after complete circumcision, *J Urol* 152:987, 1994.

165. Robinson FO, Johnston SR, Atkinson AB: Accelerated hypertension caused by severe phimosis, *J Hum Hypertens* 6:165, 1992.

166. Wright JE: The treatment of childhood phimosis with topical steroid, *Aust N Z J Surg* 64:327, 1994.

167. Zhou XH: Balloon dilation treatment of phimosis in boys, *Chi Med J (Engl)* 104:491, 1991.

168. Yaster M and Maxwell LG: The management of Acute Pain in Children. In Hoekelmann RA et al, editors: *Primary pediatric care*, ed 2, St Louis, 1992, Mosby.

169. Gonzales ET Jr: Urogenital abnormalities: Pharphimosis. In Rudolph AM et al, editors: *Rudolph's pediatrics*, ed 19, Norwalk, Conn, 1991, Appleton & Lange.

170. Barone JG and Fleisher MH: Treatment of paraphimosis using the "puncture" technique, *Pediatr Emerg Care* 9:298, 1993.

171. Zbaraschuk I, Berger RE, Hedges JR: Emergency urologic procedures. In Roberts JR and Hedges JR, editors: *Clinical procedures in emergency medicine*, ed 2, Philadelphia, 1991, WB Saunders.

Priapism

172. O'Brien WM, O'Conner KP, Lynch JH: Priapism: current concepts, *Ann Emerg Med* 18:980, 1989.

173. Ramos CE, Park JS, Ritchey ML, et al: High flow priapism associated with sickle cell disease, *J Urol* 153:1619, 1995.

174. Tarry WF, Duckett JW, Synder H: Urological complications of sickle cell disease in the pediatric population, *J Urol* 125:592, 1987.

175. Winter CC and McDowell G: Experience with 105 patients with priapism: Update review of all aspects, *J Urol* 140:980, 1988.

176. Sharpsteen JR Jr, Powars D, Johnson C, et al: Multisystem damage associated with tricorporal priapism in sickle cell disease, *Am J Med* 94:289, 1993.

177. Noe HN, Williams J, Jerkins JR: Surgical management of priapism in children with sickle cell anemia, *J Urol* 126:770, 1981.

178. Macaluso JN and Sullivan JW: Priapism: review of 34 cases, *Urology* 26:233, 1985.

179. Seeler RA: Intensive transfusion therapy for priapism in boys with sickle cell anemia, *J Urol* 110:360, 1973.

180. Pohl J, Pott B, Kleinhans G: Priapism: a three-phase concept of management according to etiology and prognosis, *Br J Urol* 58:113, 1986.
181. Strothers L and Ritchie B: Priapism in the newborn, *Can J Surg* 35:325, 1992.
182. Baruchel S, Rees J, Bernstein ML, et al: Relief of sickle cell priapism by hydralazine. Report of a case, *Am J Pediatr Hematol Oncol* 15:115, 1993.

Prostatitis

183. Mann S: Prostatic abscess in the newborn, *Arch Dis Child* 35:396, 1960.
184. Mears EM and Stamey TE: The diagnosis and management of bacterial prostatitis, *Br J Urol* 44:175, 1972.
185. Daum RS: Prostatitis. In Feigin RD and Cherry JD: *Textbook of pediatric infectious disease,* ed 3, 3 vol, Philadelphia, 1992, WB Saunders.
186. Smith DR: Nonspecific infections of the urinary tract. In Smith DR, editor: *General urology,* ed 8, Los Altos, California, 1975, Lange Medical Publications.
187. Middleton RG and Dahl DS: Urogenital tract. In Wolcott MW, editor: *Ambulatory surgery and the basics of emergency surgical care,* Philadelphia, 1988, JP Lippincott.
188. Peter G, editor: *1994 Red Book: Report of the Committee on Infectious Diseases,* ed 23, Elk Grove Village, Il, 1994, American Academy of Pediatrics.
189. Pai MG and Bhat HS: Prostatic abscess. *J Urol* 108:599, 1972.
190. Chodak GW: Prostatitis, epididymitis, and balanoposthitis. In Kass ES and Platt R, editors: *Current therapy in infectious diseases,* ed 3, Burlington, Ontario, 1990, BC Decker.
191. Govan DE and Kessler R: Urologic problems in the adolescent male, *Pediatr Clin North Am* 27:109, 1980.
192. Sanford JP, editor: *The Sanford guide to antimicrobial therapy,* Dallas, 1994, Antimicrobial Therapy.
193. Stamey TA: Prostatitis, *J Royal Society of Med* 74:22, 1981.
194. Naber KG: Use of quinolones in urinary tract infections and prostatitis, *Rev of Infect Dis,* 2 suppl:S1321, 1989.

Renal Failure, Acute

195. Ellis D, et al: Acute renal failure in infants and children diagnosis, complications, and treatment, *Crit Care Med* 9:607, 1981.
196. Badr K and Ichikawa I: Prerenal failure: a deleterious shift from renal compensation to decompensation, *N Engl J Med* 319:623, 1988.
197. Reid B and Bender T: Radiographic evaluation of children with urinary tract infections, *Radiol Clin North Am* 26:463, 1988.
198. Kallen R, et al: Fluid resuscitation of acute hypovolemic hypoperfusion status in pediatrics, *Pediatr Clin North Am* 37:287, 1990.
199. Sehic A and Chesney RW: Acute renal failure: therapy, *Pediatr Rev,* 16:137, 1995.
200. Abramowicz M, editor: Drugs for hypertensive emergencies, *Med Lett* 31:789, 1989.
201. Parra G, et al: Short-term treatment with captopril in hypertension due to acute glomerulonephritis, *Clin Nephrol* 29:58, 1988.
202. Prisant LM, et al: Treating hypertensive emergencies. Controlled reduction of blood pressure and protection of target organs, *Postgrad Med* 93:92, 1993.
203. Wells T: The pharmacology and therapeutics of diuretics in the pediatric patient, *Pediatr Clin North Am* 37:463, 1990.
204. Feld L, Chachero S, Springte J: Fluid needs in acute renal failure, *Pediatr Clin North Am* 37:337, 1990.
205. Berry P and Belsha C: Hyponatremia, *Pediatr Clin North Am* 37:351, 1990.
206. Warshaw B, et al: Long-term outcome of patients with obstructive uropathy, *Pediatr Clin North Am* 29:815, 1982.
207. Winberg J, et al: Clinical pyelonephritis and focal renal scarring, a selected review of pathogenesis, prevention and prognosis, *Pediatr Clin North Am* 29:801, 1982.

Renal Failure, Chronic

208. Fine R, Salusky I, Ettenger R: The therapeutic approach to the infant, child and adolescent with end-stage renal disease, *Pediatr Clin North Am* 34:789, 1987.
209. Chantler C and Holliday M: Progressive loss of renal function. In Holliday M, editor: *Pediatric nephrology,* ed 2, Baltimore, 1987, Williams & Wilkins.

210. Foreman J and Chan J: Chronic renal failure in infants and children, *J Pediatr* 113:793, 1988.
211. Kallen R: Paleonephrology and reflux nephropathy, *Am J Dis Child* 145:860, 1991.
212. Weiss R: Management of chronic renal failure, *Pediatr Ann* 17:584, 1988.
213. Fine R: Recombinant human growth hormone treatment of children with chronic renal failure: update 1990, *Acta Paediatr Scand Suppl* 370:44, 1990.
214. Johansson G, et al: Recombinant human growth hormone treatment in short children with chronic renal disease before transplantation or with functioning renal transplants: an interim report on five European studies, *Acta Pediatric Scand Suppl* 370:36, 1990.
215. Koch V, et al: Accelerated growth after recombinant human growth hormone treatment of children with chronic renal failure, *J Pediatr* 115:365, 1989.
216. Ridgens S, Rees L, Chantler C: Growth and endocrine function in children with chronic renal failure, *Acta Paediatr Scand Suppl* 380:20, 1990.
217. Fine R: Recent advances in the management of the infant child and adolescent with chronic renal failure, *Pediatr Rev* 11:277, 1990.
218. Scharer K: Growth and development of children with chronic renal failure: study group on pubertal development in chronic renal failure, *Acta Paediatr Scand Suppl* 366:90, 1990.
219. Hellerstein S, et al: Nutritional management of children with chronic renal failure; summary of the task force on nutritional management of children with chronic renal failure, *Pediatr Nephrol* 1:195, 1987.
220. Chandra M, Clemons G, McVicar M: Relation of serum erythropoietin levels to renal excretory function: evidence for lowers set point for erythropoietin production in chronic renal failure, *J Pediatr* 113:1015, 1988.
221. Montini G, et al: Benefits and risks of anemia correction with recombinant human erythropoietin in children maintained by hemodialysis, *J Pediatr* 117:556, 1990.
222. Nolph K, Lindblad M, Novak J: Continuous ambulatory peritoneal dialysis, *N Engl J Med* 318:1595, 1988.
223. Ettenger R and Fine R: Renal transplantation. In Holliday M, editor: *Pediatric nephrology,* ed 2, Baltimore, 1987, Williams & Wilkins.
224. Sheldon C, Najarian J, Mauer S: Pediatric renal transplantation, *Surg Clin North Am* 65:1589, 1985.
225. Trompeter R: Renal transplantation, *Arch Dis Child* 65:143, 1990.
226. Tejani A, et al: Steady improvement in renal allograft survival among North American Children: A five year appraisal by the North American Pediatric Renal Transplant Cooperative Study, *Kidney Int* 48:551, 1995.

Testicular Torsion

227. Kass EJ, Stone KT, et al: Do all children with an acute scrotum require exploration?, *J Urol* 150:667, 1993.
228. Hastie KJ and Charlton CA: Indications for conservative management of acute scrotal pain in children, *Br J Surg* 77:309, 1990.
229. Costabile RA, et al: Variability of ischemia during spermatic cord torsion in the rat, *J Urol* 151:1070, 1994.
230. Sawchuk T, et al: Spermatic cord torsion in an infant receiving human chorionic gonadotropin, *J Urol* 150:1212, 1993.
231. Cos LR and Rabinowitz R: Trauma-induced testicular torsion in children, *J Trauma* 22(3):244, 1982.
232. Tryfonas G, et al: Late postoperative results in males treated for testicular torsion during childhood, *J Pediatr Surg* 29(4):553, 1994.
233. Barkley C, et al: Testicular torsion and its effects on contralateral testicle, *Urology* 41(2):192, 1993.
234. Cilento BG, et al: Cryptorchidism and testicular torsion, *Ped Clin North Am, Pediatr Surg,* 40(6):1133, 1993.
235. Middleton WD, et al: Acute scrotal disorders: prospective comparison of color Doppler US and testicular scintigraphy, *Radiology* 177:177, 1990.
236. Patriquin HB, Yazbeck S, Trinh B, et al: Testicular torsion in infants and children: diagnosis with Doppler ultrasonography, *J Radiol* 188:781, 1993.
237. Meza MP, Amundson GM, Aquilina JW, et al: Color flow imaging in children with clinically suspected testicular torsion, *Pediatr Radiol* 22:370, 1992.

238. Lerner RM, Mevorach RA, Hulbert WC, et al: Color Dop US in the evaluation of acute scrotal disease, *Radiology* 176:355, 1990.

239. Steinhardt GF, Boyarsky S, Mackey R: Testicular torsion: pitfalls of color Doppler sonography, *J Urol* 150:461, 1993.

240. Palmer LS: Testicular torsion, *Abstract Pediatr Rev,* 15(11):455, 1994.

241. Atkinson GO, Patrick EL, et al: The normal and abnormal scrotum in children: evaluation with color Doppler sonography, *AJR* 158:613, 1992.

242. Akgur FM, Kiling K, Aktug T, et al: The effect of allopurinol pretreatment before detorting testicular torsion, *J Urol* 151:1715, 1994.

243. Betts JM, Norris M, et al: Testicular detorsion using Doppler ultrasound monitoring, *J Pediatr Surg* 18(5):607, 1983.

Urinary Tract Infection

244. Hellerstein S, et al: *Urinary tract infections in children,* Chicago, 1982, Year Book Medical Publishers.

245. Elerian LF and Adelman RD: Urinary tract infections in children. In Burg FD, Ingelfinger JR, Wald ER, editors: *Gellis and Kagan's current pediatric therapy,* Philadelphia, 1993, WB Saunders.

246. Harmon W and Mandell J: Urinary tract infections in pediatric medicine. In Avery ME and First LR, editors: *Pediatric medicine,* Baltimore, 1994, Williams & Wilkins.

247. Edelmann CM: Urinary tract infection and vesicoureteral reflux, *Pediatr Ann* 17:568, 1988.

248. Todd JK: Management of urinary tract infections: children are different. *Pediatr Rev* 16:90, 1995.

249. Hoberman A, Chao HP, Keller DM, et al: Prevalance of urinary tract infection in febrile infants, *J Pediatr* 123:17, 1993.

250. Wiswell TE and Roscelli JD: Corroborative evidence for the decreased incidence of urinary tract infections in circumcised male infants, *Pediatrics* 78:96, 1986.

251. Wiinberg J: Clinical aspects of urinary tract infection. In Holliday MA, Barratt TM, Vernier RL, editors: *Pediatric nephrology,* ed 2, Baltimore, 1987, Williams & Wilkins.

252. Hoberman A, Wald ER, et al: Pyuria and bacteriuria in urine specimens obtained by catheter from young children with fever, *J Pediatr* 124:513, 1994.

253. Heldrich FJ: Pinning down the diagnosis of UTI, *Contemp Pediatr* 5:51, 1988.

254. Kher KK and Lachter HE: Urinary tract infection. In Kher KK and Makker SP, editors: *Clinical pediatric nephrology,* New York, 1992, McGraw-Hill.

255. Majad M and Rushton HG: Renal cortical scintigraphy in the diagnosis of acute pyelonephritis, *Semin Nucl Med* 22:98, 1992.

256. McCracken GH, Ginsberg CM, Namasonthi V, et al: Evaluation of short term antibiotic therapy in children with uncomplicated urinary tract infection, *Pediatrics* 67:796, 1981.

257. Madrigal G, Odio CM, Mohs E, et al: Single dose antibiotic therapy is not as effective as conventional regimens for management of acute urinary tract infections in children, *Pediatr Infect Dis J* 7:316, 1988.

258. Moffat M, Embree J, Grimm P, et al: Short course antibiotic therapy for urinary tract infections in children: A methodological review of the literature, *Am J Dis Child* 142:57, 1988.

Urolithiasis

259. Sinno K, Boyce WH, Resnick MI: Childhood urolithiasis, *J Urol* 121:662, 1979.

260. Noe NH, et al: Clinical experience with pediatric urolithiasis, *J Urol* 129:1166, 1983.

261. Walther PC, Lamm D, Kaplan GW: Pediatric urolithiasis: A ten-year review, *Pediatrics* 65:1068, 1980.

262. Polinsky MS, et al: Renal stones and hypercalciuria, *Adv Pediatr* 40:353, 1993.

263. Fleisch H: Inhibitors and promoters of stone formation, *Kidney Int* 13:361, 1978.

264. Polinsky MS, Kaiser BA, Baluarte HJ: Urolithiasis in childhood, *Pediatr Clin North Am* 34:683, 1987.

265. Seftel A and Resnick MI: Metabolic evaluation of urolithiasis, *Urol Clin North Am* 17:159, 1990.

266. Hymes LC and Warshaw BL: Idiopathic hypercalciuria: Renal and absorptive subtypes in children, *Am J Dis Child* 138:176, 1984.

267. Santos F, et al: Idiopathic hypercalciuria in children: pathophysiologic considerations of renal and absorptive subtypes, *J Pediatr* 110:238, 1987.

268. Danpure CJ and Purdue PE: Primary hyperoxaluria. In Scriver CR, Beaudet AL, Valle D, editors: *The metabolic basis of inherited disease,* 7th edition, 3 vols, New York, 1995, McGraw-Hill.

269. Dobbins JW: Nephrolithiasis and intestinal disease, *J Clin Gastroenterol* 7:21, 1985.

270. Miller LA and Stapleton FB: Urinary citrate excretion in children with hypercalciuria, *J Pediatr* 107:263, 1985.

271. Evans WP, Resnick MI, Boyce WH: Homozygous cystinuria—evaluation of 35 patients, *J Urol* 127:707, 1982.

272. Barratt TM: Urolithiasis and nephrocalcinosis. In Holliday MA, Barratt TM, Vernier RL, editors: *Pediatric nephrology,* ed 2, Baltimore, 1987, Williams & Wilkins.

273. Arsdalem KNV, Banner MP, Pollack HM: Radiologic imaging and urologic decision making in the management of renal and ureteral calculi, *Urol Clin North Am* 17:171, 1990.

274. Drach GW: Metabolic evaluation of pediatric patients with stones, *Urol Clin North Am* 22:95, 1995.

275. Cheah WK, King PA, Tan HL: A review of pediatric cases of urinary tract calculi, *J Pediatr Surg* 29:701, 1994.

APPENDIX A: Reference Standards

Appendix A-1: Growth Curves (Boys)

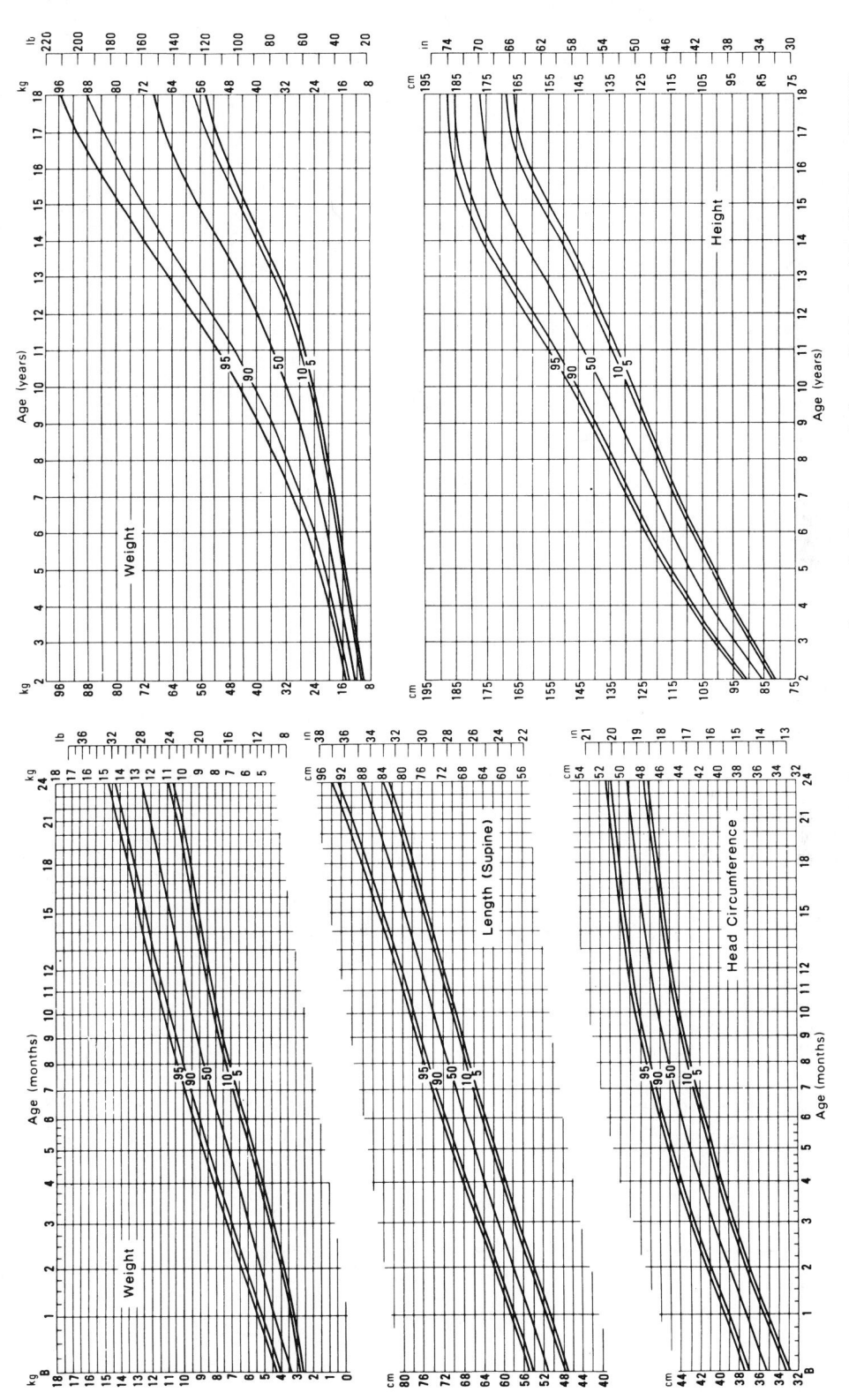

Percentile standards for growth: boys (2-18 yr). (Modified from NCHS growth charts, 1976.)

Percentile standards for growth: boys (birth-24 mon). (Modified from National Center for Health Statistics [NCHS] growth charts, 1976.)

Appendix A-1: Growth Curves (Girls)

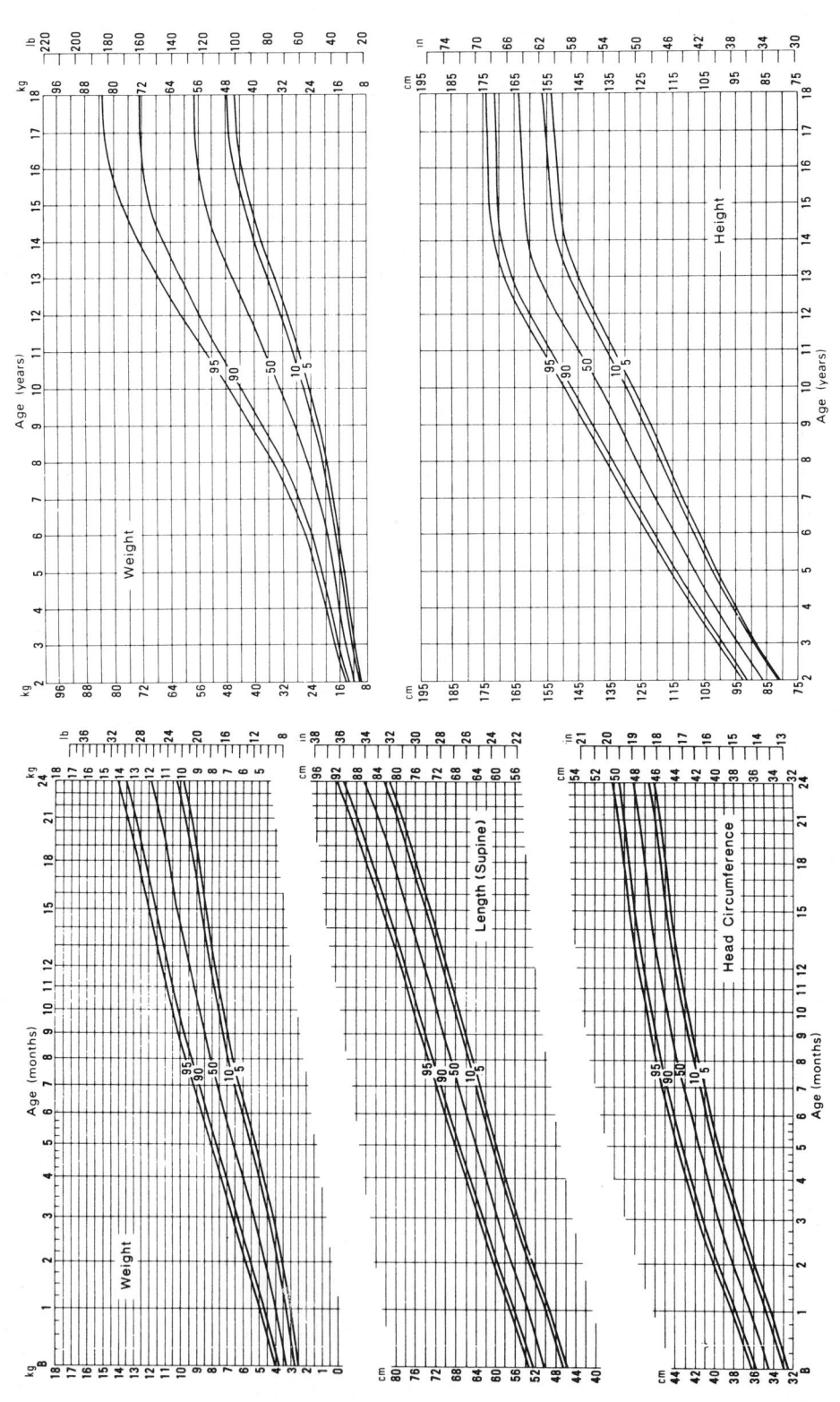

Percentile standards for growth: **girls (2-18 yr)**. (*Modified from NCHS growth charts, 1976.*)

Percentile standards for growth: **girls (birth-24 mon)**. (*Modified from NCHS growth charts, 1976.*)

Appendix A-2: Vital Signs and Ancillary Ventilatory Support

Age	Weight (kg)	Heart rate (average/min)	Respiratory rate (mean ± SD)	Blood pressure (mean ± 2 SD) Systolic	Diastolic*	ET tube ID† (mm)	Length (cm)	Suction catheter (Fr)	Chest tube (Fr)	Laryngoscopy blade
Premature	1	145	>40	42 ± 10	21 ± 8	2.5	10	6	10	0 st
Newborn	1-2	135		50 ± 10	28 ± 8	3.0	11	6-8	10-12	1 st
Newborn	2-3	125		60 ± 10	37 ± 8	3.5	12			
1 mo	4	120	38 ± 10	80 ± 16	46 ± 16	3.5	13	8		
6 mo	7	130		89 ± 29	60 ± 10	3.5-4.0	14			
1 yr	10	125	39 ± 11	96 ± 30	66 ± 15	4.0-4.5	15	8-10	16-20	1 st
2-3 yr	12-14	115	28 ± 4	99 ± 25	64 ± 25	4.5	16	10	20-24	
4-5 yr	16-18	100	27 ± 6	99 ± 20	65 ± 20	5.0-5.5	17		20-28	2
6-8 yr	20-26	100	24 ± 6	See Figs. 60-1 to 60-6		5.5-6.0	18			
10-12 yr	32-42	75	21 ± 4			5.5-7.0	20	12	28-32	2-3
>14 yr	>50	70	20 ± 4			7.5-8.5	24		32-42	3

Modified from Nadas A: *Pediatric cardiology,* ed 3, Philadelphia, 1976, WB Saunders Co.; Vesmond HT, et al: *Pediatrics* 67:607, 1981; Hooker EA et al: *J Emerg Med* 10:407, 1992.
*Point of muffling (Nadas).
†Variability of 0.5 mm is common. Estimate: $\dfrac{16 + age\ (yr)}{4}$

Appendix A-3: Surface Area Nomograms

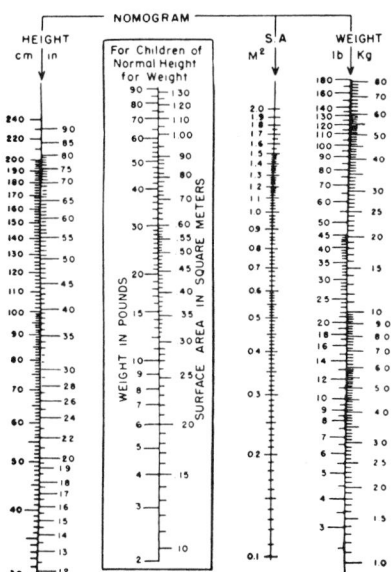

Nomogram for estimation of surface area. The surface area is indicated where a straight line that connects the height and weight levels intersects the surface area column; or the patient is roughly of average size, from the weight alone (enclosed area). (*Modified from data of E Boyd by CD West.*)

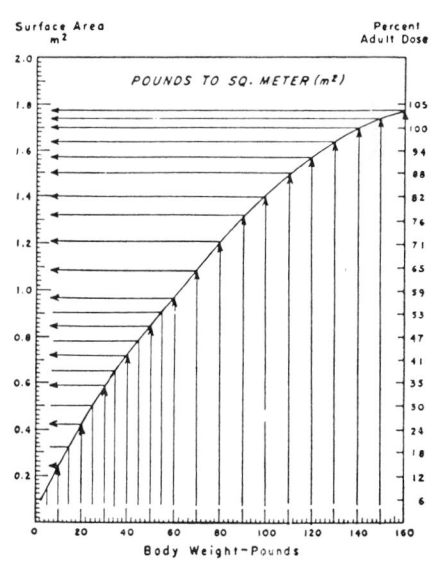

Relations between body weight in pounds, body surface area, and adult dosage. The surface area values correspond to those set forth by Crawford et al (1950). Note that the 100% adult dose is for a patient weighing about 140 pounds and having a surface area of about 1.7 square meters. (*From Talbot NB, et al:* Metabolic hemostasis—a syllabus for those concerned with the care of patients, *Cambridge, 1959, Harvard University Press.*)

(*From Vaughn VC, Behrman RE:* Nelson textbook of pediatrics, *ed 12, Philadelphia, 1991, WB Saunders Co.*)

Appendix A-4: Electrocardiographic Criteria

Age	Heart rate (/min)	QRS axis (degrees)	PR interval (sec)	QRS duration* (sec)
0-1 mo	100-180 (120)†	+75 to +180 (+120)	.08-.12 (.10)	.04-.08 (.06)
2-3 mo	110-180 (120)	+35 to +135 (+100)	.08-.12 (.10)	.04-.08 (.06)
4-12 mo	100-180 (150)	+30 to +135 (+60)	.09-.13 (.12)	.04-.08 (.06)
1-3 yr	100-180 (130)	0 to +110 (+60)	.10-.14 (.12)	.04-.08 (.06)
4-5 yr	60-150 (100)	0 to +110 (+60)	.11-.15 (.13)	.05-.09 (.07)
6-8 yr	60-130 (100)	−15 to +110 (+60)	.12-.16 (.14)	.05-.09 (.07)
9-11 yr	50-110 (80)	−15 to +110 (+60)	.12-.17 (.14)	.05-.09 (.07)
12-16 yr	50-100 (75)	−15 to +110 (+60)	.12-.17 (.15)	.05-.09 (.07)
>16 yr	50-90 (70)	−15 to +110 (+60)	.12-.20 (.15)	.05-.10 (.08)

	QT interval			T-wave orientation		
Rate/min	R-R interval (sec)	QT interval (sec)	Age	V1, V2	AVF	I, V5, V6
40	1.5	.38-.50 (.45)†	0-5 days	Variable	Upright	Upright
50	1.2	.36-.48 (.43)	6 days-2 yr	Inverted	Upright	Upright
60	1.0	.34-.46 (.41)	3 yr-adolescent	Inverted	Upright	Upright
70	0.86	.32-.43 (.37)	Adult	Upright	Upright	Upright
80	0.75	.29-.40 (.35)				
90	0.67	.27-.37 (.33)				
100	0.60	.26-.35 (.30)				
120	0.50	.24-.32 (.28)				
150	0.40	.21-.28 (.25)				
180	0.33	.19-.27 (.23)				
200	0.30	.18-.25 (.22)				

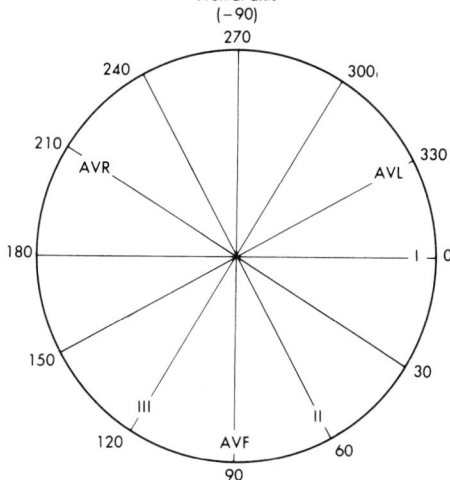

Adapted from Garson A, Jr, Gillette PC, and McNamara DG: *A guide to cardiac dysrhythmias in children,* New York, 1980, Grune & Stratton, Inc.; Guntheroth WGS: *Pediatric electrocardiography,* Philadelphia, 1965, WB Saunders Co.
*If QRS duration is normal, add R + R′ and compare total (R + R′) with standards; R/S undefined because S can be equal to 0.
†Minimum-maximum (mean).

Lead V1			Lead V6			
R-wave amplitude (mm)	S-wave amplitude (mm)	R/S ratio	R-wave amplitude (min)	S-wave amplitude (mm)	R/S ratio	Age
4-25 (15)	0-20 (10)	0.5 to ∞ (1.5)	1-21 (6)	0-12 (4)	0.1 to ∞ (2)	0-1 mo
2-20 (11)	1-18 (7)	0.3 to 10.0 (1.5)	3-20 (10)	0-6 (2)	1.5 to ∞ (4)	2-3 mo
3-20 (10)	1-16 (8)	0.3 to 4.0 (1.2)	4-20 (13)	0-4 (2)	2.0 to ∞ (6)	4-12 mo
1-18 (9)	1-27 (13)	0.5 to 1.5 (0.8)	3-24 (12)	0-4 (2)	3.0 to ∞ (20)	1-3 yr
1-18 (7)	1-30 (14)	0.1 to 1.5 (0.7)	4-24 (13)	0-4 (1)	2.0 to ∞ (20)	4-5 yr
1-18 (7)	1-30 (14)	0.1 to 1.5 (0.7)	4-24 (13)	0-4 (1)	2.0 to ∞ (20)	6-8 yr
1-16 (6)	1-26 (16)	0.1 to 1.0 (0.5)	4-24 (14)	0-4 (1)	4.0 to ∞ (20)	9-11 yr
1-16 (5)	1-23 (14)	0 to 1.0 (0.3)	4-22 (14)	0-5 (1)	2.0 to ∞ (9)	12-16 yr
1-14 (3)	1-23 (10)	0 to 1.0 (0.3)	4-21 (10)	0-6 (1)	2.0 to ∞ (9)	>16 yr

Chamber enlargement ("hypertrophy")

Right ventricular
1. RV1 >20 mm (>25 mm under 1 mon)
2. SV6 >6 mm (>12 mm under 1 mon)
3. Abnormal R/S ratio (V1 >2 after 6 mon)
4. Upright TV3R, RV1 after 5 days
5. QR pattern in V3R, V1

Left ventricular
1. RV6 >25 mm (>21 mm under 1 yr)
2. SV1 >30 mm (>20 mm under 1 yr)
3. RV6 + SV1 >60 mm (Use V5 if RV5 >RV6)
4. Abnormal R/S ratio
5. SV1 >2 × RV5

Combined
1. RVH and SV1 or RV6 exceed mean for age
2. LVH and RV1 or SV6 exceed mean for age

Right atrial
1. Peak P valve >3 mm (<6 mo), >2.5 mm (≥6 mo)

Left atrial
1. PII >0.09 sec
2. PV1 late negative deflection >0.04 sec and >1 mm

Maximal PR interval (sec)

Rate/min	<1 mo	1 mo-1 yr	1-3 yr	3-8 yr	8-12 yr	Adult
<60					0.18	0.21
60-80				0.17	0.17	0.21
80-100	0.12			0.16	0.16	0.20
100-120	0.12		0.16	0.16	0.15	0.19
120-140	0.11	0.14	0.14	0.15	0.15	0.18
140-160	0.11	0.13	0.14	0.14		0.17
>160	0.11	0.11				

Appendix A-5: Normal Laboratory Values*

Acid-base Measurements (B)

pH: 7.38-7.42
P_{O_2}: 65-76 mm Hg
P_{CO_2}: 36-38 mm Hg
Base excess: -2 to $+2$ mEq/L

Acid Phosphatase (S, P)

Newborns: 7.4-19.4 IU/L
2-13 yr: 6.4-15.2 IU/L
Adult males: 0.5-11 IU/L
Adult females: 0.2-9.5 IU/L

Alanine Aminotransferase (SGPT) (S)

Newborns (1-3 days): 1-25 IU/L
Adult males: 7-46 IU/L
Adult females: 4-35 IU/L

Alkaline Phosphatase (S)

Age	IU/L
Newborns (1-3 days)	95-368
2-24 mo	115-460
2-7 yr	115-460
8-9 yr	115-345
10-11 yr	115-437
12-13 yr	92-403
14-15 yr	78-446
16-18 yr	35-331
Adults	39-137

Ammonia (P)

Newborns: 9-150 µg/dl (53-88 µmol/L); higher in premature and jaundiced infants
Thereafter: 0-60 µg/dl (0-35 µmol/L) when blood is drawn correctly.

Amylase (S)

Neonates: undetectable
2-12 mo: levels increase to adult levels
Adults: 28-108 IU/L

Aspartate Aminotransferase (SGOT) (S)

Newborns (1-3 days): 16-74 IU/L
Adult males: 8-46 IU/L
Adult females: 7-34 IU/L

Bicarbonate (P)

18-25 mEq/L

Bilirubin (S)

After 1 mon are:
Conjugated: 0-0.3 mg/dl
Unconjugated: 0.1-0.7 mg/dl

Bleeding Time

4-9 min

Calcium (S)

Premature infants: 3.5-4.5 mEq/L
Full-term infants: 4-5 mEq/L
Infants and thereafter: 4.4-5.3 mEq/L

Carboxyhemoglobin (B)

5% of total hemoglobin

Cation-Anion Gap (S, P)

5-15 mEq/L

Chloride (S, P)

96-116 mEq/L

Cholesterol (S, P)

Full-term newborns: 45-167 mg/dl
3 days-1 yr: 69-174 mg/dl
2-14 yr: 120-205 mg/dl
14-19 yr: 120-210 mg/dl
20-29 yr: 120-240 mg/dl
30-39 yr: 140-270 mg/dl
40-49 yr: 150-310 mg/dl
50-59 yr: 160-330 mg/dl

Cholinesterase (S)

2.5-5 µmol/min/ml of serum (pseudocholinesterase)
2.3-4 µmol/min/ml of red cells

Complement (S)

C3: 96-195 mg/dl
C4: 15-20 mg/dl

Creatinine (S, P)

Values in mg/dl

Age	Males	Females
Newborns (1-3 days)	0.3-0.7	0.3-0.7
1-3 yr	0.2-0.7	0.2-0.6
4-10 yr	0.2-0.9	0.2-0.8
11-17 yr	0.3-1.2	0.3-1.1
>18 yr	0.5-1.3	0.3-1.1

Creatinine Clearance

Newborns (1 day): 5-50 ml/min/1.73 m² (mean, 18 ml/min/1.73 m²)
Newborns (6 days): 15-90 ml/min/1.73 m² (mean, 36 ml/min/1.73 m²)
Adult males: 85-125 ml/min/1.73 m²
Adult females: 75-115 ml/min/1.73 m²

Glucose (S, P)

Premature infants: 20-80 mg/dl
Full-term infants: 30-100 mg/dl
Children and adults (fasting): 60-105 mg/dl

γ-Glutamyl Transpeptidase (S)

0-1 mo: 12-27 IU/L
1-2 mo: 9-159 IU/L
2-4 mo: 7-98 IU/L
4-7 mo: 5-45 IU/L
7-15 mo: 3-30 IU/L
Adult males: 9-69 IU/L
Adult females: 3-33 IU/L

Glycohemoglobin (Hemoglobin A_{1C}) (B)

Normal: 6.3%-8.2% of total hemoglobin
Well-controlled diabetic patients ordinarily
    have levels <10%

Hematocrit (B) (see pp. 898 and 1182)

At birth: 44%-64%
14-90 days: 35%-50%
6 mon-1 yr: 35%-36%
4-10 yr: 38%-40%

Hemoglobin Electrophoresis (B)

A_1 hemoglobin: 96%-98.5% of total hemoglobin
A_2 hemoglobin: 1.5%-4% of total hemoglobin

Fetal hemoglobin

At birth: 50%-85% of total hemoglobin
At 1 yr: <15% of total hemoglobin
1-2 yr: up to 5% of total hemoglobin
>2 yr: <2% of total hemoglobin

Immunoglobins (S)

Age	IgG (mg/dl)	IgA (mg/dl)	IgM (mg/dl)
2 wk-3 mo	299-852	3-66	15-149
3-6 mo	142-988	4-90	18-118
6-12 mo	418-1142	14-95	43-223
1-6 yr	356-1381	13-209	37-239
6-12 yr	625-1598	29-384	50-278
>12 yr	660-1548	81-252	45-256

Iron (S, P)

Newborns: 20-157 μg/dl
6 wks-3 yr: 20-115 μg/dl
3-9 yr: 20-141 μg/dl
9-14 yr: 21-151 μg/dl
14-16 yr: 20-181 μg/dl
Adults: 44-196 μg/dl

Iron-Binding Capacity (S, P)

Newborns: 59-175 μg/dl
Children and adults: 275-458 μg/dl

Lactate Dehydrogenase (LDH) (S, P)

Newborns (1-3 days): 40-348 IU/L
1 mo-5 yr: 150-360 IU/L
5-12 yr: 130-300 IU/L
12-16 yr: 130-280 IU/L
Adult males: 70-178 IU/L
Adult females: 42-166 IU/L

Lactate Dehydrogenase Isoenzymes (S)

LDH_1 (heart): 24%-34%
LDH_2 (heart, red cells): 35%-45%
LDH_3 (muscle): 15%-25%
LDH_4 (liver [trace], muscle): 4%-10%
LDH_5 (liver, muscle): 1%-9%

Magnesium (S, P)

Newborns: 1.5-2.3 mEq/L
Adults: 1.4-2 mEq/L

Partial Thromboplastin Time (PTT) (P)

Children: 42-54 seconds (varies with control)

Phosphorus, Inorganic (S, P)

Full-term infants:
    At birth: 5-7.8 mg/dl
    3 days: 5.8-9 mg/dl
    6-12 days: 4.9-8.9 mg/dl
1-10 yr: 3.6-6.2 mg/dl
Adults: 3.1-5.1 mg/dl

Potassium (S, P)

Premature infants: 4.5-7.2 mEq/L
Full-term infants: 3.7-5.2 mEq/L
Children and adults: 3.5-5.8 mEq/L

Prothrombin Time (P)

Children: 11-15 seconds (varies with control)

Sedimentation Rate (Micro) (B)

<2 yr: 1-5 mm/hr
>2 yr: 1-8 mm/hr

Sodium (S, P)

Children and adults: 135-148 mEq/L

Urea Nitrogen, Blood (BUN) (S, P)

<2 yr: 5-15 mg/dl
>2 yr: 10-20 mg/dl

Protein (S)

Age	Total protein	Albumin	α_1 globulin (g/dl)	α_2 globulin	β globulin	γ globulin
Birth	4.6-7.0	3.2-4.8	0.1-0.3	0.2-0.3	0.3-0.6	0.6-1.2
3 mo	4.5-6.5	3.2-4.8	0.1-0.3	0.3-0.7	0.3-0.7	0.2-0.7
>1 yr	5.4-8.0	3.7-5.7	0.1-0.3	0.4-1.1	0.4-1.0	0.2-1.3

*Values may vary with laboratory, technique, determination, underlying conditions, etc.
B, whole blood; S, serum; P, plasma.

Normal Peripheral Blood Values at Various Ages

	1st Day	2nd Day	6th Day	2 Weeks	1 Mo	2 Mo	3 Mo
Red blood cells (millions/μ/L)	5.9 (4.1-7.5)	6 (4.0-7.3)	5.4 (3.9-6.8)	5 (4.5-5.5)	4.7 (4.2-5.2)	4.1 (3.6-4.6)	4 (3.5-4.5)
Hemoglobin (gm/dl)	19 (14-24)	19 (15-23)	18 (13-23)	16.5 (15-20)	14 (11-17)	12 (11-14)	11 (10-13)
White blood cells (per mm³)	17,000 (8-38)		13,500 (6-17)	12,000 (5-16)	11,500 (5-15)	11,000 (5-15)	10,500 (5-15)
PMNs (%)	57	55	50	34	34	33	33
Eosinophils (total/μL)	20-1000				150-1150		70-550
Lymphocytes (%)	20	20	37	55	56	56	57
Monocytes (%)	10	15	9	8	7	7	7
Immature white cells (%)	10	5	0-1	0	0	0	0
Platelets (per mm³)	350,000		325,000	300,000			260,000
Nucleated red cells/100 white cells	0-10		0-0.3	0	0	0	0
Reticulocytes (%)	3 (2-8)	3 (2-10)	1 (0.5-5)	0.4 (0-2)	0.2 (0-0.5)	0.5 (0.2-2)	2 (0.5-4)
Mean diameter of red cells (μm)	8.6				8.1		5-7
MCV (fL)	85-125		89-101	94-102	90		80
MCHC (%)	36		35	34			
MCH (pg)	35-40		36	31	30		27
Hematocrit (%)	54 ± 10		51	50	40		35

	6 Mo	1 Yr	2 Yr	5 Yr	8-12 Yr	Adults Males	Adults Females
Red blood cells (millions/μ/L)	4.5 (4-5)	4.6 (4.1-5.1)	4.7 (4.2-5.2)	4.7 (4.2-5.2)	5 (4.5-5.4)	5.4 (4.6-6.2)	4.8 (4.2-5.4)
Hemoglobin (gm/dl)	11.5 (10.5-14.5)	12 (11-15)	13 (12-15)	13.5 (12.5-15)	14 (13-15.5)	16 (13-18)	14 (11-16)
White blood cells (per mm³)	10,500 (5-15)	10,000 (5-15)	9,500 (5-14)	8,000 (5-13)	8,000 (5-12)	7,000 (5-10)	
PMNs (%)	36	39	42	55	60	57-68	
Eosinophils (total/μL)	70-550					100-400	
Lymphocytes (%)	55	53	49	36	31	25-33	
Monocytes (%)	6	6	7	7	7	3-7	
Immature white cells (%)	0	0	0	0	0	0	
Platelets (per mm³)			260,000		260,000	260,000	
Nucleated red cells/100 white cells	0	0	0	0	0	0	
Reticulocytes (%)	0.8 (0.2-1.5)	1 (0.4-1.8)	1 (0.4-1.8)	1 (0.4-1.8)	1 (0.4-1.8)	1 (0.5-2)	
Mean diameter of red cells (μm)		7.4		7.4		7.5	
MCV (fL)	78	78	80	80	82	82-92	
MCHC (%)	33		32	34	34	34	
MCH (pg)	26	25	26	27	28	27-31	
Hematocrit (%)	35	36	37	38	40	40-54	37-47

Modified from Merenstein GB, et al: *Handbook of pediatrics*, ed 16, Norwalk, Conn, 1991, Appleton & Lange.
Usual or average values; considerable individual variation may occur.
Total nucleated red cells: first day, <1000/μL.
MCV, Mean corpuscular volume; *MCHC*, mean corpuscular hemoglobin concentration; *MCH*, mean corpuscular hemoglobin.

Appendix A-6: Conversions and Estimates

Temperature

To convert centigrade to Fahrenheit: (⅘ × temperature) + 32
To convert Fahrenheit to centigrade: (temperature − 32) × ⅝

Centigrade (Celsius)	Fahrenheit	Centigrade (Celsius)	Fahrenheit
34.2	93.6	38.6	101.4
34.6	94.3	39.0	102.2
35.0	95.0	39.4	102.9
35.4	95.7	39.8	103.6
35.8	96.4	40.2	104.3
36.2	97.1	40.6	105.1
36.6	97.8	41.0	105.8
37.0	98.6	41.4	106.5
37.4	99.3	41.8	107.2
37.8	100.0	42.2	108.0
38.2	100.7	42.6	108.7

Weight

To change pounds to grams, multiply by 454
To change kilograms to pounds, multiply by 2.2

Growth Patterns

Birth weight (avg): 3.3 kg (7 lb 5 oz)
A newborn loses up to 10% of birth weight but should be up to birth weight again by 10 days
An infant gains 30 g (1 oz)/day for the first 1-2 months
5 mo: birth weight should be doubled
12 mo: birth weight should be tripled
2 yr: birth weight should be quadrupled

Estimates of Weight

4- to 8-year-old: 6 × Age + 12 = Weight (lb)
8- to 12-year-old: 7 × Age + 5 = Weight (lb)

Length

To convert inches to centimeters, multiply by 2.54
To convert centimeters to inches, multiply by 0.394

Growth Patterns

Birth length (avg): 50 cm (20 in)
12 mon: birth length should be doubled

Head Circumference
Growth Patterns

Birth head circumference (avg): 35 cm (14 in)
12 mo head circumference (avg): 47 cm (19 in)
Head circumference grows 1 cm/mo during first 9 mo

Blood Pressure (estimate)

Systolic BP (mm Hg) = 2 × Age (yr) + 80
Diastolic BP (mm Hg) = ⅔ systolic

Other Conversion Factors

To convert	To	Multiply by
1 mm Hg	PSI	0.0193
1 cm H$_2$O	mm Hg	0.735
1 mm Hg	cm H$_2$O	1.259
1 cm	inch	0.3937
1 inch	cm	2.54
1 kg	pound	2.204
1 pound	kg	0.4536
1 Fr size	mm	0.33

Weight Conversion Table (Pounds and Ounces to Grams)

Ounces	0 lb	1 lb	2 lb	3 lb	4 lb	5 lb	6 lb	7 lb	8 lb	9 lb
0		454	907	1361	1814	2268	2722	3175	3629	4082
1	28	482	936	1389	1843	2296	2750	3204	3657	4111
2	57	510	964	1418	1871	2325	2778	3232	3686	4139
3	85	539	992	1446	1899	2353	2807	3260	3714	4168
4	113	567	1020	1474	1928	2382	2835	3289	3742	4196
5	142	595	1049	1503	1956	2410	2863	3317	3771	4224
6	170	624	1077	1531	1984	2438	2892	3345	3799	4253
7	198	652	1106	1559	2013	2467	2920	3374	3827	4281
8	227	680	1134	1588	2041	2495	2948	3402	3855	4309
9	255	709	1162	1616	2070	2523	2977	3430	3884	4338
10	284	737	1191	1644	2098	2552	3005	3459	3912	4366
11	312	765	1219	1673	2126	2580	3034	3487	3940	4394
12	340	794	1247	1701	2155	2608	3062	3516	3969	4423
13	369	822	1276	1729	2183	2637	3090	3544	3997	4451
14	397	850	1304	1758	2211	2665	3119	3572	4026	4479
15	425	879	1332	1786	2240	2693	3147	3601	4054	4508

If patient weighs ≥ 10 lb, the following are used, adding the intermediate value in pounds and ounces to determine the final conversion:

10 lb	4.53 kg	110 lb	49.89 kg
20 lb	9.07 kg	120 lb	54.43 kg
30 lb	13.60 kg	130 lb	58.96 kg
40 lb	18.14 kg	140 lb	63.50 kg
50 lb	22.68 kg	150 lb	68.04 kg
60 lb	27.21 kg	160 lb	72.57 kg
70 lb	31.75 kg	170 lb	77.11 kg
80 lb	36.28 kg	180 lb	81.64 kg
90 lb	40.82 kg	190 lb	86.18 kg
100 lb	45.36 kg	200 lb	90.72 kg

Appendix A-7: Denver Developmental Screening Test

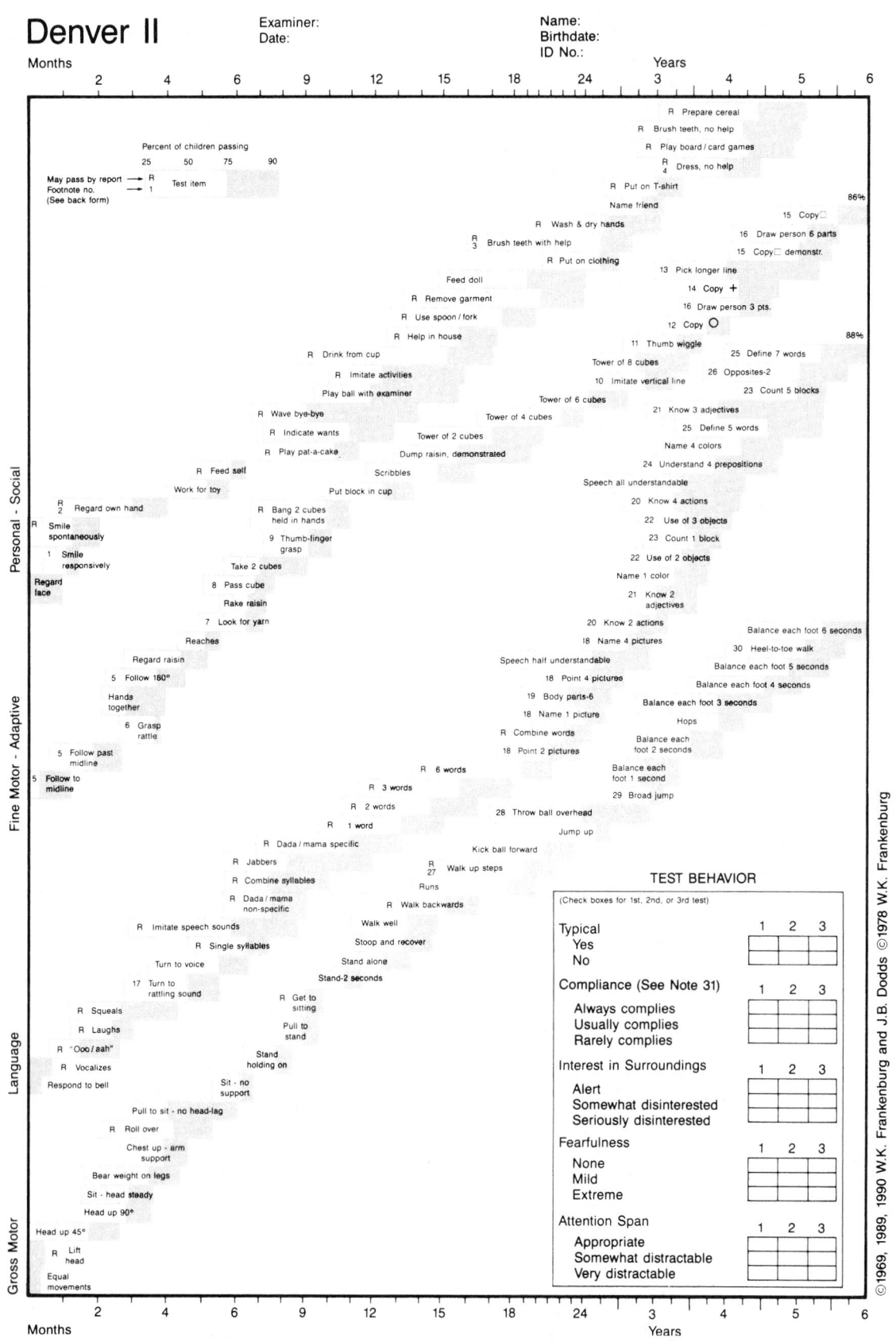

(From Frankenburg WK, Fandal AW, Sciarillo W, et al: J Pediatr 99:995, 1981.)

Appendix A-8: Immunizations and Preventive Care of Normal Infants and Children

1. **DTP** (diphtheria, tetanus toxoid, and pertussis vaccine: 0.5 ml IM). Contraindicated if, with previous administration, seizures, CNS disorder, shock, or thrombocytopenia occurred or if patient experienced excessive somnolence, screaming, or temperature over 40.5° C. Generally not recommended in children with seizure disorders or evolving or progressive neurologic disease. It is important to evaluate concurrent condition. (DT or Td may be given.) Do not give during an acute illness. Available in combination with HIB.

    Do not give to patients >6 years of age. Prophylactic antipyretics (acetaminophen) at time of administration are indicated and decrease the reaction rate. Do not give to children in whom it is important to monitor fevers over the ensuing 24-48 hr. An acellular pertussis vaccine associated with less reactions is available for boosters at 15-18 mo and 4 yr and will soon be approved for administration during the primary series.

    a. **Td** (tetanus and diphtheria toxoid, adult type: 0.5 ml IM). For those >6 yr of age, Td is given. This product contains less diphtheria antigen than pediatric DT and may be given to younger children if pediatric DT is unavailable. If primary immunization is begun after 6 yr of age, a series of only 3 Td immunizations is necessary.

    b. **Booster.** Td is recommended every 10 yr, the first one usually being given at 11-12 yr. For contaminated wounds, an additional booster dose is given if >5 yr has elapsed since the last dose. Human tetanus immune globulin (TIG) is indicated if the injured patient has had fewer than 2 previous immunizations of tetanus toxoid or has a serious wound that has been unattended for >24 hr. Prophylactic dose is 250-500 units/dose IM given concurrently with tetanus toxoid in separate sites and syringes (see Chapter 55).

2. **TOPV** (trivalent oral polio virus vaccine: 2 drops PO). This recommendation is suitable for breast-fed as well as bottle-fed infants. Infants should not be fed for 30 min after administration to prevent spitting up. Vaccination at 6 mo of age is optional.

    Inactivated polio vaccine is indicated for adults at risk of exposure to wild polio virus (travelers to endemic areas, health care workers in contact with patients with wild virus), unvaccinated adults in households with children receiving TOPV, children in households with an immunocompromised adult, and immunocompromised adults or children. Recommendations for routine use are being studied as an alternative or substitute to TOPV in a sequential schedule.

3. **Interruption of schedule.** Regardless of the time interval between doses of DTP and TOPV, continue where the patient left off.

4. **MMR** (measles, mumps, rubella vaccine: unit dose SC). The combined vaccine (MMR) is equivalent to the protection achieved when the antigens are given separately. It is maximally effective when administered at 15 mo of age or older. It may be administered at the same time as DTP, HIB, or TOPV, if necessary.

    Reimmunization for measles is currently recommended at either 4-6 yr or 11-12 yr of age. Infants under 12 mo of age who are exposed to measles may be treated with immune serum globulin within 6 days to reduce the severity of disease.

5. **Rubella vaccine.** Not to be administered to any female after the onset of menses without obtaining appropriate informed consent. The woman should be vaccinated only if she understands that it is imperative to avoid becoming pregnant in the subsequent 2 mo.

6. **H. influenzae (HIB) vaccine.** *H. influenzae* type B conjugate vaccine is indicated for children at 2, 4, 6 (optional), and 15 mo of age. If immunization is not given as an infant, one administration should be given at 15-60 mo. One dose (0.5 ml) is given IM.

7. **Pneumococcal vaccine.** Recommended for children over 2 years of age who are at risk of severe pneumococcal infection. This group includes children with autosplenectomy from SS disease, anatomic or functional asplenia, or nephrotic syndrome. The single dose is 0.5 ml.

8. *Influenzae vaccine* (inactivated). Recommended in high-risk patients, including those with renal, metabolic, cardiac, or pulmonary disease, as well as immunocompromised hosts. The recommendation is reassessed annually but, in general, children 6-35 mo receive 0.25 ml (split virus) twice given 4 weeks apart, those 3-12 yr receive 0.5 ml (split virus) twice, and children >12 year should be given 0.5 ml (whole or split virus) once.

9. *Hepatitis B vaccine.* Vaccine is administered to infants born to HBsAg-*negative* mothers; should receive the first dose within 12 hr of delivery and again at 1-4 mo and 6-18 mo of age on a routine basis. Infants born to HBsAg-*positive* mothers should receive Hep B within 12 hr of birth and 0.5 ml of Hepatitis B immune globulin. The second dose of vaccine is recommended at 1 mo of age and the third dose at 6 mo of age.

    Administered to those with exposure to blood known to be HBsAg positive. Exposure may be percutaneous, ocular, or through mucosal membrane. A single dose of HBIG (0.06 ml/kg or 5.0 ml for adults) is given IM after exposure. Hep B vaccine 1 ml (children under 10 yr: 0.5 ml) should be given IM within 7 days of exposure, with a second and third dose at 1 mo and 6 mo after the first.

10. **Varicella zoster virus vaccine.** Can be administered to susceptible children any time after 12 mo of age. Unvaccinated children who have a reliable history of chickenpox should be vaccinated at the 11-12 yr visit.

11. **General contraindications for vaccine:** (a) anaphylaxis to a vaccine or a vaccine substance, (b) moderate or severe illness, with or without fever. Factors that are not true contraindications include mild-to-moderate local reactions, mild acute illness, prematurity, or current antimicrobial therapy.

	Routine schedule
Birth	Hep B
2 mo	DTP, TOPV, HIB, Hep B
4 mo	DTP, TOPV, HIB
6 mo	DTP, (HIB), Hep B
12 mo	Tuberculin test
15 mo	Measles, mumps, and rubella, HIB
18 mo	DTP, TOPV
4-6 yr	DTP, TOPV
14-16 yr	Td and thereafter every 10 yr*

Modified Report of the Committee on Infectious Diseases, American Academy of Pediatrics, Elk Grove Village, Ill, 1994.
*Hep B (initial series if not given as infant) and MMR booster should be given at early adolescence or before.

12. **Egg allergy.** Very rare anaphylactic reactions in children allergic to eggs have been reported from the administration of vaccines produced in chick or duck fibroblast tissues (measles, mumps, rubella). Patients with impressive histories for egg-white anaphylaxis may be skin tested with vaccine before administration, but the immunization may usually be administered.

13. **Tuberculin test.** A tuberculin test is optimally given before or simultaneously with the administration of measles (or MMR) vaccine if there is a history of TB exposure or a high rate of endemicity. Routine skin testing on a biennial basis is recommended in high-risk populations.

14. **Immune serum globulin.** Indicated in individuals exposed to measles who are <1 yr of age (0.25 ml/kg IM) or immunocompromised (0.5 ml/kg IM); viral hepatitis type A contact within 14 days of exposure (0.02 ml/kg IM); and selected immunodeficiency diseases. *Hepatitis B immune globulin (HBIG)* is used with significant exposure to HBsAg-positive blood within 24 hr and 1 mo later (0.06 ml/kg/dose, or 5 ml for adult, IM). Immune serum globulin intravenously is indicated for replacement in antibody deficiency disorder (300-400 mg/kg every month with dosage being individualized), Kawasaki disease, and low birth weight infants (controversial). Zoster immune globulin (ZIG) is recommended for high-risk patients following exposure (see Appendix 55A).

15. **Intramuscular (IM) administration.** The ideal IM site is the upper outer mass of the gluteus maximus and distal from the central region of the buttock. The needle is directed anteriorly.

16. **Informed consent.** Parents and patients should be informed about the benefits and risks of immunizing procedures. Consent forms facilitate the presentation of this information and should state the benefits and risks, including adverse reactions. Information and forms are available from the American Academy of Pediatrics, Elk Grove, Illinois.

17. **Specific reporting mechanisms** are required by federal regulations, including recording of the date of vaccine administration, manufacturer and lot of vaccine, and the clinician. Adverse reactions following vaccination may be reported to 1-800-822-7267.

References

Plotkin SA and Mortimer EA: *Vaccines*, Philadelphia, 1988, WB Saunders.

Report of the committee on infectious diseases, Elk Grove, Ill, 1994, American Academy of Pediatrics.

APPENDIX B: Parental Instruction Sheets for Common Illnesses*

Appendix B-1: General Information for Parents

Medication

1. Your medication is _____ .
   Give _____ teaspoon/tablet/capsule _____ times per day.
   Give every dose, even if your child begins to feel better.
   a. If a liquid, use a measuring spoon.
   b. Store medication in refrigerator if indicated.
   c. If your child goes to school or a babysitter, arrange for someone to give the medicine if necessary.
2. Call physician if your child refuses to take the medicine or you think your child is having a reaction to the medicine.

Fever

1. For children over 3 months of age, give fever medicine if the temperature is over 101.5° F (38.6° C), if your child is very uncomfortable, or if any fever is present at bedtime. If your child is acting normally, fever medicines may be delayed until the temperature is 102.2° F (39° C). Acetaminophen (Tylenol or equivalent) is recommended every 4-6 hours. Ibuprofen in a dose similar to acetaminophen may also be used.
2. Dress your child lightly. Push fluids.
3. Do **not** use aspirin if your child has chickenpox or an influenza-like (flu) illness.

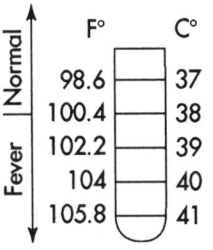

4. Call your physician if
   a. The fever goes above 105° F (40.5° C)
   b. The fever lasts beyond 48-72 hours
   c. Your child is under 3 months of age and has a fever over 100.4° F (38° C).
   d. Your child has a seizure (convulsion); develops abnormal movements of the face, arms, or legs; stiff neck; fullness of the soft spot, purple spots, difficulty breathing, burning on urination, decreased urination, or abdominal pain; marked change in behavior, level of consciousness, or level of activity; looks sicker than expected.

	Dose of fever medicine							
Brand	**0-3 mo**	**4-11 mo**	**12-23 mo**	**2-3 yr**	**4-5 yr**	**6-8 yr**	**9-10 yr**	**11-12 yr**
Acetaminophen drops (80 mg/0.8 ml)	0.4 ml	0.8 ml	1.2 ml	1.6 ml	2.4 ml	—	—	—
Acetaminophen elixir (160 mg/tsp)	—	½ tsp	¾ tsp	1 tsp	1½ tsp	2 tsp	2½ tsp	—
Chewable acetaminophen or aspirin (80 mg)	—	—	1½	2	3	4	5	6
Junior swallowable tablet (160 mg)	—	—	—	1	1½	2	2½	3
Adult tablet acetaminophen or aspirin (325 mg)	—	—	—	—	—	1	1	1½
Ibuprofen suspension (100 mg/5 ml)	½ tsp	¾ tsp	1 tsp	1½ tsp	1¾ tsp	2 tsp	—	—
Ibuprofen capsule (200 mg)	—	—	—	—	—	1	1½	2

*This section consists of material designed for reproduction and distribution. It is also useful for telephone triage and advice. Similar formats may be developed to accommodate specific facility requirements.

Appendix B-2: Respiratory Tract Problems

Ear Infection

1. Fever medicines may make your child feel better. Give other medication as indicated.
2. A return appointment in 2-3 weeks should be made to be certain the infection has cleared up and further treatment is not necessary.
3. Your child can return to school or day care when he or she is feeling better and the fever is down. Swimming is permitted if there is no hole in the eardrum.
4. Call your physician if
   a. There is no improvement in 36 hours
   b. The fever is not gone in 72 hours
   c. Your child is increasingly irritable or listless
   d. Your child develops vomiting or diarrhea

Sore Throat

1. Gargle with warm salt water (1 tsp salt in 8 ounces of water) or suck hard candy.
2. Fever medicines may make your child feel better. Give other medication, as indicated.
3. Call your physician if
   a. Your child develops severe pain or drooling
   b. Swallowing or breathing becomes difficult
   c. Your child develops big swollen lymph nodes (glands) in the neck
   d. The fever lasts over 48 hours.

Strep Throat

1. See *Sore throat.*
2. Your child may return to school or day care 24 hours after beginning antibiotics.
3. Family members who are symptomatic with fever, sore throat, or other symptoms suggestive of a strep throat should have a throat culture.

Cold

1. Children with a dry or stuffy nose will benefit from placing 2-3 drops of water in each nostril. For the younger child use a soft rubber suction bulb to clear discharge. Have older children blow their nose.
2. Fever medicines may make your child feel better.
3. A humidifier (cool mist) may be useful in maximizing comfort.
4. Call your physician if
   a. The fever lasts more than 24-48 hours
   b. Your child has fever at less than 3 months of age or has underlying heart or lung problems
   c. Evidence of infection elsewhere is present, such as red eye, ear pain, or breathing problems, including wheezing or croup
   d. The skin under the nose becomes crusty.

Cough

1. Sucking on cough drops or hard candy may be useful. A good cough medicine can be made at home by mixing equal amounts of honey (corn syrup for child under 1 year of age), lemon concentrate, and liquor, such as scotch or bourbon. Omit the liquor for younger children.
2. Cough syrups rarely are useful. Stronger cough medicines containing dextromethorphan (DM) or codeine must be prescribed by a physician, and they have the danger of reducing the cough reflex that protects the lungs.
3. Call your physician if
   a. Difficulty breathing, shortness of breath, or blue color of skin or around mouth develops

   b. The cough lasts over 2 weeks
   c. The cough changes to croup ("barking seal" cough) or wheezing
   d. Your child develops a fever that lasts over 72 hours
   e. Coughing spasms occur that cause choking, passing out, or bluish lip color
   f. There is blood in the mucus
   g. Chest pain develops

Eye Infection (Conjunctivitis)

1. Before using topical medicine, clean the eye by removing the yellow discharge and dried matter with a wet cotton ball and warm water.
2. Put 2 drops of medicine in each eye every 2 hours (or as often as possible) while your child is awake. Once the infection is improving, the drops may be given 4 times per day.
3. For younger children, you may receive only an ointment that may be used 4 times per day but stays in the eye longer. It is also useful for older children before bedtime.
4. Continue medication until your child has awakened for two mornings without a discharge in the eyes.
5. Your child may infect other people. Separate towels and washcloths; careful handwashing may be useful.
6. Call your physician if
   a. The infection has not improved in 72 hours
   b. The eyelid is red, swollen, warm, tender, or painful
   c. The eyeball is cloudy or sores develop on it
   d. Vision is blurred
   e. The eye becomes painful or develops photophobia

Nosebleed

1. If bleeding occurs, apply pressure for a full 10 minutes, compressing the soft and bony parts of the nose, pressing downward toward the cheeks with the thumb and forefinger. Preceding this, blow the nose if possible.
2. Increase home humidity. Minimize nose trauma and picking.
3. Apply Vaseline daily to the interior nose for 4-5 days.
4. Call your physician if
   a. Unexplained bruising occurs
   b. Large amounts of blood are lost
   c. Bleeding cannot be controlled by pressure

Croup

1. Keep your child's room humidified. A cool mist humidifier is best.
2. Push fluids. Try to keep the child calm.
3. Fever medicine may make your child feel better.
4. If your child worsens and develops increased difficulty breathing:
   a. Take your child outside into the cold air for 5 minutes
   b. Try to get your child to relax
   c. Arrange to go to the hospital
5. Call your physician immediately if
   a. Your child has great difficulty breathing
   b. The lips or skin turns blue
   c. Drooling or difficulty swallowing develops
   d. Your child does not improve with cold air
   e. Agitation or listlessness develops
   f. The cough does not improve in 4-5 days

Asthma

1. Give all doses of medication. Continue until there has been no wheezing for 48 hours. If your child wheezes often, your care provider may want to give the medicine for a long period.
2. Push clear liquids. Warm fluids are particularly helpful. Keep your child quiet and calm.

3. Try to identify substances that trigger attacks and avoid them. Typically, animals, feather pillows, dust, and pollens are involved. Pollutants and smoke may contribute to the problem.
4. Many patients with asthma will develop wheezing in response to an infection. If this is a trigger in your child, you should start medicine at the first sign of a cold or cough.
5. Call your physician immediately if
   a. Breathing difficulty recurs or worsens or the child has difficulty speaking
   b. The lips or skin turns blue
   c. Restlessness or sleeplessness is present
   d. Fluid intake decreases
   e. Nausea, vomiting, or irritability develops because of medicine or inability to take medication
   f. Cough or wheezing persists or chest pain or fever develops

Appendix B-3: Trauma

Head Injury

1. Limit activities and restrict to light diet. With recent injury, apply ice pack to swelling.
2. Waken your child every 2 hours and observe.
3. Aspirin or acetaminophen may be given for pain.
4. Call your physician immediately if
   a. Increasing sleepiness, drowsiness, or inability to awaken patient develops
   b. Change in equality of pupils (black center of eye) or blurred vision, peculiar movements of the eyes, or difficulty focusing develops
   c. Stumbling, unusual weakness, or problem using arms or legs develops
   d. Change in normal gait or crawl develops
   e. Seizures occur
   f. Change in personality or behavior occurs, such as increasing irritability, confusion, unusual restlessness, or inability to concentrate
   g. Persistent vomiting (more than three times) occurs
   h. Drainage of blood or fluid from the nose or ear occurs
   i. Severe headache occurs

Care of Sutured Wounds

1. Mild bleeding and some discomfort may occur after suturing as the anesthesia wears off.
2. Keep the wound clean and dry for 2 days, then begin gentle cleansing of the wound twice daily with soap and water.
3. Try to keep the area elevated.
4. Call your physician if
   a. The wound becomes red or swollen or drains pus, or if red streak appears
   b. The wound becomes more painful
5. Change the dressing in _____ days.
6. Return in _____ days for suture removal or wound check.

Sprains and Fractures

1. Elevate the injured limb to lessen swelling and pain. Ice packs may be useful for 12-24 hours.
2. If your child is wearing an elastic Ace bandage, rewrap it if it becomes too loose or tight.
3. If your child has a *cast*, keep it dry.
4. Call your physician immediately if
   a. Severe pain or pressure within the cast (if present) develops
   b. Increasing coldness or blueness of the fingers or toes occurs
   c. Excessive swelling or decreased motion of toes or fingers is present

Burns

1. Keep the wound clean and dry.
2. Change the dressing in _____ days. Wash the burn gently, apply cream, and dress as directed.
3. Call your physician if
   a. Increasing redness or discoloration of the normal tissue around the burn site develops
   b. Red streaks radiating from the burn area develop
   c. Fever or chills occur
   d. Swelling or progressive inability to use fingers and toes (if extremity) develops
   e. Shortness of breath or increased cough develops
   f. Blurred vision (if face is involved) develops
   g. Swallowing difficulty (if neck is involved) develops

Animal Bites and Scratches

1. Take medication _____ for _____ days. Give every dose. Call your physician if your child refuses the medicine or appears to have a reaction.
2. Call your physician if
   a. The wound becomes red or swollen, drains pus, or becomes more painful, or if red streaks develop
   b. A tender lump appears in the groin or under the arm
   c. Fever or chills are present

Appendix B-4: Other Pediatric Problems

Diarrhea

1. Give only clear liquids; give as much as your child wants. The following may be used during the first 24 hours:
   a. Rehydralyte, Pedialyte, or Lytren
   b. Defizzed, room-temperature soda or Gatorade for older children (over 2 years) if diarrhea is only mild
2. If your child is vomiting, give clear liquids *slowly*. In younger children, start with a teaspoonful and slowly increase the amount. If vomiting occurs, let your child rest for a while and then try again. About 8 hours after vomiting has stopped, the child can return gradually to a normal diet.
3. After 24 hours, your child's diet may be advanced if the diarrhea has improved. If only formula is being taken, mix the formula with twice as much water to make up half-strength formula, which should be given over the next 24 hours. Applesauce, bananas, and strained carrots may be given if the child is eating solids once fluids are being taken without difficulty.

   If this is tolerated, your child may be advanced to a regular diet over the next 2-3 days.
4. If your infant has had a prolonged course of diarrhea, it may be helpful in the younger child to advance from clear liquids to a soy formula (Isomil, ProSobee, or Soyalac) for 1-2 weeks.
5. Do not use boiled milk. Kool-Aid and soda are not ideal liquids, particularly in younger infants, because they contain few electrolytes.
6. Call your physician if
   a. The diarrhea or vomiting is increasing in frequency or amount

b. The diarrhea does not improve after 24 hours of clear liquids or resolve entirely after 3-4 days

c. Vomiting continues for more than 24 hours

d. The stool has blood or the vomited material contains blood or turns green

e. Signs of dehydration develop, including decreased urination, less moisture in diapers, dry mouth, no tears, weight loss, lethargy, or irritability.

Vomiting

1. Clear liquids only should be given slowly and may include defizzed soda pop (cola, ginger ale), Pedialyte, Lytren, Gatorade, etc. In younger children, start with a teaspoon and slowly advance the amount. If vomiting occurs, let your child rest for a while and then try again.

2. About 8 hours after your child has stopped vomiting, he or she can gradually return to a normal diet. For older infants and children, bland items (toast, crackers, clear soup) may be given slowly.

3. Call your physician if
   a. Vomiting increases in frequency or amount
   b. Vomiting continues for more than 24 hours
   c. Your child develops signs of dehydration, including decreased urination, less moisture in diapers, dry mouth, no tears, weight loss, lethargy, or listlessness

d. Your child becomes sleepy, difficult to awaken, or irritable

e. Vomited material has blood in it or turns green

Urinary Tract Infections

1. A urine culture has been obtained.

2. Two days after your child begins antibiotics, you should contact your care provider about the urine culture to be sure that your child is taking the correct medicine and feeling better.

3. Two weeks after your initial visit, your physician will want to see your child again for another urine culture. Arrangements also will be made for periodic urine checks over the next year.

4. Several steps may help prevent repeat infections, particularly in girls.
   a. Teach your child to wipe correctly from front to back
   b. Do not use bubble bath or let the soap float around in the bath

5. Call your physician if
   a. Fever or pain with urination is not gone 48 hours after beginning antibiotics
   b. Your child gets worse or does not tolerate the medication

APPENDIX C

Formulary

Appendix C-1: Common Medications

Drugs	Dosages	Comments
Acetaminophen (Tylenol, Tempra) Drop: 80 mg/0.8 ml Elix: 160 mg/5 ml Tab: 80 (chew), 160 (junior), 325 mg Supp. 120, 325 mg	10-15 mg/kg/dose q 4-6 hr PO (adult: 10 grains/dose); (maximum: 3.6 gm/24 hr)	May give aspirin/ibuprofen for synergistic antipyretic effect; also see Codeine Tox: hepatic: overdose
Acetazolamide (Diamox) Tab: 125, 250 mg Cap (SR): 500 mg Vial: 500 mg/5 ml	Diuretic: 5 mg/kg/24 hr q 6-24 hr PO, IV (adult: 250-375 mg/24 hr) Epilepsy: 8-30 mg/kg/24 hr q 6-8 hr PO, IM, IV (maximum: 1 gm/24 hr)	Carbonic anhydrase inhibitor; IM painful; half-life: 4-10 hr Tox: hypokalemia, acidosis (long-term therapy), paresthesias
Acetylcysteine (Mucomyst) Soln: 10% (100 mg/ml) 20% (200 mg/ml)	Acetaminophen OD: load 140 mg/kg PO, then 70 mg/kg q 4 hr PO × 17 doses Nebulizer: 2-20 ml (10%) or 1-10 ml (20%) soln q 2-6 hr	Primary treatment for acetaminophen overdose: pulmonary mucolytic; IV preparation available Tox: mucosal irritant, bronchospasm
Acyclovir (Zovirax) Tab: 800 mg Cap: 200 mg Vial: 500 mg/10 ml Susp: 200 mg/5 ml Ointment: 5%	Herpes genitalis: 200 mg q 4 hr (5 doses/24 hr) PO × 5-10 days Herpes neonatorum: 30 mg/kg/24 hr q 8 hr IV × 10 days Varicella: 80 mg/kg/24 hr q 6 hr PO × 5 days (maximum 3,200 mg/24 hr) Encephalitis: 30 mg/kg/24 hr q 8 hr IV × 10 days	IV therapy indicated in immunocompromised patient; effective in newborn; modified dose for recurrent episode; reduce with renal failure Tox: diaphoresis, hematuria, phlebitis (IV)
Adenosine (Adenocard) Vial: 3 mg/ml	50-100 μg/kg IV rapid (1-2 min) bolus Adult: 6 mg IV as rapid (1-2 min) bolus; repeat 12 mg IV up to two times if no response in 2 min	No controlled studies in children but is commonly used for paroxysmal supraventricular tachycardia Tox: facial flushing, dyspnea, nausea, metallic taste
Albumin 25% salt-poor albumin (25 gm/dl) 5% with 0.9% NS (5 gm/dl)	0.5-1 gm/kg/dose IV repeated prn	Salt-poor albumin has 0.6 mEq Na$^+$/gm; caution with hypervolemia, CHF
Albuterol (Proventil, Ventolin) Syr: 2 mg/5 ml Soln (inhalation) 0.5%: 5 mg/ml Tab: 2, 4 mg	Inhalation: 0.03 ml (0.15 mg)/kg/dose to maximum of 0.5-1.0 ml/dose diluted in 2 ml 0.9% NS; may repeat q 20 min × 3 or as needed Oral: 0.1-0.2 mg/kg/dose q 6-8 hr PO (maximum: 4 mg/dose)	Beta$_2$ agonist with little cardiac effect; in child <2 yr, give 0.15-0.40 ml/dose; children 2-5 yr, give 0.30-0.50 ml; 5-10 yr, give 0.50 ml; and adults, 0.5-1.0 ml; available as MDI

Many oral drugs may be given 3-4 times per day with more flexibility than implied by the specific intervals noted. Adult dose provided as a guideline for maximum dose. *NB,* Newborns <7 days of age; *Pen,* penicillin; *SR,* sustained release; *Tox,* toxicity of drug.

Drugs	Dosages	Comments
Allopurinol (Zyloprim) Tab: 100, 300 mg	10 mg/kg/24 hr q 6 hr PO (<6-yr-old: 150 mg/24 hr; 6- to 10-yr-old: 300 mg/24 hr) (maximum: 600 mg/24 hr)	Titrate to serum uric acid level; reduce dose with renal failure Tox: rash, hepatic, cataract
Aluminum hydroxide (Amphogel) Tab: 300, 600 mg Susp: 320 mg/5 ml **Maalox** (also magnesium hydroxide) Tab: 200/200, 400/400 mg Susp: 225/200 mg/5 ml	Peptic ulcer: 5-15 ml (adult: 15-45 ml) 1 and 3 hr after meals and before bed PO Prophylaxis GI bleeding Infant: 2-5 ml/dose q 1-2 hr PO Child: 5-15 ml/dose (adult: 30-60 ml) q 1-2 hr PO	Should be initiated early for prophylaxis. Alternative includes cimetidine
Amantidine (Symmetrel) Syr: 50 mg/5 ml Cap: 100 mg	4.4-8.8 mg/kg/24 hr q 12 hr PO (>9 yr and adult: 100 mg q 12 hr PO or 200 mg q 24 hr PO)	Continue for at least 10 days and longer in unprotected high-risk patient with on- going exposure to influenza A; only chil- dren >1 yr Tox: depression, CHF, psychosis, seizures
Amikacin (Amikin) Vial: 50, 250 mg/ml	15 mg/kg/24 hr q 8 hr IM, IV slowly over 30 min (maximum: 1.0 gm/24 hr) (NB: 15 mg/kg/24 hr q 12 hr)	Therapeutic peak level: <35 μg/ml: cau- tion in renal failure (reduce dose) Tox: renal, VIII nerve
Aminocaproic acid (Amicar) Syr: 250 mg/ml Tab: 500 mg Vial: 250 mg/ml	Load: 200 mg/kg PO (maximum: 6 gm); then 100 mg/kg/dose (maximum: 6 gm/dose) q 6 hr PO for 2-5 days or until healing occurs Load: 100 mg/kg IV; then 33.3 mg/kg/hr IV up to 30 gm/24 hr	Useful for oral bleeding; also available for IV use; Chapter 54 Tox: thrombosis, rash, hypotension
Aminophylline	Load: 7.5 mg/kg PO; maint: 5 mg/kg/dose q 6 hr PO Load: 6 mg/kg IV slowly, maint: 0.8-1.2 mg/kg/hr IV Neonatal apnea load: 5 mg/kg; then 2-3 mg/kg q 12 hr PO	85% theophylline: therapeutic level: 10-20 μg/ml; neonatal apnea (Chapters 43 and 59) Tox: nausea, vomiting, irritability, seizures, dysrhythmias
Amiodarone (Cardarone) Tab: 200 mg	10 mg/kg/24 hr q 12 hr PO for 7-10 days, then reduce to 5 mg/kg/24 hr (maximum: 15 mg/kg/24 hr for 2-3 wk) (adult: load with 800-1,600 mg/24 hr for 1-3 wks, then 600-800 mg/24 hr × 1 mon, then 200-400 mg/24 hr	Little experience in children
Amoxicillin (Amoxil, Larotid) Susp: 125, 250 mg/5 ml Cap: 125, 250 mg	30-100 mg (avg: 50 mg)/kg/24 hr q 8 hr PO (adult: 250-500 mg q 8 hr)	Do not use for *Shigella* Tox: similar to ampicillin but less diarrhea; see Penicillin G
Amoxicillin (AMX)-clavulanic acid (CLA) (Augmentin) Susp: 125 mg AMX/31.25 CLA/5 ml, 250 mg AMX/62.50 CLA/5 ml Tab: 250 mg AMX/125 CLA, 500 mg AMX/125 CLA Tab (chew): 125 mg AMX/31.25 CLA, 250 mg AMX/62.5 CLA	30-50 mg AMX/kg/24 hr q 8 hr PO (adult: 250-500 mg AMX q 8 hr PO)	Dosage is based on amount of amoxicillin; 2 tab 250 mg are not equivalent to 500 mg tab; beta-lactamase inhibitor Tox: diarrhea, similar to amoxicillin

Drugs	Dosages	Comments
Amphotericin (Fungizone) Vial: 50 mg	0.6 mg/kg/24 hr IV over 1-4 hours; begin at 0.2 mg/kg/24 hr and increase dose	May also be given intrathecal; only for severe fungal infection; initial 0.1 mg/kg test dose over 20-60 min Tox: fever, chills, bone marrow suppression
Ampicillin (Omnipen, Polycillin) Susp: 125, 250 mg/5 ml Cap: 250, 500 mg Vial: 250, 500, 1,000 mg	50-100 mg/kg/24 hr q 6 hr PO (adult: 250-500 mg/dose PO); 100-400 mg/kg/24 hr q 4-6 hr IV (NB: 50-100 mg/kg/24 hr q 12 hr IV) (adult: 4-12 gm/24 hr IV)	Higher parenteral doses with severe infection: 3 mEq Na$^+$/gm Tox: rash (esp. with infectious mononucleosis), diarrhea, superinfection; see Penicillin G
Ampicillin (AMP)/Sulbactam (SUL) (Unasyn) Vial: 1.5 gm	Adult: 1 gm AMP/0.5 gm SUL q 6 hr IV	Intraabdominal, gynecologic infections; semisynthetic beta-lactamase inhibitor Little experience in children <12 yr
Aspirin (salicylate, ASA) Tab: 81 (chew), 325 mg Supp: 65, 130, 195, 325 mg	10-15 mg/kg/dose q 4-6 hr PO (adult: 10 grains/dose) Rheumatoid: 60-100 mg/kg/24 hr q 4-6 PO (maximum: 3.6 gm/24 hr PO)	Synergistic antipyretic effect with acetaminophen; avoid with chickenpox or influenza-like illness Therapeutic level: 15-30 mg/dl Tox: GI irritation, tinnitus, platelet dysfunction; overdose (Chapter 43)
Atenolol (Tenormin) Tab: 50, 100 mg	Hypertension: 1-2 mg/kg/dose q 24 hr PO (adult: 50 mg q 24 hr PO up to 100 mg q 24 hr PO)	Little experience in children; response seen in 1 week; also available for IV use
Atropine Vial: 0.1, 0.4, 1 mg/ml	0.01-0.03 mg/kg/dose IV (minimum: 0.1 mg/dose) (adult: 0.6-1.0 mg/dose; maximum total dose 2 mg) q 5 min prn; may also be given ET	Infants require higher dose (0.03 mg/kg); organophosphate poisoning (0.05 mg/kg) (Chapter 43) Tox: dysrhythmias, anticholinergic
Azithromycin Tab: 250 mg Pack: 1 gm	Otitis media: 10 mg/kg/24 hr q 24 hr PO followed by half dose days 2-5 Pharyngitis: 12 mg/kg/24 hr q 24 hr PO Uncomplicated genital chlamydia: 1 gm PO Adult: 250-500 mg/day PO	Pharyngitis relapse high
Beclomethasone (Beclovent, Vanceril) MDI (inhalation: 42 μg/dose)	6-12 yr: 1-2 puffs QID >12 yr: 2 puffs QID	
Benztropine (Cogentin) Tab: 0.5, 1, 2 mg Vial: 1 mg/ml	>3 yr: 0.02-0.05 mg/kg/dose q 12-24 hr PO, IV Adult: 1-4 mg/dose IV	Pediatric dose not well established
Bethanechol (Urecholine)	0.6 mg/kg/24 hr q 8 hr PO (adult: 10-30 mg QID PO) 0.15-0.2 mg/kg/24 hr SC (adult: 2.5-5 mg/24 hr)	
Bicarbonate, sodium (NaHCO$_3$) Vial: 8.4% (50 mEq/50 ml) 7.5% (44 mEq/50 ml)	1 mEq/kg/dose q 10 min prn	Monitor ABG: dilute 1:1 with D5W or sterile water; incompatible with calcium, catecholamines Tox: alkalosis, hyperosmolality, hypernatremia
Bretylium (Bretylol) Vial: 50 mg/ml	5 mg/kg/dose IV followed prn by 10 mg/kg/dose q 15 min IV up to maximum total dose of 30 mg/kg	Table 12-3; limited experience in children Tox: nausea, vomiting, hypotension, bradycardia

Many oral drugs may be given 3-4 times per day with more flexibility than implied by the specific intervals noted. *NB*, Newborns <7 days of age; *Pen*, penicillin; *SR*, sustained release; *Tox*, toxicity of drug.

Drugs	Dosages	Comments
Calcium chloride Vial: 10% (100 mg/ml-1.36 mEq Ca^{++}/ml)	20-30 mg/kg/dose IV (slow) (maximum: 500 mg/dose) q 10 min prn; 250 mg/kg 24 hr q 6 hr PO (mix 2% solution)	Monitor heart, avoid extravasation; caution in digitalized patient; incompatible with NaHCO$_3$ Tox: bradycardia, hypotension
Calcium gluconate Vial: 10% (100 mg/ml-0.45 mEq Ca^{++}/ml) Tab: 1 gm	100 mg/kg dose IV (slow) (maximum: 1 gm/dose) q 10 min prn: 500 mg/kg/24 hr q 6 hr PO	See Calcium chloride
Captopril (Capoten) Tab: 12.5, 25, 50, 100 mg	1-6 mg/kg/24 hr q 6-12 hr PO (maximum: 450 mg/24 hr)	Tables 13-8 and 47-13 Tox: renal, proteinuria, neutropenia, rash
Carbamazepine (Tegretol) Tab: 100 mg (chewable), 200 mg	15-30 mg/kg/24 hr q 8-12 hr PO (adult: 1200 mg/24 hr; begin 100-200 mg/dose q 12 hr PO with 100 mg/24 hr increments)	Therapeutic level: 4-14 µg/ml: Table 56-13 Tox: hepatic, nystagmus, nausea, aplastic anemia
Carbenicillin (Geopen, Geocillin) Vial: 1, 2, 5, 10 gm Tab: 382 mg	400-600 mg/kg/24 hr q 4-6 hr IV: 30-50 mg/kg/24 hr q 6 hr PO (NB: 200 mg/kg/24 hr q 12 hr IV) (adult: 40 gm/24 hr IV; 2 gm/24 hr PO)	Used in combination therapy with aminoglycoside; 5.2-6.5 mEq Na$^+$/gm Tox: platelet dysfunction, rash; adjust dose with renal failure; see Penicillin G
Cefaclor (Ceclor) Susp: 125, 250 mg/5 ml Cap: 250, 500 mg	20-40 mg/kg/24 hr q 8 hr PO (adult: 250-500 mg q 8 hr)	Active against ampicillin-resistant *H. influenzae*; second-generation cephalosporin Tox: renal, diarrhea, vaginitis; cross-reacts with pen
Cefadroxil (Duricef) Susp: 125, 250, 500 mg/5 ml Cap: 500 mg Tab: 1 gm	30 mg/kg/24 hr q 12 hr PO (maximum: 2 gm/24 hr)	Relatively long half-life; first-generation cephalosporin Tox: diarrhea, pruritus; cross-reacts with pen
Cefamandole (Mandol) Vial: 0.5, 1, 2 gm	50-150 mg/kg/24 hr q 4-6 hr IM, IV (adult: 4-12 gm/24 hr)	Second-generation cephalosporin Tox: bleeding, renal, hepatic, rash, neutropenia; cross-reacts with pen; adjust dose with renal failure
Cefazolin (Ancef, Kefzol) Vial: 0.25, 0.5, 1 gm	25-100 mg/kg/24 hr q 6-8 hr IM, IV (NB: 40 mg/kg/24 hr q 12 hr) (adult: 2-12 gm/24 hr)	First-generation cephalosporin Tox: renal, hepatic, rash, phlebitis; cross-reacts with pen; adjust dose with renal failure
Cefixime (Suprax) Syr: 100 mg/5 ml Tab: 200, 400 mg	8 mg/kg/24 hr q 12-24 hr PO (adult: 400 mg/24 hr)	Third-generation cephalosporin
Cefoperazone (Cefobid) Vial: 1, 2 gm	Adult: 2-12 gm/24 hr q 6-12 hr IV slowly, IM	Third-generation cephalosporin; limited experience in children; half-life 2 hr Tox: diarrhea, hypersensitivity
Cefotaxime (Claforan) Vial: 1, 2 gm	50-150 mg/kg/24 hr q 4-6 hr IV, IM (neonatal meningitis: 100-150 mg/kg/24 hr q 8-12 hr) (adult: 1-2 gm q 4-6 hr up to maximum 12 gm/24 hr)	Third-generation cephalosporin; excellent broad-spectrum coverage; meningitis, UTI, bacteremia, pneumonia, skin infection; half-life 1 hr Tox: hypersensitivity (cross-reacts with pen), phlebitis, pain (IM), diarrhea, colitis, renal, hepatic

Drugs	Dosages	Comments
Cefoxitin (Mefoxin) Vial: 1, 2 gm	80-160 mg/kg/24 hr q 4-6 hr IV (maximum: 12 gm/24 hr)	Second-generation cephalosporin; good anaerobic coverage Tox: pain at site if IM injection, nausea, vomiting; adjust dose with renal failure
Cefpodoxime (Vantin) Susp: 50, 100 mg/5 ml Tab: 100, 200 mg	10 mg/kg/24 hr q 12 hr PO (maximum: 800 mg/24 hr)	Third-generation cephalosporin
Cefprozil (Cefzil) Susp: 125, 250 mg/5 ml Tab: 250, 500 mg	15-30 mg/kg/24 hr q 24 hr PO	Second-generation cephalosporin
Ceftazidime (Fortaz) Vial: 0.5, 1, 2 gm	100-150 mg/kg/24 hr q 8 hr IV (adult: 3-6 gm/24 hr)	Third-generation cephalosporin; limited CNS data Tox: diarrhea; cross-reacts with pen
Ceftizoxime (Cefizox) Vial: 1, 2 gm	100-200 mg/kg/24 hr q 6-8 hr IV (neonatal meningitis: 100-200 mg/kg/24 hr q 8-12 hr IV) (adult: 6-12 gm/24 hr)	Third-generation cephalosporin Tox: diarrhea; cross-reacts with pen
Ceftriaxone (Rocephin) Vial: 0.25, 0.5, 1, 2 gm	50-100 mg/kg/24 hr q 12-24 hr IV, IM (adult: 1-2 gm/dose q 12-24 hr IV, IM)	Third-generation cephalosporin; usually children >1 mon of age; excellent broad-spectrum coverage; half-life 5-8 hr Reports of delayed CNS sterilization, gall bladder disease; use lidocaine with IM administration Tox: diarrhea, abnormal liver function, cholecyititis
Cefuroxime (Zinacef, Ceftin) Vial: 750, 1,500 mg Tab: 125, 250, 500 mg	50-240 mg/kg/24 hr q 6-8 hr IV (adult: 4.5-9.0 gm/24 hr q 6-8 hr IV) 30 mg/kg/24 hr q 12 hr PO; >12 yr (250-500 mg q 12 hr PO)	Second-generation cephalosporin; oral formulation; higher dose IV for meningitis; useful for *H. influenzae* disease; do not use for neonatal meningitis, sepsis; oral form for nontoxic child with respiratory, skin, or urinary infections
Cephalexin (Keflex) Susp: 125, 250 mg/5 ml Cap: 250, 500 mg	25-50 mg/kg/24 hr q 6 hr PO (adult: 250-500 mg/dose q 6 hr)	First-generation cephalosporin Tox: nausea, vomiting, renal, hepatic; cross-reacts with pen; adjust dose with renal failure
Cephalothin (Keflin) Vial: 1, 2, 4 gm	75-125 mg/kg/24 hr q 4-6 hr IM, IV (NB: 40 mg/kg/24 hr q 12 hr) (adult: 4-12 gm/24 hr)	First-generation cephalosporin Tox: renal, hepatic, phlebitis, neutropenia; cross-reacts with pen; adjust dose with renal failure
Cephradine (Anspor, Velosef) Susp: 125, 250 mg/5 ml Cap: 250, 500 mg Vial: 0.25, 0.5, 1 gm	25-50 mg/kg/24 hr q 6 hr PO; 50-100 mg/kg/24 hr q 6 hr IM (deep), IV (maximum: 4 gm/24 hr)	First-generation cephalosporin Tox: renal, hepatic, nausea, vomiting, neutropenia, vaginitis, phlebitis, cross-reacts with pen; adjust dose with renal failure
Charcoal, activated	1 gm/kg or 15-50 gm PO (adult: 50-100 gm/dose)	First dose may be mixed with 35%-70% sorbitol; often requires NG tube for administration
Chloral hydrate (Noctec) Syr: 500 mg/5 ml Cap: 250, 500 mg	Hypnotic: 50-75 mg/kg/24 hr q 6-8 hr PO (maximum: 1 gm/dose) Sedative: ½ hypnotic dose	Hypnotic dose often needed for sedation; do not use with renal, hepatic disease

Many oral drugs may be given 3-4 times per day with more flexibility than implied by the specific intervals noted. *NB*, Newborns <7 days of age; *Pen*, penicillin; *SR*, sustained release; *Tox*, toxicity of drug.

Drugs	Dosages	Comments
Chloramphenicol (Chloromycetin)		
Susp: 150 mg/5 ml	50-100 mg/kg/24 hr q 6 hr IV	Tox: bone marrow suppression (reversible)
Cap: 250 mg	(NB: 25 mg/kg/24 hr q 12 hr IV) (adult:	and aplastic anemia; therapeutic level:
Vial: 1 gm (100 mg/ml)	maximum 2-4 gm/24 hr)	10-25 µg/ml
Chlorothiazide (Diuril)		
Susp: 250 mg/5 ml	10-20 mg/kg/24 hr q 12 hr PO	Table 47-12
Tab: 250, 500 mg	(NB: 30 mg/kg/24 hr PO) (adult: 500-1,000	Tox: hyponatremia, hypokalemia, alkalosis;
	mg q 12-24 hr PO)	reduce dose with renal failure
Chlorpheniramine		
(Chlor-Trimeton)		
Syr: 2 mg/5 ml	0.35 mg/kg/24 hr q 6 hr PO (adult: 4 mg	OTC antihistamine
Tab: 4 mg	q 4-6 hr)	Tox: drowsiness, anticholinergic (Chapter
Tab/cap (SR): 8, 12 mg	Sustained release in children >12 yr:	43), hypotension (IM)
	16-24 mg/kg/24 hr q 8-12 hr PO	
Chlorpromazine (Thorazine)		
Syr: 10 mg/5 ml	0.5 mg/kg/dose q 6-8 hr PO, IM, IV prn	Only children >6 mon old
Tab: 10, 25, 50, 100 mg	(adult: 25-50 mg/dose)	Tox: phenothiazine-extrapyramidal, anticho-
Cap (SR): 30, 75, 150 mg	1.0 mg/kg/dose q 6-8 hr PR prn (adult: 50-	linergic (Chapter 43); often mixed with
Supp: 25, 100 mg	100 mg/dose PR)	meperidine and promethazine (see meperi-
Vial: 25 mg/ml		dine)
Cimetidine (Tagamet)		
Susp: 300 mg/5 ml	20-30 mg/kg/24 hr q 6 hr PO,	Tox: diarrhea, renal, neutropenia; reduce
Tab: 200, 300 mg	IV (maximum: 2.4 gm/24 hr) (adult: 300	dose with renal failure
Vial: 150 mg/ml	mg/dose q 6 hr PO)	
Ciprofloxacin (Cipro)		
Tab: 250, 500, 750 mg	Adult: 250-750 mg q 12 hr PO	Should not be used in children <12 yrs
		because it probably causes arthropathy;
		reduce dose with renal impairment
Clarithromycin (Biaxin)		
Susp: 125, 250 mg/5 ml	15 mg/kg/24 hr q 12 hr PO	Increases theophylline and carbamazepine
Tab: 250, 500 mg	Adult: 250-500 mg q 12 hr PO	levels; do not refrigerate oral suspension
Clindamycin (Cleocin)		
Soln: 75 mg/5 ml	10-25 mg/kg/24 hr q 6 hr PO (adult: 600-	Caution in renal, hepatic disease
Cap: 75, 150 mg	1,800 mg/24 hr PO)	Tox: colitis, rash, diarrhea, phlebitis; only
Amp: 300, 600 mg	15-40 mg/kg/24 hr q 6-8 hr IM, IV	for child >1 mo
	(NB: 15-20 mg/kg/24 hr q 6-8 hr IV)	
	(maximum: 4.8 gm/24 hr IV)	
Clonazepam (Klonopin)		
Tab: 0.5, 1, 2 mg	0.05-0.2 mg/kg/24 hr q 8 hr PO; start at	Therapeutic level: 0.013-0.072 µg/ml; cau-
	0.01 mg/kg/24 hr and add 0.25-0.5 mg/24 hr	tion in renal disease; titrate dose slowly
	q 3 days until control (adult: 1.5-2.0 mg/24	every third day; Table 56-13; previously
	hr) (maximum total dose: 20 mg/24 hr)	Clonopin
		Tox: drowsiness, ataxia, personality change
Clonidine (Catapres)		
Tab: 0.1, 0.2, 0.3 mg	0.005-0.01 mg/kg/24 hr q 8-12 hr PO	May be used acutely in hypertension;
	(maximum: 0.8 mg/24 hr) (adult: 0.1 mg q	widely used for ADDH
	12 hr PO initially; increase 0.1-0.2 mg/24	Tox: drowsiness, headache
	hr up to 2.4 mg/24 hr PO)	
Cloroquine phosphate (Aralen)		
Tab: 500 mg (300 mg base)	10 mg base/kg/24 hr q 24 hr PO initially	Several forms available; see Table 55-3
Clotrimazole (Gyne-Lotrimin,		
Mycelex)		
Tab (vag): 100 mg	1 tablet or applicator-full vaginally nightly	Tox: local irritation
Cream (vag): 1%	× 7-14 days	
Cloxacillin (Tegopen)		
Soln: 125 mg/5 ml	50-100 mg/kg/24 hr q 6 hr PO (maximum:	Administer on empty stomach
Cap: 250, 500 mg	4 gm/24 hr)	Tox: GI irritant, see Penicillin G

Drugs	Dosages	Comments
Codeine Elix: 10 mg/5 ml (with antitussive) Tab: 15, 30, 60 mg Vial: 30, 60 mg/ml	Analgesic: 0.5 mg/kg/dose q 4-6 hr PO, IM (adult: 30-60 mg/dose) Antitussive: 1.0 mg/kg/24 hr q 4-6 hr PO (adult: 10-20 mg/dose)	Also available combined with acetaminophen 120 mg with 12 mg codeine/5 ml and tablets (acetaminophen 300 mg with 7.5 mg codeine [#1], 15 mg codeine [#2], or 30 mg codeine [#3]) Tox: dependence, CNS, and respiratory depression (Chapter 43)
Cortisone Tab: 5, 10, 25 mg Vial: 25, 50 mg/ml	Maintenance: 0.25 mg/kg/24 hr q 12-24 hr IM; 0.50-0.75 mg/kg/24 hr q 6-8 hr PO	Table 50-1
Cromolyn (Intal) Vial: 20 mg powder/soln	20 mg TID by nebulization	Spinhaler may be used to administer powder; for ongoing management of bronchospasm
Cyproheptadine (Periactin) Syr: 2 mg/5 ml Tab: 4 mg	0.25 mg/kg/24 hr q 8-12 hr PO (adult: 12-16 mg/24 hr)	
Dantrolene (Dantrium) Cap: 25 mg Vial: 20 mg	0.5 mg/kg/dose q 12 hr PO, then increase to 0.5 mg/kg/dose q 6-8 hr PO and increase up to a max of 3 mg/kg/dose	Little information about use in children <5 yr; IV solution for surgical prophylaxis for malignant hyperthermia
Deferoxamine (Desferal) Amp: 500 mg	If no shock: 90 mg/kg/dose q 8 hr IM (adult: 1-2 gm/dose × 1; titrate; maximum: 6 gm/24 hr) If shock: 15 mg/kg/hr IV	Urine turns rose colored if SI >TIBC in iron overdose; Chapter 43 Tox: urticaria, hypotension
Dexamethasone (Decadron) Vial: 4, 24 mg Elix: 0.5 mg/5 ml Tab: 1.5, 4, 6 mg	Croup: 0.25-0.6 mg/kg/dose q 6 hr IM, IV, PO Cerebral edema: 0.25-0.5 mg/kg/dose q 6 hr IM, IV Meningitis: 0.15 mg/kg/dose q 6 hr IV × 16 doses	Table 50-1; efficacy in cerebral edema controversial
Dextrose D50W (0.5 gm/ml)	0.5-1.0 gm (2-4 ml D25W)/kg/dose IV	Dilute D50W 1 : 1 to avoid hypertonicity; draw glucose
Diazepam (Valium) Tab: 2, 5, 10 mg Vial: 5 mg/ml	Status epilepticus: 0.2-0.3 mg/kg/dose IV (<1 mg/min) q 2-5 min prn (maximum total dose: child, 10 mg; adult, 30 mg) Sedation, muscle relaxation: 0.1-0.8 mg/kg/24 hr q 6-8 hr PO	If used for status epilepticus, must initiate additional drug; may be given rectally; dose 0.5 mg/kg/dose PR (Chapter 56) Tox: drowsiness, respiratory depression (increased with second drug)
Diazoxide (Hyperstat) Vial: 15 mg/ml	1-3 mg/kg/dose q 4-24 hr IV (fast); repeat in 30 min if no effect; may use intermittent smaller dose	Vasodilator: prompt (3-5 min) response (Table 13-8); also used to treat hyperinsulinemic hypoglycemia
Dicloxacillin (Dynapen) Susp: 62.5 mg/5 ml Cap: 125, 250, 500 mg	25-100 mg/kg/24 hr q 6 hr PO (adult: 125-500 mg/dose)	Do not use for NB; although optimally given on empty stomach, may have to use open capsule mixed with food Tox: GI irritant, see Penicillin G
Dicyclomine (Bentyl) Syr: 10 mg/5 ml Cap: 10, 20 mg	Children (>6 mo): 5-10 mg/dose q 6-8 hr PO; adult: 20-40 mg/dose q 6-8 hr PO	
Digoxin	See Table 47-10 and Chapters 43 and 47	

Many oral drugs may be given 3-4 times per day with more flexibility than implied by the specific intervals noted. *NB*, Newborns <7 days of age; *Pen*, penicillin; *SR*, sustained release; *Tox*, toxicity of drug.

Drugs	Dosages	Comments
Dimercaprol (BAL in oil) Amp: 100 mg/ml	Mild gold or arsenic poisoning: 2.5 mg/kg q 6 hr IM for 2 days, q 8 hr for 1 day, then q 24 hr for 10 days Severe arsenic or gold poisoning: 3 mg/kg q 4 hr for 2 days, q 6 hr for 1 day, then q 12 hr for 10 days Mercury poisoning: 5 mg/kg initially, then 2.5 mg/kg q 12-24 hr for 10 days Lead encephalopathy: 4 mg/kg, then q 4 hr in combination with edetate calcium disodium for 2-7 days; if less severe use 3 mg/kg	
Diphenhydramine (Benadryl) Elix: 12.5 mg/5 ml Cap: 25, 50 mg Vial: 10, 50 mg/ml	5 mg/kg/24 hr q 6 hr PO, IM, IV (maximum: 300 mg/24 hr) Anaphylaxis or phenothiazine overdose: 1-2 mg/kg/dose q 6 hr PO, IM, IV	Antihistamine: over the counter Tox: sedation, anticholinergic (Chapter 43); may inhibit breast milk
Diphenoxylate with atropine (Lomotil) Tab: 2.5 mg DPL/0.025 ATP Liq: 2.5 mg DPL/0.025 ATP/5 ml	0.3-0.4 mg/kg/24 hr q 6 hr PO (adult: 2 tab QID PO)	Not recommended in children <2 yr; use liquid in children <13 yr; reduce dosage or discontinue after control; avoid accidental ingestion
Dobutamine (Dobutrex) Vial: 250 mg	2-15 μg/kg/min IV infusion (maximum: 40 μg/kg/min IV) **Dilute:** 6 mg × weight (kg) in 100 ml D5W. Rate of infusion in μg/kg/min = ml/hr (1 ml/hr delivers 1 μg/kg/min); **or** 250 mg (1 vial) in 500 ml D5W = 500 μg/ml	Table 13-7
Docusate (Colace) Syr: 20 mg/5 ml Cap: 50, 100 mg	3-5 mg/kg/24 hr TID PO; (adult: 50-400 mg/24 hr)	
Dopamine (Intropin) Amp: 40 mg/ml Vial: 80 mg, 160 mg/ml	Low: 2-5 μg/kg/min IV drip Mod: 5-20 μg/kg/min IV drip High: >20 μg/kg/min IV drip **Dilute:** 6 mg × weight (kg) in 100 ml D5W. Rate of infusion in μg/kg/min = ml/hr (1 ml/hr delivers 1 μg/kg/min) **or** 200 mg (1 amp of 5 ml) in 500 ml D5W = 400 μg/ml	Table 13-7
Doxycycline (Vibramycin) Syr/susp: 25, 50 mg/5 ml Cap: 50, 100 mg Vial: 100, 200 mg	5 mg/kg/24 hr q 12 hr PO or IV slowly over 2-4 hr (adult: 100-200 mg/24 hr)	Do not use in children <9 yr of age Tox: GI irritant, hepatic, photosensitization, superinfection; adjust dose with renal failure
Droperidol (Inapsine) Vial: 2.5 mg/ml	0.1 mg/kg/dose IM, IV for anesthetic premedication; (adult: 1.25-5 mg/dose IM, IV); 0.05 mg/kg/dose q 4-6 hr prn for nausea, vomiting	Limited experience in children; monitor respirations

Drugs	Dosages	Comments
Edrophonium (Tensilon) Vial: 10 mg/ml	Test for myasthenia gravis: 0.2 mg/kg/dose and if no response in 1 min, give 1 mg increments up to maximum total dose of 5-10 mg IV (adult test dose: 2 mg) (NB: 1 mg single dose IV)	Have atropine available; may precipitate cholinergic crisis
Ephedrine Syr: 10, 20 mg/5 ml Tab/cap: 25, 50 mg	2-3 mg/kg/24 hr q 4-6 hr PO (adult: 25-50 mg q 4-6 hr PO)	Poor decongestant; potentiates side effects of theophylline without much therapeutic benefit (Chapter 59)
Epinephrine (Adrenalin) Vial (1 : 1,000-1 mg/ml) (1 : 10,000-0.1 mg/ml) Sus-Phrine (1 : 200-5 mg/ml in oil)	Asthma: 0.01 ml (1 : 1,000)/kg/dose (maximum: 0.35 ml/dose) q 15-20 min SC prn × 3: Sus-Phrine 0.005 ml/kg/dose (maximum: 0.15 ml) SC × 1 Asystole: 0.1 ml (1 : 10,000)/kg/dose (maximum: 5 ml/dose); subsequent dose and initial ET dose is 0.1 mg/kg or 0.1 ml/kg of 1:1000 solution Shock: 0.05-0.5 µg/kg/min IV infusion **Dilute** (for infusion in *shock*): 0.6 mg × weight (kg) in 100 ml D5W. Rate of infusion in 0.1 µg/kg/min = ml/hr (1 ml/hr delivers 0.1 µg/kg/min) **or** 1 mg in 500 ml D5W = 2 µg/ml	Inhalation (albuterol, terbutaline); therapy preferred for asthma; Sus-Phrine unreliable in dosing unless using single dose vial Use in shock only after isoproterenol and dopamine are ineffective; not effective with acidotic patient; Table 13-7 Tox: tachycardia, dysrhythmia, tremor, hypertension
Epinephrine, Racemic (Vaponefrin) Soln: 2.25%	0.25-0.75 ml in 2.5 ml of sterile water or saline administered by nebulizer	Rebounds, always admit patient; steroids often given with croup
Erythromycin (Pediamycin, E.E.S., Erythrocin, E-Mycin, ERYC) Susp: 200, 400 mg/5 ml Tab: 200 (chew), 250, 400, 500 mg	20-50 mg/kg/24 hr q 6 hr PO (adult: 250-1,000 mg/dose)	Also available as combination: erythromycin 200 mg + sulfisoxazole 600 mg/5 ml (Pediazole) Tox: GI irritant, rash
Ethambutol (Myambutol) Tab: 100, 400 mg	Initial TB treatment: 15 mg/kg q 24 hr PO Retreatment: 25 mg/kg q 24 hr PO	Multiple drug treatment indicated; monthly eye examination advised
Ethanol 100% (1 ml = 790 mg)	Methanol, ethylene glycol overdose: 1 ml/kg over 15 min, then 0.16 ml (125 mg)/kg/hr IV	Maintain ethanol level at ≥ 100 mg/dl; Table 43-1
Ethosuximide (Zarontin) Syr: 250 mg/5 ml Cap: 250 mg	20-40 mg/kg/24 hr q 24 hr PO; begin 250 mg q 24 hr (3-6 yr old) and increase 250 mg/24 hr at 4-7 day interval; maximum: 1 gm/24 hr	Therapeutic level: 40-100 µg/ml; Table 55-13 Tox: GI irritant, neutropenia, drowsiness, dizziness, headache
Factor VIII, IX	Tables 54-9 and 54-10	
Famciclovir (Famvir) Tab: 125, 250 mg	Adult: 500 mg/dose q 8 hr for 7 days	Preferably begin within 12 hr of onset of rash; not studied in < 18 yr old
Famotidine (Pepcid) Tab: 20, 40 mg Susp: 40 mg/5 ml Vial: 10 mg/ml	1-2 mg/kg/24 hr q 12-24 hr IV, PO; adult: 20-40 mg q 24 hr PO; 20 mg q 12 hr IV	Safety and effectiveness in children not established.

Many oral drugs may be given 3-4 times per day with more flexibility than implied by the specific intervals noted. *NB*, Newborns <7 days of age; *Pen*, penicillin; *SR*, sustained release; *Tox*, toxicity of drug.

Drugs	Dosages	Comments
Fentanyl (Sublimaze) Amp: 50 µg/ml	2-4 µg/kg/dose IV slowly (adult: 50-100 µg/dose)	Narcotic; half-life: 20 min; monitor oxygenation
Fluconazole (Diflucan) Susp: 10, 40 mg/ml Tab: 50, 100, 200 mg	*Oral candidiasis:* Load, 6 mg/kg; then 3 mg/kg/24 hr PO	Usually treat 2-3 weeks
Fludrocortisone (Florinef) Tab: 0.1 mg	0.05-0.1 mg/24 hr q 24 hr PO	Table 50-1
Flumazenil (Mazicon) Vial: 0.1 mg/ml	0.01 mg/kg initially, repeating 0.01 mg/kg q min up to max total dose of 1 mg; adult: 0.2 mg IV initially; 0.2-0.3 mg IV further dose if no initial response up to cumulative dose of 1-3 mg	Management of suspected benzodiazepine overdose; little experience in children
Folic acid	0.2-1.0 mg/24 hr PO (adult: 10-15 mg/24 hr)	
Furazolidone (Furoxone) Liq: 50 mg/15 ml Tab: 100 mg	*Giardia:* 6 mg/kg/24 hr q 6 hr PO (adult: 100 mg q 6 hr)	Do not use in children <1 mon; avoid alcohol; see Table 55-3 Tox: nausea, vomiting, rash
Furosemide (Lasix) Soln: 10 mg/ml Tab: 20, 40, 80 mg Amp: 10 mg/ml	1 mg/kg/dose q 6-12 hr IV initially (may repeat q 2 hr IV prn); 2 mg/kg/dose q 2-12 hr PO initially; may increase dose by 1 mg/kg increments (maximum: 6 mg/kg/dose PO, IM, IV)	Rapid acting; Table 47-12 Tox: hypokalemia, hyponatremia, alkalosis, prerenal azotemia; ototoxicity
Gentamicin (Garamycin) Vial: 10, 40 mg/ml	5.0-7.5 mg/kg/24 hr q 8 hr IM, IV (maximum: 300 mg/24 hr) (NB: 5 mg/kg/24 hr q 12 hr) (adult: 3-5 mg/kg/24 hr q 8 hr)	Therapeutic peak level: 6-12 µg/ml; caution in renal failure (adjust dose); slow IV infusion Tox: renal, VIII nerve
Glucagon Amp: 1 mg (1 unit)/ml	0.03-0.1 mg/kg/dose q 20 min SC, IM, IV prn (NB: 0.1-0.2 mg/kg/dose q 4 hr prn) (adult: 0.5-1.0 mg/dose)	Hypoglycemia: not adequate as only glucose support, esp in NB; treatment of propranolol (beta-blocker) overdose
Glucose (see Dextrose) **Griseofulvin** Microsize (Grisactin, Grifulvin V) Susp: 125 mg/5 ml Tab/cap: 125, 250, 500 mg Ultramicrosize (Gris-PEG, Fulvicin P/G) Tab: 125, 250, 330 mg	Microsize: 10 mg/kg/24 hr q 24 hr PO (adult: 500-1,000 mg q 12-24 hr PO) Ultramicrosize: 5 mg/kg/24 hr q 24 hr PO (adult: 250-500 mg/24 hr q 12-24 hr PO)	Give with meals; either formulation is adequate; treatment period of 4-6 wk Tox: renal, hepatic, neutropenia, rash, headache
Haloperidol (Haldol) Tab: 1, 2, 5, 10 mg Soln: 2 mg/ml Amp: 5 mg/ml	Psychosis: 0.05-0.15 mg/kg/24 hr q 8-12 hr PO. Begin at 0.5 mg/24 hr and increase Nonpsychotic behavior: 0.05-0.075 mg/kg q 8-12 hr PO Adult: initial 0.5-2.0 mg (max: 5 mg) q 8-12 hr PO	
Heparin (Liquaemin, Panheprin) Vial: 100, 1,000, 5,000, 10,000, 20,000, 40,000 units/ml	Load: 50-75 units/kg IV bolus Maint: 10-25 units/kg/hr IV infusion **or** 100 units/kg/dose q 4 hr IV Adult: load (5,000 units) with maint (20,000-30,000 unit over 24 hr IV continuous infusion **or** 5,000-10,000 q 4 hr)	Titrate to maintain PTT at 2 times control; antidote: protamine Tox: bleeding, allergy rash, wheezing, anaphylaxis

Drugs	Dosages	Comments
Hydralazine (Apresoline) Tab: 10, 25, 50, 100 mg Amp: 20 mg/ml	Crisis: 0.1-0.2 mg/kg/dose (1.7-3.5 mg/kg/24 hr) q 4-6 hr IM, IV prn (adult: 10-40 mg/dose) Maint: 0.75-3 mg/kg/24 hr q 6-12 hr PO (adult: 10-75 mg/dose q 6 hr PO)	Vasodilator, prompt (10-30 min response if IV) decrease BP; Tables 13-8 and 47-13 Tox: tachycardia, angina, SLE-like syndrome; reduce dose with renal failure
Hydrochlorothiazide (Esidrix, HydroDiuril) Tab: 25, 50, 100 mg	1-2 mg/kg/24 hr q 12 hr PO (NB: 2-3 mg/kg/24 hr PO) (adult: 25-100 mg q 12-24 hr)	Table 47-12 Tox: hyponatremia, hypokalemia, alkalosis; reduce dose with renal failure
Hydrocortisone (Solu-Cortef) Susp: 10 mg/5 ml Tab: 5, 10, 20 mg Vial: 100, 250, 500, 1,000 mg	Maintenance: 0.5 mg/kg/24 hr q 8 hr PO Septic shock: 50 mg/kg/dose (maximum: 500 mg/dose) IV Asthma: 4-5 mg/kg/dose q 6 hr IV	Table 50-1; efficacy in shock controversial
Hydroxyzine (Atarax, Vistaril) Syr/susp: 10, 25 mg/5 ml Tab (Atarax): 10, 25, 50 mg Cap (Vistaril): 25, 50, 100 mg Vial (Vistaril): 25, 50 mg/ml	2 mg/kg/24 hr q 6 hr PO (adult: 200-400 mg/24 hr q 6 hr PO) 0.5-1 mg/kg/dose q 4-6 hr IM prn (adult: 25-100 mg/dose q 4-6 hr IM prn)	Antihistamine, potentiates meperidine, barbiturates Tox: sedation, anticholinergic (Chapter 43); may inhibit breast milk
Ibuprofen (Motrin) Tab: 300, 400, 600, 800 mg Chewable: 50, 100 mg Susp: 100 mg/5 ml	40 mg/kg/24 hr q 6-8 hr PO (adult: 1.2 gm/24 hr)	Available over the counter (Nuprin, Advil 200 mg Tab) (adult: 200-400 mg q 4-6 hr PO; maximum: 1.2 gm/24 hr) Tox: GI irritant, keratopathy, hematuria, retinopathy, rash
Imipenem (IMP)-Cilastatin (CIL) (Primaxin) Vial: 250 mg IMP/250 mg CIL, 500 mg IMP/500 mg CIL	60 IMP + 60 mg CIL/kg/24 hr q hr IV (adult: 250-1,000 mg IMP + 250-1,000 mg CIL/dose) (maximum: 50 mg/kg/24 hr **or** 4 gm/24 hr of each agent)	Limited experience in children Tox: phlebitis, diarrhea, renal
Imipramine (Tofranil) Tab: 10, 25, 50 mg	Enuresis: 25-75 mg at bedtime PO	
Immune serum globulin	Exposure to measles <1 yr of age (0.25 ml/kg IM) or immunocompromised (0.5 ml/kg IM); viral hepatitis type A contact within 14 days of exposure (0.02 ml/kg IM); and selected immune deficiency disease. Hepatitis B immune globulin (HBIG) is used with significant exposure to HBsAg-positive blood within 24 hr and 1 mo later (0.06 ml/kg/dose IM) (see Chapter 55)	
Indomethacin (Indocin) Cap: 25, 50 mg	1-3 mg/kg/24 hr q 6-8 hr PO (maximum: 100-200 mg/24 hr)	Not approved in children <14 yr; may be used to close PDA (with CHF) in neonate; 0.1-0.2 mg/kg/dose q 12 hr up to maximum 0.6 mg/kg IV Tox: nausea, vomiting, headache, corneal opacity
Insulin	Chapter 50	
Iodoquinol	See Table 55-3	
Ipecac, syrup of	6-12 mon (10 ml/dose PO) 12 mon (15 ml/dose PO) Adult (30 ml/dose PO) Give initial dose and may repeat × 1	Do not use in children <6 mo; push fluids; contraindicated in caustic ingestions and patients who are comatose or having seizures; Chapter 42
Ipratropium (Atrovent) MDI (18 μg/dose) Soln (0.02%): 500 μg/2.5 ml	Adult: Inhalation (MDI): 2 inhalations q 4-6 hr prn; solution (500 μg/2.5 ml) by nebulization q 6 hr prn Child: Administer partial dose	Efficacious as nebulization solution; dose in children not well defined but useful as adjunct to Albuterol; see Chapter 59

Many oral drugs may be given 3-4 times per day with more flexibility than implied by the specific intervals noted. *NB*, Newborns <7 days of age; *Pen*, penicillin; *SR*, sustained release; *Tox*, toxicity of drug.

Drugs	Dosages	Comments
Iron, elemental (Fe) (Fer-In-Sol, Feosol) Drop: 75 mg (15 mg Fe)/0.6 ml Syr: 90 mg (18 mg Fe)/5 ml Tab: 200 mg (40 mg Fe), 325 mg (65 mg Fe)	Therapeutic: 6 mg elemental Fe/kg/24 hr q 8 hr PO Prophylactic: 1-2 mg elemental Fe/kg/24 hr q 8-24 hr PO (maximum: 15 mg elemental Fe/24 hr)	Ferrous sulfate is 20% elemental iron (Fe) (Chapter 54) Tox: GI irritant (reduce by giving with food); overdose (Chapter 43)
Isoetharine (Bronkosol, Bronko-meter) Soln: 1% (10 mg/ml) Aerosol	Nebulizer: 0.25-0.5 ml diluted in 2.5 ml saline q 4 hr prn Aerosol: 1-2 puffs q 2-4 hr prn	Administer by nebulizer with or without IPPB; limited use Tox: tachycardia, hypertension
Isoniazid (INH) Syr: 50 mg/5 ml Tab: 50, 100, 300 mg	10-20 mg/kg/24 hr q 12-24 hr PO (adult: 300 mg/24 hr)	Supplemental pyridoxine (10 mg/100 mg INH) needed in adolescents, adults Tox: peripheral neuropathy, hepatitis, seizure, acidosis
Isoproterenol (Isuprel) Amp: 200 µg/ml Neb: 1:100, 200 Aerosol	Shock: 0.05-1.5 µg/kg/min IV infusion; begin at 0.05 µg/kg/min and increase by 0.1 µg/kg/min increments (maximum: 1.5 µg/kg/min) Nebulizer: 0.5 ml diluted in 2.5 ml saline q 4 hr prn Aerosol: 1-2 puffs q 2-4 hr prn **Dilute:** (for infusion in shock) 0.6 mg × weight (kg) in 100 ml D5W. Rate of infusion in 0.1 µg/kg/min = ml/hr (1 ml/hr delivers 0.1 µg/kg/min); **or** 200 µg (1 ml) in 200 ml D5W = 1 µg/ml	Table 13-7 Rarely used as bronchodilator
Ivermectin	See Table 55-3	
Kanamycin (Kantrex) Vial: 37.5, 250, 333 mg/ml	15 mg/kg/24 hr q 8 hr IM, IV (maximum: 1 gm/24 hr) (NB: 15 mg/kg/24 hr q 12 hr)	Therapeutic peak level: 25-30 µg/ml; caution in renal failure (adjust dose); infusion IV slowly Tox: renal, hearing
Ketamine Vial: 10, 50, 100 mg/dl	2-4 mg/kg/dose IV 4 mg/kg/dose IM	Administer slowly; half-life 2½ hr, redistribution half-life 10-15 min
Ketorolac (Toradol) Syringe: 15, 30, 60 mg Tab: 10 mg	Adult: 30 mg IV slow or 60 mg IM initially up to total daily dose of 120 mg; 10-20 mg/dose q 6 hr PO	Limited experience in children < 16 yr, do not give if patient hypovolemic
Levothyroxine (Synthroid) Tab: 25, 50, 100, 200, 300 µg Vial: 500 µg	Infancy: 7-9 µg/kg/24 hr PO; thereafter 100 µg/m²/24 hr PO (child: 3-5 µg/kg/24 hr PO)	Monitor T4 and thyroid-stimulating hormone
Lidocaine (Xylocaine) Vial (IV): 10, 20 mg/ml Vial (anesthetic): 10 mg (1%), 20 mg (2%), 40 mg (4%)/ml	Load 1 mg/kg dose q 5-10 min IV prn to maximum of 5 mg/kg Maintenance: 20-50 µg/kg/min IV infusion Adult: load same; maintenance: 2-4 mg/min **Dilute** 150 mg × weight (kg) in 250 ml D5W. Rate of infusion in µg/min = 10 × ml/hr	Antidysrhythmic; therapeutic level: 1.5-5 µg/ml; may be given ET (dilute 1:1); Table 12-3 Tox: seizures, drowsiness, euphoria, muscle twitching, dysrhythmias, and titrate dose
Loperamide (Imodium) Cap: 2 mg Liq: 1 mg/5 ml	Children (>2 yr): 1 mg q 8 hr PO (adult: 2 mg q 8 hr PO)	Limited efficacy, liquid over the counter

Drugs	Dosages	Comments
Lorazepam (Ativan) Vial: 2, 4 mg/ml	0.05-0.10 mg/kg/dose IV (adult: 2.5-10 mg/dose)	May consider repeating × 1 dose in 15-20 min if necessary
Magnesium hydroxide (see aluminum hydroxide) (Maalox)		
Magnesium sulfate Crystal: Epsom salt Vial: 10%, 12.5%, 25%, 50%	Catharsis: 250 mg/kg/dose PO (adult: 30 gm/dose PO) Hypomagnesemia: 25-50 mg/kg/dose q 4-6 hr × 3-4 doses IM or IV (adult: 1-4 gm/24 hr) Anticonvulsant: 1 gm 10% soln IV or 25%/50% soln IM	Caution in renal failure; follow magnesium and calcium levels; Chapter 42 Tox: hypotension
Mannitol Vial: 20% (200 mg/ml) 25% (250 mg/ml)	Diuretic: 750 mg/kg/dose IV: do not repeat with persistent oliguria (adult: 300 mg/kg/dose) Cerebral edema: 0.25-0.5 gm/kg IV slowly over 10-15 min q 3-4 hr prn (maximum: 1 gm/kg/dose IV)	Maintain serum osmolality <320 mOsm/L; may get CNS rebound, intracranial monitor indicated Tox: hypovolemia, volume overload, hyperosmolality
Mebendazole (Vermox) Tab (chew): 100 mg	Pinworm: 100 mg PO, repeat in 1 wk Ascaris, hookworm: 100 mg q 12 hr PO for 3 days	Not studied in children <2 yr; see Table 55-3 Tox: diarrhea
Meperidine (Demerol) Syr: 50 mg/5 mg Tab: 50, 100 mg Vial: 25, 50, 100 mg/ml	1-2 mg/kg/dose q 3-4 hr PO, IM, IV prn (adult: 50-150 mg/dose) (maximum: 100 mg/dose in children)	75 mg meperidine = 10 mg morphine DPT, sedative cocktail (ratio 4 : 1 : 1) Meperidine (Demerol) 1-2 mg/kg/dose (maximum: 50 mg/dose) Promethazine (Phenergan) 0.25-0.5 mg/kg/dose (maximum: 12.5 mg/dose) Chlorpromazine (Thorazine) 0.25-0.5 mg/kg/dose (maximum: 12.5 mg/dose) Also potentiated by hydroxyzine Tox: CNS, respiratory depression, seizure, overdose (Chapter 43)
Metaraminol (Aramine) Vial: 10 mg/ml	0.01 mg/kg/dose IV prn **or** 1-4 µg/kg/min IV infusion	Tox: tachycardia, dysrhythmia, local tissue slough
Methicillin (Staphcillin) Vial: 1, 4, 6 gm	100-200 mg/kg/24 hr q 4-6 hr IM, IV (maximum: 12 gm/24 hr) (NB: 50-75 mg/kg/24 hr q 8-12 hr)	Equivalent to nafcillin, oxacillin Tox: interstitial nephritis (hematuria), bone marrow suppression; see Penicillin G
Methsuximide (Celontin) 150, 300 mg	Adult: 300 mg/24 hr q 24 hr PO × 1 wk; 300 mg/24 hr/wk increments q 3 wk as necessary (maximum: 1.2 gm/24 hr)	Petit mal seizures Tox: CNS symptoms, behavioral change, caution in liver, renal disease
Methyldopa (Aldomet) Tab: 125, 250, 500 mg Vial: 50 mg/ml Susp: 250 mg/5 ml	Crisis: 2.5-5 mg/kg/dose q 6-8 hr IV (maximum: 20-40 mg/kg/24 hr or 500 mg/dose IV) Chronic: 10 mg/kg/24 hr q 6-12 hr PO (maximum: 40 mg/kg/24 hr or total dose 2 gm/24 hr)	Tox: somnolence, hemolytic disease, ulcerogenic; reduce dose with renal failure
Methylene blue Vial: 1% (10 mg/ml)	1-2 mg/kg/dose IV q 4 hr prn	Use for methemoglobinemia

Many oral drugs may be given 3-4 times per day with more flexibility than implied by the specific intervals noted. *NB*, Newborns <7 days of age; *Pen*, penicillin; *SR*, sustained release; *Tox*, toxicity of drug.

Drugs	Dosages	Comments
Methylphenidate (Ritalin) Tab: 5, 10, 20 mg	Initial dose (>6 yr): 5 mg in AM/PM PO; titrate; maximum: 60 mg/24 hr	
Methylprednisolone (Solu-Medrol) Vial: 40, 125, 500, 1,000 mg	Septic shock: 30-50 mg/kg/dose IV Asthma: 1-2 mg/kg/dose q 6 hr IV	Table 50-1; efficacy in shock controversial; different preparation for intraarticular route
Metoclopramide (Reglan) Syr: 5 mg/5 ml Tab: 5, 10 mg Vial: 5 mg/ml	0.1 mg/kg/dose q 6 hr PO Adult: 10-15 mg QID PO	For gastroesophageal reflux, nausea, and vomiting
Metolazone (Zaroxolyn, Diulo) Tab: 2.5, 5, 10 mg Susp: 1 mg/ml	0.2-0.4 mg/kg/24 hr q 12-24 hr Adult: 2.5-10 mg/24 hr PO	Little experience in children; useful when no response to other diuretics and glomer- ular filtration rate; Table 47-12 Tox: azotemia, ↓ K$^+$, hypotension, leth- argy, coma
Metronidazole (Flagyl) Tab: 250, 500 mg	*Gardnerella vaginalis* vaginitis: 500 mg q 8 hr PO for 7-10 day *Trichomonas vaginalis:* 5 mg/kg/dose q 8 hr PO for 7 days (adult: 250 mg q 8 hr for 7 days) *Giardia lamblia:* 5 mg/kg/dose q 8 hr PO for 5 days (adult: 250 mg q 8 hr for 5 days) Amebiasis: 35-50 mg/kg/24 hr q 8 hr PO for 10 days (adult: 750 mg q 8 hr for 10 days)	IV form available for severe anaerobic infections Tox: nausea, diarrhea, neutropenia, urticaria, do not give to pregnant patient
Miconazole (Monistat) Vag cream (2%) Supp: 200 mg (Monistat 3)	*Candida (Monilia)* vaginitis: 1 applicator-full before bed for 7-14 days; supp: 200 mg before bed × 3 days	Systemic form available
Midazolam (Versed) Vial: 1 mg/ml	Conscious sedation: 0.035-0.1 mg/kg/dose IV (maximum: 5 mg)	Often used in combination with narcotic; intranasal administrations possible; (Chapter 7)
Minoxidil (Loniten) Tab: 2.5, 10 mg	0.2-1.0 mg/kg/24 hr q 24 hr PO (adult: 10-40 mg q 24 hr PO) (maximum: 100 mg/24 hr)	Peripheral vasodilator; limited experience in children
Morphine Vial: 5, 8, 10, 15 mg/ml	0.1-0.2 mg/kg/dose (maximum: 15 mg/dose) q 2-4 hr IM, IV	Antidote, naloxone (Chapters 7 and 43) Tox: CNS, respiratory depression, hypo- tension
Nafcillin (Unipen) Vial: 0.5, 1, 2 gm	50-200 mg/kg/24 hr q 4-6 hr IM, IV (maximum: 12 gm/24 hr) (NB: 40 mg/kg/24 hr q 12 hr)	Equivalent to methicillin, oxacillin; IM painful; oral form available Tox: allergy, see Pen; low renal toxicity
Naloxone (Narcan) Amp: 0.4, 1.0 mg/ml	0.1 ml/kg/dose (maximum: 0.8 mg) IV; if no response in 10 min and opiate suspected, give 2 mg IV	Narcotic antagonist; propoxyphene (Darvon) and pentazocine (Talwin) require very large doses to reverse; Chapters 42 and 43; may have role in septic shock
Naproxen (Naprosyn) Tab: 250, 375, 500 mg Susp: 125 mg/5 ml	2.5-5 mg/kg/dose q 8 hr PO (adult: 250-375 mg q 8-12 hr PO) (maximum: 15 mg/kg or 1,250 mg for adult/24 hr) Dysmenorrhea: load 500 mg PO, then 250 mg q 8-12 hr PO	Nonsteroidal antiinflammatory; children >2 yr Tox: GI irritant, vertigo, headache, platelet dysfunction; not approved for children <2 yr

Drugs	Dosages	Comments
Nitrite, Amyl	Inhale pearl q 60-120 sec	For cyanide poisoning, follow with sodium nitrite and sodium thiosulfate
Nitrite, Sodium (3%)	0.27 ml (8.7 mg)/kg (adult: 10 ml [300 mg]) IV slowly if Hgb is 10 gm	For cyanide poisoning, precede with amyl nitrite and follow with sodium thiosulfate
Nitrofurantoin (Furadantin, Macrodantin) Susp: 25 mg/5 ml Tab: 50, 100 mg Cap: 25, 50, 100 mg	5-7 mg/kg/24 hr q 6 hr PO; chronic: 2.5-5 mg/kg/24 hr (adult: 50-100 mg/dose q 6 hr PO; chronic: 50-100 mg before bed PO)	Do not use for renal disease, G6PD deficiency, child <1 mo, pregnancy Tox: hypersensitivity
Nitroprusside (Nipride) Vial: 50 mg	0.5-10 μg (avg: 3 μg)/kg/min IV infusion **Dilute** 6 mg × weight (kg) in 100 ml D5W. Rate of infusion in μg/kg/min = ml/hr **or** 50 mg (1 vial) in 100 ml of D5W = 500 μg/ml	Precise, rapid (1-2 min) BP control; requires constant monitoring; light sensitive; Tables 12-3 and 13-8 Tox: hypotension, cyanide poisoning (monitor thiocyanate level)
Norepinephrine (Levophed) Vial: 1 mg/ml	0.1-1.0 μg/kg/min IV infusion **Dilute:** 0.6 mg × weight (kg) in 100 ml D5W. Rate of infusion in 0.1 μg/kg/min = ml/hr (1 ml/hr delivers 0.1 μg/kg/min); **or** 1 mg (1 ml) in 100 ml of D5W = 10 μg/ml	Table 13-7; titrate response
Norfloxacin (Noroxin) Tab: 400 mg	Adult: 400 mg q 12 hr PO	Quinolone antibiotic No pediatric recommendation because of risk of arthropathy
Nystatin (Mycostatin) Cream: 100,000 unit/g Susp: 100,000 unit/ml Tab (vag): 100,000 unit	Thrush: 1 ml in each side of the mouth q 4-6 hr PO Diaper rash (**Candida**): apply with diaper changes (q 2-6 hr) Vaginitis: 1 tab in vagina before bed for 10 days	Continue oral and topical therapy for 2-3 days after clearing
Oxacillin (Prostaphin) Soln: 250 mg/5 ml Cap: 250, 500 mg Vial: 0.5, 1, 2, 4 gm	50-100 mg/kg/24 hr q 6 hr PO (adult: 500-1,000 mg q 6 hr PO); 50-200 mg/kg/24 hr q 4-6 hr IM, IV (maximum: 8 gm/24 hr) (NB: 25-50 mg/kg/24 hr q 8-12 hr IM, IV)	Equivalent to methicillin, nafcillin; oral form optimally given on empty stomach Tox: see Penicillin G
Pancuronium (Pavulon) Vial: 1, 2 mg/ml	Load: 0.04-0.1 mg/kg/dose IV (intubation: 0.06-0.1 mg/kg/dose IV) (NB: 0.02 mg/kg/dose IV) Maint: 0.01-0.02 mg/kg/dose q 20-40 min IV prn (NB: adjust on basis of loading dose)	Peak effect in 2-3 min; duration 40-60 min; must be able to support respirations
Paraldehyde Soln: 1 gm/ml Amp: 1 gm/ml	Sedative: 0.15 ml (150 mg)/kg/dose PO, IM Anticonvulsant: 0.3 ml (300 mg)/kg/dose q 4-6 hr PR prn (NB: 0.1-0.2 ml [100-200 mg]/kg/dose diluted in 0.9% NS q 4-6 hr PR prn; 0.15 ml/kg/dose q 4-6 hr IM, IV prn)	For PR, dissolve 1:1 in cottonseed, olive, or mineral oil; for IM, give deep; IV must be given slowly (5 min) after mixing 0.15 ml/kg/dose diluted 1 : 20 with saline in glass syringe and infused; may repeat IV dose in 20-40 min (avoid extravasation); do not give if hepatic or pulmonary disease is present Tox: IV (pulmonary edema, CHF), IM (sterile abscess), PR (proctitis), respiratory depression

Many oral drugs may be given 3-4 times per day with more flexibility than implied by the specific intervals noted. *NB*, Newborns <7 days of age; *Pen*, penicillin; *SR*, sustained release; *Tox*, toxicity of drug.

Drugs	Dosages	Comments
Penicillin G (sodium or potassium salt) Susp: 125, 250 mg/5 ml Tab: 125, 250, 500 mg Vial: 1, 5, 20 million units	25-50 mg (40,000-80,000 units)/kg/24 hr q 6 hr PO (adult: 300,000-1.2 million units/24 hr PO); 50,000-250,000 units/kg/24 hr q 4 hr IM, IV (NB: 50,000-150,000 units/kg/24 hr q 8-12 hr IM, IV)	1 mg = 1600 units; salt content (1 million units contain 1.68 mEq Na^+ or K^+); PO erratically absorbed, give on empty stomach Tox: allergy (anaphylaxis, rash, urticaria), superinfection (*Candida*), hemolytic anemia, interstitial nephritis; adjust dose with renal failure

Penicillin G benzathine and **Penicillin G procaine** (Bicillin C-R 900/300) 900,000 units benz and 300,000 units proc/2 ml		
		Benzathine pen G			*Benzathine/procaine pen G*
	Weight (lb)	*(Bicillin L-A)*	*(Bicillin C-R 900/300)*
	<30	300,000 units	300,000 : 100,000
	31-60	600,000 units	600,000 : 200,000
	61-90	900,000 units	900,000 : 300,000
	>90	1,200,000 units	Not available

Drugs	Dosages	Comments
Penicillin V (Pen-Vee K, V-Cillin K) Susp: 125 mg (200,000 units), 250 mg (400,000 units/5 ml) Tab: 125, 250, 500 mg	25-50 mg (40,000-80,000 units)/kg/24 hr q 6 hr PO (adult: 250-500 mg q 6 hr PO)	More resistant to destruction by gastric acid Tox: see Penicillin G
Pentamidine (Pentam) Vial: 300 mg	4 mg/kg/24 hr q 24 hr IM	May be given IV slowly
Pentobarbital (Nembutal) Elix: 20 mg/5 ml Cap: 30, 50, 100 mg Supp: 30, 60, 120, 200 mg Vial: 50 mg/ml	Sedation: 6 mg/kg/24 hr q 8 hr PO, PR, IM, IV (adult: 30 mg q 6-8 hr) Cerebral edema: load: 3-5 (up to 20) mg/kg slow IV; maint: 1-2 mg/kg/hr IV	Short-acting barbiturate; treatment of increased intracranial pressure must include monitor Pentobarbital to maintain intracranial pressure <15 mm Hg and barbiturate level 25-40 µg/ml; support respirations, monitor BP Tox: CNS excitement, respiratory depression, hypotension (Chapter 43)
Phenazopyridine (Pyridium) Tab: 100, 200 mg	6-12 yr of age: 100 mg q 8 hr PO (adult: 200 mg q 8 hr PO) for 1-3 days	Use until dysuria gone and diagnosis made; urine color orange/red; avoid with G6PD deficiency Tox: hemolytic anemia, methemoglobinemia
Phenobarbital (Luminal) Elix: 20 mg/5 ml Tab: 8, 15, 30, 60, 90, 100 mg Vial: 65, 130 mg/ml	Seizures: load: 15-20 mg/kg PO, IM (erratic absorption), IV (<1 mg/kg/min); with status epilepticus and no response in 20-30 min, repeat 10 mg/kg IV (adult: 100 mg/dose IV q 20 min prn × 3) Maint: 3-5 mg/kg/24 hr q 12-24 hr PO (adult: 200-300 mg/24 hr PO) Sedation: 2-3 mg/kg/dose PO q 8 hr prn	May be used as first-line drug in status epilepticus (IV) or after seizures controlled by diazepam (Valium); Chapter 56 and Table 56-13 Therapeutic level: 10-35 µg/ml Tox: drowsiness, irritability, learning problems, CNS and respiratory depression with high doses (Chapter 40) Reduce dose with renal failure
Phentolamine (Regitine) Vial: 5 mg/ml	0.05-0.1 mg/kg/dose q 1-4 hr IV (adult: 2.5-5 mg/dose IV)	Specific for pheochromocytoma and MAO-induced hypertension; rapid onset; dose, esp PO, must be individualized; may be given as continuous infusion Tox: dysrhythmia, hypotension

Drugs	Dosages	Comments
Phenytoin (Dilantin, diphen-ylhydantoin) Susp: 30, 125 mg/5 ml Tab (chew): 50 mg Cap: 30, 100 mg Amp: 50 mg/ml	Seizures: load: 15-20 mg/kg PO, IV (<0.5 mg/kg/min); maint: 5-10 mg/kg/24 hr q 12-24 hr PO (adult: 200-400 mg/24 hr PO) Dysrhythmia load: 5 mg/kg IV (<0.5 mg/kg/min) (adult: 100 mg/dose q 5 min prn up to 1 gm IV); maint: 6 mg/kg/24 hr q 12 hr PO (adult: 300 mg/24 hr PO)	Therapeutic level: 10-20 μg/ml: good for digoxin- and tricyclic antidepressant-induced dysrhythmias; Chapters 43 and 56 Tox: nystagmus, ataxia, hypotension, gingival hyperplasia, SLE-like syndrome, hirsutism
Physostigmine (Antilirium) Vial: 1 mg/ml	Child: 0.5 mg IV (over 3 min) q 10 min prn (maximum total dose: 2 mg) Adult: 1-2 mg IV (over 3 min) q 10 min prn (maximum total dose: 4 mg in 30 min)	Anticholinesterase; use in life-threatening anticholinergic overdose (Chapter 43) Tox: neurologic, dysrhythmias
Piperacillin (Pipracil) Vial: 2, 3, 4 gm	200-300 mg/kg/24 hr q 4-6 hr IV (maximum: 24 gm/24 hr) (NB: 100 mg/kg/dose q 12 hr IV)	Good *Pseudomonas* coverage Tox: neurologic, gastrointestinal
Polystyrene sodium sulfonate (Kayexalate) Powder: 450 gm	1 gm/kg/dose q 6 hr PO or q 2-6 hr PR (adult: 15 gm PO or 30-60 gm PR q 6 hr)	1 level tsp = 3.5 gm; 4.1 mEq Na$^+$/gm: exchanges 1 mEq K$^+$ for 1 gm resin, which delivers 1 mEq Na$^+$ for each 1 mEq K$^+$ removed; mix 30%-70% suspension in D10W, 1% methylcellulose, or 10% sorbitol Tox: electrolyte problems, constipation
Pralidoxime (Protopam, 2-PAM) Vial: 1 gm	20-50 mg/kg/dose (maximum: 2 gm/dose) IV slow (<50 mg/min) q 8 hr prn × 3	Cholinesterase reactivator; use after atropine in organophosphate overdose (Chapter 43); oral preparation for prophylaxis
Praziquantel (Biltricide)	See Table 55-3	
Prazosin (Minipress) Cap: 1, 2, 5 mg	Initial: 5 μg/kg/dose PO; then up to 25 μg/kg/dose q 6 hr PO Adult: 1 mg q 8-12 hr PO; may increase slowly to 20 mg/24 hr	Little experience in children; Table 47-13
Prednisolone (Prelone) Soln: 15 mg/5 ml	Asthma: 1-2 mg/kg/24 hr q 6 hr PO	Palatable, liquid steroid preparation
Prednisone Tab: 5, 10, 20 mg Susp: 5 mg/5 ml	Maintenance: 0.1-0.15 mg/kg/24 hr q 12 hr PO Asthma: 1-2 mg/kg/24 hr q 6 hr PO	Table 50-1
Primidone (Mysoline) Susp: 250 mg/5 ml Tab: 50, 250 mg	10-25 mg/kg/24 hr q 6-8 hr PO; start at 125-250 mg, increase in 125-250 increments at 1-wk intervals (adult: initial 250 mg/24 hr PO; maintenance 750-1,500 mg/24 hr q 6 hr PO)	Therapeutic level: 6-12 μg/ml (or phenobarbital 10-25 μg/ml) Table 56-13 Tox: sedation, nausea, vomiting, diplopia: reduce dose with renal failure; see Phenobarbital
Probenecid (Benemid) Tab: 500 mg	Load: 25 mg/kg PO; maint: 40 mg/kg/24 hr q 6 hr PO (adult: 2 gm/24 hr); 25 mg/kg (adult: 1 gm) PO before ampicillin or penicillin treatment of *Neisseria gonorrhoeae*	Not recommended for children <2 yr Tox: GI irritant

Many oral drugs may be given 3-4 times per day with more flexibility than implied by the specific intervals noted. *NB,* Newborns <7 days of age; *Pen,* penicillin; *SR,* sustained release; *Tox,* toxicity of drug.

Drugs	Dosages	Comments
Procainamide (Pronestyl) Tab/cap: 250, 375, 500 mg Vial: 100, 500 mg/ml	Load: 2-6 mg/kg/dose IV slow (<50 mg/min) (adult: 100 mg/dose IV slow q 10 min prn up to total load of 1 gm IV) Maint: 20-80 µg/kg/min IV (adult: 1-3 mg/min IV) or 15-50 mg/kg/24 hr q 4-6 hr PO (adult: 250-500 mg/dose q 4-6 hr PO)	IV must be given slowly at concentration <100 mg/ml; do not use with heart block Tox: GI irritant, SLE-like syndrome dysrhythmias
Prochlorperazine (Compazine) Syr: 5 mg/5 ml Tab: 5, 10, 25 mg Supp: 2.5, 5, 25 mg Amp: 5 mg/ml	0.4 mg/kg/24 hr q 6-8 hr PO, PR (adult: 5-10 mg q 6-8 hr PO or 25 mg q 12 hr PR) 0.2 mg/kg/24 hr q 6-8 hr IM (adult: 5-20 mg/dose IM) (maximum: 40 mg/24 hr)	Only children >2 yr and >10 kg Tox: phenothiazine (extrapyramidal, anticholinergic) (Chapter 43)
Promethazine (Phenergan) Syr: 6.25, 25 mg/5 ml Tab: 12.5, 25, 50 mg Supp: 12.5, 25, 50 mg Amp: 25, 50 mg/ml	Nausea, vomiting: 0.25-0.5 mg/kg/dose q 4-6 hr PO, PR, IM prn (adult: 12.5-25 mg/dose) Sedation: 0.5-1 mg/kg/dose q 6 hr PO, PR, IM prn (adult: 25-50 mg/dose)	Often mixed with meperidine and chlorpromazine for DPT cocktail (see DPT cocktail — Meperidine) Tox: phenothiazine (sedation, extrapyramidal, anticholinergic) (Chapter 43)
Propantheline (Pro-Banthine)	1-2 mg/kg/24 hr QID PO (adult: 15-30 mg QID)	
Propranolol (Inderal) Tab: 10, 20, 40, 80 mg Vial: 1 mg/ml	Dysrhythmias: load: 0.01-0.1 mg/kg/dose (maximum: 1 mg/dose) IV over 10 min (adult: 1 mg/dose IV q 5 min up to total of 5 mg); maint: 0.5-1 mg/kg/24 hr q 6 hr PO (adult: 10-30 mg/dose q 6-8 hr PO) Hypertension: 0.5-1.0 mg/kg/24 hr q 6-12 hr PO (maximum: 320 mg/24 hr PO) Tetralogy spells: 0.1-0.2 mg/kg/dose IV repeated in 15 min prn Migraine prophylaxis: 10-60 mg q 8 hr PO Thyrotoxicosis: 10-20 mg q 6-8 hr PO	Beta-blocker; contraindicated in patient with asthma or CHF; Table 13-8 Tox: dysrhythmias, hypoglycemia, hypotension, cardiac failure, bronchospasm, weakness; overdose treated with glucagon 0.1 mg/kg/dose IV
Propylthiouracil (PTU) Tab: 50 mg	Load: 5 mg/kg/24 hr q 6-8 hr PO (adult: 300 mg/24 hr); maint: ⅓-½ of loading dose once patient is euthyroid (adult: 100-150 mg/24 hr)	Tox: blood dyscrasia, hepatic, dermatitis, urticaria, neuritis
Protamine Amp: 10 mg/ml	1 mg IV for each 100 units of heparin given concurrently; 0.5 mg IV for each 100 units of heparin given in previous 30 min, and so on; maximum: 50 mg/dose	Heparin antidote Tox: hypotension, bradycardia, flushing
Pseudoephedrine (Sudafed) Syr: 30 mg/5 ml Tab: 30, 60 mg	4-6 mg/kg/24 hr q 4-6 hr PO (adult: 60 mg q 4-6 hr PO)	Tox: irritability; use with caution in hypertensive patient
Pyrantel (Antiminth) Susp: 250 mg/5 ml	11 mg (~0.2 ml)/kg/dose PO once (maximum: 1 gm/dose); repeat in 1 wk	Do not use with preexisting liver disease, pregnancy Tox: nausea, vomiting, hepatic
Pyrvinium (Povan) Tab: 50 mg Susp: 50 mg/ml	5 mg/kg/dose PO once; repeat in 2 wks	
Quinacrine (Atabrine) Tab: 100 mg	Giardiasis: 6 mg/kg/24 hr q 8 hr PO for 5 days (adult: 100 mg q 8 hr PO)	Tox: GI irritant, bone marrow depression; skin transiently turns yellow; caution in G6PD deficiency

Drugs	Dosages	Comments
Quinidine Tab: 100, 200, 300, 202 (SR), 300 (SR) mg Cap: 200, 300 mg	15-60 mg/kg/24 hr q 6 hr PO (adult: 300-400 mg q 6 hr PO)	Tox: GI irritant dysrhythmias, hypotension, blood dyscrasia
Racemic epinephrine (Vaponefrin) Soln: 2.25%	<20 kg: 0.25 ml in 2 ml saline nebulizer; 20-40 kg: 0.5 ml; >40 kg: 0.75 ml	Rebound; prolonged observation of child with croup following treatment
Ranitidine (Zantac) Tab: 150 mg Vial: 25 mg/ml	2-4 mg/kg/24 hr q 12 hr PO (adult: 150 mg q 12 hr PO; 50 mg q 6-8 hr IV; maximum: 400 mg/24 hr IV)	Little experience in children; similar to cimetidine, less drug interactions
Reserpine (Serpasil) Elix: 0.25 mg/5 ml Tab: 0.1, 0.25, 0.5, 1 mg	0.02 mg/kg/dose q 12 hr PO (adult: 0.1-0.25 mg/24 hr)	Usually used in combination with another drug; rarely used; Table 13-8 Tox: severe depression, bradycardia, ulcerogenic
Ribavirin (Virazole) Vial: 6 gm/100 ml	20 mg/ml delivered as 190 µg/l in air for 12-18 hr/24 hr for 3 days	Use Viratek Small Particle Aerosol Generator
Rifampin (Rimactane, Rifadin) Cap: 150, 300 mg	10-20 mg/kg/24 hr q 12-24 hr PO (maximum: 600 mg/24 hr) Meningococcal prophylaxis: 10 mg/kg q 12 hr PO for 2 days (adult: 600 mg q 12 hr) *H. influenzae* prophylaxis: 20 mg/kg q 24 hr for 4 days (adult: 600 mg q 24 hr × 4)	Tox: hepatic, GI irritant, hemolytic anemia; turns urine red; lower dose in children <1 mo
Rimantadine (Flumadine) Syringe: 50 mg/5 ml Tab: 100 mg	>10 yr: 100 mg/dose q 12 hr PO <10 yr: 5 mg/kg/dose up to 150 mg/24 hr as single dose PO	Prophylaxis for influenza A; begin within 24-48 hr onset of symptoms and continue for 48 hr after resolution
Secobarbital (Seconal) Cap: 30, 50, 100 mg Vial: 50 mg/ml	2-6 mg/kg/24 hr q 8 hr PO (adult: 60-120 mg/24 hr q 8-12 hr PO)	Short-acting barbiturate Tox: drowsiness, respiratory depression
Spectinomycin (Trobicin) Vial: 400 mg/ml	40 mg/kg/dose IM × 1 (adult: 2 gm IM × 1)	*N. gonorrhoeae* treatment; not good for syphilis Tox: dizziness, vertigo
Spironolactone (Aldactone) Tab: 25, 50, 100 mg	1-3 mg/kg/24 hr q 8-12 hr PO (adult: 25-100 mg/24 hr)	Useful adjunctive diuretic to maintain potassium; reduce dose with renal failure; Table 47-12
Succinylcholine (Anectine) Amp: 20 mg/ml Vial: 0.5, 1 gm	1 mg/kg/dose IV (NB: 2 mg/kg/dose IV); maint: 0.3-0.6 mg/kg/dose q 5-10 min IV	Must be able to control airway; optimally premedicate with atropine
Sulfisoxazole (Gantrisin) Susp: 500 mg/5 ml Tab: 500 mg	Load: 75 mg/kg PO; maint: 120-150 mg/kg/24 hr q 6 hr PO (adult: 500-1,000 mg q 6 hr PO) (maximum: 4-6 gm/24 hr)	Do not use in children <2 mo old: maintain good urine flow Tox: rash, Stevens-Johnson, neutropenia; reduce dose with renal failure
Sumatriptan (Imitrex) Syringe: 6 mg/0.5 ml Tab: 25, 50 mg	Adult: initial dose 25 mg PO; may give up to 100 mg after 2 hr for maximum daily dose of 300 mg PO; 6 mg initial dose SC and may repeat ≤6 mg SC up to 12 mg/24 hr SC	Subsequent treatment should reflect initial doses; limited experience in children

Many oral drugs may be given 3-4 times per day with more flexibility than implied by the specific intervals noted. *NB*, Newborns <7 days of age; *Pen*, penicillin; *SR*, sustained release; *Tox*, toxicity of drug.

Drugs	Dosages	Comments
Terbutaline (Brethine) Vial: 1 mg/ml	*Parenteral:* 0.01 ml (0.01 mg)/kg/dose (maximum: 0.25 ml/dose) q 15-20 min SC prn *Aerosol:* 0.03-0.05 mg (0.03-0.05 ml)/kg in 1-2.5 ml saline given q 4 hr (adult: 0.5-1.0 mg/dose)	Beta agonist for reactive airway disease; may have more prolonged effect than epi- nephrine Tox: sympathomimetic
Terfenadine (Seldane) Tab: 60 mg	7-12 Adult: 60 mg q 12 hr PO	Antihistamine without sedation
Tetracycline (Achromycin, Tetracyn) Syr: 125 mg/5 ml Tab/cap: 250, 500 mg Vial: 250, 500 mg (IM has lidocaine)	25-50 mg/kg/24 hr q 6 hr PO (adult: 250- 500 mg q 6 hr PO) 15-25 mg/kg/24 hr q 8-12 hr IM (adult: 200-300 mg/24 hr q 8-12 hr IM) 20-30 mg/kg/24 hr q 8-12 IV over 2 hr (adult: 250-500 mg/dose q 8-12 hr IV over 2 hr)	Do not use in children <9 yr Tox: GI irritant, hepatic, photosensitization, superinfection
Theophylline	Load: 6 mg/kg PO; maint: 4-5 mg/kg/dose q 6 hr PO Load: 5 mg/kg IV slowly: maint: 0.6-0.9 mg/kg/hr IV	Therapeutic level: 10-20 μg/ml; Chapter 59 Tox: nausea, vomiting, irritability, seizures, dysrhythmias
Thiabendazole (Mintezol)	See Table 55-3	
Thiopental (Pentothal) Vial: 0.5, 1 gm	Anesthesia: 2 mg/kg/dose IV (adult: 3-5 mg/kg/dose IV)	Respiratory support imperative; use 2.5% soln
Thioridazine (Mellaril) Susp: 25, 100 mg/5 ml Tab: 10, 15, 25, 50, 100 mg	1-2.5 mg/kg/24 hr q 8-12 hr PO (adult: 75- 300 mg/24 hr q 8-12 hr PO) (maximum: 800 mg/24 hr)	Do not use in children <2 yr; titrate dose to response Tox: phenothiazine (Chapter 43)
Thiosulfate, sodium (25%)	1.35 ml (325 mg)/kg (adult: 12.5 gm) IV slowly if Hgb is 10 gm	
Ticarcillin (Ticar) Vial: 1, 3, 6 gm	200-300 mg/kg/24 hr q 4-6 hr IM, IV (maximum: 18-24 gm/24 hr) (NB: 150-225 mg/kg/24 hr q 8-12 hr)	Similar to carbenicillin; adjust dose in renal failure; used in combination therapy
Tobramycin (Nebcin) Vial: 10, 40 mg/ml	6-7.5 mg/kg/24 hr q 8 hr IM, IV (maximum: 300 mg/24 hr) (NB: 4 mg/kg/24 hr q 12 hr)	Therapeutic peak level: 6-10 μg/ml: caution in renal failure (reduce dose); slow IV in- fusion Tox: renal, VIII nerve
Trimethadione (Tridione) Soln: 200 mg/5 ml Cap: 300 mg Tab (chew): 150 mg	10-40 mg/kg/24 hr q 12 hr PO (adult: 900- 2,400 mg/24 hr q 6-8 hr PO)	Therapeutic peak level: 600-1,000 μg/ml Tox: sedation, vision, headache
Trimethaphan (Arfonad) Vial: 50 mg/ml	50-150 μg/kg/min IV infusion (adult: 0.5-1 mg/min)	Constant monitoring required; tachyphy- laxis Tox: ganglionic blocker (paralysis of pupils, bladder, bowels)
Trimethobenzamide (Tigan) Supp: 100, 200 mg Vial: 100 mg/ml	Adult: 200 mg/dose q 6-8 hr PR, IM	Limited experience in children; do not use in patients with acute onset vomiting

Drugs	Dosages	Comments
Trimethoprim(TMP)-sulfamethoxazole(SMX) (Bactrim, Septra) Susp: 40 mg TMP/200 mg SMX/5 ml Tab: 80 mg TMP/400 mg SMX: 160 mg TMP/800 mg SMX Amp: 80 mg TMP/400 mg SMX/5 ml	6-12 mg TMP/30-60 mg SMX/kg/24 hr q 12 hr PO (adult: 80-160 mg TMP/400-800 mg SMX q 12 hr PO) *Pneumocystis:* 15-20 mg TMP/75-100 mg SMX/kg/24 hr q 6-8 hr PO, IV *Severe UTI, Shigella:* 8-10 mg TMP/40-50 mg SMX/kg/24 hr q 6-8 hr PO, IV	Do not use in children <2 mon; rare indications for IV route; reduce dose in renal failure Tox: bone marrow suppression, GI irritation
Valproic acid or valproate (Depakene) Syr: 250 mg/5 ml Cap: 250 mg	15-60 mg/kg/24 hr q 8-24 hr PO (adult: 1-3 gm/24 hr q 8-24 hr PO)	Therapeutic level: 50-100 μg/ml; Table 56-13; use in acute management of seizures is controversial; bioavailability of generic preparations variable Tox: sedation, vomiting, rash, headache, hepatotoxic; increases phenobarbital level (20%) and decreases phenytoin level (50%-100%)
Vancomycin (Vancocin) Vial: 500 mg Soln: 1, 10 gm Pulvule: 125, 250 mg	30-45 mg/kg/24 hr q 6 hr IV (<500 mg/30 min) (meningitis: up to 60 mg/kg/24 hr q 6 hr IV) (maximum: 2 gm/24 hr) (NB: 30 mg/kg/24 hr q 12 hr) For *C. difficile* or pseudomembranous colitis: 125-500 mg q 6 hr PO	Reduce dosage if renal impairment; also available in oral preparation for staphylococcal enterocolitis and pseudomembranous colitis and *C. difficile* Tox: ototoxic, renal, rash, peripheral neuropathy
Verapamil (Isoptin, Calan) Amp: 2.5 mg/ml	0.1-0.2 mg/kg/dose IV over 2 min repeated in 10-30 min prn (adult: 5 mg/dose IV)	Table 12-3; do not use if <1 yr old Tox: bradycardia, hypotension
Vitamin K (Aquamephyton) Vial: 2, 10 mg/ml	NB, infant: 1-2 mg/dose IM, IV Child, adult: 5-10 mg/dose IM, IV	May give IV (<1 mg/min) but associated with hypotension and anaphylaxis
Warfarin (Coumadin) Tab: 2, 5, 7.5, 10 mg	0.1 mg/kg/24 hr Adult: 2-10 mg/24 hr q 24 hr PO after loading with 10-15 mg/24 hr PO for 2-3 days	Adjust dose to maintain PT at 2 times normal; antidote is vitamin K Tox: dermatitis

Many oral drugs may be given 3-4 times per day with more flexibility than implied by the specific intervals noted. *NB,* Newborns <7 days of age; *Pen,* penicillin; *SR,* sustained release; *Tox,* toxicity of drug.

Appendix C-2: Simplified Schedule for Administration of Pediatric Resuscitation Drugs

Drug (availability)	Single dose	Route	Dose (ml) administered by weight (kg) (ml/kg)									
			5 kg	10 kg	15 kg	20 kg	25 kg	30 kg	35 kg	40 kg	45 kg	50 kg
Epinephrine (1 : 10,000) (0.1 mg/ml)	0.01 mg/kg 0.1 ml/kg	IV, ET	0.5	1	1.5	2	2.5	3	3.5	4	4.5	5
Epinephrine (1 : 1,000) (1 mg/ml)	0.1 mg/kg 0.1 ml/kg	Second dose: IV ET	0.5	1	1.5	2	2.5	3	3.5	4	4.5	5
Sodium bicarbonate (1 mEq/ml)	1 mEq/kg 1 ml/kg	IV	5	10	15	20	25	30	35	40	45	50
Atropine (0.1 mg/ml)	0.02 mg/kg 0.2 ml/kg	IV, ET	1	2	3	4	5	6	7	8	9	10
Calcium chloride 10% (100 mg/ml)	20 mg/kg 0.2 ml/kg	IV	1	2	3	4	5	5	5	5	5	5
Lidocaine (20 mg/ml)*	1 mg/kg 0.05 ml/kg	IV, ET	0.25	0.5	0.75	1.0	1.25	1.5	1.75	2.0	2.25	2.5
Furosemide (Lasix) (10 mg/ml)	1 mg/kg 0.1 ml/kg	IV	0.5	1	1.5	2	2.5	3	3.5	4	4.5	5
Diazepam (Valium) (5 mg/ml)	0.2 mg/kg 0.04 ml/kg	IV	0.2	0.4	0.6	0.8	1	1.2	1.4	1.6	1.8	2

Before using this schedule, it is essential to be certain that the concentration used is identical to that cited here. Clinical response and patient condition may modify this schedule (see Table 12-3).

*Also available as 10 mg/ml.

MIXING EMERGENCY DRUGS FOR CONTINUOUS INFUSION

There are several alternative approaches to preparing medication for continuous infusion, and these are outlined on the following pages.

	Rule of 6s	Drug specific
Dopamine	6 × body wt (kg) equals mg of drug to be added to IV solution to make 100 ml D5W. Infusion of 1 ml/hr will deliver 1 μg/kg/min	150 mg added to 250 ml D5W (600 μg/ml). Infusion of 1 ml/kg/hr delivers 10 μg/kg/min
Dobutamine	Same as dopamine	Same as dopamine
Nitroprusside	Same as dopamine	45 mg added to 250 ml D5W (180 μg/ml). Infusion of 1 ml/kg/hr delivers 3 μg/kg/min
Isoproterenol	0.6 × body wt (kg) equals mg of drug to be added to IV solution to make 100 ml D5W. Infusion of 1 ml/hr will deliver 0.1 μg/kg/min	1.5 mg added to 250 ml D5W (6 μg/ml). Infusion of 1 ml/kg/hr delivers 0.1 μg/kg/min

EMERGENCY RESUSCITATION MEASURES FOR 10 KG CHILD*

WEIGHT: 10 kg (22 lbs)
ET SIZE: 4.0
LARYNGOSCOPE BLADE: 1-2
SUCTION CATHETER: 8 Fr.
DEFIBRILLATION: 20 joules

AGE: 1 yr.
PULSE: 130 beats/min.
RESPIRATORY RATE: 20-30 resp/min.
BP: 96 ± 30 mm Hg
NG TUBE: 8 Fr.
FOLEY: 8 Fr.

EMERGENCY MEDICATIONS

Drug (concentration)	Therapy dose range	Route	Comments	Single dose (mg)	Dose administer (ml)
Epinephrine Syringe (1 : 10,000 = 0.1 mg/ml)	0.01 mg/kg (0.1 ml/kg)	IV	maximum dose: 5 ml	0.1 mg	1 ml
Epinephrine (1 : 1,000 = 1 mg/ml)	0.1 mg/ml (0.1 ml/kg)	Second dose: IV ET	maximum dose: 5 ml	1 mg	1 ml
Bicarbonate, Sodium (1 mEq/ml)	1 mEq/kg (1 ml/kg)	IV	<1 yr dilute 1 : 1 with nonbacteriostatic H_2O	10 mEq	10 ml
Atropine (0.1 mg/ml)	0.02 mg/kg (0.2 ml/kg)	IV ET	minimum dose: 0.1 mg; maximum dose: 2 mg; IV slowly	0.2 mg	2 ml
Calcium Cl 10% (100 mg/ml)	20 mg/kg (0.2 ml/kg)	IV	maximum dose: 500 mg	200 mg	2 ml
Lidocaine 2% (20 mg/ml)	1 mg/kg (0.05 ml/kg)	IV ET	maximum total dose: 5 mg/kg	10 mg	0.5 ml
Furosemide (Lasix) (10 mg/ml)	1 mg/kg (0.1 ml/kg)	IV	maximum dose: 6 mg/kg	10 mg	1 ml
Diazepam (Valium) (5 mg/ml)	0.2 mg/kg (0.04 ml/kg)	IV ET	maximum total dose: child 10 mg; adult 30 mg	2 mg	0.4 ml
Albuterol (Soln: 5 mg/ml)	0.03 ml (0.15 mg)/kg/dose	NEB	may give frequently; monitor response	1.5 mg	0.3 ml
Bretylium (50 mg/ml)	5 mg/kg (0.1 ml/kg)	IV	increase by 5 mg/kg q 10-15 min; maximum dose: 30 mg/kg	50 mg	1 ml
Naloxone (Narcan) (1 mg/ml)	0.1 mg/kg (0.1 ml/kg)	IV ET	if no response in 10 min may give up to 2 mg IV	1 mg	1 ml
Adenosine (3 mg/ml)	0.1 mg/kg (0.03 ml/kg)	IV	IV rapid bolus; maximum dose: 12 mg	1 mg	0.33 ml
Dextrose 50% (0.5 gm/ml)	0.5 gm/kg (1 ml/kg)	IV	<1 yr dilute to D25W with nonbacteriostatic H_2O	5 gm	10 ml
Phenytoin (Dilantin) (50 mg/ml)	LOAD: (seizure) 15 mg/kg (0.3 ml/kg)	IV PO	NOT IM: IV give slowly in saline only; maximum dose: 1250 mg: DYSRHYTHMIA: 5 mg/kg/dose q 5-20 min prn × 2 IV	150 mg	3 ml
Phenobarbital (65 mg/ml)	LOAD: 10 mg/kg (0.15 ml/kg)	IV IM PO	maximum dose: 300 mg; maint: 3-5 mg/kg/day	100 mg	1.5 ml
Methylprednisolone (Solu Medrol) (62.5 mg/ml)	ASTHMA: 1-2 mg/kg q 6 hr IV	IV	maximum dose: 500 mg	300 mg	4.8 ml

MEDICATION DRIPS

Drug (concentration)	Therapy range	Conversion mixture	Add D5W (ml)	Add drug (ml)	Initial average dose (pump required)
Dopamine (40 mg/ml)	5-20 μg/kg/min IV drip	150 mg in 250 ml D5W = 600 μg/ml; 1 ml/kg/hr = 10 μg/kg/min	250 ml	3.75 ml	10 ml/hr
Dobutamine (25 mg/ml when mixed with 10 ml)	2-15 μg/kg/min IV drip	150 mg in 250 ml D5W = 600 μg/ml; ml/kg/hr = 10 μg/kg/min	250 ml	6 ml	10 ml/hr
Nitroprusside (25 mg/ml)	0.5-10 (avg 3 μg) μg/kg/min IV drip	45 mg in 250 ml D5W = 180 μg/ml; 1 ml/kg/hr = 3 μg/kg/min	250 ml	1.8 ml	10 ml/hr
Isoproterenol (Isupel) (0.2 mg/ml)	0.05-1.5 μg/kg/min IV drip	1.5 mg in 250 ml D5W = 6 μg/ml; 1 ml/kg/hr = 0.1 μg/kg/min	250 ml	7.5 ml	10 ml/hr

*This sample layout may provide a useful format for developing age-specific drug dosing information.

Index